TEXTBOOK OF DIAGNOSTIC SONOGRAPHY

TEXTBOOK OF DIAGNOSTIC SONOGRAPHY

9TH EDITION

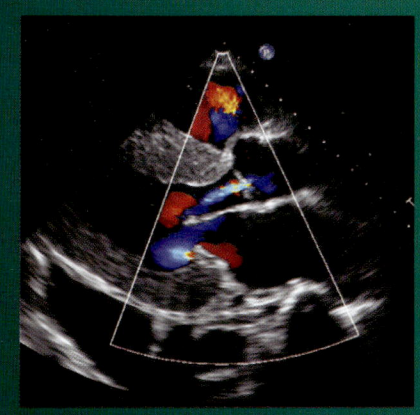
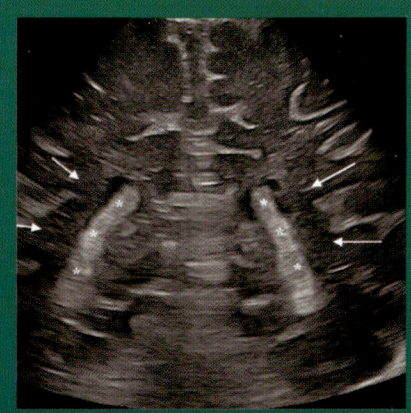
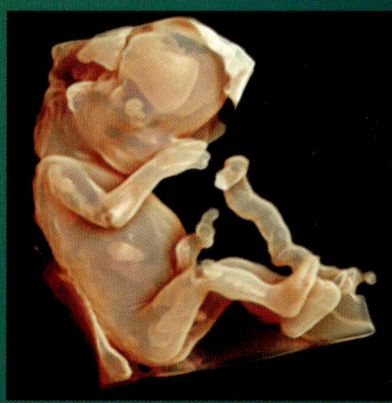

SANDRA L. HAGEN-ANSERT,
MS, RDMS, RDCS, FASE, FSDMS (RETIRED)

Cardiology Department Manager, Echo Labs
Scripps Clinic & Hospitals—La Jolla, California

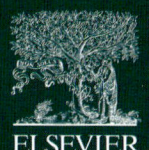

ELSEVIER

ELSEVIER
3251 Riverport Lane
St Louis, Missouri 63043

TEXTBOOK OF DIAGNOSTIC SONOGRAPHY, NINTH EDITION ISBN: 978-0-323-82646-4
 Volume 1 ISBN: 978-0-323-82761-4
 Volume 2 ISBN: 978-0-323-82762-1

Copyright © 2023 by Elsevier Inc. All rights reserved.
No part of this publication may be reproduced or transmitted in any form or by any means, electronic or mechanical, including photocopying, recording, or any information storage and retrieval system, without permission in writing from the publisher. Details on how to seek permission, further information about the Publisher's permissions policies and our arrangements with organizations such as the Copyright Clearance Center and the Copyright Licensing Agency, can be found at our website: www.elsevier.com/permissions.

This book and the individual contributions contained in it are protected under copyright by the Publisher (other than as may be noted herein).

Notices

Knowledge and best practice in this field are constantly changing. As new research and experience broaden our understanding, changes in research methods, professional practices, or medical treatment may become necessary.

Practitioners and researchers must always rely on their own experience and knowledge in evaluating and using any information, methods, compounds, or experiments described herein. In using such information or methods they should be mindful of their own safety and the safety of others, including parties for whom they have a professional responsibility.

With respect to any drug or pharmaceutical products identified, readers are advised to check the most current information provided (i) on procedures featured or (ii) by the manufacturer of each product to be administered, to verify the recommended dose or formula, the method and duration of administration, and contraindications. It is the responsibility of practitioners, relying on their own experience and knowledge of their patients, to make diagnoses, to determine dosages and the best treatment for each individual patient, and to take all appropriate safety precautions.

To the fullest extent of the law, neither the Publisher nor the authors, contributors, or editors, assume any liability for any injury and/or damage to persons or property as a matter of products liability, negligence or otherwise, or from any use or operation of any methods, products, instructions, or ideas contained in the material herein.

Previous editions copyrighted 2018, 2012, 2006, 2001, 1995, 1989, 1983, and 1978.

Executive Content Strategist: Meg Benson
Content Development Manager: Danielle Frazier
Publishing Services Manager: Catherine Jackson
Senior Project Manager/Specialist: Carrie Stetz
Design Direction: Amy Buxton

Printed in India
Last digit is the print number: 9 8 7 6 5 4 3 2 1

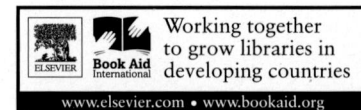

To my family,
Art, Aly, Kati, Becca and Eric, Adeline and Osborne,
who mean the world to me

CONTRIBUTORS

Alicia Armour, MA, ACS, RDCS, FASE
Health Center Administrator
Duke Triangle Heart Associates
Duke University Health System
Durham, North Carolina

Joan P. Baker, MSR, RDMS, FSDMS
President, Sound Ergonomics, LLC
Kenmore, Washington

Carolyn T. Coffin, MPH, RDMS, RVT, RDCS
CEO and Consultant
Sound Ergonomics LLC
Kenmore, Washington

M. Robert DeJong, RDMS, RDCS, RVT, FSDMS, FAIUM
Bob DeJong, LLC
Ultrasound Educational Services
Rosedale, Maryland;
Former Radiology Technical Manager–Ultrasound
Russell H. Morgan Department of Radiology and Radiological Science
Johns Hopkins Hospital
Baltimore, Maryland

Kelsey Doyle, MEd, RDMS, RVT
Education and Outreach Coordinator
Center for Perinatal Care
UnityPoint Health-Meriter/University of Wisconsin–Madison
Madison, Wisconsin

John Eisenbrey, PhD
Associate Professor of Radiology
Department of Radiology
Thomas Jefferson University
Philadelphia, Pennsylvania

Kathryn Gill, MS, RDMS, RVT, FSDMS
Sonographer
Program Director
Institute of Ultrasound Diagnostics & Medscan Clinic
Spanish Fort, Alabama

Joy Guthrie, PhD, ACS, RDMS, RDCS, RVT, FSDMS, RCS, RCCS, RVS
Advanced Practice Sonographer
Program Director, Diagnostic Medical Sonography
Researcher, Community Regional Medical Center
Fresno, California

Sandra L. Hagen-Ansert, MS, RDMS, RDCS, FASE, FSDMS (Retired)
Cardiology Department Manager, Echo Labs
Scripps Clinic & Hospitals
La Jolla, California

Talisha M. Hunt, BSRT, RDMS, RDCS, RVT
Lead Sonographer
Assistant Professor of Radiology
Mayo Clinic
Rochester, Minnesota

Mariana Kozirovsky, MS, RDMS, RDCS
Assistant Professor
Long Island University
Brooklyn, New York;
Research Scientist
NYU Grossman School of Medicine
New York, New York

Frederick W. Kremkau, PhD, RACR, RAIMBE, FAIUM, FASA
Professor of Radiologic Sciences
Director, Program for Medical Ultrasound
Center for Experiential and Applied Learning
Wake Forest University School of Medicine
Winston Salem, North Carolina

Dan Lebovic, MD
Professor
Department of Obstetrics and Gynecology
Washington University in St. Louis
St. Louis, Missouri

Daniel Merton, BS, RDMS, FSDMS, FAIUM
Diagnostic Ultrasound Specialist and Principal Project Officer
Health Devices Group
ECRI Institute
Plymouth Meeting, Pennsylvania

Carol Mitchell, PhD, ACS, RDMS, RDCS, RVT, RT(R), FASE, FSDMS
Associate Professor
Department of Medicine
School of Medicine and Public Health
University of Wisconsin–Madison
Madison, Wisconsin

Tanya Nolan, EdD, RDMS, RT(R)(ARRT)
Associate Professor
Director, Diagnostic Medical Sonography
Director, MSRS Innovation and Improvement
School of Radiologic Sciences
Weber State University
Ogden, Utah

Cindy A. Owen, RDMS, RVT, RT, FSDMS
Former Director, Clinical Insights and Development
GE Healthcare, Point of Care Ultrasound
Milwaukee, Wisconsin

Mitzi Roberts, EdD, RDMS, RDCS, FSDMS, RT(R)
Associate Professor
Baptist Health Sciences University;
Clinical Sonographer
Mid-South Maternal-Fetal Medicine
Memphis, Tennessee

Jean Lea Spitz, MPH, RDMS
Executive Director
Perinatal Quality Foundation
Oklahoma City, Oklahoma

Christina Taff, BS, RDMS
Lead Clinical Coordinator
Mid-South Maternal Fetal Medicine
Memphis, Tennessee

Shpetim Telegrafi, MD
Research Professor
Director of Diagnostic Ultrasound
Department of Urology
NYU Grossman School of Medicine
New York, New York

Barbara Trampe, BA, RN, RDMS
Education and Outreach Coordinator
Maternal-Fetal Medicine
University of Wisconsin/UnityPoint Health Meriter
Madison, Wisconsin

Kevin R. Volz, PhD, RVT
Research Lab Manager
Laboratory for Investigative Imaging
Former Instructor/Vascular Technology Clinical Coordinator
School of Health and Rehabilitation Sciences
Division of Radiologic Sciences and Therapy
The Ohio State University College of Medicine
Columbus, Ohio

Kelsi Weakley, MS, RDMS
Clinical Coordinator
Maternal-Fetal Medicine
Regional One Health
Memphis, Tennessee

Kerry Weinberg, PhD, MPA, MA, RDMS, RDCS, RT(T), FSDMS
Associate Professor and Program Director
Diagnostic Medical Sonography
Long Island University
Brooklyn, New York

Michelle Wilson, EdD, RDMS, RDCS, FSDMS
Former Clinical Sonographer and Educator
Kaiser Permanente Medical Center and Kaiser School of Allied Health
Napa, California;
Adjunct Associate Professor
DMS Program
University of Southern Indiana
Evansville, Indiana

Kathryn Zale, MS, RDMS, RVT
Faculty Instructor
Diagnostic Medical Sonography
Pennsylvania College of Health Sciences
Lancaster, Pennsylvania;
Sonographer
Department of Radiology
Children's Hospital of Philadelphia
King of Prussia, Pennsylvania

PREFACE

INTRODUCING THE NINTH EDITION

The ninth edition of *Textbook of Diagnostic Sonography* continues the tradition of excellence that began when the first edition was published in 1978. Like other medical imaging fields, diagnostic sonography has seen dramatic changes and innovations since its first clinical experimental days. Phenomenal strides in transducer design, instrumentation, three-dimensional (3D) and four-dimensional (4D) imaging, image processing, tissue harmonics, elastoraphy, and contrast agents continue to improve image resolution and the diagnostic clinical value of sonography. The ninth edition has kept abreast of advancements in the field by inviting new contributors currently working in different areas of medical sonography throughout the country. The critiques and suggestions from multiple reviewers have helped ensure that this edition includes the most complete and up-to-date information needed to meet the requirements of the modern student of sonography.

Distinctive Approach

This textbook can serve as an in-depth resource both for students of sonography and for practitioners in any number of clinical settings, including hospitals, clinics, and private practices. Care has been taken to cultivate readers' understanding of the patient's total clinical picture even as they study sonographic examination protocol and technique. To this end, each chapter covers the following:
- Key terminology
- Normal anatomy (including cross-sectional anatomy)
- Normal physiology
- Laboratory data and values
- Pathology
- Sonographic evaluation of an organ
- Sonographic findings
- Pitfalls in sonography
- Clinical findings
- Differential considerations
- "Key Pearls"

The full-color art program is of great value to the student of anatomy and pathology for sonography. Detailed line drawings illustrate the anatomic information a sonographer must know to successfully perform specific sonographic examinations. Multiple color photographs of gross pathology help the reader visualize some of the pathology presented, with 3D and color Doppler illustrations included where relevant.

To make important information easy to find, key points are pulled out into numerous boxes; tables throughout the chapters summarize the pathology under discussion and break down the information into Clinical Findings, Sonographic Findings, and Differential Considerations.

Sonographic findings for particular pathologic conditions are always preceded in the text by the following special heading:

▶ **Sonographic Findings**

This icon makes it very easy for students and practicing sonographers to locate this clinical information quickly.

Study and Review Opportunities

Study and review are also essential to gaining a solid grasp of the concepts and information presented in this textbook. Learning objectives, chapter outlines, "Key Pearls" that summarize the chapter highlights, comprehensive glossaries of key terms, and full references for cited material all help students learn the material in an organized and thorough manner.

Scope and Organization of Topics

The *Textbook of Diagnostic Sonography* is divided into eight parts:

Part I introduces the reader to the foundations of sonography and patient care and includes the following:
- Foundations of sonography, which include the basic principles of ultrasound physics and medical sonography
- Terminology frequently encountered by the sonographer
- Patient care for the sonographer
- Ergonomics and musculoskeletal issues for practitioners
- Anatomic and physiologic relationships within the abdominopelvic cavity
- Comparative sectional anatomy of the abdominopelvic cavity
- Imaging and Doppler artifacts

Part II presents the abdomen in depth. The following topics are discussed:
- Anatomic relationships and physiology
- Abdominal scanning techniques and protocols
- Abdominal applications of ultrasound contrast agents
- Ultrasound-guided interventional techniques
- Emergent abdominal ultrasound procedures
- Sonographic techniques in the transplant patient
- Separate chapters for the vascular system, liver, gallbladder and biliary system, spleen, pancreas, gastrointestinal tract, urinary system, retroperitoneum, peritoneal cavity, and abdominal wall

Part III focuses on the superficial structures of the body, including the breast, thyroid and parathyroid glands, scrotum, and musculoskeletal system.

Part IV is completely updated and explores sonographic examination of the neonate and pediatric patient, including abdomen, adrenal and urinary system, neonatal head, neonatal hip, and neonatal spine.

Part V focuses on the thoracic cavity and includes the following topics:
- Anatomic and physiologic relationships within the thoracic cavity
- Hemodynamics
- Echocardiographic evaluation and techniques
- Introduction to clinical echocardiography
- Fetal echocardiography
- Congenital heart disease

Part VI is composed of four updated chapters on extracranial and intracranial cerebrovascular imaging and peripheral arterial and venous sonographic evaluation.

Part VII is devoted to gynecology and includes the following topics:
- Normal anatomy and physiology of the female pelvis
- Sonographic and Doppler evaluation of the female pelvis
- Separate chapters on the pathologic conditions of the uterus, ovaries, and adnexa
- Updated chapter on the role of sonography in evaluating female infertility

Part VIII takes a thorough look at obstetric sonography. The following topics are discussed:
- The role of sonography in obstetrics
- Clinical ethics for obstetric sonography
- Normal first-trimester findings and first-trimester complications
- Sonography of the second and third trimesters
- Obstetric measurements and gestational age and fetal growth assessment
- Sonography in the high-risk pregnancy
- Prenatal diagnosis of congenital anomalies
- Chapters are devoted to the placenta, umbilical cord, amniotic fluid and fetal membranes, fetal face and neck, neural axis, thorax, anterior abdominal wall, abdomen, urogenital system, and skeleton

New to This Edition

Eight new contributors joined the ninth edition to update and expand existing content, bringing with them a fresh perspective and an impressive knowledge base. They also helped contribute the more than 1000 images new to this edition, including color Doppler, 3D and 4D, and contrast-enhanced images. More than 30 new line drawings complement the new chapters found in the ninth edition.

As the reader proceeds through each chapter, terminology is introduced to lay the foundation for the reader as they study the specific chapters. Information that may seem repetitive to the experienced sonographer is reinforcement for student sonographers as they build their understanding of the many concepts that must be mastered for their clinical experience.

Foundations of Ultrasound (Chapter 1) introduces the reader to the field of sonography, including the role of the sonographer, historical overview of the development of ultrasound, as well as an introduction to basic ultrasound principles and terminology.

Essentials of Patient Care for the Sonographer (Chapter 2) covers all aspects of patient care the sonographer may encounter, including obtaining and understanding vital signs, handling patients on strict bed rest, patients with tubes and oxygen, patient transfer techniques, infection control, isolation techniques, emergency medical situations, assisting patients with special needs, and patient rights.

Ergonomics and Musculoskeletal Issues in Sonography (Chapter 3) outlines the importance of proper technique and positioning throughout the sonographic examination as a way to avoid long-term disability problems that may be acquired with repetitive scanning.

Anatomic and Physiologic Relationships Within the Abdominopelvic Cavity (Chapter 4) introduces the reader to body systems and anatomic relationships, which include membranes and ligaments and potential spaces in the body.

Comparative Sectional Anatomy of the Abdominopelvic Cavity (Chapter 5) is an introduction to sectional anatomy incorporating gross anatomy with comparative ultrasound and computed tomography sectional images. This chapter provides the groundwork for understanding sectional anatomy.

Basic Ultrasound Imaging: Techniques, Terminology, and Tips (Chapter 6) describes scanning techniques, terminology, abdominal ultrasound protocol, and abdominal Doppler technique.

Imaging and Doppler Artifacts (Chapter 7) is an outstanding review of all the artifacts commonly encountered by sonographers. There are numerous examples of the various artifacts and detailed explanations of how these artifacts are produced and how to avoid them.

The abdominal chapters (Chapter 8-19) have all been updated with new images that include ultrasound, CT, and MRI.

Sonographic Techniques in the Transplant Patient (Chapter 20) has been updated to focus on criteria required for organ transplantation, including liver transplant, renal transplant, and pancreatic transplant.

The Breast (Chapter 21) has been updated by a new contributor with new techniques and images.

The Musculoskeletal System (Chapter 24) has been updated by a new contributor with beautiful illustrations and a comprehensive bibliography.

The entire pediatrics section (Chapters 25 to 29) has been fully updated with exquisite new illustrations for each chapter.

Understanding Hemodynamics (Chapter 31) introduces the student to blood flow dynamics, intracardiac pressures and volumes, Doppler basics, and quantification of intracardiac pressures by ultrasound.

Introduction to Clinical Echocardiography: Left-Sided Valvular Heart Disease (Chapter 33) and *Introduction to Clinical Echocardiography: Pericardial Disease, Cardiomyopathies, and Tumors* (Chapter 34) have been included in this edition to provide a basic understanding of significant cardiac findings that may be encountered by the general sonographer or clinician. The fetal echocardiography chapters (Chapters 35 and 36) have been updated to include current protocol and image acquisition.

The entire cerebrovascular section (Chapters 37 to 40) has been updated with new images and current techniques for the sonographer.

Several new contributors have provided their expertise in the obstetrics section (Chapters 47 to 65). *Sonography of the Second and Third Trimesters, Prenatal Diagnosis of Congenital Anomalies, The Placenta, Fetal Face and Neck, Fetal Neural Axis,* and *Fetal Skeleton* chapters have all been updated with new images and references.

Student Resources

Workbook. Available for separate purchase, the *Workbook for the Textbook of Diagnostic Sonography* has also been completely updated. This resource gives the learner ample opportunity to practice and apply the information presented in the textbook.
- Each workbook chapter covers all the material presented in the textbook.
- Each chapter includes exercises on image identification, anatomy identification, key term definitions, and sonographic technique.
- Case studies using images from the textbook invite students to test their skills at identifying key anatomy and pathology and describing and interpreting sonographic findings.
- Students can also test their knowledge with the hundreds of multiple-choice questions found in the four examinations covering different content areas: General Sonography, Pediatric, Cardiovascular Anatomy, and Obstetrics and Gynecology.

Evolve. On the Evolve site, students will find review questions for each chapter.

Instructor Resources

Resources for instructors are also provided on the Evolve site to assist in the preparation of classroom lectures and activities.
- Extensive PowerPoint lectures for each chapter that include illustrations
- Test bank of 1500 multiple-choice questions in Exam View and Word
- Electronic image collection that includes all the images from the textbook both in PowerPoint and in .jpeg format

Evolve Online Course Management. Evolve is an interactive learning environment designed to work in coordination with the *Textbook of Diagnostic Sonography*. Instructors may use Evolve to include an Internet-based course component that reinforces and expands on the concepts delivered in class. Evolve may be used to do all of the following:
- Publish the class syllabus, outlines, and lecture notes
- Set up virtual office hours and email communication
- Share important dates and information on the online class calendar
- Encourage student participation with chat rooms and discussion boards
- Post examinations and manage grade books
- For more information, visit http://www.evolve.elsevier.com/HagenAnsert/diagnostic/ or contact an Elsevier sales representative.

ACKNOWLEDGMENTS

I would like to express my gratitude and appreciation to a number of individuals who have served as mentors and guides throughout my years in sonography. It all began with Dr. George Leopold at UCSD Medical Center. His quest for knowledge and his perseverance for excellence have been the mainstay of my career in sonography. I would also like to recognize Drs. Dolores Pretorius, Nancy Budorick, Wanda Miller-Hance, and David Sahn for their encouragement throughout the years at the UCSD Medical Center in both Radiology and Pediatric Cardiology.

I would also like to acknowledge Dr. Barry Goldberg for the opportunity he gave me to develop countless numbers of educational programs in sonography in an independent fashion and for his encouragement to pursue advancement. I would also like to thank Dr. Daniel Yellon for his early-hour anatomy dissection and instruction; Dr. Carson Schneck, for his excellent instruction in gross anatomy and sections of "Geraldine"; and Dr. Jacob Zutuchni, for his enthusiasm for the field of cardiology.

I am grateful to Dr. Harry Rakowski for his continued support in teaching fellows and students while I was at the Toronto General Hospital. Dr. William Zwiebel encouraged me to continue writing and teaching while I was at the University of Wisconsin Medical Center, and I appreciate his knowledge, which found its way into the liver physiology section of this textbook.

My good fortune in learning about and understanding the total patient must be attributed to a very dedicated cardiologist, James Glenn, with whom I had the pleasure of working while I was at MUSC in Charleston, South Carolina. It was through his compassion and knowledge that I grew to appreciate the total patient beyond the transducer, and for this I am grateful.

For their continual support, feedback, and challenges, I would like to thank and recognize all the students I have taught in the various diagnostic medical sonography programs: Episcopal Hospital, Thomas Jefferson University Medical Center, University of Wisconsin-Madison Medical Center, UCSD Medical Center, and Baptist College of Health Science. These students continually work toward the development of quality sonography techniques and protocols and have given back to the sonography community tenfold.

The continual push towards excellence has been encouraged on a daily basis by our Scripps Clinic Medical Director of the Echo Lab, Dr. David Rubenson, and outstanding staff of Scripps Clinic Cardiologists.

The Cardiac Sonographers at Scripps Clinic Anderson Medical Pavillion have been invaluable in their excellent image acquisition. Special thanks to Kristen Billick for her excellent echocardiographic images. The general sonographers at Scripps Clinic have been invaluable in providing the outstanding images for the obstetrics and gynecology chapters.

I would like to thank the very supportive and capable staff at Elsevier who have guided me though yet another edition of this textbook. Danielle Frazier, Carrie Stetz, and the staff at Elsevier are to be commended on their perseverance to make this an outstanding textbook.

I would like to thank my family, Art, Becca, Aly, and Kati, for their patience and understanding, as I thought this edition would never come to an end. My recent retirement and the pandemic lockdown provided an excellent opportunity for total undivided dedication to this edition.

I think that you will find the 9th Edition of the *Textbook of Diagnostic Sonography* reflects the contribution of so many individuals with attention to detail and a dedication to excellence. I hope you will find this educational experience in sonography as rewarding as I have throughout the past 50 years.

Sandra L. Hagen-Ansert,
MS, RDMS, RDCS, FASE, FSDMS (Retired)

CONTENTS

VOLUME ONE

PART I Foundations of Sonography

1. Foundations of Clinical Sonography, 3
2. Essentials of Patient Care for the Sonographer, 29
3. Ergonomics and Musculoskeletal Issues in Sonography, 68
4. Anatomic and Physiologic Relationships Within the Abdominopelvic Cavity, 80
5. Comparative Sectional Anatomy of the Abdominopelvic Cavity, 102
6. Basic Ultrasound Imaging: Techniques, Terminology, and Tips, 123
7. Imaging and Doppler Artifacts, 147

PART II Abdomen

8. Vascular System, 169
9. The Liver, 218
10. The Gallbladder and the Biliary System, 281
11. The Spleen, 325
12. The Pancreas, 355
13. The Gastrointestinal Tract, 389
14. The Peritoneal Cavity and Abdominal Wall, 413
15. Urinary System, 435
16. The Retroperitoneum, 491
17. Abdominal Applications of Ultrasound Contrast Agents, 511
18. Ultrasound-Guided Interventional Techniques, 528
19. Emergent Ultrasound Procedures, 561
20. Sonographic Techniques in the Transplant Patient, 583

PART III Superficial Structures

21 Breast, 643

22 The Thyroid and Parathyroid Glands, 682

23 Scrotum, 708

24 Musculoskeletal System, 733

PART IV Pediatrics

25 Neonatal and Pediatric Abdomen, 761

26 Neonatal and Pediatric Adrenal and Urinary System, 791

27 Neonatal and Infant Head, 813

28 Infant and Pediatric Hip, 850

29 Neonatal and Infant Spine, 871

Glossary, G-1 to G-12

VOLUME TWO

PART V The Thoracic Cavity

30 Anatomic and Physiologic Relationships Within the Thoracic Cavity, 891

31 Understanding Hemodynamics, 908

32 Introduction to Echocardiographic Techniques, Terminology, and Tips, 916

33 Introduction to Clinical Echocardiography: Left-Sided Valvular Heart Disease, 953

34 Introduction to Clinical Echocardiography: Pericardial Disease, Cardiomyopathies, and Tumors, 980

35 Fetal Echocardiography: Beyond the Four Chambers, 1007

36 Fetal Echocardiography: Congenital Heart Disease, 1031

PART VI Cerebrovascular

37 Extracranial Cerebrovascular Evaluation, 1069

38 Intracranial Cerebrovascular Evaluation, 1087

39 Peripheral Arterial Evaluation, 1110

40 Peripheral Venous Evaluation, 1129

PART VII Gynecology

41 Normal Anatomy and Physiology of the Female Pelvis, 1157

42 Sonographic and Doppler Evaluation of the Female Pelvis, 1176

43 Pathology of the Uterus, 1202

44 Pathology of the Ovaries, 1230

45 Pathology of the Adnexa, 1260

46 Role of Ultrasound in Evaluating Female Infertility, 1272

PART VIII Obstetrics

47 The Role of Sonography in Obstetrics, 1283

48 Clinical Ethics for Obstetric Sonography, 1294

49 The Early Embryonic Stage of the First Trimester, 1300

50 First-Trimester Complications, 1319

51 Sonography of the Second and Third Trimesters, 1343

52 Obstetric Measurements and Gestational Age, 1378

53 Fetal Growth Assessment by Sonography, 1395

54 Sonography and High-Risk Pregnancy, 1406

55 Prenatal Diagnosis of Congenital Anomalies, 1426

56 Placenta, 1442

57 The Umbilical Cord, 1460

58 Amniotic Fluid and Fetal Membranes, 1474

59 Fetal Face and Neck, 1492

60 Fetal Neural Axis, 1522

61 The Fetal Thorax, 1545

62 The Fetal Anterior Abdominal Wall, 1560

63 The Fetal Abdomen, 1572

64 Fetal Urogenital System, 1592

65 Fetal Skeleton, 1622

Glossary, G-13 to G-24

Illustration Credits, C-1 to C-10

Index, I-1 to I-40

PART I

Foundations of Sonography

Chapter 1 Foundations of Clinical Sonography
Chapter 2 Essentials of Patient Care for the Sonographer
Chapter 3 Ergonomics and Musculoskeletal Issues in Sonography
Chapter 4 Anatomic and Physiologic Relationships Within the Abdominopelvic Cavity
Chapter 5 Comparative Sectional Anatomy of the Abdominopelvic Cavity
Chapter 6 Basic Ultrasound Imaging: Techniques, Terminology, and Tips
Chapter 7 Imaging and Doppler Artifacts

CHAPTER 1

Foundations of Clinical Sonography

Sandra L. Hagen-Ansert

OBJECTIVES

On completion of this chapter, you should be able to:
- Describe the role of the sonographer and the career path
- Know the historical developments in medical ultrasound
- List the basic principles and terminology of medical ultrasound
- Identify the transducers necessary for specific ultrasound applications
- Explain the multiple display modes on ultrasound instrumentation
- State the Doppler effect

OUTLINE

Role of the Sonographer 4
  Advantages and Disadvantages of a Sonography Career 5
Historical Overview of Sound Theory and Medical Ultrasound 6
Introduction to Basic Ultrasound Principles 10
  Acoustics 10
  Transducer Selection in a Clinical Imaging Practice 14
  Pulse-Echo Display Modes 17
  Harmonic Imaging 18
  Three-Dimensional and Four-Dimensional Ultrasound 20
  System Controls for Image Optimization 21
  Doppler Ultrasound 22

KEY TERMS

Absorption
Acoustic impedance
Aliasing
Amplitude
Angle of incidence
Angle of reflection
Attenuation
Axial resolution
Azumithal resolution
Color flow Doppler
Compression
Continuous wave Doppler (CW)
Cycle
Decibel (dB)
Depth gain compensation (DGC)
Doppler angle
Doppler shift
Dynamic range

Focal zone
Frame rate
Frequency shift
Gain
Gray scale
Hertz (Hz)
Gate
Intensity
Interface
Kilohertz (kHz)
Laminar
Lateral resolution
Megahertz (MHz)
Nyquist sampling limit
Power
Pulse duration
Pulsed wave (PW) Doppler
Pulse repetition frequency (PRF)

Rarefaction
Real time
Reflection
Refraction
Resistance
Resolution
Scattering
Slice thickness
Spectral analysis
Spectral broadening
Spatial pulse length
Temporal resolution
Time gain compensation (TGC)
Transducer
Turbulent
Velocity
Wave
Wavelength

The primary purpose of this chapter is to introduce the sonographer to the fascinating field of diagnostic medical ultrasound. Historians will tell us that we cannot know where we are going until we know where we have been. Therefore a brief background into the historical development of ultrasound is presented to enable the sonographer to understand the progress that has been made with technology in the medical application of ultrasound. It is important for sonographers to understand their role in the health care field and to have a global concept of anatomic reconstruction. An introduction into the terminology of the basic principles of ultrasound is critical for the student to understand how and why an anatomic image appears as it does on the ultrasound monitor.

The words *diagnostic medical ultrasound, ultrasound,* and *ultrasonography* have all been used to describe the instrumentation used in ultrasound. *Sonography* is the term used to describe a specialized imaging technique to visualize soft tissue structures in the body. The term *echocardiography*, or simple *"echo,"* refers to an ultrasound examination of only the cardiac structures.

A *sonographer* is a member of the allied health profession who has received specialized education in diagnostic medical sonography and has successfully completed the national boards given by the American Registry of Diagnostic Medical Sonography. A *sonologist* is a physician who has received specialized training in ultrasound and has successfully completed the national boards granted by their respective specialty (e.g., radiology, cardiology, obstetrics).

The field of diagnostic medical ultrasound has grown to become a well-respected and valuable addition to diagnostic imaging by providing pertinent clinical information to the physician and to the patient. The applications of ultrasound are extensive; they include, but are not limited to, the following areas:

- General ultrasound (abdominal, renal, retroperitoneal, chest)
- Superficial ultrasound (breast, thyroid, scrotum)
- Neonatal and pediatric ultrasound (abdomen, renal, hips, brain, spine)
- Echocardiography (adult, pediatric, neonatal, fetal)
- Interventional and therapeutic guided ultrasound
- Obstetric and gynecologic ultrasound
- Intraoperative ultrasound
- Musculoskeletal ultrasound
- Ophthalmologic ultrasound
- Point of care ultrasound

Extensive research has verified the safety of ultrasound as a diagnostic procedure. No harmful effects of ultrasound have been demonstrated at power levels used for diagnostic studies when performed by qualified and nationally certified sonographers, under the direction of qualified and board-certified sonologists, using appropriate equipment and techniques.

Diagnostic ultrasound has developed into a valuable imaging technique for many reasons. First is the lack of ionizing radiation for the ultrasound procedure compared with the various other imaging modalities such as computed tomography (CT) or nuclear medicine. The second reason is the portability of the ultrasound equipment. Even the high-end equipment may be moved into the intensive care unit, emergency department, operating room, cardiac catheterization lab, or physician's office. The low-end systems are now so portable they can fit into the physician's lab coat to be used at the bedside as an *initial quick look* evaluation of the patient physical examination.

Ultrasound is unique in other ways as well. The ultrasound image is presented in a real-time cine clip format, which makes it possible to see the image transition from one cardiac structure to another, or from one organ system to another. The flexible multiplanar imaging capability allows the sonographer to "follow" the path of a tortuous vessel, a moving cardiac structure, or a moving fetus to capture the necessary images. Moreover, Doppler techniques allow the qualitative and quantitative evaluation of blood flow hemodynamics within a vessel. Finally, the cost analysis of an ultrasound system is superior compared with other imaging diagnostic systems.

Currently nearly all hospitals and medical clinics have access to some form of ultrasound instrumentation to provide the clinician with an inside look at the soft tissue structures within the body. Ultrasound manufacturers continue their research to improve image acquisition, develop efficient transducer functionality and design, and create software to improve computer assessment of the acquired information. Two-dimensional (2D) ultrasound information can be recreated in a 3D or 4D (real-time) format to provide an "en face" surface rendering of the specific area. Color Doppler, harmonics, tissue characterization, elastography, strain, and spectral analysis have greatly expanded the utility of ultrasound imaging. The development of specialized contrast agents for use with ultrasound has enabled the clinicians to make specific diagnoses with greater precision.

To obtain even more information from the ultrasound image, various medical centers and manufacturers continue their work towards the development of effective contrast agents that may be ingested or administered intravenously into the bloodstream to facilitate the detection and diagnosis of specific pathologies. Early attempts at producing a contrast effect with ultrasound imaging involved administration of aerated saline or carbon dioxide. Currently research is focused on the development of gas microspheres, which are injected into the patient to provide visual contrast during the ultrasound study. Specific applications of ultrasound contrast are found in Chapter 17.

ROLE OF THE SONOGRAPHER

The sonographer is an allied health professional who has received specific training in diagnostic medical sonography (general applications) or cardiovascular technology (cardiac and vascular applications). The sonographer performs ultrasound procedures and gathers diagnostic data under the direct or indirect supervision of a physician. Sonographers are known as "image makers" who have the ability to create images of soft tissue structures and organs inside the body, such as the liver, pancreas, biliary system, kidneys, heart, vascular system, muscular skeletal system, uterus, and fetus. In addition, sonographers can record hemodynamic information with velocity measurements through the use of color Doppler and spectral analysis to determine if a vessel or cardiac valve is patent (open) or restricted.

Sonographers work directly with physicians and patients as a team member in a medical facility. They also interact with nurses and other medical staff as part of the health care team. The sonographer must be able to review the patient's records to assess clinical history and clinical symptoms, interpret laboratory values, and review other pertinent diagnostic examinations. The sonographer is required to understand and operate complex ultrasound instrumentation using the basic principles of ultrasound physics.

To produce the highest-quality sonographic image for interpretation, the sonographer must possess an in-depth understanding of anatomy and pathophysiology and be able to evaluate a patient's problem specific to the examination ordered. Sonographers use their knowledge and skills to provide physicians with clinical information such as the rapid **FAST** scan evaluation of a trauma victim's injury, visualization of detailed fetal anatomy, and measurement and evaluation of fetal growth and progress or even to evaluate the patient for cardiac abnormalities or injury. In addition to technical expertise and knowledge of anatomy and pathophysiology, several other qualities contribute to the sonographer's success (Box 1.1).

What makes the sonographer distinct from the other health care professionals? The sonographer:

- Reviews the clinical chart and speaks directly with patients to identify symptoms that relate directly to the ultrasound examination.
- Explains the procedure to the patient and performs the examination using the protocol established by the department.
- Analyses each image and correlates the information with patient information.
- Uses independent judgment in recognizing the need to make adjustments with the sonographic protocol to answer the clinical question.
- Reviews the previous sonograms and provides an oral or written summary of the technical findings to the physician for the medical diagnosis.
- Alerts the physician if critical findings or new changes are found on the sonographic examination.

Advantages and Disadvantages of a Sonography Career

Advantages. Sonographers with specialized education in ultrasound obtained from a nationally accredited diagnostic medical sonography or cardiovascular technology program have demonstrated their ability to analyze the clinical situation and to produce high-quality sonographic images, thereby earning the respect of other allied health professionals and clinicians. Every day, sonographers are faced with varied human interactions and opportunities to solve problems. These experiences give sonographers an outlet for their creativity by requiring them to come up with innovative ways to meet the challenges of performing quality sonographic examinations on difficult patients. Sonographers must have the creative ability to alter their normal protocol as difficult situations arise (i.e., trauma patient, immobile patient, postoperative surgical patient with multiple bandages). New applications in ultrasound and improvements in instrumentation create a continual challenge for the sonographer. Flexible schedules and variety in examinations and equipment, not to mention patient personalities, make each day interesting and unique. Certified sonographers find that employment opportunities are abundant, schedule flexibility is high, and salaries are attractive.

Disadvantages. Some sonographers find their position to be stressful and demanding, with the constant changes in medical care and decreased staffing causing increased workloads. Hours of continual scanning may lead to tendinitis, arm and shoulder pain, and back strain. (Chapter 3 focuses on ergonomics and musculoskeletal issues in sonography.)

Sonographers may become frustrated when dealing with terminally ill patients, which can lead to fatigue and depression.

Employment. The field of sonography continues to expand. The demand for certified sonographers exceeds the supply nationwide. Sonographers may find employment in the traditional setting of a hospital or medical clinic. Staffing positions within the hospital or medical setting may include the following: Director of Imaging, Technical Director, Manager, Supervisor, Chief Sonographer, Sonographer Educator, Clinical **S**taff Sonographer, Research Sonographer, or Clinical Instructor. Clinical research opportunities may be found in the major medical centers throughout the country.

BOX 1.1 | Qualities of a Sonographer

The sonographer must possess the following qualities and talents:

Intellectual curiosity to keep abreast of developments in the field

Perseverance to obtain high-quality images and the ability to differentiate an artifact from structural anatomy

Ability to conceptualize two-dimensional (2D) images into a 3D format; ability to reconstruct a 2D image into a 3D format to produce an "en face" image

Quick and analytical mind to continually analyze image quality while keeping the clinical situation in mind

Technical aptitude to produce diagnostic-quality images

Good physical health because continuous scanning may cause strain on back, shoulder, or arm. Equipment is mobile; thus the sonographer must be able to manipulate equipment weighing greater than 250 pounds. Doppler is audible; thus sonographers must have adequate hearing to interpolate the returning Doppler audible sound

Independence and initiative to analyze the patient, the history, and the clinical findings and tailor the examination to answer the clinical question

Emotional stability to deal with patients in times of crisis; this means the ability to understand the patient's concerns without losing objectivity

Communication skills for interactions with peers, clinicians, and patients; this includes the ability to clearly communicate ultrasound findings to physicians and the ability *not* to disclose or speculate on findings to the patient during the examination

Dedication because a willingness to go beyond the "call of duty" is often required of the sonographer

Sonographers with advanced degrees (e.g., BS, MS, or PhD) may serve as faculty in diagnostic medical sonography programs as Program Director, Department Head, or Dean of Allied Health. Many sonographers have entered the commercial world as Clinical Application Specialists or Director of Education/Continuing Education Director, marketing specialist, product design/engineering, sales, service, or quality control. Other sonographers have become independent business partners in medicine by offering mobile ultrasound services to smaller community hospitals.

Resource Organizations. Specific organizations are devoted to developing standards and guidelines for ultrasound:

- American Institute of Ultrasound in Medicine (AIUM), www.aium.org. This organization represents all facets of ultrasound to include physicians, sonographers, biomedical engineers, scientists, and commercial researchers.
- American Society of Echocardiography (ASE), www.asecho.org. This very active organization represents physicians, sonographers, and scientists involved with cardiovascular applications of sonography.
- Society of Diagnostic Medical Sonography (SDMS), www.sdms.org. This is the principal organization for more than 25,000 sonographers. The website contains information regarding the SDMS position statement on the code of ethics for the profession of diagnostic medical ultrasound; the nondiagnostic use of ultrasound, the scope of practice for the diagnostic ultrasound professional, and diagnostic ultrasound clinical practice standards.
- Society for Vascular Ultrasound (SVU), www.svunet.org. This is the principal organization representing physicians, sonographers, and scientists in vascular sonography.

Certification. The National Certification Examination for Ultrasound is provided by the American Registry for Diagnostic Medical Sonography (ARDMS), www.ardms.org. This is the primary organization offering international credentials for sonographers once their training has been completed.

Joint Review Committee. The national review boards for educational programs in sonography are provided by two groups:

- Joint Review Committee on Education in Diagnostic Medical Sonography (JRC-DMS) (includes general ultrasound, echocardiography, and vascular technology), www.jrcdms.org.
- Joint Review Committee on Education in Cardiovascular Technology (JRC-CVT) (includes noninvasive cardiology (echocardiography), invasive cardiology (cardiac catheterization), and vascular technology), www.jrccvt.org.

HISTORICAL OVERVIEW OF SOUND THEORY AND MEDICAL ULTRASOUND

A complete history of sound theory and the development of medical ultrasound is beyond the scope of this textbook. The following is a brief overview designed to provide readers a sense of the extensive history and exciting developments in this area of study. For a more detailed outline of historical data, the reader is referred to Dr. Joseph Woo's excellent article "A Short History of the Development of Ultrasound in Obstetrics and Gynecology" and other resources listed in the Selected Bibliography at the end of this chapter.

The story of acoustics began with the Greek philosopher **Pythagoras** (6th century BC), whose experiments on the properties of vibrating strings led to the invention of the sonometer, an instrument used to study musical sounds. Several hundred years later, in 1500 AD, **Leonardo da Vinci** (1452–1519) discovered that sound traveled in waves and discovered that the **angle of reflection** is equal to the **angle of incidence**. **Galileo Galilei** (1564–1642) is said to have started modern studies of acoustics by elevating the study of vibrations to scientific standards. In 1638, he demonstrated that the frequency of sound waves determined the pitch. **Sir Isaac Newton** (1643–1727) studied the speed of sound in air and provided the first analytic determination of the speed of sound. **Robert Boyle** (1627–1691), an Irish natural philosopher, chemist, physicist, and inventor, demonstrated the physical characteristics of air, showing that it is necessary in combustion, respiration, and sound transmission. **Lazzaro Spallanzani** (1729–1799), an Italian biologist and physiologist, essentially discovered echolocation. Spallanzani is famous for extensive experiments on bat navigation, from which he concluded that bats use sound and their ears for navigation in total darkness. **Augustin Fresnel** (1788–1827) was a French physicist who contributed significantly to the establishment of the theory of wave optics, forming the theory of wave diffraction named after him. **Sir Francis Galton** (1822–1911) was an English Victorian scholar, explorer, and inventor. One of his numerous inventions was the Galton whistle used for testing differential hearing ability. This is an ultrasonic whistle, also known as a dog whistle or a silent whistle. **Christian Johann Doppler** (1803–1853) was an Austrian mathematician and physicist. He is most famous for what is now called the "Doppler effect," which is the apparent change in frequency and wavelength of a wave as perceived by an observer moving relative to the wave's source. In 1880, **Paul-Jacques Curie** (1856–1941) and his brother **Pierre Curie** (1859–1906) discovered *piezoelectricity*, whereby physical pressure applied to a crystal resulted in the creation of an electric potential. **John William Strutt (Lord Rayleigh)** (1842–1919) wrote *The Theory of Sound*. The first volume, on the mechanics of a vibrating medium which produces sound, was published in 1877; the second volume on acoustic wave propagation was published the following year. **Paul Langevin** (1872–1946) was a French physicist and is noted for his work on paramagnetism and diamagnetism. He devised the modern interpretation of this phenomenon in terms of spins of electrons within atoms. His most famous work was on the use of ultrasound using Pierre and Jacques Curie's piezoelectric effect. During World War I, he began working on the use of these sounds to detect submarines through echolocation.

Sonar is an acronym for *sound navigation and ranging*. Sonar is a technique that uses sound propagation, usually underwater, to navigate, communicate with, or detect other vessels. Sonar may be used as a means of acoustic location and measurement of the echo characteristics of "targets" in the water. The term *sonar* is also used for the equipment necessary to generate and receive the sound. The acoustic frequencies used in sonar systems vary from very low (infrasonic) to extremely high (ultrasonic). World War II brought sonar equipment to the forefront of military defense, and medical ultrasound was influenced by the advances in sonar instrumentation.

In the 1940s, **Dr. Karl Dussik** (1908–1968) made one of the earliest applications of ultrasound to medical diagnosis when he used two transducers positioned on opposite sides of the head to measure ultrasound transmission profiles (Fig. 1.1). He discovered that tumors and other intracranial lesions could be detected by this technique. **Dr. William Fry**, an electrical engineer whose primary research was in the field of ultrasound, is credited with being the first to introduce the use of computers in diagnostic ultrasound. Around this same time, he and **Dr. Russell Meyers** performed craniotomies and used ultrasound to destroy parts of the basal ganglia in patients with parkinsonism.

Between 1948 and 1950, three investigators, **Drs. Douglass Howry**, a radiologist, **John Wild**, a clinician interested in tissue characterization, and **George Ludwig**, who was interested in reflections from gallstones, each demonstrated independently that when ultrasound waves generated by a piezoelectric crystal transducer are transmitted into the body, ultrasound waves of different acoustic impedances are returned to the transducer.

One of the pioneers in the clinical investigation and development of ultrasound was **Dr. Joseph Holmes** (1902–1982). A nephrologist by training, Dr. Holmes' initial interest in ultrasound involved its ability to detect bubbles in hemodialysis tubing. Holmes began work in ultrasound at the University of Colorado Medical Center in 1950, in collaboration with a group headed by **Douglass Howry**. In 1951, supported by Joseph H. Holmes, Douglass Howry, along with **William Roderic Bliss** and **Gerald J. Posakony**, both engineers, produced the "immersion tank ultrasound system," the first 2D B-mode (or plan position indicator [PPI] mode) linear compound scanner (Fig. 1.2). 2D cross-sectional images, published in 1952, demonstrated that interpretable 2D images of internal organ structures and pathologies could be obtained with ultrasound. The *Pan Scanner*, created by the Holmes, Howry, Posakony, and **Richard Cushman** team in 1957, was a landmark invention in the history of B-mode ultrasonography. With the Pan Scanner, the patient sat on a modified dental chair strapped against a plastic window of a semicircular pan filled with saline solution while the transducer rotated through the solution in a semicircular arc (Fig. 1.3).

In 1954, echocardiographic ultrasound applications were developed in Sweden by Drs. **Hellmuth Hertz** and **Inge Edler**, who first described the M-mode (motion) display (Fig. 1.4).

An early obstetric contact compound scanner was built by **Tom Brown** and **Dr. Ian Donald** (1910–1987) in Scotland in 1957. Dr. Donald went on to discover many fascinating image patterns in the obstetric patient; his work is still referred to today. Meanwhile, in the early 1960s in Philadelphia, **Dr. J Stauffer Lehman** designed a real-time water path obstetric ultrasound system (Fig. 1.5A).

In 1959 the Ultrasonic Institute was formed at the National Acoustic Laboratory in Sydney, Australia. **George Kossoff** and his team, including **Dr. William Garrett** and **David Robinson**, developed diagnostic B-scanners with the use of a water bath to improve resolution of the image

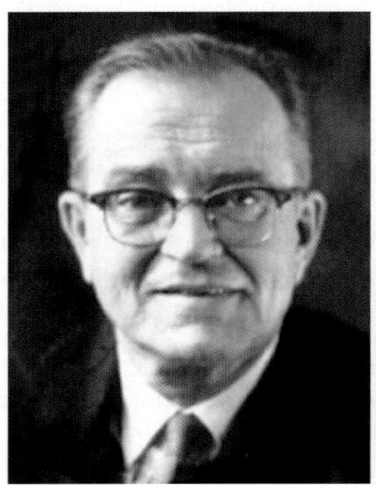
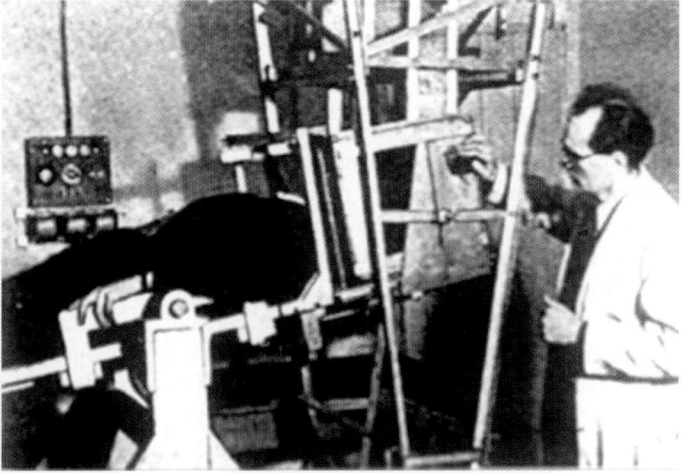

FIG. 1.1 In the 1940s, Dr. Karl Dussik (1908–1968) made one of the earliest applications of ultrasound to medical diagnosis when he used two transducers positioned on opposite sides of the head to measure ultrasound transmission profiles. He discovered that tumors and other intracranial lesions could be detected by this technique.

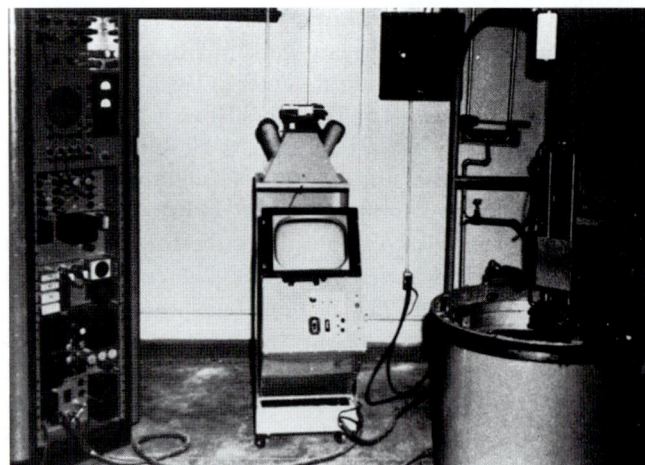

FIG. 1.2 Douglass Howry, along with William Roderic Bliss and Gerald J. Posakony, both engineers, produced the "immersion tank ultrasound system," the first two-dimensional B-mode (or plan position indicator mode) linear compound scanner.

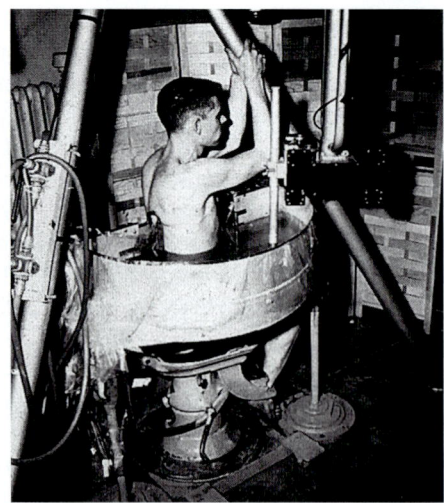

FIG. 1.3 The *Pan Scanner*, put together by the Holmes, Howry, Posakony, and Richard Cushman team in 1957, was a landmark invention in the history of B-mode ultrasonography. With the Pan Scanner, the patient sat on a modified dental chair strapped against a plastic window of a semicircular pan filled with saline solution while the transducer rotated through the solution in a semicircular arc.

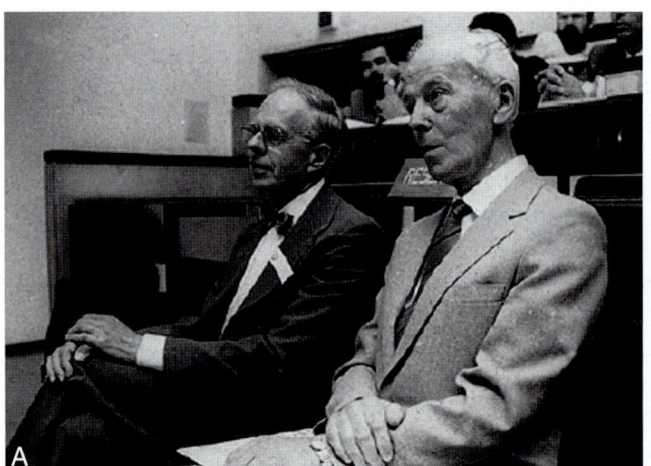
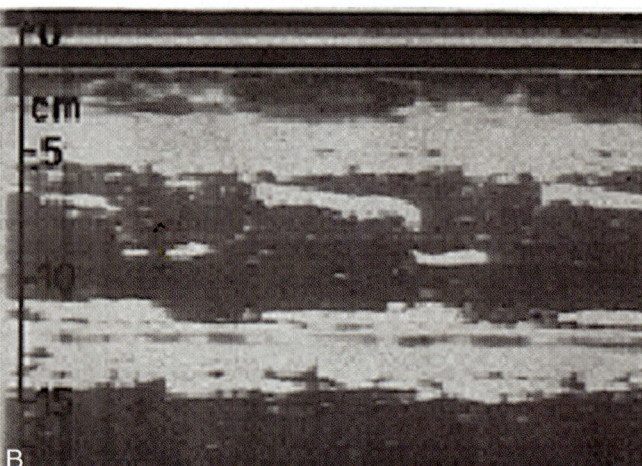

FIG. 1.4 (A) In 1954, echocardiographic ultrasound applications were developed in Sweden by Drs. Hellmuth Hertz and Inge Edler, who first described the M-mode (motion) display. (B) M-mode display of mitral stenosis.

(Figs. 1.5 and 1.6). This group was also responsible for introducing gray-scale imaging in 1972. Kossoff and his colleagues were pioneers in the development of large-aperture, multitransducer technology in which the transducers were automatically programmed to operate independently or as a whole to provide high-quality images without operator intervention, as was required with the contact static scanner that had been developed in 1962 at the University of Colorado.

The advent of real-time scanners changed the face of ultrasound scanning. The first real-time scanner (initially known as a fast B-scanner) was developed by **Walter Krause** and **Richard Soldner**. It was manufactured as the Vidoscan by Siemens Medical Systems of Germany in 1965. The Vidoscan used three rotating transducers housed in front of a parabolic mirror in a water coupling system and produced 15 images per second. The image was made up of 120 lines with basic gray scale. The use of fixed-focus, large-face transducers produced a narrow beam to ensure good resolution and a good image. Fetal life and motions could be demonstrated clearly. In 1973 **James Griffith** and **Walter Henry** at the National Institutes of Health produced a mechanical oscillating real-time scanning device that could produce clear 30-degree sector real-time cardiac images with good resolution. The phased-array scanning mechanism was first described by **Jan Somer** at the University of Limberg in the Netherlands and was in use from 1968, several years before the appearance of linear-array systems.

Medical applications of ultrasonic Doppler techniques were first implemented by **Shigeo Satomura** and **Yasuhara Nimura**

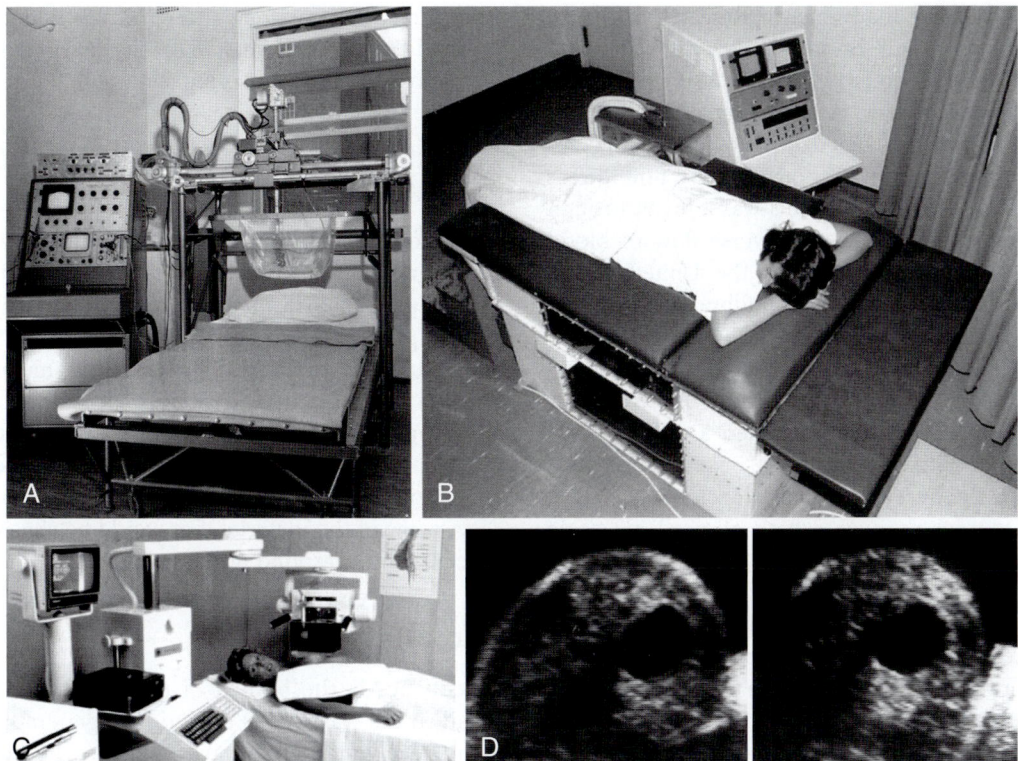

FIG. 1.5 (A) Dr. J. Stauffer Lehman designed a real-time water bath obstetric ultrasound system in Philadelphia. The weight of the water path compressed the mother's inferior vena cava and caused her to become lightheaded. (B–C) Further developments of the water path system show the patient prone with the breast suspended in water or the patient supine with the water path compressing the breast. (D) Images of a breast cyst imaged with the breast suspended.

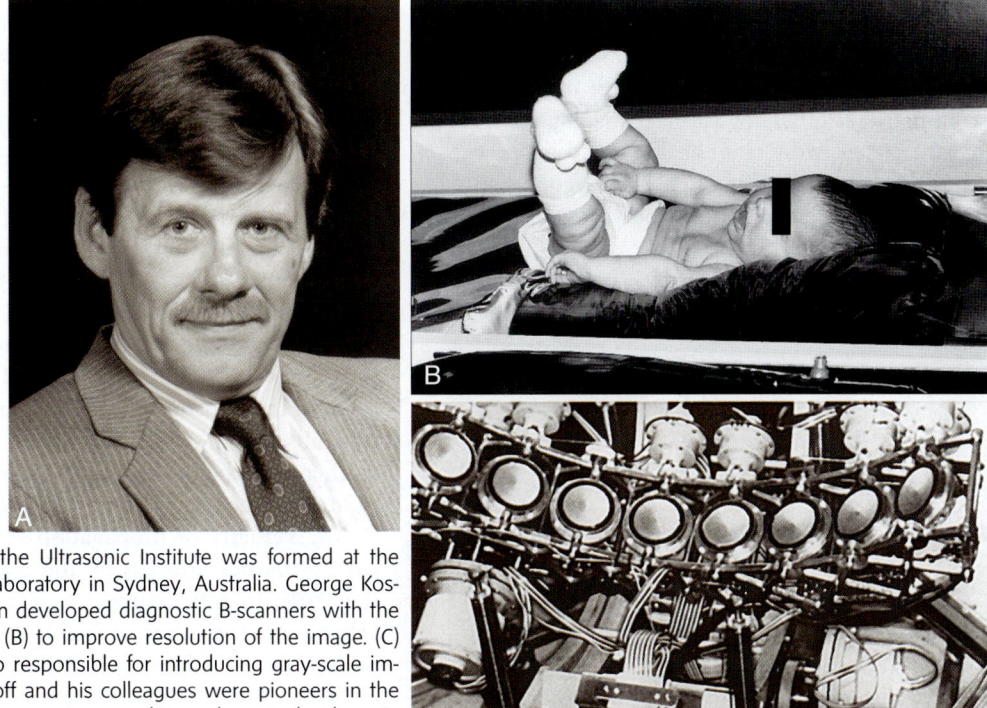

FIG. 1.6 In 1959 the Ultrasonic Institute was formed at the National Acoustic Laboratory in Sydney, Australia. George Kossoff (A) and his team developed diagnostic B-scanners with the use of a water bath (B) to improve resolution of the image. (C) This group was also responsible for introducing gray-scale imaging in 1972. Kossoff and his colleagues were pioneers in the development of large-aperture, multitransducer technology in which the transducers were automatically programmed to operate independently or as a whole to provide high-quality images without operator intervention.

at the Institute of Scientific and Industrial Research in Osaka, Japan, in 1955 for the study of cardiac valve motion and pulsations of peripheral blood vessels. This team pioneered transcutaneous Doppler flow measurements in 1959. In 1966 **Kato** and **T. Izumi** pioneered the directional flowmeter using the local oscillation method whereby flow directions were detected and displayed. This was a breakthrough in Doppler instrumentation because reverse flow in blood vessels could now be documented. In the United States, **Robert Rushmer** and his team did groundbreaking work in Doppler instrumentation, beginning in 1958. They pioneered transcutaneous continuous wave (CW) flow measurements and spectral analysis in 1963. **Donald Baker**, a member of Rushmer's team, introduced a pulsed-Doppler system in 1970 (Fig. 1.7). In 1974 Baker, along with **John Reid**, **Frank Barber**, and others, developed the first duplex pulsed-Doppler scanner, which allowed 2D scale imaging to be used to guide placement of the ultrasound beam for Doppler signal acquisition. In 1985 a work entitled "Real-Time Two-Dimensional Blood Flow Imaging Using an Autocorrelation Technique" by **Chihiro Kasai**, **Koroku Namekawa**, and **Ryozo Omoto** was published in English. The autocorrelation technique described in this publication could be applied to estimating blood velocity and turbulence in color flow imaging. The autocorrelation technique is a method for estimating the dominating frequency in a complex signal, as well as its variance. The algorithm is both computationally faster and significantly more accurate compared with the Fourier transform because the resolution is not limited by the number of samples used. This provided the rapid means of frequency estimation to be performed in real time that is still used currently.

In 1987 The Center for Emerging Cardiovascular Technologies at **Duke University** started a project to develop a real-time volumetric scanner for cardiac imaging. In 1991 they produced a matrix array scanner that could image cardiac structures in real time and in 3D. By the second half of the 1990s, many other centers throughout the world were working on laboratory and clinical research into 3D ultrasound (3DU). Currently, 3DU has developed into a clinically effective diagnostic imaging technique.

INTRODUCTION TO BASIC ULTRASOUND PRINCIPLES

To produce high-quality images that are free of artifacts, the sonographer must have a firm understanding of the basic principles of ultrasound. This section introduces the basic principles of acoustics, measurement units, instrumentation, real-time sonography, 3DU, harmonic imaging, and optimization of gray-scale and Doppler ultrasound to reinforce the sonographer's understanding of scanning techniques. The student sonographer needs to understand a new language and terminology with ultrasound physics. This serves as a brief overview of the material that would be covered in depth in a dedicated ultrasound physics textbook.

Acoustics

Acoustics is the branch of physics that deals with sound and sound waves. It is the study of generating, propagating, and receiving sound waves. Within the field of acoustics, *ultrasound* is defined as sound frequencies that are beyond (ultra-) the range of normal human hearing. Most human hearing ranges between 20 **hertz (Hz)** and 20 **kilohertz (kHz)** (Fig. 1.8). Thus ultrasound refers to sound frequencies greater than 20 kHz.

Sound is the result of mechanical energy that produces alternating **compression** and **rarefaction** of the conducting medium as it travels as a wave (Fig. 1.9). (A **wave** is a propagation of energy that moves back and forth or vibrates at a steady rate.) Diagnostic ultrasound uses short sound pulses at frequencies of 1 to 20 million **cycles**/sec (**megahertz [MHz]**) that are transmitted into the body to examine soft tissue anatomic structures (Table 1.1). In medical ultrasound, the piezoelectric vibrating source within the transducer is a ceramic element that vibrates in response to an electrical signal. The vibrating motion of the ceramic element in the transducer causes the particles in the surrounding tissue to vibrate. In this way the ultrasound transducer converts electrical energy into mechanical energy as the sonographic imaging is produced. As the sound beam is directed into the body by the transducer at various angles to the organs, reflection, absorption, and scatter cause the returning signal to be weaker than the initial impulse. Over a short period of time, multiple anatomic images are acquired in a real-time format.

The **velocity** of propagation is constant for a given tissue and is not affected by the frequency or wavelength of the pulse. In soft tissues, the assumed average propagation velocity is 1540 m/sec (Table 1.2). It is the stiffness and the density of a medium that determine how fast sound waves will travel through the structure. The more closely packed the molecules, the faster is the speed of sound.

The velocity of sound differs greatly among air, bone, and soft tissue, although the velocity of sound varies by only a little

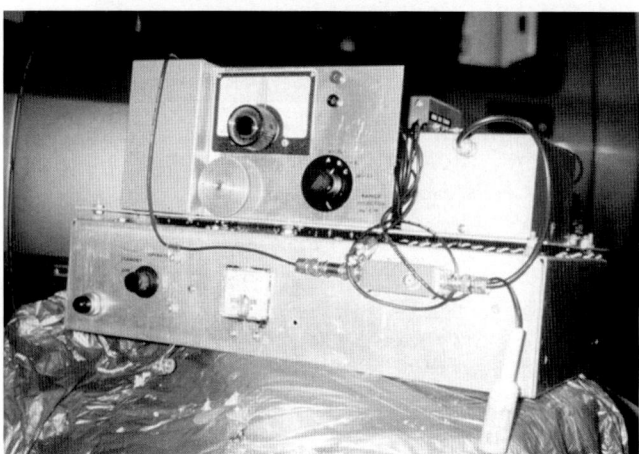

FIG. 1.7 Donald Baker, a member of Rushmer's team, introduced a pulsed-Doppler system in 1966.

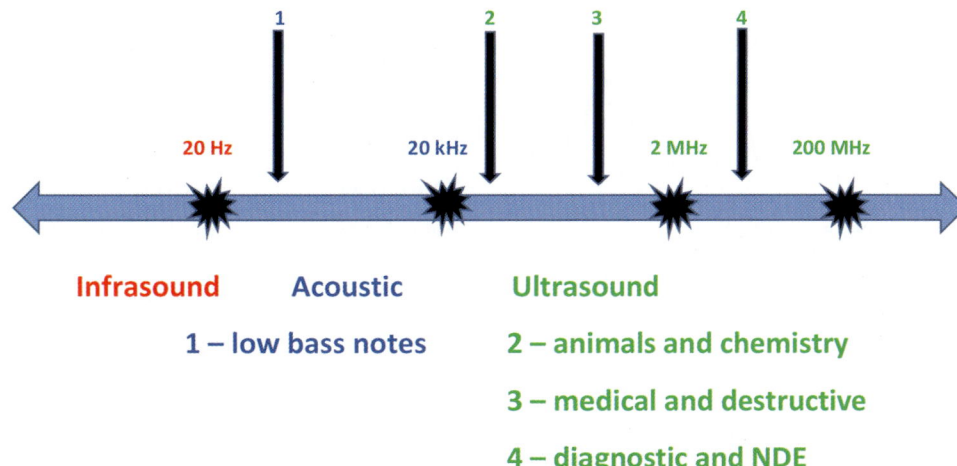

FIG. 1.8 Acoustics is the branch of physics that deals with sound and sound waves. Within the field of acoustics, ultrasound is defined as sound frequencies that are beyond (ultra-) the range of normal human hearing. Most human hearing ranges between 20 hertz (Hz) and 20 kilohertz (kHz). Thus ultrasound refers to sound frequencies greater than 20 kHz.

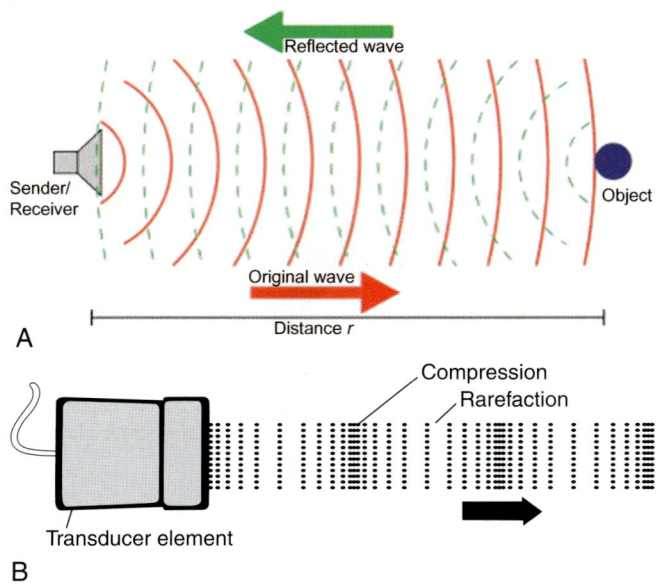

FIG. 1.9 (A) Ultrasound waves are created by a vibrating crystal within a ceramic probe. Waves travel through the tissue and are partly reflected at each tissue interface. (B) As the transducer element vibrates, waves undergo compression and expansion, or rarefaction, by which the molecules are pulled apart.

TABLE 1.1	Applications of Sound Frequency Ranges	
Frequency Range	Manner of Production	Application
Infrasound		
0–25 Hz	Electromagnetic vibrators	Vibration analysis of structures
Audible		
20 Hz–20 kHz	Electromagnetic vibrators, musical instruments	Communications, signaling
Ultrasound		
20–100 kHz	Air whistles, electric devices	Biology, sonar
100 kHz–1 MHz	Electric devices	Flaw detection, biology
1–20 MHz	Electric devices	Diagnostic ultrasound

Hz, Hertz; *kHz*, kilohertz; *MHz*, megahertz.

from one soft tissue to another. Sound waves travel slowly through gas (air), at intermediate speed through liquids, and quickly through solids (metal). Air-filled structures, such as the lungs and stomach, or gas-filled structures, such as the bowel, impede the sound transmission, and sound is attenuated through most bony structures. Small differences among fat, blood, and organ tissues that are seen on an ultrasound image may be better delineated with higher-frequency transducers that improve resolution but lose the depth penetration.
Measurement of Sound. The **decibel (dB)** unit is used to measure the intensity (strength), amplitude, and power of an ultrasound wave. Decibels allow the sonographer to compare

TABLE 1.2	Characteristic Acoustic Impedance and Velocity of Ultrasound	
Material	Acoustic Impedance (g/cm/sec × 10)	Velocity
Air	0.0001	331
Fat	1.38	1450
Water	1.50	1430
Blood	1.61	1570
Kidney	1.62	1560
Liver	1.65	1550
Muscle	1.70	1580
Skull	7.80	4080

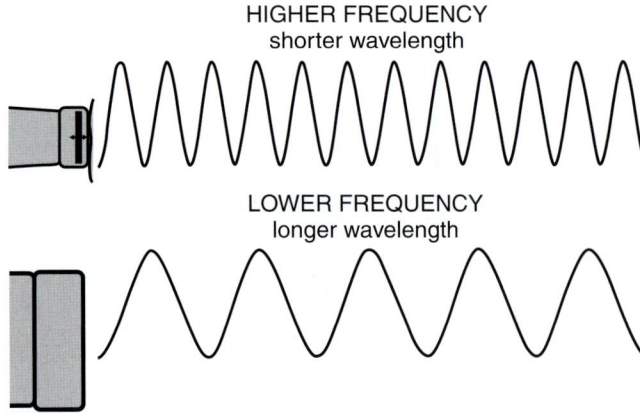

FIG. 1.10 Wavelength is inversely related to frequency. The higher the frequency, the shorter is the wavelength and the less is the depth of penetration. The longer wavelength has a lower frequency and a greater depth of penetration.

the intensity or **amplitude** of two signals. **Power** refers to the rate at which energy is transmitted. Power is the rate of energy flow over the entire beam of sound and is often measured in watts (W) or milliwatts (mW). **Intensity** is defined as power per unit area. It is the rate of energy flow across a defined area of the beam and can be measured in watts per square meter (W/m²) or milliwatts per square centimeter. Power and intensity are directly related: If you double the power, the intensity also doubles.

Frequency. Sound is characterized according to its frequency (Fig. 1.10). Frequency may be explained by the following analogy: If a stick were moved into and out of a pond at a steady rate, the entire surface of the water would be covered with waves radiating from the stick. If the number of vibrations made in each second were counted, the frequency of vibration could be determined. In ultrasound, **frequency** describes the number of oscillations per second performed by the particles of the medium in which the wave is propagating:

1 oscillation/sec = 1 cycle/sec = 1 **hertz (1 Hz)**
1000 oscillations/sec = 1 kilocycle/sec = 1 **kilohertz (1 kHz)**
1,000,000 oscillations/sec = 1 megacycle/sec = 1 **megahertz (1 MHz)**

The sonographer should be familiar with the units of measurement commonly used in ultrasound (Table 1.3).

Propagation of Sound Through Tissue. Once sound pulses are transmitted into a body, they can be reflected, scattered, refracted, or absorbed. **Reflection** occurs whenever the pulse encounters an **interface** between tissues with different acoustic impedances (Fig. 1.11). **Acoustic impedance** is the measure of a material's **resistance** to the propagation of sound. The strength of the reflection depends on the difference in acoustic impedance between the tissues, as well as the size of the interface, its surface characteristics, and its orientation with respect to the transmitted sound pulse. The greater the acoustic mismatch, the greater is the backscatter or reflection (Fig. 1.12). Large, smooth interfaces are called *specular reflectors*. If specular reflectors are aligned perpendicular to the direction of the transmitted pulse, they reflect sound

TABLE 1.3	Units Commonly Used in Ultrasound	
Quantity	**Unit**	**Abbreviation**
Amplifier gain	Decibels	dB
Area	Meters squared	m²
Attenuation	Decibels	dB
Attenuation coefficient	Decibels per centimeter	dB/cm
Frequency	Hertz (cycles per second)	Hz
Intensity	Watts per square meter	W/m²
Length	Meter	m
Period	Microseconds	μsec
Power	Watts	W
Pressure amplitude	Pascals	Pa
Relative power	Decibels	dB
Speed	Meters per second	m/sec
Time	Seconds	sec
Volume	Meters cubed	m³

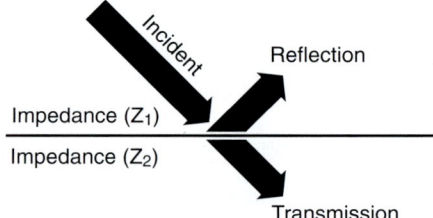

FIG. 1.11 Reflection occurs when a sound wave strikes an interface between two objects with different acoustic impedances, causing some of the energy to be transmitted across the interface and some of it to be reflected.

directly back to the active crystal elements in the transducer and produce a strong signal. Specular reflectors that are not oriented perpendicular to the sound produce a weaker signal. **Scattering** refers to the redirection of sound in multiple directions. This produces a weak signal and occurs when the pulse encounters a small acoustic interface or a large interface that is rough (Fig. 1.13). **Refraction** is a change in the direction of sound that occurs when sound encounters an interface between two tissues that transmit sound at different speeds. Because the sound frequency remains constant, the **wavelength** changes to accommodate differences in the speed of sound in the two tissues. The result of this change in wavelength is a redirection of the sound pulse as it passes through the interface. **Absorption** describes the loss of sound energy secondary to its conversion to thermal energy. This is greater in soft tissues than in fluid and greater in bone than in soft tissues. Absorption is a major cause of acoustic shadowing.

Piezoelectric Crystals. The piezoelectric effect is a method by which ultrasound is generated. An ultrasound transducer, consisting of an array of piezoelectric crystals, is used to

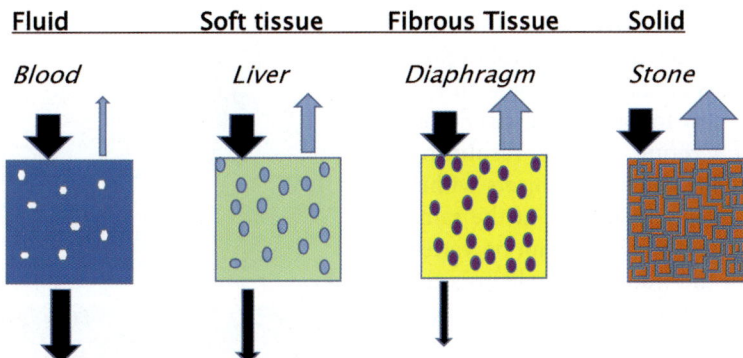

FIG. 1.12 Acoustic impedance is the measure of a material's resistance to the propagation of sound. The strength of the reflection depends on the difference in acoustic impedance between the tissues, as well as the size of the interface, its surface characteristics, and its orientation with respect to the transmitted sound pulse. The greater the acoustic mismatch, the greater is the backscatter or reflection.

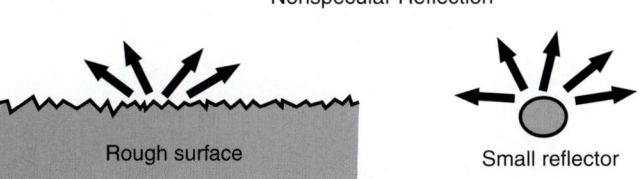

FIG. 1.13 Scattering. Nonspecular reflectors reflect, or scatter, the sound wave in many directions.

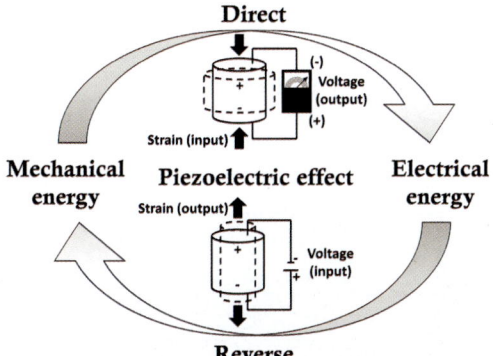

FIG. 1.14 Piezoelectric effect. When a ceramic crystal is electronically stimulated, it deforms and vibrates to produce the sound pulses used in diagnostic sonography. If the organ or structure is exposed to an electric shock, it will begin to vibrate and transmit a sound wave back to the crystal.

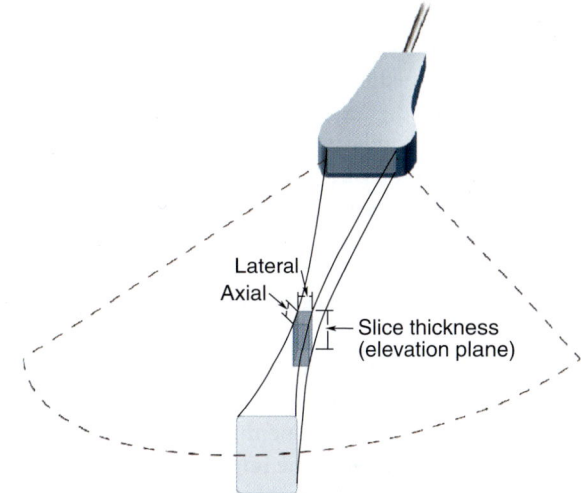

FIG. 1.15 Axial resolution refers to the ability to resolve objects within the imaging plane that are located at different depths along the direction of the sound pulse. Lateral resolution refers to the ability to resolve objects within the imaging plane that are located side by side at the same depth from the transducer. Azimuthal (elevation) resolution refers to the ability to resolve objects that are the same distance from the transducer but are located perpendicular to the plane of imaging.

generate and detect (or receive) ultrasound waves (Fig. 1.14). An ultrasound transducer converts electrical energy to a mechanical vibration and vice versa. Because ultrasound is a mechanical wave in a longitudinal direction, it is transmitted in a straight line and it can be focused. These waves obey laws of reflection and refraction.

Pulse duration is the time that a piezoelectric element vibrates after electrical stimulation. Each pulse consists of a band of frequencies referred to as *bandwidth*. The center frequency produced by a transducer is the resonant frequency of the crystal element and depends on the thickness of the crystal. The echoes that return to the transducer distort the crystal elements and generate an electric pulse that is processed into an image. The higher-amplitude echoes produce a greater crystal deformation and generate a larger electronic voltage, which is displayed as a brighter pixel. These 2D images are known as *B-mode*, or brightness mode, images.

Image Resolution. **Resolution** is the ability of an imaging process to distinguish adjacent structures in an object and is an important measure of image quality. The resolution of the ultrasound image is determined by the size and configuration of the transmitted sound pulse. Resolution is always considered in three dimensions: axial, lateral, and azimuthal (elevation). **Axial resolution** (Fig. 1.15) refers to the ability to resolve objects within the imaging plane that are located at different depths along the direction of the sound pulse. This depends on the direction of the sound pulse, which, in turn, depends on the wavelength. Because wavelength is inversely proportional to frequency, the higher-frequency probes produce shorter pulses and better axial resolution but with less penetration. These probes are best for superficial structures such as thyroid, breast, and scrotum. **Lateral resolution** (see Fig. 1.15) refers to the ability to resolve objects within the imaging plane that are located side by side at the same depth from the transducer. Lateral resolution can be varied by adjusting the **focal zone** of the transducer, which is the point at which the beam is the narrowest. **Azimuthal** (elevation) **resolution** (see Fig. 1.15) refers to the ability to resolve objects that are the same distance from the transducer but are located perpendicular to the plane of imaging. Azimuthal resolution is also related to the thickness of the tomographic slice. **Slice thickness** is usually determined by the shape of the crystal elements or the characteristics of fixed acoustic lenses.

Attenuation. Attenuation is the sum of acoustic energy loss resulting from absorption, scattering, and reflection. It refers to the reduction in intensity and amplitude of a sound wave as it travels through a medium as some of the energy is absorbed, reflected, or scattered (Fig. 1.16A). Thus, as the sound beam travels through the body, the beam becomes progressively weaker. In human soft tissue, sound is attenuated at the rate of 0.5 dB/cm per million hertz. If air or bone is coupled with soft tissue, more energy will be attenuated. Attenuation through a solid calcium interface, such as a gallstone, will produce a posterior shadow to the ultrasound beam with sharp borders on the ultrasound image (see Fig. 1.16B).

With the exception of air-tissue and bone interfaces, the differences in acoustic impedance in biologic tissues are so slight that only a small component of the ultrasound beam is reflected at each interface. The lung and bowel have a detrimental effect on the ultrasound beam, causing poor transmission of sound. Therefore anatomy beyond these two areas cannot be imaged because of air interference. Bone conducts sound at a much faster speed (4080 m/sec) than soft tissue. Recall the normal transmission of sound through soft tissue travels at 1540 m/sec. Much of the sound beam is absorbed or scattered as it travels through the body, undergoing progressive attenuation. The sound is reflected according to the acoustic impedance, which is related to tissue density. Most of the sound is passed into tissues deeper in the body and is reflected at other interfaces. Because acoustic impedance is the product of the velocity of sound in a medium and the density of that medium, acoustic impedance increases if the density or propagation speed increases.

Transducer Selection in a Clinical Imaging Practice

Many different types of ultrasound probes are available for the sonographer to become familiar with and understand which probe is best for a specific application. The probes are available in different frequencies with different physical dimensions, footprints, and shapes to provide specific image formats.

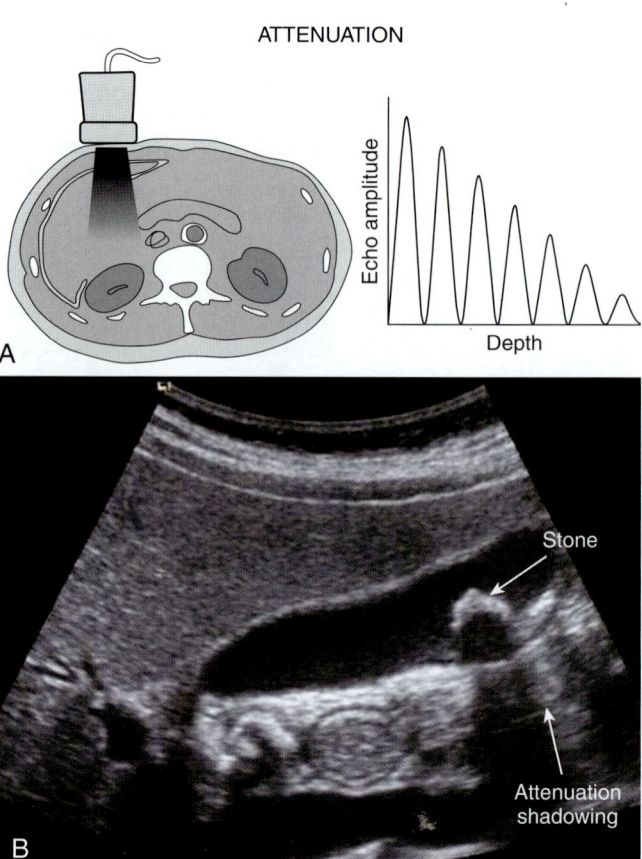

FIG. 1.16 (A) Attenuation. As the sound travels through the abdomen, it becomes attenuated, as some of it is reflected, scattered, and absorbed. (B) Large gallstone causing attenuation (shadowing) beyond the calcified stone.

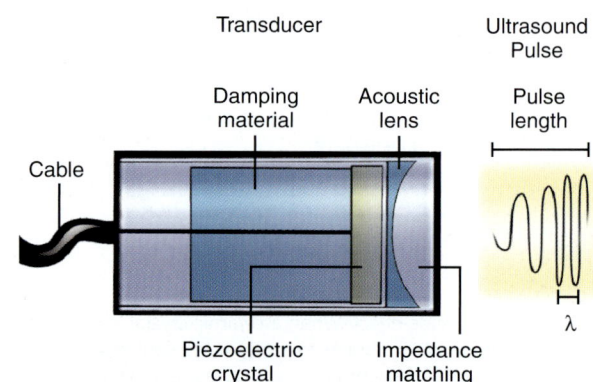

FIG. 1.17 A transducer is a device that converts energy from one form to another. Most of the transducers used currently are not a single element but rather a combination of elements that form an array. The transducer array scan head contains multiple small piezoelectric elements, each with its own electrical circuitry. These elements are very small in diameter, which greatly reduces beam divergence. A reduction in beam divergence leads to beam steering and focusing. The focus of the array transducers occurs on reception and on transmission.

A **transducer** is a device that converts energy from one form to another. Fig. 1.17 illustrates the single-element transducer design. Most of the transducers used currently are not a single element but rather a combination of elements that form an array. The transducer array scan head contains multiple small piezoelectric elements, each with its own electrical circuitry. These elements are very small in diameter, which greatly reduces beam divergence. A reduction in beam divergence leads to beam steering and focusing. The focus of the array transducers occurs on reception and on transmission (Fig. 1.18). The focusing is done dynamically during reception. Shortly after pulse transmission, the received focus is set close to the transducer. As time elapses and the echoes from the distant targets return, the focal distance is gradually lengthened. Some instruments have multiple transmit focal zones to allow better control of the resolution of the beam at certain depths of field in the image.

Very high-frequency (7 to 15 MHz) linear array probes are generally used for smaller structures (carotids, leg veins, thyroid, scrotum, breast, musculoskeletal, and peripheral vascular structures) that are superficial in nature and therefore do not require depth of view (Fig. 1.19). The footprint of the linear array may be small with small element sizes. The fine detail of the breast and thyroid uses very high frequencies (14 MHz), whereas the imaging of the peripheral vascular structures remains lower at 3 to 11 MHz.

The abdomen is usually scanned with a curved or convex array and/or a sector array; the frequency will depend on the size of the patient. Most abdominal probes are multifrequency (broadband) probes, allowing the sonographer to select the low frequency for technically difficult patients. The key factors for the selection of the convex array include the footprint, the field of view (FOV), and the radius of the curvature. The footprint describes the contact area of the area imaged and may be displayed as a rectangle, circle, or ellipse. The radius of curvature and FOV are related to the image extent and coverage. For 3D imaging in the abdomen, the fully electronic convex 2D arrays are used with two FOVs given for the orthogonal scan directions. The phased array sector probe is also available to image specific areas in the abdomen. The small footprint of the sector probe is also useful to scan in between the intercostal spaces in the abdomen.

Obstetric and gynecologic scans are usually performed with a multifocused linear or mechanically scanned convex array transducer. Matrix or fully populated 2D arrays are also available to image the fetus in real time. The endocavity probe is used to scan intercavity areas in the pelvis. The end-fire arrays are located at the end of the probe and are convex or curved arrays with wide FOVs. In addition, phased arrays in an endo-array package may be used. The frequencies are usually 5 MHz and higher.

Neonatal and pediatric probes have smaller footprints than those used for the adult. The higher frequencies (7 MHz) are used because the FOV is much less than the adult. The arrays useful in this population include the static and, for 3D,

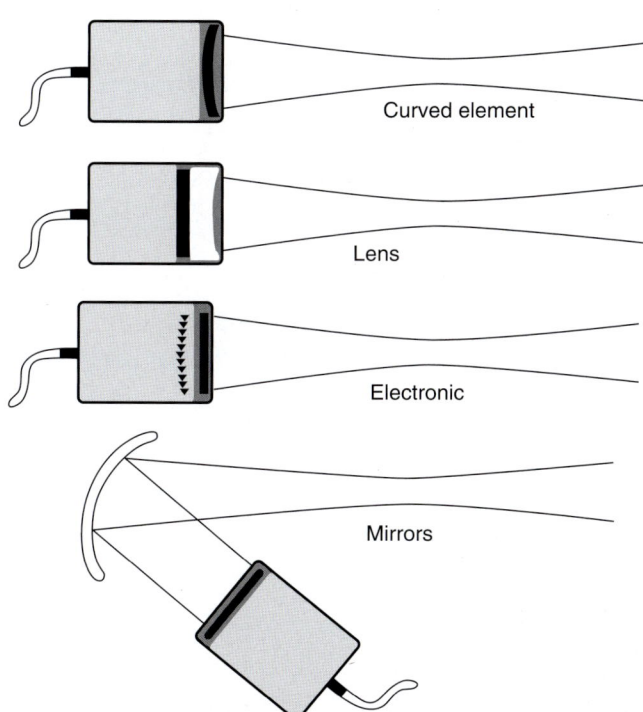

FIG. 1.18 Focusing effectively narrows the ultrasound beam. Multiple methods may be used to achieve this effect.

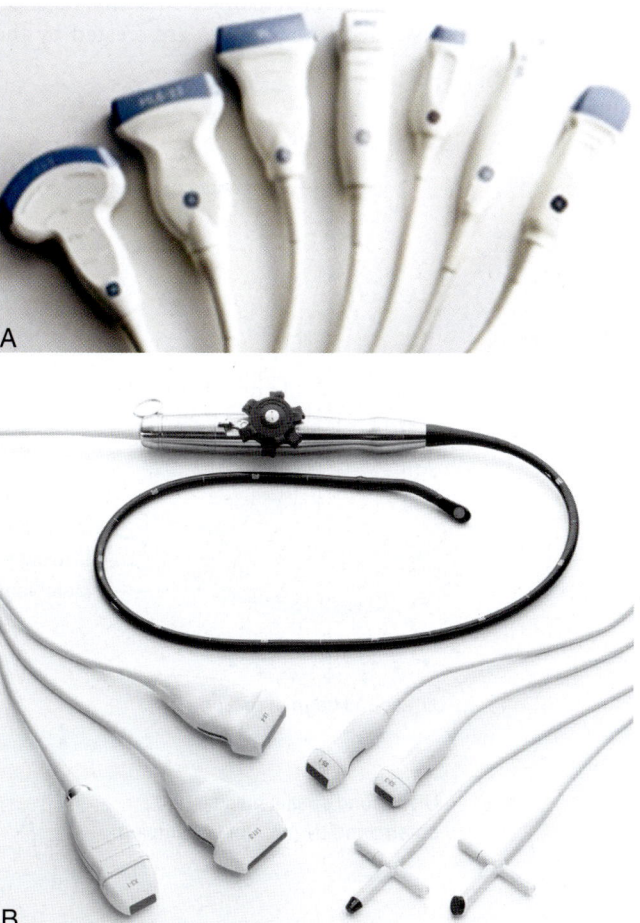

FIG. 1.19 (A) The type of transducer selected for a particular examination depends on several factors: the type of examination, size of the patient, and amount of fatty or muscular tissue present. (B) Transducers vary in size from the small Pedof transducer to the larger diameter transducers.

the mechanically swept linear array and convex probe. The cardiac images use a higher frequency phased array for 2D and 3D imaging.

The transesophageal studies are obtained with the specialized smaller transesophageal probe, which is inserted into the patient's esophagus to image detailed anatomy of the cardiac structures. This phased array or matrix probe uses high frequencies (5 MHz) and are implemented with manipulators and motors to adjust the orientation of the transducer by the physician. These probes are available in both adult and pediatric sizes.

A smaller intracardiac phased array probe with very high frequencies (20 MHz) may be used during specialized cardiac catheterization procedures to image the coronary arteries. Other surgical intracavity probes may be used during laparoscopic surgery to image vessels or specific areas in the abdomen.

An echocardiographic examination is performed with a multifocused broadband fully populated 2D or matrix arrays containing thousands of elements. This allows the sonographer to produce real-time (4D) depiction of pyramidal volumes, visualization of arbitrary cut planes, and 4D cardiac imaging and color flow mapping.

Multielement Transducer. These transducers contain groups of small crystal elements arranged in a sequential fashion (Fig. 1.20). The transmitted sound pulses are created by the summation of multiple pulses from many different elements. The timing and sequence of activation are altered to steer the transmitted pulses in different directions while focusing at multiple levels.

Sector Phased-Array Transducer. With this transducer, every element in the array participates in the formation of each transmitted pulse. The sound beams are steered at varying angles from one side of the transducer to the other to produce a sector format (Fig. 1.21). The transducer is smaller and is better able to scan in between ribs (especially useful in echocardiography). The transducer permits a large, deep FOV. The limitations of this transducer are a reduced near field focus and a small superficial FOV.

Linear-Array Transducer. The linear-array transducer activates a limited group of adjacent elements to generate each pulse. The pulses travel in the same direction (parallel) and are oriented perpendicular to the transducer surface, resulting in a rectangular image. The pulses may also be steered to produce a trapezoidal image (see Fig. 1.21). This transducer provides high resolution in the near field. The transducer is quite large and cumbersome for accessing all areas and is used more often in obstetric ultrasound.

Curved-Array Transducer. The curved-array transducer uses the linear-array transducer with the surface of the transducer re-formed into a curved convex shape to produce a moderately sized sector-shaped image with a convex apex. This

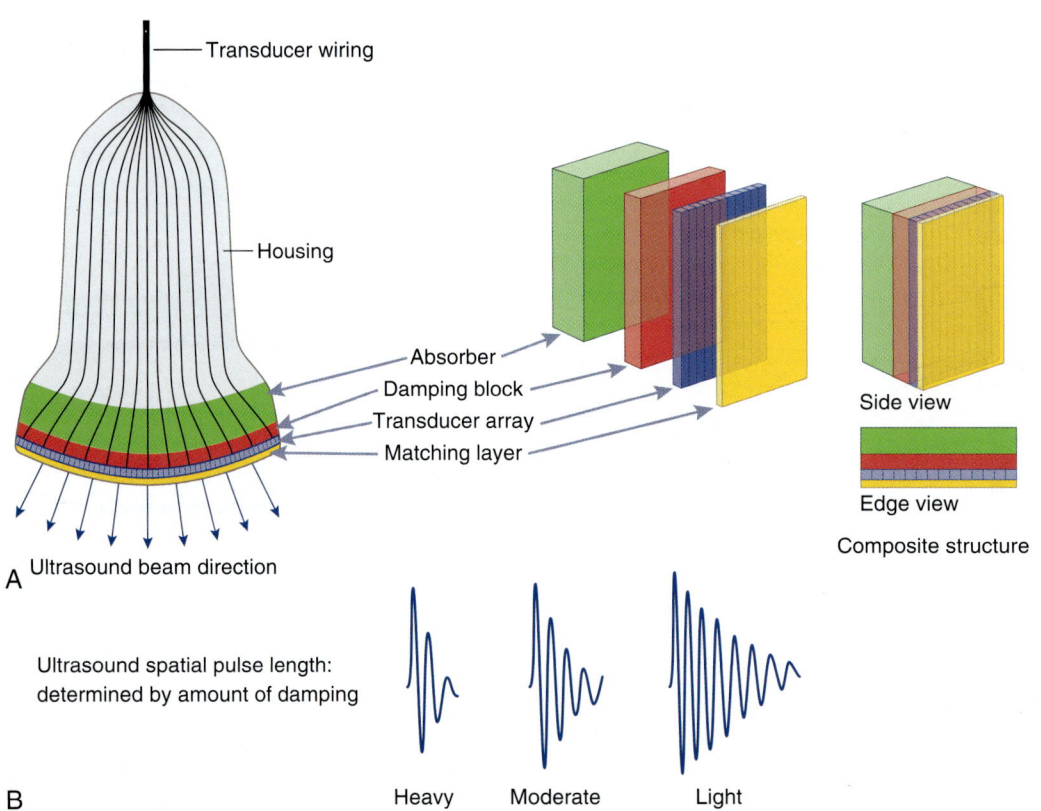

FIG. 1.20 (A) The multielement transducer contains groups of small crystal elements arranged in a sequential fashion. The transmitted sound pulses are created by the summation of multiple pulses from many different elements. (B) The timing and sequence of activation are altered to steer the transmitted pulses in different directions while focusing at multiple levels.

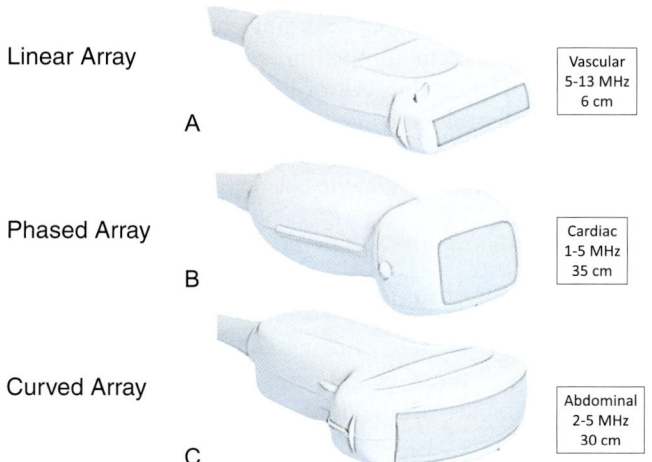

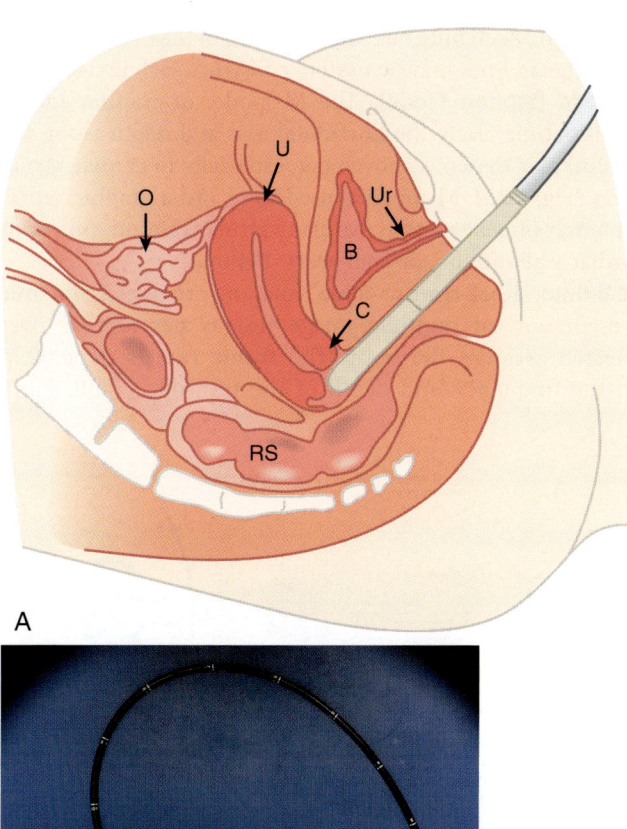

FIG. 1.21 (A) The linear-array transducer activates a limited group of adjacent elements to generate each pulse. The pulses travel in the same direction (parallel) and are oriented perpendicular to the transducer surface, resulting in a rectangular image. The pulses may also be steered to produce a trapezoidal image. (B) With the sector phased array transducer, every element in the array participates in the formation of each transmitted pulse. The sound beams are steered at varying angles from one side of the transducer to the other to produce a sector format (Fig. 1.21). The transducer is smaller and is better able to scan in between ribs (especially useful in echocardiography). The transducer permits a large, deep field of view. (C) The curved-array transducer uses the linear-array transducer with the surface of the transducer re-formed into a curved convex shape to produce a moderately sized sector-shaped image with a convex apex. This allows for a wider far field of view, with slightly reduced resolution. This type of probe can be formatted into many different applications with varying frequencies for use in the abdomen and in obstetrical ultrasound.

allows for a wider far FOV, with slightly reduced resolution. This type of probe can be formatted into many different applications with varying frequencies for use in the abdomen and in obstetrical ultrasound (see Fig. 1.21).

Intraluminal Transducer. These transducers are very small and can be placed into different body lumens that are close to the organ of interest. Much higher frequencies are used with high resolution. Elimination of the body adipose tissue greatly enhances image quality. The drawback of a high-frequency transducer is a limited depth of field. These transducers have been labeled as transvaginal and endorectal when used to image the female organs and rectum, respectively (Fig. 1.22A). Cardiologists have used the transesophageal probe to produce exquisite views of the cardiac valvular apparatus (Fig. 1.22B). Interventional physicians have used the tiny intracardiac echocardiography (ICE) probes that fit onto the end of a catheter in order to see intracoronary and intravascular detail.

Pulse-Echo Display Modes

A-Mode (Amplitude Modulation). A-mode, or amplitude modulation, produces a 1D image that displays the amplitude strength of the returning echo signals along the vertical axis and the time (distance) along the horizontal axis. The amplitude display represents the time or distance it takes the beam

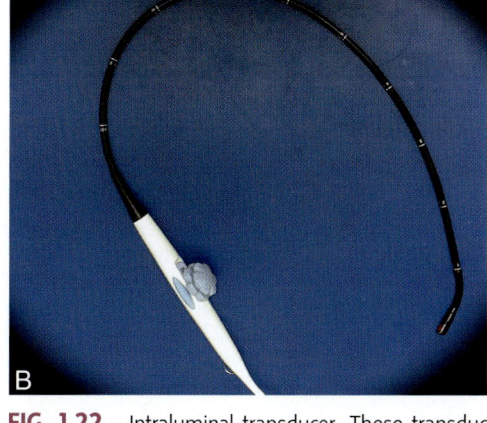

FIG. 1.22 Intraluminal transducer. These transducers are very small and can be placed into different body lumens that are close to the organ of interest. Much higher frequencies are used with high resolution. Elimination of the body adipose tissue greatly enhances image quality. The drawback of a high-frequency transducer is a limited depth of field. A transvaginal probe (A) is used for the pelvis and a transesophageal probe (B) is used for a cardiac procedure.

to strike an interface and return the signal to the transducer. The greater the reflection at the interface, the taller the amplitude spike will appear (Fig. 1.23).

B-Mode (Brightness Modulation). The B-mode, or brightness modulation, method displays the intensity (amplitude) of an echo by varying the brightness of a dot to correspond to echo strength. **Gray scale** is an imaging technique that assigns to each level of amplitude a particular shade of gray to visualize the different echo amplitudes. The B-mode is the basis for all real-time imaging in ultrasound (Fig. 1.24). In B-mode imaging, the ultrasound beam is sent in various directions into the region of interest to be scanned. Each beam interrogates the reflectors along a different line. The echo data picked up along the beam line are displayed in a B-mode format. The B-mode display "tracks" the ultrasound beam line as it scans the region, "sketching out" the 2D image of the body. As many as 200 beam lines may be used to construct each image.

M-Mode (Motion Mode). The M-mode, or motion mode, displays time along the horizontal axis and depth along the vertical axis to depict movement, especially in cardiac structures (Fig. 1.25). M-mode is used to record a graphic representation of wall motion, cardiac valvular motion, posterior cardiac wall motion, or fetal heart rhythm.

Real-time. Real-time or **"cine"** imaging provides a dynamic presentation of multiple image frames per second over selected areas of the body. The **frame rate** is dependent on the frequency and depth of the transducer and depth selection. Typical frame rates are 30 frames/sec or less. The principal barrier to higher scanning speeds is the speed of sound in tissue, dictating the time required to acquire echo data for each beam line. All of ultrasound imaging now is acquired with real-time acquisition. These images may be stored in a cine loop or single frame image. The **temporal resolution** refers to the ability of the system to accurately depict motion.

Harmonic Imaging

Sound waves contain many component frequencies. Harmonics are those components whose frequencies are integral multiples of the lowest frequency (the "fundamental" or "first harmonic"). Harmonic imaging involves transmitting at frequency f and receiving at frequency $2f$, the second harmonic. Because of the finite bandwidth constraints of transducers, the transducer insonates at half of its nominal frequency (e.g., 3 MHz for a 6-MHz transducer) in harmonic mode and then receives at its nominal frequency (6 MHz in this example). The harmonic beams generated during pulse propagation are narrower and have lower sidelobe artifacts than the fundamental beam. The strength of the harmonics generated depends on the amplitude of the incoming beam. Therefore the image-degrading portions of the fundamental beam (i.e., scattered echoes, reverberations, and slice-thickness side lobes) are much weaker than the on-axis portions of the beam and generate weaker harmonics (Fig. 1.26).

Harmonic formation increases with depth, with few harmonics being generated within the near field of the body wall. Therefore filtering out the fundamental frequency and creating an image from the echoes of the second harmonic should

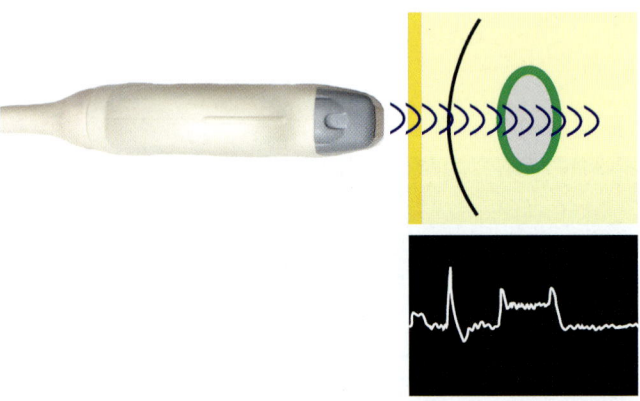

FIG 1.23 A-mode, or amplitude modulation, produces a one-dimensional image that displays the amplitude strength of the returning echo signals along the vertical axis and the time (distance) along the horizontal axis. The amplitude display represents the time or distance it takes the beam to strike an interface and return the signal to the transducer. The greater the reflection at the interface, the taller the amplitude spike will appear.

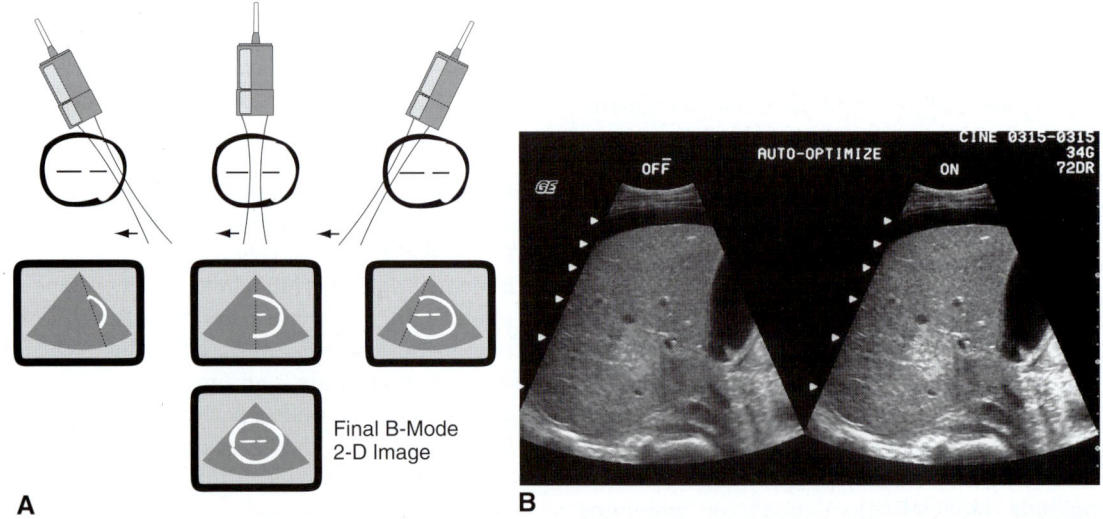

FIG 1.24 (A) Acquisition of multiple image planes over a period of time is made to produce a B-mode image. (B) B-mode image of the liver with a hemangioma in the center of the right lobe. The auto-optimize control is used in the right-hand display to show improved focus.

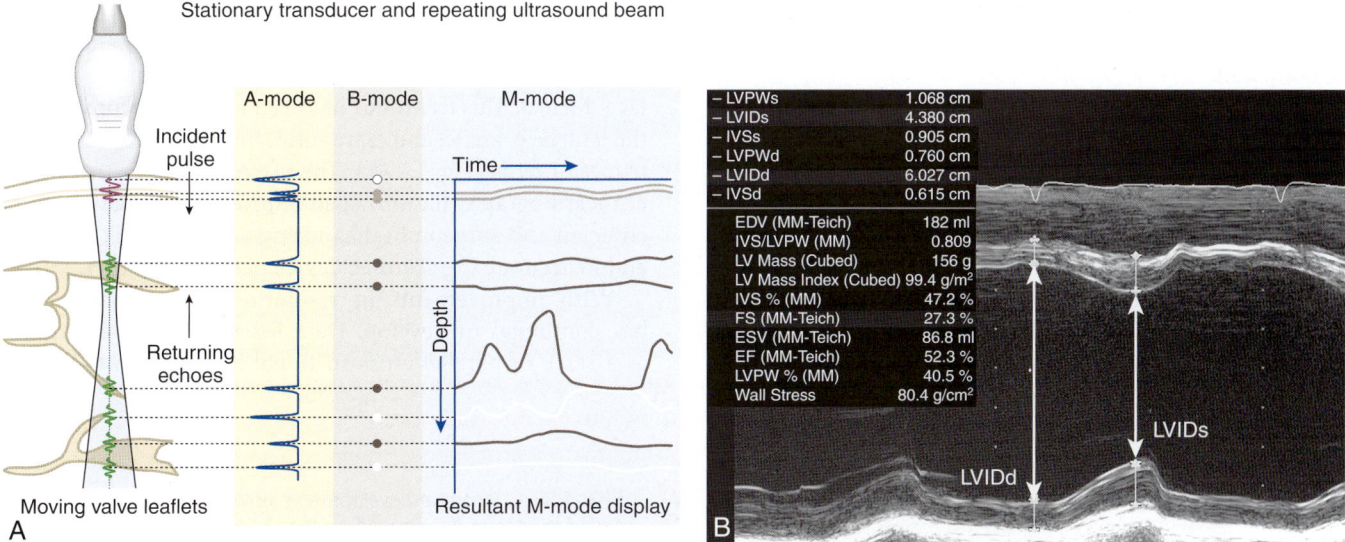

FIG. 1.25 (A) The M-mode, or motion mode, displays time along the horizontal axis and depth along the vertical axis to depict movement, especially in cardiac structures. M-mode is used to record a graphic representation of wall motion, cardiac valvular motion, posterior cardiac wall motion, or fetal heart rhythm. The diagram displays A-mode, B-mode, and M-mode. (B) The M-mode image is taken of the left ventricle. *LV*, Left ventricle; *PW*, posterior wall; *S*, septum.

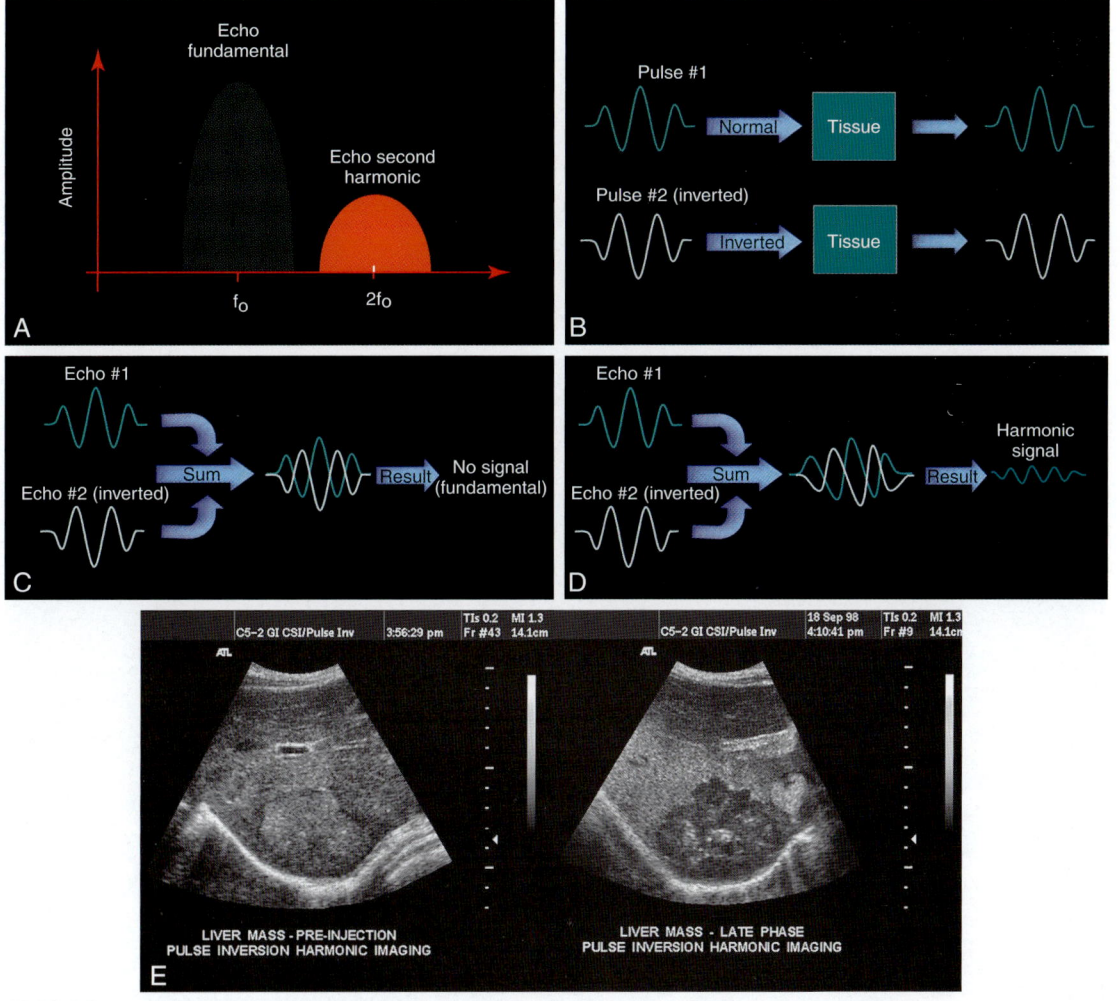

FIG 1.26 (A–D) Harmonic formation increases with depth, with few harmonics being generated within the near field of the body wall. Therefore filtering out the fundamental frequency and creating an image from the echoes of the second harmonic should result in an image that is relatively free of the noise formed during the passage of sound through the distorting layers of the body wall. (E) The liver mass is better visualized with harmonic imaging.

result in an image that is relatively free of the noise formed during the passage of sound through the distorting layers of the body wall.

Three-Dimensional and Four-Dimensional Ultrasound

Conventional ultrasound offers a 2D visualization of anatomic structures with the flexibility of visualizing images from different orientations or "windows" in real-time. The sonographer acquires these 2D images in at least two different scanning planes and then forms a 3D image in his or her head. Technical developments in technology now allow ultrasound images to be acquired on their x, y, and z axes, manually realigned, and then reconstructed into a 3D "en face" format. This technique has been useful in reconstructing the fetal face, ankle, and extremities in the second- and third-trimester fetus (Fig. 1.27A). The use of 3D reconstruction in echocardiography has provided improved information to the clinician and surgeon in diagnosing valvular heart problems and in accurate intracardiac device placement (Fig. 1.27B).

With improvements in resolution and accuracy, 3DU has continued to develop. Data for the 3DU are acquired as a stack of parallel cross-sectional images with the use of

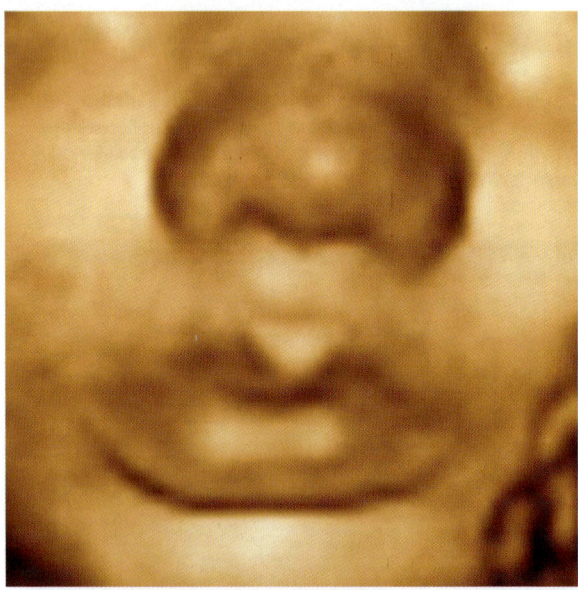
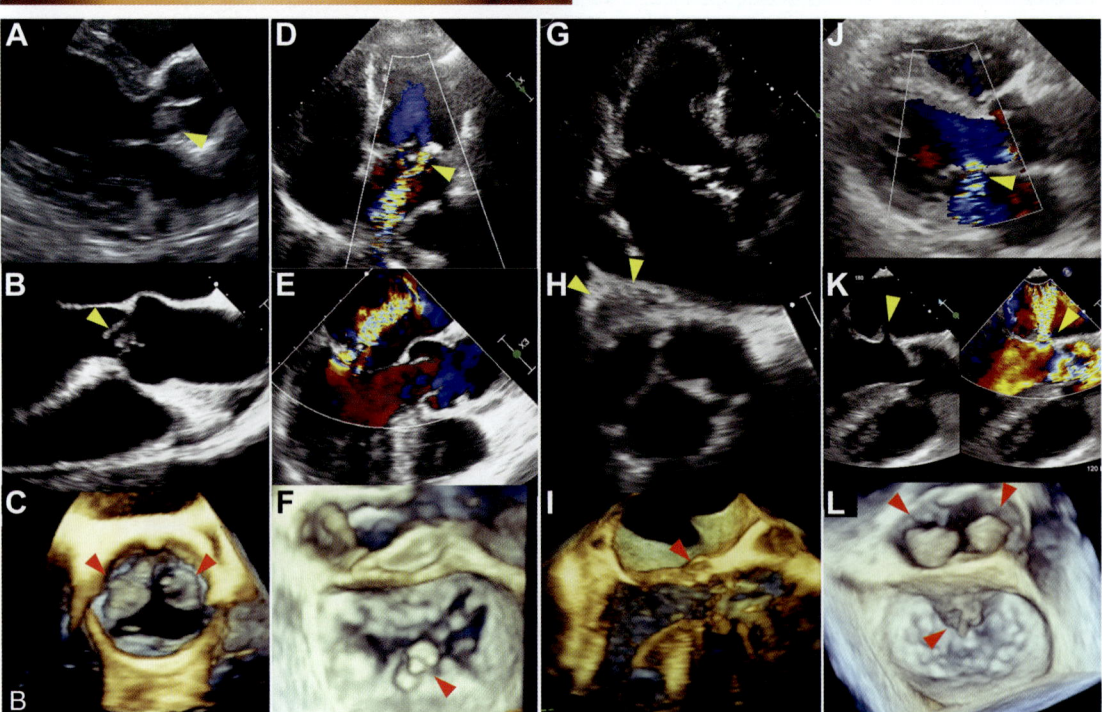

FIG. 1.27 Technical developments now allow ultrasound images to be acquired on their x, y, and z axes, manually realigned, and then reconstructed into a three-dimensional (3D) "en face" format. (A) This technique has been useful in reconstructing the fetal face, ankle, and extremities in the second- and third-trimester fetus. (B) 3D reconstruction of the aortic valve (A–F) and mitral valve (G–L).

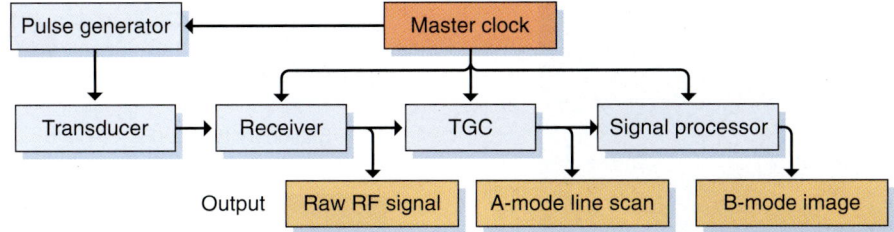

FIG. 1.28 The critical component of the pulse-echo instrument is the B-mode (two-dimensional) imager. The beam former includes the electronic transmitter and the receiver. The transmitter supplies electrical signals to the transducer for producing the sound beam. The transducer may be connected to the transmitter and receiver through a beam-former system. Echoes picked up by the transducer are applied to the receiver. At this point, the echoes are amplified and processed into a suitable format for display. An image memory (scan converter) retains data for viewing or storage on digital media.

a conventional ultrasound system or as a volume with the use of an electronic array probe. These images can be reconstructed in a variety of formats to produce the desired image. In addition, 4DU is the real-time motion of the 3DU image.

System Controls for Image Optimization

Pulse-Echo Instrumentation. The critical component of the pulse-echo instrument is the B-mode (2D) imager. The beam former includes the electronic transmitter and the receiver. The transmitter supplies electrical signals to the transducer for producing the sound beam. The transducer may be connected to the transmitter and receiver through a beam-former system. Echoes picked up by the transducer are applied to the receiver. At this point, the echoes are amplified and processed into a suitable format for display. An image memory (scan converter) retains data for viewing or storage on digital media (Fig. 1.28).

Power Output. The power output determines the strength of the pulse that is transmitted into the body. The returning echoes are stronger when the transmitted pulse is stronger, and thus the image is "brighter." The power output is displayed as a dB or as a percentage of maximum.

Gain. Once the sound wave strikes the body, sound attenuation occurs with each layer the beam transverses, causing an interface in the deep tissues to produce a weaker reflection and less distortion of the crystal than a similar interface in the near tissues. To compensate for this attenuation of sound in the deeper tissues, the sound is "electronically amplified" after the sound returns to the transducer. The receiver **gain** allows the sonographer to amplify or boost the echo signals. It may be compared with the volume control on a radio—as one increases the volume, the sound becomes louder. The acoustic exposure to the patient is not changed when the receiver gain is increased. If the gain is set too high, artifactual low level "echo noise" will be displayed throughout the image. Fluid or normal vascular structures should be anechoic (without echoes); if the gain is set too high, low level artifactual echoes will be noted in these structures.

Recall the discussion of how the signal is absorbed, reflected, and attenuated as the beam traverses the body. The depth of the interface is determined by the amount of time it takes for the transmitted sound pulse to return to the transducer. The **time gain compensation (TGC)** control, sometimes referred to as **depth gain compensation (DGC)**, allows the sonographer to manually amplify the receiver gain gradually at specific depths (Fig. 1.29). Thus the echoes well seen in the near field may be reduced in amplitude, while the echoes in the far field may be amplified or increased with changing the TGC controls. The TGC control will be continually

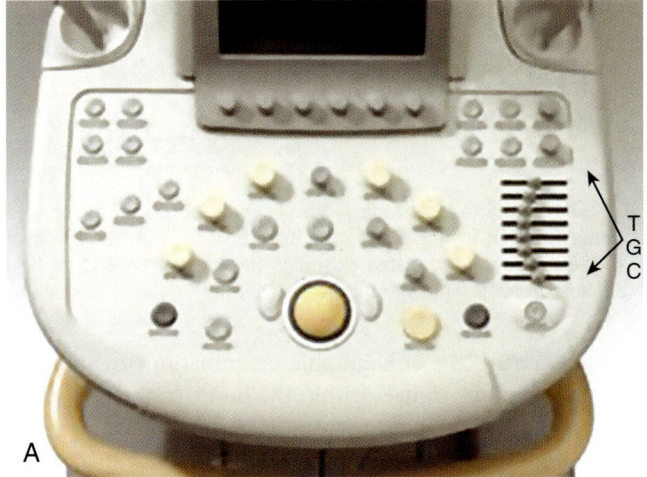

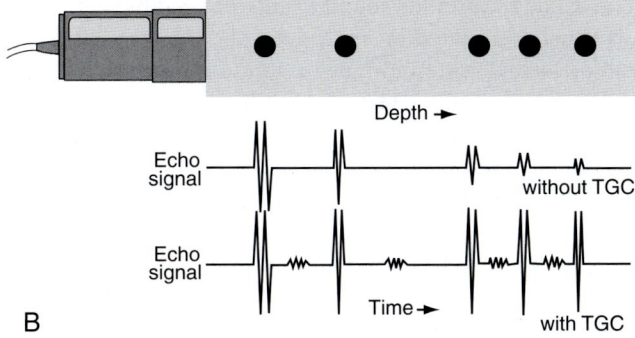

FIG. 1.29 (A) Ultrasound control panel that shows the time gain compensation (TGC) controls along the right side of the panel. (B) The TGC allows the sonographer to amplify the receiver gain gradually at specific depths to adjust for attenuation.

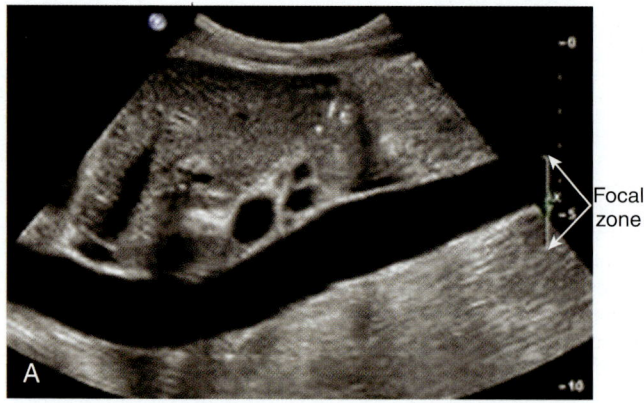
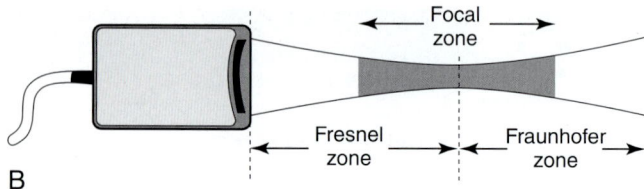

FIG. 1.30 (A) The focal zone *(arrows)* should be placed at the area of interest, which in this case is the inferior vena cava. (B) The near field (Fresnel zone) is the area closest to the transducer. The far field (Fraunhofer zone) is farthest from the transducer.

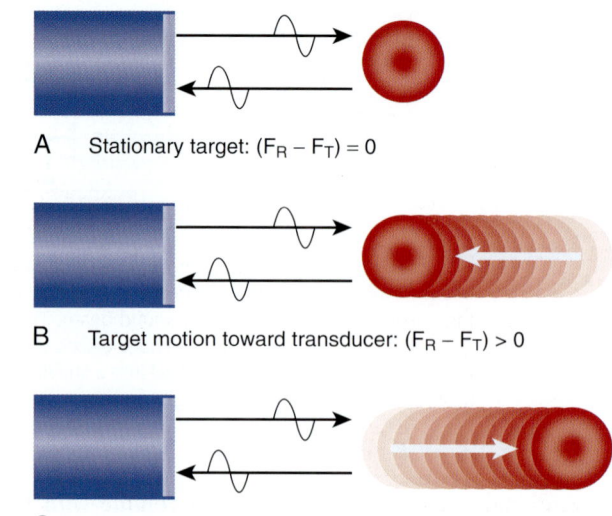

FIG. 1.31 (A–C) The Doppler effect is the apparent change in frequency of sound or light waves emitted by a source as it moves away from or toward an observer. Sound that reflects off a moving object undergoes a change in frequency. Objects moving toward the transducer reflect sound at a higher frequency than that of the incident pulse, and objects moving away reflect sound at a lower frequency. The difference between the transmitted and the received frequency is called the Doppler frequency shift.

adjusted during the sonographic examination to highlight or display various signals within the body. In the abdomen, the liver is a great organ to set the TGC controls because the organ should be homogeneous from the near field (close to the transducer) to the far field (furthest from the transducer).

Focal Zone. The focal zone control allows the transducer to focus the transmitted sound at different depths (Fig. 1.30). It is usually indicated on the side of the image as single or multiple arrowheads and may be adjusted in depth to focus on specific areas of interest. As multilevel focusing is used, a decrease in the frame rate will occur.

Field of View. This control allows the sonographer to adjust the depth and width of the image. The larger or deeper FOV will directly cause the frame rate to decrease. Depth is displayed as centimeters on the side of the image. Width adjusts the horizontal axis of the image and may be used to reduce side-lobe artifacts.

Reject. The reject control eliminates both electronic noise and low-level echoes from the display. This control is important to understand; as the sonographer attempts to "clean up" the image artifacts, one must be careful not to eliminate important low-level information that may be significant in the clinical diagnosis.

Dynamic Range. The **dynamic range** of a device is the range of input signal levels that produce noticeable changes in the output of the device. The dynamic range capabilities vary among different ultrasound machines. The sonographer usually notes the low dynamic range as one of high contrast (echocardiography and peripheral vascular), whereas the high dynamic range shows more shades of gray and lower contrast (abdominal and obstetric).

Doppler Ultrasound

Two basic modes of transducer operation are used in medical diagnostic applications: continuous wave (CW) and pulsed wave (PW). Real-time 2D instrumentation uses only the pulse-echo amplitude of the returning echo to generate gray-scale information, whereas Doppler instrumentation uses both continuous and pulsed wave operations.

Doppler Effect. The Doppler effect is the apparent change in frequency of sound or light waves emitted by a source as it moves away from or toward an observer (Fig. 1.31). Sound that reflects off a moving object undergoes a change in frequency. Objects moving toward the transducer reflect sound at a higher frequency than that of the incident pulse, and objects moving away reflect sound at a lower frequency. The difference between the transmitted and the received frequency is called the Doppler **frequency shift**. This Doppler effect is applied when the motion of laminar or turbulent flow is detected within a vascular structure. When the source moves toward the listener, the perceived frequency is higher than the emitted frequency, thus creating a higher-pitched sound. If the sound moves away from the listener, the perceived frequency is lower than the transmitted frequency, and the sound will have a lower pitch.

In the medical application of the Doppler principle, the frequency of the reflected sound wave is the same as the frequency transmitted only if the reflector is stationary. If the red blood cell (RBC) moves along the line of the ultrasound beam (parallel to flow), the Doppler shift is directly proportional to the velocity of the RBC. If the RBC moves away from the transducer in the plane of the beam, the fall in frequency is directly proportional to the velocity and direction of RBC movement (Fig. 1.32). The frequency of the echo will be higher than the transmitted frequency if the reflector is moving toward the transducer, and lower if the reflector is moving away.

Doppler Shift. The difference between the receiving echo frequency and the frequency of the transmitted beam is called the **Doppler shift**. This change in the frequency of a reflected wave is caused by relative motion between the reflector and the transducer's beam. In general, the Doppler shift is only a small fraction of the transmitted ultrasound frequency.

The Doppler shift frequency is proportional to the velocity of the moving reflector or blood cell. The frequency at which a transducer transmits ultrasound influences the frequency of the Doppler shift. The higher the original, or transmitted, frequency, the greater is the shift in frequency for a given reflector velocity. The returning frequency increases if the RBC is moving toward the transducer and decreases if the blood cell is moving away from the transducer. The Doppler effect produces a shift that is the reflected frequency minus the transmitted frequency. When interrogating the same blood vessel with transducers of different frequencies, the higher-frequency transducer will generate a larger Doppler shift frequency.

The angle that the reflector path makes with the ultrasound beam is called the **Doppler angle**. As the Doppler angle increases from 0 to 90 degrees, the detected Doppler frequency shift decreases. At 90 degrees, the Doppler shift is zero, regardless of flow velocity. The frequency of the Doppler shift is proportional to the cosine of the Doppler angle. The beam should be parallel to flow to obtain the maximum velocity. *The closer the Doppler angle is to zero, the more accurate is the flow velocity* (see Fig. 1.32). If the angle of the beam to the reflector exceeds 60 degrees, velocities will no longer be accurate.

Spectral Analysis. Blood flow through a vessel may be laminar or turbulent (Fig. 1.33). **Laminar** flow is the normal pattern of vessel flow, which occurs at different velocities, because flow in the center of the vessel is faster than it is at the edges. When the range of velocities increases significantly, the flow pattern becomes turbulent. The audio of the Doppler signal enables the sonographer to distinguish laminar flow from turbulent flow patterns. **Turbulent** flow is the abnormal pattern of vessel flow that occurs when there is a narrowing in the vessel that causes a high velocity flow profile. The process of **spectral analysis** allows the instrumentation to break down the complex multifrequency Doppler signal into individual frequency components.

The spectral display shows the distribution of Doppler frequencies versus time (Fig. 1.34). This is displayed as velocity on the vertical axis and time on the horizontal axis. Flow toward the transducer is displayed above the baseline, and flow away from the transducer is displayed below the baseline.

When the area of the vessel that is examined contains RBCs moving at similar velocities, they will be represented on the spectral display by a narrow band. This area under the band is called the "window." As flow becomes more turbulent or disturbed, the velocity increases, producing **spectral broadening** on the display. A very stenotic (high-flow velocity) lesion would cause the window to become completely filled in.

Continuous Wave Doppler. Continuous wave (CW) Doppler uses two piezoelectric elements: one for sending and one for receiving. The sound is transmitted continuously rather than in short pulses. CW is used to record the higher-velocity flow patterns, usually greater than 2 m/sec, and is especially useful in cardiology (Fig. 1.35). Unlike PW Doppler, CW cannot pinpoint exactly where along the beam axis flow is occurring because it samples all of the flow along its path. In the example of a five-chamber view of the heart, a sample volume placed in the left ventricular outflow tract will sample all the flow along that "line" to include the flows in the outflow tract and in the ascending aorta.

Pulsed Wave Doppler. Pulsed wave (PW) Doppler is used for lower-velocity flow and has one crystal that pulses to transmit the signal while also listening or receiving the returning signal (see Fig. 1.35). The PW Doppler uses brief bursts of sound like those used in echo imaging. These bursts are usually of a longer duration and produce well-defined frequencies. The sonographer may set the **gate** or Doppler window to a specific area of interest in the vascular structure so interrogated. This

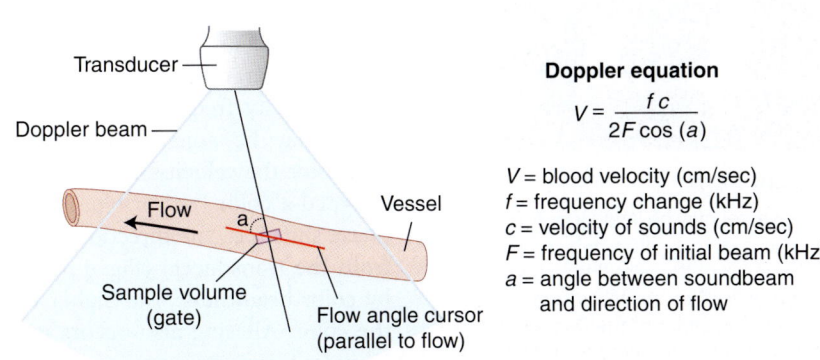

Doppler equation

$$V = \frac{f\,c}{2F\cos(a)}$$

V = blood velocity (cm/sec)
f = frequency change (kHz)
c = velocity of sounds (cm/sec)
F = frequency of initial beam (kHz)
a = angle between soundbeam and direction of flow

FIG 1.32 In the medical application of the Doppler principle, the frequency of the reflected sound wave is the same as the frequency transmitted only if the reflector is stationary. If the red blood cell (RBC) moves along the line of the ultrasound beam (parallel to flow), the Doppler shift is directly proportional to the velocity of the RBC. If the RBC moves away from the transducer in the plane of the beam, the fall in frequency is directly proportional to the velocity and direction of RBC movement.

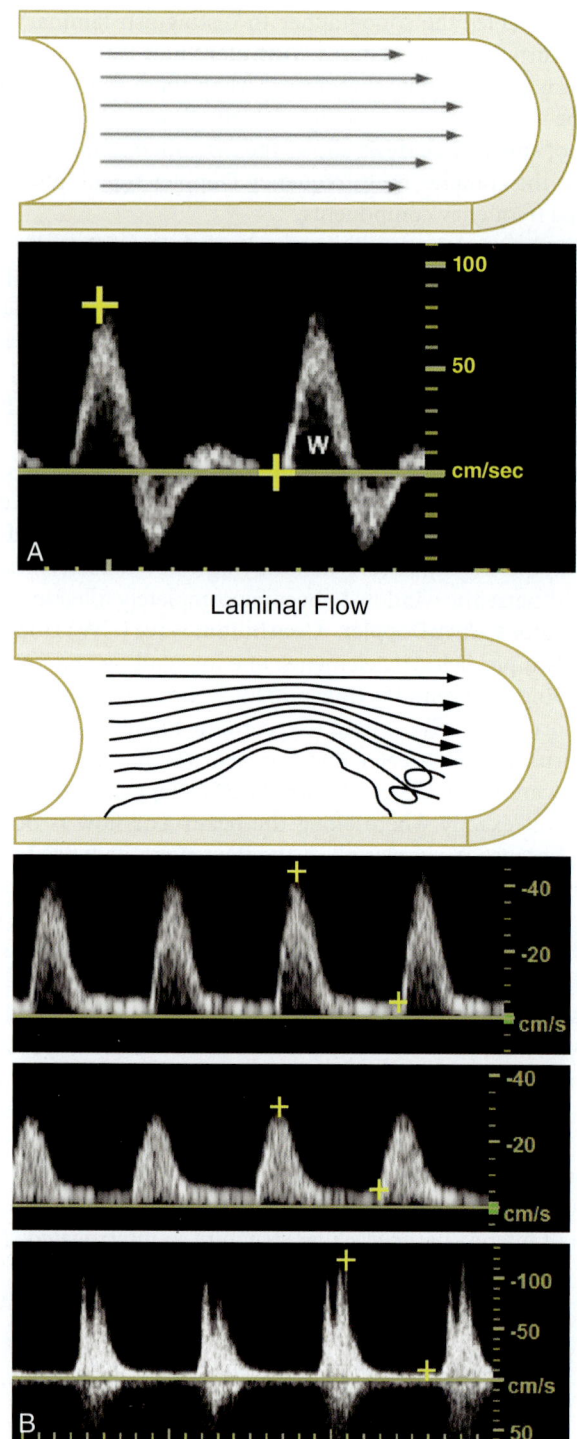

FIG. 1.33 Blood flow through a vessel may be laminar or turbulent. (A) Laminar flow is the normal pattern of vessel flow, which occurs at different velocities, as flow in the center of the vessel is faster than it is at the edges. When the range of velocities increases significantly, the flow pattern becomes turbulent. The audio of the Doppler signal enables the sonographer to distinguish laminar flow from turbulent flow patterns. (B) Turbulent flow is the abnormal pattern of vessel flow that occurs when there is a narrowing in the vessel that causes a high velocity flow profile.

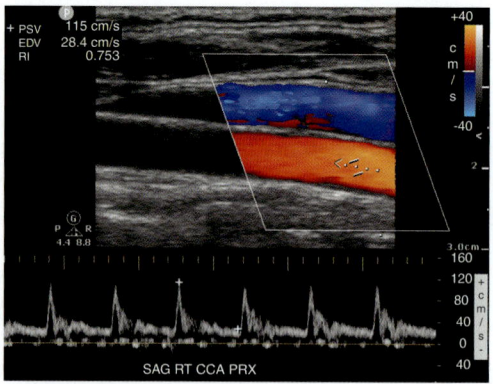

FIG. 1.34 The spectral display shows the distribution of Doppler frequencies versus time. This is displayed as velocity on the vertical axis and time on the horizontal axis. Flow toward the transducer is displayed above the baseline, and flow away from the transducer is displayed below the baseline.

means that a specific area of interest may be examined at the point the gate or sample volume is placed. For example, in a longitudinal view of the abdominal aorta, the sample volume may be placed directly in the middle of the aortic flow, and recordings only from that particular area "within the gate or window" will be measured (see Fig. 1.34).

With pulsed Doppler, for accurate detection of Doppler frequencies to occur, the Doppler signal must be sampled at least twice for each cycle in the wave. This phenomenon is known as the **Nyquist sampling limit**. When the Nyquist limit is exceeded, an artifact called aliasing occurs. **Aliasing** presents on the spectral display as an apparent reversal of flow direction and a "wrapping around" of the Doppler spectral waveform. Therefore the highest velocity may not be accurately demonstrated when aliasing occurs; this usually happens when the flows are greater than 2 m/sec. One can avoid aliasing by changing the Doppler signal from PW to CW to record the higher velocities accurately.

Color Doppler. Color Doppler is sensitive to Doppler signals throughout an adjustable portion of the area of interest. A real-time image is displayed with both gray scale and **color flow** in the vascular structures. Color Doppler is able to analyze the phase information, frequency, and amplitude of returning echoes.

Velocities are quantified by allocating a pixel to flow toward the transducer and flow away from the transducer. Each velocity frequency change is allocated a color. Color maps may be adjusted to obtain different color assignments for the velocity levels; signals from moving RBCs are assigned a color (red or blue) based on the direction of the phase shift (i.e., the direction of blood flow toward or away from the transducer) (Fig. 1.36). Flow velocity is indicated by color brightness: The higher the velocity, the brighter is the color. Aliasing also occurs in color flow imaging when Doppler frequencies exceed the Nyquist limit, just as in spectral Doppler. This appears as a wrap-around of the displayed color. The velocity scale pulse repetition frequency (PRF) may

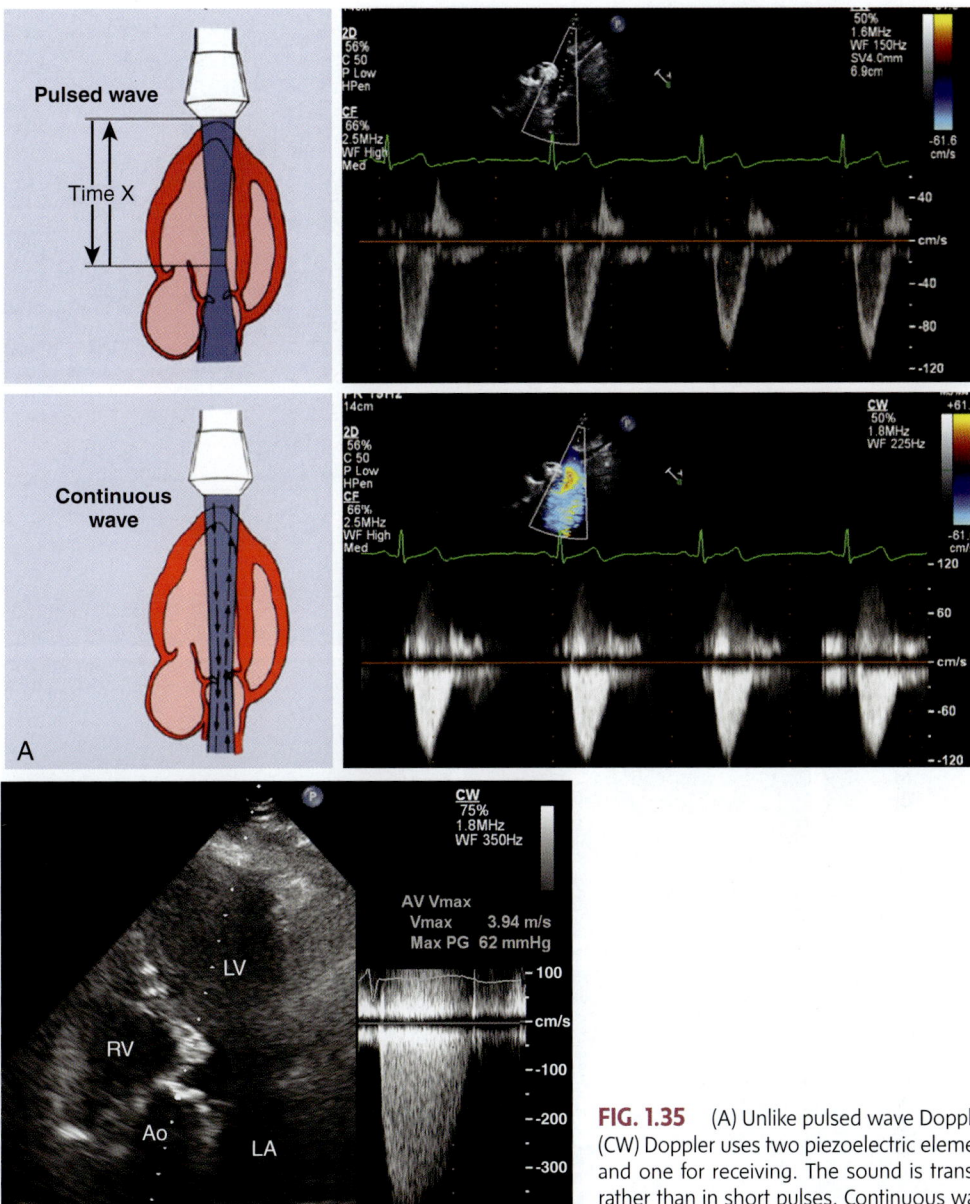

FIG. 1.35 (A) Unlike pulsed wave Doppler, continuous wave (CW) Doppler uses two piezoelectric elements: one for sending and one for receiving. The sound is transmitted continuously rather than in short pulses. Continuous wave is used to record the higher velocity flow patterns, usually greater than 2 m/sec, and is especially useful in cardiology. (B) CW example of the turbulent high flow of aortic stenosis.

be adjusted to avoid aliasing. Color arising from sources other than moving blood is referred to as flash artifact or ghosting.
Power Doppler. Power Doppler estimates the power or strength of the Doppler signal rather than the mean frequency shift. Although the Doppler detection sequence used in power Doppler is the same as that used in frequency-based color Doppler, once the Doppler shift has been detected, the frequency components are ignored in lieu of the total energy of the Doppler signal. The color and hue relate to the moving blood volume rather than to the direction or the velocity of flow (Fig. 1.37).

This principle provides power Doppler several advantages over color Doppler imaging. In power Doppler, low-level noise is assigned as a homogeneous color background, even when the gain is increased. With color Doppler, the higher gains produce noise in the signal that obscures the image. The Doppler angle is not affected in power Doppler; with color Doppler the angle is critical in determining the exact flow velocity. The downside of power Doppler is that it provides no information about the direction or velocity of blood flow, and it is susceptible to flash artifact (zones of intense color that results from motion of soft tissues and motion of the transducer).
Doppler Optimization.
Transducer Frequency. The Doppler frequency shift is proportional to the transmitted frequency. Therefore

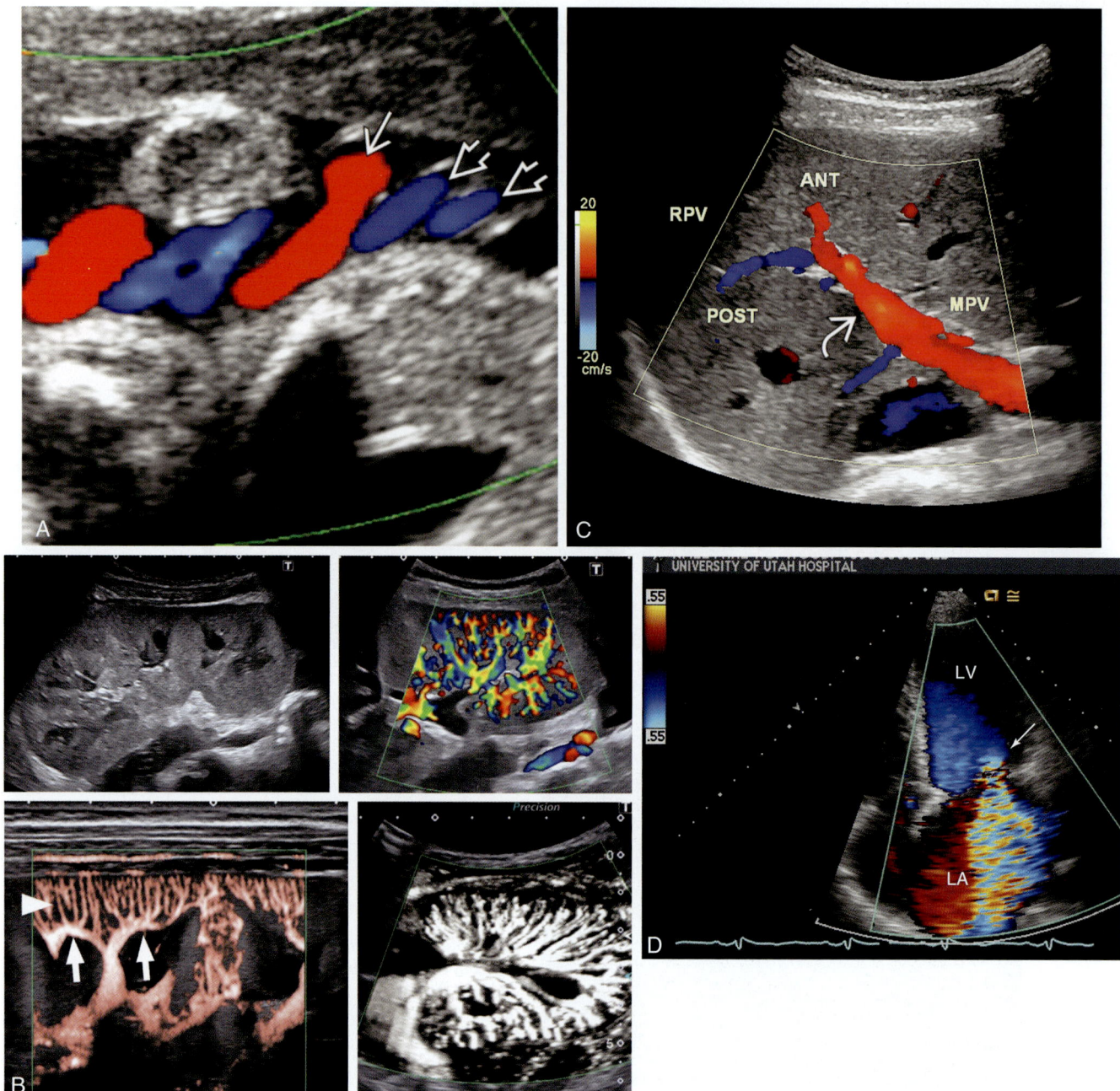

FIG. 1.36 Color Doppler is sensitive to Doppler signals throughout an adjustable portion of the area of interest. A real-time image is displayed with both gray scale and color flow in the vascular structures. Color Doppler is able to analyze the phase information, frequency, and amplitude of returning echoes. (A) Normal three-vessel umbilical cord. (B) Normal renal vasculature. (C) Normal portal vein flow. (D) Abnormal flow from the mitral regurgitation into the left atrial cavity.

higher-frequency transducers cause a higher Doppler frequency shift that is easier to detect. Higher-frequency probes also result in stronger reflections from RBCs. Remember that the higher-frequency probes are not sensitive to deeper structures; therefore multiple probes may be necessary, depending upon the type of ultrasound examination.

Gain. Doppler gain is the receiver end amplification of the Doppler signal. This can be applied to either the waveform itself or to the color Doppler image. The Doppler gain is usually increased to the maximum limit where "noise" scatter is seen in the background. The gain is then slowly decreased until that noise disappears. The Doppler gain is independent of the gray scale gain.

Scale. Scale allows the sonographer to expand or reduce the range of depth of the returning signal.

Baseline. The baseline may be moved up or down to image the maximal velocity of the returning signal.

Power. Power refers to the strength of the transmitted ultrasound pulse. The stronger pulse will produce stronger reflections that are more easily detected. Power will affect both gray-scale and Doppler images. Increasing the power may be helpful in the deeper structures, but increasing power

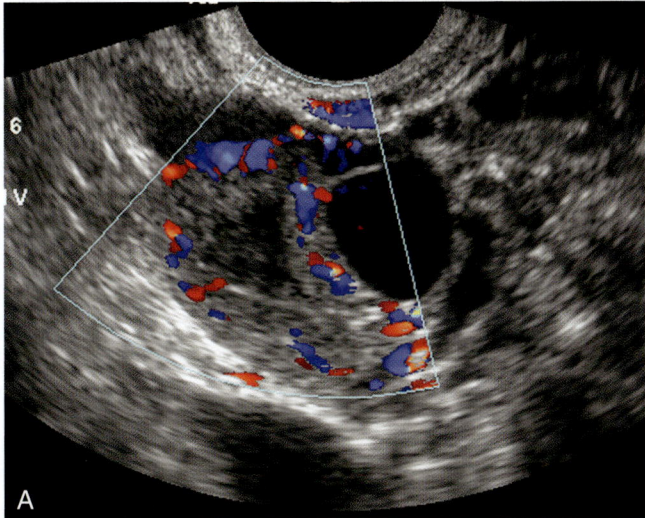

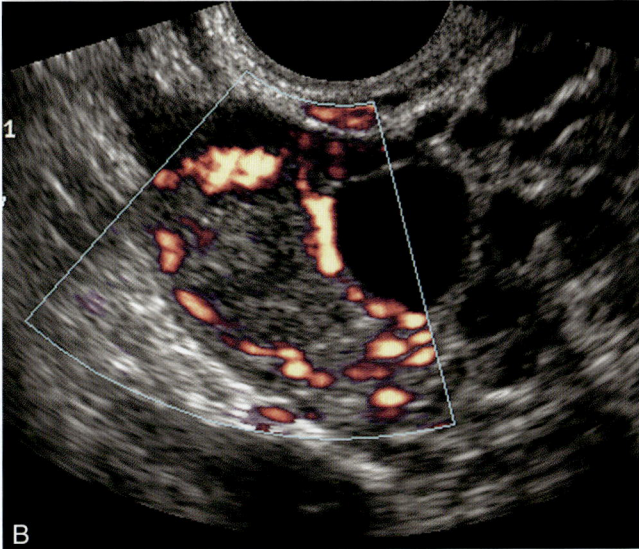

FIG. 1.37 Color Doppler (A) and power Doppler (B). Power Doppler estimates the power or strength of the Doppler signal rather than the mean frequency shift. Although the Doppler detection sequence used in power Doppler is the same as that used in frequency-based color Doppler, once the Doppler shift has been detected, the frequency components are ignored in lieu of the total energy of the Doppler signal. The color and hue relate to the moving blood volume rather than to the direction or the velocity of flow.

increases patient exposure and may cause increased artifacts. For these reasons, power controls generally are not modified as frequently by the sonographer as the other controls.

Pulse Repetition Frequency. The **pulse repetition frequency (PRF)** refers to the number of sound pulses transmitted per second. A high PRF results in a high Doppler scale (to record higher velocities, i.e., aortic stenosis), whereas a lower PRF results in a lower Doppler scale (to record lower velocities, i.e., venous return or low-flow states). The PRF is adjusted for the higher flows to eliminate aliasing.

Wall Filter. The wall filter allows the sonographer to eliminate artifactual or unwanted signals arising from pulsating vessel walls or moving soft tissues. This filter allows frequency shifts above a certain level to be displayed while lower-frequency shifts are not displayed.

Key Pearls

- Ultrasound refers to instrumentation; sonography refers to the imaging technique; echocardiography refers to cardiac imaging.
- A sonographer is a member of the allied heath profession who has received specialized education in diagnostic medical sonography and has successfully completed the national boards given by the American Registry of Diagnostic Medical Sonography.
- A sonologist is a physician who has received specialized training in ultrasound and has successfully completed the national boards granted by their respective specialty.
- Diagnostic ultrasound is portable and economical and does not use radiation.
- Diagnostic ultrasound uses short sound pulses at frequencies of 1–20 million cycles/sec that are transmitted into the body to examine soft tissue anatomic structures.
- Velocity of propagation is constant for a given tissue and not affected by the frequency or wavelength of the pulse.
- Sound waves travel slowly through gas, at intermediate speed through liquids, and quickly through solids.
- The decibel unit is used to measure the intensity, amplitude, and power of an ultrasound wave.
- Power is measured in watts or milliwatts.
- Frequency describes the number of oscillations per second performed by the particles of the medium in which the wave is propagating.
- Once sound pulses are transmitted into a body, they can be reflected, scattered, refracted, or absorbed.
- Acoustic impedance is the measure of a material's resistance to the propagation of sound.
- Resolution is the ability of an imaging process to distinguish adjacent structures in an object and is an important measure of image quality (axial, lateral, and azimuthal resolution).
- Attenuation is the sum of acoustic energy loss resulting from absorption, scattering, and reflection.
- Transducers are selected for a particular examination. (multielement, phased array, sector array, linear-array, curved-array, intraluminal)
- Pulsed echo display modes include A-mode, M-mode, B-mode, real-time, harmonics, and three and four dimensional.
- Systems controls for image optimization: power output, gain, time gain compensation, focal zone, field of view, reject, dynamic range.
- Doppler effect is the apparent change in frequency of sound or light waves emitted by a source as it moves away from or toward an observer.
- The difference between the receiving echo frequency and the frequency of the transmitted beam is called the Doppler shift.
- Doppler may be measured using either continuous wave or pulsed wave analysis.
- Color Doppler is able to analyze the phase information, frequency, and amplitude of returning echoes.
- Power Doppler estimates the power or strength of the Doppler signal rather than the mean frequency shift.
- Doppler optimization is controlled by transducer frequency, gain, scale, baseline, power, pulse repetition frequency, wall filter.

BIBLIOGRAPHY

American College of Radiology: ACR-SPR-SRU practice guideline for performing and interpreting diagnostic ultrasound examinations. Revised 2017. www.acr.org.

Baker DW, Watkins D: A phase coherent pulse doppler system for cardio-vascular measurement. In Proceedings of the 20th Annual Conference of Engineering Medicine Biologists 1967;27:2.

Bom N, Lance CT, Honkoop J, Hugenholtz PG. Ultrasonic viewer for cross-sectional analyses of moving cardiac structures. *BioMed Eng.* 1971;6:500.

Curie JP. Développement par pression de l'électricite polaire dans les cristaux hémièdres à faces inclinées. *CR Acad Sci (Paris).* 1880;91:294.

Donald I. Clinical applications of ultrasonic techniques in obstetrical and gynaecological diagnosis. *Br J Obstet Gynaecol.* 1962;69:1036.

Dussik KT. On the possibility of using ultrasound waves as a diagnostic aid. *Neurol Psychiat.* 1942;174:153–168.

Edler I, Hertz CH. The use of ultrasonic reflectoscope for the continuous recording of the movements of heart walls. *K Fysiogr Sallsk Lund Forh.* 1954;24:40.

Firestone FA. The supersonic reflectoscope, an instrument of inspecting the interior of solid parts by means of sound waves. *J Acoust Soc Am.* 1945;17:287–299.

Griffith JM, Herny WL. A sector scanner for real-time two-dimensional echocardiography. *Circulation.* 1974;49:1147.

Holmes JH, Howry DH, Posakony GJ, Cushman CR. The ultrasonic visualization of soft tissue structures in the human body. *Trans Am Clin Climatol Assoc.* 1954;66:208–223.

Howry DH. Development of an ultrasonic diagnostic instrument. *Am J Phys Med.* 1958;37:234.

Kossoff G, Carpenter D, Robinson D, Garrett WJ: A new multi-transducer water coupling echoscope. In Proceedings of the 2nd European Congress on Ultrasonics in Medicine, May 12-16, 1975, Munich, Germany.

Langévin MP. Les ondes ultrasonores. *Rev Gen Elect.* 1928;23:626.

Ludwig GD, Bolt RH, Hueter TF, Ballantine HT. Factors influencing the use of ultrasound as a diagnostic aid. *Trans Am Neurol Assoc.* 1950;51:225–228.

Nelson TR, Downey DD, Pretorius DH, et al. *Three-dimensional ultrasound.* Philadelphia. : Lippincott Williams & Wilkins; 1999.

Omoto R, Namekawa K, Kasai C. A prototype device incorporating a new technology for visualizing intracardiac flow. *Jpn Circ J.* 1983;47:191.

Reid JM, Spencer MP. Ultrasonic Doppler technique for imaging blood vessels. *Science.* 1972;176:1235–1236.

Robinette WB. Ultrasound contrast agents: an overview. *J Diagn Med Sonogr.* 1997;13:29S.

Szabo TL, Lewin PA. Ultrasound Transducer Selection in Clinical Imaging Practice. *J Ultrasound Med.* 2013;32:573–582.

von Ramm OT, Thurstone FL. Cardiac imaging using a phased array system (I. System design). *Circulation.* 1976;53:258–262.

Wild JJ, French LA, Neal D. Detection of cerebral tumours by ultrasonic pulses. *Cancer.* 1950;4:705.

Woo JSK: A short history of the development of ultrasound in obstetrics and gynecology. www.ob-ultrasound.net/history.html.

Zagzebski J, Parks J: Ultrasound physics and instrumentation, advanced ultrasound seminars, 1997.

CHAPTER 2

Essentials of Patient Care for the Sonographer

M. Robert De Jong

OBJECTIVES

On completion of this chapter, the reader should be able to:
- Discuss nonscanning aspects of being a sonographer
- Define patient-centered care
- Describe patient transfer techniques
- Demonstrate proper placement of a blood pressure cuff on the arm
- Discuss the importance of proper disinfection of the transducer and ultrasound equipment
- Discuss Spaulding's classification system and how it relates to ultrasound
- List various types of patient isolation

OUTLINE

Introduction 30
A Sonographer's Commitments 30
   Patient-Centered Care 30
Basic Patient Care 35
   Vital Signs 35
Patient Transfer Techniques 38
   Body Mechanics 38
   Stretcher and Wheelchair Transfer 39
   Moving Patients Onto a Scan Bed From a Wheelchair 39
   Moving Patients Up Toward the Head of a Stretcher 39
   Turning Patients 40
   Assisting Patients From the Scanning Stretcher Into The Wheelchair 40
Patients With Tubes 40
   Intravenous Therapy 41
   Nasogastric Tubes 43
   Urinary Catheter 43
   Oxygen Therapy 45
   Wounds, Drains, and Dressings 46
   Colostomies and Ileostomies 47
Safety in the Patient Care Environment 47
Patients on Strict Bed Rest 48
   Bedpans and Urinals 48
   Emesis Basins and Bags 49

Standard Precautions and Infection Prevention 49
   Spaulding's Classification System 51
   Hand Washing 52
Isolation Precautions 53
   Standard Precautions for All Patient Care 53
   Additional Precautions 54
   Airborne Precautions 54
   Droplet Precautions 54
   Contact Precautions 54
   Blood-Borne Precautions 55
   Reverse Isolation 55
   Strict Isolation 55
   Enteric Isolation 55
Personal Protective Equipment/Gear 55
   Basic Personal Protective Equipment Protocols 55
   How to Don Personal Protective Equipment 55
   How to Take Off Personal Protective Equipment 56
   Personal Protective Equipment 56
   Wash Your Hands 57
Patient Care Equipment 57
Environment Cleanliness 57

Assisting Patients With Special Needs 57
   Crying/Upset Patients 57
   Elderly Patients 57
   Adolescent Patients 58
   Pediatric Patients 58
   Multicultural World We Live In 59
   When a Patient Cannot Communicate 59
Understanding a Patient's Reaction to Their Illness 60
   Terminal Patients 60
The Patient Care Partnership 61
Professional Attitudes and Behaviors 61
   Reestablishing Patient-Focused Care 61
   Addressing the Patient 62
Health Insurance Portability and Accountability Act 62
Bedside Ultrasound 63
Emergency Medical Situations 65
   Choking 65
   Cardiopulmonary Resuscitation 66
Sonographer Exposure to Body Fluids 67

CHAPTER 2 Essentials of Patient Care for the Sonographer

KEY TERMS

Arrhythmia
Body mechanics
Bradycardia
Consent
Cyanosis
Dyspnea
Heimlich maneuver
Nasal cannula

Nosocomial infections
Oximetry
Oxygen therapy
Patient-centered care
Pulse
Refusal
Respiration
Standard precautions

Tachycardia
Urinary catheters
Vital signs
White coat hypertension

INTRODUCTION

Sonography is a profession that is more than just creating diagnostic images. A sonographer will have a patient under their care while they are performing the exam and will need to know some basic patient care skills as well as understand how to keep the patient, as well as themselves, safe. Understanding and mastering these nonscanning skills will make you a well-rounded sonographer. The goal of this chapter is to provide you with the knowledge needed to provide care and a safe environment for patients under your care.

A SONOGRAPHER'S COMMITMENTS

A good sonographer understands their commitments to their patient, the sonologist, their employer, their coworkers, to the sonography profession, and to themselves. What exactly are these commitments? Our patients expect us to have the skills and knowledge to produce a diagnostic sonographic exam, to keep them safe while in our care, and to be understanding of their needs.

The sonologist is the interpreting physician of the sonographic study. There are a variety of sonologists but the most common physicians that a sonographer will work with are radiologists, cardiologists, vascular surgeons, and obstetricians. Sonography is a very unique imaging modality as it involves trust between the sonographer and the sonologist. Breaking this trust (by too often missing pathology or frequently trying to cover up your mistakes) can take a long time to repair before the sonologist gains confidence in your studies. The commitment of the sonographer to the sonologist is to produce diagnostic studies, to be trustworthy, and to have good interpersonal and communication skills.

The commitment to the employer will enable the sonographer to be seen as a valuable employee. Such commitments include punctuality, protecting and respecting the work environment, adhering to policies and guidelines, being a positive representative of the institution to the outside world, and taking care of the patient.

The commitments to your coworkers are important to promote a healthy work environment. This includes maintaining good work habits, following and adhering to both the policies and guidelines of the ultrasound department, supporting each other during difficult times as well as celebrating the good times, and being respectful to one another.

As a sonographer, there is a need to educate our patients about the profession of sonography, to follow the SDMS Sonographer Code of Ethics, to support the ultrasound community and its professional organizations with our membership, and to attain national registration in the field of ultrasound in which you are practicing.

We should have the desire to help all people; to use our skills and knowledge to obtain the best diagnostic exam on every patient; to be a good team player; to constantly advance our knowledge of anatomy, physiology, and pathology; to utilize ergonomics; and to maintain good physical and mental health. A positive attitude brings with it a sense of pride in your work.

Patient-Centered Care

Florence Nightingale advocated focusing on the patient, rather than on the disease, as a way to recognize the patient's basic needs by improving hygiene practices. By distinguishing patient care from medicine, Nightingale established the value of nurses and created the earliest patient advocates.

Patient-centered care ensures that the patient and/or their family is involved in all clinical decisions for their care and treatment. To a sonographer this means being respectful if the patient refuses the exam, or part of the exam, such as the endovaginal aspect of a pelvic sonogram, or wants the exam terminated early. As a sonographer, you should not force the patient to do anything they are uncomfortable with; however, it would be appropriate to ask the question "Why?" Ask the patient why they are refusing the exam or want the exam stopped early. You may discover their fears or concerns, which may help you understand their **refusal**. You may be able to address their concerns, and they will consent to the exam or to finish the exam. For example, the patient may say that they do not want the ultrasound as they just had a CT scan, that they feel like a "guinea pig" and the hospital is just trying to make money off of them. Discussing the differences between these two imaging modalities may be enough to relieve their concerns and allow you to perform the exam.

Due to the ultrasound imaging from the entertainment industry, many patients believe that a physician will be performing their exam and may get upset when you tell them that you will be taking care of them. This situation should lead to a conversation about the roles and misconceptions of sonography, sonographers, and sonologists. Allowing the patient to voice their concerns and to ask you questions shows that you respect them. Be sure that you address their concerns and answer their questions and not brush them off.

The most important facet of being a sonographer is seeing the patient as a person, not as an appointment or a type of study. We need to treat the patient with respect, empathy, and compassion. You must put aside personal feelings and prejudices and be considerate of many factors such as patient's age, sex, gender identification, sexual orientation, race, religious beliefs, ethnicity, language spoken, occupation, disabilities, and socioeconomic status. Good patient care is more than your sonography skills and includes open communication with the patients, which will allow them to express their concerns, fears, and frustrations.

The patient-centered approach encourages sonographers to relate to patients as people with needs, who are to be respected and cared for in a mature and dignified manner. They should be listened to and their concerns not dismissed. A common phrase a sonographer may hear is, "But it hurts here. Aren't you going to look there?" The knee-jerk reaction is to say, "I can only scan the area ordered by the physician" instead of explaining things such as referred pain or the limitations of ultrasound. A good solution is to place the transducer over the area of pain and take a few images labeled as "area of pain." This makes the patient feel heard and their concerns addressed. I remember being called in to do a right upper quadrant sonogram on a patient with an indication of right-sided pain. The patient asked if I could scan where she felt the pain. I put the transducer there and found a 20 cm complex ovarian mass despite a normal pelvic exam a few days earlier. I called the emergency department physician and told them of my findings and if they would order a pelvic ultrasound, to which they agreed. The surgeon came to see me the next day and told me that I had saved her life as the mass was ready to rupture any moment and would have spread the cancer throughout her body. You can imagine how I felt especially when the patient and her husband came and thanked me for saving her life when she was being discharged. (A few tears of joy were shed by all.) This is one of many joys of being a sonographer, and I will never forget that patient. Just think of the consequences if I had refused to put the transducer where she had pain.

Sonographers must remember that the patients' needs come first, despite how it will affect you personally. You cannot let the patient know how upset and frustrated you are for having to stay over to do their exam. This frustration may manifest itself as being curt with the patient or maybe even treating them a little rough. Never take your frustrations out on the patient. After all, the patient did not ask to have a swollen leg at 5 PM on a Friday. You are working in a profession in which you may need to put yourself second to the needs of the patient. Remember, they are the reason that we have a job.

You have chosen a profession that is challenging in many ways. It will test you technically, physically, mentally, and even emotionally. As a student or staff sonographer, you will need to focus on many things at once as you are scanning including your knowledge of anatomy, physiology, pathology, imaging protocols, and techniques. You may be faced with pressures from physicians, time restraints, challenging personalities, or even your own personal issues. What is important is to provide caring attention to your patient who is not focused on the same things as you. They are worried about what you are going to do to them, will it hurt, and what the results are going to be. As a sonographer, you need to constantly provide a level of care similar to that which you would want provided to you or a loved one. You have to challenge yourself to make every patient experience one in which your patient can sense that you really care. You can do this through the practice of compassion, sympathy, and empathy.

Empathy is the ability to understand and share the feelings of another usually as a result of you having experienced similar circumstances. Sympathy refers to your ability to feel sorry about their situation even though you have not had a similar experience. In health care, empathy or sympathy toward your patient will enable you to understand what they need from you as you perform their exam. For example, maybe you had a urinary tract infection (UTI) in the past, and you remember how cold you were from the fever caused by the UTI. This might cause you to get the patient a blanket without them asking for one. This may surprise the patient at your thoughtfulness. This is an example of empathy as you have experienced something similar. By contrast, if you had never had a UTI, you would show sympathy to the patient by asking if them if they would like a blanket.

Compassion is when we are moved by someone's pain or suffering and are motivated to help them. Compassion for your patient is what drives you to do something for them. Maybe your patient has had other tests that have not diagnosed why they are in pain. This may motivate you to go that extra mile to try to find the cause of their pain, if it can be seen with ultrasound. You can show compassion by asking the patient if they need to talk when you sense that they are upset. Even if they do not want to talk, the patient will sense your compassion for them.

Explain the Ultrasound Exam. There is so much misinformation out there about sonography thanks to the entertainment industry. Some patients will assume that a doctor will perform their exam and are surprised and maybe even concerned to discover that you will be performing the sonogram. This is an educational moment to correct any misconceptions that the patient might have. Ask them if they have ever had an ultrasound before. If not, you can help patients understand how ultrasound works by saying something like, "I will be using soundwaves to create images of your uterus and ovaries," followed by a variation on the following explanation, "I will be exposing your stomach area and will be putting some gel on your skin to help the soundbeam get into your body. There is no radiation, and it should be painless. If you feel any pain, please let me know." Let them know if they will need to be in different positions: "I will start you out on your back and will also have you turn up on your side facing away from me." Do not forget to tell them that they will need to hold their breath if needed. I used to say, "Sometimes I get involved scanning and may forget to tell you to breathe. When you need to breathe, please go ahead and breathe." Always give an idea on how long they will be with you: "The ultrasound should take about 30 minutes. I then need to have the images checked by the radiologist before you leave to make sure that they don't want any additional images. The whole process takes about 40 minutes from start to finish." At the end of the exam explain that their physician will be the one giving them the results. Give them an estimation of the typical time it takes the physician to obtain the results. In this electronic world physicians typically have their patients' ultrasound results in 8 to 24 hours. Before you start, it is important to ask the patient if they have any questions. You have your spiel that you usually tell patients, but every patient is different, and you may need to address any specific questions that that patient may have.

Patient Consent and Refusal. **Consent** means giving permission to have something done, in this case an ultrasound study. Hopefully, the patient's physician has already informed the patient that they need to have an ultrasound exam, the reason why, and that the patient has verbally consented to their physician to have the test. If the patient is awake, alert, and legally responsible for their own health decisions, you will obtain their permission to perform the ultrasound exam through verbal communication. This is called *verbal consent* and typically is not documented. This is the case for any ultrasound whether it is external or internal, although some places may require a written consent for a transvaginal study. Transvaginal ultrasounds will always require the consent of the patient or the person that is legally responsible for their health care decisions, when the patient is unable to give consent or when the patient is a minor. When another person gives consent on behalf of the patient it may need to be in the form of a *written consent*, or the name of the person documented in the patient's medical records. If it is a medical emergency the physician taking care of the patient may give consent, based on hospital policy which may require two doctors to give consent. This would need to be documented as per hospital policy. As a staff sonographer you will need to know and follow these policies. For a written consent it is appropriate for the sonographer to witness the signature on the consent form. If you are asked to witness a consent when you did not see the patient sign it, show the patient the consent form and ask them to verify that that is their signature before you sign.

Consent is mandatory when the patient is having any invasive procedure such as a biopsy or fluid tap. The consent needs to list the benefits, potential complications, and alternative options to the procedure which might include doing nothing. The patient or a person legally responsible for the patient must sign the consent form, which will become part of the patient's permanent record. The consent must be witnessed and signed (which can be the sonographer as previously discussed) (Fig. 2.1). A student typically is not allowed to witness the consent since they are not an employee of the hospital. Some hospitals are transitioning into electronic consents with everyone signing on an electronic signature capture pad which will transfer everything into the patient's electronic medical record.

As discussed, an ultrasound should not be performed if the patient refuses the exam or asks you to stop. If you cannot persuade the patient to finish their exam, then the reading physician or the ordering physician should talk to the patient and address their concerns. If the patient agrees, you may finish the exam; if not, the exam will be terminated. Whatever the reason, you should remain respectful to the patient and not be rude or condescending to them.

Patient Privacy. Performing an ultrasound study will involve exposure of part of the patient's body, and you should assume everyone is modest. In fact, you may come across some cultures or religions where people cannot expose their skin in public, especially to someone they perceive as the opposite sex. The sonographer must honor if a patient specifically requests a male or female to perform their study. Before beginning each ultrasound examination, be sure to close the door and pull any curtains for the patient's privacy. Inform the patient that you are going to be lifting their shirt or gown, uncovering only the parts of the body that are necessary to perform the exam. You will want to explain to the patient why you are tucking a towel into their pants or shirt to protect their clothes from the gel. Sometimes the patient will put the gown on with the opening in the front. This can make it difficult to keep their breasts covered so place a towel, sheet, or another gown across their chest explaining that you want to keep their chest covered.

Always allow the patient privacy when they are changing their clothes. Knock on the door before entering, crack it just a little and ask if they are finished changing before entering. Do not assume that they are finished changing and barge into the room.

If you need to go into a room where a patient is being scanned, for example, looking for a certain transducer, always knock on the door and ask for permission to enter. Be respectful when entering the room, maintaining the privacy of the patient. Just imagine the patient's embarrassment if the door is flung open while they are having a vaginal, scrotal, or breast ultrasound, and have now been exposed to "the world."

Another aspect of privacy is to not discuss the patient's information in public places such as an elevator or in the hallway. Do not ask questions about their medical history where others can easily overhear you. Not only can this make the patient uncomfortable but it is also a violation of their protected health information. Your place of employment or ultrasound program will train you about the Health Insurance Portability and Accountability Act (HIPAA) of 1996, which established national standards for protection of patient medical information (or as it is commonly called, PHI). You must comply with the regulations involved with this act and be aware of ways that patient information can be compromised, especially in social media. A student may be excited when they see pathology or perform a good exam or a sonographer when they have unusual findings. However, writing about your patient on your social media account even though their name is not mentioned can be considered a violation of HIPAA. People have lost their jobs talking about patients on their social media accounts.

Who Can Be in the Room? Some patients may want a friend or family member with them for support and at other times

1. INDICATIONS FOR THE OPERATION OR OTHER PROCEDURE ARE:
   Mass/lesion, fluid, oher:_____
   _____

2. MAJOR RISKS AND PROBABILITY OF SUCCESS OF THE OPERATION OR OTHER PROCEDURE (including such items as failure to obtain the desired result, discomfort, injury, additional therapy and death):
   - Pain
   - Vasovagal reaction/allergic reaction
   - Bleeding/inadvertent injury to other organs
   - Inadequate specimen
   - Other:_____

3. DISCUSSIONS OF ALTERNATIVES TO THE PROPOSED OPERATION OR OTHER PROCEDURE **including risks, benefits and side effects as well as possible outcome of not receiving the procedure:**
   - Do nothing
   - Biopsy without imaging guidance
   - Surgery

4. IN INSTANCES WHERE A DISCUSSION OF THE ABOVE IS DEEMED UNWISE MEDICAL PRACTICE, THERE SHOULD BE DOCUMENTED A STATEMENT TO THIS EFFECT BELOW, STATING THE REASON FOR THIS DECISION. (This space may also be used for explanatory diagrams.)
   _____
   _____
   _____

_____   _____
Signature of Patient   *Signature of Witness*

_____
Signature of Physician/Health Care Provider Securing Consent

IF PATIENT IS UNABLE TO SIGN OR IS A MINOR, COMPLETE THE FOLLOWING:

Patient is a minor (___ years of age) or is unable to sign because: _____
_____

_____   _____
Signature of Parent, Surrogate, Health Care Agent or Legal Guardian   *Signature of Witness*

*****TIME OUT VERIFICATION***** – Please document the names of the participants below:

_____   _____   _____
Surgeon/Physician/Licensed Health Care Provider   *Nurse*   *Anesthesiologist/CRNA*

DATE_____   **TIME**_____**AM/PM**

FIG. 2.1 Sample basic consent form that also includes the time out documentation.

they may want privacy during their exam. The preference of the patient, whether an inpatient or outpatient, must always be considered. In a patient's hospital room, if the patient would like visitors or family members to stay with them, you should try to honor this request. Depending on the situation, you will communicate that it is either fine for them to stay, or that it is preferred that they wait somewhere else and the reason why. At times you may get more cooperation if you allow their visitors to stay.

When performing a portable ultrasound, the nurse is another person that may be in the room. The nurse in the room can also help make your job easier by providing you with information about the patient, helping to position the patient, providing comfort to the patient during the exam, and communicating as needed with the patient and their visitors. There may be times that the nurse or other hospital staff will have to interrupt the ultrasound to address a patient care issue, such as giving important meds. Usually, you can manage to work around each other but if not, you should step away from the bed until they have finished.

When a patient comes to the ultrasound department you have a little more control over who comes into the room with the patient. Consider their wishes on deciding if the visitor should wait outside. If the patient is a minor, in most cases you will have the parent come into the ultrasound room with you. A teenager may be uncomfortable having their parent in the room for an ultrasound, especially if it is a breast, pelvic, or testicular exam. A good solution is to ask the patient if they prefer to have their parent with them or to wait outside. This may be a difficult conversation with the parent explaining the reason why they should wait outside. If they are going to stay, try and position the parent so that they cannot see their child.

There may be times when you need to leave a patient alone in a room. This can be a concern for a very ill patient or someone with a risk of falling. If you need to leave the patient alone in a room, be sure to lower the bed height, raise the bedrails, and leave your patient with a call button (Fig. 2.2). If necessary, find someone to sit with your patient until you return or move them into a place where they can be observed. If a family member is waiting outside, invite them in to stay with the patient. Remember patient safety first.

Certain types of ultrasound exams may require a chaperone. A chaperone is an employee that is present during a sensitive clinical exam or procedure in which a patient may feel uncomfortable. A chaperone also protects the sonographer from being falsely accused of inappropriate behavior by the patient. A chaperone is required for a vaginal ultrasound, even if the sonographer is female since a variety of sonographers have been successfully sued. This is a serious subject, and you need to know the policy of the institution and question if they do not require a chaperone for a female sonographer performing an endovaginal exam. The legal department can be a good resource as usually there is a blanket policy that involves any employee, including doctors, who is performing any type of vaginal exam. Having a chaperone protects not only the patient's concerns, but legally protects the sonographer from any false accusations of sexually molesting or abusing the patient. The name of the chaperone is documented in the patient's medical record. If a patient ever makes a legal claim that a sonographer acted unprofessionally, the documented chaperone will serve as a witness. Sometimes you may want a chaperone to protect you if you feel threatened or perceive unwanted advances from the patient. For example, a patient may keep exposing their penis, which has an erection, to the sonographer while they are scanning their scrotum, despite multiple attempts to keep the penis covered. If you feel threatened, you need to have another person in the room. You never want to put yourself at risk, either physically, emotionally, or legally.

Efficiency in Patient Care. Timing of the ultrasound is a very important aspect of patient care. When speaking to the nurse before the exam, you will want to ask if it is a good time to perform the ultrasound. The patient may have other tests ordered that may have priority over the ultrasound, such as an endoscopy. At times you will need to work with the nurse to find the best time to get the ultrasound done, especially if it is a portable exam. Communication and planning with the nurse are crucial for efficiency and good patient care.

A patient should be off of their unit for a limited amount of time in order to receive the best care. They will typically have other tests that need to be performed, need to be available to see doctors, and will have visitors. This will require being prepared for the patient's arrival by having the room ready, inputting their identification information into the ultrasound unit, and investigating the pertinent patient history before they arrive to the department. Working efficiently will help your patients have good experiences.

Unfortunately, there will be times when the patient will need to wait. Emergent situations will happen that will need to be addressed immediately, causing patients to wait. Here communication is vital. The patient should be informed as to the reason for the wait and the expected amount of time that they will have to wait. Inpatients should be given the option to return to their unit to be called later and outpatients the chance to reschedule, especially if the wait time may exceed 30 minutes. Patients should be offered any comfort that you can provide while they wait. Any further delays will also need to be communicated to the patient. For safety, do not leave an inpatient alone for an extended period of time. They should be where other employees can watch or help them as needed. Leaving a patient alone increases the risk of the patient trying to get out of their wheelchair or off of their stretcher causing them to fall, pull out their IV, or even wander off. Critically ill patients should never be left alone. What if they code and no one is around to call the code and start cardiopulmonary resuscitation (CPR)? It is important that all safety measures

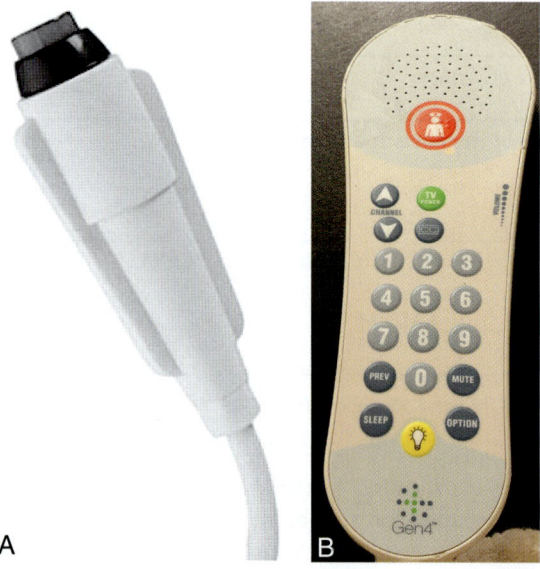

FIG. 2.2 (A) A simple call button. Pressing the button will cause an alarm to go off. This is usually the type of call bell found in an ultrasound department. (B) A call button that can also control the television in a patient's room. Pressing the red button on top with the nurse icon will notify someone that the patient needs help, causing a light to flash and an audible signal. The cancel button is typically in the patient's room, requiring a staff visit when it is pressed.

are being used when a patient has to wait, which includes but is not limited to having the brakes applied, side rails up, and that they have a call button. Failure to do so may cause the patient to harm themselves and for you to be disciplined.

BASIC PATIENT CARE

Vital Signs

Vital signs are a group of measurements that give an idea of the body's life-sustaining functions. They are used to help assess the general physical health of a person and to potentially alert the possibility of a disease process. The four most common vital signs that are taken are pulse rate, respiratory rate, body temperature, and blood pressure. The readings of the vital signs will vary with the age, sex, weight of the patient, and their overall health. The normal range for vital signs is constantly being evaluated, and these values may change. The reader is encouraged to be familiar with current normal values.

Sonographers do not routinely assess the vital signs of a patient unless performing specific ultrasound studies, such as an ankle-brachial index (ABI) or assessing for a subclavian steal. Vital signs are always part of a complete echocardiogram procedure. It is possible to be asked to help in an emergency situation, so learning how to properly take a pulse, count respirations, or to properly put on a blood pressure cuff can be helpful for the care of the patient. Automatic blood pressure pumps may have a pulse oximeter attached and the sonographer may have to place the sensor on the patient's finger so that the oxygen levels can be determined as well.

Pulse. The **pulse** is used to measure the heart rate, or the number of times the heart beats per minute. When the heart pumps, blood is forced into the arteries during contraction of the left ventricle. The amount of force that is created when the blood hits the arterial walls will produce an advancing pressure wave that causes the arterial walls to expand. This expansion produces the feeling of a pulse. The pulse can be felt in the wrists (radial artery), the neck (carotid artery), the inside of the elbow (brachial artery), the ankles (posterior tibial artery), the top of the foot (dorsalis pedis), behind the knee (popliteal artery), and in the groin (femoral artery). The place where the pulse is measured is named after the artery that is palpated, with the radial and carotid arteries being the most common places to assess the patient's pulse.

The pulse offers an easy and effective way to measure heart rate and is recorded as beats per minute. The beat of the pulse should be evaluated for rate, rhythm, and regularity, as well as for strength. Normal adult pulse rates should be between 60 and 100 beats/min with a regular rhythm. However, there are some normal variations. For example, rates in children, women, and the elderly are slightly higher, whereas rates in athletes are slightly lower.

A normal pulse will have strong palpitations, whereas a weak pulse will feel faint. No discernible pulse is suggestive of arterial occlusion. An irregular pulse and therefore heartbeat is termed an **arrhythmia** or dysrhythmia. Among the most common arrhythmias are tachycardia and bradycardia.

Tachycardia is defined as a heart rate of more than 100 beats/min. This finding may only be temporary, caused by exertion or nervousness, or it may be secondary to disease.

A heart rate of fewer than 60 beats/min is **bradycardia** and may arise from disease in the heart's electrical conduction system or with the sinoatrial node. These patients may have a sinus node dysfunction or heart block. Remember that athletes can have heart rates less than 60 beats/min, which would be normal for them.

When taking a pulse, first explain the procedure to the patient and then have them place their arm straight palm side up. The radial artery can be located by placing the index and middle fingers at the base of the wrist on the thumb side. Never use your thumb to take the patient's pulse, as the strong pulse within your own thumb may be confused with that of the patient's. Using your finger, gently feel for the radial artery on the inner side of the wrist (Fig. 2.3). If no abnormalities are detected, the pulse should be counted for 30 seconds and multiplied by 2. If irregularities are noted, the pulse should be counted for a full minute. Record the pulse rate and anything you notice about the pulse, such as its being weak, strong, or missing beats. If an irregularity is detected, determine whether it occurs in a pattern or is random. If the radial pulse is difficult to palpate, try the carotid artery. To find the carotid artery, place your fingers just below the angle of the patient's mandible (Fig. 2.4).

In the vascular lab the vascular sonographer may assess the pulses at the ankles to evaluate the legs for arterial disease. As part of a lower extremity arterial evaluation the pulse rate is typically not measured but the quality and strength of the pulse is assessed using a number from 0 to 2 with a normal strong pulse written as 2⁺, a weak pulse that is barely felt as a 1, and no pulse as a 0.

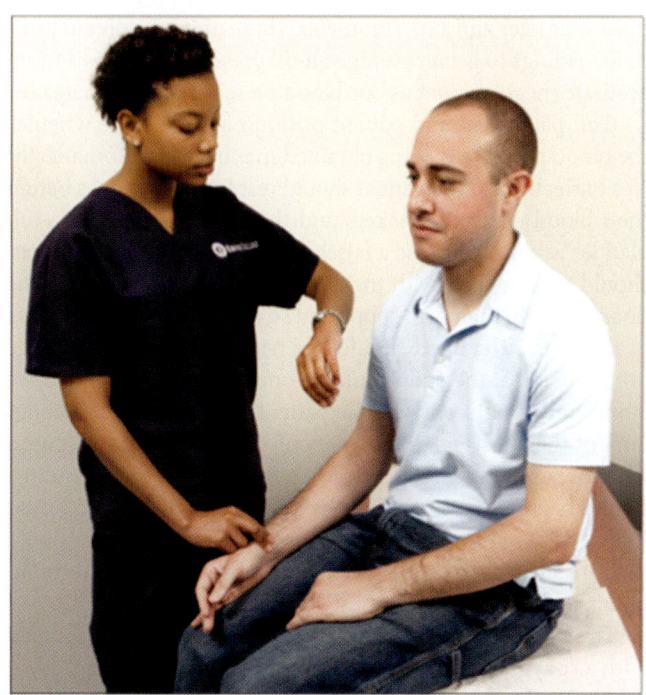

FIG. 2.3 Properly taking a radial pulse.

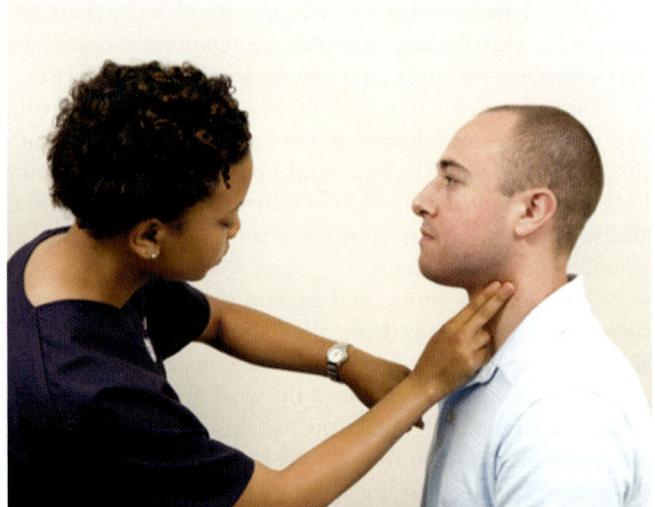

FIG. 2.4 Properly taking a carotid pulse.

Blood Pressure. One of the most important and common vital signs assessed is blood pressure. Blood pressure is the pressure or force exerted by circulating blood against the walls of the arteries. Blood pressure is expressed as two numbers. The first number is the systolic measurement, when the pressure is at its highest when the heart beats, and the second number is the diastolic measurement, when the pressure is at its lowest as the heart relaxes between beats. Blood pressure is written as follows, 120/80, and would be expressed verbally as 120 over 80. Although these numbers appear to be a fraction, they are not nor are these numbers a ratio. Blood pressure is measured in millimeters of mercury (mm Hg).

The blood pressure is typically obtained from the brachial artery in the arm. Blood pressure may be taken manually or with an automatic unit. Typically, the automatic units will also measure the pulse, and some will have accessories such as a pulse oximeter and a thermometer. These units can obtain multiple readings to get an average blood pressure, which is a more accurate measurement as our blood pressure can fluctuate.

Cuff placement and patient position are the same whether the blood pressure is being obtained manually or automatically. In a perfect world the patient should rest for five minutes before their blood pressure is taken, and they should not have a full bladder as this can cause a falsely elevated reading. The patient should sit in a chair with their back supported, feet flat on the floor and with their arm supported so that the cuff is at the level of the heart. The hand should not be clenched (Fig. 2.5). The bottom edge of the cuff should be one to two inches above the elbow and should encircle the patient's upper arm with about 80% of the cuff (Fig. 2.6). If the cuff is too small it will give a higher reading, and if it too large it will produce a lower reading. Before beginning, verify that the patient has not crossed their legs as this will increase the blood pressure. The patient should be instructed not to talk while their pressure is being taken. To obtain a manual blood pressure follow the steps in Box 2.1.

The manual measurement of blood pressure is performed with a sphygmomanometer, blood pressure cuff, and a stethoscope. The blood pressure cuff consists of an air pump, a pressure gauge, and a rubber cuff (Fig. 2.7).

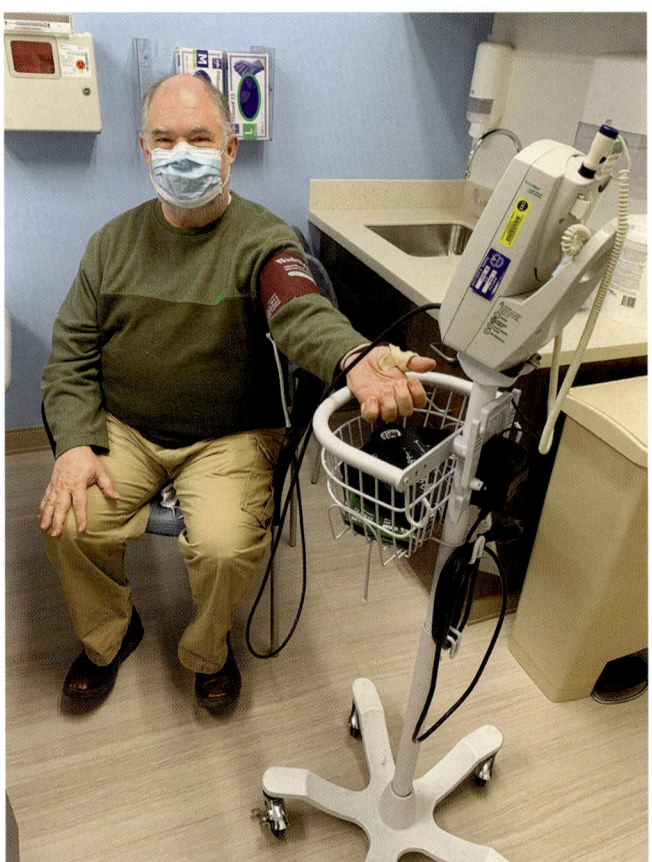

FIG. 2.5 A patient getting a blood pressure measurement with an automatic device. Notice how the patient's arm is resting on the holder to keep it at the proper height, the level of the heart, with the palm up. Both feet are flat on the floor. This unit also measures the patient's pulse simultaneously. The thermometer is stored in its holder on the back of the unit. The wire holder holds the various sized cuffs.

Blood pressure readings can be affected by a variety of factors, including cardiac disease, nervousness about seeing the doctor (called **white coat hypertension**), obesity, smoking, stress, drinking alcohol or caffeine 30 minutes before the reading, being cold or chilly, and some medications and herbal supplements. The reader is encouraged to do a search on medications and herbs that affect the blood pressure. If the first blood pressure reading is higher than normal, a second reading should be taken after 2 to 3 minutes allowing the patient time to relax.

The vascular sonographer may use a manual system for taking brachial and ankle pressures required to determine the ABI. To measure the ABI, the systolic readings are obtained using Doppler, as opposed to a stethoscope. The cuff is placed above the ankle for the ankle readings and above the elbow for the brachial reading. A reading is obtained from both arms and ankles using the brachial, dorsalis pedis, and posterior tibial arteries. Find the artery with the continuous wave Doppler transducer. Inflate the cuff until the Doppler signal is no longer heard. When the signal returns take note of the reading as this is the systolic number. Repeat for the other arteries. Note that the Doppler signal will always be present, so a diastolic reading cannot be obtained.

Pulse Oximetry. **Oximetry** is a convenient, noninvasive method of monitoring blood oxygen levels. This information is useful to

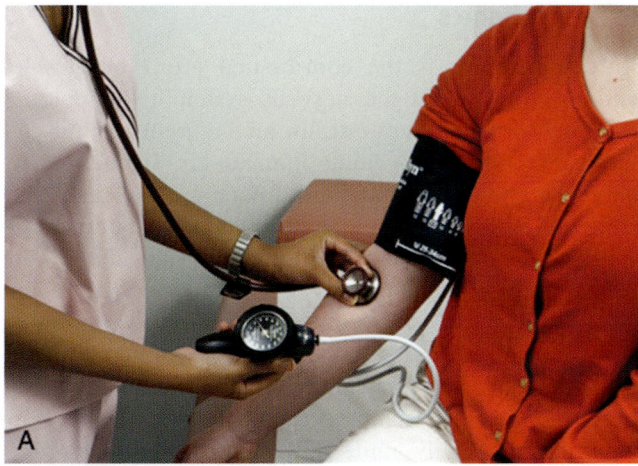

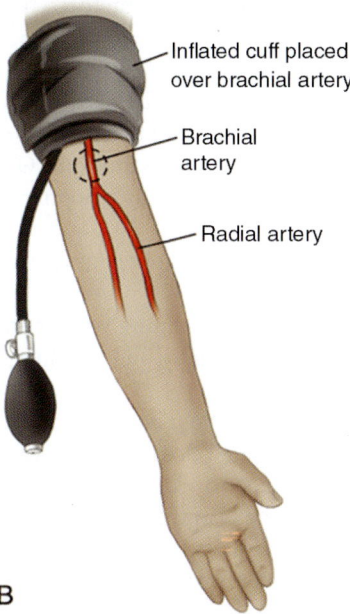

FIG. 2.6 (A) Taking a blood pressure with a manual device. (B) Proper cuff size and placement.

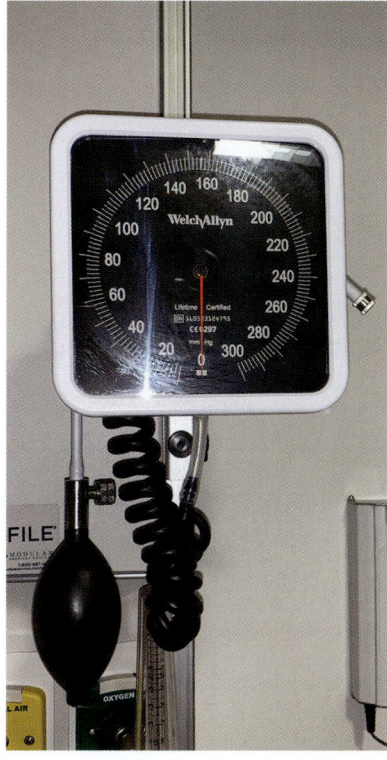

FIG. 2.7 Manual blood pressure device in a patient's room showing the pump, display, and hose to connect to the cuff.

determine whether the heart, lungs, and blood are working synchronously to deliver oxygen to various parts of the body. A low blood oxygen reading can be a sign of an illness or injury.

The test is performed by using an oximeter, a specially designed photoelectric device, which measures the difference between levels of the red pigment hemoglobin, which carries oxygen in the blood. The most commonly used oximeters are called pulse oximeters because they respond to the pulsations of the capillaries in the area to be tested. One end of the device is attached like a clothespin to the end of the patient's index finger (Fig. 2.8). The other end of the oximeter is attached to a monitor so that the patient's oxygen level can be seen at all times.

The amount of oxygen in the blood is given as a percentage. A normal reading for a person breathing room air is in the high 90 s. A reading of 90% or less will trigger visual and audible alarms, requiring immediate action. Asking the patient to take in a couple of deep breaths will help raise the oxygen levels. If the levels keep falling, the patient will be given oxygen to help maintain good levels. The oximeter acts as an indicator that something is interfering with the oxygenation of blood levels and that further investigation is required. It does not diagnose what is interfering with the patient's oxygen levels.

A patient that is having a lung or chest biopsy under ultrasound guidance will have their pulse ox monitored as a sudden drop can be a sign that the lung has been punctured.

Respiration. **Respiration**, or breathing, is the process of inhaling and exhaling air. Its primary function is to obtain oxygen for use by the body's cells and to eliminate carbon dioxide. Normal breathing is quiet, effortless, and has a regular rhythm. In an adult at rest, respiration occurs at a rate of

---

BOX 2.1 Taking a Manual Blood Pressure

- Have the patient sit with their arm supported and with the arm at the level of the chest or heart.
- The bottom edge of the cuff should be one to two inches above the elbow and should encircle the patient's upper arm with about 80% of the cuff.
- Squeeze the pump to rapidly inflate the cuff to about 200 mm Hg, or until no sound is heard with the stethoscope over the brachial artery.
- Loosen the valve slowly, about 5 mm Hg/sec, to let out air while listening for the sound of the return of the heartbeat. When it returns check the measurement on the manometer as this is the systolic reading.
- Continue deflating the cuff slowly until you can no longer hear the heartbeat. This last audible sound is the diastolic reading.
- Record both readings as a fraction (e.g., 136/88).

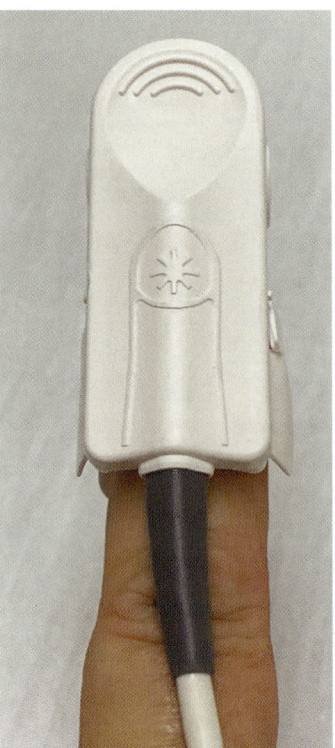

FIG. 2.8 Proper placement of the pulse oximeter sensor device on the patient's index finger.

12 to 20 breaths/min. Measuring respiration for less than a full minute may lead to inaccuracies.

When assessing a patient's respiratory rate, the rhythm, depth, and character of the respiration should be noted. Any injuries to the lungs, chest muscles, or diaphragm will affect breathing. Note whether the patient needs to sit up to breathe easily as opposed to lying down. Any difficulty in breathing, **dyspnea**, or changes in the patient's color, pallor, or **cyanosis**, should be noted.

To count respirations, note the number of inhalations per minute. Counting respirations is often done while continuing to hold the patient's wrist, after the pulse has been counted, to prevent patients from being aware that you are monitoring their breathing, as sometimes the patient may change how they are breathing in response to being observed.

It is uncommon for a sonographer to measure and qualify respirations. However, the sonographer should be aware of the patient's breathing and quality, reporting any sudden changes while performing the ultrasound exam.

PATIENT TRANSFER TECHNIQUES

Patient safety is a prime component of patient care. Equally important is sonographer safety. Some of the most common injuries among members of the health care team are musculoskeletal (MSK) strains or injuries. Sonographers can avoid injuries with a conscious use of body mechanics in their everyday activities, work activities, and especially when performing patient **transfers**. By protecting themselves from injury, they are also protecting their patients.

Body Mechanics

Body mechanics is the coordinated effort of muscles, tendons, joints, and the nervous system to complete a task safely without undue strain on any joints or muscles. Because back pain or joint injuries are frequent complaints among sonographers, you must prevent self-injury while positioning, lifting, and transferring patients as well as while performing an ultrasound study. Good body mechanics protects you from injury, reduces fatigue, and allows you to use your body more effectively. An added bonus is that the use of good body mechanics also protects patients from injury. Initially, sonographers may find that it requires a conscious effort to maintain proper body alignment especially while scanning, but when practiced on a daily basis, it will become second nature. When the sonographer is exposed to ergonomic risk factors, they become fatigued and risk MSK injury.

Lifting should be done using the strong leg muscles and not the muscles of the back, lifting straight upward in one smooth motion. When reaching, stand directly in front of the object and avoid any twisting or stretching motions. One of the most common causes of MSK injuries is stooping by bending at the waist.

The following are suggestions for sonographers on the use of good body mechanics:

- Maintain a stable center of gravity by keeping your center of gravity low, keeping your back straight, and bending at the hips and knees.
- Maintain a center of gravity by keeping your back straight and keeping any objects that are being lifted close to your body.
- Maintain a strong base of support by keeping your feet apart, placing one foot slightly ahead of the other with toes pointed in the direction of activity, and then flexing your knees and turning with your feet, instead of your hips.
- Maintain proper body alignment through good posture: Tuck in your buttocks, pull your abdomen in and up, keep your back flat, your head up, and your chin in as you keep your weight forward and supported on the outside of your feet.

Sonographers benefit greatly from using correct body mechanics when lifting and reaching. Their first consideration should be whether the object or patient is too heavy to lift alone. The potential for injury to themselves and their patients can be avoided by enlisting the help of another person.

- Always evaluate a situation and whether help is needed.
- Remove any objects or hazards before moving or during the transfer of patients.
- Be sure your feet are a shoulder width apart to provide a strong base of support. Distribute your weight evenly, standing with one foot slightly forward for balance.
- Never bend sideways from the waist or hip for any activity.
- When turning, always pivot your feet and never twist your body.
- Do not attempt to lift a heavy load alone.
- Always position yourself as closely as possible to whatever is being lifted and never reach for a load.
- Lift smoothly and avoid jerky movements.

- If lifting with the help of another person, prearrange a signal, such as lifting on the count of three.
- Always lower your body to the object being lifted by bending your knees, not your back.
- Straighten your legs while lifting the object.
- If you must start a lift with a slightly curved back, the large muscles of your legs should take over.
- Whenever possible, push, pull, or roll an object instead of lifting it.

Stretcher and Wheelchair Transfer

It is important to know the method of transport for patients who will be coming to the ultrasound department. Ask the nurse if the patient is able to get up on a stretcher on their own or with minimal assistance. This will help determine if the patient should come to the department on a stretcher or in a wheelchair. When a patient is not able to get in and out of a wheelchair with minimal assistance, it is not only a potential risk to the patient for falling, but it also poses a threat to the safety of the sonographer. If it is difficult for two people to get the patient onto the stretcher, the patient should be sent back to the unit to be put onto a stretcher. Inform the floor that you are sending the patient back to the unit to be put on a stretcher and why. Some nurses may give you a hard time as they were able to get the patient in a wheelchair by themselves. Tell them that it is a patient safety issue as you need the patient to step up on a step stool with minimal assistance, turn 180 degrees while on the step stool, and then sit on the stretcher. Some stretchers may lower to the floor in which case it may be possible to get them onto the stretcher. Do not jeopardize the patient or yourself and get help when needed.

When working with patients in wheelchairs, the sonographer should make it a practice to lock the brakes and lift the footrests. Use proper body mechanics when transferring patients to and from wheelchairs and the scan bed. If the patient has limited mobility and came to the department in a wheelchair, it may require two people to safely get the patient onto the scan bed. If the patient has a very difficult time standing or is "dead weight," do not risk injuring the patient or yourself by trying to physically lift them up onto the stretcher. As stated previously, it may not be ideal, but send the patient back to their floor to be sent back on a stretcher. If you do succeed in getting the patient up on the scan bed, consider sending the patient back on the stretcher if possible, for both the patient's and your own safety.

If a patient is transported to the department on a stretcher or in their bed, they do not need to be moved to the scan bed. If the patient has arrived by stretcher, the wheels should be locked, and the side rails should be in an upright position until the examination commences. If the patient needs to get off of the stretcher, you and possibly a coworker will need to assist the patient off of the stretcher. If they need to use the restroom and require too much assistance, offer them a bedpan or urinal. Preventing injury and falls should be your primary concern.

For patients who arrive by wheelchair, lower the scanning stretcher to its lowest position so that the patient can easily get up onto the stretcher. Have the side rails up on the opposite side of the stretcher. Be careful with any IV lines, tubes, drains, or the urinary catheter and bag when helping your patient in and out of the wheelchair. Always be next to the patient to be there to support them as needed when moving from wheelchair to the scanning stretcher and vice versa. Only use step stools that have a handle for the patient to grip (Fig. 2.9).

Moving Patients Onto a Scan Bed From a Wheelchair

When moving a patient onto a scanning stretcher from a wheelchair try using the following strategies to ensure a safe outcome for you and the patient:
- Make sure that the table is locked so that it will not slide.
- Adjust the bed to the lowest position.
- Relate what you plan to do and give instructions on how the patient can help.
- Lock the wheels on the wheelchair and lift the feet rests.
- On your count of three, ask the patient to push with their feet to stand while you support them with one hand in their armpit and your other arm around their back (Fig. 2.10).
- Help the patient to turn around and sit down on the stretcher.
- Help them to lie on their back by lifting their legs.
- Make the patient comfortable and begin the examination.
- If the patient is unable to cooperate or has mobility issues, ask a colleague for help.

Moving Patients Toward the Head of a Stretcher

- First assess the patient's size and condition. If the patient is alert and cooperative and you are confident that you do not need help, follow these steps:

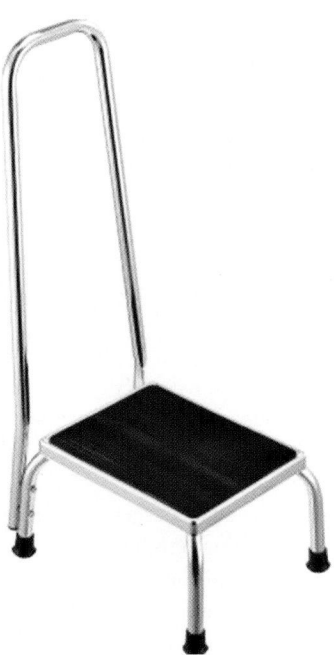

FIG. 2.9 Step stool with a handle.

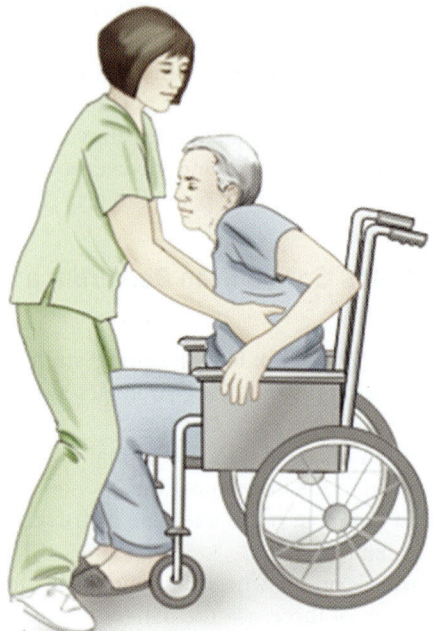

FIG. 2.10 Proper technique for assisting a patient out of the wheelchair. Notice that the patient's feet are between the legs of the sonographer.

- Explain to the patient that on the count of 3, you are going to shift them up in bed.
- Lower the side rails to the level of the patient's shoulders.
- Move close to the side of the bed, keeping your back straight, knees bent, and one foot forward to provide a base of support.
- Ask the patient to bend their knees with feet placed firmly on the stretcher.
- Place your hand under their shoulder.
- Count to 3 and help pull the patient up to the head of the bed, while they push with their feet.

Another method would be to slide the patient by using the sheet they are lying on and the help of another person:

- Grasp the sheet, pointing one of your feet in the direction in which you are moving the patient.
- Lean in the direction of the move, using your legs and body weight.
- On the count of 3, both of you slide the sheet toward the head of the stretcher.
- Reposition the patient comfortably and raise the bedside rails.

Turning Patients

Turning patients can lead to injury if proper body mechanics are not observed. To turn patients toward you, perform the following:

- Stand as close to the stretcher as possible.
- Check to see that the patient has ample space to turn.
- Ask the patient to bend the knees slightly by placing their far leg over the one nearest to you. Now place one of your hands on the patient's far shoulder and the other on their far hip and pull the patient toward you. For patients who are able to pull themselves up, raise the side rails for them to hold onto.
- If the patient has difficulty in turning on their side, get a coworker to stand on the other side of the stretcher to pull the sheet under the patient toward them as you try to turn the patient on their side.
- Maintain the patient's position by placing a pillow or a wedge behind their back to prevent them from rolling back.

To turn patients away from you, perform the following:

- Raise the side rails on the side of the bed that the patient will turn toward.
- Stand at the side that the patient is turning from with the side rails down on this side. Ask the patient to bend their knees slightly, placing one leg over the other so that their feet point away from you.
- Slip one of your arms under the patient's back and shoulder farthest from you. Your other arm should be placed on the patient's hips nearest you. Gently push the patient's hip while pulling their shoulder toward you until the patient is on their side.
- For patients who can turn themselves, raise the side rails so that the patient can grab onto them to turn.
- Maintain the patient's position by placing a pillow or a wedge behind their back to prevent them from rolling back.

Assisting Patients From the Scanning Stretcher Into the Wheelchair

- Sit the patient up by putting one arm under the patient's neck, with your hand supporting their shoulder blade and putting your other hand under the patient's knees.
- Swing the patient's legs over the edge of the bed, helping them to sit up, instructing them to "dangle" their legs over the side.
- Always stand facing the patient, while supporting your weight evenly on both feet. Ask the patient to slide to the edge of the stretcher with their feet flat on the floor or on the step stool. Allow the patient a few seconds to adjust to this upright position.
- Ask the patient to hold onto your shoulders or your arms. Place your hands under the patient's arms, and on the count of three, pull the patient forward, while shifting your weight from the forward foot to the backward foot (Fig. 2.11). The wheelchair should be parallel or at a slight angle to the stretcher, with wheels locked and footrests up and out of the way.
- Help the patient to turn and sit in the wheelchair.
- Lower the footrests and help place the patient's feet on them.
- Do not attempt to transfer patients who are unable to bear any of their own body weight; instead, ask for help.

PATIENTS WITH TUBES

The most common types of tubing that the sonographer will encounter when working with hospital patients are the following:

- Intravenous (IV) tubing (Fig. 2.12)
- Nasogastric

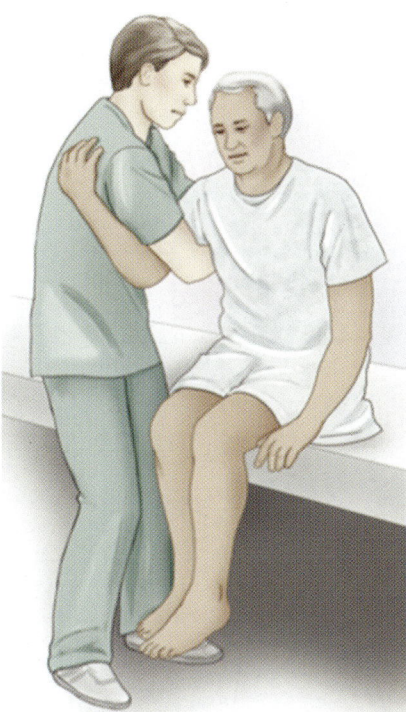

FIG. 2.11 Proper technique for helping the patient to get down from the scanning stretcher. If the patient's legs are too far away from the floor, a step stool should be provided. The handle will be on the opposite side of the sonographer.

- Urinary catheter
- Oxygen

Sonographers need to know how to properly move and care for patients who have tubes in place.

Intravenous Therapy

The intravenous (IV) therapy route is the fastest way to deliver fluids and medications. IV tubing connects a plastic bag that contains fluid to infuse into the patient's body via a catheter inserted into a vein. The chief components of a gravity IV infusion set are a prefilled, sterile plastic bag of fluids, an attached drip chamber (Fig. 2.13) that makes it easy to see the flow rate and that the IV is working, a clamp to shut off flow (Fig. 2.14), a regulator to adjust the flow rate (Fig. 2.15), and a long sterile tube that leads from the drip chamber to the insertion site of the IV. A gravity IV uses the pull of gravity to deliver the fluids to the patient, so it is important to keep the IV bag above the patient's arm. Blood will flow back into the tubing when the bag is lower than the patient's arm and if the bag is not raised above the patient's arm there is a risk that the IV will form a clot and will need to be replaced. For adult patients, arm and hand veins are commonly used and for newborn infants, the scalp veins are usually used. While moving the patient up on or down from the stretcher, it is important to take care that the tubing is not pulled as this could cause the IV to

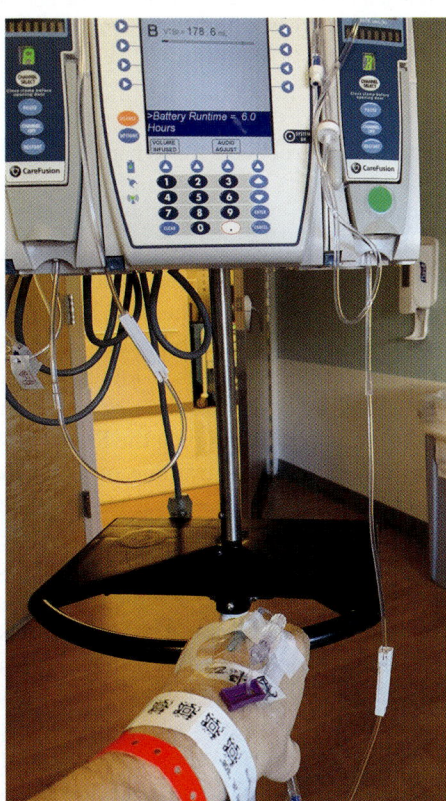

FIG. 2.12 A patient with an IV in the back of their left hand. The patient can hold on to the handle when walking or being escorted in a wheelchair.

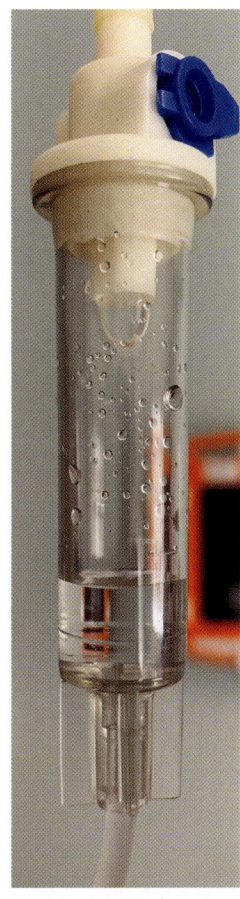

FIG. 2.13 A close-up view of the drip chamber. Notice the drop that is ready to fall at the top of the chamber. The sonographer should look at the drip chamber periodically to make sure that it is still dripping. If it stops the sonographer should see if the bag is empty or the line is accidentally pinched off. If the bag is empty the sonographer should notify the patient's nurse for instructions.

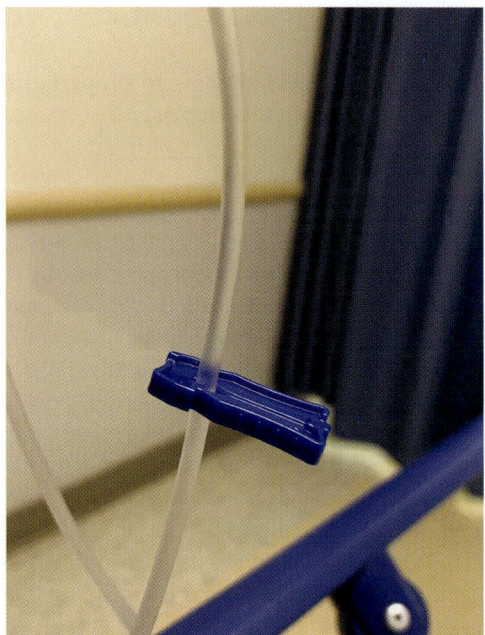

FIG. 2.14 A close-up view of the clip that can shut off the flow from the bag. It is currently in the open position. The flow may be stopped on one side so that the other side can deliver medications.

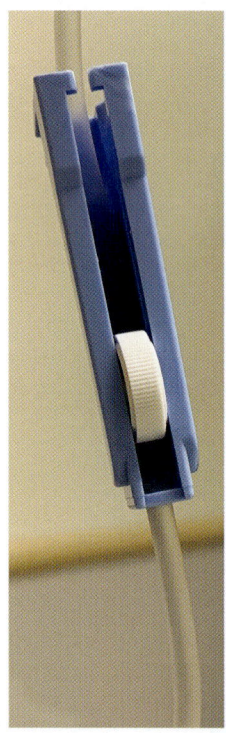

FIG. 2.15 A close-up view of the regulator that controls flow rate. When the wheel is at the top, the rate is at its fastest. When the wheel is at the bottom, the flow is stopped.

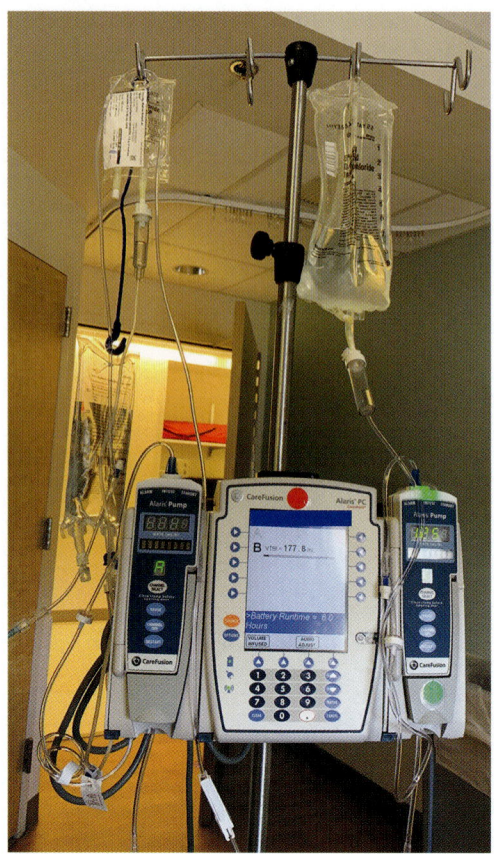

FIG. 2.16 An automatic intravenous pump with two channels marked A and B. Modern infusion pumps can deliver a precise controlled rate of fluid to the patient through an intravenous line. These pumps have state-of-the-art safety features to ensure that any failure is detected, causing an audible alarm to sound.

come out of the vein. If the needle is accidentally dislodged, the IV fluid may enter the surrounding tissue rather than the vein, which is called infiltration. The patient may complain of discomfort, and you may observe swelling or redness or discoloration of the tissues around the IV site. Clamp off the flow and notify the nursing staff for instructions. If this happens before you start the study, call the patient's nurse to determine whether you can continue the study.

Modern infusion pumps are computerized and can regulate the drip rate so that a measured amount of fluid is given over a period of time (Fig. 2.16). They also have alarms to alert that a problem has occurred, such as the bag is empty, infiltration within the patient's tissues, a low battery, or there is obstruction to flow. To minimize the risk of the battery running out while scanning, always plug the IV into a wall outlet. A sonographer does not have training on these devices and should only press the silence button when an alarm goes off. The patient's nurse should be notified and given any messages, such as infusion complete. If the pump has two chambers, A and B, make sure to tell the nurse which side .has the error (Fig. 2.17). If it is a simple fix, they may walk you through what to do. If you have to change the fluid bag, make sure you read back to the nurse accurately what type of fluid is in the bag. It is easy not to pay attention to the percent of the product in the fluid such as dextrose 10% versus 20% and administer the incorrect fluid type. If the fluid type that is needed is not available ask the nurse what can be used to keep the IV open until the patient returns to the floor, such as normal saline. If there is a nurse that works out of the area, it would be appropriate

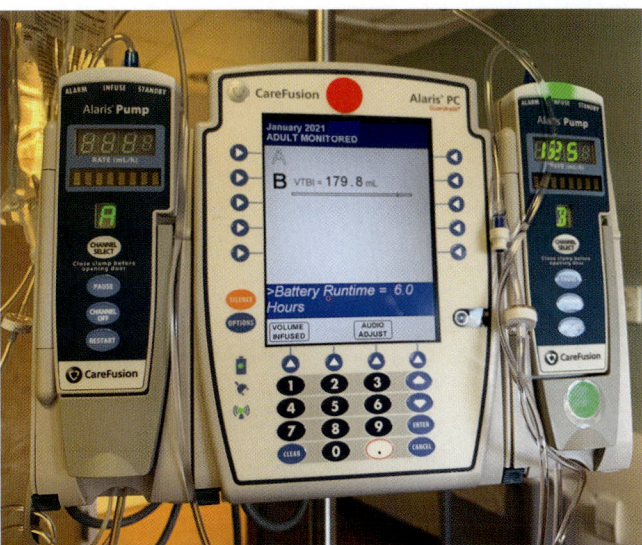

FIG. 2.17 A close-up view of the main panel. Notice the green light on the battery symbol when the unit is unplugged. There is also a message displaying battery runtime left. The B channel is delivering a rate of 179.8mL/h. The silence button is in red.

to get them to help. If the warning is "tube occluded" follow the tubing from the unit to the patient as it is possible to pinch the tubing when lowering the side rail. If the problem is because the patient has bent their arm and obstructed flow, help them straighten out their arm to resume flow. Usually once the obstruction is cleared the alarm will stop. If flow does not resume, talk to their nurse. Unless you are familiar with the type of pump that the patient has do not press any button unless you know what it does. It is possible that a nurse will write someone up for jeopardizing patient care for attempting to fix an IV pump alarm without proper training. Do not just keep pressing the silence alarm button until you are finished with the exam, as the problem could cause the line to clot and the patient to lose their IV and they will need a new IV to be placed. This is not good patient care and a good reason to be written up. As a sonographer you can be trained to perform some basic functions as well as learn to troubleshoot issues so that you can better communicate with the nurse.

The following guidelines should help in working with patients with IVs:
- If the needle has been inserted in the patient's elbow, help the patient keep the arm straight.
- Watch for and immediately report any of the following:
- No solution is passing from the bottle into the tubing, even though solution is still in the bottle.
- Blood appears in the tubing at the insertion site.
- The bag is empty. On gravity drip IVs there is no alarm, so the sonographer needs to keep an eye on the bag especially if there was less than one-third to one-half volume of fluid remaining.
- The needle has accidentally been pulled out.
- The patient complains of pain or tenderness at the needle insertion site, which may be a sign that the solution is infiltrating into the adjacent tissues.
- The tubing becomes disconnected, and the patient is bleeding freely from the connection site. Wear gloves and reconnect the line.

You will need to help your patient maneuver around the IV pump as they get up from the wheelchair and onto the scanning stretcher and vice versa. Have them turn so that they do not become tangled in the tubing. Usually this would be counterclockwise if the IV is in the patient's left hand and clockwise if it is in the right arm. Another way to think of how to turn the patient is that the patient should turn toward the IV pump. Beware of tubing that is shorter in length than usual, because you could accidentally pull the IV out of the patient's hand or arm.

Nasogastric Tubes

A nasogastric tube, commonly called an NG tube, is a flexible tube inserted through their nostril, down the nasopharynx, and terminating in the patient's stomach or duodenum (Fig. 2.18). The NG tube is taped to the nose and attached to the patient's gown to prevent the tube from moving, coming out, or ending up in a lung. NG tubes can be used for feeding or to remove gastric contents to prevent vomiting or gastric distension, or to wash the stomach of toxins. The tube may be connected to a suction device to empty the contents. The tube can be disconnected from the suction machine and attached to the patient's gown with a clamp or catheter tip syringe so that fluid does not leak out. Some patients may come to the department with their suction machine which will need to be plugged in. It is important to be conscious of the tube as you move the patient as it can be uncomfortable or painful when the tube is moved as it irritates the nasal mucosa. These patients cannot lie flat, and any scans will need to be performed with the bed or stretcher raised to at least 30 degrees. If the patient while under your care begins to have respiratory symptoms such as coughing, choking, or the pulse ox alarm goes off, immediately contact their nurse as this is an emergent situation.

Urinary Catheter

A **urinary catheter** is inserted through the patient's urethra and into their bladder to provide temporary drainage of urine. A common indwelling catheter is the Foley catheter, which is a specially designed catheter with two tubes, one inside the other. One tube ends at a small balloon which will be inflated to keep the catheter from slipping out. The other tube is open on both ends to drain the urine. Catheters are available in different sizes according to their diameter and are described in French units, which is a gauge system. The number assigned to the catheter corresponds to its diameter and goes from a 6 French catheter, the smallest diameter at 2 mm, to a 26 French catheter, the largest diameter at 8.7 mm. After the catheter has been inserted, the balloon is filled with fluid so that the catheter cannot be pulled out through the patient's urethra (Fig. 2.19). If the balloon is filled with air, it will cause artifacts and obscure the patient's

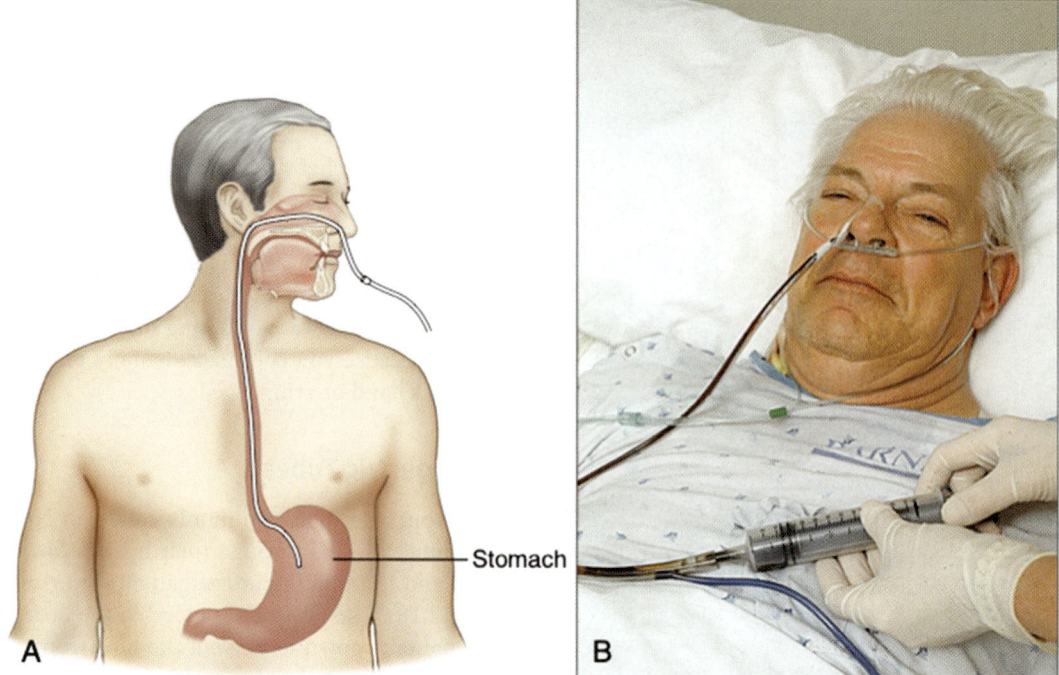

FIG. 2.18 (A) Nasogastric tube placement. (B) A patient with a nasogastric tube. Notice how the tube is secured to the side of the nose. A catheter syringe is used to drain or administer fluid.

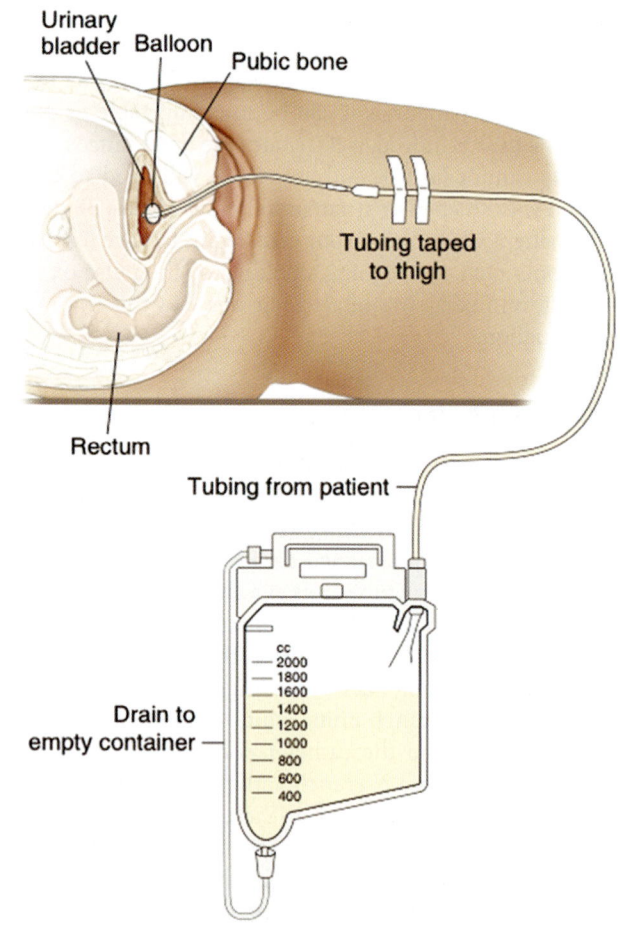

FIG. 2.19 Different parts of a Foley catheter in a female patient.

pelvic anatomy on an ultrasound exam. The sonographer should ask the nurse to remove the air from the balloon and fill it with fluid. Urine drains from the bladder and collects in a container attached to the patient's bed or table. The catheter bag must always be positioned at a level lower than the patient's urinary bladder. The catheter may be taped to the inner thigh to prevent accidentally pulling on the catheter. When moving the patient, get the wheelchair as close to the stretcher as possible and move the bag from the chair to the stretcher before moving the patient. The patient should turn to avoid getting tangled in the tubing. When the examination is finished move the bag first and then the patient, always being careful not to pull on the catheter as this will cause some discomfort. Although difficult to do, the catheter may be pulled out with enough force. Catheters left in too long can cause the patient to have a UTI. Some men will have a Texas catheter if they are incontinent. This type of catheter has a condom-like sheath that goes over the penis with an opening that leads to the tube. This type of catheter needs to be changed frequently, as often as daily.

When a catheter has been inserted into the bladder but is not draining urine, the sonographer may be called on to scan the bladder to assess the location of the tip of the catheter and the balloon, especially in male patients, where the insertion of the catheter may be impeded by an enlarged prostate gland. The balloon is usually found in the urethra that is going through the prostate. The nurse or physician will deflate the balloon, insert the catheter more, inflate the balloon and have the sonographer verify that the balloon is located in the bladder.

Oxygen Therapy

Oxygen is vital to human life. **Oxygen therapy** is used on any patient that cannot get enough oxygen on their own, usually due to a lung condition, or that has a constant low reading of below 90% on the pulse ox. The goal of oxygen therapy is to help supplement the room oxygen on a patient that has a low-oxygen concentration in their blood and to also help decrease the workload of the respiratory system. Oxygen is treated as a drug, and the concentration and its rate, in liters per minute (L/min), is ordered by a physician and may be initiated without a physician order in emergency situations. Oxygen may be contained in large tanks or small cylinders. Large tanks are used for patients requiring high flow rates or oxygen use over an extended period of time. Small cylinders are used during patient transportation or for short duration needs (Fig. 2.20). The sonographer should be familiar with reading how much oxygen is left in the tank and the rate of oxygen being delivered to the patient. Some ambulatory patients need continuous oxygen and may use over-the-shoulder slings or rolling stands to hold the tank when ambulating. The ultrasound room should be equipped with an in-room piping system, with oxygen and suction being provided through wall outlets (Fig. 2.21). For patients on oxygen, the sonographer should hook the patient up to the wall outlet so that their cylinder does not run out. The sonographer should note the flow rate, turn the cylinder off, hook the tubing onto the wall unit, and set it at the patient's rate. When transporting a patient, the sonographer should make sure that the tank is properly secured. The Joint Commission requires that there be a universal system to identify full tanks from empty tanks.

The delivery of oxygen to the patient may involve the use of either high- or low-flow devices. Among the low-flow devices are the **nasal cannula** or simple oxygen masks. The nasal cannula is used when a patient has mild hypoxia. The prongs are inserted into the patient's nostrils and held in place by an elastic band around the patient's head (Fig. 2.22). They are connected to the oxygen source by a length of plastic tubing with a rate of 1 to 6 L/min.

Several different types of oxygen masks can be used. A simple mask is a transparent mask that fits over the nose, mouth, and chin and has holes in the side of the mask through which the exhaled carbon dioxide can escape (Fig. 2.23). It is used when a moderate amount of oxygen is needed with flow

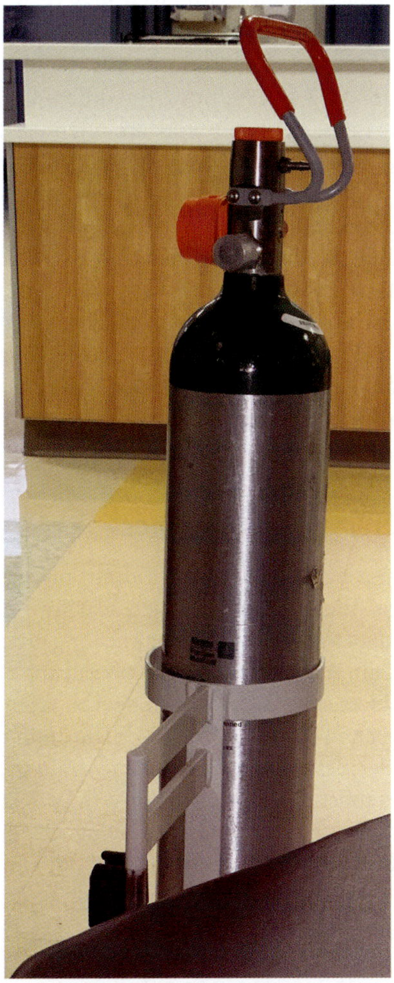

FIG. 2.20 A portable oxygen tank attached to the side of the stretcher. The red cap on the side of the tank indicates that the tank is full. There is also a handle to easily remove and carry the tank.

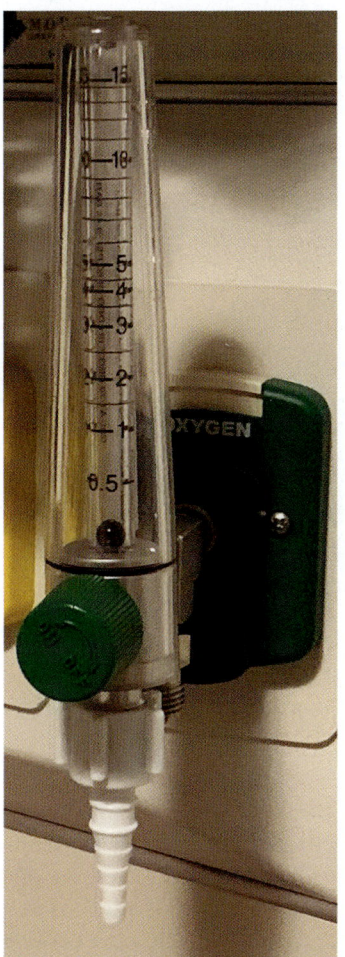

FIG. 2.21 A wall oxygen unit in a sonography room. The sonographer would attach the tubing to the white cone-shaped part and then turn the green knob until the ball is floating at the proper rate of oxygen delivery.

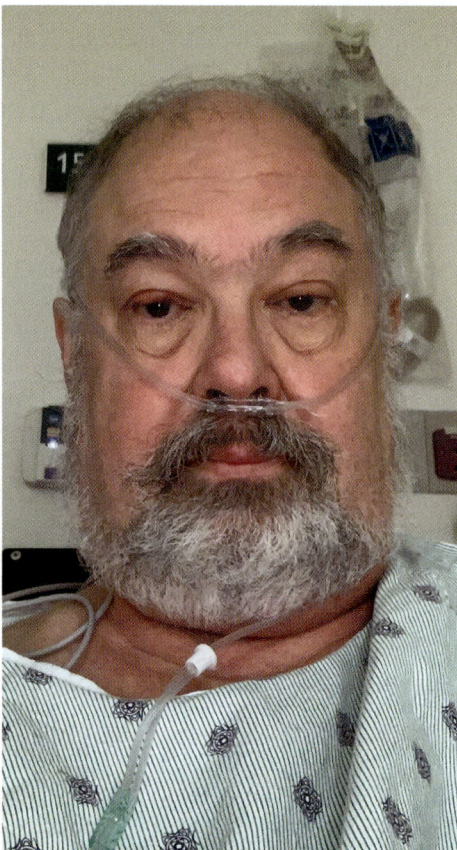

FIG. 2.22 A patient with a nasal catheter. The prongs are just inside the nasal cavity. The tubing goes around the ears and is adjusted with the white cap under the patient's chin.

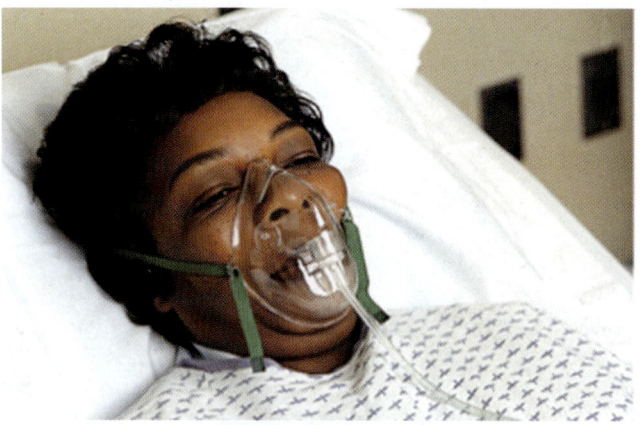

FIG. 2.23 A patient with a face mask when a higher rate of oxygen is needed as opposed to the nasal cannula.

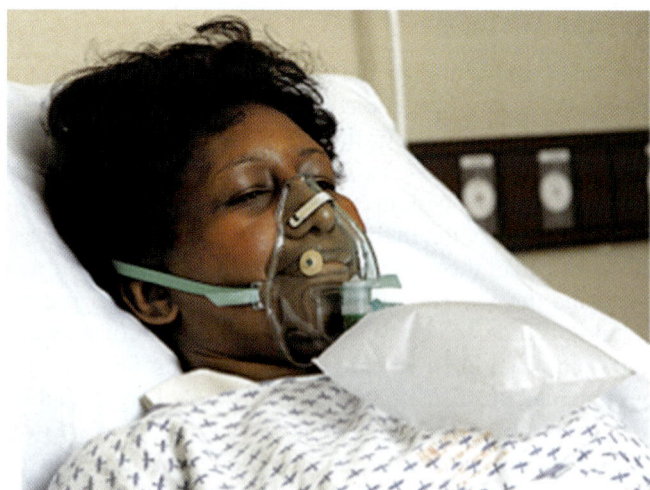

FIG. 2.24 A patient with a nonrebreather type of mask. This type of mask uses a reservoir bag to deliver a higher concentration of oxygen.

rates between 5 and 10 L/min. A partial rebreather mask is a low-flow device identified by the presence of an attached bag called the reservoir bag, which is attached to the oxygen tube (Fig. 2.24). It contains a two-way valve between the mask and the reservoir bag with a flow rate between 10 and 12 L/min. This allows the patient's breath back into the reservoir bag so that the expired air mixes with the inhaled air. Both masks cover the nose and mouth of the patient and are attached with an elastic band around the patient's head. These masks have an attached reservoir bag that should always be partially inflated. The Venturi mask is a high-flow mask designed to administer precisely controlled oxygen concentrations at a constant oxygen concentration regardless of breathing rate. This is accomplished by a Venturi device, which is a color-coded hard plastic adapter that controls the flow rate, which can be as high as 12 to 15 L/min. The different colors deliver different flow rates. Venturi masks are often used on patients with chronic obstructive pulmonary disease (COPD).

To prevent the nasal passages from becoming dry, a humidifier can be placed on the wall outlet with the tubing attached to the humidifier so that humidified oxygen is delivered to the patient. Although oxygen itself cannot burn, it does support combustion meaning that some materials can readily catch fire and burn in the presence of oxygen. The cylinders should be kept away from heat sources and objects that can cause a spark, and the room should be checked for electrical hazards and that no one is smoking.

Wounds, Drains, and Dressings

After surgery, a patient may have a drain placed to allow for fluid drainage. These drains provide a way for fluid, blood, or air to drain out of the body and aid the healing process. One end of a wound drain is placed within the wound and the other may be connected to a suction collection device. Wound drains are evaluated daily and emptied as needed. The drain remains until the surgeon decides that it is safe for the drain to be removed. Sonographers must be cautious to avoid the possibility of pulling or dislodging the drain when moving or positioning the patient. Some drains can be easily pulled out while others are stitched into place. Some wounds may only be covered with a gauze pad that is taped over the wound.

If a wound with dressing is situated within the scanning field, the patient's nurse should be contacted to see if it is permissible to remove the dressing. There may be times when just removing the tape gives you enough access to the area, and the dressing itself does not need to be removed. If not, remove the dressing when permitted and throw it away in the trash can. Wipe any gel off and use sterile gel to scan near the wound. When finished scanning that area, wipe off the gel and cover the wound with a sterile pad. Notify the patient's nurse that you had to remove the dressing to access the area and you are sending them back to the unit with a temporary cover. Explain that because of the gel the tape would not stick to the skin. If you have the proper supplies and training you could redress the wound yourself, but still let the nurse know what you did. If the dressing cannot be removed, try angling under the dressing from multiple sides. A sector transducer, because of its small footprint, may allow better access than a curved array.

Colostomies and Ileostomies

Surgical treatment of patients with disorders of the intestinal tract may result in the construction of a colostomy, an opening of the colon to the skin surface, or an ileostomy, which is an opening of the ileum to the skin surface. In such patients, a loop of intestine is brought out of the body through a surgical incision on the abdominal wall which will allow for drainage of feces. The colostomy or ileostomy opening, called a stoma, will protrude above the skin, be pink to red in color, round, and covered by a plastic disposable bag or pouch held in place by double-faced adhesive tape or special glue. This disposable pouching system consists of a plastic bag and a skin barrier, called a flange, which sits against the patient's skin. Some bags are equipped with a clamp to keep the bag closed between emptying while others will require that the bag be removed to be emptied. Care should be taken when scanning around the colostomy or ileostomy bag so that you do not dislodge the bag and cause leakage. The proper person, usually the patient's nurse, should be contacted when any assistance is needed in emptying or replacing the bag. If the patient is an outpatient, they will know how to take care of their **ostomy** and will have the needed supplies with them.

SAFETY IN THE PATIENT CARE ENVIRONMENT

Patient safety is a prime component of patient care. Equally important is sonographer safety. Often sonographers become so focused on performing the ultrasound examination and caring for their patients that they overlook the obvious need to provide safety for themselves. Consider the following suggestions to help keep everyone safe:
- Use good **body mechanics** and be sure to obtain adequate help for lifting or moving patients.
- Ensure that electrical equipment is properly grounded.
- Periodically inspect transducer for cracks and electrical cords for fraying.
- Use only safety-inspected and approved devices for warming scanning gel.
- Make sure to dispose of all sharps in a sharp container (Fig. 2.25).
- Secure oxygen or other gas containers to prevent them from falling.

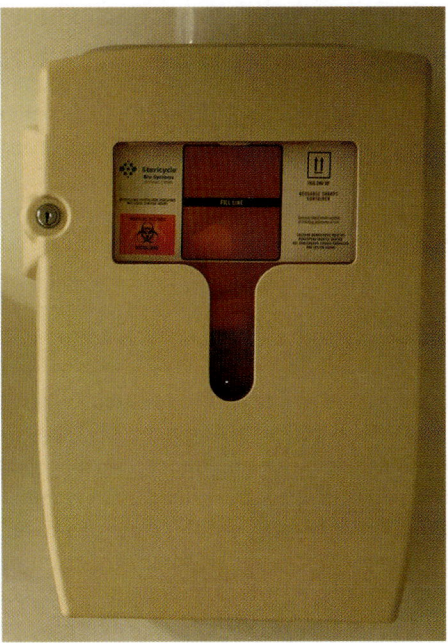

FIG. 2.25 A sharps disposal system in the ultrasound room. All used needles, scalpels, and any other sharp object that has been used must be deposited in this container. Notice that a key is needed to open the device to remove a full container. The department responsible for the safe disposal of the container usually has the key.

In January 2003, the Joint Commission issued the first National Patient Safety Goals (NPSGs) to promote specific improvements in patient safety. These goals highlight problem areas in health care and describe solutions. Accredited health organizations are evaluated for continuous compliance with the requirements of the NPSGs, which are revised every year.

Although not every aspect of the NPSGs will apply to ultrasound, it is important for sonographers to know which ones they need to follow, both past and present. Important goals include identifying patients correctly, getting important findings to the right staff person quickly, preventing infections, identifying patients at risk for suicide, and performing a "time out" before an invasive procedure. Both students and sonographers may need to address questions about the NPSGs to The Joint Commission surveyors during accreditation visits.

To learn more about NPSGS and to see the current version, visit The Joint Commission at https://www.jointcommission.org/standards_information/npsgs.aspx.
- Know where a fire alarm is located and how to report a fire. The sonographer should know the location of the crash cart and other emergency equipment for patient safety as any patient could code unexpectedly. Recognizing the fact that unconscious or sedated patients are not responsible for their own safety should prompt sonographers to use side rails. Double-checking that you have the right patient by matching their identification bracelets to the requisition or order ensures that you are performing the ultrasound on the correct patient. Do not rely on just verbal communication because the patient may misunderstand the name you

are saying or have a similar name. If an inpatient does not have an ID band on, it is usually against hospital policy to perform a test on that patient until someone from the floor comes down and places an ID band on the patient. Before calling the floor, check to see if the ID band is around their ankle as sometimes that is where it is placed. Besides an ID band, inpatients may have additional bands on their wrist such as allergy, fall risk, Do Not Resuscitate (DNR), or isolation (Fig. 2.26).

PATIENTS ON STRICT BED REST

Patients on strict bed rest usually have their ultrasound exam done bedside. Occasionally, patients on bed rest are brought to the ultrasound department for certain ultrasound studies such as a pelvic ultrasound with an endovaginal, prostate ultrasound, contrast studies, and biopsies or procedures. The patient may have to travel in their bed. This can make endovaginal and prostate exams difficult and the sonographer should discuss with the ordering physician if the patient can be transported via stretcher. Unless they have bathroom privileges, the patient should always stay in their bed or on the stretcher while in the ultrasound area.

Bedpans and Urinals

When a patient is unable to leave their bed or stretcher and needs to use the restroom, the sonographer should offer the patient a bedpan or urinal and assist as needed. It is important not to forget to give the patient some tissues so that they can clean themselves. There are two types of bedpans. Fracture pans have a flat lip in the front allowing them to slide easily under a patient who has problems lifting their pelvis for bedpan placement. The regular bedpan is somewhat larger and deeper, with a rounded lip designed to support the buttocks (Fig. 2.27A). Be sure to wear gloves when assisting the patient on or off the bedpan. When helping female patients with a bedpan, the upper torso needs to be slightly elevated to prevent urine from running up the patient's back. Single-use disposable bed pans are now available. Bedpans usually are made of plastic and should be stocked in the room or centrally in the ultrasound department. The use of a fracture bedpan may be a better option as it is smaller, easier to position under the patient, and more comfortable for the patient.

When handling used bedpans always wear gloves and if afraid of spillage a gown to protect your clothes. If the patient is possibly pregnant and experiencing heavy vaginal bleeding, inspect the contents for the presence of any products of conception which should be reported to the patient's nurse or physician. Always talk to the patient's nurse before flushing the contents to make sure that they do not need it for testing or need to know the amount of the urine. If not, empty the contents into a toilet and rinse the bedpan before disposal.

Constructed of plastic, urinals have a cap on the top and a hook-like handle (Fig. 2.27B). The patient should stand, if possible, to urinate. Otherwise, they can sit on the side of the scanning table with their feet on a step stool. Just make sure the wheels on the stretcher are locked. If the patient cannot sit up, you may need to place their penis inside the urinal for them. Always remember to use gloves when touching the penis. I would usually hold onto the urinal making sure that it tipped back so that the urine did not spill out. Always talk to the patient's nurse before disposing of the urine to make

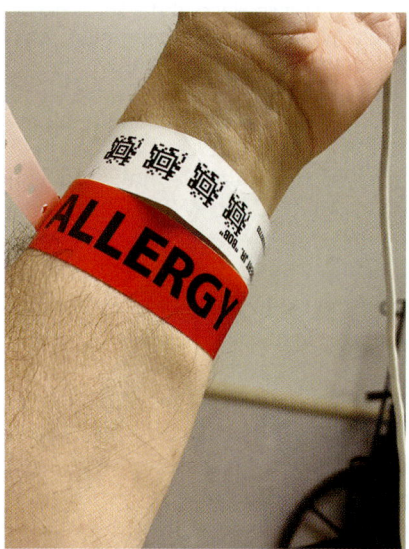

FIG. 2.26 A patient with a white ID bracelet and a red allergy bracelet. Notice the QR codes on the white band. These are used to accurately identify the patient, charge the patient for consumables, and track medications.

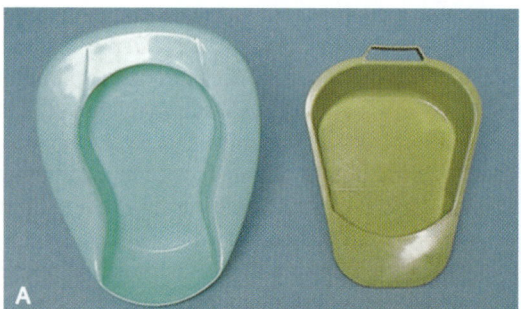 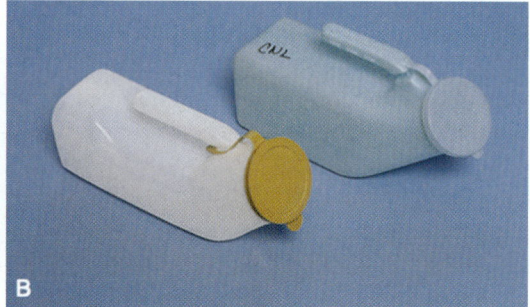

FIG. 2.27 (A) The normal bed pan is in blue and the fracture bedpan is in yellow. (B) The clear urinal is a one-time use while the blue urinal has a higher capacity needed for collecting urine for measurement.

sure that they do not need it for testing or need to know the amount of the urine. If not, empty the urine into a toilet and rinse the urinal before disposal. Male patients that are on input and output usually will travel with a urinal. If the patient uses it securely seal the top of the urinal and hang it back on the side of the wheelchair or stretcher.

Remember to always respect the patient's privacy and their dignity. Pull curtains, but remain on the other side to assist the patient as needed. If you need to go into a public hallway to dispose of the contents in a restroom, cover the bedpan with something disposable such as an underpad. Some departments may have a dirty utility room where bedpans and urinals can be emptied into a hopper or disposable sink. These units will have a water spray hose to facilitate cleaning. Be professional and do not make any comments about the smell, even if you think they cannot hear you. Discretely use any air sanitizer or freshener as needed. Many patients will be embarrassed by the situation, so it is important to be reassuring and understanding. Unfortunately, some patients cannot control their body functions and will come down in adult diapers. They may have a bowel movement while they are in your care and although it may be an unpleasant task, find someone to help you clean up the patient and put a clean diaper on them. Adults can develop "diaper" rash if left lying in their waste products for an extended period of time. Even if the patient is not conscious or seems not to be aware of their surroundings, do not discuss the incident in a negative way or complain about cleaning up the patient. Always treat the patient with respect.

Emesis Basins and Bags

Vomiting often accompanies illness, severe pain, or injury. Emesis basins are kidney-shaped with markers to measure the amount of the vomit as needed (Fig. 2.28). If the patient feels nauseated, turn their head well to one side to prevent aspiration of vomit. Place an emesis basin under the patient's chin and provide the patient with water and tissues to cleanse their mouth when finished. Some places have switched to emesis bags. These biodegradable bags catch the vomitus better, reduce potential contact risk to the health care worker, and can be tied off at the ring, which helps prevent spillage and reduce any odors (Fig. 2.29). Often the feeling to vomit may come on suddenly and you might not have time to grab an

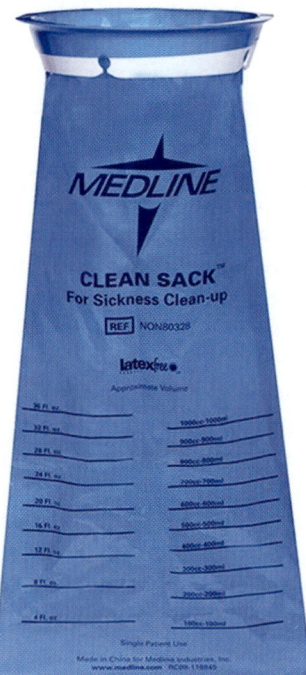

FIG. 2.29 An emesis sack or bag. Notice the markings on the outside of the bag to measure the contents as needed.

emesis basin, so just grab the trash can and allow the patient to throw up in that. When the patient is finished, help clean them up, get into a fresh gown if needed, and place clean sheets on the stretcher as needed. It is a good idea to have an emesis basin handy in case the patient needs to vomit again. You can throw the emesis basin in the trash can and change the bag after the patient has left the room. Again, discretely spray air freshener if needed. Have emesis basins handy for patients from the emergency department that are referred to evaluate for acute cholecystitis or kidney stones, as this group of patients have a higher incidence of nausea and vomiting.

STANDARD PRECAUTIONS AND INFECTION PREVENTION

In the early 1800s, people believed that fresh air and sunlight were all that was needed to kill germs, and those working in the medical profession were not much more enlightened. Physicians spent little time washing their hands, and a patient's skin was seldom cleansed before surgery. Instruments were simply rinsed off between operations and sponges were reused. That all changed when Joseph Lister decided to spray carbolic acid on wounds, dressings, and surgical instruments. This one simple act significantly reduced postsurgical deaths. Not until the early 1900s would nurses begin to wear gloves, not to protect the patients but to protect their hands against the harsh chemicals used during surgery. Often the surgeons operated without wearing any gloves. It would take many years for the medical profession to realize that wearing gloves also protects patients and to begin routinely using them as barriers to infection.

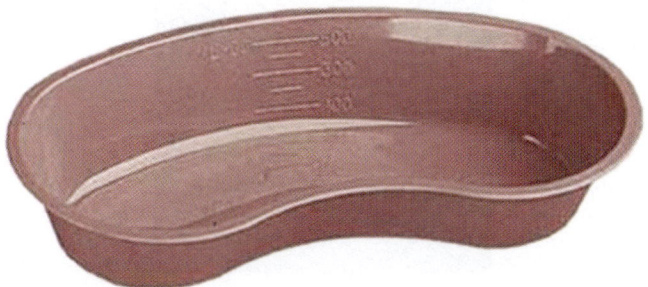

FIG. 2.28 An emesis basin. Notice the markings inside to measure the contents as needed.

The symptoms of a **nosocomial infection** should be suspected when patients develop fever and other symptoms not associated with their primary complaint. Prevention of nosocomial infections relies on following stringent quality infection prevention procedures.

There is a lot of emphasis today on nosocomial infections, also called hospital-acquired infections (HAIs), which are infections that a patient acquires during their hospital stay. These infections are costly to the health care financial burden and can be fatal. If a patient develops an HAI, the hospital cannot bill the insurance company or the patient for any costs associated with the HAI. HAIs can be reduced by adhering to and practicing good standard precautions.

Microorganisms grow best wherever they find sufficient food, moisture, and warmth. They can enter the body through the nose, mouth, eyes, or breaks in the skin. Organisms can be transported on soiled equipment and supplies, discarded tissues and linens, and from the hands. **Standard precautions** are infection-control guidelines used to reduce the risks of spreading an infection. As a sonographer, it is important to always follow standard precautions to protect yourself and your patient by practicing proper hand hygiene and appropriately disinfecting the transducer and ultrasound equipment between patients.

Standard precautions are the basic infection prevention guidelines that are used to reduce the risks of infection spread via the three transmission modes of airborne, droplet, and contact. Standard precautions will include the practice of wearing personal protective gear (PPG), also called personal protective equipment (PPE), to prevent contact with potentially infectious body fluids. This gear includes nonporous gloves, masks, gowns, and sometimes eye protection, which can be your own prescription glasses or use of goggles (Fig. 2.30) or a face shield (Fig. 2.31). Special masks or ventilators will be required if the patient has a known airborne contagious illness, such as tuberculosis (TB). The protective gear mandated will depend on the type of infectious process; however, the sonographer should always wear gloves when scanning any patient. Some patients may wear protective gear to protect themselves from others since they are immunocompromised, which means that they have a weakened immune system and cannot easily fight off infections.

There are departments in a hospital to help the staff understand infection prevention. The first department can go by various names such as Infection Prevention, Infection Control, Infection Prevention and Control, or Department of Hospital Epidemiology and Infection Control. Whatever their name, this department's job is to keep current on infection prevention techniques; update the hospital's policies and guidelines and evaluate departments for compliance; and investigate when a patient becomes infected, among other duties. They can be a wealth of knowledge and are there to help the department and not criticize. They may be willing to come to a staff meeting to discuss infection prevention as it relates to ultrasound.

Another department is the Department of Health, Safety, and Environment. This department will evaluate the products

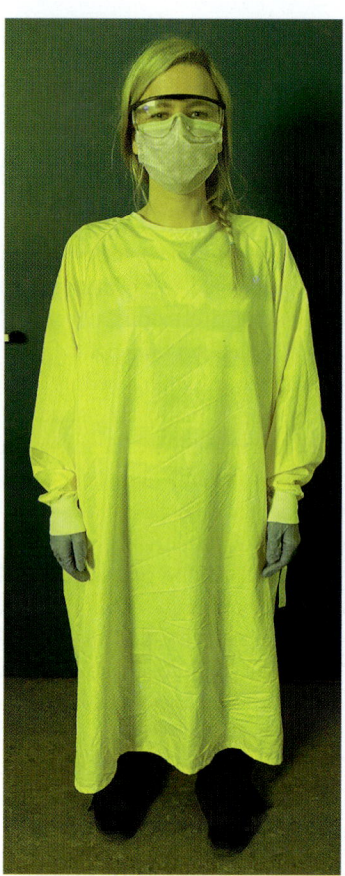

FIG. 2.30 A sonographer wearing personal protective equipment that includes goggles. (Courtesy Tara Cielma.)

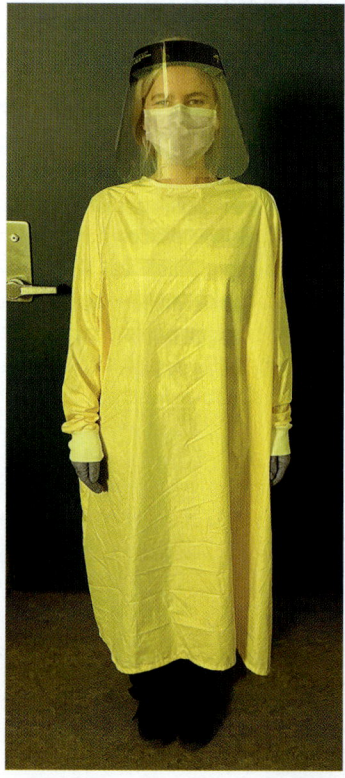

FIG. 2.31 A sonographer wearing personal protective equipment that includes a face shield. Goggles are not typically worn with a face shield. (Courtesy Tara Cielma.)

used for disinfection to ensure that the product is not harmful to the employee or that the area has what is needed to protect the employee, for example, proper ventilation. They will also make sure that the staff knows how to use the product properly and effectively and how to protect themselves as needed. They are also involved with fire safety, biological safety, and chemical safety, and have employee safety programs, among other responsibilities to ensure a safe and healthy workplace.

The disinfection of ultrasound machines and transducers is an important part of patient safety as microbes and bacteria can enter the body from the equipment. Any equipment that is used on a patient must be properly cleaned or disinfected. The protocol for disinfecting equipment in ultrasound may vary with your place of employment and the level of disinfection required. The disinfection products that can be used safely on the ultrasound machines and transducers will be found on the manufacturer's web site and can include disinfection wipes (Fig. 2.32), soaking agents, automated closed systems, as well as other devices and methods. The goal of disinfection is to eliminate pathogens from the prior patient to prevent transmission of them to the next patient.

Spaulding's Classification System

The level of disinfection needed is governed by the three levels of the Spaulding's classification system (Table 2.1).

The first level is for "noncritical" devices and includes equipment like blood pressure cuffs and transducers used on intact skin. This level requires low-level disinfection (LLD) which can be achieved with the use of the proper wipe. It is important that the proper type of disinfection product is used, or any warranties may become void. Check the ultrasound manufacturer's web site to determine the correct product to use on both their transducers and equipment, which may be different products. Then check the product's web site on how to properly use the product to achieve LLD.

The next level of disinfection includes equipment that contacts mucous membranes, such as the vagina, rectum, or nonintact skin, such as an open wound or a skin ulcer. Items in this category are termed *semicritical* and include transvaginal, transrectal, transesophageal, any transducer that is used in an ultrasound guided procedure, and any transducer that is contaminated with body fluid, such as blood. Semicritical items require high-level disinfection (HLD), which is defined as the complete elimination of microorganisms on an instrument, except for a small number of bacterial spores. HLD is accomplished with the use of automated devices or by soaking the transducer in an approved liquid chemical. Automated HLD methods include sonically activated hydrogen peroxide mist devices (Fig. 2.33) and liquid soak devices. An automated process is preferable due to the reduced risk of operator error, and the process can be easily documented. Some automated disinfection units can interface with the hospital's electronic patient record so that the sonographer, the transducer used, the disinfecting start and stop times, and if the process was successful are automatically documented in the patient's record. Again, the manufacturer's web site must be consulted to ensure that the proper device and/or method is used as well as the product's web site to make sure that the product will not harm the transducer while performing HLD. The

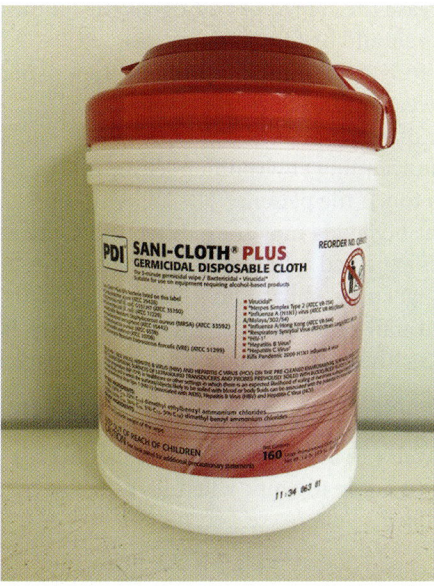

FIG. 2.32 A container of wipes for low-level disinfection. This brand of disinfection wipes has many different types, and each has its own color lid. The type of wipe is typically referred to by the color of the lid. This example would be called the "red top container."

TABLE 2.1	Spaulding Classification System		
Patient Contact	**Transducer Type**	**Device Classification**	**Disinfection Level**
Intact skin	Normal surface transducers	Noncritical	Low-level disinfection (LLD) Wipes can be used per manufacturer's instructions
Mucous membranes or nonintact skin such as wounds, ulcers, post-surgical, burns	Endovaginal, endorectal	Semicritical	High-level disinfection (HLD) Automated devices such as the Trophon, ASTRA VR system, or systems that use ultraviolet rays
Sterile areas of the body, contact with blood	Transducers used in the operating room; transducers used in procedures	Critical	HLD with a sterile probe cover

approved method for each transducer must be determined as sometimes the same method cannot be used on all transducers on the same model of an ultrasound machine.

Instruments and devices that enter sterile body cavities, such as in the operating room, or the vascular system, need to be sterilized. These devices are categorized as "critical" and must be free of all microbial life. It is very difficult to sterilize an ultrasound transducer. Fortunately, HLD is suitable for a critical transducer as long as the transducer is used with a sterile transducer cover.

Transducers need to be disinfected to prevent the spread of an infection, maintain a high standard of patient care, keep patients safe, and maintain the trusted reputation of sonography. Infections transmitted by contaminated transducers can lead to serious consequences. Multiple studies have shown that patients have been infected from incorrectly reprocessed transducers. There have been studies that have shown that ultrasound transducers have remained contaminated even after disinfection with low-level disinfectant wipes. Other studies have shown the need to disinfect the handles of intercavitary transducers. Deadly bacteria, such as vancomycin-resistant enterococcus (VRE) and methicillin-resistant *Staphylococcus aureus* (MRSA), can live on surfaces for weeks, so it is important to have a good disinfection protocol for the ultrasound room and equipment.

The reader is encouraged to learn more about Spaulding's Classification System and proper disinfection techniques for ultrasound transducers, the ultrasound unit, and any other equipment in the room. The reader is also encouraged to learn more about HAIs, how to prevent them, their effect on the health care system, and about the different pathogens that can infect the patient.

Recently there has been concern about the ultrasound transducers stored in an open wall bracket. It is recommended only to have the necessary transducers to perform the study on the ultrasound unit and all other transducers should be kept in an enclosed cabinet and marked as clean. Another concern is the use of gel bottles because the gel provides a warm environment in which to grow bacteria. Single-use gel packets are being encouraged. Many places have banned the refilling of ultrasound bottles and the empty bottle is discarded. To help protect patients a regularly scheduled cleaning and disinfection of the ultrasound console, tables, transducer holders, gel bottle warmers, cords, and transducer cables should be implemented.

To decrease the spread of pathogens the following general precautions should be followed.
- Wash hands before and after each direct patient contact, even if wearing gloves.
- Dispose of used linens in a hamper.
- Keep the scanning environment clean, allowing only clean items to touch the patient.

Different hospitals may have different guidelines that the employee is expected to follow. Here are a few examples:
- Keep fingernails short and clean underneath the nails. Chipped nail polish and artificial nails may not be permitted as they can harbor and spread bacteria to the patient.
- Wear clean uniforms or laboratory coats.
- Keep jewelry to a minimum as they can harbor germs.
- Try not to come to work when ill, especially with a communicable disease.

Hand Washing

Germs can spread from other people or from surfaces to a person by the following methods.
- Touching the eyes, nose, and mouth with unwashed hands which will allow germs to enter the body.
- Preparing or eating food with unwashed hands which can allow germs to contaminate the food and enter the body.
- Touching contaminated surfaces which will then contaminate your hands and allow germs to enter your body when you touch your face, or you eat without washing your hands first.
- Hand washing should be performed:
- After getting contaminated by blood, body fluids, or contaminated items, whether or not gloves are worn.
- After removing gloves, between patient contacts, and whenever indicated, to avoid transfer of microorganisms to other patients or the environment.

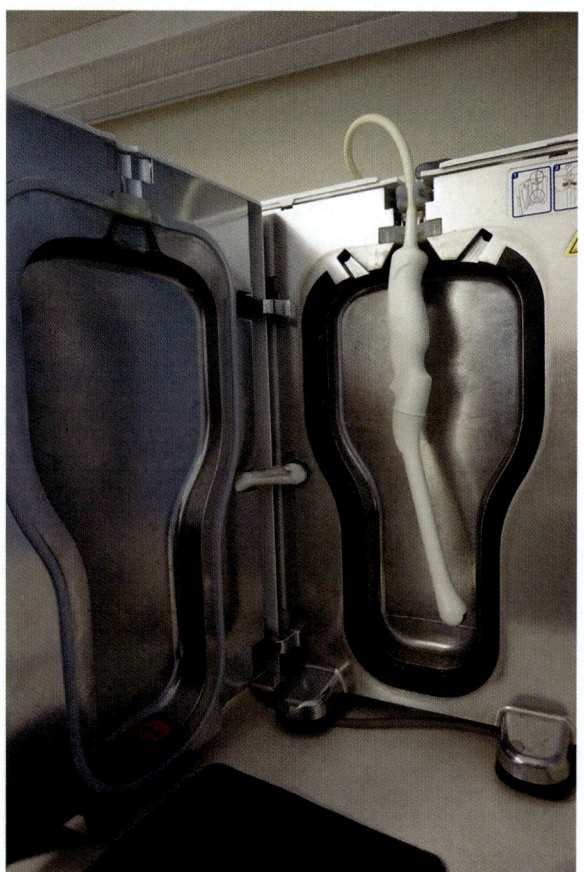

FIG. 2.33 A high-level disinfection automated device that uses sonically activated hydrogen peroxide mist to disinfect. The red disk will turn orange if the disinfection process was successful.

- It may be necessary to wash hands between tasks and procedures on the same patient to prevent cross-contamination of different body sites.
- Before and after eating.
- After using the restroom including men that only used the restroom to urinate. It is best to use soap and water and not a hand sanitizer as a hand sanitizer will not be effective against *Clostridium difficile* (*C. difficile*).
- Washing hands with soap and water is the best way to get rid of germs in most situations and should be used when hands are visibly dirty.
- If soap and water is not readily available, use an alcohol-based hand sanitizer that contains at least 60% alcohol.

How to Properly Wash Your Hands With Soap and Water. Box 2.2 describes the recommended method of washing your hands by the Centers for Disease Control and Prevention (CDC).

The reader is encouraged to read https://www.cdc.gov/handwashing/when-how-handwashing.html to understand the necessity of hand washing as well as to stay up to date on the proper ways to wash your hands using both soap and water and a hand sanitizer. There is a link to "Show Me the Science—How to Wash Your Hands" on that web page (https://www.cdc.gov/handwashing/show-me-the-science-handwashing.html) that includes the below points:

- Turning off the faucet after wetting hands saves water, and there is little data to prove whether significant numbers of germs are transferred between hands and the faucet.
- Using soap to wash hands is more effective than using water alone because the surfactants in soap lift soil and microbes from the skin, and people tend to scrub hands more thoroughly when using soap, which further removes germs.
- While some recommendations include using a paper towel to turn off the faucet after hands have been rinsed, this practice leads to increased use of water and paper towels, and there are no studies to show that it improves health.

However, you will always follow the procedures of your place of employment which has to be at least as strict as the CDC guidelines.

How to Properly Use Hand Sanitizers. Box 2.3 reviews the proper way to use a hand sanitizer. Remember if your patient has *C. difficile*, you must use soap and water.

ISOLATION PRECAUTIONS

The goal of isolation is to prevent the spread of communicable diseases and microorganisms among patients, personnel, and visitors. Because sonographers may be requested to perform bedside examinations on patients in isolation or to care for patients with impaired immunity, they must understand and follow isolation guidelines or policies. Institutional policies may vary, so the following suggestions are simply general guidelines (Box 2.4). Be familiar with your institution's policy. A student should not assume that every hospital has the same guidelines, and they should inquire about their isolation techniques.

Standard Precautions for All Patient Care

The CDC has recommended the following as **Standard Precautions** for all patient care:
- Perform hand hygiene.
- Use PPE whenever there is an expectation of possible exposure to infectious material.

BOX 2.2 How to Wash Your Hands Per the CDC

- Wet your hands with clean, running water (warm or cold), turn off the tap, and apply soap. Do not use hot water as that will open up your pores.
- Lather your hands by rubbing them together with the soap. Lather the backs of your hands, between your fingers, and under your nails.
- Scrub your hands for at least 20 seconds. Need a timer? Hum the "Happy Birthday" song from beginning to end twice.
- Rinse your hands well under clean, running water. Soap and friction will help to lift dirt and microbes, including disease-causing germs, from the skin so they can then be rinsed off of the hands.
- Dry your hands using a clean towel or air dry them.

BOX 2.3 How to Properly Use Hand Sanitizers

- Apply the gel product to the palm of one hand (read the label to learn the correct amount).
- Rub your hands together.
- Rub the gel over all the surfaces of your hands and fingers until your hands are dry. This should take around 20 seconds.

BOX 2.4 Isolation Technique Checklist

- Organize all necessary supplies before entering the isolation area. Working under isolation precautions can be time-consuming and frustrating; thus it is particularly important to avoid leaving the area for forgotten supplies.
- Clean ultrasound equipment before entering the isolation unit.
- Wash hands before and after each patient contact, even when wearing gloves. This is the most effective means of preventing the spread of infection.
- Discard all gloves used during an examination in an appropriate container before leaving the isolation area.
- Discard gowns in a designated hamper before leaving the isolation area.
- Masks should cover the nose and mouth. Put the mask on before entering the isolation area and remove or discard it before leaving the isolation room.
- Use masks only once. Never lower a mask around one's neck and then reuse it.
- Properly disinfect all equipment after use before leaving the area. Do not assume the needed products will be on the unit. Always bring them with you.

- Follow respiratory hygiene/cough etiquette principles.
- Properly handle and properly clean and disinfect patient care equipment and instruments/devices.
- Clean and disinfect the environment appropriately.
- Handle textiles and laundry carefully.
- Ensure health care worker safety including proper handling of needles and other sharps.

This is just a partial list; the reader is encouraged to visit the CDC at www.cdc.gov to learn more.

Additional Precautions

Recognizing that some patients require more than basic methods of infection control, the CDC developed extra guidelines known as additional precautions. These are divided into disease categories related to specific transmission patterns. After performing the ultrasound exam, the unit and transducer will need to be disinfected. This usually will occur outside the patient's room. Since the floor may not have the appropriate type of LLD needed, the sonographer should bring the necessary products. If possible, since the transducer had intimate contact with the patient, consider a HLD of the transducers used upon returning to the department. For any questions about the type of isolation that the patient is on and the proper PPG/PPE to wear, the nurse of the patient is a great resource. Patients that can leave their room should be wearing an isolation bracelet that specifies the type of isolation.

Airborne Precautions

Germs are capable of floating airborne for long periods of time and are often very contagious and can travel long distances. This type of isolation is used to protect others from germs in the patient's nose, mouth, throat, and lungs. It is used for disease spread by droplets that are coughed, sneezed, or breathed into the air. A private room is indicated. If a portable exam needs to be performed the sonographer needs to wash their hands before entering and when leaving the room, put on a fit-tested N-95 mask before entering the room, remove mask after leaving the room and closing the door. Gowns are not usually indicated but can still be worn to protect clothing from contamination. Hands must be washed after touching the patient. Depending on the reason for isolation, these patients may be able to travel to the department and will need to keep their mask on at all times. Some diseases that spread by airborne transmission include TB, measles, and chickenpox.

Droplet Precautions

Droplet precautions are for patients with a pathogen transmitted by respiratory droplets that can be transmitted when the patient coughs, sneezes, or talks. Because droplets are too heavy to float, they usually do not travel more than 3 feet and can land on surfaces. Infection can occur touching an infected surface and then your face. Droplets are defined as being larger than 5 μm in size. Anything smaller than this will follow airborne precautions. Patients on droplet precautions should be placed in private rooms and wear a mask. The sonographer should wear gloves, mask, goggles, and a gown when scanning these patients. They will need to wash their hands before entering and leaving the room. Face protection should be removed before room exit. Diseases spread via droplet transmission include pertussis (whopping cough), influenza or the flu, meningitis, and pneumonia.

Contact Precautions

Patients on contact precautions have bacteria, parasites, or viruses that are spread via contact, either directly or indirectly. Contamination can occur by touching an infected person and their dirty items such as their gown. Patients should be in a private room. The sonographer will need to use gloves and wear a gown donning PPE upon room entry and properly discarding before exiting the patient room to contain pathogens. Hands need to be washed before entering and when leaving the room. Diseases spread through contact include MRSA, *Escherichia coli*, VRE, *C. difficile*, respiratory syncytial virus, norovirus, draining wounds, impetigo, hepatitis A, shingles, conjunctivitis, and scabies.

One of the most serious of these diseases is MRSA, which is a form of staph bacteria that lives on the skin and in the nasal passages of a third of the world's population. MRSA infections can be divided into two categories which are community-acquired infections and HAIs. Community-acquired MRSA is defined as individuals in the community, who are generally healthy and are not receiving health care in a hospital or in an outpatient facility. Community-acquired MRSA can happen when there are groups of people that spend time in close quarters. Examples include gyms, athletic teams, people in prison or the military, and children in daycare. The primary differences between them are that community-acquired forms typically produce skin infections, whereas the hospital-acquired forms can develop into more serious lung and bloodstream infections. MRSA is primarily spread on the hands of health care workers and infected persons. Draining wounds and infected discharge are other methods of transmission.

It is not possible to eliminate MRSA in health care settings, because new patients, visitors, and employees will reintroduce the infection. The best defense against MRSA is hand washing and the proper use of barrier devices. Risk factors for MRSA are greatest among health care workers and patients in a hospital or in an assisted living facility. MRSA skin infections resemble pimples, boils, or spider bites that are painful and red with a swollen ring of skin surrounding the bite. These red bumps can quickly turn into deep, painful abscesses that require surgical draining. The bacteria can burrow deep into the body, causing potentially life-threatening infections in bones, joints, surgical wounds, the bloodstream, the heart valves, and the lungs. Community-acquired MRSA is often treated with oral antibiotics, while hospital-acquired MRSA frequently requires intravenous antibiotic therapy.

Blood-Borne Precautions

Blood-borne diseases are spread when the blood of an infected person comes in contact with the blood of another person. HIV/AIDS and hepatitis C are two of the most common diseases spread by blood-borne transmission. For a sonographer, especially one that is involved in procedures, they may become infected if stuck by a dirty needle. If stuck with a dirty needle it is important to act quickly. Wash the area right away with running water and soap even if you do not think that the needle pierced your skin. Do not wash the area with antiseptics or bleach. If the hospital has a number to call when stuck by a needle call it for further instructions. Your workplace will have guidelines that tell you what to do if you are stuck. Fortunately, the chance of catching a disease from a needle stick is usually very low. Look at the CDC guidelines for needle-stick injury and postexposure prophylaxis treatment for their recommendations.

Reverse Isolation

A special type of isolation where the sonographer is not at risk is called reverse isolation. This type of isolation is used to protect patients with neutropenia, on anticancer chemotherapy, steroid therapy, and/or severely immunocompromised from becoming infected. Wash hands before entering the room. If the patient is wearing a gown and mask you might not need to wear a gown or mask. Sometimes these patients will come to the ultrasound department and will be wearing a mask and gown. Cleansing of the ultrasound equipment and transducer before the patient is scanned will help reduce the risk of passing along an infection.

Strict Isolation

This type of isolation is designed to protect others from the patients' germs. It is used to prevent the spread, by air or contact, of highly contagious or virulent diseases. A private room is required, and gowns, gloves, and masks must be worn before entry. Hands must be washed after leaving the room, and any contaminated articles must be disinfected or disposed of properly. In some cases, protective eyewear and/or face shields may be required. Sometimes special respiratory equipment must be worn. The ultrasound machine and transducer need to be wiped down before leaving the patient's area.

Enteric Isolation

Enteric precautions are used to prevent infections transmitted by direct or indirect contact with feces. Diarrheal viruses, hepatitis A, and enteroviruses are included in this category. A private room is indicated. Handwashing and wearing gowns and gloves for direct contact are necessary. Wearing a mask is not. For diarrhea patients with *C. difficile*, strict handwashing only with soap and water is required before and after patient contact as hand sanitizers have no effect on *C. difficile*.

PERSONAL PROTECTIVE EQUIPMENT/GEAR

Do not underestimate the importance of personal protective equipment or PPE, which can also be referred to as personal protective gear or PPG, to help keep you safe from communicable disease exposure. PPE is specialized clothing and equipment that is worn to help prevent contact with body fluids and infectious materials. It is an integral part of infection control and prevention measures to protect health care workers, including sonographers. PPE provides physical barriers that prevent the hands, skin, clothing, eyes, nose, and mouth from coming in contact with infectious agents. PPE is used to reduce transmission of communicable diseases. PPE helps to reduce the risk of exposure, but to ensure maximum protection it is important to know the proper order in which PPE should be donned and removed. The CDC recommends the following:

- Put on PPE before entering the patient's room.
- Once PPE is on, use it properly to avoid contamination.
- Keep your hands away from your face.
- Work from clean to dirty areas.
- Limit the surfaces you touch.
- Change the PPE when torn or heavily contaminated.

Basic Personal Protective Equipment Protocols

There is more than one way to put on or don and take off PPE/PPG. Use your health care facility's policy.

How to Don Personal Protective Equipment

1. Identify and gather the proper PPE to don. Ensure choice of gown size is correct.
2. Perform hand hygiene.
3. Put on isolation gown. Gowns should cover your clothing or uniform and be snug around the neck. Wear the gown overlapped at the back and snugly tied at both the neck and the back. You may need some help from another employee to help tie the gown.
4. Facemask: Do not touch the part of the mask that will touch your face. Tie the upper strings in back, over the ears, and toward the top of your head. Tie the lower strings in back, under the ears. Fit the top of the mask snugly over your nose. If glasses are worn, the mask should fit under the bottom edge of the glasses to help prevent fogging of the lens.
5. Put on face shield or goggles. If required select the proper eye protection. Face shields provide full face coverage. Goggles provide excellent protection for eyes.
6. Put on gloves. Gloves should cover the cuff of the gown.
7. You may now enter the patient's room.

Note that there will be some patients, such as those with TB or severe acute respiratory syndrome, that will require special masks, such as fit tested N-95 masks or powered air-purifying respirators (PAPRs), and pronounced pampers, as a standard mask will not provide the protection needed. Put them on and remove them as instructed by the hospital.

How to Take Off Personal Protective Equipment

While removing PPE the goal is to avoid contaminating yourself or the environment. The outside of the gloves and masks are considered contaminated, regardless of their appearance. The outside front and sleeves of a gown are considered contaminated.

1. Remove gloves. Ensure glove removal does not cause additional contamination of hands. To remove gloves, grasp the outer edge near the wrist. Peel the glove away from the hand, turning the glove inside out. Hold it in the opposite glove, then slide an ungloved finger under the wrist of the remaining glove and peel it off from the inside, creating a "bag" for both used gloves
2. Remove gown. Untie all ties being careful not to touch the outside of the gown. Some gown ties can be broken rather than untied. Reach up to the shoulders and carefully pull gown down and away from the body turning it inside out as it is removed. Holding the inside shoulder seams of the gown, bring your arms together and roll the gown away from you, while keeping it inside out. Dispose in trash receptacle.
3. You may now exit the patient's room.
4. Perform hand hygiene.
5. Remove face shield or goggles. Carefully remove face shield or goggles by grabbing the strap and pulling upwards and away from head. Do not touch the front of face shield or goggles.
6. Facemask. First, untie the bottom strings, followed by the top strings. Holding the top strings, remove the mask and bring the strings together so that the inside of the mask folds together.
7. Perform hand hygiene after removing facemask.

Personal Protective Equipment

Gloves. Gloves are worn as protection from the patient's germs and to protect the patient from any germs on the sonographer's hands. Clean, disposable gloves should be worn when there is a possibility of direct contact with blood, body fluids, mucous membranes, nonintact skin, or any other potentially infectious material. The gloves must not be damaged when they are put on. At times you may need to wear sterile gloves when scanning postoperative transplant patients or those with a wound from a recent surgery. Long fingernails, rings, or carelessness can cause pinpricks, cuts, or tears and allow blood or body fluids to enter the glove and contaminate your hand. Disposable gloves are available in latex, vinyl, and nitrile materials but many places no longer have latex gloves due to people that have latex allergies. When doing a portable exam there will be gloves in the patient's room usually stored in some type of storage unit that is hanging on the wall (Fig. 2.34).

- Hands should be dry before putting on gloves.
- Any glove that is punctured, torn, or cut should be discarded and replaced.
- Gloves should cover the wrists. If wearing a gown, gloves must cover the cuffs.

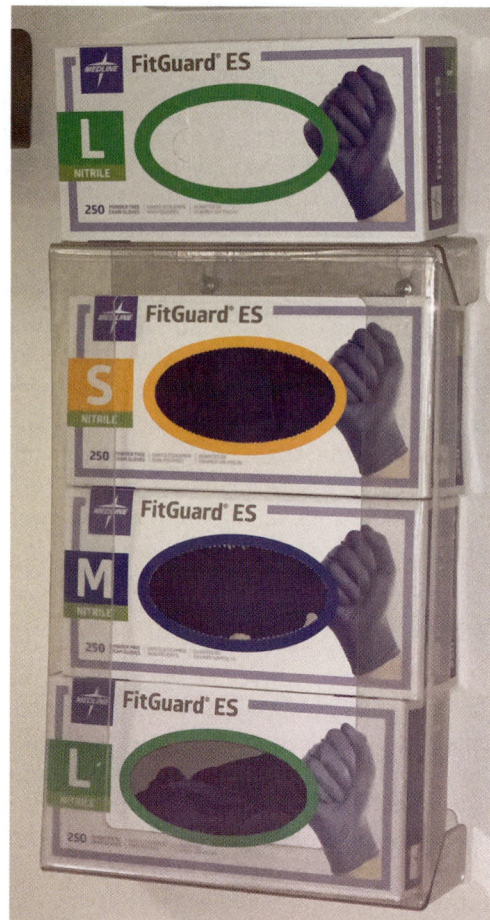

FIG. 2.34 Different size gloves stored on a wall rack in a patient's room.

- Gloves should be used only once and discarded after use.
- Whenever gloves are exposed to blood, bodily fluids, secretions, or excretions, sonographers must put on a new pair of gloves.
- When removing gloves, ensure that the inside part is on the outside, because the inside is considered clean.
- Wash hands immediately after removing gloves.

Eye Protection and Face Shields. Wear eye protection and/or face shields whenever there is a risk of body fluids splashing into your eyes or possibly acquiring infectious diseases through the mucous membranes of the eye. Once your work with the patient is finished, discard any disposable eyewear and clean any reusable eyewear with soap, water, and a disinfectant before using them again. Depending on the situation, your personal glasses may be sufficient for protection or you may have to wear goggles that fit over your eyeglasses.

Masks. Masks are used for airborne particle and droplet protection and are used to protect health care workers from people who may have a respiratory infection. They are also used to protect the wearer's mouth and nose. A mask only provides barrier protection against large-particle droplets and does not effectively filter small particles, fumes, or vapors. Always put on the mask before gowning.

Gowns. A gown is used to protect the skin and clothing when there is a possibility of getting contaminated by body fluids. The following are guidelines concerning gowns. Wear gowns that are long and large enough to completely cover your clothing. Any gown that becomes wet is contaminated and should be removed and replaced. The inside and neck of the gown are clean; the outside and waist ties are dirty.

Wash Your Hands

By now you are tired of reading to wash your hands. However, it is so important for the sonographer to have a good understanding of infection prevention so as not to bring these microorganisms home, contaminating the home environment and possibly infecting family members. Remember some of these microorganisms can live for weeks on surfaces.

PATIENT CARE EQUIPMENT

Handle used patient care equipment, including linens, that is soiled with blood, body fluids, secretions, and excretions in a way that prevents skin and mucous membrane exposure, contamination of clothing, and transfer of microorganisms to other patients and environments. If disposable items are used, they must be disposed of properly and not used again. Ensure that reusable equipment is not used for another patient until it has been properly reprocessed. A patient's used linens should not be shaken but rolled up and placed into a laundry hamper or bag for cleaning. Always hold the used linens away from your clothes. Thoroughly clean the transducer and ultrasound panel after every patient with the proper level of disinfection as per manufacturer's guidelines.

ENVIRONMENT CLEANLINESS

- Keep the work environment as clean as possible, especially after any spills.
- Be sure your institution has adequate procedures for routine care, cleaning, and disinfection of the ultrasound room.
- Know who to call if the patient vomits or if urine or feces is spilled onto the floor to get it properly disinfected. The next patient cannot come into the room until it is cleaned.
- Know who to call if the bathroom needs cleaning or has plumbing issues.

ASSISTING PATIENTS WITH SPECIAL NEEDS

Although much of your focus as a sonographer is on the art and science of creating diagnostic images, another important aspect of being a sonographer is that of assessing any special needs that the patient may have while in your care. This section provides suggestions on how to deal with many types of patients, including the elderly, those with sensory challenges, and culturally diverse patients whose religious and ethnic backgrounds are different from your own.

Crying/Upset Patients

People respond to news in many different ways. Part of being a sonographer is to offer comfort to our patients. You may not have to do anything if your patient is crying but be present and offer emotional support. Let them know that it is all right to cry and be upset. Sharing a burden with someone else can make bad news a little more tolerable. If you acknowledge the situation in a calm manner, you communicate to the patient that you are concerned about them and that although there may be nothing you can do to fix the situation, you would like to offer what help you can. If you do not know what to do, ask the patient what would be most helpful at that moment. It may be to leave them in private for a few minutes. Do not try to hurry them out of the room or appear impatient with them. Ask them to let you know when they feel they are ready to leave. As I write this the world is in the middle of the Covid-19 pandemic. This is causing our patients to have to be alone in the ultrasound room and therefore have no support when they receive "bad" news until they either get to their car or back home. This is emotionally difficult for our pregnant patients who cannot even celebrate this joyous moment with their spouse or significant other or have their support if there is something wrong with the fetus. Although this is an unusual situation, there will be times postpandemic when a patient will not have anyone with them for a variety of reasons. In these emotional situations, the sonographer has an opportunity to help their patients.

Elderly Patients

Patients in this age group are not really much different from those from any other group, but because of the physical and social changes associated with aging, their ability to cope and maintain a positive outlook might be challenging. The losses experienced by aged patients are numerous and wide ranging and include loss of spouse, family, friends, job, familiar environment, pets, health, and vigor. Most elderly persons can cope and adapt if losses come gradually. However, when losses come too rapidly, they become overwhelming and create feelings of loneliness and thoughts of loss of independence and privacy.

Sensory changes of diminished vision and hearing that occur with age can lead to an inability to respond to the environment. Eventually such a lack of sensory stimulation leads to confusion and withdrawal that can be common in elderly patients. By demonstrating concern and preparing elderly patients for their sonograms, the sonographer can help these patients increase their feelings of control and help to decrease their levels of stress. As you assist them onto the scan bed, they may tell you that they do not need any help as they try to demonstrate their independence. Make a joke, if appropriate, that you help every patient no matter their age as the paperwork is unreal when someone falls. Boosting their self-esteem and independence can make elderly patients more cooperative and feel better about themselves.

Some memory loss is common with aging, producing slower reactions to questions, directions, and decision-making. Sonographers can overcome this problem by slowing the rate at which they give instructions, communicating in a quiet environment, and providing extra time for response. Do not show signs of impatience and repeat the question. Make sure that your body language and tone of voice remain caring. Do not speak in a louder voice unless the patient states that they cannot hear you. While scanning, turn your head toward the patient for any instructions you need the patient to hear such as "hold your breath." When not scanning look at them and maintain eye contact. Respecting these patients and treating them as adults and not children is very important.

Adolescent Patients

Working with adolescent patients can be challenging and will require creativity, flexibility, and openness. Young adolescents often try to act like adults, while hiding the fact that they are confused or frightened. In this age group, modesty and privacy are very important. This age group can be very moody, sullen, and withdrawn, sometimes making it a challenge to communicate with them. You can earn the adolescent patient's trust by adopting a friendly and nonjudgmental approach and being sensitive to their concerns about privacy and confidentiality. Ice breakers may be talking about their favorite bands or movies. Sometimes asking about school can make them become withdrawn and even angry. Make sure that they are comfortable having someone in the room with them even if it is their parents. They are at an age where their body is changing, and they may not want their parents to see their genitals or see them "naked." If the parent stays in the room, try to have them sit where they can see the monitor but not the patient. Make sure that you only expose the area of the body being scanned at that moment. For example, if doing a bilateral breast ultrasound, keep the breast not being scanned covered. For a scrotal ultrasound give the patient a towel that they can hold to keep their penis covered. Periodically ask them how they are doing. When finished with the exam wipe off the gel and cover them up. Pull the curtain and have the parent stand on the other side with you while they finish cleaning the gel off of them and get dressed.

Pediatric Patients

It takes a very special sonographer to work with pediatric patients, especially from birth to about 4 to 5 years of age. Many of these patients are scared and assume that you will cause them pain as they perceive that they get shots or have blood drawn every place they go in the hospital. Gaining their trust can lead to a more cooperative patient. Sometimes this is easy and other times it is difficult to win their trust. Unfortunately, you may need to begin the examination with a crying child. With babies or kids, do not be rigid with the protocol but obtain images as they present themselves. Basically, get what you can when you see it. Be creative; for example, obtain images of the gallbladder and bile ducts immediately, and then allow the child to eat, as the crying may be the result of hunger. Consider having the parent hold the child at shoulder level as this may help in obtaining images of the kidneys from a prone view and the spine in spine ultrasound examinations. Sometimes you can get liver and spleen images from a coronal plane. Allow the parent to lie on the scanning stretcher next to the child to provide some comfort.

If your department performs ultrasound examinations on a large volume of pediatric patients, consider having a monitor and a DVD player with kid-friendly movies. Try to have the room decorated and inviting for children. Allow the child to play on a phone or tablet that they have brought with them. Ask them about the game they are playing or the show that they are watching. Do not make negative remarks about their choices. Try and make a positive comment or ask them to tell you about the character they are watching or game that they are playing. Sometimes they will listen to the same song a few times in a row. Even if you're sick of hearing "Let it Go," just grin and bear it. If you scan a lot of pediatric patients try to learn about the latest television shows, games, and music so you can impress them with your knowledge. Have books that a parent can read to the child as you scan.

Sometimes it can be helpful to demonstrate the examination on the parent. Consider allowing the child to hold the transducer and scan their parent or maybe even your arm. Sometimes just leaving the room for a few minutes will allow the parent to calm the child down. Because most children equate a laboratory coat with a needle, remove your laboratory coat before approaching the child. If your dress code allows wear cartoon or child-friendly scrubs. Engage the parents to help you gain the cooperation of their child. Assure them that this is common behavior that you are used to and to not be upset with their child. It is important that you as the sonographer do not lose patience with the child or develop an attitude. Even older children may cry and be uncooperative, and it is important to respect their fears. Usually once they realize that you are not going to hurt them, they will stop crying and begin to cooperate. Younger children and infants may cry themselves to sleep. Try turning on color Doppler and showing them some crazy colors to distract them. Warn the child before obtaining a Doppler signal because the noise may startle them causing them to cry again. Here you can engage the child by saying something like "Let's listen to some funny noises that your body can make."

When talking to a child get down on their level and do not tower over them. Talk to the child about school, video or computer games, favorite songs and artists, or a favorite movie or television show. Getting them to talk about themselves or things that they like will help take their mind off of the ultrasound examination and you will start to develop rapport. At the end of the examination praise the child and congratulate them for finishing the test, no matter how uncooperative the child was during the examination. Try to have goodie bags or stickers to give the child. If there are siblings present, make sure that you give them something too. There is nothing like getting a hug from a child that was very upset in the beginning of the exam and during the exam became your friend.

Multicultural World We Live In

With the arrival of increasing numbers of immigrants and refugees, America has become even more multicultural. The world is getting smaller, and sonographers will interact with patients from diverse cultural backgrounds from all over the world. To best serve these patients, health care professionals may need access to resources to help them understand cultural differences. Consequently, sonographers must develop an understanding of the beliefs and cultural differences of their patients. It may not be acceptable for a male sonographer to perform an ultrasound on a woman from certain cultures. A request for a female sonographer must be respected. In an emergent situation in which only a male sonographer is on site, they may need to work with the patient, their family, and the ordering physician on how to get the ultrasound performed, especially if a transvaginal examination is needed. Do not stare at their attire or clothes, especially women who wear a head scarf. Never make derogatory comments or make fun of the patient to your coworkers. The patient, their family, or other patients may hear your remarks, and it shows your insensitivity and immaturity. Learn about the beliefs and culture of your patient. If you sense that the patient or their family member would be willing to talk to you, ask them about their culture or where they are from. Most people like to educate others about their beliefs and customs. This may help us realize that we have things in common. In some cultures, the patient will reward the person performing a service to them. If they offer you a gift, which could be money, accept the gift because the person may be offended if you refuse. It is important to let your supervisor know about the gift as soon as possible, as typically hospital policies do not allow employees to accept gifts from a patient. If it is money, consider buying treats or lunch for everyone.

Studies have shown that patients from other cultures feel alienated by language and communication barriers. Any alienation they feel in their daily life is carried over into their perceptions of the health care system. You may need the services of an interpreter to help with communication.

Culturally appropriate care respects individuality, creates mutual understanding, caters to spiritual and cultural needs, and maintains the dignity of the patient. Recognize any potential conflict between your personal and institutional values and the patient's cultural or religious requirements. This will allow you to understand their needs and expectations before beginning the study. The following suggestions are intended to help both you and your patients:

- Document any request to be treated by only male or female staff.
- Thoroughly explain the procedure that you need to conduct, including which body parts you will need to touch and the reason for examining them.
- Understand that there may be a cultural reluctance to discuss certain topics, particularly if you or an interpreter are not of the same gender as the patient.
- Use words, not gestures, to convey your meaning. Gestures acceptable in one culture may be offensive in other cultures.
- Be aware of the personal wishes of patients regarding their condition. In some cultures, medical decisions are made by the family unit.
- Respect the patient's privacy at all times. Some patients may prefer to converse or pray in private with family members while in your department.
- Respect the patient's dietary requirements and be aware that some patients may be fasting for religious reasons at certain times.
- Respect the patient's dress requirements as decreed by the individual's faith.

Interacting with others from different cultures gives the sonographer the chance to learn about them and to appreciate the similarities that we share. There is no good substitute for receptiveness to others, good observation skills, effective questions, and plain common sense.

As stated at the beginning of the chapter, as a sonographer it is important to respect all of your patients regardless of your own personal beliefs. Refusing to do their study or treating the patient in an undignified manner is not acceptable. Along with religious and cultural differences, patients may be open about their sexual or gender identity. Respect extends past the patients and to our coworkers as well. Many hospitals offer training to help staff overcome their prejudices and biases so that they can interact in a positive and accepting manner with patients and coworkers. The more we learn about one another, the more accepting we will be of our differences as we see what we have in common.

When a Patient Cannot Communicate

There will be situations when a patient is not able to communicate with you easily or not at all. This may be because of a condition the patient has, such as having a tracheostomy or being deaf. A language barrier, including sign language, may make communication difficult. Some departments have laminated papers with common ultrasound phrases in a variety of languages. It can also be possible to use a translation app or website, understanding that the translation is not always 100% accurate. Whatever the reason, it is important to find a way to communicate with the patient before you start the exam. This can be by using an approved interpreter or arranging for an interpreter using a computer or tablet. If no help is available, sometimes communicating by showing the patient the transducer, the gel, and mimicking scanning yourself, will let the patient know what you are going to do. You could use paper and a pen or pencil with a patient who cannot talk, or by asking yes or no questions, as they then can communicate their answers by shaking their head. The patient needs to fully understand when having a transvaginal, transrectal, or any invasive procedure using ultrasound. With these types of exams clear understanding is important before proceeding as you do not want to scare or upset them.

A family member or guardian cannot be used to help obtain consent for a procedure or one that requires written consent. An approved interpreter must be used. This is to ensure that the correct information is being given and that the radiologist is receiving the correct responses. Before a procedure can begin the patient needs to understand what will happen, any potential risks, and any alternate options.

Communication difficulties may arise when working with patients who have speech impairments or have lost the ability to talk. Various reasons exist for speech loss such as a stroke, brain damage, or removal of the larynx. For patients who have difficulty speaking, provide ample time for them to organize what they want to say. Do not hurry or pressure them into speaking before they are ready. Watch for gestures as they may try to use them to help with their communication. Above all, be patient and do not try to speak for them but give them a chance to try to say the words. It is not their fault that this has happened to them, and they are trying to cope with their loss. Stroke patients may know what they want to say but be unable to communicate properly. Remember that sudden speech loss can be depressing and frustrating to the patient. Patients with brain damage may be able to speak but unable to find the right words and may become frustrated. A patient whose larynx has been removed will use a special device to speak, which can sometimes be difficult to understand. Communicating with these patients will take a lot of patience on your part. It is important that you do not show any signs of frustration or irritation with the patient as this will only make the patient become more upset with their situation.

UNDERSTANDING A PATIENT'S REACTION TO THEIR ILLNESS

Some patients will come to the ultrasound department with a known diagnosis. For example, the patient knows that they have pancreatic cancer and that they are having the ultrasound exam to look for liver pathology. There will be times when you will be the person to support a patient as they learn the results of their sonogram. This can be especially challenging when it is an obstetric patient with a fetal death.

When patients are sick, they will have a variety of emotions such as fear, anger, hopelessness, and self-pity, among others. Being able to recognize how the patient is coping is essential to providing effective care. Besides concerns about themselves, patients will have worries about how their illness may affect relationships, create financial problems, and how it will affect their quality of life. Patients will go through many emotional and psychological changes with regard to personal illness:

- Denial or disbelief. Patients may avoid accepting or talking about their illness.
- Acceptance. Some patients may become dependent on the health care team as they focus attention on their symptoms, illness, and treatment.
- Recovery. The patient will eventually begin to recover, rehabilitate, or convalesce.

The patient will go through a process of resolving and accepting perceived loss or impairment of normal function and how it will affect them on a daily basis.

With a diagnosis of a disease process most patients will experience fear and anxiety. Am I going to die? What does my future look like? Will I lose my job? Fear and anxiety can affect the body and cause insomnia, difficulty in concentrating and listening, loss of appetite, headaches, frequent urination, rapid heart pain, chest pain, nausea, digestive issues, excessive perspiration, decreased libido, and other symptoms. These feelings will eventually turn into stress and the patient may develop high blood pressure, ulcers, body aches and pains, diarrhea and constipation, appetite changes, sleeping problems, sexual issues, and depression, among other problems.

As a sonographer you will interact with patients exhibiting all these emotions and more. While with the patient they may want to talk out their fears and anxieties or not want to talk at all. They may be upset and crying as this is one more test to see how bad the disease is or help determine how much time they have left to live. Some patients may be angry, and it is important to not allow their anger and maybe even the way they treat you to affect how you treat the patient. You will learn that kindness, courtesy, and understanding will help most of your patients have a positive experience while under your care. I have had patients apologize for their behavior toward me at the end of the exam. My response would be something like, "No need to apologize. You're going through a lot right now and I understand that." This is why it is so important to understand what our patients are going through and how it affects their behavior so that we can help give them a positive experience, despite their circumstances. It is easy to be empathetic if you have had a family member diagnosed with a fatal disease. If you have not had these experiences, use sympathy skills to support the patient.

Terminal Patients

As a sonographer we will be scanning patients that are terminally ill. We may be scanning them to help these patients have some comfort by draining fluid from their chest or abdomen or to look for a venous thrombosis. We may not understand why, but we may be scanning them for further progression of their disease such as evaluating the liver for metastatic disease when they develop right upper quadrant pain or have abnormal liver function tests.

Scanning these patients can be uncomfortable as we are not sure what to say or talk about. We do not want to come across as cold and clinical to the patient as this can make them more upset. Some patients may want to talk about themselves, their life, their regrets, their illness, and even give you advice on life. Here we need to be a really good listener and find verbal ways to let the patient know that we are listening to them. We might say, "I am so sorry that you are going through this," or "It sounds like you have a great support team." Never give the patient false hope for a cure as that only makes us feel better. Be careful saying something like, "You're in God's hands now." You cannot assume the religion of the patient and you may offend them or upset them, especially if the patient does not believe in your God or they may be angry with God. Unless the patient brings up their faith it is best to not discuss religion. I would try to end my encounter with the patient by telling them to try and stay positive even though it will be difficult at times. It is easy to develop a bond with these patients especially if they are returning periodically for a procedure like a large volume ascites drainage. During these procedures the patient may grow to depend on you to help them get through the procedure and request that you be involved with their ultrasound studies. While this makes us feel appreciated it may not always be possible. If you cannot be there, reassure the patient that the other sonographer is excellent and will take just as good care of them.

The emotional aspect of being a sonographer is not often discussed. Scanning critically ill patients may remind us of a loved one who died, especially if it was recent. We can also develop a "friendship" with the patient we scan often and become attached to them. We may become upset to learn a patient has died. Both of these situations can cause us to become visibly upset and maybe even cry. This is OK and is where our coworkers can help us heal. (So, if you see or sense that your fellow sonographer is upset, take them aside and see if they need or want to talk.)

THE PATIENT CARE PARTNERSHIP

When patients seek health care, they expect that they have certain rights, including the right to open and honest communication, respect for their values, and sensitivity to any differences between them and you. In 2004 the American Hospital Association replaced an earlier Patients' Bill of Rights with a plain-language brochure called "The Patient Care Partnership: Understanding Expectations, Rights and Responsibilities." This document is available in a variety of different languages, including English, Arabic, Chinese, Russian, Spanish, Tagalog, and Vietnamese. The brochure informs the patient what to expect during their hospital stay and defines the following expectations:

1. High-quality patient care
2. A clean and safe environment
3. Involvement in their care
4. Protection of their privacy
5. Help when leaving the hospital
6. Help with billing claims

This brochure can be supplied by the hospital or downloaded from https://www.aha.org/system/files/2018-01/aha-patient-care-partnership.pdf.

PROFESSIONAL ATTITUDES AND BEHAVIORS

Professionalism is composed of attitudes and behaviors. Often, we behave in a manner to achieve optimal outcomes in our professional tasks and interactions. Whether it is attitudes or behaviors, how we interact with patients will have a significant effect on their reactions to us and their willingness to work together to perform their ultrasound study.

The first step in caring for our patients is in how we communicate with them. Accurate communication is essential not only for the immediate situation but also for ongoing patient care. The way to establish rapport with our patients is by showing respect and by listening and responding to them, as well as by giving instructions. Nonverbal communication is a process of communicating by sending and receiving wordless messages through body language, gesture, facial expression, eye contact, physical proximity, and touching. Patients will not entirely trust information given them when the body language and the verbal language of the speaker are not harmonious. The three parts of communication are the words, body language, and tone of voice. Interestingly the words are the least important aspect, with body language being the most important, followed by tone of voice. The following suggestions are helpful in making sure that your patients fully understand you:

- Make eye contact with the patients to demonstrate that they have your full attention and to see that they are listening to you attentively.
- Sit rather than stand. Looking down on patients when communicating with them is intimidating. Sitting also will make the conversation seem less rushed and more respectful.
- Maintain a relaxed posture when speaking to patients. Do not cross your arms over your chest, as that gesture can indicate negativity.
- Use a calm, steady voice whenever communicating sensitive or important information. Patients will be more receptive to a lower, softer voice than a shrill one.
- Do not speak rapidly or use medical jargon because it will overwhelm your patient.
- Ask comprehensive questions that require a mixture of responses from the patient rather than just a yes or a no.
- If you give instructions, be sure to ask if the patient understands. Many patients will say yes, but after additional conversation, you should be able to determine whether they really do understand.

Reestablishing Patient-Focused Care

A patient is someone in need. Patients come to us because they have health problems, and our job is to assist them. The move toward patient-focused care comes at a time when it is important to stem the tide against the trend of turning health care into a business by treating patients as clients and focusing primarily on cost-cutting and maximizing productivity. The term *patient* should be defended. It implies suffering over time. Patients should be treated with dignity and as individuals, and they should be empowered to make choices about their own care. This can only be done if they are not hurried along, if they are provided information in a form they can understand, and if their views are listened to. It is hoped that among all health professionals and administrators, the return to this kind of focus will rekindle the long-admired traits of caring, compassion, and respect and encourage a sharing of skills to enhance the patient's existence.

Addressing the Patient

How you address the patient will show respect. For outpatients, because of HIPAA, it is now acceptable to call for the patient by their first name. To make sure you have the right patient, ask them for their full name and date of birth. For an inpatient, ask the patient their name and then check their ID bracelet. For every patient, unless you are familiar with them, the encounter should begin with "How should I address you?" Do not assume that an adult patient wants to be called using the traditional Mrs., Ms., or Mr. They may want to be addressed with the gender neutral Mx., pronounced mix or mux. Some patients, especially those around your age or younger, may prefer to be called by their first name. With pediatric patients ask them (if they are old enough), "What would you like to be called?" or if it is a young child ask a parent what the child likes to be called. Get down on the child's level when you talk to them either by stooping or sitting on a stool or scanning chair. Do not tower over them as this can be intimidating to the child.

As we strive to be inclusive and use gender-neutral pronouns, it will not be uncommon to forget and use traditional terms in error. The traditional terms of Mr., Mrs., and Ms. may offend some patients and they will correct you on how they prefer to be addressed. If you think you have offended the patient, apologize and thank them for correcting you. This could open up a dialog with the patient helping you to understand gender-neutral pronouns, showing the patient that you want to be respectful to them as well as to future patients. As stated above, the preferred method is by asking the patient how they would like to be addressed using something like, "How should I address you?" being careful not to add "sir" or "ma'am" at the end of the question.

If you are not sure which pronoun to use for the patient, ask the patient for their preferred pronouns. Although you may not use them in front of the patient, there is a possibility that you will need to know their preference when going over the exam with the sonologist. This will show respect for the patient as well as respect to your coworkers that use gender-neutral pronouns. For example, instead of saying, "He or she presented to the ED with RUQ pain." you would say, "Ze presented to the ED with RUQ pain." or "They presented to the ED with RUQ pain." Some people use the pronoun "they," which can be used for a single person or for multiple people. This takes some getting used to, as using "they" for a single person may sound grammatically incorrect. For a pediatric patient, ask the parent which pronouns to use as some parents will become upset if you assume it is OK to use traditional pronouns for their child. Again, this shows respect. Of note: some people are putting at the bottom of their emails or other written forms of communication their preferred pronouns. For example, under my name would be (he, him, his) while someone else may have the gender-neutral pronouns (they, them, their or ze, zim, zir) (Table 2.2).

Every patient you encounter deserves to be treated with respect no matter their age, sex, gender identification, sexual orientation, race, religious beliefs, ethnicity, language spoken, disability, or socioeconomic status. Creating a welcoming environment for all patients will create a nonbiased, healthy, and respectful atmosphere. Everyone should be sensitive to others and use gender-neutral pronouns. Even foreign languages, like French, which assign a gender to each noun, are moving toward gender-neutral words.

It is beyond the scope of this chapter to fully educate the reader on gender identity, sexual orientation, and associated topics. The reader is encouraged to learn more to better educate themselves. Consider having an outside speaker at a staff meeting. Remember using and understanding gender-neutral language is not just being respectful to the patient but also being respectful to your coworkers as well as helping to create an inclusive environment.

TABLE 2.2	Gender Pronouns[a]		
Subjective	Objective	Possessive	Reflexive
She	Her	Hers	Herself
He	Him	His	Himself
They	Them	Theirs	Themself
Ze	Hir/Zir	Hirs/Zirs	Hirself/zirself

[a]This list may change over time, and new pronouns may be added. Always ask someone for their pronouns. Remember that "they" can refer to a single individual or a group of people.

HEALTH INSURANCE PORTABILITY AND ACCOUNTABILITY ACT

The HIPAA of 1996 established new standards for the uses of health care information. HIPAA created standards that affect the day-to-day functioning of the nation's hospitals, medical providers, and medical community. HIPAA affects virtually every department of every entity that provides or pays for health care. It also created national standards to protect individuals' medical records and other personal health information called PHI. HIPAA does the following:

- Gives patients more control over their health information
- Sets boundaries on the use and release of health records
- Establishes appropriate safeguards that health care providers and others must achieve to protect the privacy of health information
- Holds violators accountable with civil and criminal penalties that can be imposed if they violate a patients' privacy rights
- Being able to make informed choices when seeking care and reimbursement for care, based on how personal health information may be used
- Generally, obtaining the right to examine and obtain a copy of their own health records and request corrections
- Empowering individuals to control certain uses and disclosures of their health information
- For sonographers, the HIPAA act affects us as follows:
- Putting patient information away when finished with it

- Setting screensavers on computers for the shortest time possible
- Not having the worklist on the monitor so that other patients' names are visible
- Taking care that other patients do not overhear any conversations, including phone conversations
- Honoring patient requests that students, other observers, medical personnel, and families leave the room during their sonography examination
- Explaining to patients the hospital or department policies regarding the rights of friends and family to view their ultrasound examination and to know the results
- Removing any patient identification from any scans that will be used for publication or a presentation or case study

This can be challenging with patients having an obstetrical ultrasound. Understand that if someone watching the scan asks a question, you need to ask the patient if you can give them an answer. It is acceptable to correct someone that blurts out incorrect information. I have had people say, "It's a boy!" or my favorite, "That's my son!" when they were looking at the umbilical cord. (This last statement is ironic when you know that the fetus is female.) I would respond with, "That is the umbilical cord you are seeing so that doesn't mean it is a girl or a boy." A big challenge is when the husband or significant other wants to know the sex of the fetus and the person being scanned does not. Remember that the patient's wants are be respected, and you may need to explain to the other person that you cannot legally give them an answer. This can really create some tension in the room, especially as the two of them argue. Be sure to meet the patient's expectation of a pleasant physical and emotional environment where comfort, safety, and respect as an individual are ensured.

The following link to HIPAA should be reviewed for any updates: http://www.hhs.gov/ocr/privacy/hipaa/understanding/consumers/index.html.

BEDSIDE ULTRASOUND

Ultrasound should be done portably only if it is not possible to bring the patient to the department. Reasons for this may include the patient needs continuous monitoring, they are intubated, on dialysis, receiving blood products, or they are too unstable to be off the floor. Bedside monitors are extremely helpful in quickly identifying changes in the patient's condition. These monitors can evaluate different vital signs, displaying them on the screen, and if any one of the values becomes abnormal an alarm will sound (Fig. 2.35). If the patient came down to the department there would be a large gap in monitoring these vital signs with potential to miss an important change to one or more vital signs. It is important to not take your frustrations of having to do their study bedside out on the patient. It may appear that they could come down to the department but there is a good reason why the patient needs to be in their room. If the patient is not conscious talk to them as if they

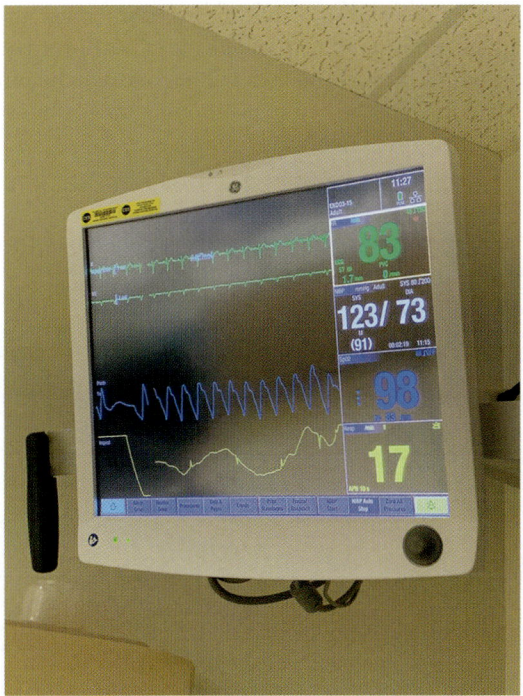

FIG. 2.35 A monitor used to track the patient's vital signs. The green line at the top is an electrocardiogram tracing, the blue line represents oxygen levels, the yellow line represents respirations, 83 represents the heart rate, 123/73 is the blood pressure, 98 is the oxygen level, and 17 is the respiration rate.

were as there is clinical evidence that some patients can hear us, even though they cannot respond.

When you are going to do an ultrasound bedside you will need to call the patient's nurse to see if it is a good time to come up and perform the study as you could be turned away because the patient is having another test, eating, bathing, has visitors, or may be off of the unit for another test. Because the patient is off the unit for another test does not mean they could come down to the ultrasound department. Some tests cannot be done bedside such as endoscopy, nuclear medicine, CT, or a procedure that requires sedation. If it is nighttime, the patient care team may not want the patient woken up. Now you have wasted 10 to 15 minutes of your time as well as delayed the care of another patient. Communication and planning with the nurse are crucial for efficiency and good patient care.

Portable ultrasound will be an ergonomic challenge for the sonographer. In some instances, it may require two sonographers to scan the patient. A good example is a child on extracorporeal membrane oxygenation (ECMO), as these machines are very big, cannot be moved, and take up a lot of space in the room, thus giving the sonographer very little space for the ultrasound unit and themselves (Fig. 2.36). It may be necessary for one sonographer to scan the brain while the other sonographer manipulates controls and captures the images.

When performing a portable ultrasound, you will need to be aware of the other equipment in the room such as IV poles, central or arterial lines, pulse oximeter, electrocardiogram leads or other monitoring wires, drains, ventilators, and urinary catheters. Some machines that are used in a patient's room cannot be moved and you will need to ask the nurse to assist you in moving the bed or positioning the patient so that you can reach them. This is especially true in the intensive care units. Often you will have to arrange chairs, tables, and other items in the room to make a space for the ultrasound unit (Fig. 2.37). Sometimes you will also need to move or angle the patient's bed so that there is enough room for the ultrasound machine to perform the ultrasound study. These situations where there is not enough space for the unit and for you to be able to scan can be an ergonomic nightmare.

You may need to remove an ECG lead or a bandage to get access to the skin to scan. Always inform the patient's nurse and let them know what you need to do. If you remove the ECG lead without telling anyone, you will set off the alarm and the nurse will come running into the room to investigate. They will not be too happy to learn that it was a false alarm due to you removing the lead. Warn the nurse so they can temporarily turn off the ECG alarm.

Always return the room in the condition that you found it in or better. Be careful as you unplug the ultrasound machine that you do not accidentally unplug other equipment. If you do, plug it back in and if the machine does not start up again, or resets itself, immediately notify the nurse. Make sure that the patient does not need anything before you leave. Ask them about lights, window shades, and if they want their door open or closed. When you are finished, inform the nurse so that they can replace any leads or dressings that were removed as well as know the status of their patient to continue care.

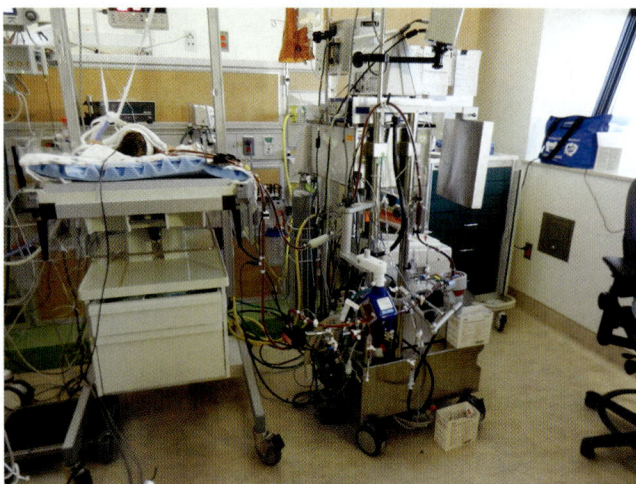

FIG. 2.36 A patient on extracorporeal membrane oxygenation. Notice that there is hardly any room to place the ultrasound machine next to the patient. This patient had to be scanned with the unit placed by their head. (Courtesy Tara Cielma.)

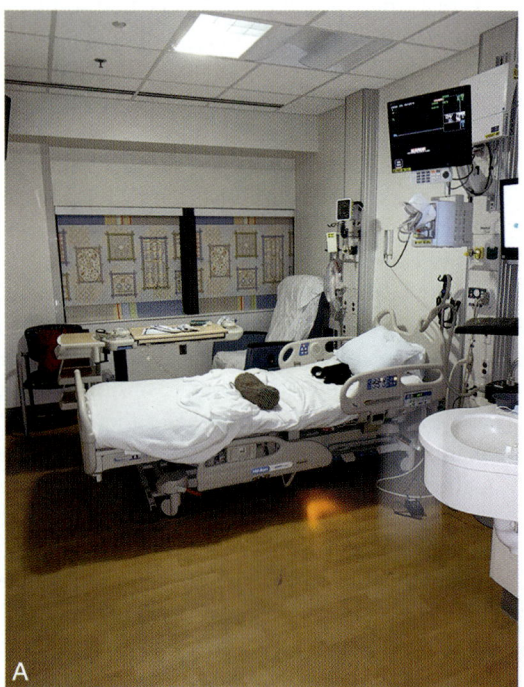
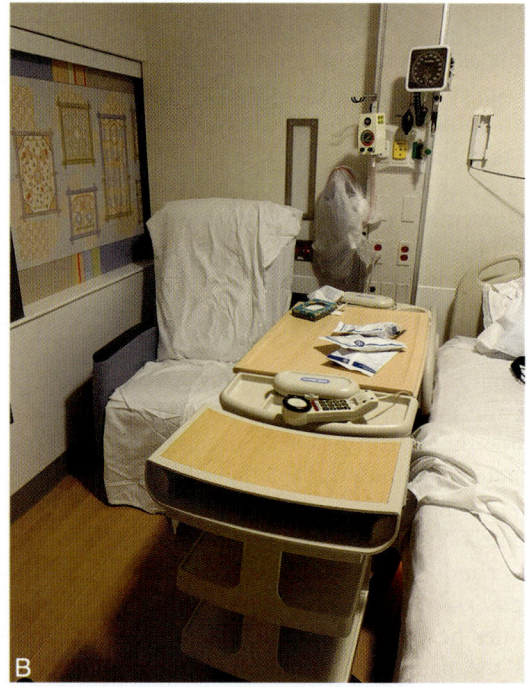

FIG. 2.37 (A) A patient's room. Upon entering the room there looks to be a lot of space, but unfortunately it is on the wrong side of the bed. (B) The space where the ultrasound machine should be placed. To get the unit in that space, the patient's tray would need to be moved, and the extra chair and the reclining chair would need to be turned sideways. Because of the chair, the bottom of the bed may need to be moved away from the unit. You may need to plug the ultrasound unit in before moving the unit into its final position in order not to have to climb over the machine and the recliner to get to the wall socket. Another option is to ask the patient, if able, to turn around so that their head is at the foot of the bed. This position will allow easy access to the patient without having to move all the furniture. After the exam is finished, any objects that have been moved must be returned to their original positions.

EMERGENCY MEDICAL SITUATIONS

Heart attacks and choking because of obstructed airways are frequent causes of accidental death. Choking is especially prevalent in children, who are known to put "everything" into their mouths. Although most sonographers perform their examinations in a medically supervised setting, familiarity with basic lifesaving measures may be helpful as they await the arrival of the code team. If working in a hospital, you may be required to have and maintain CPR certification. Letting it expire may cause you to be disciplined, and you may not be allowed to work with patients until it is renewed.

The American Heart Association and the American Red Cross are two organizations that have long been involved in establishing and teaching basic lifesaving procedures in practice today. Throughout the years, these procedures have changed in response to medical advances and experience gained. Consequently, sonographers must stay current, and one of the best ways to do so is to routinely check the websites of these organizations. The best way to learn and master these lifesaving techniques is to take a formal CPR course. Check with your hospital or facility to see if they offer courses or have a partnership with an organization that teaches the appropriate lifesaving courses required for your place of employment. By knowing these techniques, you might not only save a patient, but possibly a friend, family member, or even a stranger.

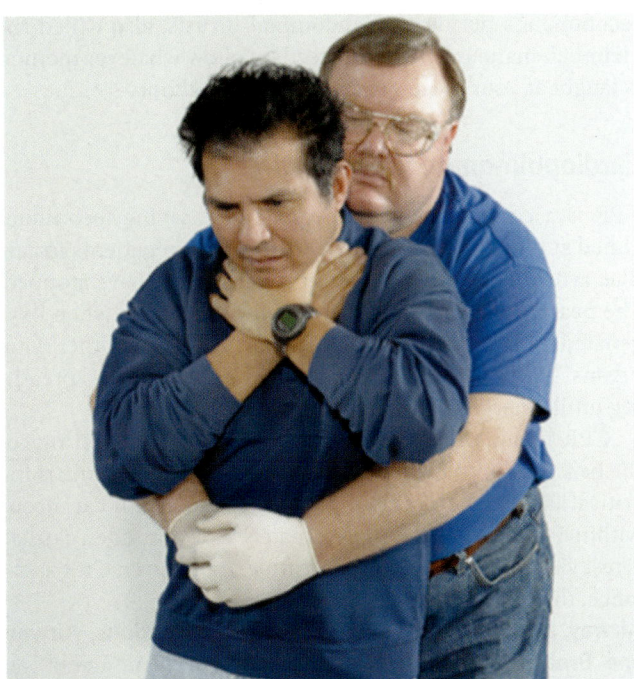

FIG. 2.38 A person demonstrating the universal sign for choking. The rescuer is demonstrating good technique for performing the Heimlich maneuver. As this can occur anywhere the rescuer typically does not wear gloves.

Choking

Choking results from a blockage of the upper airway by food or other objects, preventing normal breathing. Sometimes the person can dislodge the object by coughing; however, if they do not, choking becomes a medical emergency requiring fast, appropriate action. When someone with a completely blocked airway begins to choke, no oxygen can enter the lungs. Brain cells, which are extremely sensitive to oxygen deprivation, will begin to die within 4 to 6 minutes. If first aid is not initiated quickly, brain death can occur in as little as 10 minutes.

The universal sign of choking is that of clutching the throat (Fig. 2.38). At times, the person's attempts to inhale may produce a high-pitched sound. The symptoms can rapidly progress to **cyanosis** and loss of consciousness.

First ask, "Are you choking?" Do not perform first aid if the person is coughing forcefully and is able to speak. A strong cough can often dislodge the object.

If the person is choking, perform abdominal thrusts, also known as the **Heimlich maneuver** (Box 2.5). According to The American Heart Association:

- Stand behind the person. Place one foot slightly in front of the other for balance. Wrap your arms around the waist. Tip the person forward slightly. If a child is choking, kneel down behind the child.
- Make a fist with one hand. Position it slightly above the person's navel.
- Grasp the fist with the other hand. Press hard into the abdomen with a quick, upward thrust, as if trying to lift the person up.

BOX 2.5	How to Perform the Heimlich Maneuver

- Stand behind the person. Place one foot slightly in front of the other for balance. Wrap your arms around the waist. Tip the person forward slightly.
- Make a fist with one hand. Position it slightly above the person's navel.
- Grasp the fist with the other hand. Press hard into the abdomen with a quick, upward thrust, as if trying to lift the person up.
- Perform between 6 and 10 abdominal thrusts until the blockage is dislodged.

- Perform between 6 and 10 abdominal thrusts until the blockage is dislodged.

You may need to repeat the procedure several times before the object is dislodged. If repeated attempts do not free the airway, call 911.

Alternatively, if the person cannot stand up, help them to lie on the floor and straddle their waist, facing toward their head. Push your fist inward and upward in the same manner as you would if they were standing.

Currently there is a disagreement about back blows between the American Red Cross, which recommends back blows, and The American Heart Association and the Heimlich family, which do not recommend back blows. The American Red Cross advises bending the patient over and giving five back blows between the shoulder blades with the heel of your hand followed by five abdominal thrusts, alternating until the object is dislodged. The American Heart Association only recommends performing abdominal thrusts, also called the Heimlich maneuver. You will need to follow whatever method is taught at your place of employment or school.

Cardiopulmonary Resuscitation

CPR is a combination of emergency life-saving techniques aimed at restarting lung and heart function in patients in cardiac arrest where breathing and the heartbeat have stopped. The heart is a muscle that can rapidly deteriorate when oxygenated blood stops flowing to the brain and other vital organs. The goal of CPR is to maintain circulation and breathing until emergency help arrives.

CPR includes chest compressions to pump blood out of the heart and into the body and rescue breathing. Time is the critical factor when initiating CPR because death can occur within 8 to 10 minutes. Approximately 95% of sudden cardiac arrest victims will die without treatment, but given CPR assistance, the survival rate triples.

Airway, Breathing, and Circulation to Compressions, Airway, and Breathing. In the past, CPR for a cardiac arrest was guided by ABC, airway, breathing, and circulation. In 2010 the American Heart Association changed ABC to CAB, compressions, airway, and breathing. First 30 compressions are given, then the airway is opened and two rescue breaths are given, allowing a victim to receive chest compressions much faster and only delaying the rescue breaths by around 20 seconds. For unconscious patients with a pulse but are not breathing, the ABC guidelines should still be followed.

The first step in administering CPR is to evaluate the situation and check the patient for consciousness by tapping or gently shaking the patient's shoulder and loudly asking, "Are you OK?" Do not shake the person if there is a possibility of a neck or spinal injury. If there is no response call 911 for assistance using the speakerphone function of your mobile phone. This will allow you to communicate with medical professionals who will guide you while performing CPR. In the hospital setting when finding a nonresponsive person, yell for help and call the number for a code. If you are using your cell phone, make sure you know the full 10-digit number as you will not be able to dial just the extension from your personal phone. If someone is around have them get the AED. Check for breathing and the carotid pulse simultaneously for no more than 10 seconds. If no pulse is found begin CPR. The current ratio is 30 compressions followed by 2 breaths. Hands should be placed on the lower half of the breastbone using your body weight to administer the compressions. Do not compress over the xiphoid process as it is possible to fracture it. The new guidelines call for the person performing CPR to push hard, with compressions at a depth of 2 to 2.4 inches, 5 to 6 cm, and push fast at a rate of 100 to 120 compressions per minute. This rate can be achieved by singing aloud or in your head or humming the classic Bee-Gees song "Staying Alive." It is important to allow for complete chest recoil between compressions. The two breaths should take no more than a few seconds as it is recommended to interrupt chest compressions for no more than 10 seconds. The new guidelines strongly advise 911 dispatchers to guide untrained bystanders in "compression-only" CPR. A new rescuer if present should take over compressions after 2 minutes as the person performing CPR will tire quickly. CPR should continue until an AED arrives (Fig. 2.39). Never use an AED on a person who is breathing and has a pulse. Before using an AED unit, make sure the surroundings are safe. Tell people to step back, and then follow the prompts given by the AED machine.

- Place one pad on the upper right side of the victim's chest and one on the lower left. The AED unit will diagnose the heart rhythm and indicate if a shock is needed (Fig. 2.40). Only apply shock if there is no pulse and the unit instructs you to do so.
- Continue CPR until another shock command is issued. If only one shock was needed, simply follow the unit's commands until help arrives.

The reader is advised to follow the CPR practice and methods of their place of employment. The reader is also encouraged to check the web sites of the American Heart

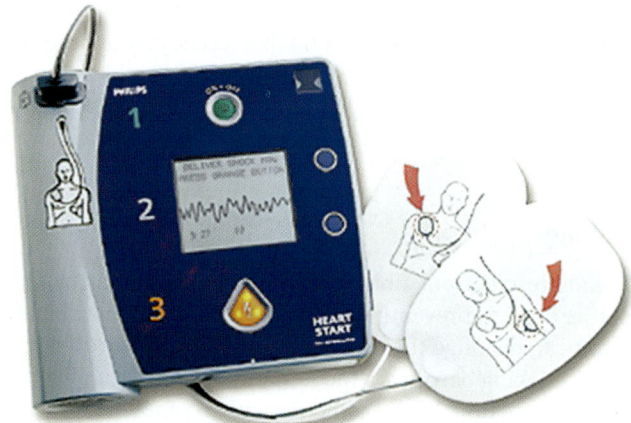

FIG. 2.39 An automated external defibrillation device.

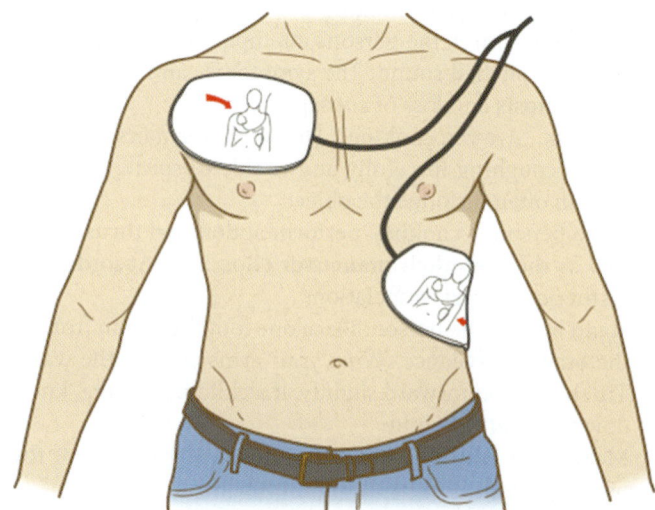

FIG. 2.40 Proper pad placement for an automated external defibrillation device. The pads indicate where they should be placed.

Association and the American Red Cross for current CPR, assisted breathing, and choking guidelines. Your place of employment may require you to maintain CPR certification and not to let it lapse, as policy may be that you cannot scan or interact with patients until you are certified again.

SONOGRAPHER EXPOSURE TO BODY FLUIDS

If you suffer an injury, such as a needle stick, or exposure to blood, semen, vaginal secretions, or any type of body fluid, you must follow the recommendations, depending on the body part affected, of your place of employment. Your chances of catching a disease from a needle stick are usually very low. For needle sticks wash the area with soap and water thoroughly immediately. If fluid is splashed into your eyes, follow the instructions of the eye wash. You need to learn your facility's procedures regarding who to report to and how to get help and care. You should never ignore it or say it was nothing as you never know what disease the person had. You want to be diagnosed and start treatment as soon as possible especially for hepatitis and HIV exposure. For current recommendations on bloodborne pathogens visit https://www.cdc.gov/niosh/topics/bbp/emergnedl.html.

CONCLUSION

Providing competent and excellent patient care in today's health care environment has never been more challenging because the majority of patients are better educated and more demanding. Some are newcomers to the United States with preconceived notions on how they should be treated. Patients expect sonographers to be proficient and empathetic and to focus on them as human beings. Patients expect reliable care, prompt responses to their requests, and assurances that they will be safe while under your care. Today's sonographers must connect with a diverse group of patients and meet their needs while competently and efficiently performing their diagnostic studies.

As a sonographer you must be aware of the importance of being professional, patient, and kind to every person you scan, even when the patient is difficult. Never forget that you chose to be there, but the patient did not necessarily make that choice, and many are ill and anxious. In addition, patient care education must continue after graduation. Sonographers should continue learning everything they can about their profession. Do not make this a 9 to 5 job. Become credentialed in every specialty you practice. Sonography is a growing field and lifelong learning is simply a part of being a sonographer. It is important to continue learning on non-ultrasound-related topics such as CPR, dealing with patients from different cultures and beliefs, keeping up with changes in infection prevention, how to keep yourself and your patient safe, and developing basic skills in taking vital signs and dealing with IVs and other types of tubes. As you have just learned, there is more to being a sonographer than performing sonographic exams.

Key Pearls

- Patient is the primary focus of the sonographer.
- Vital signs are the observable and measurable signs of life and include the following: pulse, respiratory rate, body temperature, and blood pressure.
- The sonographer should be aware of how to meet the patient's needs: bedpans and urinals, emesis basins, tubes and tubing management, and oxygen.
- Body mechanics is essential to performing the daily routine in a health care environment.
- Infection control is a standard precaution to preventing the spread of disease.
- The sonographer should have a working knowledge of basic life support and be able to react to any emergent situation.
- Empathy, understanding, and compassion are essential to care for the variety of patients.
- The sonographer must be compliant with the Patient's Bill of Rights and HIPAA requirements.

BIBLIOGRAPHY

DeJong MR. *Craig's Essentials of Sonography and Patient Care.* 4th ed. St. Louis: Elsevier; 2018.

Diversity Inc. Cultural and religious consideration to competent healthcare. https://www.diversityinc.com/cultural-religious-consideration-competent-healthcare.

Ehman J. Religious diversity: practical points for health care providers. http://www.uphs.upenn.edu/pastoral/resed/diversity_points.html.

Harvard Health Publishing. Reading the new blood pressure guidelines. http://www.health.harvard.edu/blog/new-guidelines-published-for-managing-high-blood-pressure-201312186953.

Medisound. Cross-infection risks in ultrasound examinations. https://medisound.com.au/knowledge/cross-infection-risks-in-ultrasound-examinations-5bj6k?rq=cross%20infection.

Medline Plus. Pulse. https://medlineplus.gov/ency/article/003399.htm.

OneView Healthcare. The eight principles of patient-centered care. http://www.oneviewhealthcare.com/the-eight-principles-of-patient-centered-care/.

U.S. Department of Health and Human Services. Summary of the HIPAA security rule. https://www.hhs.gov/hipaa/for-professionals/security/laws-regulations/index.html.

University of Milwaukee Lesbian, Gay, Bisexual, Transgender, Queer Plus (LGBTQ+) Resource Center. Gender pronouns. https://uwm.edu/lgbtrc/support/gender-pronouns.

Zimlichman E, Henderson D, Tamir O, et al. Health care-associated infections: a meta-analysis of costs and financial impact on the US health care system. *JAMA Intern Med.* 2013;173(22):2039–2046. http://jamanetwork.com/journals/jamainternalmedicine/fullarticle/1733452.

CHAPTER 3

Ergonomics and Musculoskeletal Issues in Sonography

Carolyn T. Coffin and Joan P. Baker

OBJECTIVES

On completion of this chapter, you should be able to:
- Discuss the history of work-related musculoskeletal disorders in sonography
- Define Occupational Safety and Health Administration and discuss its role in sonography
- Define common types of work-related injury for sonographers and know what causes them
- Describe and apply "best practices" in sonography
- Outline the costs of occupational injury to yourself and your employer
- Discuss the ultrasound workstation setup and how it can help minimize injury risk

OUTLINE

History of Ergonomics 68
   History of Work-Related Musculoskeletal Disorders in Sonography 69
   History of the Occupational Safety and Health Administration's Involvement in Sonography 69
Injury Data in Sonography 70
   Definitions 70
   Surveys 70

Risk Factors 70
Mechanisms of Injury 70
Types of Injury 72
Industry Awareness and Changes 72
   Ergonomically Designed Ultrasound Systems 73
   Administrative Controls 73
Work Practice Changes 74
   Gripping the Transducer 74

Wrist Flexion and Extension 75
Twisting Your Neck 75
Abduction of Your Scanning Arm 76
Transducer Cable Management 76
Reaching 77
Exercise 77
Economics of Ergonomics 77
Workstation Setup 78

KEY TERMS

Bursitis
Carpal tunnel
Cubital tunnel
de Quervain disease
Epicondylitis (lateral and medial)
Ergonomics

"Magic triangle"
Occupational Safety and Health (OSH) Act
Rotator cuff injury
Spinal degeneration
Tendonitis

Tenosynovitis
Thoracic outlet syndrome
Trigger finger
Work-related musculoskeletal disorder (WRMSD)

HISTORY OF ERGONOMICS

Broadly defined, **ergonomics** is the science of designing a job to fit the individual worker. One of its primary goals is increasing productivity and decreasing injury by modifying products, tasks, and environments to better fit people.

The term *ergonomics* comes from the Greek words *ergon*, meaning *work*, and *nomos*, meaning *study of* or *natural laws*. The word first entered the modern lexicon when Wojciech Jastrzebowski used it in his 1857 philosophical tract titled *The Science of Work, Based on the Truths Taken from the Natural Science*. The association between work activities and musculoskeletal injuries has been documented for centuries. Bernardino Ramazinni (1633–1714) was the first physician to write about work-related injuries and illnesses in his 1700 publication *De Morbis Artificum (Diseases of Workers)*, which he researched by visiting the workplaces of his patients.[1]

In the early 1900s, industrial production was still largely dependent on human power and motion, rather than on machines, and ergonomic concepts were developing to improve worker productivity. Frederick Winslow Taylor pioneered the "scientific management" method, which sought to improve worker efficiency by discovering the optimum way to do any task. Frank and Lillian Gilbreth expanded upon Taylor's methods in the early 1900s with their time and motion studies aimed at improving efficiency by eliminating unnecessary steps and motion.

The emerging field of ergonomics heavily influenced the assembly line developed by Ford Motor Company between 1908 and 1915. In assembly line manufacturing, parts are added to a product in a set sequential, well-planned manner to create a finished product much faster than with handcrafting-type methods. Although assembly line production improved productivity in the Ford Motor Company, it also reduced the need for workers to move throughout their workday and thus resulted in static work postures.

World War II brought about a greater interest in human-machine interaction, a natural result of developing new and complex machines and weaponry. It was observed that the machine's success depended on its operator and that the design of the machine influenced how successful its operator was. Equipment needed to fit the size of the soldier and controls had to be logical and easy to understand. After World War II, the equipment design focus expanded to include worker safety as well as productivity.

In the decades since the war, the field of ergonomics has continued to flourish and diversify with the advent of the Space Age and the Computer Age.

History of Work-Related Musculoskeletal Disorders in Sonography

Awareness of pain and discomfort associated with the occupation of sonography surfaced around 1980, just before the widespread use of real-time scanners. The most common complaint was shoulder pain in the sonographer's scanning arm. The increasing number of complaints reached the attention of Marveen Craig, a well-known sonographer, educator, and author. Craig published an article in 1985 summarizing the results of a survey done of 100 sonographers who had between 5 and 20 years of scanning experience.[2] The survey respondents complained of stress and burnout, vision problems that improved when images switched from black on white to white on black, infections, and allergies. Electric shock was not uncommon, especially when doing bedside studies and removing transducers from static scanners' articulated arms. Muscle strain involving the wrist, base of the thumb, and shoulder was also reported. Sonographers complained of heavy transducers and cables, and carpal tunnel syndrome claimed its first victim. The term *sonographer's shoulder* came into use.

In the early 1980s, ultrasound systems underwent a complete redesign to real-time two-dimensional scanners, and although articulated arm scanners were used for many more years, real-time scanners were slowly introduced to most facilities.

As more real-time systems came into use, the sonographer's shoulder appeared to diminish. However, this decline lasted only 10 years, and by 1995 the Society of Diagnostic Medical Sonography (SDMS) started receiving increasingly more and varied complaints. In 1997 an extensive 125-question survey was developed by the Health Care Benefit Trust of Vancouver Canada (HBT), in collaboration with the SDMS, the Canadian Society of Diagnostic Medical Sonography (CSDMS), and the British Columbia Ultrasound Society (BCUS). Through this survey, the incidence of work-related musculoskeletal disorder (WRMSD) was found to be 81% in the United States and 87% in Canada, for a combined average incidence in North America of 84%.[3,4]

In 2008 a follow-up survey was conducted, and the incidence increased from 81% to 90% in the United States. Several variables may account for this increase: an aging workforce, increased awareness of WRMSD among sonographers, and increased willingness by sonographers to report an injury.

History of the Occupational Safety and Health Administration's Involvement in Sonography

In 1970 Congress passed the federal **Occupational Safety and Health (OSH) Act**. The purpose of the OSH Act is to ensure, as far as possible, that every working man and woman in the nation has safe and healthful working conditions. Employers may be subjected to civil and sometimes criminal penalties if they violate this act.[5]

The OSH Act is administered by the Occupational Safety and Health Administration (OSHA) of the U.S. Department of Labor, although individual states could create their own agency to enforce the act. Approximately 50% of the states opted to be regulated by the federal OSHA. The other states created their own agencies, which operate under a "state plan." For example, California has a state plan and created its own agency, Cal/OSHA, to enforce safety regulations within that state.[5]

Where industry-specific guidelines do not exist within the OSH Act, the general duty clause can be used. Lawyers representing injured sonographers seeking legal recourse refer to this clause. The criteria for applying the general duty clause are as follows:
- No acceptable standard for an industry
- Exposure to hazard that causes serious physical harm
- Hazard is recognized by the industry
- Feasible abatement method exists to correct the hazard

Section 5B of the general duty clause states that each employee shall comply with occupational safety and health standards and all rules, regulations, and orders issued pursuant to this act that are applicable to his or her own actions and conduct.[6]

It is under the provisions of paragraph 5 A (1) that the OSH Act addresses ergonomic disorders. The language in paragraph 5B gives the impression that the employee holds significant responsibility for complying with health and safety standards; however, the employer bears most of the responsibility for compliance in the eyes of OSHA.[6]

Over the years, OSHA has used many different labels for occupational injury:
- Cumulative trauma disorder (CTD)
- Repetitive motion injury (RMI)
- Overuse syndrome
- Repetitive strain injury (RSI)
- Musculoskeletal strain injury (MSI)

The term **work-related musculoskeletal disorder (WRMSD)** is currently in use. WRMSD incidents are defined as injuries that result in (1) restricted work, (2) days away from work, (3) symptoms of musculoskeletal disorder (MSD) that remain for 7 or more days, and (4) MSD requiring medical treatment beyond first aid.

According to Liberty Mutual, which collects data on WRMSD and the associated costs, repetitive motion injuries cost U.S. industries $2.3 billion per year. Ultrasound examination specialties such as echocardiography, high-risk obstetrics, and to a lesser extent, vascular sonography involve repetitive motion.

Liberty Mutual also reports that 95% of chief executive officers support workplace safety. Benefits include improved employee health. Indirect costs such as morale, productivity, and hiring of replacement staff are significantly reduced, whereas direct costs such as wage replacement and medical expenses are avoided.[7]

Over the years, the Department of Labor received numerous requests from workers' unions to create a way for employees to deal with their WRMSDs. This resulted in an Alliance Program, which enables organizations to work with OSHA to prevent workplace injuries by educating and leading employers and their employees in advancing workplace safety and health.

In May 2003, an International Ultrasound Industry Consensus Conference was hosted by the SDMS to develop injury risk-reducing standards to address the problem of WRMSDs in sonography. Twenty-six organizations represented by 32 participants attended the conference to discuss designing new platforms and procedures that incorporate better ergonomics. The industry standards address the role of employees and employers, educators, medical facilities, and equipment manufacturers in reducing the impact of these injuries on the workforce and are intended to assist all stakeholders in making informed decisions.

Separately, but at the same time, administrators addressed the issues of workload, scheduling, and room size, while sonographers discussed best practices, education, and training. The need for accredited programs to include curricula related to ergonomics and injury prevention and certifying bodies testing knowledge of risk factors was covered.

INJURY DATA IN SONOGRAPHY

Definitions

WRMSDs are injuries of muscles, tendons, and joints caused by or aggravated by workplace activities. These injuries are the main reason for long-term absence among health care workers,[8] accounting for up to 60% of all workplace illnesses. Survey data have shown that more than 80% of sonographers have some form of MSD that can be attributed to their work activities.

Surveys

Table 3.1 outlines the numerous surveys that have been conducted on the incidence of this injury in sonography. These surveys have produced other data relevant to the study of occupational injury in ultrasound, and their results support the presence of risk factors in the sonography profession. Several other factors contribute to reported injury rates, including worker awareness, unwillingness to work in pain, busier patient schedules, job dissatisfaction, an aging workforce, and workplace computerization.

A positive relationship has been demonstrated between the severity of WRMSDs and the performance of repetitive work tasks or tasks that require forceful movements, with or without repetitive motion.[9] Increased use of technology has resulted in workers' accomplishing the same work tasks with fewer movements. Thus the relationship between the user and the workstation equipment has become "frozen," and the worker is often forced into a static posture. This combination of repetitive motions and prolonged static postures results in musculoskeletal discomfort and eventually injury.

Risk Factors

Risk factors include forceful exertions, awkward postures, prolonged static postures, repetitive motions, "pinch" grip, and exposure to environmental factors such as extreme heat, cold, humidity, or vibrations (Fig. 3.1). The accumulated exposure to one or more of these risk factors over time leads to injury because repeated exposure interferes with the ability of the body to recover. WRMSDs cause pain, inflammation, swelling, deterioration of tendons and ligaments, and spinal degeneration. Muscles and joints are further stressed once their support structures are weakened.

Mechanisms of Injury

Sustained awkward postures can cause imbalances between the muscles that move and the muscles that stabilize. Repeatedly rotating the head, neck, and trunk causes one set of muscles to become stronger and shorter and the opposing muscles to become weaker and elongated. Asymmetric forces are exerted on the spine, causing misalignment (see Fig. 3.1). Nerve entrapment syndromes can result from increased muscle and tendon pressure on major nerves that run behind tightened muscles. Tasks requiring the worker to lean forward continually or bend the head down or laterally are examples of these types of postures. Prolonged static postures, whether sitting or standing, increase the load on soft tissues and the compressive forces in the spine

CHAPTER 3 Ergonomics and Musculoskeletal Issues in Sonography

TABLE 3.1 Surveys of Work-Related Musculoskeletal Disorders

Author	Year	Number Surveyed	Number Responded	Incidence (%)	Scope
Vanderpool	1993	225	101	86	Random, ARDMS
BCUS	1994	232	211	91	BC, Canada
SDMS	1995	3000	983	81	Random, ARDMS
CSDMS	1995	Unknown	427	87	Canada
Smith	1997	220	113	80	ASE
Wihlidal	1997	156	96	89	Alberta, Canada
Gregory	1998	Unknown	197	77.8	Australia
Magnavita	1999	2670	2041	74	Italy
McCullough	2002	Unknown	295	82	United States
Ransom	2002	Unknown	300	89	United Kingdom
Sound Ergonomics	2008	5800	3244	90	United States

ASE, American Society of Echocardiography; *ARDMS*, American Registry for Diagnostic Medical Sonography; *BCUS*, British Columbia Ultrasound Society; *CSDMS*, Canadian Society of Diagnostic Medical Sonography; *SDMS*, Society of Diagnostic Medical Sonography.

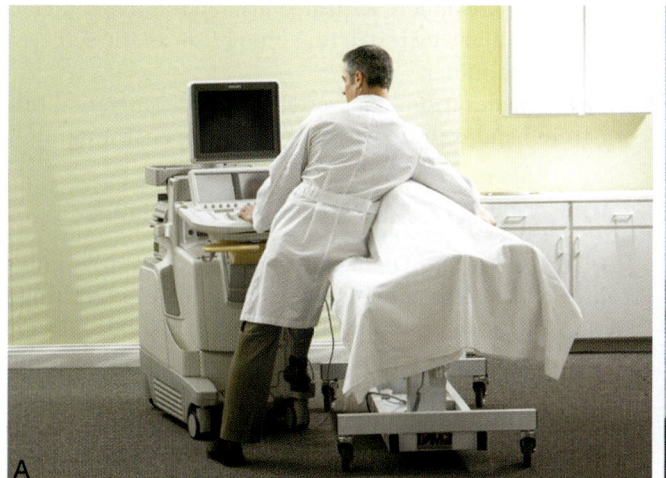
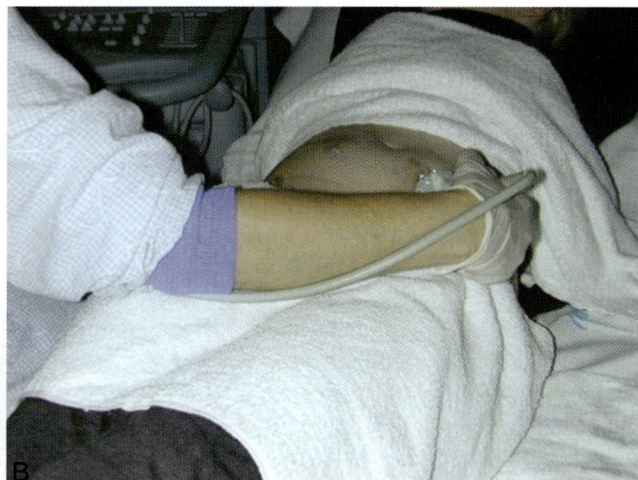
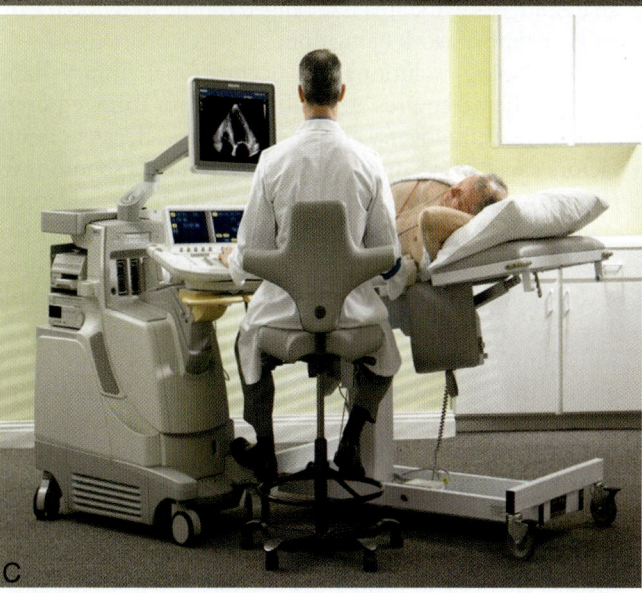

FIG. 3.1 (A) Bad ergonomics. Right-handed cardiac scanning is likely to cause injury to the sonographer because of the abduction of the arm over the patient's back, the hyperflexion of the right wrist, and the need to lean to the right and twist the neck to view the monitor. (B) Hyperflexion of the right wrist. In addition, the amount of stretching and twisting is often increased when scanning obese patients. (C) Good ergonomics. It is difficult to reduce these risk factors, but turning the patient around to perform the study is one way. (A, Courtesy Philips Healthcare, Ultrasound North America.)

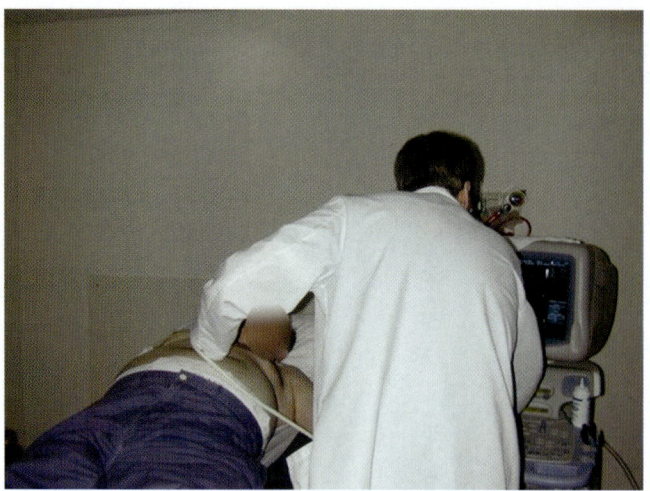

FIG. 3.2 Tasks requiring the worker to lean forward continually or bend the head down or laterally result in incorrect postures. Prolonged static postures, whether sitting or standing, increase the load on soft tissues and the compressive forces on the spine.

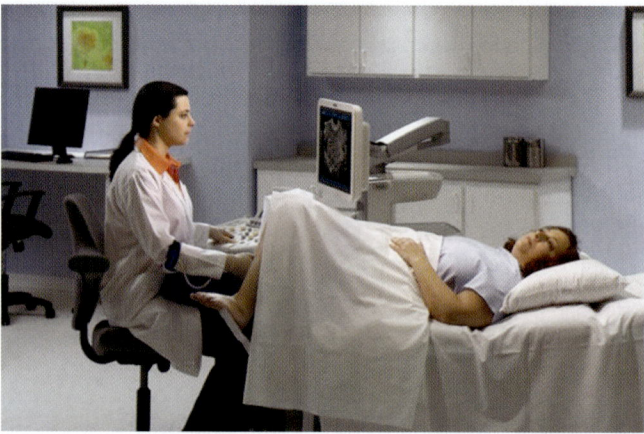

FIG. 3.3 Epicondylitis (lateral and medial). Inflammation of the periosteum in the area of the insertion of the biceps tendon into the distal humerus. This can result from repeated twisting of the forearm, which can occur when performing an endovaginal scan.

(Fig. 3.2). Additionally, the contraction of more than 50% of the body's muscles is required to maintain static postures.[10] Human physiology depends on movement, which promotes normal muscle contraction and relaxation. Muscle activity circulates blood to carry nutrients to and remove toxins from muscles. Awkward and static postures cause muscles to be contracted continuously; therefore they cannot receive oxygen or get rid of toxins.[11]

Types of Injury

Tendonitis and **tenosynovitis**. Inflammation of the tendon and the sheath around the tendon. These often occur together.

de Quervain disease. Specific type of tendonitis involving the thumb that can result from gripping the transducer.

Carpal tunnel. Entrapment of the median nerve as it runs through the carpal bones of the wrist. This results from repeated flexion and extension of the wrist and from mechanical pressure against the wrist.

Cubital tunnel. Entrapment of the ulnar nerve as it runs through the elbow. This can result from repeated twisting of the forearm and mechanical pressure against the elbow when you rest it on the examination table while scanning.

Epicondylitis (lateral and medial). Inflammation of the periosteum in the area of the insertion of the biceps tendon into the distal humerus. This can result from repeated twisting of the forearm (Fig. 3.3).

Thoracic outlet syndrome. Nerve entrapment can occur at different levels, resulting in a variety of symptoms.

Trigger finger. Inflammation and swelling of the tendon sheath in a finger entrap the tendon and restrict motion of the finger.

Bursitis (shoulder). Inflammation of the shoulder bursa from repeated motion.

Rotator cuff injury. Repeated motion results in fraying of the rotator cuff muscle tendons. This injury increases with age and is even more prevalent when work-related stresses are added. Repeated arm abduction contributes to this injury by restricting blood flow to the soft tissues of the shoulder.

Spinal degeneration. Intervertebral disc degeneration results from bending and twisting and improper seating.

INDUSTRY AWARENESS AND CHANGES

The increase in MSDs in industry led to research into the causes and to legislation in the United States regulating the design of office furniture and duration of video terminal work. Appropriate ergonomic adaptations have been found to reduce the risk of MSD symptoms effectively. Adapting a workstation to each person and their work requirements ensures that it functions as intended. Productivity increases if an employee's work area is arranged for the individual worker and the type of work being done.

Developing solutions to occupational injury among sonographers requires a combined effort from equipment companies, employers, and sonographers. Because multiple factors cause MSD, injury prevention requires solutions from many sources as well. By taking a multidisciplinary approach, significant improvements can be made in the risk for work-related injury in the sonography profession.

Mitigating risk for injury involves a strategy for control. The first solutions to consider are engineering solutions, which involve a change in the physical features of a workplace. This is the preferred method for control because it can effectively eliminate the workplace hazard. However, these solutions also tend to be the most expensive initially.[7]

When engineering controls are not feasible or cost prohibitive, administrative controls can be implemented. These solutions are not as effective as engineering controls and include changes in workplace policies, patient scheduling and sonographer rotations, and the implementation of rest breaks. Administrative controls lessen the duration and frequency of exposure to an injury risk.[7]

The least effective control is the use of personal protective equipment (PPE) or professional practices. This method addresses best practices and the use of arm support devices. The sonographer is still exposed to the risk factor, but the exposure is somewhat reduced.[7]

Over the years, the major ultrasound equipment manufacturers addressed the issue of occupational injury by redesigning the platform of their systems. This involved changing the aspects of the system's control panel, monitors, and transducers. As a result, many features of today's ultrasound systems are designed with ergonomics in mind.

Ergonomically Designed Ultrasound Systems

The well-designed ultrasound system should be easily mobile and have brakes. The control panel should be height adjustable and should swivel. The monitor should also be height adjustable, independent of the control panel, and should turn and tilt. Controls should be easy to access without overreaching. Transducers should not be too wide, which causes stretching of the fingers, or too narrow, which causes a "pinch grip." Transducer cables should be thin, flexible, and lightweight, and the transducer cable should be supported during an examination. In addition, transducers should be easy to activate with readily accessible connecting ports and storage.

Other engineering controls involve the workstation, which includes the examination table and the chair and accessories (Fig. 3.4). An electronically height-adjustable examination table is an important component of an ergonomically designed workstation. It should be specialty specific by providing options that adapt it for use in certain procedures. Examples would be a drop section for apical cardiac views or stirrups for obstetric/gynecologic examinations. If the sonographer sits to scan, a height-adjustable chair with an appropriate height range is equally as important as the examination table. The sonographer also should be able to support their arms while scanning and have an examination room that is large enough to allow for a flexible setup. The room must have appropriate lighting to avoid glare on the monitor and reduce eyestrain.

Administrative Controls

Patient examinations should be carefully scheduled to prevent repeating the same type of examination back to back. It is important to perform a variety of examinations, allowing different muscles to fire. The schedule should allow enough time between examinations for muscle recovery. Examination gloves should have textured fingers to prevent the need to grip the transducer too tightly. Take short "mini" breaks during examinations to relax muscles, especially in the shoulder and neck. If it is necessary to perform bedside examinations, make sure that the ultrasound system can be moved easily and has a small footprint. Try to share bedside examinations with other staff and do these examinations only when absolutely necessary, not because it is more convenient. Bedside examinations should be reserved for those patients whose condition prohibits transporting them.

Provide separate monitors so that the patient and the sonographer do not have to share the monitor mounted on the system. Provide ergonomically designed scanning rooms to reduce the risk of injury to the sonographer, including appropriately adjustable ancillary equipment.

Personal Protective Equipment/Professional Controls. You are the only person who can control your work postures and behaviors, some of which may be injury producing (Fig. 3.5). You must take responsibility for your postural alignment and take the time to arrange the examination room equipment to suit you and the study you are performing. Best practices address how to prevent or reduce your exposure to known risk factors. Be aware of what causes pain and make changes in technique and postures immediately:

- Minimize sustained bending, twisting, reaching, lifting, and transducer pressure.
- Avoid awkward postures (see Figs. 3.1 and 3.5A).
- Alternate sitting and standing throughout examinations.
- Vary scanning techniques and transducer grips (Fig. 3.6C).
- Adjust all equipment to suit each user's size (see Fig. 3.1C).
- Have accessories on hand before beginning the examination.
- Use appropriate measures to reduce arm abduction (Fig. 3.7).
- Avoid forward and backward reach (see Fig. 3.5).
- Instruct the patient to move as close to you as possible.
- Adjust the height of the table and chair (see Fig. 3.5B).
- Use support for your arms.
- Relax your muscles periodically throughout the day.
- Stretch your hand, wrist, shoulder muscles, and spine.
- Take mini breaks during the procedure.

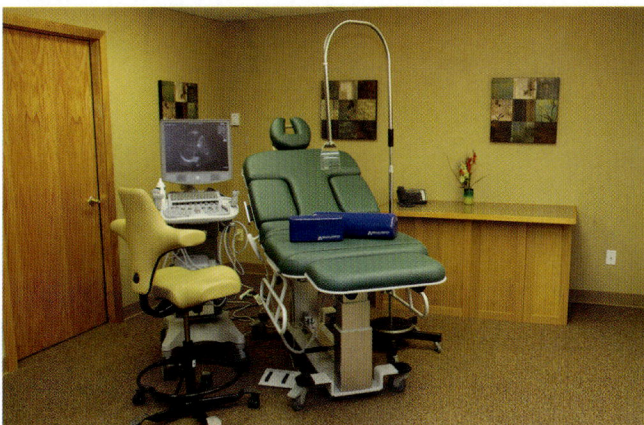

FIG. 3.4 An ultrasound workstation with an ergonomically designed table and chair. You must take responsibility for your postural alignment and take the time to arrange the examination room equipment to suit you and the study you are performing. (Courtesy Oakworks Medical, Inc., New Freedom, PA.)

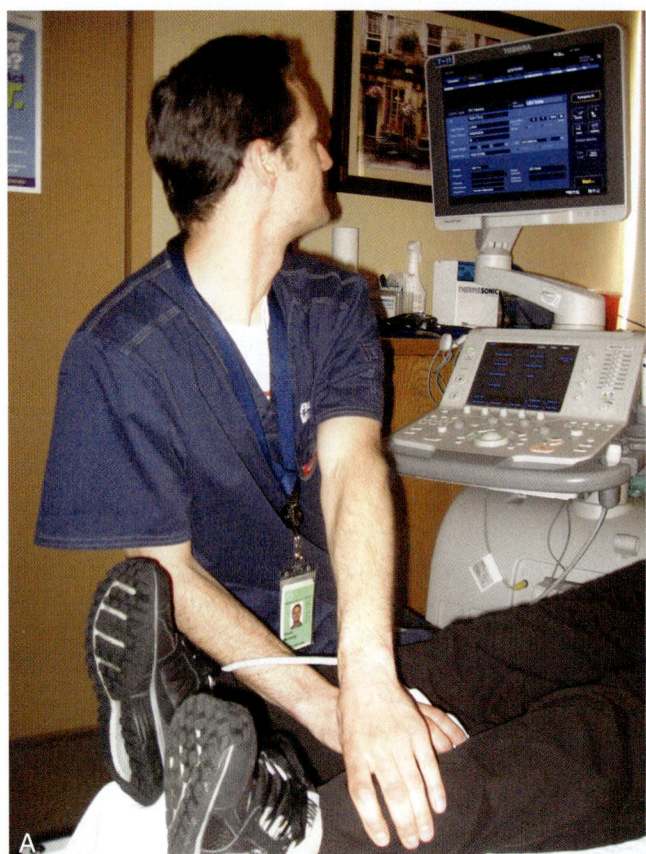
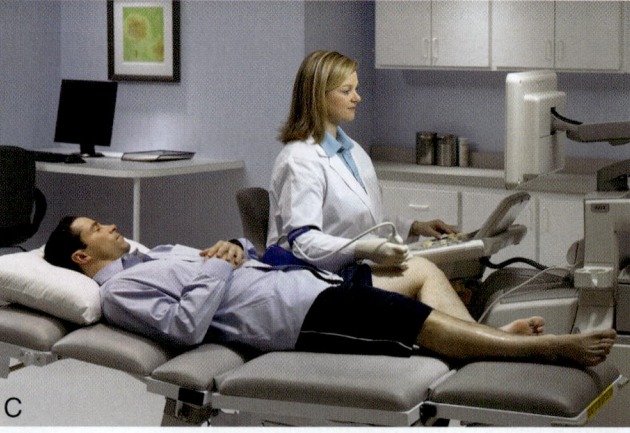
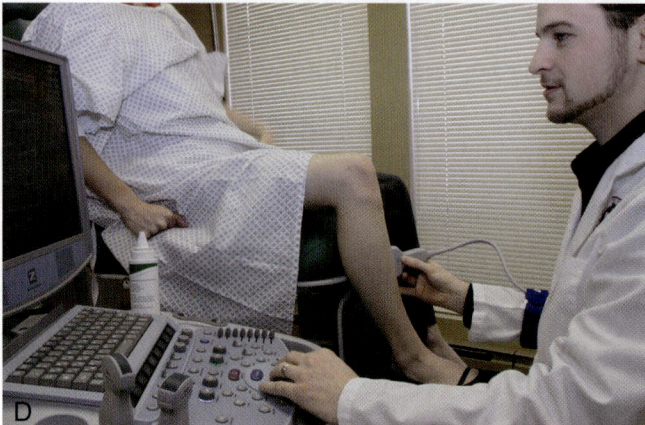
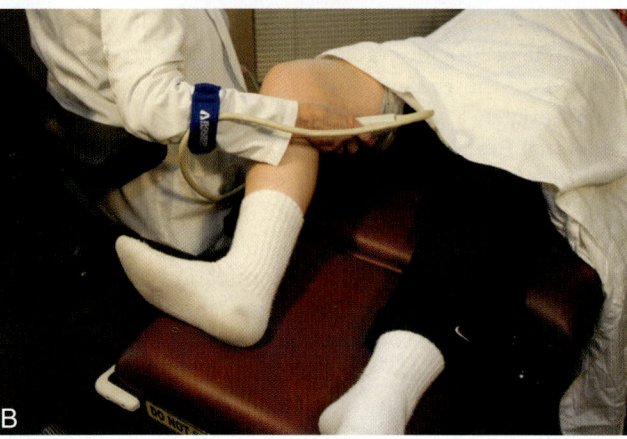

FIG. 3.5 (A) Ultrasound performed to evaluate deep vein thrombosis (DVT) can be very injury producing if not performed correctly. (B) The best augmentation is self-augmentation, where the patient moves their foot similar to pumping the gas pedal of a car. (C) When scanning the patient's left leg, turn the patient so that the left leg is closest to you. (D) This is the most ergonomic way to perform a scan to evaluate DVT if you have a mobile patient. (C, Courtesy Siemens Healthcare Ultrasound, USA Division.)

- Take meal breaks separate from work-related tasks.
- Using the 20-20-20 rule, refocus your eyes every 20 minutes on an object about 20 feet from you for 20 seconds.
- Vary procedures, tasks, and skills as much as reasonably possible.
- Use correct body mechanics when moving patients, wheelchairs, beds, stretchers, and ultrasound systems.
- Report and document any persistent pain to your employer and seek competent medical advice.
- Maintain a good level of physical fitness to perform the demanding work tasks required.
- Collaborate with employers on staffing solutions that allow sufficient time away from work.

WORK PRACTICE CHANGES

Gripping the Transducer

Use mild transducer pressure. Avoid the temptation to be "image driven"—sacrificing your body for a "pretty picture" that does not affect the diagnosis. It is unnecessary to grip the transducer tightly. This might be no more than a bad habit, and you may be unaware that you are doing it. This is also a difficult habit to break, as it is as natural as holding a pen.

Manufacturer improvements, such the lightweight, flexible cables, can reduce the weight and torque that the transducer produces on the scanning hand. If they are available in your

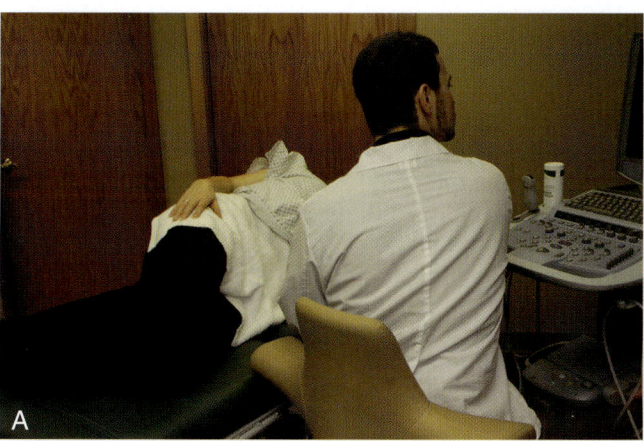 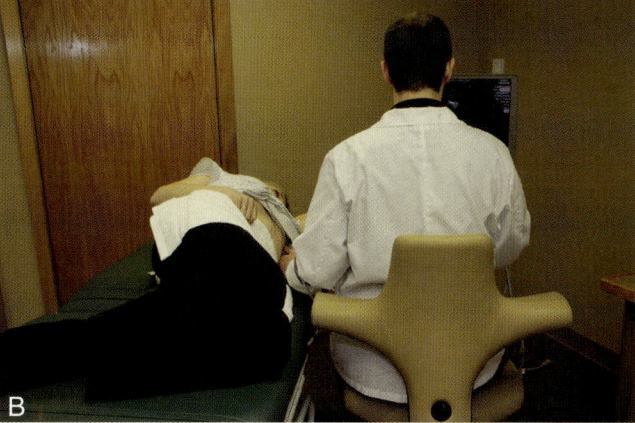

FIG. 3.6 You are the only person who controls your work posture. (A) Bad ergonomic practice in left-handed cardiac scanning. (B) Good ergonomics. In left-handed cardiac scanning, it is easy to adjust the height of the chair up and the table down to reduce the angle of abduction to 30 degrees or less. This often requires that you bring the patient to the edge of the table.

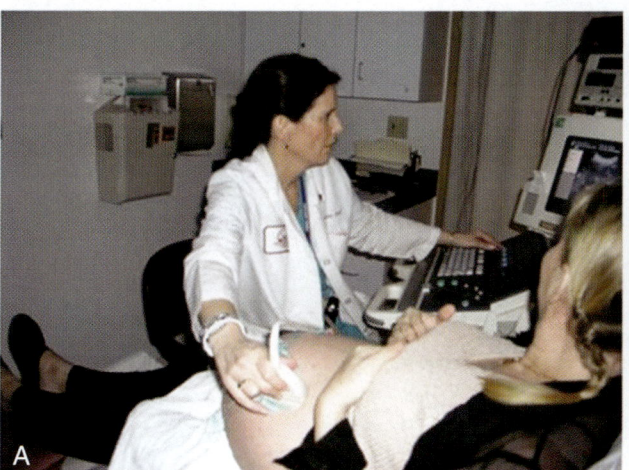 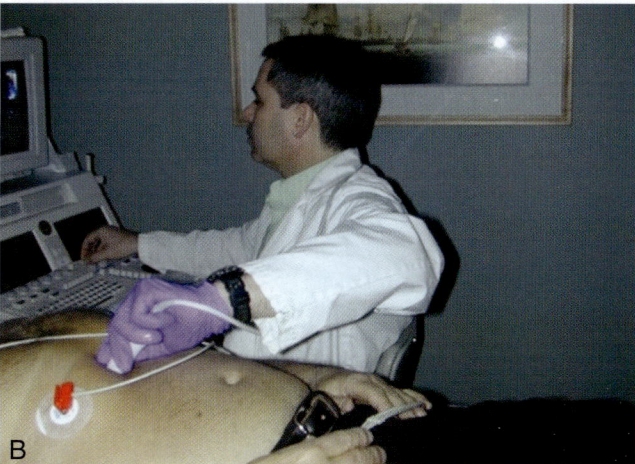

FIG. 3.7 (A) The main reason for shoulder pain associated with right-handed scanning is due to the abduction of the shoulder. Shoulder abduction must be reduced to 30 degrees or less. (B) Bad ergonomic practice in left-handed cardiac scanning. Shoulder pain can often be experienced on the nonscanning side or in both shoulders because leaning to the right as a means to reduce the pain arising from the abduction on that side results in overreaching on the left side to reach the controls.

department, use lightweight transducers. Keeping the transducer handle free of excess gel will also reduce the amount of force needed to grip the transducer. It is also important to use gloves that fit properly. Gloves that are too large require more muscle force to grip than gloves that fit (Fig. 3.8C). Additionally, it takes 40% more effort to hold a transducer in a pinch grip versus a power grip. Therefore it is important to learn different ways to hold the transducer to use more of your hand than your fingers.

Wrist Flexion and Extension

It is important to keep the wrist in a neutral or "normal" position. Dorsiflexion of the wrist can lead to pressure and resultant injury in the carpal tunnel. This position requires the muscles of the forearm to fire continuously (see Fig. 3.8A).

When transporting the equipment, push from the legs, not the arms and wrists, keeping your wrists in a neutral position (see Fig. 3.8B). Avoid resting your wrist on the keyboard while scanning or typing. Be sure to support your forearm while scanning to reduce muscle fatigue of the forearm, neck, and shoulder.

Twisting Your Neck

This position produces increased pressure on the intervertebral discs and should be minimized as much as possible. Position the ultrasound system so that it is as close to the examination table as possible with the monitor facing you to reduce neck twisting. Do not share the monitor with the patient. An external monitor for patient viewing is strongly recommended. Also remember to keep your shoulders

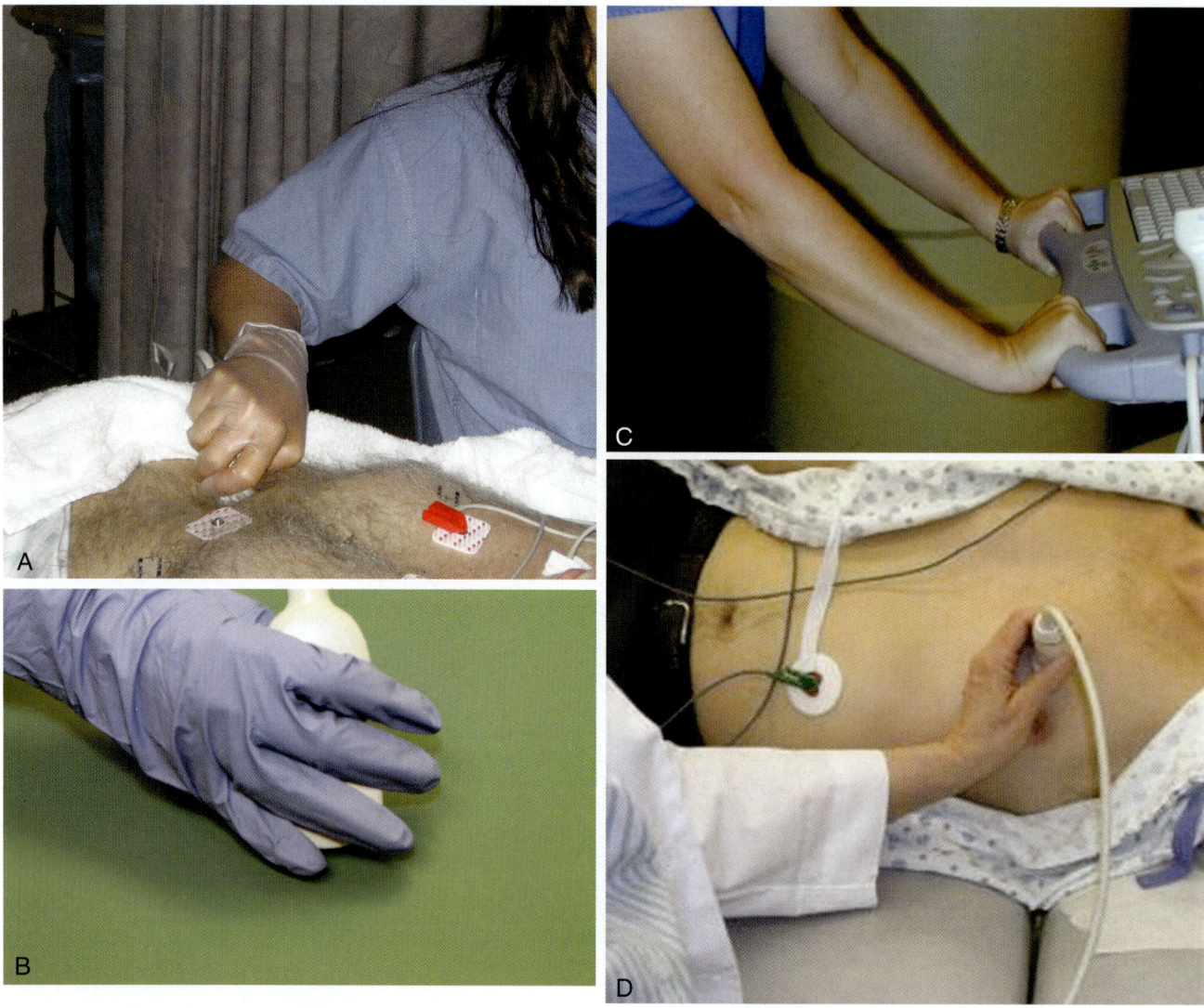

FIG. 3.8 (A) If you can see your knuckles through your gloves, you are gripping the transducer too tightly. (B) Gloves that are too big require increased strength to scan. (C) When transporting the equipment, avoid wrist extension as shown here. Push from the legs, not the arms and wrists. (D) Support your forearm while scanning; an arm support cushion elevates the forearm and reduces wrist extension.

relaxed as much as possible, rolling them periodically during the scan to release your neck muscles (see Fig. 3.6A).

Abduction of Your Scanning Arm

The main reason for shoulder pain associated with right-handed scanning is due to the abduction of the shoulder. Shoulder abduction must be reduced to 30 degrees or less (see Figs. 3.1 and 3.3). Lower the examination table or elevate the chair to achieve the correct posture. The sonographer must also position the patient by having them move to the edge of the examination table so that the patient's side is touching the sonographer's right hip to reduce abduction further and reach. One study showed that decreasing the angle of abduction from 75 to 30 degrees and supporting the forearm on support cushions could reduce up to 88% in muscle activity of the shoulder. Sonographers who are short in stature may have to stand to scan. It may also be helpful to sit for part of the scan and stand for other parts, as long as the equipment is readjusted to suit the two different positions. Support your scanning arm by placing support cushions or a rolled-up towel under your elbow.

Transducer Cable Management

Current transducers inherently create torque on the wrist forcing the muscles of the hand and forearm to fire constantly to counteract the drag. Cable braces can be used to hold and support the cable of ultrasound transducers. This takes the strain off the operator's hand and forearm created by the imbalance of the transducer and cable, significantly reducing torque on the wrist. Additionally, cable braces can alleviate the need to grip as tightly or the need to put the cable around your neck or between your hip and the table. This latter position creates issues of spinal alignment and weight imbalance trunk-twisting.

Trunk-twisting is often necessary for small rooms where equipment cannot be optimally positioned to reduce twisting. Sonographers with poor scanning technique also exhibit this posture (see Fig. 3.3). If you stand to scan, have your weight evenly distributed over both feet so that your spine remains straight. If you are uncertain as to whether you have the habit of leaning on one leg, ask a colleague to watch you scan and observe your spine position. When seated, use your abdominal muscles to support your trunk, and sit upright with good postural alignment. This often takes some practice but can be more readily achieved by using a specially designed chair that puts you into a more natural position (see Fig. 3.6). These chairs have a saddle-type seat and are ideal for maintaining the natural lordosis of the spine. Another option is an air-filled cushion, which forces you to maintain a stable, more neutral position by engaging your abdominal muscles to help you balance on the cushion.

Reaching

Reaching occurs when you reach for the controls while scanning with the opposite hand. To reduce reach, the ultrasound system must be brought as close as possible to you. Frequently used controls should be in the middle of the control panel so that regardless of the hand used to manipulate them, they can be adjusted without causing strain. If you sit to scan, you must be able to fit your legs under the control panel to position the system close enough. Be sure your feet are fully supported when sitting, either on the system, the floor, the chair, or a footstool. If this is not possible, it may be better to stand while scanning. Do not get into the habit of leaving your non-scanning arm in an extended position over the control panel, especially over the freeze-frame control (see Fig. 3.3).

These work practices also apply to your computer workstation and the Picture Archiving and Communication Systems (PACS) station. These environments are part of your workday and can be another source of injury. The heights of the computer monitor, work desk, and chair should all be adjustable. The keyboard should be positioned to minimize reach and maximize a neutral wrist posture.

Exercise

Sonographers should also learn and perform a regular maintenance exercise program designed to strengthen and stretch the shoulders, arms, hands, and trunk (Fig. 3.9).

ECONOMICS OF ERGONOMICS

The cost of occupational injury to both the employer and the employee is phenomenal. The losses to the employer encompass not only the medical costs of an injury but also the cost of replacement staff, workers' compensation, and loss of revenue. The loss of experienced professionals and a skilled, stable workforce also affects productivity. The cost to the worker includes not only monetary hardship but also the possibility of permanent injury, chronic pain, and loss of profession.

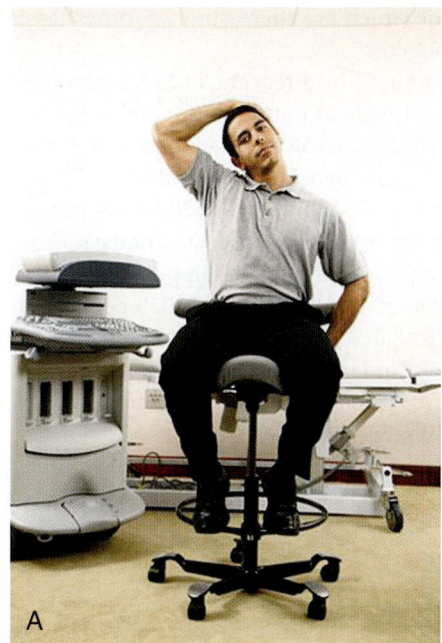

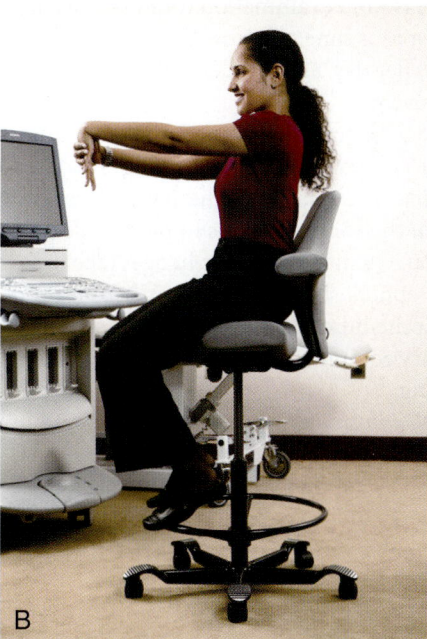

FIG. 3.9 (A–B) Simple stretches and exercises performed for a few minutes at intervals throughout the day can make a significant difference to your health and well-being. (Courtesy Siemens Healthcare Ultrasound, USA Division.)

Acute and chronic MSDs are the most prevalent workplace injury in all industries. The Bureau of Labor Statistics states that more than 300,000 MSDs are reported annually. They account for 56% of the work-related illnesses reported to OSHA and are responsible for 640,000 lost workdays. MSDs are also the costliest of all occupational problems, accounting for the majority of workers' compensation costs. The costs related to occupational MSDs are both direct and indirect. MSDs cost $60 billion overall per year and $5 billion to $20 billion per year in direct costs to businesses. These costs include workers' compensation and medical expenses, the latter of which are increasing 2.5 times faster than any other benefit cost.

In sonography, the direct and indirect costs have been estimated at $771,500 per injured sonographer.[12]

- Approximately $1 of every $3 of workers' compensation costs are spent on occupational MSDs.
- Employers pay $15 billion to $20 billion per year in workers' compensation costs for lost workdays.
- The mean cost per cause of upper extremity WRMSD is $8070 versus a mean cost of $4075 per case for all types of work-related injury. Regarding incurred claim costs (which include indemnity and medical payments), the average for all claims is $10,105, but for carpal tunnel syndrome, it is $13,263.
- Indirect costs are 3 to 5 times higher, reaching approximately $150 billion per year. These include absenteeism, staff replacement and retraining, and loss of productivity or quality.
- The cost of hiring temporary replacement staff is between $130,000 and $166,000 per year. The estimated average cost to find and hire a new sonographer is $10,000.
- If an ultrasound examination room is down because of the loss of worker time, the loss of chargeable income is equal to $4500 per day, $22,500 per week, or $1,170,000 per year in lost revenue.

The cost of equipping a sonography examination room is minimal compared with addressing a workers' compensation injury. The quality of the patient's examination may also suffer if the sonographer is in pain while performing the examination. Quality diagnostic images take time to produce, and sonographers should not feel rushed to produce images because of scheduling conflicts or pain.

Accessory equipment that can mitigate injury risk includes the following:

- *A height-adjustable stool.* Cost: $950 reimbursement on two to three patient studies.
- *Arm support cushions.* Cost: $100 each reimbursement on one patient study.
- *An ergonomic examination table.* Cost: $9000 reimbursement from 2 to 3 days' work.

Work-related injuries must be reported immediately to occupational health or risk management departments. These injuries should be recorded on OSHA logs. Failure to do this may result in denial of claims.

WORKSTATION SETUP

The ultrasound room has received truly little attention regarding design or the arrangement of the equipment (see Fig. 3.4). However, the room should be large enough for the workers to change the position of the ultrasound system or exam table, especially when different sonographers use the room throughout the day. An ideal exam room would be at least 150 square feet, have no windows, have only lower storage cabinets and adjustable lighting, preferably within reach of the sonographer while scanning. The room size should allow the sonographer to move the ultrasound system completely around the exam table. This enables the sonographer to bring the ultrasound system to the foot of the exam table for endocavitary exams or to accommodate the necessary equipment for stress echocardiograms and the ultrasound system.

Since older, heavier ultrasound systems had fixed monitors and control panels, it was best to position them parallel to the exam table. In this configuration, the monitor and control panel were directly in front of the sonographer. It was not conducive to patient interaction during the exam, and, anecdotally, patients have commented that they felt ignored or left out after the exam began.

Today's systems are easily moved and repositioned, and the control panels can be rotated into many different positions. The monitors can be positioned independent of the control panel, thus allowing each sonographer to set up the system in a more comfortable configuration and with more patient interaction. The sonographer can access the keys without reaching too far forward or across their body by positioning the control panel off-center and to the left (right for left-handed cardiac exams). Then the monitor can be positioned more toward the patient so that the sonographer can view it and still see and talk with the patient. This takes the sonographer out of the "silo" and puts them into a patient-engagement, sonographer-neutral position, a position referred to as the **magic triangle** (Fig. 3.10).

Key Pearls

- The term work-related musculoskeletal disorder (WRMSD) incidents are defined as injuries that result in (1) restricted work, (2) days away from work, (3) symptoms of musculoskeletal disorder (MSD) that remain for 7 or more days, and (4) MSD requiring medical treatment beyond first aid.
- WRMSDs are injuries of muscles, tendons, and joints that are caused by or aggravated by workplace activities.
- Risk factors include forceful exertions, awkward postures and prolonged static postures, repetitive motions, "pinch" grip, and exposure to environmental factors such as extreme heat, cold, humidity, or vibrations.
- Sustained awkward postures can cause imbalances between the muscles that move and the muscles that stabilize.
- Adapting a workstation to each person and their work requirements ensures that it functions as intended. Productivity is increased if an employee's work area is arranged for the individual worker and the type of work being done.
- You are the only person who can control your work postures and behaviors, some of which may be injury producing.
- Best practices address how to prevent or reduce your exposure to known risk factors.
- Be aware of what causes pain and make changes in technique and postures immediately.
- The cost of occupational injury to both the employer and the employee is phenomenal. The losses to the employer encompass not only the medical costs of an injury but also the cost of replacement staff, workers' compensation, and loss of revenue.

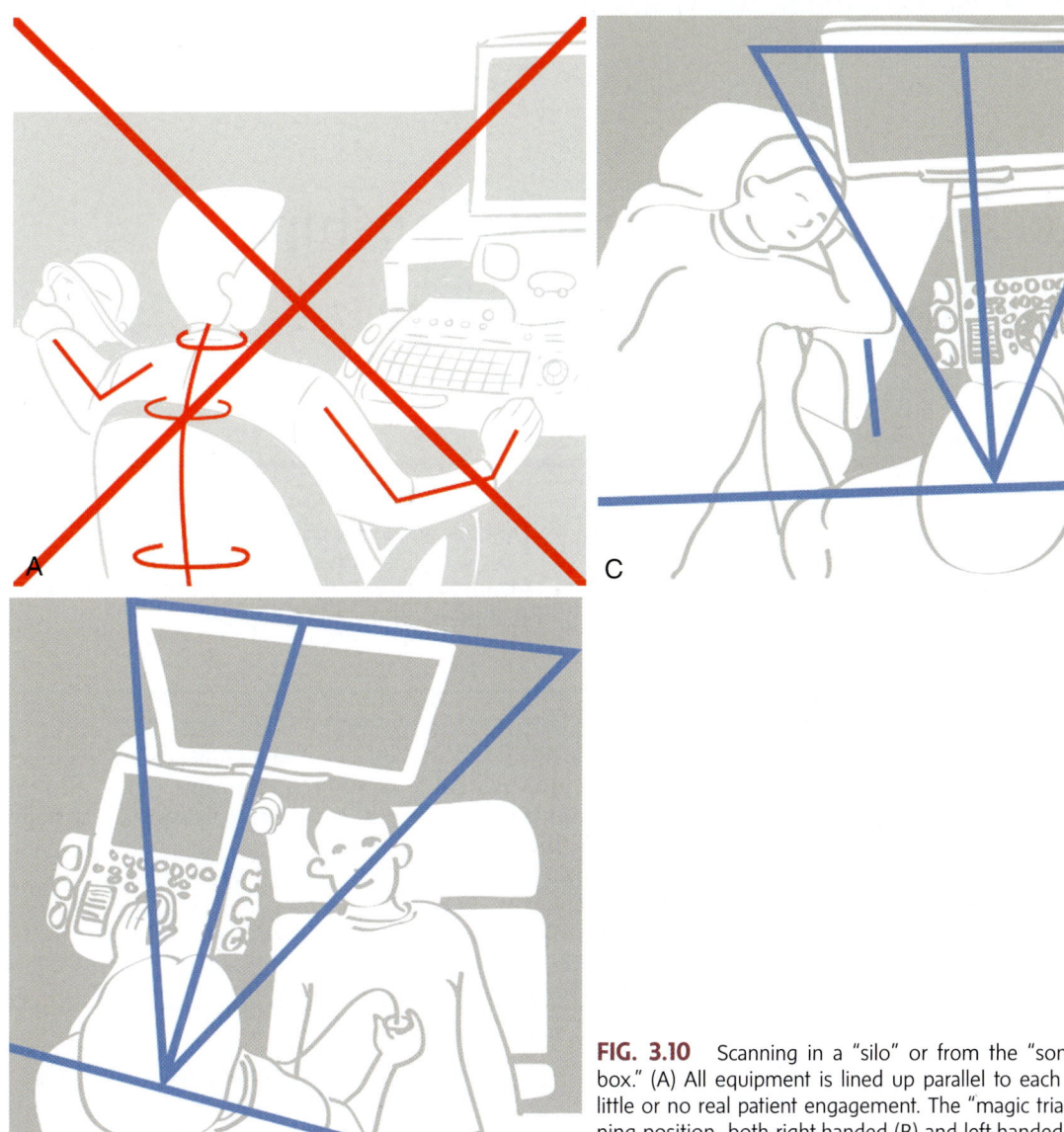

FIG. 3.10 Scanning in a "silo" or from the "sonographers' box." (A) All equipment is lined up parallel to each other with little or no real patient engagement. The "magic triangle" scanning position, both right-handed (B) and left-handed (C), results in more patient engagement and a sonographer neutral posture.

REFERENCES

1. Ergoweb: History of Ergonomics. 2017. Availanle at: www.ergoweb.com/history-of-ergonomics/.
2. Craig M. Sonography: an occupational health hazard? *J Diagnost Med Sonogr.* 1985;1(3):121–126.
3. Pike I, Russo A, Berkowitz J, et al. The prevalence of musculoskeletal disorders among diagnostic medical sonographers. *J Diagnost Med Sonogr.* 1997;13(5):219–227.
4. Murphy C, Russo A. *An Update on Ergonomic Issues in Sonography.* Healthcare Benefit Trust; 2000.
5. U.S. Department of Labor: The Occupational Safety and Health Administration: a history of its first thirteen years, 1971-1984. https://www.dol.gov/general/aboutdol/history/mono-osha13introtoc.
6. U.S. Department of Labor, Occupational Safety and Health Administration. OSH Act of 1970. Sec. 5. Duties. www.osha.gov/pls/oshaweb/owadisp.show_document?p_id=3359&p_table=OSHACT.
7. Society of Diagnostic Medical Sonography. *Industry Standards for the Prevention of Work-Related Musculoskeletal Disorders in Sonography,* May 2003. www.sdms.org/pdf/wrmsd2003.pdf.
8. Bongers PM, deWinter CR, Kompier MAJ, Hildebrandt VH. Psychosocial factors at work and musculoskeletal disease. *Scand J Work Environ Health.* 1993;19(5):297–312.
9. Barr AE, Safadi FF, Gorzelany I, et al. Repetitive, negligible force reaching in rates induces pathological overloading of upper extremity bones. *J Bone Miner Res.* 2003;18(11):2023–2032.
10. Valachi B, Valachi K. Mechanisms leading to musculoskeletal disorders in dentistry. *J Am Dent Assoc.* 2003;134:1344–1350.
11. Kroemer K, Grandjean E. *Fitting the Task to the Human.* ed 5. Philadelphia: Taylor & Francis; 2000.
12. Ergoweb: Ergonomics Software and Services. https://ergoweb.com/about-ergoweb/.

CHAPTER 4

Anatomic and Physiologic Relationships Within the Abdominopelvic Cavity

Sandra L. Hagen-Ansert

OBJECTIVES

On completion of this chapter, you should be able to:
- Define and use terms for anatomic directions
- Discuss the body systems and their functions
- Know the terms for the body planes
- Describe and locate the abdominal quadrants and regions
- List the organs located in each major body cavity
- Identify and locate the abdominal viscera and other abdominal structures and spaces

OUTLINE

From Atom to Organism 81
   Metabolism 81
   Homeostasis 81
   Vital Signs 81
Body Systems 81
   The Circulatory System: Blood Composition 81

The Gastrointestinal System 83
The Genitourinary Systems 86
Anatomic Relationships Within the Abdominopelvic Cavities 88
   The Abdominal Cavity 88
   The Retroperitoneal Cavity 92
   The Pelvic Cavity 92

Abdominopelvic Membranes and Ligaments 95
Potential Spaces in the Body 98

KEY TERMS

Acidic
Acidosis
Aklaline
Alkalosis
Anterior pararenal space
Ascites
Bile
Buffer
Diaphragm
Dorsal cavity
Dysuria
Erythrocyte
Erythropoiesis
Formed element
Hematochezia
Hematocrit

Hemoglobin
Homeostasis
Hypertension
Hypotension
Inguinal ligament
Lateral arcuate ligament
Left crus of the diaphragm
Leukocyte
Leukopoiesis
Linea semilunaris
Medial arcuate ligament
Metabolism
Morison's pouch
Organism
Parietal peritoneum
Pelvic cavity

Perirenal space
Peritoneal cavity
Peritoneal recesses
Plasma
Rectourterine pouch
Rectus abdominus muscle
Right crus of the diaphragm
Scrotal cavity
Superficial inguinal ring
Tachycardia
Thrombocyte
Urinary incontinence
Ventral cavity
Vesicouterine pouch
Viscera
Visceral peritoneum

To understand the complexity of the human body and how the parts work together to function as a whole truly is to gain an appreciation of anatomy and physiology. The science of body structure (anatomy) and the study of body function (physiology) are intricately related, for each structure of the human body system carries out a specific function. Anatomy and physiology can take many forms: gross anatomy studies the body by dissection of tissues, histology studies parts of body tissues under the microscope, embryology studies development before birth, and pathology is the study of disease processes.

FROM ATOM TO ORGANISM

A review of the composition of the human body begins with an understanding that all materials consist of chemicals. The basic units of all matter are tiny invisible particles called *atoms*. An atom is the smallest component of a chemical element that retains the characteristic properties of that element. Atoms can combine chemically to form larger particles called *molecules*. For example, two atoms of hydrogen combine with one atom of oxygen to produce a molecule of water.

The next level of complexity in the human body is a microscopic unit called a *cell*. Although they share common traits, cells can vary in size, shape, and specialized function. In the human body, atoms and molecules associate in specific ways to form cells, and trillions of different types of cells are found within the body. All cells have specialized tiny parts called *organelles*, which carry on specific activities. These organelles consist of aggregates of large molecules, including those of such substances as proteins, carbohydrates, lipids, and nucleic acids. One organelle, the *nucleus*, serves as the information and control center of the cell.

Cells that are organized into layers or masses that have common functions are known as *tissue*. The four primary types of tissue in the body are muscle, nervous, connective, and epithelial tissues. Groups of different tissues combine to form *organs*—complex structures with specialized functions, such as the liver, pancreas, or kidneys. One organ may have more than one type of tissue (i.e., the heart mainly consists of muscle tissue, but it is also covered by epithelial tissue and contains connective and nervous tissue).

A coordinated group of organs are arranged into organ or *body systems*. For example, the digestive system consists of the mouth, esophagus, stomach, intestines, liver, gallbladder, and pancreas. Body systems make up the total part or *organism* that is the human body.

Metabolism

All physical and chemical changes that occur within the body are referred to as **metabolism**. The metabolic process is essential to digestion, growth and repair of the body, and conversion of food energy into forms useful to the body. Other metabolic processes maintain the routine operations of the nerves, muscles, and other body parts.

Homeostasis

The anatomic structures and functions of all body parts are directed toward maintaining the life of the organism. To sustain life, an organism must have the proper quantity and quality of water, food, oxygen, heat, and pressure. Maintenance of life depends on the stability of these factors. **Homeostasis** is the ability to maintain a steady and stable internal environment. Stressful stimuli, or *stressors*, disrupt homeostasis.

Vital Signs

Vital signs are medical measurements used to ascertain how the body is functioning. These measurements include body temperature and blood pressure and rates and types of pulse and breathing movements. A close relationship has been noted between these signs and the homeostasis of the body because vital signs are the result of metabolic activities.

BODY SYSTEMS

A body system consists of a group of tissues and organs that work together to perform specific functions. Each system contributes to the dynamic, organized, and carefully balanced state of the body. The sonographer should be familiar with at least the integumentary, lymphatic, skeletal, endocrine, muscular, respiratory, and nervous systems of the body. The remaining systems—circulatory, digestive, urinary, and reproductive—should be thoroughly understood by the sonographer. Table 4.1 lists the components and functions of human body systems.

The Circulatory System: Blood Composition

Knowledge of the circulatory system is fundamental to understanding human physiology. The circulation of blood throughout the body serves as a vital connection to the cells, tissues, and organs to maintain a relatively constant environment for cell activity. Blood is composed of **plasma** and **formed elements**. The formed elements comprise platelets, leukocytes (neutrophils, lymphocytes, monocytes, eosinophils, and basophils), and erythrocytes.

Blood Composition. Plasma makes up 55% of the total blood volume and consists of approximately 91% water (Fig. 4.1). The remaining 9% comprises numerous substances suspended or dissolved in this water. Hemoglobin of the red cells accounts for two thirds of the blood proteins, with the remaining consisting of plasma proteins that include serum albumin, globulin, fibrinogen, and prothrombin.

Serum album constitutes 53% of the total plasma proteins. It is produced in the liver and serves to regulate blood volume. A high level of albumin in the blood is symptomatic of dysfunction within the body. Globulin can be separated into alpha, beta, and gamma globulin. Gamma globulin is involved in immune reactions in the body's defense against infection. Fibrinogen is concerned with coagulation of blood. Prothrombin is produced in the liver and participates in blood coagulation. Vitamin K is essential for prothrombin production.

Functions of the Blood. The blood is responsible for a variety of functions, including transportation of oxygen and nutrients, defense against infection, and maintenance of pH. The red blood cells (RBCs), white blood cells (WBCs), and

TABLE 4.1 Systems in the Human Body

System	Components	Functions
Integumentary	Skin, hair, nails, sweat glands	Covers and protects tissues, regulates body temperature, supports sensory receptors
Skeletal	Bones, cartilage, joints, ligaments	Supports the body, provides framework, protects soft tissues, provides attachments for muscles, produces blood cells, stores inorganic salts, provides calcium storage
Muscular	Skeletal, cardiac, smooth muscle	Moves parts of skeleton, provides locomotion, pumps blood, aids movement of internal materials, produces body heat
Nervous	Nerves and sense organs, brain, and spinal cord	Receives stimuli from external and internal environment, conducts impulses, integrates activities of other systems
Endocrine	Pituitary, adrenal, thyroid, pancreas, parathyroid, ovaries, testes, pineal, and thymus gland	Regulates body chemistry and many body functions
Lymphatic	Lymph nodes	Returns tissue fluid to the blood, carries specific absorbed food molecules, defends the body against infection
Circulatory	Heart, blood vessels, blood, lymph and lymph structures	Moves the blood through the vessels and transports substances throughout the body
Respiratory	Lungs, bronchi, and air passageways	Exchanges gases between blood and external environment
Digestive	Mouth, tongue, teeth, salivary glands, pharynx, esophagus, stomach, liver, gallbladder, pancreas, small and large intestines	Receives, breaks down, and absorbs food and eliminates unabsorbed material from the body
Urinary	Kidney, bladder, ureters	Excretes waste from the blood, maintains water and electrolyte balance, and stores and transports urine
Reproductive	Testes, scrotum, spermatic cord, vas deferens, ejaculatory duct, penis, epididymis, prostate, uterus, ovaries, fallopian tubes, vagina, breast	Reproduction; provides for continuation of the species

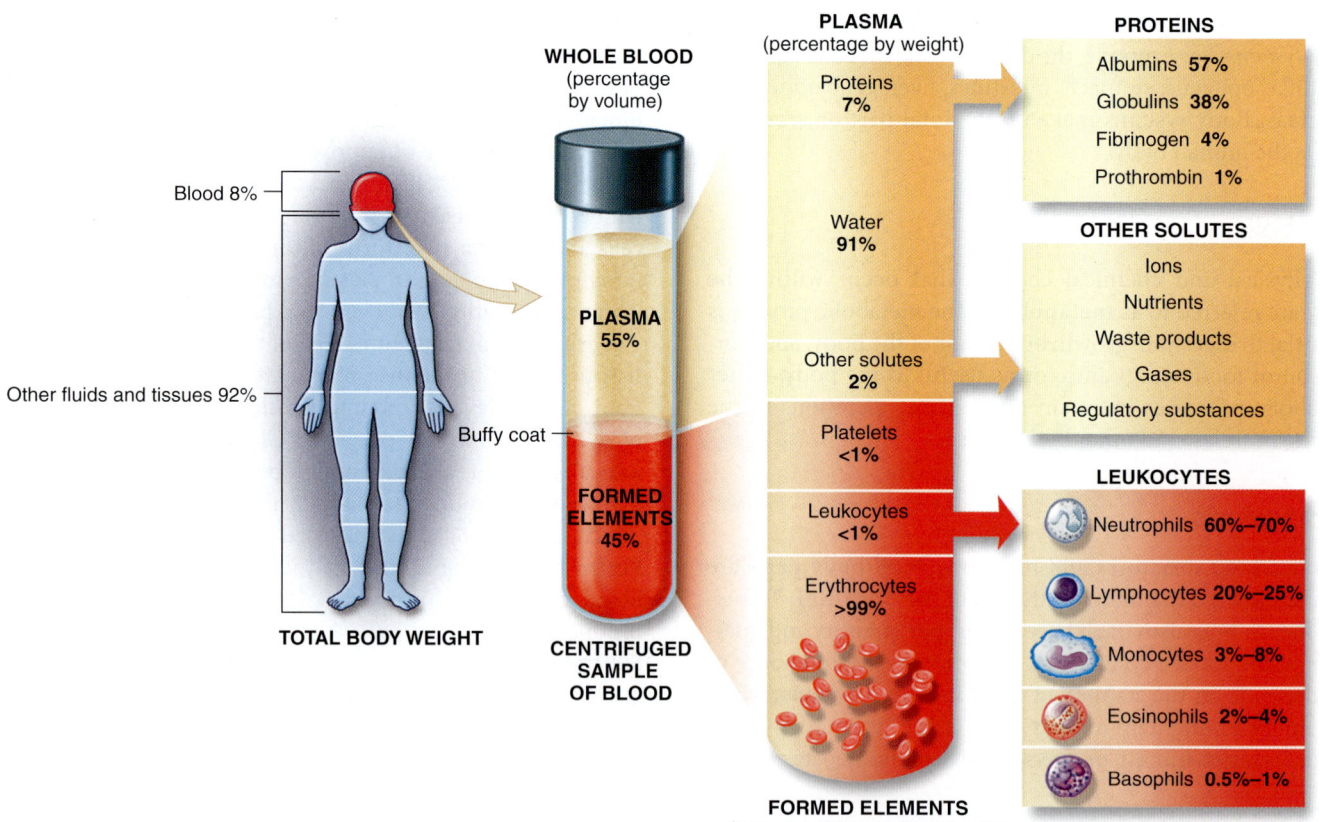

FIG. 4.1 Components of blood. Approximate values for the components of blood in a typical adult.

platelets are continually being destroyed so the body must make new ones to replace the destroyed cells every second. There are two kinds of connective tissue that make blood cells for the body: myeloid tissue (red bone marrow) and lymphatic tissue (lymph nodes, thymus, spleen). The formation of new blood cells is called hemopoiesis. As the blood cells mature, they move into the circulatory vessels.

Acidic Versus Alkaline. Blood is thicker than water and therefore flows more slowly than water. The specific gravity of blood may be calculated by comparing the weight of blood versus water; with water being 1.00, blood is in the range of 1.045 to 1.065. The hydrogen ion and the hydroxyl ion are found within water. When a solution contains more hydrogen than hydroxyl ions, it is called an **acidic** solution. Likewise, when it contains more hydroxyl ions than hydrogen ions, it is referred to as an **alkaline** solution. This concentration of hydrogen ions in a solution is called the pH, with the scale ranging up to 14.0.

In water, an equal concentration of both ions exists; water is thus a neutral solution, or 7.0 on the pH scale. Human blood has a pH of 7.34 to 7.44, being slightly alkaline. A blood pH less than 6.8 is a condition called *acidosis;* blood pH greater than 7.8 is known as *alkalosis.* Both conditions can lead to serious illness and eventual death unless proper balance is restored. To help in this process, blood plasma is supplied with chemical compounds called *buffers*. These buffers can act as weak acids or bases to combine with excess hydrogen or hydroxyl ions to neutralize the pH. Plasma is the basic supporting fluid and transporting vehicle of the blood.

The volume of blood in the body depends on the body surface area; however, the total volume may be estimated as approximately 9% of total body weight. Most adults have a blood volume between 5 and 6 liters.

The RBCs (**erythrocytes**), the WBCs (**leukocytes**), and the platelets (**thrombocytes**) make up the remainder of the blood. The percentage of the total blood volume containing these three elements is called the **hematocrit**. Normally, the hematocrit is 45% of the total blood volume, with plasma accounting for the remaining 55%.

Complete Blood Count. The differential complete blood count (CBC) is a laboratory blood test that evaluates and states specific values for all these subgroups of WBCs.

Red Blood Cells. RBCs are disk-shaped, biconcave cells without a nucleus. They are formed in the bone marrow and are the most prevalent of the formed elements in the blood. Their primary role is to carry oxygen to the cells and tissues of the body. Oxygen is picked up by a protein in the red cell called **hemoglobin**. Hemoglobin releases oxygen in the capillaries of the tissues. The function of *erythrocytes* is to provide oxygen and carbon dioxide transport.

The production of RBCs is called **erythropoiesis**. Their life span is approximately 120 days. Vitamin B_{12} is necessary for complete maturity of the RBCs. The inner mucosal lining of the stomach secretes a substance called the intrinsic factor, which promotes absorption of vitamin B_{12} from ingested food.

As old RBCs are destroyed in the liver, part of the hemoglobin is converted to bilirubin, which is excreted by the liver in the form of **bile**. When excessive amounts of hemoglobin are broken down or when biliary excretion is decreased by liver disease or biliary obstruction, the plasma bilirubin level rises. This rise in plasma bilirubin results in a yellow-skin condition known as jaundice.

White Blood Cells. WBCs are the body's primary defense against infection. WBCs lack hemoglobin, are colorless, contain a nucleus, and are larger than RBCs. White cells are extremely active and move with an ameboid motion, often against the flow of blood. They can pass from the bloodstream into intracellular spaces to phagocytize foreign matter found between the cells. A condition called *leukopoiesis* is WBC formation stimulated by the presence of bacteria.

Leukocytes. Neutrophils, lymphocytes, monocytes, eosinophils, and basophils are in the group of leukocytes. Their function is to ingest and destroy bacteria with the formation of pus. The function of the specific leukocytes are:
- Neutrophil and monocyte: immune defense—phagocytosis
- Lymphocyte: antibody production and cellular immune response
- Eosinophil: defense against irritants that cause allergies; phagocytosis
- Basophil: inflammatory response; contains heparin and controls clotting

Lymphocytes and Monocytes. The lymphocytes are WBCs formed in lymphatic tissue. They enter the blood by way of the lymphatic system and contain antibodies responsible for delayed hypersensitivity reactions. Monocytes are large white cells capable of phagocytosis and are quite mobile. Their numbers are few, and they are produced in the bone marrow.

White Blood Cells. White cells have two main sources: (1) red bone marrow (granulocytes) and (2) lymphatic tissue (lymphocytes). When an increase in the white cells arises from a tumor of the bone marrow, it is called *myelogenous leukemia* and is noted as an increase in granulocytes. On the other hand, an increase in WBCs caused by overactive lymphoid tissue is called *lymphatic leukemia*, with an increase in lymphocytes. In bacterial infections, the white cells increase in number (leukocytosis), with most of the increase noted in the neutrophils. A decrease in the total white cell count (leukopenia) is a result of a viral infection.

Thrombocytes. Thrombocytes, or blood platelets, are formed from giant cells in the bone marrow. They initiate a chain of events involved in blood clotting together with a plasma protein called fibrinogen. Thrombocytes are destroyed by the liver and have a life span of 8 days.

The Gastrointestinal System

The gastrointestinal (GI) system consists of two major divisions: the GI tract and the accessory organs. The GI tract is a hollow tube that begins at the mouth and ends at the anus.

Approximately 25 feet long, the GI tract includes the pharynx, esophagus, stomach, small intestine, and large intestine (Fig. 4.2). Accessory GI organs include the liver, pancreas, gallbladder, and bile ducts and will be discussed in detail in their respective chapters. The abdominal aorta and the portal venous system also aid the GI system.

Major functions of the GI system include ingestion and digestion of food and elimination of waste products. GI complaints can be especially difficult to assess and evaluate because the abdomen has so many organs and structures that may influence pain and tenderness.

Normal Findings for the Gastrointestinal System.
Visual Inspection.
- Skin is free from vascular lesions, jaundice, surgical scars, and rashes.
- Faint venous patterns (except in thin patients) are apparent.
- Abdomen is symmetric, with a flat, round, or scaphoid contour.
- Umbilicus is positioned midway between the xiphoid process and the symphysis pubis, with a flat or concave hemisphere.
- No variations in the color of the patient's skin are detectable.
- No bulges are apparent.
- The abdomen moves with respiration.

Guidelines for Gastrointestinal Assessment.
Temperature. Fever may be a sign of infection or inflammation.

Pulse. **Tachycardia** may occur with shock, pain, fever, sepsis, fluid overload, or anxiety. A weak, rapid, and irregular pulse may point to hemodynamic instability, such as that caused by excessive blood loss. Diminished or absent distal pulses may signal vessel occlusion from embolization associated with prolonged bleeding.

Respirations. Altered respiratory rate and depth can result from hypoxia, pain, electrolyte imbalance, or anxiety. Respiratory rate also increases with shock. Increased respiratory rate with shallow respirations may signal fever and sepsis. Absent or shallow abdominal movement on respiration may point to peritoneal irritation.

Blood Pressure. Decreased blood pressure may signal compromised hemodynamic status, perhaps from shock caused by GI bleed. Sustained severe **hypotension** results in diminished renal blood flow, which may lead to acute renal failure. Moderately increased systolic or diastolic pressure may occur with anxiety or abdominal pain, and such **hypertension** can result from vascular damage caused by renal disease or renal artery stenosis. A blood pressure decrease of greater than 30 mm Hg when the patient sits up may indicate fluid volume depletion.

Common Signs and Symptoms of Gastrointestinal Diseases and Disorders.
The most significant signs and symptoms related to GI diseases and disorders are abdominal pain, diarrhea, bloody stools, nausea, and vomiting (Table 4.2).

Abdominal Pain. Abdominal pain usually results from a GI disorder, but it can be caused by a reproductive, genitourinary, musculoskeletal, or vascular disorder; use of certain drugs; or exposure to toxins.
- Constant, steady abdominal pain suggests organ perforation, ischemia, inflammation, or blood in the peritoneal cavity.
- Intermittent and cramping abdominal pain suggests the patient may have obstruction.
- Ask if the pain radiates to other areas or if eating relieves the pain.
- Abdominal pain may arise from the abdominopelvic viscera, the parietal peritoneum, or the capsule of the liver, kidney, or spleen and may be acute or chronic, diffuse or localized.
- Visceral pain develops slowly into a deep, dull, aching pain that is poorly localized in the epigastric, periumbilical, or hypogastric region.
- Mechanisms that produce abdominal pain, including stretching or tension of the gut wall, traction on the peritoneum or mesentery, vigorous intestinal contraction, inflammation, or ischemia, may cause sensory nerve irritation.

Diarrhea. Diarrhea is usually a primary sign of intestinal disorder. Diarrhea is an increase in the volume, frequency, and liquidity of stools compared with the patient's normal bowel habits. It varies in severity and may be acute or chronic.

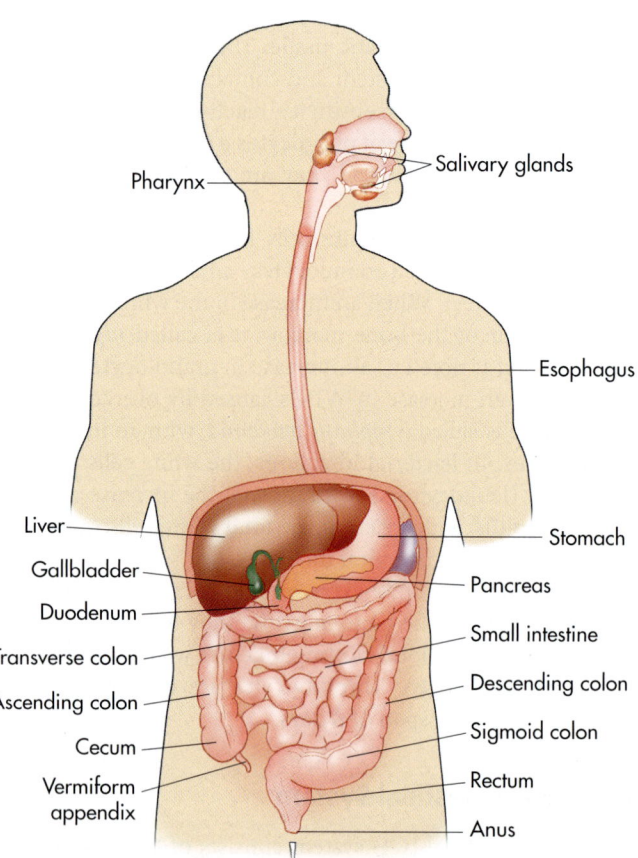

FIG. 4.2 The digestive system includes the mouth, pharynx, esophagus, stomach, small intestine, large intestine, rectum, and anus.

TABLE 4.2 Signs and Probable Indications of Gastrointestinal Diseases and Disorders

Signs or Symptoms	Probable Indication
Abdominal Pain	
Localized abdominal pain, described as steady, gnawing, burning, aching, or hunger-like; high in the mid-epigastrium slightly off center, usually on the right	Duodenal ulcer
Pain begins 2–4 h after a meal	
Ingestion of food or antacids brings relief	
Changes in bowel habits	
Heartburn or retrosternal burning	
Pain and tenderness in the right or left lower quadrant, may be sharp and severe on standing or stooping	Ovarian cyst
Abdominal distention	
Mild nausea and vomiting	
Occasional menstrual irregularities	
Slight fever	
Referred, severe upper abdominal pain, tenderness, and rigidity that diminish with inspiration	Pneumonia
Fever, shaking, chills, aches, and pains	
Blood-tinged or rusty sputum	
Dry, hacking cough	
Dyspnea	
Diarrhea	
Occurs within several hours of ingesting milk or milk products	Lactose intolerance
Abdominal pain, cramping, and bloating	
Flatus	
Recurrent bloody diarrhea with pus or mucus	Ulcerative colitis
Hyperactive bowel sounds	
Cramping lower abdominal pain	
Occasional nausea and vomiting	
Hematochezia	
Moderate to severe rectal bleeding	Coagulation disorders
Epistaxis (nosebleed)	
Purpura (skin rash resulting from bleeding into the skin from small blood vessels)	
Bright-red rectal bleeding with or without pain	Colon cancer
Diarrhea or ribbon-shaped stools	
Stools may be grossly bloody	
Weakness and fatigue	
Abdominal aching and dull cramps	
Chronic bleeding with defecation	Hemorrhoids
Painful defecation	
Nausea and Vomiting	
May follow or accompany abdominal pain	Appendicitis
Pain progresses rapidly to severe, stabbing pain in the right lower quadrant (McBurney sign)	
Abdominal rigidity and tenderness	
Constipation or diarrhea	
Tachycardia	
Nausea and vomiting of undigested food	Gastroenteritis
Diarrhea	
Abdominal cramping	
Hyperactive bowel sounds	
Fever	
Headache with severe, constant, throbbing pain	Migraine headache
Fatigue	
Photophobia	
Light flashes	
Increased noise sensitivity	

- Acute diarrhea may result from acute infection, stress, fecal impaction, or use of certain drugs.
- Chronic diarrhea may result from chronic infection, obstructive and inflammatory bowel disease, malabsorption syndrome, an endocrine disorder, or GI surgery.
- The fluid and electrolyte imbalance may precipitate life-threatening arrhythmias or hypovolemic shock.

Hematochezia. Hematochezia is the passage of bloody stools and may be a sign of GI bleeding below the ligament of Treitz. It may also result from a coagulation disorder, exposure to toxins, or a diagnostic test. It may lead to hypovolemia.

Nausea and Vomiting. Nausea is a sensation of profound revulsion to food or of impending vomiting. Vomiting is the forceful expulsion of gastric contents through the mouth that is often preceded by nausea.

- Nausea and vomiting may occur with fluid and electrolyte imbalance, infection, metabolic, endocrine, cardiac disorders, use of certain drugs, surgery, or radiation.
- Nausea and vomiting may also arise from severe pain, anxiety, alcohol intoxication, overeating, or ingestion of distasteful food or liquids.

The Genitourinary System

It is important to recognize that a disorder of the genitourinary system can affect other body systems. For example, ovarian dysfunction can alter endocrine balance, or kidney dysfunction can affect the production of certain hormones that regulate RBC production.

The urinary system consists of the kidneys, ureters, bladder, and urethra (Fig. 4.3). The primary functions of the urinary system are the formation of urine and the maintenance of homeostasis. These functions are performed by the kidneys. Kidney dysfunction can cause trouble with concentration, memory loss, or disorientation. Progressive chronic kidney failure can also cause lethargy, confusion, disorientation, stupor, convulsions, and coma. Observation of the patient's vital signs may give indication of hypertension, which may be related to renal dysfunction if the hypertension is uncontrolled.

Kidneys. The kidneys are highly vascular organs that function to produce urine and maintain homeostasis in the body. The two bean-shaped organs of the kidneys are located in the retroperitoneal cavity along either side of the vertebral column. The peritoneal fat layer protects the kidneys. The right kidney lies slightly lower than the left because it is displaced by the liver. Each kidney contains approximately 1 million nephrons. Urine gathers in the collecting tubules and ducts and eventually drains into the ureters, then the bladder, and through the urethra (via urination).

Ureters. The ureters are 25 to 30 cm long. The narrowest part of the ureter is at the ureteropelvic junction. The other two constricted areas occur as the ureter leaves the renal pelvis and at the point it enters into the bladder wall. The ureters carry urine from the kidneys to the bladder by peristaltic contractions that occur one to five times per minute.

Bladder. The bladder is the vessel where urine collects. Bladder capacity ranges from 500 to 1000 mL in healthy adults. Children and older adults have less bladder capacity. When the bladder is empty, it lies behind the symphysis pubis; when it is full, it becomes displaced under the peritoneal cavity and serves as an excellent "window" for the sonographer to view the pelvic structures.

Urethra. The urethra is a small duct that carries urine from the bladder to the outside of the body. It is only 2.5 to 5 cm long and opens anterior to the vaginal opening. In the male, the urethra measures approximately 15 cm as it travels through the penis.

Common Signs and Symptoms Related to Urinary Dysfunction. The most common symptom of urinary dysfunction for both women and men is urinary incontinence. For women, a common symptom is dysuria, which often means a urinary tract infection (UTI). For men, common signs of urinary dysfunction include urethral discharge and urinary hesitancy. Tables 4.3 and 4.4 summarize the most common symptoms and probable causes of urinary dysfunction for women and men, respectively.

Dysuria. Dysuria is painful or difficult urination and is commonly accompanied by urinary frequency, urgency, or hesitancy. This symptom usually reflects a common female disorder of a lower UTI. Pertinent questions for the patient would include how long the patient has noticed the symptoms, whether anything precipitates them, if anything aggravates or alleviates them, and where exactly the discomfort is felt. You might also ask if the patient has undergone a recent invasive procedure such as a cystoscopy or urethral dilation.

Urinary Incontinence. Urinary incontinence is the uncontrollable passage of urine. Incontinence results from a bladder abnormality or a neurologic disorder. A common urologic sign may involve large volumes of urine or dribbling. This condition would be important for the sonographer if a full bladder were required. It may be difficult for the patient to hold large enough volumes of fluid to fill the bladder for proper visualization.

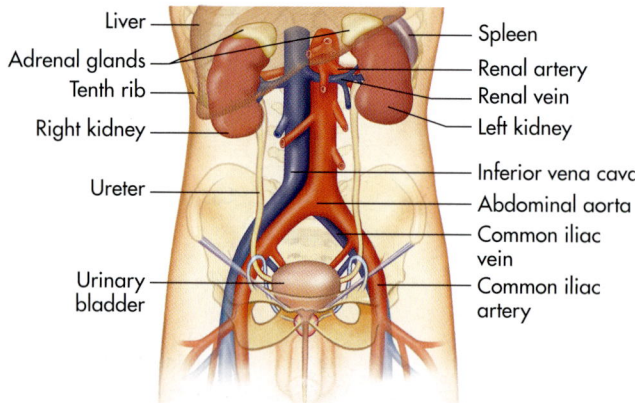

FIG. 4.3 The urinary system includes the kidneys, ureters, bladder, and urethra.

TABLE 4.3	Signs and Probable Indications of Urinary Dysfunction in Women
Signs or Symptoms	**Probable Indication**
Dysuria	
Urinary frequency	Cystitis
Nocturia	
Straining to void	
Hematuria	
Perineal or low-back pain	
Fatigue	
Low-grade fever	
Dysuria throughout voiding	Urinary system obstruction
Bladder distention	
Diminished urinary stream	
Urinary frequency and urgency	
Sensation of bloating or fullness in the lower abdomen or groin	
Urinary urgency	Urinary tract infection
Hematuria	
Cloudy urine	
Bladder spasms	
Feeling of warmth or burning during urination	
Urinary Incontinence	
Urge or overflow incontinence	Bladder cancer
Hematuria	
Dysuria	
Nocturia	
Urinary frequency	
Suprapubic pain from bladder spasms	
Palpable mass on bimanual examination	
Overflow incontinence	Diabetic neuropathy
Painless bladder distention	
Episodic diarrhea or constipation	
Orthostatic hypotension	
Syncope	
Dysphagia	
Urinary urgency and frequency	Multiple sclerosis
Visual problems	
Sensory impairment	
Constipation	
Muscle weakness	

TABLE 4.4	Signs and Probable Indications of Urinary Dysfunction in Men
Signs or Symptoms	**Probable Indication**
Scrotal Swelling	
Swollen scrotum that is soft or unusually firm	Hernia
Bowel sounds may be heard in the scrotum	
Gradual scrotal swelling	Hydrocele
Scrotum may be soft and cystic or firm and tense	
Painless	
Round, nontender scrotal mass on palpation	
Glowing when transilluminated	
Scrotal swelling with sudden and severe pain	Testicular torsion
Unilateral elevation of the affected testicle	
Nausea and vomiting	
Urethral Discharge	
Purulent or milky urethral discharge	Prostatitis
Sudden fever and chills	
Lower back pain	
Myalgia (muscle pain)	
Perineal fullness	
Arthralgia	
Urinary frequency and urgency	
Cloudy urine	
Dysuria	
Tense, boggy, very tender, and warm prostate palpated on digital rectal examination	
Opaque, gray, yellowish, or blood-tinged discharge that is painless	Urethral neoplasm
Dysuria	
Eventual anuria	
Scant or profuse urethral discharge that is thin and clear, mucoid, or thick and purulent	Urethritis
Urinary hesitancy, frequency, and urgency	
Dysuria	
Itching and burning around the meatus	
Urinary Hesitancy	
Reduced caliber and force of urinary stream	Benign prostatic hyperplasia
Perineal pain	
Feeling of incomplete voiding	
Inability to stop the urine stream	
Urinary frequency	
Urinary incontinence	
Bladder distention	
Urinary frequency and dribbling	Prostate cancer
Nocturia	
Dysuria	
Bladder distention	
Perineal pain	
Constipation	
Hard, nodular prostate palpated on digital rectal examination	
Dysuria	Urinary tract infection
Urinary frequency and urgency	
Hematuria	
Cloudy urine	
Bladder spasms	
Costovertebral angle tenderness	
Suprapubic, low back, pelvic, or flank pain	
Urethral discharge	

Male Urethral Discharge. Male urethral discharge is discharge from the urinary meatus that may be purulent, mucoid, or thin; sanguineous or clear. It usually develops suddenly. The patient may have other signs of fever, chills, or perineal fullness. Previous history of prostate problems, sexually transmitted disease, or UTIs may be associated with this condition.

Male Urinary Hesitancy. Male urinary hesitancy is a condition that usually arises gradually with a decrease in urinary stream. When the bladder becomes distended, the discomfort increases. Often prostate problems, previous UTI or obstruction, or neuromuscular disorders are associated with this condition.

ANATOMIC RELATIONSHIPS WITHIN THE ABDOMINOPELVIC CAVITIES

The human body includes many cavities. These body cavities contain the internal organs, or **viscera**. The two principal body cavities are the **dorsal cavity** and the **ventral cavity** (Fig. 4.4). The bony dorsal cavity may be subdivided into the *cranial cavity*, which holds the brain, and the *vertebral* or *spinal canal*, which contains the spinal cord. The ventral cavity is located near the anterior body surface and is subdivided into the *thoracic cavity* and the *abdominopelvic cavity*.

The thoracic and abdominopelvic cavities are separated by a broad muscle called the **diaphragm**. The diaphragm forms the floor of the thoracic cavity. Divisions of the thoracic cavity are the pleural sacs, each containing a lung, with the mediastinum between them. Within the mediastinum lie the heart, the thymus gland, and part of the esophagus and trachea. The heart is surrounded by another cavity called the *pericardial sac*.

The *retroperitoneal space* lies on the posterior abdominal wall behind the parietal peritoneum. It extends from the twelfth thoracic vertebra and the twelfth rib to the sacrum and the iliac crests.

The Abdominal Cavity

The abdominal cavity is a cavity within the abdomen that is lined with serous membrane, the *peritoneum*. It is bounded superiorly by the diaphragm, anteriorly by the abdominal wall muscles, posteriorly by the vertebral column, ribs, and iliac fossa, and inferiorly by the pelvis. It is continuous with the pelvic cavity to form the abdominopelvic cavity.

To identify specific abdominal structures or to refer to an area of pain, the abdominopelvic cavity may be divided into four quadrants. The quadrant is determined by a midsagittal plane and a transverse plane that passes through the umbilicus. The four quadrants include the right upper quadrant (RUQ), left upper quadrant (LUQ), right lower quadrant (RLQ), and left lower quadrant (LLQ) (Fig. 4.5).

Visceral Organs of the Abdominal Cavity. The visceral organs within the abdominal cavity include the liver, gallbladder, spleen, pancreas, adrenal glands, kidneys and ureters, stomach, small and large intestines (except sigmoid colon and rectum), bladder, and uterus or prostate gland (Fig. 4.6). Throughout the ultrasound examination, the sonographer will observe respiratory and positional variations in the abdominal viscera as they occur from patient to patient.

Liver. The liver lies posterior to the lower ribs, with most of the right lobe in the right hypochondrium and epigastrium; the left lobe lies in the epigastrium/left hypochondrium.

Gallbladder. The fundus of the gallbladder usually lies opposite the tip of the right ninth costal cartilage.

Spleen. The spleen lies in the left hypochondrium under cover of the ninth, tenth, and eleventh ribs. Its long axis corresponds to the tenth rib, and in adults it usually does not project forward of the midaxillary line.

Pancreas. The pancreas lies in the epigastrium. The head usually lies inferior and to the right (in the lap of the duodenum), the neck lies on the transpyloric plane, and the body and tail lie superior and to the left (hilum of the spleen).

Adrenal Glands. The adrenal glands lie along the superior medial border of the kidneys.

Kidneys and Ureters. The right kidney lies slightly lower than the left. Each kidney moves approximately 2 cm in a vertical direction during full respiratory movement of the diaphragm. The hilus of the kidney lies on the transpyloric plane, approximately three finger-widths from the midline.

Stomach. The stomach usually lies in the LUQ transpyloric plane between the esophagus and the small intestine.

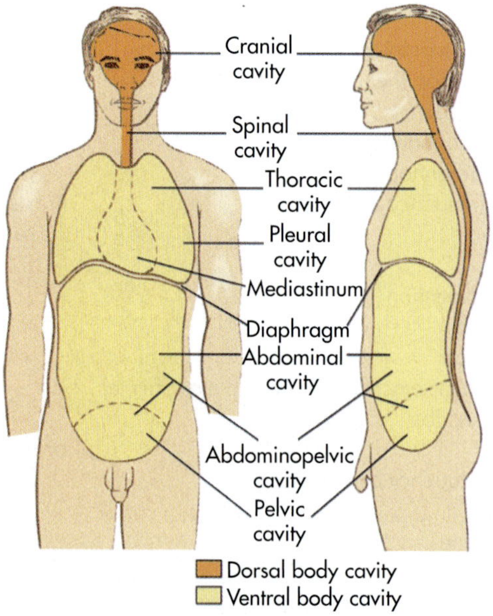

FIG. 4.4 **Body cavities.** Locations and divisions of the dorsal and ventral body cavities in the anterior and lateral views.

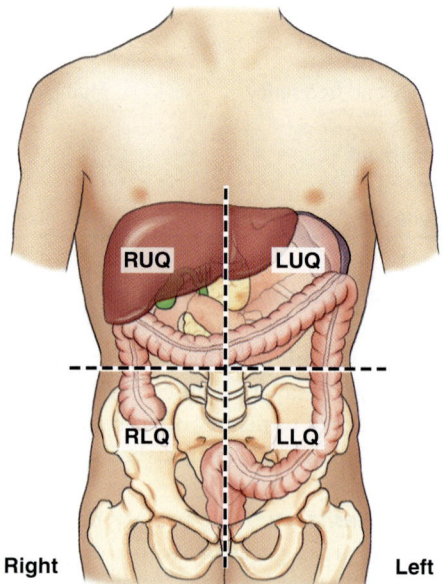

FIG. 4.5 The four abdominal quadrants include the right upper quadrant (RUQ), left upper quadrant (LUQ), right lower quadrant (RLQ), and left lower quadrant (LLQ).

CHAPTER 4 Anatomic and Physiologic Relationships Within the Abdominopelvic Cavity

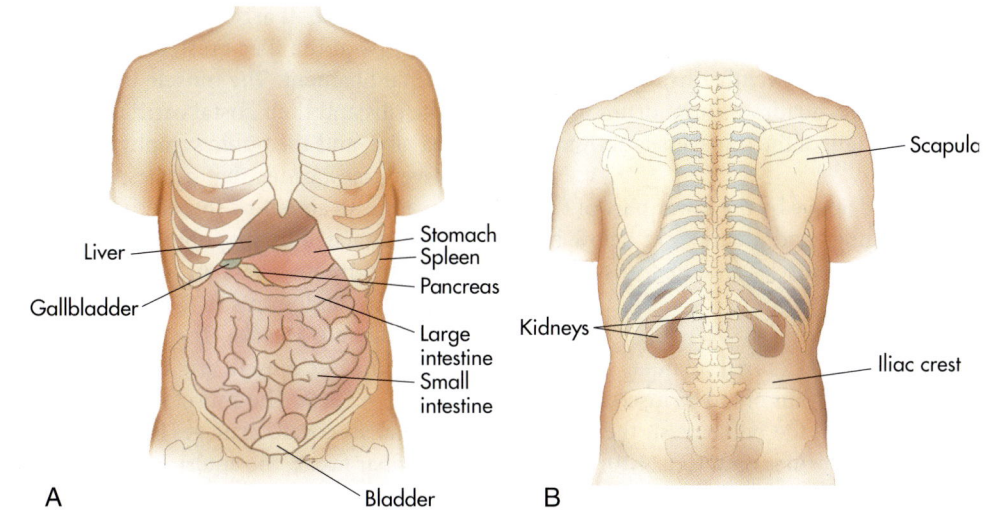

FIG. 4.6 (A) Basic abdominal landmarks and viscera viewed from anterior. (B) Landmarks of the posterior torso.

Small Intestine. This tubular organ extends from the pyloric sphincter to the beginning of the large intestine.

Large Intestine. The large intestine extends from the small intestine to the anal canal.

Bladder and Uterus. The bladder and uterus lie in the lower pelvis in the hypogastric plane.

Prostate Gland. The prostate gland lies in the lower pelvic in the hypogastric plane between the neck of the bladder above and the urogenital diaphragm below.

Other Abdominal Structures.

Diaphragm. The diaphragm is a dome-shaped muscle that separates the thorax from the abdominal cavity (Fig. 4.7). Its muscular component arises from the margins of the thoracic outlet. The **right crus of the diaphragm** arises from the sides of the bodies of the first three lumbar vertebrae; the **left crus of the diaphragm** arises from the sides of the bodies of the first two lumbar vertebrae.

Lateral to the crura, the diaphragm arises from the medial and lateral arcuate ligaments. The **medial arcuate ligament** is the thickened upper margin of the fascia covering the anterior surface of the psoas muscle. It extends from the side of the body of the second lumbar vertebra to the tip of the transverse process of the first lumbar vertebra. The medial arcuate ligament connects the medial borders of the two crura as they cross anterior to the aorta.

The **lateral arcuate ligament** is the thickened upper margin of the fascia covering the anterior surface of the quadratus lumborum muscle (Fig. 4.7A). It extends from the tip of the transverse process of the first lumbar vertebra to the lower border of the twelfth rib.

The diaphragm inserts into a *central tendon* (Fig. 4.7B). The superior surface of the tendon is partially fused with the inferior surface of the fibrous pericardium. Fibers of the right crus surround the esophagus to act as a sphincter to prevent regurgitation of gastric contents into the thoracic part of the esophagus.

Abdominal Wall. Superiorly, the abdominal wall is formed by the diaphragm. Inferiorly, it is continuous with the pelvic

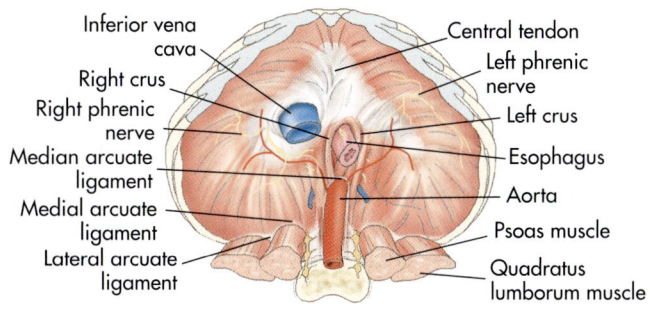

FIG. 4.7 Inferior (A) and anterior (B) views of the diaphragm. Note the posterolateral extension of the diaphragm along the rib cage.

cavity through the pelvic inlet. Anteriorly, the wall is formed above by the lower part of the thoracic cage and below by several layers of muscles: rectus abdominis, external oblique, internal oblique, and transversus abdominis (Fig. 4.8).

Posteriorly, the abdominal wall is formed at the midline by five lumbar vertebrae and their disks (Fig. 4.9). Posterolaterally, it is formed by the twelfth ribs, upper part of the bony pelvis, psoas muscles, quadratus lumborum muscles, and aponeuroses of the origin of the transversus abdominis muscles.

Laterally, the wall is formed above by the lower part of the thoracic wall, including the lungs and pleura, and below by the external and internal oblique muscles and the transversus abdominis muscles.

Abdominal Muscles.

External Oblique Muscle. The external oblique muscle arises from the lower eight ribs and fans out to be inserted into the xiphoid process, the linea alba, the pubic crest, the pubic tubercle, and the anterior half of the iliac crest (Fig. 4.10A).

The **superficial inguinal ring** is a triangular opening in the external oblique aponeurosis and lies superior and medial to the pubic tubercle. The spermatic cord or the round ligament of the uterus passes through this opening.

The **inguinal ligament** (see Fig. 4.10) is formed between the anterior superior iliac spine and the pubic tubercle, where the lower border of the aponeurosis is folded backward on itself. The lateral part of the posterior edge of the inguinal ligament gives origin to part of the internal oblique and transverse abdominal muscles.

Internal Oblique Muscle. The internal oblique muscle lies very deep to the external oblique muscle (see Fig. 4.10B). Most of its fibers are aligned at right angles to the external oblique muscle. It arises from the lumbar fascia, the anterior two thirds of the iliac crest, and the lateral two thirds of the inguinal ligament. The muscle inserts into the lower borders of the ribs and their costal cartilages, the xiphoid process, the linea alba, and the pubic symphysis. The internal oblique has a lower free border that arches over the spermatic cord or the round ligament of the uterus and then descends behind it to be attached to the pubic crest and the pectineal line. The lowest tendinous fibers are joined by similar fibers from the transversus abdominis to form the conjoint tendon.

Transversus Muscle. The transversus muscle lies deep to the internal oblique muscle, and its fibers run horizontally forward (see Fig. 4.10C). The muscle arises from the deep surface of the lower six costal cartilages (interlacing with the diaphragm), the lumbar fascia, the anterior two thirds of the iliac crest, and the lateral third of the inguinal ligament. It inserts into the xiphoid process, the linea alba, and the pubic symphysis.

Rectus Sheath. The **rectus abdominis muscle** is a sheath formed by the aponeuroses of the muscles of the lateral group (see Figs. 4.8 and 4.11). The rectus muscle arises from the front of the symphysis pubis and from the pubic crest. It inserts into the fifth, sixth, and seventh costal cartilages and the xiphoid process. On contraction, the lateral margin forms a palpable curved surface, termed the **linea semilunaris**, which extends

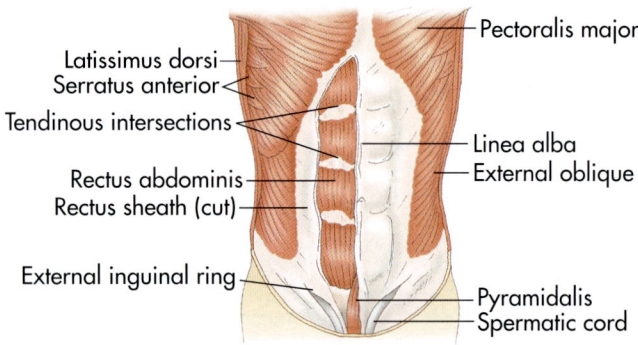

FIG. 4.8 Anterior view of the abdominal muscles.

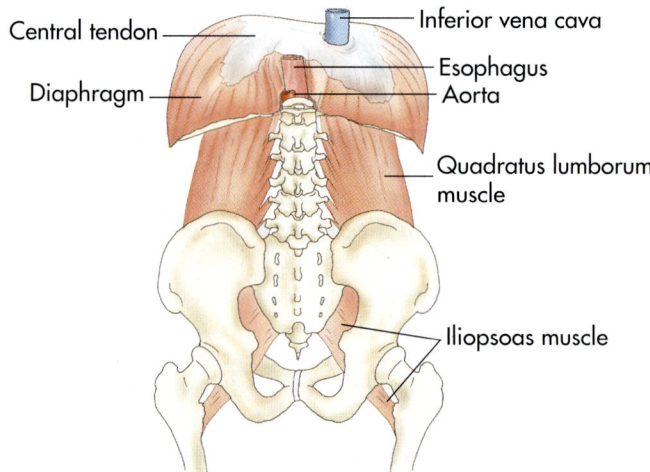

FIG. 4.9 Posterior view of the diaphragm and abdominal muscles.

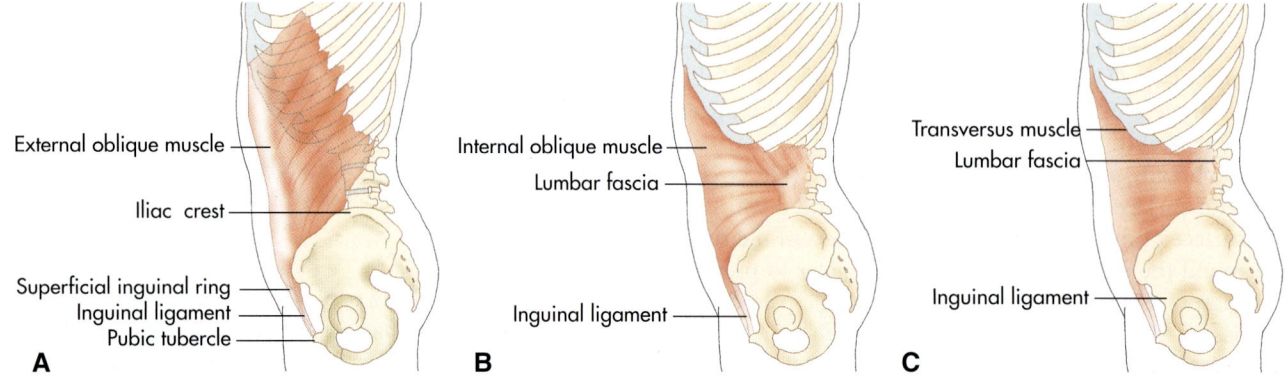

FIG. 4.10 (A) External oblique muscle of the anterior and lateral abdominal wall. (B) Internal oblique muscle of the anterior and lateral abdominal wall. (C) Transversus muscle of the anterior and lateral abdominal wall.

CHAPTER 4 Anatomic and Physiologic Relationships Within the Abdominopelvic Cavity

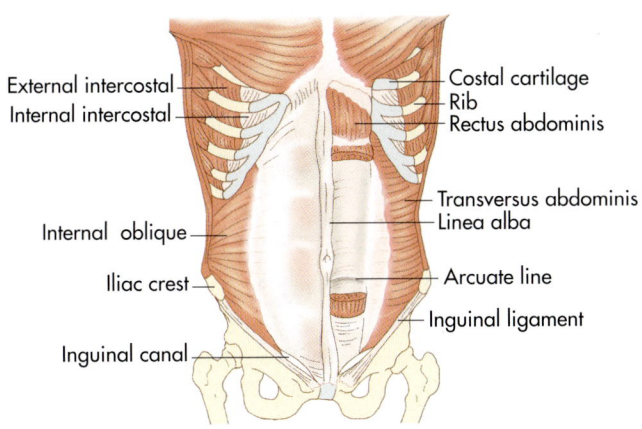

FIG. 4.11 Anterior view of the rectus abdominis muscle and rectus sheath.

from the ninth costal cartilage to the pubic tubercle. The anterior surface of the rectus muscle is crossed by three tendinous intersections and is firmly attached to the anterior wall of the rectus sheath.

Linea Alba. The linea alba is a fibrous band stretching from the xiphoid to the symphysis pubis (see Fig. 4.8). It is wider above than below and forms a central anterior attachment for the muscle layers of the abdomen. It is formed by the interlacing of the aponeuroses of the right and left oblique muscles and transversus abdominis muscles.

Back Muscles. The deep muscles of the back help to stabilize the vertebral column. They also influence the posture and curvature of the spine. These muscles have the ability to extend, flex laterally, and rotate all or part of the vertebral column.

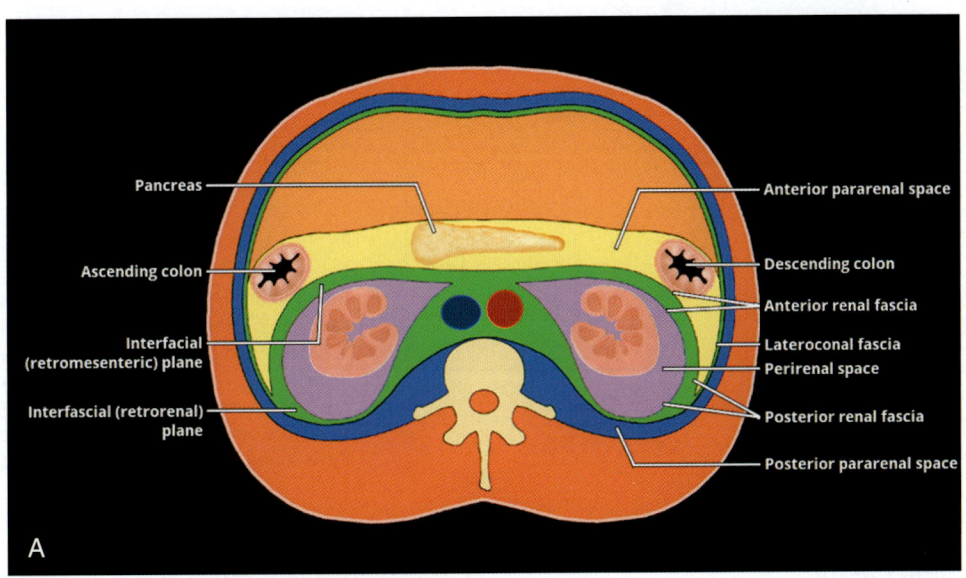

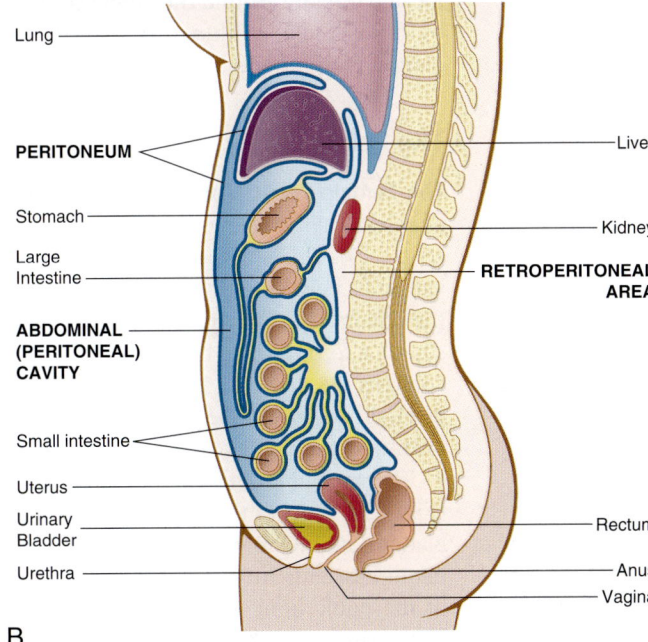

FIG. 4.12 (A) There are three retroperitoneal spaces: anterior pararenal, posterior pararenal, and perirenal. (B) The retroperitoneal cavity contains the pancreas, kidneys, ureters, adrenal glands, aorta, inferior vena cava, bladder, uterus, and prostate gland. The ascending and descending colon and most of the duodenum are also located in the retroperitoneum.

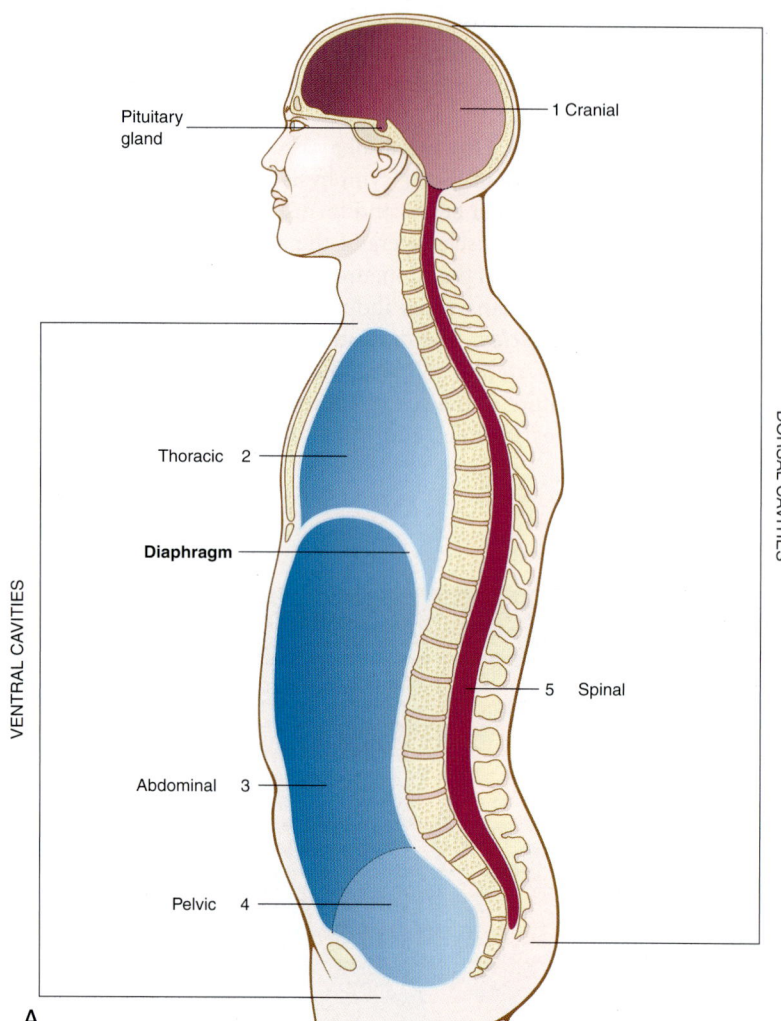
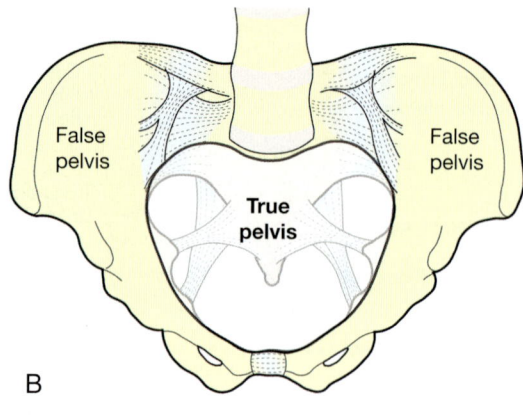

FIG. 4.13 (A) The lower portion of the abdominopelvic cavity below the pelvic brim is the pelvic cavity. (B) The pelvis is divided into a pelvis major (false pelvis) and a pelvis minor (true pelvis). The pelvis major is part of the abdominal cavity proper and lies between the iliac fossae, superior to the pelvic brim. The pelvis minor (which actually contains the pelvic cavity) is found inferior to the brim of the pelvis.

The Retroperitoneal Cavity

The retroperitoneal cavity contains the pancreas, kidneys, ureters, adrenal glands, aorta, inferior vena cava, bladder, uterus, and prostate gland (Fig. 4.12). The ascending and descending colon and most of the duodenum are also located in the retroperitoneum.

Aorta. The aorta lies anterior to the spine, slightly to the left of the midline in the abdomen. The distal abdominal aorta bifurcates into the right and left common iliac arteries opposite the fourth lumbar vertebra on the intercristal plane.

Inferior Vena Cava. The inferior vena cava is formed by the confluence of the right and left common iliac veins. The inferior vena cava lies to the right of the spine to empty blood from the abdominopelvic cavity and lower extremities into the right atrium.

Retroperitoneal Spaces. The **anterior pararenal space** (see Fig. 4.12) is located between the anterior surface of the renal fascia (Gerota's fascia) and the posterior area of the peritoneum. Within this area are the ascending and descending colon, the pancreas, and the duodenum. The **posterior pararenal space** is found between the posterior renal fascia and the muscles of the posterior abdominal wall. Only fat and vessels are found within this space. The **perirenal space** is located directly around the kidney and is completely enclosed by renal fascia. Within this space lie the kidneys, adrenal glands, lymph nodes, blood vessels, and perirenal fat.

The Pelvic Cavity

The Female Pelvic Cavity. The lower portion of the abdominopelvic cavity below the pelvic brim is the **pelvic cavity** (Fig. 4.13). The pelvis is divided into a pelvis major (false pelvis) and a pelvis minor (true pelvis). The pelvis major is part of the abdominal cavity proper and lies between the iliac fossae, superior to the pelvic brim. The pelvis minor (which actually contains the pelvic cavity) is found inferior to the brim of the pelvis. The cavity of the pelvis minor is continuous at the pelvic brim with the cavity of the pelvis major.

The female pelvic cavity contains several pelvic organs (Fig. 4.14): part of the large intestine, the rectum, the urinary bladder, and the reproductive organs. In the female, the peritoneum descends from the anterior abdominal wall to the level of the pubic bone onto the superior surface of the bladder. The peritoneum covers the fundus and body of the uterus and extends over the posterior fornix and the wall of the vagina.

CHAPTER 4 Anatomic and Physiologic Relationships Within the Abdominopelvic Cavity

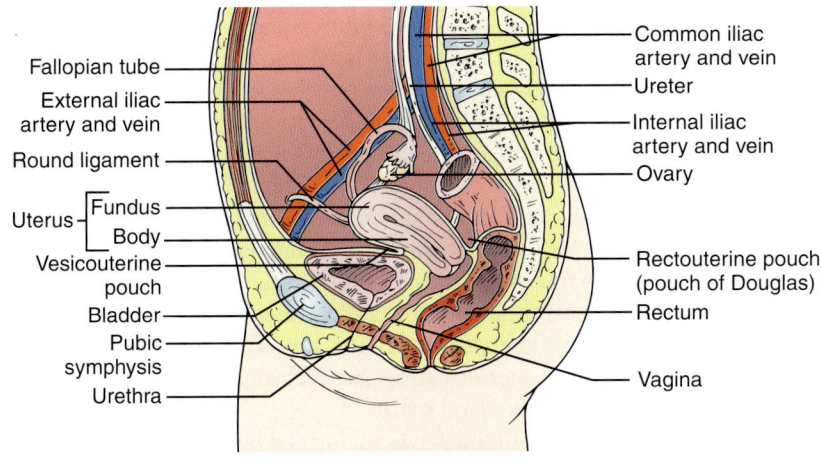

FIG. 4.14 The female pelvic cavity contains several pelvic organs: part of the large intestine, the rectum, the urinary bladder, and the reproductive organs. In the female, the peritoneum descends from the anterior abdominal wall to the level of the pubic bone onto the superior surface of the bladder. The peritoneum covers the fundus and body of the uterus and extends over the posterior fornix and the wall of the vagina.

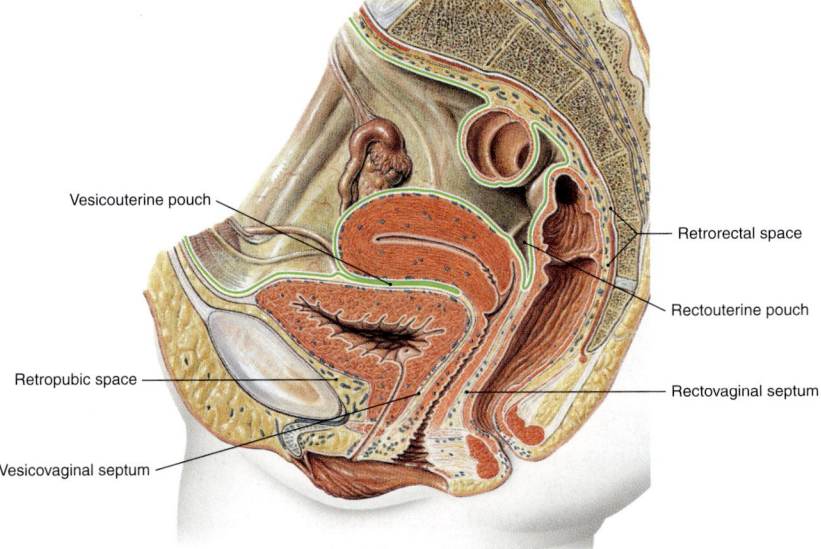

FIG. 4.15 The uterus lies anterior to the rectum and posterior to the bladder and divides the pelvic peritoneal space into anterior and posterior pouches. The anterior pouch is termed the *vesicouterine pouch*, and the posterior pouch is called the *rectouterine pouch*, or the pouch of Douglas. The rectouterine pouch is a common location for accumulation of fluids, such as pus or blood.

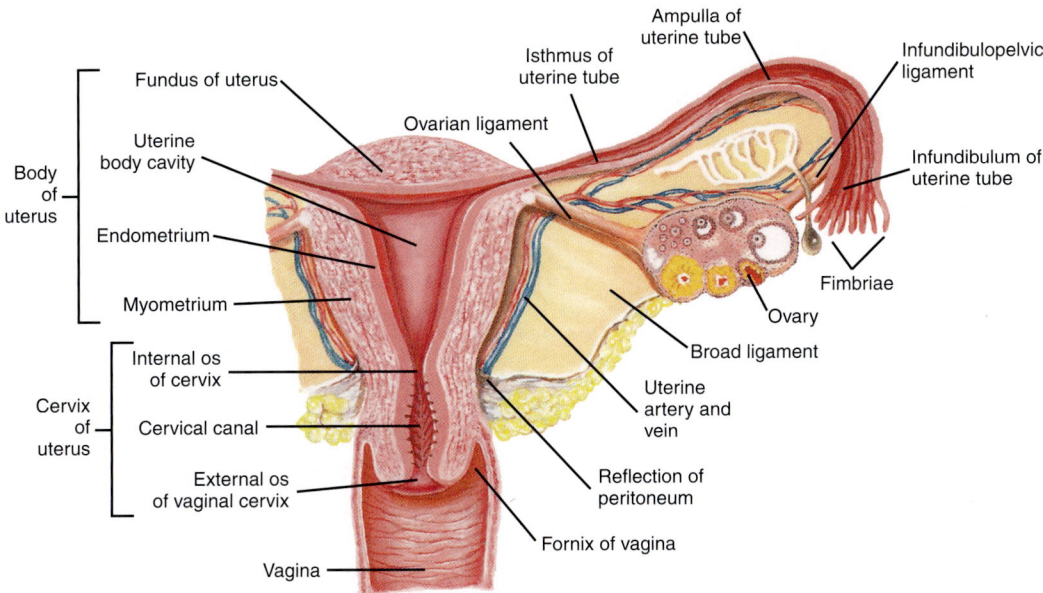

FIG. 4.16 The fallopian tubes extend laterally from the fundus of the uterus and are enveloped by a fold of peritoneum known as the broad ligament. This ligament arises from the floor of the pelvis and contributes to the division of the peritoneal space into anterior and posterior pouches.

False Pelvis. The false pelvis is bound posteriorly by the lumbar vertebrae, laterally by the iliac fossae and iliacus muscles, and anteriorly by the lower anterior abdominal wall. The sacral promontory and the iliopectineal line form the boundary between the false pelvis and the true pelvis to delineate the boundary of the abdominal and pelvic cavities.

The uterus lies anterior to the rectum and posterior to the bladder and divides the pelvic peritoneal space into anterior and posterior pouches (Fig. 4.15). The anterior pouch is termed the **vesicouterine pouch**, and the posterior pouch is called the **rectouterine pouch**, or the pouch of Douglas. The rectouterine pouch is a common location for accumulation of fluids, such as pus or blood.

The fallopian tubes extend laterally from the fundus of the uterus and are enveloped by a fold of peritoneum known as the broad ligament (Fig. 4.16). This ligament arises from the floor of the pelvis and contributes to the division of the peritoneal space into anterior and posterior pouches.

True Pelvis. The true pelvis protects and contains the lower parts of the intestinal and urinary tracts and the reproductive organs. The true pelvis has an inlet, outlet, and cavity and is bounded posteriorly by the sacrum and coccyx (Fig. 4.17). The anterior and lateral margins are formed by the pubis, the ischium, and a small portion of the ilium. A muscular "sling" consisting of the coccygeus and levator ani muscles forms the inferior boundary of the true pelvis and separates it from the perineum.

The true pelvis is divided into anterior and posterior compartments. The anterior compartment contains the bladder and reproductive organs. The posterior compartment contains the posterior cul-de-sac, rectosigmoid muscle, perirectal fat, and presacral space.

The walls of the pelvis are formed by bones and ligaments, which are partially lined by muscles covered with fascia and parietal peritoneum. The pelvis has anterior, posterior, and lateral walls and an inferior floor. The obturator internus muscle lines the lateral pelvic wall. These muscles are symmetrically aligned along the lateral border of the pelvis with a concave medial border (see Fig. 4.17).

The psoas and iliopsoas muscles lie along the posterior and lateral margins of the pelvis major (Fig. 4.18). The fan-shaped iliacus muscles line the iliac fossae in the false pelvis. The psoas and iliacus muscles merge at their inferior portions to form the iliopsoas complex. The posterior border of the iliopsoas lies along the iliopectineal line and may be used as a separation landmark of the true pelvis from the false pelvis.

The piriformis muscles form the posterior pelvic wall (Fig. 4.19). The pelvic floor stretches across the pelvis and divides it into the main pelvic cavity, which contains the pelvic viscera, and the perineum below.

Perineum. The pelvic diaphragm is formed by the levator ani and coccygeus muscles. The coccygeus muscles are rounded, concave muscles that lie more posterior than the obturator internus muscles. The perineum has the following surface relationships: The pubic symphysis is anterior, posterior is the tip of the coccyx, and lateral are the ischial tuberosities. The region is divided into two triangles formed by joining the ischial tuberosities with an imaginary line. The posterior triangle is the anal triangle, and the anterior triangle is the urogenital triangle.

Male Pelvic Cavity. In the male, the peritoneum is reflected onto the upper part of the posterior surface of the bladder and the seminal vesicles, forming the rectovesical pouch (Fig. 4.20). Also in the male, the pelvic cavity has a small outpocket called the **scrotal cavity**, which contains the testes. The essential organs

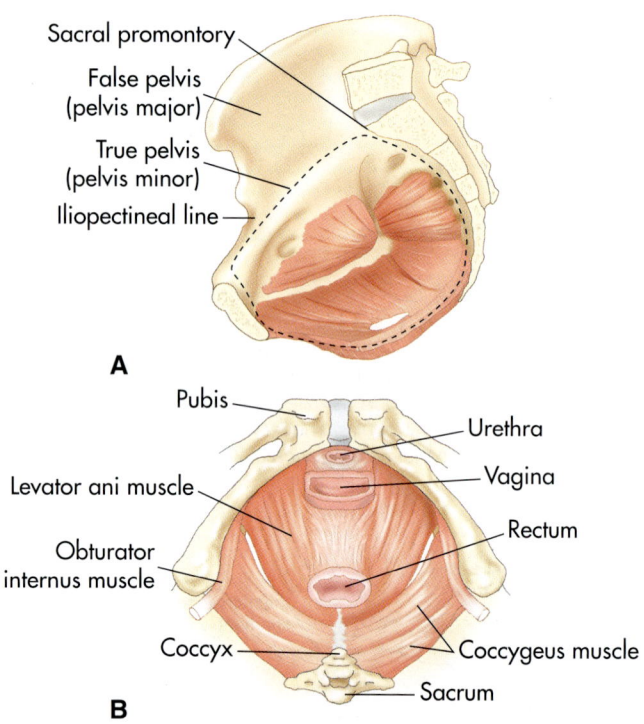

FIG. 4.17 (A) Lateral view of the pelvis demonstrating the true pelvis and the false pelvis. (B) Inferior view of the pelvic diaphragm muscles.

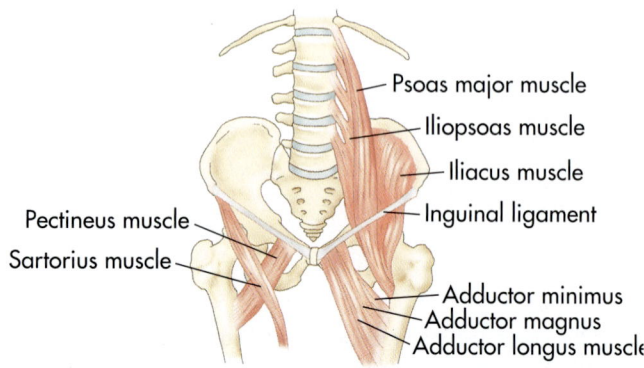

FIG. 4.18 Anterior view of the psoas and iliopsoas muscles.

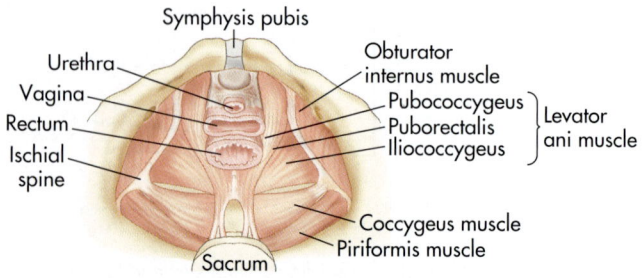

FIG. 4.19 View of the female pelvic floor shows the levator ani, coccygeus, and piriformis muscles.

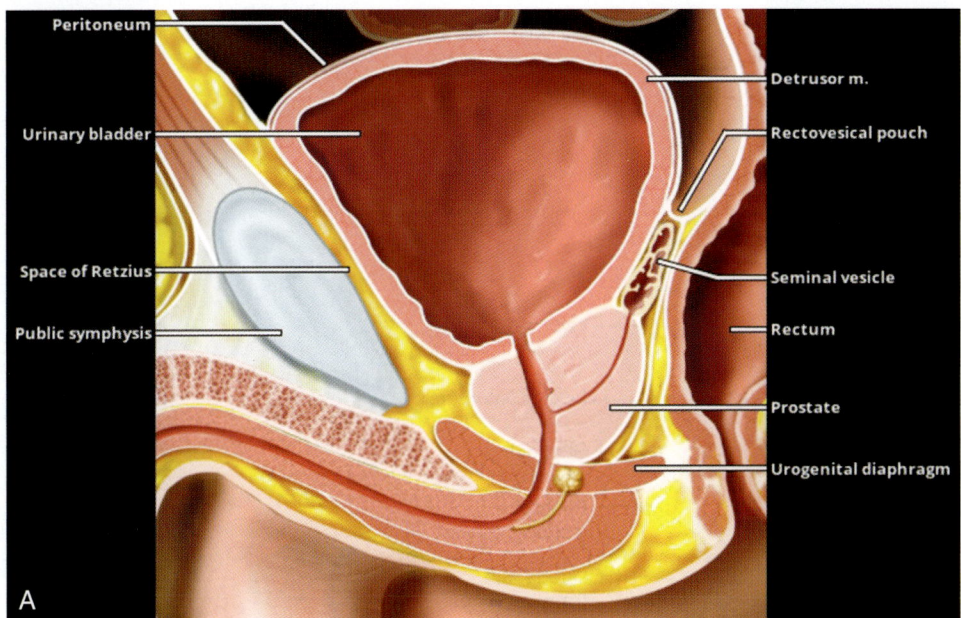

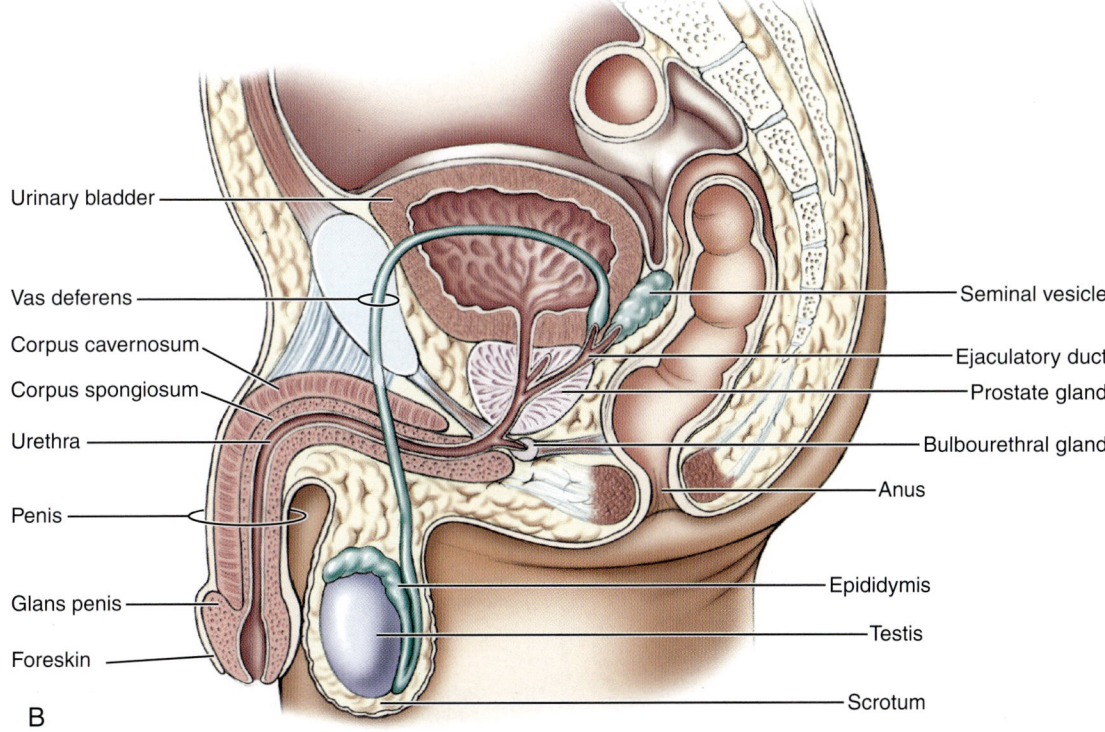

FIG. 4.20 (A) In the male, the peritoneum is reflected onto the upper part of the posterior surface of the bladder and the seminal vesicles, forming the rectovesical pouch. (B) Also in the male, the pelvic cavity has a small outpocket called the *scrotal cavity*, which contains the testes.

in the male are the gonads, which consist of a pair of main sex glands called the testes. The accessory organs include the epididymis, vas deferens, ejaculatory duct, and urethra. Also included are the seminal vesicles, Cowper glands, and prostate gland. The external genitals include the scrotum and penis.

Abdominopelvic Membranes and Ligaments

The major membranes and ligaments within the abdominopelvic cavity include the peritoneum, the mesentery, omentum, greater and lesser sacs, epiploic foramen, and peritoneal ligaments.

Peritoneum. The peritoneum is a serous membrane lining the walls of the abdominal cavity and clothing the abdominal viscera (Fig. 4.21). The peritoneum is formed by a single layer of cells called the mesothelium, which rests on a thin layer of connective tissue. If the mesothelium is damaged or removed in any area (e.g., in surgery), the danger is that two layers of peritoneum may adhere to each other and form an adhesion. This adhesion may interfere with the normal movements of the abdominal viscera.

The peritoneum is divided into two layers. The **parietal peritoneum** is the portion that lines the abdominal wall but does not cover a viscus; the **visceral peritoneum** is the portion

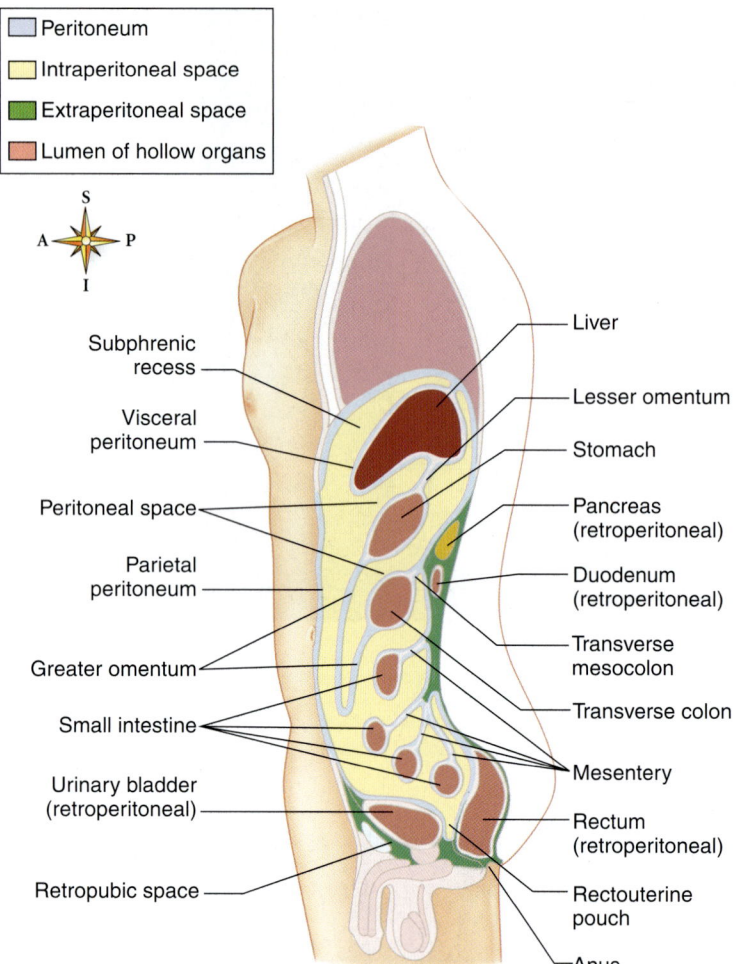

FIG. 4.21 The peritoneum is a serous membrane lining the walls of the abdominal cavity and covering the abdominal viscera.

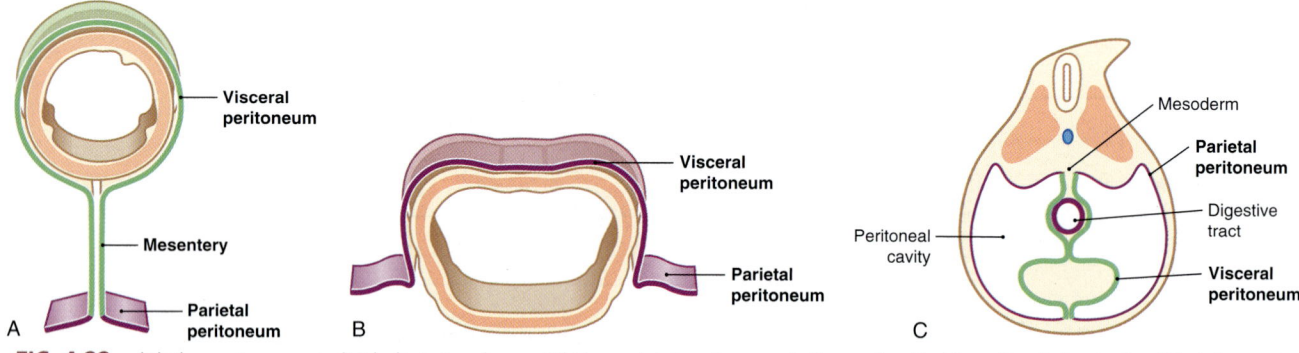

FIG. 4.22 (A) The peritoneum is divided into two layers. (B) The parietal peritoneum is the portion that lines the abdominal wall but does not cover a viscus. (C) The visceral peritoneum is the portion that covers an organ.

that covers an organ (Fig. 4.22). The **peritoneal cavity** is the potential space between the parietal and visceral peritonea. This cavity contains a small amount of lubricating serous fluid to help the abdominal organs move on one another without friction. With certain pathologies, the potential space of the peritoneal cavity may be distended into an actual space containing several liters of fluid. This accumulation of fluid is known as **ascites**. Other fluid substances, such as blood from a ruptured organ, bile from a ruptured duct, or fecal matter from a ruptured intestine, also may accumulate in this cavity.

The peritoneal cavity forms a completely closed sac in the male; in the female, communication with the exterior occurs through the fallopian tubes, uterus, and vagina. Retroperitoneal organs and vascular structures remain posterior to the cavity and are covered anteriorly with peritoneum. These include the urinary system, aorta, inferior vena cava, colon, pancreas, uterus, and bladder. The other abdominal organs are located within the peritoneal cavity.

Mesentery. A mesentery is a two-layered fold of peritoneum that attaches part of the intestines to the posterior abdominal wall and includes the mesentery of the small intestine, the transverse mesocolon, and the sigmoid mesocolon (Fig. 4.23).

Omentum. The omentum is a two-layered fold of peritoneum that attaches the stomach to another viscous organ. The greater omentum is attached to the greater curvature of the stomach and hangs down like an apron in the space between the small intestine and the anterior abdominal wall (Fig. 4.24). The greater omentum is folded back on itself and is attached to the inferior border of the transverse colon. The lesser omentum slings the lesser curvature of the stomach to the undersurface of the liver (see Fig. 4.24B). The gastrosplenic omentum ligament connects the stomach to the spleen.

Greater and Lesser Sacs. The peritoneal cavity may be divided into two parts known as the greater and lesser sacs (Fig. 4.25). The greater sac is the primary compartment of the peritoneal cavity and extends across the anterior abdomen and from the diaphragm to the pelvis. The lesser sac is an extensive peritoneal pouch located behind the lesser omentum and stomach. It extends upward to the diaphragm and inferior between the layers of the greater omentum. The left margin is formed by the spleen and the gastrosplenic and lienorenal ligaments. The right margin of the lesser sac opens into the greater sac through the epiploic foramen.

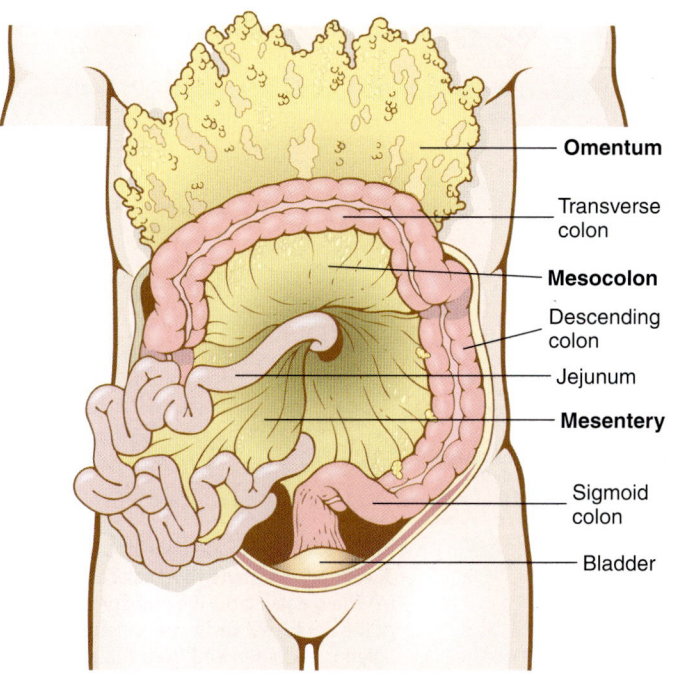

FIG. 4.23 The mesentery is a two-layered fold of peritoneum that attaches part of the intestines to the posterior abdominal wall and includes the mesentery of the small intestine, the transverse mesocolon, and the sigmoid mesocolon.

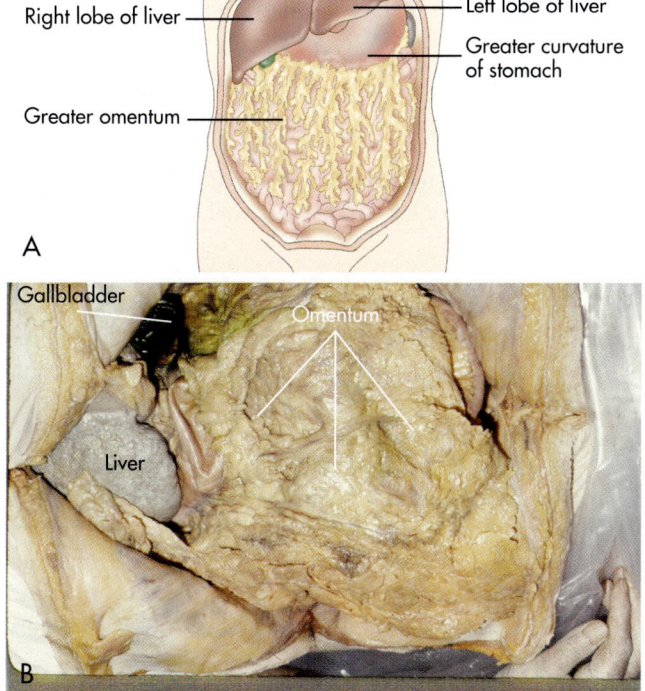

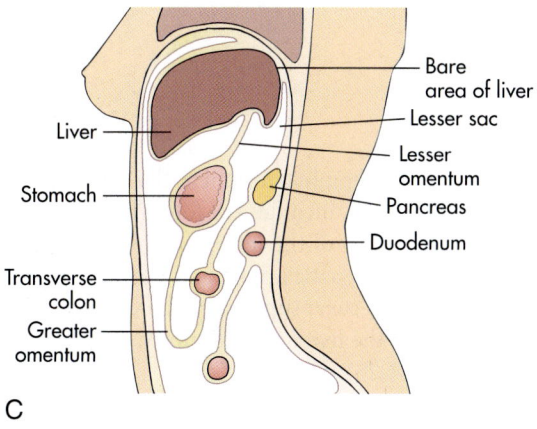

FIG. 4.24 (A) Anterior view of the greater omentum. (B) Gross anatomy with the anterior abdominal flap open to demonstrate the extent of the omentum. (C) Sagittal view of the lesser omentum.

CHAPTER 4 Anatomic and Physiologic Relationships Within the Abdominopelvic Cavity

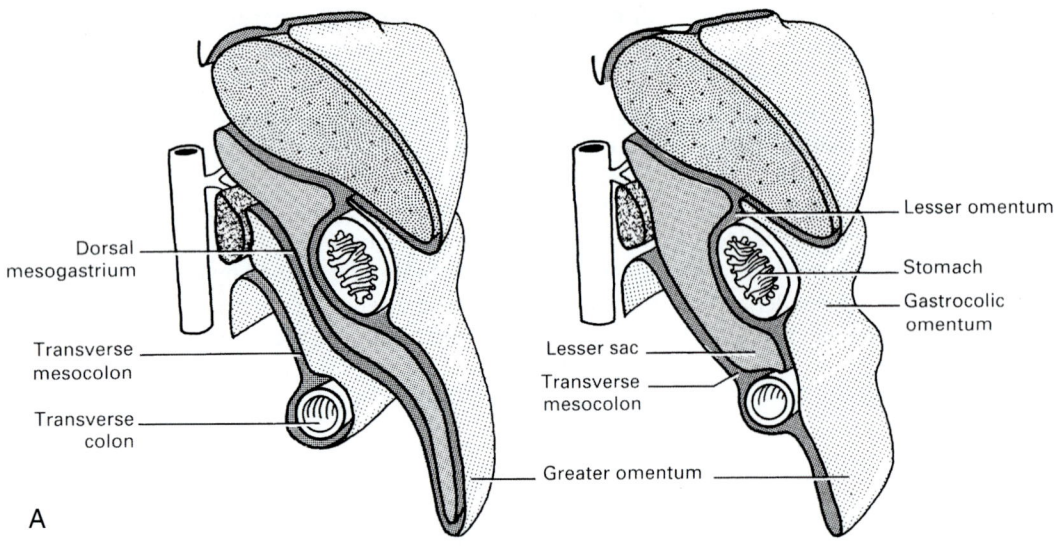

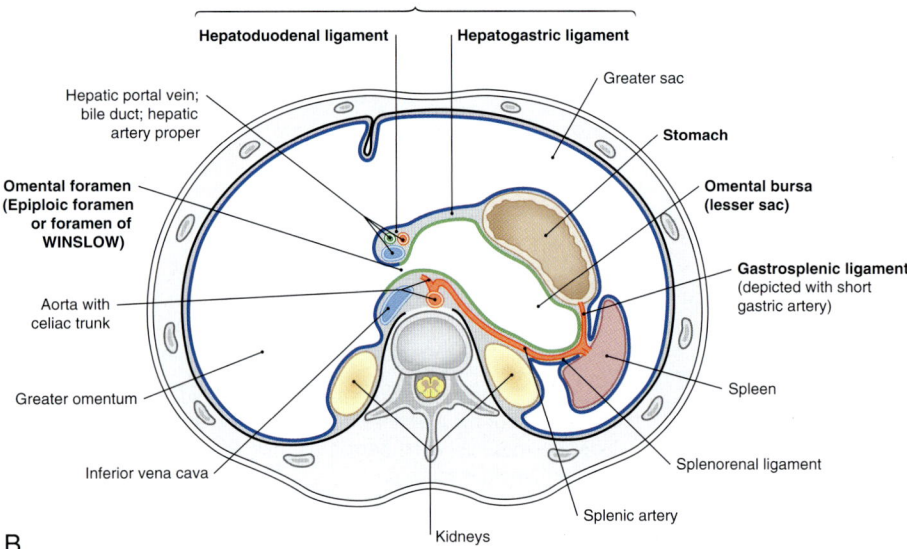

FIG. 4.25 The peritoneal cavity may be divided into two parts: the greater and lesser sacs. (A) The greater sac is the primary compartment of the peritoneal cavity and extends across the anterior abdomen and from the diaphragm to the pelvis. (B) The lesser sac is an extensive peritoneal pouch located behind the lesser omentum and stomach.

Epiploic Foramen. The epiploic foramen, the opening to the lesser sac in the abdomen, includes the following boundaries: anteriorly, the free border of the lesser omentum containing the common bile duct, hepatic artery, and portal vein; posteriorly, the inferior vena cava; superiorly, the caudate process of the caudate lobe of the liver; and inferiorly, the first part of the duodenum (Fig. 4.26).

Ligament. The peritoneal ligaments are two-layered folds of peritoneum that attach the lesser mobile solid viscera to the abdominal walls. For example, the liver is attached by the falciform ligament to the anterior abdominal wall and to the undersurface of the diaphragm (Fig. 4.27). The ligamentum teres lies in the free borders of this ligament. The peritoneum leaves the kidney and passes to the hilus of the spleen as the posterior layer of the lienorenal ligament. The visceral peritoneum covers the spleen and is reflected onto the greater curvature of the stomach as the anterior layer of the gastrosplenic ligament.

Potential Spaces in the Body

Subphrenic Spaces. The subphrenic spaces are the result of the complicated arrangement of the peritoneum in the region of the liver (Fig. 4.28). The right and left anterior subphrenic spaces lie between the diaphragm and the liver, one on each side of the falciform ligament. The sonographer should become very familiar with the right posterior subphrenic space that lies between the right lobe of the liver, the right kidney, and the right colic flexure. This is also called **Morison's pouch**. It is a frequent location for fluid collections, such as ascites, blood, and infection, to accumulate.

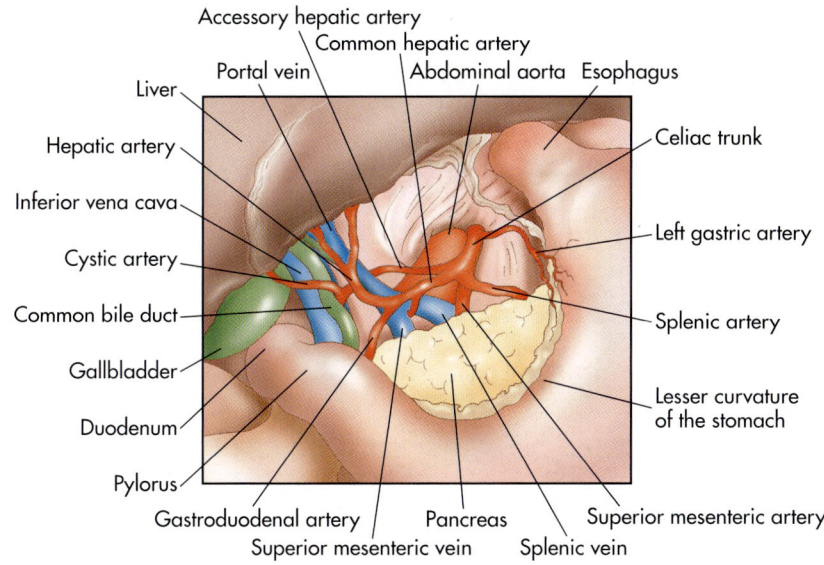

FIG. 4.26 Upper abdominal dissection, with part of the left lobe of the liver and the lesser omentum removed to show the area of the epiploic foramen. Posterior to the foramen lie the celiac trunk, portal vein, bile duct, and related structures; this is one of the most important regions in the abdomen.

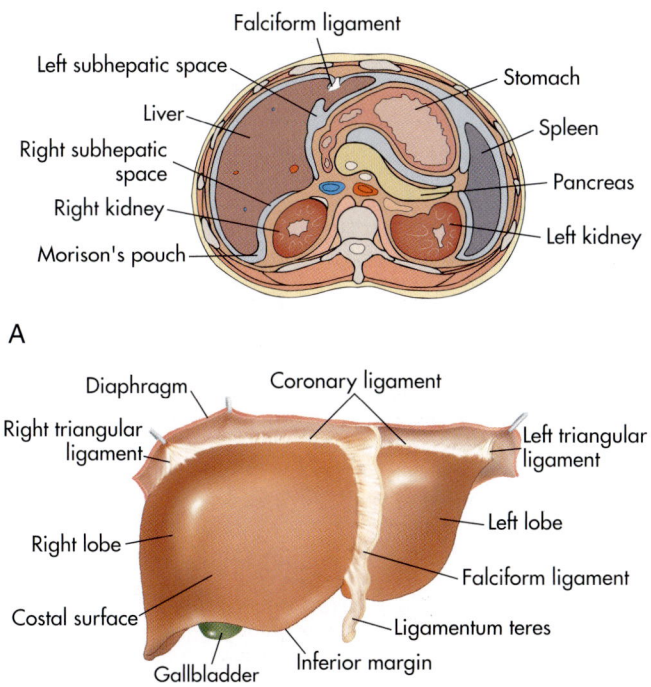

FIG. 4.27 (A) Transverse view of the falciform ligament. (B) Anterior view of the falciform ligament.

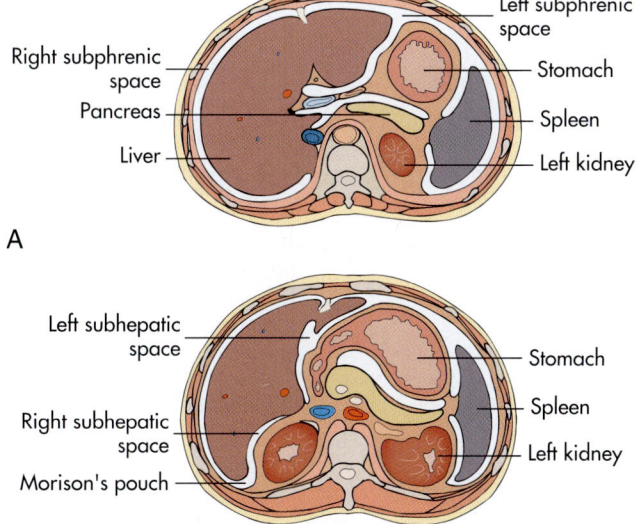

FIG. 4.28 The supracolic compartment is located above the transverse colon and contains the right and left subphrenic spaces and the right and left subhepatic spaces. (A) Transverse view of the subphrenic spaces. (B) Transverse view of the subhepatic spaces.

Peritoneal Recesses. The omental bursa normally has some empty places. Parts of the peritoneal cavity near the liver are so slitlike that they are also isolated. These areas, known as **peritoneal recesses**, are clinically important because infection may collect in them. Two common sites are where the duodenum becomes the jejunum and where the ileum joins the cecum (Fig. 4.29).

Paracolic Gutters. The arrangement of the ascending and descending colon, the attachments of the transverse mesocolon, and the mesentery of the small intestine to the posterior abdominal wall results in the formation of four paracolic gutters (see Fig. 4.29). The clinical significance of these gutters is their ability to conduct fluid materials from one part of the body to another. Materials such as abscess, ascites, blood, pus, bile, or metastases may be spread through this network.

The gutters are on the lateral and medial sides of the ascending and descending colon. The right medial paracolic

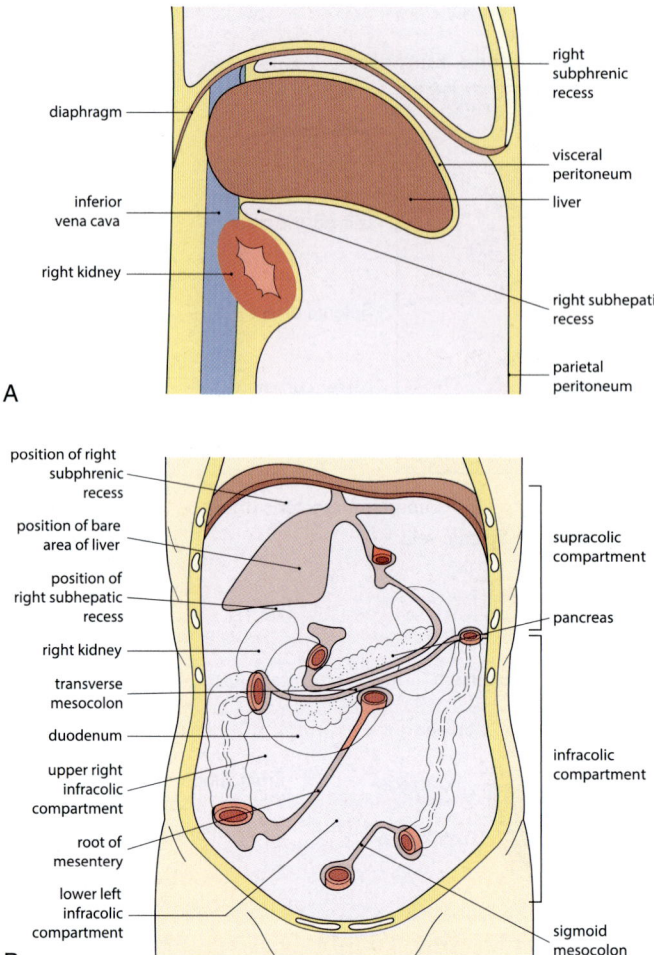

FIG. 4.29 (A) Peritoneal recesses are clinically important because infection or fluid may collect in them. (B) Two common sites are where the duodenum becomes the jejunum and where the ileum joins the cecum. The arrangement of the ascending and descending colon, the attachments of the transverse mesocolon, and the mesentery of the small intestine to the posterior abdominal wall result in the formation of four paracolic gutters.

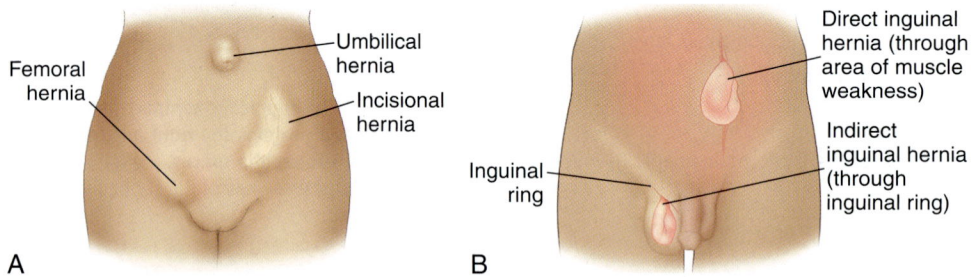

FIG. 4.30 The inguinal canal is an oblique passage through the lower part of the anterior abdominal wall. The inguinal canal in the female (A) is narrower than in the male (B). The canal permits passage of the round ligament of the uterus from the uterus to the labium major.

gutter is closed off from the pelvic cavity inferiorly by the mesentery of the small intestine. The other gutters are in free communication with the pelvic cavity. The right lateral paracolic gutter communicates with the right posterior subphrenic space. The left lateral gutter is separated from the area around the spleen by the phrenicocolic ligament.

Inguinal Canal. The inguinal canal is an oblique passage through the lower part of the anterior abdominal wall. In the male, it allows structures to pass to and from the testes to the abdomen (Fig. 4.30). In the female, the inguinal canal is narrower than the male canal. The canal permits passage of the round ligament of the uterus from the uterus to the labium majora.

CHAPTER 4 Anatomic and Physiologic Relationships Within the Abdominopelvic Cavity

Key Pearls

- The body is comprised of atoms, molecules, cells, organs, and body systems.
- All physical and chemical changes that occur within the body are referred to as metabolism.
- Homeostasis is the ability to maintain a steady and stable internal environment.
- Vital signs are medical measurements used to ascertain how the body is functioning.
- The circulation of blood throughout the body serves as a vital connection to the cells, tissues, and organs to maintain a relatively constant environment for cell activity.
- Blood is composed of plasma and hemoglobin.
- The blood is responsible for a variety of functions, including transportation of oxygen and nutrients, defense against infection, and maintenance of pH.
- The GI system consists of two major divisions: the GI tract (pharynx, esophagus, stomach, small intestine, and large intestine) and the accessory organs.
- Major functions of the GI system include ingestion and digestion of food and elimination of waste products.
- The most significant signs and symptoms related to GI diseases and disorders are abdominal pain, diarrhea, bloody stools, nausea, and vomiting.
- The urinary system consists of the kidneys, ureters, bladder, and urethra.
- The primary functions of the urinary system are the formation of urine and the maintenance of homeostasis.
- The two principal body cavities are the dorsal cavity and the ventral cavity.
- The ventral cavity is located near the anterior body surface and is subdivided into the *thoracic cavity* and the *abdominopelvic cavity*.
- The *retroperitoneal space* lies on the posterior abdominal wall behind the parietal peritoneum.
- The abdominal cavity is a cavity within the abdomen that is lined with serous membrane, the peritoneum.
- The visceral organs within the abdominal cavity include the liver, gallbladder, spleen, pancreas, adrenal glands, kidneys and ureters, stomach, small and large intestines (except sigmoid colon and rectum), bladder, and uterus or prostate gland.
- The retroperitoneal cavity contains the pancreas, kidneys, ureters, adrenal glands, aorta, inferior vena cava, bladder, uterus, and prostate gland. The ascending and descending colon and most of the duodenum are also located in the retroperitoneum.
- The pelvis is divided into two parts: a pelvis major (false pelvis) and a pelvis minor (true pelvis).
- The major membranes and ligaments within the abdominopelvic cavity include the peritoneum, the mesentery, omentum, greater and lesser sacs, epiploic foramen, and peritoneal ligaments.
- The subphrenic spaces are the result of the complicated arrangement of the peritoneum in the region of the liver.
- The sonographer should become very familiar with the right posterior subphrenic space that lies between the right lobe of the liver, the right kidney, and the right colic flexure. This is also called Morison's pouch.
- The omental bursa normally has some empty places, known as peritoneal recesses; these are clinically important because infection may collect in them.
- The arrangement of the ascending and descending colon, the attachments of the transverse mesocolon, and the mesentery of the small intestine to the posterior abdominal wall results in the formation of four paracolic gutters.

BIBLIOGRAPHY

McMinn RMH, Gaddum-Rosse P, Hutchings RT, Logan BM. *McMinn's Functional and Clinical Anatomy*. St. Louis: Mosby; 1995.

The Netter Collection of Medical Illustrations: Digestive System, vol. 2. Philadelphia: Elsevier; 2016.

Snell RS. *Clinical Anatomy*. 7th ed. Baltimore: Lippincott Williams & Wilkins; 2004.

Swobodnik W, Herrmann M, Altwein J. *Atlas of Ultrasound Anatomy: Normal Anatomy as the Basis of Sonographic Diagnosis*. New York: Thieme; 1991.

CHAPTER 5

Comparative Sectional Anatomy of the Abdominopelvic Cavity

Sandra L. Hagen-Ansert

OBJECTIVES

On completion of this chapter, you should be able to:
- Know the abdominal quadrants and regions of the body
- List the body planes in the abdomen
- Identify the abdominal structures in the transverse and sagittal planes
- Discuss the difference between a coronal image and a sagittal image
- Compare and contrast computed tomography and magnetic resonance to ultrasound

OUTLINE

Comparison of Ultrasound, Computed Tomography, Magnetic Resonance Imaging, and Radiography 103
   Ultrasound 103
   Computerized Tomography 103
   Magnetic Resonance Imaging 104
   Radiography 104

Abdominal Quadrants, Planes, and Regions 104
Planes or Body Sections 105

Sectional Anatomy 105
   Transverse Plane 106
   Sagittal/Longitudinal Plane 108

KEY TERMS

Aorta (Ao)
Caudate lobe
Coronal
Falciform ligament
Gastroduodenal artery
Hepatic artery
Iliac arteries
Iliac vein
Inferior mesenteric artery

Inferior vena cava (IVC)
Left gastric artery
Left renal artery
Left renal vein
Ligamentum venosum
Longitudinal
Morison's pouch
Portal confluence
Psoas major muscles

Right renal artery
Right renal vein
Sagittal
Splenic artery
Splenic hilum
Splenic vein
Superior mesenteric artery (SMA)
Superior mesenteric vein
Transverse

Sonographers should understand other imaging modalities, especially computed tomography (CT) and magnetic resonance imaging (MRI), which most frequently complement sonography. No longer does each of the various imaging modalities operate within a "silo," independent of each other. Instead, many diagnostic algorithms may require two or more imaging modalities to be employed, and diagnosis requires specific comparisons between them. In this way, ultrasound now interacts extensively with CT and other imaging methods to optimize the workup of a patient. Understanding what each modality offers is of prime importance in crafting the multimodality imaging workup for any particular problem.

Physicians may utilize ultrasound to follow up an abnormality that has been previously diagnosed with CT or MRI. Ultrasound is often the primary imaging tool as it provides rapid access with good soft tissue and vascular analysis. Depending on the clinical problem, it may be preferred over CT, which involves ionizing radiation, or MRI, both time-consuming and costly. To effectively meet the patient's needs, the sonographer must tailor their exam appropriately to exploit the unique strengths of ultrasound and minimize its limitations. The sonographer must also understand how the ultrasound examination in each setting may be influenced or guided by findings from previous CT, MRI, or other imaging studies.

The various imaging modalities have the ability to ultimately depict and evaluate the same abnormalities, and they are generally equivalent in identifying the physical size and shape of pathologic lesions. However, each modality approaches the problem from a different standpoint, using differing physical properties of the normal tissue and pathologic lesions to derive image contrast and resolve important details. As previously stated, ultrasound and MRI both have a safety advantage in that they do not use ionizing radiation. On the other hand, CT scanning and general diagnostic (radiographic) imaging both image the body using ionizing radiation, often in significant doses. The radiation for both CT and radiography is produced by an external source and tends to produce sharp images with high anatomic detail.

The purpose of this chapter is to introduce the sonographer to sectional anatomy as compared with CT, MRI, and ultrasound images (Table 5.1).

COMPARISON OF ULTRASOUND, COMPUTED TOMOGRAPHY, MAGNETIC RESONANCE IMAGING, AND RADIOGRAPHY

Ultrasound

Recall that ultrasound utilizes high-frequency sound waves by manually placing a transducer with a piezoelectric crystal on or inside the body. The various acoustic interfaces reflect the transmission of the sound waves to create an image. Ultrasound images may be quickly produced in real-time cine loops so movement may be easily seen and advantageous in emergent situations. Ultrasound technology is an excellent diagnostic tool for seeing live images of the working structures of the body. Ultrasound is the "eyes" for helping physicians obtain a closer look into the body to make an accurate diagnosis. The quality of the ultrasound images is produced based on the reflection of the waves off of the body structures. The strength or amplitude of the sound signal and the time it takes for the wave to travel through the body provide the information necessary to produce an image.

The advantages of ultrasound are numerous. The system is portable, ranging in size from hand-held pocket devices to high-end larger equipment. It is nonionizing and therefore is excellent to image the neonatal, pediatric, and adult patients, the pregnant patient, and the fetus. Ultrasound may be able to characterize the internal composition of a mass to distinguish cystic from solid components. The definition of soft tissue structures, internal organs, causes for abdominal pain, emergency department trauma "FAST" evaluations, and evaluation of muscles and tendons is well documented with ultrasound. Ultrasound is useful to document the site and depth of the mass for biopsy procedures. Its portability makes it invaluable for the physician in the emergency department and operating room. Ultrasound may be used in the neonatal nursery to provide daily evaluations of the premature neonate.

The disadvantage is that ultrasound does not transmit through bone or gas (lungs and bowel).

Computerized Tomography

The CT system combines both x-rays and a computer to create 360-degree pictures of the spine and internal organs. During the CT examination, the technician acquires a series of radiographic images from many different angles. The computer then processes and assembles the series of images to create multiple cross-sectional or coronal images of the bones, blood vessels, and soft tissue. Computerized tomography

TABLE 5.1	Comparison of Ultrasound, Computed Tomography, and Magnetic Resonance Imaging		
	Ultrasound	**CT**	**MRI**
Exam cost	$100–$1200	$1200–$3200	$2400–$6400
Scan time	5 min (FAST exam) to 45 min	5 min	20–40 min
Portability	Yes	No	No
Radiation exposure	No	Yes	No
Contrast use	Under evaluation	Nephrotoxic/adverse reaction to iodinated contrast agent	Gadolinium (may cause side effects in patients with impaired renal function)
Image detail/contrast	Good detail, but less than CT, MRI	Good spatial resolution/ detail	Good detail; Better contrast
Image planes	All planes	Transverse; after helical scan with multiplanar function, operator can construct any plane	All planes
Contraindications	None	Not applicable for pregnant patients	Implanted metal devices
Visualization of bony structures	No	Good detail	Good detail
Visualization of soft tissue structures	Detailed evaluation of soft tissues and blood vessels with hemodynamic data	Detailed soft tissue and blood vessels	Detailed soft tissue and blood vessels

CT, Computed tomography; *MRI*, magnetic resonance imaging.

technology was designed for taking detailed pictures of the brain. Now it is more advanced and is used for taking pictures of virtually any part of the body, such as internal organs, bones, soft tissue, and blood vessels. CT images are more detailed than conventional radiograph. CT is utilized for acute injuries and chronic vascular conditions and detecting abnormalities in organ systems. With the combined fusion technique, CT is used to determine the exact size and location of tumors, which enables the interventionalist to provide needle guidance for procedures.

The image detail CT may provide advantages as it offers higher contrast images between the tissue types. Computer manipulation allows the operator to zoom in on specific structures or areas within the body, thus eliminating possible obstructions by other organs, bones, or tissues. With reconstruction, the clinicians can review different angles and planes to increase diagnostic clarity. In the emergency department, the CT is utilized frequently to evaluate for head trauma.

The disadvantage of CT is that it does use radiation, which has an increased risk of cancer, although the newer CT systems use a lower dose of radiation for shorter periods. The radiation risk cautions the use of CT with pregnant and pediatric patients. The contrast agents used to enhance visibility may have potentially serious long-term effects on renal function.

Magnetic Resonance Imaging

MRI uses a powerful magnetic field combined with specific radio frequencies to create detailed images of internal body structures with a sophisticated computing system. The body is composed mainly of water, which has magnetic polarity. The fluid in the body contains atoms that spin at a specific rate. Atoms in some tissues spin faster than atoms in other tissues. In some cases, the atoms in the diseased tissue spin at a different rate than atoms in healthy tissue. MRIs use magnets to spin the atoms and radio waves that detect how fast the atoms spin. A computer transforms the information into images. The movement of the magnets is extremely loud and can be annoying for the patient.

MRI provides excellent detail, but images are time consuming and are typically static. Patients may require gadolinium contrast to obtain better-detailed images. This agent may cause side effects in patients with impaired renal function and may not be used with pregnant patients.

The disadvantage of MRI is its limited access and expense. Specific building requirements are needed to install such a system. MRI is not readily available in all areas. The magnet is generally in an enclosed tubular capsule, and once activated, the loud pounding noise of the magnet is not acceptable for many patients. Open scanners are scarce. MRI is affected by movement, and with the length of each scan, some patients are unable to tolerate this component.

Radiography

Radiography uses radiation (x-rays) to create images. During a radiographic examination, radiation passes through the body onto an x-ray film. Radiation passes right through fluid and thin tissues to cause a dark area on the x-ray film. Bones and other dense tissues stop the x-rays from passing, so these areas show up as light areas on the x-ray film. Radiographs are utilized to diagnose lung and bone disease, fractures, dislocations, and tumors.

ABDOMINAL QUADRANTS, PLANES, AND REGIONS

The ability of the sonographer to understand anatomy as it relates to cross-sectional, coronal, oblique, and sagittal projections is critical to performing a quality sonographic examination. Normal anatomy has many variations in size and position, and the sonographer must demonstrate these findings on the sonogram. A thorough understanding of anatomy related to anteroposterior and medial-lateral relationships and variations in sectional anatomy is required and is essential in 3D analysis and reconstruction. The sonographer images the body in multiple planes, which include, but are not limited to, transverse, sagittal, longitudinal, and coronal (Fig. 5.1).

1. **Transverse**. The transverse plane is horizontal to the body. This plane divides the body or any of its parts into upper and lower portions. The orientation is viewed from the "feet up" so the liver will be on the left of the image and the spleen on the right.
2. **Sagittal**. The sagittal plane is a lengthwise plane running from front to back. It divides the body or any of its parts into right and left sides, or two halves; this is known as the midsagittal plane. The orientation with ultrasound is to orient the patient's head to the left of the image.
3. **Longitudinal**. The longitudinal plane is parallel to the long axis of the body or part. The sonographer may alter the orientation of the transducer to align with the longitudinal axis of the organ or lesion.
4. **Coronal**. The coronal plane is a lengthwise plane running from side to side, dividing the body into

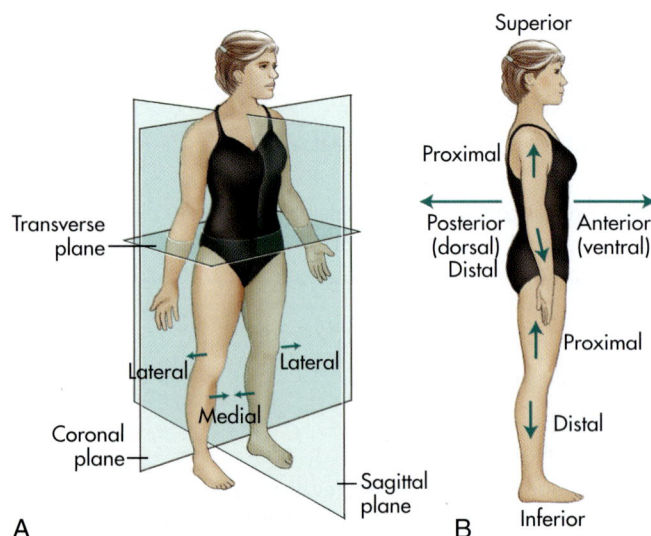

FIG. 5.1 (A) Anterior view of the body in the anatomic position. Note the directions and body planes. (B) Lateral view of the body.

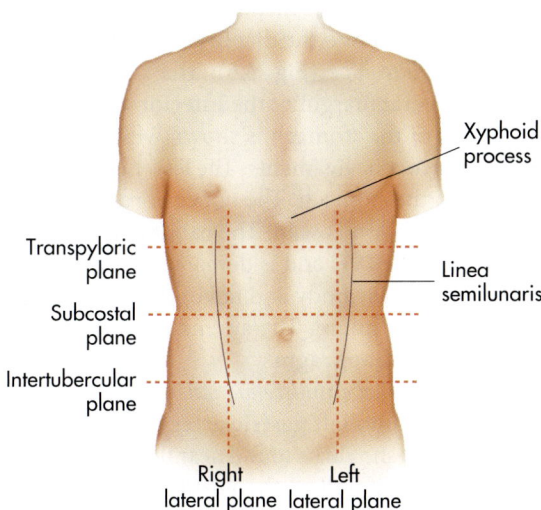

FIG. 5.2 Surface landmarks of the anterior abdominal wall.

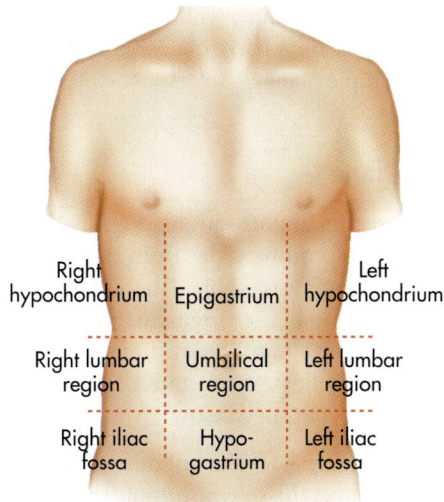

FIG. 5.3 Regions of the abdominal wall.

anterior and posterior portions. This plane is utilized in 3D reconstruction.

The abdominopelvic cavity may be divided into four quadrants and nine abdominal regions to identify specific abdominal structures or refer to an area of pain. The quadrant is determined by a midsagittal plane and a transverse plane that pass through the umbilicus. The four quadrants include the right upper quadrant, left upper quadrant (LUQ), right lower quadrant, and left lower quadrant.

PLANES OR BODY SECTIONS

The abdominopelvic cavity is commonly divided into nine regions by two vertical and two horizontal lines. The anterior abdominal wall's surface landmarks help define the specific abdominal regions (Fig. 5.2). Each vertical line passes through the mid-inguinal point (i.e., the point that lies on the inguinal ligament halfway between the pubic symphysis and the anterior superior iliac spine). The upper horizontal line, referred to as the **subcostal plane**, joins the lowest point of the costal margin on each side of the body. The lowest horizontal line, the **intertubercular plane**, joins the tubercles on the iliac crests. The **transpyloric plane** is a horizontal plane that passes through the pylorus, the duodenal junction, the neck of the pancreas, and the hilum of the kidneys.

The nine abdominal regions (Fig. 5.3) include the following: (1) upper abdomen/right hypochondrium, (2) epigastrium, (3) left hypochondrium, (4) middle abdomen/right lumbar, (5) umbilical, (6) left lumbar, (7) lower abdomen/right iliac fossa, (8) hypogastrium, and (9) left iliac fossa. Box 5.1 provides a list of additional terms that the sonographer is likely to encounter when identifying specific body regions or structures.

SECTIONAL ANATOMY

The sonographer must have a solid knowledge of gross and sectional anatomy and awareness of the many anatomic

BOX 5.1	Terms for Common Body Regions and Structures

Portion of trunk below the diaphragm
Area of armpit
Arm
Abdomen
Neck region
Ribs
Thigh; the part of the lower extremity between the hip and the knee
Depressed region between the abdomen and the thigh
Lower extremity, especially from the knee to the foot
Loin; the region of the lower back and side, between the lowest rib and the pelvis
Breasts
Pelvis; the bony ring that girdles the lower portion of the trunk
Region between the anus and the pubic arch; includes the region of the external reproductive structures
Area behind the knee
Chest; the part of the trunk below the neck and above the diaphragm

variations that may occur in the body. The sonographer should carefully evaluate organ and vascular relationships to neighboring structures, rather than memorize where in the abdomen a particular structure "should" be: It is better to recall the location of the gallbladder as anterior to the right kidney and medial to the liver than to remember than it is found 6 cm above the umbilicus. The sonographer should also reflect on the anatomical variations that are present in each individual. Such variations will be further discussed in the respective chapters.

Keep in mind the descriptors below may vary somewhat from the examples shown for CT, MRI, and ultrasound. Note on CT, the air in the stomach appears as "black" as the patient is supine and the air rises to the anterior fundus of the stomach. On ultrasound, the vascular and fluid-filled structures within the body appear as "black." Images were selected to highlight the anatomy described; CT and MRI are a composite image of the transverse plane, while most ultrasound images in this chapter focus on a particular organ and may be demonstrated in multiple planes.

Transverse Plane

The transverse sectional illustrations (Figs. 5.4 through 5.17) are presented in descending order from the dome of the diaphragm to the symphysis pubis. The sonographer should review the relationship of each organ to its neighboring structures while proceeding in a caudal direction. Specific detail is listed below each illustration, and a thumbnail sketch of expected anatomy is outlined below:

Dome of the liver (Fig. 5.4): The **splenic artery** enters as the **splenic vein** leaves the splenic hilum. The abdominal portion of the esophagus lies to the left of the midline and opens into the stomach through the cardiac orifice. The liver extends to the left mammillary line. The **falciform ligament** extends into the diaphragm.

Level of the caudate lobe (Fig. 5.5): The right **hepatic vein** enters the lateral margin of the **inferior vena cava (IVC)**. The fundus of the stomach is shown with the hepatogastric and gastrocolic ligaments. The lesser omental cavity is posterior to the stomach. The upper border of the splenic flexure of the colon is seen. The **caudate lobe** of the liver is anterior to the IVC and is demarcated by the **ligamentum venosum**. The body and tail of the pancreas are seen near the splenic hilum. The adrenal glands are lateral to the **crus of the diaphragm**.

Level of the caudate lobe and celiac axis (Fig. 5.6): The **celiac axis** (branches into **left gastric artery**, splenic artery, and **hepatic artery**) should be found near this section as it arises from the anterior wall of the **aorta (Ao)**. The transverse and descending colons are shown inferior to the splenic flexure. The caudate lobe of the liver is shown. The body

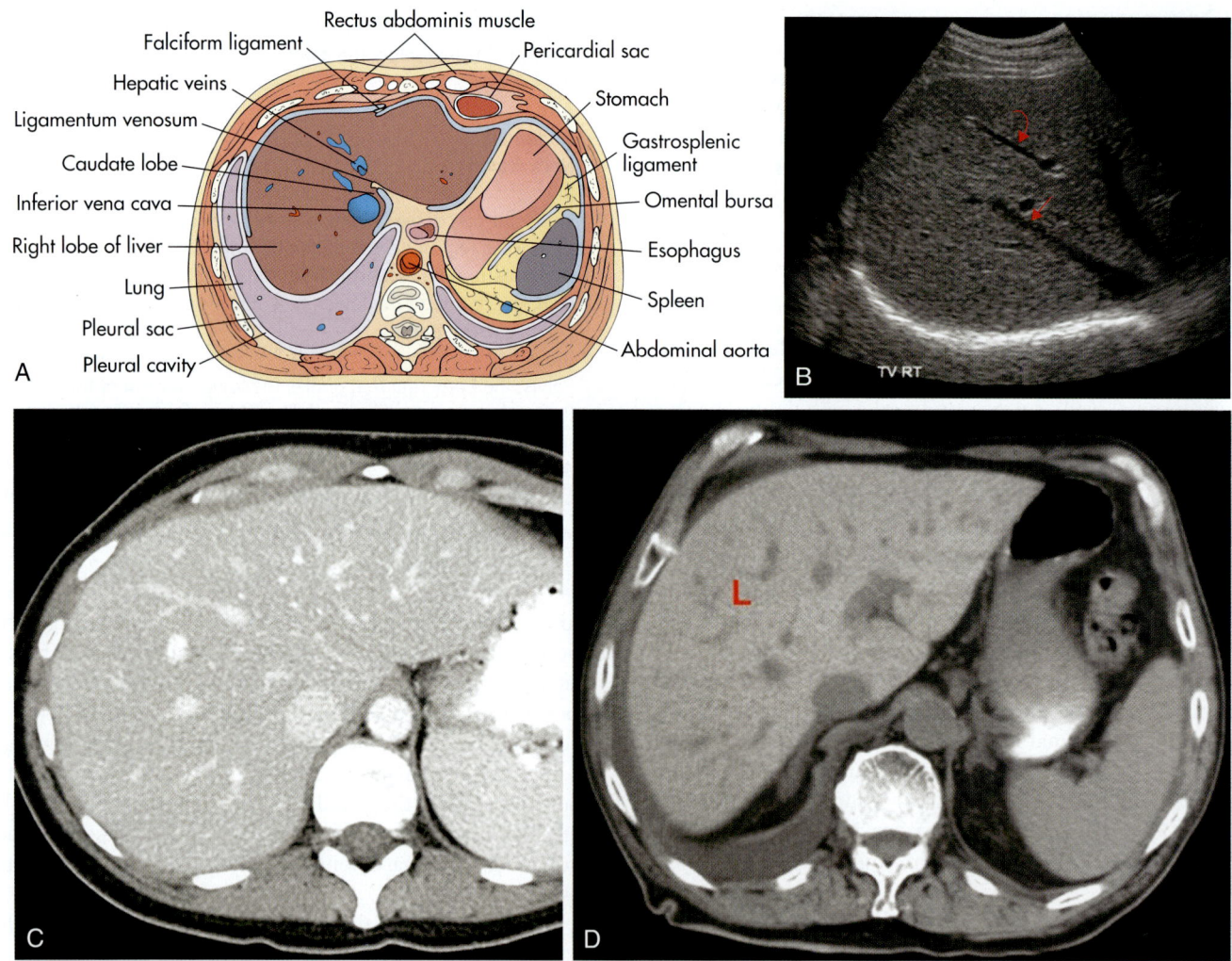

FIG. 5.4 (A) Cross section of the abdomen at the level of the tenth intervertebral disk. The lower portion of the pericardial sac is seen. The splenic artery enters the spleen, and the splenic vein emerges from the splenic hilum. The abdominal portion of the esophagus lies to the left of the midline and opens into the stomach through the cardiac orifice. The liver extends to the left mammillary line. The falciform ligament extends into the section above this. The spleen is shown to lie alongside the ninth rib. (B) Ultrasound image of the right lobe of the liver. Note the hepatic veins *(straight arrow)* and portal veins *(curved arrow)*. CT (C) and transverse section MRI (D) through the liver (L), stomach, spleen, and aorta.

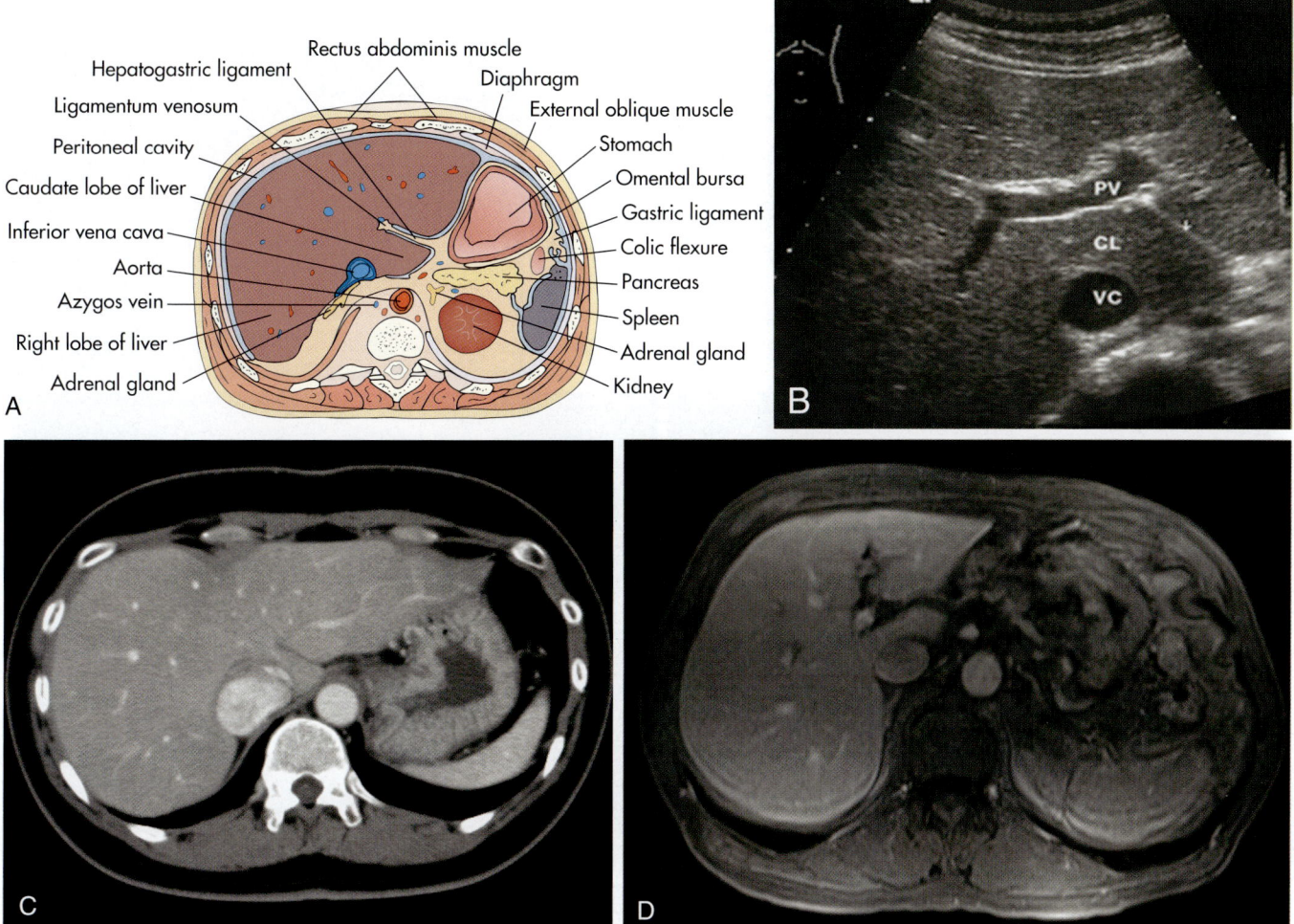

FIG. 5.5 (A) Cross section of the abdomen at the level of the eleventh thoracic disk. The right hepatic vein is shown to enter the inferior vena cava. The upper part of the stomach is shown with the hepatogastric and gastrocolic ligaments. The lesser omental cavity is posterior to the stomach. The upper border of the splenic flexure of the colon is seen. The caudate lobe of the liver is in this section. The tail and body of the pancreas are shown anterior to the left kidney. The spleen is shown to lie along the left lateral border. The adrenal glands are lateral to the crus of the diaphragm. (B) Focused transverse ultrasound image near the dome of the liver demonstrate the portal vein (PV), caudate lobe (CL), and inferior vena cava (IVC). CT (C) and transverse section MRI (D) through the liver, caudate lobe, stomach, spleen, aorta, inferior vena cava, and crus of the diaphragm.

of the pancreas is anterior to the splenic vein. Both kidneys and the adrenal glands are shown lateral to the spine and crus of the diaphragm. The IVC is shown anterior to the crus, and the Ao is posterior to the crus of the diaphragm.

Level of the superior mesenteric artery (SMA) and pancreas (Fig. 5.7): The **psoas major muscles** are lateral to the spine. The **right renal artery** is shown posterior to the IVC. The **left renal artery** would arise from the posterolateral wall of the Ao; the **right** and **left renal veins** are inferior to the renal arteries. The **portal confluence** (also called the **confluence of the splenic and portal veins**) is formed by the splenic vein and the **superior mesenteric vein**. The superior portion of the duodenum is shown posterior to the stomach. Part of the transverse colon is shown. The hepatic duct is anterior to the portal vein.

Level of the gallbladder and right kidney (Fig. 5.8): The kidneys are lateral to the psoas muscles. The **gastroduodenal artery** lies along the anterolateral border of the head of the pancreas, and the duodenum surrounds the lateral border. The stomach and transverse colon fill the LUQ, and the liver fills the right upper quadrant. The gallbladder is medial to the liver. The common bile duct is seen along the posterior lateral border of the pancreatic head.

Level of the liver, gallbladder, and right kidney (Fig. 5.9): The **inferior mesenteric artery** originates from the abdominal Ao at this level. The greater omentum is shown on the left side of the abdomen. The descending and ascending portions of the duodenum lie between the Ao and the SMA and vein. The gallbladder is seen along the medial border of the right lobe of the liver. Both lower poles of the kidneys are seen lateral to the psoas muscles.

Level of the right lobe of the liver (Fig. 5.10): The lower portion of the right lobe of the liver and the duodenum are shown.

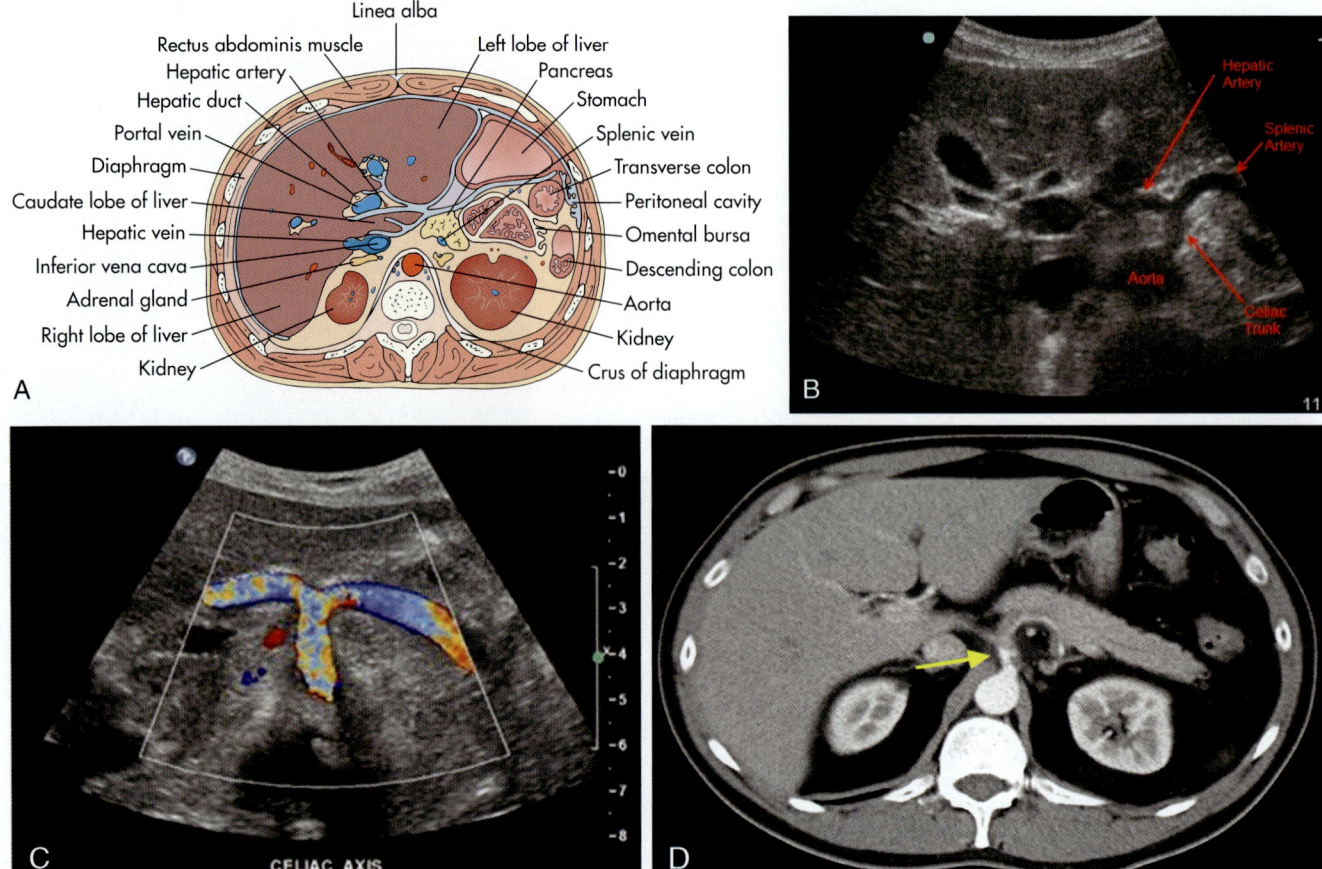

FIG. 5.6 (A) Cross section of the abdomen at the level of the twelfth thoracic vertebra. The celiac axis arises in the middle of this section from the anterior abdominal aorta. The right renal artery originates at this level. The hepatic vein is shown to enter the inferior vena cava. The greater curvature of the stomach is shown. The transverse and descending colon are shown inferior to the splenic flexure. The caudate lobe of the liver is well seen. The body of the pancreas, both kidneys, and the lower portions of the adrenal glands are shown. (B–C) Focused ultrasound images demonstrating the celiac trunk and its branches as it arises from the anterior aortic wall. The inferior vena cava is shown to the right of the aorta. (D) CT transverse image showing the liver, stomach, kidneys, aorta and celiac trunk *(arrow)*, inferior vena cava, and spine.

Level of the bifurcation of the Ao (Fig. 5.11): The psoas major muscles are lateral to the spine. The **iliac arteries** are anterior to the spine. The common **iliac veins** unite to form the IVC.

Level of the external iliac arteries (Fig. 5.12): The external iliac arteries are well seen. The ileum is seen throughout this level, and the mesentery terminates at this level.

Level of the external iliac veins (Fig. 5.13): The internal and external iliac veins have united to form the common iliac vein.

Level of the male pelvis (Fig. 5.14). The pelvic muscles are shown; the rectum is seen in the midline. The trigone of the bladder and urethral orifice is shown, and the seminal vesicles and the ampulla of the vasa deferentia can be identified. The ejaculatory ducts enter the urethra in the lower portion of this section.

Level of the male pelvis (Fig. 5.15). The rectum, prostate gland, penis, and corpus cavernosum are seen.

Level of the female pelvis (Fig. 5.16). The bladder is anterior to the uterus. The pouch of Douglas is posterior to the uterus, anterior to the rectum. The ovaries are seen along the fundal border of the uterus.

Level of the female pelvis (Fig. 5.17): The pelvic diaphragm muscles are shown.

Sagittal/Longitudinal Plane

The longitudinal sectional illustrations (Figs. 5.18 through 5.26) are presented from the right abdominal border, proceeding across the abdominal wall to the left border.

Level of the right lobe of the liver (Fig. 5.18): The right lobe of the liver, diaphragm, omentum, and muscles are shown.

Level of the liver, portal veins, and gallbladder (Fig. 5.19): The diaphragm, right lobe of the liver, gallbladder, and perirenal fat area are shown. The costodiaphragmatic recess is seen superior to the diaphragm.

Level of the liver, gallbladder, and right kidney (Fig. 5.20): The diaphragm, right lobe of the liver, gallbladder, and right kidney are seen. The perirenal fat and fascia are shown

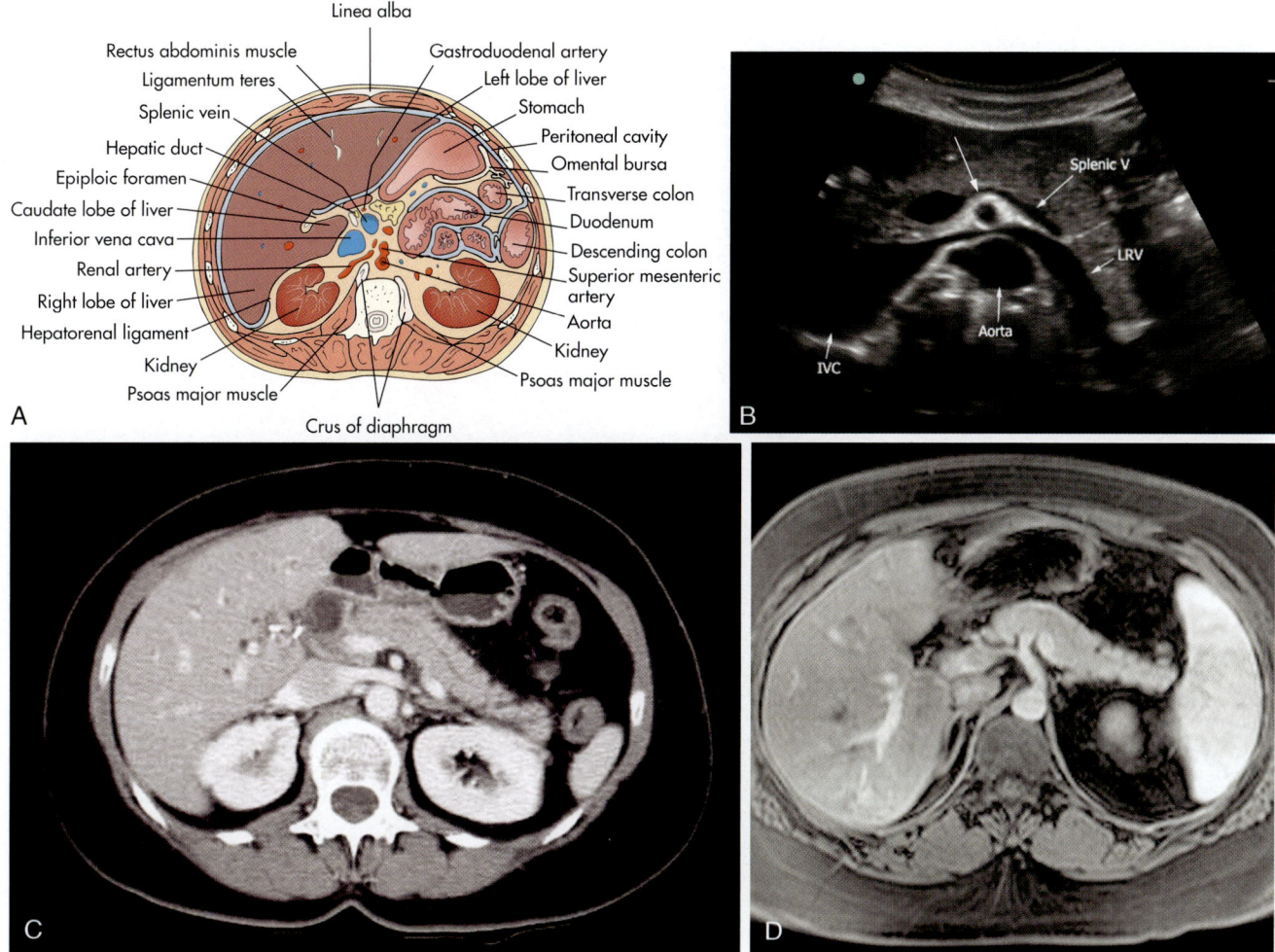

FIG. 5.7 (A) Cross section of the abdomen at the first lumbar vertebra. The psoas major muscle is seen. The crura of the diaphragm are on either side of the spine. The right renal artery is seen. The left renal artery arises from the lateral wall of the aorta. Both renal veins enter the inferior vena cava. The portal vein is seen to be formed by the union of the splenic vein and the superior mesenteric vein. The lower portions of the stomach and the pyloric orifice are seen, as is the superior portion of the duodenum. The duodenojejunal flexure and the descending and transverse colon are shown. The small, non-peritoneal area of the liver is shown anterior to the right kidney. The hepatorenal ligament of the liver and the ligamentum teres are seen. The hepatic duct lies just anterior to the cystic duct. Both kidneys are seen just lateral to the psoas muscles. (B) Focused ultrasound image demonstrating the aorta and inferior vena cava (IVC). The superior mesenteric artery (SMA) is anterior to the aorta *(arrow)*, and the splenic vein is anterior to the SMA. The left renal vein (LRV) crosses anterior to the aorta and posterior to the SMA to enter the IVC. CT (C) and transverse section MRI (D) through the right lobe of the liver, pancreas, stomach, spleen, aorta, and inferior vena cava.

surrounding the kidney. **Morison's pouch** is found anterior to the kidney and posterior to the inferior right lobe of the liver. The caudate lobe of the liver is beginning to show.

Level of the liver, caudate lobe, and psoas muscle (Fig. 5.21): The diaphragm, right lobe of the liver, caudate lobe, and neck of the gallbladder are seen.

Level of the liver, duodenum, and pancreas (Fig. 5.22): The portal vein and cystic duct are shown. The duodenum wraps around the head of the pancreas.

Level of the IVC, left lobe of the liver, and pancreas (Fig. 5.23): The IVC is shown along the posterior border of the liver. The pancreas lies anterior to the IVC and inferior to the portal vein.

Level of the hepatic vein and IVC, pancreas, and superior mesenteric vein (Fig. 5.24): The superior mesenteric vein flows anterior to the uncinate portion of the pancreas and posterior to the body. The middle hepatic vein empties into the IVC. The falciform ligament is seen along the anterior border of the abdomen.

Level of the Ao and SMA (Fig. 5.25): The **superior mesenteric artery (SMA)** arises from the anterior border of the Ao. The pancreas is seen anterior to the SMA; the splenic artery and vein form the posterior border. The left renal vein is posterior to the SMA and anterior to the Ao. The area of the lesser sac is shown.

Level of the spleen and left kidney (Fig. 5.26): The spleen is shown just below the diaphragm in the LUQ. The left kidney is inferior to the spleen. The tail of the pancreas lies anterior to the kidney and inferior to the **splenic hilum**.

110 CHAPTER 5 Comparative Sectional Anatomy of the Abdominopelvic Cavity

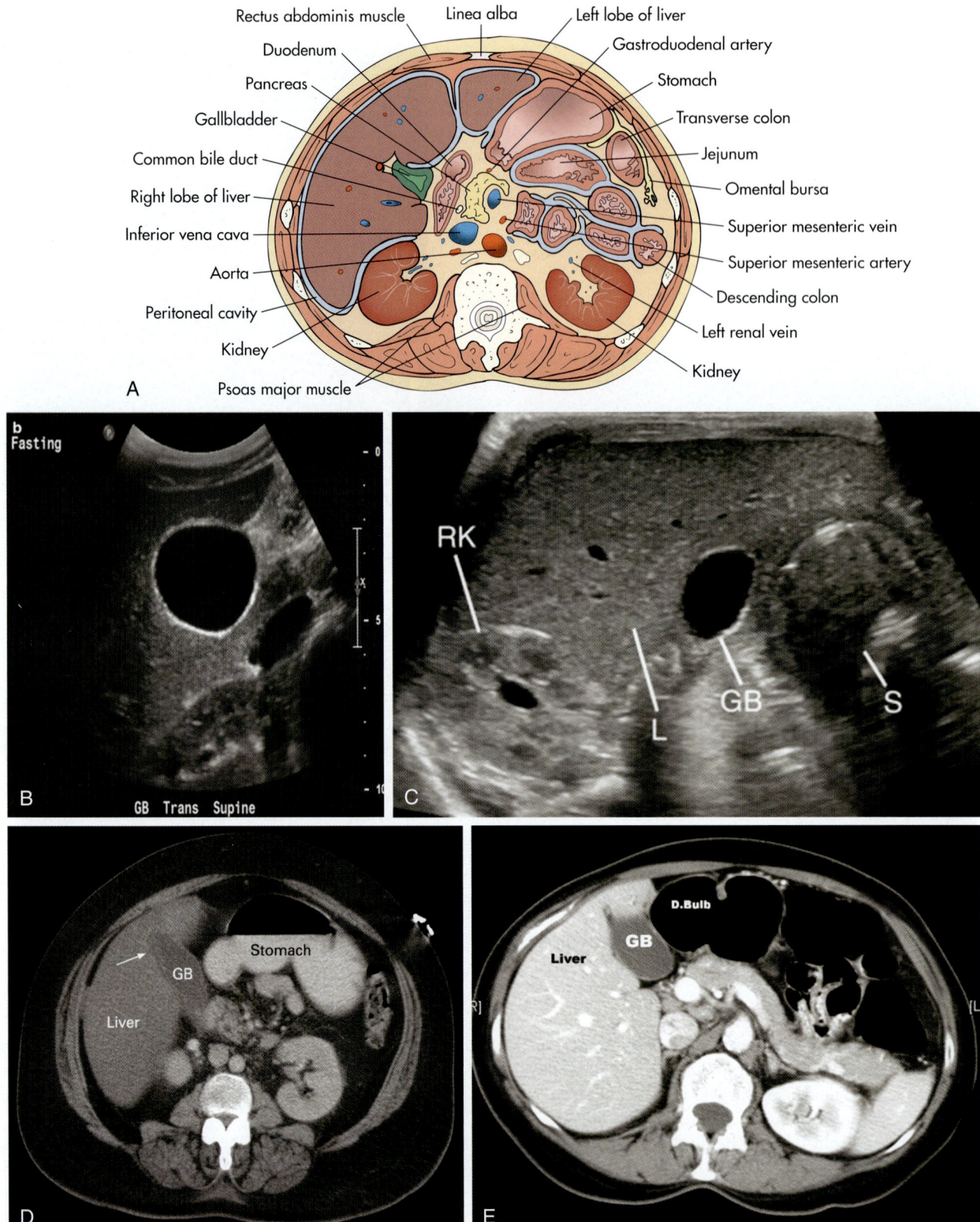

FIG. 5.8 (A) Cross section of the abdomen at the level of the second lumbar vertebra. The lower portion of the stomach is found in this section, and the descending colon is seen. The left lobe of the liver ends at this level. The head and neck of the pancreas drape around the superior mesenteric vein. Both kidneys and the psoas muscles are shown. (B–C) Focused ultrasound images of the gallbladder (GB), right kidney (RK), liver (L), and stomach (S). CT (D) and transverse section MRI (E) at the level of the liver, gallbladder, stomach, spleen, aorta, and inferior vena cava.

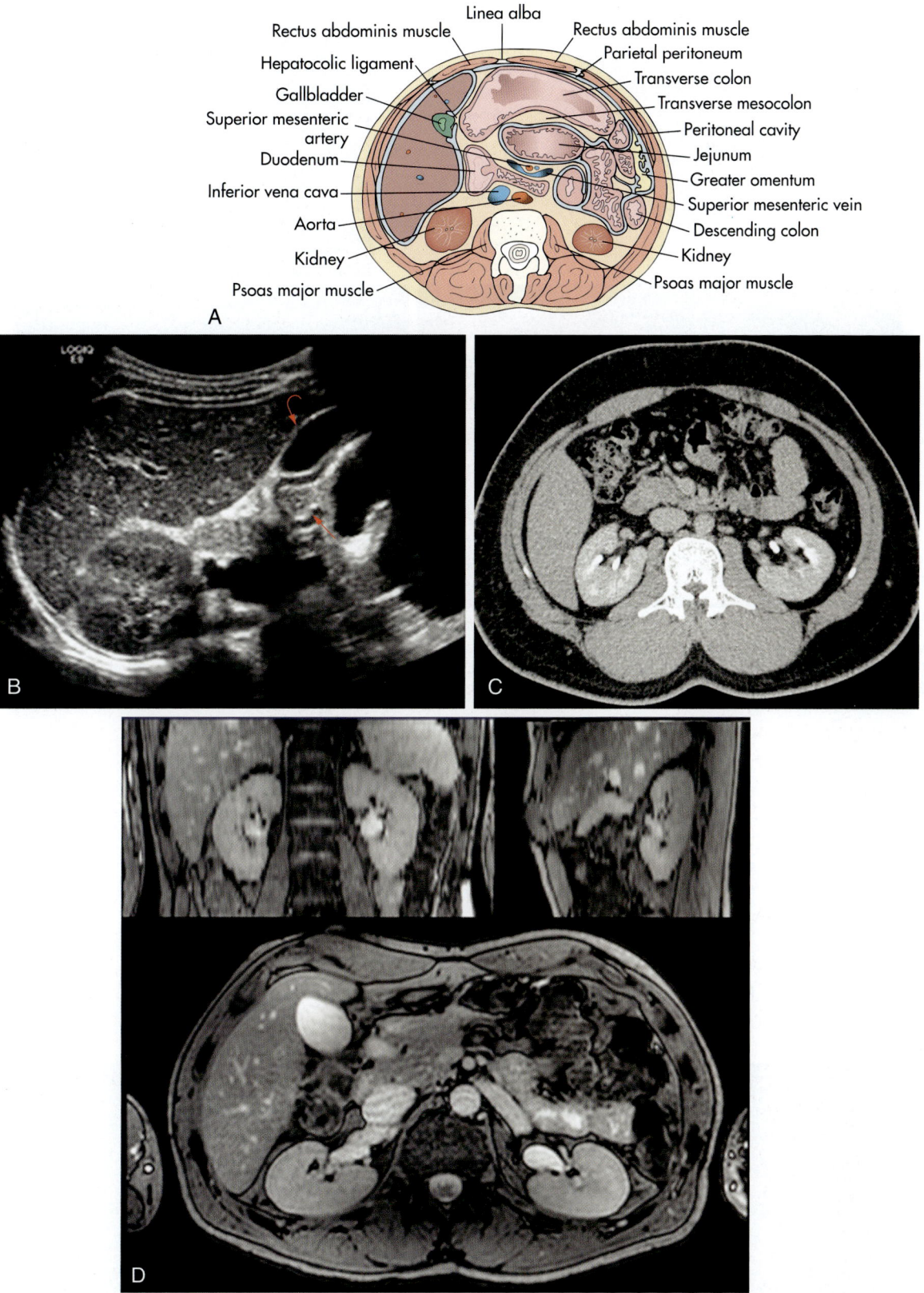

FIG. 5.9 (A) Cross section of the abdomen at the level of the third lumbar vertebra. The inferior mesenteric artery originates from the abdominal aorta at this level. The greater omentum is shown mainly on the left side of the abdomen. The descending and ascending portions of the duodenum lie between the aorta and the superior mesenteric artery and vein. The fundus of the gallbladder lies in the lower portion of this section. The lower poles of both kidneys lie lateral to the psoas muscles. (B) Focused ultrasound images at the lower right lobe of the liver, gallbladder *(curved arrow)*, duodenum *(straight arrow)*, right kidney, pancreas, and inferior vena cava. Computed tomography (C) and MRI (D) at the level of the gallbladder, liver, stomach, splenic vein, spleen, aorta, and inferior vena cava.

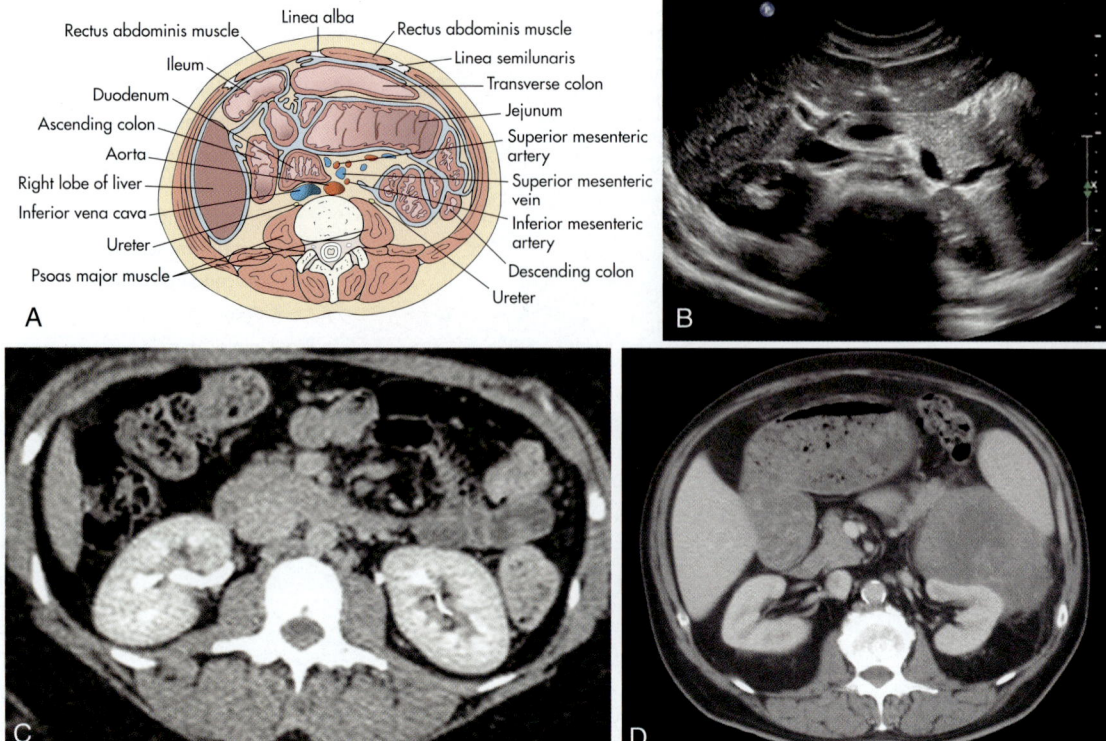

FIG. 5.10 (A) Cross section of the abdomen at the level of the third lumbar disk. The lower portion of the duodenum is shown. The lower margin of the right lobe of the liver is seen along the right lateral border. (B) Focused ultrasound of the mid-abdomen shows the left lobe of the liver, pancreas, right kidney, stomach, splenic vein, inferior vena cava. CT (C) and transverse section MRI (D) at the lower right lobe of liver, pancreas, spleen, colon, aorta, kidneys, and inferior vena cava.

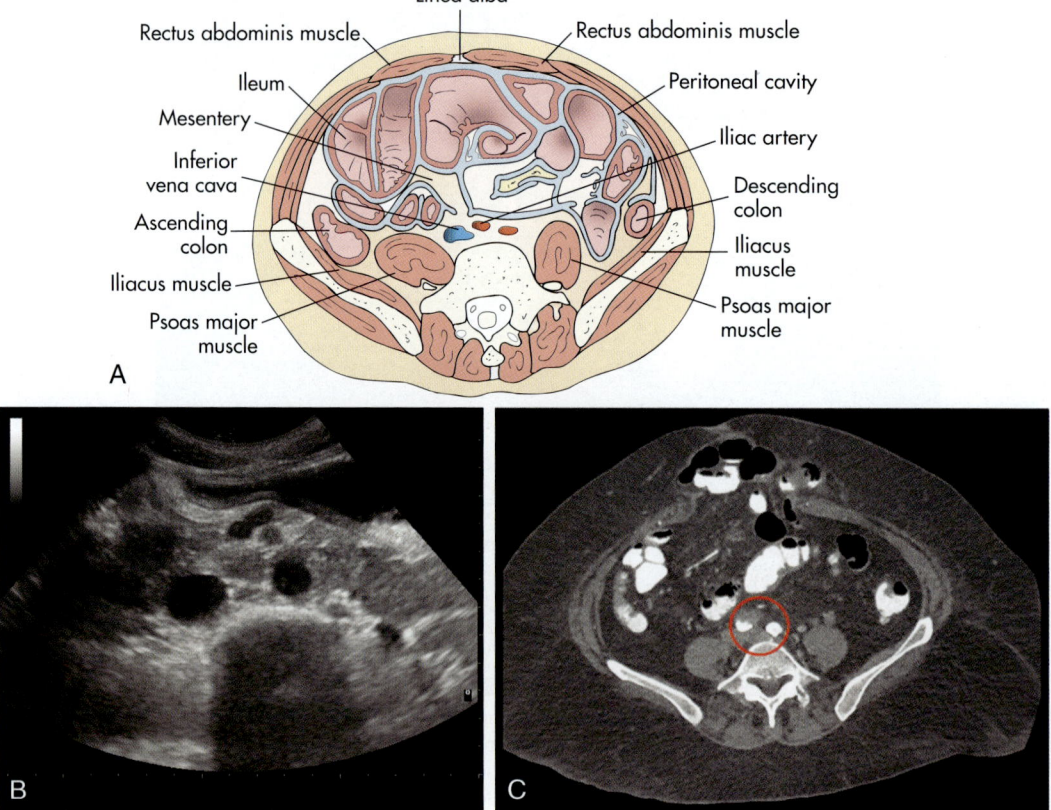

FIG. 5.11 (A) Cross section of the abdomen at the level of the fifth lumbar vertebra. It cuts the ileum through the upper part of the iliac fossa and passes just above the wings of the sacrum. The psoas and iliacus muscles are shown. The right common iliac artery bifurcates into the external and internal iliac arteries. The common iliac veins are shown to unite to form the inferior vena cava. The mesentery is shown in this section. (B) Focused ultrasound of the aorta just above the bifurcation and the inferior vena cava. (C) Transverse section CT of the bowel, iliac vessels, and psoas muscles.

CHAPTER 5 Comparative Sectional Anatomy of the Abdominopelvic Cavity

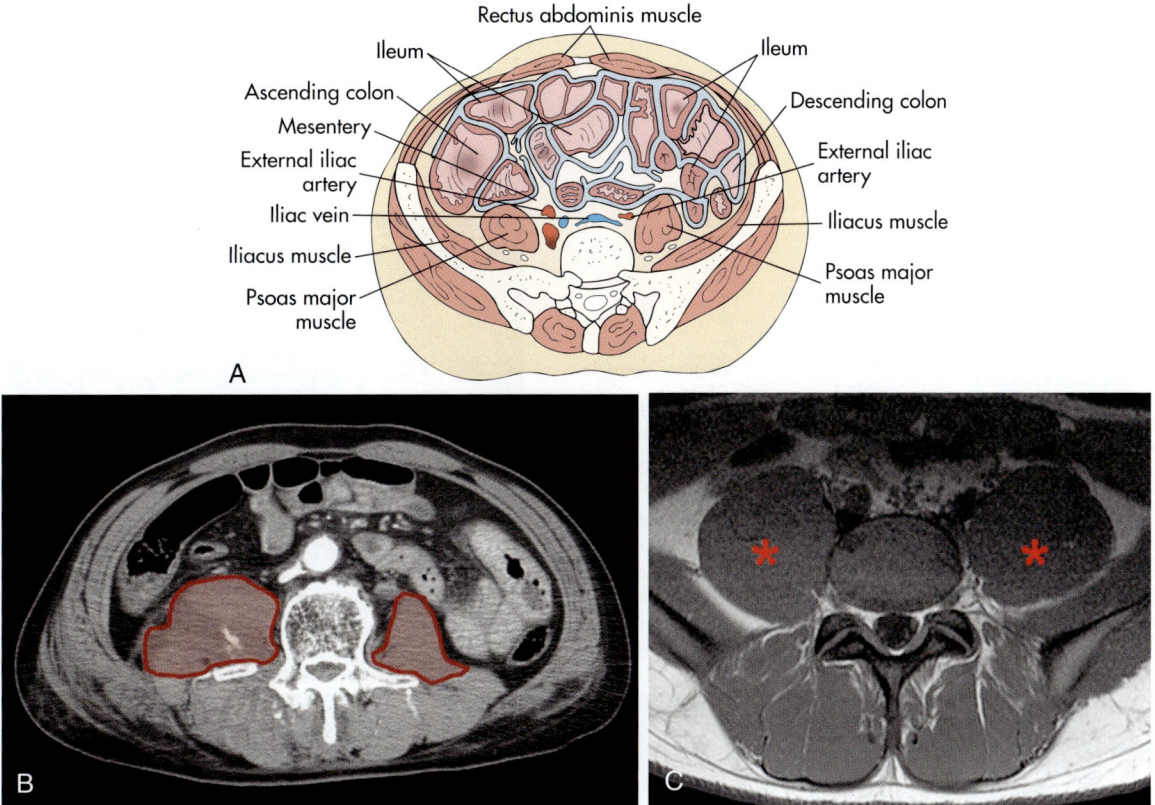

FIG. 5.12 (A) Cross section of the pelvis taken at the lower margin of the fifth lumbar vertebra and disk. The gluteus minimus muscle is shown in this section, as are the right external and internal iliac arteries. The left common iliac artery branches into the external and internal arteries. The ileum is seen throughout this level, and the mesentery terminates at this level. (B) Transverse section CT shows the aortic bifurcation, psoas muscles, and iliac wing. (C) MRI shows the psoas muscles adjacent to the iliac wing *(asterisks)*.

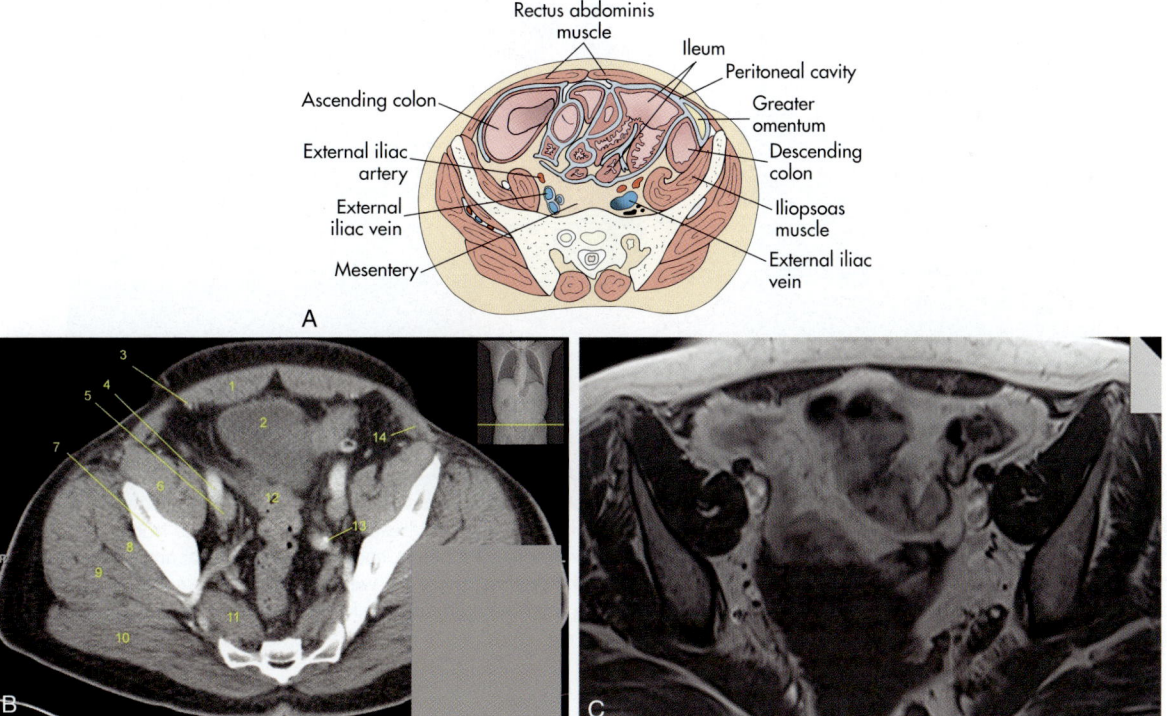

FIG. 5.13 (A) Cross section of the pelvis taken at the level of the sacrum and the anterior superior spine of the ilium. The gluteus maximus muscle appears on both sides. The internal and external iliac veins have united to form the common iliac vein. The ileum is seen throughout this section. CT (B) and transverse section MRI (C) through the lower abdomen and iliopsoas muscle. *1,* Rectus abdominis; *2,* bladder; *3,* inferior epigastric artery and vein; *4,* right external iliac artery; *5,* right external iliac vein; *6,* iliopsoas muscle; *7,* ilium; *8,* gluteus minimus muscle; *9,* gluteus medius muscle; *10,* gluteus maximus muscle; *11,* piriformis; *12,* sigmoid colon; *13,* left ureter; *14,* obliquis externus, internus, and transversus muscles.

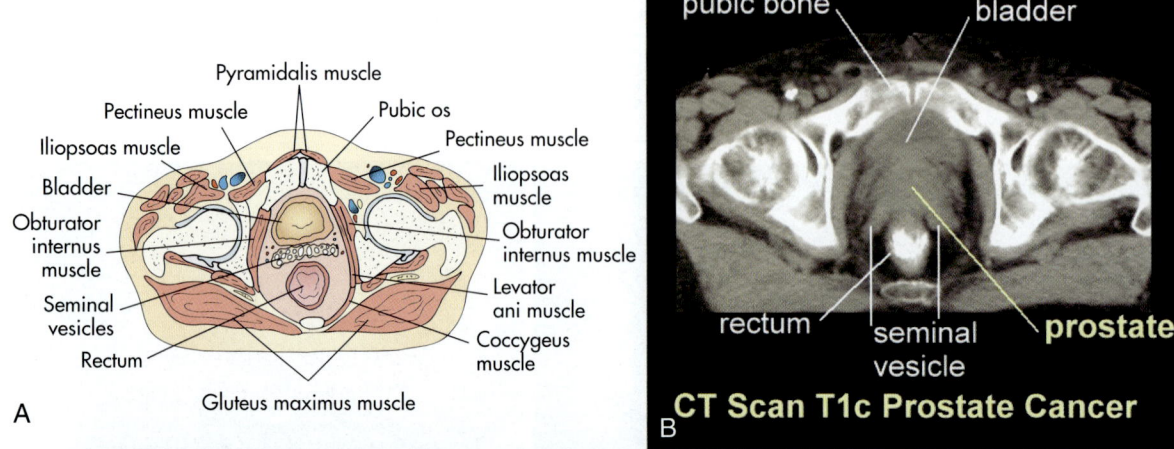
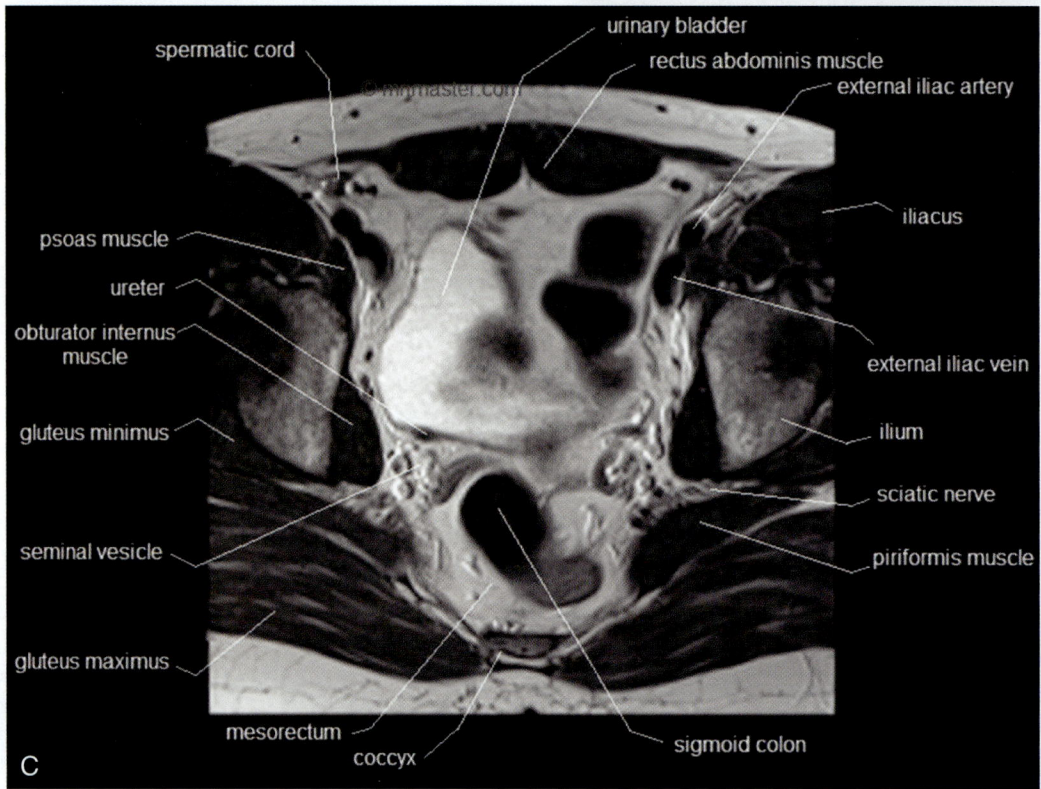

FIG. 5.14 (A) Cross section through the coccyx, spine of the ischium, acetabulum, head of the femur, greater trochanter, pubic symphysis, and upper margins of the obturator foramen. The gemellus inferior and superior, coccygeus, and levator ani muscles are shown. The rectum is seen in the midline. The trigone of the bladder and the urethral orifice are well shown, and the seminal vesicles and the ampulla of the vasa deferens can be identified. The ejaculatory ducts enter the urethra in the lower portion of this section. CT (B) and MRI (C) of the prostate, rectum, and iliopsoas muscles.

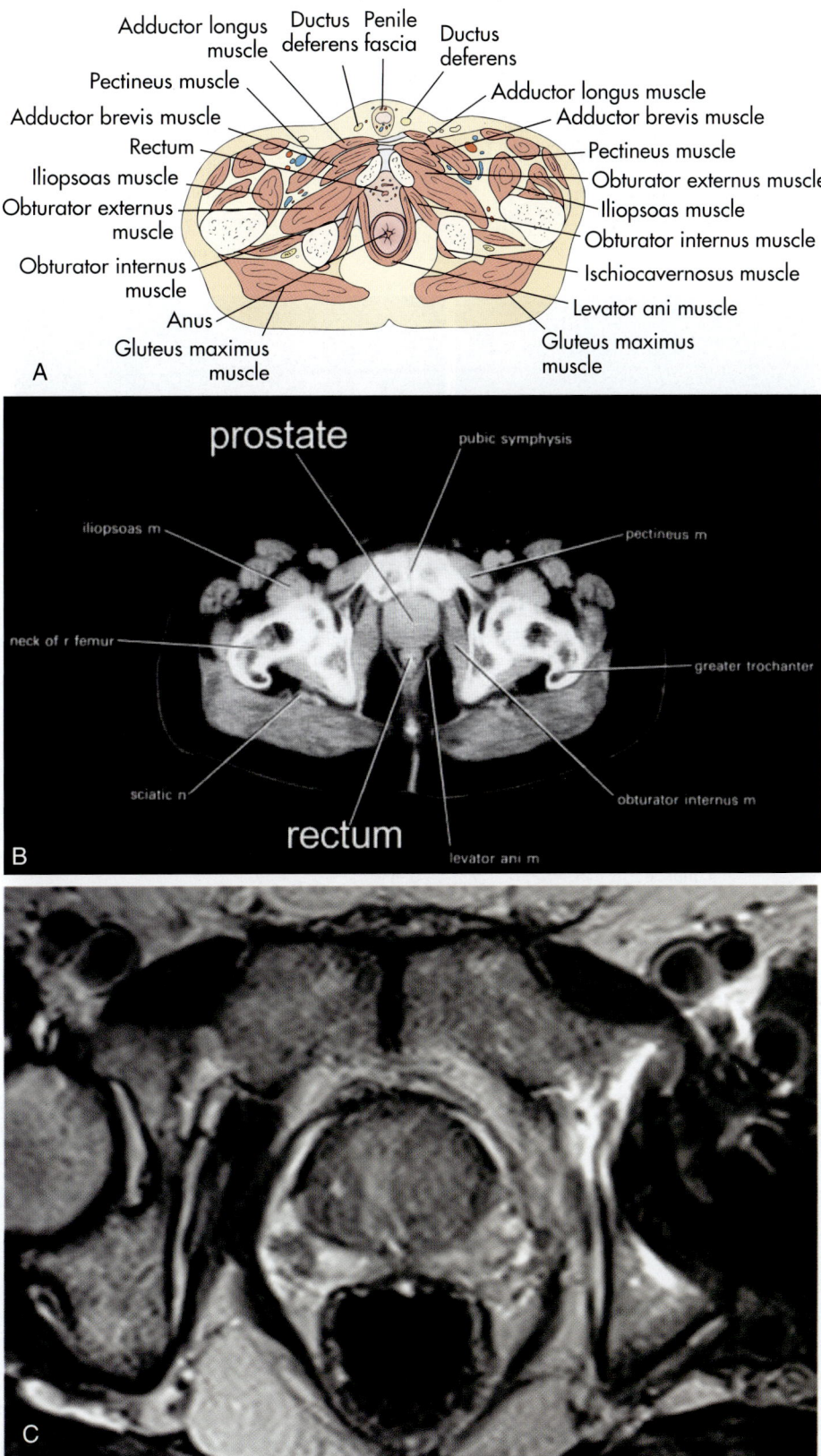

FIG. 5.15 (A) Cross section of the male pelvis at the tip of the coccyx, inferior ramus of the pubis, and neck of the femur. The rectum, penis, and corpus cavernosum are seen. Transverse computed tomography (B) and magnetic resonance imaging (C) of the prostate and rectum.

CHAPTER 5 Comparative Sectional Anatomy of the Abdominopelvic Cavity

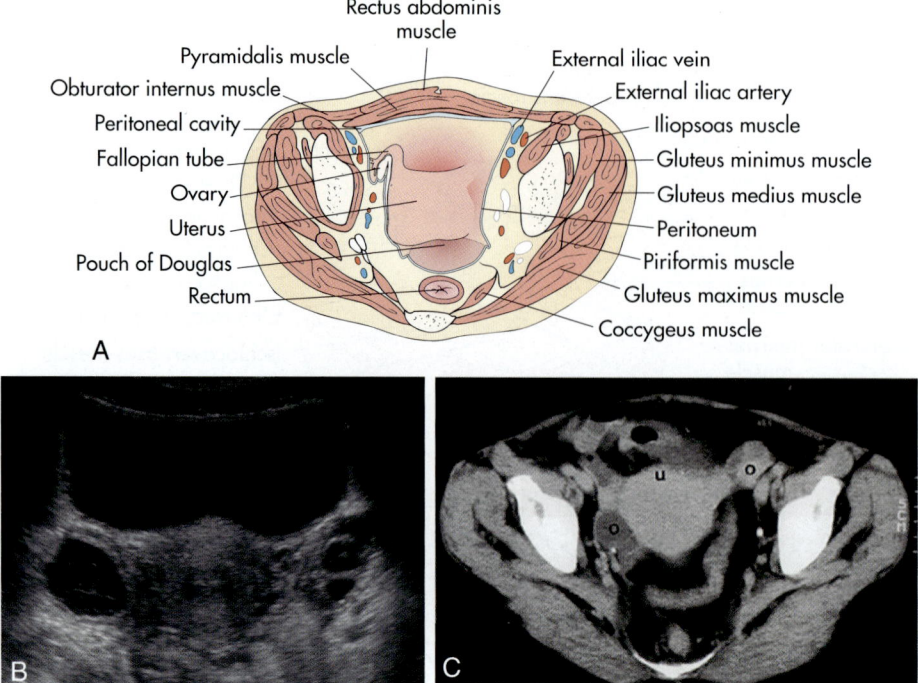

FIG. 5.16 (A) Cross section through the female pelvis just below the junction of the sacrum and coccyx, through the anterior inferior spine of the ilium and the greater sciatic notch. The uterine artery and vein and the ureter are shown dissected beyond the uterine wall. The bladder is anterior to the uterus (u). The ovaries (o) are cut through their midsections on this level. (B) Ultrasound reconstruction of the pelvic floor. (C) MRI of the pelvic diaphragm. *o*, Ovary, *u*, uterus.

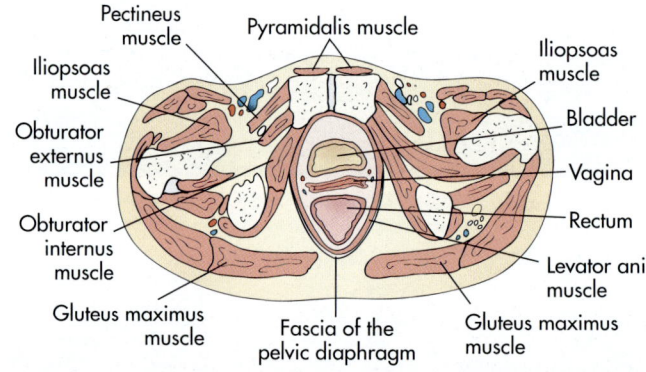

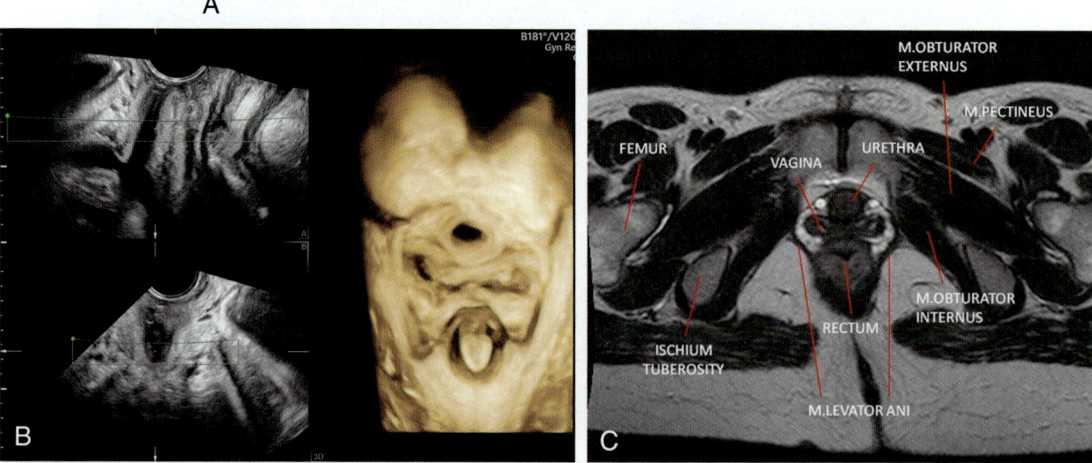

FIG. 5.17 (A) Cross section of the female pelvis taken through the lower part of the coccyx and the spine of the ischium. The pectineus muscle appears in this section, and the coccygeus muscle terminates here. The gluteus maximus, gluteus minimus, and gluteus medius muscles all begin their insertions in the lower part of this section. The external os of the cervix is shown. The ureters empty into the bladder at the base. (B) Ultrasound reconstruction of the pelvic floor. (C) MRI of the pelvic diaphragm.

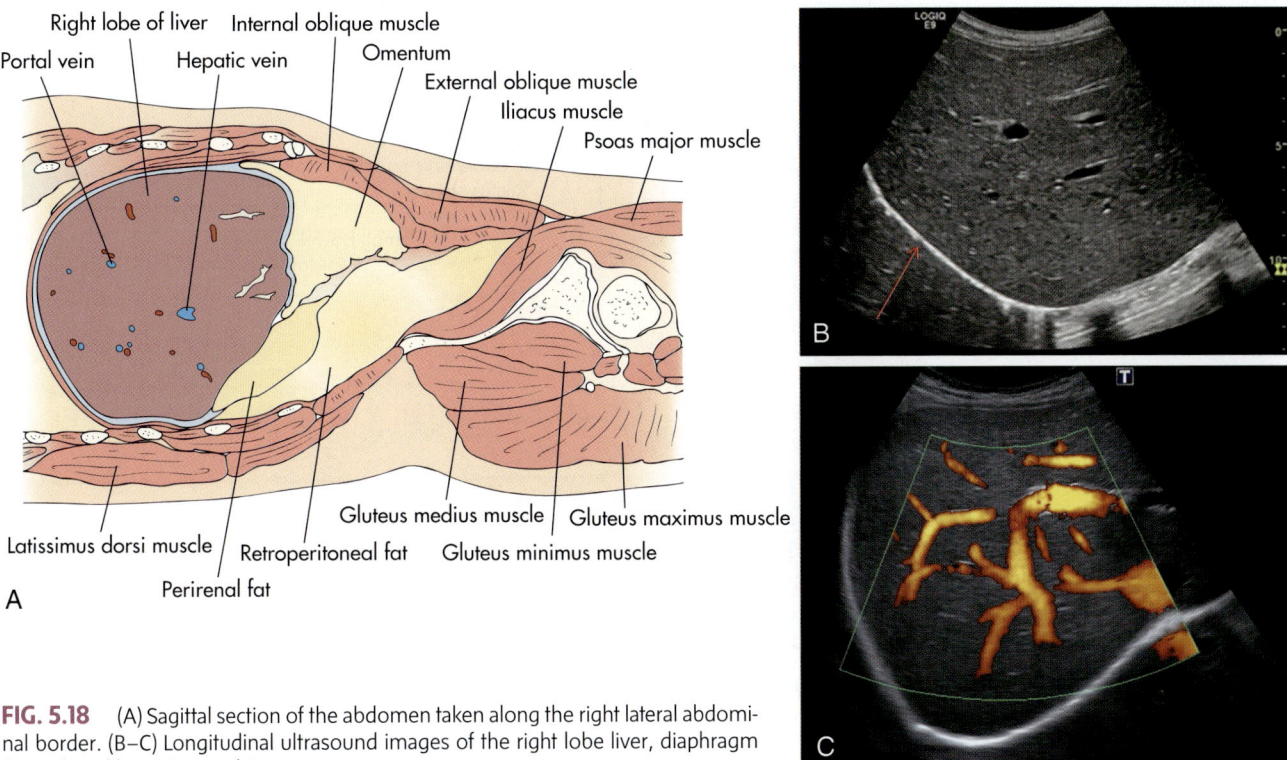

FIG. 5.18 (A) Sagittal section of the abdomen taken along the right lateral abdominal border. (B–C) Longitudinal ultrasound images of the right lobe liver, diaphragm *(arrow)*, and hepatic vasculature.

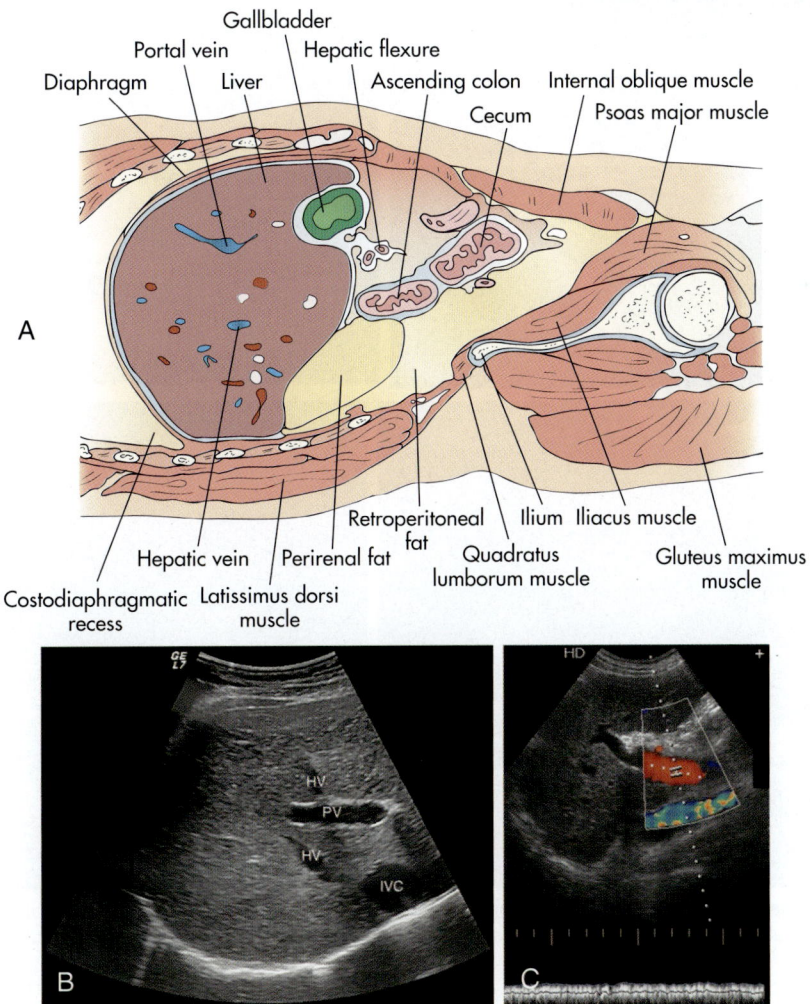

FIG. 5.19 (A) Sagittal section of the abdomen 8 cm from the midline. (B) Sagittal ultrasound image of the right lobe liver, portal vein (PV) hepatic veins (HV), and inferior vena cava (IVC). (C) Color Doppler through the portal vein.

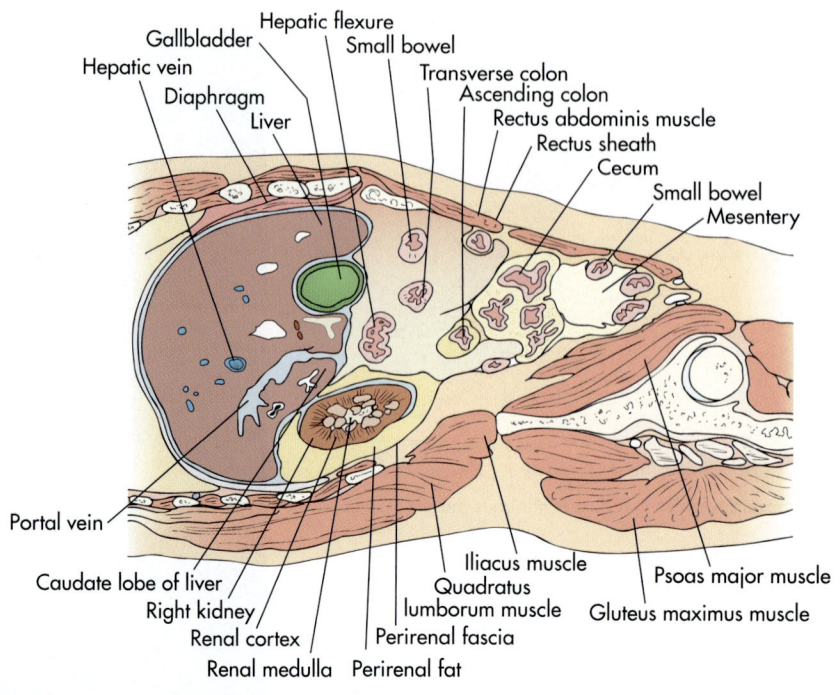
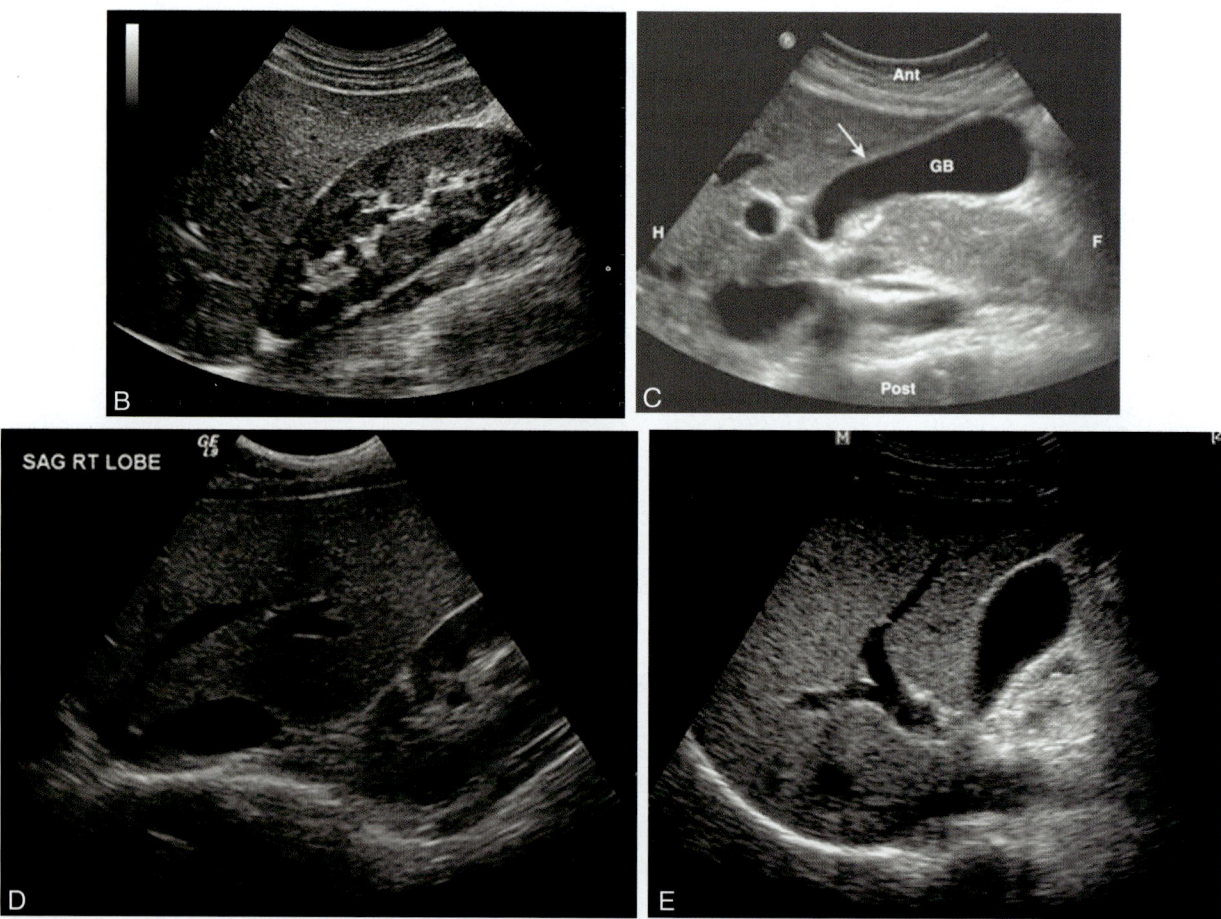

FIG. 5.20 (A) Sagittal section of the abdomen 7 cm from the midline. (B) Longitudinal ultrasound images of right lobe of the liver and right kidney, (C) gallbladder, (D) inferior vena cava, hepatic vein, portal veins, and right kidney, (E) gallbladder (GB) liver, and portal vein.

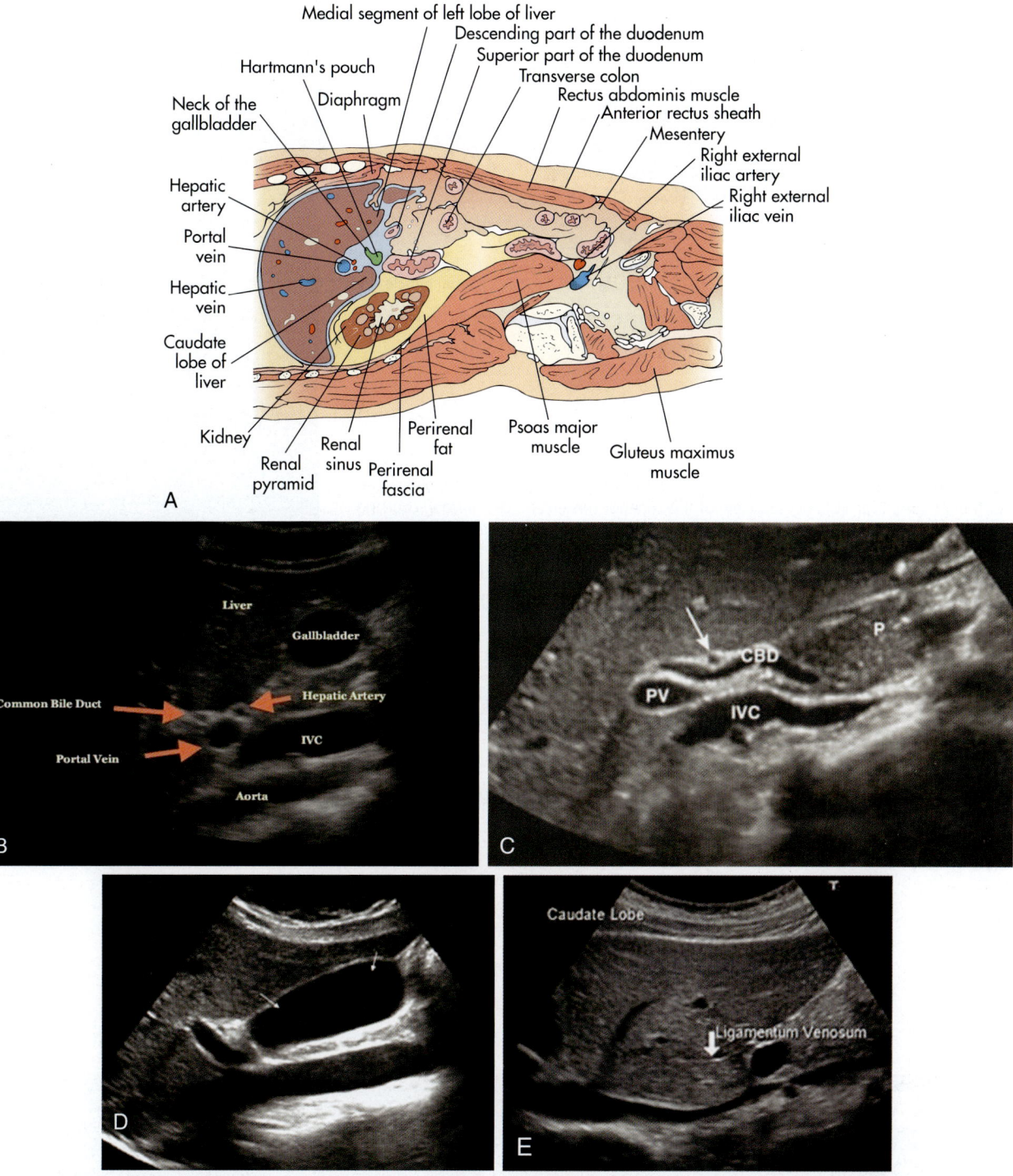

FIG. 5.21 (A) Sagittal section of the abdomen 6 cm from the midline (B) Longitudinal ultrasound of right lobe of the liver and gallbladder. (C) The pancreas (P) is anterior to the IVC. The portal vein (PV) is superior to the pancreas, and the common bile duct (CBD) is anterior to the portal vein. The *arrow* points to the hepatic artery. (D) The two smaller arrows point to the medial gallbladder as seen anterior to the aorta. (E) Note the hepatic vein draining into the inferior vena cava, which is compressed by the caudate lobe. The ligamentum venosum marks the anterior border of the caudate lobe.

120 CHAPTER 5 Comparative Sectional Anatomy of the Abdominopelvic Cavity

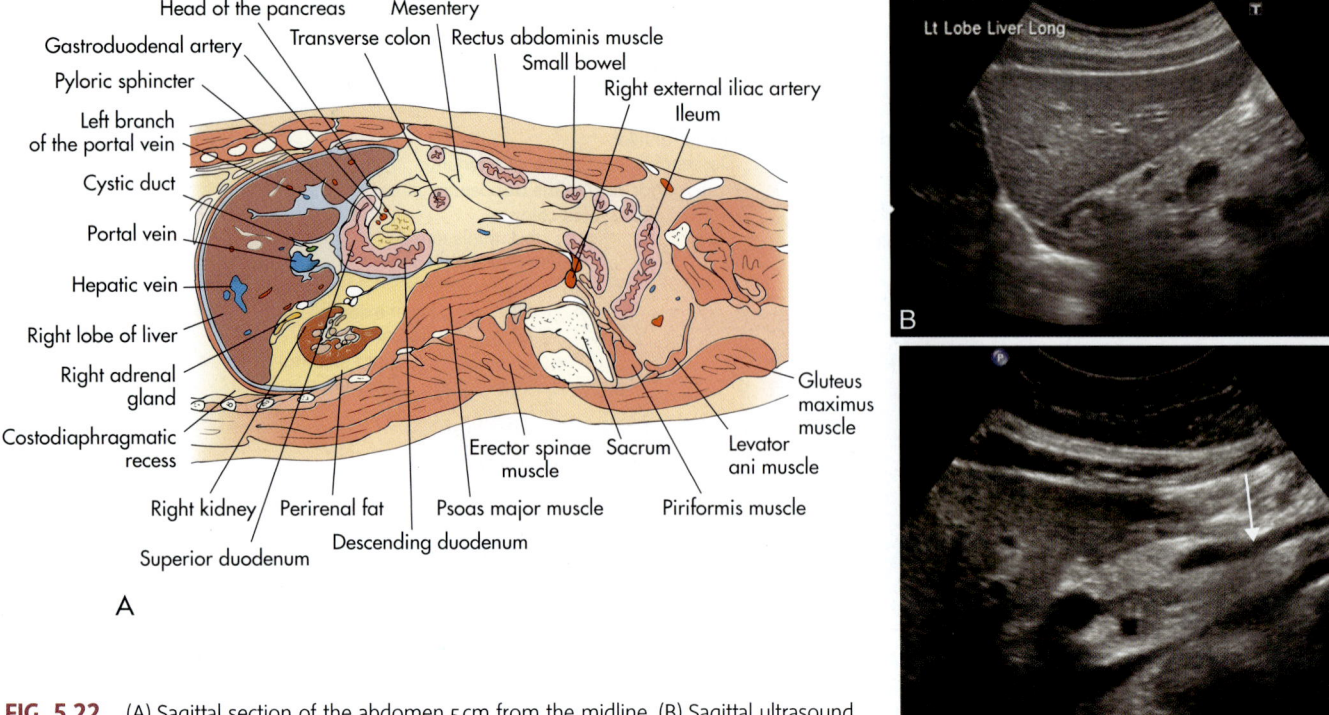

FIG. 5.22 (A) Sagittal section of the abdomen 5 cm from the midline. (B) Sagittal ultrasound image of the left lobe liver. (C) Focused view of the superior mesenteric vein *(arrow)* coursing cephalad with the uncinated process of the pancreas anterior and the body of the gland posterior.

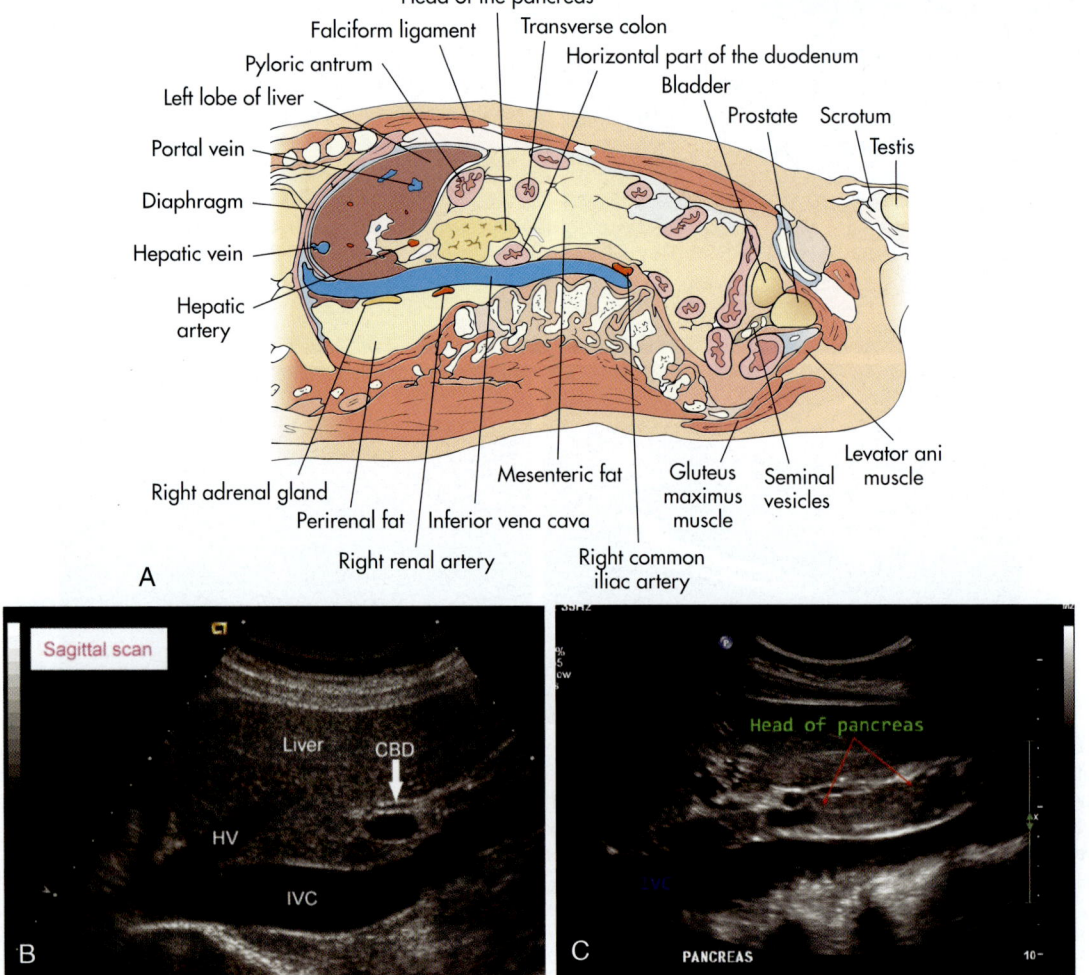

FIG. 5.23 (A) Sagittal section of the abdomen 3 cm from the midline. (B) Sagittal ultrasound image of left lobe liver, hepatic vein (HV), pancreas, inferior vena cava (IVC), and common bile duct (CBD). (C) The head of the pancreas causes hammocking of the inferior vena cava.

CHAPTER 5 Comparative Sectional Anatomy of the Abdominopelvic Cavity

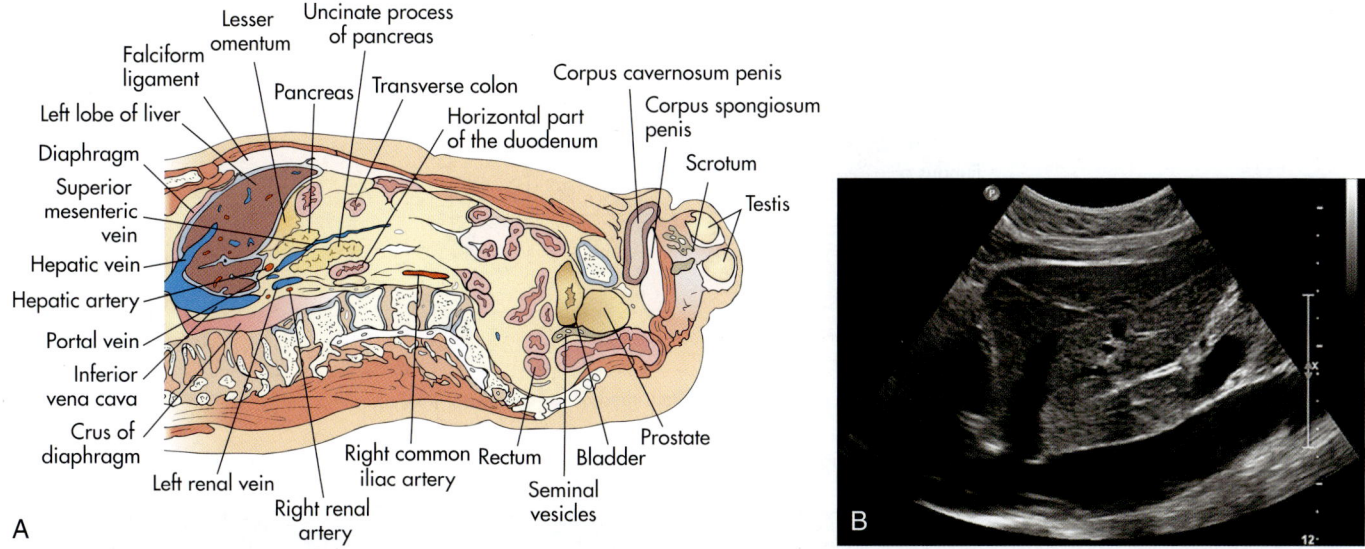

FIG. 5.24 (A) Sagittal section of the abdomen 5 cm from the midline. (B) Sagittal ultrasound image of the patient in full inspiration shows the left lobe of the liver, inferior vena cava, portal vein, and hepatic vein.

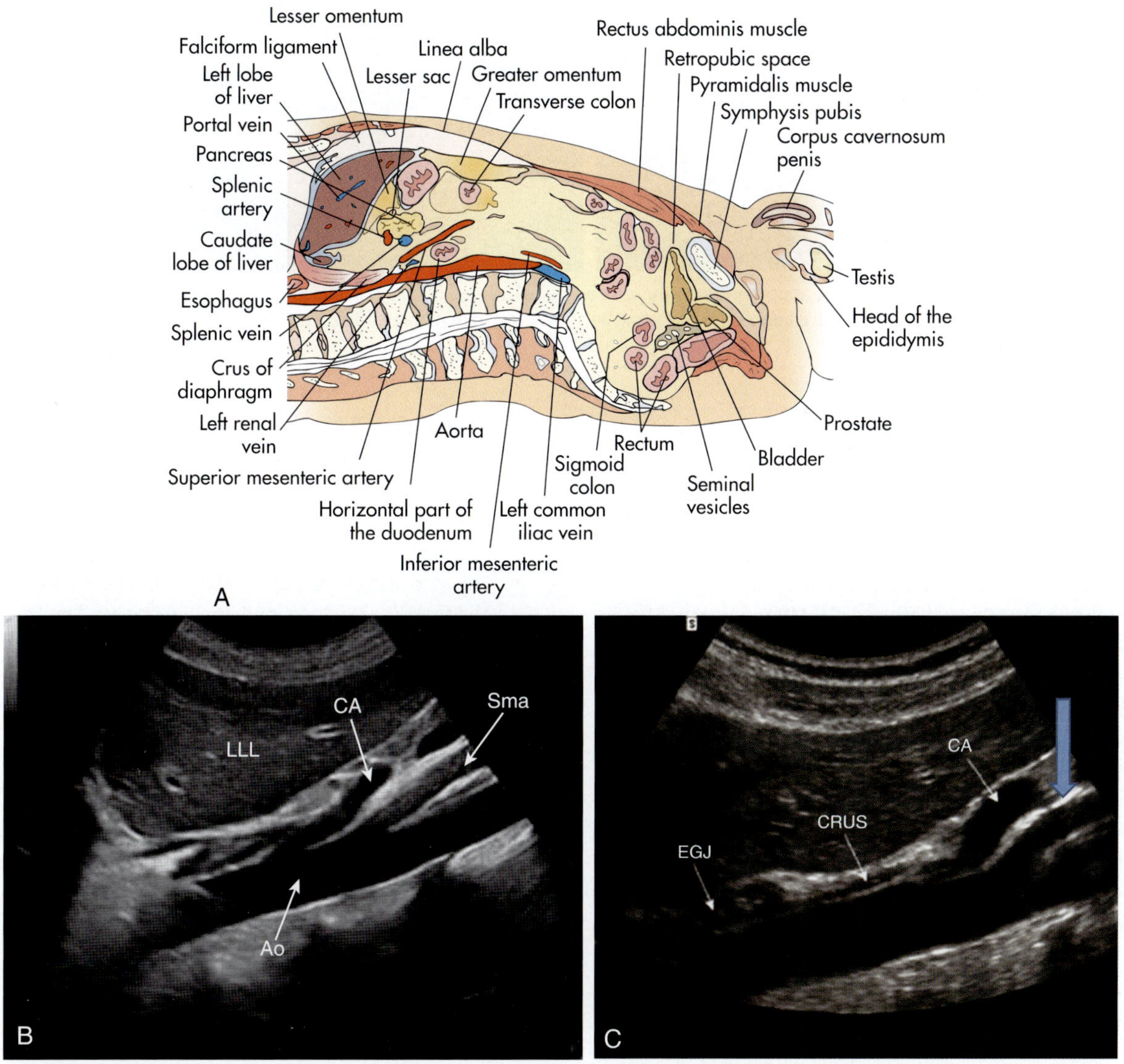

FIG. 5.25 (A) Midline sagittal section of the abdomen. (B) Sagittal ultrasound image of the left lobe of liver, aorta, celiac artery, and superior mesenteric artery (Sma). (C) The esophageal gastric junction (EGJ) and crus of the diaphragm are well seen. *CA*, Celiac artery.

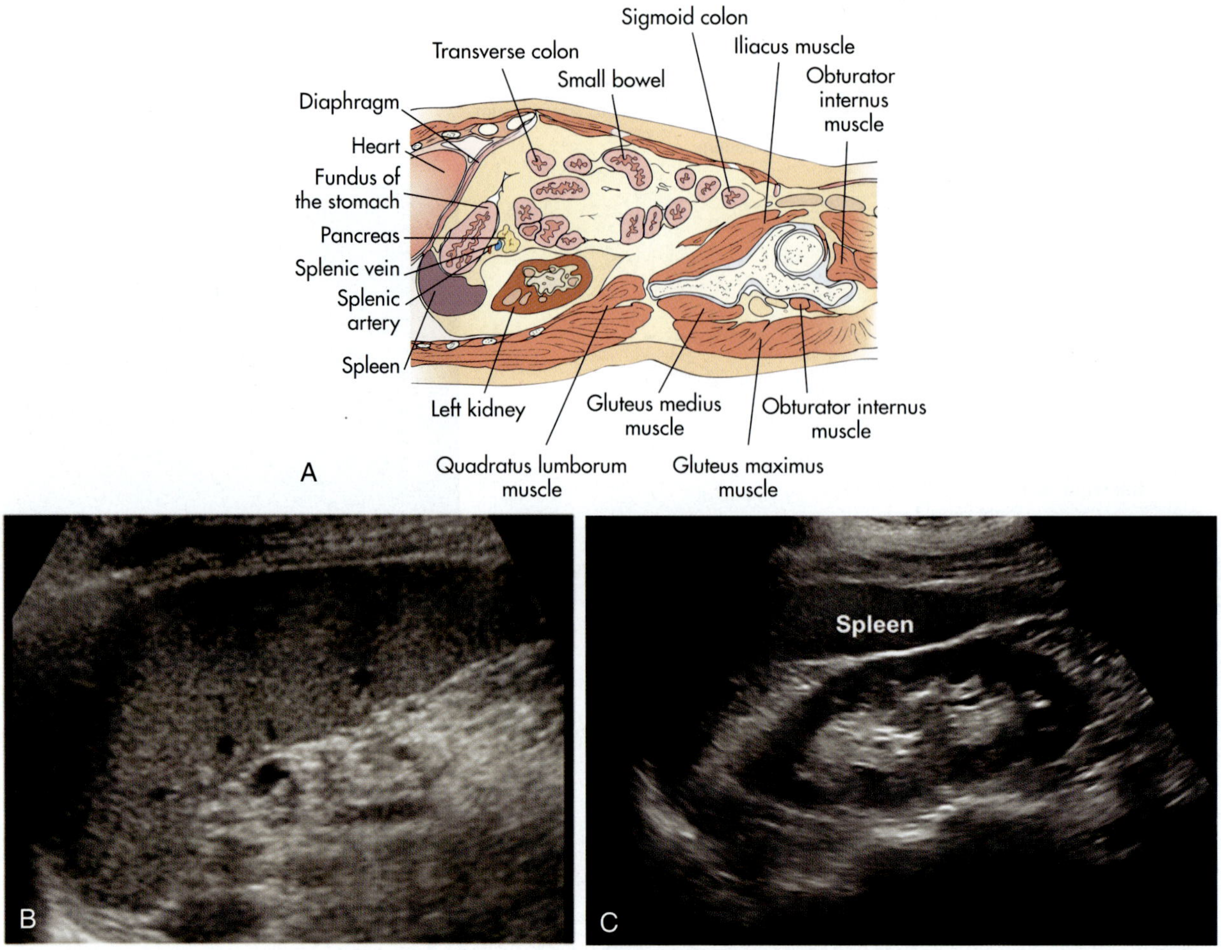

CHAPTER 5 Comparative Sectional Anatomy of the Abdominopelvic Cavity

FIG. 5.26 (A) Sagittal section of the abdomen along the left abdominal border. (B) Sagittal ultrasound image of the spleen and air-filled stomach. (C) Sagittal image with medial angulation of the probe shows the spleen and left kidney. Note the homogeneity of the spleen compared with the liver.

Key Pearls

1. Ultrasound is often preferred as a first imaging examination for nonemergent problems over computed tomography, which involves ionizing radiation, or magnetic resonance imaging (MRI), which is both time consuming and costly.
2. Each imaging modality (ultrasound, CT, MRI) approaches the problem from a specific standpoint, using differing physical properties of the normal tissue and pathologic lesions to derive image contrast and resolve important details.
3. Ultrasound and MRI both have a safety advantage in that they do not use ionizing radiation.
4. CT scanning and general diagnostic (x-ray) imaging both image the body using ionizing radiation.
5. The transverse plane is horizontal to the body. This plane divides the body or any of its parts into upper and lower portions.
6. The sagittal plane is a lengthwise plane running from front to back. It divides the body or any of its parts into right and left sides, or two halves; this is known as the midsagittal plane.
7. The longitudinal plane is parallel to the long axis of the body or part.
8. The coronal plane is a lengthwise plane running from side to side, dividing the body into anterior and posterior portions.
9. To identify specific abdominal structures or refer to an area of pain, the abdominopelvic cavity may be divided into four quadrants and nine abdominal regions.
10. The four quadrants include the right upper quadrant, left upper quadrant, right lower quadrant, and left lower quadrant.
11. The nine abdominal regions include the following: (1) upper abdomen/right hypochondrium, (2) epigastrium, (3) left hypochondrium, (4) middle abdomen/right lumbar, (5) umbilical, (6) left lumbar, (7) lower abdomen/right iliac fossa, (8) hypogastrium, and (9) left iliac fossa.

BIBLIOGRAPHY

Kelley LL, Petersen CM. *Sectional Anatomy for Imaging Professionals*. 2nd ed. St. Louis: Elsevier; 2007.

Moses KP, Banks JC, Nava PB, Petersen D. *Atlas of Clinical Gross Anatomy*. St. Louis: Elsevier; 2005.

Snell RS. *Clinical Anatomy*, 7th ed. Philadelphia: Lippincott, Williams & Wilkins; 2004.

Swobodnik W, Herrmann M, Altwein J. *Atlas of Ultrasound Anatomy: Normal Anatomy as the Basis of Sonographic Diagnosis*. New York: Thieme; 1991.

Yokochi C, Rohen JW, Weinreb EL. *Photographic Anatomy of the Human Body*. 3rd ed. New York: Igaku-Shoin; 1989.

CHAPTER 6

Basic Ultrasound Imaging: Techniques, Terminology, and Tips

Sandra L. Hagen-Ansert

OBJECTIVES

On completion of this chapter, you should be able to:
- Describe the scanning techniques used in abdominal scanning
- State how to properly label a sonogram
- List the criteria for identifying abnormalities
- Explain terminology used to describe the results of ultrasound examinations
- Define the criteria for an adequate scan
- Identify abdominal sectional anatomy in the transverse and longitudinal planes
- Describe the use of Doppler in the abdomen, including Doppler scanning techniques for abdominal vessels

OUTLINE

Before You Begin To Scan
Patients 124
   Orientation to the Clinical Laboratory 124
   Written Order for the Examination 125
   Documentation for the Ultrasound Examination 125
   Scanning Techniques 125
   Patient Preparation 125

Patient Positions 125
Transducer Selection 125
Knobology 126
Transducer Positions 126
Annotation 128
Artifacts 129
Indications For Abdominal Sonography 129
Ultrasound Terminology 129
Identifying Abnormalities 131

Anatomic Directions 132
Criteria for an Adequate Scan 134
General Abdominal Ultrasound Protocols 134
   Initial Survey of the Abdomen 134
   Transverse Scans 135
   Longitudinal Scans 140
Abdominal Doppler 141
   Doppler Scanning Techniques 145

KEY TERMS

Curved array transducer
Fan
Macro movement
Micro movement

Portal venous system Protocol
Rock
Rotate
Scan window

Sector array transducer
Slide
Sweep

The production of a high-quality sonographic image is an art that demands many talents of the sonographer: a high degree of manual dexterity and hand-eye coordination; the ability to conceptualize two-dimensional (2D) information into a three-dimensional (3D) format; and a thorough understanding of anatomy, physiology, pathology, instrumentation, artifact recognition, and transducer characteristics. The sophistication of ultrasound systems requires a greater understanding of the physical principles of ultrasound and computers than ever before. Moreover, sonographers should incorporate Doppler techniques, color flow mapping, tissue harmonics, strain analysis, and 3D imaging to understand better anatomy and physiology related to hemodynamic blood flow and reconstruction.

Although one-on-one, hands-on training in a clinical setting is an essential part of the sonographer's experience of producing high-quality scans, this chapter will take you on a journey toward mastering the foundations of abdominal scanning. Correlation of ultrasound images with sectional anatomy is critical for producing consistent, quality images. This chapter will present the approach to general abdominal ultrasound. Specific organ protocols will be presented in their respective chapters. You may find the protocol for an abdominal scan to differ slightly between ultrasound departments; the key is to develop a protocol that is within the national practice guidelines, such as the American Institute of Ultrasound in Medicine (AIUM) or American College of Radiology and to maintain such protocol for all patients consistently. The protocol presented here is generic and may be adapted to the particular laboratory situation. Also included in this chapter are special scanning techniques and specific applications of abdominal scanning.

BEFORE YOU BEGIN TO SCAN PATIENTS

Remember that your goals as a sonographer are to produce diagnostic images that the physician can interpret to answer a clinical question, to create diagnostically useful images, and to be familiar with ultrasound instrumentation and the clinical considerations of the patient examination. Clinical considerations include knowing which patient position should be used for specific examinations, transducer selection and scanning techniques, patient breathing techniques, and how to perform a sonographic survey of the abdomen.

Be sure you are very familiar with various types of ultrasound equipment. Know where the operator's manual is and how to find what you need in the manual. (Every manufacturer places the power supply in a different position, so make sure you know how to turn the machine on and off.) Become familiar with the transducers available for each machine, how to activate the transducers, and how to change transducers; some of the plug-in formats take some practice to master. Know where the critical knobs are that operate the ultrasound instrumentation (e.g., time gain compensation [TGC], power, gain, depth, angle, focus, Doppler, color flow). Know where the annotate text keys are for labeling the image. If the ultrasound equipment is new to you, it may be a good idea to use a team approach as one sonographer manipulates the controls while the other sonographer acquires the images until you become comfortable with the equipment.

It is highly recommended that the student sonographer practice in a supervised laboratory setting (away from patients) or with one of the anatomic mannequin/ultrasound models before working with patients. This way, the student sonographer can become familiar with the ultrasound equipment by scanning phantoms or even "building" their own phantoms to be scanned.

The next step should be for one student to scan the other students in the sonography laboratory. This step allows the experience of feeling how cold that gel is when applied to the abdomen and knowing what the probe feels like with different individual scan techniques. (Most laboratories are equipped with gel warmers to avoid that patient discomfort.) The student can see firsthand how a *light* touch does not make as pretty an image as a moderate touch with the transducer adjacent to the skin; also, the student may experience the agony of the *heavy hand* as the transducer scrapes across the rib cage. The student will also learn how much scanning gel is the right amount: It is too much gel if it drips down your wrist and onto your clothes.

Controlled supervised scanning should also emphasize how important it is for the patient to take a breath or suspend breathing to obtain the highest quality images. A recommended patient breathing technique tip is to have the patient inhale through the nose to reduce the amount of air going into the stomach. *Breathing is probably the weakest learning link for the student.* Careful control of respiration is critical for making a beautiful scan versus an image that is not easy to interpret.

The student sonographer should also begin to learn the specific **protocols** required for each examination. Nationally recognized protocols for all areas of ultrasound have been developed by the American College of Radiology (www.acr.org) and the AIUM (www.aium.org) for ultrasound examinations. Likewise, the American College of Obstetricians and Gynecologists (www.acog.org) has developed ultrasound protocols for the female patient. The American Society of Echocardiography (www.asecho.org) has developed extensive guidelines for all areas in echocardiography. The Society for Vascular Ultrasound (www.svt.org) has established protocols and guidelines for specific vascular examinations. Each of these protocols can be found on the websites of the respective organizations.

Students may be overwhelmed at first with the detail these protocols require and may not completely remember all the steps in the protocols when they first begin their clinical scanning experience. Some equipment manufacturers have built a Smart Examination Protocol into the equipment; once activated, the system will direct the sonographer to the next required view. Suggested steps to help the student master the protocols are included in the workbook that accompanies this textbook.

Orientation to the Clinical Laboratory

A new student in the clinical ultrasound laboratory may be overwhelmed at first with the control panel on the ultrasound system, the hand-eye coordination required to produce an image, understanding the probe orientation and translation of right from left on the monitor, and the protocol necessary for the particular examination. The following suggestions may make your entrance into the clinical world a little smoother:

- Know all the ultrasound equipment in your laboratory. This means that every free minute should be spent with the equipment, finding the correct knobs necessary to perform the examination. Know where the depth, gain, 2D, color, M-mode, harmonics, and TGC controls are located.
- Know where the operator's manuals are for each piece of equipment so you may have a reference for troubleshooting.
- Find out what protocols are used for each examination. Most departments have a Standard Manual of Protocols for all their examinations.
- Understand how to read the patient order, determine what question the ordering physician needs to have answered, and know which items in the patient records are relevant for patient identification.
- When you call for patients, be sure to check their ID with at least two identifiers (i.e., name and birth date, doctor who ordered the examination, type of examination ordered).

- Introduce yourself and briefly explain the procedure you are going to do. Also, explain the department's procedure to notify the patient's physician of the examination results.
- Know the pertinent questions to ask a patient prior to the ultrasound examination, e.g., "Is this the first imaging study?" "Do you know why your physician sent you for an ultrasound?" "Do you have any specific pain or symptoms?" "Have you had previous surgery?"
- Always keep your conversation professional. Remember that you need to focus on the examination.
- Discuss the case only with your mentor or with the physician responsible for interpreting the study.

Written Order for the Examination

An electronic or written order by the health care provider will indicate the reason for the ultrasound examination. This order should contain the appropriate clinical information relevant to the patient to provide the necessary information from the ultrasound procedure to the clinician.

Documentation for the Ultrasound Examination

Accurate documentation must be made for the ultrasound procedure. There should be a permanent record of the examination and its interpretation available on the electronic medical record or written format. The images obtained from the examination should be recorded in a retrievable format (i.e., picture archiving communication system [PACS] system or disc). Communication of the results must be maintained between the providing physician and the ordering physician.

Scanning Techniques

Ultrasound can distinguish multiple interfaces between soft tissue structures of different acoustic densities. The strength of the echoes reflected depends on the acoustic interface and the angle at which the sound beam strikes the interface. The sonographer must determine which patient "**scan window**" is best to record optimal ultrasound images and which transducer size best fits into that window. The **curved array transducer** provides a large field of view, but in some patients, this transducer may be too large to fit in between the ribs to provide adequate contact for accurate reflection of the sound wave. The smaller diameter or *footprint* transducer allows the sonographer to scan between intercostal spaces with the patient in a supine, coronal, decubitus, or upright position but limits the near field of view. It is not unusual to use multiple transducers on one patient to complete the examination, as transducers are available in multiple sizes and frequencies.

Patient Preparation

It is recommended that the patient fast for 8 hours before the ultrasound examination of the abdomen. Fasting helps to reduce the interference that may be caused by gas overlying the midline abdominal structures. It will also ensure that the gallbladder will be fully distended. If the patient has eaten, it is still possible to perform the general ultrasound examination; however, visualization of all structures may not be as clear.

Patient Positions

The general abdominal examination is performed initially with the patient in the supine position. Additional views may require the oblique, lateral decubitus, prone, and occasionally upright positions to examine specific areas of interest (Fig. 6.1). For example, the gallbladder may be examined with the patient in the supine, oblique, or lateral decubitus positions. These organ-specific positions will be discussed in more detail in their respective chapters.

Transducer Selection

Be aware of the various transducers available for each ultrasound system, and know which transducers are used for specific examinations. Transducers are available in multiple frequencies, shapes, and sizes. Fig. 6.2 illustrates the curved array, linear array, phased array, and **sector array transducers.** An *array transducer* is a transducer assembly with more than one element. Most transducers contain multiple active elements. The real-time array transducers provide rapid and dynamic imaging.

The curved array transducer (Fig. 6.3) provides a large pie sector and is used to survey the abdomen, pelvis, and obstetrical evaluation. This transducer is curved because the piezoelectric crystal arrangement is curvilinear. The curved array transducers combine advantages of the sector and linear formats and are optimally used when the sonographic window is large.

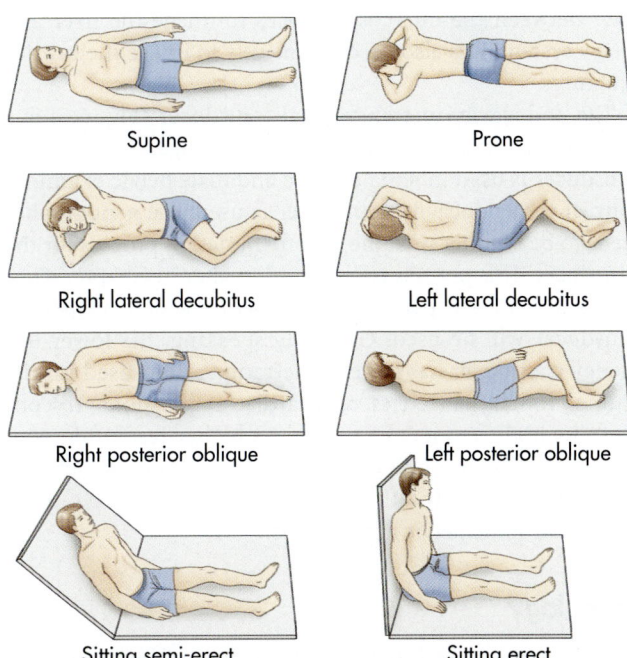

FIG 6.1 Standard patient positions for the ultrasound examination include the supine, prone, decubitus, oblique, and erect positions.

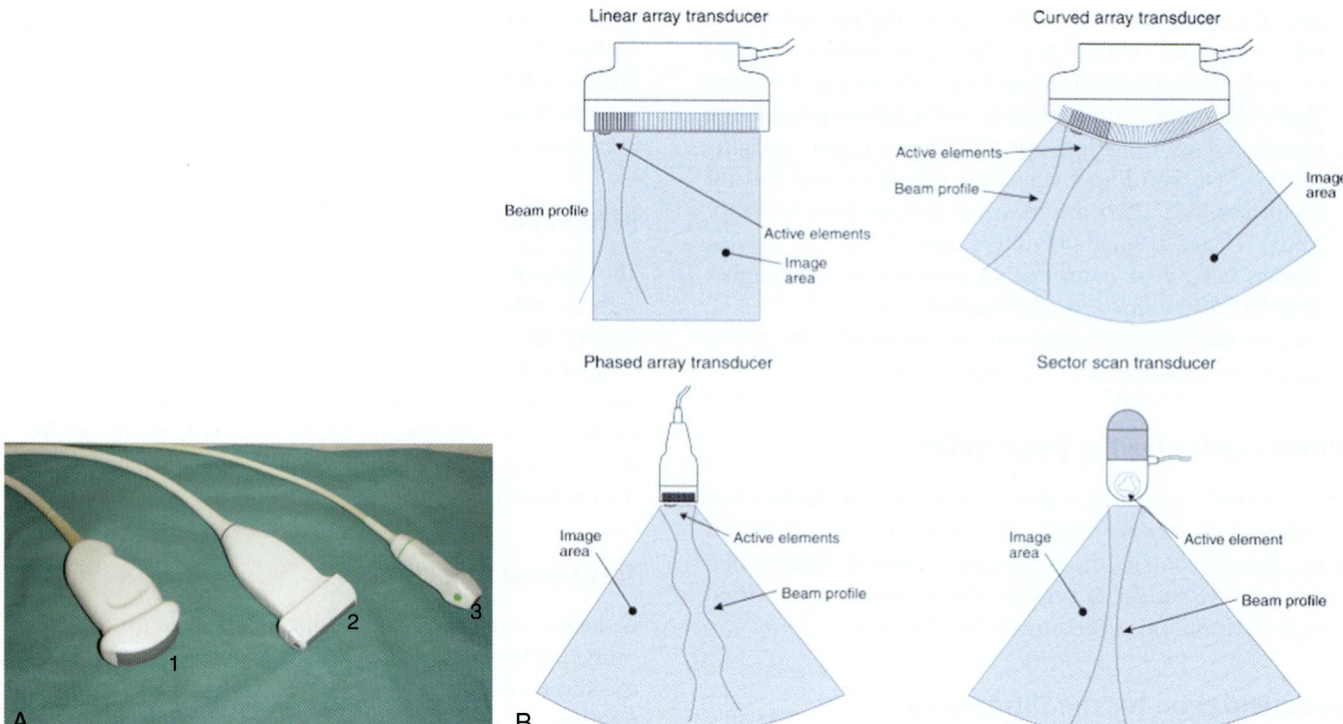

FIG 6.2 (A) *Left to right:* Curved array, linear array, and sector phased array transducers. (B) Diagram of the respective probes showing the transmission pattern.

The linear array transducer (Fig. 6.4) provides a rectangular image of the structure and offers the best overall image quality. The footprint is wide, and the frequency is high (7.5 to 11 MHz); thus, excellent imaging is available for the more superficial structures such as the vascular and musculoskeletal system. A linear, curved array transducer is also available (the piezoelectric crystal arrangement is curvilinear).

The sector phased array (Fig. 6.5) provides a small pie sector of the area. The sector array is useful for finding a "window" between the intercostal spaces to image the liver and biliary system. It is also used extensively to image the cardiac structures.

The endocavity or transvaginal transducer (Fig. 6.6) is a high-frequency crystal mounted on a longer handle. The transducer is used in female pelvic and male pelvic examinations. If the endocavity transducer is used, the sonographer needs to be familiar with the decontamination process for the transducer. This process is discussed further in Chapter 42.

The size of the patient will influence which megahertz transducer will be used. Generally speaking, the lower-frequency transducer has better penetration and is used for the adult abdomen, obstetrics, and cardiac applications. In contrast, the high-frequency probe has a higher resolution with improved axial resolution and is used for more superficial structures such as the thyroid, scrotum, breast, early pregnancy, and some pelvic applications.

Knobology

The sonographer needs to be familiar with the ultrasound control panel to produce an anatomic image (Fig. 6.7). The primary controls include the depth, gain (TGC, lateral gain), frequency, focal zone, modes (2D, M-mode, 3D, pulsed wave [PW] Doppler, continuous wave Doppler, and color Doppler), annotation, and calculation package. Each of these controls has multiple layers of software (tissue harmonics, dynamic compression range, frame rate, scale, baseline, etc.) that the sonographer will learn to manipulate to produce the high-quality image. The location of these knobs will vary with each manufacturer.

Transducer Positions

The sonographer will use multiple wrist actions throughout the study. Remember that the beam is ideally reflected when the transducer is perpendicular to the surface. However, the body has many angles, curves, and rib interferences, causing the sonographer to use intercostal spaces, subcostal windows, multiple degrees of angulation, and many rotations of the transducer to obtain anatomic images (Fig. 6.8).

There are multiple scanning motions that the sonographer needs to master throughout the examination: *sweep, slide, rock or fan, rotate, tilt,* and *compress* (Fig. 6.9). These movements may be large (macro) or small (micro). The **macro movement** of the probe is used with the sweep and slide motion in which the probe is moved greater than 1 cm. Macro movement also occurs if the fan or rock motion changes the angle of insonation by more than 15 degrees in either direction. The **micro movement** of the probe is used with the sweep and slide motion in which the probe is moved less than 1 cm. Micro movement likewise occurs if the fan or rock motion changes the angle of insonation by less than 15 degrees in either direction. It is important to perform only one motion at a time. The movement should be similar every time you have the same scanning window to produce an image consistently.

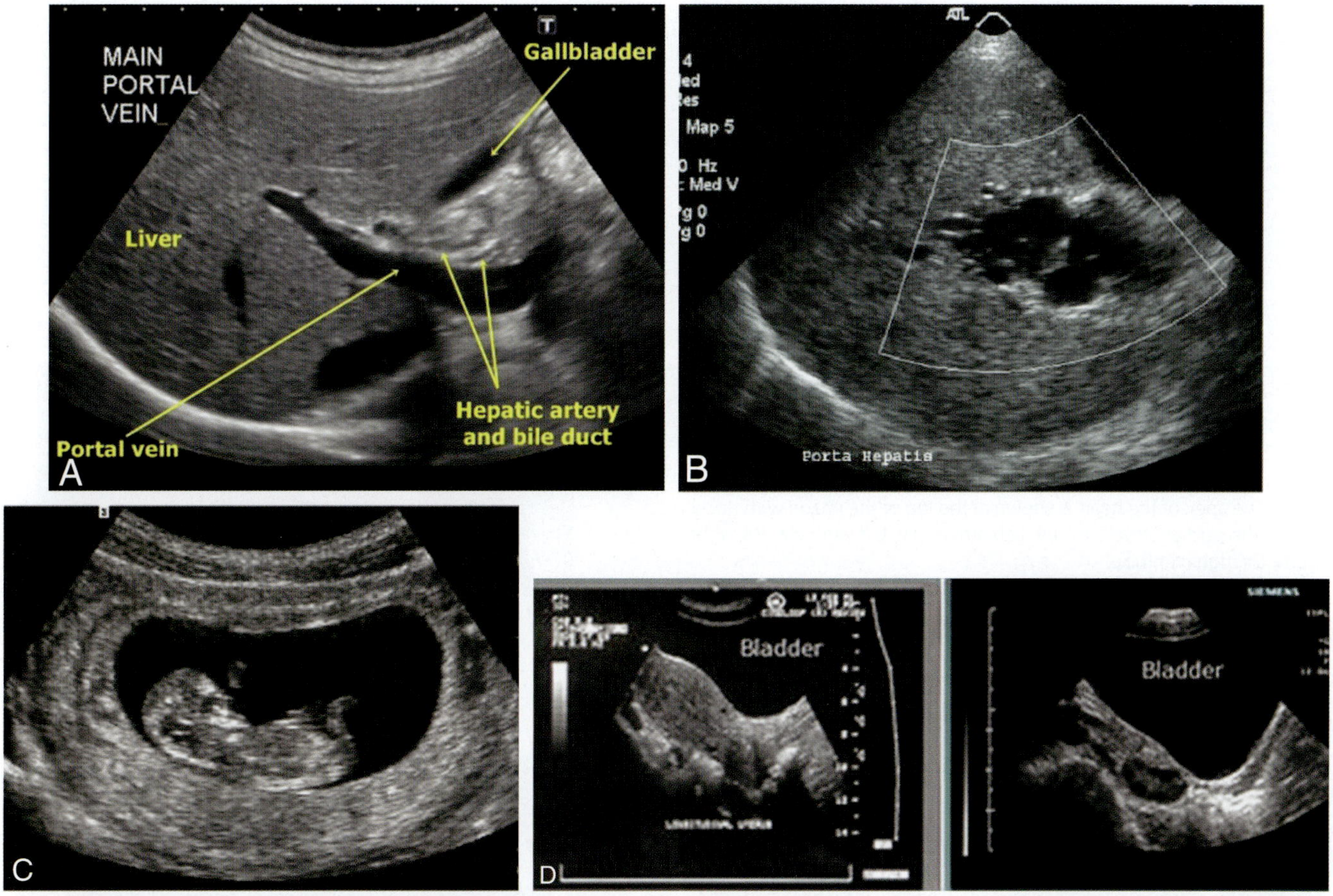

FIG 6.3 Images of the abdomen and pelvis demonstrating the difference between the curved array (A and C) and the sector array (B); note the great near field definition and larger field of view with the curved array transducer (D).

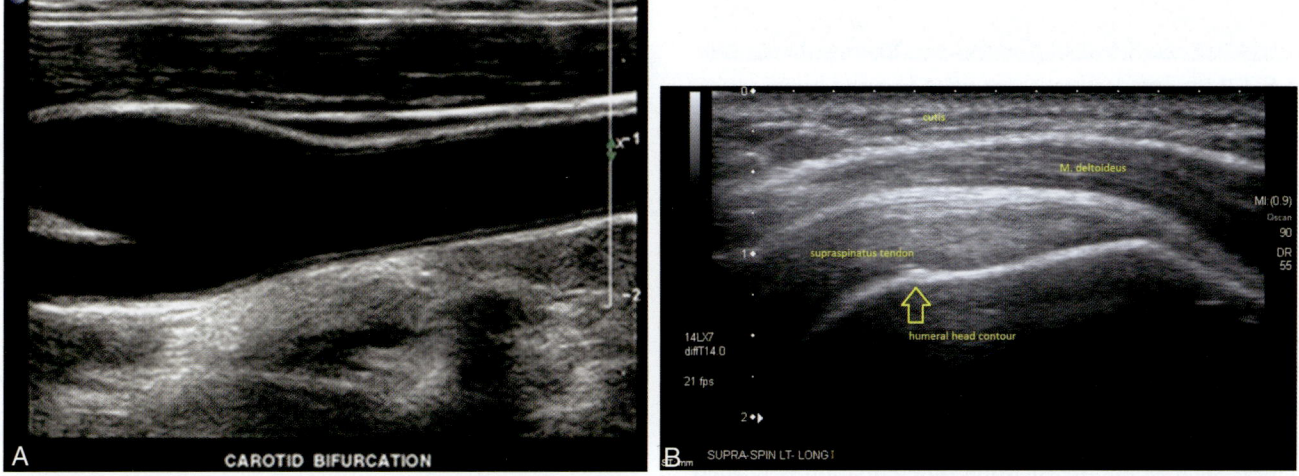

FIG 6.4 Images of the carotid artery bifurcation (A) and the shoulder muscles (B) are well demonstrated with the linear array transducer. Note the detail in the near field with the higher frequency transducer.

In a survey of the abdomen, the sonographer will initially use the **sweep** motion. This requires the transducer to remain in one area while using a large wrist motion with the probe perpendicular to the skin surface to sweep through the abdomen. It is used to locate and interrogate an area of interest or to evaluate the scan windows of abdominal structures before the scan protocol is begun.

The **slide** motion is used when the transducer is physically moved along the abdomen, such as a longitudinal movement to follow the course of the abdominal aorta into the bifurcation of the iliac arteries.

Once an area of interest is located, the sonographer may pause over the structure and slowly rock or pivot the transducer back and forth or up and down to image the area

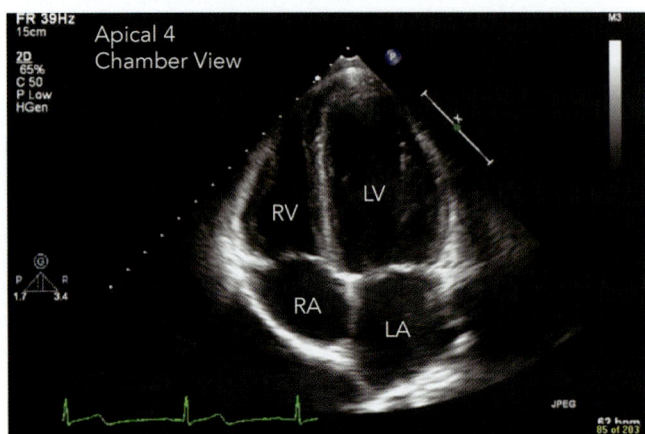

FIG 6.5 **The sector phased array is utilized in echocardiography.** The small sector footprint allows excellent visualization in the intercostal spaces. The apex of the heart is shown at the top of the image with good detail of the cardiac structures. *LA*, Left atrium; *LV*, left ventricle; *RA*, right atrium; *RV*, right ventricle.

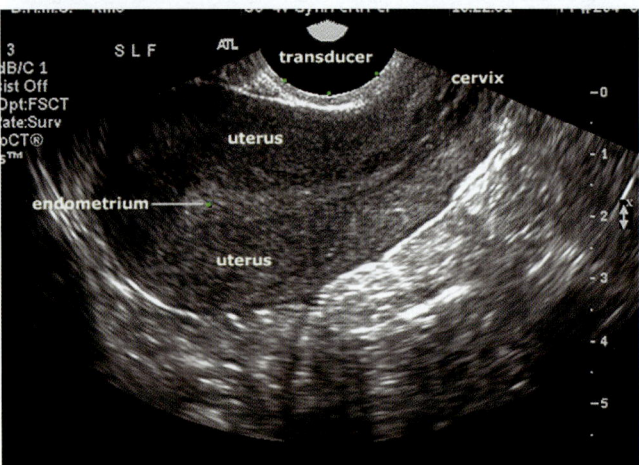

FIG 6.6 The transvaginal probe uses a high frequency to provide excellent detail of the pelvic structures.

entirely or follow the anatomic structure. This is when the "cine" frame capture is useful to record the motion. This may be used to demonstrate the junction of the common bile duct and cystic duct or to track the hepatic artery's communication as it arises from the celiac trunk.

A smaller version of the sweep motion is the **fan** or **rock** motion used when the transducer is minutely swept, pivoting on a point of interest. This may be useful in the superficial structures such as the breast when differentiation is needed between the duct and the invasive lesion within the duct.

The **rotate** motion is useful for navigating between the ribs or changing from transverse to longitudinal planes. The transducer is held in one area and rotated 90 degrees to the opposite plane. Rotate is also used in smaller increments as the transducer is slowly turned around the area of interest.

The **compress** motion is useful when evaluating vascular anatomy to see if the venous structure compresses with gentle pressure, as in a deep venous thrombosis. It may also be useful in evaluating the bowel or appendix area.

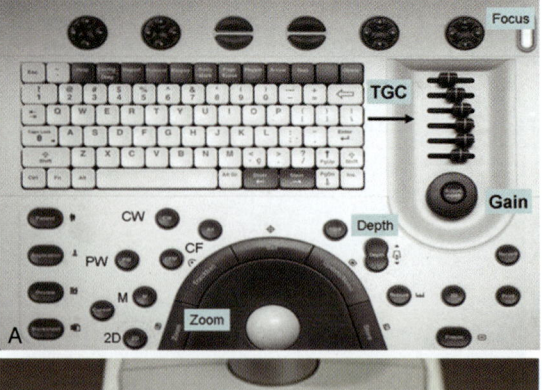

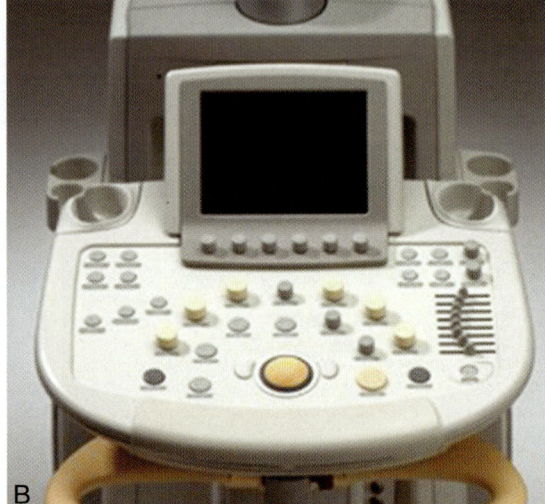

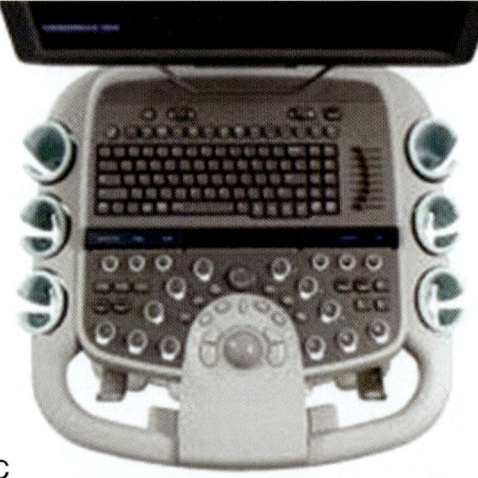

FIG 6.7 (A) The primary controls include the depth, gain (TGC, lateral gain), frequency, focal zone, modes (2D, M-mode, 3D, pulsed wave Doppler, continuous wave Doppler, and color Doppler), annotation, and calculation package. Each of these controls has multiple layers of software (tissue harmonics, dynamic compression range, frame rate, scale, baseline, etc.) that the sonographer will learn to manipulate to produce the high-quality image. (B–C) The location of these controls will vary among the various manufacturers. *PW*, Pulsed wave; *TGC*, time gain compensation.

Annotation

Ultrasound images are labeled as *transverse* or *longitudinal or coronal* for a specific organ, such as the liver, gallbladder, pancreas, spleen, or uterus (Fig. 6.10). The smaller organs that can be imaged on a single plane, such as the kidney, are labeled as

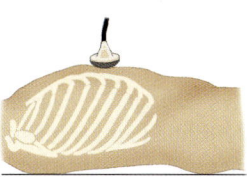

Perpendicular
The transducer is straight up and down.

Subcostal
The transducer is angled superiorly just beneath the inferior costal margin.

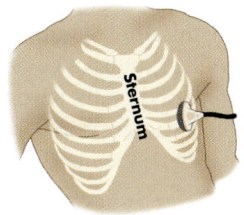

Intercostal
The transducer is between the ribs. It can be perpendicular, subcostal, or angled.

Angled
The transducer is angled superiorly, inferiorly, or right and left laterally at varying degrees.

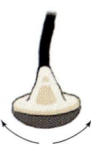

Rotated
The transducer is rotated varying degrees to oblique the scanning plane.

FIG 6.8 The sonographer must utilize a variety of different transducer positions and angulations to complete the ultrasound examination.

long-midline, *-lateral*, or *-medial*, whereas the transverse scans are labeled as *transverse-low*, *-middle*, or *-high*.

All transverse supine scans are oriented with the liver on the left of the monitor; this means that the sonographer will be viewing the body from the feet up to the head ("optimistic view") (Fig. 6.11). Longitudinal scans display the patient's head to the left (superior) and feet to the right (inferior) of the screen and use the xiphoid, umbilicus, or symphysis to denote the midline of the scan plane (Fig. 6.12).

All scans should be appropriately labeled for future reference, including the patient's name, date, and anatomic position. Body position markers are available on many ultrasound machines and may be used in place of written labels.

The patient's position should be described in relation to the scanning table (e.g., a right decubitus would mean the right side down; a left decubitus would indicate the left side down). If the scanning plane is oblique, the sonographer should merely state that it is an oblique view without specifying the exact degree of obliquity.

Artifacts

Sonographers need to learn about ultrasound artifacts early in their learning curve. Sonographers should recognize a few primary artifacts as they begin their scanning experience: reverberation, mirror, side lobe, and shadowing (Fig. 6.13). *Reverberation* artifacts occur between the transducer and a strong reflector such as the rib, causing multiple linear lines equidistant apart. A *mirror* artifact is a form of reverberation that shows structures that exist on one side of a strong reflector as being present on the other side as well; for example, the liver/diaphragm interface may show "liver" tissue in the pleural space. *Side lobe* artifacts are beams that propagate from a single transducer element in directions different from the primary beam, such as those produced by bone or gas. *Shadowing* is the reduction in echo amplitude from reflectors that lie behind a strongly reflecting or attenuating structure; for example, calcified gallstone will cause a "shadow" posterior to the stone. Artifacts found in ultrasound images are discussed in more detail in Chapter 7.

INDICATIONS FOR ABDOMINAL SONOGRAPHY

The AIUM has listed multiple indications for an abdominal sonogram that include, but are not limited to, the following:

- Signs or symptoms that may be referred from the abdominal and/or retroperitoneal regions such as jaundice or hematuria
- Generalized abdominal, flank, or back pain
- Palpable mass or organomegaly
- Abnormal laboratory values or abnormal findings on other imaging modalities
- Follow-up of known or suspected abnormalities in the abdomen or retroperitoneum
- Search for metastatic disease or occult primary neoplasm
- Evaluation of suspected congenital abnormalities
- Trauma to the abdomen or retroperitoneum
- Pretransplant and posttransplant evaluation
- Invasive procedure localization
- Localization for free or loculated peritoneal, pleural, or retroperitoneal fluid
- Suspicion of hypertrophic pyloric stenosis or intussusception
- Evaluation of a urinary tract infection

The request for an abdominal or retroperitoneal sonographic examination needs to provide sufficient information to demonstrate the medical necessity of the examination with allowance for proper performance and interpretation.

The documentation that must be met for medical necessity includes the following items: (1) patient signs and symptoms and (2) previous history pertinent to the examination requested. Additional information such as the specific reason for the examination or a provisional diagnosis would be helpful and may aid in the proper performance and interpretation of the examination. This will allow the sonographer to tailor the examination to answer the question from the ordering physician.

ULTRASOUND TERMINOLOGY

The sonographer is responsible for reviewing the patient's request for the ultrasound examination and for discussing any specific requests with the referring physician. Therefore a familiarity with basic medical terminology and abbreviations is necessary.

Transducer Movements

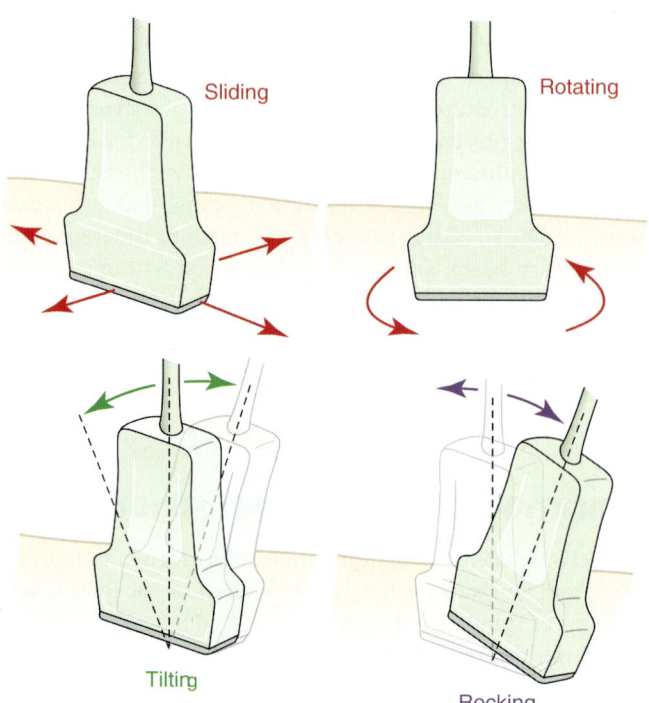

FIG 6.9 There are multiple scanning motions that the sonographer needs to master throughout the examination: *sweep, slide, rock or fan, rotate, tilt,* and *compress.*

One of the sonographer's primary responsibilities is the identification and description of normal and abnormal anatomy. The following list of terms is universally accepted and will help the sonographer describe the results obtained from various ultrasound examinations:

Anechoic or sonolucent: Opposite of echogenic; without internal echoes; the structure is fluid filled and transmits sound easily (Fig. 6.14A). Examples: vascular structures, distended urinary bladder, gallbladder, and amniotic cavity.

Echogenic or hyperechoic: Opposite of anechoic; echo-producing structure; reflects sound with a brighter intensity (Fig. 6.14B). Examples: gallstone, renal calyx, bone, fat, fissures, and ligaments.

Enhancement, increased through-transmission: Sound that travels through an anechoic (fluid-filled) substance and is not attenuated; brightness is increased directly beyond the posterior border of the anechoic structure compared with the surrounding area—this is "enhancement" (see Fig. 6.14A).

Fluid-fluid level: Interface between two fluids with different acoustic characteristics; this level will change with patient position. Example: dermoid tumor with fluid level.

Heterogeneous: Not uniform in texture or composition (Fig. 6.14C). Example: Many tumors have characteristics of both decreased and increased echogenicity.

Homogeneous: Opposite of heterogeneous; completely uniform in texture or composition (Fig. 6.14D). Example: The textures of the liver, thyroid, testes, renal parenchyma, and myometrium are generally considered homogeneous.

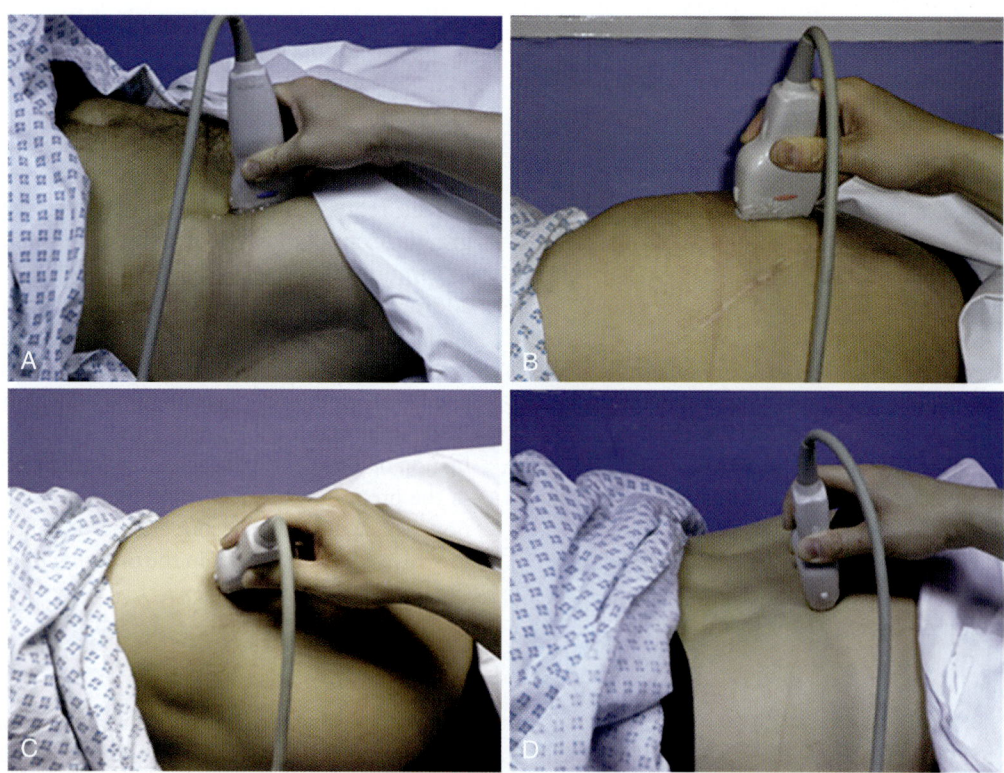

FIG 6.10 Ultrasound images are labeled as *transverse* (D), *longitudinal* (B), or *coronal* (A and C) for a specific organ, such as the liver, gallbladder, pancreas, spleen, or uterus.

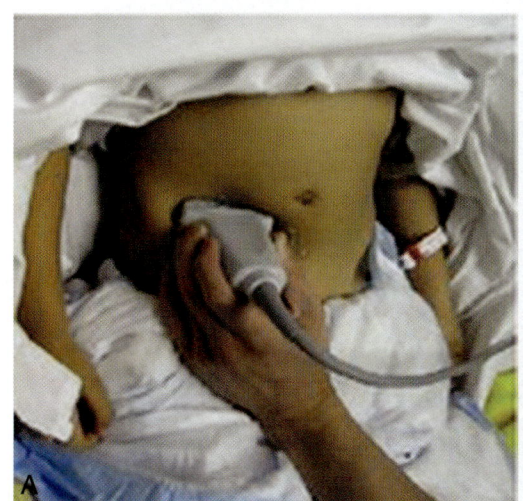
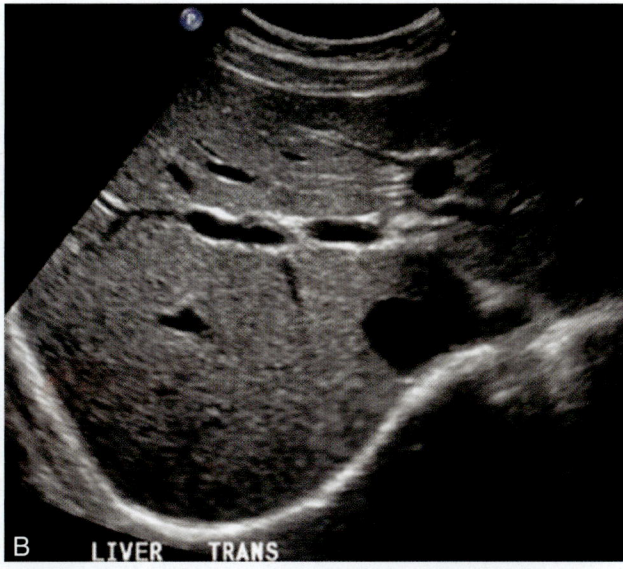

FIG 6.11 (A–B) All transverse supine scans are oriented with the liver on the left of the monitor; this means that the sonographer will view the body from the feet up to the head ("optimistic view").

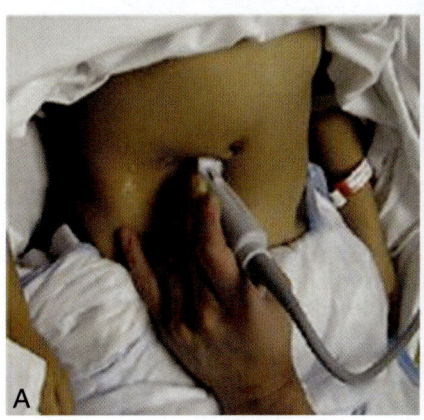
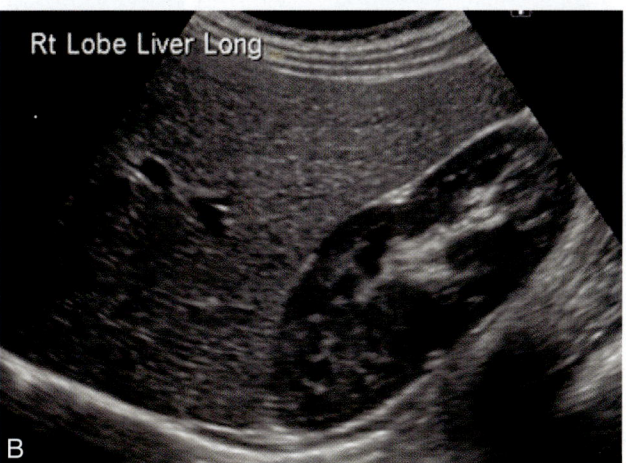

FIG 6.12 (A–B) Longitudinal scans display the patient's head to the left (superior) and feet to the right (inferior) of the screen and use the xiphoid, umbilicus, or symphysis to denote the midline of the scan plane. The notch on the transducer is pointed towards the patient's head.

Hypoechoic: Low-level echoes within a structure (Fig. 6.14E). Examples: lymph nodes and fibroma.

Infiltrating: Usually refers to a diffuse disease process or metastatic disease (Fig. 6.14F). Examples: carcinoid or sarcoid infiltration.

Irregular borders: Borders are not well defined, ill-defined, or not present (Fig. 6.14G). Examples: abscess, thrombus, and metastases.

Isoechoic: Very close to the normal parenchyma echogenicity pattern (Fig. 6.14H). Example: metastatic disease.

Loculated mass: Well-defined borders with internal echoes; the septa may be thin (likely benign) or thick (likely malignant) (Fig. 6.14I).

Shadowing: The sound beam is attenuated by a solid or calcified object. This reflection or absorption may be partial or complete; air bubbles in the duodenum may cause a "dirty shadow" to occur secondary to reflection; a stone would cause a sharp shadow posterior to its border (see Fig. 6.14B).

IDENTIFYING ABNORMALITIES

Careful evaluation for the presence of pathology is incorporated into the general abdominal protocol. The sonographer needs to be able to demonstrate the normal anatomic structures and the pathology that may invade or surround such structures. The abnormality is identified and evaluated according to several criteria, including the border definition, internal texture, tissue characteristics, and transmission of sound, which are listed in Box 6.1 and illustrated in Fig. 6.15.

The internal composition may further identify pathology as cystic, complex, or solid (Box 6.2). A cystic mass has a well-defined, smooth border; internally, the lesion is anechoic with increased through sound transmission beyond its posterior border (Fig. 6.16). A solid mass has irregular borders, internal echoes (echogenic), and decreased through-transmission (Fig. 6.17). A complex mass has characteristics of both a cyst and a solid lesion. Transmission characteristics

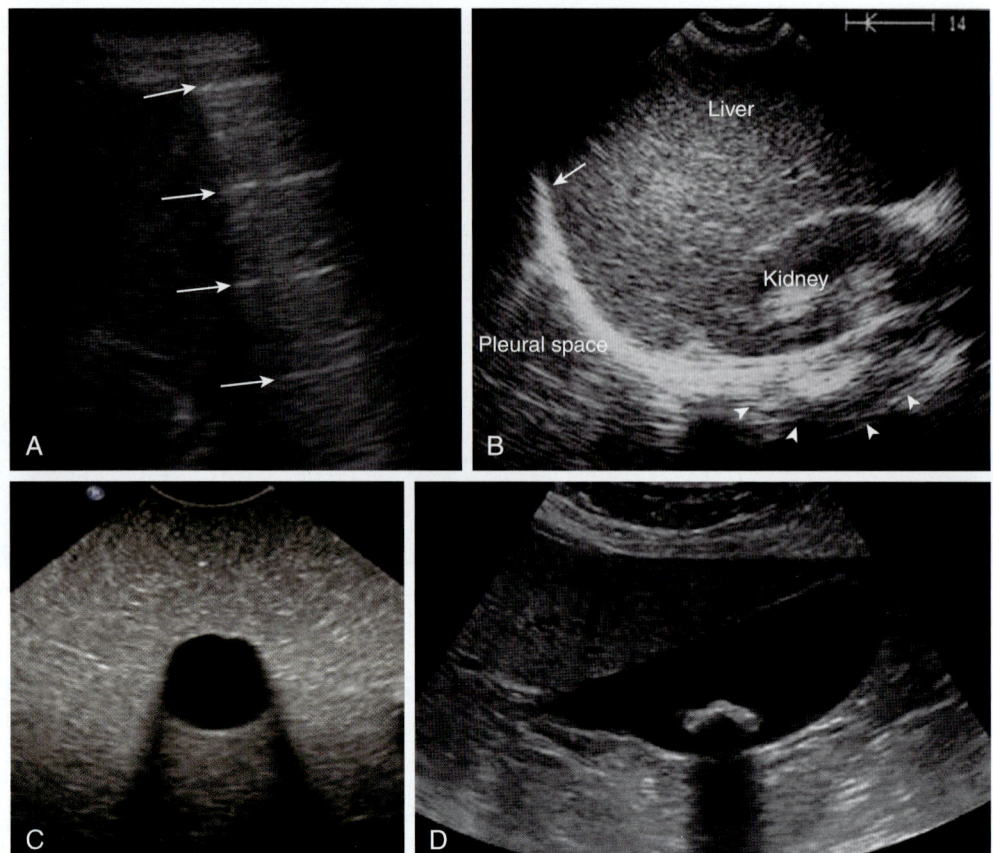

FIG 6.13 Artifacts. (A) *Reverberation* artifacts occur between the transducer and a strong reflector, such as the rib causing multiple linear lines equidistant apart *(arrows)*. (B) A *mirror* artifact is a form of reverberation that shows structures that exist on one side of a strong reflector as being present on the other side as well; for example, the liver/diaphragm interface may show "liver" tissue in the pleural space. (C) *Side lobe* artifacts are beams that propagate from a single transducer element in directions different from the primary beam, such as those produced by bone or gas. (D) *Shadowing* is the reduction in echo amplitude from reflectors that lie behind a strongly reflecting or attenuating structure; for example, calcified gallstone will cause a "shadow" posterior to the stone.

are determined by how easily the sound is able to transmit through the mass. Transmission is altered depending on what the mass is composed of pathologically. Throughout the chapters of this text, gross pathologic specimens will be included to provide the sonographer with a better understanding of these principles.

ANATOMIC DIRECTIONS

The anatomic position assumes that the body stands erect, the eyes look forward, and the arms are at the sides with the palms and toes directed forward. Refer to Fig. 6.18 for the five anatomic directions of the body discussed here.

1. **Superior/inferior.** The top of the head is the most superior point of the body. The inferior point of the body is the bottom of the feet. All anatomic structures are designated relative to these two terms. The liver is considered to be superior to the bladder because the liver is closer to the head. The gallbladder is inferior to the diaphragm because it is closer to the feet. Other terms that are interchanged with *superior* are *cephalic* and *cranial* (toward the head). *Caudal* (toward the tail) is sometimes used instead of *inferior*.
2. **Anterior/posterior.** The front (belly) surface of the body is anterior or *ventral*. The back surface of the body is posterior or *dorsal*. This concept is very important to sonographers and their understanding of sectional anatomy. If the patient is lying supine (face up), the aorta is anterior to the vertebral column. The right kidney is posterior to the head of the pancreas.
3. **Medial/lateral.** The body axis is an imaginary line from the center of the top of the head to the groin. *Medial* is described as the superior-inferior body axis as it goes right through the midline of the body. Structures are said to be medial if they are closer to the body's midline than to another structure (e.g., the hepatic artery is medial to the common duct). The structure is *lateral* if it is toward the side of the body (e.g., the adnexae are lateral to the uterus).
4. **Proximal/distal.** When a structure is closer to the body midline or point of attachment to the trunk, it is described as *proximal* (e.g., the hepatic duct is proximal to the common bile duct). *Distal* means farther from the midline or

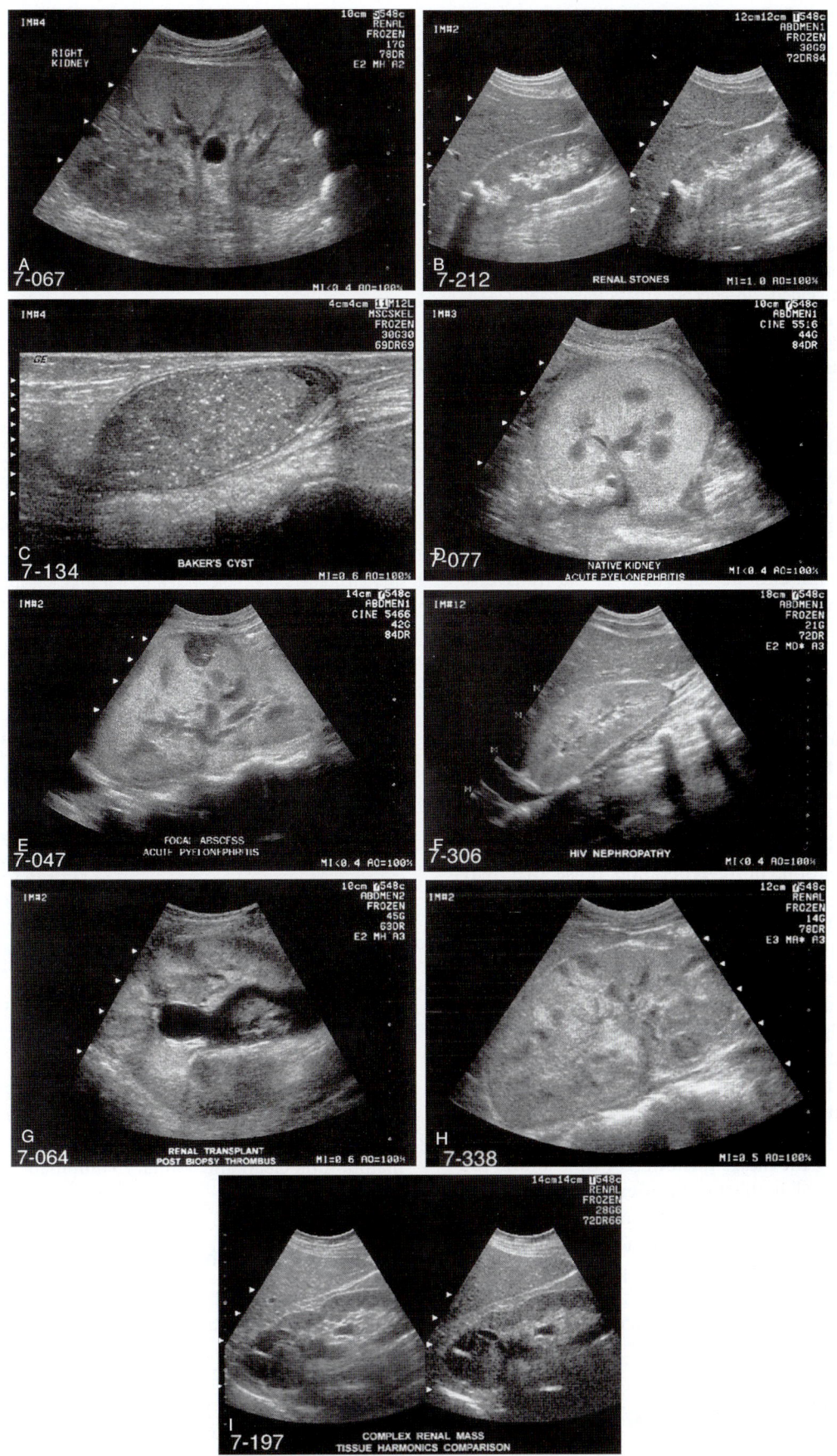

FIG 6.14 (A) Anechoic (simple cyst). (B) Echogenic (stone with shadowing). (C) Heterogeneous (Baker cyst with a mixture of fluid, debris, and bright echo reflectors). (D) Homogeneous (renal parenchyma). (E) Hypoechoic (hemorrhagic cyst). (F) Infiltrating (HIV systemic disease process involving the kidney). (G) Irregular borders (thrombus within the renal pelvis). (H) Isoechoic (one-half of renal parenchyma has lower-level echoes). (I) Loculated (complex renal mass with septations).

| BOX 6.1 | Ultrasound Criteria for Identifying Abnormal Structures |

Border. Border of the structure may be smooth and well defined or irregular.
Texture. Texture (parenchyma) of the structure may be homogeneous or heterogeneous.
Characteristic. Characteristic of an organ or a mass is said to be anechoic, hypoechoic, isoechoic, hyperechoic, or echogenic to the rest of the parenchyma.
Transmission. Transmission of sound may be increased, decreased, or unchanged. An anechoic mass (fluid-filled cyst) will show increased sound transmission, whereas a dermoid tumor (composed of muscle, teeth, and bone) will show decreased transmission.

point of attachment to the trunk (e.g., the sphincter of Oddi is distal to the common bile duct).

5. **Superficial/deep.** Additionally, structures may be identified as being superficial or deep. Structures located close to the surface of the body are *superficial*. The rectus abdominis muscles are superficial to the transverse abdominis muscles. Structures located farther inward (away from the body surface) are *deep*.

CRITERIA FOR AN ADEQUATE SCAN

With real-time ultrasound, it is sometimes difficult to become oriented to all the anatomic structures on a frozen image; it is therefore critical to obtain as many landmarks of the anatomy as possible in a single image. Make every effort to avoid rib interference to eliminate artifactual ring-down, attenuation, or reverberation noise that may distort anatomic information. Most abdominal surveys are performed with the curved array multi-hertz transducer. Although the small-footprint sector array transducer allows the sonographer to scan in between the ribs, it limits the near-field visualization. Variations in the patient's respirations may also help eliminate rib interference and improve image quality. The sonographer can easily see in real-time how much interference is caused by patient breathing and can ask the patient to take in a breath and hold it or to stop breathing at critical points to capture particular parts of the anatomy. Observing the image form in real-time allows the sonographer to see what effect respiration will have on the image. If the left upper quadrant is not adequately imaged, the patient may be given water to fill the stomach. As the patient is rolled into a right decubitus position, the fluid flows from the body of the stomach to fill the antrum and duodenum, allowing the head of the pancreas and great vessels to be imaged.

GENERAL ABDOMINAL ULTRASOUND PROTOCOLS

It is the responsibility of the sonographer to ensure that patients are afforded the highest-quality care possible during

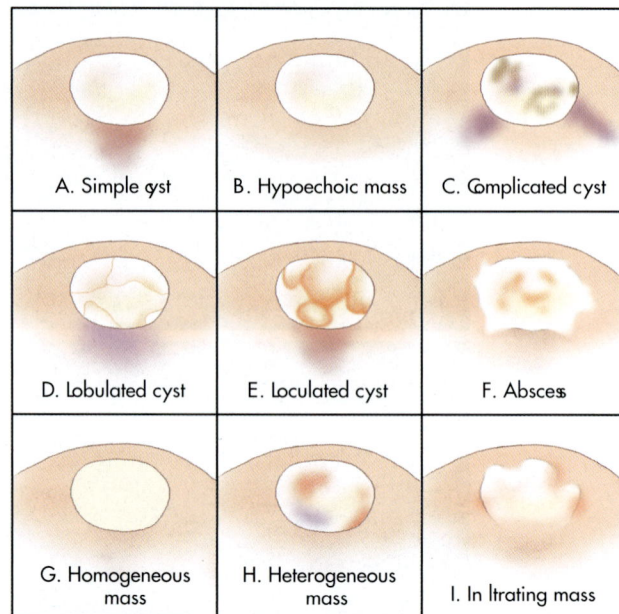

FIG 6.15 Ultrasound criteria for describing a mass. (A) Simple cyst: smooth borders, anechoic, increased transmission. (B) Hypoechoic mass: few to low-level internal echoes, smooth border, no increased transmission. (C) Complicated cyst: mixed pattern of cystic and solid, fluid, debris, and blood; transmission may or may not increase. (D) Lobulated cyst: well defined with thin septa, increased transmission. (E) Loculated cyst: well defined with thick septa. (F) Abscess: may have irregular borders, debris within, transmission may or may not be increased. (G) Homogeneous mass: uniform texture within. (H) Heterogeneous mass: nonuniform texture within. (I) Infiltrating mass: distorted architecture, irregular borders, decreased transmission.

| BOX 6.2 | Abnormal Structures That Affect Transmission |

Cyst: Has smooth, well-defined borders, anechoic, increased through-transmission.
Complex: Has characteristics of both a cyst and a solid structure.
Solid: Irregular borders, internal echoes, decreased through-transmission.

their sonographic examination. This entails identifying the patient properly, ensuring the confidentiality of information and patient privacy, providing proper nursing care, and maintaining clean and sanitary equipment and examination rooms.

Initial Survey of the Abdomen

The upper abdomen is imaged with high-resolution real-time ultrasound equipment. As discussed previously, the transducer may be a sector or curved linear array or, in many cases, a combination of the two. The frequency of the transducer used depends on the patient's size, muscle, and fat composition. Generally, a broad-bandwidth transducer is used, with variations of 2.25 to 7.5 MHz, depending on the size of the patient and the depth of field. All organs are routinely imaged in at least two planes: transverse and longitudinal.

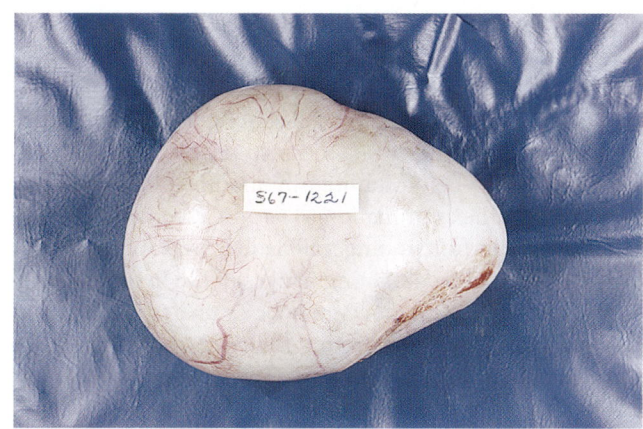

FIG 6.16 Gross pathology of a simple ovarian cyst showing well-defined smooth borders; straw-colored fluid was found inside the mass.

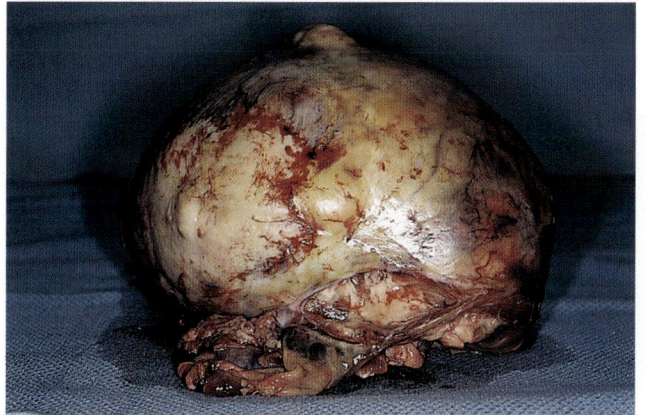

FIG 6.17 Gross pathology of a solid ovarian mass with irregular borders; the mass was filled with complex tissue.

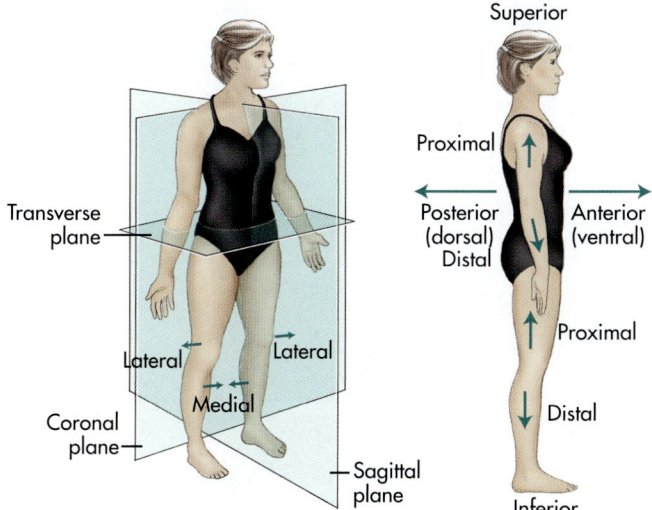

FIG 6.18 The anatomic position assumes that the body is standing erect, the eyes are looking forward, and the arms are at the sides with the palms and toes directed forward.

The baseline abdominal ultrasound examination may include the complete abdomen and/or retroperitoneal space, a single organ, or several organs. A combination of structures may be imaged because of their location or function. For example, the upper abdominal scan includes a survey of the liver and porta hepatis, vascular structures, biliary system, pancreas, kidneys, spleen, and para-aortic area. A functional focused scan may include the liver, gallbladder, and bile ducts. A follow-up or focused examination is generally performed once a complete baseline scan has been made. An established protocol (such as established by the AIUM) should be used. The baseline upper abdominal ultrasound examination includes a survey of the liver and porta hepatis, vascular structures, biliary system, pancreas, kidneys, spleen, and para-aortic area. If variations in anatomy or pathology are seen, multiple views are obtained over the area of interest.

Before you begin the protocol for the specific examination, take a minute to survey the abdomen by using the sweep motion. Remember to ask the patient to take in a deep breath for this survey. This will allow you to see how the patient images appear with "routine" instrument settings, to observe where the organs are in relationship to the patient's respiration pattern, and to see if the patient has a good scanning window in the supine position, or if the patient position needs to be moved into a decubitus or upright position.

In a general abdominal survey, ask the patient to take a deep breath; begin at the xiphoid level in the midline with the transducer angled steeply toward the patient's head (cephalic) to be perpendicular to the diaphragm. With the transducer fixed at the xyphoid, slowly angle the transducer inferiorly to sweep through the liver, gallbladder, head of the pancreas, and right kidney. The transducer may then be redirected in the same manner, only angled toward the left shoulder with a gradual angulation made inferiorly, to see the stomach, spleen, pancreas, and left kidney. Likewise, a quick survey of the abdomen may be done with the transducer in the midline sagittal position. Always remember to ask the patient to take in a breath and hold it. Image the aorta first with the vertebral column posterior to the aorta. Then slowly angle the transducer to the right to image the dilated inferior vena cava (suspended respiration allows the inferior vena cava to fill with blood returning to the heart) and liver. Continue to angle toward the right to image the right lobe of the liver, gallbladder, and right kidney. If adequate penetration is seen with balanced TGC and overall gain adjustments, you can proceed with the routine protocol for the abdominal study.

Transverse Scans

In the transverse plane, the sonographer should adjust the depth of the field of view with the depth knob on the ultrasound system control panel. The gain should be adjusted so that the homogeneous liver parenchyma is uniform in texture. The homogeneous echogenicity of the liver parenchyma should be compared with the right kidney. The echogenic horseshoe-shaped contour of the vertebral column should be well delineated to ensure adequate sound penetration is present through the abdominal structures without obstruction from bowel gas interference.

With the patient in deep inspiration, the posterior border of the liver should be imaged as the transducer is angled in a cephalic direction and slowly swept from the diaphragm/dome of the liver to its inferior edge (Fig. 6.19). This will ensure that the TGC is correctly adjusted with a gradual increase to boost the echoes of the deeper tissue along the posterior border of the liver. The overall gain should be adjusted to provide uniform homogeneous liver parenchyma throughout. If too many echoes are seen "outside the liver," the overall gain should be decreased. If the near gain or TGC is set too low, the anterior surface of the liver will not be delineated. The liver should be evaluated for focal and/or diffuse abnormalities. The vascular structures within the liver should be well demonstrated to include the hepatic veins, main portal vein with right and left branches, and inferior vena cava. The right, left, and caudate hepatic lobes should be demonstrated (Fig. 6.20). The right hemidiaphragm and pleural space may be seen posterior to the right lobe of the liver with steep cephalic angulation of the transducer.

In addition to the supine views, the gallbladder and biliary system will require additional oblique, decubitus, and upright views to demonstrate the anatomy (see Fig. 6.20E–F). The patient must be on nothing-by-mouth status for at least 8 hours before the examination to permit adequate distention of the normally functioning gallbladder. Intrahepatic ducts may be evaluated by obtaining images of the liver and portal veins. The intrahepatic ducts may be evaluated by obtaining views of the liver demonstrating the right and left branches of the portal vein; these ducts are not well seen until they are dilated.

All areas of the pancreas should be evaluated (head, body, tail). The distal common bile duct in the pancreatic head

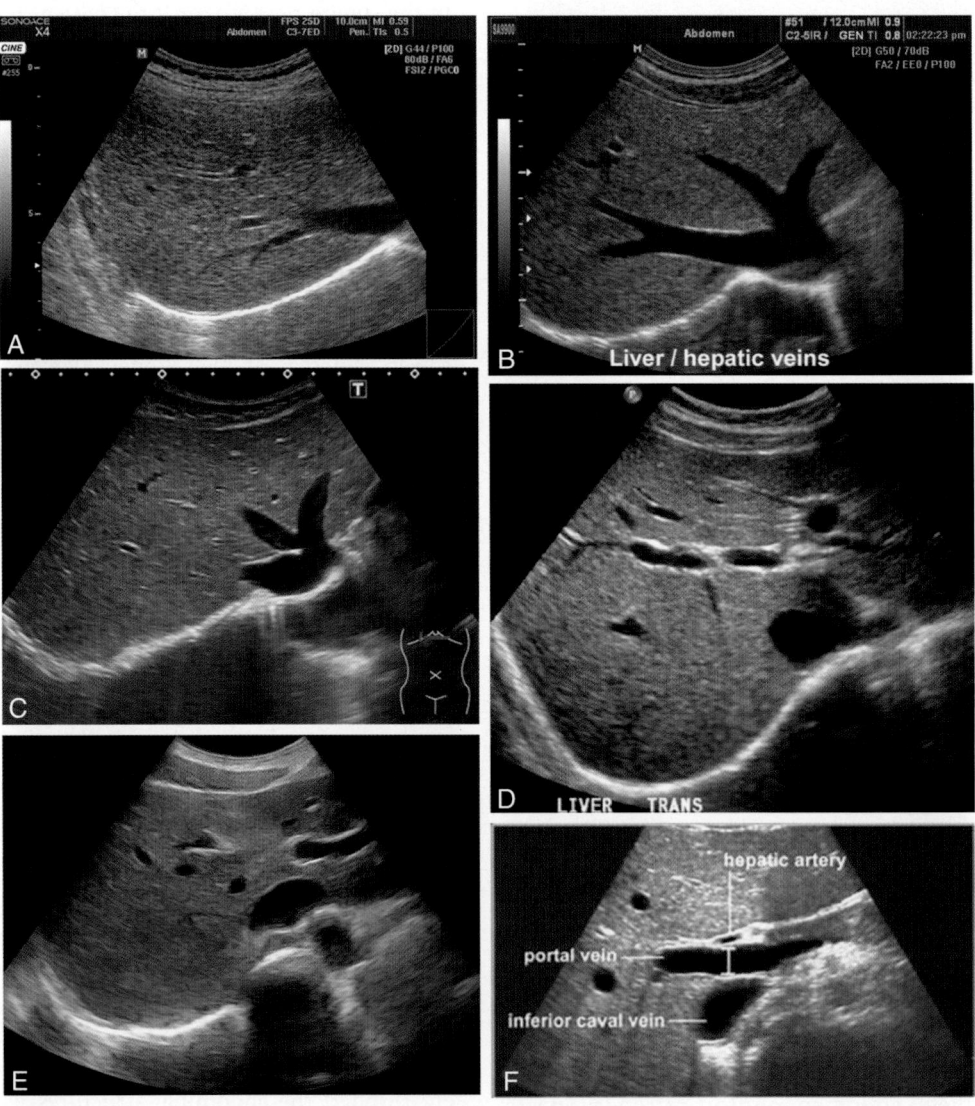

FIG 6.19 (A) Transverse image of the right lobe of the liver at the liver/lung interface. (B–C) Transverse image at the dome of the liver in full inspiration to demonstrate the hepatic veins (HV) flowing into the inferior vena cava (IVC). (D) Transverse image of the liver, main portal vein (MPV), and right portal vein with bifurcation of anterior (ARPV) and posterior (PRPV) branches. (E) Left portal vein in left lobe of liver. (F) Transverse image of liver, inferior vena cava, main portal vein, and hepatic artery.

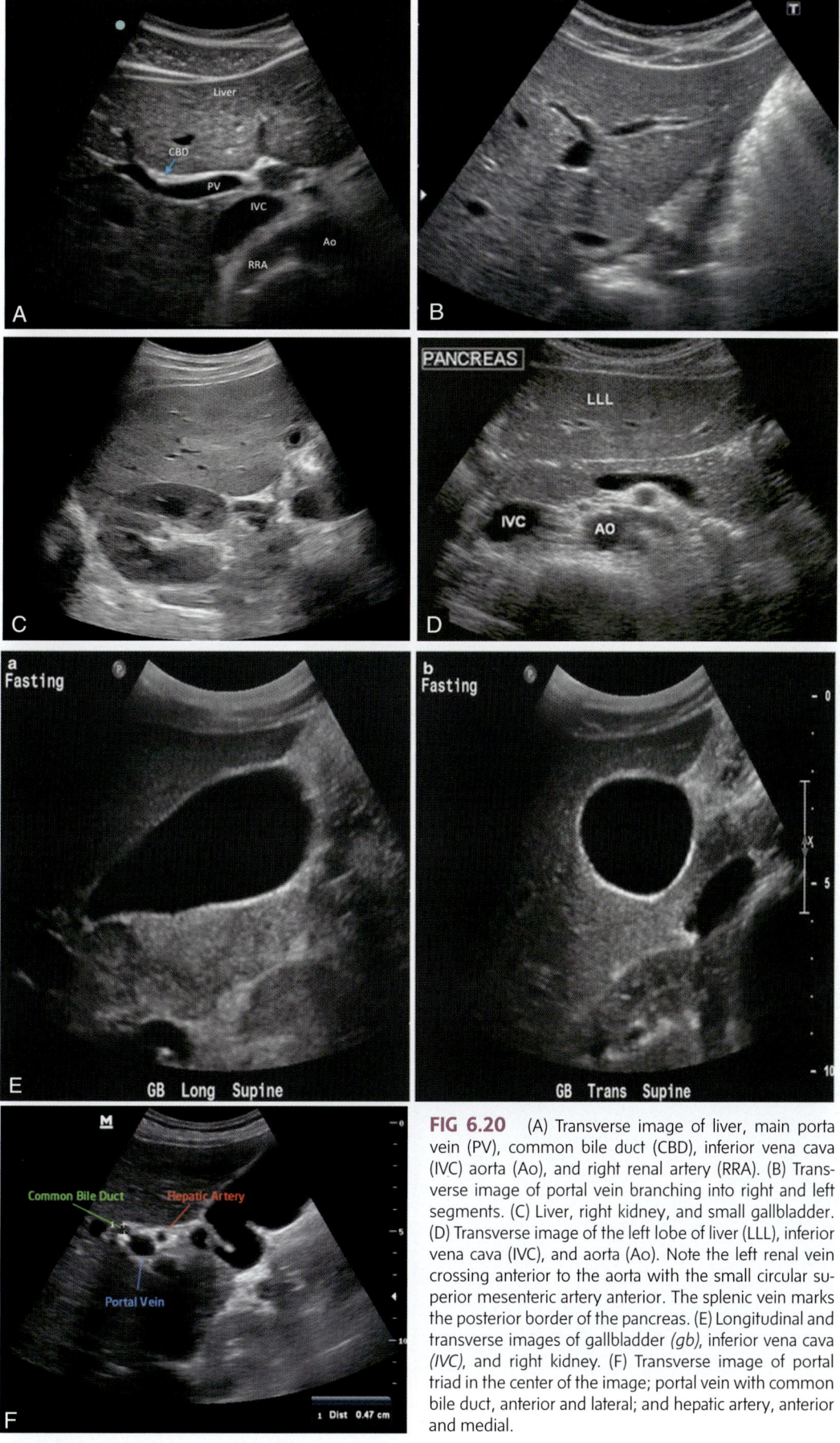

FIG 6.20 (A) Transverse image of liver, main porta vein (PV), common bile duct (CBD), inferior vena cava (IVC) aorta (Ao), and right renal artery (RRA). (B) Transverse image of portal vein branching into right and left segments. (C) Liver, right kidney, and small gallbladder. (D) Transverse image of the left lobe of liver (LLL), inferior vena cava (IVC), and aorta (Ao). Note the left renal vein crossing anterior to the aorta with the small circular superior mesenteric artery anterior. The splenic vein marks the posterior border of the pancreas. (E) Longitudinal and transverse images of gallbladder *(gb)*, inferior vena cava *(IVC)*, and right kidney. (F) Transverse image of portal triad in the center of the image; portal vein with common bile duct, anterior and lateral; and hepatic artery, anterior and medial.

should also be evaluated—this is best seen on the transverse view (Fig. 6.21). If the pancreas is not clearly seen, oral contrast agents or water may be administered to provide better visualization.

The aorta, inferior vena cava, and other vascular structures should be well seen anterior to the vertebral column as echo-free, or anechoic, structures (Fig. 6.22). The aorta is usually found as the pulsatile vessel slightly to the left of the midline.

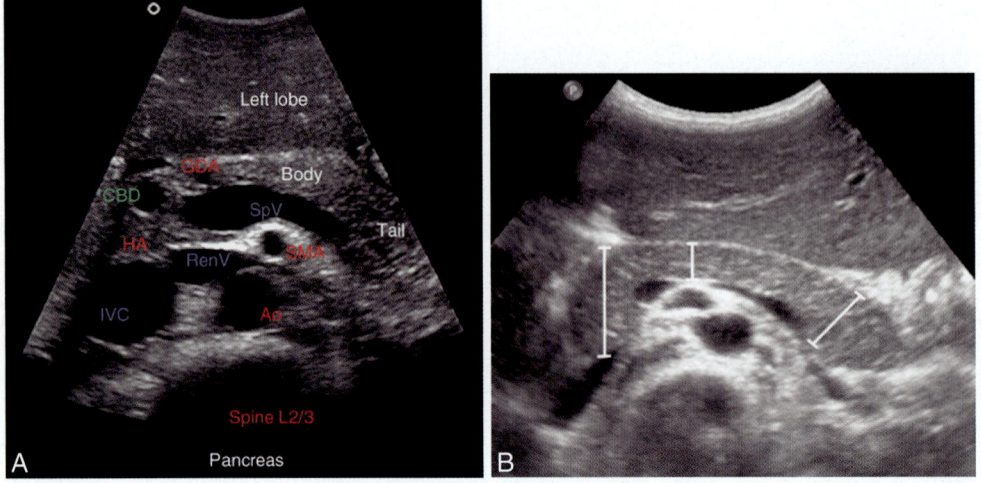

FIG 6.21 (A) Transverse image of pancreas as it lies anterior to superior mesenteric artery (SMA) and vein (SpV). The aorta (Ao) and inferior vena cava (IVC) are anterior to the horseshoe shape of the spine. The renal vein (RenV) crosses anterior to the aorta to enter the IVC. The gastroduodenal artery (GDA) is the anterolateral border of the head; the common bile duct (CBD) is the posterolateral border of the head. (B) Transverse image of head, body, and tail of the pancreas.

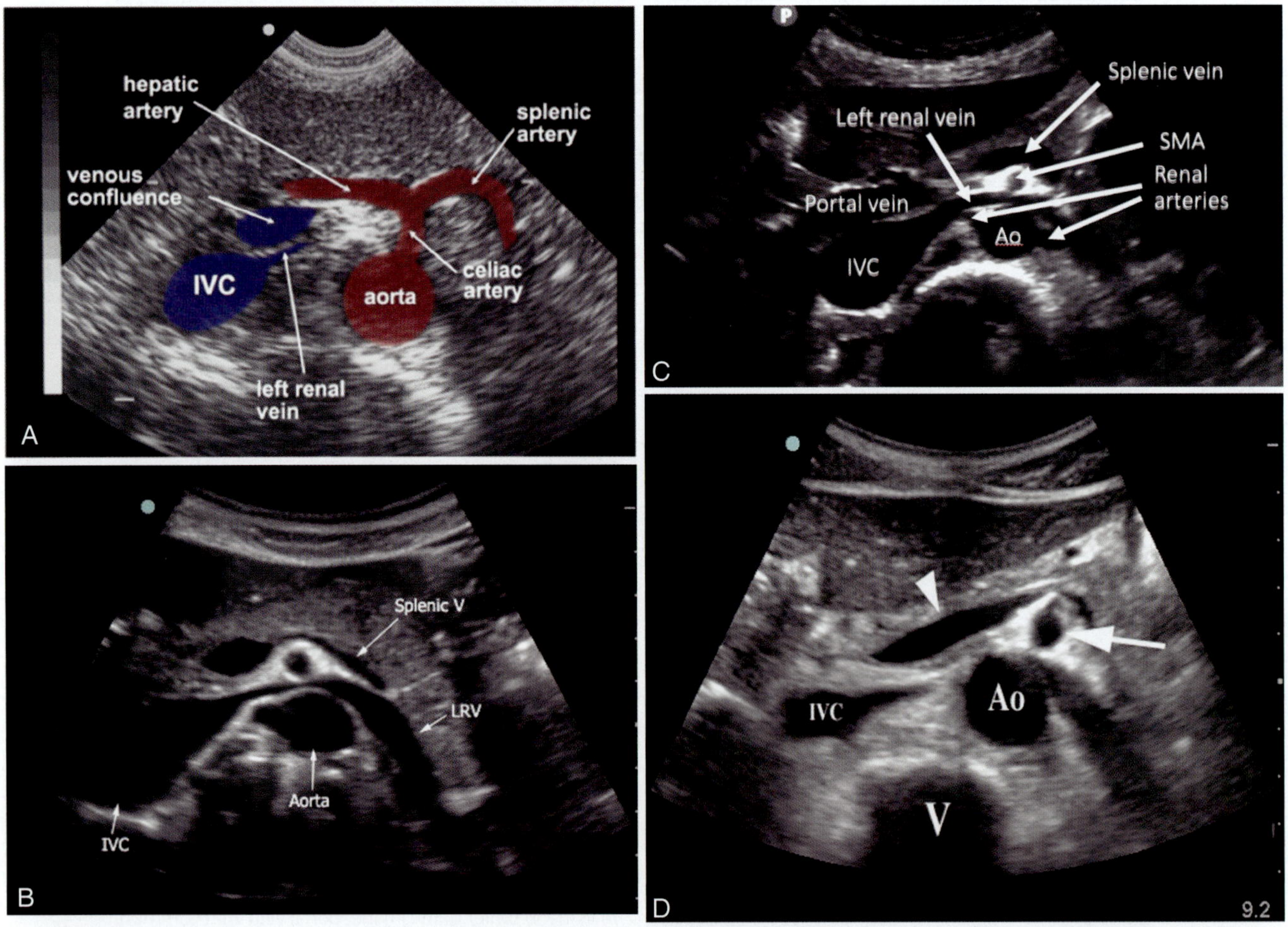

FIG 6.22 (A) Transverse image of the high abdominal aorta at the level of the celiac trunk with the bifurcation of the splenic and hepatic arteries. (B–C) Transverse image of the mid-abdominal aorta (Ao) at the level of the renal vessels. (D) The gain should be reduced to demark the normal aorta clearly. The *arrow* points to the superior mesenteric artery (SMA); the *arrowhead* points to the splenic vein. *IVC*, Inferior vena cava; *LRV*, left renal vein.

The inferior vena cava is found slightly to the right of the midline and varies with inspiration and expiration.

The spleen should be assessed with the patient in a steep decubitus position. The parenchyma of the spleen may be compared with the echogenicity of the left kidney (Fig. 6.23). With deep inspiration, the sonographer should be able to see the movement of the diaphragm and the left pleural space.

The sonographer should be aware of the fluid-filled stomach, antrum of the stomach, and duodenum in the left upper quadrant (Fig. 6.24). Bowel structures may be evaluated for wall thickening, dilation, hypertrophy, or other pathology. Normal bowel should compress with gentle pressure. The sonographer may note peristalsis within the bowel.

The kidneys, adrenals, and urinary bladder are well imaged with ultrasound. The renal cortex and renal pelvis

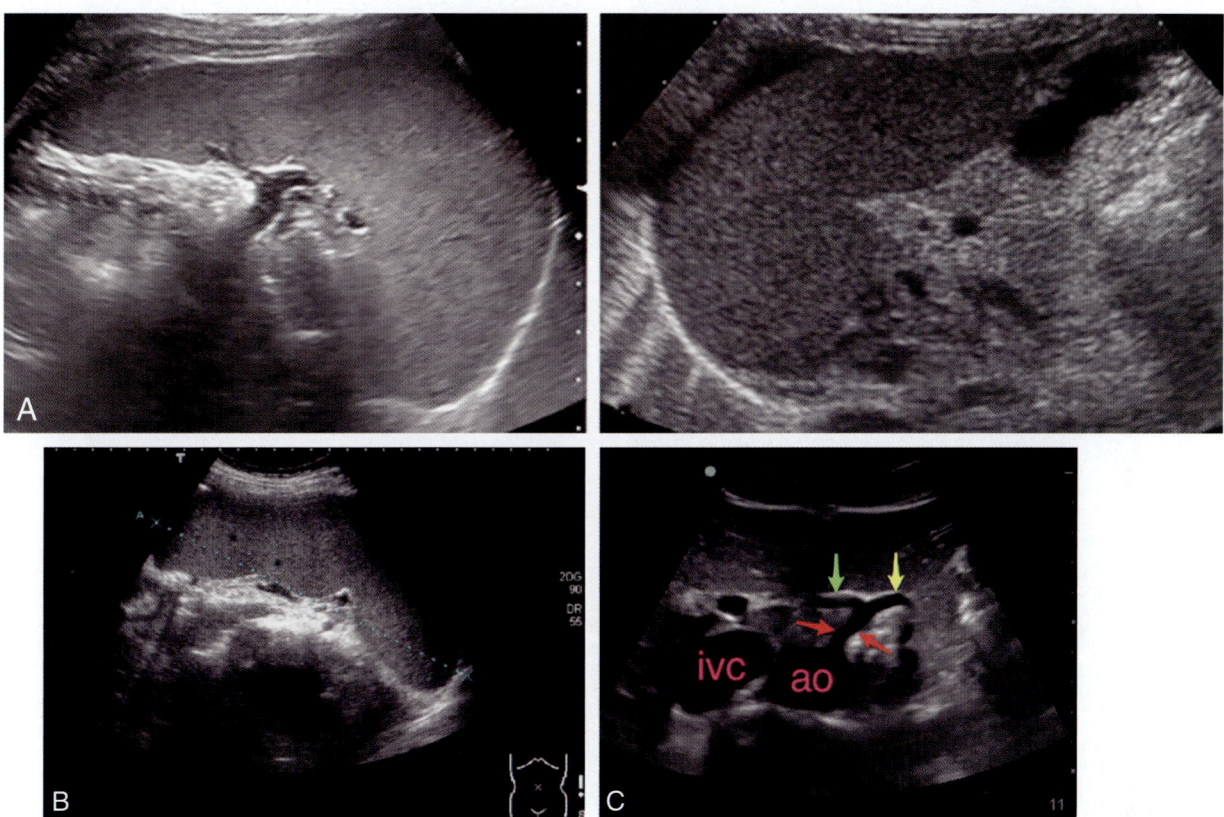

FIG 6.23 (A) Transverse image of spleen found in the left upper quadrant. (B) The normal splenic parenchyma is homogeneous like the liver. (C) Note the tortuous splenic artery *(yellow arrow)* as it arises from the celiac trunk *(red arrows)*. The *green arrow* denotes the hepatic artery. *ao*, Aorta; *ivc*, inferior vena cava.

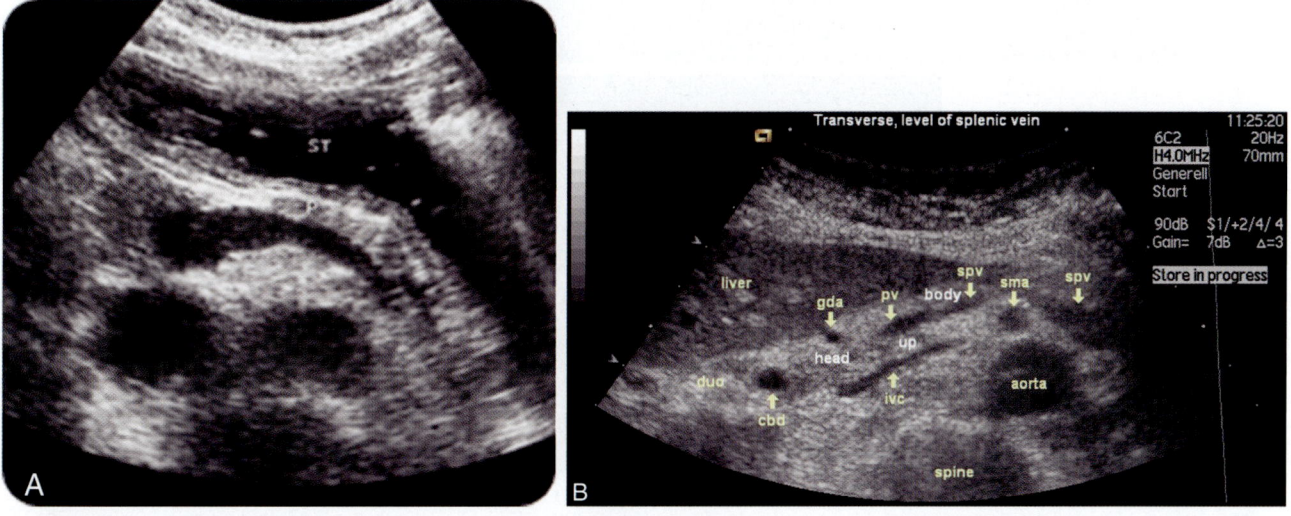

FIG 6.24 (A) The sonographer should be aware of the fluid-filled stomach, antrum of the stomach, and duodenum in the left upper quadrant. Normal bowel should compress with gentle pressure. The sonographer may note peristalsis within the bowel. (B), The duodenum serves as the lateral border to the common bile duct. *cbd*, Common bile duct; *duo*, duodenum; *gda*, gastroduodenal artery; *pv*, portal vein; *sma*, superior mesenteric artery; *smv*, superior mesenteric vein; *spv*, splenic vein; *ST*, stomach; *up*, uncinate process.

should be assessed, and the renal length recorded. Doppler velocities of the renal vascular structures may be assessed to identify stenosis or thrombosis (Fig. 6.25). The patient may be rolled into a decubitus or prone position to better image the kidneys.

Longitudinal Scans

The anatomic structures (liver and vascular structures, gallbladder, pancreas, kidneys, aorta, inferior vena cava, spleen, and gastrointestinal organs) visualized in the transverse views should also be demonstrated in the longitudinal plane.

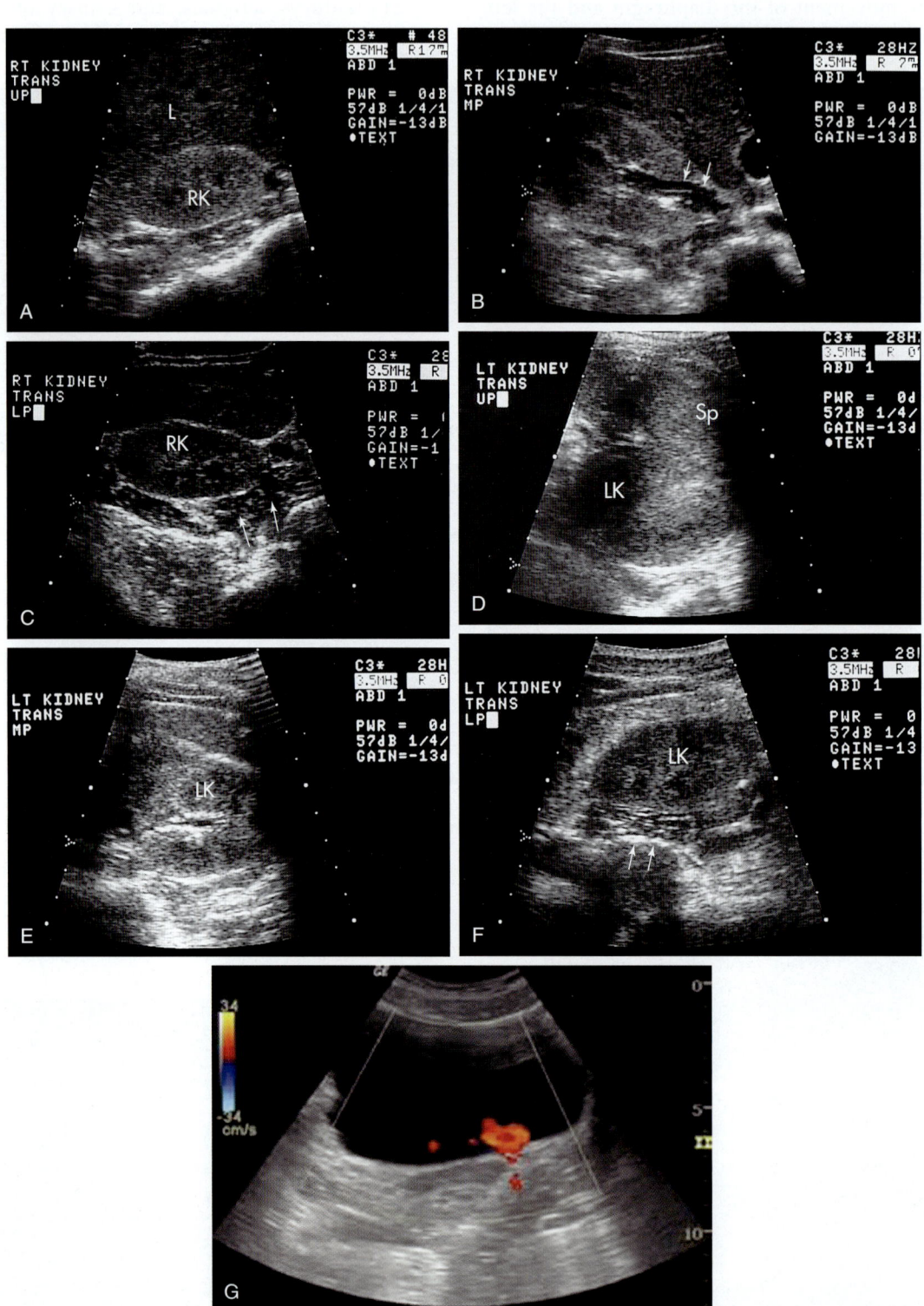

FIG 6.25 (A) Transverse image of upper pole of right kidney (RK) and liver (L). (B) Transverse image of middle of right kidney with the renal vein *(arrows)*. (C) Transverse image of lower pole of right kidney (RK). The psoas muscle is medial to the kidney *(arrows)*. (D) Transverse image of upper pole of left kidney (LK) and spleen (Sp). (E) Transverse image of middle of left kidney (LK). (F) Transverse image of lower pole of left kidney (LK) and psoas muscle *(arrows)*. (G) Transverse image of full urinary bladder with color flow of ureteral jets.

To obtain the longitudinal plane, the transducer should be rotated 90 degrees.

Liver. The diaphragm should be well defined as a bright linear line superior to the dome of the liver (Fig. 6.26). The curved array transducer will display the greatest area of the liver. To image the liver completely, the probe should be placed in the midline below the xyphoid process and slowly angled toward the right lobe of the liver as the patient takes in a deep breath (Fig. 6.27). A lower frequency setting may be selected to provide increased sensitivity if the gain is adjusted to the maximum without adequate uniform penetration. The larger vascular structures (aorta and inferior vena cava) should be well outlined as hollow tubular structures with the patient in deep inspiration. The liver parenchyma should be homogeneous and uniform throughout, except for the anechoic portal and hepatic veins. The liver should be imaged from the midline to the far-right lateral border.

Vascular Structures. The abdominal aorta and inferior vena cava may be demonstrated in their long axis with the probe in the midline of the abdomen. A slight angulation to the patient's left will demonstrate the pulsatile abdominal aorta, with the anterior branches of the celiac artery and superior mesenteric artery (Fig. 6.28). With the patient in deep inspiration, the transducer should be angled slightly to the patient's right of the midline to demonstrate the inferior vena cava as it drains the lower abdomen to empty into the right atrium of the heart.

Gallbladder and Common Bile Duct. The gallbladder and common bile duct may be seen in the right upper quadrant of the abdomen with the patient in deep inspiration (Fig. 6.29). The portal vein serves as a useful posterior landmark to locate the common bile duct.

Kidneys and Spleen. The right and left kidneys are demonstrated anterior to the psoas muscle along the flanks of the mid-abdomen with the patient in deep inspiration (Fig. 6.30). The entire organ should be demonstrated on the sonogram.

The homogeneous spleen is anatomically found lateral to the upper pole of the left kidney. Occasionally this structure may be seen with the patient in a supine position; however, the best image is with the patient in a steep lateral position on an echo bed with a drop-down door so the sonographer may image the spleen from the inferior border of the spleen to the upper border/diaphragm interface.

ABDOMINAL DOPPLER

Doppler ultrasound has been used for many decades to evaluate cardiovascular flow patterns. As in other areas of ultrasound, many improvements have been made to the technology, such as the development of PW Doppler, spectral analysis of the returning waveform, power Doppler, and color flow mapping. These advances in Doppler instrumentation, combined with high-resolution imaging of the vessels, have led to duplex scanning equipment, which combines these modalities into a single probe.

Doppler is used to ascertain the presence or absence of flow. It can be used to differentiate vessels from nonvascular structures with confusingly similar images (e.g., common duct from the hepatic artery, arterial aneurysm from a cyst). The determination and direction of flow may also be of diagnostic value. Once the presence and direction of flow have been determined, spectral analysis of the flow gives further information on flow velocity and turbulence. Increased velocity and post-stenotic turbulence may be seen in vascular stenosis. In postoperative patients, increased turbulence alone may be present at the graft anastomosis site with the native vessel. Evaluation of the shape of the waveform, with a comparison of the systolic and diastolic components, may yield information on increased vascular impedance, as is seen in renal transplant rejection. Doppler may also be useful in determining whether a mass is vascular or avascular.

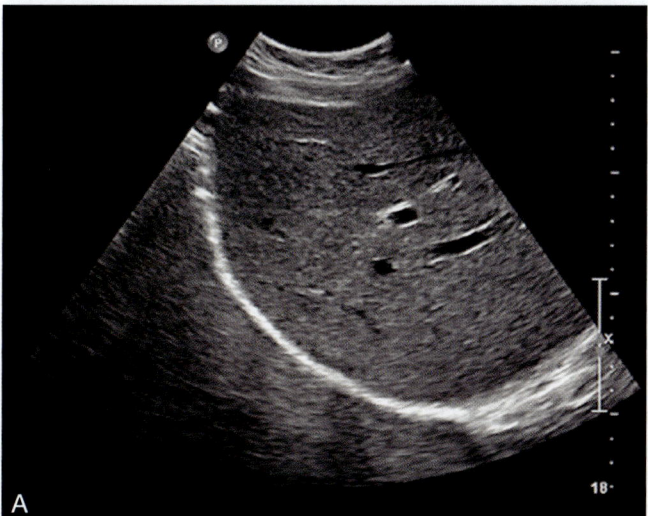 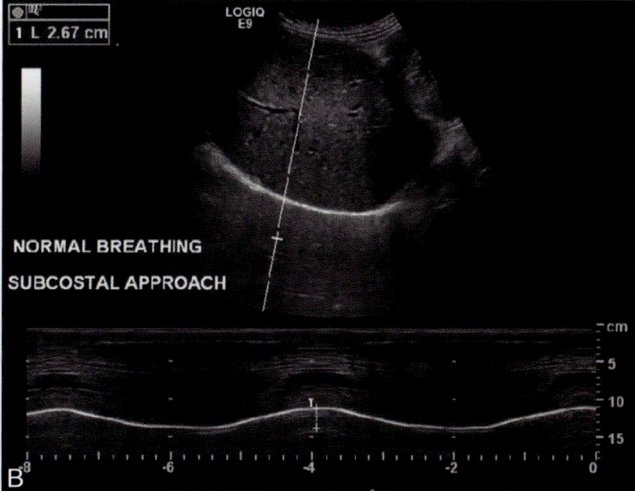

FIG 6.26 (A) The diaphragm should be well defined as a bright linear line superior to the dome of the liver. (B) The M-mode tracing of the diaphragm will denote breathing motion.

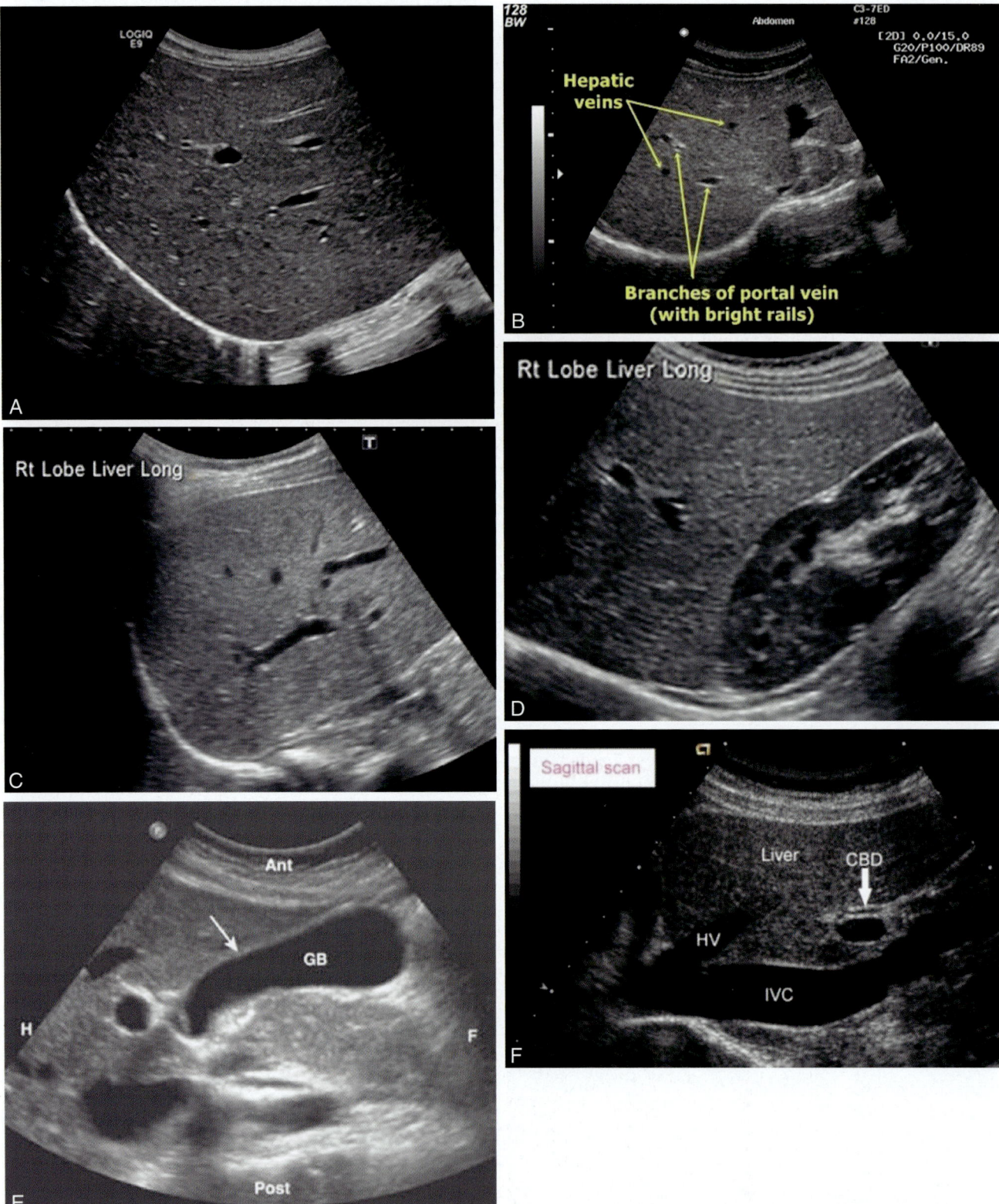

FIG 6.27 (A) Sagittal image of the right lobe of the liver and diaphragm. (B) The portal veins have more echogenic borders than do the hepatic veins. (C) Portal veins and hepatic veins in the right lobe of the liver. (D) Right lobe of liver and right kidney; notice the liver is homogeneous compared to the right kidney. (E) The gallbladder (GB) is usually seen in the midaxillary plane. (F) Sagittal image closer to the midline demonstrates the inferior vena cava (IVC) with the hepatic vein (HV) draining into the IVC. The common bile duct (CBD) is seen anterior to the portal vein.

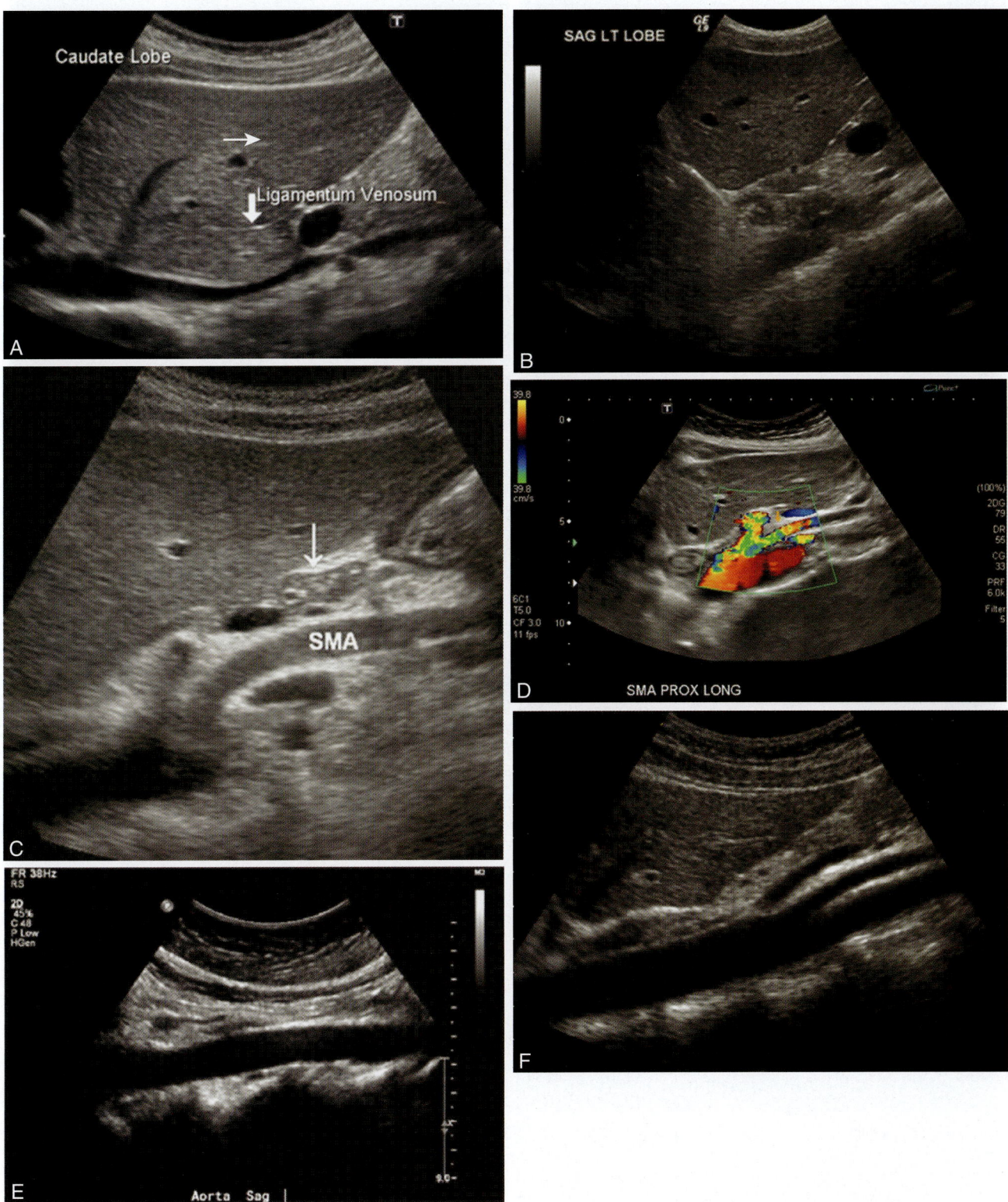

FIG 6.28 (A) Midline sagittal image of the inferior vena cava and left lobe of liver. The caudate lobe is located just posterior to the ligamentum venosum. (B) The portal vein is visible. (C) Sagittal images just left of midline show the body of the pancreas *(arrow)* with the superior mesenteric artery (SMA) posterior. (D) Color flow of the celiac trunk and superior mesenteric artery as they arise anterior from the aorta. (E) Abdominal aorta. (F) Abdominal aorta with the celiac trunk *(arrow)* and superior mesenteric artery.

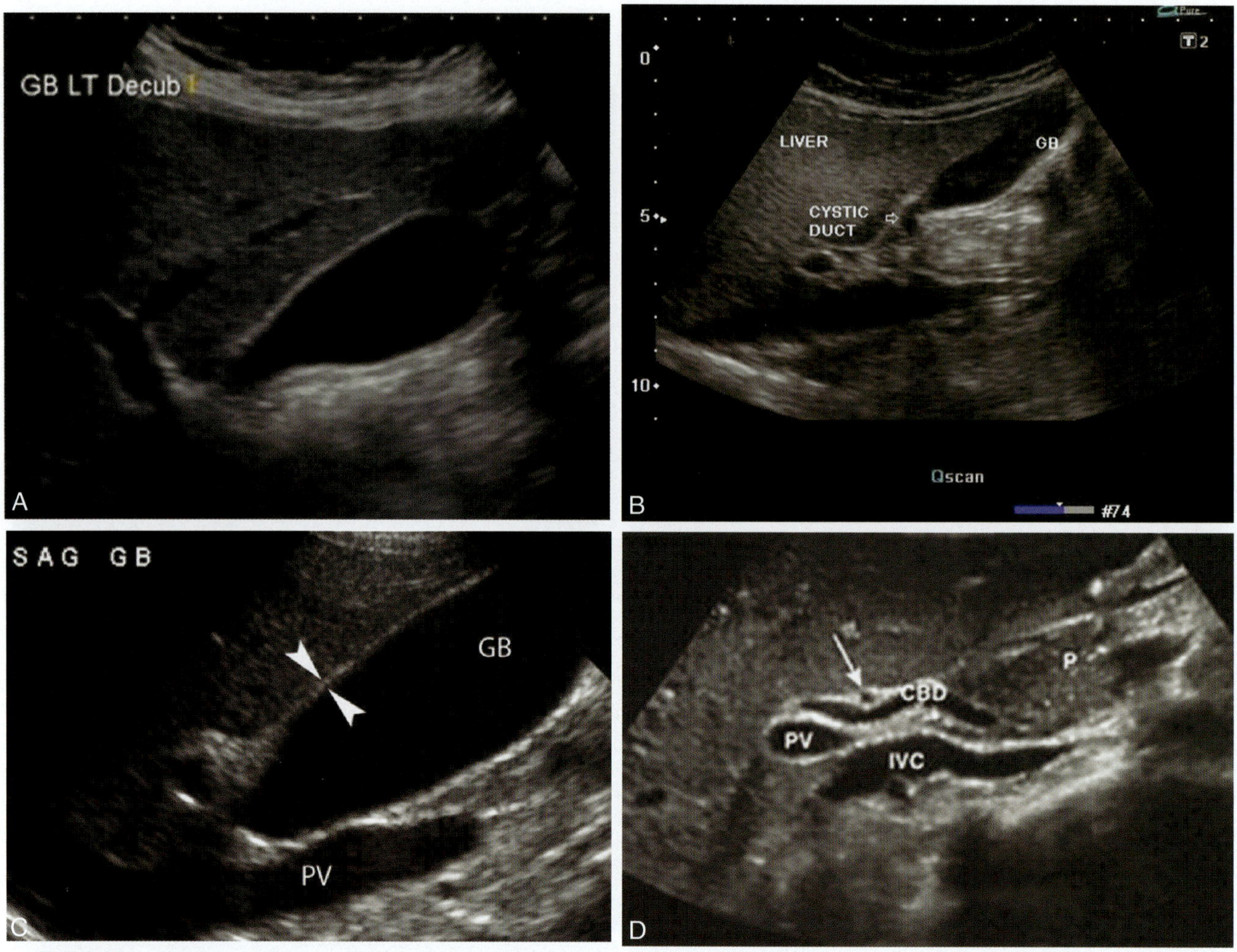

144 CHAPTER 6 Basic Ultrasound Imaging: Techniques, Terminology, and Tips

FIG 6.29 (A) Left decubitus images of the fasting gallbladder should demonstrate a sonolucent parenchyma. (B) The cystic duct may be seen arising from the neck of the gallbladder (GB). (C) The zoom feature should enlarge the image so the wall thickness may be calculated. (D) The common bile duct (CBD) is seen anterior to the portal vein (PV) and inferior vena cava (IVC) as it drains into the head of the pancreas (P).

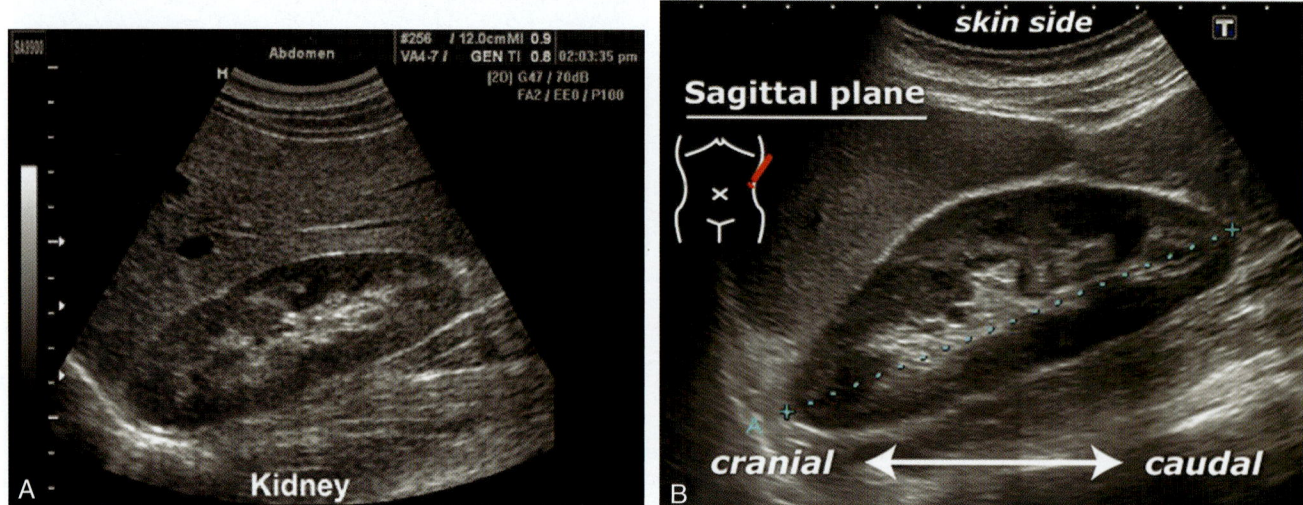

FIG 6.30 (A) Sagittal image of the right lobe of the liver and right kidney. (B) Sagittal plane along the lateral border demonstrates the spleen anterior to the left kidney.

Doppler Scanning Techniques

Normal routine longitudinal, transverse, coronal, and oblique scans of vascular structures are used to produce adequate images. Doppler techniques supplement the routine examination by permitting blood flow within those vessels to be detected and characterized. The probe should be placed parallel to the flow velocity to obtain the most accurate spectral waveforms. Flow toward the transducer is positive, or above baseline, whereas flow away from the transducer is negative, or below baseline (Fig. 6.31). Arterial flow pulsates with the cardiac cycle and shows its maximal peak during the systolic part of the cycle. Venous flow shows no pulsatility and has lower flow velocity than arterial structures. A phasic pattern may be seen in the hepatic veins (near the heart) associated with an overload of the right ventricle.

As seen in echocardiography, many abdominal vessels have characteristic waveforms. If the sample volume can be directed parallel to the flow, quantification of peak gradients can be estimated. However, given the tortuous course of most abdominal vascular structures, this can be very difficult in the abdomen.

PW Doppler is the most common instrumentation used to evaluate the lower-velocity abdominal flow patterns. PW Doppler allows placement of the small sample volume within the vascular structure of interest by means of a trackball movement. If the velocities are lower than 3 m/sec and the probe is parallel to the vascular flow profile, accurate hemodynamic information may be obtained.

Aorta. Doppler flow in the pulsatile aorta demonstrates arterial signals in the patent lumen. If the vessel were occluded, no arterial signals would be recorded (Fig. 6.32). Flow, often with two distinct patterns, can be seen in the true and false lumens by Doppler ultrasound. The development of a

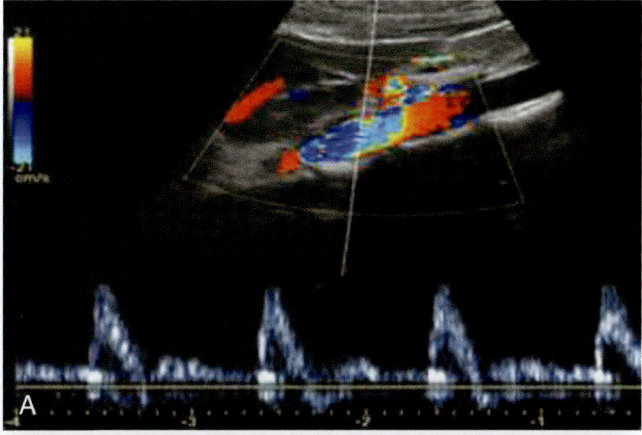
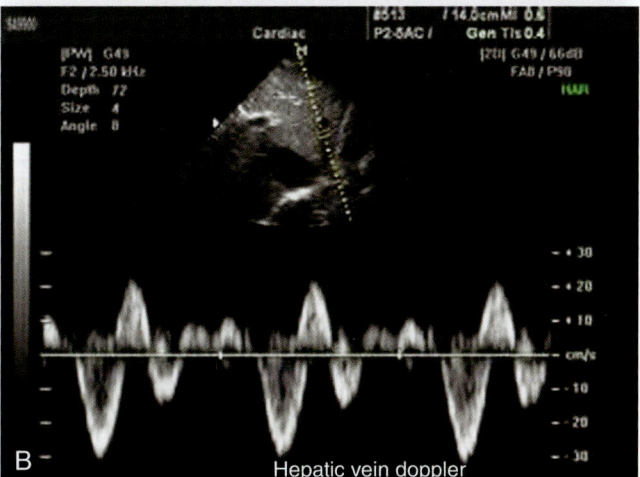

FIG 6.31 (A) Doppler tracing of the abdominal aorta demonstrates a high systolic peak with a relatively low diastolic component on the spectral tracing. (B) Pulsed wave Doppler tracing of the middle hepatic vein shows a continuous undulating low-flow profile representing blood flow from the hepatic vein into the inferior vena cava.

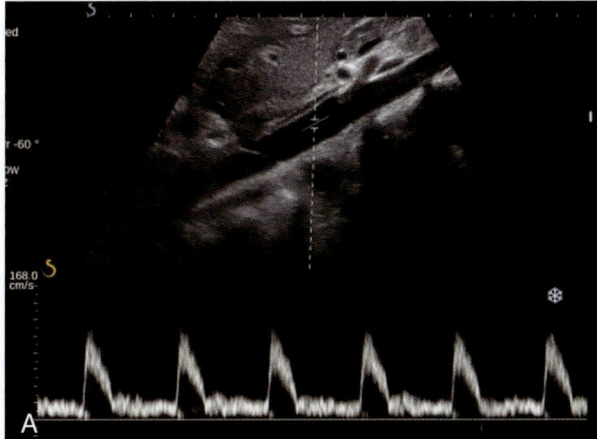
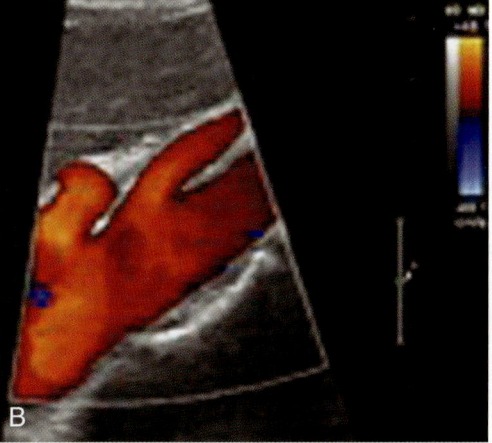

FIG 6.32 (A) The sample volume is placed in the mid-abdominal aorta to record the Doppler velocity profile. The flow is positive, above the baseline. There is a high systolic component and a small diastolic component. (B) Color Doppler of the abdominal aorta, celiac trunk, and superior mesenteric artery.

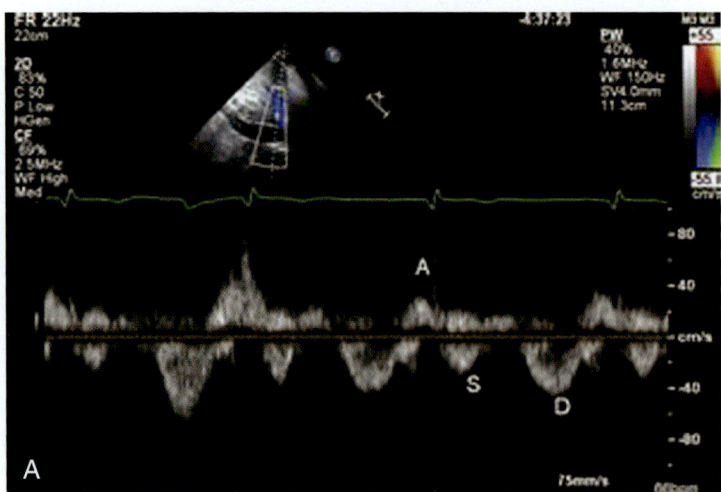
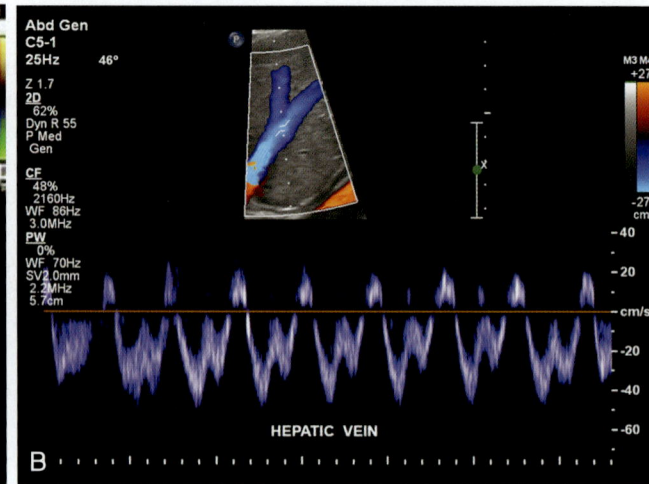

FIG 6.33 (A) The sample volume is placed in the midpoint of the inferior vena cava to record a small atrial reversal *(A)*, a systolic component *(S)*, and a diastolic component *(D)*. (B) A similar flow pattern is noted in the hepatic veins.

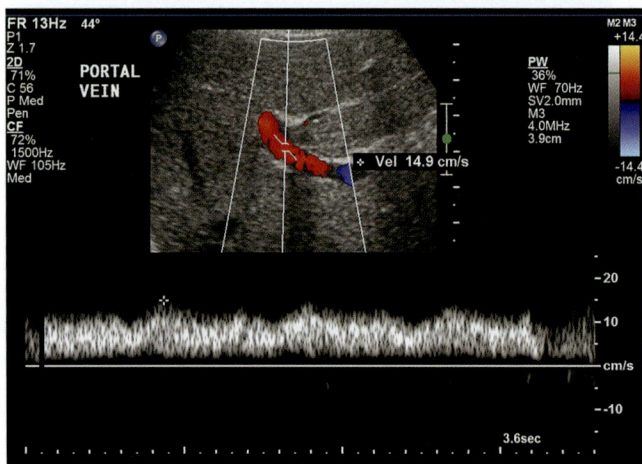

FIG 6.34 **The sample volume is placed in the portal vein.** Venous flow shows no pulsatility and has lower flow velocity than arterial structures.

pseudoaneurysm as a complication of an aortic graft procedure may be difficult to determine if pulsations are present or transmitted through the aortic wall. Doppler ultrasound may be useful to detect flow within the pseudoaneurysm.

Inferior Vena Cava and Hepatic Vein. The Doppler waveform recorded in the inferior vena cava and hepatic veins shows a lower flow than is found in arterial structures. The flow is increased in the presence of thrombus formation (Fig. 6.33).

Portal Venous System. Doppler flow patterns can be used to diagnose varices or collaterals in the **portal venous system** (Fig. 6.34). Doppler flow patterns can be used to evaluate changes in flow patterns that occur during portal hypertension. As liver function improves, normal hepatopetal flow is restored. If pressures worsen, shunting away from the liver may be increased. If a shunt is present in the porta hepatis, Doppler may be useful to determine the patency of the shunt.

Key Pearls

- Become familiar with all the ultrasound equipment in your laboratory and understand the knobology.
- Read the operator's manuals are for each piece of equipment so you may have a reference for troubleshooting.
- There are specific protocols for each examination that the sonographer should know.
- Read the patient order, find out what question the ordering physician needs to have answered, and know which items in the patient records are relevant for patient identification.
- Curved array and sector array probes have different applications that the sonographer should understand.
- Transducer scan movements affect the image.
- The indications for abdominal sonography should be understood by the sonographer.
- Become familiar with the ultrasound terminology and anatomic directions.
- The sonographer should know how to perform an initial survey of the abdomen.
- The sonographer should understand and demonstrate how to perform the general protocol for an abdominal sonographic examination.
- The sonographer should understand basic Doppler concepts, hemodynamics, and flow patterns within the abdominal vascular structures.

BIBLIOGRAPHY

American Institute of Ultrasound in Medicine. AIUM practice guideline for documentation of an ultrasound examination. *J Ultrasound Med*. 2014;33:1098–1102.

American Institute of Ultrasound in Medicine. AIUM practice parameter for documentation of an ultrasound examination. *J Ultrasound Med*. 2020;39:E1–E4.

American Institute of Ultrasound in Medicine. Ultrasound examination of the abdomen and/or retroperitoneum, 2017. www.aium.org.

Block B. *Color atlas of ultrasound anatomy*. New York: Thieme; 2004.

Kremkau F. *Diagnostic Ultrasound: Principles and Instruments*. ed 8. Philadelphia: Elsevier; 2011.

CHAPTER 7

Imaging and Doppler Artifacts*

Frederick W. Kremkau

OBJECTIVES

On completion of this chapter, you should be able to:
- List ways in which sonographic gray-scale images can present anatomic structures incorrectly
- List ways in which spectral and color Doppler displays can present motion and flow information incorrectly
- Describe how specific artifacts can be recognized
- Explain how artifacts can be handled to avoid the pitfalls and misdiagnoses that they can cause

OUTLINE

Propagation 147
   Section Thickness 148
   Speckle 148
   Reverberation 148
   Mirror Image 149
   Refraction 149
   Grating Lobes 151
   Speed Error 151
   Range Ambiguity 151

Attenuation 153
   Shadowing 153
   Enhancement 156
   Noise 156

Spectral Doppler 156
   Aliasing 156
   Nyquist Limit 156
   Range Ambiguity 159
   Mirror Image 160

Noise 160
Color Doppler 160
   Aliasing 160
   Mirror Image, Shadowing, Clutter, and Noise 160

Virtual Beam-Forming 163
Summary 163

KEY TERMS

Aliasing
Comet tail
Enhancement
Grating lobes
Mirror image
Noise

Nyquist limit
Range ambiguity
Refraction
Resonance
Reverberation
Ring-down artifact

Section thickness artifacts
Shadowing
Speckle
Speed error

In sonographic imaging, an artifact is the appearance of anything that does not properly present the structures or motion imaged. An artifact is caused by some problematic aspect of the imaging technique. Some artifacts are helpful. They should be used to advantage in the diagnostic imaging process. Others hinder proper interpretation and diagnosis. These artifacts must be avoided or handled properly when encountered.

Artifacts in sonography occur as apparent structures that are one or more of the following:
- Not real
- Missing
- Misplaced
- Of improper brightness, shape, or size

Some artifacts are produced by improper equipment operation or settings (e.g., incorrect gain and compensation settings). Others are inherent in the sonographic and Doppler methods and can occur even with proper equipment and technique.

PROPAGATION

The assumptions in the design of sonographic instruments are that sound travels in straight lines, that echoes originate from objects located on the beam axis, that the amplitudes of returning echoes are related directly to the echogenicity of the objects that produced them, and that the distance to echogenic objects is proportional to the round-trip travel time (13 µsec/cm of depth). If any of these assumptions is violated, an artifact occurs.

---

*This chapter is adapted from Kremkau FW. Artifacts. In *Sonography: Principles and Instruments*, ed 10. Philadelphia: Elsevier; 2021.

Section Thickness

Axial and lateral (detail) resolutions are artifactual because a failure to resolve means a loss of detail, and two adjacent structures may be visualized as one. These artifacts occur because the ultrasound pulse has finite length and width in the scan plane. Increasing frequency improves both resolutions, whereas focusing improves lateral (Fig. 7.1A). The beamwidth perpendicular to the scan plane (the third dimension in Fig. 7.1B) results in section thickness artifacts, for example, the appearance of false debris in what should be echo-free areas (Fig. 7.1C–D). These artifacts occur because the interrogating beam has finite thickness as it scans through the patient. Echoes are received that originate not only from the center of the beam but also from off-center. These echoes are all collapsed into a thin (zero-thickness) two-dimensional image composed of echoes that have come from a not-so-thin tissue volume scanned by the beam. Section thickness artifact is also called slice thickness or partial volume artifact.

Speckle

Apparent image resolution can be deceiving. The detailed echo pattern often is not related directly to the scattering properties of tissue (called *tissue texture*) but rather is the result of the interference effects of the scattered sound from the distribution of scatterers in the tissue. There are many scatterers in the ultrasound pulse at any instant as it travels through tissue. Their echoes can combine constructively or destructively. The result varies as the beam is scanned through the tissue, producing the pattern of bright and dark spots. This phenomenon is called acoustic **speckle** (Fig. 7.2).

Reverberation

Multiple reflection, or **reverberation**, can occur between the transducer and a strong reflector (Fig. 7.3). The multiple echoes may be sufficiently strong to be detected by the instrument and cause confusion on the display (additional echoes that do not represent additional structures). The process by which they are produced is shown in Fig. 7.3B. This results in the display of additional reflectors that are not real (Fig. 7.4). The multiple reflections are placed beneath the real reflector at separation intervals equal to the separation between the transducer and the real reflector. Each subsequent reflection is weaker than prior ones, but this diminution is counteracted at least partially by the attenuation compensation (time gain compensation) function. Reverberations can also originate between two anatomic reflecting surfaces. When closely spaced, they appear in a form called *comet tail* (Fig. 7.5). **Comet tail**, a particular form of reverberation, is a series of closely spaced, discrete echoes. Fig. 7.6 shows an artifact that appears similar but is fundamentally different. Discrete echoes cannot be identified here because continuous sound emission from the origin appears to be occurring. This continuous effect, termed **ring-down artifact**, is caused by a resonance phenomenon associated with the presence

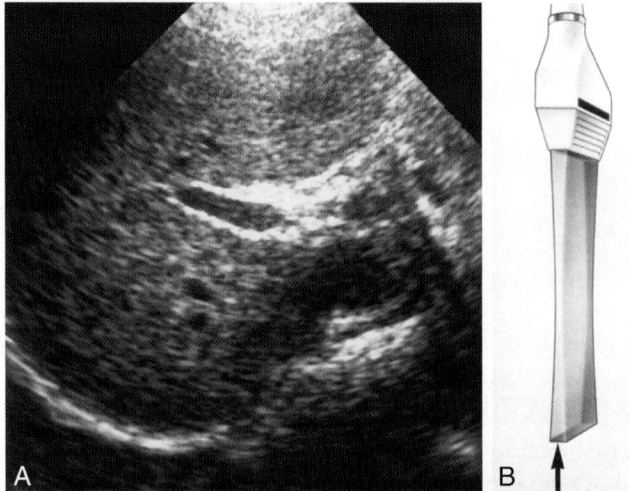

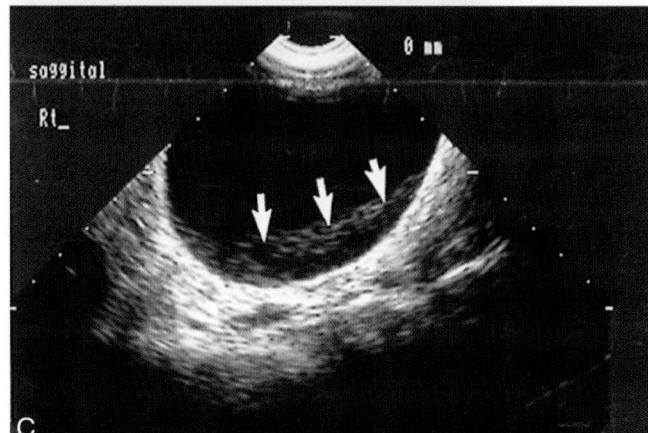

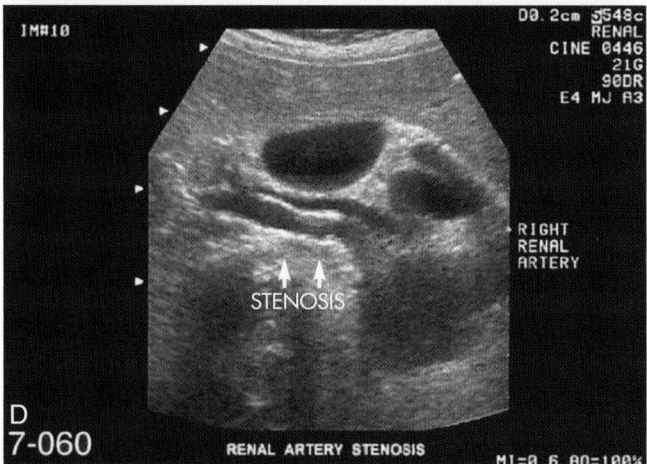

FIG. 7.1 (A) Without focusing, there is lateral smearing in this abdominal image. (B) The scan "plane" through the tissue is a three-dimensional volume. Two dimensions (axial and lateral) are in the scan plane, but there is a third dimension (called section thickness or slice thickness). The third dimension *(arrow)* is collapsed to zero thickness when the image is displayed in two-dimensional format. (C) An ovarian cyst that should be echo-free has an echogenic region *(arrows)*. These off-axis echoes are a result of scan-plane section thickness. (D) Section thickness artifact appears as low-level echoes within hypoechoic structures.

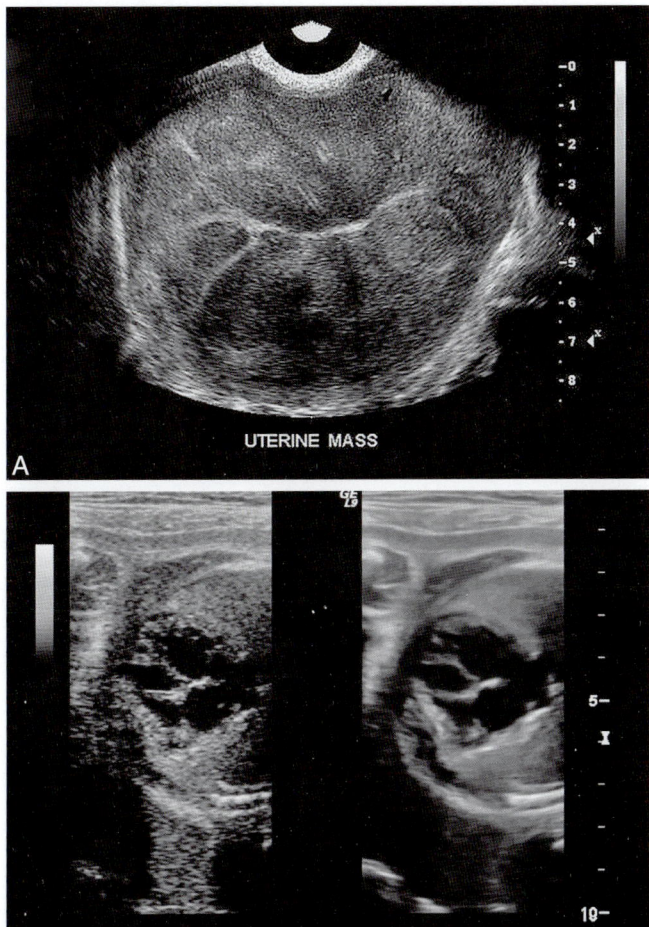

FIG. 7.2 (A) The typically grainy appearance of this ultrasound image is not primarily the result of detail resolution limitations but rather of speckle. Speckle is the interference pattern resulting from constructive and destructive interference of echoes returning simultaneously from many scatterers within the propagating ultrasound pulse at any instant. (B) Approaches to speckle reduction (*right image* compared with the *left*) are implemented in modern instruments.

of a collection of gas bubbles. **Resonance** is the condition in which a driven mechanical vibration is of a frequency similar to a natural vibration frequency of the structure. The bubbles are stimulated into vibration by the incident ultrasound pulse. They then pulsate (expand and contract) for several cycles, acting as a source of ultrasound, producing a continuous stream of ultrasound that progresses distally to the bubble collection as the echo stream returns.

Mirror Image

Mirror image, also a form of reverberation, shows structures that exist on one side of a strong reflector as being present on the other side as well. Fig. 7.7 explains how this happens and shows examples. Mirror image artifacts are common around the diaphragm and pleura because of the total reflection from the air-filled lung. They occasionally occur in other locations (Fig. 7.7C). Sometimes the mirrored structure is not in the unmirrored scan plane.

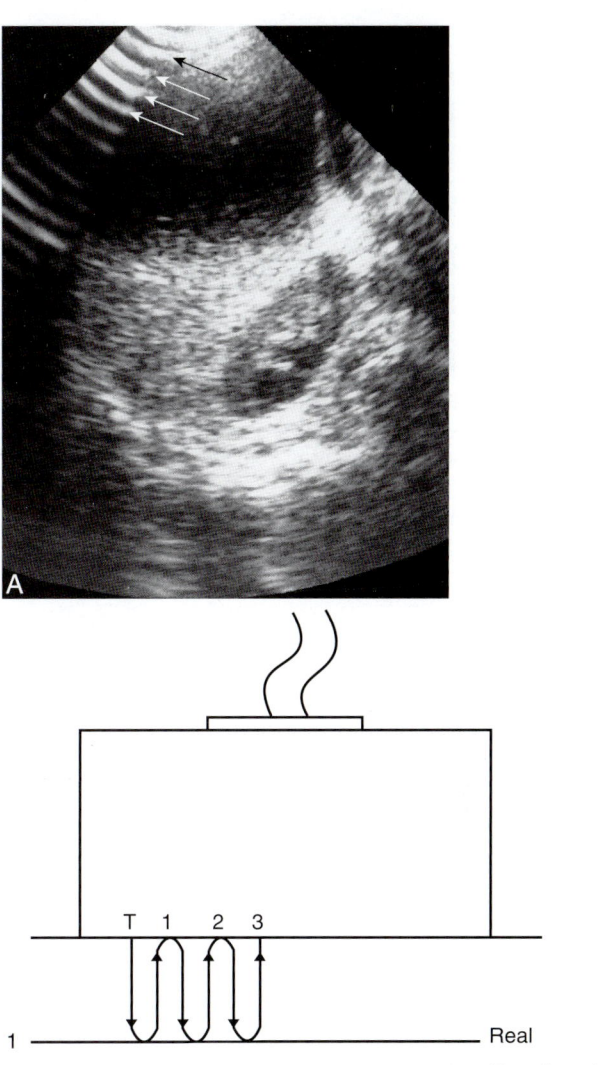

FIG. 7.3 (A) Reverberation artifact appearing as multiple presentations of a rib *(arrows)*. (B) The behavior in part A is explained as follows: A pulse (T) is transmitted from the transducer. A strong echo is generated at the rib and is received (1) at the transducer, allowing correct object imaging. However, the echo is reflected partially at the transducer so that a second echo (2) is received and a third (3) and possibly more. Because these echoes arrive later, they appear deeper on the display, where there are no reflectors. The lateral displacement of the reverberating sound path is for figure clarity. In fact, the sound travels down and back the same path repeatedly.

Refraction

Refraction of light enables lenses to focus and distorts the presentation of objects, as shown in Fig. 7.8. Refraction can cause a reflector to be positioned improperly (laterally) on a sonographic display (Fig. 7.9). Refraction is likely to occur, for example, when the transducer is placed on the abdominal midline (Fig. 7.10), producing doubling of single objects. Beneath are the rectus abdominis muscles, which are surrounded by fat. These tissues present refracting boundaries because of their different propagation speeds.

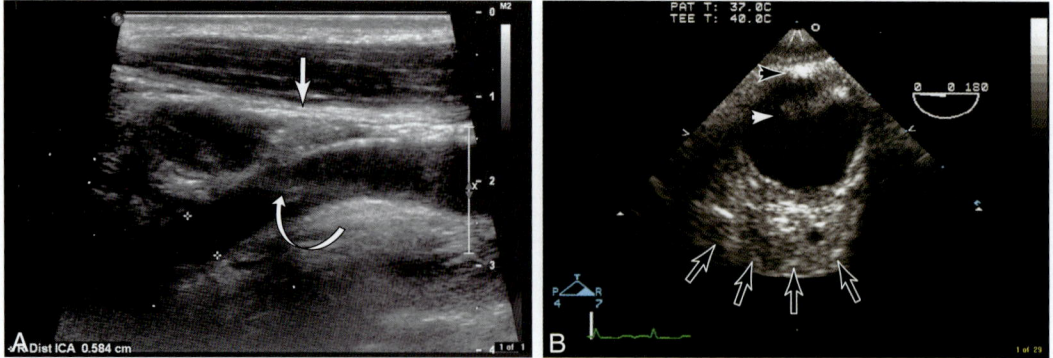

FIG. 7.4 (A) Reverberation *(curved arrow)* appearing in the carotid artery. This is a second echo from the proximal echogenic layer *(straight arrow)*. (B) Transesophageal scan of ascending aorta shows reverberation *(white arrowhead)* as the second echo from the proximal margin *(black arrowhead)*. Enhancement *(arrows)* is also evident.

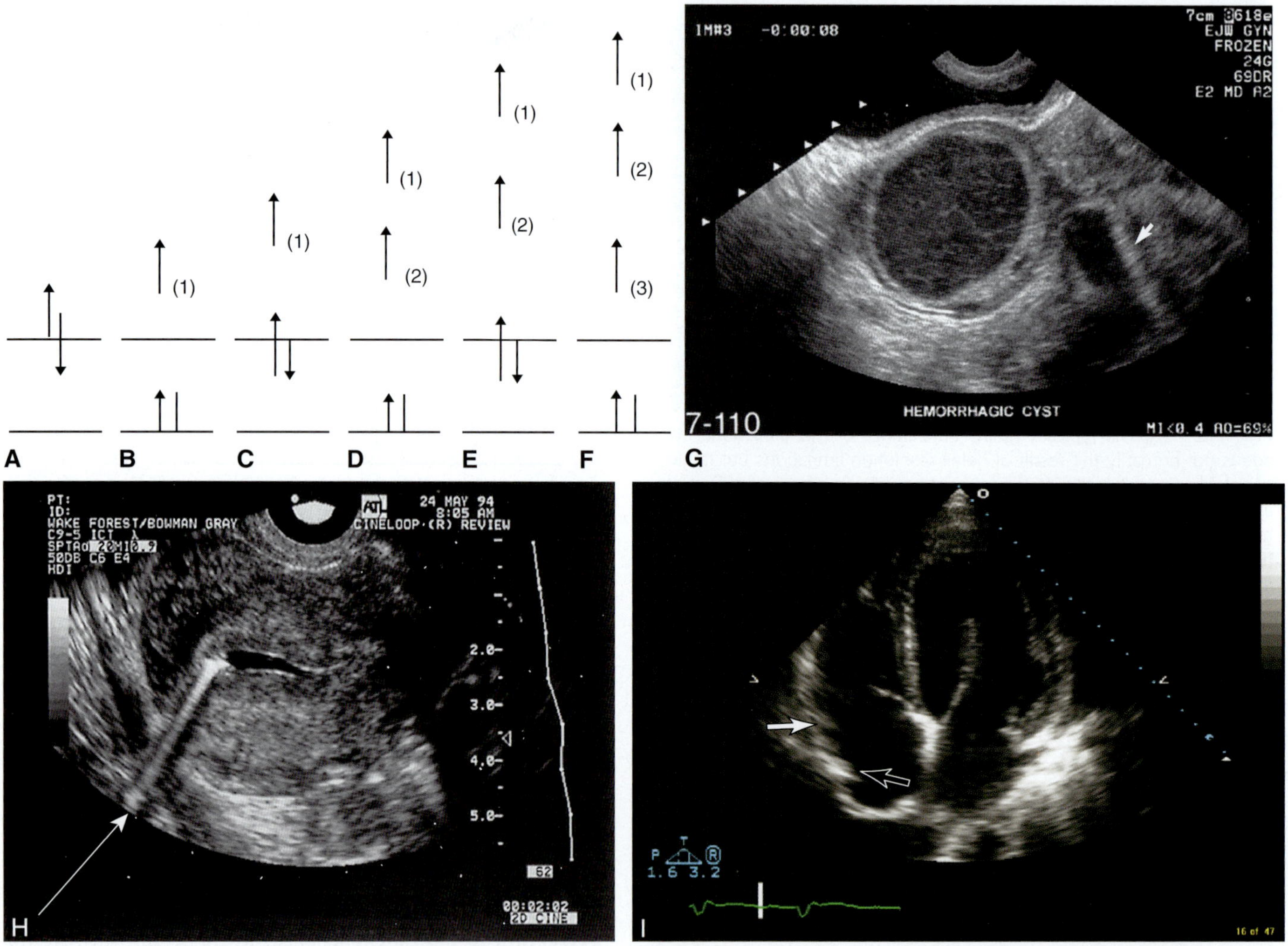

FIG. 7.5 Generation of comet-tail artifact (closely spaced reverberations). Action progresses in time from left to right. (A) An ultrasound pulse encounters the first reflector and is reflected partially and is transmitted partially. (B) Reflection and transmission at the first reflector are complete. Reflection at the second reflector is occurring. (C) Reflection at the second reflector is complete. Partial transmission and partial reflection are again occurring at the first reflector as the second echo passes through. (D) The echoes from the first (1) and second (2) reflectors are traveling toward the transducer. A second reflection (repeat of B) is occurring at the second reflector. (E) Partial transmission and reflection are again occurring at the first reflector. (F) Three echoes are now returning—the echo from the first reflector (1), the echo from the second reflector (2), and the echo from the third reflector (3)—that originated from the back side of the first reflector (C) and reflected again from the second reflector (D). A fourth echo is being generated at the second reflector (F). (G) Comet tail appears as a strong acoustic interface *(arrow)* from gas-filled bowel. (H) Comet tail *(arrow)* from bubbles in an intrauterine saline injection. (I) Apical four-chamber view of comet-tail artifact *(top left arrow)* in the left ventricle. Artifact is connected to the anterior mitral leaflet *(lower right arrow)*.

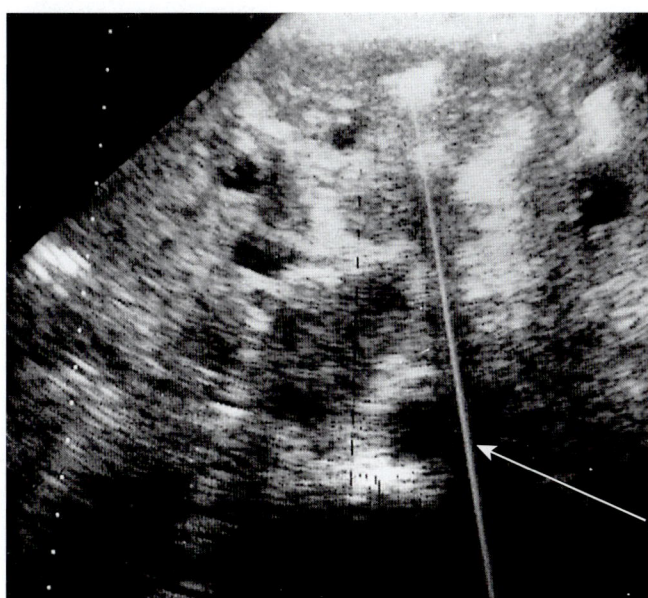

FIG. 7.6 Ring-down artifact *(arrow)* from air in the bile duct.

Grating Lobes

Side lobes are beams that propagate from a single transducer element in directions different from the primary beam. **Grating lobes** are additional beams emitted from an array transducer that are stronger than the side lobes of individual elements (Fig. 7.11). Side and grating lobes are weaker than the primary beam and normally do not produce echoes that are imaged, particularly if they fall on a normally echogenic region of the scan. However, if grating lobes encounter a strong reflector (e.g., bone or gas), their echoes may well be imaged, particularly if they fall within an anechoic region. If so, they appear in incorrect locations (Fig. 7.12).

Speed Error

Propagation **speed error** occurs when the assumed value for propagation speed (1.54 mm/μsec, leading to the 13 μsec/cm round-trip travel time rule) is incorrect. If the propagation speed that exists over a path traveled is greater than 1.54 mm/μsec, the calculated distance to the reflector is too small, and the display will place the reflector too close to the transducer (Fig. 7.13). This occurs because the increased speed causes the echoes to arrive sooner. If the actual speed is less than 1.54 mm/μsec, the reflector will be displayed too far from the transducer (Fig. 7.14) because the echoes arrive later. Refraction and propagation speed error also can cause a structure to be displayed with incorrect shape.

Range Ambiguity

In sonographic imaging, it is assumed that for each pulse, all echoes are received before the next pulse is emitted. If this were not the case, an error could result (Figs. 7.15 and 7.16). The maximum depth imaged correctly by an instrument is

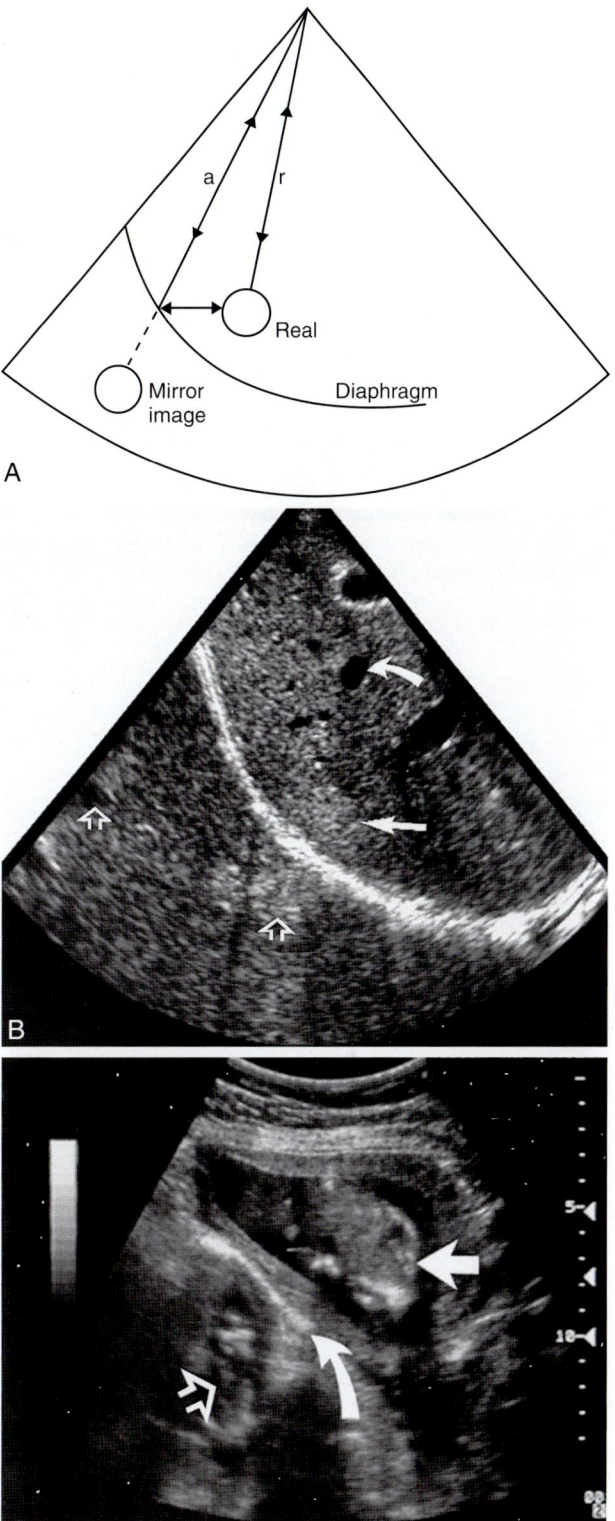

FIG. 7.7 (A) When pulses encounter a real hepatic structure directly (scan line *r*), the structure is imaged correctly. If the pulse first reflects off the diaphragm (scan line *a*) and the echo returns along the same path, the structure is displayed on the other side of the diaphragm. (B) A hemangioma *(straight arrow)* and vessel *(curved arrow)* with their mirror images *(open arrows)*. (C) A fetus *(straight arrow)* also appears as a mirror image *(open arrow)*. The mirror *(curved arrow)* is probably echogenic muscle.

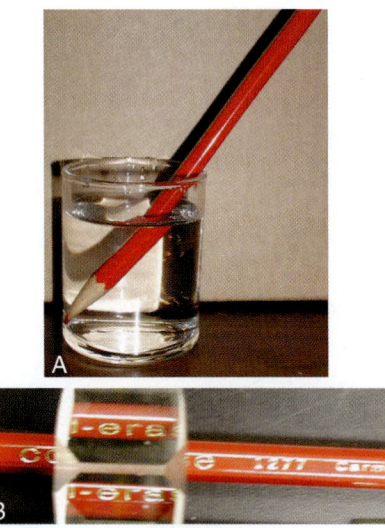

FIG. 7.8 (A) A pencil in water appears to be broken. (B) A pencil beneath a prism appears to be split into two.

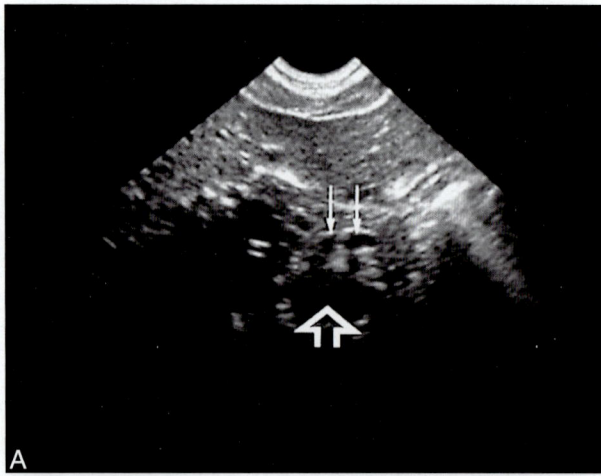

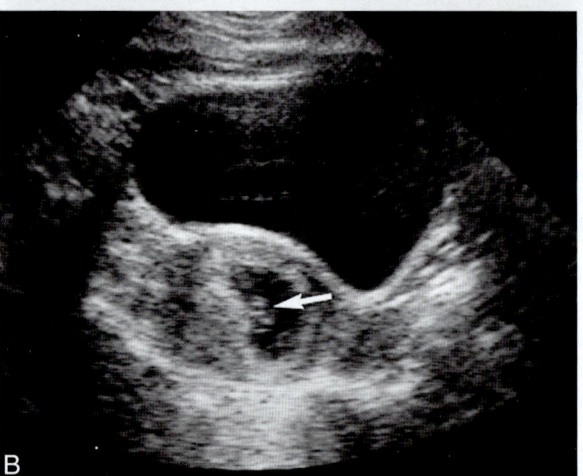

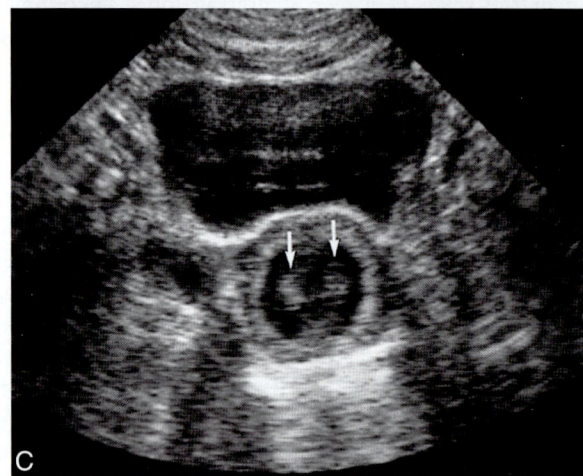

FIG. 7.10 (A) Refraction (probably through the rectus abdominis muscle) has widened the aorta *(open arrow)* and produced a double image of the celiac trunk *(arrows)*. Refraction may cause a single gestation (B) to appear as a double gestation (C).

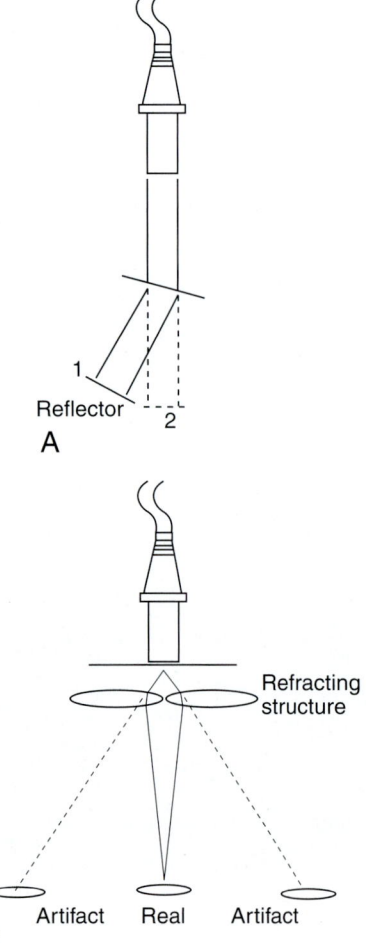

FIG. 7.9 Refraction (A) results in improper positioning of a reflector on the display. The system places the reflector at position 2 (because that is the direction from which the echo was received). The reflector is at position 1. (B) One real structure is imaged as two artifactual objects because of the refracting structure close to the transducer. A triple presentation (one correct, two artifactual) will result if unrefracted pulses can propagate to the real structure.

determined by its pulse repetition frequency (PRF). To avoid **range ambiguity**, PRF is automatically reduced in deeper imaging situations. This also causes a reduction in frame rate. Sometimes two artifacts combine to present even more challenging cases. An example involving range ambiguity is shown in Fig. 7.17.

ATTENUATION

Another assumption in anatomic imaging is that the brightness (gray level) of the displayed echo is a proportional representation of the echogenicity of the object producing the echo. If this assumption is violated, echo strengths are presented improperly on the display. This artifact occurs primarily in two forms: shadowing and enhancement.

Shadowing

Shadowing is the reduction in echo amplitude from reflectors that lie behind a strongly reflecting or attenuating structure. A strongly attenuating or reflecting structure weakens the sound distal to it, causing echoes from the distal region to be weak and thus to appear darker, like a shadow. Of course, the returning echoes also must pass through the attenuating structure, adding to the shadowing effect. Examples of

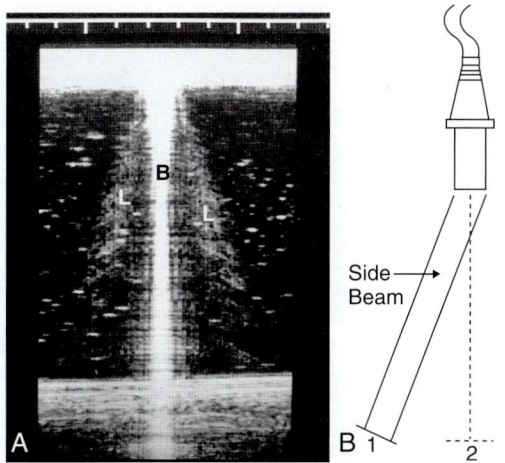

FIG. 7.11 (A) The primary beam *(B)* and grating lobes *(L)* from a linear array transducer. (B) A side lobe or grating lobe can produce and receive a reflection from a "side view."

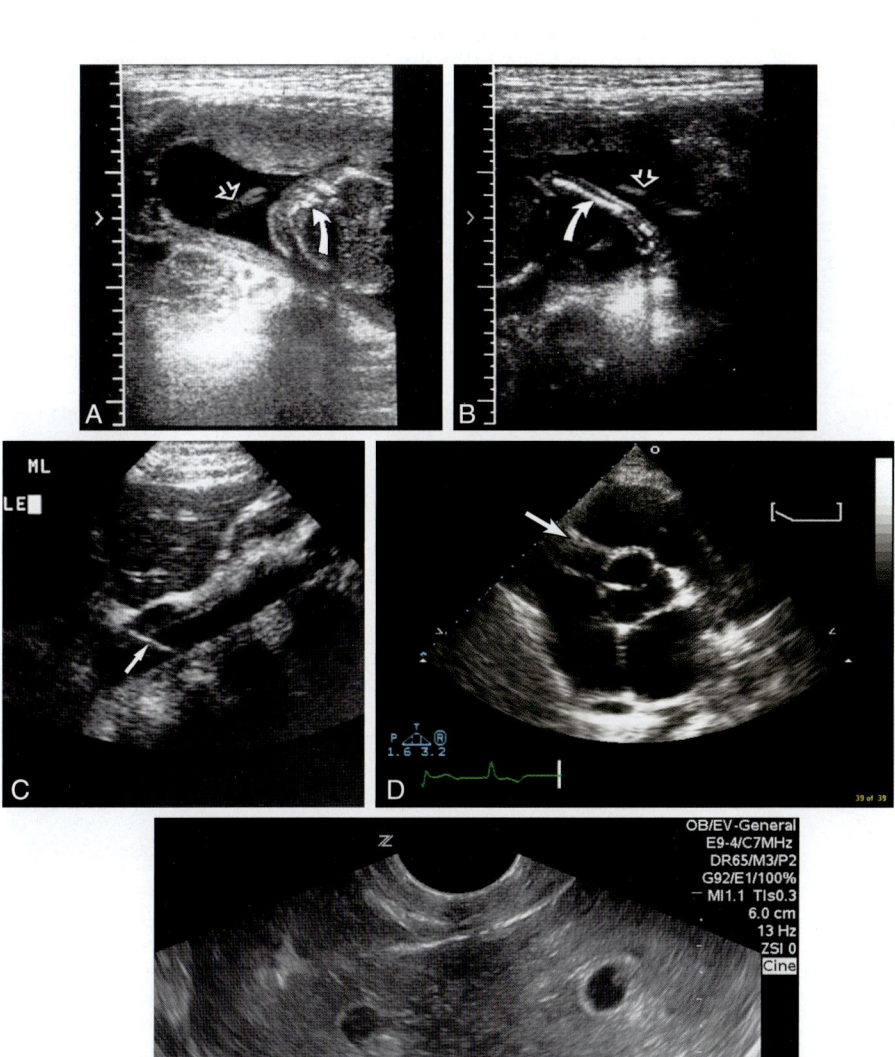

FIG. 7.12 Grating lobes in obstetric scans can produce the appearance of amniotic sheets or bands. (A–B) Grating lobe duplication *(open arrows)* of fetal bones *(curved arrows)* resembles amniotic bands or sheets. (C) Artifactual grating lobe echoes *(arrow)* cross the aorta. (D) Grating lobe *(arrow)* in the cardiac right ventricle. (E) At first glance, this seems to be a mirror image artifact, similar to what is seen in abdominal imaging (see Fig. 7.7). However, it is not for two reasons: (1) There is no apparent echogenic mirror. (2) The repeat on the left side is not horizontally reversed, as would be the case with mirroring. Rather, it is a less echogenic repeat of what is on the right. Therefore this is grating-lobe duplication. Such duplications appear laterally and with less brightness than the correct presentation. (E, Courtesy David Bahner, MD, RDMS, Ohio State University, College of Medicine.)

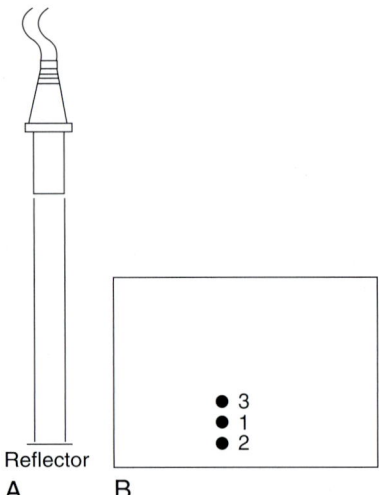

FIG. 7.13 The propagation speed over the traveled path (A) determines the reflector position on the display (B). The reflector is actually in position 1. If the actual propagation speed is less than that assumed, the reflector will appear in position 2. If the actual speed is more than that assumed, the reflector will appear in position 3.

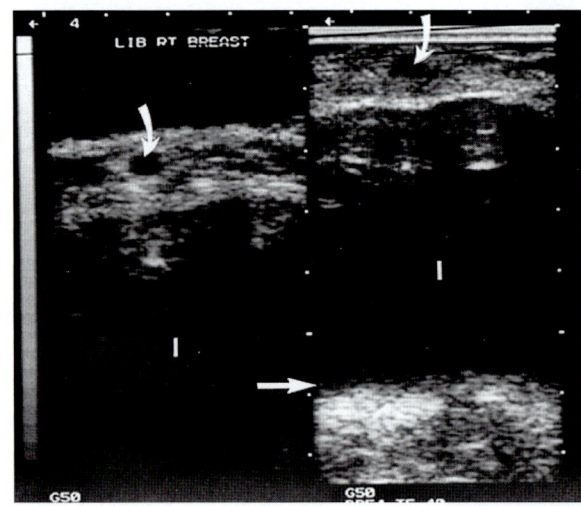

FIG. 7.14 The low propagation speed in a silicone breast implant (I) causes the chest wall *(straight arrow)* to appear deeper than it should. Note that a cyst *(curved arrows)* is shown more clearly on the left image than on the right because a gel standoff pad has been placed between the transducer and the breast, moving the beam focus closer to the cyst.

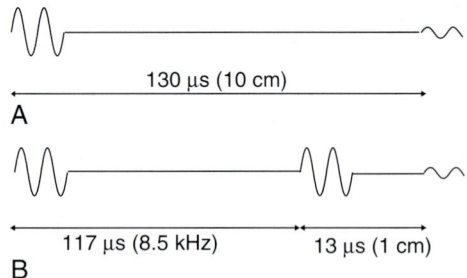

FIG. 7.15 (A) An echo (from a 10-cm depth) arrives 130 μsec after pulse emission. (B) If the pulse repetition period were 117 μsec (corresponding to a pulse repetition frequency of 8.5 kHz), the echo in (A) would arrive 13 μsec after the next pulse was emitted. The instrument would place this echo at a 1-cm depth rather than the correct value. This range location error is known as the range-ambiguity artifact.

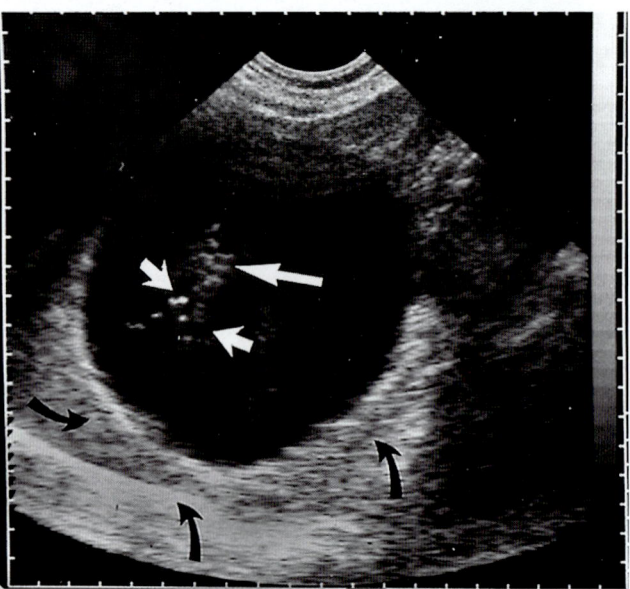

FIG. 7.16 A large renal cyst (diameter about 10 cm) has artifactual range-ambiguity echoes within it *(white arrows)*. They are generated from structure(s) below the display. These deep echoes arrive after the next pulse is emitted. Because the time from the emission of the last pulse to echo arrival is short, the echoes are placed closer to the transducer than they should be. Echoes arrive from much deeper (later) than usual in this case because the sound passes through the long, low-attenuation paths in the cyst. These echoes may have come from bone or far body wall. Low attenuation in the cyst is indicated by the strong echoes (enhancement) below it *(curved black arrows)*.

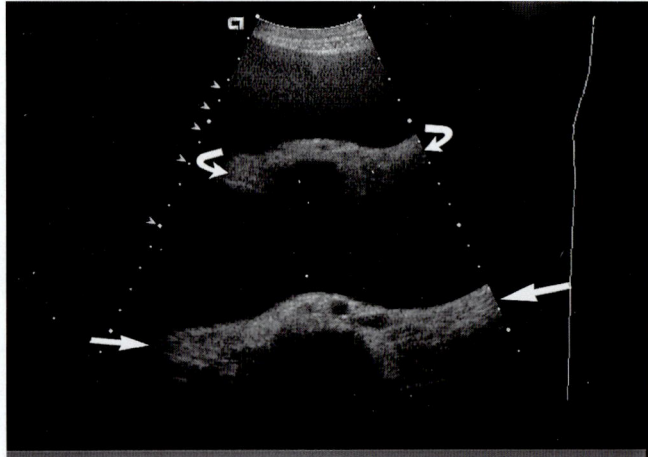

FIG. 7.17 A large pelvic cyst produces a large echo-free region in this scan. A structure is located at a depth of about 13 cm *(straight arrows)*. Located in the anechoic region at a depth of about 6 cm is a structure *(curved arrows)* shaped like that at 13 cm. How could this artifact appear closer than the actual structure, implying that these echoes arrived earlier than those from the correct location? It turns out that the artifact is a combination of two phenomena: reverberation and range ambiguity. The artifact seen is a reverberation from the deep structure and the transducer. But a reverberation should appear at twice the depth of the actual structure—that is, at about 26 cm. However, the arrival of the reverberation echoes occurs about 78 μsec after the next pulse is emitted so that they are placed at a 6-cm depth. Single artifacts are difficult enough. Fortunately, combinations like this occur infrequently.

shadowing structures include calcified plaque, bone, and stone (Fig. 7.18). Shadowing also can occur beyond the edges of objects that are not necessarily strong attenuators (Fig. 7.19). In this case, the cause may be the defocusing action of a refracting curved surface. Alternatively, it may be attributable to destructive interference caused by portions of an ultrasound pulse passing through tissues with different propagation speeds and subsequently getting

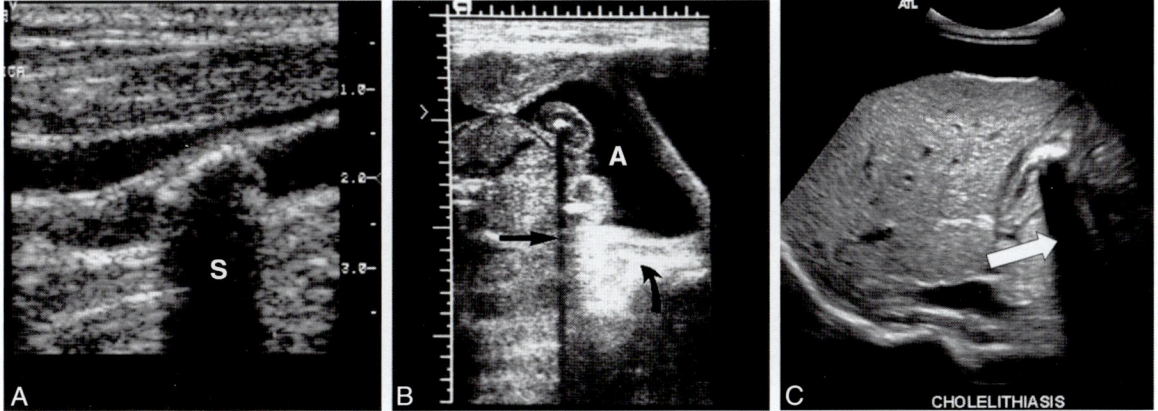

FIG. 7.18 (A) Shadowing from a high-attenuation calcified plaque in the common carotid artery. (B) Shadowing *(straight arrow)* from a fetal limb bone and enhancement *(curved arrow)* caused by the low attenuation of amniotic fluid through which the ultrasound travels. (C) Shadowing *(arrow)* from gallstones.

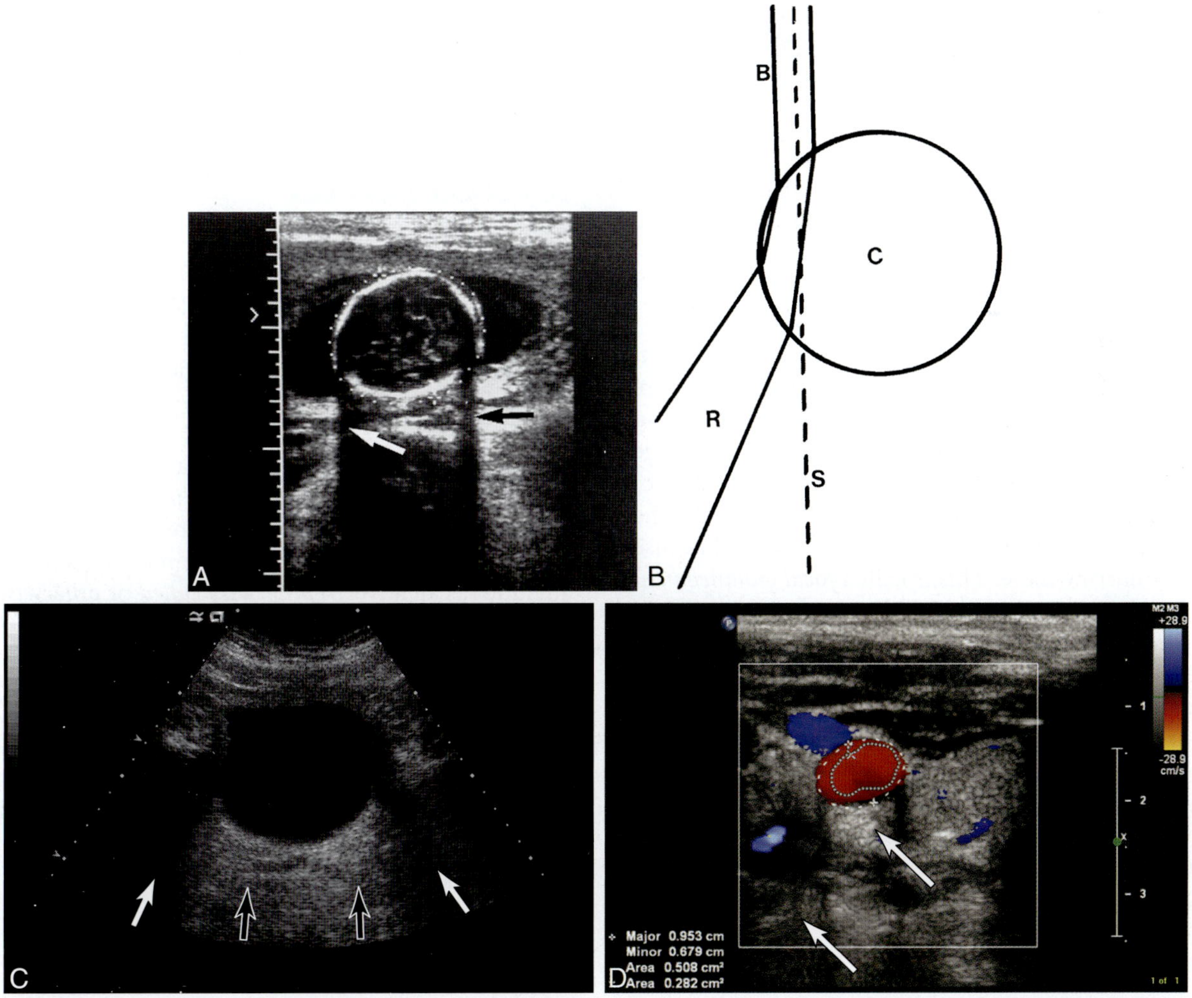

FIG. 7.19 (A) Edge shadows *(arrows)* from a fetal skull. (B) As a sound beam *(B)* enters a circular region *(C)* of higher propagation speed, it is refracted, and refraction occurs again as it leaves. This causes spreading of the beam with decreased intensity. The echoes from region R are presented deep to the circular region in the neighborhood of the dashed line. Because of beam spreading, these echoes are weak and thus cast a shadow *(S)*. (C) Enhancement (black arrows) and edge shadows (white arrows) from pediatric bladder. (D) Transverse carotid scan showing edge shadows *(arrows)*.

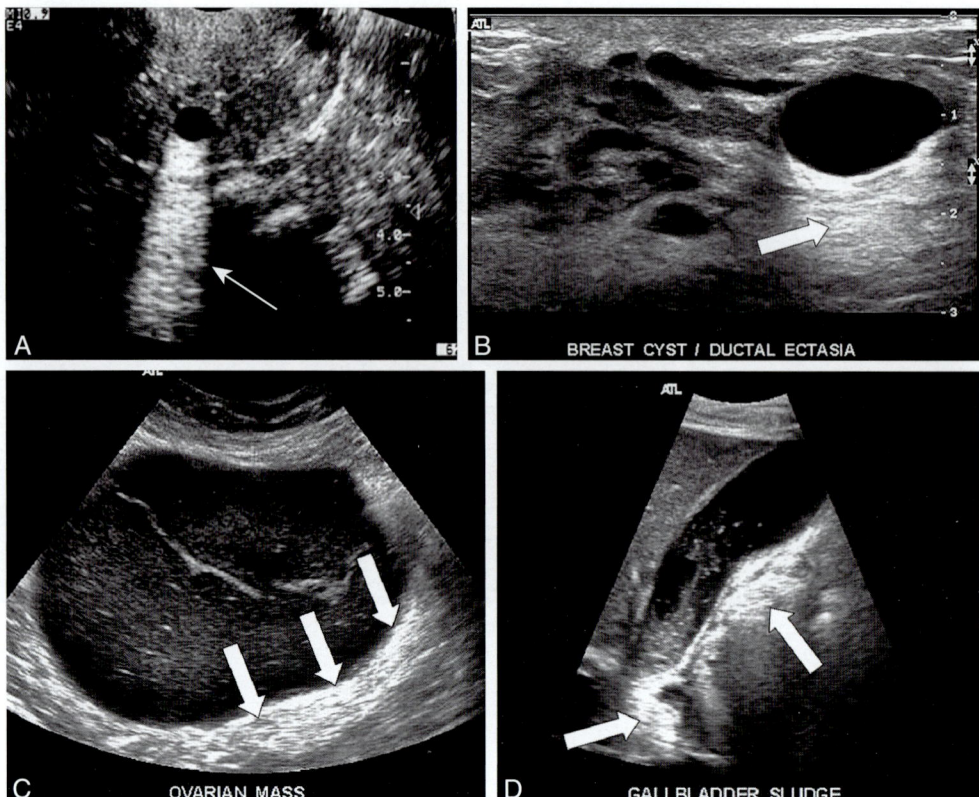

FIG. 7.20 (A) Enhancement *(arrow)* beyond a cervical cyst. (B–D) Examples of enhancement *(arrows)*.

out of phase. In either case, the beam's intensity decreases beyond the edge of the structure, causing echoes to be weakened.

Enhancement

Enhancement is the strengthening of echoes from reflectors that lie behind a weakly attenuating structure (Fig. 7.20; also see Figs. 7.16 and 7.18B). Shadowing and enhancement result in reflectors being placed on the image with amplitudes that are too low and too high, respectively. The brightening of echoes also can be caused by the increased intensity in the focal region of a beam because the beam is narrow there. This is called *focal enhancement* or *focal banding* (Fig. 7.21A). Banding can also be caused by incorrect gain and time gain compensation settings (Fig. 7.21B). Shadowing and enhancement are often useful for determining the nature of masses and structures. Shadowing is reduced with spatial compounding because several approaches to each anatomic site are used, allowing the beam to "get under" the attenuating structure. This is useful with shadowing because it can uncover structures (especially pathologic ones) that were not imaged because they were located in the shadow.

Noise

Noise, generated internally or from external influences, also can produce artifacts (Fig. 7.22).

SPECTRAL DOPPLER

Several artifacts are encountered in Doppler ultrasound, yielding incorrect presentations of Doppler flow information, either in spectral or color Doppler form. The most common of these is aliasing. Others include spectrum mirror image and those that also occur in anatomic imaging.

Aliasing

Aliasing is the most common artifact encountered in Doppler ultrasound. The word *alias* comes from Middle English *elles*, Latin *alius*, and Greek *allos*, which mean *other* or *otherwise*. Contemporary meanings for the word include (as an adverb) *otherwise called* or *otherwise known as* and (as a noun) *an assumed or additional name*. Aliasing in its technical use indicates the improper representation of information that has been sampled insufficiently. An optical form of temporal aliasing occurs in motion pictures when wagon wheels appear to rotate at various speeds and in the reverse direction. Similar behavior is observed when a fan is lighted with a strobe light. Depending on the flashing rate of the strobe light, the fan may appear stationary or rotating clockwise or counterclockwise at various speeds.

Nyquist Limit

Pulsed wave Doppler instruments are sampling instruments. Each emitted pulse yields a sample of the desired

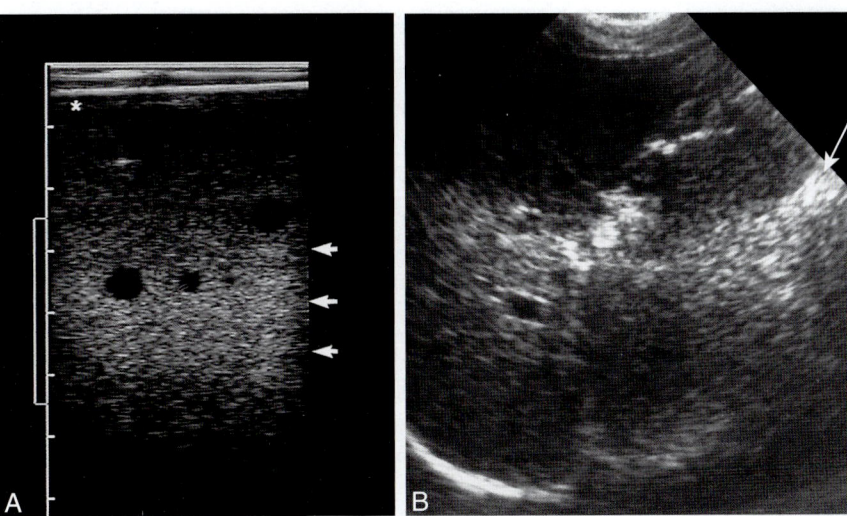

FIG. 7.21 (A) Focal banding *(arrows)* is the brightening of echoes around the focus, where intensity is increased by the narrowing of the beam. (B) Banding *(arrow)* caused by incorrect time gain compensation settings. The midfield gain is too high compared with near- and far-field gain.

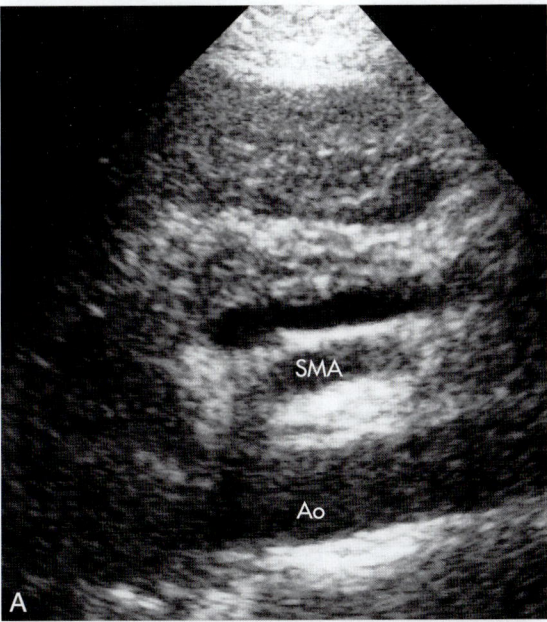

FIG. 7.22 (A) Noise is seen with "fill-in" of anechoic vascular structures. *Ao*, Aorta; *SMA*, superior mesenteric artery. (B) Interference (repeating white specks) from nearby electronic equipment.

TABLE 7.1	Aliasing and Range-Ambiguity Artifact Values	
Pulse Repetition Frequency (kHz)	Doppler Shift Above Which Aliasing Occurs (kHz)	Range Beyond Which Ambiguity Occurs (cm)
5.0	2.5	15
7.5	3.7	10
10.0	5.0	7
12.5	6.2	6
15.0	7.5	5
17.5	8.7	4
20.0	10.0	3
25.0	12.5	3
30.0	15.0	2

Doppler shift. The upper limit to Doppler shift that can be detected properly by pulsed instruments is called the **Nyquist limit**. If the Doppler-shift frequency exceeds one-half the PRF (which, for Doppler functions, is normally in the 5 to 30 kHz range), temporal aliasing occurs. Improper Doppler shift information (improper direction and improper value) results. Higher PRFs (Table 7.1) permit higher Doppler shifts to be detected but increase the chance of the range-ambiguity artifact occurring. Continuous wave Doppler instruments do not experience aliasing, but neither do they provide depth localization. Fig. 7.23 illustrates aliasing in the popliteal artery and the heart of a normal subject. This figure also illustrates how aliasing can be corrected, reduced, or eliminated (Box 7.1) by increasing PRF, increasing Doppler angle (which decreases the Doppler shift for a given flow), or by *baseline shift*. The latter is an electronic cut-and-paste technique that moves the misplaced aliasing peaks over to their proper location. The technique is successful as long as there are no legitimate Doppler shifts in the region of the aliasing. Otherwise, legitimate Doppler shifts will be moved over to an inappropriate location along with the aliasing peaks. (This would happen if the baseline were shifted farther down in Fig. 7.23E.) Baseline shifting is not helpful if the desired information (e.g., peak systolic

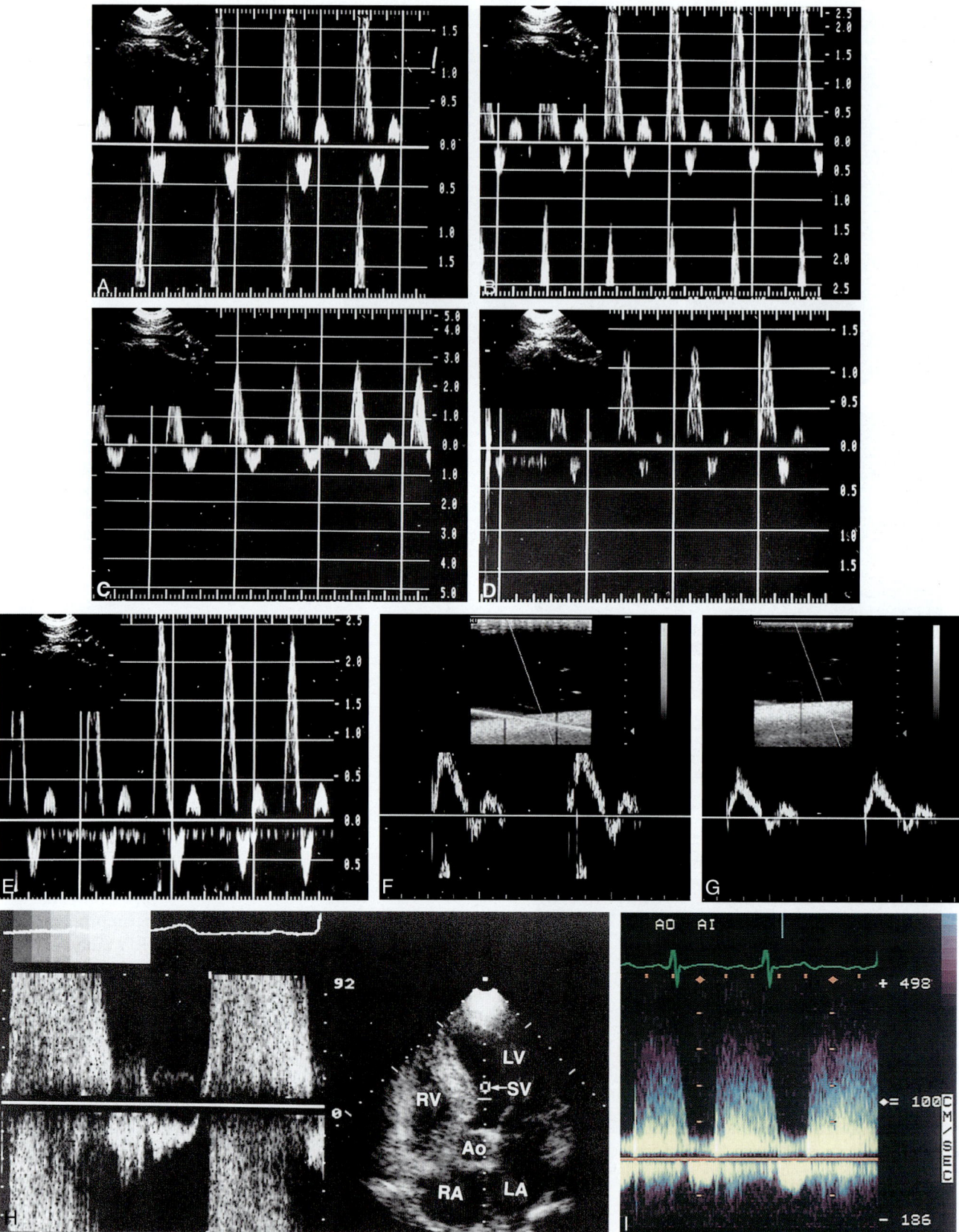

FIG. 7.23 (A) Aliasing in the popliteal artery. (B) Pulse repetition frequency (PRF) is increased. (C) The PRF is increased further. (D) Doppler angle is increased with original PRF. (E) Baseline is shifted down with original PRF. (F) Aliasing is occurring with an operating frequency of 6 MHz. (G) When operating frequency is reduced to 4 MHz, the Doppler shifts are reduced to less than the Nyquist limit, thereby eliminating the aliasing seen in (F). (H) The sample volume (SV) is placed in the left-ventricular outflow tract. There is aortic insufficiency that causes the Doppler shifts to exceed the Nyquist limit producing aliasing. (I) Using continuous wave ultrasound eliminates the aliasing because there is no sampling. *Ao*, Aorta; *LA*, left atrium, *LV*, left ventricle; *RA*, right atrium; *RV*, right ventricle.

Doppler shift) is buried in another portion of the spectral display, as in Fig. 7.23H. Other approaches to eliminating aliasing include changing to a lower-frequency Doppler transducer (Fig. 7.23F–G) or switching to continuous wave operation (Fig. 7.23H–I). The common and convenient solutions to aliasing are first shifting the baseline and then increasing PRF if necessary in extreme cases.

In Fig. 7.23A, the vertical axis is calibrated in Doppler-shift frequency units to see that aliasing occurs at Doppler shifts greater than 1.75 kHz. The aliased peaks add another 1.25 kHz of Doppler shift, so the correct peak systolic shift is 3 kHz. With the higher PRF in Fig. 7.23C, this result is confirmed. Thus at the lower PRF, the peak shift can be determined, and baseline shifting is not necessary (but is convenient). However, if the peaks were buried in other portions of the Doppler signal (as in Fig. 7.23H), baseline shifting would not help, but a higher PRF (most convenient method), a larger Doppler angle, or a lower operating frequency would. Aliasing occurs with the pulsed system because it is a sampling system; that is, a pulsed system acquires samples of the desired Doppler shift frequency from which it must be synthesized. If samples are taken often enough, the correct result is achieved. Fig. 7.24 shows the temporal sampling of a signal. Sufficient sampling yields the correct result. Insufficient sampling yields an incorrect result.

> **BOX 7.1 Methods of Correcting, Reducing, or Eliminating Aliasing**
>
> Shift the baseline[a]
> Increase the pulse repetition frequency[a]
> Increase the Doppler angle
> Use a lower operating frequency
> Use a continuous wave device
>
> [a]These are the most convenient and commonly used. Both are required in extreme cases.

The Nyquist limit, or Nyquist frequency, describes the minimum number of samples required to avoid aliasing. At least two samples per cycle of the desired Doppler shift must be obtained for the image to be presented correctly. For a complicated signal, such as a Doppler signal containing many frequencies, the sampling rate must be such that at least two samples occur for each cycle of the highest frequency present. To restate this rule, if the highest Doppler-shift frequency present in a signal exceeds one-half the PRF, aliasing will occur (see Fig. 7.24).

Lesser-used correction methods include increasing the Doppler angle (which reduces the Doppler shift), reducing the operating frequency, and switching to continuous wave operation. Continuous wave operation, because it is not pulsed, is not a sampling mode, and is thus not subject to aliasing. However, it does not have range selectivity ability.

Range Ambiguity

In attempting to solve the aliasing problem by increasing the PRF, one can encounter the range-ambiguity problem. As described previously under the propagation group, this problem occurs when a pulse is emitted before all the echoes from the previous pulse have been received. When this happens, early echoes from the last pulse are received simultaneously with late echoes from the previous pulse. The instrument is unable to determine whether an echo is an early one (superficial) from the last pulse or a late one (deep) from the previous pulse. To solve this difficulty, the instrument simply assumes that all echoes are derived from the last pulse and that these echoes have originated from depths determined by the 13 μsec/cm rule. As long as all echoes are received before the next pulse is sent out, this is true. However, with high PRFs, this may not be the case. Doppler flow information therefore may come from locations other than the assumed one (the gate location). In effect, multiple gates or sample volumes are operating at different depths. Table 7.1 lists, for various PRFs,

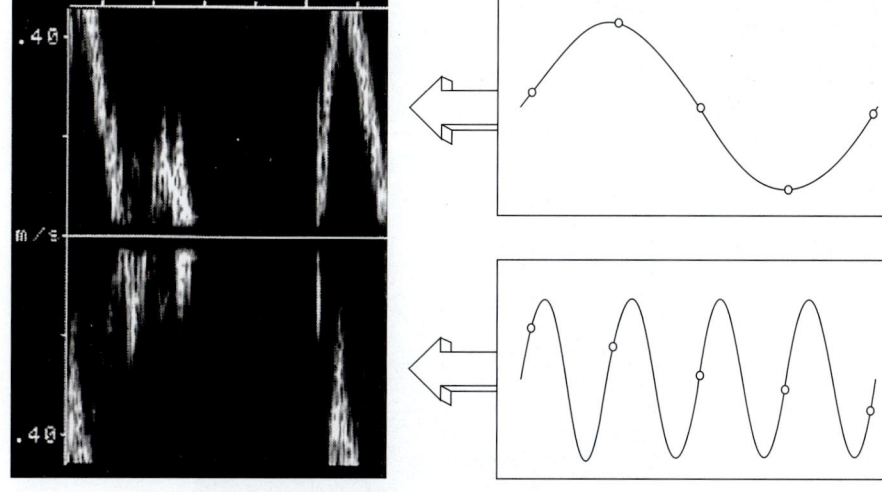

FIG. 7.24 In this spectral display, the presentation above the baseline is correct (unaliased, five samples per cycle), whereas the systolic peaks appear incorrectly below the baseline (aliased, one sample per cycle).

the ranges beyond which ambiguity occurs. Multiple sample volumes are shown on the display to indicate this condition.

Mirror Image

A mirror image of a Doppler spectrum can appear on the opposite side of the baseline when, indeed, flow is unidirectional and should appear only on one side of the baseline. This is an electronic duplication of the spectral information. The duplication can occur when Doppler gain is set too high, causing overloading in the amplifier and leakage, called *crosstalk*, of the signal from the proper-direction channel into the opposite-direction channel (Fig. 7.25).

Noise

Doppler spectra have a speckled quality to them that is similar to that observed in sonography. Internally generated electronic noise appears if Doppler gain is set too high (Fig. 7.26A). Electromagnetic interference from nearby equipment can cloud the spectral display with lines or "snow" (Fig. 7.26B–C).

COLOR DOPPLER

Artifacts observed with color Doppler imaging are two-dimensional color presentations of artifacts seen in gray-scale sonography and Doppler spectral displays. They are incorrect presentations of two-dimensional motion information, the most common of which is aliasing. However, others occur, including anatomic mirror image, Doppler angle effects, shadowing, and clutter.

Aliasing

Aliasing occurs when the Doppler shift exceeds the Nyquist limit (Fig. 7.27). The result is incorrect flow direction on the color Doppler image (Fig. 7.28). Increasing the flow speed range (which is actually an increase in PRF) can solve the problem (Fig. 7.29). However, too high a range can cause loss of flow information, particularly if the wall filter is set high (Fig. 7.29D–E). Baseline shifting can decrease or eliminate the effect of aliasing (Fig. 7.29C), as in spectral displays.

Mirror Image, Shadowing, Clutter, and Noise

In the mirror (or ghost) artifact (Fig. 7.30), an image of a vessel and source of Doppler-shifted echoes can be duplicated on the opposite side of a strong reflector (e.g., pleura or diaphragm). This is a color Doppler extension of gray-scale mirror. Shadowing is the weakening or elimination of Doppler-shifted echoes beyond a shadowing object, just as occurs with non–Doppler-shifted (gray-scale) echoes (Fig. 7.31). Clutter, also called flash artifact, results from tissue, heart wall or valve, or vessel wall motion (Fig. 7.32).

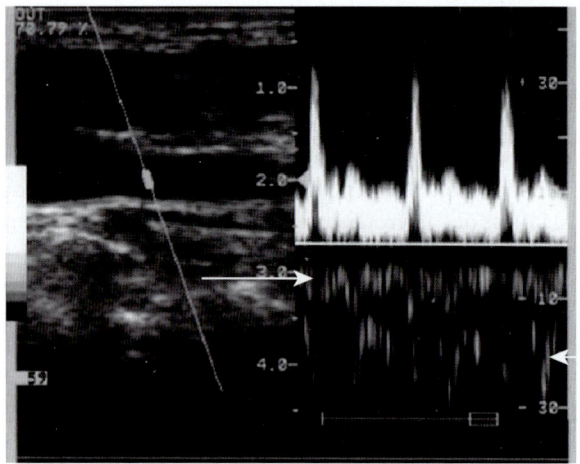

FIG. 7.25 High gain produces a mirror image *(arrows)* of the carotid artery spectrum below the baseline.

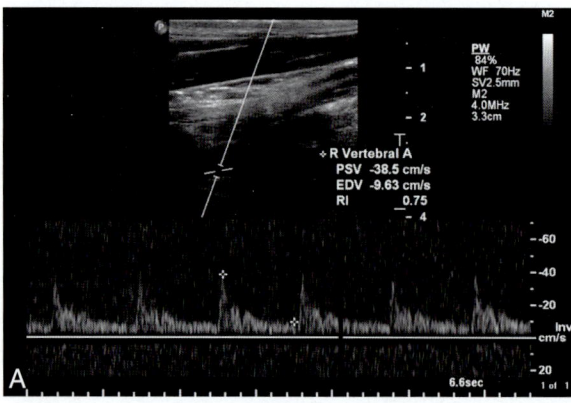

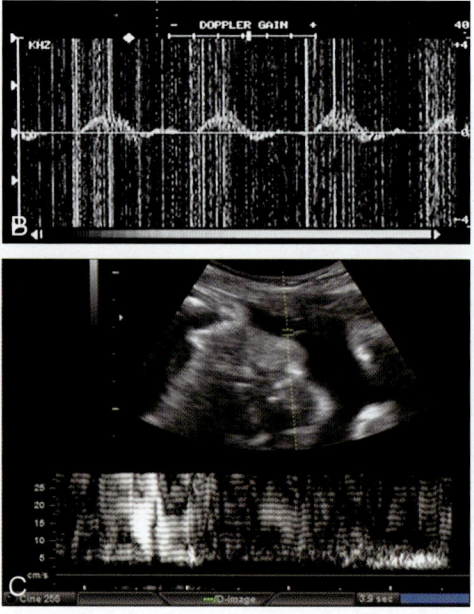

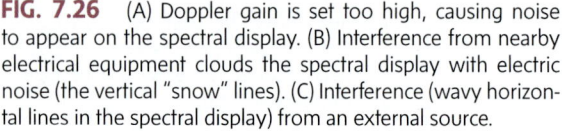

FIG. 7.26 (A) Doppler gain is set too high, causing noise to appear on the spectral display. (B) Interference from nearby electrical equipment clouds the spectral display with electric noise (the vertical "snow" lines). (C) Interference (wavy horizontal lines in the spectral display) from an external source.

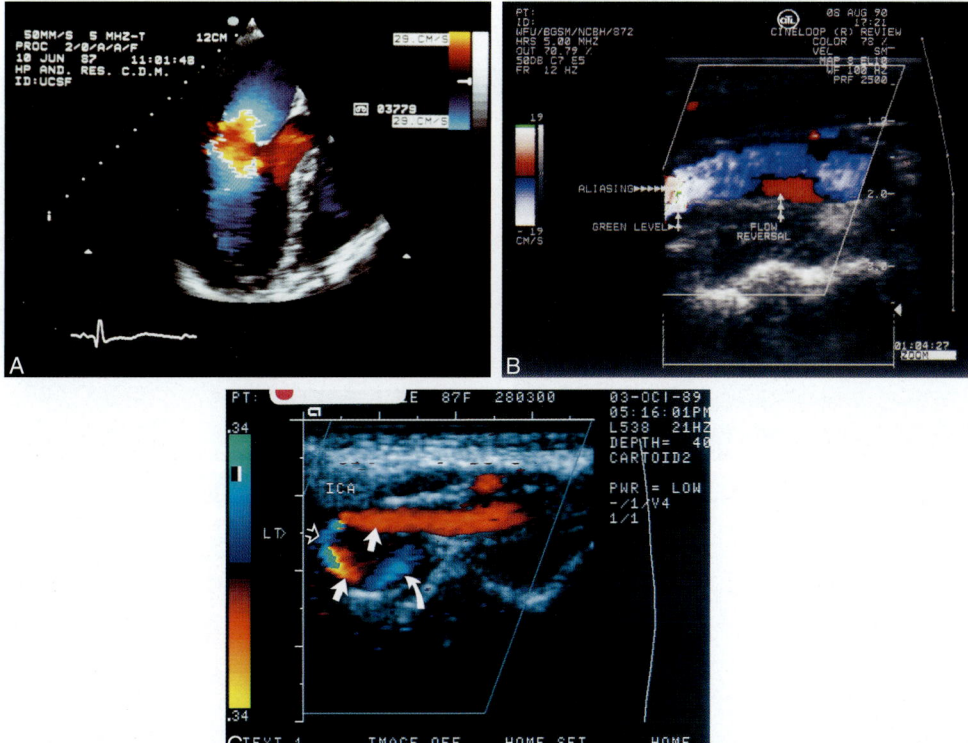

FIG. 7.27 (A) A transesophageal cardiac color Doppler image of the long axis in diastole. The blue colors in the left atrium *(upper)* and left ventricle *(lower)* represent blood traveling away from the transducer, but where the flow speeds exceed the Nyquist limit (29 cm/sec), aliasing occurs, and the yellow and orange colors have replaced the blue colors. (B) Color Doppler presentation of common carotid artery flow, including flow reversal and aliasing. The two can be distinguished because the boundary between the different directions with flow reversal passes through the baseline *(black)*, whereas the aliasing boundary passes through the upper and lower extremes of the color bar *(white)*. In this color bar assignment, the maximum positive Doppler shifts are assigned the color green so that a thin green region shows the exact boundary where aliasing occurs. The aliasing occurs in the distal portion of the vessel because it is curving down, reducing the Doppler angle between the flow and the scan lines. (C) Negative Doppler shifts in a tortuous internal carotid artery are indicated in the red regions *(solid straight arrows)*. Two regions of positive Doppler shifts *(blue)* are seen *(open arrow* and *curved arrow)*. In the latter, legitimate flow toward the transducer is indicated. In the former, the flow away from the transducer has yielded high Doppler shifts (because of a small Doppler angle, i.e., flow is approximately parallel to scan lines), which produces a color shift to the opposite side of the map because of aliasing. The boundaries from and to normal negative Doppler shifts into and out of the aliased region are bright yellow and cyan from the ends of the color bars. The transition from unaliased negative Doppler shift into unaliased positive Doppler shift (near the bottom) is black, representing the baseline of the color bar. The flow direction is counterclockwise.

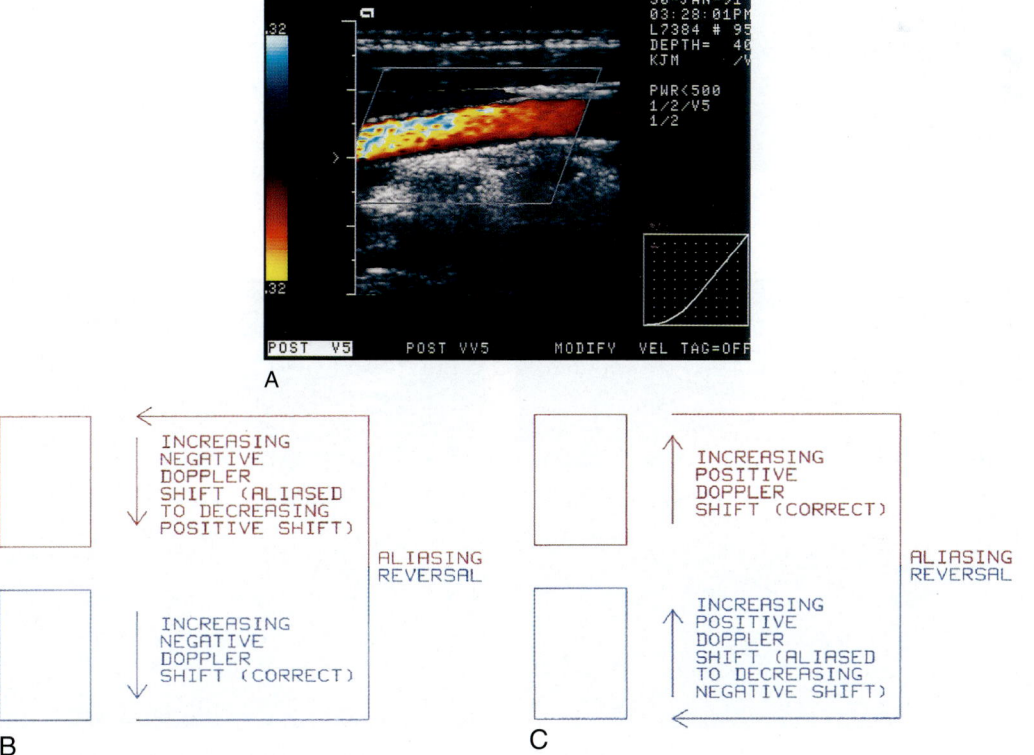

FIG. 7.28 (A) Positive *(blue)* Doppler shifts are shown in the arterial flow in this image. (B) These are negative Doppler shifts that have exceeded the lower Nyquist limit (converted here to the equivalent flow speed: −0.32 m/sec) and are wrapped around to the positive portion of the color bar (C). Positive shifts that exceed the +0.32 m/sec limit would alias to the negative side.

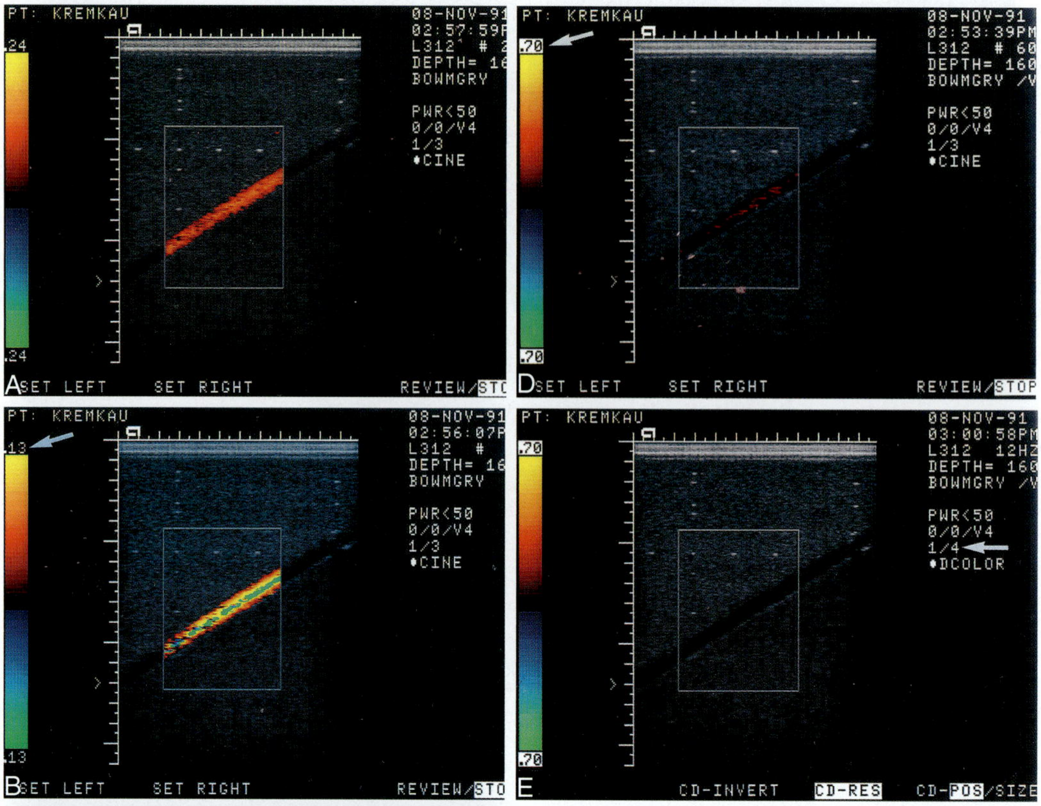

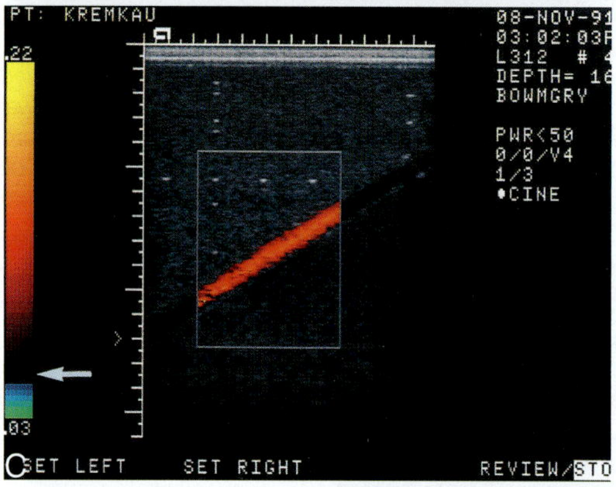

FIG. 7.29 (A) Flow is toward the upper right, producing positive Doppler shifts. (B) The pulse repetition frequency and Nyquist limit (0.13, *arrow*) are too low, resulting in aliasing (negative Doppler shifts) at the center of the flow in the vessel. (C) With the same pulse repetition frequency setting as in (B) the aliasing has been corrected by shifting the baseline *(arrow)* down 10 cm/sec below the center of the color bar. (D) The Nyquist limit setting (0.70, *arrow*) is too high, causing the detected Doppler shifts to be well down the positive scale, producing a dark red appearance. (E) With the Nyquist limit set as in part D an increase in the wall filter setting *(arrow)* eliminates what little color flow information there was in part D.

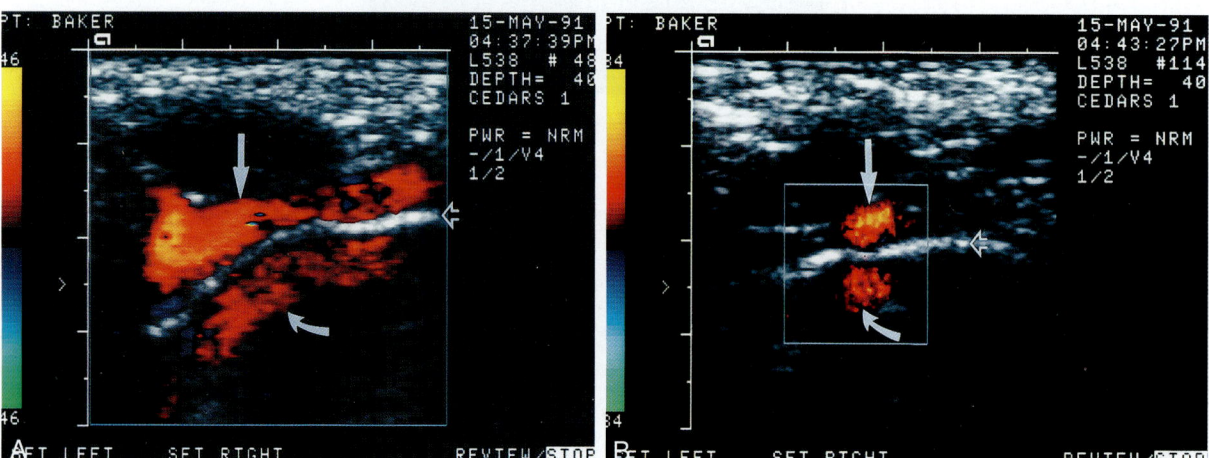

FIG. 7.30 Color Doppler imaging of the subclavian artery *(straight arrow)* in longitudinal (A) and transverse (B) views. The pleura *(open arrow)* causes the mirror image *(curved arrow)*.

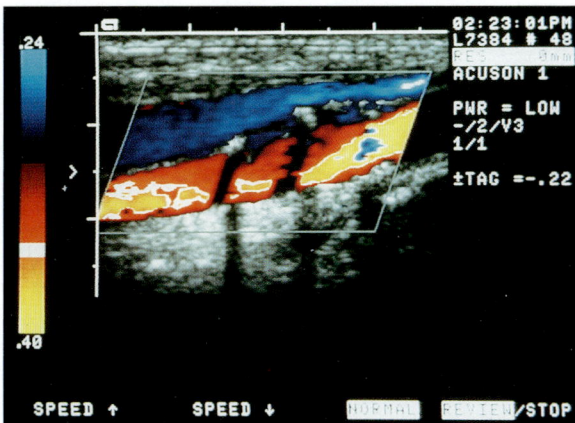

FIG. 7.31 Shadowing from calcified plaque follows the gray-scale scan lines straight down while following the angled color scan lines parallel to the sides of the parallelogram.

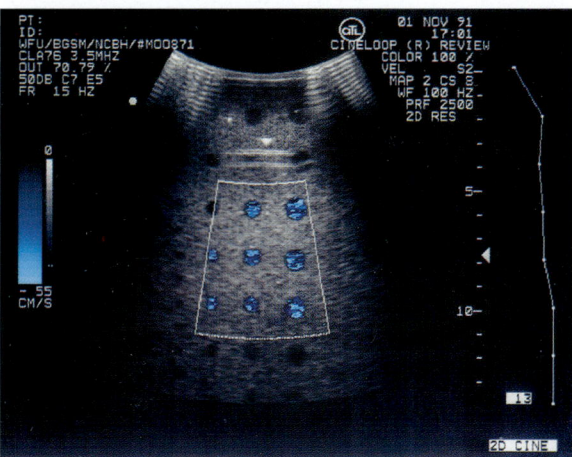

FIG. 7.33 Color appears in echo-free (cystic) regions of a tissue-equivalent phantom. The color gain has been increased sufficiently to produce this effect. The instrument tends to write color information preferentially in areas where non–Doppler-shifted echoes are weak or absent.

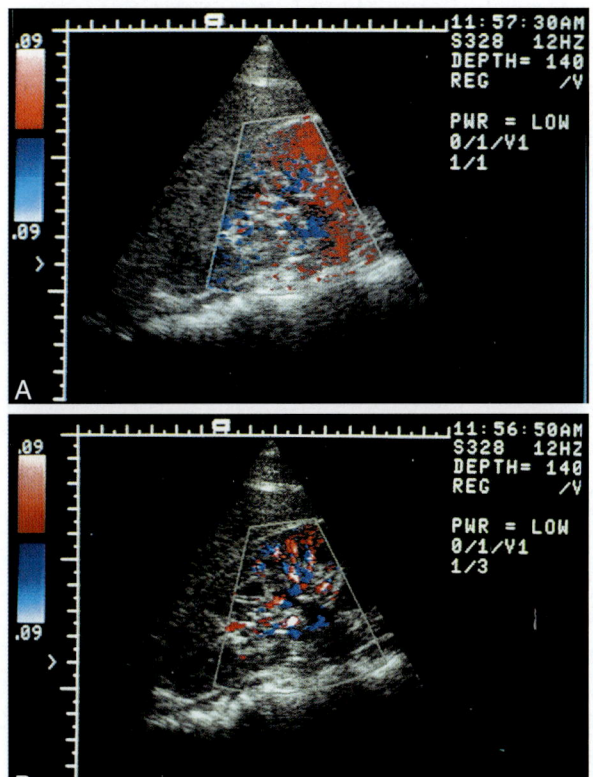

FIG. 7.32 (A) Clutter from tissue motion (caused by respiration) obscures underlying blood flow in the renal vasculature. (B) An increased wall filter setting removes the clutter, revealing the underlying flow.

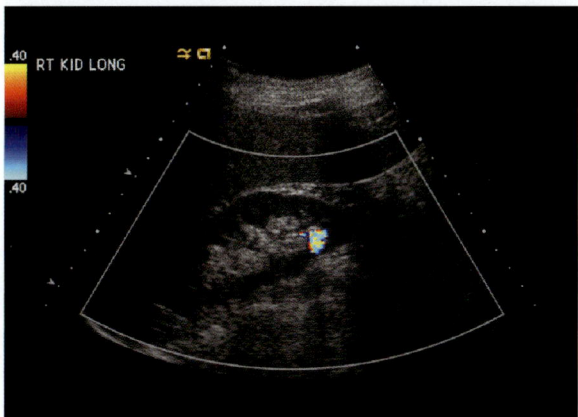

FIG. 7.34 Twinkling artifact associated with a renal stone.

VIRTUAL BEAM-FORMING

During the decades in which sonography has been applied to diagnostic medicine, the fundamental, pulse-echo principle has been operating throughout. Over those decades, there was one operating principle. Now there are two. Some current systems operate on the conventional pulse-echo principle, and others operate on the new virtual-beam principle. The examples of sonographic artifacts in this chapter involve instruments operating with the conventional pulse-echo principle. Instruments operating with the virtual beam-forming principle have several advantages, some of which impact artifacts (Boxes 7.2 and 7.3). In addition, the entrance of artificial intelligence into contemporary sonographic systems enables the automation of functions that previously were accomplished manually. Examples include automated baseline shift (and scale change if needed) to correct for spectral aliasing (Fig. 7.35) and elimination of flash artifact (Fig. 7.36).

SUMMARY

This chapter has discussed several ultrasound imaging and flow artifacts, which are listed in Table 7.2, along with their

Such clutter is eliminated by wall filters. Doppler angle effects include zero Doppler shift when the Doppler angle is 90 degrees, as well as the change of color in a straight vessel viewed with a sector transducer. Noise in the color Doppler electronics can mimic flow, particularly in hypoechoic or anechoic regions (Fig. 7.33). The "twinkling" artifact (Fig. 7.34) has been observed at strongly reflecting scattering surfaces. It is thought to occur with complications in the phase detection process of Doppler detection when a finite number of strong scatterers is encountered.

BOX 7.2 Improvements in Anatomic Imaging With Virtual Beam-Forming

- Detail resolution *improved dramatically*
  - Laser-thin virtual beam
  - Entire image in focus
- Contrast resolution *improved*
  - Section thickness reduced
- Temporal resolution *improved significantly*
  - Broad physical beam (fewer pulses required)
  - No multiple foci needed
  - Frame rates >1000/sec
  - Real-time volume imaging (4D)
  - Quantitative shear-wave elastography
- Sensitivity and penetration *improved*
- Artifacts *reduced*
  - Speed correction throughout the image
  - Section thickness reduced

BOX 7.3 Improvements in Doppler Operation With Virtual Beam-Forming

Simultaneous gray scale, color Doppler, and spectral Doppler (no time sharing)
- Color flash reduced or eliminated (see Fig. 7.35)
- Flow velocity vector mapping (see Fig. 7.36)
- Retrospective sample volume
- Automatic aliasing correction

TABLE 7.2 Artifacts and Their Causes

Artifact	Cause
Axial resolution	Pulse length
Comet tail	Reverberation
Grating lobe	Grating lobe
Lateral resolution	Pulse width
Mirror image	Multiple reflection
Refraction	Refraction
Reverberation	Multiple reflection
Ring down	Resonance
Section thickness	Pulse width
Speckle	Interference
Speed error	Speed error
Range ambiguity	High pulse repetition frequency
Shadowing	High attenuation
Edge shadowing	Refraction or interference
Enhancement	Low attenuation
Focal enhancement	Focusing
Aliasing	Low pulse repetition frequency
Spectrum mirror	High Doppler gain

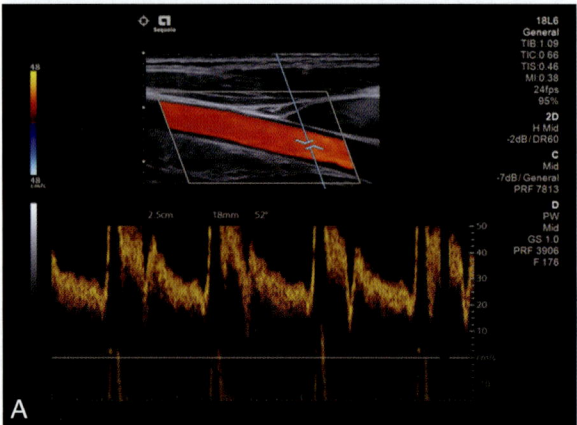

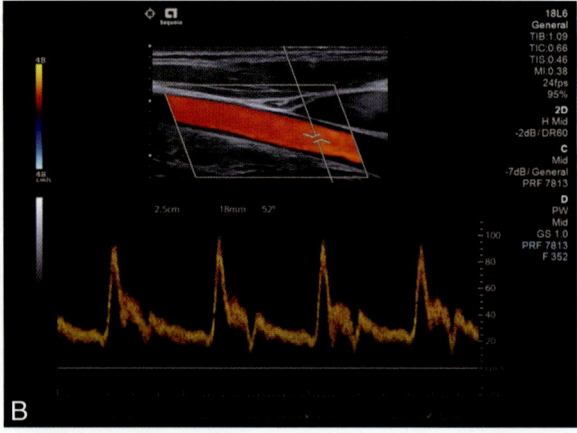

FIG. 7.35 (A) Spectral display with aliasing. (B) Aliasing recognized and corrected by artificial intelligence. Baseline was shifted down, and scale (pulse repetition frequency) doubled.

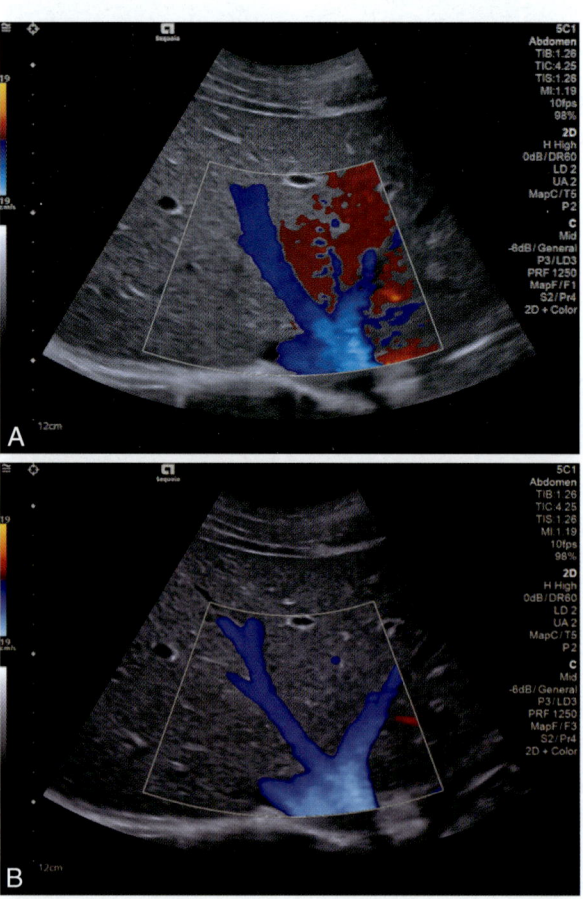

FIG. 7.36 (A) Color Doppler image with flash artifact. (B) Flash artifact automatically eliminated.

causes. In some cases, the names of the artifacts are identical to their causes.

- Shadowing and enhancement are useful in interpretation and diagnosis.
- Other artifacts can cause confusion and error.
- Artifacts seen in two-dimensional imaging are also evidenced in three-dimensional imaging, sometimes in unusual ways.
- These artifacts can hinder proper interpretation and diagnosis and so must be avoided or handled properly when encountered.
- A proper understanding of artifacts and how to deal with them when they are encountered enables sonographers and sonologists to use them to their advantage while avoiding the pitfalls that they can cause.

Key Pearls

- An artifact is the appearance of anything that does not properly present the structures or motion imaged.
- An artifact is caused by some problematic aspect of the imaging technique.
- Axial and lateral (detail) resolutions are artifactual because a failure to resolve means a loss of detail, and two adjacent structures may be visualized as one.
- The beam width perpendicular to the scan plane results in section thickness artifacts, for example, the appearance of false debris in what should be echo-free areas.
- The detailed echo pattern often is not related directly to the scattering properties of tissue (called tissue texture) but rather is the result of the interference effects of the scattered sound from the distribution of scatterers in the tissue.
- Multiple reflections are placed beneath the real reflector at separation intervals equal to the separation between the transducer and the real reflector.
- Comet tail, a particular form of reverberation, is a series of closely spaced, discrete echoes.
- Ring-down artifact is caused by a resonance phenomenon associated with the presence of a collection of gas bubbles.
- Resonance is the condition in which a driven mechanical vibration is of a frequency similar to a natural vibration frequency of the structure.
- The mirror image artifact, also a form of reverberation, shows structures that exist on one side of a strong reflector as being present on the other side as well.
- Refraction can cause a reflector to be positioned improperly (laterally) on a sonographic display.
- Side lobes are beams that propagate from a single transducer element in directions different from the primary beam.
- Grating lobes are additional beams emitted from an array transducer that are stronger than the side lobes of individual elements.
- Propagation speed error occurs when the assumed value for propagation speed (1.54 mm/μsec, leading to the 13 μsec/cm round-trip travel time rule) is incorrect.
- Shadowing is the reduction in echo amplitude from reflectors that lie behind a strongly reflecting or attenuating structure.
- Enhancement is the strengthening of echoes from reflectors that lie behind a weakly attenuating structure.
- Aliasing is the most common artifact encountered in Doppler ultrasound.
- The upper limit to Doppler shift that can be detected properly by pulsed instruments is called the Nyquist limit.
- The Nyquist limit, or Nyquist frequency, describes the minimum number of samples required to avoid aliasing.
- Clutter results from tissue, heart wall or valve, or vessel wall motion; such clutter is eliminated by wall filters.

BIBLIOGRAPHY

Campbell SC, Cullinan JA, Rubens DJ. Slow flow or no flow? Color and power Doppler US pitfalls in the abdomen and pelvis. *RadioGraphics.* 2004;24:497–506.

Kremkau FW. Instruments: Imaging anatomy, motion and flow with virtual beam-forming In: *Sonography: principles and instruments.* ed 10. Philadelphia: Elsevier; 2021.

Kremkau FW. Your new paradigm for understanding and applying sonographic principles. *J Diag Med Sonography.* 2019;35:439–446.

Mitchell C, Pozniak M, Zagzebski J, Ledwidge M. Twinkling artifact related to intravesicular suture. *J Ultrasound Med.* 2003;22:1409–1411.

Nelson TR, et al. Sources and impact of artifacts on clinical three-dimensional ultrasound imaging. *Ultrasound Obstet Gynecol.* 2000;16:374–383.

PART II

Abdomen

Chapter 8 Vascular System
Chapter 9 The Liver
Chapter 10 The Gallbladder and the Biliary System
Chapter 11 The Spleen
Chapter 12 The Pancreas
Chapter 13 The Gastrointestinal Tract
Chapter 14 The Peritoneal Cavity and Abdominal Wall
Chapter 15 Urinary System
Chapter 16 The Retroperitoneum
Chapter 17 Abdominal Applications of Ultrasound Contrast Agents
Chapter 18 Ultrasound-Guided Interventional Techniques
Chapter 19 Emergent Ultrasound Procedures
Chapter 20 Sonographic Techniques in the Transplant Patient

CHAPTER 8

Vascular System

Sandra L. Hagen-Ansert

OBJECTIVES

On completion of this chapter, you should be able to:
- Describe the anatomy of the arterial system, venous system, and portal venous system
- Understand the function of the circulatory system
- Recognize the sonographic findings and pathology found in the vascular structures
- Define the two types of aneurysm formation
- Explain the factors that may cause development of an aneurysm
- Identify the sonographic findings in aortic dissection
- Identify causes of pseudopulsatile abdominal masses
- Explain the sonographic findings and complications in portal hypertension
- Describe the Doppler flow patterns in arterial versus venous structures

OUTLINE

Function of the Circulatory System 170
Aorta 171
   Root of the Aorta 171
   Ascending Aorta 172
   Descending Aorta 172
   Abdominal Aorta and Iliac Arteries 172
   Common Iliac Arteries 178
   Abdominal Aortic Branches 179
   Pathology of the Aorta 187
Inferior Vena Cava 195
   Inferior Vena Cava Abnormalities 198
   Lateral Tributaries to the Inferior Vena Cava 199
   Anterior Tributaries to the Inferior Vena Cava 204
Portal Venous System 206
   Portal Vein 206
   Splenic Vein 206
   Superior Mesenteric Vein 207
   Inferior Mesenteric Vein 209
Abdominal Doppler Techniques 209
   Blood Flow Analysis 209
   Doppler Technique 210
   Doppler Flow Patterns in the Abdominal Arterial Vessels 212
   Doppler Flow Patterns in the Abdominal Venous Vessels 214

KEY TERMS

Abdominal aortic aneurysm
Anastomosis
Aorta
Arteries
Arteriosclerosis
Atherosclerosis
Capillaries
Cavernous transformation of the portal vein
Common hepatic artery
Common iliac arteries
Cystic medial necrosis
Dissecting aneurysm
Doppler sample volume
Fusiform aneurysm
Gastroduodenal artery
Hepatic veins

Hepatofugal
Hepatopetal
Inferior mesenteric artery
Inferior mesenteric vein
Inferior vena cava
Left gastric artery
Left hepatic artery
Left renal artery
Left renal vein
Marfan syndrome
Nonresistive
Portal vein
Portal venous hypertension
Pseudoaneurysm
Renal vein thrombosis
Resistive
Resistive index

Right gastric artery
Right hepatic artery
Right renal artery
Right renal vein
Saccular aneurysm
Spectral broadening
Splenic artery
Splenic vein
Superior mesenteric artery
Superior mesenteric vein
Tunica adventitia
Tunica intima
Tunica media
Vasa vasorum
Veins

CHAPTER 8 Vascular System

Knowledge of the vascular structures within the abdomen, retroperitoneum, and pelvis is beneficial to the sonographer as landmarks for identifying specific organ structures. To understand the origin and anatomic variations of the major arterial and venous structures, the sonographer must be able to identify the anatomy correctly on the sonographic image.

FUNCTION OF THE CIRCULATORY SYSTEM

The function of the circulatory system, along with the heart and lymphatics, is to transport gases, nutrient materials, and other essential substances to the tissues and subsequently transport waste products from the cells to appropriate sites for excretion.

Blood is carried away from the heart by the arteries and is returned from the tissues to the heart by the veins (Fig. 8.1).

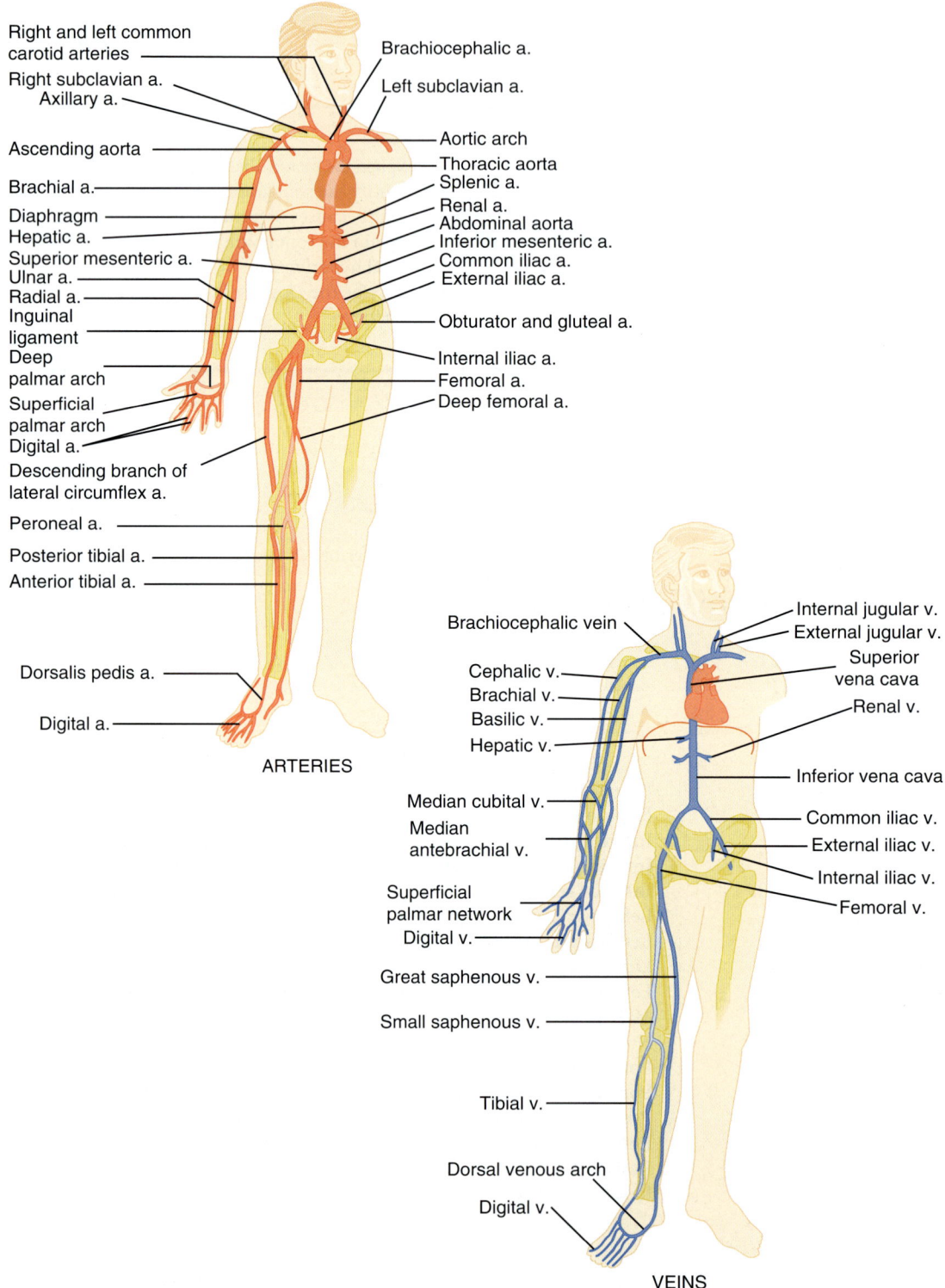

FIG. 8.1 The human vascular system. Blood is carried away from the heart by the arteries *(left)* and is returned from the tissues to the heart by the veins *(right)*.

Arteries divide into progressively smaller branches, the smallest of which are the arterioles. These lead into the capillaries, which are minute vessels that branch and form a network where the exchange of materials between blood and tissue fluid occurs. After the blood passes through the capillaries, it is collected in the small veins, or venules. These small vessels unite to form larger vessels that eventually return the blood to the heart for recirculation.

A typical artery in cross section consists of the following three layers (Fig. 8.2A):

- **Tunica intima** (inner layer) consists of the following three layers: a layer of endothelial cells lining the arterial passage (lumen), a layer of delicate connective tissue, and an elastic layer made up of a network of elastic fibers.
- **Tunica media** (middle layer) consists of elastin, smooth muscle fibers, and collagenous tissue. The media provides the strength of the aorta. Unfortunately, elastin is produced only minimally in the body. Therefore with increasing age, the elastin production is lost.
- **Tunica adventitia** (external layer) consists of loose connective tissue with bundles of smooth muscle fibers and elastic tissue and carries nerves and the vaso vasorum. The **vasa vasorum** comprises the tiny arteries and veins that supply the walls of blood vessels.

Specific differences exist between the arteries and the veins. The **arteries** are hollow elastic tubes that carry blood away from the heart. They are enclosed within a sheath that includes a vein and a nerve. The smaller arteries contain less elastic tissue and more smooth muscles than the larger arteries. The elasticity of the larger arteries is important in maintaining a steady blood flow. The abdominal aorta will not change in diameter with changes in respiration; however, pulsation of blood flow corresponding to the cardiac cycle will be noted.

The **veins** are hollow collapsible tubes with diminished tunica media that carry blood toward the heart. The veins appear collapsed because they have little elastic tissue or muscle within their walls (see Fig. 8.2B). Veins have a larger total diameter than arteries, and they move blood more slowly. The veins contain special valves that prevent backflow and permit blood to flow in only one direction—toward the heart. Numerous valves are found within the extremities, especially the lower extremities, because flow must work against gravity. Venous return is also aided by muscle contraction, overflow from capillary beds, gravity, and suction from negative thoracic pressure. The sonographer may note that the inferior vena cava should dilate slightly with suspended respiration.

The **capillaries** are microscopic vessels just wide enough to let one red blood cell squeeze through. These tiny vessels connect the arterial and venous systems. Their walls have only one layer. The body's cells and tissues receive their nutrients from fluids passing through the capillary walls; at the same time, waste products from the cells pass into the capillaries. Arteries do not always end in capillary beds; some end in anastomoses, which are end-to-end grafts between different vessels that equalize pressure over vessel length and provide alternative flow channels.

AORTA

The **aorta** is the largest principal artery of the body. It may be divided into the following five sections: (1) root of the aorta, (2) ascending aorta and arch, (3) descending aorta, (4) abdominal aorta and abdominal aortic branches, and (5) bifurcation of the aorta into iliac arteries (see Fig. 8.1B).

Root of the Aorta

The systemic circulation leaves the left ventricle of the heart by way of the aorta (Fig. 8.3). The root of the aorta arises from the left ventricular outflow tract in the heart. The aortic root has three semilunar cusps that prevent blood from flowing back into the left ventricle. These cusps open with ventricular systole to eject blood into the ascending aorta; the cusps are closed during ventricular diastole. The coronary arteries arise superiorly from the right and left coronary cusps to form the right and left coronary arteries, respectively. These coronary arteries further bifurcate to supply the vasculature of the cardiac structures. After the aorta arises from the left ventricle, it ascends posterior to the main pulmonary artery to form the ascending aorta.

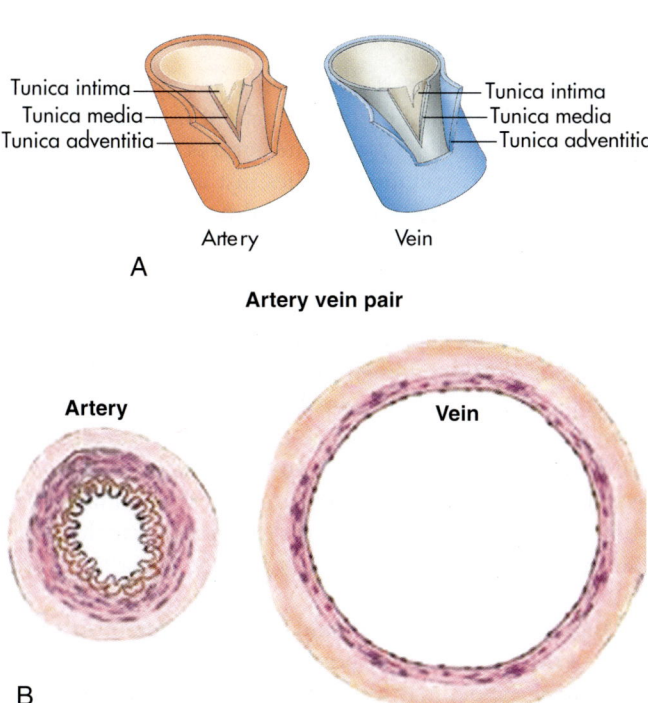

FIG. 8.2 (A) Cross section of an artery and vein showing the distinctions among the three layers of each vessel: tunica intima (inner layer), tunica media (middle layer), and tunica adventitia (external layer). (B) Specific differences exist between the arteries and the veins. The arteries are hollow elastic tubes that carry blood away from the heart. They are enclosed within a sheath that includes a vein and a nerve. The veins are hollow collapsible tubes with diminished tunica media that carry blood toward the heart. The veins appear collapsed because they have little elastic tissue or muscle within their walls.

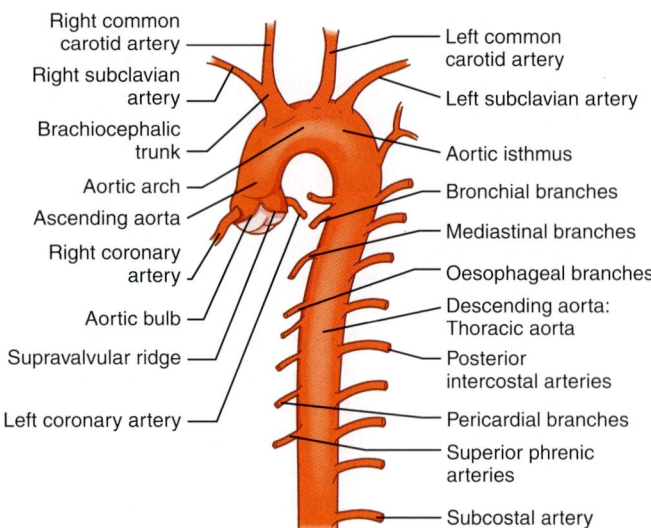

FIG. 8.3 The aorta is divided into five sections: the aortic root, the ascending aorta, the aortic arch (brachiocephalic artery, common carotid artery, and subclavian artery), the thoracic (descending) artery, and the abdominal aorta, with the bifurcation.

Ascending Aorta

The ascending aorta arises a short distance from the ventricle and arches superiorly to form the aortic arch at the level of the sternoclavicular junction. Three arterial branches arise from the superior border of the aortic arch to supply the head, neck, and upper extremities: the brachiocephalic, left common carotid, and left subclavian arteries.

Descending Aorta

From the aortic arch, the aorta descends posteriorly along the back wall of the heart through the thoracic cavity, where it pierces the diaphragm to become the abdominal aorta. The descending (thoracic) aorta enters the abdomen through the aortic opening of the diaphragm anterior to the twelfth thoracic vertebra in the retroperitoneal space.

Abdominal Aorta and Iliac Arteries

The abdominal aorta is the largest artery in the body that supplies blood to all visceral organs and the legs. The aorta continues to flow in the retroperitoneal cavity anterior and slightly left of the vertebral column. The aorta lies posterior to the left lobe of the liver, the body of the pancreas, the gastroesophageal junction, the pylorus of the stomach, and the splenic vein (Fig. 8.4). The diaphragmatic crura surrounds the proximal abdominal aorta as this vessel projects through the diaphragm into the abdominal cavity (Fig. 8.5). Many branches arise from the abdominal aorta: the celiac axis, superior mesenteric, inferior mesenteric, renal, suprarenal, and gonadal arteries (Fig. 8.6). At the level of the fourth lumbar vertebra (near the umbilicus), the aorta bifurcates into the right and left common iliac arteries. The aorta has four branches that supply other visceral organs and the mesentery: the celiac trunk, the superior and inferior mesenteric arteries, and the renal arteries.

Sonographic Findings. In most patients, the abdominal aorta is usually one of the easiest abdominal structures to image with ultrasound because of the marked change in acoustic impedance between its elastic walls and blood-filled lumen. Sonography provides the diagnostic information needed to create an image of the entire abdominal aorta, assess its diameter, and visualize the presence of thrombus, calcification, or dissection within the walls. Box 8.1 outlines the protocol to image the abdominal aorta.

Multiple acoustic windows may be utilized to image the aorta. The traditional view is performed with the patient in the supine position. Gas-filled loops of bowel may prevent adequate visualization of the aorta, but this can sometimes be overcome by applying gentle pressure with the transducer or by changing the angle of the transducer to move the gas out of the way. An alternative imaging plane is made when the patient is rolled into a right lateral decubitus position and scanned along the left lateral flank with the transducer directed slightly toward the spine. (Recall that the aorta will be seen directly anterior to the spine.) Other visualization problems encountered in the abdominal aortic ultrasound may occur with increased mesenteric fat in obese patients. Patients should wait to be imaged at least 24 hours after a barium study or an endoscopic evaluation, as barium or air may still be a residual impairment to adequate visualization.

Longitudinal Plane. To begin the sonographic evaluation of the abdominal aorta, the patient is usually imaged first in the longitudinal plane. The aorta is imaged as a long pulsatile tubular structure that lies just anterior and to the left of the spine (Fig. 8.7). The landmarks of the left lobe of the liver and the gastroesophageal junction may be seen anterior to the aorta. Longitudinal images should include the proximal, mid, and distal aorta to the bifurcation. The image acquisition should be made with the transducer perpendicular to the abdomen, beginning at the midline with a slight angulation of the transducer to the left of the spine, from the xiphoid to well below the level of bifurcation. In the average individual, the luminal dimension of the aorta gradually tapers as it proceeds distally in the abdomen. The abdominal aorta gives rise to two important branches from the anterior wall: the celiac trunk and the superior mesenteric artery (see Fig. 8.7D).

A low to medium gain should be used to demonstrate the walls of the aorta without "noisy" artifactual internal echoes. These weak echoes may result from increased gain, reverberation from the anterior abdominal wall fascia or musculature, or poor lateral resolution. These factors result in echoes being recorded at the same level as those from the soft tissue surrounding the vessel lumen, particularly if the vessels are smaller in diameter than the transducer. Try to use different techniques of breath-holding to eliminate these *artifactual* echoes. Sometimes, increased gentle pressure or change in angulation of the transducer may help displace bowel gas or

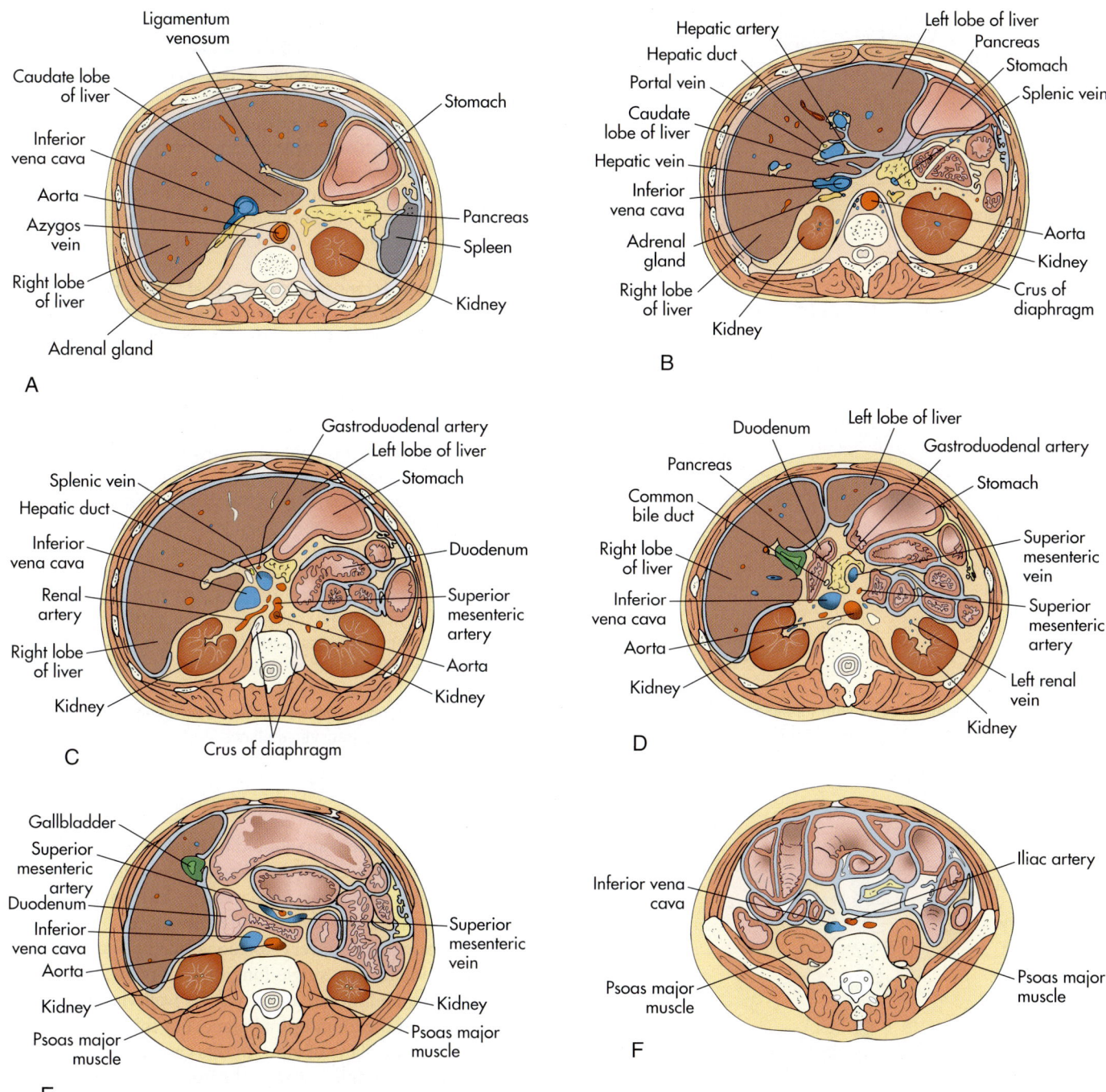

FIG. 8.4 (A–F) Cross-sectional images from the dome of the liver to the bifurcation of the aorta. The abdominal aorta is the largest artery in the body that supplies blood to all visceral organs and to the legs. The aorta continues to flow in the retroperitoneal cavity anterior and slightly left of the vertebral column. The aorta lies posterior to the left lobe of the liver, the body of the pancreas, the gastroesophageal junction, the pylorus of the stomach, and the splenic vein.

may compress fatty tissue so that the transducer will be closer to the abdominal aorta. If the abdomen is very concave, the patient may be instructed to extend his or her abdomen ("push the abdomen muscle out") to provide a better scanning plane. Color Doppler is useful to fully demonstrate the patent lumen of the aorta, from the diaphragm (celiac axis) to the bifurcation of the aorta into the iliac arteries (Fig. 8.8).

Coronal Plane. The coronal plane is useful when there is air-filled bowel obstructing the longitudinal plane. The patient may be rolled into a slight right decubitus position, and the transducer should be angled toward the midline to see the inferior vena cava and aorta. This view is excellent to image the renal arteries as they arise from the lateral wall of the aorta (Fig. 8.9).

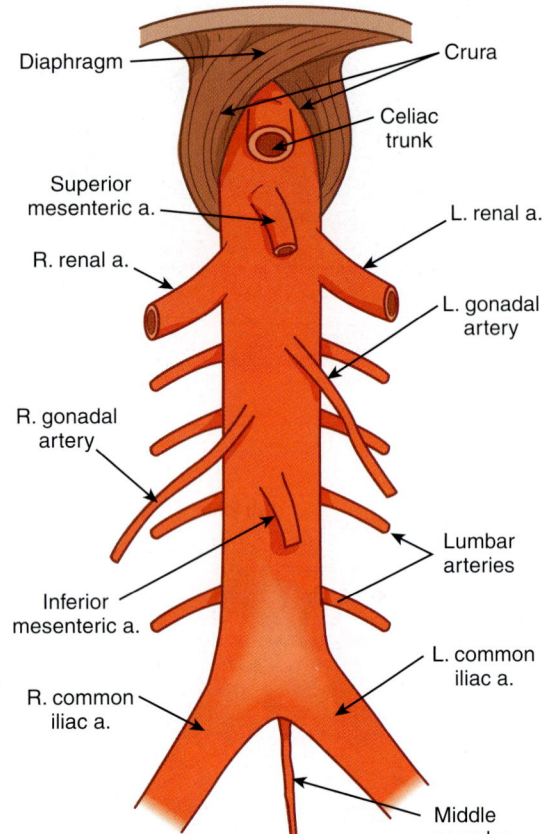

FIG. 8.5 **The abdominal aorta with multiple arterial branches.** The diaphragmatic crura surrounds the proximal abdominal aorta as this vessel projects through the diaphragm into the abdominal cavity.

> **BOX 8.1   Aorta and Iliac Artery Protocol**
>
> The aorta is examined primarily to determine the presence of aneurysmal dilation.
> 1. Patient preparation: nothing by mouth for at least 6 h.
> 2. Transducer selection: 2.5–4 MHz curvilinear.
> 3. Patient position: supine or slightly decubitus.
> 4. Images and observations should include the following:
>   - The aorta should be imaged in the longitudinal plane from the diaphragm to below the bifurcation at the iliac junction.
>   - Transverse scans should be made at the diaphragm level, superior to the renal arteries, inferior to the renal arteries, and at the bifurcation. Scans of the iliac arteries should be made.
>   - Lymphadenopathy should also be evaluated because the lymph nodes lie anterior to the vessels.
>   - The inferior vena cava is best imaged on a longitudinal plane through the right lobe of the liver with the patient in full inspiration.
>
> An alternative imaging plane is the slight decubitus view. The patient rolls onto his or her left side; the transducer is longitudinal and is sharply angled from the right lobe of the liver to the left iliac wing. This allows the sonographer to image the inferior vena cava "anterior" to the aorta. This view usually allows the sonographer to perform a shallow sweep to follow the entrance and exit of the renal veins and arteries into the great vessels and provides an excellent window to perform color flow or Doppler interrogation of the renal vessels.
>
> Outer to outer measurements should be taken of the aorta in the longitudinal and transverse planes.

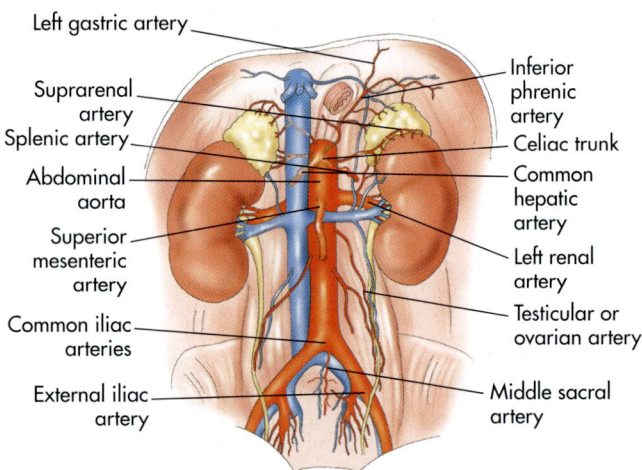

FIG. 8.6 Many branches arise from the abdominal aorta: the celiac axis, superior mesenteric, inferior mesenteric, renal, suprarenal, and gonadal arteries.

Transverse Plane. In the transverse plane, the aorta is imaged as a circular structure anterior to the spine and slightly to the left of the midline (Fig. 8.10). In some cases, the transverse diameter of the aorta (anterior-posterior and width) differs from that found in longitudinal measurements; thus it is important to identify and measure the vessel in two dimensions. Multiple scans should be made from the xiphoid to the bifurcation to record the dimensions of the aorta at the diaphragm, just above the renal vessels, just inferior to the renal vessels, and at the level of the bifurcation.

If the patient has a very tortuous aorta, scans may be difficult to obtain in a single longitudinal plane. The upper portion of the abdominal aorta may be well visualized during scanning in the longitudinal plane, but the lower portion may be out of the plane of view. In this case, the sonographer should obtain a complete scan of the upper segment and then concentrate fully on the lower segment. In some patients, the aorta may stretch from the far right of the abdomen to the far left. Transverse images of the aorta may be helpful to map the course of the vessel.

Measurement of the Aorta. The aorta follows the anterior course of the vertebral column, and it is important that the transducer also follow a perpendicular path along the entire curvature of the spine. The anterior and posterior walls of the aorta should be easily seen as two thin pulsatile parallel lines. This facilitates measuring the anteroposterior diameter of the aorta, which in most institutions is done from the leading outer edge of the anterior wall to the outer edge of the posterior wall. Measurements are made at the proximal, mid, and distal aorta in the transverse and longitudinal planes. These measurements are made with the

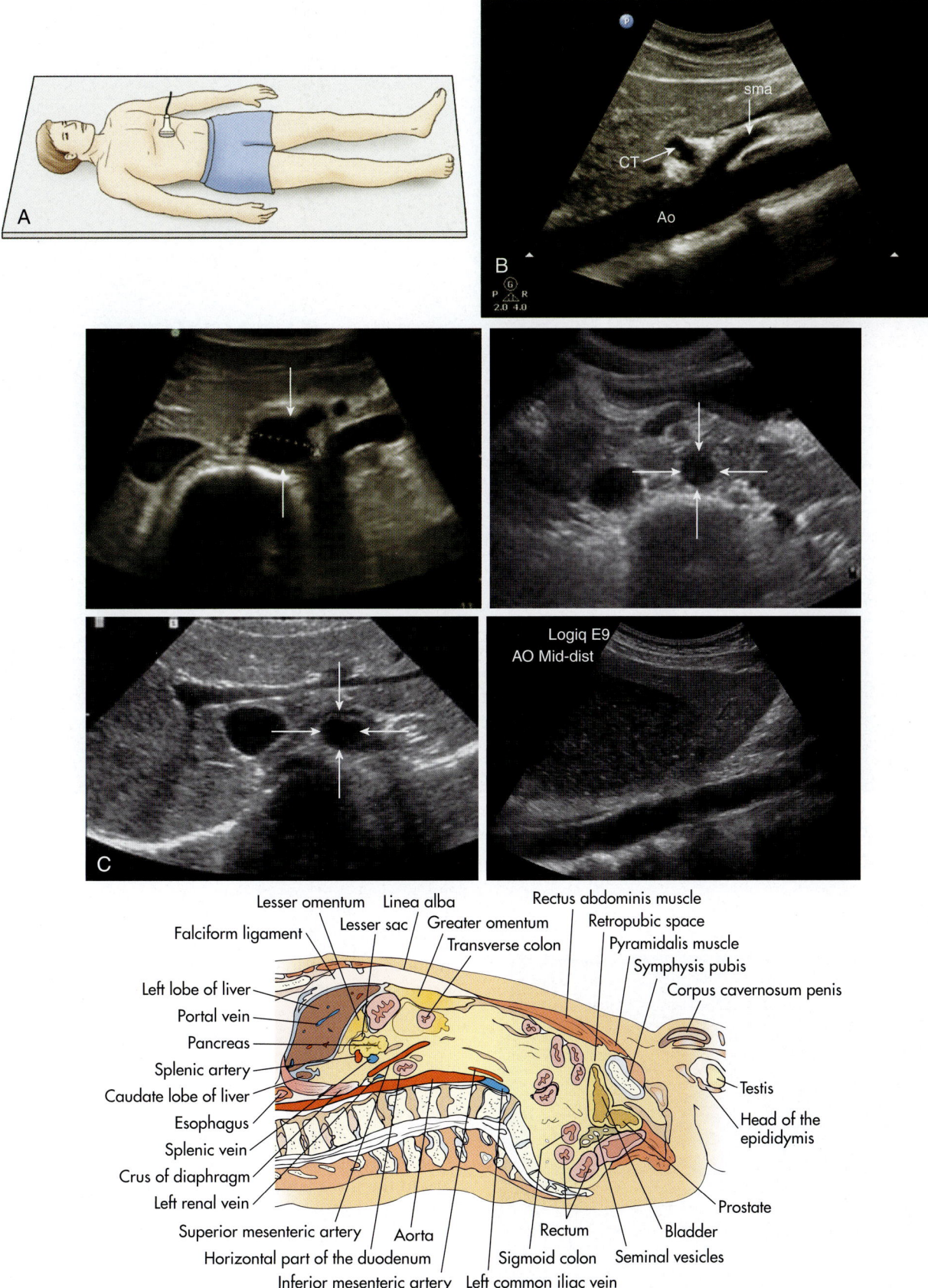

FIG. 8.7 (A) To begin the sonographic evaluation of the abdominal aorta, the patient is usually imaged first in the longitudinal plane. (B) Longitudinal image of the abdominal aorta (Ao) with the celiac trunk (CT) and superior mesenteric artery (sma) arising from the anterior wall. (C) The aorta is imaged as a long pulsatile tubular structure that lies just anterior and to the left of the spine. (D) The abdominal aorta gives rise to two important branches from the anterior wall: the celiac trunk and the superior mesenteric artery.

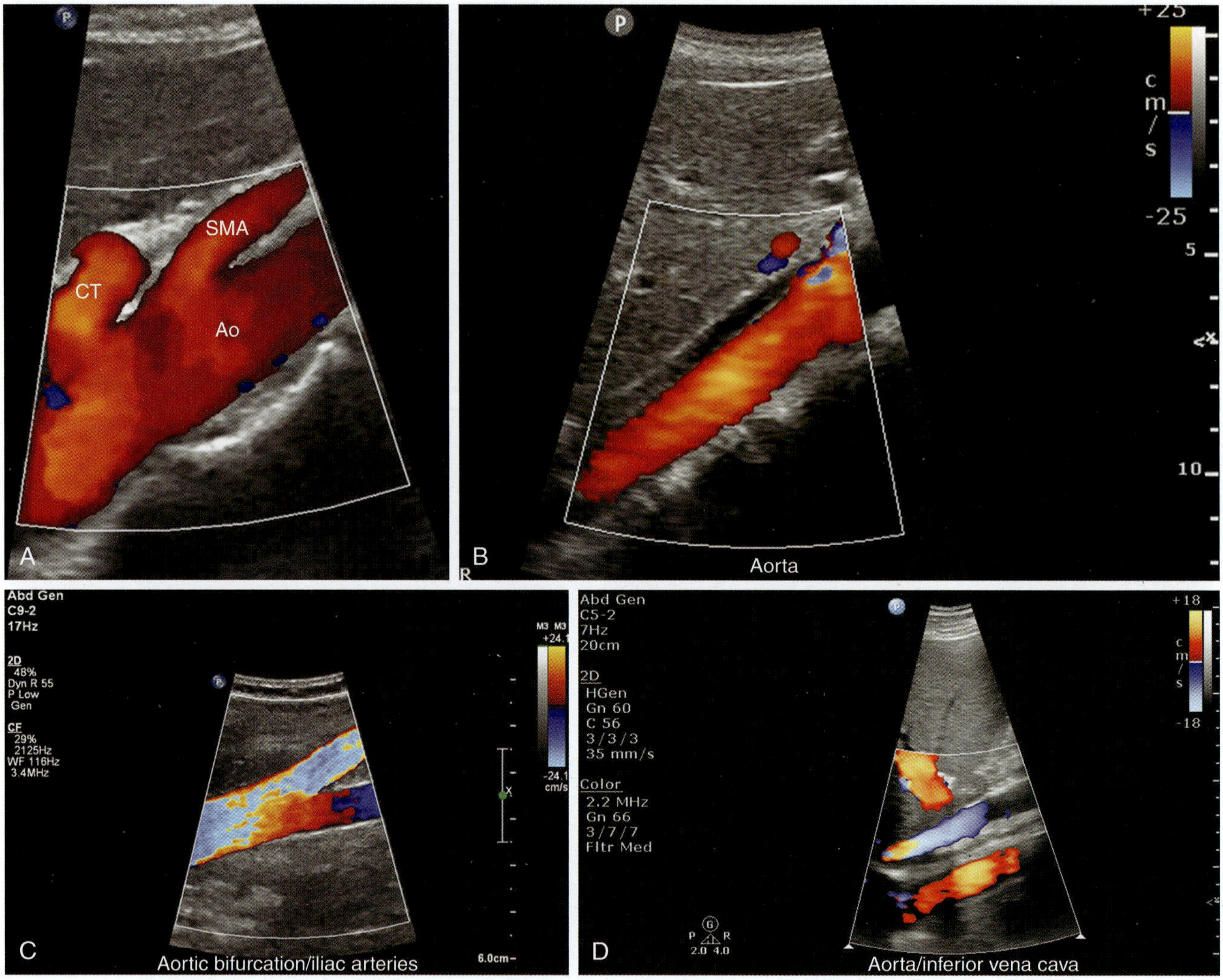

FIG. 8.8 (A) Color Doppler longitudinal image of the abdominal aorta (Ao) with the celiac trunk (CT) and superior mesenteric artery (SMA) arising from the anterior border. (B) Color Doppler of the normal aorta. (C) Color Doppler of the bifurcation of the aorta into the iliac arteries. (D) Coronal oblique view of the inferior vena cava *(blue)* anterior to the aorta *(red)*.

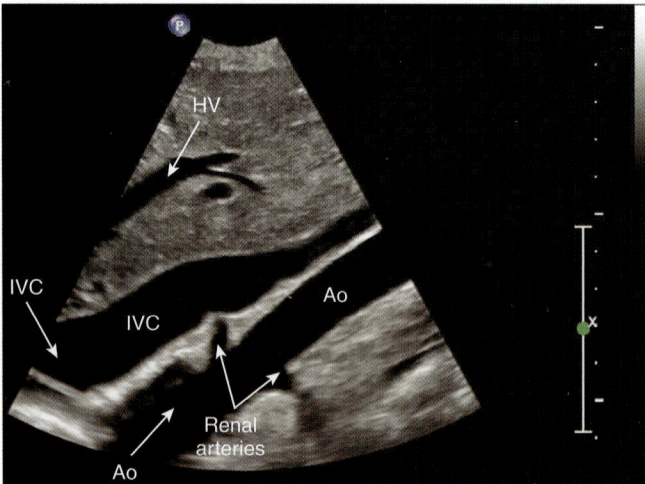

FIG. 8.9 Coronal image with the transducer slightly angled toward the midline to see the inferior vena cava (IVC) anterior to the aorta (Ao) and renal arteries. *HV*, Hepatic vein.

reduced gain setting from outer edge to outer edge at the greatest diameter (Fig. 8.11).

The sonographer should be careful to identify the posterior edge of the aorta as separate from the spine when performing the measurements. Calcification of the aorta or ossification of the spine may require careful analysis to make this measurement accurate.

The aortic diameter in men is slightly greater than in women. The proximal abdominal aorta tapers in size secondary to the three large branches (celiac, superior mesenteric, and renal arteries). In the supraceliac area, the aorta measures 2.5 to 2.7 cm in men and 2.1 to 2.3 cm in women. In the infrarenal area, the aorta measures 2.0 to 2.4 cm in men and 1.7 to 2.2 cm in women. There is gradual tapering to 1.1 to 1.5 cm in men and 1.1 to 1.3 cm in women at the bifurcation into the iliac arteries (Table 8.1). The size of the aorta will vary slightly according to body mass index; the larger the body size, the greater is the measurement of the aorta. It is also important to

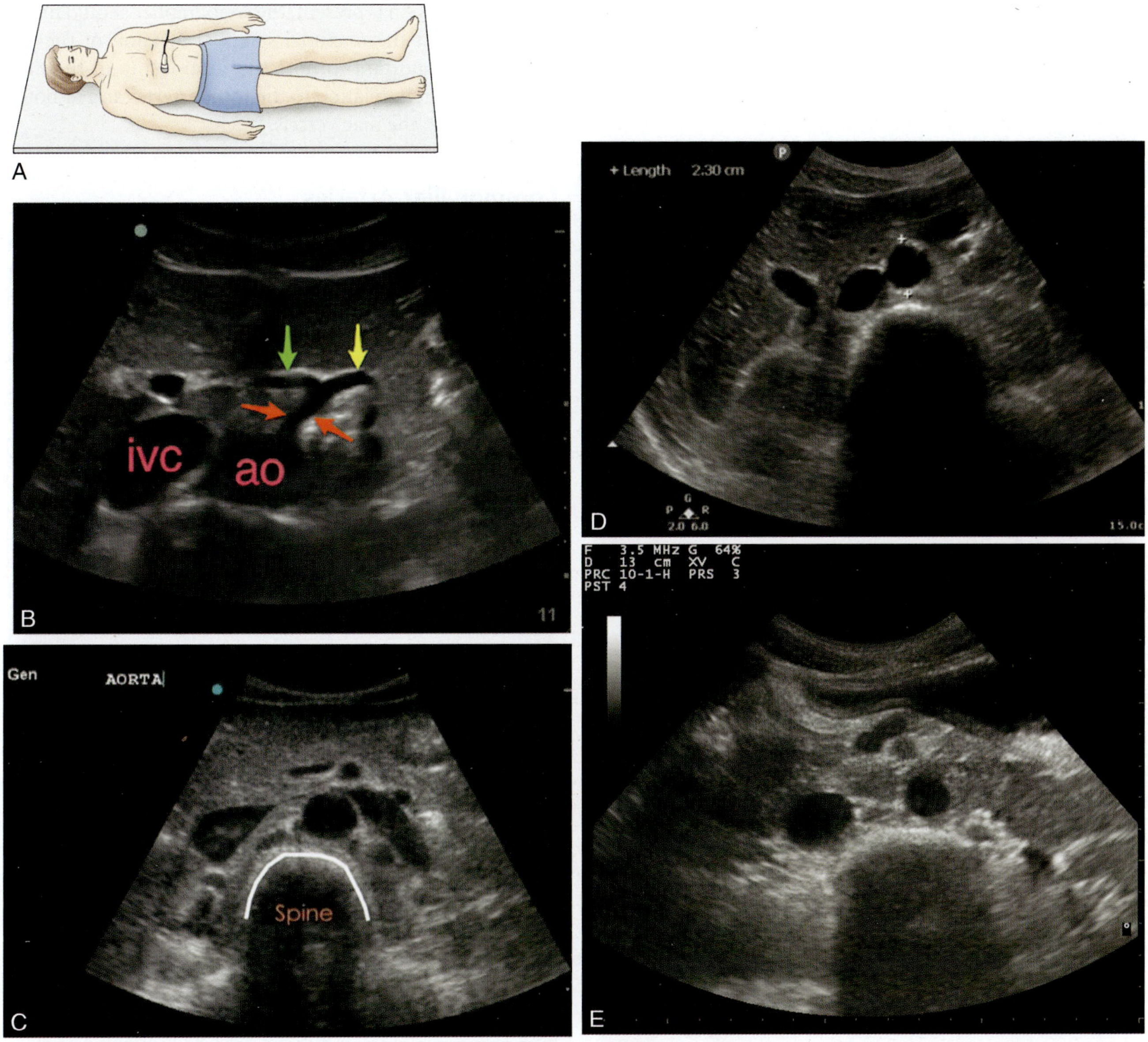

CHAPTER 8 Vascular System

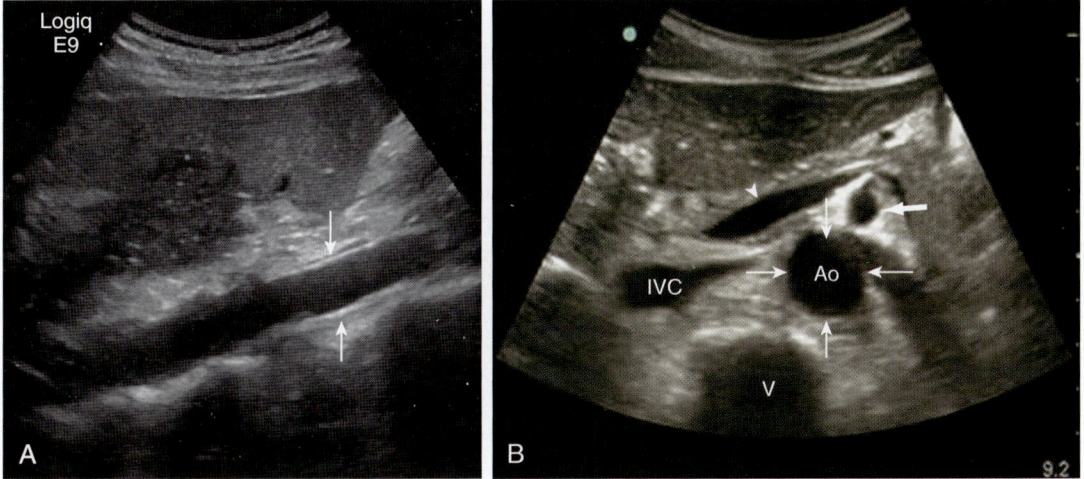

FIG. 8.10 (A) Transverse plane. Multiple scans should be made from the xiphoid to the bifurcation to record the dimensions of the aorta. (B) The celiac trunk *(orange arrows)*, hepatic artery *(green arrow)*, and splenic artery *(yellow arrow)* are a good landmark for the upper aorta. (C) The left renal vein is seen inferior to the celiac trunk image. (D) The mid-abdominal image shows the aorta (hashmarks) to the left of the inferior vena cava. (E) Inferior margin of the abdominal aorta just before the bifurcation.

FIG. 8.11 (A) Outer to outer measurements should be taken of the aorta in the longitudinal (A) and transverse (B) planes. *Ao*, Aorta; *IVC*, inferior vena cava; *thick arrow*, superior mesenteric artery; *V*, vertebra; *arrowhead*, splenic vein.

note that the aorta does change in size as one grows older; therefore an aorta in a younger adult measuring 1.8 cm may increase to 2.2 cm by the time the adult reaches 60 years of age.

If an aneurysm is present, the sonographer should measure and document the maximal size and location of the aneurysm. It is important to note the relationship of the dilated aortic segment in relation to the renal arteries and to note the extension into the iliac vessels.

Common Iliac Arteries

The **common iliac arteries** arise at the bifurcation of the abdominal aorta at the fourth lumbar vertebra (near the superior sacrum). These vessels further divide into the internal and external iliac arteries (Fig. 8.12). The internal iliac artery enters the pelvis anterior to the sacroiliac joint, at which point

TABLE 8.1	Diameter of Abdominal Aorta and Iliac Branches	
	Men	Women
Aorta supraceliac	2.5–2.7 cm	2.1–2.3 cm
Aorta infrarenal	2.0–2.4 cm	1.7–2.2 cm
Common iliac artery	1.1–1.5 cm	1.0–1.3 cm
Common femoral artery	0.9–1.2 cm	0.8–1.0 cm

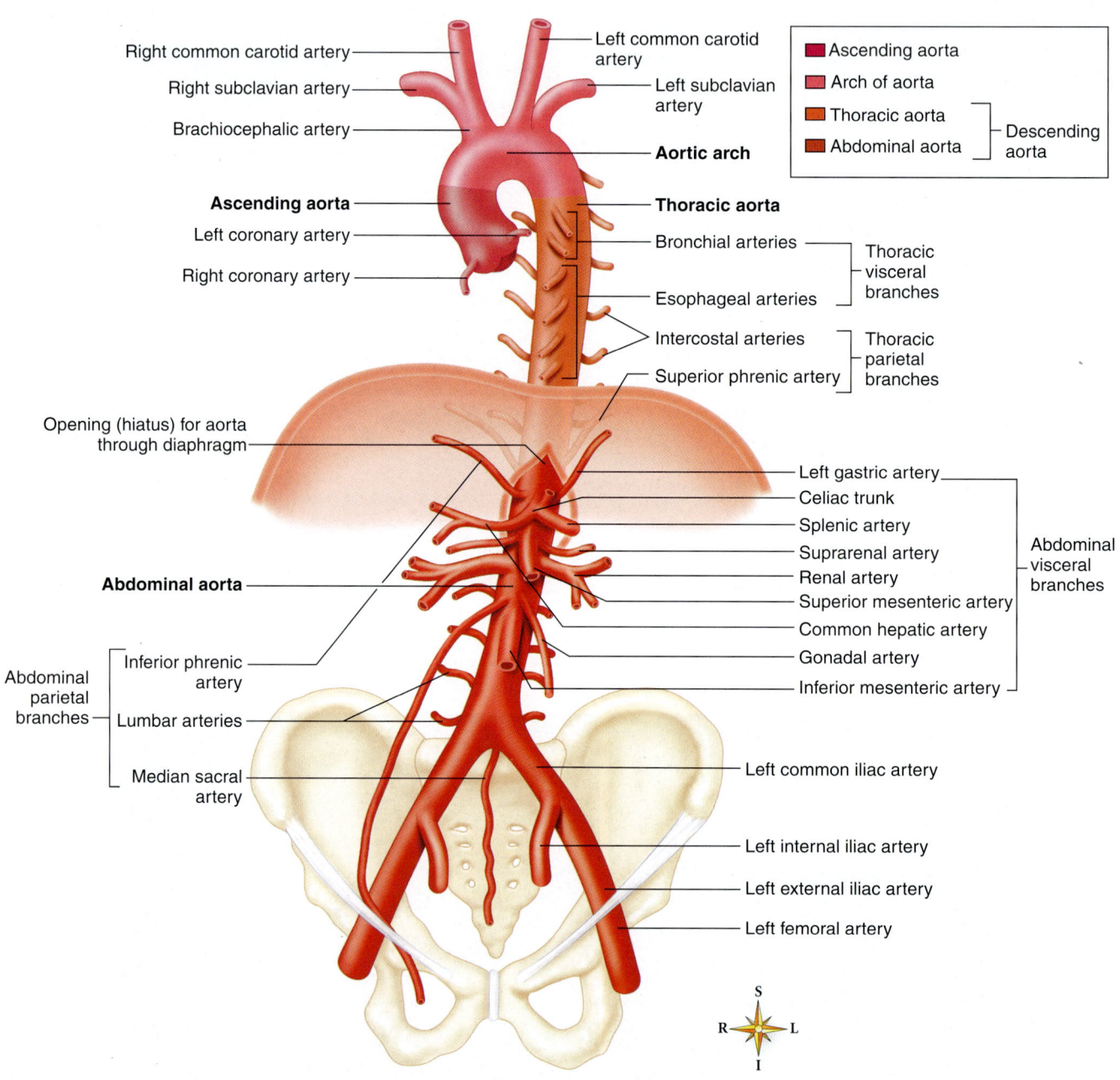

FIG. 8.12 The common iliac arteries arise at the bifurcation of the abdominal aorta at the fourth lumbar vertebra (near the superior sacrum). These vessels further divide into the internal and external iliac arteries.

it is crossed anteriorly by the ureter. It divides into anterior and posterior branches to supply the pelvic viscera, peritoneum, buttocks, and sacral canal. The external iliac artery runs along the medial border of the psoas muscle, following the pelvic brim. The inferior epigastric and deep circumflex iliac branches branch off before they pass under the inguinal ligament to become the femoral artery. The portion of the femoral artery posterior to the knee is the popliteal artery. This artery further divides into the anterior and posterior tibial arteries.

Sonographic Findings. To better visualize the iliac arteries at the aortic bifurcation, use a slight lateral decubitus position. The patient should be rotated 5 to 10 degrees from the true lateral position. The patient should be examined in deep inspiration, which projects the liver and diaphragm into the abdominal cavity and provides an acoustic window to image the vascular structures. Slight medial to lateral angulation of the transducer may be necessary to image the bifurcation in the longitudinal plane. With the patient rolled into this oblique plane, the inferior vena cava may be visualized anterior to the aorta (Fig. 8.13). The iliac arteries should measure less than 1.2 cm in the transverse anteroposterior diameter. It is common for the iliac arteries to be dilated if an aortic aneurysm is present, as most aneurysms develop inferior to the renal vessels near the bifurcation of the aorta. If the iliac artery measures greater than 3 cm, it may be considered for surgical repair.

Abdominal Aortic Branches

The small phrenic arteries arise from the lateral walls of the aorta to supply the undersurface of the diaphragm. Surgical intervention or trauma to the phrenic artery may cause limited movement of the diaphragm. The celiac trunk is the first anterior branch of the aorta, arising 1 to 2 cm inferior to the diaphragm. The median arcuate ligament surrounds the aorta and has been known to compress the celiac trunk. The short celiac trunk gives rise to three smaller vessels: the splenic, common hepatic, and left gastric arteries (see Fig. 8.12). The superior mesenteric artery is the second anterior branch, arising approximately 2 cm from the celiac trunk. The right renal artery and the left renal artery are lateral branches that arise just inferior to the superior mesenteric artery. The small inferior mesenteric artery arises anteriorly near the bifurcation. The distribution of these branch arteries is to the visceral organs and the mesentery.

Anterior Branches of the Abdominal Aorta.

Celiac Trunk. The celiac trunk originates within the first 2 cm from the diaphragm (Fig. 8.14). It is surrounded by the liver, spleen, inferior vena cava, and pancreas. After arising from the anterior wall, it immediately branches into the following three vessels: common hepatic, left gastric, and splenic arteries.

Common Hepatic Artery. The **common hepatic artery** arises from the celiac trunk and courses to the right of the abdomen at almost a 90-degree angle (see Fig. 8.14). At this point, it branches into the proper hepatic artery and the gastroduodenal artery. The gastroduodenal artery courses along the upper border of the head of the pancreas, behind the

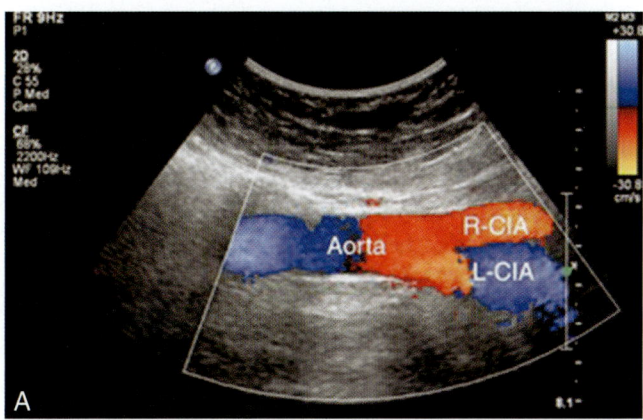
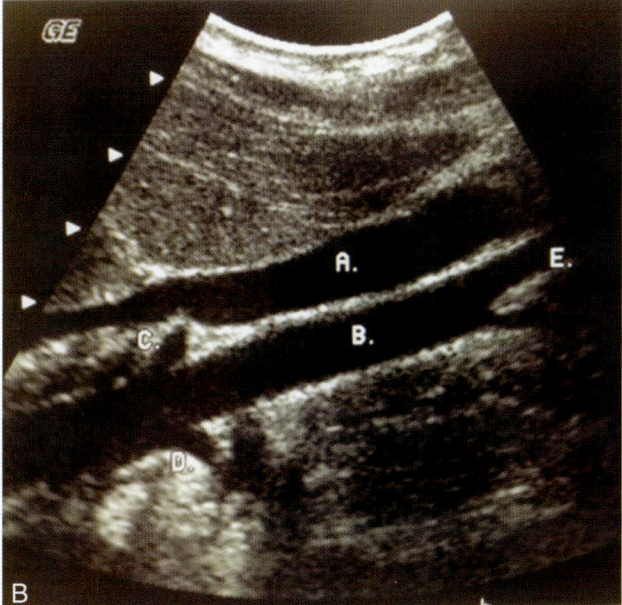

FIG. 8.13 (A) Color Doppler displays the decubitus view of the distal aorta and bifurcation of the iliac arteries. (B) Coronal view of the bifurcation of the iliac arteries. *A,* Inferior vena cava; *B,* aorta; *C,* right renal artery; *D,* left renal artery; *E,* iliac arteries.

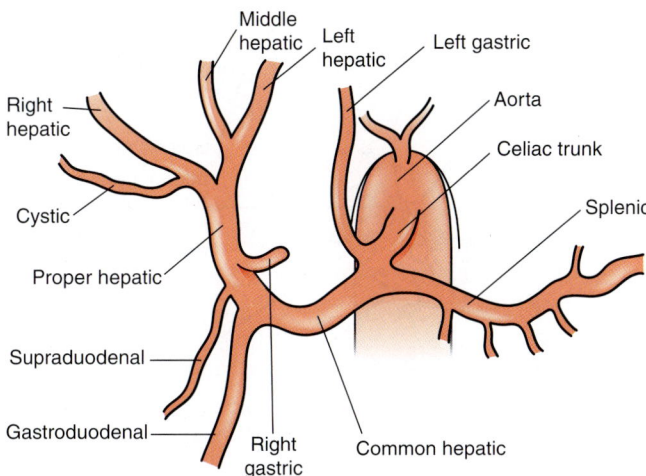

FIG. 8.14 The celiac trunk originates from the anterior abdominal aortic wall within the first 2 cm from the diaphragm and branches into the splenic artery, left gastric artery, and common hepatic artery.

posterior layer of the peritoneal bursa, to the upper margin of the superior part of the duodenum, which forms the lower boundary of the epiploic foramen (see Fig. 8.15). The duodenum and parts of the stomach are supplied by the **gastroduodenal artery** and the **right gastric artery**. Along with the hepatic duct and the portal vein, the common hepatic artery then ascends into the liver (through the porta hepatis), which divides into two branches: the right and left hepatic arteries.

Left and Right Hepatic Arteries. The **left hepatic artery** is a small branch of the proper hepatic artery supplying the caudate and left lobes of the liver. The **right hepatic artery** supplies the gallbladder via the cystic artery and the liver (see Fig. 8.14).

Left Gastric Artery. The **left gastric artery** is a small branch of the celiac trunk, passing anterior, cephalic, and left to reach the esophagus and then descending along the lesser curvature of the stomach (see Fig. 8.14). It supplies the lower third of the esophagus and the upper right of the stomach.

Splenic Artery. The **splenic artery** is the largest of the three branches of the celiac trunk (see Fig. 8.14). From its origin, the artery takes a somewhat tortuous course horizontally to the left as it forms the superior border of the pancreas. At a variable distance from the spleen, it divides into two branches. One of these branches, the left gastroepiploic artery, runs caudally into the greater omentum toward the right gastroepiploic artery. The other courses in a cephalic direction and divides into the short gastric artery, which supplies the fundus of the stomach, and into a number of splenic branches, which supply the spleen.

Several smaller arterial branches originate at the splenic artery as it courses through the upper border of the pancreas: the dorsal pancreatic, great pancreatic, and caudal pancreatic arteries. The dorsal or superior pancreatic artery originates from the beginning of the splenic artery or the hepatic artery, celiac trunk, or aorta. It runs behind and within the substance of the pancreas, dividing into right and left branches. The left branch is the transverse pancreatic artery. The right branch constitutes an anastomotic vessel to the anterior pancreatic arch and a branch to the uncinate process.

The great pancreatic artery originates from the splenic artery farther to the left and passes downward, dividing into branches that anastomose with the transverse or inferior pancreatic artery. The caudal pancreatic artery supplies the tail of the pancreas and divides into branches that anastomose with terminal branches of the transverse pancreatic artery. The transverse pancreatic artery courses behind the body and tail of the pancreas close to the lower pancreatic border. It may originate from or communicate with the superior mesenteric artery.

The distribution of the celiac trunk vessels is to the liver, spleen, stomach, pancreas, and duodenum.

Sonographic Findings. The celiac trunk may be visualized sonographically on transverse or longitudinal images (see Fig. 8.16). It is usually seen as a small vascular structure arising anteriorly from the abdominal aorta just below the diaphragm. Because it is only 1 to 2 cm long, it is sometimes challenging to record unless the area near the midline of the aorta is carefully examined. Sometimes the celiac trunk can be seen to extend in a cephalic rather than a caudal presentation. The superior mesenteric artery is just inferior to the origin of the celiac trunk. The superior mesenteric artery may be used as a landmark in locating the celiac trunk. Transversely, one can differentiate the celiac trunk as the "wings of a seagull," arising with its short trunk before dividing into the "wings" of the hepatic and splenic arteries.

The splenic artery may be seen to flow directly from the celiac trunk toward the spleen (see Figs. 8.14 and 8.16). Because it is so tortuous, it may be difficult to follow on the transverse scan. Generally, small pieces of the splenic artery are visible as the artery weaves in and out of the left upper quadrant.

The common hepatic artery (see Fig. 8.15) can be seen to branch anterior and to the right of the celiac trunk, where it then divides into the right and left hepatic arteries in the liver (see Fig. 8.17). The sonographer should be aware of the many variations in the hepatic artery branches as seen in Fig. 8.18.

The left gastric artery (see Fig. 8.14) has a very small diameter and often is difficult to visualize with ultrasound. It becomes difficult to separate from the splenic artery unless distinct structures are seen in the area of the celiac trunk branching to the left of the abdominal aorta (see Fig. 8.16).

Superior Mesenteric Artery. The **superior mesenteric artery** (SMA) arises from the anterior abdominal aortic wall approximately 1 cm inferior to the celiac trunk (see Fig. 8.12). Occasionally, the SMA may have a common origin with the celiac trunk. The SMA runs posterior to the neck of the pancreas and anterior to the uncinate process, which is anterior to the third part of the duodenum; it then branches into the mesentery and colon. The right hepatic artery is sometimes seen to arise from the superior mesenteric artery.

The SMA has the following five main branches (see Fig. 8.19): inferior pancreatic artery, duodenal artery, colic artery, ileocolic artery, and intestinal artery. These branch

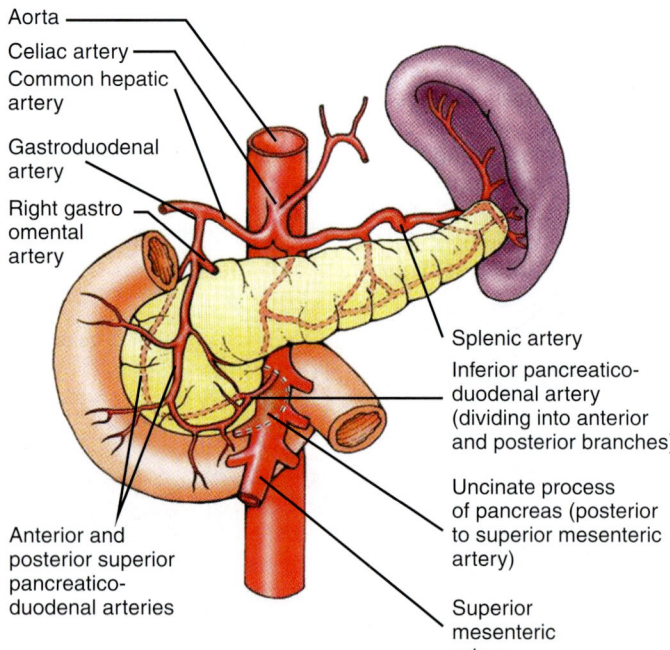

FIG. 8.15 The gastroduodenal artery courses along the upper border of the head of the pancreas, behind the posterior layer of the peritoneal bursa, to the upper margin of the superior part of the duodenum, which forms the lower boundary of the epiploic foramen.

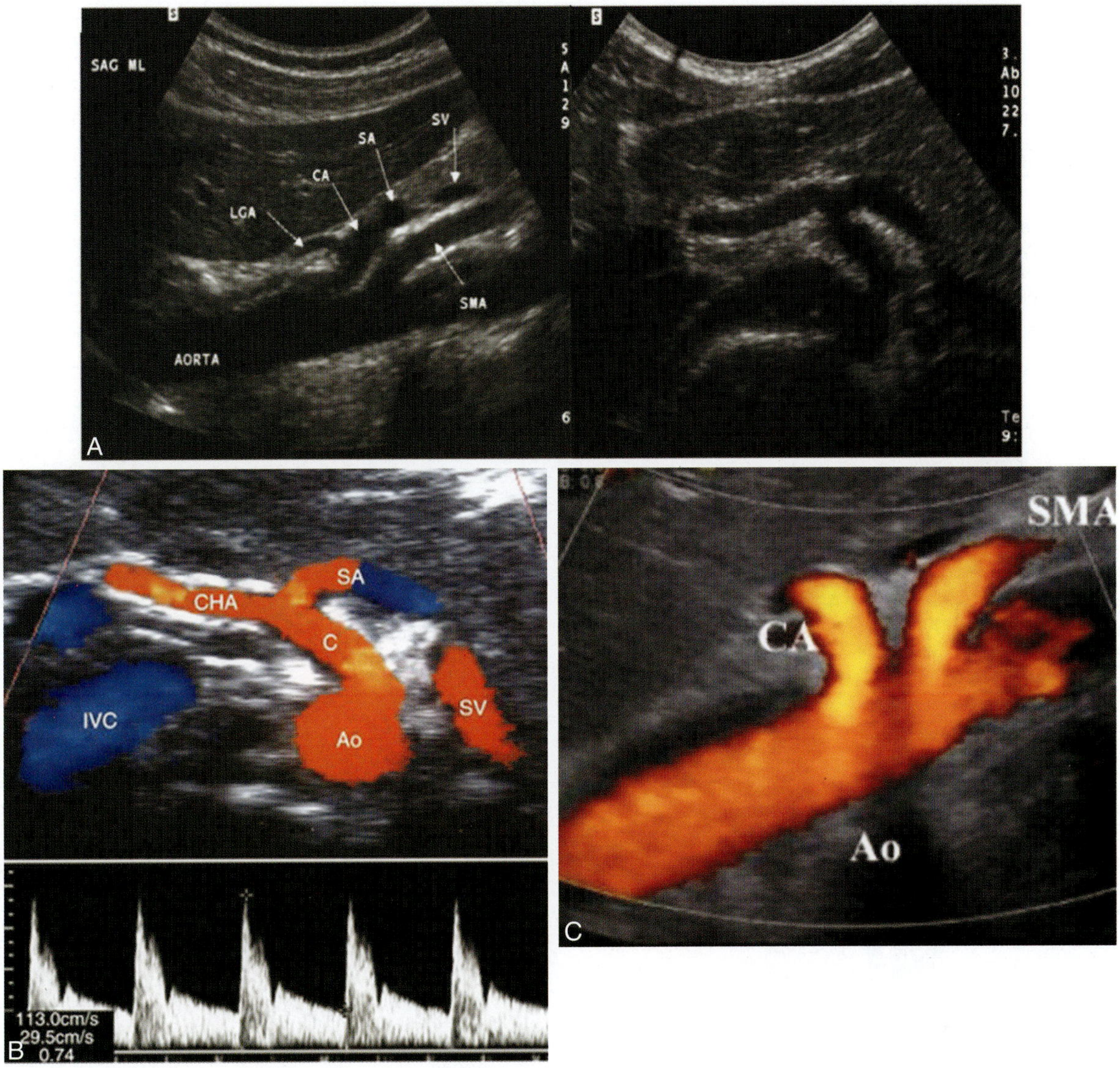

FIG. 8.16 (A–C) The celiac trunk may be visualized sonographically on transverse or longitudinal images. It is usually seen as a small vascular structure arising anteriorly from the abdominal aorta just below the diaphragm. The superior mesenteric artery is just inferior to the origin of the celiac trunk. *Ao*, Aorta; *CA*, celiac artery; *CHA*, common hepatic artery; *IVC*, inferior vena cava; *LGA*, left gastric artery; *SA*, splenic artery; *SMA*, superior mesenteric artery; *SV*, splenic vein. (C, From Zachrisson H, et al. *J Med Diagn Meth*. 2013;3:2.)

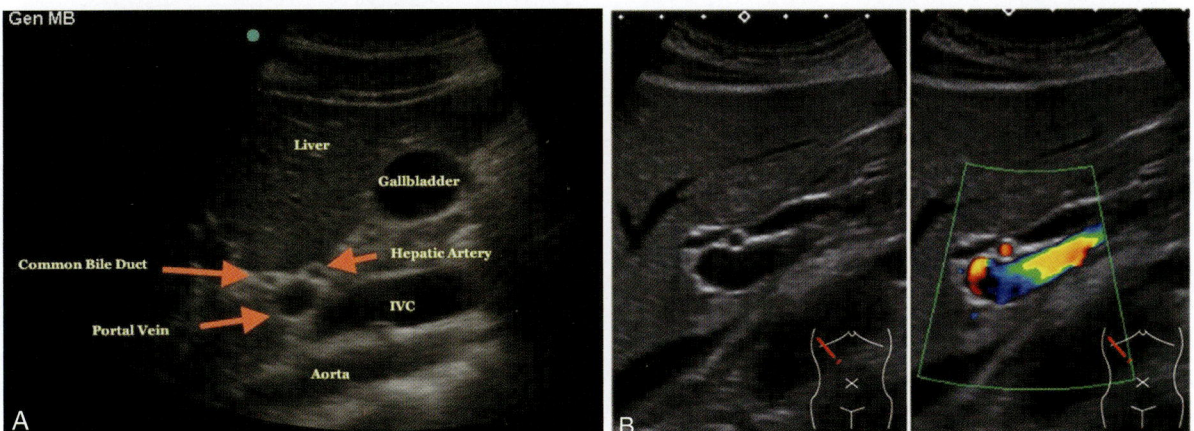

FIG. 8.17 (A) The small common hepatic artery can be seen to branch anterior and to the right of the celiac trunk, where it then divides into the right and left hepatic arteries in the liver. On transverse images, the common hepatic artery is found anterior and lateral to the portal vein. (B) On longitudinal images, the small artery may be seen anterior to the portal vein. *IVC*, Inferior vena cava.

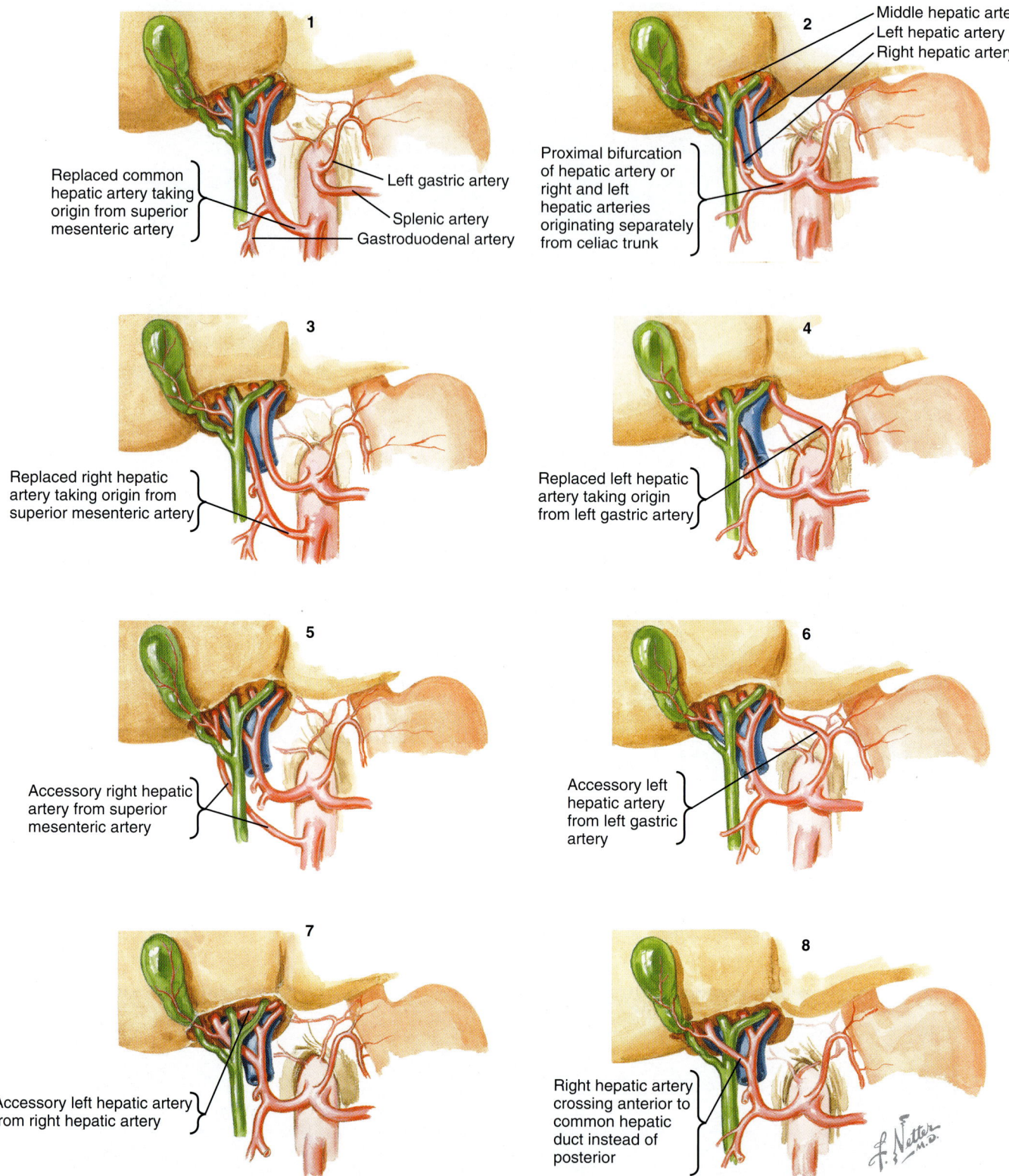

FIG. 8.18 The many variations in the hepatic artery branches. (Copyright 2017 Elsevier Inc. All right reserved. www.netterimages.com.)

arteries supply the small bowel; each consists of 10 to 16 branches arising from the left side of the superior mesenteric trunk. They extend into the mesentery, where adjacent arteries unite with them to form loops or arcades. Their distribution is to the proximal half of the colon (cecum, ascending, and transverse) and the small intestine.

Sonographic Findings. The SMA is well seen on both transverse and longitudinal scans (see Fig. 8.20). As it arises from the anterior aortic wall, the SMA branches off the anterior wall of the aorta at a slight angle and then follows a parallel course. Transversely, the artery can be seen as a separate small, circular structure anterior to the abdominal

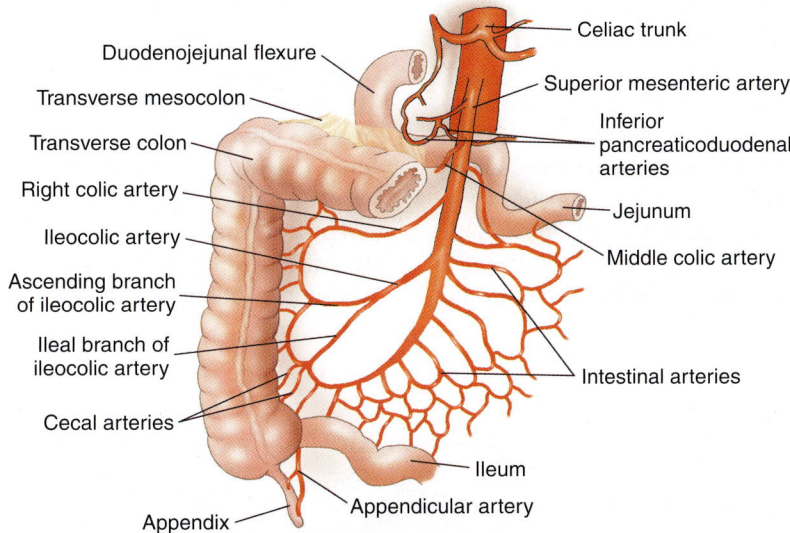

FIG. 8.19 The superior mesenteric artery arises anteriorly from the abdominal aorta approximately 1 cm below the celiac trunk. It supplies the proximal half of the colon and small intestine.

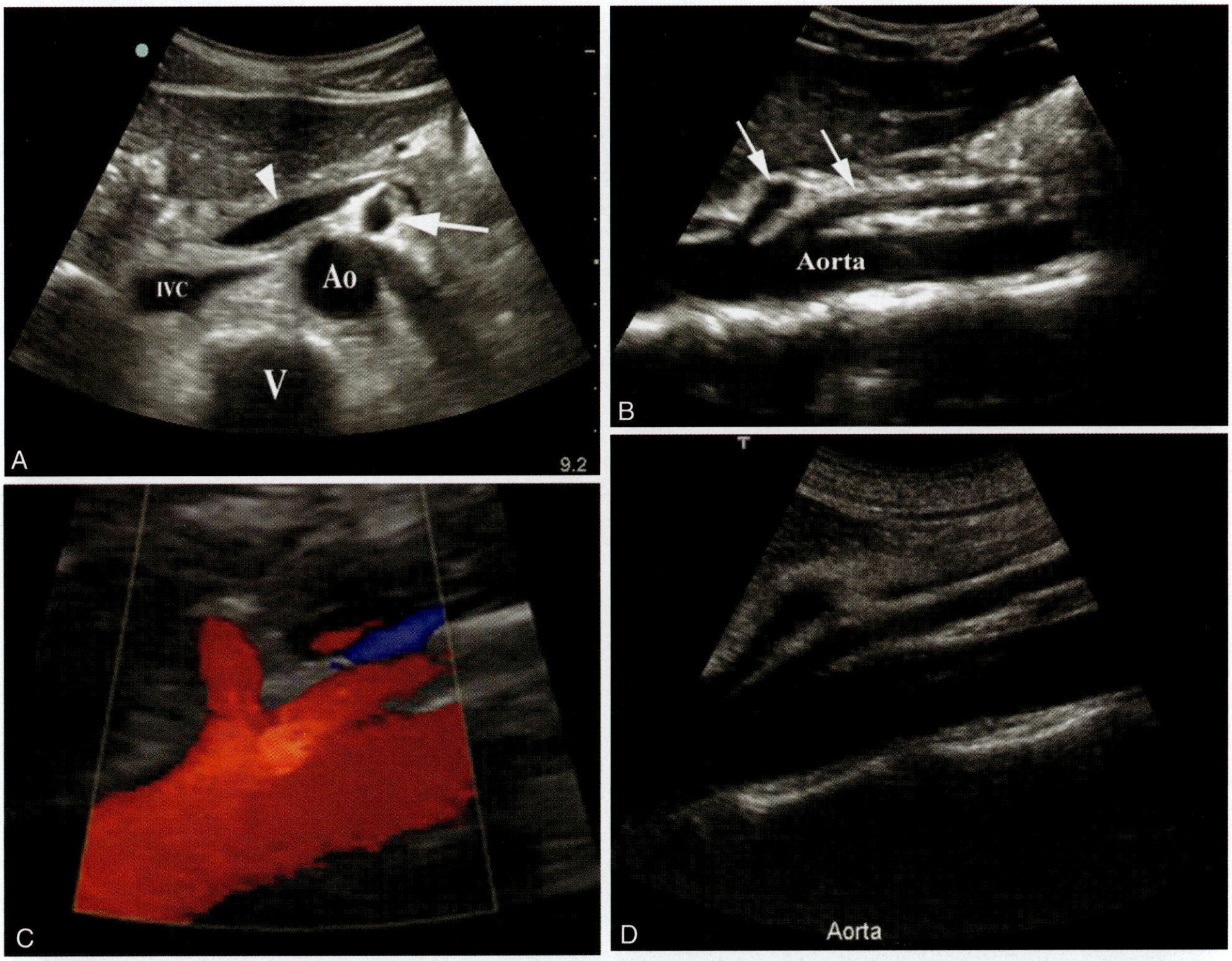

FIG. 8.20 (A–B) The superior mesenteric artery (SMA) is well seen on both transverse and longitudinal scans as it arises from the anterior aortic wall. The SMA branches off the anterior wall of the aorta at a slight angle and then follows a parallel course. Transversely, the artery can be seen as a separate small, circular structure anterior to the abdominal aorta and posterior to the pancreas. Characteristically, it is surrounded by highly reflective echoes from the retroperitoneal fascia. (C) Color Doppler in the sagittal plane shows the aorta with the celiac trunk and SMA. (D) Adenopathy should be considered if the angle of the superior mesenteric to the aorta is greater than 15 degrees. *Ao*, Aorta; *IVC*, inferior vena cava; *V*, vertebra.

aorta and posterior to the pancreas. Characteristically, it is surrounded by highly reflective echoes from the retroperitoneal fascia.

Adenopathy should be considered if the angle of the superior mesenteric to the aorta is severe (greater than 15 degrees).

Inferior Mesenteric Artery. The **inferior mesenteric artery** arises from the anterior abdominal aorta approximately at the level of the third or fourth lumbar vertebra (see Fig. 8.21). It proceeds to the left to distribute arterial blood to the descending colon, sigmoid colon, and rectum. It has the following three main branches: left colic, sigmoid, and superior rectal arteries. The distribution is to the left transverse colon, descending colon, sigmoid colon, and rectum.

Sonographic Findings. The inferior mesenteric artery is more difficult to visualize using ultrasound; it is generally on a longitudinal scan when it is seen. It is a small tubular structure inferior to the superior mesenteric artery, which originates from the anterior wall of the aorta. On transverse scans, it is difficult to separate from small loops of bowel within the abdomen.

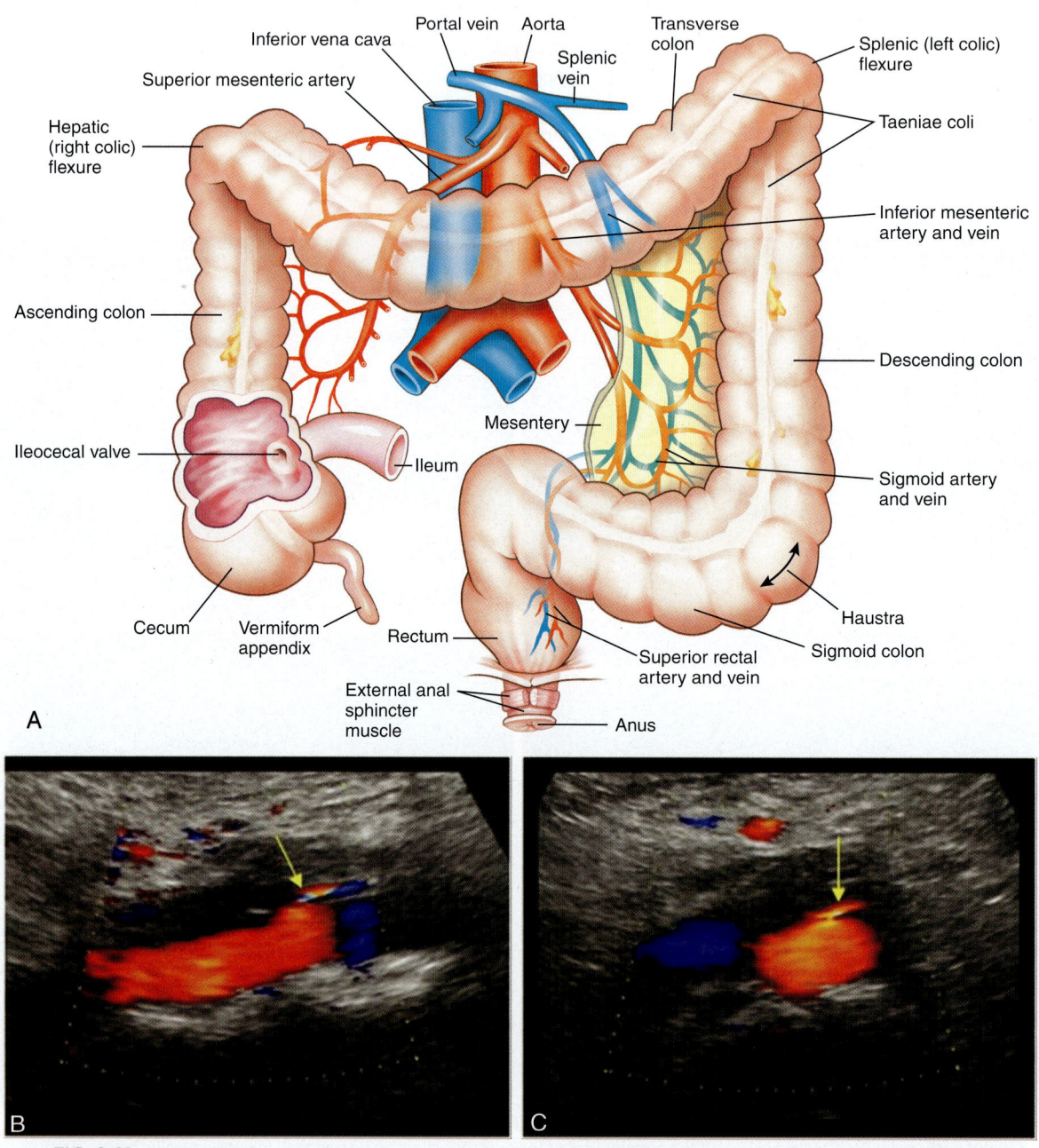

FIG. 8.21 (A) The inferior mesenteric artery arises from the anterior abdominal aorta approximately at the level of the third or fourth lumbar vertebra. It proceeds to the left to distribute arterial blood to the descending colon, sigmoid colon, and rectum. It has the following three main branches: left colic, sigmoid, and superior rectal arteries. (B) Longitudinal image of the inferior mesenteric artery. (C) Transverse image of the small inferior mesenteric artery.

Splanchnic Aneurysms. The splanchnic aneurysms may be atherosclerotic, posttraumatic, mycotic, congenital, or inflammatory (see Fig. 8.22). A small percentage of patients with chronic pancreatitis may develop these aneurysms, which may occur in the SMA, hepatic and splenic arteries, gastroduodenal arteries, or inferior mesenteric artery. They may have mural thrombus that is well demonstrated with color Doppler.

Lateral Branches of the Abdominal Aorta.

Phrenic Arteries. The phrenic arteries are paired small vessels that arise from the aorta's lateral wall to supply the diaphragm's undersurface (see Fig. 8.12).

Renal Arteries. The renal arteries arise from the lateral aspect of the aorta at the level of and anterior to the first lumbar vertebra, just inferior to the superior mesenteric artery (Fig. 8.23). Both vessels divide into the anterior and inferior suprarenal arteries. Duplication of the renal arteries is not uncommon. The **right renal artery** is a longer vessel than the left; it courses from the aorta posterior to the inferior vena cava and anterior to the vertebral column in a posterior and slightly caudal direction to enter the hilus of the right kidney. The renal artery passes posterior to the renal vein before entering the renal hilus. The **left renal artery** courses from the aorta directly into the hilus of the left kidney.

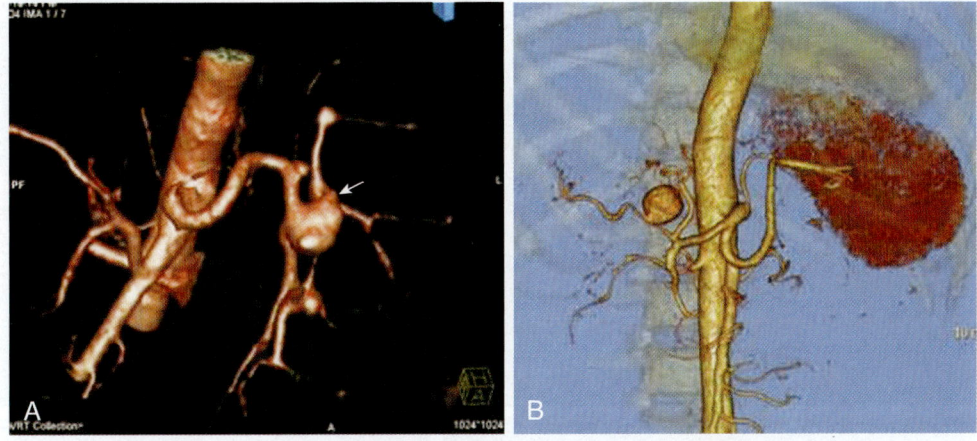

FIG. 8.22 (A) The splanchnic aneurysms may be atherosclerotic, posttraumatic, mycotic, congenital, or inflammatory. (B) Small aneurysm of the hepatic artery.

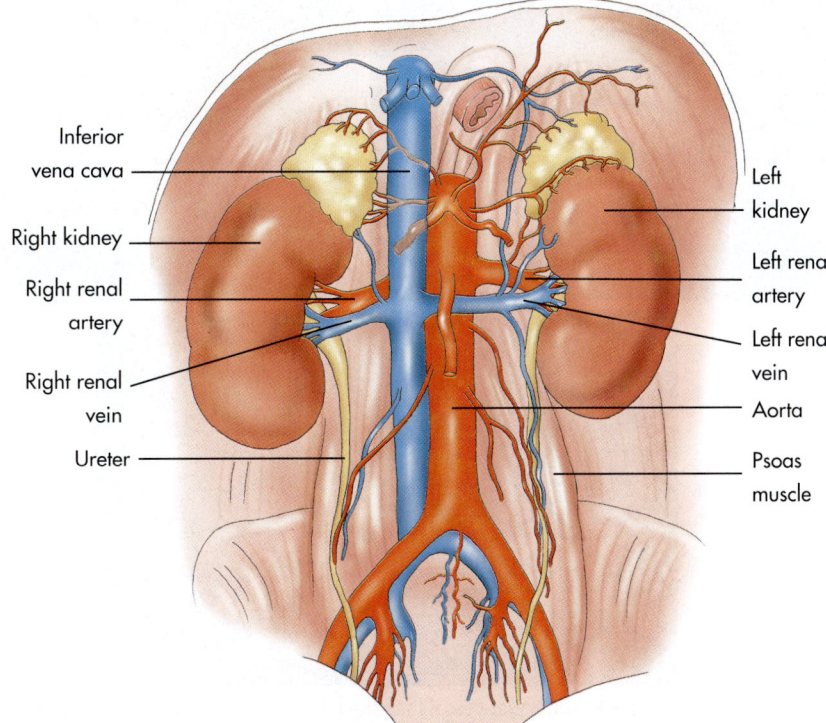

FIG. 8.23 The renal arteries arise from the lateral aspect of the aorta at the level of and anterior to the first lumbar vertebra, just inferior to the superior mesenteric artery. Both vessels divide into the anterior and inferior suprarenal arteries. The renal artery passes posterior to the renal vein before entering the renal hilus.

Sonographic Findings. Both renal arteries are best seen on transverse sonograms. The right renal artery passes posterior to the inferior vena cava and anterior to the vertebral column in a posterior and slightly caudal direction (Fig. 8.24). Occasionally, on longitudinal scans, a segment of the right renal artery is seen as a circular structure posterior to the inferior vena cava. The left renal artery takes a direct course from the aorta, anterior to the psoas muscle, to enter the renal sinus (Fig. 8.25).

The coronal oblique scan of the aorta and inferior vena cava is excellent for demonstrating the origin of the renal arteries and veins (see Fig. 8.24D). The patient is rolled into a steep decubitus position. The transducer is directed longitudinally with its axis across the inferior vena cava and aorta to see the origin of the renal vessels. The patient should be in full inspiration to dilate the venous structures for better visualization.

Gonadal Artery. The gonadal artery arises inferior to the renal arteries and courses along the psoas muscle to the respective gonadal area (see Fig. 8.12).

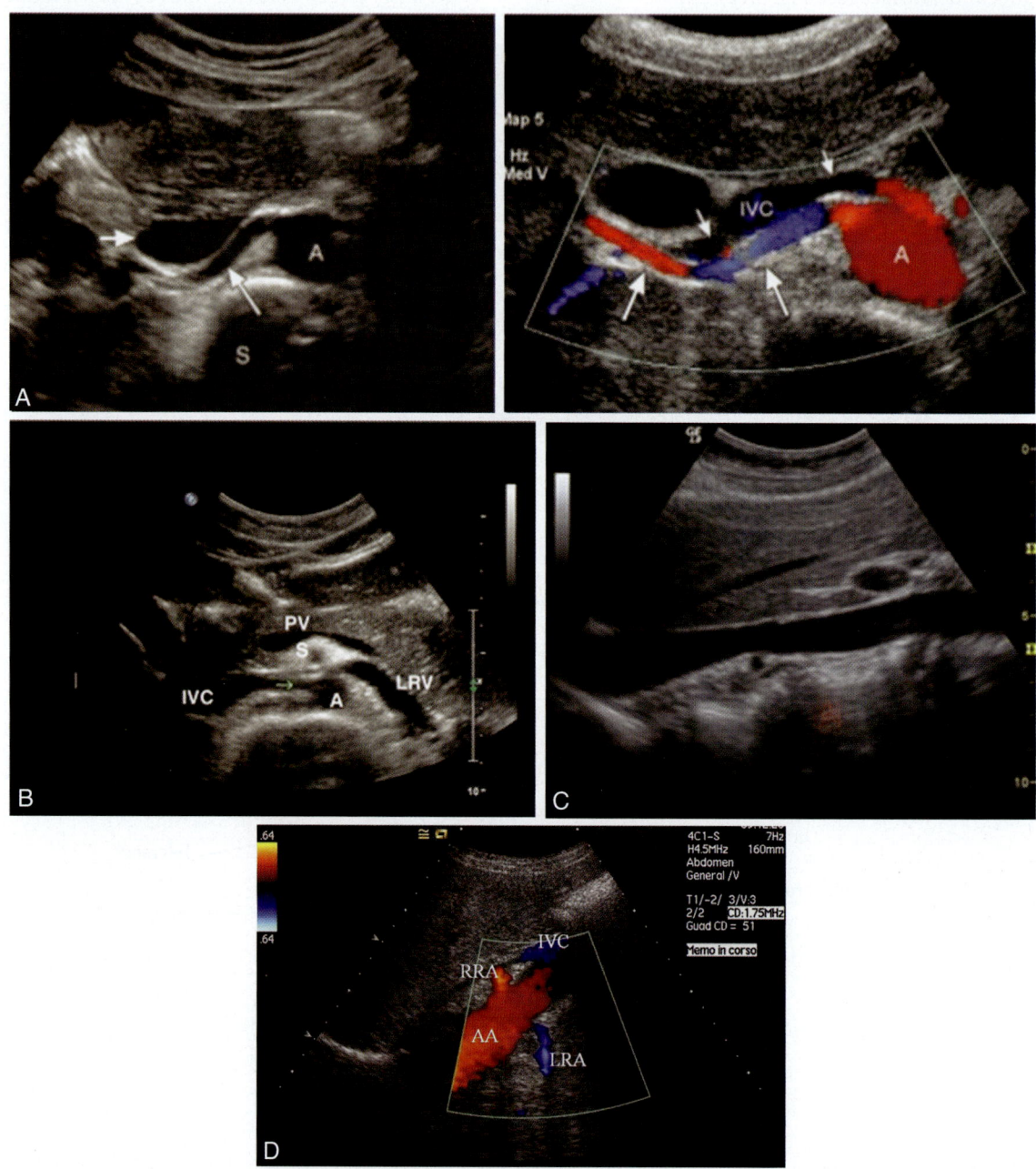

FIG. 8.24 The right renal artery (RRA) is a longer vessel than the left; it courses from the aorta posterior to the inferior vena cava (IVC) and anterior to the vertebral column in a posterior and slightly caudal direction to enter the hilus of the right kidney. (A) Transverse gray scale image *(left)* and color Doppler image *(right)* of the RRA. (B) The RRA is seen posterior to the IVC *(arrow).* (C) Longitudinal image of the RRA *(arrow)* posterior to the IVC. (D) The slight decubitus coronal view illustrates both renal arteries as they arise from the lateral wall of the aorta (A). *AA,* Abdominal aorta; *IVC,* inferior vena cava; *LRA,* left renal artery; *LRV,* left renal vein; *PV,* portal vein; *S,* spine. (A, From Moukaddam H, et al. Ultrasound Clin. 2007;2:455–475.)

Distinguishing between aortic ectasia and an aneurysm of the aorta is essential. Ectasia implies the diffuse dilation of a vessel, whereas an abdominal aortic aneurysm is a region of focal enlargement (Fig. 8.26). Ectasia occurs when the aorta increases both in transverse diameter and in vertical length, which causes the distal aorta to "kink," usually anterior and to the left. The aorta may be "folded," or tortuous, in its course, providing a challenge to the sonographer to follow the vessel in its entirety.

Arteriosclerosis Versus Atherosclerosis. Arteriosclerosis occurs when the arterial vascular system becomes thick and stiff, leading to blood flow restriction to the organs and tissues in the body. Normal healthy arteries are flexible and elastic. With the development of arteriosclerosis, the walls in the arteries can harden and stiffen, resulting in higher blood pressure. **Atherosclerosis** is a specific form of arteriosclerosis. These terms are often used interchangeably. The buildup of fats, cholesterol, and other substances within the arterial wall (known as *plaque*) can restrict blood flow (Fig. 8.27). These plaques may burst and trigger a blood clot or thrombus to form in the artery. The disease usually affects the ascending and descending aorta but can be found in any arterial vessel in the body. Atherosclerosis is preventable and treatable with medication and lifestyle changes. The disease process develops gradually so patients do not have early warning symptoms until the plaque ruptures or obstructs the blood flow.

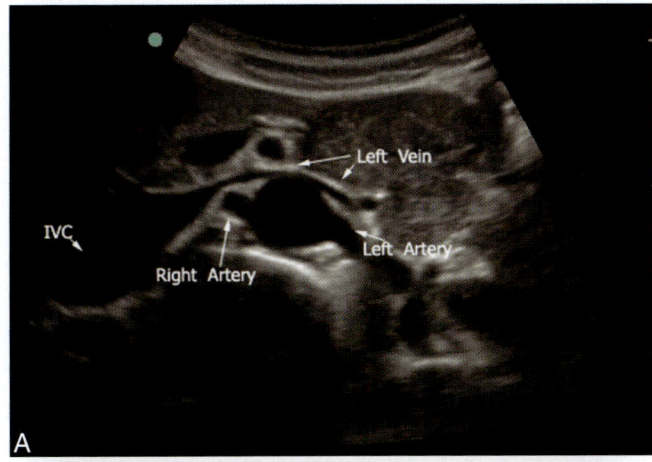
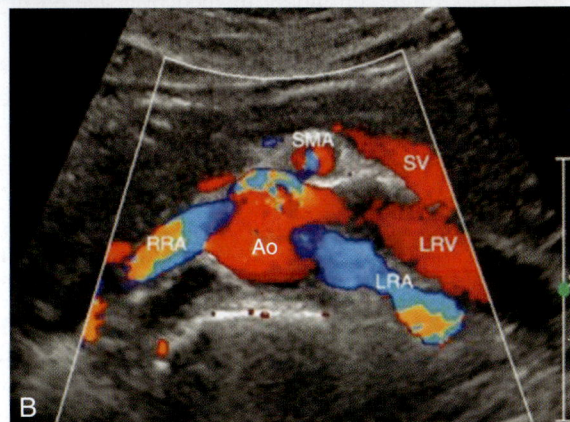

FIG. 8.25 (A–B) The left renal artery courses from the aorta directly into the hilus of the left kidney. *AO,* Aorta; *IVC,* inferior vena cava; *LRV,* left renal vein; *RRA,* right renal artery; *SV,* splenic vein; *SMA,* superior mesenteric artery.

Dorsal Aortic Branches.

Lumbar Artery. Four lumbar arteries are usually present on each side of the aorta (see Fig. 8.12). The vessels travel lateral and posterior to supply muscle, skin, bone, and spinal cord. The midsacral artery supplies the sacrum and rectum.

Pathology of the Aorta

The sonographer may be asked to evaluate the abdominal aorta for several clinical reasons: pulsatile abdominal mass, abdominal pain radiating to the back, an abdominal bruit, or hemodynamic compromise in the lower legs. The arterial system may be affected by atheroma, aneurysm, connective tissue disorder, rupture, thrombosis, or infection.

The sonographer has several objectives to meet when performing a complete evaluation of the abdominal aorta. Recall the discussion that the entire aorta should be imaged in at least two planes (transverse and longitudinal) with appropriate measurements of the aortic diameter in the proximal, mid, and distal segments. The real advantage for the sonographer is the ability to "follow" the vessel with the transducer. If the vessel is tortuous, the transducer should be rotated or angled slightly to follow the artery's course. The size of the aorta increases up to 25% in the seventh and eighth decades.

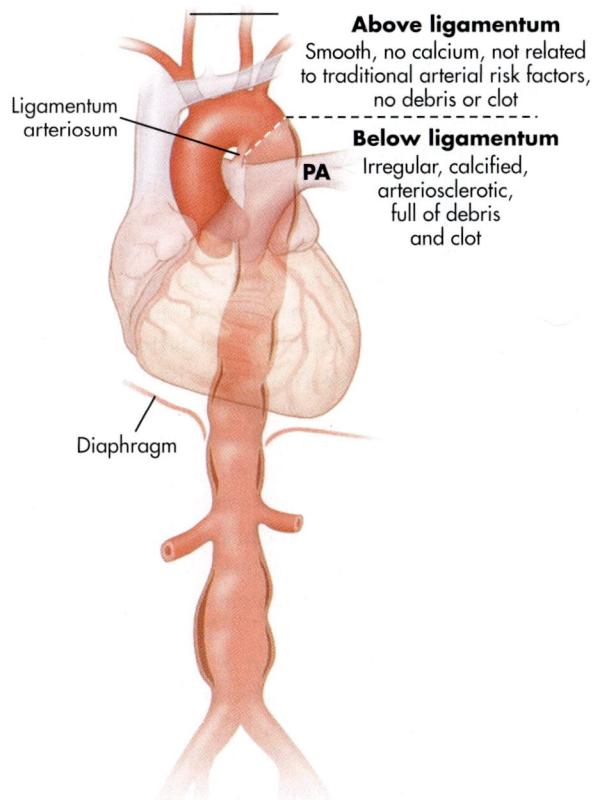

FIG. 8.26 Ectasia implies the diffuse dilation of a vessel, whereas an abdominal aortic aneurysm is a region of focal enlargement. *PA,* Pulmonary artery.

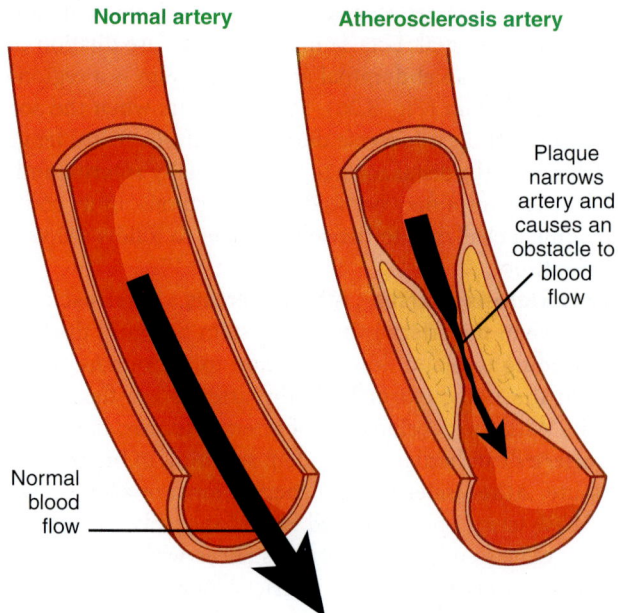

FIG. 8.27 Arteriosclerosis occurs when the arterial vascular system becomes thick and stiff, which can lead to restriction of blood flow to the organs and tissues in the body. Atherosclerosis is a specific form of arteriosclerosis.

Symptoms of moderate to severe atherosclerosis depend on which arteries are affected:
- Heart—chest pain or pressure (angina)
- Brain—sudden numbness or weakness in arms or legs, difficulty speaking or slurred speech, or drooping muscles in the face
- Arms and legs—leg pain when walking or exercising (intermittent claudication)
- Kidneys—high blood pressure or kidney failure

Atherosclerosis is a slow, progressive disease. The damage builds over the years and is caused by many factors, including elevated blood pressure, high cholesterol, high triglycerides, smoking, diabetes, inflammation from systemic diseases such as arthritis or lupus, or infections. Other risk factors include family history of heart disease and lack of exercise. Once the wall of the artery is damaged, the cells clump at the injury site to build up in the inner lining of the artery. These fatty deposits harden and cause narrowing the vessel, thus preventing the organs and tissue the proper blood supply. These fatty deposits may break off and enter the bloodstream to cause a blood clot that may embolize anywhere in the body. Arteriosclerosis is most commonly associated with the development of an aneurysm.

Abdominal Aortic Aneurysm. An **abdominal aortic aneurysm (AAA)** is a localized dilation of the abdominal aorta, usually greater than 3 cm in diameter or more than 1.5 times the diameter of the proximal aorta. The force of blood pushing against the walls of an artery combined with damage or injury to the artery's walls may cause an aneurysm. The abdominal aorta is more common than the thoracic aorta for aneurysm formation (Fig. 8.28). The aneurysm may develop over years without the patient complaining of symptoms. Symptoms may not occur until the pressure of the aneurysm compresses adjacent organs, causes a blockage of blood flow, or ruptures into the abdominal or thoracic cavity. The primary risk factors for a patient with an AAA are dissection and rupture of the vessel. Dissection occurs when the force of blood pumping splits the arterial wall layers, allowing blood to leak in between the walls. The critical condition is when the aneurysm ruptures, causing bleeding internally. Catastrophic outcomes may result from an aortic dissection or rupture. Box 8.2 summarizes the features of AAAs.

Risk factors that contribute to the development of an aneurysm include tobacco use, hypertension, and other cardiovascular diseases. Other risk factors include chronic obstructive pulmonary disease and positive family history for AAA. Genetic conditions linked to AAA include Marfan syndrome and Ehlers-Danlos syndrome (Box 8.3).

AAA occurs more commonly in men over age 65 in the United States compared with women. Visualization of the abdominal aorta has traditionally been an asset in diagnosing the clinical problem. Ultrasound is very capable of demonstrating abnormalities in the diameter, length, and extent of the AAA. The majority of AAAs occur below the kidneys (infrarenal), with the remainder occurring at the level of or above the kidneys (Fig. 8.29). The diagnosis of an aneurysm depends on comparing the aortic diameter of the suspicious area versus that of the normal area of the vessel above and below that area. The sonographer should note the relationship of the aortic aneurysm to the renal arteries. Thus the diameter and the longitudinal extent of the aneurysm as it relates to the origin of the renal vessels should be measured. Often bowel gas may impair adequate visualization of the renal arteries; therefore a more indirect method must be used to locate the origin of the superior mesenteric artery and renal arteries. The patient should be examined from both the supine and the left flank, with the patient rolled into a right lateral decubitus position. Color Doppler may be useful for producing an image of arterial flow from the lateral margins of the abdominal aorta to the kidneys.

Clinical Symptoms. Most patients with an AAA are asymptomatic. If the patient does have symptoms, they may include throbbing or deep pain in the abdomen, back, or flank area. The pain may extend into the buttocks, groin, or legs. The enlarged vessel may be found during routine physical examination or during an unrelated radiologic or surgical procedure.

Clinical symptoms of the patient with an aortic aneurysm may result from rupture or expansion of the vessel. The enlarged vessel may produce symptoms by impinging on adjacent structures, or the vessel may become occluded by direct pressure or thrombus with resulting embolism. The enlarged aneurysm may rupture into the peritoneal cavity or the retroperitoneum, causing intense back pain and a drop in hematocrit. *Grey Turner sign* may be associated with an extensive bleed in the retroperitoneal cavity. Patients may present with satiety (becoming full easily) or nausea and vomiting. Abrupt onset of severe, constant pain in the abdomen, back, or flank that is unrelieved by positional changes is characteristic of rapid expansion or rupture of an aneurysm. Other complications may include dissection, thrombosis, distal embolism, infection, and obstruction and invasion of adjacent structures. Commonly, branch artery occlusions or stenosis may be seen in the inferior mesenteric artery or renal arteries.

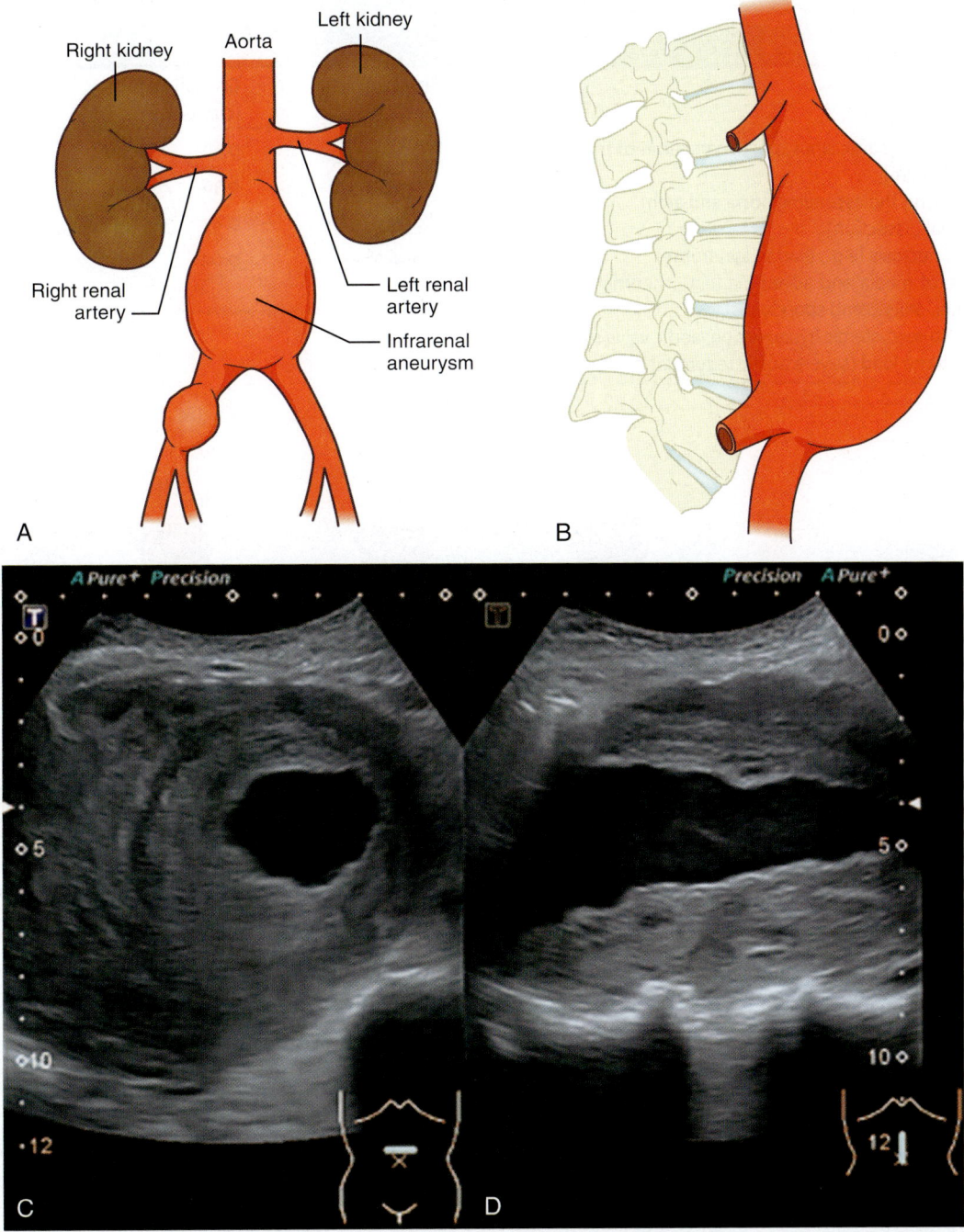

FIG. 8.28 (A–B) An aortic aneurysm is defined as that with a vessel diameter greater than 3 cm or noted focal dilation of the vessel. (C) Transverse and (D) longitudinal sonographic images of the aortic aneurysm with circumferential thrombus.

BOX 8.2	Features of Abdominal Aortic Aneurysms

- Most are true aneurysms, involving all three layers
- Approximately 85% are infrarenal
- Measure anteroposterior diameter on longitudinal views
- Mural thrombus common with larger aneurysm
- Atherosclerosis—tortuosity, folding
- Aortic pseudoaneurysm—trauma
- Mycotic aneurysm—infection
- Surgery may be considered when >5 cm

The patient with an aneurysm most likely has many other medical problems. The clinician must be able to sequentially follow the size and growth of the aneurysm noninvasively over a structured time by sonography. Therefore it is important in these cases to measure the exact location of the aneurysm so subsequent follow-up sonographic evaluations will be accurate. The patient with an AAA measurement of less than 4 cm in diameter is generally followed every 6 months with sonography; intervention may occur once the patient becomes symptomatic. In patients with aneurysms ranging from 4 to 5 cm

BOX 8.3	Factors That May Cause the Development of an Aortic Aneurysm

- Atherosclerosis
- Trauma to the chest
- Congenital defects (aortic sinus, post-coarctation of the aorta, ductus diverticulum)
- Syphilis (involving the ascending aorta and arch)
- Mycosis (fungal dissection)
- Cystic medial necrosis (e.g., Marfan syndrome)
- Inflammation of media and adventitia (e.g., rheumatic fever, polychondritis, ankylosing spondylitis)
- Increased pressure (systemic hypertension, aortic valve stenosis)
- Abnormal volume load (severe aortic regurgitation)

TABLE 8.2 Size, Growth Rate, and Risk of Rupture for Abdominal Aortic Aneurysms

Size (cm)	Growth Rate (cm/year)	Annual Rupture Risk (%)
3.0–3.9	0.39	0
4.0–4.9	0.36	0.5–5
5.0–5.9	0.43	3–15
6.0–6.9	0.64	10–20
>7.0		20–50

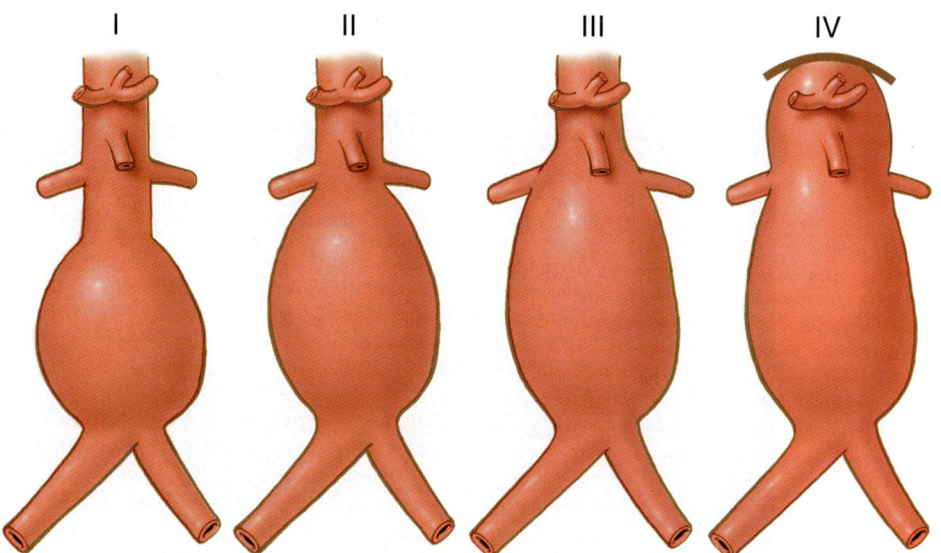

FIG. 8.29 The majority of abdominal aortic aneurysms occur below the kidneys (infrarenal), with the remainder occurring at the level of or above the kidneys. *I*, Infrarenal; *II*, juxtarenal; *III*, pararenal; *IV*, suprarenal.

in diameter, surgery or endovascular aneurysm repair may be suggested if the patient is in good health. Patients with aneurysms ranging from 5 to 6 cm may benefit from repair, especially if they have other factors for rupture (e.g., hypertension, smoking, chronic obstructive pulmonary disease). Aneurysms less than 6 cm show a very slow growth pattern (less than 0.2 to 0.5 cm/year) and may be followed annually with sonography. Patients with aneurysms measuring 6 cm may be followed at 6-month intervals. Patients at the highest risk are those with aneurysms measuring greater than 6 to 7 cm. The risk increases with age and other medical problems (Table 8.2). Three primary factors are related to the growth rate of abdominal aneurysms: the initial size of the aortic aneurysm, the presence of cardiac disease, and the presence of beta-adrenergic blockade (blood pressure–lowering medications).

Surgical intervention may be considered if associated renal and iliac involvement is present with occlusive disease or aneurysmal development. The sonographer should measure the length of the infrarenal aortic neck, which may help determine the best surgical approach (retroperitoneal vs. transabdominal) and the location of the aortic cross-clamp. Endovascular stent grafts for treatment are a less invasive approach to repairing an aneurysm as this graft is placed through two small incisions in the abdomen.

Classification of Aneurysms. Histologically, the aneurysm may be classified as a *true aneurysm* (lined by all three layers of the aorta) or as a *false aneurysm (pseudoaneurysm)* (not lined by all three layers). A true aneurysm forms when the tensile strength of the wall decreases (Fig. 8.30A). A small percentage of true aneurysms occur secondary to underlying diseases such as Marfan syndrome, Ehlers-Danlos syndrome, and familial aortic dissection.

In the **pseudoaneurysm** (see Fig. 8.30B), blood escapes through a hole in the intima of the vessel wall but is contained by the deeper layers of the aorta or by adjacent tissue. With color Doppler, blood can be seen to flow into the protuberance during systole and out during diastole. These events can occur after trauma to the vessel due to accident or surgery or after an interventional cardiac catheterization or angiography procedure. Ultrasound evaluation of the pulsatile mass is conducted, with color Doppler showing communication between the artery and the vein. Compression of the mass with a linear transducer at 20-minute compression intervals may allow the lesion to close if the communication is small.

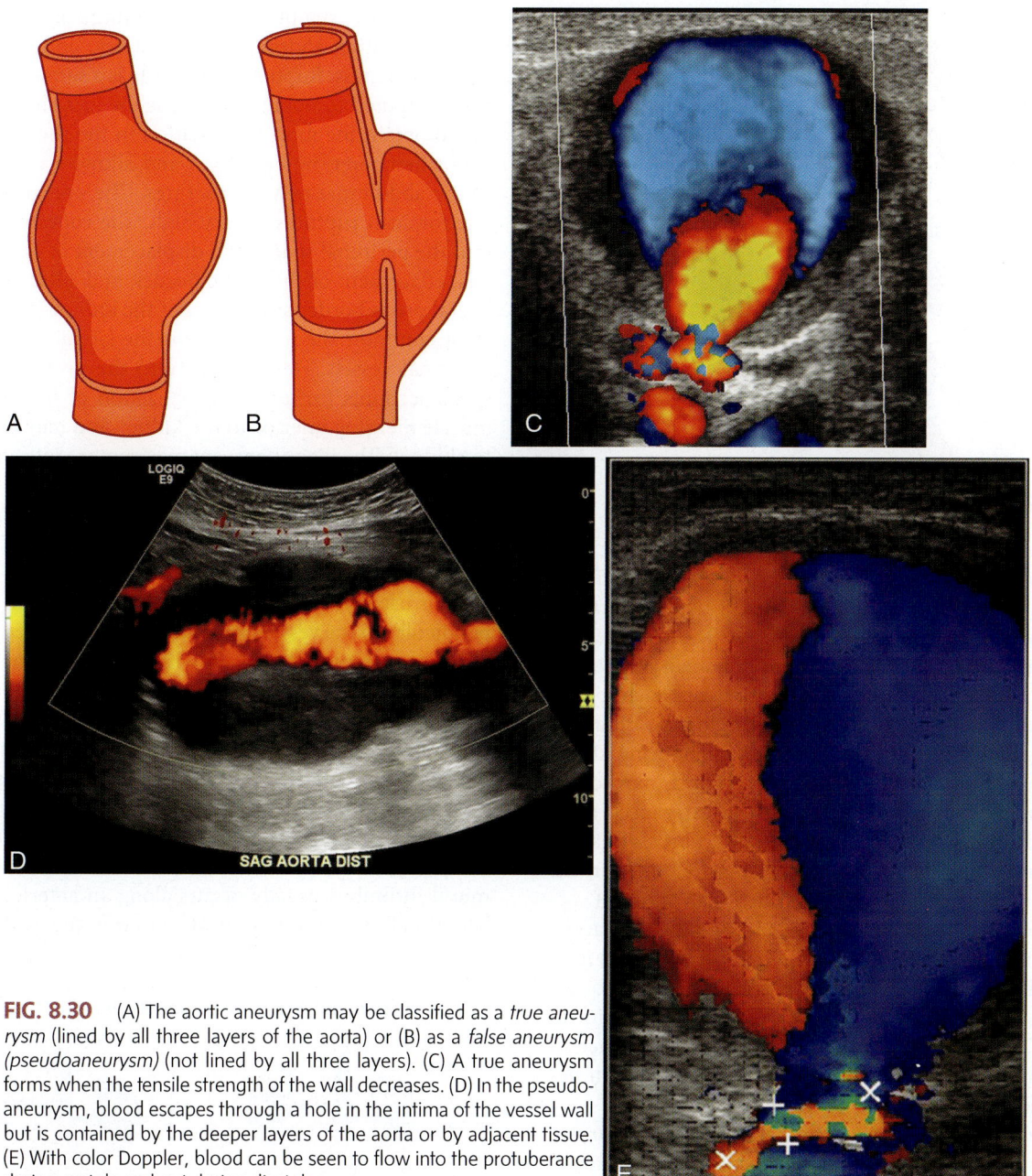

FIG. 8.30 (A) The aortic aneurysm may be classified as a *true aneurysm* (lined by all three layers of the aorta) or (B) as a *false aneurysm (pseudoaneurysm)* (not lined by all three layers). (C) A true aneurysm forms when the tensile strength of the wall decreases. (D) In the pseudoaneurysm, blood escapes through a hole in the intima of the vessel wall but is contained by the deeper layers of the aorta or by adjacent tissue. (E) With color Doppler, blood can be seen to flow into the protuberance during systole and out during diastole.

Sometimes it takes several compressions (20 minutes on and 20 minutes off) to close the communication completely. Color flow allows the sonographer to see whether the communication is closed. Pseudoaneurysms that cannot be closed with this technique may require surgical intervention, as they may become a source of emboli, the site of increased chance of infection secondary to abnormal blood flow communication, or a cause of local pressure effects. In addition, they can rupture, which may result in exsanguination.

Descriptive Terms for an Abdominal Aortic Aneurysm. An aneurysm may be described as fusiform or saccular (Fig. 8.31). The idiopathic abdominal aneurysm is a true aneurysm that most commonly develops below the renal vessels (in more than 85% of patients). It usually begins below the renal arteries (inferior to the superior mesenteric artery) and extends to the bifurcation of the aorta at the iliac arteries.

The most common presentation of an atherosclerotic aneurysm is a **fusiform aneurysm** of the distal aorta at the aortic bifurcation. The fusiform aneurysm represents a gradual transition between normal and abnormal and extends over the length of the aorta to resemble a "football-like" shape. Sonography displays atherosclerosis of the vessel as decreased pulsations of the aortic walls, with bright echoes reflecting the degree of thickening and calcification. These aneurysms often extend into the iliac vessels in the pelvis.

A **saccular aneurysm** shows a sudden transition between normal and abnormal and is somewhat spherical and larger (5 to 10 cm) than fusiform aneurysms. This type of aneurysm

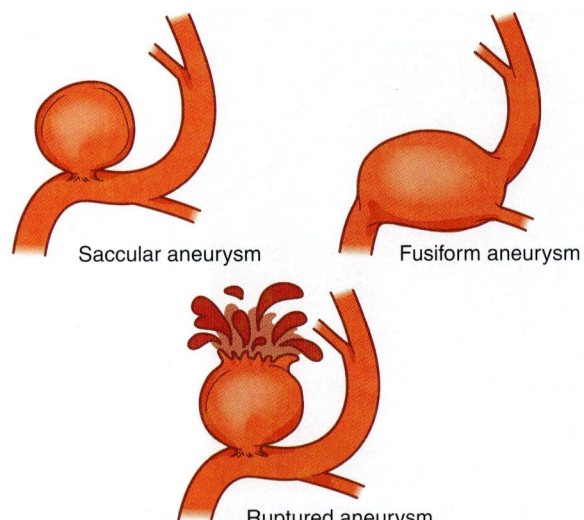

FIG. 8.31 The three types of aneurysms.

is connected to the vascular lumen by a mouth that varies in size but may be as large as an aneurysm. It may be partially or completely filled with mural thrombus. The sonographer must carefully follow the course of such an aneurysm to differentiate it from a retroperitoneal mass or lymphadenopathy. Pulsations are usually diminished secondary to clot formation.

A large aneurysm may compress its neighboring structures. Compression of the common bile duct may cause obstruction; compression of the renal artery can cause hypertension and renal ischemia. Retroperitoneal fibrosis with an aneurysm may involve the ureter, causing hydronephrosis. The left kidney is more frequently affected than the right.

The abdominal aneurysm may extend into the iliac arteries. The sonographer should examine both iliac arteries in at least two planes. At the level of the bifurcation, the iliac vessels may be seen as circular, pulsatile vessels just anterior to the spine. The oblique longitudinal scan is used to produce an image of the vessel in its entire length. Normal iliac arteries usually measure less than 1 cm in diameter.

Inflammatory Aortic Aneurysm. This type of aneurysm is a variant in which the wall of the aneurysm is thickened and surrounded by fibrosis and adhesions of a type similar to those found in retroperitoneal fibrosis. These patients present with a higher surgical risk. Clinically, they present with pain that may mimic a retroperitoneal hemorrhage. A rare condition is the development of a mycotic aneurysm secondary to infection. The most common infections result from septic emboli, streptococci, staphylococci, and *Salmonella*. The infection may produce a focal abscess that appears as a complex fluid collection with irregular borders.

Rupture of Aortic Aneurysm. The rupture of an aortic aneurysm is catastrophic, with a mortality rate of 50%. The diameter alone may not accurately predict rupture risk as smaller aortic diameters may rupture, and larger diameter aortas may remain stable. The wall stress may influence the risk of rupture (when the wall stress exceeds the wall strength). The diameter rate of change may influence the rupture risk.

The classic symptoms of a ruptured aortic aneurysm are excruciating abdominal pain, shock, and an expanding abdominal mass. Rupture of the aorta is a surgical emergency, and computed tomography (CT) is the first choice for imaging to obtain the most information in the shortest time. CT is not hampered by bowel gas and allows a rapid overview of the abdominal pelvic structures. The operative mortality rate for such ruptures is very high. The rupture may extend into the perirenal space with displacement of renal hilar vessels, effacement of the aortic border, and silhouetting of the lateral psoas border at the level of the kidney (Fig. 8.32). The most common site for rupture is the lateral wall inferior to the renal vessels. Hemorrhage into the posterior pararenal space accounts for loss of visualization of the lateral psoas muscle merging inferior to the kidney and may also displace the kidney. The iliac aneurysm may rupture into the rectosigmoid colon, iliac vein, or ureter.

Sonographic Findings. Box 8.4 outlines the protocol for ultrasound evaluation of the abdominal aorta. Recall that the normal average measurement for a male adult abdominal aorta is usually less than 3 cm, with measurement taken perpendicular to the vessel from outer layer–to–outer layer walls. (This measurement correlates with the measurement made by the surgeon.) The sonographer should search for focal dilation of the abdominal aorta or lack of normal tapering distally. The anterior and posterior borders are often better imaged than the lateral borders. The adventitia is slightly echogenic; however, with atherosclerosis, the walls may become increasingly echogenic with calcification. When an aneurysm is detected, the presence of a mural thrombus should be evaluated. A mural thrombus usually occurs along an anterior or anterolateral wall. The thrombus is often poorly attached and friable

Abdominal Aortic Aneurysm with Fatal Rupture

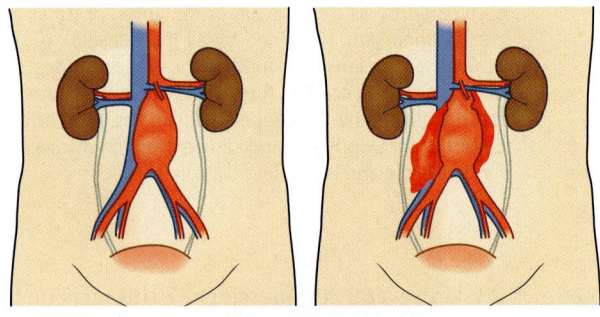

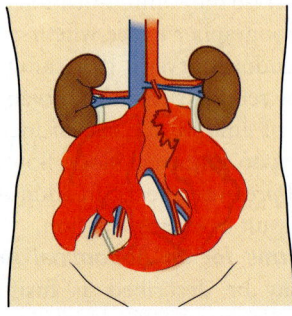

FIG. 8.32 The retroperitoneal collection of blood that may result in the retroperitoneal cavity from an abdominal aortic rupture.

and may be a source for distal emboli. Thrombus within an aneurysm is shown ultrasonically as medium- to low-level echoes (Fig. 8.33). Generally, increased sensitivity is likely to highlight the low-level echoes from the thrombus. These echoes should be seen in both planes on more than one scan to be separated from low-level reverberation echoes. A chronic thrombotic clot is easier to see with sonography because of the bright calcification that appears as thick, echogenic echoes, sometimes with posterior shadowing. The amount of thrombus in a vessel has no relation to the risk of rupture.

The sonographer should note the maximum length, width, and transverse dimension of the aortic aneurysm. Documentation of the shape (fusiform or saccular) and location of the aneurysm in relation to the renal arteries is important. Extension of the aneurysm into the iliac arteries should also be noted. Measurements of length × width × height should be included in the report. A description of wall thickening, the presence of calcification, blood flow, soft plaque, or calcified plaque should also be included in the report. Careful evaluation of the presence or absence of an aortic dissection should be noted. Because the aneurysm may often affect the renal vessels, both kidneys should be analyzed. (Measure the renal size and exclude pelvocaliectasis.) If hypertrophy of one or both kidneys occurs, a full Doppler evaluation of the renal vessels should be conducted to rule out renal artery stenosis.

Aortic Dissection. A defect in the vessel intimal wall must exist along with internal weakness for a dissection to occur. Dissection of the aorta may occur secondary to **cystic medial necrosis** (weakening of the arterial wall), to hypertension, or to the inherited disease **Marfan syndrome**. Individuals with this disorder are extremely tall, lanky, and double-jointed; a progressive stretching disorder exists in all arterial vessels,

> **BOX 8.4 Protocol to Evaluate an Abdominal Aortic Aneurysm**
>
> An *aortic aneurysm* is defined as that with a vessel diameter greater than 3 cm or noted focal dilation of the vessel. An *iliac aneurysm* is defined as a vessel with a diameter greater than 2 cm. Aneurysms larger than 5 cm and those with documented rapid rates of expansion have an increased risk of catastrophic rupture. *The physician must be made aware of these patients before they leave the department.* If an abnormal bulging of the abdominal aorta (aneurysm) is present, the sonographer should note the following additional views:
> - The aneurysm should be followed to measure the length of the dilation and to note the position of the renal arteries in relation to the aneurysm.
> - The aneurysm should be measured in both transverse (depth and width) and longitudinal planes.
> - Clot or thrombus formation should be carefully assessed.
> - Longitudinal scans of each iliac vessel from the bifurcation to the most distal segment should be taken.
> - Transverse scans of the iliacs below the bifurcation should be taken.

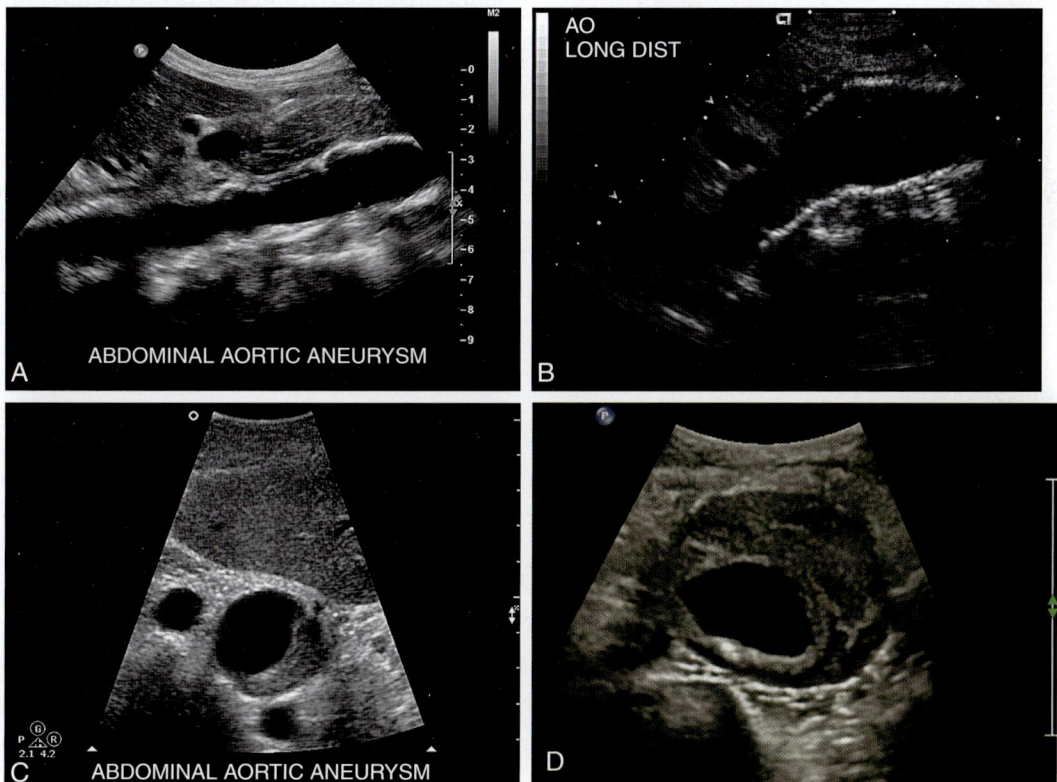

FIG. 8.33 **Abdominal aortic aneurysm.** (A) Longitudinal image of a small abdominal aortic aneurysm extending superior to the bifurcation. (B) Longitudinal image of a large abdominal aortic aneurysm; the largest diameter of the aneurysm should be measured. (C) Multiple echoes within represent thrombus formation. (D) Transverse image of a large abdominal aortic aneurysm with thrombus along the anterolateral borders. *AO*, Aorta.

especially in the aorta, causing abnormal dilation, weakened walls, and eventual dissection, rupture, or both. Color flow Doppler may be used to detect flow into the false channel.

Three classifications of aortic dissection are based on the DeBakey model (Fig. 8.34). Types I and II involve the ascending aorta and the aortic arch; type III involves the descending aorta at a level inferior to the left subclavian artery. A high incidence of mortality is associated with type I and II dissections because of possible obstruction at the origin of the coronary arteries and possible obstruction of blood into the head and neck vessels. The lowest mortality rate is associated with the type III dissection, which begins inferior to the left subclavian artery with possible extension into the abdominal aorta.

The type I dissection begins at the root of the aorta and may extend the entire length of the arch, descending to the aorta and into the abdominal aorta. This is the most dangerous, especially if the dissection spirals around the aorta, cutting off the blood supply to the coronary, carotid, brachiocephalic, and subclavian vessels. The third dissection type (type III) begins at the lower end of the descending aorta and extends into the abdominal aorta (Fig. 8.35). This may be critical if the dissection spirals around to impede blood flow into the renal vessels. Less than 5% of dissections occur primarily in the abdomen.

A **dissecting aneurysm** may be detected with sonography, although CT is generally the preferred imaging choice in emergent situations. The patient may be known to have an aortic or thoracic aneurysm and presents clinically with sudden excruciating chest pain radiating to the back that develops as the result of a dissection. These critical patients may go into shock very quickly, and CT is generally ordered to obtain the most information in the shortest amount of time. However, the patient who presents with some of these symptoms and is stable may have a slow leak aneurysm. These stable patients are appropriately imaged with sonography. The sonographer should look for a dissection "flap" or recent channel, with or without frank aneurysmal dilation. This flap is well demonstrated with M-mode as a fluttering within the lumen at different phases of the cardiac cycle. The dissection of blood occurs along the laminar planes of the aortic media with the formation of a blood-filled channel within the aortic wall. Color Doppler will demonstrate flow in both channels (true and false lumens), with the flow rate differing between the channels.

When the dissection develops, hemorrhage may occur between the middle and outer thirds of the media. An intimal tear is considered if the tear is found in the ascending portion of the arch. This type of dissection extends proximally toward the heart and distally, sometimes to the iliac and femoral arteries. A small number of dissections do not have an obvious intimal tear. Extravasation may completely encircle the aorta or may extend along one segment of its circumference, or the aneurysm may rupture into any of the body cavities.

Aortic Graft. An abdominal aortic aneurysm may be surgically repaired with a flexible graft material attached to the end of the remaining aorta. The synthetic material used for a graft produces bright textured echo reflections compared with those from typical aortic walls. After surgery, the attached walls may swell at the attachment site and form another aneurysm or pseudoaneurysm (Fig. 8.36). Other complications of prosthetic grafts include hematoma, infection, and degeneration of graft material.

Newer surgical techniques now repair the aneurysm with an endovascular graft treatment. The graft may be anastomosed in an end-to-side or end-to-end manner. These grafts would be placed within the aorta, at the level of the aorta and iliac artery, or within the femoral artery (Fig. 8.37). Further development in techniques has placed the grafts in the aortofemoral and juxtarenal positions. Complications of these grafts resulted in endoleak formations that were immediate, without outflow, and persistent. The type of graft used, the technique of graft insertion, and the aortic anatomic features all affected the endoleak rate.

The sonographer should carefully examine the upper and lower ends of the anastomoses with both real-time and color Doppler. During the evaluation of the graft, the sonographer should look for stenosis at the ends of the graft, aneurysm formation, or pseudoaneurysm development. Doppler

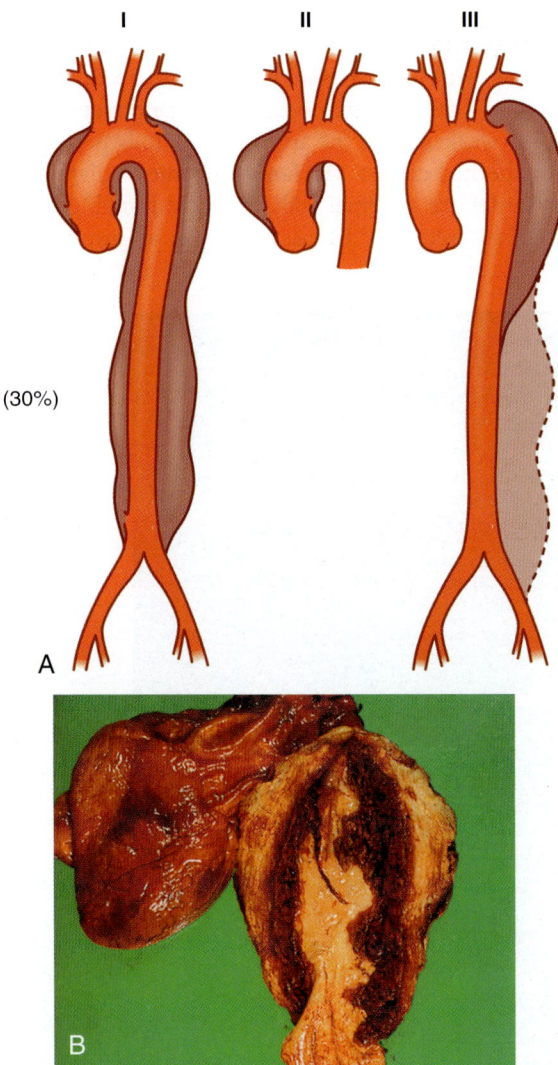

FIG. 8.34 (A) Three classifications of aortic dissection are based on the DeBakey model. Types I and II involve the ascending aorta and the aortic arch; type III involves the descending aorta at a level inferior to the left subclavian artery. (B) Dissecting aneurysm of the thoracic aorta. The blood has filled the space formed by the separation of the intima and media of the aorta.

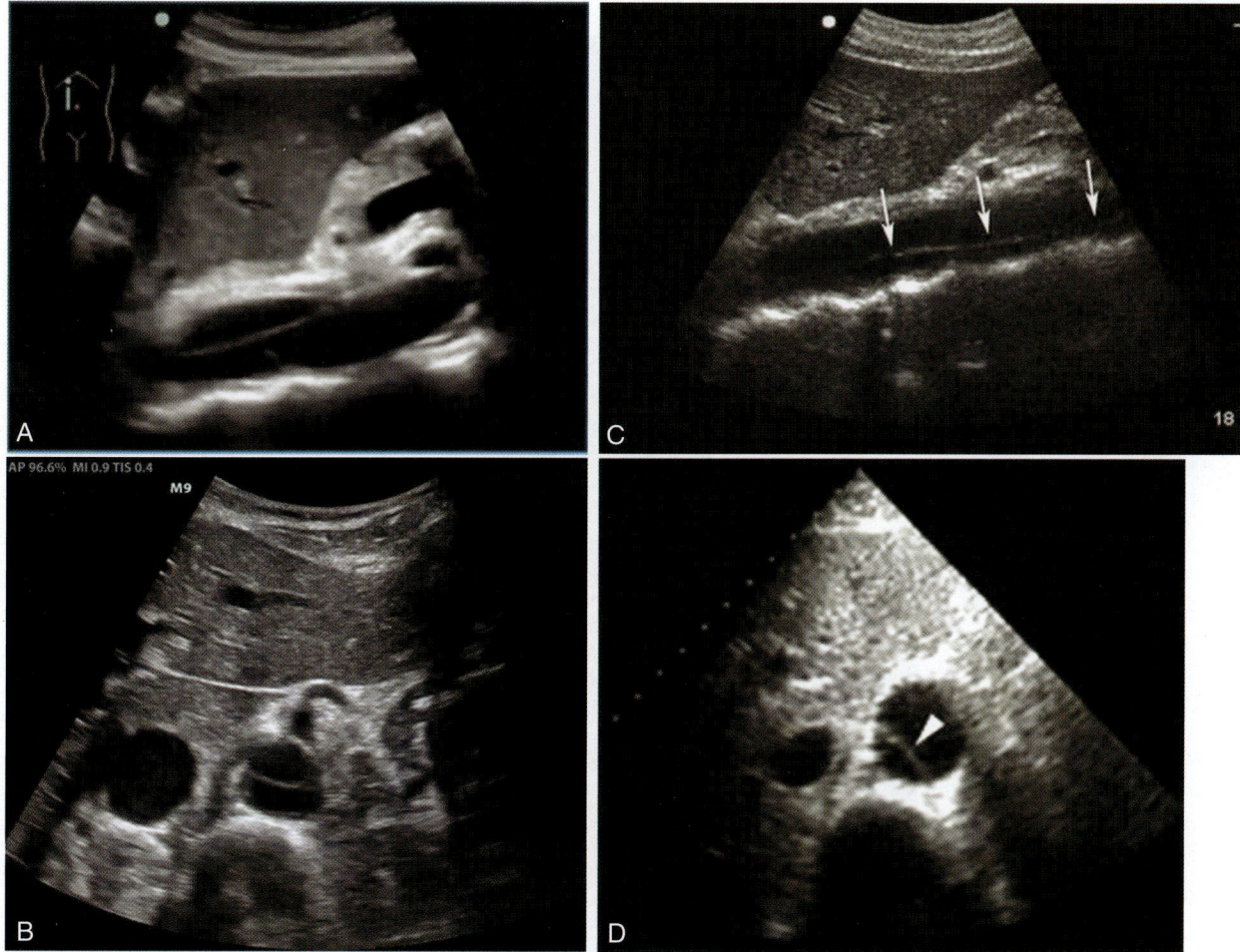

FIG. 8.35 (A–D) Type III dissection occurs in the descending aorta and extends into the abdominal aorta; the *arrows* point to the luminal flap.

evaluation of the distal vessels should be conducted to ensure that adequate blood flow is available. Fluid collections (i.e., hematoma, lymphocele, seroma, or abscess formation) may develop at the graft site.

Iliac and Thoracic Aneurysms.

Iliac Aneurysm. A very small percentage of patients (less than 5%) with an abdominal aneurysm will also have an iliac aneurysm. These may occur at the bifurcation of the common iliac artery or in the external iliac just distal to the bifurcation.

Pseudopulsatile Abdominal Masses. Masses other than an aortic aneurysm that can simulate a pulsatile abdominal mass include retroperitoneal tumor, huge fibroid uterus, or para-aortic nodes. Because the mass is adjacent to the aorta, pulsations are transmitted from the aorta to the mass. Next to an abdominal aneurysm, the most common cause for a pulsatile abdominal mass is enlarged retroperitoneal lymph nodes. This mass is usually the result of lymphoma in the middle-aged patient. On ultrasound, the nodes are homogeneous masses surrounding the aorta. The aortic wall may be poorly defined because of the close acoustic impedance of the nodes and the aorta. The sonographer should also look for splenomegaly. A retroperitoneal sarcoma may present as a pulsatile mass; it may extend into the root of the mesentery and give rise to a larger intraperitoneal component. The echodensity depends on the tissue type that predominates; fatty lesions are more echodense than fibrous or myomatous lesions.

Splanchnic Aneurysm. The splanchnic aneurysms may be atherosclerotic, posttraumatic, mycotic, congenital, or inflammatory. A small percentage of patients with chronic pancreatitis may develop these aneurysms, which may occur in the SMA, hepatic and splenic arteries, gastroduodenal arteries, or inferior mesenteric artery. They may have mural thrombus that is well demonstrated with color Doppler.

Renal Arterial Disease.

Renal Artery Stenosis. Renal artery stenosis may present clinically as hypertension. The stenosis is due to atherosclerotic disease or fibromuscular hyperplasia. Color and spectral Doppler are used to investigate the renal vessels for increased velocity flow patterns representative of obstruction of flow into the kidney (Fig. 8.38). Recall that the right renal artery arises from the kidney and travels posterior to the inferior vena cava to enter the medial wall of the abdominal aorta. The left renal artery has a more direct course from the kidney to the lateral wall of the aorta. Thus the renal arteries may be challenging to align parallel with the Doppler beam to obtain a correct velocity measurement. This is further discussed in Chapter 15.

INFERIOR VENA CAVA

The **inferior vena cava** (IVC) is formed by the union of the common iliac veins posterior to the right common iliac artery at the level of the fifth lumbar vertebra (Figs. 8.39 and 8.40).

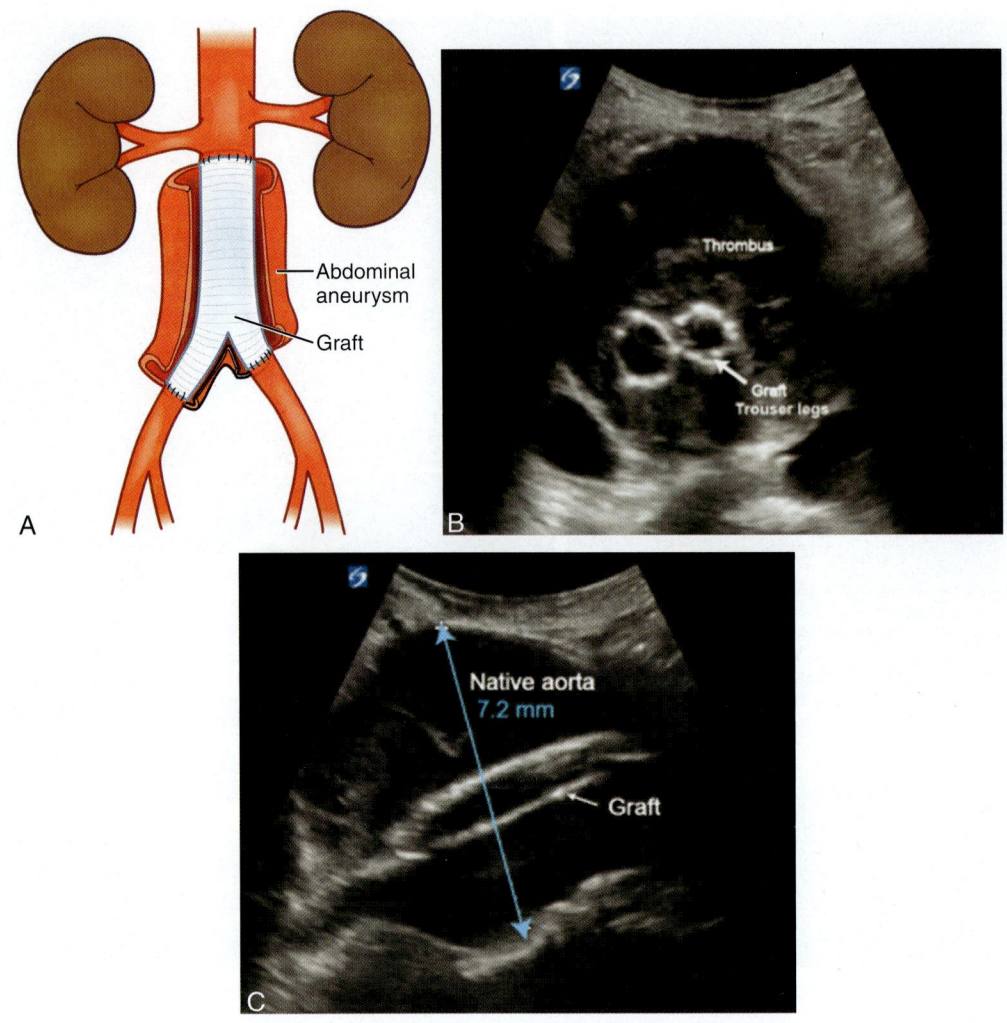

FIG. 8.36 (A) An abdominal aortic aneurysm may be surgically repaired with a flexible graft material attached to the end of the remaining aorta. (B–C) Transverse and longitudinal images of a patient with an aortic graft in place.

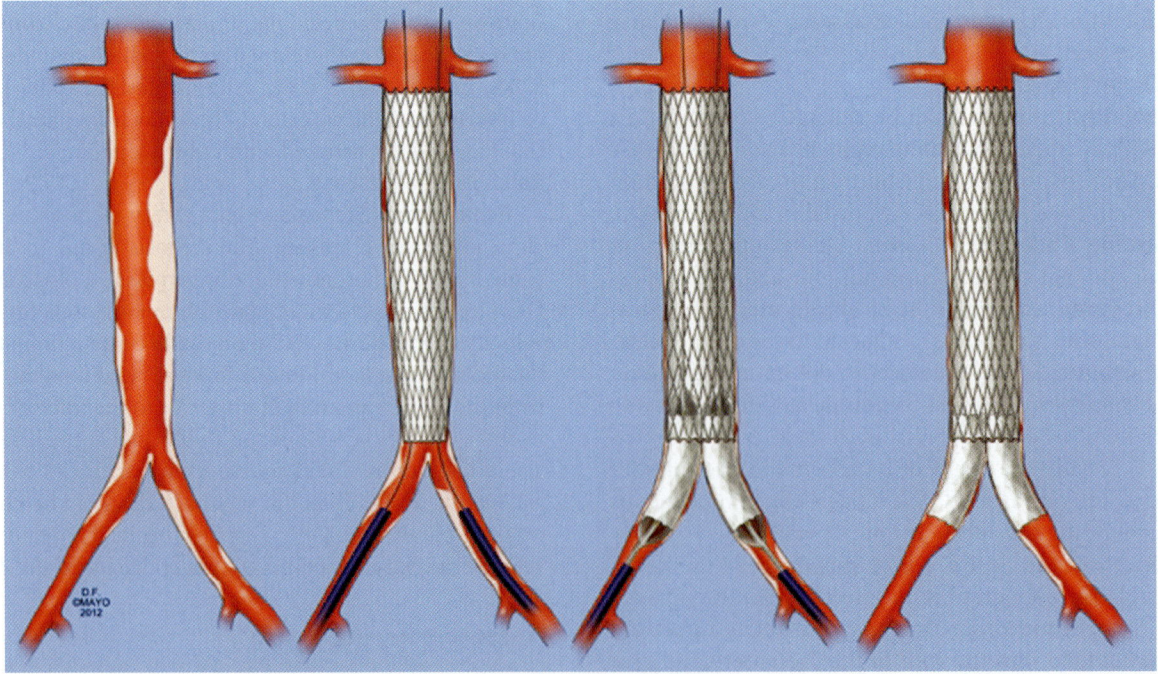

FIG. 8.37 The endovascular graft. The graft may be anastomosed in an end-to-side or end-to-end manner. These grafts would be placed within the aorta, at the level of the aorta and iliac artery, or within the femoral artery. (Courtesy Mayo Foundation for Medical Education and Research.)

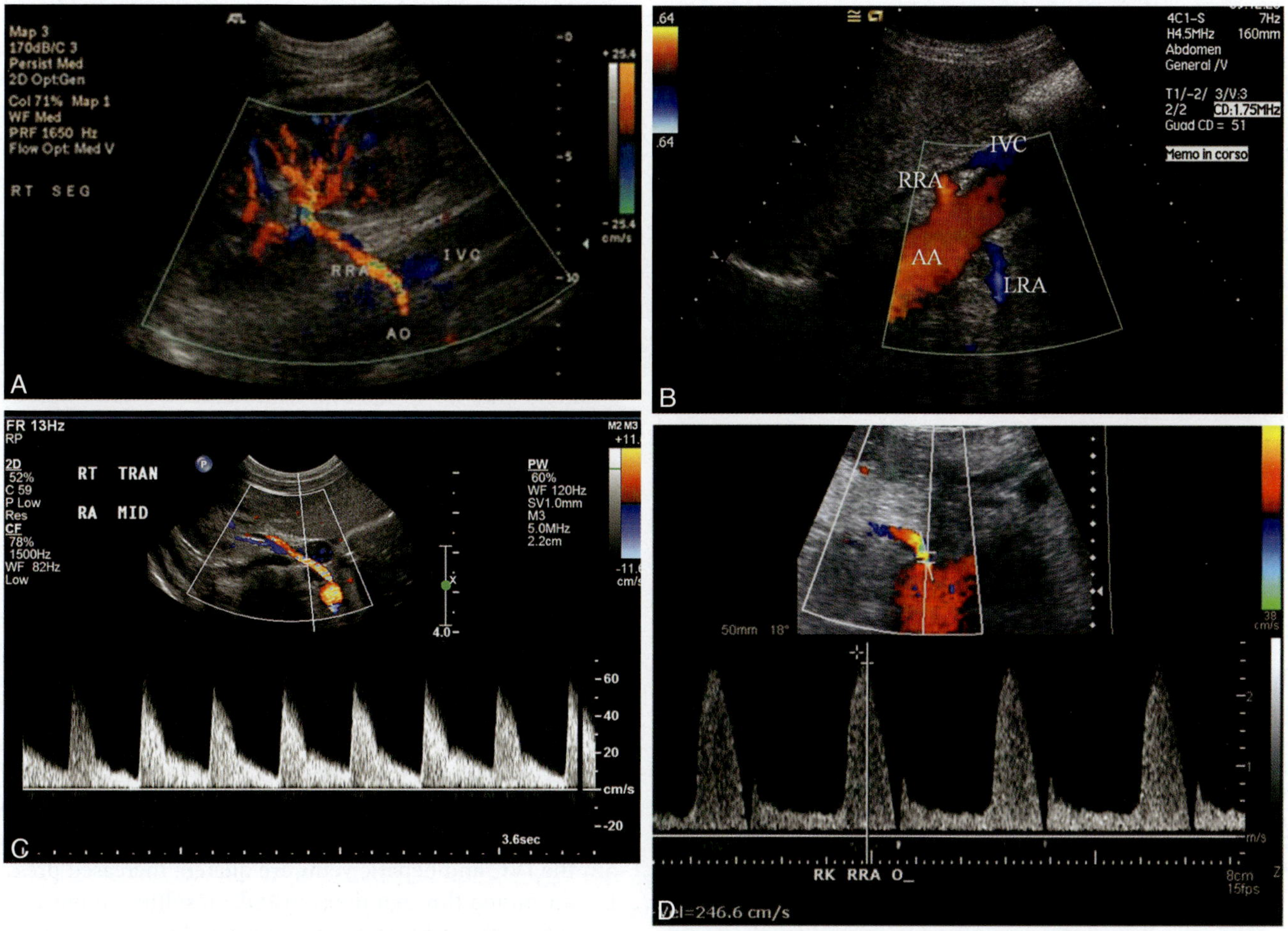

FIG. 8.38 (A–B) Color and spectral Doppler are used to investigate the renal vessels for increased velocity flow patterns representative of obstruction of flow into the kidney. (C) The Doppler sample volume is placed within the proximal right renal artery (RRA). The Doppler angle should be less than 60 degrees. (D) Renal artery stenosis presents with a high velocity flow pattern in the RRA. This shows a velocity of 246 cm/sec. *AA*, Abdominal aneurysm; *AO*, aorta; *IVC*, inferior vena cava; *LRA*, left renal artery.

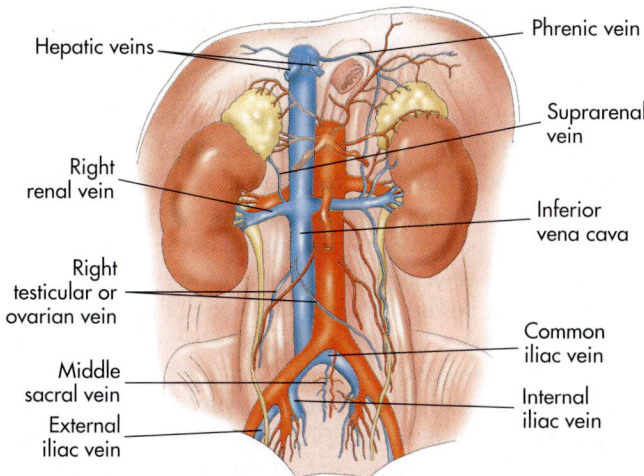

FIG. 8.39 The inferior vena cava is formed by the union of the common iliac veins posterior to the right common iliac artery at the level of the fifth lumbar vertebra.

The IVC ascends vertically through the retroperitoneal space on the right side of the aorta posterior to the liver, piercing the central tendon of the diaphragm at the level of the eighth thoracic vertebra to enter the right atrium of the heart. Its entrance into the lesser sac separates it from the portal vein. Caudal to the renal vein entrance, the IVC shows posterior "hammocking" through the bare area of the liver (Fig. 8.41).

The tributaries of the IVC include the following:
- Three anterior hepatic veins
- Three lateral tributaries: the right suprarenal vein (the left suprarenal vein drains into the left renal vein), the renal veins, and the right testicular or ovarian vein
- Five lateral abdominal wall tributaries: the inferior phrenic vein and the four lumbar veins
- Three veins of origin: the two common iliac veins and the median sacral vein

The IVC is a large, collapsible vein that returns blood from the abdomen, pelvis, and lower limbs through the system's major tributaries into the right atrium of the heart. The superior vena cava drains the head, neck, thoracic cavity, and upper extremities and is discussed in Chapter 40. The walls of the cava are much thinner than those of the aorta because the pressure of blood flow is much lower.

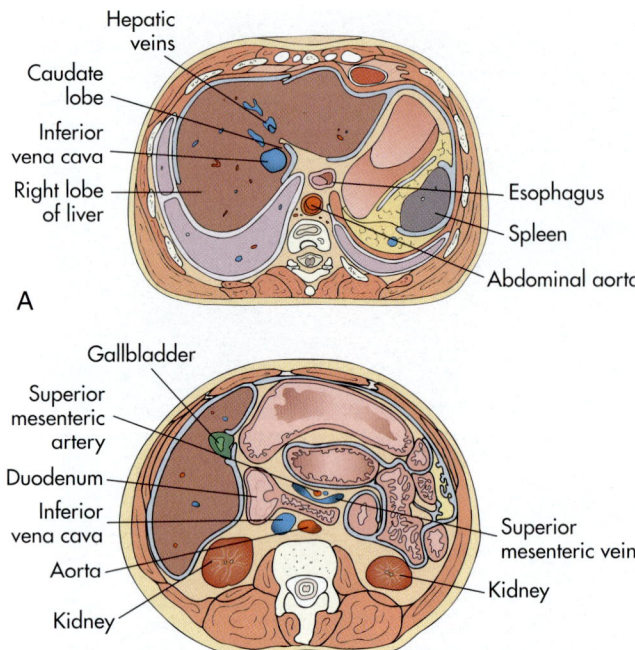

FIG. 8.40 The inferior vena cava ascends vertically through the retroperitoneal space on the right side of the aorta posterior to the liver, piercing the central tendon of the diaphragm at the level of the eighth thoracic vertebra to enter the right atrium of the heart. Its entrance into the lesser sac separates it from the portal vein. (A) Cross section of the abdomen at the level of the tenth intervertebral disk. (B) Cross section of the abdomen at the first lumbar vertebra.

Sonographic Findings. The IVC serves as a landmark for many other abdominal structures and should be routinely visualized on all examinations. The intrahepatic portion of the cava is seen by using the liver as an acoustic window (Fig. 8.42). Beyond the liver border, the cava may become obscured by overlying bowel gas. The complete IVC is imaged on a sagittal scan. Beginning at the midline of the abdomen, the transducer should be angled slightly to the right with a slight oblique tilt until the entire vessel is seen. The patient should be instructed to hold their breath; this causes the patient to perform a slight Valsalva maneuver toward the end of inspiration, which dilates the IVC. The inferior vena cava may expand to 2.5 cm in diameter with this maneuver. With expiration, venous return improves, and therefore the caval diameter decreases. Both cardiac and respiratory pulsations are transmitted in the IVC to produce a phasic pattern similar to the pattern in the peripheral veins. The diameter of the IVC will depend on the patient's age and body mass. The average adult inferior vena cava size should measure less than 2.2 cm with greater than 50% respiratory collapse.

The pulsatile aorta is easily differentiated from the IVC as the IVC travels in a horizontal course with its proximal portion curving slightly anterior as it pierces the diaphragm to empty into the right atrial cavity (Fig. 8.43). On the other hand, the aorta follows the curvature of the spine, with its distal portion lying more posterior before bifurcating into the iliac vessels. The lumen of the cava should be anechoic, although with slow-flowing blood, the lumen becomes slightly more echogenic with *swirling* of the blood seen in real-time.

On transverse scans, the almond-shaped IVC serves as a landmark for localizing the splenic vein, which is generally found anterior and slightly medial to the cava as it crosses in a horizontal path from the spleen to form the portal vein (Fig. 8.44A). On longitudinal scans, the IVC serves as a landmark for the portal vein, which is located just anterior to the anterior wall of the midpoint of the inferior vena cava (see Fig. 8.44B).

The inferior vena cava is also useful in identifying the echogenic pancreas and small common bile duct (Fig. 8.45). The head of the pancreas is seen just inferior to the portal vein and anterior to the IVC as it makes a slight impression or indentation on the anterior wall of the cava. The common duct is seen anterior to the portal vein as it dips posterior to enter the head of the pancreas.

Inferior Vena Cava Abnormalities

Inferior Vena Cava Dilation or Compression. In patients with right ventricular failure, the IVC does not collapse with inspiration or expiration. Dilation of the IVC may be noted in several pathologies, including right ventricular heart failure (Fig. 8.46), congestive heart disease, constrictive pericarditis, tricuspid disease, and right heart obstructive tumors. Tumor or thrombus may be found in the IVC and may obstruct blood returning into the right atrium. In patients with hepatomegaly, the IVC and hepatic veins are dilated; increased pressure is transmitted through the sinusoids, resulting in portal vein distention. If severe cirrhosis is present, the sinusoids may not transmit pressure, and the portal veins will not distend.

Compression of the IVC may be seen in later stages of pregnancy as the enlarged uterus compresses the vena cava. Over time, this compression will produce edema of the ankles and feet and temporary varicose veins. Other forms of caval compression may arise from malignant retroperitoneal tumors, hepatic neoplasm, or pancreatic mass. The presence of thrombus within the vessel should be evaluated, especially in patients with a known renal tumor.

Inferior Vena Cava Tumors, Thrombus, and Filters. Masses that may affect the inferior vena cava are grouped into three categories: (1) hepatic portion, (2) pancreatic portion, and (3) small bowel portion. Understanding the effect such masses have on the displacement or compression of the inferior vena cava may help distinguish the mass's location.

Hepatic Portion of Inferior Vena Cava. Masses posterior to the hepatic portion of the IVC include the right adrenal, neurogenic, and hepatic. With enlargement of the liver, the cava is compressed rather than displaced. A localized liver mass would produce posterior, lateral, or medial displacement of the IVC, whereas a mass in the posterior caudate lobe and right lobe may elevate the cava.

Pancreatic Portion of the Inferior Vena Cava. The middle, or pancreatic, portion of the IVC may elevate the cava from abnormalities of the right renal artery, right kidney, lumbar spine, or lymph node masses.

Small Bowel (Lower) Segment. Lumbar spine abnormalities or lymph nodes would elevate the IVC.

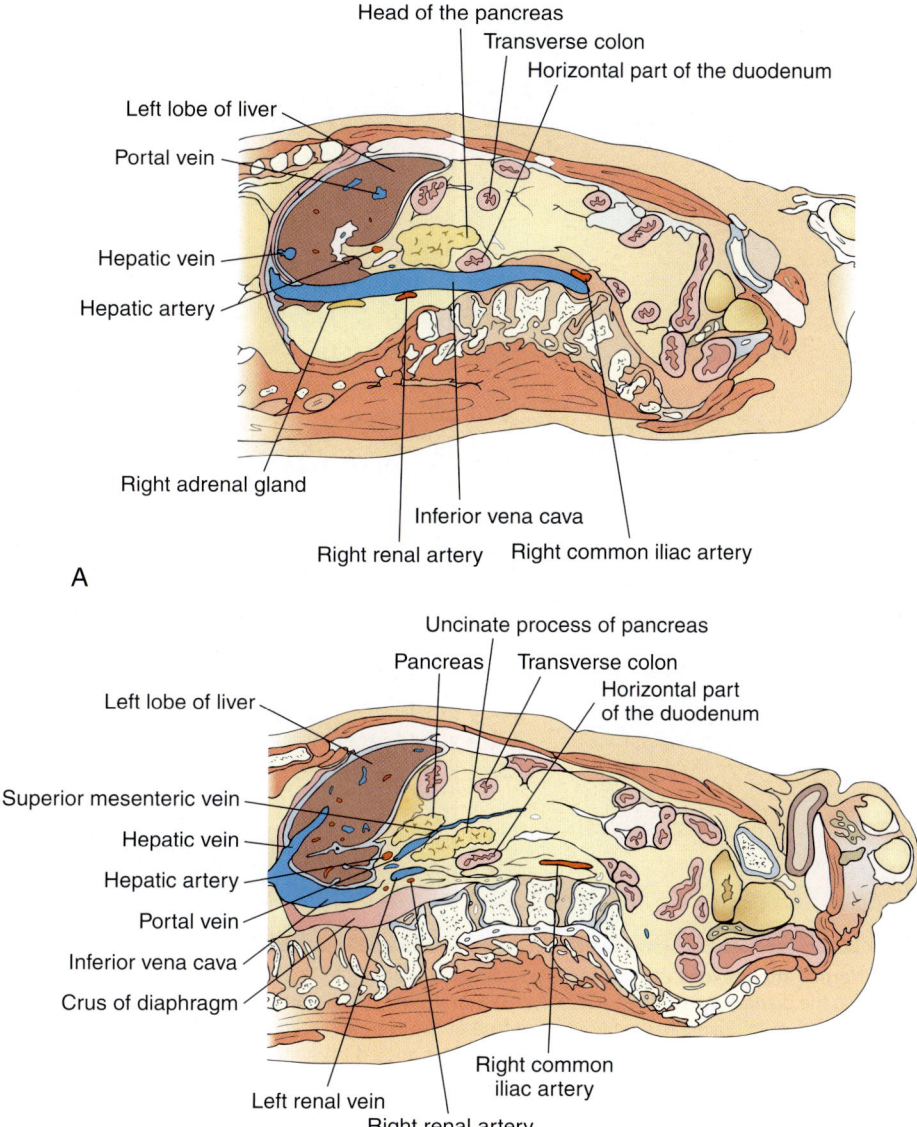

FIG. 8.41 Caudal to the renal vein entrance, the inferior vena cava shows posterior "hammocking" through the bare area of the liver. (A) Sagittal section of the abdomen 3 cm from the midline. (B) Sagittal section of the abdomen 2 cm from the midline.

Sonographic Findings. The IVC may become obstructed by tumor formation (Fig. 8.47). The ultrasound appearance of the tumor consists of single or multiple echogenic nodules along the wall. The cava may be distended and filled with a tumor. The most common tumor is renal cell carcinoma, usually from the right kidney. Wilms' tumor is also seen extending into the IVC and right atrium. Other less common tumors are retroperitoneal liposarcoma, leiomyosarcoma, pheochromocytoma, osteosarcoma, and rhabdomyosarcoma. Benign tumors, such as angiomyolipoma, can have venous involvement.

Inferior Vena Cava Thrombosis. Complete thrombosis of the IVC is life-threatening. Patients present with leg edema, low back pain, pelvic pain, gastrointestinal complaints, and renal and liver abnormalities. Thrombosis within the IVC appears as a homogeneous echo mass (Fig. 8.48). Color Doppler is useful to determine whether the vessel is occluded.

Inferior Vena Cava Filters. The most common origin of pulmonary emboli is venous thrombosis from the lower extremities. Surgical and angiographic placement of transvenous filters into the cava has been used to prevent recurrent embolization in patients who cannot tolerate anticoagulants (Fig. 8.49). The preferred location of the filter is in the iliac bifurcation below the renal veins. The filter is a tubular wire mesh implanted into the IVC to trap small emboli that may cause problems in the heart or the lungs. After placement, some filters can migrate cranially or caudally and perforate the cava, producing a retroperitoneal bleed. Filters can also perforate the duodenum, aorta, ureter, and hepatic vein.

Lateral Tributaries to the Inferior Vena Cava

Renal Veins. Five or six branches of the renal vein unite to form the main renal vein. The right and left main renal veins

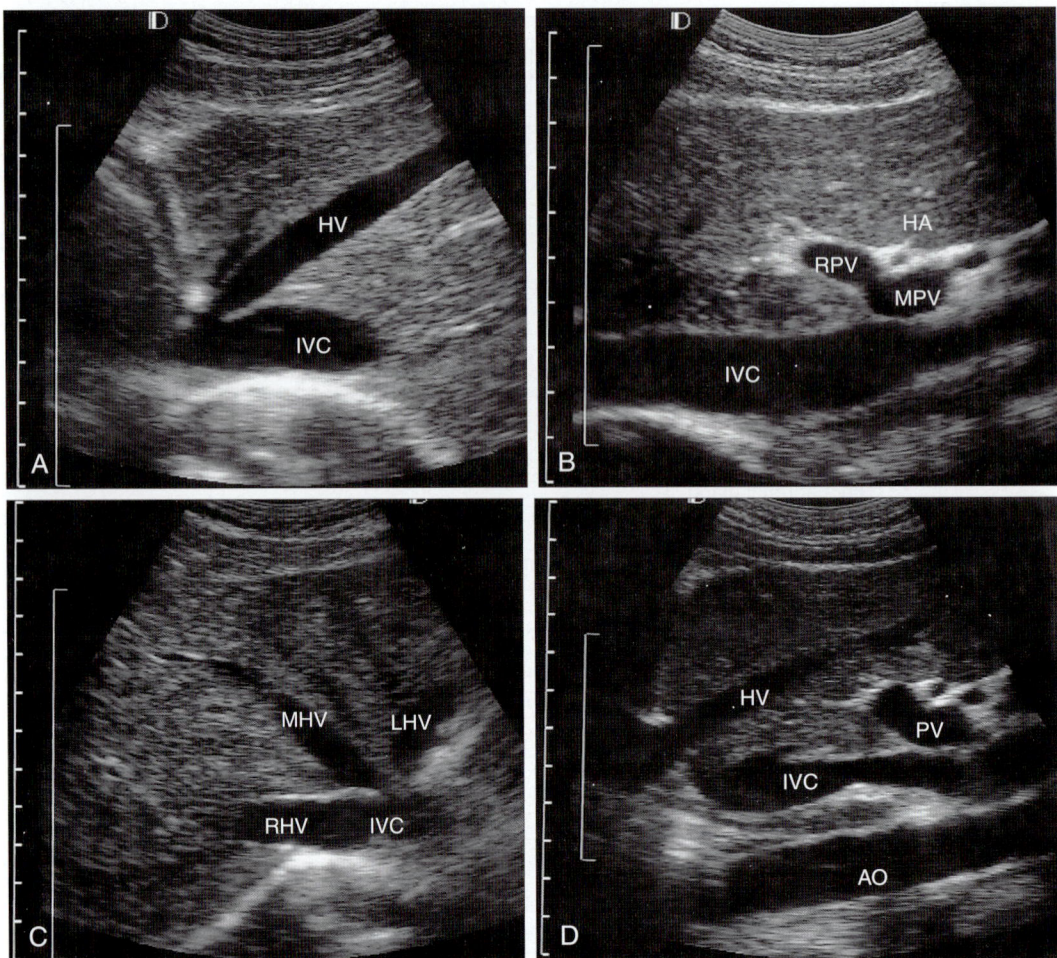

FIG. 8.42 Normal inferior vena cava protocol. Longitudinal images. (A) The hepatic vein (HV) drains into the inferior vena cava (IVC) at the diaphragm. (B) The IVC is the posterior border of the portal vein. (C) Transverse image. The three hepatic veins are shown to drain into the IVC at the dome of the liver. (D) Oblique coronal image. The patient is rolled into a slightly oblique position (right side up). The transducer is angled from the midclavicular line toward the midline of the abdomen to see the IVC "anterior" to the abdominal aorta (AO). *HA,* Hepatic artery; *LHV,* left hepatic vein; *MHV,* middle hepatic vein; *MPV,* main portal vein; *PV,* portal vein; *RHV,* right hepatic vein; *RPV,* right portal vein.

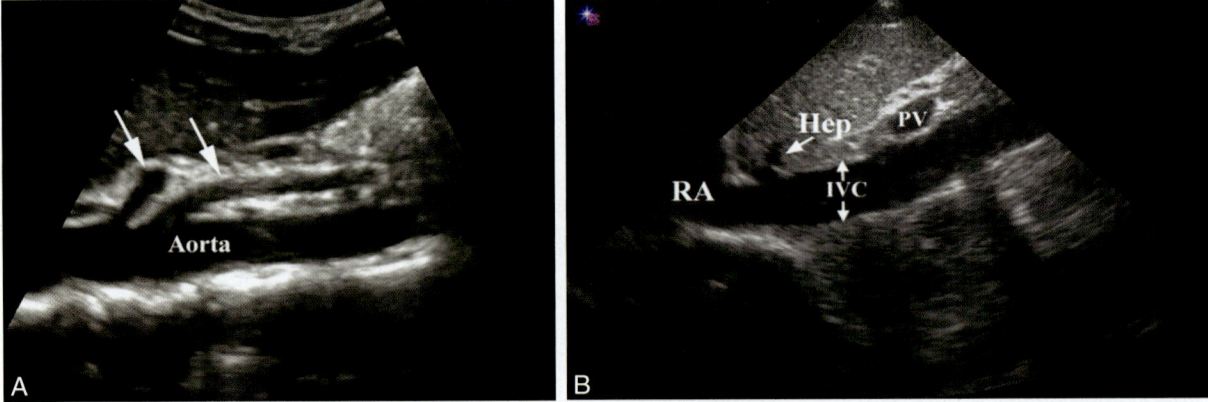

FIG. 8.43 (A) The aorta follows the curvature of the spine, with its distal portion lying more posterior, before bifurcating into the iliac vessels. The aorta has two prominent vessels (celiac trunk and superior mesenteric artery) arising from the anterior wall. (B) The inferior vena cava (IVC) travels in a horizontal course with its proximal portion curving slightly anterior as it pierces the diaphragm to empty into the right atrial (RA) cavity. *Hep,* Hepatic vein; *PV,* portal vein.

arise anterior to the renal arteries at their respective sides of the IVC at the level of L2 (Fig. 8.50).

Left Renal Vein. The **left renal vein** arises medially to exit from the hilus of the kidney. It flows from the left kidney posterior to the superior mesenteric artery and anterior to the aorta to enter the medial wall of the IVC (Fig. 8.51). Above the entry of the renal veins, the IVC enlarges because of the increased volume of blood returning from the kidneys. The left renal vein is larger than the right renal vein. It accepts branches from the left adrenal, left gonadal, and lumbar veins. Best images are

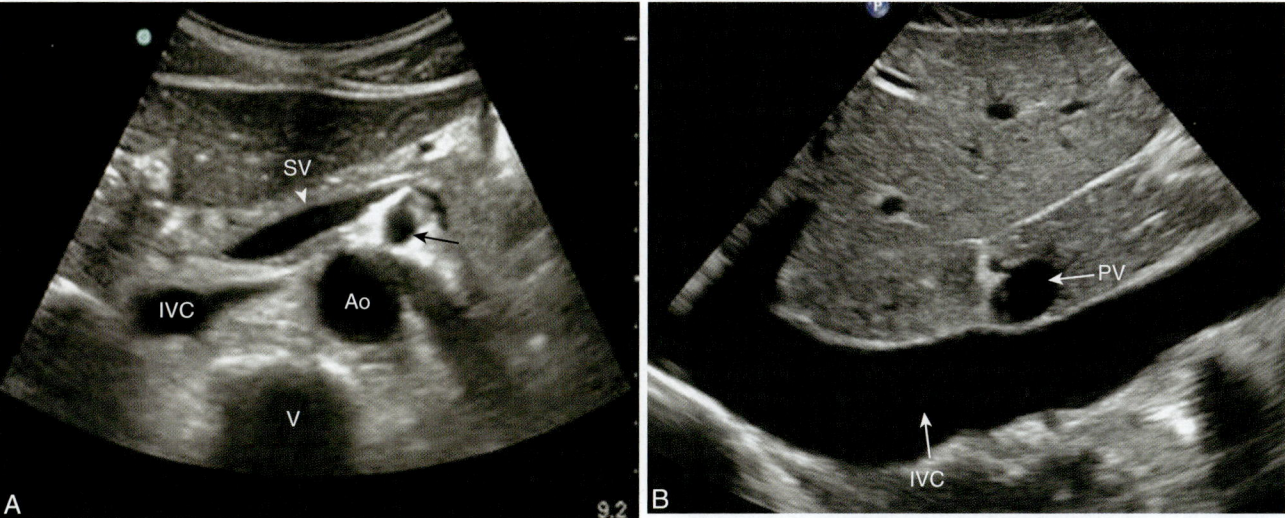

FIG. 8.44 (A) On transverse scans, the almond-shaped inferior vena cava (IVC) serves as a landmark for localizing the splenic vein (SV; *arrowhead*), which is generally found anterior and slightly medial to the cava as it crosses in a horizontal path from the spleen to form the portal vein (PV). *Arrow* denotes the superior mesenteric artery. (B) On longitudinal scans, the IVC serves as a landmark for the PV, located just anterior to the anterior wall of the midpoint of the IVC. *Ao*, Aorta; *V*, vertebral body.

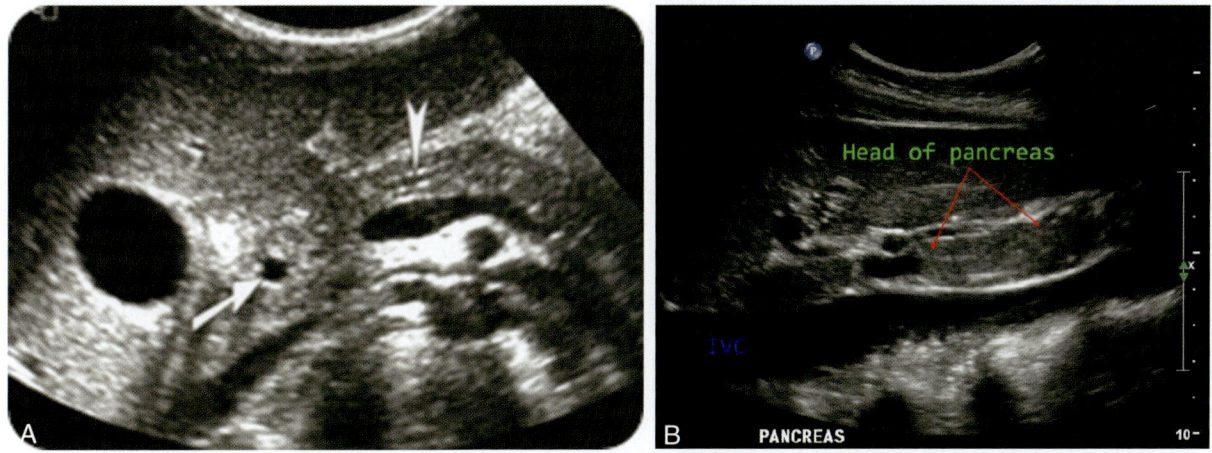

FIG. 8.45 (A) Transverse image. The inferior vena cava is also useful in identifying the echogenic pancreas and small common bile duct *(straight arrow)*. The *arrowhead* marks the pancreatic duct. (B) Longitudinal image. The head of the pancreas is seen just inferior to the portal vein and anterior to the inferior vena cava (IVC) as it makes a slight impression or indentation on the anterior wall of the cava.

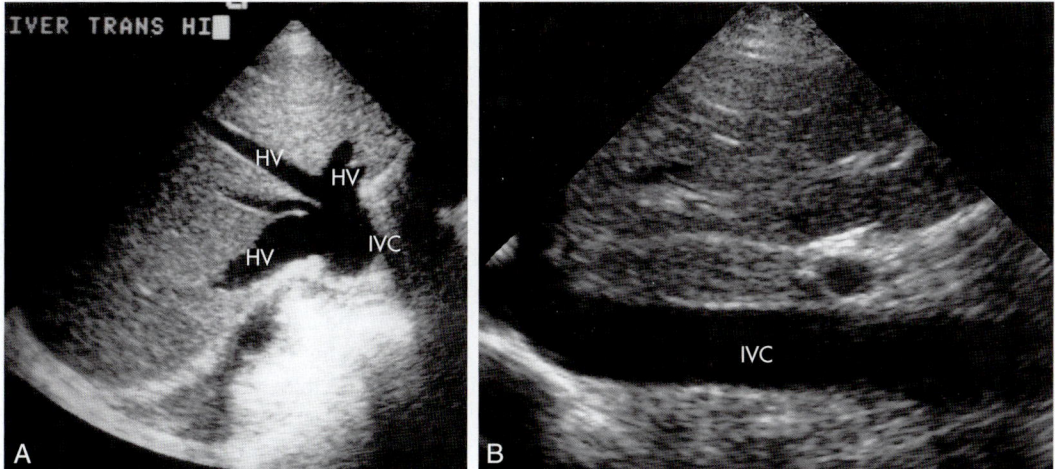

FIG. 8.46 Transverse (A) and sagittal (B) scans of a patient in right ventricular heart failure show a dilated inferior vena cava (IVC) and hepatic veins (HV).

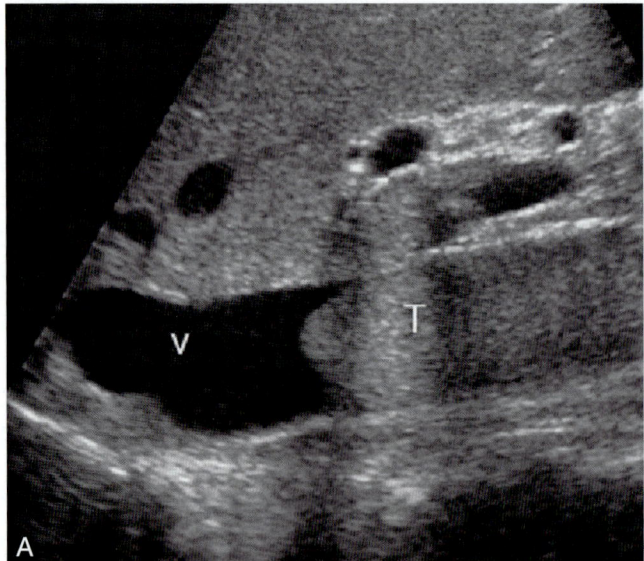

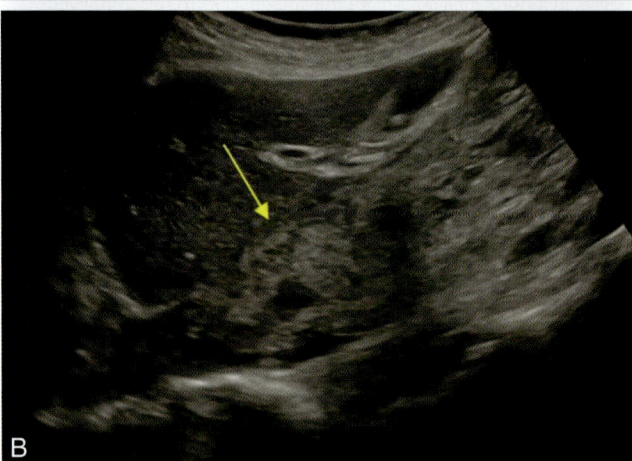

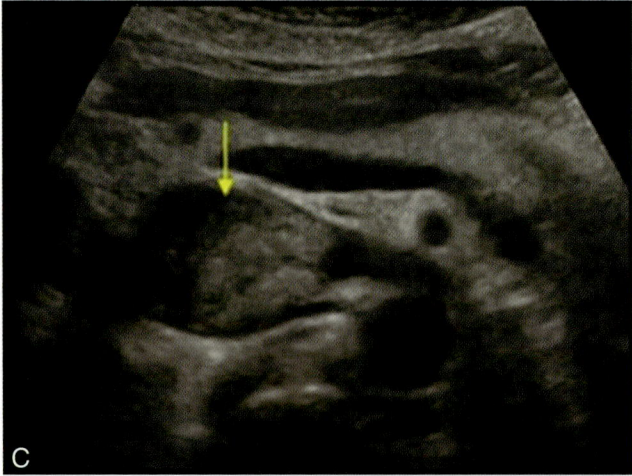

FIG. 8.47 (A) Longitudinal image of the dilated inferior vena cava (V) with a large tumor mass (T). Longitudinal (B) and transverse (C) images of the renal cell carcinoma *(arrows)* invading the inferior vena cava.

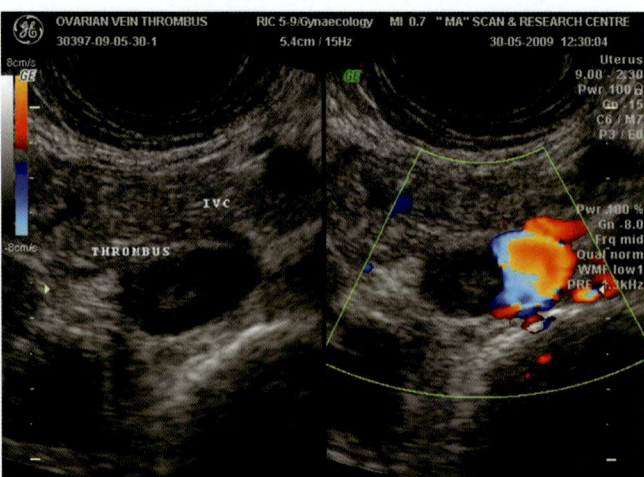

FIG. 8.48 Thrombosis within the inferior vena cava (IVC) appears as a homogeneous echo mass. Color Doppler is useful to determine whether the vessel is completely occluded.

seen on the transverse views as an anechoic tubular structure that originates from the medial hilum of the left kidney. The left renal vein is visualized as a small circular structure coursing between the SMA and the aorta on the longitudinal image.

Right Renal Vein. The **right renal vein** is best seen on transverse images as it flows directly from the hilum of the right kidney into the posterolateral aspect of the IVC (Fig. 8.52). It seldom accepts tributaries; the right adrenal and right gonadal veins enter the IVC directly.

Renal Vein Obstruction. Renal vein obstruction may be seen in the dehydrated or septic infant. It may also be seen in adults with multiple renal abnormalities (nephrotic syndrome, shock, renal tumor, kidney transplant, or trauma). Left renal vein obstruction may result from the spread of such nonrenal malignancies as carcinoma of the pancreas or lung or lymphoma. A retroperitoneal tumor can occlude the left renal vein by direct extension into the vein lumen or compression of the lumen by a contiguous mass.

Clinical Signs. The patient presents with flank pain, hematuria, flank mass, and proteinuria. The condition may be associated with maternal diabetes and transient high blood pressure.

Sonographic Findings. Sonography may be used to confirm that a palpable flank mass is kidney and to exclude hydronephrosis and multicystic kidney as causes of a nonfunctioning kidney. In infants with renal vein obstruction, enlarged kidneys without cysts are seen. Medium echoes or "clumps" of echoes may be randomly scattered within the kidney, with surrounding echo-free spaces. The parenchymal anechoic areas are the result of hemorrhage and infarcts. The renal pattern progresses to atrophy over 2 months. Late findings include increased parenchymal echoes, loss of corticomedullary junction, and decreased renal size.

Renal Vein Thrombosis. Renal vein thrombosis is the formation of a clot in the vein that drains blood from the kidneys, ultimately leading to a reduction in the drainage of one or both kidneys and the possible migration of the clot to other parts of the body (Fig. 8.53). Thrombosis most commonly affects newborns with blood clotting abnormalities or dehydration and adults with nephrotic syndrome.

If the following findings are present on sonography, renal vein thrombosis may be diagnosed:
1. Direct visualization of thrombi in the renal vein and IVC
2. Demonstrated renal vein dilation proximal to the point of occlusion
3. Loss of normal renal structure

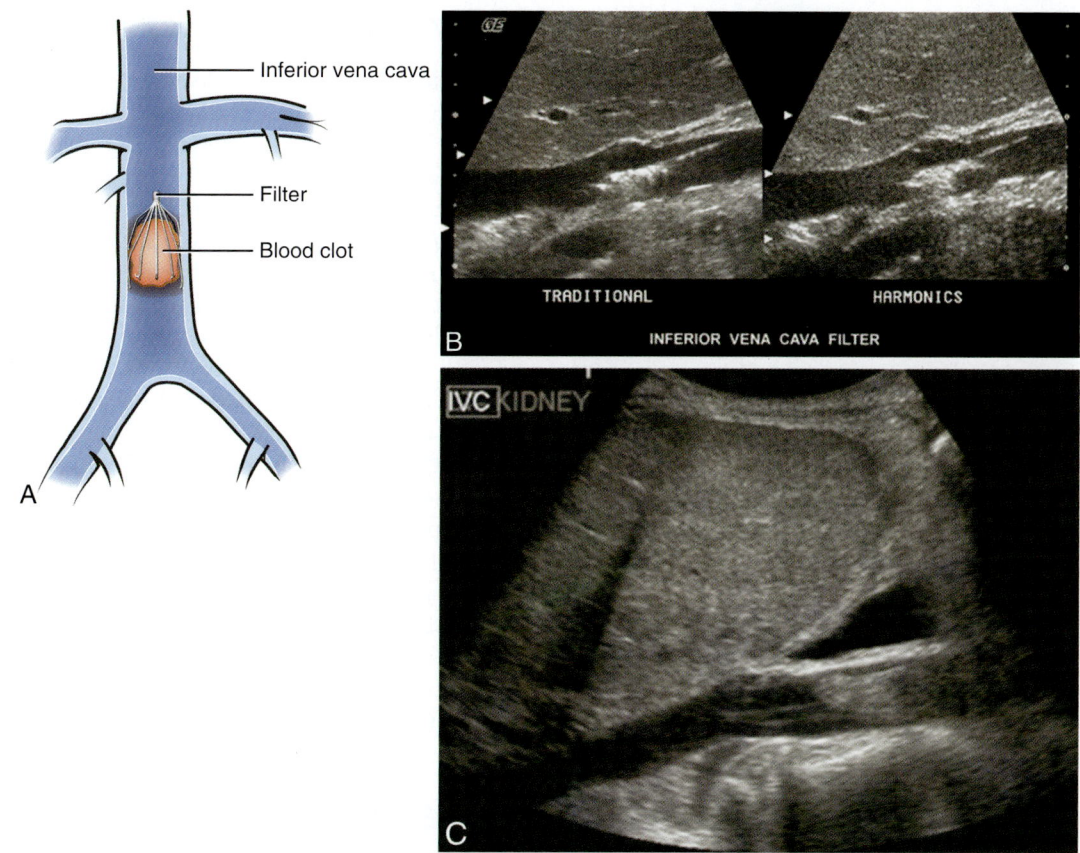

FIG. 8.49 (A–C) The inferior vena cava filter is a tubular wire mesh *(arrow)* that is implanted into the inferior vena cava to trap small emboli that may cause problems in the heart or the lungs.

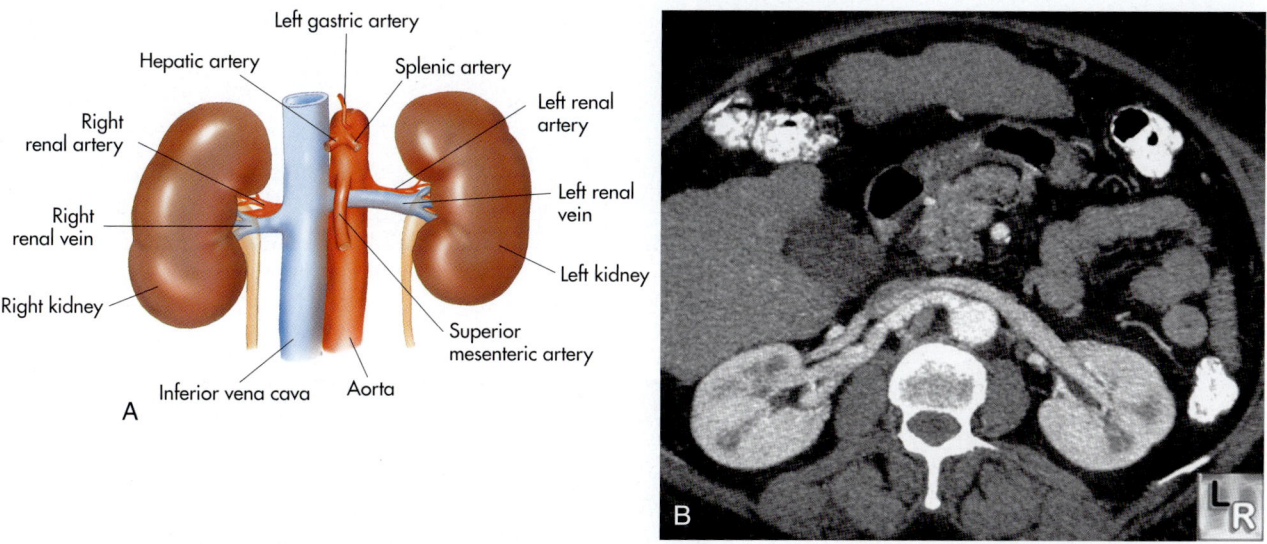

FIG. 8.50 (A) The right and left main renal veins arise anterior to the renal arteries at their respective sides of the inferior vena cava at the level of L2. (B) Transverse computed tomography of the left renal vein arising from the hilum of the kidney, crossing anterior to the aorta to enter the inferior vena cava. The right renal artery may be seen to leave the medial wall of the aorta, posterior to the left renal vein, into the right renal hilum.

4. Increased renal size (acute phase)
5. Decreased flow or no flow shown on Doppler

Clinical Signs. The patient presents with pain, nephromegaly, hematuria, or thromboembolic phenomena elsewhere in the body. A variety of lesions may be associated with this abnormality.

Gonadal Veins. The gonadal veins (testicular and ovarian) course anterior to the external and internal iliac veins and continue cranially and retroperitoneally along the psoas muscle until their terminus. The left gonadal vein usually enters the left renal vein or the left adrenal vein, which empties into

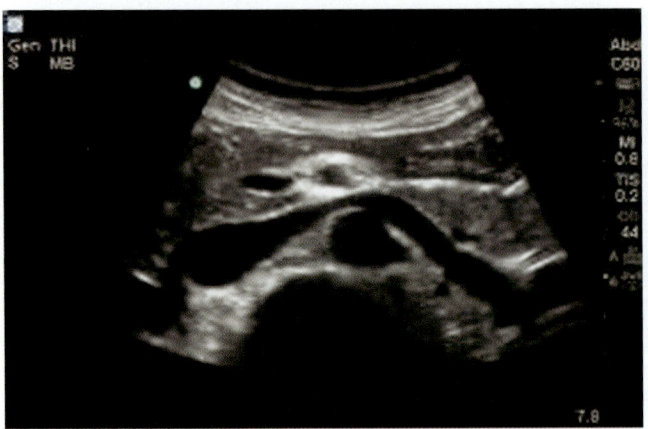

FIG. 8.51 The left renal vein is well seen as it leaves the renal hilus and flows anterior to the aorta and posterior to the superior mesenteric artery to enter the lateral wall of the inferior vena cava.

the IVC. The right gonadal vein enters the IVC on the anterolateral border above the entrance of the lumbar veins.

Suprarenal Veins. The right suprarenal vein arises from the suprarenal gland and usually drains directly into the IVC. The left arises from the suprarenal gland and drains into the left renal vein.

Anterior Tributaries to the Inferior Vena Cava

Hepatic Veins. The hepatic veins are the largest visceral tributaries of the IVC. They originate between the segments of the liver and drain posteriorly into the IVC at the level of the diaphragm (Fig. 8.54). The hepatic veins return unoxygenated blood from the liver. The veins collect blood from the three minor tributaries within the liver: the right hepatic vein drains the right lobe of the liver, the middle hepatic vein drains the caudate lobe, and the left hepatic vein drains the left lobe of the liver. The middle and left hepatic veins may fuse before emptying into the IVC.

Sonographic Findings. The hepatic veins are best visualized on longitudinal scans of the liver as they drain into the IVC at the level of the diaphragm (Fig. 8.55). Transverse scans obtained with a cephalic angle of the transducer at the level of the xiphoid often show at least two of the three veins draining into the IVC (Fig. 8.56). The hepatic veins resemble the "bunny" or "reindeer" sign on the sonogram.

Distinguishing hepatic veins from portal veins requires recognition of their anatomic patterns. (Fig. 8.57) Hepatic veins drain cephalad toward the diaphragm and then dorsomedial toward the IVC. Hepatic veins increase in caliber as they approach the

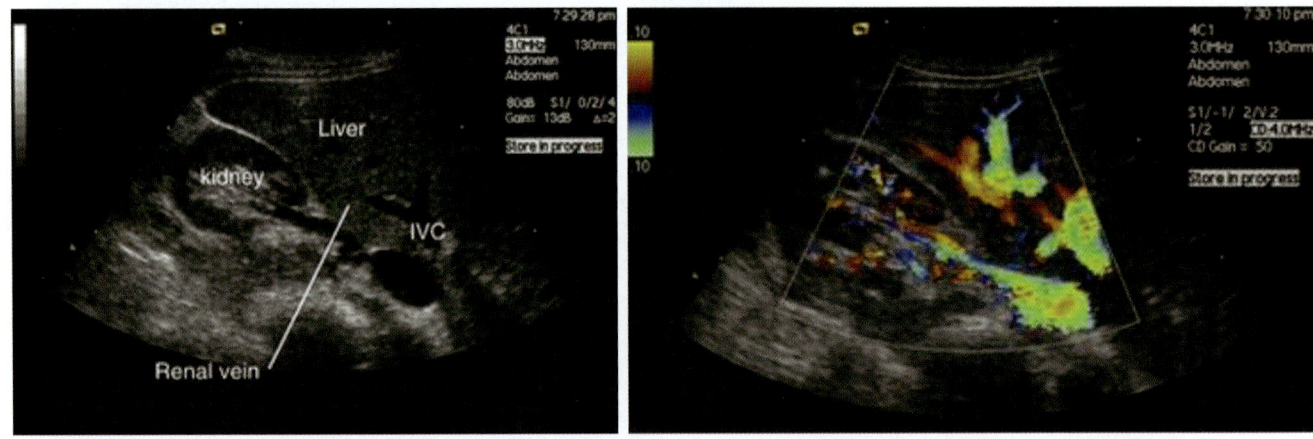

FIG. 8.52 The right renal vein is best seen on transverse images as it flows directly from the hilum of the right kidney into the posterolateral aspect of the inferior vena cava.

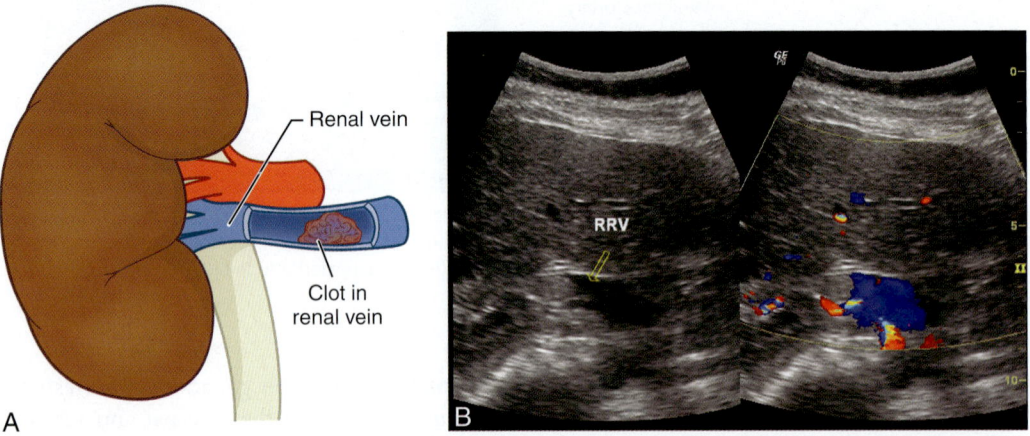

FIG. 8.53 (A) Renal vein thrombosis is the formation of a clot in the vein that drains blood from the kidneys, ultimately leading to a reduction in the drainage of one or both kidneys and the possible migration of the clot to other parts of the body. (B) Transverse images of the right renal vein (RRV) with thrombus. Note the restriction of color flow secondary to the thrombus formation.

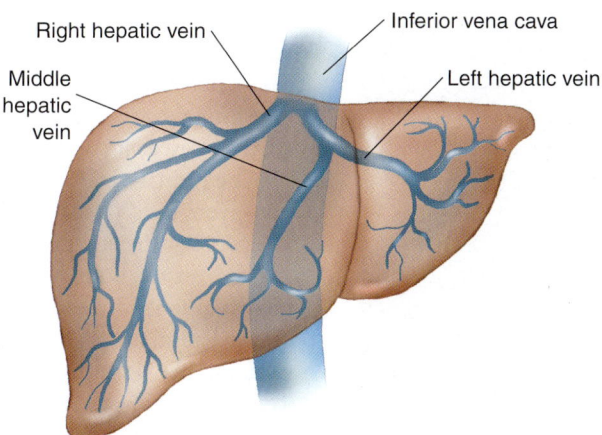

FIG. 8.54 The hepatic veins are divided into three components: right, middle, and left. They all drain into the inferior vena cava at the level of the diaphragm.

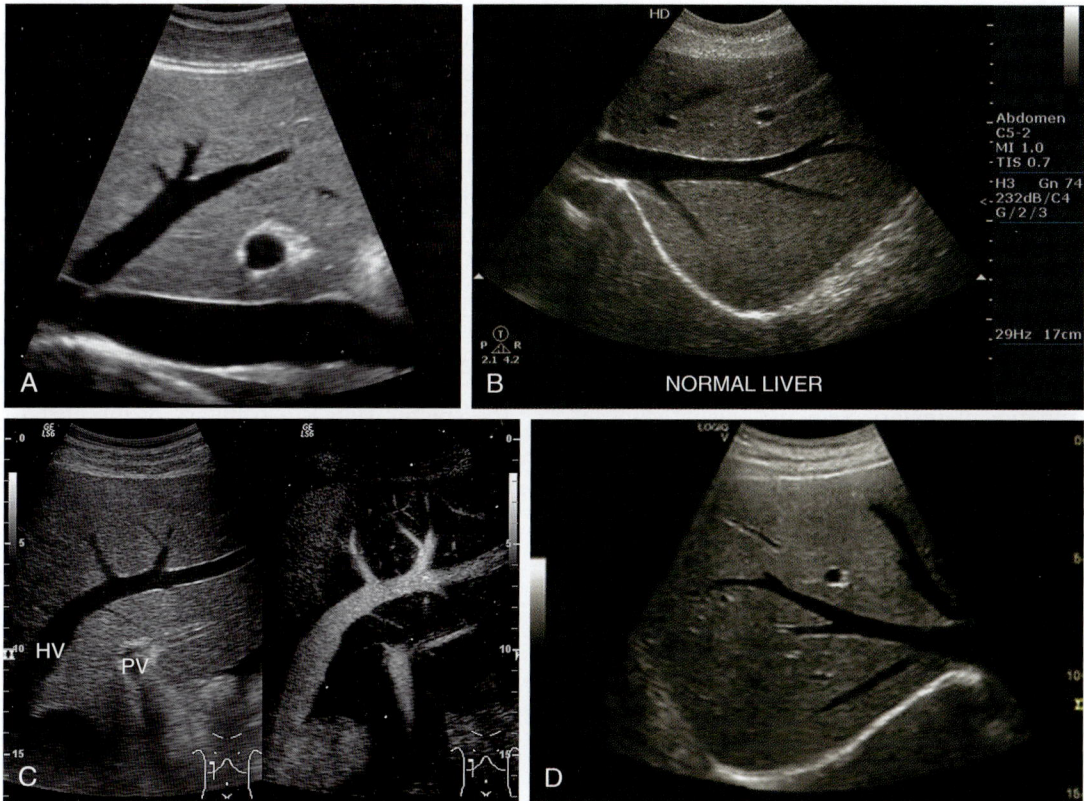

FIG. 8.55 (A–C) Longitudinal image of the hepatic vein draining into the inferior vena cava at the level of the diaphragm. (D) Transverse images of the right, middle, and left hepatic veins. *HV*, Hepatic vein; *PV*, portal vein.

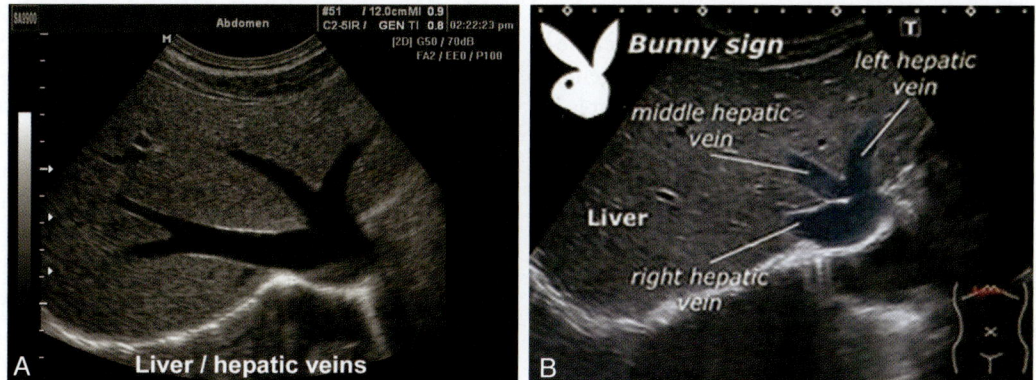

FIG. 8.56 (A) Transverse scans obtained with a cephalic angle of the transducer at the level of the xiphoid often show at least two of the three veins draining into the inferior vena cava. (B) The hepatic veins resemble the "bunny" or "reindeer" sign on the sonogram.

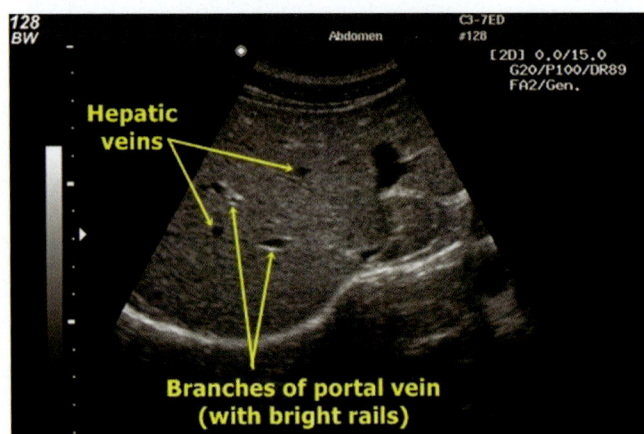

FIG. 8.57 Hepatic veins drain cephalad toward the diaphragm and then dorsomedial toward the inferior vena cava. Hepatic veins increase in caliber as they approach the diaphragm. Unlike portal veins, they are not surrounded by bright acoustic reflections, although a slight amount of acoustic enhancement may be seen along their posterior border.

diaphragm. Unlike portal veins, they are not surrounded by bright acoustic reflections, although a slight amount of acoustic enhancement may be seen along their posterior border.

PORTAL VENOUS SYSTEM

Portal Vein

The **portal vein** is formed posterior to the pancreas by the union of the superior mesenteric vein and splenic veins at the level of L2. Its trunk is 5 to 7 cm in length (Fig. 8.58). The portal vein courses posterior to the first portion of the duodenum and then between the layers of the lesser omentum to the porta hepatis, where it bifurcates into its hepatic branches. It carries blood from the intestinal tract to the liver by means of its two main branches: the right and left portal veins. It drains blood from the gastrointestinal tract, from the lower end of the esophagus to the upper end of the anal canal, and from the pancreas, gallbladder, bile ducts, and spleen. The portal vein has an **anastomosis** with the esophageal veins, rectal venous plexus, and superficial abdominal veins. The portal venous blood traverses the liver and drains into the IVC via the hepatic veins.

The liver receives a dual blood supply from the portal vein and the hepatic artery. The portal vein supplies up to one-half of the oxygen requirements of the hepatocytes because of its great flow, even though it carries incompletely oxygenated (less than 80%) venous blood from the intestines and spleen.

The portal triad contains branches of the portal vein, hepatic artery, and bile duct within a connective tissue sheath that gives the portal vein an echogenic wall, as seen on liver sonographic images.

Sonographic Findings. The portal vein is clearly seen on both transverse and sagittal scans. On transverse scans, it is often possible to record the splenic vein as it crosses the midline of the abdomen to join the superior mesenteric vein to form the main portal trunk. Portal veins become smaller as they progress into the liver from the porta hepatis. Large radicles situated near or approaching the porta hepatis are portal veins, not hepatic veins. The portal veins are characterized by high-amplitude acoustic reflections that presumably arise from the fibrous tissues surrounding the portal triad as it courses through the liver substance.

The right and left portal veins course transversely through the liver; thus transverse scans display their longest extent (Fig. 8.59). The right portal vein is most consistently demonstrated on the sonogram. Anatomically, any intraparenchymal segment of the portal venous system lying to the right of the lateral aspect of the IVC is a branch of the right portal system. The right portal vein has an anterior branch that lies centrally within the anterior segment of the right lobe and a posterior branch that lies centrally within the posterior segment of the right lobe.

The left portal vein has a narrow-caliber trunk and may be seen coursing transversely through the left hepatic lobe from a posterior to an anterior position. The main portal vein is well seen as a circular anechoic structure to the IVC. The portal radicle may have many different variations; therefore it is important to become familiar with their patterns to distinguish them from dilated biliary radicles.

On sagittal images, the portal vein is seen anterior to the inferior vena cava (Fig. 8.60). The main portal vein serves as a landmark to image the head of the pancreas, common bile duct, and hepatic artery.

Splenic Vein

The **splenic vein** is a tributary of the portal circulation. It begins at the hilum of the spleen, where it is formed by the union of several veins. It is subsequently joined by the short gastric and left gastroepiploic veins (see Fig. 8.58). The splenic vein runs along the posteromedial border of the pancreas. It joins the superior mesenteric vein posterior to the neck of the pancreas to form the portal vein. Additional veins from the pancreas and inferior mesenteric vein drain into the splenic vein. The splenic vein drains blood from the stomach, spleen, and pancreas.

Sonographic Findings. The splenic vein is best visualized in the transverse plane as it crosses the upper abdomen from the hilum of the spleen to join the superior mesenteric vein to form the portal vein slightly to the right of midline (Fig. 8.61). The splenic vein crosses anteriorly to the aorta and the IVC and generally relates to the medial and posterior borders of the pancreatic body and tail. Its course is variable, so small degrees of obliquity with the transducer may be necessary to image the vein entirely. It is usually smaller than the superior mesenteric vein and the main portal vein. (The larger diameter of the portal vein is the result of the influx of blood from the superior mesenteric vein.) An obvious widening is demonstrated at the junction of the portal and splenic veins.

On sagittal scans, the splenic vein can be visualized posterior to the left lobe of the liver and anterior to the major vascular structures. The pancreas may be seen inferior and slightly anterior to the vein (see Fig. 8.61A). When splenomegaly is present, it is often possible to identify the origin of the splenic vein at the splenic hilum.

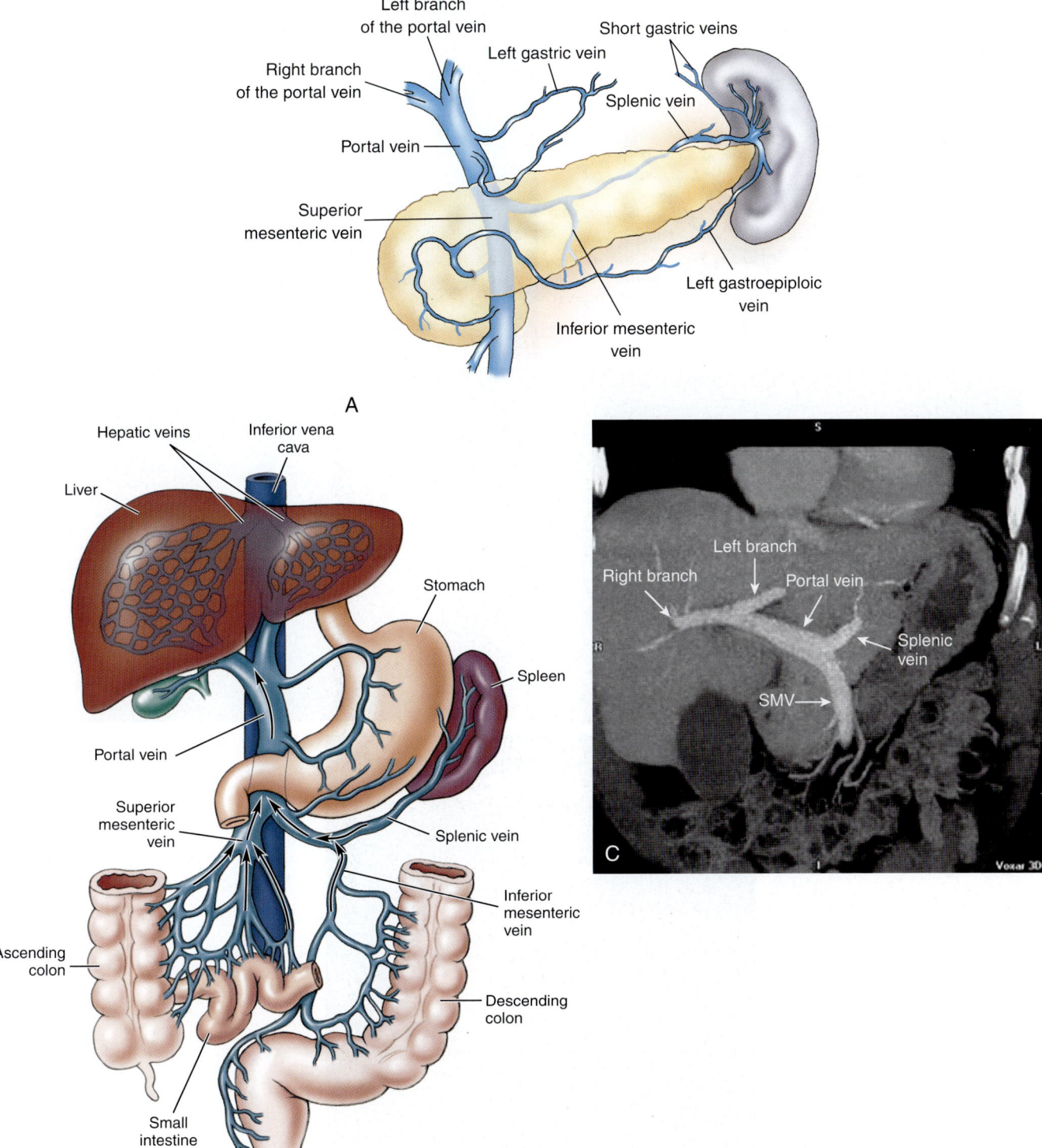

FIG. 8.58 (A) The superior and inferior mesenteric veins join the splenic vein to form the portal vein. (B) The portal vein is formed posterior to the pancreas by the union of the superior mesenteric vein (SMV) and splenic veins at the level of L2. (C) Computed tomographic contrast image of the portal system.

Superior Mesenteric Vein

The **superior mesenteric vein** is also a tributary to the portal vein (see Fig. 8.58). It begins at the ileocolic junction and runs cephalad along the posterior abdominal wall within the root of the mesentery of the small intestine to the right of the superior mesenteric artery. The superior mesenteric vein passes anterior to the third part of the duodenum and posterior to the neck of the pancreas, where it joins the splenic vein to form the main portal vein. It also receives tributaries

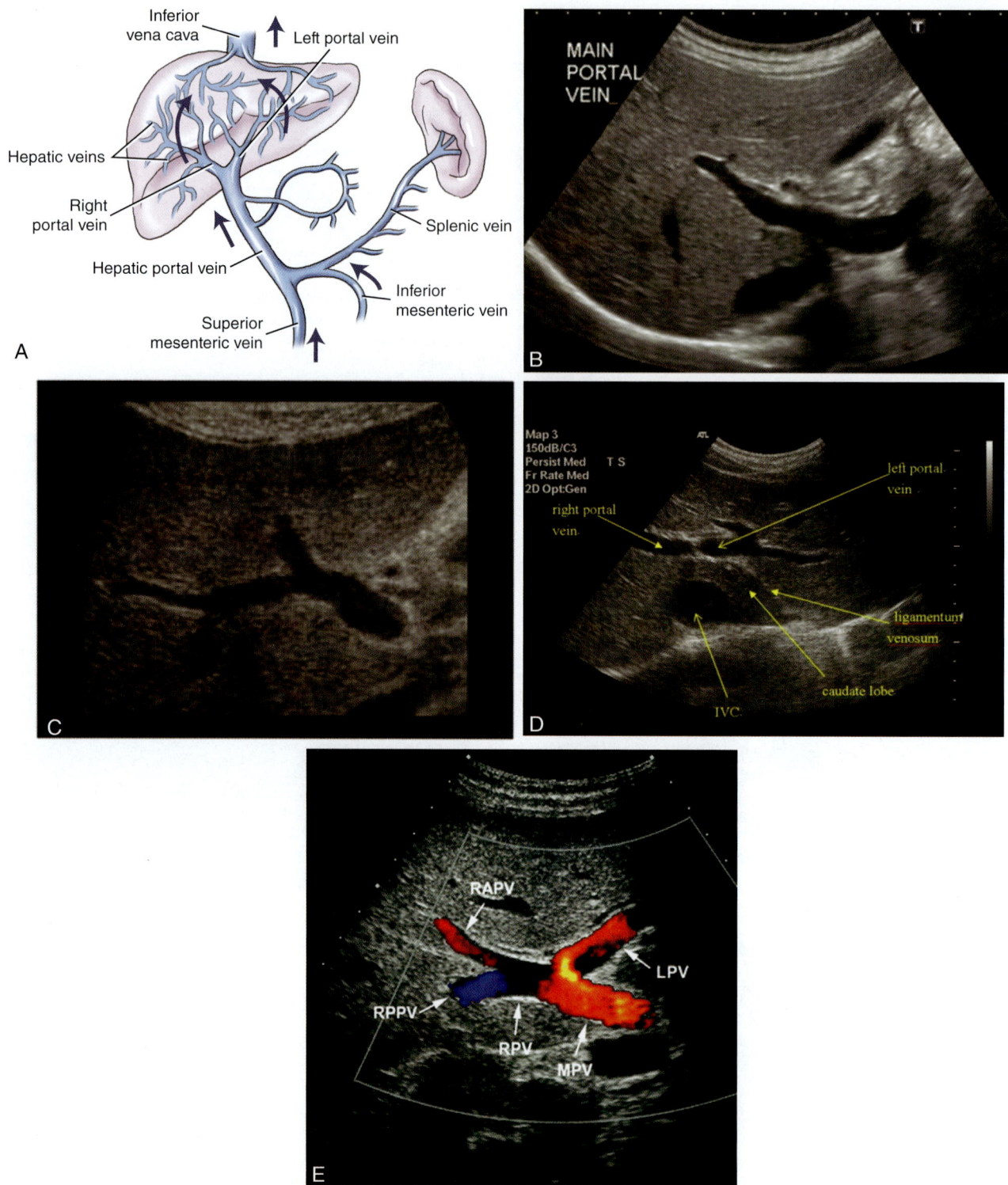

FIG. 8.59 (A–E) The right and left portal veins course transversely through the liver; thus transverse scans display their longest extent. *IVC*, Inferior vena cava; *LPV*, left portal vein; *MPV*, main portal vein; *RAPV*, right anterior portal vein; *RPV*, right portal vein; *RPPV*, right posterior portal vein.

that correspond to the branches of the superior mesenteric artery, where it is joined by the inferior pancreaticoduodenal vein to the right gastroepiploic vein from the right aspect of the greater curvature of the stomach. The superior mesenteric vein drains blood from several smaller veins: the middle colic vein (transverse colon), the right colic vein (ascending colon), and the pancreatic duodenal vein.

Sonographic Findings. The superior mesenteric vein is somewhat variable in its anatomic location. Generally, it is anterior to the IVC and to the right of the superior mesenteric

CHAPTER 8 Vascular System

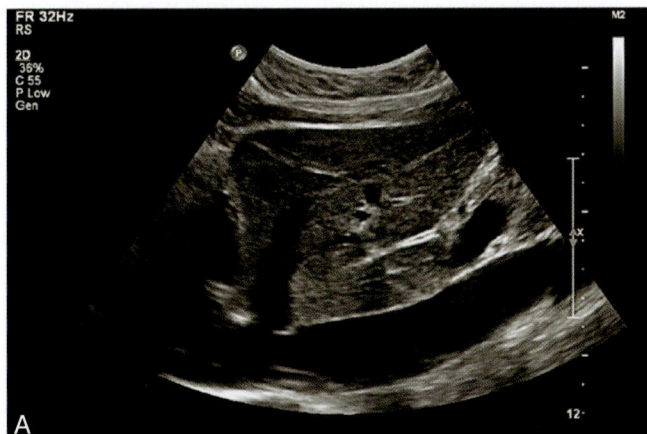

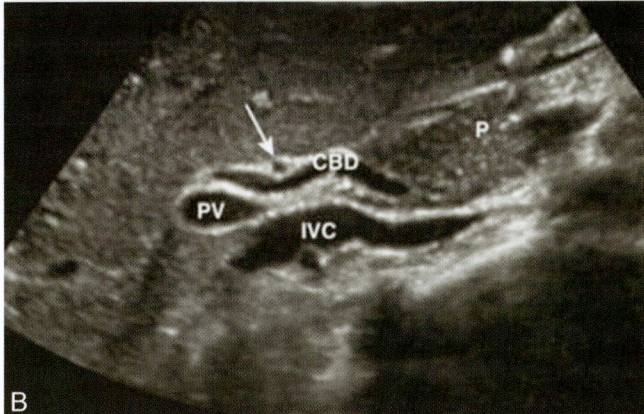

FIG. 8.60 (A) The portal vein *(arrow)* is seen anterior to the inferior vena cava (IVC) on sagittal images. (B) The main portal vein (PV) serves as a landmark to image the head of the pancreas (P), common bile duct (CBD), and hepatic artery *(arrow)*.

artery. The superior mesenteric vein drains into the main portal vein (along with the splenic vein); therefore the sonographer should not be able to demonstrate these three structures together on a single transverse scan (Fig. 8.62). The superior mesenteric vein is the posterior border of the neck of the pancreas and the anterior border of the uncinate process of the pancreatic head.

On sagittal scans, the vein is seen as a long, tubular structure anterior to the IVC. With correct oblique angulation of the transducer, the path of the superior mesenteric vein can be followed as it enters the portal system.

The following points help to distinguish the superior mesenteric artery from the vein:
- The superior mesenteric vein is of larger caliber than the artery.
- Real-time identification of the confluence of the superior mesenteric vein–portal vein or superior mesenteric artery is possible as the superior mesenteric artery originates directly from the anterior wall of the abdominal aorta.

Inferior Mesenteric Vein

The **inferior mesenteric vein** drains the left third of the colon and upper colon and ascends retroperitoneally along the left psoas muscle. It begins midway down the anal canal as the superior rectal vein (see Fig. 8.58). It runs cranially in the posterior abdominal wall on the left side of the inferior mesenteric artery and duodenojejunal junction to join the splenic vein posterior to the pancreas. It receives many tributaries along its way, including the left colic vein. The inferior mesenteric vein drains several tributaries: the left colic vein (descending colon), the sigmoid vein (sigmoid colon), and the superior rectal vein (upper rectum).

Sonographic Findings. The inferior mesenteric vein is difficult to recognize on ultrasound because of its anatomic location and small diameter. It is generally covered by the small bowel and has no major vascular structures posterior to it to aid in its recognition.

ABDOMINAL DOPPLER TECHNIQUES

Doppler ultrasound is a useful clinical tool for diagnosing normal and abnormal flow velocities. The following paragraphs present an overview of abdominal applications that have been used with color flow detection and spectral pulsed Doppler techniques. Doppler has helped detect the presence or absence of blood flow, the direction of blood flow, and flow disturbance patterns. It has also been used in tissue characterization and waveform analysis.

Blood Flow Analysis

Presence or Absence of Flow. Doppler ultrasound frequently is used to differentiate vessels from nonvascular structures. For example, to distinguish the common bile duct from the hepatic artery, look for absence of flow in the common duct; to distinguish the hepatic artery from the splenic artery, look for direction of flow; to differentiate an aneurysm from a pancreatic pseudocyst, look for slow flow in the aneurysm; to differentiate dilated intrahepatic bile ducts and prominent hepatic artery, again look for absence of flow in the bile duct.

Direction of Flow. In patients who develop **portal venous hypertension**, the portal blood flow becomes **hepatofugal** (away from the liver) instead of **hepatopetal** (toward the liver). This may occur secondary to portal venous shunts or varices. The sonographer detects a high-velocity flow pattern at the site of the shunt with a turbulent flow pattern on color Doppler.

Disturbance of Flow. A flow disturbance (increased velocity or obstruction of flow) may result from the formation of an atheroma, arteriovenous fistula, pseudoaneurysm, or aneurysmal dilation.

Tissue Characterization. Research is currently underway in the area of tissue characterization. Doppler is thought to be capable of characterizing tissue because of the specific perfusion patterns characteristic of some tissues or states of tissue activity. Hepatocellular carcinomas of the liver appear to have a specific pattern. Pseudoaneurysms of peripancreatic arteries have turbulent flow patterns. Pancreatic tumors may have specific flow patterns.

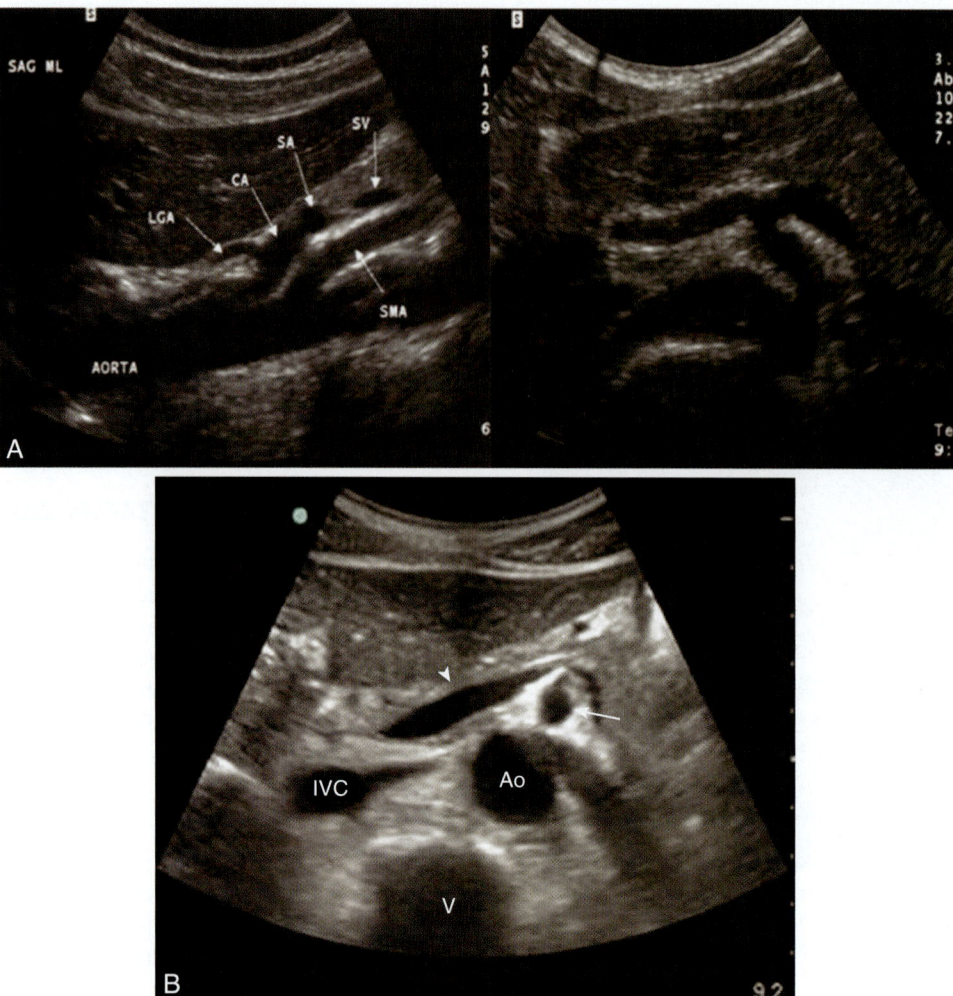

FIG. 8.61 (A) Longitudinal *(left)* and transverse *(right)* images of the splenic vein. (B) The splenic vein *(arrowhead)* is best visualized in the transverse plane as it crosses the upper abdomen from the hilum of the spleen to join the superior mesenteric vein to form the portal vein slightly to the right of midline. *Arrow* denotes the superior mesenteric artery. *Ao,* Aorta; *IVC,* inferior vena cava.

Doppler Waveform Analysis. The shape of the waveform provides information on the vascular impedance of the organ the vessel supplies. Spectral analysis tells the velocity and turbulence of blood flow.

Nonresistive Versus Resistive Vessels. **Nonresistive** vessels have a high diastolic component and supply organs that need constant perfusion, such as the internal carotid artery, the hepatic artery, and the renal artery. **Resistive** vessels have very little or even reversed flow in diastole and supply organs that do not need a constant blood supply, such as the external carotid and the iliac and brachial arteries.

Peak systole is compared with minimum diastole to quantify a vessel's impedance. This ratio is the **resistive index**.

The Spectral Doppler display shows us the following:

- x = Time is depicted on the horizontal axis.
- y = Doppler shift frequency (velocity) is on the vertical axis (flow toward the transducer equals positive shift, or above baseline; flow away from the transducer equals negative shift, or below baseline).
- z = Gray scale indicates the quantity of blood flowing at a given velocity. More red blood cells produce a brighter gray-scale assignment.

Plug flow is a pattern of blood flow, typically seen in large arteries, in which most cells are moving at the same velocity across the entire diameter of the vessel. In other vessels, the different velocities are the result of friction between the cells and arterial walls. A "clear window" under systole is typical of plug flow. When plug flow is present, the volume of blood flow can be calculated.

Doppler Technique

Unlike visualization of the heart, in which high-velocity flows are present, visualization of abdominal vessels requires very sensitive Doppler instrumentation. Abdominal vessels generally have low velocity and flow. This segment provides a brief overview of Doppler techniques the beginning student should become familiar with.

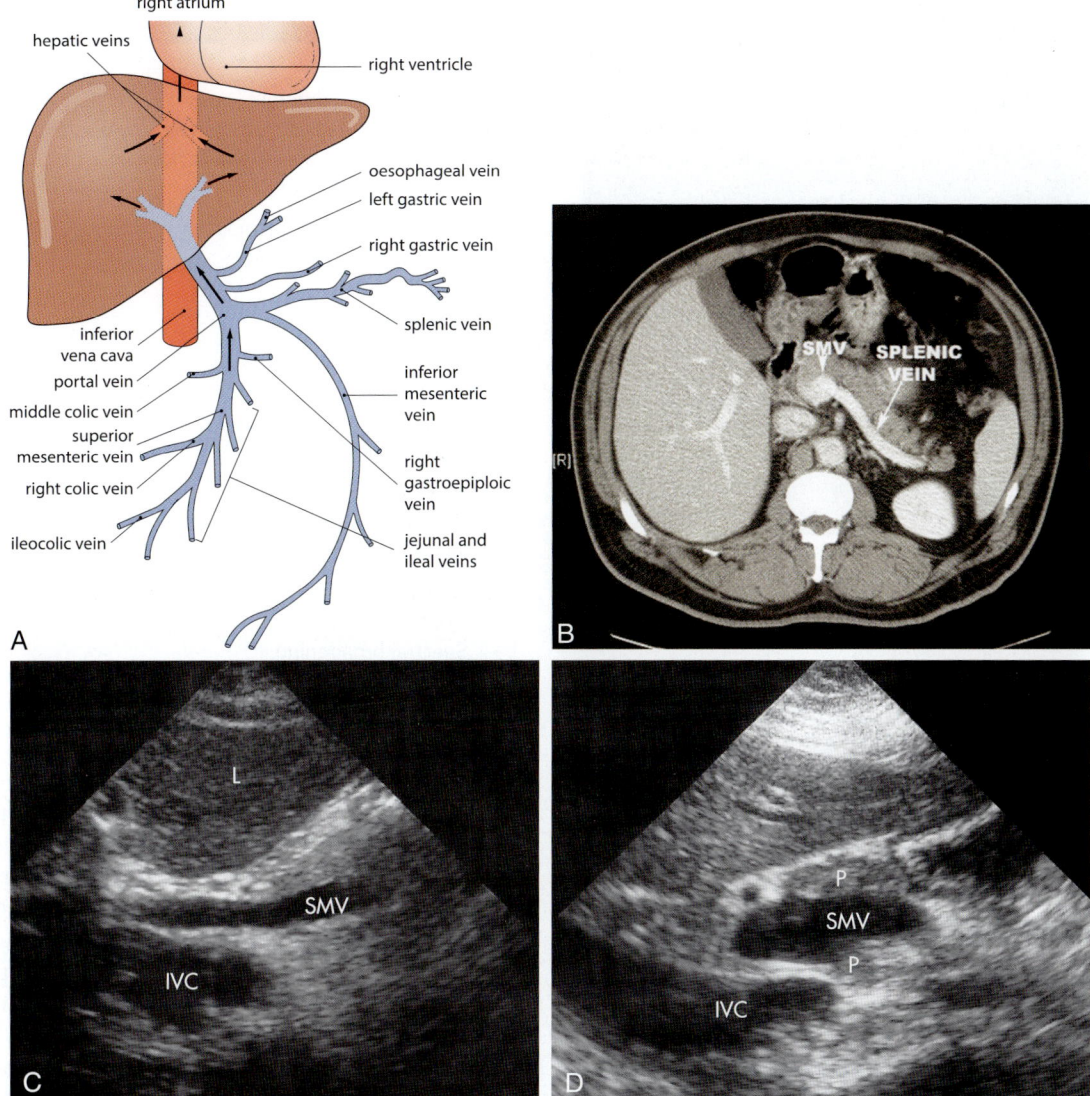

FIG. 8.62 (A) The superior mesenteric vein (SMV) drains into the main portal vein (along with the splenic vein); therefore the sonographer should not be able to demonstrate these three structures together on a single transverse scan. The superior mesenteric vein is the posterior border of the neck of the pancreas and the anterior border of the uncinate process of the pancreatic head. (B) Computed tomographic image of the splenic vein as it joins the SMV. (C–D) Sagittal images of the SMV as it lies anterior to the uncinate process of the pancreas (P) and posterior to the body. *IVC,* Inferior vena cava; *L,* liver.

Methods. Doppler is performed as part of the routine real-time examination. The patient should be fasting and should suspend respirations for the best color and pulsed **Doppler sample volume**. The Doppler sample volume (sometimes referred to as the Doppler "gate") should be adjusted to encompass but not exceed the diameter of the vessel. If the sample volume exceeds the diameter, noise and ghost echoes may appear (Fig. 8.63A). This occurs because a too wide Doppler gate causes interference from surrounding vessels and structures.

The sonographer has the ability to control the velocity of the returning echoes to prevent the alias pattern by using a lower-frequency transducer or changing from pulsed wave to continuous wave. Another feature of Doppler is that the beam records only accurate velocity patterns when the beam is parallel to the flow (the angle of flow can be changed up to 60 degrees and still be accurate). The more perpendicular the beam is to the flow, the less signal is recorded; it falls to zero velocity when the beam is directly perpendicular to the flow (see Fig. 8.63B). Thus Doppler causes the sonographer to be creative in attempting to record accurate velocity flow patterns. The patient must be rolled into various obliquities with different angulations of the transducer to be parallel to many vascular structures.

Color Doppler is a relatively new and exciting modality that makes it easier to localize and identify smaller vessels from the biliary tree, lymphadenopathy, or other pathology. Colors are arbitrarily assigned on all equipment and refer to the direction of flow. If red is assigned as a positive flow signal, all flow toward the transducer is coded in various shades of red, depending on returning velocity. If blue is assigned a negative flow signal, the flow away from the transducer is

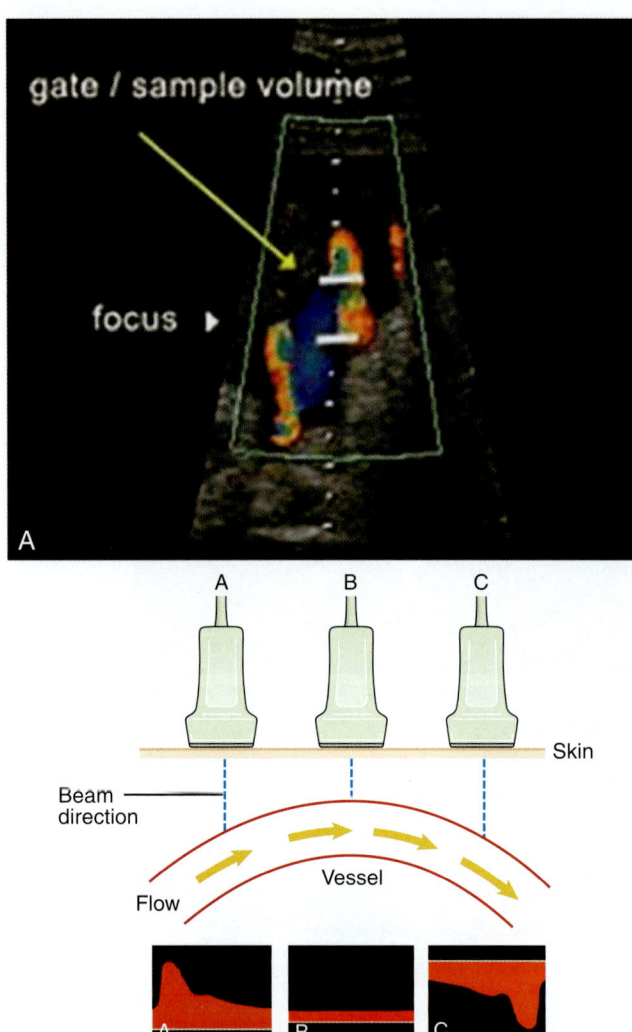

FIG. 8.63 (A) Doppler sample volume (sometimes referred to as the Doppler "gate") should be adjusted to encompass but not exceed the diameter of the vessel. If the sample volume exceeds the diameter, noise and ghost echoes may appear. (B) The Doppler records accurate velocity patterns when the beam is parallel to the flow (the angle of flow can be changed up to 60 degrees and still be accurate). The more perpendicular the beam is to the flow, the less signal is recorded; it falls to zero velocity when the beam is directly perpendicular to the flow.

| BOX 8.5 | Doppler Flow Patterns in Abdominal Arteries |

Aorta
- Flow varies at different levels
- Proximal aorta has high systolic/low diastolic flow
- Distal demonstrates triphasic flow

Celiac Axis
- Some spectral broadening
- Unchanged after meals

Hepatic Artery
- Spectral broadening
- Crucial in heart transplants

Splenic Artery
- Very turbulent flow pattern
- Very prone to aneurysm

Superior Mesenteric Artery
- Highly resistive in fasting patient
- Nonresistive in nonfasting patient

Renal Artery
- Nonresistive
- Spectral broadening

coded in various shades of blue. The sonographer may select the particular color scheme to be used; some laboratories choose to code all positive-flow patterns red and negative-flow patterns blue. Other laboratories code all arterial flows red and venous flows blue.

Doppler Flow Patterns in the Abdominal Arterial Vessels

Box 8.5 lists Doppler flow patterns in the abdominal arteries.

Aorta. The patient should be scanned in the longitudinal plane (Fig. 8.64). The flow pattern of the proximal abdominal aorta above the renal arteries shows a high systolic peak and a relatively low diastolic component. Little spectral broadening (turbulence) is evident. A clear window under systole means that plug flow is present. The distal abdominal aorta below the renal arteries shows flow with a small, reversed component present during diastole. The closer the sonographer approaches the common iliac vessels, the greater the reverse component becomes. This occurs because of the high impedance of peripheral circulation in the leg as it becomes triphasic, crossing the baseline three times.

Celiac Axis. The sonographer should scan transversely to search for the *seagull sign*, i.e., celiac trunk, hepatic artery, and splenic artery. If they cannot be seen, the sonographer should scan longitudinally. The celiac trunk's spectral analysis shows systolic flow with spectral broadening (turbulence) in diastole (Fig. 8.65A). No change in the flow pattern is observed after meals.

Hepatic Artery. The hepatic artery is the most variable of all abdominal arteries. It has been reported that 12% of the population has a replaced hepatic artery arising from the superior mesenteric artery (Fig. 8.65B). Two thirds of patients have a right hepatic artery that crosses posterior to the common bile duct or right hepatic duct, whereas the left hepatic artery crosses anterior to the left hepatic duct. Flow in diastole persists because of the low vascular impedance of the liver. Similar waveforms are seen in the main hepatic and intrahepatic arteries. Typically, more spectral broadening occurs during systole and diastole.

Splenic Artery. The splenic artery shows the greatest turbulence of all the celiac branches, probably because of its tortuosity (Fig. 8.65C). Aneurysms of the celiac branches have been described most commonly in the splenic branch.

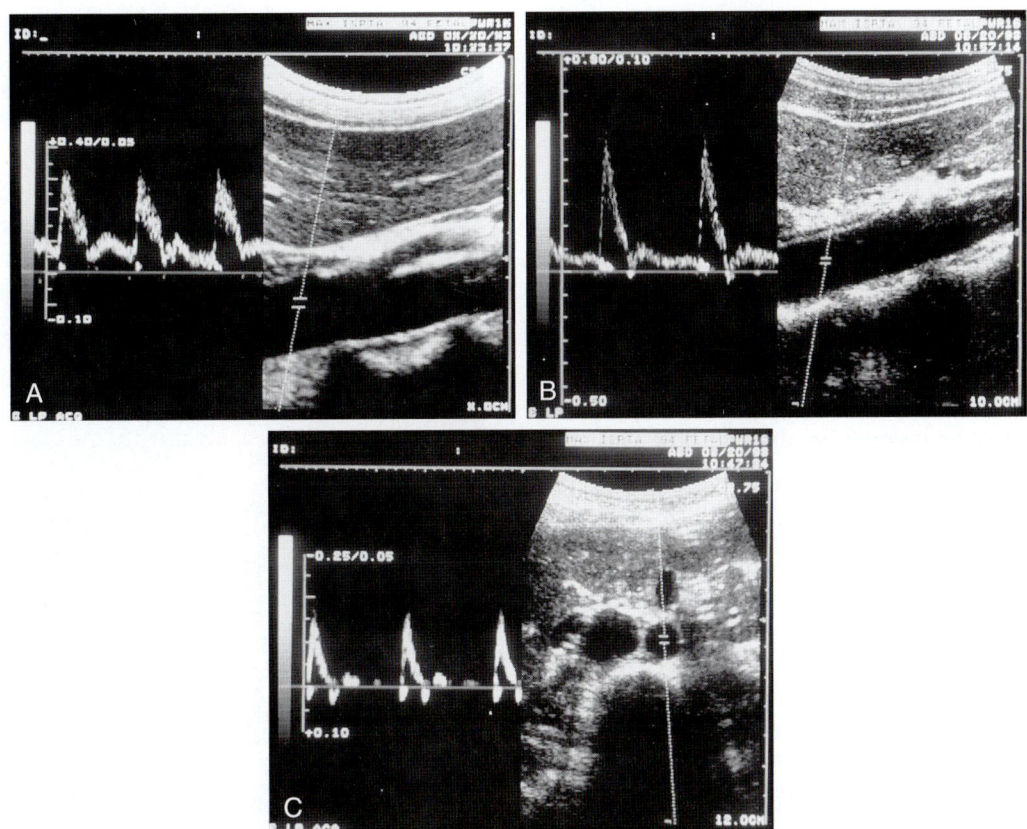

FIG. 8.64 (A) Sagittal scans of normal flow in the abdominal aorta. (B) The flow pattern of the proximal aorta above the renal arteries shows a high systolic peak and a relatively low diastolic component. (C) Transverse view.

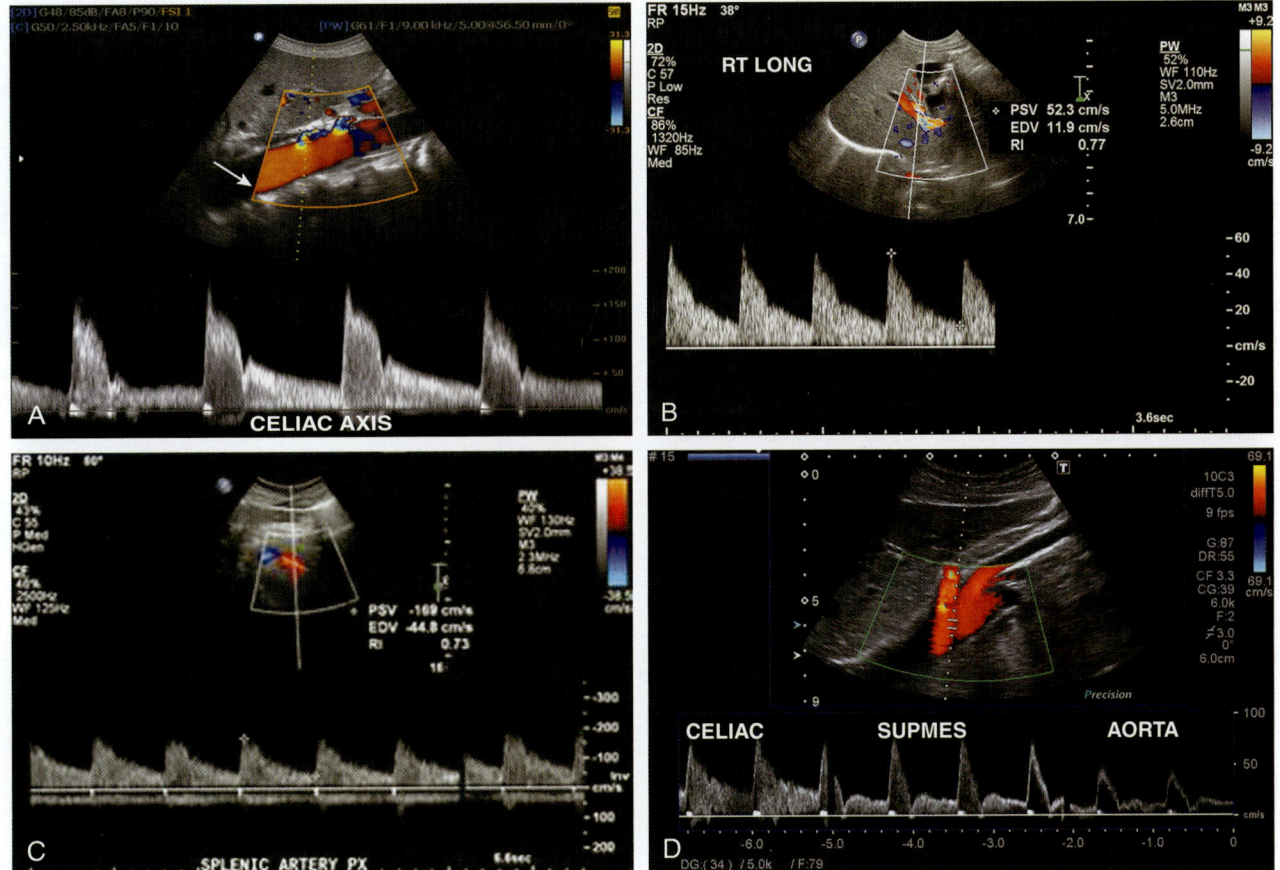

FIG. 8.65 (A) Longitudinal image of the Doppler flow obtained from the celiac axis. (B) Flow in the hepatic artery in diastole persists because of the low vascular impedance of the liver. (C) The splenic artery shows the greatest turbulence of all the celiac branches, probably because of its tortuosity. (D) The superior mesenteric artery is a highly resistive vessel (with decreased diastolic flow) in the fasting state, with little or no flow in diastole.

Patients with chronic pancreatitis are particularly prone to these. The sonographer should always apply Doppler to pancreatic pseudocysts; their appearance is very similar to that of vascular aneurysms.

Superior Mesenteric Artery. Typically, the SMA is a highly resistive vessel (with decreased diastolic flow) in the fasting state, with little or no flow in diastole (Fig. 8.65D). However, after a meal, the pattern of the SMA changes to a low-resistive waveform demonstrating enhanced diastolic flow. Doppler analysis of the SMA has the potential to diagnose mesenteric arterial occlusion and abdominal angina.

Renal Artery. The main renal artery has a low-impedance (nonresistive) pattern with significant diastolic flow—usually 30% to 50% of peak systole (Fig. 8.66). Continuous diastolic flow provides continuous perfusion of the kidneys. Spectral broadening occurs in systole and diastole. Segmental, interlobar, and arcuate arteries demonstrate a pattern similar to that of the main renal artery. However, the flow is progressively dampened in the periphery and shows reduced velocity patterns. It may be very hard to demonstrate renal artery stenosis in a native kidney because of the difficulty involved in seeing the vessel at its origin and in its entirety. Renal artery occlusion can be declared only when the artery is unquestionably imaged. The sonographer should be careful because complete obstruction of the native artery as collateral arterial pathways may be mistaken for a patent renal artery. At least 30% of the population has multiple renal arteries, making it more difficult to rule out obstruction.

Doppler Flow Patterns in the Abdominal Venous Vessels

Box 8.6 lists Doppler flow patterns in the abdominal veins.

Renal Vein. The renal vein shows a variable flow pattern similar to that found in the IVC (Fig. 8.67). The sonographer should closely evaluate the renal veins in any patient with a suspected tumor or renal obstructive lesion as this tumor may invade outside the renal capsule into the venous pathway

Inferior Vena Cava and Hepatic Veins. The IVC and hepatic veins present a complex waveform, which flows above and below the baseline, reflecting reflux of blood from the right atrium during systole and variations with the respiratory cycle (Fig. 8.68). The sonographer should always look at the cava and renal veins for tumor invasion when a renal cell carcinoma is observed.

Portal Vein. In the normal superior mesenteric vein and splenic vein, flow is hepatopetal (toward the liver) (Fig. 8.69). The portal vein shows a relatively continuous flow at low velocities, which may vary slightly with respirations. Portal vein thrombosis can be easily diagnosed with sonography. A direct sign is visualization of a thrombus. Indirect signs include the loss of normal portal venous landmarks, dilation of the superior mesenteric vein and splenic vein, and venous

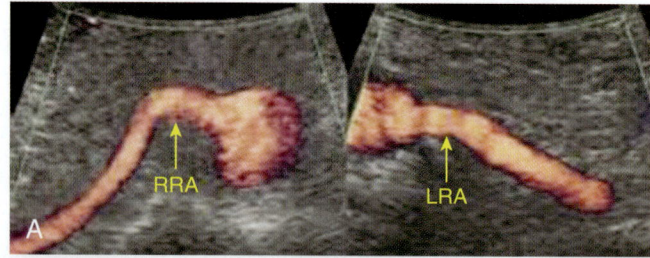
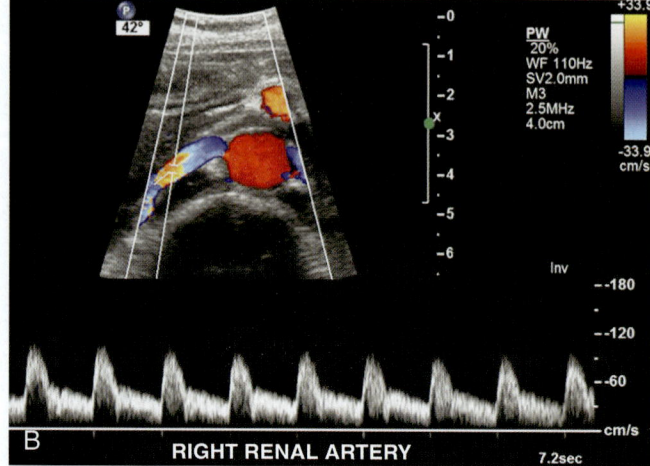
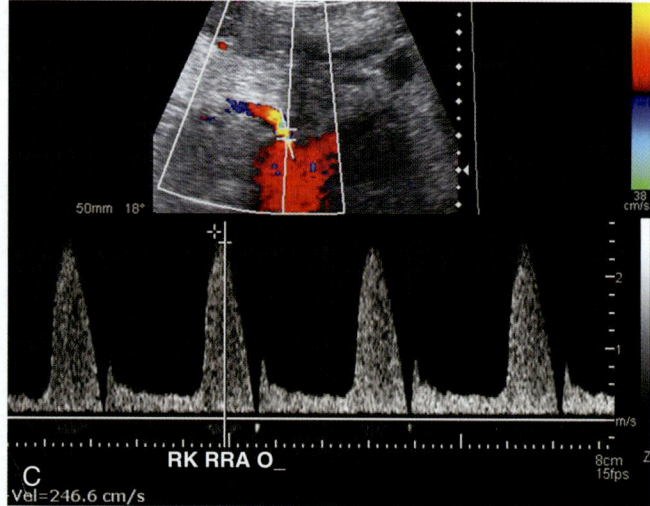

FIG. 8.66 (A) Power Doppler flow in the renal arteries. (B) Normal right renal artery flow velocity. (C) High velocity flow profile in a patient with renal artery stenosis.

BOX 8.6	Doppler Flow Patterns in Abdominal Veins

Renal Vein
- Variable flow much like the inferior vena cava
- Evaluate with transplants

Inferior Vena Cava and Hepatic Veins
- Vary with respiration
- Flow above and below the baseline, reflux from right atrium

Portal Vein
- Hepatopetal flow
- Continuous flow pattern; varies slightly with respirations

CHAPTER 8 Vascular System

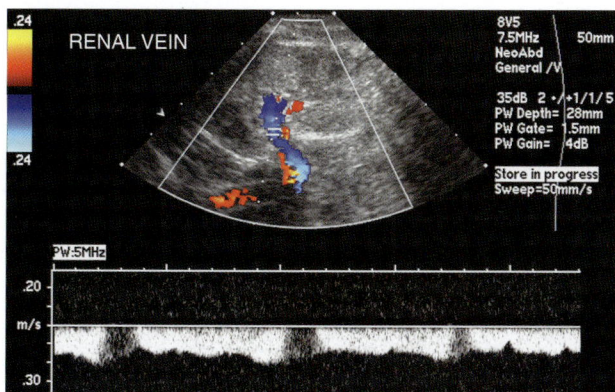

FIG. 8.67 Normal flow velocity of the renal vein.

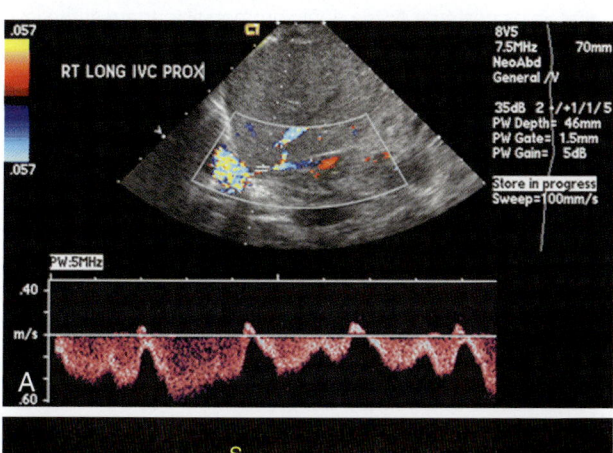

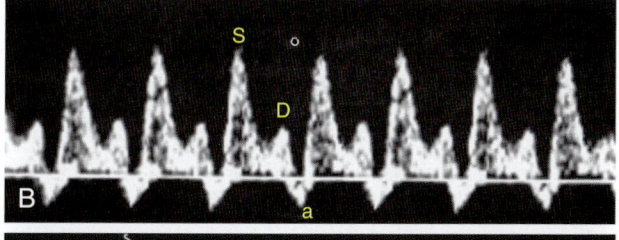

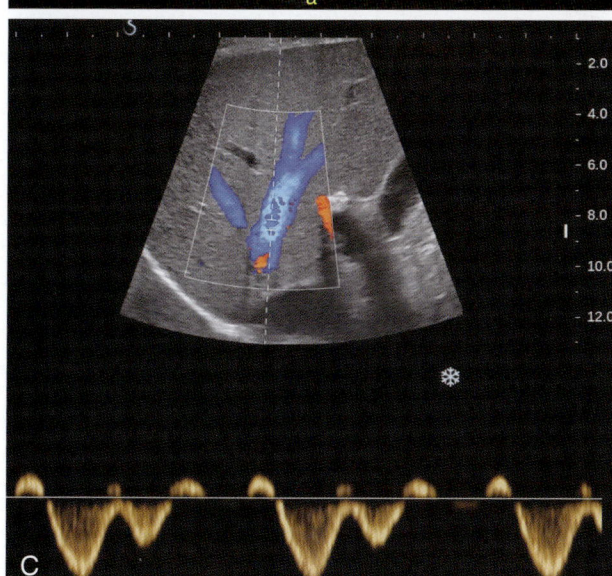

FIG. 8.68 (A) The inferior vena cava and hepatic veins present a complex waveform, which flows above and below the baseline, reflecting reflux of blood from the right atrium during systole and variations with the respiratory cycle. (B) Hepatic vein flow is triphasic, with systolic (S), diastolic (D), and atrial (a) components. (C) Color Doppler of normal hepatic vein flow.

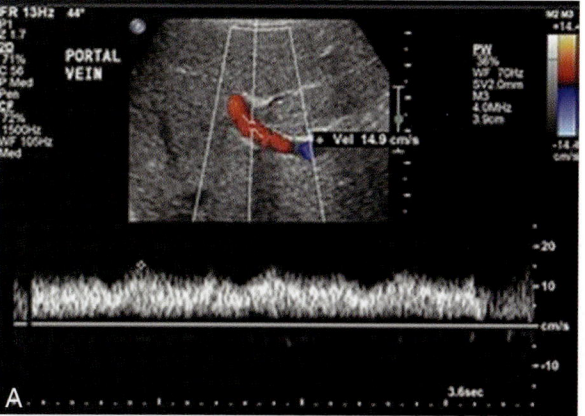

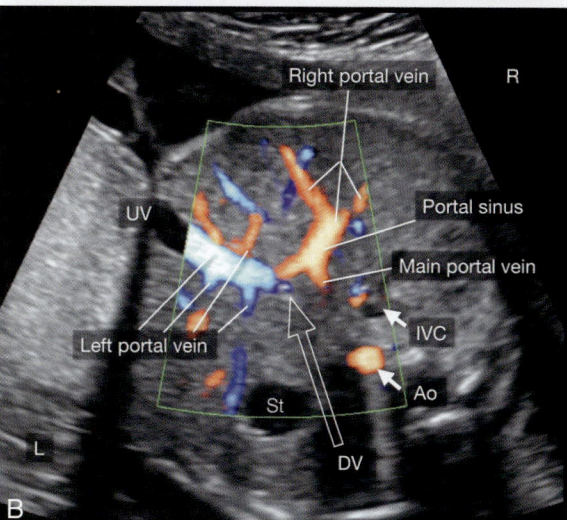

FIG. 8.69 (A) Portal vein flow is monophasic and hepatopetal (toward the liver). (B) Color Doppler of the normal portal vein flow within the liver. *Ao*, Aorta; *DV*, ductus venosus; *IVC*, inferior vena cava; *St*, stomach; *UV*, umbilical vein.

collaterals in the porta hepatis (**cavernous transformation of the portal vein**).

Pulsed Doppler adds to these findings; lack of Doppler signals from the lumen indicates absence of blood flow. In cirrhotic patients, thrombosis is often suspected when ascites suddenly worsens. Consequently, special attention must be paid to the portal vein to identify a thrombus in these patients. It is often difficult to visualize the portal vein flow in such patients.

 Key Pearls

- The function of the circulatory system, along with the heart and lymphatics, is to transport gases, nutrient materials, and other essential substances to the tissues and subsequently to transport waste products from the cells to appropriate sites for excretion.
- Blood is carried away from the heart by the arteries and is returned from the tissues to the heart by the veins.

- Veins have a diminished tunica media compared with the arteries.
- The aorta may be divided into the following five sections: (1) root of the aorta, (2) ascending aorta and arch, (3) descending aorta, (4) abdominal aorta and abdominal aortic branches, and (5) bifurcation of the aorta into iliac arteries.
- The diaphragmatic crura surrounds the proximal abdominal aorta as this vessel projects through the diaphragm into the abdominal cavity.
- The normal diameter of the abdominal aorta is evaluated at the region of the supraceliac and infrarenal locations.
- Measurements are made at the proximal, mid, and distal aorta in the transverse and longitudinal plane.
- The common iliac arteries arise at the bifurcation of the abdominal aorta at the fourth lumbar vertebra (near the superior sacrum). These vessels further divide into the internal and external iliac arteries.
- The short celiac trunk gives rise to three smaller vessels: the splenic, common hepatic, and left gastric arteries.
- The right renal artery and the left renal artery are lateral branches that arise just inferior to the superior mesenteric artery.
- The common hepatic artery branches into the proper hepatic artery and the gastroduodenal artery.
- The left hepatic artery is a small branch supplying the caudate and left lobes of the liver. The right hepatic artery supplies the gallbladder via the cystic artery and the liver.
- Several smaller arterial branches originate at the splenic artery as it courses through the upper border of the pancreas: the dorsal pancreatic, great pancreatic, and caudal pancreatic arteries.
- The superior mesenteric artery arises from the anterior abdominal aortic wall approximately 1 cm inferior to the celiac trunk.
- The right renal artery is a longer vessel than the left; it courses from the aorta posterior to the inferior vena cava and anterior to the vertebral column in a posterior and slightly caudal direction to enter the hilus of the right kidney.
- The left renal artery courses from the aorta directly into the hilus of the left kidney.
- Ectasia implies the diffuse dilation of a vessel, whereas an abdominal aortic aneurysm is a region of focal enlargement.
- Arteriosclerosis occurs when the arterial vascular system becomes thick and stiff, leading to restriction of blood flow to the organs and tissues in the body.
- An *aortic aneurysm* is defined as that with a vessel diameter greater than 3 cm or noted focal dilation of the vessel.
- The primary risk factors for a patient with an AAA are dissection and rupture of the vessel.
- Grey Turner sign may be associated with an extensive bleed in the retroperitoneal cavity.
- An aneurysm may be classified as a true aneurysm (lined by all three layers of the aorta) or as a false aneurysm (pseudoaneurysm) (not lined by all three layers).
- The fusiform aneurysm represents a gradual transition between normal and abnormal and extends over the length of the aorta to resemble a football-like shape.
- A saccular aneurysm shows a sudden transition between normal and abnormal and is somewhat spherical and larger (5 to 10 cm) than fusiform aneurysms.
- Three classifications of aortic dissection are based on the DeBakey model. Types I and II involve the ascending aorta and the aortic arch; type III involves the descending aorta at a level inferior to the left subclavian artery.
- An abdominal aortic aneurysm may be surgically repaired with a flexible graft material attached to the end of the remaining aorta.
- Masses other than an aortic aneurysm that can simulate a pulsatile abdominal mass include retroperitoneal tumor, huge fibroid uterus, or para-aortic nodes.
- The inferior vena cava is formed by the union of the common iliac veins posterior to the right common iliac artery at the level of the fifth lumbar vertebra.
- In patients with right ventricular failure, the inferior vena cava does not collapse with inspiration or expiration.
- Masses posterior to the hepatic portion of the inferior vena cava are the right adrenal, neurogenic, and hepatic.
- The middle, or pancreatic, portion of the inferior vena cava may elevate the cava from abnormalities of the right renal artery, right kidney, lumbar spine, or lymph node masses.
- The right and left main renal veins arise anterior to the renal arteries at their respective sides of the inferior vena cava at the level of L2.
- Renal vein thrombosis is the formation of a clot in the vein that drains blood from the kidneys, ultimately leading to a reduction in the drainage of one or both kidneys and the possible migration of the clot to other parts of the body.
- The hepatic veins are the largest visceral tributaries of the inferior vena cava. They originate between the segments of the liver and drain posteriorly into the inferior vena cava at the level of the diaphragm.
- The right hepatic vein drains the right lobe of the liver, the middle hepatic vein drains the caudate lobe, and the left hepatic vein drains the left lobe.
- The portal vein is formed posterior to the pancreas by the union of the superior mesenteric vein and splenic veins at the level of L2.
- The portal vein has an anastomosis with the esophageal veins, rectal venous plexus, and superficial abdominal veins.
- The liver receives a dual blood supply from the portal vein and the hepatic artery.
- The portal triad contains branches of the portal vein, hepatic artery, and bile duct within a connective tissue sheath that gives the portal vein an echogenic wall, as seen on liver sonographic images.
- Portal veins become smaller as they progress into the liver from the porta hepatis.
- The right and left portal veins course transversely through the liver; thus transverse scans display their longest extent.
- The splenic vein is a tributary of the portal circulation. It begins at the hilum of the spleen, where the union of several veins forms it.
- The superior mesenteric vein is also a tributary to the portal vein.

- Doppler ultrasound frequently is used to differentiate vessels from nonvascular structures.
- In patients who develop portal venous hypertension, the portal blood flow becomes hepatofugal (away from the liver) instead of hepatopetal (toward the liver).
- A flow disturbance (increased velocity or obstruction of flow) may result from the formation of an atheroma, arteriovenous fistula, pseudoaneurysm, or aneurysmal dilation.
- Spectral analysis tells the velocity and turbulence of blood flow.
- Nonresistive vessels have a high diastolic component and supply organs that need constant perfusion, such as the internal carotid artery, the hepatic artery, and the renal artery.
- Resistive vessels have very little or even reversed flow in diastole and supply organs that do not need a constant blood supply, such as the external carotid and the iliac and brachial arteries.
- The flow pattern of the proximal abdominal aorta above the renal arteries shows a high systolic peak and a relatively low diastolic component.
- Two thirds of patients have a right hepatic artery that crosses posterior to the common bile duct or right hepatic duct, whereas the left hepatic artery crosses anterior to the left hepatic duct.
- The splenic artery shows the greatest turbulence of all the celiac branches, probably because of its tortuosity.
- Typically, the superior mesenteric artery is a highly resistive vessel (with decreased diastolic flow) in the fasting state, with little or no flow in diastole.
- The main renal artery has a low impedance (nonresistive) pattern with significant diastolic flow—usually 30% to 50% of peak systole.
- The inferior vena cava and hepatic veins present a complex waveform, which flows above and below the baseline, reflecting reflux of blood from the right atrium during systole and variations with the respiratory cycle.
- The renal vein shows a variable flow pattern similar to that found in the inferior vena cava.
- In the normal superior mesenteric vein and splenic vein, flow is hepatopetal (toward the liver).
- The portal vein shows a relatively continuous flow at low velocities, which may vary slightly with respirations.

BIBLIOGRAPHY

Middleton WD, Kurtz AB, Hertzberg BS. *The Requisites: Ultrasound*. 2nd ed. St. Louis: Elsevier; 2004.

Rumack CM, Wilson SR, Charboneau JW, et al. *Diagnostic Ultrasound*. 4th ed. St. Louis: Elsevier; 2011.

Snell RS. *Clinical Anatomy*. 7th ed. Philadelphia: Lippincott Williams & Wilkins; 2017.

Thibodeau GA, Patton KT. *The Human Body in Health & Disease*. 2nd ed. St. Louis: Mosby; 1997.

CHAPTER 9

The Liver

Sandra L. Hagen-Ansert

OBJECTIVES

On completion of this chapter, you should be able to:
- Describe normal anatomy of the liver, including vascular supply and relational landmarks
- List the functions of the liver
- Describe the liver function tests and their relevance to hepatic disease
- Discuss the sonographic evaluation of the liver in the sagittal, transverse, and decubitus planes
- List the clinical signs, sonographic features, and differentials for the pathology discussed in this chapter

OUTLINE

Anatomy of the Liver 219
  Normal Anatomy 219
  Couinaud's System of Hepatic Nomenclature 219
  Lobes of the Liver 220
  Hepatic Vascular Supply 223
Physiology and Laboratory Data of the Hepatobiliary System 225
  Hepatic Physiology 225
  Hepatic Versus Obstructive Disease 225
  Hepatic Metabolic Functions 227
  Hepatic Detoxification Functions 229
  Bile 230
  Liver Function Tests 230
Sonographic Evaluation of the Liver 231
  Liver and Porta Hepatis Protocol 233
  Normal Sonographic Anatomy and Texture 234
  Sagittal Plane 235
  Transverse Plane 239
  Lateral Decubitus Plane 239
Pathology of the Liver 239
  Developmental Anomalies 239
  Diffuse Disease 243
  Hepatic Vascular Flow Abnormalities 249
  Diffuse Abnormalities of the Liver Parenchyma 258
  Focal Hepatic Disease 260
  Infectious Disease of the Liver 265
  Hepatic Tumors 268

KEY TERMS

Alanine aminotransferase (ALT)
Alkaline phosphatase
Aspartase aminotransferase (AST)
Bare area
Bilirubin
Bull's-eye (target) lesion
Caudate lobe
Collateral circulation
Diffuse hepatocellular disease
Epigastrium
Extrahepatic
Falciform ligament
Hepatocellular disease
Hepatocyte
Hepatofugal
Hepatopetal
Hyperglycemia
Hypoglycemia
Intrahepatic
Left hypochondrium
Left lobe of the liver
Left portal vein
Ligamentum teres
Ligamentum venosum
Liver function tests
Main lobar fissure
Main portal vein
Metastatic disease
Neoplasm
Obstructive disease
Pyogenic abscess
Right hypochondrium
Right lobe of the liver
Right portal vein
Transjugular intrahepatic portosystemic shunt (TIPS)

The liver is the largest organ in the abdominal cavity, measuring approximately 21 to 22.5 cm in its greatest transverse diameter, 13 to 17.5 cm in its greatest vertical height, and 10 to 12.5 cm in its anteroposterior depth, weighing approximately 1200 to 1600 g in the adult. The size and relative homogeneous texture of the liver parenchyma makes it very accessible to sonographic evaluation. The parenchyma of the normal liver is used to evaluate other organs and glands in the body—that is, the kidneys are equally echogenic or less echogenic than the liver, the spleen has about the same to slightly more echogenicity than the liver, and the pancreas is as echogenic as or slightly more echogenic than the liver. The size and shape of the liver determine the quality of the sonographic examination performed. For example, the prominent left lobe of the liver facilitates visualization of the pancreas, which is situated just inferior to the border of the left lobe, whereas if the right lobe extends just below the costal margin, it may facilitate visualization of the gallbladder and right kidney.

ANATOMY OF THE LIVER

Normal Anatomy

The liver occupies almost all the **right hypochondrium**, the greater part of the **epigastrium**, and the **left hypochondrium** as far as the mammillary line. The contour and shape of the liver vary according to the patient's habitus and lie. Its shape is also influenced by the lateral segment of the left lobe and the length of the right lobe of the liver. The liver lies inferior to the diaphragm. The ribs cover the greater part of the right lobe (usually a small part of the right lobe is in contact with the abdominal wall). In the epigastric region, the liver extends several centimeters below the xiphoid process. Most of the left lobe is covered by the rib cage (Fig. 9.1).

The fundus of the stomach lies posterior and lateral to the left lobe of the liver and may frequently be seen on transverse sonograms. The remainder of the stomach lies inferior to the liver and is best visualized on sagittal sonograms. The duodenum lies adjacent to the right lobe and medial segment of the left lobe of the liver. The body of the pancreas is usually seen just inferior to the left lobe of the liver. The posterior border of the liver contacts the right kidney, inferior vena cava, and aorta. The diaphragm covers the superior border of the liver (Fig. 9.2A). The liver is suspended from the diaphragm and anterior abdominal wall by the falciform ligament and from the diaphragm by the reflections of the peritoneum.

Most of the liver is covered by peritoneum, but a large area rests directly on the diaphragm; this is called the **bare area** (Fig. 9.2B). The subphrenic space between the liver (or spleen) and the diaphragm is a common site for abscess formation. The right posterior subphrenic space lies between the right lobe of the liver, the right kidney, and the right colic flexure (Fig. 9.2C). The lesser sac is an enclosed portion of the peritoneal space posterior to the liver and stomach. This sac communicates with the rest of the peritoneal space at a point near the head of the pancreas. It also may be a site for abscess formation. The right subhepatic space is located inferior to the right lobe of the liver and includes Morison pouch, which lies between the posterior aspect of the right lobe and the upper pole of the right kidney.

The posterior borders of the liver are in contact with the inferior vena cava, the gallbladder and cystic duct, the portal vein confluence, the hepatic artery, the right kidney, and the colon (Fig. 9.2D).

Projections of the liver may be altered by some disease states. Tumor infiltration, cirrhosis, or a subphrenic abscess often causes inferior displacement, whereas ascites, excessive dilation of the colon, or abdominal tumors can elevate the liver. Retroperitoneal tumors may move the liver slightly anterior.

Couinaud's System of Hepatic Nomenclature

The liver has been divided into a large right lobe and a smaller left lobe by the attachment of the peritoneum of the falciform ligament. The right lobe is further divided into a quadrate lobe and a caudate lobe by the presence of the gallbladder, the fissure for the ligamentum teres, the inferior vena cava, and the fissure for the ligamentum venosum. In actuality, the quadrate and caudate are a functional part of the left lobe of the liver. However, functional divisions have more value from a surgical perspective. The functional division between the left and right lobes is based upon the vasculature, not the falciform ligament.

Although the liver has been divided into four anatomical lobes with the falciform ligament "separating the left from the right lobe," Couinaud's system of hepatic nomenclature (Box 9.1) provides the functional division between the right and left lobes based upon the vasculature, not the falciform ligament, for hepatic surgical resections. The vascular supply

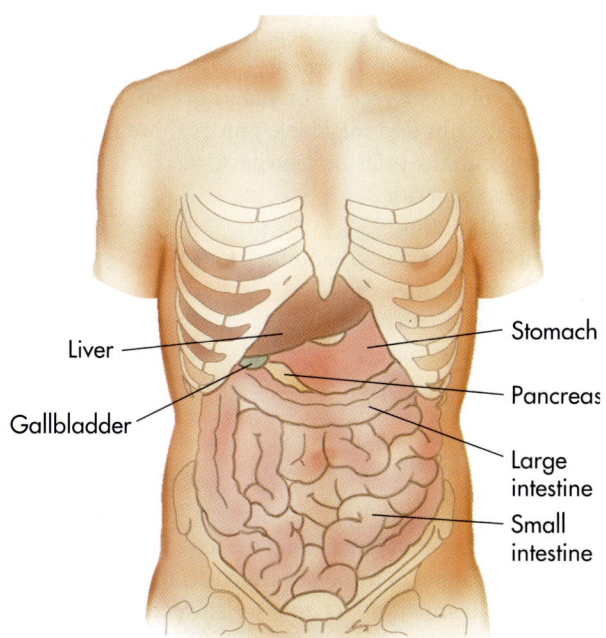

FIG. 9.1 Anteroposterior view of the abdomen shows the right lobe of the liver covered by the ribs. The left lobe of the liver lies in the midline just posterior to the tip of the sternum. The stomach lies posterior and lateral to the left lobe of the liver.

CHAPTER 9 The Liver

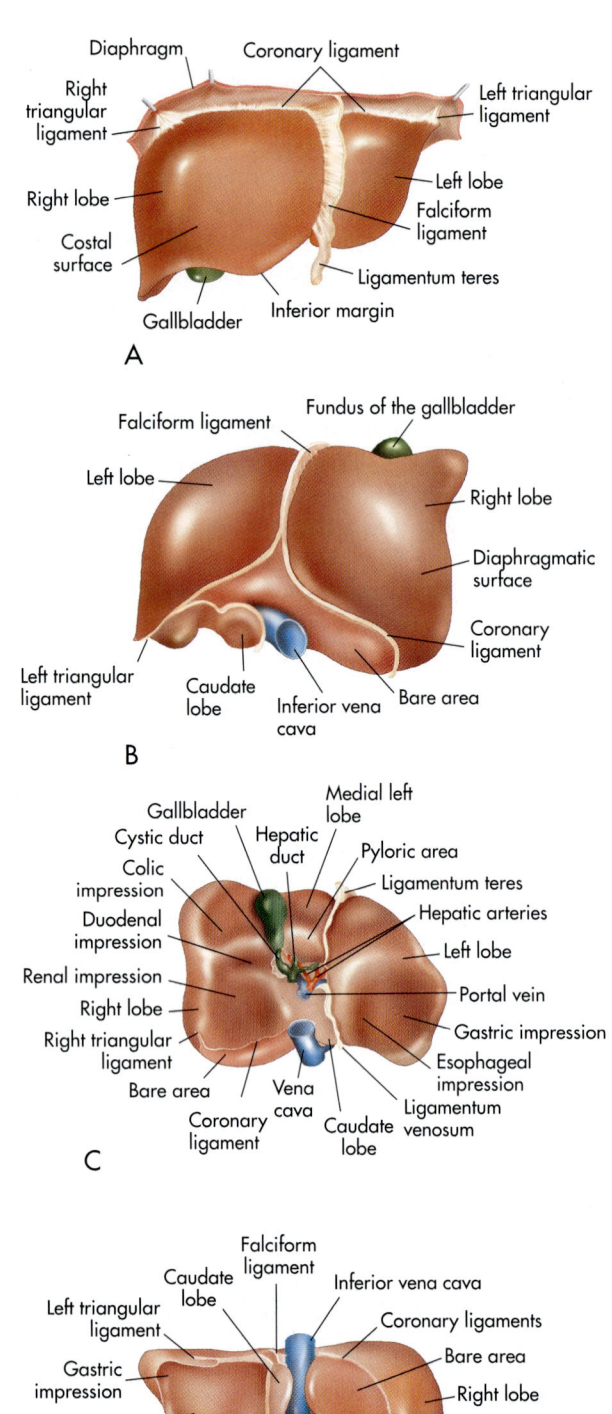

FIG. 9.2 (A) Anterior view of the liver. The right lobe is the largest of the four lobes of the liver. (B) Superior view of the liver. The left lobe of the liver lies in the epigastric and left hypochondriac regions. (C) Inferior view of the visceral surface of the liver. (D) Posterior view of the diaphragmatic surface of the liver. The caudate lobe is located on the posterosuperior surface of the right lobe, opposite the tenth and eleventh thoracic vertebrae.

> **BOX 9.1   Hepatic Segmental Anatomy**
>
> Segment I: Caudate lobe
> Segments II and III: Left superior and inferior lateral segments
> Segments IVa and IVb: Medial segments of the left lobe
> Segments V and VI: Caudal to the transverse plane
> Segments VII and VIII: Cephalad to the transverse plane

and drainage divide the liver into regions that can be resected independently. The middle hepatic vein and the ascending section of the left portal vein divide the liver, functionally, into a left lobe and a right lobe (Fig. 9.3). This dividing line tends to be near the left edge of the inferior vena cava and the gallbladder fossa. The quadrate lobe is functionally part of the medial segment of the left lobe, which lies between the middle hepatic vein and the left hepatic vein. Using these functional divisions, the falciform ligament now belongs to the left lobe, which runs along the medial left lobe, close to the border with the lateral left lobe.

Using the Couinaud system, the sonographer should be able to precisely isolate the location of a lesion for the surgical team. The description of the liver segments is based on the portal and hepatic venous segments, with each segment having its own blood supply, lymphatics, and biliary drainage. Each of the eight segments has a central branch or branches of the portal vein that is bounded by a hepatic vein. The right, middle, and left hepatic veins divide the liver longitudinally into four sections. Each of these sections is further divided transversely by an invisible plane through the right and left portal veins.

The Couinaud system divides the left lateral, right anterior, and right posterior segments into superior and inferior subsegments and maintains the caudate lobe and the medial left segment as single segments. The eight segments are divided and numbered as follows: (A separate portal venous branch supplies each of these subsegments.)

1. Caudate lobe may receive branches of both the right and left portal veins and may have one or more hepatic veins draining into the inferior vena cava.
2. Left lateral superior
3. Left lateral inferior
4. Left medial superior (a) and inferior (b)
5. Right anterior inferior
6. Right posterior inferior
7. Right posterior superior
8. Right anterior superior

Lobes of the Liver

Right Lobe. The right hypochondrium contains the right lobe, which is six times larger than the left lobe. Anatomically, the right lobe appears to be separated from the left lobe by the falciform ligament on its *anterior* surface and main lobar fissure. However, functionally the middle hepatic vein runs vertically between the left medial segment and right anterior segment. Its *inferior* and *posterior* surfaces are marked by three fossae: the porta hepatis, the gallbladder fossa, and

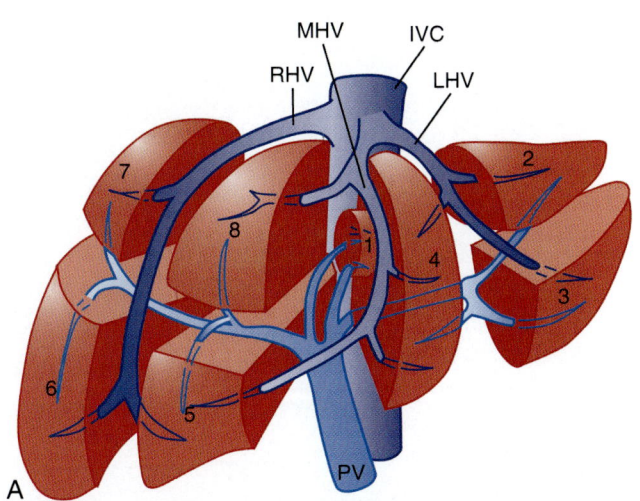 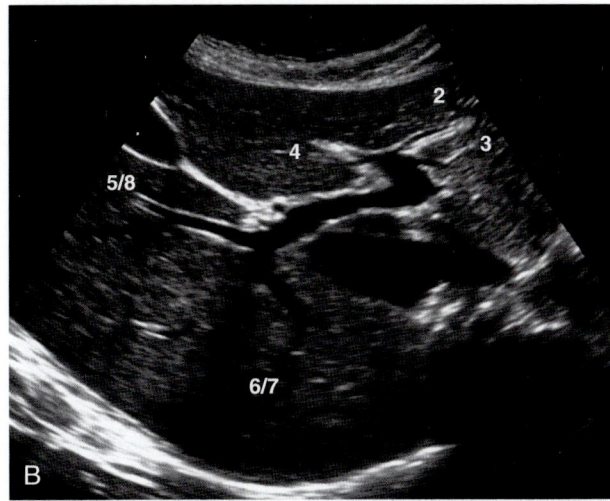

FIG. 9.3 **Couinaud's hepatic segments divide the liver into eight segments.** The three hepatic veins are the longitudinal boundaries. The transverse plane is defined by the right and left portal pedicles. The caudate lobe is situated posteriorly. Segment I includes the caudate lobe. Segments II and III include the left superior and inferior lateral segments. Segment IV includes the medial segment of the left lobe. Segments V and VI are caudal to the transverse plane. Segments VII and VIII are cephalad to the transverse plane.

the inferior vena cava fossa. The right lobe contains an anterior and posterior segment; the right hepatic vein runs horizontally between the right anterior and posterior segments. A congenital variant, Riedel lobe, can sometimes be seen as an anterior projection of the liver and may extend to the iliac crest.

Left Lobe. The **left lobe of the liver** lies in the epigastric and left hypochondriac regions. The left intersegmental fissure divides the left lobe into medial and lateral segments; the left hepatic vein runs horizontally between the medial and lateral segments. Its upper surface is convex and molded onto the diaphragm. The left lobe is bound posterior by the porta hepatis, medially by the fossa for the gallbladder, and laterally by the fossa for the umbilical vein. The size of the left lobe of the liver varies considerably; a more prominent left lobe will allow the sonographer to image the pancreas and vascular structures anterior to the spine. The left lobe has two fissures: the fissure for the ligamentum teres and the ligamentum venosum.

Caudate Lobe. The **caudate lobe** is a small lobe situated on the posterior surface of the left lobe, with the inferior vena cava as its posterior border and the fissure for the ligamentum venosum as its anterior border. The hepatic boundary of the superior recess of the lesser sac is formed by the left margin of the caudate lobe. A small papillary process that extends obliquely and laterally from the caudate lobe is called the *caudate process*. This small projection courses between the portal vein and inferior vena cava toward the right lobe of the liver. This process may appear separate from the caudate lobe and thus be mistaken for a mass such as pancreatic tumor or enlarged lymph node.

Vascular Anatomy and Intersegmental Segments. Understanding the vascular relationships within the hepatic segments is crucial for the surgical approach. It is important to note that the hepatic veins course between the lobes and interlobar/intersegmental segments. Refer to Fig. 9.4 to understand the vascular patterns within the liver. The *right hepatic vein* courses within the right intersegmental fissure to divide the right lobe into anterior and posterior segments. The *middle hepatic vein* courses within the main lobar fissure to separate the anterior segment of the right lobe from the medial segment of the left lobe. The left intersegmental fissure separates the medial segment of the left lobe from the lateral segment. This fissure is further divided into *cranial, middle*, and *caudal* sections. The *left hepatic vein* forms the boundary of the cranial third, the ascending branch of the left portal vein represents the middle third, and the fissure for the ligamentum teres forms the most caudal division of the left lobe. The main branches of the *portal veins* run centrally within the segments (intrasegmental) with the exception of the ascending portion of the left portal vein, which runs in the left intersegmental fissure.

Ligaments and Fissures. There are several important ligaments and fissures to remember in the liver: Glisson's capsule, main lobar fissure, falciform ligament, ligamentum teres (round ligament), and ligamentum venosum (Fig. 9.5). These ligaments and fissures appear echogenic or hyperechoic because of the presence of collagen and fat within and around the structures.

The liver is covered by a thin connective tissue layer called Glisson's capsule. This capsule surrounds the liver and is thickest around the inferior vena cava and porta hepatis. The hepatoduodenal ligament contains the main portal vein, the proper hepatic artery, and the common duct. The **main lobar fissure** is the boundary between the right and left lobes of the liver. On the longitudinal scan, it may be seen as a hyperechoic line extending from the portal vein to the neck of the gallbladder. The sonographer uses this ligament to find the gallbladder on the longitudinal scan, especially when it is packed with stones and not well imaged. The **falciform ligament** extends from the umbilicus to the diaphragm in a parasagittal plane and contains the ligamentum teres. In the anteroposterior axis, the falciform ligament extends from

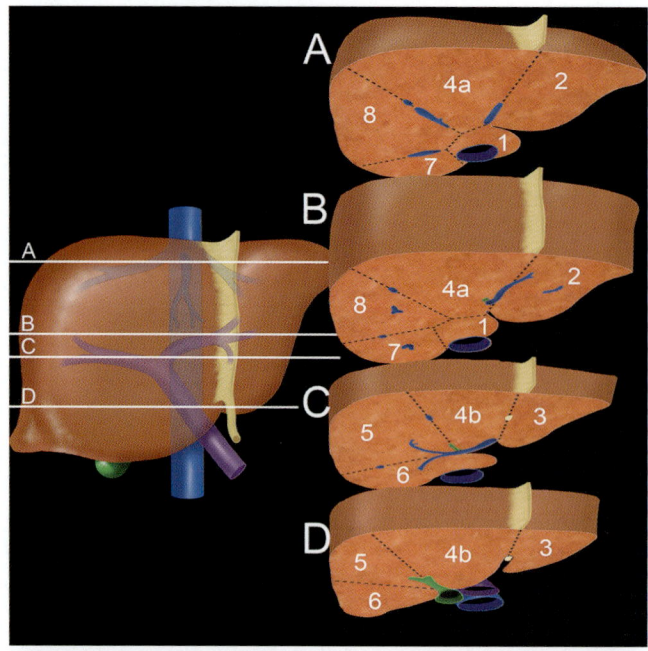

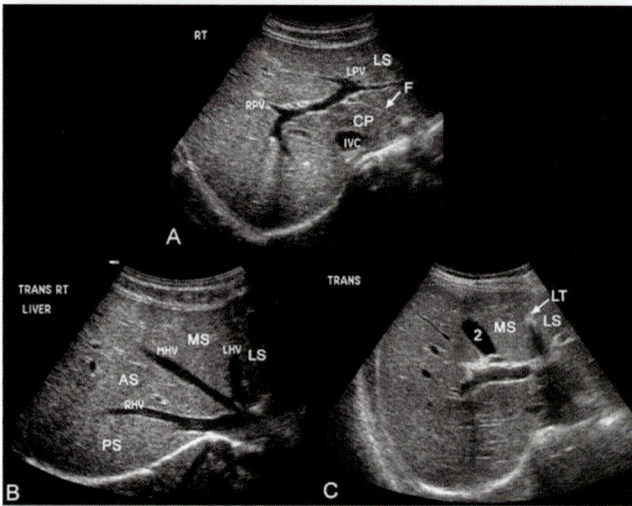

FIG. 9.4 The right hepatic vein (RHV) courses within the right intersegmental fissure to divide the right lobe into anterior segment (AS) and posterior segment (PS). The middle hepatic vein (MHV) courses within the main lobar fissure to separate the AS of the right lobe from the medial segment (MS) of the left lobe. The left hepatic vein (LHV) forms the boundary of the cranial third, the ascending branch of the left portal vein (LPV) represents the middle third, and the fissure (F) for the ligamentum teres (LT) forms the most caudal division of the left lobe. The main branches of the *portal veins* run centrally within the segments (intrasegmental) except for the ascending portion of the LPV, which runs in the left intersegmental fissure. *CP,* Caudate process; *IVC,* inferior vena cava; *LS,* lateral segment; *RPV,* right pulmonary vein.

the right rectus muscle to the bare area of the liver, where its echogenic reflections separate to contribute to the hepatic coronary ligament and attach to the undersurface of the diaphragm. The **ligamentum teres** appears as a bright echogenic focus on the sonogram and is seen as the rounded termination of the falciform ligament. The fissure for the **ligamentum venosum** separates the left lobe from the caudate lobe. On ultrasound, it may be seen just inferior to the dome of the liver as a linear horizontal line just anterior to the caudate

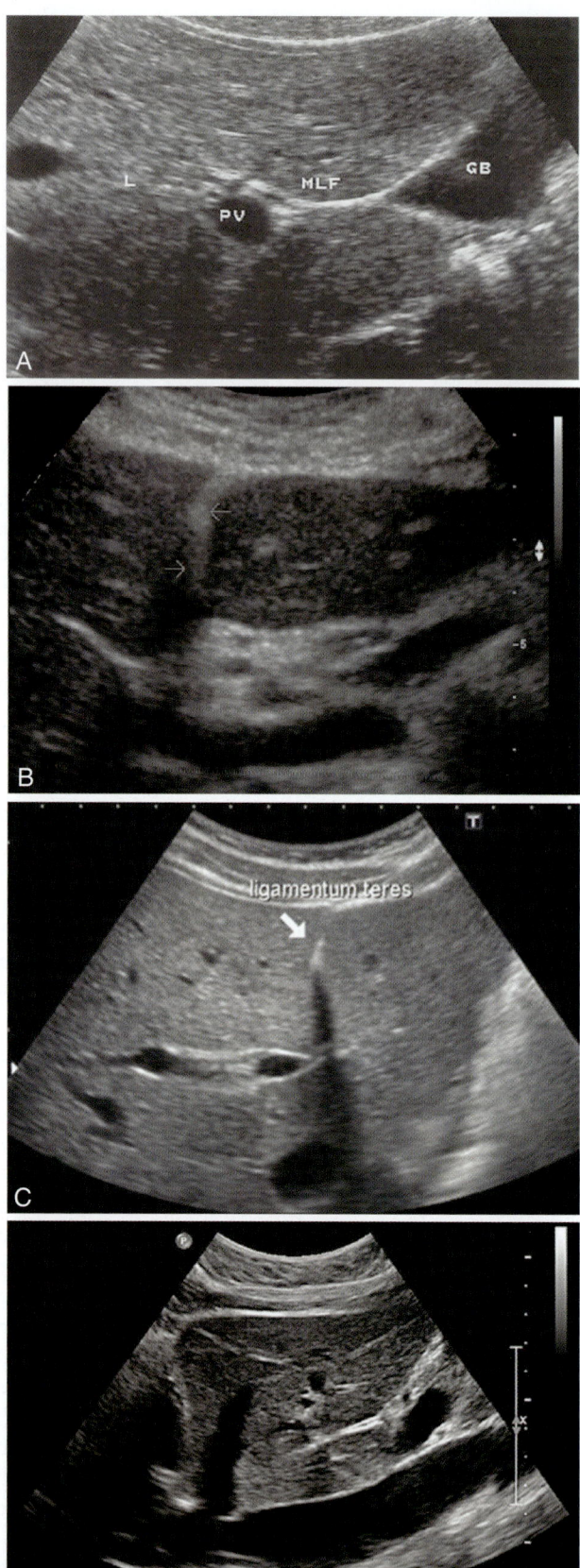

FIG. 9.5 Ligaments and fissures within the liver (L). (A) The main lobar fissure (MLF), (B) falciform ligament *(arrows)*, (C) ligamentum teres *(arrow)*, and (D) ligamentum venosum appear echogenic or hyperechoic because of the presence of collagen and fat within and around the structures. *GB,* Gallbladder; *PV,* portal vein.

lobe and inferior vena cava. The caudate lobe, ligamentum venosum, portal vein, and left lobe of the liver may be seen on the longitudinal plane over the area of the inferior vena cava.

Hepatic Vascular Supply

The liver receives blood supply from the portal veins and hepatic artery. The portal vein conveys about 70% to 80% of the blood to the liver; the remaining 20% to 30% is oxygenated blood conveyed to the liver via the hepatic artery. The right lobe of the liver receives blood primarily from the intestine, whereas the left lobe and caudate lobes receive blood from the stomach and the spleen.

The venous blood supply from the greater part of the gastrointestinal tract and its accessory organs drains into the liver through the portal venous system. The proximal tributaries drain directly into the portal vein, but the veins forming the distal tributaries correspond to the branches of the celiac artery and superior and inferior mesenteric arteries.

Hepatic Portal Vein. The portal vein drains blood from the gastrointestinal tract from the lower third of the esophagus to midway down the anal canal; it also drains blood from the spleen, pancreas, and gallbladder. The portal vein enters the liver and breaks up into sinusoids, from which blood passes into the hepatic veins that empty into the inferior vena cava. The portal venous system is a reliable indicator of various ultrasonic tomographic planes throughout the liver (Fig. 9.6).

The portal triad consists of the portal vein, hepatic artery, and bile duct. The portal vein is contained within a connective tissue sheath which provides an echogenic structure on the sonographic image to distinguish it from the hepatic vein.

Main Portal Vein. The **main portal vein** approaches the porta hepatis in a rightward, cephalic, and slightly posterior direction within the hepatoduodenal ligament. It comes in contact with the anterior surface of the inferior vena cava near the porta hepatis and serves to locate the liver hilum (Fig. 9.7A). It then divides into two branches: the right and left portal veins.

Right Portal Vein. The **right portal vein** is the larger of the two branches and requires a more posterior and more caudal transducer approach. It usually is possible to identify the anterior and posterior divisions of the right portal vein on sonography (Fig. 9.7C–D). The right portal vein has an anterior branch that lies centrally within the anterior segment of the right lobe and a posterior branch that lies within the posterior segment of the right lobe.

Left Portal Vein. The **left portal vein** lies more anterior and cranial than the right portal vein. The main portal vein is seen to elongate at the origin of the left portal vein (see Fig. 9.7D). The vessel lies within a canal containing large amounts of connective tissue, which results in the visualization of an echogenic linear band coursing through the central portion of the lateral segment of the left lobe. The left portal vein courses anterior to the caudate lobe initially and then travels anteriorly in the left intersegmental fissure to divide the medial and lateral segments of the left lobe.

Hepatic Arteries. The hepatic artery arises from the celiac trunk to supply the liver. The right and left branches of the hepatic artery accompany the portal veins (Fig. 9.8).

Hepatic Veins. The blood is perfused within the liver parenchyma through the hepatic sinusoids before it enters the terminal hepatic venules which unite to form the larger hepatic veins. There are essentially three main components of the hepatic veins–right, middle, and left—which drain into the inferior vena cava (Fig. 9.9). The right hepatic vein is the largest, courses in the right intersegmental fissure, and enters the right lateral aspect of the inferior vena cava. The right hepatic vein separates the anterior and posterior lobes of the right lobe. Often it is possible to identify a long horizontal branch of the right hepatic vein coursing between the anterior and posterior divisions of the right portal vein. The middle hepatic vein courses in the main lobar fissure and enters the anterior or right anterior surface of the inferior vena cava. The middle hepatic vein often forms a common trunk with the left hepatic vein. The left hepatic vein, which is the smallest, enters the left anterior surface of the inferior vena cava. The left hepatic vein forms the most cephalad boundary between the medial and lateral segments of the left lobe.

Distinguishing Characteristics of Portal and Hepatic Veins. The best way to distinguish the hepatic from the portal vessels is to trace their points of entry to the liver. The hepatic vessels flow into the inferior vena cava, whereas the splenic vein and superior mesenteric vein join to form the portal venous system. A continuous sector scanning sweep allows the sonographer to make this assessment within a few seconds. Hepatic veins course between the hepatic lobes and segments. The portal veins are larger at their origin as they emanate from the porta hepatis. Portal veins have more echogenic borders than the hepatic veins because they have a thicker collagenous sheath (Fig. 9.10).

Intrahepatic Vessels and Ducts. The portal veins carry blood to the liver, whereas the hepatic veins drain the blood

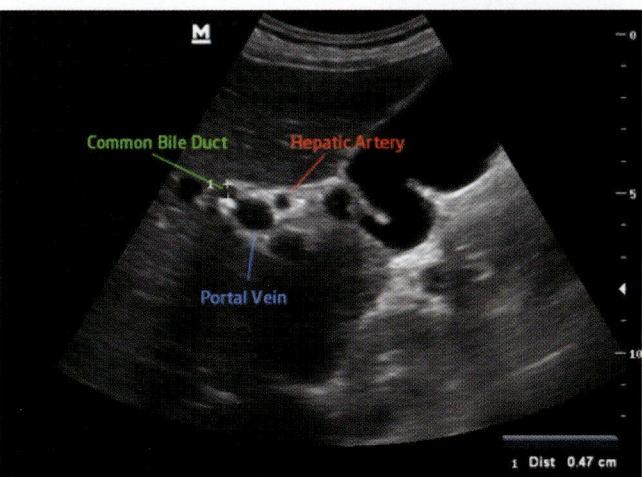

FIG. 9.6 **Vascular system of the liver.** The liver receives blood supply from the portal veins and hepatic artery. The venous blood supply from the greater part of the gastrointestinal tract and its accessory organs drains into the liver through the portal venous system. The portal triad consists of the portal vein, hepatic artery, and bile duct. There are essentially three main components of the hepatic veins—right, middle, and left—that drain into the inferior vena cava.

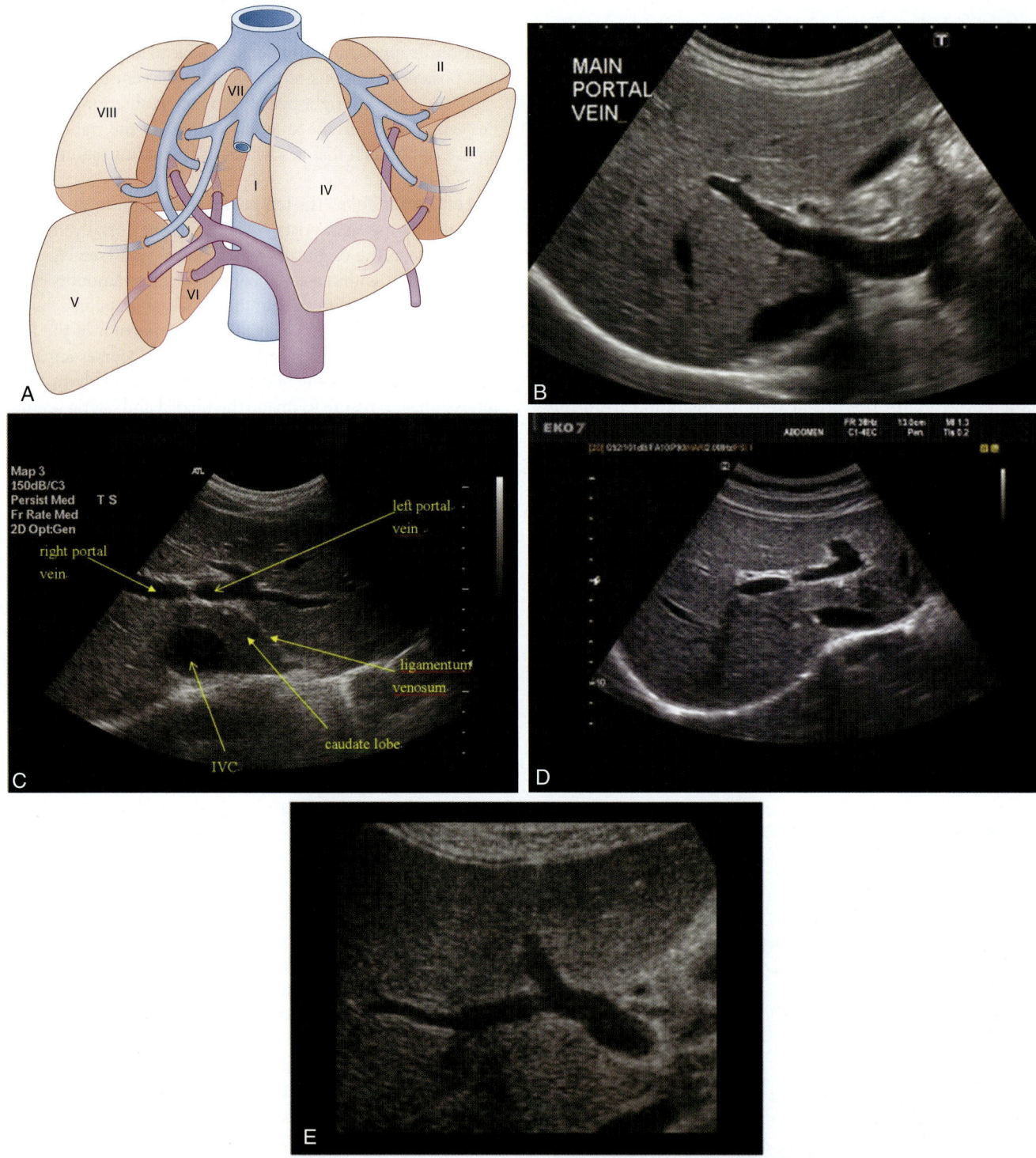

FIG. 9.7 (A) Portal venous tributaries and branches. (B) The main portal vein approaches the porta hepatis in a rightward, cephalic, and slightly posterior direction within the hepatoduodenal ligament. (C) The left portal vein lies more anterior and cranial than the right portal vein. (D) The right portal vein is the larger of the two branches and requires a more posterior and more caudal transducer approach. (E) It usually is possible to identify the anterior and posterior divisions of the right portal vein on sonography. The right portal vein has an anterior branch that lies centrally within the anterior segment of the right lobe and a posterior branch that lies within the posterior segment of the right lobe. *IVC*, Inferior vena cava.

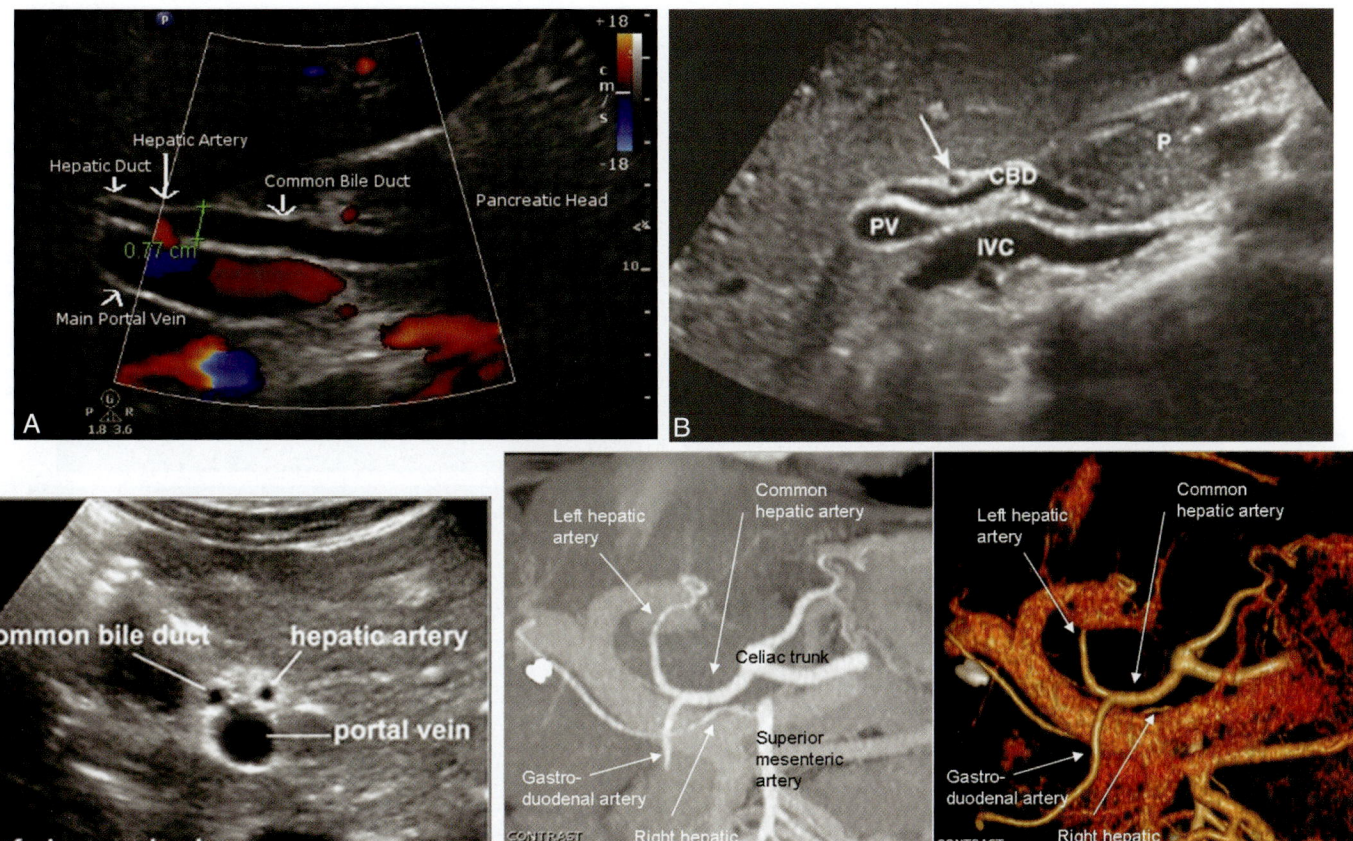

FIG. 9.8 **The hepatic artery arises from the celiac trunk to supply the liver.** The right and left branches of the hepatic artery accompany the portal veins. *CBD*, Common bile duct; *IVC*, inferior vena cava; *P*, pancreas; *PV*, portal vein.

from the liver into the inferior vena cava. The hepatic arteries carry oxygenated blood from the aorta to the liver. The bile ducts transport bile manufactured in the liver to the duodenum.

PHYSIOLOGY AND LABORATORY DATA OF THE HEPATOBILIARY SYSTEM

The liver, bile ducts, and gallbladder constitute the hepatobiliary system, which performs metabolic and excretory functions essential to physical well-being. Although sonography is an important clinical tool for detecting anatomic changes associated with hepatobiliary disease, accurate sonographic evaluation can be accomplished only when other diagnostic information (e.g., signs, symptoms, and laboratory results) are considered in conjunction with the sonographic findings. The task of correlating these clinical and ultrasound data falls primarily to the sonologist. However, the sonographer must also understand the entire clinical picture to be able to plan and properly perform the ultrasound examination. It is necessary, therefore, that the sonographer be aware of the normal and abnormal physiology of the hepatobiliary system. This section is intended as a primer of hepatobiliary physiology, with particular attention to physiologic alterations that commonly occur in hepatobiliary disease.

Hepatic Physiology

The liver has many functions, including metabolism, digestion, storage, and detoxification (Box 9.2). The liver is a significant center of metabolism, which may be defined as the physical and chemical process whereby foodstuffs are synthesized into complex elements, complex substances are transformed into simple ones, and energy is made available for use by the organism. Through the process of digestion, the liver expels these waste products from the body via its excretory product, bile, which also plays an important role in fat absorption. **Bilirubin** is a pigment released when the red blood cells are broken down. The liver is a storage site for several compounds used in a variety of physiologic activities throughout the body. In hepatobiliary disease, each of these functions may be altered, leading to abnormal physical, laboratory, and sonographic findings. Finally, the liver is also a center for detoxification of the waste products of metabolism accumulated from other sources in the body and foreign chemicals (usually drugs) that enter the body.

Hepatic Versus Obstructive Disease

Diseases affecting the liver may be classified as *hepatocellular*, when the liver cells or hepatocytes are the immediate

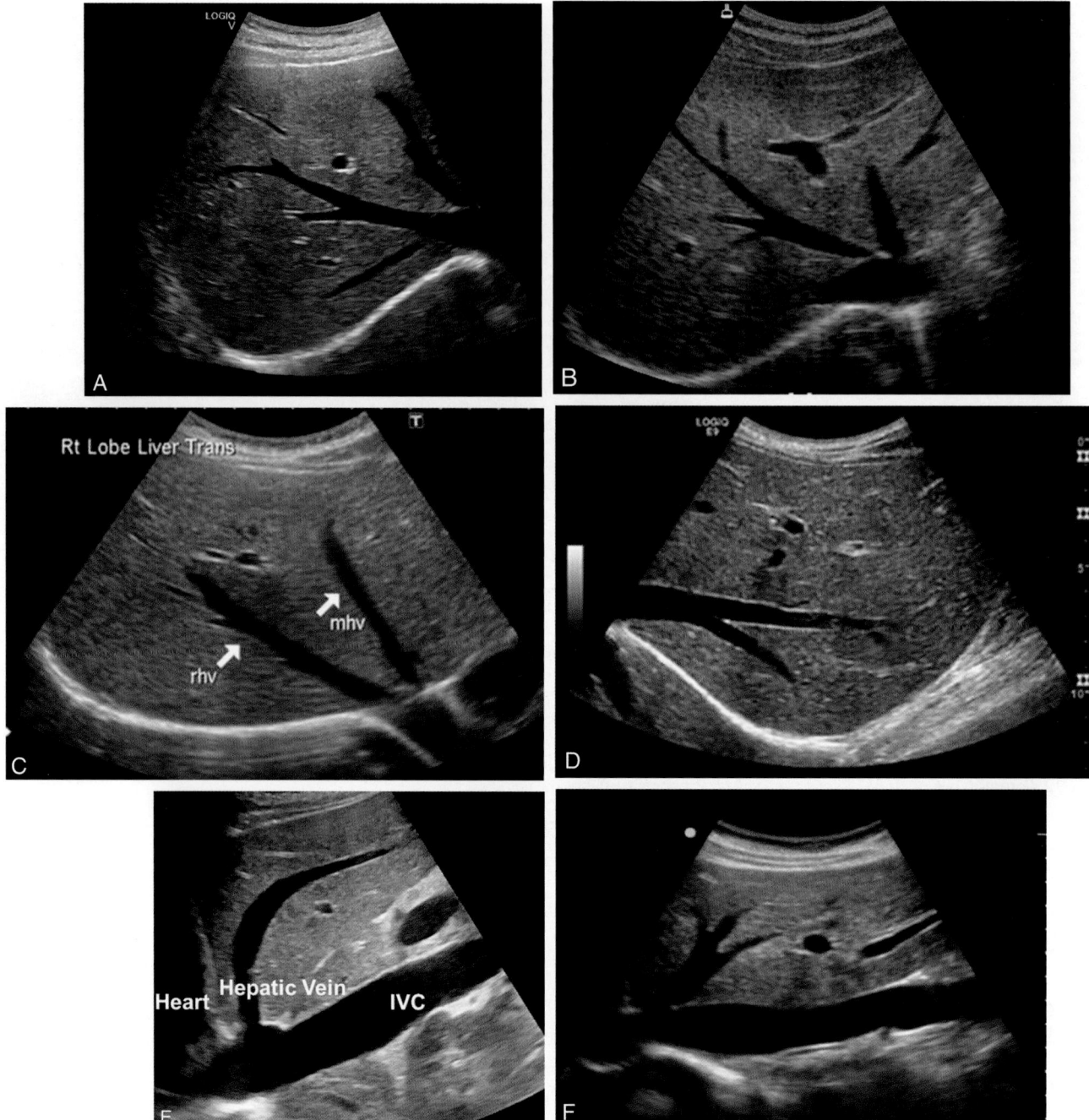

FIG. 9.9 The hepatic veins have three main components—right, middle, and left—that drain into the inferior vena cava (IVC). The right hepatic vein is the largest, courses in the right intersegmental fissure, and enters the right lateral aspect of the IVC. The middle hepatic vein courses in the main lobar fissure and enters the anterior or right anterior surface of the IVC. The left hepatic vein, which is the smallest, enters the left anterior surface of the IVC. (A–C) Transverse images. (D–F) Longitudinal images. *mhv*, Middle hepatic vein; *rhv*, right hepatic vein.

problems, or *obstructive* when bile excretion is blocked. Viral hepatitis is an example of hepatocellular liver disease: The virus attacks liver cells and damages or destroys them, resulting in altered liver function. In obstructive disorders, the flow of bile from the liver is blocked at some point, and the liver malfunctions as a secondary result of the blockage.

The differentiation between **hepatocellular disease** and **obstructive disease** is of considerable importance clinically. Hepatocellular diseases are treated medically with supportive measures and drugs; obstructive disorders are usually treated surgically. In some cases the distinction between hepatocellular and obstructive disease can be made through clinical laboratory tests, but often the laboratory findings are equivocal. Sonography has been of great benefit because it allows the physician to accurately separate hepatocellular and obstructive causes of liver disease.

Hepatic Metabolic Functions

Raw materials in the form of carbohydrates (sugars), fats, and amino acids (basic components of proteins) are absorbed from the intestine and transported to the liver via the circulatory system. In the liver, these substances are converted chemically to other compounds or are processed for storage or energy production. The following sections are brief discussions of the liver's metabolic functions and of how liver disease can disturb these functions.

Carbohydrates. Sugars may be absorbed from the blood in several forms, but only glucose can be used by cells throughout the body as a source of energy. The liver functions as a significant site for the conversion of dietary sugars into glucose, which is released into the bloodstream for general use. The body requires only a certain amount of glucose at any one time. Excess sugar is converted by the liver to glycogen (a starch), which may be stored in the liver cells or transported in the blood to distant storage sites. When dietary sugar is unavailable, the liver converts glycogen released from storage into glucose; it can also manufacture glucose directly from other compounds, including proteins or fats, when other sources of glucose have been depleted. Thus the liver helps to maintain a steady state of glucose in the bloodstream.

In severe liver disease, unless glucose is administered intravenously, the body may become glucose-deficient (**hypoglycemia**), with profound effects on the function of the brain and other organs. Uncontrolled increases in blood glucose (**hyperglycemia**) may occur in severe liver disease if a large dose of glucose is administered because the liver fails to convert the excess glucose to glycogen.

Fats. The liver is also a principal site for the metabolism of fats, which are absorbed from the intestine in the form of monoglycerides and diglycerides. Dietary fats are converted in the hepatocytes to lipoproteins, in which form fats are transported throughout the body to sites where they are stored or used by other organs. Conversely, stored fats may be transported to the liver and converted into energy, yielding glucose or other substances, such as cholesterol.

In severe liver disease, abnormally low blood levels of cholesterol may be noted because the liver is the principal site for cholesterol synthesis. Furthermore, failure of hepatic conversion of fat to glucose in liver disease may contribute to hypoglycemia. A *striking histologic* manifestation of many forms of hepatocellular disease is the so-called *fatty liver*. On gross pathologic examination, the fatty liver has a yellow color and feels greasy to the touch; on microscopic study, globules of fat (primarily triglycerides) crowd the hepatocytes. The cause of fat accumulation in the liver cells is poorly understood, but it is believed to result from failure of the hepatocytes to manufacture special proteins, called lipoproteins, that coat small quantities of fat, making the fat soluble in plasma and allowing for its release into the bloodstream. Fatty liver is a nonspecific finding that may be seen in a variety of conditions, including viral hepatitis, alcoholic

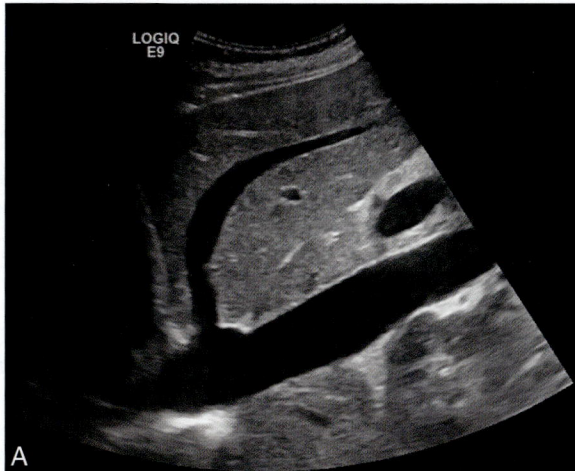
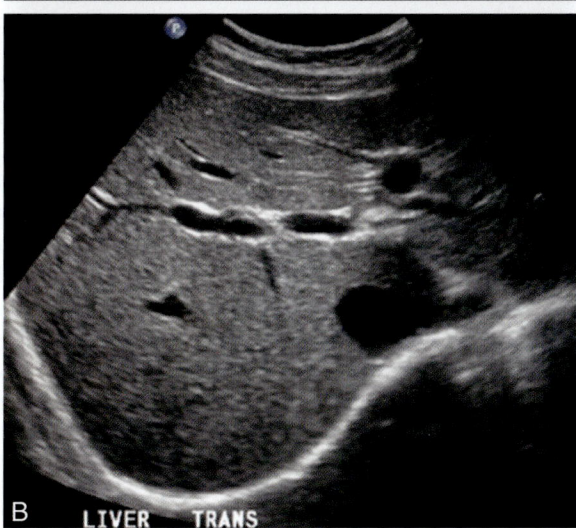

FIG. 9.10 (A) The hepatic vessels flow into the inferior vena cava, whereas the splenic vein and superior mesenteric vein join to form the portal venous system. (B) The portal veins are larger at their origin as they emanate from the porta hepatis. Portal veins have more echogenic borders than the hepatic veins because they have a thicker collagenous sheath.

BOX 9.2 Primary Functions of the Liver

Metabolism
- *Carbohydrate.* The liver converts glucose to glycogen and stores it; when glucose is needed, it breaks down the glycogen and releases glucose into the blood.
- *Protein.* The liver performs many important functions in metabolism of proteins, fats, and carbohydrates. It manufactures many of the plasma proteins found in the blood. The liver converts excess amino acids to fatty acids and urea. It also removes nutrients from the blood and phagocytizes bacteria and worn-out red blood cells.

Digestion
The liver secretes bile, which is important in the digestion of fats. Bilirubin, a pigment released when red blood cells are broken down, is excreted in the bile.

Storage
The liver stores iron and certain vitamins.

Detoxification
The liver detoxifies many drugs and poisons that enter the body.

liver disease, obesity, diabetes, pregnancy, and exposure to toxic chemicals.

Proteins. The liver produces a variety of proteins, either indirectly from amino acids absorbed from the gut or directly from raw materials stored within the body. Albumin, in particular, is produced in significant quantities. In the bloodstream, it functions as a transport medium for some kinds of molecules. Because it is nonionic, it also functions to draw water into the vascular system from tissue spaces; therefore it helps to maintain oncotic pressure within the vascular system. When the liver is chronically diseased, clinical laboratory results may reveal a significant lowering of the serum albumin, a condition called *hypoalbuminemia*. The accompanying loss of osmotic pressure in the vascular system allows fluid to migrate into the interstitial space, resulting in edema (swelling) in dependent areas, such as the lower extremities. In patients with severe liver disease, especially advanced cirrhosis, ascites also develops. Hypoalbuminemia may account in part for the ascites, but the development of ascites is principally caused by portal hypertension.

In addition to being the primary source of albumin synthesis, the liver is the principal source of proteins necessary for blood coagulation, including fibrinogen (factor I), prothrombin (factor II), and factors V, VII, IX, and X. In liver disease, decreased production of these proteins may lead to inadequate blood coagulation and uncontrollable hemorrhage. Commonly, such hemorrhages occur into the bowel after rupture of a dilated vein or development of an ulcer. These hemorrhages are often the immediate or contributing cause of death. Deficiencies of clotting factors II, VII, IX, and X also may result from failure of intestinal absorption of vitamin K, which is a precursor (raw material) required for synthesis of these factors. Vitamin K is a fat-soluble vitamin (as are vitamins D, A, and E) and is absorbed only from the intestine in solution with fat.

Fat absorption is severely limited in cases of bile duct obstruction because of the absence of bile salts (discussed later), which severely reduces the absorption of fat-soluble vitamins. Ultimately, the deficiency of vitamin K lowers the amount of the previously mentioned factors, and coagulation is retarded. Deficiency of prothrombin and other vitamin K–dependent factors can be corrected in cases of obstruction through parenteral administration of vitamin K.

In hepatocellular disease, administration of vitamin K may improve the coagulopathy but frequently does not restore normal clotting function because the primary problem is hepatocyte dysfunction.

Clotting deficiencies related to liver disease may be detected with several laboratory tests. Of particular interest are the prothrombin time (pro-time) and partial thromboplastin time tests. The results of these tests are presented as percentages of the time required for certain coagulation steps to occur in the patient's blood compared with normal blood. Longer periods (lower percentages) indicate greater degrees of abnormality in each of these tests.

Enzymes. Enzymes are protein catalysts used throughout the body in all metabolic processes. Because the liver is a major center of metabolism, large quantities of enzymes are present in hepatocytes, and these enzymes leak into the bloodstream when the liver cells are damaged or destroyed by disease. The presence of increased quantities of enzymes in the blood is a sensitive indicator of a hepatocellular disorder.

In hepatobiliary disease the enzymes **aspartate aminotransferase (AST)**, **alanine aminotransferase (ALT)**, and alkaline phosphatase are of particular interest. Serum levels of all three of these enzymes are increased in both hepatocellular disease and biliary obstruction, but the patterns of elevation may help differentiate hepatocellular from obstructive causes (Table 9.1). In biliary obstruction, elevation of AST and ALT is usually mild (serum levels typically do not exceed 300 units). However, in severe hepatocellular destruction, such as acute viral or toxic hepatitis, a striking elevation of AST and ALT may be seen (levels frequently exceed 1000 units).

Marked elevation of alkaline phosphatase, on the other hand, is typically associated with biliary obstruction or the presence of mass lesions in the liver (e.g., metastatic disease or abscesses). Low levels of alkaline phosphatase are unusual in obstruction, and high levels (greater than 15 Bodansky units) are uncommon in hepatocellular disorders. Alkaline phosphatase is such a sensitive indicator of obstruction that it may become elevated before the serum bilirubin in cases of acute obstruction. Hence, a disproportional increase of alkaline phosphatase relative to bilirubin always suggests obstruction. Elevation of serum alkaline phosphatase may be the only abnormal laboratory finding in metastatic disease.

Whereas the pattern of enzyme abnormality may strongly suggest hepatocellular disease or obstruction in some cases, it may not allow this distinction to be made in others because obstruction may be superimposed on preexisting hepatocellular disease or unrelieved obstruction may cause hepatocellular damage. Confusion in interpretation of serum enzyme abnormalities may also occur when AST, ALT, or alkaline

TABLE 9.1	Comparison of Laboratory Abnormalities in Hepatocellular Disease and Biliary Obstruction				
Condition	**Bilirubin**	**Serum Albumin**	**AST**	**ALT**	**Alkaline Phosphatase**
Hepatocellular disease	Minimal to severe increase	Decreased	Moderate to severe increase	Moderate to severe increase	Minimal to moderate increase
Obstruction	Severe increase	Normal	Mild increase	Mild increase	Severe increase

ALT, Alanine aminotrasnferase; *AST*, aspartate aminotransferase.

phosphatase is released from diseased tissues other than the liver. For example, AST and ALT increase with damage to heart and skeletal muscle, and alkaline phosphatase elevates in bone disease and in normal pregnancies. ALT is somewhat more specific for liver disease than AST; therefore elevation of ALT above AST suggests a hepatic cause.

Hepatic Detoxification Functions

The liver is a significant location for detoxification of waste products of energy production and other metabolic activities occurring throughout the body. It is also the principal site of breakdown of foreign chemicals, such as drugs. Although these functions fall under the general definition of metabolism and could therefore be grouped in the preceding section, it is useful for instructional purposes to think of these functions as separate categories of hepatic activity.

Ammonium, a toxic product of nitrogen metabolism, is converted to nontoxic urea in the liver, which is practically the only site where this conversion occurs. Urea is subsequently eliminated from the body by the kidneys. The level of urea in the blood is measured as the blood urea nitrogen (BUN), and in severe liver disease (acute or chronic) the blood urea nitrogen may be abnormally low because of falloff of urea production. The exhaled breath of patients with severe liver disease may have a fruity or pungent odor (known as *fetor hepaticus*) because of ammonium (NH_4) accumulation. More importantly, the concentration of NH_4 in the blood may rise to toxic levels and cause brain dysfunction (including confusion, coordination disturbances, tremor, and coma).

Gastrointestinal hemorrhage frequently leads to the accumulation of toxic levels of NH_4 in the blood. Blood lost into the intestine is broken down by bacteria into nitrogen-containing substances, which are absorbed into the bloodstream. The failing liver may therefore be presented with a large amount of NH_4 that it cannot detoxify; coma may result and is frequently a precursor to death if the patient does not succumb to the direct effects of blood loss. Thus failure of ammonium detoxification is a serious consequence of liver failure.

Bilirubin Detoxification. Bilirubin, the breakdown product of hemoglobin, is also an important substance detoxified in the liver. Along with detoxification, the liver also excretes bilirubin into the gut via the biliary tree. Red blood cells survive an average of 120 days in the circulatory system; they are then trapped and broken down by reticuloendothelial cells, primarily within the spleen. Hemoglobin released from the red cells is converted to bilirubin within the reticuloendothelial system and is then released into the bloodstream. The bilirubin molecules become attached to albumin in the blood and are transported to the liver where the following metabolic steps take place in the hepatocytes:

1. *Uptake.* The bilirubin is separated from albumin, probably at the cell membrane, and is taken within the hepatocytes.
2. *Conjugation.* The bilirubin molecule is combined with two glucuronide molecules, forming bilirubin diglucuronide.
3. *Excretion.* The bilirubin molecule is actively transported across the cell membrane into the bile canaliculi, which are the microscopic "headwaters" of the biliary system. Bilirubin released from the hepatocytes passes through the bile ducts with other components of bile and is delivered to the bowel, where most bilirubin diglucuronide is excreted into the feces. (A small portion is broken down into urobilinogen by intestinal bacteria, absorbed into the portal system, and re-excreted by the liver.)

Measurement of the concentration of bilirubin in the blood is a standard laboratory test for hepatocellular disease. The following two fractions of bilirubin are measured: the direct-acting fraction, which reacts chemically in an aqueous medium and consists of conjugated bilirubin, and the indirect-acting fraction, which consists of unconjugated bilirubin released from the reticuloendothelial system. Indirect bilirubin reacts only in a nonaqueous (alcohol) medium. The total bilirubin is the sum of the direct-acting and the indirect-acting fractions and typically does not exceed 1 mg/100 mL of serum. In hematologic diseases associated with an abrupt breakdown of large numbers of red blood cells (hemolytic anemias, transfusion reactions), the liver may receive more bilirubin from the reticuloendothelial system than it can detoxify. The level of indirect, or unconjugated, bilirubin, therefore, is elevated.

In biliary obstruction, the hepatocytes pick up bilirubin and conjugate it with glucuronide molecules but cannot dispose of it. The conjugated form is then regurgitated into the bloodstream, with resultant elevation of the direct-acting bilirubin fraction. The indirect-acting bilirubin may also rise slightly in biliary obstruction, but the direct bilirubin predominates.

The direct, or conjugated, form also predominates in hepatocellular disease. Excretion of bilirubin is the step most readily affected when the hepatocytes are damaged; therefore the diseased hepatocytes continue to take in and conjugate bilirubin but are unable to excrete it. As in biliary obstruction, the accumulated conjugated bilirubin is regurgitated into the blood.

The direct and indirect patterns may be summarized as in Table 9.2.

Elevation of serum bilirubin results in jaundice, a yellow coloration of the skin, sclerae, and body secretions. Jaundice is a nonspecific finding seen in massive blood breakdown, hepatocellular disease, or biliary obstruction. Chemical separation of bilirubin into direct and indirect fractions helps to specify a hepatocellular or hematologic cause for jaundice. Furthermore, if jaundice results from liver disease, the level of bilirubin may help to separate hepatocellular disease from obstruction because it is uncommon for the total bilirubin to rise above 35 mg/100 mL of serum with obstruction.

TABLE 9.2	Direct and Indirect Patterns of Bilirubin	
Condition	Direct Bilirubin Predominates	Indirect Bilirubin Predominates
Hemolysis		X
Hepatocellular disease	X	
Biliary obstruction	X	

Hormone and Drug Detoxification. The liver breaks down several hormones that otherwise would accumulate in the body. For example, failure to metabolize estrogen in men with chronic hepatocellular disease, such as cirrhosis, causes gynecomastia (breast enlargement), testicular atrophy, and changes in body-hair patterns. Reduced detoxification of the hormone glucagon, which is an insulin antagonist, occurs in liver disease and may contribute to the fluctuations in blood sugar levels seen in severe hepatic disorders. The liver is also the primary location for breakdown of medications and other foreign chemicals administered orally or parenterally. It is of particular concern that doses of medications be reduced to compensate for the loss of this function in patients with severe liver disease; otherwise, accumulation of drugs may lead to overdosage.

Bile

Bile is the excretory product of the liver. It is formed continuously by the hepatocytes, collects in the bile canaliculi adjacent to these cells, and is transported to the gut via the bile ducts (Fig. 9.11). The principal components of bile are water, bile salts, and bile pigments (primarily bilirubin diglucuronide). Other components include cholesterol, lecithin, and protein. The primary functions of bile are the emulsification of intestinal fat and the removal of waste products excreted by the liver.

Fats are absorbed into the portal blood and intestinal lymphatics in the form of monoglycerides and triglycerides by the action of the intestinal mucosa, but efficient absorption occurs only when the fat molecules are suspended in solution through the emulsifying action of bile salts. As emulsifiers, bile salts act like nonionic detergents to suspend fats in solution within the watery medium of the intestinal contents. Both hepatocellular disease and biliary obstruction affect the amount of bile salts available for fat absorption, but obstruction generally has the more profound effect. Absence of bile salts may lead to steatorrhea (fatty stools), but a more important effect is failure of absorption of the fat-soluble vitamins (D, A, K, and E). As previously noted, vitamin K is an essential precursor for hepatic production of several clotting factors; the absence of this vitamin leads to bleeding tendencies in patients with hepatobiliary disease.

Bile Pigments. Bile pigments are the principal cause of ultrasonic scattering in echogenic bile, although cholesterol crystals may also contribute to this finding. The presence of echogenic bile indicates stasis, but this stasis is not always pathologic and may simply result from prolonged fasting.

Liver Function Tests

Liver function tests are a group of laboratory tests established to analyze how the liver is performing under normal and diseased conditions. In patients with known liver disease, several laboratory tests are used to help in the diagnosis, including the following:

- Aspartate aminotransferase (AST)
- Alanine aminotransferase (ALT)
- Lactic acid dehydrogenase (LDH)
- Alkaline phosphatase (alk phos)
- Bilirubin (indirect, direct, and total)
- Prothrombin time
- Albumin and globulins

Aspartate Aminotransferase. AST is an enzyme present in tissues that have a high rate of metabolic activity, one of which is the liver. As a result of death or injury to the producing cells, the enzyme is released into the bloodstream in abnormally high levels. Any disease that injures the cells causes an elevation in AST levels. This enzyme is also produced in other high-metabolic tissues, so an elevation does not always mean liver disease is present. Significant elevations are characteristic of acute hepatitis and cirrhosis. The level is also elevated in patients with hepatic necrosis, acute hepatitis, and infectious mononucleosis.

Alanine Aminotransferase. ALT is more specific than AST for evaluating liver function. This enzyme is slightly elevated in acute cirrhosis, hepatic metastasis, and pancreatitis. There is a mild to moderate increase in obstructive jaundice. Hepatocellular disease and infectious or toxic hepatitis produce moderate to highly increased levels. In alcoholic hepatitis, AST is higher.

Lactic Acid Dehydrogenase. Lactic acid dehydrogenase is found in the tissues of several systems, including the kidneys, heart, skeletal muscle, brain, liver, and lungs. Cellular injury and death cause this enzyme to increase. This test is

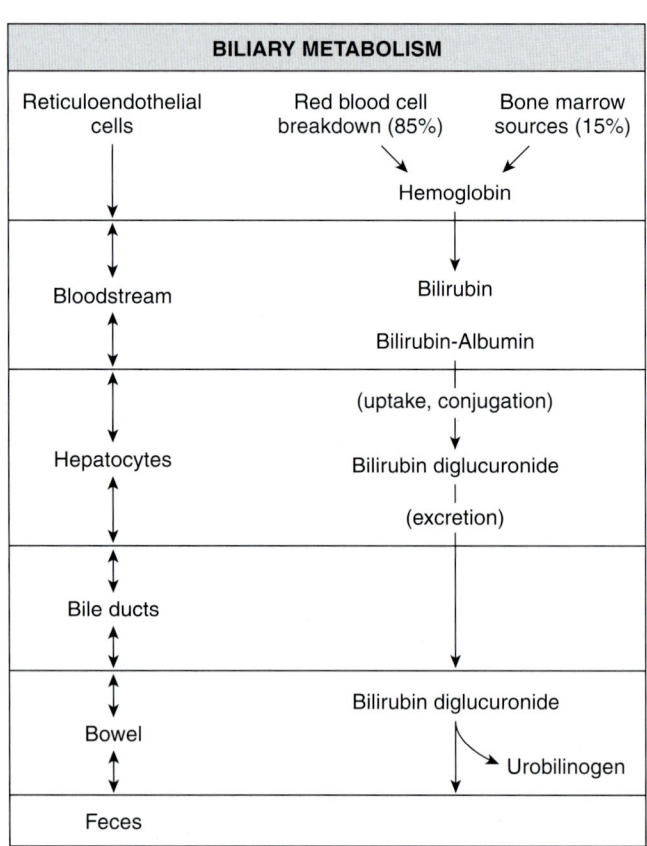

FIG. 9.11 Biliary metabolism.

moderately increased in infectious mononucleosis and mildly elevated in hepatitis, cirrhosis, and obstructive jaundice. Its primary use is in detection of myocardial or pulmonary infarction.

Alkaline Phosphatase. **Alkaline phosphatase** is produced by the liver, bone, intestines, and placenta. It may be a good indicator of intrahepatic or extrahepatic obstruction, hepatic carcinoma, abscess, or cirrhosis. In hepatitis and cirrhosis the enzyme is moderately elevated.

Bilirubin. Bilirubin is a product of the breakdown of hemoglobin in tired red blood cells. The liver converts these by-products into bile pigments, which, along with other factors, are secreted as bile by the liver cells into the bile ducts. The following are three ways this cycle can be disturbed:
- An excessive amount of red blood cell destruction
- Malfunction of liver cells
- Blockage of ducts leading from cells

These disturbances cause a rise in serum bilirubin, which leaks into the tissues and thus gives the skin a jaundiced, or yellow, coloration.

Indirect bilirubin is unconjugated bilirubin. Elevation of this test result is seen with increased red blood cell destruction (anemias, trauma from a hematoma, or hemorrhagic pulmonary infarct).

Direct bilirubin is conjugated bilirubin. This product circulates in the blood and is excreted into the bile after it reaches the liver and is conjugated with glucuronide. Elevation of direct bilirubin is usually related to obstructive jaundice (from stones or neoplasm).

Specific liver diseases may cause an elevation of both direct and indirect bilirubin levels, but the increase in the direct level is more marked. These diseases are hepatic metastasis, hepatitis, lymphoma, cholestasis secondary to drugs, and cirrhosis.

Prothrombin Time. Prothrombin is a liver enzyme that is part of the blood clotting mechanism. The production of prothrombin depends on adequate intake and use of vitamin K. The prothrombin time is increased in the presence of liver disease with cellular damage. Cirrhosis and metastatic disease are examples of disorders that cause prolonged prothrombin time.

Albumin and Globulins. Assessment of depressed synthesis of proteins, especially serum albumin and the plasma coagulation factors, is a sensitive test for metabolic derangement of the liver. In patients with hepatocellular damage, a low serum albumin suggests decreased protein synthesis. A prolonged prothrombin time indicates a poor prognosis. Chronic liver diseases commonly show an elevation of gamma globulins.

SONOGRAPHIC EVALUATION OF THE LIVER

Evaluation of the hepatic structures is one of the most important procedures in sonography for many reasons. The normal homogeneous parenchyma of the liver allows imaging of the neighboring anatomic structures in the upper abdomen. Echo amplitude, attenuation, transmission, and parenchymal textures may be sonographically assessed with proper evaluation of the hepatic structures. The patient should be instructed to fast for at least 6 to 8 hours to eliminate bowel gas and assure distention of the gallbladder. The liver is examined with the patient in a supine or right anterior oblique position, usually with deep inspiration to allow the liver to move inferior to the rib cage. The liver is then examined in a transverse, coronal, subcostal oblique, and sagittal view to completely survey the organ. The left lobe of the liver is imaged from the subxiphoid window with the transducer angled slightly cephalic. The right lobe of the liver may be imaged from both a subcostal and intercostal approach. The intercostal space is generally most effective with the patient supine with normal respiration to avoid interference from the right lung base. The patient may be instructed to place their arm above their head to help open the intercostal spaces and allow better probe connection to image the hepatic parenchyma. Rib shadowing may also be minimized by using a smaller transducer face or scanning obliquely in a plane parallel to the long axis of the intercostal spaces. If adequate windows are not available through the subxiphoid or intercostal window, the subcostal approach may be used. This approach requires the patient to be rolled slightly into a left lateral decubitus or left posterior oblique position to allow the liver to shift medial and inferior, thus providing a better window for visualization. Keep in mind the transducer should be angled in a superior enough position to fully image the dome of the liver and the diaphragm.

Within the homogeneous liver parenchyma lie the thin-walled hepatic veins, the brightly reflective portal veins, the hepatic arteries, and the hepatic duct. Color flow Doppler imaging is useful in determining the direction of flow of the portal and hepatic veins in relation to the Doppler probe (Fig. 9.12). The portal flow is shown to be **hepatopetal** (toward the liver), whereas the hepatic venous flow is **hepatofugal** (away from the liver). The portal vein serves as the landmark to locate the smaller hepatic duct and artery. Near the porta hepatis, the hepatic duct can be seen along the anterior lateral border of the portal vein, whereas the hepatic artery can be seen along the anterior medial border (Fig. 9.13). With color Doppler, the hepatic artery would show flow toward the liver, whereas the ductal system would show no flow.

The system gain should be adjusted to adequately penetrate the entire right lobe of the liver as a smooth, homogeneous echo-texture pattern (Fig. 9.14A–B). Adequate sensitivity (gain) must be adjusted to image the normal smooth liver parenchyma. If too much gain is used, the electronic "noise" or "snow" is produced that appears as low-level echoes in the background of the image (e.g., outside the liver parenchyma, above the diaphragm, or within the vascular structures). The ultrasound manufacturers have made it possible to preselect various pre -and postprocessing controls to allow the sonographer to emphasize or highlight various aspects of the liver parenchyma. This setting is automatically visible on the monitor once the equipment is turned on or the "reset" button is depressed.

The time gain compensation (TGC) should be adjusted to balance the far-gain and the near-gain echo signals. The

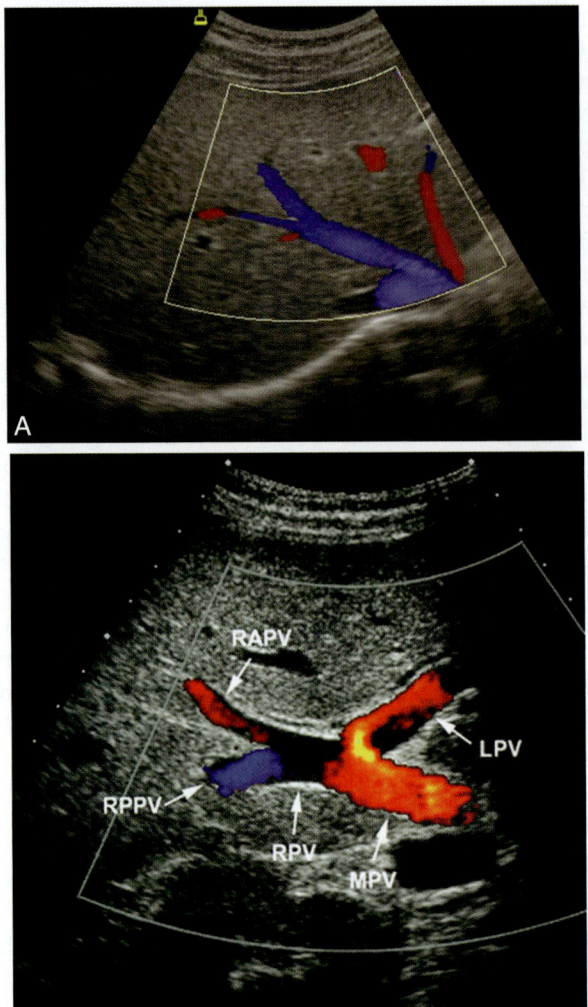

FIG. 9.12 Color flow Doppler imaging is useful in determining the direction of flow of the portal and hepatic veins in relation to the Doppler probe. (A) The hepatic vein flow is hepatofugal (away from the liver). (B) The portal flow is shown to be hepatopetal (toward the liver). *LPV*, Left portal vein; *MPV*, main portal vein; *RAPV*, right anterior portal vein; *RPPV*, right posterior portal vein; *RPV*, right portal vein.

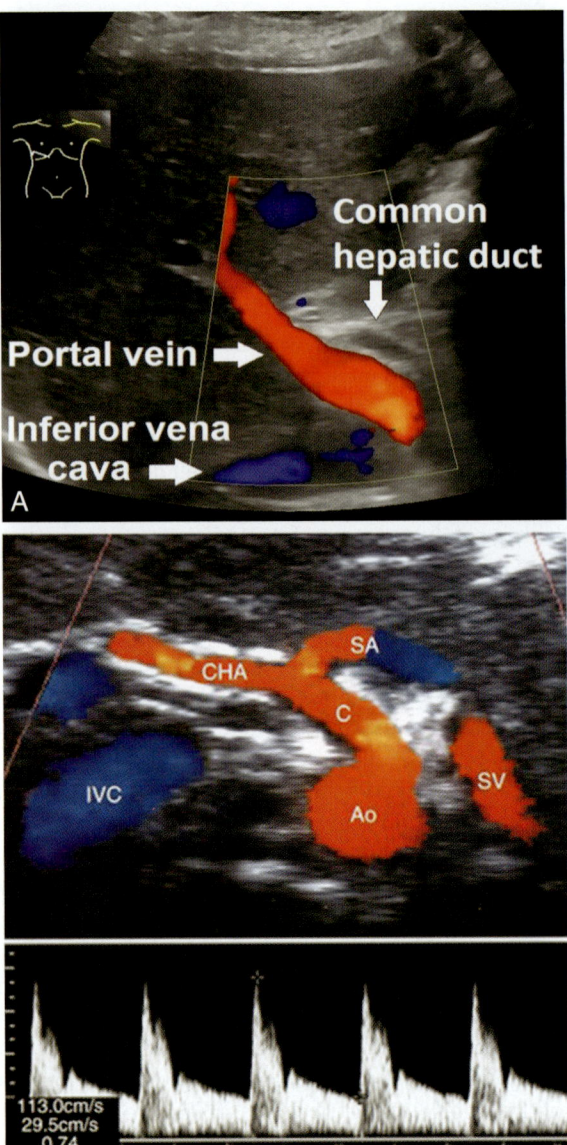

FIG. 9.13 (A) Near the porta hepatis, the hepatic duct can be seen along the anterior lateral border of the portal vein, whereas the hepatic artery can be seen along the anterior medial border (B). *Ao*, Aorta; *C*, celiac trunk; *CHA*, common hepatic artery; *IVC*, inferior vena cava; *SA*, splenic artery; *SV*, splenic vein.

easiest way to do this is to hold the transducer over a deep segment of the right lobe of the liver. The far TGC pods should gradually be increased with a smooth motion of the index finger until the posterior aspect of the liver is clearly visible. The near-field, TGC pods should be adjusted (usually decreased) to distinguish the anterior wall and muscles, the anterior hepatic capsule, and the near field of the hepatic parenchyma.

The depth should be adjusted so the posterior right lobe is positioned at the lower border of the screen (Fig. 9.14C–D). The electronic focus on the equipment is positioned near the posterior border of the liver, or the multiple focus points may be positioned equidistant throughout the liver to further enhance the hepatic parenchyma. The multifocal technique causes the frame rate to decrease and thus causes a "slower sweep" of the real-time image (Fig. 9.15). If the patient cannot take a deep breath, the sonographer may choose not to use the multiple-frequency focus with decreased frame rate. In most patients who can suspend their respiration for a variable amount of time, this multifocal technique works well because the liver is a non-dynamic organ and does not need a high frame rate to obtain a quality image.

The appropriate transducer depends on the patient's body habitus and the clinical request for the ultrasound examination. The transducer frequency depends on the body habitus and size. The average adult abdomen usually requires at least a broadband 2.5- to 5-MHz frequency, whereas the more obese adult may require a lower frequency transducer. Slender adults and young children may require a higher frequency,

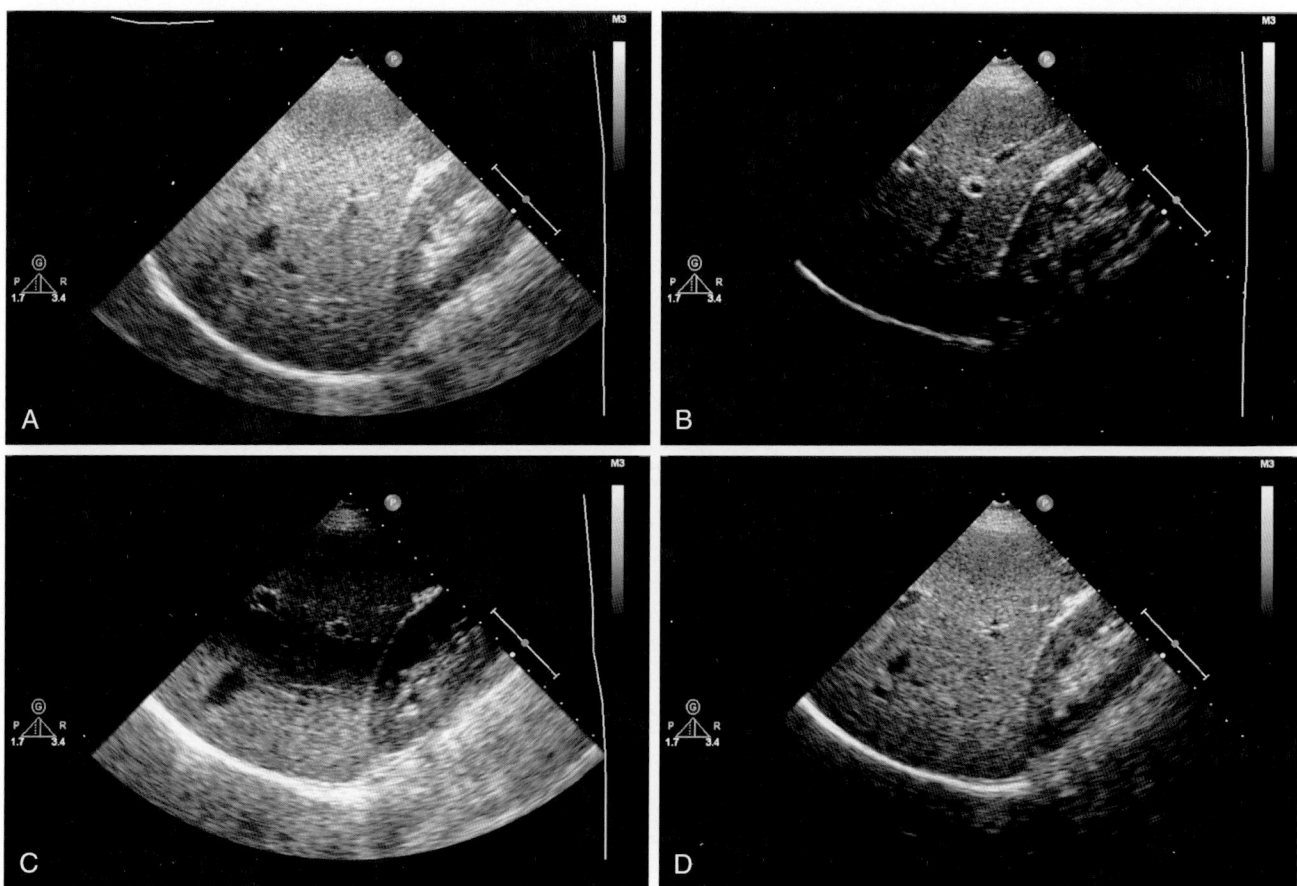

FIG. 9.14 (A) Longitudinal image of the liver shows equal distribution of echoes from anterior to posterior, which means the gain and time gain compensation settings are correct. (B) Incorrect gain settings show the lack of echoes in the distal (posterior) lobe of the liver. (C) Incorrect near field gain settings eliminate texture information in more than half of the liver. (D) Depth of field set correctly at 15 cm with a balanced time gain compensation to balance the near and far fields.

while the neonate may need an even higher frequency, 7.5- to 12-MHz transducer.

Generally, a wider "pie" sector or curved linear array transducer is the most appropriate to optimally image the near field of the abdomen (Fig. 9.16). This transducer is especially useful in detecting liver abscesses or metastases. To image the far field better, a sector or curved array transducer with a longer focal zone is used. Often the transducers are interchanged throughout the examination to obtain the ideal image pattern.

Liver and Porta Hepatis Protocol

The liver is examined as part of a comprehensive sonographic evaluation of the abdomen. Adequate scanning technique demands that each patient be examined with the following assessment criteria: The size of the liver in the longitudinal plane should measure approximately 15 cm; the liver parenchyma is homogeneous with the presence of hepatic vascular structures, ligaments, and fissures; the liver texture is usually greater than the right kidney, but less than the pancreas and spleen; the surface of the liver is smooth (Fig. 9.17).

The basic ultrasound instrumentation should be adjusted for each patient: TGC should be altered to balance the echoes in the near, mid, and far field; overall gain adjusted to see detail within the structure; change transducer frequency and type (sector, linear), and the depth and focus. Color and pulsed wave Doppler are used to assess the hepatic vascular system (Table 9.3).

1. Patient preparation: Nothing by mouth (NPO) for at least 6 to 8 hours.
2. Transducer selection: 2.5 to 4 MHz curvilinear/sector, or 3 to 5 MHz curvilinear.
3. Patient position: Supine and decubitus as necessary.
4. Images and observations should include the following:
   - Compare echogenicity of the liver parenchyma to the renal parenchyma.
   - Identify hepatic veins, portal veins, and inferior vena cava.
   - Ligamentum teres (LT) should be identified in the left lobe of the liver.
   - The dome of the right lobe of the liver should be surveyed with the patient in deep inspiration.
   - The right hemidiaphragm and right pleural gutter.
   - The main lobar fissure, as it projects from the right portal vein (RPV) to the neck of the gallbladder.
   - Liver size in a parasagittal scan demonstrating the diaphragm and tip of the right lobe of the liver should be measured.

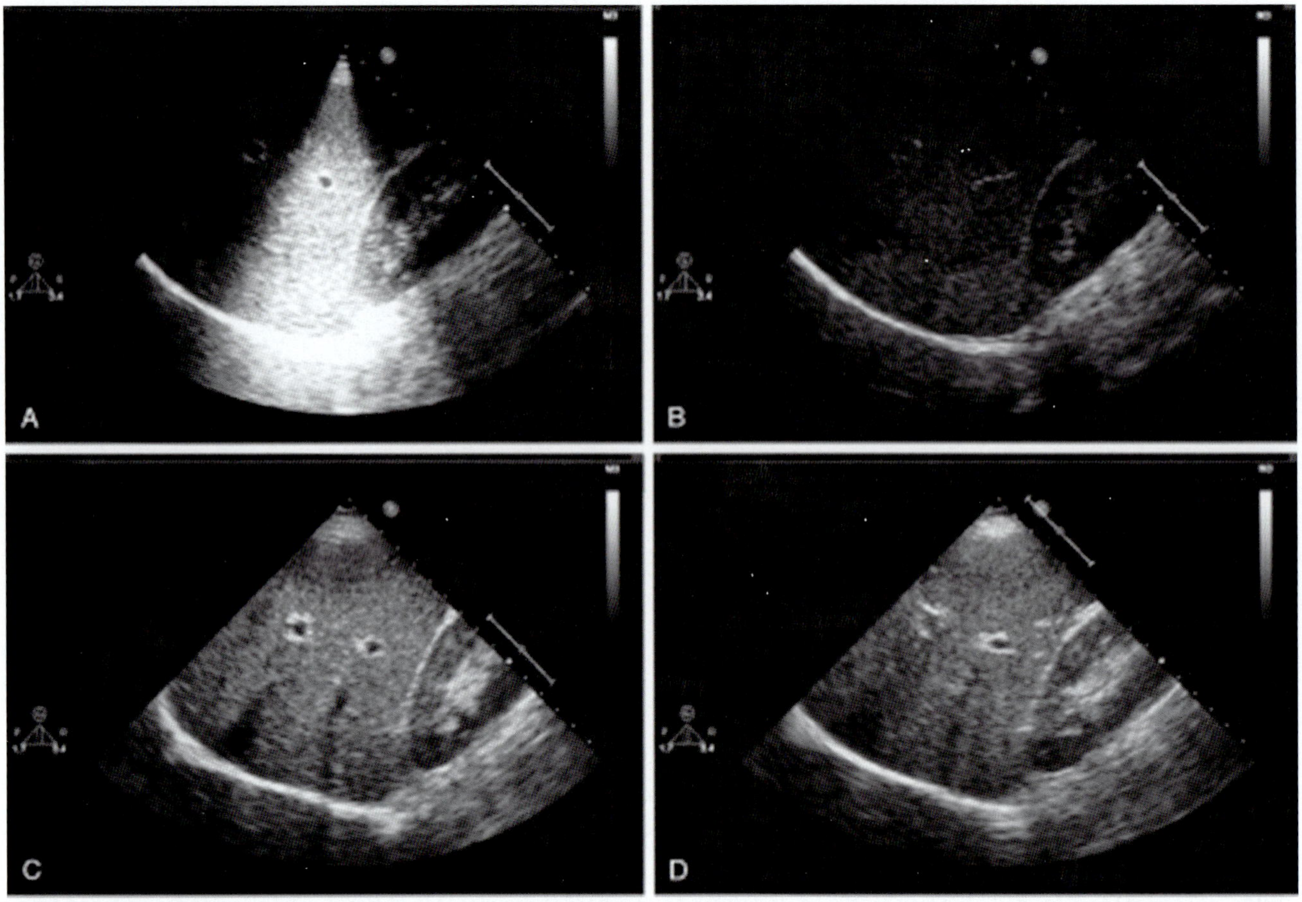

FIG. 9.15 (A–C) Examples of incorrect gain/focal zone settings (look at the line to the right of the image). The focal zone should be set to encompass the total area of interest or to "clean up" the far field echoes to increase sharpness. (D) Shadowing from the portal veins or variations in breathing may cause image distortion.

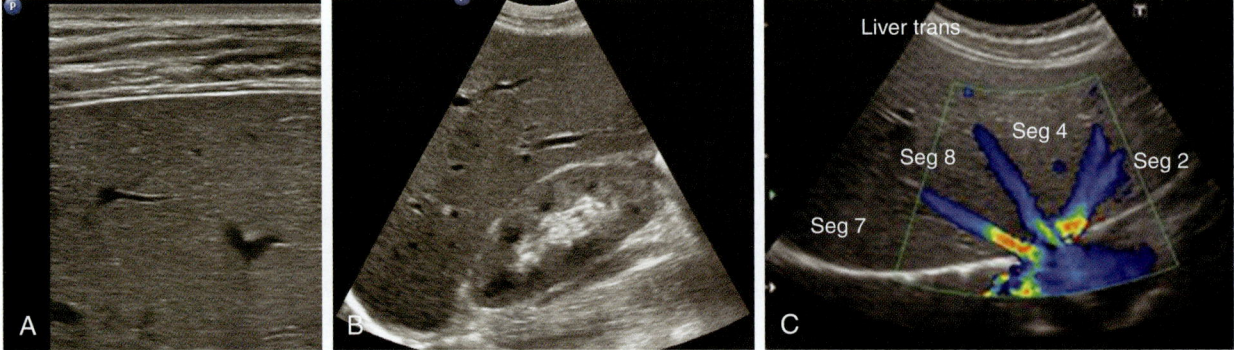

FIG. 9.16 (A) Linear array with excellent visualization of the near field of the liver. (B) Small sector probe limits the near field of view. (C) Curved array versus sector changes the near field of focus and the focal zone in the far field.

- The size of any demonstrated masses should be imaged in two planes.

Color and spectral Doppler of the vascular structures in the liver if pathology is present:
- Assessment of the patency and direction of flow of the main, right, and left portal veins.
- Assessment of the patency of the right, middle, and left hepatic veins.
- Assessment of the patency of the umbilical vein (recanalized umbilical vein) or other collateral vessels.
- Assessment of the patency of surgically or angiographically placed shunts.
- Performance of pulsed Doppler analysis of the hepatic artery with resistance measurements.

Normal Sonographic Anatomy and Texture

The upper border of the liver is usually found at the fifth intercostal space at the midclavicular line. The lower border of the liver may extend to slightly below the costal margin.

CHAPTER 9 The Liver

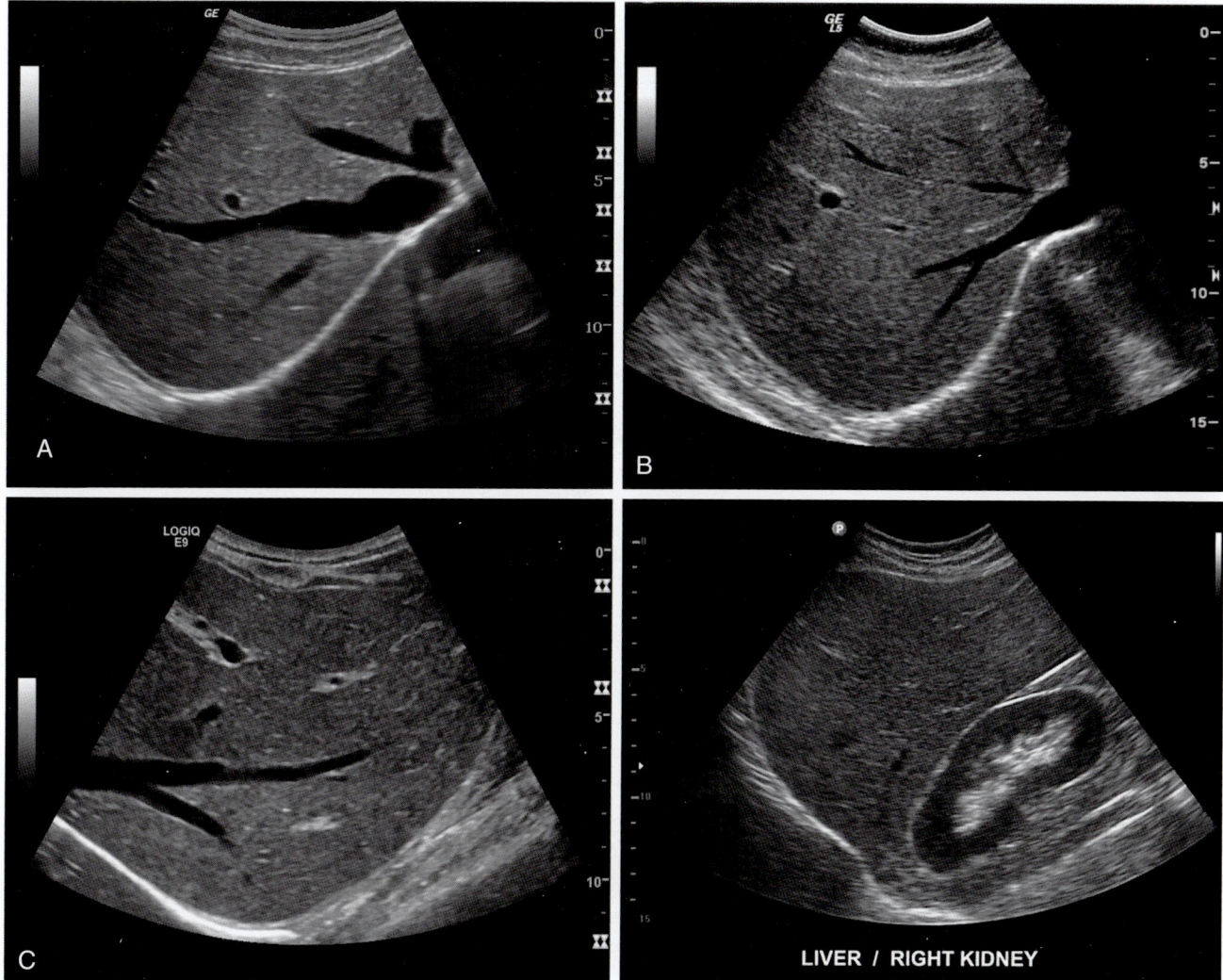

FIG. 9.17 Transverse (A–B) and longitudinal (C–D) images should show adequate gain, time gain compensation, depth, and landmarks within the liver (ligaments, vascular structures, and spine).

TABLE 9.3	Abdominal Ultrasound Protocol: Liver	
Organ	Scan Plane	Anatomy
Liver	Transverse Right lobe/ (dome) hepatic veins	Right lobe/lung Left lobe/left portal vein Left lobe/caudate lobe Right lobe/portal veins (main, right) Right lobe/gallbladder/kidney
	Longitudinal	Left lobe/aorta Left lobe/caudate lobe/IVC Right lobe/dome (diaphragm) Right lobe/lung Right lobe/portal vein Right lobe/kidney (measure right lobe)

IVC, Inferior vena cava.

The length of the liver may be assessed in the midclavicular line, usually measuring approximately 15.5 cm. On occasion, a normal tongue-like variant, Reidel lobe, may be seen as an extension of the right lobe. The normal texture of the liver is homogeneous with fine, low-level echoes. Compared to the renal cortex of the kidneys, the liver texture is minimally hyperechoic to isoechoic. Compared to the texture of the spleen, the liver is hypoechoic.

Sagittal Plane

The sagittal plane offers an excellent window to visualize the hepatic structures (Fig. 9.18). With the patient in full inspiration, the transducer may be swept from the base of the costal margin (with slight to medium pressure) in a cephalic direction to record the liver parenchyma from the anterior abdominal wall to the diaphragm.

Scan I. With the transducer perpendicular to the abdominal wall, the initial scan should be made slightly to the left of the midline to record the left lobe of the liver and the abdominal aorta. The left hepatic and portal veins may be seen as small circular structures in this view (Fig. 9.19A).

Scan II. With the probe still perpendicular, as the sonographer scans slightly to the right of midline, a larger segment of the left lobe and the inferior vena cava may be seen posteriorly.

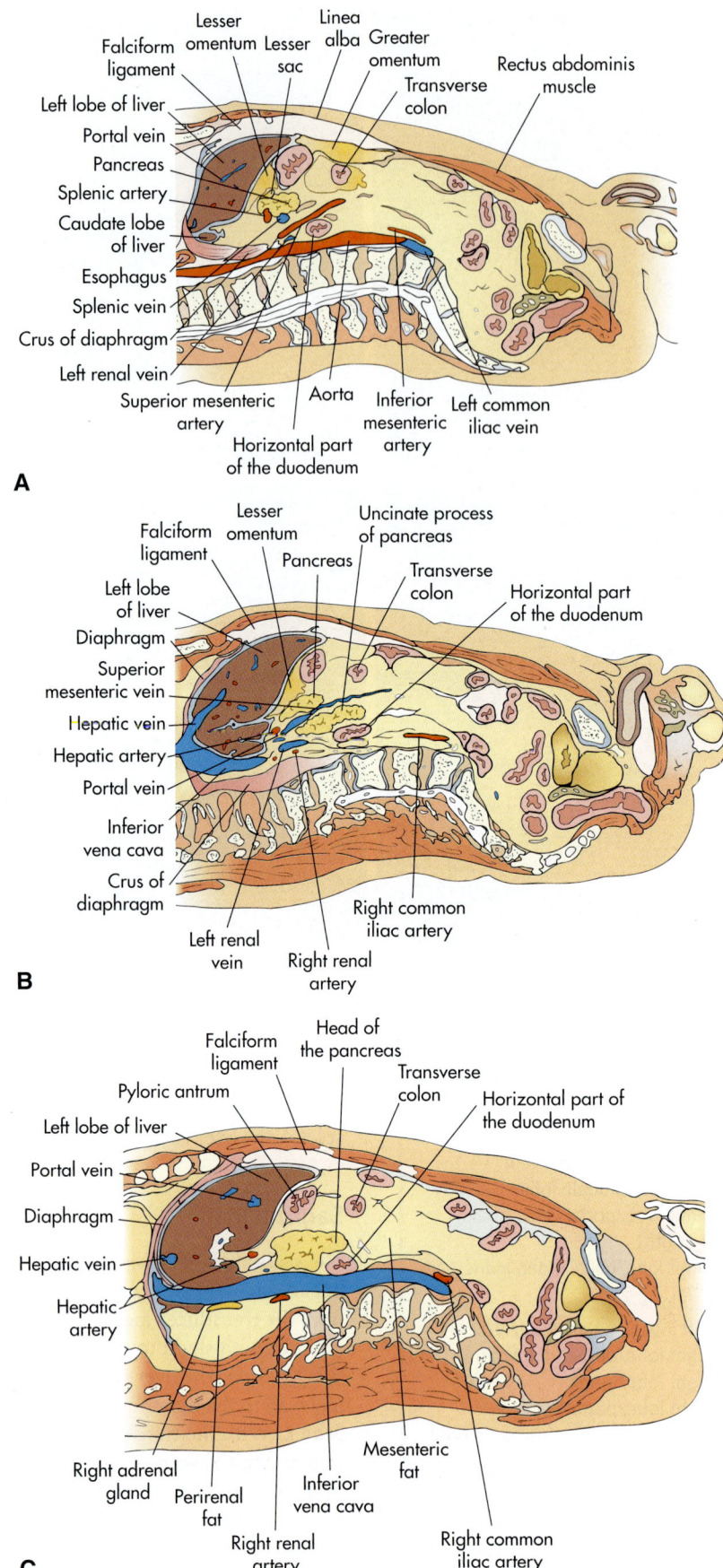

FIG. 9.18 **Longitudinal plane.** (A) Midline sagittal section of the abdomen. (B) Sagittal section of the abdomen. (C) Sagittal section of the abdomen 3 cm from the midline.

CHAPTER 9 The Liver 237

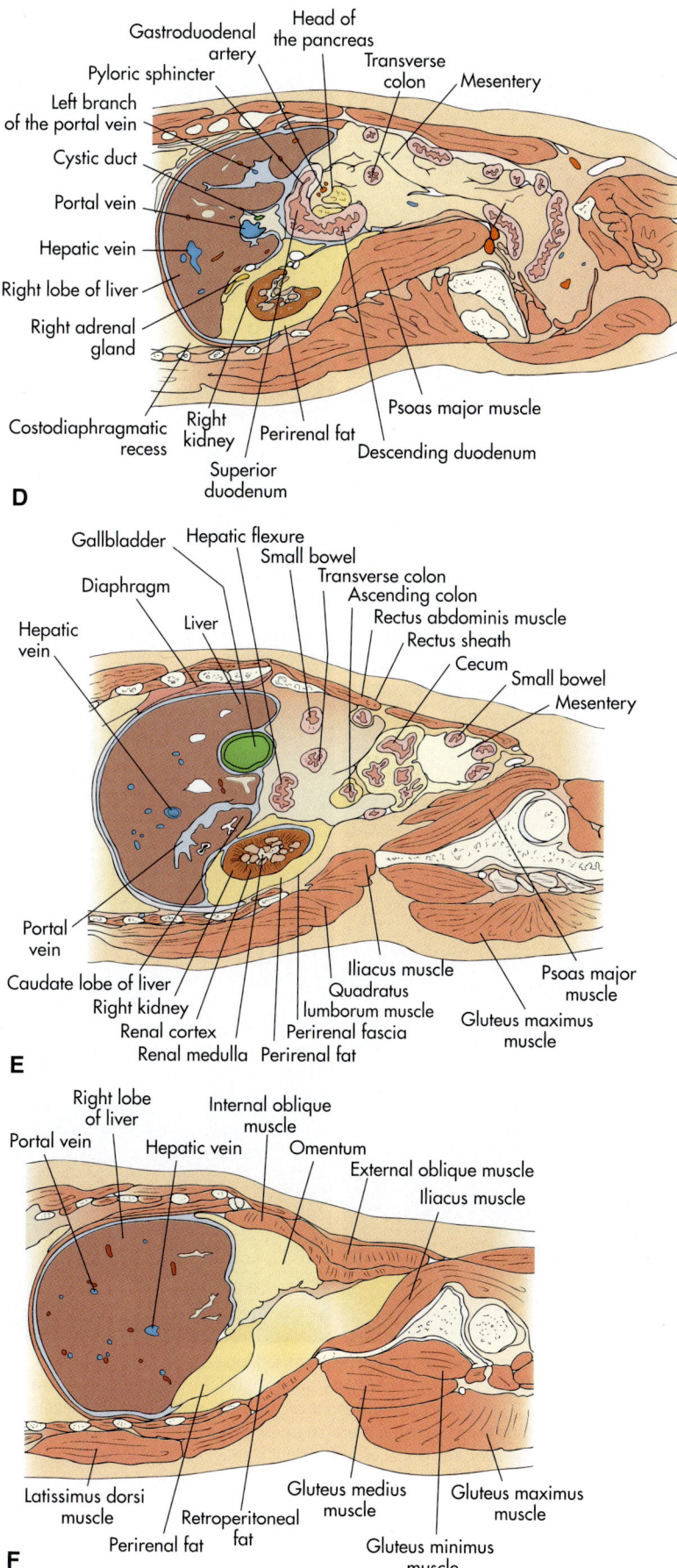

FIG. 9.18, cont'd (D) Sagittal section of the abdomen 5 cm from the midline. (E) Sagittal section of the abdomen 7 cm from the midline. (F) Sagittal section of the abdomen taken along the right abdominal border.

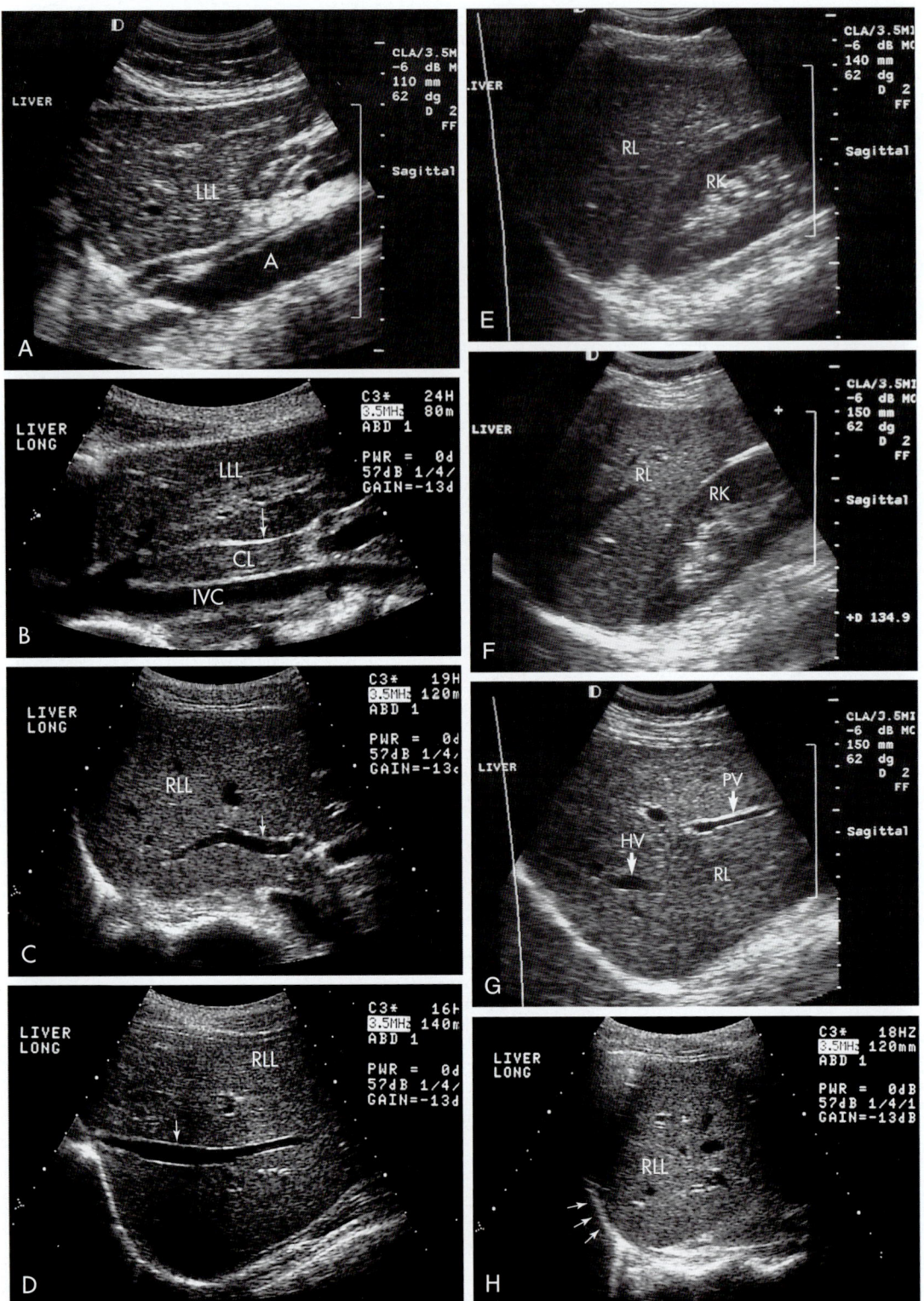

FIG. 9.19 Longitudinal images. (A) Midline left lobe liver, aorta. (B) Midline *(right)* left lobe liver, inferior vena cava, portal vein, caudate lobe. (C) *Midline with right lateral angle:* right lobe liver, right kidney. (D) *Midline with right lateral angle:* right lobe liver, hepatic vein *(arrow)*. (E) *Mid-subcostal with right lateral angle:* right lobe liver, hepatic vein, right kidney. (F) *Mid-subcostal with right lateral angle:* right lobe liver, hepatic vein, right kidney. (G) *Mid-subcostal sweep to identify hepatic and portal veins.* (H) Longitudinal image of the lateral segment of the right lobe liver (RLL), diaphragm *(arrows)*. *CL,* Caudate lobe; *HV,* hepatic veins; *IVC,* inferior vena cava; *LLL,* left lobe liver; *PV,* portal vein; *RK,* right kidney; *RL,* right lobe.

In this view, it is useful to record the inferior vena cava as it is dilated near the end of inspiration. The left or middle hepatic vein may be imaged as it drains into the inferior vena cava near the level of the diaphragm. The area of the porta hepatis is shown anterior to the inferior vena cava as the superior mesenteric vein and splenic vein converge to form the main portal vein. The common bile duct may be seen just anterior to the main portal vein. The head of the pancreas may be seen just inferior to the liver and main portal vein, and anterior to the inferior vena cava (Fig. 9.19B).

Scan III. The next image should be made slightly lateral to this sagittal plane to record part of the right portal vein and right lobe of the liver. The caudate lobe is often seen in this view (see Fig. 9.19C).

Scans IV, V, and VI. The next five scans should be made with the sweep movement of the probe (from the abdominal wall to the diaphragm) in small increments through the right lobe of the liver (Fig. 9.19D–H). The last scan is usually made to assess the right kidney and lateral segment of the right lobe of the liver. The liver texture is compared with the renal parenchyma. The normal liver parenchyma should have a softer, more homogeneous texture than the dense medulla and hypoechoic renal cortex. Liver size may be measured with the probe in the midclavicular line extending from the inferior tip of the liver to the dome/diaphragm interface. Generally this measurement is less than 15 cm, with 15 to 20 cm representing the upper limits of normal. Hepatomegaly is present when the liver measurement exceeds 20 cm.

Transverse Plane

Multiple transverse scans are made across the upper abdomen to record specific areas of the liver (Fig. 9.20). The transducer should be angled in a steep cephalic direction to be as parallel to the diaphragm as possible. The patient should be in full inspiration to obtain adequate detail of the liver parenchyma, vascular architecture, and ductal structures.

Scan I. The initial transverse image is made with the transducer inferior to the costal margin at a steep angle perpendicular to the diaphragm (Fig. 9.21A). The patient should be in deep inspiration to adequately record the dome of the liver, the inferior vena cava, and three hepatic veins as they drain into the cava. This pattern has sometimes been referred to as the "reindeer sign" or "Playboy bunny" sign.

Scan II. The probe should be steeply angled towards the diaphragm to image the dome of the liver (Fig. 9.21B).

Scan III. The transducer is then directed slightly inferior to the point described in scan I to record the left portal vein as it flows into the left lobe of the liver (Fig. 9.21C).

Scan III. The porta hepatis is seen as a tubular structure within the central area of the liver. The bifurcation of the portal vein into the left or right portal vein can be identified. The caudate lobe is shown anterior to the inferior vena cava (Fig. 9.21D).

Scan IV. The next two images should show the right portal vein as it divides into the anterior and posterior segments of the right lobe of the liver. The gallbladder may be seen in this scan as an anechoic structure medial to the right lobe and anterior to the right kidney (Fig. 9.21E–F).

Scans V and VI. These two scans are made through the lower segment of the right lobe of the liver. The right kidney is the posterior border (Fig. 9.21G). Usually intrahepatic vascular structures are not clearly identified in these views (see Fig. 9.21F).

Lateral Decubitus Plane

Left Posterior Oblique/Right Anterior Oblique. The left posterior/right anterior oblique image requires that the patient roll slightly to the left. A 45-degree sponge or pillow may be placed under the right hip to support the patient. This view allows better visualization of the lower right lobe of the liver, usually displacing the duodenum and transverse colon to the midline of the abdomen, out of the field of view. Transverse, oblique, or longitudinal scans may be made in this position.

Left Lateral Decubitus. If the previously described scans do not allow adequate visualization of the liver and vascular structures, the lateral decubitus position may be used. If the body habitus allows the transducer to image between the intercostal spaces, additional views may be obtained of the dome of the liver and medial segment of the left lobe of the liver.

PATHOLOGY OF THE LIVER

Evaluation of the liver parenchyma includes the assessment of its size, configuration, homogeneity, and contour. Liver volume may be determined from serial scans to detect subtle increases in size or hepatomegaly. The development and clinical utility of three-dimensional ultrasound in determining organ volumes is currently under clinical investigation at many academic institutions.

As in other organ systems, the hepatic parenchymal pattern changes with disease processes. Hepatocellular disease affects the hepatocytes and interferes with liver function enzymes. Cirrhosis, ascites, or fatty liver patterns may be detected with the ultrasound examination. To provide a differential diagnosis for the clinician, intrahepatic, extrahepatic, subhepatic, and subdiaphragmatic masses may be outlined and their internal composition recognized as specific echo patterns.

Subsequent sections discuss the pathology of liver disease in the following categories: developmental anomalies, diffuse disease, functional disease, infectious disease, benign disease, malignant disease, and vascular problems.

Developmental Anomalies

Agenesis. Agenesis of the liver is incompatible with life. Cases of partial agenesis of the right, left, or caudate lobes have been reported. When this occurs, hypertrophy of the other lobes develops.

Anomalies of Position. The liver may be found in other locations in two conditions: situs inversus, in which the organs are reversed, with the liver on the left and spleen on the right; or in a congenital diaphragmatic hernia or omphalocele, where varying amounts of liver tissue may herniate into the thorax or outside the abdominal cavity.

Accessory Fissures. True accessory fissures are uncommon and caused by infolding of peritoneum. The inferior accessory hepatic fissure is a true accessory fissure that stretches inferiorly from the right portal vein to the inferior surface of the right lobe of the liver.

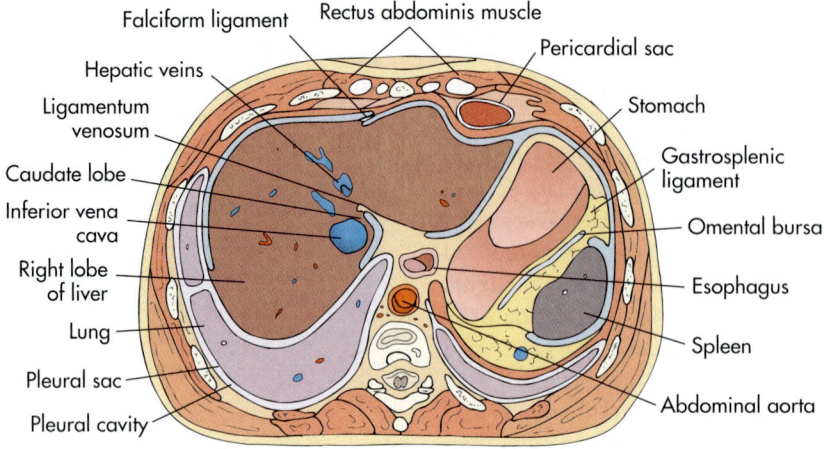

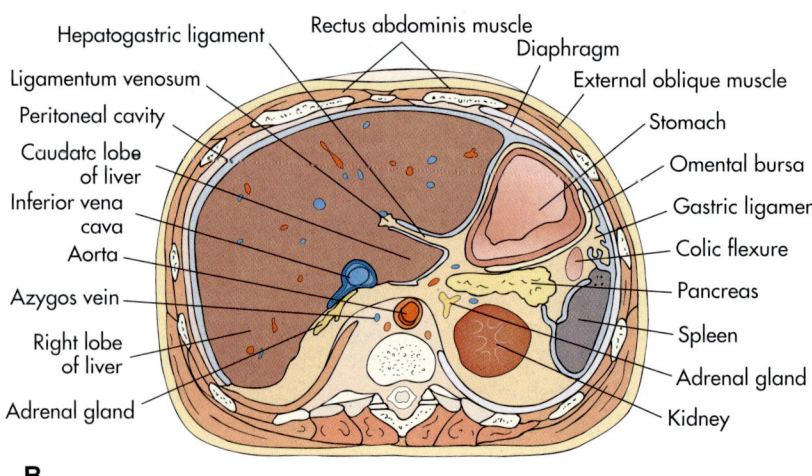

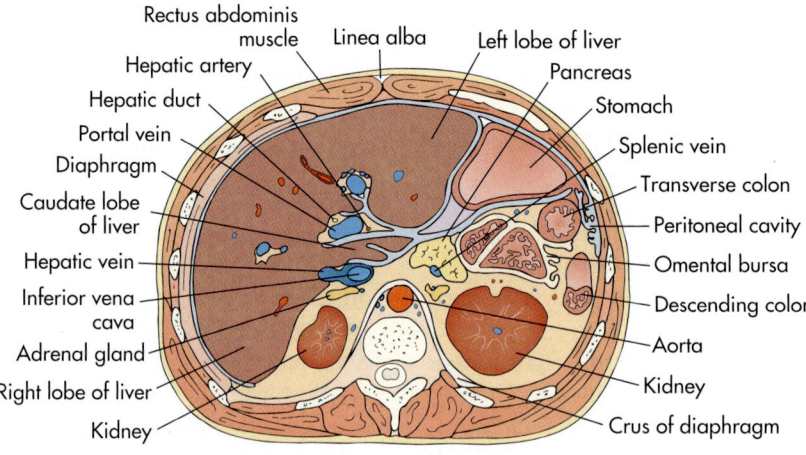

FIG. 9.20 **Transverse plane**. (A) Cross section of the abdomen at the level of the tenth intervertebral disk. (B) Cross section of the abdomen at the level of the eleventh thoracic disk. (C) Cross section of the abdomen at the level of the 12th thoracic vertebra.

CHAPTER 9 The Liver 241

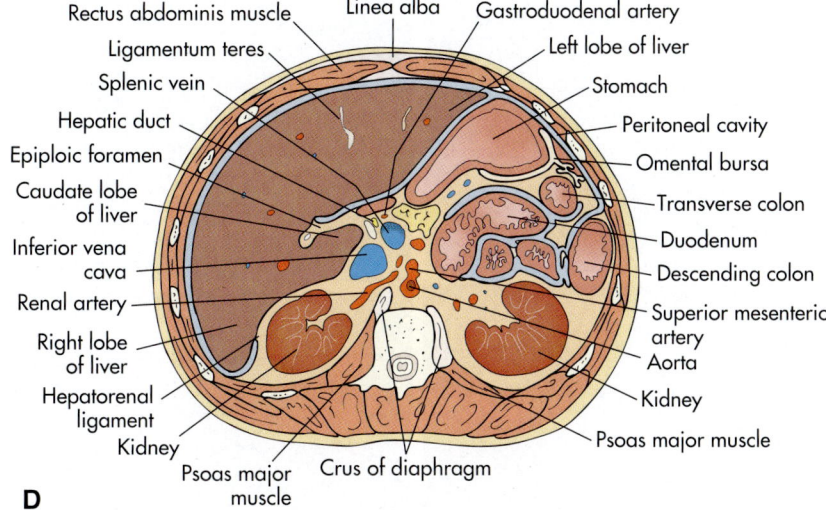

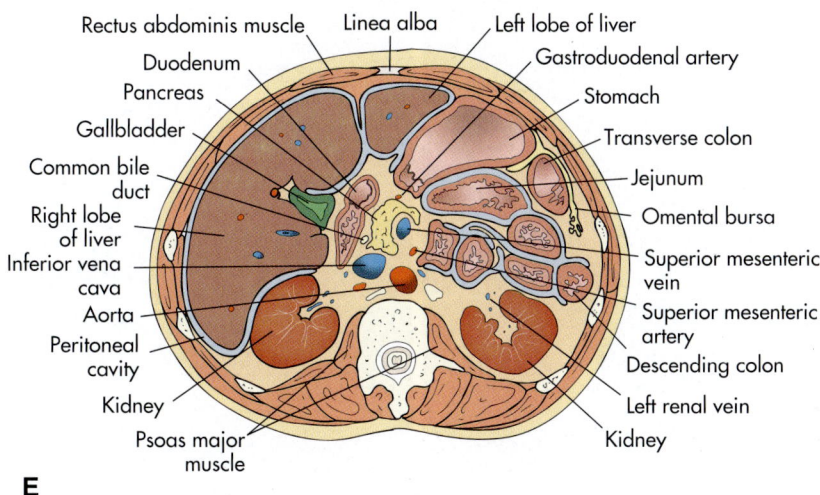

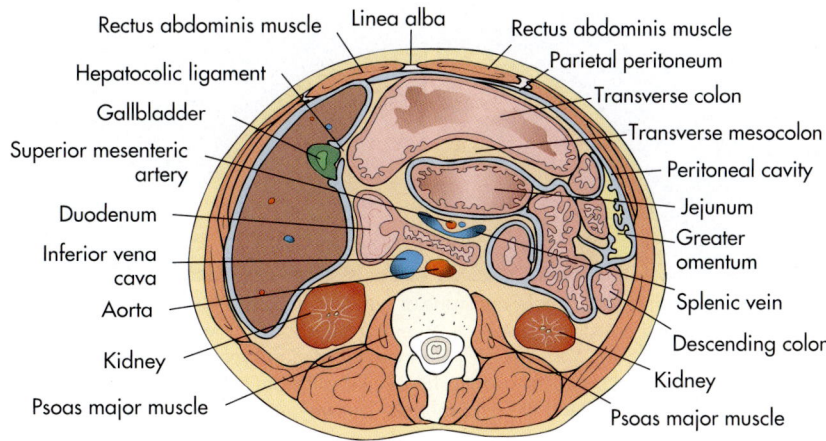

FIG. 9.20, cont'd (D) Cross section of the abdomen at the first lumbar vertebra. (E) Cross section of the abdomen at the level of the second lumbar vertebra. (F) Cross section of the abdomen at the level of the third lumbar vertebra.

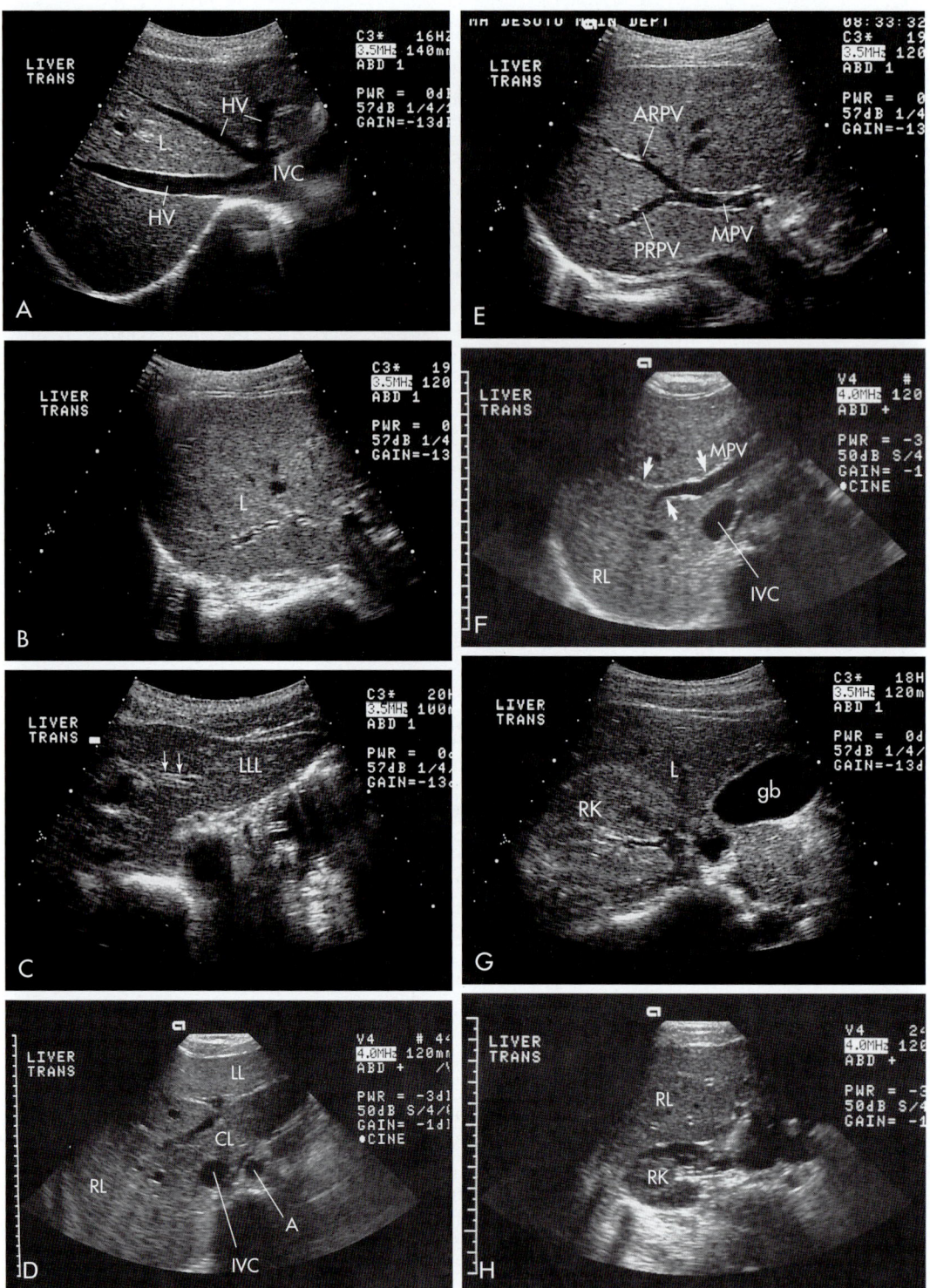

FIG. 9.21 Transverse Images. (A) *Subcostal with cephalic angle:* right lobe of liver (RL), hepatic veins (HV; *arrows*), inferior vena cava (IVC). (B) *Subcostal with steeper cephalic angle:* left lobe of liver (LL), left portal vein *(arrow),* ligamentum venosum *(arrows),* caudate lobe (CL). (C) *Slow caudal inferior sweep from dome:* CL, LL, RL, left and right portal veins, IVC, and aorta (Ao). (D) *Slow caudal inferior sweep from dome:* RL, main portal vein (MPV), right portal vein with branches (RPV), and IVC. (E) Deep inspiration, subcostal over RL. (F) Deep inspiration, subcostal over RL and right kidney (RK). (G) Slight caudal sweep through right lobe liver to area of gallbladder (gb) and RK. (H) Slight caudal sweep through RL and RK. *ARPV,* Anterior right portal vein; *PRPV,* posterior right portal vein.

Vascular Anomalies. The hepatic artery may have many variations as it arises from the celiac axis. At least 45% of patients may have the following variations: (1) replaced left hepatic artery originating from the left gastric artery, (2) replaced right hepatic artery originating from the superior mesenteric artery, and (3) replaced common hepatic artery originating from the superior mesenteric artery.

Variations in the portal venous anatomy are uncommon but include atresias, strictures, and obstructing valves. On the other hand, variations in the branching of the hepatic veins are common, with the most common being when the accessory vein drains the superoanterior segment of the right lobe. It may empty into the middle hepatic vein or join the right hepatic vein.

Diffuse Disease

Diffuse hepatocellular disease affects the hepatocytes and interferes with liver function. The **hepatocyte** is a parenchymal liver cell that performs all the functions ascribed to the liver. This abnormality is measured through the series of liver function tests. The hepatic enzyme levels are elevated with cell necrosis. With cholestasis (i.e., interruption in the flow of bile through any part of the biliary system, from the liver to the duodenum), the alkaline phosphatase and direct bilirubin levels increase. Likewise, when there are defects in protein synthesis, there may be elevated serum bilirubin levels and decreased serum albumin and clotting factor levels.

There are many subcategories of diffuse parenchymal disease, including fatty infiltration, acute and chronic hepatitis, early alcoholic liver disease, and acute and chronic cirrhosis. See Table 9.4 for clinical findings, sonographic findings, and differential considerations for diffuse hepatic disease.

Fatty Infiltration. Fatty infiltration of the liver is an acquired, reversible disorder of metabolism, resulting in an intracellular accumulation of triglycerides within hepatocytes. Fatty infiltration implies increased lipid accumulation in the hepatocytes and results from major injury to the liver or a systemic disorder leading to impaired or excessive metabolism of fat. Fatty infiltration is a benign process and may be reversible with correction of the process, although it has been shown that fatty infiltration

TABLE 9.4 Liver Findings: Diffuse Disease

Clinical Findings	Sonographic Findings	Differential Considerations
Fatty Infiltration		
Normal to ↑ hepatic enzymes ↑ Alk phos ↑ Direct bilirubin	↑ Echogenicity ↑ Attenuation Impaired visualization of borders of portal/hepatic structures (secondary to increased attenuation) Hepatomegaly May be patchy, inhomogeneous Focal sparing	Hepatitis Cirrhosis Metastases
Acute Hepatitis		
↑ AST, ALT ↑ Bilirubin Leukopenia	Nonspecific and variable Normal to slightly ↑ Echogenicity ↑ Brightness of portal vein borders Hepatosplenomegaly ↑ Thickness of gallbladder wall	Fatty liver
Chronic Hepatitis		
↑ AST, ALT ↑ Bilirubin Leukopenia	Coarse hepatic parenchyma ↑ Echogenicity ↓ Visualization brightness of portal triad Fibrosis may produce soft shadowing	Cirrhosis Fatty liver
Cirrhosis		
↑ Alk phos ↑ Direct bilirubin ↑ AST, ALT Leukopenia	Coarse liver parenchyma with nodularity ↑ Echogenicity ↑ Attenuation ↓ Vascular markings with acute cirrhosis Hepatosplenomegaly with ascites Shrunken liver with chronic cirrhosis (also ↑ nodularity) Regeneration of hepatic nodules Portal hypertension	Fatty liver Hepatitis
Glycogen Storage Disease		
Disturbance of acid-base balance	Hepatomegaly ↑ Echogenicity ↑ Attenuation von Gierke adenoma (round, homogeneous)	Focal nodular hyperplasia Fatty liver
Hemochromatosis		
↑ Iron levels in blood	↑ Echogenicity throughout liver	Cirrhosis

↑, Increased; ↓, decreased; *Alk phos,* alkaline phosphatase; *ALT,* alanine aminotransferase; *AST,* aspartate aminotransferase.

of the liver is the precursor for significant chronic disease in a percentage of patients. The patient is usually asymptomatic, although some patients may present with jaundice, nausea, vomiting, and abdominal tenderness or pain. Common causes of fatty liver include obesity, alcohol abuse, cholesterol-lowering medications, diabetes, and certain chemotherapy agents. Box 9.3 lists the common findings of fatty liver.

Sonographic Findings. Fatty infiltration of the liver appears in a variety of patterns that depend on the amount and distribution of fat in the liver parenchyma (Fig. 9.22). Fatty infiltration most commonly appears in a diffuse distribution and results in uniform increased echogenicity of the liver. Thus comparison of the liver parenchyma to the kidney is very useful in determining if fatty infiltration is present. The pancreas may also be used to judge the fatty infiltration pattern as its parenchyma is more echogenic that the liver. If the liver appears more "hyperechoic" than the pancreas, fatty infiltration should be considered. Localized enlargement of the lobe affected by fatty infiltration is evident. The portal vein structures may be difficult to visualize because of the increased attenuation of the ultrasound beam. The increased attenuation also causes a decrease in penetration of the sound beam, which may be a clue for the sonographer to think of fatty liver disease. The liver is so dense that "typical" gain settings do not allow penetration to the posterior border of the liver. It thus becomes more difficult to see the outline of the portal vein and hepatic vein borders. Authors have stated that this increase in echo texture may result from increased collagen content of the liver or increase in lipid accumulation. The following three grades of liver texture have been defined in sonography for classification of fatty infiltration:

- *Mild.* The mild form will present with minimal diffuse increase in hepatic echogenicity with normal visualization of the diaphragm and intrahepatic vascular borders (Fig. 9.23B).
- *Moderate.* Moderate fatty infiltration shows increased cchogenicity with slightly impaired visualization of the diaphragm and intrahepatic vascular borders (Fig. 9.23C).
- *Severe.* The severe form presents with a marked increase in echogenicity of the liver parenchyma, decreased penetration of the posterior segment of the right lobe of the liver and decreased to poor visualization of the diaphragm and hepatic vessels (Fig. 9.23D).

Focal Fatty Infiltration and Focal Fatty Sparing. Fatty infiltration is not always uniform throughout the liver parenchyma; in fact, regions of increased echogenicity are present within a normal liver parenchyma. Patchy distribution of hypoechoic masses (fat) within a dense, fatty infiltrated liver parenchyma, especially in the right lobe of the liver is uncommon. The fat does not displace normal intraheptic vascular architecture. The margins of the fatty tissue may appear nodular, round, or interdigitated with the normal hepatic tissue. Fatty infiltration can resolve rapidly.

The other characteristic of fatty infiltration is focal sparing. This condition should be suspected in patients who have "mass-like" hypoechoic areas in typical locations in a liver that is otherwise increased in echogenicity. The most common areas are anterior to the gallbladder or the portal vein and the periportal region of the medial segment of the left lobe of the liver (Fig. 9.24). Focal subcapsular fat may be found in diabetic patients receiving insulin in peritoneal dialysate.

Viral Hepatitis. Hepatitis is considered to result from infection by a group of viruses that specifically target the hepatocytes. Hepatitis is the general name for inflammatory and infectious disease of the liver, of which there are many causes. The disease may result from a local infection (viral hepatitis),an infection elsewhere in the body (e.g., infectious mononucleosis or amebiasis), or chemical or drug toxicity.

BOX 9.3	Causes of Fatty Liver

Obesity
Excessive alcohol intake (alcohol stimulates lipolysis)
Poorly controlled hyperlipidemia
Diabetes mellitus
Excess corticosteroids
Pregnancy
Total parenteral hyperalimentation (nutrition)
Severe hepatitis
Glycogen storage disease
Cystic fibrosis
Pharmaceutical
Chronic illness

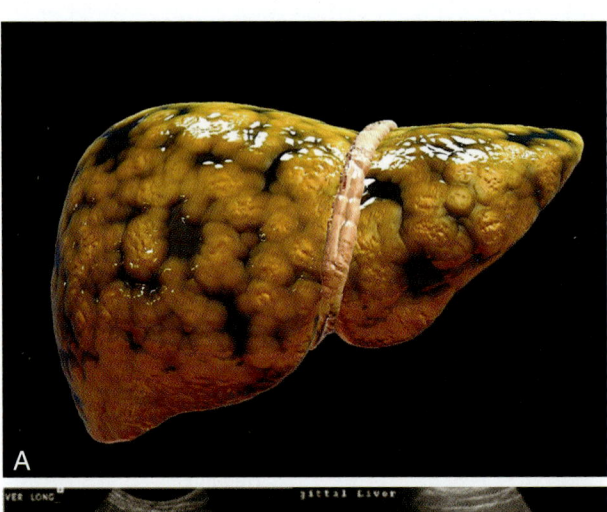
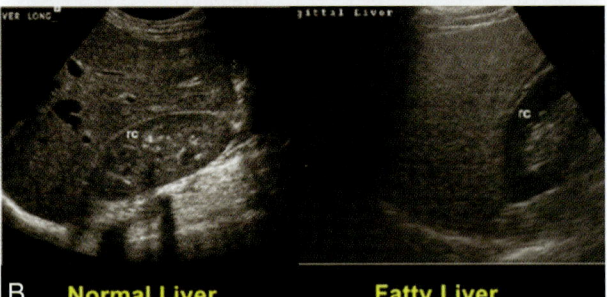

FIG. 9.22 Fatty infiltration most commonly appears in a diffuse distribution and results in uniform increased echogenicity of the liver. Thus comparison of the liver parenchyma to the kidney is very useful in determining if fatty infiltration is present. (A) Gross pathology of the diffuse fatty liver parenchyma. (B) Normal liver on left compared to the fatty liver on the right.

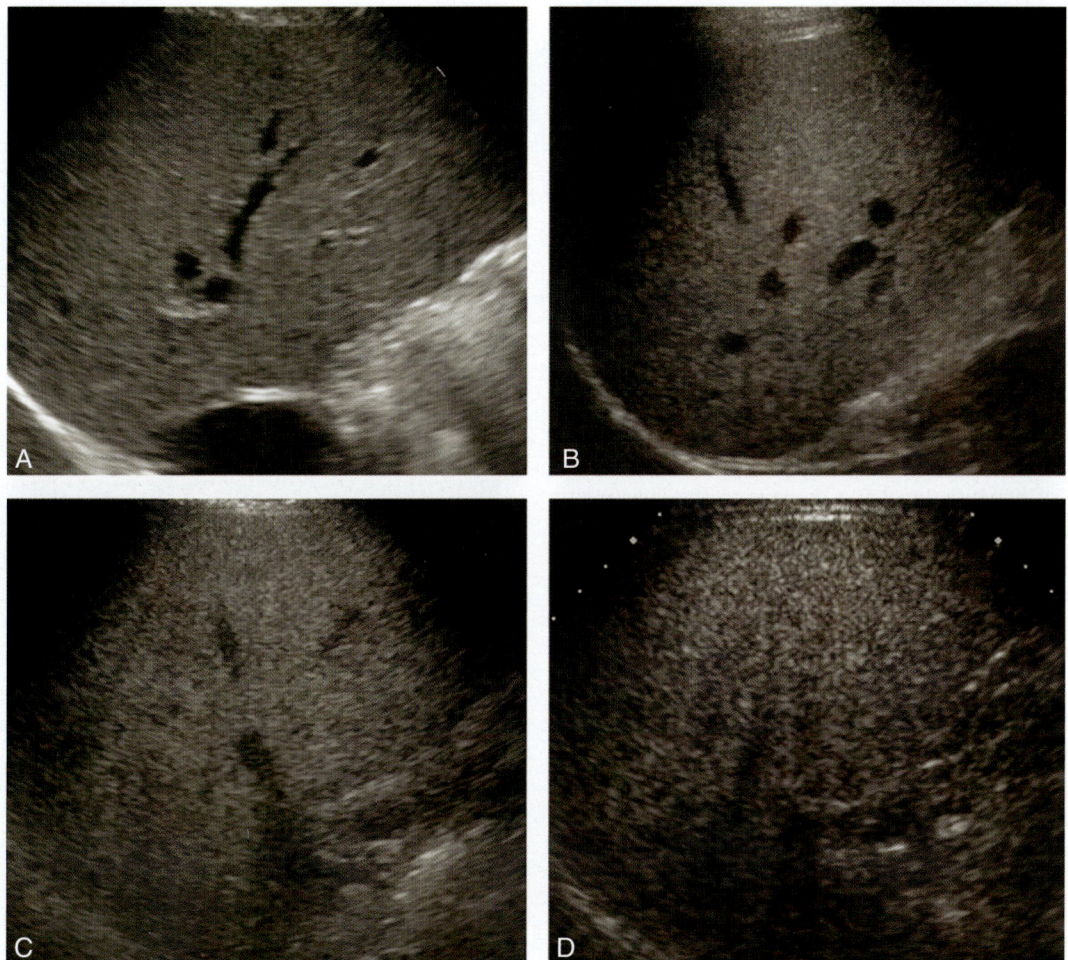

FIG. 9.23 (A) Normal liver homogeneous parenchyma. (B) The mild form of fatty liver will present with minimal diffuse increase in hepatic echogenicity with normal visualization of the diaphragm and intrahepatic vascular borders (C) Moderate fatty infiltration shows increased echogenicity with slightly impaired visualization of the diaphragm and intrahepatic vascular borders. (D) The severe form presents with a marked increase in echogenicity of the liver parenchyma, decreased penetration of the posterior segment of the right lobe of the liver, and decreased to poor visualization of the diaphragm and hepatic vessels.

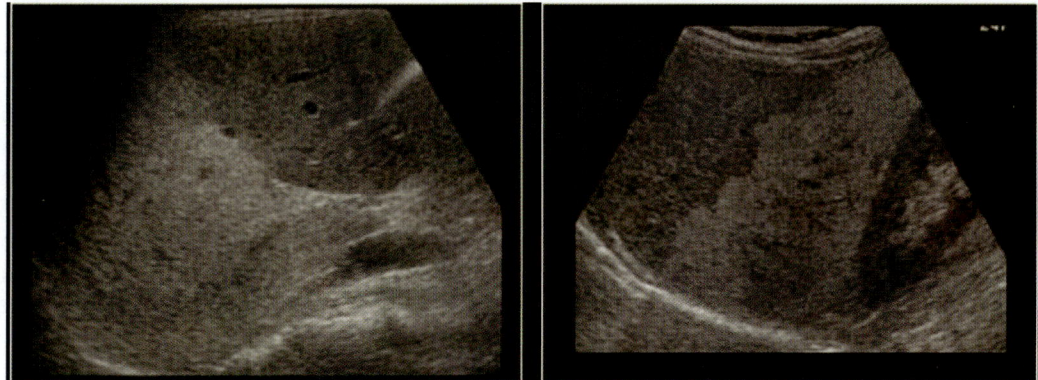

FIG. 9.24 Focal sparing is a condition that should be suspected in patients who have mass-like hypoechoic areas in typical locations in a liver that is otherwise increased in echogenicity. The most common areas are anterior to the gallbladder or the portal vein and the periportal region of the medial segment of the left lobe of the liver. (Courtesy Dr. Taco Geertsma, www.ultrasoundcases.info.)

Mild inflammation impairs hepatocyte function, whereas more severe inflammation and necrosis may obstruct blood and bile flow in the liver and impaired liver cell function.

Patients with hepatitis may initially present with flu-like and gastrointestinal symptoms, including loss of appetite, nausea, vomiting, and fatigue. Viral hepatitis may be fatal with secondary acute hepatic necrosis or chronic hepatitis, which may lead to portal hypertension, cirrhosis, and hepatocellular carcinoma (HCC).

Many distinct hepatitis viruses have been identified and are beyond the scope of this chapter. The more common hepatitis A, B, and C will be discussed. Hepatitis A is found worldwide and is spread primarily by fecal contamination because the virus lives in the alimentary tract. In developing countries, the disease is endemic, and the infection occurs very early in life. Hepatitis A is an acute infection that leads to either complete recovery or death from acute liver failure. Hepatitis B is caused by the type B virus, which exists in the bloodstream and can be spread by transfusions of infected blood or plasma or through using contaminated needles. Hepatitis B is of the greatest risk to health care workers because of the nature of transmission. This virus is also found in body fluids, such as saliva and semen, and may be spread by sexual contact. Hepatitis C is diagnosed by the presence in blood of the antibody to HCV (anti-HCV).

Acute Hepatitis. In acute hepatitis, without complications, the clinical recovery usually occurs within 4 months. Complications of hepatitis involving damage to the liver may range from mild disease to massive necrosis and liver failure. The pathologic changes seen include the following: (1) liver cell injury, swelling of the hepatocytes, and hepatocyte degeneration, which may lead to cell necrosis; (2) reticuloendothelial and lymphocytic response with Kupffer cells enlarging; and (3) regeneration.

Sonographic Findings. The liver texture may appear normal, or the sonographer may note that the portal vein borders are more echogenic than usual (known as the "starry sky" sign), the liver parenchyma is slightly more echogenic than normal, and attenuation may be present (Fig. 9.25). Hepatosplenomegaly is present, and the gallbladder wall is markedly thickened with contraction of the gallbladder lumen.

Chronic Hepatitis. Chronic hepatitis exists when there is clinical or biochemical evidence of hepatic inflammation that extends beyond 6 months. Chronic hepatitis may be viral, metabolic, autoimmune, or drug induced. Chronic active hepatitis has more extensive changes than chronic persistent hepatitis, with inflammation extending across the limiting plate, spreading out in a perilobular fashion, and causing piecemeal necrosis, which is frequently accompanied by fibrosis. Patients may present with nausea, anorexia, weight loss, tremors, jaundice, dark urine, fatigue, and varicosities. Chronic persistent hepatitis is a benign, self-limiting process. Chronic active hepatitis usually progresses to cirrhosis and liver failure.

Sonographic Findings. On ultrasound examination, the liver parenchyma is coarse with decreased brightness of the portal triads, but the degree of attenuation is not as great as is seen in fatty infiltration (Fig. 9.26). The liver does not increase in size with chronic hepatitis. Fibrosis may be evident and may produce "soft shadowing" posteriorly.

Cirrhosis. Cirrhosis is a chronic degenerative disease of the liver in which the hepatic lobes are covered with fibrous tissue, the parenchyma degenerates, and the lobules are infiltrated with fat. The essential feature is simultaneous parenchymal necrosis, regeneration, and diffuse fibrosis resulting in disorganization of lobular architecture (Fig. 9.27). Cirrhosis may be classified as micronodular (nodules 0.1 to 1 cm in diameter) or macronodular (nodules up to 5 cm in diameter). The process of cirrhosis is chronic and progressive, with liver cell failure and portal hypertension as the end

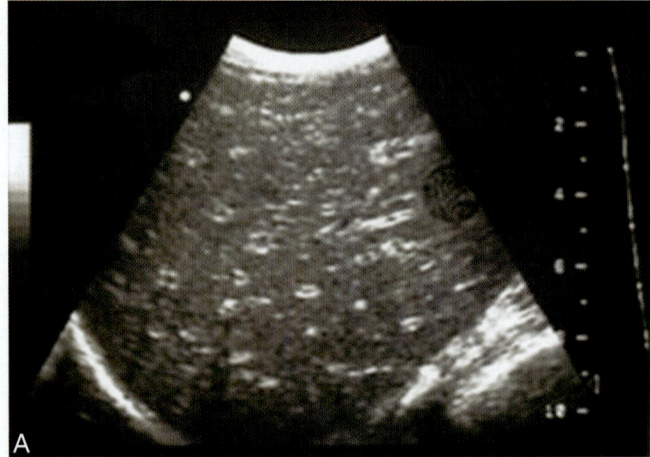
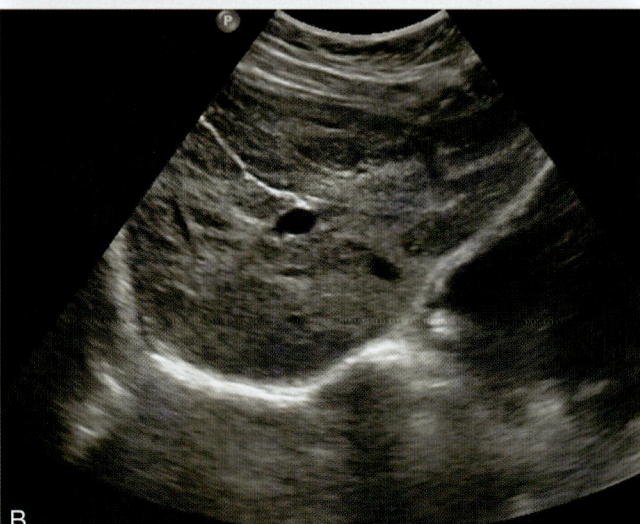

FIG. 9.25 In patients with acute hepatitis, the portal vein borders are more echogenic than usual (known as the "starry sky" sign), the liver parenchyma is slightly more echogenic than normal, and attenuation may be present.

stage. Micronodular cirrhosis is most commonly the result of chronic alcohol abuse, whereas macronodular cirrhosis is caused by chronic viral hepatitis or other infection. Other causes of cirrhosis include biliary cirrhosis, Wilson disease, primary sclerosing cholangitis, and hemochromatosis.

Patients with acute cirrhosis may seem asymptomatic or may have symptoms that include nausea, flatulence, ascites, light-colored stools, weakness, abdominal pain, varicosities, and spider angiomas. The classic clinical presentation of a patient with cirrhosis is hepatomegaly, jaundice, and ascites. Chronic cirrhosis patient symptoms include nausea, anorexia, weight loss, jaundice, dark urine, fatigue, or varicosities. Chronic cirrhosis may progress to liver failure and portal hypertension.

Sonographic Findings. The sonographic diagnosis of cirrhosis may be challenging. In the early stage of cirrhosis, hepatomegaly is the first sonographic finding. As the cirrhosis becomes more severe, the liver volume decreases in the right lobe, with enlargement of the left and caudate lobes.

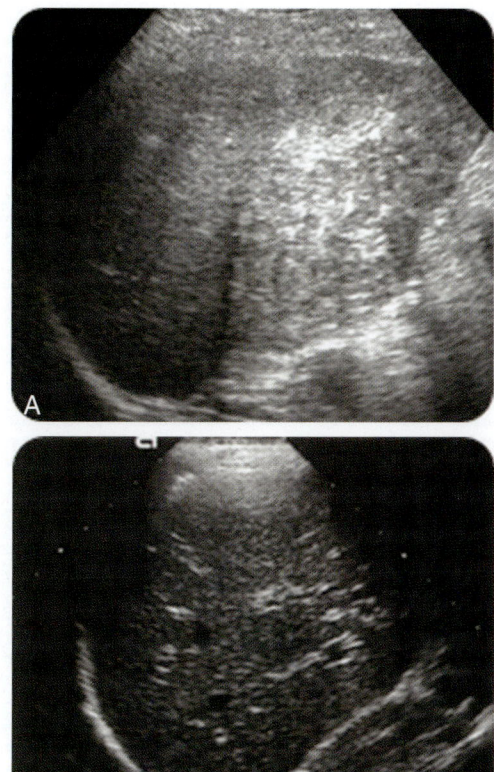

FIG. 9.26 The liver parenchyma is coarse with decreased brightness of the portal triads, but the degree of attenuation is not as great as is seen in fatty infiltration. The liver does not increase in size with chronic hepatitis. Fibrosis may be evident, which may produce "soft shadowing" posteriorly.

The evaluation of the ratio of the caudate lobe width to the right lobe width (C/RL) has been used as an indicator of cirrhosis. A C/RL value of 0.65 is considered indicative of cirrhosis. (This measurement is useful if abnormal, but not as sensitive when it is normal.)

Specific findings may include increased echogenicity and coarsening of the hepatic parenchyma secondary to fibrosis and surface nodularity (Fig. 9.28). This evaluation is subjective and depends on appropriate gain settings (both TGC and overall gain). Increased attenuation may be present with decreased vascular markings. The amount of fatty infiltration will certainly influence the amount of echogenicity and attenuation. Hepatosplenomegaly may be present with ascites surrounding the liver. In addition, there may be atrophy of the right and left medial lobes of the liver.

Chronic cirrhosis may show surface nodularity of the liver edge, especially well demonstrated if ascites is present. The use of a higher frequency, linear array transducer may allow the sonographer to demonstrate the surface of the liver. The hepatic fissures may be accentuated. The isoechoic regenerating nodules may be seen throughout the liver parenchyma. Portal hypertension may be present with or without abnormal Doppler flow patterns. Patients who have cirrhosis have an increased incidence of hepatoma tumors within the liver parenchyma.

Regenerating nodules represent regenerating hepatocytes surrounded by fibrosis septa. They are "isoechoic" to the liver parenchyma and thus may be indistinguishable from normal liver texture. Dysplastic nodules or adenomatous hyperplastic nodules are larger than the regenerating nodules and

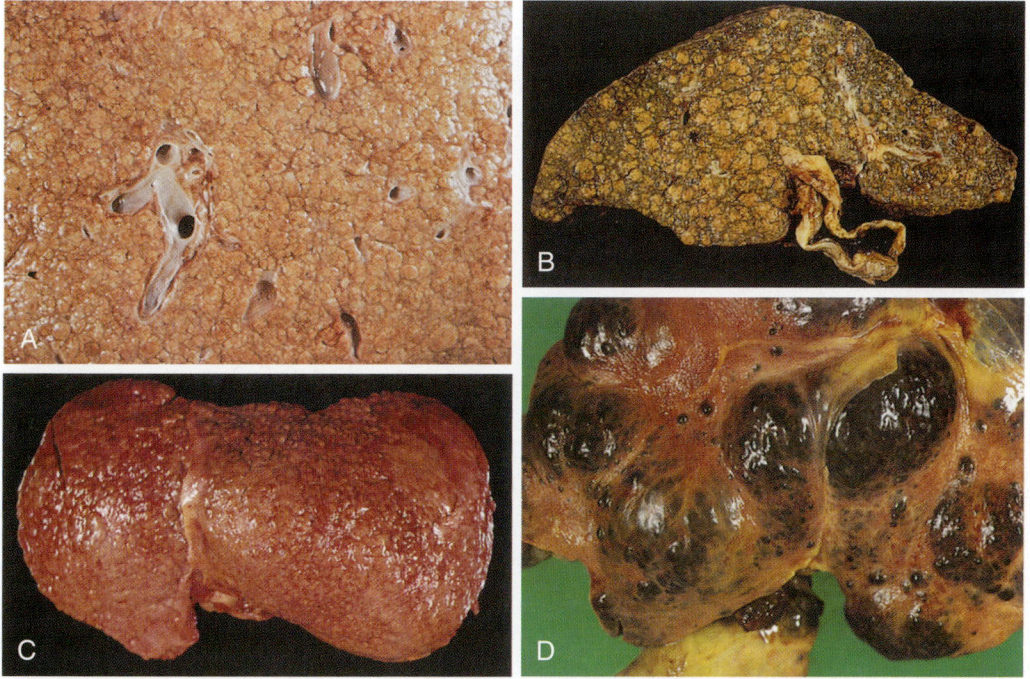

FIG. 9.27 (A) Gross pathology of alcoholic cirrhosis with high degree of fat content. (B) Biliary cirrhosis (liver is nodular). (C) Micronodular cirrhosis (nodules are small with uniform size). (D) Macronodular cirrhosis.

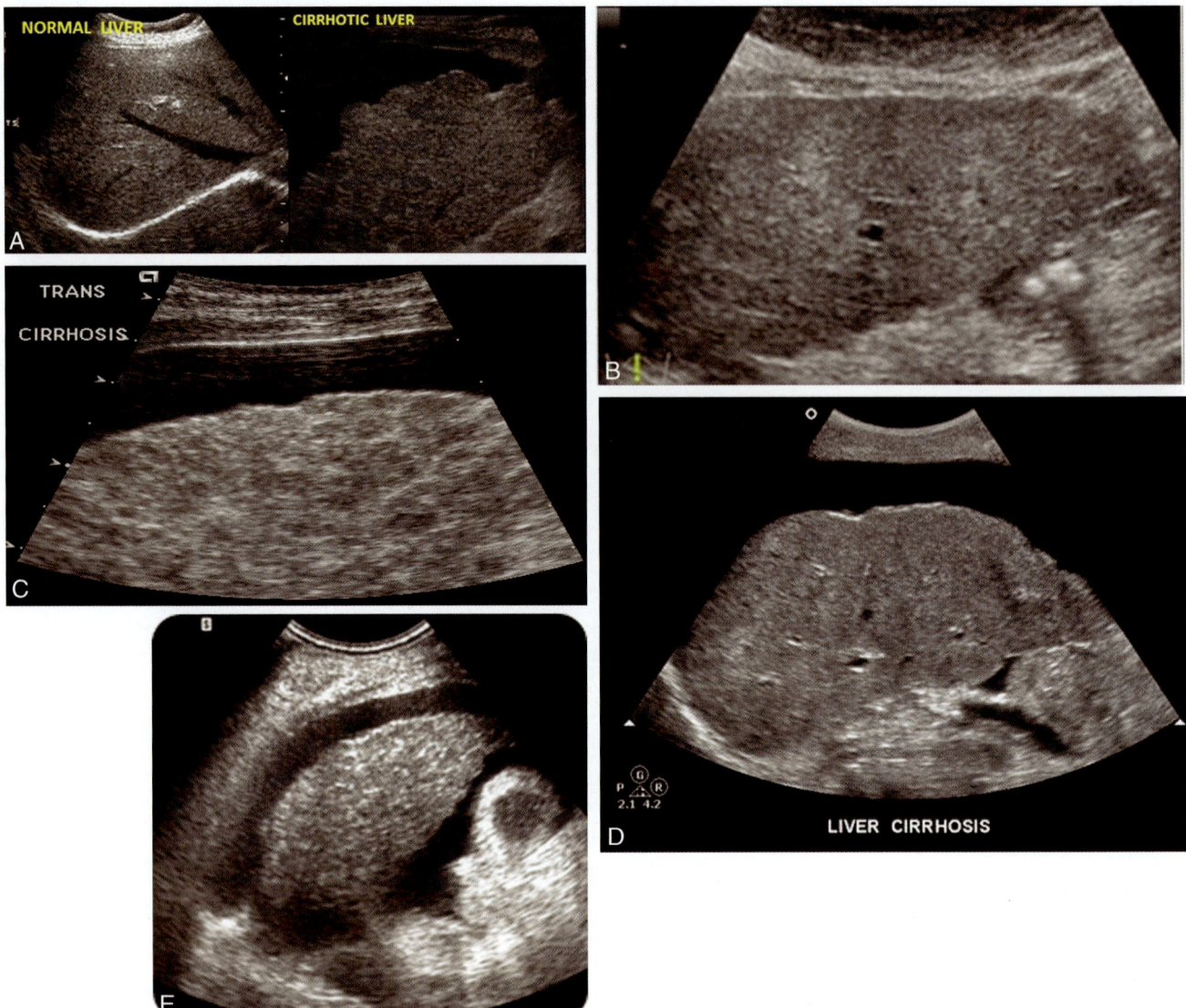

FIG. 9.28 In the early stage of cirrhosis, hepatomegaly is the first sonographic finding. As the cirrhosis becomes more severe, the liver volume decreases in the right lobe, with enlargement of the left and caudate lobes. (A) Normal liver compared to cirrhotic liver. (B) Hepatomegaly with some liver nodularity is noted. (C) The ascites demarks the surface liver nodularity. (D) Hepatomegaly with ascites is noted. (E) Shrunken liver with ascites.

are considered premalignant. These nodules contain well-differentiated hepatocytes, portal venous blood supply, and atypical or frankly malignant cells. Color Doppler is utilized to image the portal venous blood supply.

Doppler Characteristics of Cirrhosis. Doppler evaluation of the hepatic veins is useful to detect the presence of altered flow dynamics. The hepatic vein velocity waveform reflects the hemodynamics of the right atrium. This is a triphasic pattern with two large antegrade diastolic and systolic waves and a small retrograde wave corresponding to the atrial kick (from the heart). Recall that the thin walls of the hepatic veins easily receive the transfer of flow via the collaterals from the portal veins in a normal liver. In patients with compensated cirrhosis (no portal hypertension), the Doppler waveform is abnormal with decreased amplitude of phasic oscillations with loss of reversed flow and a flattened waveform. As the cirrhosis advances, the hepatic veins develop luminal narrowing with increased velocities and turbulence of the flow patterns (Fig. 9.29).

The hepatic artery waveform also shows altered flow dynamics in cirrhosis and chronic liver disease. The resistive index is blunted after a meal in patients with liver disease (Fig. 9.30).

Glycogen Storage Disease. Glycogen storage disease is an inherited disease characterized by the abnormal storage and accumulation of glycogen in the tissues, especially the liver and kidneys. There are six categories of glycogen storage disease, divided based on clinical symptoms and specific enzymatic defects. The most common is type I, or von Gierke disease. This is a form of glycogen storage disease in which abnormally large amounts of glycogen are deposited in the liver and kidneys.

Sonographic Findings. On sonography, patients with glycogen storage disease present with hepatomegaly, increased echogenicity, and slightly increased attenuation (similar to diffuse fatty infiltration). The disease is associated with hepatic adenomas, focal nodular hyperplasia (FNH), and hepatomegaly. The adenoma presents as well-demarcated, round, homogeneous,

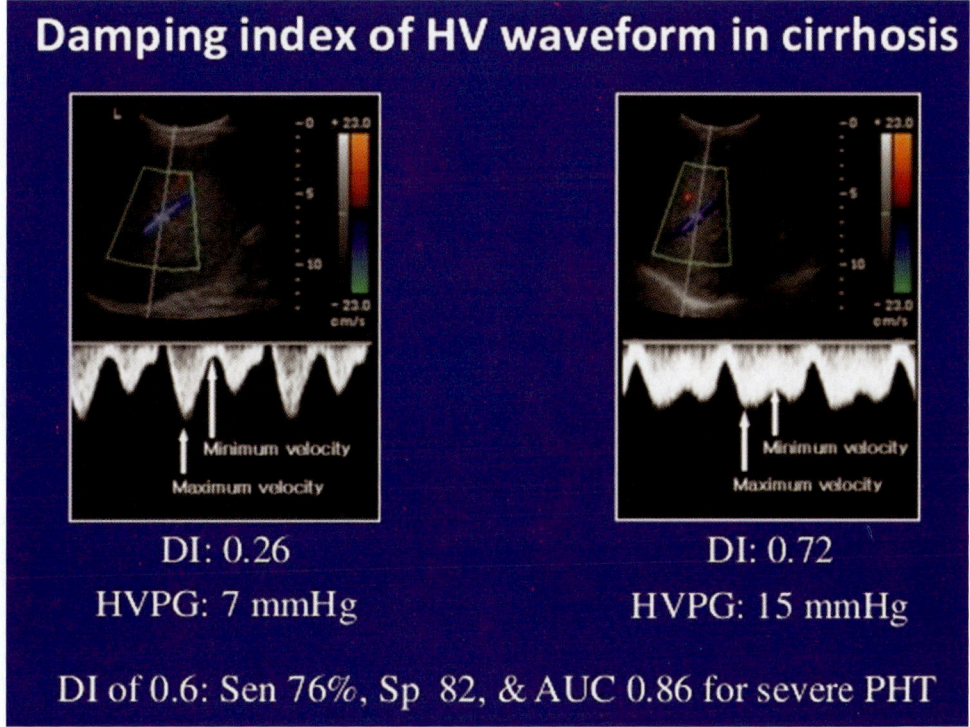

FIG. 9.29 The hepatic veins receive the transfer of flow via the collaterals from the portal veins in a normal liver. In patients with compensated cirrhosis (no portal hypertension), the Doppler waveform is abnormal with decreased amplitude of phasic oscillations with loss of reversed flow and a flattened waveform. As the cirrhosis advances, the hepatic veins develop luminal narrowing with increased velocities and turbulence of the flow patterns. *HV*, Hepatic veins. (From Kim MY, et al. Damping index of Doppler hepatic vein waveform to assess the severity of portal hypertension and response to propranolol in liver cirrhosis: a prospective nonrandomized study. *Liv Int.* 2007;27:1103–1110.)

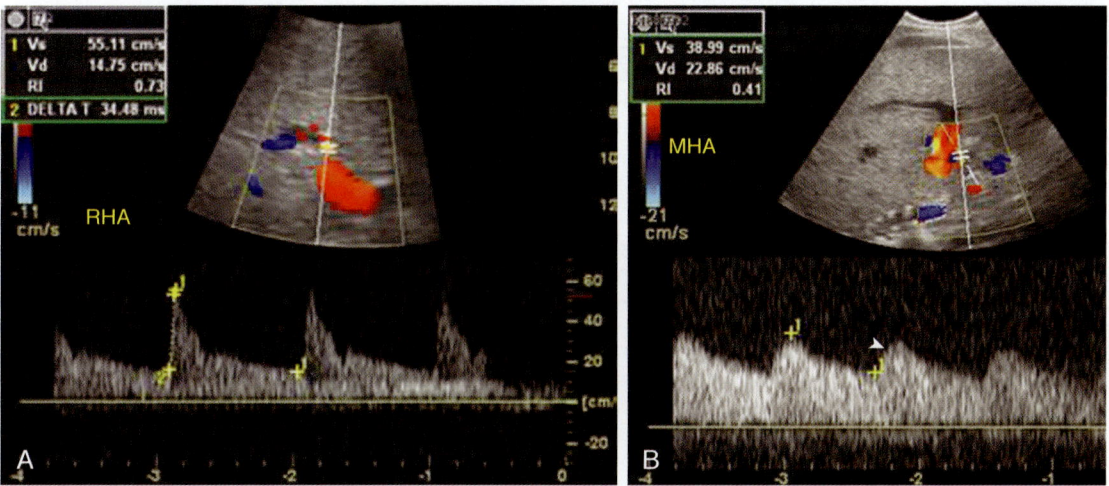

FIG. 9.30 (A) Normal hepatic arterial flow velocity. (B) High-velocity hepatic arterial flow pattern. *RHA*, Right hepatic artery.

echogenic tumors (Fig. 9.31). If the tumor is large, it may be slightly inhomogeneous.

Hemochromatosis. Hemochromatosis is a rare disease of iron metabolism characterized by excess iron deposits throughout the body. This disorder may lead to cirrhosis and portal hypertension.

Sonographic Findings. Ultrasound does not show specific findings other than hepatomegaly and cirrhotic changes. Some increased echogenicity may be seen uniformly throughout the hepatic parenchyma (Fig. 9.32).

Hepatic Vascular Flow Abnormalities

Portal Hypertension. Portal hypertension is caused by increased resistance to venous flow through the liver. It is associated with cirrhosis, hepatic vein thrombosis, portal vein thrombosis, and thrombosis of the inferior vena cava. Ultrasound findings include dilation of the portal, splenic, and mesenteric veins, reversal of portal venous blood flow, and the development of collateral vessels (e.g., patent umbilical vein, gastric varices, splenorenal shunting).

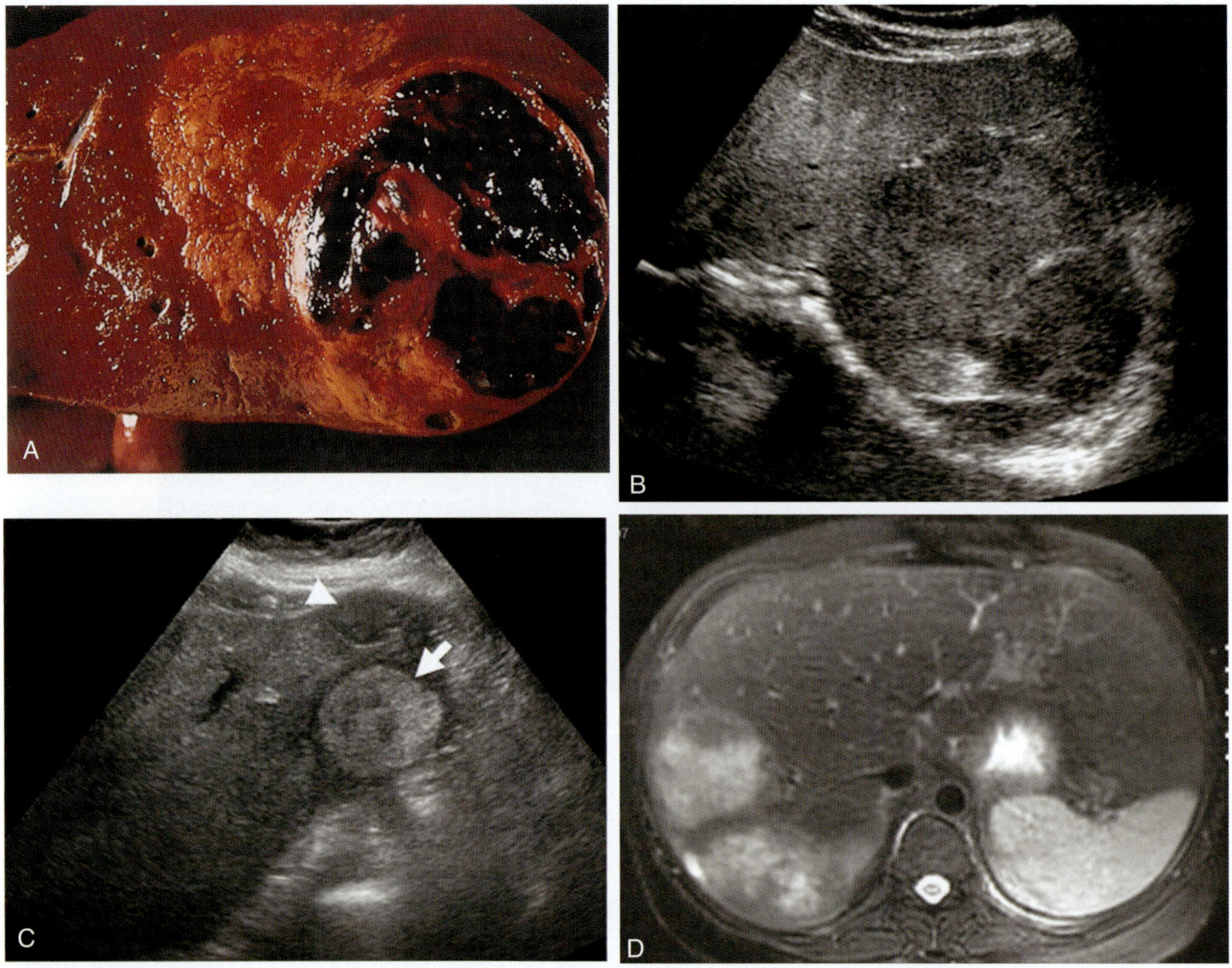

FIG. 9.31 (A) Gross pathology of hepatic adenoma with hemorrhage. (B) Glycogen storage disease on ultrasound presents with hepatomegaly, increased echogenicity, and slightly increased attenuation (similar to diffuse fatty infiltration). The disease is associated with hepatic adenomas, focal nodular hyperplasia, and hepatomegaly. The adenoma presents as a well-demarcated, round, homogeneous, echogenic tumors. (C) If the tumor is large, it may be slightly inhomogeneous. (D) Magnectic resonance image of hepatic adenomas.

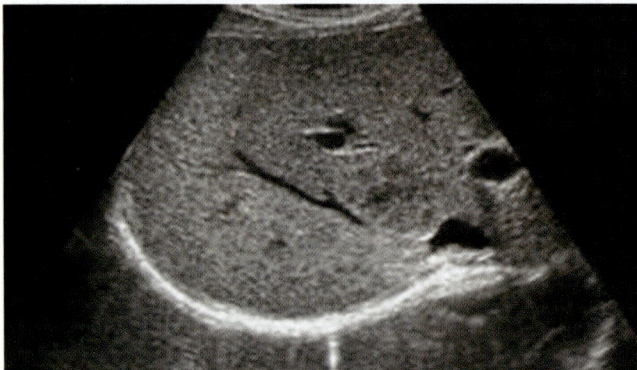

FIG. 9.32 **Hemochromatosis.** Hepatomegaly with slightly increased echogenicity throughout the liver parenchyma.

The sonographic protocol for portal hypertension includes the following:
- Perform the routine abdominal imaging protocol
- Assess for the presence of ascites
- Obtain diameter measurements of the splenic and main portal veins on inspiration and expiration
- Assess for the presence of collateral blood vessels (splenic hilum, porta hepatis, umbilical vein)
- Determine the flow direction of the portal veins (main, left, and right portal veins) and splenic and superior mesenteric veins
- Assess for the presence of splenorenal shunting
- Assess for patency of the umbilical vein
- Determine the patency and direction of flow in the inferior vena cava and hepatic veins
- Assess and document the patency of surgically placed shunts

Portal Venous Hypertension. Portal hypertension is defined as an increase in portal venous pressure or hepatic venous gradient. It exists when the portal venous pressure is above 10 mm Hg, or the hepatic venous gradient is more than 5 mm Hg. Portal hypertension may be further defined by the following:
- A wedged hepatic vein pressure or direct portal vein pressure of more than 5 mm Hg greater than the inferior vena cava pressure

- Splenic vein pressure of greater than 15 mm Hg
- Portal vein pressure of greater than 30 cm H_2O

Portal hypertension is divided into presinusoidal and intrahepatic groups, depending on whether the hepatic vein wedge pressure is normal (presinusoidal) or elevated (intrahepatic). The development of increased pressure in the portal-splenic venous system is the cause of extrahepatic portal hypertension. Acute or chronic hepatocellular disease can block the flow of blood throughout the liver, causing it to back up into the hepatic portal circulation. This causes the blood pressure in the hepatic circulation to increase, thus the development of portal hypertension. To relieve the pressure, collateral veins are formed that connect to the systemic veins. These are known as varicose veins and occur most frequently in the area of the esophagus, stomach, and rectum. Rupture of these veins can cause massive bleeding that may result in death.

Intrahepatic portal hypertension is the result of diseases that affect the portal zones of the liver like primary biliary cirrhosis, schistosomiasis, congenital hepatic fibrosis, or toxic drugs. Cirrhosis is the most common cause of intrahepatic portal hypertension. Diffuse metastatic liver disease may also produce portal hypertension as the normal architecture of the liver is replaced by the distorted vascular channels that provide increased resistance to portal venous blood flow and obstruction to hepatic venous outflow. Other causes include thrombotic diseases of the inferior vena cava and hepatic veins constrictive pericarditis or other right-sided heart failure over time will cause centrilobular fibrosis, hepatic regeneration, cirrhosis, all leading to subsequent portal hypertension.

Portal hypertension may also develop when hepatopetal flow (toward the liver) is impeded by thrombus or tumor invasion. The blood becomes obstructed as it passes through the liver to the hepatic veins and is diverted to collateral pathways in the upper abdomen. Box 9.4 lists the indications for portal hypertension.

Portal hypertension may develop along two pathways. One entails increased resistance to flow and the other increased portal blood flow. The most common mechanism for increased resistance to flow occurs in patients with cirrhosis. The disease process of cirrhosis produces areas of micronodular and macronodular regeneration, atrophy, and fatty infiltration, making it difficult for the blood to perfuse. This condition may be found in patients with liver disease or diseases of the cardiovascular system. Patients who present with increased portal blood flow may have an arteriovenous fistula or splenomegaly secondary to a hematologic disorder.

Collateral circulation develops when the normal venous channels become obstructed. This diverted blood flow causes embryologic channels to reopen; blood flows hepatofugally (away from the liver) and is diverted into collateral vessels. The collateral channels may be into the gastric veins (coronary veins), esophageal veins, recanalized umbilical vein, or splenorenal, gastrorenal, retroperitoneal, hemorrhoidal, or intestinal veins (Fig. 9.33). The most common collateral pathways are through the coronary and esophageal veins as occurs in 80% to 90% of patients with portal hypertension. Varices, tortuous dilations of veins, may develop because of increased pressure in the portal vein, usually secondary to cirrhosis. Bleeding from the varices occurs with increased pressure.

The most definitive way to diagnose portal hypertension is with arteriography. Sonography may be useful to define the presence of ascites, hepatosplenomegaly, and collateral circulation; the cause of jaundice; and the patency of hepatic vascular channels. See Table 9.5 for clinical findings, sonographic findings, and differential considerations for portal venous hypertension.

Patient Preparation and Positioning. A history should be obtained from the patient to focus on the risk factors, signs, and symptoms of hepatocellular disease. Any previous medical history relating to hepatocellular disease should be noted. Likewise, any recent surgical intervention or shunt placement within the portal venous system should be documented in the patient history worksheet. The patient is placed initially in the supine position; the patient may also be rolled into a slight left lateral decubitus position to obtain a better intercostal window. The images and Doppler evaluation may be obtained in the longitudinal, coronal, oblique, or transverse plane. Breath holding is extremely important in obtaining good Doppler color and spectral waveforms. Initially, the sonographer should image the patient in shallow respiration to set up his or her controls and depth. They then instruct the patient to stop breathing or take in a deep breath and hold it while the Doppler images are recorded. The image may be visualized on the monitor, allowing the sonographer to see which technique works best to obtain the clearest images. It is helpful to remember that a portal vein diameter greater than 13 mm has been associated with portal hypertension. As portosystemic shunts develop, the diameter of the portal vein decreases. Secondary signs of splenomegaly, alterations in liver size, ascites, and portosystemic venous collaterals should be evaluated (Box 9.5).

The sonographer should keep in mind these important technical points in evaluating the patient for portal hypertension:

- The examination is performed with both imaging and Doppler evaluation of the portal system, the hepatic veins, and the hepatic arteries.
- The transducer must be *parallel* to the vessel; the Doppler angle should be less than 60 degrees to obtain the maximum peak systolic velocity.
- The evaluation of the portal venous system, hepatic veins, and hepatic artery is performed during the Doppler imaging examination.

BOX 9.4 Indications for Portal Hypertension

- Suspected portal hypertension secondary to liver disease
- Portal vein compression or thrombosis
- Acute onset of hepatic vein occlusion (Budd-Chiari syndrome), constrictive pericarditis, or congestive heart failure with tricuspid regurgitation
- Congenital, traumatic, or neoplastic arterioportal fistula

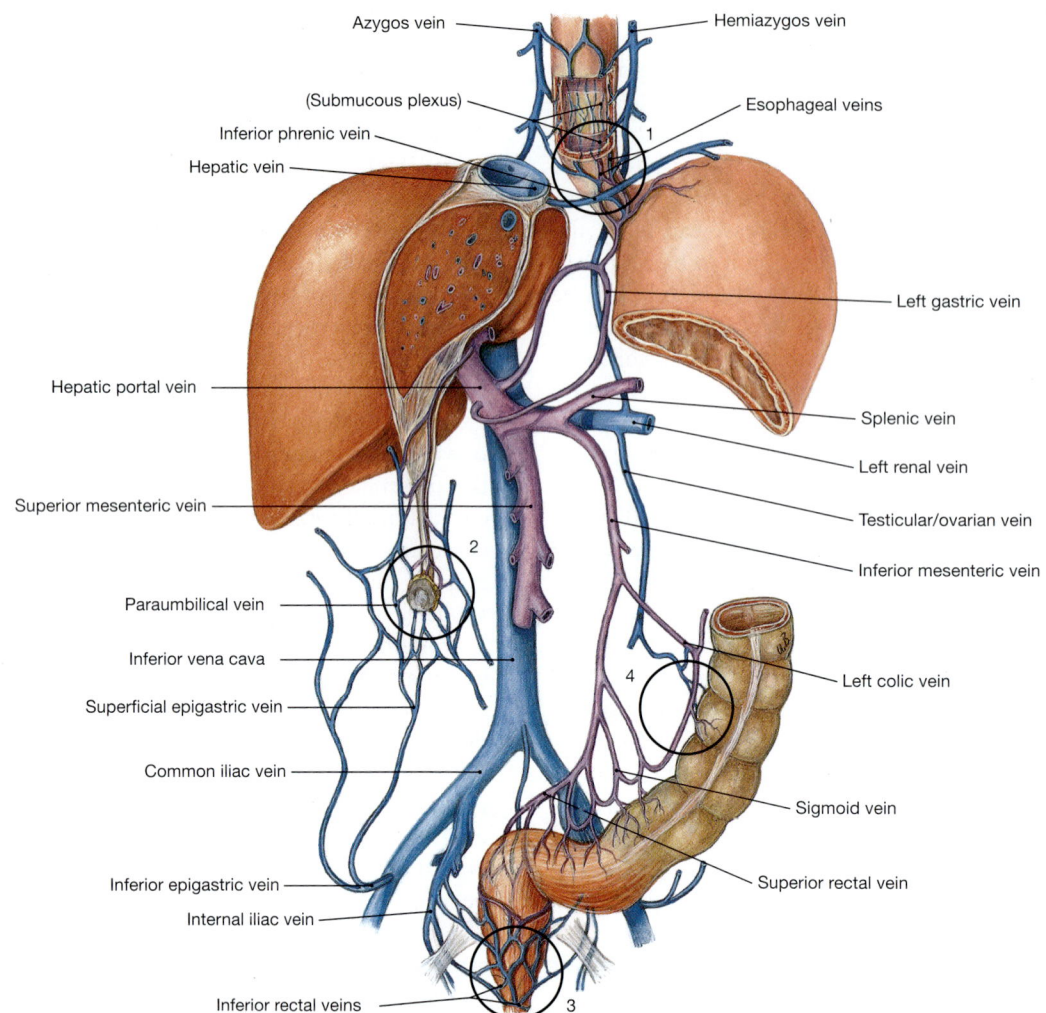

FIG. 9.33 Collateral circulation develops when the normal venous channels become obstructed. The collateral channels may be into the gastric veins (coronary veins), esophageal veins, recanalized umbilical vein, or splenorenal, gastrorenal, retroperitoneal, hemorrhoidal, or intestinal veins.

TABLE 9.5	Liver Findings: Portal Venous Hypertension	
Clinical Findings	**Sonographic Findings**	**Differential Considerations**
↑ Liver enzymes Gastrointestinal bleeding Jaundice Hematemesis	Collateral circulation/reversal of flow Ascites Hepatosplenomegaly	Occlusion of vessels

BOX 9.5 Major Sites of Portosystemic Venous Collaterals

- Gastroesophageal junction located between the coronary and short gastric veins and the systemic esophageal veins (may lead to fatal hemorrhage)
- Paraumbilical vein runs in the falciform ligament and connects the left portal vein to the systemic epigastric veins near the umbilicus
- Splenorenal and gastrorenal veins
- Intestinal veins
- Hemorrhoidal veins

- A Doppler examination should also evaluate flow in the extrahepatic portal venous system and the inferior vena cava, as well as the size of the common bile duct, liver, kidneys, and spleen.
- The pelvic cavity, flanks, and lower quadrants should be evaluated for the presence of free fluid.

Doppler Technique. Box 9.6 summarizes Doppler technique for abdominal exams.

Color Doppler Evaluation of Collateral Circulation. Under normal circumstances, the portal venous blood transverses the liver and drains into the inferior vena cava of the systemic venous circulation by way of the hepatic veins. This is the direct route. However, other smaller communications exist between the portal and systemic systems, and they become important when the direct route becomes blocked. The sonographer should be aware of these communications that include the lower third of the esophagus, the esophageal branches of the left gastric vein (portal tributary) anastomose with the esophageal veins draining the middle third of the esophagus into the azygos veins (systemic tributary). The paraumbilical veins connect the left branch of the portal

BOX 9.6 Doppler Technique

- The pulse repetition frequency (PRF) allows one to record lower velocities as the PRF is lowered; as the PRF is increased, the lower velocities are filtered out to record only the higher velocity signal.
- The PRF may be changed with the scale control on the Doppler panel (look at the color bar on the left side of the monitor; the PRF will change as the "scale" on the Doppler control is changed).
- The PRF increases as imaging depth increases and decreases as depth decreases. Flow within the normal hepatic venous system is low; therefore a lower PRF is necessary to record the flow pattern. As the flow increases beyond 40 cm/sec, the PRF should be increased to prevent aliasing. (Aliasing may also be reduced by scanning at a lower frequency.)
- The Doppler sample volume should be smaller than the diameter of the lumen. One who has difficulty finding the vessel should increase the width of the sample volume to locate the flow, and then reduce the volume width to clear up the spectral waveform.
- The Doppler angle correction should be less than 60 degrees to display the peak spectral velocity.
- Wall filters help to eliminate "noise" or low-level Doppler shifts seen within the vessel.
- Pulsed wave Doppler provides quantitative information from a selected location.
- Color Doppler velocity is dependent on the direction of flow, velocity, and angle to flow. A positive Doppler shift is toward the transducer; negative shift shows flow away from the transducer. The laminar flow is distinguished from turbulent flow by varying the shades of color on the color map.
- Doppler measurements: peak systolic velocity (calculated highest velocity in cm/sec); Resistive Index (RI): subtract the end diastolic velocity from the peak systolic velocity and divide by the peak systolic velocity. Normal or low resistive RI measures <0.7.

vein with the superficial veins of the anterior abdominal wall (systemic tributaries). The paraumbilical veins travel in the falciform ligament and accompany the ligamentum teres. The veins of the ascending colon, descending colon, duodenum, pancreas, and liver (portal tributary) anastomose with the renal, lumbar, and phrenic veins (systemic tributaries).

The dilated venous structures near the superior mesenteric-splenic vein confluence, the main portal vein, and the gastric veins should be evaluated (Fig. 9.34). As the sonographer scans in the longitudinal plane, medial to the superior mesenteric and splenic vein confluence, the right and left gastric veins may be seen as collateral circulation. If the gastric veins are serving as collateral circulation, their diameter should be enlarged to 4 to 5 mm. The Doppler signals should be obtained from the imaging plane that allows the beam to be as parallel to the vessel as possible.

The umbilical vein may become recanalized secondary to portal hypertension. This vessel is best seen on the longitudinal plane near the midline as a tubular structure coursing posterior to the medial surface of the left lobe of the liver (Fig. 9.35). On transverse scans, a bull's-eye is seen within the ligamentum teres as the enlarged umbilical vein. Color Doppler helps the sonographer identify this vascular structure. Table 9.6 summarizes hepatic vasculature technique.

The collateral esophageal vessels are best seen in the midline transverse plane as the transducer is angled in a cephalic direction through the left lobe of the liver. The dilated gastrorenal, splenorenal, and short gastric veins are appreciated in the transverse and longitudinal planes near the splenic hilum.

As discussed earlier, the normal portal venous blood flows toward the liver, with the main portal vein flowing in a hepatopetal direction into the liver. Color Doppler will show this flow as a red or positive color pattern. The portal branches coursing posteriorly, or away from the transducer, will appear as blue, or negative, flow. The normal portal vein waveform is monophasic with low velocity (15 to 18 cm/sec) and varies with the patient's respiration and cardiac pulsation. The flow should be smooth and laminar. The normal diameter of the portal vein is 1.0 to 1.2 cm. With the development of portal hypertension, the flow in the portal vein loses its undulatory pattern and becomes monophasic. With severe portal hypertension, the flow becomes biphasic and finally hepatofugal (away from the liver). At this point, intrahepatic arterial-portal venous shunting may also be seen.

The superior mesenteric vein and splenic vein are more influenced by respiration and patient position; thus, if they appear larger, it may not be because of portal hypertension. Flow reversal is seen both with spectral waveform patterns below the baseline in the main portal vein and with reversed color direction. Obstruction of the portal venous system is recognized by turbulence within the vessel. Table 9.7 summarizes observations important in abdominal Doppler exams.

Doppler Interrogation. The hepatic vessels should be imaged at four anatomic locations:

1. Midline, beneath the xiphoid for the left hepatic vein, left hepatic artery, and left portal vein
2. Midclavicular and intercostals at the porta hepatis for the middle hepatic artery and main portal vein
3. Lateral and intercostals at the right lobe for the right hepatic artery and right portal vein
4. Subcostal and midclavicular for the right hepatic vein and middle hepatic vein

Portal Hypertension Secondary to Portal Vein Thrombosis. The invasion of the portal system with tumor or thrombosis may cause portal hypertension if the vessel is significantly occluded, preventing blood flow into the liver. The clinical symptoms are very different from those of intrahepatic disease; ascites is the primary complaint. The patient does not have jaundice or a tender enlarged liver. Splenomegaly and bleeding varices may be present. Portal vein thrombosis (Fig. 9.36) may develop secondary to trauma, sepsis, cirrhosis, or HCC. The definitive diagnosis is made with a liver biopsy and positive findings of portal hypertension.

Sonographic Findings. Portal vein thrombosis shows absence of portal flow with echogenic thrombus within the lumen of the vein, the development of portal vein collaterals, expansion of the caliber of the vein, and cavernous transformation of the vessels. The cavernous transformation of

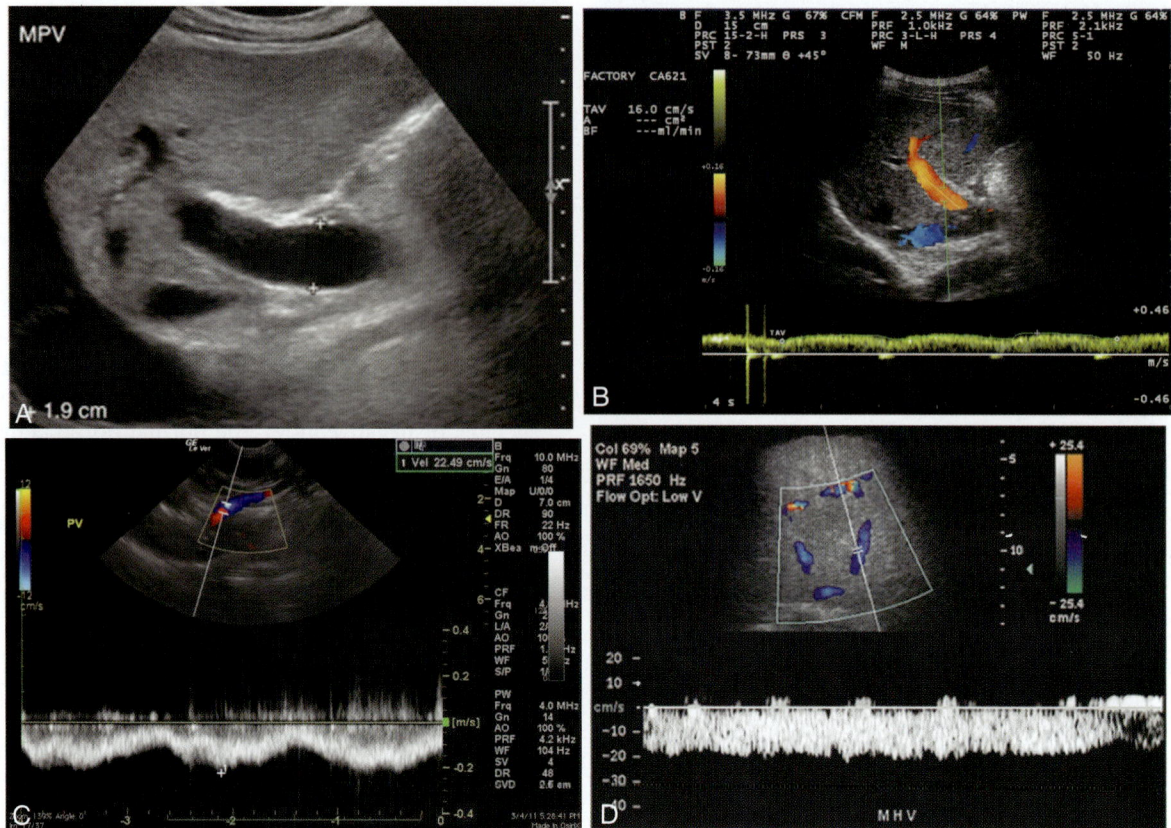

FIG. 9.34 (A) The dilated venous structures near the superior mesenteric-splenic vein confluence, the main portal vein, and the gastric veins should be evaluated. (B) Color Doppler is useful to assess the direction of blood flow within the vascular structures. Spectral Doppler shows the abnormal flow patterns of the portal vein (C) and hepatic vein (D).

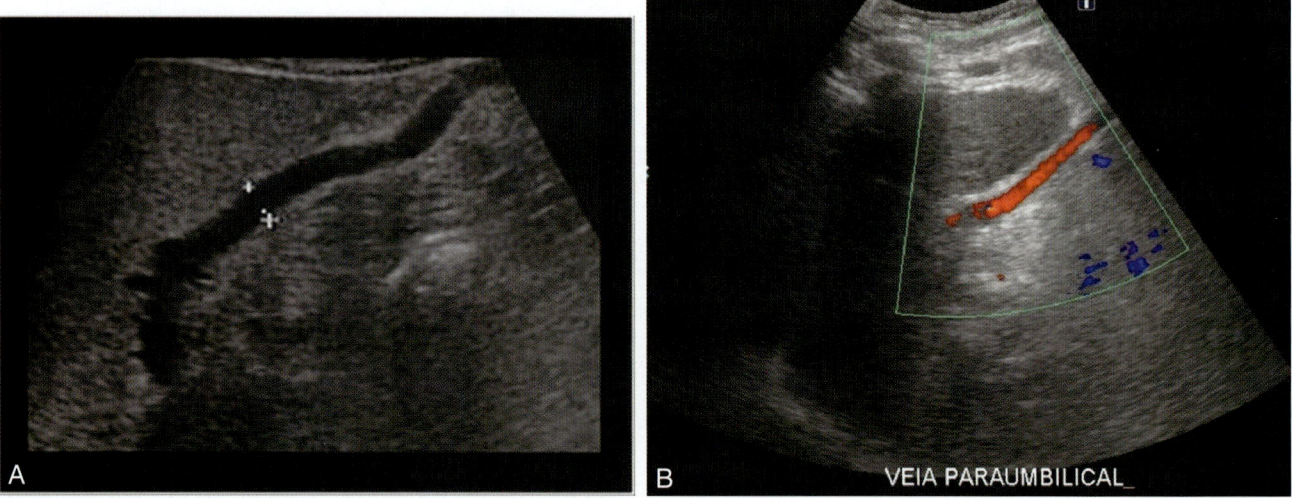

FIG. 9.35 (A) The umbilical vein may become recanalized secondary to portal hypertension. (B) This vessel is best seen on the longitudinal plane near the midline as a tubular structure coursing posterior to the medial surface of the left lobe of the liver.

the portal vein appears as a *wormlike* structure in the porta hepatis that completely fills with color representing the periportal collateral circulation. Acute thrombus may appear anechoic and thus be missed by the sonographer if Doppler interrogation is not performed. Malignant thrombosis of the portal vein is closely associated with HCC and is often expansive.

Portal Vein Hypertension and Portal Caval Shunts. If portal hypertension becomes extensive, the portal system can be decompressed by shunting blood to the systemic venous system. Portalcaval shunts for the treatment of portal hypertension may involve the anastomosis of the portal vein because it lies within the lesser omentum, to the anterior wall of the inferior vena cava behind the entrance into the lesser sac.

TABLE 9.6	Hepatic Vasculature Technique	
Vessel	**Image Plane**	**Technique**
LHV	Transverse/longitudinal	• Locate the left lobe of the liver. • Identify the IVC and angle steeply toward the diaphragm. • The LHV and MHV should be seen as they drain into the IVC.
LPV, LHA	Transverse, coronal, intercostal, decubitus Transverse	• Locate horizontal segment of LPV, adjust transducer to obtain steepest angle for Doppler (parallel to the vessel), and zoom in on the LPV. • Usually found posterior to horizontal segment of LPV. • After interrogating the LPV, look for LHA with color Doppler (expand color box to cover the LPV and adjacent liver tissue). • Place PW cursor/sample volume in area of LHA (suspend respiration); watch for "flashing" of signal as it comes in and out of view with respiration. • Look for LHA on deep inspiration. • If you cannot get the signal in the periphery of the liver, move to another location closer to the main portal vein.
Common HA	Longitudinal—porta hepatis	• Use same technique as described for LHA. • Transplant recipient patients: usually only able to Doppler HA at the porta hepatis. • Include extrahepatic and intrahepatic segments of HA. • Difficult to image site of anastomosis.
MPV, IVC	Longitudinal—porta hepatic Longitudinal, coronal—slightly to right of midline; suspend breath. Angle transducer in cephalad to caudal sweep to record flow.	• If shunt is present, anastomosis site easier to identify (more prone to thrombosis); be sure to investigate the MPV proximal, within, and distal to anastomosis. • May be difficult to obtain good angle because of horizontal location on transverse plane. • If shunt is present, evaluate site of anastomosis carefully (proximal, within, and distal). • Look carefully for presence of internal echoes that represent thrombosis. • If you suspect thrombus is present, and the Doppler signal is very "choppy" with high velocity and little phasicity, the likelihood of thrombus is good. • Be sure to follow the IVC all the way into the right atrium of the heart.
SV, RHA	Transverse Transverse, anterior to right posterior portal branch	• Examine SV from the splenic hilum to the portal-splenic confluence. • Use same techniques as mentioned to Doppler the RPV and RHA. • If you are unable to locate the RHA in the periphery of the liver, move closer to the trunk of the adjacent PV. • If you cannot find the RHA at the right posterior portal branch, try looking for it at the level of the right anterior PV branch.
RPV	Anterior, intercostal approach; one rib space away from window for porta hepatis	• To locate the right posterior branch of RPV, begin with the MPV at the porta hepatis. • Follow the MPV into the liver until you see the RPV. • The posterior branch extends posteriorly into the right lobe. It is easier to obtain a good Doppler angle if you use a more anterior intercostal approach.
RHV	Transverse, subcostal	• Place the probe just below the level of the xiphoid with a steep angulation toward the diaphragm. • Locate the IVC; the RHV will be seen in the right lobe of the liver in a horizontal plane as it empties into the IVC.
MHV	Transverse, subcostal	• Place the probe just below the level of the xiphoid with a steep angulation toward the diaphragm. • Locate the IVC; the MHV will be seen in a vertical plane as it separates the right lobe from the left lobe of the liver as it empties into the IVC.

HA, Hepatic artery; *IVC*, inferior vena cava; *LHA*, left hepatic artery; *LHV*, left hepatic vein; *LPV*, left portal vein; *MHV*, middle hepatic vein; *MPV*, middle portal vein; *RHA*, right hepatic artery; *RHV*, right hepatic vein; *RPV*, right portal vein; *SV*, splenic vein.

TABLE 9.7 Doppler Observations

Hepatic Artery

LHA, RHA, CHA
- Low resistance waveform; forward flow in diastolic above baseline.
- Vessel is tortuous; flow may appear to move toward and away from the transducer.
- Systolic window with narrow bandwidth with parabolic flow profile.
- Spectral fill-in of systolic window because of small vessel diameter.
- High-resistance waveforms may indicate veno-occlusive disease.

Portal Venous System

LPV, RPV, MPV
- Continuous, low-velocity phasic signal (phasic means that the velocity increases and decreases with respiration, giving the signal a smooth wavelike appearance).
- Normal flow is termed *hepatopetal* (toward the liver).
- Reversed flow is *hepatofugal* (away from the liver).
- Portal venous thrombosis or postoperative anastomosis from a liver transplant can cause an abnormal portal vein signal. This results from decreased vessel lumen size, which reduces the pressure and consequently increases the velocity of flow through the narrowed region, giving a "choppy" appearance as a result of increased velocities.
- *Note:* The hepatic artery and portal vein flow should be in the same direction since the hepatic artery runs parallel with the portal vein.

Hepatic Venous System

LHV, RHV, MHV
- Multiphasic pulsatile flow pattern secondary to proximity of the right atrium with flow above and below the baseline caused by proximity to the right atrium, which results in hemodynamic changes.
- Right-sided heart failure may cause the hepatic veins to become pulsatile and dilated.
- Increased intrahepatic pressure or venous obstruction demonstrates a more continuous or monophasic signal.

Inferior Vena Cava
- Continuous waveform with respiratory variations; becomes more pulsatile as it empties into the right atrium.
- Best imaged with a slight cranial-caudal sweep in the longitudinal plane with the patient in deep inspiration.
- Anastomosis from surgical transplantation may alter the normal flow into the inferior vena cava.
- Thrombosis can cause the inferior vena cava waveform to appear monophasic with high velocities ("choppy" appearance). Examine for thrombus in the renal veins as well.
- If a surgical shunt is present, be sure to check the patient's history to find out if the specific type of shunt (portal/cava or mesenteric/cava) is in place.

CHA, Common hepatic artery; *LHA*, left hepatic artery; *LHV*, left hepatic vein; *LPV*, left portal vein; *MHV*, middle hepatic vein; *MPV*, middle portal vein; *RHA*, right hepatic artery; *RHV*, right hepatic vein; *RPV*, right portal vein.

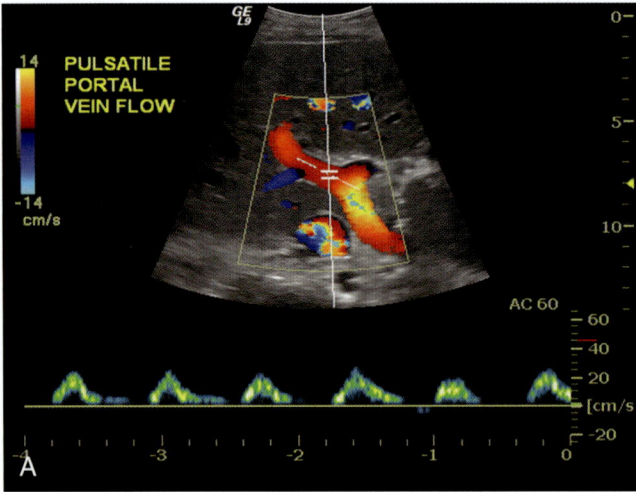 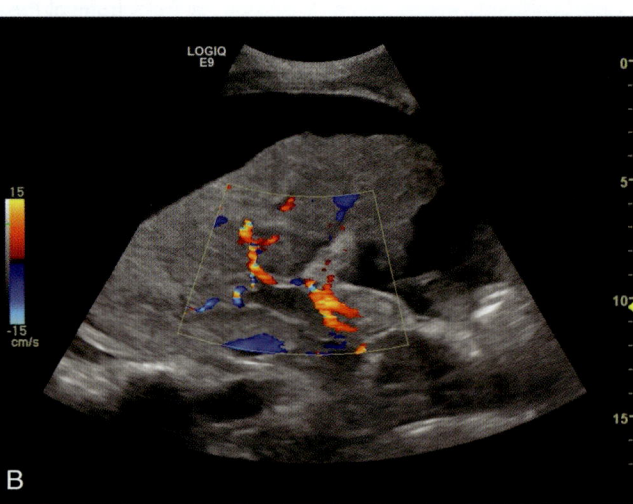

FIG. 9.36 (A) Normal portal vein flow. (B) Portal vein thrombosis.

The splenic vein may be anastomosed to the left renal vein after removing the spleen. Basically, the three types of shunts are portacaval, mesocaval, and splenorenal. It is the responsibility of the sonographer to know specifically which type of shunt the patient has in place to image the flow patterns correctly.

The portacaval shunt attaches the main portal vein at the superior mesenteric vein-splenic vein confluence to the

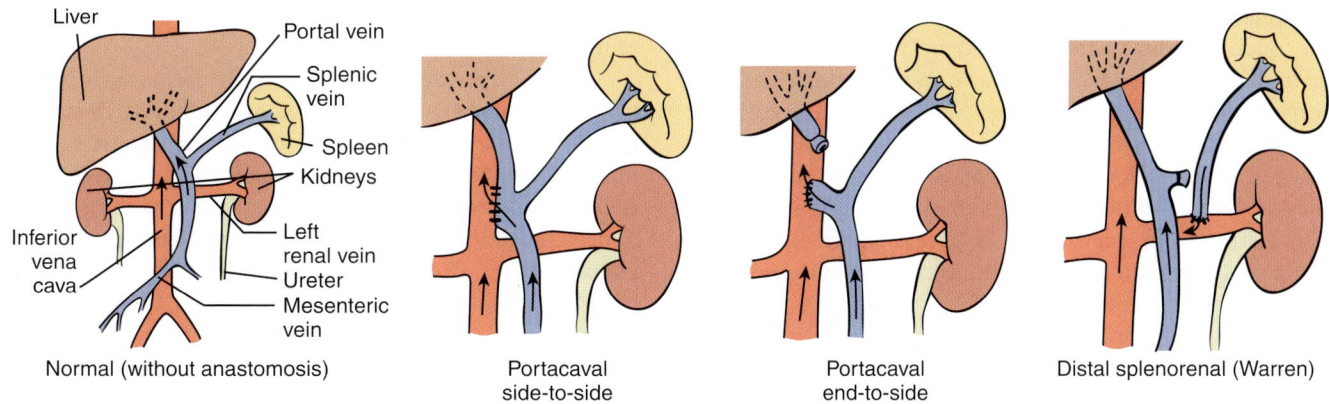

FIG. 9.37 Portocaval shunt attaches the main portal vein at the superior mesenteric vein-splenic vein confluence to the anterior aspect of the inferior vena cava. Mesocaval shunt attaches the mid-distal superior mesenteric vein to the inferior vena cava.

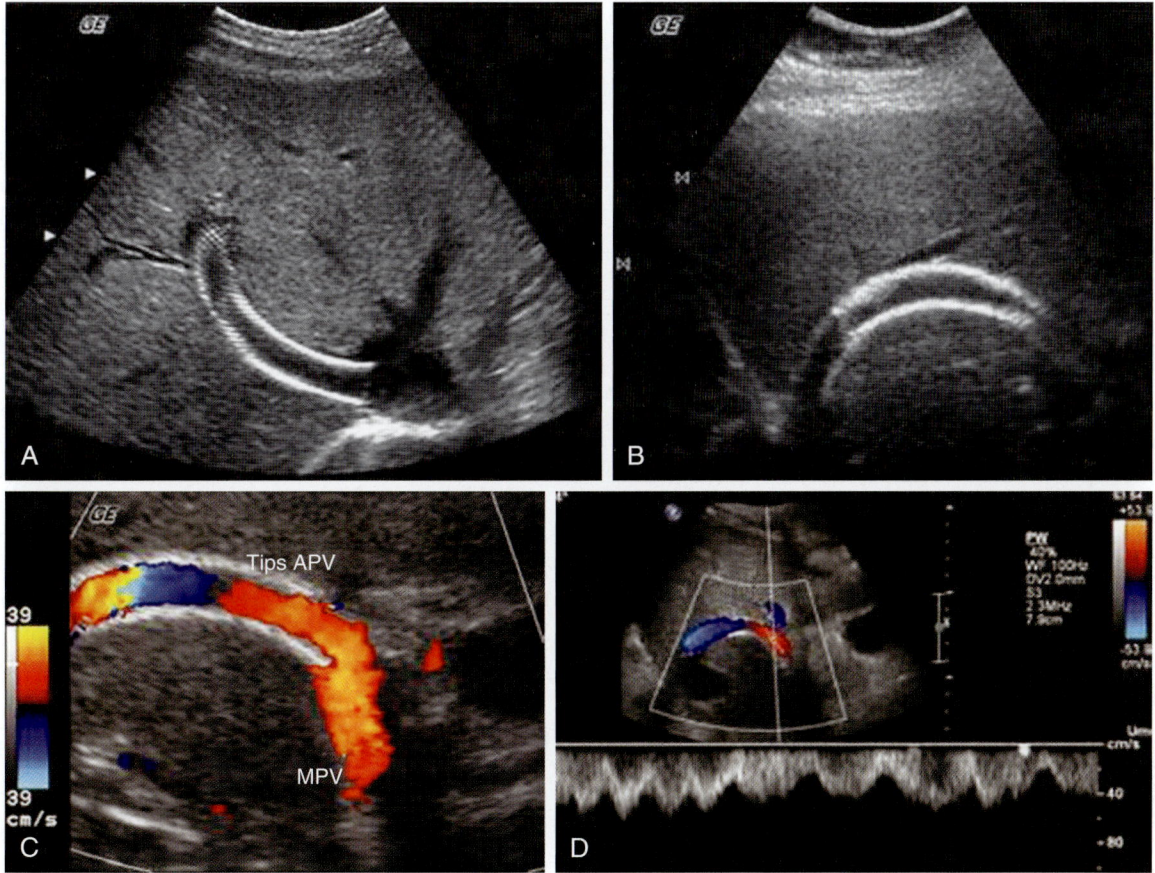

FIG. 9.38 Transjugular intrahepatic portosystemic shunt (TIPS). (A–D) Images of a 50-year-old man after TIPS procedure shows patency of the stent and normal flow from the portal vein to the inferior vena cava without evidence of thrombus. *APV,* Anterior portal vein; *MPV,* main portal vein.

anterior aspect of the inferior vena cava (Fig. 9.37). The mesocaval shunt attaches the mid-distal superior mesenteric vein to the inferior vena cava. This shunt may be difficult to image if overlying bowel gas is present. The splenorenal shunt attaches the splenic vein to the left renal vein. The shunt and connecting vessel should be documented with pulsed wave Doppler and color Doppler to determine flow patterns and patency.

Intrahepatic shunts are created percutaneously with the use of metallic expandable stents, which can be seen on ultrasound. This type of shunt is the **transjugular intrahepatic portosystemic shunt (TIPS)** (Fig. 9.38). The TIPS shunt is evaluated for patency by viewing the liver in an acoustic window to image the flow velocity pattern within the shunt. Baseline studies are performed with color and spectral Doppler so variations in flow patterns may be monitored before clinical symptoms are apparent. Stenosis may occur at the hepatic vein level or within the shunt.

Budd-Chiari Syndrome. Budd-Chiari syndrome is an uncommon, often dramatic illness caused by thrombosis of the hepatic veins or inferior vena cava. It was first described by George Budd in 1846 and by Hans Chiari in 1899. The patient with Budd-Chiari syndrome has a poor prognosis and is characterized by abdominal pain, massive ascites, and hepatomegaly. This condition may present acutely or as a chronic illness lasting from a few weeks to several years. Extensive hepatic vein occlusion is usually fatal within weeks or months of the onset of symptoms.

Budd-Chiari syndrome may be classified as primary or secondary based on its pathophysiology. The primary type is caused by congenital obstruction of the hepatic veins or inferior vena cava by membranous webs across the upper vena cava at or just above the entrance of the left and middle hepatic veins. This lesion has been found to be most common in Asia.

The secondary type results from thrombosis in the hepatic veins or inferior vena cava. It often occurs in patients with predisposing conditions, such as prolonged use of oral contraceptives, pregnancy tumors (HCC, renal cell carcinoma, adrenal carcinoma, leiomyosarcoma of the inferior vena cava), infections, and in rare cases, trauma. In approximately 25% to 30% of all cases, the exact cause is never determined.

Ascites is the most characteristic clinical feature of Budd-Chiari syndrome. Other symptoms are abdominal pain, hepatosplenomegaly, jaundice, vomiting, and diarrhea. Rarely, patients present with acute illness with abdominal pain, hepatomegaly, and shock. More commonly, patients have a vague illness and abdominal distress weeks or months in duration, followed by the appearance of ascites and hepatomegaly. Jaundice is mild or absent. As portal hypertension increases, the spleen becomes palpable. When thrombus is found in the inferior vena cava, edema of the legs is gross, and there is venous distention over the abdomen, flanks, and back. Albuminuria may be found.

Routine biochemical determinations of aminotransferases and alkaline phosphatase indicate mild or moderate impairment of hepatic function, depending on the stage of disease. See Table 9.8 for clinical findings, sonographic findings, and differential considerations for Budd-Chiari syndrome.

Sonographic Findings. Sonography is useful in imaging patients with hepatic vein thrombosis. The caudate lobe of the liver, seen in longitudinal and transverse scans, has an independent vascular supply. In Budd-Chiari syndrome, the caudate lobe becomes enlarged, and there is often atrophy of the right hepatic lobe, probably because of sparing of caudate lobe hepatic veins when there is thrombosis of the right, middle, and left hepatic veins.

The liver appears hypoechoic in the early stages of acute thrombosis; it appears hyperechoic and inhomogeneous, with fibrosis in later stages. The middle and left hepatic veins are imaged in the transverse plane at the level of the xiphoid. The transducer is angled in a cephalad position with the patient in deep inspiration. This allows the veins to be parallel to the Doppler beam. The right hepatic vein is evaluated from a right intercostal approach. With thrombosis, the hepatic veins become enlarged. In chronic cases of Budd-Chiari syndrome, the hepatic veins are usually not visualized. Demonstration of at least one major vein may show abnormalities in the vessel suggestive of this syndrome, including stenosis, dilation, thick wall echoes, abnormal course, extrahepatic anastomoses, and thrombosis (Fig. 9.39).

Doppler sonography may show altered blood flow patterns in the hepatic veins and inferior vena cava. In normal subjects, the Doppler signal in the hepatic veins is phasic in response to both the cardiac and respiratory cycles, with wide variations in flow velocity and direction. In Budd-Chiari syndrome, flow in the inferior vena cava or hepatic veins changes from phasic to absent, reversed, turbulent, or continuous. Abnormal Doppler patterns with slow, continuous flow may indicate partial obstruction. The absence of flow signals suggests subtotal or total occlusion. Turbulent flow may be observed beyond the area of stenosis. The portal venous flow pattern may also be affected with decreased velocities or reversal of flow.

Color flow Doppler is an excellent technique for evaluating the hepatic venous system. Flow direction and velocities, and areas of turbulent flow can be demonstrated with color. Patency of the hepatic veins and inferior vena cava can be determined with color flow Doppler, which compares very favorably with angiography.

Diagnostic Criteria for Hepatic Vascular Imaging. See Table 9.9 for the diagnostic criteria for hepatic vascular imaging, including grayscale, Doppler, and color Doppler.

Diffuse Abnormalities of the Liver Parenchyma

Abnormalities—such as biliary obstruction, common duct stones and stricture, extrahepatic mass, and passive hepatic congestion—are discussed as each lesion is seen on the ultrasound. See Table 9.10 for clinical findings, sonographic findings, and differential considerations of diffuse abnormalities of the liver parenchyma.

Biliary Obstruction: Proximal. Biliary obstruction proximal to the cystic duct can be caused by gallstones, carcinoma of the common bile duct, or metastatic tumor invasion of the porta hepatis (Fig. 9.40). Clinically, the patient may be jaundiced and have pruritus (itching). Liver function tests show an elevation in the direct bilirubin and alkaline phosphatase levels.

Sonographic Findings. Sonographically, carcinoma of the common duct presents as a tubular branching with dilated intrahepatic ducts best seen in the periphery of the liver.

TABLE 9.8	Liver Findings: Budd-Chiari Syndrome	
Clinical Findings	Sonographic Findings	Differential Considerations
Ascites, right upper quadrant pain, hepatomegaly	Enlarged caudate lobe Atrophy in right lobe of the liver	Portal hypertension

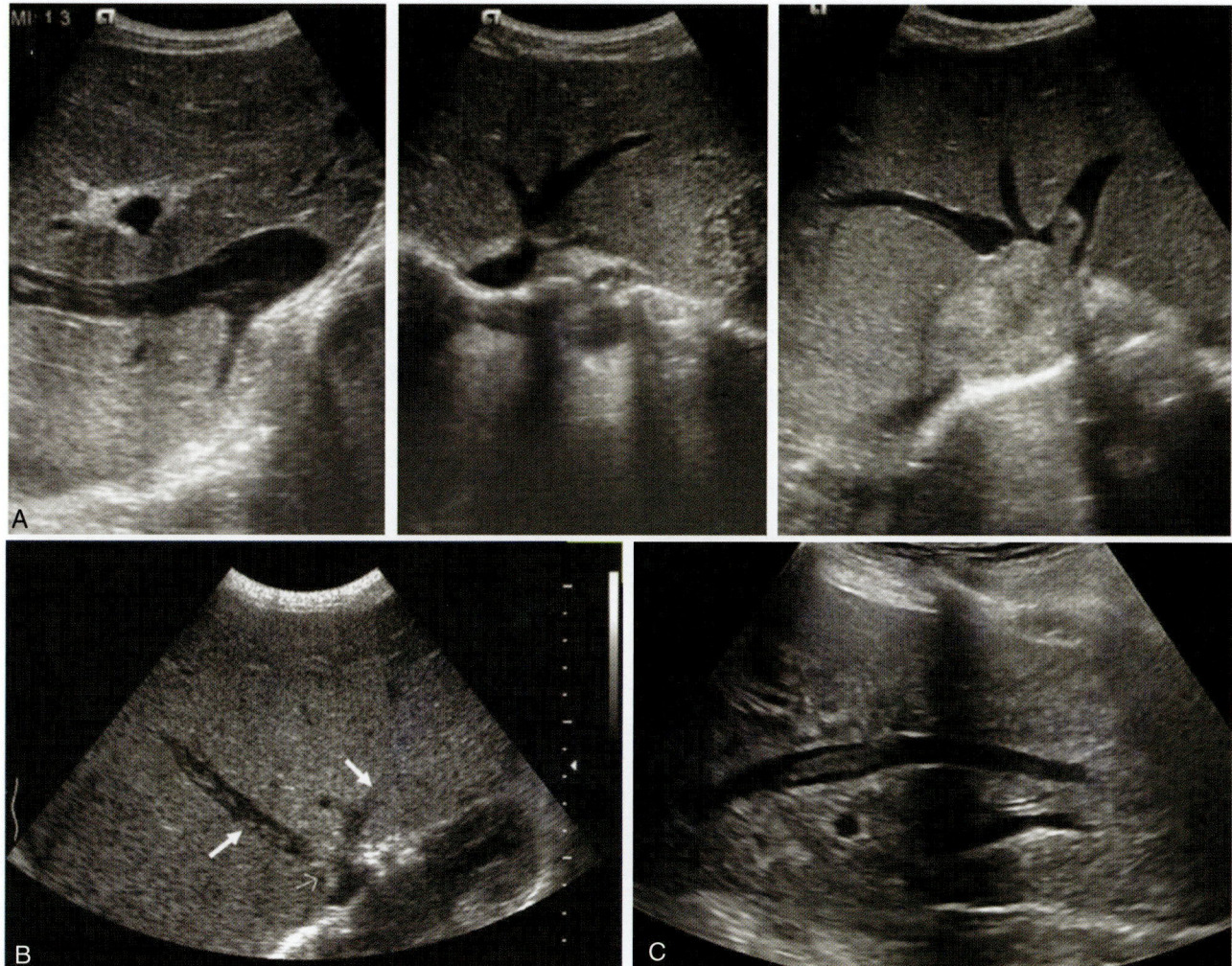

FIG. 9.39 (A) In Budd-Chiari syndrome, the caudate lobe becomes enlarged, and there is often atrophy of the right hepatic lobe, probably as a result of sparing of caudate lobe hepatic veins when there is thrombosis of the right, middle, and left hepatic veins. (B) *Arrows* point to thrombosis in the middle and left hepatic veins. (C) Longitudinal image of thrombosis in the right hepatic vein.

Gallstones lodged in the common bile duct will cause dilation (Fig. 9.41). It may be difficult to image a discrete mass lesion. The gallbladder is of normal size, even after a fatty meal is administered.

Biliary Obstruction: Distal. A biliary obstruction distal to the cystic duct may be caused by stones in the common duct, an extrahepatic mass in the porta hepatis, or stricture of the common duct. Clinically, common duct stones cause right upper quadrant pain, jaundice, and pruritus, as well as an increase in direct bilirubin and alkaline phosphatase.

Sonographic Findings. On ultrasound examination, the dilated intrahepatic ducts are seen in the periphery of the liver (Fig. 9.42). The gallbladder size is variable, usually small. Gallstones are often present and appear as hyperechoic lesions along the posterior floor of the gallbladder with a sharp posterior acoustic shadow. Careful evaluation of the common duct may show shadowing stones within the dilated duct.

Extrahepatic Mass. An extrahepatic mass in the area of the porta hepatis causes the same clinical signs as seen in biliary obstruction. The lesion may arise from the lymph nodes, pancreatitis, pseudocyst, or carcinoma in the head of the pancreas.

Sonographic Findings. On ultrasound examination, an irregular, ill-defined, hypoechoic, and inhomogeneous mass lesion may be seen in the area of the porta hepatis (Fig. 9.43).

There is intrahepatic ductal dilation with a hydropic gallbladder.

Common Duct Stricture. Clinically, the patient is jaundiced and has had a previous cholecystectomy. Laboratory values show an increase in the direct bilirubin and alkaline phosphatase levels.

Sonographic Findings. On ultrasound examination, common duct stricture presents as dilated intrahepatic ducts with absence of a mass in the porta hepatis.

Passive Hepatic Congestion. Passive hepatic congestion develops secondary to congestive heart failure with signs of hepatomegaly. Laboratory data indicate normal to slightly elevated liver function tests.

TABLE 9.9 Diagnostic Criteria for Hepatic Vascular Imaging

Interpretation	Gray Scale	Doppler	Color Doppler
Portal Veins			
Normal	No intraluminal echoes; bright, echogenic borders	Low-velocity signal with respiratory variation	Smooth fill-in of color
Thrombus	Enlarged or normal portal venous system with low-level echoes within the lumen; may appear isoechoic with the liver	Decreased low velocity to absent Doppler waveform; look for hepatofugal flow	Decreased to absent color flow
Portal hypertension	Enlargement of the portal venous system Recanalization of the umbilical vein	Look for hepatofugal flow in portal venous system	Hepatofugal flow with good color fill of lumen
Cavernous transformation	Multiple vascular channels near the porta hepatis and/or splenic hilum Thrombosis of the extrahepatic portal vein (may be difficult to image) Look for recanalized umbilical vein	Continuous low-velocity flow	Color fills dilated collateral vessels; portal vein is difficult to fill with color
Hepatic Artery (HA)			
Normal	Follow course of portal vein to image hepatic artery anterior Enlarge image size to visualize artery Proximal HA best seen at level of celiac axis Distal HA seen in intercostal coronal view at level of main portal vein and common bile duct	Low-resistance waveform with systolic and diastolic component	Increase gain slightly to fill in vessel lumen with color
Thrombus	Increased low-level echoes within the lumen	Obstruction would cause increased velocity waveforms	Turbulence or absence of flow if complete obstruction is present
Inferior Vena Cava (IVC)			
Normal	Low-level intraluminal echoes within the lumen returning to right atrium; changes size with respiration	Continuous triphasic waveform with respiratory variations	Color fills lumen
Thrombosis	Increased echogenicity of low-level echoes filling lumen Examine renal veins for extension of thrombus	Decreased Doppler waveform secondary to degree of thrombus	Decreased color within lumen; color will outline the area of thrombus/obstruction
Right-sided heart failure	Dilation of lumen that does not change with respiration	Multiphasic, pulsatile flow	Color fills lumen of hepatic veins and inferior vena cava
Thrombosis/Budd-Chiari	Low-level echoes within the lumen of the hepatic veins; may completely restrict blood flow into the inferior vena cava Caudate lobe enlargement may be suspicious of thrombosis of hepatic veins	Decreased flow signal	Decreased color fill-in of hepatic veins; IVC may appear collapsed with decreased blood return

Sonographic Findings. On ultrasound examination, dilation of the inferior vena cava, superior mesenteric, hepatic, portal, and splenic veins is noted (Fig. 9.44). The inferior vena cava normally decreases in size with expiration and increases with inspiration; however, with congestion, there is little change in the size.

Focal Hepatic Disease

Few hepatic lesions have specific sonographic features. Therefore knowing the patient's clinical history and the sonographic patterns associated with various lesions is important. The knowledge of laboratory values in liver function tests also helps determine the hepatic lesions. The differential diagnosis for focal diseases of the liver includes cysts, abscess, hematoma, primary tumor, and metastases. See Table 9.11 for clinical findings, sonographic findings, and differential considerations for focal hepatic disease.

The sonographer should be able to differentiate whether the mass is **extrahepatic** or **intrahepatic**. Intrahepatic masses may cause the following findings on ultrasound: displacement of the hepatic vascular radicles, external bulging of the liver capsule, or a posterior shift of the inferior vena cava.

TABLE 9.10	Liver Findings: Diffuse Abnormalities of the Liver Parenchyma	
Clinical Findings	**Sonographic Findings**	**Differential Considerations**
Biliary Obstruction: Proximal		
↑ Direct bilirubin ↑ Alk phos	Carcinoma of common bile duct shows tubular branching with dilated intrahepatic ducts Gallbladder small to normal size; gallstones	Obstruction to distal duct Extrahepatic metastases
Biliary Obstruction: Distal		
↑ Direct bilirubin ↑ Alk phos	Carcinoma of common bile duct shows tubular branching with dilated intrahepatic ducts Gallbladder small; gallstones and common duct stones	Obstruction to proximal duct Extrahepatic metastases
Extrahepatic Mass		
↑ Direct bilirubin ↑ Alk phos	Irregular, ill-defined hypoechoic, heterogeneous lesion in area of porta hepatic Intrahepatic ductal dilation Hydropic gallbladder	Proximal or distal obstruction to the cystic duct Metastases
Common Duct Stricture		
↑ Direct bilirubin ↑ Alk phos ↑ Previous cholecystectomy	Dilated intrahepatic ducts Absence of mass in porta hepatis	Extrahepatic mass Passive hepatic congestion
Passive Hepatic Congestion		
↑ LFT	↑ IVC, HV, PV	N/A

Alk phos, Alkaline phosphatase; *IVC*, inferior vena cava; *HV*, hepatic vein; *LFT*, liver function test; *N/A*, not applicable; *PV*, portal vein.

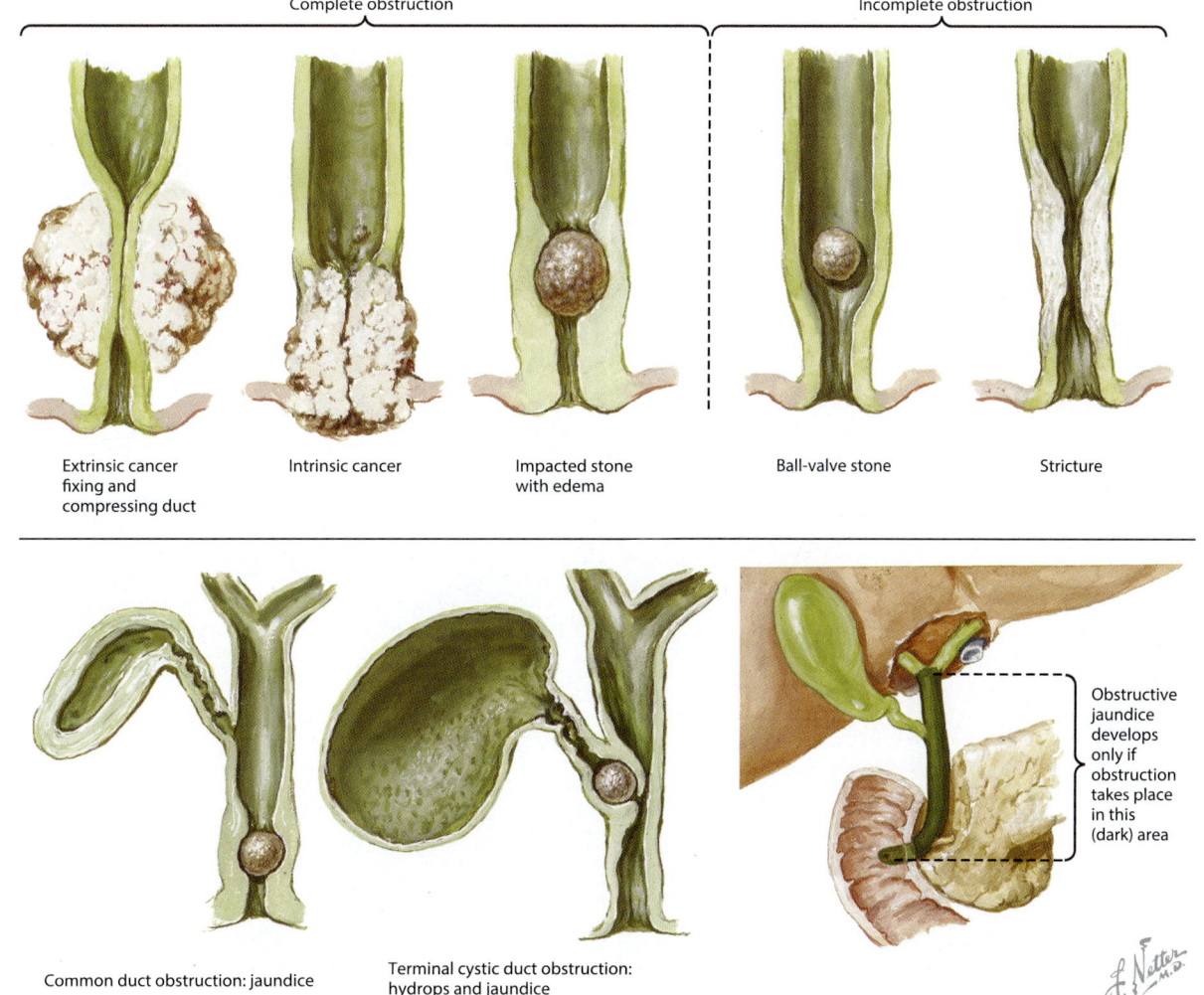

FIG. 9.40 Biliary obstruction proximal to the cystic duct can be caused by gallstones, carcinoma of the common bile duct, or metastatic tumor invasion of the porta hepatis.

An extrahepatic mass may show internal invagination or discontinuity of the liver capsule, formation of a triangular fat wedge, anteromedial shift of the inferior vena cava, or anterior displacement of the right kidney.

Cystic Lesions. *Hepatic cyst* usually refers to a solitary nonparasitic cyst of the liver. The cyst may be solitary or multiple. Cystic lesions within the liver include the following: simple or congenital hepatic cysts, traumatic cysts, parasitic cysts, inflammatory cysts, polycystic disease, and pseudocysts.

Patients are often asymptomatic and require no treatment. When the cysts become large, pain may develop as the lesion compresses the hepatic vasculature or ductal system. Fever may be present if the cyst hemorrhages and becomes infected. Once the cyst becomes infected, septations and internal echoes from the debris replace the anechoic properties. The wall may become thickened.

Simple Hepatic Cysts. The sonographic finding of a simple hepatic cyst is usually incidental because most patients are asymptomatic. As the cyst grows, it may cause pain or a mass effect to suggest a more serious condition, such as infection, abscess, or necrotic lesion. Hepatic cysts occur more often in females than in males.

Sonographic Findings. On ultrasound examination, the cyst walls are thin, with well-defined borders, and anechoic, with distal posterior enhancement (Fig. 9.45A). Infrequently, cysts contain fine linear internal septa. Complications, such as hemorrhage, may occur and cause pain (Fig. 9.45B). Calcification may be seen within the cyst wall and may cause shadowing.

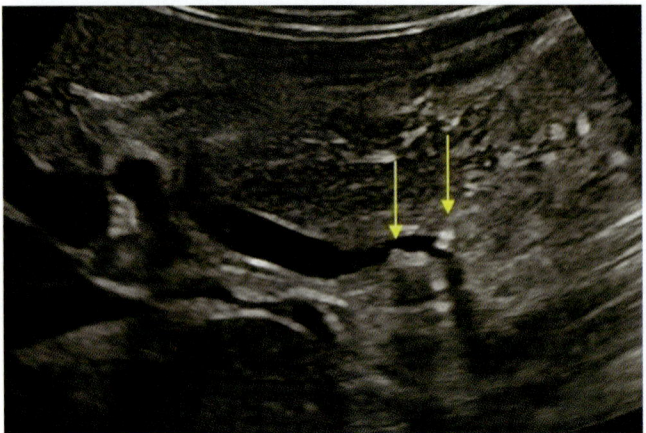

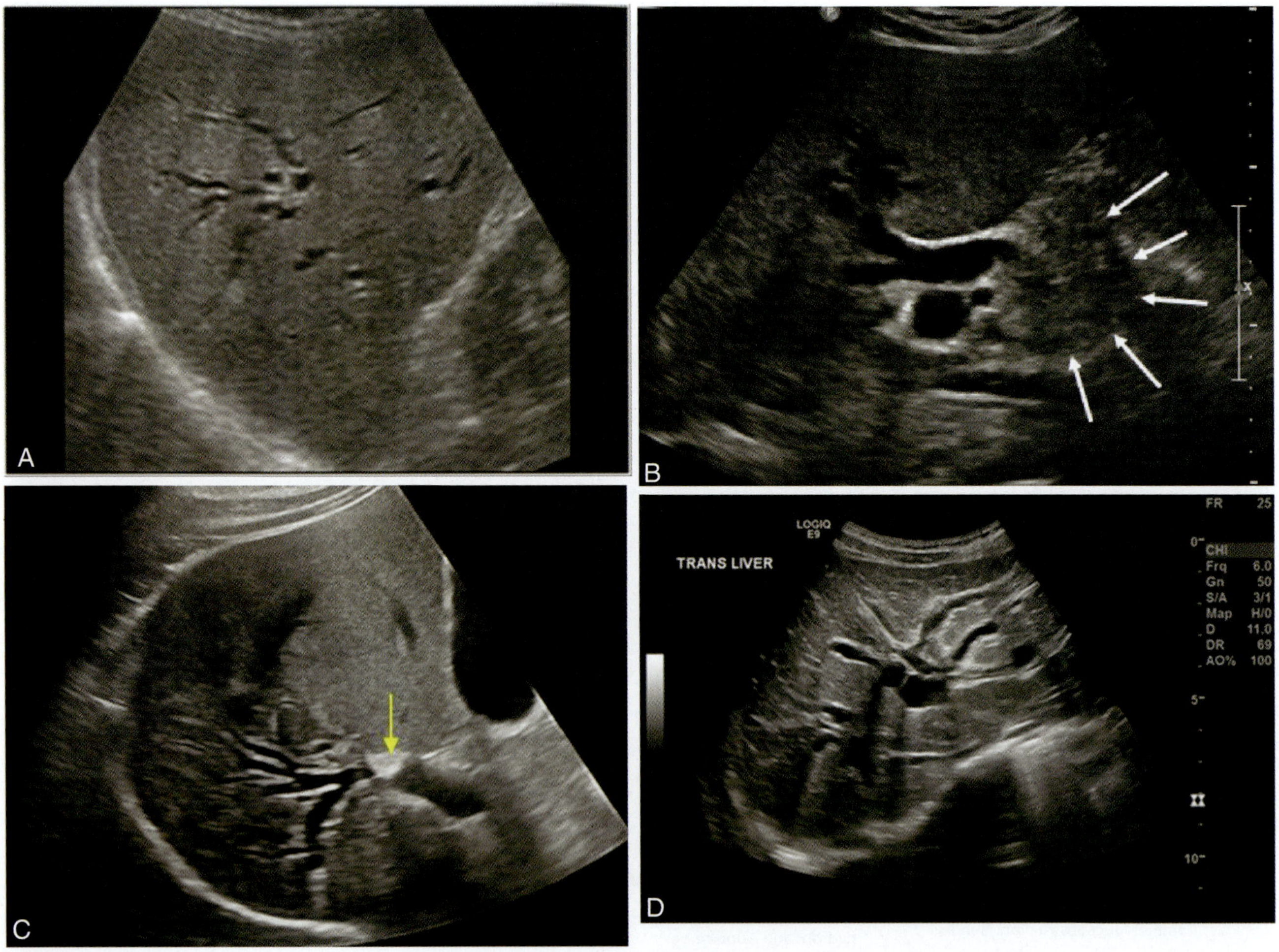

FIG. 9.41 Gallstones lodged in the common bile duct will cause dilation.

FIG. 9.42 (A–D) A biliary obstruction distal to the cystic duct may be caused by stones in the common duct, an extrahepatic mass in the porta hepatis, or stricture of the common duct. On ultrasound examination, the dilated intrahepatic ducts are seen in the periphery of the liver.

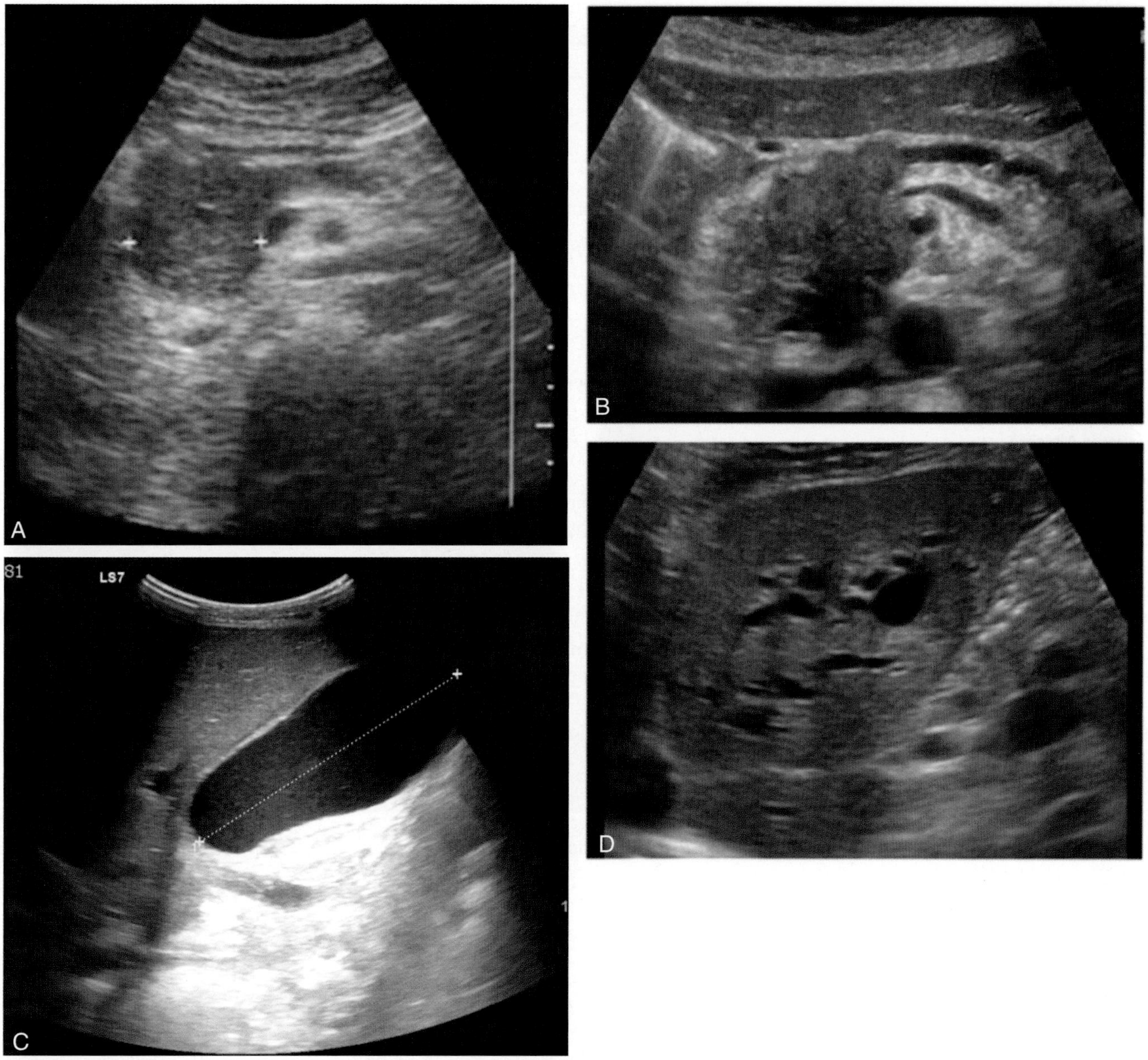

FIG. 9.43 An extrahepatic mass, such as a tumor in the head of the pancreas (A–B), may cause hydrops of the gallbladder (C) and intrahepatic biliary duct dilation (D).

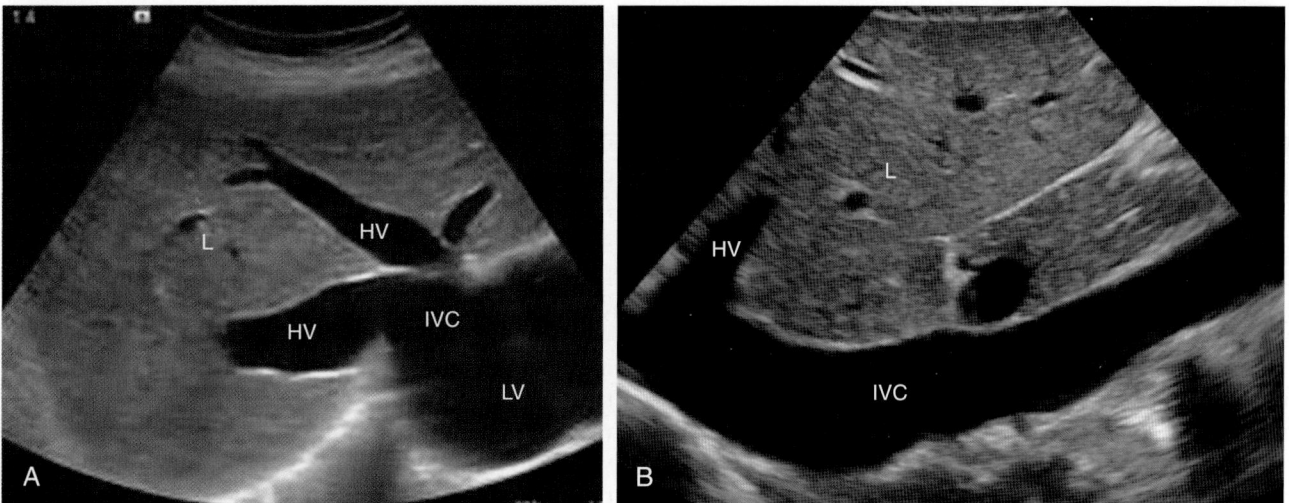

FIG. 9.44 (A) Transverse and (B) longitudinal images of a patient in congestive liver failure. The inferior vena cava (IVC) and hepatic veins (HV) are dilated without respiratory collapse. *L*, liver.

TABLE 9.11 Liver Findings: Focal Disease

Clinical Findings	Sonographic Findings	Differential Considerations
Simple Hepatic Cysts		
N/A	Anechoic Thin walls Well-defined borders Distal posterior enhancement May have calcification	Congenital Hematoma Necrotic tumor
Polycystic Liver Disease		
Autosomal dominant 25%–50% of patients with polycystic kidney disease have hepatic cysts 60% of patients with polycystic liver disease have associated PKD	Anechoic Well-defined borders ↑ Acoustic enhancement Multiple cysts throughout liver parenchyma	Necrotic metastasis Echinococcal cyst Hematoma Abscess Hepatic cystadenocarcinoma
Pyogenic Abscess		
↑ White cell count Abnormal LFT Anemia	Variable appearance Right central lobe most common site Hypoechoic to complex to hyperechoic when fluid level present Round to oval or irregular Complex	Amebic abscess Echinococcal cyst Hepatic candidiasis
Hepatic Candidiasis		
↑ WBC Fever	Multiple small hypoechoic masses with echogenic central core "bulls-eye" lesions "wheel-within-wheel" pattern	Abscess Echinococcal cyst Metastases
Chronic Granulomatous Disease		
N/A	Poorly marginated Hypoechoic Posterior enhancement May have calcification/shadowing	Abscess
Amebic Abscess		
↑ Leukocytes Low fever Abdominal pain and diarrhea	Mass is variable Round or oval; lack notable borders Hypoechoic with debris	Pyogenic abscess Echinococcal cyst Hepatic candidiasis
Echinococcal Cyst		
↑ WBC History of sheep-farming exposure	Simple to complex cysts Acoustic enhancement Oval or spherical Calcification Honeycomb appearance/"water lily" sign	Polycystic liver disease Amebic abscess Pyogenic abscess

LFT, Liver function test; *N/A*, not applicable; *PKD*, polycystic kidney disease; *WBC*, white blood cell count.

Congenital Hepatic Cysts. A solitary congenital cyst of the liver is rare and usually is an incidental lesion. This abnormality arises from developmental defects in the formation of bile ducts.

Sonographic Findings. The mass is usually solitary and may vary in size from tiny to as large as 20 cm. The cyst is usually found on the anterior undersurface of the liver. It usually does not cause liver enlargement and is found in the right lobe of the liver more often than the left lobe.

Peribiliary Cysts. These tiny cysts (which range in size from 0.2 to 2.5 cm) are more commonly found in patients with severe liver disease. They are located centrally within the porta hepatis at the junction of the right and left hepatic ducts. Obstruction may occur if the cyst becomes large enough to cause biliary obstruction.

Sonographic Findings. These small cysts are seen as discrete, clustered tubular-appearing cysts with thin septae that parallel the bile ducts and portal veins in the central area of the liver (Fig. 9.46).

Polycystic Liver Disease. Polycystic liver disease is inherited in an autosomal dominant pattern that affects 1 in 500 individuals. At least 50% to 74% of patients with polycystic renal disease have one to several hepatic cysts. Of patients with polycystic liver disease, 60% have associated polycystic renal disease. The cysts are small, less than 2 to 3 cm, and multiple throughout the hepatic parenchyma. Cysts within

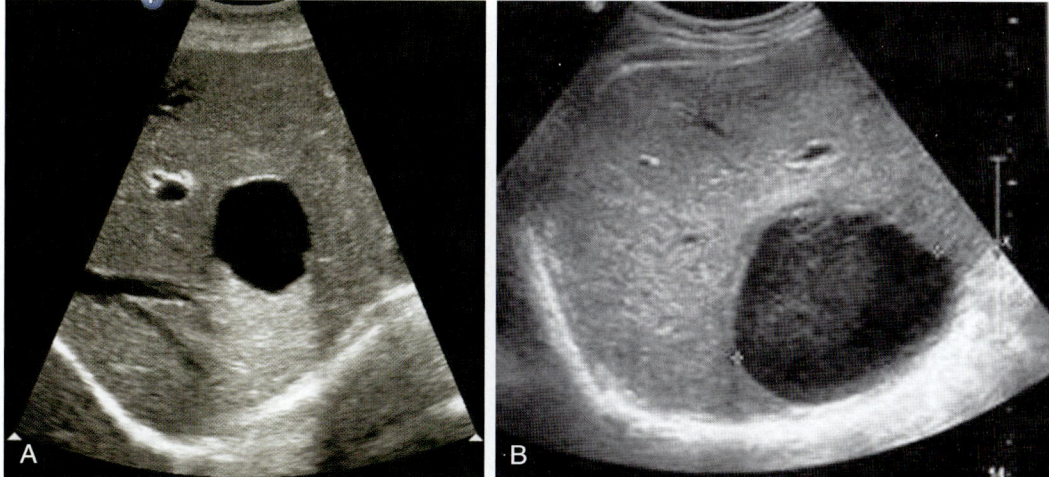

FIG. 9.45 (A) Solitary hepatic cyst in the left lobe of the liver shows increased through-transmission and well-defined borders. (B) Liver cyst appears complex secondary to the hemorrhage.

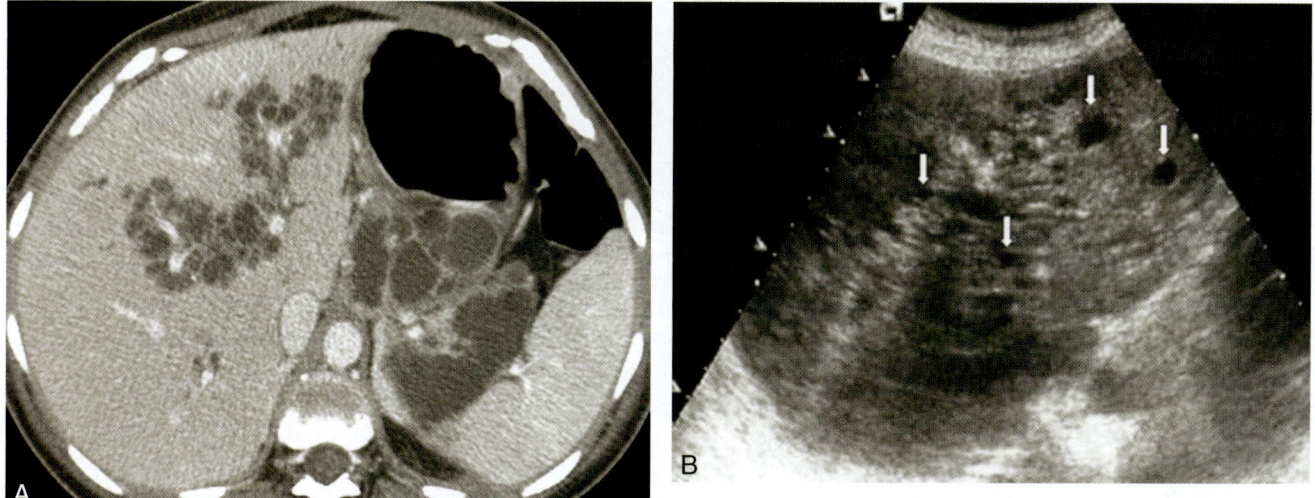

FIG. 9.46 Peribiliary cysts are located centrally within the porta hepatis at the junction of the right and left hepatic ducts. They are seen as discrete, clustered tubular-appearing cysts with thin septae that parallel the bile ducts and portal veins in the central area of the liver.

the porta hepatis may enlarge and cause biliary obstruction. Histologically, they appear similar to simple hepatic cysts. It may be difficult to assess an abscess formation or neoplastic lesion in a patient with polycystic liver disease. Liver function tests are usually normal.

Sonographic Findings. On ultrasound examination, the cysts generally present as anechoic, well-defined borders with acoustic enhancement (Fig. 9.47A–D). The differential diagnosis for a cystic lesion includes the following: necrotic metastasis, echinococcal cyst, hematoma, hepatic cystadenocarcinoma, and abscess. Ultrasound may be used to direct the needle if percutaneous aspiration is necessary to obtain specific diagnostic information.

Infectious Disease of the Liver

Hepatic abscesses occur most often as complications of biliary tract disease, surgery, or trauma. The following three basic types of abscess formation occur in the liver: intrahepatic, subhepatic, and subphrenic. Clinically the patient presents with fever, elevated white cell count, and right upper quadrant pain. The search for an abscess must be made to locate solitary or multiple lesions within the liver or to search for abnormal fluid collections in Morison pouch or in the subdiaphragmatic or subphrenic space. The following infectious processes are discussed: pyogenic abscess, hepatic candidiasis, chronic granulomatous disease, amebic abscess, and echinococcal disease.

Pyogenic Abscess. A **pyogenic abscess** is a pus-forming abscess. There are many routes for bacteria to gain access to the liver: through the biliary tree, the portal vein, or the hepatic artery; through a direct extension from a contiguous infection; or, rarely, through hepatic trauma. Sources of infection include cholangitis; portal pyemia secondary to appendicitis, diverticulitis, inflammatory disease, or colitis; direct spread from another organ; trauma with direct

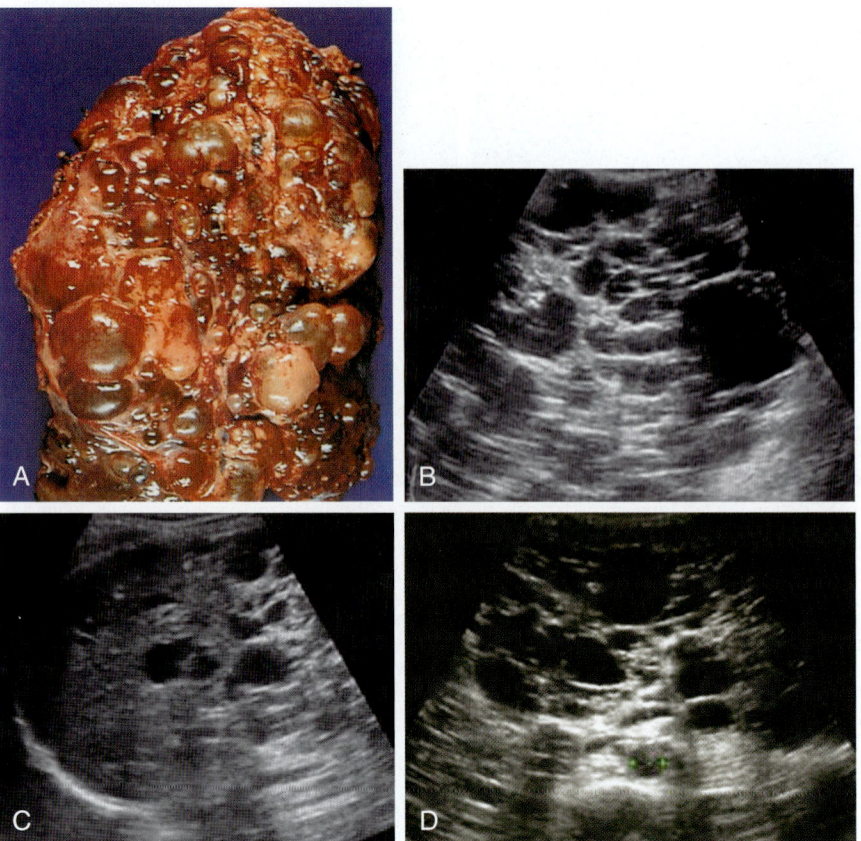

FIG. 9.47 (A) Gross pathology of polycystic liver disease. There are numerous large cysts throughout the liver parenchyma. (B–D) Images of a liver parenchyma filled with multiple cystic lesions in patients with hepatic polycystic disease.

contamination; or infarction after embolization or from sickle cell anemia.

Clinically the patient presents with fever, pain, pleuritis, nausea, vomiting, and diarrhea. Elevated liver function tests, leukocytosis, and anemia are present. The abscess formation is multiple in 50% to 67% of patients. The most frequent organisms are *Escherichia coli* and anaerobes.

Sonographic Findings. The ultrasound appearance of a pyogenic abscess may be variable, depending on the internal consistency of the mass. The size varies from 1 cm to very large. The right central lobe of the liver is the most common site for abscess development. The abscess may be hypoechoic with round or ovoid margins and acoustic enhancement, or it may be complex, with some debris along the posterior margin and irregular walls (Fig. 9.48A–B). It may have a fluid level; if gas is present, it can be hyperechoic with dirty shadowing.

Hepatic Candidiasis. Hepatic candidiasis is caused by a species of *Candida*. It usually occurs in immunocompromised hosts, such as patients undergoing chemotherapy, organ transplant recipients, or individuals with human immunodeficiency infection. The candidal fungus invades the bloodstream and may affect any organ, with the more perfused kidneys, brain, and heart affected the most. Clinically the patient may present with nonspecific findings, such as persistent fever in a neutropenic patient whose leukocyte count is returning to normal. Localized pain may also be present.

Sonographic Findings. Candidiasis within the liver may present as multiple small hypoechoic masses with echogenic central cores, referred to as **bull's-eye** or **target lesions** (Fig. 9.48C–D). The hyperechoic center (containing inflammatory cells) with a hypoechoic rim is present when the neutrophil counts return to normal. Other sonographic patterns have been described as "wheel-within-wheel" patterns or multiple small hypoechoic lesions. A peripheral hypoechoic zone with an inner echogenic wheel and central hypoechoic focal necrosis may be found. The most common finding is uniformly hypoechoic. As scar formation develops, the pattern becomes echogenic. Specific diagnosis can only be made with fine-needle aspiration.

Chronic Granulomatous Disease. Chronic granulomatous disease is a genetic disorder in which phagocytes are unable to kill certain bacteria and fungi. It occurs mostly in children, with a more frequent occurrence in boys because it is a recessive trait. A pediatric patient may have recurrent respiratory infections.

Sonographic Findings. A poorly marginated, hypoechoic mass is seen with posterior enhancement. Calcification may be present with posterior shadowing (Fig. 9.49). Aspiration is necessary to specifically classify the mass as granulomatous disease.

Amebic Abscess. Amebic abscess is a collection of pus formed by disintegrated tissue in a cavity, usually in the liver, caused by the protozoan parasite *Entamoeba histolytica*. The infection is primarily a disease of the colon, but it can also spread to the liver, lungs, and brain. The parasites reach the liver parenchyma via the portal vein. Amebiasis is contracted by ingesting the cysts in contaminated water and food. The

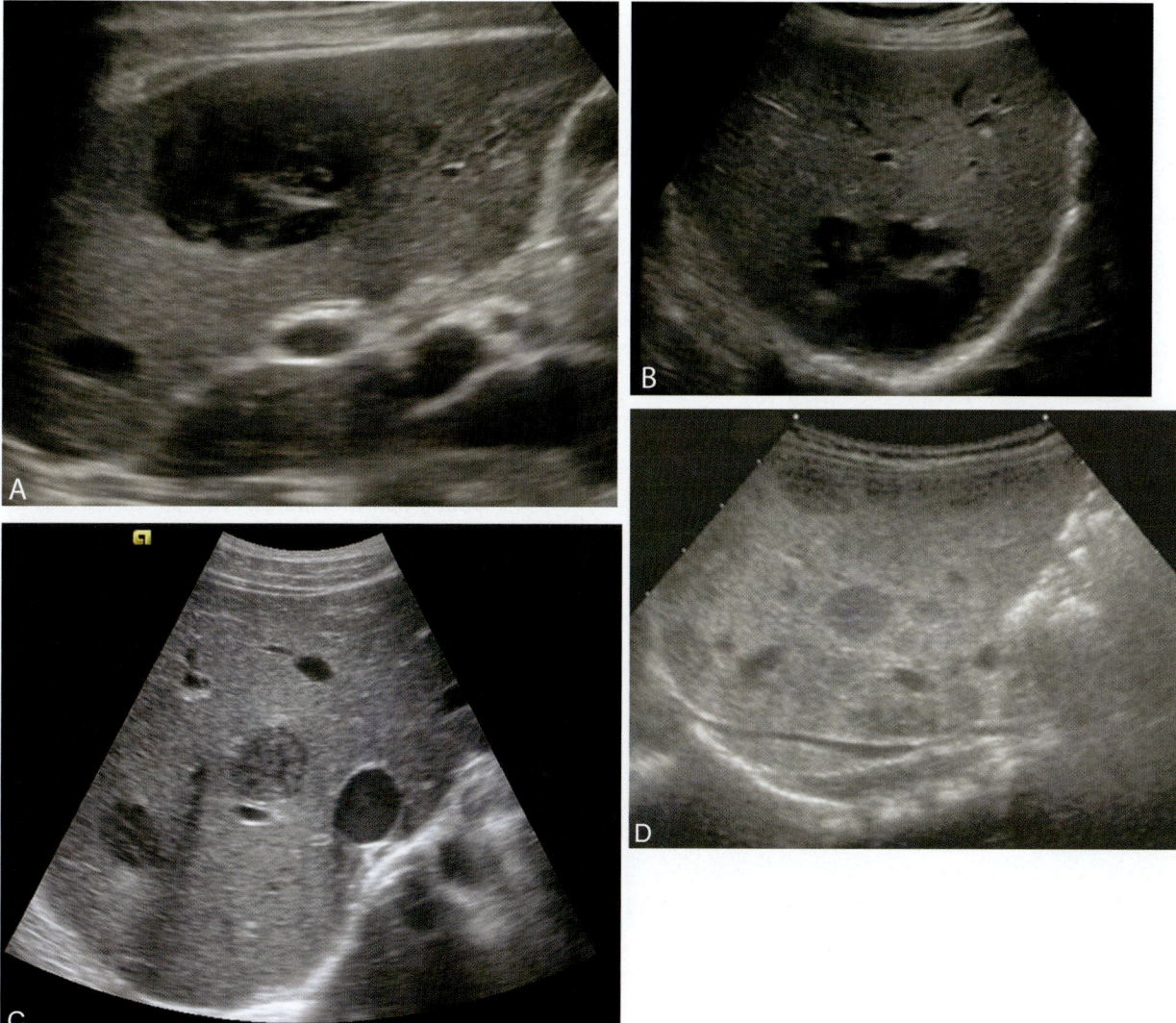

FIG. 9.48 (A–B) The right central lobe of the liver is the most common site for a pyogenic abscess to occur. The abscess may be hypoechoic with round or ovoid margins and acoustic enhancement, or it may be complex, with some debris along the posterior margin and irregular walls. (C–D) *Candidiasis* within the liver may present as multiple small hypoechoic masses with echogenic central cores, referred to as bull's-eye or target lesions.

ameba usually affects the colon and cecum, and the organism remains within the gastrointestinal tract. If the organism invades the colonic mucosa, it may travel to the liver via the portal venous system. Patients may be asymptomatic or may show the gastrointestinal symptoms of abdominal pain, diarrhea, leukocytosis, and low fever.

Sonographic Findings. The sonographic appearance of amebic abscess is variable and nonspecific. The abscess may be round or oval and lack notably defined wall echoes. The lesion is hypoechoic compared with normal liver parenchyma, with low-level echoes at higher sensitivity. There may be some internal echoes along the posterior margin secondary to debris (Fig. 9.50). Distal enhancement may be seen beyond the mass lesion. Some organisms may rupture through the diaphragm into the hepatic capsule.

Echinococcal Cyst. Hepatic echinococcosis is an infectious cystic disease common in sheep-herding areas of the world but seldom encountered within the United States. The echinococcus is a tapeworm that infects humans as the intermediate host. The worm resides in the small intestine of dogs. The ova from the adult worm are shed through canine feces into the environment, where the intermediate hosts ingest the eggs. After entering the proximal portion of the small intestine in humans, the larvae burrow through the mucosa, enter the portal circulation, and travel to the liver.

The echinococcal cyst has two layers: the inner layer and the outer, or inflammatory, reaction layer. The smaller daughter cysts may develop from the inner layer. The cysts may enlarge and rupture. The cysts may also impinge on the blood vessels and lead to vascular thrombosis and infarction.

Sonographic Findings. Several patterns may occur, from a simple cyst to a complex mass with acoustic enhancement. The shape may be oval or spherical, with regularity of the walls. Calcifications may occur. Septations are frequent and include honeycomb appearance with fluid collections; "water lily" sign, which shows a detachment and collapse of the germinal layer; or "cyst within a cyst." Sometimes the liver contains multiple parent cysts in both lobes of the liver; the cyst

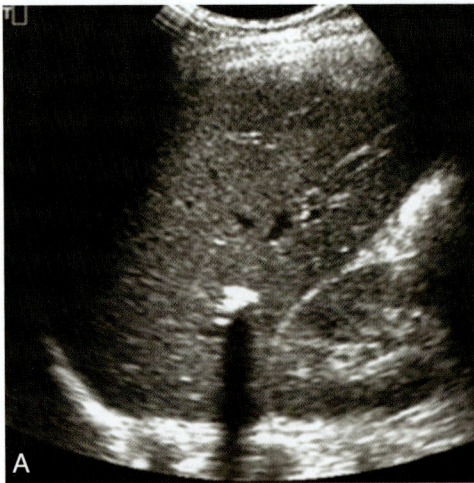

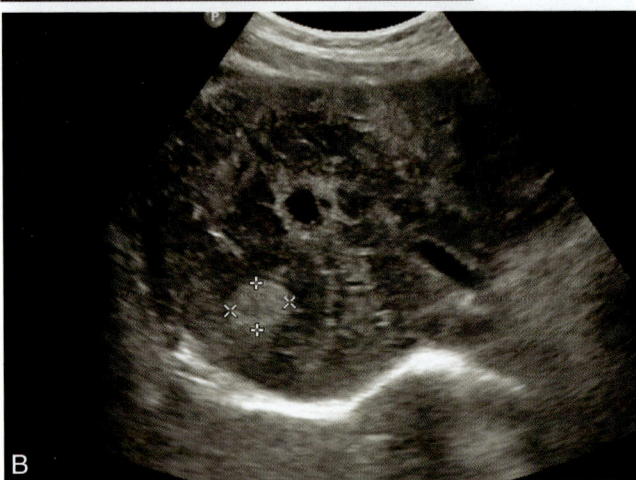

FIG. 9.49 In chronic granulomatous disease a poorly marginated, hypoechoic mass is seen with posterior enhancement. Calcification may be present with posterior shadowing.

with the thick walls occupies a different part of the liver (Fig. 9.51). The tissue between the cysts indicates that each cyst is a separate parent cyst and not a daughter cyst. If a daughter cyst is found, it is specific for echinococcal disease.

Pneumocystis carinii. *Pneumocystis carinii* is the most common organism causing opportunistic infection in patients with acquired immunodeficiency syndrome. Pneumocystis pneumonia is a common life-threatening infection in patients with human immunodeficiency virus. *P. carinii* affects patients undergoing bone marrow and organ transplantation or patients receiving chemotherapy.

Sonographic Findings. The pattern ranges from diffuse, tiny, nonshadowing echogenic foci to extensive replacement of the liver parenchyma by various echogenic clumps of calcification (Fig. 9.52).

Hepatic Tumors

A **neoplasm** is any new growth of new tissue, either benign or malignant. A benign growth occurs locally but does not spread or invade surrounding structures. It may push surrounding structures aside or adhere to them. A malignant mass is uncontrolled and is prone to metastasize to nearby or distant structures via the bloodstream and lymph nodes. Thus it is important not only to recognize the tumor mass itself but also to appreciate which structures the malignancy may invade. See Table 9.12 for clinical findings, sonographic findings, and differential considerations for hepatic tumors.

Benign Hepatic Tumors.

Cavernous Hemangioma. A cavernous hemangioma is the most common benign neoplasm of the liver. This spongelike tumor consisting of large, blood-filled cystic spaces is found more frequently in females. Patients are usually asymptomatic, although a small percentage may bleed, causing right upper quadrant pain. Hemangiomas enlarge slowly and undergo degeneration, fibrosis, and calcification. They are found in the subcapsular hepatic parenchyma or in the posterior right lobe more than the left lobe of the liver.

Sonographic Findings. The appearance is typically a homogeneous, hyperechoic mass that is usually less than 3 cm in size with acoustic enhancement (Fig. 9.53). Within the tumor are found multiple, small, blood-filled spaces separated by fibrous septations and lined with endothelial cells. The lesions are round, oval, or slightly lobulated with sharp, well-defined borders. The larger hemangiomas are more likely to appear with an atypical pattern because of fibrosis, thrombosis, and necrosis. Hemangiomas may become more heterogeneous as they undergo degeneration and fibrous replacement. Calcifications may occur but are unusual. The atypical hemangioma may have a hyperechoic periphery with a hypoechoic central core producing a "reverse" target echo pattern. There is low-velocity blood flow that is too low to be detected by color Doppler. This diminished blood flow pattern may help to distinguish the hemangioma from a malignant mass. Intravenous contrast has demonstrated peripheral puddling in the mass. Hemangiomas are generally stable over time; however, some will show regression, and others may show a decrease in echogenicity; rarely will the mass enlarge. The differential considerations for hemangioma should include metastases, hepatoma, focal fatty infiltration, and adenoma.

Focal Nodular Hyperplasia. FNH is the second most common benign liver mass after hemangioma. FNH is a benign tumor of the liver composed of Kupffer cells, hepatocytes, and biliary structures but lacks the typical normal lobular hepatic features of portal triads and central veins. The mass is thought to arise from developmental hyperplastic lesions related to an area of congenital vascular formation. Hormonal influence may be present as FNH is found more commonly in women under forty than in men. The mass is usually found as an incidental finding as the patient is asymptomatic. There is typically one well-circumscribed lesion, but there may be more than one mass; many are located along the subcapsular area of the liver, some are pedunculated, and many have a central scar from the bile ducts and prominent thick-walled arterial vessels. Bands of fibrous tissue separate the multiple nodules. The size of the mass is usually less than 5 cm in diameter. The mass may displace the normal blood vessels within the liver parenchyma.

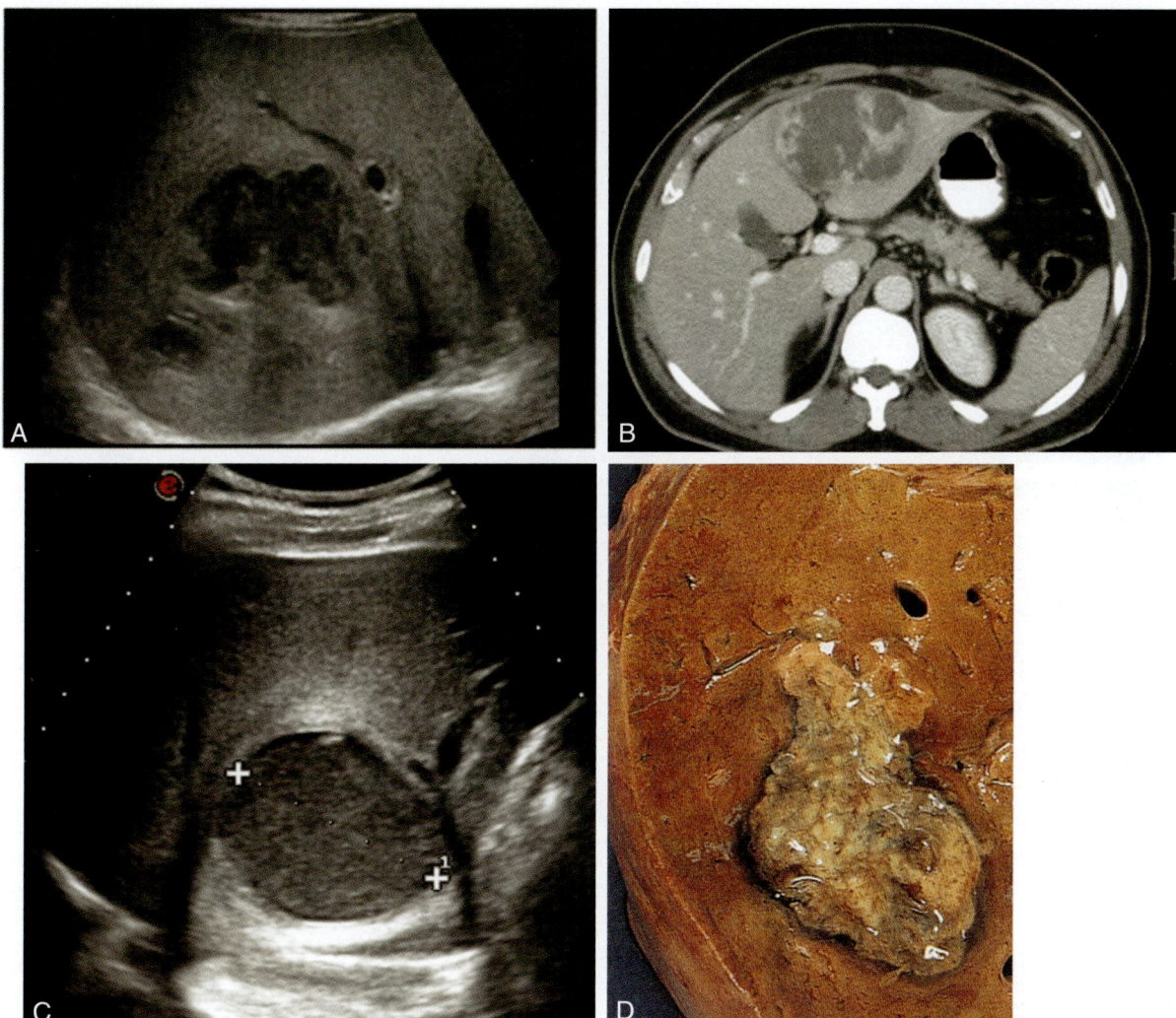

FIG. 9.50 (A–C) The *amebic abscess* may be round or oval and lack notable defined wall echoes. The lesion is hypoechoic compared with normal liver parenchyma, with low-level echoes at higher sensitivity. There may be some internal echoes along the posterior margin secondary to debris. (D) Gross pathology of an amebic abscess. The intracavitary lesion is filled with yellow necrotic material and does not contain pus.

Sonographic Findings. FNH is a subtle liver mass that may be difficult to differentiate in echogenicity from the liver parenchyma. The mass is usually isoechoic or nearly isoechoic when compared to the liver parenchyma. The sonographer may note subtle contour abnormalities and displacement of the vascular structures secondary to the mass. The central scar may be identified as a hypoechoic linear or stellate area within the center of the mass (Fig. 9.54). The internal linear echoes may be seen within the lesions if multiple nodules occur together. Color Doppler may show the well-developed peripheral and central blood vessels that feed into the FNH lesion, known as the "*spoke-wheel*" pattern. Contrast agents may help to define the hypervascular arterial phase and the presence of stellate vessels with the tortuous feeding artery.

The differential diagnosis of FNH includes fibrolamellar carcinoma, hepatic adenoma, HCC, hemangioma, and vascular metastases.

Hepatic Adenoma. An adenoma is a rare benign tumor that consists of normal or slightly atypical hepatocytes, frequently containing areas of bile stasis and focal hemorrhage or necrosis. Tumors capsules are absent or incomplete. The lesion is found more commonly in women and has been related to oral contraceptive usage. The adenoma has also been found in men taking anabolic steroids. The presence of multiple adenomas is increased in patients with type I glycogen storage disease or von Gierke disease. Patients may present with right upper quadrant pain secondary to rupture with bleeding into the tumor. Adenomas have a low but real risk of malignant degeneration.

Sonographic Findings. The mass may have varied and nonspecific findings. The echogenicity may be hyperechoic, hypoechoic, isoechoic, or mixed. With hemorrhage, a fluid component may be seen within or around the lesion. This lesion is usually hyperechoic with a central hypoechoic area caused by hemorrhage (Fig. 9.55). The lesion may be solitary and well encapsulated or multiple. If the lesion ruptures, fluid should be found in the peritoneal cavity. A hepatic adenoma may be difficult to distinguish sonographically from FNH.

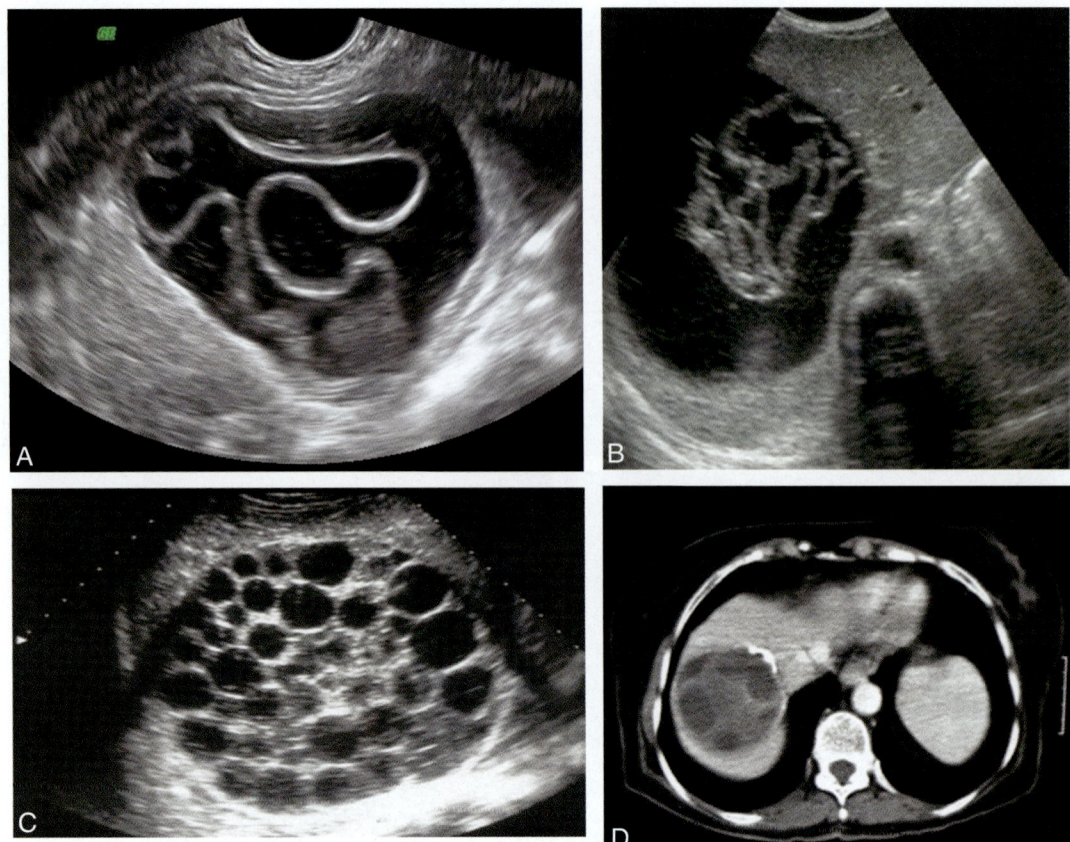

FIG. 9.51 (A–B) The shape of the echinococcal cyst may be oval or spherical, with regularity of the walls. Calcifications may occur. (C) Septations are frequent and include honeycomb appearance with fluid collections; "water lily" sign, which shows a detachment and collapse of the germinal layer, or "cyst within a cyst" (D).

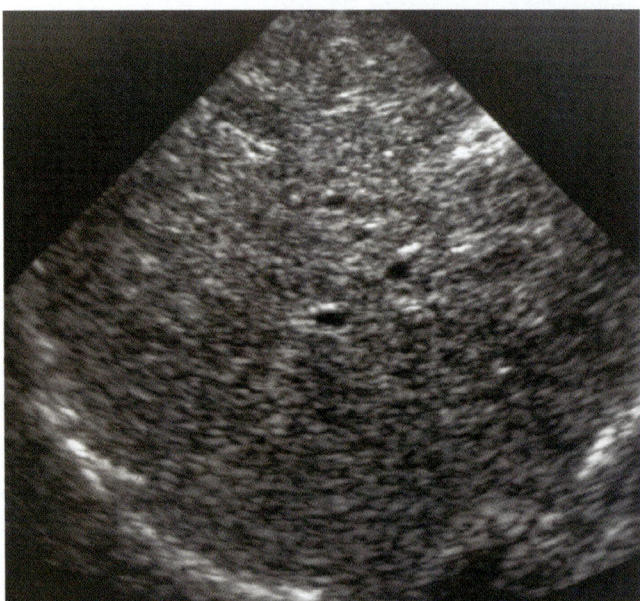

FIG. 9.52 The pattern of *pneumocystic carinii* ranges from diffuse, tiny, nonshadowing echogenic foci to extensive replacement of the liver parenchyma by various echogenic clumps of calcification.

Malignant Hepatic Neoplasms. Primary malignant tumors are relatively rare in the liver. The most common tumor is HCC, sometimes referred to as hepatoma. Tumors may also result from prolonged exposure to carcinogenic chemicals.

Sonography has the advantage over other imaging modalities in defining liver texture in many different planes. This technique is especially useful in the diagnosis of malignant hepatic disease.

The clinical signs of liver cancer are similar to those of other hepatocellular diseases. These symptoms include nausea and vomiting, fatigue, weight loss, and hepatomegaly. Portal hypertension and splenomegaly are common.

Hepatocellular Carcinoma. As noted, HCC is the most common primary malignant neoplasm. While HCC can occur in patients with normal livers, it is strongly associated with chronic liver disease. The prevalence varies, depending on predisposing factors such as hepatitis B and C infection and cirrhosis. There is a high incidence of HCC in Africa, Japan, Greece, Italy, and Southeast Asia, secondary to the prevalence of hepatitis and aflatoxin ingestion. In the non-Asian population, cirrhosis is the most important condition predisposing to HCC; other predisposing conditions include hemochromatosis, Wilson disease, and type I glycogen storage disease.

The pathogenesis of HCC is related to cirrhosis (80% of patients with preexisting cirrhosis develop HCC), chronic hepatitis B virus infection, and hepatocarcinogens in foods. The tumor occurs more frequently in men. Clinically, patients with HCC usually present with a previous history of cirrhosis or hepatitis B and C, a palpable mass, hepatomegaly, appetite disorder, and fever.

TABLE 9.12	Liver Findings: Tumors	
Clinical Findings	**Sonographic Findings**	**Differential Considerations**
Cavernous Hemangioma		
Small percentage may bleed; right upper quadrant pain More frequent in women	Most are hyperechoic with enhancement Round or oval, well defined Larger masses may show necrosis, degeneration, calcification	Metastasis Hepatoma (HCC) Adenoma Focal nodular hyperplasia
Liver Cell Adenoma		
RUQ pain when mass bleeds	Hyperechoic with central echogenic area caused by hemorrhage Solitary or multiple Fluid may be present	Hemangioma Focal nodular hyperplasia Hepatoma (HCC)
Focal Nodular Hyperplasia		
More frequent in women <40 years	Multiple, well defined with hyperechoic to isoechoic patterns Frequently found in right lobe of liver	Hemangiomas Hepatoma (HCC) Metastases Adenoma
Hepatocellular Carcinoma		
70% of patients have ↑ alpha-fetoprotein level Abnormalities in liver function tests, with the indications of cirrhosis	Solitary, multiple Infiltrative, diffuse Hypoechoic, isoechoic, or hyperechoic May invade hepatic veins Thrombus	Hemangioma Metastases
Metastatic Disease		
Abnormal LFTs Jaundice Hepatomegaly Weight loss Decreased appetite	Hypoechoic or echogenic mass Diffuse distortion of bull's-eye pattern Solitary or multiple Well to ill-defined	Abscess Hemangioma Hepatoma (HCC) Adenoma
Lymphoma		
Abnormal LFT	Hypoechoic or diffuse patterns Target or echogenic lesions Intrahepatic and lucent multiple small, discrete solid lesions without enhancement	Hemangioma HCC Metastases

HCC, Hepatocellular carcinoma; *LFT*, liver function test.

The HCC may present in one of three patterns: solitary massive tumor, multiple nodules throughout the liver, or diffuse infiltrative masses in the liver. Pathologically, the tumor may present as a focal lesion, an invasive lesion with necrosis and hemorrhage, or a poorly defined lesion (Fig. 9.56). The carcinoma can be very invasive and has been known to invade the hepatic veins to produce Budd-Chiari syndrome. The portal venous system may also be invaded with tumor or thrombosis. Hepatocellular carcinoma tends to destroy the portal venous radicle walls, with invasion into the lumen of the vessel.

Sonographic Findings. A variable sonographic appearance is noted with discrete lesions, either solitary or multiple, that are usually hypoechoic or hyperechoic. Sometimes the lesions may be isoechoic, and a thin, peripheral hypoechoic halo may surround the lesion (Fig. 9.57). Another pattern presents as diffuse parenchymal involvement with inhomogeneity throughout the liver without distinct masses. Over time the mass becomes more complex and inhomogeneous, with resulting fibrosis and necrosis. The last pattern is a combination of discrete and diffuse echoes. Hepatocellular carcinoma cannot be differentiated from metastases on ultrasound.

Internal echoes within the portal veins, hepatic veins, or inferior vena cava indicate tumor invasion or thrombosis within the vessel. The evaluation of the vascular structures with color Doppler helps to rule out the presence of clot or tumor invasion. Hepatic flow is abnormal if an obstruction is present. Obstruction of the portal vein may be present with thrombosis and well demonstrated with color Doppler.

Metastatic Disease. The most common form of neoplastic involvement of the liver is **metastatic disease** (see Fig. 9.57).

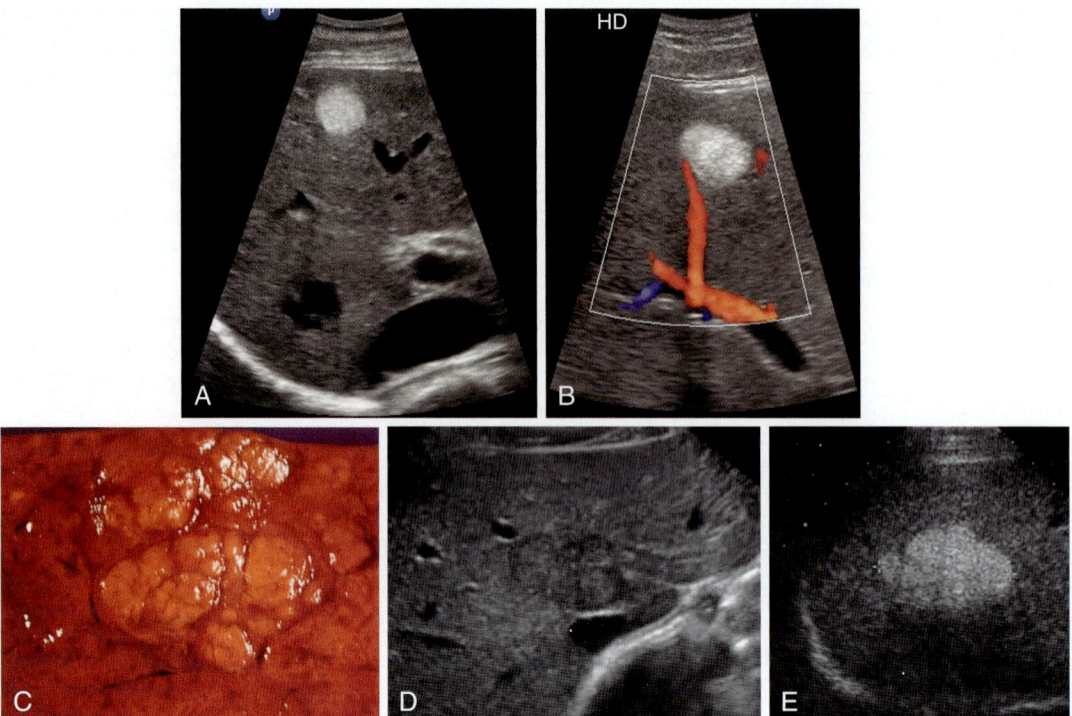

FIG. 9.53 (A–B) Cavernous hemangioma. The appearance is typically a homogeneous, hyperechoic mass that is usually less than 3 cm in size. (C) Gross pathology of focal nodular hyperplasia with a lobular mass with a central fibrotic scar. (D) Focal nodular hyperplasia is a subtle liver mass that may be difficult to differentiate in echogenicity from the liver parenchyma. The mass is usually isoechoic or nearly isoechoic when compared to the liver parenchyma. (E) Hepatic adenoma. This lesion is usually hyperechoic with a central hypoechoic area caused by hemorrhage.

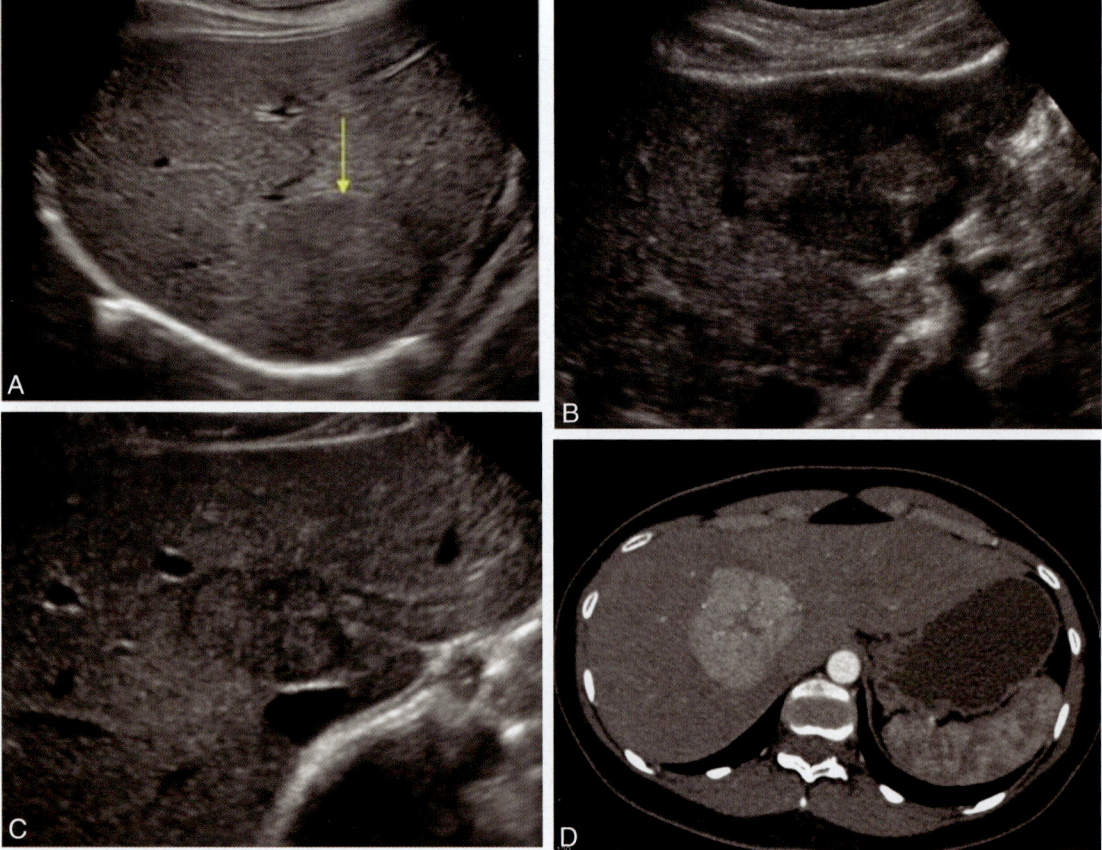

FIG. 9.54 (A–C) Focal nodular hyperplasia is a subtle liver mass that may be difficult to differentiate in echogenicity from the liver parenchyma. The mass is usually isoechoic or nearly isoechoic when compared to the liver parenchyma. The sonographer may note subtle contour abnormalities and displacement of the vascular structures secondary to the mass. (D) The central scar may be identified as a hypoechoic linear or stellate area within the center of the mass.

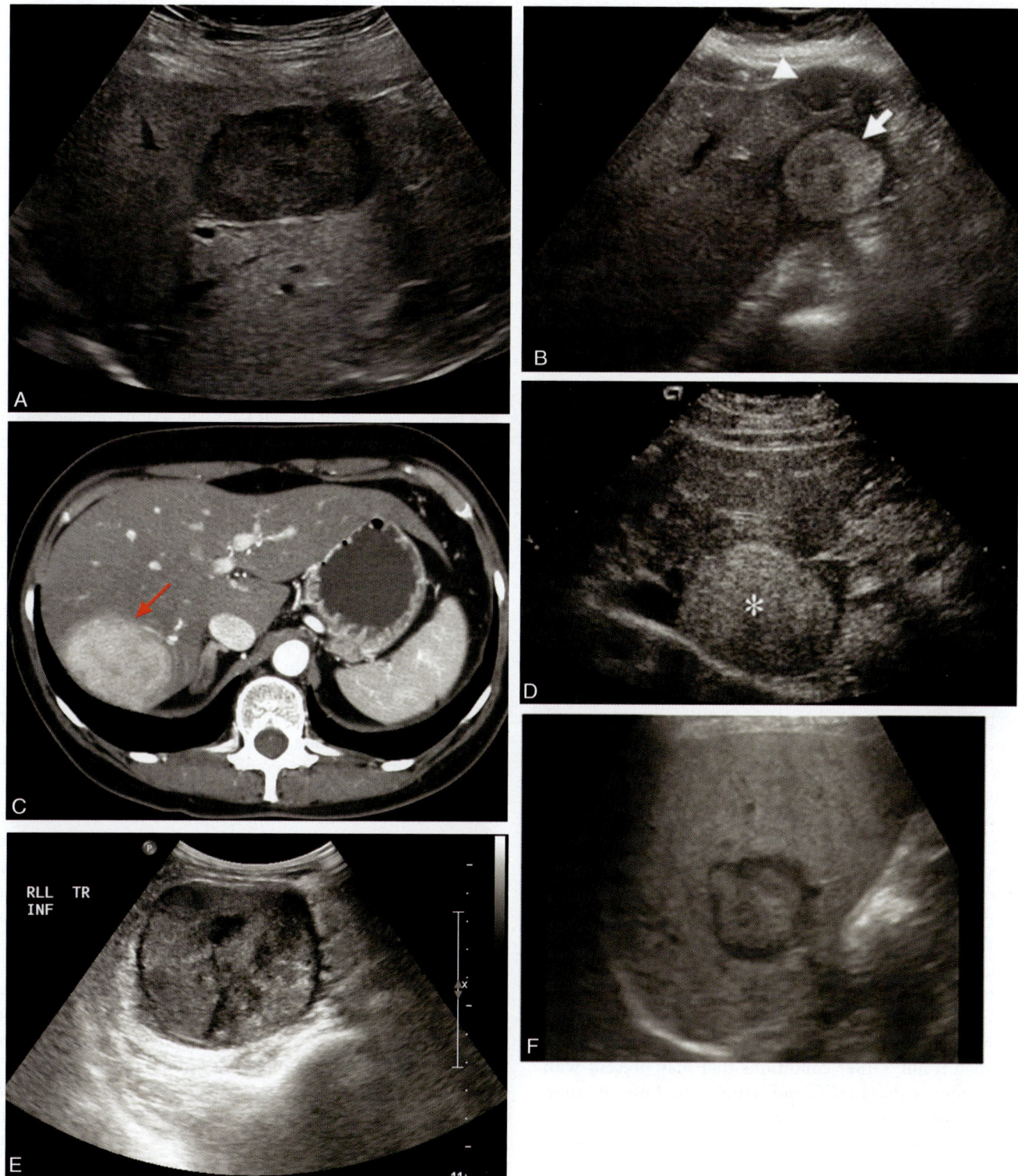

FIG. 9.55 The echogenicity of a hepatic adenoma may be hyperechoic, hypoechoic, isoechoic, or mixed. This lesion is usually hyperechoic with a central hypoechoic area caused by hemorrhage. Echogenicity examples: (A) hypoechoic, (B) hyperechoic with hypoechoic central hemorrhage, (C) computed tomographic image of adenoma, (D) hyperechoic, (E) mixed, and (F) hyperechoic with central hemorrhage.

The lungs and the liver are the most frequent sites of distant metastatic disease. The primary sites are the colon, breast, and lung, with the majority of metastases arising from a primary colonic malignancy or a hepatoma. The incidence of hepatic metastases depends on the type of tumor and its stage at initial detection. Patients with short survival rates after initial detection of liver metastases are those with HCC and carcinoma of the pancreas, stomach, and esophagus. Patients with a more prolonged survival are those with head and neck carcinoma and carcinoma of the colon. Metastatic spread to the

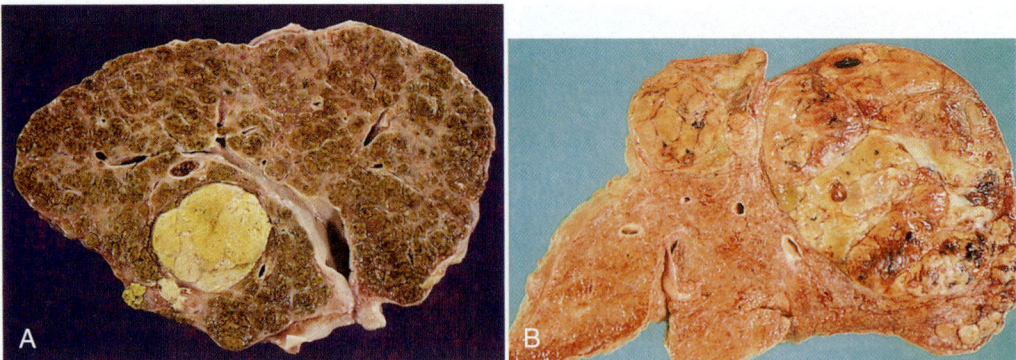

FIG. 9.56 Gross pathology of hepatocellular carcinoma. (A) The cirrhotic liver contains a solitary malignant nodule. (B) The huge tumor is poorly demarcated from the remaining liver.

liver occurs as the tumor erodes the wall and travels through the lymphatic system or through the bloodstream to the portal vein or hepatic artery to the liver.

Sonographic Findings. The sonographic patterns of metastatic tumor involvement in the liver vary. It is typical to have multiple nodes throughout both lobes of the liver. The following three specific patterns have been described: (1) a well-defined hypoechoic mass, (2) a well-defined echogenic mass, and (3) diffuse distortion of the normal homogeneous parenchymal pattern without a focal mass (Fig. 9.58). The hypovascular lesions produce hypoechoic patterns in the liver because of necrosis and ischemic areas from neoplastic thrombosis. Most cases of hypervascular lesions correspond to hyperechoic patterns.

The echogenic lesions are common with primary colonic tumors and may present with calcification. Target types of metastases or *bull's-eye* patterns are the results of edema around the tumor or necrosis or hemorrhage within the tumor. Thus on sonography, the target lesion has an appearance with an echogenic or isoechoic center with a hypoechoic halo (see Fig. 9.58C). The appearance may vary; when the halo is thin, it may represent dilated peritumoral sinusoids or compressed liver parenchyma. The proliferating tumor demonstrates a thick halo surrounding the echogenic center. As the nodules increase rapidly in size and outgrow their blood supply, central necrosis and hemorrhage may result. Other conditions that may present with target lesions include HCC and lymphoma. Less common target lesions are seen in abscesses, adenomas, and FHN, and rarely hemangioma.

Hyperechoic metastases are found to occur more frequently with gastrointestinal lesions, most commonly from the colon, and neuroendocrine tumors. Calcified metastases are most common from the colon; however, metastasis from the ovary, breast, and stomach may also calcify. Cystic hepatic metastases are less frequent; these have a thick wall, thick septations, or obvious solid components.

Various combinations of these patterns can be seen simultaneously in a patient with metastatic liver disease. The first abnormality is hepatomegaly or alterations in contour, especially on the lateral segment of the left lobe. The lesions may be solitary or multiple, be variable in size and shape, and have sharp or ill-defined margins. Metastases may be extensive or localized to produce an inhomogeneous parenchymal pattern.

Ultrasound may be useful to follow patients after surgery. After a baseline hepatic ultrasound has been performed, the sonographer can assess any regression or progression of tumor and change in parenchymal pattern.

Lymphoma. Lymphomas are malignant neoplasms involving lymphocyte proliferation in the lymph nodes. The two main disorders, Hodgkin lymphoma and non-Hodgkin lymphoma, are differentiated by lymph node biopsy. No specific cause is known. Hepatic lymphoma usually presents in the setting of advanced disease elsewhere and is of the non-Hodgkin variety. Primary hepatic lymphoma occurs most often in the setting of an immunocompromised state such as AIDS or post-transplantation. Patients with lymphoma have hepatomegaly with a normal or diffuse alteration of parenchymal echoes. A focal hypoechoic mass is sometimes seen. The patient may present with enlarged, nontender lymph nodes, fever, fatigue, night sweats, weight loss, bone pain, or an abdominal mass. The presence of splenomegaly or retroperitoneal nodes may help confirm the diagnosis of lymphadenopathy.

Sonographic Findings. Hodgkin lymphoma shows up as diffuse parenchymal changes in the liver. Non-Hodgkin lymphoma may appear with target hypoechoic mass lesions. Burkitt lymphoma lesions may appear intrahepatic and lucent. Patients with leukemia have multiple small, discrete hepatic masses that are solid with no acoustic enhancement (Fig. 9.59). A bull's-eye appearance with a dense central core may be present as a result of tumor necrosis.

In the pediatric population, the most common malignancies are neuroblastomas, Wilms tumor, and leukemia. The neuroblastoma presents as a densely reflective echo pattern with liver involvement similar to that of a hepatoma. In patients with a Wilms tumor, metastases generally invade the lung; however, the liver may be a secondary site. These lesions present as a densely reflective pattern with lucencies resulting from necrosis.

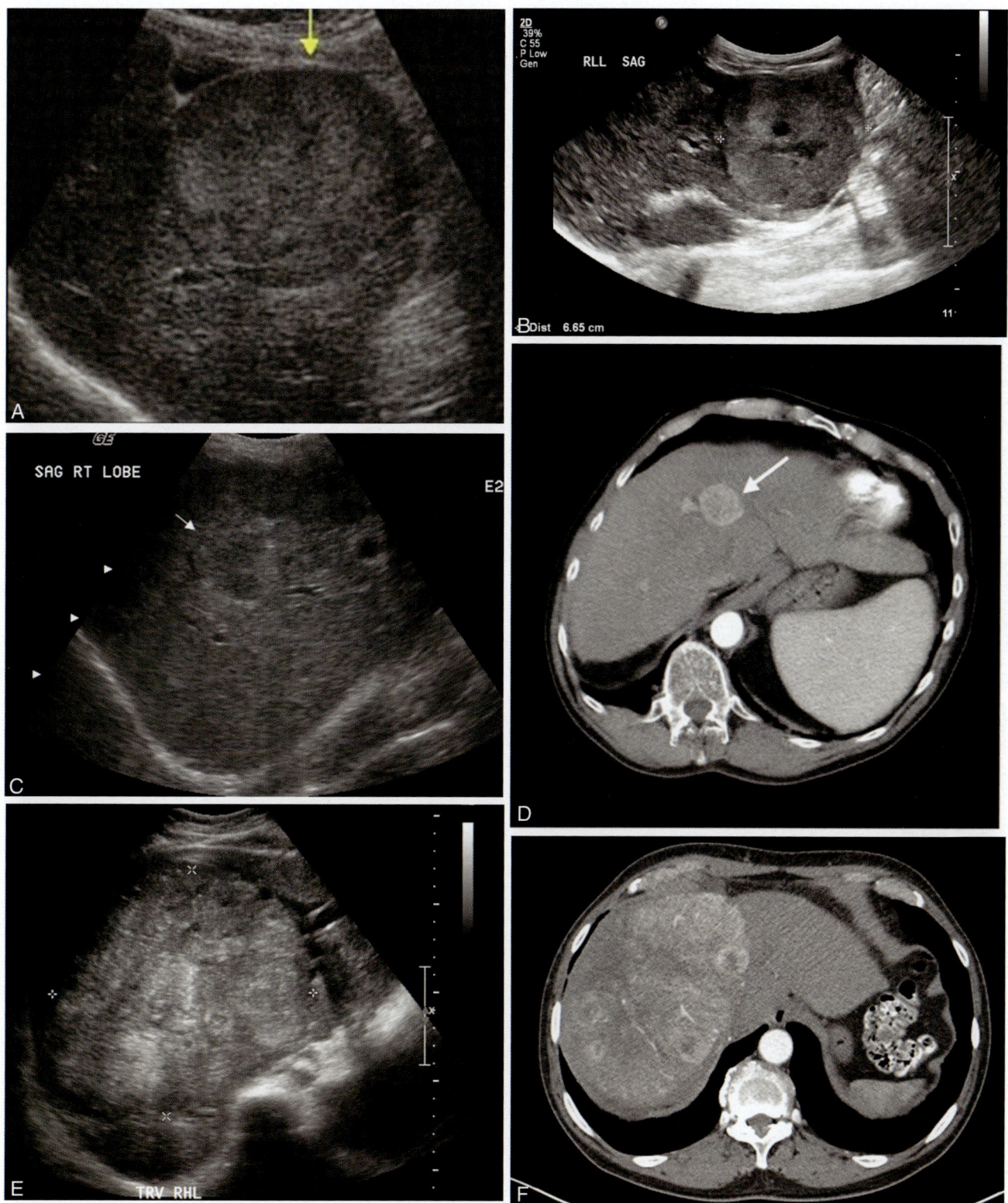

FIG. 9.57 A variable sonographic appearance is noted in hepatocellular carcinoma with discrete lesions, either solitary or multiple, that are usually hypoechoic or hyperechoic. (A–C) The lesions may be isoechoic, and a thin, peripheral hypoechoic halo may surround the lesion. (D) CT image of a discrete hepatic lesions, (E) Another pattern presents as diffuse parenchymal involvement with inhomogeneity throughout the liver without distinct masses; over time the mass becomes more complex and inhomogeneous with resulting fibrosis and necrosis. (F) The last pattern is a combination of discrete and diffuse echoes.

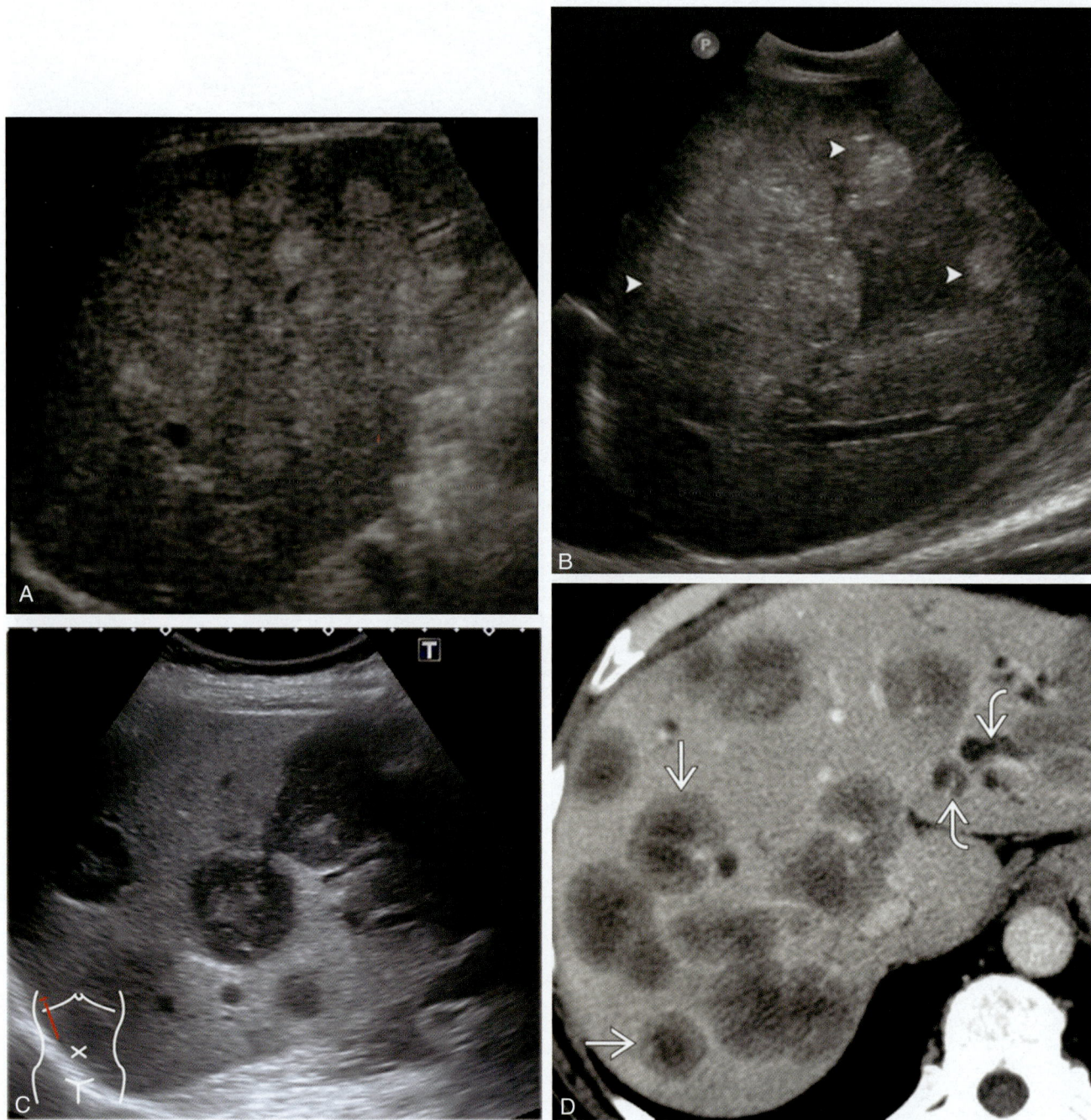

FIG. 9.58 The sonographic patterns of metastatic tumor involvement in the liver vary. It is typical to have multiple nodes throughout both lobes of the liver. (A–C) The mass is well defined with varying texture from homogeneous to isoechoic to echogenic. (D) CT image of the metastatic liver disease.

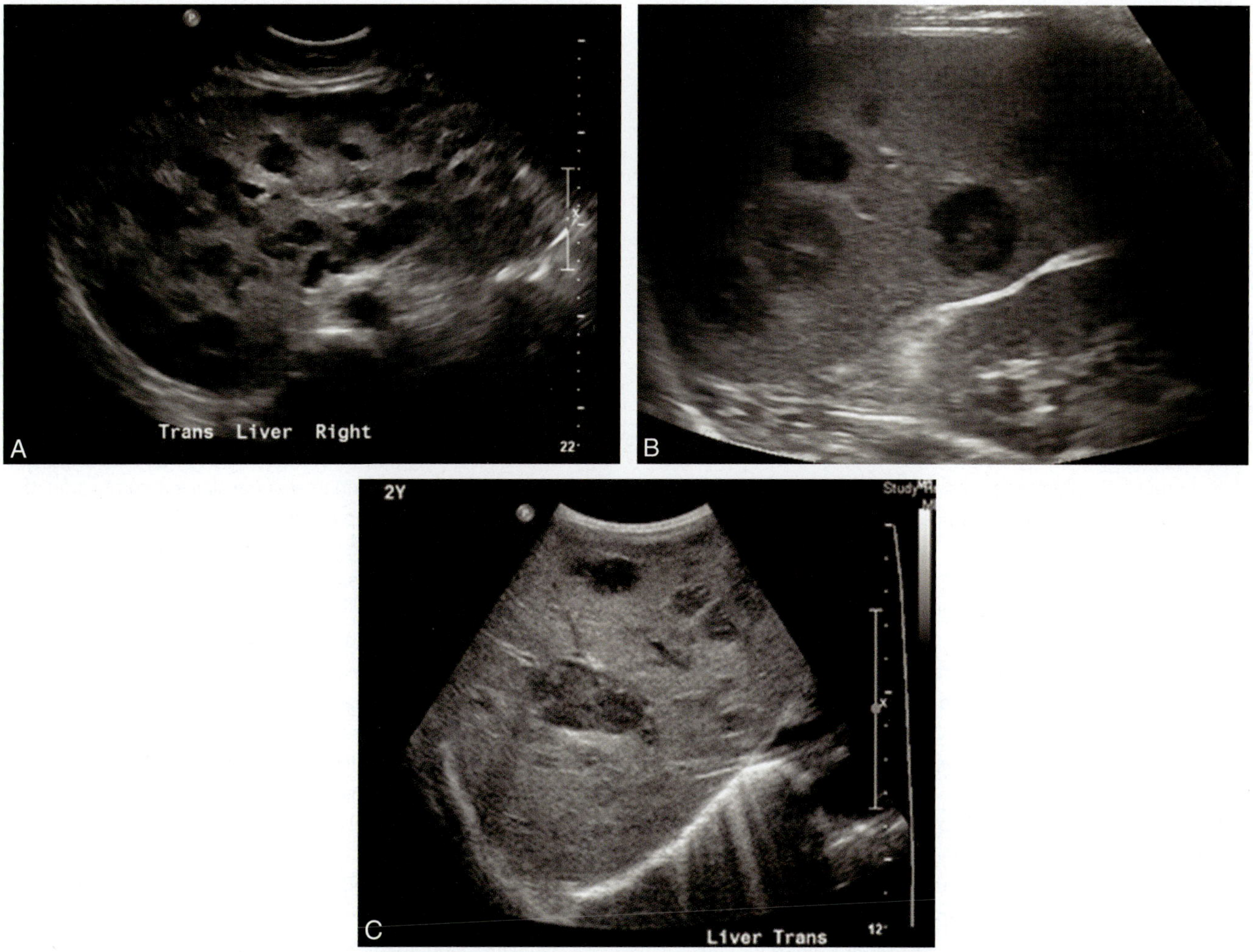

FIG. 9.59 (A) Hodgkin lymphoma shows up as diffuse parenchymal changes in the liver. (B) Non-Hodgkin lymphoma may appear with target hypoechoic mass lesions. (C) Burkitt lymphoma lesions may appear intrahepatic and lucent.

Key Pearls

- The liver is the largest organ in the abdominal cavity, measuring approximately 21 to 22.5 cm in its greatest transverse diameter, 13 to 17.5 cm in its greatest vertical height, and 10 to 12.5 cm in its anteroposterior depth.
- The liver occupies almost all the right hypochondrium, the greater part of the epigastrium, and the left hypochondrium as far as the mammillary line.
- Most of the liver is covered by peritoneum, but a large area rests directly on the diaphragm; this is called the bare area.
- The subphrenic space between the liver (or spleen) and the diaphragm is a common site for abscess formation.
- The right posterior subphrenic space lies between the right lobe of the liver, the right kidney, and the right colic flexure.
- The right subhepatic space is located inferior to the right lobe of the liver and includes Morison pouch, which lies between the posterior aspect of the right lobe and the upper pole of the right kidney.
- Tumor infiltration, cirrhosis, or a subphrenic abscess often causes inferior displacement, whereas ascites, excessive dilation of the colon, or abdominal tumors can elevate the liver; retroperitoneal tumors may move the liver slightly anterior.
- The liver has been divided into four anatomical lobes: the left, right, quadrate, and caudate, with the falciform ligament separating the left from the right lobe; however, functional divisions have more value from a surgical perspective (Couinaud's system of hepatic nomenclature).
- The right hypochondrium contains the right lobe, which is six times larger than the left lobe.
- The middle hepatic vein and the ascending section of the left portal vein divide the liver functionally into a left lobe and a right lobe.
- Using these functional divisions, the falciform ligament now belongs to the left lobe; it runs vertically along the medial left lobe close to the border with the lateral left lobe.
- The left intersegmental fissure divides the left lobe into medial and lateral segments; the left hepatic vein runs horizontally between the medial and lateral segments.

- There are two fissures in the left lobe: the fissure for the ligamentum teres and the ligamentum venosum.
- The caudate lobe is a small lobe situated on the posterior surface of the left lobe, with the inferior vena cava as its posterior border and the fissure for the ligamentum venosum its anterior border.
- Note the hepatic veins course between the lobes and interlobar/intersegmental segments.
- The major branches of the *portal veins* run centrally within the segments (intrasegmental) except for the ascending portion of the left portal vein, which runs in the left intersegmental fissure.
- The Couinaud system divides the left lateral, right anterior, and right posterior segments into superior and inferior subsegments and maintains the caudate lobe and the medial left segment as single segments.
- The liver is covered by a thin connective tissue layer called Glisson's capsule.
- The main lobar fissure is seen on sonography as a hyperechoic line extending from the portal vein to the neck of the gallbladder.
- The falciform ligament extends from the umbilicus to the diaphragm in a parasagittal plane and contains the ligamentum teres.
- The fissure for the ligamentum venosum separates the left lobe from the caudate lobe.
- The portal vein conveys about 70% to 80% of the blood to the liver, and the remaining 20% to 30% is oxygenated blood conveyed to the liver via the hepatic artery.
- The venous blood supply from the greater part of the gastrointestinal tract and its accessory organs drains into the liver through the portal venous system.
- The portal triad consists of the portal vein, hepatic artery, and bile duct.
- The blood is perfused within the liver parenchyma through the hepatic sinusoids before it enters the terminal hepatic venules which unite to form the larger hepatic veins.
- The best way to distinguish the hepatic from the portal vessels is to trace their points of entry to the liver.
- The liver has many functions, including metabolism, digestion, storage, and detoxification.
- Through the process of digestion, the liver expels these waste products from the body via its excretory product, bile, which also plays an important role in fat absorption.
- Diseases affecting the liver may be classified as *hepatocellular* when the liver cells or hepatocytes are the immediate problems, or *obstructive* when bile excretion is blocked.
- The liver is a major location for detoxification of waste products of energy production and other metabolic activities occurring throughout the body.
- Along with detoxification, the liver also excretes bilirubin into the gut via the biliary tree.
- Elevation of serum bilirubin results in jaundice, which is a yellow coloration of the skin, sclerae, and body secretions.
- Bile is the excretory product of the liver and is formed continuously by the hepatocytes, collects in the bile canaliculi adjacent to these cells, and is transported to the gut via the bile ducts.
- Liver function tests are a group of laboratory tests established to analyze how the liver is performing under normal and diseased conditions.
- Evaluation of the liver parenchyma includes the assessment of its size, configuration, homogeneity, and contour.
- Hepatocellular disease affects the hepatocytes and interferes with liver function enzymes.
- The hepatocyte is a parenchymal liver cell that performs all the functions ascribed to the liver.
- There are many subcategories of diffuse parenchymal disease, including fatty infiltration, acute and chronic hepatitis, early alcoholic liver disease, and acute and chronic cirrhosis.
- Fatty infiltration of the liver is an acquired, reversible disorder of metabolism, resulting in an intracellular accumulation of triglycerides within hepatocytes.
- Fatty infiltration most commonly appears in a diffuse or patchy distribution and results in uniformly increased echogenicity of the liver.
- Fatty infiltration is not always uniform throughout the liver parenchyma; in fact, regions of increased echogenicity are present within a normal liver parenchyma.
- Focal sparing should be suspected in patients who have *masslike* hypoechoic areas in typical locations in a liver that is otherwise increased in echogenicity.
- Hepatitis is the general name for inflammatory and infectious diseases of the liver.
- Complications of hepatitis involving damage to the liver may range from mild disease to massive necrosis and liver failure.
- On ultrasound, the patient with acute hepatitis may demonstrate a normal liver texture, or the portal vein borders may be more echogenic than usual (known as the "starry sky" sign); the liver parenchyma is slightly more echogenic than normal, and attenuation may be present.
- With chronic hepatitis, the liver parenchyma is coarse with decreased brightness of the portal triads, but the degree of attenuation is not as great as is seen in fatty infiltration.
- Cirrhosis is a chronic degenerative disease of the liver in which the hepatic lobes are covered with fibrous tissue, the parenchyma degenerates, and the lobules are infiltrated with fat.
- The process of cirrhosis is chronic and progressive, with liver cell failure and portal hypertension as the end stage.
- With sonography, cirrhosis may appear as hepatomegaly, increased echogenicity, and coarsening of the hepatic parenchyma secondary to fibrosis and surface nodularity.
- Chronic cirrhosis may show surface nodularity of the liver edge, especially well demonstrated if ascites is present.
- Doppler evaluation of the hepatic veins is useful to detect the presence of altered flow dynamics.
- Glycogen storage disease is an inherited disease characterized by the abnormal storage and accumulation of glycogen in the tissues, especially the liver and kidneys.
- The most common glycogen storage disease is type I, or von Gierke disease. On sonography, patients with glycogen storage

- disease present with hepatomegaly, increased echogenicity, and slightly increased attenuation.
- Hemochromatosis is a rare disease of iron metabolism characterized by excess iron deposits throughout the body. Some increased echogenicity may be seen uniformly throughout the hepatic parenchyma.
- Portal hypertension is caused by increased resistance to venous flow through the liver. It is associated with cirrhosis, hepatic vein thrombosis, portal vein thrombosis, and thrombosis of the inferior vena cava.
- Portal hypertension is divided into presinusoidal and intrahepatic groups, depending on whether the hepatic vein wedged pressure is normal (presinusoidal) or elevated (intrahepatic).
- The development of increased pressure in the portal-splenic venous system is the cause of extrahepatic portal hypertension. Acute or chronic hepatocellular disease can block the flow of blood throughout the liver, causing it to back up into the hepatic portal circulation.
- Intrahepatic portal hypertension is the result of diseases that affect the portal zones of the liver, like primary biliary cirrhosis, schistosomiasis, congenital hepatic fibrosis, or toxic drugs. Cirrhosis is the most common cause of intrahepatic portal hypertension.
- Portal hypertension may also develop when hepatopetal flow (toward the liver) is impeded by thrombus or tumor invasion.
- Collateral circulation develops when the normal venous channels become obstructed.
- If portal hypertension becomes extensive, the portal system can be decompressed by shunting blood to the systemic venous system.
- Portacaval shunts for the treatment of portal hypertension may involve the anastomosis of the portal vein because it lies within the lesser omentum, to the anterior wall of the inferior vena cava behind the entrance into the lesser sac.
- The mesocaval shunt attaches the mid-distal superior mesenteric vein to the inferior vena cava.
- The splenorenal shunt attaches the splenic vein to the left renal vein.
- Intrahepatic shunts are created percutaneously with the use of metallic expandable stents, which can be seen on ultrasound. This type of shunt is the transjugular intrahepatic portosystemic shunt (TIPS).
- Budd-Chiari syndrome is uncommon and caused by thrombosis of the hepatic veins or inferior vena cava.
- Biliary obstruction proximal to the cystic duct can be caused by gallstones, carcinoma of the common bile duct, or metastatic tumor invasion of the porta hepatis.
- A biliary obstruction distal to the cystic duct may be caused by stones in the common duct, an extrahepatic mass in the porta hepatis, or stricture of the common duct.
- An extrahepatic mass in the area of the porta hepatis causes the same clinical signs as seen in biliary obstruction.
- Passive hepatic congestion develops secondary to congestive heart failure with signs of hepatomegaly and dilation of the inferior vena cava, superior mesenteric, hepatic, portal, and splenic veins.
- The differential diagnosis for focal diseases of the liver includes cysts, abscess, hematoma, primary tumor, and metastases.
- Intrahepatic masses may cause the following findings on ultrasound: displacement of the hepatic vascular radicles, external bulging of the liver capsule, or a posterior shift of the inferior vena cava.
- An extrahepatic mass may show internal invagination or discontinuity of the liver capsule, formation of a triangular fat wedge, anteromedial shift of the inferior vena cava, or anterior displacement of the right kidney.
- *Hepatic cyst* usually refers to a solitary nonparasitic cyst of the liver. The cyst may be congenital or acquired, solitary or multiple.
- Patients with polycystic liver disease may also have polycystic renal disease.
- Hepatic abscesses occur most often as complications of biliary tract disease, surgery, or trauma.
- The following three basic types of abscess formation occur in the liver: intrahepatic, subhepatic, and subphrenic.
- A pyogenic abscess is a pus-forming abscess. There are many routes for bacteria to gain access to the liver: through the biliary tree, the portal vein, or the hepatic artery; through a direct extension from a contiguous infection; or, rarely, through hepatic trauma.
- Hepatic candidiasis is caused by a species of *Candida*. It usually occurs in immunocompromised hosts, such as patients undergoing chemotherapy, organ transplant recipients, or individuals with human immunodeficiency infection.
- Amebic abscess is a collection of pus formed by disintegrated tissue in a cavity, usually in the liver, caused by the protozoan parasite *Entamoeba histolytica*.
- Hepatic echinococcosis is an infectious cystic disease common in sheep-herding areas of the world but seldom encountered within the United States.
- The echinococcal cyst has two layers: the inner layer and the outer, or inflammatory, reaction layer. The smaller daughter cysts may develop from the inner layer. The cysts may enlarge and rupture.
- A neoplasm is any new growth of new tissue, either benign or malignant.
- A benign growth occurs locally but does not spread or invade surrounding structures. It may push surrounding structures aside or adhere to them.
- A malignant mass is uncontrolled and is prone to metastasize to nearby or distant structures via the bloodstream and lymph nodes.
- Cavernous hemangioma is typically a homogeneous, hyperechoic mass that is usually less than 3 cm in size with acoustic enhancement.
- Focal nodular hyperplasia is a subtle liver mass that may be difficult to differentiate in echogenicity from the liver parenchyma (isoechoic or nearly isoechoic when compared to the liver parenchyma).
- An adenoma is a rare benign tumor that consists of normal or slightly atypical hepatocytes, frequently containing areas of bile stasis and focal hemorrhage or necrosis.

- Hepatocellular carcinoma (HCC) is the most common primary malignant neoplasm.
- The HCC may present in one of three patterns: solitary massive tumor, multiple nodules throughout the liver, or diffuse infiltrative masses in the liver.
- The most common form of neoplastic involvement of the liver is metastatic disease.
- The primary sites are the colon, breast, and lung, with the majority of metastases arising from a primary colonic malignancy or a hepatoma.
- On sonography, the following three specific patterns are seen in metastatic disease: (1) a well-defined hypoechoic mass, (2) a well-defined echogenic mass, and (3) diffuse distortion of the normal homogeneous parenchymal pattern without a focal mass.
- Hodgkin lymphoma shows up as diffuse parenchymal changes in the liver.
- Non-Hodgkin lymphoma may appear with target hypoechoic mass lesions.
- Burkitt lymphoma lesions may appear intrahepatic and lucent.
- Patients with leukemia have multiple small, discrete hepatic masses that are solid with no acoustic enhancement.

BIBLIOGRAPHY

Abdalla EK, Vauthey JN, Couinaud C. The caudate lobe of the liver: implications of embryology and anatomy for surgery. *Surg Oncol Clin North Am.* 2002;11:835–848.

Bertolotto M, Catalano O. Contrast-enhanced ultrasound: past, present, and future. *Ultrasound Clin.* 2009;4:339–367.

Carr CE, Tuite CM, Soulen MC, et al. Role of ultrasound surveillance of transjugular intrahepatic portosystemic shunts in the covered stent era. *J Vasc Interv Radiol.* 2006;17:1297–1305.

Castroagudin JF, Molina E, Abdulkader I, et al. Sonographic features of liver involvement by lymphoma. *J Ultrasound Med.* 2007;26:791–796.

Feigin RD, Glickson M, Varstending A. Familial Budd-Chiari syndrome due to membranous obstruction of the hepatic vein treated with transluminal angioplasty. *Am J Gastroenterol.* 1990;85(1):94.

Fratzer W, Fritz V, Mason RA, et al. Factors affecting liver size. *J Ultrasound Med.* 2003;22:1155–1161.

Li D, Hann LE. A practical approach to analyzing focal lesions in the liver. *Ultrasound Quarterly.* 2005;21:187–200.

Middleton WD, Kurtz AB, Hertzberg BS. *Ultrasound: The Requisites.* ed 2 St Louis: Elsevier; 2004.

Ong JP, Sands M, Younossi ZM. Transjugular intrahepatic portosystem shunts (TIPSS) a decade later. *J Clin Gastroenterol.* 2000;30(1):14–28.

Robinson KA, Middleton WD, Al-Sukaiti R, et al. Doppler sonography of portal hypertension. *Ultrasound Quarterly.* 2009;25:3–13.

Rumack CM, Wilson SB, Charboneau JW, et al. ed 4 *Diagnostic Ultrasound.* vol 1 St Louis: Elsevier; 2011.

Sabih DE, Sabih Z, Khan A. "Congealed waterlily" sign: a new sonographic sign of hydatid cyst. *J Clin Ultrasound.* 1996;24:297–303.

Shin DS, Jeffrey RB, Desser TS. Pearls and pitfalls in hepatic ultrasonography. *Ultrasound Quarterly.* 2010;26:17–25.

Smith D. Sonographic demonstration of Couinaud's liver segments. *J Ultrasound Med.* 1998;17:375.

Snell RT. *Clinical Anatomy.* ed 7. Lippincott Williams & Wilkins; 2004.

Sugiura N. Portosystemic collateral shunts originating from the left portal veins in portal hypertension: demonstration by color Doppler flow imaging. *J Clin Ultrasound.* 1992;20:427.

Tchelepi H, Ralls PW, Radin R, Grant E. Sonography of diffuse liver disease. *J Ultrasound Med.* 2002;21:1023–1032.

Wilson SR, Jang HJ, Kim TK, Burns PN. Diagnosis of focal liver masses on ultrasonography. *J Ultrasound Med.* 2007;26:775–787.

CHAPTER 10

The Gallbladder and the Biliary System

Sandra L. Hagen-Ansert

OBJECTIVES

On completion of this chapter, you should be able to:
- Describe the internal, surface, and relational anatomies of the gallbladder
- Explain the function of the gallbladder
- Differentiate the sectional anatomy of the hepatobiliary system and adjacent structures
- Describe the normal sonographic pattern of the gallbladder, cystic duct, hepatic ducts, and common bile duct
- Differentiate the sonographic appearances of the gallbladder and biliary system pathologies discussed in this chapter

OUTLINE

Anatomy of the Biliary System 281
    Normal Anatomy 281
    Vascular Supply 285
Physiology and Laboratory Data of the Gallbladder and Biliary System 285
    Removal of the Gallbladder 285
Sonographic Evaluation of the Biliary System 285
    Biliary System Protocol 285
    Gallbladder 287
    Bile Ducts 289
Pathology of the Gallbladder and Biliary System 289

Clinical Symptoms of Gallbladder Disease 290
Wall Thickness 293
Cholecystitis 293
Torsion of the Gallbladder 299
Porcelain Gallbladder 303
Hyperplastic Cholecystosis 303
Gallbladder Carcinoma 306
Pathology of the Biliary Tree 308
    Choledochal Cysts 308
    Dilated Biliary Ducts 311
    Biliary Obstruction 312

Extrahepatic Biliary Obstruction 312
Choledocholithiasis 313
Hemobilia 315
Pneumobilia 315
Cholangitis: Bile Duct Wall Thickening 315
Ascariasis 318
Intrahepatic Biliary Neoplasms 318
Cholangiocarcinoma 318

KEY TERMS

Adenomyomatosis
Ampulla of Vater
Bilirubin
Cholangitis
Cholecystectomy
Cholecystitis
Cholecystokinin
Choledochal cyst
Choledocholithiasis
Cholelithiasis
Cholesterolosis

Common bile duct
Common hepatic duct
Cystic duct
Gallbladder
Hartmann's pouch
Heister valve
Hydrops
Jaundice
Junctional fold
Klatskin tumor
Main portal vein (MPV)

Murphy sign
Pancreatic duct
Phrygian cap
Polyp
Porcelain gallbladder
Porta hepatis
Sludge
Sphincter of Oddi
Wall echo shadow (WES) sign

Together with the liver and pancreas, the biliary system plays a role in the digestive process. The gallbladder serves as a reservoir for bile that is drained from the hepatic ducts within the liver. Sonographic evaluation of the gallbladder and biliary system is used as a primary diagnostic tool and has proven effective in diagnosing various types of gallbladder disease, including the more common problems of cholelithiasis, cholecystitis, and dilation of the ductal system.

ANATOMY OF THE BILIARY SYSTEM

Normal Anatomy

The biliary apparatus consists of the right and left hepatic ducts, the common hepatic duct, the common bile duct, the pear-shaped gallbladder, and the cystic duct (Fig. 10.1). The bile ducts are divided into intrahepatic and extrahepatic segments. The intrahepatic ducts run in the portal triads along with the portal veins and hepatic arteries (Fig. 10.2). The peripheral intrahepatic ducts run parallel and adjacent to the hepatic arteries and portal veins. The anterior and posterior relationship of the three structures is more variable than that of the extrahepatic ducts.

Hepatic Ducts. The extrahepatic portion of the bile ducts includes the common hepatic duct, common bile duct, and a portion of the central right and left ducts (see Fig. 10.1). The right and left hepatic ducts emerge from the right lobe of the liver in the **porta hepatis** and unite to form the common hepatic duct, which then passes caudally and medially.

The hepatic duct runs parallel with the portal vein. Each duct is formed by the union of bile canaliculi from the liver lobules.

The common hepatic duct is approximately 4 mm in diameter and descends within the edge of the lesser omentum. The common hepatic duct is the segment above the cystic duct, and the common bile duct is the segment below. The cystic duct may be difficult to image on sonography; therefore, the sonographer may use the general term as the *proximal or distal* segments of the "common duct." The **common hepatic duct** is the bile duct system that drains the liver into the common bile duct.

Common Bile Duct. The normal **common bile duct** has a diameter of up to 6 mm. The first part of the duct lies in the right free edge of the lesser omentum (Fig. 10.3). The second part of the duct is situated posterior to the first part of the duodenum. The third part of the duct lies in a groove on the posterior surface of the head of the pancreas. It ends by piercing the medial wall of the second part of the duodenum about halfway down the duodenal length. The main pancreatic duct joins the common bile duct, and together they open through a small ampulla (the **ampulla of Vater**) into the duodenal wall. The end parts of both ducts (common bile duct and

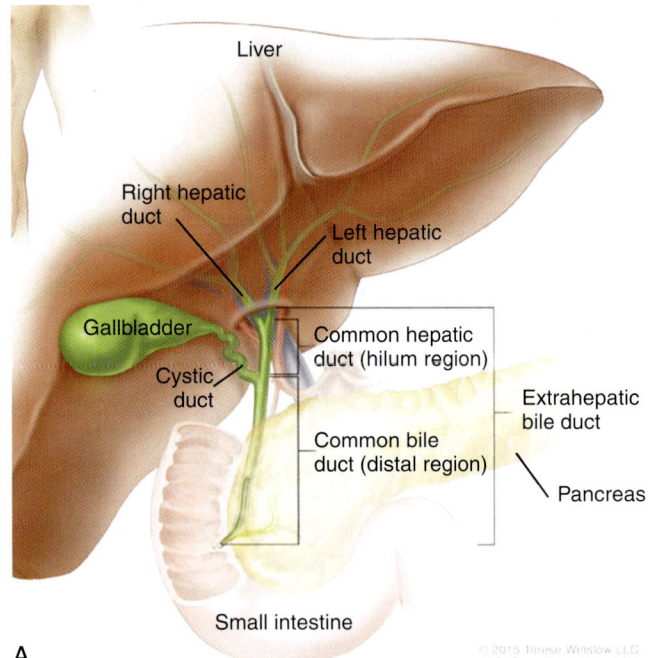

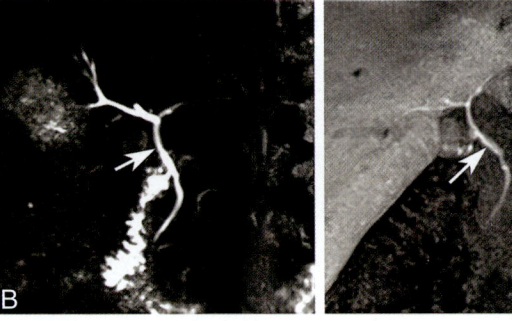

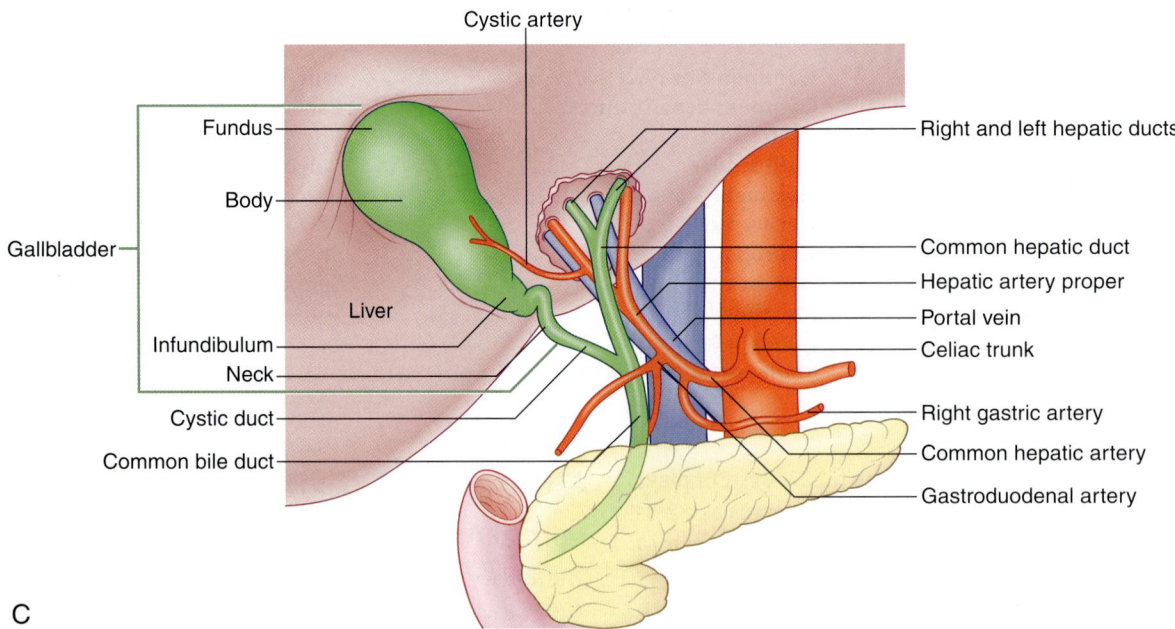

FIG. 10.1 (A) The biliary apparatus consists of the right and left hepatic ducts, the common hepatic duct, the common bile duct, the pear-shaped gallbladder, and the cystic duct. (B) Magnetic resonance imaging of the biliary system. (C) The common bile duct measures 8 cm, the cystic duct measures 3 to 4 cm, and the hepatic duct measures 3 cm.

main **pancreatic duct**) and the ampulla are surrounded by circular muscle fibers known as the **sphincter of Oddi**.

The proximal portion of the common bile duct is lateral to the hepatic artery and anterior to the portal vein. The duct moves more posterior after it descends behind the duodenal bulb and enters the pancreas. The distal duct lies parallel to the anterior wall of the vena cava.

Within the liver parenchyma, the bile ducts follow the same course as the portal venous and hepatic arterial branches. The hepatic and bile ducts are encased in a common collagenous sheath, forming the portal triad. The hepatic artery arises from the celiac axis and travels in the hepatoduodenal ligament anterior to the portal vein and medial to the common duct. On transverse views, this is known as the "Mickey Mouse" sign with the portal vein as the head, the hepatic artery the left ear, and the bile duct the right ear. In most patients, the right hepatic artery passes between the common duct and the portal vein; however, in a small percentage, the hepatic artery passes either anterior to the common duct, or there may be a variant of two hepatic arteries anterior and/or posterior to the duct. The hepatic artery can be quite tortuous, so only a small segment is usually imaged. A replaced right hepatic artery that arises from the superior mesenteric artery is a normal variant that alters the anatomy of the porta hepatis. Color Doppler and tracing the vessel to its point of origin help to define the vessel.

Cystic Duct. The **cystic duct** is about 4 cm long and connects the neck of the gallbladder with the common hepatic duct to form the common bile duct. It is usually somewhat S-shaped and descends for a variable distance in the right free edge of the lesser omentum.

The Gallbladder. The **gallbladder** is a pear-shaped organ found on the inferior margin of the liver between the right and left lobes of the liver (Fig. 10.4). Two useful anatomical landmarks are utilized to locate the gallbladder. The middle hepatic vein is in alignment with the gallbladder fossa. The interlobar fissure extends from the right portal vein to the gallbladder fossa. The gallbladder lies in the intrahepatic position, but as it migrates to the surface of the liver during embryologic development, it acquires a peritoneal covering over most of its surface (Fig. 10.5). The remainder of the gallbladder surface is covered with adventitial tissue that merges with the connective tissue with the liver. This potential space between the liver and the gallbladder is an area for infection or inflammation to collect. If this migration does not occur, the gallbladder remains intrahepatic, or it may be enveloped in the visceral peritoneum, hanging into the lower abdomen. The gallbladder has been found to lie in various ectopic positions (suprahepatic, suprarenal, within the anterior abdominal wall, or in the falciform ligament). Failure of the gallbladder to develop is rare; this failure is known as *agenesis* of the gallbladder. These patients may still have the biliary ductal system, which can become inflamed or filled with stones.

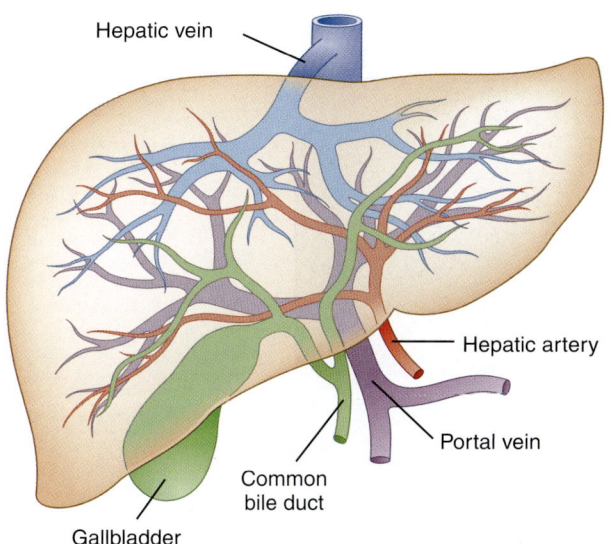

FIG. 10.2 **Vascular and ductal system of the liver and gallbladder.** The *green* represents the biliary ductal system, the *blue* represents the portal venous system, the *pink* represents the hepatic arterial system, and the *purple* represents the hepatic venous system (portal vein).

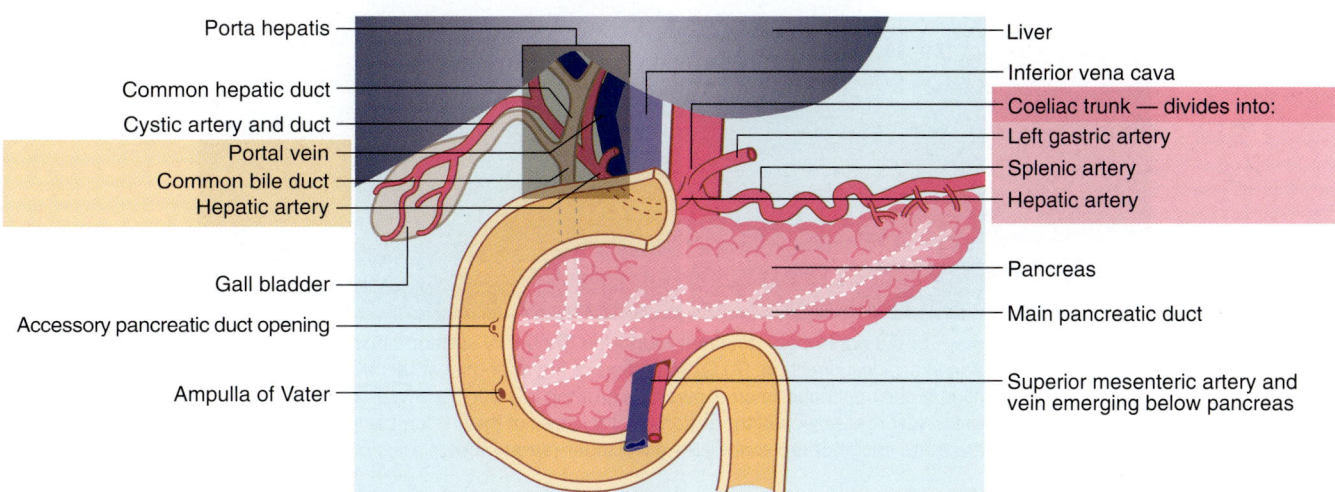

FIG. 10.3 **Relationships within the porta hepatis.** Note the relationship of the pancreas, duodenum, and colon to the biliary system.

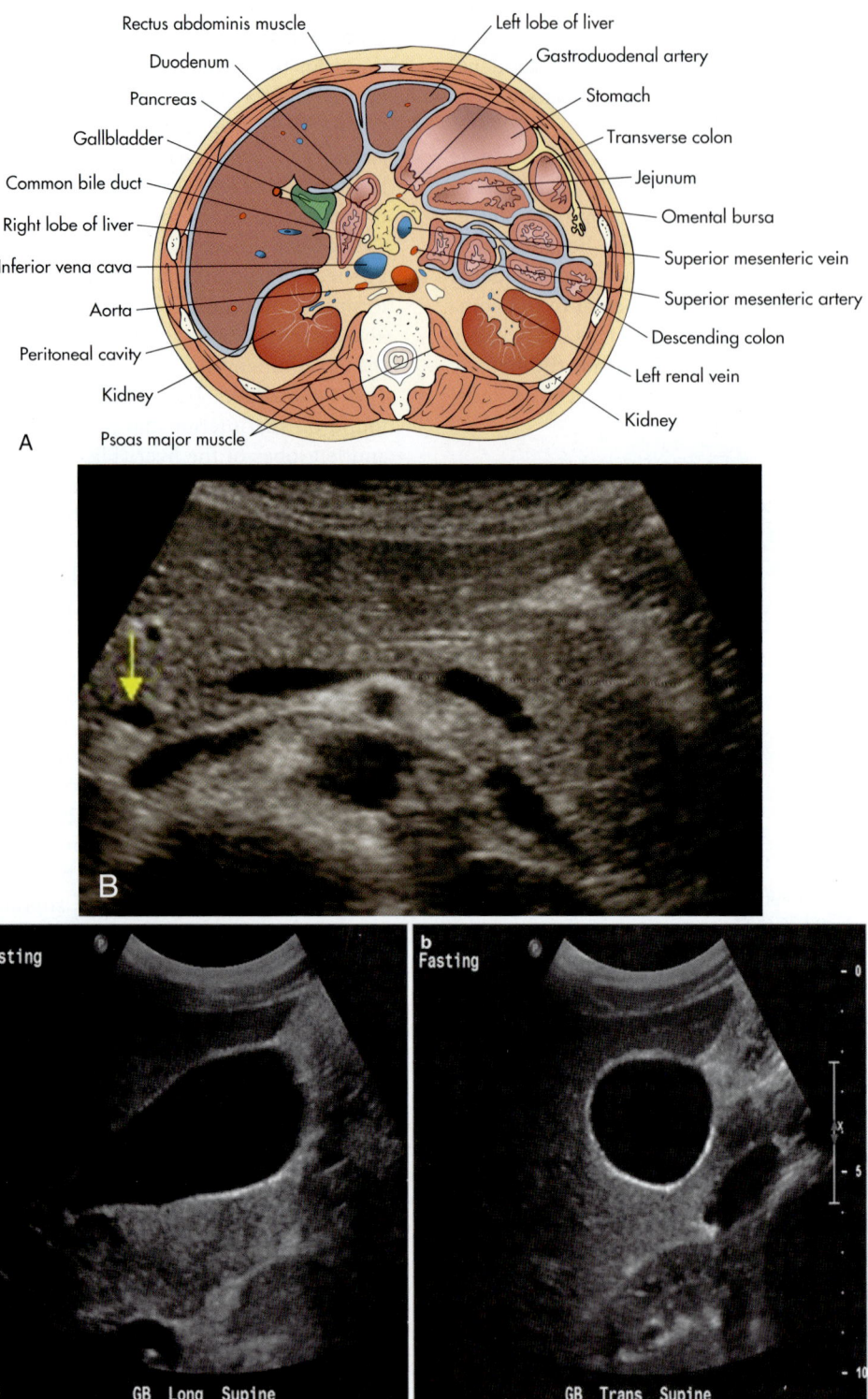

FIG. 10.4 Transverse views of the right upper quadrant to include the biliary system, beginning at the level of the caudate lobe and proceeding in a caudal direction. (A) Cross section of the abdomen at the level of the second lumbar vertebra. (B) Transverse image of the upper abdomen shows the common bile duct *(arrow)* as a circular structure posterior to the head of the pancreas. (C) Cross section of the abdomen at the level of the first lumbar vertebra. (D) Longitudinal and transverse "zoom" ultrasound image of the sonolucent gallbladder *(arrow)* shown anterior to the right kidney and medial to the liver.

The gallbladder is divided into the *fundus, body*, and *neck* (Fig. 10.6A). The rounded fundus usually projects below the inferior margin of the liver, where it comes into contact with the anterior abdominal wall at the level of the ninth right costal cartilage. The body generally lies in contact with the visceral surface of the liver and is directed upward, backward, and to the left. The neck becomes continuous with the cystic duct, which turns into the lesser omentum to join the right side of the common hepatic duct to form the common bile duct. The neck of the gallbladder is oriented posteromedially toward the porta hepatis. The fundus is situated lateral, caudal, and anterior to the neck.

The size and shape of the gallbladder are variable. Generally, the normal gallbladder measures approximately 2.5 to 4 cm in diameter and 7 to 10 cm in length. The walls are less than 3 mm thick. Dilation of the gallbladder is known as **hydrops**.

Several anatomic variations may occur within the gallbladder to give rise to its internal echo pattern on the sonogram. The gallbladder may have a small outpouch, also known as the infundibulum, forming **Hartmann's pouch**; this is significant as gallstones may collect in this pouch (see Fig. 10.6B). Other anomalies include partial septation, complete septation (double gallbladder), and folding of the fundus (**Phrygian cap**) (Fig. 10.7).

With a capacity of 50 mL, the gallbladder serves as a reservoir for bile. It also has the ability to concentrate the bile. To aid this process, its mucous membrane contains folds that unite with each other, giving the surface a honeycomb appearance. **Heister valve** in the neck of the gallbladder helps prevent kinking of the duct (see Fig. 10.6A).

Vascular Supply

The arterial supply of the gallbladder is from the cystic artery, which is a branch of the right hepatic artery (see Fig. 10.3). The cystic vein drains directly into the portal vein. Smaller arteries and veins run between the liver and the gallbladder.

PHYSIOLOGY AND LABORATORY DATA OF THE GALLBLADDER AND BILIARY SYSTEM

The primary functions of the extrahepatic biliary tract are (1) the transportation of bile from the liver to the intestine and (2) the regulation of its flow. These are important functions as the liver secretes approximately 1 to 2 L of bile per day. When the gallbladder and bile ducts are functioning normally, they respond in a fairly uniform manner in various phases of digestion. Concentration of bile in the gallbladder occurs during a state of fasting. It is forced into the gallbladder by an increased pressure within the common bile duct, which is produced by the action of the sphincter of Oddi at the distal end of the gallbladder.

During the fasting state, very little bile flows into the duodenum. Stimulation produced by the influence of food causes the gallbladder to contract, resulting in an outpouring of bile into the duodenum. When the stomach is emptied, duodenal peristalsis diminishes, the gallbladder relaxes, the tonus of the sphincter of Oddi increases slightly, and thus very little bile passes into the duodenum. Small amounts of bile secreted by the liver are retained in the common duct and forced into the gallbladder. The contracted gallbladder appears on sonography as a thick-walled structure with a slit for the bile. It is nearly impossible to see luminal or wall abnormalities when the gallbladder is contracted.

Removal of the Gallbladder

When the gallbladder is removed, the sphincter of Oddi loses tonus, and pressure within the common bile duct drops to that of intraabdominal pressure. Bile is no longer retained in the bile ducts but is free to flow into the duodenum during fasting and digestive phases. Dilation of the extrahepatic bile ducts (usually less than 1 cm) occurs after **cholecystectomy**.

Secretion is largely caused by a bile salt–dependent mechanism, and ductal flow is controlled by secretion. Bile is the principal medium for excretion of **bilirubin** and cholesterol. The products of steroid hormones are also excreted in the bile, as are drugs and poisons (e.g., salts of heavy metals). The bile salts from the intestine stimulate the liver to make more bile. Bile salts activate intestinal and pancreatic enzymes.

SONOGRAPHIC EVALUATION OF THE BILIARY SYSTEM

Biliary System Protocol

Ultrasound examinations of the gallbladder and bile ducts are performed to determine cholelithiasis, changes secondary to acute and chronic cholecystitis, obstruction, and primary or metastatic tumor involvement. The examination is performed as part of a comprehensive general abdominal evaluation (Table 10.1).

1. Patient preparation: NPO for at least 6 hours.
2. Transducer selection: broadband curvilinear or section probe 2.5 to 5 MHz.
3. Patient position: Supine and decubitus (see Fig. 10.8 A–C).
4. Images and observations should include the following (Fig. 10.9):
   - The fundus, body, and neck should be surveyed.
   - Gallbladder wall thickness (normal is less than 3 mm) should be recorded. If thickened, the wall should be measured from the anterior wall to the posterior wall with the transducer perpendicular to the anterior wall.
   - The presence of echogenic foci (e.g., stones, polyps) within the gallbladder lumen should be evaluated. If echogenic foci are present, the sonographer should attempt to demonstrate acoustic shadowing and mobility with change in patient position.
   - The common bile duct should be imaged in at least the oblique long-axis plane as it lies anterior to the **main portal vein (MPV)** before coursing posterior to the head of the pancreas.
   - The transverse scan of the porta hepatis may help delineate the portal vein from the common duct

286 CHAPTER 10 The Gallbladder and the Biliary System

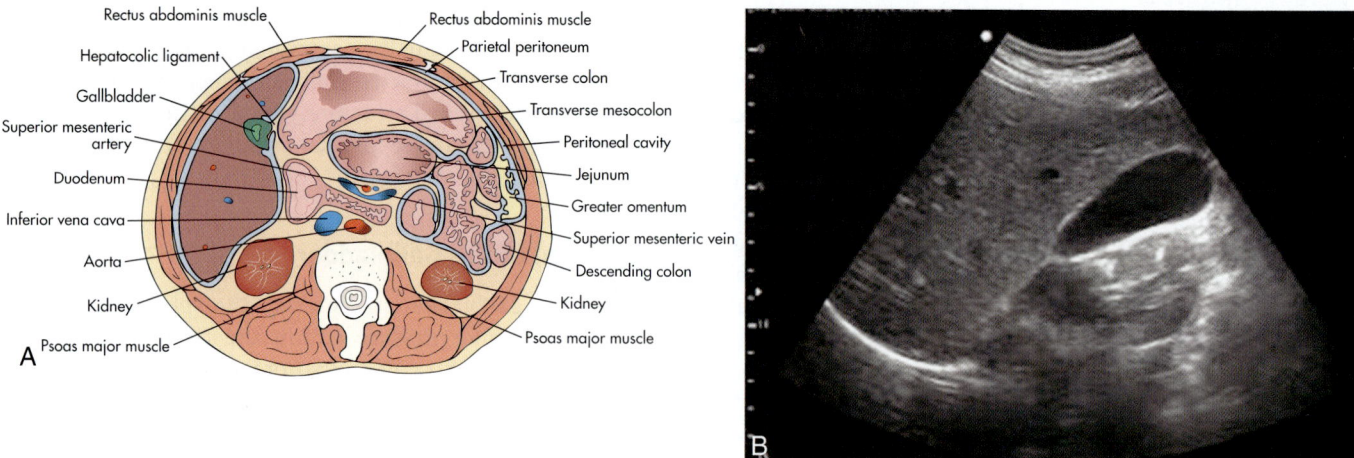

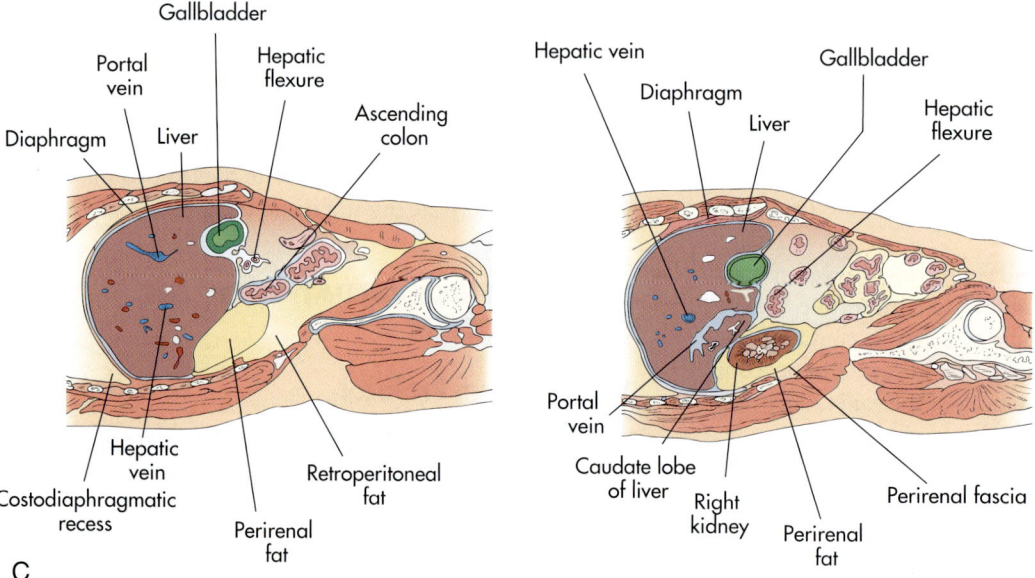

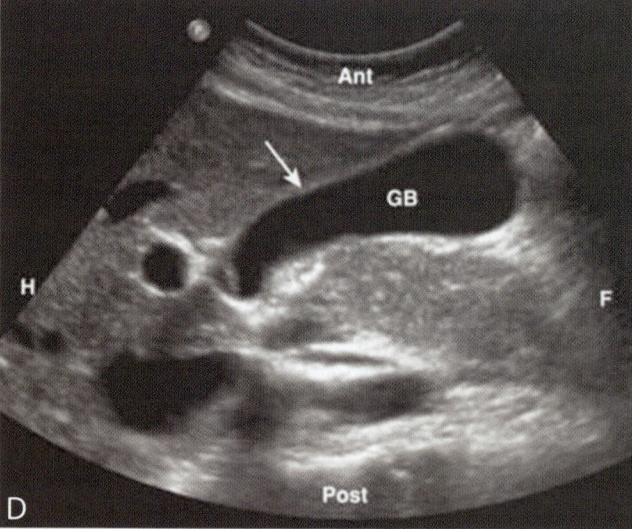

FIG. 10.5 **Sagittal views of the right upper quadrant to include the biliary system beginning near the midclavicular line and moving toward the midline.** (A) Sagittal view of the right upper quadrant near the midclavicular line. (B) Longitudinal ultrasound image of the normal sonolucent gallbladder. (C) Sagittal view of the right upper quadrant between the midclavicular line and the midline. (D) Longitudinal ultrasound image of the normal gallbladder (GB; *arrow*).

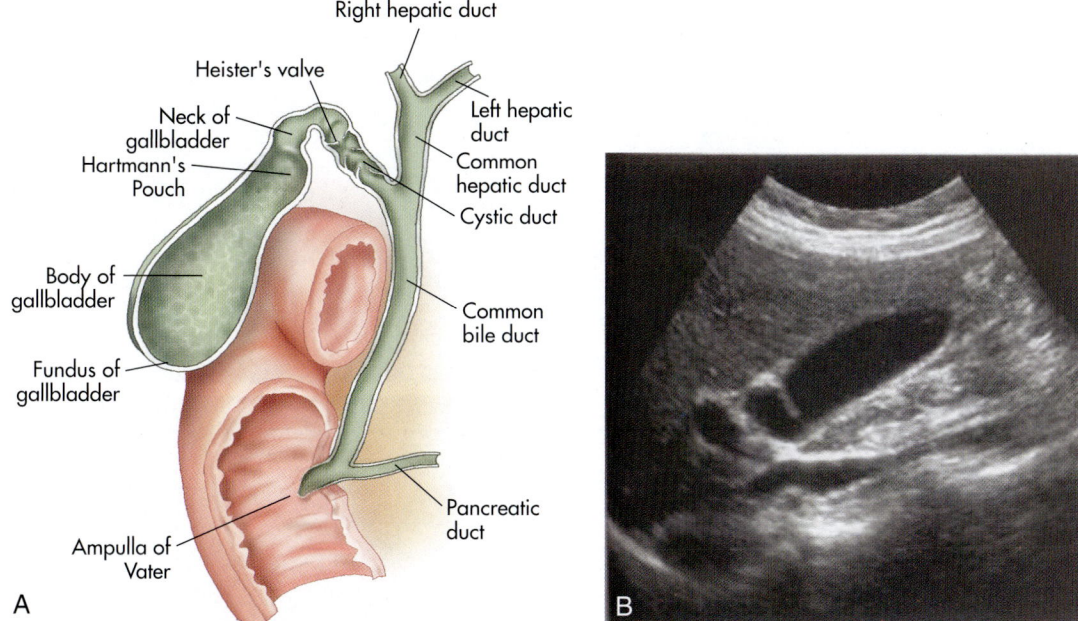

FIG. 10.6 (A) Gallbladder and biliary ducts. The first part of the duct lies in the right free edge of the lesser omentum. The second part of the duct is situated posterior to the first part of the duodenum. The third part lies in a groove on the posterior surface of the head of the pancreas. The common bile duct is joined by the main pancreatic duct, and together they open through the ampulla of Vater into the duodenal wall. (B) Hartmann's pouch may be seen near the neck of the gallbladder *(arrow)*.

(anterior and to the right) and hepatic artery (anterior and to the left).
- Visualization of the intrahepatic ducts may be difficult unless dilation is present. Ductal dilation may be seen as the liver is scanned, demonstrating right and left branches of the portal vein as the hepatic ducts follow a parallel course.
- To examine gallstones, the focal point of the transducer is placed at the region of the posterior gallbladder wall, and the gain reduced. This facilitates demonstration of acoustic shadowing.

Gallbladder

To ensure maximum dilation of the gallbladder, the patient should be given nothing to eat for at least 6 hours prior to the ultrasound examination. The patient is initially examined in the supine position in full inspiration. Transverse, sagittal, and oblique scans are made over the upper abdomen to identify the gallbladder, biliary system, liver, right kidney, and head of the pancreas. The oblique scans are made with the transducer in the subcostal position with a slight cephalic angulation. The probe sweep is aligned between the right shoulder and left hip of the patient. If stones or polyps are suspected, the patient should also be rolled into a steep decubitus or upright position (to ensure there are no stones within the gallbladder) in an attempt to separate small stones from the gallbladder wall or cystic duct (Fig. 10.10).

The gallbladder may be identified as a sonolucent oblong structure located anterior to the right kidney, lateral to the head of the pancreas and duodenum. The gallbladder fossa causes a slight indentation on the posterior surface of the medial aspect of the right lobe of the liver. The sagittal scans may show the right kidney posterior to the gallbladder when the probe is angled toward the right hip. The fundus is generally oriented slightly more anterior and, on sagittal scans, often reaches the anterior abdominal wall. Box 10.1 lists the sonographic characteristics of the normal gallbladder.

The middle hepatic vein lies in the same anatomic plane and may prove to be a useful landmark in locating the gallbladder. A sweep from cephalad to caudad shows the interlobar fissure (a structure that separates the right and left hepatic lobes) as a bright linear echo within the liver connecting the gallbladder fossa and the right portal vein. The neck of the gallbladder usually comes into contact with the main segment of the portal vein near the origin of the left portal vein. The gallbladder commonly resides in a fossa on the medial aspect of the liver. Because of fat or fibrous tissue within the main lobar fissure of the liver (which lies between the gallbladder and the right portal vein), this bright linear reflector is a reliable indicator of the location of the gallbladder. The gallbladder lies in the posterior and caudal aspect of the fissure. The caudal aspect of the linear echo "points" directly to the gallbladder. If the gallbladder has been removed, the fossa appears as an echogenic line as a result of the remaining connective tissues.

A small echogenic fold has been reported to occur along the posterior wall of the gallbladder at the junction of the body/neck. It may be very small (3 to 5 mm) but may give rise to an acoustic shadow in the supine position. It is not duplicated

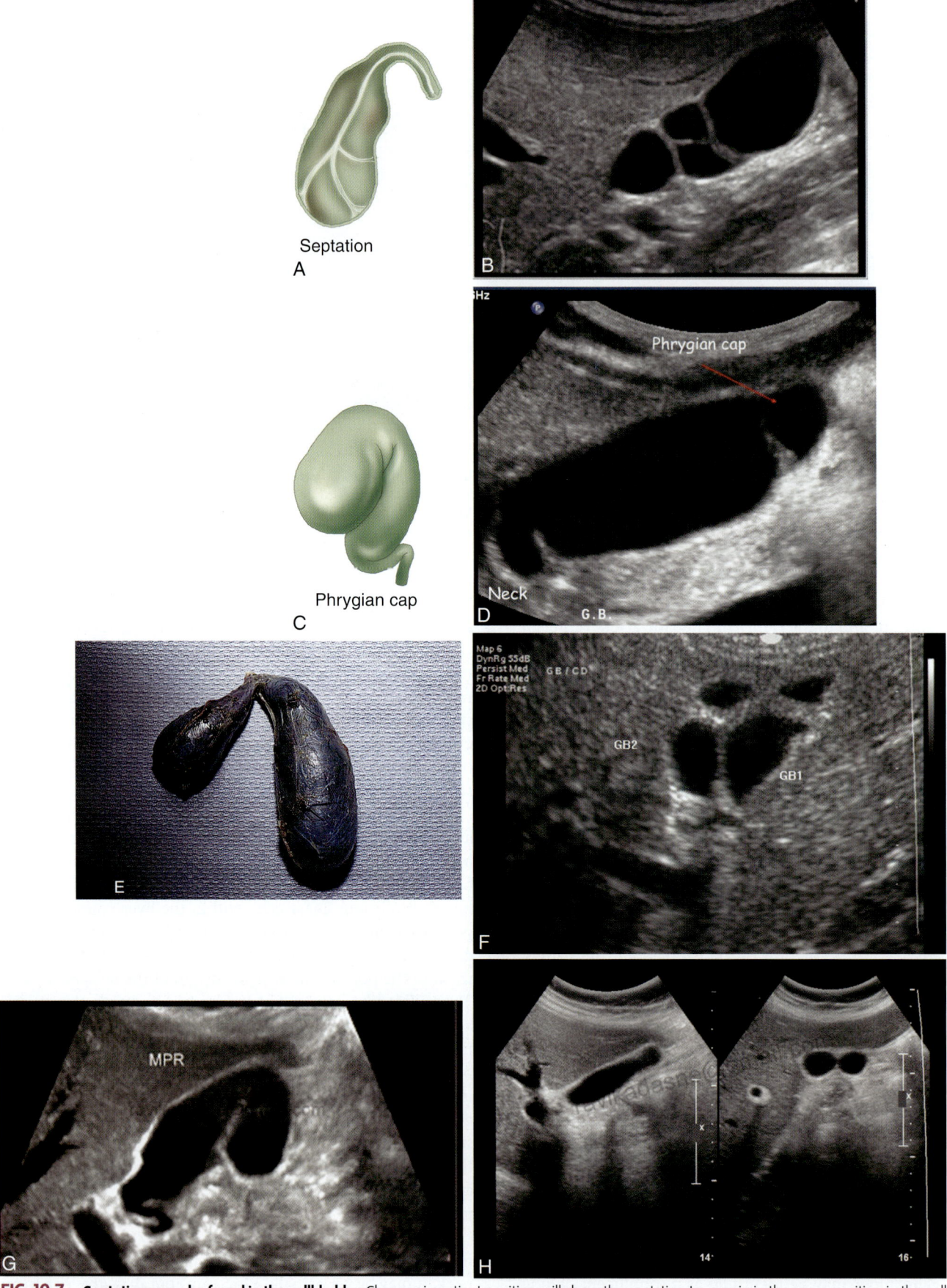

FIG. 10.7 Septations may be found in the gallbladder. Changes in patient position will show the septation to remain in the same position in the gallbladder. (A–B) Septated gallbladder shows a prominent gallbladder with multiple septations within the body. (C–D) The Phrygian cap is a variant in which part of the fundus of the gallbladder is bent back on itself. (E–F) The double gallbladder is seen infrequently; the recognition of two distinct sacs will confirm the diagnosis. (G–H) The folded gallbladder wall is seen in these longitudinal *(left)* and transverse *(right)* images.

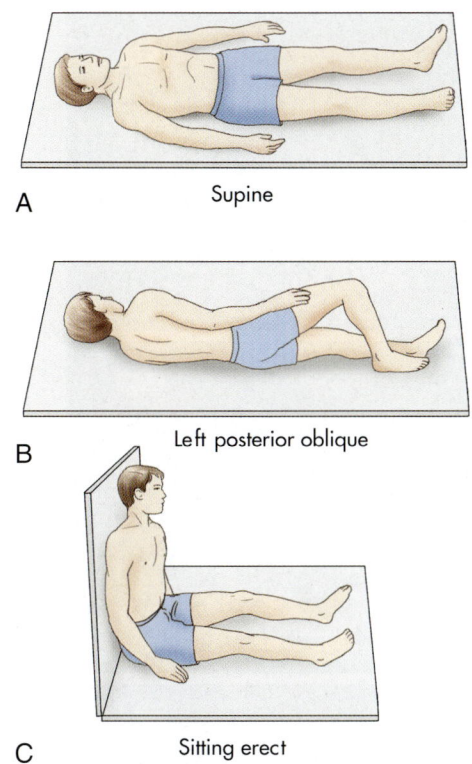

FIG. 10.8 (A–C) The gallbladder should be examined with the patient in the supine (A), left posterior oblique (B), and sometimes upright positions (C).

TABLE 10.1	Abdominal Ultrasound Protocol: Gallbladder	
Organ	Scan Plane	Anatomy
GB (supine and LLD)	Long	Body/fundus
	Trv	Body/neck (measure wall) Body/neck
CBD	Trv	Portal triad
	Long	Measure duct

CBD, Common bile duct; *GB*, gallbladder; *LLD*, left lateral decubitus; *Long*, longitudinal; *Trv*, transverse.

in the oblique position. The cause for such a **junctional fold** is the indentation between the body/neck or Heister valve, a spiral fold beginning in the neck of the gallbladder and lining the cystic duct (see Fig. 10.6).

A prominent gallbladder may be normal in some individuals secondary to their fasting state (Fig. 10.11). A large gallbladder has also been detected in patients with diabetes, patients bedridden with protracted illness or pancreatitis, and patients taking anticholinergic drugs. A large gallbladder may even fail to contract after a fatty meal or intravenous **cholecystokinin**; other studies may be needed before making a diagnosis of obstruction.

If a gallbladder appears abnormally enlarged, a fatty meal may be administered and further sonographic evaluation made to detect whether the enlargement is abnormal or normal. If the gallbladder fails to contract during the examination, the pancreatic area should be investigated further. Courvoisier sign indicates an extrahepatic mass compressing the common bile duct, which can produce an enlarged gallbladder (Fig. 10.12). In addition, the liver should be carefully examined for the presence of dilated bile ducts.

In a well-contracted gallbladder, the wall changes from a single to a double concentric structure with the following three components: (1) a strongly reflective outer contour, (2) a poorly reflective inner contour, and (3) a sonolucent area between both reflecting structures.

Bile Ducts

Sonographically, the common duct lies anterior and to the right of the portal vein in the region of the porta hepatis and gastrohepatic ligament. The hepatic artery lies anterior and to the left of the portal vein. On a transverse scan, the common duct, hepatic artery, and portal vein have been referred to as the portal triad or "Mickey Mouse sign" (Fig. 10.13). The portal vein serves as Mickey's face, with the lateral ear the common duct and the medial ear the hepatic artery. To obtain such a cross-section, the transducer must be directed in a slightly oblique path from the left shoulder to the right hip.

On sagittal scans, the right branch of the hepatic artery usually passes anterior to the common duct (Figs. 10.14 and 10.15). The common duct is seen just anterior to the portal vein before it dips posteriorly to enter the head of the pancreas. The patient may be rotated into a slight (45-degree) or steep (90-degree) right anterior oblique position, with the beam directed posteromedially to visualize the duct. This enables the examiner to avoid cumbersome bowel gas and to use the liver as an acoustic window.

When the right subcostal approach is used, the main portal vein may be seen as it bifurcates into the right and left branches. As the right branch continues into the right lobe of the liver, it can be followed laterally in a longitudinal plane. The portal vein appears as an almond-shaped sonolucent structure anterior to the inferior vena cava. The common hepatic duct is seen as a tubular structure anterior to the portal vein. The right branch of the hepatic artery can be seen between the duct and the portal vein as a small circular structure.

The small cystic duct is generally not identified. Because this landmark is necessary to distinguish the common hepatic duct from the common bile duct, the more general term *common duct* is used to refer to these structures (Fig. 10.16).

PATHOLOGY OF THE GALLBLADDER AND BILIARY SYSTEM

See Table 10.2 for clinical findings, sonographic findings, and differential considerations for gallbladder and biliary diseases and conditions.

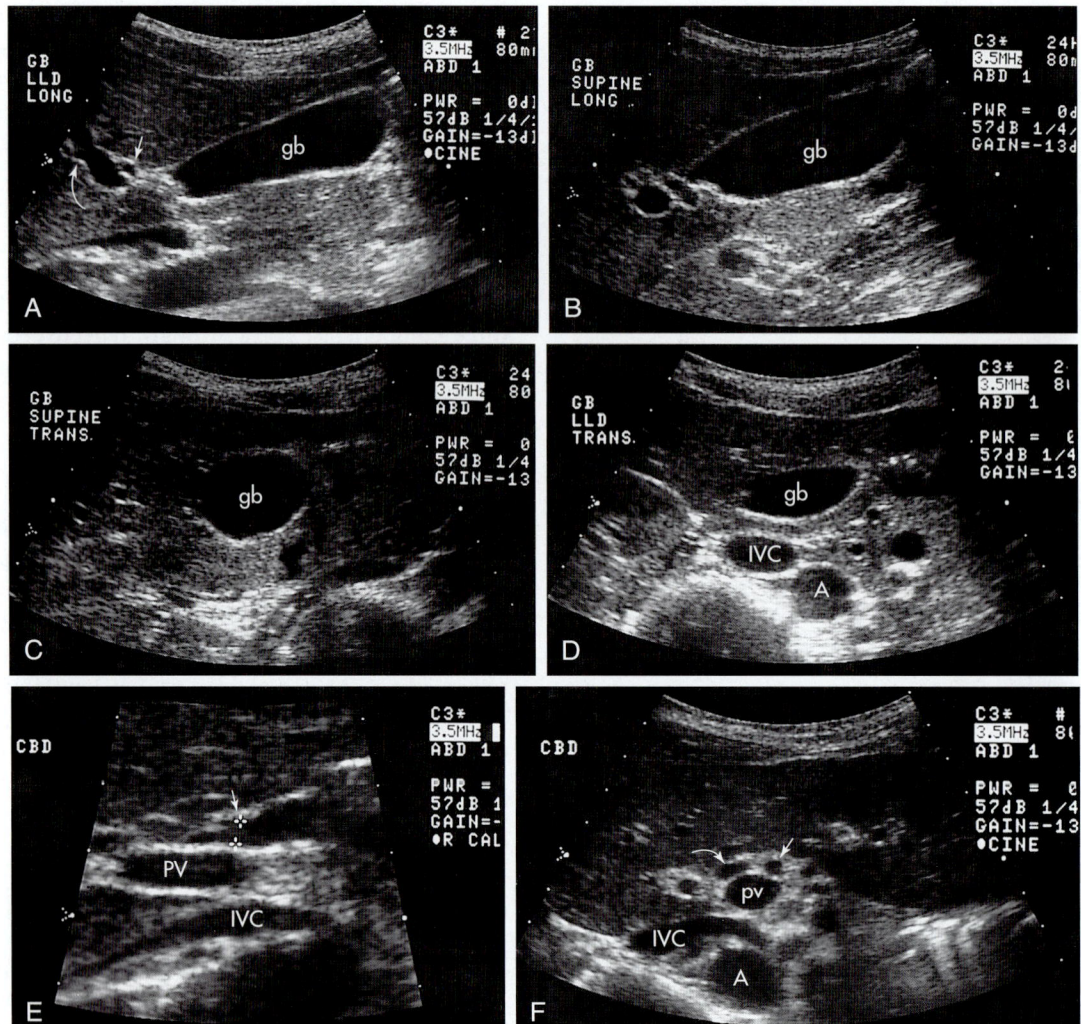

FIG. 10.9 (A) Longitudinal images of the gallbladder (gb), main lobar fissure *(arrow)*, and portal vein *(curved arrow)*. (B) Longitudinal image of gallbladder, including the neck. (C) Transverse image of gallbladder. (D) Transverse image of gallbladder, inferior vena cava (IVC), and aorta (A). (E) Longitudinal image of common bile duct *(arrow)* anterior to portal vein (PV) that lies anterior to the inferior vena cava. (F) Transverse image of portal tried in the center of the image: portal vein with common bile duct *(curved arrow)* anterior and lateral; hepatic artery *(arrow)* anterior and medial; inferior vena cava and aorta.

Clinical Symptoms of Gallbladder Disease

Pain. The most classic symptom of gallbladder disease is right upper quadrant abdominal pain, usually occurring after ingestion of greasy foods. Nausea and vomiting sometimes occur and may indicate the presence of a stone in the common bile duct. A gallbladder attack may cause referred pain to the right shoulder, with inflammation of the gallbladder often causing referred pain in the right shoulder blade.

BOX 10.1	Sonographic Characteristics of the Normal Gallbladder

- Size: ≤4 cm transverse; ≤10 cm longitudinal
- Wall thickness: <3 mm
- Lumen: anechoic
- Landmarks: right upper quadrant, between right and left lobes of liver, right kidney, main lobar fissure, and portal vein

Jaundice. Jaundice is characterized by the presence of bile in the tissues with resulting yellow-green color of the skin. It may develop when a tiny gallstone blocks the bile ducts between the gallbladder and the intestines, producing pressure on the liver and forcing bile into the blood.

Sludge. Sludge, or thickened bile, frequently occurs from bile stasis. Sludge may be seen in patients with prolonged fasting, hyperalimentation therapy, or with obstruction of the gallbladder. Some gallbladders may be so packed with this thickened bile that the gallbladder is isoechoic and difficult to distinguish from the liver parenchyma. Occasionally sludge is also found in the common duct. Sludge is gravity dependent; therefore with alterations in the patient's position, the sonographer may be able to separate sludge from occasional artifactual echoes found in the gallbladder. Sludge will slowly resettle as the patient changes their position. Sludge should be considered an abnormal finding because either a functional or a pathologic abnormality exists when calcium bilirubin or cholesterol precipitates

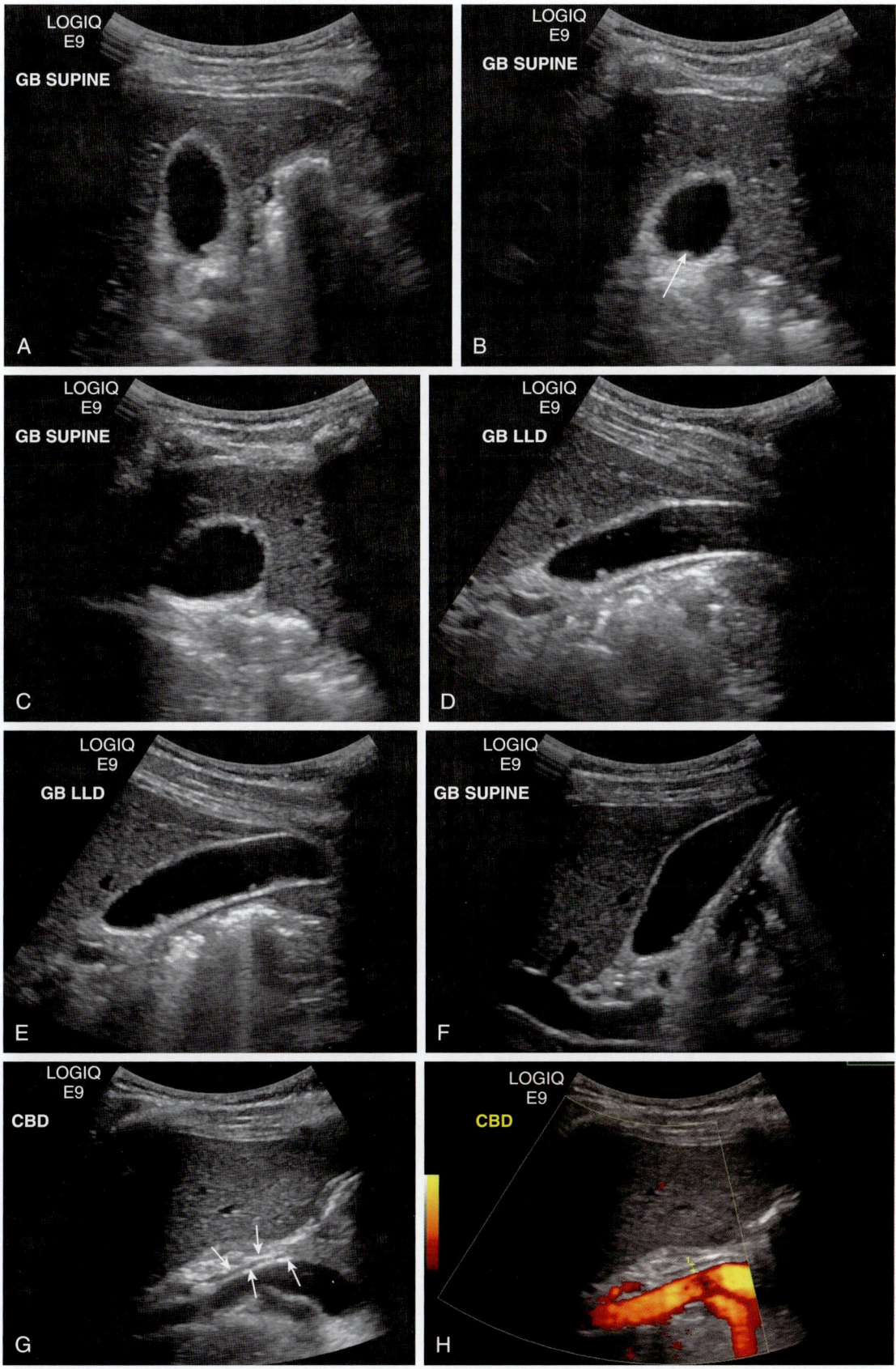

FIG. 10.10 (A–C) Supine transverse images of the gallbladder. Note the small echogenic adenoma attached to the posterior wall *(arrow)*. This does not move with alterations in patient position. (D–E) Left lateral decubitus images of the long axis of the gallbladder. (F–H) Supine longitudinal images of the gallbladder and common bile duct *(arrows)*.

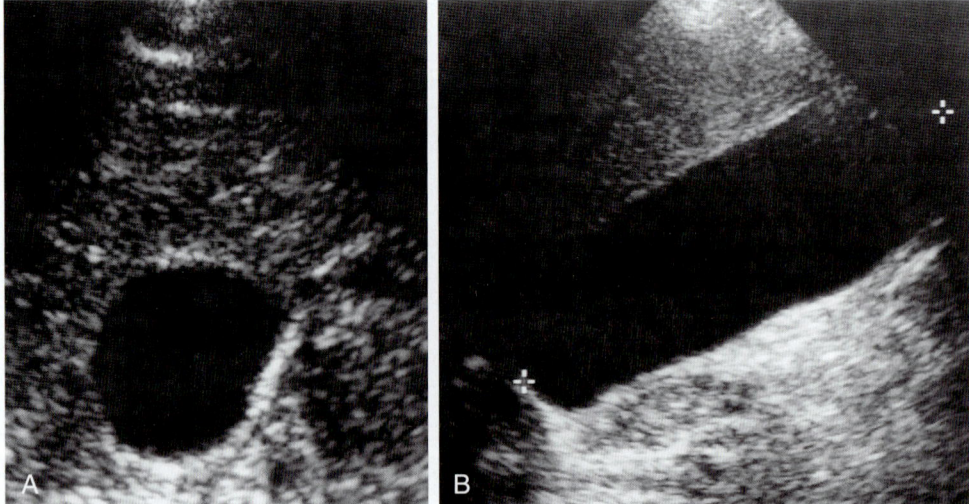

FIG. 10.11 (A) Transverse and (B) longitudinal scans of the distended gallbladder. The gallbladder size may be quite variable from patient to patient. A good rule of thumb is to compare the size of the gallbladder with the transverse view of the right kidney. The width should always be smaller ≤4 cm.

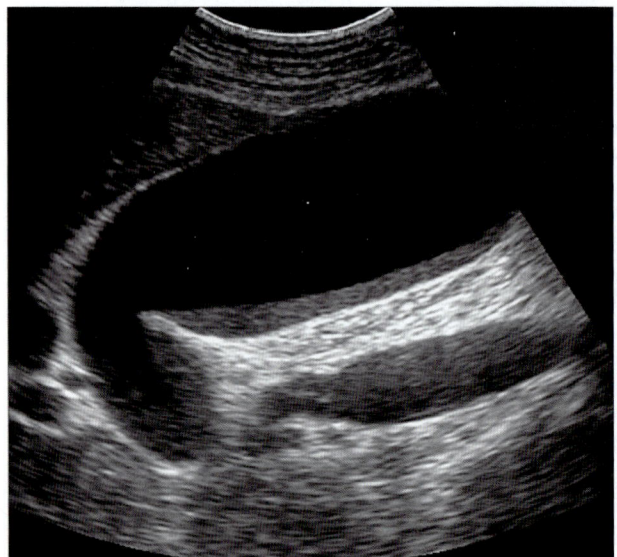

FIG. 10.12 Distention (hydrops) of the gallbladder may be found in patients who have been on intravenous fluids for several days or may be secondary to a mass or enlarged lymph nodes compressing the common bile duct.

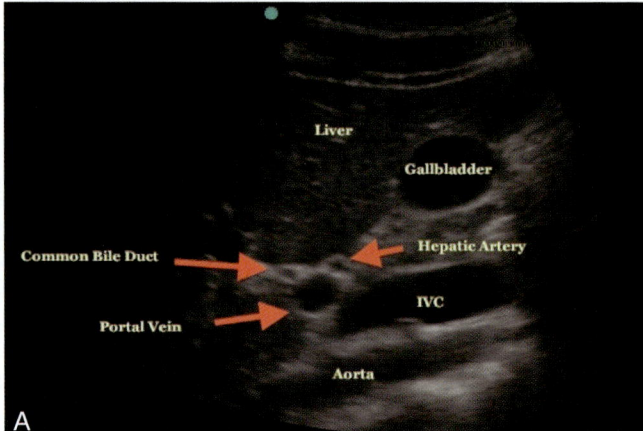

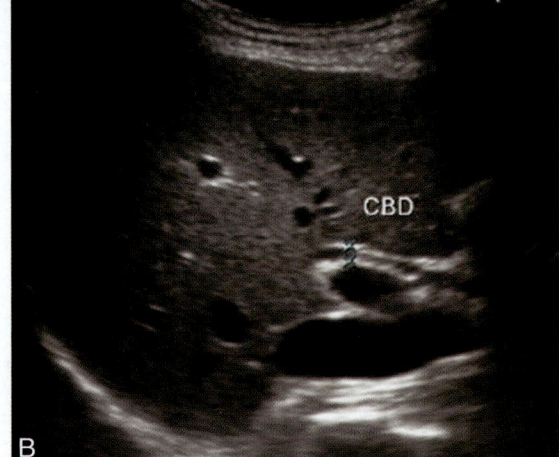

FIG. 10.13 Transverse oblique (A) and sagittal (B) views of the common bile duct. The transverse oblique view shows the portal triad with the portal vein posterior, the common duct anterior and lateral, and the hepatic artery anterior and medial. The sagittal view shows the common duct anterior to the main portal vein and tubular inferior vena cava.

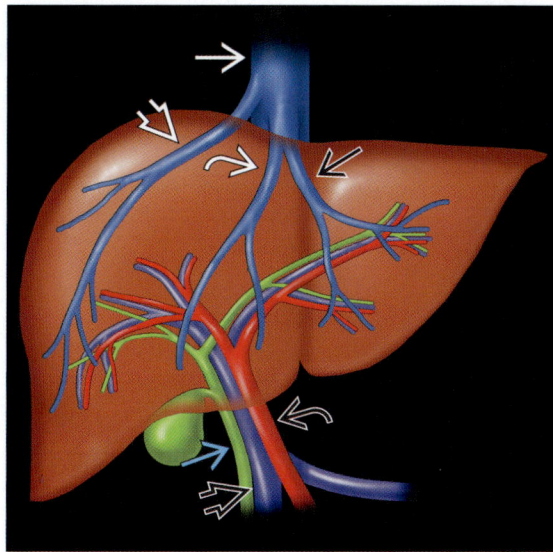

FIG. 10.14 Anatomical relationship of the cystic duct, cystic artery, and common bile duct. The right branch of the hepatic artery usually passes anterior to the common duct. The common duct is seen just anterior to the portal vein.

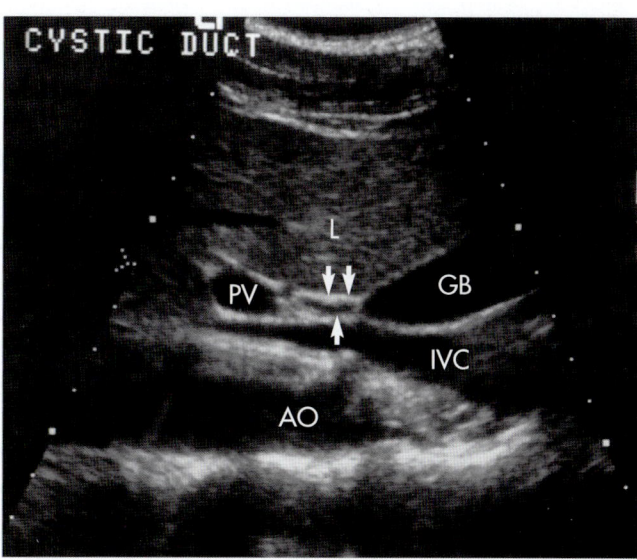

FIG. 10.16 The cystic duct is sometimes seen to arise from the neck of the gallbladder *(arrows)*. This coronal decubitus view shows the aorta (AO), inferior vena cava (IVC), gallbladder (GB), portal vein (PV), and liver (L).

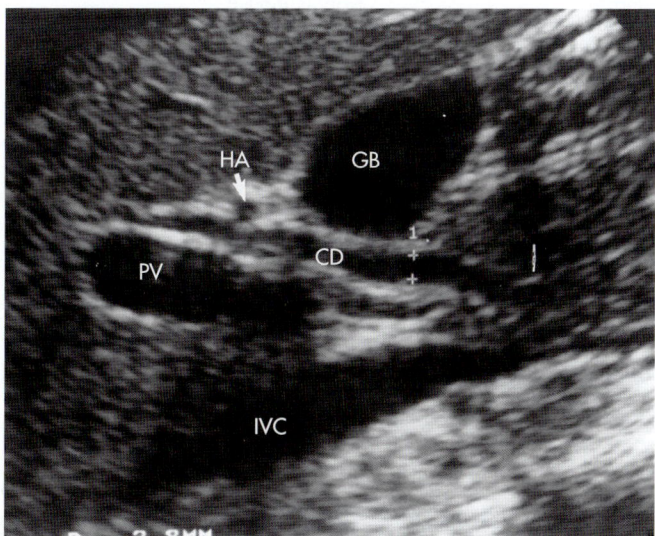

FIG. 10.15 On this sagittal image, the hepatic artery (HA) is shown anterior to the common duct (CD). The portal vein (PV) is anterior to the inferior vena cava (IVC). *GB*, Gallbladder.

in bile. Complications of biliary sludge are stone formation, biliary colic, acalculous cholecystitis, and pancreatitis.

Sonographic Findings. Occasionally a patient presents sonographically with a prominent gallbladder containing amorphous, low-level internal echoes without acoustic shadowing, which may be attributed to thick or inspissated bile. The source of echoes in biliary sludge is thought to be particulate matter (predominantly pigment granules with lesser amounts of cholesterol crystals). The viscosity does not appear to be important in the generation of internal echoes in fluids. The particles can be small and still produce perceptible echoes (Fig. 10.17). Sludge may mimic polypoid tumors (tumefactive sludge). Sludge will not present with gallbladder wall thickening or internal vascularity as tumor would. Sludge may also be seen in combination with cholelithiasis, cholecystitis, and other biliary diseases.

Wall Thickness

The normal wall thickness of the gallbladder is less than 3 mm. Biliary causes of gallbladder wall thickening include cholecystitis, adenomyomatosis, cancer, acquired immunodeficiency syndrome, cholangiopathy, severe hypoalbuminemic state, and sclerosing cholangitis (Box 10.2). Nonbiliary causes include diffuse liver disease (cirrhosis and hepatitis), pancreatitis, portal hypertension, and heart failure. A thickened wall is a nonspecific sign and is not necessarily related to gallbladder disease.

Sonographic Findings. The gallbladder wall thickness should be measured when the transducer is perpendicular to the anterior gallbladder wall. This is usually done in the transverse plane, but in some cases, the longitudinal plane allows a better alignment. The gain should be reduced and the focal zone aligned to the gallbladder area to clearly demarcate the anterior wall. The anterior wall is measured from outer to outer margins. Sonographically the gallbladder wall may be underestimated when the wall has extensive fibrosis or is surrounded by fat (Fig. 10.18).

Cholecystitis

Cholecystitis is an inflammation of the gallbladder that may have one of several forms: acute or chronic, acalculous, emphysematous, or gangrenous (Box 10.3).

Acute Cholecystitis. The most common cause of acute cholecystitis occurs from persistent obstruction of the cystic duct or gallbladder neck by an impacted gallstone. When stones become impacted in the cystic duct or the neck of the gallbladder (Hartmann's pouch), obstruction results with distention of the lumen, ischemia, and infection (cholecystitis) with eventual necrosis of the gallbladder (Fig. 10.19). If the impacted stone does not spontaneously disimpact, the gallbladder may become necrotic and perforate. Even though

TABLE 10.2 The Gallbladder and the Biliary System

Clinical Findings	Sonographic Findings	Differential Considerations
Sludge		
May be asymptomatic	Low-level internal echoes layering in dependent part of GB Prominent GB size Changes with patient position	Pseudosludge Empyema of GB Hemobilia Neoplasm
Acute Cholecystitis		
↑ Serum amylase Abnormal LFTs	Dilation and rounding of GB + Murphy sign Thick GB wall with irregular wall (edema) Stones Pericholecystic fluid	Chronic cholecystitis Nonfasting GB Acute pancreatitis GB carcinoma
Chronic Cholecystitis		
↑ Serum amylase Abnormal LFTs Transient RUQ pain	Contraction of GB Stones WES sign	Cholelithiasis Nonfasting GB Acute pancreatitis GB carcinoma
Acalculous Cholecystitis		
↑ Serum amylase Abnormal LFTs	Dilation of GB + Murphy sign Thick GB wall with irregular wall (edema) Sludge Pericholecystic fluid Subserosal edema	Chronic cholecystitis Nonfasting GB Acute pancreatitis GB carcinoma
Emphysematous Cholecystitis		
Gas-forming bacteria in GB Abnormal LFTs	Bright echo in area of GB with "ring down" or "comet tail" artifact May appear as WES	Chronic cholecystitis GB carcinoma
Gangrenous Cholecystitis		
Abnormal LFTs	Medium to coarse echogenic densities that fill GB lumen in absence of duct obstruction No shadow Not gravity dependent Does not layer	GB carcinoma
Cholelithiasis		
Check bilirubin levels Acute ↑ amylase Abnormal LFTs (increased alkaline phosphatase); AST and ALT may be normal	Dilated GB with thick wall Hyperechoic intraluminal echoes with posterior acoustic shadowing WES sign Gravity-dependent calcifications in GB	Duodenal gas Porcelain GB Sludge
Choledochal Cysts		
Jaundice Possibly increased bilirubin	True cysts in RUQ with or without communication with biliary system Classified by anatomy: 1. Localized dilated cystic CBD 2. Diverticulum of CBD 3. Invagination of CBD into duodenum 4. Dilated CBD and CHD	Hepatic cyst Hepatic artery aneurysm Pancreatic pseudocyst
Adenoma of the Gallbladder		
	Occurs as flat elevations located in the body of the GB, almost always near the fundus Does not change with position No shadow produced	Adenomyomatosis

Continued

CHAPTER 10 The Gallbladder and the Biliary System

TABLE 10.2	The Gallbladder and the Biliary System		
Clinical Findings		**Sonographic Findings**	**Differential Considerations**
Adenomyomatosis of the Gallbladder			
		Papillomas may occur singly or in groups and may be scattered over a large part of the mucosal surface of the GB Does not move with position changes "Comet-tail" artifact	Adenoma
Porcelain Gallbladder			
Female predominance Found in patients >60 years		GB wall thickly calcified with shadowing	Gallstones with emphysematous cholecystitis
Choledocholithiasis			
Increased direct bilirubin Abnormal liver enzymes Leukocytosis Increased alkaline phosphatase		Echogenic structure in extrahepatic duct Dilated biliary tree	Surgical clips Artifact from right hepatic artery Cystic duct remnant

ALT, Alanine aminotransferase; *AST*, aspartate aminotransferase; *CBD*, Common bile duct; *CHD*, common hepatic duct; *GB*, gallbladder; *LFTs*, liver function tests; *RUQ*, right upper quadrant; *WES*, wall echo shadow.

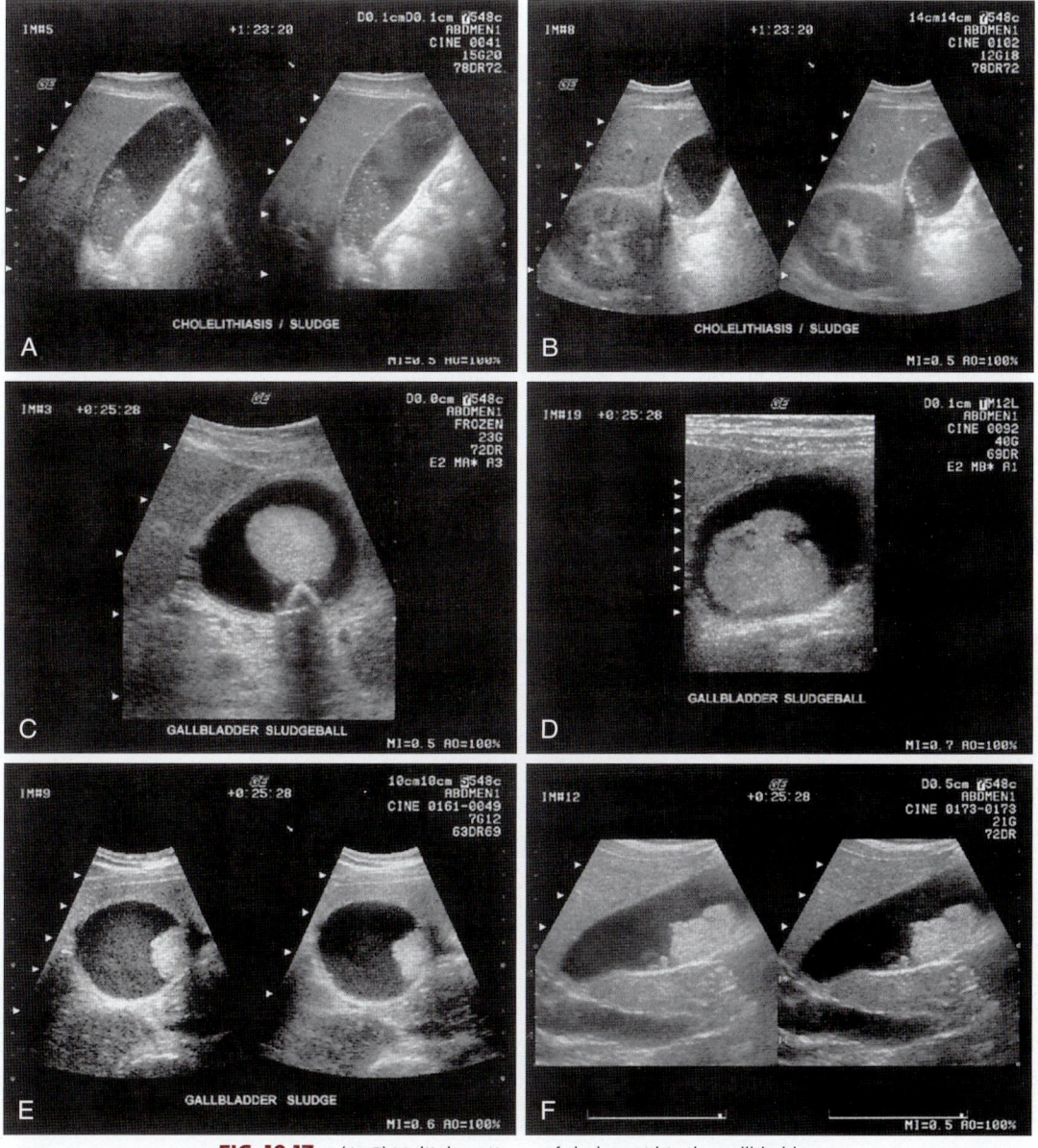

FIG. 10.17 (A–F) Multiple patterns of sludge within the gallbladder.

it may be difficult to visualize the actual stone causing the obstruction, other gallstones may be seen.

Acute cholecystitis is found three times more frequently in females than males over 50, but it has a similar incidence in higher age groups. Clinically the patient with acute cholecystitis presents with acute right upper quadrant pain (positive **Murphy sign**—inspiratory arrest upon palpation of gallbladder area; may be false positive in a small percentage of patients), fever, and leukocytosis; increased serum bilirubin and alkaline phosphatase levels may be present.

Cholecystectomy surgery is the treatment of choice. Antibiotics may be administered to reduce the inflammation prior to surgery. Complications of acute cholecystitis may be serious to include empyema, emphysematous or gangrenous cholecystitis, and perforation.

Sonographic Findings. Acute cholecystitis has very specific findings on sonography. The patient will have a positive Murphy sign, making the area of the gallbladder extremely sensitive to touch. The gallbladder wall is thickened to greater than 3 mm. This should be measured at the anterior wall with the wall parallel to the transducer (Fig. 10.20). A distended gallbladder lumen greater than 4 cm is present. Gallstones are usually present, and the sonographer should search for an impacted stone in Hartmann's pouch or cystic duct. Increased color Doppler flow will be present secondary to the inflammation of the gallbladder wall. Pericholecystic fluid collection around the gallbladder bed may be present.

The sonographic appearance of acute cholecystitis is identified as a gallbladder with an irregular outline of a thickened wall (Fig. 10.21). A sonolucent area likely caused by edema has been found within the thickened wall. If the irregular gallbladder wall shows striated sonolucencies, a more advanced case of cholecystitis may be present. Some walls will be thicker because of a pericholecystic abscess (Fig. 10.22). Occasionally a thickened gallbladder wall is seen in normal individuals, related to the degree of contraction of a normal gallbladder. Enlargement of the gallbladder is another important sign of acute cholecystitis, with the width dimension more relevant than the length.

The sonographic *Murphy sign* is positive when tenderness is demonstrated over the area of the gallbladder when the sonographer touches the right upper quadrant with the transducer, and gentle compression is applied. When the patient takes in a deep breath, the gallbladder is displaced below the protective costal margin. This positive sign may not be present if the patient has been given analgesics before the study or if the condition has been prolonged with resultant gangrenous cholecystitis.

Color Doppler velocities (with low PRF setting) are increased in the cystic artery, which encompasses the inflamed gallbladder wall. Power Doppler may better demonstrate this increased flow because the transducer does not need to be parallel to flow as it does with color Doppler.

The sonographer should assess the presence or absence of pericholecystic fluid (Fig. 10.23). The wall may become inflamed and edematous with subsequent leakage into the pericholecystic space surrounding the gallbladder.

If the thickened wall is localized and irregular, an abscess, cholecystosis, or carcinoma of the gallbladder should be considered.

Complications of Acute Cholecystitis

Emphysematous Cholecystitis. This is a rare complication of acute cholecystitis. This occurs more frequently in elderly men and diabetic patients; often, gallstones may not be present. This

BOX 10.2	Common Causes of Thickening of the Gallbladder Wall (≥3 mm)
Intrinsic	**Extrinsic**
Cholecystitis	Hepatitis/cirrhosis
Gallbladder perforation	Hypoalbuminemia
Sepsis	Renal failure
Hyperplastic cholecystosis	Right heart failure
Gallbladder carcinoma	Ascites
AIDS cholangiography	Multiple myeloma
Sclerosing cholangitis	Portal node lymphatic obstruction

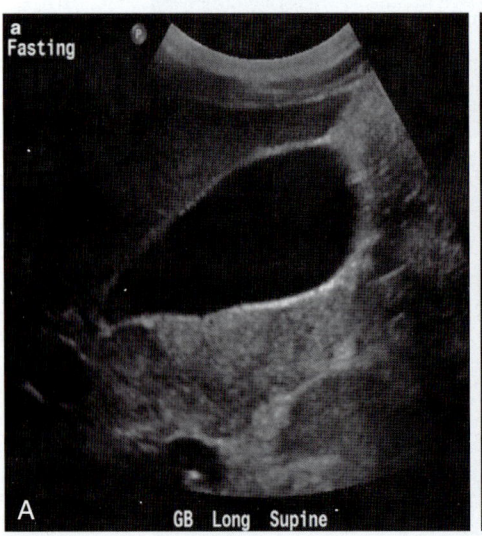
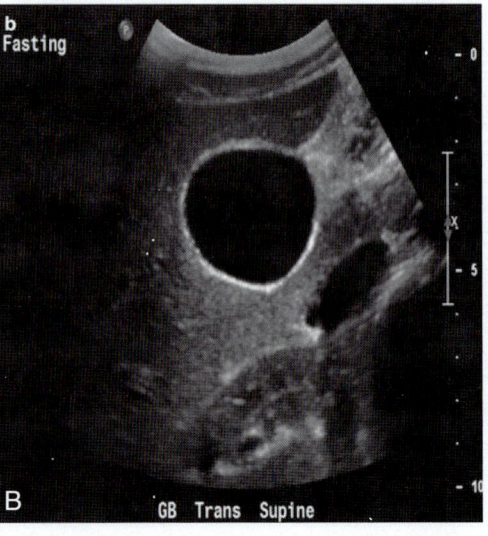

FIG. 10.18 (A) The sagittal image of the gallbladder is often at an angle to the transducer and may be used to measure the wall thickness when the sonographer can achieve a perpendicular angle. (B) The gallbladder wall should be measured on the transverse image at the anterior wall that is perpendicular to the transducer.

d0isease is associated with the presence of gas-forming bacteria in the gallbladder wall and lumen with extension into the biliary ducts. Perforation of the gallbladder is more likely to occur with emphysematous cholecystitis than with gallstone-induced cholecystitis. This condition is a surgical emergency.

Sonographic Findings. The sonographic appearance will depend on the amount of gas within the wall of the gallbladder. If the gas is intraluminal, the sonographer should look for a prominent bright echo along the anterior wall with ring down or comet-tail artifact directly posterior to the echogenic structure (Fig. 10.24). If a large amount of gas is present, the appearance may simulate a packed bag or Wall echo shadow (WES) sign with a curvilinear echogenic area with complete posterior fuzzy shadowing.

Gangrenous Cholecystitis. Another serious, painful complication of acute cholecystitis that may lead to perforation is gangrenous cholecystitis. This process may occur after a prolonged infection, which causes the gallbladder to undergo necrosis. The gallbladder wall may be thickened and edematous, with focal areas of exudate, hemorrhage, and necrosis. In addition, there may be ulcerations and perforations resulting in pericholecystic abscesses or peritonitis. Gallstones or fine gravel occur in 80% to 95% of patients.

Sonographic Findings. The common echo features of gangrene are the presence of diffuse medium to coarse echogenic densities filling the gallbladder lumen in the absence of bile duct obstruction. This echogenic material has the following three characteristics: (1) it does not cause shadowing, (2) it is not gravity dependent, and (3) it does not show a layering effect (Fig. 10.25). The lack of layering is attributed to increased viscosity of the bile. In addition, the gallbladder wall becomes irregular, with edematous pockets within the wall representing hemorrhage or abscess collections. The wall may become so inflamed with hemorrhage that a hemorrhagic cholecystitis develops. Pericholecystic fluid may be present in the area surrounding the gallbladder bed.

Acalculous Cholecystitis. This uncommon condition is an acute inflammation of the gallbladder in the absence of acute cholecystitis. This condition may develop secondary to gallbladder wall infection, ischemia, chemical toxicity to the gallbladder wall, and cystic duct obstruction. It is most likely caused by decreased blood flow through the cystic artery. Conditions that produce depressed motility (trauma, burns, postoperative patients, HIV, etc.) may preclude the development of

---

BOX 10.3　Sonographic Findings in Cholecystitis

- Thickened gallbladder wall >3 mm
- Distended gallbladder lumen >4 cm
- Gallstones
- Impacted stone in Hartmann's pouch or cystic duct
- Positive Murphy sign
- Increased color Doppler flow
- Pericholecystic fluid collection

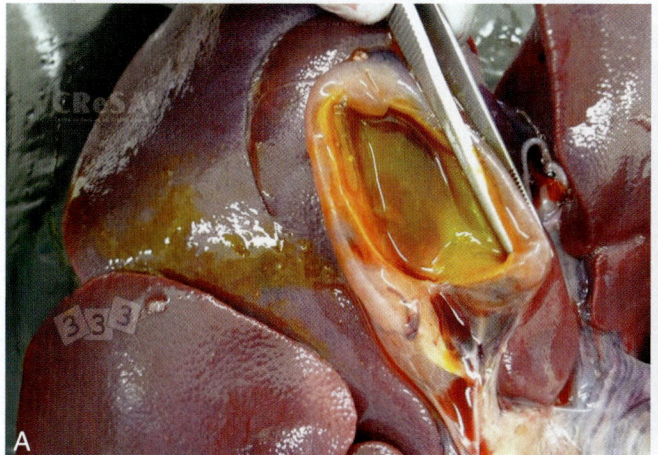
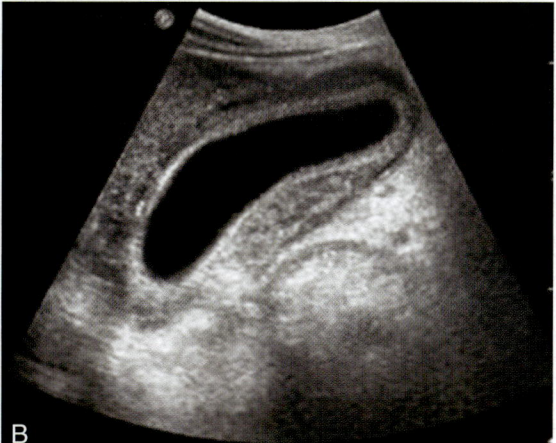
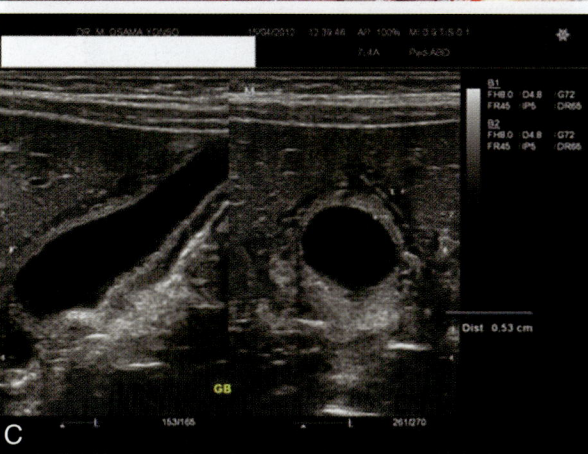

FIG. 10.19 (A) Gross pathology of acute cholecystitis; the gallbladder wall was thick and swollen. (B) Longitudinal image of the edematous gallbladder wall in a patient with acute cholecystitis. (C) Longitudinal *(left)* and transverse *(right)* images of a patient with acute cholecystitis show the thickened, edematous wall.

298 CHAPTER 10 The Gallbladder and the Biliary System

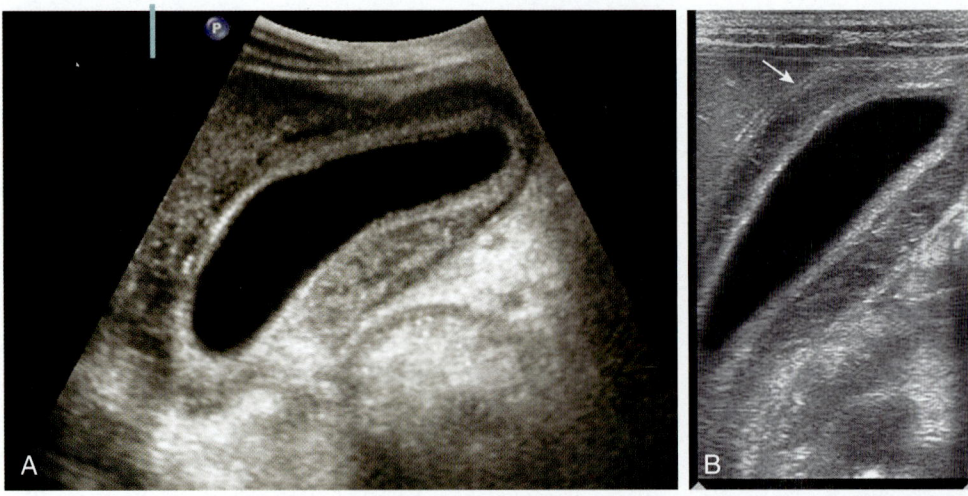

FIG. 10.20 (A–B) Acute cholecystitis. Inflammation of the gallbladder wall >3 mm. This should be measured at the anterior wall with the wall parallel to the transducer.

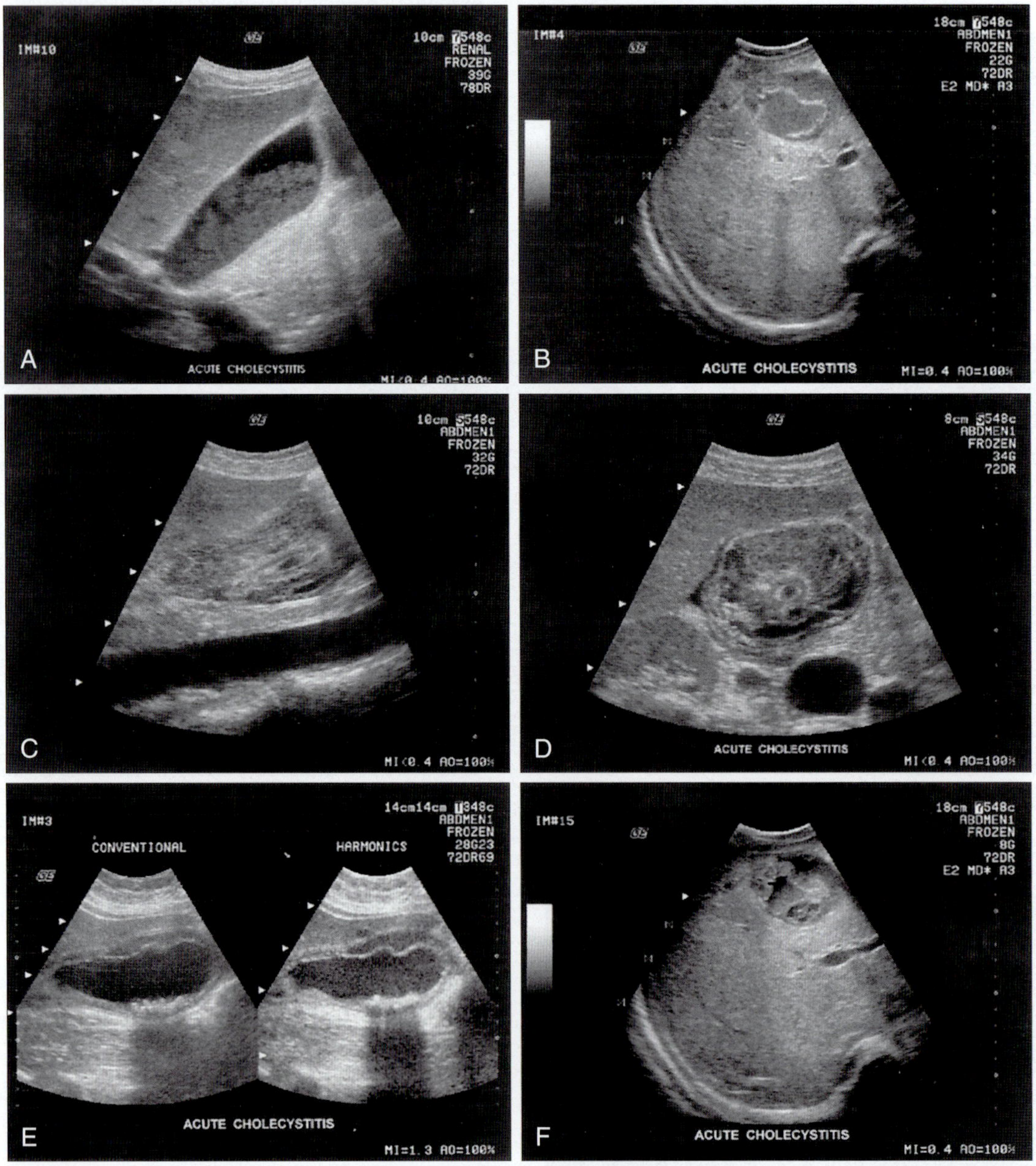

FIG. 10.21 (A–F) Multiple patterns of acute cholecystitis. Note the irregular gallbladder wall with edema. Striations may be seen in the more advanced form of the disease.

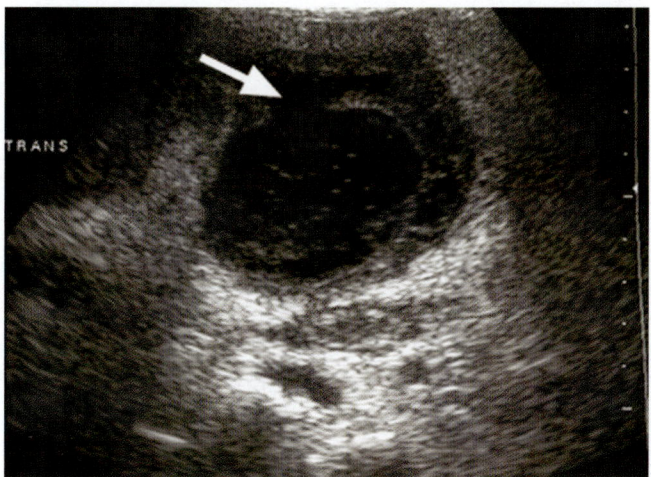

FIG. 10.22 Irregularity of the gallbladder wall in acute cholecystitis may indicate development of a pericholecystic abscess or, in this case, rupture of the gallbladder wall *(arrow)*.

acalculous cholecystitis. Extrinsic compression of the cystic duct by a mass or lymphadenopathy may also cause this condition. Clinically the patient has a positive Murphy sign.

Sonographic Findings. The gallbladder wall is extremely thickened (greater than 4 to 5 mm), and echogenic sludge is seen within a dilated gallbladder. The sonographer should look for the presence of pericholecystic fluid within ascites or subserosal edema (Fig. 10.26).

Torsion of the Gallbladder

Torsion of the gallbladder is a rare condition that is found more in elderly females and is associated with a mobile gallbladder with a long suspensory mesentery. Symptoms present typical of acute cholecystitis.

Sonographic Findings. The gallbladder becomes massively inflamed and distended. The cystic artery and cystic duct may also become twisted. If the gallbladder becomes twisted

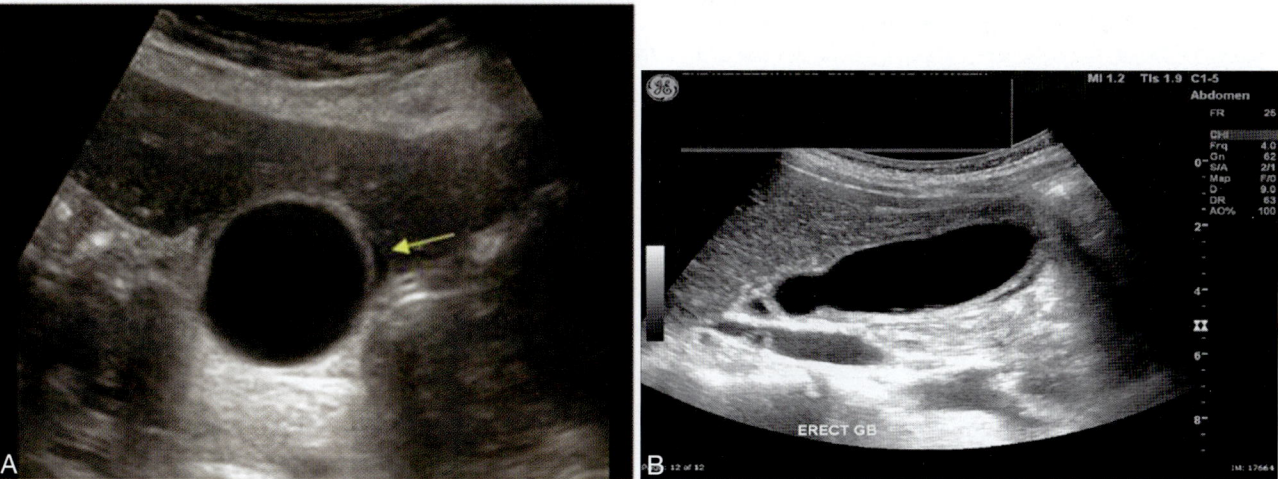

FIG. 10.23 (A–B) Transverse and longitudinal images of a patient with acute cholecystitis. A small fluid collection is noted at the fundus of the gallbladder.

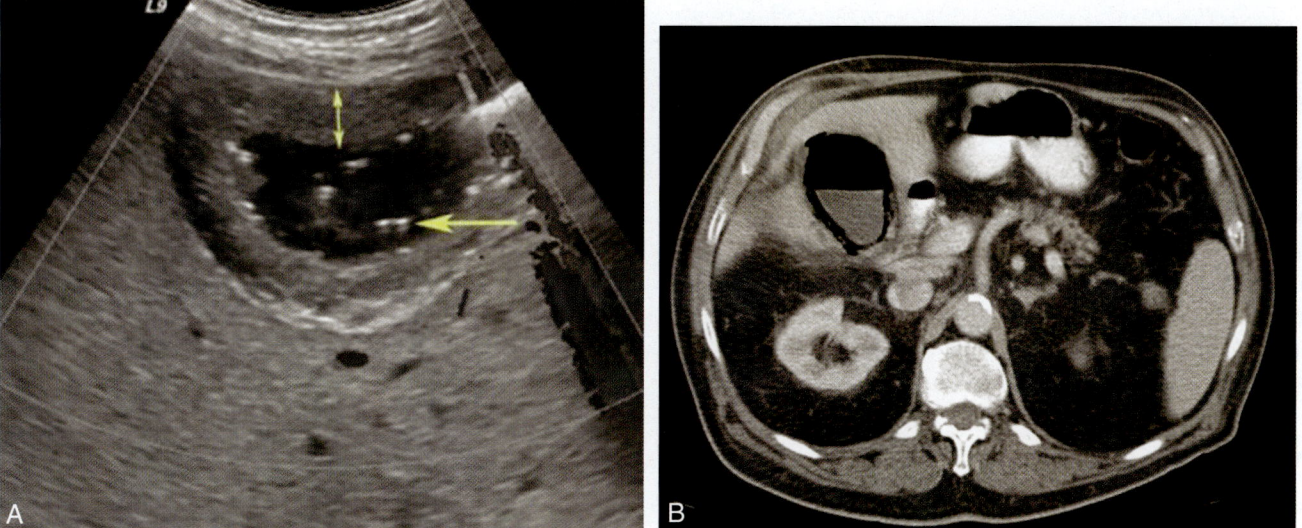

FIG. 10.24 (A) Emphysematous cholecystitis. If the gas is intraluminal, the sonographer should look for a prominent bright echo along the anterior wall with ring down or comet-tail artifact directly posterior to the echogenic structure *(arrow)*. The thickened gallbladder wall is denoted by the double arrow. (B) Contrast computed tomographic image of the emphysematous gallbladder.

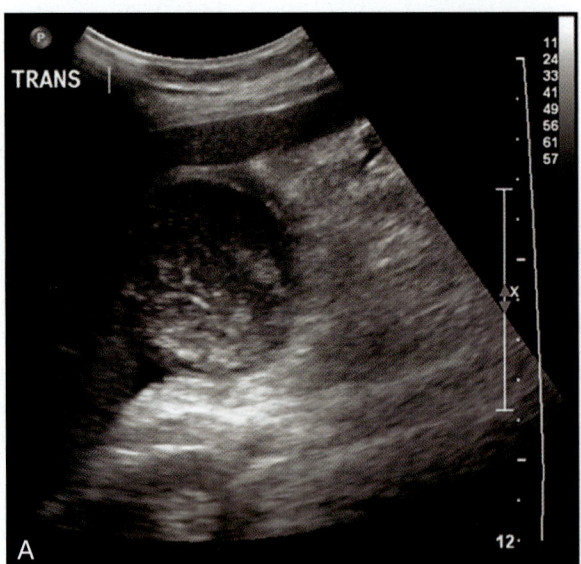
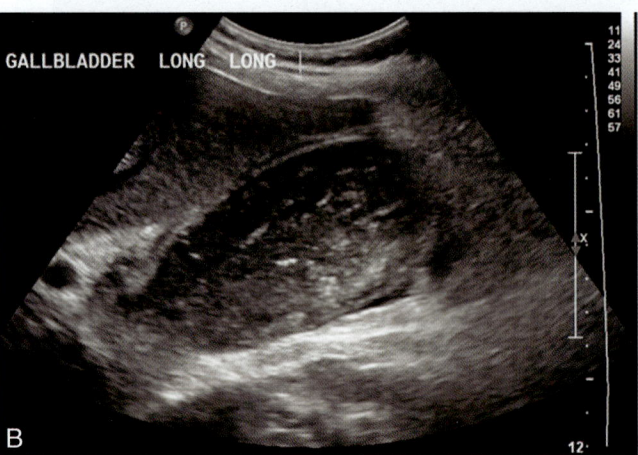

FIG. 10.25 **Gangrenous cholecystitis.** Transverse (A) and longitudinal (B) images show the common echo features of gangrene that include the presence of diffuse medium to coarse echogenic densities filling the gallbladder lumen in the absence of bile duct obstruction.

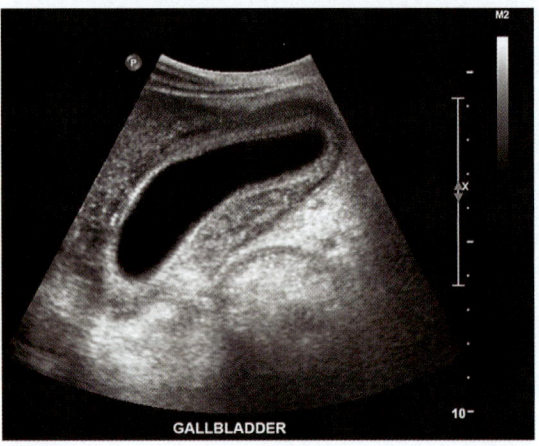

FIG. 10.26 Acalculous cholecystitis with thickening of the gallbladder wall secondary to edema and inflammation.

more than 180 degrees, the risk of gangrene may develop. Surgical intervention is the treatment for this condition.

Chronic Cholecystitis

Chronic cholecystitis is the most common form of gallbladder inflammation. This is the result of numerous attacks of acute cholecystitis with subsequent fibrosis of the gallbladder wall. Clinically the patients may have some transient right upper quadrant pain, but not the tenderness as experienced with acute cholecystitis.

Cholelithiasis

Wall Echo Shadow Sign. The WES sign (wall, echo, shadow) is described as a contracted bright gallbladder with posterior shadowing caused by a packed bag of stones (Fig. 10.27). When the gallbladder is completely packed full of stones, the sonographer will only be able to image the anterior border of the gallbladder, with the stones casting a distinct acoustic shadow known as the **wall echo shadow (WES)** sign. This WES sign consists of three arc-shaped lines followed by a shadow. The first line is echogenic and represents the pericholecystic fat as well as the interface between the gallbladder wall and the liver. The second line is hypoechoic and represents the gallbladder. The third line is echogenic, reflecting the packed bag of stones within the gallbladder. The acoustic shadow is seen posterior to this third line.

Cholelithiasis. Cholelithiasis is the most common disease of the gallbladder. In cholelithiasis, there may be a single large gallstone or hundreds of tiny ones (Fig. 10.28). The tiny stones are the most dangerous because they can enter the bile ducts and obstruct the outflow of bile. After a fatty meal, the gallbladder contracts to release bile; if gallstones block the outflow tract, pain results. As the bile is being stored in the gallbladder, small crystals of bile salts precipitate and may form gallstones varying from pinhead size to the size of the organ itself.

The five "F" risk factors for the patient with cholelithiasis are fat, female, forty, fertile, and fair. In addition, many other factors lead to the development of gallstones that include pregnancy, diabetes, oral contraceptive use, hemolytic diseases, diet-induced weight loss, and total parenteral nutrition. Patients may be asymptomatic until a stone lodges in the cystic or common duct, which causes biliary colic. Acute right upper quadrant or epigastric pain with radiation to the shoulder after a high-fat meal, nausea, and vomiting is a typical presentation for cholelithiasis. This pain may last for up to six hours and only ends when the stone disimpacts from the gallbladder neck or passes completely through the cystic duct.

Sonographic Findings. The evaluation of gallstones with sonography has proven to be an extremely useful procedure in patients who show symptoms of cholelithiasis. The gallbladder is evaluated for increased wall thickness, presence of internal reflections within the lumen with posterior acoustic shadowing (Fig. 10.29). Gallstones appear as mobile,

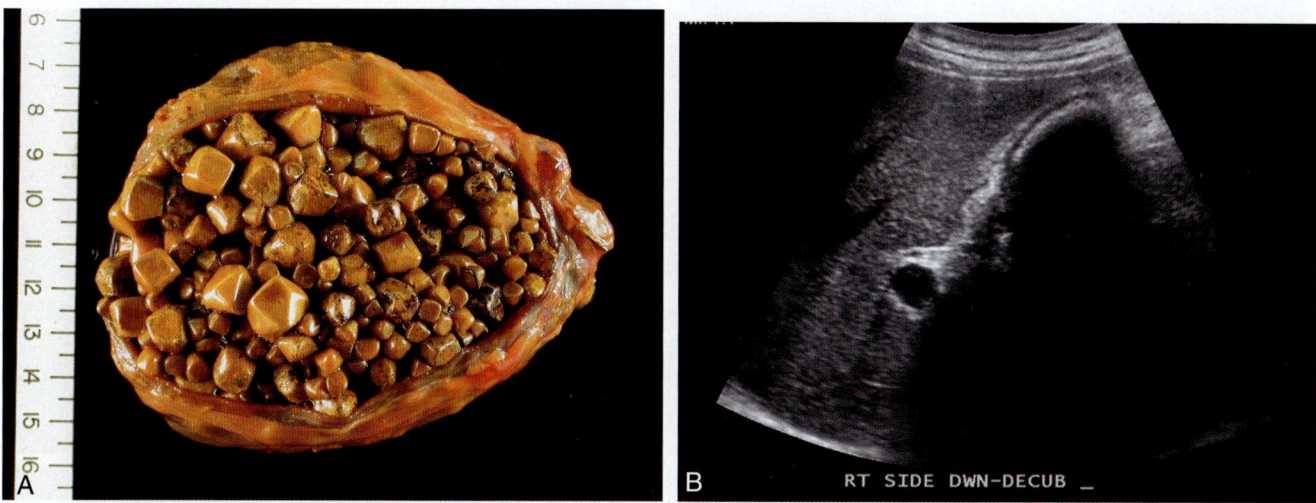

FIG. 10.27 (A) Gross specimen of a "packed bag" gallbladder filled with stones. (B) The ultrasound shows the gallbladder is filled with stones. Note the dramatic shadow posterior to the packed bag.

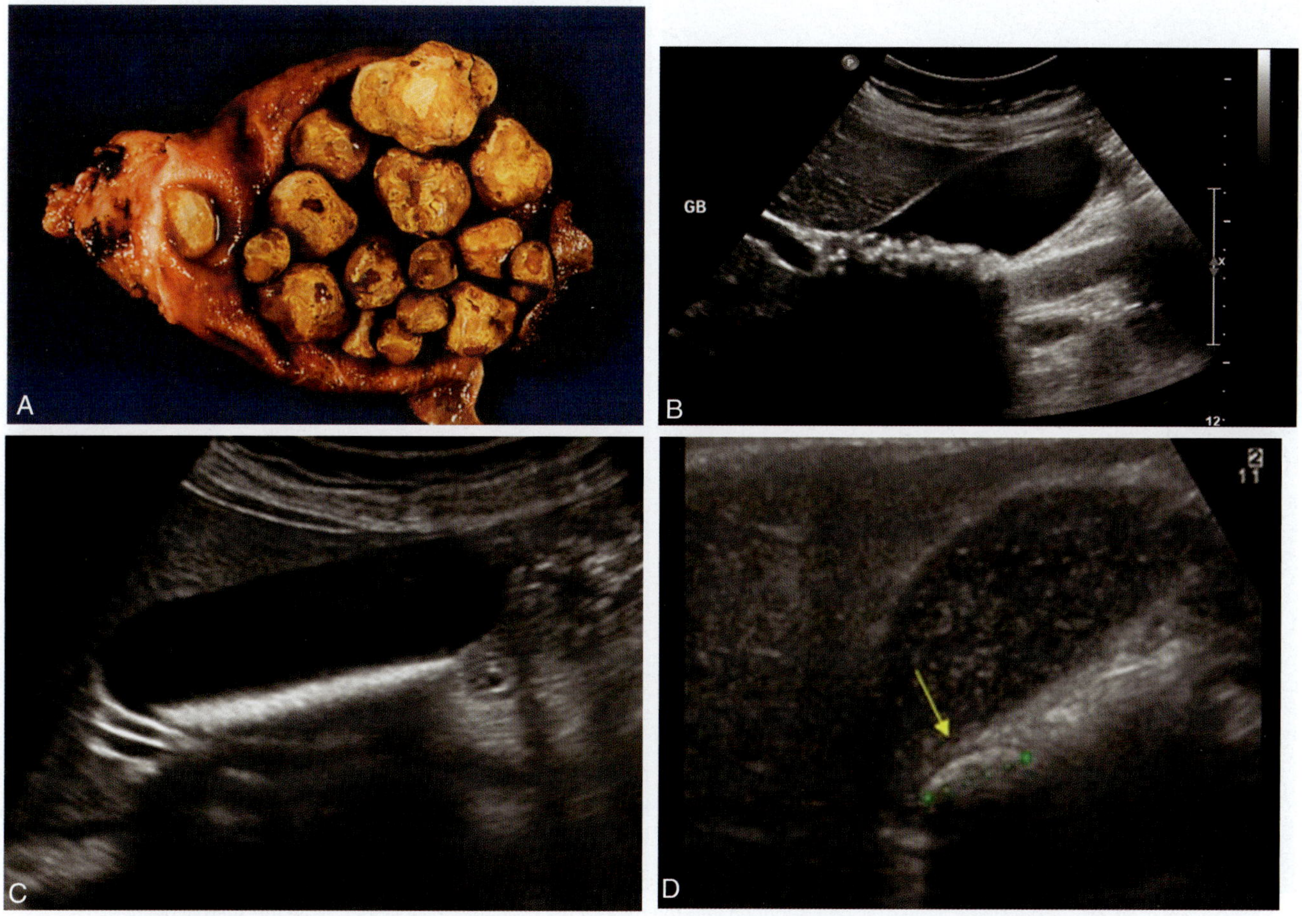

FIG. 10.28 (A) Gross pathology of multiple gallstones within the gallbladder. (B) Transverse oblique view of the gallbladder filled with stones that show a distinct shadow posterior to the stones. (C) Longitudinal view of the prominent gallbladder with a layer of stones along the posterior border casting a shadow beyond. (D) Longitudinal view of the gallbladder filled with a soft echogenic sludge and a large gallstone near the neck of the gallbladder *(arrow)*.

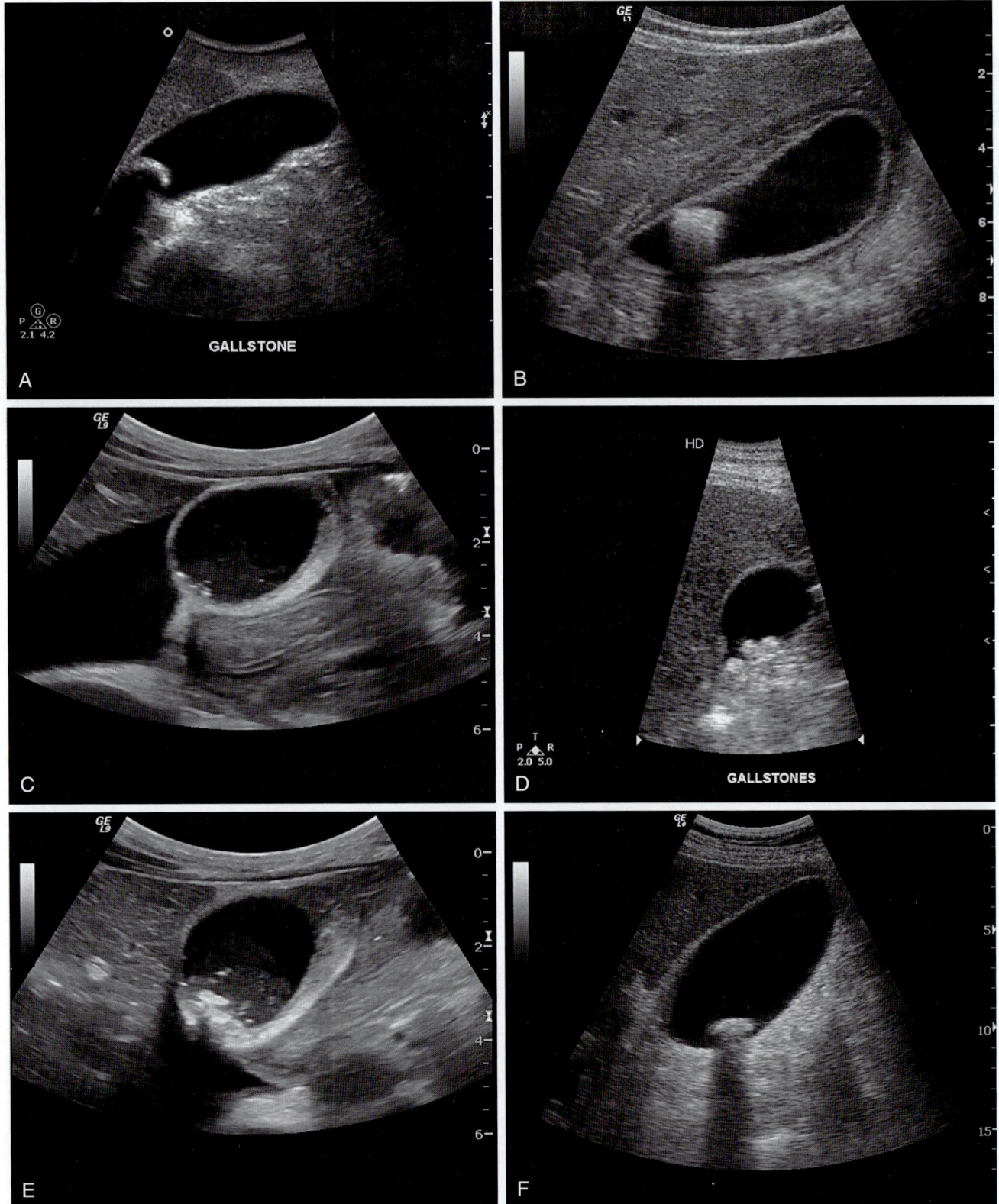

FIG. 10.29 (A) A single large gallstone is lodged into the neck of the distended gallbladder. Note the sharply defined shadow. (B) A single large gallstone near the neck of the gallbladder. Note the thickening of the gallbladder wall. (C) Tiny gallstones are seen within the sludge layered along the posterior margin of the gallbladder. (D) Several medium-sized stones (without a shadow) are seen along the posterior margin of the gallbladder. The patient should be rolled into a decubitus position to watch the movement of these stones. (E) Multiple stones with posterior shadow. (F) Solitary stone with posterior shadow.

echogenic intraluminal structures that cast acoustic shadows. Frequently, patients with gallstones have an enlarged gallbladder lumen. Stones that are less than 1 to 2 mm may be difficult to separate from one another by ultrasound evaluation (Fig. 10.30). A high-frequency transducer should be used to better delineate the stones and their shadowing characteristics. The curved array probe will allow a broader view of the near field to image the gallbladder completely. The focal zone should be adjusted to the level of the gallstone.

The patient's position should be shifted during the procedure to demonstrate the presence of movement of the stones. Patients should be scanned in the left decubitus, right lateral, or upright position. The stones should shift to the most dependent area of the gallbladder. In some cases, the bile has a thick consistency, and the stones remain near the top of the gallbladder. Thus the density of the stones and the posterior shadow will be the sonographic evidence for stones.

Regarding acoustic shadowing, scattered reflections do not affect shadowing as much as specular reflections. The factors that produce a shadow are attributed to acoustic impedance of the gallstones; refraction through them or diffraction around them; their size, central or peripheral location, and position in relation to the focus of the beam; and the intensity of the beam (Fig. 10.31).

All stones cast acoustic shadows regardless of the specific properties of the stones. The size of the stone is important. Stones greater than 3 mm always cast a shadow. Any stone scanned two or more times with the same transducer and machine settings may or may not generate a shadow even when the scans are made within seconds of each other. The shadow is highly dependent on the relationship between the stone and the acoustic beam. If the central beam is aligned on the stone, a shadow appears. Thus some critical ratio between the stone diameter and the beam width must be achieved before shadowing is seen.

Some stones are seen to float ("floating gallstones") when contrast material from an oral cholecystogram is present because the contrast material has a higher specific gravity than the bile and indicates the floating stones are composed of cholesterol. The gallstones seek a level at which their specific gravity equals that of the mixture of bile and contrast material (Fig. 10.32).

Differential diagnoses of cholelithiasis include gallbladder polyps and sludge balls. Polyps are tiny soft tissue structures that adhere to the gallbladder wall. They do not move or shadow. Sludge balls are larger than most gallstones and move, although they do not produce an acoustic shadow.

Porcelain Gallbladder

A **porcelain gallbladder** is a rare occurrence that is defined as calcium incrustation of the gallbladder wall. It is associated with gallstones in most patients and may represent a form of chronic cholecystitis and inflammation. It occurs more often in elderly female patients. The patient is generally asymptomatic, and the diagnosis is generally made as an incidental finding or when a mass is found on physical examination. The clinical significance of a porcelain gallbladder is the increased risk of gallbladder carcinoma.

Sonographic Findings. On sonography, a bright echogenic echo is seen in the region of the gallbladder with shadowing posterior (Fig. 10.33). The differential will include a packed bag or WES sign. The entire gallbladder wall may not be completely calcified; thus the appearance will vary with the amount of calcification present.

Hyperplastic Cholecystosis

Hyperplastic cholecystosis is represented by a variety of degenerative and proliferative changes of the gallbladder characterized by hyperconcentration, hyperexcitability, and hyperexcretion. Cholesterolosis and adenomyomatosis of the gallbladder are two types of this condition.

Cholesterolosis. **Cholesterolosis** is a condition in which cholesterol is deposited within the lamina propria of the gallbladder. The disease process is often associated with

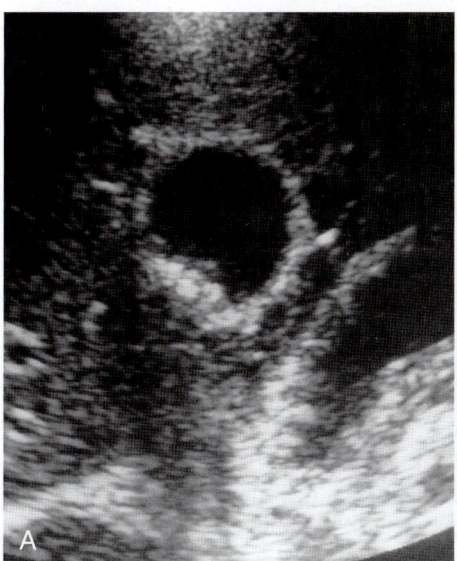 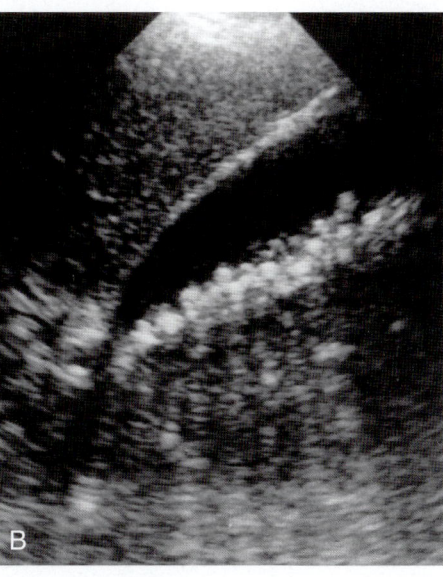

FIG. 10.30 (A) Multiple small stones are layered along the posterior wall of the gallbladder. These bright echogenic foci give acoustic shadowing beyond. (B) A higher-frequency transducer would outline the stones and the shadowing even more clearly.

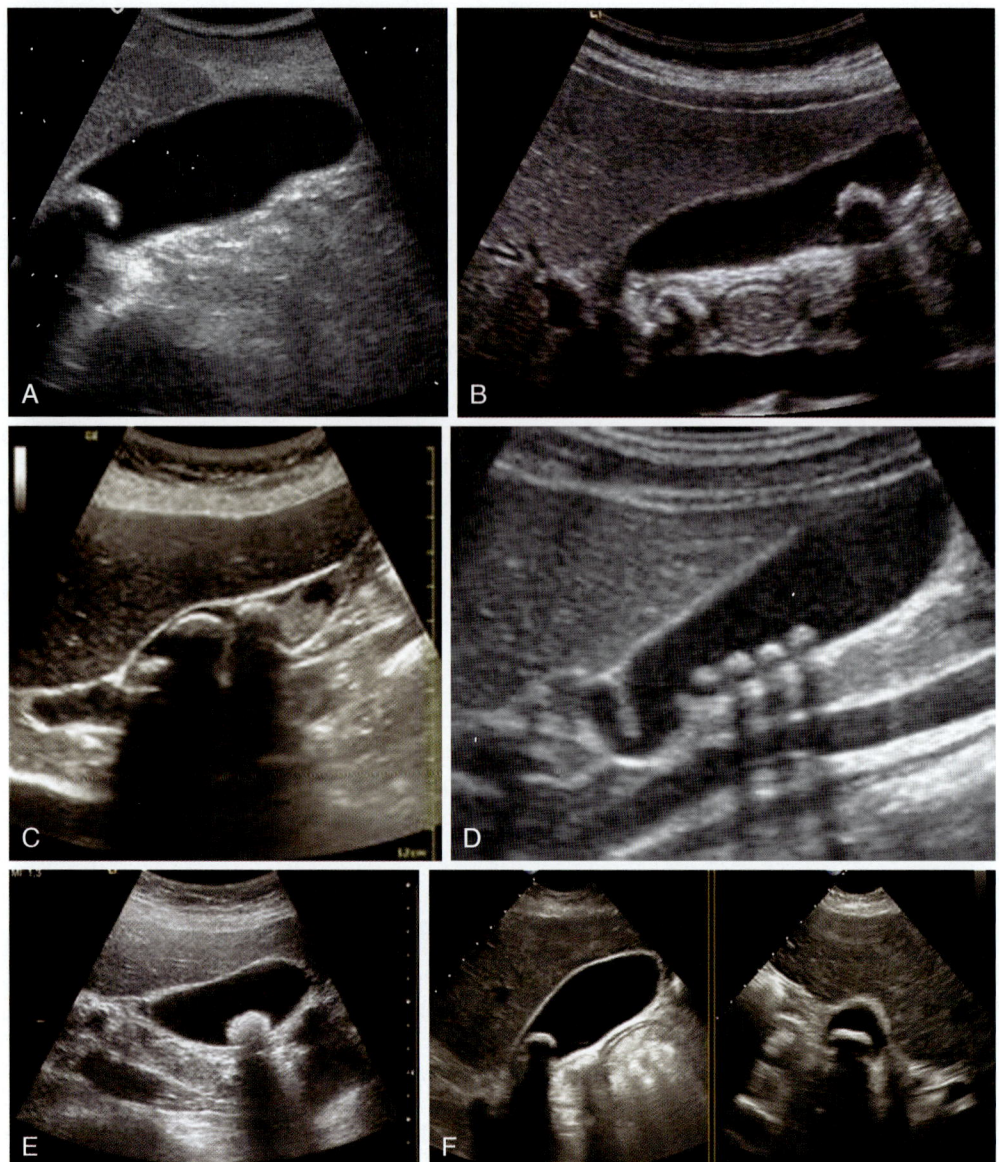

FIG. 10.31 (A–F) Multiple images of gallstones. The factors that produce a shadow are attributed to acoustic impedance of the gallstones; refraction through them or diffraction around them; their size, central or peripheral location, and position in relation to the focus of the beam; and the intensity of the beam.

cholesterol stones. It is often referred to as a "strawberry gallbladder" because the mucosa resembles the surface of a strawberry (Fig. 10.34).

Most patients with cholesterolosis do not show thickening of the gallbladder wall on imaging studies; a small percentage of patients with this condition will show cholesterol polyps, which may be detected with ultrasound. **Polyps of the gallbladder** are small, well-defined soft tissue projections from the gallbladder wall (Fig. 10.35). The cholesterol polyp is a small structure covered with a single layer of epithelium and is attached to the gallbladder with a delicate stalk. These polyps usually are found in the middle third of the gallbladder and are less than 10 mm in diameter. Cholesterol polyps are the most common pseudotumor of the gallbladder. Other masses that occur are mucosal hyperplasia, inflammatory polyps, mucous cysts, and granulomata (resulting from parasitic infections).

Sonographic Findings. Cholesterol polyps are small, smooth ovoid wall projections seen to arise from the gallbladder wall (Fig. 10.36). The polyps usually are multiple, do not shadow, and remain fixed to the wall with changes in patient position. The "comet tail" artifact may be present, emanating from the cholesterol polyps, and this may be indistinguishable from adenomyomatosis.

Adenomyomatosis. **Adenomyomatosis** is a benign condition that demonstrates a hyperplastic change in the gallbladder wall. This condition is caused by exaggeration of the normal invaginations of the luminal epithelium (Rokitansky-Aschoff sinuses) with associated smooth muscle proliferation. The cholesterol crystals may settle within these sinus pockets. This condition is characterized by mucosal hyperplasia and thickening of the muscular layer of the gallbladder wall. Papillomas may occur alone or in groups and may be scattered over a

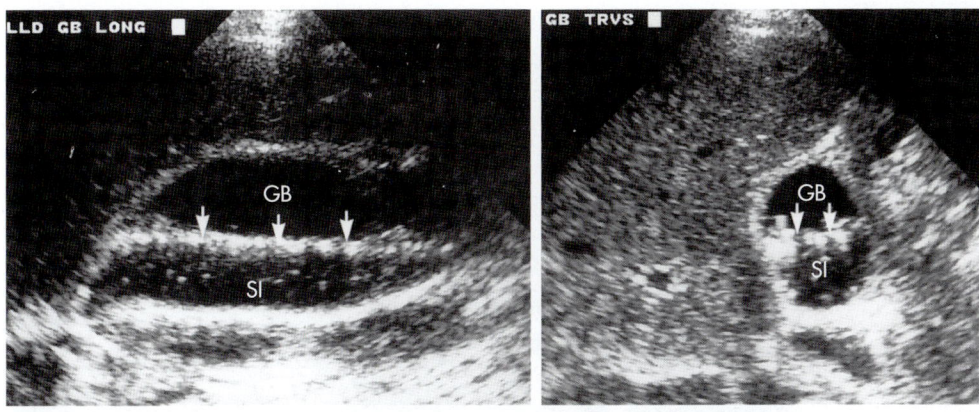

FIG. 10.32 Longitudinal and transverse scans of the gallbladder (GB), with a layer of stones "floating" (arrows) along the thick bile layer of sludge (Sl).

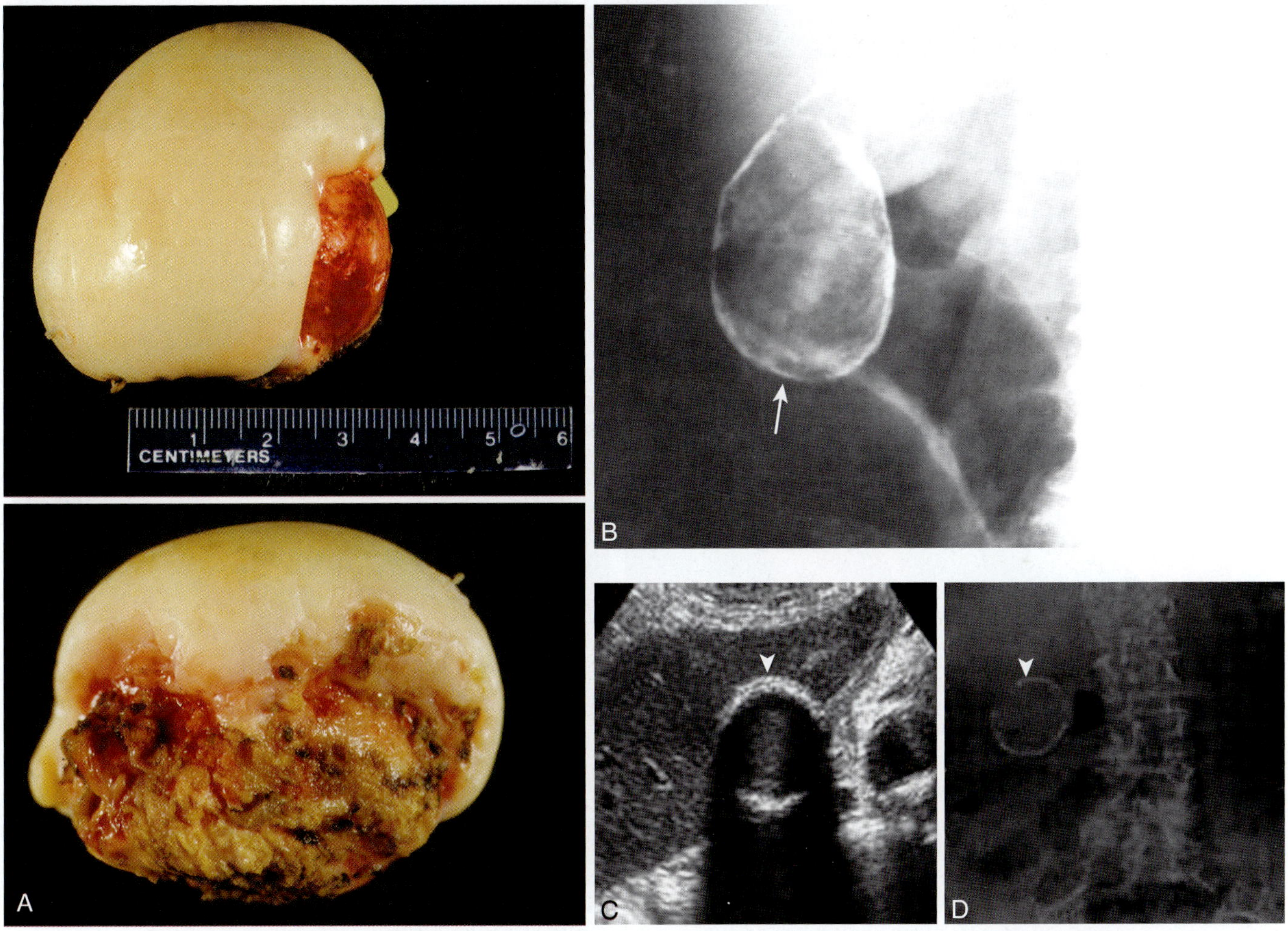

FIG. 10.33 **Porcelain gallbladder.** (A) Gross specimen of a porcelain gallbladder. Note the calcification within the wall. (B) Radiograph of the calcified porcelain gallbladder. On sonography (C), with corresponding radiograph (D), a bright echogenic echo (arrowhead) is seen in the region of the gallbladder with shadowing posterior.

large part of the mucosal surface of the gallbladder. These papillomas are not precursors to cancer.

Sonographic Findings. Benign tumors appear as small elevations in the gallbladder lumen. The affected areas show thickening of the gallbladder wall with internal cystic spaces. The adenomyomatosis may be focal or diffuse. Commonly small echogenic foci are seen in the gallbladder wall that create a very specific comet tail artifact. Various patient positions and compression show the lesion to be immobile within the gallbladder. No acoustic shadow is seen posterior to this papillomatous elevation (Fig. 10.37).

Adenoma. Adenomas are benign neoplasms of the gallbladder with a premalignant potential much lower than colonic adenomas. This condition usually occurs as a solitary lesion. The smaller lesions are pedunculated, whereas the larger lesions may contain foci of malignant transformation

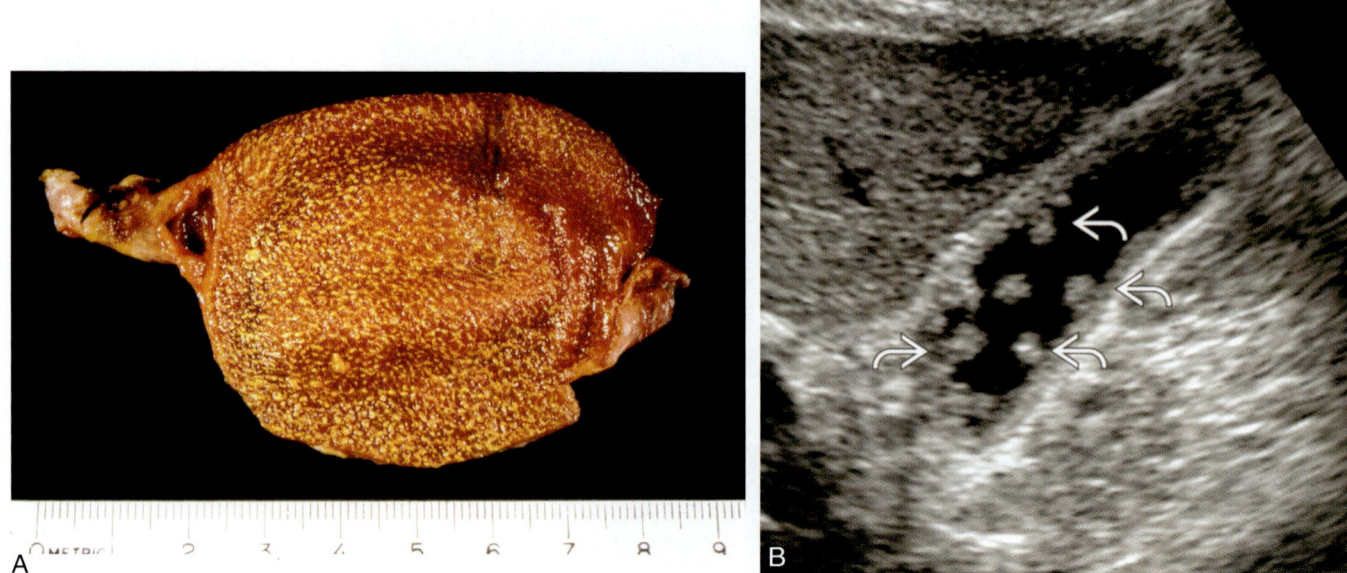

FIG. 10.34 (A) Gross pathology of cholesterolosis, a "strawberry gallbladder." (B) Ultrasound image of cholesterolosis.

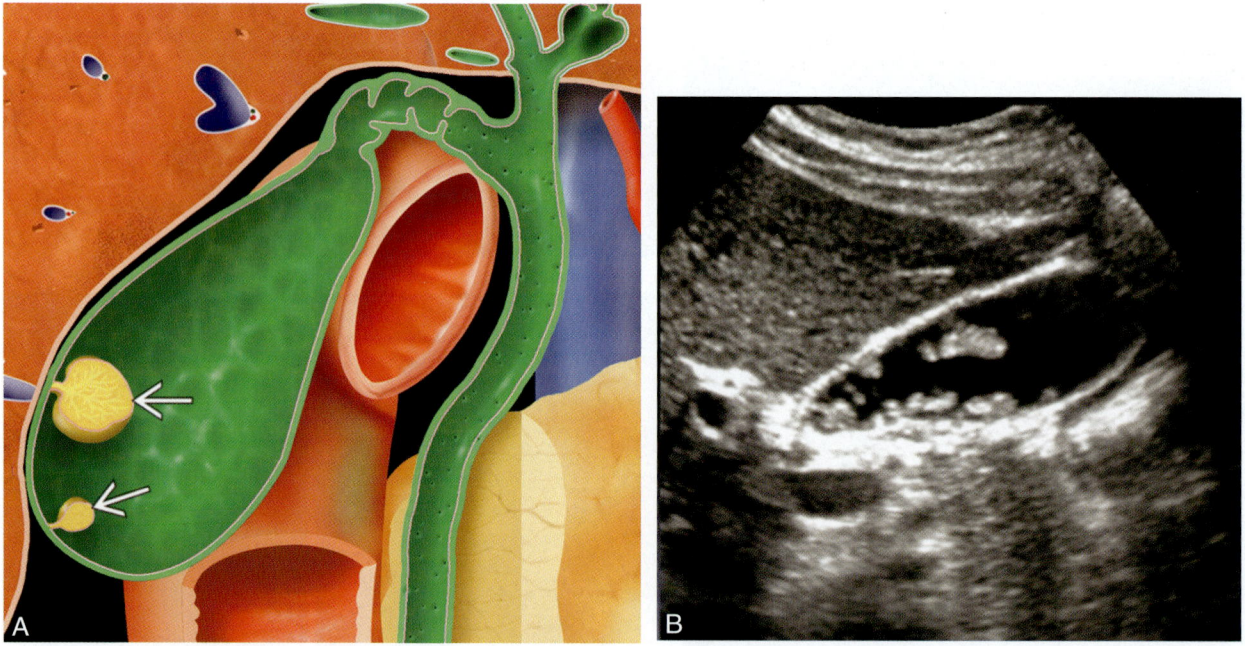

FIG. 10.35 (A) Pathology of the various abnormalities of the gallbladder. (B) The sonographic appearance of cholesterol polyps is multiple ovoid, nonshadowing lesions attached to the gallbladder wall.

(Fig. 10.38). The adenomas tend to be homogeneously hyperechoic but become more heterogeneous as they grow. If the gallbladder wall is thickened adjacent to the adenoma, then malignancy should be suspected.

Gallbladder Carcinoma

Primary carcinoma of the gallbladder is rare and is nearly always a rapidly progressive disease, with a mortality rate approaching 100%. It is associated with cholelithiasis in about 80% to 90% of cases (although there is no direct proof that gallstones are the carcinogenic agent). It is twice as common as cancer of the bile ducts and occurs most frequently in women 60 years of age and older. The tumor arises in the body of the gallbladder or rarely in the cystic duct (Fig. 10.39). The tumor infiltrates the gallbladder locally or diffusely and causes thickening and rigidity of the wall. The adjacent liver is often invaded by direct continuity

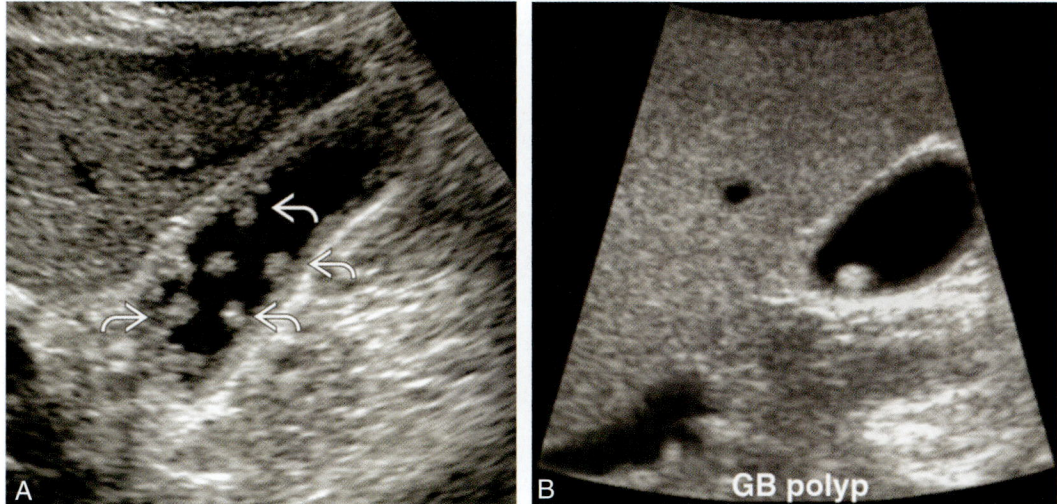

FIG. 10.36 (A) Multiple polyps are seen within the gallbladder. Cholesterol polyps are small, smooth, ovoid projections seen to arise from the gallbladder wall and do not move with change in patient position. (B) Longitudinal view of a single polyp within the gallbladder. Note the polyp does not produce a shadow.

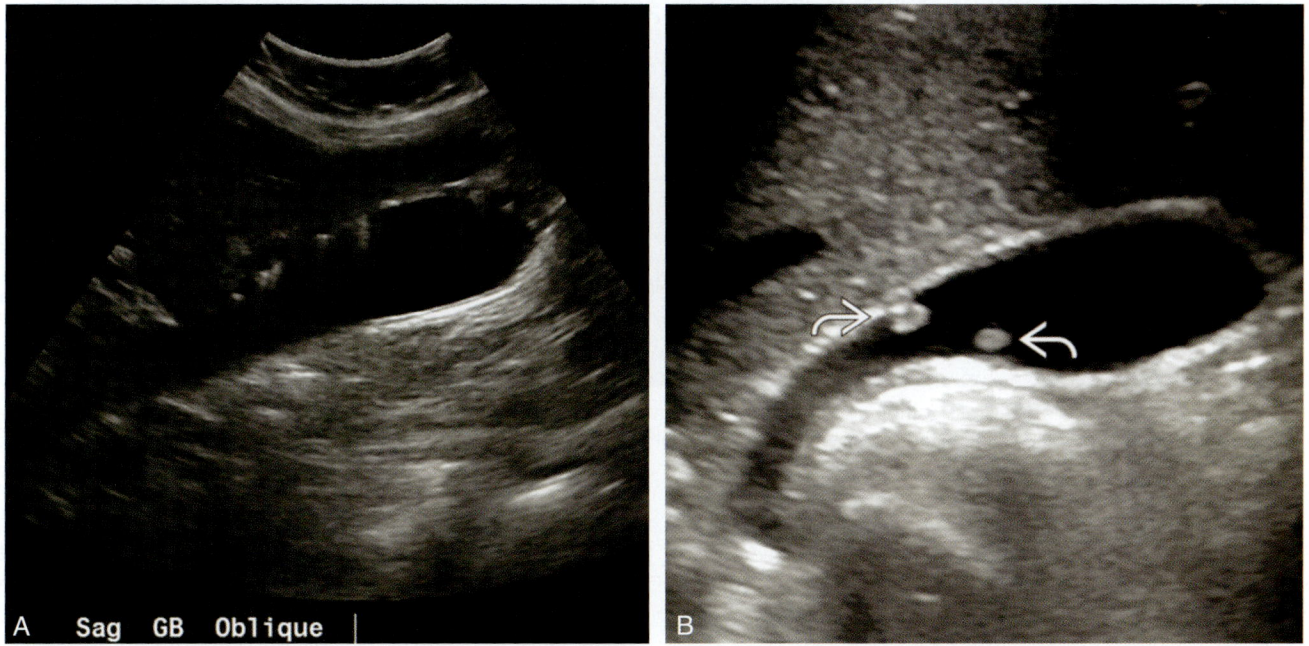

FIG. 10.37 (A) Adenomyomatosis seen within the gallbladder wall may be a single or diffuse foci that produce a characteristic "comet tail" artifact. (B) Compare this longitudinal image of a gallbladder polyp which projects as a smooth, oval foci that remain attached to the gallbladder wall.

extending through tissue spaces, the ducts of Luschka, the lymph channels, or some combination of these. Obstruction of the cystic duct results from direct extension of the tumor or extrinsic compression by involved lymph nodes (this obstruction occurs early).

The gallbladder tumor is usually columnar cell adenocarcinoma, sometimes mucinous in type (Fig. 10.40). Squamous cell carcinoma occurs but is unusual. Metastatic carcinoma in the gallbladder may occur secondary to melanoma. It usually is accompanied by liver metastases. Most patients have no symptoms that relate to the gallbladder unless there is complicating acute cholecystitis.

Sonographic Findings. The most common sonographic appearance of the soft tissue mass is a heterogeneous solid or semisolid echo texture. The mass is centered in the gallbladder fossa that completely or partially obliterates the lumen. The gallbladder wall is markedly abnormal and thickened. This thickening may be focal or diffuse but is usually irregular and asymmetric. The identification of gallstones within the area helps identify the mass as part of the gallbladder (Fig. 10.41). The adjacent liver tissue in the hilar area is often heterogeneous because of direct tumoral spread. There may be dilated biliary ducts within the liver parenchyma, causing the "shotgun" sign (a "double-barrel" appearance of portal veins and dilated ducts).

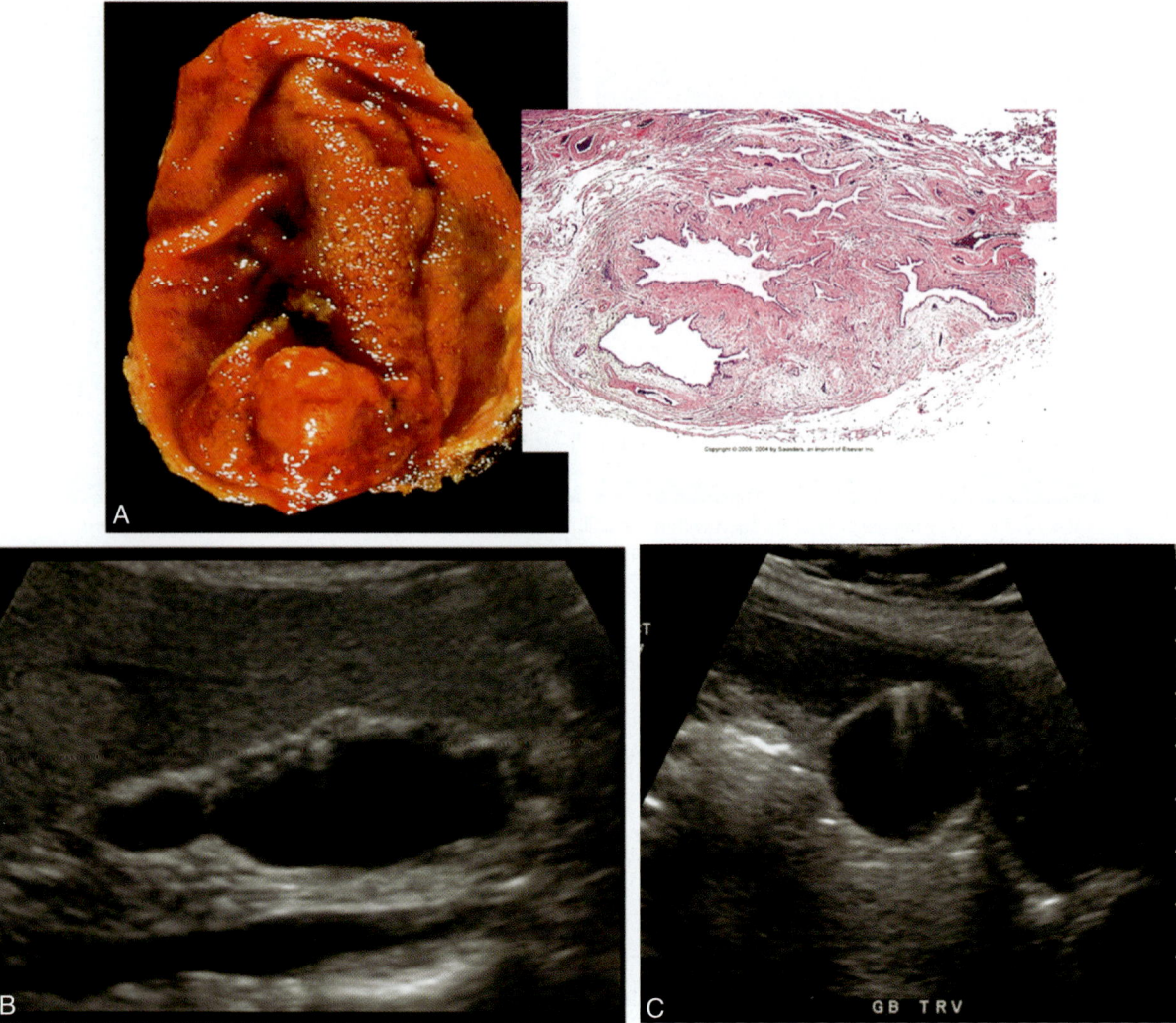

FIG. 10.38 (A) Gross pathology of an adenomyoma of the gallbladder. Longitudinal (B) and transverse (C) images of the gallbladder adenoma with the "comet tail" artifact.

Carcinoma of the gallbladder is seldom detected at a resectable stage. Obstruction of the cystic duct by the tumor or lymph nodes occurs early in the course of the disease and causes nonvisualization of the gallbladder on oral cholecystogram. Differential diagnoses for gallbladder masses included tumefactive sludge, inflammatory wall thickening, polyps, metastases, and focal adenomyomatosis.

PATHOLOGY OF THE BILIARY TREE

Choledochal Cysts

Choledochal cysts are an unusual, diverse group of diseases that may manifest as congenital, focal, or diffuse cystic dilation of the biliary tree. The choledochal cyst may result from pancreatic juices refluxing into the bile duct because of an anomalous junction of the pancreatic duct into the distal common bile duct, causing duct wall abnormality, weakness, and outpouching of the ductal walls. These cysts are rare; the incidence is more common in females than males (4:1), with an increased incidence in infants (the condition may occur in less than 20% of adults). Choledochal cysts may be associated with gallstones, pancreatitis, or cirrhosis. The patient presents with an abdominal mass, pain, fever, or jaundice. The diagnosis may be confirmed with a nuclear medicine hepatobiliary scan. The majority of cases are thought to be congenital and result from bile reflux. The mass presents as a cystic dilation of the biliary system.

The classification of choledochal cysts is divided into five types:

Type I cysts are a fusiform dilation of the common bile duct.

Type II cysts are true diverticular outpouching of the bile ducts.

Type III cysts (choledochoceles) are a dilation of the distal mural portion of the CBD that protrudes into the duodenum.

Type IV cysts are multifocal biliary dilations of the intra- and extrahepatic ducts.

Type V cysts have been classified as Caroli disease.

Sonographic Findings. Choledochal cysts appear as true cysts in the right upper quadrant with or without

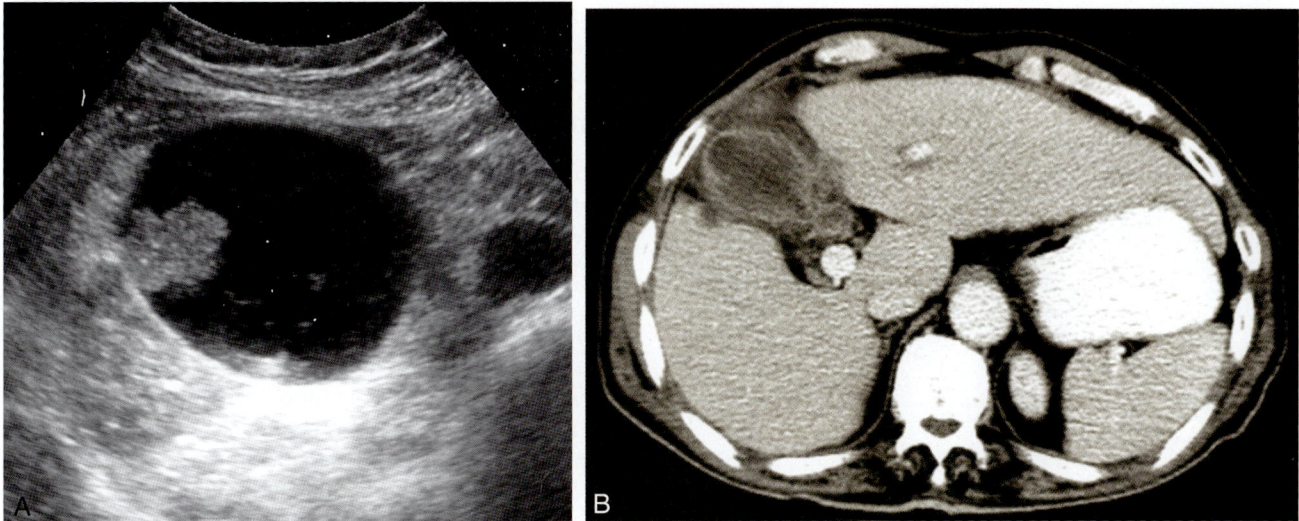

FIG. 10.39 (A) Gross specimen of gallbladder carcinoma. (B) Contrast computed tomographic image of gallbladder carcinoma.

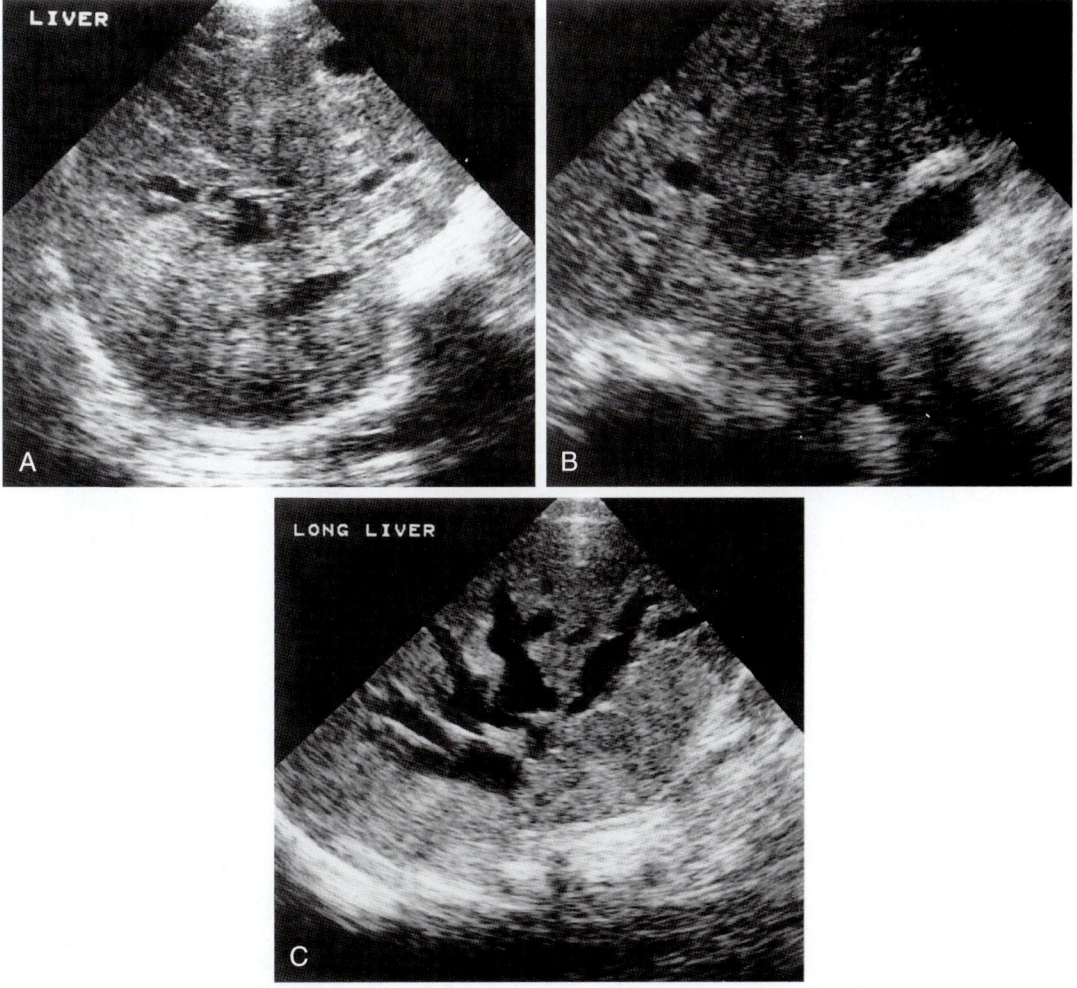

FIG. 10.40 Carcinoma of the gallbladder may extend into the cystic duct either by direct extension of the tumor or by extrinsic compression by the involved lymph nodes. (A) Transverse scan of the liver shows dilated ducts with an inhomogeneous liver parenchyma. (B) Transverse scan of the inhomogeneous liver parenchyma. (C) Transverse scan of the dilated ducts within the liver.

an apparent communication with the biliary system (Fig. 10.42). The cystic structure may contain internal sludge, stones, or solid neoplasm. If the cyst is very large, the connection to the bile duct may be difficult to distinguish on sonography.

Caroli Disease

Caroli disease is a rare congenital abnormality that is most likely inherited in an autosomal recessive fashion. This condition is a communicating cavernous ectasia of intrahepatic ducts characterized by congenital segmental saccular cystic dilation of major intrahepatic bile ducts (Fig. 10.43). It is usually found in the young adult or pediatric population and may be associated with renal disease or congenital hepatic fibrosis. Patient symptoms include recurrent cramping upper abdominal pain secondary to biliary stasis, ductal stones, cholangitis, and hepatic fibrosis. Cystic disease of the kidney (medullary sponge kidney) is strongly associated with Caroli disease. Renal failure may be a dominant feature. There are two types of Caroli disease: the simple classic form and the more common form associated with periportal hepatic fibrosis.

FIG. 10.41 Transverse images of inhomogeneous gallbladder carcinoma (*arrow*).

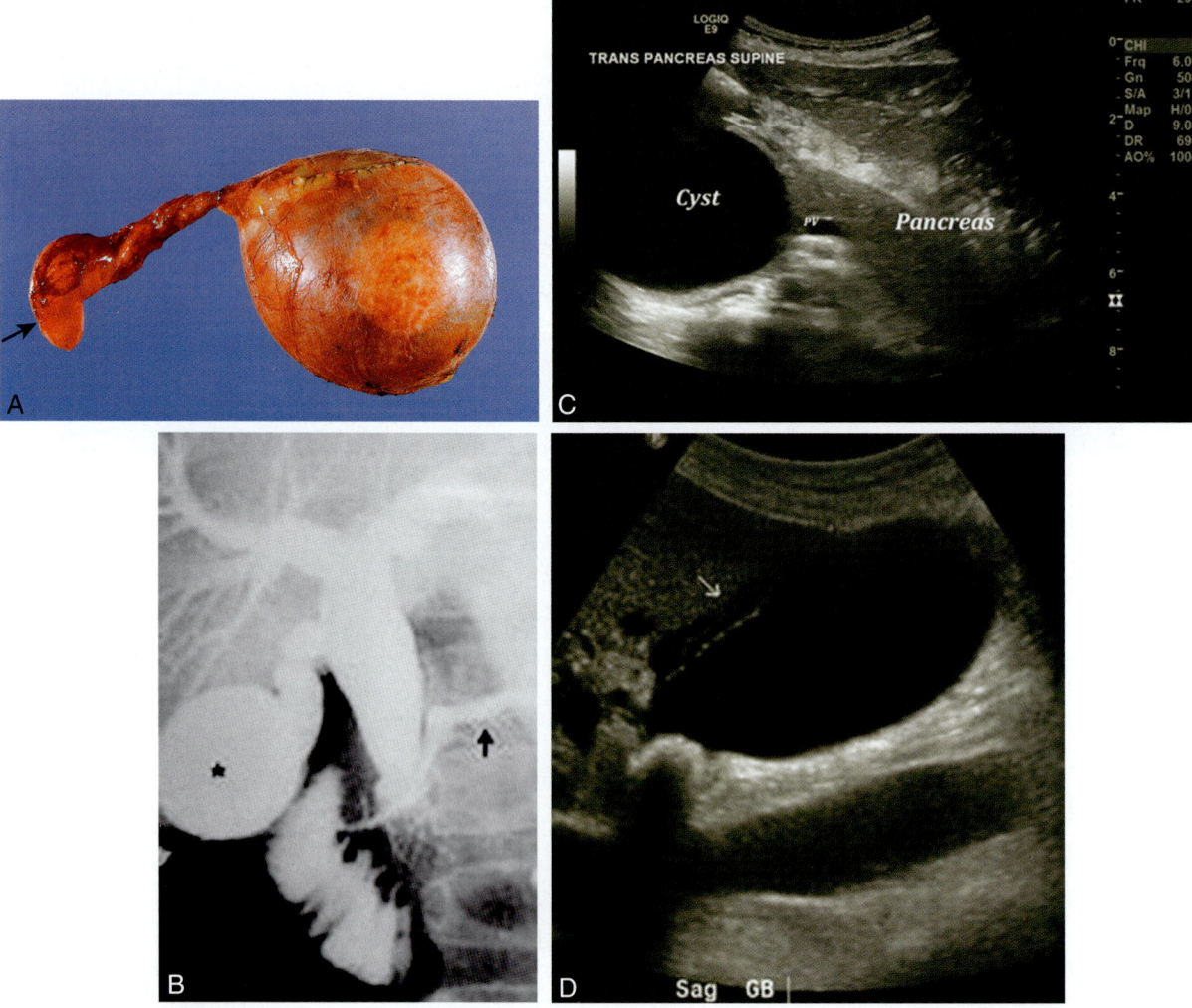

FIG. 10.42 (A) Gross specimen of a choledochal cyst. (B) Radiographic image of a choledochal cyst. Transverse (C) and longitudinal (D) images of a large sonolucent choledochal cyst that lies adjacent to the pancreas.

Sonographic Findings. On sonographic examination, multiple cystic structures in the area of the ductal system converge toward the porta hepatis (Fig. 10.44). These masses may be seen as localized or diffusely scattered cysts that communicate with the bile ducts. The differential will include cystic liver disease or biliary obstruction. In addition to the abnormality in the porta hepatis, the ducts may show a beaded appearance as they extend into the periphery of the liver. Ectasia of the extrahepatic and common bile ducts may be present. In addition, sludge or calculi may reside in the dilated ducts. Secondary signs of portal hypertension may occur. The "central dot" sign is classic for Caroli disease and is caused by the dilated duct surrounding the adjacent hepatic artery and portal vein.

Dilated Biliary Ducts

The small size of the peripheral intrahepatic bile ducts (normal <2 mm) implies that sonography cannot image the ducts routinely until their size dilates to greater than 4 mm. Evaluation of the portal structures will allow the sonographer to search for the dilated ducts as they parallel the course of the portal veins. The common hepatic duct has an internal diameter of less than 4 mm. A duct diameter of 5 mm is borderline, and one of 6 mm requires further investigation. A patient may have a normal-size hepatic duct and still have distal obstruction. The distal duct is often obscured by gas in the duodenal loop. The common bile duct has an internal diameter slightly greater than that of the hepatic duct. Generally, a duct more

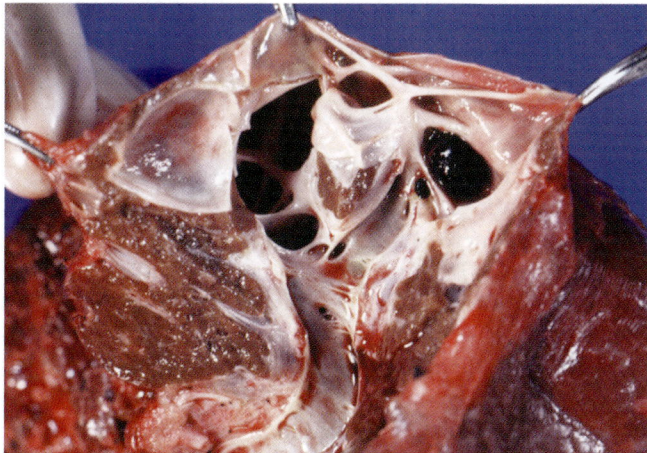

FIG. 10.43 Caroli disease. Gross anatomy of the multiple cystic structures within the liver.

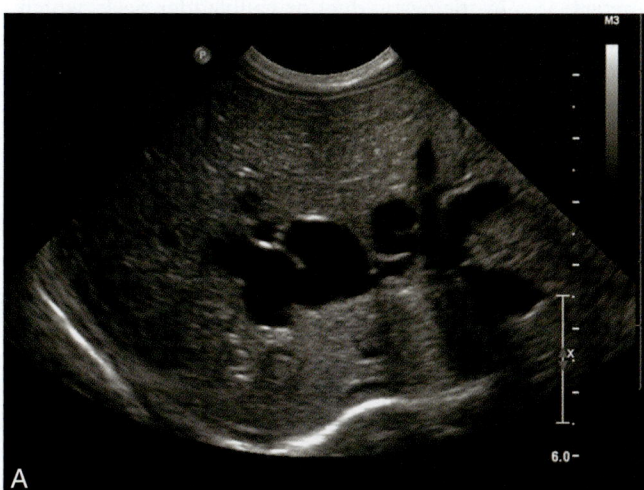

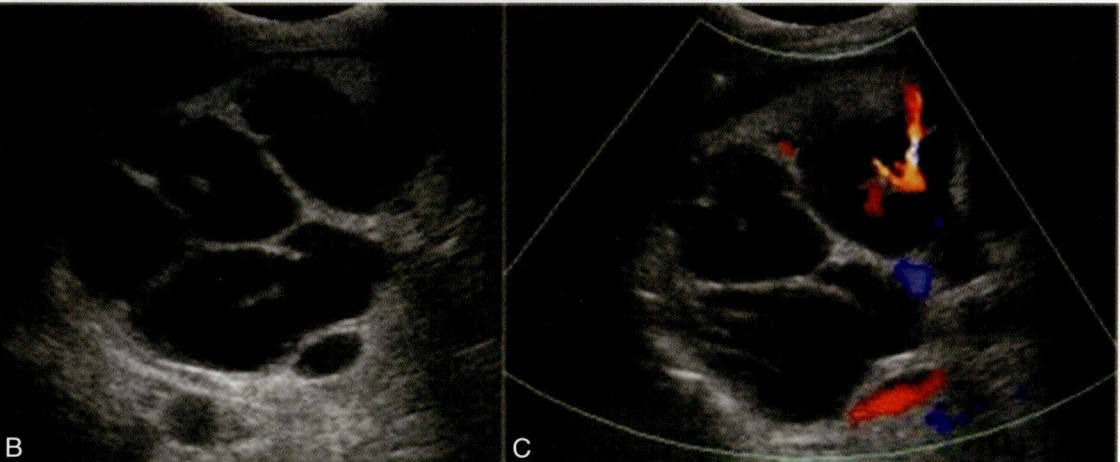

FIG. 10.44 (A–C) Transverse images of Caroli disease with multiple cystic structures in the area of the ductal system that converge towards the porta hepatis; the masses may be localized or diffusely scattered cysts that communicate with the bile ducts. Note the central dot sign *(arrow)* as seen in patients with the dilated ducts.

than 6 mm in diameter is considered borderline, and more than 10 mm is dilated (Fig. 10.45). The dilated duct is distinguished from the portal vein by its tortuosity, increased through transmission and central stellate configuration.

Biliary Obstruction

The most common cause of biliary ductal system obstruction is the presence of a tumor or thrombus within the ductal system (Fig. 10.46). The process may be found in the extrahepatic or intrahepatic ductal pathway. Obstruction of the biliary ductal system is diagnosed by ultrasound when the sonographer finds the presence of ductal dilation. This finding has been termed on sonography as "too many tubes" or "shotgun" sign when intrahepatic ducts are dilated. These dilated intrahepatic ducts can be seen as parallel channels adjacent to the portal veins. The normal intrahepatic ducts should not be more than 40% of the diameter of the adjacent portal vein. Likewise, the peripheral ducts should not be more than 2 mm in diameter.

Bile ducts expand centrifugally from the point of obstruction. Therefore, extrahepatic dilation occurs before intrahepatic dilation. In patients with obstructive jaundice, isolated dilation of the extrahepatic duct may be present. Fibrosed or infiltrative disease of the liver may prevent intrahepatic dilation because of lack of compliance of the hepatic parenchyma.

Clinically the elevation of cholestatic liver parameters may present as jaundice. Painful jaundice is seen with acute obstruction or infection that may invade the biliary tree.

Extrahepatic Biliary Obstruction

The job of the sonographer is to localize the level and cause of the obstruction. The least restrictive segment of the bile duct is the midsegment between the right hepatic artery and the pancreas, so this segment dilates first in obstruction. Dilation is present when the common duct is more than 7 mm in diameter. The sonographer should keep in mind that the duct does increase in size with age and after cholecystectomy.

Another assessment of extrahepatic ductal dilation is to measure the proximal duct at the point it crosses the right hepatic artery. A duct more than 4 mm is abnormal at this intersection. This segment may not dilate as early as the midduct. Also, there may be a partial or intermittent obstruction of the duct.

There are three primary areas for obstruction to occur: (1) intrapancreatic, (2) suprapancreatic, and (3) porta hepatic (see Fig. 10.46).

Intrapancreatic Obstruction. Three primary conditions cause the majority of biliary obstruction at the level of the distal duct and cause the extrahepatic duct to be entirely dilated: (1) pancreatic carcinoma, (2) choledocholithiasis, and (3) chronic pancreatitis with stricture formation (Fig. 10.47A).

Suprapancreatic Obstruction. This obstruction originates between the pancreas and the porta hepatis. The head of the pancreas, the intrapancreatic duct, and pancreatic duct are normal with ultrasound. The most common cause for this obstruction is malignancy or adenopathy at this level.

Porta Hepatic Obstruction. This area of obstruction is usually due to a neoplasm. In patients with obstruction at the level of the porta hepatis, ultrasound will show intrahepatic ductal dilation and a normal common duct (see Fig. 10.47B). Hydrops of the gallbladder may be present.

Mirizzi syndrome is an uncommon cause for extrahepatic biliary obstruction resulting from an impacted stone in the cystic duct or gallbladder neck, which creates extrinsic mechanical compression of the common hepatic duct (see Fig. 10.47C). The patient presents with painful jaundice. This stone may penetrate the common hepatic duct or the gut, which results in a cholecystobiliary or cholecystenteric fistula. In this case, the cystic duct inserts unusually low into the common hepatic duct, and thus the two ducts have parallel alignment, which allows for the development of this syndrome. Using sonography, an intrahepatic ductal dilation is seen with a normal-size common duct and a large stone in the neck of the gallbladder or cystic duct.

Sonographic Findings. Minimal dilation may be seen in nonjaundiced patients with gallstones or pancreatitis or jaundiced patients with a common duct stone or tumor

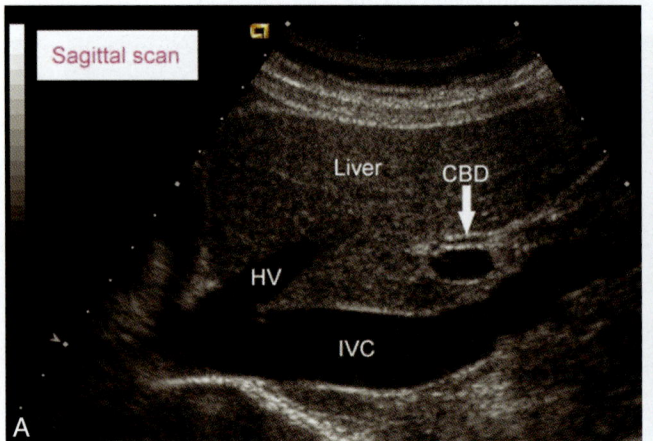
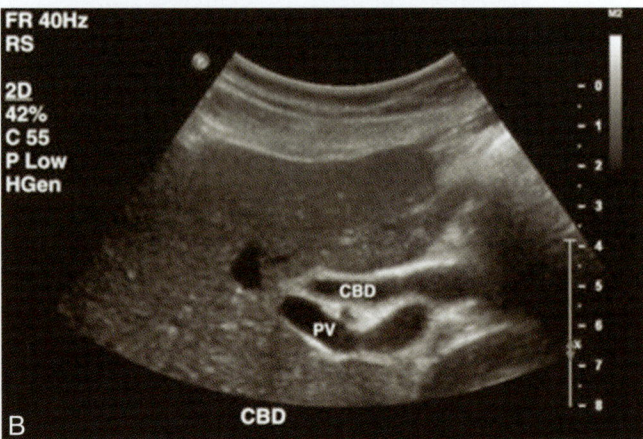

FIG. 10.45 The normal common bile duct (CBD) should measure <3 mm *(arrow)*. Note the dilation of the CBD on the right. *IVC*, Inferior vena cava; *HV*, hepatic vein; *PV*, portal vein.

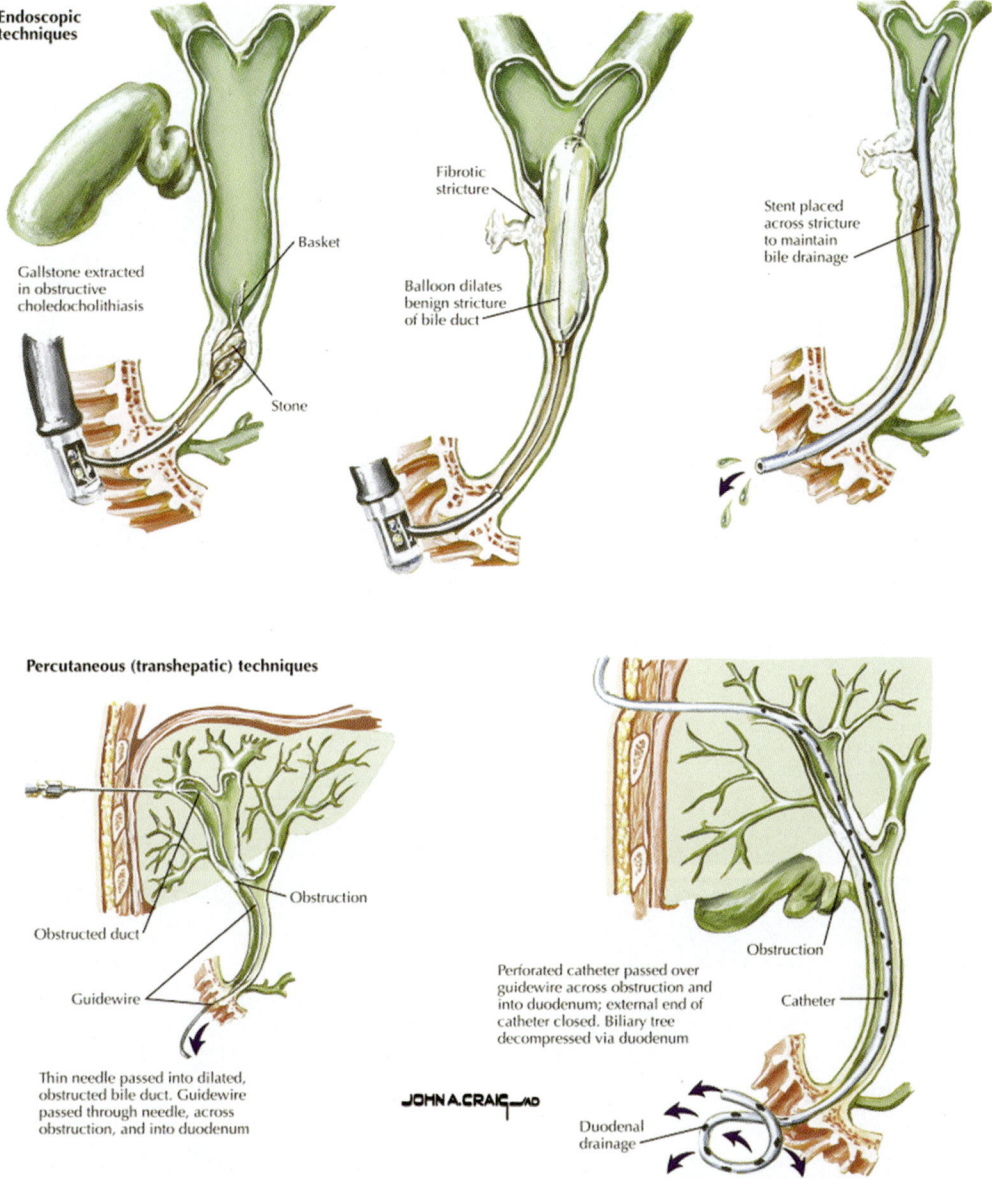

FIG. 10.46 **Levels of obstruction.** Obstruction of the biliary tree may occur in any of three sites: intrapancreatic, suprapancreatic, and porta hepatic.

(Fig. 10.48). However, a diameter of more than 11 mm suggests obstruction by stone or tumor of the duct or pancreas or some other source (Fig. 10.49).

Dilated ducts may also be found in the absence of jaundice. The patient may have biliary obstruction involving one hepatic duct, an early obstruction secondary to carcinoma, or gallstones causing intermittent obstruction resulting from a ball-valve effect (Fig. 10.50).

Choledocholithiasis

Choledocholithiasis is classified into primary and secondary forms. Primary choledocholithiasis is the de novo formation of calcium stones in the bile duct. These stones may result from disease-causing strictures or dilation of the bile ducts leading to stasis, as seen in sclerosing cholangitis, Caroli disease, parasitic infections, chronic hemolytic diseases, and prior biliary surgery. The secondary form denotes that most stones in the common bile duct have migrated from the gallbladder. Common duct stones are usually associated with calculous cholecystitis.

Sonographic Findings. Stones tend to become impacted in the distal portion of the intrahepatic duct of the ampulla of Vater and may project into the duodenum (Fig. 10.51). This is the reason it is important for the surgeons to check the common bile duct when removing the gallbladder. The sonographer should look for a dilated duct with a ductal stone that appears hyperechoic and casts a posterior shadow. Not all ductal stones may shadow, nor will they show mobility. Alterations in the patient position ranging from the right posterior oblique to upright scanning may help distinguish the impacted ductal stone from the duodenum.

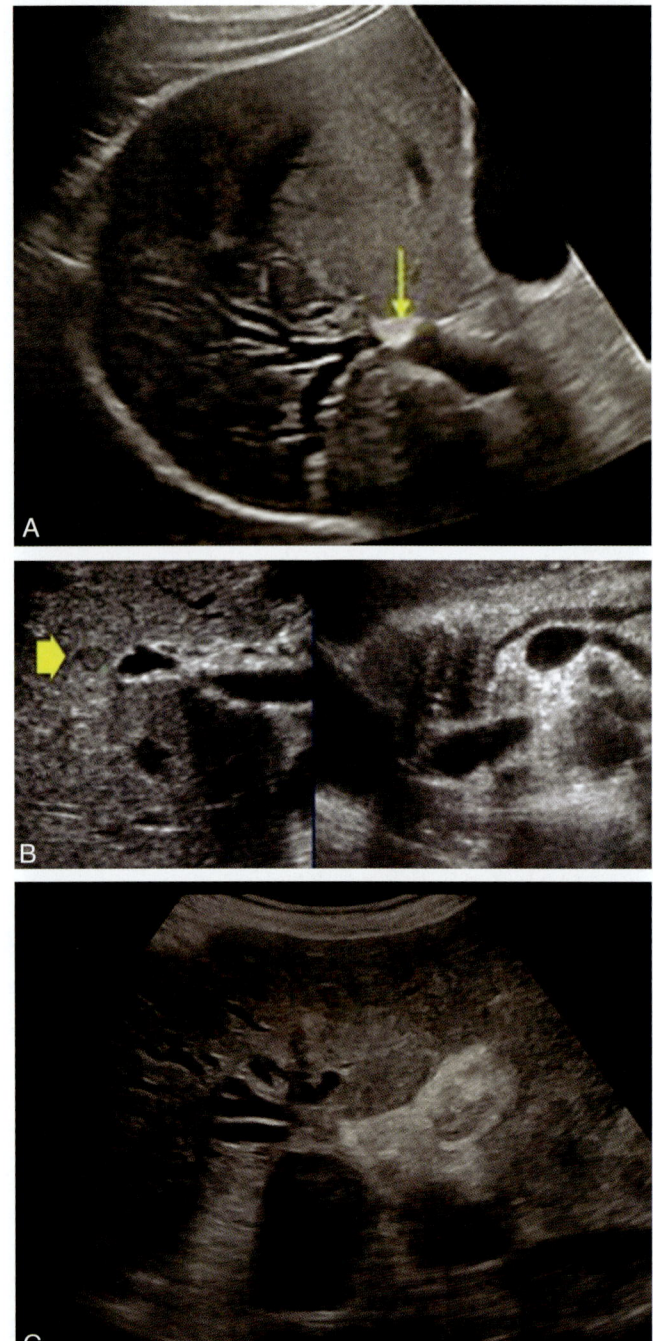

FIG. 10.47 (A) Intrapancreatic obstruction secondary to a stone *(arrow)*. (B) Suprapancreatic obstruction. The *arrow* denotes the dilated duct, secondary to a mass in the head of the pancreas. (C) Porta hepatic obstruction. Note the dilated ducts within the liver.

Other Causes of Shadowing. The sonographer should be aware that structures or conditions other than stones may lead to attenuation of the ultrasound beam or shadowing. Calcifications in the hepatic artery and pancreatic head may cause shadowing to occur in the area of the gallbladder and be misinterpreted as stones. Air or gas within the duodenum may also give rise to a dirty shadow in the right upper quadrant. Intrabiliary gas is sometimes difficult to separate from stones, although the gas usually produces a brighter reflection with a

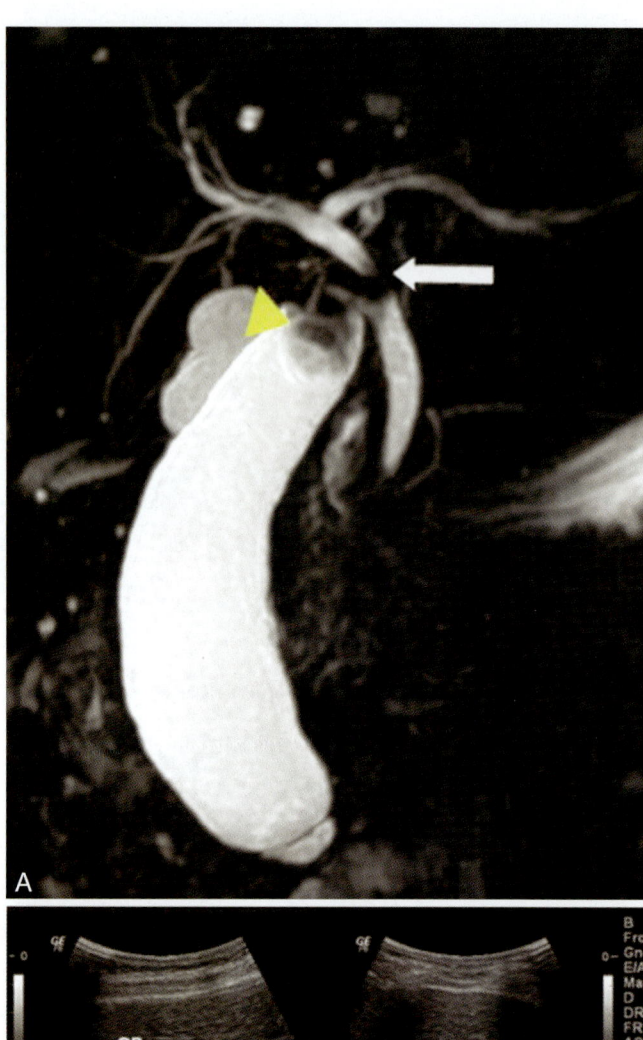
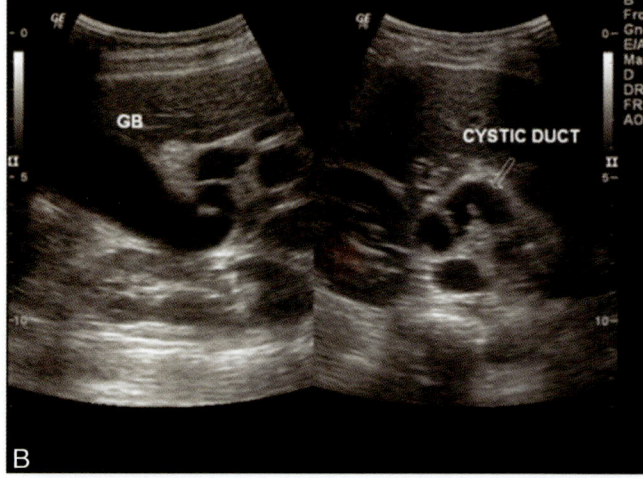

FIG. 10.48 (A) Mirizzi syndrome occurs when the gallstone is impacted at the gallbladder neck, causing chronic inflammation and fibrosis that results in obstruction of erosion of the common duct. (B) Mirizzi syndrome is an uncommon cause for extrahepatic biliary obstruction resulting from an impacted stone in the cystic duct or gallbladder neck.

ring down artifact and dirtier shadow versus the clean, sharp shadow from a stone (Fig. 10.52). Another cause of shadowing in the right upper quadrant is gas in the biliary tree. This is a spontaneous occurrence resulting from the formation of a biliary enteric fistula in chronic gallbladder disease.

Intrahepatic duct stones are less common than common bile duct stones. The intrahepatic duct stones tend to form

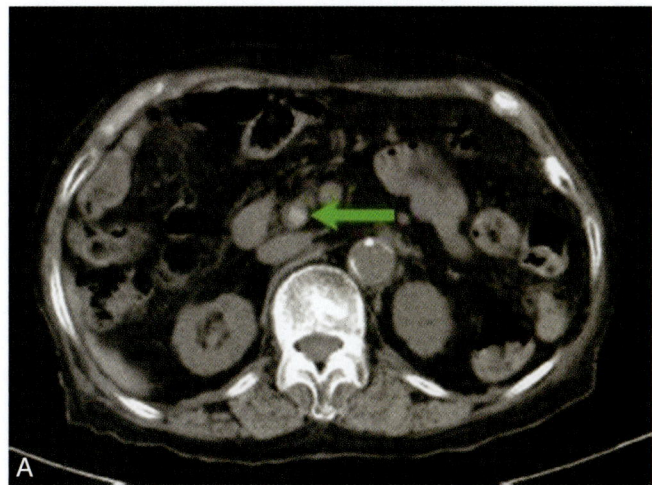
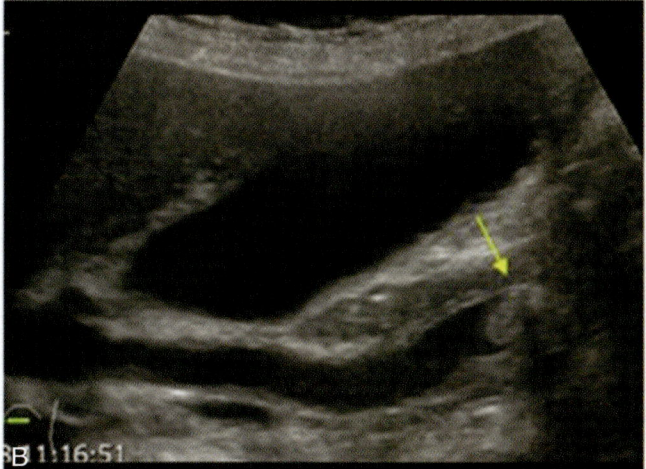

FIG. 10.49 (A) Computed tomographic image of a stone in the distal common bile duct *(arrow)*. (B) Ultrasound of the dilated duct secondary to the distal stone *(arrow)*.

primarily in the bile ducts and typically are a complication of another biliary tract abnormality.

Hemobilia

Biliary trauma secondary to percutaneous biliary procedures or liver biopsies accounts for the majority of hemobilia cases. Other causes include cholangitis, cholecystitis, vascular malformations, abdominal trauma, and malignancies. The usual clinical findings are pain, bleeding, and jaundice. The sonographic appearance of blood in the biliary tree will depend on the length of time the blood has been present (Fig. 10.53). Acute hemorrhage will appear as fluid with low-level internal echoes. Look for blood clots that may move in the duct with extension into the gallbladder.

Pneumobilia

Pneumobilia is air within the biliary tree secondary to biliary intervention, biliary-enteric anastomoses, or common bile duct stents. In the patient with an acute abdomen, pneumobilia may be caused by emphysematous cholecystitis, inflammation from an impacted stone in the common bile duct, or prolonged acute cholecystitis, which may lead to erosion of the bowel. On sonography, the air in the bile ducts presents as bright, echogenic linear structures that follow the portal triads (Fig. 10.54). The posterior dirty shadow and reverberating artifact are seen. The sonographer should look for the movement of tiny air bubbles with a change in the patient's position.

Cholangitis: Bile Duct Wall Thickening

Cholangitis is an inflammation of the bile ducts (Fig. 10.55). It may present as acute bacterial cholangitis, recurrent pyogenic cholangitis, or primary sclerosing cholangitis. The cause of cholangitis is dependent on the type of disease, but the obstruction may include ductal strictures, parasitic infestation, bacterial infection, stones, choledochal cysts, or neoplasm.

Cholangitis may be identified as recurrent pyogenic cholangitis (seen more frequently in the United States with immigration from Southeast Asia). Other forms of cholangitis include AIDS cholangitis and acute obstructive suppurative cholangitis. Clinically the patient presents with malaise and fever, followed by sweating and shivering. They may have right upper quadrant pain and jaundice. In severe cases, the patient is lethargic, prostrate, and in shock. Elevated lab values show leukocytosis as well as elevation of serum alkaline phosphatase and bilirubin.

Cholangitis is a medical emergency as it develops increasing pressure in the biliary tree with pus accumulation. Decompression of the common bile duct is necessary. More than half of the patients with sclerosing cholangitis have ulcerative colitis. Both sclerosing and AIDS cholangitis can have intrahepatic biliary changes that are nearly identical on ultrasound.

Sonographic Findings. The sonographer needs to determine the cause and level of obstruction and exclude other diseases such as cholecystitis or hepatitis. The biliary tree is dilated, and the common bile duct wall may show a smooth or irregular thickening (Fig. 10.56). There may be choledocholithiasis with sludge. The ductal wall may be so thickened that it is difficult to recognize on sonography without careful evaluation. Cholangitis usually involves the bile duct in a more generalized manner. Careful evaluation of the liver parenchyma should also be made to look for hepatic abscesses.

The subcostal oblique imaging of the porta hepatis to image the portal venous system is the landmark to find the biliary tree. The common bile duct may or may not be enlarged, but the walls may become slightly irregular and thickened. The stones are usually lodged in the distal common bile duct or must be mobile to cause intermittent obstruction.

In patients with oriental cholangitis, the lateral segment of the left lobe of the liver is most often involved. In the acute septic phase, the patient may need urgent percutaneous biliary decompression or surgery. Atrophy of the affected duct develops with chronic stasis and inflammation followed by biliary cirrhosis and cholangiocarcinoma. Ultrasound is excellent for following these patients. As the biliary tree dilates, the internal

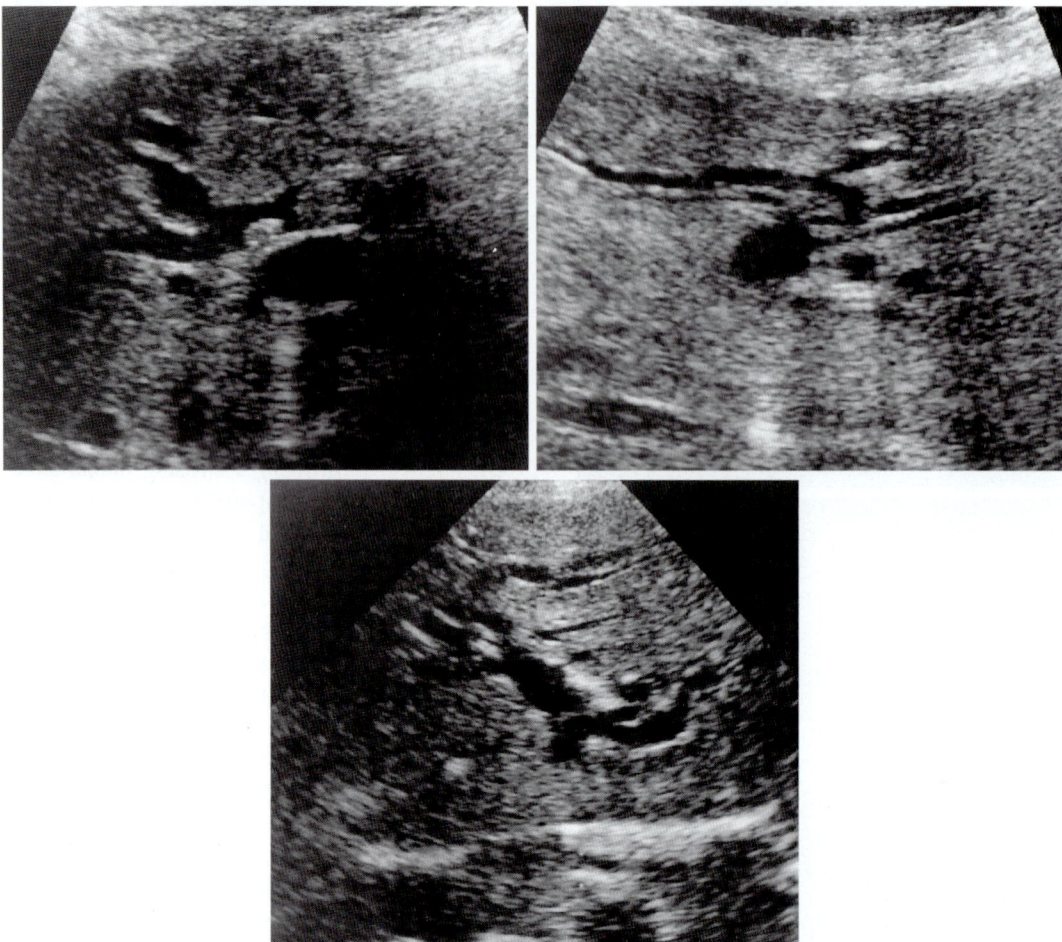

FIG. 10.50 A 60-year-old woman with a history of cholecystectomy several years previously. The patient was known to have had previous hepatic calculi and now has right upper quadrant pain. Moderate diffuse dilation of the right and left intrahepatic ducts is present. Echogenic ovoid structures seen in the distal right hepatic and left hepatic ducts represent calculi or sludge balls. The intrahepatic duct was minimally dilated.

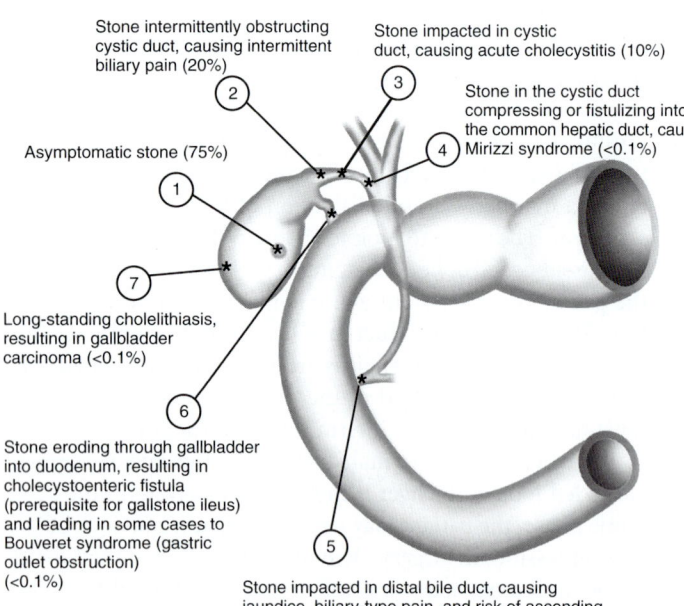
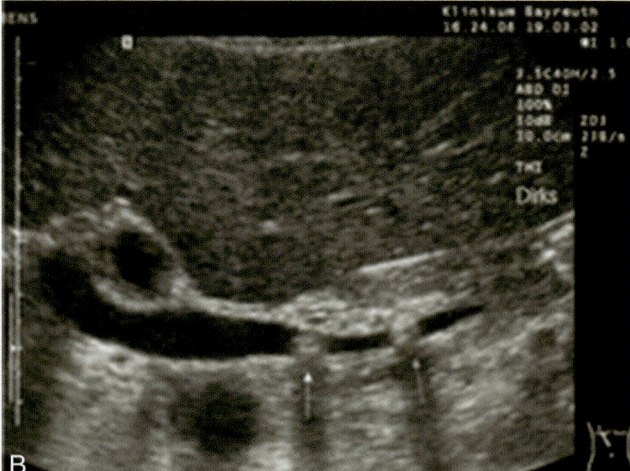

FIG. 10.51 (A) Stones tend to become impacted in the distal portion of the intrahepatic duct of the ampulla of Vater and may project into the duodenum. (B). The *arrows* point to the stones in the common bile duct. Note the dilation of the mid to proximal duct.

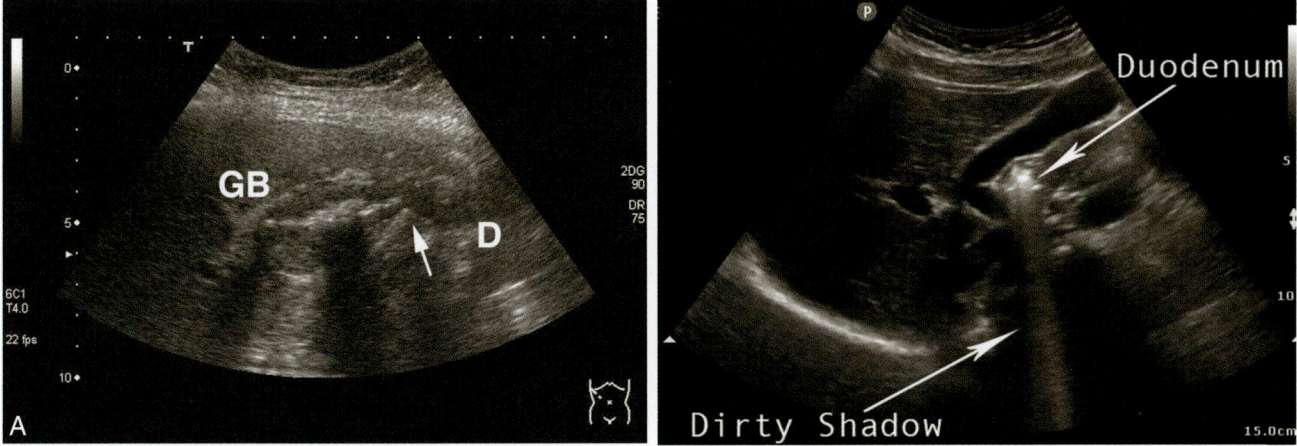

FIG. 10.52 Air in the duodenum may obstruct visualization of the gallbladder or cause confusion with a dirty shadow beyond the gallbladder wall.

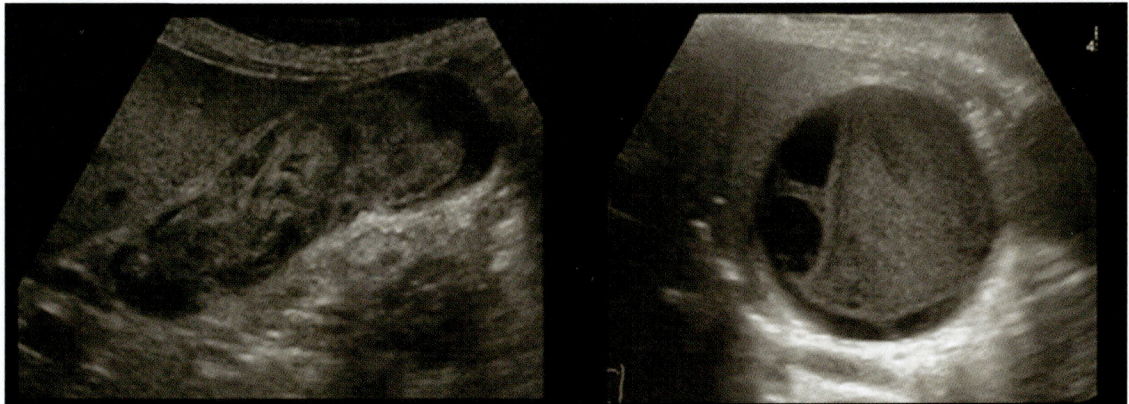

FIG. 10.53 Hemobilia. Longitudinal and transverse images of the gallbladder filled with inhomogeneous echoes that represent blood. (Courtesy Taco Geertsma, www.ultrasoundcases.info.)

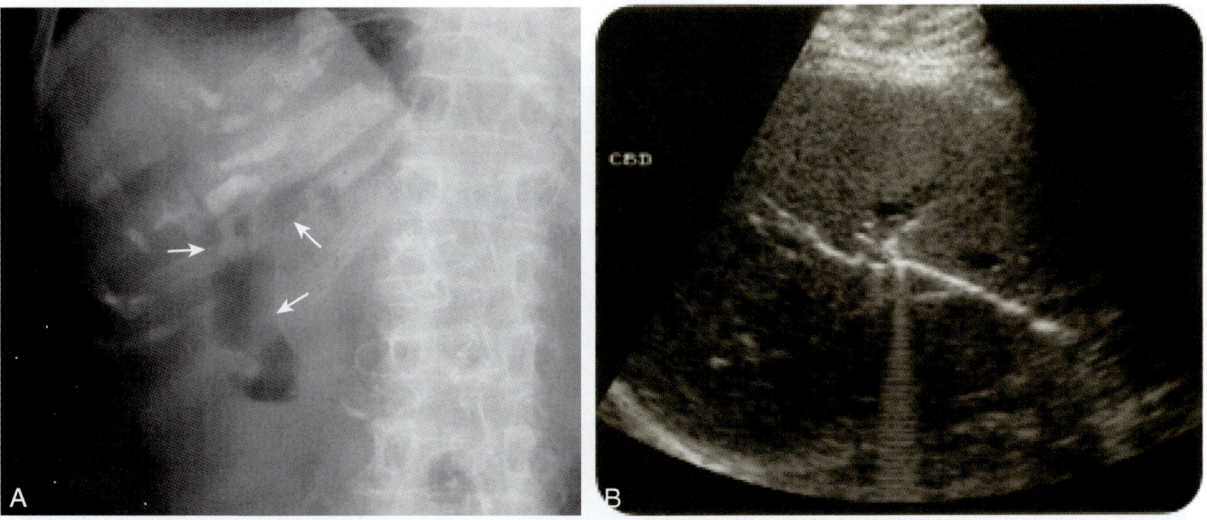

FIG. 10.54 (A) Radiograph depicts air in the biliary tree *(arrows)*. (B) The air within the biliary tree generally produces a brighter reflection within the ring-down artifact.

lumen may be hypoechoic or echogenic with stones; these stones may not shadow, especially if they are tiny.

Ascariasis

This is a parasitic roundworm *(Ascaris lumbricoides)* that uses a fecal-oral route of transmission. The worm may be 20 to 30 cm long and 6 cm in diameter. It grows in the small bowel before entering the biliary tree through the ampulla of Vater. These worms cause acute biliary obstruction and are dramatic when seen on sonography. Clinically the patient may be asymptomatic or present with biliary colic, pancreatitis, or biliary symptoms.

Sonographic Findings. On sonography, the sonographer may denote an enlarged duct with a moving "tube" or parallel echogenic lines within the biliary ducts. As the transducer is rotated into the transverse position, the worm is surrounded by the duct wall and gives a target appearance. If the transducer is held in place over the area, small discrete movements may be seen on the image. The worm may fold over itself, or there may be multiple worms that present as an amorphous echogenic filling defect in the right upper quadrant (Fig. 10.57).

Intrahepatic Biliary Neoplasms

Changes in the intrahepatic biliary ducts occur secondary to extrahepatic bile duct obstruction in most cases. Occasionally intrahepatic lesions are responsible for the changes in the duct. Intrahepatic biliary tumors are rare and are primarily limited to cystadenoma and cystadenocarcinoma. The tumors are more frequently found in middle-aged women who clinically present with abdominal pain or mass or jaundice (if the mass is near the porta hepatis). The sonographic appearance is a cystic mass with multiple septa and papillary excrescences. The mass may show variations in this pattern and present as unilocular, calcified, or multiple. The lesion may be associated with dilation of the intrahepatic ducts. The differential includes a hemorrhagic cyst or infection, echinococcal cyst, abscess, or cystic metastasis.

Cholangiocarcinoma

Cholangiocarcinoma is a rare malignancy that originates within the larger bile ducts, which is usually the common duct or common hepatic duct (Fig. 10.58). The incidence is uncommon, and the frequency increases with age. The most common risk factor in the Western world is primary sclerosing cholangitis. The classification of the tumor is based on the anatomic location: intrahepatic (peripheral), hilar (Klatskin's), and distal (Fig. 10.59). Most cholangiocarcinomas are adenocarcinomas, followed by squamous carcinomas. The tumors are further divided into subtypes: sclerosing, nodular, and papillary. Nodular sclerosing tumors are the most common. Hilar cholangiocarcinoma is a nodular sclerosing tumor, a firm mass surrounding and narrowing the affected duct with a nodular intraductal component. Papillary cholangiocarcinomas are found in the distal common bile duct.

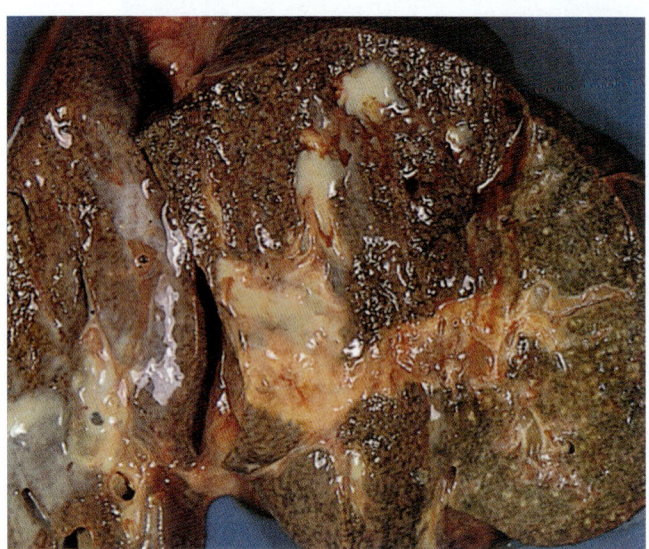

FIG. 10.55 Gross pathology of bacterial cholangitis with pus in the bile ducts.

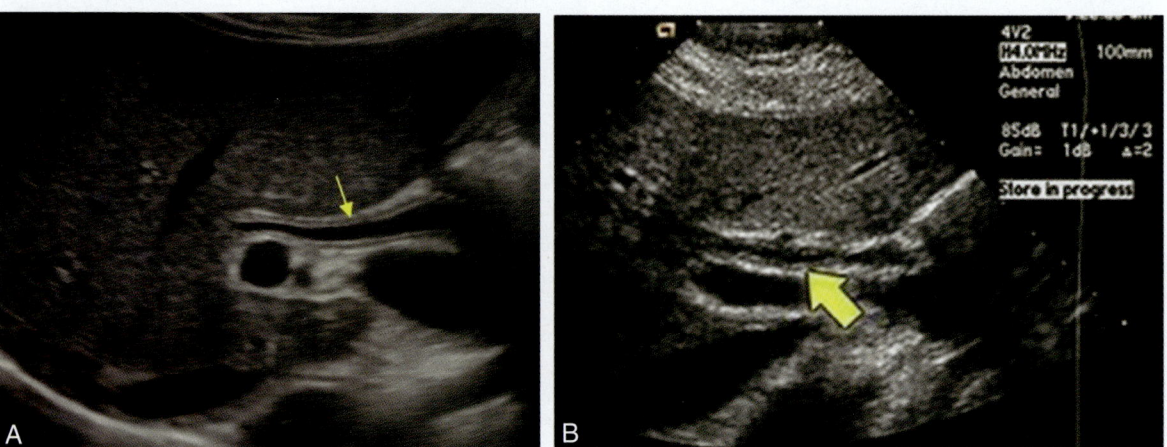

FIG. 10.56 Sclerosing cholangitis. Transverse oblique images of the prominent inflamed bile duct with thickening along the walls *(arrows)*.

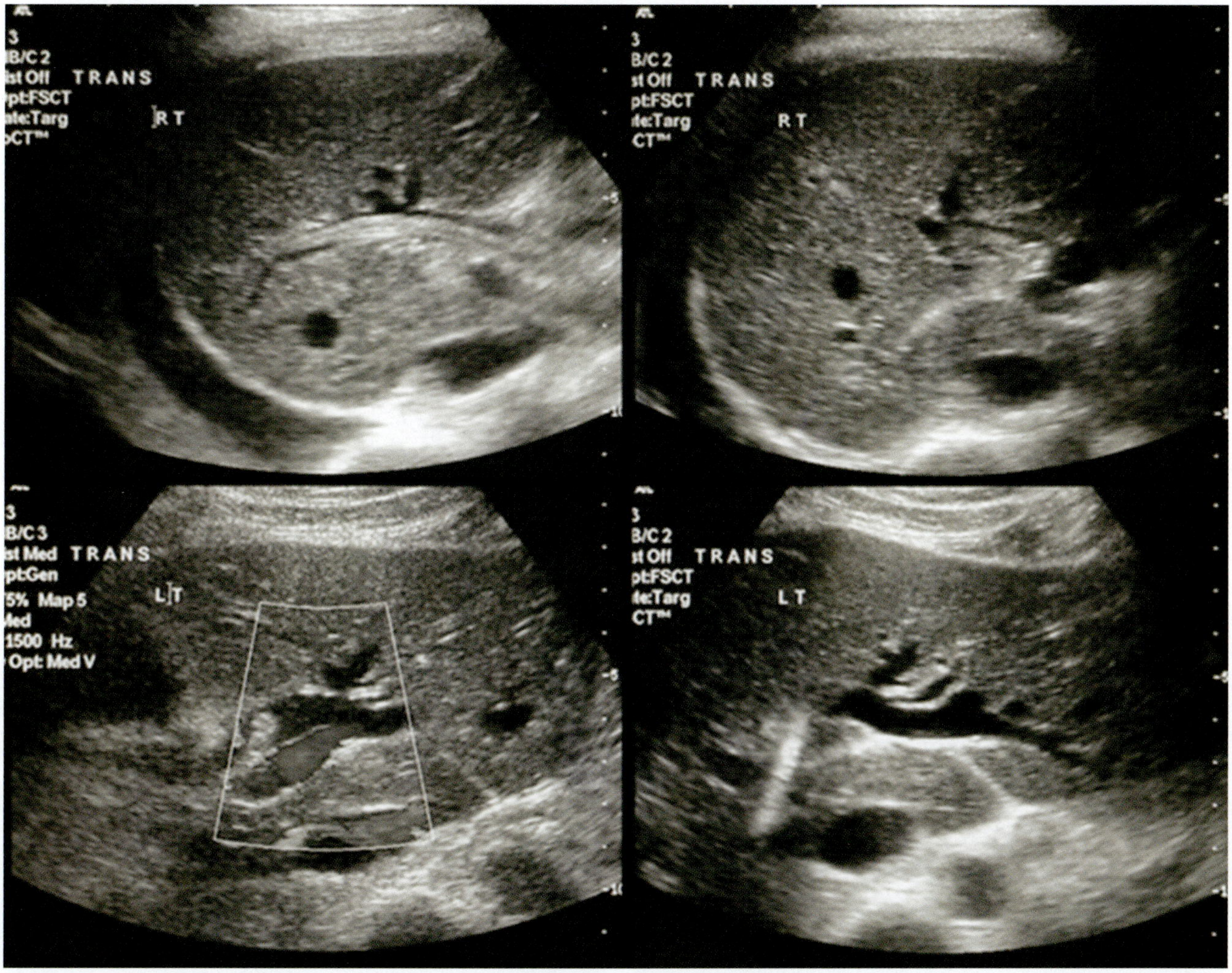

FIG. 10.57 **Ascariasis.** On sonography, the sonographer may denote an enlarged duct with a moving "tube" or parallel echogenic lines *(arrows)* within the biliary ducts.

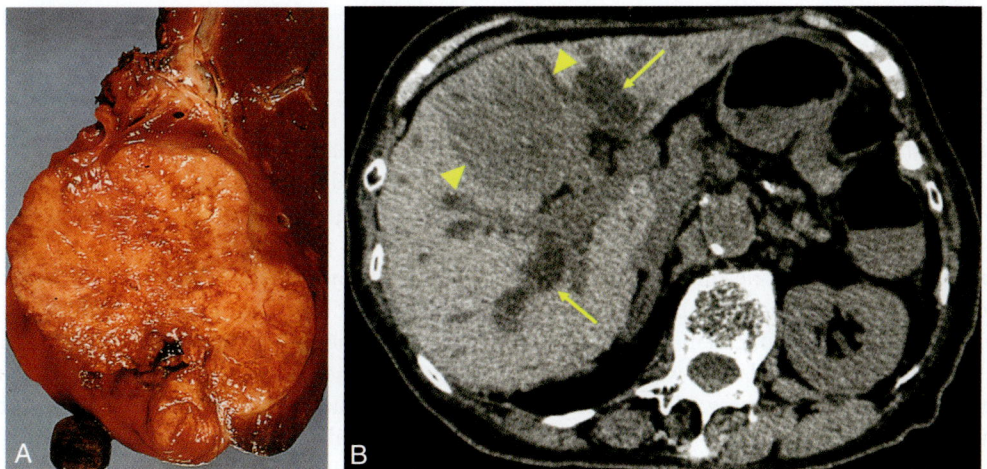

FIG. 10.58 (A) Gross pathology of cholangiocellular carcinoma. (B) Computed tomographic image of a patient with cholangiocarcinoma, *(arrows)*.

Intrahepatic Cholangiocarcinoma. Although this is the least common location for cholangiocarcinomas, it represents the second most common primary malignancy of the liver. An increased incidence of this tumor has risen over the past two decades, secondary to an increasing number of patients with liver cirrhosis and hepatitis C infection. These tumors are often unresectable, with a poor prognosis.

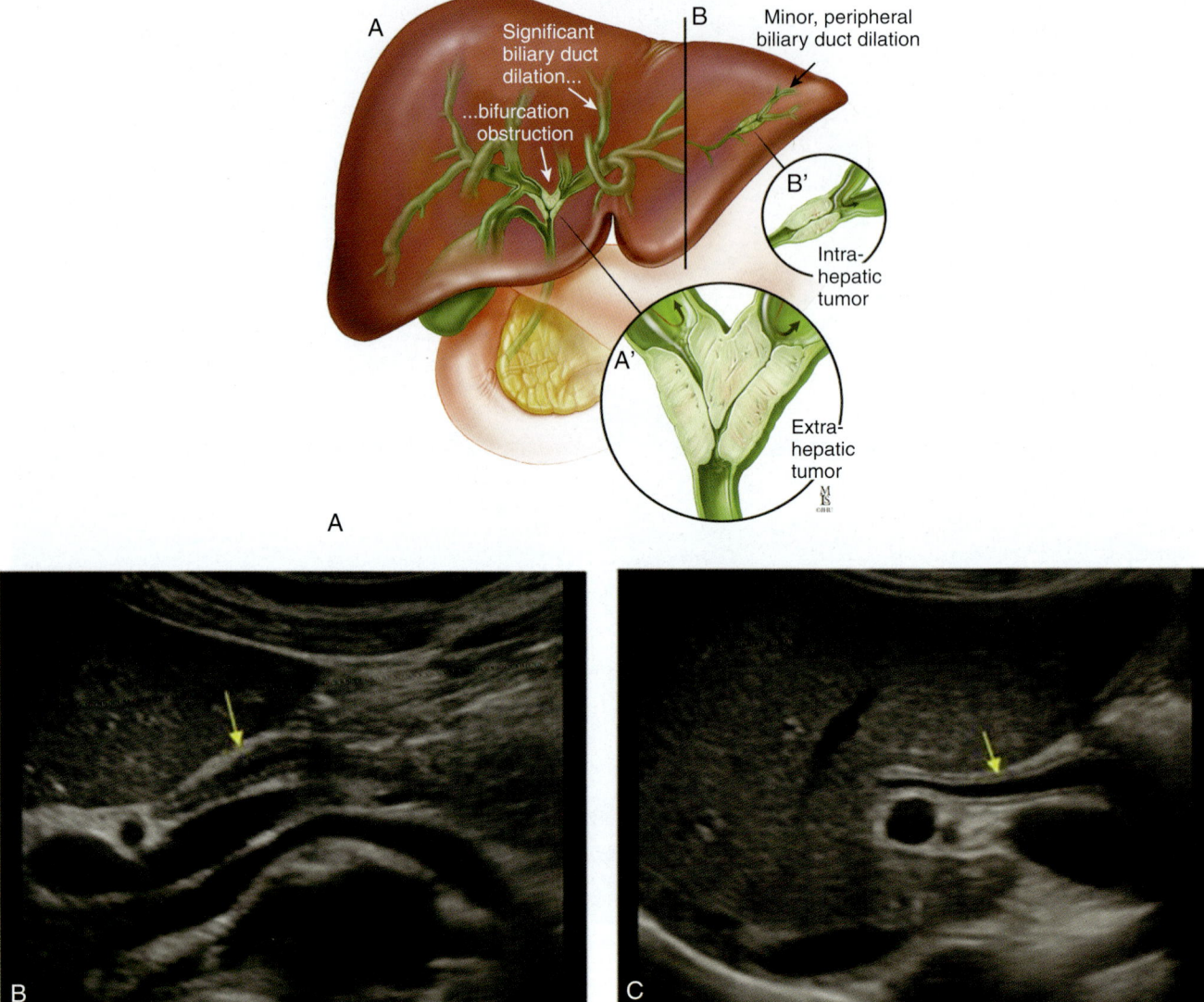

FIG. 10.59 (A) Cholangiocarcinoma is a rare malignancy that originates within the larger bile ducts, usually the common duct or common hepatic duct. Transverse (B) and longitudinal (C) sclerosing cholangitis with a thick bile duct wall.

Sonographic Findings. On sonography, a large hepatic mass may be seen. The appearance is varied, from hypoechoic to hyperechoic. A heterogeneous texture or hypovascular solid mass may be present. Biliary ductal dilation is associated with these obstructive masses in one-third of cases (Fig. 10.60). Uncommonly, an intrahepatic cholangiocarcinoma presents as one or more polypoid intraductal masses. Another uncommon form may present as a solid mass within a cystic structure representing a tumor within a very dilated duct that does not communicate with the biliary tree.

Hilar Cholangiocarcinoma. A **Klatskin tumor** is a specific type of cholangiocarcinoma that can occur at the bifurcation of the common hepatic duct, with involvement of both the central left and right duct. The most suggestive sonographic feature to indicate cholangiocarcinoma is isolated intrahepatic duct dilation. Even though the obstructing mass may not be imaged, a nonunion of the right and left ducts is characteristic of a Klatskin tumor.

This tumor is challenging for most imaging modalities. The patient clinically presents with jaundice, pruritus, and elevated cholestatic liver parameters. This disease usually begins in the right or left bile duct and then extends into the proximal duct and distally into the common hepatic duct and contralateral bile ducts. The tumor may extend outside the ducts to involve the adjacent portal vein and arteries. Chronic obstruction leads to atrophy of the involved lobe. The nodal disease originates in the porta hepatis and extends to the celiac axis with subsequent metastases to the liver. Although

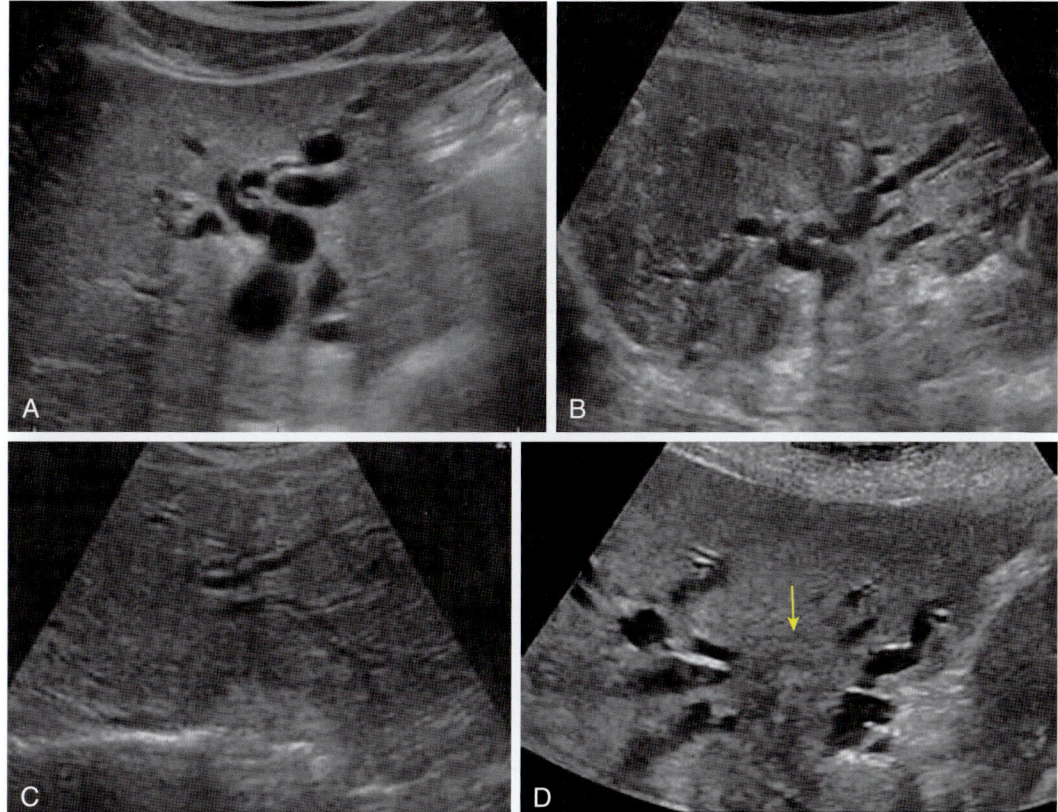

FIG. 10.60 (A–B) Intrahepatic cholangiocarcinoma. A large heterogeneous or hypovascular solid hepatic mass may be seen with a variable texture that ranges from hypoechoic to hyperechoic. Biliary ductal dilation may also be associated with these obstructive masses. (C–D) Klatskin tumor is a specific type of cholangiocarcinoma that can occur at the bifurcation of the common hepatic duct, with involvement of both the central left and right duct. The most suggestive sonographic feature to indicate cholangiocarcinoma is isolated intrahepatic duct dilation.

surgical resection is utilized, the majority of patients die within a year of diagnosis.

With sonography, careful attention is directed to the porta hepatis region (Fig. 10.61). The sonographer should assess the level of the obstruction, the presence of a mass, lobar atrophy, and the patency of main, right, and left portal veins; the sonographer should also evaluate the encasement of the hepatic artery and look for local and distant adenopathy and metastases.

If the ducts are dilated, the sonographer should follow their course centrally toward the hepatic hilum to determine which order of branching is involved with the tumor. Resection is precluded once the tumor extension is found in the segmental ducts.

Evaluation of the portal system is critical. The narrowing of the right or left portal vein leads to compensatory increased flow in the hepatic artery. Tumor narrowing or encasing that obliterates the main portal vein, or proper hepatic artery makes the tumor unresectable.

Distal Cholangiocarcinoma. This tumor is difficult to distinguish from hilar cholangiocarcinoma, although progressive jaundice is seen in the majority of patients. The tumor mass may be sclerosing or polypoid. Evaluation of tumor spread in the superior ductal system, and extrahepatic area should be carefully evaluated. The tumor may extend into the adjacent lymph nodes.

▸ **Sonographic Findings.** On sonography, the sclerosing tumor is nodular with focal irregular ductal constriction and wall thickening (Fig. 10.62). The tumor is hypoechoic and hypovascular with poorly defined margins. The more common polypoid tumor is seen as a hypovascular well-defined mass found within the distal ductal system.

Metastases to the Biliary Tree. The most common tumor sites that can spread to the biliary system are from the breast, colon, or melanoma. These metastases can affect the intrahepatic and extrahepatic ductal systems. On sonography, the appearance of metastases is similar to that of cholangiocarcinoma, with the tumor presenting as hyperechoic or hypoechoic and hypovascular with poorly defined margins.

CHAPTER 10 The Gallbladder and the Biliary System

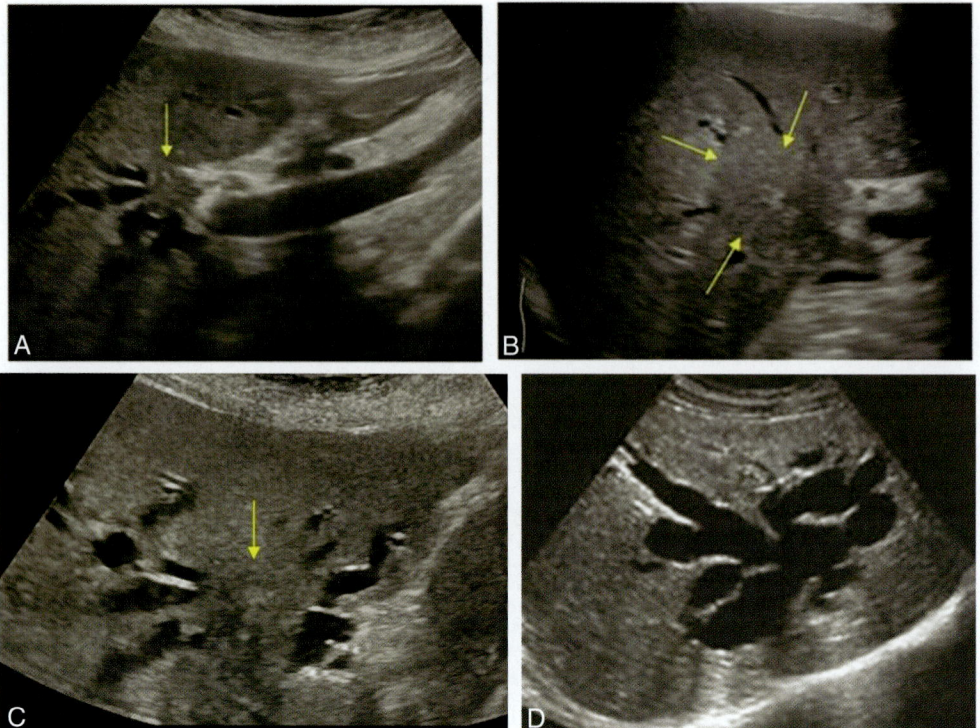

FIG. 10.61 Klatskin tumor in the porta hepatis *(arrows)* with dilated intrahepatic ducts.

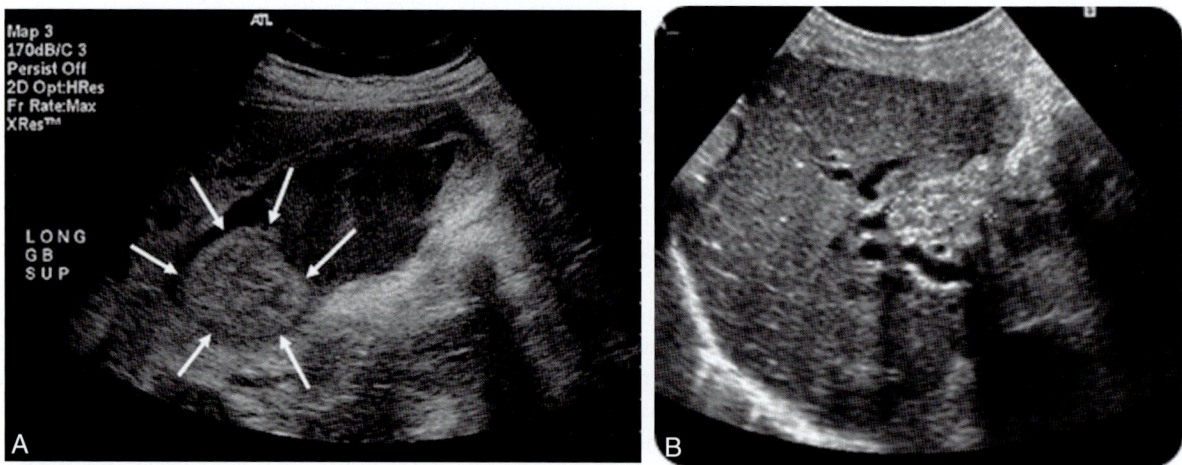

FIG. 10.62 Distal cholangiocarcinoma on sonography shows a sclerosing tumor as nodular with focal irregular ductal constriction and wall thickening.

Key Pearls

- The biliary apparatus consists of the right and left hepatic ducts, the common hepatic duct, the common bile duct, the pear-shaped gallbladder, and the cystic duct.
- The bile ducts are divided into intrahepatic and extrahepatic segments. The intrahepatic ducts run in the portal triads along with the portal veins and hepatic arteries. The peripheral intrahepatic ducts run parallel and adjacent to the hepatic arteries and portal veins.
- The extrahepatic portion of the bile ducts includes the common hepatic duct, common bile duct, and a portion of the central right and left ducts.
- The right and left hepatic ducts emerge from the right lobe of the liver in the porta hepatis and unite to form the common hepatic duct, which then passes caudally and medially.

- The common bile duct is joined by the main pancreatic duct, and together they open through a small ampulla (the ampulla of Vater) into the duodenal wall.
- The middle hepatic vein is in alignment with the gallbladder fossa. The interlobar fissure extends from the right portal vein to the gallbladder fossa.
- The gallbladder is divided into the *fundus, body*, and *neck*.
- The primary functions of the extrahepatic biliary tract are (1) the transportation of bile from the liver to the intestine and (2) the regulation of its flow.
- The common duct lies anterior and lateral to the portal vein in the region of the porta hepatis and gastrohepatic ligament. The hepatic artery lies anterior and medial to the portal vein.
- The most classic symptom of gallbladder disease is right upper quadrant abdominal pain, usually occurring after ingestion of greasy foods.
- Jaundice is characterized by the presence of bile in the tissues with resulting yellow-green color of the skin.
- Sludge, or thickened bile, frequently occurs from bile stasis.
- Biliary causes of gallbladder wall thickening include cholecystitis, adenomyomatosis, cancer, acquired immunodeficiency syndrome, cholangiopathy, severe hypoalbuminemic state, and sclerosing cholangitis.
- Nonbiliary causes of gallbladder wall thickening include diffuse liver disease (cirrhosis and hepatitis), pancreatitis, portal hypertension, and heart failure.
- Cholecystitis is an inflammation of the gallbladder that may have one of several forms: acute or chronic, acalculous, emphysematous, or gangrenous.
- The patient with acute cholecystitis presents with acute right upper quadrant pain (positive Murphy sign—inspiratory arrest upon palpitation of the gallbladder area, fever, and leukocytosis.
- Chronic cholecystitis results from numerous attacks of acute cholecystitis with subsequent fibrosis of the gallbladder wall.
- When the gallbladder is completely packed full of stones, the sonographer will only be able to image the anterior border of the gallbladder, with the stones casting a distinct acoustic shadow known as the wall echo shadow (WES) sign.
- Cholelithiasis is the most common disease of the gallbladder.
- A porcelain gallbladder is associated with gallstones in most patients and may represent a form of chronic cholecystitis and inflammation.
- Cholesterolosis is a condition in which cholesterol is deposited within the lamina propria of the gallbladder and is often associated with cholesterol stones.
- Polyps of the gallbladder are small, well-defined soft tissue projections from the gallbladder wall.
- Adenomyomatosis is a benign condition that demonstrates a hyperplastic change in the gallbladder wall.
- Adenomas are benign neoplasms of the gallbladder with a premalignant potential much lower than colonic adenomas.
- Primary carcinoma of the gallbladder is rare and is nearly always a rapidly progressive disease and is associated with cholelithiasis.
- Choledochal cysts are an unusual, diverse group of diseases that may manifest as congenital, focal, or diffuse cystic dilation of the biliary tree.
- The most common cause of biliary ductal system obstruction is the presence of a tumor or thrombus within the ductal system.
- There are three primary areas for obstruction to occur: (1) intrapancreatic, (2) suprapancreatic, and (3) porta hepatic.
- Cholangitis is an inflammation of the bile ducts that may present as acute bacterial cholangitis, recurrent pyogenic cholangitis, or primary sclerosing cholangitis.
- Cholangiocarcinoma is a rare malignancy that originates within the larger bile ducts, usually the common duct or common hepatic duct.
- A Klatskin tumor is a specific type of cholangiocarcinoma that can occur at the bifurcation of the common hepatic duct, with involvement of both the central left and right duct.

BIBLIOGRAPHY

Ahrendt AS, Nakeeb A, Pitt HA. Cholangiocarcinoma. *Clin Liver Dis*. 2001;5:191–218.

Bachar GN, Cohen M, Belenky A, et al. Effect of aging on the adult entrahepatic bile duct: a sonographic study. *J Ultrasound Med*. 2003;22:879–882.

Collett JA. Gallbladder polyps: prospective study. *J Ultrasound Med*. 1998;17:207.

Dobbins JM, Rao PM, Novelline RA. Posttraumatic hemobilia. *Emerg Radiol*. 1997;4:180.

Ghersin E, Soudack M, Galtini D. Twinkling artifact in gallbladder adenomyomatosis. *J Ultrasound Med*. 2003;22:229–231.

Gore RM, Yaghmai V, Newmark GM, et al. Imaging benign and malignant disease of the gallbladder. *Radiol Clin North Am*. 2002;40:1307–1323.

Gremmels JM, Kruskal JB, Parangi S, Kane RA. Hemorrhagic cholecystitis simulating gallbladder carcinoma. *J Ultrasound Med*. 2004;23:993–995.

Hann LE. Cholangiocarcinoma at the hepatic hilus: sonographic findings. *Am J Roentgenol*. 1997;168:985.

Harvey RT, Muller Jr. WT. Acute biliary disease: initial CT and follow-up US versus initial US and follow-up CT. *Radiology*. 1999;213:831–836.

Indar AA, Beckingham IJ. Acute cholecystitis. *BMJ*. 2002;325:639–643.

Kao EY, Desser TS, Jeffrey RB. Sonographic diagnosis of traumatic gallbladder rupture. *J Ultrasound Med*. 2002;21:1295–1297.

Kim HC, Yang DM, Jin W, et al. Large fibrous polyps of the gallbladder simulating gallbladder carcinoma. *J Ultrasound Med*. 2009;28:537–540.

Klatskin G. Adenocarcinoma of the hepatic duct at its bifurcation within the porta hepatis: an unusual tumor with distinctive clinical and pathologic features. *Am J Med*. 1965;38:241.

Konno K, Ishida H, Sato M, et al. Gallbladder perforation: color Doppler findings. *Abdom Imaging*. 2002;27:47–50.

Kurtz AB, Middleton W. *The Gallbladder in Ultrasound: The Requisites*. St Louis: Elsevier; 2004.

Lim JH. Anatomic relationship of intrahepatic bile ducts to portal veins. *J Ultrasound Med*. 1990;9:137.

Mittelstaedt CA. Ultrasound of the bile ducts. *Semin Roentgenol*. 1997;832:161.

Pandey M. Carcinoma of the gallbladder: role of sonography in the diagnosis and staging. *J Clin Ultrasound*. 2000;28:227–232.

Pinto A, Reginelli A, Cagini L, et al. Accuracy of ultrasonography in the diagnosis of acute calculous cholecystitis: review of the literature. *Crit Ultrasound J.* 2013;5:S11.

Rumack CM, Wilson SR, Charboneau JW, Levine D. Diagnostic Ultrasound. ed 4, vol 1 St Louis: Elsevier; 2011.

Simmons MZ. Pitfalls in ultrasound of the gallbladder and biliary tract. *Ultrasound Q.* 1998;14:2.

Smith EA, Dillman JR, Elsayes KM, et al. Cross-sectional imaging of acute and chronic gallbladder inflammatory disease. *AJR Am J Roetgenol.* 2009;192:188–196.

Ueno N, Togo S. Bleeding from the gallbladder: novel ultrasonographic features. *J Ultrasound Med.* 2006;25:111–113.

Van Breda Vriesman AC, Engelbrecht MR, Smithuis RH, Puylaert JB. Diffuse gallbladder wall thickening: differential diagnosis. *AJR Am J Roentgenol.* 2007;188:495–501.

CHAPTER 11

The Spleen

Sandra L. Hagen-Ansert

OBJECTIVES

On completion of this chapter, you should be able to:
- List the normal anatomy and relational landmarks of the spleen
- Discuss the size and primary functions of the spleen
- Describe the normal sonographic pattern of the spleen
- Explain the sonographic findings and differential diagnoses for the pathologies discussed in this chapter

OUTLINE

Anatomy of the Spleen 326
   Normal Anatomy 326
   Size 326
   Vascular Supply 326
   Relational Anatomy 326
   Displacement of the Spleen 326
Congenital Anomalies 327
   Splenic Agenesis 327
   Accessory Spleen 329
Physiology and Laboratory Data of the Spleen 329
Sonographic Evaluation of the Spleen 333
   Spleen Protocol 333
   Normal Texture and Patterns 333
   Patient Position and Technique 334
   Nonvisualization of the Spleen 336

Pathology of the Spleen 336
Splenomegaly 336
Congestion of the Spleen 339
Storage Disease 339
   Amyloidosis 339
   Gaucher Disease 340
   Niemann-Pick Disease 340
Diffuse Disease 340
   Sickle Cell Anemia 340
   Congenital Spherocytosis 340
   Hemolytic Anemia 341
   Autoimmune Hemolytic Anemia 341
   Polycythemia Vera 341
   Thalassemia 341
   Myeloproliferative Disorders 342

   Granulocytopoietic Abnormalities 342
   Reticuloendotheliosis 342
   Letterer-Siwe Disease 342
   Hand-Schüller-Christian Disease 342
Splenic Abscess and Infection 342
   Splenic Abscess 342
   Splenic Infection 344
Splenic Infarction 344
Splenic Trauma 345
Splenic Cysts 348
Benign Primary Neoplasms 349
   Hemangioma 349
   Hamartoma 349
   Lymphangioma 351
   Malignant Primary Neoplasms 351

KEY TERMS

Accessory spleen
Amyloidosis
Autoimmune hemolytic anemia
Culling
Erythrocyte
Gastrosplenic ligament
Gaucher disease
Hematopoiesis
Hemoglobin
Hemolytic anemia
Hemosiderin
Hodgkin lymphoma
Infarction

Intraperitoneal
Leukopenia
Lienorenal ligament
Lymph
Mononucleosis
Non-Hodgkin lymphoma
Phagocytosis
Phrenicocolic ligament
Pitting
Polycythemia
Polycythemia vera
Polysplenia
Red pulp

Reticuloendothelial
Sickle cell anemia
Sickle cell crisis
Spherocytosis
Splenic agenesis
Splenic artery
Splenic hilum
Splenic vein
Splenomegaly
Thalassemia
Wandering spleen
White pulp

The spleen is the largest single mass of lymphoid tissue in the body. It is part of the **reticuloendothelial** system and has a role in the synthesis of blood proteins. The spleen is active in blood formation (**hematopoiesis**) during the initial part of fetal life. This function decreases gradually by the fifth or sixth month when the spleen assumes its adult characteristics and discontinues its hematopoietic (blood-producing) activities. The spleen plays a vital role in defense of the body. Although it is often affected by systemic disease processes, the spleen is rarely the primary disease site.

The left upper quadrant may be rapidly assessed with sonography in patients with palpable splenomegaly or trauma to the left upper quadrant. The normal texture of the spleen is homogeneous, being slightly more echogenic than the texture of the liver; therefore, pathology or blood collection secondary to a splenic rupture is usually easily identified.

ANATOMY OF THE SPLEEN

Normal Anatomy

The spleen is an **intraperitoneal** organ covered with peritoneum over its entire extent, except for a small area at its hilum, where the vascular structures and lymph nodes are located. The spleen lies in the posterior left hypochondrium between the fundus of the stomach and the diaphragm. The splenic axis is along the shaft of the eighth to tenth ribs with the lower pole extending forward as far as the midaxillary line (Fig. 11.1). The inferomedial surface of the spleen comes into contact with the stomach, left kidney, pancreas, and splenic flexure of the colon (Fig. 11.2). The *splenorenal ligament* extends between the hilum of the spleen and the anterior aspect of the left kidney. The splenic vessels lie within this ligament, as does the tail of the pancreas (Fig. 11.3). This ligament is in contact with the posterior peritoneal wall, the **phrenicocolic ligament**, and the **gastrosplenic ligament**. The gastrosplenic ligament is significant in that it is composed of a double layer of peritoneum that connects the fundus of the stomach to the hilum of the spleen. In this double layer of the peritoneum are the short gastric and left gastroepiploic vessels. This dorsal mesentery separates the lesser sac posteriorly from the greater sac anteriorly. A protective capsule covers the spleen with the peritoneum. In most adults, a portion of the splenic capsule is firmly adherent to the fused dorsal mesentery anterior to the upper pole of the left kidney, which produces a "bare area" of the spleen. This bare area can help distinguish intraperitoneal from pleural fluid collections.

Size

The spleen is of variable size and shape (e.g., "orange segment," tetrahedral, triangular) but generally is considered to be ovoid with smooth, even borders and a convex superior and concave inferior surface (Fig. 11.4). The spleen is normally measured with ultrasound on a longitudinal image from the upper margin (near the diaphragm) to the inferior margin at the long axis. Normal measurements for the average adult should be 8 to 13 cm in length, 7 cm in width, and 3 to 4 cm in thickness. The spleen decreases slightly in size with advancing age. The size of the spleen may vary in size in accordance with the nutritional status of the body.

Vascular Supply

Blood is supplied to the spleen by the tortuous **splenic artery** that travels horizontally along the superior border of the pancreas (Fig. 11.5). Upon entering the **splenic hilum**, the splenic artery immediately branches into six smaller arteries to supply the organ with oxygenated blood to profuse the splenic parenchyma. Color Doppler imaging allows the sonographer to image the vascularity of the spleen; gray-scale imaging will show small echogenic lines throughout the spleen that represent the arterial system. The splenic arteries are subject to **infarction** because adequate anastomoses between the vessels are lacking.

The **splenic vein** is formed by multiple branches within the spleen and leaves the hilum in a horizontal direction to join the superior mesenteric vein. The superior mesenteric vein returns unoxygenated blood from the bowel to form the main portal vein (Fig. 11.6). The splenic vein usually travels along the posteromedial border of the pancreas.

The **lymph** vessels emerge from the splenic hilum, pass through other lymph nodes along the course of the splenic artery, and drain into the celiac nodes. The nerves to the spleen accompany the splenic artery and are derived from the celiac plexus.

Relational Anatomy

The spleen lies between the left hemidiaphragm and the stomach. The diaphragm may be seen as a bright, curvilinear, echogenic structure close to the proximal superolateral surface of the spleen. Posteriorly, the diaphragm, left pleura, left lung, and ribs are in contact with the spleen. The medial surface is related to the stomach and lesser sac (Fig. 11.7). The fundus of the stomach may contain gas or fluid, which may cause confusion in the left upper quadrant during attempts to demonstrate the spleen. Alteration in the patient's position or ingestion of fluids may help to separate the stomach from splenic tissue. The tail of the pancreas lies posterior to the stomach and lesser sac as it approaches the hilum of the spleen and splenic vessels. The spleen may serve as a good acoustic window to image the tail of the pancreas. The left kidney lies inferior and medial to the spleen.

Displacement of the Spleen

The spleen is held in place by the **lienorenal**, gastrosplenic, and phrenocolic ligaments (see Fig. 11.3). These ligaments are derived from the layers of the peritoneum that form the greater and lesser sacs. A mass in the left upper quadrant may displace the spleen inferiorly. Caudal displacement may occur secondary to a subclavian abscess, splenic cyst, or left pleural effusion. Cephalic displacement may result from volume loss in the left lung, left lobe pneumonia, paralysis of the left hemidiaphragm, or a large intra-abdominal mass. A normal spleen with medial lobulation between the pancreatic tail and the left kidney may be confused with a cystic mass in the tail of the pancreas.

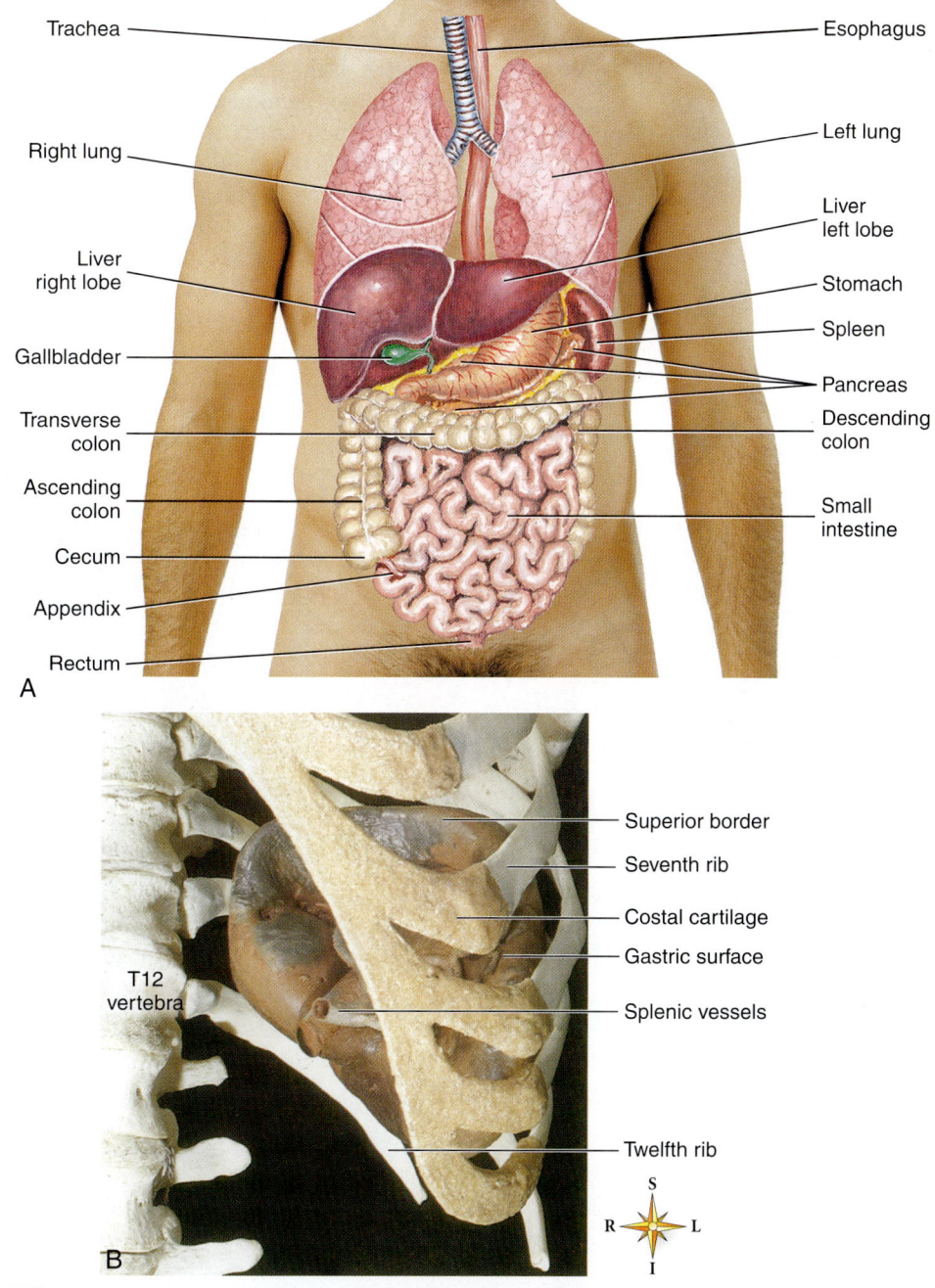

FIG. 11.1 The spleen lies between the left hemidiaphragm and the stomach. Posteriorly, the diaphragm, left pleura, left lung, and ribs are in contact with the spleen. The medial surface is related to the stomach and lesser sac. The tail of the pancreas lies posterior to the stomach and lesser sac as it approaches the hilum of the spleen and splenic vessels. The left kidney lies inferior and medial to the spleen. (A) Anterior view of the upper abdomen shows the posterior position of the spleen in the left upper quadrant. (B) The normal spleen should not extend beyond the 12th rib.

The term **wandering spleen** describes a spleen that has migrated from its normal location in the left upper quadrant. It results from an embryologic anomaly of the dorsal mesentery that fails to fuse with the posterior peritoneum without supporting ligaments of the spleen. The patient may present with an abdominal or pelvic mass, intermittent pain, and volvulus, that is, splenic torsion. The sonographer should use color Doppler to map the vascularity within the spleen. When torsion is complete, the vascular pattern shows decreased velocity.

CONGENITAL ANOMALIES

Splenic Agenesis

Complete absence of the spleen (asplenia), or **splenic agenesis**, is rare, and by itself, causes no difficulties. However, it may occur as part of a significant congenital abnormality. Visceral heterotaxy is the common name that consists of a spectrum of anomalies. Asplenic or **polysplenia** syndromes are associated with complex cardiac malformations, bronchopulmonary

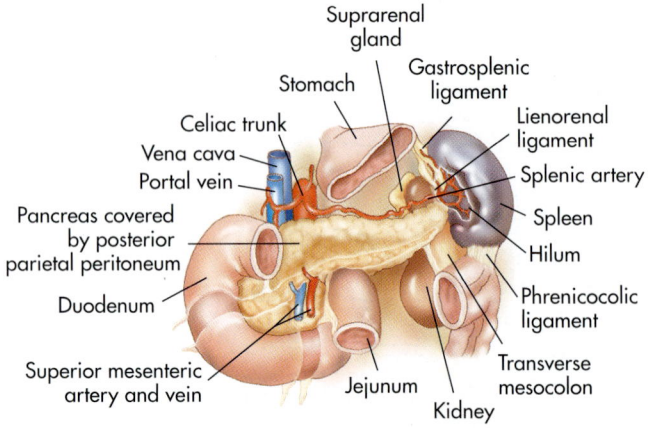

FIG. 11.2 **Anterior view of the spleen as it lies in the left hypochondrium.** Note the relational anatomy, ligament attachments, and vascular landmarks.

abnormalities, or visceral heterotaxis (anomalous placement of organs or major blood vessels, including a horizontal liver, malrotation of the gut, and interruption of the inferior vena cava with azygos continuation). The typical arrangement of asymmetrical body parts is called *situs solitus*. The mirror image condition is called *situs inversus*. The term *situs ambiguous* is used when the anatomy falls in between these two conditions.

Patients with polysplenia may have bilateral left-sidedness (two morphologic left lungs, left-sided azygous continuation of an interrupted inferior vena cava, biliary atresia, absence of the gallbladder, gastrointestinal malrotation, and cardiovascular abnormalities). On the other hand, patients with asplenia may have bilateral right-sidedness (two morphologic right lungs, midline location of the liver, reversed position of the abdominal aorta and inferior vena cava, anomalous pulmonary venous return, and horseshoe kidneys). Patients

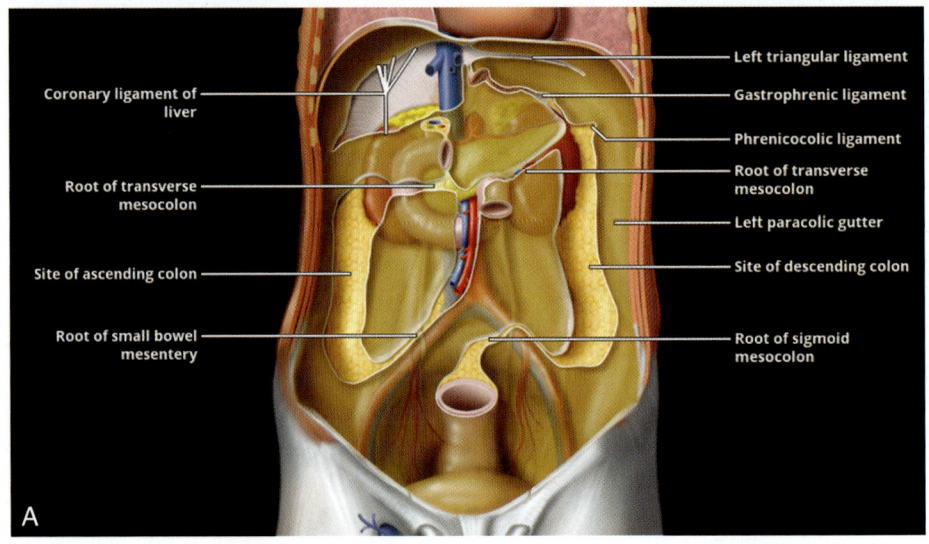

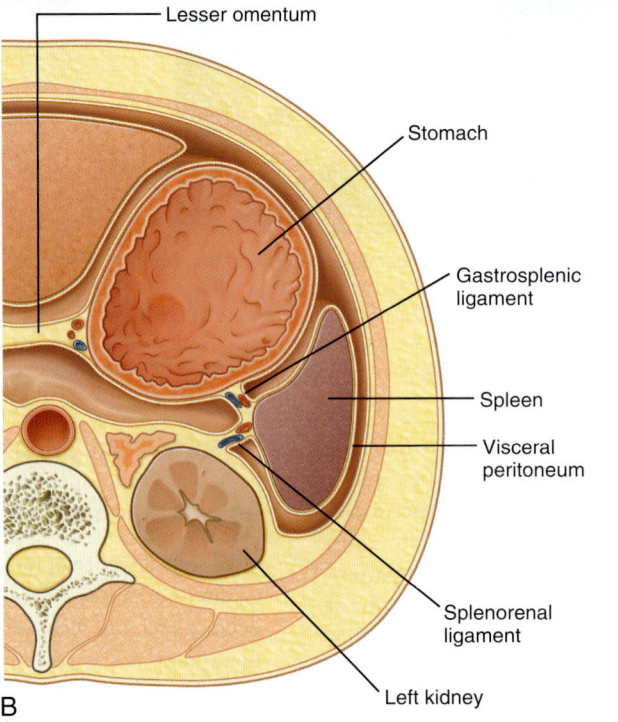

FIG. 11.3 The splenorenal ligament that extends between the hilum of the spleen and left kidney, the phrenicocolic ligament, and the gastrosplenic ligament that connects the fundus of the stomach to the hilum of the spleen.

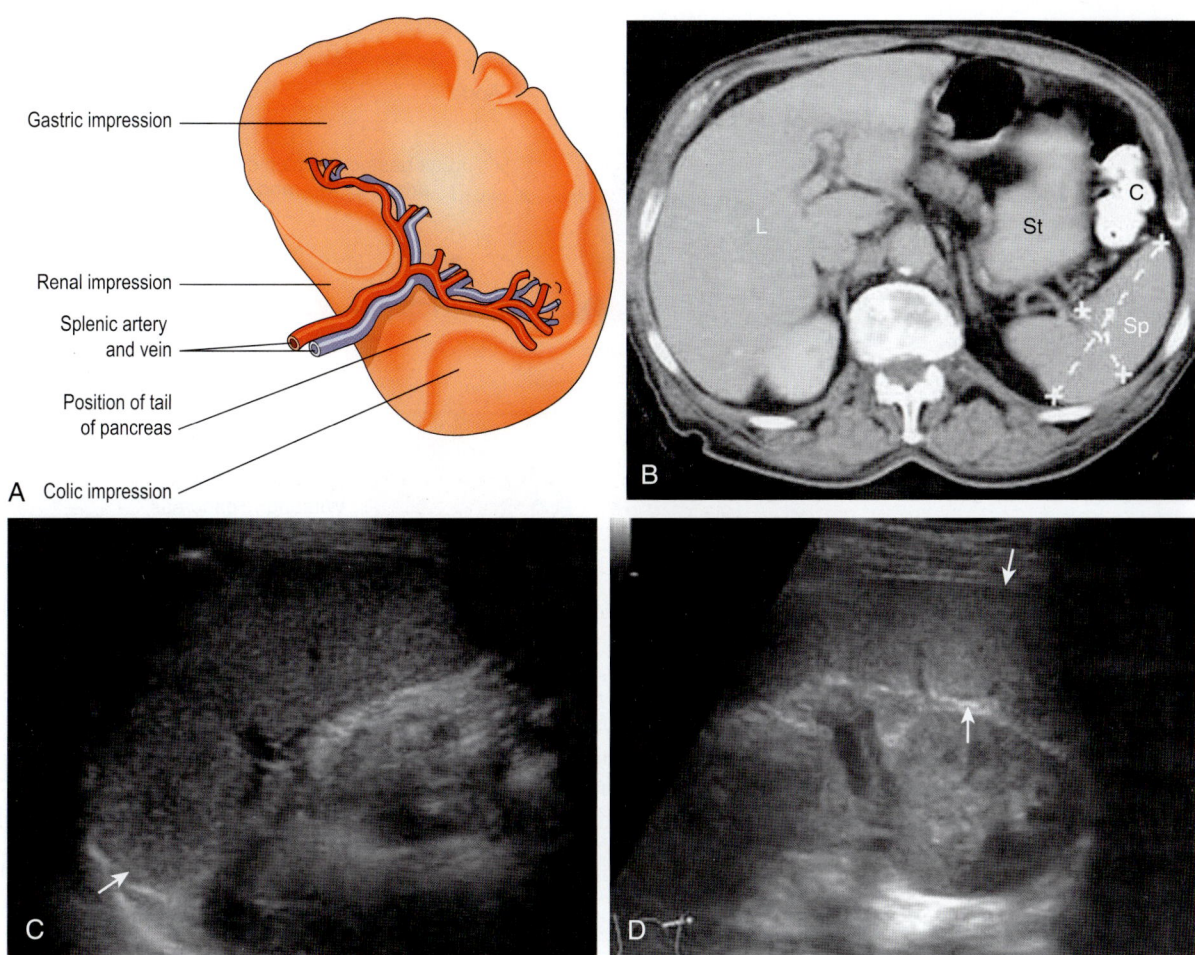

FIG. 11.4 (A) The spleen is variable in size and shape: "orange segment," tetrahedral, or triangular. (B) Transverse computed tomographic image of the upper left quadrant demonstrates the posterior position of the spleen. Longitudinal image of the spleen with measurement of its length (C) and transverse image with measurement of the A–P dimension of the spleen (D). *C*, Colon; *L*, liver; *Sp*, spleen; *St*, stomach.

with agenesis of the spleen have significant problems with severe infection as their immune response is absent.

Splenic agenesis may be ruled out by demonstrating a spleen on ultrasound. The sonographer should be careful not to confuse the spleen with the bowel, which may lie in the area usually occupied by the spleen. Color Doppler helps determine the splenic vascular pattern and thus helps to separate it from the colon.

Accessory Spleen

An **accessory spleen**, or splenunculus, is a more common congenital anomaly that may be found in up to 30% of patients (Fig. 11.8). The accessory spleen may be difficult to demonstrate by sonography if it is very small. However, when it is seen, it appears as a homogeneous pattern similar to that of the spleen. It usually is found near the hilum or inferior border of the spleen but has been reported elsewhere in the abdominal cavity. Lesions affecting the normal spleen would also affect the accessory spleen. An accessory spleen results from failure of fusion of separate splenic masses forming on the dorsal mesogastrium; it is most commonly located in the splenic hilum or along the splenic vessels or associated ligaments. The location of the accessory spleen has been reported anywhere from the diaphragm to the scrotum, and it is usually solitary. It usually remains small and does not present as a clinical problem. The accessory spleen may simulate enlarged lymph nodes in the spleen area or a tumor of the pancreatic, suprarenal, or retroperitoneal structures. As the spleen enlarges, so does the accessory spleen.

PHYSIOLOGY AND LABORATORY DATA OF THE SPLEEN

The spleen is part of the reticuloendothelial system and is rarely the site of primary disease. It is commonly involved in metabolic, hematopoietic, and infectious disorders. Blunt abdominal trauma to the spleen may result in splenic laceration and rupture. The spleen is active in the body's defense against disease; its primary function is to filter the peripheral blood.

The spleen is a soft organ with elastic properties that allow it to distend as blood fills the venous sinuses. These characteristics are related to the function of the spleen as a blood reservoir. Within the lobules of the spleen are tissues called

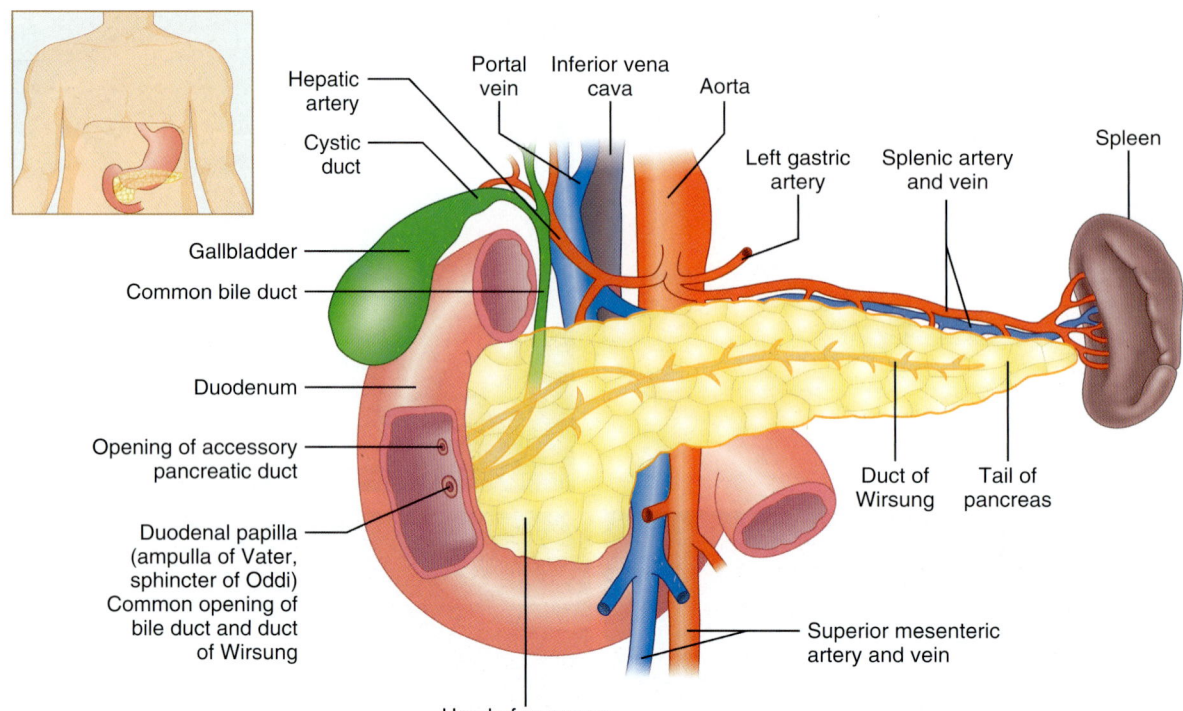

FIG. 11.5 **The splenic hilum with the splenic artery and vein.** The splenic artery *(red)* flows from the celiac axis into the splenic hilum, while the splenic vein *(blue)* empties the spleen into the main portal vein.

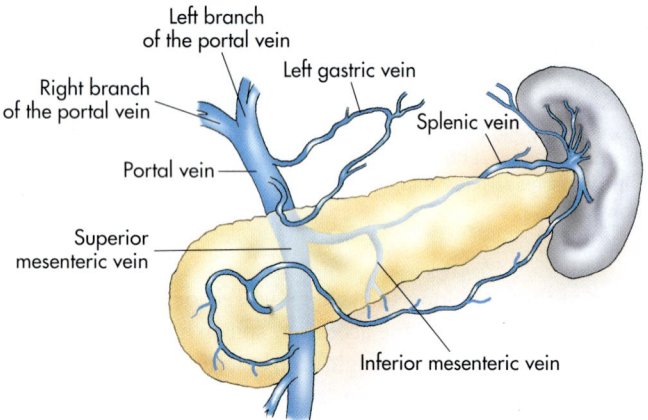

FIG. 11.6 The splenic vein leaves the hilum of the spleen to join the main portal vein posterior to the head of the pancreas.

pulp. Two components are found within the spleen: red pulp and white pulp (Fig. 11.9). *White pulp* is distributed throughout the spleen in tiny islands. This tissue consists of splenic nodules, similar to those found in lymph nodes, and contains large numbers of lymphocytes. *Red pulp* fills the remaining spaces of the lobules and surrounds the venous sinuses. The pulp contains relatively large numbers of red blood cells, which are responsible for its color, along with many lymphocytes and macrophages.

The **red pulp** of the spleen consists of splenic sinuses alternating with splenic cords. The blood capillaries within the red pulp are quite permeable. Red blood cells can squeeze through the pores in these capillary walls and enter the venous sinuses. The older, more fragile red blood cells may rupture as they make this passage, and the resulting cellular debris is removed by phagocytic macrophages located within the splenic sinuses. The macrophages engulf and destroy foreign particles, such as bacteria, that may be carried in the blood as it flows through the sinuses. The lymphocytes of the spleen help to defend the body against infection. The blood that leaves the splenic sinuses to enter the reticular cords passes through a complex filter. The venous drainage of the sinuses and cords is not well defined, but it is assumed that tributaries of the splenic vein connect with sinuses of the red pulp.

The **white pulp** of the spleen consists of the malpighian corpuscles, small nodular masses of lymphoid tissue attached to the smaller arterial branches. Extending from the splenic capsule inward are the trabeculae, which contain blood vessels and lymphatics. The lymphoid tissue or malpighian corpuscles have the same structure as the follicles in the lymph nodes; however, they differ in that the splenic follicles surround arteries so that on cross section, each contains a central artery. These follicles are scattered throughout the organ and are not confined to the peripheral layer or cortex, as are lymph nodes.

As part of the reticuloendothelial system, the spleen plays an important role in the defense mechanisms of the body and is also implicated in pigment and lipid metabolism. It is not essential to life and can be removed with no ill effects. The functions of the spleen may be classified under two general headings: those that reflect the functions of the reticuloendothelial system and those that are characteristic of the organ itself (Box 11.1). The role of the spleen as an immunologic organ involves the production of cells capable of making antibodies (lymphocytes and plasma cells); however, antibodies are also produced at other sites.

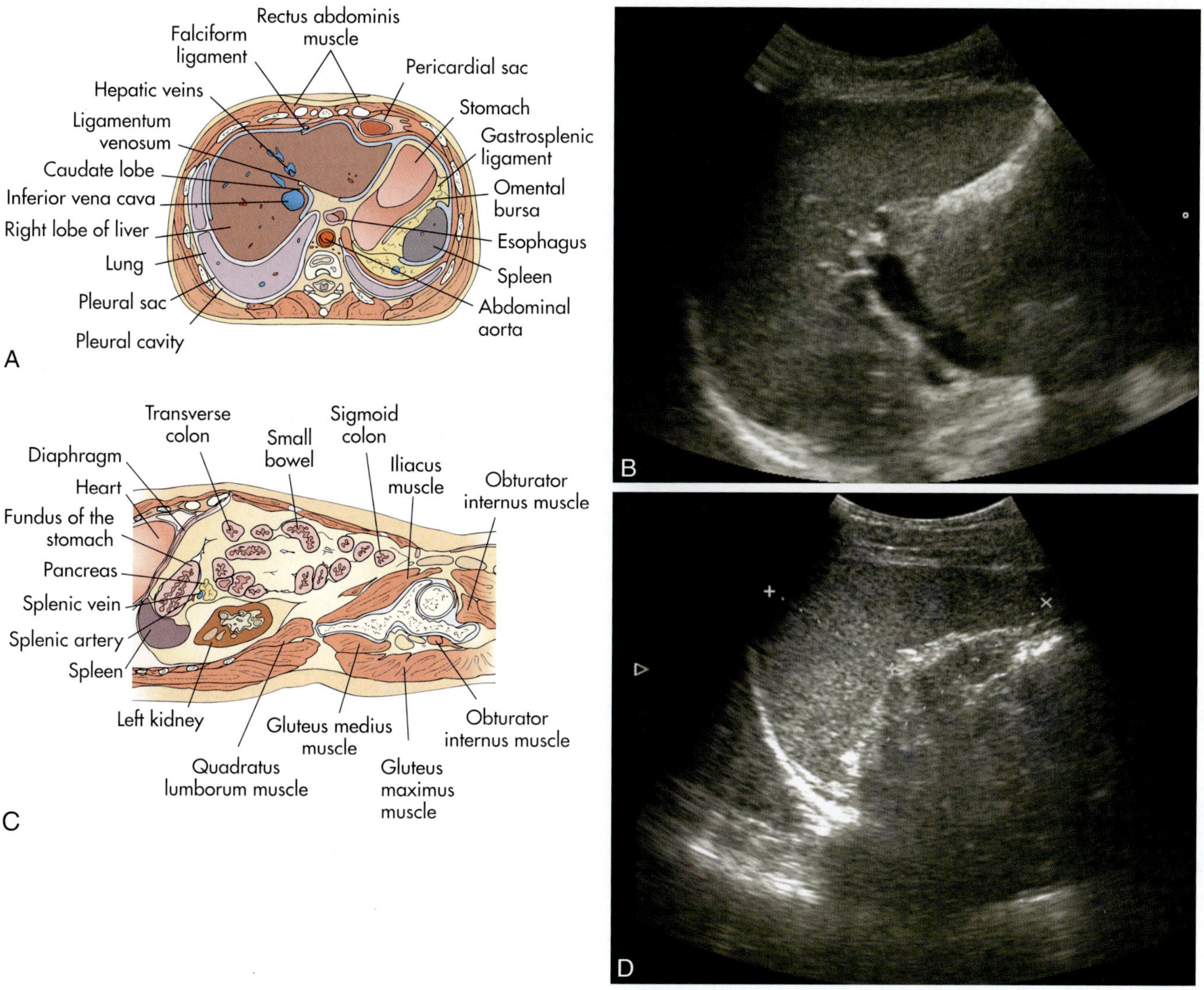

FIG. 11.7 (A–B) Transverse section of the diaphragm and spleen with the corresponding sonographic image. (C–D) Longitudinal cross-section of the spleen with corresponding sonographic image.

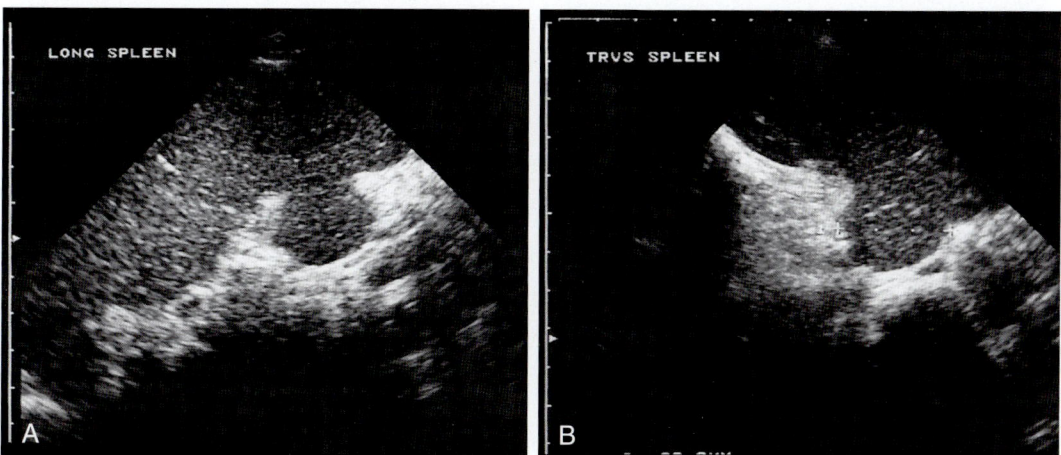

FIG. 11.8 Accessory spleen. Longitudinal (A) and transverse (B) images of the small accessory spleen as it projects from the hilum of the spleen.

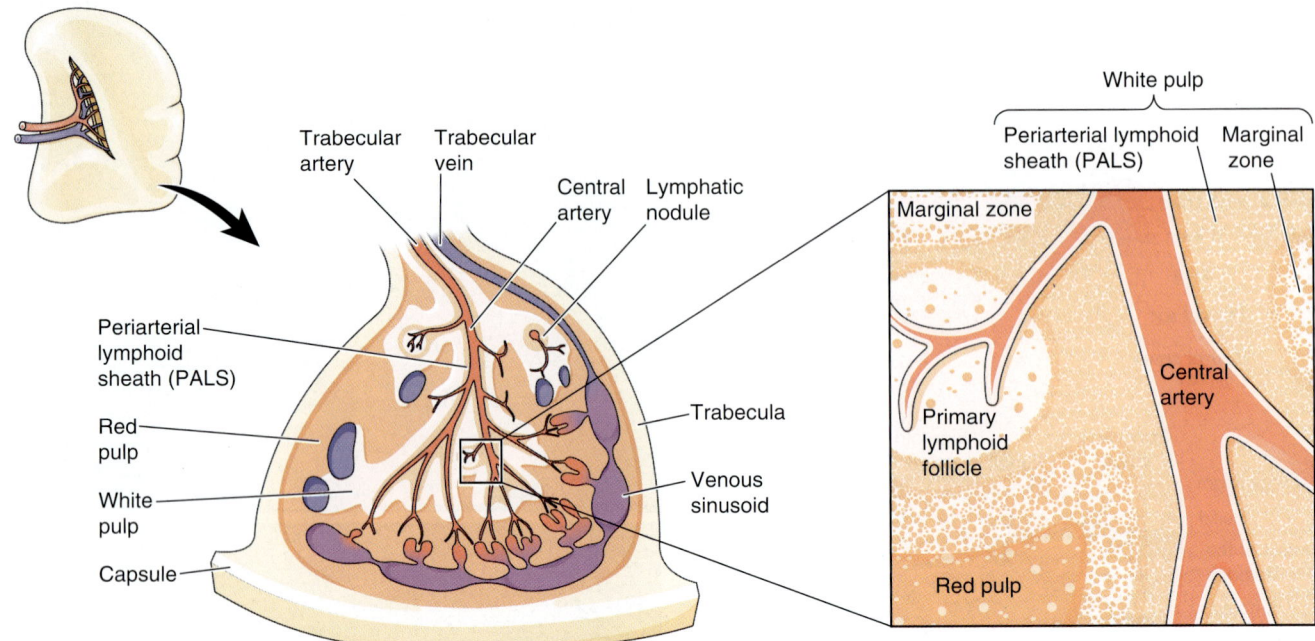

FIG. 11.9 Within the lobules of the spleen are tissues called red pulp and white pulp. *White pulp* is distributed throughout the spleen in tiny islands. This tissue consists of splenic nodules, similar to those found in lymph nodes, and contains large numbers of lymphocytes. *Red pulp* fills the remaining spaces of the lobules and surrounds the venous sinuses. The pulp contains relatively large numbers of red blood cells, which are responsible for its color, along with many lymphocytes and macrophages.

BOX 11.1 Functions of the Spleen as an Organ of the Reticuloendothelial System

Functions as an Organ of the Reticuloendothelial System
Production of lymphocytes and plasma cells
Production of antibodies
Storage of iron
Storage of other metabolites

Characteristic Functions
Maturation of the surface of erythrocytes
Reservoir
Culling
Pitting function
Disposal of senescent or abnormal erythrocytes
Functions related to platelet and leukocyte life span

Phagocytosis of **erythrocytes** and the breakdown of **hemoglobin** occur throughout the entire reticuloendothelial system, but roughly half the catabolic activity is localized in the normal spleen. In splenomegaly, the major portion of hemoglobin breakdown occurs in the spleen. The iron that is liberated is stored in the splenic phagocytes. In anomalies such as the hemolytic anemias, the splenic phagocytes become engorged with **hemosiderin** when erythrocyte destruction is accelerated. In addition to storing iron, the spleen is subject to storage diseases such as Gaucher disease and Niemann-Pick disease. Abnormal lipid metabolites accumulate in all phagocytic reticuloendothelial cells but may also involve the phagocytes in the spleen, producing gross splenomegaly.

Functions of the spleen that are characteristic of the organ relate primarily to the circulation of erythrocytes through it. In a normal individual, the spleen contains only about 20 to 30 mL of erythrocytes. In splenomegaly, the reservoir function is significantly increased, and the abnormally enlarged spleen contains many times this volume of red blood cells. Transit time is lengthened, and the erythrocytes are subject to destructive effects for a long time. In part, ptosis causes glucose consumption, on which the erythrocyte depends to maintain normal metabolism, and the erythrocyte is destroyed. Selective destruction of abnormal erythrocytes is also accelerated by splenic pooling.

As erythrocytes pass through the spleen, the organ inspects them for imperfections and destroys those it recognizes as abnormal or senescent. **Pitting** is the process of removing the nuclei from the red blood cells. **Culling** is the process by which the spleen removes abnormal red blood cells. The normal function of the spleen keeps the number of circulating erythrocytes with inclusions at a minimum.

The spleen also pools platelets in large numbers. Entry of platelets into the splenic pool and their return to the circulation are extensive. In splenomegaly, the splenic pool may be so large that it produces thrombocytopenia. Sequestration of leukocytes in the enlarged spleen may produce leukopenia.

Laboratory data include the following:
- **Hematocrit**. The hematocrit indicates the percentage of red blood cells per volume of blood. Abnormally low readings indicate hemorrhage or internal bleeding within the body.
- **Bacteremia**. The test for bacteremia indicates the presence of bacteria within the body. The term *sepsis* indicates

bacteria in the bloodstream. Typical symptoms of fever and chills, along with other medical conditions, may indicate the presence of an infection.
- **Leukocytosis.** An increase in the number of white cells present in the blood is usually a typical finding in infection. This finding may also occur after surgery, in malignancies, or the presence of leukemia.
- **Leukopenia.** Abnormal decrease in white blood corpuscles may be secondary to certain medications or bone marrow disorder.
- **Thrombocytopenia.** Thrombocytopenia is an abnormal decrease in platelets, which may be due to internal hemorrhage.

SONOGRAPHIC EVALUATION OF THE SPLEEN

Spleen Protocol

Ultrasound examinations are performed to assess overall splenic architecture, examine or detect intrasplenic masses, examine the splenic hilum and vasculature, and determine splenic size (Fig. 11.10 and Box 11.2).
1. Patient preparation: NPO for at least 6 hours.
2. Transducer selection: broadband (2.5 to 4 MHz) curvilinear or sector.
3. Patient position: Supine or decubitus; use steep left lateral if echo bed with a drop-leaf component is available
4. Images and observations include the following:
   - Coronal scans of the long axis of the spleen should be performed.
   - The left hemidiaphragm, splenic hilus, and upper and lower borders of the spleen should be demonstrated.
   - The splenic length should be measured.
   - The texture of the spleen should be compared with that of the liver. The splenic parenchyma should be homogeneous with the liver.
   - Transverse scans of the spleen at the level of the splenic hilus should be performed. The sonographer should look for increased vascularity or splenic nodes with a sweep from the superior to inferior borders.

Normal Texture and Patterns

Sonographically, the splenic parenchyma should have a fine uniform homogeneous mid- to low-level echo pattern and be slightly more echogenic than the liver parenchyma (Fig. 11.11). As the spleen enlarges, echogenicity further increases. The shape of the spleen has considerable variation. The spleen has two components joined at the hilum: a superomedial component and an inferolateral component. Transverse scans have a crescent-shaped "inverted comma"

BOX 11.2	Abdominal Protocol: Spleen

Scan Plane Anatomy
Long spleen/left kidney; measure length; color Doppler
Transverse splenic hilum/measure width; color Doppler

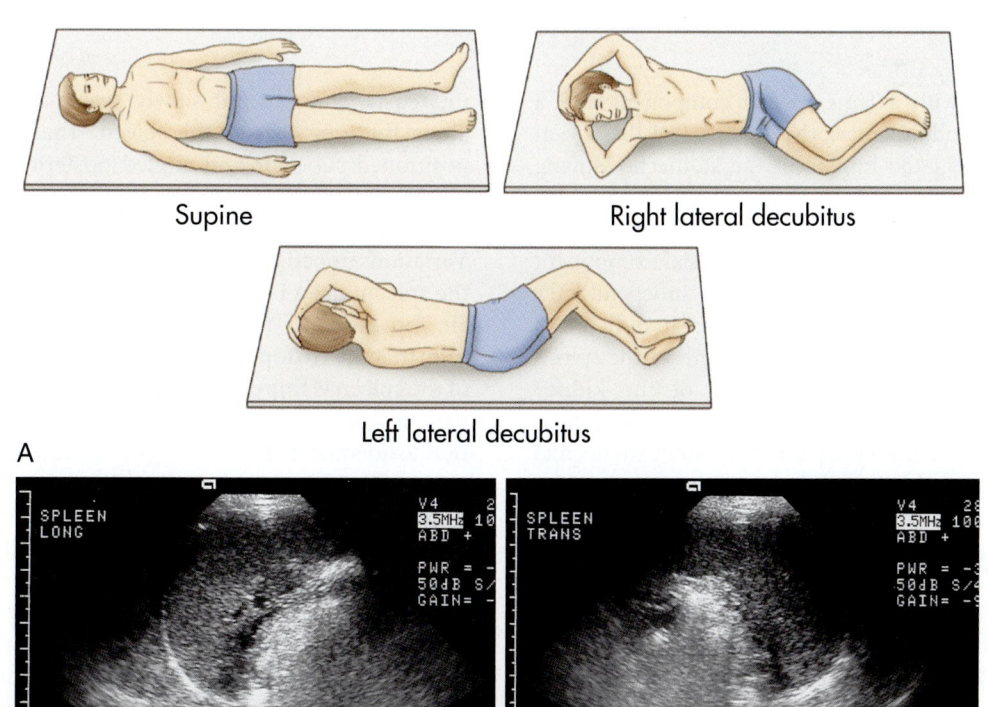

FIG. 11.10 (A) Positions to image the spleen include supine and decubitus. Longitudinal (B) and transverse (C) images of the normal spleen. The parenchyma is homogeneous throughout except for the area of the hilum where the vascular structures enter and leave the spleen.

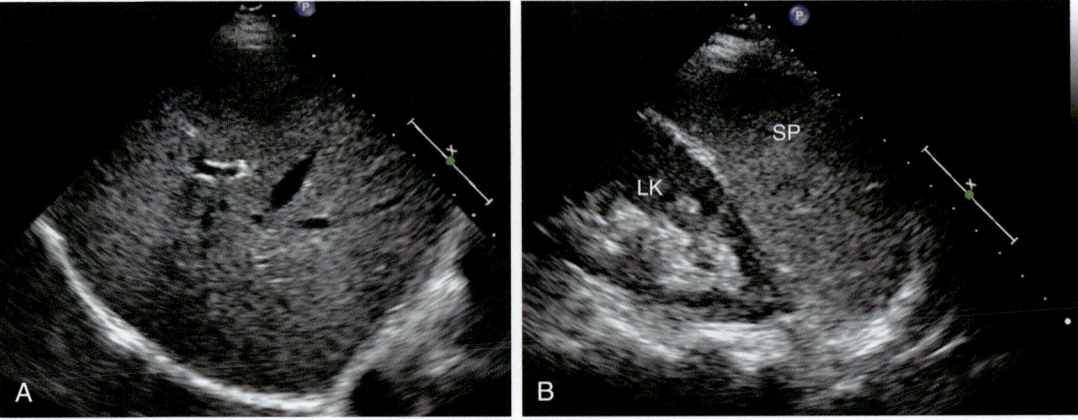

FIG. 11.11 The splenic parenchyma should have a fine uniform homogeneous mid-to-low level echo pattern, which is slightly more echogenic than the liver. Liver (A) and spleen (B). *LK*, Left kidney; *SP*, spleen.

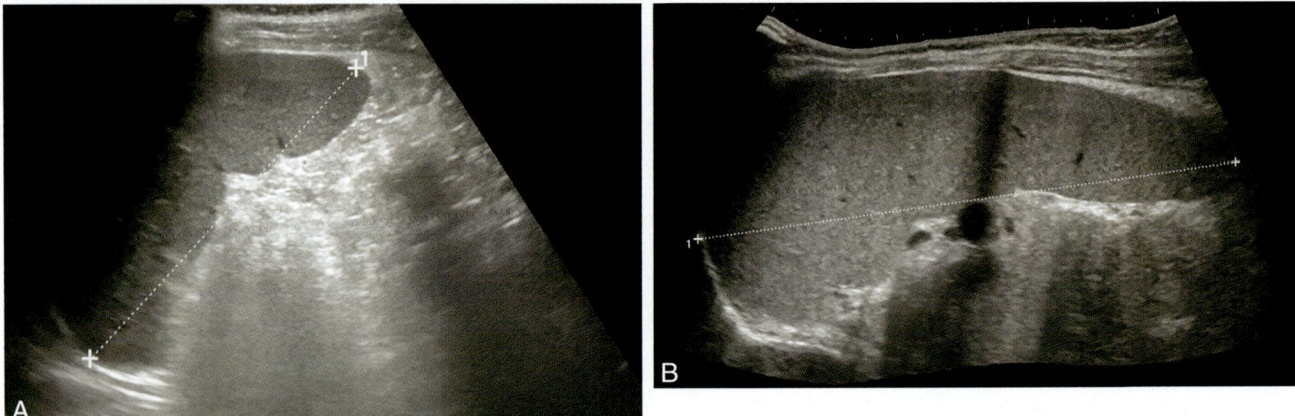

FIG. 11.12 (A) The length of the spleen should measure less than 13 cm. (B) Splenomegaly shows the length of the spleen to measure over 20 cm.

appearance, usually with a large medial component and a thin component extending anteriorly. This part of the spleen may be seen to indent the fundus of the stomach. Moving inferiorly, only the lateral component is imaged. On longitudinal scans, the superior component extends more medially than the inferior component. The superomedial component or the inferolateral component may enlarge independently. The irregularity of these components makes it difficult to assess mild splenomegaly accurately. The length of the spleen usually measures greater than the length of the kidney (Fig. 11.12). Splenomegaly is diagnosed when the spleen measures more than 13 cm in the adult patient or more than normal length in the respective child.

Patient Position and Technique

The left upper quadrant may be imaged as the sonographer carefully manipulates the transducer between intercostal margins to image the left kidney, spleen, and diaphragm. The sector transducer may fit between the intercostal margins better than the larger curved-array transducer. The spleen generally lies in an oblique pathway in the posterior left upper quadrant; therefore, with the patient supine, the transducer should be placed in the superior left upper quadrant intercostal margin and slowly sweep anterior to posterior along the long axis of the spleen. The transducer must be positioned superior and angled posterior enough to image the spleen (Fig. 11.13). A deep inspiration may help to bring the spleen into the field of view from the subcostal approach. Variations in patient respiration may also facilitate imaging of the spleen; deep inspiration causes the lungs to expand with air and displaces the diaphragm; the lungs may expand so fully that the costophrenic angle is obscured and visualization of the spleen is impeded. The sonographer should observe the patient's breathing pattern and modify the amount of inspiration to adequately image the spleen without interference from the air-filled lungs.

When the patient is lying supine, the problem of overlying air-filled stomach or bowel anterior to the spleen may interfere with adequate visualization. The steep right decubitus position with the intercostal approach is not recommended as this causes the spleen to fall away from the abdominal wall and allows aerated lung to migrate inferiorly and obscure the acoustic window. If the ultrasound laboratory has an echo bed with a drop-leaf component, the patient should be rolled onto their left side and the transducer directed along the left intercostal margin to image the spleen. Excellent visualization is achieved because the spleen will lie flush against the patient's abdominal wall.

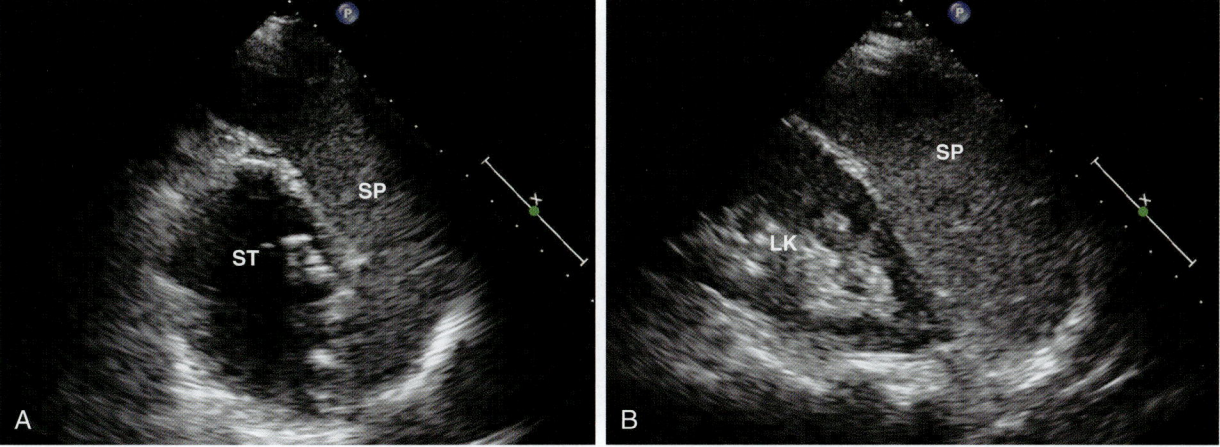

FIG. 11.13 Normal images of the spleen. (A) Transverse image of the spleen (SP) and fluid-filled stomach (ST). (B) Longitudinal image of the spleen and left kidney (LK).

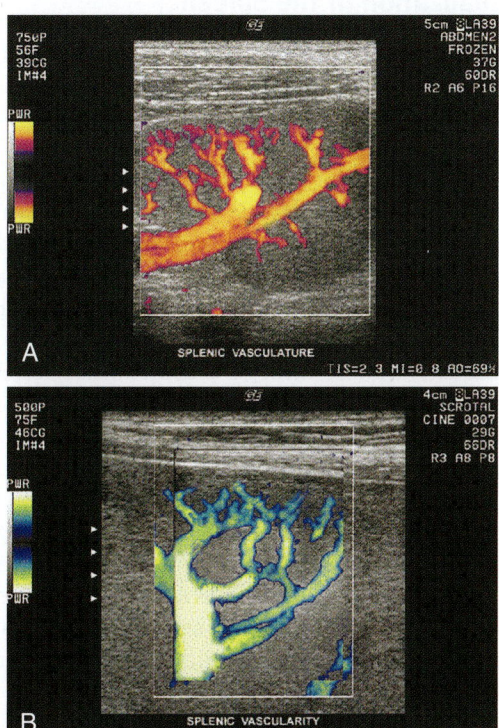

FIG. 11.14 (A) Color Doppler shows the splenic arterial system within the spleen. (B) The splenic venous system is well demarcated with color Doppler.

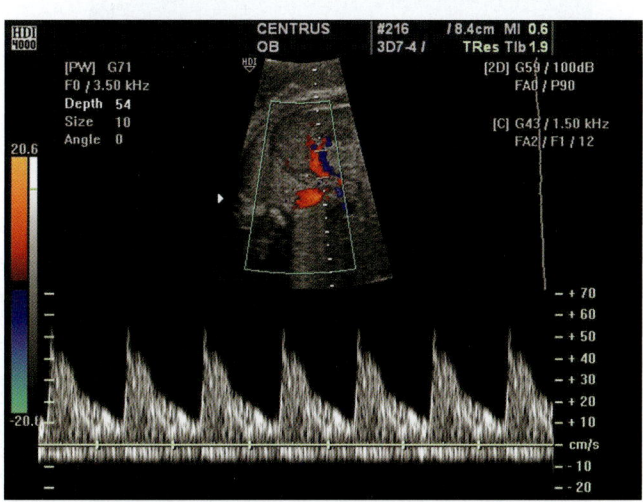

FIG. 11.15 Forward (positive to the baseline) pulsatile arterial flow should be seen entering the main splenic artery.

In a routine abdominal examination, the spleen should be surveyed to ensure that the parenchyma is uniform with a homogeneous texture, except for the splenic hilum, which shows normal tubular vascular structures (Fig. 11.14) At least two images of the spleen should be recorded in the longitudinal and transverse planes. The longitudinal plane, the image should demonstrate the left hemidiaphragm, the superior and inferior margins of the spleen, and with medial angulation, the upper pole of the left kidney. The sonographer should look at the left pleural space superior to the diaphragm to see if fluid is present in the lower costal margin. The long axis of the spleen is measured from its superior-to-inferior border.

After the longitudinal oblique scan is completed, the transducer is rotated 90 degrees to survey the spleen in a transverse plane. The sonographer should obtain at least one transverse image at the hilum of the spleen. The sonographer should observe the flow of the splenic artery and vein with color Doppler. Forward (positive to the baseline) pulsatile arterial flow should be seen entering the main splenic artery as it bifurcates into multiple branches to supply the splenic parenchyma (Fig. 11.15). Conversely, returning flow (negative to the baseline) from the multiple splenic venous branches enters into the splenic vein. The splenic vein leaves the hilum of the spleen to transverse horizontally across the abdomen before joining the superior mesenteric vein, which leads into the main portal vein anterior to the inferior vena cava (Fig. 11.16).

Increased hypoechoic structures in the area of the splenic hilum may indicate portal hypertension with collateral vessels or enlarged lymph nodes. A correlation has been noted between the caliber of splenic arteries and the size

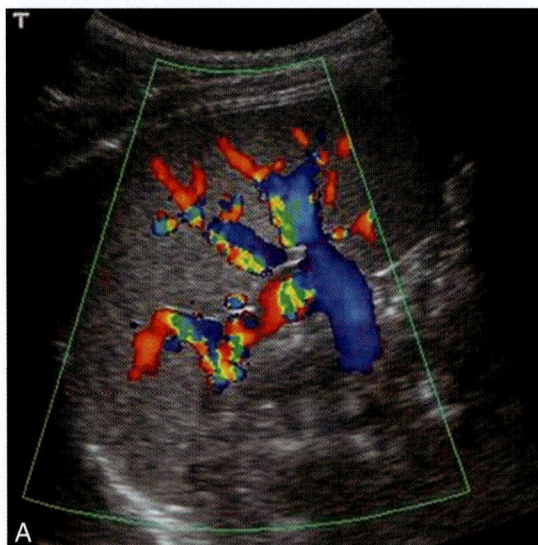

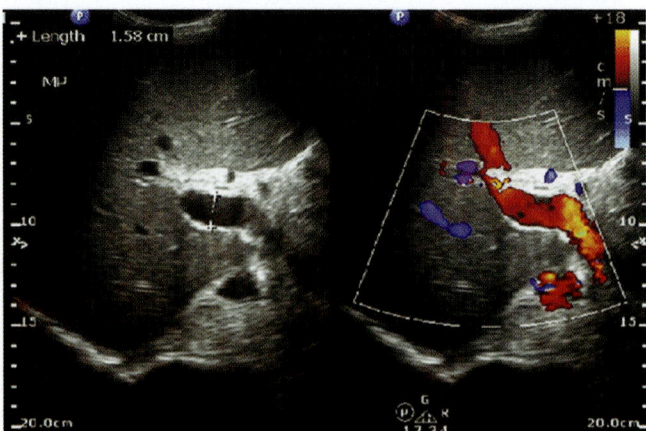

FIG. 11.17 Color Doppler shows the dilated splenic vessels that may be seen with portal hypertension and varices.

Nonvisualization of the Spleen

The inability to image the spleen in its standard location may result from one of several conditions (e.g., asplenia syndrome, polysplenia syndrome, traumatic fragmentation of the spleen, wandering spleen).

Atrophy. Atrophy of the spleen may occur in average individuals. It may also occur in wasting diseases. Chronic hemolytic anemias, particularly sickle cell anemia, involve excessive loss of pulp, increasing fibrosis, scarring from multiple infarcts, and encrustation with iron and calcium deposits. In the final stages of atrophy, the spleen may be so small that it is hardly recognizable. Advanced atrophy is sometimes referred to as autosplenectomy.

PATHOLOGY OF THE SPLEEN

Table 11.1 and Box 11.3 list the clinical findings, sonographic findings, and differential considerations for selected splenic diseases and conditions to include splenomegaly, infection, infarction, trauma, cystic disease, and primary tumors. The sonographic appearance of splenic disorders is found in Table 11.2.

SPLENOMEGALY

As the largest unit of the reticuloendothelial system, the spleen is involved in all systemic inflammations and generalized hematopoietic disorders and much metabolic disturbance (Box 11.4). Whenever the spleen is involved in systemic disease, splenic enlargement, or **splenomegaly**, usually develops (Fig. 11.18).

Obvious gross splenomegaly is easily defined with sonography. If mild splenomegaly is present, sonographic findings may be more challenging to obtain. Volume measurements of the spleen are necessary to determine the exact size. Although splenomegaly is the most common

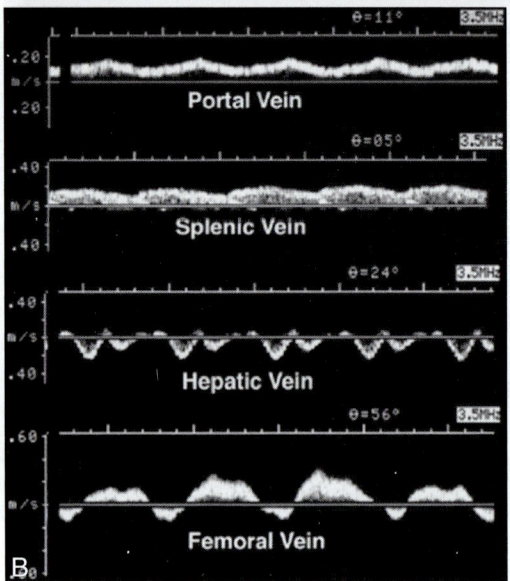

FIG. 11.16 (A) Returning flow (negative to the baseline) from the multiple splenic venous branches enters into the splenic vein, shown in blue. (B) The pulsatile Doppler represents the biphasic flow pattern of the splenic vein.

of the spleen in cirrhotic patients with esophageal varices. The splenic artery is larger in patients with splenomegaly (patients with cirrhosis with esophageal varices and patients with hematologic malignancies). The use of color Doppler imaging will help the sonographer determine whether the structures are vascular or nonvascular in composition (Fig. 11.17).

Care should be taken when hepatomegaly is present with a prominent left lobe of the liver. The homogeneous texture of the liver may be confused as the spleen, especially if the left lobe extends to the left upper quadrant. The sonographer should evaluate the patient in multiple planes to separate the splenic tissue from the hepatic structures.

TABLE 11.1	Splenic Findings	
Clinical Findings	**Sonographic Findings**	**Differential Considerations**
Splenomegaly		
Depends on cause	Long axis ≥13 cm Look for liver anomalies (e.g., cirrhosis, diffuse disease)	
Splenic Abscess		
Fever Leukocytosis	Splenomegaly Irregular, ill-defined borders May have internal septa	Hematoma Necrotic neoplasm Lymphoma Leukemia
Splenic Infarction		
Related to primary diagnosis	Acute: wedge-shaped, hypoechoic area Chronic: wedge-shaped, echogenic area (base points to periphery) Look for splenic atrophy	Infection Hemorrhage Neoplasm Lymphoma
Splenic Trauma		
↓ Hematocrit	Spleen may appear enlarged Hematoma may form later along subcapsular area or internally	
Splenic Cysts		
Asymptomatic	Solitary Anechoic ↑ transmission Well-defined walls Look for tissue compression	Hematoma Lymphangioma Echinococcal cyst
Primary Tumors		
Depends on primary	Splenomegaly May be diffuse, single, or multiple Hypoechoic to hyperechoic	Infection

> **BOX 11.3 Pathologic Classification of Splenic Disorders**
>
> **Hematopoiesis**
> Granulocytopoiesis
> - Reactive hyperplasia to acute and chronic infection (low sonodensity)
>
> Noncaseous granulomatous inflammation
> Myeloproliferative syndromes (normal)
> Chronic myelogenous leukemia
> Acute myelogenous leukemia
> Lymphopoiesis (low sonodensity or focal sonolucent)
> Chronic lymphocytic leukemia
> - Lymphoma
> - Hodgkin disease
>
> Erythropoiesis (normal)
> Sickle cell disease
> - Hereditary spherocytosis
> - Hemolytic anemia
> - Chronic anemia
> - Myeloproliferative syndrome
>
> Other
> - Multiple myeloma (low sonodensity)
>
> **Reticuloendothelial Hyperactivity (Normal)**
> Still disease
> Wilson disease
> Felty syndrome
> Reticulum cell sarcoma
>
> **Congestion (Normal or Low Sonodensity)**
> Hepatocellular disease
>
> **Nonspecific**
> Neoplasm-metastasis (focal sonodense)
> Cyst (focal sonolucent)
> Abscess (focal sonolucent)
> Malignant neoplasm (focal sonolucent)
> - Hodgkin disease
> - Lymphoma
>
> Benign neoplasm (focal sonolucent)
> - Lymphangiomatosis
>
> Hematoma (perisplenic)

TABLE 11.2	Sonographic-Pathologic Classification of Splenic Disorders				
	Uniform Splenic Sonodensity			**Focal Defects**	
Normal Sonodensity	**Low Sonodensity**	**Sonodense**		**Sonolucent**	**Perisplenic Defects**
Erythropoiesis (including myeloproliferative disorders) Reticuloendothelial Congestion Hyperactivity	Granulocytopoiesis (excluding myelo disorders) Lymphopoiesis Other (multiple myeloma) Congestion	Nonspecific (metastasis)		Nonspecific (benign primary neoplasm, cyst, abscess, malignant neoplasm [lymphopoietic])	Nonspecific (hematoma)

From Mittelstaedt CA, Partain CL. Ultrasonic-pathologic classification of splenic abnormalities: gray-scale patterns. *Radiology*. 1980;134:697.

disease process encountered by the sonographer when evaluating this organ, careful evaluation of splenic contour and homogeneity should be undertaken to determine whether a disease process involves the spleen. Assessment of the splenic parenchyma and vascular patterns may demonstrate changes in the size, texture, and vascularity of the organ, which could be helpful in the patient's clinical evaluation to rule out the presence of a diffuse disease process or focal lesion. The spleen may grow to enormous size with extension into the iliac fossa. The medial segment may cross the midline of the abdomen to mimic a mass inferior to the left lobe of the liver. Splenomegaly has multiple causes, as noted in Box 11.5. Table 11.3 lists possible causes, depending on the degree of enlargement.

BOX 11.4	Causes of Splenomegaly

Collagen-vascular disease
Congestion
Extramedullary hematopoiesis
Hemolytic anemia
Infection
Neoplasm
Storage disease
Trauma

BOX 11.5	Causes of Congestive Splenomegaly

Heart failure
Portal hypertension, portal or splenic vein thrombosis
Leukemia
Lymphoma
Mononucleosis
Generalized infections
Hemolytic anemias
Glycogen storage disease
Malaria
Myelofibrosis

TABLE 11.3	Causes of Splenomegaly
Degree of Splenomegaly	**Possible Causes**
Mild to moderate	Infection
	Portal hypertension
	AIDS
Moderate	Leukemia
	Lymphoma
	Infectious mononucleosis
Massive	Myelofibrosis
Focal lesions	Lymphomatous involvement
	Metastatic disease
	Hematomas

Clinical signs of splenomegaly may include left upper quadrant pain (secondary to stretching of the splenic capsule or ligaments) or fullness. Enlargement of the spleen may encroach upon surrounding organs, such as the left kidney, pancreas, stomach, and intestines (Fig. 11.19).

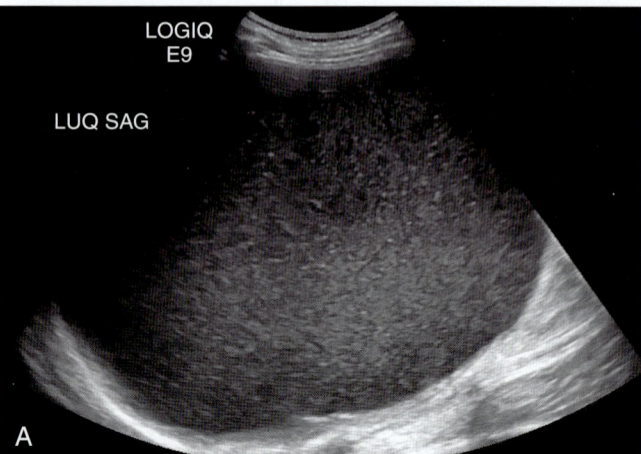

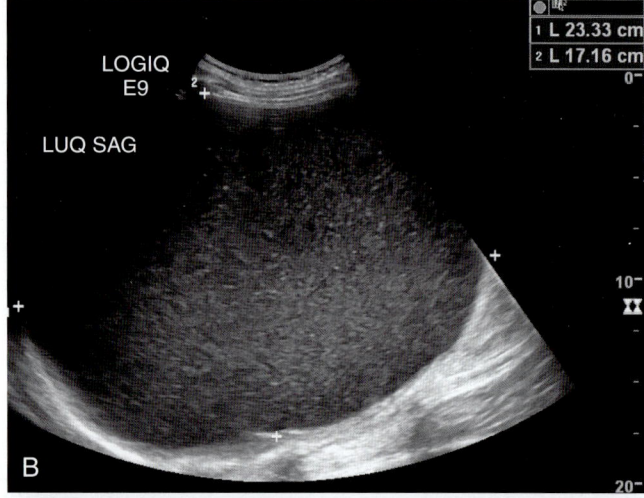

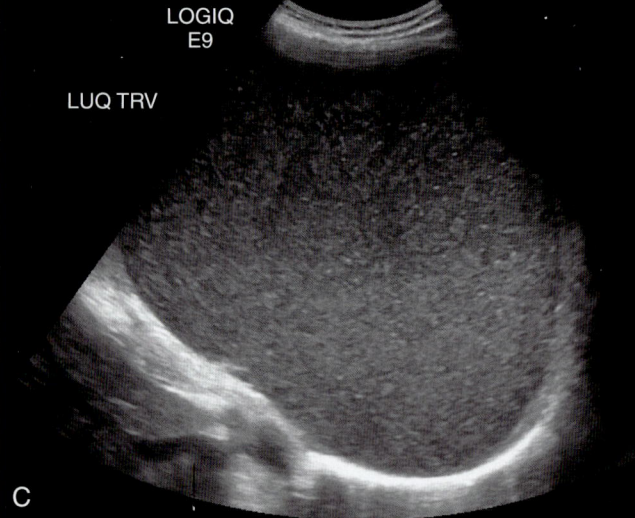

FIG. 11.18 (A–B) The enlarged spleen consumes the left upper quadrant in this patient with splenomegaly. (C) Transverse image of the enlarged spleen.

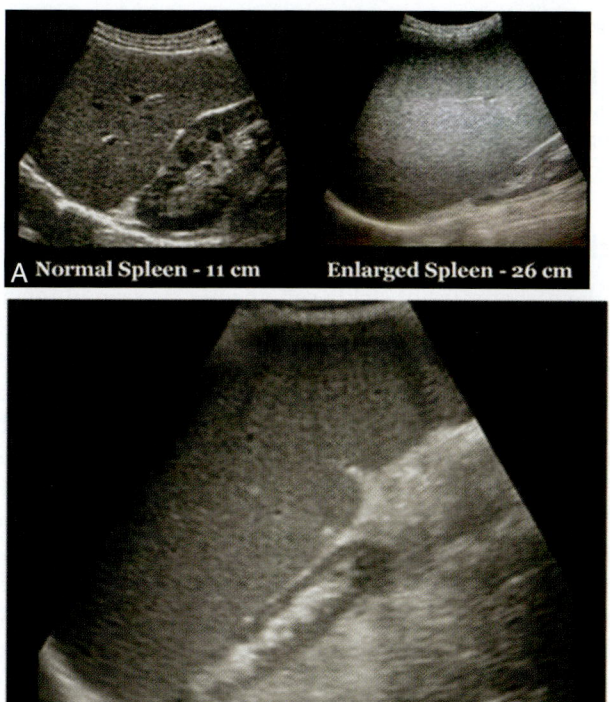

FIG. 11.19 (A) Normal spleen and left kidney. (B) As splenomegaly becomes more advanced, the left kidney appears compressed. (A, Courtesy University Medical Imaging Group, www.universalmedicalimaging.com.)

CONGESTION OF THE SPLEEN

Two types of splenic congestion are known: acute and chronic. In acute congestion, active hyperemia accompanies the reaction in the moderately enlarged spleen. In chronic venous congestion, diffuse enlargement of the spleen occurs. The venous congestion may be of systemic origin, caused by intrahepatic obstruction to portal venous drainage or obstructive venous disorders in the portal or splenic veins. Systemic venous congestion is found in cardiac decompensation involving the right side of the heart. It is particularly severe in tricuspid or pulmonary valvular disease and in chronic cor pulmonale. The most common causes of striking congestive splenomegaly are the various forms of cirrhosis of the liver. It is also caused by obstruction to the extrahepatic portal or splenic vein (e.g., spontaneous portal vein thrombosis) (see Box 11.5).

STORAGE DISEASE

Amyloidosis

In systemic diseases leading to **amyloidosis**, the spleen is the most frequently involved organ. Two types of involvement are seen: nodular and diffuse. In the nodular type, amyloid is found in the walls of the sheathed arteries and within the follicles, but not in the red pulp (Fig. 11.20). In the diffuse type, the follicles are not involved, the red pulp is prominently involved, and the spleen is usually greatly enlarged and firm. On sonography, the

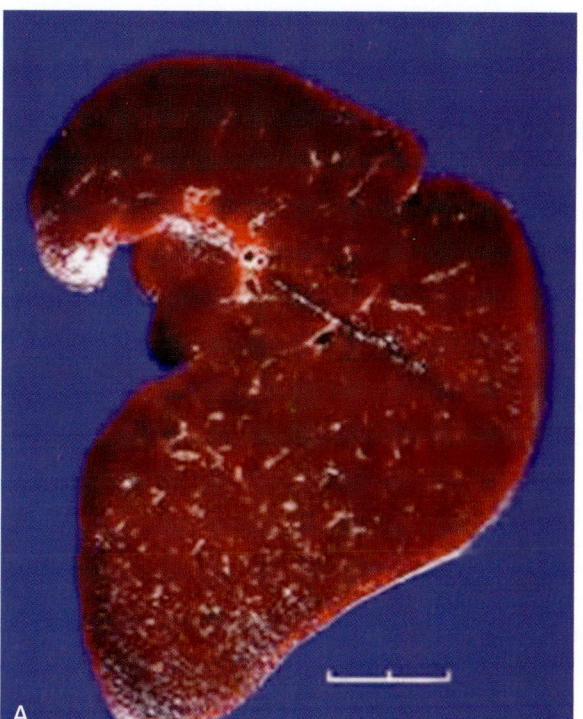

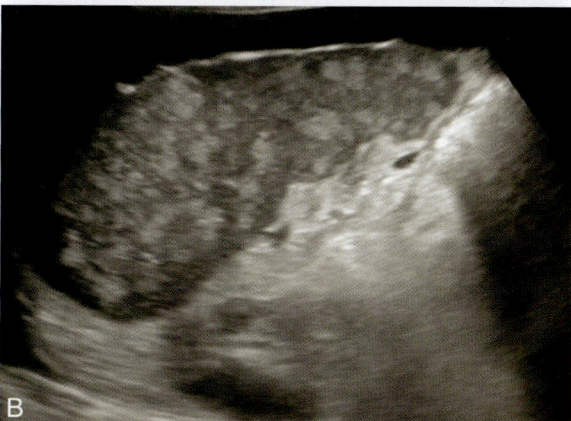

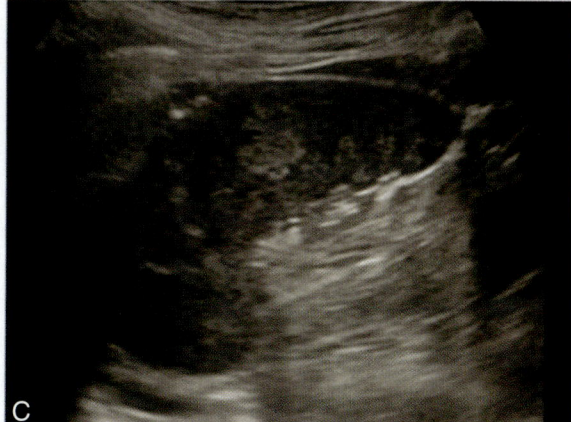

FIG. 11.20 (A) Gross pathology of the enlarged spleen in a patient with amyloidosis; note the diffuse involvement of the red pulp. (B–C) Sonographic images of two patients with amyloidosis. The inhomogeneous echogenic spread of the disease is seen throughout the parenchyma.

spleen may be of normal size or decidedly enlarged, depending on the amount and distribution of amyloid.

Gaucher Disease

All age groups can be affected by **Gaucher disease**. About 50% of patients are younger than 8 years, and 17% are younger than 1 year. Clinical features follow a chronic course, with bone pain and changes in skin pigmentation. Sonographic findings show splenomegaly, diffuse inhomogeneity, and multiple splenic nodules (well-defined hypoechoic lesions) are seen (Fig. 11.21). These nodules may be irregular, hyperechoic, or mixed. They represent focal areas of Gaucher cells associated with fibrosis and infarction.

Niemann-Pick Disease

Niemann-Pick disease is a rapidly progressing fatal disease that predominantly affects female infants. Clinical features consist of hepatomegaly, digestive disturbances, and lymphadenopathy.

DIFFUSE DISEASE

Erythropoietic abnormalities include the following: sickle cell, hereditary spherocytosis, hemolytic anemia, chronic anemia, polycythemia vera, thalassemia, and myeloproliferative disorders.

Sickle Cell Anemia

In the earlier stage of **sickle cell anemia**, as seen in infants and children, the spleen is enlarged with marked congestion of the red pulp (Fig. 11.22). Later, the spleen undergoes progressive infarction and fibrosis and decreases in size until, in adults, only a small mass of fibrous tissue may be found (autosplenectomy). It is generally believed that these changes result when sickle cells plug the vasculature of the splenic substance, effectively producing ischemic destruction of the spleen. Sonographic findings for sickle cell disease have different sonographic appearances, depending on its disease state (Fig. 11.23). An acute **sickle cell crisis** commonly occurs in children with homozygous sickle cell disease with splenomegaly and a sudden decrease in hematocrit. In addition, these patients may develop a subacute hemorrhage that appears as a hypoechoic area in the periphery of the spleen.

Congenital Spherocytosis

In congenital or hereditary **spherocytosis**, an intrinsic abnormality of the red cells gives rise to erythrocytes that are small and spheroid rather than normal, flattened, biconcave disks. The two results of this disease are production by the bone marrow of spherocytic erythrocytes and increased destruction of these cells in the spleen (Fig. 11.24). The spleen destroys spherocytes selectively. On sonography, splenomegaly may be seen.

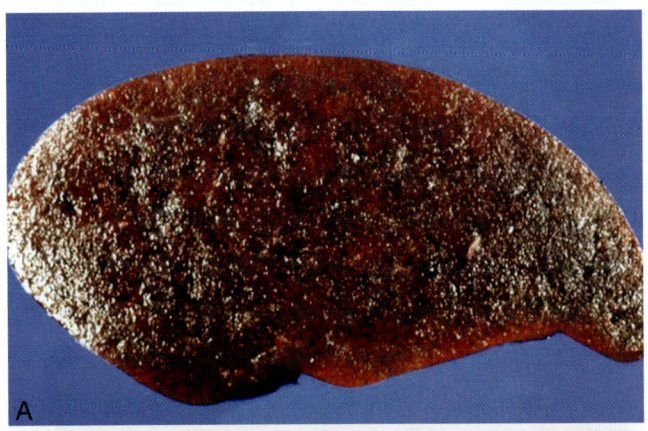

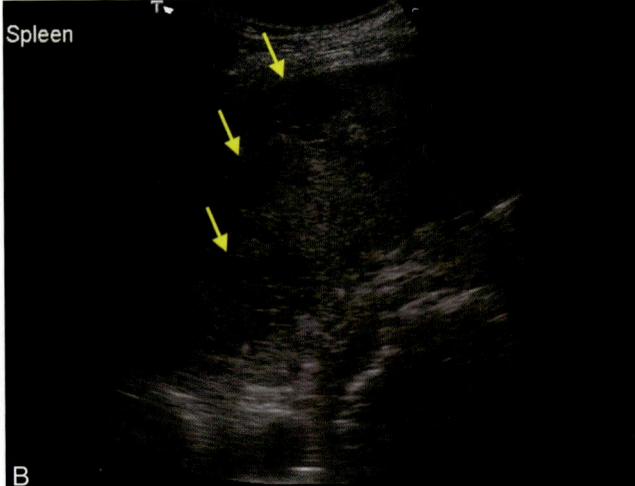

FIG. 11.21 (A) Gross pathology of Gaucher disease, noting multiple splenic nodules. (B) Sonographic findings of Gaucher disease with multiple well-defined hypoechoic nodules *(arrows)*.

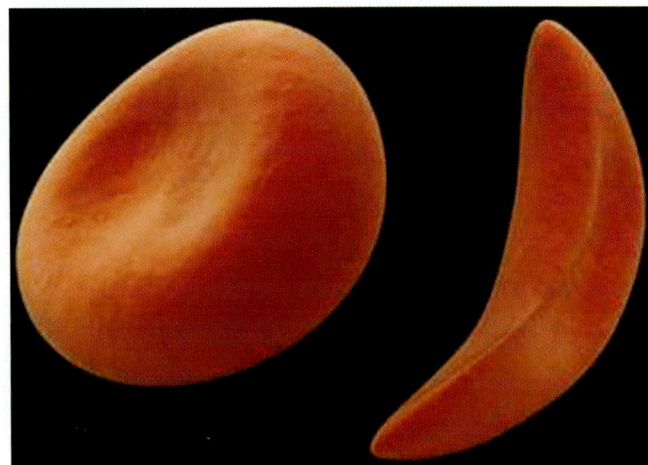

FIG. 11.22 Gross pathology of a patient with sickle cell anemia *(right)* compared to the normal spleen *(left)*.

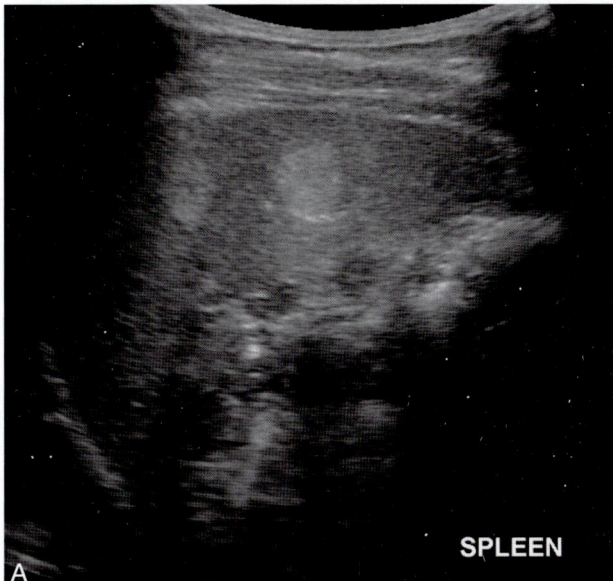
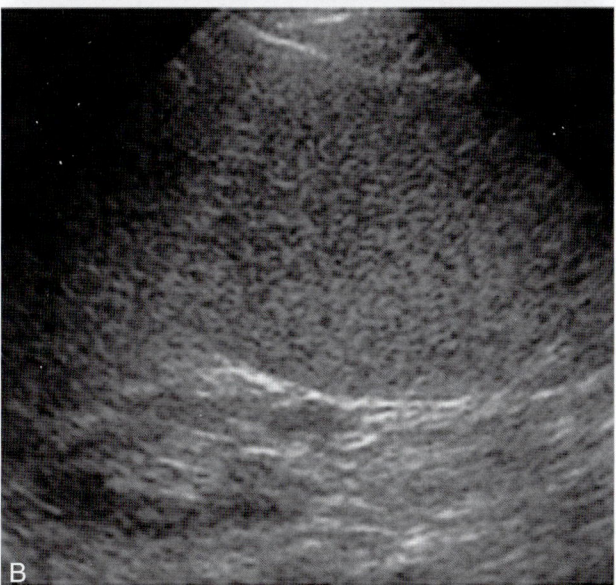
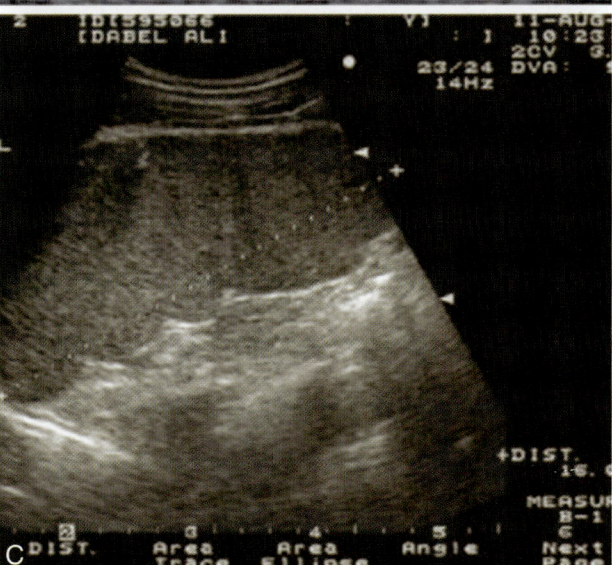

FIG. 11.23 Sonographic patterns of sickle cell anemia. An acute sickle cell crisis commonly occurs in children with homozygous sickle cell disease with splenomegaly and a sudden decrease in hematocrit.

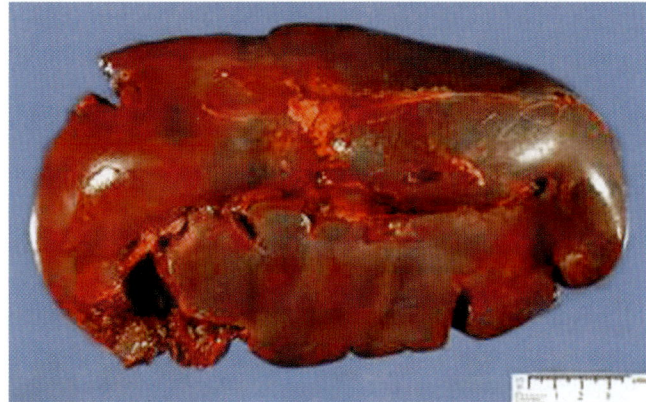

FIG. 11.24 Gross pathology of an enlarged spleen in a patient with congenital spherocytosis.

Hemolytic Anemia

Hemolytic anemia is the general term applied to anemia linked to decreased life of the erythrocytes. When the rate of destruction is greater than what the bone marrow can compensate for, anemia results.

Autoimmune Hemolytic Anemia

Autoimmune hemolytic anemia can occur in its primary form without underlying disease, or it may be seen as a secondary disorder in patients already suffering from some disorder of the reticuloendothelial or hematopoietic system, such as lymphoma, leukemia, or infectious **mononucleosis.** Splenomegaly may be present.

Polycythemia Vera

Polycythemia is an excess of red blood cells. **Polycythemia vera** is a chronic disease of unknown cause that involves all bone marrow elements. It is characterized by an increase in red blood cell mass and hemoglobin concentration. Clinical symptoms include weakness, fatigue, vertigo, tinnitus, irritability, splenomegaly, flushing of the face, redness and pain in the extremities, and blue-and-black spots. Splenomegaly is present (Fig. 11.25). Infarcts and thromboses are common in polycythemia vera.

Thalassemia

The spleen is severely involved in **thalassemia.** This hemoglobinopathy differs from the others in that an abnormal molecular form of hemoglobin is not present. Instead, suppression of synthesis of beta or alpha polypeptide chains occurs, resulting in deficient synthesis of normal hemoglobin. Not only are the erythrocytes deficient in normal hemoglobin, but they are also abnormal in shape; many are target cells, whereas others vary considerably in size and shape. Their life span is short because the spleen destroys them in large numbers. The disease ranges from mild to severe. Changes in the spleen are most significant in thalassemia

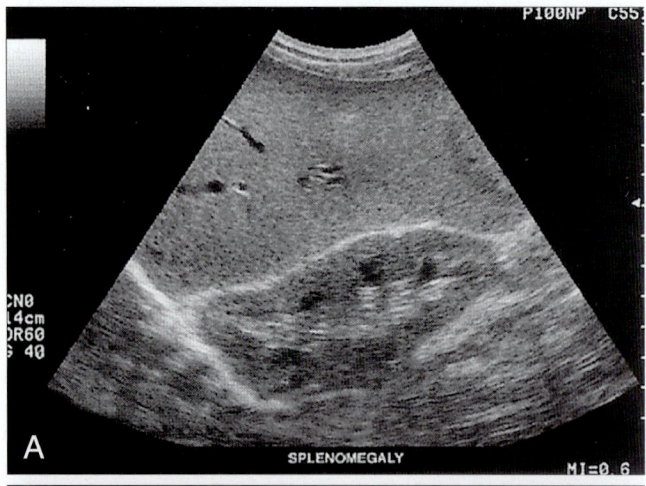

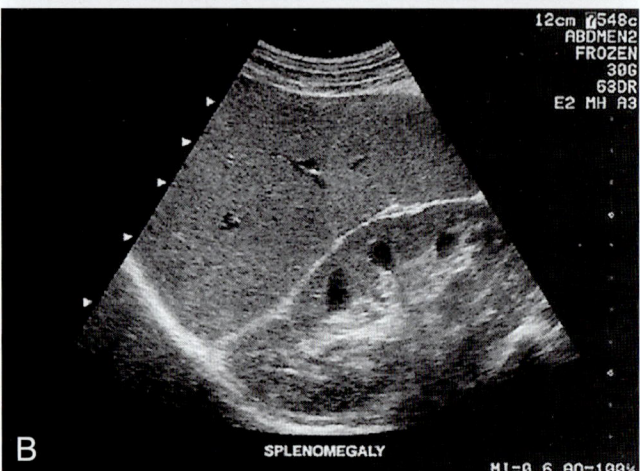

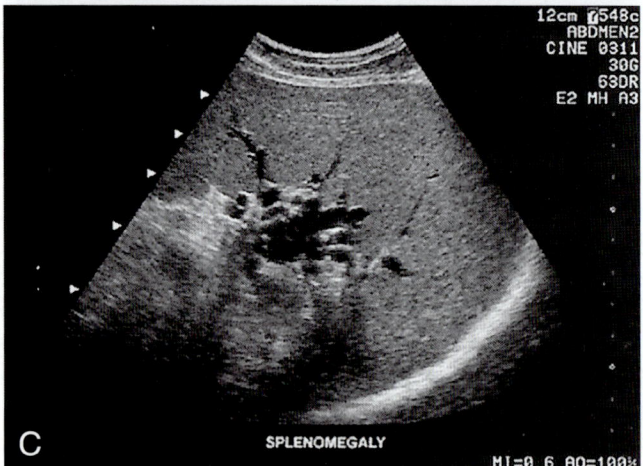

FIG. 11.25 **Patterns of splenomegaly.** (A–B) The tip of the enlarged spleen covers the lower pole of the kidney. (C) The dilated splenic hilum is secondary to portal hypertension, with hepatosplenomegaly.

major (Fig. 11.26). Splenomegaly is present, often filling the entire abdominal cavity.

Myeloproliferative Disorders

Myeloproliferative disorders include acute and chronic myelogenous leukemias, polycythemia vera, myelofibrosis, megakaryocytic leukemia, and erythroleukemia (Fig. 11.27). An isoechoic sonographic pattern is seen in this condition because the parenchyma is hypoechoic compared with the liver.

Granulocytopoietic Abnormalities

Granulocytopoietic abnormalities include reactive hyperplasia resulting from acute or chronic infection (e.g., splenitis sarcoid, tuberculosis). On sonographic examination, splenomegaly is seen with a diffusely hypoechoic pattern (less dense than the liver). Patients who have had a previous granulomatous infection may have bright echogenic lesions on sonography, with or without shadowing (Fig. 11.28). Histoplasmosis and tuberculosis are the most common causes; sarcoidosis is rare. The sonographer may also find calcium in the splenic artery.

Reticuloendotheliosis

Diseases characterized by reticuloendothelial hyperactivity and varying degrees of lipid storage in phagocytes are included in the category of reticuloendotheliosis. On ultrasound, the spleen appears isoechoic.

Letterer-Siwe Disease

In Letterer-Siwe disease, sometimes called *nonlipid reticuloendotheliosis*, proliferation of reticuloendothelial cells occurs in all tissues, but particularly in the splenic lymph nodes and bone marrow. This disease is generally found in children younger than 2 years. Clinical features include hepatosplenomegaly, fever, and pulmonary involvement. It is rapidly fatal. Usually, the spleen is only moderately enlarged, although the change may be more severe in affected older infants.

Hand-Schüller-Christian Disease

Hand-Schüller-Christian disease is benign and chronic, despite many features similar to those of Letterer-Siwe disease. It usually affects children older than 2 years. Clinical features include a chronic course, diabetes, and moderate hepatosplenomegaly.

SPLENIC ABSCESS AND INFECTION

Splenic Abscess

The phagocytic activity of the spleen's efficient reticuloendothelial system and leukocytes help to prevent abscess formation within the spleen. However, the spleen may be infected by the following: subacute bacterial endocarditis, septicemia, decreased immunologic states, drug abuse, splenic trauma and infarcts. In the majority of patients, the infection is spread from distant foci in the abdomen, or an inflammatory process extends directly from adjacent organs. Extrinsic processes (i.e., perinephric or subphrenic abscess, perforated gastric or colonic lesions, or pancreatic abscess) may invade the splenic parenchyma.

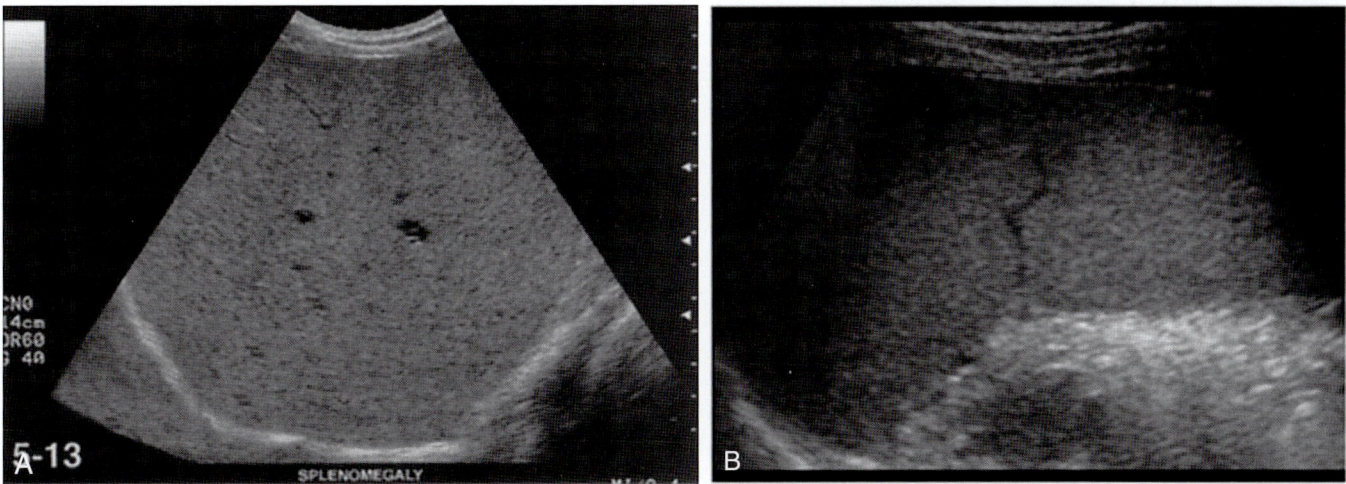

FIG. 11.26 Massive enlargement of the spleen is noted in patients with thalassemia.

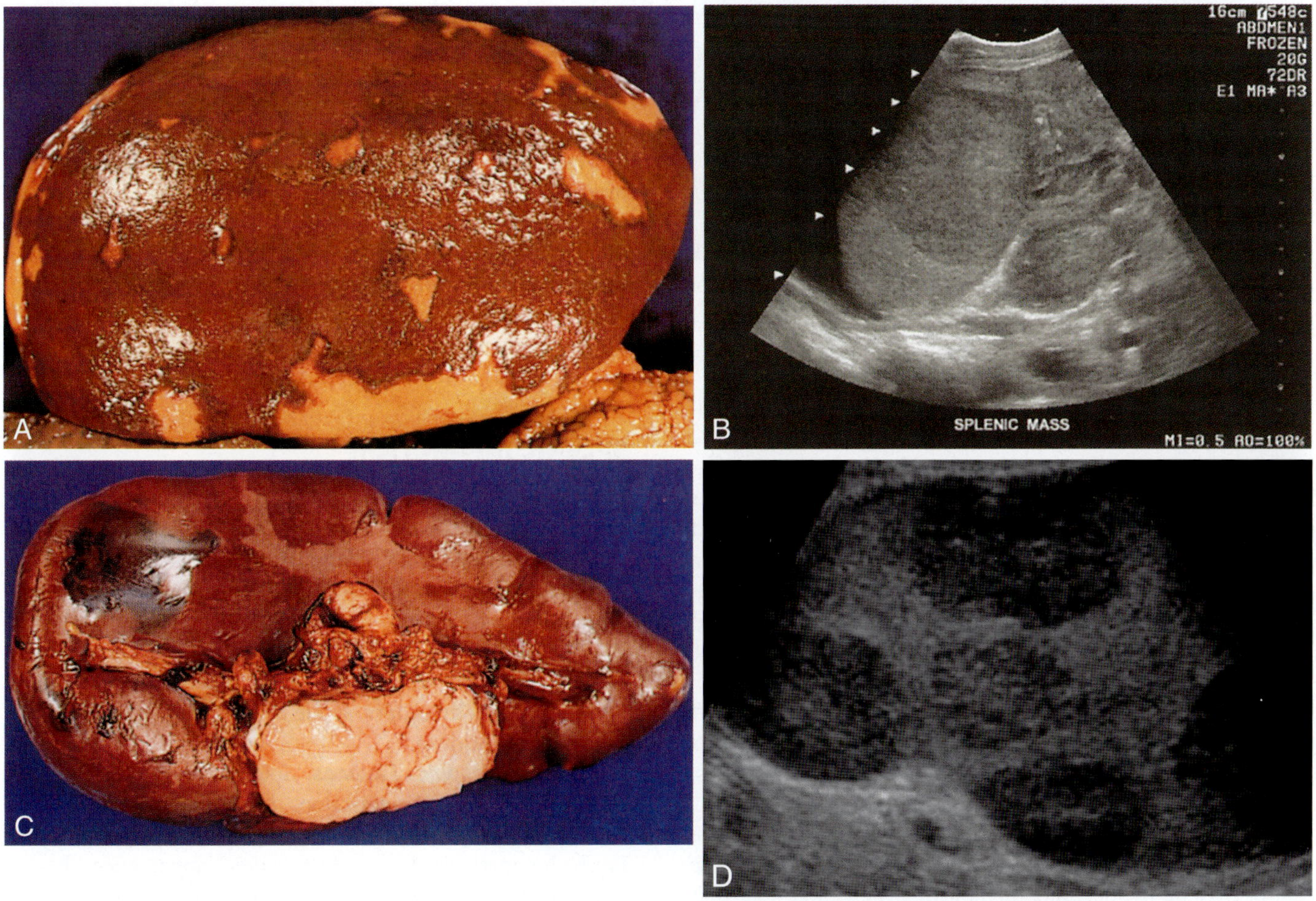

FIG. 11.27 (A) Chronic myeloid leukemia shows infarcts in a gross specimen with splenomegaly. (B) Patient with acute myelogenous leukemia shows a large mass within the splenic parenchyma and enlarged nodes in the hilum. (C) Lymphoblastic lymphoma. Tumor cells form a discrete mass in the spleen. (D) On sonography, an enlarged spleen is seen with an inhomogeneous texture in this patient with lymphoma.

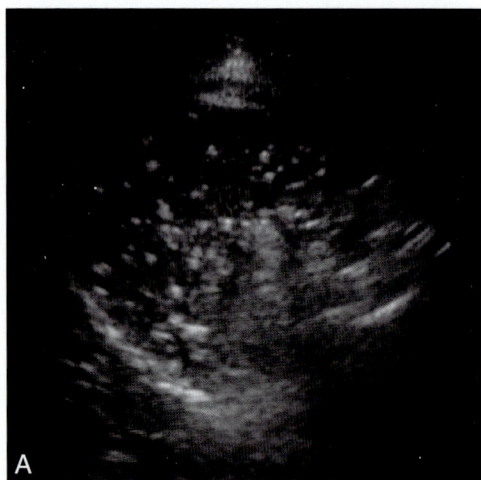

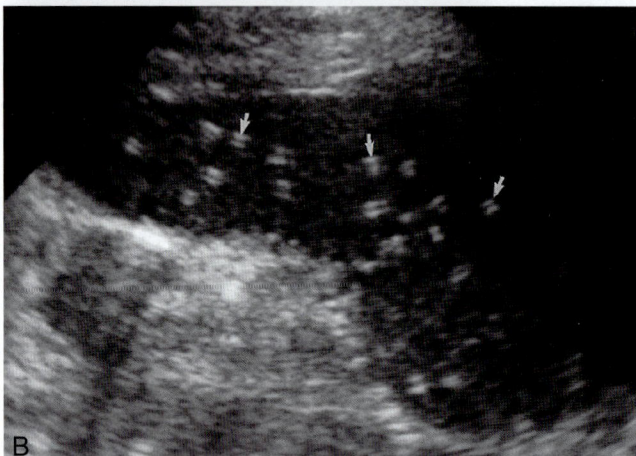

FIG. 11.28 Patient with granulomatous infection presents with bright echogenic lesions on sonography (arrows).

An abscess may be difficult to distinguish from an infarct, neoplasm, or hematoma, and clinical correlation is necessary (Fig. 11.30).

Splenic Infection

Many infections can affect the spleen. The most prominent feature is splenomegaly. Many immunocompromised patients also have multiple nodules within the spleen.

Hepatosplenic candidiasis on ultrasound may show irregular masses within the spleen, the "wheels-within-wheels" pattern, with the outer wheel representing the ring of fibrosis surrounding the inner echogenic wheel of inflammatory cells and a central hypoechoic area. Other patterns seen include bull's eye (hypoechoic rim with an echogenic central core), hypoechoic nodule, or hyperechoic nodule.

Patients with mycobacterial infections show tiny, diffuse echogenic foci throughout the spleen. Active tuberculosis shows echo-poor or cystic masses, representing abscess lesions (Fig. 11.31). These small punctate areas may show increased echogenicity with calcification.

In patients with acquired immunodeficiency syndrome (AIDS), the most common finding is splenomegaly. There can be multiorgan involvement (i.e., liver, spleen, and kidneys). Focal lesions include *Candida, Pneumocystis jiroveci* pneumonia, *Mycobacterium*, disseminated *Pneumocystis*, Kaposi sarcoma, and lymphoma. Sonographic findings may demonstrate focal splenic lesions displaying small round lesions that may be multiple, hypoechoic, and well defined. Many of these lesions are caused by disseminated *Mycobacterium tuberculosis* infection, *Candida, P. jiroveci*, or *Mycobacterium avium*. In addition, hepatomegaly with focal lesions, retroperitoneal lymphadenopathy, and ascites may be seen.

SPLENIC INFARCTION

Splenic infarction is the most common cause of focal splenic lesions resulting from occlusion of the major splenic artery or any of its branches. They are almost always the result of emboli that arise in the heart, produced from mural thrombi or from vegetation on the valves of the left side of the heart. Other causes include septic emboli and local thrombosis in patients with pancreatitis, leukemia, lymphomatous disorders, sickle cell anemia, sarcoidosis, or polyarteritis nodosa.

Sonographic Findings. Splenomegaly is not present with a splenic infarction. Sonography may show a localized hypoechoic area, depending on the time of onset. Fresh hemorrhage has a hypoechoic appearance; healed infarctions appear as echogenic, peripheral wedge-shaped lesions with their base toward the subcapsular surface of the spleen (Fig. 11.32). The infarction may become nodular or hyperechoic with time. The entire spleen or focal segmental areas may be affected. The infarcted segment will be avascular.

The abscess formations may be typical pyogenic, atypical pyogenic, of microabscess collections. The typical pyogenic abscess is a focal collection of pus within the splenic parenchyma. The appearance is hypoechoic with internal septations with low-level echoes representing pus or debris. Decreased acoustic enhancement may be present. The atypical pyogenic abscess demonstrates reverberation artifacts from gas; therefore, the image is echogenic. The microabscess formation demonstrates a target or bull's eye appearance on sonography, similar to that seen in the liver.

Clinical findings may be subtle and may include fever, left upper quadrant tenderness, and splenomegaly. Lab results would demonstrate positive blood cultures and leukocytosis, depending on the type of infection present.

Sonographic Findings. Sonography may demonstrate a simple cystic pattern to mixed echo pattern (Fig. 11.29). The lesion may be hypoechoic, often with hyperechoic foci that represent debris or gas. Other findings include the following: thick or shaggy walls, anechoic (without echoes within a mass) appearance, poor definition of the lesion, and increased to decreased transmission (depending on the presence of gas).

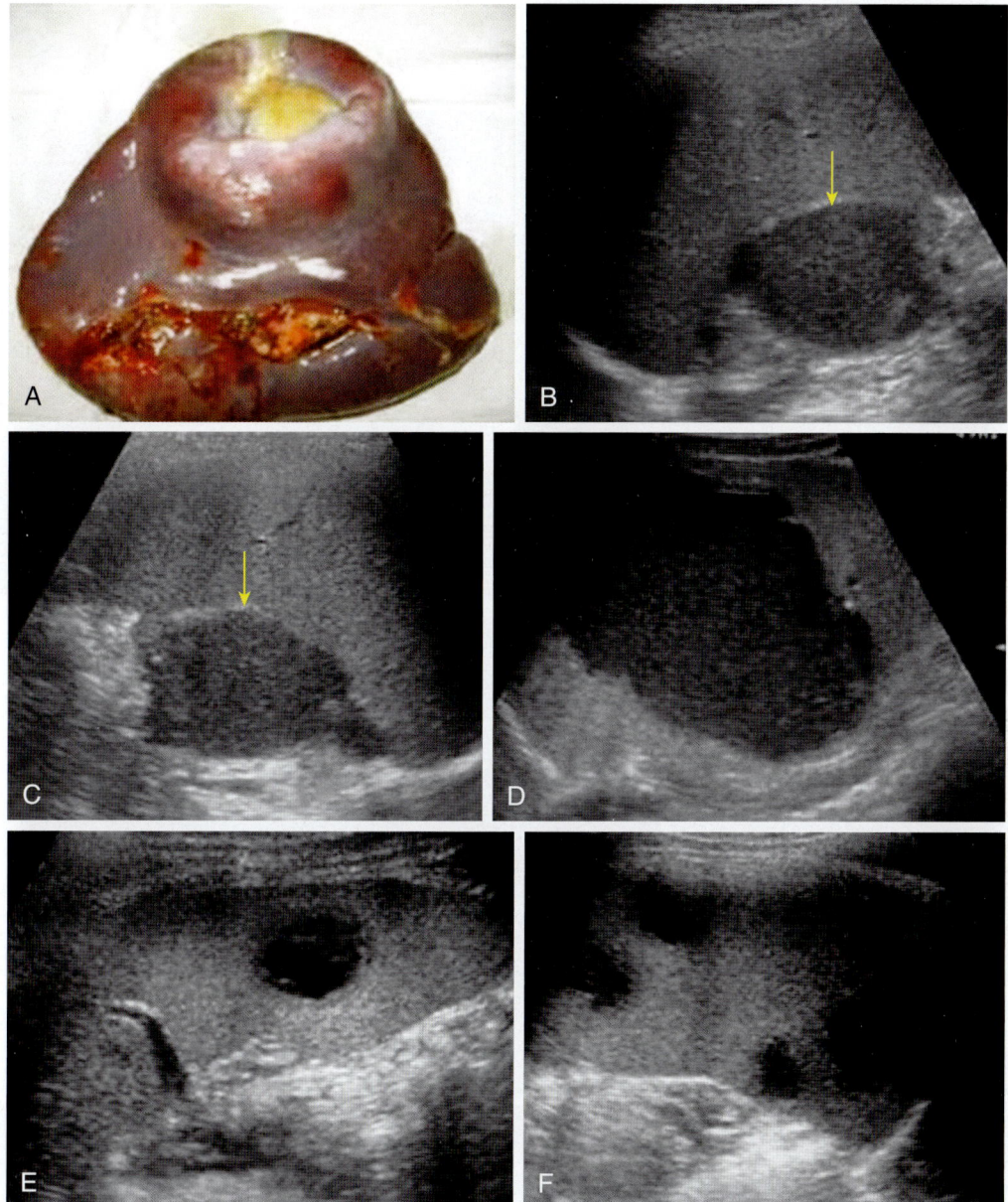

FIG. 11.29 (A) Gross pathology of a large splenic abscess. (B–C) Transverse and longitudinal images of a patient with a splenic abscess. (D) Sonography of a patient with a large splenic abscess. (E) Sonography of a small splenic abscess with debris within. (F) Sonography of the spleen with multiple areas of abscess formation.

SPLENIC TRAUMA

The spleen is most commonly injured as a result of blunt abdominal trauma. If the patient has severe left upper quadrant pain secondary to trauma, a splenic hematoma or subcapsular hematoma should be considered. The tear may result in linear or stellate lacerations or capsular tears, puncture wounds from foreign bodies or rib fractures, or subcapsular hematomas. Blunt trauma has two outcomes. If the capsule is intact, the outcome may be intraparenchymal or subcapsular hematoma; if the capsule ruptures, a focal or free intraperitoneal hematoma may form (Fig. 11.33). In delayed rupture, a subcapsular hematoma may develop with subsequent rupture. Quick assessment of free fluid that may surround the splenic capsule in blunt abdominal trauma can lead to a life-saving diagnosis for the patient.

Sonographic Findings. Sonography is a sensitive and specific test used to examine trauma patients for abdominal injury requiring surgery (Fig. 11.34). Routine abdominal ultrasound examination can be performed at the bedside in the trauma center. The use of screening ultrasound can improve clinical decision-making for the benefit of emergency laparotomy.

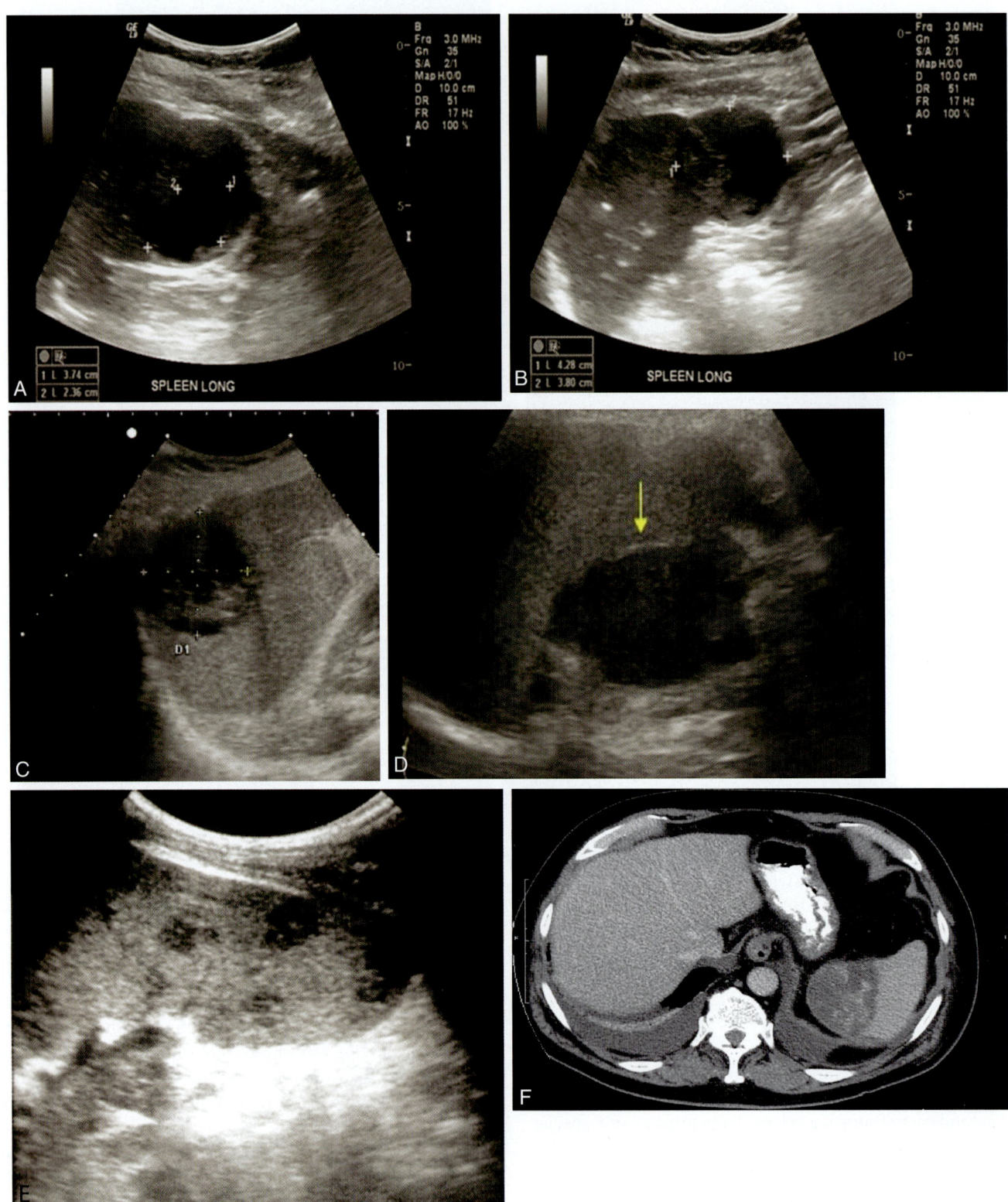

FIG. 11.30 (A–E) Multiple sonographic patterns of splenic abscess. (F) Contrast computed tomographic image of complex splenic abscess.

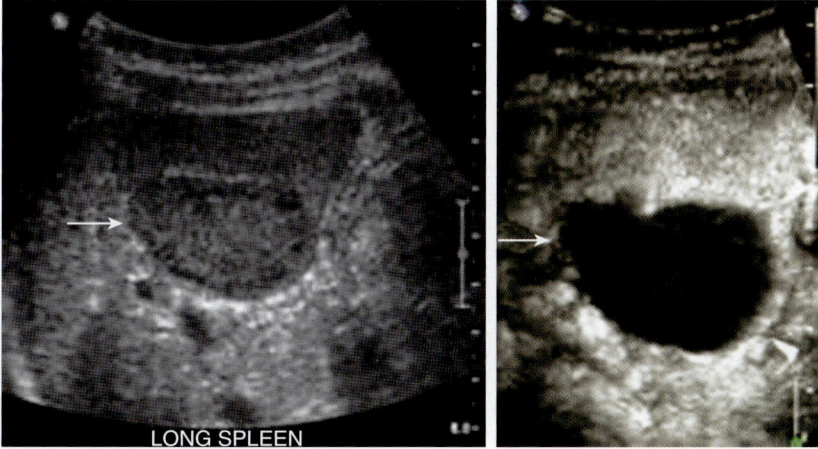

FIG. 11.31 Sonography of a tuberculous abscess of the spleen; these collections may show echo-poor or cystic masses.

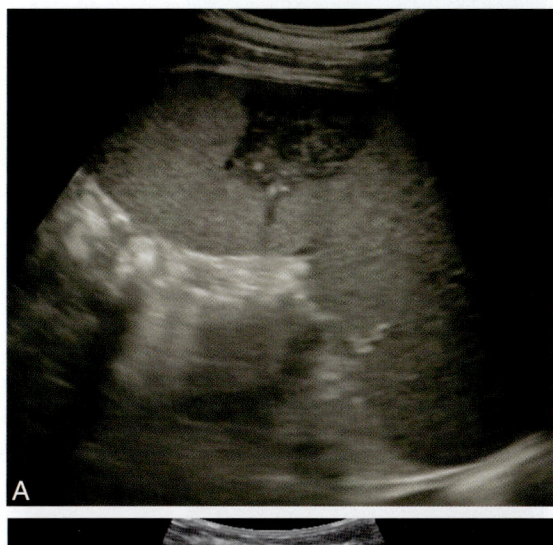

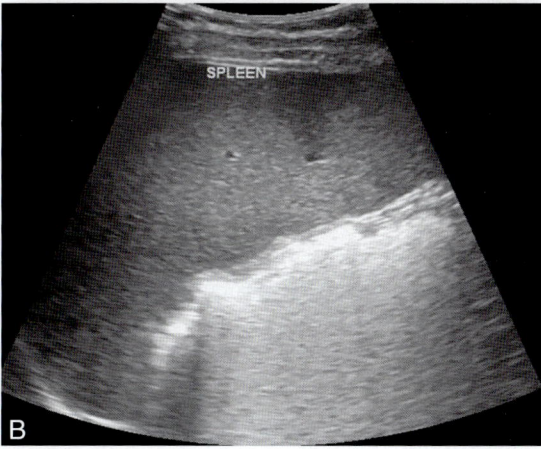

FIG. 11.32 A fresh hemorrhage has a hypoechoic appearance; healed infarctions appear as echogenic, peripheral wedge-shaped lesions with their base toward the subcapsular surface of the spleen.

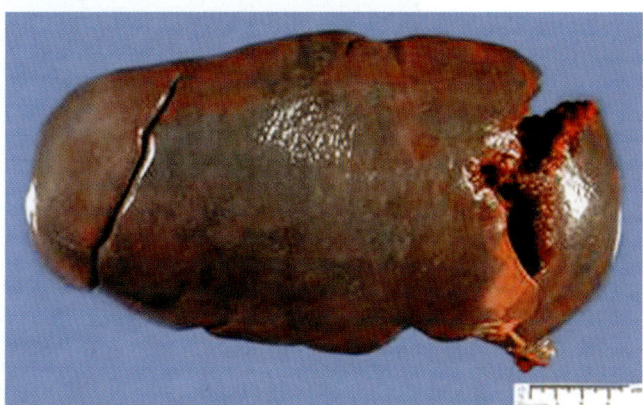

FIG. 11.33 Gross pathology demonstrating a large tear in the splenic parenchyma from blunt trauma.

The patient typically presents with left upper quadrant pain, left shoulder pain, left flank pain, or dizziness. On clinical evaluation, the patient may have tenderness over the left upper quadrant, hypotension, and decreased hemoglobin, indicating a bleed. A timely response to this emergent situation may save the patient undergoing peritoneal lavage or exploratory surgery. The sonographer should quickly examine the four abdominopelvic quadrants: the area surrounding the kidneys (Morison pouch), the subdiaphragmatic areas, the liver and splenic capsule, and the bladder and anterior rectal area to determine whether free fluid is present. The patient's bladder may be filled retrograde to help serve as a window in the pelvic cavity. The entire screening examination should take less than 5 minutes and may be video recorded.

If the spleen has been lacerated and blood is contained within the splenic capsule, the most prominent ultrasound finding is splenomegaly, with progressive enlargement as the bleeding continues. In addition, an irregular splenic border, hematoma, contusion (splenic inhomogeneity), subcapsular and pericapsular fluid collections, free intraperitoneal blood, or left pleural effusion may be present.

Focal hematomas may have intrasplenic fluid collections. Perisplenic fluid is seen in patients with subcapsular hematomas. The sonographer should be aware that blood exhibits various echo patterns, depending on the time that has passed since the trauma. Fresh hemorrhage may appear hypoechoic

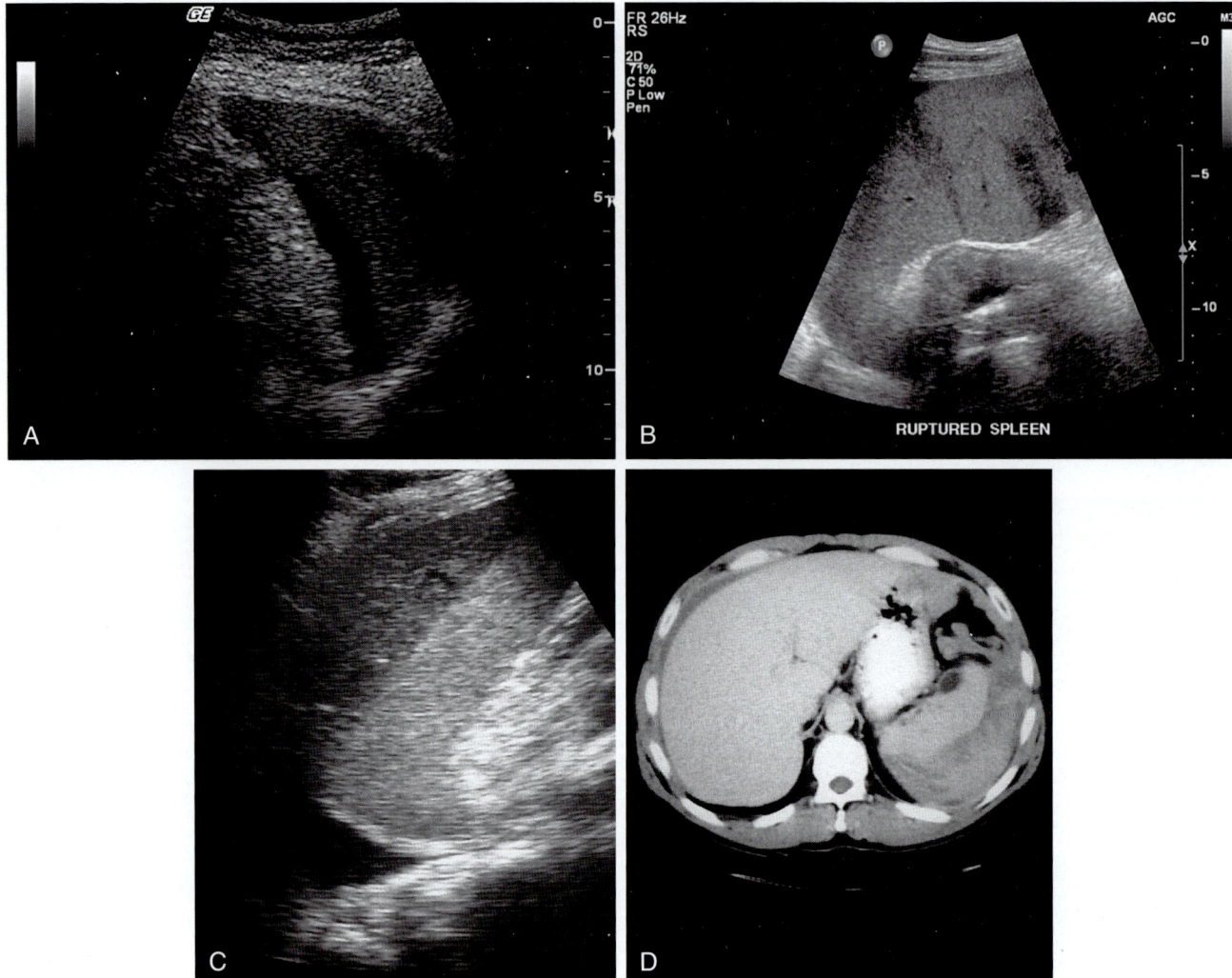

FIG. 11.34 **Splenic hematoma.** (A) Small hypoechoic separation medial to the splenic capsule represents a splenic hematoma. (B) Inhomogeneity of the splenic texture represents a laceration in the spleen. (C) Separation of the splenic capsule from the spleen secondary to a large hematoma resulting from an automobile accident. (D) Computed tomography demonstrates the splenic hematoma along the posterolateral wall of the abdomen.

and may be difficult to distinguish from normal splenic tissue. The sonographer should look for a double-contour sign depicting the hematoma as separate from the spleen (Fig. 11.35). As the protein and cells resorb the hematoma, the fluid becomes organized, hyperechoic, and similar to splenic tissue. In focal areas, tiny splenic lacerations give rise to small collections of blood interspersed with disrupted splenic pulp (contusion). Over time, the hematoma becomes more fluid or appears lucent.

The echo-free, intraperitoneal fluid is probably blood mixed with peritoneal transudate. Healing of the lesion often takes months. The free fluid disappears more quickly because the fluid is moved across the pleural and peritoneal membranes rapidly (2 to 4 weeks). Intrasplenic hematomas and contusions take longer because the fluid, protein, and necrotic debris must be resorbed from within a solid organ in which the blood supply has already been focally disrupted. When the spleen returns to normal, small irregular foci may remain, or the parenchyma may be normal.

SPLENIC CYSTS

Cystic masses do not commonly occur in the spleen. Splenic cysts may be classified as congenital or acquired in origin. The congenital cyst has an endothelial lining present. These cysts present on ultrasound as an anechoic, smooth bordered mass without septations or nodules (Fig. 11.36). If they are complicated cysts, there may be septations with internal echoes, a thickened wall, and usually do not have calcifications. Simple congenital cysts can have internal echoes at an increased gain. Hemorrhage within the cyst may produce a fluid level.

The acquired cyst is considered "post-traumatic" or "pseudo" cyst as the inner cellular wall is absent, but a fibrous wall if present. Most acquired cysts are considered secondary cysts caused by trauma, infection, or infarction. These acquired cysts on sonography appear as small anechoic or mixed homogeneity. The wall may be echogenic (calcified) (Fig. 11.37). *Echinococcus* is the only parasite that forms splenic cysts; it is uncommon in the United States. Parasitic cysts appear as anechoic lesions with possible daughter cysts and calcification or as solid masses with fine internal echoes and poor distal enhancement. Infectious cysts of *Echinococcus* and hydatid cysts may show calcifications within their walls. Post-traumatic cysts that have no cellular lining are called pseudocysts. These cysts may develop calcifications in their walls.

BENIGN PRIMARY NEOPLASMS

Generally speaking, primary tumors of the spleen are rare. The tumors may be divided into two groups: benign and malignant. With benign primary tumors, splenomegaly is the first indication of an abnormality. The tumor appearance may be solid or cystic, and they may be solitary or multiple. Most of these tumors appear isoechoic compared with the normal splenic parenchyma. Benign primary tumors include hemangioma, hamartoma, and lymphangioma.

Hemangioma

The hemangioma is the most common benign tumor of the spleen. It is usually an isolated inhomogeneous echogenic mass with multiple small hypoechoic areas (Fig. 11.38). The patient displays no symptoms and becomes symptomatic only when the size of the spleen increases and it compresses other organs. Complications occur when the tumor increases in size to cause a splenic rupture with peritoneal symptoms. The sonographic appearance is variable, from a well-defined echogenic appearance to a complex mixed pattern; infarction with coagulated blood or fibrin in the cavities may be seen but is nonspecific. Hydatid cyst, abscess, dermoid cyst, and metastasis should be considered in the differential diagnosis.

Hamartoma

The patient with a rare hamartoma is asymptomatic. The tumor may be solitary or multiple and is considered well defined but not encapsulated. The hamartoma consists of lymphoid tissue or a combination of sinuses and structures equivalent to pulp cords of normal splenic tissue. Symptomatic splenic hamartomas are rare in the pediatric age group. The hamartoma has both solid and cystic components and is generally hyperechoic on sonography (Fig. 11.39).

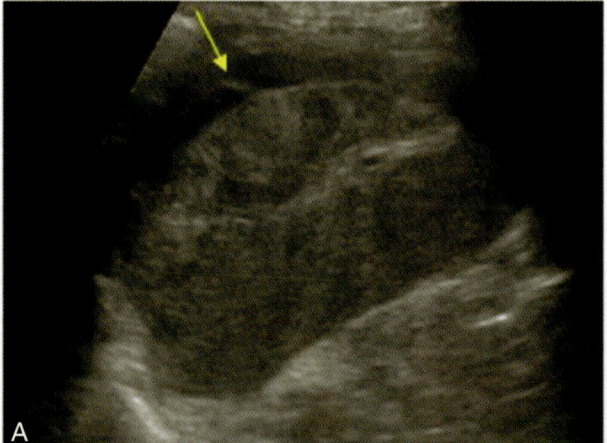
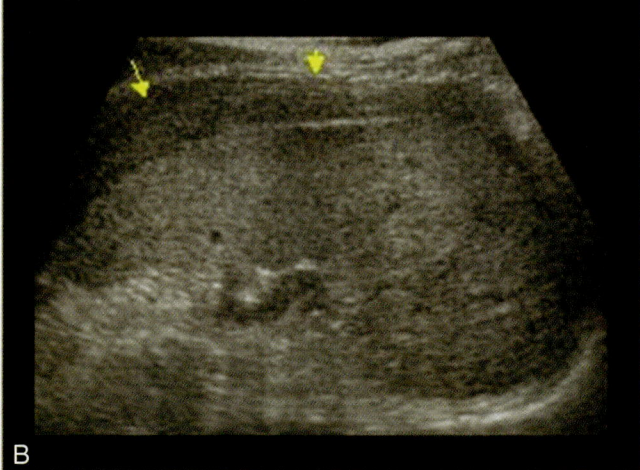

FIG. 11.35 Perisplenic Fluid is seen in patients with subcapsular hematomas. The sonographer should be aware that blood exhibits various echo patterns, depending on the time that has passed since the trauma, and should look for a double-contour sign depicting the hematoma as separate from the spleen.

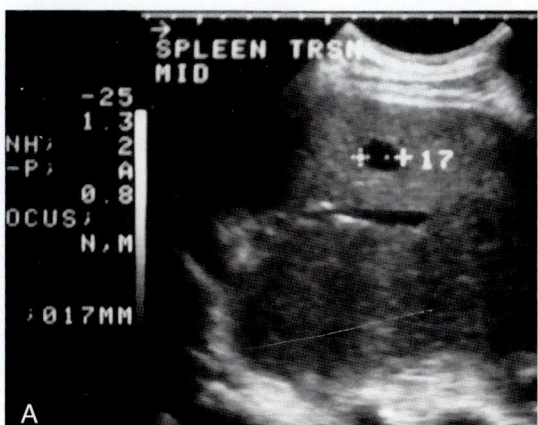
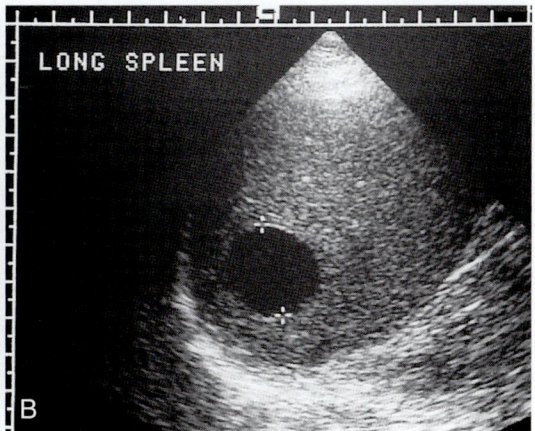

FIG. 11.36 Splenic cyst. (A) Tiny anechoic mass found within the splenic parenchyma as an incidental finding. (B) Well-defined anechoic mass found within an asymptomatic young woman.

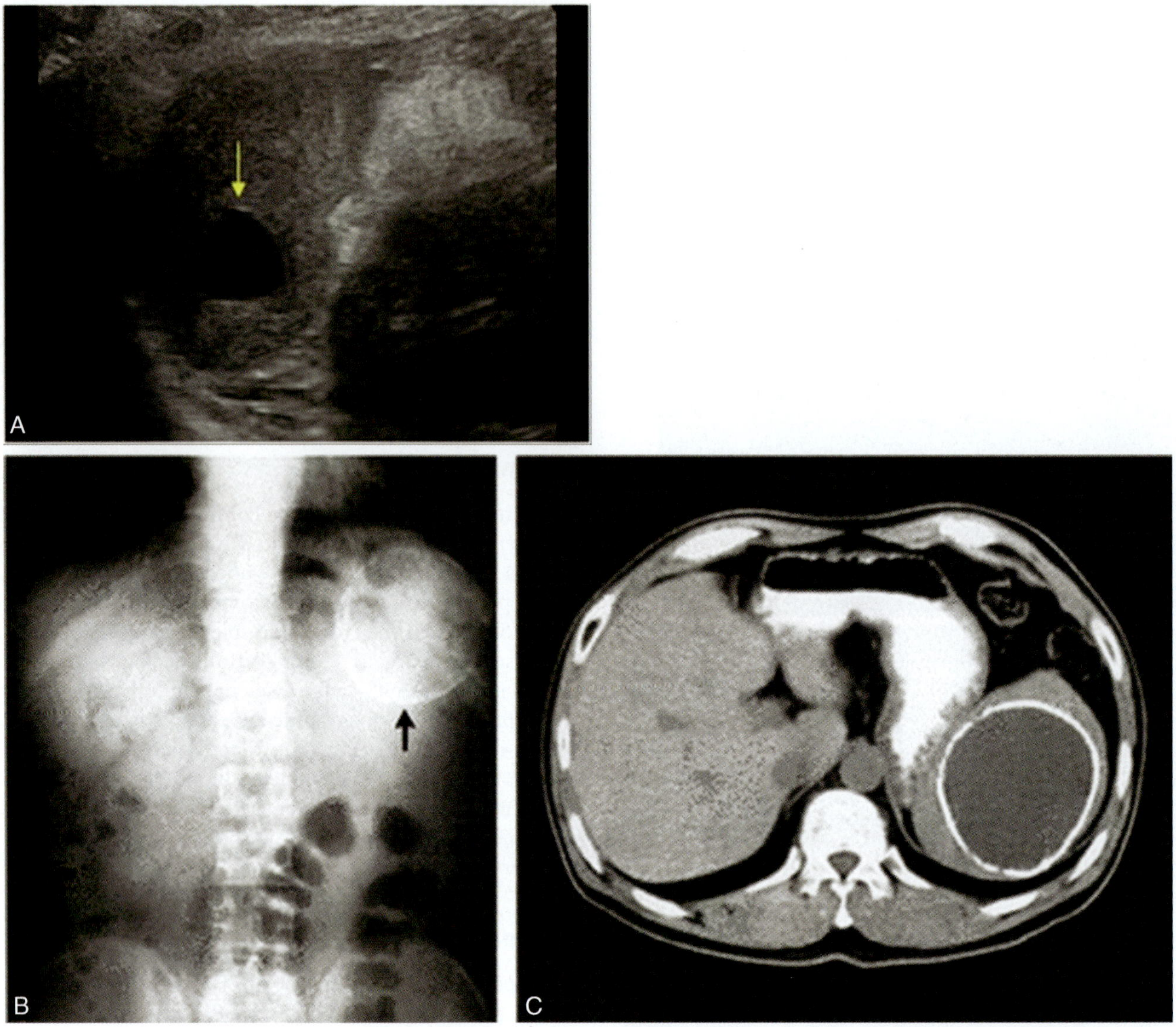

350 CHAPTER 11 The Spleen

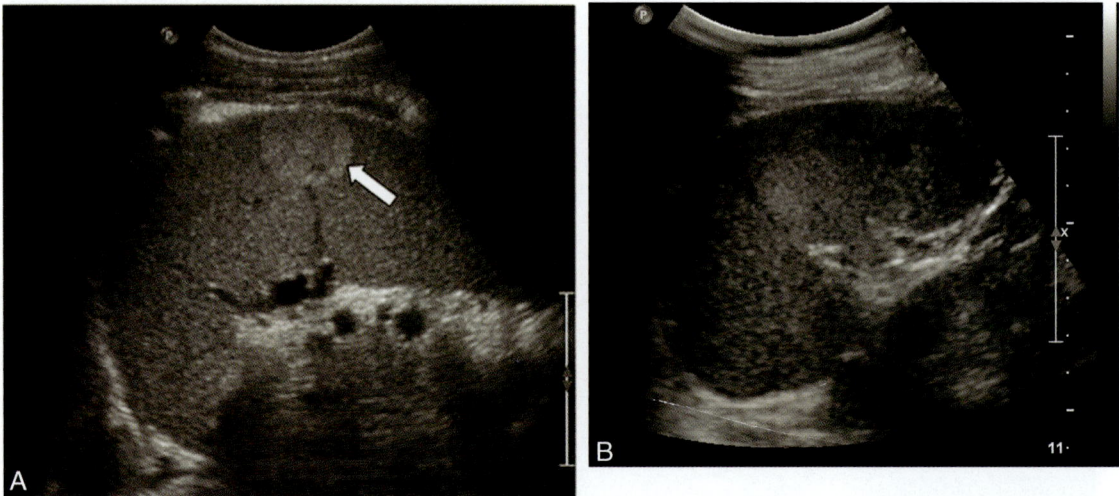

FIG. 11.37 Most acquired cysts are considered secondary cysts caused by trauma, infection, or infarction. (A) On sonography they appear as small anechoic or mixed homogeneity. The wall may be echogenic (calcified) as seen on radiography (B) and computed tomography (C).

FIG. 11.38 The hemangioma on sonography appears as an isolated inhomogeneous echogenic mass with multiple small hypoechoic areas *(arrow)*.

Lymphangioma

Lymphangioma is a rare benign malformation of lymphatics, consisting of endothelium-lined cystic spaces that vary in size. If the cysts are large enough, they may appear anechoic; however, if the cysts are multiple and grouped closely together, they may appear as a solid lesion. This condition may involve multiple organ systems or may be confined to solitary organs, such as the liver, spleen, kidney, or colon. Cystic lymphangioma appears as a mass with extensive cystic replacement of splenic parenchyma (Fig. 11.40).

Malignant Primary Neoplasms

Malignant tumors of the spleen are uncommon. Primary tumors found in the spleen include lymphoma and hemangiosarcoma. Very rare splenic tumors include malignant fibrous histiocytoma, leiomyosarcoma, and fibrosarcoma.

Lymphoma. The spleen is commonly involved in lymphoma. The lesions may be focal or diffuse. Splenomegaly may or may not be present. The most common malignant tumors are **Hodgkin lymphoma** and **non-Hodgkin lymphoma**. It may be challenging to detect splenic lymphoma by sonography. When it is seen, however, it appears to be typically hypoechoic. Four different sonographic patterns have been reported in patients with malignant lymphoma: (1) diffuse involvement, (2) focal small nodular lesions, (3) focal large nodular lesions, and (4) bulky disease (Fig. 11.41). The diffuse or small nodular pattern was seen predominantly in low-grade lymphomas and in Hodgkin disease.

AIDS lymphoma shows a uniform decreased echogenicity or focal hypoechoic lesions in the spleen.

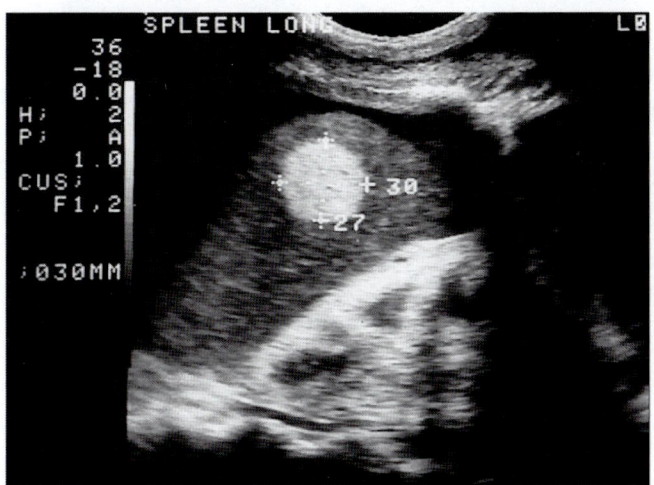

FIG. 11.39 **Hamartoma of the spleen.** Small, solitary hyperechoic lesion within the spleen was seen in a young patient with ascites.

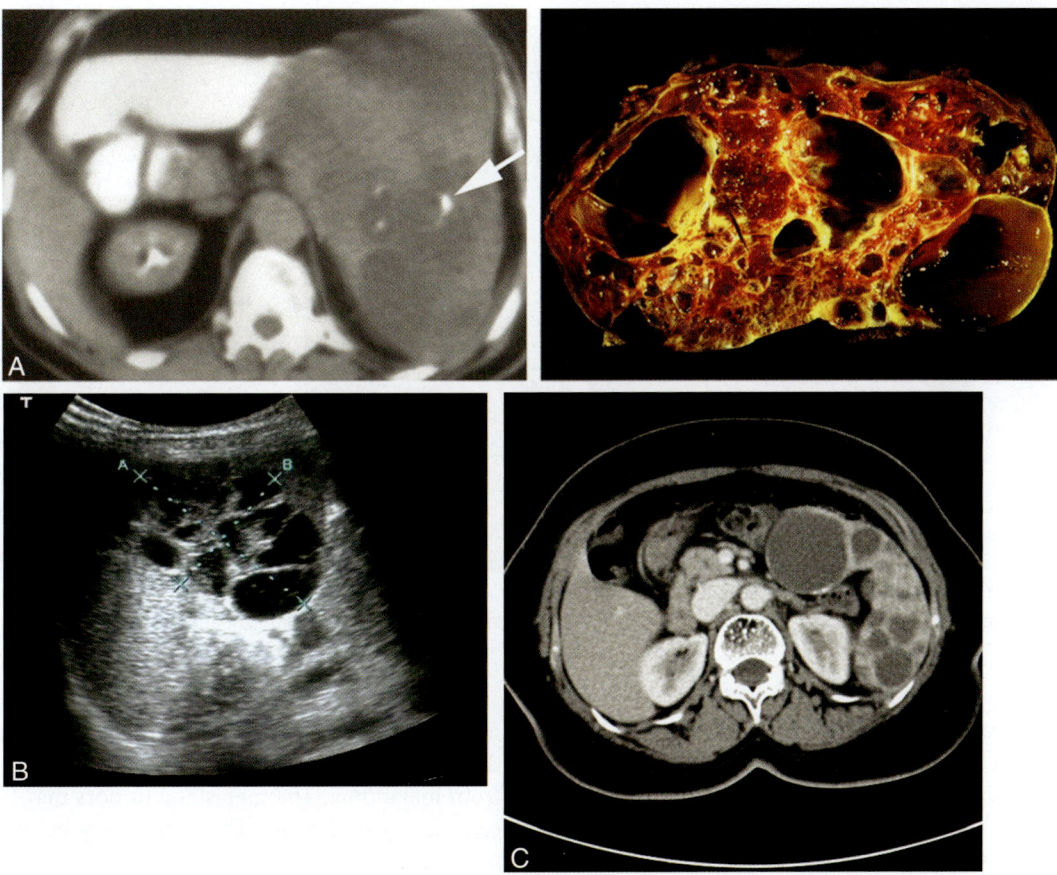

FIG. 11.40 (A) Gross pathology of splenic lymphangioma. (B) Sonography shows extensive cystic replacement of the splenic parenchyma. (C) Computed tomographic image of the cystic replacement of the splenic parenchyma.

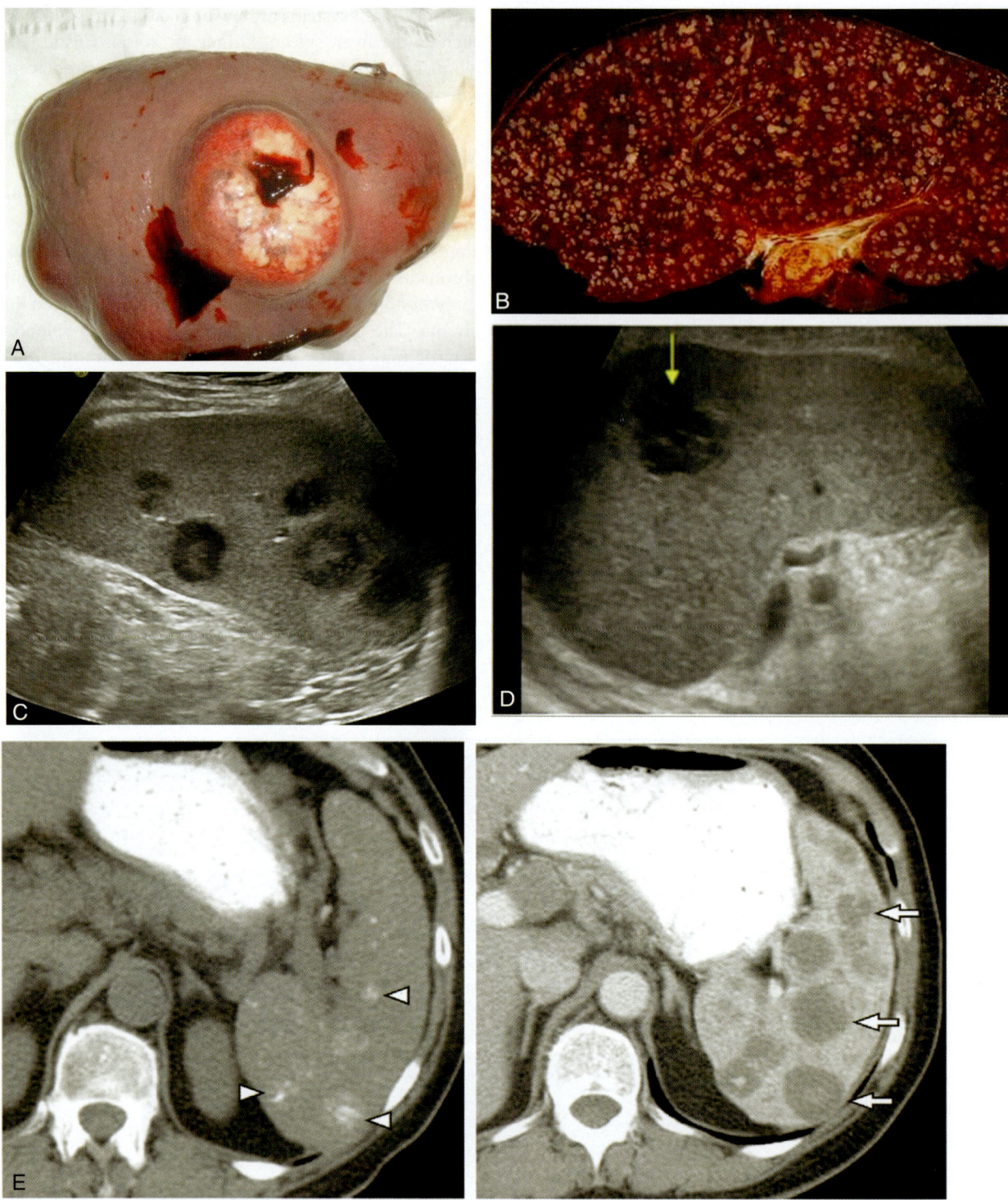

FIG. 11.41 (A–B) Gross pathology of non-Hodgkin lymphoma, focal and diffuse patterns. (C–D) Sonographic patterns of diffuse and focal lymphoma. (E) Contrast computed tomography shows diffuse pattern of lymphoma.

Hemangiosarcoma. Hemangiosarcoma is a very rare malignant neoplasm arising from the vascular endothelium of the spleen. The mixed cystic sonographic pattern of hemangiosarcoma resembles that of a cavernous hemangioma, but the tumor can also be hyperechoic.

Metastases. Metastases are the result of a hematogenous spread from another primary site. The spleen is the tenth most common site of metastases, which may originate from the breast, lung, ovary, stomach, colon, kidney, or prostate, or from melanoma. The metastatic tumors may be microscopic, causing no symptoms. The tumor may be multiple, solitary, nodular, or diffuse.

Sonographic Findings. The sonographer should carefully examine the splenic parenchyma to detect abnormalities

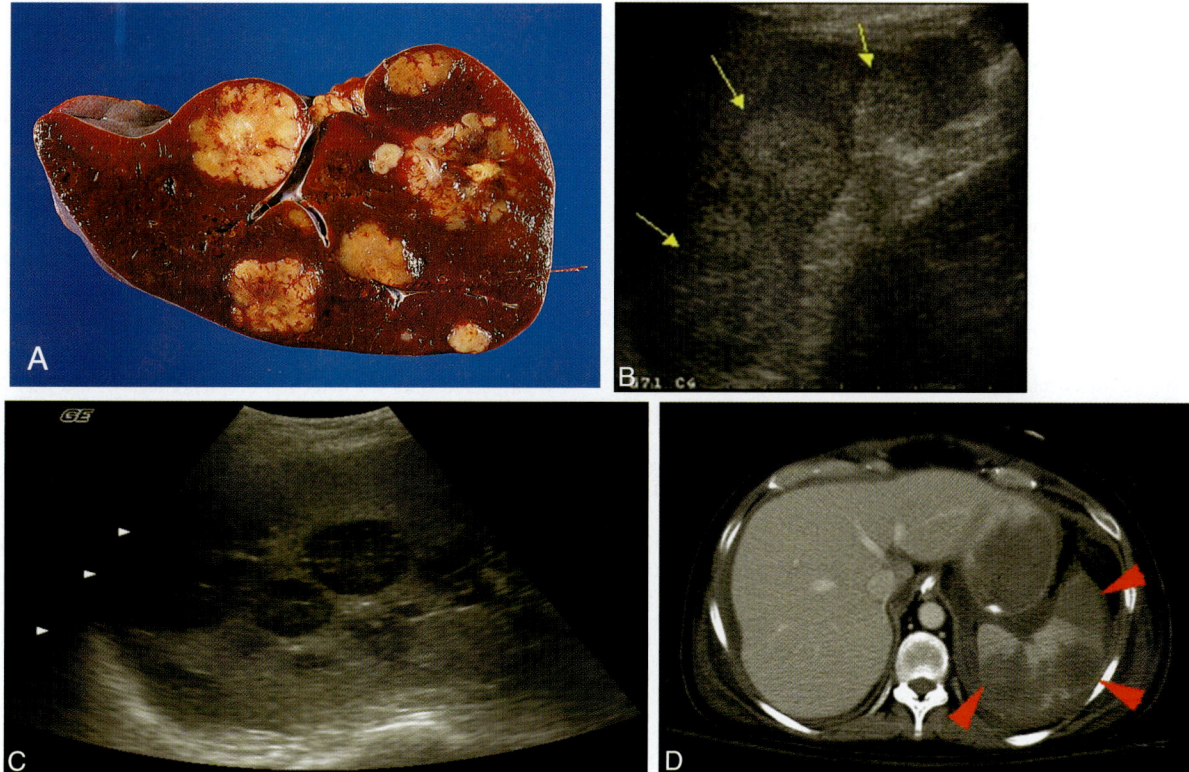

FIG. 11.42 (A) Gross pathology of splenic metastases. (B) Sonographic image of three slightly hyperechoic masses within the spleen. (C) Multiple target lesions are noted within the enlarged spleen. (D) Computed tomographic contrast image of multiple splenic metastases.

of the splenic parenchyma. The tumors are usually well-defined lesions that may appear isoechoic, hypoechoic, hyperechoic, target lesions, or halo lesions (Fig. 11.42). The larger lesions appear more complex. *Melanoma* deposits appear hypoechoic but are of higher echo amplitude than lymphoma; some are echodense.

Key Pearls

- The spleen, as part of the reticuloendothelial system, is the largest single mass of lymphoid tissue in the body.
- Splenic functions include hematopoiesis and the body's defense against disease.
- The normal texture of the spleen is homogeneous, being slightly more echogenic than the texture of the liver.
- The spleen is of variable size and shape (e.g., "orange segment," tetrahedral, triangular) but generally is considered to be ovoid with smooth, even borders and a convex superior and concave inferior surface.
- The splenic hilum contains both the splenic artery and vein.
- Variations of the spleen include wandering spleen, agenesis, accessory spleen, asplenia, and polysplenia.
- Significant laboratory data related to the spleen include hematocrit, bacteremia, leukocytosis, and leukopenia.
- On sonography, the spleen should be evaluated with longitudinal, transverse, and coronal views from the supine or decubitus position.
- Splenic enlargement, or splenomegaly, usually develops whenever the spleen is involved in systemic disease.
- Splenic congestion: (1) In acute congestion, active hyperemia accompanies the reaction in the moderately enlarged spleen; (2) In chronic venous congestion, diffuse enlargement of the spleen occurs.
- Storage diseases include amyloidosis, Gaucher disease, Niemann-Pick disease.
- Erythropoietic abnormalities include the following: sickle cell, hereditary spherocytosis, hemolytic anemia, chronic anemia, polycythemia vera, thalassemia, and myeloproliferative disorders.
- The spleen may be infected by the following: subacute bacterial endocarditis, septicemia, decreased immunologic states, drug abuse, splenic trauma, and infarcts.
- The spleen is most commonly injured due to blunt abdominal trauma; the tear may result in linear or stellate lacerations or capsular tears, puncture wounds from foreign bodies or rib fractures, or subcapsular hematomas.
- Cystic masses do not commonly occur in the spleen; splenic cysts may be classified as congenital or acquired in origin.
- Primary tumors of the spleen are rare; they include hemangioma, hamartoma, and lymphangioma.
- Malignant tumors of the spleen are uncommon; primary tumors found in the spleen include lymphoma and hemangiosarcoma, and very rare splenic tumors include malignant fibrous histiocytoma, leiomyosarcoma, and fibrosarcoma.

BIBLIOGRAPHY

Akhan O, Koroglu M. Hydatid disease of the spleen. *Semin Ultrasound CT, MR*. 2007;28:28–34.

Al-Salem AH, Qaisaruddin S, Al-Jams A, et al. Splenic abscess and sickle cell disease. *Am J Hematol*. 1998;58:2–8.

Cessford T, Meneilly GS, Arishenkoff S, et al. Comparing physical examination with sonographic versions of the same examination techniques for splenomegaly. *JUM*. 2017;37:1621–1629.

Changchien CS. Sonographic patterns of splenic abscess: an analysis of 34 proven cases. *Abdom Imaging*. 2002;27:739–745.

Danaci M, Belet U, Yalin T, et al. Power Doppler sonographic diagnosis of torsion in a wandering spleen. *J Clin Ultrasound*. 2000;28:246–248.

Fitoz S, Atasoy C, Düsünceli E, et al. Post-traumatic intrasplenic pseudoaneurysms with delayed rupture: color Doppler sonographic and CT findings. *J Clin Ultrasound*. 2001;29:102–104.

Gamblin TC, Wall Jr CE, Royer GM, et al. Delayed splenic rupture: case reports and review of the literature. *J Trauma*. 2005;59:1231–1234.

Goldberg BB, McGahan JP. *Atlas of Ultrasound Measurements*. St. Louis: Elsevier; 2006.

Gorg C, Weide R, Schwek W. Malignant splenic lymphoma: sonographic patterns, diagnosis and follow-up. *Clin Radiol*. 1997;52:7–12.

Kamaya A, Weinstein S, Desser TS. Multiple lesions of the spleen: differential diagnosis of cystic and solid lesions. *Semin Ultrasound CT MR*. 2006;27:389–403.

Kessler A, Miller E, Keidar S, et al. Mass at the splenic hilum: a clue to torsion of a wandering spleen located in a normal left upper quadrant position. *J Ultrasound Med*. 2003;22:527–530.

Lamb PM, Lund A, Kanagasaby RR, et al. Spleen size: how well do linear ultrasound measurements correlate with 3D CT volume assessments? *Br J Radiol*. 2002;75:573–577.

Middleton WB, Kurtz AB, Hertzberg BS. *Ultrasound: The Requisites*. 2nd ed. St Louis: Elsevier; 2004.

Perez Fontan FJ, Soler R, Santos M, et al. Accessory spleen torsion: US, CT and MR findings. *Eur Radiol.*. 2001;11:509–512.

Stewart KR, Derck AM, Long KL, et al. Diagnostic accuracy of clinical tests for the detection of splenomegaly. *Phys Ther Rev*. 2013;18:173–184.

Thibodeau GA, Patton KT. *The Human Body in Health & Disease*. 7th ed. St Louis: Elsevier; 2017.

Warshauer DM, Hall HL. Solitary splenic lesions. *Semin Ultrasound CT MR*. 2006;27:370–388.

Wilcox TM, Speer RW, Schlinkert RT, et al. Hemangioma of the spleen: presentation, diagnosis, and management. *J Gastrointest Surg*. 2000;4:611–613.

CHAPTER 12

The Pancreas

Sandra L. Hagen-Ansert

OBJECTIVES

On completion of this chapter, you should be able to:
- Describe the normal anatomy and relational landmarks of the pancreas
- Name the exocrine and endocrine functions of the pancreas
- Describe the laboratory tests used to detect pancreatic disease
- Describe the sonographic technique and patterns of the normal pancreas
- Define the clinical signs and symptoms of pancreatic disease
- Name the congenital anomalies of the pancreas
- List the sonographic findings and differential diagnoses of the following diseases: pancreatitis, pancreatic cyst, and pancreatic tumors

OUTLINE

Anatomy of the Pancreas 356
   Normal Anatomy 356
   Size of the Pancreas 359
   Vascular Supply 359
   Vascular and Ductal Landmarks to the Pancreas 359
   Congenital Anomalies 359
Physiology and Laboratory Data of the Pancreas 360
   Physiology 360
   Laboratory Tests 361

Sonographic Evaluation of the Pancreas 362
   Pancreas Protocol 362
   Normal Pancreatic Texture 363
   Sonographic Scan Technique 363
Pathology of the Pancreas 368
   Pancreatitis 368
   Complications of Pancreatitis 373
   Benign Cystic Lesions of the Pancreas 377
   Cystic Pancreatic Neoplasms 377

Endocrine Pancreatic Neoplasms 381
Metastatic Disease to the Pancreas 386
Parapancreatic Neoplasms 386

KEY TERMS

Acini cells
Amylase
Body of the pancreas
Caudal pancreatic artery
C-loop of the duodenum
Common hepatic artery
Courvoisier sign
Dorsal pancreatic artery
Duct of Santorini

Duct of Wirsung
Endocrine
Exocrine
Glucagon
Head of the pancreas
Hypercalcemia
Hyperlipidemia
Insulin
Islets of Langerhans

Lipase
Neck of the pancreas
Pancreatic ascites
Pancreatic pseudocyst
Pancreatitis
Serum amylase
Tail of the pancreas
Uncinate process

The pancreas continues to be a technical challenge for the sonographer because this gland is in the retroperitoneal cavity posterior to the stomach, duodenum, and proximal jejunum of the small bowel. In addition, the transverse colon may obstruct visualization of the pancreas as it runs horizontally across the abdominal cavity.

Other noninvasive procedures were unsuccessful in visualization of the pancreas before the development of computed tomography (CT), magnetic resonance imaging (MRI), and ultrasound. Plain film of the abdomen may lead to a diagnosis of pancreatitis if calcification is visible in the pancreatic area, but calcification does not occur in all cases. Localized ileus, dilated loops of bowel without peristalsis ("paralyzed gut") caused by gas and fluid accumulation near the area of inflammation, may be shown on the plain radiograph in patients with pancreatitis. The upper gastrointestinal test series provides indirect information about the pancreas when the widened duodenal loops are visualized.

CT and MRI have become the primary modalities to image the patient with pancreatic disease because of their improved resolution of the retroperitoneal structures. However, the normal pancreas can be visualized in most gas-free patients with sonography by using the neighboring organs and vascular landmarks to aid in localization. The gland appears sonographically isoechoic to more hyperechoic than the hepatic parenchyma. Variations in patient positioning or ingestion of water to fill the stomach (that serves as a window to image the pancreas) is used routinely in many laboratories to further aid in visualizing the entire gland. In addition, clinicians performing the endoscopic retrograde cholangiopancreatography (ERCP) examination of the pancreatic duct are incorporating endoscopic ultrasound as an aid in visualizing the detailed anatomy of the pancreatic area.

Sonography is readily accessible and less expensive than other imaging modalities. The primary tasks of the sonographer are to distinguish the normal gland from an abnormal process, image the ductal system, and separate inflammation of the gland from malignancies. Sonography may also aid in percutaneous fine needle aspiration when a lesion is found.

ANATOMY OF THE PANCREAS

Normal Anatomy

The pancreas lies anterior to the first and second lumbar bodies located deep in the epigastrium and left hypochondrium, behind the lesser omental sac (Fig. 12.1). The major posterior vascular landmarks of the pancreas are the aorta and inferior vena cava. The pancreas most commonly extends in a horizontal, oblique lie extending from the second portion of the duodenum to the splenic hilum. Other variations in the lie of the pancreas include transverse, horseshoe, sigmoid, L-shaped, and inverted V. When a variation occurs, the transducer may be angled or rotated to obtain a composite image of the pancreatic gland as the tail may be in a different plane than the body and the head.

It may be surprising that most of the pancreas lies within the retroperitoneal cavity, except for a small portion of the head that is surrounded by peritoneum. Posterior to the pancreas are the connective prevertebral tissues, the portal-splenic confluence, the superior mesenteric vessels, the aorta, the inferior vena cava, and the lower border of the diaphragm (Fig. 12.2). The stomach, duodenum, and transverse colon form the superior and lateral borders of the pancreas, which makes visualization of the pancreas by ultrasound difficult (air and gas interference).

The pancreas is divided into the following four areas: head, neck, body, and tail (see Fig. 12.1). Each area is discussed as it relates to its surrounding anatomy.

Head. The **head of the pancreas** is the most inferior portion of the gland. It lies anterior to the inferior vena cava, to the right of the portal-splenic confluence, inferior to the main portal vein and caudate lobe of the liver, and medial to the duodenum as it "lies in the lap" of the **C-loop of the duodenum** (see Fig. 12.1). The splenic vein forms the posterior medial border of the pancreas, where the superior mesenteric vein joins it to form the main portal vein, thus forming the portal-splenic confluence (Fig. 12.3). The superior mesenteric vein crosses anterior to the uncinate process of the head of the gland and posterior to the neck and body of the pancreas.

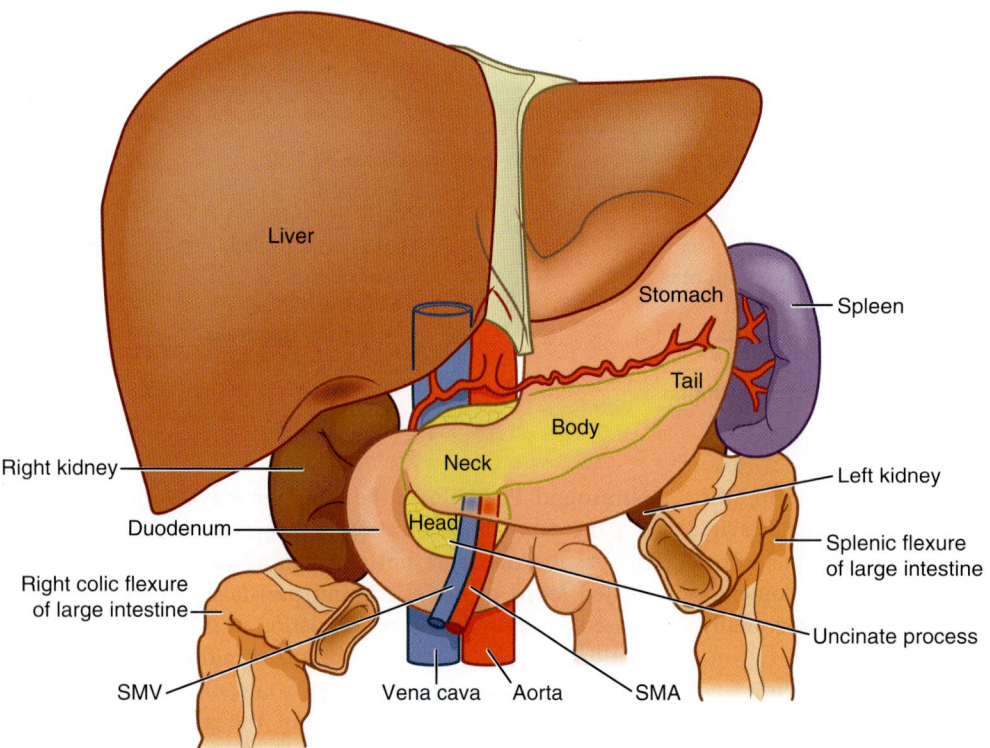

FIG. 12.1 The aorta and inferior vena cava are the posterior landmarks of the pancreas; the stomach is the anterior border. The tail of the pancreas is directed toward the upper pole of the left kidney and hilum of the spleen. The body and head lie anterior to the prevertebral vessels. The four major areas of the pancreas are the head (with the uncinate process), the neck, the body, and the tail. The superior mesenteric vein (SMV) is anterior to the uncinate process. The superior mesenteric artery (SMA) is posterior to the neck/body.

CHAPTER 12 The Pancreas   357

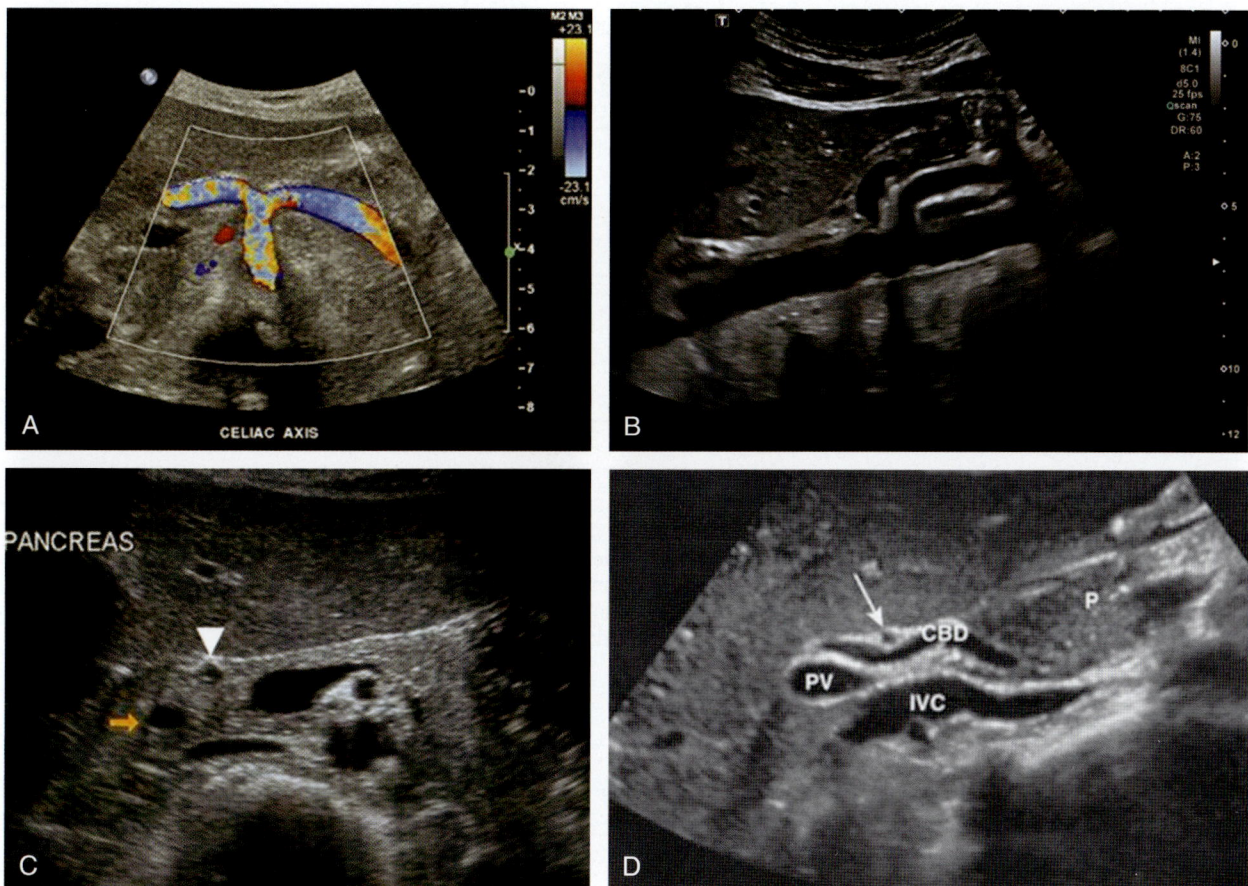

FIG. 12.2 Transverse (A) and sagittal (B) views of the celiac axis with common hepatic and splenic arteries. (C) Gastroduodenal artery *(arrowhead)* is anterior and medial to the common bile duct *(arrow)*. These structures help to define the head of the pancreas. (D) On sagittal views, the portal vein (PV) lies superior to the pancreas (P) and posterior to the common bile duct (CBD). The inferior vena cava (IVC) is the most posterior border.

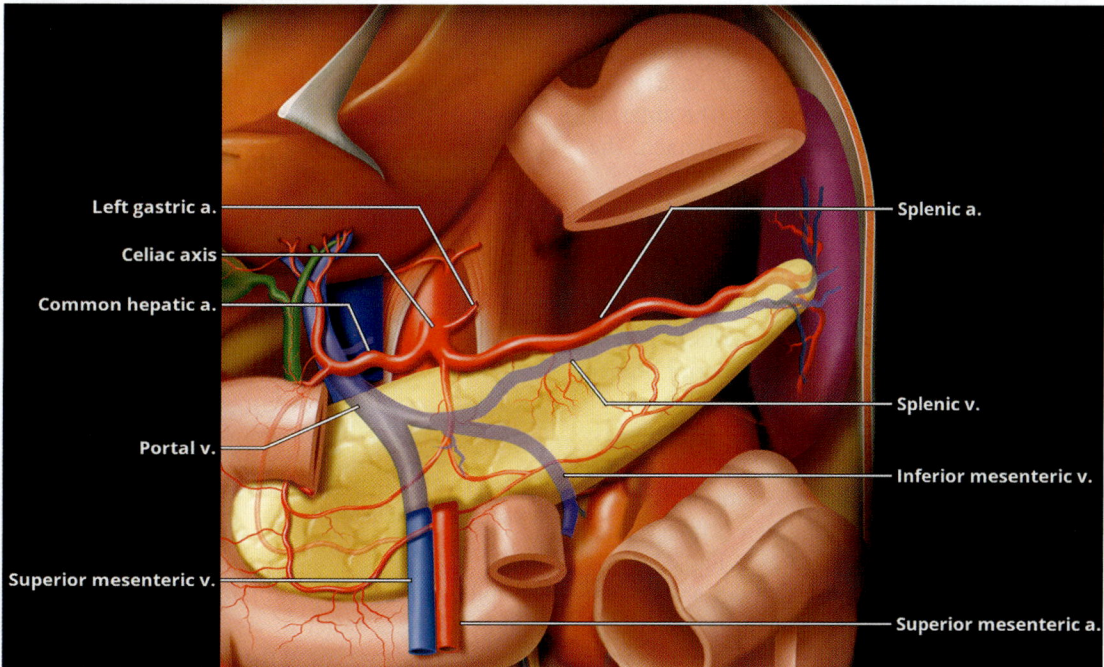

FIG. 12.3 The splenic vein forms the posterior medial border of the pancreas, where it is joined by the superior mesenteric vein to form the main portal vein, thus forming the portal-splenic confluence.

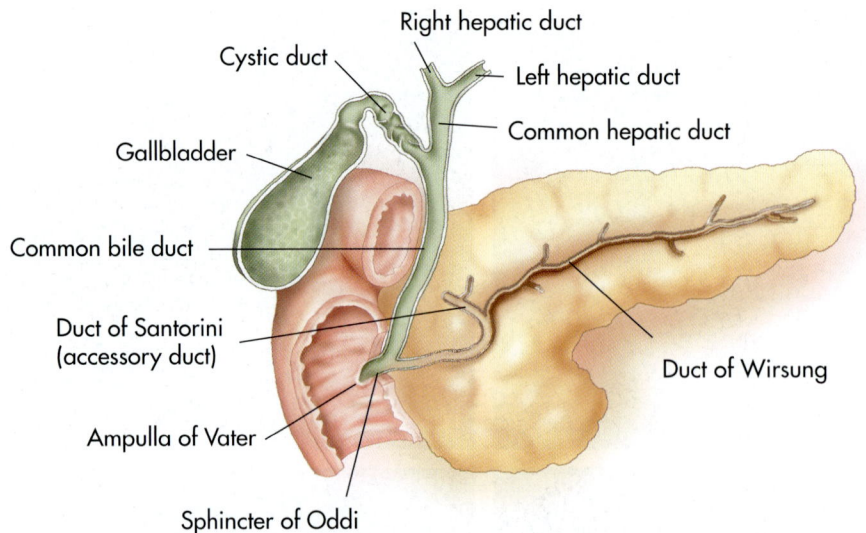

FIG. 12.4 **The head of the pancreas lies in the C-loop of the duodenum.** The common bile duct passes posterior to the first part of the duodenum and courses through a groove posterior to the pancreatic head, where it meets the pancreatic duct to enter the duodenum through the ampulla of Vater. This opening is guarded by the sphincter of Oddi.

The **uncinate process** is the small, curved tip at the end of the head of the pancreas. It lies anterior to the inferior vena cava and posterior to the superior mesenteric vein. As Fig. 12.4 shows, the common bile duct passes posterior to the first part of the duodenum and courses through a groove posterior to the pancreatic head, whereas the gastroduodenal artery forms the anterolateral border (Fig. 12.5).

Neck. The neck is located between the pancreatic head and body and is often included as "part of the body" of the gland. It is found directly anterior to the portal-splenic confluence/superior mesenteric vein (see Fig. 12.1).

Body. The **body of the pancreas** is the largest section of the pancreas. It lies anterior to the aorta and celiac axis, left renal vein, adrenal gland, and kidney. The tortuous splenic artery is the superior border of the gland (see Fig. 12.5). The anterior border is the posterior wall of the antrum of the stomach. The **neck of the pancreas** forms the right lateral border.

Tail. The **tail of the pancreas** is more difficult to image because it lies anterior to the left kidney and posterior to the left colic flexure and transverse colon. The tail begins to the left of the lateral border of the aorta and extends toward the splenic hilum (see Fig. 12.5). The splenic vein is the posterior border of the body and tail. The splenic artery forms the superior border of the tail, whereas the stomach is the anterior border.

Pancreatic Ducts. Two ducts are seen within the pancreas: the duct of Wirsung and the duct of Santorini. To aid in the transport of pancreatic fluid, the ducts have smooth muscle surrounding them. The **duct of Wirsung** is a primary duct extending the entire length of the gland (see Fig. 12.4). It receives tributaries from lobules at right angles and enters the medial second part of the duodenum with the common bile duct at the ampulla of Vater (guarded by the sphincter of Oddi). The **duct of Santorini** is a secondary duct that drains the upper anterior head. It enters the duodenum at the minor

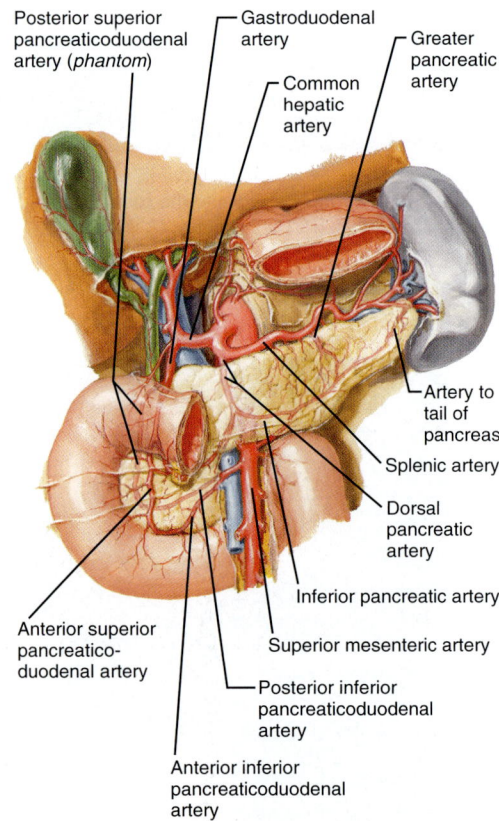

FIG. 12.5 The blood supply for the pancreas is the splenic artery and pancreaticoduodenal arteries.

papilla about 2 cm proximal to the ampulla of Vater. The duct of Wirsung is easier to visualize on ultrasound as it courses through the midline of the gland's body. It appears as an echogenic line or lucency bordered by two echogenic lines. The duct should measure less than 2 mm, tapering as it reaches the tail. Color Doppler imaging may help distinguish the dilated pancreatic duct from the vascular structures (splenic vein and artery) in the area.

Common Bile Duct. The common bile duct runs inferiorly in the free edge of the lesser omentum to the level of the duodenum (see Fig. 12.4). Then it travels posterior to the first portion of the duodenum and the head of the pancreas to the right of the main pancreatic duct. The common bile duct opens into the duodenum after forming a common trunk with the pancreatic duct.

Size of the Pancreas

The average length of the pancreas (head to tail) is about 15 cm, with the range extending between 12 and 18 cm. The head is the thickest part of the gland, measuring 2 to 3 cm in its anterior-to-posterior dimension. The neck measures 1.5 to 2.5 cm, the body measures 2 to 2.5 cm, and the tail measures 1 to 2 cm. The sonographer should evaluate the total size, contour, and texture of the gland to determine enlargement. The gland appears larger or thicker in children than in adults and decreases in size with advancing age.

Vascular Supply

The blood supply for the pancreas is the splenic artery and pancreaticoduodenal arteries (see Fig. 12.5). The anterior and inferior pancreaticoduodenal arteries supply the head and part of the duodenum. The splenic artery supplies the body and tail of the pancreas through four smaller branches: (1) suprapancreatic (rises from the celiac axis/splenic artery), (2) pancreatic, (3) prepancreatic (before leaving the pancreas), and (4) prehilar (before leaving the spleen) and hepatic artery (gastroduodenal artery). The **dorsal pancreatic artery** rises from the suprapancreatic section, the pancreatica magna artery rises from the pancreatic section, and the **caudal pancreatic artery** rises from the prepancreatic or prehilar section. Venous drainage is through tributaries of the splenic and superior mesenteric veins.

Vascular and Ductal Landmarks to the Pancreas

Celiac Axis and Branches. The celiac axis originates from the anterior abdominal aorta and serves as the superior border of the pancreas. It gives rise to three branches: the left gastric, common hepatic, and splenic arteries (see Fig. 12.5).

Splenic Artery. The splenic artery follows a tortuous course along the superior border of the pancreatic body and tail as it crosses horizontally toward the splenic hilum (see Fig. 12.5).

Common Hepatic Artery. The common hepatic artery rises from the celiac axis and courses along the superior margin of the first portion of the duodenum to divide into the proper hepatic artery and gastroduodenal artery, usually when it crosses anterior to the portal vein (see Fig. 12.5). The **common hepatic artery** forms the right superior border of the body and head of the gland and gives rise to the gastroduodenal artery. In some patients, the right hepatic artery rises from the superior mesenteric artery and courses posterior to the medial portion of the splenic vein.

Gastroduodenal Artery. The gastroduodenal artery is seen along the anterolateral border of the pancreas as it travels a short distance along the anterior aspect of the pancreatic head just to the right of the neck before it divides into the superior pancreaticoduodenal branches; they join with the inferior pancreaticoduodenal branches, which rise from the superior mesenteric artery (see Fig. 12.5).

Superior Mesenteric Artery. The superior mesenteric artery rises from the aorta inferior to the celiac axis and posterior to the lower portion of the pancreatic body and courses anterior to the third portion of the duodenum to enter the small bowel mesentery (see Fig. 12.5).

Portal Vein and Tributaries. The main portal vein is formed posterior to the neck of the pancreas by the junction of the superior mesenteric vein and splenic vein (see Fig. 12.3). The splenic vein runs from the splenic hilum along the posterior aspect of the pancreas. The superior mesenteric vein runs posterior to the neck of the pancreas and anterior to the uncinate process, which forms the small, curved tip of the pancreatic head.

Common Bile Duct. The common bile duct crosses the anterior aspect of the portal vein to the right of the proper hepatic artery (Fig. 12.6). The portal vein is anterior to the inferior vena cava. The duct passes along the anterior border of the portal vein and travels posterior to the first portion of the duodenum to course inferior and somewhat posterior in the parenchyma of the head of the pancreas. It joins the pancreatic duct close to the ampulla of Vater.

Congenital Anomalies

Congenital abnormalities of the pancreas are uncommon. The following abnormalities are presented: agenesis, pancreas divisum, ectopic pancreatic tissue, and annular pancreas.

Agenesis. Agenesis of the body and tail, with hypertrophy of the pancreatic head, is a congenital defect.

Pancreas Divisum. This rare condition is caused by the lack of fusion of the dorsal and ventral pancreatic buds. The drainage of the dorsal pancreas is through the minor papilla, with the ventral part draining through the major papilla. On sonography, this diagnosis is challenging. A persistent dorsal pancreatic duct in the head may be identified, but communication with the ventral duct is difficult to ascertain with sonography (Fig. 12.7).

Ectopic Pancreatic Tissue. Ectopic pancreatic tissue is the most common pancreatic anomaly, usually in the form of intramural nodules. The ectopic tissue may be found in various places in the gastrointestinal tract. Frequent sites are the stomach, duodenum, small bowel, and large bowel. On palpation, these lesions may seem polypoid, and they characteristically have a central dimple. They consist of elements of the pancreas, usually the acinar and ductal structures, and less frequently, the islets of Langerhans. They are generally small (0.5 to 2 cm), and acute pancreatitis or tumor may occur within these elements.

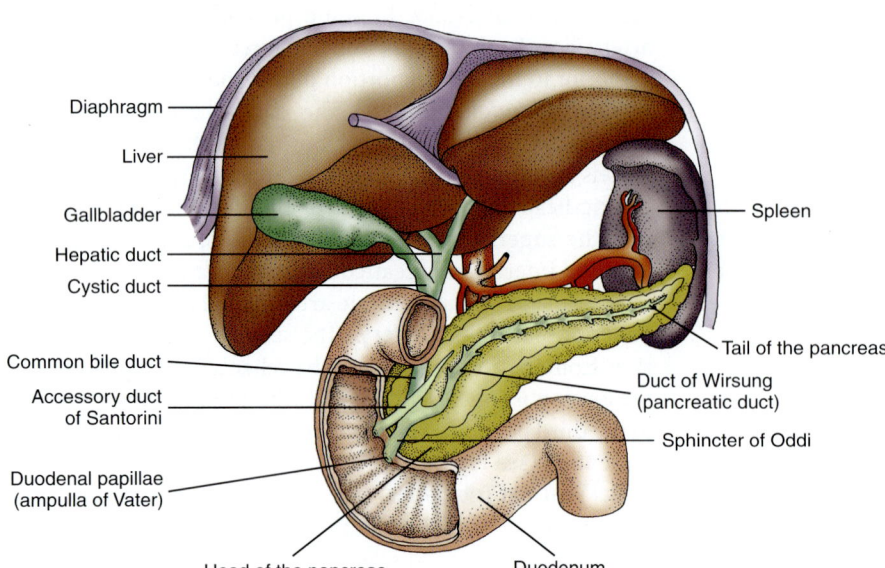

FIG. 12.6 The common bile duct crosses the anterior aspect of the portal vein to the right of the proper hepatic artery. The portal vein is anterior to the inferior vena cava. The duct passes along the anterior border of the portal vein and travels posterior to the first portion of the duodenum to course inferior and somewhat posterior in the parenchyma of the head of the pancreas. It joins the pancreatic duct close to the ampulla of Vater.

Annular Pancreas. Annular pancreas is a rare anomaly in which the head of the pancreas surrounds the second portion of the duodenum (Fig. 12.8). It is more common in males than in females, and all grades (from an overlapping of the posterior duodenal wall to a complete ring) may be found. It may be associated with complete or partial atresia of the duodenum and is susceptible to any of the diseases of the pancreas.

PHYSIOLOGY AND LABORATORY DATA OF THE PANCREAS

Physiology

The pancreas is both a digestive (**exocrine**) and hormonal (**endocrine**) gland. The primary exocrine function is to produce pancreatic juice, which enters the duodenum together with bile. The exocrine secretions of the pancreas and those of the liver, which are delivered into the duodenum through duct systems, are essential for normal intestinal digestion and absorption of food. Pancreatic secretion is under the control of the vagus nerve and two hormonal agents, secretin and pancreozymin, that are released when food enters the duodenum. The endocrine function controls the secretion of glucagons and insulin into the blood. Failure of the pancreas to furnish sufficient insulin leads to diabetes mellitus.

Exocrine Function. Exocrine function is performed by **acini cells** of the pancreas, producing up to 2 L of pancreatic juice per day. These cells are arranged in saclike clusters (acini) connected by small, intercalated ducts to larger excretory ducts. The excretory ducts converge into one or two main ducts, which deliver the exocrine secretion of the pancreas into the duodenum. The enzymes of the pancreatic juice that aid in digestion include **lipase**, which digests fats; **amylase**, which digests carbohydrates; carboxypeptidase, trypsin, and chymotrypsinogen, which digest proteins; and nucleases, which digest nucleic acids (Table 12.1).

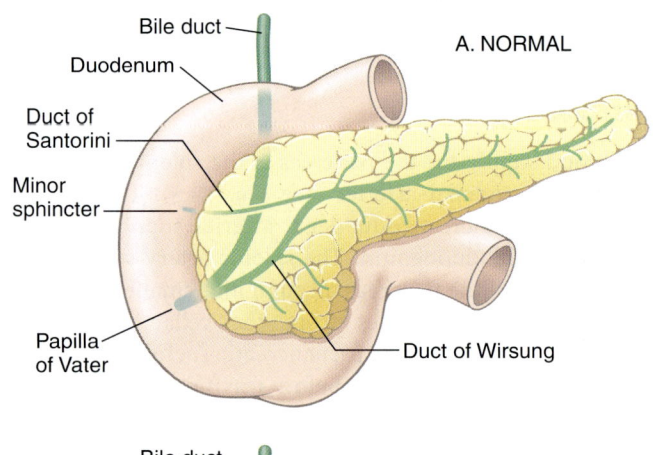
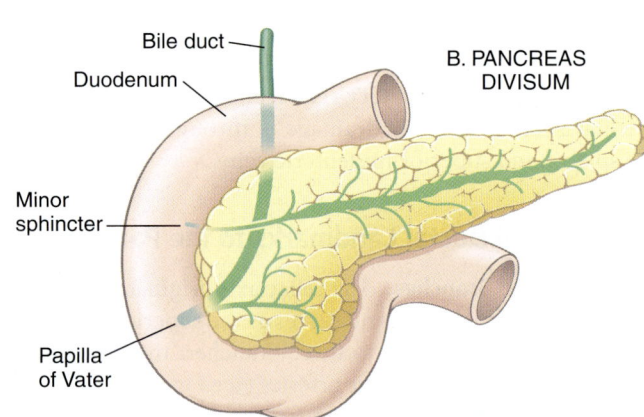

FIG. 12.7 **Pancreas divisum.** The drainage of the dorsal pancreas is through the minor papilla, with the ventral part draining through the major papilla.

Pancreatic juice is the most versatile and active of the digestive secretions. Its enzymes are capable of nearly completing the digestion of food in the absence of all other digestive secretions. Because the digestive enzymes that are secreted into the lumen of the small intestine require an almost neutral pH for best activity, the acidity of the contents entering the duodenum must be reduced. Thus the pancreatic juice contains a relatively high concentration of sodium bicarbonate, and this alkaline salt is largely responsible for the neutralization of gastric acid.

The nervous secretion of pancreatic juice is thick and rich in enzymes and proteins. The chemical secretion, resulting from pancreozymin activity, also is thick, watery, and rich in enzymes. Pancreatic juice is alkaline and becomes more so with increasing rates of secretion. This is because of a simultaneous increase in bicarbonates and decrease in chloride concentration.

The proteolytic enzyme trypsin may hydrolyze protein molecules to polypeptides. Chymotrypsinogen is activated by trypsin. Amylase causes hydrolysis of starch with the production of maltose, which is further hydrolyzed to glucose. Lipase is capable of hydrolyzing some fats to monoglycerides and some to glycerol and fatty acids. Although the small intestine also secretes lipases, what is secreted by the pancreas accounts for 80% of all fat digestion. Thus, impaired fat digestion is an important indicator of pancreatic dysfunction.

Partially digested food, or chyme, in the duodenum stimulates the release of hormones that act on pancreatic juice formation. These hormones include gastrin, cholecystokinin, acetylcholine (all digestive enzymes), and secretin (stimulates production of sodium bicarbonate).

The pancreatic juice enters the duodenum through the duct of Wirsung. This duct joins the common bile duct as it drains bile from the liver, and both enter the duodenum through the ampulla of Vater. The sphincter of Oddi is a muscle surrounding the ampulla of Vater that relaxes to allow pancreatic juice and bile to empty into the duodenum.

Endocrine Function. The endocrine function is in the **islets of Langerhans** in the pancreas. Specialized cells within the islets are called *alpha, beta,* and *delta* cells. The beta cells are most prevalent and produce **insulin**, which causes glycogen formation from glucose in the liver. It also enables cells within insulin receptors to take up glucose (to decrease blood sugar). Alpha cells produce **glucagon**, a hormone that causes the cells to release glucose to meet the body's energy needs. Glucagon stimulates the liver to convert glycogen to glucose to increase sugar levels. Delta cells are the smallest component of endocrine tissue and produce somatostatin. This hormone inhibits the production of both insulin and glucagon. All the hormones are released into the bloodstream (Table 12.2).

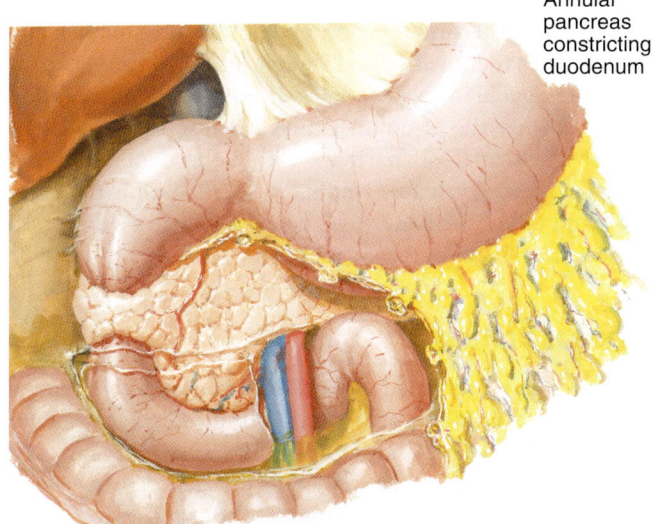
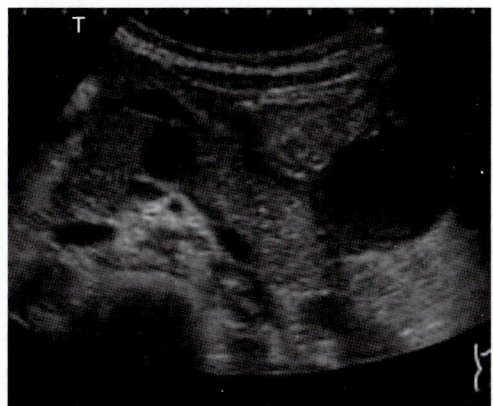
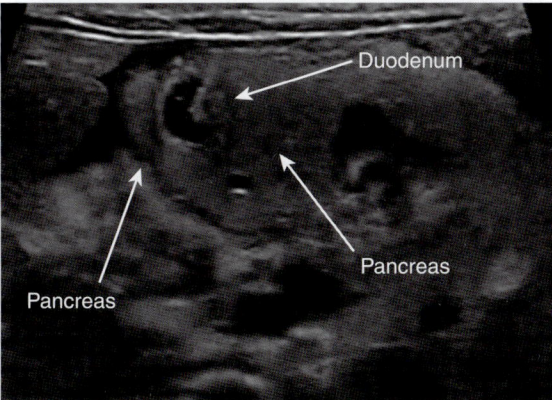

FIG. 12.8 Annular pancreas occurs when the ventral bud fails to rotate with the duodenum and instead surrounds it. This may result in duodenal obstruction.

TABLE 12.1	Pancreatic Exocrine Function
Enzymes of Pancreatic Juice	**Digestive Action**
Lipase	Fats
Amylase	Carbohydrates
Trypsin, chymotrypsinogen, carboxypeptidase	Proteins
Nucleases	Nucleic acids

Laboratory Tests

Specific enzymes of the pancreas may become altered in pancreatic disease, namely amylase and lipase. Increased glucose levels may indicate abnormalities of the pancreas (Table 12.3).

TABLE 12.2	Pancreatic Endocrine Function	
Pancreatic Hormone	**Cell Type**	**Action**
Insulin	Beta	Glucose to glycogen
Glucagon	Alpha	Glycogen to glucose
Somatostatin	Delta	Alpha and beta inhibitor

TABLE 12.3	Laboratory Values for Pancreatic Disease
Condition	**Amylase Level**
Acute pancreatitis	Twice normal
Chronic pancreatitis	No change
Mumps, ischemic bowel disease, pelvic inflammatory disease	↑
	Lipase Level
Acute pancreatitis	↑
Carcinoma of the pancreas	↑
	Blood Glucose Level
Severe diabetes	↑
Chronic liver disease	↑
Overactive endocrine glands	↑
Tumor in islet of Langerhans	↓

↑, Increased; ↓, decreased.

Amylase. Amylase is a digestive enzyme for carbohydrates. It is secreted by the pancreas, parotid glands, gynecologic system, and bowel. In certain types of pancreatic disease, the digestive enzymes of the pancreas escape into the surrounding tissue, producing necrosis with severe pain and inflammation. Under these circumstances, **serum amylase** increases. A serum amylase level of twice normal usually indicates acute pancreatitis.

Other conditions that may cause an increase in amylase include chronic pancreatitis, obstruction of the pancreatic duct, perforated peptic ulcer, acute cholecystitis, and alcohol poisoning. Less common conditions include mumps, ischemic bowel disease, and pelvic inflammatory disease.

Urine Amylase. Urine amylase may be elevated in pancreatitis. Diseases not affecting the pancreas may cause the elevation of serum amylase without elevation of urine amylase.

Lipase. Lipase is an enzyme that is excreted specifically by the pancreas and parallels the elevation in amylase levels. The lipase test is performed to assess damage to the pancreas. The pancreas secretes lipase, and small amounts pass into the blood. The lipase level rises in acute pancreatitis and carcinoma of the pancreas. Both amylase and lipase rise at the same rate, but the elevation in lipase concentration persists for a longer period. Lipase may also be elevated with obstruction of the pancreatic duct, pancreatic carcinoma, and acute cholecystitis.

Glucose. Glucose controls the blood sugar level in the body. The glucose tolerance test is performed to discover whether there is a disorder of glucose metabolism. An increased blood glucose level is found in severe diabetes, chronic liver disease, and overactivity of several endocrine glands. A decreased blood sugar level may occur in tumors of the islets of Langerhans in the pancreas.

SONOGRAPHIC EVALUATION OF THE PANCREAS

The pancreas is one of the most challenging abdominal organs to image with sonography because it lies posterior to the stomach and sometimes the transverse colon. To help visualize the pancreas, the patient should fast for 6 to 8 hours; this decreases the amount of air and fluid in the stomach and colon that may impede visualization. It also promotes dilation of the gallbladder and ducts. If fluid is administered to better visualize the gland, real-time visualization of peristaltic movement of food particles within the duodenum and stomach can be a valuable landmark to help outline the head, body, and tail of the pancreas. This process will be discussed in more detail later in the chapter.

Pancreas Protocol

The pancreas is examined as part of a comprehensive general abdominal study (Table 12.4). Specific indications for pancreatic scanning include abdominal pain, clinically manifested acute or chronic pancreatitis, abnormal laboratory values, cholecystitis, or obstructive jaundice. The examination determines the presence of cystic and solid masses, biliary and ductal dilation, and the presence of extrapancreatic masses and fluid collections.

1. Patient preparation: NPO for at least 6 hours; may need to give water to fill the stomach as a window to image the pancreas.
2. Transducer selection: broadband 2.5 to 5 MHz curvilinear.
3. Patient position: supine, oblique, or upright.
4. Images and observations should include the following:
   - The head, neck/body, and tail should be well delineated once the celiac axis, superior mesenteric artery and vein, aorta, and inferior vena cava are identified. (Often, the lie of the pancreas makes it challenging to image the gland in one plane; the tail may be seen on an image that is more superior than the head of the gland.)
   - Transverse scans along the region of the splenic vein should be performed to demonstrate the body and tail of the pancreas.
   - The pancreatic duct may be seen on the transverse scan as it courses through the body of the gland.
   - The longitudinal view of the pancreatic head lies anterior to the inferior vena cava and inferior to the portal vein.
   - The superior mesenteric vein may be seen to course anterior to the uncinate process of the head and posterior to the body.
   - The pancreatic tail may be seen as gentle, but firm, pressure is applied to the abdomen to displace overlying gas in the antrum of the stomach or transverse colon. The tail

TABLE 12.4	Abdominal Ultrasound Protocol: Pancreas
Scan Plane	**Anatomy**
Transverse	Head/IVC/SMV
	Body and tail/SMV/SMA
Longitudinal	Head/portal vein/IVC
	Body and tail/aorta

IVC, Inferior vena cava; *SMA*, superior mesenteric artery; *SMV*, superior mesenteric vein.

may also be seen with the patient in a right decubitus position, as the transducer is angled through the spleen and left kidney; the pancreatic tail is anterior to the left kidney.
- The presence of dilated pancreatic or biliary ducts should be assessed, and their size measured.
- The presence of cystic or solid masses should be assessed.
- The presence of peripancreatic nodes should be assessed.
- The presence of peripancreatic fluid collections (e.g., pseudocysts) should be assessed.
- The presence of any pancreatic calcifications detected should be recorded.

Normal Pancreatic Texture

The echogenicity of the pancreas is discussed in terms of how it relates to the liver's homogeneous soft echo pattern. The normal pancreas has an echo pattern that is slightly more hyperechoic and finer in texture than that of the surrounding retroperitoneum. The echo intensity of the pancreas is usually slightly less than that of surrounding soft tissue and slightly greater than that of the liver (Fig. 12.9).

The parenchymal texture of the pancreas depends on the amount of fat between the lobules and, to a lesser extent, on the interlobular fibrous tissue. The internal echoes of the pancreas consist of closely spaced elements of the same intensity with uniform distribution throughout the gland. Fat is strongly echogenic, and the extensive fatty infiltrations of the pancreas are difficult to visualize by ultrasound because the pancreas blends in with the surrounding retroperitoneal fat. A lesser degree of fatty infiltration may not render the pancreas invisible but may raise the amplitude of returning pancreatic echoes, resulting in the clinical observation that the pancreas returns stronger echoes than the liver. Fibrous tissue may also account for the portion of increased echogenicity. Box 12.1 lists the sonographic characteristics of the normal pancreas.

Sonographic Scan Technique

The patient is usually examined in the supine, oblique, and sometimes upright position (Fig. 12.10). Sonographic techniques vary according to the patient's body habitus. For adult patients, use a low-frequency broadband transducer with a midfocal zone; for pediatric patients, use at least a 5- to 7.5-MHz transducer. The curved array transducer allows for a better near field of view than the sector transducer allows. The time gain compensation and overall gain should be adjusted so that the pancreatic tissue has the same echo brightness or slightly greater than the normal liver. The texture of the pancreas will appear coarser than the liver, depending on the amount of fibrous/fatty tissue interfaces within the gland. The younger pediatric patients tend to have less echogenicity of the pancreas than the older patients do (i.e., more fatty interfaces in the gland of the older patient). The diabetic patient may be challenging to image through the fatty liver texture; therefore, a lower frequency transducer may be useful. With the patient in deep inspiration, gentle pressure on the abdomen with the transducer allows the sonographer to get as close as possible to the pancreatic tissue to improve visualization.

Box 12.2 summarizes the typical pancreatic landmarks. The sonographer should identify the head, neck, body, and tail in the transverse and longitudinal planes (Figs. 12.11 and 12.12). The sonographer should evaluate the shape, contour, lie, and texture of the pancreas (compared with the liver parenchyma). The oblique or upright position of the patient may improve visualization of the pancreas and peripancreatic

> **BOX 12.1   Normal Characteristics of the Pancreas**
>
> *Size:* Head ≤3 cm; neck ≤2.5 cm; body ≤2.5 cm; tail ≤2 cm
> *Echogenicity:* >liver < or > spleen (depends on fatty/fibrous texture)
> *Echotexture:* Homogeneous
> *Surface:* Smooth to slightly lobular (islets of Langerhans)

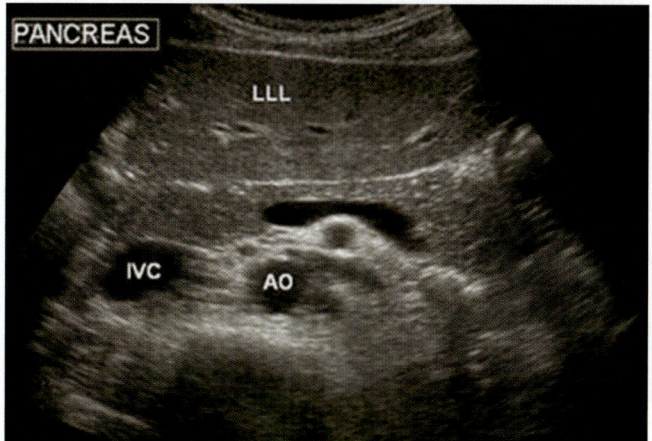

FIG. 12.9 The echo intensity of the pancreas is usually slightly less than that of surrounding soft tissue and slightly greater than that of the liver. *AO*, Aorta; *IVC*, inferior vena cava; *LLL*, left lobe of liver.

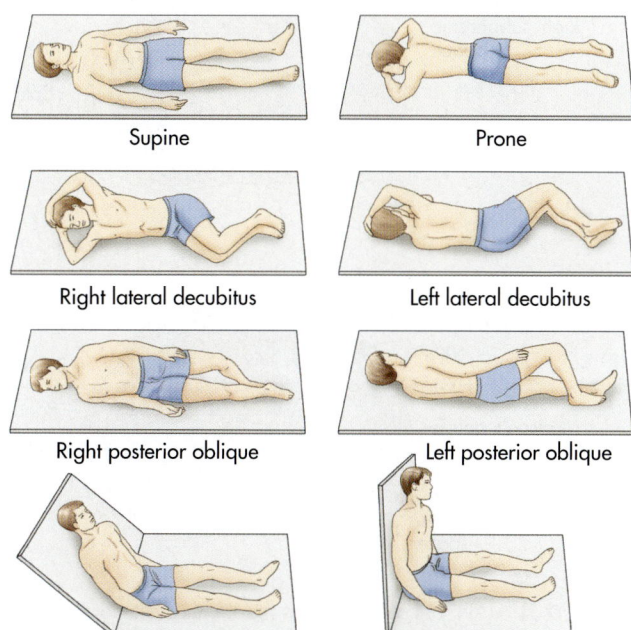

FIG. 12.10 Patient positions to image the pancreas include the supine, decubitus, and semi-upright.

region. The following surrounding structures should be identified: superior mesenteric artery and vein, portal and splenic veins, aorta and inferior vena cava, common bile duct, gastroduodenal artery, left renal vein, duodenal bulb, posterior wall of the stomach, and pancreatic duct.

Windows for Visualization. Difficulties in visualization of the pancreas may result from bowel gas, a transverse stomach obscuring the anatomy, or a small left lobe of the liver. A left lobe measuring at least 2 to 2.5 cm makes an excellent sonic window for imaging the pancreatic area. The subcostal view can be used with a slight caudal angle of the transducer (15 to 20 degrees) as the transducer is directed from the midabdomen (at the level of the xiphoid process) through the left lobe of the liver and angled through the pancreatic area with the prevertebral vessels demarcating its posterior border.

The patient should be in full inspiration to image the pancreas well. This causes the liver to be inferiorly displaced and provides a better scanning window. If the patient has a concave abdomen, ask the patient to take a deep breath and push out the abdomen to provide a better scanning window.

If the sonographer cannot image the pancreas, the water ingestion technique may be an effective window to image the gland. The initial scans of the biliary system should be made before asking the patient to drink 32 to 300 mL of fluid through a straw (to prevent swallowing of air) in the erect or right lateral decubitus position. In the upright position, the stomach can be used as an acoustic window; if the patient cannot sit up, the examination can be done in the right lateral decubitus position. This water method fills the body and antrum of the stomach initially to help outline the body and tail of the pancreas (Fig. 12.13). The fluid then fills the duodenal cap to outline the lateral margin of the head of the pancreas. The upright position allows the air to move from the gastric antrum to the fundus of the stomach and causes the upper viscera to move downward for a better sonic window. The upright position also results in distention of the venous structures, which further aids in the localization of the pancreas (see Box 12.2).

Transverse Plane. Generally, the pancreas is imaged first in the transverse plane (Fig. 12.14). The patient should be in full inspiration to distend the venous structures that serve as posterior landmarks to visualize the pancreas. As previously mentioned, the sonographer should use the left lobe of the liver at the level of the xiphoid and angle the transducer slightly toward the feet to image the aorta and celiac axis. This is near the superior border of the pancreas (remember that the tortuous splenic artery may be seen rising from the

---

BOX 12.2 Normal Pancreatic Landmarks

Head: Anterior to inferior vena cava, lateral to duodenum; gastroduodenal artery is anterolateral border; common bile duct is posterior medial border. On sagittal plane, portal vein is superior to head of the pancreas.
Uncinate process: Anterior to inferior vena cava, posterior to superior mesenteric vein.
Body: Anterior to superior mesenteric artery and vein, aorta, splenic vein; posterior to stomach, inferior to splenic artery.
Tail: Medial to hilum of spleen; superior to left kidney.
Pancreatic duct: Runs through mid portion of body of pancreas.

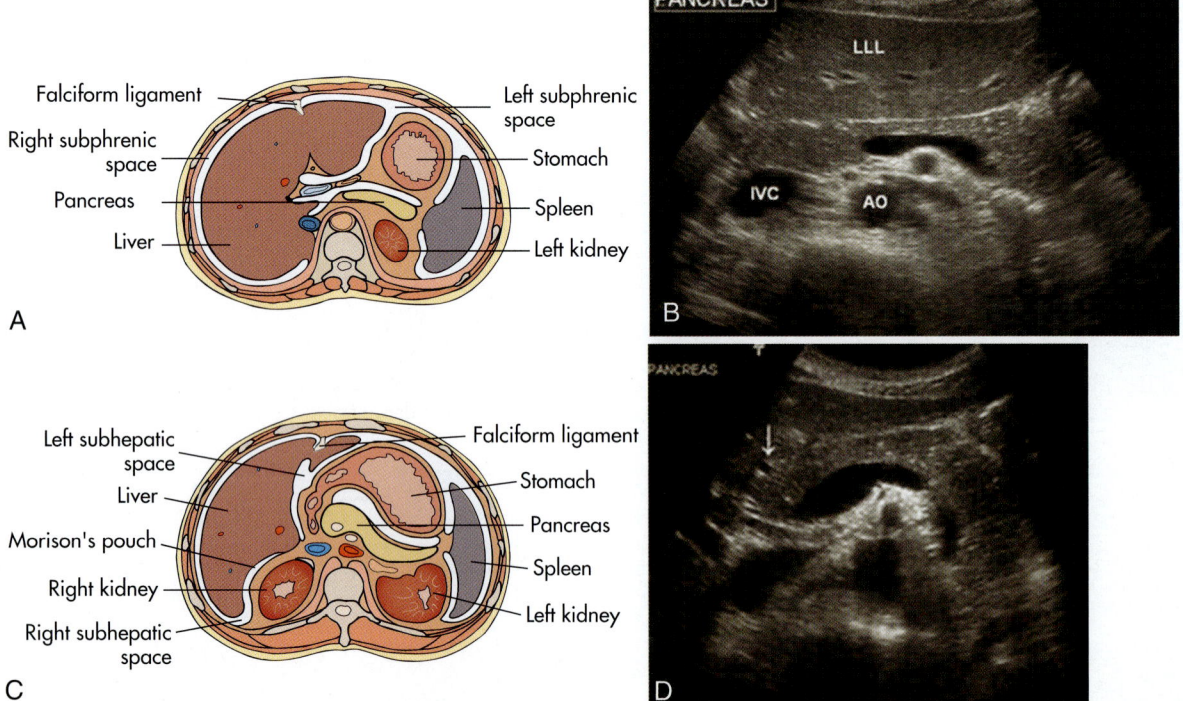

FIG. 12.11 (A) Cross section shows the stomach anterior to the body and tail of the pancreas; the posterior structures to the gland are the superior mesenteric artery, aorta (AO) and inferior vena cava (IVC), and left kidney. (B) Sonographic transverse image demonstrates the left lobe of the liver (LLL) anterior to the pancreas. The splenic vein is posterior, and the superior mesenteric artery, aorta, and IVC are inferior. (C) Cross section of the abdomen just inferior to part A. (D) Sonographic transverse image of the pancreas. The *arrow* points to the gastroduodenal artery.

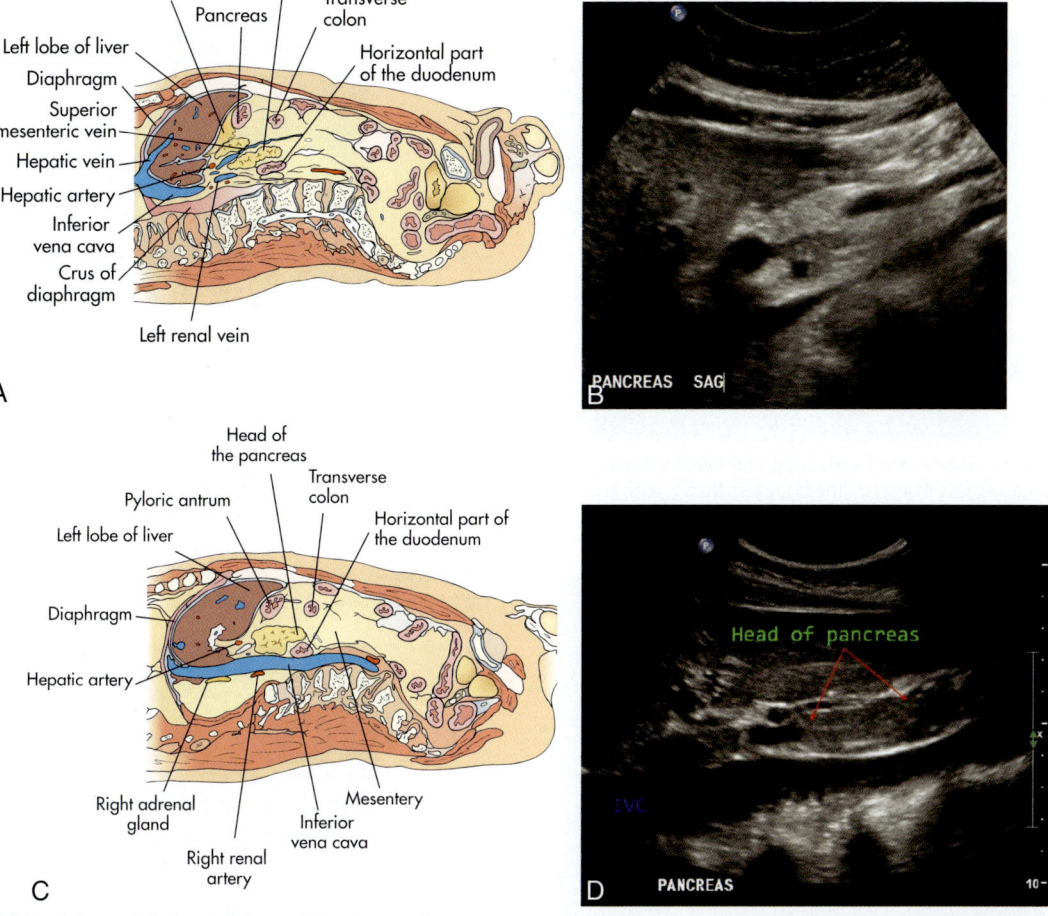

FIG. 12.12 (A) Sagittal plane of the pancreas. Note the superior mesenteric vein is posterior to the neck and anterior to the uncinated process of the pancreas. (B) Sagittal image of the superior mesenteric vein demarcating the body/head of the pancreas. (C) Sagittal plane of the pancreas. The head of the pancreas lies anterior to the inferior vena cava and inferior to the portal vein. (D) Head of the pancreas is compressing the inferior vena cava. The portal vein *(curved arrow)* is seen superior to the head. *IVC*, Inferior vena cava.

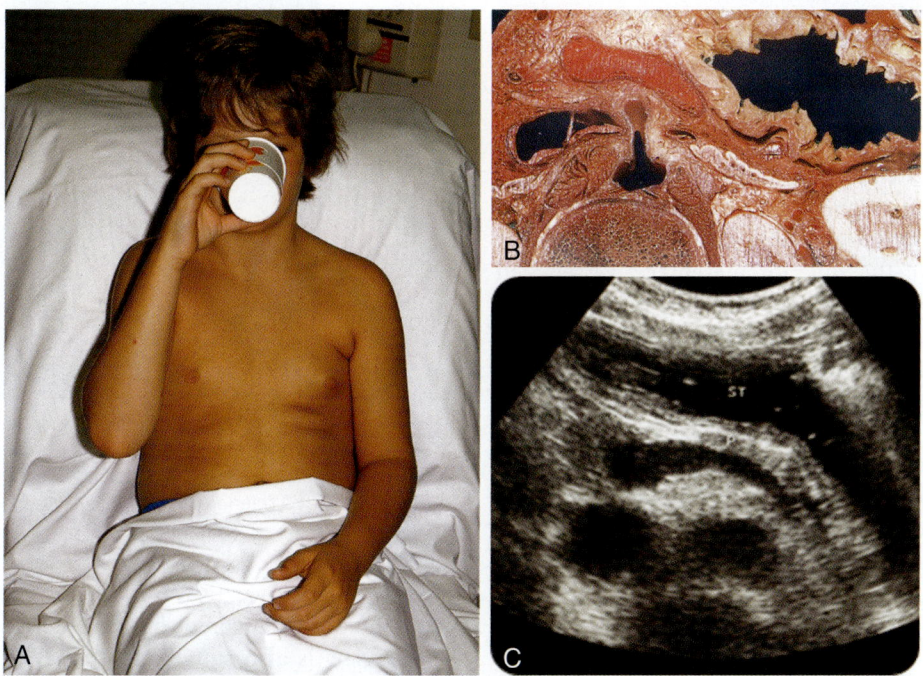

FIG. 12.13 (A) To better visualize the pancreas, the patient should drink more than 16 ounces of water and be imaged in the semiupright position. (B) Gross anatomy of the midepigastrium at the level of the superior mesenteric artery. The body of the pancreas is clearly seen anterior to the superior mesenteric artery and posterior to the stomach. (C) A fluid-filled stomach (ST) may serve as a window to visualize the pancreas.

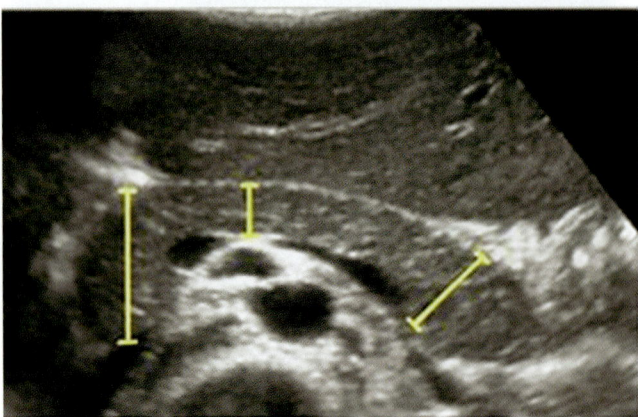

FIG. 12.14 Transverse view of the head, body, and tail of the pancreas. The head should measure less than 3 cm, the body less than 2.5 cm, and the tail less than 2 cm.

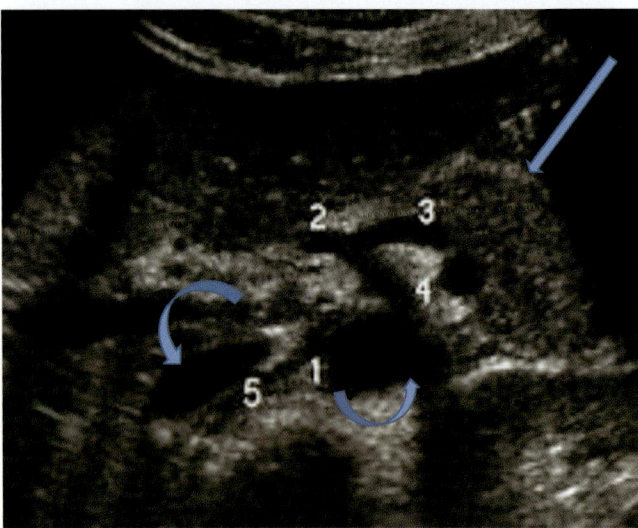

FIG. 12.15 Transverse image of vascular landmarks for the pancreas (arrows). 1, Aorta. 2, Hepatic artery. 3, Splenic artery. 4, Celiac trunk. 5, Inferior vena cava.

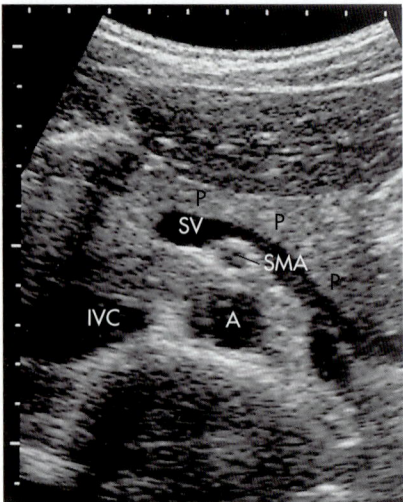

FIG. 12.16 Transverse scan of the normal pancreas and its vascular landmarks. *A,* Aorta; *IVC,* inferior vena cava; *P,* pancreas; *SMA,* superior mesenteric artery; *SV,* splenic vein.

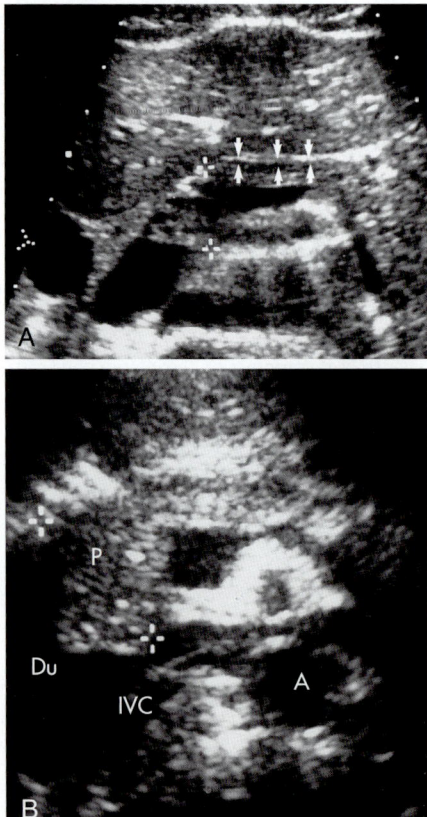

FIG. 12.17 (A) The collapsed wall of the stomach *(arrows)* may be seen as two parallel lines anterior to the body of the pancreas. (B) The fluid-filled duodenum (Du) marks the lateral border of the head of the pancreas (P). *A,* Aorta; *IVC,* inferior vena cava.

celiac axis to demarcate the superior border of the pancreas) (Fig. 12.15). The body and tail of the gland should be imaged as the transducer is slowly angled inferiorly from the celiac axis. Visualization of the superior mesenteric vessels, left renal vein, and inferior vena cava also helps delineate the borders of the body of the pancreas (Fig. 12.16). The stomach may be seen as the walls are collapsed because it lies anterior to the pancreas (Fig. 12.17). The duodenum, gastroduodenal artery, and common bile duct are useful landmarks in identifying the lateral margin of the pancreatic head (Fig. 12.18). The sonographer may watch for peristalsis or fluid to pass through the second part of the duodenum as it forms the C-loop around the lateral border of the head.

Sagittal Plane. The initial scan should be made slightly to the right of midline with the patient in full inspiration. The dilated inferior vena cava is seen as the posterior border (Fig. 12.19). The main portal vein or right branch of the portal vein is the next landmark seen anterior to the cava. The pancreas lies just inferior to the portal vein and anterior to the inferior vena cava. As the pancreas enlarges, a slight indentation is apparent on the anterior border of the cava. This view is also suitable for visualizing the common bile duct because it lies anterior to the portal vein before dropping posterior to enter the head of the pancreas (Fig. 12.20). The hepatic artery is sometimes visible as a circular tube

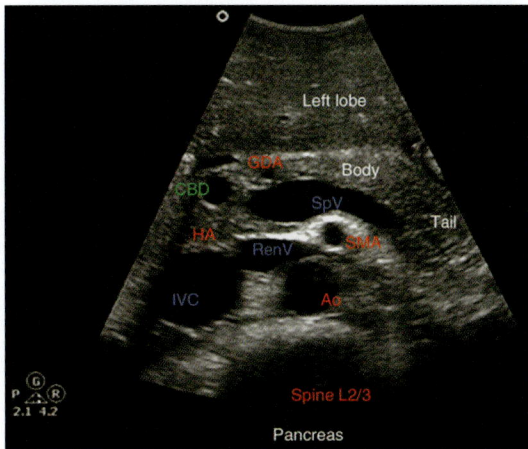

FIG. 12.18 The duodenum, gastroduodenal artery, and common bile duct are useful landmarks in identifying the lateral margin of the pancreatic head. *Ao*, Aorta; *CBD*, common bile duct; *GDA*, gastroduodenal artery; *HA*, hepatic artery; *IVC*, inferior vena cava; *RenV*, renal vein; *SMA*, superior mesenteric artery; *SpV*, splenic vein.

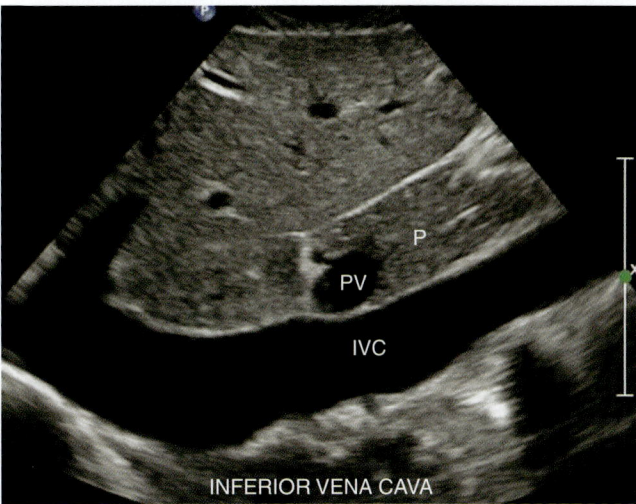

FIG. 12.19 Sagittal image of the dilated inferior vena cava (IVC) as it demarcates the posterior border of the pancreas (P). The portal vein (PV) is seen anterior to the IVC and cephalad to the pancreas.

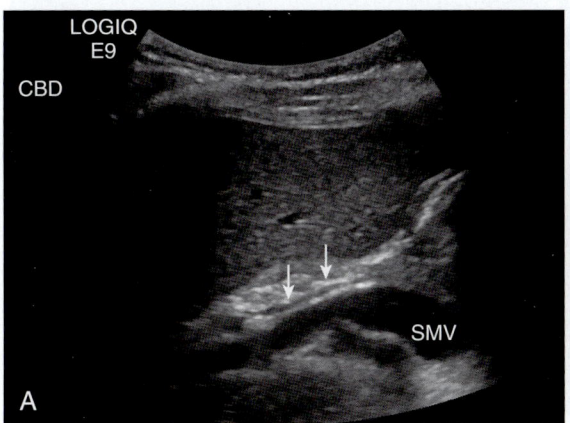
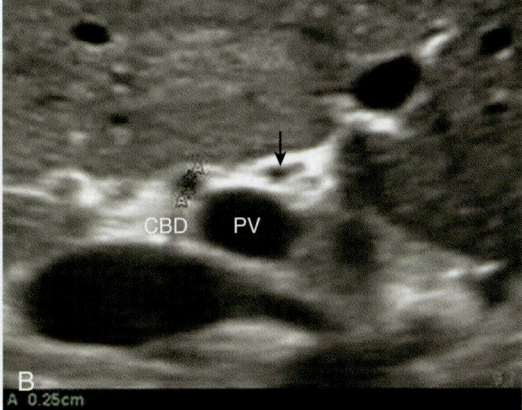

FIG. 12.20 (A) Sagittal scan of the common bile duct *(white arrows)* and its surrounding vascular landmarks. (B) The common bile duct (CBD, *open arrows*) is seen anterior and lateral to the portal vein (PV), while the hepatic artery *(black arrow)* is anterior medial with the patient in a decubitus position. *CBD*, Common bile duct; *SMV*, superior mesenteric vein/portal vein confluence.

when the common duct is seen. The use of color Doppler may help the sonographer separate the hepatic artery from the common duct.

Subsequent scans are made slightly to the left of the midline to image the aorta and superior mesenteric artery and vein because they form the posterior border of the body of the pancreas (Fig. 12.21). The superior mesenteric vein flows cephalad to join the portal vein and may be seen as a long, tubular structure posterior to the neck of the pancreas and anterior to the uncinate process. The tail of the pancreas is more difficult to see, but it may be imaged as the sonographer angles slightly to the left of the aorta. The patient may be rolled into a steep right decubitus position to image the tail of the gland as it lies in the hilum of the spleen near the left kidney.

The antrum of the stomach appears as a collapsed bull's-eye and may be identified anterior and slightly caudal to the body of the pancreas (Fig. 12.22). The splenic vein is a circular sonolucent structure posterior to the cephalic portion of the gland. The left renal vein is a slitlike sonolucency between the aorta and the superior mesenteric artery.

Pancreatic Duct. The main pancreatic duct may be visualized best on the transverse image as it courses through the body of the gland (Fig. 12.23). The sonographer should be sure to identify pancreatic tissue on both sides of the duct to avoid confusing it with vascular structures that may lie near it. The splenic vein is usually too posterior and the hepatic artery too anterior to be confused with the duct. Color Doppler may be used to help distinguish a dilated duct from vascular structures. The duct appears as an echo-free area sharply marginated by two parallel echogenic lines. A thin strip of retroperitoneal fat may underlie the anterior aspect of the pancreas. This sonolucent linear pattern should not be mistaken for duct. On transverse scans, the posterior wall of the antrum can be seen overlying the pancreas. Care should be taken to distinguish the antrum of the collapsed stomach from the small pancreatic duct.

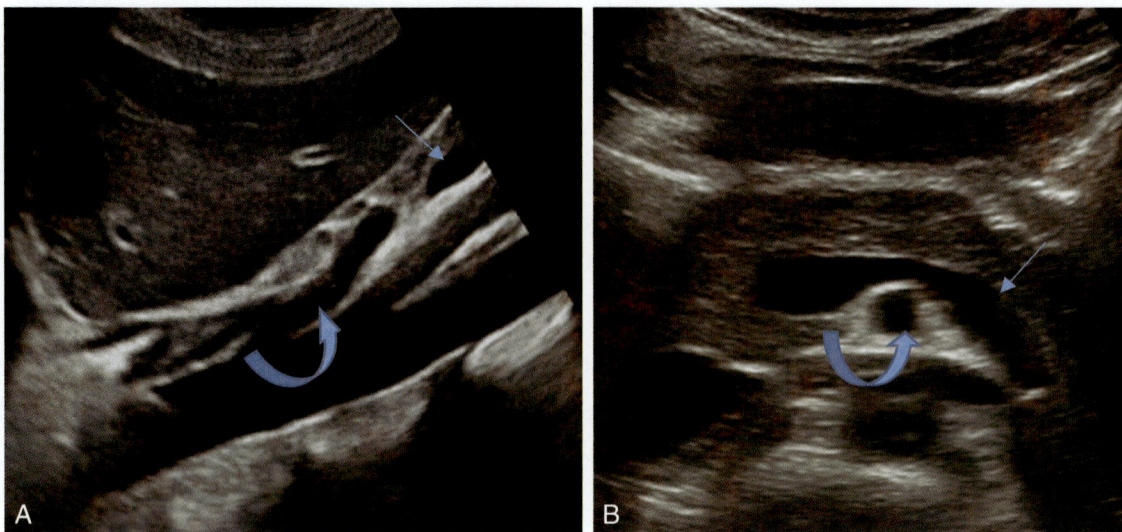

FIG. 12.21 Sagittal (A) and transverse (B) images of the superior mesenteric artery *(curved arrow)* and vein *(straight arrow)* that form the posterior border of the pancreas.

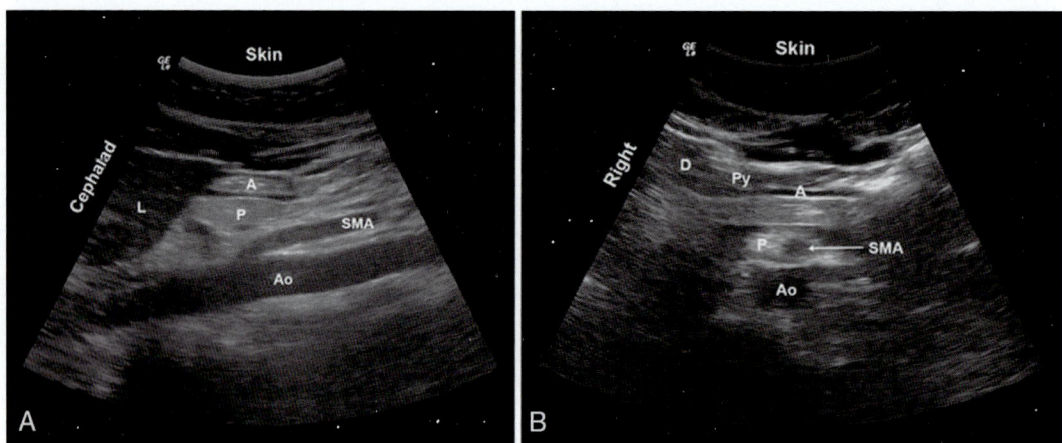

FIG. 12.22 Sagittal (A) and transverse (B) images. The antrum (A) of the stomach appears as a collapsed bull's-eye and may be identified anterior and slightly caudal to the body of the pancreas (P). *Ao,* Aorta; *D,* duodenum; *L,* liver; *Py,* pylorus; *SMA,* superior mesenteric artery.

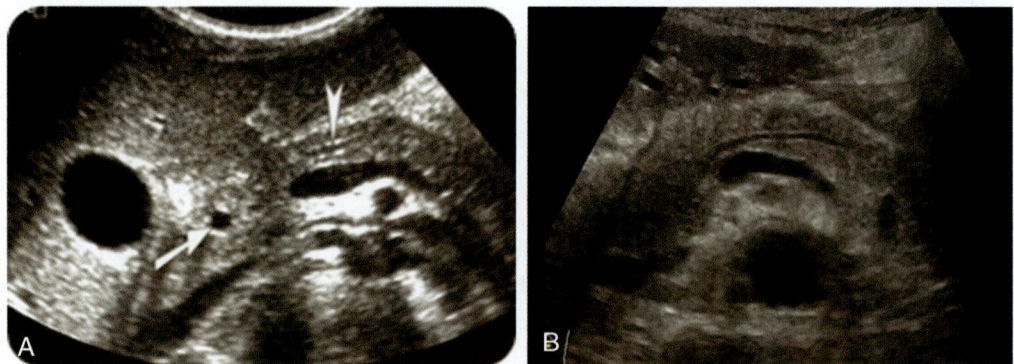

FIG. 12.23 (A) Transverse images of the normal pancreatic duct *(arrowhead).* The common bile duct is denoted by the *arrow.* (B) Transverse image of the pancreas. The small tubular structure is the pancreatic duct. The splenic vein is seen just posterior to the duct.

PATHOLOGY OF THE PANCREAS

Pancreatitis

Pancreatitis is inflammation of the pancreas; this condition may be chronic or acute. Pancreatitis occurs when the pancreas becomes damaged and malfunctions as a result of increased secretion and blockage of ducts. When this occurs, the pancreatic tissue may be digested by its own enzymes. Pancreatitis may be classified as acute or chronic with a further subdescription of mild to severe. In patients with acute pancreatitis, ultrasound may not always be the first imaging performed because often ileus is associated with this condition. Therefore, the optimal imaging procedure is the dynamic intravenous and oral contrast-enhanced computed tomography. Table 12.5 provides clinical findings, sonographic findings, and differential considerations for pancreatitis.

Acute Pancreatitis. Acute pancreatitis is an inflammation of the pancreas caused by the inflamed acini releasing pancreatic enzymes into the surrounding pancreatic tissue (Fig. 12.24). Usually, these enzymes do not become active until they reach the duodenum, enabling the breakdown of food in the system. The classification of acute pancreatitis is further divided into the following three categories: (1) mild acute pancreatitis, characterized by the absence of organ failure and local or systemic complications, (2) moderately severe acute pancreatitis, characterized by transient organ failure and local or systemic complications without persistent organ failure, and (3) severe acute pancreatitis, characterized by persistent organ failure that may involve one or multiple organs.

The clinical features of acute process of pancreatitis usually do not last more than several days. Most patients present with acute onset of persistent, severe mid-epigastric pain accompanied by nausea and vomiting. In patients with gallstone pancreatitis, the pain is well localized, and the onset of pain is rapid, reaching maximum intensity in 10 to 20 minutes. In

TABLE 12.5 Pancreatitis Findings

Clinical Findings	Sonographic Findings	Differential Considerations
Acute Pancreatitis		
• Sudden onset of moderate to severe abdominal pain with radiation to back • Nausea and vomiting • History of gallstones (localized) or alcoholism • Mild fever • ↑ Pancreatic enzymes in blood (amylase, lipase) • Leukocytosis (↑ white blood cells) • Abdominal distention	• Ranges from normal size to focal/diffuse enlargement • Hypoechoic texture (edema) • Borders distinct but irregular • Enlargement of head causes depression on inferior vena cava • 40%–60% have gallstones • Pancreatic duct may be enlarged • Parapancreatic fluid collections	• Hemorrhagic pancreatitis • Pancreatic neoplasm • Lymphoma • Retroperitoneal neoplasm
Hemorrhagic Pancreatitis		
• ↓ Hematocrit and serum calcium level • Intense, severe pain radiating to back, with subsequent shock and ileus • Hypotension despite volume replacement, with metabolic acidosis and adult respiratory distress syndrome	• Depends on age of hemorrhage • Well-defined homogeneous mass in area of pancreas	• Chronic hemorrhage
Phlegmonous Pancreatitis		
See acute pancreatitis	• Hypoechoic, ill-defined mass	• Chronic hemorrhage
Pancreatic Abscess		
• Fever, chills • ↑ Leukocytosis • Hypotension • Tender abdomen	• Hypoechoic mass with smooth borders • Thick walls • Echo-free to echogenic	• Acute pancreatitis • Chronic pancreatitis
Chronic Pancreatitis		
• Severe abdominal pain radiating to back • Malabsorption • Fatty stools • Signs of diabetes • Weight loss • Jaundice • ↑ Amylase and lipase	• Gland is small and fibrotic • Irregular borders • Mixed echogenicity • Dilated pancreatic duct (string of pearls sign with dilated duct) • Look for calculi within duct	• Acute pancreatitis • Thrombosis of portal system • Pancreatic pseudocyst • Dilated common bile duct
Pancreatic Pseudocyst		
• Asymptomatic unless large enough to put pressure on other organs • ↑ Amylase and lipase • ↑ Alkaline phosphatase if obstruction develops	• Well-defined mass, usually in area of pancreas • ↑ Through-transmission • Variable size (round or oval) • May have debris at bottom	• True cyst • Fluid-filled cystadenoma

↑, Increased; ↓, decreased.

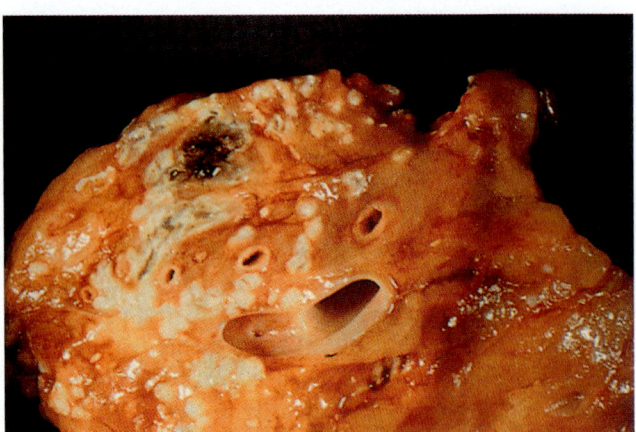

FIG. 12.24 Gross pathology of acute pancreatitis. The foci of fat necrosis appear as white opaque patches.

contrast, the pain is usually not as abrupt and is poorly localized in patients with pancreatitis secondary to alcohol, metabolic, or hereditary causes. The pain may radiate to the back and persist for several hours to days. The patient may be at risk for abscess and hemorrhage secondary to the pancreatitis.

An acute attack of pancreatitis is commonly related to biliary tract disease and alcoholism. The most common cause of pancreatitis in the United States is biliary tract disease. Gallstones are present in 40% to 60% of patients, and 5% of patients with gallstones have acute pancreatitis. Gallstone pancreatitis causes a relatively sudden onset of constant biliary pain. As the pancreatic parenchyma is further damaged, the pain becomes more severe, and the abdomen becomes rigid and tender.

Alcohol abuse is the second most common cause of pancreatitis. Other less common causes include trauma, inflammation from adjacent peptic ulcer or abdominal infection, pregnancy, mumps, tumors, congenital causes, vascular thrombosis or embolism, and drugs.

The laboratory analysis of pancreatic enzymes is the key to pancreatic destruction (see Table 12.5). Serum amylase rises within 6 to 12 hours of the onset of acute pancreatitis. Amylase has a short half-life of approximately 10 hours and, in uncomplicated attacks, returns to normal within three to five days. Serum lipase rises within 4 to 8 hours of the onset of symptoms, peaks at 24 hours, and returns to normal within 8 to 14 days. Lipase elevations occur earlier and last longer than elevations in amylase and are therefore especially useful in patients who present greater than 24 hours after the onset of pain. Serum lipase is also more sensitive compared with amylase in patients with pancreatitis secondary to alcohol abuse.

Acute pancreatitis may be mild to severe. Damage to the acinar tissue and ductal system results either in exudation of pancreatic juice into the gland's interstitium, leakage of secretions into the peripancreatic tissues, or both. After the acini or duct disrupts, the secretions migrate to the surface of the gland. The common course is for fluid to break through the pancreatic connective tissue layer and thin posterior layer of the peritoneum and enter the lesser sac. The mild form of pancreatitis demonstrates interstitial edema within the gland with little or no peripancreatic inflammation. Small areas of acinar cell necrosis may be within the pancreas. As the process becomes more severe, fat necrosis, parenchymal necrosis, and necrosis of the blood vessels develop with subsequent hemorrhage and peripancreatic inflammation within 1 to 2 days. With time, this necrotic tissue is replaced by diffuse or focal fibrosis, calcifications, and irregular ductal dilations. The formation of a pseudocyst may develop secondary to acute pancreatitis.

The pancreatic juice enters the anterior pararenal space by breaking through the thin layer of the fibrous connective tissue, or the fluid may migrate to the surface of the gland and remain within the confines of the fibrous connective tissue layer.

Collections of fluid in the peripancreatic area generally retain communication with the pancreas. A dynamic equilibrium is established so that fluid is continuously absorbed from the collection and replaced by additional pancreatic secretions. The drainage of juices may cease as the pancreatic inflammatory response subsides and the rate of pancreatic secretions returns to normal. The collections of extrapancreatic fluid should be reabsorbed or, if drained, should not recur with recovery of proper drainage through the duct.

Sonographic Findings. The sonographic description of acute pancreatitis may be defined by distribution (focal or diffuse) and by severity (mild, moderate, or severe). In the early stages of acute pancreatitis, the gland may not show swelling on sonography (Fig. 12.25). When swelling does occur, the gland is hypoechoic to anechoic and is less echogenic than the liver because of the increased prominence of lobulations and congested vessels. The borders may be somewhat indistinct but smooth. On a longitudinal scan, the anterior compression of the inferior vena cava by the swollen head of the pancreas may be apparent. Thus pancreatic enlargement and decreased pancreatic echogenicity are sonographic landmarks for acute pancreatitis.

If localized enlargement is present, it may be difficult to separate from neoplastic involvement of the gland. Analysis of patient history and laboratory values should enable the clinician to make the distinction. If the serum amylase level is normal and the patient is asymptomatic, the mass is likely to represent a neoplasm. However, if the patient has severe abdominal pain, tender to the touch, this focal hypoechogenicity is more likely caused by pancreatitis than by a neoplastic growth. If the mass has calcification within an enlarged ductal system, a neoplasm is more likely suspected. The evaluation by ERCP may provide better resolution of the pancreatic head and ductal system to further delineate neoplastic growth from pancreatitis.

The pancreatic duct may be obstructed in acute pancreatitis due to inflammation, spasm, edema, swelling of the papilla, or pseudocyst formation (Fig. 12.26). The detection of biliary obstruction is important as many of the patients have coexisting liver disease. Obstruction of the biliary system may be due to stricture in the distal common duct or to compression of the common bile duct by a pseudocyst or inflammation of the head of the pancreas.

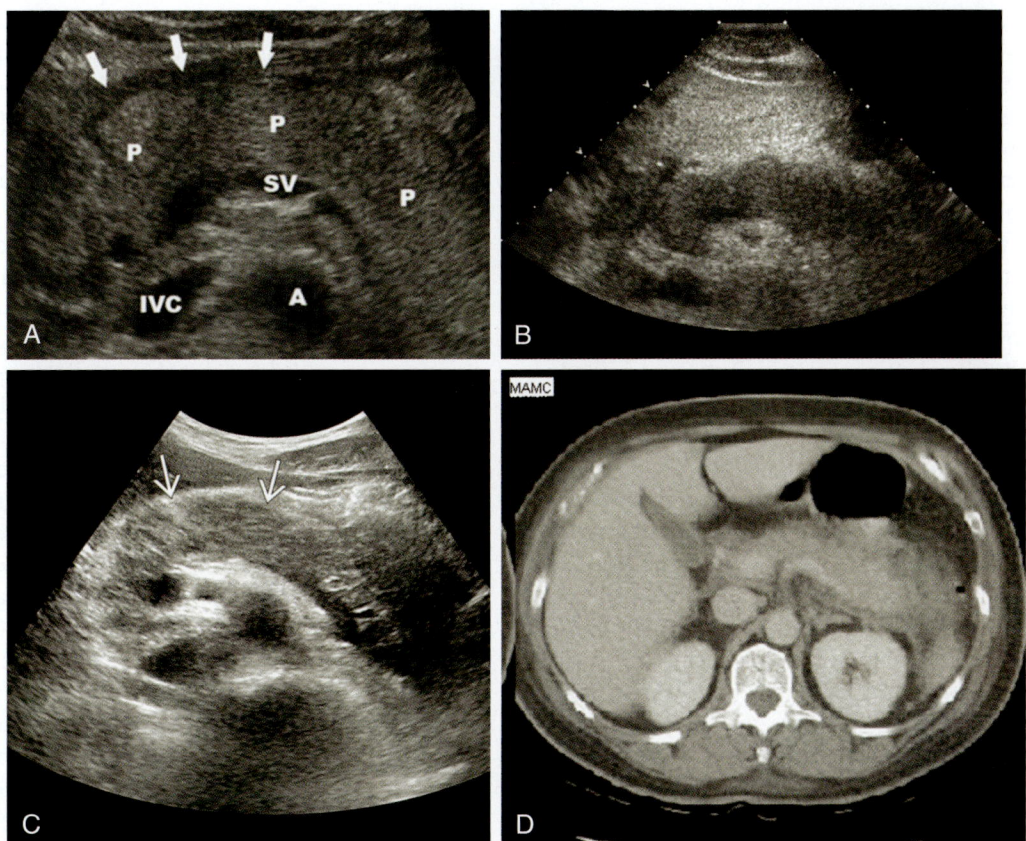

FIG. 12.25 Sonographic (A–C) and computed tomographic (D) patterns seen in patients with acute pancreatitis. The mild form of pancreatitis demonstrates interstitial edema within the gland with little or no peripancreatic inflammation. *A*, Aorta; *IVC*, inferior vena cava; *P*, pancreas; *SV*, splenic vein. *Arrows* denote the inflamed pancreas.

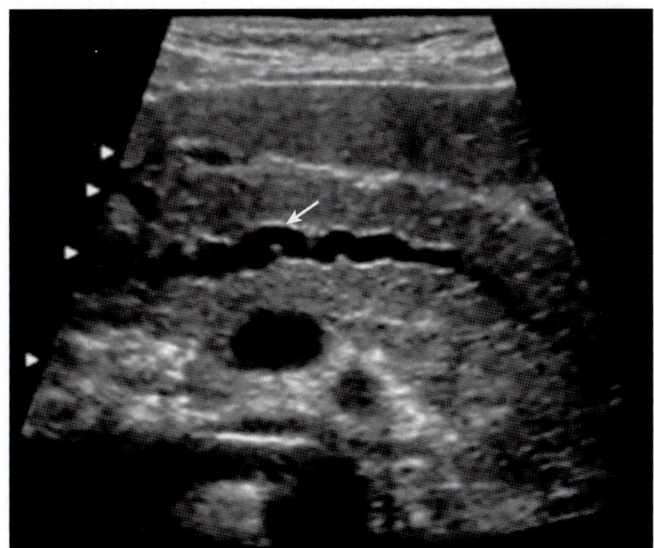

FIG. 12.26 Dilation of the pancreatic duct *(arrow)* secondary to pancreatitis and inflammation in the head of the pancreas.

In diffuse pancreatitis, the pancreas enlarges, and the texture becomes hypoechogenic compared with the "normal" liver texture. Because alcohol is a frequent cause of pancreatitis, the development of a hyperechoic diffuse fatty liver makes this comparison invalid. As the disease progresses, the decreased echogenicity and enlargement are readily seen secondary to increased fluid content in the interstitium caused by the inflammation. The pancreas may be diffusely inhomogeneous. The pancreatic duct may be either compressed by the edema or dilated (from the focal pancreatic inflammation or obstruction of the stone or tumor).

Sonography is not as effective as CT in the early stages of pancreatitis, as CT is more specific in its ability to demonstrate the detail of the pancreas and the retroperitoneal structures, regardless of bowel interference. CT can detect necrosis and acute fracture of the pancreas. Sonographic detection of pancreatitis is effective when ileus is not present to obstruct the visualization of the pancreatic area.

Complications of acute pancreatitis include hemorrhage, pseudocyst formation, inflammatory mass, and intrapancreatic and extrapancreatic fluid collections. Sonography may directly guide the interventionalist for needle aspiration to help differentiate between an infected and noninfected inflammatory mass and pseudocyst collection.

Extrapancreatic Fluid Collections and Edema. The findings of fluid collections and edema are frequent in patients with severe acute pancreatitis. The most common sites for fluid collection are found in the lesser sac, anterior pararenal spaces, mesocolon, perirenal spaces, and peripancreatic soft tissue spaces (Fig. 12.27).

For the sonographer, the fluid in the lesser sac that is found between the stomach and the pancreas is easily imaged. Fluid in the superior recess of the lesser sac is seen to surround the caudate lobe with visualization of the gastrohepatic ligament. Fluid that lies in the perirenal space may also be demonstrated on sonography. As fluid collects in the anterior pararenal space, it is best demonstrated on the sagittal sonographic image. The fluid may be anechoic or contain fine linear lines within that represent septations secondary to infection or hemorrhage. The more solid composition of the retroperitoneal or intraperitoneal fluid collections is most difficult to image with sonography because of bowel interference. These extrapancreatic fluid collections occur within 4 weeks from the acute onset of the pancreatitis and may resolve spontaneously. The formation of a pseudocyst occurs when the fluid collection develops into a well-defined, walled-off fluid collection of amylase. Other sonographic findings may include ascites, thickened wall of the gallbladder, and thickening of the adjacent gastrointestinal tract.

Chronic Pancreatitis. Chronic pancreatitis results from recurrent attacks of acute pancreatitis and causes continuing destruction of the pancreatic parenchyma that results in permanent structural damage, which can lead to impairment of exocrine and endocrine function (see Table 12.5). There are several features to distinguish chronic from acute pancreatitis. Patients with chronic pancreatitis may be asymptomatic over long periods, may present with a fibrotic mass, or may have symptoms of pancreatic insufficiency without pain. In contrast, acute pancreatitis is almost always associated with epigastric pain. The lab values of serum amylase and lipase are usually typical in chronic pancreatitis, almost always elevated in patients with acute disease. Chronic pancreatitis presents with patchy focal fibrotic disease, whereas acute pancreatitis usually involves the entire gland.

Clinical findings in patients with chronic pancreatitis include epigastric abdominal pain radiating to the back, which may be associated with nausea and vomiting. Patients with severe pancreatic exocrine dysfunction cannot properly digest complex foods or absorb partially digested breakdown products. Glucose intolerance may develop in patients with chronic pancreatitis.

Chronic pancreatitis is generally associated with chronic alcoholism or biliary disease, although patients with **hypercalcemia** (elevated calcium levels) and **hyperlipidemia** (elevated fat levels) are more predisposed to chronic pancreatitis. In chronic alcoholic pancreatitis, the alcoholic intake causes increased pancreatic protein secretion with subsequent ductal obstruction resulting in chronic calcifying pancreatitis. The fibrous connective tissue rapidly grows around the ducts and between the lobules with resultant scarring that leads to a nodular, irregular surface of the pancreas. The pancreatic ducts become obstructed with a build-up of protein plugs with resultant calcifications along the duct. The less common type is chronic obstructive pancreatitis with a nonlobular distribution, less ductal epithelial damage, and rarely calcified stones. This form is usually caused by stenosis of the sphincter of Oddi by cholelithiasis or pancreatic tumor.

Patients with chronic pancreatitis may develop pseudocysts, a dilated common bile duct, or thrombosis of the splenic vein with extension into the portal vein. Patients with chronic pancreatitis have an increased risk of developing pancreatic cancer.

On pathologic examination, the pancreas shows an increase in the interlobular fibrous tissue and chronic inflammatory infiltration changes. Stones of calcium carbonate may be found inside the ductal system, and pseudocysts are common (Fig. 12.28). Calcification of the gland occurs in 20% to 40% of the patients.

> **Sonographic Findings.** Chronic pancreatitis appears as a mixed pattern. The tissue affected may appear as a diffuse or localized involvement of the gland (Fig. 12.29). Echogenicity of the pancreas is usually increased beyond normal because of fibrotic and fatty changes, with a mixture of hypoechoic (from inflammation) and hyperechoic foci. The size of the gland is reduced, and the borders are irregular, and the pancreatic duct may be irregular and dilated secondary to stricture or as the result of an extrinsic stone moving from a smaller pancreatic duct into a major duct. The classic sonographic finding is calcifications. With pancreatic ductal lithiasis, shadowing may be present, with the most common site of obstruction at the papilla. Chronic pancreatitis is more highly suspected when the duct contains calcification, and no obstructing mass lesion is seen, whereas carcinoma is suggested when a parenchymal mass lesion is identified at the site of obstruction of the pancreatic duct.

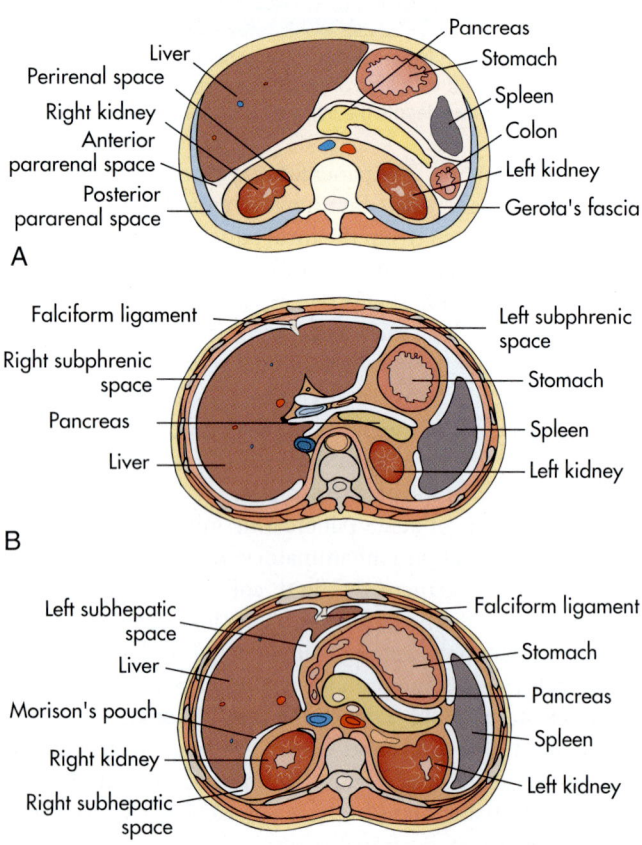

FIG. 12.27 (A) The pancreas lies in the anterior pararenal space. (B) The stomach is anterior to the body and tail of the gland, whereas the aorta and inferior vena cava, superior mesenteric artery, and vein lie posterior to the gland. (C) The head of the pancreas lies in the lap of the duodenum.

A focal mass or enlargement may be seen in the pancreas secondary to perilobular scarring with edema and inflammation. The presence of calcification is useful to differentiate such focal enlargements from neoplasms. Pseudocysts over 5 cm in size that persist beyond 6 weeks require decompression with significant risk of complications. Decompression may also be required in smaller pseudocysts that compress adjacent structures to cause persistent symptoms or if significant complications arise such as infection, hemorrhage, or perforation.

Complications of Pancreatitis

Pancreatitis may be associated with a variety of complications. These include walled-off pancreatic fluid collections, bile duct or duodenal obstruction, pancreatic ascites or pleural effusion, splenic vein thrombosis, pseudoaneurysms, and pancreatic cancer. Pancreatic and parapancreatic fluid collections are most often complications of pancreatitis.

Walled-off Pancreatic Fluid Collections. The inflammatory pancreatic fluid collections include acute peripancreatic fluid collections, pseudocysts, acute necrotic collections, and walled-off pancreatic necrosis. The acute peripancreatic fluid collections occur in the setting of acute interstitial pancreatitis within 4 weeks of the onset of pancreatitis. They typically are extra-pancreatic and do not have a definable wall (Fig. 12.30). The fluid contains no solid material, and no pancreatic necrosis is present. The pseudocyst represents a more mature fluid collection located outside the pancreas, has a well-defined wall, no solid internal material or necrosis. Acute necrotic collections occur in necrotizing pancreatitis, may be adjacent to or involve the pancreas, have no definable wall, and may contain liquid and solid material. The walled-off pancreatic necrosis is a mature mass that may be intra- or extra-pancreatic with an encapsulated collection of necrosis with liquid and solid components. Walled-off pancreatic fluid collections include pseudocysts and

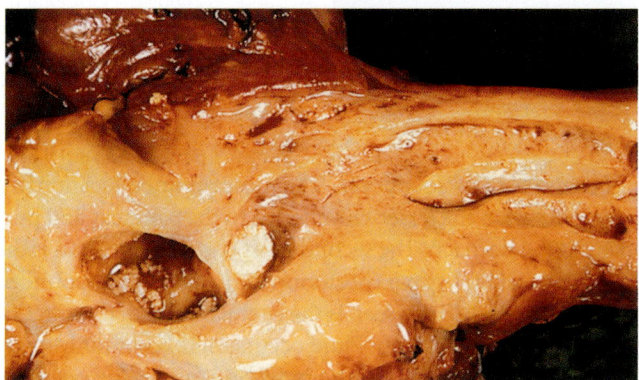

FIG. 12.28 Gross pathology of chronic pancreatitis. The main pancreatic duct is dilated and contains calculi. The pancreatic acini have been replaced by fibrous tissue.

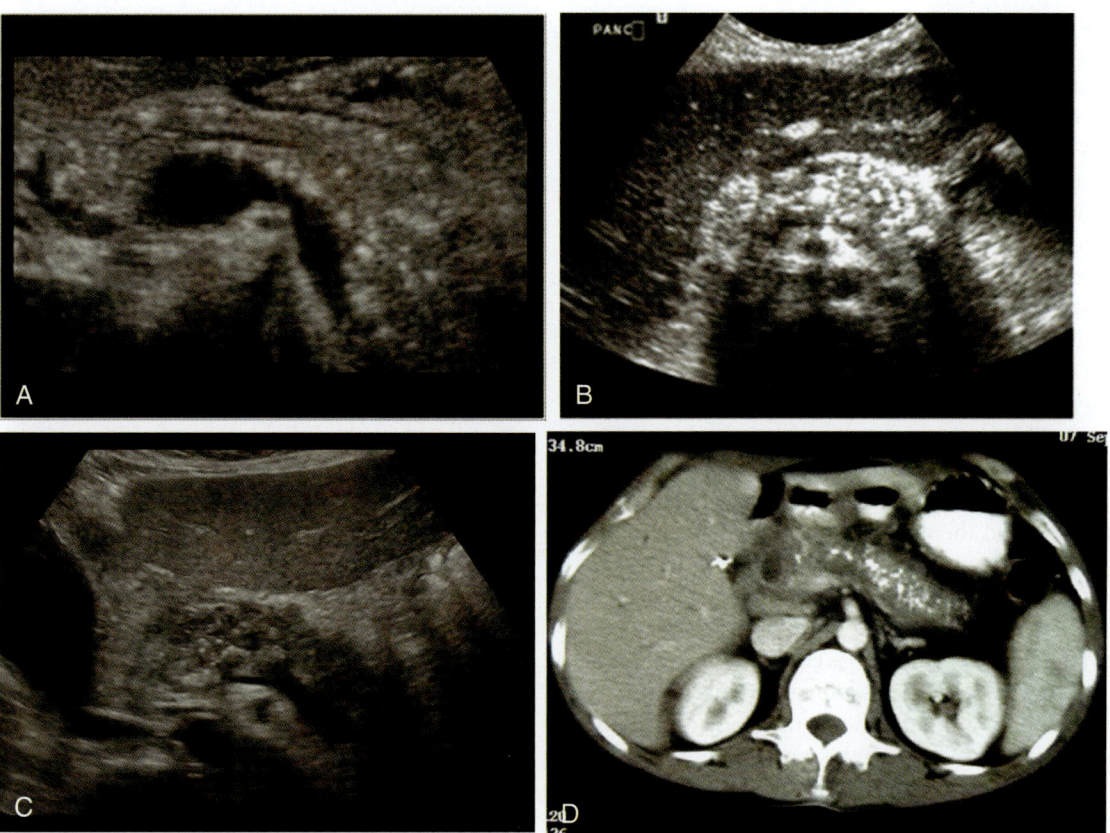

FIG. 12.29 Patterns of chronic pancreatitis. Chronic pancreatitis appears as a mixed pattern. The tissue affected may appear as a diffuse or localized involvement of the gland. Echogenicity of the pancreas is usually increased beyond normal because of fibrotic and fatty changes, with a mixture of hypoechoic (from inflammation) and hyperechoic foci.

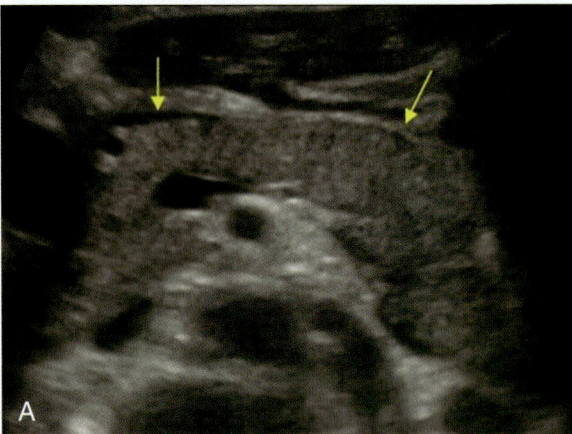 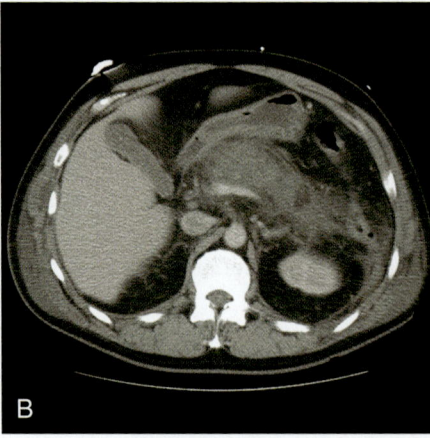

FIG. 12.30 Transverse sonogram (A) and computed tomographic cross section (B) show the acute pancreatitis with peripancreatic fluid collections *(arrows)*.

walled-off pancreatic necrosis. Most walled-off pancreatic fluid collections are now classified as walled-off pancreatic necrosis rather than pseudocysts.

Although many of these walled-off pancreatic fluid collections resolve without intervention, a variety of clinical problems may develop depending on the location and extent of the fluid collection and if the collection becomes infected. The expansion of the fluid collection may produce abdominal pain, duodenal or biliary obstruction, vascular occlusion, or fistula formation into adjacent viscera, the pleural space, or pericardium. If an adjacent vessel is digested by the pancreatic enzymes, a pseudoaneurysm can develop, which can produce sudden, painful expansion of the cyst or gastrointestinal bleeding due to the bleeding into the pancreatic duct. Pancreatic ascites or pleural effusion may result from disruption of the pancreatic duct with fistulization to the abdomen or chest.

The walled-off pancreatic fluid collection known as the pseudocyst may be defined as a collection of fluid that arises from the loculation of inflammatory processes, necrosis, trauma, or hemorrhage. Pseudocysts are always acquired; they result from trauma to the gland or acute or chronic pancreatitis (see Table 12.5). In approximately 10% to 20% of patients with acute pancreatitis, a pseudocyst develops over four to six weeks after the onset of pancreatitis. This collection is formed when pancreatic enzymes escape from the gland and break down tissue to form a sterile abscess somewhere in the abdomen. Its walls are not true cyst walls; hence the name *pseudo-*, or false, cyst. Pseudocysts generally take on the contour of the available space around them and therefore are not always spherical, as are normal cysts. There may be more than one pseudocyst, so the sonographer should search for daughter collections.

The patient does not experience symptoms as a result of the pseudocyst until it becomes large enough to cause pressure on the surrounding organs. Pseudocysts usually develop through the lesser omentum, displacing the stomach or widening the duodenal loop. Although the most common association of pseudocyst development is in patients with alcoholic or biliary disease, it may also develop after blunt trauma or secondary to pancreatic malignancy. Clinically the patient may present with a history of pancreatitis, persistent pain, and elevated amylase levels.

Locations of a Pseudocyst. The most common location of a pseudocyst is in the lesser sac anterior to the pancreas and posterior to the stomach. The second most common location is the anterior pararenal space (posterior to the lesser sac, bounded by Gerota fascia). The spleen is the lateral border of the anterior pararenal space on the left. Fluid occurs more commonly in the left pararenal space than in the right. Sometimes the posterior pararenal space is fluid-filled; fluid spreads from the anterior pararenal space to the posterior pararenal space on the same side. Fluid may enter the peritoneal cavity via the foramen of Winslow or by disrupting the peritoneum in the anterior surface of the lesser sac. It may extend into the mediastinum by extending through the esophageal or aortic hiatus, or it may extend into small bowel mesentery or down into the retroperitoneum into the pelvis and groin.

Sonographically, the walled-off pseudocyst usually appears as well-defined mass with essentially sonolucent, echo-free interior. Debris seen within the collection may occur from complications of infection or hemorrhage; scattered echoes may be seen at the bottom of the cysts, and increased through-transmission is present (Fig. 12.31). The borders are very echogenic, and the cysts usually are thicker than other simple cysts. Calcification may develop within the walls of the pseudocyst. When a suspected pseudocyst is located near the stomach, the stomach should be drained so the cyst is not mistaken for a fluid-filled stomach. If the patient has been on continual drainage before the ultrasound examination, this problem is eliminated. Spontaneous rupture is the most common complication of a **pancreatic pseudocyst**, occurring in 5% of patients. In 3% of these patients, drainage is directly into the peritoneal cavity. Clinical symptoms are sudden shock and peritonitis. The mortality rate is 50%.

Walled-off Necrotic Intra- or Extrapancreatic Fluid Collections. The walled-off necrotic intra- or extrapancreatic fluid collection appears as a heterogeneous collection with liquid and solid components with varying degrees of loculation. This necrosis is well-defined and completely encapsulates the fluid collection.

Pancreatic ascites occurs when the pancreatic pseudocyst ruptures into the abdomen. Pancreatic ascites that develops as a consequence of spontaneous rupture may be differentiated from pancreatic ascites associated with cirrhosis in patients

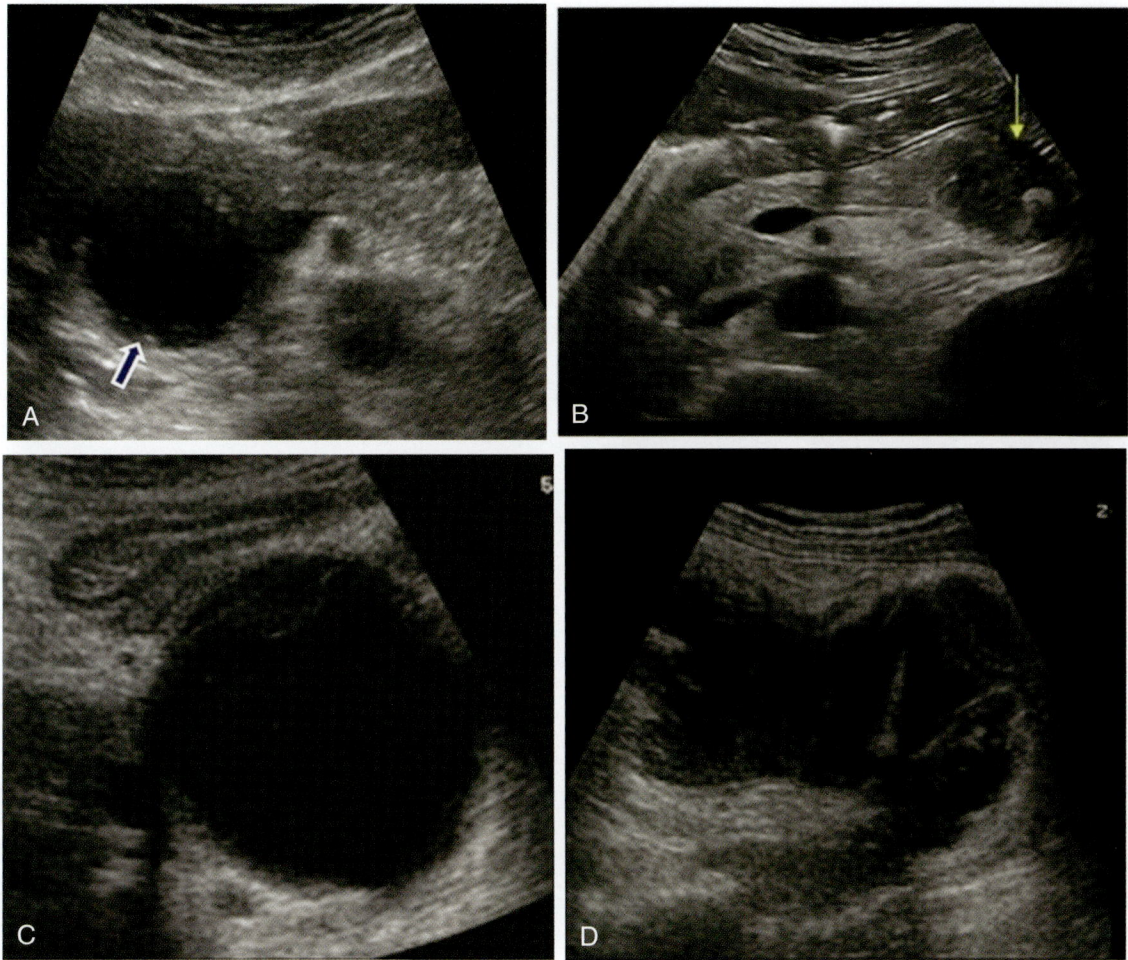

FIG. 12.31 Pseudocyst of the pancreas. The walled-off pancreatic fluid collection known as the *pseudocyst* may be defined as a collection of fluid that arises from the loculation of inflammatory processes, necrosis, trauma, or hemorrhage.

who have known rupture of a pseudocyst by analysis of the fluid for elevated amylase and protein content (Fig. 12.32). In 2% of patients, the rupture is into the gastrointestinal tract. Such patients may present a confusing picture sonographically. The initial scan shows a typical pattern for a pseudocyst formation, but the patient may have intense pain develop secondary to the rupture, and consequent examination shows the disappearance of the mass.

Hemorrhagic Pancreatitis. Hemorrhagic pancreatitis is a rapid progression of acute pancreatitis with rupture of pancreatic vessels and subsequent hemorrhage (see Table 12.5). In hemorrhagic pancreatitis, there is diffuse enzymatic destruction of the pancreatic substance caused by a sudden escape of active pancreatic enzymes into the glandular parenchyma (Fig. 12.33). These enzymes cause focal areas of fat necrosis in and around the pancreas, which leads to rupture of pancreatic vessels and hemorrhage. Nearly half of these patients have sudden necrotizing destruction of the pancreas after an alcoholic binge or an excessively large meal.

Specific sonographic findings depend on the age of the hemorrhage. A well-defined homogeneous mass in the area of the pancreas may be seen with areas of fresh necrosis. Foci of extravasated blood and fat necrosis are also seen. Further necrosis of the blood vessels results in the development of hemorrhagic areas referred to as Grey Turner sign (discoloration of the flanks). At 1 week, the mass may appear cystic with solid elements or septation. After several weeks the hemorrhage may appear cystic.

Phlegmonous Pancreatitis. A phlegmon is an inflammatory process that spreads along fascial pathways, causing localized areas of diffuse inflammatory edema of soft tissue that may proceed to necrosis and suppuration. Extension outside the gland occurs in 18% to 20% of patients with acute pancreatitis. The phlegmonous tissue appears on ultrasound as hypoechoic texture with good through-transmission (Fig. 12.34). The phlegmon usually involves the lesser sac, left anterior pararenal space, and transverse mesocolon. Less commonly, it involves the small bowel mesentery, lower retroperitoneum, and pelvis. See Table 12.5 for sonographic findings and differential considerations for phlegmonous pancreatitis.

Pancreatic Abscess. Pancreatic abscess has a low incidence, although it is a serious complication of pancreatitis; the condition is related to the degree of tissue necrosis (see Table 12.5). The majority of patients develop abscesses secondary to pancreatitis that develops from postoperative procedures. A very high mortality rate is associated with this condition if left untreated. An abscess may rise from a neighboring infection, such as a

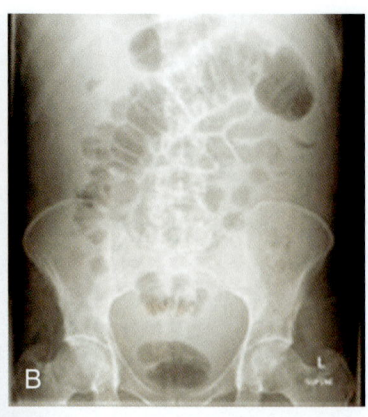

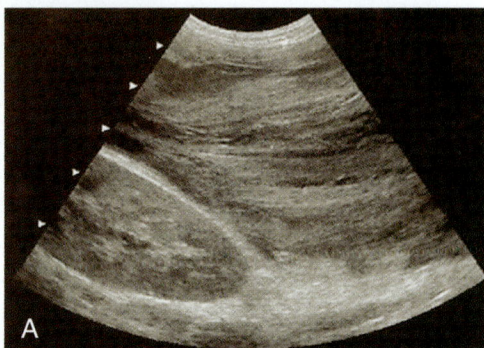

FIG. 12.32 (A) Gross pathology of a pancreatic pseudocyst rupture. (B) Radiograph of a patient with ascites pushing the bowel into the central abdominal cavity.

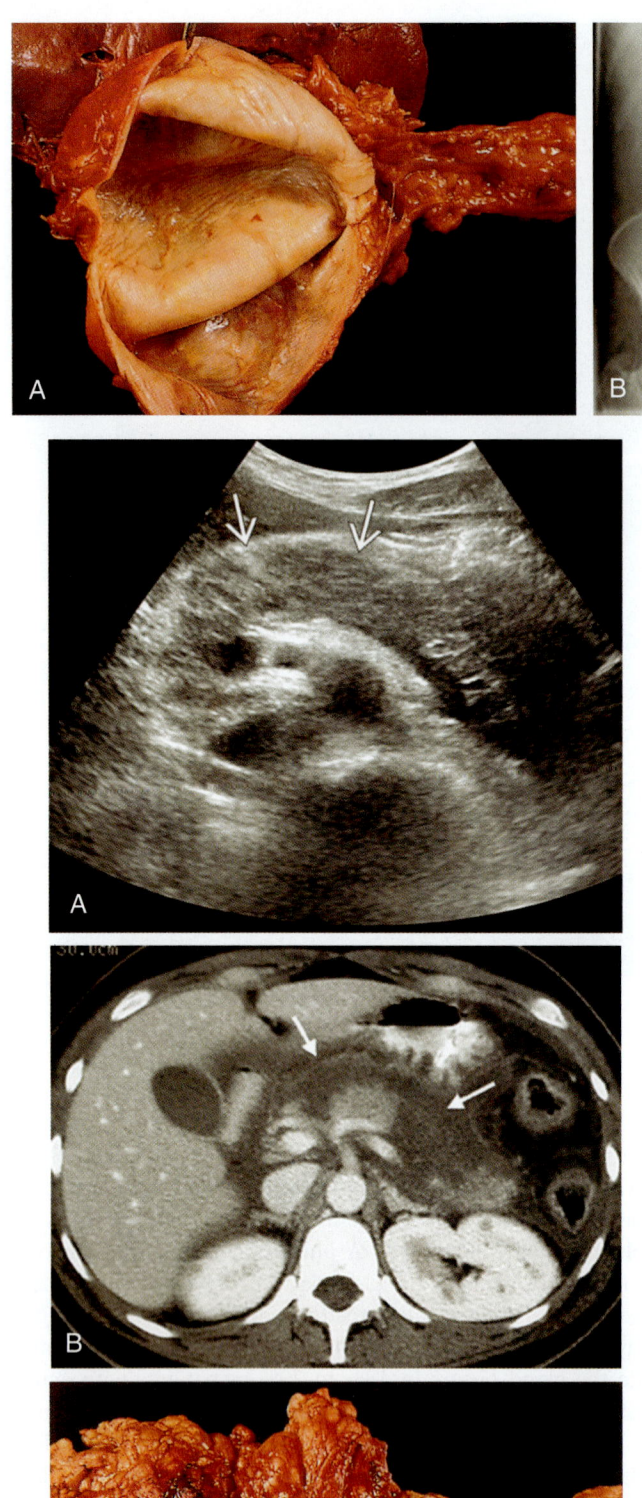

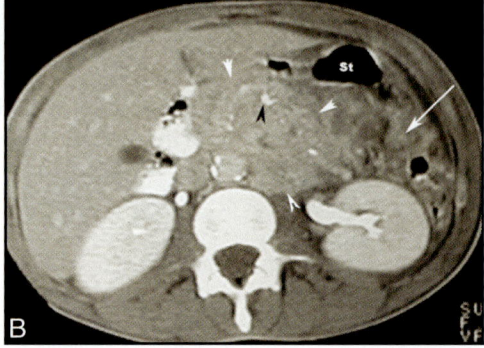

FIG. 12.34 A phlegmon is an inflammatory process that spreads along fascial pathways, causing localized areas of diffuse inflammatory edema of soft tissue that may proceed to necrosis and suppuration. Sonographic (A) and computed tomographic sagittal view (B) of the left kidney and phlegmon.

FIG. 12.33 Hemorrhagic pancreatitis *(arrows)* denoted in both the sonographic (A) and computed tomographic (B) images. (C) Gross pathology of acute hemorrhagic pancreatitis.

perforated peptic ulcer, acute appendicitis, or acute cholecystitis. A pancreatic abscess may be unilocular or multilocular and can spread superiorly into the mediastinum, inferiorly into the transverse mesocolon, or down the retroperitoneum into the pelvis. Acute peritonitis may develop as the pseudocyst ruptures into the peritoneal cavity.

Sonographic Findings. A pancreatic abscess is imaged with sonography (Fig. 12.35). The sonographic appearance depends on the amount of debris present. If air bubbles are present, an echogenic region with a shadow posterior is imaged. A pseudocyst that forms during acute necrotizing pancreatitis has a higher likelihood of spontaneous regression, whereas a pseudocyst that forms secondary to chronic pancreatitis and develops calcification in its walls usually does not resolve on its own.

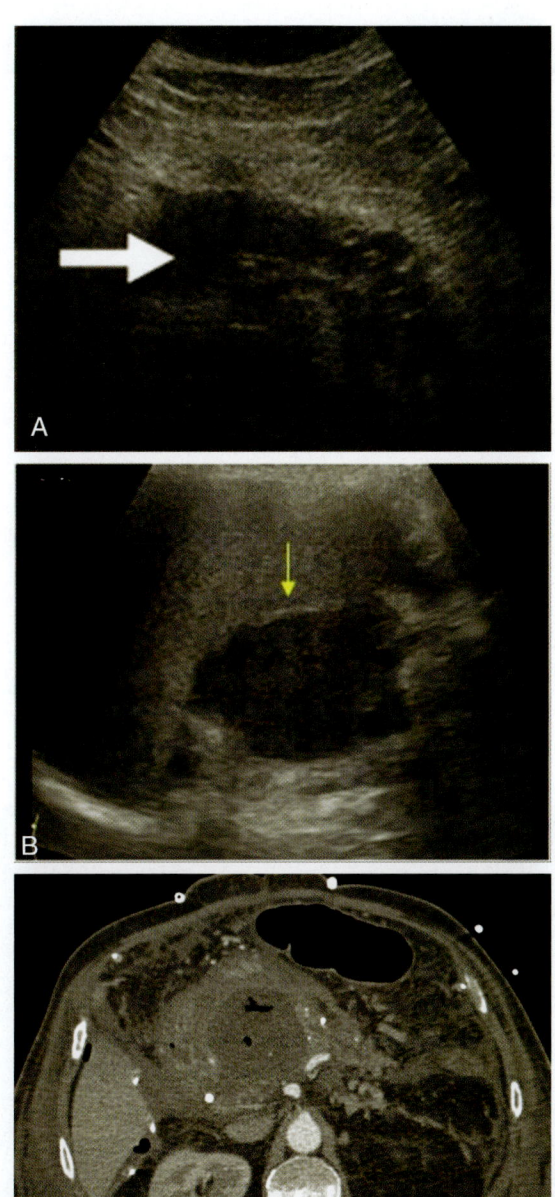

FIG. 12.35 (A–B) Sonographic images of the poorly defined hypoechoic mass with smooth or irregular thick walls, causing few internal echoes; it may be echo-free to echo-dense. (C) Computed tomographic image of the large focal abscess in the head of the pancreas.

Benign Cystic Lesions of the Pancreas

A wide variety of cystic lesions of the pancreas may be seen on imaging studies of the abdomen. Pancreatic cysts may be neoplastic or non-neoplastic. Ultrasound, CT, MRI, and ERCP are imaging modalities that are used to help narrow the differential diagnosis to aid the clinician in arriving at a diagnosis when correlated with clinical, pathologic, and laboratory findings. See Table 12.6 for clinical findings, sonographic findings, and differential considerations for pancreatic cysts.

Multiple Pancreatic Cysts.

Autosomal Dominant Polycystic Disease. This disease is characterized by the presence of multiple small cysts in the kidney and liver, with rare extension into the pancreas. These cysts vary from microscopic to several centimeters in diameter and, with increasing size, may destroy the normal pancreatic tissue.

von Hippel–Lindau Syndrome. von Hippel–Lindau syndrome is an inherited disorder characterized by the formation of tumors and fluid-filled sacs (cysts) in many different parts of the body (Fig. 12.36). The tumors may be either noncancerous or cancerous and most frequently appear during young adulthood; however, the signs and symptoms of von Hippel–Lindau syndrome can occur throughout life. Tumors called hemangioblastomas are characteristic of von Hippel–Lindau syndrome. These growths are made of newly formed blood vessels. Although they are typically noncancerous, they can cause serious or life-threatening complications. People with von Hippel–Lindau syndrome commonly develop cysts in the kidneys, pancreas, and genital tract. They are also at an increased risk of developing a type of pancreatic cancer called a pancreatic neuroendocrine tumor.

Cystic Fibrosis. Cystic fibrosis is a hereditary disease that causes excessive production of thick mucus by the endocrine glands. The most common pancreatic abnormality found is fatty replacement of the pancreas, sometimes with calcifications. The cysts develop from inspissated mucin that obstructs the pancreatic ducts. The cysts are either single or multiple (Fig. 12.37). Most are microscopic, but they can also be several centimeters in diameter.

Cystic Pancreatic Neoplasms

There are four subtypes of pancreatic cystic neoplasms with varying malignant potential: serous cystic tumors, mucinous cystic neoplasms, intraductal papillary mucinous neoplasms, and solid pseudopapillary neoplasms (Table 12.7). The cystic neoplasms of the pancreas account for between 10% and 15% of all pancreatic cysts and less than 1% of all pancreatic malignancies.

Serous Cystic Tumors. Serous cystadenoma is a rare, benign well-circumscribed tumor with multiple tiny cysts found more often in elderly females (Fig. 12.38). This lesion is the least likely to develop malignant potential. The sonographic appearance depends on the number and size of the cysts. The lesions may appear cystic, solid, or even echogenic if the cysts are very small and more numerous along the periphery. The coarsely lobulated cystic tumors sometimes present sonographically with cyst walls thicker than the membranes between multilocular cysts (Figs. 12.39 and 12.40). A minority of the cysts have an echogenic central stellate scar that may have calcification. The pseudocapsule and septa of the mass tend to be hypervascular and seen well with color Doppler. The mass usually does not cause obstruction of the pancreatic duct. Differentiating between a serous cystadenoma and a malignant mucinous cystic tumor is difficult without pathologic confirmation.

Mucinous Cystic Neoplasms. Mucinous cystadenoma/cystadenocarcinoma is an uncommon, slow-growing tumor that rises from the ducts as a cystic neoplasm. The tumor may be either malignant or benign with a significant "malignant potential." It occurs predominantly in both middle- and elderly females, usually in the body or tail. Clinically patients

TABLE 12.6 Congenital Pancreatic Lesions

Clinical Findings	Sonographic Findings	Differential Considerations
Autosomal Dominant Polycystic Kidney Diseases		
• Asymptomatic, often found in patients with polycystic renal disease	• Well-defined mass with serous fluid • Size varies from microscopic to several centimeters	• Pseudocyst • Other cystic lesions of the pancreas
von Hippel–Lindau Disease		
• Asymptomatic • Patients may have central nervous system and retinal hemangioblastomas, visceral cysts, pheochromocytomas, and renal cell carcinoma	• Well-defined mass with thick fluid; calcifications • Single or multiple • Size varies from microscopic to several centimeters	• Pseudocyst • Other cystic lesions of the pancreas
Cystic Fibrosis		
• Asymptomatic	• Well-defined mass with serous fluid • Size varies from microscopic to several centimeters	• Pseudocyst • Other cystic lesions of the pancreas
True Pancreatic Cysts		
• Asymptomatic, often found in infants	• Well-defined mass with serous fluid • Unilocular or multilocular	• Pseudocyst • Other cystic lesions of the pancreas

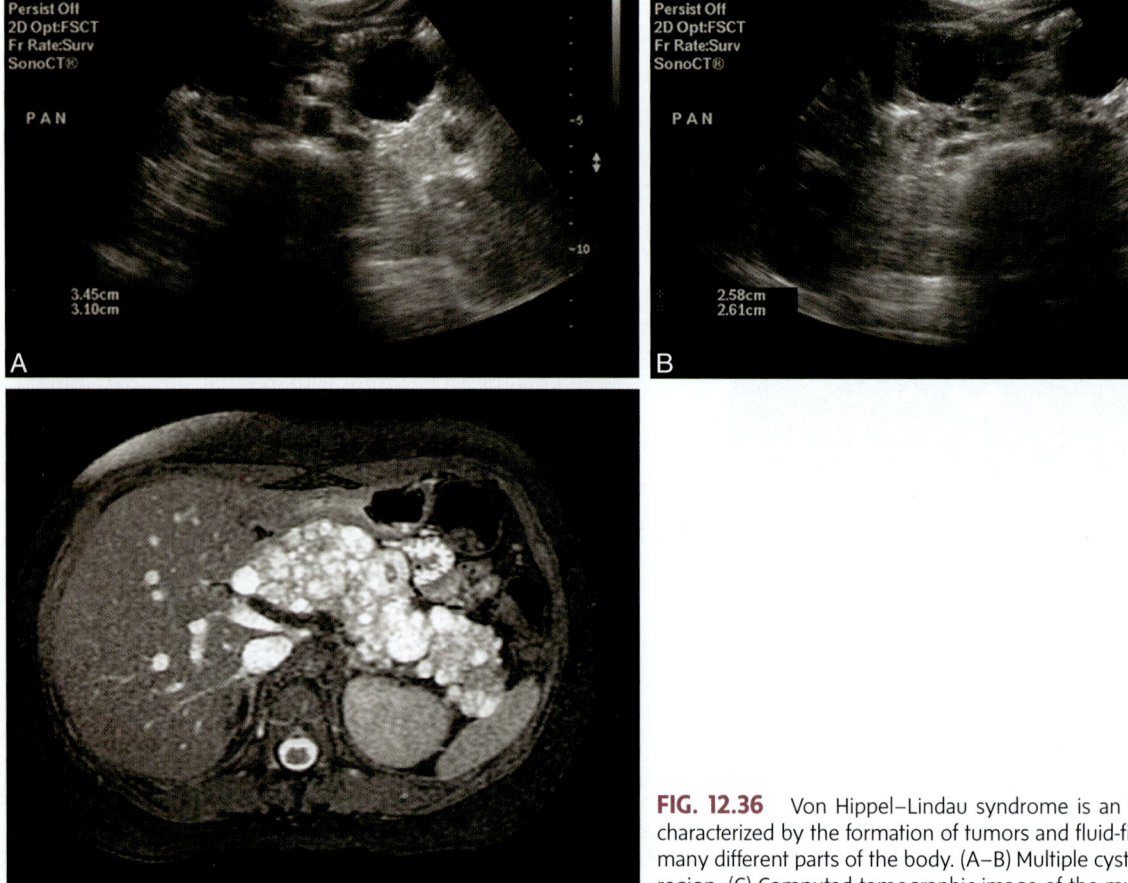

FIG. 12.36 Von Hippel–Lindau syndrome is an inherited disorder characterized by the formation of tumors and fluid-filled sacs (cysts) in many different parts of the body. (A–B) Multiple cysts in the pancreatic region. (C) Computed tomographic image of the multiple cysts within the pancreas.

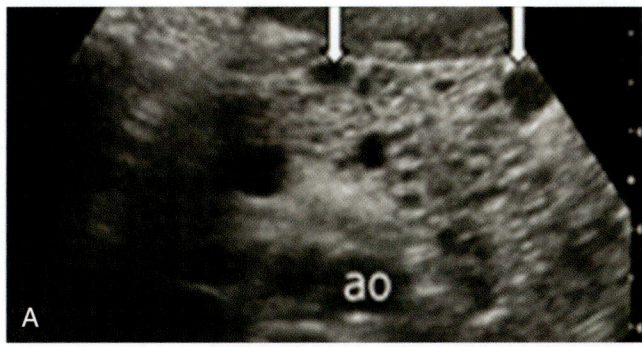
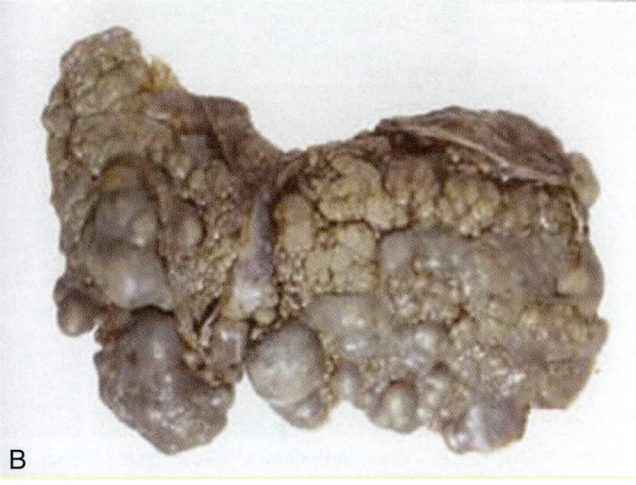

FIG. 12.37 **Cystic fibrosis of the pancreas.** (A) The *arrows* point to two of the larger cysts within the pancreas. (B) Gross pathology of cystic fibrosis.

TABLE 12.7	Pancreatic Tumor Findings	
Clinical Findings	**Sonographic Findings**	**Differential Considerations**
Adenocarcinoma		
• Depends on size and location of tumor (symptoms occur late if located in body or tail) • Weight loss • Decreased appetite • Nausea, vomiting • Stool changes • Pain radiating to back • Painless jaundice if tumor is in the head (hydrops of GB—Courvoisier sign) • Metastasizes to lymph nodes, liver, lungs, bone, duodenum, peritoneum, and adrenal glands	• Loss of normal pancreatic parenchyma • Hypoechoic poorly defined mass • Focal mass with irregular border • Enlargement of pancreas • If mass is in head of pancreas, look for hydrops, compression of inferior vena cava, and dilated ducts	• Pseudocyst • Cystadenoma • Lymphoma
Cystadenoma		
• ↑ Amylase	• Anechoic mass with posterior enhancement • May have internal septa • Thick walls • Small size of tumor makes it difficult to image • Single or multiple • Occur in body and tail • Hypoechoic	• Pseudocyst • Metastases
Cystadenocarcinoma		
• Epigastric pain or palpable mass • Abdominal pain	• Irregular lobulated cystic tumor • Thick walls • Hypoechoic mass	• Pseudocyst • Cystadenoma • Adenocarcinoma • Islet cell tumor

↑, Increased; ↓, decreased.

present with epigastric pain or a palpable mass, weight loss, abdominal mass, or jaundice. Many patients have concurrent diseases: diabetes, calculous disease of biliary tract, or arterial hypertension.

This lesion presents as well-circumscribed, smooth-surfaced, thin- or thick-walled, unilocular, or multilocular cystic lesions of variable sizes (usually more than 20 mm in diameter and less than six in number) on sonography. The tumor is typically composed of well-defined cysts containing thick mucinous fluid, internal septations, or mural nodules (Fig. 12.41). The large cyst (greater than 5 cm) with or without septations, irregular wall, and calcification of the cyst wall has a significant malignant potential, and compared to adenocarcinoma of the pancreas, the survival is better with cystadenocarcinoma if the lesion is intact. Frequently, foci of calcification may be seen within the pancreas.

Intraductal Papillary Mucinous Neoplasms. The intraductal papillary mucinous tumor is a form of mucinous cystic

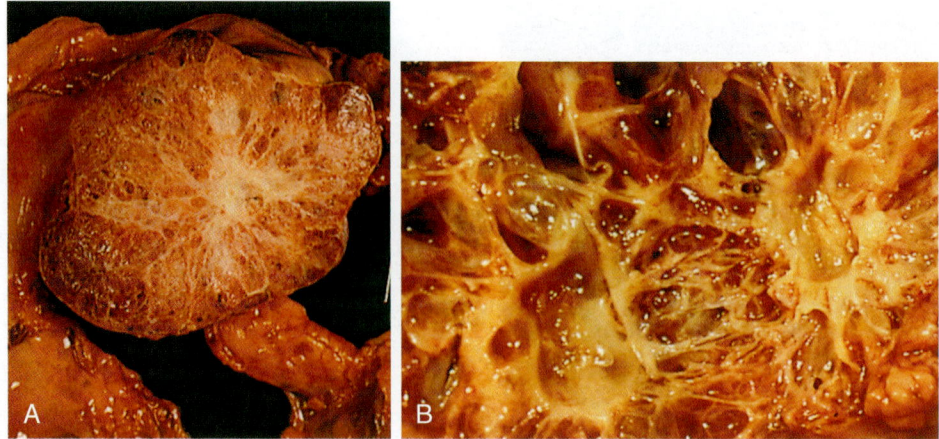

FIG. 12.38 **Gross pathology of serous cystadenoma.** (A) Well-circumscribed tumor. (B) Tumor appears microcystic.

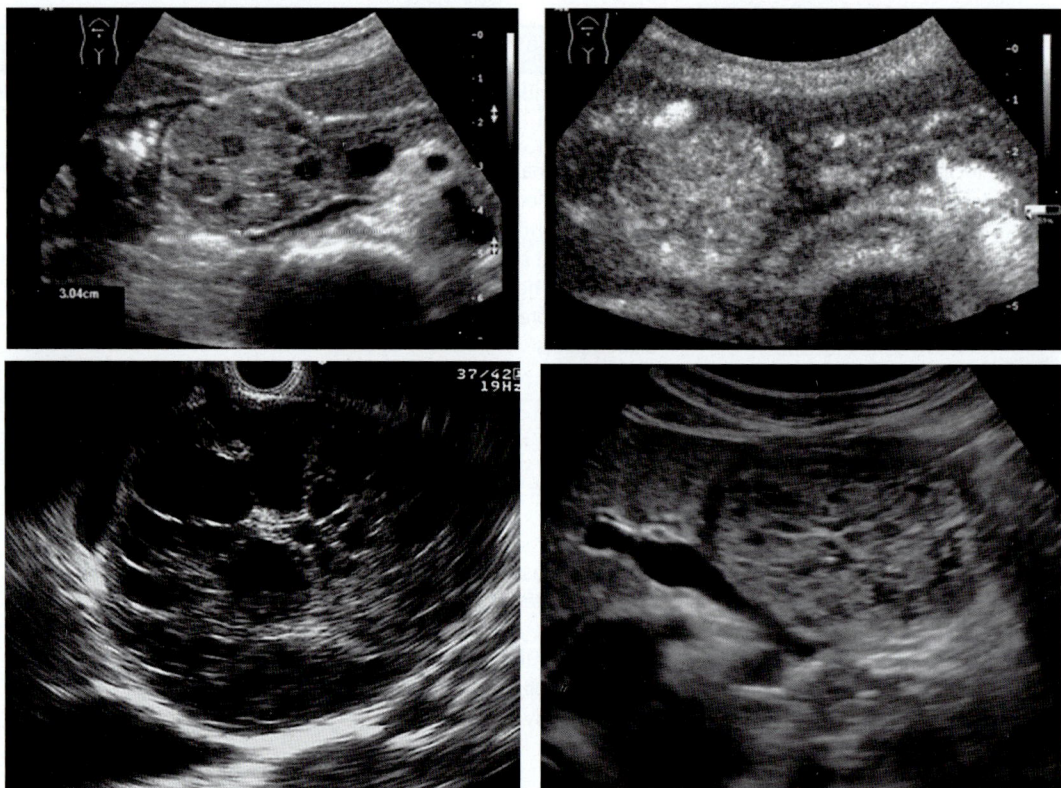

FIG. 12.39 **Serous cystadenoma of pancreas.** The sonographic appearance depends on the number and size of the cysts. The lesions may appear cystic, solid, or even echogenic if the cysts are very small and more numerous along the periphery.

neoplasm. The tumor originates from the main pancreatic duct or its branches. This slow-growing lesion affects both elderly men and women. The histology ranges from benign to malignant. Many patients with intraductal papillary mucinous neoplasms are asymptomatic. However, some patients have a recurrent history of acute pancreatitis or symptoms suggestive of chronic pancreatitis, which result from intermittent obstruction of the pancreatic duct with mucus plugs. The presence of back pain, jaundice, weight loss, anorexia, steatorrhea, and diabetes may be precursors to malignancy.

The ductal tumors demonstrate specific patterns on abdominal imaging. The main pancreatic duct type presents as segmental or diffuse dilation of the duct with or without side branch dilation. The branch type shows a single or multicystic mass with a microcystic or macrocystic appearance (Fig. 12.42). Careful demonstration of the mass should show communication with the pancreatic duct, usually best seen with ERCP. The tumors may present as nonvascular nodules within the dilated ducts. The presence of vascular nodules and a thick wall differentiates the mass benign from malignant.

Solid Pseudopapillary Neoplasms. The finding of a heterogeneous sonographic pattern with solid and cystic components in young women suggests a solid pseudopapillary neoplasm. This tumor has a lower incidence of malignancy.

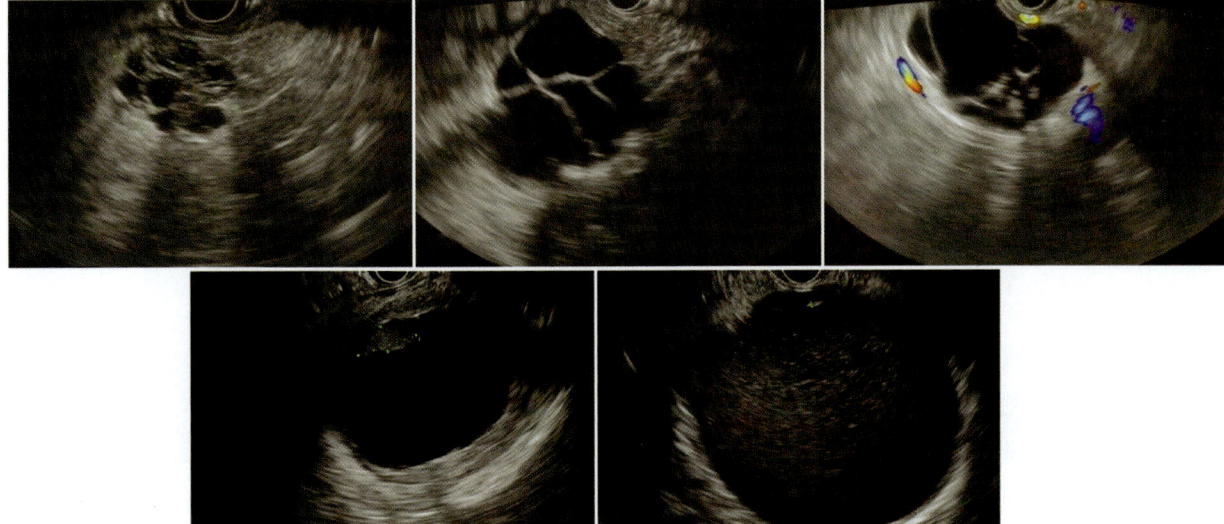

FIG. 12.40 The coarsely lobulated cystic tumors sometimes present sonographically with cyst walls thicker than the membranes between multilocular cysts. A minority of the cysts have an echogenic central stellate scar that may have calcification.

Patients with pseudopapillary neoplasm are usually symptomatic with abdominal pain, nausea, vomiting, and weight loss. Additional symptoms of abdominal mass, gastrointestinal obstruction, anemia, jaundice, and pancreatitis may also be present. These tumors are usually smaller in size, and thus MRI is more specific.

This tumor occurs most frequently in the tail of the pancreas. The tumors are usually round, encapsulated masses with variable amounts of necrotic, cystic-appearing areas and soft tissue foci (Fig. 12.43). These masses are necrotic masses containing blood and debris. A small number may have central and rim calcifications.

Endocrine Pancreatic Neoplasms

The endocrine tumors rise from the islet cells of the pancreas. There are several types of islet cell tumors; they may be functional or nonfunctional and may be classified as benign adenomas or malignant tumors. Nonfunctioning islet cell tumors comprise one third of all islet cell tumors, with the majority (85%) classified as adenocarcinoma.

Functional Endocrine Pancreatic Neoplasm. The most common functioning islet cell tumor is insulinoma (60%), followed by gastrinoma (18%). The tumor size is small (1 to 2 cm) and is well encapsulated with a good vascular supply. A large percentage of insulinoma tumors occur in patients with hyperinsulinism and hypoglycemia. Most gastrinomas are malignant, with up to 40% appearing with metastatic disease at the time of diagnosis.

Insulinoma (B-Cell Tumor). Insulinoma is the most common functioning islet cell tumor. The clinical triad is found in patients in their fourth to sixth decades of life with hypoglycemic symptoms with immediate relief of symptoms after the administration of IV glucose. Clinical symptoms include palpitations, headache, confusion, pallor, sweating, slurred speech, and coma. This tumor is usually benign. A small percent of insulinomas are multiple, 10% are malignant, and 10% of patients have hyperplasia rather than neoplasia. Most of the insulinomas are small, well encapsulated, and hypervascular. Some of the lesions contain calcification (Fig. 12.44).

Gastrinoma (G-Cell Tumor). Gastrinoma is the second most common functioning islet cell tumor and produces the Zollinger-Ellison syndrome. This condition is caused by non-insulin-secreting pancreatic tumors, which secrete excessive amounts of gastrin. This stimulates the stomach to secrete significant amounts of hydrochloric acid and pepsin, leading to peptic ulceration of the stomach and small intestine. These lesions usually affect young adults with peptic ulcer disease (when ulcers are recurrent, intractable, multiple, or in unusual locations). Diarrhea is common because of the increased gastrin on the small bowel. Gastrinomas are frequently multiple, extrapancreatic, difficult to locate, and 60% are malignant. Total gastrectomy and local excision of the pancreatic tumor may be performed if metastases have not appeared. Most gastrinomas are found in the pancreas, with a small amount (10% to 15%) arising in the duodenum. These tumors are frequently hypervascular and best imaged on CT (Fig. 12.45).

Nonfunctioning Islet Cell Tumors. These tumors comprise 33% of all islet cell neoplasms. These tumors tend to present as large tumors in the head of the pancreas with a high incidence of malignancy. Adenocarcinoma is the most common malignant tumor

Adenocarcinoma. The most common primary neoplasm of the pancreas is adenocarcinoma. This fatal tumor involves the exocrine portion of the gland (ductal epithelium) and accounts for greater than 90% of all malignant pancreatic tumors (Fig. 12.46). Pancreatic carcinoma accounts for approximately 3% of all cancers in the United States and about 7% of all cancer deaths. Carcinoma of the pancreas is rare before the age of 40; the majority of patients present after the age of 60. Clinical symptoms depend on the location of the tumor. Tumors in the pancreatic head present symptoms early, causing obstruction of the common bile

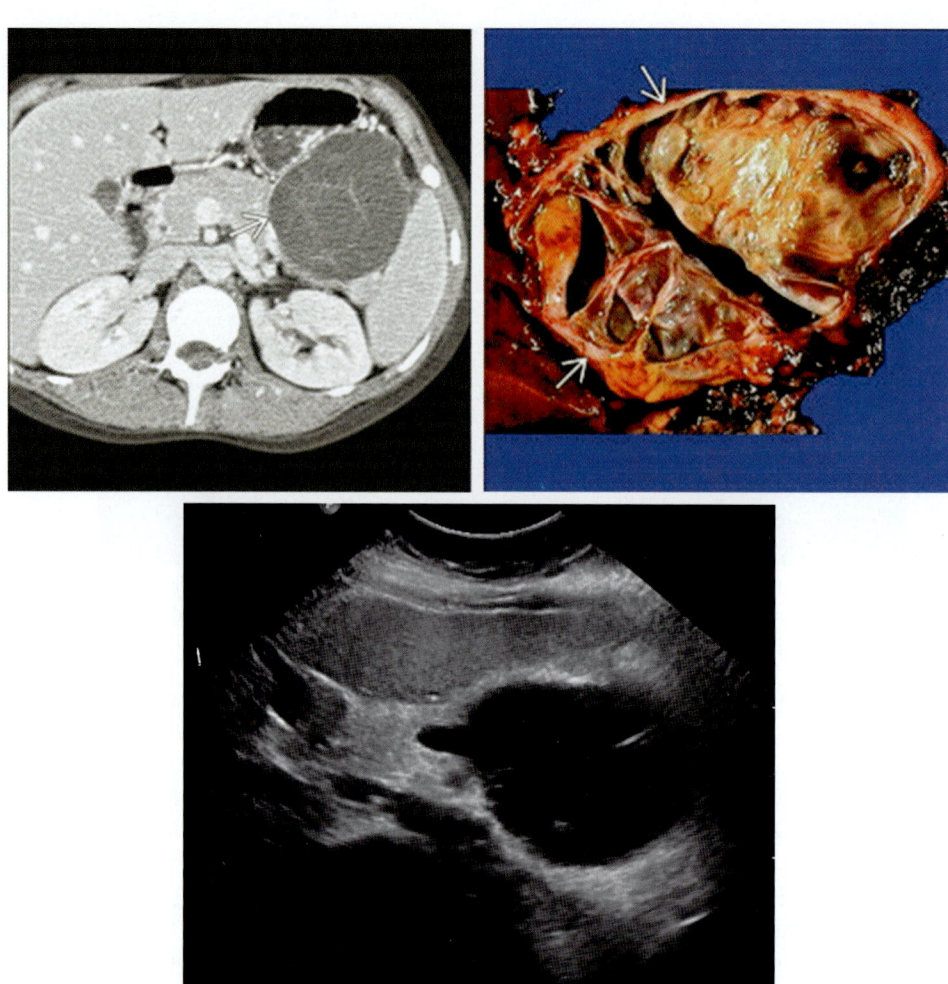

FIG. 12.41 **Mucinous cystadenoma of pancreas.** The tumor is typically composed of well-defined cysts containing thick mucinous fluid, internal septations, or mural nodules.

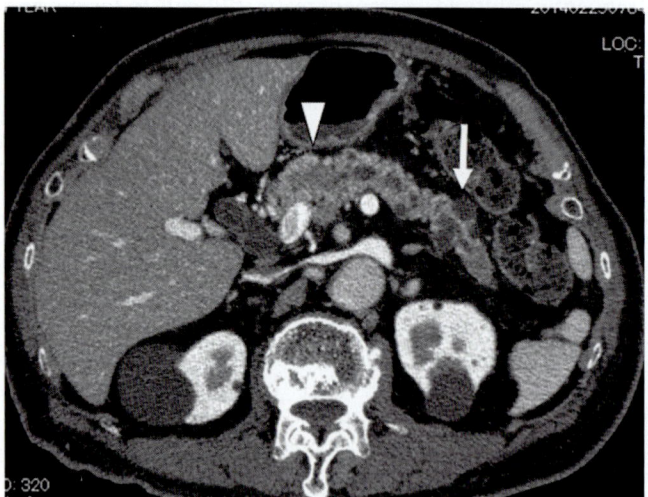

FIG. 12.42 **Intraductal mucinous neoplasm of pancreas.** On computed tomography, the branch type shows a single or multicystic mass with a microcystic or macrocystic appearance.

duct with subsequent jaundice and hydrops of the gallbladder (**Courvoisier sign**). A palpable, nontender gallbladder accompanied by jaundice is present in 25% of patients with pancreatic carcinoma. Tumors in the body and tail of the gland present with less specific symptoms, most commonly weight loss, pain, jaundice, and vomiting as the gastrointestinal tract becomes invaded by tumor. The tumors in the body and tail are more frequently larger and tend to invade the adjacent organs such as the stomach, transverse colon, spleen, and adrenal gland. These organs tend to present with metastases more often than tumors in the head. Metastases to the liver, regional lymph nodes, lungs, peritoneum, and adrenal glands have been reported. Peripancreatic, gastric, mesenteric, omental, and portohepatic nodes have been identified with adenocarcinoma.

On pathology, nearly all adenocarcinomas of the pancreas originate in the ductal epithelium, with less than 1% arising in the acini. The tumor may be either mucinous or nonmucinous. The most frequent site of occurrence is in the head of the gland (60% to 70%), with 20% to 30% in the body and 5% to 10% in the tail. One fifth of the tumors are diffuse.

Sonographic Findings. The sonographic appearance of adenocarcinoma is the loss of the normal pancreatic parenchymal pattern (Fig. 12.47). The most common finding on sonography is a poorly defined mass in the

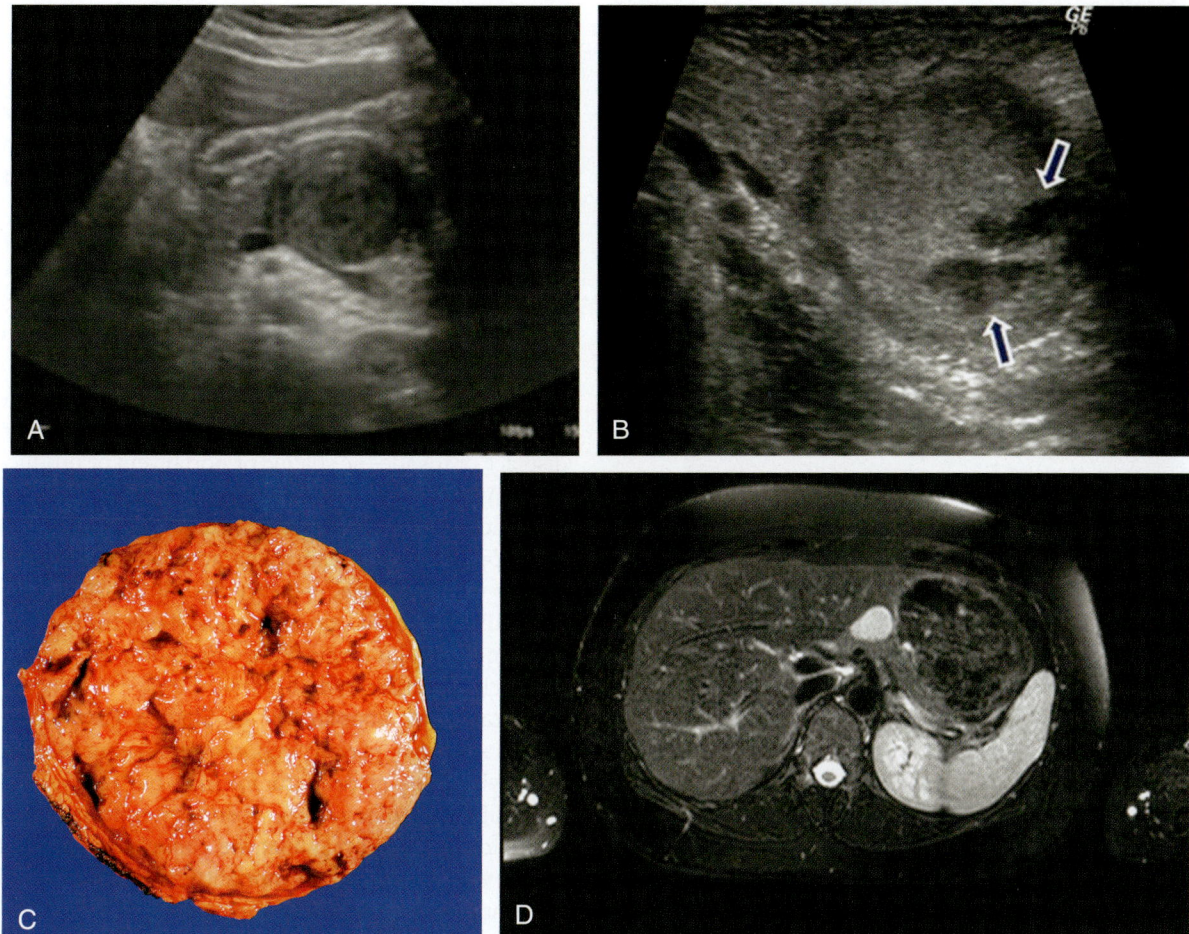

FIG. 12.43 Solid pseudopapillary Neoplasm of Pancreas. The tumors are usually round, encapsulated masses with variable amounts of necrotic, cystic-appearing areas and soft tissue foci. (A–B) Sonographic images of the necrotic tumor. (C) Gross pathology of the pseudopapillary tumor. (D) Computed tomographic image of the large solid tumor in the tail of the pancreas.

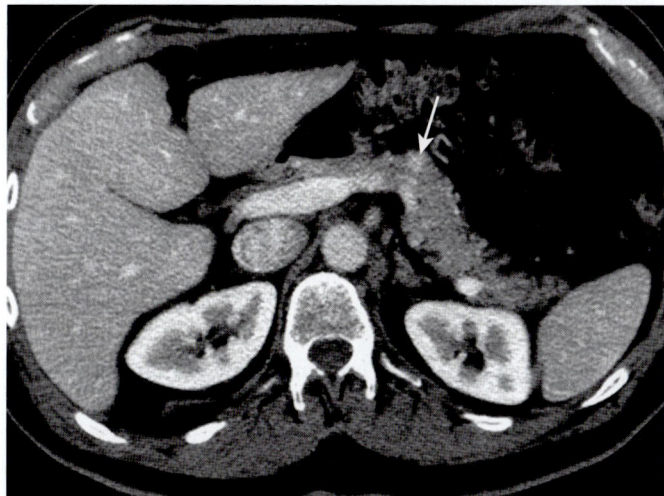

FIG. 12.44 Insulinoma. Computed tomographic image of a small calcified insulinoma *(arrow)*.

region of the pancreas. The lesion represents localized change in the echogenicity of the pancreas texture. The echo pattern is hypoechoic or isoechoic, with a texture less dense than the pancreas or liver. (The hypoechoic or isoechoic ill-defined tumor is better identified when the pancreatic texture is more echogenic.) Rarely, necrosis will be seen as a cystic area within the mass. The borders of the gland become irregular, and the pancreas may be enlarged. There may be secondary enlargement of the common duct resulting from edema or tumor invasion of the pancreatic head. If the mass obstructs the duct, look for dilation of the pancreatic duct (>2 to 3 mm). If the tumor is located within the head, look for biliary duct dilation. Remember, the level of the obstruction may be in the head, above the head, or in the porta hepatis, depending on the size of the lesion. The distinction of echogenic sludge within the common bile duct may be difficult to separate from tumor extension. Dilation of both the pancreatic and common bile duct may be seen in chronic pancreatitis as well as pancreatic adenocarcinoma.

There may be expansion or compression of the adjacent structures. The formation of a pseudocyst secondary to associated pancreatitis may be seen adjacent to the carcinoma. A diffuse spread of the tumor throughout the pancreas may appear as edematous pancreatitis. The sonographer should carefully evaluate the gland for the vague appearance of a lobulated mass and correlate with clinical symptoms.

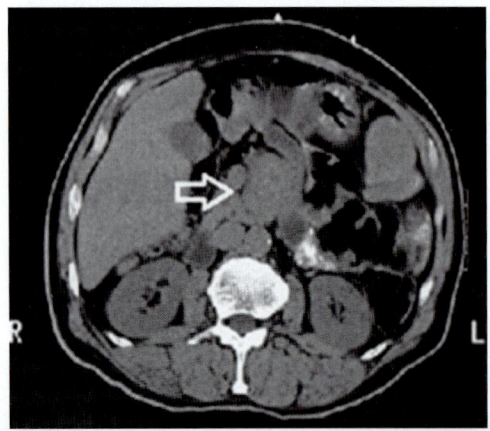
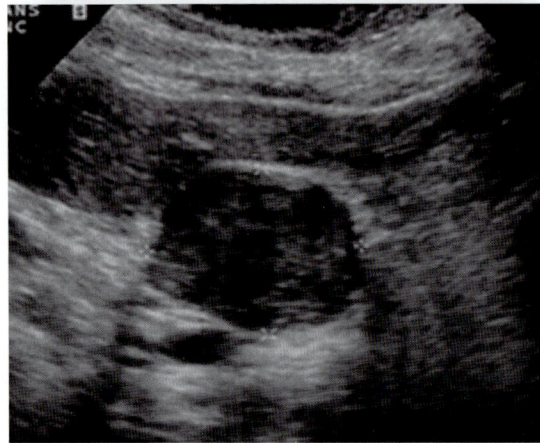

FIG. 12.45 **Gastrinoma.** These hypervascular tumors are frequently found in the pancreatic head near the duodenum and best imaged on computed tomography.

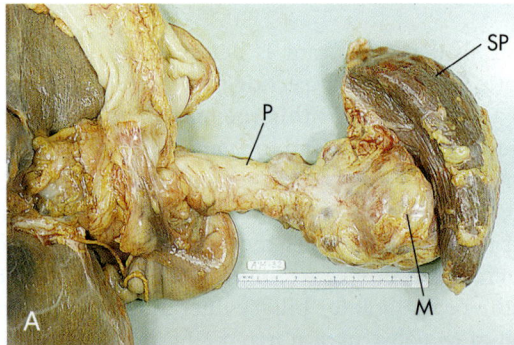
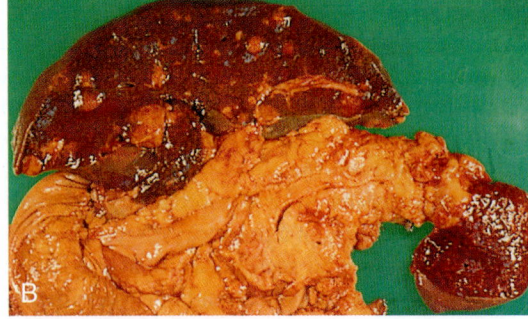

FIG. 12.46 (A) Gross specimen of a pancreatic mass (M) in the tail of the gland. (B) Carcinoma of the body of the pancreas. The tumor has metastasized to the liver. *P*, Pancreas; *SP*, spleen.

The sonographer should look for metastatic spread into the liver, lymph nodes (abnormal displacement of the superior mesenteric artery), or portal venous system. The superior mesenteric vessels may be displaced posteriorly by the pancreatic mass; anterior displacement is present when the carcinoma is in the uncinate process, and posterior displacement is present when the tumor is in the head or body. A soft tissue thickening caused by neoplastic infiltration of perivascular lymphatics may be seen surrounding the celiac axis, or superior mesenteric artery may be seen more with carcinoma of the body and tail.

Many patients with a mass in the head of the gland will have obstructive jaundice and anterior wall compression of the inferior vena cava. A tumor in the tail may compress the splenic vein, producing secondary splenic enlargement. A tumor may displace or invade the splenic or portal vein or produce thrombosis. Atrophy of the gland proximal to an obstructing mass in the head may appear hypoechoic or hyperechoic.

Doppler patterns feature characteristics of other malignant lesions with increased velocity and diminished flow impedance. The increased velocity is most likely from arteriovenous shunting and the diminished impedance to vascular spaces that lack muscular walls.

Significance of Sonography in Staging Pancreatic Tumors. Sonography may play an important screening role not only in identifying the pancreatic tumor mass but also in assessing the possibility of tumor resection. Surgery remains the treatment of choice in carcinomas that are considered resectable, but it comes with a high rate of mortality and morbidity. The ability to identify the extension of the carcinoma beyond the border of the pancreas—including invasion of the carcinoma into the lymph nodes, surrounding venous structures and organs, retroperitoneal fat, and liver metastases—precludes the feasibility of surgery. This abdominal/pelvic imaging survey has been more effective with CT evaluation. The demonstration of anatomical structures by sonography will be determined by the adequate image quality. The retroperitoneal structures are often precluded by bowel gas interference and thus inadequate image quality results. However, if the pancreas can be adequately imaged in its entirety and has a normal appearance, pancreatic carcinoma can be excluded with a high degree of certainty.

The sonographer should strive to carefully evaluate the vascular structures surrounding the pancreas. The gland lies in the middle of a significant vascular highway, namely the celiac plexus, and if a mass is present in the pancreas, it may easily travel to adjacent organs. It may be difficult to distinguish between compression and invasion of the venous structures. Secondary signs should be noted, such as interruption of a vein, organomegaly, or collateral formation in the peripancreatic and periportal region and along the stomach wall. Enlargement of the lymph nodes in the pancreatic area may lead to encasement of the celiac axis or superior mesenteric artery.

Differential Diagnosis for Pancreatic Carcinoma. The primary differential diagnosis of pancreatic carcinoma is focal pancreatitis or a focal mass associated with chronic pancreatitis. Calcification may be seen in patients with pancreatitis to help delineate the gland. However, it is possible to have concurrent neoplastic growth in the presence

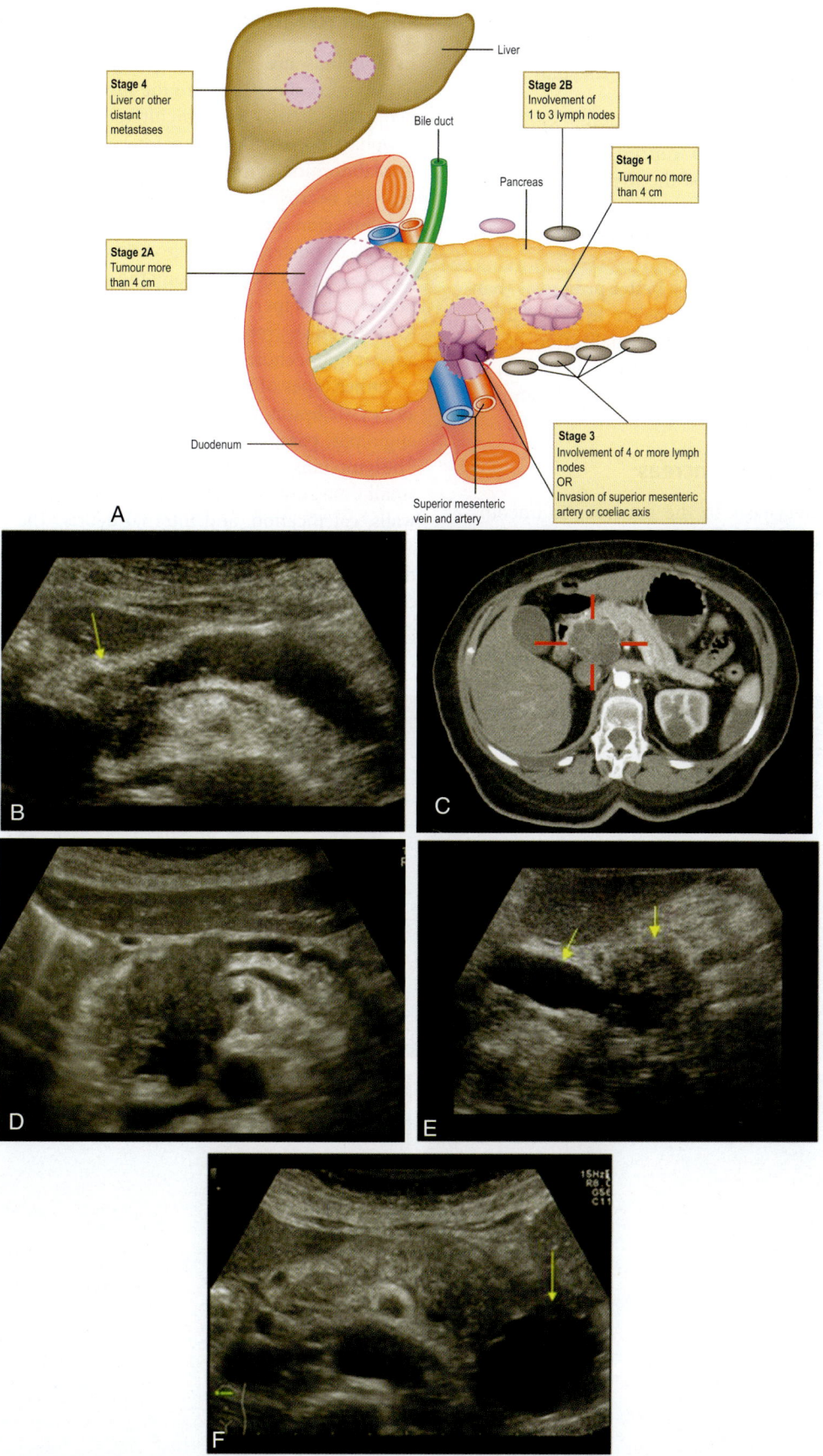

FIG. 12.47 Adenocarcinoma of pancreas. (A) Illustration of the tumor occurring in the head of the pancreas, causing obstruction to the common bile duct. (B) Transverse sonogram shows a large mass in the head of the pancreas *(arrow)*. Computed tomography (C) and ultrasound (D) show a large mass in the head of the pancreas. (E) Sagittal sonogram of the pancreatic mass causing obstruction to the common bile duct. (F) Transverse sonogram shows a large mass in the tail of the pancreas *(arrow)*.

of pancreatitis. Comparative imaging with CT and ERCP may be necessary to evaluate the texture of the gland and retroperitoneal area and to further assess the pancreatic duct.

Enlarged lymph nodes in the peripancreatic area may be differentiated from pancreatic cancer by identifying the echogenic septa between each of the hypoechoic nodes. The absence of jaundice in the presence of a mass near the head of the pancreas favors the presence of lymphadenopathy over pancreatic carcinoma.

Ampullary adenocarcinomas have a better prognosis than pancreatic adenocarcinoma when lesions are less than 2 cm. Endoscopic ultrasound has allowed the visualization of the pancreatic duct to stage this neoplastic growth. Dilation of the pancreatic and common duct is common with the ampullary tumor.

Metastatic Disease to the Pancreas

Generally speaking, metastasis to the pancreas is uncommon but has been reported to be found in 10% of patients with cancer. Primary tumors that can metastasize to the pancreas include melanomas, breast, gastrointestinal, and lung tumors.

Parapancreatic Neoplasms

Lymphomas are malignant neoplasms that rise from the lymphoid tissues. They are the most frequent parapancreatic neoplasm. It may be difficult to separate a parapancreatic lymphadenopathy from a primary lesion in the pancreas. An intraabdominal lymphoma may appear as a hypoechoic mass or, with necrosis, a cystic mass in the pancreas (Fig. 12.48). The superior mesenteric vessels may be displaced anterior instead of posterior as seen with a primary pancreatic mass. Multiple nodes are seen along the pancreas, duodenum, porta hepatis, and superior mesenteric vessels; they may be difficult to distinguish from a pancreatic mass. The enlarged nodes appear hypoechoic and well defined.

Other types of retroperitoneal neoplasms that may appear as a cystic lesion near the area of the pancreas include lymphangiomas, paragangliomas, cystic teratomas, and metastases. The lymphangiomas are most often thin-walled, homogeneous, small cysts, but they have also been seen to have septa, thick walls, calcification, and internal debris. The paragangliomas are usually found near the inferior mesenteric artery or near the kidney. The cystic teratomas are found more frequently in children and young adults. Their appearance is a mixed sonographic pattern of cystic, solid, fat, and calcifications.

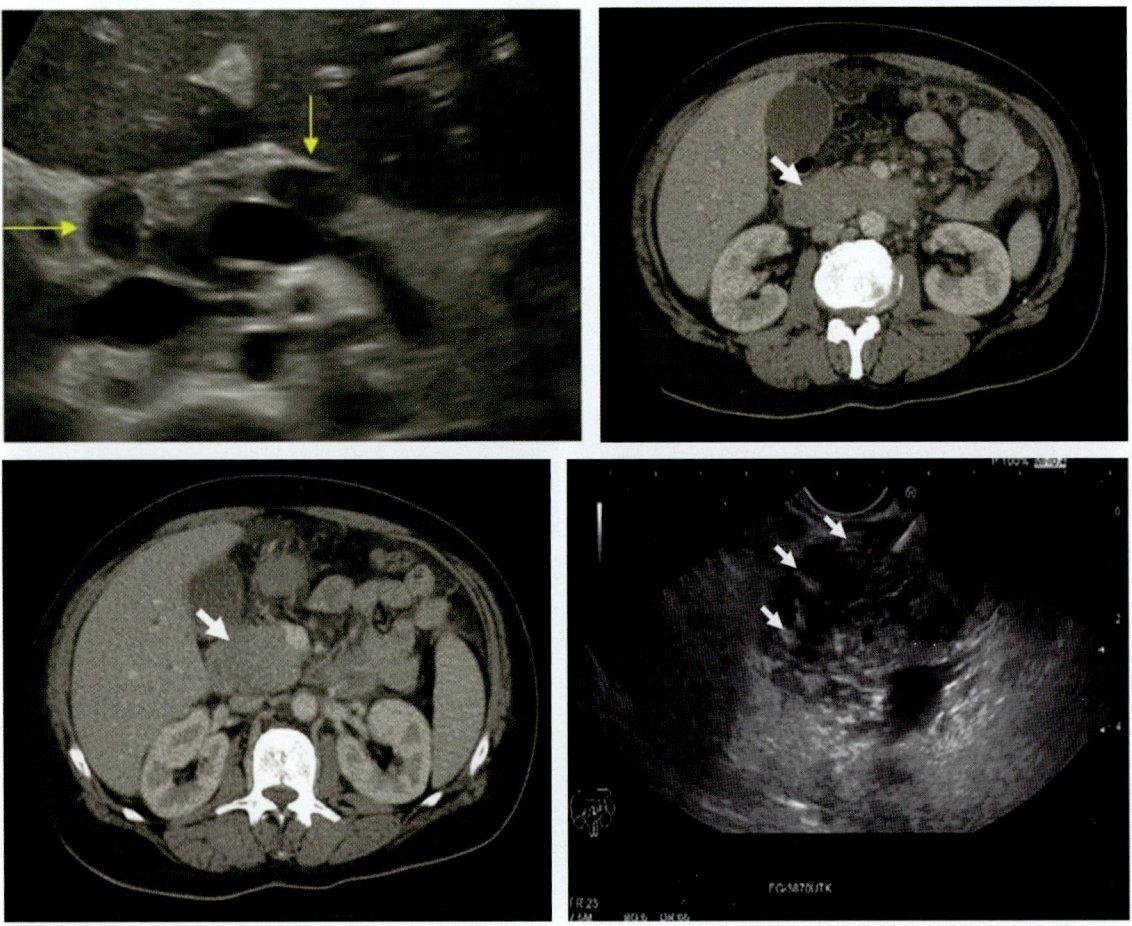

FIG. 12.48 Lymphoma. An intraabdominal lymphoma may appear as a hypoechoic mass or, with necrosis, a cystic mass in the pancreas. The superior mesenteric vessels may be displaced anterior instead of posterior as seen with a primary pancreatic mass. The *arrows* denote the hypoechoic enlarged lymph nodes.

Key Pearls

- The pancreas lies anterior to the first and second lumbar bodies located deep in the epigastrium and left hypochondrium, behind the lesser omental sac
- The majority of the pancreas lies within the retroperitoneal cavity, except for a small portion of the head that is surrounded by peritoneum.
- The pancreas is divided into the following four areas: head, neck, body, and tail.
- Two ducts are seen within the pancreas: the duct of Wirsung and the duct of Santorini.
- The blood supply for the pancreas is the splenic artery and pancreaticoduodenal arteries.
- The splenic artery supplies the body and tail of the pancreas through four smaller branches: (1) suprapancreatic (rises from the celiac axis/splenic artery), (2) pancreatic, (3) prepancreatic (before leaving the pancreas), and (4) prehilar (before leaving the spleen) and hepatic artery (gastroduodenal artery).
- The gastroduodenal artery is seen along the anterolateral border of the pancreas as it travels a short distance along the anterior aspect of the pancreatic head just to the right of the neck before it divides into the superior pancreaticoduodenal branches.
- Annular pancreas is a rare anomaly in which the head of the pancreas surrounds the second portion of the duodenum.
- The pancreas is both a digestive (exocrine) and hormonal (endocrine) gland.
- The primary exocrine function is to produce pancreatic juice, which enters the duodenum together with bile.
- Exocrine function is performed by acini cells of the pancreas, which can produce up to 2 L of pancreatic juice per day.
- The endocrine function controls the secretion of glucagons and insulin into the blood.
- The endocrine function is in the islets of Langerhans in the pancreas.
- There are specific enzymes of the pancreas that may become altered in pancreatic disease, namely amylase and lipase.
- Lipase is an enzyme that is excreted specifically by the pancreas and that parallels the elevation in amylase levels.
- Glucose controls the blood sugar level in the body.
- The normal pancreas has an echo pattern that is slightly more hyperechoic and finer in texture than that of the surrounding retroperitoneum.
- The echo intensity of the pancreas is usually slightly less than that of surrounding soft tissue and slightly greater than that of the liver.
- Pancreatitis is inflammation of the pancreas; this condition may be chronic or acute.
- Pancreatitis occurs when the pancreas becomes damaged and malfunctions as a result of increased secretion and blockage of ducts.
- Acute pancreatitis is an inflammation of the pancreas caused by the inflamed acini releasing pancreatic enzymes into the surrounding pancreatic tissue.
- An acute attack of pancreatitis is commonly related to biliary tract disease and alcoholism.
- Collections of fluid in the peripancreatic area generally retain communication with the pancreas.
- The pancreatic duct may be obstructed in acute pancreatitis as a result of inflammation, spasm, edema, swelling of the papilla, or pseudocyst formation.
- The alteration in the size and echogenic texture of the pancreas may be subtle; therefore, the diagnosis of pancreatitis may be based on the visualization of peripancreatic fluid collections in a patient with abnormal pancreatic enzymes and clinical history suggestive of pancreatitis.
- Complications of acute pancreatitis include hemorrhage, pseudocyst formation, inflammatory mass, and intrapancreatic and extrapancreatic fluid collections.
- Complications of acute pancreatitis include hemorrhage, pseudocyst formation, inflammatory mass, and intrapancreatic and extrapancreatic fluid collections.
- Chronic pancreatitis results from recurrent attacks of acute pancreatitis and causes continuing destruction of the pancreatic parenchyma that results in permanent structural damage, which can lead to impairment of exocrine and endocrine function.
- Chronic pancreatitis is generally associated with chronic alcoholism or biliary disease, although patients with hypercalcemia (elevated calcium levels) and hyperlipidemia (elevated fat levels) are more predisposed to chronic pancreatitis.
- The most common location of a pseudocyst is in the lesser sac anterior to the pancreas and posterior to the stomach.
- A phlegmon is an inflammatory process that spreads along fascial pathways, causing localized areas of diffuse inflammatory edema of soft tissue that may proceed to necrosis and suppuration.
- Benign cystic lesions of the pancreas include autosomal dominant polycystic disease, Von Hippel–Lindau syndrome, and cystic fibrosis.
- There are four subtypes of pancreatic cystic neoplasms with varying malignant potential: serous cystic tumors, mucinous cystic neoplasms, intraductal papillary mucinous neoplasms, and solid pseudopapillary neoplasms.
- The endocrine tumors rise from the islet cells of the pancreas.
- There are several types of islet cell tumors; they may be functional or nonfunctional and may be classified as benign adenomas or malignant tumors.
- The most common functioning islet cell tumor is insulinoma, followed by gastrinoma.
- The most common primary neoplasm of the pancreas is adenocarcinoma.
- Many patients with a mass in the head of the gland will have obstructive jaundice and anterior wall compression of the inferior vena cava.
- Primary tumors that can metastasize to the pancreas include melanomas, breast, gastrointestinal, and lung tumors.
- Lymphomas are malignant neoplasms that rise from the lymphoid tissues; they are the most frequent parapancreatic neoplasm.
- Other types of retroperitoneal neoplasms that may appear as a cystic lesion near the area of the pancreas include lymphangiomas, paragangliomas, cystic teratomas, and metastases.

REFERENCES

Banks PA, Bollen TL, Dervenis C, et al. Classification of acute pancreatitis-2012; revision of the Atlanta classification and definitions by international consensus. *Gut*. 2013;62:102.

Bang UC, Benfield T, Hyldstrup L, et al. Mortality, cancer, and comorbidities associated with chronic pancreatitis: a Danish nationwide matched-cohort study. *Gastroenterology*. 2014;146:989.

Barge JU, Lopera JE. Vascular complications of pancreatitis: role of interventional therapy. *Korean J Radiol*. 2012;13(Suppl 1):S45.

Bergman S, Melvin WS. Operative and nonoperative management of pancreatic pseudocysts. *Surg Clin North Am*. 2007;87:1447.

Carpenter SL, Scheiman JM. Pancreatic imaging. *Curr Opin Gastroenterol*. 1996;12:442.

Demos TC, Posniak HV, Harmath C, et al. Cystic lesions of the pancreas. *Am J Roentgenol*. 2002;179:1375–1388.

Dietrich CF, Chichakli M, Hirche TO, et al. Sonographic findings of the hepatobiliary-pancreatic system in adult patients with cystic fibrosis. *J Ultrasound Med*. 2002;21:409–416.

Goodman M, Willmann JK, Jeffrey RB. Incidentally discovered solid pancreatic masses: imaging and clinical observations. *Abdom Imaging*. 2012;37:91.

Grogan JR, Saeian K, Taylor AJ, et al. Making sense of mucin-producing pancreatic tumors. *Am J Roentgenol*. 2001;176:921–929.

Grube J. Epigastric pain. In: Henningsen C, ed. *Clinical Guide to Ultrasonography*. St Louis: Elsevier; 2004.

Gumaste VV, Pitchumoni CS. Pancreatic pseudocyst. *Gastroenterologist*. 1996;4:33.

Jung-Hee Y, Han SS, Cha SS, Lee SJ. Color Doppler ultrasonography of a pancreatic arteriovenous malformation. *J Ultrasound Med*. 2005;24:113–117.

Khalid A, Brugge W. ACG practice guidelines for the diagnosis and management of neoplastic pancreatic cysts. *Am J Gastroenterol*. 2007;102:2339.

Lim JH, Lee G, Oh YL. Radiologic spectrum of intraductal papillary mucinous tumor of the pancreas. *RadioGraphics*. 2001;21:323–337.

Lundstedt C, Dawiskiba S. Serous and mucinous cystadenomas/cystadenocarcinomas of the pancreas. *Abdomn Imaging*. 2000;25:201–206.

Megibow AJ, Lavelle MT, Rofsky NM. Cystic tumors of the pancreas: the radiologist. *Surg Clin North Am*. 2001;81:489–495.

Middleton WD, Kurtz AB, Hertzberg BS. *Ultrasound: The Requisites*. 2nd ed. St Louis: Elsevier; 2004.

Morgan DE, Baron TH. Practical imaging in acute pancreatitis. *Semin Gastrointest Dis*. 1998;9:41.

Neumyer MM. Ultrasonographic assessment of renal and pancreatic transplants. *J Vasc Technol*. 1995;19:321.

Nicolau C, Torra R, Bianchi L, et al. Abdominal sonographic study of autosomal dominant polycystic disease. *J Clin Ultrasound*. 2000;28:277–282.

Ocampo C, Oria A, Zandalazini H, et al. Treatment of acute pancreatic pseudocysts after severe acute pancreatitis. *J Gastrointest Surg*. 2007;11:357.

Porta M, Fabregat X, Malats N, et al. Exocrine pancreatic cancer: symptoms at presentation and their relation to tumour site and stage. *Clin Transl Onocol*. 2005;7:189.

Rumack CM, Wilson SR, Charboneau JW, Johnson J. *Diagnostic Ultrasound*. ed 3 St Louis: Elsevier; 2005.

Ryan DP, Hong TS, Bardeesy N. Pancreatic adenocarcinoma. *N Engl J Med*. 2014;371:1039.

Scott J, Martin I, Redhead D. Mucinous cystic neoplasm of the pancreas: imaging features and diagnostic difficulties. *Clin Radiolol*. 2000;55:187–192.

Sharma A. Tumors of the pancreas. In: Blumberg RS, Burakoff R, Greenberger NJ, eds. *Current Diagnosis & Treatment: Gastroenterology, Hepatology & Endoscopy*. New York: McGraw-Hill; 2009.

Siegel RL, Miller KD, Jemal A. Cancer statistics, 2015. *CA Cancer J Clin*. 2015;65:5.

Tseng JF, Warshaw AL, Sahani DV, et al. Serous cystadenoma of the pancreas: tumor growth rates and recommendations for treatment. *Ann Surg*. 2005;242:413.

Yoon SH, Lee JM, Cho JY, et al. Small (<20 mm) pancreatic adenocarcinomas: analysis of enhancement patterns and secondary signs with multiphasic multidetector CT. *Radiology*. 2011;259:442.

CHAPTER 13

The Gastrointestinal Tract

Sandra L. Hagen-Ansert

OBJECTIVES

On completion of this chapter, you should be able to:
- Describe the anatomy and relational landmarks of the gastrointestinal system
- Discuss the size of wall thickness and diameters of the gastrointestinal tract
- Describe the sonographic technique used to image the gastrointestinal tract and appendix
- Differentiate the sonographic appearances of the pathologies covered in this chapter

OUTLINE

Anatomy of the Gastrointestinal Tract 389
   Normal Anatomy 389
   Vascular Anatomy 392
Physiology and Laboratory Data of the Gastrointestinal Tract 393

Sonographic Evaluation of the Gastrointestinal Tract 394
   Stomach 395
   Duodenum 396
   Small Bowel 397
   Appendix 398
   Colon 398

Pathology of the Gastrointestinal Tract 399
   Upper Gastrointestinal Tract 399
   Lower Gastrointestinal Tract 402

KEY TERMS

Absorption
Alimentary tract
Appendicolith
Ascites
Cardiac orifice
Cholecystokinin
Crohn disease
Diverticulum
Duodenal bulb
Fecalith
Gastrin
Gastrohepatic ligament
Gastrophrenic ligament
Gastrosplenic ligament

Greater omentum
Haustra
Hepatic flexure
Lesser omentum
Lienorenal ligament
Lymphoma
McBurney's point
McBurney's sign
Meckel's diverticulum
Mesentery
Mucin
Mucocele
Mucosa
Muscularis

Paralytic ileus
Peristalsis
Polyp
Pseudomyxoma peritonei (PMP)
Pyloric canal
Rugae
Secretin
Serosa
Splenic flexure
Submucosa
Target sign
Valvulae conniventes
Villi

Sonography is not the primary imaging tool utilized to investigate the gastrointestinal system due to the limited visualization of many structures. However, some patients present with nonspecific complaints related to the gastrointestinal tract that sonography may help direct the further workup of the patient. The gastrointestinal tract may be difficult to image with ultrasound in most patients unless they ingest fluids or some other acoustic transmittable contrast agent. Many laboratories have begun to investigate various contrast agents in pursuit of the ideal medium for imaging the stomach, duodenum, small bowel, and colon. The retrograde infusion of water can also be used to distend the colon to evaluate for abnormalities.

ANATOMY OF THE GASTROINTESTINAL TRACT

Normal Anatomy

The digestive tract, also known as the **alimentary tract**, is a tube about 8 m long extending from the mouth to the anus (Fig. 13.1). The gastrointestinal tract is that part of the digestive system

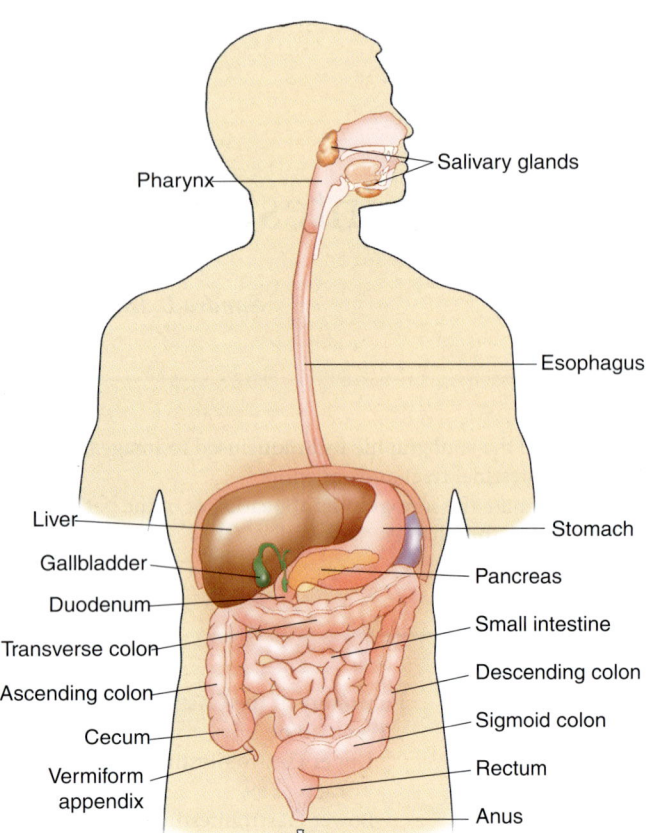

FIG. 13.1 The digestive tract, also known as the alimentary tract, is a tube about 8 m long extending from the mouth to the anus. The gastrointestinal tract is that part of the digestive system below the diaphragm. The sequential parts of the digestive system include the mouth, pharynx, esophagus, stomach, small intestine, and large intestine.

below the diaphragm. Together, the digestive tract and gastrointestinal tract comprise the digestive system. The sequential parts of the digestive system include the mouth, pharynx, esophagus, stomach, small intestine, and large intestine. Three types of accessory digestive glands—the salivary glands, liver, and pancreas—secrete digestive juices into the digestive system.

Esophagus. The esophagus extends from the pharynx through the thoracic cavity, then passes through the diaphragm and empties into the stomach (see Fig. 13.1). The lower end of the esophagus is a circular muscle that acts as a sphincter, constricting the tube so that the entrance to the stomach, at the **cardiac orifice**, is generally closed. This helps to prevent gastric acid from moving up into the esophagus.

Stomach. The stomach is a large, smooth, muscular organ with two surfaces: the lesser curvature and the greater curvature (Fig. 13.2). The stomach is divided into three parts: The *fundus* is found in the superior aspect, the *body* makes up the major central axis, and the *pylorus* is the lower aspect. The pylorus is further subdivided into the antrum, the pyloric canal, and the pyloric sphincter (Fig. 13.3). The **pyloric canal** is a muscle that connects the stomach to the proximal duodenum.

Supporting ligaments of the greater curvature of the stomach include the **greater omentum**, the **gastrophrenic ligament**, the **gastrosplenic ligament**, and the **lienorenal ligament** (see Fig. 13.2). Ligaments that support the lesser curvature of the stomach include the **gastrohepatic ligament** of the **lesser omentum**. Folds of the **mucosa** and **submucosa** are called **rugae**.

Small Intestine. The small intestine is a long, coiled tube about 5 m long by 4 cm in diameter (see Fig. 13.1). The first 22 cm is the duodenum, which is curved like the letter *C*. The duodenum is subdivided into four segments: (1) superior, (2) descending, (3) transverse, and (4) ascending (Fig. 13.4). The first part of the duodenum is not attached to the mesentery; the remainder of the small intestine, including the rest of the duodenum, is attached to the mesentery. The **mesentery** projects from the parietal peritoneum and attaches to the small intestine to anchor it to the posterior abdominal wall.

The first part of the duodenum, the **duodenal bulb**, begins at the pylorus and terminates at the neck of the gallbladder, posterior to the left lobe of the liver and medial to the gallbladder. The duodenal bulb is peritoneal, supported by the hepatoduodenal ligament, and passes anterior to the common bile duct, gastroduodenal artery, common hepatic artery, hepatic portal vein, and head of the pancreas. This is an important point for sonographers to recognize: if there is air in the duodenal bulb, it will be more difficult to image the common bile duct and smaller vessels that help to define the head of the pancreas (Fig. 13.5). This is avoided by changing patient position (decubitus or upright) or giving the patient water to fill the duodenal loop and serve as an acoustic window to image these structures.

The second part (descending) of the duodenum is retroperitoneal and runs parallel, posterior, and to the right of the spine. The transverse colon crosses anterior to the middle third of the descending duodenum. The pancreatic head is medial to the duodenum at this point. The common bile duct joins the pancreatic duct to enter the ampulla of Vater.

The third part (transverse) of the duodenum begins just to the right of the fourth lumbar vertebra and passes anterior to the aorta, inferior vena cava, and crura of the diaphragm. The superior mesenteric vessels course anterior to the duodenum.

The fourth part (ascending) of the duodenum ascends superiorly to the left of the spine and aorta to the second lumbar vertebra, where it joins the proximal jejunum (duodenojejunal flexure). This portion lies on the left crus of the diaphragm. It is held in place by the ligament of Treitz (which courses from the left toward the right crus of the diaphragm).

As the duodenum turns downward, it is called the jejunum. The jejunum extends for about 2 m before becoming the ileum. The inner wall of the small intestine is marked by circular folds of the mucous membrane, the **villi** (Fig. 13.6). The **valvulae conniventes** are large folds of mucous membrane that project into the lumen of the bowel and help retard the passage of food to provide greater absorption. The lower part of the small intestine is the ileum. The ileocecal orifice marks the entry into the large intestine and prevents food from reentering the small intestine.

Large Intestine. This is the last part of the digestive system. The large intestine is larger in diameter and shorter in

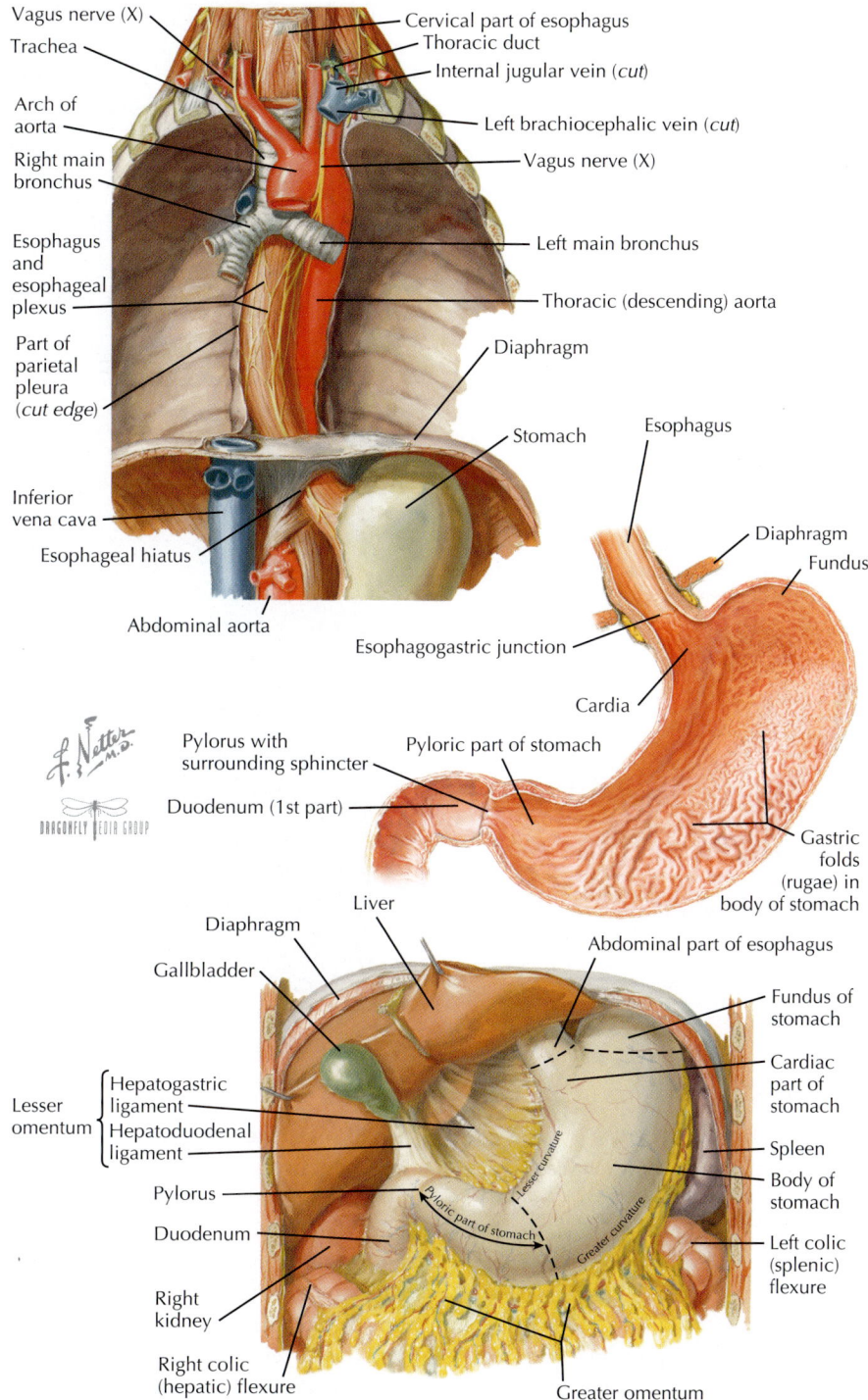

FIG. 13.2 The stomach is a large, smooth, muscular organ that has two surfaces: the lesser curvature and the greater curvature. The stomach is divided into three parts: The *fundus* is found in the superior aspect, the *body* makes up the major central axis, and the *pylorus* is the lower aspect.

length than the small intestine. The cecum and vermiform appendix, ascending colon, transverse colon, and descending colon, sigmoid colon, and rectum all make up the large intestine (Fig. 13.7). The **haustra** of the colon are the small pouches caused by sacculation, which give the colon its segmented appearance (Fig. 13.8). The ascending colon extends from the cecum vertically to the lower part of the liver. It turns horizontally at the **hepatic flexure** and moves to become the transverse colon. On the left side of the abdomen, at the **splenic flexure**, it then descends vertically to become the descending colon and eventually the sigmoid colon, which empties into the rectum. The rectum is 12 cm long, terminating at the anus. The mucosa of the large intestine lacks villi and produces no digestive enzymes. The surface epithelium consists of cells specialized for absorption and goblet cells that secrete mucus.

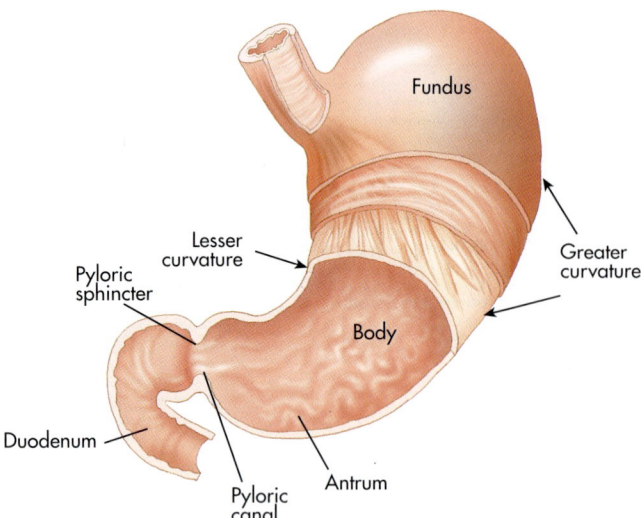

FIG. 13.3 The pylorus is further subdivided into the antrum, the pyloric canal, and the pyloric sphincter. The pyloric canal is a muscle that connects the stomach to the proximal duodenum.

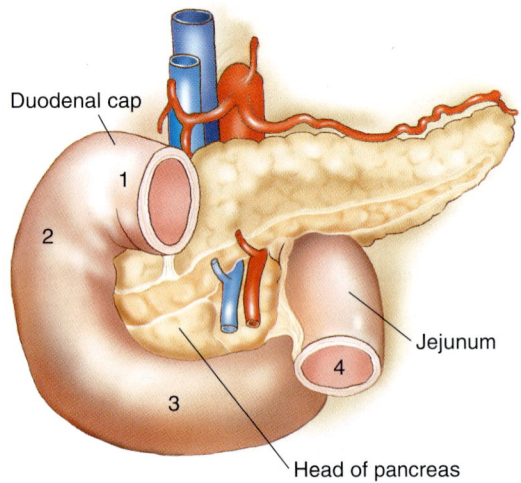

FIG. 13.4 The duodenal cap is an excellent landmark for the head of the pancreas. The duodenum is divided into four sections. See text for explanation. (The fourth part of the duodenum is posterior to the jejunum.)

Vascular Anatomy

Esophagus. The arteries that supply the esophagus rise from the high, mid, and lower sections of this muscular tube. The inferior thyroid branch of the subclavian artery supplies the upper esophagus, the descending thoracic aorta supplies the mid-esophagus, and the gastric branch of the celiac axis and the left inferior phrenic artery of the abdominal aorta supply the lower end of the esophagus. Varices may be seen to rise from the gastroesophageal arteries (Fig. 13.9).

Stomach. The vascular supply to the stomach is provided by the right gastric arterial branch, pyloric and right gastroepiploic branches of the hepatic artery, left gastroepiploic branch and vasa brevia of the splenic artery, and left gastric artery (see Fig. 13.8). The venous system of the stomach is parallel to the arterial vessels, which drain into the portal venous system.

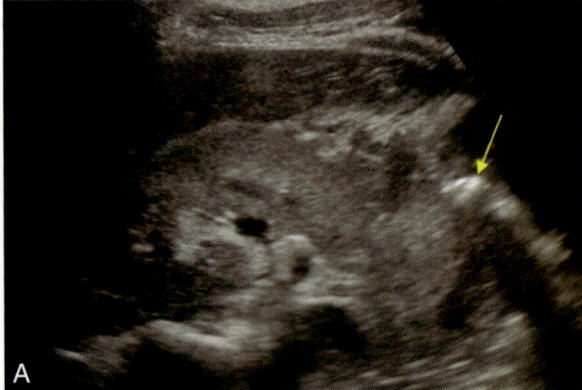

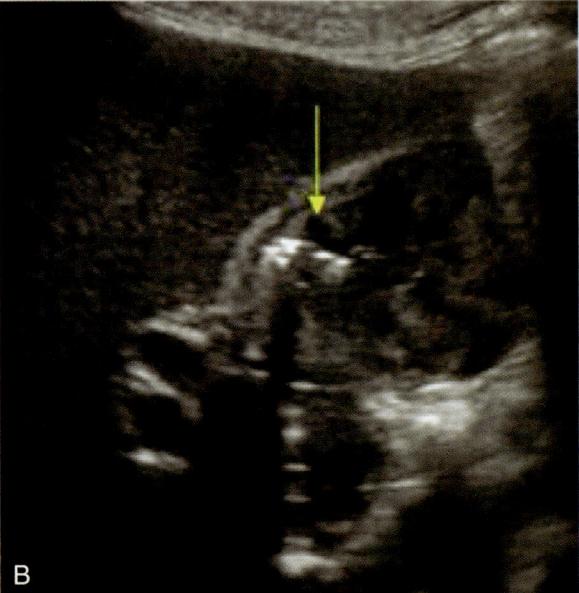

FIG. 13.5 (A) Transverse sonogram of the air-filled pylorus and duodenum. (B) The *arrow* points to fluid and air bubbles in the duodenum.

Small Intestine. The mesentery outlines the small intestine and contains superior mesenteric vessels, nerves, lymphatic glands, and fat between its two layers. The celiac axis supplies the duodenum through its right gastric, gastroduodenal, and superior pancreaticoduodenal branches (Fig. 13.10). The superior mesenteric artery has multiple branches to the small bowel, including the inferior pancreaticoduodenal, jejunal, and ileal arteries. The venous system parallels the arterial system and empties into the portal venous system.

Large Intestine. The celiac, superior mesenteric, and inferior mesenteric arteries supply both the small and the large intestine. The superior mesenteric arterial branches include the ileocolic, right colic, and middle colic arteries (Fig. 13.11). The inferior mesenteric artery supplies the intestine from the left border of the transverse colon to the rectum, rising from the anterior surface of the abdominal aorta at the level of the third lumbar vertebra and descending retroperitoneally. Branches of the inferior mesenteric artery include the left colic, sigmoid, and superior rectal arteries. The venous system parallels the arterial system and empties into the portal venous system.

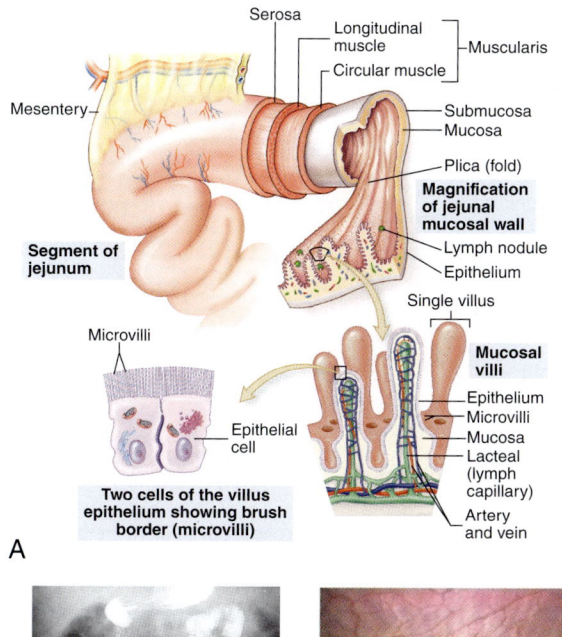
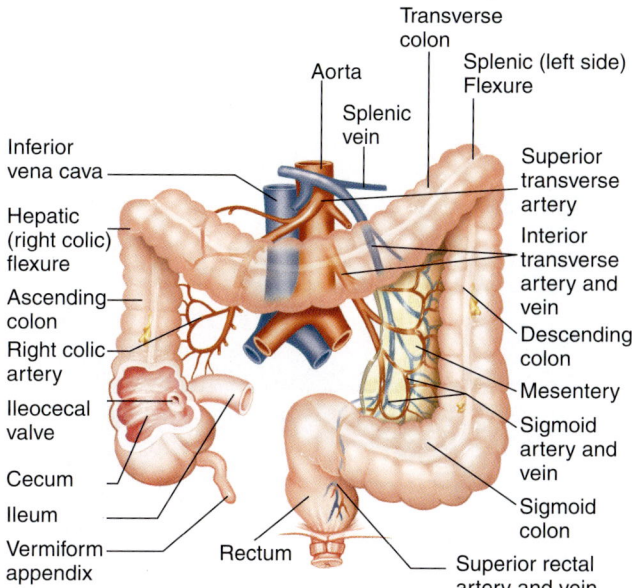

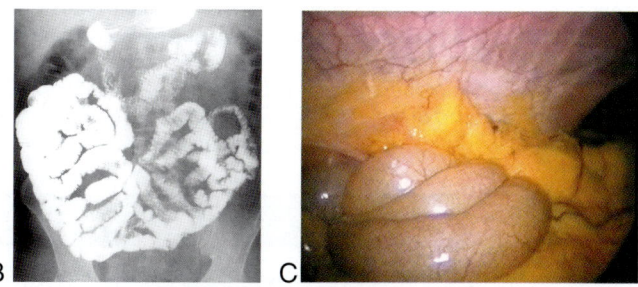

FIG. 13.6 **The small intestine.** (A) The folds of mucosa are covered with villi; each villi is covered with epithelium, which increases the surface area for absorption of food. (B) Anteroposterior radiograph obtained during a contrast (barium enhanced) study of the small intestine. The individual is lying supine on the x-ray table. (C) Laparoscopic view of the small intestine.

FIG. 13.7 Divisions of the large intestine include the cecum, vermiform appendix, ascending colon, transverse colon, descending colon, sigmoid colon, and rectum.

PHYSIOLOGY AND LABORATORY DATA OF THE GASTROINTESTINAL TRACT

Digestion and absorption are the primary functions of the gastrointestinal tract. Food is ingested through the mouth, chewed, and swallowed. The molecules of food must be further digested or mechanically broken down and chemically split into small molecules. The chemical digestion of food breaks down long-chain organic molecules (i.e., polysaccharides or proteins). Each reaction is carried on with the help of a specific enzyme produced by cells of the digestive tract or its accessory glands. When these particles are small enough, nutrient molecules pass through the wall of the intestine into the blood or lymph system by **absorption**.

Nutrients are transported to the liver after they are absorbed by the blood; the liver processes and stores nutrients. The remaining nutrients in the blood are transported to cells throughout the body. Undigested and unabsorbed food is eliminated from the digestive tract by the process of defecation.

When food enters the stomach, the rugae gradually smooth out, causing the stomach to stretch and increase its capacity for food intake. Contractions of the stomach help to mix the food. The three layers of smooth muscle in the wall enable the stomach to mash and churn food and move it along through **peristalsis**. Large amounts of mucus are secreted in the stomach. Gastric glands secrete gastric juice containing hydrochloric acid and enzymes. Over a 3- to 4-hour period, food is converted into chyme. This soupy mixture is moved toward the pylorus and into the small intestine. Small quantities of water, salts, and lipid-soluble substances, such as alcohol, are absorbed through the stomach mucosa. The pyloric sphincter is a strong band of muscle that relaxes when necessary to release the food.

Villi within the small intestine increase its surface area for digestion and absorption of nutrients. If the villi were not present, food would move quickly through the intestine without time for absorption. The intestinal glands are found between the villi and secrete large amounts of fluid that serve as a medium for digestion and absorption of nutrients. The hormone **gastrin**, which is released by the stomach mucosa, stimulates the gastric glands to secrete. Most digestion occurs within the duodenum. Bile and enzymes from the liver and pancreas are secreted into the duodenum to act on the chyme and break down the food particles for absorption. The intestinal glands are stimulated to release their fluid mainly by local reflexes initiated when the small intestine is distended by chyme.

Other gastrointestinal hormones include **cholecystokinin** and **secretin**. Cholecystokinin is released by the presence of fat in the intestine and regulates gallbladder contraction and gastric emptying. Secretin is released from the small bowel to stimulate the secretion of bicarbonate to decrease the acid content of the intestine.

A period of 1 to 3 days or longer may be required for the journey through the large intestine. Undigestible chime becomes stool within the large intestine as most of the

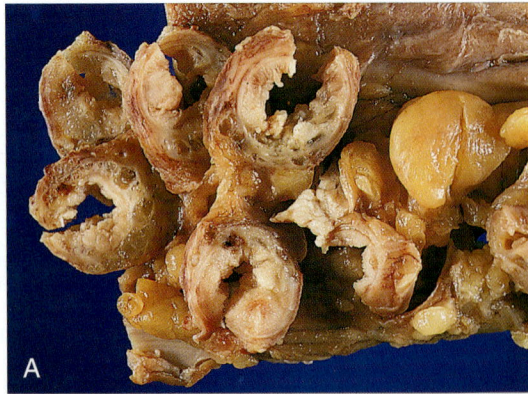
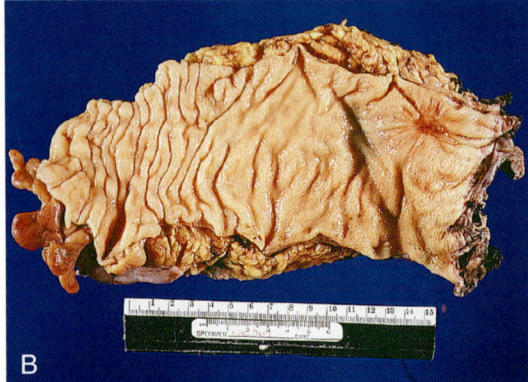
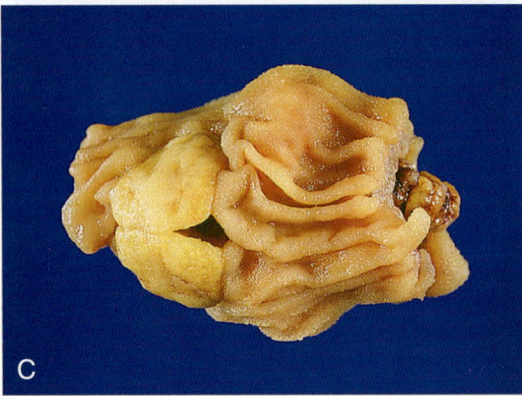

FIG. 13.8 (A) Gross specimen of the small intestine. (B–C) Gross specimens of the large intestine.

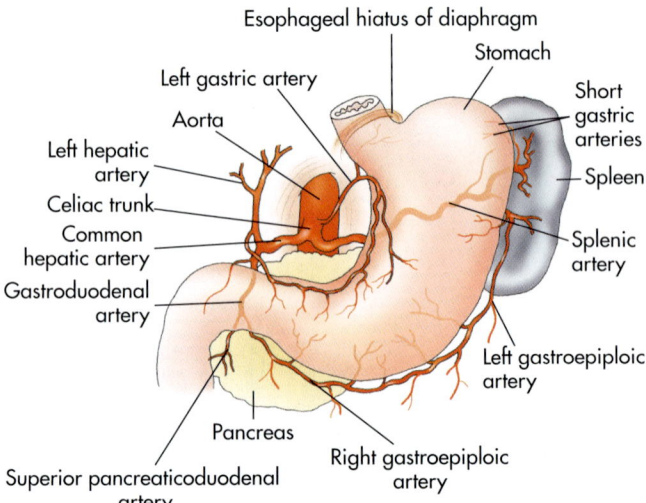

FIG. 13.9 Vascular supply to the stomach is received from the branches of the celiac axis. The left gastric artery supplies the lower third of the esophagus and the upper right part of the stomach. The right gastric artery supplies the lower right part of the stomach. The short gastric arteries supply the fundus. The left gastroepiploic artery supplies the upper part of the greater curvature of the stomach, and the right gastroepiploic artery supplies the lower part of the greater curvature of the stomach.

BOX 13.1 Layers of Bowel

Mucosa: directly contacts the intraluminal contents; lined with epithelial folds; echogenic
Submucosa: contains blood vessels and lymph channels
Muscularis: contains circular and longitudinal bands of fiber
Serosa: thin, loose layer of connective tissue
Mesothelium: covers intraperitoneal bowel loops

SONOGRAPHIC EVALUATION OF THE GASTROINTESTINAL TRACT

Visualizing the gastrointestinal tract with ultrasound may be difficult because intraluminal air produces an echogenic shadow, which prevents the sound beam from penetrating structures posteriorly. The scattering and reflection effect of gas in the gastrointestinal tract often produces an incomplete or mottled distal acoustic shadow. The rim of lucency represents the wall (i.e., intima, media, and serosa), and its periserosal fat produces the outer echogenic border of the tract wall.

The bowel wall consists of five layers (Box 13.1). The odd-numbered walls (first, third, and fifth) are echogenic, and the even-numbered walls (second and fourth) are hypoechoic, with an average total thickness of 3 mm if distended and 5 mm if undistended.

The technique used to observe the upper gastrointestinal tract is for the patient to drink 10 to 40 oz of water through a straw after a baseline ultrasound study of the upper abdomen is completed. The straw helps prevent ingestion of excess air when the water is consumed. The patient should be in an upright position for the examination; this causes air in the stomach to rise to the fundus of the stomach and not interfere with the ultrasound beam (Fig. 13.12). The lower

remaining sodium and water are reabsorbed. Some of the indigestible remains of the chime are devoured by gut bacteria. Most of the absorption process of sodium and water occurs in the cecum.

The most common laboratory data the sonographer may come across in a patient with gastrointestinal disease relates to blood in the stool. If chronic, this blood loss can lead to anemia. Blood in the stool indicates the presence of a bleed somewhere in the gastrointestinal system. Infection would show elevation of the white blood count. An increase in the carcinoembryonic antigen is found in patients with inflammatory bowel disease.

Clinical signs and symptoms of nausea, vomiting, and diarrhea are common with gastrointestinal problems. Abdominal pain and fever may also be present with gastrointestinal conditions, such as colitis, bowel abscess, acute diverticulitis, and appendicitis.

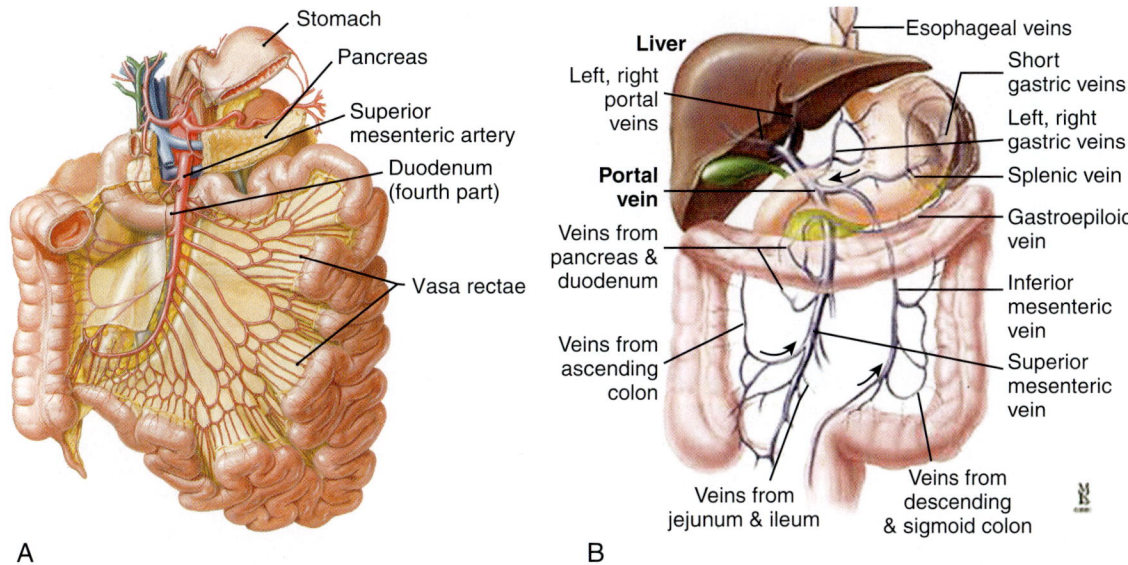

FIG. 13.10 (A) Arterial supply for the small intestine. (B) Venous supply for the gastrointestinal system.

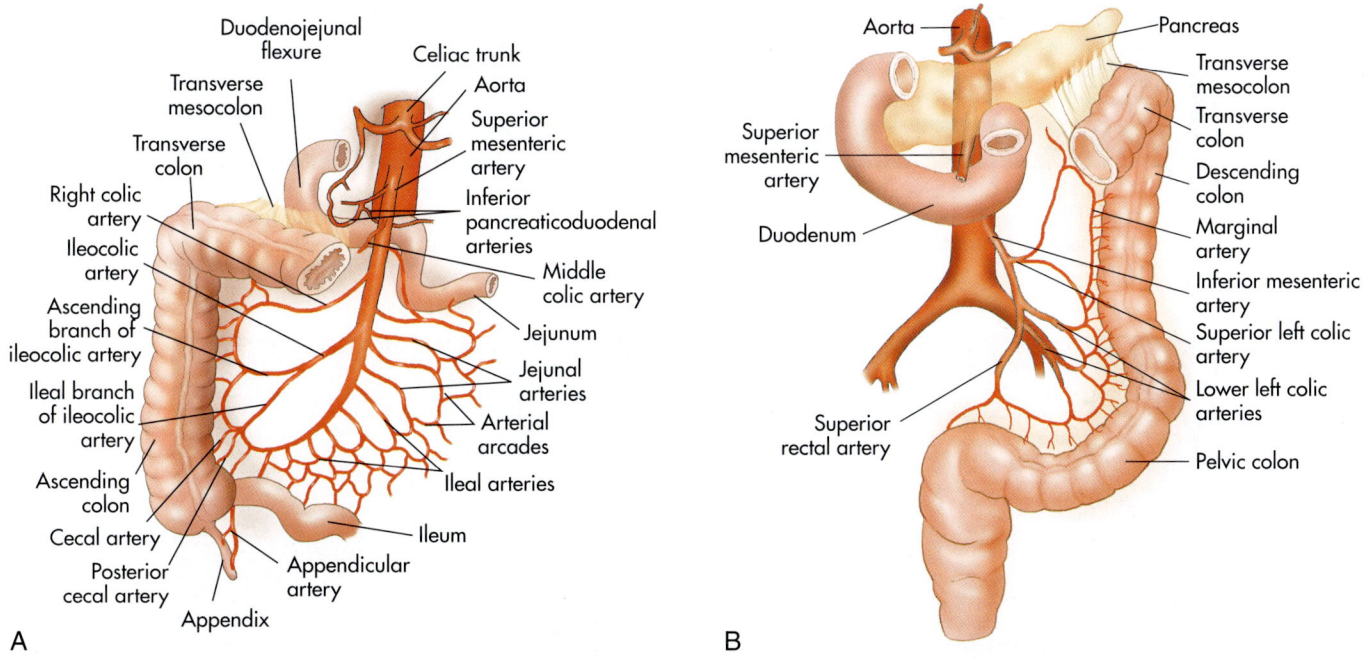

FIG. 13.11 (A) The superior mesenteric artery supplies the gut from halfway down the second part of the duodenum to the distal third of the transverse colon. (B) The inferior mesenteric artery supplies the large bowel from the distal third of the transverse colon to halfway down the anal canal. It forms an anastomosis with the middle colic branch of the superior mesenteric artery.

gastrointestinal tract requires no preparation. When imaging the lower colon, it may be useful to give the patient a water enema to better delineate the colon.

Stomach

The gastroesophageal junction is seen on the sagittal scan to the left of the midline as a bull's eye or target-shaped structure anterior to the aorta, posterior to the left lobe of the liver, and inferior to the hemidiaphragm (Fig. 13.13). The left lobe of the patient's liver must be large enough to allow imaging of the gastroesophageal junction. The gastric antrum can be seen as a target shape in the midline (Fig. 13.14). The remainder of the stomach usually is not visualized well unless dilated with fluid (Fig. 13.15).

When pathology is present, the serosal layer of the normal gastric wall is seen running toward the serous side of a tumor, which allows differentiation of intramural from extraserosal tumors. If a serosal bridging layer (three layers are seen on the mucosal side of the tumor, and at least two of them are continuous with the first and second layers of the normal gastric wall) is present, the tumor lies within the gastric wall. If mucosal bridging is continuous with the mucosal layers of the normal gastric wall, is intramucosal, or is deeply infiltrated, carcinoma can be excluded. The

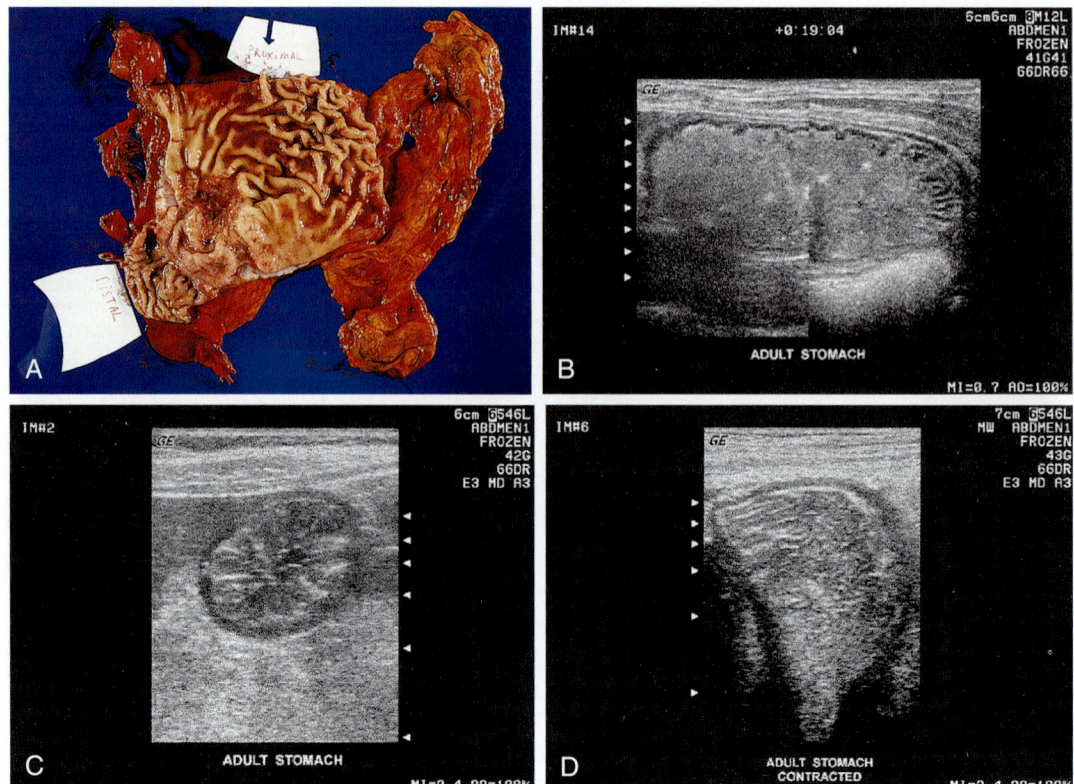

FIG. 13.12 (A) Gross specimen of the stomach showing the internal rugae of the wall. (B) Sagittal image of the fluid-filled stomach. Rugae may be seen along the peripheral margins of the wall. (C) Transverse image of the prominent stomach and rugae. (D) Contracted stomach after fluid has passed through the pylorus.

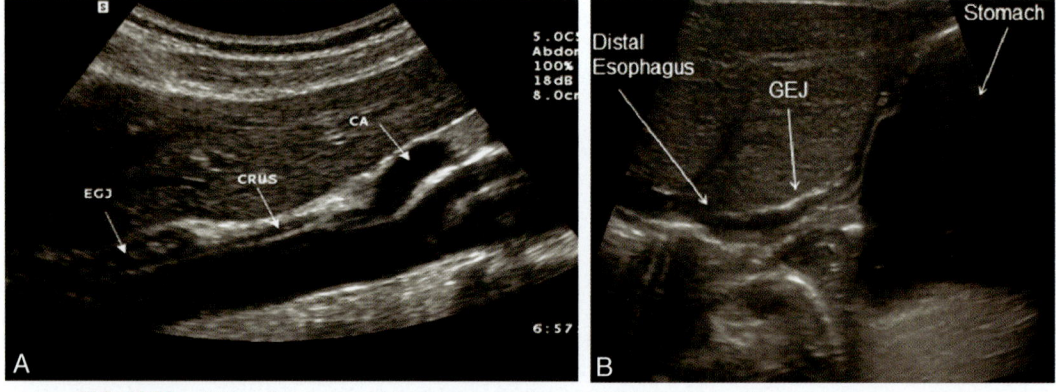

FIG. 13.13 (A) Sagittal image of the gastroesophageal (EGJ) junction, which is shown as a small bull's eye shape anterior to the aorta and posterior to the left lobe of the liver. (B) Transverse image of the gastroesophageal junction (GEJ) just medial to the fluid-filled stomach. *CA,* Celiac axis.

sonographer should orient the transducer vertical to the area of transition between the lesion and the stomach wall to show their relationship.

Cystic Mass in the Left Upper Quadrant. If a patient has a cystic mass in the left upper quadrant, several measurements can be taken to determine whether the mass is the fluid-filled stomach or another mass arising from adjacent organs. The sonographer may give the patient a carbonated drink to see bubbles in the stomach, ask the clinician to place a nasogastric tube for drainage, watch for a change in the shape or size of the "stomach" mass with ingestion of fluids, alter the patient's position by scanning in an upright or left or right lateral decubitus position, watch for peristalsis, or ask the patient to drink water to see the swirling effect.

Duodenum

Usually, only the gas-filled duodenal cap is seen to the right of the pancreas. As discussed previously, the duodenum is divided into the following four segments: (1) superior, (2) descending, (3) transverse, and (4) ascending.

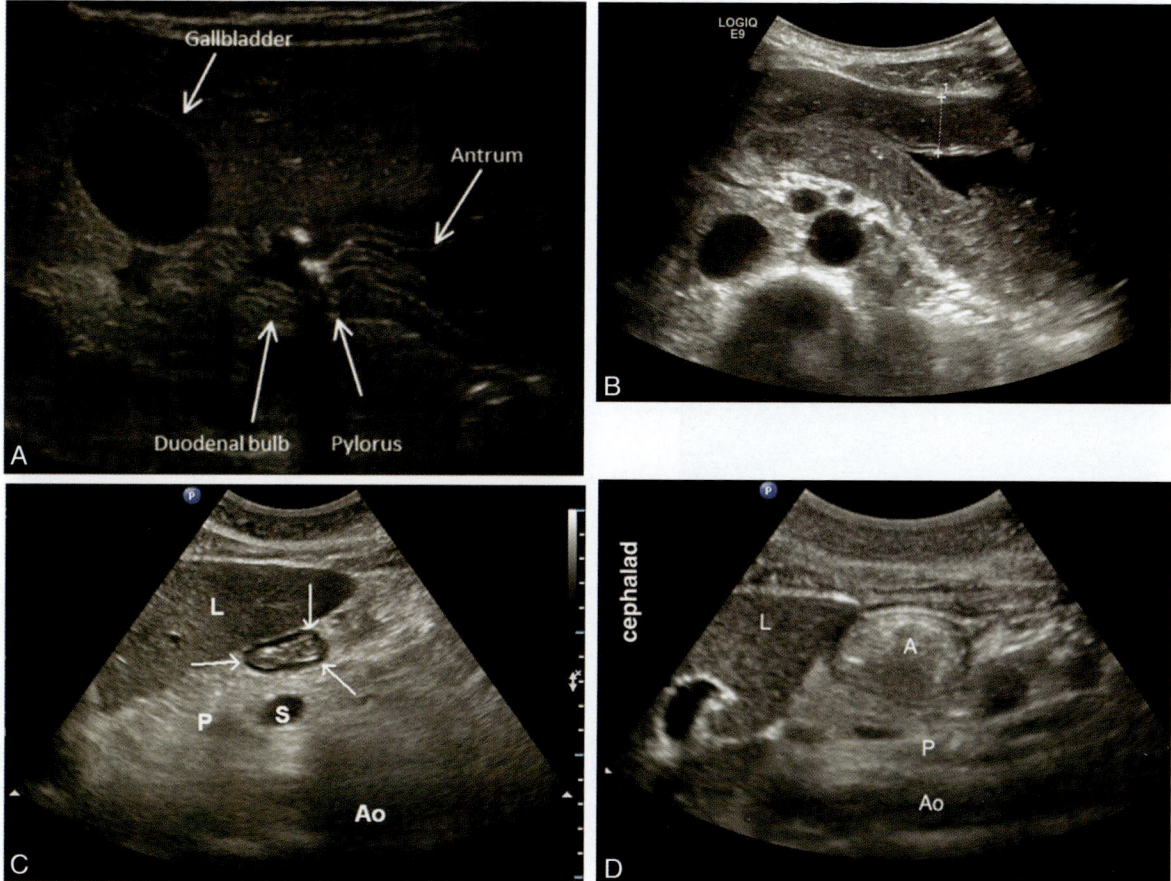

FIG. 13.14 (A) Transverse image of the antrum, pylorus, and duodenal bulb. (B) Note the thickness of the wall of the antrum. (C) Sagittal image of the "target" antrum of the stomach *(arrows)*. (D) Sagittal image of the full antrum of the stomach. *Ao*, Aorta; *L*, liver; *P*, pancreas, *S*, splenic vein.

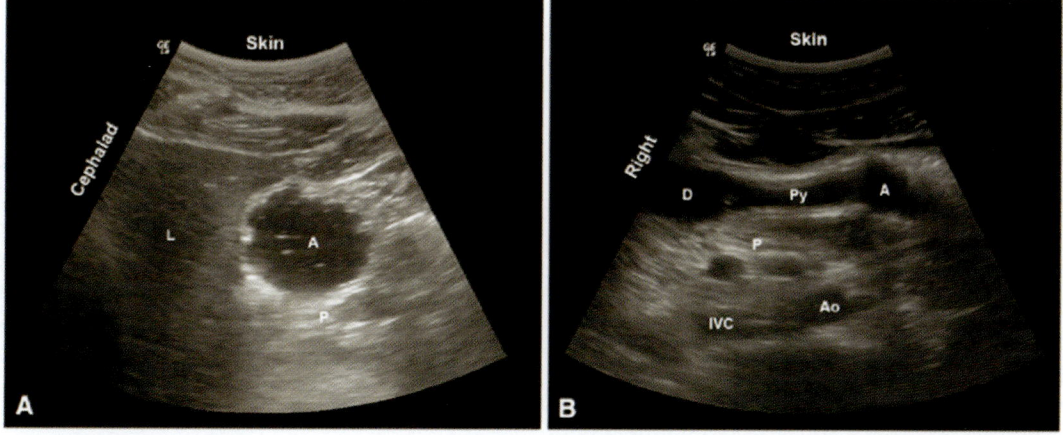

FIG. 13.15 Sagittal (A) and transverse (B) images of the fluid-filled antrum (A), pylorus (Py), and duodenal bulb (D). *Ao*, Aorta; *IVC*, inferior vena cava; *P*, pancreas.

The duodenum can be outlined easily with water ingestion or a change in position (see Fig. 13.15). Generally, the right lateral decubitus position allows the fluid to drain from the antrum of the stomach into the duodenum. Observation of peristalsis is useful to delineate the duodenum.

Small Bowel

The sonographer usually cannot see the small bowel with sonography; the valvulae conniventes may be seen as linear echo densities spaced 3 to 5 mm apart (Fig. 13.16). This is called the "keyboard sign" and can be seen in the duodenum

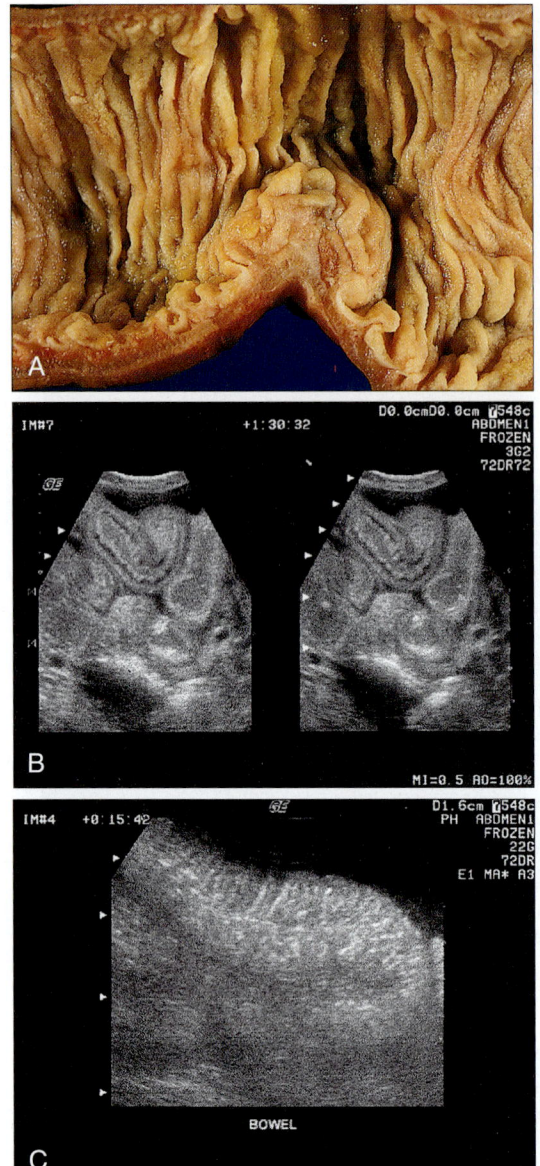

FIG. 13.16 (A) Gross specimen showing the valvulae conniventes within the small bowel lumen. (B–C) Ultrasound images of prominent small bowel with valvulae conniventes.

and jejunum. The ileum is smooth walled, and the small bowel wall is less than 3 mm thick. The small bowel is more difficult to image unless contrast or fluid is present. When fluid is present in the bowel loops, the sonographer may be able to look for peristalsis, air movement, or movement of intraluminal fluid contents to rule out obstruction.

Appendix

The vermiform appendix is a remnant of what was originally the apex of the cecum. It is a long, tubular structure extending from the cecum in one of several directions; it may lie superiorly behind the cecum, medially behind the ileum and mesentery, or downward and medial into the true pelvis (see Fig. 13.7). The appendix is located on the abdominal wall under McBurney's point.

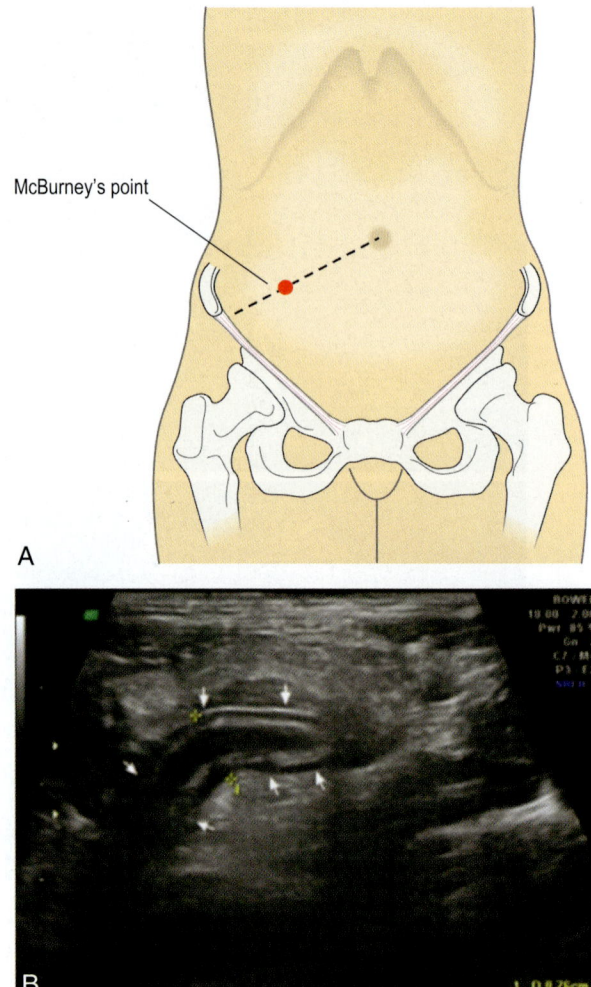

FIG. 13.17 (A) McBurney's point is located by drawing a line from the right anterosuperior iliac spine to the umbilicus. (B) At approximately the midpoint of this line lies the root of the appendix.

McBurney's point is located by drawing a line from the right anterosuperior iliac spine to the umbilicus (Fig. 13.17). At approximately the midpoint of this line lies the root of the appendix.

The appendix varies from 2 to 20 cm in length. It is retained in position by a fold of the peritoneum that forms a mesentery for the appendix. This triangular structure covers two-thirds of the appendix, leaving the distal one-third completely uncovered by the peritoneum. A branch of the ileocolic artery, the artery of the appendix, lies between the layers of this mesentery. This artery runs the entire length of the appendix.

The small canal of the appendix communicates with the cecum by an orifice that is below and behind the ileocecal opening. The cellular layers that make up the appendix are the **serosa** or adventitia, muscularis propria, submucosa, and mucosa—the same layers as in the intestine. An abundant amount of retiform tissue is found in the mucosa layer, especially at younger ages. The appendix has no known physiologic significance.

Colon

A prominent fluid-filled colon may present as a mass (Fig. 13.18). The water enema technique should be used to help

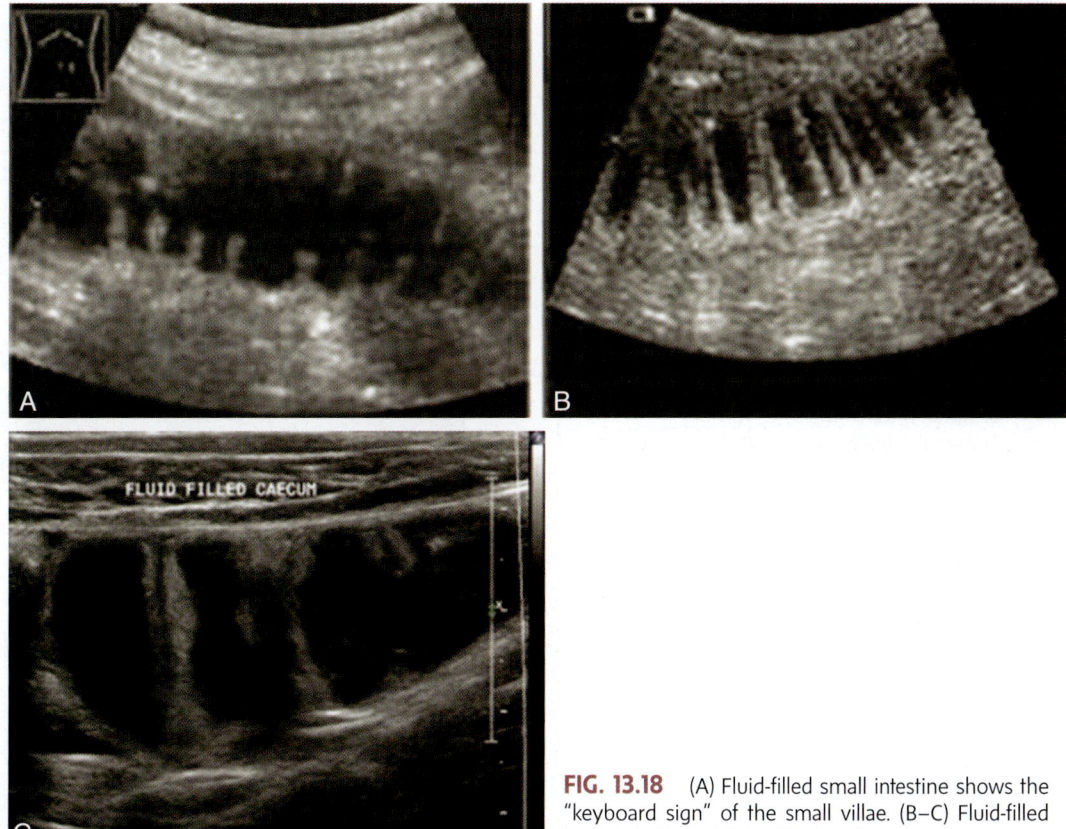

FIG. 13.18 (A) Fluid-filled small intestine shows the "keyboard sign" of the small villae. (B–C) Fluid-filled large intestine outlining the haustra valves.

delineate if the mass is within the colon, separate from the colon, or just the colon itself. The patient should have a full bladder when scanned to help push the small bowel out of the pelvis. The water in the enema should be lukewarm, and the patient rolled into the left lateral decubitus position. Only a small amount of water needs to be given as the sonographer follows the rectum and rectosigmoid colon with the endoluminal probe. The normal wall thickness measures 4 mm. The colon consists of five layers: From innermost to outermost, the first two layers are mucosa, the third is submucosa, the fourth is muscularis propria, and the fifth is subserosal fatty tissue. If the colon is dilated, the sonographer should measure from the fluid to the outside of the wall. Distention is considered adequate if the lower bowel is larger than 5 cm; the entire halo should measure less than 2 cm (target sign).

PATHOLOGY OF THE GASTROINTESTINAL TRACT

Upper Gastrointestinal Tract

Table 13.1 lists the clinical findings, sonographic findings, and differential considerations for upper gastrointestinal tract diseases and conditions.

Duplication Cyst. Duplication cysts are embryologic mistakes. They may cause symptoms, depending on their size, location, and histology (see Table 13.1). The criteria for a duplication cyst are as follows: (1) The cyst is lined with alimentary tract epithelium, (2) the cyst has a well-developed muscular wall, and (3) the cyst is contiguous with the stomach. These cysts may come from the pancreas or duodenum and occur more often in females than in males. They usually are found on the greater curvature of the stomach. Clinical symptoms include high intestinal obstruction-distention, vomiting, and abdominal pain; hemorrhage and fistula formation may also occur. Differential considerations include mesenteric or omental cyst, pancreatic cyst or pseudocyst, enteric cyst, renal cyst, splenic cyst, congenital cyst of the left lobe of the liver, and gastric distention.

Sonographic Findings. On ultrasound examination, duplication cysts appear anechoic with a thin inner echogenic rim (mucosa) and a wider outer hypoechoic rim (muscle layer) (Fig. 13.19).

Gastric Bezoar. A gastric bezoar is an intragastric mass composed of accumulated ingested material. Bezoars are divided into the following three categories: (1) trichobezoars—hairballs in young women, (2) phytobezoars—vegetable matter (e.g., unripe persimmons), and (3) concretions—inorganic materials (e.g., sand, asphalt, shellac). Gastric bezoars are movable intraluminal masses of congealed ingested materials that are seen on upper gastrointestinal radiographs. Clinically, patients may present with nausea, vomiting, crampy epigastric pain, or signs of bowel obstruction (see Table 13.1). Differential diagnoses would include gastric carcinoma, postprandial food, or intramural mass.

Sonographic Findings. Radiography or CT is the imaging modality of choice; however, with sonographic evaluation, a complex mass is seen with internal mobile echogenic components (Fig. 13.20). In the fasting patient, the

TABLE 13.1	Upper Gastrointestinal Tract Findings		
	Clinical Findings	Sonographic Findings	Differential Considerations
Duplication Cysts	↓ Hematocrit with hemorrhage	Anechoic mass with thin inner echogenic rim; Wide outer hypoechoic rim	Mesenteric or omental cyst; Pancreatic cyst; Enteric cyst; Renal cyst; Splenic cysts; Hepatic cyst in LLL
Gastric Bezoar	Nausea; Vomiting; Pain	Complex mass with internal mobile components; Hyperechoic curvilinear dense strip at anterior margin	Tumor; Cyst
Polyps	Abdominal pain	Echogenic; Heterogeneous	Leiomyoma
Leiomyomas	N/A	Hypoechoic and contiguous with muscular layer of stomach; Solid with cystic areas (necrosis)	Carcinoma; Polyp
Gastric Carcinoma	↑ LFTs; Abdominal pain	Target or pseudokidney sign; Gastric wall thickening	Leiomyoma; Lymphoma; Metastatic disease
Lymphoma	Nausea, vomiting; Weight loss	Large, hypoechoic mass; Thickened gastric walls; Spoke-wheel pattern	Gastric carcinoma; Leiomyosarcoma; Metastatic disease
Leiomyosarcoma	N/A	Target lesion with variable pattern; Irregular echoes; Cystic cavity	Lymphoma; Gastric carcinoma; Metastatic disease
Metastatic Disease	Secondary to other cancers	Target pattern; Circumscribed thickening; Uniform widening of wall without layering	Lymphoma; Gastric carcinoma; Leiomyosarcoma

LFTs, Liver function tests; *LLL*, left lobe of the liver; *N/A*, not applicable.

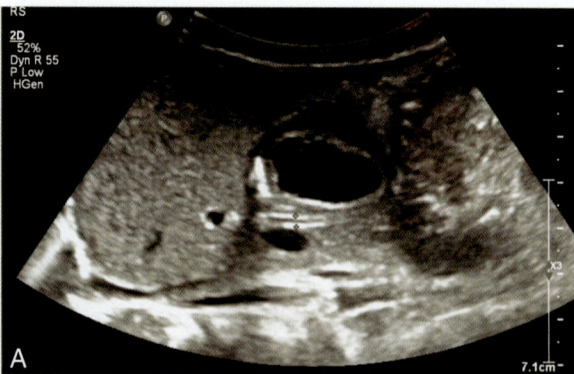

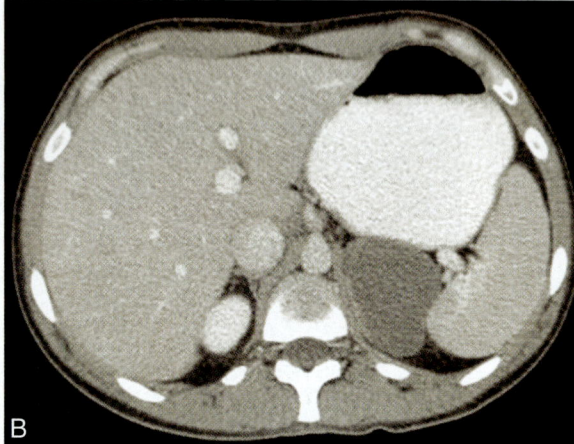

FIG. 13.19 (A) On ultrasound examination, duplication cysts appear anechoic with a thin inner echogenic rim (mucosa) and a wider outer hypoechoic rim (muscle layer). (B) Computed tomographic contrast image of the gastric duplication cyst.

clinical findings, sonographic findings, and differential considerations for upper gastrointestinal tract polyps.

Sonographic Findings. Polyps may be seen as an incidental finding with fluid distention of the stomach and appear as solid masses that adhere to the gastric wall. The polyp has variable echogenicity. A large polyp may be inhomogeneous; its contours may be sharply defined, depending on the nature of the surface; a pedicle may be detected.

Intramural Benign Gastric Tumors. These tumors are defined as a benign mass composed of one or more tissue elements of the gastric wall. There are many different types of benign tumors, that is, gastrointestinal stromal tumor, leiomyoma, leiomyoblastoma, schwannoma, neurofibroma, lipoma, hemangioma, and lymphangioma.

Leiomyoma is the most common tumor of the stomach. Leiomyoma is seen as a small mass similar to carcinoma. Clinically the patient is asymptomatic (see Table 13.1). Differential diagnosis includes gastric carcinoma, gastric metastases and lymphoma, ectopic pancreatic tissues, and gastric or duodenal ulcer.

Sonographic Findings. On sonography, the mass is seen as hypoechoic and continuous with the muscular layer of the stomach (Fig. 13.22). It may also be seen as a circular or oval space-occupying lesion with a homogeneous echo pattern and hemispheric bulging into the lumen, frequently separated from the lumen by two or three layers continuous

sonographer would see a broad band of high-amplitude echoes or a hyperechoic curvilinear dense strip at the anterior margin.
Benign Tumors.
Polyp. A **polyp** is a protruding, space-occupying, epithelial lesion within the stomach. A gastric polyp is an outgrowth of tissue from the gastric wall (Fig. 13.21). Patients are asymptomatic when the polyp is small. As the polyp grows, abdominal pain may be present. See Table 13.1 for

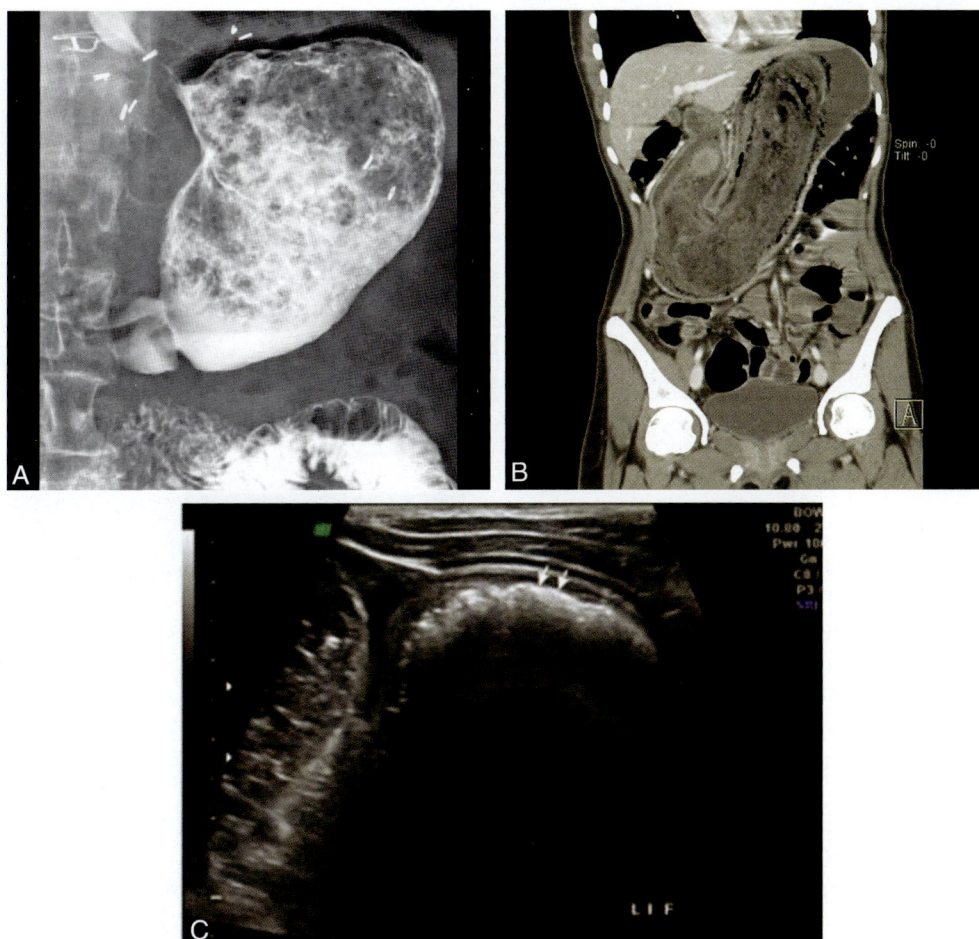

FIG. 13.20 Gastric bezoar. Radiography (A) or computed tomography (B) is the imaging modality of choice; however, with sonographic evaluation, a complex mass is seen with internal mobile echogenic components. (C) The sonographer would see a broad band of high-amplitude echoes in the fasting patient or a hyperechoic curvilinear dense strip at the anterior margin *(arrows)*.

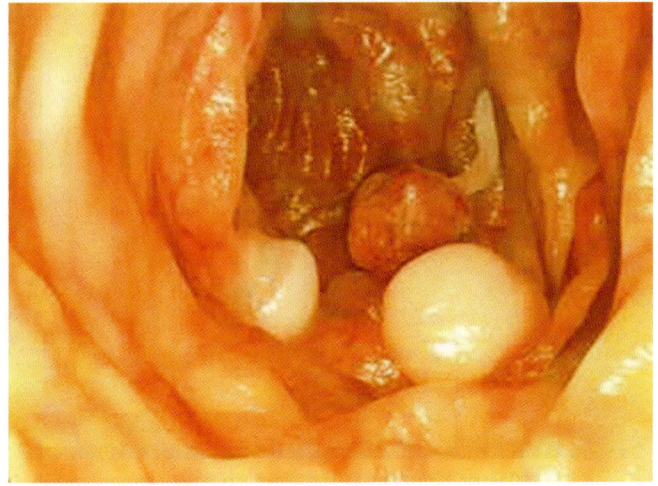

FIG. 13.21 Endoscopic view of a polyp in the gastrointestinal tract.

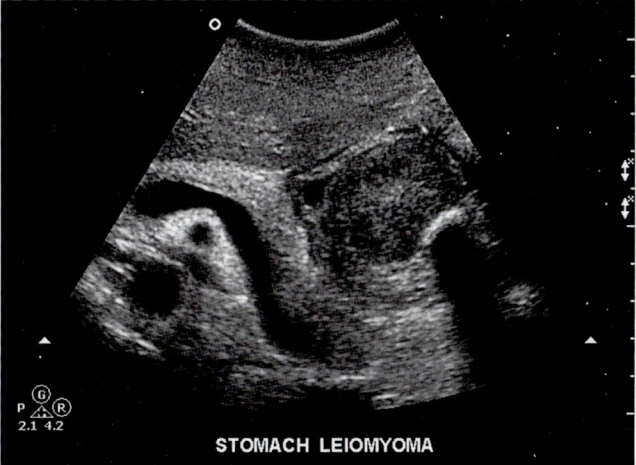

FIG. 13.22 Transverse image of the left upper quadrant demonstrates a complex tumor in the region of the stomach, which was diagnosed as a leiomyoma.

with those of normal wall. The mass may appear as a solid with cystic areas that represent necrosis.

Malignant Tumors.

Gastric Carcinoma. Stomach cancer or gastric cancer develops from the lining of the stomach. Gastric carcinoma is the fifth leading cause of cancer and the third leading cause of death from cancer; it occurs twice as often in males than females and is more common in Eastern Asia and Eastern

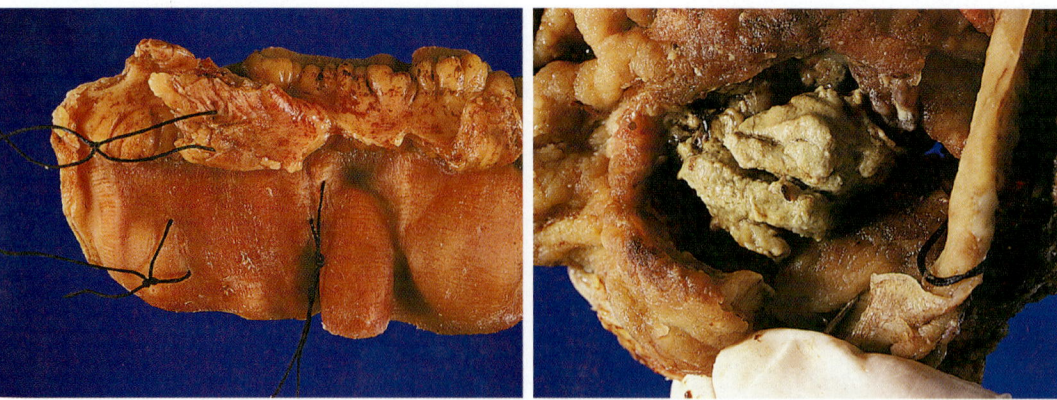

FIG. 13.23 Gross specimens of adenocarcinoma of the stomach.

Europe. Clinical symptoms range from asymptomatic to nonspecific. Patients may experience indigestion or a burning sensation, loss of appetite, and abdominal discomfort. One-half of these tumors occur in the pylorus, and one fourth occur in the body and fundus of the stomach. The lesions may be ulcerated, diffuse, polypoid, superficial, or some combination of these (see Table 13.1 and Fig. 13.23).

Sonographic Findings. The sonographer should look for the target or pseudokidney sign; the patient may have gastric wall thickening. The mass will be polypoid or circumferential with no peristalsis throughout the lesion. Polypoid cancer can be lobulated or fungating (Fig. 13.24). Gastric outlet obstruction may be present secondary to the mass.

Lymphoma. Lymphoma can occur as a primary tumor of the gastrointestinal tract with 3% comprising stomach tumors. In patients with disseminated lymphoma, a primary tumor occurs as a multifocal lesion in the gastrointestinal tract. The stomach has enlarged and thickened mucosal folds, multiple submucosal nodules, ulceration, and a large extraluminal mass. Clinical symptoms include nausea and vomiting with weight loss (see Table 13.1).

Sonographic Findings. The sonographer will note a large and poorly echogenic (hypoechoic) mass, thickening of the gastric walls, and a "spoke-wheel" or "bull's-eye" pattern within the mass (Fig. 13.25).

Leiomyosarcoma. The second most common malignant tumor is the leiomyosarcoma gastric sarcoma comprising 1% to 5% of tumors. The mass is generally globular or irregular; it may become huge, outstripping its blood supply, with central necrosis leading to cystic degeneration and cavitation (see Table 13.1).

Sonographic Findings. A target-shaped hypoechoic lesion is visible on sonography. Although the pattern is variable, hemorrhage and necrosis may occur, causing irregular echoes or a cystic cavity (Fig. 13.26).

Metastatic Disease. Metastatic disease to the stomach is rare; it may result from a melanoma or lung or breast cancer. The tumor is found in the submucosal layer, forming circumscribed nodules or plaques (see Table 13.1).

Sonographic Findings. A target pattern with circumscribed thickening or uniform widening of the stomach wall without layering is visible (Fig. 13.27).

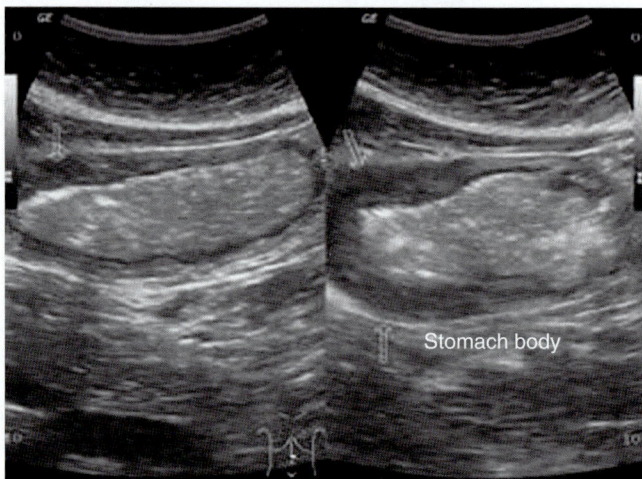

FIG. 13.24 Sonographic images of a large heterogeneous cancerous mass within the stomach.

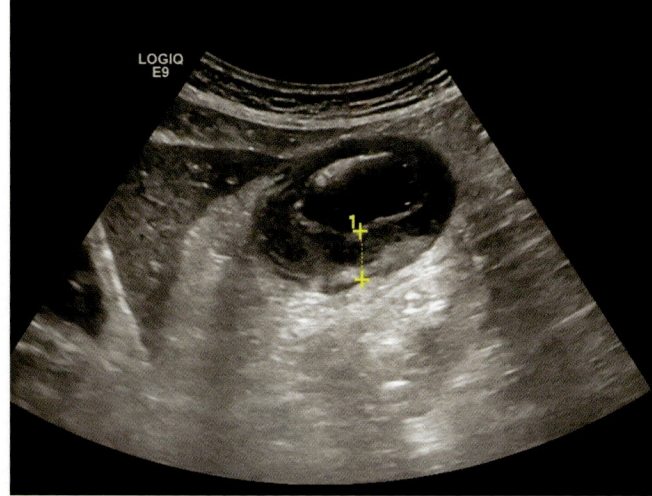

FIG. 13.25 Gastric lymphoma. The stomach has enlarged and thickened mucosal folds, multiple submucosal nodules, ulceration, and a large extraluminal mass.

Lower Gastrointestinal Tract

Table 13.2 lists the clinical findings, sonographic findings, and differential diagnoses for lower gastrointestinal tract diseases and conditions.

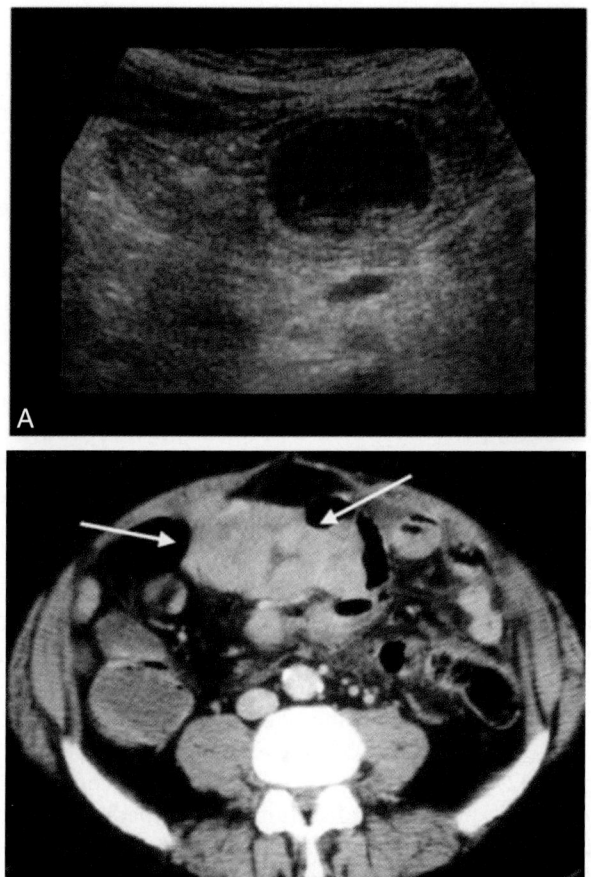

FIG. 13.26 **Leiomyosarcoma.** (A) A target-shaped hypoechoic lesion is visible on sonography. Although the pattern is variable, hemorrhage and necrosis may occur, causing irregular echoes or a cystic cavity. (B) Computed tomographic contrast image of the tumor.

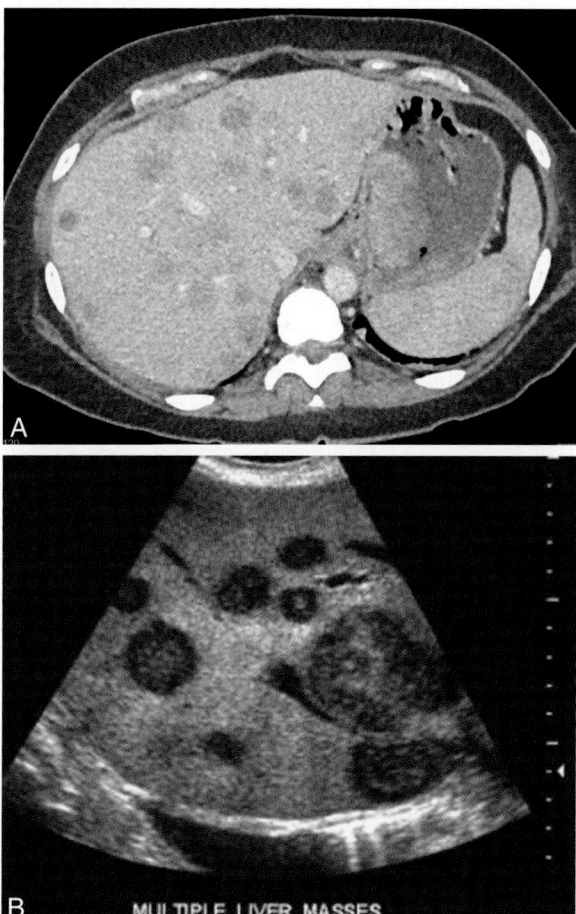

FIG. 13.27 Computed tomographic (A) and ultrasound (B) images of gastric adenocarcinoma with liver metastases.

Obstruction and Dilation. A small bowel obstruction is associated with dilation of the bowel loops proximal to the site of obstruction (Fig. 13.28). In 6% of cases, the dilated loops are fluid-filled and can be mistaken for a soft tissue mass on x-ray examination (see Table 13.2).

Sonographic Findings. The dilated loops have a tubular or round echo-free appearance. In adynamic ileus, the dilated bowel has normal to somewhat increased peristaltic activity and less distention than in dynamic ileus. In dynamic ileus, the loops are round, with minimal deformity at the interfaces with adjacent loops of distended bowel; valvulae conniventes and peristalsis are seen. The fluid loops are not always associated with obstruction; they can occur with gastroenteritis and **paralytic ileus** or in dilated, fluid-filled bowel loops without peristalsis. The sonographer should demonstrate pliability and compressibility of the bowel wall (Fig. 13.29). With volvulus (closed-loop obstruction), the involved loop is doubled back on itself abruptly so that a U-shaped appearance is seen on sagittal scan, and a C-shaped anechoic area with a dense center is seen on a transverse scan. The dense center represents the medial bowel wall and mesentery.

Abnormalities of the Appendix.

Acute Appendicitis. Acute appendicitis results from luminal obstruction and inflammation, leading to ischemia of the vermiform appendix (Fig. 13.30). This may produce necrosis, perforation, and subsequent abscess formation and peritonitis. The appendix lumen may be obstructed by fecal material, a foreign body, carcinoma of the cecum, stenosis, inflammation, kinking of the organ, or even lymphatic hypertrophy resulting from systemic infection. Obstruction results in edema, which can compromise the vascular supply to the appendix. Subsequently, the permeability of the mucosa increases, and bacterial invasion of the wall of the appendix results in infection and inflammation. Increased intraluminal pressure may cause occlusion of the appendicular end artery. If the condition persists, the appendix may necrose, leading to gangrene, rupture, and subsequent local or generalized peritonitis. Periappendiceal abscess or peritonitis does not necessarily mean perforation; the organism may permeate the wall in the absence of perforation to cause these extra-appendiceal complications.

The symptoms of acute appendicitis are pain and rebound tenderness, which is usually localized over the right lower quadrant (**McBurney's sign**). Typically, the pain is followed by nausea and vomiting, diarrhea, and systemic signs of inflammation, such as leukocytosis and fever (see Table 13.2). Acute appendicitis can occur at any age but is more prevalent at younger ages.

TABLE 13.2	Lower Gastrointestinal Findings	
Clinical Findings	Sonographic Findings	Differential Considerations
Obstruction and/or Dilation		
Epigastric pain	Tubular, round, echo-free lesion Compressibility of bowel	Appendicitis
Acute Appendicitis		
Pain rebound tenderness over McBurney's point Diarrhea Fever Nausea, vomiting	Thickened muscular wall and ↑ appendiceal diameter (6 mm) Lack of peristalsis Not compressible ↑ Blood flow (Doppler)	Ruptured ectopic pregnancy Fluid-filled colon Inflammation of Meckel's diverticulum
Mucocele		
↑ Leukocytes RLQ pain Asymptomatic	Variable: anechoic, hypoechoic, complex	Appendicitis
Meckel's Diverticulitis		
Rectal bleeding Tenderness	Loop pattern	Acute appendicitis
Crohn Disease		
Diarrhea Fever RLQ pain	Symmetrically swollen bowel Target pattern with preserved parietal layers around stenotic and hyperdense lumen ↑ Wall thickening Rigidity to pressure Peristalsis absent or sluggish	Appendicitis Meckel's diverticulum Diverticulitis
Lymphoma		
Abdominal pain Palpable mass Weight loss Blood loss	Large, discrete mass Exoenteric pattern	Pseudokidney Leiomyosarcoma
Leiomyosarcoma		
Abdominal pain Palpable mass	Large, solid mass Contained in necrotic areas	Lymphoma

RLQ, Right lower quadrant.

Progression of acute appendicitis to frank perforation is more rapid in the younger child, sometimes occurring within 6 to 12 hours. The perforation rate in the preschool child can be as high as 70% compared with the overall figure of 30% for children and 21% to 22% for adults. Women aged 20 to 40 years are at high risk for misdiagnosis of the condition on initial physical examination.

Diagnosis of even the classic case of appendicitis is complicated because many disorders present with a similar clinical picture of an acute condition in the abdomen. Differential diagnosis may include the following: (1) acute gastroenteritis, (2) mesenteric lymphadenitis in children, (3) ruptured ectopic pregnancy, (4) mittelschmerz, (5) inflammation of Meckel's diverticulum, (6) regional enteritis, and (7) right ovarian torsion.

Sonographic Findings. The normal appendix occasionally can be visualized with gradual compression sonography (Fig. 13.31). The maximal outer diameters of the normal appendix can measure up to 6 mm. The inflamed appendix will show edema of the wall measuring greater than 2 mm thick; perforation may be present when asymmetrical wall thickening is seen. In inflamed specimens, both the integrity and the stratification of wall layers are altered. The distinction of layers is impaired, and each layer is sonographically inhomogeneous.

Wall appearance should not be the only criterion for confirmation of appendicitis. The ultrasound pattern of acute appendicitis is characterized by a target-shaped appearance of the appendix in a transverse view. Views of the appendix in the transverse plane should demonstrate a thickened muscular wall and increased appendiceal diameter (Fig. 13.32). The typical target-shaped lesion consists of a hypoechoic, fluid-distended lumen, a hyperechoic inner ring representing mainly the mucosa and the submucosa, and an outer hypoechoic ring representing the **muscularis externa.** The inflamed appendix is further characterized by lack of peristalsis and compressibility and by demonstration of its "blind end tip." It is important to carefully survey the entire length of the appendix to prevent a false-negative examination.

Retrocecal appendicitis is seen in approximately 28% of pediatric appendicitis patients and is easy to diagnose by ultrasound. No bowel loops are interposed between the appendix and the lateral wall of the abdomen. The inflamed appendix is identified on cross section as a **target sign** underneath the abdominis muscle. The incidence of complex masses is greater in retrocecal appendicitis, reflecting a higher incidence of perforation. The sonographic appearance of an appendiceal abscess is a complex mass. Sometimes the sonographer can recognize the appendix inside the mass. The omentum wrapping the appendix is seen as an echogenic band and bowel loops.

The initial inflammatory changes in appendicitis are more pronounced in the distal half of the appendix and may be focally confined to the appendiceal tip. Ulcerations and necrosis may cause loss of the echogenic submucosal layer in the tip of the appendix. The appendix should be compressed to the tip and visualized longitudinally and transversely to its blind termination. **Appendicoliths** are **fecaliths** or calculi in the appendix. They are seen as intraluminal foci of high-amplitude echoes with acoustic shadowing (Fig. 13.33).

In infancy and childhood, the appendix frequently becomes decompressed after perforation, and the inflammatory process may not wall off or form a well-defined abscess,

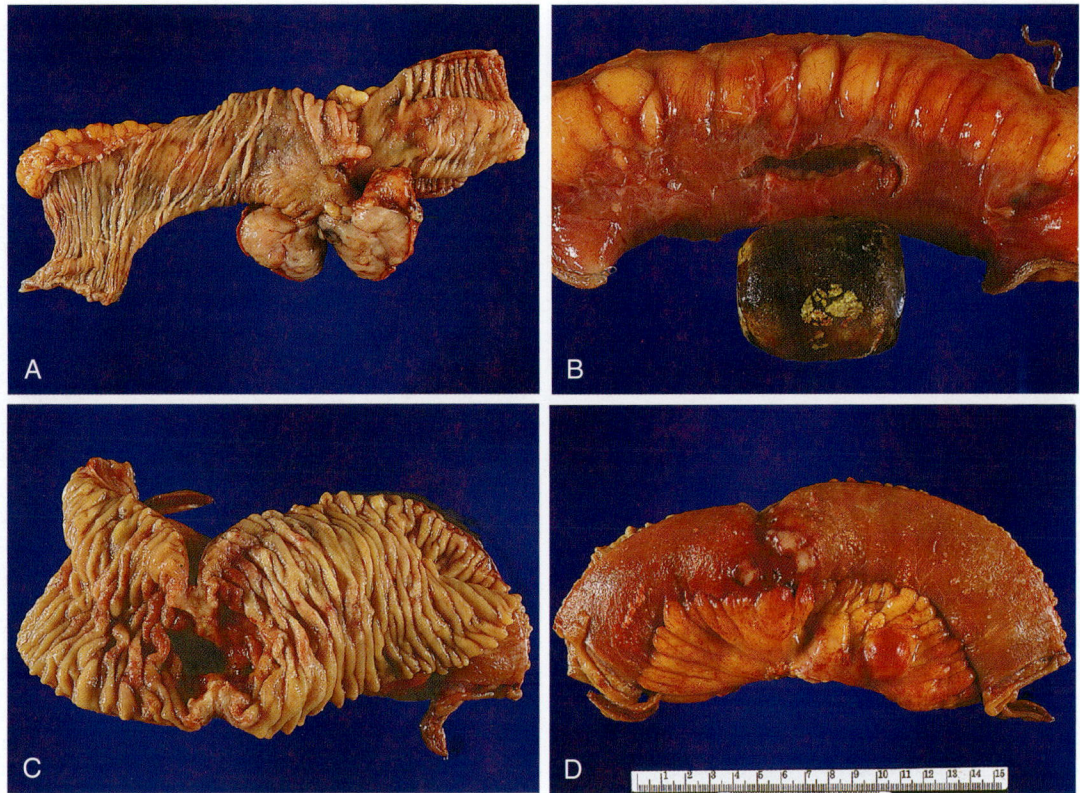

FIG. 13.28 (A) Gross specimen example of small bowel obstruction. (B) Small bowel obstruction secondary to gallstones. (C–D) Small bowel adenocarcinoma. The tumor may cause obstruction of the small bowel.

as is typically seen in adults. With perforation and decompression and an abnormally thickened wall, a collapsed appendix may still be identified. In some patients, however, no appendix may be found, and only questionable remnants remain. Supplemental findings, such as free abdominal fluid with debris or thickening of the adjacent abdominal wall, may suggest the diagnosis. However, the possibility of appendicitis cannot be ruled out even in a patient who lacks an abnormal appendix or a well-defined abscess. Radiographic contrast studies may help diagnosis.

Gas collections within the appendix may be a pitfall in ultrasound evaluation. Gas within the appendix is diagnosed based on sonographic findings of high-amplitude echogenic foci, causing distal reverberation artifacts (i.e., "comet tails" or "dirty" acoustic shadowing). Although this is a relatively rare finding, its importance lies in the fact that it may be misconstrued as a normal bowel loop or a gas-forming appendiceal abscess. Gas collections from within the bowel loops should be distinguished from an inflamed appendix. The inflamed appendix is noncompressible and demonstrates other specific anatomic features.

Graded compression ultrasound is an alternative technique for diagnosing appendicitis; it has a sensitivity of 88% and a specificity of 96%. Color Doppler ultrasound imaging can be used to detect increased flow, demonstrating hyperperfusion associated with inflammation (Fig. 13.34). Vessels can be seen coursing through the periphery of the dilated appendix. The addition of color Doppler alone does not increase the sensitivity for detecting appendicitis compared with ultrasound alone. Color Doppler is a simple means of confirming gray scale sonographic findings.

Mucocele. Mucocele of the appendix is a rare pathologic entity. This term designates gross enlargement of the appendix from accumulation of mucoid substance within the lumen. Scarring or fecalith after an appendectomy is the most common cause of mucocele, although proximal obstruction of the lumen by inflammatory fibrosis, cecal carcinoma, carcinoid polyp, and even endometriosis has been reported. Mucoceles have been classified into three distinct entities: mucosal hyperplasia (an innocuous hyperplastic process), mucinous cystadenoma (a benign neoplasm), and mucinous cystadenocarcinoma (a malignant tumor).

Several classifications of mucoceles are known. If the tumor remains encapsulated and no malignant cells are present, this lesion is called a mucocele. If the mucus spreads through the abdominal cavity without evidence of malignant cells, this condition is called pseudomyxoma peritonei. Pseudomyxoma assumes a malignant potential only when epithelial cells occur within the gelatinous peritoneal fluid in association with carcinoma.

Appendiceal mucoceles reportedly show a female-to-male predominance of 4:1, with an average age at presentation of 55 years. The most common clinical complaint is right lower quadrant pain (see Table 13.2). About 25% of cases are asymptomatic. Other symptoms include right iliac fossa mass, sepsis, and urinary symptoms. Bloating of the abdomen is specific to patients with pseudomyxoma peritonei. Laboratory values

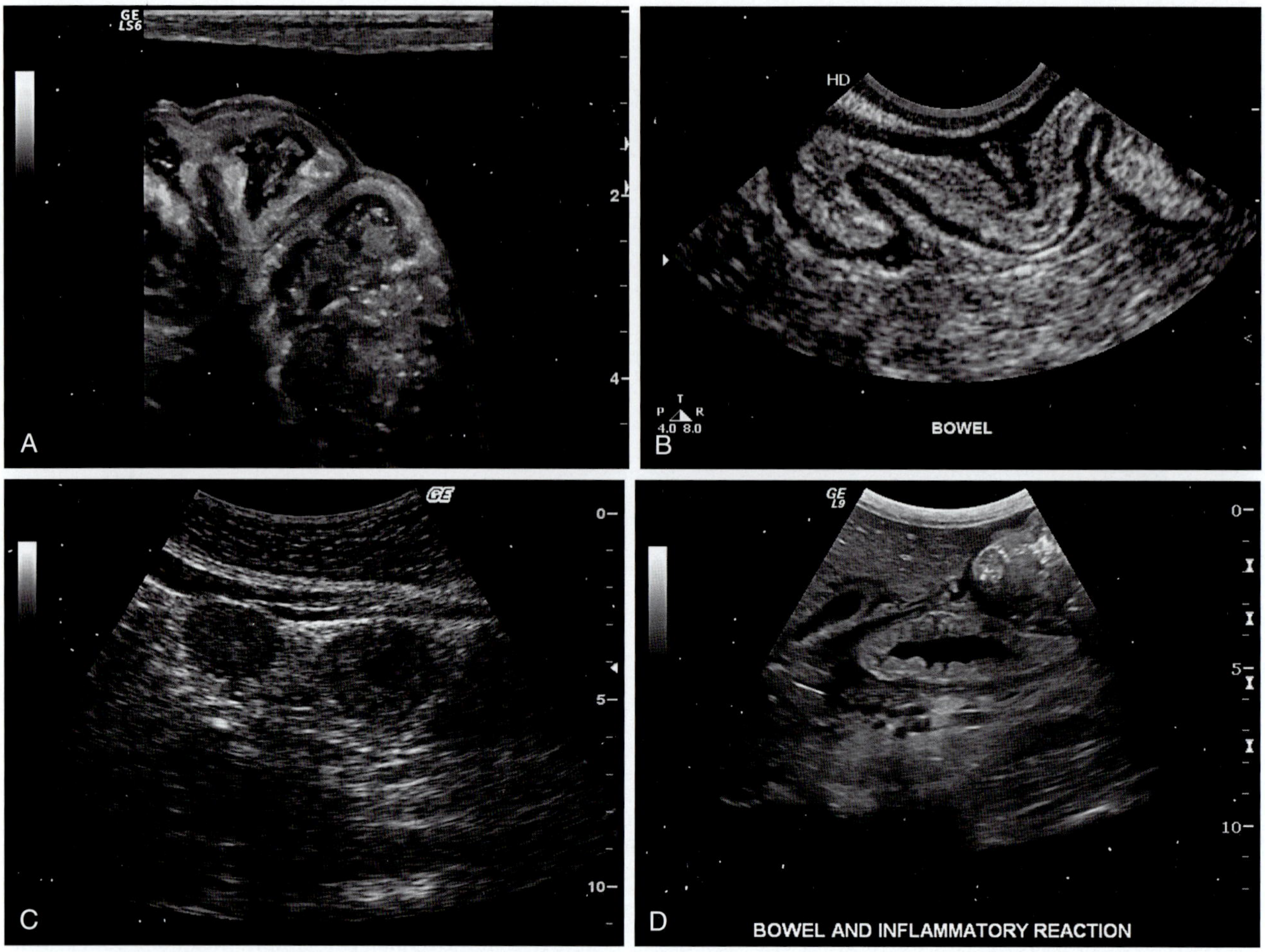

FIG. 13.29 (A) Transverse image of prominent fluid-filled bowel loops. (B) The bowel is surrounded by ascitic fluid. (C) Inflammation of the bowel demonstrates prominent dilated loops of bowel shown as circular bull's eye or target structures in the lower abdomen. (D) Inflammatory reaction of the bowel.

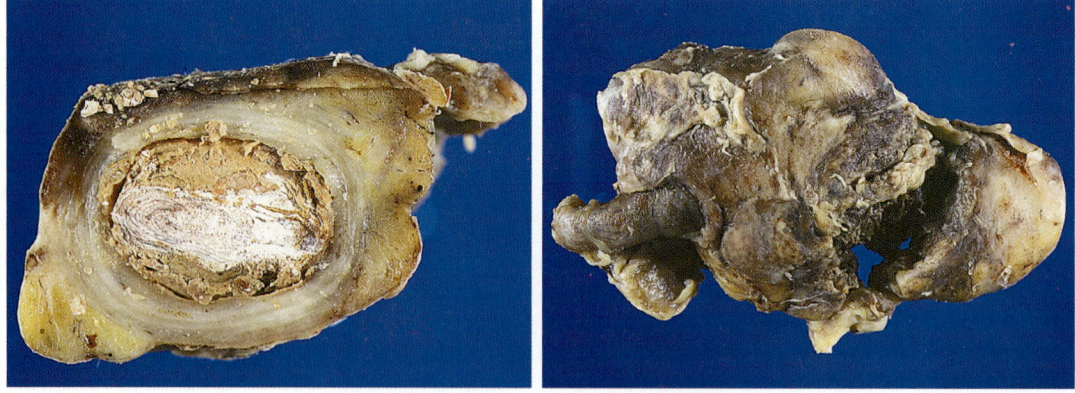

FIG. 13.30 Gross specimens of appendicitis.

show an increased erythrocyte sedimentation rate and an elevated leukocyte count. Also, elevated levels of carcinoembryonic antigen have been reported. Pseudomyxoma peritonei significantly decreases survival of patients with appendiceal cystadenocarcinomas.

Sonographic Findings. The sonographer should locate the appendix in the right lower quadrant, referencing the psoas muscle and iliac vessels. The image varies according to the content of the mucocele, which may be anechoic when mucoid material is more fluid. The following patterns have been defined: (1) a purely cystic lesion with anechoic fluid; (2) a hypoechoic mass containing fine internal echoes; and (3) a complex mass with high-level echoes (Fig. 13.35). As it enlarges, inspissation of the mucoid material creates this

CHAPTER 13 The Gastrointestinal Tract   407

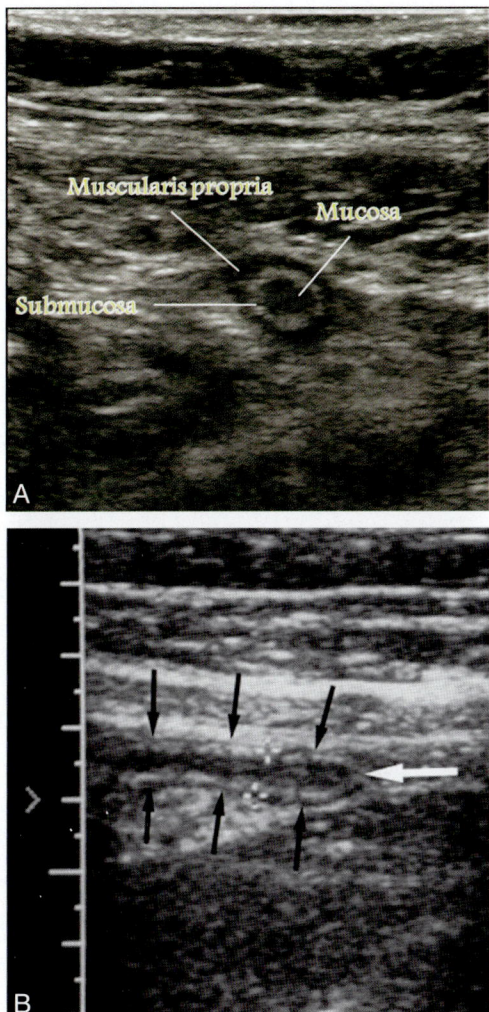

FIG. 13.31 Normal transverse (A) and sagittal (B) views of the appendix.

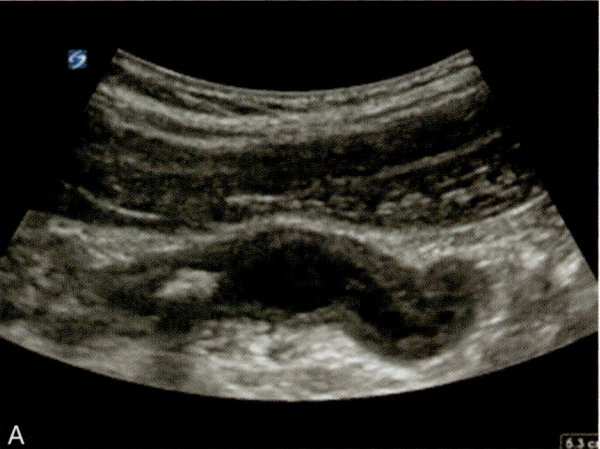

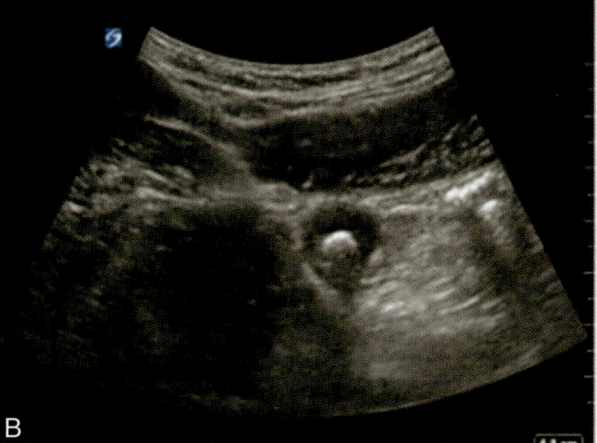

FIG. 13.33 Sagittal (A) and transverse (B) images of an appendicolith seen as intraluminal foci of high-amplitude echoes with acoustic shadowing.

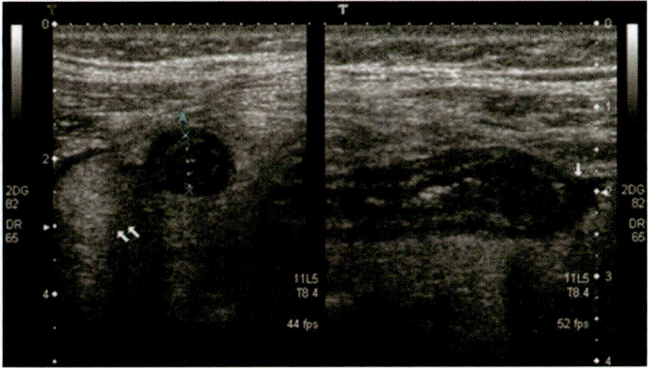

FIG. 13.32 Transverse *(left)* and sagittal *(right)* images of the inflamed appendix with marked wall thickening.

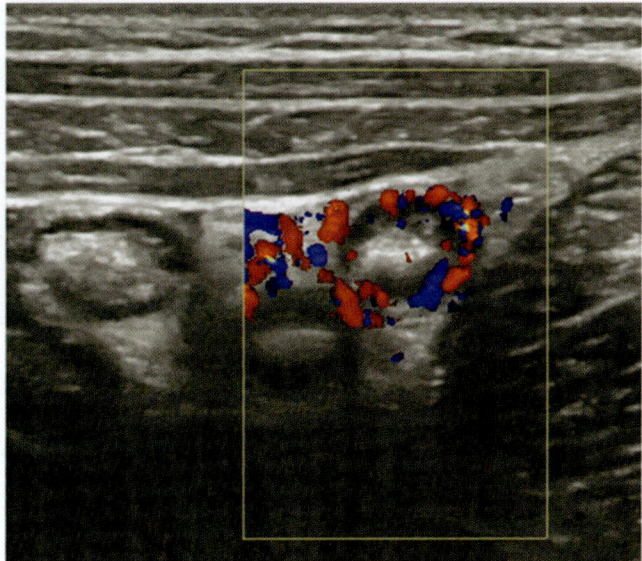

FIG. 13.34 Color Doppler shows increased flow around the inflamed appendix.

internal echo pattern. This mass has an irregular inner wall caused by mucinous debris with varying degrees of epithelial hyperplasia. Calcification of the rim can produce acoustic shadowing. Internal, thin septations have been seen along with variable degrees of mucosal atrophy and ulceration.

Pseudomyxoma peritonei (PMP) is a clinical condition caused by cancerous cells (mucinous adenocarcinoma) that produce abundant mucin or gelatinous ascites. The tumors cause fibrosis of tissues and impede digestion or organ function, and if left untreated, the tumors and mucin they produce will fill the abdominal cavity. This will result in the

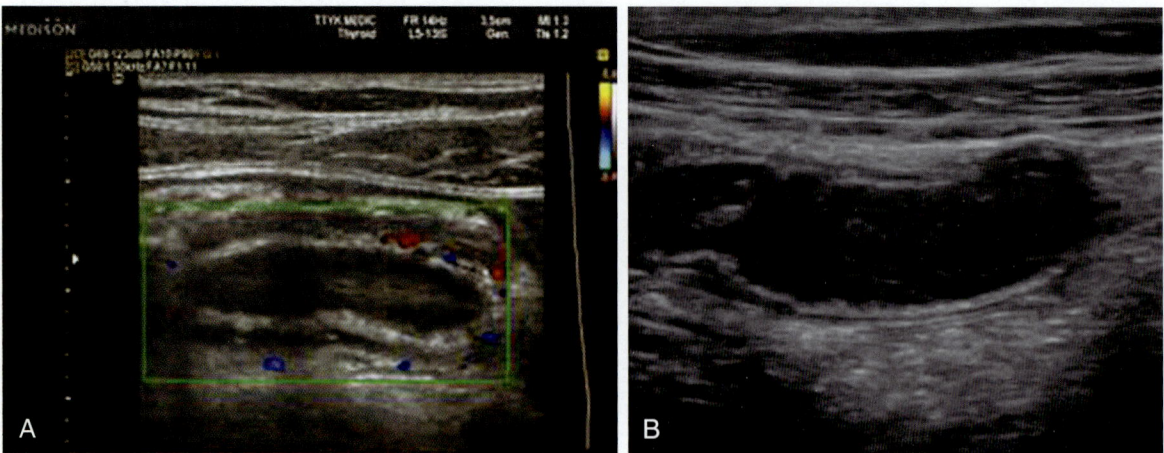

FIG. 13.35 **Mucocele.** (A–B) The sonographic image varies according to the content of the mucocele, which may be anechoic when mucoid material is more fluid.

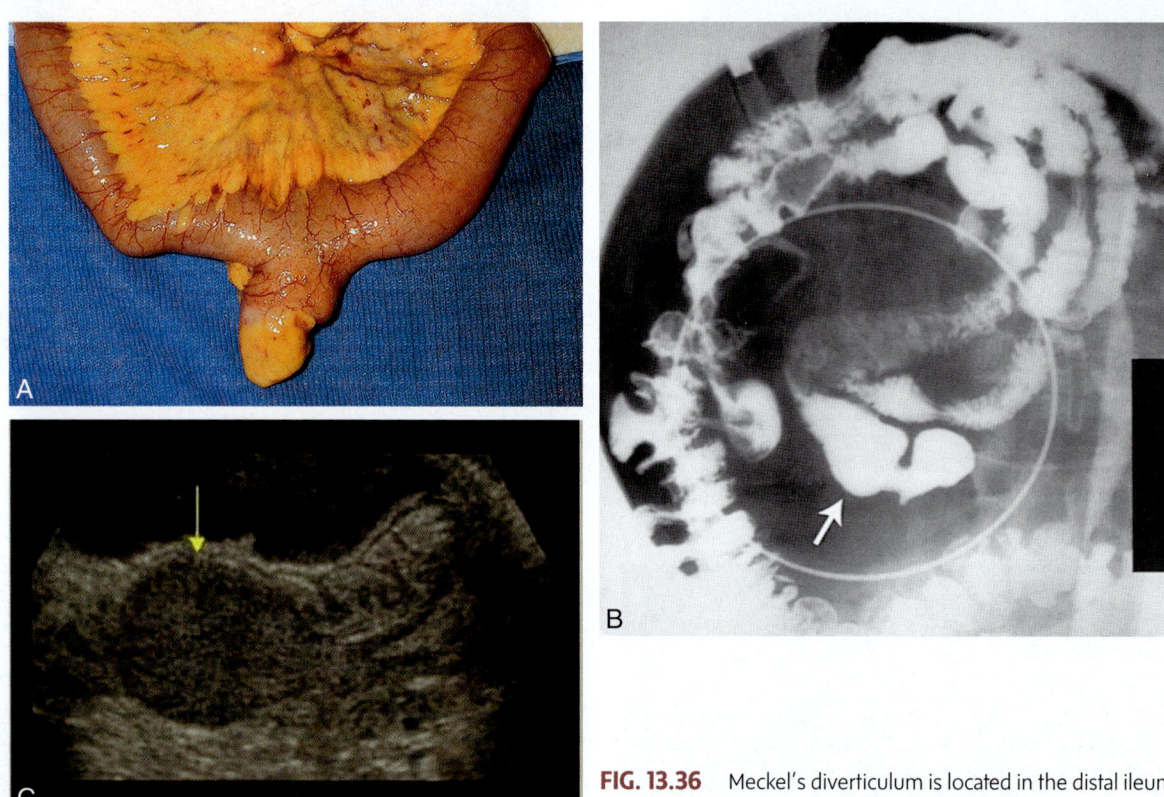

FIG. 13.36 Meckel's diverticulum is located in the distal ileum, usually within 60 to 100 cm of the ileocecal valve.

compression of organs and will destroy the function of the colon, small intestine, stomach, or other organs. Prognosis with treatment in many cases optimistic, but the disease is lethal if untreated, with death by cachexia, bowel obstruction, or other types of complications.

This disease is most commonly caused by an appendiceal primary cancer (cancer of the appendix); mucinous tumors of the ovary have also been implicated, although in most cases, ovarian involvement is favored to be a metastasis from an appendiceal or other gastrointestinal source. Disease is typically classified as low- or high-grade (with signet ring cells). When disease presents with low-grade histologic features, the cancer rarely spreads through the lymphatic system or through the bloodstream.

With sonography, the disease is seen as septated **ascites** (fluid in the abdomen) with numerous suspended echoes that do not mobilize as the patient changes position. When combined with ultrasound, paracentesis may accurately establish the diagnosis of gelatinous ascites.

Meckel's Diverticulitis. A **diverticulum** is a pouchlike herniation through the muscular wall of a tubular organ that occurs in the stomach, the small intestine, or, most commonly, the colon. **Meckel's diverticulum** is located in the distal ileum, usually within 60 to 100 cm of the ileocecal valve.

This blind segment or small pouch is about 3 to 6 cm long and may have a greater lumen diameter than that of the ileum. It runs antimesenterically and has its own blood supply. It is a remnant of the connection from the yolk sac to the small intestine present during embryonic development. It is a true diverticulum consisting of all three layers of the bowel wall, which are **mucosa**, **submucosa**, and **muscularis propria**.

As the vitelline duct consists of pluripotent cell lining, Meckel's diverticulum may harbor abnormal tissues containing embryonic remnants of other tissue types. Jejunal, duodenal mucosa, or Brunner tissue were each found in 2% of ectopic cases. Heterotopic rests of gastric mucosa and pancreatic tissue are seen in 60% and 6% of cases, respectively. Heterotopic means the displacement of an organ from its normal anatomic location. Inflammation of this Meckel's diverticulum may mimic appendicitis. Therefore during appendectomy, the ileum should be checked for Meckel's diverticulum; if it is found to be present, it should be removed along with the appendix.

In Meckel's diverticulitis, adults may present with intestinal obstruction, rectal bleeding, or diverticular inflammation (see Table 13.2). Acute appendicitis and acute Meckel's diverticulitis may not be distinguished clinically.

Sonographic Findings. The wall of Meckel's diverticulum consists of mucosal, muscular, and serosal layers. Noncompressibility of the obstructed, inflamed diverticulum indicates that intraluminal fluid is trapped (Fig. 13.36). The area of maximal tenderness is evaluated along with its distance from the cecum.

Crohn Disease. **Crohn disease** is regional enteritis, a recurrent granulomatous inflammatory disease that affects the terminal ileum, colon, or both at any level (Fig. 13.37). The reaction involves the entire thickness of the bowel wall. Clinical symptoms include diarrhea, fever, and right lower quadrant pain (see Table 13.2).

Sonographic Findings. A symmetrically swollen bowel target pattern with preserved parietal layers around the stenotic and echogenic lumen is seen on sonography (Fig. 13.38). Findings are most prominent in ileocolonic disease, with uniformly increased wall thickness involving all layers, especially the mucosa and submucosa. A matted-loop pattern is found in the late stages. Patients with Crohn disease show rigidity to pressure exerted with the transducer. Peristalsis is absent or sluggish.

Tumors of the Colon.

Lymphoma. Lymphoma is a tumor that usually occurs late in life, near the sixth decade; it is also the most common tumor of the gastrointestinal tract in children younger than 10 years of age. Intraperitoneal masses frequently involve the mesenteric vessels that encase them. Clinical signs include intestinal blood loss, weight loss, anorexia, and abdominal pain (see Table 13.2). The patient may have an intestinal obstruction or a palpable mass.

Sonographic Findings. The sonographer may see a large, discrete mass with a target pattern, an exoenteric pattern with a large mass on the mesenteric surface of the bowel, and a small anechoic mass representing subserosal nodes or mesenteric nodal involvement (Fig. 13.39).

Lymphomatous involvement of the intestinal wall may lead to pseudokidney or hydronephrotic pseudokidney. The

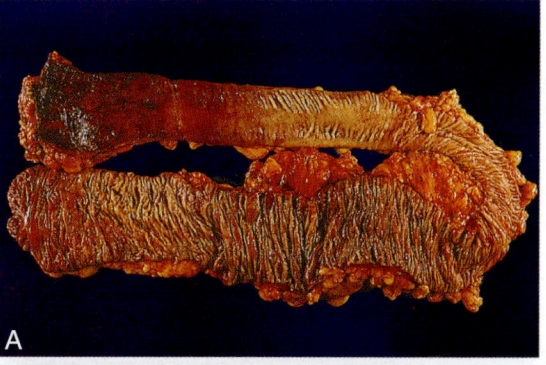
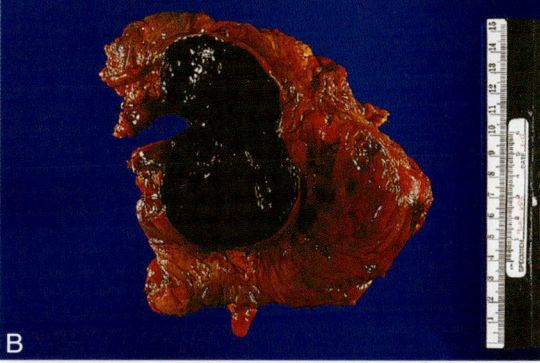
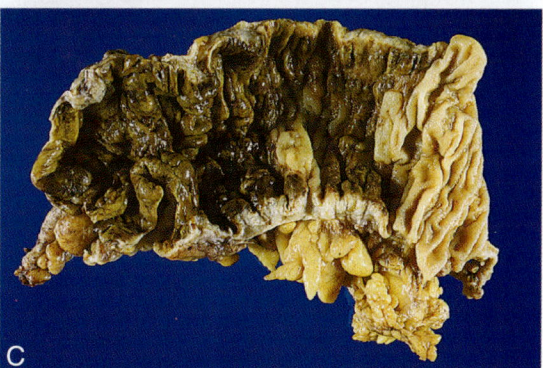

FIG. 13.37 (A) Gross specimen of ulcerative colitis. Gross specimens show complications of colitis. (B) Hematoma in the colon. (C) Gangrenous colon.

lumen may be dilated with fluid and may demonstrate a lack of peristalsis. The bowel wall is uniformly thickened, with homogeneous low echogenicity between the well-defined mucosal and serosal surfaces that contain a persistent, echo-free, wide, and long lumen.

Leiomyosarcoma. Leiomyosarcoma is a rare, malignant (cancerous) smooth muscle tumor. It must not be confused with leiomyoma, which is a benign tumor originating from the same tissue. Leiomyosarcomas can be very unpredictable. They can remain dormant for long periods of time and recur after years. It is a resistant cancer, meaning generally not very responsive to chemotherapy or radiation. The best outcomes occur when it can be removed surgically with wide margins early, while small and still in situ.

Smooth muscle cells make up the involuntary muscles, which are found in most parts of the body, including the uterus, stomach and intestines, the walls of all blood vessels,

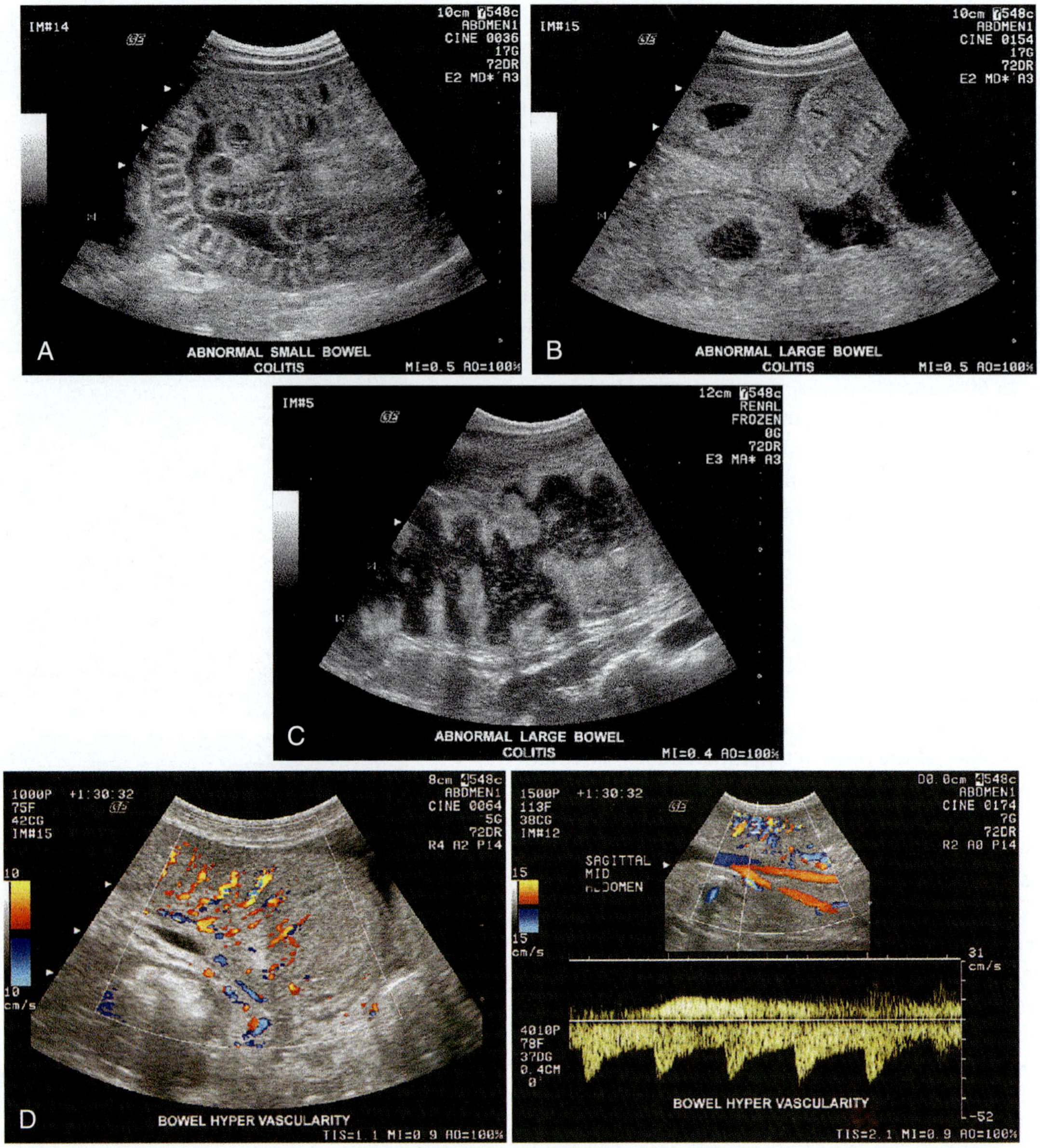

410 CHAPTER 13 The Gastrointestinal Tract

FIG. 13.38 **Ulcerative colitis.** (A) Small bowel colitis. (B–C) Dilated colon with colitis. (D) Prominent colon with increased vascularity.

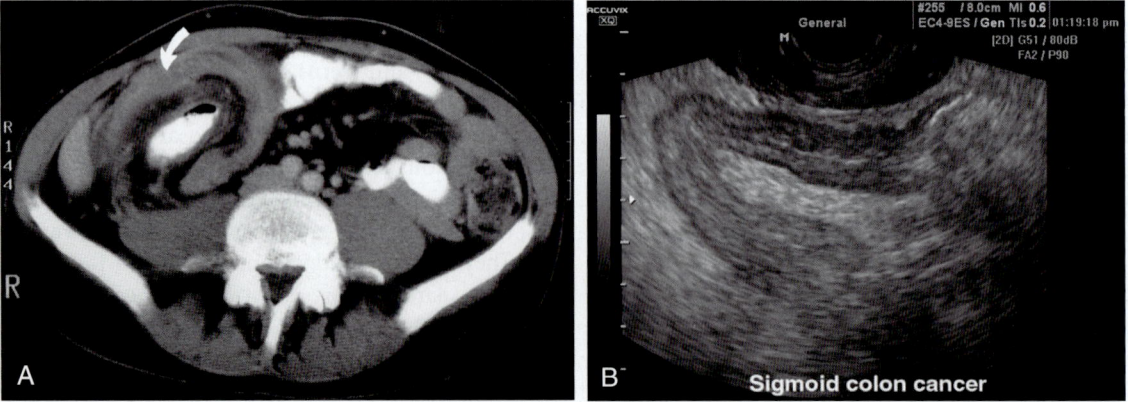

FIG. 13.39 Lymphoma of the sigmoid colon seen with wall thickening *(arrow)* in the computed tomographic (A) and ultrasound (B) images.

and the skin. It is therefore possible for leiomyosarcomas to appear at any site in the body (including the breasts); they are most commonly found in the uterus, stomach, small intestine, and retroperitoneum. This tumor can have a primary site of origin anywhere in the body where there is a blood vessel. Leiomyosarcoma represents 10% of primary small bowel tumors. Approximately 10% to 30% of these occur in the duodenum, 30% to 45% in the jejunum, and 35% to 55% in the ileum. Patients are in their fifth to sixth decade of life.

Sonographic Findings. A large solid mass containing necrotic areas anterior to the solid viscus may be found. Color Doppler will demonstrate a low-velocity flow within the mass (Fig. 13.40).

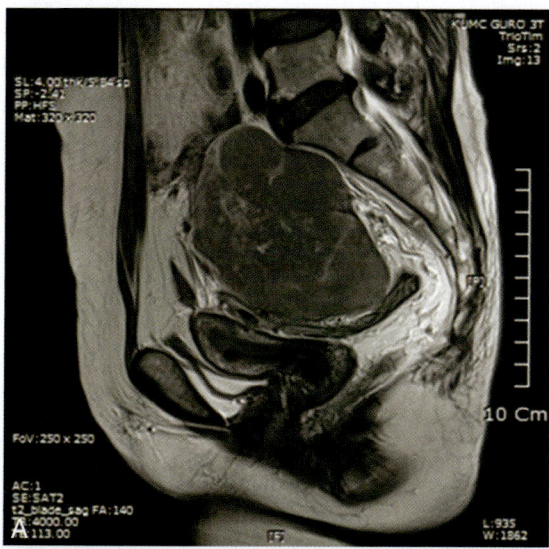
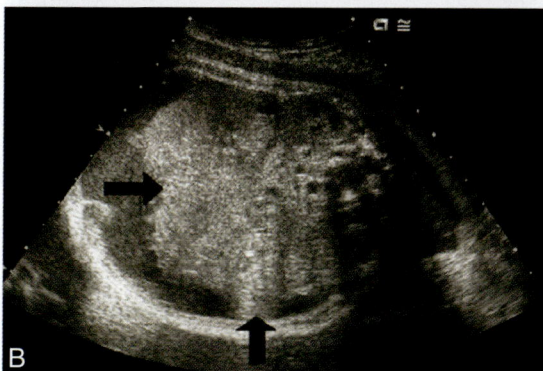

FIG. 13.40 Leiomyosarcoma is a rare, malignant smooth muscle tumor that represents 10% of small bowel tumors.

Key Pearls

- The digestive tract and gastrointestinal tract comprise the digestive system.
- The stomach is divided into three parts: The *fundus* is found in the superior aspect, the *body* makes up the major central axis, and the *pylorus* is the lower aspect.
- The duodenum is subdivided into four segments: (1) superior, (2) descending, (3) transverse, and (4) ascending.
- The valvulae conniventes of the small intestine are large folds of mucous membrane that project into the lumen of the bowel and help retard the passage of food to provide greater absorption.
- The haustra of the colon are the small pouches caused by sacculation, which give the colon its segmented appearance.
- The arteries that supply the esophagus rise from the high, mid, and lower sections of this muscular tube.
- Varices may be seen to rise from the gastroesophageal arteries.
- The celiac axis supplies the duodenum through its right gastric, gastroduodenal, and superior pancreaticoduodenal branches.
- The celiac, superior mesenteric, and inferior mesenteric arteries supply both the small and the large intestine.
- Digestion and absorption are the primary functions of the gastrointestinal tract.
- Visualization of the gastrointestinal tract with ultrasound may be difficult because intraluminal air produces an echogenic shadow, which prevents the sound beam from penetrating structures posteriorly.
- The bowel wall consists of five layers: the odd-numbered walls (first, third, and fifth) are echogenic, and the even-numbered walls (second and fourth) are hypoechoic, with an average total thickness of 3 mm if distended, and 5 mm if undistended.
- The gastroesophageal junction is seen on the sagittal scan to the left of the midline as a bull's eye or target-shaped structure anterior to the aorta, posterior to the left lobe of the liver, and inferior to the hemidiaphragm.
- The duodenum can be outlined easily with water ingestion or a change in position.
- The sonographer usually cannot see the small bowel with sonography; the valvulae conniventes may be seen as linear echo densities spaced 3 to 5 mm apart.
- The vermiform appendix is a remnant of what was originally the apex of the cecum.
- The appendix is located on the abdominal wall under McBurney's point, located by drawing a line from the right anterosuperior iliac spine to the umbilicus: the appendix lies at the midpoint of this line.
- The criteria for a duplication cyst are as follows: (1) The cyst is lined with alimentary tract epithelium, (2) the cyst has a well-developed muscular wall, and (3) the cyst is contiguous with the stomach.
- A gastric bezoar is an intragastric mass composed of accumulated ingested material.
- A polyp is a protruding, space-occupying, epithelial lesion within the stomach.
- Leiomyoma is the most common tumor of the stomach.
- Gastric carcinoma is the fifth leading cause of cancer and the third leading cause of death from cancer.
- A small bowel obstruction is associated with dilation of the bowel loops proximal to the site of obstruction.
- Acute appendicitis results from luminal obstruction and inflammation, leading to ischemia of the vermiform appendix.
- The symptoms of acute appendicitis are pain and rebound tenderness, which is usually localized over the right lower quadrant.
- The inflamed appendix will show edema of the wall measuring greater than 2 mm thick; perforation may be present when asymmetrical wall thickening is seen.

- Mucocele of the appendix is a gross enlargement of the appendix from accumulation of mucoid substance within the lumen.
- Meckel's diverticulum is a pouchlike herniation through the muscular wall of a tubular organ that occurs in the stomach, the small intestine, or, most commonly, the colon. Diverticulum.
- Crohn disease is regional enteritis, a recurrent granulomatous inflammatory disease that affects the terminal ileum, colon, or both at any level.
- Lymphomatous involvement of the intestinal wall may lead to pseudokidney or hydronephrotic pseudokidney.

REFERENCES

Birnbaum BA, Jeffrey Jr. RB. CT and sonographic evaluation of acute right lower quadrant abdominal pain. *Am J Roentgenol*. 1998;170:361–371.

Chaubal N, Manjiri D, Shah M, Chaubal J. Sonography of the gastrointestinal tract. *J Ultrasound Med*. 2006;25:87–97.

Curry R, Tempkin B, eds. *Sonography: Introduction to Normal Anatomy and Structure*. ed 3 Philadelphia: Elsevier; 2010.

Khaja M, Kilani R, Jacobson W, Hiett AK. Gastrointestinal stromal tumor presenting as a mass on pelvic sonography. *J Ultrasound Med*. 2007;26:117–120.

Liu JB, Miller LS, Bagley DH, Goldberg BB. Endoluminal sonography of the genitourinary and gastrointestinal tracts. *J Ultrasound Med*. 2002;21:323–337.

Lorentzen T, Nolsoe CP, Khattar SC, et al. Gastric and duodenal wall thickening on abdominal ultrasonography: positive predictive value. *J Ultrasound Med*. 1993;12:633–637.

Rapp CL, Stavros AT, Meyers PR. Ultrasound of the normal appendix: the how and why. *J Diagn Med Sonogr*. 1998;14:195.

Rumack C, Wilson S, Charboneau W, Johnson J. *Diagnostic Ultrasound*. ed 4 St Louis: Elsevier; 2011.

Stavros AT, Rapp CL, Thickman D. Sonography of inflammatory conditions. *Ultrasound Q*. 1995;13:1.

Tarantino L, Nocera V, Perrotta M, et al. Primary small bowel melanoma: color Doppler ultrasonographic, computed tomographic, and radiological findings with pathologic correlations. *J Ultrasound Med*. 2007;26:121–127.

Worrell JA, Drolshagen LF, Kelly TC, et al. Graded compression ultrasound in the diagnosis of appendicitis: a comparison of diagnostic criteria. *J Ultrasound Med*. 1990;9:145.

Yacoe ME, Jeffrey Jr. RB. Sonography of appendicitis and diverticulitis. *Radiol Clin North Am*. 1994;32:899–912.

CHAPTER 14

The Peritoneal Cavity and Abdominal Wall

Sandra L. Hagen-Ansert

OBJECTIVES

On completion of this chapter, you should be able to:
- Describe the normal anatomy of the abdominal wall
- List the peritoneal and retroperitoneal organs
- Compare and contrast the different locations of fluid and their sonographic appearances
- Discuss the pathology and sonographic findings of the peritoneal cavity, mesentery, omentum, peritoneum, and abdominal wall

OUTLINE

Anatomy and Sonographic Evaluation of the Peritoneal Cavity and Abdominal Wall 413
    Peritoneal Cavity 413
    Determination of Intraperitoneal Location 414
    Intraperitoneal Compartments 417
    Lower Abdominal and Pelvic Compartments 418
    Abdominal Wall 419
Pathology of the Peritoneal Cavity 419
    Ascites 419
    Inflammatory or Malignant Ascites 420
    Hepatorenal Recess 420

Abscess Formation and Pockets in the Abdomen and Pelvis 420
    Gas-Containing Abscess 421
    Peritonitis 422
    Lesser Sac Abscess 423
    Subphrenic Abscess 423
    Subcapsular Collections 424
    Biloma Abscess 425
    General Abdominal Abscess 425
Pathology of the Mesentery, Omentum, and Peritoneum 426
    Cysts 426
    Urachal Cyst 427
    Urinoma 427
    Peritoneal Metastases 427

Lymphomas of the Omentum and Mesentery 428
Tumors of the Peritoneum, Omentum, and Mesentery 428
Pathology of the Abdominal Wall 428
    Abdominal Wall Masses 428
    Lymphoceles 428
    Extraperitoneal Hematoma 430
    Bladder Flap Hematoma 430
    Subfascial Hematoma 430
    Inflammatory Lesion (Abscess) 430
    Neoplasm or Peritoneal Thickening 432
    Hernias 432

KEY TERMS

Abscess
Ascites
Bare area
Biloma
Greater sac
Gutters
Hemorrhage
Lesser sac
Leukocytosis

Lymphocele
Mesentery
Morison's pouch
Omentum
Parietal peritoenum
Peritonitis
Pyogenic
Retrovesical space
Sandwich sign

Subcapsular
Sepsis
Septicemia
Subhepatic
Subphrenic
Supravesical space
Urinoma
Visceral peritoneum

ANATOMY AND SONOGRAPHIC EVALUATION OF THE PERITONEAL CAVITY AND ABDOMINAL WALL

Peritoneal Cavity

The peritoneal cavity is comprised of multiple peritoneal ligaments and folds that connect the viscera to each other and the abdominopelvic walls. Within the cavity are the lesser and greater **omentum**, the mesenteries, the ligaments, and multiple fluid spaces (lesser sac, perihepatic and **subphrenic** spaces). The peritoneum is a smooth membrane that lines the entire abdominal cavity and is reflected over the contained organs. The section that lines the cavity walls is the **parietal peritoneum**, whereas the part covering the abdominal organs to a greater or lesser extent is the **visceral peritoneum**

(Fig. 14.1). In the male, the peritoneum forms a closed cavity; in the female, there is a "communication" outside the peritoneum through the uterine tubes, uterus, and vagina. In reality, however, the complex linings of the uterus and fallopian tubes tend to close off any potential space and prohibit the entrance of air into the peritoneal cavity.

The relationship of the peritoneum to the abdominal structures may be understood with the visualization of an inflated balloon (the peritoneum) within an empty box (the abdominal cavity) (Fig. 14.2). If one were to place objects within the box, yet outside the balloon, these objects might impinge on the balloon shape. This is the same condition that the kidneys and the ascending and descending colon have on the peritoneal cavity. Because these structures lie along the posterior surface of the peritoneal cavity, they are considered "retroperitoneal," and they are overlaid by the visceral peritoneum. If an object bulges so far into the balloon that it loses contact with the box, the object will become surrounded by a fold of the balloon. This is the situation with the small intestine, transverse colon, and the sigmoid colon; they are suspended from the posterior abdominal wall by a double fold of peritoneum called the **mesentery**. Thus the peritoneal cavity is really empty of abdominal organs, as they bulge into or are covered by the cavity but are not located within the cavity.

The general peritoneal cavity is known as the **greater sac** of the peritoneum. With the development of the stomach and the spleen, a smaller sac, called the **lesser sac** (omental bursa), is the peritoneal recess posterior to the stomach (Fig. 14.3). This sac communicates with the greater sac through a small vertical opening known as the epiploic foramen. The epiploic foramen is just inferior to the liver and superior to the first part of the duodenum; the inferior vena cava is posterior, and the portal vein is anterior (Fig. 14.4).

The attachments of the peritoneum to the abdominal walls and organs help determine the way abnormal collections of fluid within the peritoneal cavity can collect or move (Fig. 14.5). When the patient is lying supine, the lowest part of the body is the pelvis. On a transverse view, the flanks are lower than the midabdomen. Fluid will accumulate in the lowest parts of the body; therefore, the pelvis and lateral flanks (**gutters**) should be carefully examined for pathologic collections of fluid.

The lesser omentum is a double layer of peritoneum, extending from the liver to the lesser curvature of the stomach. This structure acts as a sling for the stomach, suspending it from the liver. (Fig. 14.6).

The greater omentum is an apron-like fold of the peritoneum that hangs from the greater curvature of the stomach (Fig. 14.7). The omentum lies freely over the intestine except for the upper part, which is fused with the transverse colon and mesocolon. The greater omentum can adhere to diseased organs, which in turn helps prevent further spread of infected fluid by essentially "walling it off" from the rest of the body. The greater omentum is profusely supplied with blood vessels by the epiploic branches of the gastroepiploic vessels and thus can bring masses of blood phagocytes to the areas it adheres to, which in turn helps combat infection.

Determination of Intraperitoneal Location

The determination of intraperitoneal fluid from pleural, subdiaphragmatic, subscapular, or retroperitoneal fluid is necessary to determine a differential diagnosis or to locate a fluid pocket for aspiration or a biopsy.

Pleural Versus Subdiaphragmatic. Because of the coronary ligament attachments, collections in the right posterior subphrenic space cannot extend between the bare area of the liver and the diaphragm. On the other hand, because the right pleural space extends medially to the attachment of the right superior coronary ligament, pleural collections may appear apposed to the bare area of the liver (Fig. 14.8). Unless it is loculated, the pleural fluid tends to distribute posteromedially in the chest (Fig. 14.9).

Subcapsular Versus Intraperitoneal. Subcapsular liver and splenic collections are seen when they are inferior to the diaphragm unilaterally, and they conform to the shape of an organ capsule (Fig. 14.10). They may extend medially to the attachment of the superior coronary ligament.

Retroperitoneal Versus Intraperitoneal. A mass is confirmed to be within the retroperitoneal cavity when anterior renal displacement or anterior displacement of the dilated ureters can be documented. The mass interposed anteriorly or superiorly to kidneys can be located either intraperitoneally or retroperitoneally (Fig. 14.11).

Fatty and collagenous connective tissues in the perirenal or anterior pararenal space produce echoes that are best demonstrated on sagittal scans. Retroperitoneal lesions displace echoes ventrally and cranially; hepatic and **subhepatic** lesions produce inferior and posterior displacement.

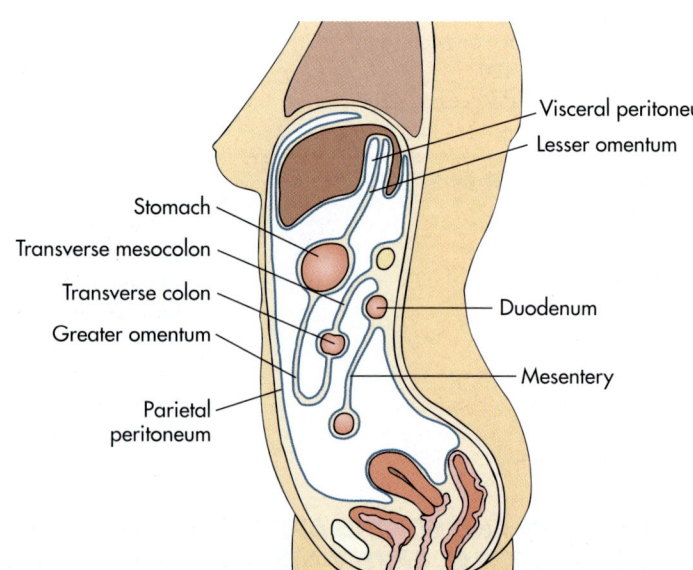

FIG. 14.1 (A) The peritoneum that lines the walls of the cavity is the parietal peritoneum, whereas the part covering the abdominal organs to a greater or lesser extent is the visceral peritoneum.

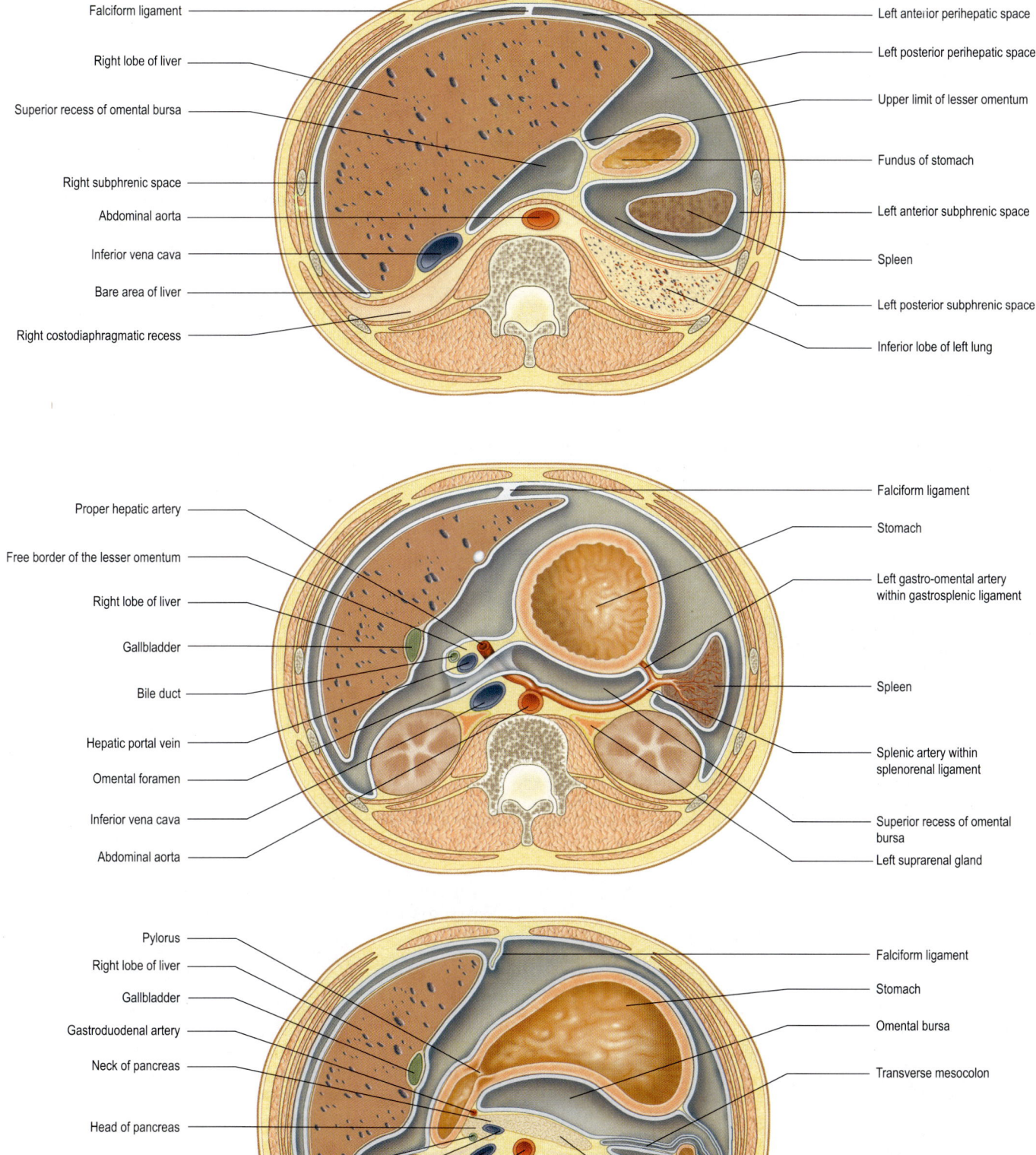

B
FIG. 14.1 Cont'd (B) Transverse view of the abdomen illustrates the parietal and visceral peritoneum and the splenorenal, gastrosplenic, and hepatogastric ligaments.

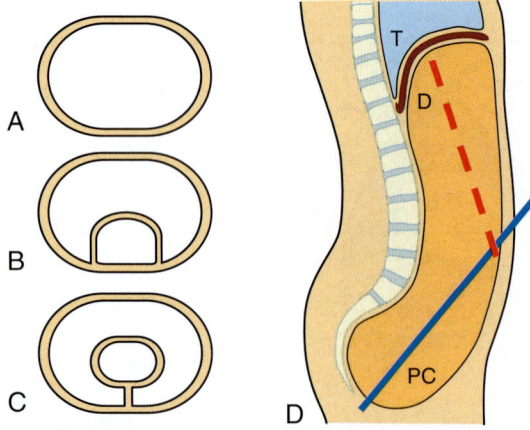

FIG. 14.2 (A) The "abdominal cavity" containing a "balloon" (peritoneum). (B) An organ inside the abdomen and partly covered by peritoneum, such as the kidney, which is said to be in the retroperitoneal cavity. (C) An organ suspended from the abdominal wall by a fold of peritoneum, such as the small intestine suspended by its mesentery. (D) When supine, the backward tilt of the pelvis makes it the lowest part of the peritoneal cavity. *D,* Diaphragm; *dashed line,* long axis of abdomen; *PC,* pelvic part of peritoneal cavity; *solid line,* long axis of pelvis; *T,* thorax.

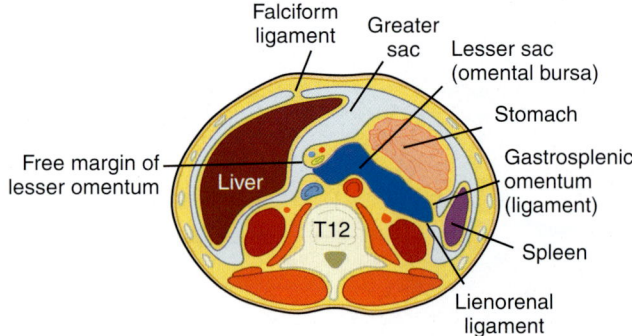

FIG. 14.3 The general peritoneal cavity is known as the greater sac of the peritoneum. With the development of the stomach and the spleen, a smaller sac, called the lesser sac (omental bursa), is the peritoneal recess posterior to the stomach.

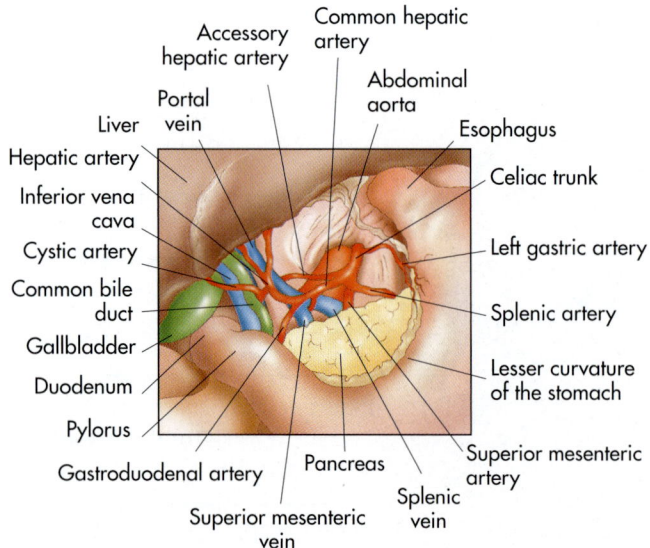

FIG. 14.4 Upper abdominal dissection, with part of the left lobe of the liver and the lesser omentum removed to show the celiac trunk, portal vein, bile duct, and related structures.

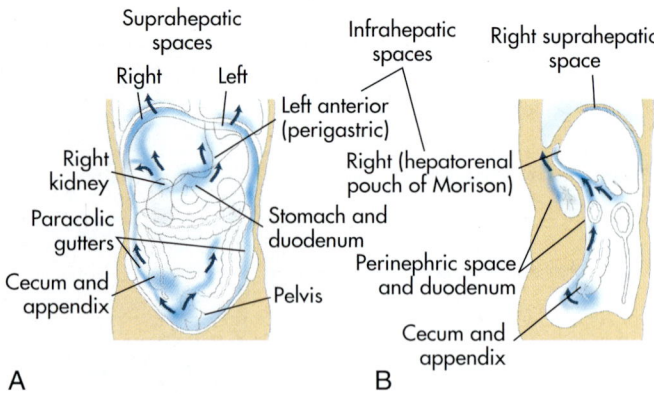

FIG. 14.5 (A) Anterior view of the collection of fluid in the abdominal and pelvic cavities. (B) Sagittal view of the right abdomen shows how the fluid collects in the most dependent areas of the abdomen and pelvis.

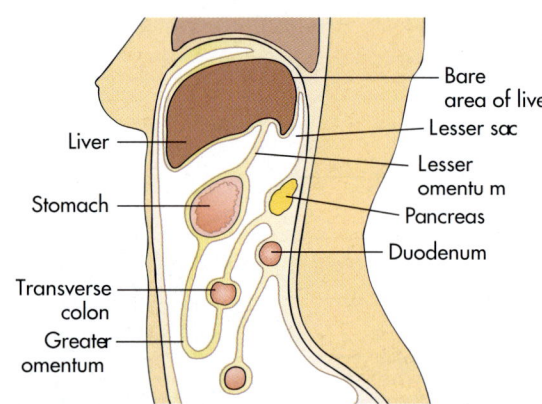

FIG. 14.6 The lesser omentum is a double layer of peritoneum, extending from the liver to the lesser curvature of the stomach; this structure acts as a sling for the stomach, suspending it from the liver.

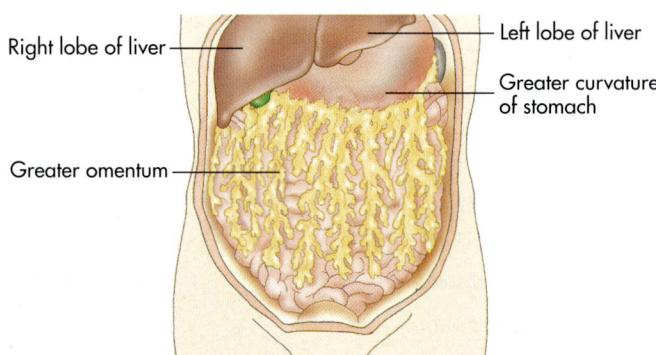

FIG. 14.7 The greater omentum is an apron-like fold of peritoneum that hangs from the greater curvature of the stomach.

The anterior displacement of the superior mesenteric vessels, splenic vein, renal vein, and inferior vena cava excludes an intraperitoneal location. A large, right-sided retroperitoneal mass rotates the intrahepatic portal veins to the left. This causes the left portal vein to show reversed flow. Right posterior hepatic masses of similar dimensions may produce minor displacement of the intrahepatic portal vein. Primary liver masses should move simultaneously with the liver.

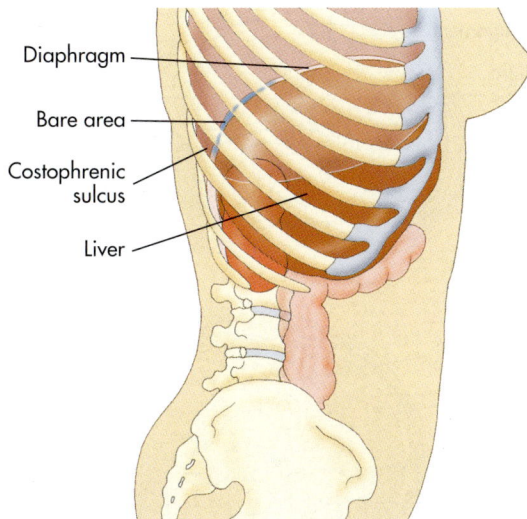

FIG. 14.8 Sagittal plane of the body shows the diaphragm and liver with the highlighted "bare" area of the liver. The costophrenic sulcus forms the sharp border posterior to the liver and may be identified when fluid is present.

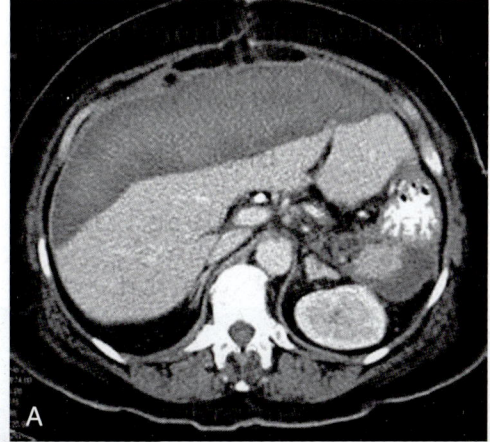

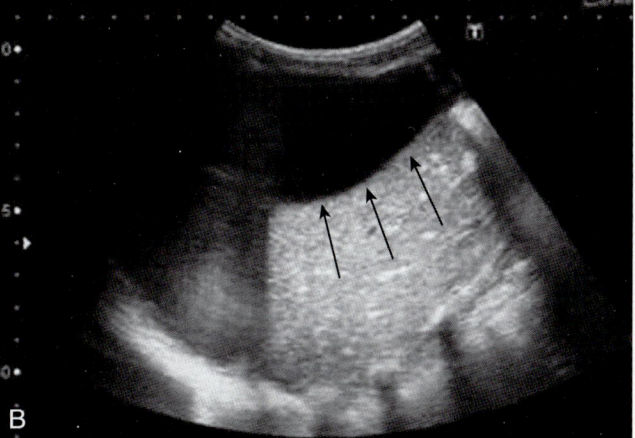

FIG. 14.10 (A) Computed tomographic image of a patient with a large subcapsular hematoma. (B) Ultrasound image of the subcapsular hematoma *(arrows)*.

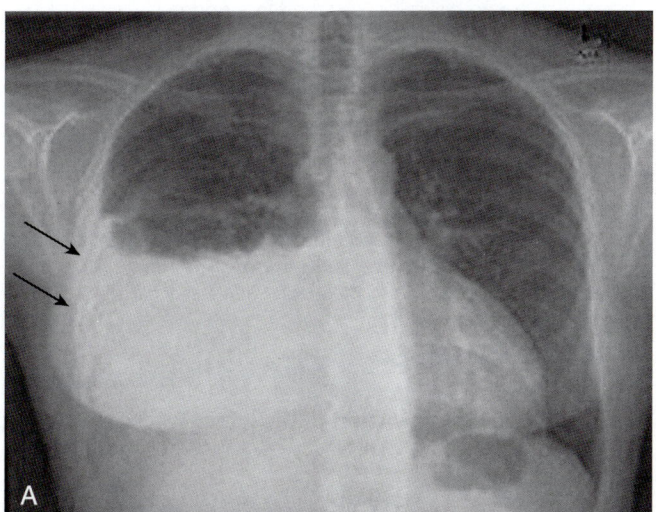

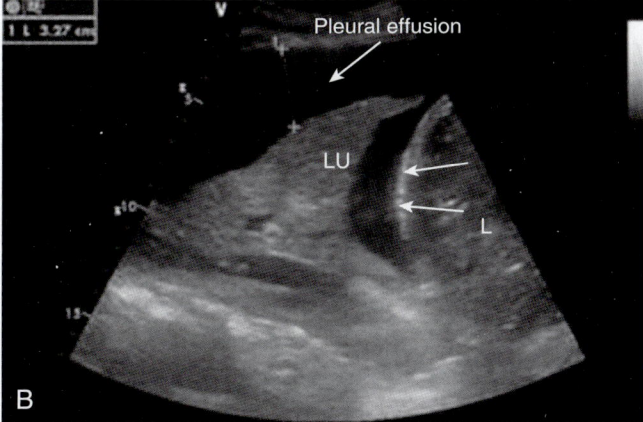

FIG. 14.9 (A) Chest radiography demonstrating a large right pleural effusion with blunting of the costophrenic sulcus *(arrrows)*. (B) Sonogram of the right pleural space demonstrating a large right pleural effusion above the diaphragm *(pair of arrows)*. *L*, liver; *LU*, lung.

Intraperitoneal Compartments

Perihepatic and Upper Abdominal Compartments. Ligaments on the right side of the liver form the **subphrenic** and **subhepatic spaces**. The falciform ligament divides the subphrenic space into right and left components. The ligamentum teres hepatis ascends from the umbilicus to the umbilical notch of the liver within the free margin of the falciform ligament before coursing within the liver (Fig. 14.12).

The **bare area** is delineated by the right superior and inferior coronary ligaments, which separate the posterior subphrenic space from the right superior subhepatic space **(Morison's pouch)**. Lateral to the bare area and right triangular ligament, the posterior subphrenic and subhepatic spaces are continuous.

A single large and irregular perihepatic space surrounds the superior and lateral aspects of the left lobe of the liver, with the left coronary ligaments anatomically separating the subphrenic space into anterior and posterior compartments. The left subhepatic space is divided into an anterior compartment (the gastrohepatic recess) and a posterior compartment (the lesser sac) by the lesser omentum and stomach (Fig. 14.13). The lesser sac lies anterior to the pancreas and

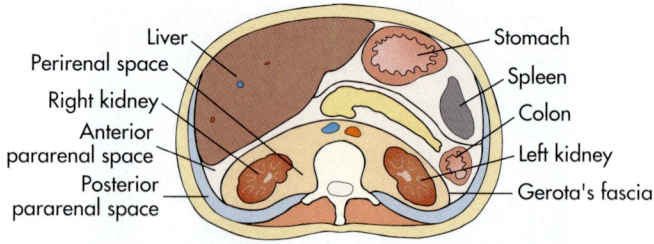
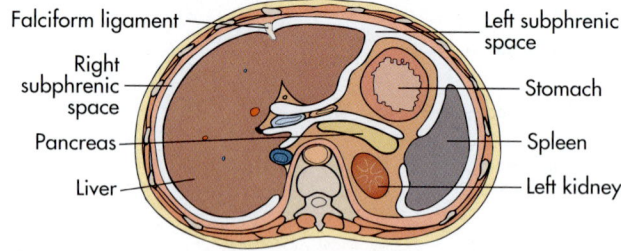
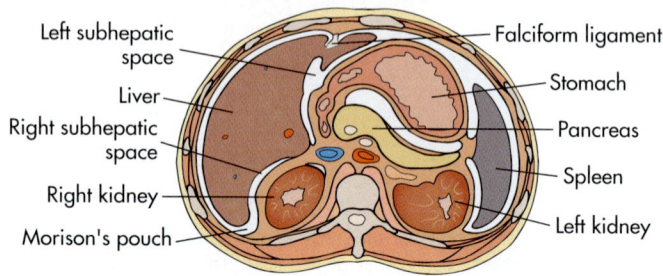
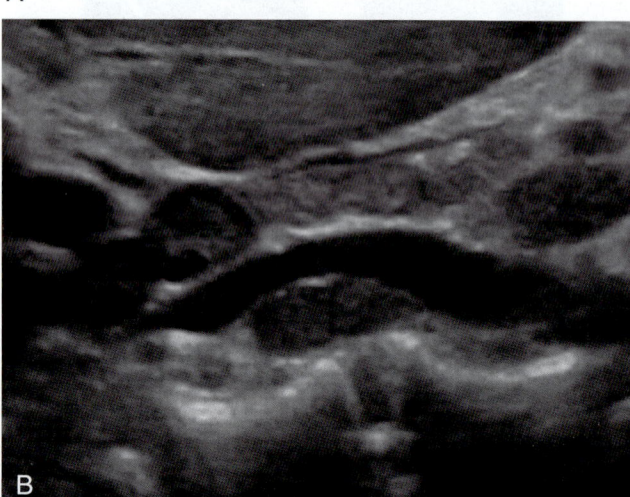
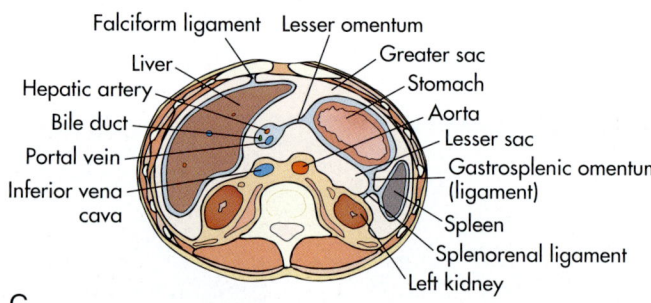
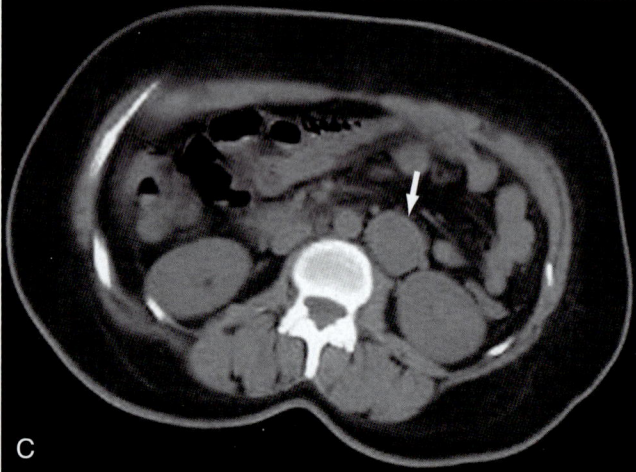

FIG. 14.11 (A) Transverse view of the retroperitoneal space. (B) Enlarged lymph nodes surrounding the inferior vena cava. (C) Computed tomographic presentation of an enlarged node *(arrow)*.

FIG. 14.12 (A) Transverse view of the subphrenic spaces. (B) Transverse view of the subhepatic spaces and Morison's pouch. (C) Transverse view of the abdomen showing the greater and lesser sac, the falciform ligament, the gastrosplenic ligament, and the splenorenal ligament.

posterior to the stomach. With fluid in the lesser and greater omental cavities, the lesser omentum may be seen as a linear, undulating echodensity extending from the stomach to the porta hepatis.

Gastrosplenic Ligament. The gastrosplenic ligament is the left lateral extension of the greater omentum that connects the gastric greater curvature to the superior splenic hilum and forms a portion of the left lateral border of the lesser sac (see Fig. 14.12C).

Splenorenal Ligament. The splenorenal ligament is formed by the posterior reflection of the peritoneum of the spleen and passes inferiorly to overlie the left kidney (see Fig. 14.12C). It forms the posterior portion of the left lateral border of the lesser sac and separates the lesser sac from the renosplenic recess.

Lesser Omental Bursa. The lesser omental bursa is subdivided into a larger lateroinferior and a smaller mediosuperior recess by the gastropancreatic folds, which are produced by the left gastric and hepatic arteries (Fig. 14.14). The lesser sac extends to the diaphragm. The superior recess of the bursa surrounds the anterior, medial, and posterior surfaces of the caudate lobe, making the caudate a lesser sac structure. The lesser sac collections may extend a considerable distance below the plane of the pancreas by inferiorly displacing the transverse mesocolon or extending into the inferior recess of the greater omentum.

Lower Abdominal and Pelvic Compartments

The **supravesical space** and the medial and lateral inguinal fossae represent intraperitoneal paravesical spaces formed by indentation of the anterior parietal peritoneum by the bladder, obliterated umbilical arteries, and inferior epigastric

CHAPTER 14 The Peritoneal Cavity and Abdominal Wall

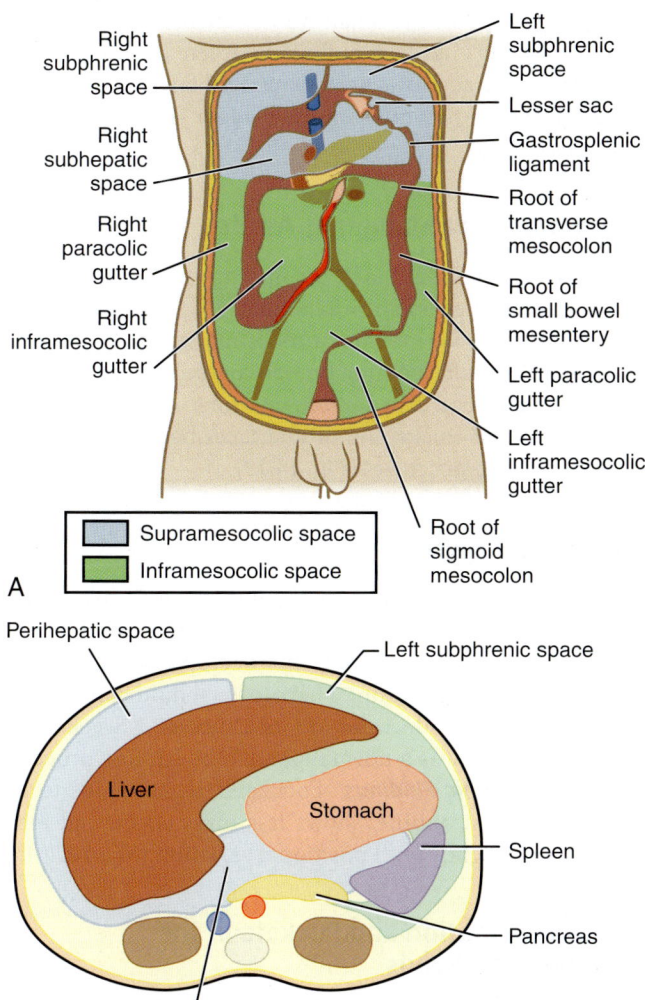

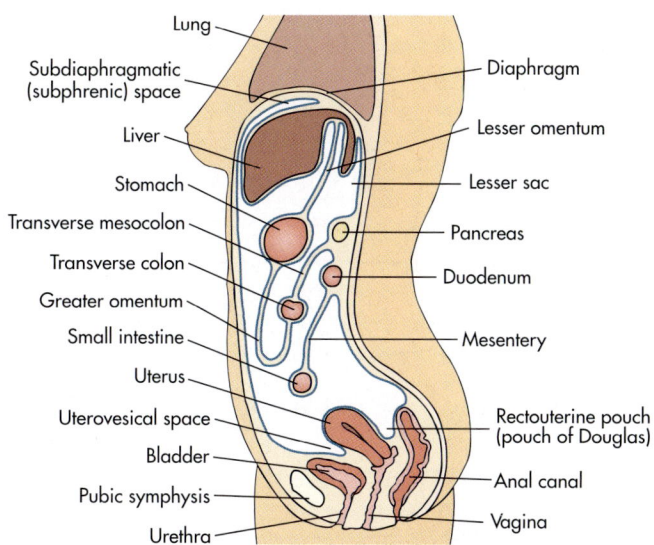

FIG. 14.14 Sagittal view of the abdomen delineating the peritoneal cavity.

FIG. 14.13 (A) The supramesocolic space lies above the root of the transverse mesocolon, and the inframesocolic space lies below the root of the mesocolon. (B) The lesser sac lies anterior to the pancreas and posterior to the stomach.

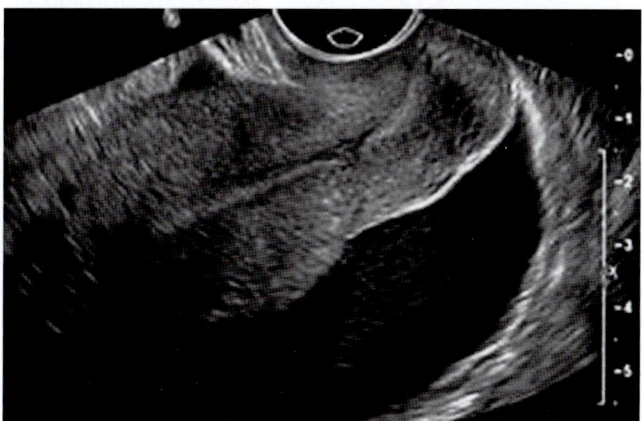

FIG. 14.15 Transvaginal image of fluid in the extraperitoneal prevesical space displacing the uterus anteriorly.

vessels. The **retrovesical space** is divided by the uterus into an anterior vesicouterine recess and a posterior rectouterine sac (pouch of Douglas) (see Fig. 14.14). The peritoneal reflection over the dome of the bladder may have an inferior recess extending anterior to the bladder. Ascites displaces the distended urinary bladder inferiorly but not posteriorly. Intraperitoneal fluid compresses the bladder from its lateral aspect in cases of loculation. Fluid in the extraperitoneal prevesical space has a "dumbbell" configuration, displacing the bladder posteriorly and compressing it from the sides along its entire length (Fig. 14.15).

Abdominal Wall

The paired rectus abdominis muscles are delineated medially in the midline of the body by the linea alba (Fig. 14.16). Laterally the aponeuroses of external oblique, internal oblique, and transversus abdominis muscles unite to form a band-like vertical fibrous groove called the linea semilunaris

or spigelian fascia. The sheath of the three anterolateral abdominal muscles invests the rectus both anteriorly and posteriorly. Midway between the umbilicus and symphysis pubis, the aponeurotic sheath passes anteriorly to the rectus.

Below the peritoneal line, the rectus muscle is separated from the intraabdominal contents only by the transversalis fascia and the peritoneum. The rectus muscles are seen as a biconvex muscle group delineated by the linea alba and linea semilunaris. The peritoneal line is seen as a discrete linear echogenicity in the deepest layer of the abdominal wall.

PATHOLOGY OF THE PERITONEAL CAVITY

Ascites

Ascites is the accumulation of serous fluid in the peritoneal cavity. The amount of intraperitoneal fluid depends on the location, volume, and patient position. Factors other than fluid volume that affect the distribution of intraperitoneal

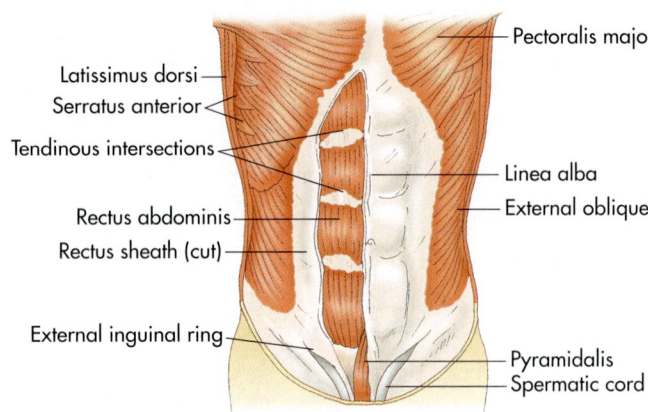

FIG. 14.16 (A) The rectus abdominis muscle rises from the front of the symphysis pubis and the pubic crest. (B) The muscles of the anterior and lateral abdominal walls include the external oblique, internal oblique, transversus, rectus abdominis, and pyramidalis.

fluid include peritoneal pressure, the area from which fluid originates, rapidity of fluid accumulation, presence or absence of adhesions, density of fluid with respect to other abdominal organs, and degree of bladder fullness.

▸ **Sonographic Findings.** Serous ascites appears as echo-free fluid regions indented and shaped by the organs and viscera it surrounds or between where it is interposed (Fig. 14.17). The fluid first fills the pouch of Douglas, then the lateral paravesical recesses, before it ascends to both paracolic gutters. The major flow from the pelvis is via the right paracolic gutter. Small volumes of fluid in the supine patient first appear around the inferior tip of the right lobe in the superior portion of the right flank and in the pelvic cul-de-sac, then in the paracolic gutters, before moving lateral and anterior to the liver.

The small bowel loops, sinks, or floats in the surrounding ascitic fluid, depending on relative gas content and amount of fat in the mesentery (Fig. 14.18). The middle portion of the transverse colon usually floats on top of fluid because of its gas content, whereas the ascending portions of the colon, which are fixed retroperitoneally, remain in their normal location with or without gas.

Floating loops of the small bowel, anchored posteriorly by the mesentery and with fluid between the mesenteric folds, have a characteristic anterior convex fan shape or arcuate appearance. An overdistended bladder may mask small quantities of fluid.

Inflammatory or Malignant Ascites

The sonographer should look for findings within the ascitic fluid that may suggest an inflammatory or malignant process. In searching for inflammatory or malignant ascites, the sonographer should look for fine or coarse internal echoes; loculation; unusual distribution, matting, or clumping of bowel loops; and thickening of interfaces between the fluid and neighboring structures (Fig. 14.19).

Hepatorenal Recess

Generalized ascites, inflammatory fluid from acute cholecystitis, fluid resulting from pancreatic autolysis, or blood from a ruptured hepatic neoplasm or ectopic gestation may contribute to the formation of hepatorenal fluid collections. Abdominal fluid collections do not persist 1 week after abdominal surgery as a normal part of the healing process.

▸ **Sonographic Findings.** Loculated ascites tends to be more irregular in outline, shows less mass effect, and may change shape slightly with positional variation (Fig. 14.20).

Abscess Formation and Pockets in the Abdomen and Pelvis

An **abscess** is a cavity formed by necrosis within a solid tissue or a circumscribed collection of purulent material. The sonographer is frequently asked to evaluate a patient to rule out an abscess formation. The patient may present with a fever of unknown origin or with tenderness and swelling from a postoperative procedure. Other clinical signs include chills, weakness, malaise, and pain at the localized site of infection. Laboratory findings include normal liver function values, increased white blood cell count (**leukocytosis**), generalized **sepsis**, and bacterial cultures (if superficial).

▸ **Sonographic Findings.** Abscess collections can appear quite varied in their texture depending on the length of time the abscess has been forming and the space available for the abscess to localize. Therefore, many collections appear predominantly fluid filled with irregular borders; they can also be complex, with debris floating within the cystic mass, or they may show a more solid pattern (Fig. 14.21). If the collection is in the pelvis, careful analysis of bowel patterns and peristalsis should be made in an attempt to separate the bowel from the abscess collection.

Classically an abscess appears as an elliptical sonolucent mass with thick and irregular margins. The margins tend to be under tension and displace surrounding structures. A septated appearance may result from previous or developing adhesions. Necrotic debris produces low-level internal echoes that may be seen to float within the abscess. Fluid

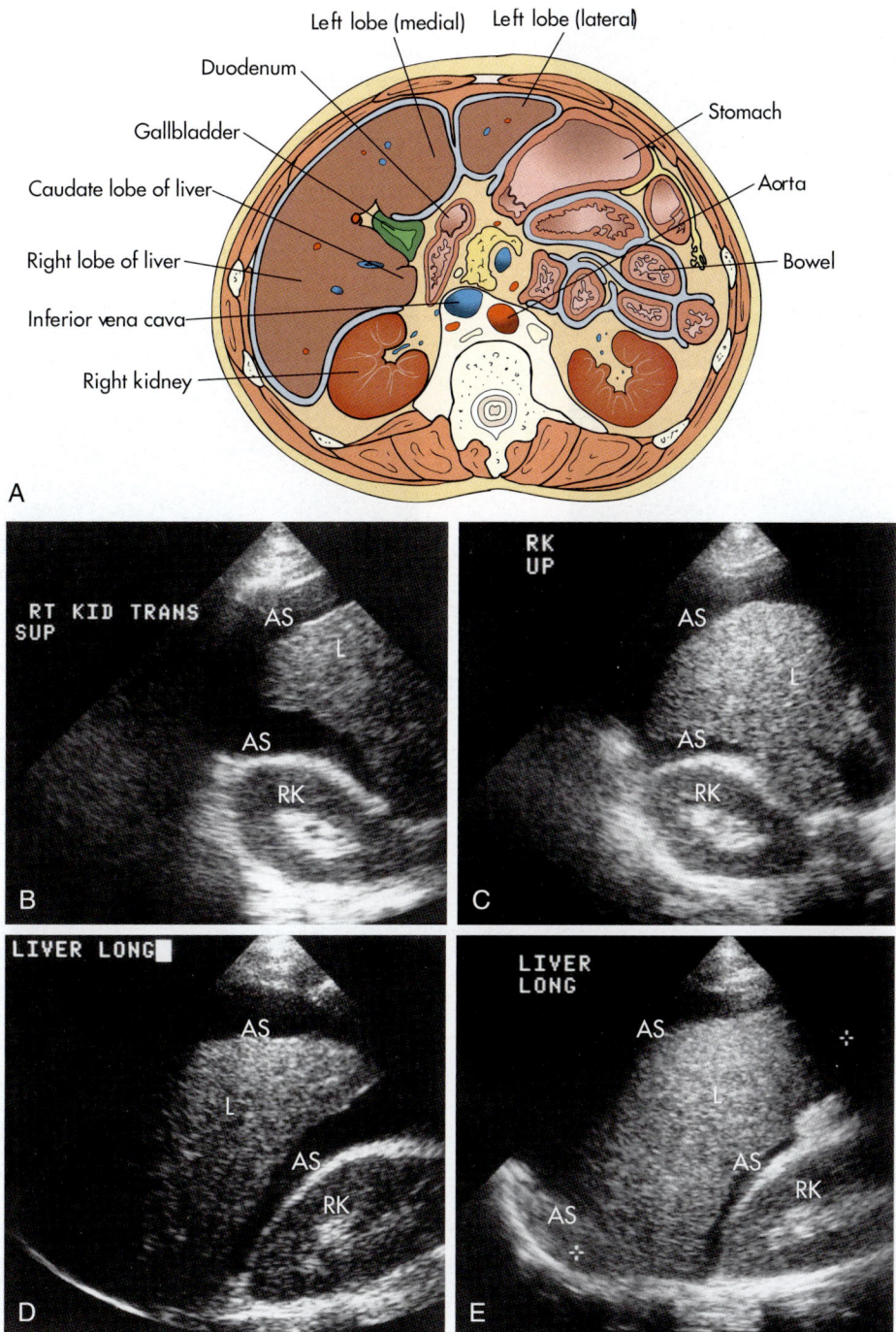

FIG. 14.17 (A) Transverse view of the posterior pararenal space. This space is located between the posterior renal fascia and the transversalis fascia. It communicates with the peritoneal fat, lateral to the lateroconal fascia. The space merges inferiorly with the anterior pararenal space and retroperitoneal tissue of the iliac fossa. Ascites may fill the peritoneal cavity. Small volumes of fluid in the supine position first appear around the inferior tip of the right lobe of the superior portion of the right flank. (B–C) Transverse views show ascitic fluid in the pararenal and subhepatic spaces. (D–E) Longitudinal views with ascitic fluid in the pararenal space (Morison's pouch) and subhepatic space. *AS,* Ascites; *L,* liver; *RK,* right kidney.

levels are secondary to layering, probably because of the settling of debris.

Gas-Containing Abscess

Scattered air reflectors may be the sonographer's clue in a gas- or air-filled abscess collection.

Sonographic Findings. Gas-containing abscesses have varying echo patterns. Generally, they appear as a densely echogenic mass with or without acoustic shadowing and otherwise increased through-transmission (Fig. 14.22). A teratoma may mimic the pattern of a gas-containing abscess, but clinical history and x-rays exclude this tumor from the

422 CHAPTER 14 The Peritoneal Cavity and Abdominal Wall

diagnosis. A gas-containing abscess may be confused with a solid lesion because it can be difficult to determine the presence of through-transmission.

Peritonitis

Peritonitis and the resultant abscess formation may be a generalized or localized process. Multiloculated abscesses or multiple collections should be recorded and their size

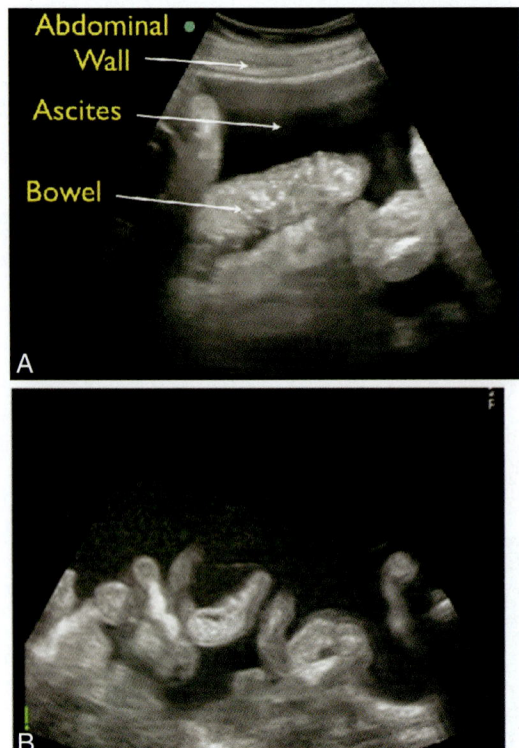

FIG. 14.18 The small bowel loops, sinks, or floats in the surrounding ascitic fluid, depending on relative gas content and amount of fat in the mesentery.

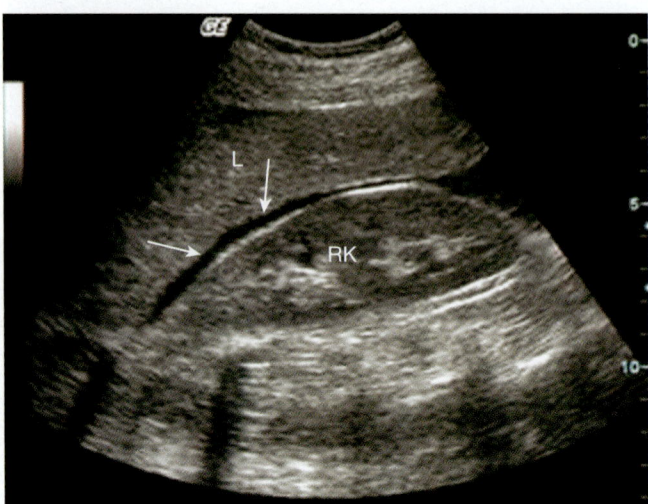

FIG. 14.20 Fluid in Morison's pouch seen anterior to the right kidney in this sagittal view. *Arrows*, Fluid; *L*, liver; *RK*, right kidney.

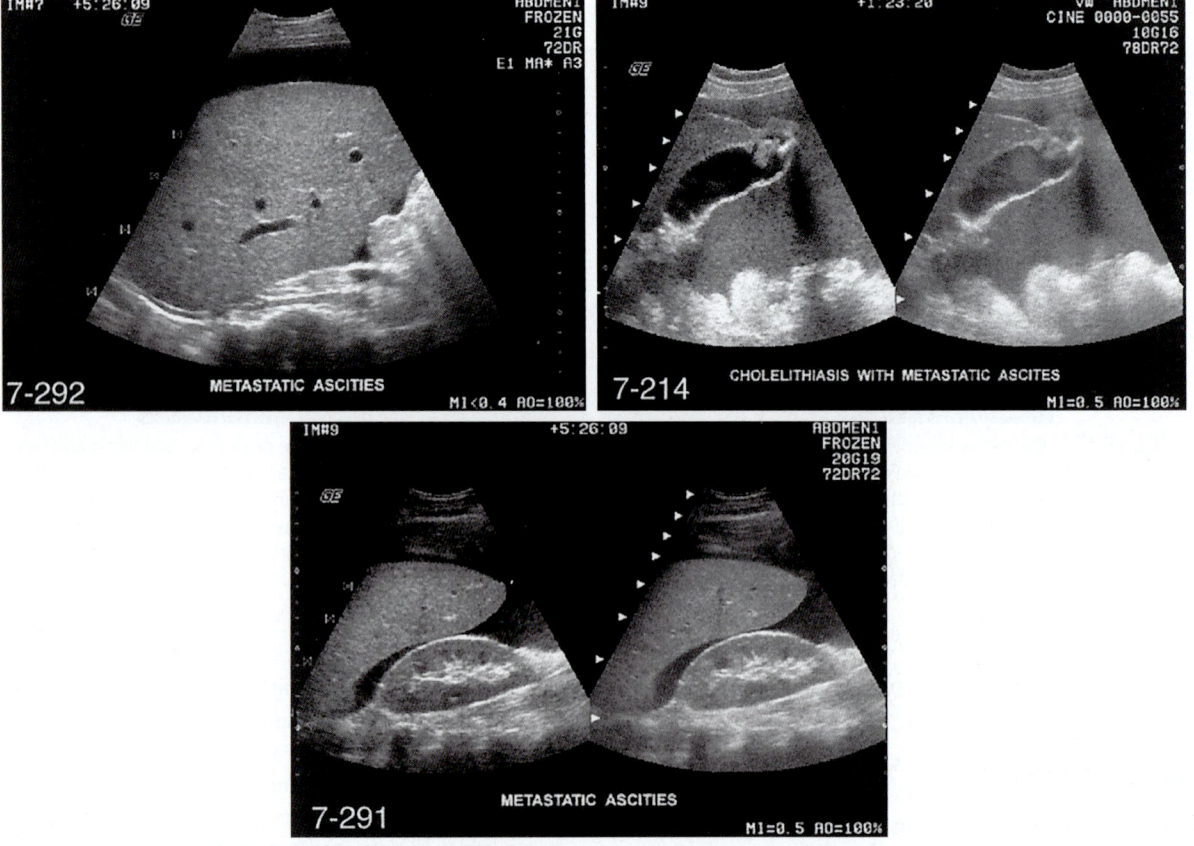

FIG. 14.19 **Malignant ascites.** Fine internal echoes are seen within the ascitic fluid.

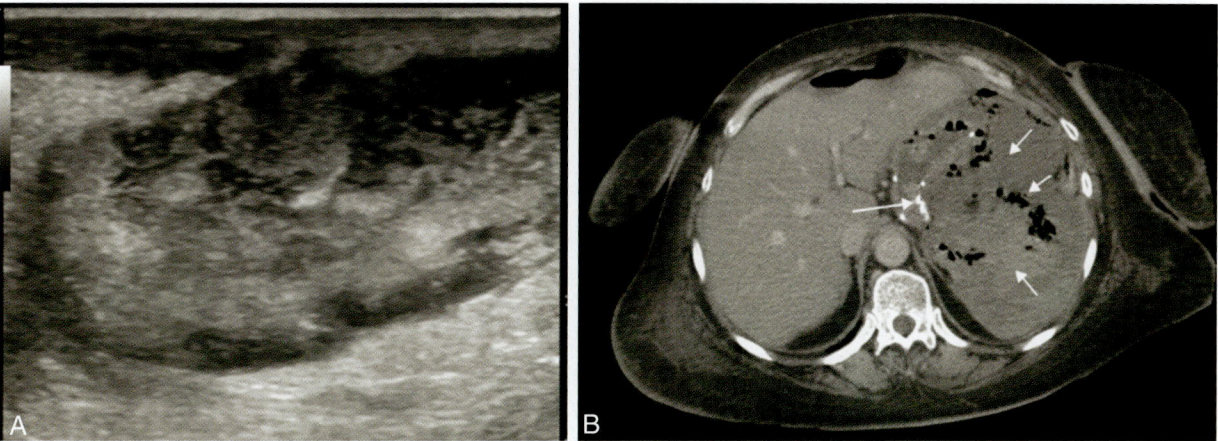

FIG. 14.21 Ultrasound (A) and computed tomographic (B) images of a complex abscess in the abdominal cavity. Abscess collections may appear predominantly fluid filled with irregular borders; they can also be complex, with debris floating within the cystic mass, or they may show a more solid pattern.

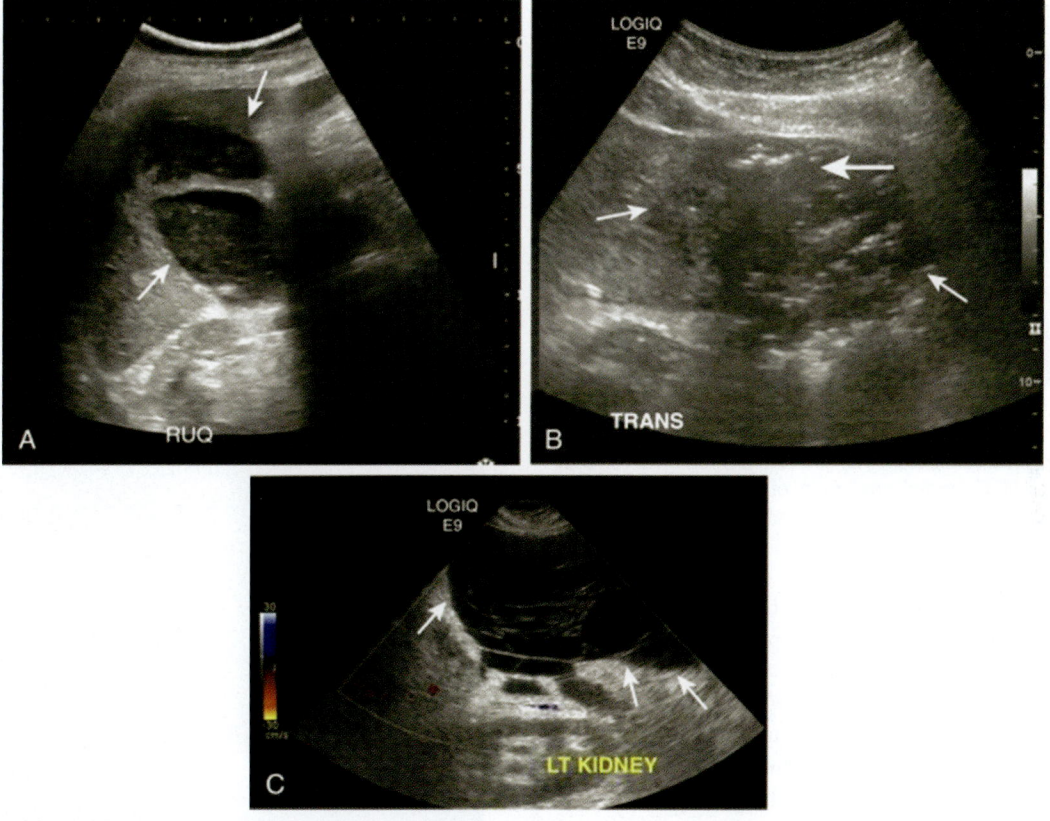

FIG. 14.22 Gas-containing abscesses have varying echo patterns. In general, they appear as a densely echogenic mass with or without acoustic shadowing and otherwise increased through-transmission.

determined as accurately as possible to help plan drainage and improve accuracy in follow-up studies.

Lesser Sac Abscess

The small slit-like epiploic foramen usually seals off the lesser sac from inflammatory processes extrinsic to it. If the process begins within the lesser sac, such as with a pancreatic abscess, the sac may be involved along with other secondarily affected peritoneal and retroperitoneal spaces (Fig. 14.23).

Differential diagnoses should include pseudocyst, pancreatic abscess, gastric outlet obstruction, and fluid-filled stomach.

Subphrenic Abscess

The left upper quadrant may be difficult to examine because of the air interference. The sonographer may alter the patient's position to a right lateral decubitus position to scan along the coronal plane of the body, or prone, to use the spleen as a window. A sonographer must decide if the fluid collection

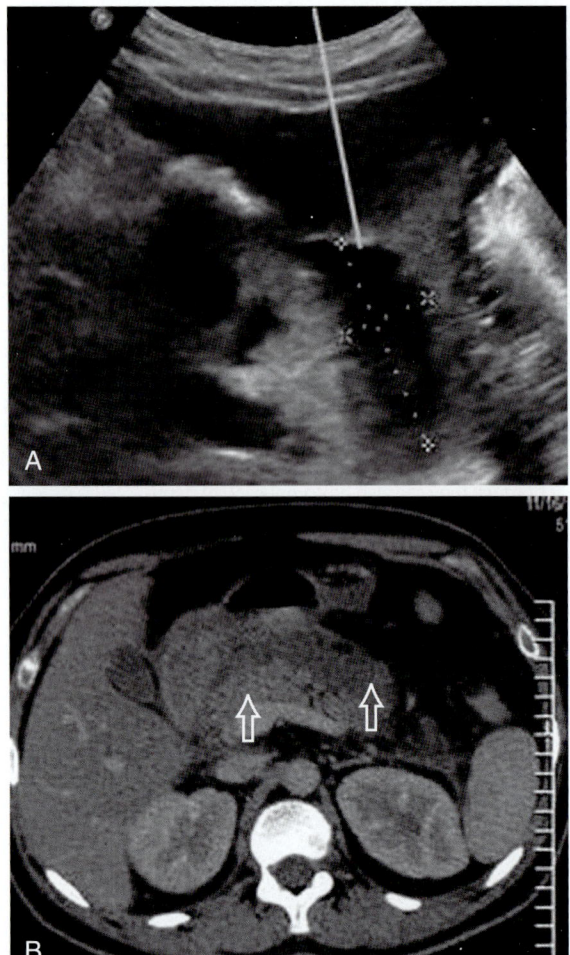

FIG. 14.23 If the process begins within the lesser sac, such as with a pancreatic abscess, the sac may be involved along with other secondarily affected peritoneal and retroperitoneal spaces. (A) Small localized collection of complex fluid in the lesser sac. (B) Computed tomography of the upper abdomen that shows a complex fluid in the lesser sac *(arrows)* near the pancreas.

is above or below the diaphragm. With the patient in a right lateral decubitus position, the probe is placed at the midaxilla line over the dome of the liver. As the patient takes in a breath, the diaphragm moves, and the distinction of the fluid collection may be seen either below the diaphragm or above the diaphragm, extending into the costal phrenic sulcus (Fig. 14.24). The sonographer may also perform the scan with the patient upright to better demonstrate the pleural and subdiaphragmatic areas.

Subcapsular Collections

Intraabdominal fluid may be differentiated by its smooth border and its tendency to conform to the contour of the liver. It displaces the liver medially rather than indenting the border locally, as subcapsular fluid might. A tense subphrenic abscess can displace the liver. The subcapsular fluid collections may be the result of a traumatic injury or other abscess formation. The sonographic pattern is usually heterogeneous (Fig. 14.25).

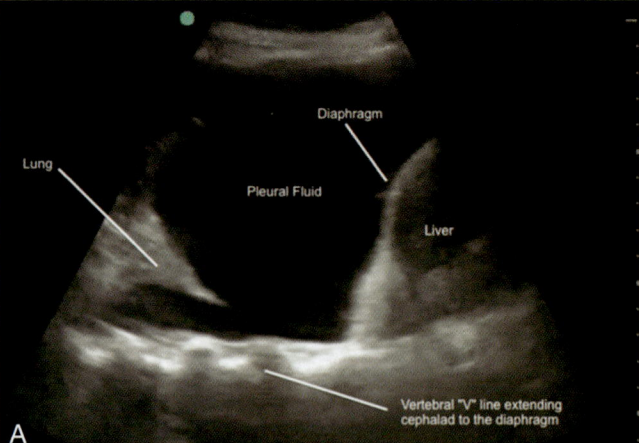
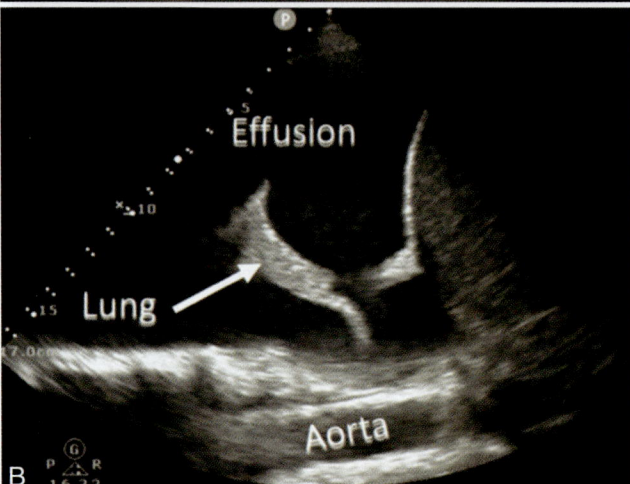
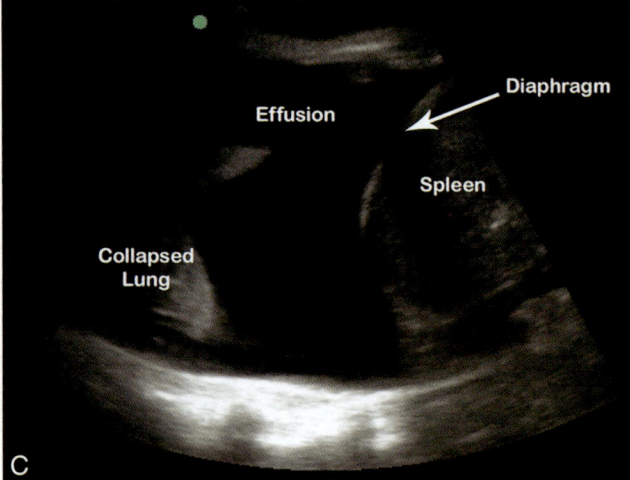

FIG. 14.24 (A) Sagittal image shows the large pleural effusion superior to the diaphragm and liver as the transducer is angled in a cephalic direction. (B) Sagittal images of a patient with a moderate pleural effusion shown superior to the liver. (C) Left pleural effusion with a collapsed lung.

It may be difficult to distinguish a subphrenic abscess from ascites. To do so, the sonographer can look at the margins of the fluid collection or look for other collections of fluid (in the pelvis) to distinguish ascites from abscess. Preperitoneal fat anterior to the liver may mimic a localized fluid collection. An abscess collects in the most dependent area of the body; therefore, all the gutters should be examined,

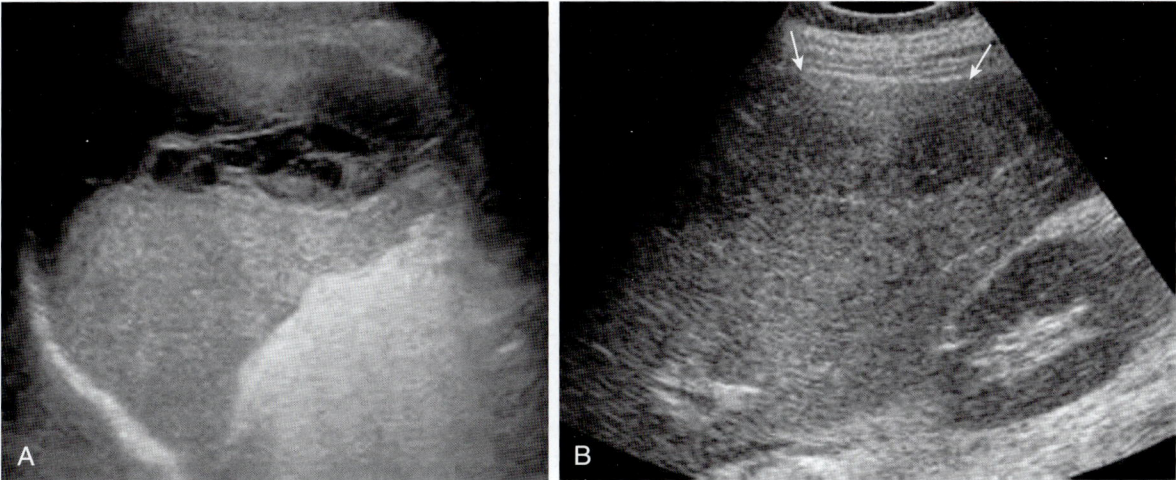

FIG. 14.25 Subcapsular collections of fluid within the liver can mimic loculated subphrenic fluid. (A) Sonogram of a moderate size subcapsular heterogeneous collection in the right upper quadrant. (B) Isoechoic subcapsular hematoma of the liver *(arrows)*.

> **BOX 14.1 Sonography of Abscesses**
>
> If an abscess is suspected (e.g., the patient has a fever of unknown origin), the sonographer should evaluate the following areas:
> - Subdiaphragmatic area (liver and spleen)
> - Splenic recess and borders
> - Hepatic recess and borders
> - Pericolic gutters
> - Lesser omentum
> - Transverse mesocolon
> - Morison's pouch
> - Gastrocolic ligament
> - Phrenicosplenic ligament
> - Recesses between intestinal loops and colon
> - Extrahepatic falciform ligament
> - Pouch of Douglas
> - Broad ligaments (female)
> - The area anterior to the urinary bladder

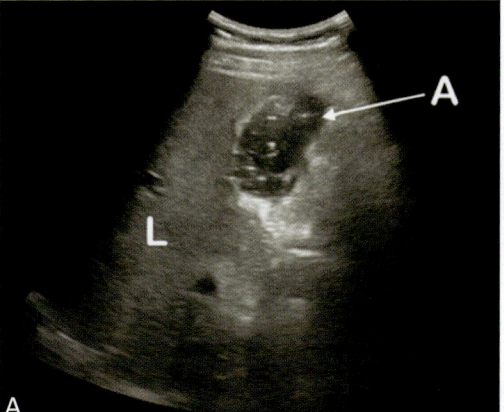

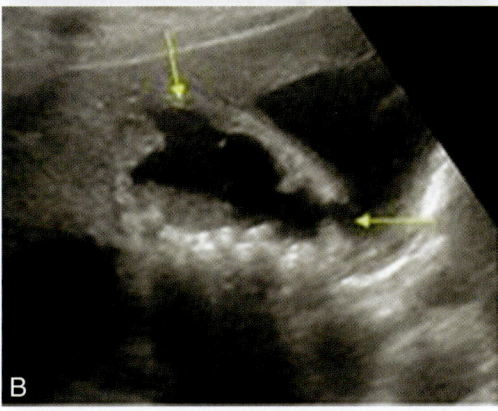

FIG. 14.26 (A) On sonography, a biloma abscess may appear cystic with weak internal echoes (A) or (B) show a fluid-fluid level if clots or debris are not present (B). *A*, Abscess; *L*, liver.

including the "pockets" and "pouches" and the spaces above and around the various organs (Box 14.1).

Biloma Abscess

Bilomas are extrahepatic loculated collections of bile that may develop because of iatrogenic, traumatic, or spontaneous rupture of the biliary tree. On sonography, a biloma abscess may appear cystic with weak internal echoes or a fluid-fluid level if clots or debris are not present (Fig. 14.26). They usually have sharp margins. The extrahepatic bilomas are usually crescentic, surrounding and compressing structures with which they come in contact.

General Abdominal Abscess

A high percentage of abdominal and pelvic abscesses appear after surgery or trauma. The hepatic recesses and perihepatic spaces are the most common sites for abscess formation (Fig. 14.27). The pelvis is another common site. Free fluid below the transverse mesocolon often flows into the pouch of Douglas and perivesical spaces. An abscess may form in the right subhepatic space. The fluid ascends the right pericolic gutter into Morison's pouch. When the fluid fills Morison's pouch, it spreads past the coronary ligament over the dome of the liver. The presence of a right subhepatic abscess generally implies previous contamination of the right subhepatic space.

PATHOLOGY OF THE MESENTERY, OMENTUM, AND PERITONEUM

A mass or lesion within the mesentery and omentum may have solid or cystic characteristics, whereas a mass within the peritoneum may show an infiltrative pattern (Table 14.1). With an omental mass, at least one-third of these lesions are malignant, and secondary neoplasms are more frequent than primary. In the mesentery, a benign primary tumor is more common than a malignant tumor, and secondary neoplasms are more frequent than primary. A cystic mass is more common than a solid mass. Malignant solid tumors are more likely found near the root of the mesentery, whereas benign solid tumors are found in the periphery near the bowel.

Cysts

Abdominal cysts may have (1) embryologic, (2) traumatic or acquired, (3) neoplastic, or (4) infective and degenerative origins. It is important to determine the organ of origin of the mass. If the mass is adherent to the mesentery or small intestine, it may be difficult for an ultrasound to distinguish the anatomic landmarks necessary to determine the point of origin; therefore, many patients will have a CT or MRI of the abdomen to better define these borders. **Hemorrhage** into omental or mesenteric cysts may cause rapid distention and clinically mimic ascites. Peritoneal inclusion cysts are considered in the differential diagnosis when large adnexal cystic structures are identified in a young woman. Fungal infections present as peritoneal cystic lesions.

Sonographic Findings. Mesenteric and omental cysts may be uniloculated or multiloculated with smooth walls and thin internal septations (Fig. 14.28). The internal echoes

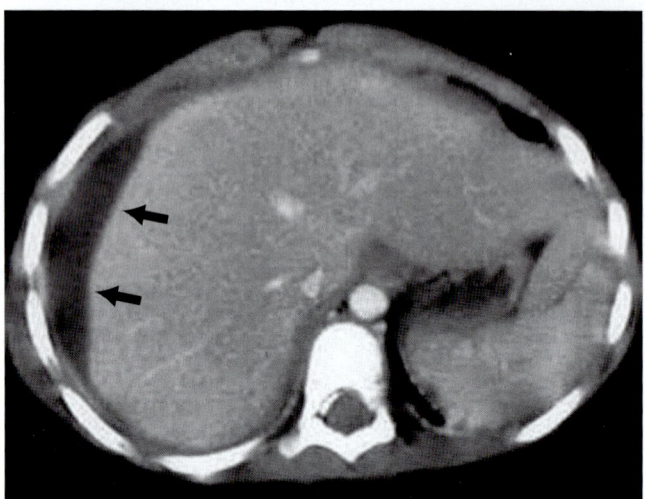

FIG 14.27 The hepatic recesses and perihepatic spaces are the most common sites for abscess formation. Computed tomographic image of the upper abdomen shows a fluid collection along the right lateral margin of the liver.

TABLE 14.1	Description of Peritoneal, Omental, and Mesenteric Masses		
Solid		**Cystic**	**Infiltrative**
Peritoneal Mass			
• Peritoneal mesothelioma • Peritoneal carcinomatosis		• Cystic mesothelioma • Pseudomyxoma peritonei • Bacterial/mycobacterial infection	• Peritoneal mesothelioma
Omental Mass			
• Benign: leiomyoma, lipoma, neurofibroma • Malignant: leiomyosarcoma, liposarcoma, fibrosarcoma, lymphoma, peritoneal mesothelioma, hemangiopericytoma, metastases • Infection: tuberculosis		• Hematoma	
Round		**Loculated Cystic**	**Ill-Defined/Stellate**
Mesenteric Mass			
• Metastases, especially from colon, ovary • Lymphoma • Leiomyosarcoma • Neural tumor • Lipoma, lipomatosis, liposarcoma • Fibrous histiocytoma • Hemangioma		• Cystic lymphangioma • Pseudomyxoma • Peritonei • Cystic mesothelioma • Mesenteric cyst • Mesenteric hematoma • Benign cystic teratoma • Cystic spindle cell tumor	• Metastases (ovary) • Lymphoma • Fibromatosis • Fibrosing mesenteritis • Lipodystrophy • Mesenteric panniculitis • Stellate: peritoneal mesothelioma, retractile mesenteritis, fibrosis reaction of carcinoid, desmoid tumor, tuberculous peritonitis, metastases, diverticulitis, pancreatitis

are correlated with fat globules, debris, superimposed hemorrhage, or infection. They may follow the contour of the underlying bowel and conform to the anterior abdominal wall rather than produce distention.

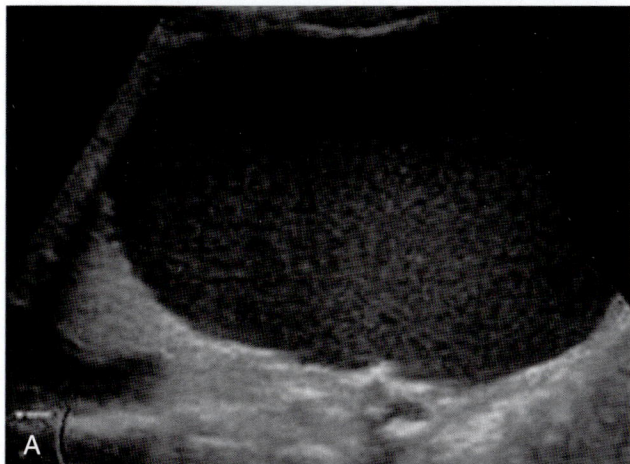
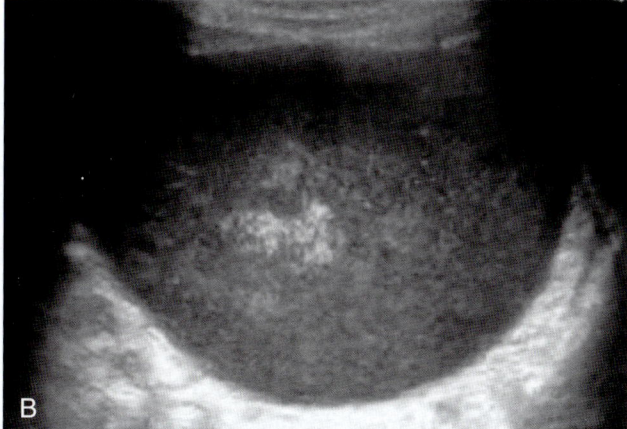

FIG. 14.28 Mesenteric and omental cysts may be uniloculated or multiloculated with smooth walls and thin internal septations.

Urachal Cyst

A urachal cyst is an incomplete regression of the urachus during development. The apex of the bladder is continuous with the allantois, which becomes obliterated and forms a fibrous core, the urachus. The urachus persists throughout life as a ligament that runs from the apex of the bladder to the umbilicus and is called the median umbilical ligament.

Sonographic Findings. On sonography, the sonographer may see a cystic mass between the umbilicus and the bladder (Fig. 14.29). The mass may be small or giant, multiseptated, and extend into the upper abdomen.

Urinoma

A **urinoma**, an encapsulated collection of urine, may result from a closed renal injury or surgical intervention or may develop spontaneously secondary to an obstructing lesion. The extraperitoneal extravasation may be subcapsular or perirenal: the latter collections are sometimes termed uriniferous pseudocysts. The extravasation may leak around the ureter, where the perinephric fascia is weakest, or into adjoining fascial planes and peritoneal cavity.

Sonographic Findings. Cystic masses are most often oriented inferomedially, with upward and lateral displacement of the lower pole of the kidney along with medial displacement of the ureter. They usually present on ultrasound as anechoic or contain low-level echoes (Fig. 14.30).

Peritoneal Metastases

Peritoneal metastases develop from cellular implantation across the peritoneal cavity. The most common primary sites are the ovaries, stomach, and colon. Other less common sites are the pancreas, biliary tract, kidneys, testicles, and uterus.

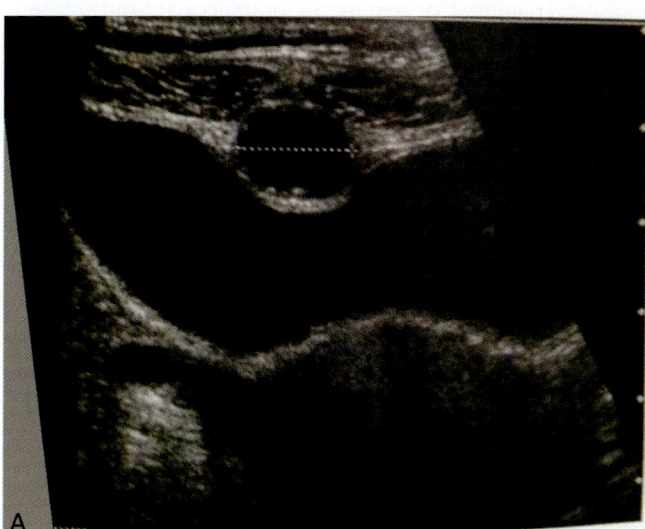
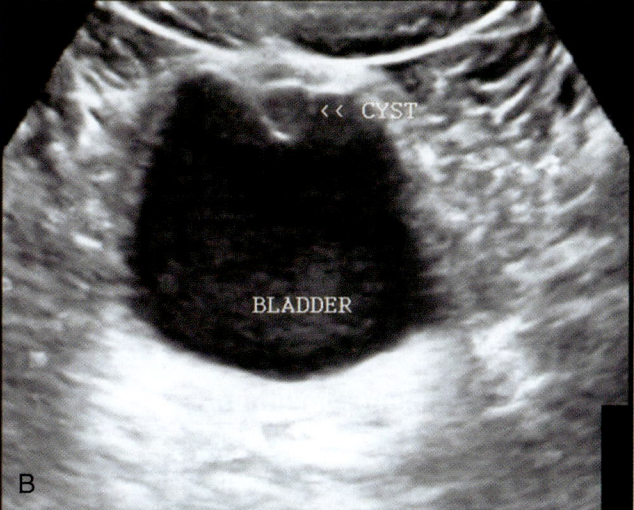

FIG. 14.29 The urachal cyst may appear as a cystic mass found between the umbilicus and anterior to the bladder.

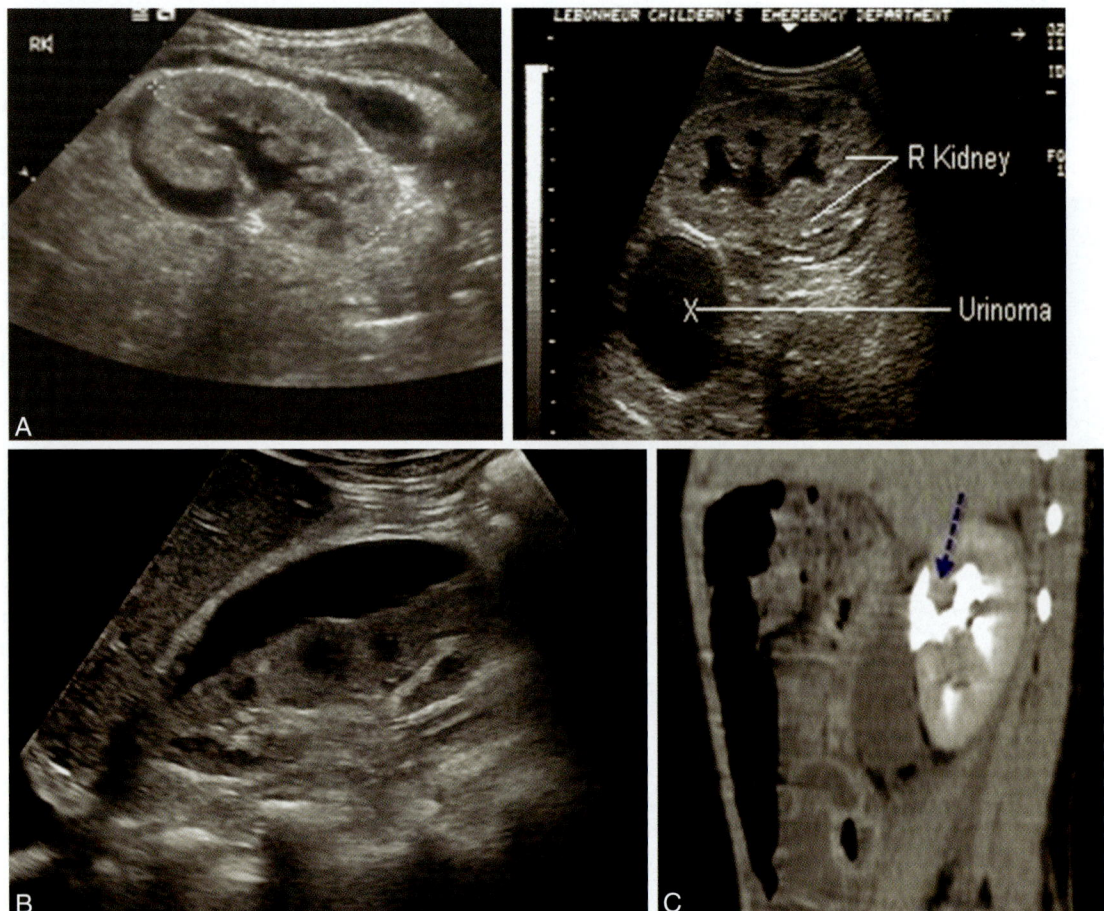

FIG. 14.30 (A–B) A urinoma may result from a closed renal injury or surgical intervention or may develop spontaneously secondary to an obstructing lesion. (C) Coronal computed tomography image shows small urinoma (*arrow*).

Metastases may arise from tumors, such as sarcomas, melanomas, teratomas, or embryonic tumors.

▶ **Sonographic Findings.** The metastases form a nodular, sheetlike, irregular configuration. Multiple small nodules are seen along the peritoneal line. The larger masses obliterate the line and cause adhesion to bowel loops (Fig. 14.31).

Lymphomas of the Omentum and Mesentery

Lymphoma presents as a uniformly thick, hypoechoic, band-shaped structure that follows the convexity of the anterior and lateral abdominal wall, creating the omental band.

▶ **Sonographic Findings.** On ultrasound examination, omental and mesenteric lymphomas present as a lobulated, confluent, hypoechoic mass surrounding a centrally positioned echogenic area. The "**sandwich sign**" represents a mass infiltrating the mesenteric leaves and encasing the superior mesenteric artery (Fig. 14.32).

Tumors of the Peritoneum, Omentum, and Mesentery

Secondary tumors and lymphoma are neoplasms that most commonly involve the peritoneum and mesentery. Peritoneal and omental mesotheliomas most often occur in middle-aged men as the result of exposure to asbestos. The common symptoms are abdominal pain, weight loss, and ascites.

▶ **Sonographic Findings.** The tumor may present as a large mass with discrete smaller nodes scattered over large areas of the visceral and parietal peritoneum, or it may present as diffuse nodes and plaques that coat the abdominal cavity and envelope and mat together in the abdominal viscera (Fig. 14.33).

PATHOLOGY OF THE ABDOMINAL WALL

Abdominal Wall Masses

Lesions found within the superficial abdominal wall include inflammatory lesions, hematomas, neoplasms, hernias, and postsurgical lesions. Symmetry of the rectus sheath muscles is a key factor in determining if an abdominal wall mass is present. The higher-resolution transducers may help the sonographer distinguish between the amount of fat and muscle present and an abnormal lesion.

Lymphoceles

A **lymphocele** is a collection of fluid that occurs after surgery in the pelvis, retroperitoneum, or recess cavities.

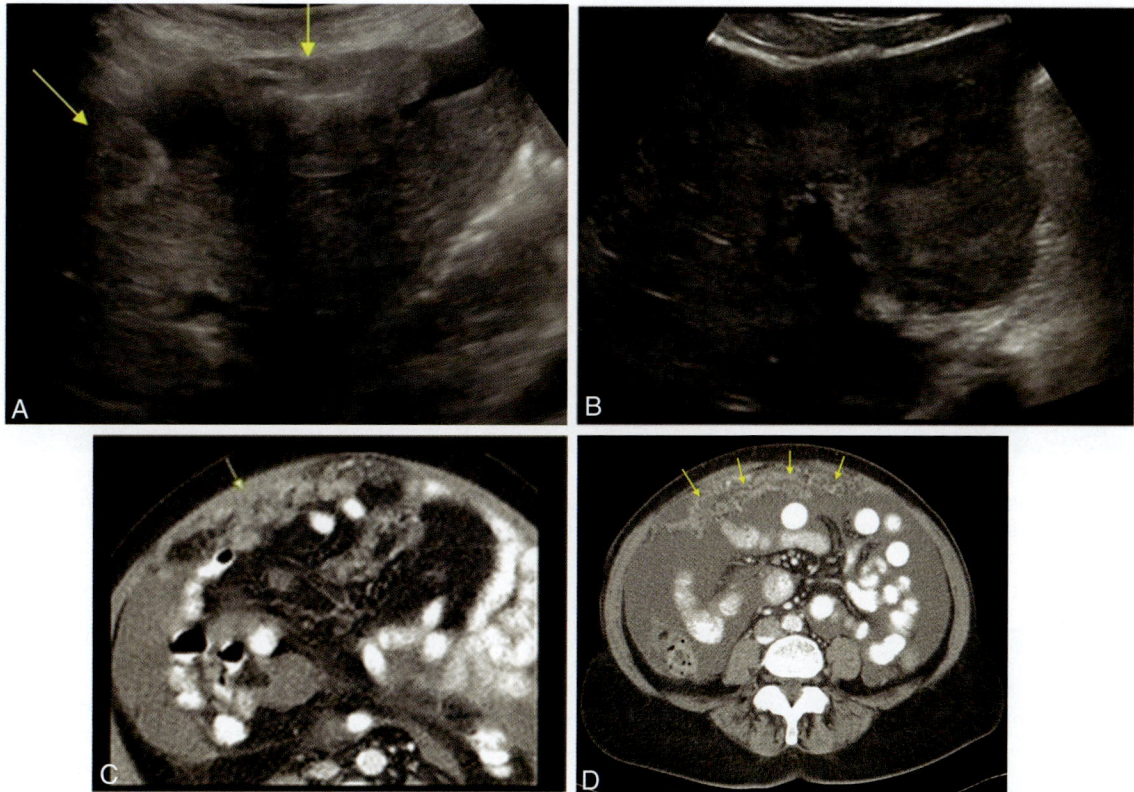

FIG. 14.31 Peritoneal metastases form a nodular, sheet-like, irregular configuration. Multiple small nodules are seen along the peritoneal line. The larger masses obliterate the line and cause adhesion to bowel loops. (A–B) Sonographic images of the peritoneal metastases. (C–D) Computed tomographic images of the peritoneal metastases *(arrows)*.

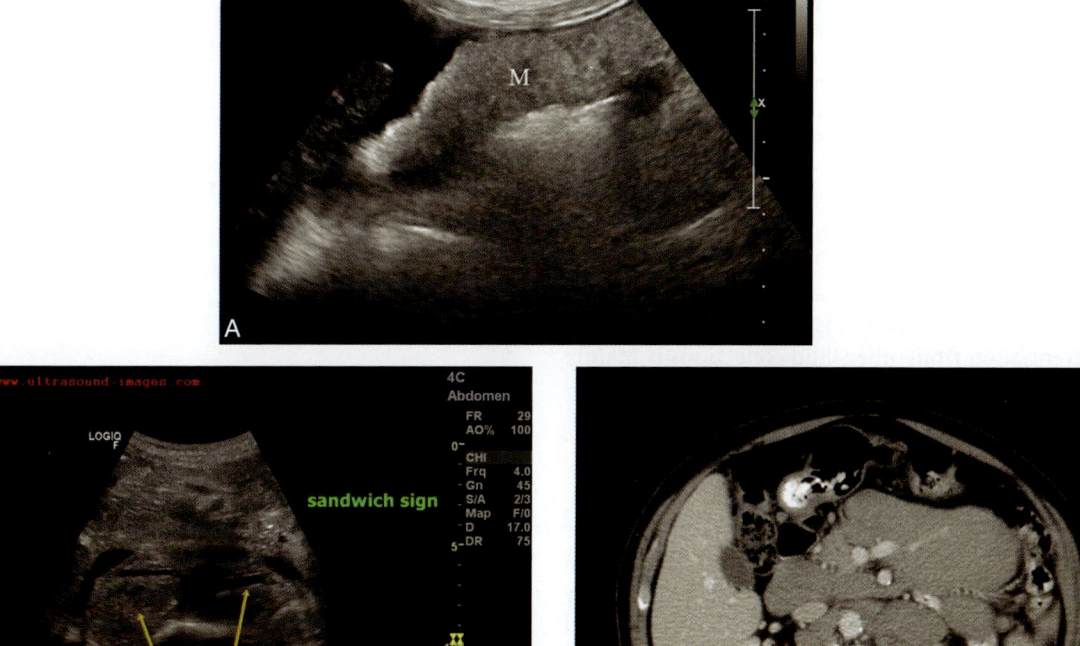

FIG. 14.32 (A) On ultrasound examination, omental and mesenteric lymphomas present as a lobulated, confluent, hypoechoic mass surrounding a centrally positioned echogenic area. (B–C) The "sandwich sign" of lymphoma or enlarged nodes represents a mass infiltrating the mesenteric leaves and encasing the superior mesenteric artery.

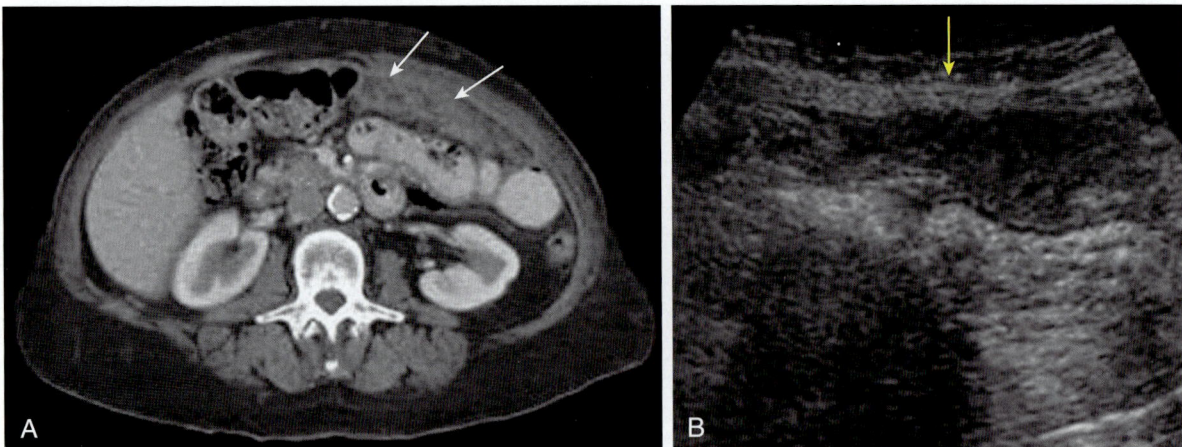

FIG. 14.33 The secondary tumor may present as a mass with discrete smaller nodes scattered over large areas of the visceral and parietal peritoneum, or it may present as diffuse nodes with plaques that envelope and mat together in the abdominal viscera to coat the abdominal cavity. Computed tomography (A) and ultrasound (B).

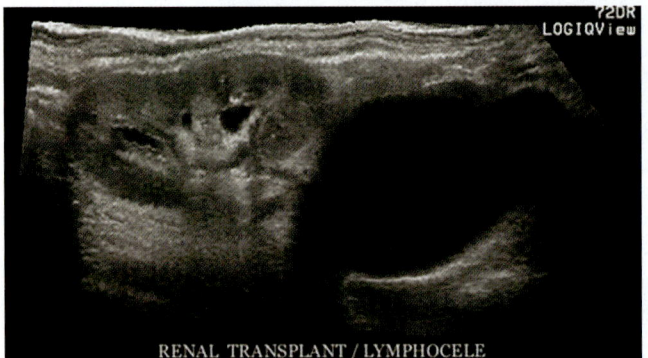

FIG. 14.34 A lymphocele is a collection of fluid that occurs after surgery in the pelvis, retroperitoneum, or recess cavities. Lymphoceles generally look like loculated, simple fluid collections, although they may have a more complex, usually septated, morphology.

Lymphoceles generally look like loculated, simple fluid collections, although they may have a more complex, usually septated, morphology (Fig. 14.34). Differentiation from loculated ascites is usually possible because the mass effect of a lymphocele that is under tension displaces the surrounding organs. Differentiation from other fluid collections is mainly made by aspiration.

Extraperitoneal Hematoma

Extraperitoneal rectus sheath hematomas are acute or chronic collections of blood lying either within the rectus muscle or between the muscle and its sheath (Fig. 14.35). They occur due to direct trauma, pregnancy, cardiovascular and degenerative muscle diseases, surgical injury, anticoagulation therapy, steroids, or extreme exercise. Clinically the patient may present with acute, sharp, persistent nonradiating pain.

Hematomas are caused by surgical injury to tissue or by blunt trauma to the abdomen. Laboratory values may show a decrease in hematocrit and red blood cell count; the patient may go into shock.

Sonographic Findings. On ultrasound examination, the sonographer notices an asymmetry between the rectus sheath muscles. The hematoma may appear as an anechoic mass with scattered internal echoes (Fig. 14.36). The sonographic appearance depends on the stage of the bleed. Acute bleeds are primarily cystic, with some debris and blood clots; as the blood begins to organize and clot, the mass becomes more solid in appearance. Newly formed clots may be very homogeneous. Hematomas can become infected and, at any stage, may be sonographically indistinguishable from abscesses. They may mimic subphrenic fluid.

Bladder Flap Hematoma

A bladder flap hematoma is a collection of blood between the bladder and lower uterine segment, resulting from a lower uterine transverse cesarean section and bleeding from the uterine vessels.

Subfascial Hematoma

A subfascial hematoma is found in the prevesicular space and is caused by a disruption of the inferior epigastric vessels or their branches during a cesarean section.

Inflammatory Lesion (Abscess)

An abscess or inflammation in the abdominal wall may occur after surgery. The sonogram may show cystic, complex, or solid characteristics. Generally, the masses are superficial and are easy to locate and needle aspirate with ultrasound guidance if necessary. A high-frequency, linear array transducer should be used to image the superficial area. The patient may

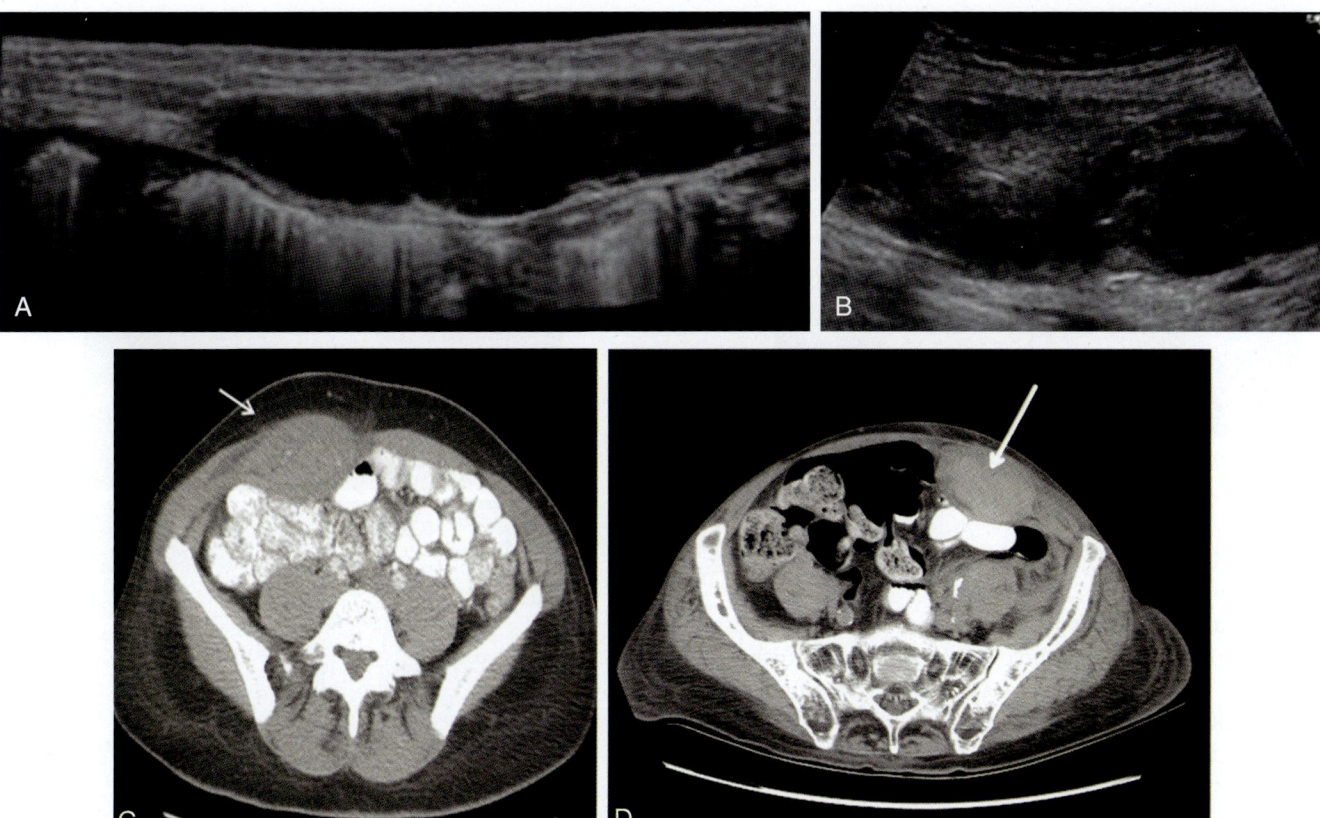

FIG. 14.35 (A–B) The rectus sheath hematoma may appear as an anechoic mass with scattered internal echoes. (C–D) Computed tomographic images of the rectus sheath hematoma *(arrows)*.

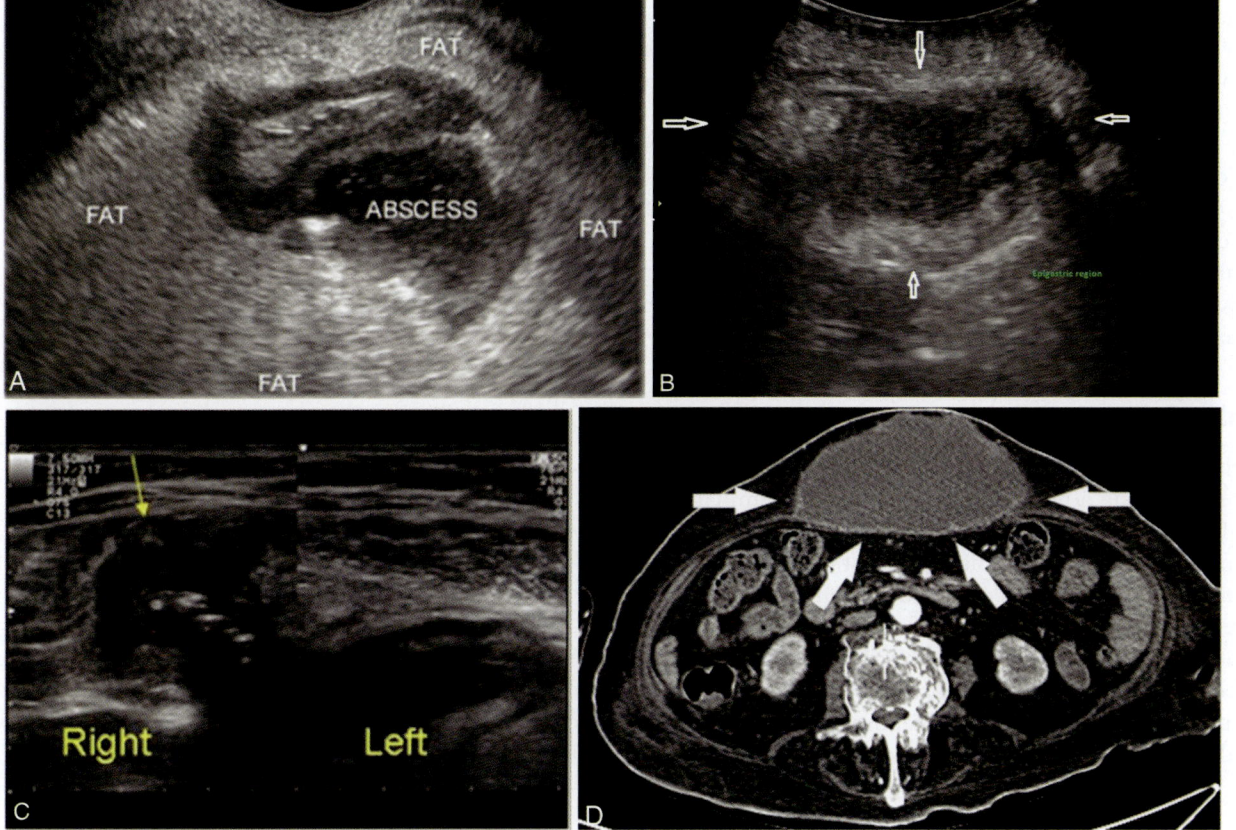

FIG. 14.36 An abdominal wall abscess presents as an anechoic or echoic mass with internal echoes from debris. (A–C) Ultrasound examples of the abscess show an irregular shape with heterogeneous texture. (D) Computed tomographic image of an anterior abdominal wall abscess.

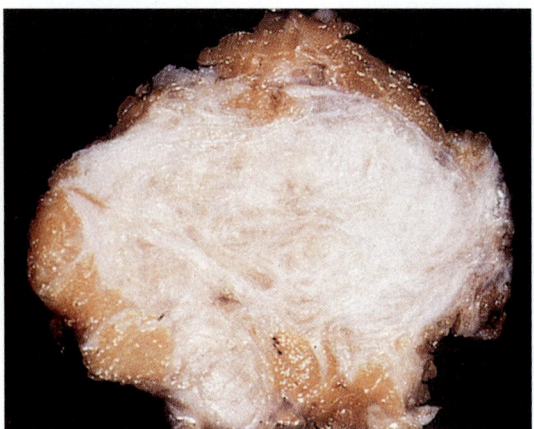

FIG. 14.37 Gross pathology of a desmoid tumor of the abdominal wall.

present with leukocytosis, **septicemia**, or a previous history of **pyogenic** infection.

▸ *Sonographic Findings.* An abdominal wall abscess presents as an anechoic or echoic mass with internal echoes from debris. The mass usually has irregular margins and shape (see Fig. 14.36). It may have gas bubbles within that show shadowing on the ultrasound image.

Neoplasm or Peritoneal Thickening

Neoplasms of the abdominal wall include lipomas, desmoid tumors, or metastases. The desmoid tumor is a benign fibrous neoplasm of aponeurotic structures. It most commonly occurs in relation to the rectus abdominis and its sheath (Fig. 14.37). The tumor may present as hypoechoic to cystic (except lipomas).

▸ *Sonographic Findings.* A desmoid tumor presents as anechoic to hypoechoic, with smooth and sharply defined walls (Fig. 14.38). The peritoneal lining is not seen as a distinct structure during sonography unless it is thickened. This is usually secondary to metastatic implants or direct extension of the tumor from the viscera or mesentery. Primary mesotheliomas occur rarely.

Hernias

An abdominal hernia is the protrusion of a peritoneal-lined sac through a defect in the weakened abdominal wall (Fig. 14.39). The viscera beneath the weakened tissue may protrude, resulting in a hernia. The most common areas of weakness are the umbilical area and the femoral and inguinal rings. (The inguinal hernia is discussed in Chapter 23.) An incarcerated hernia is one that cannot be "reduced" or pushed back into the abdominal cavity. Complications may arise if edema develops or if the opening constricts so much that the protrusion cannot be placed back into position.

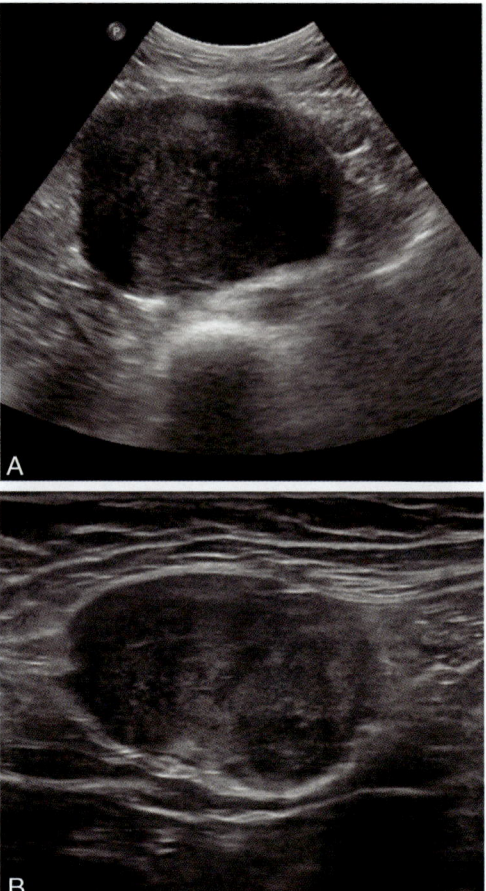

FIG. 14.38 A desmoid tumor presents as anechoic to hypoechoic, with smooth and sharply defined walls.

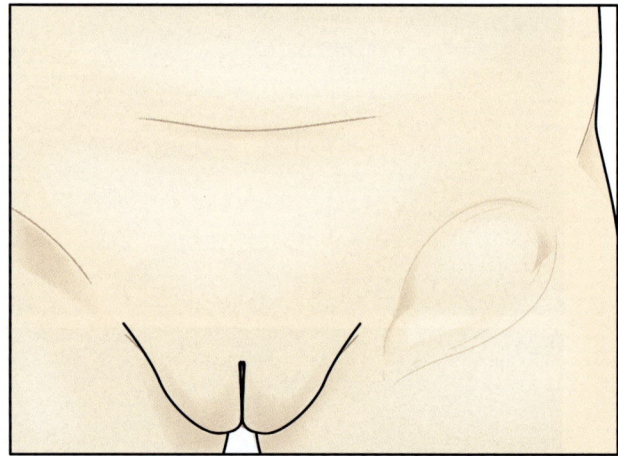

FIG. 14.39 Femoral hernia causing a bulging enlargement of the femoral canal.

Strangulation (interruption of the blood supply) of the bowel can also occur in an incarcerated hernia that is not surgically repaired promptly. This bowel can become necrotic and require resection.

The abdominal wall hernia consists of three parts: the sac, the contents of the sac, and the covering of the sac. Common locations for hernias are umbilical (congenital or acquired), epigastric, inguinal, femoral, and at the separation of the rectus abdominis (Fig. 14.40). The hernia may involve the omentum only, or it may mimic other masses. The hernia commonly originates near the junction of the linea semilunaris and arcuate line in the paraumbilical area.

Epigastric hernias are found in the widest part of the linea alba between the xiphoid process and the umbilicus. This hernia is usually filled with fat, which over the years may carry a piece of omentum along with it.

A spigelian hernia is a variant of the ventral hernia, which is found more laterally in the abdominal wall.

Sonographic Findings. Many hernias are palpable and do not require sonographic evaluation. However, if the mass is not well defined on physical examination, ultrasound evaluation may be helpful. If a hernia is present, the sonographer will note an interruption of the peritoneal line separating the muscles and abdominal contents.

Sonography may outline the contents of the mass where it is fluid-filled or contains peristaltic bowel or mesenteric fat. The sonographer should look for bowel peristalsis within the mass, although the peristalsis may be absent with incarceration (Fig. 14.41). If the hernia is not readily apparent, the patient may be asked to lift the head or strain (Valsalva maneuver) to see if the mass moves or changes shape. The sonographic criteria for a hernia include (1) demonstration of an abdominal wall defect, (2) presence of bowel loops or mesenteric fat within a lesion, (3) exaggeration of the lesion with strain (Valsalva), and (4) reducibility of the lesion by gentle pressure.

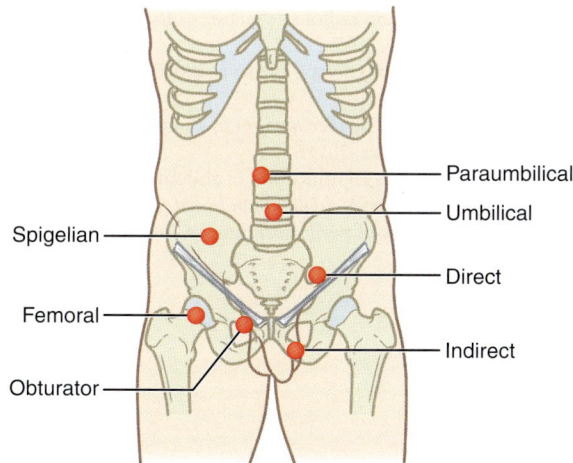

FIG. 14.40 Common locations of hernias in the abdominal and pelvic cavities.

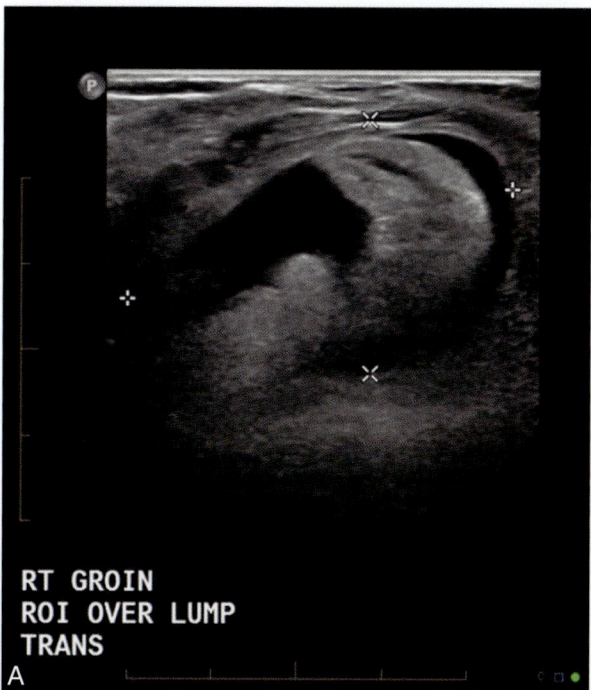

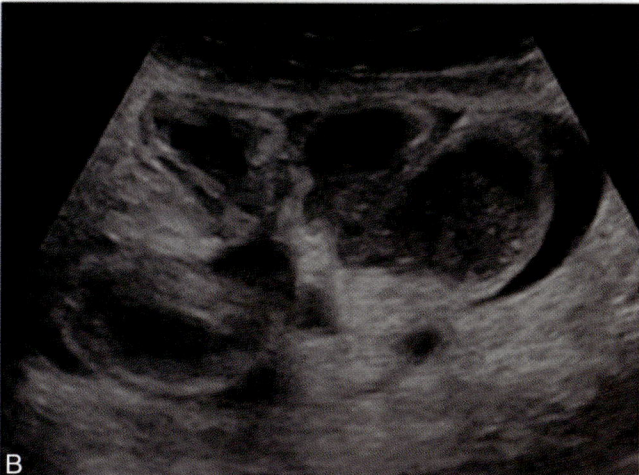

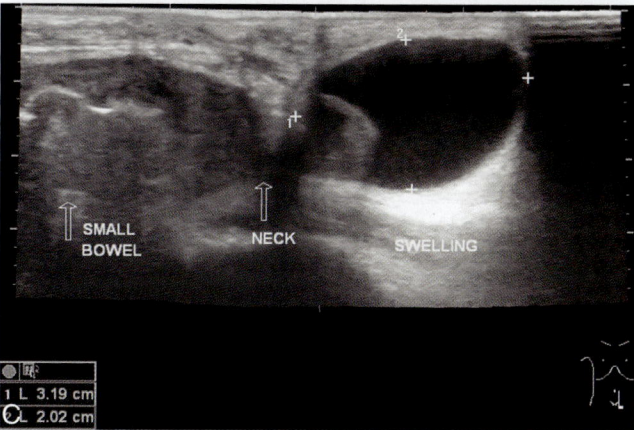

FIG. 14.41 Sonography may outline the contents of the mass where it is fluid-filled or contains peristaltic bowel or mesenteric fat. The sonographer should look for bowel peristalsis within the mass, although the peristalsis may be absent with incarceration. If the hernia is not readily apparent, the patient may be asked to lift the head or to strain (Valsalva maneuver) to see if the mass moves or changes shape.

Key Pearls

- The peritoneal cavity is made up of multiple peritoneal ligaments and folds that connect the viscera to each other and the abdominopelvic walls.
- Within the cavity are the lesser and greater omentum, the mesenteries, the ligaments, and multiple fluid spaces (lesser sac, perihepatic and subphrenic spaces).
- The section that lines the walls of the cavity is the parietal peritoneum, whereas the part covering the abdominal organs to a greater or lesser extent is the visceral peritoneum.
- The general peritoneal cavity is known as the greater sac of the peritoneum. With the development of the stomach and the spleen, a smaller sac, called the lesser sac (omental bursa), is the peritoneal recess posterior to the stomach.
- The attachments of the peritoneum to the abdominal walls and organs help determine how abnormal collections of fluid within the peritoneal cavity can collect or move.
- Because of the coronary ligament attachments, collections in the right posterior subphrenic space cannot extend between the bare area of the liver and the diaphragm.
- Ligaments on the right side of the liver form the subphrenic and subhepatic spaces.
- The *bare area* is delineated by the right superior and inferior coronary ligaments, which separate the posterior subphrenic space from the right superior subhepatic space (Morison's pouch).
- A single large and irregular perihepatic space surrounds the superior and lateral aspects of the left lobe of the liver, with the left coronary ligaments anatomically separating the subphrenic space into anterior and posterior compartments.
- The retrovesical space is divided by the uterus into an anterior vesicouterine recess and a posterior rectouterine sac (pouch of Douglas).
- Ascites is the accumulation of serous fluid in the peritoneal cavity.
- An abscess is a cavity formed by necrosis within a solid tissue or a circumscribed collection of purulent material.
- A mass or lesion within the mesentery and omentum may have solid or cystic characteristics, whereas a mass within the peritoneum may show an infiltrative pattern.
- With an omental mass, at least one-third of these lesions are malignant, and secondary neoplasms are more frequent than primary.
- In the mesentery, a benign primary tumor is more common than a malignant tumor, and secondary neoplasms are more frequent than primary.
- A cystic mass is more common than a solid mass in the mesentery.
- A urachal cyst is an incomplete regression of the urachus during development.
- A urinoma, an encapsulated collection of urine, may result from a closed renal injury or surgical intervention or may develop spontaneously secondary to an obstructing lesion.
- Lymphoma presents as a uniformly thick, hypoechoic, band-shaped structure that follows the convexity of the anterior and lateral abdominal wall, creating the omental band.
- Secondary tumors and lymphoma are neoplasms that most commonly involve the peritoneum and mesentery.
- Lesions found within the superficial abdominal wall include inflammatory lesions, hematomas, neoplasms, hernias, and postsurgical lesions.
- A lymphocele is a collection of fluid that occurs after surgery in the pelvis, retroperitoneum, or recess cavities.
- Extraperitoneal rectus sheath hematomas are acute or chronic collections of blood lying either within the rectus muscle or between the muscle and its sheath.
- Neoplasms of the abdominal wall include lipomas, desmoid tumors, or metastases.
- An abdominal hernia is the protrusion of a peritoneal-lined sac through a defect in the weakened abdominal wall.

BIBLIOGRAPHY

Abrahams PH, Boon J, Spratt JD. *McMinn's Clinical Atlas of Human Anatomy with DVD*. St Louis: Elsevier; 2008.
Damjanov I. *Pathology for the Health Professions*. 3rd ed. Philadelphia: Elsevier; 2006.
Damjanov I, Linder J. *Pathology: A Color Atlas*. St Louis: Mosby; 2000.
Fakuda T, Sakamoto I, Kohzaki S, et al. Spontaneous rectus sheath hematomas: clinical and radiologic features. *Abdom Imaging*. 1996;21:58–61.
Gould BE, Dyer R. *Pathophysiology for the Health Professions*. 4th ed. Philadelphia: Elsevier; 2011.
Hanbidge AE, Wilson SR. *The Peritoneum in Diagnostic Ultrasound*. 4th ed. St Louis: Elsevier; 2011.
Sudheer G. Sonography in identification of abdominal wall lesions presenting as palpable masses. *J Ultrasound Med*. 2006;25:1199–1209.
Yeh HC. Ultrasonography of peritoneal tumors. *Radiology*. 1979;133:419–424.

CHAPTER 15

Urinary System

Kerry Weinberg, Shpetim Telegrafi, and Mariana Kozirovsky

OBJECTIVES

On completion of this chapter, you should be able to:
- Discuss normal anatomic location, function, and sonographic appearance of urinary system organs
- Discuss normal physiology of the urinary system
- Describe the sonographic scanning technique to image the urinary system
- Define and discuss the pathologies discussed in this chapter
- Identify and define the sonographic appearance of pathologies included in this chapter
- Describe the clinical signs and symptoms of urinary tract problems and the laboratory tests that are used to evaluate them

OUTLINE

Anatomy of the Urinary System 435
   Normal Anatomy 435
   Vascular Supply 437
Physiology and Laboratory Data of the Urinary System 438
   Excretion 438
   Laboratory Tests for Renal Disease 438
Sonographic Evaluation of the Urinary System 439
   Kidneys 439
   Renal Variants 444

Renal Anomalies 445
Evaluation of a Renal Mass 449
Aspiration of Renal Masses 449
Lower Urinary Tract 450
Bladder 451
Pathology of the Urinary System 453
   Renal Cystic Disease 453
   Medullary Cystic Disease 462
   Renal Neoplasms 463
   Renal Disease 468
   Renal Failure 473
   Hydronephrosis 474

Renal Infections 478
Urinary Tract Calcifications 479
Renal Artery Stenosis 480
Renal Infarction 481
Arteriovenous Fistulas and Pseudoaneurysm 482
Kidney Stone (Urolithiasis) 483
Bladder Diverticulum 485
Bladder Inflammation (Cystitis) 485
Bladder Tumors 486

KEY TERMS

Afferent arteriole
Arcuate arteries
Blood urea nitrogen (BUN)
Bowman capsule
Calyx
Columns of Bertin
Cortex
Creatinine (Cr)
Dromedary hump
Ectopic kidney
Efferent arteriole
Gerota fascia
Glomerulus

Hilus
Homeostasis
Horseshoe kidney
Hydronephrosis
Loop of Henle
Major calyces
Medulla
Minor calyces
Morison's pouch
Nephron
Renal agenesis
Renal capsule
Renal corpuscle

Renal ectopia
Renal hilum
Renal hypoplasia
Renal pelvis
Renal pyramids
Renal sinus
Retroperitoneum
Specific gravity
Ureter
Urethra
Urinary bladder
Urolithiasis

The urinary system has two principal functions: excreting wastes and regulating the composition of blood. Blood composition must not be allowed to vary beyond tolerable limits, or the conditions in tissue necessary for cellular life will be lost. Regulating blood composition involves not only removing harmful wastes but also conserving water and metabolites in the body.

ANATOMY OF THE URINARY SYSTEM

Normal Anatomy

Kidneys. The urinary system is located posterior to the peritoneum lining the abdominal cavity in an area called the

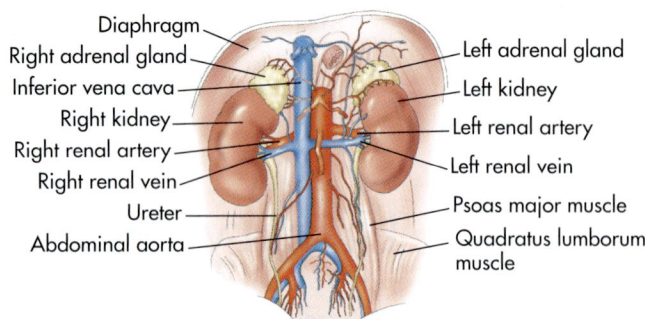

FIG. 15.1 Relationships of the kidneys, suprarenal glands (adrenal), and vascular structures to one another.

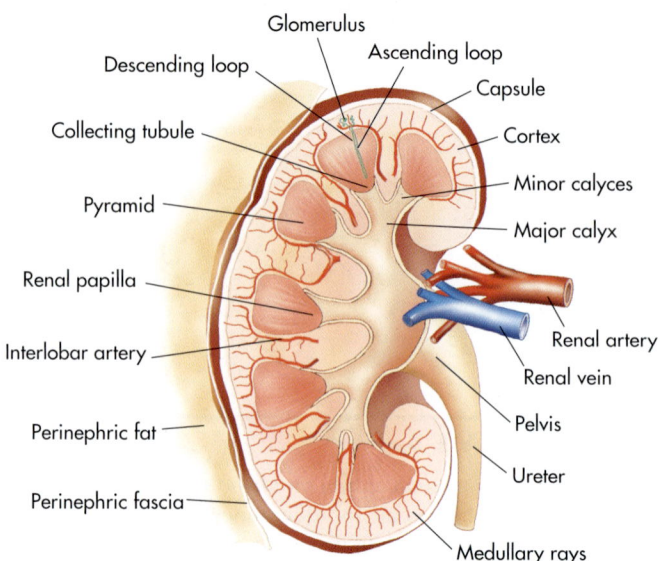

FIG. 15.2 The kidney cut longitudinally to show the internal structure.

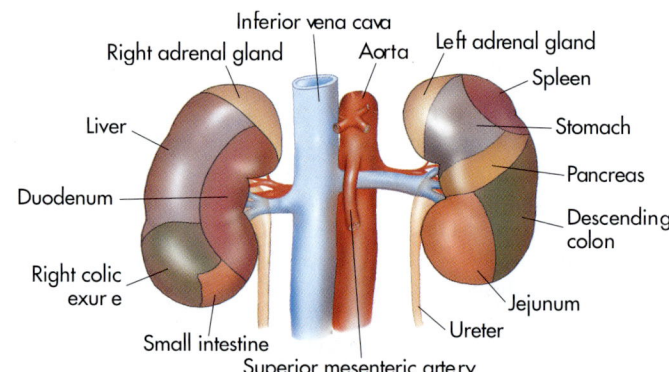

FIG. 15.3 Anatomic structures related to the anterior surfaces of the kidneys.

retroperitoneum. The kidneys lie in the retroperitoneal cavity near the posterior body wall, just below the diaphragm (Fig. 15.1). The lower ribs protect both kidneys. The right kidney lies slightly inferior to the left kidney because the large right lobe of the liver pushes it inferiorly. The kidneys move readily with respiration; on deep inspiration, both kidneys move downward approximately 1 inch.

The kidneys are dark red, bean-shaped organs that measure 9 to 12 cm long, 5 cm wide, and 2.5 cm thick. The outer **cortex** of the kidney is darker than the inner **medulla** because of the increased perfusion of blood. The inner surface of the medulla is folded into projections called **renal pyramids**, which empty into the renal calyces. The **arcuate arteries** are located at the base of the pyramids and separate the medulla from the cortex. Numerous collecting tubules bring the urine from its sites of formation in the cortex to the pyramids. The renal tubules, or **nephrons**, are the functional units of the kidney.

On the medial surface of each kidney is a vertical indentation called the **renal hilum**, where the renal vessels and ureter enter and exit. Within the **hilus** of the kidney are other vascular structures, a ureter, and the lymphatics. The renal artery is posterior and superior to the renal veins. The two branches of the renal vein are anterior to the renal artery (Fig. 15.2). The ureter is located slightly inferior to the renal artery. When present, the third branch of the renal artery may be seen to arise from the hilus. The lymph vessels and sympathetic fibers also are found within the renal hilus.

Three layers of tissue surround and protect the kidneys. The inner layer that surrounds the kidney is a fibrous capsule called the true capsule. The next layer, which covers the fibrous capsule, is perinephric fat. The outer most layer is the perinephric fascia, which surrounds the perinephric fat and encloses the kidneys and adrenal glands. The perinephric fascia is a condensation of areolar tissue that is continuous laterally with the fascia transversalis. The renal fascia, known as **Gerota fascia**, surrounds the true capsule and perinephric fat.

Anterior to the right kidney are the right adrenal gland, liver, **Morison's pouch**, second part of the duodenum, and right colic flexure (Fig. 15.3). Anterior to the left kidney are the left adrenal gland, spleen, stomach, pancreatic tail, left colic flexure, and coils of jejunum.

Posterior to the right kidney are the diaphragm, costodiaphragmatic recess of the pleura, twelfth rib, psoas muscle, quadratus lumborum, and transversus abdominis muscles. The subcostal (T12), iliohypogastric, and ilioinguinal (L1) nerves run downward and laterally. Posterior to the left kidney are the diaphragm, costodiaphragmatic recess of the pleura, eleventh and twelve ribs, psoas muscle, quadratus lumborum, and transversus abdominis muscles. The same nerves are seen near the left kidney as in the right.

Within the kidney, the upper expanded end of the ureter, known as the **renal pelvis** of the ureter, divides into two or three **major calyces**, each of which divides further into two or three **minor calyces** (see Fig. 15.2). The apex of a medullary pyramid, called the renal papilla, indents each minor **calyx**. The kidney consists of an internal medullary portion and an external cortical substance. The medullary substance consists of a series of striated conical masses, called the renal pyramids. The pyramids vary from 8 to 18 in number, and their bases are directed toward the outer circumference of the kidney. Their apices converge toward the **renal sinus**, where their prominent papillae project into the lumina of the minor calyces. Spirally arranged muscles surround the calyces and may exert a milking action on these tubes, aiding in the flow of urine into the renal pelvis. As the pelvis leaves the renal sinus, it rapidly becomes smaller and ultimately merges with the ureter.

Nephron. The nephrons are in the renal parenchyma and consist of two main structures: a renal corpuscle and a renal tubule. Nephrons filter the blood and produce urine. Blood is filtered in the renal corpuscle. The filtered fluid passes through the renal tubule. As the filtrate moves through the tubule, substances needed by the body are returned to the blood. Waste products, excess water, and other substances not needed by the body pass into the collecting ducts as urine.

The **renal corpuscle** consists of a network of capillaries called the **glomerulus**, which is surrounded by a cup-like structure known as **Bowman capsule**. Blood flows into the glomerulus through a small **afferent arteriole** and leaves the glomerulus through an **efferent arteriole**. This arteriole conducts blood to a second set of capillaries, the peritubular capillaries, which surround the renal tubule.

Filtrate passes into the renal tubule through an opening in the bottom of Bowman capsule. The first part of the renal tubule is the coiled proximal convoluted tubule. After passing through the proximal convoluted tubule, filtrate flows into the **loop of Henle** and then into the distal convoluted tubule. Urine from the distal convoluted tubules of several nephrons drains into a collecting duct. A portion of the distal convoluted tubule curves upward and contacts the afferent and efferent arterioles. Some cells of the distal convoluted tubule and some cells of the afferent arteriole are modified to form the juxtaglomerular apparatus, a structure that helps regulate blood pressure in the kidney.

The renal corpuscle, the proximal convoluted tubule, and the distal convoluted tubule of each nephron are located within the renal cortex. The loops of Henle dip down into the medulla.

Ureter. The **ureter** is a 25-cm tubular structure whose proximal end is expanded and continuous with the funnel shape of the renal pelvis. The renal pelvis lies within the hilus of the kidney and receives major calyces. The ureter emerges from the hilus of the kidney and runs vertically downward behind the parietal peritoneum along the psoas muscle, which separates it from the tips of the transverse processes of the lumbar vertebrae. It enters the pelvis by crossing the bifurcation of the common iliac artery anterior to the sacroiliac joint. The ureter courses along the lateral wall of the pelvis to the region of the ischial spine and turns forward to enter the lateral angle of the bladder. The ureter from the ureteropelvic junction to the bladder is not routinely visualized on a sonogram. The ureters are in the retroperitoneal cavity with the superior and distal ends of the ureters more readily visualized than the midsection due to overlying bowel gas.

Constrictions can occur along three areas of the ureter's course: (1) where the ureter leaves the renal pelvis, (2) where it crosses the pelvic brim, and (3) where it pierces the bladder wall.

Urinary Bladder. The **urinary bladder** is a large muscular bag located above and behind the pubic bone. It has a posterior and lateral opening for the ureters and an anterior opening for the urethra. The interior of the bladder is lined with highly elastic transitional epithelium. When the bladder is full, the lining is smooth and stretched; when it is empty, the lining is a series of folds. In the middle layer, a series of smooth muscle coats distend as urine collects and contract to expel urine through the urethra. Urine is produced almost continuously and accumulates in the bladder until the increased pressure stimulates the organ's nervous receptors to relax the urethra's sphincter and urine is released from the urinary bladder. The urinary bladder is visualized sonographically when it is distended with fluid.

Urethra. The **urethra** is a membranous tube that passes from the anterior part of the urinary bladder to the outside of the body. It includes two sphincters: the internal sphincter and the external sphincter. The urethra is not routinely visualized sonographically.

Vascular Supply

The main renal artery supplies blood to the kidney. When a person is at rest, approximately 1.2 liters of blood per minute is pumped to the kidneys. The renal arteries are lateral branches of the aorta that are located just inferior to the superior mesenteric artery (Fig. 15.4). The branches of the renal artery may vary in size and number. In most cases, the renal artery is divided into two primary branches: a larger anterior and a smaller posterior. These arteries break down into smaller segmental arteries, then into interlobar arteries, and finally into tiny arcuate arteries.

Five to six veins join to form the main renal vein. This vein emerges from the renal hilus anterior to the renal artery. The renal vein drains into the lateral walls of the inferior vena cava (see Fig. 15.4). The left renal vein courses transversely across the body going anterior to the aorta and posterior to the superior mesenteric artery.

The lymphatic vessels follow the renal artery to the lateral aortic lymph nodes near the origin of the renal artery. Nerves originate in the renal sympathetic plexus and are distributed along the branches of the renal vessels.

Blood supply to nephrons begins at the renal artery. The artery subdivides within the kidneys. A small vessel (afferent

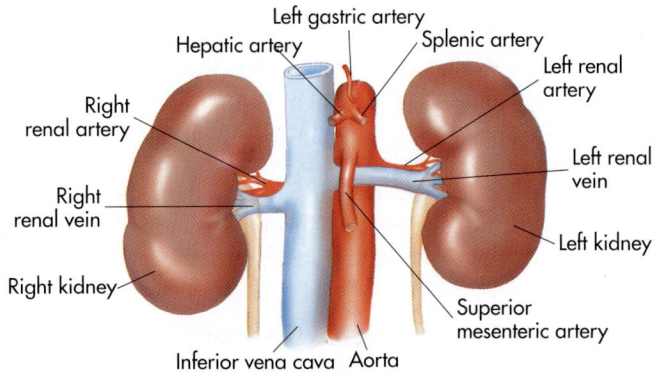

FIG. 15.4 Vascular relationships of the great vessels and their tributaries to the kidneys.

arteriole) enters Bowman capsule, where it forms a tuft of capillaries, the glomerulus, which entirely fills the concavity of the capsule. Blood leaves the glomerulus via the efferent arteriole, which subdivides into a network of capillaries that surround the proximal and distal tubules and eventually unite as veins, which become the renal vein.

The renal vein returns the cleansed blood to the general circulation. Movements of substances between the nephron and the capillaries of the tubules change the composition of the blood filtrate moving along in the tubules. From the nephrons, the fluid moves to collecting tubules and into the ureter, leading to the bladder, where urine is stored.

The arterial supply to the ureter is provided by the following three sources: the renal artery, the testicular or ovarian artery, and the superior vesical artery.

PHYSIOLOGY AND LABORATORY DATA OF THE URINARY SYSTEM

The urinary system consists of two kidneys, which remove wastes from the blood and produce urine, and two ureters, which act as tubal ducts leading from the hilus of the kidneys and drain into the urinary bladder. The bladder collects and stores urine, which is eventually discharged through the urethra. The urinary system is located posterior to the peritoneum lining the abdominal cavity in an area called the retroperitoneum.

The function of the kidneys is to excrete urine. More than any other organ, the kidneys regulate the amounts of water and electrolytes leaving the body so that these equal the amounts of substances entering the body. The formation of urine involves the following three processes: glomerular filtration, tubular reabsorption, and tubular secretion.

Excretion

Cells in the body continually carry on metabolic activities that produce waste products. If permitted to accumulate, metabolic wastes eventually reach toxic concentrations and threaten **homeostasis**. To prevent this, metabolic wastes must be quickly excreted. The process of excretion entails separating and removing substances harmful to the body. The skin, lungs, liver, large intestine, and kidneys carry out excretion.

The principal metabolic waste products are water, carbon dioxide, and nitrogenous wastes, including urea, uric acid, and **creatinine (Cr)**. Nitrogen is derived from amino acids and nucleic acids. Amino acids break down in the liver, and the nitrogen-containing amino group is removed. The amino group is then converted to ammonia, which is chemically converted to urea. Uric acid is formed from the breakdown of nucleic acids. Both urea and uric acid are carried away from the liver into the kidneys by the vascular system. Creatinine is nitrogenous waste produced from phosphocreatine in the muscles.

Laboratory Tests for Renal Disease

The clinical symptoms of a patient with specific renal pathology may be nonspecific. Therefore a patient with symptoms of renal infection, renal insufficiency, or disease may undergo several laboratory tests to help the clinician determine the cause of the problem.

A patient's history of infection, previous urinary tract problems (renal stones), or hypertension or family history of renal cystic disease is useful information. A patient with a renal infection or disease process may have any of the following symptoms: flank pain, hematuria, polyuria, oliguria, fever, urgency, weight loss, or general edema.

Urinalysis. Urinalysis is essential to detect urinary tract disorders in patients whose renal function is impaired or absent. Most renal inflammatory processes introduce a characteristic exudate for a specific type of inflammation into the urine. The presence of an acute infection causes *hematuria* (red blood cells in the urine), which may be microscopic, or *pyuria*, pus in the urine.

Urine pH. Urine pH is very important in managing diseases such as bacteriuria and renal calculi. The pH refers to the strength of the urine as a partly acidic or alkaline solution. The abundance of hydrogen ions in a solution is called pH. If urine contains an increased concentration of hydrogen ions, the urine is acidic. The formation of renal calculi depends in part on the pH of urine. Other conditions, such as renal tubular acidosis and chronic renal failure, are associated with alkaline urine.

Specific Gravity. The **specific gravity** is the measurement of the kidney's ability to concentrate urine. The concentration factor depends on the quantity of dissolved waste products. Excessive intake of fluids or decreased perspiration may cause a large output of urine and a decrease in the specific gravity. Low fluid intake, excessive perspiration, or diarrhea can cause the output of urine to be low and the specific gravity to increase. The specific gravity is especially low in cases of renal failure, glomerular nephritis, and pyelonephritis. These diseases cause renal tubular damage, which affects the ability of the kidneys to concentrate urine.

Blood. Hematuria is the appearance of blood cells in the urine; it can be associated with early renal disease. An abundance of red blood cells in the urine may suggest renal trauma, neoplasm, calculi, pyelonephritis, or glomerular or vascular inflammatory processes, such as acute glomerulonephritis and renal infarction.

Leukocytes may be present whenever inflammation, infection, or tissue necrosis originates from anywhere in the urinary tract.

Hematocrit. The hematocrit is the relative ratio of plasma to packed cell volume in the blood. Decreased hematocrit occurs with acute hemorrhagic processes secondary to disease or blunt trauma.

Hemoglobin. Hemoglobin is present in urine whenever extensive damage or destruction of the functioning erythrocytes occurs. This condition injures the kidney and can cause acute renal failure.

Protein. When glomerular damage is evident, albumin and other plasma proteins may be filtered in excess, allowing the overflow to enter the urine, which lowers the blood serum albumin concentration. Albuminuria is commonly found with benign and malignant neoplasms, calculi, chronic infection, and pyelonephritis.

Creatinine Clearance. Specific measurements of creatinine concentrations in urine and blood serum are considered an accurate index for determining the glomerular filtration rate. Creatinine is a by-product of muscle energy metabolism; it is normally produced at a constant rate if the body muscle mass remains relatively constant. Creatinine normally goes through complete glomerular filtration without being reabsorbed by the renal tubules. Decreased urinary creatinine clearance indicates renal dysfunction because creatinine blood levels are constant, and only decreased renal function prevents the normal excretion of creatinine.

Blood Urea Nitrogen. The **blood urea nitrogen (BUN)** is the concentration of urea nitrogen in blood and is the end product of cellular metabolism. Urea is formed in the liver and is carried to the kidneys through the blood to be excreted in urine. Impairment of renal function and increased protein catabolism result in BUN elevation that is relative to the degree of renal impairment and the rate of urea nitrogen excretion by the kidneys.

Serum Creatinine. Renal dysfunction also results in serum creatinine elevation. Blood serum creatinine levels are said to be more specific and more sensitive in determining renal impairment than BUN.

SONOGRAPHIC EVALUATION OF THE URINARY SYSTEM

Kidneys

Sonographic evaluation of the kidneys is a noninvasive, relatively inexpensive, reproducible diagnostic test used to evaluate renal anatomy and pathology. In patients with renal colic without a history of renal stones, a noncontrast computed tomography (NCCT) is typically performed. NCCT requires no patient preparation and is not operator or patient dependent. The main disadvantages of NCCT are cost and the use of ionizing radiation. Patients with a history of renal stones require a plain film x-ray, and a renal sonogram with Doppler is usually the first diagnostic test performed.

Magnetic resonance imaging (MRI) using magnetic resonance urography (MRU) is currently being investigated for diagnosing renal disease. MRU can assess renal function, in addition to diagnosing obstructive uropathy. MRI can assess other abdominal organs for disease.

A renal sonogram can identify the presence and location of both kidneys, image renal congenital anomalies, determine renal size, show parenchymal detail, and delineate an abnormal lie of a kidney resulting from an extrarenal mass. In addition, sonography can demonstrate the acoustic properties of a mass, or determine whether hydronephrosis is secondary to renal stones. Sonography can also define perirenal fluid collections, such as a hematoma, lymphocele, urinoma, or an abscess, and detect dilated ureters and **hydronephrosis**.

Normal Texture and Patterns. The normal sonographic appearance of the kidneys includes a smooth thin border due to the reflected echoes of perirenal fat. The renal parenchyma surrounds the fatty central renal sinus, which contains

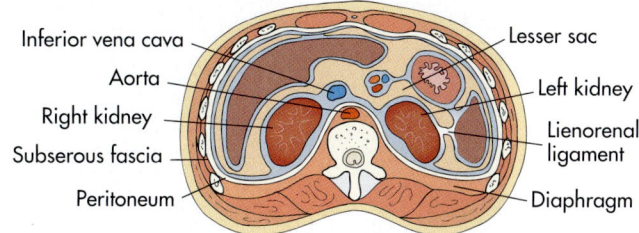

FIG. 15.5 Transverse section of the abdominal cavity through the epiploic foramen.

the calyces, infundibula, pelvis, vessels, and lymphatics (Fig. 15.5). Because of the fat interface, the renal sinus is imaged as an area of intense echoes with variable contours. If two separate collections of renal sinus fat are identified, a double collecting system should be suspected.

Generally, patients are given nothing by mouth before a sonogram or other imaging examinations are performed. This state of dehydration causes the infundibula and renal pelvis to be collapsed and thus indistinguishable from the echo-dense renal sinus fat. If, on the other hand, the bladder is distended from rehydration, the intrarenal collecting system also will become distended. If an extrarenal pelvis is present it may be seen as a fluid-filled structure medial to the kidney on transverse scans extending outside the renal border. The normal variant from obstruction is differentiated by noting the absence of a distended intrasinus portion of the renal pelvis and infundibula. Dilation of the collecting system has also been noted in pregnant patients. (The right kidney is generally involved with a mild degree of hydronephrosis. This distention returns to normal shortly after delivery.)

Patient Position and Technique. The patient should be in a supine and/or decubitus position using the liver as a window to image the right kidney (Figs. 15.6 and 15.7) or through the spleen for the left kidney (Fig. 15.8). Several alternative scanning windows can be used to image the kidney. These include the right posterior oblique, right lateral decubitus, and left lateral decubitus views. Having the patient take in a deep breath will move the liver and spleen distally, which may create a better window to enhance visualization of the kidneys. A subcostal or intercostal transducer approach may be used for visualization of the upper and lower poles of the kidneys.

Proper adjustment of time gain compensation (TGC) with adequate sensitivity settings allows a uniform acoustic pattern throughout the image. The renal cortical echo amplitude should be compared with the normal liver parenchymal echo amplitude at the same depth to effectively set the TGC and sensitivity.

If the patient has a substantial amount of perirenal fat, a high-frequency transducer may not provide the penetration necessary to optimally visualize the area. The deeper areas of the kidney may appear hypoechoic. Renal detail may also be obscured if the patient has hepatocellular disease, gallstones, rib interference (Figs. 15.9 and 15.10), or other abnormal collections between the liver and kidney. The use of harmonic imaging or tissue contrast enhancement technology (Fig. 15.11) may help to optimize visualization of the kidneys.

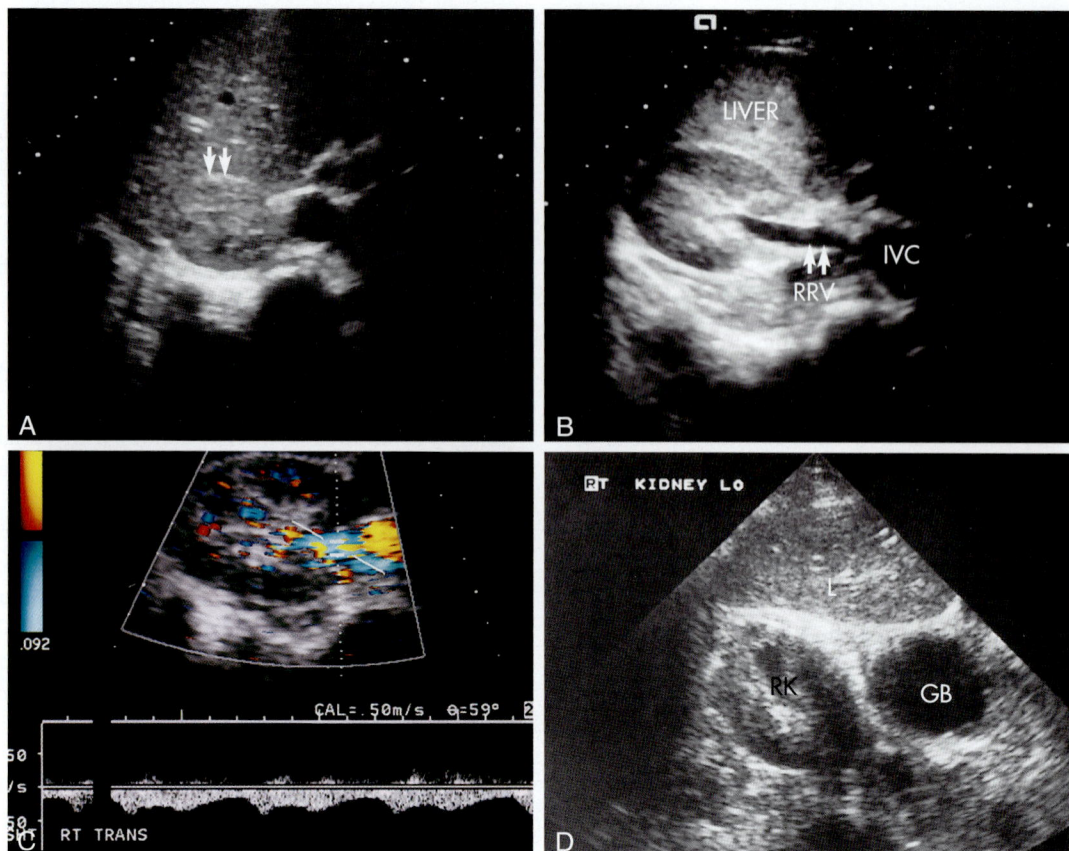

FIG. 15.6 (A–B) Transverse scan of the normal upper pole of the right kidney imaged through the homogeneous liver. Scans are made from the upper pole, from the mid pole to include the right renal vein (RRV), and from the inferior vena cava (IVC) to the lower pole. (C) Normal blood flow is seen through the right renal vein to the IVC. (D) A slight decubitus position allows the liver (L) to roll anterior to the right kidney (RK) and gallbladder (GB) for better visualization.

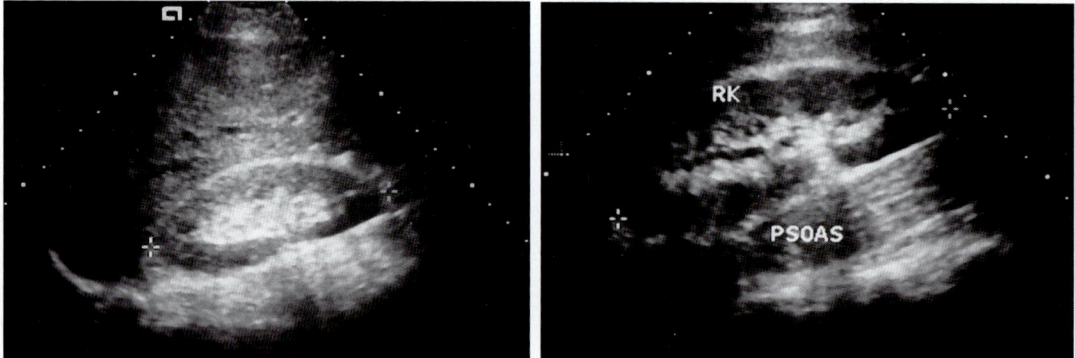

FIG. 15.7 Longitudinal scans through the long axis of the right kidney (RK) and psoas muscle. Measurements are made along the maximum length of the right kidney from upper pole to lower pole.

Renal Parenchyma. The parenchyma is the area from the renal sinus to the outer renal surface (Fig. 15.12). The arcuate arteries and interlobar vessels are found within and are best demonstrated as intense specular echoes in cross section or oblique section at the corticomedullary junction.

The cortex generally is mid-level echo producing (Fig. 15.13A) (although its echoes are less echogenic than those from normal liver), whereas the medullary pyramids are hypoechoic (Fig. 15.13B). The two are separated from each other by bands of cortical tissue, called columns of Bertin, which extend inward to the renal sinus.

Diseases of the renal parenchyma are those that accentuate cortical echoes but preserve or exaggerate the corticomedullary junction (type I) and those that distort the normal anatomy, obliterating the corticomedullary differentiation in a focal or diffuse manner (type II).

Criteria for type I changes include the following: (1) The echo intensity in the cortex must be equal to or greater than

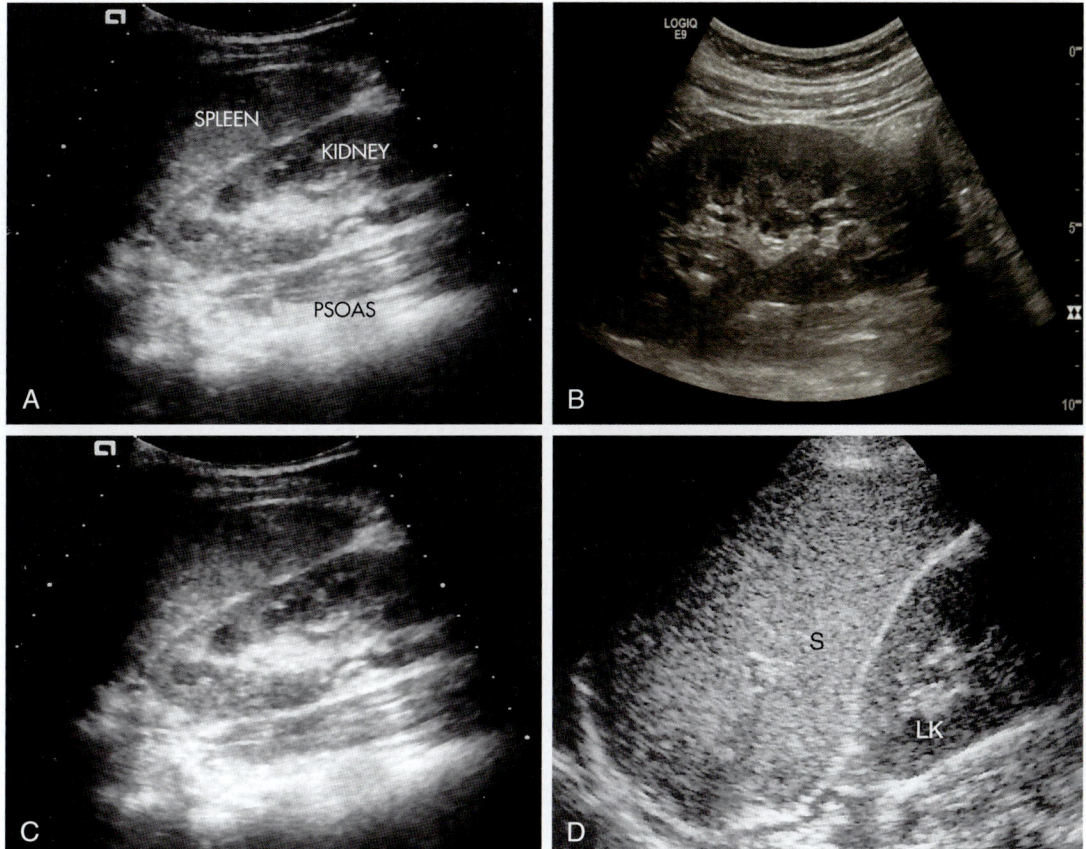

FIG. 15.8 (A) Longitudinal scan of the normal left kidney as imaged through the homogeneous spleen. The psoas muscle is the posterior medial border of the kidney. (B) Measurements are made along the maximum length of the kidney from the upper pole to the lower pole. (C) The patient may be rolled into a right lateral decubitus position for better visualization of the renal medullary pyramids and parenchyma. (D) Splenomegaly (S) aids in visualization of the upper pole of the left kidney (LK).

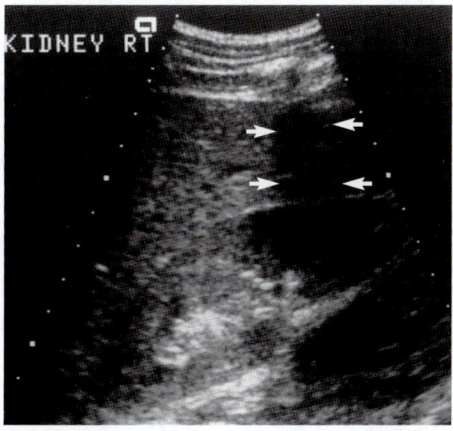

FIG. 15.9 The ribs may interfere with uniform visualization of the kidney. Variations in respiration help the sonographer find the best window through which to image the renal parenchyma without rib interference.

that in the adjacent liver or spleen, and (2) the echo intensity in the cortex must be equal to that in the adjacent renal sinus. Minor signs would include the loss of identifiable arcuate vessels and the accentuation of corticomedullary definition.

Type II changes can be seen in focal disruption of normal anatomy with any mass lesion, including cysts, tumors, abscesses, and hematomas.

Renal Vessels. The arteries are best seen with the supine and left lateral decubitus views (right side up). The right renal artery extends from the lateral wall of the aorta to enter the central renal sinus (Figs. 15.14 and 15.15). On the longitudinal scan, the right renal artery can be seen as a round anechoic structure posterior to the inferior vena cava. The right renal vein extends from the central renal sinus directly into the inferior vena cava (Fig. 15.16). Both vessels appear as tubular structures in the transverse plane.

The renal arteries have an echo-free central lumen with highly echogenic borders that consist of a vessel wall and surrounding retroperitoneal fat and connective tissue. They lie posterior to the veins and can be demonstrated with certainty if their junction with the aorta is seen.

The left renal artery flows from the lateral wall of the aorta to the central renal sinus (Fig. 15.17). The left renal vein flows from the central renal sinus, anterior to the aorta and posterior to the superior mesenteric artery, to join the inferior vena cava (Fig. 15.18). It is seen as a tubular structure on the transverse scan.

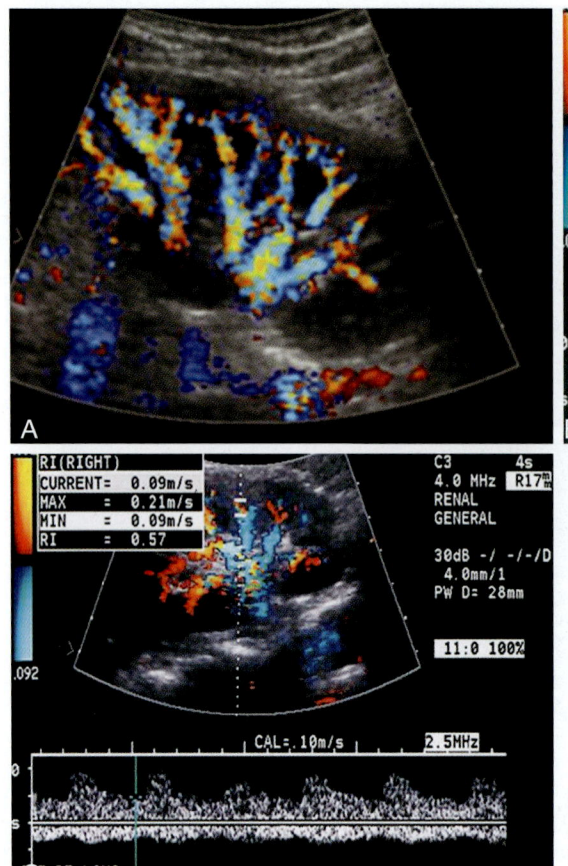

FIG. 15.10 (A) Longitudinal scan of the interlobar arteries facing the renal pyramids and the peripheral arcuate arteries. (B) Spectral arterial waveform of the interlobar arteries. (C) Spectral waveform of the arcuate arteries.

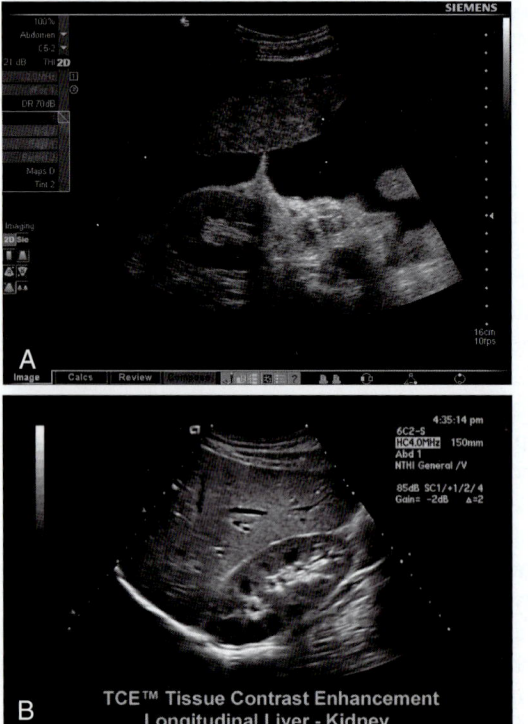

FIG. 15.11 (A) Transverse view of right kidney with ascites in Morison's pouch. (B) Sagittal view of normal liver/kidney using tissue contrast enhancement technology. (Courtesy Siemens Medical Solutions USA, Inc.)

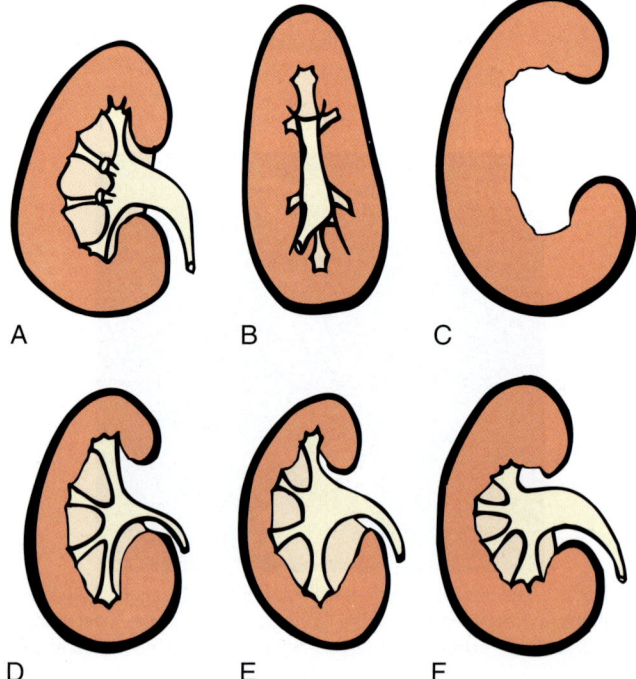

FIG. 15.12 (A) Thickness of the renal substance. (B) Medial plane showing the pelvis emerging through the hilum and minimal thickness anteriorly and posteriorly. (C) Hypertrophy. (D) Normal adult proportions of the renal substance. (E) Senile atrophy. (F) Normal appearance in a 2-year-old child.

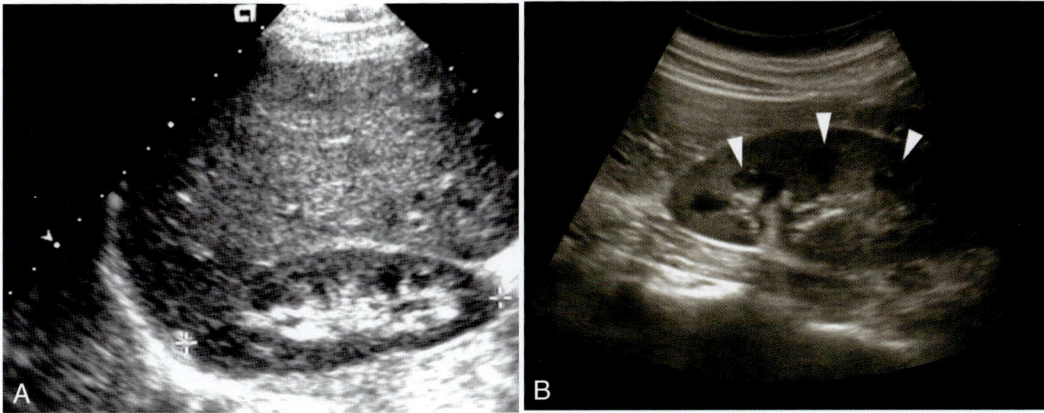

FIG. 15.13 Sagittal scan of the normal kidney. The cortex is the brightest of the echoes within the renal parenchyma. The medullary pyramids are echo free. The pyramids are separated from the cortex by bands of cortical tissue and the columns of Bertin that extend inward to the renal sinus. (A) Echogenic renal cortex. (B) Hypoechoic renal pyramids.

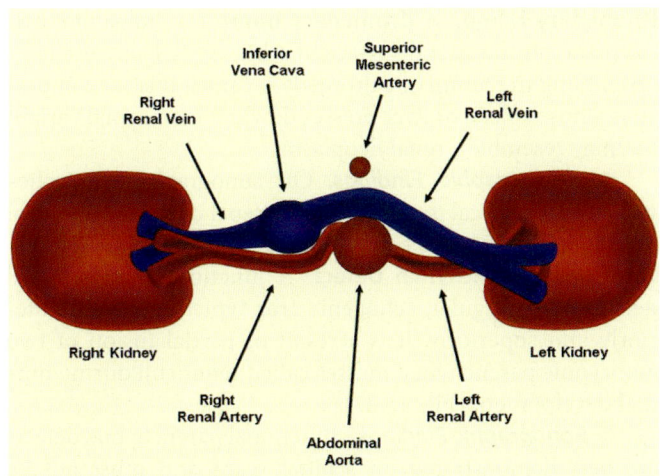

FIG. 15.14 The right renal artery extends from the lateral wall of the aorta to enter the central renal sinus.

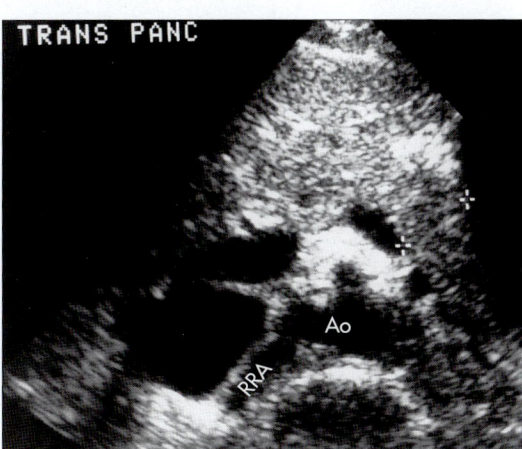

FIG. 15.15 Transverse image of the right renal artery (RRA) as it extends from the posterior lateral wall of the aorta (Ao) to enter the central renal sinus.

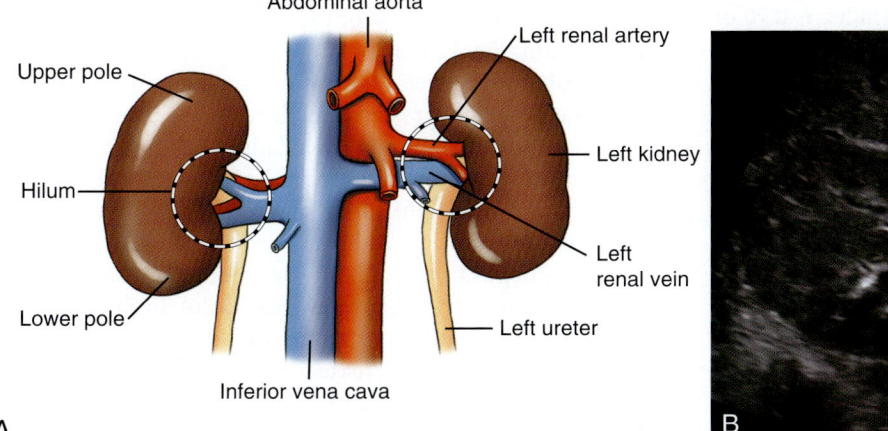
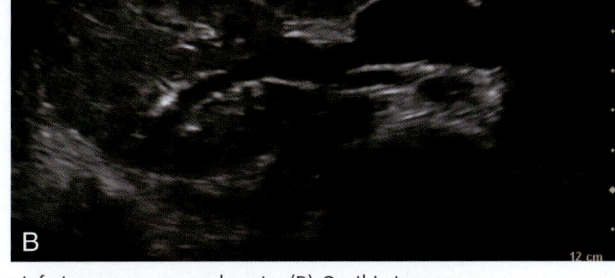

FIG. 15.16 (A) The relationship of the renal vessels to the inferior vena cava and aorta. (B) On this transverse image, the right renal vein extends from the central renal sinus directly into the inferior vena cava.

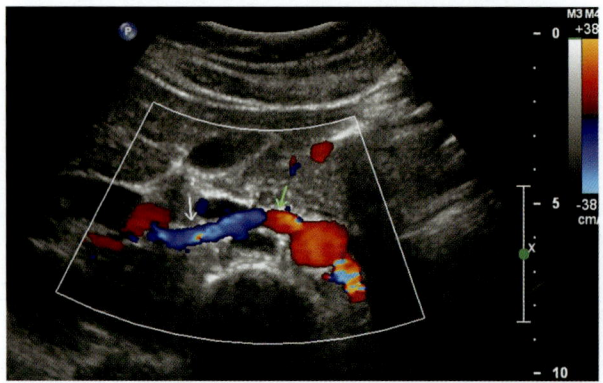

FIG. 15.17 The right and left renal arteries arise from the lateral wall of the aorta.

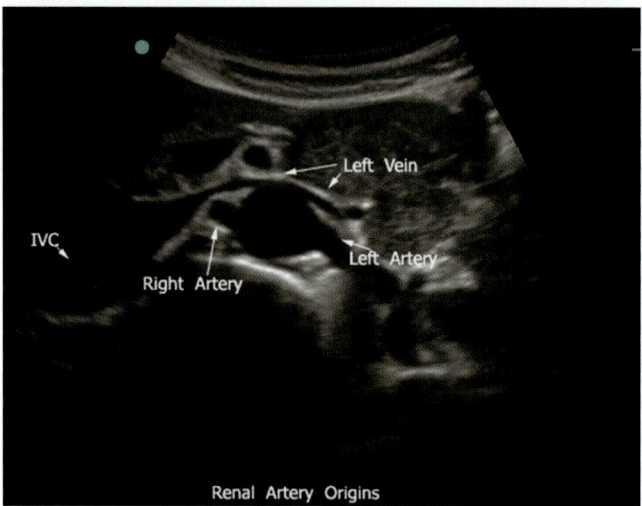

FIG. 15.18 The left renal artery *(arrows)* flows from the posterior lateral wall of the aorta to the central renal sinus. The left renal vein flows from the central renal sinus, anterior to the aorta and posterior to the superior mesenteric artery, to join the inferior vena cava.

The normal arterial renal spectral waveforms have an early systolic peak with a rapid systolic rise time. The peak velocity is less than 160 cm/sec, with an overall waveform shape of a normal low-resistance pattern. The resistive index is 0.70 or less (Fig. 15.19).

The diaphragmatic crura run transversely in the paraaortic region. The crura lie posterior to the renal arteries and should be identified by their lack of pulsations and absence of Doppler flow (Fig. 15.20). They vary in echogenicity, depending on the amount of surrounding retroperitoneal fat. They may appear hypoechoic, as lymph nodes do.

Renal Medulla. The renal medulla consists of hypoechoic pyramids dispersed in a uniform distribution, separated by bands of intervening parenchyma that extend toward the renal sinus. The pyramids are uniform in size, shape (triangular), and distribution. The apex of the pyramid points toward the sinus, and the base lies adjacent to the renal cortex. The interlobar arteries lie alongside the pyramids, and arcuate vessels lie at the base of the pyramids (see Fig. 15.2).

Renal Variants

Renal variants include slight alterations in anatomy that may lead the sonographer to suspect an abnormality is present when it really is a normal variation. See Table 15.1 for a description of renal variants and anomalies.

Columns of Bertin. The **columns of Bertin** are prominent invaginations of the cortex located at varying depths within the medullary substance of the kidneys. Hypertrophied columns of Bertin contain renal pyramids and may be difficult to differentiate from an avascular renal neoplasm. The columns are most exaggerated in patients with complete or partial duplication (Fig. 15.21).

Sonographic Findings. Sonographic features of a renal mass effect produced by a hypertrophied column of Bertin include the following: a lateral indentation of the renal sinus, a clear definition from the renal sinus, or a maximum dimension that does not exceed 3 cm. Contiguity with the renal cortex is evident, and overall echogenicity is similar to that of the renal parenchyma.

Dromedary Hump. A **dromedary hump** is a bulge of cortical tissue on the lateral surface of a kidney (usually the left), resembling the hump of a dromedary camel. It is seen in persons whose spleen or liver presses down. It is a normal variant but may resemble a renal neoplasm.

Sonographic Findings. On sonography, the echogenicity is identical to the rest of the renal cortex, and a renal pseudotumor needs to be considered (Fig. 15.22).

Junctional Parenchymal Defect. A junctional parenchymal defect is a triangular, echogenic area typically located anteriorly and superiorly. It is a result of partial fusion of two embryonic parenchymal masses called renunculi during normal development (Fig. 15.23).

Sonographic Findings. Junctional parenchymal defects are best demonstrated on sagittal scans and must not be confused with pathologic processes such as parenchymal renal scars and angiomyolipoma. A lobar dysmorphism is a lobar fusion variant in which malrotation of the renal lobe occurs. The middle and upper calyces may be splayed and displaced, and the lower calyx is deviated posteriorly. The dysmorphic lobe may resemble a mass or prominent column of Bertin on a sonogram (Fig. 15.24).

Fetal Lobulation. Fetal lobulation is developmental variation that is usually present in children up to 5 years old and may be persistent in up to 51% of adults. The surfaces of the kidneys are generally indented in between the calyces, giving the kidneys a slightly lobulated appearance (Fig. 15.25).

Sinus Lipomatosis. Sinus lipomatosis is a condition characterized by deposition of a moderate amount of fat in the renal sinus with parenchymal atrophy (Fig. 15.26). In sinus lipomatosis, the abundant fibrous tissue may cause enlargement of the sinus region with increased echogenicity and regression toward the center of the parenchymal. Occasionally, a fatty mass is localized in only one area; this is called lipomatosis circumscripta.

Extrarenal Pelvis. The normal renal pelvis is a triangular structure. Its axis points inferiorly and medially. The

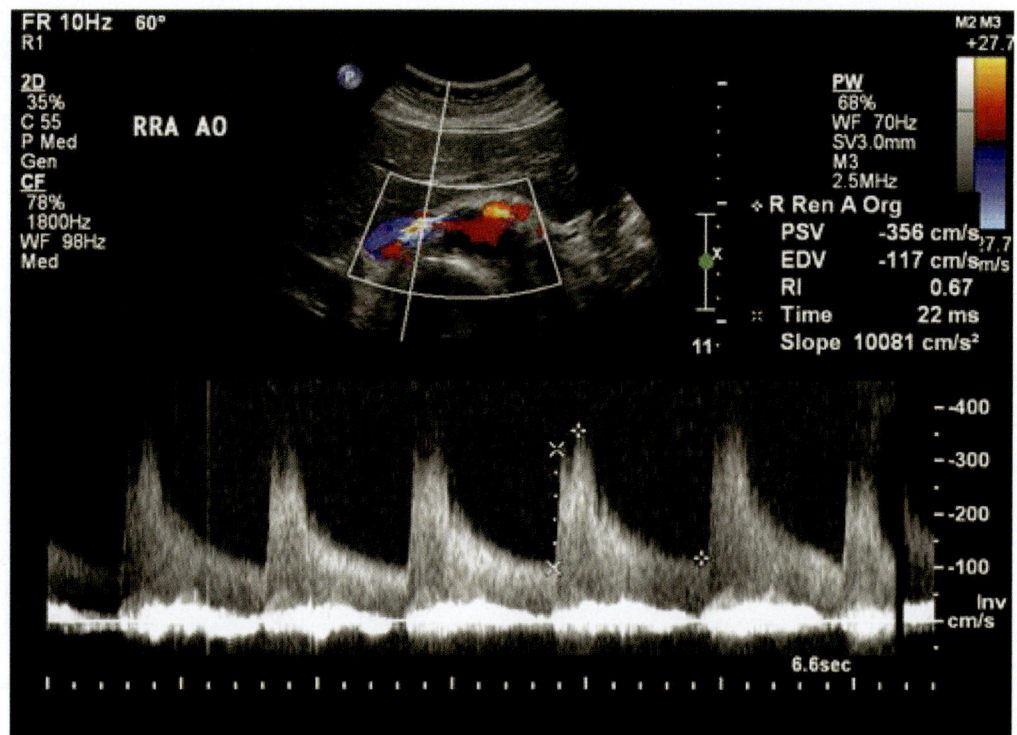

FIG. 15.19 The normal arterial renal spectral waveforms have an early systolic peak with a rapid systolic rise time. The peak velocity is less than 160 cm/sec, with an overall waveform shape of normal low-resistance pattern. The resistive index is ≤0.70.

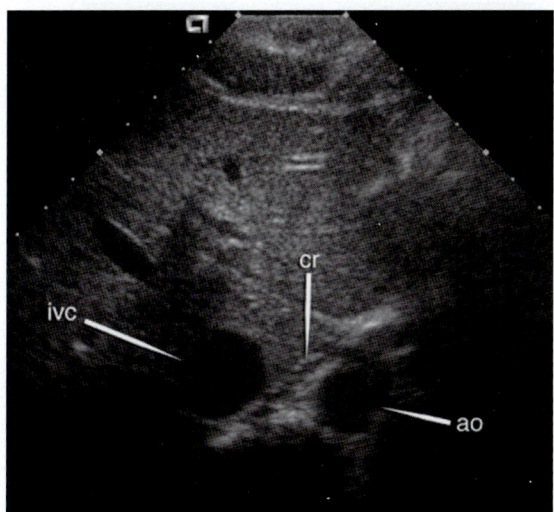

FIG. 15.20 The crura of the diaphragm lie posterior to the renal arteries and should be identified by their lack of pulsations and lack of Doppler flow *(arrows)*.

intrarenal pelvis lies almost completely within the confines of the central renal sinus. This is usually small and foreshortened. The extrarenal pelvis tends to be larger with long major calyces.

Sonographic Findings. On sonography, the pelvis appears as a central cystic area that may be partially or entirely beyond the confines of the bulk of the renal substance. Transverse views are best for viewing continuity with the renal sinus. The dilated extrarenal pelvis will usually decompress when the patient is placed in the prone position (Fig. 15.27).

Renal Anomalies

Renal anomalies comprise abnormalities in number, size, position, structure, or form (Figs. 15.28 and 15.29) (see Table 15.1). Anomalies in number include agenesis, dysgenesis (defective embryonic development of the kidney), and supernumerary kidney. Supernumerary kidney is an additional kidney to the number usually present, which is two. In some cases, separation of the reduplicated organ is incomplete (fused supernumerary kidney). *Bifid* means *cleft*, or *split into two parts*. Bifid renal pelvis is a common anomaly and is considered a normal variant. The renal pelvis may appear to be more prominent on sonography. A pseudotumor is an overgrowth of cortical tissue that indents the echogenic renal sinus and may be mistaken for a renal tumor on sonography.

Renal Agenesis. Renal agenesis is absence of the kidney or failure of the kidney to form; it may be bilateral or unilateral. Bilateral renal agenesis is very rare and is incompatible with life. Unilateral renal agenesis results in a solitary kidney. Congenital absence of one kidney is rare and is commonly associated with other congenital anomalies such as seminal vesical cyst, vaginal agenesis, or bicorn uterus. Renal compensatory hypertrophy (enlargement) generally occurs with a solitary kidney (Fig. 15.30).

Renal hypoplasia is incomplete development of the kidney, usually with fewer than five calyces. Functionally and

TABLE 15.1 Renal Anomalies and Variants

Type	Location	Sonographic Appearance	Differential Considerations	Distinguishing Characteristics
Column of Bertin	Medulla	Indentation of the renal sinus	Renal mass effect	Similar to renal parenchyma; contiguous with cortex
Dromedary hump	Lateral border of the kidney	Identical to the renal cortex	Mass effect	Usually seen on the left kidney
Junctional parenchymal defect	Upper pole of renal parenchyma	Echogenic triangular area	Mass effect	Best seen on sagittal scans
Fetal lobulation	Surface of the kidney	Indentations between the calyces	Mass effect	Best seen on sagittal scans
Lobar dysmorphism	Middle and upper calyces	Elongation of upper and middle calyces	Column of Bertin	Best seen on sagittal scans
Duplex collecting (complete) system	Central renal sinus	Two echogenic regions separated by moderately echogenic parenchymal tissue	Mass effect	"Faceless"; no echogenic renal pelvis seen on transverse view at the level of the midpole
Bifid renal pelvis (incomplete duplication)	Central renal sinus	Middle calyces, two echogenic regions	Pseudomass effect	One ureter entering the bladder on each side of the bladder
Extrarenal pelvis	Long renal pelvis that extends outside the renal border	Central cystic region that extends beyond the medial renal border	Renal aneurysm, dilated proximal ureter	Best seen on a transverse view at the level of the midpole
Horseshoe kidney	Kidneys seen more medial and anterior to the spine	Fusion of the polar region, usually the lower poles	Inferior poles lie more medial, associated with pyelocaliectasis, anomalous extrarenal pelvis, urinary calculi	

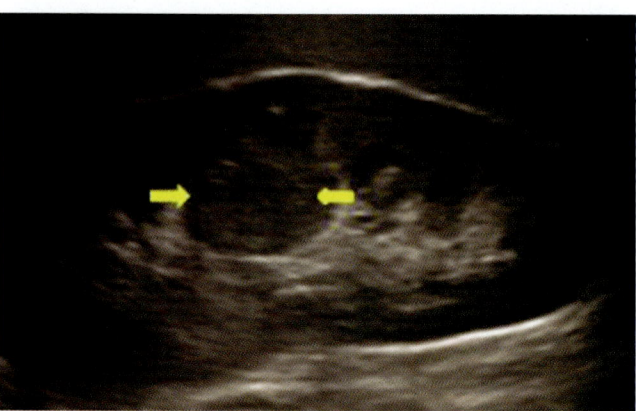

FIG. 15.21 Longitudinal scan of the kidney with arrows pointing to a prominent column of Bertin.

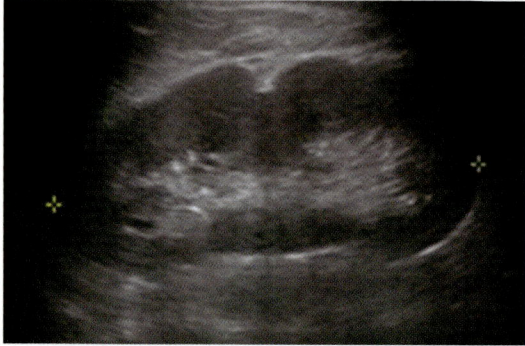

FIG. 15.23 The junctional parenchymal defect *(arrows)* is a triangular area in the upper pole of the renal parenchyma.

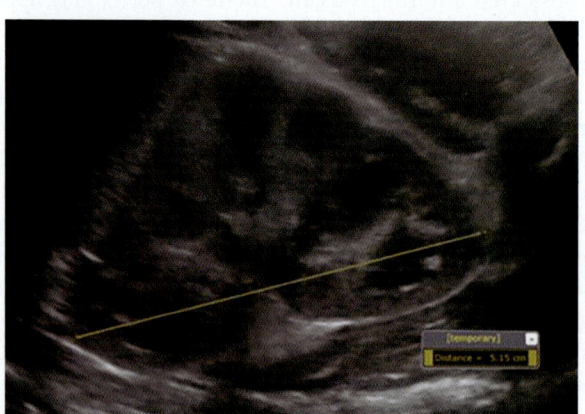

FIG. 15.22 Coronal view of the left kidney. The dromedary hump is a cortical bulge that occurs on the lateral border of the kidney, typically on the left more than on the right.

morphologically, the kidney is normal and should be differentiated from an atrophy kidney secondary to pyelonephrosis or renal artery stenosis. Usually, the pyelonephritic kidney is scarred and echogenic, and the small kidney that results from renal artery stenosis has abnormal Doppler parameters (tardus and parvus waveform).

Bifid Renal Pelvis. A common renal anomaly with a duplication of the renal pelvis and one ureter is considered a normal variant.

Incomplete Duplication. Incomplete, or partial, duplication is the most frequently occurring congenital anomaly in the neonate. Duplication consists of two collecting systems and two ureters, with a single ureter entering into the urinary bladder. The two ureters join and form a single ureter anywhere between the kidney and the bladder.

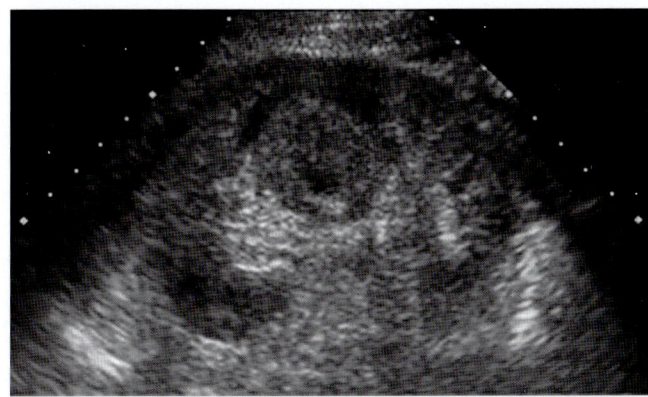
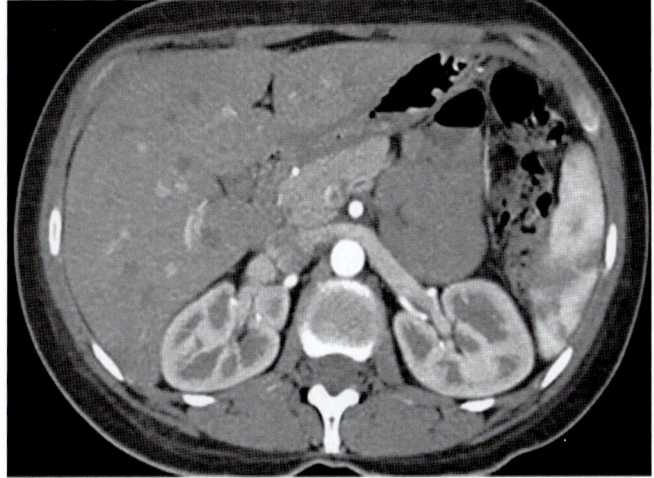

FIG. 15.24 Contrast renal computed tomography lobar dysmorphism, confirming the absence of renal mass.

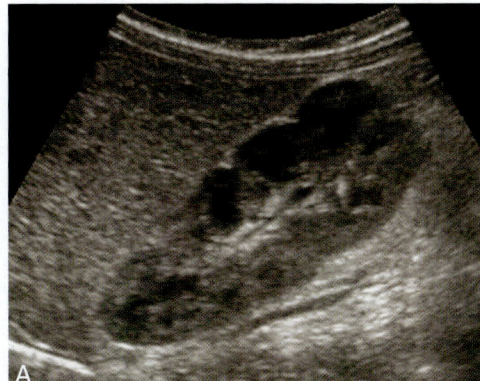
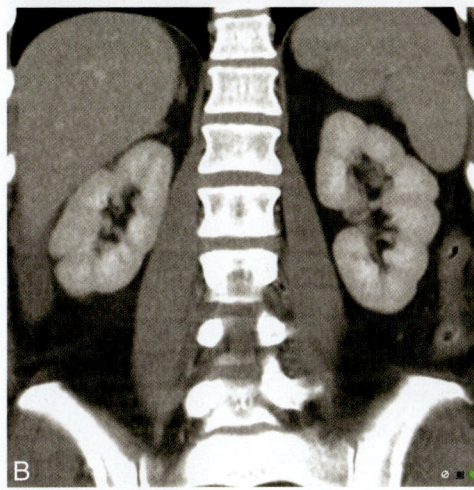

FIG. 15.25 Remnant fetal renal lobulations (an irregularly shaped renal border) kidneys originate as distinct lobules which fuse as they develop and grow. Ultrasound (A) and magnetic resonance (B) images.

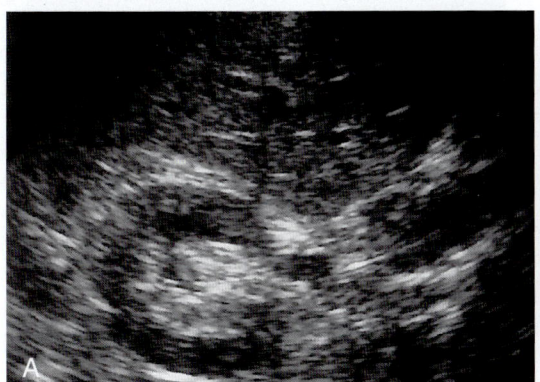
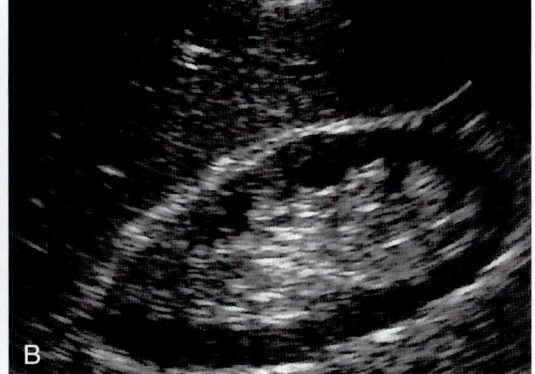

FIG. 15.26 Transverse (A) and longitudinal (B) scans of a patient with renal sinus lipomatosis.

Complete Duplication. Complete duplication is the rare condition of a duplex collecting system. This anomaly results in two separate collecting systems, each with its own ureter that enters the bladder. In cases of double ureter, the ureter from the upper pole of the kidney usually opens below and medial to the one from the lower pole (rule of Weigert-Meyer). The ureter of the lower calyx inserts into the bladder more superiorly and laterally to the normal location of the vesicoureteral orifice, with a short intramural portion. This short intramural portion of the ureter increases the chance of a prevesicoureteral reflux. The ureter from the upper pole calyx inserts into the bladder medially and distally to the normal location of the vesicoureteral orifice. The low insertion of the ureter into the bladder causes an ectopic posterior insertion of the urethra with posterior displacement of the vagina, which increases the chance of urethral obstruction by a stricture or ureterocele, vesicoureteral reflux, or both.

Sonographic Findings. The way to confirm a complete collecting system is to demonstrate two ureteral jets entering the bladder on the same side. The duplex kidney is usually enlarged with smooth margins. The central renal sinus appears as two echogenic regions separated by a cleft of

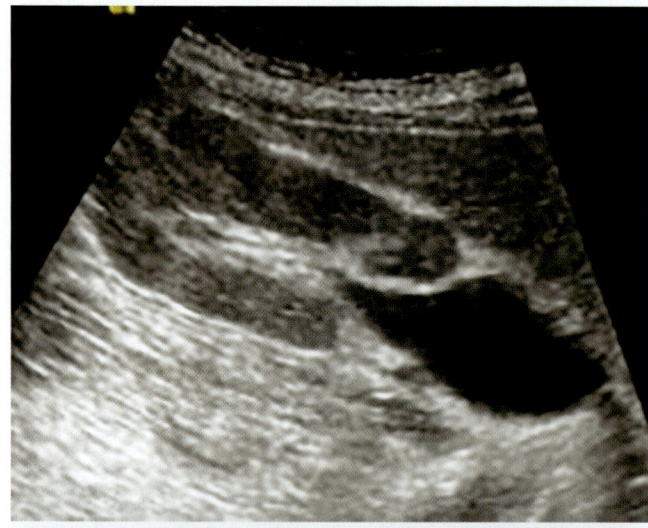
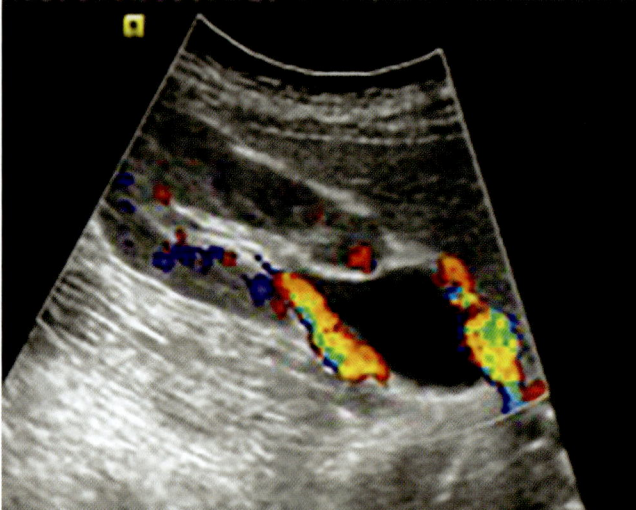

FIG. 15.27 **Extrarenal pelvis.** Scan of the right kidney with a large extrarenal pelvis appearing as a cystic area that extends beyond the confines of the renal borders.

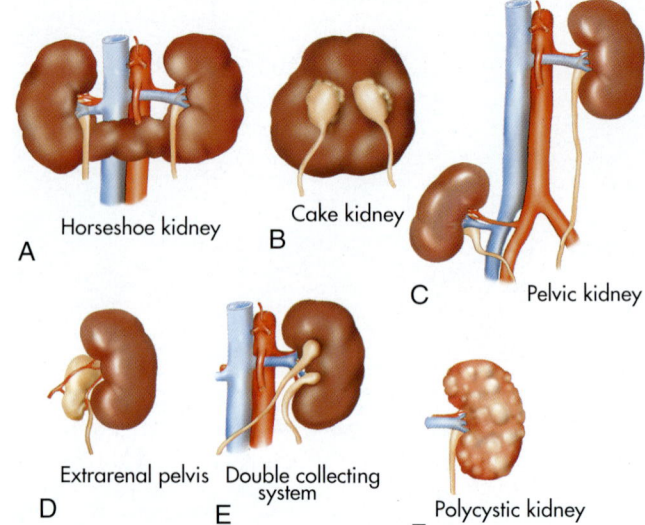

FIG. 15.28 **Variations of renal anatomy, position within the retroperitoneal cavity, and pathology.** (A) Horseshoe kidney shown as two kidneys connected by an isthmus anterior to the great vessels and inferior to the inferior mesenteric artery. (B) Cake kidney with a double collecting system. (C) Pelvic kidney with one kidney in the normal retroperitoneal position. (D) Extrarenal pelvis. (E) Double collecting system in a single kidney. (F) Polycystic kidney.

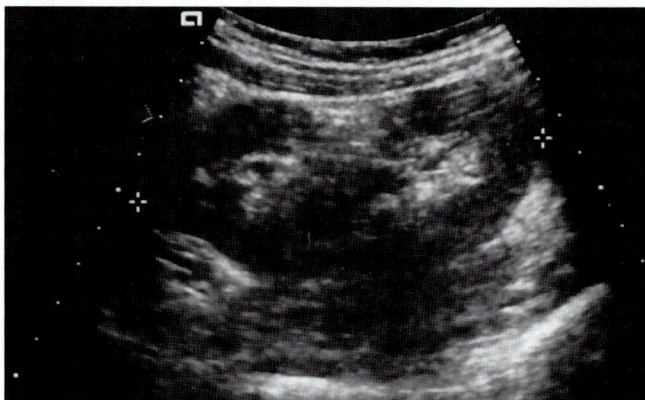

FIG. 15.29 Longitudinal view of a malrotated right kidney, with the renal pelvis facing anteriorly.

moderately echogenic tissue similar in appearance to the normal renal parenchyma. On the transverse view, the area separating the renal pelvis is called "faceless" because the tissue is homogenous, with no central echogenic renal pelvis. Hydronephrosis of the upper pole with a ureterocele, or hydronephrosis of the upper pole and lower pole calyces, may be present (Figs. 15.31 and 15.32).

Renal Ectopia. **Renal ectopia**, or **ectopic kidney**, describes a kidney that is not located in its usual position, the renal fascia. It results when the kidney fails to ascend from its origin in the true pelvis or from a superiorly ascended kidney located in the thorax. Pelvic kidney, also called sacral kidney, is the most common renal ectopia and should not be misdiagnosed as a primary pelvic tumor. It is almost always malrotated; the renal pelvis faces anteriorly and is predisposed to reflux, infection, ureteropelvic junction (UPJ) obstruction, and stone formation (Fig. 15.33). Pelvic kidney may be bilateral, but this is very rare. A thoracic kidney migrates through the diaphragm into the thoracic cavity. It is a rare finding and is not easily diagnosed with ultrasound. Other renal ectopias include intrathoracic kidney and abdominal (iliac crest) kidney.

Two types of crossed renal ectopia can occur: fused and nonfused. Both are associated with malrotation. Fused crossed renal ectopia occurs more frequently than nonfused and most often on the right side. In most cases of crossed renal ectopia, the ureters are not ectopic. Cystoscopy reveals a normal trigone, and the incidence of associated congenital anomalies is low. Renal calculi are the most common complication. Sonography shows both kidneys located on the same side, with most demonstrating fusion (Fig. 15.34).

Horseshoe Kidney. **Horseshoe kidney** is the most common anomaly of renal fusion. Fusion of the lower poles occurs in 96% of cases, with ureters passing anterior to the renal parenchyma and variation of arterial land venous blood

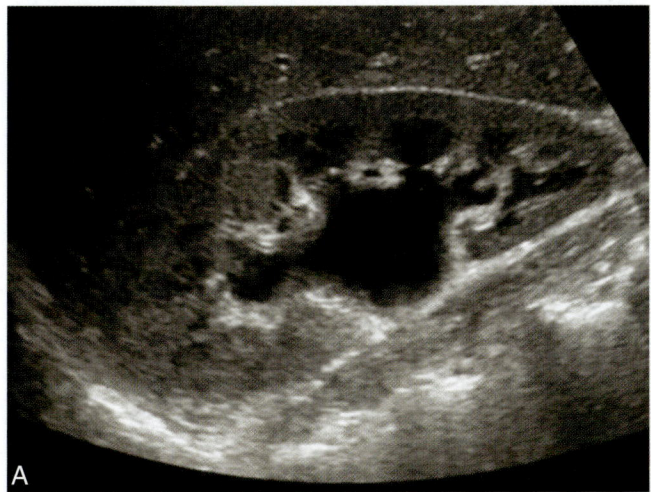
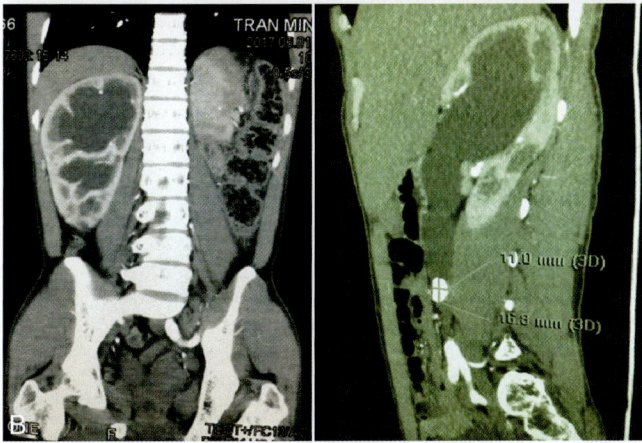

FIG. 15.30 Unilateral renal agenesis. (A) Enlarged (compensatory hypertrophy) solitary right kidney. (B) Computed tomography images of the solitary hydronephrotic kidney.

Renal masses are categorized as cystic, solid, or complex by a sonographic evaluation. A cystic mass sonographically displays several characteristic features: (1) smooth, thin, well-defined border; (2) round or oval shape; (3) sharp interface between the cyst and the renal parenchyma; (4) no internal echoes (anechoic); and (5) increased posterior acoustic enhancement.

A solid lesion projects as a nongeometric shape with irregular borders, a poorly defined interface between the mass and the kidney, low-level internal echoes, a weak posterior border caused by increased attenuation of the mass, and poor through-transmission.

Areas of necrosis, hemorrhage, abscess, or calcification within the mass may alter the classification and cause the lesion to fall into the complex category. This means the mass shows characteristics associated with both cystic and solid lesions.

Sonography allows the sonographer to carefully evaluate the renal parenchyma in many stages of respiration. If the mass is very small, respiratory motion may cause it to move in and out of the field of view. Careful evaluation of the best respiratory phase combined with use of the cine-loop feature will allow the sonographer to adequately image most renal masses to determine their characteristic composition.

Aspiration of Renal Masses

Most renal masses that have met the criteria for a simple cystic mass do not require needle aspiration. The Bosniak classification of cysts is used to determine the appropriate workup for a cystic mass (Table 15.2). A needle aspiration may be recommended to obtain fluid from the lesion to evaluate its internal composition.

The patient should be placed in a prone position with sandbags or rolled sheets under the abdomen to help push the kidneys toward the posterior abdominal wall and provide a flat scanning surface. Sterile technique is used for aspiration and biopsy procedures. The transducer must be gas sterilized. Sterile lubricant is used to couple the transducer to the patient's skin.

The renal mass should be located in the transverse and longitudinal planes, with scans performed at midinspiration. Hold the transducer lightly over the scanning surface so as not to compress the subcutaneous tissue. The depth of the mass should be noted from its posterior to anterior borders, so the exact depth can be given to aid in placement of the needle. Compression of the subcutaneous tissue results in an inaccurate depth measurement. When the area of aspiration is outlined on the patient's back, the distance is measured from the posterior surface to the middle of the lesion.

A beveled needle causes multiple echoes within the walls of the lesion. If the needle is slightly bent, many echoes appear until the bent needle is completely out of the transducer's path. The larger the needle gauge, the stronger the reflection.

The patient's skin is painted with tincture of benzalkonium (Zephiran), and sterile drapes are applied. A local anesthetic agent is administered over the area of interest,

supply. The isthmus, or connecting bridge, typically consists of renal parenchymal tissue; rarely is it fibrotic tissue. The most common complications associated with horseshoe kidney are kidney malrotation, urolithiasis, UPJ obstruction, and infection. The isthmus of the kidney lies anterior to the spine and may simulate a solid pelvic mass or enlarged lymph nodes (Fig. 15.35).

Evaluation of a Renal Mass

Before starting the sonographic examination for the evaluation of a renal mass, the sonographer should review the patient's chart, including the laboratory findings and previous diagnostic examinations, which may include a plain radiograph of the abdomen, computed tomography (CT), or MRI. Whenever possible, these films should be obtained before the sonogram is done, so the examination can be tailored to address the clinical problem. The sonographer should evaluate the sonographic images to determine the shape and size of the kidney and the location of the mass lesion, to observe distortion of the renal or ureter structure, and to look for calcium stones or gas within the kidney.

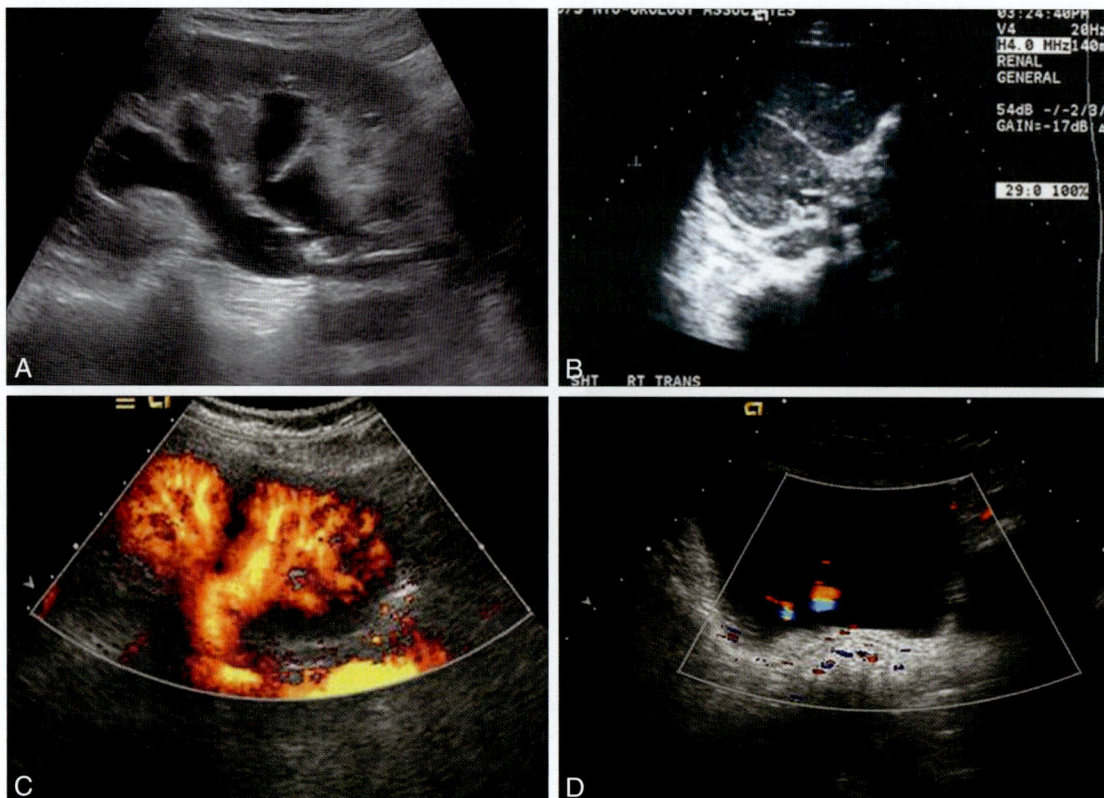

FIG. 15.31 (A) Bifid kidney. (B) The central sinus appears as two echogenic regions separated by a cleft of moderate hypoechoic tissue similar to the normal renal parenchyma. (C) Transverse view of the echogenic tissue that separates the renal sinus ("faceless"). (D) Power Doppler of duplex collecting system. (E) Double right ureteral jets confirm a complete duplex collecting system.

and the sterile transducer is used to relocate the lesion. The needle is inserted into the central core of the cyst. The needle stop helps ensure that the needle does not go through the cyst. The fluid is then withdrawn according to volume calculations. The volume of the cyst may be determined by measuring the radius of the mass and using the following formula: $V = 4/3\pi r^3$.

The diameter of the mass can be applied to the formula $V = d^3/2$.

Lower Urinary Tract

Ureters

Stricture. Ureteral narrowing due to fibrosis is a common form of ureteral stricture. Ureteral strictures may also result from inflammatory disease, tuberculosis, localized periureteral fibrosis, impacted ureteral stone, schistosomiasis, iatrogenic ureteral injury, or radiation therapy. Other causes include amyloidosis, adjacent malignancies, metastases, extrinsic compression due to primary retroperitoneal tumors, enlarged lymph nodes, and medial lower pole renal masses (Box 15.1).

Ureterocele. A ureterocele is a cystlike enlargement of the lower end of the ureter (Fig. 15.36) caused by congenital or acquired stenosis of the distal end of the ureter. Ureteroceles are usually small and asymptomatic, although they may cause obstruction and infection of the upper urinary system. If large, a ureterocele may cause bladder outlet obstruction. Ureteroceles are found more often in adults than in children and may be unilateral or bilateral. On sonography, a "cobra head" appearance is seen in sagittal view.

Sonographic Findings. A large ureterocele may fill the urinary bladder and have the same sonographic appearance as diverticula. If the patient can partially empty the bladder, a better diagnostic-quality image will be produced, as the ureterocele will be empty. One of the advantages of ultrasound is dynamic imaging; alternate filling and emptying of the ureterocele as the result of peristalsis may be demonstrated. Calculi may also be present.

Ectopic Ureterocele. Ectopic ureteroceles are rare and are found more commonly in children and young adults, especially in females. They usually are associated with complete ureteral duplication. The ureter, which empties the upper pole, inserts low in the bladder by the bladder neck, urethra, or lower genital tract. The ectopic ureter may become stenotic and cause ureteral obstruction, which is associated with hydroureter and hydronephrosis. The ureterocele sac may obstruct the bladder outlet or may prolapse through the urethra.

Sonographic Findings. An ectopic ureterocele appears on sonography as a round, thin-walled cystic structure that may contain debris protruding into the bladder.

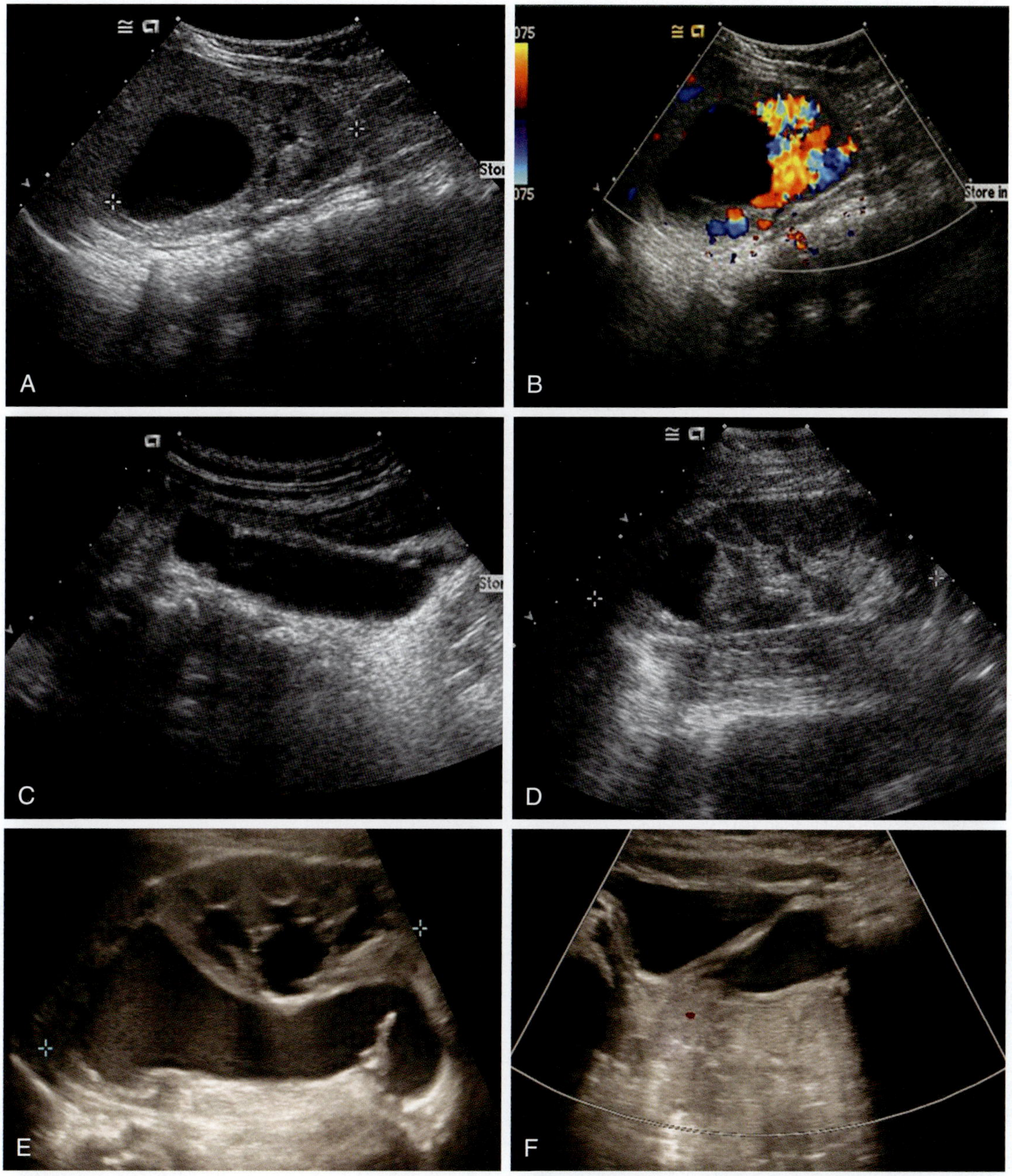

FIG. 15.32 (A) Longitudinal scan of a duplicated right collecting system with severe hydronephrosis of upper moiety. (B) Ectopic right distal ureter. (C) Longitudinal scan of a duplicated right collecting system with moderate hydronephrosis of the upper moiety. (D) Ureterocele of the distal right ureter (rule of Weigert-Meyer). (E–F) Longitudinal scan of a left collecting system with severe upper moiety, hydronephrosis, and ectopic ureter.

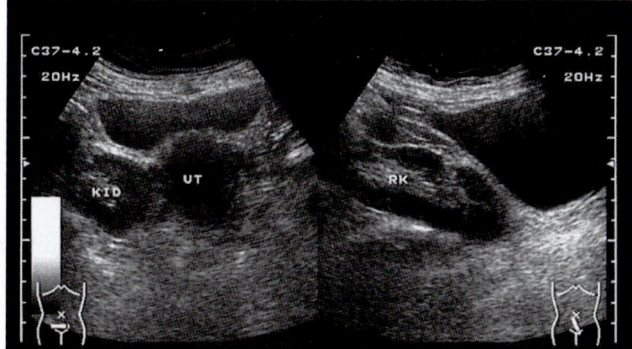

FIG. 15.33 Transverse *(left)* and sagittal *(right)* images of ectopic kidney found in the pelvis, just posterior to the distended urinary bladder.

Bladder

Ultrasound is not the imaging modality of choice to examine the bladder. Cystoscopy is usually used to examine the bladder because of its ability to diagnose early neoplasms. Transabdominal sonography will allow visualization of most lesions greater than 5 mm. A transurethral intravesicular sonographic approach has been used to evaluate bladder tumors.

The urinary bladder should be examined at the same time as the upper urinary tract. A complete review of the patient's chart, including previous diagnostic imaging procedures, should be conducted before a sonographic examination of the bladder is begun.

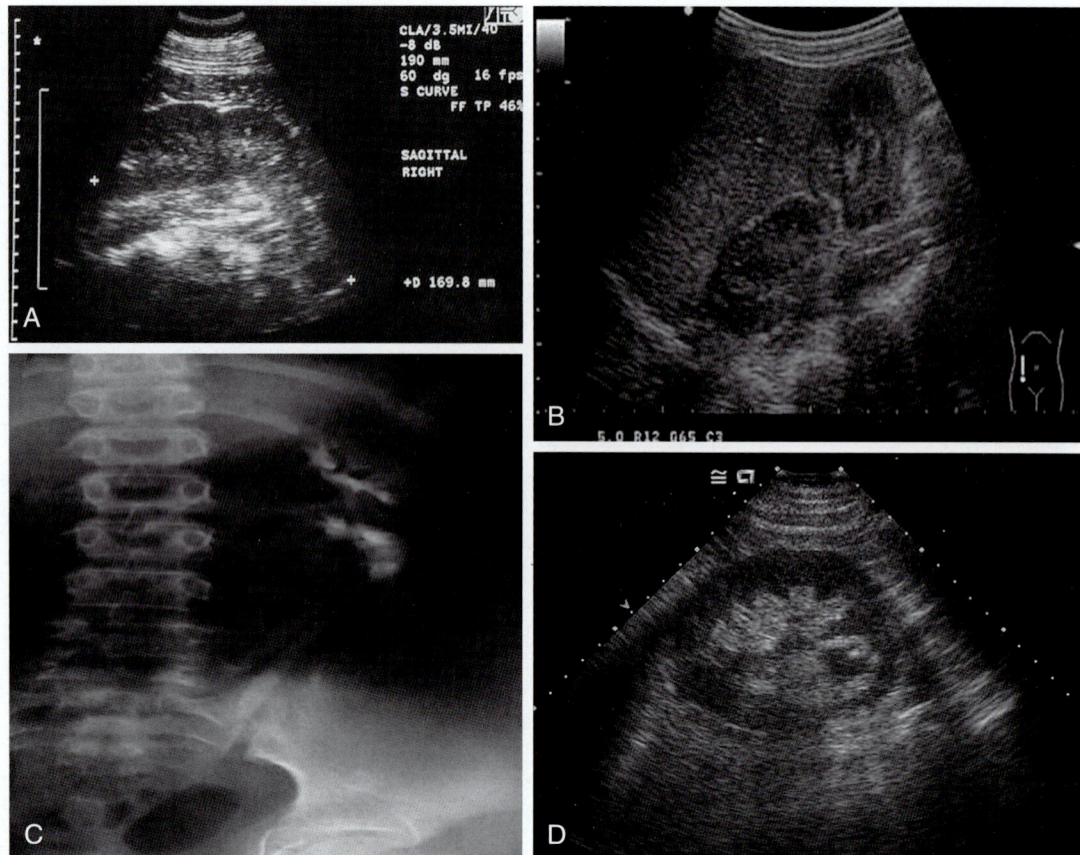

FIG. 15.34 (A) Crossed kidney on the right side of the body. Sonogram (B) and intravenous pyelogram (C) of the left crossed fused kidney. (D) Cake kidney.

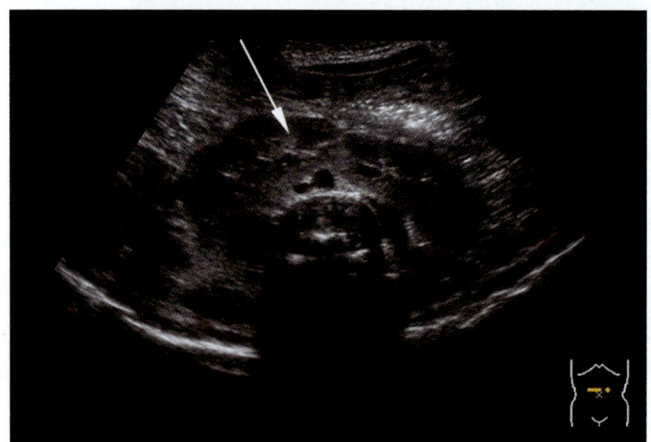

FIG. 15.35 Transverse scan of a horseshoe kidney with isthmus connecting each pole.

TABLE 15.2	Bosniak Cyst Categories, Criteria, and Workup	
Category	Criteria	Workup
Simple cyst (I)	Thin smooth wall, anechoic, round or oval in shape; increased through-transmission	None
Mildly complex cyst (II)	Thin septation or calcified wall	2–3-month follow-up with CT or sonogram
Mildly complex (IIF)	Atypical features; does not fall into category II	6–12-month follow-up
Indeterminate lesion (III)	Multiple septa, thickened septa, internal echoes	Biopsy or partial nephrectomy—increased risk for malignancy
Malignant lesion (IV)	Solid component, irregular walls	Nephrectomy

CT, Computed tomography.

A sonogram of the bladder is obtained with a distended bladder. The patient lies in a supine position. A right or left decubitus position may be used to demonstrate movement of calculi. Proper adjustment of the TGC allows for minimization of anterior wall reverberations and anechoic bladder, with posterior acoustic enhancement. The depth of the image should be set to visualize any structure that may lie posterior or caudal to the bladder. A 3.5-MHz transducer is usually used. In very thin patients, a 5-MHz transducer may be used. If evaluation of the anterior bladder wall is indicated, a high-frequency, curved linear-array transducer or linear transducer will give a larger anterior field if view.

The transducer should be placed in the middle of the filled urinary bladder and angled laterally, inferiorly, and superiorly. The bladder walls should be smooth and thin (3 to 6 mm).

BOX 15.1	Causes of Narrowing of the Ureter

Internal causes
  Fibrosis
  Inflammatory disease
  Tuberculosis
  Localized periureteral fibrosis
  Impacted ureteral stone
  Schistosomiasis
  Iatrogenic ureteral injury
  Radiation therapy
  Amyloidosis
Extrinsic compression
  Adjacent malignancies
  Metastases
  Primary retroperitoneal tumors
  Enlarged lymph nodes
Medial lower renal pole mass

BOX 15.2	Conditions That Cause Incomplete Emptying of Bladder

Bladder calculi
Diabetes mellitus
Foley catheter
Inflammation
Neoplasms—benign or malignant
Neurogenic bladder
Postsurgical intervention
Pregnancy
Radiation therapy
Rectal or vaginal fistulas
Renal disease
Sexual intercourse
Trauma (blood clot)
Tuberculosis (lower ureteric stricture)
Urethral stricture

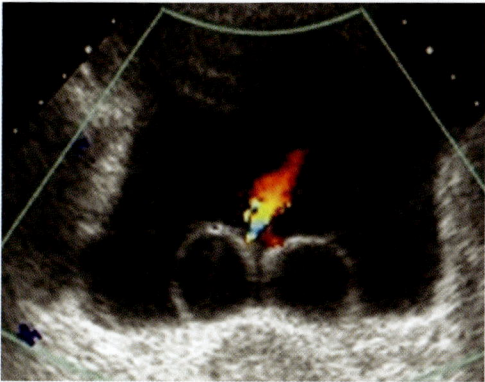

FIG. 15.36 Bilateral ureteroceles on color Doppler "candle sign" showing tiny continuous ureteral jets.

The bladder should be midline and should not be deviated to either side or have any irregular or asymmetric indentations.

Sonography is used to evaluate residual bladder volume in patients with outflow obstruction. The postvoid bladder is scanned in two planes: anteroposterior and transverse. Measurements are obtained in three planes: anteroposterior, transverse, and longitudinal. Images and measurements are obtained at the largest dimensions. Because bladder shape varies, any volume measurement can be used to approximate volume. A residue of less than 20 mL of urine is considered normal in an adult.

Ureteral jets should be identified as flashes of Doppler color entering the bladder from the lateral posterior border of the bladder and coursing superior and medial.

An enlarged prostate, enlarged uterus, pelvic mass, or filled loop of bowel may indent and displace the urinary bladder. Box 15.2 lists the conditions under which the bladder may not empty completely.

PATHOLOGY OF THE URINARY SYSTEM

See Table 15.3 for clinical findings, sonographic findings, and differential considerations for various renal diseases and conditions. Box 15.3 lists the main signs and symptoms of common renal diseases.

Renal Cystic Disease

Simple renal cystic disease encompasses a wide range of disease processes, which may be typical, complicated, or atypical. The disease may be acquired (nongenetic) or inherited (genetic) (e.g., von Hippel–Lindau disease, tuberous sclerosis). Cystic disease may occur in the renal cortex, medulla, or renal sinus (see Table 15.3).

Simple Renal Cyst. The most common renal mass lesion is a simple cortical renal cyst. Although the origin is unknown, these cysts are considered acquired lesions, probably arising from obstructed ducts or tubules. It is estimated that they occur in 50% of the population older than 50 years of age. Most patients with a simple cyst are asymptomatic, and the cyst is detected as an incidental finding in the kidney. A renal simple cyst can be solitary or multiple, involving one or both kidneys. Rarely, several simple cysts may involve only one kidney or a localized portion of a kidney. In rare cases, a large lower pole cyst may obstruct the collecting system and cause hydronephrosis and/or hypertension. Local pain and hematuria may be caused by distention of the cyst wall or spontaneous bleeding into the cyst. Occasionally, a simple cyst can be complicated by hemorrhage, infection, or calcification, which causes it to become a complex cyst. Renal cysts are unusual in children, with an overall frequency of less than 1%. A cyst in a child must be examined carefully to differentiate a benign cyst from a cystic form of nephroblastoma (Wilms tumor).

Sonographic Findings. Sonography is the most efficient imaging modality for confirming the presence of a simple cyst that is poorly seen during CT and/or MRI. Classical sonographic criteria used to diagnose a simple renal cyst include a round or oval shape, anechoic, thin walls, and posterior acoustic enhancement. No further evaluation is required for a simple renal cyst (Fig. 15.37).

TABLE 15.3 Renal Findings

Clinical Findings	Sonographic Findings	Differential Considerations
Simple Cysts		
Usually asymptomatic Usually normal laboratory findings	Found anywhere in the kidney, but usually in cortex Round or ovoid in shape, anechoic Thin, well-defined walls No color flow or Doppler in mass	Hemorrhagic cyst, infected cyst, necrotic cyst, malignant cyst, obstruction of upper pole, calyceal diverticula, pseudoaneurysm, arteriovenous malformation
Parapelvic Cysts		
Usually asymptomatic May present with hypertension or obstruction (hilum cyst) Pain Usually normal laboratory findings	Found in the renal hilum or renal sinus Well-defined sonolucent mass with regular or irregular borders Good through-transmission Not connected to the renal collecting system	Hydronephrosis
von Hippel–Lindau Cysts		
Flank pain General discomfort Involves many body systems Usually presents in third to fifth decade Initial clinical symptoms caused by cerebellar or spinal cord hemangioblastomas, not abdominal If renal involvement occurs, there is an ↑ chance of renal carcinoma No hypertension or renal failure	Bilateral cysts and masses Other organs are affected Masses may develop within the cysts Hyperplastic linings of cysts Pancreatic cysts	Multiple cysts Renal adenoma
Tuberous Sclerosis		
Involves several body systems Patient usually presents with mental retardation, seizures, and cutaneous lesions	Multiple cysts or angiomyolipomas Multiple organs involved Multiple angiomyolipomas that may become large	Angiomyolipomas
Acquired Cystic Disease of Dialysis		
Usually occurs in patients on renal dialysis for ≥ 3 years Flank pain	Found in cortex Simple cysts Atypical because of hemorrhage Normal or small echogenic kidneys with a decrease in corticomedullary distinction with simple or atypical cysts	Renal cyst Adenoma Renal cell carcinoma
Autosomal Dominant Polycystic Kidney Disease (ADPKD), Also Known as Adult Polycystic Kidney Disease		
Hypertension Renal failure Abdominal, flank pain Fever, chills (infection) Uremia Palpable mass Polycythemia Hematuria	Bilateral enlarged kidneys with multiple cysts of varied size Kidneys lose their reniform shape; in the late stages, no normal renal parenchyma may be identified Cysts may be atypical because of infection or hemorrhage Cysts may be found in liver, spleen, testes, pancreas	Cortical cysts Localized hydronephrosis Renal tuberculosis Multilocular cyst
Autosomal Recessive Polycystic Kidney Disease (ARPKD), Also Known as Infantile Polycystic Kidney Disease		
May be seen in utero Renal insufficiency Lung hypoplasia, usually fatal depending on the amount of renal function In juvenile form: Portal hypertension Hepatic fibrosis GI hemorrhage	Bilateral enlarged echogenic kidneys Cysts too small to be seen No distinction between the corticomedullary region	In utero: ADPKD, dysplasia, glomerulocystic kidney disease

TABLE 15.3	Renal Findings—cont'd		
Clinical Findings	**Sonographic Findings**	**Differential Considerations**	
Multicystic Dysplastic Kidney			
Most common palpable mass in neonates Restricted growth in children Polyuria Hypertension Infection Usually unilateral; bilateral is incompatible with life	Multiple cysts of varying size No renal parenchyma surrounding the cyst Enlarged kidneys in children Small kidneys in adults Absence of renal vascularity	Hydronephrosis	
Medullary Sponge Kidney			
Usually asymptomatic unless calculus is present, then hematuria and infections Pain Hydronephrosis Infection	Normal or small kidneys with echogenic parenchyma (cysts too small to be resolved on a sonogram), or Small cysts in medulla and corticomedullary region with increased echogenicity	Papillary necrosis Nephrocalcinosis Renal cystic disease Pyelonephritic cysts	
Medullary Cystic Disease			
Normal renal function Anemia Salt loss Progressive azotemia Polyuria Pain Infection	Normal or small echogenic kidneys with Widening of the renal sinus after 2 cm in the medulla or corticomedullary junction	Medullary sponge kidney small cysts <2 cm	
Renal Cell Carcinoma			
Hematuria Weight loss Fatigue Fever Flank pain Palpable mass Hypertension	Cystic or complex mass that may have areas of calcifications May displace renal pyramids and invade renal architecture Irregular margins Hypervascular Renal vein or IVC thrombosis	Angiomyolipoma Transitional cell carcinoma Lymphoma Oncocytoma Column of Bertin Renal vein or IVC thrombus	
Transitional Cell Carcinoma			
Hematuria Weight loss Fatigue Fever Flank pain	Solid hypoechoic mass Not well defined within the renal sinus May be multiple	Squamous cell tumor Renal cell carcinoma Adenoma Blood clot Fungus ball	
Squamous Cell Carcinoma			
Gross hematuria History of chronic irritation Palpable kidney if severe hydronephrosis is present	Large bulky mass Invasion of the renal vein and IVC	Transitional cell carcinoma	
Renal Lymphoma			
Not a primary site; usually caused by adjacent lymph involvement More common in patients with non-Hodgkin lymphoma Usually no renal symptoms Asymptomatic Pain Hematuria	Hypoechoic mass may be bilateral Enlarged kidney	Renal cell carcinoma Cyst	

Continued

TABLE 15.3   Renal Findings—cont'd

Clinical Findings	Sonographic Findings	Differential Considerations
Wilms Tumor		
Palpable abdominal mass in children Abdominal pain Nausea and vomiting Hematuria	Usually unilateral, may be bilateral Heterogeneous Look for extension into renal vein and inferior vena cava	Nephroblastoma Renal cell carcinoma Mesoblastoma Multicystic kidney Retroperitoneal sarcoma
Benign Renal Tumor		
Usually asymptomatic May cause painless hematuria	Well-defined mass—hyperechoic to hypoechoic	Angiomyolipoma Transitional cell carcinoma Oncocytoma Lymphoma Column of Bertin
Adenoma		
Asymptomatic	Well-defined mass with calcifications	Renal cell carcinoma
Angiolipoma		
Usually asymptomatic Possible flank pain Normal laboratory values Hematuria if tumor hemorrhages	Usually echogenic homogeneous mass with well-defined borders Hemorrhagic neoplasm	Oncocytoma Renal cell carcinoma
Lipoma		
Usually asymptomatic Normal laboratory values	Well-defined echogenic mass	Fibromas Adenoma
Oncocytoma		
Asymptomatic	Well-defined mass with spoke-wheel patterns of enhancement and central scar	Renal abscess
Acute Glomerulonephritis		
Nephrotic syndrome Hypertension Anemia Peripheral edema	Increased cortical echoes	Chronic glomerulonephritis Acute tubular nephrosis AIDS Lupus nephritis Acute interstitial nephritis
Acute Interstitial Nephritis		
Uremia Hematuria Rash Fever Eosinophilia	Enlarged kidneys with increased cortical echoes	Acute glomerulonephritis Chronic glomerulonephritis Acute tubular necrosis AIDS Lupus nephritis
Lupus Nephritis		
Hematuria Proteinuria Renal vein thrombus Renal insufficiency	Increased cortical echoes and renal atrophy	Acute glomerulonephritis Chronic glomerulonephritis Acute tubular necrosis AIDS Acute interstitial nephritis
Acquired Immunodeficiency Syndrome (AIDS)		
Renal dysfunction	Kidneys are normal or enlarged Echogenic parenchyma Increased cortical echoes	Acute glomerulonephritis Chronic glomerulonephritis Acute tubular necrosis Lupus nephritis Acute interstitial nephritis

TABLE 15.3 Renal Findings—cont'd

Clinical Findings	Sonographic Findings	Differential Considerations
Sickle Cell Nephropathy		
Hematuria Renal vein thrombosis	Varies—patients with acute renal vein thrombosis: enlarged kidneys with decreased echogenicity Subacute: enlarged kidneys with increased cortical echogenicity	Lupus nephritis
Hypertensive Nephropathy		
Uncontrolled hypertension	Small kidneys with smooth borders may have distortion of intrarenal anatomy	Hypoplasia
Papillary Necrosis		
Hematuria Flank pain Hypertension Dysuria Acute renal failure	Fluid-filled spaces at the corticomedullary junction Round or triangular Mimics calculi	Congenital megacalyces Hydronephrosis Postobstruction atrophy
Renal Atrophy		
Renal failure	Small echogenic kidneys	Renal hypoplasia Chronic renal failure
Renal Sinus Lipomatosis		
Asymptomatic	Enlarged kidneys with increased echogenicity of renal sinus Hyperechoic areas decreased renal parenchyma	Infection Atrophy Hydronephrosis
Acute Renal Failure		
Renal insufficiency Decreased urine output	Hydronephrosis Enlarged hypoechoic kidneys Renal artery stenosis	Prerenal, renal, or postrenal causes
Obstructive Hydronephrosis		
Renal insufficiency Decreased urine output Hypertension	Fluid-filled renal collecting system Thin parenchyma Hydroureter Decreased or absent ureteral jets	Extrarenal collecting system Parapelvic cyst Reflux Renal artery aneurysm Transient diuresis Congenital megacalyces Papillary necrosis Arteriovenous malformation
Renal Infarction		
Asymptomatic	Irregular triangle masses in the renal parenchyma Lobulated renal contour	Renal lobulations Dromedary hump
Acute Tubular Necrosis		
Renal insufficiency Hematuria	Bilaterally enlarged kidneys with hyperechoic pyramids	Nephrocalcinosis
Chronic Renal Failure		
Renal failure Hypertension	Bilateral small echogenic kidneys	Multiple causes AIDS Chronic parenchymal infection
Pyonephrosis		
Renal insufficiency Hematuria	Dilated collecting system with low-level echoes or decreased through-transmission	Hydronephrosis Hemorrhage Blood clot Uroepithelial tumors

Continued

TABLE 15.3 Renal Findings—cont'd

Clinical Findings	Sonographic Findings	Differential Considerations
Xanthogranulomatous Pyelonephritis		
Multiple infections Nonfunctioning kidneys	"Staghorn appearance" Destruction of renal parenchyma Increased echogenicity Increased renal size Dilated calyces	Hydronephrosis Renal calculi

GI, Gastrointestinal; *IVC*, inferior vena cava.

BOX 15.3 Signs and Symptoms of Renal Disease

Renal Cystic Disease
Inflammatory or necrotic cysts
- Flank pain
- Hematuria
- Proteinuria
- White blood cells in urine
- ↑ Protein

Renal subcapsular hematoma
- Hematuria
- ↓ Hematocrit

Renal Inflammatory Processes
Abscess
- Acute onset of symptoms
- Fever
- Palpable mass
- ↑ White blood cell count
- Pyuria

Acute focal bacterial nephritis
- Fever
- Flank pain
- Pyuria
- ↑ Blood urea nitrogen
- ↑ Albumin
- ↑ Total plasma proteins

Acute tubular necrosis
- Moderate to severe intermittent flank pain (caused by renal calculi)
- Vomiting (caused by renal calculi)
- Hematuria
- Infection
- Leukocytosis with infection

Chronic renal failure
- ↑ Concentration of urea in blood
- High urine protein excretion
- ↑ Creatinine
- Presence of granulocytes

Renal cell carcinoma
- Erythrocytosis may occur
- Leukocytosis
- Red blood cells in urine
- Pyuria
- ↑ Lactic acid dehydrogenase

Complex Cyst. If a renal cyst does not meet all of the criteria for a simple cyst, it is termed *complex* and must be considered malignant until proven otherwise. Complex cysts may contain septations, thick walls, calcifications, internal echoes, and mural nodularity.

Sonographic Findings. Thick walls: Anything thicker than 1 mm is considered abnormal, and the cystic form of a renal carcinoma often presents in this manner (Fig. 15.38). Most of the time, internal echoes within a cyst are the result of protein content, hemorrhage, and/or infection. Any irregularity at the base of the cyst should be considered a malignant growth (Box 15.4). Thin septations can be detected by sonography, and their presence alone does not suggest malignancy. If irregularity of septa (thicker than 1 mm) showing vascularity on color or power Doppler is seen, the lesion must be presumed malignant. Fine, thin linear calcification in the cyst wall or in a septum without associated soft tissue mass or enhancement on CT likely represents a complex cyst, rather than a malignancy.

Bosniak classification of cysts was introduced in 1986, before CT or MRI was used for diagnosing renal cystic disease. In 2005 the Bosniak classification was updated from four categories—I, II, III, and renal cyst IV—to five categories:

- **Category I** lesions are simple benign cysts: anechoic, thin walls, no calcifications or septations; no atypical features; and no further evaluation is needed.
- **Category II** lesions are cystic lesions with one or two thin (≤1 mm thick) septations, fine calcifications in the walls or septa (wall thickening >1 mm advances the lesion into surgical category III), and hyperdense benign cysts with all features of category I cysts, except for being homogeneously hyperechoic. A benign category II lesion must be 3 cm or less in diameter, must have one-quarter of its wall extending outside the kidney so the wall can be assessed, and must show no vascularity (must be nonenhancing after contrast material is administered on CT) on color Doppler.
- **Category IIF** comprises minimally complicated cysts that need follow-up. This is a group not well defined by Bosniak, but it consists of lesions that do not fall neatly into category II. These lesions have some atypical features

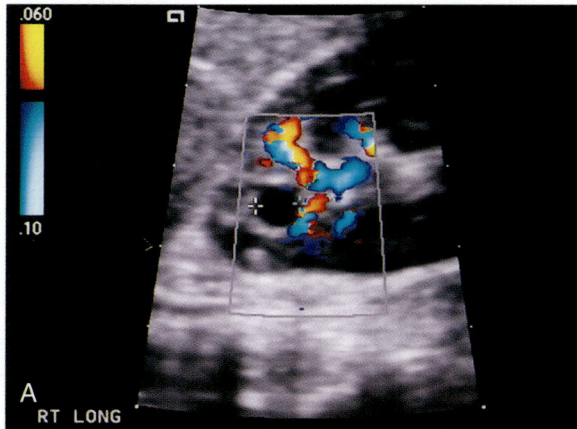
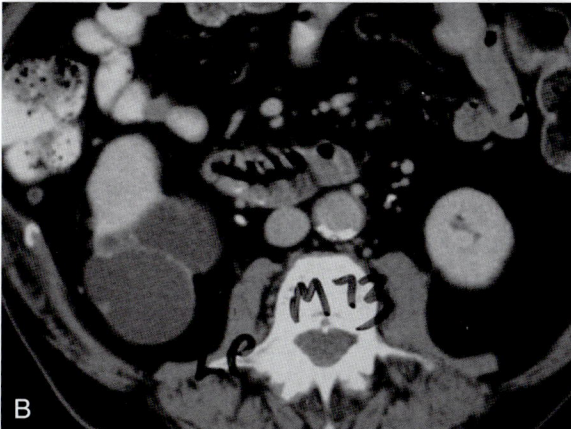
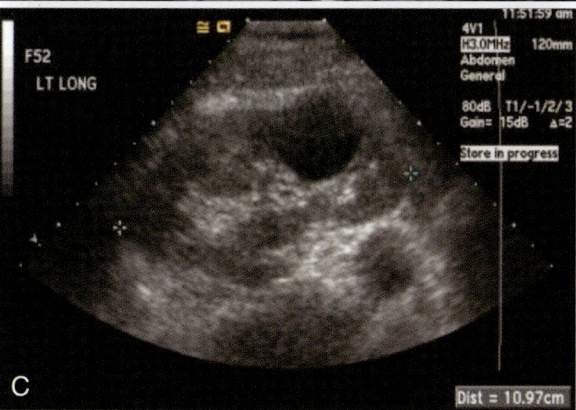

FIG. 15.37 (A) Upper pole renal cyst with no blood flow to the cyst. (B) Computed tomography scan of a lower pole complicated cyst. (C) Sagittal view of the left kidney with a cystic mass.

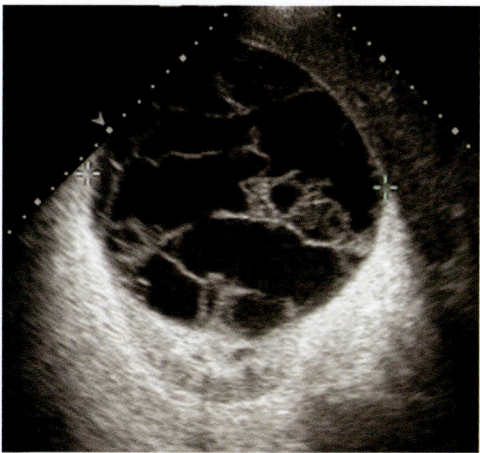

FIG. 15.38 Right hemorrhagic cyst.

| BOX 15.4 | What to Do When a Renal Mass Is Discovered |

- If the renal mass is solid, it must be considered malignant, unless fat is present within the mass.
- The presence of calcifications in a renal mass is always a sign of malignancy.
- If a cystic renal mass does not meet the sonographic criteria for a simple renal cyst, it must be considered malignant.
- A renal pseudotumor needs to be considered when a renal mass is discovered.
- Metastasis rate is 10%–15% at time of diagnosis.

Sonographic Considerations
- Evaluate the renal vein and inferior vena cava into the right atrium to look for thrombus/tumor.
- Evaluate the contralateral kidney, liver, and retroperitoneum for metastases.

and are most likely benign. Six months to 1 year follow-up is required.
- **Category III** consists of true indeterminate cystic masses showing uniform wall thickening, nodularity (especially in the base of the cyst), thick or irregular peripheral calcification, or a multilocular nature with multiple vascular (enhancing) septa. These cysts cannot be distinguished from malignancies and require a biopsy and/or surgery for evaluation. The distinction between some categories, especially IIF and III, is not clear, and variability in how the cysts in these two categories are classified may occur.
- **Category IV** cysts have diffuse wall thickening and may include areas with increased vascularity, or large nodules in the wall, or clearly solid vascular components in the cystic lesion—all features that strongly suggest malignancy. The cystic masses are presumed to be renal cell carcinoma, and the same treatment is followed, typically a nephrectomy.

Sonographically, it is difficult to differentiate between a septated cyst and small, adjacent cortical cysts known as "kissing" cysts (Fig. 15.39). A cyst may also have a cyst or mass within it (Fig. 15.40). Sometimes small sacculations or infoldings of the cystic wall produce wall irregularity; a cyst puncture or aspiration may be recommended to ascertain the pathology of the fluid within the mass.

Low-level echoes within a renal cyst may be artifacts (sensitivity too high or transducer frequency too low) or may result from infection, hemorrhage (Figs. 15.41 and 15.42), or a necrotic cystic tumor, or, in rare cases, malignancy.

Renal Sinus Parapelvic Cysts. The parapelvic cyst originates from the renal sinus and is most likely lymphatic in origin. These small cysts do not communicate with the collecting system. Most often, patients with parapelvic cysts are asymptomatic. Clinical symptoms are infrequent, but

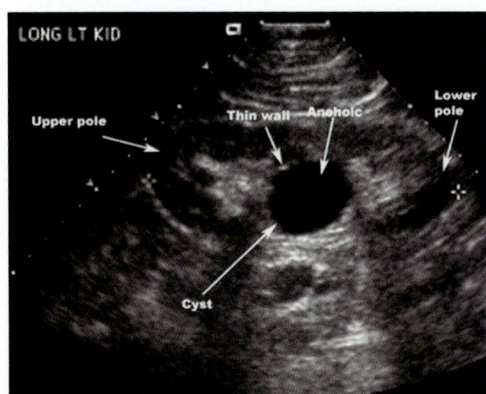

FIG. 15.39   A single upper-pole cortical cyst with a thin septation.

occasionally the cyst may cause pain, hematuria, hypertension, or obstruction.

Sonographic Findings. The sonogram shows a well-defined mass with no internal septations. The cyst can have irregular borders because it may compress adjacent renal sinus structures. Parapelvic cysts (especially those located in the medial lower portion of the kidney) may cause obstruction; peripelvic cysts do not. The sonographer should be able to differentiate the parapelvic cyst from hydronephrosis by trying to connect the dilated renal pelvis centrally. A transverse view is very useful. The dilated renal pelvis may present a cauliflower-like appearance, whereas the parapelvic cyst is more spherical in appearance.

Renal Cysts Associated With Renal Neoplasms

von Hippel–Lindau. Von Hippel–Lindau disease is an autosomal dominant genetic disorder. Several areas of the body may be affected. Predominant abnormalities include retinal angiomas, cerebellar hemangioblastomas, and a variety of abdominal cysts and tumors, including renal and pancreatic cysts, renal adenomas, and frequent multiple and bilateral renal adenocarcinoma tumors. Renal cell carcinoma in patients with this disease is multifocal and bilateral. A high incidence of renal cysts is found in patients with Von Hippel–Lindau disease, usually of cortical origin.

Tuberous Sclerosis. Tuberous sclerosis is an autosomal dominant genetic disorder characterized by mental retardation, seizures, and adenoma sebaceum. Associated renal lesions include multiple renal cysts or angiomyolipomas and/or cutaneous, retinal, and cerebral hamartomas. This disease may be difficult to separate from adult polycystic kidney disease.

Acquired Cystic Kidney Disease. This condition is found in native kidneys of patients with renal failure who need to undergo renal dialysis or peritoneal dialysis. Patients with this condition have been shown to have a slightly increased incidence of renal cysts, adenomas, and renal carcinoma. It is theorized that epithelial hyperplasia caused by tubular obstruction that occurs as a result of toxic substances plays a role in the development of these masses. Incidence increases

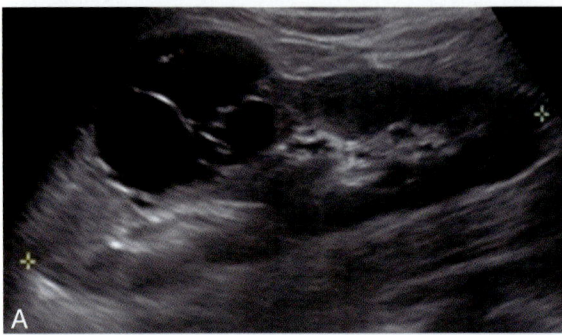
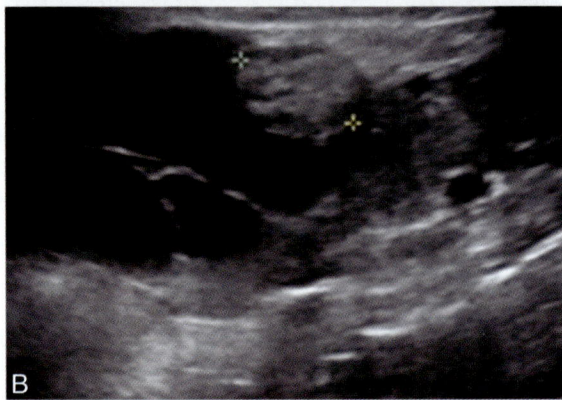

FIG. 15.40   (A) A 3-cm complex cyst. (B) A 1-cm solid nodule within the cyst.

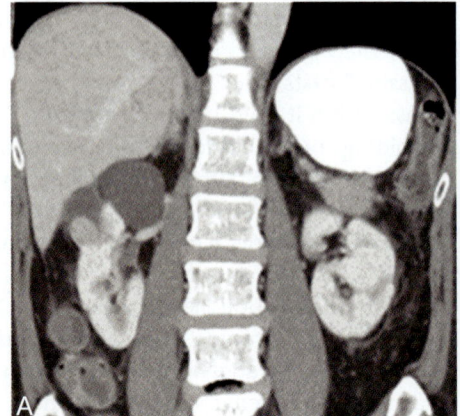
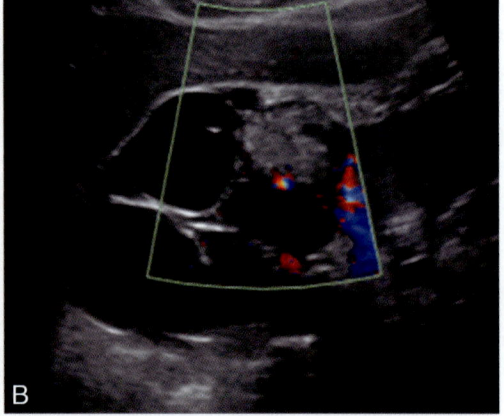

FIG. 15.41   (A) Contrast computed tomography confirmation enhancing nodule. (B) Color Doppler shows presence of nodule vascularity.

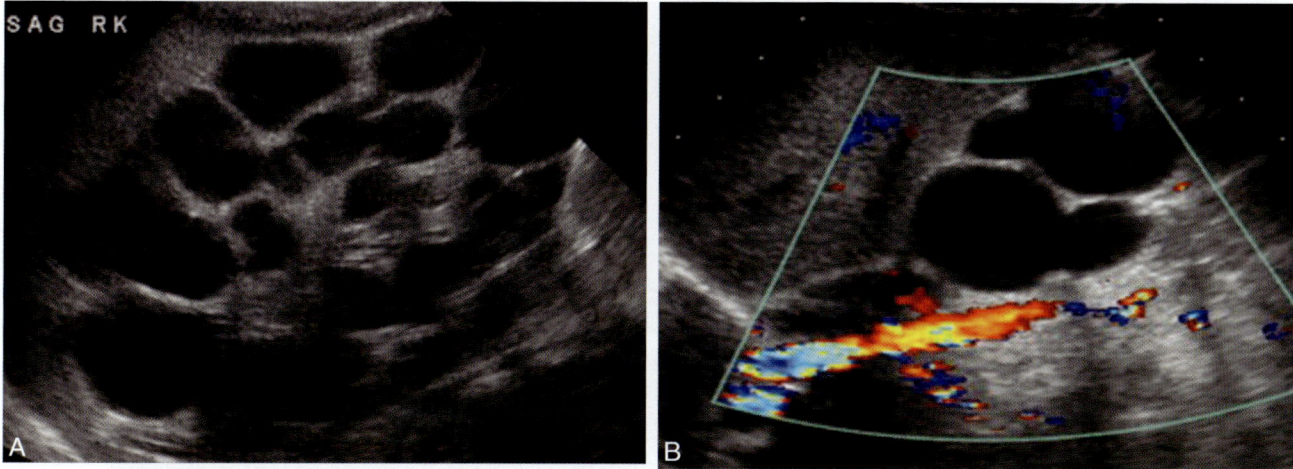

FIG. 15.42 Multicystic dysplastic kidney. (A) Multiple cysts of varying sizes with no normal parenchyma. (B) Atretic ureter absent renal pedicle.

with time, particularly after the first 3 years of dialysis. It increases up to 90% after 5 years of dialysis. Renal cysts can show spontaneous bleeding and hemorrhage, causing pain and flank discomfort. Solid tumors, including adenomas, oncocytomas, and renal cell carcinomas, are seen in up to 7% of patients.

Sonographic Findings. On a sonogram, the native kidneys are small and echogenic with several small cysts. In a patient with chronic renal failure, three to five cysts in each kidney are diagnostic. The incidence of hemorrhage into the renal cysts is increased; this will reveal internal echoes within the cyst or hyperechoic cysts. Renal masses with internal echoes, mural nodularities, and increased vascularity on color Doppler, with no posterior acoustic enhancement, are likely to be renal carcinoma.

Polycystic Kidney Disease. Polycystic renal disease may present in one of two forms: the infantile autosomal recessive form and the adult autosomal dominant form.

Autosomal Recessive Polycystic Kidney Disease. Autosomal recessive polycystic kidney disease (ARPKD) was previously called infantile polycystic disease and is a fairly rare genetic disorder. The gene that causes this disorder has two gene alterations. Dilation of the renal collecting tubules causes renal failure, and in later forms of the disease, liver involvement is seen. Four forms of ARPKD are classified according to the age of the patient at the onset of clinical signs: perinatal, neonatal, infantile, and juvenile. The perinatal form is found in utero and usually progresses to renal failure, causing pulmonary hypoplasia and intrauterine demise. On the perinatal sonogram, oligohydramnios, hypoplastic lungs, and massively enlarged echogenic kidneys may be visualized.

The juvenile form may present with hypertension, renal insufficiency, nephromegaly, hepatic cysts, bile duct proliferation, and Caroli disease, which may be associated with periportal fibrosis (which causes portal hypertension and esophageal varices). Renal function is usually decreased secondary to hepatic problems when ARPKD appears later in life. In older children, the kidneys are enlarged with an echogenic cortex and medulla and lack of corticomedullary differentiation. Microscopic or small cysts (1 to 2 mm) may be located in the medulla, often associated with hepatic fibrosis and splenomegaly.

Autosomal Dominant Polycystic Kidney Disease. Autosomal dominant polycystic kidney disease (ADPKD) (previously known as adult polycystic renal disease) is a common genetic disease that occurs in both men and women. The severity of the disease varies depending on the genotype. The most common type is ADPKD1 (located on the short arm of the sixteenth chromosome), which affects the kidneys more severely than ADPKD2 (located on the long arm of the fourth chromosome). Some people have no known genetic disposition to ADPKD, but it may result from spontaneous mutations. It is a bilateral disease that is characterized by enlarged kidneys with multiple asymmetric cysts varying in size and location in the renal cortex and medulla. The disease is progressive and does not usually clinically manifest until the fourth or fifth decade when hypertension or hematuria develops. By age 60, approximately 50% of patients will have end-stage renal disease (ESRD). Clinical symptoms include pain (common complaint), hypertension, palpable mass, hematuria, headache, urinary tract infection, and renal insufficiency. There is a high incidence of urolithiasis. Complications may include infection, hemorrhage, rupture of cyst, and renal obstruction.

Associated abnormalities include cysts in the liver, spleen, pancreas, thyroid, ovary, testes, or breast; cerebral berry aneurysm; and abdominal aortic aneurysm. Patients who are on renal dialysis have an increased incidence of renal cell carcinoma.

Sonographic Findings. The sonographic appearance of ADPKD is similar to the autosomal recessive form of polycystic disease. In the neonate, sonography demonstrates diffusely enlarged kidneys, due to multiple interfaces of the small cysts. This appearance is not unique to ADPKD, but further screening is warranted when noted on prenatal sonographic examination. Diagnosis is based on family history and tissue sampling.

In the adult patient, bilateral renal enlargement occurs with multiple asymmetric cysts of varying size in both cortex and medulla. In the most advanced cases, the normal renal parenchyma is replaced bilaterally with multiple cysts (Figs. 15.43 and 15.44) and the kidneys lose their reniform shape. The cysts may grow large enough to obliterate the renal sinus. They may become infected or hemorrhagic, which is characterized

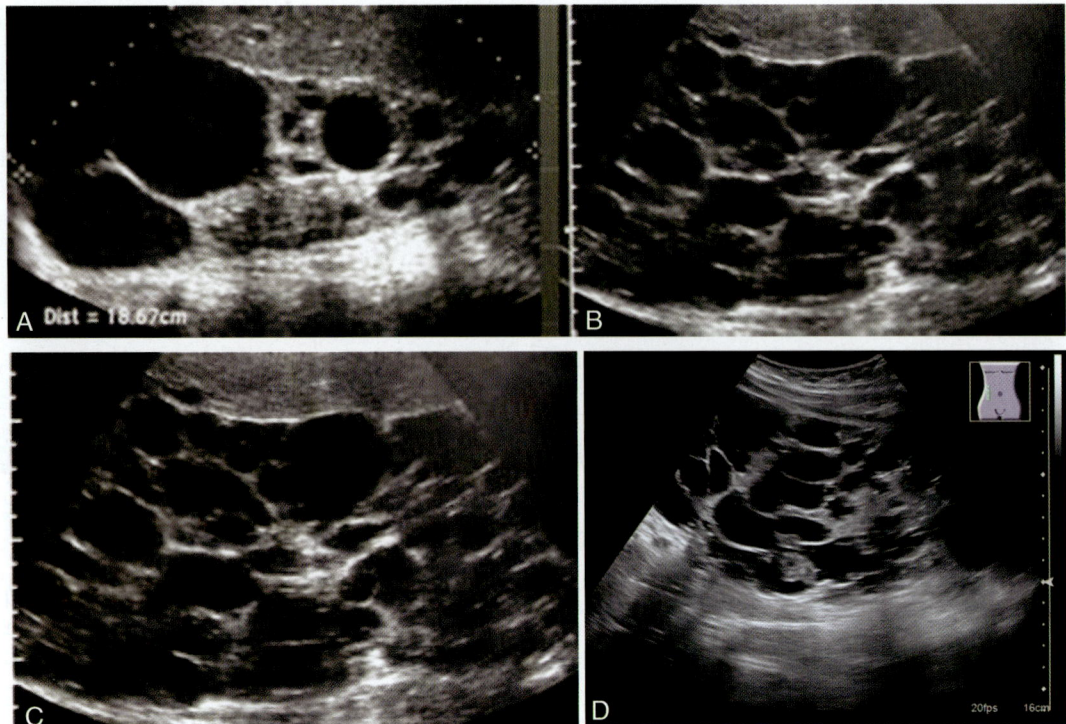

FIG. 15.43 (A–B) Images of a young adult male with polycystic renal disease. Longitudinal scans of both kidneys show enlarged kidneys (right kidney 15.2 cm and left kidney 17.4 cm) with a variety of cyst sizes. (C) Polycystic kidney with stone. (D) Approximately one-third of patients with polycystic renal disease also have cysts on the liver or other organs.

sonographically by internal debris within the cysts or thickened walls. The walls of the cysts may be calcified, or stones may form. A complicated cyst may result in spontaneous bleeding, causing flank pain for the patient (see Table 15.3).

Multicystic Dysplastic Kidney. Multicystic dysplastic kidney (MCDK) disease is a common nonhereditary renal dysplasia that usually occurs unilaterally, with the kidney functioning poorly, if at all. MCDK is the most common form of cystic disease in neonates and is believed to be the consequence of early in utero urinary tract obstruction. Dysplastic changes usually involve the entire kidney but, rarely, may be segmental or focal. Bilateral MCDK is incompatible with life. Complications arising from a multicystic dysplastic kidney that is not removed include hypertension, hematuria, infection, and flank pain. A slightly increased risk of malignant transformation can occur if the kidney is not removed.

Sonographic Findings. In neonates and children, the kidneys are multicystic, with absence of renal parenchyma, renal sinus, and atretic renal artery. In adults, the kidneys may be small (atrophic and calcified) and echogenic. Other possible findings include ureteral atresia (failure of the ureter to develop from the calyceal system), contralateral ureteropelvic obstruction (in 30% of patients) (development of the ureter from the bladder with retrograde filling), and a nonfunctioning kidney.

Medullary Cystic Disease

Medullary Sponge Kidney. Medullary sponge kidney (MSK) is a development anomaly that occurs in the medullary pyramids and consists of cystic or fusiform dilation of the distal collecting

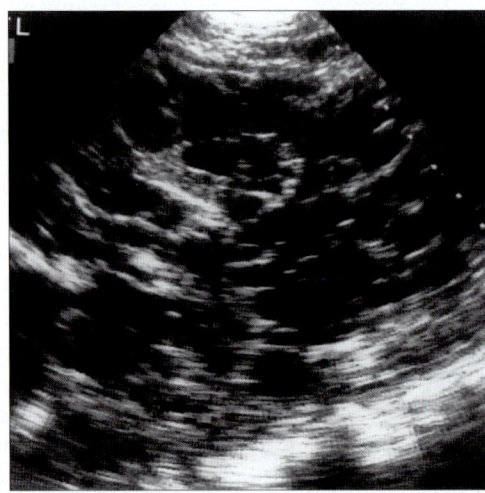

FIG. 15.44 A 30-year-old man with a solitary left polycystic kidney and hematuria underwent imaging to rule out obstruction. It is very difficult to rule out obstruction with so many small cysts.

ducts (ducts of Bellini), causing stasis of urine and stone formation. Because the medullary sponge kidney is an anatomic rather than a metabolic defect, the pathologic process may be unilateral or segmental. The cause is unknown. Many patients remain asymptomatic, but patients with hematuria, infection, and renal stones should be evaluated for medullary sponge kidney.

MSK may be associated with a variety of other congenital and inherited disorders, including Beckwith-Wiedemann syndrome, polycystic kidney disease (PKD) (about 3% of patients with autosomal dominant polycystic kidney disease have evidence of MSK), Caroli disease, and congenital hepatic fibrosis.

Medullary Cystic Kidney Disease and Nephronophthisis. Nephronophthisis and medullary cystic kidney disease are inherited disorders that eventually lead to ESRD. They are grouped together because they share many features. Pathologically, they cause cysts restricted to the renal medulla or corticomedullary border, as well as a triad of tubular atrophy, tubular basement membrane disintegration, and interstitial fibrosis.

Medullary cystic kidney disease (MCKD) is very similar to the childhood disease familial juvenile nephronophthisis (NPH). Both lead to scarring of the kidney and formation of fluid-filled cavities (cysts) in the deeper parts of the kidney. In these conditions, the kidneys do not concentrate the urine enough, leading to excessive urine production and loss of sodium and other chemical changes in the blood and urine.

MCKD occurs in older patients and is inherited in an autosomal dominant pattern. NPH occurs in young children and is usually due to autosomal recessive inheritance.

Sonographic Findings. The patient presents with small echogenic kidneys, with loss of corticomedullary differentiation, and multiple small medullary cysts (<2 cm). With MCKD, sonography shows hyperechoic calyces, with or without stones (Figs. 15.45 and 15.46).

Renal Neoplasms

Sonography is often the first imaging modality that detects renal masses. Often these masses are incidental findings. Even though ultrasound may not be as sensitive as CT or MRI in finding small masses, ultrasound is able to accurately differentiate cysts from solid masses, especially in cases where CT and MRI fail to do so. The sonographic appearance of most renal masses is nonspecific. Very often, the sonographic characteristic patterns of benign and malignant tumors cannot be differentiated from one another. In the study of the solid renal masses the role of sonography has been focused on the differentiation of renal cell carcinoma and angiomyolipoma, the most common malignant and benign solid renal tumors.

Research in using contrast-enhanced sonography along with Doppler in identifying tumor vascularity to differentiate between a benign and malignant mass has provided encouraging results. The use of contrast agents in sonography has not, however, been approved by the Food and Drug Administration in the United States. If a solid mass is detected, renal cell carcinoma, oncocytoma, angiomyolipoma, transitional cell carcinoma, or secondary neoplasms (e.g., metastasis, lymphoma) must be considered (see Box 15.4).

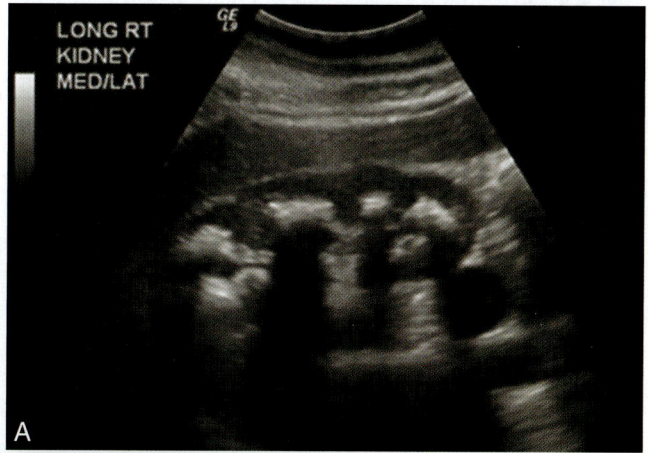

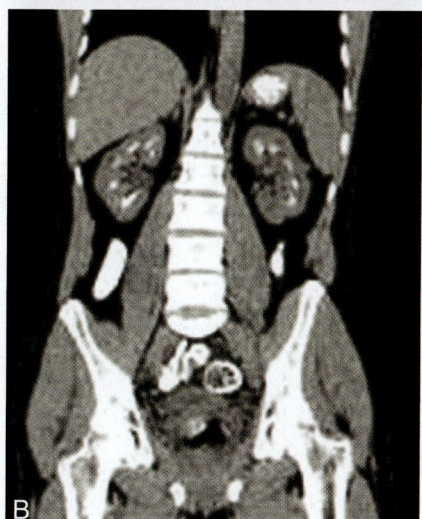

FIG. 15.46 (A) Longitudinal view of the right kidney with hyperechoic calyces and stones. (B) Tiny medullary calculi are detected on computed tomography.

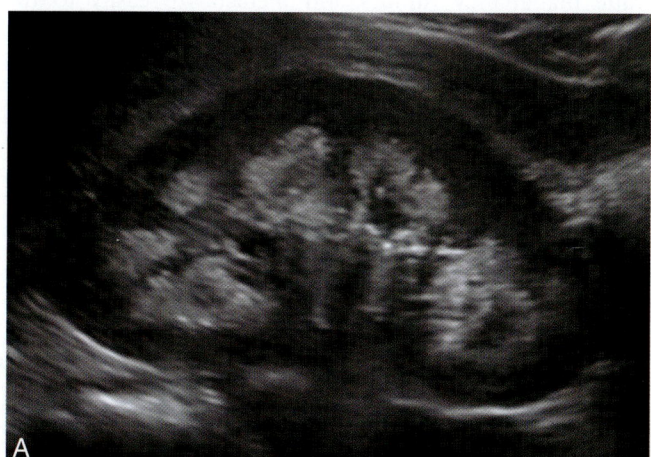

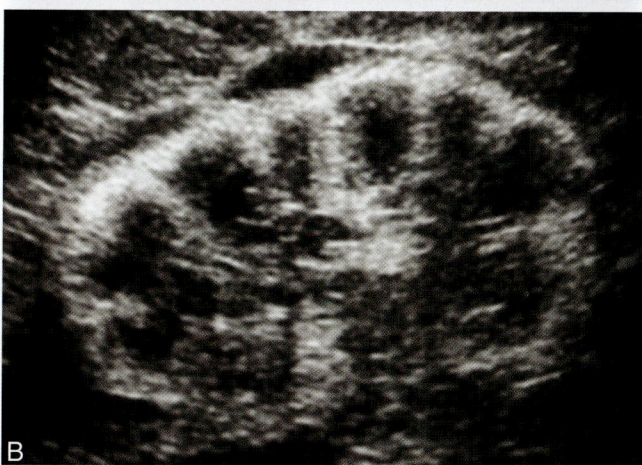

FIG. 15.45 (A) Medullary nephrocalcinosis. (B) Cortical nephrocalcinosis.

Renal Cell Carcinoma. Renal cell carcinoma (RCC), also called hypernephroma, or Grawitz tumor, is the most common of all renal neoplasms and represents 85% of all kidney tumors. It is twice as common in males as in females, usually in the sixth to seventh decade of life. The classical clinical presentation is nonspecific; however, the patient may report hematuria, flank pain, and a palpable mass. The tumor appears bilaterally in 0.1% to 1.5% of patients, and is multifocal in 13% of cases. An association with von Hippel–Lindau disease, acquired cystic disease (dialysis patients), and tuberous sclerosis is reported. Regardless of histologic subtype, the sonographic appearance of most RCCs is solid with no predilection for left or right kidney or location in the organ. One to two percent of RCCs are predominantly cystic, and very rarely the tumor may be entirely cystic.

Sonographic Findings. Most RCCs are isoechoic, but they may also present as hyperechoic (Fig. 15.47). Usually, large tumors have a heterogeneous echotexture, caused by intratumoral hemorrhage and necrosis. Small tumors (<3 cm in diameter) have the same hyperechoic appearance as fat-containing tumors, such as angiomyolipomas. A hypoechoic rim, which represents a vascular pseudocapsule on color Doppler, may be very helpful in making the diagnosis of RCC. The presence of intratumoral calcifications is considered specific for RCC. In cases in which renal cell carcinoma is represented as cystic, a variety of types, such as unilocular, multilocular, completely necrotic, and tumor originating in a cyst, may be demonstrated on sonography.

Use of color Doppler for the detection of tumor vascularity shows high sensitivity for malignant renal tumors, especially RCC. In RCC, tumor vascularity can be demonstrated in up to 92% of cases, and the most common vascular patterns include a "basket sign" and/or "vessels within the tumor." High systolic and high end-diastolic arterial flow with low resistive index is the most typical flow pattern in spectral Doppler waveforms. Renal vein and inferior vena cava invasion occurs in 5% to 24% of RCCs at the time of diagnosis, and metastasis from renal malignancies is seen in lungs, mediastinum, other nodes, liver, bone, adrenal glands, and the opposite kidney. CT and MRI with contrast are the most sensitive radiographic examinations for the detection and characterization of renal masses (Figs. 15.48–15.50). Box 15.5 summarizes the sonographic characteristics of malignant renal tumors.

Transitional Cell Carcinoma. Transitional cell carcinoma (TCC) accounts for 90% of malignancies that involve the renal pelvis, ureter, and bladder, and for up to 7% to 10% of all renal tumors. The tumor is often multifocal, with a 40% to 80% incidence. TCC occurs twice as often in men as in women, with a peak occurrence in the seventh decade. TCC of the renal pelvis is 2 to 3 times more common than ureteral neoplasm, and is almost 50 times less common than TCC of the urinary bladder. The TCC may be papillary or flat. Papillary TCCs are more common, with an exophytic polypoid appearance attached to mucosa. They usually are low-grade malignancies and tend to have a more benign course. Small TCCs tend to be flat and are difficult to detect with any type of imaging. Small TCCs are generally high-grade malignancy tumors and metastasize easily to the other tissues and organs. Clinically, the patient may present with gross or microscopic hematuria and flank pain. The

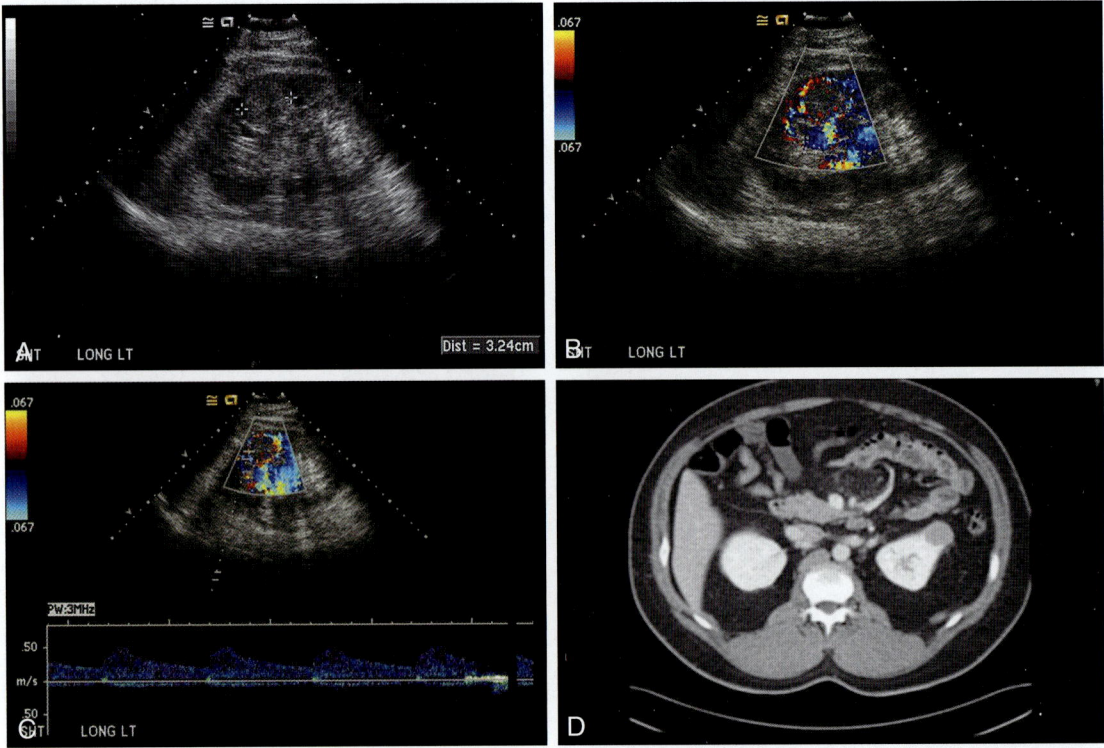

FIG. 15.47 (A) Longitudinal view of a small hyperechoic renal cell carcinoma. (B–C) Color Doppler demonstrates peripheral vascularity of the tumor ("basket sign"). (D) Contrast computed tomography confirms a small enhancing renal tumor; pathology confirmed cell carcinoma.

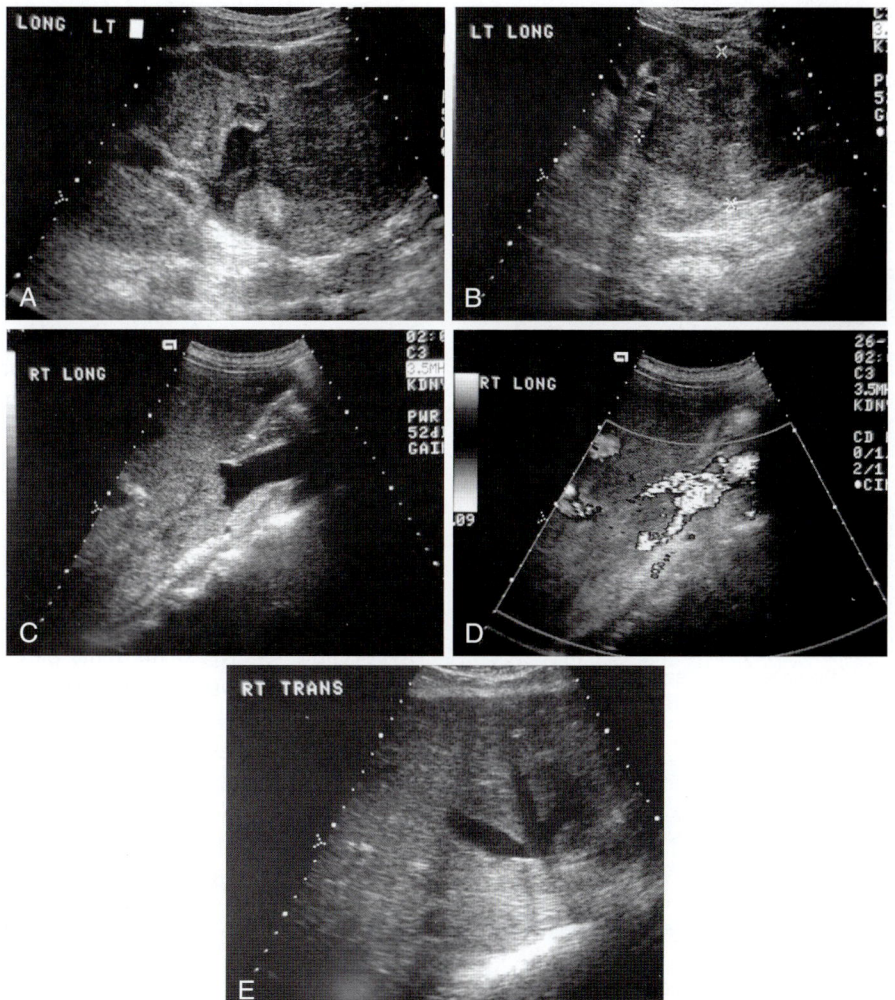

FIG. 15.48 Stage III renal cell carcinoma with invasion into the inferior vena cava. (A) Longitudinal scan shows lower pole mass with no normal renal parenchyma. (B) Measurement of the lower pole mass. (C) Longitudinal scan demonstrating the thrombus-filled inferior vena cava (IVC). (D) Longitudinal scan of IVC with color flow showing obstruction. (E) Transverse view of the dome of the liver with patent hepatic veins and nonvisualization of the IVC.

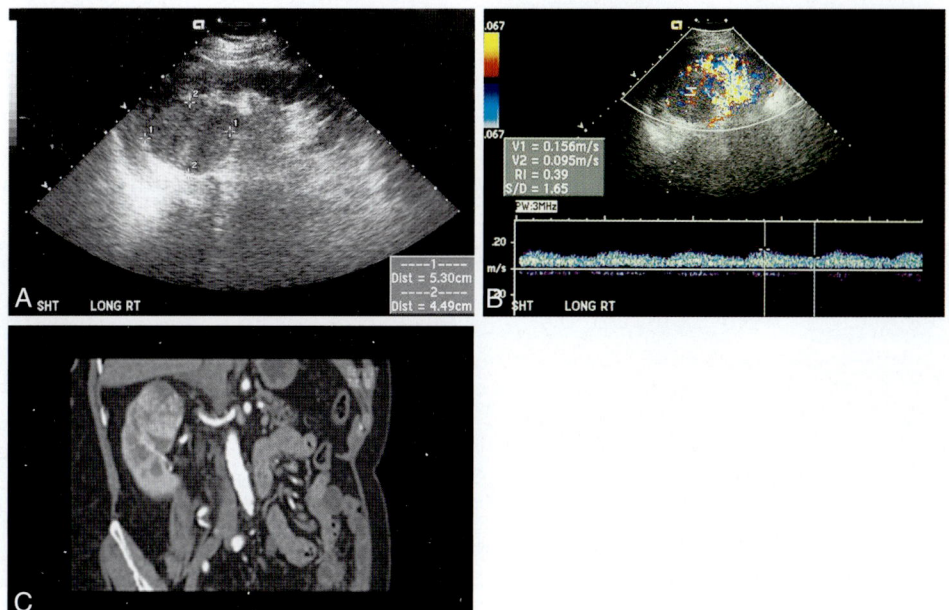

FIG. 15.49 (A–B) Longitudinal scan of the right kidney showing a large (5.30 × 4.49 cm) hypoechoic vascular mass with low resistive index (RI). (C) Contrast computed tomography confirms a highly enhancing renal tumor; pathology confirmed renal cell carcinoma.

differential diagnosis includes other tumors of the renal pelvis, such as squamous cell tumor, adenoma, a blood clot, or a fungus ball (see Table 15.2).

Sonographic Findings. The typical appearance is that of a hypoechoic mass within the collecting system, with low vascularity on color Doppler and, extremely rarely, calcifications. TCC may invade adjacent renal parenchyma and form an infiltrating mass, which usually preserves the renal contour.

Squamous Cell Carcinoma. Squamous cell carcinoma is a rare, highly invasive tumor with a poor prognosis. Clinically, the patient usually has a history of chronic irritation and gross hematuria, with a palpable kidney secondary to severe hydronephrosis.

Sonographic Findings. The sonographic finding is usually a large mass in the renal pelvis. Obstruction from kidney stones may also be present (Figs. 15.51 and 15.52).

Renal Lymphoma. Primary lymphomatous involvement of the kidneys is rare, with a 3% occurrence. The secondary form is more common. This form of lymphoma may occur as a hematogenous spread (90%) or as direct extension via the retroperitoneal lymphatic channels with a contiguous spread from the retroperitoneum (see Table 15.2). Non-Hodgkin lymphoma is more common than Hodgkin lymphoma. Lymphoma is more common as a bilateral invasion with multiple nodules.

Sonographic Findings. The kidneys are enlarged and hypoechoic relative to the renal parenchyma (the mass may simulate a renal cyst without posterior acoustic enhancement). The mass rarely demonstrates a sonographic halo of hypoechoic mass in the perinephric regions (Fig. 15.53). The sonographer should be careful of highly hypoechoic renal tumors with poorly defined margins without posterior enhancement, as they may be mistaken initially for "renal cysts."

Secondary Malignancies of the Kidneys. Metastases to the kidneys are relatively common, occurring late in the course of the disease. Secondary malignancies are bilateral in one-third of cases and multiple in more than 50%. The most common primary malignancies that metastasize to the kidneys include carcinoma of the lung or breast and RCC of the contralateral kidney. On sonography, the lesion usually presents as multiple, poorly marginated hypoechoic masses. Renal enlargement without a discrete mass also may occur.

Sonographic Findings. The tumor may spread beyond the **renal capsule** and invade the renal vein. The tumor cells can extend into the inferior vena cava to the right atrium and can eventually metastasize into the lungs. The tumor may be multifocal in a small percentage of patients.

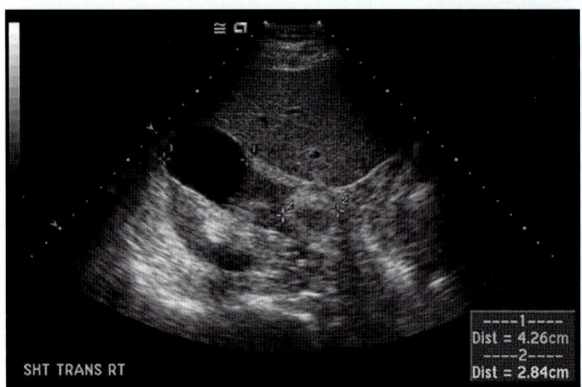

FIG. 15.50 Transverse view of the right kidney demonstrating a cyst and a small hyperechoic mass, which is consistent with renal cell carcinoma.

BOX 15.5 Sonographic Characteristics of a Malignant Renal Tumor

- Renal cell carcinomas (RCCs) less than 2–3 cm in diameter are always hyperechoic.
- The bigger the tumor, the more heterogeneous is its echotexture.
- Hypoechoic rim represents a vascular pseudocapsule.
- In up to 92% of RCCs, peripheral (basket sign) and/or central (vessel within the tumor) vascularity can be demonstrated on color Doppler.
- Invasion of the renal vein and/or inferior vena cava occurs in 5%–24% of cases.

In Cases With Cystic Appearance
- Thick wall >1 mm
- Irregularity at the base of the cyst
- Septations
- Calcifications
- Presence of vascularity in the septa and/or cystic wall

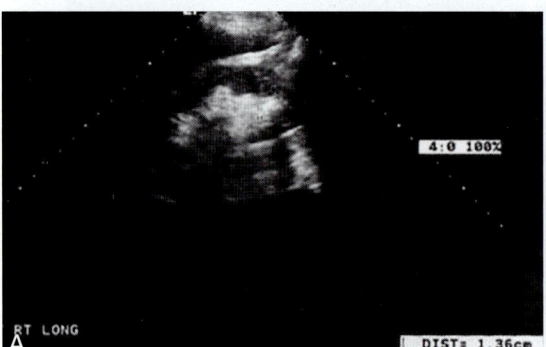 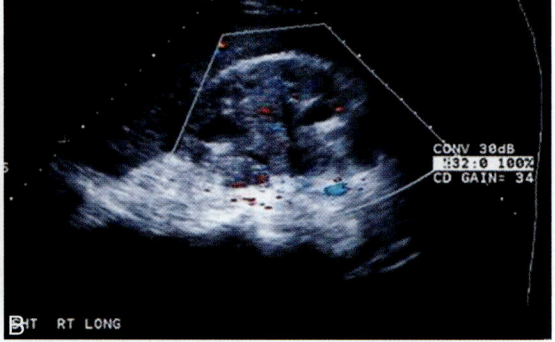

FIG. 15.51 (A) Longitudinal scan of the right kidney with a small hypoechoic mass (transitional cell carcinoma) in the mid-upper collection system and a 1.36 cm nonobstructing stone in the lower pole. (B) A large vascular hypoechoic mass occupying most of the collection system and causing an obstruction.

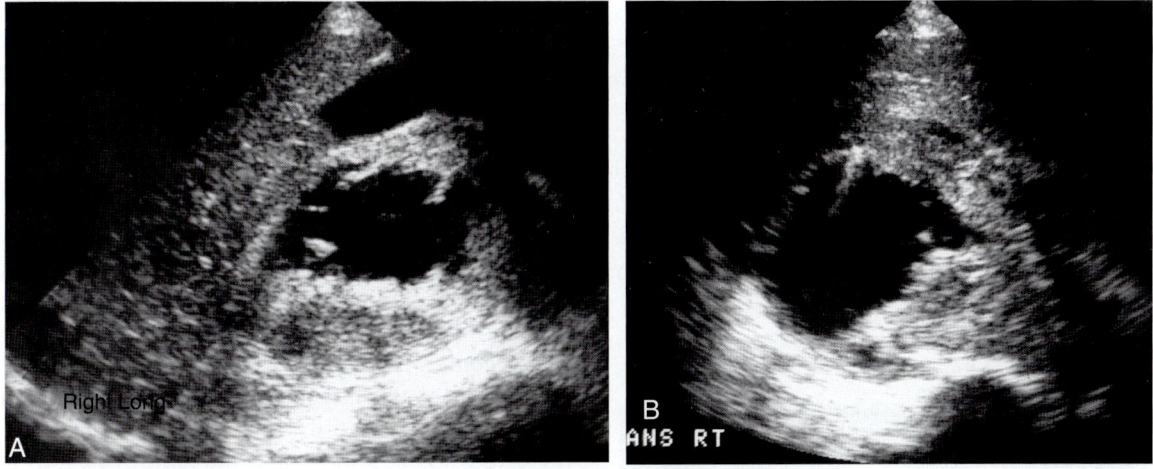

FIG. 15.52 Sixty-year-old patient with metastatic disease. (A) Sagittal image of right kidney shows irregularly shaped mass filling the renal sinus. (B) Transverse image of the squamous cell carcinoma.

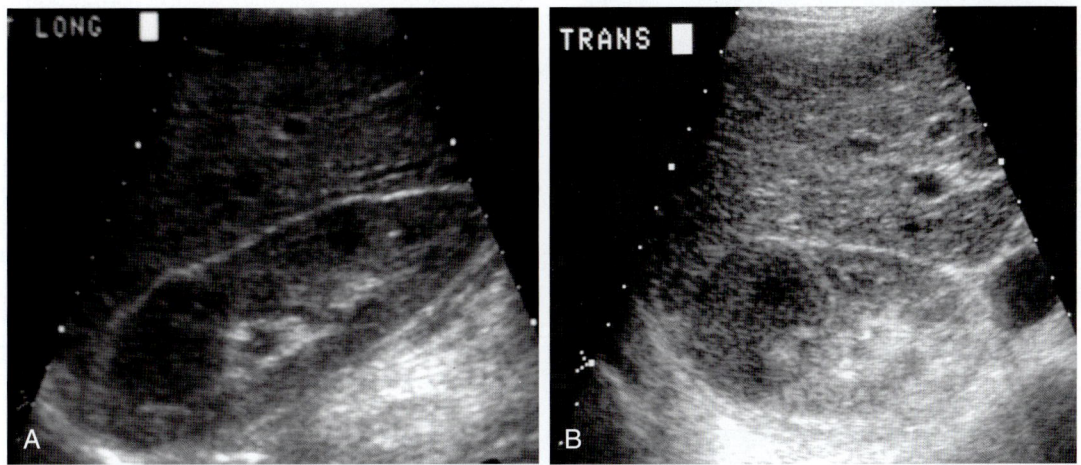

FIG. 15.53 Sixty-year-old patient with bilateral renal lymphomas. (A) Sagittal image of right kidney with hypoechoic upper pole mass. (B) Transverse image of upper pole of right kidney with hypoechoic lymphoma.

Nephroblastoma. Nephroblastoma, or Wilms tumor, is the most common abdominal malignancy in children and the most common solid renal tumor in pediatric patients 1 to 8 years old. Peak incidence is seen at 2.5 to 3 years of age; 90% of patients are younger than 5 years, and 70% are younger than 3 years. Nephroblastoma is 2 to 8 times more common in patients with horseshoe kidney. Clinical signs may include abdominal flank mass, hematuria, fever, and anorexia.

Sonographic Findings. The mass varies from hypoechoic to moderately echogenic. A 5% to 10% incidence of bilateral tumors has been reported, so careful evaluation of both kidneys is crucial. Up to 40% of patients with Wilms tumor have renal vein thrombosis and/or vena cava or atrial thrombus by the time of diagnosis. Venous obstruction may result, with findings of leg edema, varicocele, or Budd-Chiari syndrome (Figs. 15.54–15.56).

Benign Renal Tumors. Benign renal tumors are rare. All renal tumors are treated as malignant until proven otherwise. The patient usually is asymptomatic and presents with flank pain only if the mass is large or if hemorrhage from the mass occurs. Adenomas and oncocytomas are two common benign renal tumors (see Table 15.3).

Renal Angiomyolipoma. Renal angiomyolipoma (AML) is the most common benign renal tumor. It is composed of varying proportions of fat, muscle, and blood vessels. AML has an incidence of 0.07% to 0.3% in the general population; 80% of cases occur in females, and 80% in the right kidney. The tumor is found in 80% of patients with tuberous sclerosis. Tumor size varies between 1 and 20 cm and may be multifocal.

Sonographic Findings. The echo pattern of AML is usually hyperechoic, depending on the proportions of fat, muscle, and vessels within the mass. Intratumoral hemorrhage and organ displacement are the primary complications. Differential diagnosis is made with small (<3 cm) renal cell carcinomas, which are also hyperechoic in echotexture and may simulate AML in up to 33% of cases. A hypoechoic rim, presented as a basket sign on color Doppler, favors renal cell carcinoma. Color Doppler shows no intratumoral vascularity. On angiography, the tumor is highly vascular; CT is determinant in the diagnosis of AML because of its sensitivity in detecting intratumoral fat (Figs. 15.57 and 15.58).

Renal Adenomatous Tumors. Renal adenomatous tumors can be seen as nephrogenic adenofibroma or embryonal adenoma. Patients are usually asymptomatic. Incidental findings may be noted if the mass is large or if intratumoral hemorrhage occurs. In some cases, these tumors may cause hematuria.

▸ ***Sonographic Findings.*** These tumors appear as solid masses on sonography, are hyperechoic to hypoechoic in echotexture, and are hypovascular on color Doppler (Fig. 15.59). As with oncocytomas, renal adenomatous tumors may be indistinguishable from RCC.

Oncocytoma. Oncocytoma is another uncommon renal tumor that is usually benign. Incidence is increased in the middle-aged or elderly patient. This lesion represents 3.1% to 6% of all renal tumors. Tumor size varies, with an average size of 6 cm. The patient is typically asymptomatic, but the tumor may cause pain and hematuria.

▸ ***Sonographic Findings.*** In more than 50% of cases, the mass is hypoechoic in echotexture. Oncocytomas resemble "spoke-wheel" patterns of enhancement with a central scar. It is practically impossible to differentiate them from RCC; 5% of oncocytomas are initially diagnosed as RCC (Fig. 15.60).

Lipomas. A lipoma consists of fat cells and is the most common of the mesenchymal type of tumors. This tumor is found more often in females than in males. The patient is typically asymptomatic, but the tumor has been reported to cause hematuria.

▸ ***Sonographic Findings.*** Lipomas appear as well-defined echogenic masses within the kidney (Fig. 15.61).

Renal Disease

Intrinsic renal disease can be identified by examining the renal parenchyma with ultrasound. Two classifications of disease processes have been described. One group produces a generalized increase in cortical echoes, believed to result from deposition of collagen and fibrous tissue. This group includes interstitial nephritis, acute tubular necrosis, amyloidosis, diabetic nephropathy, systemic lupus erythematosus, and myeloma. The second group of diseases may cause loss of normal anatomic detail, resulting in inability to distinguish the cortex and medullary regions of the kidneys. This group

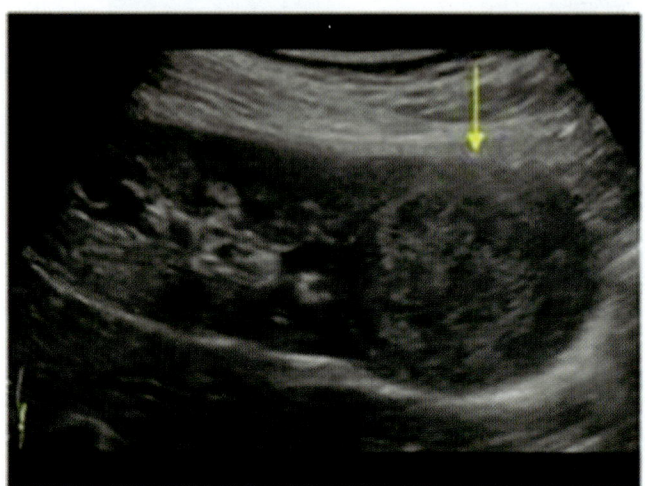

FIG. 15.54 Eight-year-old with hematuria and large palpable right renal mass disrupting the normal renal architecture.

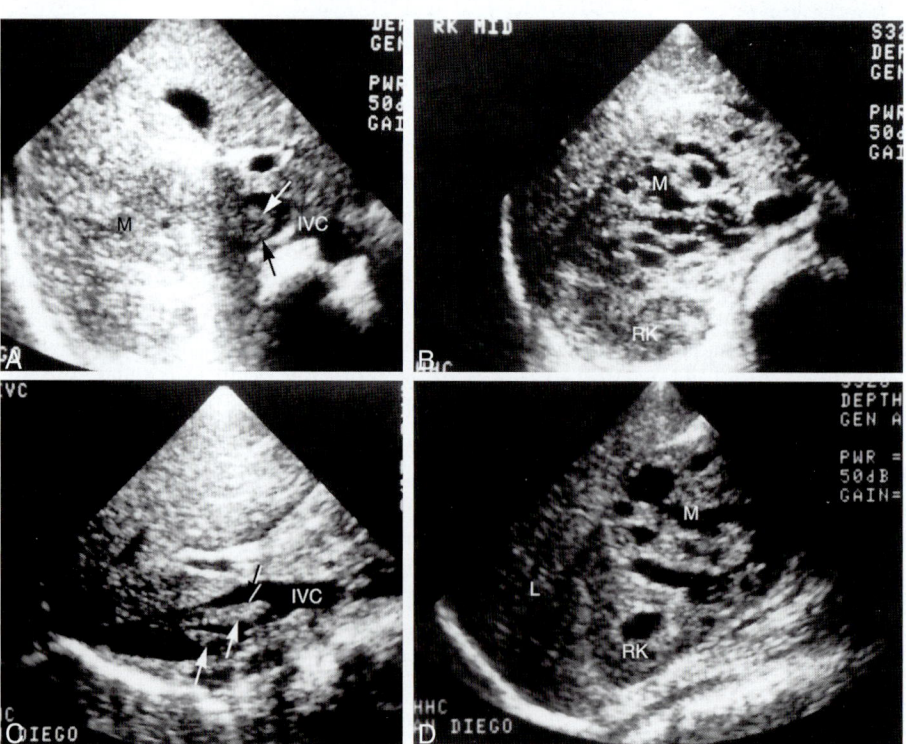

FIG. 15.55 (A) One of the complications of a Wilms tumor (M) is spread beyond the renal capsule into the renal vein and inferior vena cava (IVC). (B) This 18-month-old child had a large, complex tumor with extension into the IVC *(arrows)*. (C–D) Longitudinal scan, showing the dilated inferior vena cava with tumor echoes along the posterior border. The tumor may extend into the right atrium of the heart. *L,* Liver; *RK,* right kidney.

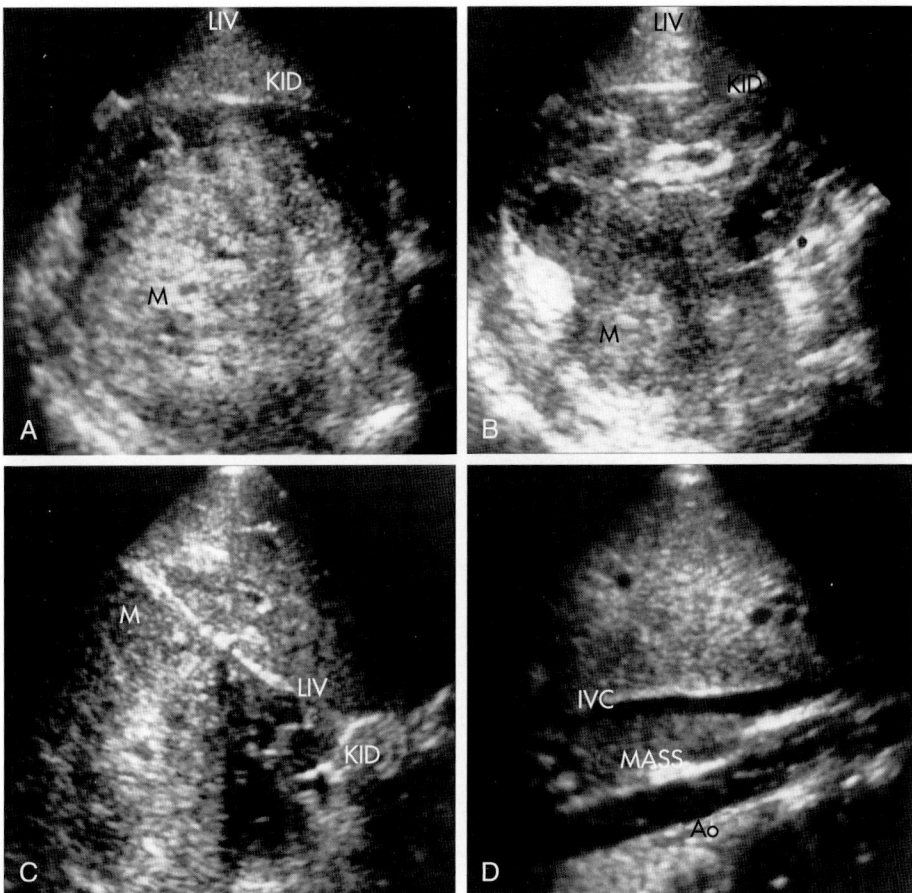

FIG. 15.56 A 14-month-old child with a large Wilms tumor (M) extending from the right kidney (KID) into the inferior vena cava (IVC). On coronal scan (D), the tumor mass is seen within the IVC. The patient is rolled into a slight decubitus position for better imaging of the IVC and aorta (Ao). *LIV*, Liver.

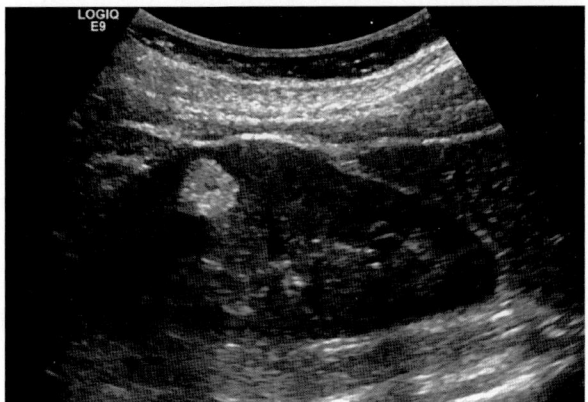

FIG. 15.57 Angiomyolipoma appears as an echogenic focal mass in the renal parenchyma.

of diseases includes chronic pyelonephritis, renal tubular ectasia, and acute bacterial nephritis (see Table 15.3).

The end stage of many of these disease processes is renal atrophy, which can be identified on a sonogram by measuring renal length and cortical thickness. Some acute renal disorders produce exactly the opposite findings—decreased parenchymal echogenicity and renal enlargement. Examples include acute renal vein thrombosis, acute pyelonephritis, and acute renal transplant rejection. Interstitial edema is believed to be the most likely cause of these findings.

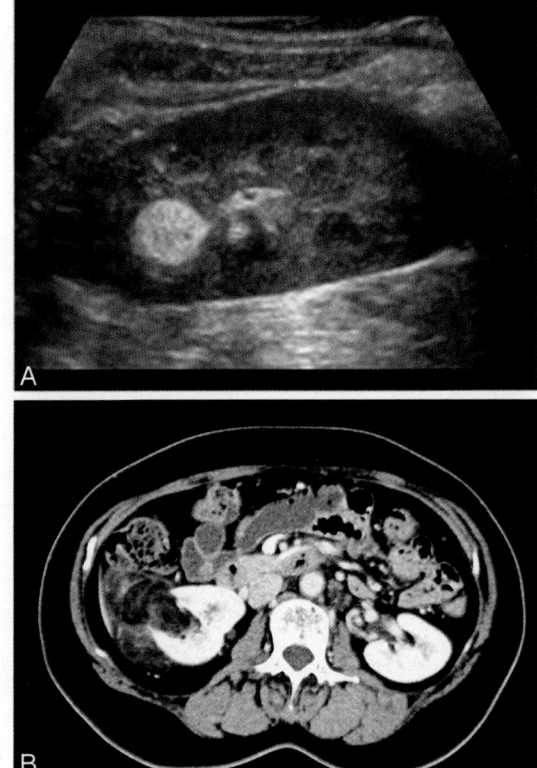

FIG. 15.58 (A) Angiolipomas are common benign tumors that usually appear as unilateral solitary or multiple echogenic masses in middle-aged women. (B) Computed tomography image of the tumor.

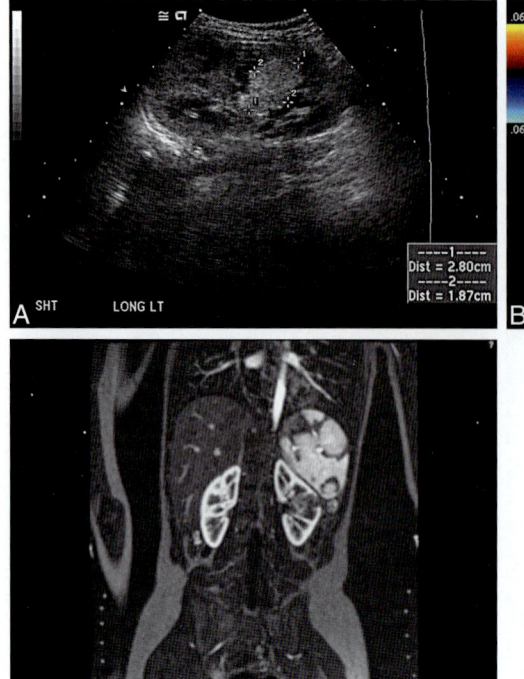

FIG. 15.59 (A–B) Left kidney mid-lower pole 3-cm hyperechoic vascular mass. (C) On magnetic resonance imaging, the mass shows a homogeneous low signal on T1 phase images.

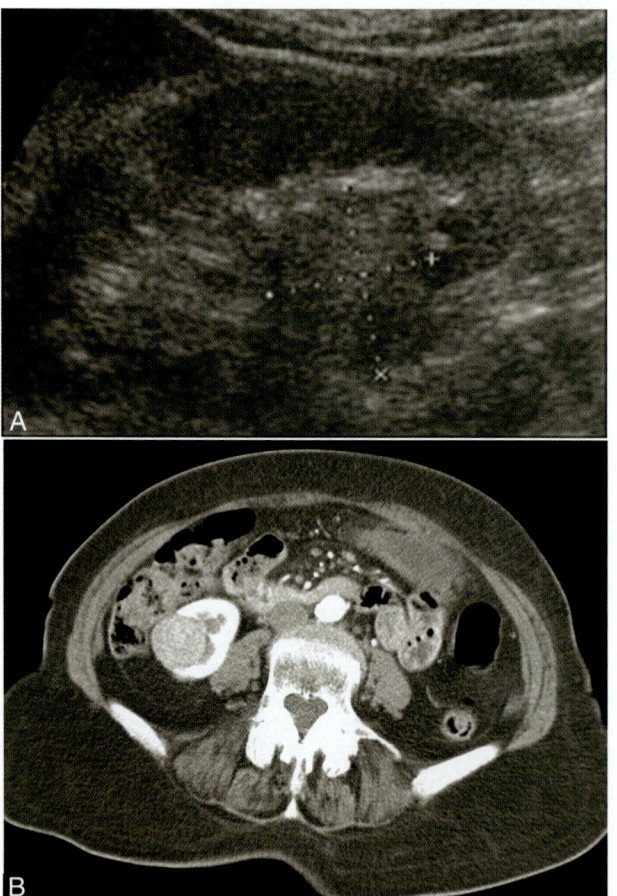

FIG. 15.60 (A) Longitudinal view of the left kidney shows large exophytic heterogeneous mass. (B) Computed tomographic transverse view of the kidneys shows enhancement of the mass with a central scar. Mass proved to be oncocytoma.

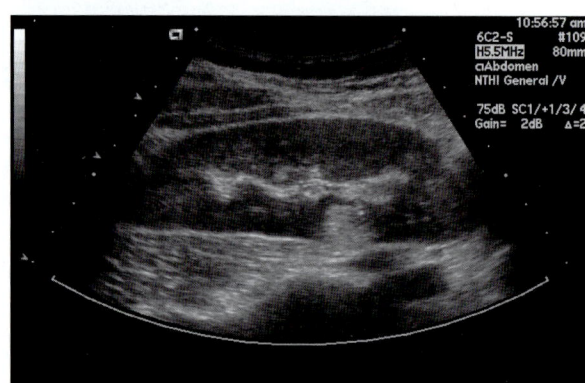

FIG. 15.61 Sagittal view of left kidney with lipoma. (Courtesy Siemens Medical Solutions USA, Inc.)

Acute Glomerulonephritis. In acute glomerulonephritis, necrosis or proliferation of cellular elements (or both) occurs in the glomeruli. The vascular elements, tubules, and interstitium become secondarily affected; the end result is enlarged, poorly functioning kidneys.

Sonographic Findings. Different forms of glomerulonephritis, including membranous, idiopathic, membranoproliferative, rapidly progressive, and poststreptococcal, can be associated with abnormal echo patterns from the renal parenchyma on a sonogram (Fig. 15.62). Increased cortical echoes probably result from changes within the glomerular, interstitial, tubular, and vascular structures. Patients have many symptoms, including nephrotic syndrome, hypertension, anemia, and peripheral edema.

Acute Interstitial Nephritis. Acute interstitial nephritis has been associated with the infectious processes of scarlet

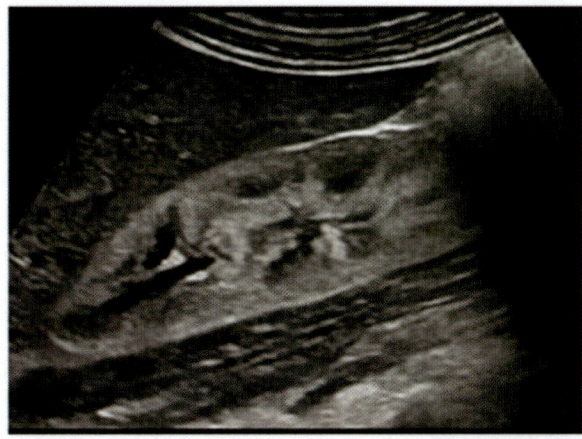

FIG. 15.62 Acute glomerulonephritis may be suspected when the echogenicity of the renal parenchyma exceeds that of the liver.

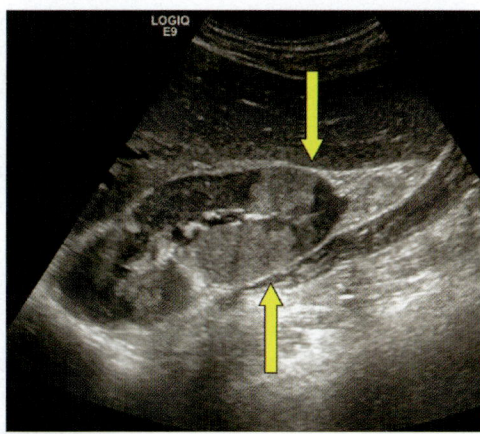

FIG. 15.63 Patients with lupus nephritis demonstrate a highly echogenic renal parenchymal pattern compared with the liver. Renal atrophy is usually present.

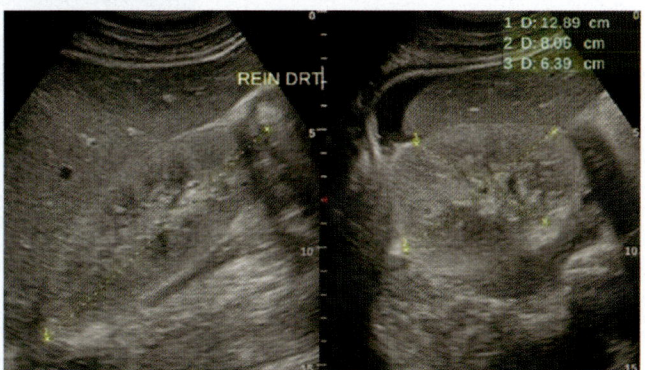

FIG. 15.64 Longitudinal *(left)* and transverse *(right)* scans in a patient with AIDS show cortical echogenicity with normal to slightly increased renal size.

fever and diphtheria. It may be a manifestation of an allergic reaction to certain drugs. Patient signs and symptoms include uremia, proteinuria, hematuria, rash, fever, and eosinophilia.

Sonographic Findings. The kidneys are enlarged and mottled. On a sonogram, renal cortical echogenicity is increased. The increase in echogenicity is greatest in cases of diffuse active disease. This increase is less apparent in diffuse scarring.

Lupus Nephritis. Systemic lupus erythematosus is a connective tissue disorder believed to result from an abnormal immune system. Females are affected more often than males, and incidence peaks between 20 and 40 years of age. The kidneys are involved in more than 50% of patients. Renal manifestations include hematuria, proteinuria, hypertension, renal vein thrombosis, and renal insufficiency.

Sonographic Findings. Sonographic appearance is increased cortical echogenicity and renal atrophy (Fig. 15.63).

Acquired Immunodeficiency Syndrome. Acquired immunodeficiency syndrome (AIDS) is a highly contagious disease, spread mainly by unprotected sexual activity or infected needles. The virus destroys T cells and then replicates rapidly within the body. It affects many organs. Patients have various symptoms (see Table 15.2).

Unexplained uremia or azotemia may indicate renal dysfunction resulting from AIDS; it is usually a late finding. Causes of renal dysfunction in AIDS patients include acute tubular necrosis, nephrocalcinosis, interstitial nephritis, and focal segmental glomerulosclerosis.

Sonographic Findings. An echogenic parenchymal pattern is evident on a sonogram. Cortical echogenicity is increased. Kidneys are normal in size or enlarged (Figs. 15.64–15.66). If AIDS-related lymphoma or Kaposi sarcoma occurs, the kidneys appear enlarged and hypoechoic on a sonogram.

Sickle Cell Nephropathy. Renal involvement is common in patients with sickle cell disease. Abnormalities include glomerulonephritis, renal vein thrombosis, and papillary necrosis. Hematuria is common.

Sonographic Findings. The sonographic appearance depends on the type of disorder. In acute renal vein thrombosis, the kidneys are enlarged with decreased echogenicity secondary to edema. In patients with subacute cases, renal enlargement is present with increased cortical echoes.

Hypertensive Nephropathy. Uncontrolled hypertension can lead to progressive renal damage and azotemia.

Sonographic Findings. Sonographically, the kidneys are small with smooth borders. Superimposed scars of pyelonephritis or lobar infarction may distort the intrarenal anatomy. Bilateral small kidneys occur secondary to end-stage disease as a result of hypertension, inflammation, or ischemia.

Papillary Necrosis. Renal papillary necrosis (RPN) is not a pathologic entity, but rather a descriptive term for a condition—necrosis of the papillae. The renal papillae (the apex of the renal pyramid that projects into the minor calyx) are vulnerable to ischemic necrosis. Diabetes is the most frequent condition associated with RPN in adults. Other conditions that cause RPN include analgesic abuse, sickle cell disease, obstructive uropathy, renal vein thrombosis, tuberculosis, pyelonephritis, and renal transplant. Necrosis may develop within weeks or months after renal transplantation, especially in patients previously treated for rejection and those with cadaveric kidney. Ischemia is believed to have an important role in necrosis.

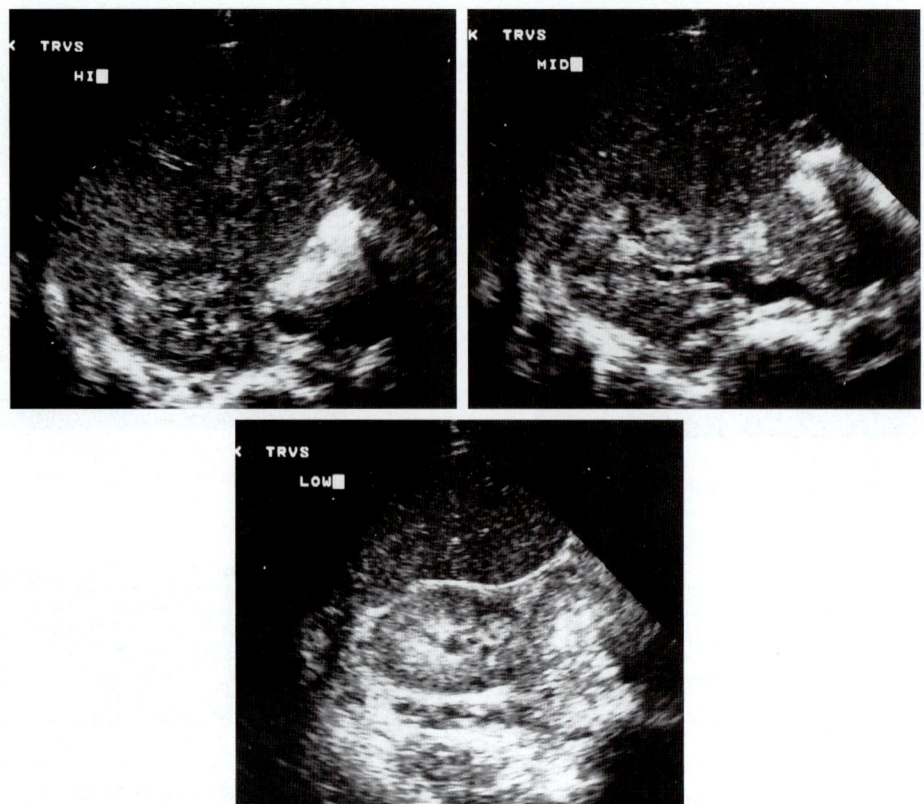

FIG. 15.65 Transverse scans of a young man with AIDS show a mildly echogenic renal parenchyma.

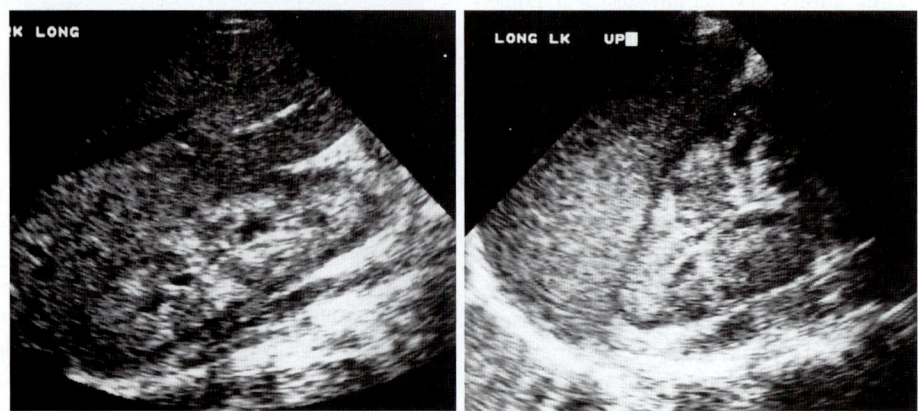

FIG. 15.66 Longitudinal scans of a 26-year-old man with AIDS.

Symptoms depend on the etiology of RPN and most of the time complications suggest calculus or an inflammatory process. Complaints include hematuria, flank pain, dysuria, fever, hypertension, and acute renal failure. Differential considerations include congenital megacalyces, hydronephrosis, and postobstructive atrophy.

Sonographic Findings. Sonographic findings include one or more fluid spaces at the corticomedullary junction that correspond to the distribution of the renal pyramids. The cystic spaces may be round or triangular. Sloughed papillae may appear as echogenic material within the necrotic medullary cavities. Correlation with clinical and laboratory findings help distinguish renal papillary necrosis from other renal abnormalities that have similar features on sonography and that are associated with areas of increased echogenicity (e.g., nephrocalcinosis).

Renal Atrophy. Renal atrophy results from numerous disease processes. Intrarenal anatomy is preserved with uniform loss of renal tissue. Renal sinus lipomatosis occurs secondary to renal atrophy. More severe lipomatosis results from a tremendous increase in renal sinus fat content in cases of marked renal atrophy caused by hydronephrosis and chronic calculus disease.

Sonographic Findings. The kidneys appear enlarged with a highly echogenic, enlarged renal sinus and a thin cortical rim. Renal sinus fat is easily seen on a sonogram as highly echogenic reflections (Fig. 15.67).

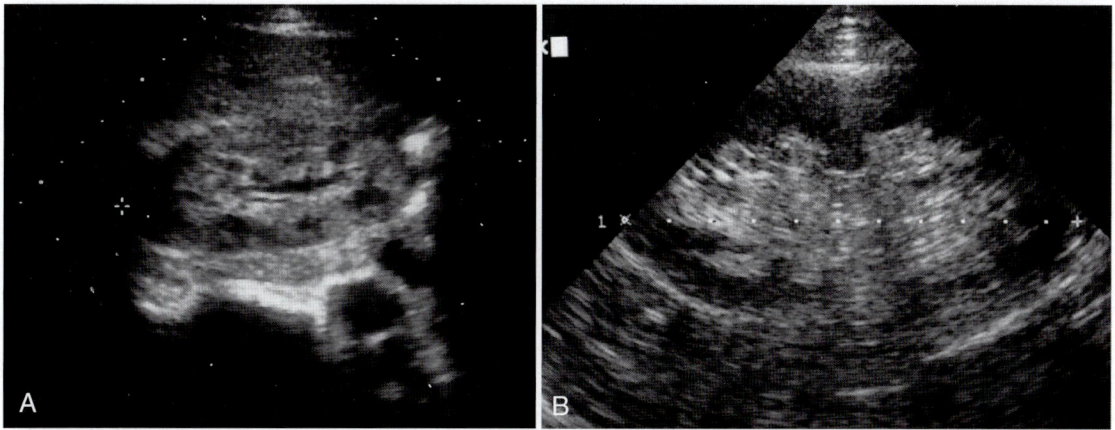

FIG. 15.67 (A) A 73-year-old man with chronic renal disease. Small echogenic kidney with inability to distinguish the medulla from the cortex region of the kidney. (B) Renal sinus lipomatosis appears as enlarged kidneys with an echogenic, enlarged renal sinus and a thin cortical rim. Renal sinus fat is easily seen on ultrasound as highly echogenic reflections.

> **BOX 15.6 Causes of Renal Failure**
>
> Prerenal
>   Hypoperfusion
>   Hypotension
>   Congestive heart failure
> Renal
>   Infection
>   Nephrotoxicity
>   Renal artery occlusion
>   Renal mass or cyst
> Postrenal
>   Lower urinary tract obstruction (ureter, bladder)
> Retroperitoneal fibrosis

Renal Failure

The excretory and regulatory functions of the kidneys are decreased in acute and chronic renal failure. Acute renal failure (ARF) is a common medical condition that can be caused by numerous medical diseases or pathophysiologic mechanisms. ARF is typically an abrupt transient decrease in renal function often heralded by oliguria. Pathophysiologic states that cause varying degrees of renal malfunction have been categorized as prerenal, renal, and postrenal (Box 15.6). Decreased perfusion of the kidneys can cause prerenal failure (e.g., renal vein thrombus, congestive heart failure, renal artery occlusion) and can be diagnosed by clinical and laboratory data and also by color Doppler. Renal causes of acute azotemia include parenchymal disease (e.g., acute glomerulonephritis, acute interstitial nephritis, acute tubular necrosis) and hydronephrosis. Major postrenal causes of acute renal failure include bladder, pelvic, or retroperitoneal tumor, and calculi. Prompt diagnosis and treatment of postrenal failure is crucial; the condition is potentially reversible.

Chronic renal failure may be caused by obstructive nephropathies, parenchymal diseases, renovascular disorders, or any process that progressively destroys nephrons. See Table 15.3 for clinical findings, sonographic findings, and differential considerations for malfunctioning kidney conditions.

Numerous studies have previously documented that sonography is extremely sensitive in diagnosing hydronephrosis. Patients for whom laboratory test results indicate compromised renal function should receive rule-out obstruction studies. Most agree that sonography is the initial procedure of choice in evaluating all patients with known or suspected renal failure. See Table 15.3 for clinical findings, sonographic findings, and differential considerations for renal failure.

Acute Renal Failure. ARF may occur in prerenal, renal, or postrenal failure stages (see Box 15.6). The prerenal stage is secondary to hypoperfusion of the kidney. The renal stages may be caused by parenchymal diseases (i.e., acute glomerulonephritis, acute interstitial nephritis, or acute tubular necrosis). They may also be caused by renal vein thrombosis or renal artery occlusion. In postrenal failure, radiologic imaging plays a major role. This condition is usually the result of outflow obstruction and is potentially reversible. Postrenal failure is usually increased in patients with malignancy of the bladder, prostate, uterus, ovaries, or rectum. Less frequent causes include retroperitoneal fibrosis and renal calculi.

Sonographic Findings. The cause of acute renal disease urinary outflow obstruction can be differentiated from parenchymal disease. The kidneys may appear normal in size or enlarged and may be hypoechoic with parenchymal disease. Obstruction is responsible for approximately 5% of cases of ARF. The most important issue is the presence or absence of urinary tract dilation. The degree of dilation does not necessarily reflect the presence or severity of an obstruction. A sonographer should try to determine the level of obstruction. A normal sonogram does not totally exclude urinary obstruction. In the clinical setting of acute obstruction secondary to calculi, a nondistended collecting system can be present.

Acute Tubular Necrosis. Acute tubular necrosis is the most common medical renal disease to produce acute renal failure, although it can be reversible.

Sonographic Findings. The sonogram shows bilaterally enlarged kidneys with hyperechoic pyramids; this can revert

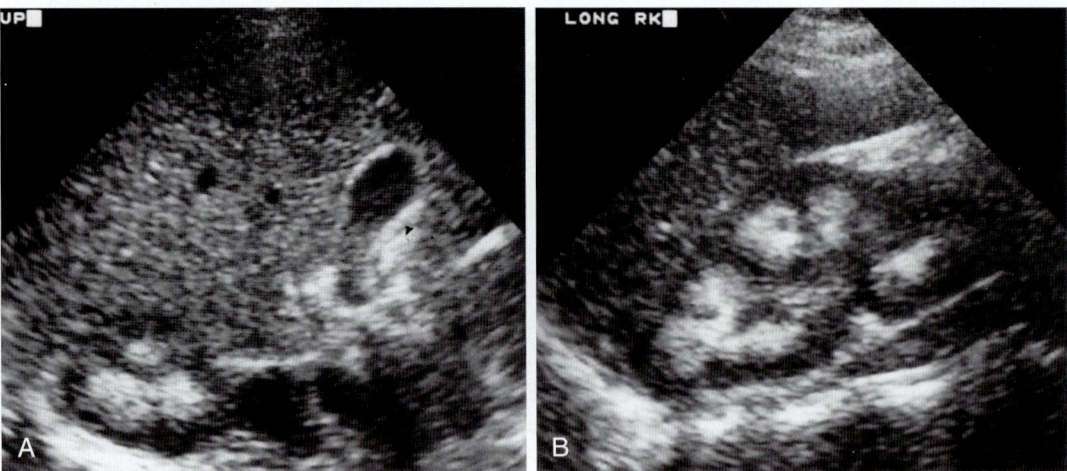

FIG. 15.68 Transverse (A) and longitudinal (B) scans of the pediatric patient with acute tubular necrosis and nephrocalcinosis. The echogenic renal pyramids are well seen.

to a normal appearance. Differential considerations include nephrocalcinosis. In pediatric patients, the renal pyramids are highly echogenic without shadowing. The calculi may be too small to cause dilation and shadowing of the pyramids (Fig. 15.68). As renal function improves, echogenicity decreases. This can occur in the medulla or the cortex. If the condition reverses, it is probably acute tubular necrosis.

Chronic Kidney Disease. Chronic kidney disease (CKD) is the loss of renal function as a result of disease, most commonly parenchymal disease. Three primary types of chronic renal failure are known: nephron, vascular, and interstitial abnormalities. Glomerulonephritis, chronic pyelonephritis, renal vascular disease, and diabetes are a few of the diseases that lead to renal failure.

Intrarenal fibrosis is a final common pathway for all CKD, and the degree of fibrosis correlates with disease severity. Nonfocal renal biopsy is the only method in current clinical use for the evaluation of intrarenal fibrosis. However, nonfocal renal biopsy has significant disadvantages: it is invasive, with risk of major complications; it is expensive; and it is subject to sampling error, as the biopsy cores comprise a small fraction of the renal parenchyma, and highly fibrotic kidneys often have insufficient glomerular tissue on biopsy samples to permit accurate histopathologic diagnosis.

There is an increased incidence of CKD in individuals with diabetes and hypertension-related nephropathies. CKD causes end-stage renal failure with high morbidity and mortality rates. In most types of kidney diseases, the progressive fibrotic processes may first involve either glomeruli (glomerulosclerosis) or the interstitial spaces (interstitial fibrosis), depending on the initial nephropathy. In renal transplantation the development of interstitial fibrosis and tubular atrophy is the major determinant of renal allograft failure.

Sonographic Findings. Chronic renal disease is a diffusely echogenic kidney with loss of normal anatomy. It is a nonspecific sonographic finding; chronic renal disease can have multiple causes (AIDS can produce echogenic kidneys). If chronic renal disease is bilateral, small kidneys are identified. This may result from hypertension, chronic inflammation, or chronic ischemia.

Shear wave elastography (SWE) is an emerging ultrasound technique that permits the noninvasive measurement of tissue stiffness. SWE uses focused acoustic energy pulses to produce microscopic tissue displacement, which induces perpendicular shear waves that are sonographically tracked as they progress through tissue. Stiffer tissues have been shown to have increased shear wave velocities. SWE may be a low-cost way to provide additional diagnostic information in CKD. Further studies are required to determine the relationship between estimated renal stiffness and renal fibrosis severity. Whereas native kidneys are quite deep within the abdomen and hardly compressible, renal transplants are much more superficial, located in the iliac fossa.

Hydronephrosis

Hydronephrosis–Urinary Tract Obstruction. Hydronephrosis is the separation of renal sinus echoes by interconnected fluid-filled calyces. Box 15.7 lists the causes of hydronephrosis. Dilation of the pelvocalyceal system is called hydronephrosis. In 1988 the Society for Fetal Urology proposed the following classification of grading hydronephrosis:
- Grade 1: small fluid-filled separation of the renal pelvis
- Grade 2: dilation of some but not all of the calyces; calyx orientation still concave
- Grade 3: complete pelvocaliectasis; calyx orientation changed in convex; echogenic line separating collecting system from renal parenchyma can be demonstrated (Fig. 15.69)
- Grade 4: prominent dilation of the collecting system, thinning of renal parenchyma, and no differentiation between collecting system and renal parenchyma

Urinary tract obstruction is not synonymous with dilation; in almost 35% of cases with acute urinary obstruction, no dilation is seen. Nonobstructive dilation is also seen in childhood during vesicoureteral reflux (see Box 15.7).

BOX 15.7 Causes of Hydronephrosis

Acquired
Bladder tumors
Calculi
Carcinoma of the cervix
Neurogenic bladder
Normal pregnancy
Pelvic mass
Prostatic enlargement
Retroperitoneal fibrosis

Intrinsic
Bladder neck obstruction
Calculus
Congenital
Inflammation
Posterior urethral valves
Pyelonephritis
Stricture
Ureterocele
Ureteropelvic junction obstruction

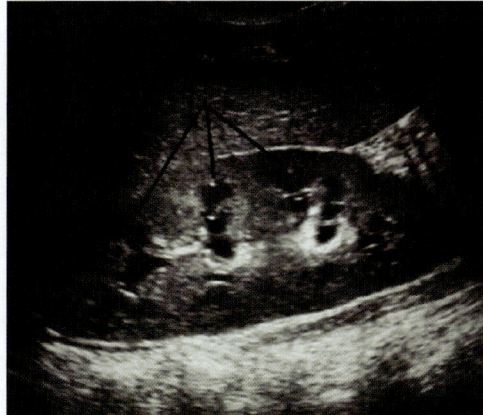

FIG. 15.70 A longitudinal left kidney scan with dilation of the proximal ureter caused by a stone *(arrows)*.

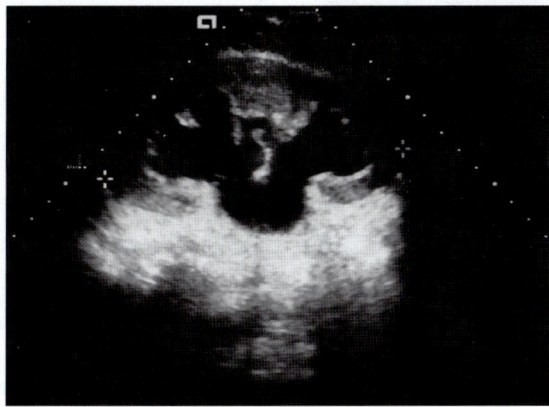

FIG. 15.69 **Hydronephrosis of the kidney.** The dilated pyelocaliceal system appears as separation of the renal sinus echoes by fluid-filled areas that conform anatomically to the infundibula, calyces, and pelvis.

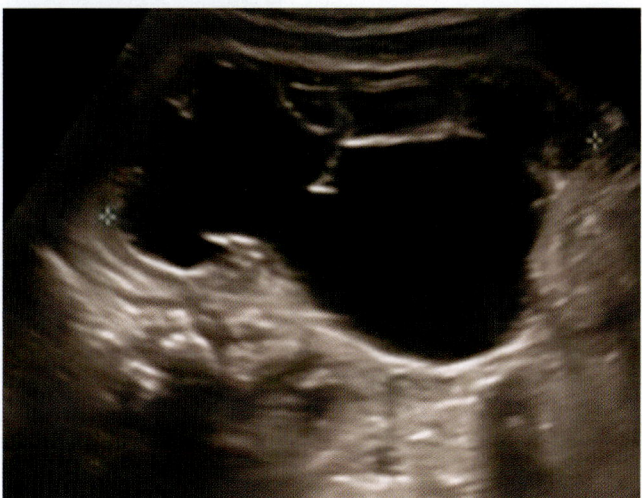

FIG. 15.71 Severe left hydronephrosis ureteral pelvic junction obstruction with no evidence of dilated ureter.

Sonographic Findings. Whenever the renal collecting system is dilated, the ureters and bladder are scanned to locate the level of obstruction. It is possible to identify the site of obstruction by using sonography. A congenital obstruction of the ureteropelvic junction can be seen in utero and in infants. The collecting system will be dilated without dilation of the ureter. Localized hydronephrosis occurs as a result of strictures, calculi, focal masses, or a duplex collecting system (Figs. 15.70 and 15.71). Hydronephrosis with a dilated ureter indicates obstruction of the ureterovesical junction; hydroureteronephrosis with a dilated bladder indicates obstruction of the posterior urethra (posterior urethral valves).

A mildly distended collecting system can be caused by overhydration, a normal variant of extrarenal pelvis, or by a previous urinary diversion procedure (Fig. 15.72). Postvoid scanning techniques are helpful in preventing these errors.

If hydronephrosis is suspected, the sonographer should examine the bladder. If it is full, a postvoid longitudinal scan of each kidney should be done to show that hydronephrosis has disappeared or remains the same. At the level of obstruction, the sonographer should sweep the transducer back and forth in two planes to see if a mass or stone can be distinguished. The sonographer must be able to rule out a parapelvic cyst (septations may be numerous) or a crossing renal vessel in the peripelvic area (color flow Doppler is extremely useful). An extrarenal pelvis would protrude outside of the renal area, and the sonographer probably would not confuse this pattern with hydronephrosis.

In evaluating the patient for hydronephrosis, the sonographer must be sure to look for a dilated ureter, an enlarged prostate, or an enlarged bladder (which may occur secondary to an enlarged prostate). Bladder carcinoma may obstruct the pathway of the urethra, causing urine to back into both ureters and renal pelvis. A ureterocele may also block urine output. This condition occurs with an anomalous insertion of the ureter into the bladder wall. The ureter can turn inside out and obstruct the orifice.

Obstructive Hydronephrosis. Dilation of the renal pelvis is just one factor present in patients with obstructive hydronephrosis.

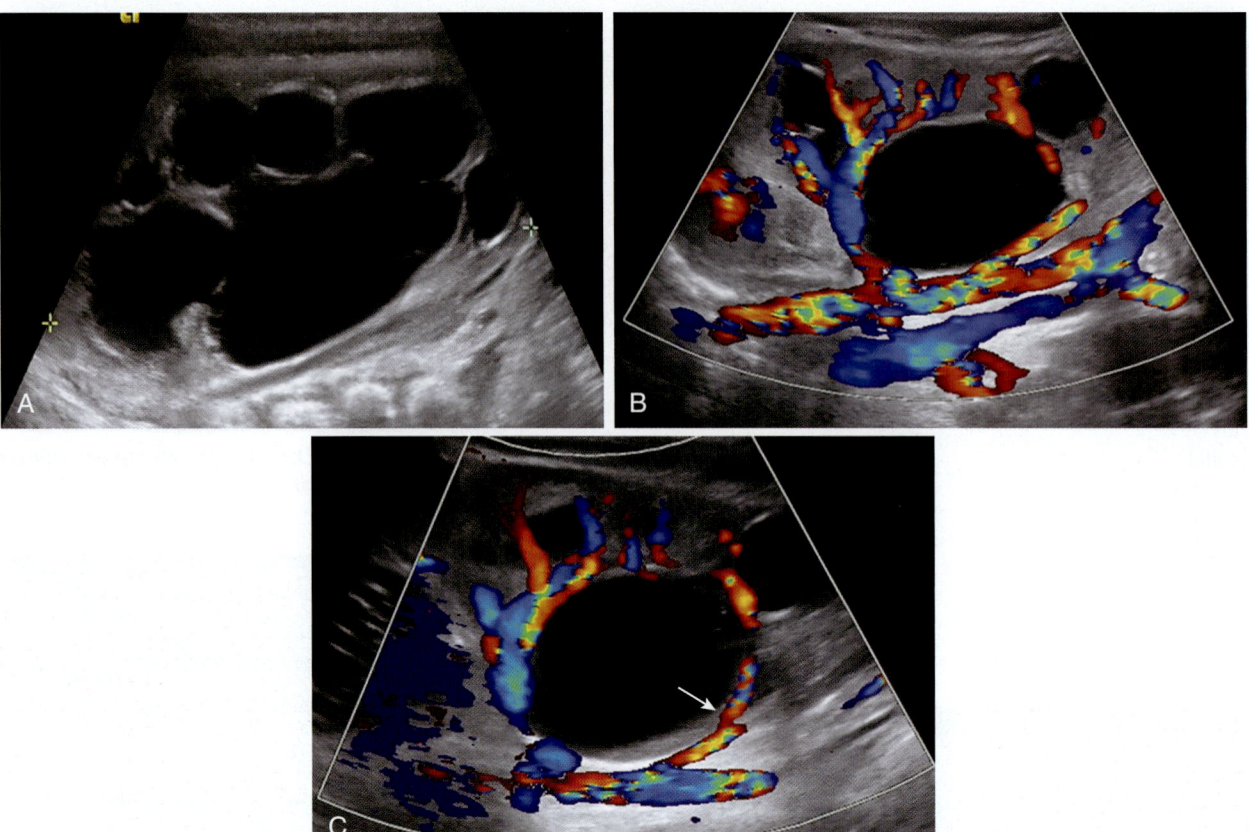

FIG. 15.72 (A) Severe left pelvocaliectasis. Note the absence of a dilated ureter after the ureteral pelvic junction (UPJ). (B) Severe left pelvocaliectasis without a dilated ureter after UPJ. (C) Color Doppler demonstrates the crossing vessel causing UPJ obstruction.

(See Table 15.3 for clinical findings, sonographic findings, and differential considerations for obstructive hydronephrosis.)

Sonographic Findings. In cases of acute urinary tract obstruction (UTO), the resistive index (RI) of the interlobar and arcuate intrarenal vessels may be greater than 0.70, starting 6 hours after acute onset and for up to 72 hours (Fig. 15.73). The RI returns to normal value after 120 hours of obstruction. The value of the RI may be higher than 0.70 in some normal conditions, as in neonates and infants up to 6 years old and in elderly patients, and in some pathologic conditions related to intrinsic renal disease, diabetes, and/or hypertension. Use of nonsteroidal antiinflammatory drugs may lower the value of the RI on the affected side, which decreases the sensitivity of Doppler ultrasound in identifying UTO. Level of obstruction is another important factor in elevation of the RI value. The resistive index is greater in patients with an obstruction in the proximal ureter or in the distal intramural ureteral portion.

It is very important to measure and compare the RI in both kidneys, because a ΔRI is more useful for diagnosis of UTO than a solid value for RI. No ureteral jet will be seen on the affected side if the obstruction is complete, or the jet may be noted if obstruction is partial.

Classical sonographic findings in the diagnosis of UTO include the following: grade I or II hydronephrosis; Doppler showing elevated RI or difference of ΔRI; absence of the respective ureteral jet; and visualization of the dilated ureter and/or stone. Sonography can be normal in up to 50% of cases in the first 6 hours after acute onset, which means that the normal sonogram does not exclude acute urinary obstruction, and a noncontrast CT will be necessary.

Ureteral Jet Phenomenon. The ureteral jet phenomenon picked up by gray scale or color Doppler is caused by the difference in density between urine in the bladder and urine coming from the ureter (kidney). The frequency and size (velocity) of the ureteral jet range from 0.2 to 1.7 m/sec. Duration of the jets is 0.6 to 4.1 seconds, with a 30-second interval jet time. The jets are directed upward and toward the contralateral side, and the shape of the spectral Doppler curve varies with the amount of urine produced. Complete obstruction shows absence of the respective ureteral jet; partial obstruction may show a low-level jet on the side of obstruction and/or asymmetry of the ureteral jets.

Urine fills the bladder at a rate of up to 2 mL/min. Patients who have voided before the renal examination and are rehydrated may have a false-positive absence of ureteral jets. This occurs because the concentration of urine in the recently distended bladder is similar in density to that of urine entering the bladder. Comparison of the two ureteral jets is necessary to confirm that nonvisualization of the symptomatic side is not related to the fact that the density of urine in the ureter is similar to that in the bladder (Figs. 15.74 and 15.75).

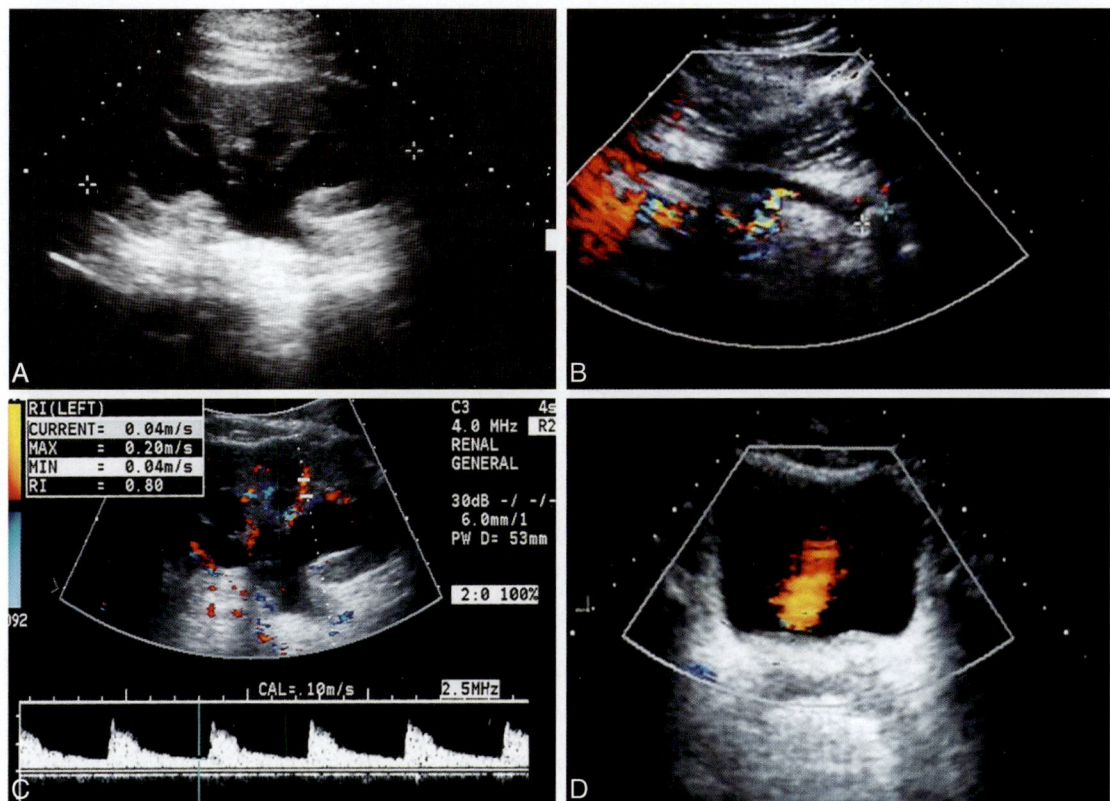

FIG. 15.73 (A) Grade 2 to 3 left ureterohydronephrosis. (B) A 1 cm obstructing stone in the lower portion of the left ureter. (C) High resistive index (RI = 0.80) documenting an acute urinary obstruction. (D) Absence of the left ureteral jet.

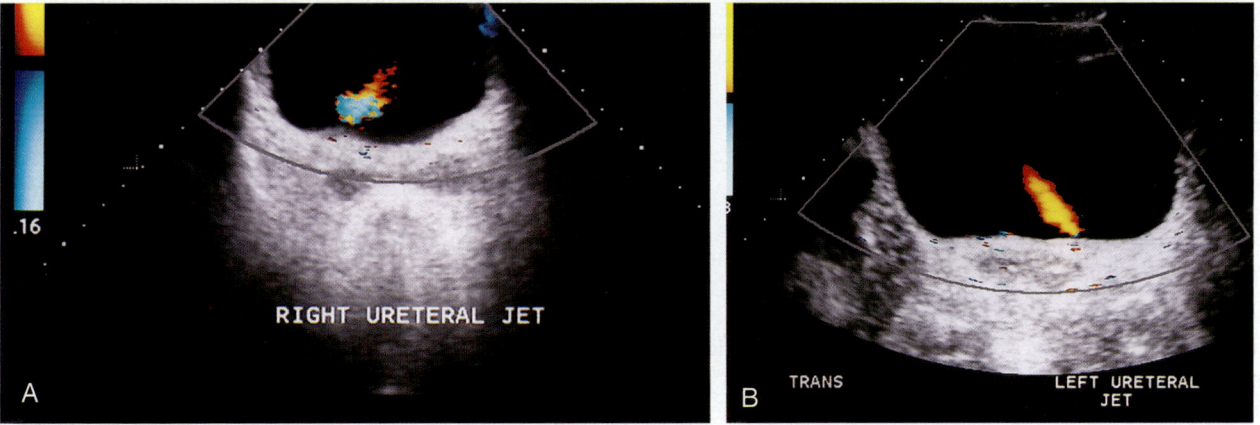

FIG. 15.74 Normal right (A) and left (B) ureteral jets seen in the fluid-filled bladder.

Nonobstructive Hydronephrosis. Dilation of the renal pelvis does not always mean that obstruction is present. Several other factors, such as reflux, infection, large extrarenal pelvis, high-flow states (polyuria), distended renal bladder, atrophy after obstruction, or pregnancy dilation, may cause the renal pelvis to be dilated. (The enlarged uterus can compress the ureter; this usually occurs more frequently on the right during the third trimester, causing the so-called *hydronephrosis of pregnancy* with normal RI.)

False-Positive Hydronephrosis. Many conditions may mimic hydronephrosis (Box 15.8); these include extrarenal pelvis, parapelvic cyst, reflux, multicystic kidney, central renal cyst, transient diuresis, congenital megacalyces, papillary necrosis, renal artery aneurysm (color can help distinguish that this enlargement, not the renal pelvis, is vascular), or an arteriovenous malformation (color can distinguish this abnormality).

Localized hydronephrosis may occur secondary to strictures, calculi, or focal masses (transitional). It may also be seen in a duplex system when one of the systems can be obstructed by an ectopic insertion of the ureter. In females, the ureter can insert below the external urinary sphincter, causing dribbling.

False-Negative Hydronephrosis. A dilated renal pelvis may be distinguished from other conditions by the use of other techniques. In patients with retroperitoneal fibrosis or necrosis, give liquids to see if the renal pelvis dilates. In patients with distal calculi, no obstruction can be seen unless the

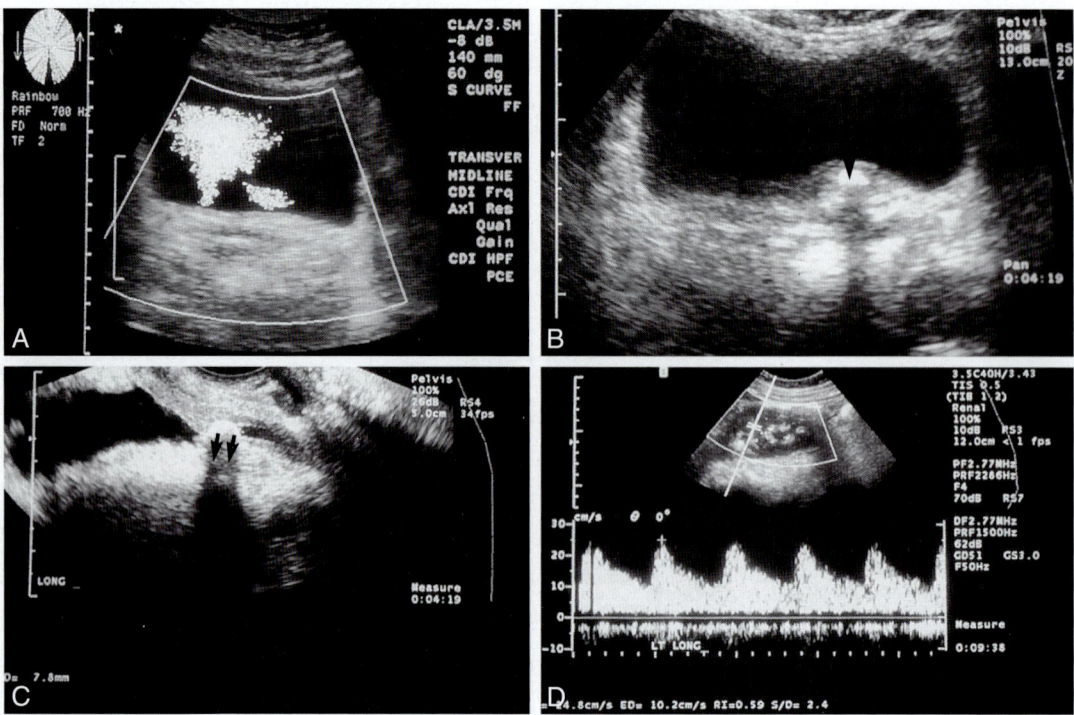

FIG. 15.75 (A) Transverse scan of a fluid-filled bladder with a normal right ureteral jet. A partially obstructed left ureter with decreased flow. (B) Transverse scan of a partially obstructed distal left ureter. *Arrows* indicate the stone and shadowing posterior to the stone. (C) Transvaginal scan of the dilated distal ureter with a ureteral stone. (D) Normal resistive index of 0.59 for left kidney.

BOX 15.8 Conditions That Mimic Hydronephrosis

Arteriovenous malformation
Congenital megacalyces
Extrarenal pelvis
Papillary necrosis
Parapelvic cysts
Persistent diuresis
Reflux
Renal artery aneurysm

---

calculi have been there for several days. A staghorn calculus can mask an associated dilation.

The conditions of adult polycystic disease and multicystic renal disease with severe hydronephrosis may be confused. In patients with severe hydronephrosis, the image shows dilated calyces as they radiate from a larger central fluid collection in the renal pelvis. The kidney usually retains a normal shape. The sonographer sees fluid-filled sacs in a radiating pattern or cauliflower configuration. In patients with adult polycystic renal disease or multicystic renal disease, the renal cysts are randomly distributed, the contour is disturbed, and the cysts are variable in size. Once obstruction has been ruled out, consider renal medical disease, which is the leading cause of ARF.

Renal Infections

A spectrum of severity is possible in renal infection. The disease can progress from pyelonephritis to focal bacterial nephritis to an abscess. An abscess can be transmitted through the parenchyma into the blood. Most renal infections stay in the kidney and are resolved with antibiotics. A perirenal abscess may occur from direct extension. (See Table 15.3 for clinical findings, sonographic findings, and differential considerations for renal infections.)

Pyonephrosis. Pyonephrosis occurs when pus is found within the collecting renal system. It is often associated with severe urosepsis and represents a true urologic emergency that requires urgent intravenous antibiotic therapy and/or percutaneous drainage. It usually occurs secondary to long-standing ureteral obstruction resulting from calculus disease, stricture, or a congenital anomaly.

Sonographic Findings. Sonographic findings include the presence of low-level echoes with a fluid-debris level (Fig. 15.76). The sonographer should be aware that an anechoic dilated system may be found. (Sonographic guided aspiration or CT may be necessary.)

Emphysematous Pyelonephritis. Emphysematous pyelonephritis occurs when air is present in the parenchyma (diffuse gas-forming parenchymal infection). It may be caused by *Escherichia coli* bacteria. When this occurs in diabetic patients, they become very sick. It generally is found unilaterally and may be cause for an emergency nephrectomy.

Sonographic Findings. On a sonogram, the enlarged kidneys appear hypoechoic and inflamed (Fig. 15.77).

Xanthogranulomatous Pyelonephritis. Xanthogranulomatous pyelonephritis is an uncommon renal disease associated with chronic obstruction and infection. It involves destruction of renal parenchyma and infiltration of lipid-laden histiocytes. Clinically, the patient presents with a large nonfunctioning kidney, staghorn calculus, and multiple infections (Fig. 15.78). The disease is more common in females and is poorly understood.

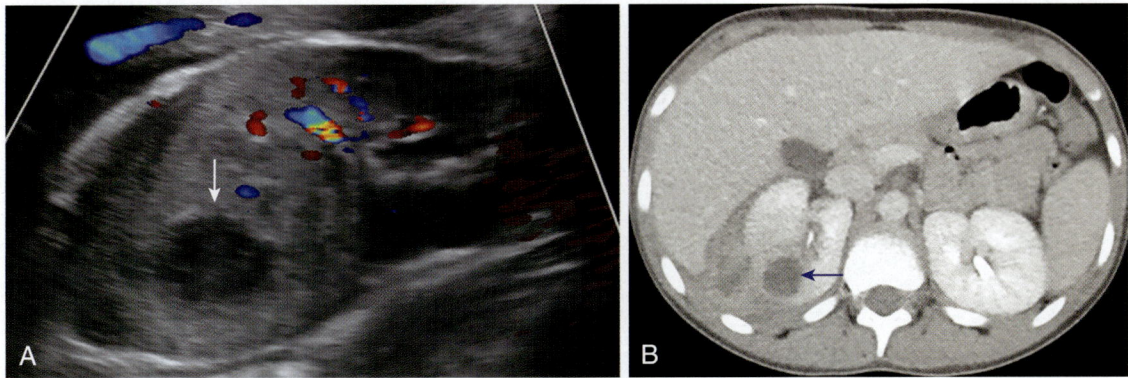

FIG. 15.76 Renal infection. This patient presented with an elevated white blood cell count and spiking fever. (A) Supine sagittal scan reveals a homogeneous, slightly irregular mass arising from the upper pole of the right kidney. (B) Computed tomography confirms right renal abscess extending into posterior pararenal space.

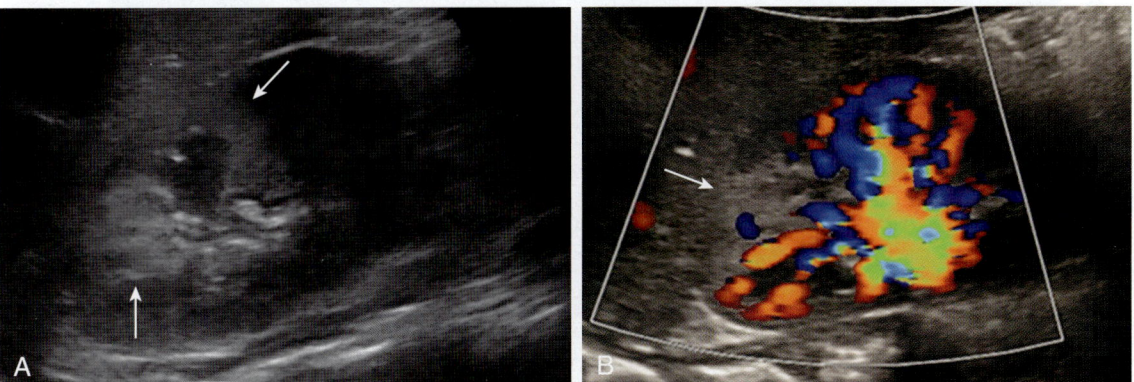

FIG. 15.77 (A) Right upper pole focal pyelonephritis. (B) Longitudinal view right kidney shows slightly hyperechoic, avascular area consistent with focal pyelonephritis.

It is thought to represent an impaired host response to infection in a chronically obstructed and infected kidney.

Sonographic Findings. The sonographic appearance may show bright echogenicity from the staghorn calculus. (Peripelvic fibrosis can prevent the staghorn from shadowing.) The renal parenchyma is replaced by cystic spaces. Overall renal size is increased. The disease process may be diffuse or segmental.

Urinary Tract Calcifications

Renal Calcifications. Renal calcifications may be seen as localized parenchymal calcifications, resulting from scar tissue caused by bacterial infection, renal abscess, infected hematoma, urinoma, lymphocele, tuberculosis, or infarction, or post–percutaneous renal procedures. Malignant solid and/or cystic masses often demonstrate calcifications, but benign renal masses may also calcify. Linear vascular calcifications commonly are associated with renal artery atherosclerosis and/or vascular malformation.

Most of the intraluminal renal calcifications seen on sonography are renal calculi. Milk of calcium cyst and obstructed calyceal diverticulum are rare conditions with suspension of small, calcified crystals and/or small stones in layers within the renal cystic structure.

Medullary Sponge Kidney. As was previously discussed, medullary sponge kidney (MSK), or intratubular renal calcification, is a developmental anomaly that occurs in the medullary pyramids and consists of cystic or fusiform dilation of the distal collecting ducts (ducts of Bellini), causing stasis of the urine and stone formation. Because MSK is an anatomic rather than a metabolic defect, the pathologic process may be unilateral or segmental. The cause is unknown. Many patients remain asymptomatic, but patients with hematuria, infection, and renal stones should be evaluated for MSK. Sonographically, MSK appears as hyperechoic calyces, with or without stones (Fig. 15.79).

Nephrocalcinosis. Nephrocalcinosis, or parenchymal calcification, involves diffuse foci of calcium deposits, which usually are located in the medulla but infrequently can be seen in the renal cortex. Both kidneys are affected. Calcification may be dystrophic from devitalized tissues, ischemia, and/or necrosis, or from hypercalcemic states, hyperparathyroidism, renal tubular acidosis, and renal failure.

Metastatic nephrocalcinosis is based on location and is classified as cortical or medullary. Cortical nephrocalcinosis is most commonly seen with chronic glomerulonephritis, chronic hypercalcemic states, sickle cell disease, and rejected renal transplants. Medullary nephrocalcinosis occurs more often with disorders such as hyperparathyroidism (40%), renal tubular acidosis (20%), MSK, chronic pyelonephritis, hyperthyroidism, sickle cell disease, and renal papillary necrosis.

Sonographic Findings. Sonographically, cortical nephrocalcinosis appears as increased cortical echogenicity with

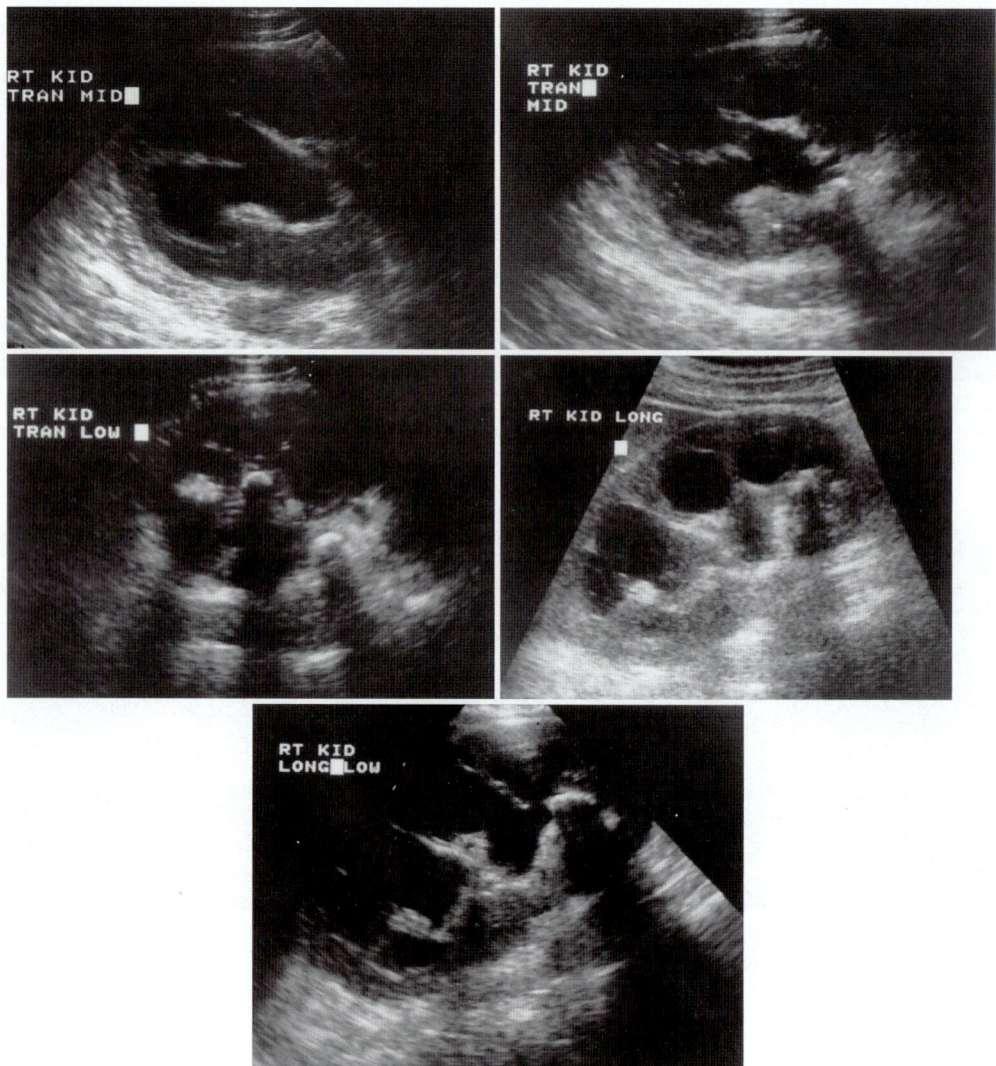

FIG. 15.78 Patient with xanthogranulomatous pyelonephritis shows a large, nonfunctioning right kidney secondary to a stone. Multiple areas of shadowing are seen within the renal parenchyma from the renal stones.

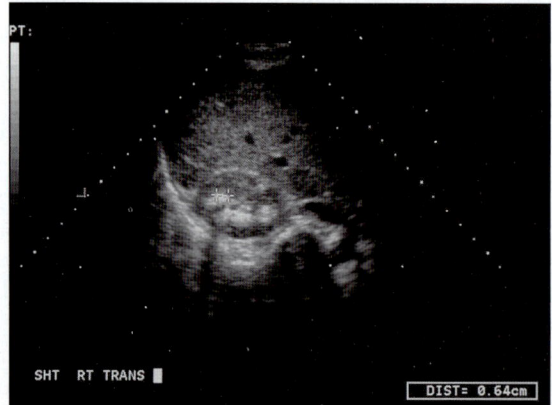

FIG. 15.79 Transverse view of the right kidney for measuring the renal stone.

spared pyramids (Fig. 15.80). In cases of medullary nephrocalcinosis, the pyramids become more echogenic than the adjacent cortex. A combination corticomedullary form exists, which shows both renal cortex and medulla as echogenic.

Renal Artery Stenosis

Renal artery stenosis (RAS) is the most common correctable cause of hypertension. Only 1% to 5% of hypertensive patients have a renovascular origin; most patients have essential hypertension. Renovascular hypertension is renin mediated and occurs as a response to renal ischemia, and later as a response to high circulating levels of angiotensin II. The most common causes of renal artery stenosis are atherosclerosis and fibromuscular dysplasia (Box 15.9).

Atherosclerosis is associated with hypertension, which is more common in older patients, and accounts for one-third of cases of RAS. It occurs more frequently in males. Atherosclerosis usually occurs within the first 2 cm of the renal artery, and because this is a generalized process, it may be multifocal, or both renal arteries may be affected.

Fibromuscular dysplasia accounts for approximately two-thirds of renal artery stenosis cases and is seen in younger patients. Fibromuscular dysplasia may involve any layer of the renal artery wall and is classified as intimal, medial, or adventitial,

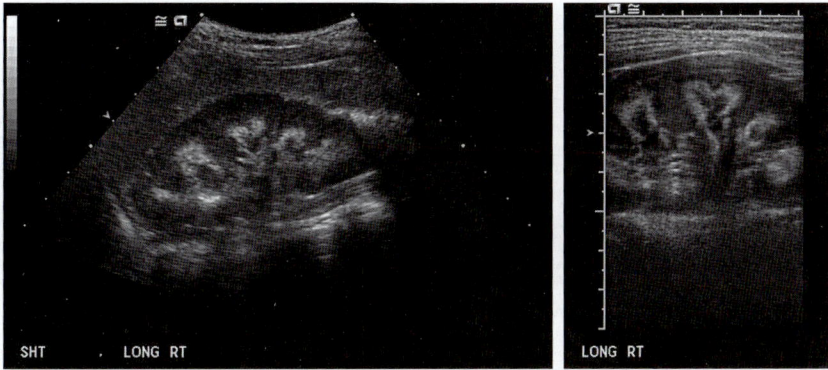

FIG. 15.80 Longitudinal scans of the right kidney show hyperechoic pyramids, consistent with nephrocalcinosis.

> **BOX 15.9 Sonographic Characteristics of Renal Artery Stenosis**
>
> Kidney smaller than contralateral side
> Absence of early systolic peak
> Overall waveform shape: "tardus and parvus" waveform
> Delayed systolic rise time: ΔT <0.1 sec
> Peak systolic velocity: PSV >160/180 cm/sec
> Resistive index: RI = (S − D)/S ≥ 0.70

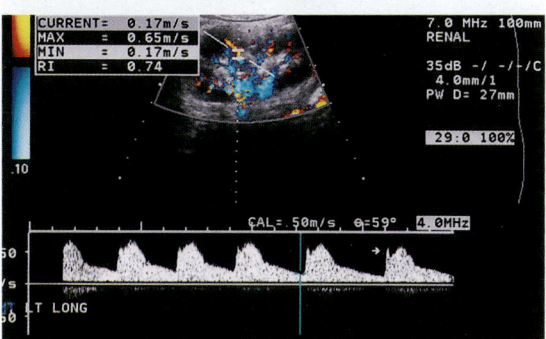

FIG. 15.81 Normal resistive index of 0.74 in a 4-year-old girl. The *arrow* indicates an early systolic peak.

creating a smooth stenosis, usually in the midportion of the renal artery. Involvement of the medial layer is seen in the most common subtype of fibromuscular dysplasia, accounting for more than 90% of cases. Medial dysplasia consists of the replacement of smooth muscle by collagen, forming thick ridges and alternating with areas of small aneurysm formation, which results in the classic "string of beads" appearance on arteriography or CT angiography. Fibromuscular dysplasia is most commonly seen in young women. It is progressive and may be seen not only in renal arteries but also in cephalic, visceral, and peripheral arteries.

Sonographic Findings. Selective renal arteriography is the gold standard for visualizing renal artery stenosis. Color Doppler sonography was developed as a noninvasive alternative to detect RAS in hypertensive patients. Direct evaluation of the main renal artery and indirect evaluation via the arcuate and intralobar renal arteries are the two methods used. Accuracy rate depends on operator hand, patient body habitus, and adequacy of the technique.

The most reliable signs for diagnosing RAS using the main renal artery are (1) increased velocity through the stenotic area greater than 150 to 190 cm/sec and (2) turbulence distal to the narrowing. Use of peak systolic velocity has not proved accurate because of overestimation caused by suboptimal angles of incidence. The use of frequency ranges has been shown to be of little value because of the tortuosity of the renal artery, which causes varied frequencies throughout the vessel.

A problem that occurs when the main renal artery is used to evaluate renal blood flow is that more than one renal artery may be found. The main renal artery may have normal blood flow and a stenotic accessory renal artery, causing hypertension. Evaluating the entire course of the main renal arteries is a long and tedious study and one that sonographers and sonologists try to avoid. Several technical factors (body habitus, tortuosity of the vessel, overlying bowel gas, respiratory motion, and underlying arteriosclerotic disease) may prohibit visualization of the entire length of the renal artery. The proximal portion of the renal arteries may be difficult to evaluate because of cardiac or aortic pulse frequencies.

Evaluating the segmental and intralobar renal vessels is an indirect method of evaluating for RAS. They are easier to see than the main renal artery with the use of convergent color or power color (Figs. 15.81–15.83). It is very difficult to obtain a 60-degree angle of the renal vessels. Convergent color and power color are not angle dependent.

Studies have used various Doppler parameters to assist in the evaluation of RAS. The normal intrarenal Doppler signal has a rapid systolic upstroke and an early systolic peak (Figs. 15.84 and 15.85). The absence of early systolic peak and a prolonged systolic upstroke or acceleration time, together with decreased peak systole and dampening of the distal waveform, are indications of RAS. The term *tardus-parvus* is used to describe the decreased acceleration time and the decreased peak (Fig. 15.86).

Clinical studies with contrast agents are continuing to improve the use of sonography and Doppler for evaluation of renal vascularity. The use of three-dimensional imaging to demonstrate the renal vasculature is also being investigated (Fig. 15.87).

Renal Infarction

A renal infarction occurs when part of the tissue undergoes necrosis after cessation of the blood supply, usually as a result of artery occlusion. Renal function is usually normal. This may result from a thrombus, a tumor infiltration, or

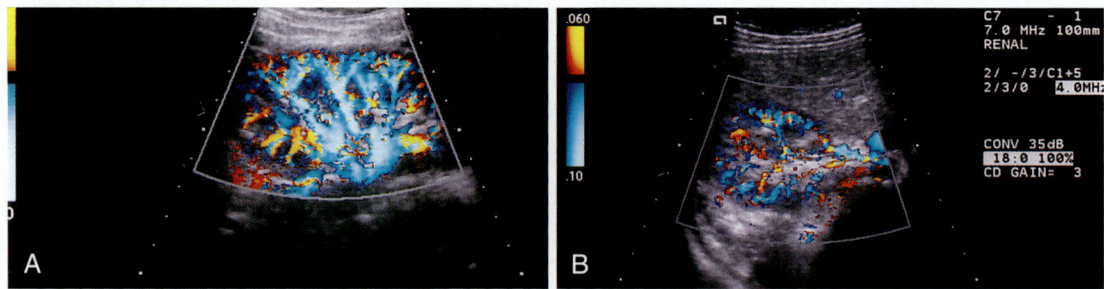

FIG. 15.82 Longitudinal (A) and transverse (B) color Doppler of normal intrarenal vessels with vascular flow throughout the renal cortex.

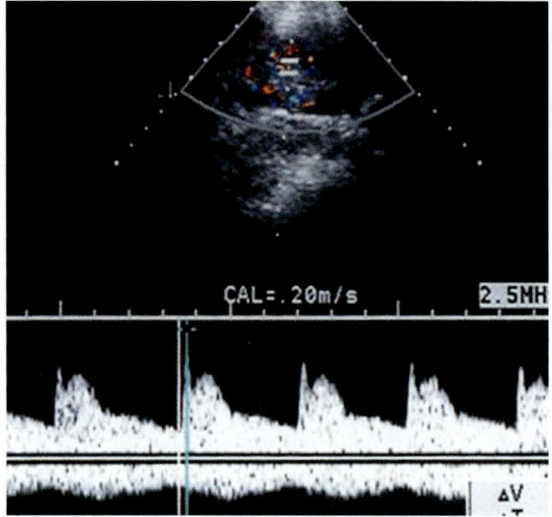

FIG. 15.83 Normal renal spectral waveform taken at the interlobar arteries.

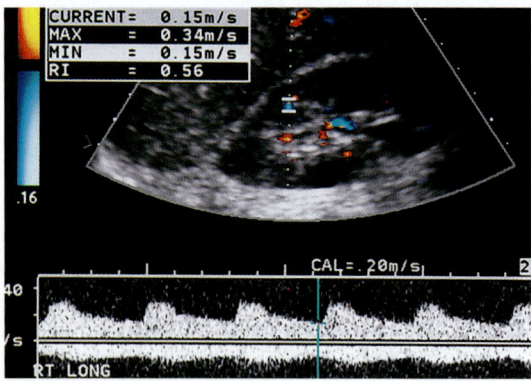

FIG. 15.84 **Normal arcuate vessel Doppler spectral signal.** A rapid systolic rise with a resistive index of 0.56. A gradual decrease into diastole.

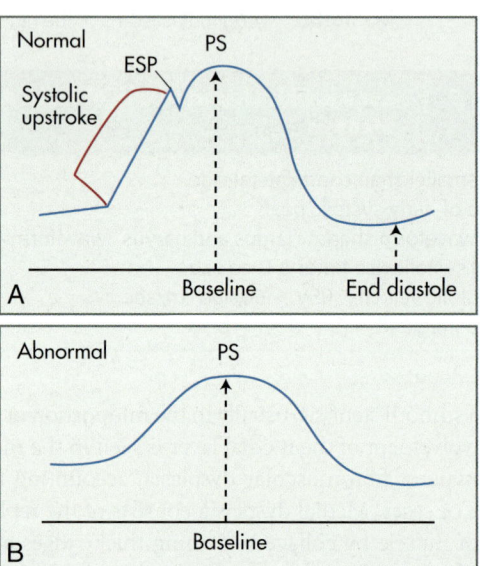

FIG. 15.85 (A) A normal renal artery spectral waveform with early systolic peak (ESP) and a rapid systolic upstroke followed by peak systole (PS) and a gradual decrease into diastole. (B) An abnormal renal artery spectral waveform with absence of early systolic peak and a long systolic upstroke.

Arteriovenous Fistulas and Pseudoaneurysm

Arteriovenous fistulas (AVFs) are most often acquired rather than congenital. AVFs may be due to renal biopsies, complications from partial nephrectomies, or trauma. Gray-scale sonography shows no abnormalities in the kidney, but color Doppler easily depicts the arteriovenous malformation. The diagnosis is based on detection of a perivascular artifact that reflects local tissue vibration produced by the arteriovenous shunt. Because power Doppler usually demonstrates a larger, artifactual area of uniform color signal that is more pronounced than on conventional color Doppler imaging, it has the potential to facilitate detection of small, low-flow AVF. No abnormalities or small cystic lesions are evident on gray scale. Spectral Doppler shows increased flow velocities, decreased resistive indexes, and arterialization of the draining vein, regardless of the cause of arteriovenous malformation.

Pseudoaneurysm may develop following graft anastomosis, renal biopsy, or intratumoral hemorrhage (angiomyolipomas), or it may occur after renal surgery (partial nephrectomies) or after trauma; as with AVF, it is very rarely congenital. Color flow Doppler sonographic patterns associated with pseudoaneurysm have been well described in the literature. Sonography

obstruction, or it may be iatrogenic. (See Table 15.3 for clinical findings, sonographic findings, and differential considerations for renal infarction.)

Sonographic Findings. Infarcts within the renal parenchyma appear as irregular areas, somewhat triangular in shape, along the periphery of the renal border. The renal contour may be somewhat "bumpy." Remember that lobulations in the pediatric patient may be normal, except for the dromedary hump variant. In the adult patient, the renal contour should be smooth. In a patient with a renal infarct, the irregular area may be slightly more echogenic than the renal parenchyma.

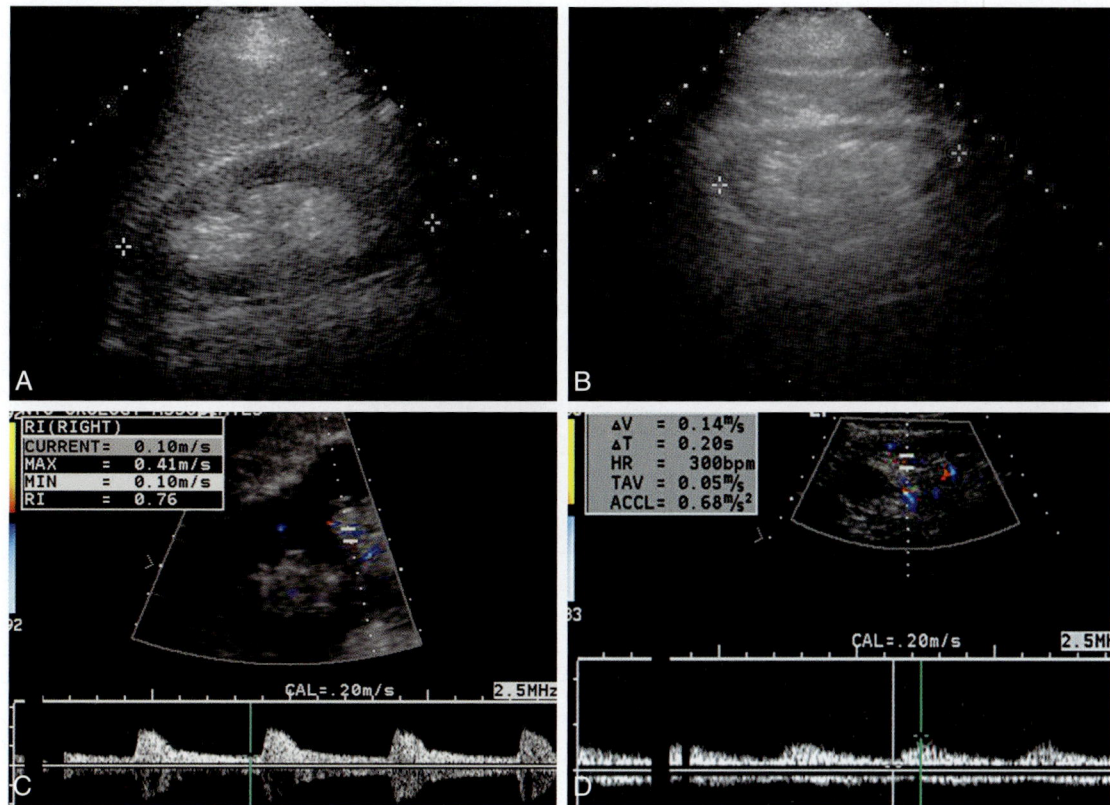

FIG. 15.86 (A) Longitudinal scan of normal size of right kidney. (B) Longitudinal scan of small (shrunken) left kidney with cortical atrophy. (C) Normal spectral waveform right kidney. (D) Parvus-tardus (delayed systolic rise time) left kidney consistent with renal artery stenosis.

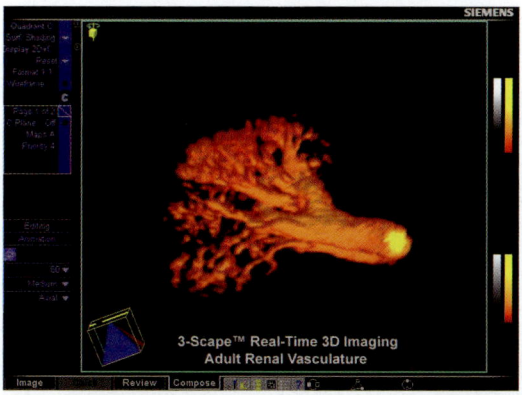

FIG. 15.87 Adult renal vasculature demonstration using 3-Scape real-time three-dimensional imaging. (Courtesy Siemens Medical Solutions USA, Inc.)

shows a round hypoechoic or cystic mass in the renal parenchyma that fills with color signal on color flow Doppler imaging. Spectral analysis performed at the level of the communicating channel shows a typical pattern known as the to-and-fro sign, which signifies both systolic feeding arterial flow and diastolic draining arterial flow—in other words, bidirectional flow occurs (Figs. 15.88 and 15.89).

Kidney Stone (Urolithiasis)

A stone located in the urinary system is called **urolithiasis**. Most urinary tract stones are formed in the kidney and course down the urinary tract. Stones consist of a combination of chemicals that precipitate out of urine. The most common chemical found in stones is calcium, along with oxalate or phosphate. Uric acid, cystine, and xanthine can also be found in kidney stones. Kidney stones are one of the most common kidney problems that can occur; they may cause obstruction, and this obstruction can be extremely painful. Most kidney stones are small and can travel through the urinary system without treatment or with increased hydration. Stones that are large and fill the renal collecting system are called staghorn calculi. Kidney stones that travel down the urinary system may obstruct the ureter in constricted areas.

The number of people with kidney stones in the United States has increased in the past 20 years. Kidney stones are more common in men. Some people are more likely to form kidney stones than others, and once a kidney stone has formed, the person is at increased risk of getting stones in the future. Kidney stones are associated with renal acidosis (a rare hereditary disorder); people taking the protease inhibitor indinavir are at increased risk for developing kidney stones. The initial clinical sign of a kidney stone is extreme pain, typically followed by cramping on the side on which the stone is located; nausea and vomiting may also occur. The pain may subside while the stone is traveling down the ureter.

Treatment for stones that cause obstruction varies depending on the size and location of the stone. Treatment can include extracorporeal shockwave lithotripsy (ESWL), percutaneous nephrolithotomy, and ureteroscopic stone removal. ESWL uses ultrasound or x-ray to locate the stone, and shockwaves are used

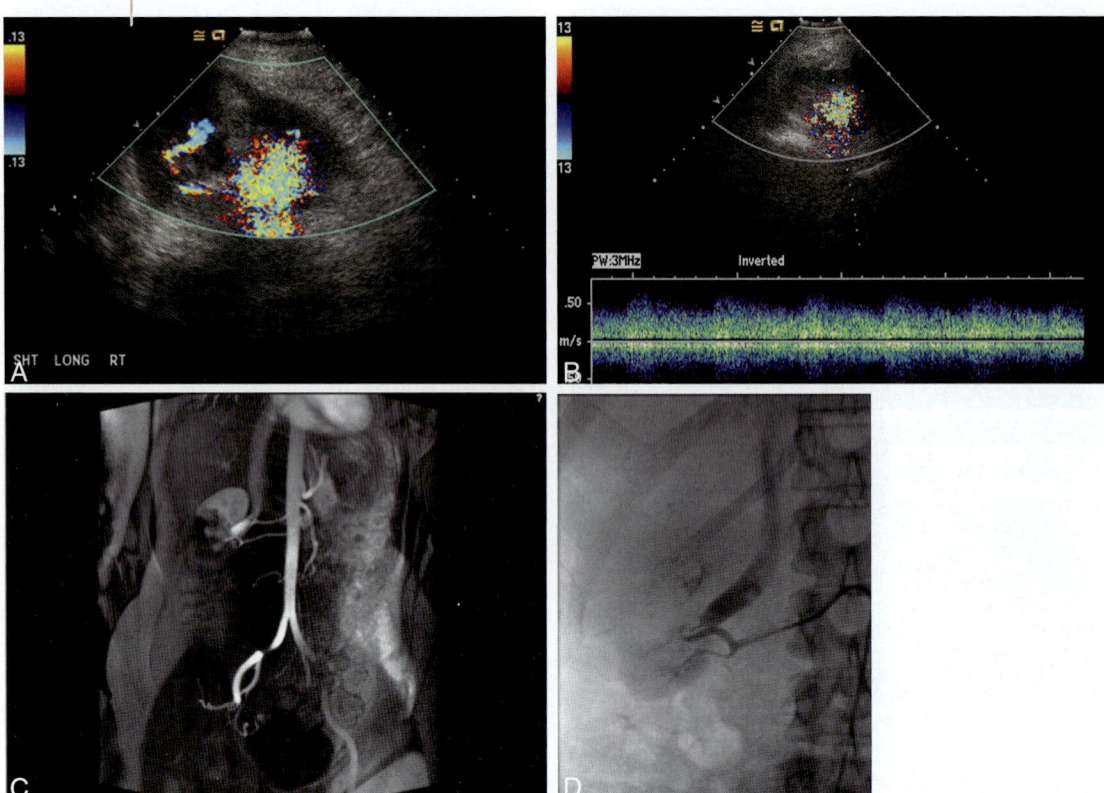

FIG. 15.88 (A) Color duplex Doppler with a pulsating vascular malformation in the right renal hilum. (B) Arterialization of renal venous flow. (C) Coronal view magnetic resonance imaging with simultaneous visualization of the renal artery (aorta) and the inferior vena cava consistent with an arteriovenous fistula. (D) Renal angiogram shows early visualization of the inferior vena cava.

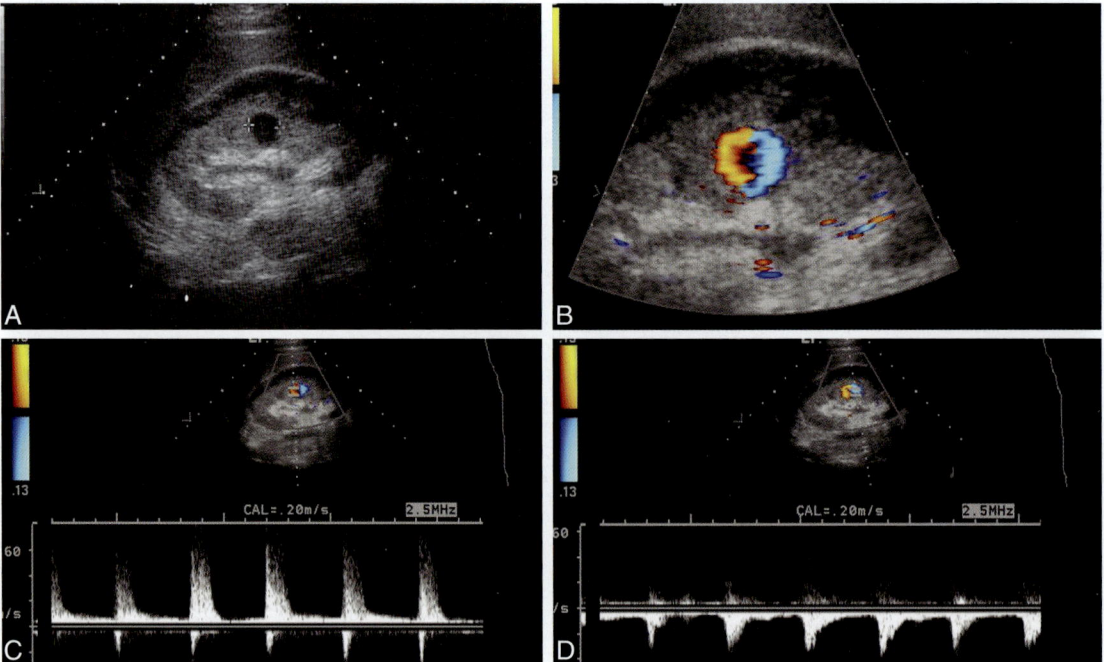

FIG. 15.89 (A) Longitudinal scan of the right kidney 1 week post–ureteroscopic laser treatment for a mid-calyx stone with a perinephric fluid collection and a newly discovered 1.8 cm cystic structure. (B) Color Doppler shows a typical "yin-yang" or swirling appearance consistent with a renal artery pseudoaneurysm. (C–D) Spectral arterial waveform demonstrates clean bidirectional arterial blood flow above and below baseline, consistent with a renal pseudoaneurysm.

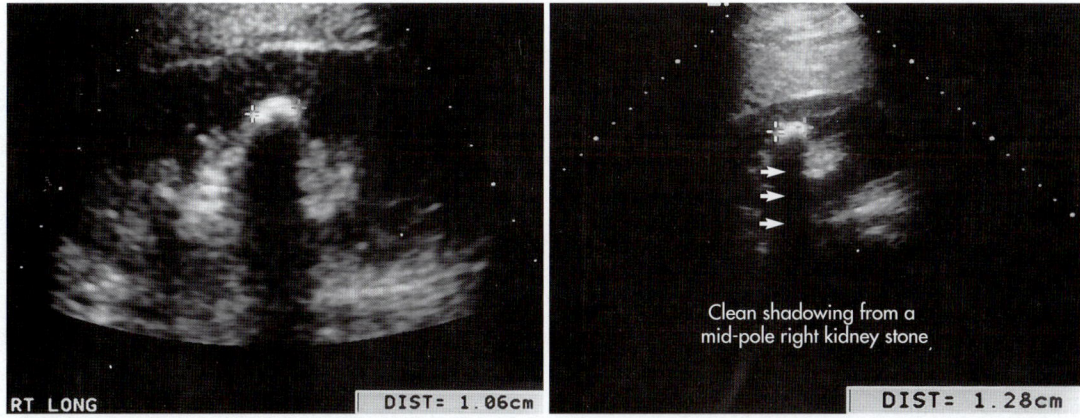

FIG. 15.90 A 69-year-old man presented with right flank pain. A mid-pole echogenic structure with indicating posterior shadowing *(arrows)*, representative of a renal stone.

to break up the stone into smaller particles, which can readily pass through the urinary system. Percutaneous nephrolithotomy is a surgical procedure in which an opening is made in the kidney, and a nephroscope is used to remove the stone from the kidney. For mid and lower urinary tract stones, a ureteroscope (which has a basket-like end) can be placed through the urethra and bladder and guided up to the level of the stone to capture and remove the stone. Early treatment of stones that cause obstruction is important to reverse any renal damage that the obstruction may cause.

Sonographic Findings. Renal stones are highly echogenic foci with posterior acoustic shadowing (Fig. 15.90). When searching for renal stones, the sonographer should scan along the lines of renal fat; usually, stones smaller than 3 mm may not shadow with the use of traditional B-mode. Prominent renal sinus fat, mesenteric fat, and bowel have high attenuation and may appear as an indistinct echogenic focus with questionable posterior acoustic shadowing, making it difficult to differentiate from stones. The use of tissue harmonics can demonstrate the shadowing of small stones measuring millimeters in size (Fig. 15.91). Color and power Doppler have increased the sensitivity of confirming the presence of stones. Color and power Doppler cause a twinkling artifact posterior to the stone. This artifact is referred to as the *twinkling sign* and is imaged as a rapidly changing mixture of red and blue colors posterior to the stone (Fig. 15.92). Color and power Doppler are more sensitive when an "all-digital" processing technology is used because of its increased color sensitivity and acoustic power.

If the stone causes obstruction, hydronephrosis will be noted, and depending on the location of the stone, the ureter may be dilated superior to the level of obstruction (Fig. 15.93). The ureter—from the ureteropelvic junction to the bladder—is not routinely visualized on a sonogram unless dilated. The superior and distal ends of the ureters are more readily visualized than the midsection. The ureters lie in the retroperitoneal cavity and are obscured by bowel gas. Stones can also be imaged when the urinary bladder is distended with fluid (Figs. 15.94 and 15.95).

Bladder Diverticulum

A bladder diverticulum is a herniation of the bladder wall. These outpouchings may be singular or multiple and are thinner than the normal bladder wall (Fig. 15.96). Diverticula can

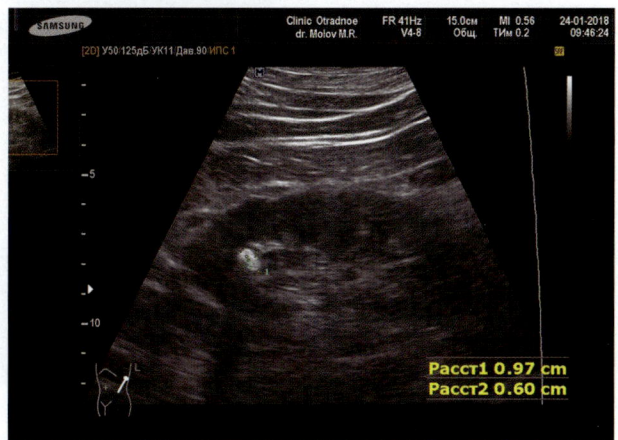

FIG. 15.91 A small (3.1 mm) right renal stone detected using tissue harmonics.

be congenital or acquired. An acquired bladder diverticulum is an outpouching of bladder mucosa between muscle bundles caused by increased intravesical pressure. A diverticulum lacks a muscular layer and has a neck, which usually is narrow. Acquired diverticula are commonly associated with calculi and are more prevalent in patients with chronic bladder outlet obstruction or neurogenic bladder.

Congenital bladder diverticula are rare. They originate at the posterior angle of the bladder trigone and contain all components of the bladder wall.

Sonographic Findings. The sonographic finding is a neck of varying size connecting the adjacent fluid-filled structure to the bladder. The diverticulum may still be filled with fluid after the patient empties the bladder. Urine stasis leads to recurrent infection and stone formation (Fig. 15.97).

Bladder Inflammation (Cystitis)

Inflammation of the bladder has several infectious and noninfectious causes. Cystitis is usually secondary to another condition that causes stasis of urine in the bladder. Conditions that cause incomplete emptying of the bladder include urethral stricture, benign and malignant neoplasms, bladder calculi, trauma (blood clot), tuberculosis (lower ureteric strictures), pregnancy, neurogenic bladder, and radiation therapy. Other causes of

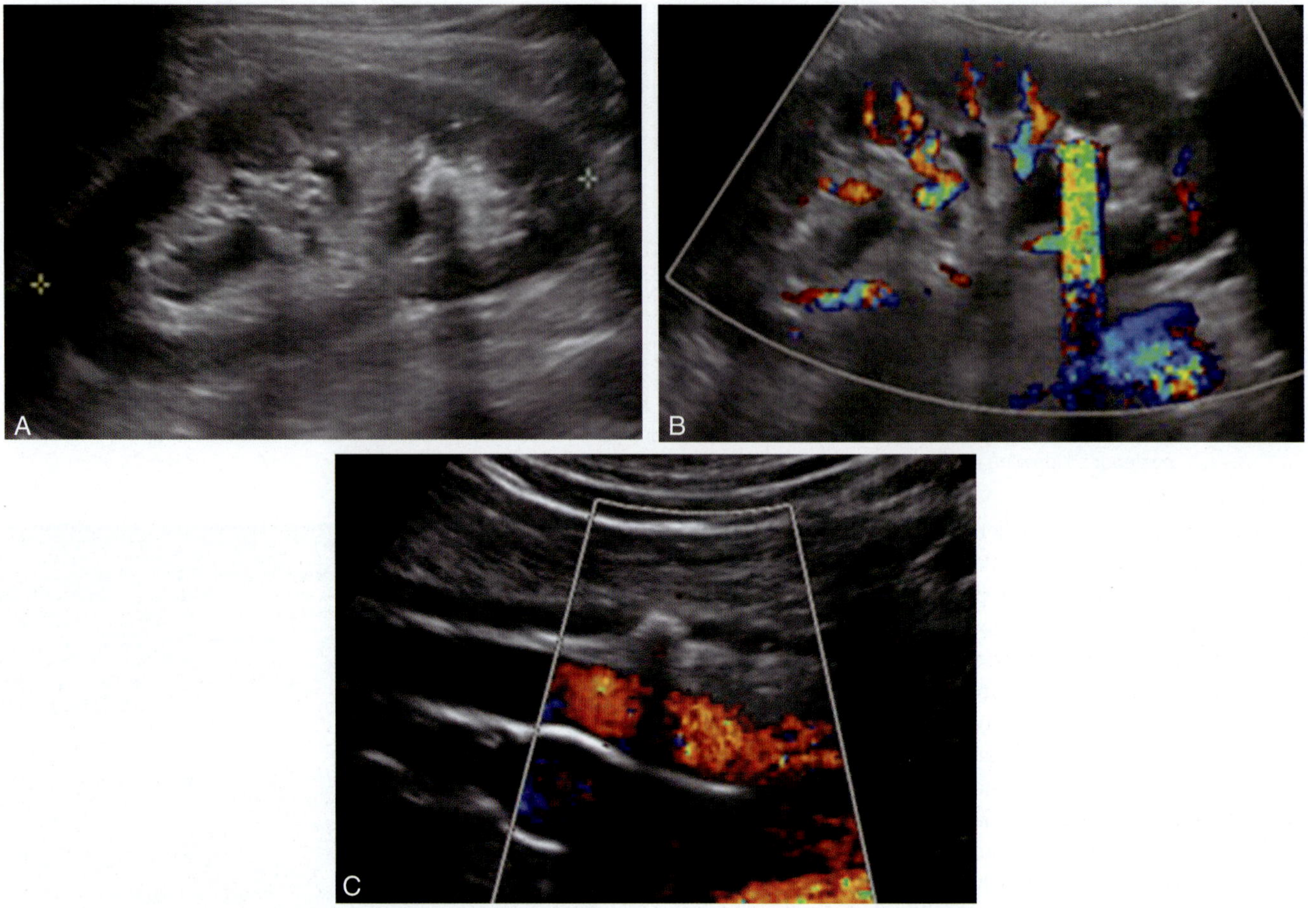

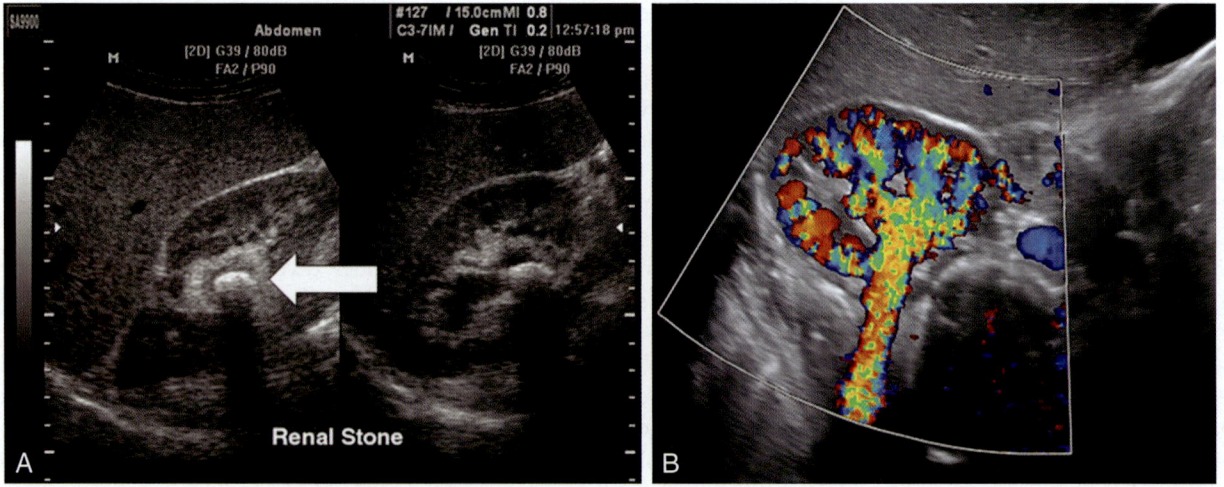

FIG. 15.92 Color Doppler twinkling artifacts occur frequently with urolithiasis and can be generated independently from stone formation. (A) Renal and ureteral stone on the same patient. (B) Full twinkling artifact on the stone. (C) Absent twinkle artifact on the ureteral stone. Twinkling artifact is positive almost 80% of the time with urolithiasis.

FIG. 15.93 (A–B) Right mid-pole obstructing ureteral stone.

cystitis include Foley catheter, common rectal or vaginal fistulas, renal disease, sexual intercourse, poor hygiene, diabetes mellitus, and inflammation following surgical intervention.

Sonographic Findings. Sonographically, the bladder wall may appear normal in the early stages of inflammatory disease. As the duration of inflammation increases, the smooth bladder wall will become diffuse or nondiffuse with hypoechoic thickening. As the inflammatory process progresses, the bladder wall will become fibrotic and scarred. The bladder wall will appear more echogenic on a sonogram.

Bladder Tumors

Most bladder tumors in adults (95%) are transitional cell carcinoma. Bladder tumors usually are not detected until

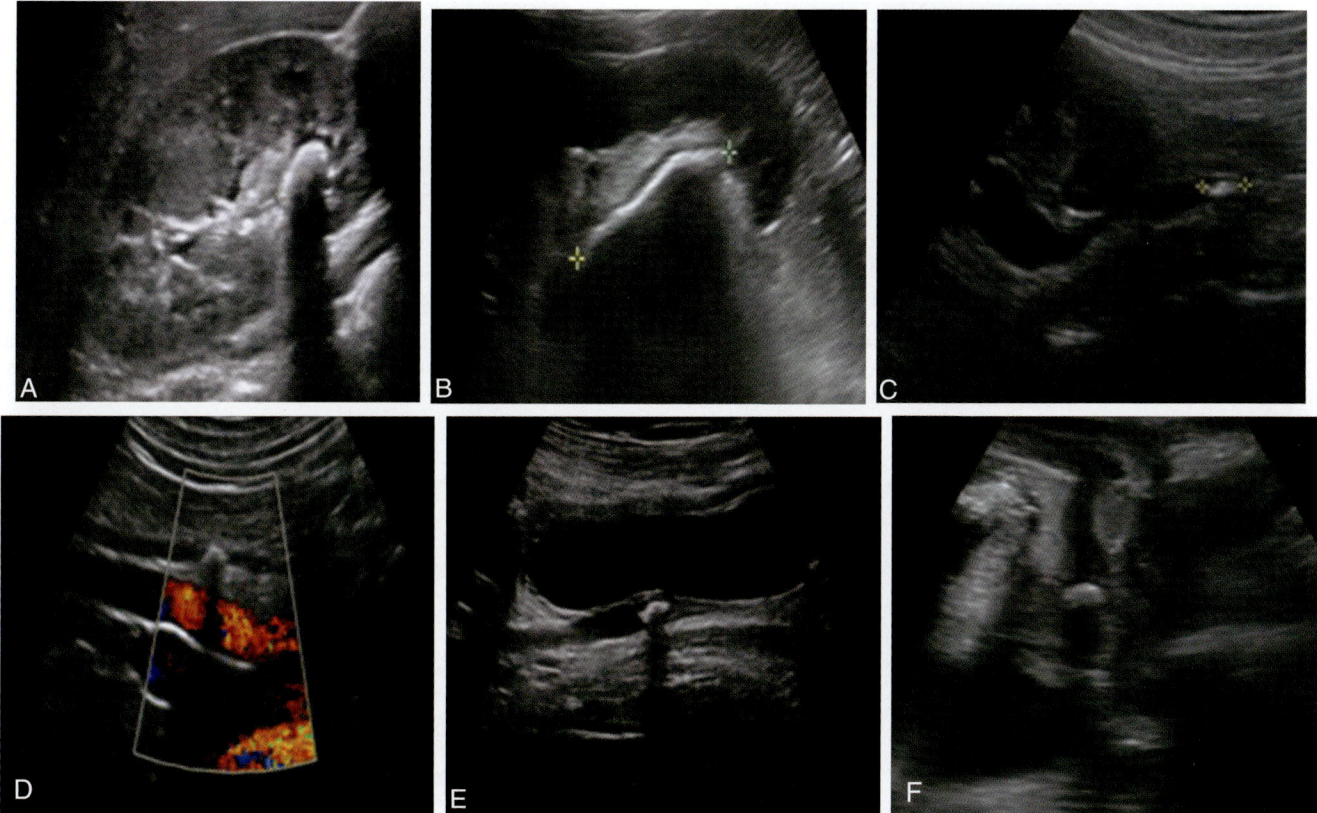

FIG. 15.94 **Ultrasound and urolithiasis.** (A) A 1-cm left renal pelvis stone. (B) A 3.5-cm partial staghorn stone. (C) An 8-mm partially obstructed proximal left ureteral stone. (D) A 5-mm left ureteral stone at iliac crossing point. (E) A 9-mm stone at the right ureteral vesical junction level. (F) A 6-mm stone stuck in the male proximal urethra.

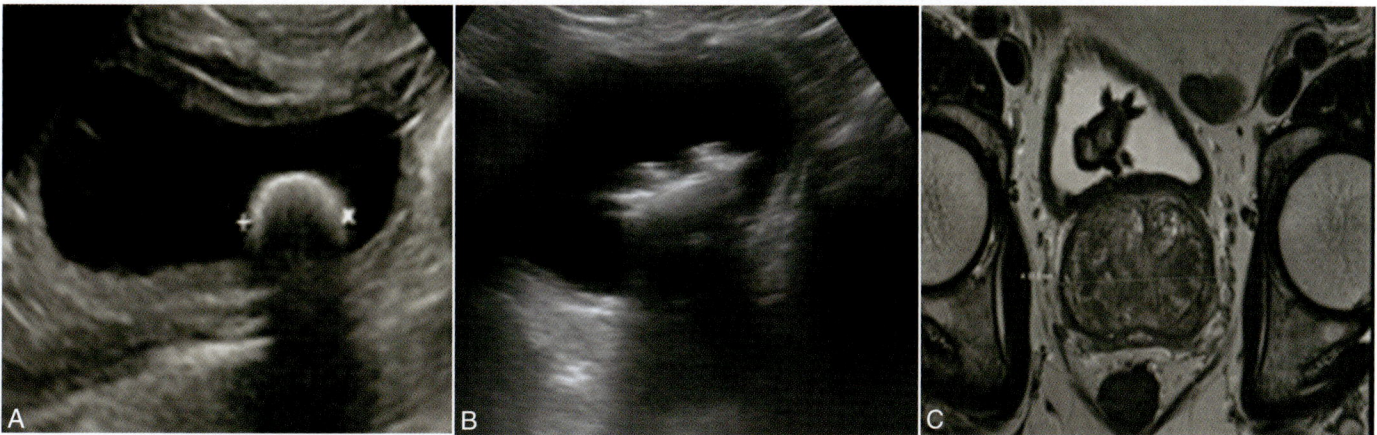

FIG. 15.95 (A) Transverse scan of the shadowing bladder stone measuring 1.5 cm in diameter. (B) Ultrasound of "jack stone" in the bladder. (C) T1-weighted magnetic resonance imaging of the stone.

they have become advanced. Patients usually present with gross hematuria and may also present with dysuria, urinary frequency, or urinary urgency. Sonography cannot distinguish between benign and malignant masses. A cystoscopy or a biopsy may allow differentiation between a benign and a malignant neoplasm. The bladder may be the secondary site of malignancy. The most common site is the prostate. Invasion of the bladder may result from colon, uterine, or ovarian carcinoma or endometriosis.

Sonographic Findings. The sonographic appearance of bladder masses varies; they commonly appear as a focal bladder wall thickness. Sonography, CT, or MRI may be used to perform staging of bladder carcinoma. A transabdominal sonographic approach can detect intravesical lesions as small as 3 to 4 mm. Sonography is limited and is unable to detect a perivesical extension and pelvic wall involvement. A transrectal approach can be used to detect intravesicular involvement.

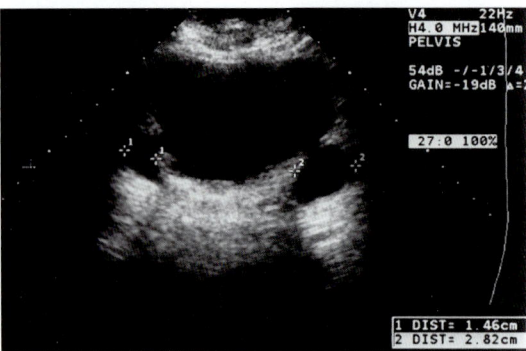

FIG. 15.96 Congenital bladder diverticulae originate posterior to the bladder and contain all the components of the bladder wall. A stone is present in 50% of cases.

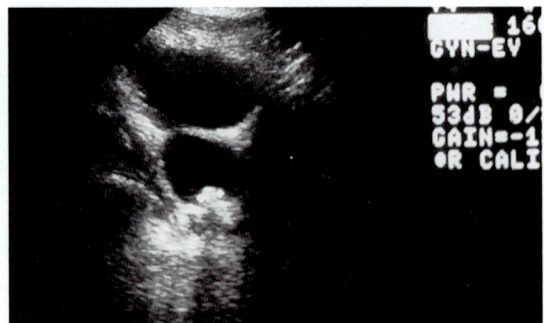

FIG. 15.97 Acquired bladder diverticulum in an outpouching of bladder mucosa between muscle bundles caused by increased intravesical pressure.

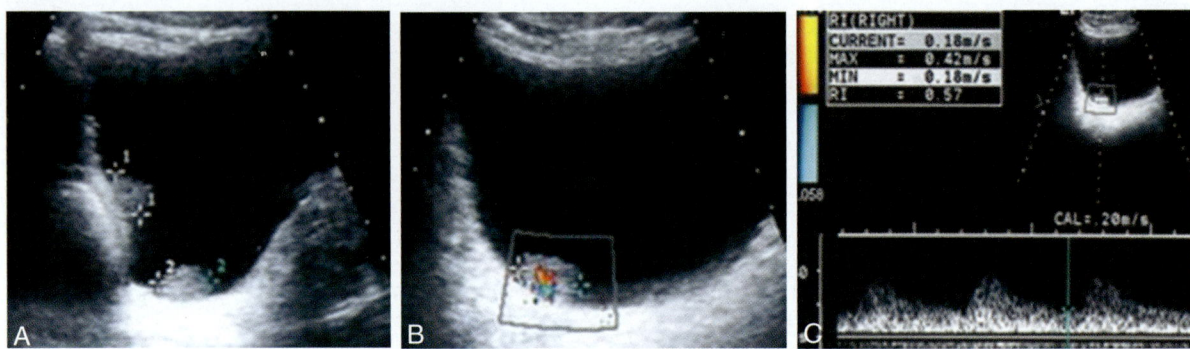

FIG. 15.98 (A) Carcinoma of the urinary bladder which is multifocal in up to 40% of cases. (B) Color Doppler demonstrates intratumoral vascularity. (C) Continuous blood flow.

Benign tumors are typically hypoechoic compared with malignant bladder tumors, but they may have the same echogenicity. All primary bladder tumors—squamous cell carcinoma, adenocarcinoma, and rhabdomyosarcoma in children—have the same sonographic appearance: an irregular echogenic mass that projects into the lumen of the bladder. Color Doppler can be used to determine increased vascularity (Fig. 15.98). Any bladder mass may cause outflow obstruction, and the kidneys should be evaluated for hydronephrosis.

Key Pearls

- The normal urinary system has two principal functions: excreting wastes and regulating the composition of blood.
- The urinary system is located posterior to the peritoneum lining the abdominal cavity in an area called the retroperitoneum.
- Within the kidney, the upper expanded end of the ureter, known as the renal pelvis of the ureter, divides into two or three major calyces, each of which divides further into two or three minor calyces.
- The renal corpuscle consists of a network of capillaries called the glomerulus, which is surrounded by a cuplike structure known as Bowman capsule. Blood flows into the glomerulus through a small afferent arteriole and leaves the glomerulus through an efferent arteriole.
- Three constrictions occur along the ureter's course: (1) where the ureter leaves the renal pelvis, (2) where it is kinked as it crosses the pelvic brim, and (3) where it pierces the bladder wall.
- The renal arteries are lateral branches of the aorta that are located just inferior to the superior mesenteric artery.
- Five to six veins join to form the main renal vein. This vein emerges from the renal hilus anterior to the renal artery.
- Hematuria is the appearance of blood cells in the urine; it can be associated with early renal disease.
- Leukocytes may be present whenever inflammation, infection, or tissue necrosis originates from anywhere in the urinary tract.
- The blood urea nitrogen (BUN) is the concentration of urea nitrogen in blood and is the end product of cellular metabolism.
- The columns of Bertin are prominent invaginations of the cortex located at varying depths within the medullary substance of the kidneys.

- A dromedary hump is a bulge of cortical tissue on the lateral surface of a kidney (usually the left), resembling the hump of a dromedary camel.
- A junctional parenchymal defect is a triangular, echogenic area typically located anteriorly and superiorly.
- Sinus lipomatosis is a condition characterized by deposition of a moderate amount of fat in the renal sinus with parenchymal atrophy.
- Renal hypoplasia is incomplete development of the kidney, usually with fewer than five calyces.
- Incomplete, or partial, duplication is the most frequently occurring congenital anomaly in the neonate. Duplication consists of two collecting systems and two ureters, with a single ureter entering into the urinary bladder.
- Complete duplication is the rare condition of a duplex collecting system. This anomaly results in two separate collecting systems, each with its own ureter that enters the bladder. In cases of double ureter, the ureter from the upper pole of the kidney usually opens below and medial to the one from the lower pole (rule of Weigert-Meyer).
- Renal ectopia (ectopic kidney) describes a kidney that is not located in its usual position, the renal fascia.
- Horseshoe kidney is the most common anomaly of renal fusion. Fusion of the lower poles occurs in 96% of cases, with ureters passing anterior to the renal parenchyma and variation of arterial land venous blood supply.
- A cystic mass sonographically displays several characteristic features: (1) smooth, thin, well-defined border; (2) round or oval shape; (3) sharp interface between the cyst and the renal parenchyma; (4) no internal echoes (anechoic); and (5) increased posterior acoustic enhancement.
- Complex cysts may contain septations, thick walls, calcifications, internal echoes, and mural nodularity.
- Polycystic renal disease may present in one of two forms: the infantile autosomal recessive form and the adult autosomal dominant form.
- Autosomal recessive polycystic kidney disease, also called infantile polycystic disease, is a fairly rare genetic disorder.
- Multicystic dysplastic kidney (MCDK) disease is a common nonhereditary renal dysplasia that usually occurs unilaterally, with the kidney functioning poorly, if at all. MCDK is the most common form of cystic disease in neonates and is believed to be the consequence of early in utero urinary tract obstruction.
- Medullary sponge kidney is a development anomaly that occurs in the medullary pyramids and consists of cystic or fusiform dilation of the distal collecting ducts (ducts of Bellini), causing stasis of urine and stone formation.
- A solid lesion projects as a nongeometric shape with irregular borders, a poorly defined interface between the mass and the kidney, low-level internal echoes, a weak posterior border caused by increased attenuation of the mass, and poor through-transmission.
- Renal cell carcinoma, also called hypernephroma, or Grawitz tumor, is the most common of all renal neoplasms and represents 85% of all kidney tumors.
- Transitional cell carcinoma accounts for 90% of malignancies that involve the renal pelvis, ureter, and bladder, and for up to 7%–10% of all renal tumors.
- Metastases to the kidneys are relatively common, occurring late in the course of the disease. Secondary malignancies are bilateral in one-third of cases and multiple in more than 50%. The most common primary malignancies that metastasize to the kidneys include carcinoma of the lung or breast and renal cell carcinoma of the contralateral kidney.
- Nephroblastoma, or Wilms tumor, is the most common abdominal malignancy in children and the most common solid renal tumor in pediatric patients 1–8 years old.
- Renal angiomyolipoma is the most common benign renal tumor. It is composed of varying proportions of fat, muscle, and blood vessels.
- A ureterocele is a cystlike enlargement of the lower end of the ureter caused by congenital or acquired stenosis of the distal end of the ureter.
- Different forms of glomerulonephritis, including membranous, idiopathic, membranoproliferative, rapidly progressive, and poststreptococcal, can be associated with abnormal echo patterns from the renal parenchyma on a sonogram.
- Acute interstitial nephritis has been associated with the infectious processes of scarlet fever and diphtheria.
- Systemic lupus erythematosus is a connective tissue disorder believed to result from an abnormal immune system. Females are affected more often than males, and incidence peaks between 20 and 40 years of age.
- Renal involvement is common in patients with sickle cell disease. Abnormalities include glomerulonephritis, renal vein thrombosis, and papillary necrosis.
- Renal papillary necrosis is not a pathologic entity, but rather a descriptive term for a condition—necrosis of the papillae. The renal papillae (the apex of the renal pyramid that projects into the minor calyx) are vulnerable to ischemic necrosis.
- The excretory and regulatory functions of the kidneys are decreased in acute and chronic renal failure.
- Acute renal failure is a common medical condition that can be caused by numerous medical diseases or pathophysiologic mechanisms.
- Acute tubular necrosis is the most common medical renal disease to produce acute renal failure, although it can be reversible.
- Chronic kidney disease is the loss of renal function as a result of disease, most commonly parenchymal disease. Three primary types of chronic renal failure are known: nephron, vascular, and interstitial abnormalities.
- Hydronephrosis is the separation of renal sinus echoes by interconnected fluid-filled calyces.
- Pyonephrosis occurs when pus is found within the collecting renal system.
- Emphysematous pyelonephritis occurs when air is present in the parenchyma (diffuse gas-forming parenchymal infection).
- Renal calcifications may be seen as localized parenchymal calcifications, resulting from scar tissue caused by bacterial infection, renal abscess, infected hematoma, urinoma,

- lymphocele, tuberculosis, or infarction, or post–percutaneous renal procedures.
- A renal infarction occurs when part of the tissue undergoes necrosis after cessation of the blood supply, usually as a result of artery occlusion.
- Arteriovenous fistulas (AVFs) are most often acquired rather than congenital. AVFs may be due to renal biopsies, complications from partial nephrectomies, or trauma.
- Kidney stones are one of the most common kidney problems that can occur; they may cause obstruction, and this obstruction can be extremely painful.
- Stones that are large and fill the renal collecting system are called staghorn calculi.
- A bladder diverticulum is a herniation of the bladder wall. These outpouchings may be singular or multiple and are thinner than the normal bladder wall.
- Inflammation of the bladder has several infectious and noninfectious causes. Cystitis is usually secondary to another condition that causes stasis of urine in the bladder.
- Most bladder tumors in adults (95%) are transitional cell carcinoma.

BIBLIOGRAPHY

Abed A, El-Nahas AR, Al-Kandari AM, Shokeir AA. *Percutaneous nephrolithotomy (PCNL) in the treatment of stones within horseshoe kidneys and in patients with autosomal dominant polycystic kidney disease. Difficult cases in endourology*. London: Springer; 2013:115–121.

Bajwa ZH, Gupta S, Warfield CA, et al. Pain management in polycystic kidney disease. *Int Soc Nephrol*. 2001;60:1631–1644.

Brun M, Maugey-Laulom B, Eurin D, et al. Prenatal sonographic patterns in autosomal dominant polycystic kidney disease: a multicenter study. *Ultrasound Obstet Gynecol*. 2004;24:55–61.

Buturovic-Ponikvar J, Visnar-Perovic A. Ultrasonography in chronic renal failure. *Eur J Radiol*. 2003;46:115–122.

Cai Y, Lianfang D, Li F, Jiying G. Quantification of enhancement of renal parenchymal masses with contrast-enhanced ultrasound. *Ultrasound Med Biol*. 2014;40(7):1387–1393.

Gordon D. Imaging in cystic renal disease. *Arch Dis Child*. 2000;83:533.

Hélénon O, Correas JM, Balleyguier C, et al. Ultrasound of renal tumors. *Euro Radiol*. 2001;11:1890–1901.

Hennerici M, Neuerbrug-Hensler D. *Vascular diagnosis with ultrasound*. New York: Thieme; 1998.

Henningsen C. *Clinical guide to ultrasonography*. St Louis: Mosby; 2004.

Kamaya A, Tuthill T, Rubin J. Twinkling artifact on color Doppler sonography: depending on machine parameters and underlying cause. *Am J Roentgenol*. 2003;180:215–222.

Lee HY, Grant EG. Sonography in renovascular hypertension. *J Ultrasound Med*. 2002;21:431–441.

Lee JY, Kim AH, Cho JY, et al. Color and power Doppler twinkling artifacts from urinary stones. *Am J Roentgenol*. 2001;176:1441–1445.

Lucisano G, Comi N, Pelagi E, et al. Can renal sonography be a reliable diagnostic tool in the assessment of chronic kidney disease? *J Ultrasound Med*. 2015;34(2):299–306.

Mostbeck GH, Gossinger HD, Mallek R. Effect of heart rate on Doppler measurements of RI in renal arteries. *Radiology*. 1990;175:511.

Nicolau C, Torra R, Bianchi L, et al. Abdominal sonographic study of autosomal dominant polycystic kidney disease. *J Clin Ultrasound*. 2000;22:277–282.

Oei T, Hedgire S, Harisinghan M. Advanced cross-sectional imaging techniques for the detection and characterization of renal masses. *Imaging Med*. 2001;3(2):207–218.

Pepe P, Motta L, Pennisi M, et al. Functional evaluation of the urinary tract by color-Doppler ultrasonography (CDU) in 100 patients with renal colic. *Eur Radiol*. 2005;53:131–135.

Pickerwell D. Elastography: imaging of tomorrow? *J Diagn Medical Sonography*. May 2010:1–5.

Redmond A, McDevitt M, Barnes S. Acute renal failure: recognition and treatment in ward patients. *Nurs Stand*. 2004;18:46–55.

Shokeir AA. Renal colic: new concepts related to pathophysiology, diagnosis and treatment. *Curr Opin Urol*. 2002;12:263–269.

Tempkin B. *Ultrasound scanning: principles and protocols*. ed 3 Philadelphia: Elsevier; 2009.

Wolf Jr SJ. State of the art article evaluation and management of solid and cystic renal masses. *J Urol*. 1998;159:1120.

CHAPTER 16

The Retroperitoneum

Sandra L. Hagen-Ansert

OBJECTIVES

On completion of this chapter, you should be able to:
- Identify the retroperitoneal anatomy
- List the adrenal gland hormones and describe the syndromes associated with hypersecretion and hyposecretion
- Describe the sonographic appearance and clinical findings of adrenal tumors, retroperitoneal fibrosis, and retroperitoneal fluid collections
- Explain the role that sonography plays in the evaluation of para-aortic nodes and describe the sonographic technique used to visualize them

OUTLINE

Anatomy of the Retroperitoneum 491
- Normal Anatomy 491
- Vascular Supply 496

Physiology and Laboratory Data of the Retroperitoneum 497
- Cortex 497
- Medulla 497

Sonographic Evaluation of the Retroperitoneum 497
- Adrenal Glands 497
- Sonography Pitfalls 498
- Diaphragmatic Crura 498
- Para-aortic Lymph Nodes 498

Pathology of the Retroperitoneum 499
- Adrenal Cortical Syndromes 499
- Adrenal Cysts 502
- Adrenal Hemorrhage 503
- Adrenal Tumors 503
- Adrenal Medulla Tumors 505
- Retroperitoneal Fat 506
- Primary Retroperitoneal Tumors 506
- Secondary Retroperitoneal Tumors 508
- Retroperitoneal Fluid Collections 508
- Retroperitoneal Fibrosis (Ormond Disease) 509

KEY TERMS

Addison disease
Adenoma
Adrenocorticotropic hormone (ACTH)
Cortex
Cushing syndrome
False pelvis
Hyperplasia
Lymphadenopathy
Lymphoma
Medulla
Neuroblastoma
Neuroectodermal tissue
Pheochromocytoma

ANATOMY OF THE RETROPERITONEUM

Normal Anatomy

The retroperitoneal space is the area between the posterior portion of the parietal peritoneum and the posterior abdominal wall muscles. It extends from the diaphragm to the pelvis. Laterally, the boundaries extend to the extraperitoneal fat planes within the confines of the transversalis fascia, and medially the space encloses the great vessels. It is subdivided into the following three categories: anterior pararenal space, perirenal space, and posterior pararenal space (Fig. 16.1).

Box 16.1 lists the respective organs in the retroperitoneal space. The perirenal space (Fig. 16.2) surrounds the kidney, adrenal, and perirenal fat. The anterior pararenal space includes the duodenum, pancreas, and ascending and transverse colon. The posterior pararenal space includes the iliopsoas muscle, ureter, and branches of the inferior vena cava (IVC) and aorta and their lymphatics.

The retroperitoneum is protected by the spine, ribs, pelvis, and musculature and has been a difficult area to assess clinically by sonography. Computerized tomography (CT) imaging is better to outline the retroperitoneal cavity. Occasionally, however, the sonographer is asked to rule out a fluid collection, hematoma, urinoma, or ascitic fluid in the retroperitoneal space.

The retroperitoneum is delineated anteriorly by the parietal peritoneum, posteriorly by the transversalis fascia, and laterally by the lateral borders of the quadratus lumborum muscles and peritoneal leaves of the mesentery (Fig. 16.3A). Proceeding from a superior to inferior direction,

CHAPTER 16 The Retroperitoneum

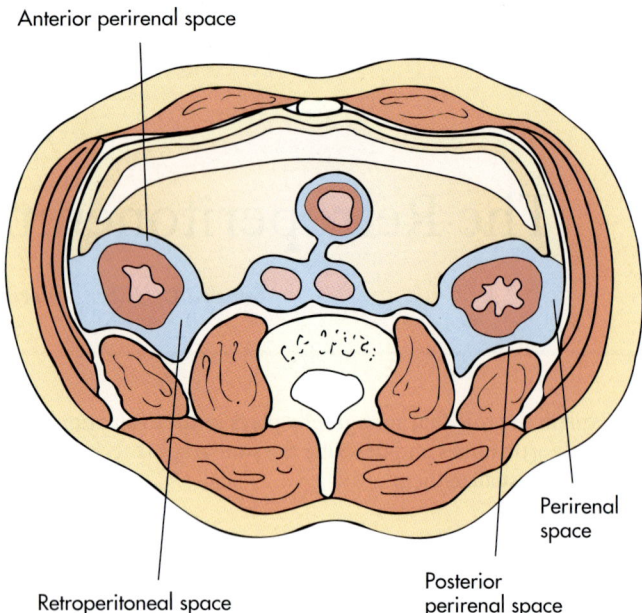

FIG. 16.1 Transverse illustration of the anterior pararenal space, perirenal space, and posterior perirenal space. The retroperitoneal space is outlined in *blue*.

BOX 16.1 Organs in the Retroperitoneal Spaces

Anterior Pararenal Space
- Pancreas
- Duodenum
- Ascending and transverse colon

Perirenal Space
- Adrenal glands
- Kidneys
- Ureter
- Great vessel

Posterior Pararenal Space
- Blood
- Lymph nodes

Iliac Fossa
- Ureter
- Major branches of great vessels
- Lymphatics

Retrofascial Space (Three Compartments)
- Psoas
- Lumbar (quadratus lumborum)
- Iliacus

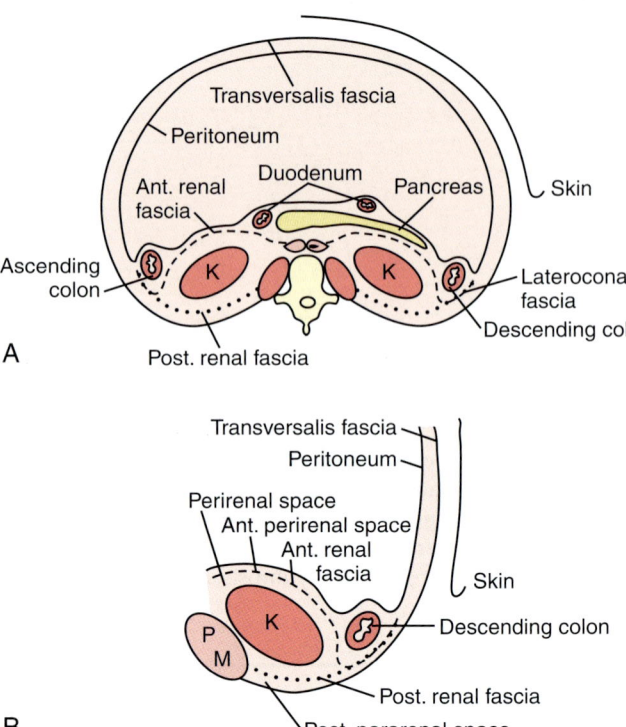

FIG. 16.2 **Retroperitoneal space.** Anterior *(dashed lines)* and posterior *(dotted lines)* perirenal fascia join to form lateroconal fascia. These fasciae divide the retroperitoneum into (1) the anterior pararenal space, which contains the duodenum, pancreas, and right and left colon, (2) the perirenal space, which contains the kidney and adrenal gland, and (3) the posterior pararenal space, which contains fat. (A) Axial section of the pancreas. (B) Axial section of the left upper quadrant just caudal to the pancreatic tail. The anterior pararenal space is subtended ventrally by the posterior peritoneum and dorsolaterally by the anterior renal fascia and lateroconal fascia. The posterior pararenal space is demarcated ventrally by the posterior perirenal fascia and lateroconal fascia and dorsolaterally by transversalis fascia.

the retroperitoneum extends from the diaphragm to the pelvic brim. Superior to the pelvic brim, the retroperitoneum can be partitioned into the lumbar and iliac fossae. The pararenal and perirenal spaces are included in the lumbar fossa (Fig. 16.3B).

Pathologic processes can stretch from the anterior abdominal wall to the subdiaphragmatic space, mediastinum, and subcutaneous tissues of the back and flank. The retrofascial space, which includes the psoas, quadratus lumborum, and iliacus muscles (muscles posterior to the transversalis fascia), is often the site of extension of retroperitoneal pathologic processes.

Anterior Pararenal Space. The anterior pararenal space is bound anteriorly by the parietal peritoneum and posteriorly by the anterior renal fascia (see Fig. 16.3A). It is bound laterally by the lateroconal fascia formed by the fusion of the anterior and posterior leaves of the renal fascia. (This space merges with the bare area of the liver by the coronary ligament.) The pancreas, duodenum, and ascending and transverse colon are included in the anterior pararenal space (see Fig. 16.2).

Perirenal Space. The perirenal space is surrounded by the anterior and posterior layers of the renal fascia (Gerota fascia), attaching to the diaphragm superiorly. They are united loosely at their inferior margin at the iliac crest level or superior border of the **false pelvis**. Collections in the perinephric space can communicate within the iliac fossa of the retroperitoneum (see Fig. 16.2).

The lateroconal fascia (the lateral fusion of the renal fascia) proceeds anteriorly as the posterior peritoneum (Fig. 16.4). The posterior renal fasciae fuse medially with the psoas or quadratus lumborum fascia. The anterior renal fascia fuses medially with connective tissue surrounding

CHAPTER 16 The Retroperitoneum   493

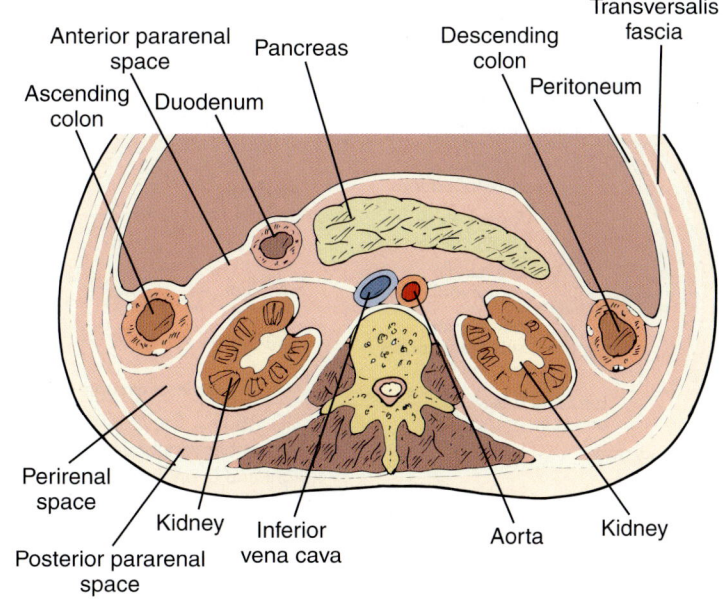

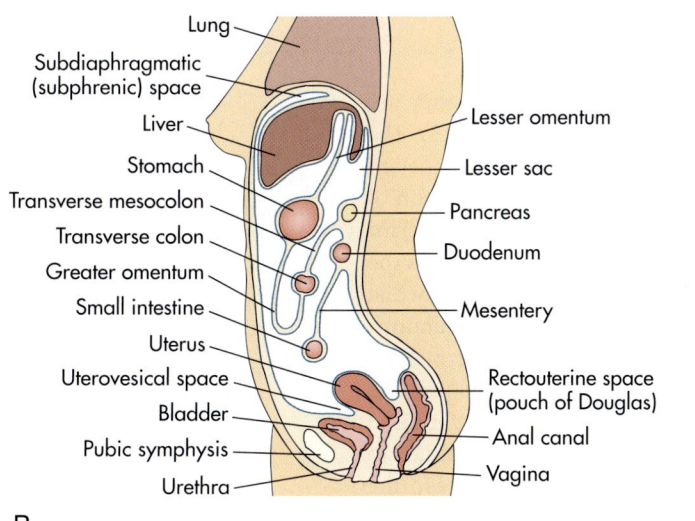

FIG. 16.3 (A) The retroperitoneum is delineated anteriorly by the parietal peritoneum, posteriorly by the transversalis fascia, and laterally by the lateral borders of the quadratus lumborum muscles and peritoneal leaves of the mesentery. (B) Proceeding from a superior to inferior direction, the retroperitoneum extends from the diaphragm to the pelvic brim. Superior to the pelvic brim, the retroperitoneum can be partitioned into the lumbar and iliac fossae. The pararenal and perirenal spaces are included in the lumbar fossa.

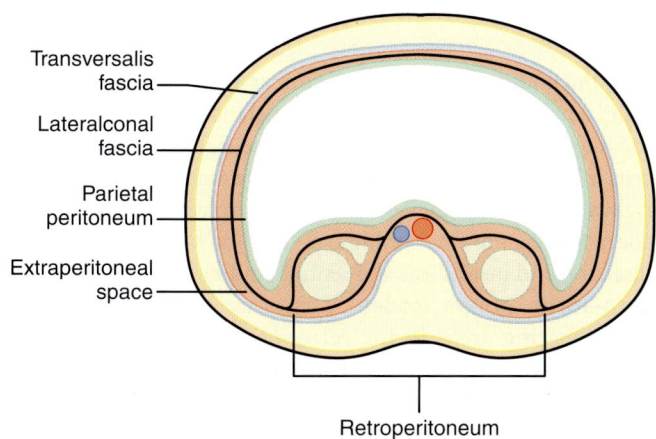

FIG. 16.4 The lateroconal fascia.

the great vessels. (This space contains the adrenal gland, kidney, and ureter; the great vessels, also within this space, are largely isolated within their connective tissue sheaths; see Fig. 16.3.) The perirenal space contains the adrenal gland and kidney (in a variable amount of echogenic perinephric fat, the thickest portion of which is posterior and lateral to the kidney's lower pole). The kidney is anterolateral to the psoas muscle, anterior to the quadratus lumborum muscle, and posteromedial to the ascending and descending colon.

The second portion of the duodenum is anterior to the renal hilum on the right. On the left, the kidney is bounded by the stomach anterosuperiorly, the pancreas anteriorly, and the spleen anterolaterally.

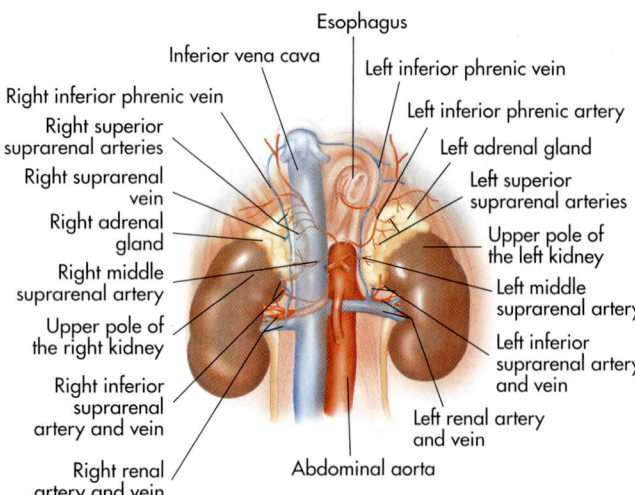

FIG. 16.5 The adrenal glands are retroperitoneal organs that lie on the upper pole of each kidney. They are surrounded by perinephric fat. The right adrenal gland is triangular and caps the upper pole of the right kidney. It extends medially behind the inferior vena cava and rests posteriorly on the diaphragm. The left adrenal gland is semilunar and extends along the medial borders of the left kidney. It lies posterior to the pancreas, the lesser sac, and the stomach and rests posteriorly on the diaphragm.

Adrenal Glands. In the adult patient, the adrenal glands are anterior, medial, and superior to the kidneys (Fig. 16.5). The right adrenal is more superior to the kidney, whereas the left adrenal is more medial to the kidney. The medial portion of the right adrenal gland is immediately posterior to the inferior vena cava (above the level of the portal vein and lateral to the crus). The lateral portion of the gland is posterior and medial to the right lobe of the liver and posterior to the duodenum.

The left adrenal gland is lateral or slightly posterolateral to the aorta and lateral to the crus of the diaphragm. The superior portion is posterior to the lesser omental space and posterior to the stomach. The inferior portion is posterior to the pancreas. The splenic vein and artery pass between the pancreas and the left adrenal gland.

The adrenal glands vary in size, shape, and configuration; the right adrenal is triangular and caps the upper pole of the right kidney. The left adrenal is semilunar in shape and extends along the medial border of the left kidney from the upper pole to the hilus. The internal texture is medium in consistency; the cortex and medulla are not distinguished.

The adrenal gland is a distinct hypoechoic structure; sometimes, highly echogenic fat is seen surrounding the gland. The normal size is usually smaller than 3 cm.

Neonatal Adrenal. The neonatal adrenal glands are characterized by a thin echogenic core surrounded by a thick transonic zone. This thick rim of transonicity represents the hypertrophied adrenal cortex, whereas the echogenic core is the adrenal medulla. An infant adrenal gland is proportionally larger than an adult adrenal gland (one third the size of the kidney; in adults it is one-thirteenth the size).

Diaphragmatic Crura. The diaphragmatic crura begins as tendinous fibers from the lumbar vertebral bodies, disks, and transverse processes of L3 on the right and L1 on the left (Fig. 16.6). The right crus is longer, larger, and more lobular and is associated

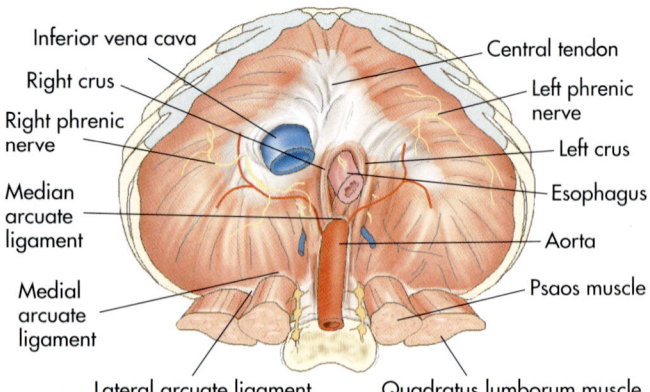

FIG. 16.6 The crura of the diaphragm begin as tendinous fibers from the lumbar vertebral bodies, disks, and transverse processes of L3 on the right and L1 on the left.

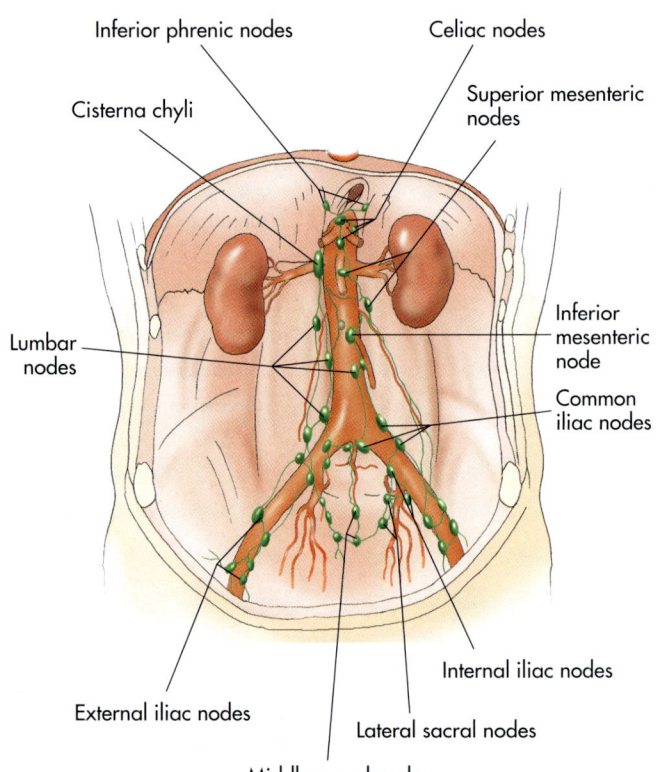

FIG. 16.7 The lymphatic chain follows the course of the aorta and iliac arteries.

with the anterior aspect of the lumbar vertebral ligament. The right renal artery crosses anterior to the crus and posterior to the inferior vena cava at the level of the right kidney. The right crus is bounded by the inferior vena cava anterolaterally and the right adrenal and right lobe of liver posterolaterally. The left crus courses along the anterior lumbar vertebral bodies in a superior direction and inserts into the central tendon of the diaphragm.

Para-aortic Lymph Nodes. There are two major lymph-node-bearing areas in the retroperitoneal cavity: the iliac and hypogastric nodes within the pelvis and the para-aortic group in the upper retroperitoneum. The lymphatic chain follows the course of the thoracic aorta, abdominal aorta, and iliac arteries (Fig. 16.7). Common sites are the para-aortic and paracaval areas near the great vessels, peripancreatic area, renal hilar area, and mesenteric region. Normal nodes are smaller than the tip of a finger, less than 1 cm, and are not imaged on a sonogram. However, if these nodes enlarge because of infection or tumor, they can be seen on a sonogram.

Posterior Pararenal Space. The posterior pararenal space is located between the posterior renal fascia and the transversalis fascia. It communicates with the peritoneal fat, lateral to the lateroconal fascia. The posterior pararenal space merges inferiorly with the anterior pararenal space and retroperitoneal tissues of the iliac fossa (see Fig. 16.3).

The psoas muscle, the fascia of which merges with the posterior transversalis fascia, makes up the medial border of this posterior space. This space is open laterally and inferiorly. The blood and lymph nodes embedded in fat may be found in the posterior pararenal space.

Iliac Fossa. The iliac fossa is the region extending between the internal surface of the iliac wings, from the crest to the iliopectineal line. This area is known as the false pelvis and contains the ureter and major branches of the distal great vessels and their lymphatics. The transversalis fascia extends into the iliac fossa as the iliac fascia.

Retrofascial Space. The retrofascial space is made up of the posterior abdominal wall, muscles, nerves, lymphatics, and areolar tissue behind the transversalis fascia. It is divided into the following three compartments:

1. The psoas compartment: a muscle that spans from the mediastinum to the thigh (Fig. 16.8). The fascia attaches to the pelvic brim.
2. The lumbar region consists of the quadratus lumborum, a muscle that originates from the iliolumbar ligament, the adjacent iliac crest, and the superior borders of the transverse process of L3 and L4 and inserts into the margin of the 12th rib (Fig. 16.9). It is adjoining and posterior to the colon, kidney, and psoas muscle.
3. The iliac area, which is made up of the iliacus and extends the length of the iliac fossa. The psoas passes through the iliac fossa medial to the iliacus and posterior to the iliac fascia (see Fig. 16.8). These two muscles merge as they extend into the true pelvis. The iliopsoas takes on a more anterior location caudally to lie along the lateral pelvic sidewall.

Pelvic Retroperitoneum. The pelvic retroperitoneum lies between the sacrum and pubis from back to front, between the pelvic peritoneal reflection above and pelvic diaphragm (coccygeus and levator ani muscles) below, and between the obturator internus and piriformis muscles. There are four subdivisions: (1) prevesical, (2) rectovesical, (3) presacral, and (4) bilateral pararectal (and paravesical) spaces (Fig. 16.10).

Prevesical and Rectovesical Spaces. The prevesical space spans from the pubis to the anterior margin of the bladder. It is bordered laterally by the obturator fascia. The connective tissue covering the bladder, seminal vesicles, and prostate is continuous with the fascial lamina within this space. The space is an extension of the retroperitoneal

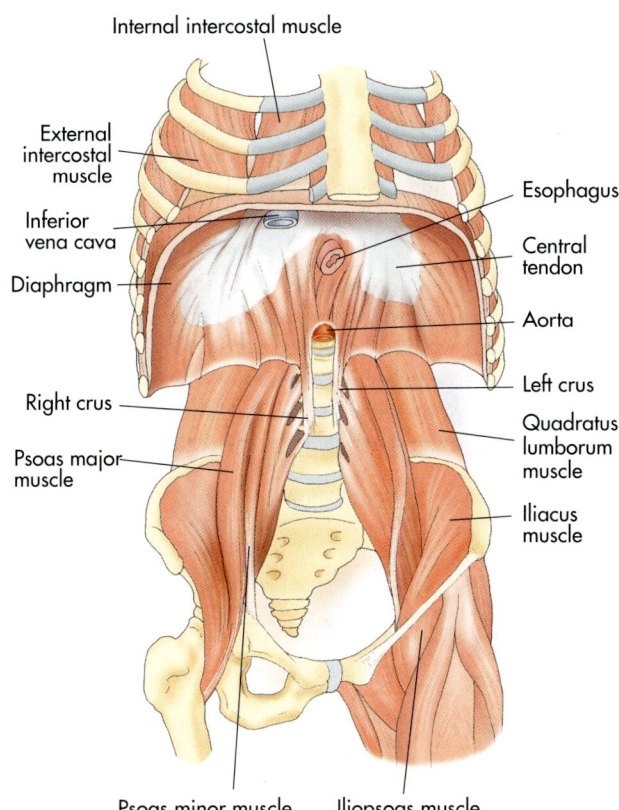

FIG. 16.8 The psoas compartment consists of a muscle that spans from the mediastinum to the thigh. The fascia attaches to the pelvic brim.

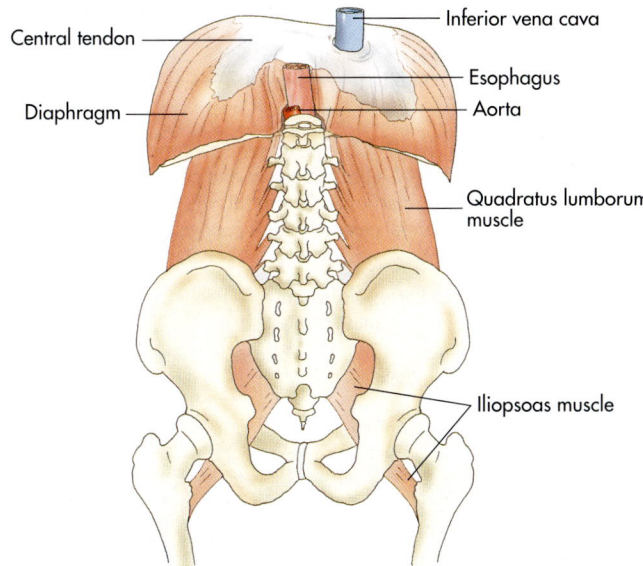

FIG. 16.9 The lumbar region consists of the quadratus lumborum, a muscle that originates from the iliolumbar ligament, the adjacent iliac crest, and the superior borders of the transverse process of L3 and L4 and inserts into the margins of the 12th rib. It is adjoining and posterior to the colon, kidney, and psoas muscle.

space of the anterior abdominal wall deep to the rectus sheath, which is continuous with the transversalis fascia. The space between the bladder and rectum is the rectovesical space.

Presacral Space. The presacral space lies between the rectum and fascia, covering the sacrum and posterior pelvic floor musculature.

Bilateral Pararectal Space. The pararectal space is bounded laterally by the piriformis and levator ani fascia and medially by the rectum. It extends anteriorly from the bladder, medially to the obturator internus, and laterally to the external iliac vessels (Fig. 16.11).

The paravesical and pararectal spaces are traversed by the two ureters. The pelvic wall muscles, iliac vessels, ureter, bladder, prostate, seminal vesicles, and cervix are retroperitoneal structures within the true pelvis. The obturator internus muscle lines the lateral aspect of the pelvis. Posteriorly the piriformis muscle is seen extending anterolaterally from the region of the sacrum.

Vascular Supply

Aorta. The aorta enters the abdomen posterior to the diaphragm at the level of L1 and passes posterior to the left lobe of the liver. The aorta has a straight horizontal course to the level of L4, where it bifurcates into the common iliac arteries. A slight anterior curve of the aorta is the result of lumbar lordosis.

Inferior Vena Cava. The inferior vena cava extends from the junction of the two common iliac veins to the right of L5 and travels cephalad. Unlike the aorta, it curves anterior toward its termination into the right atrial cavity.

Adrenal Glands. Three arteries supply each adrenal gland: the suprarenal branch of the inferior phrenic, the suprarenal branch of the aorta, and the suprarenal branch of the renal

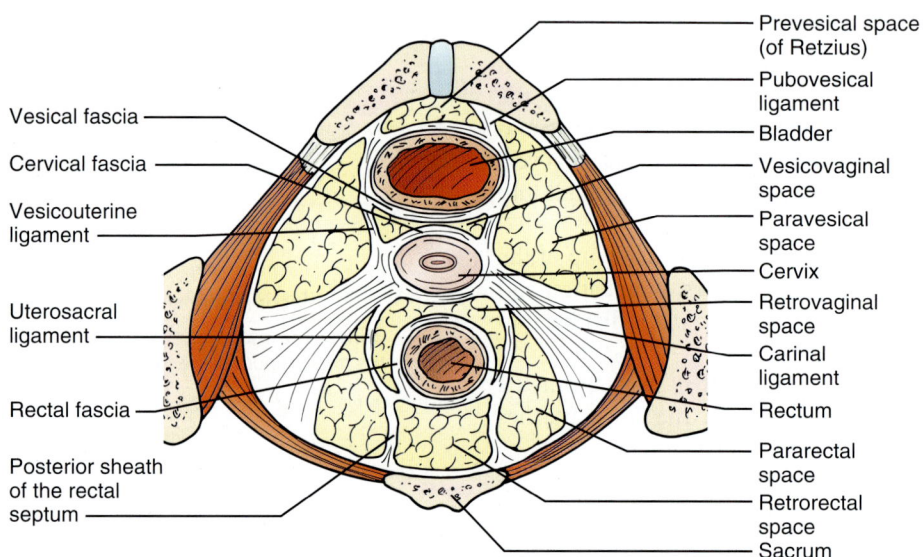

FIG. 16.10 The pelvic retroperitoneum lies between the sacrum and pubis from back to front, between the pelvic peritoneal reflection above and pelvic diaphragm (coccygeus and levator ani muscles) below, and between the obturator internus and piriformis muscles. There are four subdivisions: (1) prevesical, (2) rectovesical, (3) presacral, and (4) bilateral pararectal (and paravesical) spaces.

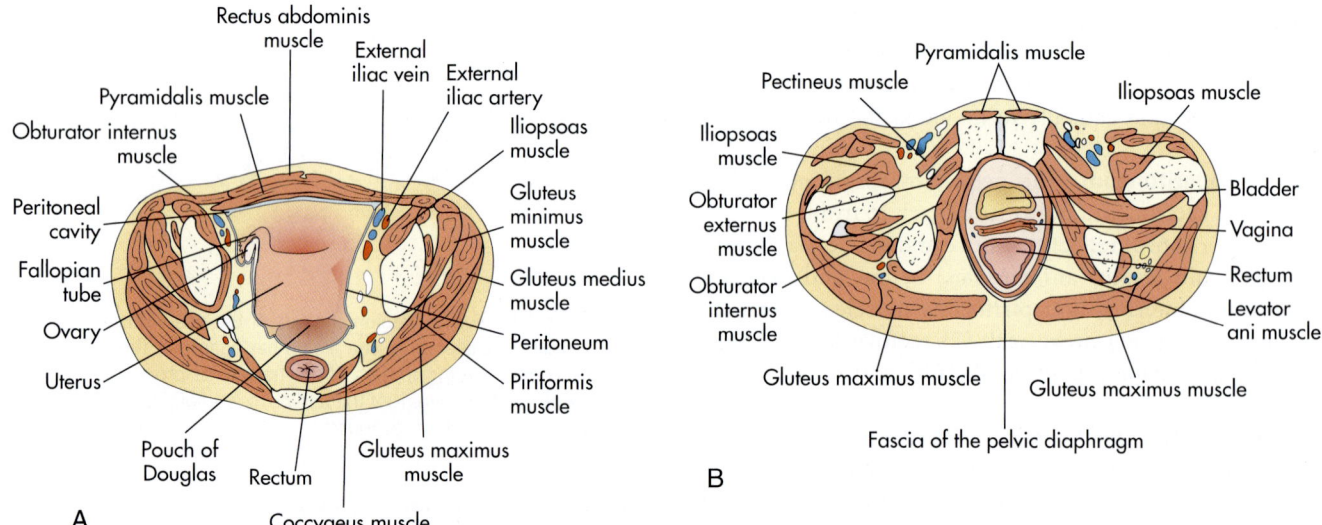

FIG. 16.11 (A) The pararectal space is bounded laterally by the piriformis and levator ani fascia and medially by the rectum. (B) The pararectal space extends anteriorly from the bladder, medially to the obturator internus, and laterally to the external iliac vessels.

artery. A single vein from the hilum of each gland drains into the inferior vena cava on the right, and on the left, the vein drains into the left renal vein.

PHYSIOLOGY AND LABORATORY DATA OF THE RETROPERITONEUM

Each adrenal gland is made up of two endocrine glands. The **cortex**, or outer part, secretes a range of steroid hormones; the **medulla**, or core, secretes epinephrine and norepinephrine.

Cortex

The steroids secreted by the adrenal cortex fall into the following three main categories: mineralocorticoids, glucocorticoids, and sex hormones (androgen and estrogen).

Mineralocorticoids. Mineralocorticoids regulate electrolyte metabolism. Aldosterone is the principal mineralocorticoid. It has a regulatory effect on the relative concentrations of mineral ions in the body fluids and therefore on the water content of the tissue. An insufficiency of this steroid leads to increased excretion of sodium and chloride ions and water into the urine. This is accompanied by a fall in sodium, chloride, and bicarbonate concentrations in the blood, resulting in a lowered pH or acidosis.

Glucocorticoids. Glucocorticoids play a principal role in carbohydrate metabolism. They promote deposition of liver glycogen from proteins and inhibit use of glucose by the cells, thus increasing blood sugar level. Cortisone and hydrocortisone are the primary glucocorticoids. They diminish allergic response, especially the more serious inflammatory types (rheumatoid arthritis and rheumatic fever).

Sex Hormones. Androgens are the male sex hormones, and estrogens are the female sex hormones. The adrenal gland secretes both types of hormones regardless of the patient's gender. Normally these are secreted in minute quantities and have almost insignificant effects. With oversecretion, however, a marked effect is seen. Adrenal tumors in women can promote secondary masculine characteristics. Hypersecretion of the hormone in prepubertal boys accelerates adult masculine development and the growth of pubic hair. The adrenal cortex is controlled by **adrenocorticotropic hormone (ACTH)** from the pituitary. A diminished glucocorticoid blood concentration stimulates the secretion of ACTH. Consequent increase in adrenal cortex activity inhibits further ACTH secretion.

Hypofunction of the adrenal cortex in humans is called **Addison disease**. Symptoms and signs include hypotension, general weakness, fatigue, loss of appetite and weight, and a characteristic bronzing of the skin (hyperpigmentation).

Oversecretion of the adrenal cortex may be caused by an overproduction of ACTH resulting from a pituitary tumor, **hyperplasia**, or a tumor in the cortex itself. Hypersecretion of the cortical hormones produces distinct syndromes. The features of the syndromes often overlap and can be either acquired or congenital. Adrenal hyperfunction can cause Cushing syndrome, Conn syndrome, or adrenogenital syndrome.

Medulla

The adrenal medulla makes up the core of the gland in which groups of irregular cells are located amid veins that collect blood from the sinusoids. The adrenal medulla produces epinephrine and norepinephrine. Both of these hormones are amines, sometimes referred to as catecholamines. They elevate the blood pressure, the former working as an accelerator of the heart rate and the latter as a vasoconstrictor. The two hormones together promote glycogenolysis, the breakdown of liver glycogen to glucose, which causes an increase in blood sugar concentration.

The adrenal medulla is not essential for life and can be removed surgically without causing untreatable damage. An increase in the production of the medulla hormones may be caused by a **pheochromocytoma**.

SONOGRAPHIC EVALUATION OF THE RETROPERITONEUM

No specific patient preparation is necessary to image the retroperitoneal cavity, although 6 to 8 hours of fasting may help to eliminate bowel gas. To image the retroperitoneum, scans should be made in the longitudinal and transverse planes from the diaphragm to the iliac crest, with the patient in a supine, decubitus, or prone position, and from the crest to the symphysis, with the patient in a supine position and having a full bladder. The upper abdomen may also be scanned with the patient in a decubitus position. All scans should include the kidneys and retroperitoneal muscles.

Adrenal Glands

Although sonography has proven useful in evaluating soft tissue structures within the abdominal cavity, visualizing the adrenal glands has been difficult because of their small size, medial location, and surrounding perirenal fat. Sonography is not the imaging modality of choice for evaluation of an adrenal mass. If the adrenal gland becomes enlarged secondary to disease, it is easier to image and separate from the upper pole of the kidney.

Visualization of the adrenal area depends on several factors: the size of the patient and the amount of perirenal fat surrounding the adrenal area, the presence of bowel gas, and the ability to move the patient into multiple positions.

With the patient in the decubitus position, the sonographer should attempt to align the kidney and ipsilateral paravertebral vessels (inferior vena cava or aorta). The right adrenal gland has a "comma" or triangular shape in the transaxial plane (Fig. 16.12). The best visualization is obtained by a transverse scan with the patient in a left lateral decubitus position. When the patient assumes this position, the inferior vena cava moves forward, and the aorta rolls over the crus of the diaphragm, offering a good window to image the upper pole of the right kidney and adrenal gland. If the patient is obese, it may be difficult to recognize the triangular- or crescent-shaped adrenal gland. The adrenal should not appear rounded; if it does, the

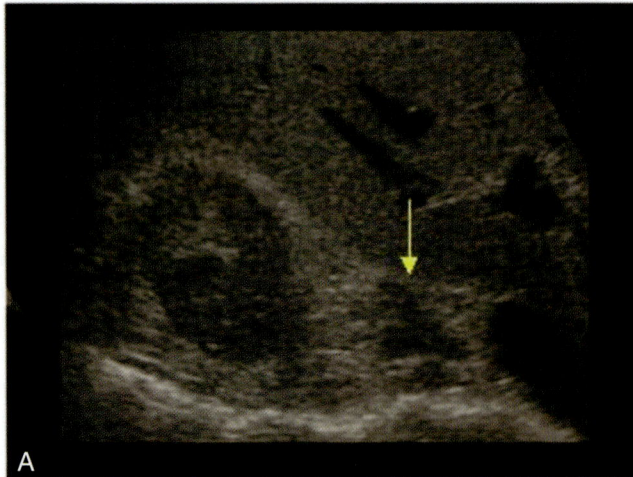
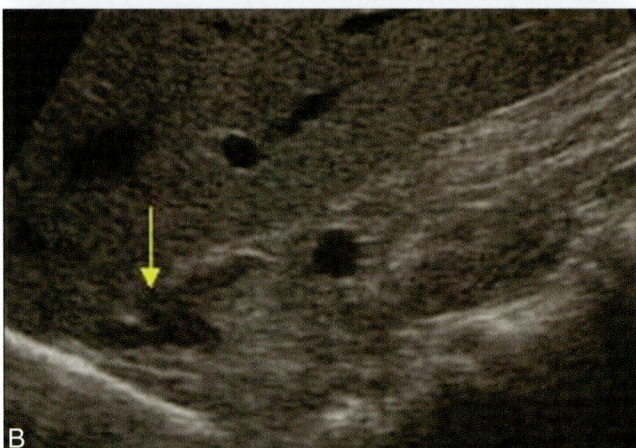

FIG. 16.12 (A) The right adrenal gland has a "comma" or triangular shape in the transaxial plane. (B) Computed tomographic coronal image of the left adrenal gland.

- Medial lobulations of the spleen
- Splenic vasculature
- Body-tail region of the pancreas
- Fourth portion of the duodenum

Diaphragmatic Crura

The crus of the diaphragm may be imaged in the transverse or longitudinal coronal plane. The right crus is seen in a plane that passes through the right lobe of the liver, kidney, and adrenal gland (Fig. 16.15). The left crus is seen using the spleen and left kidney as a window, with the crus to the left of the aorta.

Para-aortic Lymph Nodes

Sonography patterns associated with nodes include rounded, focal, echo-poor lesions (1 to 3 cm in size and larger) and confluent, echo-poor masses, which often displace the kidney laterally. The sonographer may also detect a "mantle" of nodes in the paraspinal location, a "floating" or anteriorly displaced aorta secondary to the enlarged nodes, or the mesenteric "sandwich" sign representing the anterior and posterior node masses surrounding mesenteric vessels (Fig. 16.16).

The lymph nodes lie along the lateral and anterior margins of the aorta and inferior vena cava (see Fig. 16.7); thus the best scanning is done with the patient in the supine or decubitus position. A left coronal view using the left kidney as a window may be used to discover paraaortic nodes. It is always important to examine the patient in two planes because in only one plane, the enlarged nodes may mimic an aortic aneurysm or tumor.

Longitudinal scans may be made first to outline the aorta and to search for enlarged lymph nodes (Fig. 16.17). The aorta provides an excellent background for the hypoechoic nodes. Scans should begin at the midline, and the transducer should be angled both to the left and right at small angles to image the anterior and lateral borders of the aorta and inferior vena cava.

Transverse scans are made from the level of the xiphoid to the symphysis. Careful identification of the great vessels, organ structures, and muscles is important. Patterns of a fluid-filled duodenum or bowel may make it difficult to outline the great vessels or may cause confusion in diagnosing **lymphadenopathy**.

Scans below the umbilicus are more difficult because of interference from the small bowel. Careful attention should be given to the psoas and iliacus muscles within the pelvis, where the iliac arteries run along their medial border. Both muscles serve as a hypoechoic marker along the pelvic sidewall. Enlarged lymph nodes can be identified anterior and medial to these margins. A smooth sharp border of the muscle indicates no nodal involvement. The bladder should be filled to help push the small bowel out of the pelvis and serve as an acoustic window to better image the vascular structures. Color Doppler may be used to help delineate the vascular structures.

finding suggests a pathologic process. The longitudinal scan is made through the right lobe of the liver, perpendicular to the linear right crus of the diaphragm. The retroperitoneal fat must be recognized as separate from the liver, crus of the diaphragm, adrenal gland, and great vessel (Fig. 16.13).

The left adrenal gland is closely related to the left crus of the diaphragm and the anterior-superior-medial aspect of the upper pole of the left kidney. It may be more difficult to image the left adrenal gland because of the stomach gas interference. The patient should be placed in a right lateral decubitus position and transverse scans made in an attempt to align the left kidney and the aorta. The left adrenal gland is seen by scanning along the posterior axillary line (Fig. 16.14). The patient should be in deep inspiration to bring the adrenal and renal areas into better view.

Sonography Pitfalls

- Right crus of the diaphragm
- Second portion of the duodenum
- Gastroesophageal junction (cephalad to the left adrenal gland)

CHAPTER 16 The Retroperitoneum

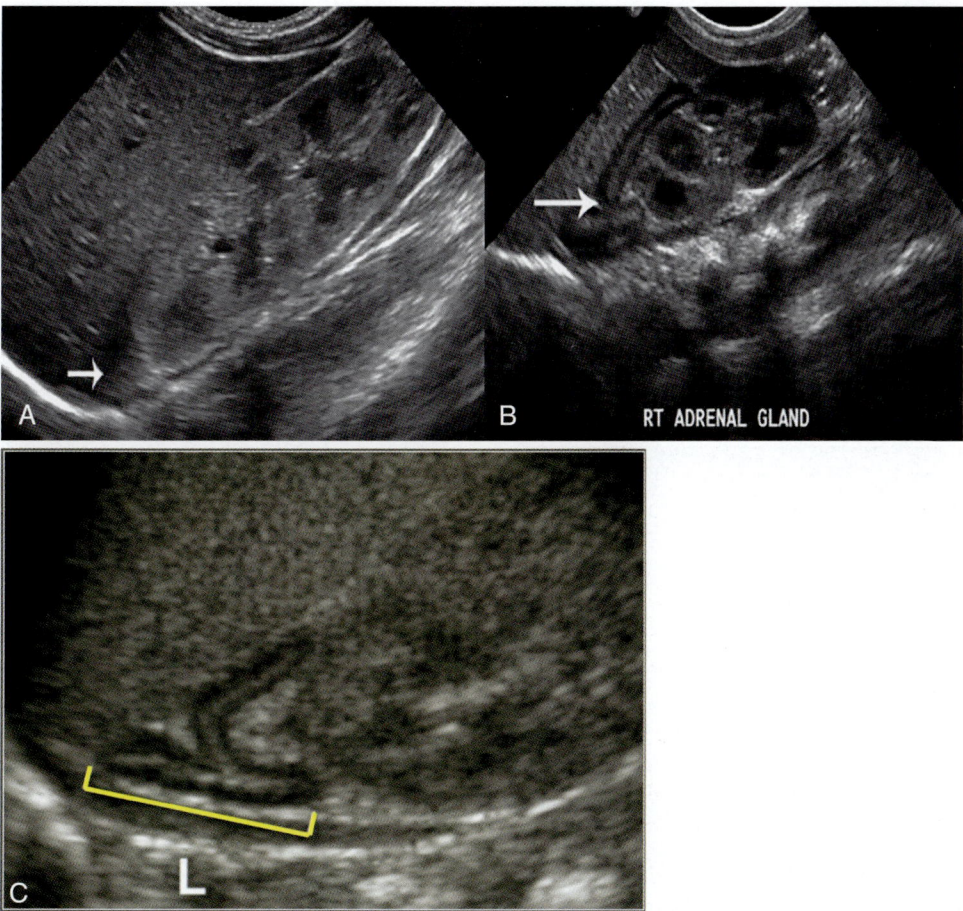

FIG. 16.13 (A–C) The longitudinal scan is made through the right lobe of the liver, perpendicular to the linear right crus of the diaphragm. The retroperitoneal fat must be recognized as separate from the liver, crus of the diaphragm, adrenal gland, and great vessel.

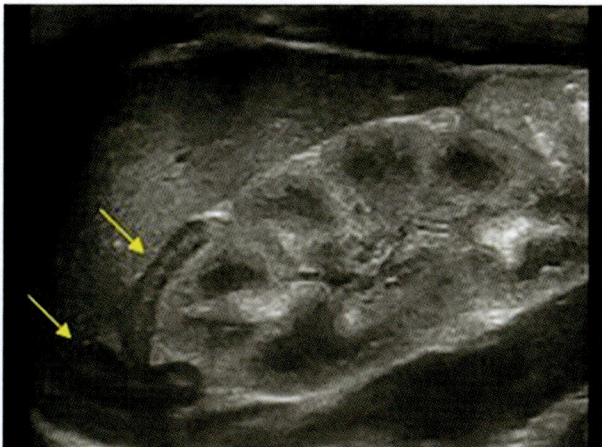

FIG. 16.14 The left adrenal gland is closely related to the left crus of the diaphragm and the anterior-superior-medial aspect of the upper pole of the left kidney.

Splenomegaly should also be evaluated in patients with lymphadenopathy. As the sonographer moves caudal from the xiphoid, attention should be on the splenic size and great vessel area to detect nodal involvement near the hilus of the spleen (Fig. 16.18).

Lymph nodes remain consistent patterns, whereas bowel and the duodenum display changing peristaltic patterns when imaged with a sonogram. As gentle pressure is applied with the transducer to displace the bowel, the lymph nodes remain constant in shape. The echo pattern posterior to each structure is different. Lymph nodes are homogeneous and thus transmit sound easily; the bowel presents a more complex pattern with dense central echoes from its mucosal pattern. Often the duodenum has air within its walls, causing a shadow posteriorly. Enlarged lymph nodes should be reproducible on a sonogram in two projections. After the abdomen is completely scanned, repeat sections over the enlarged nodes should demonstrate the same pattern as on the earlier scan.

PATHOLOGY OF THE RETROPERITONEUM

Adrenal Cortical Syndromes

The cortical syndromes that the sonographer may encounter while scanning for an adrenal mass are as follows:
- *Addison disease (adrenocortical insufficiency).* Affects males and females equally and can be diagnosed in any age group. It is characterized by atrophy of the adrenal

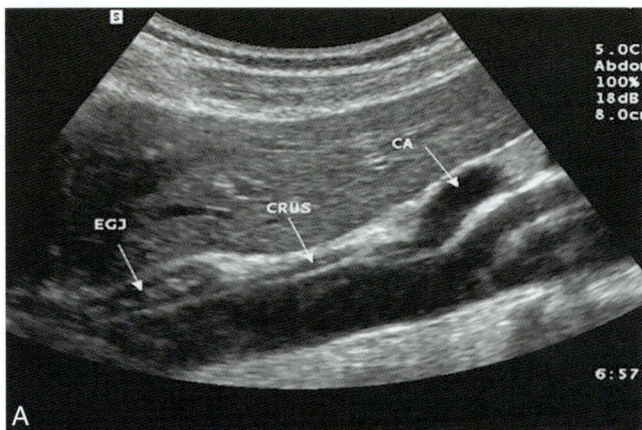

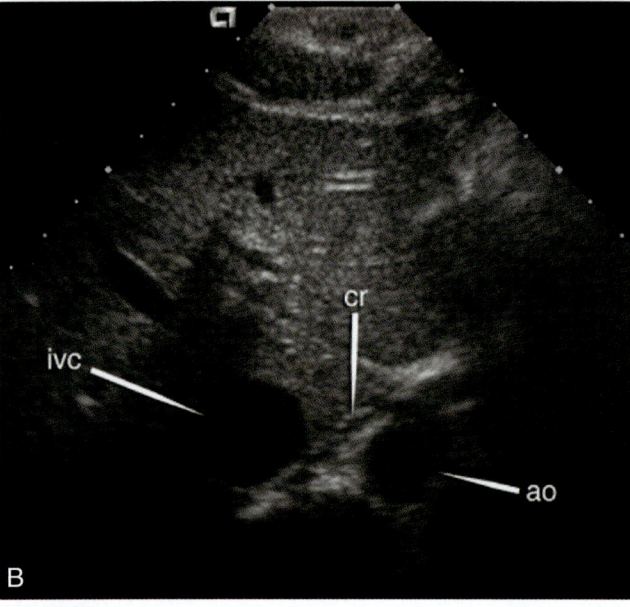

FIG. 16.15 Longitudinal (A) and transverse (B) images of the crus (cr) of the diaphragm. *ao*, aorta; *CA*, celiac axis; *EGJ*, esophagogastric junction; *ivc*, inferior vena cava.

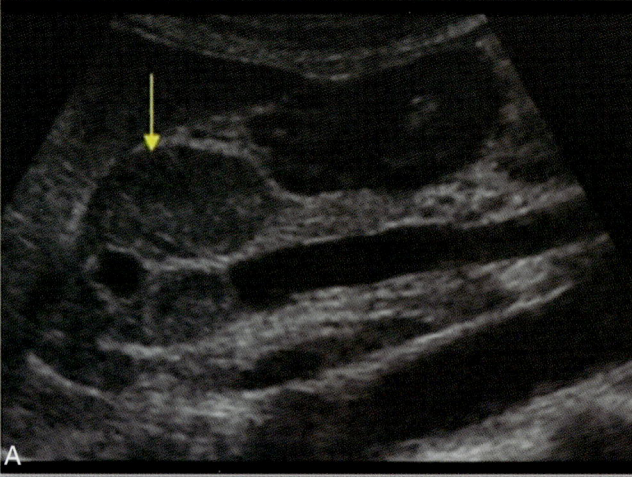

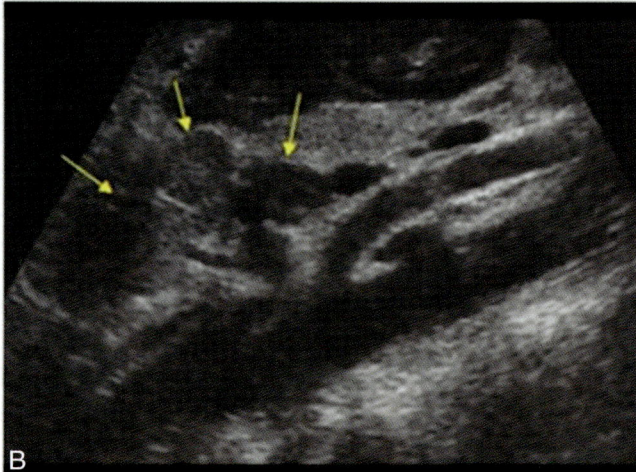

FIG. 16.16 Sonographic patterns associated with nodes include rounded, focal, echo-poor lesions and confluent, echo-poor masses. The enlarged nodes may present as a "mantle" of nodes in the paraspinal location or anteriorly displaced aorta secondary to the enlarged nodes, or the mesenteric "sandwich" sign representing the anterior and posterior node masses surrounding mesenteric vessels.

cortex with decreased production of cortisol and sometimes aldosterone. Usually, the majority of the cortical tissue is destroyed before adrenal insufficiency is diagnosed. Primary causes of reduced adrenal cortical tissue include an autoimmune process, tuberculosis (TB), an inflammatory process, a primary neoplasm, or metastases. Secondary adrenal insufficiencies are caused by pituitary dysfunction and a decrease in production of the pituitary hormone ACTH (adrenocorticotropic hormone). The clinical signs and symptoms usually manifest during metabolic stress or trauma. Symptoms include increased sodium retention, which leads to tissue edema; increased plasma volume; increased potassium excretion; hyperpigmentation; and a mild alkalosis. Fatigue and muscle and bone weakness are common. Prognosis is good with steroid replacement therapy.

- *Adrenogenital syndrome (adrenal virilism).* Results from the excessive secretion of the sex hormones and adrenal androgens. It is caused either by an adrenal tumor or by hyperplasia. The symptoms and clinical signs vary depending on the age and sex of the person. In a newborn, there may be ambiguous genitalia with or without adrenal hyperplasia. (Things other than adrenal hyperplasia can also cause ambiguous genitalia.) Adrenal virilism has masculinizing effects on adult women. The clinical signs and symptoms in a female adult include hirsutism, baldness, and acne; deepening of the voice; atrophy of the uterus; decreased breast size; clitoral hypertrophy; and increased muscularity. Prepubescent males will have signs of masculine development, deepening voice, and an increase in body hair. The imaging modality of choice to confirm the presence or absence of an adrenal tumor is computerized tomography (CT) and magnetic resonance imaging scan.

- *Conn syndrome (aldosteronism).* Conn syndrome occurs in 0.5% of patients with sustained hypertension and is caused by excessive secretion of aldosterone, usually because of a cortical **adenoma** of the glomerulosa cells or less frequent causes, including adrenal hyperplasia or adrenal carcinoma. Hyperplasia is more common in males, and adrenal

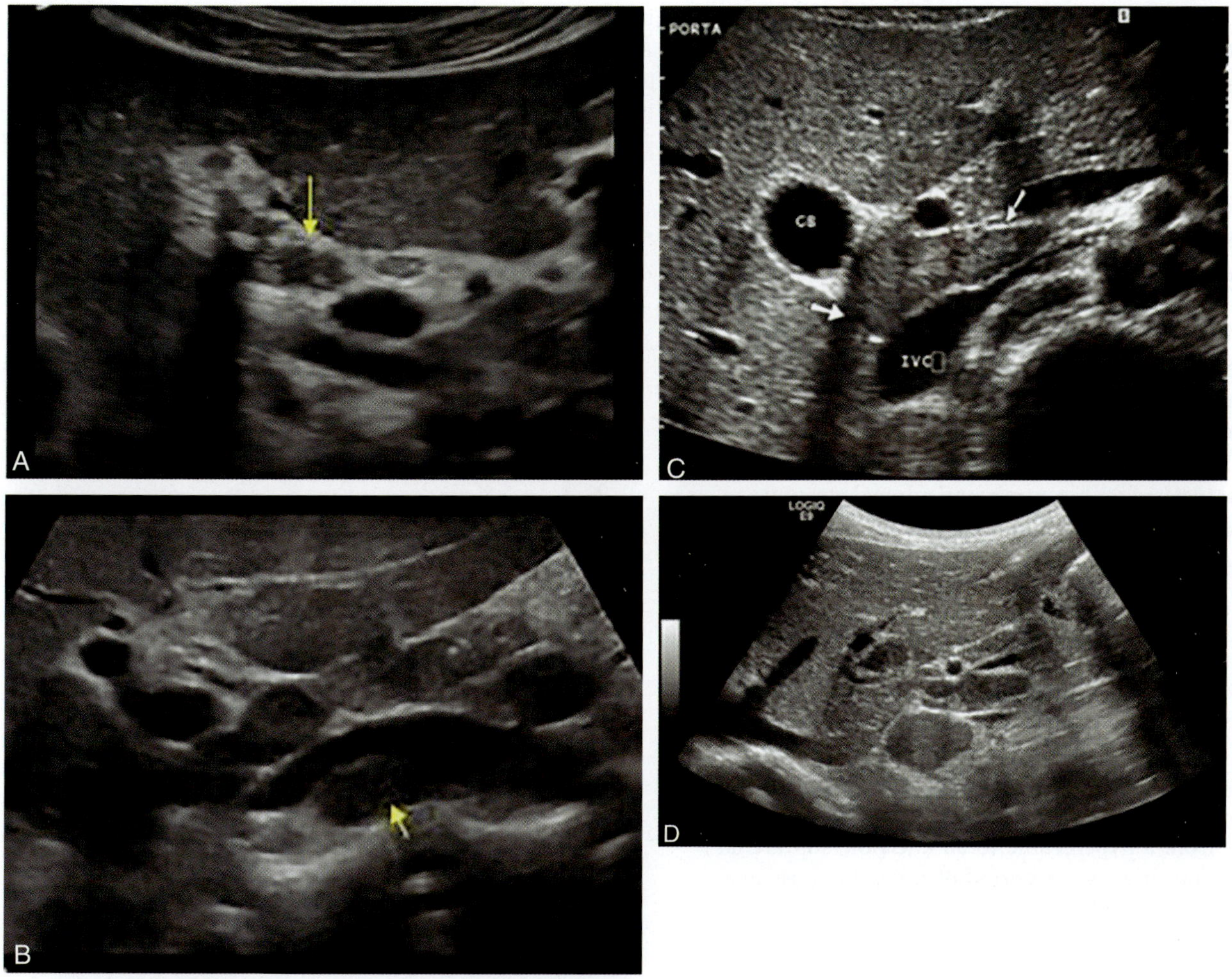

CHAPTER 16 The Retroperitoneum

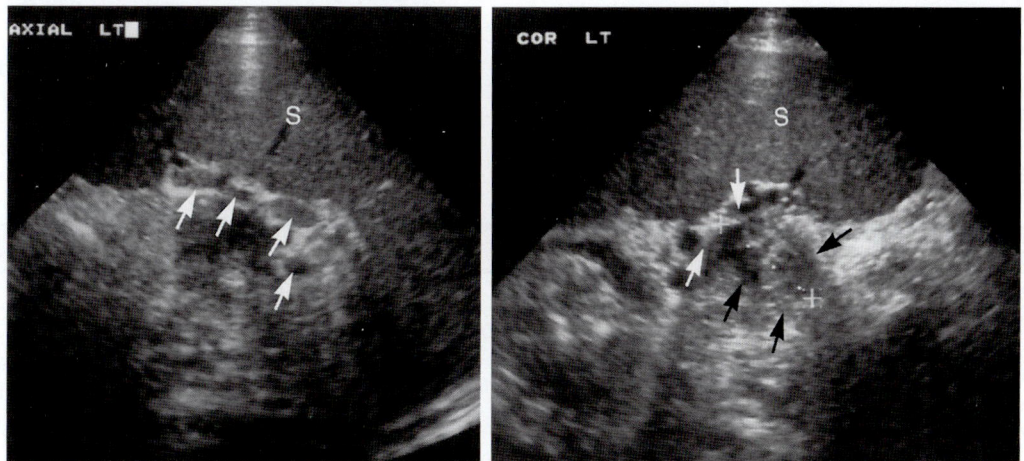

FIG. 16.17 Longitudinal (A) and transverse (B) images of the enlarged lymph nodes *(arrows)* adjacent to the aorta. The lymph nodes lie along the lateral and anterior margins of the aorta and inferior vena cava (IVC). Transverse (C) and longitudinal (D) images of the enlarged lymph nodes adjacent to the IVC. *GB*, Gallbladder.

FIG. 16.18 Axial *(left)* and coronal *(right)* scans of a patient with splenomegaly and enlarged nodes *(arrows)* in the area of the splenic hilus. Color flow imaging should be used to document that the lesions are nodes and not dilated vascular structures. *S*, Spleen.

adenomas are more common in females. Adenomas measure 0.5 to 3 cm in diameter, and contralateral adrenal atrophy is identified. Clinical signs and symptoms include muscle weakness, hypertension, and abnormal electrocardiogram.

If an adenoma is causing the hyperaldosteronism, removal of the adenoma is performed. In rare cases, a bilateral adrenalectomy is necessary. In cases of secondary aldosteronism, the hypertension may be caused by renal artery disease.

- *Cushing syndrome.* **Cushing syndrome** is caused by excessive secretion of cortisol resulting from adrenal hyperplasia, cortical adenoma, adrenal carcinoma, or elevated ACTH resulting from a pituitary adenoma. Cushing syndrome symptoms include truncal obesity, pencil-thin extremities, "buffalo hump," "moon face," hypertension, renal stones, irregular menses in females, and psychiatric disturbances. If an adrenal tumor is present, the secretion of androgens may increase and cause masculinizing effects in women. Cushing syndrome can also be caused by an anterior pituitary tumor. Treatment to decrease the production of cortisol varies depending on the cause of the hypersecretion. If an adrenalectomy is performed, the patient will require replacement steroids for life. Functioning adrenal adenomas are usually small 2 to 5 cm and hypoechoic. They typically are associated with contralateral adrenal atrophy.
- *Waterhouse-Friderichsen syndrome.* With Waterhouse-Friderichsen syndrome, there is a fulminant bacterial sepsis, shock, and necropsy with evidence of bilateral adrenal hemorrhage complicated with acute adrenocortical insufficiency in up to 25% of severely traumatized patients. Adrenal hemorrhage may occur 20% bilateral, which most often is caused by severe meningococcal infection. It is characterized by acute adrenal gland insufficiency, which is fatal if not treated immediately. With sonography, depending on the stage of hemorrhage, the echo pattern can range from a hyperechoic to an anechoic suprarenal mass. Subsequently, over a period of time, the mass may shrink, and calcifications may appear as focal hyperechoic areas with acoustic shadowing (Table 16.1).

Adrenal Cysts

Adrenal cysts are uncommon lesions that produce no clinical symptoms when the lesion is small. The cysts affect females more often than males (3:1). Adrenal cysts are usually unilateral and tend to be found incidentally. They may vary in size and can be unilocular or multilocular.

Sonographic Findings. Sonographically, adrenal cysts present a typical cystic pattern, with a strong posterior wall, no internal echoes, and good through-transmission (Fig. 16.19). Adrenal cysts have the tendency to become calcified, which gives them the sonographic appearance of a somewhat sonolucent solid mass appearing with a sharp posterior border and poor through-transmission (Fig. 16.20). Hemorrhage within

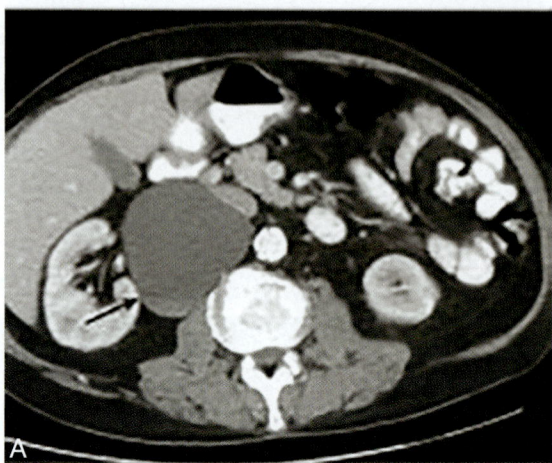
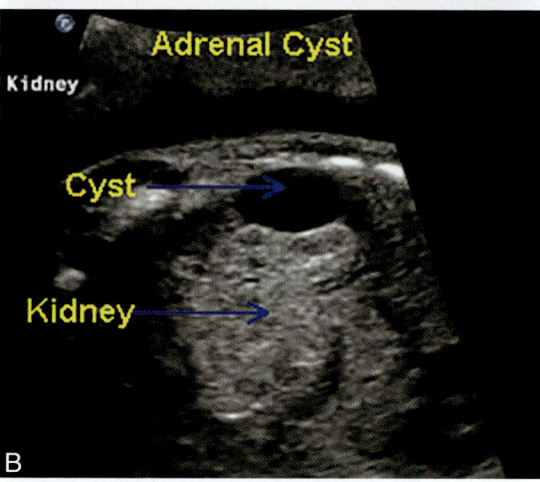

FIG. 16.19 (A) Computed tomographic contrast image of a large adrenal cyst adjacent to the right kidney with anterior displacement of the inferior vena cava. (B) Sonographically, adrenal cysts present a typical cystic pattern, with a strong posterior wall, no internal echoes, and good through-transmission.

TABLE 16.1	Adrenal Pathology	
Adrenal Diseases	**Hormone Secreted**	**Distinguishing Characteristics**
Addison disease	Hyposecretion of cortisol, aldosterone	Increases when there is stress or trauma Hypotension, general weakness, loss of appetite, bronzing of skin (hyperpigmentation), may have renal failure
Adrenogenital syndrome	Excessive secretion of androgens (male) Excessive secretion of estrogen (female)	Prepubertal males accelerate adult masculine development and growth of pubic hair Female: masculine characteristics
Conn syndrome	Excessive secretion of aldosterone	Cortical adenoma, carcinoma
Cushing syndrome	Excessive secretion of glucocorticoids	Hyperplasia, benign tumor, carcinoma
Waterhouse-Friderichsen syndrome		Bilateral hemorrhage into adrenal glands
Medulla tumor, pheochromocytoma	Excessive secretion of epinephrine and norepinephrine	Intermittent hypertension; large tumor with varied sonographic pattern (cystic, solid, calcified components)

the cyst would appear like a complex mass with multiple internal echoes and good through-transmission.

Adrenal Hemorrhage

Adrenal hemorrhage in adults is rare and is usually caused by severe trauma or infection. Posttraumatic hemorrhage is usually unilateral and does not cause any major clinical problems. A bilateral hemorrhage may cause adrenal insufficiency. Adrenal hemorrhages are more common in neonates who experience a traumatic delivery with stress, asphyxia, and septicemia. The adrenal glands in a neonate are very vascular, and the glands are proportionally larger than in an adult. Clinical signs and symptoms include abdominal mass, anemia, and hyperbilirubinemia.

Sonographic Findings. The sonographic appearance of an adrenal hemorrhage will vary depending on the age of the hemorrhage. The adrenal gland will appear as a solid mass initially, and over time the mass will have a more cystic or complex appearance. As the hemorrhage resolves, the mass will decrease in size. The adrenal gland may go back to a normal size with focal areas of calcification (Fig. 16.21).

Adrenal Tumors

Sonography can detect 90% of known adrenal masses that were first detected by CT. Sonography is used to characterize a known adrenal mass as cystic or solid, evaluate the position and patency of the IVC and draining veins, evaluate tumor invasion into adjacent structures, and determine the origin of a large retroperitoneal mass. Sonography is also used to follow an adrenal mass that is not surgically removed.

Adrenal Adenoma. Benign nonfunctioning adenoma is the most common primary adrenal tumor. Adrenal nodules are usually less than 2.5 cm. There is a high incidence of adrenal adenomas in older patients with diabetes or hypertension. A significant percentage of the malignant adrenal adenomas may be due to metastases.

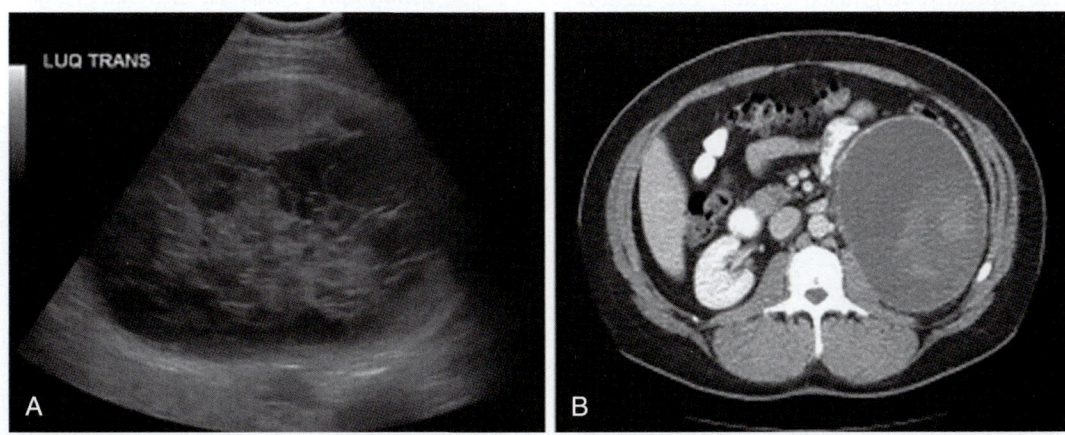

FIG. 16.20 Ultrasound (A) and computed tomography (B) images of a calcified adrenal cyst. Adrenal cysts have the tendency to become calcified, which gives them the sonographic appearance of a somewhat sonolucent solid mass appearing with a sharp posterior border and poor through-transmission.

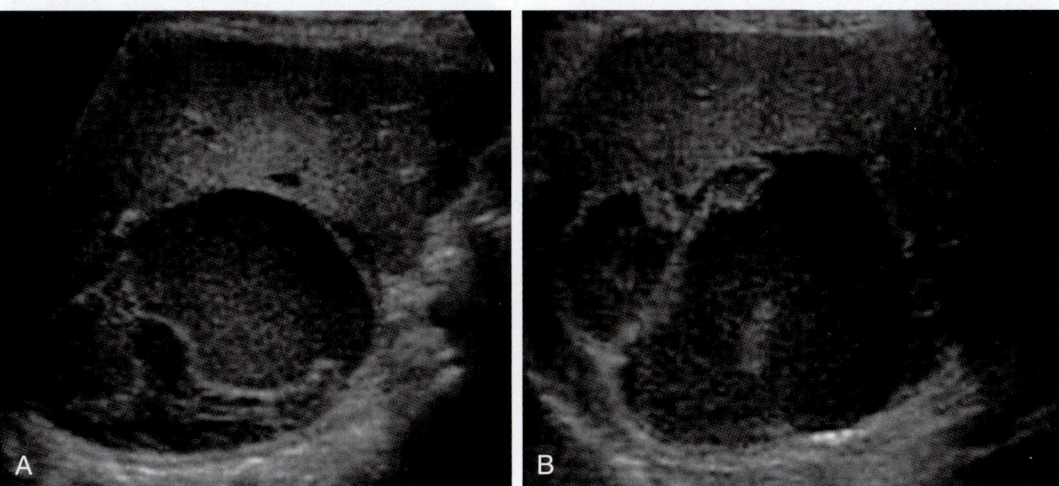

FIG. 16.21 The sonographic appearance of an adrenal hemorrhage will vary depending on the age of the hemorrhage. The adrenal gland will appear as a solid mass initially, and over time the mass will have a more cystic or complex appearance.

Sonographic Findings. In nonfunctioning adenomas, sonographic findings demonstrate a well-defined, round, slightly hypoechoic homogeneous mass (Fig. 16.22). Almost always, the mass is detected as an incidental finding. On rare occasions, the mass may be so large that it may compress the adjacent structures.

Further pathology of the adrenal glands is related to the tumors arising within them and their hyposecretion or hypersecretion of hormones. Rare nonfunctional adrenal tumors include myelolipomas, hemangiomas, teratomas, lipomas, and fibromas. These tumors are typically not seen on a sonogram and are more frequently imaged with CT or magnetic resonance imaging.

Adrenal Malignant Tumors. Primary adrenal carcinomas are rare and may be hyperfunctional or nonfunctional. Hyperfunctional malignant tumors are more common in females. Adrenal malignant tumors may cause Cushing syndrome, Conn syndrome, or adrenogenital syndrome. The origin of the tumor should be clearly defined. Functional tumors tend to be smaller than nonfunctional tumors because they are typically diagnosed earlier. The tumors are homogeneous with the same echogenicity as the renal cortex. The larger neoplasms tend to be nonfunctional and heterogeneous, with a central area of necrosis and hemorrhage.

Sonographic Findings. If the mass is small (2 to 6 cm), it is well defined and homogeneous. If the mass is larger, it tends to have necrosis with central hemorrhage and often calcifies. In color Doppler, the tumor is hypervascular with a high incidence of invasion of the adrenal or renal vein, IVC, hepatic veins, and lymph nodes (Fig. 16.23). The sonographic appearance of a mass cannot be used to differentiate between a benign or malignant tumor, as this is a histologic diagnosis.

Metastasis. Adrenals glands are the fourth most common site in the body for metastasis, after the lung, liver, and the bones. Primarily there are metastases from lung in 33%, breast carcinomas in 30%, followed by melanoma, gastric carcinoma, colon, kidney, and thyroid. Bilateral involvement is seen in more than half of the patients. Metastases to the adrenal gland typically cause adrenal insufficiency.

Sonographic Findings. Adrenal glands vary in size and echogenicity. Metastatic lesions have a nonspecific appearance.

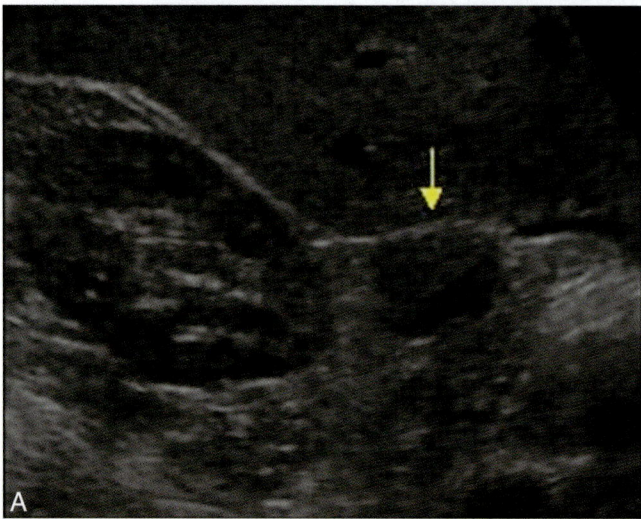
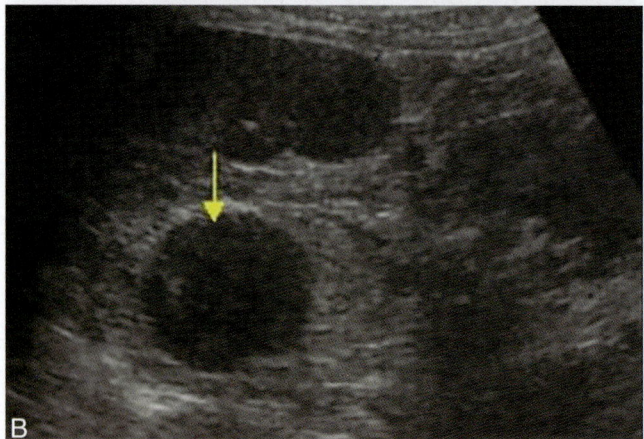

FIG. 16.22 In nonfunctioning adenomas, sonographic findings demonstrate a well-defined, round, slightly hypoechoic homogeneous mass.

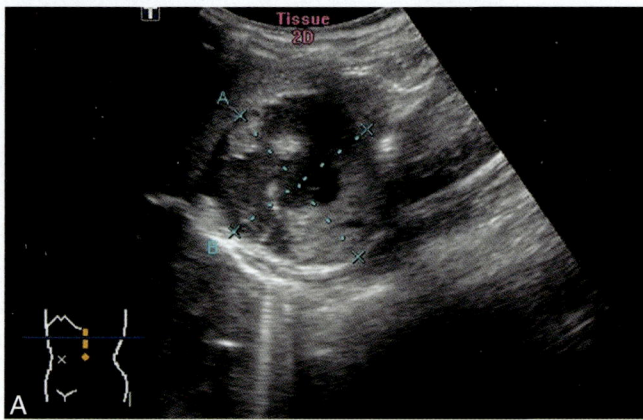
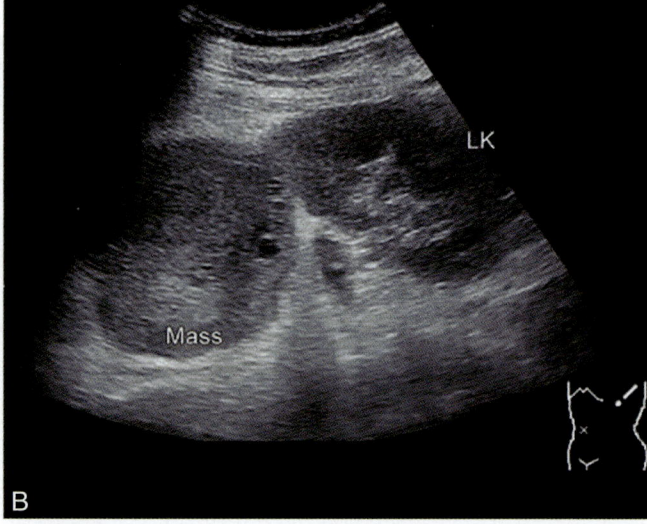

FIG. 16.23 If the mass is small (2 to 6 cm), it is well defined and homogeneous. If the mass is larger, it tends to have necrosis with central hemorrhage and often calcifies.

Large masses may contain areas of necrosis and hemorrhage. Sometimes differentiation of a common benign adenoma from a metastatic lesion is difficult when there is no other evidence of metastatic disease, and the adrenal mass is unilateral (Fig. 16.24). Often central necrosis causes sonolucent areas within the tumor.

Adrenal Medulla Tumors

Pheochromocytoma. The pheochromocytes of the adrenal medulla may produce a tumor called a **pheochromocytoma**, which secretes epinephrine and norepinephrine in excessive quantities. A small percentage of patients will have ectopic adrenal pheochromocytomas rising from the **neuroectodermal tissue**; these tumors tend to be malignant. The clinical symptoms include intermittent hypertension, severe headaches, heart palpitations, and excess perspiration. Treatment usually is removal of the tumor.

▸ **Sonographic Findings.** The tumor has a homogeneous pattern that can be differentiated from a cyst by its weak posterior wall and poor through-transmission (Fig. 16.25). Pheochromocytomas are usually unilateral and may be large, bulky tumors with various sonographic patterns, including cystic, solid, and calcified components.

Adrenal Neuroblastoma. The adrenal **neuroblastoma** is the most common malignancy of the adrenal glands in childhood and the most common tumor of infancy, representing 30% of all neonatal tumors. Neuroblastoma is a well-encapsulated tumor that usually displaces the kidney inferiorly and laterally and elevates levels of the vanillylmandelic acid (VMA) and homovanillic acid (HVA). More than 90% of fetal neuroblastomas are located in the adrenal glands, and 50% of these have cystic components. Generally, the tumor develops within the adrenal medulla. Although children are usually asymptomatic, some do present with a palpable abdominal mass that must be differentiated from a neonatal hemorrhage and hydronephrosis. It is known to be one of the most common tumors of childhood. Spontaneous regression is common before the age of one. Otherwise, it has a poor prognosis and is not responsive to either irradiation or chemotherapy.

▸ **Sonographic Findings.** Lesions generally are heterogeneously echogenic with poorly defined margins. A small

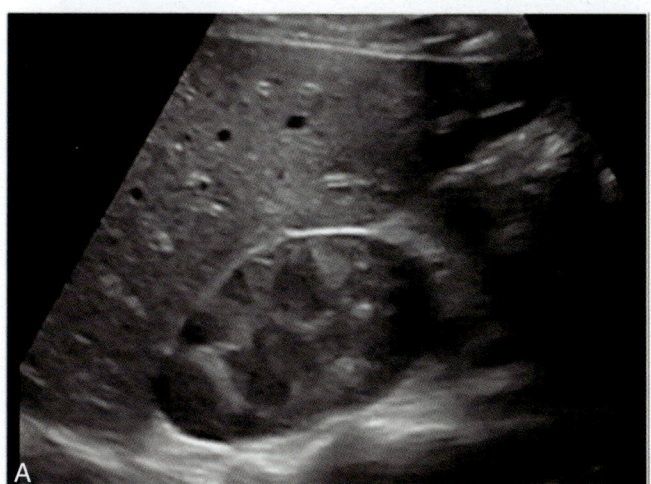
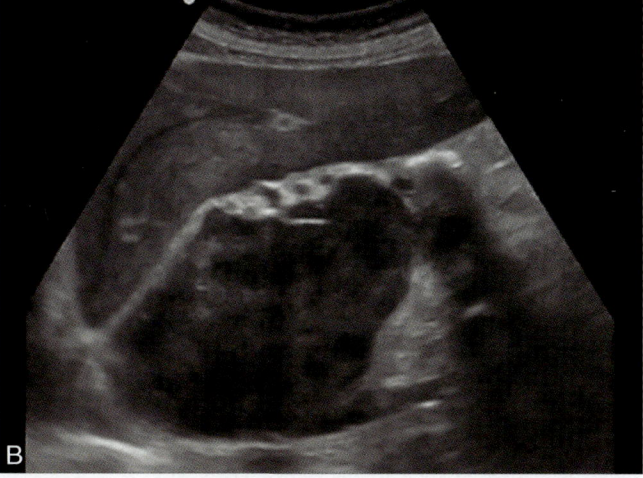

FIG. 16.24 Adrenal metastatic lesions have a nonspecific appearance. Large masses may contain areas of necrosis and hemorrhage.

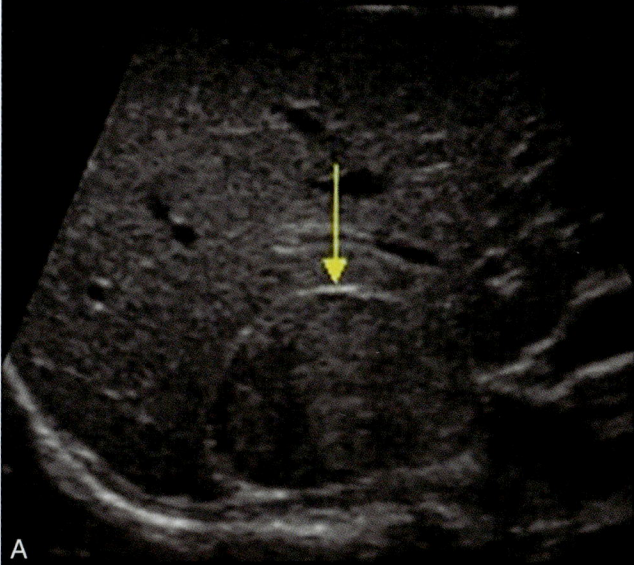
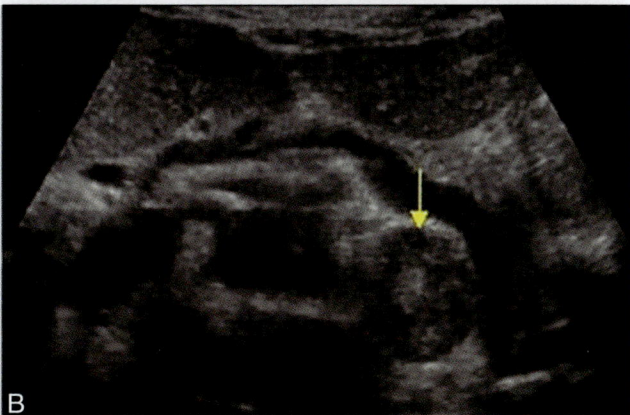

FIG. 16.25 Pheochromocytomas are usually unilateral and may be large, bulky tumors with various sonographic patterns, including cystic, solid, and calcified components.

percentage of neuroblastomas demonstrate internal calcifications with anechoic "cystic" areas. The "ultrasound lobule" (an area of increased echogenicity in the tumor) seems to be characteristic of neuroblastomas (Fig. 16.26). The use of color Doppler may be helpful in demonstrating capsular flow and low-resistance arterial waveforms. Evaluation of the surrounding retroperitoneum and liver should be made to rule out metastases. When a large, solid, upper abdominal mass is identified in an infant or young child, the differential diagnosis should include neuroblastoma, Wilms' tumor (nephroblastoma), and hepatoblastoma.

Retroperitoneal Fat

The anatomic origin of the right upper quadrant mass may be difficult to determine. The reflection produced by the retroperitoneal fat is displaced in a characteristic manner by masses originating from this area. This pattern of displacement helps to localize the origin of the mass. Retroperitoneal lesions cause ventral and often cranial displacement of the lesion.

Sonographic Findings. The lesions in the liver or in Morison pouch displace the echoes posterior and inferior, whereas renal and adrenal lesions cause anterior displacement of structures. An extrahepatic mass may shift the inferior vena cava anteromedially (anterior displacement of right kidney).

Primary Retroperitoneal Tumors

A primary retroperitoneal tumor (PRT) is one that originates independently within the retroperitoneal space. Primary malignancies are more common than benign neoplasms, but both are rare.

Lymphoma is the most common PRT. Sonographic evaluation for abdominal lymphoma is performed to determine the presence or absence of lymphadenopathy, and the primary areas to be evaluated include the hepatic and splenic hilum, origin of celiac, and superior mesenteric artery (peripancreatic, mesenteric), para-aortic, and renal hilar areas. Accuracy of sonographic detection is close to 90% when the lymph nodes are

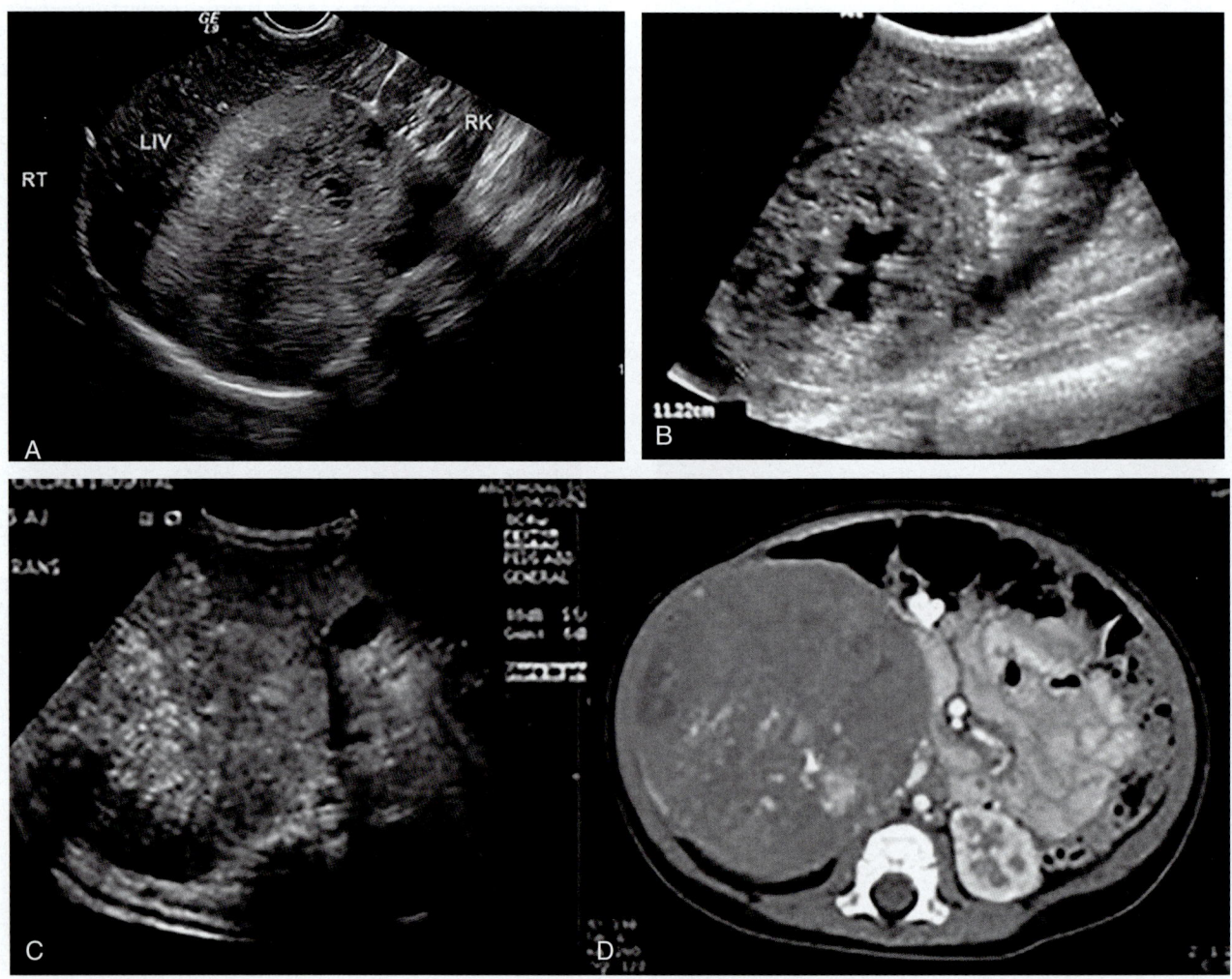

FIG. 16.26 A small percentage of neuroblastomas demonstrate internal calcifications with anechoic "cystic" areas. (A-C) The "ultrasound lobule" (an area of increased echogenicity in the tumor) seems to be characteristic of neuroblastomas. (D) Computed tomographic image of a large neuroblastoma.

larger than 2 cm in diameter. The sonographic appearance varies from round, hypoechoic masses to anechoic masses with good posterior enhancement (Fig. 16.27).

Color Doppler shows increased intranodal vascularity. The primary criteria for differentiating a malignant from a benign lymph node are size greater than 2 cm; shape, round; and resistive index greater than 0.70. The other PRT can develop anywhere, with most tumors proving to be malignant. The tumor is derived either from mesenchymal or neurogenic tissues. Mesenchymal tumors develop within connective tissues of the retroperitoneum, and most fat-containing tumors are liposarcomas, which is the third most common malignant tumor of soft tissues. More than one third of the tumors originate from perirenal fat, including malignant fibrous histiocytomas, fibrosarcomas, and desmoid tumors. All of these tumors are nonspecific by sonography.

Neurogenic tumors are usually encountered in the paravertebral region, where they rise from nerve roots or sympathetic chain ganglia. They extend into the retroperitoneum and may be classified as benign or malignant tumors. The sonographic patterns of neurogenic tumors are quite variable.

Tumors of Muscle Origin. Leiomyosarcoma is the second most common PRT. This tumor may originate from smooth muscles of small blood vessels or within gastrointestinal tract and extend into the retroperitoneum (Fig. 16.28). On sonography, leiomyosarcomas generally present as a large complex mass with areas of necrosis and cystic degeneration.

Fibrosarcomas and rhabdomyosarcomas may be quite invasive and may infiltrate widely into muscles and adjoining soft tissue. They often extend across the midline and appear similar to lymphomas. Sonographically, they are highly reflective tumors.

Germ Cell Tumors. Germ cell tumors can be either benign or malignant, and the retroperitoneal space is the fourth most frequent site (ovaries, testes, anterior mediastinum,

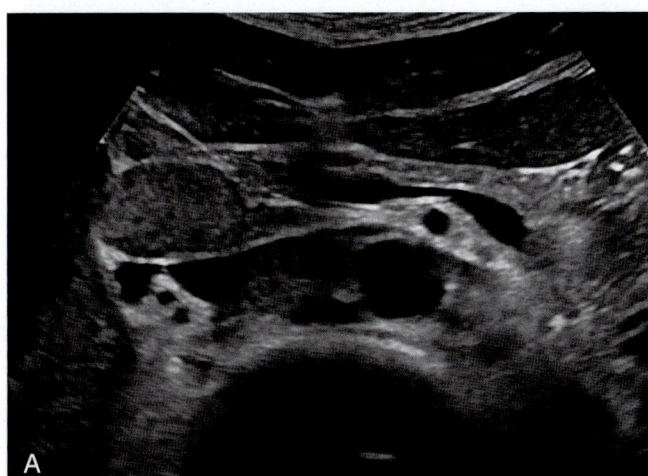

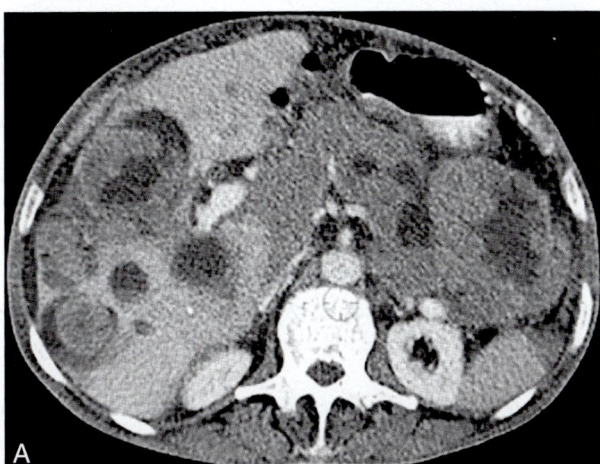

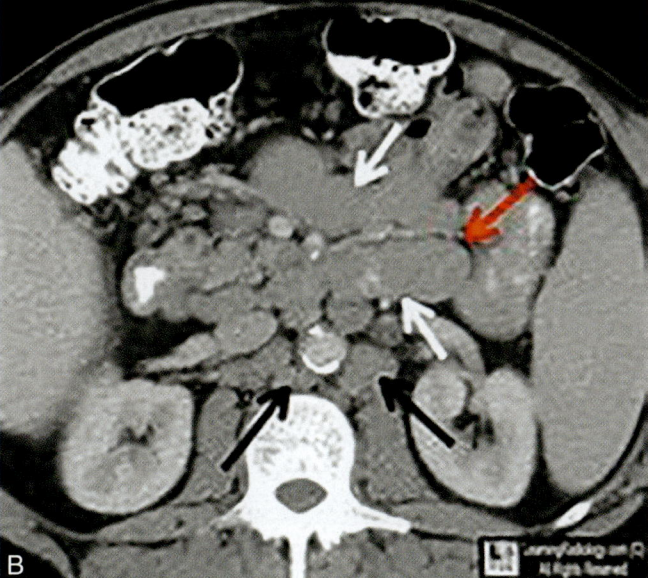

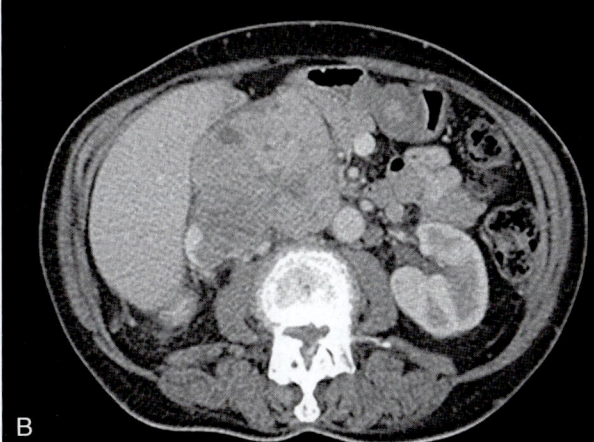

FIG. 16.27 Sonographic evaluation for abdominal lymphoma is performed to determine the presence or absence of lymphadenopathy, and the primary areas to be evaluated include the hepatic and splenic hilum, origin of celiac, and superior mesenteric artery (peripancreatic, mesenteric), para-aortic, and renal hilar areas. The sonographic appearance varies from round, hypoechoic masses to anechoic masses with good posterior enhancement. (A) Transverse sonographic image of lymphoma. (B) Computed tomographic image of multiple enlarged lymph nodes.

FIG. 16.28 Leiomyosarcoma may originate from smooth muscles of small blood vessels or within gastrointestinal-tract and extend into the retroperitoneum, as shown on these computed tomographic images.

retroperitoneum, and sacrococcygeal region). Teratomatous tumors may arise within the upper retroperitoneum and the pelvis. They may contain calcified echoes from bones, cartilage, teeth, and soft tissue elements.

Teratomas are seen more commonly in childhood and are usually located in the upper pole of the left kidney. Sonographically they are heterogeneous tumors with solid areas, calcifications, and cystic spaces.

Secondary Retroperitoneal Tumors

Metastatic disease may occur anywhere in the retroperitoneum, secondary to hematogenous, or lymphatic spread, or by direct extension. The most common primary malignancies that spread into the retroperitoneum are from the breast, lung, testis, or the recurrence of previously resected urologic or gynecologic tumor.

Ascitic fluid, along with a retroperitoneal tumor, usually indicates seeding or invasion of the peritoneal surface. Evaluation of the para-aortic region should be made for extension to the lymph nodes. The liver should also be evaluated for metastatic involvement.

Retroperitoneal Fluid Collections

Urinoma. A urinoma is a walled-off collection of extravasated urine that develops spontaneously after trauma, surgery, or a subacute or chronic urinary obstruction. Urinomas usually collect around the kidney or upper ureter in the perinephric space. Occasionally urinomas dissect into the pelvis and compress the bladder.

▶ **Sonographic Findings.** Generally, the sonographic pattern of urinomas is sonolucent unless they become infected.

Hemorrhage. A retroperitoneal hemorrhage may occur in a variety of conditions, including trauma, vasculitis, bleeding diathesis, a leaking aortic aneurysm, or a bleeding neoplasm.

▶ **Sonographic Findings.** Sonographically the hemorrhage may be well localized and produce displacement of other organs, or it may present as a poorly defined infiltrative process. Fresh hematomas present as sonolucent areas, whereas an organized thrombus with clot formation shows echo densities within the mass (Fig. 16.29). Calcification may be seen in long-standing hematomas.

Abscess. Abscess formation may result from surgery, trauma, or perforation of the bowel or duodenum.

▶ **Sonographic Findings.** Sonographically the abscess usually has a complex pattern with debris (Fig. 16.30). Gas within the abscess causes a "reflective" pattern on sonography and casts an acoustic shadow. The sonographer should be careful not to mistake a gas-containing abscess for "bowel" patterns. The radiograph should be evaluated in this case. The abscess frequently extends along or within the muscle planes, is of an irregular shape, and lies in the most dependent portion of the retroperitoneal space.

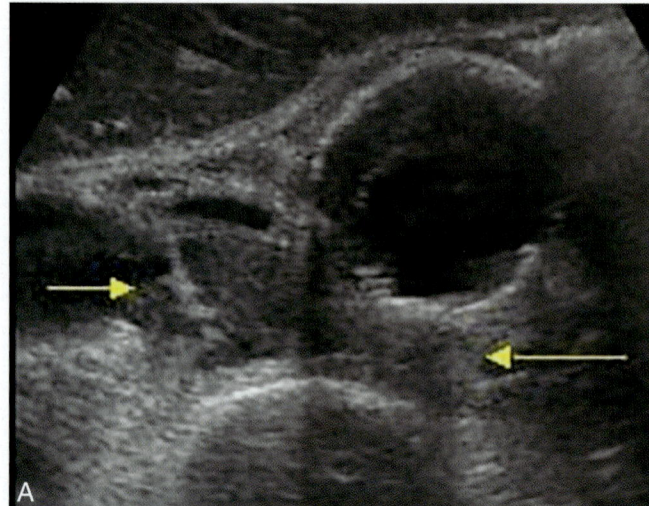
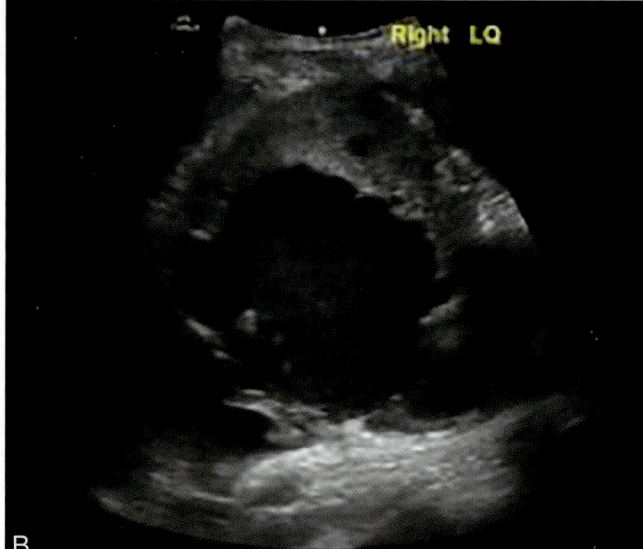
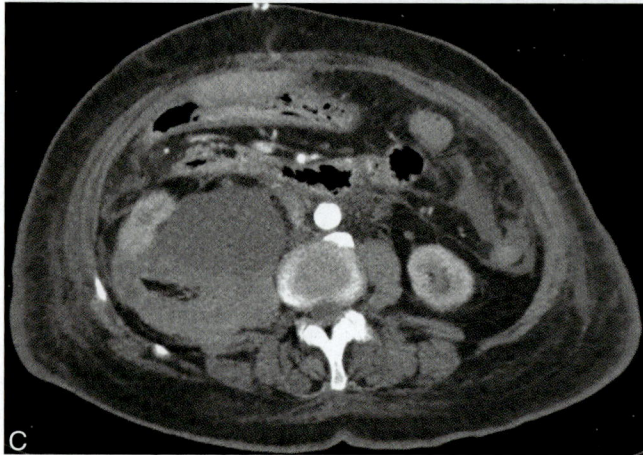

FIG. 16.29 Sonographically the hemorrhage may be well localized and produce displacement of other organs such as the inferior vena cava (A), or it may present as a poorly defined infiltrative process. Fresh hematomas present as sonolucent areas (B), whereas an organized thrombus with clot formation shows echo densities within the mass. (C) Computed tomographic image of a retroperitoneal hematoma displacing the right kidney anterior and lateral, secondary to a sports injury.

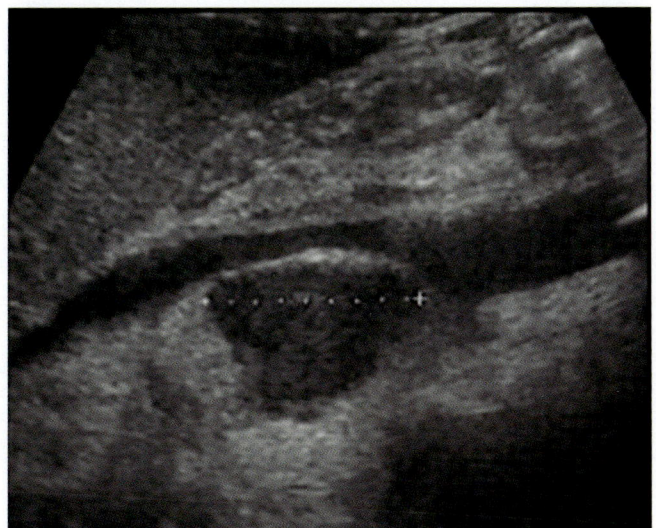

FIG. 16.30 Sonographically the abscess usually has a complex pattern with debris.

Retroperitoneal Fibrosis (Ormond Disease)

Retroperitoneal fibrosis (RPF) is an idiopathic condition characterized by thick sheets of fibrous tissue in the retroperitoneal cavity. The fibrosis may encase and obstruct the ureters and vena cava, with resultant hydronephrosis. RPF can also be associated with infiltrating neoplasms, acute immune diseases (Crohn disease), ulcerative colitis, sclerosing cholangitis, and so on. Clinically the patient may present with abdominal pain, hypertension, and oligo-anuria. Radiographically, an intravenous pyelogram shows medial displacement and bilateral (one-third are unilateral) hydronephrosis. Sonography may demonstrate abnormal hypoechoic tissue surrounding the anterolateral aspect of the aorta or IVC (Fig. 16.31). Sonography may also be useful to evaluate the kidneys, as well as fibrosis regression in response to steroids. Further imaging with CT may be necessary to establish whether there is a benign or malignant disease process.

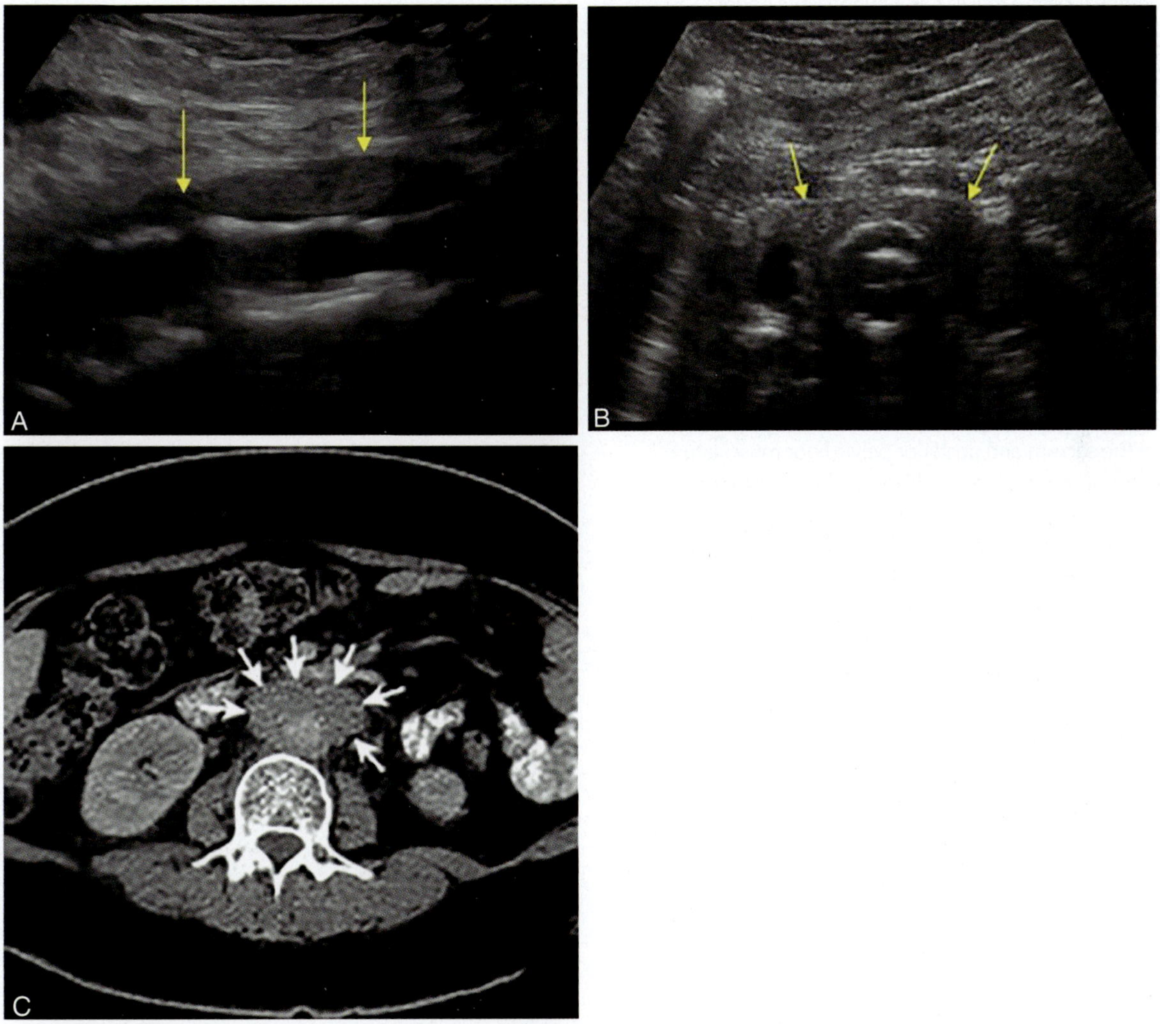

FIG. 16.31 (A–B) Sonography may demonstrate abnormal hypoechoic tissue surrounding the anterolateral aspect of the aorta or inferior vena cava. (C) Computed tomographic image of the retroperitoneal fibrosis surrounding the aorta *(arrows)*.

Key Pearls

- The retroperitoneal space is the area between the posterior portion of the parietal peritoneum and the posterior abdominal wall muscles. It extends from the diaphragm to the pelvis.
- Laterally, the boundaries extend to the extraperitoneal fat planes within the confines of the transversalis fascia, and medially the space encloses the great vessels.
- It is subdivided into the following three categories: anterior pararenal space, perirenal space, and posterior pararenal space.
- The perirenal space surrounds the kidney, adrenal, and perirenal fat.
- The anterior pararenal space includes the duodenum, pancreas, and ascending and transverse colon.
- The posterior pararenal space includes the iliopsoas muscle, ureter, and branches of the inferior vena cava and aorta and their lymphatics.
- The right adrenal is more superior to the kidney, whereas the left adrenal is more medial to the kidney.
- There are two major lymph-node-bearing areas in the retroperitoneal cavity: the iliac and hypogastric nodes within the pelvis and the para-aortic group in the upper retroperitoneum.
- The retrofascial space is made up of the posterior abdominal wall, muscles, nerves, lymphatics, and areolar tissue behind the transversalis fascia.
- The pelvic retroperitoneum lies between the sacrum and pubis from back to front, between the pelvic peritoneal reflection above and pelvic diaphragm (coccygeus and levator ani muscles) below, and between the obturator internus and piriformis muscles.
- The prevesical space spans from the pubis to the anterior margin of the bladder. It is bordered laterally by the obturator fascia.
- The presacral space lies between the rectum and fascia, covering the sacrum and posterior pelvic floor musculature.
- The pararectal space is bounded laterally by the piriformis and levator ani fascia and medially by the rectum. It extends anteriorly from the bladder, medially to the obturator internus, and laterally to the external iliac vessels.
- Sonography patterns associated with nodes include rounded, focal, echo-poor lesions (1–3 cm in size and larger) and confluent, echo-poor masses, which often displace the kidney laterally.
- The sonographer may also detect a "mantle" of nodes in the paraspinal location, a "floating" or anteriorly displaced aorta secondary to the enlarged nodes, or the mesenteric "sandwich" sign representing the anterior and posterior node masses surrounding mesenteric vessels.
- Adrenal hemorrhages are more common in neonates who experienced a traumatic delivery with stress, asphyxia, and septicemia.
- Benign nonfunctioning adenoma is the most common primary adrenal tumor.
- Adrenal glands are the fourth most common site in the body for metastasis, after the lung, liver, and the bones.
- The pheochromocytes of the adrenal medulla may produce a tumor called a pheochromocytoma, which secretes epinephrine and norepinephrine in excessive quantities.
- The adrenal neuroblastoma is the most common malignancy of the adrenal glands in childhood and the most common tumor of infancy, representing 30% of all neonatal tumors.
- Lymphoma is the most common primary retroperitoneal tumor.
- Metastatic disease may occur anywhere in the retroperitoneum, secondary to hematogenous, or lymphatic spread, or by direct extension.
- A urinoma is a walled-off collection of extravasated urine that develops spontaneously after trauma, surgery, or a subacute or chronic urinary obstruction.
- A retroperitoneal hemorrhage may occur in a variety of conditions, including trauma, vasculitis, bleeding diathesis, a leaking aortic aneurysm, or a bleeding neoplasm.
- Retroperitoneal fibrosis is an idiopathic condition characterized by thick sheets of fibrous tissue in the retroperitoneal cavity.

BIBLIOGRAPHY

Bertino RE, Saucier NA, Barth DJ. The retroperitoneum. ed 4. In: Rumack CM, Wilson SR, Charboneau JW, eds. *Diagnostic Ultrasound*. vol 1 St Louis: Elsevier; 2011:447–485.

Choyke PL, Glenn G, Walther M. Von Hippel-Lindau disease: genetic, clinical and imaging features. *Radiology*. 1996;194:629.

Dalrymple NC, John R, Leyendecker JR, Oliphant M. *imagingProblem Solving in Abdominal Imaging*. St Louis: Elsevier; 2009:464–566.

Fried AM. Spleen and retroperitoneum: the essentials. *Ultrasound Q*. 2005;21:275–286.

Heinz-Peer G, Memarsadeght M, Niederle B. Imaging of adrenal masses. *Curr Opin Urol*. 2007;17:32–38.

Ishikawa K, Idoguchi K, Tanaka H, et al. Classification of acute pancreatitis based on retroperitoneal extension: application of the concept of interfascial planes. *Eur J Radiol*. 2006;60:445–452.

Lee SL, Ku YM, Rha SE. Comprehensive reviews of the interfascial plane of the retroperitoneum: normal anatomy and pathologic entities. *Emerg Radiol*. 2010;17:3–11.

Little AF. Adrenal gland and renal sonography. *World J Surg*. 2000;24:171.

Moussavian B, Horrow NM. Retroperitoneal fibrosis. *Ultrasound Q*. 2009;25:89–91.

Rosenblatt GS, Takesita K, Fuch G, et al. Adrenal metastasis with inferior vena cava tumor thrombus through adrenal vein. *Clin Urol*. 2009;74:290–291.

CHAPTER 17

Abdominal Applications of Ultrasound Contrast Agents

Daniel A. Merton and John R. Eisenbrey

OBJECTIVES

On completion of this chapter, you should be able to:
- List the current limitations of ultrasound imaging that may be overcome by the use of ultrasound contrast agents
- Describe the properties that an ultrasound contrast agent must have to be clinically accepted
- Describe the difference between tissue-specific ultrasound contrast agents and vascular agents
- Describe how nonlinear contrast imaging modes improve the clinical capabilities of ultrasound contrast agents
- Describe the current clinical applications of contrast agents

OUTLINE

Types of Ultrasound Contrast Agents 511
    Vascular Ultrasound Contrast Agents 511
    Tissue-Specific Ultrasound Contrast Agents 514

Ultrasound Imaging Modes 515
Clinical Applications 517
    Hepatic Applications 517
    Renal Applications 521
    Splenic Applications 522
    Pancreatic Applications 523

Organ Transplants 523
Other Applications 524
Conclusion 524

KEY TERMS

Acoustic emission (AE)
Contrast-enhanced ultrasound imaging (CEUS)
Harmonic imaging (HI)
Liver Imaging Reporting and Data Systems (LI-RADS)
Mechanical index (MI)
Molecular imaging agents
Tissue-specific ultrasound contrast agent
Ultrasound contrast agents (UCAs)

Since the 1980s, a significant amount of research has been conducted toward the development of **ultrasound contrast agents (UCAs)**.[1] Most of the work has centered on developing agents that can be administered intravenously to evaluate blood vessels, blood flow, tumors, and solid organs.

The clinical utilization of **contrast-enhanced ultrasound imaging (CEUS)** has been shown to reduce or eliminate some of the current limitations of ultrasound imaging and Doppler blood flow detection. These include limitations of spatial and contrast resolution on B-mode ultrasound and the detection of low-velocity blood flow and flow in smaller vessels using Doppler flow detection modes, including color flow imaging and pulsed wave Doppler with spectral analysis. Advances in ultrasound technology following the development of UCAs have resulted in contrast-specific imaging modes, which allow detection, display, and quantification of blood flow without the limitations of Doppler. The use of CEUS is growing around the world, and published clinical guidelines describe the most appropriate use of CEUS for a variety of abdominal, retroperitoneal, and other applications.[2-4] Ultrasound contrast agents (UCA) are increasingly being used to improve the sensitivity and specificity of ultrasound diagnoses and are expanding sonography's already broad range of clinical applications.[5]

TYPES OF ULTRASOUND CONTRAST AGENTS

Vascular Ultrasound Contrast Agents

Sonographic detection of blood flow is limited by factors including the depth and size of a vessel, the attenuation properties of intervening tissue, or low-velocity flow. Limitations of ultrasound equipment sensitivity and the operator dependence of Doppler ultrasound are also factors that may affect the results of a vascular examination. UCA are gas microbubbles encapsulated by an outer shell for stability.[5] When injected intravenously, the agents are small enough (<8 μm) to pass through the pulmonary capillary beds but large enough to remain trapped within the vasculature. Vascular or blood-pooling UCAs can enhance Doppler (color and spectral) flow signals by adding more and better acoustic scatterers to the bloodstream (Figs. 17.1 and 17.2). The use of these UCAs improves the color flow imaging detection of blood flow from vessels that are often difficult to assess without their use, such as the renal arteries, intracranial vessels, and small capillaries within organs (i.e., tissue perfusion) (Fig. 17.3). However, contrast-specific imaging modes, which utilize the nonlinear scattering properties of UCAs, provide substantial improvements in contrast-to-tissue signal and improved detection of smaller vessels relative to contrast-enhanced Doppler.[5] These

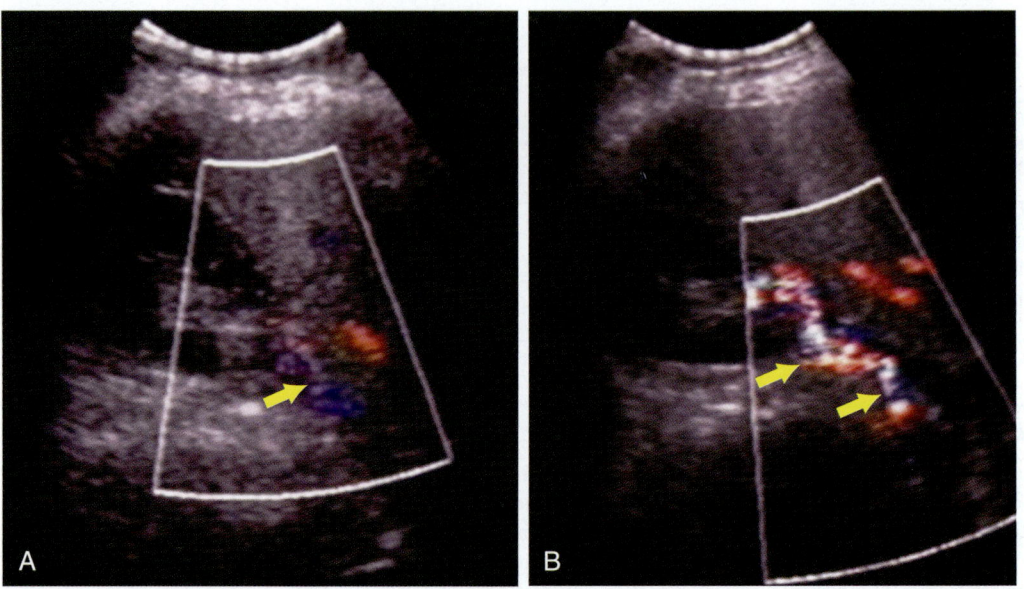

FIG. 17.1 Color Doppler imaging of a patient's right renal artery before (A) and after (B) administration of a vascular ultrasound contrast agent. Note the increased visualization of flow in the renal artery (*arrows*) after intravenous injection of contrast. In this case, no vascular abnormality was detected.

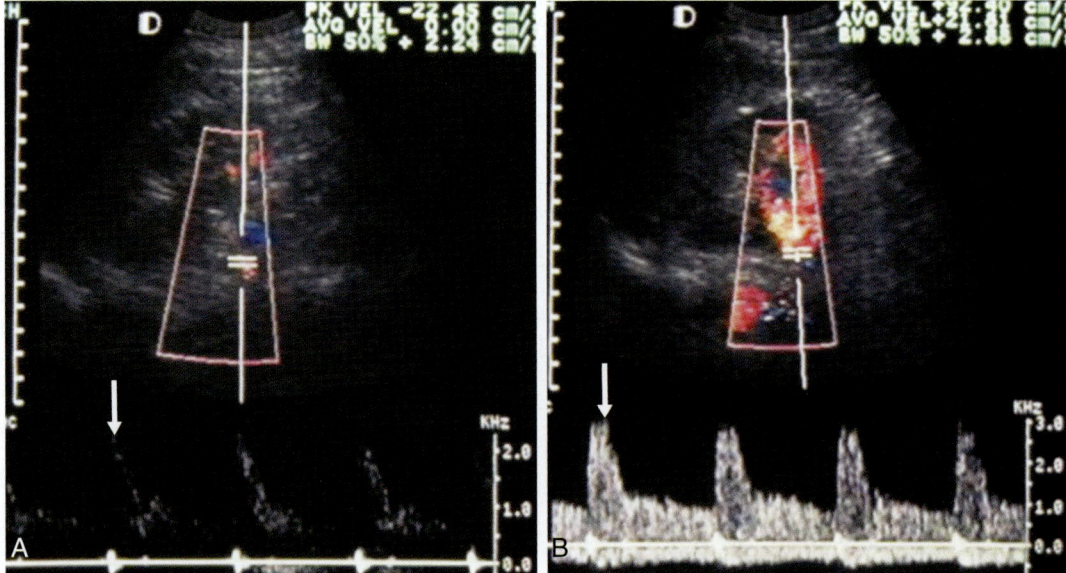

FIG. 17.2 Color flow imaging and spectral Doppler analysis of renal artery flow. (A) Before contrast, the spectral waveforms are weak, and there is minimal color flow information. (B) After intravenous administration of a contrast, the spectral wave forms have a higher signal intensity, and additional color flow information is provided.

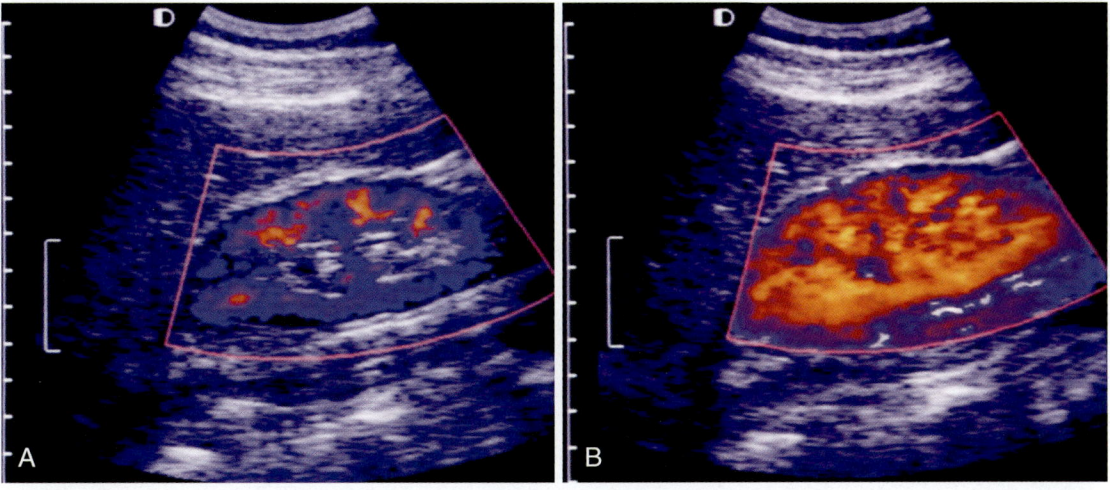

FIG. 17.3 Power Doppler imaging of a normal right kidney before (A) and after (B) injection of a vascular ultrasound contrast agent. Note the improved demonstration of flow in the renal parenchyma after intravenous injection of contrast.

modes are the preferred approach for CEUS imaging and are now available on most mid- to high-end commercial ultrasound scanners.[6]

The concept of a UCA was first introduced by Gramiak and Shah in 1968, who, in their initial work, injected agitated saline directly into the ascending aorta and cardiac chambers during echocardiographic examinations.[7] The microbubbles formed by agitation resulted in strong reflections arising from within the normally echo-free lumen of the aorta and chambers of the heart. Eventually, other solutions were discovered that could produce similar effects. However, microbubbles produced by simple agitation are nonuniform in size, relatively large, and quickly diffuse, which makes them unsuitable for sonographic evaluations of the left heart and systemic circulation because the microbubbles do not persist through passage of the pulmonary and cardiac circulations. Furthermore, to provide contrast enhancement, agitated saline required direct injection into the vessel under evaluation (e.g., the aorta), and a more clinically practicable administration method, such as intravenous (IV) injection, was desired.

For a UCA to be clinically useful, it should be nontoxic, have microbubbles or microparticles that are small enough to traverse the pulmonary capillary beds (i.e., less than 8 microns in size), and be stable enough to provide multiple recirculations.[5] Furthermore, the contrast agent should be administered via IV injection and provide enhancement of ultrasound signals. A number of agents possess these desirable traits, and presently several microbubble-based UCAs are commercially available worldwide (Tables 17.1 and 17.2). Specific UCA properties and their instructions for reconstitution and administration are provided in the product package insert.

The specific type of gas contained within a UCA microbubble and its shell composition influence the microbubble's acoustic behavior (e.g., reflectivity and elasticity), method

TABLE 17.1	Ultrasound Contrast Agents Commercially Available in the United States and Their FDA-Approved Indications
Agent	**Approved Indications**
Optison, GE Healthcare	LVO/EBD
Definity, Lantheus Medical Imaging	LVO/EBD
Lumason, Bracco International	LVO/EBD, characterization of focal hepatic tumors in adult and pediatric patients, ultrasonography of the urinary tract for the evaluation of suspected or known vesicoureteral reflux in pediatric patients

EBD, Endocardial border definition; *FDA*, US Food and Drug Administration; *LVO*, left ventricular opacification.

of metabolism, and stability within the blood.[8,9] In 1998, Optison (FSO 69; GE Healthcare) was approved by the United States Food and Drug Administration (FDA) for cardiac applications. The microbubbles of Optison are composed of a shell of 5% sonicated human serum albumen that contains a high-molecular-weight gas (perfluoropropane), which extends the stability and plasma longevity of the agent. Optison has shown potential for use with nonlinear harmonic imaging and Doppler modes for echocardiography, as well as systemic vascular, tumor characterization, and abdominal applications.[10–15]

Similarly, Definity (Lantheus Medical Imaging; marketed as Luminity in some countries) is composed of octafluoropropane microbubble encapsulated in an outer lipid shell. The agent was cleared by the US Food and Drug Administration in 2001 and is indicated for patients with

TABLE 17.2	Ultrasound Contrast Agents Commercially Available Outside the United States and Their Approved Indications	
Agent Name	**Countries**	**Approved Indications**
Definity, Lantheus Medical Imaging (marketed as Luminity in some countries)	Canada, Mexico, Israel, New Zealand, India, Australia, European Union, South Korea, Singapore, United Arab Emirates[a]	LVO/EBD, liver, kidney
Optison, GE Healthcare	European Union	LVO/EBD
Sonazoid, GE Healthcare AS	Japan, China, South Korea, and Norway	Focal liver lesions Focal breast lesions
SonoVue, Bracco International, Milan, Italy	European Union, Norway, Switzerland, China, Singapore, South Korea, Iceland, India, Canada[b]	LVO/EBD, breast, liver, portal vein, extracranial carotid, peripheral arteries (macrovascular and microvascular)

[a]Approved in these countries only for LVO/EBD.
[b]Approved in Canada for LVO/EBD and diagnostic assessment of vessels.
EBD, Endocardial border definition; *LVO*, left ventricular opacification.

suboptimal echocardiograms to opacify the left ventricular chamber and to improve the delineation of the left ventricular endocardial border. Definity is approved for numerous other applications worldwide[5] and can be used off-label for improved visualization of the vasculature in a variety of clinical applications.[16-18]

SonoVue (Bracco Diagnostics; marketed as Lumason within the United States) is an aqueous suspension of phospholipid-stabilized sulfur hexafluoride microbubbles which have a low solubility in blood.[19] SonoVue enhances the echogenicity of blood and provides opacification of the cardiac chambers resulting in improved left ventricular endocardial border definition. In clinical trials, it has been shown to increase ultrasound's accuracy in detection or exclusion of abnormalities in intracranial, extracranial carotid, and peripheral arteries. SonoVue also increases the quality of Doppler flow signals and the duration of clinically useful signal enhancement in portal vein assessments. SonoVue improves the detection of liver and breast lesion vascularity resulting in more specific lesion characterization.[5,20,21] SonoVue has been approved for use in Europe for echocardiography and macrovascular applications. In the United States, SonoVue is marketed as Lumason, and it received FDA approval for echocardiography applications in 2014.[19] Lumason has also been studied for liver lesion characterization,[22,23] and in April 2016, it became the first UCA to gain FDA approval for a radiologic application with the indication for the characterization of focal liver lesions in both adult and pediatric patients.[19] It is also FDA approved for ultrasonography of the urinary tract for the evaluation of suspected or known vesicoureteral reflux in pediatric patients.[19]

Tissue-Specific Ultrasound Contrast Agents

The kinetics of UCA microbubbles following IV injection is complex, and each agent has its own unique characteristics.[24] In general, after IV administration, blood-pool UCAs are contained exclusively in the body's vascular spaces. Once a vascular agent's microbubbles are ruptured or otherwise destroyed, the microbubble shell products are metabolized or eliminated by the body, and the gas is exhaled.[9]

Tissue-specific ultrasound contrast agents differ from vascular agents in that the microbubbles of these agents are removed from the blood pool and taken up by, or have an affinity toward, specific tissues, for example, the reticuloendothelial system (RES) in the liver and spleen, or thrombi in blood vessels.[25,26] Over time the presence of contrast microbubbles within or attached to the target tissue changes its sonographic appearance. By changing the signal impedance (or other acoustic characteristics) of normal and abnormal tissues, these agents improve the detectability of abnormalities and permit more specific sonographic diagnoses. Tissue-specific UCAs are typically administered by IV injection. Most tissue-specific UCAs also enhance the sonographic detection of blood flow and are therefore potentially multipurpose. Because tissue-specific UCAs passively target specific types of tissues and their behavior is predictable, they can be considered in the category of **molecular imaging agents**.[25,26]

Sonazoid is a tissue-specific UCA that contains microbubbles of perfluorobutane gas in a stable lipid shell.[5] Sonazoid is currently approved for use in Japan, China, Korea, Taiwan, and Norway.[5] After being injected intravenously, Sonazoid behaves as a vascular agent (i.e., enhances the detection of flowing blood) and, over time, the microbubbles are phagocytosed by the RES (macrophage Kupffer cells) of the liver and spleen. The intact microbubbles may remain stationary in the tissue for several hours. When insonated after uptake, the stationary contrast microbubbles increase the reflectivity of the contrast-containing tissue. If an appropriate level of acoustic energy is applied to the tissue, the microbubbles first oscillate (emitting harmonic signals that can be detected with gray-scale CHI) and then

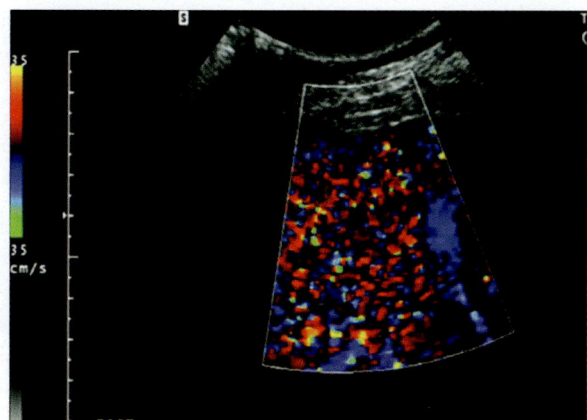

FIG. 17.4 Color Doppler imaging display of acoustic emission after intravenous injection of a tissue-specific ultrasound contrast agent. The rupture of contrast microbubbles present within the reticuloendothelial system cells of the liver results in the characteristic random color display.

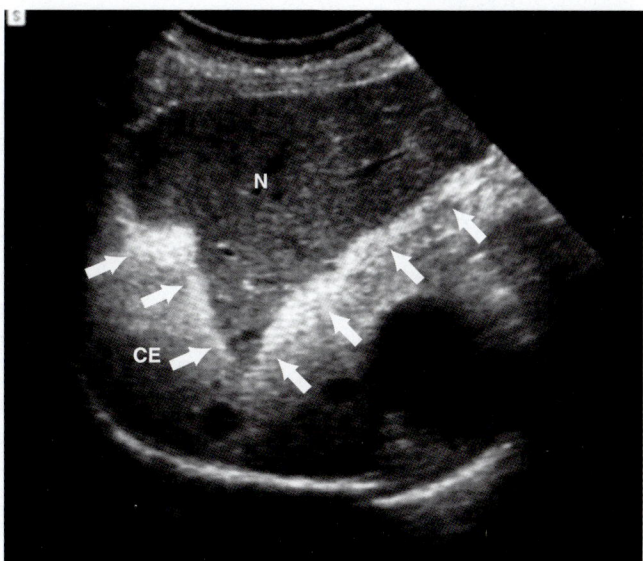

FIG. 17.5 Gray-scale contrast harmonic imaging display of the acoustic emission effect after intravenous injection of a tissue-specific ultrasound contrast agent. As the acoustic energy traverses through the liver parenchyma, it causes the contrast microbubbles to rupture, resulting in a characteristic wave of intense echoes *(arrows)*. The normal echogenicity of the liver parenchyma in the near field (N) is restored after the microbubbles have ruptured, whereas deep to the acoustic emission wave, the contrast-enhanced tissue (CE) remains echogenic because of the presence of intact microbubbles. This effect is dramatic when visualized in real time.

rupture. The rupture of the microbubbles results in random Doppler shifts appearing as a transient mosaic of colors on a color Doppler display (Fig. 17.4). This effect has been termed induced acoustic emission (IAE), stimulated acoustic emission (SAE), or simply **acoustic emission (AE)**.[27,28] By exploiting the color Doppler–depicted AE phenomenon, masses that have destroyed or replaced the normal Kupffer cells will be displayed as color-free areas and thus become more sonographically conspicuous. These same AE effects can also be demonstrated using gray-scale CHI (see the CHI discussion below) (Fig. 17.5).[28,29] Improvements in contrast-specific ultrasound imaging technologies have obviated the use of Doppler modes with UCAs for the majority of applications.[2–4,30]

ULTRASOUND IMAGING MODES

Microbubble-based UCAs enhance the detection of blood flow when used with conventional ultrasound imaging techniques, including gray-scale ultrasound and Doppler techniques (i.e., color flow imaging and pulsed wave Doppler with spectral analysis). However, research and experience have led to a better understanding of the nonlinear interactions between acoustic energy (i.e., the ultrasound beam) and UCA microbubbles, which in turn has led to contrast-specific imaging modes that greatly improve the clinical utility of CEUS and obviate the need to use conventional imaging modes with UCAs.[30] Contrast imaging features and capabilities vary by manufacturer, but all utilize proprietary technologies designed to maximize the signal intensity of echoes arising from UCA microbubbles while suppressing echoes from surrounding tissue.

Harmonic imaging (HI) uses the same broadband transducers used for conventional ultrasound, but in HI mode, the system is configured to receive only echoes at the second harmonic frequency, which is twice the transmit frequency (e.g., 7.0 MHz for a 3.5-MHz transducer).[31] When using a microbubble-based UCA, the microbubbles oscillate (i.e., they get larger and smaller) when subjected to the acoustic energy present in the ultrasound field. The reflected echoes from the oscillating microbubbles contain energy components at the fundamental frequency and at the higher and lower harmonics (i.e., subharmonics). Contrast harmonic imaging (CHI) allows detection of UCA microbubbles by imaging the nonlinear harmonics. The use of CHI for CEUS avoids many of the limitations and artifacts encountered when using Doppler techniques and UCAs, such as angle dependence and "color blooming" artifacts.[32] In CHI mode, the echoes from the oscillating microbubbles have a higher signal-to-noise ratio than would be provided by using conventional ultrasound so that regions with microbubbles (e.g., blood vessels and organ parenchyma) are more easily appreciated visually. Advanced CHI technology (e.g., coded-pulse HI, wideband HI, phase-inversion HI, and pulse-inversion HI) employ either image processing algorithms to subtract echoes arising from body tissues while echoes arising from contrast microbubbles are preferentially displayed or nonlinear pulses to maximize the generation of harmonic signal.[33] Thus, CHI provides a way to better differentiate areas with and without contrast and has the potential to demonstrate real-time grayscale blood-pool imaging (i.e., perfusion imaging). Similarly, techniques using a combination of phase and amplitude pulse modulation, such as cadence contrast pulse sequencing (CPS), are commercially available to maximize nonlinear signals while reducing linear tissue signal. The benefits of using nonlinear imaging techniques for CEUS (e.g., higher frame rates, improved contrast resolution, reduced artifacts) are so great that conventional color flow imaging is neither necessary nor advised.

When using microbubble-based UCAs, the energy present within the acoustic field can have a detrimental effect on the contrast microbubbles.[8] A significant number of the microbubbles can be destroyed by the acoustic pressure even though the actual pressure contained within the ultrasound field is relatively low. Once the microbubble is destroyed, contrast enhancement is no longer provided, which reduces the clinical utility and duration of contrast enhancement. Several approaches have been used to minimize this problem. One relatively easy technique is to use a low acoustic output power as defined by the **mechanical index (MI)**.[34] However, reducing the MI also limits tissue penetration, so this is not always an adequate solution. Furthermore, the MI may be an imprecise predictor of the effect of acoustic energy on contrast microbubbles.[35] Current scanners that have CEUS packages provide exam presets that use low (<0.2) MI values to avoid microbubble destruction during continuous imaging.

Some equipment manufacturers have incorporated *intermittent imaging* (also referred to as *interval delay imaging*) capabilities on their systems to provide an additional option to the user seeking to reduce microbubble destruction during CEUS examinations.[36,37] In this mode, the system is gated to only transmit and receive data at predetermined intervals. The gating may be triggered on a specific portion of the electrocardiogram (e.g., the r-wave) or a time interval such as once or twice per second.

A manual approach to intermittent imaging can also be used to reduce the exposure of contrast microbubbles to the acoustic energy and prolongs the duration of contrast enhancement. This approach is especially useful for evaluating late tumor washout as described in the hepatic applications below. Using this approach, scanning is paused for a duration (generally 20 to 30 seconds) with short clips of the area of interest obtained at set time intervals. A disadvantage to intermittent imaging is its lack of a real-time display of data, which can cause technical challenges, but this technique is helpful in detecting low levels of contrast enhancement and for prolonging the duration of contrast enhancement.

Other contrast-specific technologies include advanced three-dimensional (3D) and four-dimensional (4D) imaging (Figs. 17.6 and 17.7). Furthermore, a number of contrast-specific measurements and calculations can be performed, including onboard video densitometry, calculation of the integrated backscatter from contrast, measurement of the transit time of contrast-containing blood through normal and diseased tissue, estimations of blood volume, and assessment of tissue perfusion differences in solid organs.[38,39] Systems have been developed that allow onboard calculation of the unique data provided by the use of UCAs (Fig. 17.8).

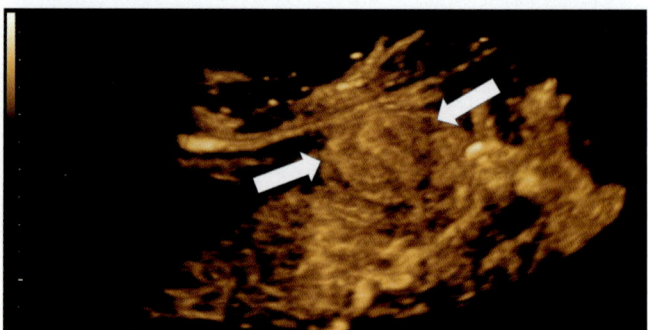

FIG. 17.6 Contrast-enhanced 4D coded harmonic imaging of hepatocellular carcinoma *(arrows)* prior to locoregional treatment. Volume data image reconstruction software is used to better appreciate the mass and feeding vasculature.

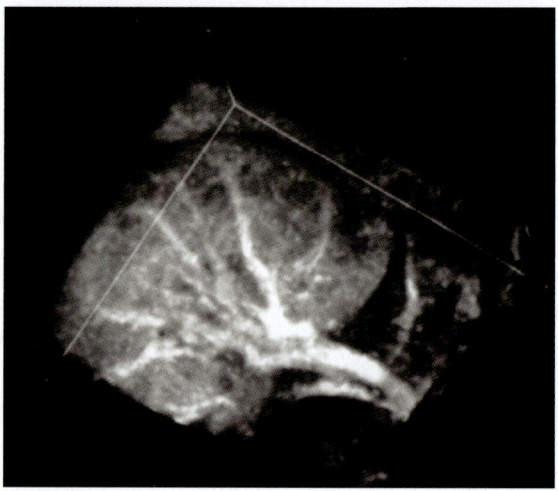

FIG. 17.7 The combination of 3D gray-scale harmonic imaging and administration of a vascular ultrasound contrast agent results in an "ultrasound angiogram."

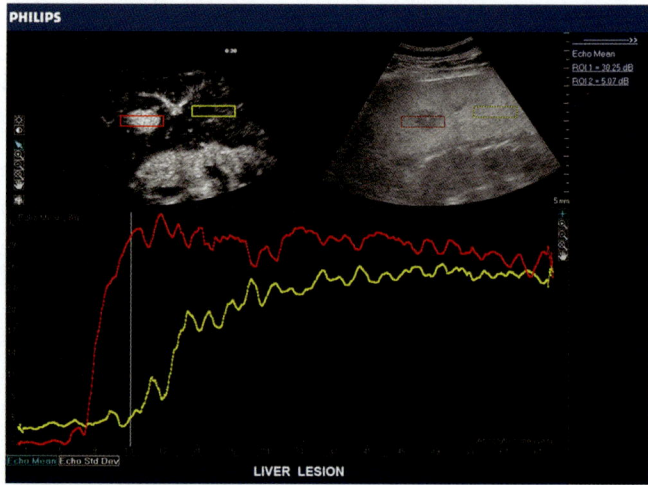

FIG. 17.8 Contrast-specific quantification of changes in signal intensity within a liver tumor compared with the normal liver. Time-intensity curves generated after intravenous administration of contrast from regions of interest placed over the tumor *(red box)* and the normal liver *(yellow box)*. The graphic displays time on the *x*-axis and signal intensity on the *y*-axis. Note that the signal intensity on the tumor *(red tracing)* demonstrates more rapid uptake of contrast and higher signal intensity as compared to the normal liver *(yellow tracing)*. Contrast enhancement can also be seen in the right kidney deep to the liver. (Courtesy Philips Healthcare, Bothell, WA.)

CLINICAL APPLICATIONS

Hepatic Applications

There are limitations to the sonographic evaluation of hepatic lesions and other hepatic abnormalities. Although ultrasound is usually sensitive for the detection of medium to large hepatic lesions, it is limited in its ability to detect small (less than 10 mm), isoechoic, or peripherally located lesions, particularly in obese patients or patients with diffuse liver disease. Furthermore, characterization of hepatic tumors cannot be performed without evaluating the enhancement kinetics of the mass.

Hepatic ultrasound blood flow studies are limited by low-velocity blood flow, such as in cases of portal hypertension (PHT) or for the detection of flow in the intrahepatic artery branches. UCA have shown the potential to improve the accuracy of hepatic sonography, including enhanced detection and characterization of hepatic masses and improved detection of intrahepatic and extrahepatic blood flow.

Hepatic Blood Flow. Vascular UCAs have been shown to improve the assessment of hepatic blood flow in normal subjects, as well as in patients with liver disease and PHT.[40,41]

Most sonographic examinations for PHT include a qualitative assessment of blood flow with color flow imaging to identify the presence and direction of flow in the splenic and superior mesenteric veins, as well as the main portal vein and the intrahepatic portal and hepatic veins. When scanning patients with PHT, slow-moving portal flow can be difficult to detect using conventional Doppler techniques. Studies have found that the increased reflectivity of contrast-containing blood allows the detection of abnormal blood flow in the portal and hepatic veins, as well as in portal-systemic collaterals.[41,42] Contrast-enhanced sonography has also been used effectively in the assessment of flow through transjugular intrahepatic portosystemic shunts (TIPS).[42] A technique using the subharmonic (half the transmit frequency) amplitude from UCA has recently been validated in a multicenter trial for the diagnosis of portal hypertension.

Published reports have also described CEUS-detectable alterations in blood flow transit time through the livers of patients with diffuse hepatic disease compared with normal controls.[40,41] In cases of cirrhosis, there is often reduced portal venous flow and a compensatory increase in hepatic artery flow. Zhou and colleagues[43] examined blood flow in the hepatic arteries and hepatic veins of 52 patients with metastases and 23 normal control subjects after bolus injections of SonoVue. The results of this study suggest that CEUS assessment of changes in the hemodynamic parameters of the hepatic artery and vein can be used to improve diagnosis of liver metastases, possibly before sonographic detection of focal lesions.

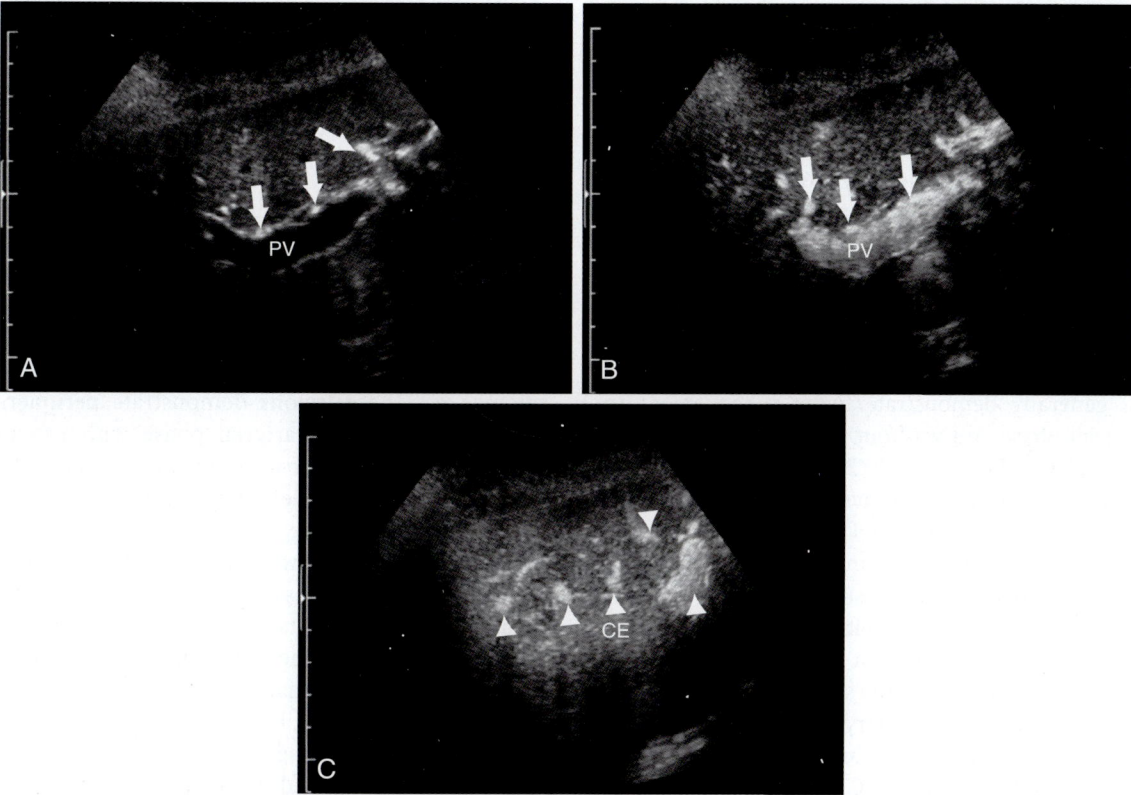

FIG. 17.9 Contrast-enhanced demonstration of the various phases of hepatic blood flow. (A) Twenty-five seconds after IV injection of an ultrasound contrast agent, the first vessels to demonstrate contrast enhancement in the liver are the hepatic arteries *(arrows)*, whereas the portal vein (PV) remains anechoic in the arterial phase. (B) In this patient, the portal venous phase occurred 37 seconds after injection, with contrast seen in the portal vein. (C) In the late vascular phase, at 71 seconds after injection, the liver parenchyma is becoming echogenic (i.e., contrast-enhanced; CE) and there is persistent enhancement of the major hepatic vessels *(arrowheads)*.

Hepatic Tumors. Liver lesion characterization is recognized around the world as one of the most important applications of CEUS. CEUS has established itself as an important diagnostic tool for the evaluation of patients with focal liver lesions of unknown origin and has the potential to reduce the use of competing imaging modalities for this application. Many patients who have hepatic tumors first identified sonographically eventually require a contrast-enhanced CT or MRI examination to better determine the extent of disease and to more accurately characterize the lesions. However, using CEUS, it is possible to distinguish the various phases of blood flow to and within the liver.[44,45] In normal situations after IV administration of a UCA, contrast-enhanced flow in the hepatic artery is identified first (arterial phase), followed by enhanced portal venous flow (portal venous phase). Detection of flow in the hepatic capillaries is identified later (late phase) as a parenchymal blush (Fig. 17.9). If an RES-specific agent is used, identification of the delayed enhancement phase representing the enhancement from the stationary microbubbles that have been phagocytosed by the RES is possible.[44] Diagnostic criteria used for the characterization of focal liver lesions on CEUS in cirrhotic patients have recently been incorporated into the American College of Radiology's **Liver Imaging Reporting & Data Systems (LI-RADS)** system (Fig. 17.10).[45] This system of standardization requires defining the lesion enhancement during the arterial phase and washout kinetics relative to the surrounding liver tissue in order to classify the risk of malignancy.[45,46] The use of CEUS for characterization of focal liver lesions has been shown to be a useful problem solver, particularly in patients with contradictory or equivocal findings on cross-sectional imaging or in whom MRI or CT with contrast is contraindicated.[47–50] In fact, CEUS, because of its ability to image dynamic events in real time, may prove to be better than CT or MRI in the evaluation of hemodynamics that occur in the various hepatic vascular phases, and thus more accurate for the characterization of focal liver lesions. Numerous published reports confirm the diagnostic potential of CEUS for the detection and characterization of liver lesions.[49–52]

Using the LI-RADS system, hepatocellular carcinoma (HCC) will generally demonstrate hyper-enhancement in the early arterial phase and washout of contrast in the later portal venous phase (Fig. 17.11).[45–50] When using an RES-specific agent, HCC lesions can have a similar appearance to focal nodular hyperplasia (FNH) in the early arterial phase. However, on delayed phase imaging, the HCC tumor will be hypoechoic relative to the surrounding liver tissue because of the lack of Kupffer cells within the tumor, whereas FNH tumors, because they contain abundant amounts of Kupffer cells, will be isoechoic to the surrounding liver tissue (Fig. 17.12). The central feeding artery and spoke-wheel radiating branches that are characteristic of FNH on dynamic CT angiography can also be depicted by CEUS and can be used to differentiate HCC from FNH.[46–48]

Additionally, CEUS can be used to avoid biopsy in some indeterminate (on unenhanced sonography) lesions with hallmarks of benign lesions on CEUS. Cavernous hemangiomas are common benign solid neoplasms of the liver and

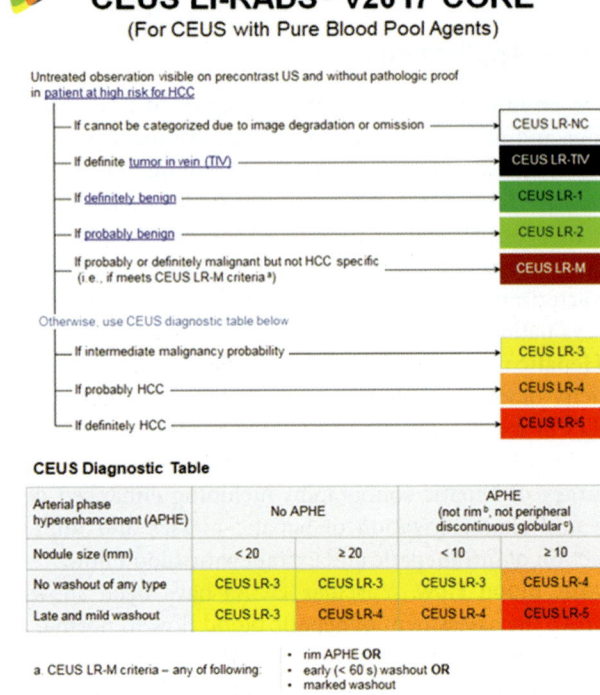

FIG. 17.10 Contrast-enhanced ultrasound imaging Liver Imaging Reporting and Data Systems (LI-RADS) criteria for the classification of indeterminate liver lesions in patients with high risk of hepatocellular carcinoma. (From American College of Radiology Committee on LI-RADS. CEUS LI-RADS v2017. https://www.acr.org/Clinical-Resources/Reporting-and-Data-Systems/LI-RADS/CEUS-LI-RADS-v2017.)

are frequently detected during hepatic sonography examinations. Not all hemangiomas have the classic sonographic appearance of a rounded, homogeneously hyperechoic mass that has well-defined margins, nor can they be accurately characterized sonographically (Fig. 17.13). Several reports indicate that CEUS can improve the assessment of hemangiomas.[49,53] These lesions demonstrate peripheral globular enhancement in the arterial phase with progressive centripetal filling without washout lasting from 5 to 7 minutes and are classified as "definitely benign" (LR-1) on the CEUS LI-RADS system.

CEUS has been shown to improve the detection and delineation of liver metastases (Fig. 17.14).[42,53] However, accurate characterization of metastatic liver tumors with CEUS can be problematic because the degree of vascularity in these lesions is related to the primary cancer.[54] Therefore, some metastatic liver lesions will be hypervascular, whereas others are hypovascular. One imaging characteristic of liver metastases that has been identified during delayed phase imaging is an echogenic rim around the tumor.[45–47] Early (<60 seconds after UCA injection) washout is also often indicative of metastatic liver disease, and the presence of either rim hyper-enhancement during the arterial phase or early washout is classified as LR-M in the CEUS LI-RADS system.[45]

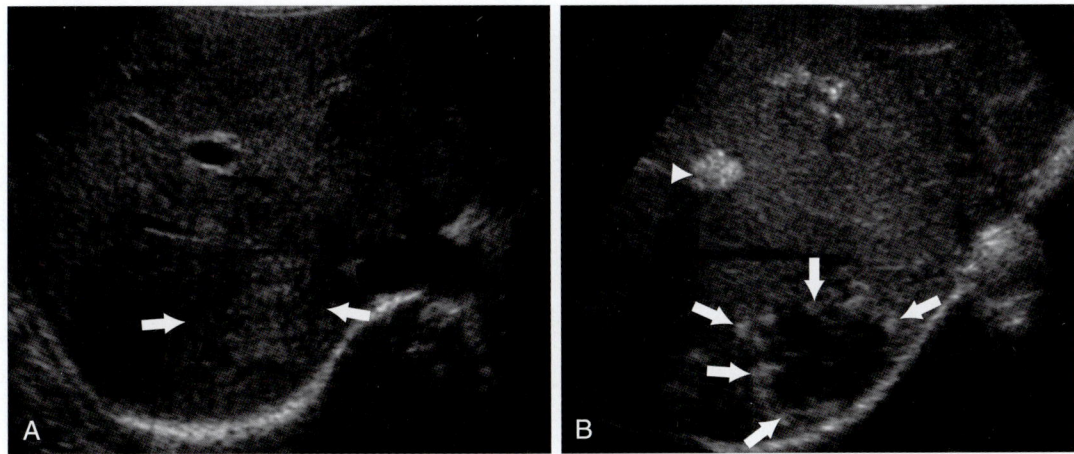

FIG. 17.11 Improved detection and characterization of a liver hemangioma. (A) A conventional ultrasound examination identified a poorly demarcated mass *(arrows)* in the right posterior lobe of the liver. (B) After contrast administration using contrast harmonic imaging, there is pooling of contrast-containing blood at the periphery of the lesion and increased echogenicity of the normal liver parenchyma. This pattern is characteristic of hemangiomas.

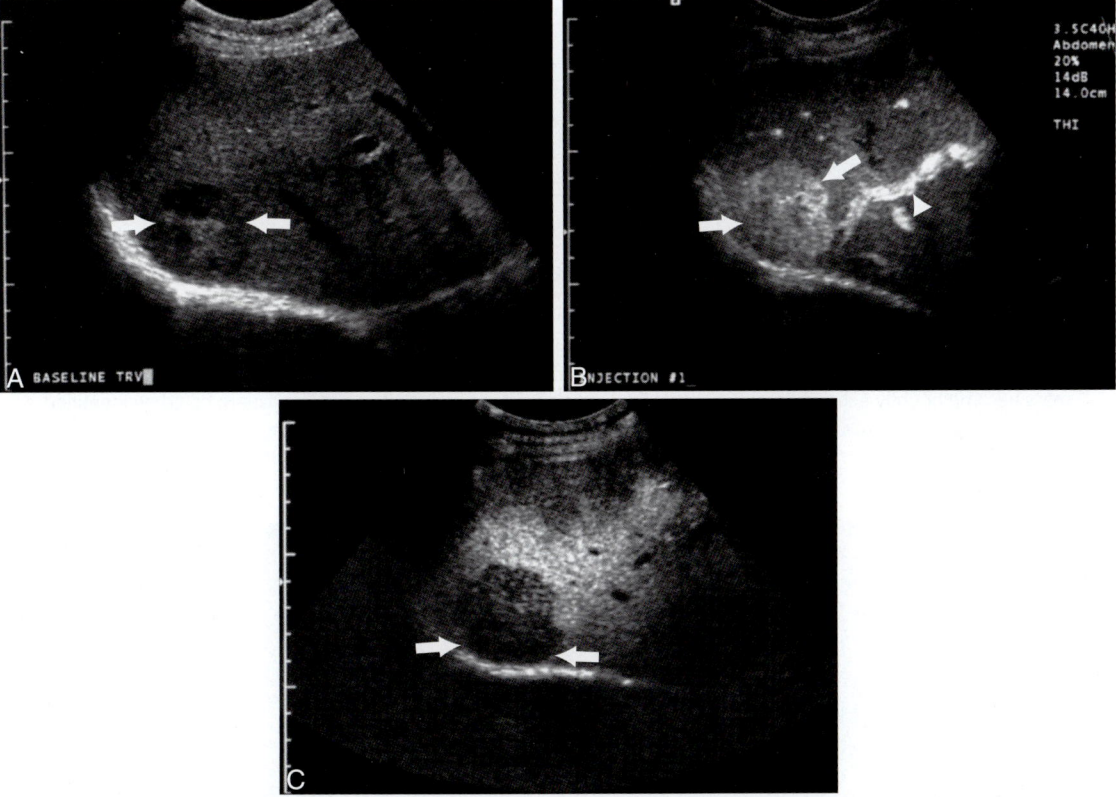

FIG. 17.12 Improved characterization of hepatocellular carcinoma (HCC) using a reticuloendothelial system-specific ultrasound contrast agent. (A) A conventional ultrasound examination identified a mass *(arrows)* in the right posterior lobe of the liver having mixed echogenicity. (B) After contrast administration using contrast harmonic imaging, the hepatic artery and portal veins filled with contrast *(arrowheads)*, and the mass became brightly echogenic compared with the surrounding liver tissue in the arterial and portal venous phases. (C) On delayed imaging, the lesion was hypoechoic compared with the surrounding liver tissue. This contrast-enhanced sonographic pattern is characteristic of HCC.

The role of CEUS for monitoring HCC response to locoregional therapies has also been well established.[55] Locoregional therapies for HCC include ablation (alcohol, microwave, radiofrequency, or cryo), transarterial embolization, or transarterial radioembolization, and these treatments are also iterative following identification of residual disease. For percutaneous ablation, CEUS has demonstrated value in both guiding probe placement and monitoring treatment response.[56-58] Serial monitoring of patients following transarterial chemoembolization (Fig. 17.15) can also be improved by CEUS, which can provide shorter follow up times and improved accuracy by providing real-time imaging with fewer artifacts from

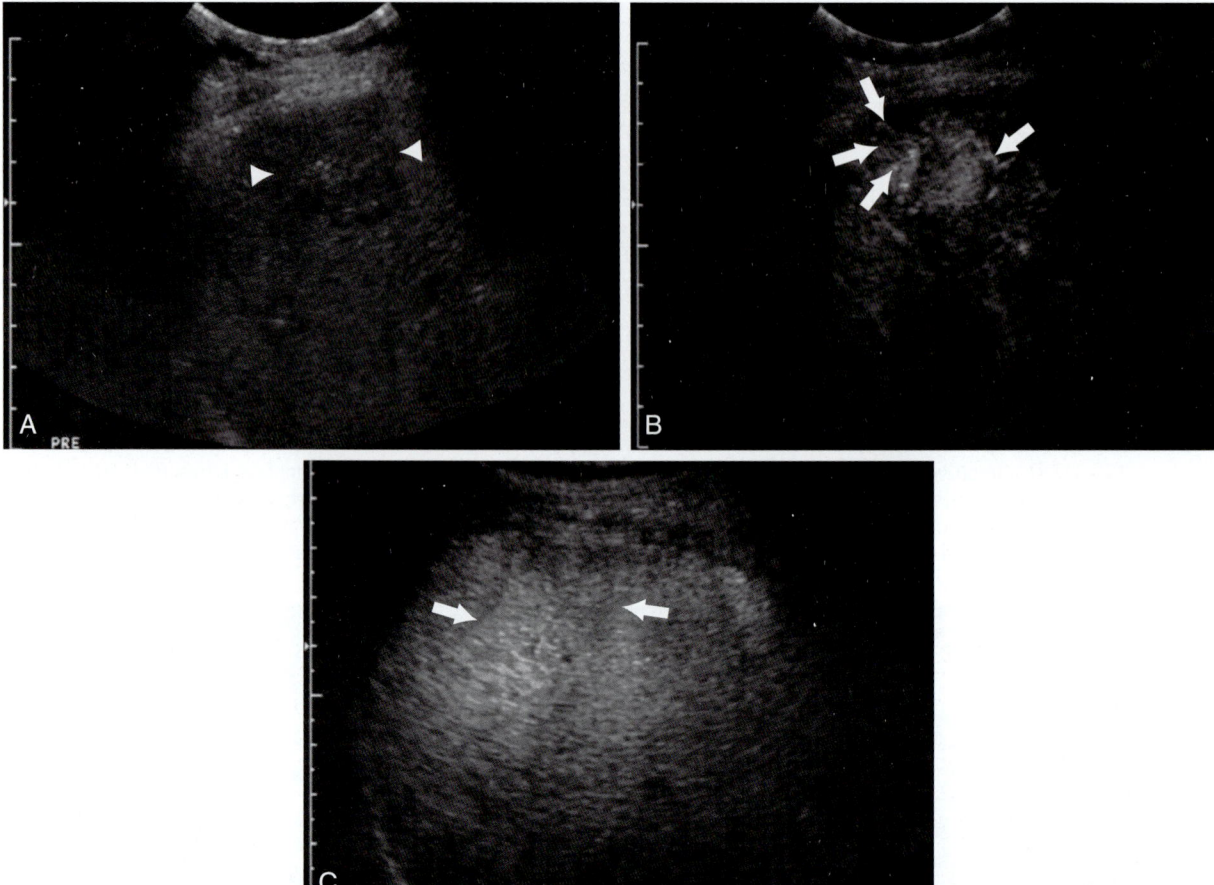

FIG. 17.13 Improved characterization of focal nodular hyperplasia (FNH) using an reticuloendothelial system-specific ultrasound contrast agent. (A) A conventional ultrasound examination identified a hypoechoic mass *(arrowheads)* in the right anterior lobe of the liver. (B) After contrast administration using contrast harmonic imaging, the mass became brightly echogenic, and intratumoral vessels having a radiating spoke-like pattern could be identified *(arrows)*. A central hypoechoic area within the mass that did not enhance represents a scar. (C) On delayed imaging, the lesion was isoechoic compared with the surrounding liver tissue. This contrast-enhanced sonographic pattern is characteristic of FNH.

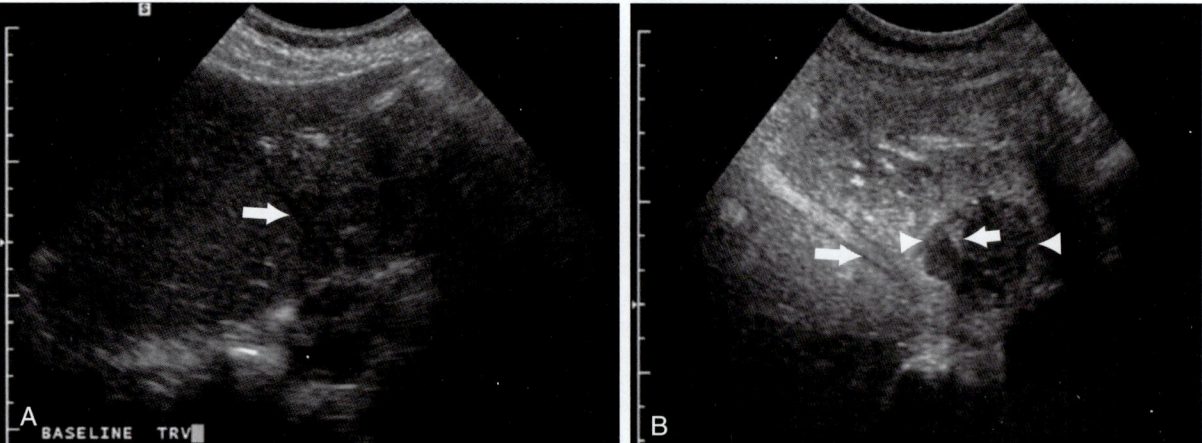

FIG. 17.14 Improved detection and delineation of a colorectal carcinoma liver metastasis. (A) A transverse conventional ultrasound image at the level of the middle hepatic vein *(arrow)* did not identify the mass, which had been detected on a prior computed tomographic examination. (B) After ultrasound contrast agent administration using contrast harmonic imaging in the portal venous phase, there was increased echogenicity of the surrounding liver parenchyma that resulted in improved delineation of the tumor *(arrowheads)*. Contrast-enhanced blood flow could also be identified in the hepatic vein *(arrow)* and small vessels within the mass *(short arrow)*. In this case, the patient was being evaluated for possible ultrasound-guided radiofrequency ablation of this nonresectable tumor, and the contrast-enhanced sonographic results enhanced the ability to identify the location of the tumor, as well as its size and margins.

tumoral inflammation and the embolic materials compared to MRI or CT.[59-61] Therefore, CEUS has the potential to provide clinical value across the full spectrum of HCC management, spanning lesion detection, characterization, treatment planning, and monitoring of therapeutic response.

Renal Applications

CEUS is frequently used for renal applications, including the evaluation of suspected renal masses and renal artery stenosis.[62-65] This is an ideal patient population for CEUS, as compromised renal function may prohibit the use of MRI or CT contrast agents. Several recent reports describe the increased use and clinical utility of renal CEUS, including its ability to obviate the use of alternative imaging modalities and its impact on patient management.

Renal Artery Stenosis. The sonographic evaluation of the main and intrarenal renal arteries in patients with suspected renal artery stenosis is fraught with problems. Because the main renal arteries are retroperitoneal in location, these vessels are typically difficult to evaluate sonographically, particularly in the obese patient. A significant number of patients will have anatomic variations of the renal vasculature, including duplicate or accessory renal arteries, and these variations can be difficult to identify using conventional ultrasound. Furthermore, ultrasound examinations for RAS are often time consuming and are extremely operator dependent. These factors likely contribute to the wide variability reported in the accuracy of ultrasound when used for RAS examinations.[66,67] Although not a common clinical application of CEUS, it has been investigated as a salvage tool employed when conventional ultrasound RAS examinations are nondiagnostic (Fig. 17.16).[68]

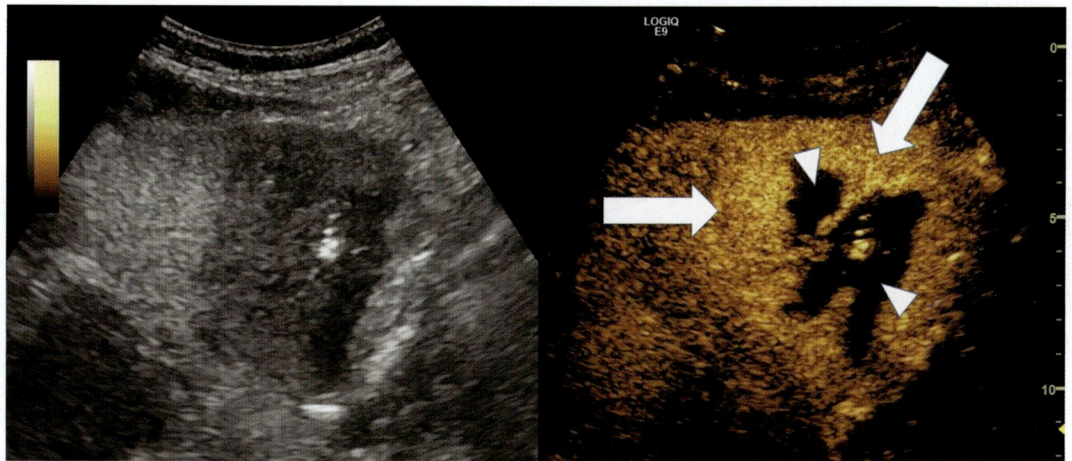

FIG. 17.15 The use of contrast-enhanced ultrasound imaging (CEUS) to monitor the response of hepatocellular carcinoma (HCC): Two weeks post–transarterial chemoembolization, conventional B-mode imaging *(left)* demonstrates an 8 cm HCC. CEUS *(right)* demonstrates pockets of areas without enhancement *(arrowheads)* representing effective embolization; however, enhancement is still evident at the tumor periphery *(arrows)*, indicating a need for additional therapy.

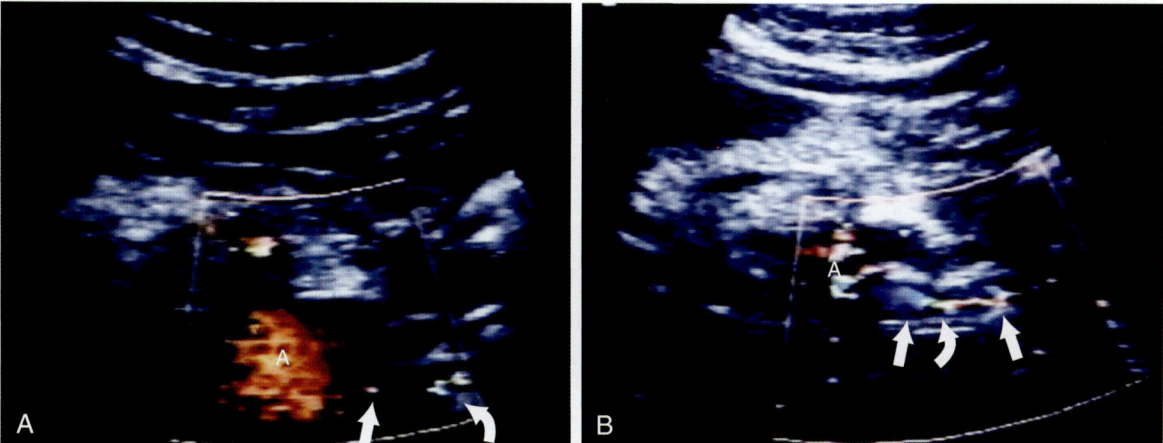

FIG. 17.16 Transverse color Doppler images of the abdominal aorta and proximal left renal artery in a patient with suspected renal artery stenosis. (A) Before intravenous administration of contrast, flow in the aorta *(A)* and proximal-most renal artery *(arrow)* are visualized, and there is aliasing of the color flow display *(curved arrow)*. (B) After injection of contrast, the stenotic vessel lumen *(arrows)* can be clearly visualized. Advances in contrast imaging modes have obviated the use of color flow imaging modes when performing contrast-enhanced examinations.

Renal Masses. Diagnostic sonography has been a reliable method of evaluating patients with renal masses, particularly in the differentiation of cystic from solid lesions, and this is now used routinely as part of clinical practice. Sonography is usually accurate in its ability to identify large (greater than 2 cm) renal cell carcinomas (RCCs) and to identify tumor thrombus in the renal veins or inferior vena cava. However, in a small percentage of cases, sonography cannot identify small neoplasms or differentiate solid hypoechoic renal lesions from hemorrhagic cysts or other benign processes (Fig. 17.17). Large, retrospective studies have shown CEUS has exceptional accuracy for the characterization of indeterminate renal masses and that RCC can be ruled out in a large percentage of these patients.[69,70] Direct impact of renal CEUS on patient management has also been shown, resulting in decreased cost and image wait time and clearance for renal transplants.[71–73] In rare cases, RCC may mimic oncocytomas on sonography.

The use of CEUS allows detection of normal renal blood flow using a non-Doppler mode (Fig. 17.18) and improves the ability to identify the normal renal vasculature and detect the presence of lesions that distort the vascular architecture.[71]

Similar to HCC, CEUS may be useful for guiding and monitoring locoregional therapies for RCC; CEUS has been shown to be effective for detecting both residual and recurrent RCC following percutaneous ablation therapy (Fig. 17.19).[74–76] This is an important alternative to patients with chronic kidney disease as post-RCC ablation monitoring typically requires serial CE-MRI assessments for up to 3 years despite nephrotoxicity concerns in patients with compromised glomerular filtration rates.

Splenic Applications

Several reports have described the clinical value of CEUS for the evaluation of the spleen.[20,77–79] Picardi and colleagues[79] compared CEUS to CT and fluorodeoxyglucose positron

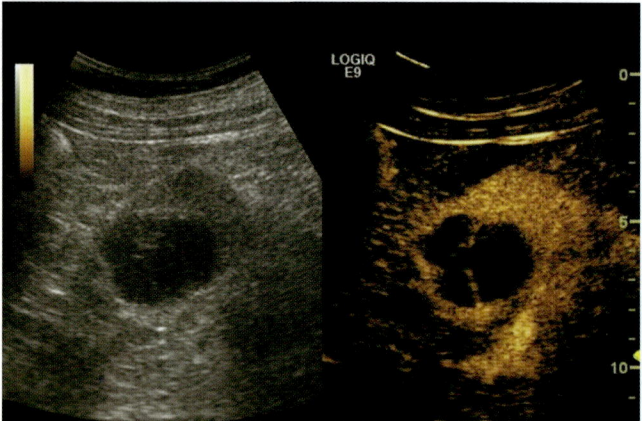

FIG. 17.17 Improved characterization of a cystic renal mass. Dual imaging displays conventional B-mode *(left)* and contrast harmonic imaging *(right)*. On B-mode, characterization of the mass is difficult as the low-level echoes in the mass could represent tumor tissue or debris in the cystic areas. On contrast-enhanced ultrasound imaging, the septations appear fine with smooth margins, and no other internal enhancement is observed, confirming internal echoes seen on B-mode are debris within the cyst. This information allowed the clinician to rule out the risk of malignancy.

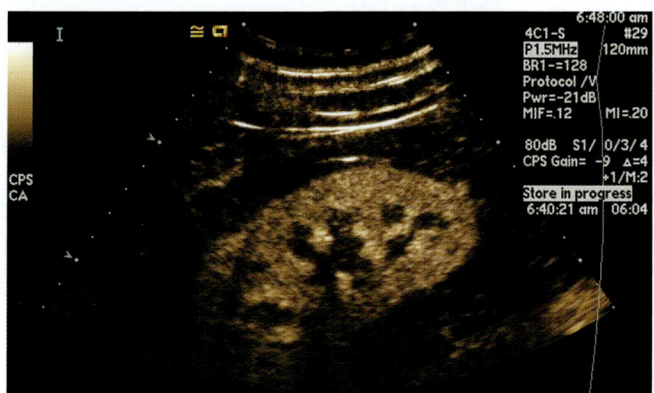

FIG. 17.18 Contrast harmonic imaging after intravenous administration of contrast demonstrates a uniform increase in the signal intensity within a normal kidney.

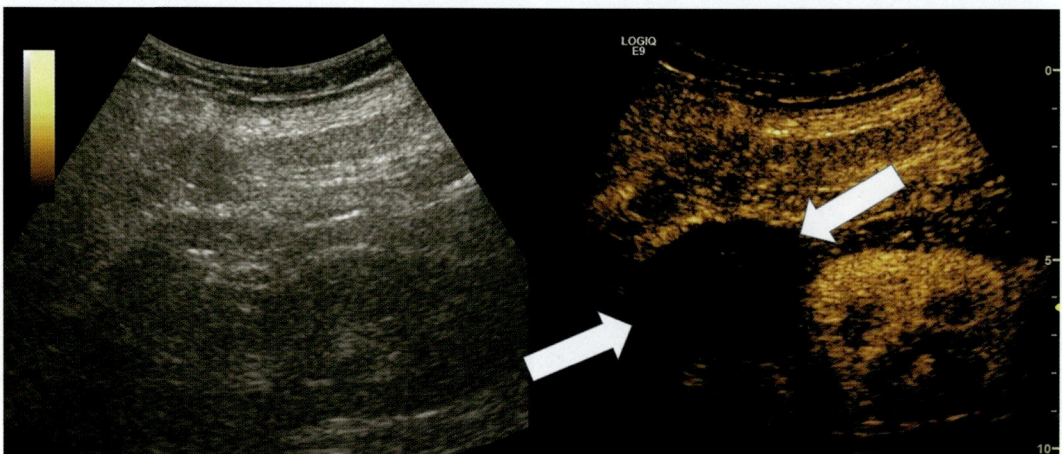

FIG. 17.19 Use of contrast-enhanced ultrasound imaging to rule out renal cell carcinoma recurrence following percutaneous ablation. Two years post–focal ablation, B-mode imaging *(left)* is used to identify the kidney and prior ablation cavity at the upper pole *(arrows)*. Coded harmonic imaging *(right)* shows no internal enhancement within the previously ablated tumor, indicating effective ablation of the mass.

emission tomography (PET) for the detection of nodular infiltration in the spleen of 100 patients with newly diagnosed Hodgkin lymphoma. Malignant nodules were detected with CT in 13 patients, with PET in 13 patients, and with CEUS in 30 patients. The authors concluded that CEUS provides a higher sensitivity than does CT or PET in the detection of splenic involvement by Hodgkin lymphoma.

Catalano and colleagues studied 55 patients with a variety of suspected splenic abnormalities, including traumatic injuries and tumors.[80] CEUS results were compared with baseline (noncontrast) ultrasound, CT, or MRI. In this series, parenchymal injuries were detected with a sensitivity of 63% on baseline ultrasound, whereas the sensitivity improved to 89% after CEUS. Parenchymal injuries included posttraumatic infarctions that were not identified on baseline ultrasound but were identified with CEUS. CEUS also identified 35 of 39 proven focal lesions in patients with Hodgkin disease, whereas baseline ultrasound detected only 23 lesions. The use of CEUS is particularly attractive for the assessment of pediatric patients to obviate the use of CT and radiation exposure.[77,81]

Pancreatic Applications

Visualization of the pancreas using transabdominal ultrasound is often hampered by the gland's deep location within the retroperitoneum and the presence of overlying bowel. Advances in ultrasound technology (e.g., endoscopic ultrasound), combined with UCAs, have led to a significant improvement in the diagnostic potential of ultrasound for a range of pancreatic disorders.[82] Several published reports describe the ability of UCAs to improve pancreatic ultrasound evaluations.[83–89]

Kersting and colleagues evaluated the value of transabdominal CEUS for differential diagnosis of pancreatic ductal adenocarcinoma (PDAC) and focal inflammatory masses resulting from chronic pancreatitis.[86] Of the 60 patients examined, histology revealed 45 PDACs and 15 inflammatory masses. The time-dependent parameters (arrival time and time-to-peak) were significantly longer in PDACs compared with focal masses. The authors concluded that PDAC and focal inflammatory masses exhibit different perfusion patterns that can be visualized with CEUS. Additionally, the contrast quantification software provided objective criteria that could be used to facilitate pancreatic lesion diagnoses.

Organ Transplants

Sonography is routinely used to evaluate kidney, liver, and pancreas transplants. The modality is often employed as a first-line examination tool in the immediate postsurgical period, as well as for serial studies to confirm organ viability. After organ transplantation, sonography is used to detect postsurgical fluid collections, to identify urinary or bile obstructions, and to assess blood flow to and from the transplanted organ. Conventional sonography is also useful in the evaluation of blood flow within the organ, but it does not have an adequate level of sensitivity to detect flow at the microvascular level (i.e., tissue perfusion).

The enhanced detection of blood flow provided by CEUS improves the assessment of blood flow in the arteries and veins that supply the transplanted organ and the vessels to which these vessels are anastomosed. CEUS has also been found to improve the ability to detect the lack of flow within transplanted organs (i.e., ischemic regions) within renal and pancreatic grafts.[90–94] Reports also suggest that CEUS is useful for the evaluation of liver transplant recipients.[95,96]

For renal transplants, CEUS can permit better differentiation of regions that have decreased perfusion from true vascular defects resulting from a renal artery branch occlusion or

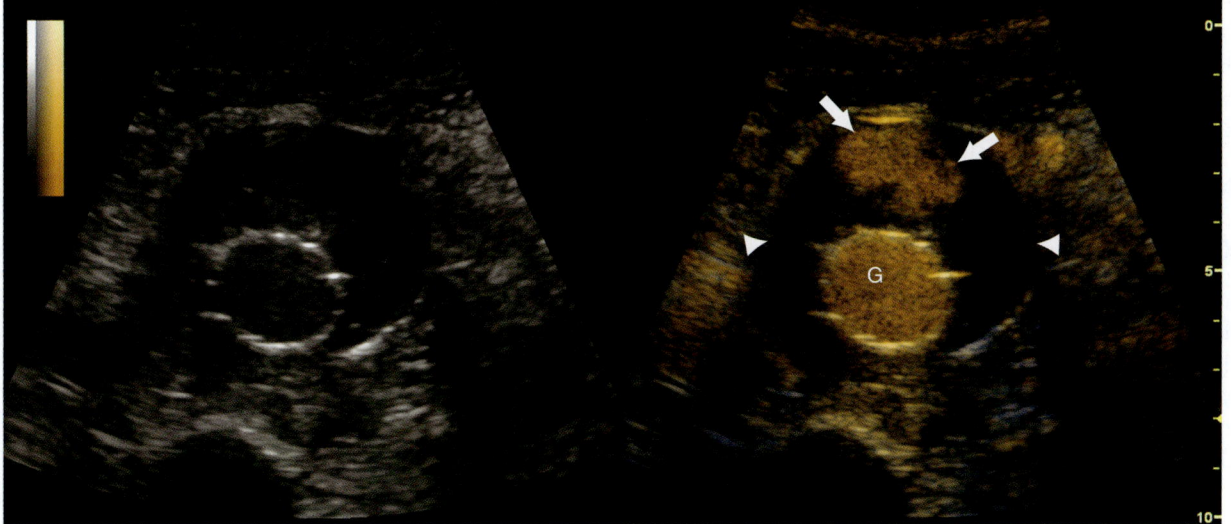

FIG. 17.20 Contrast-enhanced ultrasound imaging detection of an endovascular aortic aneurysm graft leak. This transverse contrast harmonic imaging image using a dual display (conventional gray-scale image at *left;* contrast-specific imaging mode at *right*) demonstrates the aneurysmal sack *(arrowheads)* and contrast-enhanced blood flow in the graft (G). Contrast-containing blood *(arrows)* is identified in the aneurysmal sack consistent with an endoleak. (Courtesy Dirk Clevert, MD, University of Munich, Germany.)

acute rejection.[13] The use of CEUS has also been investigated as a means to detect early organ rejection.[97]

Contrast-enhanced sonography has also been found to be superior to conventional sonography for differentiating parenchymal abnormalities in renal transplants, such as acute tubular necrosis (ATN), from other abnormalities.[90,98]

Other Applications

Other common abdominal/retroperitoneal applications of ultrasound include assessment of flow in the mesenteric arteries (for mesenteric ischemia), as well as the aorta and iliac arteries for aneurysms, stenoses, endovascular leaks, or dissections. Often these examinations are limited by the presence of overlying bowel and bowel gas, or the effects of signal attenuation resulting from the deep location of the vessels. Vascular UCAs have been used with success to improve the assessment of the abdominal vasculature and blood flow.[99,100]

A promising application for CEUS is for surveillance of patients after endovascular aneurysm repair (EVAR) of abdominal aortas (Fig. 17.20).[99–101] Postsurgical surveillance of these patients is required to detect endoleaks, and patients commonly are followed for months or even years after EVAR. Administration of a UCA provides several minutes of contrast enhancement, thereby allowing time to assess the graft for both fast-flowing and slow-flowing endoleaks. This is an advantage over CE-CT, which may only use one or a few phases (to limit ionizing radiation exposure).

Finally, nonvascular CEUS has shown to be advantageous in many clinical applications. Lumason is approved for CEUS of the urinary tract for the evaluation of suspected or known vesicoureteral reflux in pediatric patients and has shown excellent safety and high diagnostic accuracy.[102,103] This is an important alternative to CT imaging which requires the use of ionizing radiation in a particularly vulnerable patient population.

CEUS has also been shown to have the potential to improve the assessment of lymph nodes and tumor staging. UCA can be injected peri-tumorally or subcutaneously to image the lymphatics (termed lymphosonography).[104,105] The feasibility of this work was initially demonstrated in animal models, but recent clinical trials have shown the ability of lymphosonography to detect sentinel lymph nodes to direct node biopsy and ultimately guide cancer management.[106–108]

CONCLUSION

Several UCAs are currently marketed in the United States, and their use in radiologic applications continues to expand. Vascular agents have been shown to improve the detection of blood flow in small and deep vessels throughout the body. The ability of UCAs to improve the sonographic detection and characterization of tumors and other abnormalities within the abdomen is well documented. Clinical guidelines have been developed to standardize how CEUS examinations are performed and reported. Data showing the usefulness and accuracy of CEUS for hepatic and renal mass characterization is robust, and these approaches are becoming the standard of care in many medical centers.

The enhancement capabilities of UCAs have been shown to have the ability to salvage nondiagnostic ultrasound examinations and render them diagnostic. The use of UCAs has also resulted in new ultrasound applications that were not possible without their use. Improvements in ultrasound technology designed to exploit the acoustic behavior of contrast microbubbles complement the use of UCAs. Advances in both ultrasound instrumentation and the development of UCAs will continue to have a positive impact on the future of diagnostic sonography.

> ### Key Pearls
>
> - The clinical utilization of contrast-enhanced ultrasound imaging (CEUS) has been shown to reduce or eliminate some of the current limitations of ultrasound imaging and Doppler blood flow detection.
> - Sonographic detection of blood flow is limited by factors including the depth and size of a vessel, the attenuation properties of intervening tissue, or low-velocity flow.
> - The use of UCAs improves the detection of blood flow from vessels that are often difficult to assess without their use, such as the renal arteries, intracranial vessels, and small capillaries within organs (i.e., tissue perfusion).
> - For a UCA to be clinically useful, it should be nontoxic, have microbubbles or microparticles that are small enough to traverse the pulmonary capillary beds (i.e., less than 8 microns in size), and be stable enough to provide multiple recirculations.
> - Once a vascular agent's microbubbles are ruptured or otherwise destroyed, the microbubble shell products are metabolized or eliminated by the body, and the gas is exhaled.
> - Tissue-specific ultrasound contrast agents differ from vascular agents in that the microbubbles of these agents are removed from the blood pool and taken up by, or have an affinity toward, specific tissues, for example, the reticuloendothelial system in the liver and spleen, or thrombi in blood vessels.
> - Nonlinear contrast imaging technologies such as harmonic imaging use the same broadband transducers used for conventional ultrasound but are configured to maximize nonlinear signals arising from UCA microbubbles while suppressing linear signals from tissue.
> - Contrast-enhanced ultrasound has been well validated for the characterization of hepatic and renal tumors.
> - Established guidelines and specific classification criteria for CEUS exams are now available.

REFERENCES

1. Ophir J, Gobuty A, McWhirt RE, Maklad NF. Ultrasonic backscatter from contrast producing collagen microspheres. *Ultrasound Imaging*. 1980;2:67–77.
2. Lee JY, Minami Y, Choi BI, et al. The AFSUMB Consensus Statements and Recommendations for the Clinical Practice of Contrast-Enhanced Ultrasound Using Sonazoid. *J Med Ultrasound*. 2020;28(2):59–82.

3. Dietrich CF, Nolsøe CP, Barr RG, et al. Guidelines and Good Clinical Practice Recommendations for Contrast-Enhanced Ultrasound (CEUS) in the Liver-Update 2020 WFUMB in Cooperation with EFSUMB, AFSUMB, AIUM, and FLAUS. *Ultrasound Med Biol*. 2020;46(10):2579–2604.
4. Sidhu PS, Cantisani V, Dietrich CF, et al. The EFSUMB Guidelines and Recommendations for the Clinical Practice of Contrast-Enhanced Ultrasound (CEUS) in Non-Hepatic Applications: Update 2017 (Short Version). *Ultraschall Med*. 2018;39(2):154–180.
5. Lyshchik A. *Specialty Imaging: Fundamentals of CEUS*. Philadelphia: Elsevier; 2019.
6. Gummadi S, Eisenbrey J, Li J, et al. Advances in modern clinical ultrasound. *Advanced Ultrasound in Diagnosis and Therapy*. 2018;2(2):51–63.
7. Gramiak R, Shah PM. Echocardiography of the aortic root. *Invest Radiol*. 1968;3:356–366.
8. Chomas JE, Dayton PA, Allen J, Ferrara KW. Optical and acoustical observation of contrast-agent destruction. In: Goldberg BB, Raichlen JS, Forsberg F, eds. *Ultrasound Contrast Agents*. 2nd ed. London: Martin Dunitz; 2001, pp. 259–266.
9. Wheatley MA. Composition of contrast microbubbles: basic chemistry of encapsulated and surfactant-coated bubbles. In: Goldberg BB, Raichlen JS, Forsberg F, eds. *Ultrasound Contrast Agents*. 2nd ed. London: Martin Dunitz; 2001, pp. 3–13.
10. Forsberg F, Liu JB, Merton DA, et al. Tumor detection using an ultrasound contrast agent. *J Ultrasound Med*. 1995;4:S8.
11. Forsberg F, Liu JB, Rawool NM, et al. Gray-scale and color Doppler flow harmonic imaging with proteinaceous microspheres. *Radiology*. 1995;197(2):403.
12. Kono Y, Mattrey RF, Pinnell SP, et al. Contrast-enhanced B-mode harmonic imaging for the evaluation of HCC viability after therapy in cirrhotic patients. *J Ultrasound Med*. 2001;20:S10.
13. von Herbay A, Vogt C, Haussinger D. Pulse inversion sonography in the early phase of the sonographic contrast agent Levovist: differentiation between benign and malignant focal liver lesions. *J Ultrasound Med*. 2002;21:1191–1200.
14. Eisenbrey JR, Shaw CM, Lyshchik A, et al. Contrast-enhanced subharmonic and harmonic ultrasound of renal masses undergoing percutaneous cryoablation. *Acad Radiol*. 2015;22(7):820–826.
15. Eisenbrey JR, Forsberg F, Wessner CE, et al. US-triggered microbubble destruction for augmenting hepatocellular carcinoma response to transarterial radioembolization: a randomized pilot clinical trial. *Radiology*. 2021;298(2):450–457.
16. Mihalik JE, Smith RS, Toevs CC, et al. The use of contrast-enhanced ultrasound for the evaluation of solid abdominal organ injury in patients with blunt abdominal trauma. *J Trauma Acute Care Surg*. 2012;73(5):1100–1105.
17. Erlichman DB, Weiss A, Koenigsberg M, Stein MW. Contrast enhanced ultrasound: a review of radiology applications. *Clin Imaging*. 2020;60(2):209–215.
18. Dave JK, Mc Donald ME, Mehrotra P, Kohut AR, Eisenbrey JR, Forsberg F. Recent technological advancements in cardiac ultrasound imaging. *Ultrasonics*. 2018;84:329–340.
19. Bracco. Lumason package insert. https://imaging.bracco.com/us-en/lumason.
20. Allard CB, Coret A, Dason S, et al. Contrast-enhanced ultrasound for surveillance of radiofrequency-ablated renal tumors: a prospective, radiologist-blinded pilot study. *Urology*. 2015;86(6):1174–1178.
21. Catalano O, Aiani L, Barozzi L, et al. CEUS in abdominal trauma: multi-center study. *Abdom Imaging*. 2009;34(2):225–234.
22. Quaia E, De Paoli L, Angileri R, et al. Indeterminate solid hepatic lesions identified on non-diagnostic contrast-enhanced computed tomography: assessment of the additional diagnostic value of contrast-enhanced ultrasound in the non-cirrhotic liver. *Eur J Radiol*. 2014;83(3):456–462.
23. Ryu SW, Bok GH, Jang JY, et al. Clinically useful diagnostic tool of contrast enhanced ultrasonography for focal liver masses: comparison to computed tomography and magnetic resonance imaging. *Gut Liver*. 2014;8(3):292–297.
24. Blomley MJK, Harvey CJ, Eckersley RJ, Cosgrove DO. Contrast kinetics and Doppler intensitometry. In: Goldberg BB, Raichlen JR, Forsberg F, eds. *Ultrasound Contrast Agents: Basic Principles and Clinical Applications*. 2nd ed. London: Martin Dunitz; 2001, pp. 81–89.
25. Postema M, Gilja OH. Contrast-enhanced and targeted ultrasound. *World J Gastroenterol*. 2011;17(1):28–41.
26. Thumar Vishal, Liu Ji-Bin, Eisenbrey John. Applications in molecular ultrasound imaging: present and future. *Advanced Ultrasound in Diagnosis and Therapy*. 2019;3(3):62–75.
27. Goldberg BB, Forsberg F, Fitzts T, et al. Induced acoustic emission as a contrast mechanism for detection of hepatic abnormalities. *J Ultrasound Med*. 1995;14:S7.
28. Harvey CJ, Blomley MJK, Cosgrove DO. Acoustic emission imaging. In: Goldberg BB, Raichlen JS, Forsberg F, eds. *Ultrasound Contrast Agents*. 2nd ed. London: Martin Dunitz; 2001, pp. 71–80.
29. Forsberg F, Liu JB, Merton DA, et al. Gray scale second harmonic imaging of acoustic emission signals improves detection of liver tumors in rabbits. *J Ultrasound Med*. 2000;19:557–563.
30. Porter TR, Xie F. Contrast echocardiography: latest developments and clinical utility. *Curr Cardiol Rep*. 2015;17(3):569.
31. Forsberg F, Goldberg BB, Liu JB, et al. On the feasibility of real-time, in vivo harmonic imaging with proteinaceous microspheres. *J Ultrasound Med*. 1996;15:853–860.
32. Forsberg F, Liu JB, Burns PN, Merton DA, Goldberg BB. Artifacts in ultrasound contrast agent studies. *J Ultrasound Med*. 1994;13:357–365.
33. Kono Y, Mattrey RT. Harmonic imaging with contrast microbubbles. In: Goldberg BB, Raichlen JS, Forsberg F, eds. *Ultrasound Contrast Agents*. 2nd ed. London: Martin Dunitz; 2001, pp. 37–46.
34. Porter TR, Xie F. Accelerated intermittent harmonic imaging. In: Goldberg BB, Raichlen JS, Forsberg F, eds. *Ultrasound Contrast Agents*. 2nd ed. London: Martin Dunitz; 2001, pp. 67–70.
35. Forsberg F, Shi WT, Merritt CRB, et al. Does the Mechanical Index predict destruction rates of contrast microbubbles? *J Ultrasound Med*. 2001;20:S12.
36. Merton DA. An easily implemented method to improve detection of ultrasound contrast in body tissues: frame one imaging. *J Diag Med Sonography*. 2000;16(1):14–20.
37. Sirlin CB, Girard MS, Baker K, et al. Effect of gated US acquisition on liver and portal vein contrast enhancement. *Radiology*. 1996;201(1):158.
38. Wei K, Le E, Bin JP, et al. Quantification of renal blood flow with contrast-enhanced ultrasound. *J Am Coll Cardiol*. 2001;37(4):1135–1140.
39. Blomley MJ, Lim AK, Harvey CJ, et al. Liver microbubble transit time compared with histology and Child-Pugh score in diffuse liver disease: a cross sectional study. *Gut*. 2003;52(8):1188–1193.
40. Cocciolillo S, Parruti G, Marzio L. CEUS and Fibroscan in non-alcoholic fatty liver disease and non-alcoholic steatohepatitis. *World J Hepatol*. 2014;6(7):496–503.
41. Kim MY, Suk KT, Baik SK, et al. Hepatic vein arrival time as assessed by contrast-enhanced ultrasonography is useful for the assessment of portal hypertension in compensated cirrhosis. *Hepatology*. 2012;56(3):1053–1062.
42. Micol C, Marsot J, Boublay N, et al. Contrast-enhanced ultrasound: a new method for TIPS follow-up. *Abdom Imaging*. 2012;37(2):252–260.
43. Zhou JH, Li AH, Cao LH, et al. Haemodynamic parameters of the hepatic artery and vein can detect liver metastases: assessment using contrast-enhanced ultrasound. *Br J Radiol*. 2008;81(962):113–119.

44. Sugimoto K, Shiraishi J, Moriyasu F, et al. Improved detection of hepatic metastases with contrast-enhanced low mechanical-index pulse inversion ultrasonography during the liver-specific phase of Sonazoid: observer performance study with JAFROC analysis. *Acad Radiol.* 2009;16(7):798–809.
45. American College of Radiology Committee on LI-RADS (2017) CEUS LI-RADS v2017. https://www.acr.org/Clinical-Resources/Reporting-and-Data-Systems/LI-RADS/CEUS-LI-RADS-v2017.
46. Lyshchik A, Kono Y, Dietrich CF, et al. Contrast-enhanced ultrasound of the liver: technical and lexicon recommendations from the ACR CEUS LI-RADS working group. *Abdom Radiol (NY).* 2018;43(4):861–879.
47. Kim TK, Noh SY, Wilson SR, et al. Contrast-enhanced ultrasound (CEUS) liver imaging reporting and data system (LI-RADS) 2017 - a review of important differences compared to the CT/MRI system. *Clin Mol Hepatol.* 2017;23(4):280–289.
48. Barr RG, Wilson SR, Lyshchik A, et al. Contrast-enhanced ultrasound: state of the art in North America. *Ultrasound Q.* 2020;36(3):206–217.
49. Piscaglia F, Wilson SR, Lyshchik A, et al. American College of Radiology Contrast Enhanced Ultrasound Liver Imaging Reporting and Data System (CEUS LI-RADS) for the diagnosis of hepatocellular carcinoma: a pictorial essay. *Ultraschall Med.* 2017;38(3):320–324. English.
50. Hu J, Bhayana D, Burak KW, Wilson SR. Resolution of indeterminate MRI with CEUS in patients at high risk for hepatocellular carcinoma. *Abdom Radiol (NY).* 2020;45(1):123–133.
51. Wang JY, Feng SY, Yi AJ, et al. Comparison of contrast-enhanced ultrasound versus contrast-enhanced magnetic resonance imaging for the diagnosis of focal liver lesions using the Liver Imaging Reporting and Data System. *Ultrasound Med Biol.* 2020;46(5):1216–1223.
52. Trillaud H, Bruel JM, Valette PJ, et al. Characterization of focal liver lesions with SonoVue® enhanced sonography: international multicenter-study in comparison to CT and MRI. *World J Gastroenterol.* 2009;15(30):3748–3756.
53. Strobel D, Seitz K, Blank W, et al. Tumor-specific vascularization pattern of liver metastasis, hepatocellular carcinoma, hemangioma and focal nodular hyperplasia in the differential diagnosis of 1,349 liver lesions in contrast-enhanced ultrasound (CEUS). *Ultraschall Med.* 2009;30(4):376–382.
54. Wilson SR, Burns PN, Muradali D, et al. Harmonic hepatic US with microbubble contrast agent: initial experience showing improved characterization of hemangioma, hepatocellular carcinoma, and metastasis. *Radiology.* 2000;215:153–161.
55. Gummadi S, Eisenbrey JR, Lyshchik A. Contrast-enhanced ultrasonography in interventional oncology. *Abdom Radiol (NY).* 2018;43(11):3166–3175.
56. Francica G, Meloni MF, Riccardi L, et al. Ablation treatment of primary and secondary liver tumors under contrast-enhanced ultrasound guidance in field practice of interventional ultrasound centers. A multicenter study. *Eur J Radiol.* 2018;105:96–101.
57. Meloni MF, Andreano A, Zimbaro F, et al. Contrast enhanced ultrasound: roles in immediate post-procedural and 24-h evaluation of the effectiveness of thermal ablation of liver tumors. *J Ultrasound.* 2012;15:207–214.
58. Qu P, Yu X, Liang P, et al. Contrast-enhanced ultrasound in the characterization of hepatocellular carcinomas treated by ablation: comparison with contrast-enhanced magnetic resonance imaging. *Ultrasound Med Biol.* 2013;39:1571–1579.
59. Kono Y, Lucidarme O, Choi SH, Rose SC, Hassanein TI, Alpert E, Mattrey RF, et al. Contrast-enhanced ultrasound as a predictor of treatment efficacy within 2 weeks after transarterial chemoembolization of hepatocellular carcinoma. *J Vasc Interv Radiol.* 2007;18(1 Pt 1):57–65.
60. Shaw CM, Eisenbrey JR, Lyshchik A, et al. Contrast-enhanced ultrasound evaluation of residual blood flow to hepatocellular carcinoma after treatment with transarterial chemoembolization using drug-eluting beads: a prospective study. *J Ultrasound Med.* 2015;34:859–867.
61. Watanabe Y, Ogawa M, Kumagawa M, et al. Utility of contrast-enhanced ultrasound for early therapeutic evaluation of hepatocellular carcinoma after transcatheter arterial chemoembolization. *J Ultrasound Med.* 2020;39:431–440.
62. Bertelli E, Palombella A, Sessa F, et al. Contrast-enhanced ultrasound (CEUS) imaging for active surveillance of small renal masses. *World J Urol.* 2021;39(8):2853–2860.
63. Barr RG. Is there a need to modify the Bosniak renal mass classification with the addition of contrast-enhanced sonography? *J Ultrasound Med.* 2017;36(5):865–868.
64. Correas J, Claudon M, Tranquart F, Helenon O. Contrast-enhanced ultrasonography: renal applications. *J Radiol.* 2003;84:2041–2054.
65. Robbin ML, Lockhart ME, Barr RG. Renal imaging with ultrasound contrast: current status. *Radiol Clin North Am.* 2003;41(5):963–978.
66. Berland LL, Koslin DB, Routh WD, Keller FS. Renal artery stenosis: prospective evaluation of diagnosis with color duplex US compared with angiography. *Radiology.* 1990;174:421–423.
67. Olin JW, Piedmonte MR, Young JR, et al. The utility of duplex ultrasound scanning of the renal arteries for diagnosing significant renal artery stenosis. *Ann Intern Med.* 1995;122:833–838.
68. Missouris CG, Allen CM, Balen FG, et al. Non-invasive screening for renal artery stenosis with ultrasound contrast enhancement. *J Hypertens.* 1996;14(4):519–524.
69. Zarzour JG, Lockhart ME, West J, et al. Contrast-enhanced ultrasound classification of previously indeterminate renal lesions. *J Ultrasound Med.* 2017;36(9):1819–1827.
70. Barr RG, Peterson C, Hindi A. Evaluation of indeterminate renal masses with contrast-enhanced US: a diagnostic performance study. *Radiology.* 2014;271(1):133–142.
71. Kazmierski B, Deurdulian C, Tchelepi H, Grant EG. Applications of contrast-enhanced ultrasound in the kidney. *Abdom Radiol (NY).* 2018;43(4):880–898.
72. Streb JW, Tchelepi H, Malhi H, Deurdulian C, Grant EG. Retrospective analysis of contrast-enhanced ultrasonography effectiveness in reducing time to diagnosis and imaging-related expenditures at a single large United States county hospital. *Ultrasound Q.* 2019;35(2):99–102.
73. Eisenbrey JR, Kamaya A, Gummadi S, et al. Effects of contrast-enhanced ultrasound of indeterminate renal masses on patient clinical management: retrospective analysis from 2 institutions. *J Ultrasound Med.* 2021;40(1):131–139.
74. Li X, Liang P, Yu J, et al. Role of contrast-enhanced ultrasound in evaluating the efficiency of ultrasound guided percutaneous microwave ablation in patients with renal cell carcinoma. *Radiol Oncol.* 2013;47(4):398–404.
75. Calio BP, Lyshchik A, Li J, et al. Long term surveillance of renal cell carcinoma recurrence following ablation using 2D and 3D contrast-enhanced ultrasound. *Urology.* 2018;121:189–196.
76. Chen CN, Liang P, Yu J, et al. Contrast-enhanced ultrasound-guided percutaneous microwave ablation of renal cell carcinoma that is inconspicuous on conventional ultrasound. *Int J Hyperthermia.* 2016;32(6):607–613.
77. Oldenburg A, Hohmann J, Skrok J, Albrecht T. Imaging of paediatric splenic injury with contrast-enhanced ultrasonography. *Pediatr Radiol.* 2004;34(4):351–354.
78. Manetta R, Pistoia ML, Bultrini C, et al. Ultrasound enhanced with sulphur-hexafluoride-filled microbubbles agent (SonoVue) in the follow-up of mild liver and spleen trauma. *Radiol Med.* 2009;114(5):771–779.
79. Picardi M, Soricelli A, Pane F, et al. Contrast-enhanced harmonic compound US of the spleen to increase staging accuracy in patients with Hodgkin lymphoma: a prospective study. *Radiology.* 2009;251(2):574–582.
80. Catalano O, Lobianco R, Sandomenico F, et al. Realtime contrast-enhanced ultrasound of the spleen: examination technique and preliminary clinical experience. *Radiol Med.* 2003;106(4):338–356.

81. Armstrong LB, Mooney DP, Paltiel H, et al. Contrast enhanced ultrasound for the evaluation of blunt pediatric abdominal trauma. *J Pediatr Surg.* 2018;53(3):548–552. https://doi.org/10.1016/j.jpedsurg.2017.03.042. Epub 2017 Mar 20.
82. Martínez-Noguera A, Montserrat E, Torrubia S, et al. Ultrasound of the pancreas: update and controversies. *Eur Radiol.* 2001;11(9):1594–1606.
83. Boggi U, Morelli L, Amorese G, et al. Contribution of contrast-enhanced ultrasonography to nonoperative management of segmental ischemia of the head of a pancreas graft. *Am J Transplant.* 2009;9(2):413–418.
84. Faccioli N, Crippa S, Bassi C, D'Onofrio M. Contrast-enhanced ultrasonography of the pancreas. *Pancreatology.* 2009;9(5):560–566.
85. Karamehic J, Scoutt LM, Tabakovic M, Heljic B. Ultrasonography in organ transplantation. *Med Arh.* 2004;58(1 Suppl 2):107–108.
86. Kersting S, Konopke R, Kersting F, et al. Quantitative perfusion analysis of transabdominal contrast-enhanced ultrasound of pancreatic masses and carcinomas. *Gastroenterology.* 2009;137(6):1903–1911.
87. Numata K, Yutaka O, Noritoshi K, et al. Contrast-enhanced sonography of autoimmune pancreatitis: comparison with pathologic findings. *J Ultrasound Med.* 2004;23(2):199–206.
88. Krishnan K, Bhutani MS, Aslanian HR, et al. Enhanced EUS imaging (with videos). *Gastrointest Endosc.* 2021;93(2):323–333.
89. Itonaga M, Kitano M, Kojima F, et al. The usefulness of EUS-FNA with contrast-enhanced harmonic imaging of solid pancreatic lesions: A prospective study. *J Gastroenterol Hepatol.* 2020;35(12):2273–2280.
90. Benozzi L, Cappelli G, Granito M, et al. Contrast-enhanced sonography in early kidney graft dysfunction. *Transplant Proc.* 2009;41(4):1214–1215.
91. Mueller-Peltzer K, Negrão de Figueiredo G, Fischereder M, et al. Contrast-enhanced ultrasound (CEUS) as a new technique to characterize suspected renal transplant malignancies in renal transplant patients in comparison to standard imaging modalities. *Clin Hemorheol Microcirc.* 2018;69(1-2):69–75.
92. Goyal A, Hemachandran N, Kumar A, Sharma R, Shamim SA, et al. Evaluation of the graft kidney in the early postoperative period: performance of contrast-enhanced ultrasound and additional ultrasound parameters. *J Ultrasound Med.* 2021;40(9):1771–1783.
93. Como G, Da Re J, Adani GL, Zuiani C, Girometti R. Role for contrast-enhanced ultrasound in assessing complications after kidney transplant. *World J Radiol.* 2020;12(8):156–171.
94. Hai Y, Chong W, Liu JB, Forsberg F, Eisenbrey J. The Diagnostic Value of contrast-enhanced ultrasound for monitoring complications after kidney transplantation: a systematic review and meta-analysis. *Acad Radiol.* 2021;28(8):1086–1093.
95. Sidhu PS, Shaw AS, Ellis SM, et al. Microbubble ultrasound contrast in the assessment of hepatic artery patency following liver transplantation: role in reducing frequency of heaptic artery arteriography. *Eur Radiol.* 2004;14(1):21–30.
96. Como G, Montaldo L, Baccarani U, et al. Contrast-enhanced ultrasound applications in liver transplant imaging. *Abdom Radiol (NY).* 2021;46(1):84–95.
97. Correas J, Helenon O, Moreau JF. Contrast-enhanced ultrasonography of native and transplanted kidney diseases. *Eur Radiol.* 1999;9 (Suppl 3):S394–S400.
98. Zeisbrich M, Kihm LP, Drüschler F, et al. When is contrast-enhanced sonography preferable over conventional ultrasound combined with Doppler imaging in renal transplantation? *Clin Kidney J.* 2015;8(5):606–614.
99. Giannoni MF, Palombo G, Sbarigia E, et al. Contrast-enhanced ultrasound for aortic stent-graft surveillance. *J Endovasc Ther.* 2003;10(2):208–217.
100. Iezzi R, Cotroneo AR, Basilico R, et al. Endoleaks after endovascular repair of abdominal aortic aneurysm: value of CEUS. *Abdom Imaging.* 2010;35(1):106–114.
101. Yang X, Chen YX, Zhang B, et al. Contrast-enhanced ultrasound in detecting endoleaks with failed computed tomography angiography diagnosis after endovascular abdominal aortic aneurysm repair. *Chin Med J (Engl).* 2015;128(18):2491–2497.
102. Papadopoulou F, Ntoulia A, Siomou E, Darge K. Contrast-enhanced voiding urosonography with intravesical administration of a second-generation ultrasound contrast agent for diagnosis of vesicoureteral reflux: prospective evaluation of contrast safety in 1,010 children. *Pediatr Radiol.* 2014;44(6):719–728.
103. Darge K, Moeller RT, Trusen A, et al. Diagnosis of vesicoureteric reflux with low-dose contrast-enhanced harmonic ultrasound imaging. *Pediatr Radiol.* 2005;35(1):73–78.
104. Goldberg BB, Merton DA, Liu JB, Murphy G, Forsberg F. Contrast-enhanced sonographic imaging of lymphatic channels and sentinel lymph nodes. *J Ultrasound Med.* 2005;24(7):953–965.
105. Mattrey RF, Kono Y, Baker K, Peterson T. Sentinel lymph node imaging with microbubble ultrasound contrast material. *Acad Radiol.* 2002;9(Suppl 1):S231–235.
106. Machado P, Stanczak M, Liu JB, et al. Subdermal Ultrasound Contrast Agent Injection for Sentinel Lymph Node Identification: An Analysis of Safety and Contrast Agent Dose in Healthy Volunteers. *J Ultrasound Med.* 2018;37(7):1611–1620.
107. Hao Y, Sun Y, Lei Y, Zhao H, Cui L. Percutaneous aonazoid-enhanced ultrasonography combined with in vitro verification for detection and characterization of sentinel lymph nodes in early breast cancer. *Eur Radiol.* 2021;31(8):5894–5901.
108. Lowes S, Leaver A, Cox K, et al. Evolving imaging techniques for staging axillary lymph nodes in breast cancer. *Clin Radiol.* 2018;73(4):396–409.

CHAPTER 18

Ultrasound-Guided Interventional Techniques

M. Robert DeJong

OBJECTIVES

On completion of this chapter, you should be able to:
- Describe the advantages of ultrasound-guided procedures
- Describe the benefits of sonographer involvement in procedures
- Discuss the advantages and disadvantages of free-hand and needle-guided techniques
- List potential complications of ultrasound-guided interventional techniques
- Discuss techniques for finding the needle tip
- Discuss indications and contraindications for the procedures discussed in this chapter

OUTLINE

Ultrasound-Guided Procedures 529
Indications for a Biopsy 530
Contraindications for a Biopsy 531
Laboratory Tests 531
Ultrasound-Guided Biopsy Equipment and Techniques 532
Ultrasound Guidance Methods 535
Cytopathology 538
   Inconclusive Specimens 539
Biopsy Complications 539
Fusion Technology 540
Ultrasound-Guided Biopsy Equipment and Process 543

The Sonographer's Role in Interventional Procedures 548
Finding the Needle Tip 550
What to Do When the Needle Deviates 551
Biopsies and Procedures by Organ 552
   Liver 552
   Pancreas 553
   Kidney 554
   Renal Transplants 555
   Retroperitoneal Lymph Nodes 555
   Lung 556

Thyroid Gland 557
Neck Nodes and Masses 557
Musculoskeletal Biopsies 557
Pelvis 558
Prostate Gland 558
Fluid Collections and Abscesses 559
   Pleural Fluid 559
   Ascites 559
   Abscess Drainage 559
New Applications 559

KEY TERMS

Alpha-fetoprotein (AFP)
Biopsy gun
Coagulopathy
Consent form
Core biopsy

Fine-needle aspiration (FNA)
International normalized ratio (INR)
Partial thromboplastin time (PTT)
Pneumothorax

Prostate-specific antigen (PSA)
Prothrombin time (PT)
Thoracentesis
Vasovagal reaction

Ultrasound has been used to assist in interventional procedures since the 1970s by means of specially designed A-mode and B-mode transducers (Fig. 18.1). Ultrasound-guided procedures have come a long way since those early days of A-mode and static B-scan units with the development of real time imaging and color Doppler. Ultrasound is being used to guide a variety of invasive procedures on various organs and masses located in the neck, chest, abdomen, retroperitoneum, musculoskeletal (MSK) system, and pelvis and on the fetus and gravid uterus. Ultrasound is also being used to drain a variety of fluid collections and abscesses.

The use of ultrasound to guide procedures continues to grow, with procedures being performed by a wide variety of medical personnel. Besides radiologists and maternal fetal medicine physicians, other health care providers have started to use ultrasound to help them in their practice. Anesthesiologists place ultrasound-guided intravenous (IV) lines and perform nerve blocks, the orthopedic department performs ultrasound-guided joint and nerve injections as well as tap joint effusions, some physical therapists do ultrasound-guided dry needling, urologists perform prostate biopsies, pain management physicians perform

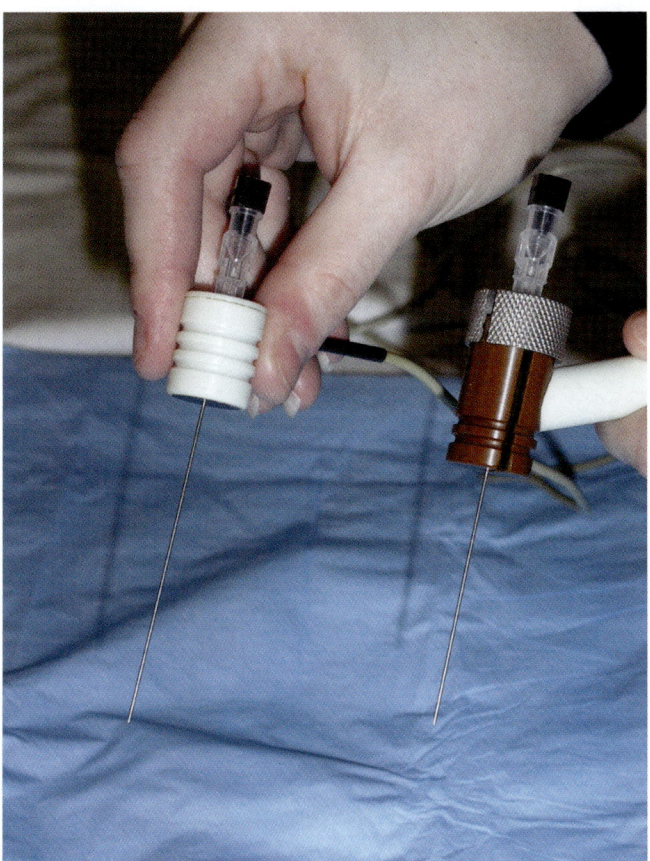

FIG. 18.1 The white transducer is an A-mode transducer. The brown transducer is a B-mode transducer.

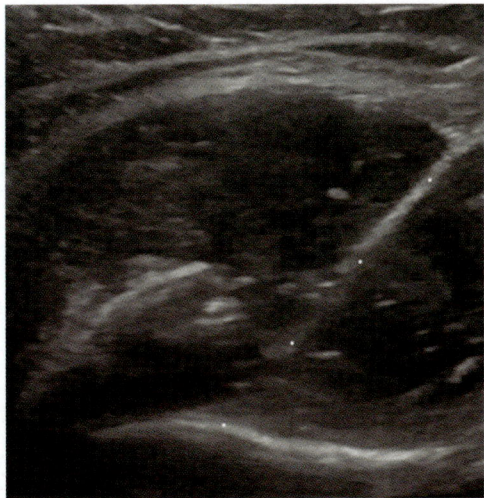

FIG. 18.2 Chondrosarcoma of the rib.

ultrasound-guided nerve blocks, the IV team does ultrasound-guided IV placement, hospitalists use ultrasound-guided aspiration techniques to tap ascites and pleural effusion, and endocrinologists as well as cytopathologists perform thyroid and neck node biopsies. There are other medical practices that use ultrasound for procedures, and there are other uses for ultrasound-guided procedures that these specialties may perform that are not listed. There are multiple factors contributing to this growth: the development of low-cost compact and laptop units, hands-on training with simulated biopsy phantoms provided by the ultrasound vendors, and training offered by various medical societies.

ULTRASOUND-GUIDED PROCEDURES

In recent years, there has been a movement to perform more and more procedures under ultrasound guidance. Retroperitoneal masses, pleural-based masses, deep masses in the liver, and MSK masses that were once typically biopsied with computed tomography (CT) guidance or in open surgical biopsies are now being successfully performed using ultrasound guidance (Fig. 18.2).

Ultrasound can be used to:
- Biopsy malignant or benign masses.
- Biopsy organs for parenchymal disease or transplant rejection.
- Drain various fluid collections, including cysts, joint effusions, ascites, or pleural fluid.
- Drain or obtain samples of abscesses to determine the type of organism, especially on patients who are not responding well to antibiotic therapy.
- Mark spots for fluid taps to be performed without direct sonographic guidance.
- Guide needles for nerve injections.
- Help place IV lines, especially on patients that are difficult sticks.

The main advantage of using ultrasound for guidance is that it has continuous real-time visualization of the needle, which allows adjustment of the needle as needed during the procedure. When used to guide biopsies, the needle tip can be watched in real time to ensure that it does not slip outside the mass. This is especially important for small masses or if the patient has trouble holding their breath. Ultrasound also has the advantage over CT of allowing different patient positions and approaches to be considered. The patient may be turned into a decubitus or oblique position to allow safe access to the mass (Fig. 18.3). Liver masses in the dome of the liver can be accessed by a subcostal approach using a steep angle with the needle directed cephalad, reducing the risk of a **pneumothorax**, which could happen with an intercostal approach. Using ultrasound, the patient can be placed in a comfortable position. For example, the patient's head may be slightly elevated, or the patient can move slightly between passes to relieve back or joint pain. Another benefit is the ability to comfort and reassure the patient, because the sonologist, sonographer, and nurse are with the patient during the entire procedure. Even the most anxious patients can be coached to cooperate when the team is by their side and not constantly in and out of the room. Other advantages include the ability to perform the biopsy in a single breath hold, portability, lack of radiation, and shorter procedure times.

Despite all its benefits, ultrasound guidance does have some limitations. Not all masses can be visualized with ultrasound, because the mass may be isoechoic to the normal

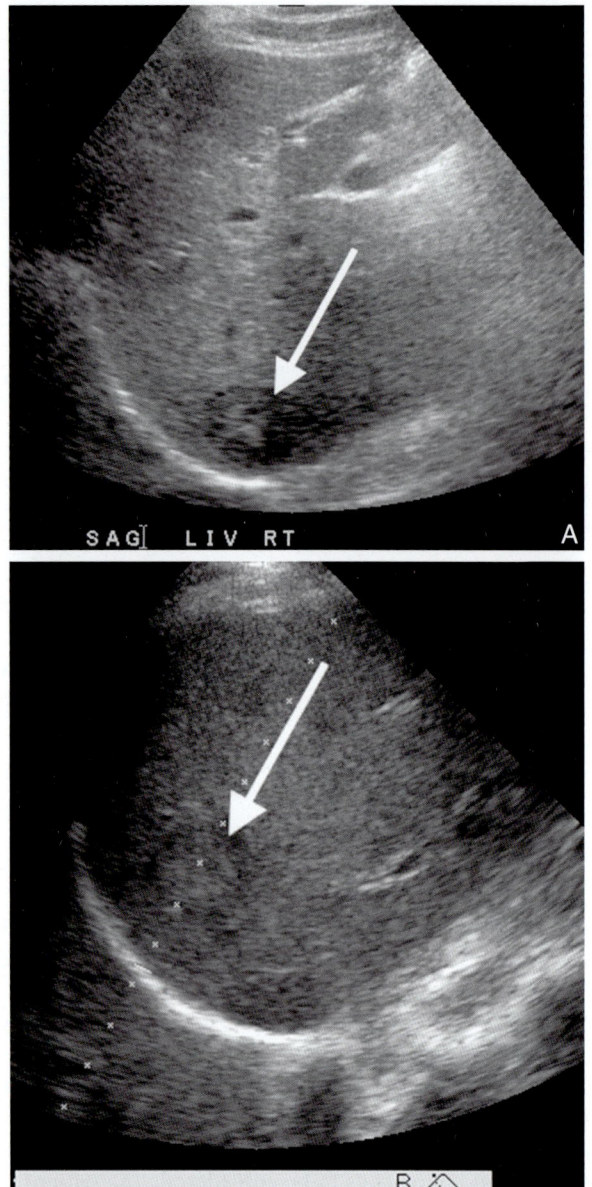

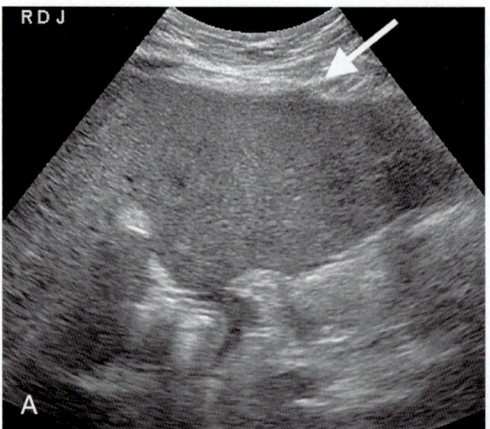

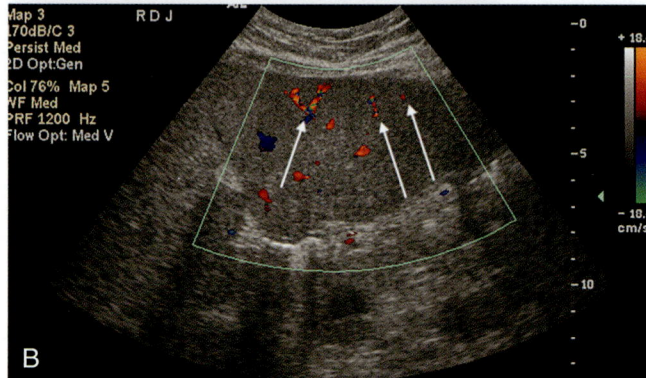

FIG. 18.3 (A) With the patient supine, the liver mass *(arrow)* is 15 cm deep. (B) The patient is now in the left lateral decubitus position, the liver has fallen forward, and the same mass *(arrow)* is now only 7 cm deep. An easy, successful biopsy showed metastatic disease from a pancreas primary.

FIG. 18.4 (A) Although a mass was seen on a contrast magnetic resonance imaging (MRI), it was not appreciated by ultrasound. Using the MRI as a guide and looking for indirect signs, the area was identified. The arrow is pointing to a bulge in the capsule. (B) Color Doppler found areas of abnormal flow in the area of the bulge *(arrows)*. A successful biopsy diagnosed infiltrative hepatocellular carcinoma.

tissue. When this is the case, the sonographer should look for indirect signs of the presence of a mass, such as displaced vessel capsule bulges or the presence of tumor vessels (Fig. 18.4). These isoechoic masses may potentially be biopsied using fusion technology or contrast imaging. Abdominal masses may be obscured by bowel gas, or gas may move during the procedure, causing difficulty in seeing the mass. The sonographer can try to press the gas out of the way with the transducer. If this does not work, the biopsy may be canceled under ultrasound and either performed under CT or rescheduled for another day. There may be issues seeing the needle tip, especially if it deviates from the projected path. This problem relies on the sonographer's scanning skills to maneuver the transducer to find the needle tip or to correct for needle deviation. By understanding the cause of the deviation, the sonographer can determine how to correct for it, allowing for a successful biopsy (Fig. 18.5). It sometimes felt like some of our best samples occurred when we could not see the needle tip. A major limitation can be the comfort level of both the sonographer and the sonologist. Without proper training, they both can feel intimidated and not confident, especially if the radiologist has a comfort level using CT guidance.

INDICATIONS FOR A BIOPSY

The most common indication for a biopsy is to confirm if a mass is malignant. The mass may be a primary tumor in a patient or a metastatic mass in a patient with an unknown primary. The liver is a common place for metastatic disease, and these masses can be easily biopsied using ultrasound. With a biopsy of the metastatic tumor, the primary tumor can be determined. Other indications include the need to differentiate between a metastatic mass and a second primary, to differentiate recurrent tumor from postoperative or therapy scarring, to differentiate malignancy from inflammatory or infectious disease, to determine metastatic lymph adenopathy from lymphoma, or to characterize a benign mass. Procedures that are not mass related include obtaining a sample of the parenchyma of an organ to determine the severity or progression of a disease such as fatty liver, hepatitis, or renal failure or to obtain a sample of tissue to determine the cause of rejection in a transplanted organ (Fig. 18.6).

CONTRAINDICATIONS FOR A BIOPSY

Contraindications of ultrasound-guided procedures are few because of the procedure's minimally invasive nature. Most contraindications include an uncorrectable bleeding disorder, the lack of a safe needle pathway (Fig. 18.7), or an uncooperative patient. Patient cooperation is needed so that the mass may be biopsied safely. If the patient will not hold still, is jumpy, or cannot control their breathing, the risk of a complication for the patient increases significantly, as does the risk to the sonographer or sonologist of being stuck by a contaminated needle.

LABORATORY TESTS

With the exception of bleeding times, blood or urine tests are not needed before an ultrasound-guided procedure. An abnormal laboratory value will be part of the patient's work-up that led to the biopsy. Some abnormal values that may trigger a request for a biopsy or aspiration include elevated **alpha-fetoprotein (AFP)** in the presence of a liver lesion, elevated **prostate-specific antigen (PSA)** to evaluate the prostate for cancer, changes in thyroglobulin levels

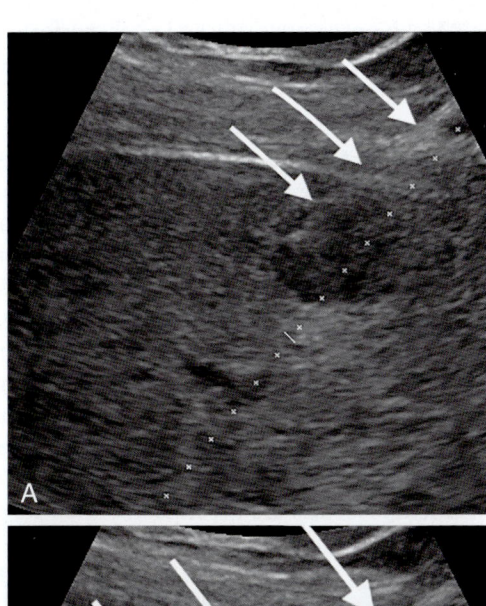

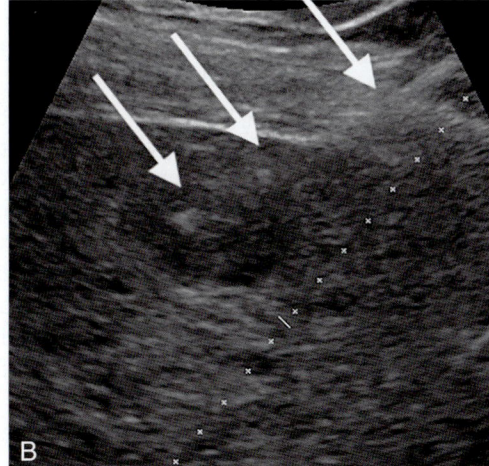

FIG. 18.5 (A) The needle *(arrows)* deviated from the projected path of the guide *(dotted line)*. (B) Because of the constant deviation of the needle from the projected path, the sonographer had to compensate by moving the transducer laterally so that the needle would pass through the center of the mass. Note that the projected path does not even go through the mass. A diagnosis of hepatocellular carcinoma was obtained.

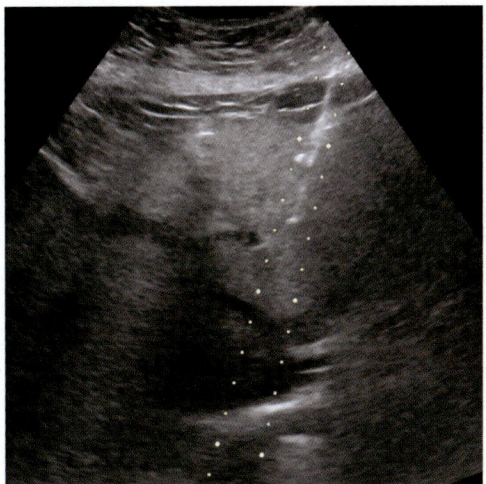

FIG. 18.6 A liver core on a fatty liver.

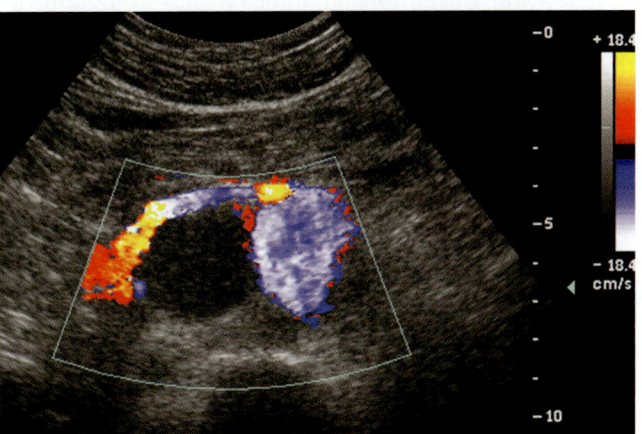

FIG. 18.7 This retroperitoneal lymph node could not be biopsied under ultrasound because of the vessels that surrounded it.

in a patient with a history of thyroid cancer, and increased white blood cell count, leukocytosis, when an abscess is suspected.

It is important to know that the patient will stop bleeding after the needle is removed and does not have a blood clotting problem. Therefore blood tests that determine the patient's bleeding times should be reviewed before most procedures. These tests measure the time it takes the blood to form a clot. This is especially needed for patients who are on blood thinners such as warfarin or Coumadin, heparin, or aspirin therapy. Because vitamin K is essential in the blood clotting process, patients with liver disease can be at a risk for prolonged bleeding times. To eliminate patient rescheduling or cancellation, test results should be obtained as close to the date of the procedure as possible, although results may be acceptable up to 3 to 4 weeks before the scheduled procedure, depending on the type of procedure and the guidelines of the lab where the procedure is being performed.

At least a dozen factors are needed to form a blood clot to stop bleeding; they all interact through a complex series of reactions called the coagulation cascade. There are three pathways in the blood clotting process: intrinsic, extrinsic, and common. To evaluate all three pathways, both **prothrombin time (PT)** and **partial thromboplastin time (PTT)** may be evaluated. PTT measures the time it takes a clot to form and is also used to evaluate the effects of heparin therapy. PTT evaluates factors found in the intrinsic and common pathways. PTT values may vary depending on the method and activators used, with normal values typically between 30 and 45 seconds. PT also tells the physician how likely the patient is to have a bleeding or clotting problem during or after surgery and is used to evaluate factors found in the extrinsic pathway, which may be affected by patients on Coumadin. Normal values are typically between 10 and 13 seconds. Because of the variability of PT results between laboratories, a method of standardization was developed called the **international normalized ratio (INR)**. The INR test was created in 1983 by the World Health Organization (WHO) to account for the various thromboplastin reagents used to determine PT. The INR is a calculation that adjusts for the variations in PT processing and values so that test results from different laboratories can be compared. The INR is expressed as a number. Values of less than 1.4 are needed to ensure a safe procedure. The INR/PT is not used on patients with liver disease or on heparin. It is evaluated on patients taking anticoagulants, especially Coumadin. In addition to PT, PTT, and INR, the patient's platelet count may be required. Patients with a defect in their blood clotting mechanism, **coagulopathy**, will need to have a platelet transfusion just before and during the procedure to ensure that their body can form a blood clot to stop any bleeding. Some departments may not require a hemostatic evaluation for fluid aspirations and superficial biopsies with a low risk of bleeding such as of the thyroid, neck nodes, or prostate.

Anticoagulants should be discontinued before the biopsy to reduce the risk of postprocedural bleeding. Patients should be off their blood thinners before the procedure as follows: 4 to 6 hours for heparin, 5 days for Coumadin, and 5 days for aspirin, although these values can be different for different hospitals or imaging centers. Patients need to discuss stopping these drugs with their physician. Recent studies have shown that patients taking omega-3 and fish oils do not have an increased risk for postprocedural bleeding and that they may be actually beneficial, so stopping them is no longer required. The reader is encouraged to stay current on medicines and supplements that might put the patient at an increased risk of prolonged bleeding after a procedure.

ULTRASOUND-GUIDED BIOPSY EQUIPMENT AND TECHNIQUES

Biopsies are used to confirm if a mass is benign, malignant, or infectious. Most biopsies are easily and safely performed as an outpatient procedure. Good success rates have been reported using ultrasound for biopsy guidance. Cell type is often needed to determine treatment type and options, as specific tumors respond better to certain types of chemotherapy or to radiation therapy. **Fine-needle aspiration (FNA)** uses thin-gauge needles to obtain cells from within the mass. FNAs are performed using a 20- to 25-gauge needle with a cutting tip, such as a Franseen, Chiba, or spinal needle (Fig. 18.8). These types of needles have the least risk associated with their use, allowing multiple passes as needed. The number of the gauge corresponds to the diameter of the needle, the higher the number, the smaller the diameter, and refers to the inner measurement or opening of the needle. For example, a 20-gauge needle has a 0.6-mm internal diameter, and an 18 gauge has a 0.8 mm internal diameter. Needles are described by their length and gauge. For example, if the physician asks for a 20 × 15 needle, they want a 20-gauge needle that is 15 cm in length. If different types of needles are available, the physician might ask for a specific type of needle for that procedure. For example, they may ask for a Franseen 20, 15 meaning they want a Franseen style needle that is 20 gauge and 15 cm long. The needles are color coded so that by looking at the color of the hub you know the needle size. 25 Gauge needles are blue, 22 gauge are black, 20 gauge are yellow, and 18 gauge are pink (see Fig. 18.8A). This is a universal coloring system. Seeing the length of the needle may cause a patient to become quite apprehensive. The sonographer should explain to the patient that most of the needle will be inside the needle guide and not in their body. I would also tell the patient that it is the diameter of the needle that causes pain and not the length, and we usually use needles that are smaller than used to take their blood. The specimen is obtained by using a capillary action technique. This involves a steady, quick up-and-down motion of the needle, after the stylet is removed, which obtains the needed cells through a scraping or cutting action. As the needle is removed from the body, the physician will place their thumb over the open hub

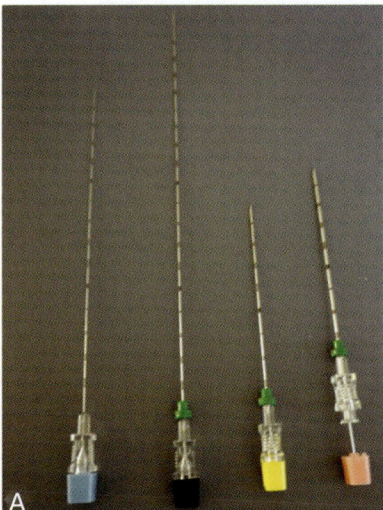

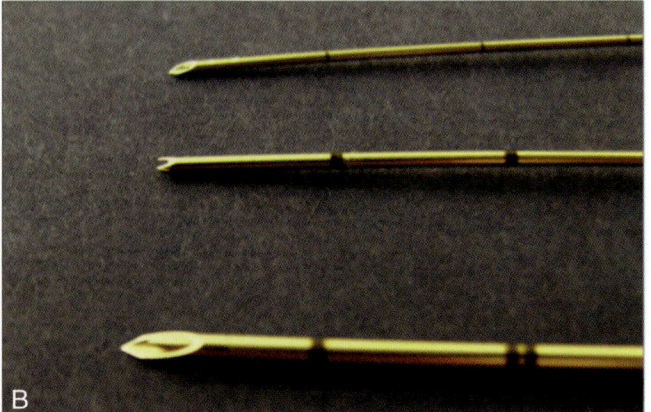

FIG. 18.8 (A) Different types of needles and gauges used for fine-needle aspiration biopsies. Blue: 25 gauge × 15 cm; black: 22 gauge × 20 cm; yellow: 20 gauge × 9 cm; pink: 18 gauge × 9 cm. (B) Different types of needle tips. *From top:* Chiba, Franseen, Spinal.

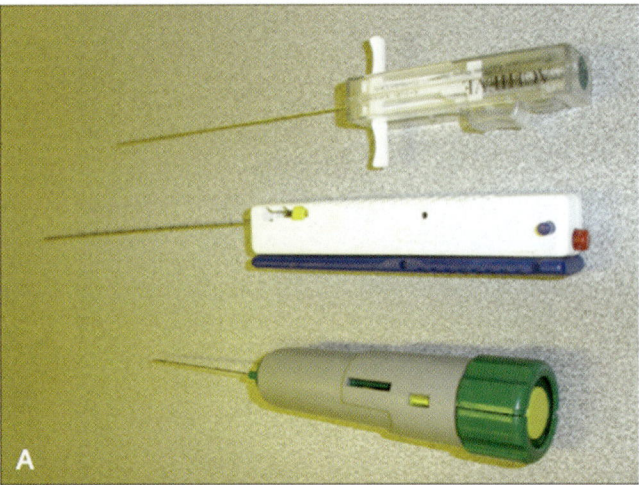

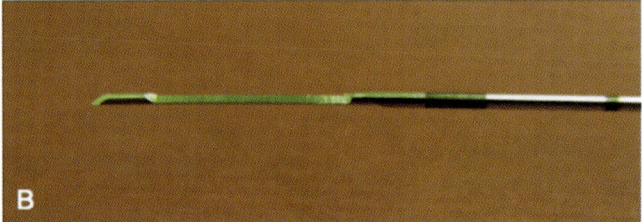

FIG. 18.9 (A) Biopsy devices used for core biopsies. (B) Close-up of a core needle where the specimen is deposited.

so that the cells are not sucked back into the body. An FNA technique reduces the trauma to the cells and decreases the amount of background blood. If the sample is scant, suction techniques can be used. Suction technique involves using a syringe and tubing attached to the needle. As the needle is being moved up and down, suction is applied to draw up the cells into the needle. Once the needle is removed, the physician will place the tip of the needle over the slide to deposit the cells so that they can be smeared for staining and evaluation. The physician may also express the cells into a container holding special fluid to preserve the cells. Because of its thin size, this type of needle can safely go through the gastrointestinal tract and near vascular structures. FNA in conjunction with onsite cytopathology can help ensure that the procedure is diagnostic and minimize the number of passes.

A **core biopsy** uses an automated, spring-loaded device, termed a **biopsy gun**, to obtain a core of tissue for histologic analysis (Fig. 18.9). The biopsy device is cocked, and the needle tip is placed just inside the mass or on the outside edge of the mass. For a biopsy of an organ for parenchymal disease, the needle tip can be placed just inside the organ itself. Sometimes if the needle tip is just on the outside of the organ and then fired, going through the capsule could sometimes deflect the needle as the capsule offers some resistance. The Glisson capsule is a good example because you can see the needle pushing the capsule out of the way but never piercing it when positioning the needle. This is called tenting (Fig. 18.10). The button is then pushed, and the cutting needle is thrown, obtaining a core of tissue, which is deposited into the slot on the inner needle (see Fig. 18.9B). Various throw lengths are available, ranging from 10 to 23 mm, which will correspond to the length of the specimen that is obtained. The throw length is the distance that the cutting needle will advance when fired. The inner needle that receives the specimen is stationary. The proper throw distance needs to be determined so that the needle does not go through the back wall of the mass and damage underlying structures or vessels (Fig. 18.11). The snapping sound that the device makes can be startling to the patient, and it is advised to let the patient hear the sound before obtaining the specimen. This also ensures that the device is not defective. Core biopsy needles are larger in diameter and range in size from 14 to 20 gauge. A core biopsy can be used in conjunction with FNA techniques, especially if a definitive diagnosis could not be determined from the FNA or if the cytopathologist requires more tissue for special stains to confirm or make the diagnosis. Core biopsies are used to diagnose diffuse parenchymal disease of the liver, kidney, and transplanted organs (Fig. 18.12), as well as masses in the breast and prostate.

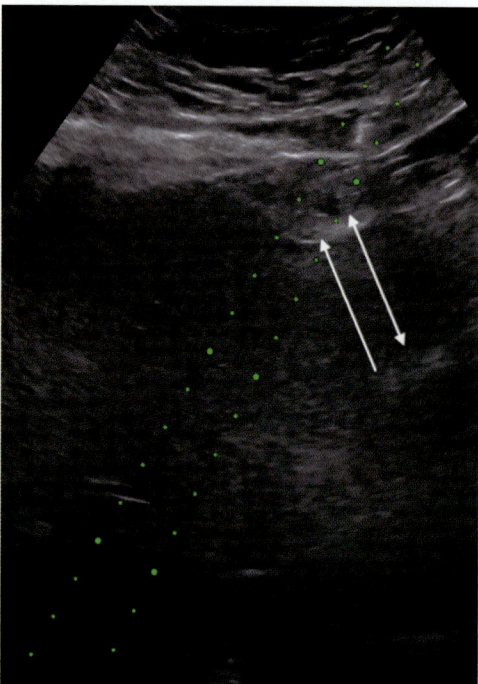

FIG. 18.10 *Arrow* shows where the needle is tenting the capsule. The *double arrow* points to the needle tip.

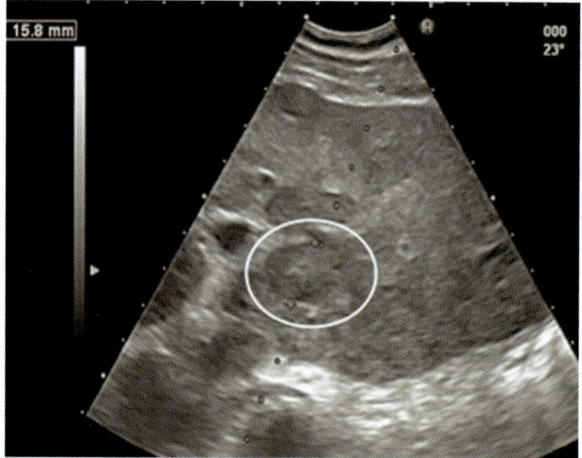

FIG. 18.11 The sonographer measured the lesion (calipers in circle) to determine the size of the core needle to be used. The diameter of the lesion along the needle path is 15.8 mm, so a 15-mm throw is needed to stay within the lesion.

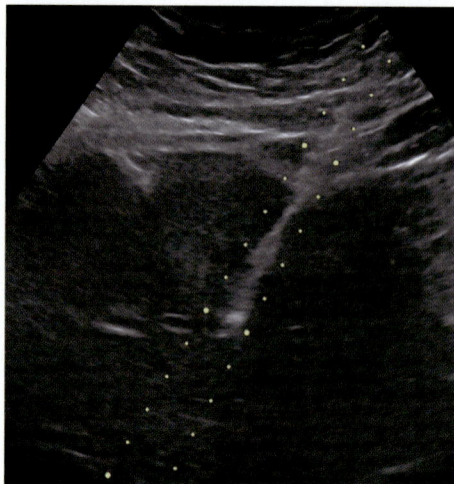

FIG. 18.12 A core biopsy to stage a patient with a fatty liver.

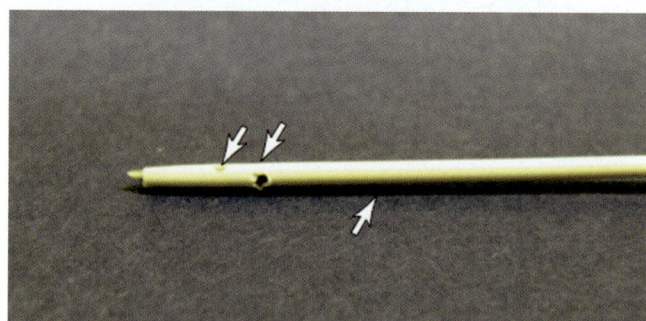

FIG. 18.13 A centesis catheter. The arrows point to the side holes.

Ultrasound is routinely used to guide needle placement to drain or obtain samples from ascites or pleural effusions. Usually, these procedures are performed without the use of a needle guide unless the fluid is multiloculated, is only a small amount, or is unsafe to drain by free-hand techniques. If a small amount of fluid is needed, a 22- or 20-gauge needle may be used. If the fluid is viscous, an 18- or a 16-gauge needle may be required. If the goal is to drain as much fluid as possible, a special catheter, called a centesis catheter, is used (Fig. 18.13). After the needle is properly placed, the stylet is removed, leaving the catheter which will have multiple side holes to drain the fluid. For large volume drainage, a 1-L vacuum bottle is used to drain the fluid as the vacuum pressure will draw the fluid out. As the bottle gets full, it is replaced with another empty bottle. This continues until no more fluid is draining into the bottle. If the vacuum becomes broken, the fluid will not drain. This will occur if the draining tubing is not closed off when inserting the spike into the collection jar. Ultrasound can be used periodically to check the amount of fluid remaining or when the fluid stops draining to help reposition the catheter or to free it from bowel that may have been sucked against the wall of the catheter (Fig. 18.14). The sonographer can usually scan outside the sterile field on these exams (Fig. 18.15). In a patient with massive ascites, a large volume of fluid may be drained for patient comfort. It is usually recommended that no more than 4 to 6 L be drained because draining more than that can place the patient at risk for electrolyte imbalance, hypovolemia, hypotension, and hepatorenal syndrome. If more than 5 L are to be removed, the patient is usually given IV albumin to decrease the chance of these complications.

Fluid or abscess collections are usually performed using a needle guide. Abscess or fluid collections may be located in or around the liver, in the peripancreatic, perinephric, intra-abdominal, pelvic, or intramuscular regions, or in the prostate gland. The needle gauge used to drain the fluid depends on the thickness of the fluid. For pelvic collections, depending on their location, an endovaginal approach can be considered and endorectal approaches in both men and women. For prostatic abscess drainage, an endorectal technique is used. Fluid is obtained to determine the type of organism present, so that the correct antibiotics can be administered to the patient. For a large abscess, catheters may be left in place to drain the collection. Patients may have follow-ups to monitor that the cavity is getting smaller and to check that the catheter is still in the correct position. These follow-up examinations are performed under fluoroscopy in a procedure called a sinogram, which uses iodinated contrast media to outline the cavity. It can be common for the person calling to schedule the patient's exam incorrectly as a sonogram as opposed to a sinogram because the names are only one letter different and sound similar. Asking the reason for the exam will uncover that a sinogram is needed and not a sonogram.

Ultrasound is used in the radiology interventional lab to guide placements of catheters and lines in various vessels, including the subclavian, jugular, brachial, and femoral vessels, to assist in transjugular intrahepatic portosystemic shunt procedures, and to place nephrostomy tubes in obstructed kidneys.

ULTRASOUND GUIDANCE METHODS

There are three different methods to perform an ultrasound-guided procedure: in-plane and out-of-plane free-hand techniques and using needle guides. The free-hand technique is performed without the use of a needle guide on the transducer. The transducer is placed in a sterile cover, and the radiologist, or the physician who performs the biopsy, will hold the transducer in one hand and the needle in the other hand. The in-plane technique is similar to using a guide in that the needle will approach from the short end of the transducer so that the shaft of the needle can be seen as it advances through the tissue (Fig. 18.16). Care must be taken to align the needle with the soundbeam, using the transducer as a guide, or else the needle tip will not be seen as it traverses the soundbeam. If the needle tip disappears while advancing the needle on the image, the transducer should be repositioned in alignment with the needle path to bring the needle tip back into view (Fig. 18.17). If this causes the area of interest to no longer be seen, the

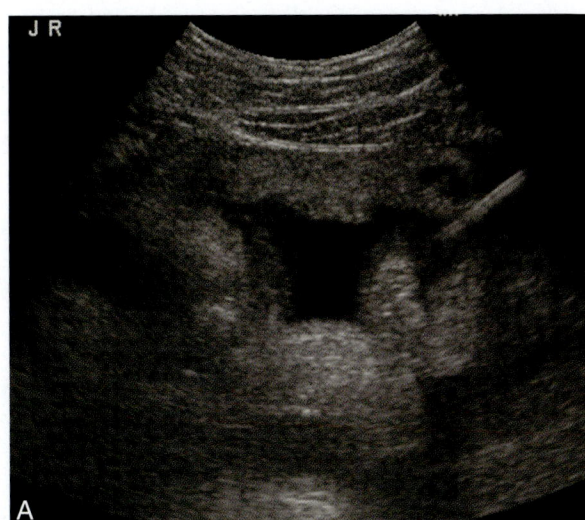
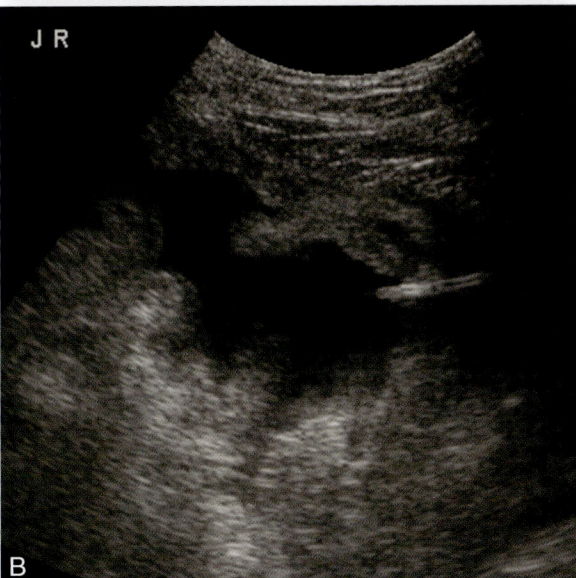

FIG. 18.14 (A) Bowel has been sucked up against the catheter, obstructing the flow of fluid. (B) By having the patient roll into an oblique position, the fluid collected to the dependent portion and the bowel loop floated away from the catheter, allowing drainage to continue.

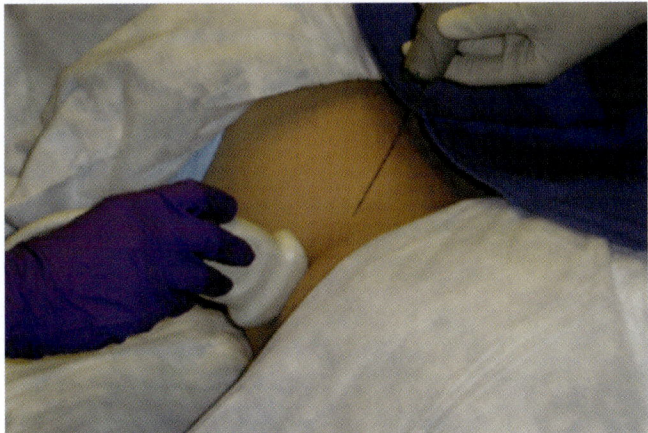

FIG. 18.15 Two-person free-hand technique with the sonographer scanning outside the sterile field.

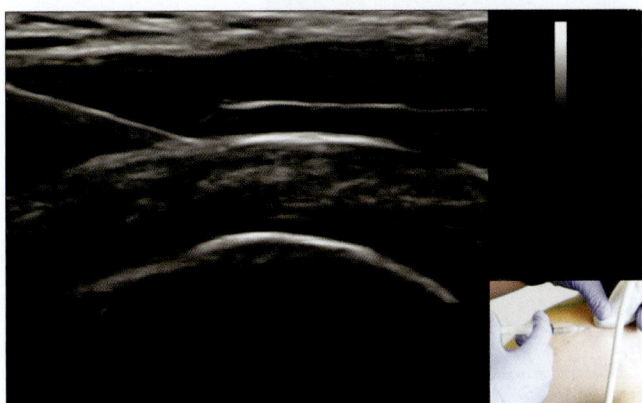

FIG. 18.16 A corticosteroid injection of the shoulder using an in-plane technique. (Courtesy Colin Rigney PT, DPT, OCS, RMSK.)

needle should be withdrawn and inserted again. It is important to remember that to see the needle tip, the transducer must be aligned to the needle path. If deviation continues to be an issue, the last resort would be to attach a needle guide.

The out-of-plane technique is favored for superficial procedures in which the needle would not be seen until it is in the area of interest, such as starting an IV line. With this technique the needle approaches the long side of the transducer and the needle is not visualized until the tip intercepts the soundbeam, causing a bright white echo to appear (Fig. 18.18). It is important that the needle approaches the transducer at a perpendicular angle and stays on course for a successful procedure. If the needle approaches the transducer at a slight angle, the needle will miss the target area and be either lateral or medial to the target. Although the needle may start out perpendicular to the transducer before it pierces the skin, it is easy to slightly angle the needle while shifting your focus to observe the monitor. This is a drawback of this approach because you cannot see that the needle is not heading to the target until it has missed it.

The third method involves using a needle guide that is attached to the transducer. Each transducer type will have its own needle guide (Fig. 18.19). The predicted needle path is displayed on the screen either as a single line or as two parallel lines (Fig. 18.20). The mass is then lined up along the path, either on the single line or between the two lines. Some transducers offer a choice of angles, usually a steep angle, a shallow angle, and one or three angles in between (Fig. 18.21).

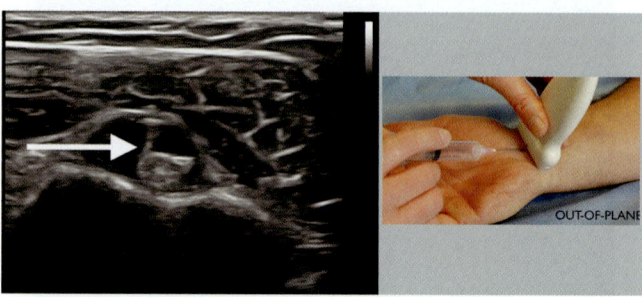

FIG. 18.18 A bicep sheath injection using an out-of-plane technique. (Courtesy Colin Rigney PT, DPT, OCS, RMSK.)

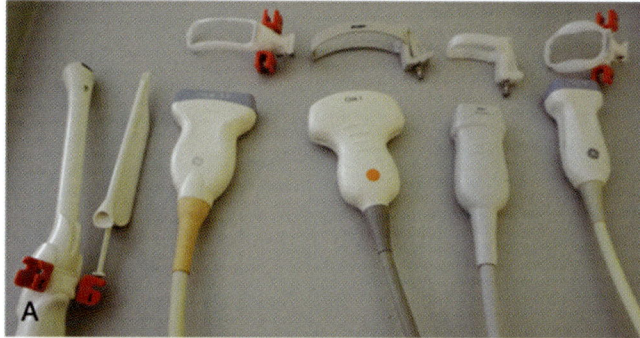

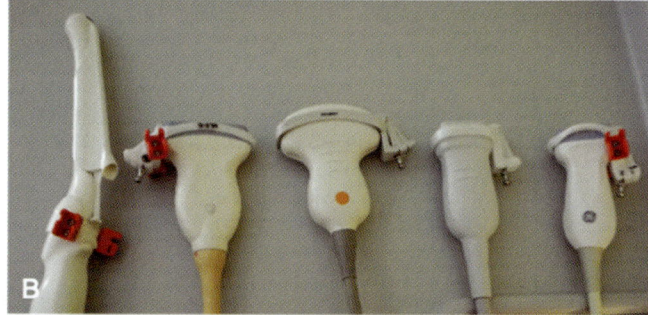

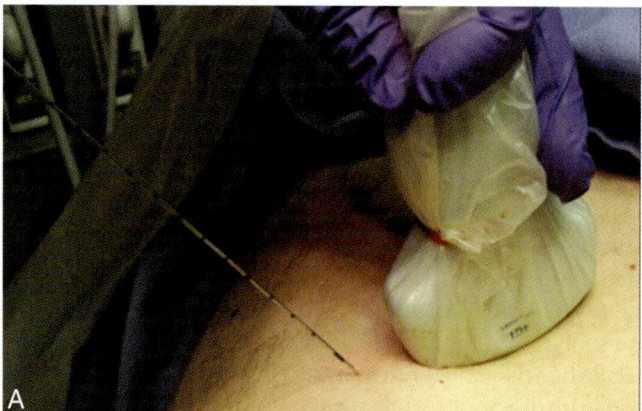

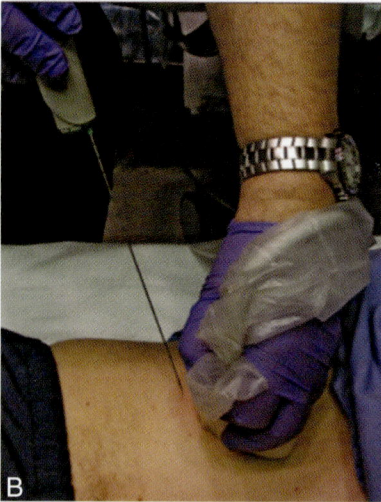

FIG. 18.17 One-person free-hand technique. (A) The needle is not in plane with the transducer, and the needle tip could not be seen. (B) The transducer has now been moved to be in line with the needle.

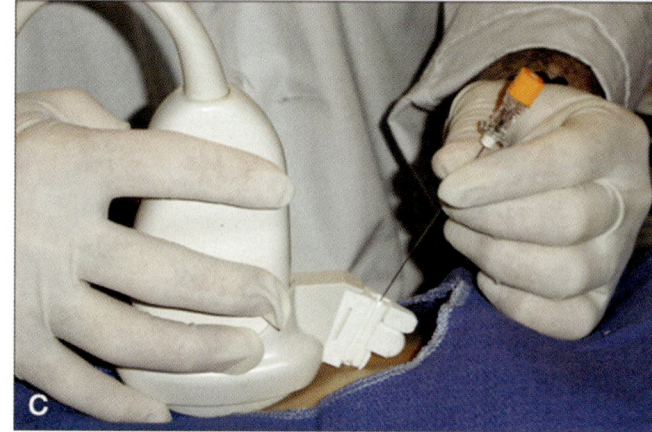

FIG. 18.19 (A) Various types of transducers and their guides. (B) Same transducers with their guides attached. (C) Biopsy using a needle guide.

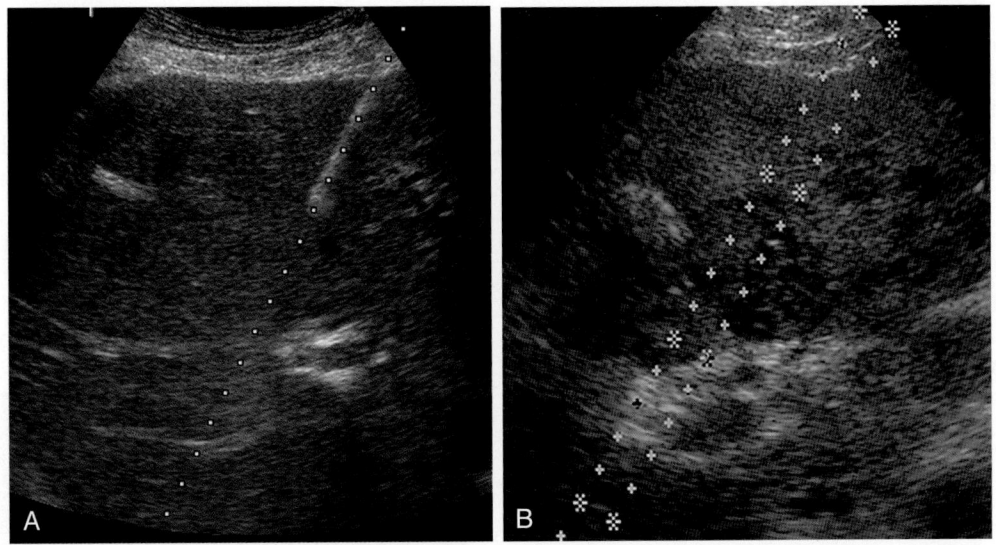

FIG. 18.20 (A) A single line predicted needle path on a liver core biopsy. (B) An example of two lines for the predicted needle path on a patient with metastatic pancreatic liver cancer.

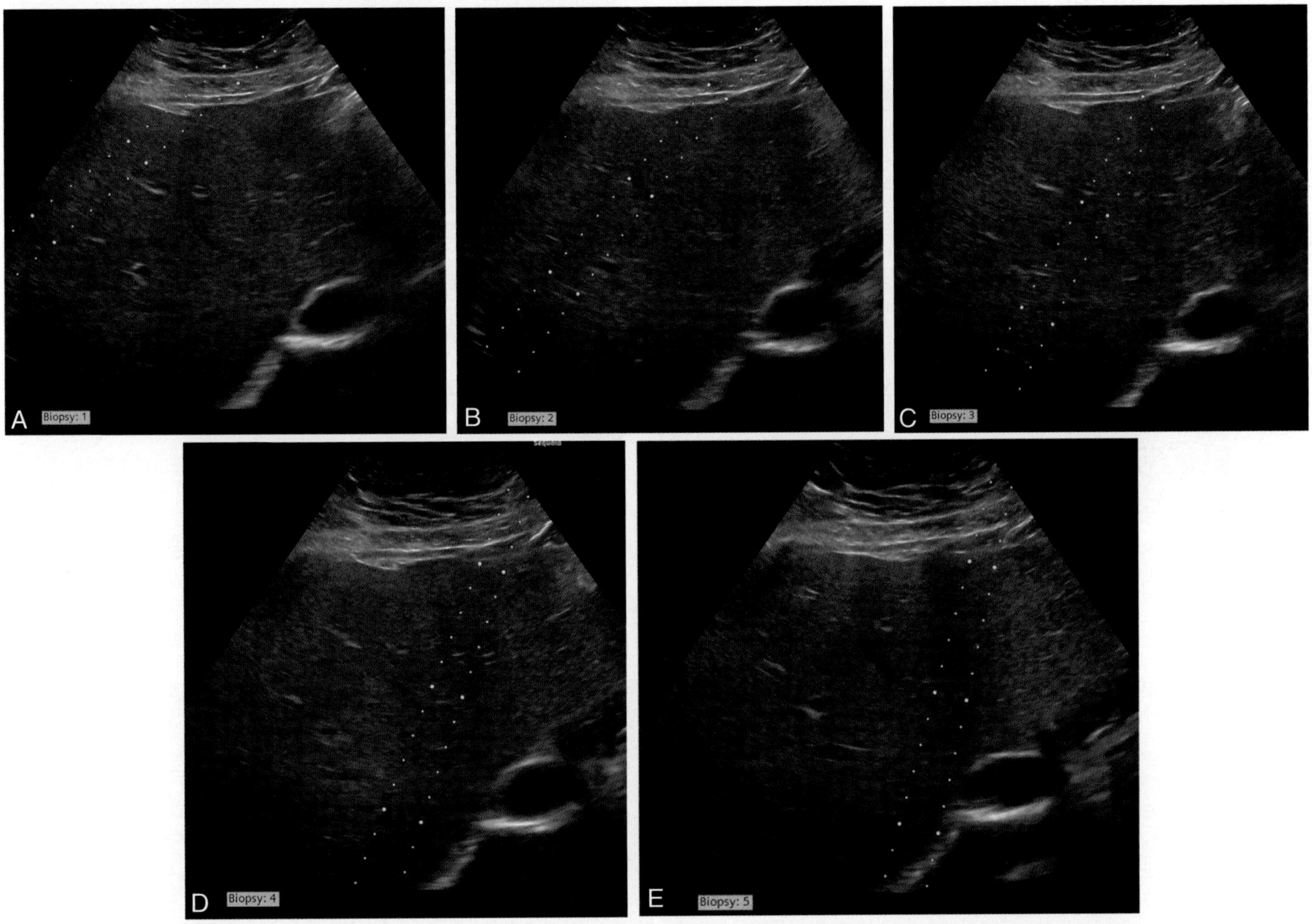

FIG. 18.21 This system offers a choice of five different angles. Biopsy 3 (C) or biopsy 4 (D) would be used for this liver core biopsy.

This gives some flexibility for finding the best approach and to avoid vessels and other structures as needed. There are many benefits to using a needle guide, which may include a faster learning curve especially for the sonologist, more accurate placement of the needle, and the ability to keep the needle going through the anesthetized area when multiple passes are required. The use of needle guides has expanded the role of ultrasound-guided procedures by allowing biopsies of pleural-based lung lesions (Fig. 18.22), deep retroperitoneal lesions, and small masses. When the sonographer attaches the needle guide to the transducer, it is important to attach it correctly and set the angle on the guide to the same angle as on the screen (Fig. 18.23). The needle guides are precision-made devices and need to be handled with care and attached properly. If the angle that is set on the transducer is not the same angle as on the screen, the needle will appear to deviate, as it is not following the projected path on the screen; if the guide is put on backward, the needle will come in from the opposite side of the guide (Fig. 18.24).

All methods have their pros and cons, and the physician performing the biopsy or procedure will decide which technique is the best and offers the safest approach.

CYTOPATHOLOGY

Some ultrasound departments collaborate with the cytopathology department by having the cytopathology team present during the procedure. Usually, one to three passes are made, placed on the sterile slides, and stained in the ultrasound room. The cytopathologist looks at the slides to determine if the material is diagnostic. This can ensure that enough diagnostic material is obtained and helps to minimize the number of passes. If it is a necrotic mass, the cytopathologist can determine the best area to obtain good material. They might say "pass number 3 was good," so the sonographer should try to remember the areas biopsied so that they can return to that location. The cytopathologist may request additional material for special stains and flow cytometry. (Flow cytometry may be needed when lymphoma is suspected.) The cytopathologist may also request that a core sample be obtained to enhance the chances of obtaining a diagnosis for the patient. It typically takes 3 to 5 minutes to stain and

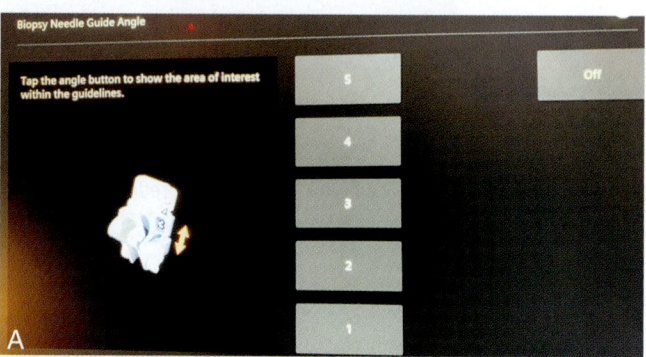

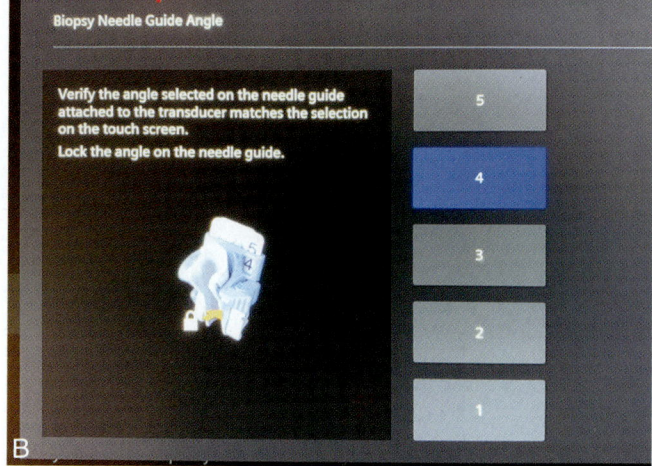

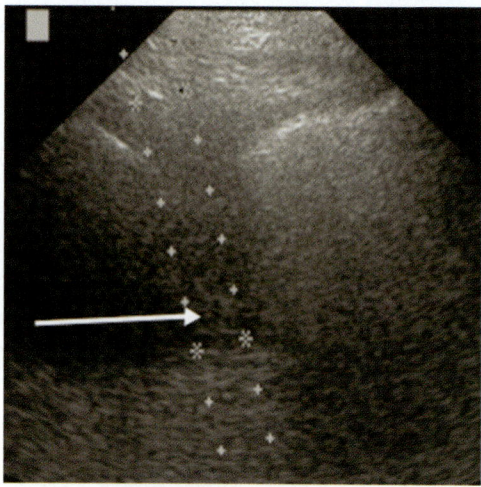

FIG. 18.22 Biopsy of a pleural-based lung mass. Although a noisy image, the break in the white line, which represents the pleura, helps to locate the mass. The *arrow* points to the needle tip. This was an adenocarcinoma.

FIG. 18.23 (A) The screen to set the chosen angle. "Off" will turn off the biopsy guide. (B) Four has been selected as the best angle. The unit reminds the sonographer to verify the angle on the guide.

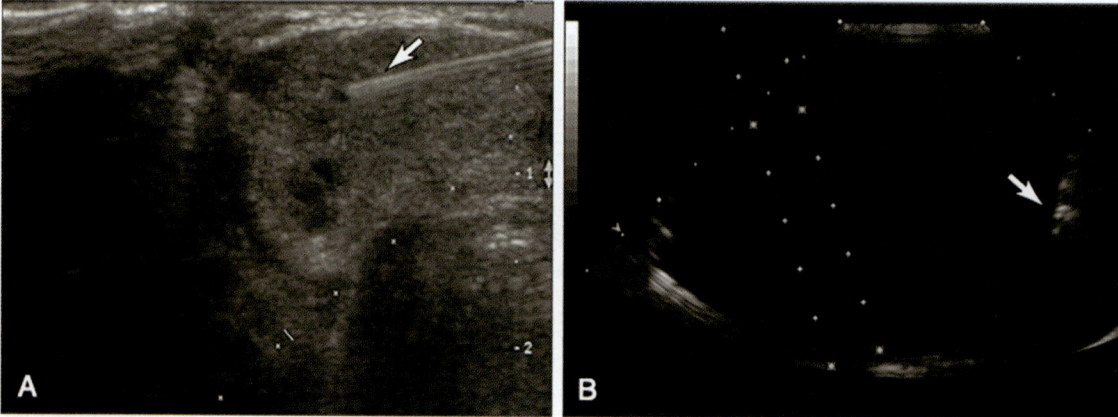

FIG. 18.24 (A) The *arrow* points to the needle, which appears to be deviating. In fact, the guide setting on the transducer does not match the setting on the unit. (B) The bracket was attached backward. When the needle is inserted *(arrow)*, it appears from the opposite side of the screen.

evaluate the slides per pass or group of passes. It is important to tell the patient why the radiologist is waiting before the next pass. The benefit of having cytopathology onsite is that it increases the percentage of successful biopsies, helps to minimize the number of passes, and possibly reduces overall procedure time. For some biopsies, such as a thyroid biopsy, only a cytopathology technician may be present to evaluate the specimen. They will not give a diagnosis but have the skills to determine if the pass is diagnostic. With the changes in health care, having a cytopathologist or even a cytopathology technician in the room is now a rare occurrence.

Inconclusive Specimens

Unfortunately, not all biopsies yield sufficient material to provide a diagnosis. There are multiple reasons that can lead to an inconclusive result, including insufficient material, necrotic areas in the lesion making it difficult to find viable cells, and not sampling the area where there are malignant cells. The possibility of an inconclusive result should have been explained to the patient during the consent process. The patient should be given the option of a repeat biopsy. The radiologist may prefer to repeat the biopsy with CT, although that is not a guarantee of a successful outcome.

BIOPSY COMPLICATIONS

Complications from an ultrasound-guided biopsy are usually minor and may include postprocedural pain or discomfort, vasovagal reaction, and hematoma. Serious complications, although rare, include hemorrhage, pneumothorax, pancreatitis, infection, and possibly death. Another complication is tumor seeding of the needle track, allowing tumor dissemination outside of the biopsied mass. If this occurs, it can change the staging of the tumor or cause metastatic disease. It is estimated to occur in approximately 1 in 20,000 patients. These potential complications must be explained to the patient during the consent process. It is important for the sonographer to look for any sign of a complication by observing the patient and scanning the area where the biopsy took place. The sonographer should scan after every pass to look for any sonographic sign of bleeding both with gray scale and color Doppler (Fig. 18.25). The sonographer should observe the patient for any indication of a vasovagal reaction or active bleeding from the biopsy site. Any complication should be reported to the physician immediately. Applying pressure with the transducer over the area of bleeding can treat both internal and external bleeding. For bleeding from the skin at the biopsy site, cover the puncture site with a sterile 4 × 4 gauze and press with

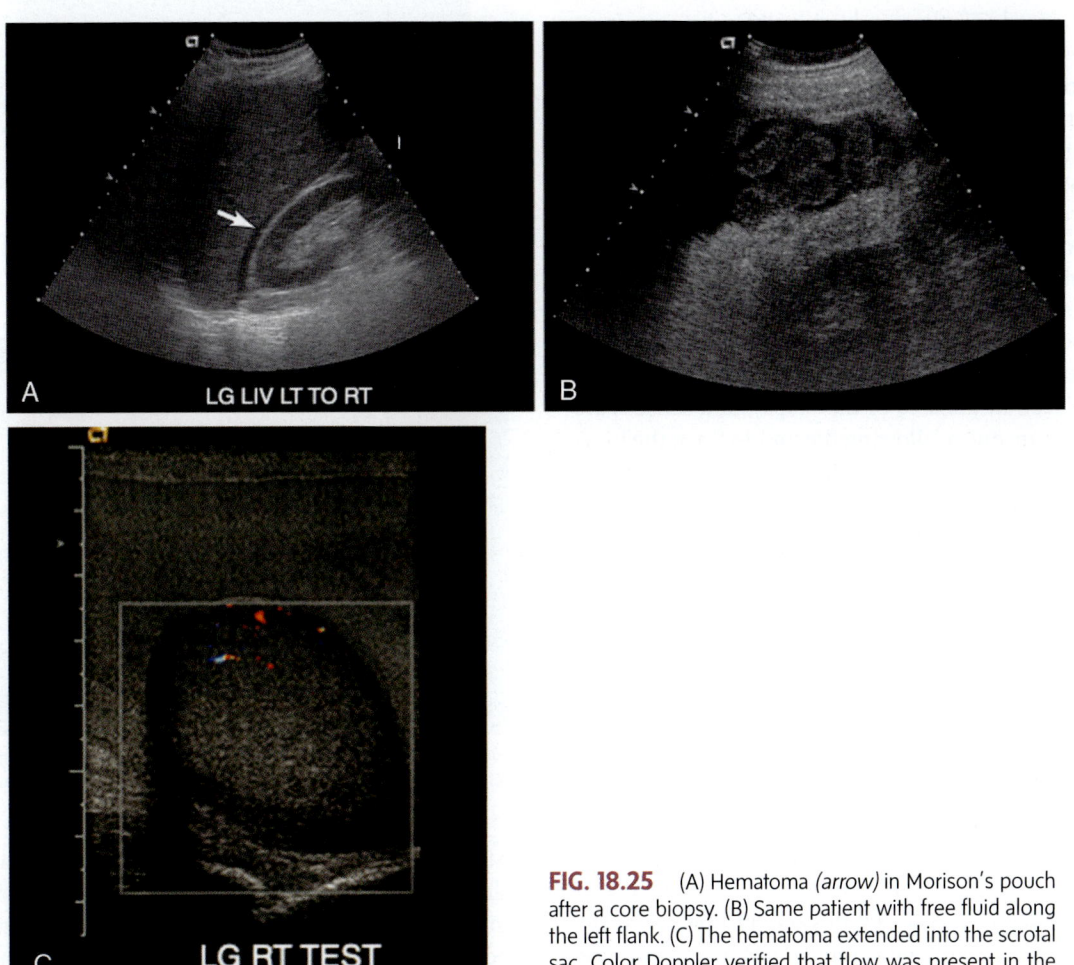

FIG. 18.25 (A) Hematoma *(arrow)* in Morison's pouch after a core biopsy. (B) Same patient with free fluid along the left flank. (C) The hematoma extended into the scrotal sac. Color Doppler verified that flow was present in the testicle.

the transducer. The sterile 4 × 4 gauze will absorb the blood so that it does not drip down the patient's side and will lend stability to the transducer so that it does not slide. Vasovagal symptoms include paleness, profuse sweating, complaining of feeling faint or lightheaded, passing out, and nausea. The vasovagal syncope occurs as a reaction to something and causes the heart rate and blood pressure to drop suddenly. It is thought that this can occur during a biopsy due to the stress of the situation or the body's reaction to pain even though the patient does not feel any. A vasovagal reaction causes reduced blood flow to the brain, causing the patient to lose consciousness. The patient should be placed in a Trendelenburg position or have their feet elevated with a stack of sheets to help restore blood back to the brain. A cold cloth or compress can also be placed on the forehead to help cool the patient down. After these feelings pass, the biopsy may continue.

FUSION TECHNOLOGY

Newer technologies have expanded the ability to perform ultrasound-guided procedures. Harmonic and compound imaging have improved resolution and decreased artifacts in the image, improving visualization of subtler lesions as well as the needle tip (Fig. 18.26). However, there are still some lesions that cannot be seen by ultrasound because they are isoechoic, especially in the liver. These lesions are usually seen only on a contrast-enhanced CT, thus making it difficult to perform the biopsy even under CT guidance. Some ultrasound systems have an option called fusion technology. Fusion will allow the ultrasound unit to import the patient's CT or magnetic resonance imaging (MRI) images directly into the ultrasound unit. This technology allows the CT/MRI images to be in sync with the active ultrasound images as the sonographer scans. Thus the same anatomy is seen in real time on both the ultrasound and the CT/MRI images, allowing the sonographer to compare the two sets of images in side-by-side format (Fig. 18.27).

This technology has evolved over the years and is now much easier and quicker to set up. An electromagnetic field generator is placed in the area of the biopsy, and sensors are attached to the transducer, allowing the unit to track the location of the transducer. Newer transducers have these sensors built into the transducer. Some systems also allow the ability to use special needles that will track the needle tip or a sensor to be placed on the hub of the needle to track the needle.

To begin, the MRI or CT data set, usually CT, must be imported into the ultrasound unit. This can either be done via the network or uploaded from a DVD. Next is the fusing process. The sonographer obtains a sweep through the organ of interest, such as the liver. Then the ultrasound unit performs an autoregistration that finds the anatomic information within the CT/MRI volume and automatically matches it with the ultrasound volume. This process usually takes less than 1 minute to perform. In some scenarios the sonographer may have to find and mark common anatomic points that can be identified on both the ultrasound image and the CT/MRI image. This technique is more challenging and time consuming. As the ultrasound transducer is moved, the CT/

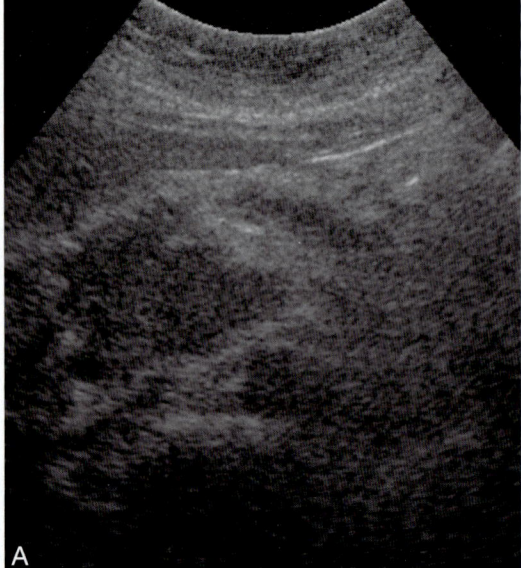

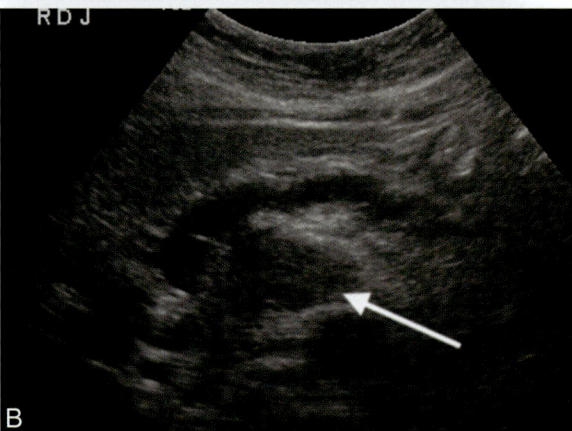

FIG. 18.26 (A) A biopsy was requested of the pancreatic head mass. (B) Because there was a lot of noise in the image, compound imaging was activated. The mass *(arrow)* is now well defined.

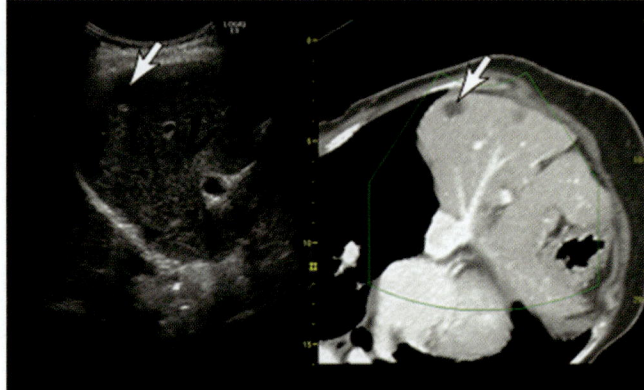

FIG. 18.27 Fused studies of an ultrasound and computed tomography demonstrating a simple liver cyst in the dome of the liver (arrows).

MRI images will also move displaying the same anatomic slice. The images can then be displayed either side by side or in a blended, overlapping format. The ultrasound image can be removed, allowing the sonographer to scan and see only the CT/MRI image. This can be helpful in allowing the sonographer to "scan" and locate the lesion on the CT/MRI images. Once the area of concern is located, the ultrasound side is activated, and the sonographer can scan in a side-by-side format. Another option allows superimposing the two images on top of one another with controls that allow the ultrasound image or CT/MRI image to be emphasized. For example, while locating the mass, the CT/MRI image is emphasized, whereas the ultrasound image will be emphasized during the actual biopsy (Fig. 18.28). Once the lesion is seen on the CT/MRI scan, it will be displayed on the ultrasound image. If the area is not well seen by ultrasound, a marker can be placed on the MRI or CT image and a corresponding marker will appear on the ultrasound image (Fig. 18.29). When the mass is not seen on the ultrasound image well enough to perform the biopsy, the two modalities are superimposed, the biopsy guidelines displayed, and the biopsy is performed using the CT image to guide the needle and the ultrasound image to see the needle (Fig. 18.30).

Another use for marking the mass is to quickly locate the mass when the transducer needs to be removed from the patient's skin. When the area that has been marked is on the screen, the marker will appear as a small square. As the sonographer scans away from the area, the marker grows larger. Marking the area on the image allows the sonographer to rest their arm between passes or before the procedure begins, thus helping to reduce MSK strain from prolonged holding of the transducer in one place. The sonographer can place the transducer back on the patient when the biopsy is ready to proceed, look for the marker, and scan the area

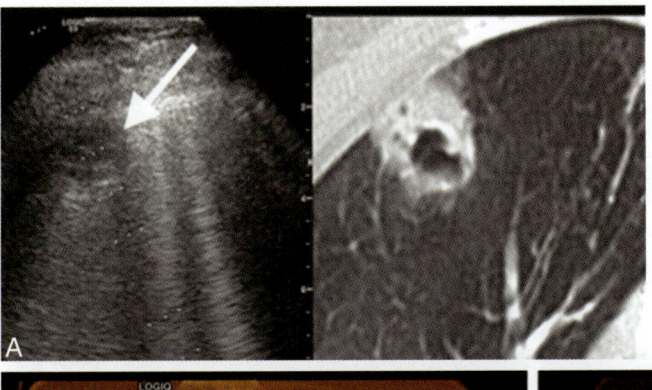
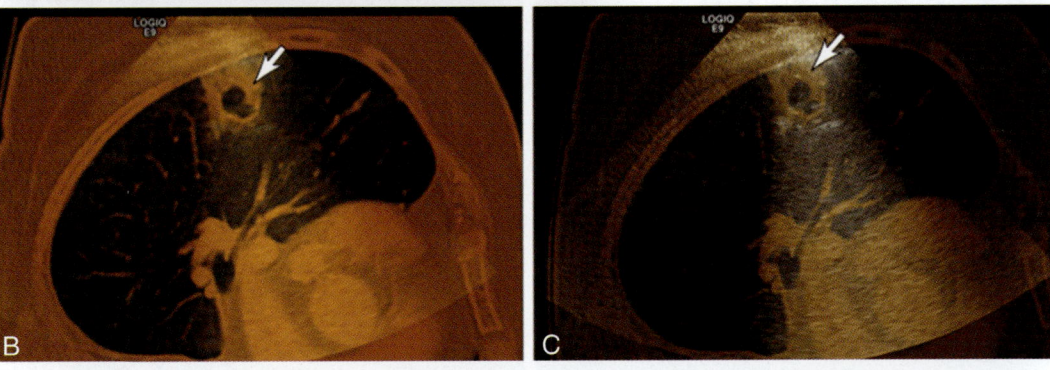

FIG. 18.28 (A) Fusion with chest computed tomography (CT) with side-by-side images used to guide the biopsy. The *arrow* points to the mass. (B) Fused images of the chest CT and ultrasound. The *arrow* points to the mass. In this image, the CT has preference over the ultrasound image. (C) Same two images, but this time the ultrasound has preference over the CT image. This patient had adenocarcinoma of the lung.

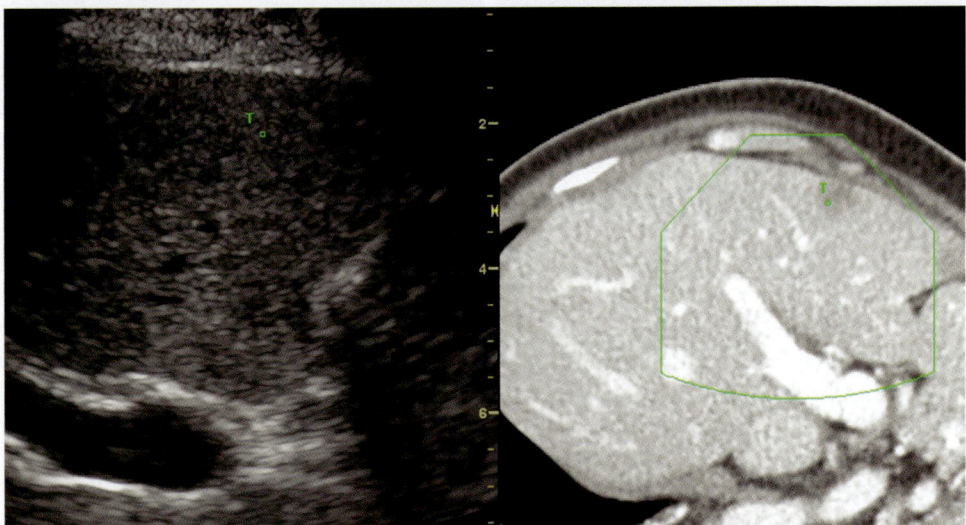

FIG. 18.29 The mass could not be seen on ultrasound. By placing the letter "T" on the magnetic resonance imaging, it automatically appears on the ultrasound image marking the area of the mass.

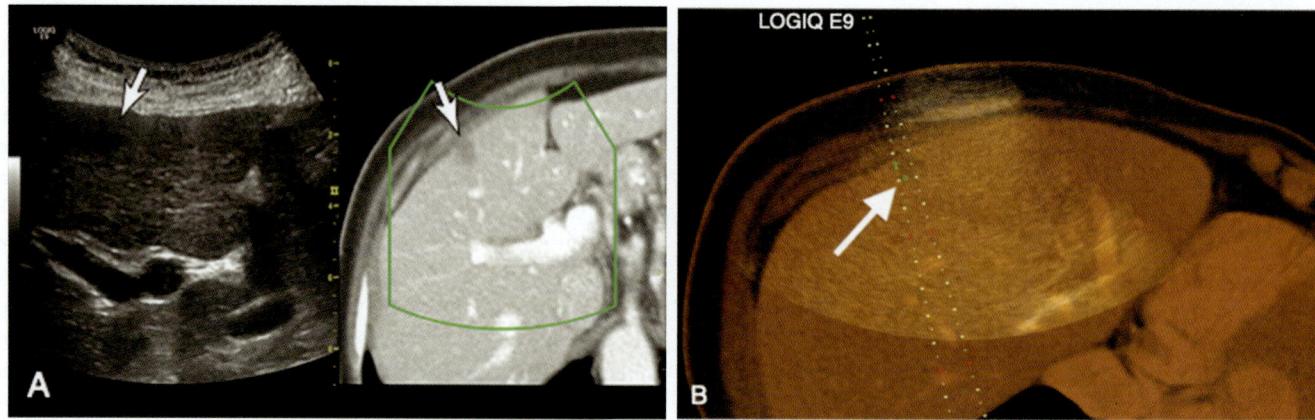

FIG. 18.30 (A) A very subtle liver mass *(arrow)* found on ultrasound with the aid of fusing the ultrasound with the imported computed tomography scan. (B) The biopsy was performed in a fused mode. The small green box *(arrow)* marks the liver mass. The biopsy specimen came back positive for metastatic colon cancer.

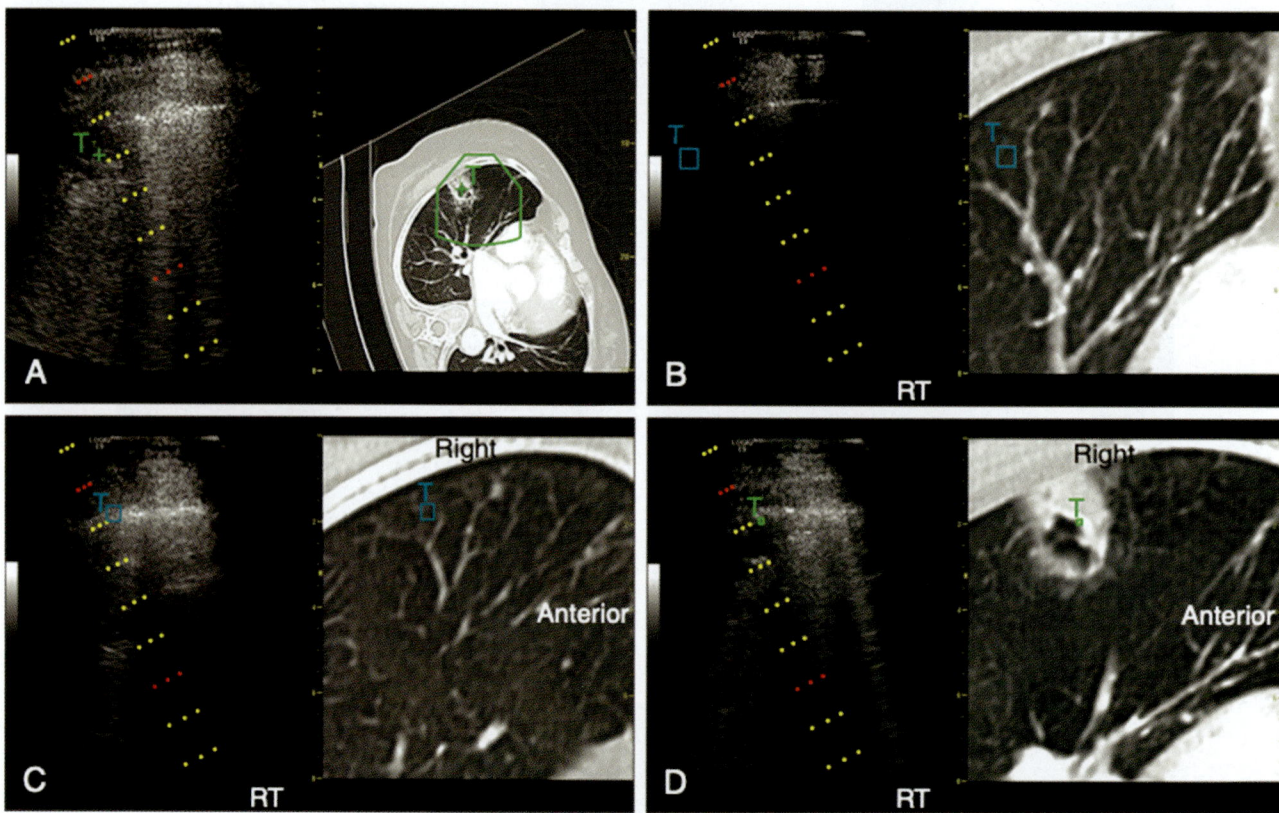

FIG. 18.31 (A) The lung lesion is found with the help of the computed tomography (CT) and the biopsy path determined. A target marker was placed on the CT image and is duplicated on the ultrasound image (small green T+). (B) The sonographer removed the transducer to rest their arm while waiting for the procedure to begin. Upon placing the transducer back on the patient, the blue box and T appeared on both the CT and ultrasound image. This denotes that the lesion is close. (C) As the sonographer scans closer to the lesion, the blue box gets smaller. (D) The box is small and has turned green because the site marked on part A is now in view.

until the marker is small and the area of interest is displayed (Fig. 18.31). This can be a time-saver to quickly find difficult to see lesions when the transducer is removed, because the tracking box will help the sonographer quickly return to the lesion with confidence. Fusion techniques are also helpful if multiple lesions are visible on the MRI or CT and there is a specific lesion that the clinician wants biopsied.

Fusion technology allows needles to use a stylet with electromagnetic sensors. By using this system, the radiologist will know exactly where the needle tip is at all times. This is helpful if the needle keeps deviating, if the biopsy is difficult or "tricky," and to ensure that the needle is in the proper place for a small or difficult to access mass or when a certain part of the mass needs to be sampled such as when the mass is very necrotic. This technology will help the radiologist always know where the needle tip is during the insertion stage. Once the needle tip is in the proper location, the stylet with the sensor is removed, and the biopsy performed.

ULTRASOUND-GUIDED BIOPSY EQUIPMENT AND PROCESS

1. Before beginning the procedure, the patient's medical history, laboratory values, and imaging studies should be reviewed. If the patient's PT, PTT, and INR are normal, the procedure can safely begin. The radiologist should review the CT or MRI study and the location of the mass with the sonographer.
2. A physician involved with the biopsy will obtain the patient's consent for the biopsy to be performed. During the consent process, the patient will be informed of any potential risks, if there are any alternative methods of obtaining the same information, and what might happen if the biopsy is not performed. The procedure itself should be explained in detail and any potential complications discussed, including the possibility of a nondiagnostic procedure. The patient is informed of all the personnel in the room and their roles because the room can become crowded with people, which could include any or all of the following: the sonographer, attending radiologist, any fellows or residents, the nurse, and the cytopathology team. Time should be allowed for the patient to ask questions. A common question asked by patients is whether they can be "put to sleep." Most patients are anxious about having needles stuck in odd places like their "stomach," and the process is frightening to them. It should be explained that they need to be awake so that they can hold their breath as needed, but local numbing will be used. After all questions and concerns are addressed, the **consent form** is then signed and witnessed. The sonographer may serve as the witness. If the sonographer did not see the patient sign the form, they should show the signature to the patient and verify that it is the patient's signature. Some hospitals now have the ability to capture an electronic signature, replacing the paper consent form.
3. The patient's vital signs are taken by the nurse and the preprocedural checklist completed. Any additional equipment that is needed, such as a pulse oximeter, can be attached to the patient.
4. The sonographer performs a limited ultrasound to localize the mass and choose the best approach. The best transducer type and frequency should be determined (Fig. 18.32). It is important to realize with a biopsy that the diagnostic process is complete and that the transducer needed for the biopsy might not be the same as the one that would be used for a diagnostic examination. For example, it may be necessary to use a high-frequency linear array for a superficial liver or abdominal mass, a phased array transducer for intercostal approaches, or even an endocavitary transducer for a subclavicular mass (Fig. 18.33). As a sonographer, we will use our critical thinking skills and think outside the box to determine how to best see and approach the mass. When appropriate, older units can be used for biopsies, freeing up newer machines for diagnostic studies. This is especially true for low-resolution procedures such as a paracentesis, **thoracentesis**, renal and liver cores, and transplants. The sonographer will review the approach with the radiologist to make sure that they are comfortable with it. An X or a dot is marked on the skin with a marker at the site where the needle will pierce the skin. If a marker is used, it must be a one-time use marker and discarded at the end of the procedure. Because the mark is usually erased as the skin is cleansed, the sonographer needs to remember the location of the spot. Another option is to take a retractable pen or a needle cap and gently press it into the skin so that it leaves an indentation of a circle. You should tell the patient what you are doing and why before pressing the cap into their skin, because it can be slightly uncomfortable. I would also draw a line next to the transducer so that I knew where to place the transducer edge because it can be difficult to see the spot marked for the biopsy (Fig. 18.34). This can be helpful because that line is on the border of the sterile field and usually does not get erased as the skin is prepped. The minimal length of the needle needed to reach the mass needs to be determined. This is usually calculated by the ultrasound unit when the biopsy guideline is activated (Fig. 18.35). Common needle lengths are 6, 9, 15, and 20 cm. Usually, it is best to

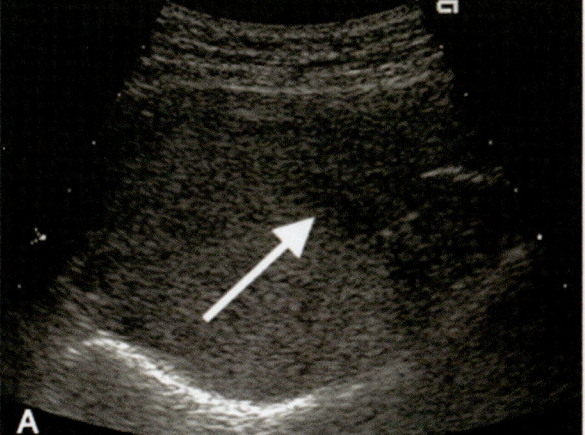
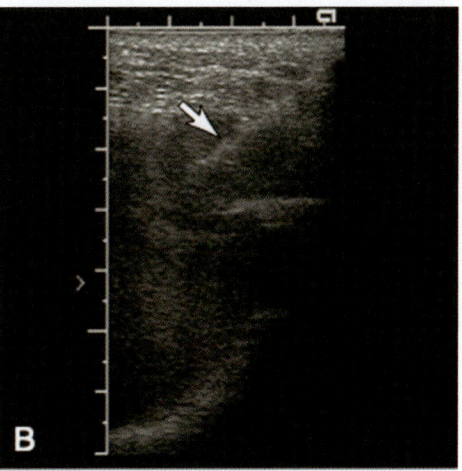

FIG. 18.32 (A) A large mediastinal mass is seen with a 5-MHz curved array transducer. (B) The same patient is biopsied using a 7-MHz linear array because the hypoechoic area in the mass (*arrow* on A) was better appreciated. The *arrow* is pointing to the needle. This is the area from which positive cells were found. Lymphoma was diagnosed.

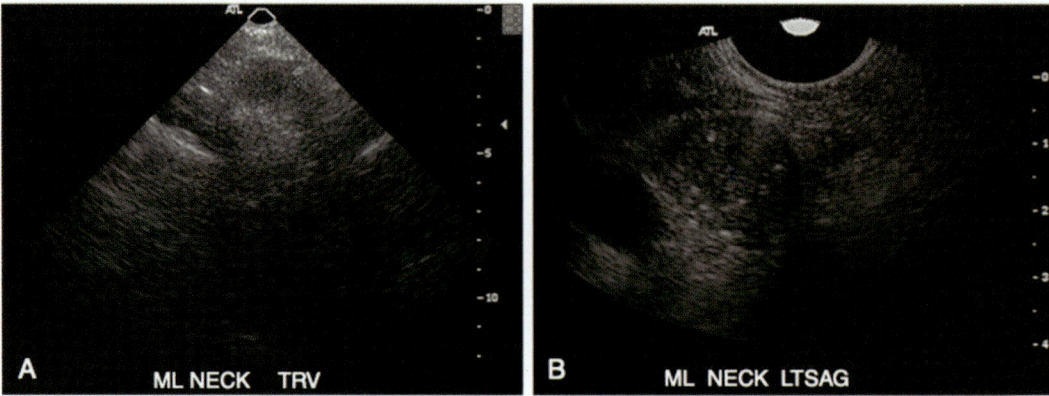

FIG. 18.33 (A) Viewing this neck mass around the clavicle using a linear array transducer was difficult. To angle under the clavicle, a phased array transducer was first used. (B) The same patient evaluated with an endocavity transducer. This proved to be the best transducer, allowing an easy and safe path to the lymph node as well as the resolution to see the small calcifications. Metastatic thyroid cancer was diagnosed.

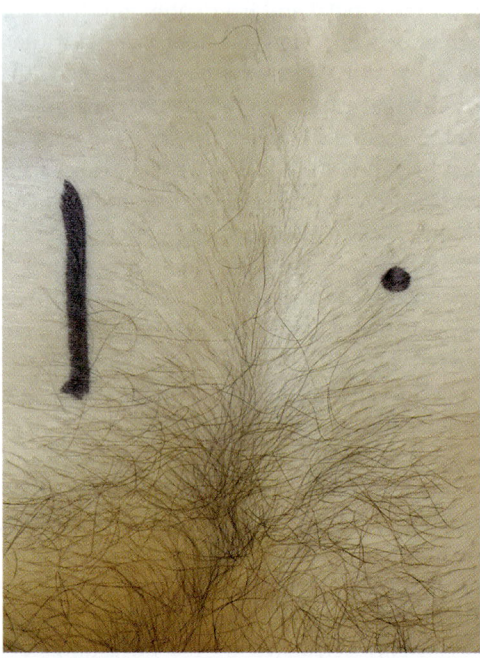

FIG. 18.34 A patient marked for a biopsy. The dot is where superficial numbing should be given. The line is where the edge of the transducer should be placed.

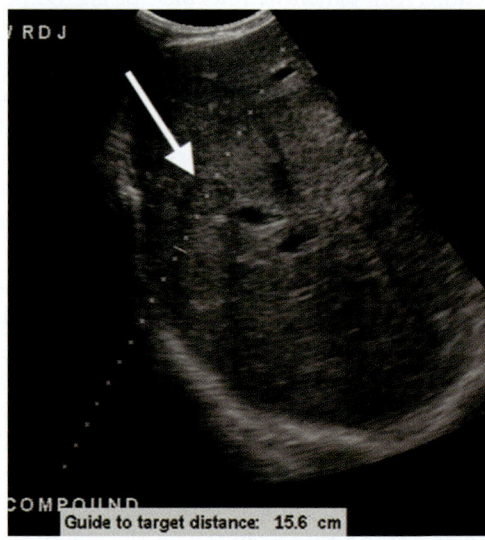

FIG. 18.35 The line on the needle path guideline is the distance to the needle guide bracket. A 20-cm length needle is needed to get to this lesion (arrow).

have the sonographer on one side of the patient next to the ultrasound machine and the physician on the other side of the patient. Sometimes both the sonographer and physician will need to be on the same side of the patient. If this is the situation, the two of them will need to determine the best position so that they both can see the ultrasound monitor. One solution is for the sonographer to sit on a stool so that they are shorter than the radiologist. This allows the sonographer to have access to the controls and still be able to see the monitor. Good ergonomics should try to be maintained. The sonographer could also consider rearranging the relationship of the stretcher and machine to accommodate both the sonographer and the physician being on the same side of the patient.

5. The national patient safety standards mandate that a "time-out" be performed before beginning any procedure. A member of the biopsy team should ask the patient to recite their full name and the reason that they are there. The patient's ID or history number is confirmed, as is the type and location of the procedure. The time-out needs to be documented, which may be part of the consent form or filled out in the patient's electronic record. The words "time-out" can be typed on the screen, and an image documented as part of the ultrasound examination (Fig. 18.36). This is not a legal documentation of a time-out but can be helpful if documentation did not occur, thus allowing the proper time to be recorded.

6. The radiologist may start prepping the skin, after the time-out, while the sonographer preps and bags the transducer. Prepping the transducer may require the assistance of another person such as a nurse, a sonography student, or even another sonographer, to help maintain sterility of the transducer, although it can be done by one person. The sonographer assisting with the study puts the needle guide bracket on the transducer (Fig. 18.37) and then opens the outside wrapper of the needle guidance kit exposing the sterile package inside (Fig. 18.38). The sonographer puts on

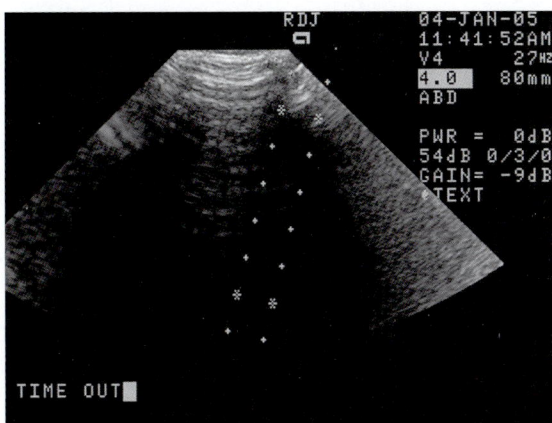

FIG. 18.36 The time-out was performed on January 4, 2005, at 11:41 AM; This image can be used as a reference if the time was not recorded.

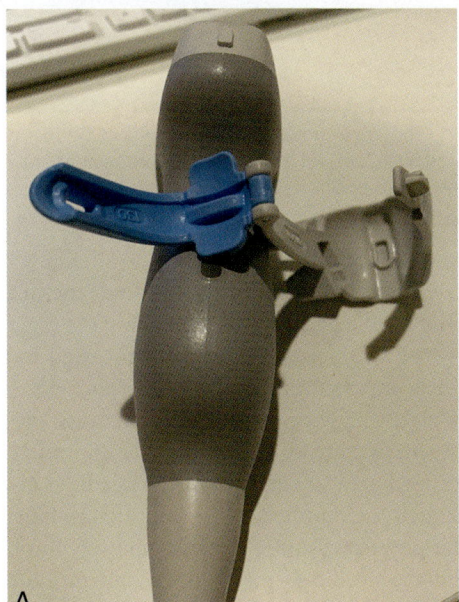

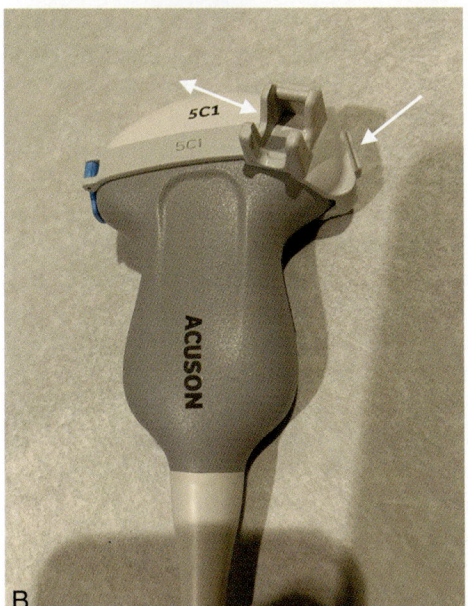

FIG. 18.37 (A) The needle guide bracket for this transducer. The slot in the blue area attaches to the raised area on the transducer. This ensures that the bracket is attached properly. (B) The bracket is attached to the transducer. The *arrow* points to where the guide attachment will be placed. The *double arrow* points to where the sensor would be placed for needle tracking.

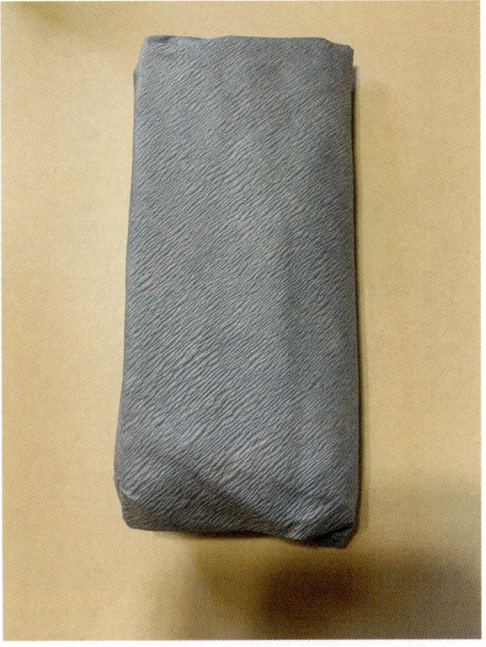

FIG. 18.38 The biopsy kit removed from its wrapping. The inside is sterile but the outside is not.

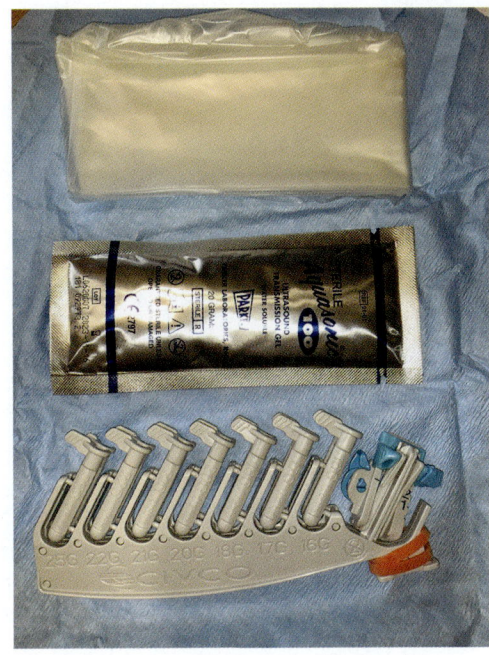

FIG. 18.39 The inside of the kit shown in Fig. 18.38. *Top to bottom:* the sterile transducer and cord cover, sterile gel, needle inserts (ranging from 25 to 16 gauge), biopsy guide attachment, and sterile rubber bands.

sterile gloves and opens the kit separating the items inside (Fig. 18.39). The sterile sonographer holds the sterile cover with the opening facing up while the other person places normal scanning gel on the transducer and places it in the sterile cover. The sterile sonographer pulls the probe cover down over the cable and then places a sterile rubber band, which is part of the kit, beneath the head of the transducer to secure the bag. Next, the device that holds the insert is attached over the sterile cover onto the needle guide bracket (Fig. 18.40). If there is a choice of angles, the correct angle is chosen (Fig. 18.41) and the correct size sterile insert is

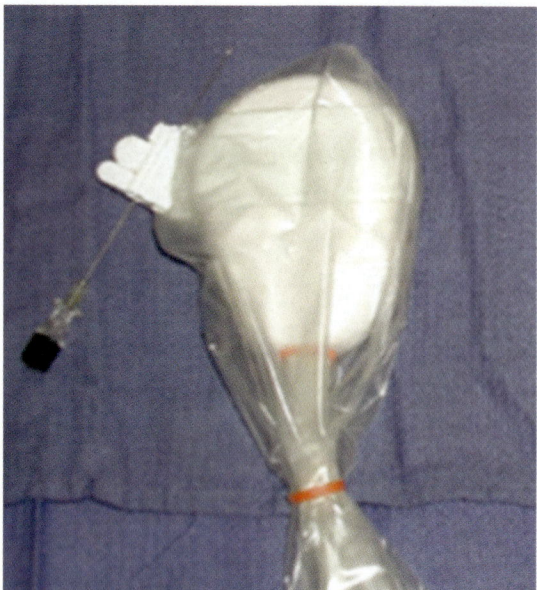

FIG. 18.40 A properly prepped transducer with the needle guide on the outside of the sterile cover. Notice the rubber band that secures the transducer cover.

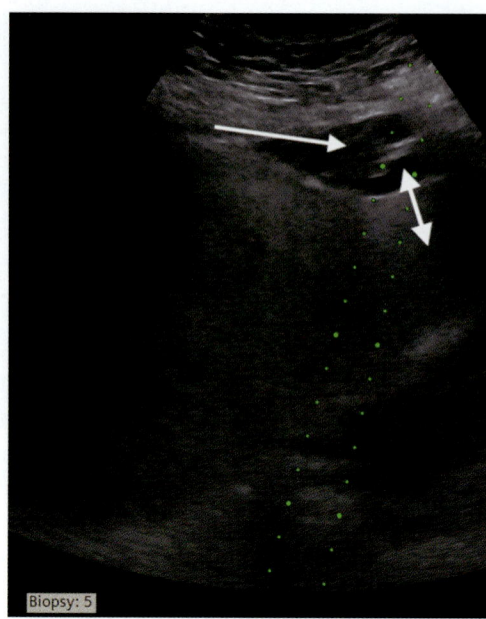

FIG. 18.42 The *arrow* points to a pool of lidocaine that was injected adjacent to the liver capsule. It is important for the sonographer to keep the transducer in this position so that the biopsy needle goes through the anesthetized area. The *double arrow* points to the needle tip.

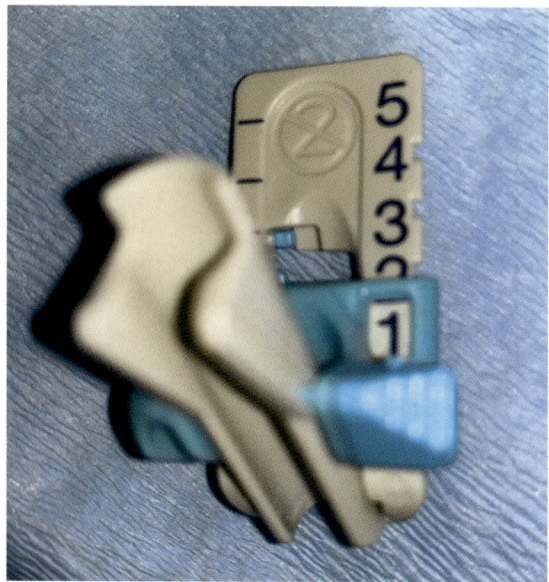

FIG. 18.41 A needle guide that offers five choices, as shown in Fig. 18.21. This guide is set up for angle 1. The needle is inserted in the curved aspect.

attached based on the gauge of the needle being used. The needle gauge inserts may need to be changed during the procedure. For example, a 22-gauge insert may be used during the FNA but will need to be changed to an 18-gauge insert for the core. If the needle seems very tight in the slot, going up an insert size can help. The use of sterile bags for certain procedures can vary among practices. For example, one practice may bag the transducer and guide keeping it sterile for a thyroid biopsy, whereas another institution may use the transducer and guide in a clean but not sterile fashion.

7. After the patient and transducer are prepped, sterile gel is used to rescan and check the mark. Once the area of the biopsy has been rechecked, local skin anesthesia is given, usually with a 25-gauge needle.

8. Next, deeper numbing is given through the needle guide along the needle path with a 9-cm, 22-gauge spinal needle. The proper size needle insert does not need to be on the transducer for the numbing needle. This helps for patient comfort, especially on liver masses, because the liver capsule is very sensitive. The transducer should stay on the anesthetized area to ensure that the needle is always passing through the numbed tissue (Fig. 18.42). It is important that the physician squirt the lidocaine or numbing agent through the needle to push out any air inside the needle shaft before inserting the needle into the patient. Otherwise, air will be injected into the patient's tissue which may cause an issue seeing the mass (Fig. 18.43). Patients should be told that they should not feel any sharp pain but that they may feel pressure as some patients will complain of "pain" during the procedure when what they are really feeling is the pressure of the needle passing through their tissue. It is a good idea to let patients know that they may feel some pressure from the transducer itself as it is held steadily in place.

9. When a sonographer assists with the procedure, they will have one sterile hand, which is holding the transducer, while the other hand will be dirty because it will be optimizing the controls and documenting the needle tip. The needle should be advanced in a steady motion while it is being tracked. Echogenic tip needles should be used because the tip of the needle has been scored to produce an increase in scattered echoes, causing it to be more echogenic and easier to find. The shaft of the needle is echogenic because it is a specular reflector (Fig. 18.44), whereas the tip of the needle is more echogenic because of the scored tip. Some needles have the stylet scored to enhance visualization of the needle (Fig. 18.45).

10. For chest, abdominal, and retroperitoneal biopsies, the patient is asked to stop breathing while the needle is

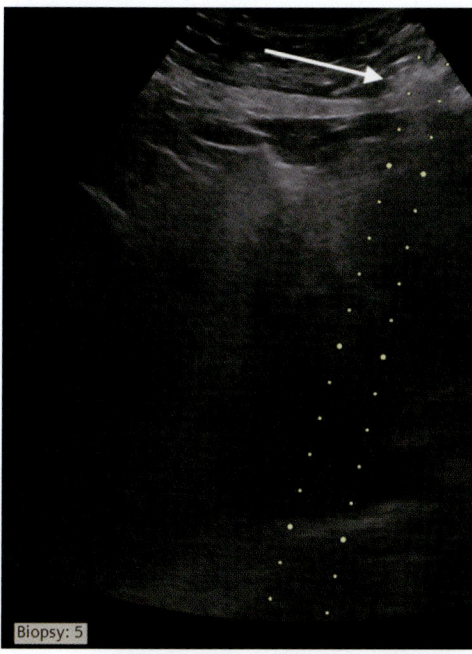

FIG. 18.43 Air was not cleared out of the needle and was injected into the patient, obscuring the needle tip and the liver. Fortunately this was a liver core biopsy and, as the air dissipated, enough of the needle path could be seen to perform the biopsy.

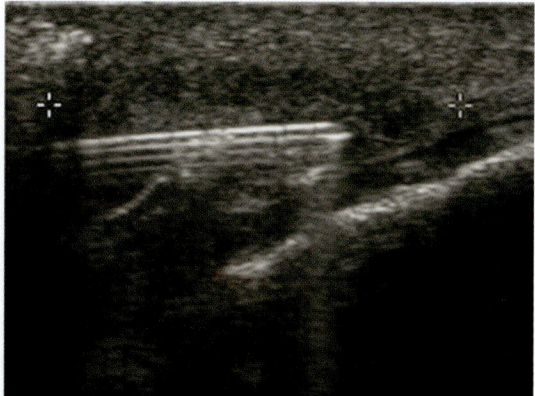

FIG. 18.44 A needle demonstrating a nice reverberation artifact.

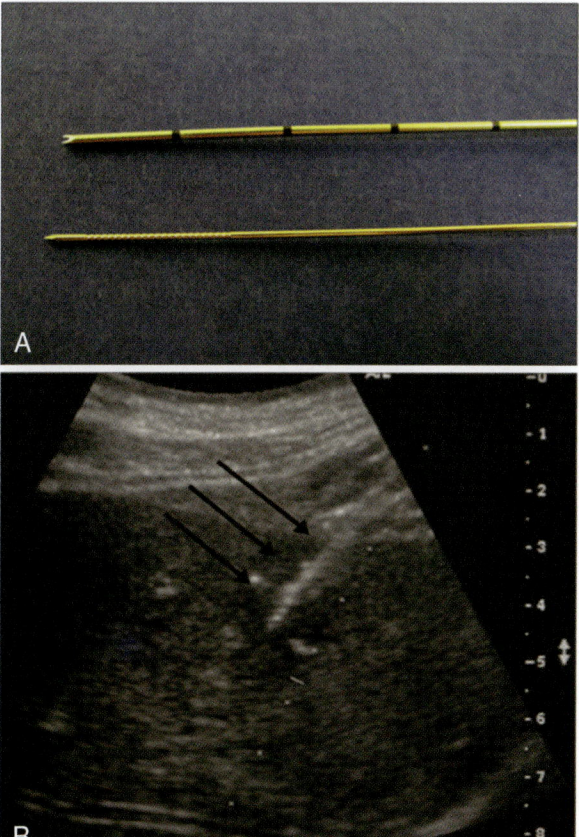

FIG. 18.45 (A) A biopsy needle with a scored stylet. (B) Needle with an echogenic stylet (arrows) allowing easy visualization of the needle. The arrows denote a hypoechoic mass determined to be a metastatic lesion from the colon.

inserted. A typical FNA pass lasts from 15 to 30 seconds. Patients who cannot hold their breath for this long should be instructed to breathe shallowly until the needle is removed, because deep breaths may cause the needle to bend. The sonographer can be helpful by coaching and encouraging patients with their breathing and breath holding. When locating the mass, try to let patients breathe normally as much as possible, having them hold their breath to verify the selected path. This will allow the patient to be "fresh" for the biopsy and not out of breath already from the pre-biopsy scans. For masses that move a lot with breathing, it can be helpful to show the patient the mass and biopsy line and how their breathing affects the location of the mass.

11. After the procedure is finished, the patient's skin is cleaned off and a bandage placed over the biopsy site. A cold compress can also be placed over the biopsy site to reduce swelling and pain as needed. The bag should be placed over the patient's gown, or it can be wrapped in a towel or a paper towel because direct skin contact may be uncomfortable for the patient.
12. The sterile bag and needle guide are removed from the transducer. Care should be taken not to accidentally throw the reusable needle guide bracket in the garbage, because these guides are expensive. Any parts that were from the kit are disposable such as the insert. The sonographer should scan the area to look for any postprocedural bleeding or hematoma (Fig. 18.46). Color or power Doppler can be used to ensure that there is no active bleeding. This is especially useful in renal biopsies. If an active bleed is discovered, the sonographer can use the transducer to apply pressure over the area to stop the bleeding. Usually, the bleeding can be stopped within 5 to 10 minutes.
13. Before the patient leaves the room, the nurse will assess the patient's pain level and check vital signs. The sonographer should take the transducer and bracket, remove the gel and any blood, and perform high-level disinfection according to the hospital's infection control policies and the recommendations of the transducer manufacturer.

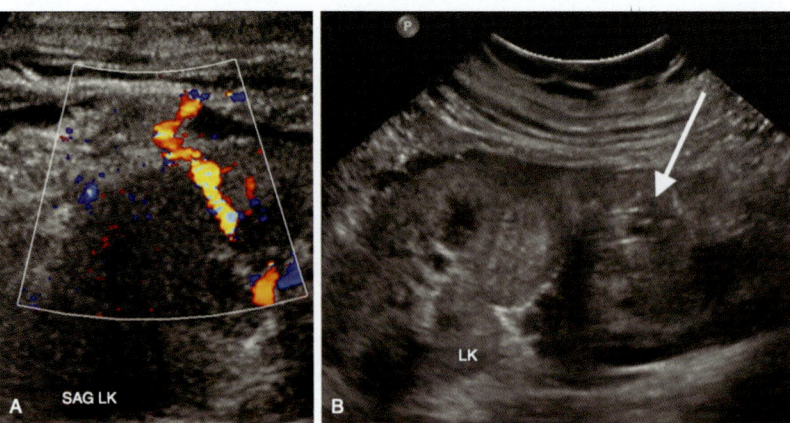

FIG. 18.46 (A) A color Doppler image during a renal biopsy showing blood, called a *jet*, leaving the kidney. The sonographer applied pressure which stopped the "leak." (B) The *arrow* points to the resulting hematoma.

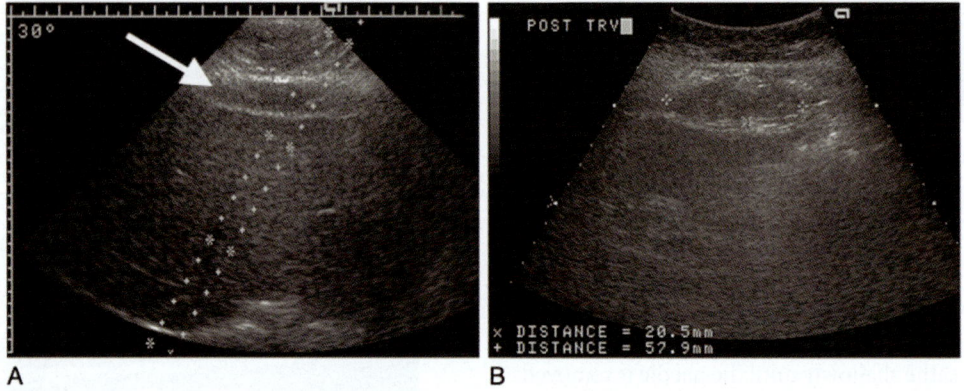

FIG. 18.47 (A) A liver core biopsy. The *arrow* points to the rectus muscle. (B) One hour after the biopsy the patient started to complain of epigastric pain. A sonogram shows a hematoma. Notice the similar appearance to the rectus abdominis muscle, which can be mistaken for a hematoma. It is recommended that a prebiopsy image be taken for comparison to avoid this mistake.

14. The patient is then taken to a holding or observation area if needed. Depending on the type of procedure, the patient may remain in this area between 15 and 120 minutes. If the patient develops increasing pain, the sonographer should rescan to look for a hematoma (Fig. 18.47). Stable patients can be discharged with appropriate instructions. Patients who have had chest procedures or procedures near the lungs will be sent for a chest x-ray to make sure that there is no pneumothorax.
15. Typically, the nurse makes a follow-up phone call within the next 24 to 48 hours to ensure that the patient did not experience any complications.

THE SONOGRAPHER'S ROLE IN INTERVENTIONAL PROCEDURES

A sonographer who has an interest in interventional ultrasound can be a valuable asset to the interventional team. Sonographers may work closely with a radiologist, sonologist, or other physicians such as a nephrologist in native kidney biopsies, surgeons in kidney or liver transplant biopsies, or other clinicians. Sonographer involvement has many benefits because they can locate the pathology and determine various approaches, offering recommendation for the best and safest needle path to the mass.

The different transducer types (linear, curved linear, phased array) should be evaluated as they offer different angles and approaches to the mass. Remember we are not evaluating the image for its resolution, because that has already occurred, but trying to determine the safest approach to the mass.

Using their scanning skills, sonographers can optimize the image to locate subtle masses and use Doppler to ensure that there are no vessels in the needle path (Fig. 18.48). The sonographer can place the patient in a variety of positions to determine the best approach. For example, by placing the patient in a left posterior oblique or left lateral decubitus position, the liver may drop into a more subcostal position or a mass may roll away from a vessel. Placing the patient in a prone position may give better access to a renal mass. Knowledge of technologies such as harmonic and compound imaging may facilitate finding or better defining the borders of the mass (Fig. 18.49).

Using their Doppler skills, the sonographer can locate vessels that may potentially traverse the needle path or be in close proximity to the mass. The sonographer can help guide the needle safely to deep retroperitoneal masses that may be near major vessels. Using color or power Doppler, the sonographer can locate vessels in a mass, which may represent areas of viable tumor tissue, because getting a good sample can be a challenge in masses that have areas of necrosis (Fig. 18.50).

Sonographers will need to discuss and determine solutions to problems such as needle deviation (Fig. 18.51). If

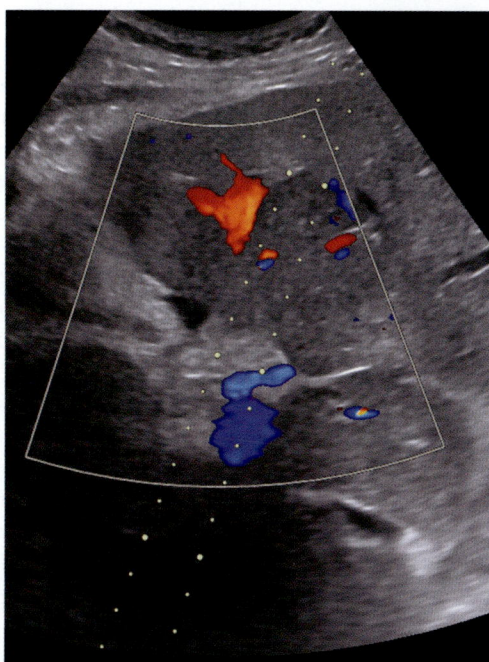

FIG. 18.48 A biopsy of a liver mass was diagnosed as a hepatocellular carcinoma. Color Doppler was used to find an area with no vessels. Although vessels are present, there is a path that is vessel free.

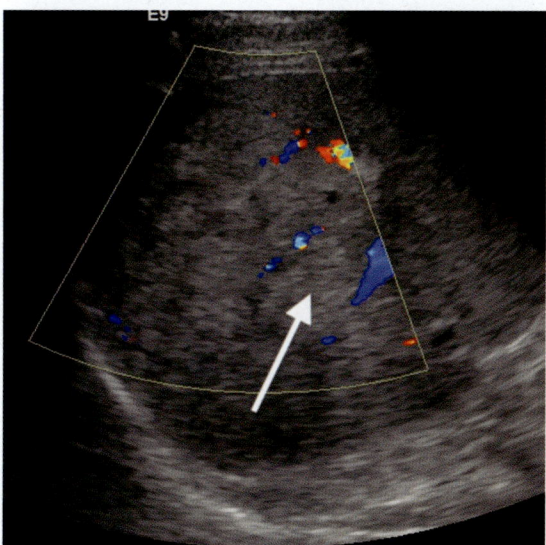

FIG. 18.50 After several unsuccessful passes that showed necrotic tissue, the sonographer investigated the mass with color Doppler. The arrow points to where a successful sample obtained cells that showed the mass to be a hepatocellular carcinoma.

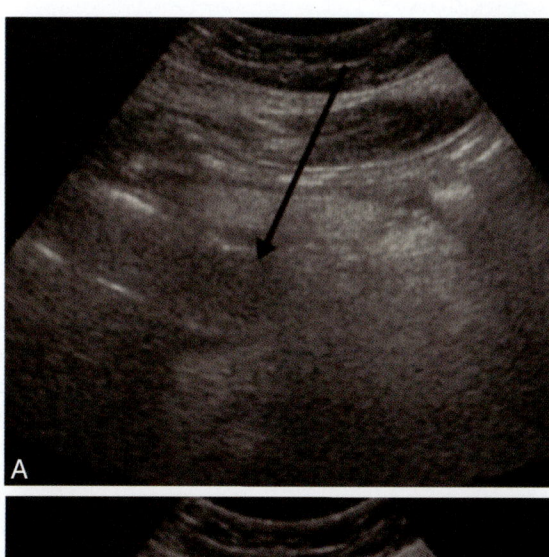

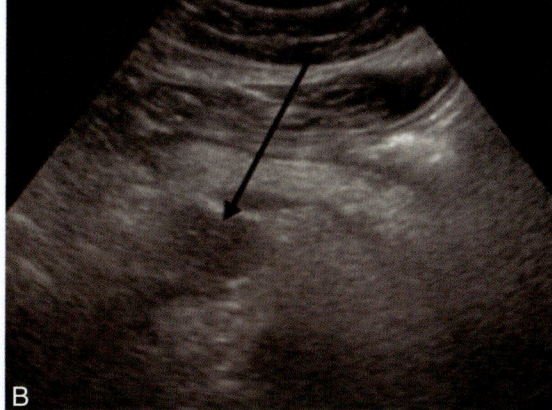

FIG. 18.49 With compound imaging and harmonics, this pancreatic head mass *(arrow)* is better defined, leading to a successful biopsy with a diagnosis of adenocarcinoma of the pancreas.

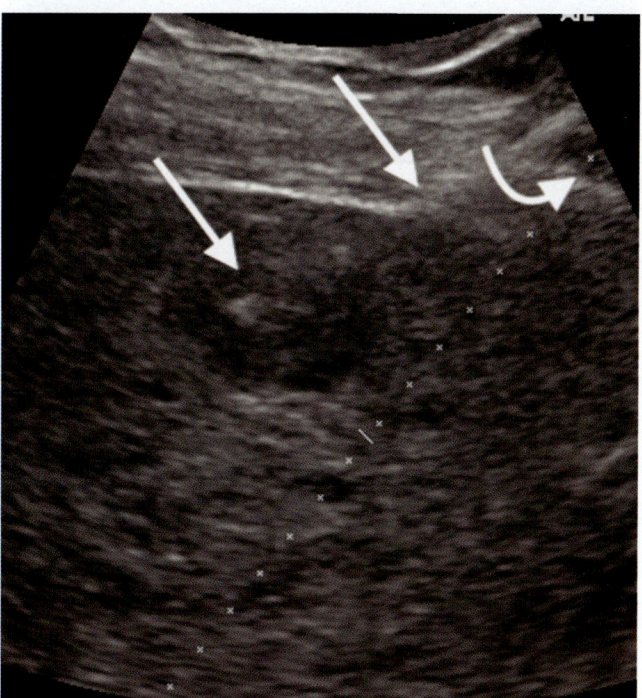

FIG. 18.51 The *arrows* point to a needle that greatly deviated from the projected path. The sonographer adjusted for the deviation and a successful biopsy was performed on this patient with a hepatocellular carcinoma. The *curved arrow* points to the rectus muscle, which was believed to be causing the deviation.

they realize that the guide is on wrong or the angle on the transducer is not the same as the angle on the screen, they should correct the error and confess what happened after the procedure is over (Fig. 18.52).

When using biopsy guides, the sonographer can hold the transducer, freeing the physician's hands. This can be especially helpful when aspiration techniques are used. The sonographer can use the transducer to press bowel out of the way, allowing the mass to be seen. This increased transducer pressure needs to be maintained while obtaining the specimen. This technique can also be used to minimize the distance between the skin and deep lesions (Fig. 18.53).

The sonographer can assist and encourage the patient during the procedure. They can support the patient emotionally, allowing the physician to concentrate on the procedure or discuss the specimen with the cytopathologist, if they are present. While the radiologist and nurse are busy with the specimen, the sonographer can talk to the patients and make sure that they are doing okay, assure the patient that they are doing a great job, and communicate to the patient what the next step will be. Talking to the patient during these down times can help the patient get through the procedure. Patients tend to talk to the sonographer more, and their questions or fears can then be relayed to the physician.

Experienced sonographers may find being involved with procedures a welcome change from routine scanning. It allows them to interact with the patient in a different way, be part of an important team, and bring into play all their scanning skills and knowledge.

FINDING THE NEEDLE TIP

The needle tip should appear as an echogenic dot on the ultrasound image. The needle tip may not be seen despite the shaft being seen. This is caused by the needle approaching the sound beam at an angle so that part of the shaft is in the sound beam while the tip has passed through it. Visualizing the needle tip depends on several factors, including the type of needle because specially designed echogenic needles are better seen than normal needles, the gauge of the needle because larger gauge needles cause brighter reflections, and the echogenicity of the mass because hypoechoic masses allow easier visualization of the needle than echogenic masses (Fig. 18.54).

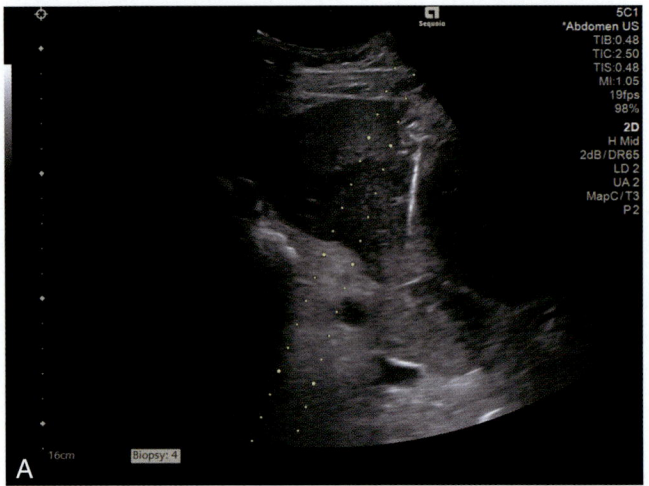
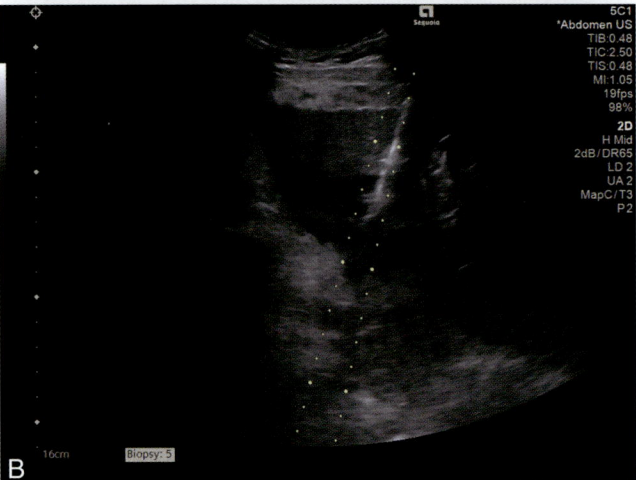

FIG. 18.52 (A) The needle is deviating from the projected path. The sonographer realized that the angle chosen on the guide was 5, but the needle path was on angle 4. (B) Changing the guide to 5 resulted in the needle going through the correct path.

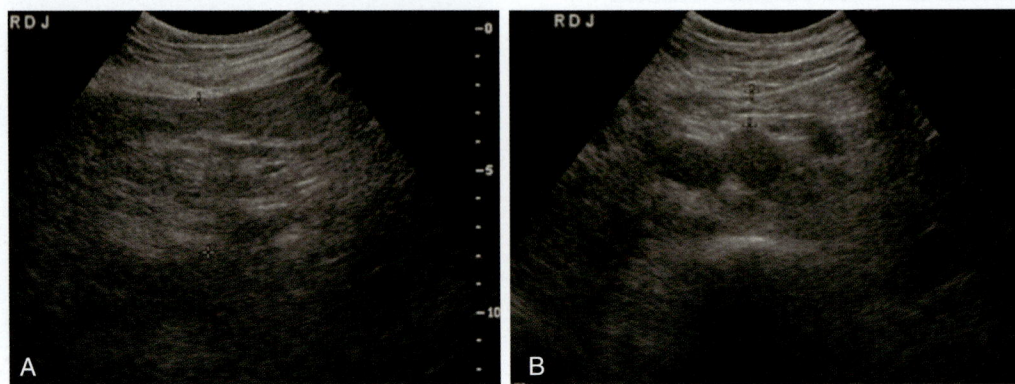

FIG. 18.53 (A) Deep retroperitoneal lymph nodes are difficult to see with normal scanning techniques. There is approximately 8 cm of tissue between the abdominal wall and the anterior surface of the nodes. (B) By applying pressure with the transducer, the distance from the abdominal wall and the nodes has decreased to approximately 3 cm, allowing visualization of the nodes. This amount of pressure was applied during the biopsy, allowing a successful biopsy and a diagnosis of lymphoma.

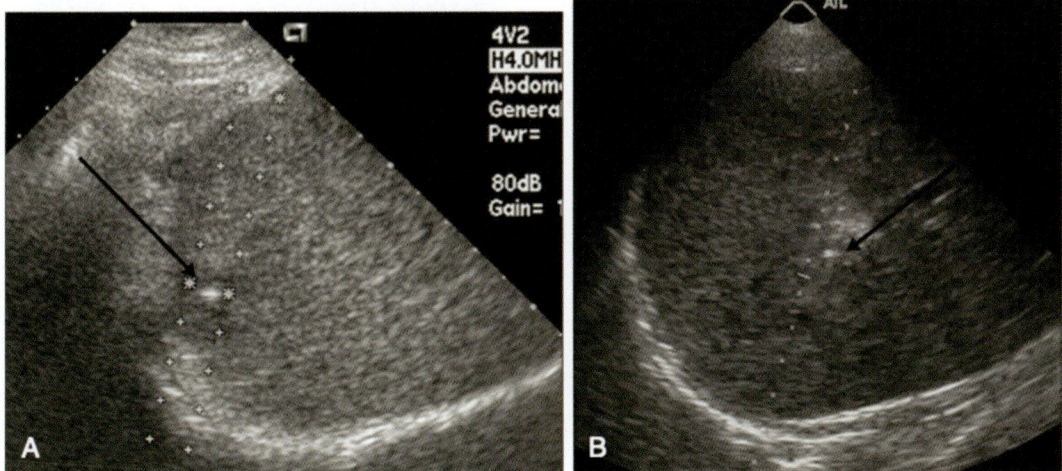

FIG. 18.54 (A) The needle tip is easily seen *(arrow)* in this patient with a hypoechoic metastatic lesion. (B) The needle tip is hard to see *(arrow)* in this patient with a hyperechoic metastatic lesion.

The needle should be followed as it advances toward the mass. The needle may deviate out of the projected path and away from the ultrasound beam, causing loss of visualization of the needle tip. This deviation of the needle can be caused by the physician bending or tilting the needle as it is being advanced or by the tissue and muscle planes it is traversing. Sometimes the needle's path is influenced depending on if the needle is bevel up or bevel down.

Tricks to try to see the needle tip include the following:
1. Moving the needle up and down in a bobbing motion.
2. Bobbing or jiggling the stylet inside the needle.
3. Scanning and angling the transducer in a superior and inferior motion. This is helpful when the needle is bent out of the plane of the soundbeam. Note that these will be very small movements.
4. Using harmonics or compound imaging.
5. A last resort is to remove the needle and start again, closely watching the displacement of the tissue as the needle advances.

At times the patient may move or breathe at the time that the biopsy core is fired, preventing the needle path from being visible for documentation. In these instances, the sonographer can scan the area and look for the needle track. This will be seen as an echogenic line caused by the air that is introduced into the tissue during the firing process (Fig. 18.55).

WHAT TO DO WHEN THE NEEDLE DEVIATES

Deviation of the needle from the projected path can be an issue and a challenge for the sonographer. The tissue and organs between the skin and the mass are usually the cause of this problem. For example, in pancreatic biopsies, the needle is often deflected as it passes through the posterior wall of the stomach. If it is a constant problem, the sonographer can overcorrect (i.e., move the transducer more lateral or medial so that the path that the needle is following will intersect the mass) (Fig. 18.56). It is important that the sonographer verify that the correct size needle guide insert was used, because if the guide is

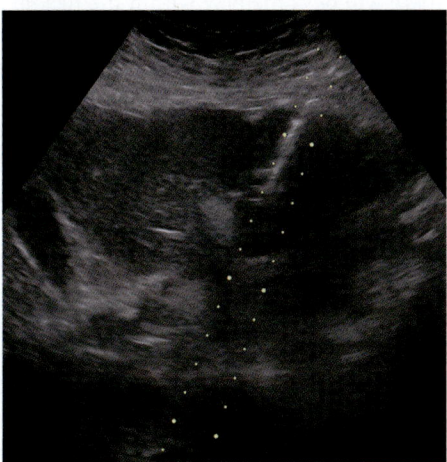

FIG. 18.55 At the time of the biopsy the needle documentation image was missed. Fortunately, when using a core needle, as the needle advances it pushes some air along the tract, which can be used to document the needle.

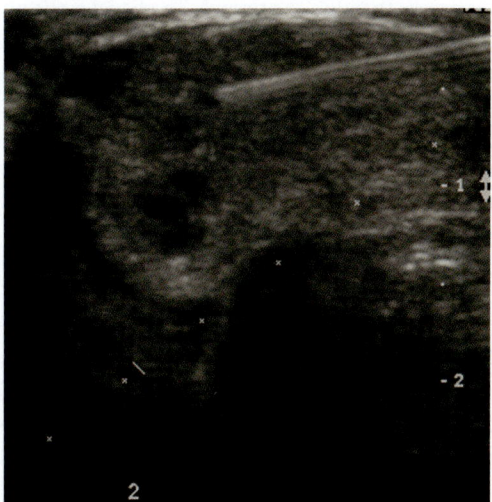

FIG. 18.56 The needle consistently deviated so the sonographer moved the transducer so that the biopsy line is lateral to the mass, resulting in a successful biopsy. Sometimes the cause of needle deviation cannot be determined.

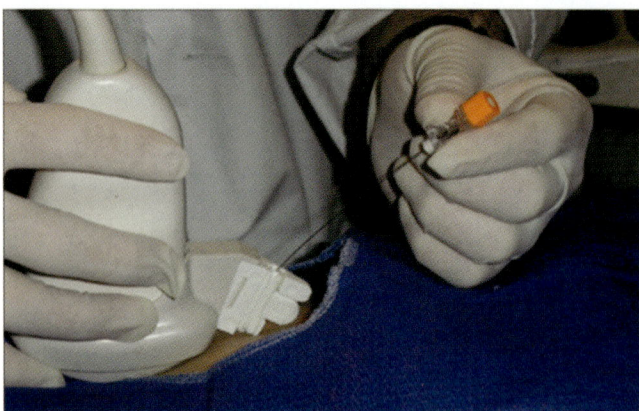

FIG. 18.57 Notice the bending of the needle as it is being inserted. This will cause the needle to deviate and not follow the biopsy guideline.

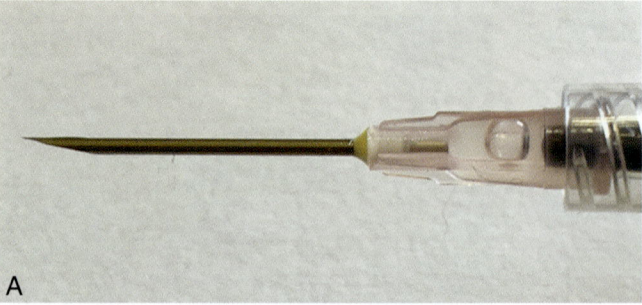

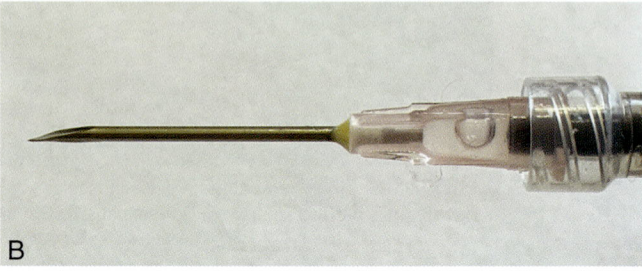

FIG. 18.58 (A) The needle bevel shown up so the point easily goes through the tissue. (B) The needle bevel shown down. Notice how the opening of the needle could cause impedance or bending as it "fights" to get through the tissue.

too large, there will be some play within the needle guide that can cause this problem. As previously discussed, the sonographer should ensure that the guide on the transducer is set to the correct angle. The sonographer should make sure that the transducer and needle guide are in the proper relationship with the patient's skin for that needle guide. Usually this is with the exit point of the needle guide touching the patient's skin. It is vital that the sonographer become familiar with the various transducers and guides, how they should be placed on the body, and how to correct or adjust the transducer position as needed. If the problem persists, sometimes using a 20-gauge as opposed to a 22-gauge needle may correct the situation because the larger-gauge needle is sturdier and does not bend as easily. In extreme cases, another pathway may need to be determined. The sonographer can watch how the physician is inserting the needle to make sure that the needle is not bending as it is being inserted into the skin (Fig. 18.57). Finally, the position of the tip of the needle can influence deviation on certain types of needles. When the needle is inserted with the tip of the needle at the top, called bevel-up, the needle will encounter less resistance as it passes through the tissues. The bevel is the angled tip of the needle. Inserting the needle into the patient's skin with the bevel up allows the sharp tip of the needle to pierce the skin first, paving the way for the rest of the needle. With the needle tip bevel down, the needle has some impedance with the tissue, causing a possible deviation (Fig. 18.58). Another problem is when a mass is pushed out of the way by the needle. This can be a problem with small nodes and masses. The sonographer needs to understand how to counter these situations. Applying firm pressure with the transducer against the mass can stabilize the mass and allow the needle to enter it. Trying to get the needle to approach the center of the mass, so that it does not push the mass to the left or to the right, is another possible solution. The physician can try to quickly insert the needle or try to rotate the bevel of the needle into a different position. Sometimes another approach may be needed, which may require breaking down the sterile field and starting again. When any of these situations arise, the sonographer should be thinking of possible solutions to suggest.

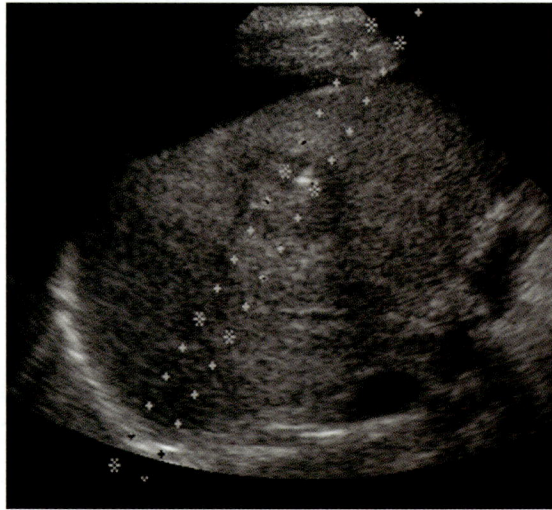

FIG. 18.59 Biopsy of a hypoechoic lesion in a cirrhotic liver. Pathology showed this to be a regenerating nodule.

BIOPSIES AND PROCEDURES BY ORGAN

Liver

The liver is one of the most common organs for which a biopsy is requested. It may be to characterize a mass, drain a fluid collection, or evaluate or stage parenchymal disease in patients with hepatitis or a fatty liver. Various types of liver lesions are amenable to ultrasound-guided biopsy and include metastatic masses, hepatocellular carcinoma or other primary cancer, benign lesions, or abscesses. A biopsy of a hypoechoic area in a cirrhotic liver may be requested, especially if the patient has an elevated alpha-fetoprotein, to differentiate between an hepatocellular carcinoma and a regenerating nodule (Fig. 18.59). The inability to biopsy a liver mass can be due to a lack of a safe approach or the failure to visualize the mass. However, with the approval of ultrasound contrast, these isoechoic masses can now be visualized and biopsied using ultrasound contrast (Fig. 18.60). This can be a simpler solution than using fusion; however, the ultrasound unit will need to have contrast software. It is easier to upgrade to contrast, because it is typically just a software upgrade, than it is for fusion capabilities, which will need not only a software upgrade but also special equipment. Patients that need to have their biopsy with contrast will need to have an IV line placed to administer the contrast. Unlike CT or MRI contrast, ultrasound contrast is not nephrotoxic. Whenever possible, a subcostal approach should be used to biopsy a liver mass to avoid the possibility of a pneumothorax or damage to the intercostal arteries (Fig. 18.61). Intercostal biopsies also tend to be more painful to the patient due to the numerous intercostal nerves. Masses at the dome of the liver are easier to biopsy under ultrasound than CT, although a steep angle approach is often required. In some cases, performing a biopsy in a sagittal plane may offer the best approach. Core biopsies may be obtained on patients with hepatitis, cirrhosis, fatty livers, or unexplained elevated liver function tests. An ultrasound-guided biopsy in this group of patients is easier to perform and more comfortable for the patient than the traditional blind approach through the ribs of the right lobe. Specific complications of liver biopsies include pneumothorax for masses near the dome of the liver, bile leak, and hematomas (Fig. 18.62). Consider multiple patient positions to try to decrease the distance to the mass and to avoid intercostal approaches.

Pancreas

Most pancreatic biopsies are performed to confirm the diagnosis of adenocarcinoma in the presence of a mass, evaluate pancreatic cysts, or in patients with unusual imaging findings. Over the years, percutaneous ultrasound-guided biopsies of the pancreas have decreased even under CT. Currently most

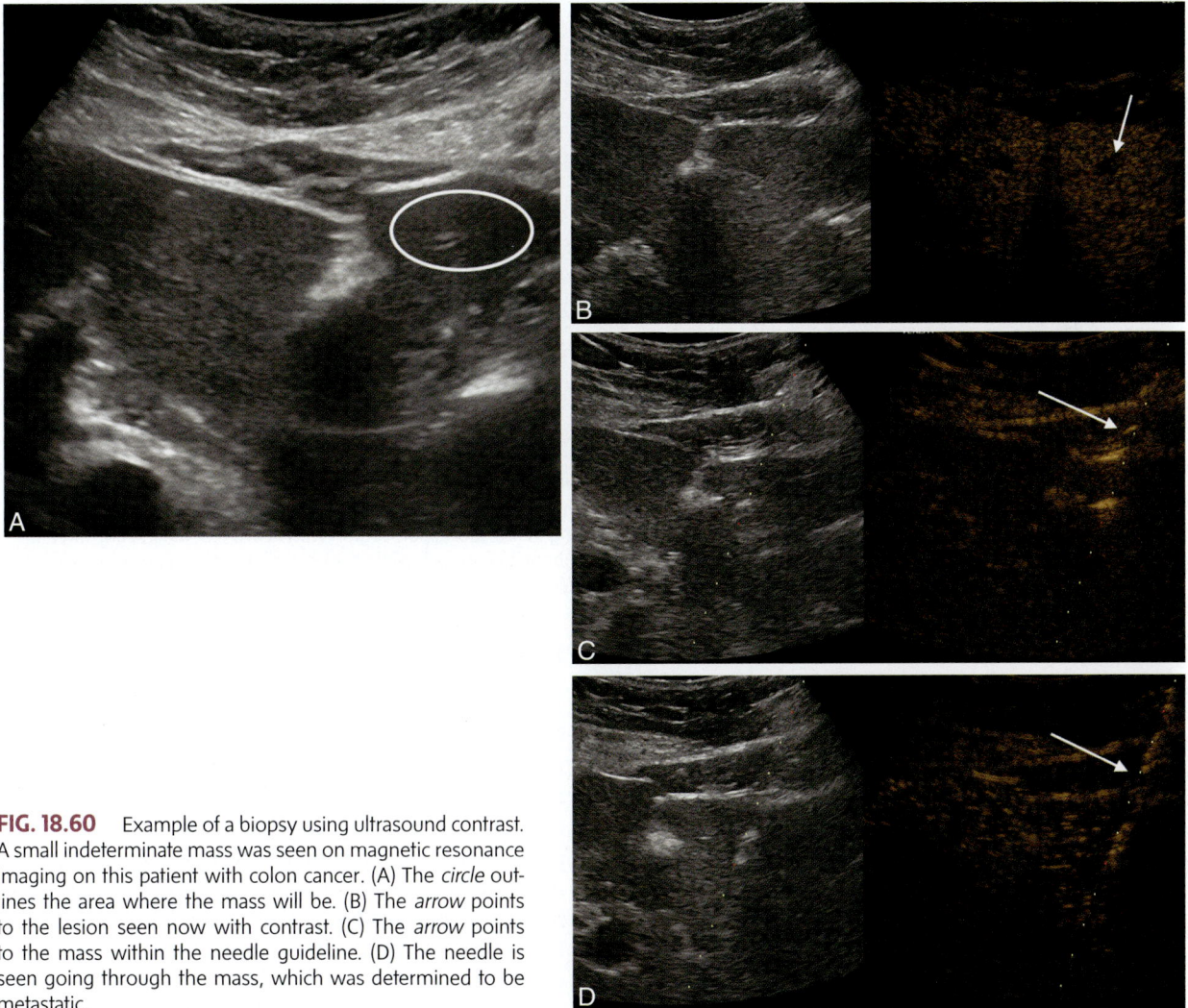

FIG. 18.60 Example of a biopsy using ultrasound contrast. A small indeterminate mass was seen on magnetic resonance imaging on this patient with colon cancer. (A) The *circle* outlines the area where the mass will be. (B) The *arrow* points to the lesion seen now with contrast. (C) The *arrow* points to the mass within the needle guideline. (D) The needle is seen going through the mass, which was determined to be metastatic.

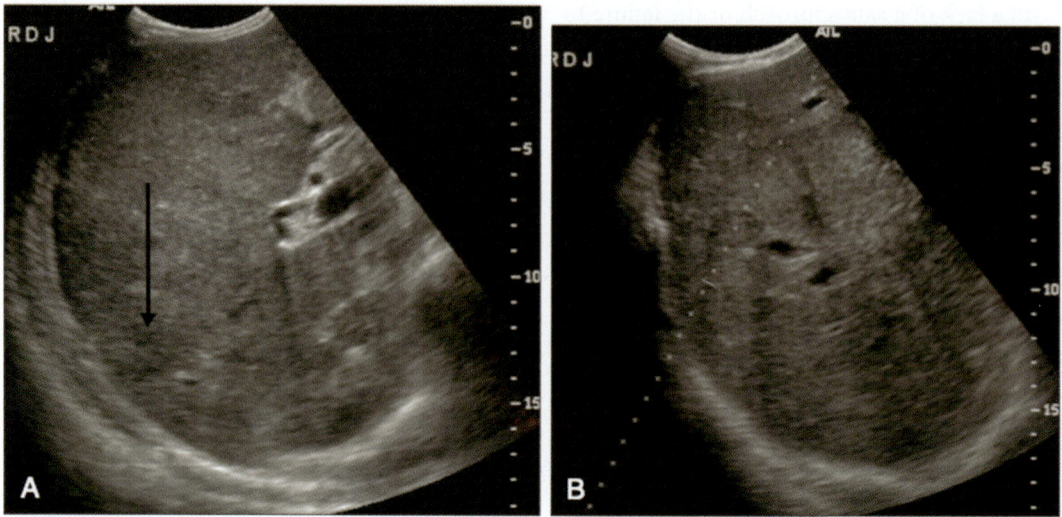

FIG. 18.61 (A) This liver lesion *(arrow)* could be seen only along the intercostal margin with the patient supine. (B) With the patient in a right posterior oblique position, the liver rolled out from under the ribs, allowing better visualization of the mass, and a subcostal approach could be used to view this metastatic mass.

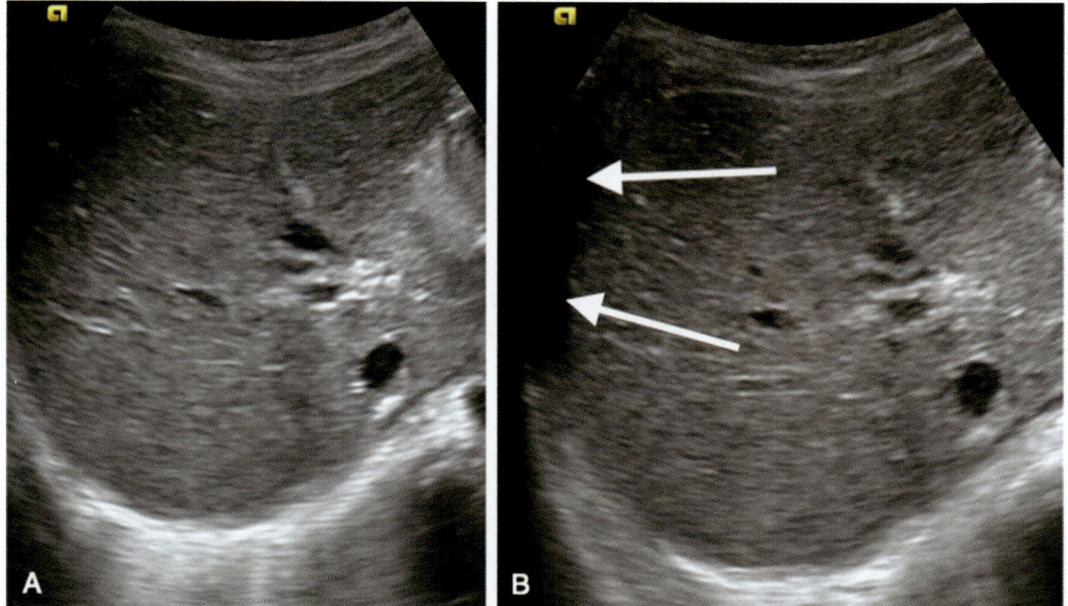

FIG. 18.62 (A) Prebiopsy image to evaluate for liver fibrosis in a pediatric patient with short gut syndrome. (B) Immediately after this, intercostal biopsy fluid was seen collecting in the subcapsule region with active bleeding seen. The sonographer applied pressure with the transducer in a subcostal approach while the physician applied pressure from an intercostal approach. Ten minutes later the bleeding had stopped and the patient was fine.

pancreatic mass biopsies are performed in the endoscopy suite using endoscopic ultrasound (EUS). With the increased resolution offered by EUS, masses are better visualized, and with an endoscopic approach there is no issues with gas. EUS has similar potential complications as percutaneous biopsies, which include bleeding, infection, or acute pancreatitis. Some patients are put on an antibiotic before an EUS biopsy to reduce the risk of an infection. An EUS biopsy will also carry the risks of general anesthesia. In patients who have a pancreatic mass with liver masses, usually a biopsy of the liver masses is performed but not of the pancreatic mass; this will confirm the pancreatic mass is adenocarcinoma and will help in staging.

Kidney

It is rare to biopsy a solid renal mass. This is because even if it is a benign mass, with the exception of an angiomyolipoma, it will need to be excised because there is potential for the mass to turn malignant. However, a biopsy of a renal mass may be needed to differentiate an incidental renal cell carcinoma (RCC) from a renal metastasis in a patient with a known primary cancer or if the patient has a prior history of RCC. For biopsies of renal masses, various patient positions should be evaluated, including supine, decubitus, oblique, and prone (Fig. 18.63). Atypical cysts, especially those with thick septations, will be biopsied to differentiate between a cystic RCC and a benign complex cyst.

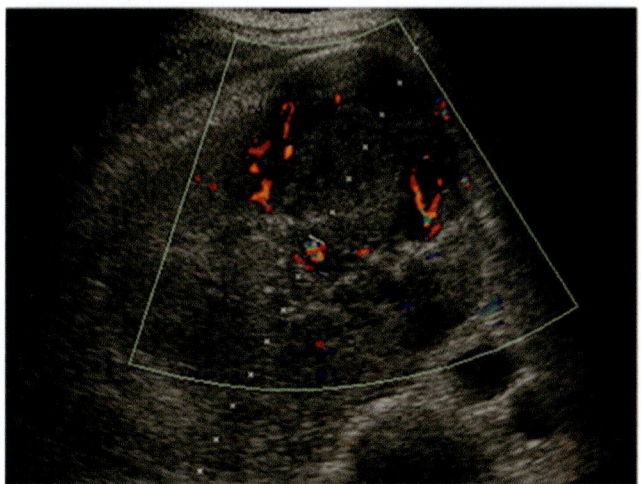

FIG. 18.63 Biopsy of a right renal mass with the patient in the left lateral decubitus position; the mass was diagnosed as metastatic disease from melanoma.

The most common biopsy on the kidney is a parenchymal biopsy on patients with increasing blood urea nitrogen (BUN) and creatinine to help determine the cause so that the proper treatment may be determined. Because the disease process affects both kidneys, either kidney can be biopsied; however, the left kidney is preferred because it offers a safer approach than the right because the spleen is well above the left kidney. These biopsies are performed with the patient prone, and the biopsy is taken from the lower pole of the left kidney, usually with an 18-gauge core needle. The needle tip is placed on the kidney capsule because cortical tissue is needed to make the diagnosis. Specific complications of renal biopsies include perinephric hematoma and hematuria. The sonographer should evaluate the needle track area with color Doppler immediately after the biopsy to ensure that there is no active bleeding. A hematoma will form with active bleeding. Fresh hematomas are echogenic. To help stop bleeding, press over the area of the jet until it stops. Keep pressing for 5 to 10 minutes until it stops. To reduce shoulder injury, stand on a step stool and use your body weight to apply pressure. If the bleeding cannot be stopped, interventional radiology should be contacted immediately because these patients are at risk of bleeding to death.

Renal Transplants

Ultrasound is used to guide biopsies when there is elevation of the creatinine or when the cause of rejection needs to be determined for treatment. Typically, the upper pole of the kidney is biopsied to avoid possible lacerations of the main renal vessels and ureter. After each pass, check for any evidence of a hematuria forming (Fig. 18.64). It is also recommended that a color Doppler image of the entire kidney be obtained at the end of the biopsy to use as a baseline in case there are complications such as an arteriovenous fistula or pseudoaneurysm formation of intrarenal vessels. Specific complications include hematomas, hematuria, pseudoaneurysm, and arteriovenous fistula (Fig. 18.65).

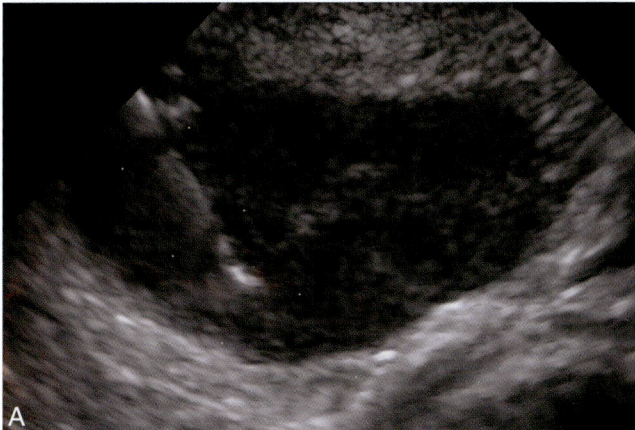

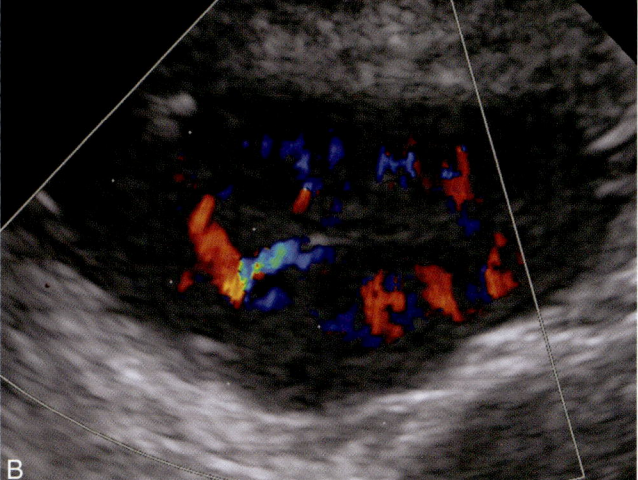

FIG. 18.64 (A) Biopsy on a renal transplant. (B) Color Doppler image showing no active bleeding.

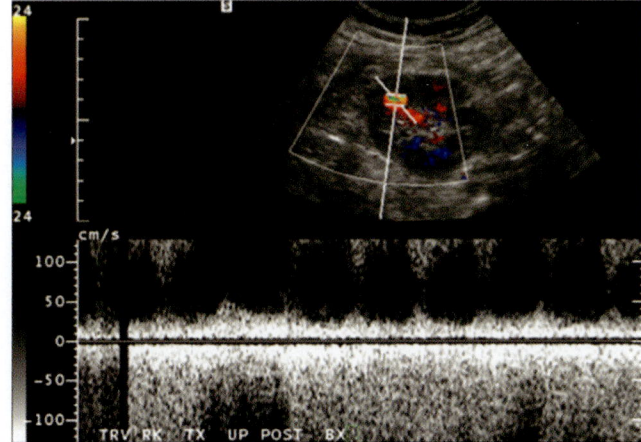

FIG. 18.65 Post-biopsy image of a renal transplant demonstrates an arteriovenous fistula. Notice the mosaic color and turbulent Doppler flow.

Retroperitoneal Lymph Nodes

Most retroperitoneal masses, including para-aortic and pericaval lymph nodes, are amenable to ultrasound guidance. These can be technically challenging, especially with small masses and in larger patients, so the use of a needle guide is essential (Fig. 18.66). To avoid major vessels and other

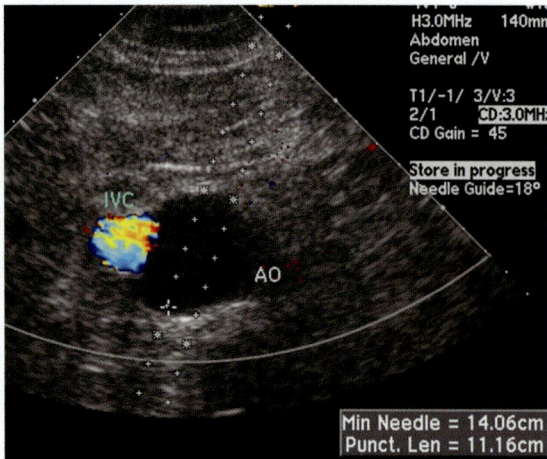

FIG. 18.66 Biopsy of an enlarged node on a patient with a yolk sac testicular cancer that was located between the inferior vena cava and aorta. The node came back positive.

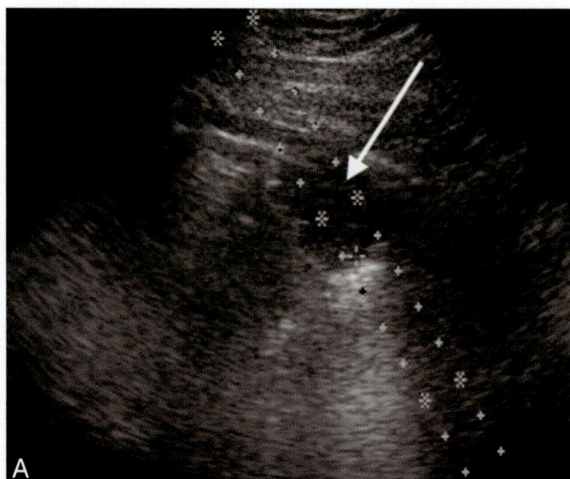

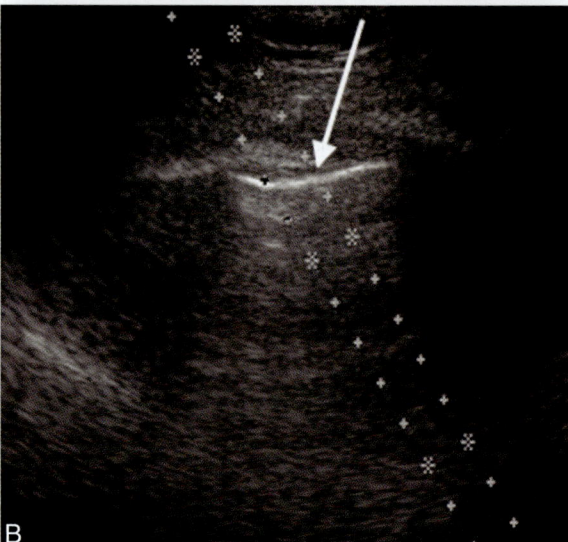

FIG. 18.67 (A) Pleura-based lung lesion *(arrow)*. (B) Unfortunately, the needle nicked the lung, causing a small pneumothorax, and the biopsy had to be rescheduled. A repeat biopsy was successful, with a diagnosis of adenocarcinoma of the lung.

structures, multiple biopsy transducers and guides may need to be evaluated to determine the safest path. Usually an anterior approach is preferred, and by applying a firm and steady pressure with the curved linear array transducer, overlying bowel loops and intra-abdominal fat can be displaced (see Fig. 18.53). This technique also reduces the depth at which the needle needs to be placed. Because the sonographer may have to apply transducer pressure, the patient may feel more discomfort than usual from the increased pressure. The sonographer should explain this to the patient. In addition, this increased pressure can add fatigue to the sonographer's wrist, hand, and shoulder joints. Therefore sonographers should relax the pressure and their grip on the transducer to reduce MSK strain between passes. Real time monitoring of the needle tip ensures that the needle excursions during the biopsy stay within the node. In patients with suspected lymphoma, tissue needs to be obtained not only to diagnose lymphoma but also to determine the subtype, because this is critical for treatment. Usually, part of the sample is sent for flow cytometric studies, and a core may be required. Specific complications include retroperitoneal hematomas.

Lung

Ultrasound guidance has been shown to be a safe alternative to CT for biopsy of pleural, parenchymal, or mediastinal masses that touch the chest wall. This technique is associated with a high success rate and lower complications than CT and is particularly valuable for small peripheral masses in close proximity to a rib and diaphragmatic masses where slight respiratory excursion can affect the position of the mass. The transducer is placed parallel to the intercostal space, and the needle is advanced in a single breath hold to minimize trauma to the pleura. The tip is monitored to ensure it does not slip out of the mass into normal aerated lung, causing a pneumothorax (Fig. 18.67). Intraparenchymal tumors are generally not amenable to ultrasound guidance, unless they are within an area of consolidation or if the patient has a large pleural effusion that can be used as an acoustic window. Lung lesions can be challenging by ultrasound, and it is always helpful to have the CT films present for guidance. Fusion technology can assist in finding these masses quickly and accurately. These lesions are usually small and mobile with respiration. Creative positioning may be needed to get between ribs and around the scapula. The patient may need to be placed in a variety of positions, including oblique, decubitus, or prone. A pillow or sponge may be placed under the patient to help spread the ribs apart. The patient's arm may also need to be adjusted to get the scapula out of the way in apical lesions. Transducer type also needs to be evaluated because sometimes a phased array transducer provides better access than a linear array transducer. Remember that resolution is not as much an issue as is accessibility. Start with a small footprint phased array transducer because it helps to image between the ribs and allows the sonographer to angle through the rib space. Once the lesion is located, the linear array transducer can be evaluated for path access. In lung biopsies, patient breathing is crucial because the lesion will move with respirations. The sonographer will need to evaluate the patient in various degrees of inspiration and expiration. These lesions can be challenging for the sonographer to find because there are few landmarks to use. Specific complications include pneumothorax. If the patient starts to cough up blood, hemoptysis, the biopsy needs to stop immediately for patient safety.

Thyroid Gland

Thyroid biopsy is one of the most common biopsies performed under ultrasound guidance. Because of the low risk, these biopsies are performed in private offices by endocrinologists and outpatient radiology centers. A thyroid biopsy is performed to distinguish malignant masses from goiters or adenomas. Biopsies should be taken in various portions of the mass to confirm colloid or abnormal cells. The sonographer should look for small calcifications because there is a higher percentage of positive cells in these areas (Fig. 18.68). The sonographer should evaluate if the thyroid gland moves with respiration. If it does, the patient should be told to hold their breath as the needle is inserted. Usually, the patient can breathe shallowly during the biopsy process. Specific complications include neck pain and hematomas. Elastography may prove beneficial in finding areas of suspicion to improve biopsy results.

Neck Nodes and Masses

Biopsies of neck masses can easily be performed with ultrasound guidance. In a patient with a history of thyroid cancer, it is important to differentiate between malignant and benign lymph nodes. Round, homogeneous lymph nodes are usually suspicious for cancer as opposed to oval nodes with echogenic centers from a fatty hilum. Other causes of neck masses include lymphoma and submandibular gland tumors. Masses of the parotid gland can also be biopsied under ultrasound guidance. Large masses seen in a supraclavicular location may be difficult to access using a linear array transducer. High-frequency curved arrays, phased arrays, or even an endocavitary transducer may give more access to these masses.

Musculoskeletal Biopsies

Procedures in MSK applications are growing and being performed by radiologists and orthopedic physicians and physician assistants (PAs). Most masses are typically biopsied with a radiologist, whereas joint effusions are drained by the orthopedic department. Masses may be muscular in origin, such as a leiomyosarcoma or rhabdomyosarcoma, or from nerves, such as a schwannoma or neurofibroma (Fig. 18.69). If a bony lesion has broken through the cortex, ultrasound can be used to guide the biopsy (Fig. 18.70). Ewing sarcoma,

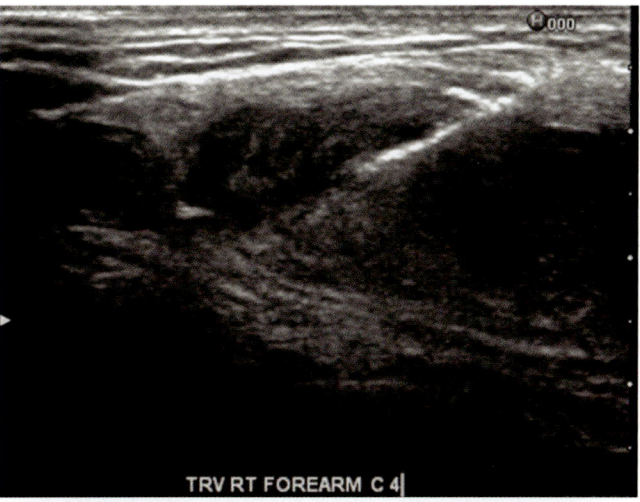

FIG. 18.69 Biopsy of a mass in the forearm that was diagnosed as rhabdomyosarcoma.

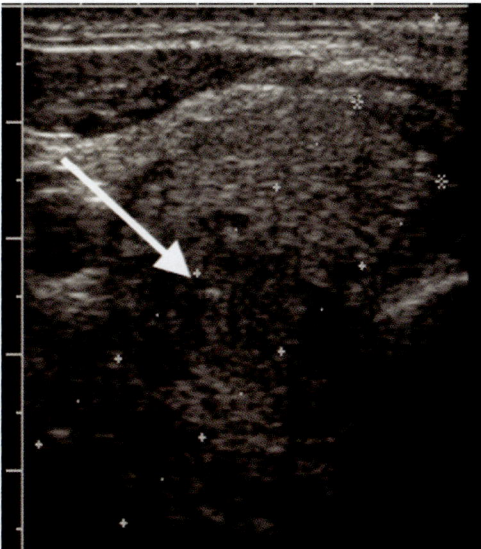

FIG. 18.68 After several negative passes in this large thyroid nodule, positive cells were obtained in the area of the small calcifications *(arrow)*.

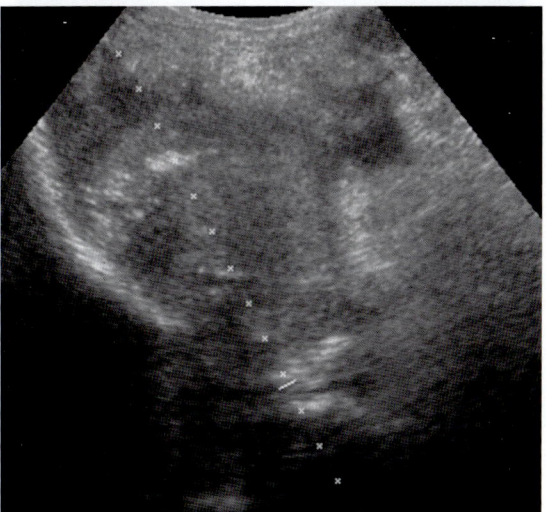

FIG. 18.70 Biopsy of a mass in the right iliac crest that had broken through the cortex, allowing it to be biopsied using ultrasound. The pathology came back as a chondrosarcoma.

osteosarcoma, and metastatic disease from prostate cancer are some examples of bone cancers. Ultrasound is being widely used to perform nerve blocks and drain effusions and give corticosteroid injections in various joints (Fig. 18.71). Typically, a cocktail of Kenalog or Depo-Medrol and lidocaine is used for joint injections to help reduce inflammation and pain.

Pelvis

Pelvic masses can be biopsied with a transabdominal, transvaginal, or transrectal approach. The approach used will depend on the location of the mass. With a biopsy of pelvic lymph nodes, color Doppler is used to identify the location of the iliac vessels. Transvaginal biopsies are usually performed with the patient in stirrups. Because of the sensitivity of the vaginal wall, the patient may need something more than a local anesthetic, such as conscious sedation.

Prostate Gland

Prostate biopsies are being performed more and more by urologists, especially with ultrasound equipment designed especially for prostate fusion. Men with elevated prostate-specific antigen levels or palpable nodules found on a rectal digital examination may be referred for a prostate biopsy. If a full scan is needed before the biopsy, the biopsy guide should be placed on the transducer so that the probe does not need to be removed and reinserted. The patient is biopsied in the left lateral decubitus position. Because the biopsy is through the rectal wall, the patient should be placed on a broad-spectrum antibiotic the day before and usually 2 days after the biopsy to reduce the chance of infection. Some institutions may require a urine sample before the biopsy, to evaluate for a urinary tract infection (UTI) because a UTI can become a urosepsis after biopsy, which may be life threatening. Because of the possibility of postbiopsy infections, some institutions have started having their patients have a rectal swab to look for drug-resistant organisms. These are usually performed 5 to 14 days before the procedure. Transrectal prostate biopsies are considered clean procedures, not sterile procedures. Random samples are taken from the apex, mid, and base of the peripheral zone and the central gland on both the right and left sides of the gland. The number of passes in each region will vary between practices. For the peripheral zone area, the needle tip is placed on the edge of the prostate gland and fired. For central gland passes, the needle tip is placed inside the prostate gland, just inside the central gland. MRI fused biopsies are performed on men with persistent elevating PSA levels and a history of a normal traditional prostate biopsy. The MRI will demonstrate suspicious nodules that can be biopsied (Fig. 18.72). On the patient for whom a rectal approach is not feasible because of rectal surgery, a transperineal biopsy can be performed (Fig. 18.73). The best transducer is typically a phased array transducer because a small footprint is required. The patient is placed in stirrups, with the perineum exposed. The penis and scrotum need to be positioned out of the biopsy field and held in place with towels and tape. The patient is usually given IV sedation in addition to plenty of local numbing because of the sensitivity of this area. Because of the lack of resolution, two to three random specimens are obtained from both the right and left sides of the prostate gland.

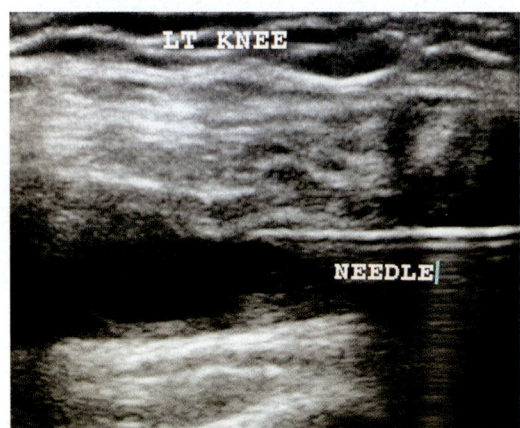

FIG. 18.71 Ultrasound-guided aspiration of fluid in the left knee.

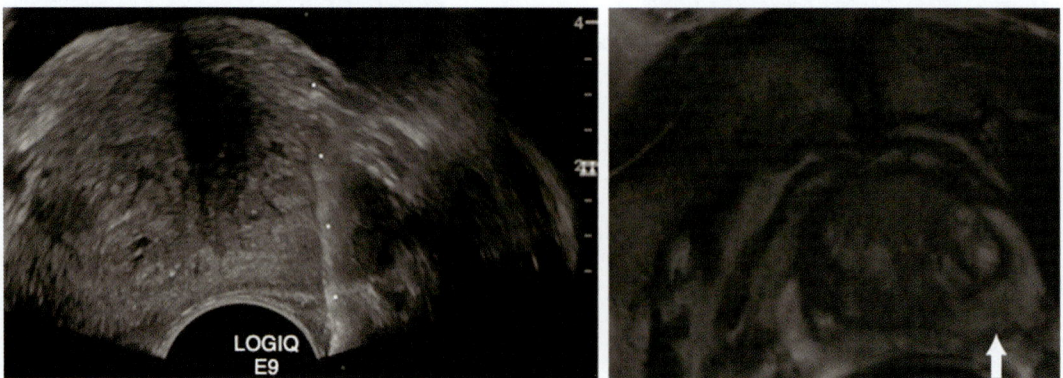

FIG. 18.72 Prostate guided biopsy using magnetic resonance imaging (MRI) fusion technique. The patient's previous biopsies were normal, yet his prostate-specific antigen kept rising. MRI demonstrated a suspicious lesion *(arrow)*. Biopsy through this area found the prostate cancer with a Gleason grade of 5.

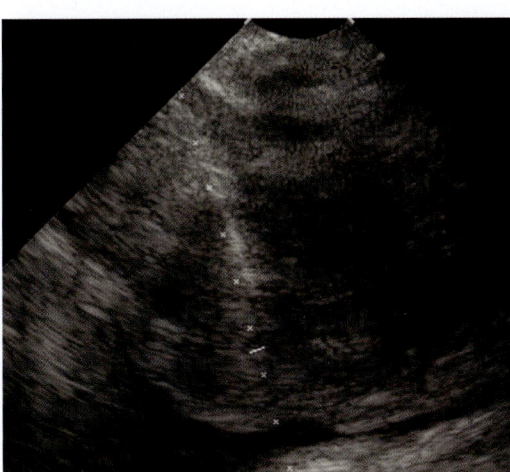

FIG. 18.73 This patient had a prostate-specific antigen of 4.1 but had a history of rectal cancer that prevented transrectal ultrasound. A transperineal biopsy was ordered. The samples came back negative for cancer.

FLUID COLLECTIONS AND ABSCESSES

Pleural Fluid

Many hospitals have hospitalists who use compact ultrasound units to perform thoracentesis studies at bedside, so these procedures are now rarely performed by the ultrasound department. However, when performed by the ultrasound department, the patient should be scanned in an upright position, through the back, usually with a small footprint transducer such as a curved linear array or phased array transducer. While the fluid is being drained, the patient may start to cough as the lung expands with air. After the procedure the patient may be sent for a chest radiograph to make sure that there is no pneumothorax. If unable to see any fluid in an upright position, the patient should be scanned supine to see if there really is any fluid above the diaphragm. This will help to determine if it is a very small effusion that is not amenable to draining.

Ascites

Just like thoracentesis, procedures on inpatients with ascites that needs to be drained are usually performed by the hospitalist. Outpatient procedures or large volume drains are performed in the ultrasound department. The entire abdomen and pelvis should be evaluated for the extent of fluid and to locate the largest area or "pocket" of fluid. To pool the fluid in the pelvis, the patient may be scanned in a reverse Trendelenburg position of 30 to 45 degrees. If the fluid is septated, the pocket is small, or there are organs or bowel loops in the way, a guide may need to be used. During the procedure, the patient may be rolled into an oblique position so that the fluid drains to the dependent portion where the needle or centesis catheter is located. A postprocedural image should be taken to document any remaining fluid.

Abscess Drainage

Drainage of abscess collections is typically performed by the interventional lab because typically drains will be placed and the patient will need follow-up. The ultrasound department may be used to obtain a small amount of fluid to determine the type of organism that is causing the infection so that the proper type of antibiotic can be used. Infected fluid is typically complex and may contain low-level echoes. Larger-bore needles from 16 to 18 gauge may be needed to remove the viscous fluid.

NEW APPLICATIONS

As elastography and ultrasound contrast continue to evolve and get approval, they will have an impact on biopsies. Liver elastography may replace or greatly reduce the need for liver core biopsies in patients with parenchymal liver disease. Elastography may also help to identify abnormal tissue to aid in determining where to biopsy in such organs as the prostate and thyroid. Contrast may help in reducing the need to biopsy masses with clear benign flow patterns, especially in the liver and kidney. These new technologies may help solve current issues so that more patients may have their procedure under ultrasound guidance, thus improving patient care and reducing costs to the health system.

> **Key Pearls**
>
> - The main advantage of using ultrasound for guidance is to have continuous real time visualization of the biopsy needle, which allows adjustment of the needle as needed during the procedure.
> - The sonographer should look for indirect signs of the presence of a mass, such as displaced vessels, capsule bulges, or the presence of tumor vessels.
> - Biopsies are used to confirm if a mass is benign, malignant, or infectious.
> - Other indications include the need to differentiate between a metastatic and a second primary mass, to determine the cause of metastases in a patient with multiple primaries, to differentiate recurrent tumor from postoperative or therapy scarring, to differentiate malignancy from inflammatory or infectious disease, to determine metastatic lymph adenopathy from lymphoma, and to characterize a benign mass.
> - Other common reasons for a biopsy are to obtain a sample of the parenchyma in an organ to determine the severity or progression of a disease process such as hepatitis or renal failure or to determine the cause of rejection in a transplanted organ.
> - Complications from an ultrasound-guided biopsy are usually minor and may include postprocedural pain or discomfort, vasovagal reactions, and hematomas.
> - Serious complications, although rare, include bleeding, hemorrhage, pneumothorax, pancreatitis, biliary leakage, peritonitis, infection, and possibly death.

BIBLIOGRAPHY

Bhairvi SJ, et al. Endoscopic ultrasound-guided fine-needle aspiration of pancreatic lesions: a systematic review of technical and procedural variables. *N Am J Med Sci.* 2016;8(1):1–11.

Brugge WR. Pancreatic fine needle aspiration: to do or not to do? *J Pancreas (Online).* 2004;5(4):282–288.

Carberry GA, et al. Percutaneous biopsy in the abdomen and pelvis: a step-by-step approach. *Abdom Radiol.* 2016;41:720–742.

Elmageed MKA, et al. Ultrasound and CT guided biopsy of suspicious musculoskeletal lesions: diagnostic performance and implications for the management. *Int J Radiology & Radiat Ther.* 2020;7(1).

Kawamura DM, Lunsford BM, eds Rybynski AJ: Sonography-guided interventional procedures. Abdomen and Superficial Structures (Diagnostic Medical Sonography Series). Philadelphia: Lippincott Williams & Wilkins; 2012. ed 4.

Khosia R, et al. Ultrasound-guided versus computed tomography-scan guided biopsy of pleural-based lung lesions. *Lung India.* 2016;33(5):487–492.

Kim SY, Chung HW, Oh TS, et al. Practical guidelines for ultrasound-guided core needle biopsy of soft-tissue lesions: transformation from beginner to specialist. *Korean J Radiol.* 2017;18(2):361–369.

Kliewer M, Sheafor D, Hertzberg B, et al. Percutaneous liver biopsy: a cost-benefit analysis comparing sonographic and CT guidance. *Am J Roentgenol.* 1999;173(5):1199–1202.

Malanga G, Mautner K. *Atlas of Ultrasound-Guided Musculoskeletal Injections (Atlas Series)*: McGraw-Hill; 2014.

Marks L, et al. MRI–ultrasound fusion for guidance of targeted prostate biopsy. *Curr Opin Urol.* 2013;23(1):43–50.

MedlinePlus. Prothrombin time test and INR (PT/INR). https://medlineplus.gov/lab-tests/prothrombin-time-test-and-inr-ptinr/

Potretzke TA et al: Ultrasound-Guided Biopsy of Chest, Abdomen and Pelvis, Chapter in Rumack CM, Levine D: Diagnostic Ultrasound, 5th Edition Elsevier; 2017.

Radiology Key. Percutaneous biopsy. https://radiologykey.com/percutaneous-biopsy-2/

Radiopaedia. Liver biopsy (percutaneous). https://radiopaedia.org/articles/liver-biopsy-percutaneous?lang=us

Radiopaedia. Percutaneous renal biopsy. https://radiopaedia.org/articles/percutaneous-renal-biopsy-1?lang=us

Shyamala K, et al. Risk of tumor cell seeding through biopsy and aspiration cytology. *Int J Radiology & Radiat Ther.* 2020;7(1).

Uppot RN, et al. Imaging-guided percutaneous renal biopsy: rationale and approach. *AJR.* 2010;194(6).

Wikipedia. Partial thromboplastin time. https://en.wikipedia.org/wiki/Partial_thromboplastin_time

Wikipedia. Prothrombin time: International Normalized Ratio. https://en.wikipedia.org/wiki/Prothrombin_time#International_normalized_ratio

Winter TC, et al. Ultrasound-guided biopsies in the abdomen and pelvis. *Ultrasound Q.* 2008;24:45Y68.

CHAPTER 19

Emergent Ultrasound Procedures

Sandra L. Hagen-Ansert

OBJECTIVES

On completion of this chapter, you should be able to:
- Discuss the advantages and disadvantages of sonography for the trauma patient
- Define the goal of sonography in the assessment of blunt trauma
- Describe the protocol for focused assessment with sonography for trauma (FAST)
- Describe the sonographic findings for aortic dissection, right upper quadrant pain, free fluid in the abdominopelvic region, acute pelvic pain, and scrotal trauma and torsion
- Identify the modalities commonly used to evaluate flank pain

OUTLINE

Assessment of Abdominal Trauma 561
   Diagnostic Peritoneal Lavage 562
   Computed Tomography 562
   Ultrasound 562
Focused Assessment with Sonography for Trauma 563
   Assessment of Blunt Trauma With Ultrasound 563
   Parenchymal Injury 566

Right Upper Quadrant Pain 567
   Acute Cholecystitis Versus Cholelithiasis 567
   Biliary Dilation 568
Epigastric Pain 568
   Pancreatitis 568
   Abdominal Aortic Aneurysm 569
Extreme Shortness of Breath 570
   Pericardial Effusion 570
Chest Pain 572

Thoracic Aortic Dissection 572
Flank Pain 573
   Urolithiasis 573
Right Lower Quadrant Pain 574
   Appendicitis 574
Paraumbilical Hernia 575
Acute Pelvic Pain 578
   Sonography of Pelvic Structures 578
Scrotal Trauma and Torsion 579
Extremity Swelling and Pain 579

KEY TERMS

Blunt abdominal trauma (BAT)
Diagnostic peritoneal lavage (DPL)
Focused assessment with sonography for trauma (FAST) exam

Hemoperitoneum
Incarcerated hernia
Intravenous urography (IVU)
Pseudodissection

Reducible hernia
Strangulated hernia

Sonography is well recognized as a powerful and efficient tool for the diagnosis and evaluation of the patient in the emergency department (ED). The development of smaller ultrasound equipment and improvement in transducer technology have enabled the sonographic examination to extend beyond the imaging departments and be especially prevalent in the ED. The implementation of educational curriculum changes in specialized residency programs and specialty practice has facilitated the integration of focused ultrasound into specific emergent settings. In emergent and critical situations, the ED team must be able to efficiently and accurately assess the patient's problem, and sonography is a tool that allows the team to quickly evaluate the patient.

The most common reasons people go to the ED include trauma, acute chest pain, shortness of breath, hypotensive events, acute abdominal or pelvic pain, syncope, extreme nausea and vomiting, lacerations, and broken bones.

The primary focus of this chapter is to cover the more common emergent abdominal procedures that the sonographer is likely to encounter in a call-back situation from the ED. The ED resident or emergency physician may have already performed a rapid survey of the area of interest and may call for a "formal or complete" ultrasound evaluation if further information is needed. Potential life-threatening emergencies such as abdominal emergencies, internal hemorrhage following blunt trauma, ectopic pregnancy, pericardial tamponade, and ruptured aortic aneurysm may be rapidly assessed with sonography.

ASSESSMENT OF ABDOMINAL TRAUMA

The assessment of the abdomen for possible sustained abdominal injury caused by blunt abdominal trauma is a common clinical challenge for physicians and emergency medicine physicians. The physical findings may be unreliable because of the state of patient consciousness, neurologic deficit, medication, or other associated injuries.

Diagnostic Peritoneal Lavage

Diagnostic peritoneal lavage (DPL) was used to sample the intraperitoneal space for evidence of damage to the viscera and blood vessels in patients with blunt abdominal trauma to decide which patients needed exploratory laparotomy. For this procedure the patient is placed in the supine position and the urinary bladder is emptied by catheterization. The patient's stomach is emptied by a nasogastric tube because the distended stomach may extend to the anterior abdominal wall. The skin is anesthetized, and a small vertical incision is made. The incision is made either in the midline or at the paraumbilical site, with multiple layers of tissue penetrated before the parietal peritoneum is located (Fig. 19.1). Although peritoneal lavage has been used successfully to assess abdominal injuries, it is an invasive procedure that takes at least 10 to 15 minutes and that carries a risk of bowel perforation, bladder penetration, vascular laceration, and wound complications. This procedure has been inappropriate for alert patients in stable condition, who represented the majority of patients with blunt abdominal trauma. Peritoneal lavage decreases the specificity of subsequent ultrasonography or computed tomography (CT) because of the introduction of intraperitoneal fluid and air.

Computed Tomography

CT remains the radiology standard for investigating the injured abdomen but requires patient transfer and inevitable delay (bowel preparation). CT is usually performed in patients in whom intra-abdominal injury is strongly suspected. Other indications for CT include equivocal findings of abdominal examination in stable patients, persistent abdominal pain, and decreasing hematocrit. CT is unsuitable for patients who are clinically unstable. The time required to complete a CT scan is variable; however, the sensitivity and specificity is high to detect fluid collections.

Ultrasound

The clinical utilization of sonography in the evaluation of **blunt abdominal trauma (BAT)** has existed in Europe and Asia since the 1970s (Box 19.1) North America and the United Kingdom did not incorporate its use until the 1990s. The development of smaller ultrasound systems and improved transducer technology have made this application grow. Using sonography as a screening procedure involves many factors that will be fast, accurate, portable, and noninvasive. A rapid survey with sonography may be made in less than 4 minutes. Disadvantages include the presence of subcutaneous or intra-abdominal air and obesity. Sonography is now well established as a noninvasive and easily repeatable tool to image many areas of the body.

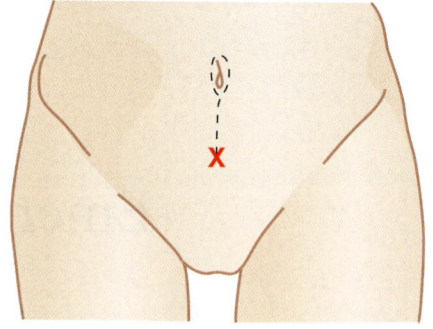

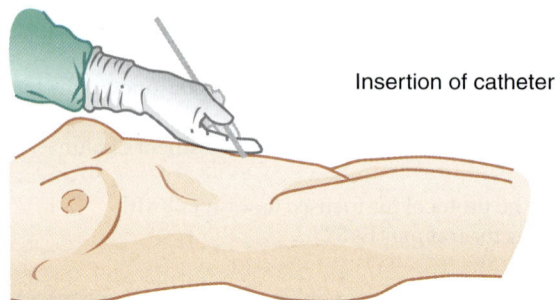

Insertion of catheter

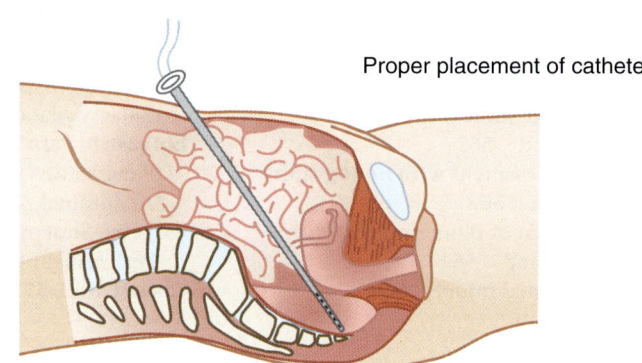

Proper placement of catheter

After infusion of lavage fluid, the bag is dropped below the patient to allow fluid to drain out

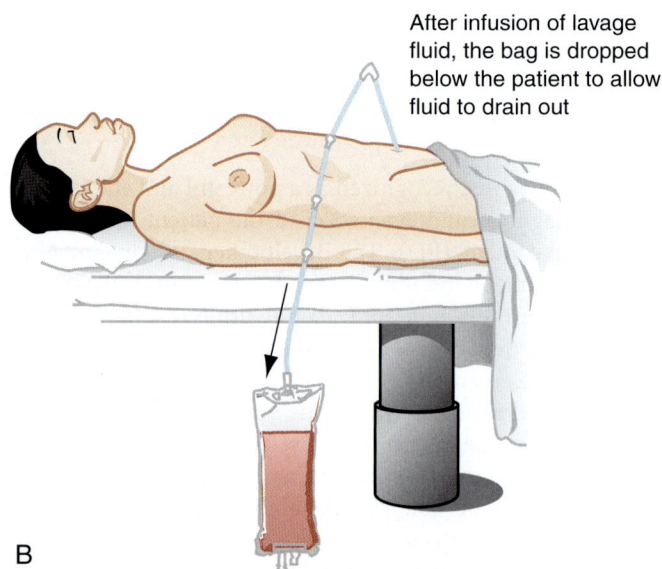

B

FIG. 19.1 Peritoneal lavage. The incision is made either in the midline or at the paraumbilical site with multiple layers of tissue penetrated before the parietal peritoneum is located.

| BOX 19.1 | Blunt Abdominal Trauma |

Hemodynamically Unstable Patient
FAST examination
Determine if intraperitoneal fluid is present
Exploratory laparotomy is indicated for patients with positive DPL or FAST exam
Consider other sites of blood loss or nonhemorrhagic shock (repeat FAST or DPL)

Hemodynamically Stable Patient
Surveillance studies and clinical observation
- FAST examination to determine presence of intraperitoneal fluid
- CT scan

CT, Computed tomography; *DPL*, diagnostic peritoneal lavage; *FAST*, focused assessment with sonography for trauma.

FOCUSED ASSESSMENT WITH SONOGRAPHY FOR TRAUMA

Focused assessment with sonography for trauma (FAST) has become an extension of the physical examination of the trauma patient. This is a focused survey examination of the abdomen, pelvis, and pericardium to evaluate free fluid or pericardial fluid (Fig. 19.2). The FAST exam is performed in the ED by properly trained and credentialed staff. In the context of traumatic injury, the timely diagnosis of potentially life-threatening hemorrhage found during the FAST exam is a decision-making tool to help determine the transfer to the operating room, CT scanner, or angiography suite.

FAST Survey
- Perihepatic and hepatorenal space (right upper quadrant)
- Perisplenic (left upper quadrant)
- Pelvis: cul-de-sac (bladder)
- Pericardium (cardiac)

The FAST ultrasound evaluation survey is widespread, extending from the pericardial sac to the urinary bladder and includes the perihepatic area (including Morison's pouch), perisplenic region (including splenorenal recess), paracolic gutters, and cul-de-sac (Fig. 19.3). The visceral organs are assessed for heterogeneity and evaluated with color Doppler if necessary.

Accessibility and speed of performance are critical in the trauma setting. Onsite personnel who are educated in performing the ultrasound examination provide the highest success rate. Limitations of ultrasound include its dependence on operator skill and patient body habitus, which becomes particularly important if surgeons or emergency physicians with limited training perform the studies. Although CT remains the standard of reference for intraperitoneal and retroperitoneal assessment, this application is not available at the bedside.

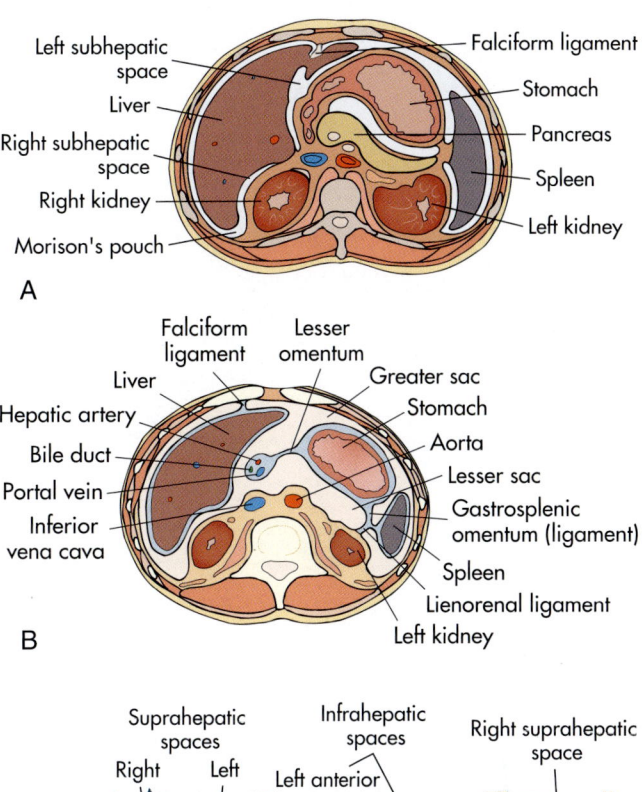

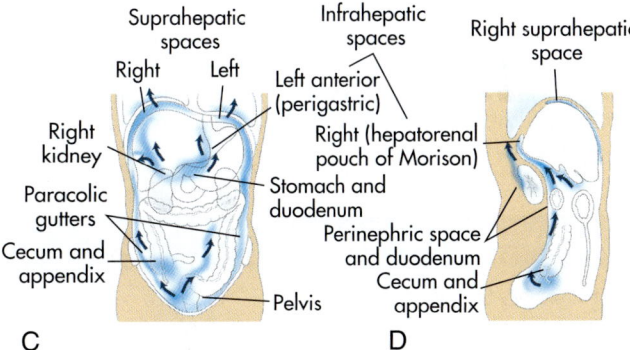

FIG. 19.2 (A) Transverse view of the perihepatic space and Morison's pouch. (B) Transverse view of the perisplenic area and the splenorenal ligament. (C) Anterior view of the collection of fluid in the abdomen and pelvic cavities. (D) Sagittal view of the right abdomen shows how the fluid collects in the most dependent areas of the abdomen and pelvis.

Assessment of Blunt Trauma With Ultrasound

Ultrasound of the abdomen and pelvis is performed simultaneously with the physical assessment, resuscitation, and stabilization of the trauma patient. The examination usually takes less than 4 minutes. The goal is to scan the four quadrants, pericardial sac, and cul-de-sac for the presence of free fluid or **hemoperitoneum**. Ultrasound has been found to be highly sensitive for the detection of free intraperitoneal fluid, but it is not sensitive for the identification of organ injuries. If the patient is hemodynamically stable, the value of ultrasound is limited by the large percentage of organ injuries that are not associated with free fluid.

Protocol for Focused Assessment With Sonography for Trauma. The ultrasound examination is performed with the proper transducer selection according to the patient size. The patient is usually in the supine position. The right and left upper quadrants of the abdomen, epigastrium, paracolic

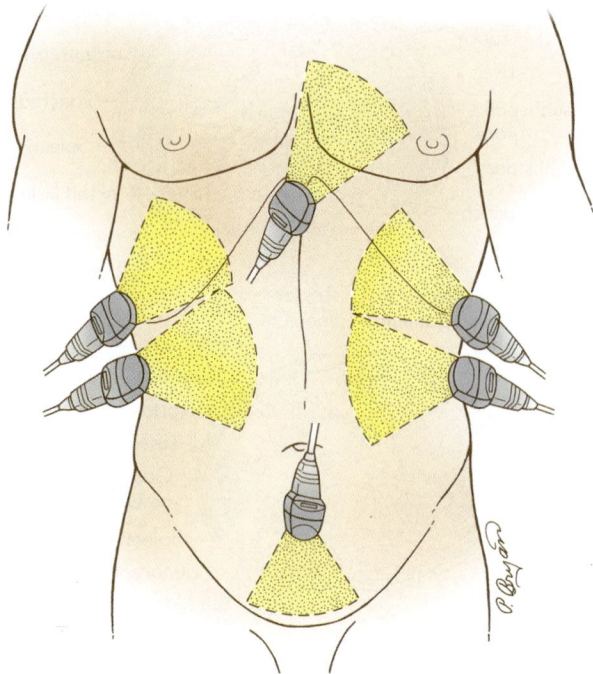

FIG. 19.3 The focused assessment with sonography for trauma ultrasound evaluation survey is widespread, extending from the pericardial sac to the urinary bladder and includes the perihepatic area (including Morison's pouch), perisplenic region (including splenorenal recess), paracolic gutters, and cul-de-sac.

BOX 19.2	FAST Scan Protocol

- Fill urinary bladder
- Scan subxiphoid to look for pericardial effusion
- Evaluate RUQ: diaphragm, subhepatic space/Morison's pouch, right kidney, right flank
- Evaluate liver for texture abnormalities
- Evaluate epigastrium
- Evaluate LUQ: diaphragm, spleen, left kidney, left flank
- Evaluate RLQ
- Evaluate LLQ

FAST, Focused assessment with sonography for trauma; *LLQ*, left lower quadrant; *LUQ*, left upper quadrant; *RLQ*, right lower quadrant; *RUQ*, right upper quadrant.

gutters, retroperitoneal space, and pelvis are evaluated with ultrasound (Box 19.2). If there is no contraindication to catheterization, the empty bladder is filled with 200 to 300 mL of sterile saline through a Foley catheter to ensure bladder distention to allow adequate visualization of the pelvic cavity. The examination is focused to look for the presence of free fluid, the texture of the visceral organs, and the pericardial sac around the heart.

The initial survey is directed in the subcostal plane with the transducer angled in a cephalic direction toward the four-chamber view of the heart to image the pericardial sac (Fig. 19.4). The right upper quadrant is then evaluated, including the diaphragm, dome of the liver, subhepatic space (Morison's pouch), right kidney, and right flank (Fig. 19.5).

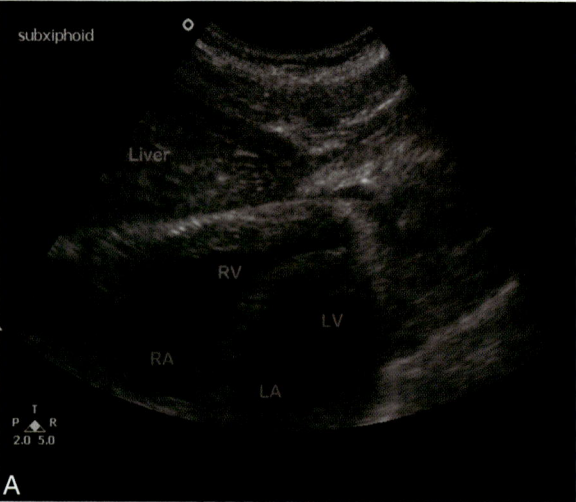

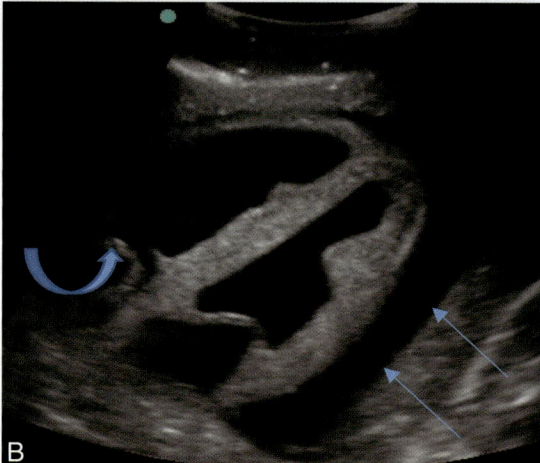

FIG. 19.4 The initial survey is directed in the subcostal plane with the transducer angled in a cephalic direction toward the four-chamber view of the heart to image the pericardial sac. (A) Subcostal view shows no evidence of pericardial fluid. (B) Moderate pericardial fluid seen within the pericardial sac *(arrows)*, as well as right atrial collapse *(curved arrow)* that indicates impending tamponade. *LA*, Left atrium; *LV*, left ventricle; *RA*, right atrium, *RV*, right ventricle.

The liver is quickly scanned to look for free fluid or hematoma. The epigastrium is briefly examined. The transducer is then moved to the left upper quadrant to observe the diaphragm, spleen, left kidney, and left flank and to search for the presence of fluid (Fig. 19.6). The pelvic cavity (with the bladder distended) is evaluated for the presence of free fluid in the cul-de-sac (Fig. 19.7).

Sonographic Findings. In the trauma setting, free fluid usually represents hemoperitoneum, although it may also represent bowel, urine, bile, or ascitic fluid. Hemorrhage in the peritoneal cavity collects in the most dependent area of the abdomen. The fluid is usually hypoechoic or hyperechoic, with scattered internal echoes representing the blood, and conforms to the anatomic site it occupies (Fig. 19.8). The most common site of fluid accumulation is the subhepatic space (Morison's pouch), regardless of the site of the injury (Fig. 19.9). The next most common space is the pelvis. The blood in the pelvis may collect centrally in

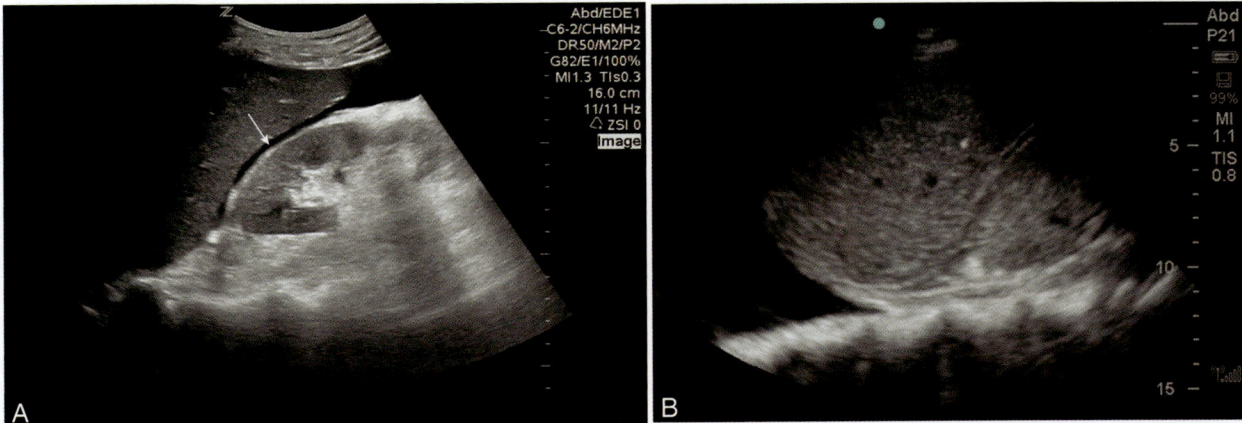

FIG. 19.5 The right upper quadrant is evaluated, including the diaphragm, dome of the liver, subhepatic space (Morison's pouch), right kidney, and right flank. (A) Note the fluid in Morison's pouch *(arrow)* between the right lobe of the liver and right kidney. (B) Pleural effusion is seen in the costophrenic angle.

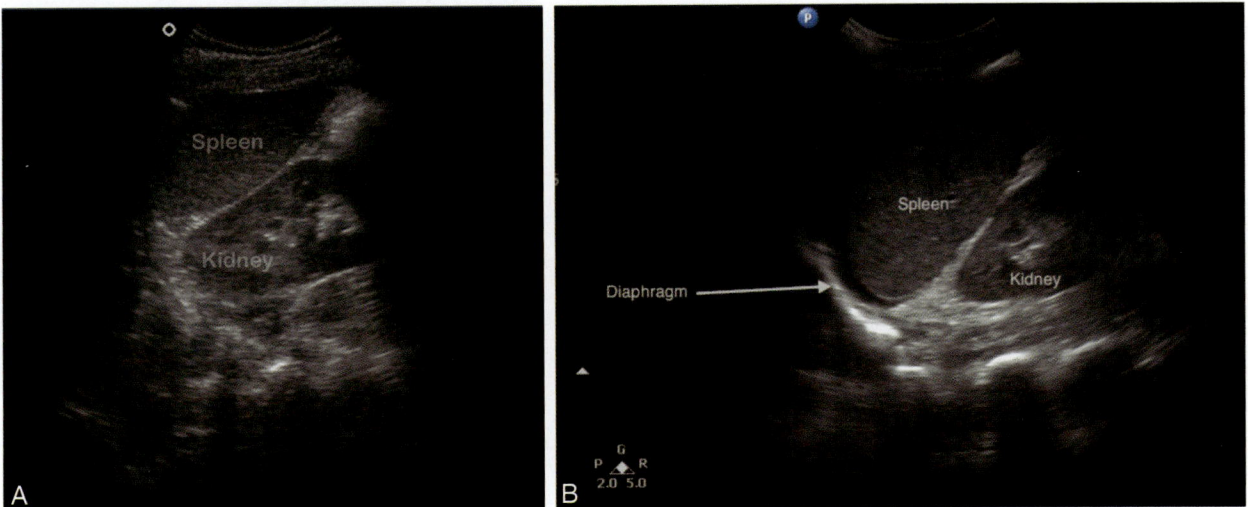

FIG. 19.6 The transducer is moved to the left upper quadrant to observe the diaphragm, spleen, left kidney, and left flank and to search for the presence of fluid. (A) Normal spleen and left kidney. (B) Fluid surrounds the splenic capsule.

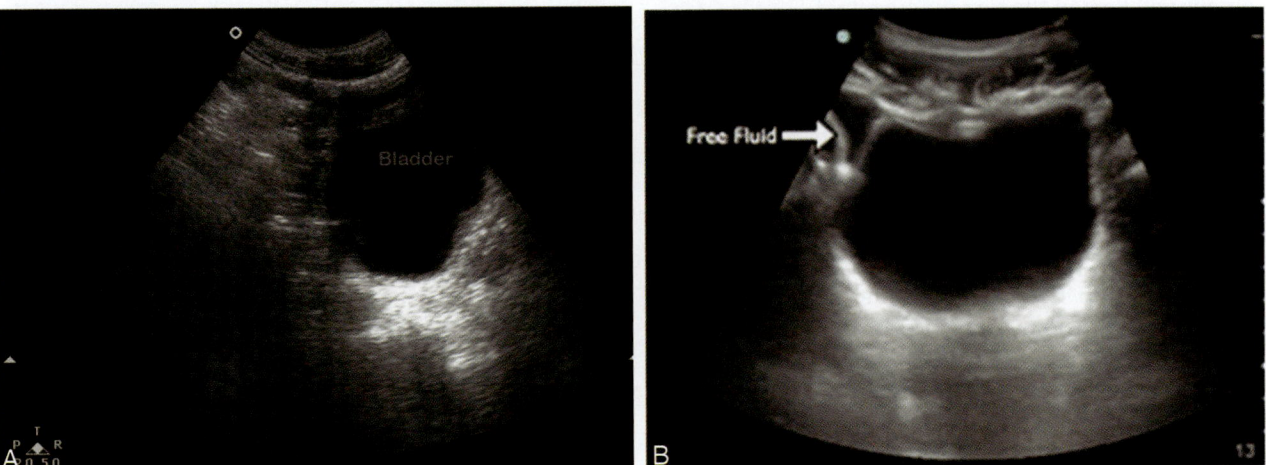

FIG. 19.7 The bladder is filled via a urinary catheter to image the pelvic region for the presence of free fluid. (A) Suprapubic image in the longitudinal axis on a male. (B) Transverse image of the distended bladder with free fluid outside the wall.

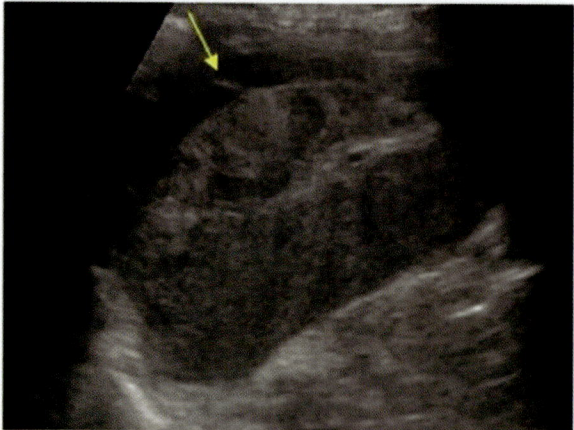

FIG. 19.8 **Subcapsular hematoma of the spleen.** The fluid is usually hypoechoic or hyperechoic, with scattered internal echoes representing the blood, and conforms to the anatomic site it occupies.

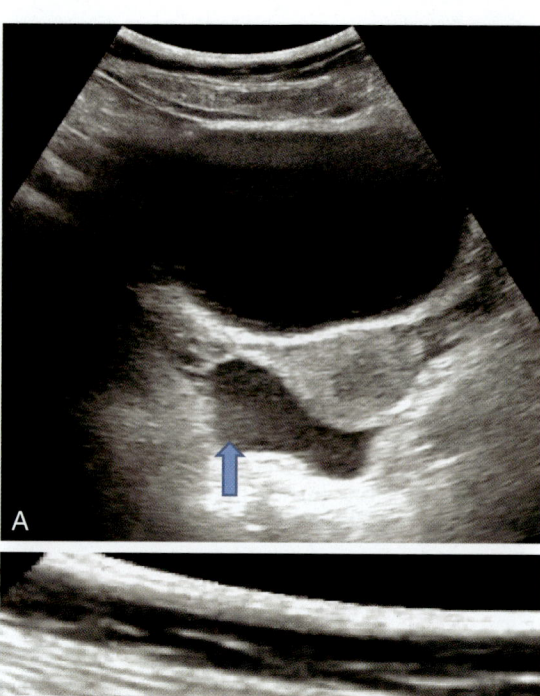

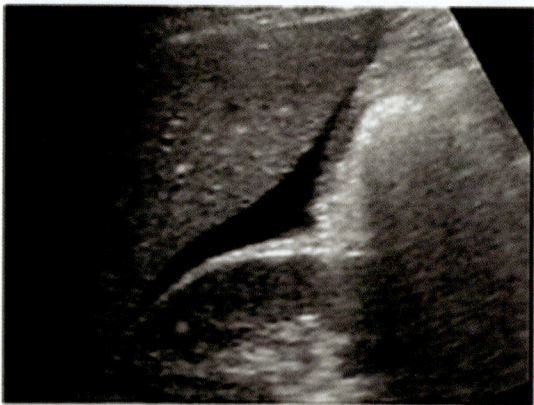

FIG. 19.9 The most common site of fluid accumulation is the subhepatic space (Morison's pouch), regardless of the site of the injury.

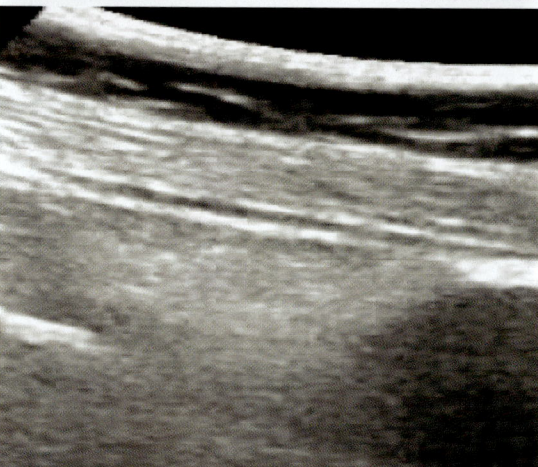

FIG. 19.10 Transverse (A) and longitudinal (B) images of free fluid in the pouch of Douglas *(arrows)*. The blood in the pelvis may collect centrally in the pouch of Douglas or laterally in the paravesical space.

the pouch of Douglas or laterally in the paravesical space (Fig. 19.10). When fluid is present, the poorly visualized loops of bowel are separated by triangular collections of fluid. If there is a massive hemoperitoneum, the intraperitoneal organs will float in the surrounding fluid.

If the collection of fluid is small, the surgeon may not want to do an immediate laparotomy. Close monitoring of the patient with either ultrasound or CT imaging may help to define the further extent of the injury after the patient stabilizes.

Parenchymal Injury

The ultrasound appearance of hepatic and splenic injury will vary with both the type and time of injury. Liver lacerations or contusions are more easily detected with ultrasound than any other visceral abdominal injury (Fig. 19.11). Such injuries appear as heterogeneous or hyperechoic. Hematomas and localized lacerations will appear initially hypoechoic with low-level echoes generated from the red blood cells, or echogenic, as the blood begins to coagulate, which over time will become more anechoic with the onset of hemolysis. Pitfalls of abdominal ultrasound include failure to show contained solid-organ injuries; injuries to the diaphragm, pancreas, and adrenal gland; and some bowel injuries. Therefore a negative ultrasound does not exclude an intraperitoneal injury, and close clinical observation or CT is warranted.

A brisk intraparenchymal hemorrhage may be identified as an anechoic region within the abnormal parenchyma, whereas a global parenchymal injury may project in the liver as a widespread architectural disruption with absence of the normal vascular pattern. An extensive splenic injury presents as a diffusely heterogeneous parenchymal pattern with both hyperechoic and hypoechoic regions.

The early diagnosis of parenchymal injury can affect patient treatment. The clinically stable patient with a hemoperitoneum and an obvious splenic injury seen on ultrasound can be taken directly to surgery. However, if extensive hepatic disruption is demonstrated, the surgeon may want further investigation with CT or even angiography before the surgery is performed.

Free Pelvic Fluid in Women. In female patients of reproductive age with trauma, free fluid isolated to the cul-de-sac is

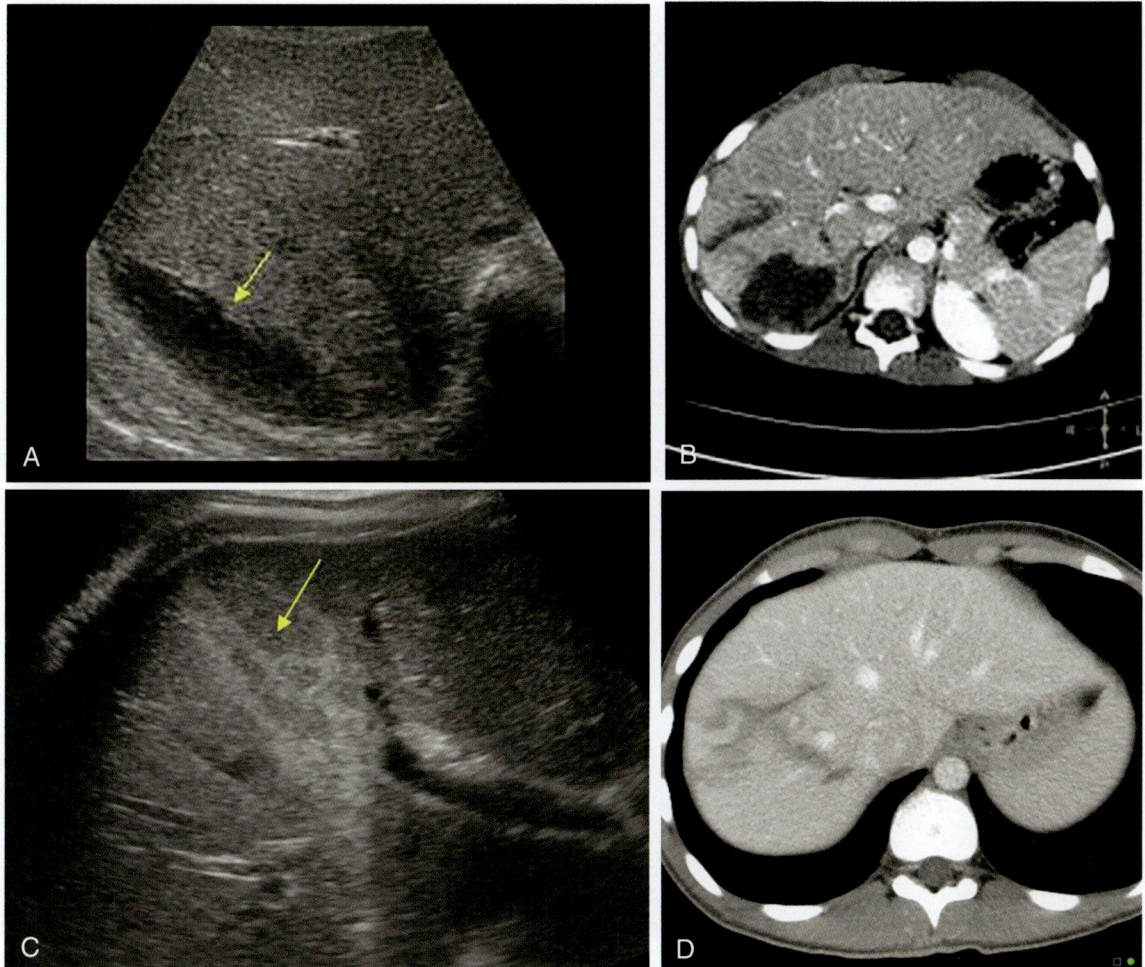

FIG. 19.11 Liver lacerations or contusions are more easily detected with ultrasound than any other visceral abdominal injury. Hematomas and localized lacerations will appear initially hypoechoic with low-level echoes generated from the red blood cells, or echogenic, as the blood begins to coagulate, which over time will become more anechoic with the onset of hemolysis. (A–B) Transverse images with ultrasound and computed tomography show a fluid collection along the posterior border from a liver laceration. (C–D) The liver laceration is located within the right lobe of the liver.

likely physiologic and clinical follow-up should suffice. Female patients with fluid elsewhere usually have a clinically important injury and require further evaluation.

Pitfalls and Limitations. As in other ultrasound procedures, obesity may prevent adequate visualization of the anatomic structures. In some cases the presence of subcutaneous emphysema precludes adequate ultrasound views. The presence of subcutaneous air from a pneumothorax that dissects into the abdominal cavity may collect over the liver or spleen.

An intraperitoneal clot is usually hyperechoic relative to the neighboring structures; however, occasionally, it is isoechoic, and intraperitoneal bleeding or parenchymal injury may go unrecognized.

Contained parenchymal injuries of the liver and spleen, as well as bowel injuries, may not be accompanied by hemoperitoneum and may therefore be missed if screening ultrasound alone is used to evaluate for blunt trauma. Ultrasound may not depict injuries to the diaphragm, the pancreas, the adrenal gland, and bone.

RIGHT UPPER QUADRANT PAIN

Acute Cholecystitis Versus Cholelithiasis

One of the most frequent complaints in the ED is the onset of severe right upper quadrant pain. The patient may have other medical conditions, such as diabetes or peptic ulcer disease, which may contribute to the pain. A myocardial infarction may also present with radiating right upper quadrant pain. Thus a clinically focused physical examination in conjunction with historical and laboratory information should provide the information necessary for decision making. If the patient is female with symptoms of right upper quadrant pain with point tenderness, fever, and leukocytosis, acute cholecystitis should be ruled out. The most common cause of acute cholecystitis is cholelithiasis with a cystic duct obstruction.

Sonographic Findings. Sonographic findings of acute cholecystitis include an irregular, thickened gallbladder wall, a positive sonographic Murphy sign, sludge, pericholecystic fluid, and a dilated gallbladder greater than

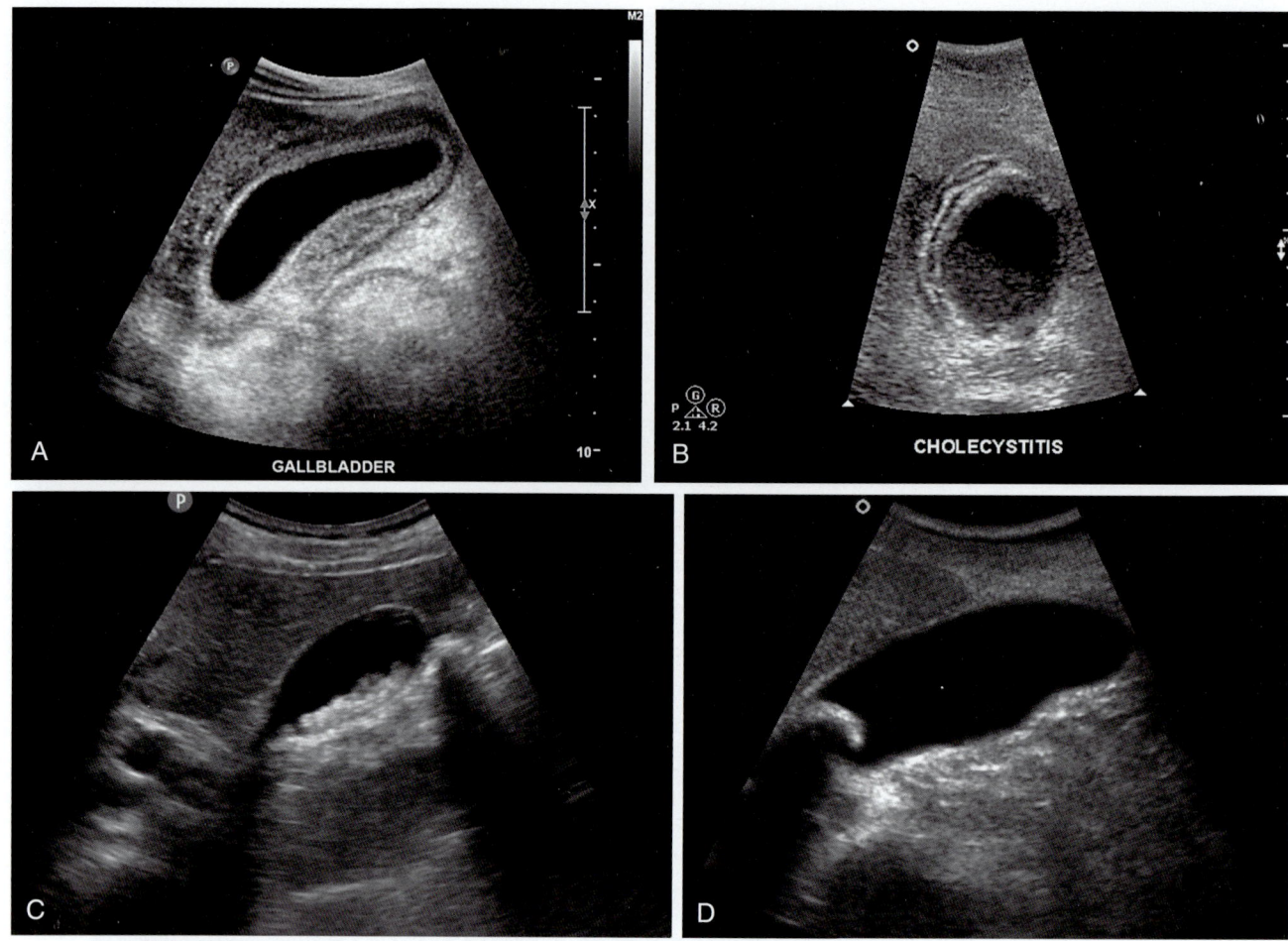

FIG. 19.12 Sagittal (A) and transverse (B) images of the distended gallbladder with edema and wall thickening secondary to acute cholecystitis and sludge. (C) Patient with chronic cholelithiasis shows an edematous thick-walled gallbladder with multiple small stones and (D) a single large gallstone within the fundus of the gallbladder. This stone may obstruct the bile in the area of Hartmann's pouch, causing extreme right upper quadrant pain.

5 cm in transverse diameter (Fig. 19.12). The presence of biliary stones within the inflamed gallbladder is recognized as tiny echogenic foci collected along the posterior wall with a well-demarcated acoustic shadowing in at least two planes. The sonographer must be careful to make sure the shadowing is secondary to gallstones and not to surrounding bowel gas. By holding the transducer carefully over the area of interest, the presence of peristalsis in the bowel may cause shifting of the dirty shadow. Alterations in the patient position will cause movement of the gallstones, with resultant movement of the acoustical shadow. If the stones are very small, they have a chance of becoming lodged within the neck of the gallbladder and may be too small to render an acoustical shadow. The gallbladder will show signs of inflammation. Cholesterol stones are usually smaller than the biliary stones and on sonography are less echogenic. They may be seen to "float" within the thick bile and demonstrate a "comet tail" artifact on sonography.

Biliary Dilation

The common bile duct (CBD) is demonstrated on sonography by identifying the portal vein. The duct is seen anterior and to the right of the portal vein on a transverse image and does not fill in with color Doppler. Recall the hepatic artery is anterior and medial of the portal vein. The normal upper limit of the CBD is 6 mm, although with age this diameter may extend up to 10 mm in size. The presence of stones within the duct should be carefully assessed. The sonographer should look for echogenic foci with acoustical shadowing beyond the foci (Fig. 19.13). Adjustment of gains should be made to delineate the CBD, and alterations in patient position may allow the visualization of the duct to be separated from bowel gas interference.

EPIGASTRIC PAIN

Pancreatitis

Midepigastric pain that radiates to the back is characteristic of acute pancreatitis. Pancreatitis occurs when the toxic enzymes escape into the parenchymal tissue of the gland, causing obstruction of the acini, ducts, small blood vessels, and fat with extension into the peripancreatic tissue. Clinical findings of fever and leukocytosis are found along with elevated enzymes.

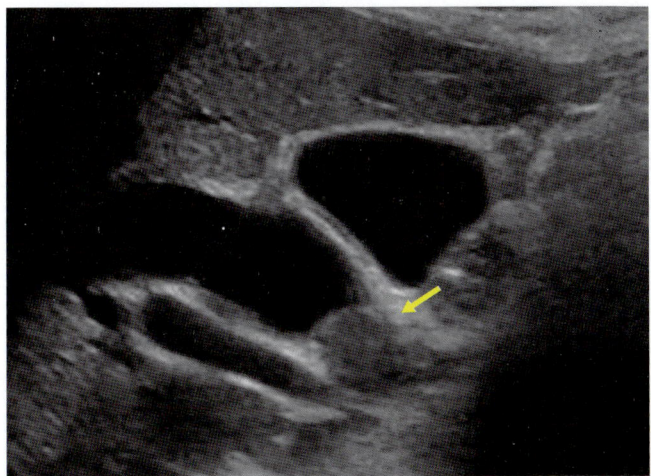

FIG. 19.13 Prominent common bile duct is seen anterior to the portal vein in this sagittal image. Careful sweep of the transducer should demonstrate echo density *(arrow)* with shadowing if stones are present and large enough to be detected with sonography.

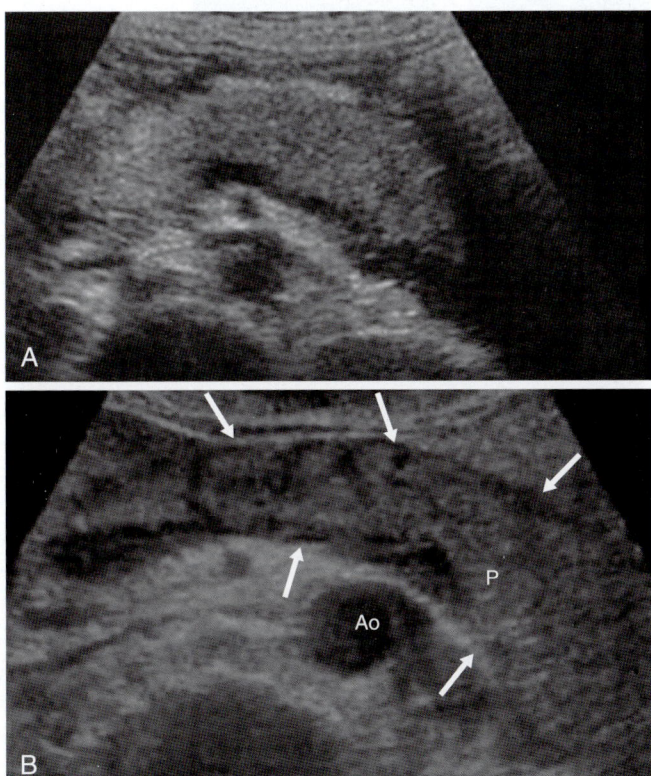

FIG. 19.14 (A) Acute epigastric pain may be secondary to pancreatitis with an enlarged pancreatic duct. (B) Patient with diffuse pancreatitis shows the gland to be enlarged and edematous. *Ao,* Aorta; *P,* pancreas.

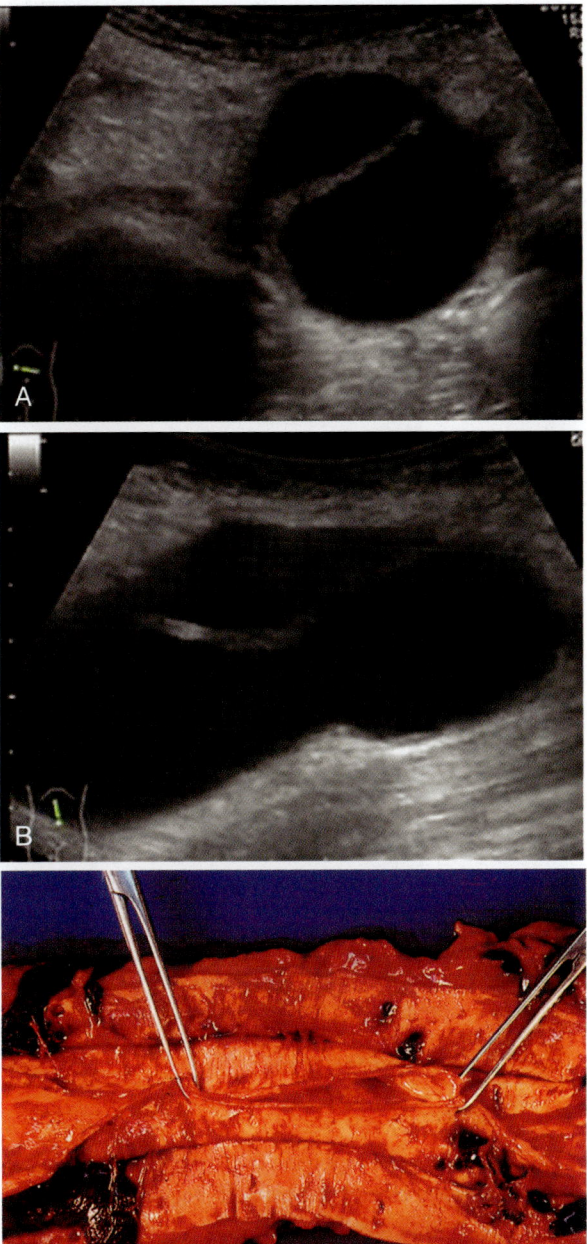

FIG. 19.15 Dissection of the abdominal aortic aneurysm. (A) This transverse image of the abdominal aorta demonstrates an enlarged aortic aneurysm just superior to the bifurcation of the vessel with a fine line within that represents the dissection. (B) Sagittal image of the dilated aorta with the linear line representing the dissection. (C) Gross pathology of a dissecting aortic aneurysm demonstrates the layers of the aortic wall separated by the blood.

The serum amylase levels increase within the first 24 hours of onset but fall rather quickly, whereas the lipase levels take longer to elevate (as much as 72 hours) and remain elevated for a longer period of time. Sonographic findings in acute pancreatitis show a normal to edematous gland that is somewhat hypoechoic to normal texture (Fig. 19.14). The borders are irregular secondary to the inflammation. Increased vascular flow may be apparent because of the inflammatory nature of the disease.

Abdominal Aortic Aneurysm

The patient who presents with classic abdominal pain radiating to the back, with hypotension and a pulsatile abdominal mass, is not a diagnostic dilemma in the ED (Fig. 19.15). Sonography

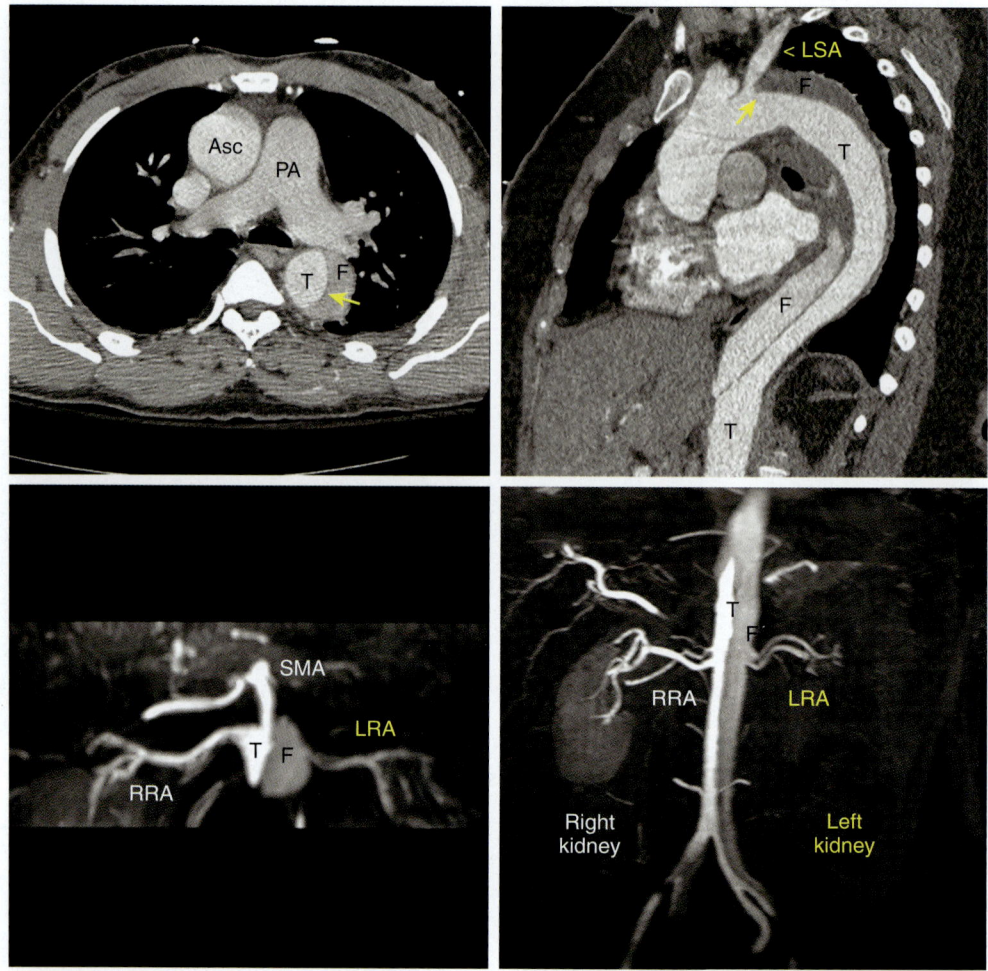

FIG. 19.16 If a dissection is suspected, computed tomography with contrast is generally more specific than sonography because the full length of the aorta may be clearly imaged in a matter of minutes without bowel gas interference. *Asc,* Ascending aorta; *F,* false lumen; *LRA,* left renal artery; *PA,* pulmonary artery; *RRA,* right renal artery; *T,* true lumen.

can rapidly separate the emergent patient with a possible aortic dissection from the elderly patient with vague abdominal complaints or the middle-aged patient with symptoms that mimic nephrolithiasis. If a dissection is suspected, CT with contrast is generally more specific than sonography, because the full length of the aorta may be clearly imaged in a matter of minutes without bowel gas interference (Fig. 19.16). Sonography may identify the abdominal aortic aneurysm in relation to the renal vessels, which is important because in the event a dissection occurs, extension may extend into the renal arteries. Recall that the aorta and iliac arteries are measured from the outside margin of the wall on one wall to the outside margin on the other wall. This measurement should be performed in two planes, transverse and longitudinal. Most aneurysms occur at the level of the umbilicus, at the junction of the bifurcation into the iliac vessels. Aneurysms may expand in the transverse diameter as well as in the anteroposterior diameter. The sonographic examination may be inhibited by obesity, bowel gas interference, or extreme abdominal tenderness.

The sonographer should be aware of several pitfalls when scanning the abdominal aorta. If bowel gas precludes adequate visualization of the aorta from the anterior wall, the transducer may be directed from the lateral abdominal wall, using the liver or spleen as an acoustic window to image both the aorta and inferior vena cava. Alternately, the patient could be rolled into a decubitus position and imaged from the lateral wall. The true diameter of the aorta should be measured with the transducer perpendicular to the vessel; an oblique or angled image would exaggerate the true aortic diameter. A small aneurysm does not preclude rupture. The sonographer should also assess for free intraperitoneal fluid when a patient with an acute abdominal aortic aneurysm is examined. Paraaortic nodes may be confused with the aorta, mimicking an aneurysm. These nodes often are anterior to the aorta, but they can be found posterior as well, encasing the aorta and displacing it from the vertebral body. The nodes are irregular in shape without luminal flow.

EXTREME SHORTNESS OF BREATH

Pericardial Effusion

The primary application of cardiac ultrasound in an emergent situation is to rule out the presence of pericardial effusion or to

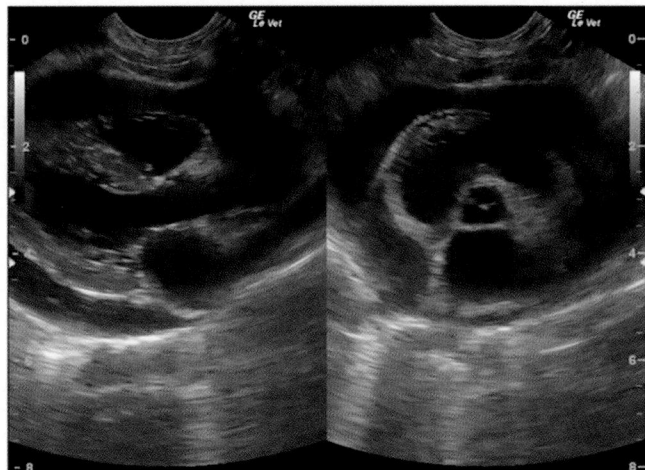

FIG. 19.17 The pericardial effusion usually appears as an anechoic or hypoechoic fluid collection within the pericardial space. Parasternal long axis (left) and short axis (right) views of the heart demonstrate a moderate pericardial effusion.

evaluate cardiac function in patients with sudden cardiac arrest. Body habitus and underlying pathologic conditions will affect the accessibility of the heart to sonographic evaluation. Patients with pulmonary hyperinflation have poor parasternal windows but generally have adequate apical and subcostal windows.

The sonographer should be aware that when a pericardial effusion is demonstrated, several observations should be made. The pericardial effusion usually appears as an anechoic or hypoechoic fluid collection within the pericardial space (Fig. 19.17). With inflammatory, malignant, or hemorrhagic etiologies, this fluid may have a more complex echogenic texture. Fluid usually initially collects dependently. The size of the effusion is important to document. In the parasternal long axis view, the fluid is demonstrated within the pericardial sac beyond the epicardial border of the left ventricle. If the fluid collection is small (<1 cm between the epicardium and posterior border of the fluid in diastole), it may be seen only in the posterior of the heart. As the fluid increases, it becomes circumferential, reflecting off the great vessels and not extending beyond the atrial appendage. A moderate size effusion measures between 1 to 2 cm in diastole and is usually circumferential. Beyond 2 cm in diastole, the fluid is considered large. The fluid should be assessed in multiple planes, short axis, apical four chamber, and subcostal views.

Care should also be taken not to confuse pleural effusions with a pericardial effusion (Fig. 19.18). Patients with congestive heart failure who present with acute failure may have both pericardial and pleural effusion. Again in a long axis view of the heart, the pericardial effusion will be seen posterior to the epicardial border of the left ventricular and anterior to the descending aorta. The pleural effusion will also be found in that similar area but will be seen posterior to the descending aorta.

Other emergent situations such as cardiac tamponade involve a more complex evaluation of the cardiac structures that require high-end ultrasound equipment that is not commonly found in the ED. The diastolic collapse of right heart chambers in the presence of a moderate to large effusion may be indicative of

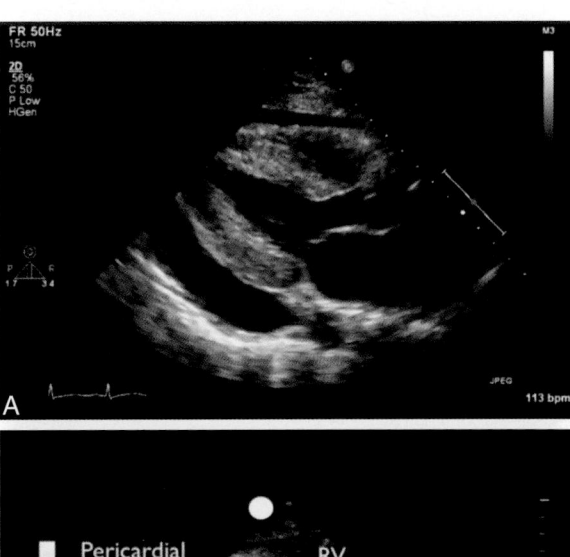

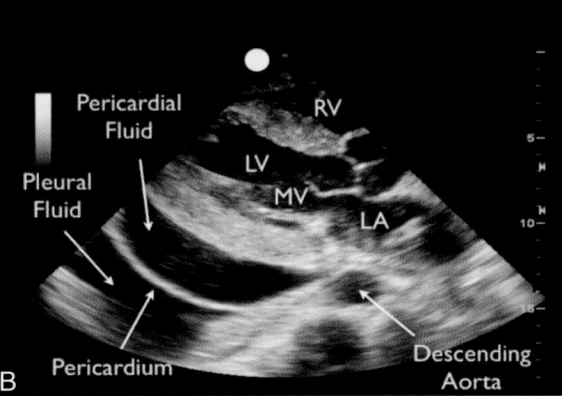

FIG. 19.18 (A) In the parasternal long axis view, the fluid is demonstrated within the pericardial sac beyond the epicardial border of the left ventricle. (B) In addition to the pericardial fluid, there may also be pleural fluid. Pleural fluid is seen posterior to the descending aorta while the pericardial effusion is anterior to the descending aorta. *LA*, Left atrium; *LV*, left ventricle; *MV*, mitral valve; *RV*, right ventricle.

tamponade (Fig. 19.19). This is usually seen in the right atrial collapse or right ventricular collapse. Further Doppler evaluation of both the tricuspid and mitral valve inflow patterns with a respirator monitor is made to look for alterations of flow secondary to cardiac tamponade. The inferior vena cava should be assessed for dilation without respiratory collapse in patients with tamponade. Clinically, the presence of the pulsus tardus should be present in the setting of tamponade.

Acute right ventricular dysfunction or acute pulmonary hypertension in the clinical setting of acute and unexplained chest pain, dyspnea, or hemodynamic instability is best evaluated by the high-end ultrasound equipment. In this case, patients with suspected pulmonary embolism are usually referred for a rapid CT scan to demonstrate the presence of clot or thrombus lodged within the pulmonary arteries.

In the acute hemopericardium trauma patient with clotted blood, the fluid may have a soft echogenic to isoechoic texture as compared with the myocardial texture which would represent blood within the pericardial space. Hypoechoic fatty tissue found in the epicardial layer surrounding the heart may sometimes mimic pericardial effusion. It is important to note that a small rapidly forming effusion may lead to tamponade, whereas extremely large, slowly forming effusions may be tolerated with minimal symptoms.

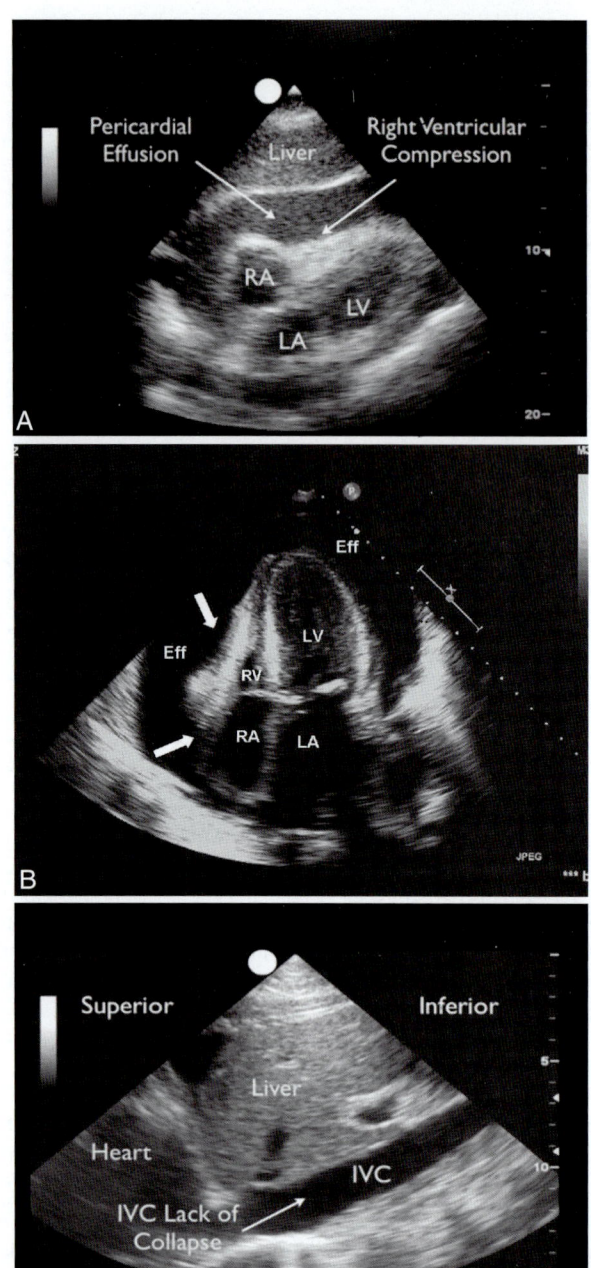

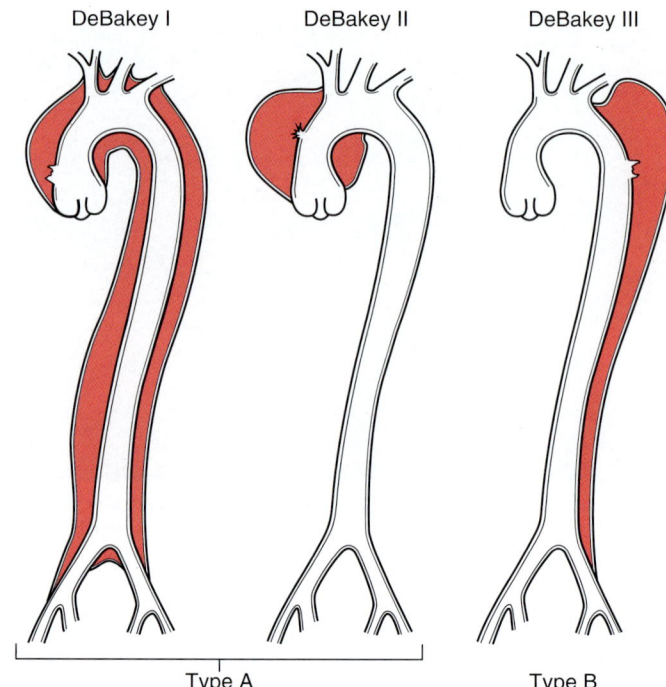

FIG. 19.19 (A–B) Subcostal and apical four-chamber images of a large pericardial effusion. Note the compression of the right ventricular wall indicating signs of tamponade. (C) Evaluation of the inferior vena cava may be made with the "sniff test" to see if the cava collapses after the patient takes three to four sniffs through the nose. *Eff*, Effusion; *IVC*, inferior vena cava; *LA*, left atrium; *LV*, left ventricle; *RA*, right atrium; *RV*, right ventricle.

FIG. 19.20 Most aortic dissections will occur at one of three sites: (1) at the root of the aorta with possible extension into the arch, descending aorta, and abdominal aorta; (2) at the level of the left subclavian artery, with extension into the descending aorta or abdominal aorta; and (3) only at the level of the ascending aorta.

BOX 19.3	Causes of Aortic Dissection

- Hypertension (70%–90%)
- Marfan syndrome (16%)
- Pregnancy
- Acquired or congenital aortic stenosis
- Coarctation of the aorta
- Trauma
- Iatrogenic (cardiac catheterization, aortic valve replacement)

aortic media. At this point, blood surges into the media, separating the intima from the adventitia. This channel is called the *false lumen*. This blood in the false lumen can reenter the true lumen anywhere along the course of the dissection (Fig. 19.20).

Approximately 70% of dissections are located in the ascending aorta, 10% to 20% in the aortic arch, and 20% in the abdominal aorta. Most often, the dissection will propagate distally in the aorta into the iliac vessels, although proximal extension can occur.

Clinical Findings for Aortic Dissection. The typical presentation for an aortic dissection is that of a sudden onset of severe, tearing chest pain radiating to the arms, neck, or back (Box 19.3). Syncope occurs in a small percentage of patients. The complexity of the symptoms will depend on the extension of the dissection, the specific branches of the aorta involved, and the location of external rupture if present (Table 19.1). If the carotid artery is affected, hemiplegia may result. Involvement of the subclavian or iliac vessels will appear with decreased or absent pulses in the arms or legs.

CHEST PAIN

Thoracic Aortic Dissection

A dissecting aortic aneurysm is a condition in which a propagating intramural hematoma actually dissects along the length of the vessel, stripping away the intima and, in some cases, part of the media. The resultant aortic dissection is a defect or tear in the aortic intima with concomitant weakness of the

TABLE 19.1 Common Emergency Conditions

Clinical Findings	Sonographic Findings
RUQ Pain: Cholecystitis	
RUQ pain	Thickened GB wall
Fever	+ Murphy sign
Nausea, vomiting	Pericholecystic fluid
Leukocytosis	Dilated GB
Epigastric Pain: Pancreatitis	
Midepigastric pain radiating to back	Normal to edematous gland
Fever	Hypoechoic texture
Leukocytosis	Irregular borders
↑ Amylase	Increased vascular flow
↑ Lipase	
Flank Pain: Urolithiasis	
Spasmodic flank pain	Echogenic foci with shadowing
Pain may radiate into pelvis	Hydronephrosis may be present
Hematuria	Look for ureteral jets in bladder
Fever	
Leukocytosis	
Thoracic or Abdominal Pain: Aortic Dissection	
Sudden onset of severe chest pain with radiation to arms, neck, or back	Aneurysm
	Look for flap at site of dissection
Syncope may be present	Look for false lumen
RLQ Pain: Appendicitis	
Intense RLQ pain	Distended, noncompressible appendix
Nausea, vomiting	↑ Color flow
Fever	McBurney sign
Leukocytosis	
Lower Abdominal Pain: Paraumbilical Hernia	
Asymptomatic to mild discomfort	Lower abdominal mass; look for peristalsis of bowel in hernia
Palpable mass	
Valsalva: shows exaggeration of mass	
Reduce sac with gentle pressure	

GB, Gallbladder; *RLQ*, right lower quadrant; *RUQ*, right upper quadrant.

The location of the pain may be a clue to the site of the dissection. If the pain centers in the anterior thorax, a proximal dissection may be present; severe pain in the interscapular area is more common with distal involvement. However, the majority of patients with distal dissection of the aorta have back pain. Occlusion of the visceral arteries may appear with abdominal pain.

Sonographic Findings. In an acute aortic dissection time is of the essence, and therefore magnetic resonance imaging or contrast-enhanced CT is the imaging modality of choice for evaluating aortic dissections. In the stabilized patient with a suspected dissection, sonography may be performed. Because most dissections are seen in the ascending aorta, transesophageal echocardiography will be performed by the cardiology department. If the dissection is suspected in the abdomen, an abdominal ultrasound may be requested.

On sonography, the classic finding is the visualization of the flap at the site of the dissection. An echogenic intimal membrane within the aorta or the iliac arteries may be seen to move freely with arterial pulsations on sonography if both the true and false lumen are patent (Fig. 19.21). However, if the membrane is thick and the lumen is thrombosed, the membrane may not move. Color Doppler may demonstrate slow flow in both the true and false lumen. The flow is decreased or reversed in the false lumen. The sonographer should look for the presence of the intimal membrane with concomitant clotting in the iliac, celiac, and superior mesenteric arteries.

A **pseudodissection** on color flow demonstrates a turbulent blood flow pattern, indicating a hypoechoic thrombus near the outer margin of the aorta with an echogenic laminated clot. No intimal flap is seen with a pseudodissection.

FLANK PAIN

Urolithiasis

Flank pain caused by urolithiasis is a common problem in patients coming to the ED. Radiology plays a vital role in the evaluation of these patients through the use of **intravenous urography (IVU)**, ultrasonography, and limited noncontrast helical CT studies. The most sensitive and specific for the presence of stones are the IVU and helical CT. Traditional evaluation of the patient with flank pain consisted of conventional radiography followed by IVU with noniodinated contrast. In those patients unable to undergo IVU safely (i.e., patients with dye allergies, renal insufficiency, congestive heart failure, or suspected pregnancy), ultrasound was used to evaluate for secondary signs of obstruction, namely hydronephrosis. CT has largely replaced these other modalities with its ability to identify calculi and their location, determine the size, and guide the management.

Clinical Findings for Urolithiasis. Acute ureteral obstruction usually manifests as renal colic, a severe pain that is often spasmodic, that increases to a peak level of intensity, and then decreases before increasing again. The pain can also manifest as steady and continuous. The pain usually begins abruptly in the flank and increases rapidly to a level of discomfort that often requires narcotics for adequate pain control. Over time, the pain may radiate to the lower abdomen and into the scrotum or labia as the stone moves into the more distal portion of the ureter.

Urinalysis is the initial laboratory examination. Hematuria is the common finding in 85% of the patients. However, if the stone completely obstructs the ureter, no hematuria will be

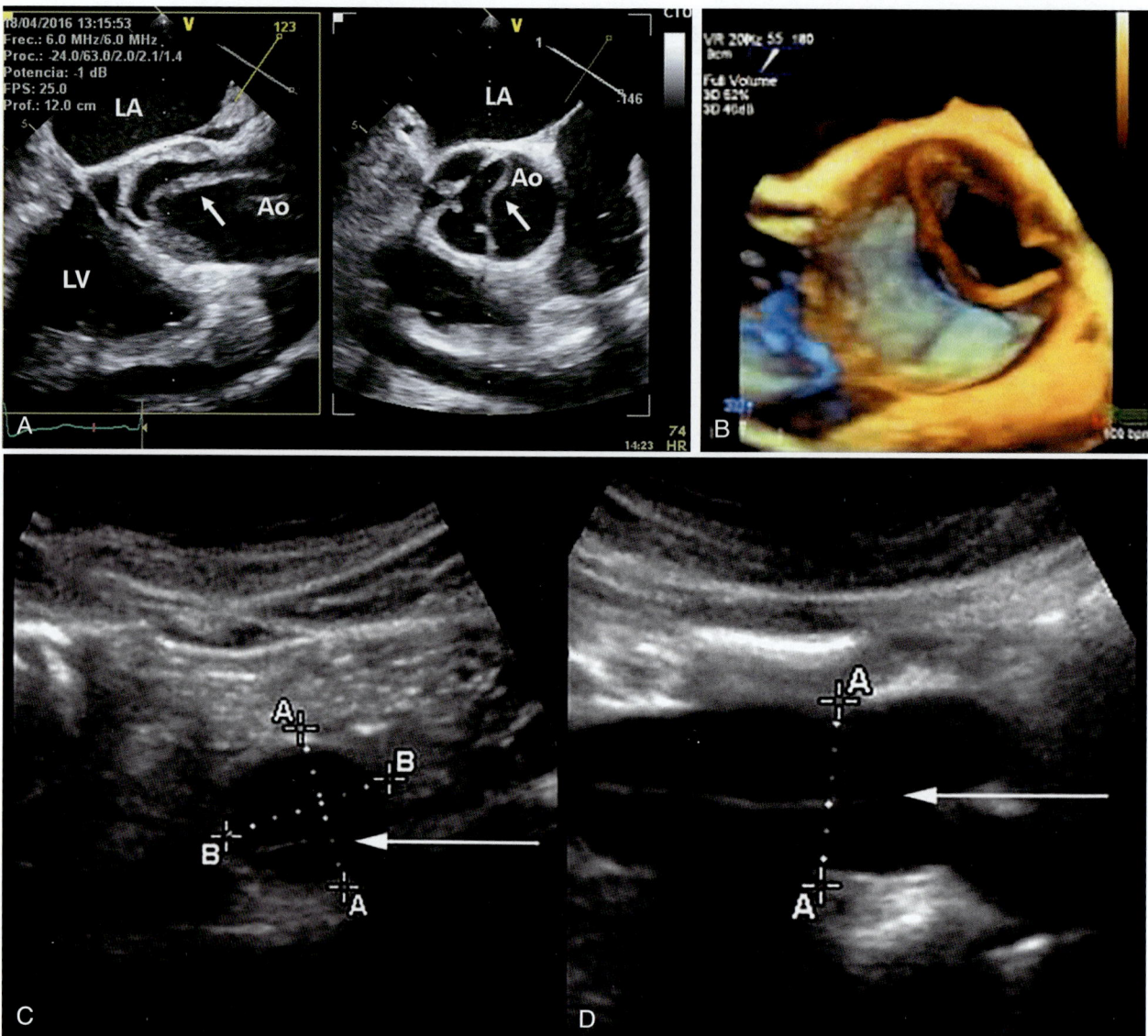

FIG. 19.21 Aortic dissection. (A) Transesophageal images of the aortic dissection which begins at the root of the aorta and extends into the aortic arch. (B) Three-dimensional rendering of the dissection. The abdominal aortic dissection on both transverse (C) and longitudinal views (D; flap of dissection, *arrow*). *Ao,* Aorta; *LA,* left atrium; *LV,* left ventricle.

present. Clinical symptoms such as fever, leukocytosis, and urine gram staining can help to identify a superimposed urinary tract infection.

Sonographic Findings. The calculi imaged with sonography are highly echogenic foci with distinct acoustic shadowing. Stones as small as 0.5 mm may be seen. When obstruction occurs, ultrasound is effective in demonstrating the secondary sign of hydronephrosis (Fig. 19.22). Overlying bowel gas in the pelvis may obscure the evaluation of the distal ureters. The pulse repetition frequency should be decreased to assess the low velocity of the ureteral jet flow. The color gain should be turned up just enough to barely see color in the background. Usually within 2 to 3 minutes the jet will light up with color as the urine drains into the bladder (Fig. 19.23). Be sure to look for the presence of both the right and left ureteral jet with this technique. Power Doppler may also be used to image the ureteral jets and is very effective.

The presence of hydronephrosis in a pregnant patient may be more problematic because it is not uncommon for the kidneys to become slightly hydronephrotic during the latter stage of pregnancy because the uterus enlarges and causes pressure on the ureter. This is seen especially in the right kidney because it lies lower than the left and is more likely to show minimal hydronephrosis. Therefore the appearance of ureteral jets may help to rule out the presence of obstruction secondary to calculi.

RIGHT LOWER QUADRANT PAIN

Appendicitis

Acute appendicitis is one of the most common diseases that necessitates emergency surgery and is the most common atraumatic surgical abdominal disorder in children 2 years of

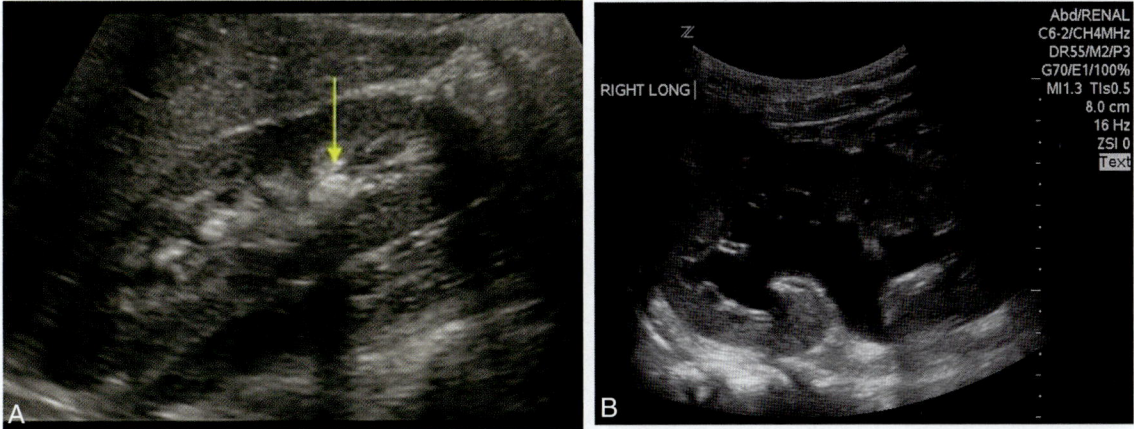

FIG. 19.22 (A) The calculi imaged with sonography are highly echogenic foci with distinct acoustic shadowing. Stones as small as 0.5 mm may be seen. (B) When obstruction occurs, ultrasound is effective in demonstrating the secondary sign of hydronephrosis.

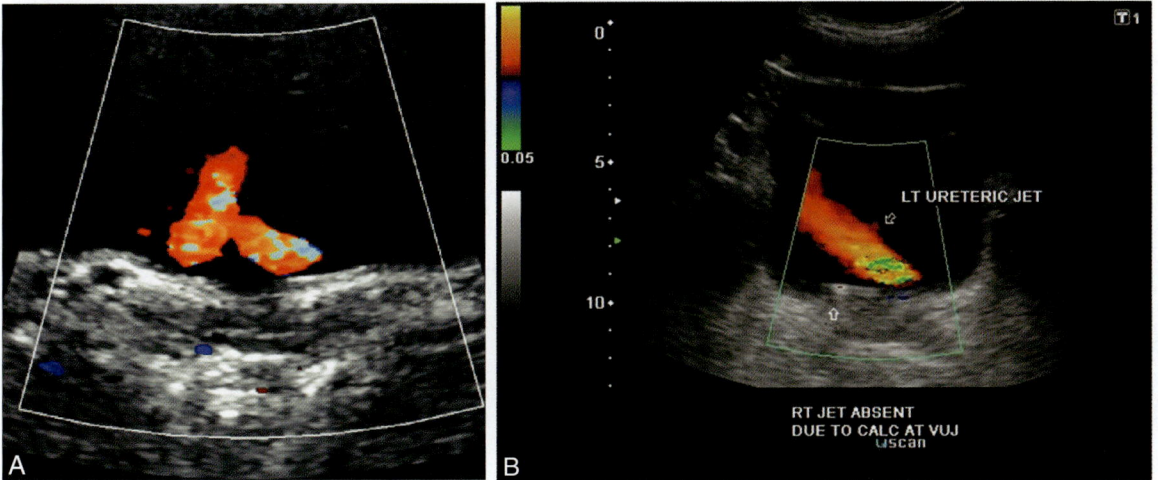

FIG. 19.23 (A) With the bladder distended, color Doppler is an excellent tool to image the presence of ureteral jets in the bladder. The transducer should be angled in a cephalic presentation through the distended urinary bladder. Color Doppler is turned on and the probe is held stationary to watch for the appearance of ureteral jets. (B) Right jet is absent due to calculi at the vesicouteral junction.

age and older. Appendicitis is the result of luminal obstruction and inflammation, leading to ischemia of the vermiform appendix. The early diagnosis of acute appendicitis is essential in the prevention of perforation, abscess formation, and postoperative complications. The classic clinical symptoms include exquisite lower abdominal pain, nausea, vomiting, fever, and leukocytosis. The quick release maneuver is performed by applying pressure with the fingertips directly over the area of the appendix and then quickly letting go. With appendicitis, the patient will usually have rebound tenderness (McBurney sign) associated with peritoneal irritation.

The sonographer should use a high-frequency linear transducer to image the right lower quadrant. Careful explanation of the technique to the patient with care over the tender abdomen is essential in performing an adequate examination. The inflamed appendix will demonstrate a thickened edematous wall greater than 2 mm thick (Fig. 19.24). If the wall is asymmetric, perforation may have occurred and the search for fluid collections around the appendiceal area should be made. The inflamed appendix may also demonstrate a target lesion on transverse images demonstrating a hypoechoic, fluid-distended lumen, with a hyperechoic inner ring, and an outer hypoechoic ring representing the muscularis externa. There is a lack of peristalsis and compressibility of the inflamed appendix. Gradual pressure with the transducer is placed over the point of tenderness in an effort to displace the bowel to image the area of inflammation (see Table 19.1).

PARAUMBILICAL HERNIA

Another cause of abdominal pain and intestinal obstruction is the presence of an abdominal wall hernia. The hernia may be classified into one of three types: (1) **reducible hernia** is one in which the visceral contents can be returned to the normal intra-abdominal location; (2) **incarcerated hernia** means the visceral contents cannot be reduced; and (3) **strangulated hernia** is an incarcerated hernia with vascular compromise.

A hernia forms when the abdominal wall muscles are weakened, which allows the viscera to protrude into the weakened abdominal wall. The weakest area of the abdomen

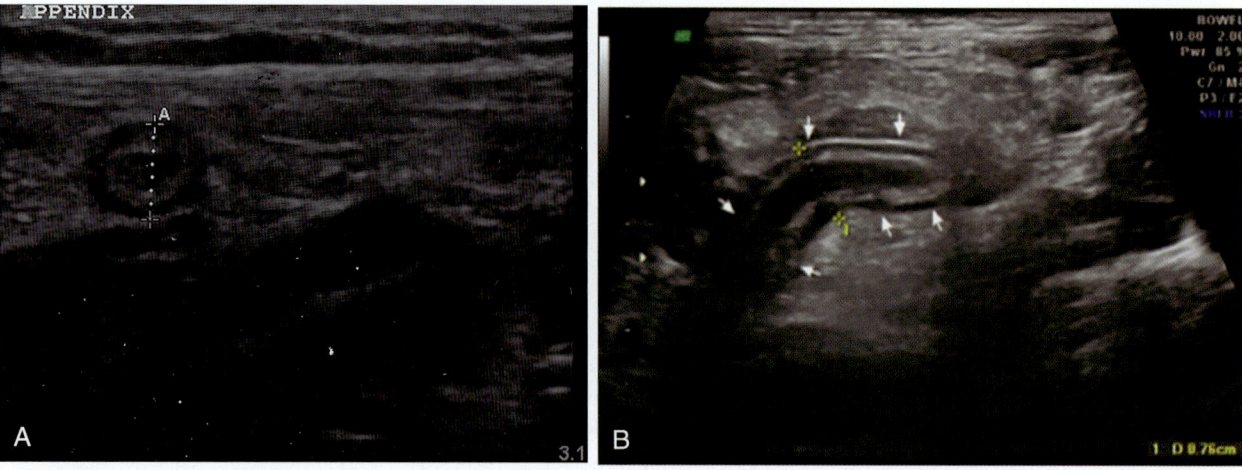

FIG. 19.24 (A) In acute appendicitis, the inflamed appendix will demonstrate a thickened edematous wall greater than 2 mm thick. (B) The inflamed appendix may also demonstrate a "target" lesion on transverse images demonstrating a hypoechoic, fluid-distended lumen, with a hyperechoic inner ring, and an outer hypoechoic ring representing the muscularis externa.

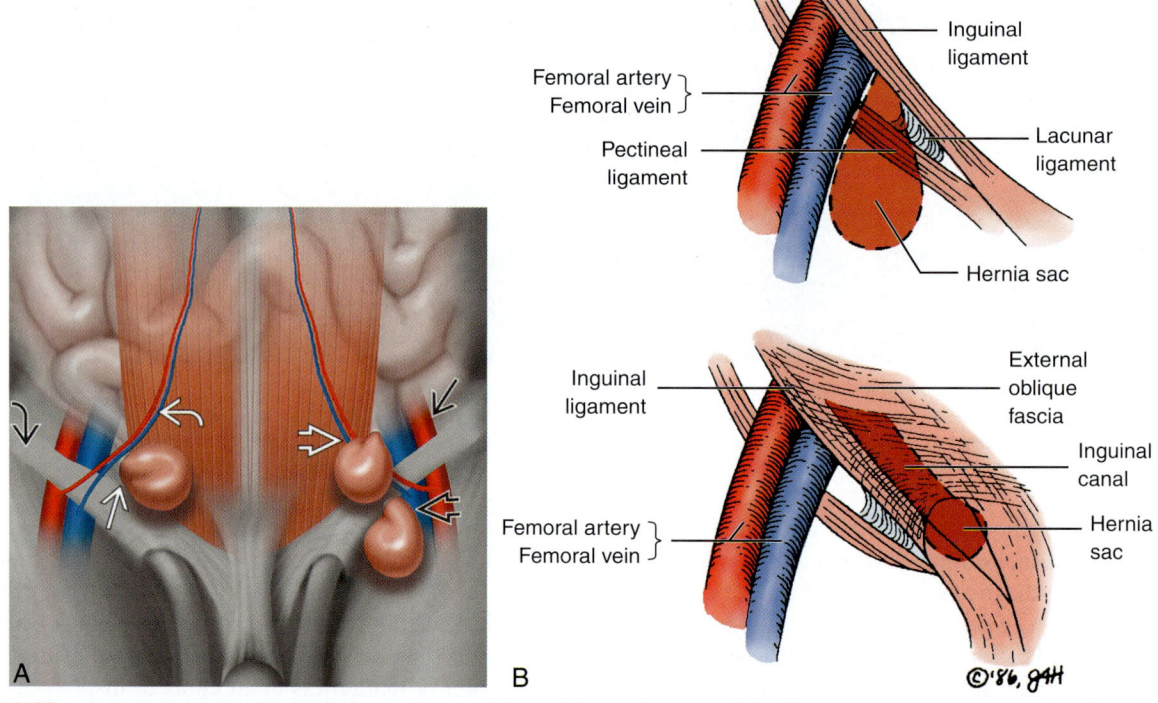

FIG. 19.25 The weakest area of the abdomen is the site of the umbilicus. The paraumbilical hernia occurs more often in females, whereas the inguinal hernia is more common in males. The hernia may be classified into one of three types: reducible hernia, incarcerated hernia, and strangulated hernia. (A-B) The arrows point to the hernial sac.

is the site of the umbilicus, and this paraumbilical hernia occurs more often in females, whereas the inguinal hernia is more common in males (see Fig. 19.24).

Common causes of herniation include congenital defect or weakening of the abdominal wall, increased abdominal pressure secondary to ascites, abdominal mass, bowel obstruction, obesity, and repeated pregnancy. Strangulation of the colon and omentum is a complication of the hernia. Another complication of a hernia is rupture of the abdominal wall in severe chronic ascites.

Sonographic Findings. The real-time visualization of the bowel within the hernia provides critical information for the clinician. Sonography allows visualization of the peristaltic movement of the bowel during Valsalva maneuvers and determines the presence or absence of vascular flow within the defect. The sonographic criteria for a paraumbilical hernia include (1) demonstration of an anterior wall defect, (2) presence of bowel loops within the sac, (3) exaggeration of the sac during the Valsalva maneuver, and (4) reducibility of the sac with gentle pressure (Fig. 19.25). Most paraumbilical hernias contain colon, omentum, and fat. The large intestine will display a complex pattern of fluid, gas, and peristalsis. Of course, the mesenteric fat is very echogenic. The high-frequency linear array transducer allows the sonographer to demonstrate a wide area of the abdominal wall. Reduced gain is necessary to demonstrate the layers of the abdominal wall and will be useful to see the distinction between the hernia, bowel, and muscular layers of tissue. Color flow will be required to determine the vascular flow within the hernia sac. The patient should be instructed to perform a Valsalva maneuver to determine the site of wall defect and confirm the presence of the protruding hernia. It is important to visualize the peristalsis of the bowel loops within the hernia to confirm the diagnosis (see Table 19.1).

The inguinal hernia may be indirect or direct. The indirect hernia follows the same course as the spermatic cord. It traverses the inguinal canal and enters the canal at the deep inguinal ring. It is found lateral to the inferior epigastric vessels. It is either congenital or a result of injury.

The direct hernia bulges through the weakened fascia of the abdominal wall directly behind the superficial inguinal ring (Fig. 19.26D). It is medial to the inferior epigastric vessels and rarely enters the scrotum. This is more common in elderly men with weak abdominal muscles.

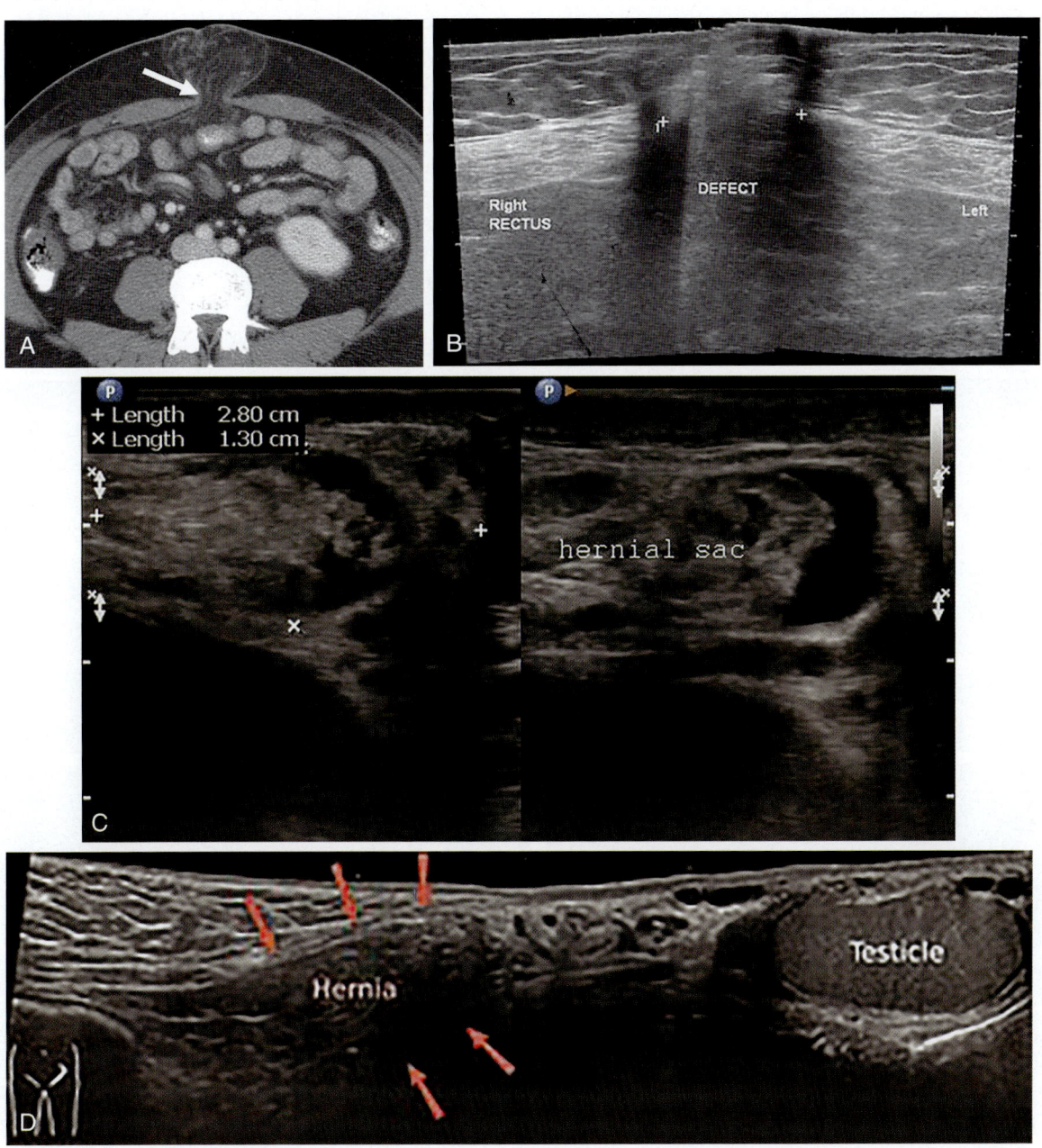

FIG. 19.26 **Sonographic patterns of inguinal hernias.** Sonography allows visualization of the peristaltic movement of the bowel during Valsalva maneuvers and determines the presence or absence of vascular flow within the defect. Computed tomography (A) and ultrasound (B) images of the paraumbilical hernia. (C) Presence of bowel loops within the sac. (D) Direct inguinal hernia is seen as it bulges through the fascia of the abdominal wall.

ACUTE PELVIC PAIN

The evaluation of the patient in acute pelvic pain can be challenging for the sonographer in the middle of the night. These patients usually appear in the ED when the pain is so intense that they cannot bear it any longer. The sonographer must rule out acute pathology such as tubo-ovarian abscess, ruptured ovarian cyst, or ectopic pregnancy. Ovarian torsion is likewise an emergent situation for the patient with severe pelvic pain.

Sonography of Pelvic Structures

Sonography of the pelvic structures should include evaluation in at least two planes of the uterus, cul-de-sac, ovaries, fallopian tubes, and adnexal area. Transabdominal imaging with a full bladder will provide an overview of the entire pelvic area, whereas transvaginal imaging requires the bladder to be empty and allows exquisite detail of the uterus, ovaries, and fallopian tubes.

Uterus. On sonography the uterus should appear as a homogeneous structure with an echogenic line in the center representing the endometrial canal (Fig. 19.27). The long axis plane should demonstrate the uterus from fundus to cervix with the endometrial cavity well demonstrated. The entire uterus should be evaluated to look for inhomogeneity in texture that may represent degenerating fibroids or an interstitial pregnancy. Fibroids may cause significant pain and bleeding. A pregnancy that is within 5 to 7 mm from the edge of the myometrium is at risk for becoming an interstitial ectopic pregnancy. The presence of a normal gestational sac implanted high in the uterine cavity is the sign of an intrauterine pregnancy. Viability may be assessed with transvaginal ultrasound with demonstration of the fetal heart rate.

Cul-de-Sac. This area may normally contain a small amount of fluid in the healthy female that is dependent on her point in the menstrual cycle. However, large amounts of fluid are abnormal. An ectopic pregnancy that has ruptured may lead to increased amounts of fluid in the cul-de-sac. A pelvic inflammatory disease may also expand with pus into the cul-de-sac. Ascites or other free fluid secondary to trauma will accumulate in this dependent area of the pelvis.

Ovaries. The ovaries are best imaged with transvaginal sonography. Careful evaluation of the texture of the ovary should separate an enlarged ovarian cyst, ectopic pregnancy, or other ovarian masses that may lead to pelvic pain. Torsion of the ovary shows an enlarged edematous with severe reduction of flow on color Doppler.

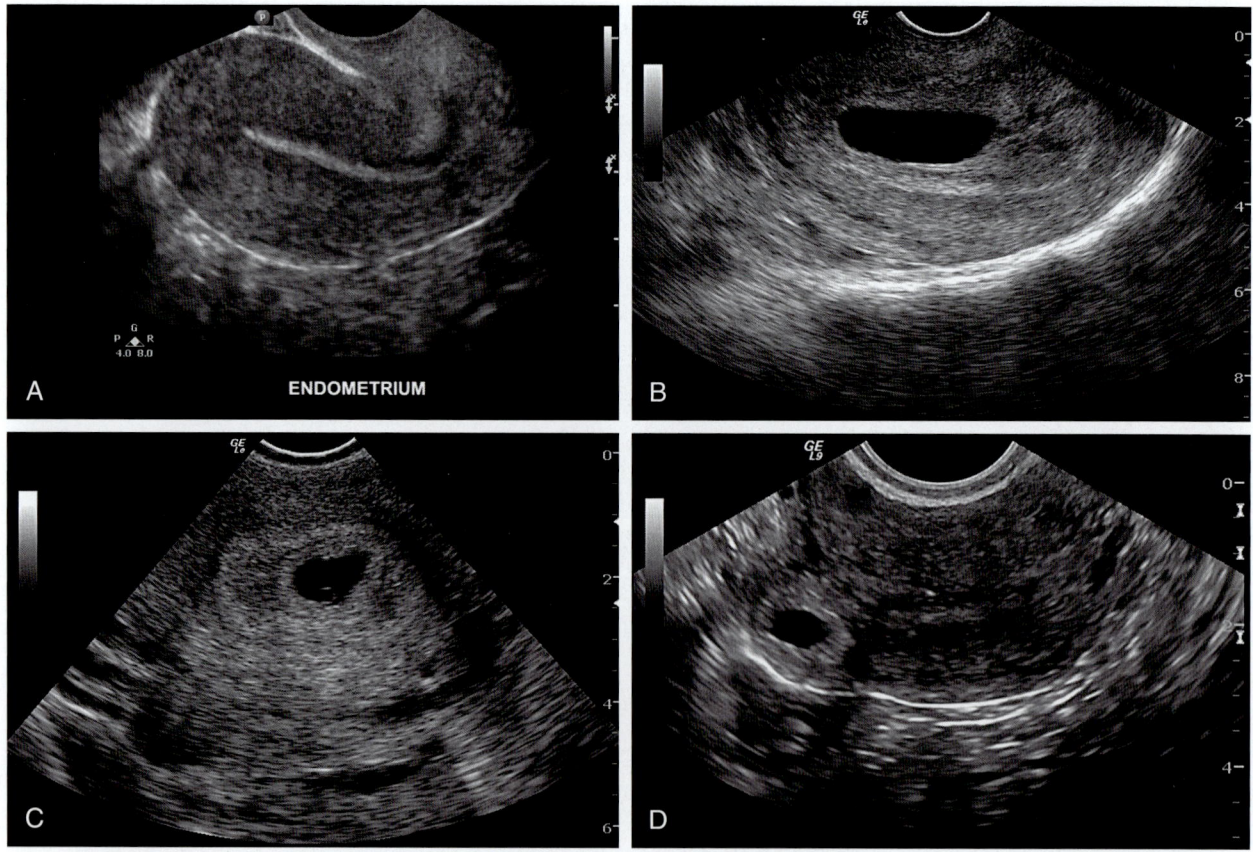

FIG. 19.27 (A) Transvaginal image of the normal uterus with the endometrial stripe. (B) Blighted ovum shows dilation of the endometrium without products of conception. (C) Tiny yolk sac is seen within the endometrial cavity in this very early pregnancy. (D) The uterine cavity is normal; however, the gestational sac is lying outside the uterine cavity in the adnexa.

Fallopian Tubes. Again, the fallopian tubes are best imaged with transvaginal ultrasound because they originate from the cornua of the uterus. The presence of enlarged anechoic to slightly heterogeneous tubes may signify hydrosalpinx or the presence of a tubo-ovarian abscess.

SCROTAL TRAUMA AND TORSION

Scrotal trauma presents a challenge to the sonographer because the scrotum is often painful and swollen. The trauma may be the result of a motor vehicle accident, athletic injury, direct blow to the scrotum, or a straddle injury. The most important goal of the sonographic examination is to determine if a rupture has occurred. Rupture of the testis is a surgical emergency requiring a prompt diagnosis. If surgery is performed within 72 hours following injury, at least 90% of testes can be saved; this number decreases to 45% after 72 hours. Hydrocele and hematocele are both complications of trauma. Hematoceles contain blood and are also found in advanced cases of epididymitis or orchitis (Fig. 19.28).

On sonography, findings associated with scrotal rupture include a focal alteration of the testicular parenchymal pattern, interruption of the tunica albuginea, irregular testicular contour, scrotal wall thickening, and hematocele. These findings may also be associated with abscess, tumor, or other clinical conditions; however, when combined with a history of trauma, they suggest rupture.

Torsion of the spermatic cord occurs as a result of abnormal mobility of the testis within the scrotum. Torsion is a surgical emergency, and it is important to obtain diagnostic images as soon as possible. The abnormality is seen more frequently in the adolescent and young adult. The patient presents with a sudden onset of pain and swelling on the affected side. On sonography, the early stages of torsion may show the testis to have a normal homogeneous pattern (Fig. 19.29). After 4 to 6 hours, the testis becomes swollen and hypoechoic. The lobes within the testis are well identified during this time secondary to interstitial and septal edema. After 24 hours, the testis becomes heterogeneous as a result of hemorrhage, infarction, necrosis, and vascular congestion. The epididymal head appears enlarged and may have decreased echogenicity or become heterogeneous. Color Doppler is useful to differentiate torsion from epididymo-orchitis. An absence of perfusion in the symptomatic testis with normal perfusion demonstrated in the asymptomatic side is considered to be diagnostic of torsion.

EXTREMITY SWELLING AND PAIN

The evaluation of deep venous thrombosis in the patient with swelling of the proximal lower extremities may be made in the ED. There are essentially two types of evaluation: one is a superficial "compression" of the venous structures to see if there is an obstruction in the venous system, and the other is the thorough examination of the entire lower venous structures with gray scale, color, and spectral Doppler evaluation. The thrombosis may be acute, chronic, distal, or superficial in the venous system. Other causes of extremity pain and swelling include Baker cyst (posterior swelling of the knee with extension into the lower calf), cellulitis, abscess, muscle hematoma, and fasciitis (Fig. 19.30). Often the patient with extremity swelling presents with a swollen, tender extremity that is painful to the touch. Care must be taken to adequately evaluate the leg with gentle compression. The use of color and spectral Doppler allows the sonographer to determine the arterial from venous flow patterns to avoid the false-negative or false-positive result. In the obese patient, the large superficial veins may be mistaken for the deep veins and may prevent adequate compression of the venous structures. The unclotted thrombus may be isoechoic to slightly hypoechoic and thus not well seen in the lower-level equipment.

The proximal deep veins of the lower extremity are those in which thrombus poses a significant risk of pulmonary embolization. These veins include the common femoral, superficial femoral, and popliteal veins. (Note the superficial femoral vein is part of the deep system, not the superficial system.) The deep femoral vein is not considered to be a source of embolizing thrombi and is not included in the evaluation for deep venous thrombosis.

The sonographic evaluation is performed with a high-frequency linear array transducer using both real time imaging and compression of the venous structures. The compression should be made with the vein directly under the transducer while watching for complete apposition of the anterior and posterior walls. If thrombus is present, complete compression will not be possible.

Other structures may be inflamed next to the venous structures as in cases of lymphadenopathy. The enlarged lymph nodes are hypoechoic with a small echogenic center and will not compress; these may be mistaken for thrombus within the venous structures.

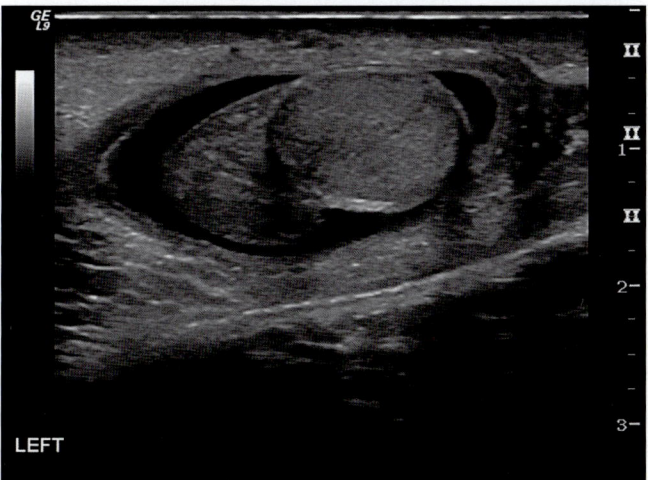

FIG. 19.28 Acute scrotal pain with hydrocele and epididymitis.

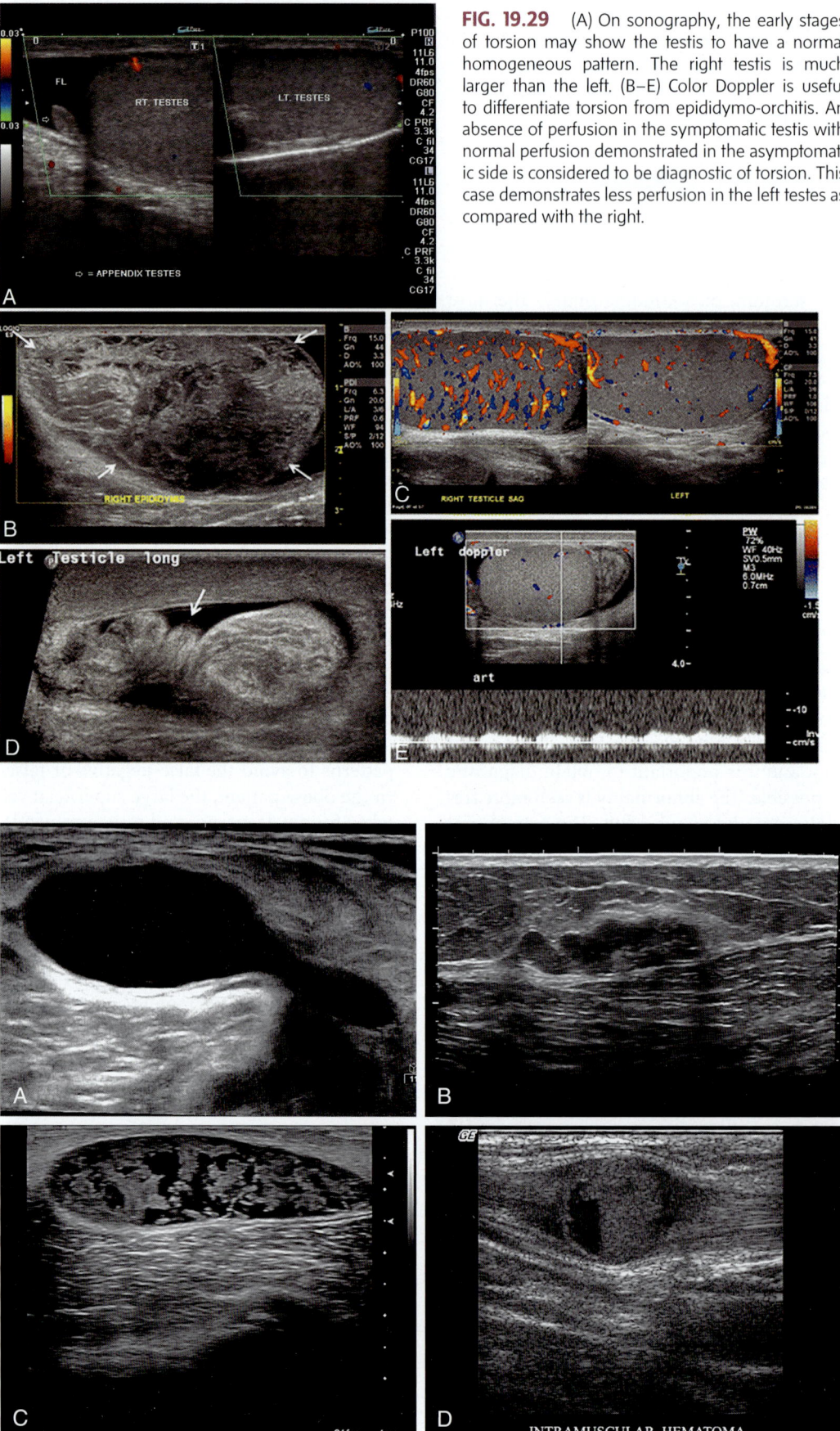

FIG. 19.29 (A) On sonography, the early stages of torsion may show the testis to have a normal homogeneous pattern. The right testis is much larger than the left. (B–E) Color Doppler is useful to differentiate torsion from epididymo-orchitis. An absence of perfusion in the symptomatic testis with normal perfusion demonstrated in the asymptomatic side is considered to be diagnostic of torsion. This case demonstrates less perfusion in the left testes as compared with the right.

FIG. 19.30 (A) Baker cyst. (B) Musculofascitis. (C) Large Baker cyst with complex echo pattern. (D) Intramuscular hematoma.

The inferior vena cava and iliac veins should also be assessed for a possible source of emboli or thrombi, causing lower extremity pain and swelling.

Key Pearls

- Diagnostic peritoneal lavage (DPL) was used to sample the intraperitoneal space for evidence of damage to the viscera and blood vessels in patients with blunt abdominal trauma to decide which patients needed exploratory laparotomy.
- The focused assessment with sonography for trauma (FAST) scan in the emergency department has become an extension of the physical examination of the trauma patient.
- The FAST exam is a focused survey examination of the abdomen, pelvis, and pericardium to evaluate free fluid or pericardial fluid.
- The FAST evaluation survey is widespread, extending from the pericardial sac to the urinary bladder and includes the perihepatic area (including Morison's pouch), perisplenic region (including splenorenal recess), paracolic gutters, and cul-de-sac.
- Liver lacerations or contusions are more easily detected with ultrasound than any other visceral abdominal injury.
- Pitfalls of abdominal ultrasound include failure to show contained solid-organ injuries; injuries to the diaphragm, pancreas, and adrenal gland; and some bowel injuries.
- One of the most frequent complaints in the emergency department is the onset of severe right upper quadrant pain.
- Midepigastric pain that radiates to the back is characteristic of acute pancreatitis.
- Most aneurysms occur at the level of the umbilicus (at the junction of the bifurcation into the iliac vessels). Aneurysms may expand in the transverse diameter as well as in the anteroposterior diameter.
- The primary application of cardiac ultrasound in an emergent situation is to rule out the presence of pericardial effusion or to evaluate cardiac function in patients with sudden cardiac arrest.
- A dissecting aortic aneurysm is a condition in which a propagating intramural hematoma actually dissects along the length of the vessel, stripping away the intima and, in some cases, part of the media.
- Most aortic dissections will occur at one of three sites: (1) at the root of the aorta with possible extension into the arch, descending aorta, and abdominal aorta; (2) at the level of the left subclavian artery, with extension into the descending aorta or abdominal aorta; and (3) only at the level of the ascending aorta.
- The typical presentation for an aortic dissection is that of a sudden onset of severe, tearing chest pain radiating to the arms, neck, or back.
- Flank pain caused by urolithiasis is a common problem in patients coming to the emergency department.
- Acute appendicitis is one of the most common diseases that necessitates emergency surgery and is the most common atraumatic surgical abdominal disorder in children 2 years of age and older.
- Appendicitis is the result of luminal obstruction and inflammation, leading to ischemia of the vermiform appendix.
- A less common cause of abdominal pain and intestinal obstruction is the presence of an abdominal wall hernia.
- Acute pelvic pain may indicate acute pathology such as tubo-ovarian abscess, ruptured ovarian cyst, ectopic pregnancy, or ovarian torsion.
- Scrotal trauma may lead to formation of a hydrocele or hematocele.
- Torsion of the spermatic cord occurs as a result of abnormal mobility of the testis within the scrotum. Torsion is a surgical emergency, and it is important to obtain diagnostic images as soon as possible.
- Swelling in the extremity may be acute, chronic, distal, or superficial in the venous system. Other causes of extremity pain and swelling include Baker cyst (posterior swelling of the knee with extension into the lower calf), cellulitis, abscess, muscle hematoma, and fasciitis.

BIBLIOGRAPHY

AIUM Practice Parameter for the Performance of Point-of-Care Ultrasound Examinations *J Ultra Med.* 2019;38:833–849.

American College of Emergency Physicians Policy Statement: Emergency Ultrasound Imaging Crtieria. *Compendium*. October 2014:1–55.

American Society of Echocardiography. Focused cardiac ultrasound in the emergent setting: consensus statement of the ASE, Morrisville, NC: 2010.

Bahner D, Blaivas M, Cohen HL, et al. AIUM practice guideline for the performance of the focused assessment with sonography for trauma (FAST) examination. *J Ultrasound Med*. 2008;27(2):313–318.

Branney SW, Moore EE, Cantrill SV, et al. Ultrasound based key clinical pathway reduces the use of hospital resources for the evaluation of blunt abdominal trauma. *Journal of Trauma*. 1997;42(6):1086–1090.

Cha JY, Kashuk JL, Sarin EL, et al. Diagnostic peritoneal lavage remains a valuable adjunct to modern imaging techniques. *J Trauma*. 2009;67(2):330–334. discussion 334-6.

Durston W, Carl ML, Guerra W, et al. Comparison of quality and cost-effectiveness in the evaluation of symptomatic cholelithiasis with different approaches to ultrasound availability in the ED. *The American Journal of Emergency Medicine*. 2001;19(4):260–269.

Gonzalez RP, Ickler J, Gaschassin P. Complementary roles of diagnostic peritoneal lavage and computed tomography in the evaluation of blunt abdominal trauma. *J Trauma*. 2001;51:1128–1136.

Griffin XL, Pullinger R. Are diagnostic peritoneal lavage or focused abdominal sonography for trauma safe screening investigations for hemodynamically stable patients after blunt abdominal trauma? A review of the literature. *J Trauma*. 2007;62(3):779–784.

Heller M, Melanson S, Patterson J, Raftis J. Impact of emergency medicine resident training in ultrasonography on ultrasound utilization. *The American Journal of Emergency Medicine*. 1999;17(1):21–22.

Hussain ZJ, Figueroa R, Budorick NE. How much free fluid can a pregnant patient have? Assessment of pelvic free fluid in pregnancy patients without antecedent trauma. *J Trauma*. 2011;70(6):1420–1423.

Korner M, Krotz MM, Degenhart C, et al. Current role of emergency US in patients with major trauma. *Radiographics*. 2008;28(1):225–242.

Labovitz AJ, Noble VE, Bierig M, et al. Focused Cardiac Ultrasound in the Emergent Setting. *A Concensus Statement of the American Society of Echocardiography and the American College of Emergency Physicians*. 2010

Ma OJ, Gaddis G, Steele MT, et al. Prospective analysis of the effect of physician experience with the FAST examination in reducing the use of CT scans. *Emergency Medicine Australasia*. 2005;17(1):24–30.

Marx J, Isenhour J. Abdominal trauma. In: Marx JA, Hockberger RS, Walls RM, eds. *Rosen's Emergency Medicine Concepts and Clinical Practice*. 5th ed. St. Louis: Elsevier; 2006.

Moore CL, Molina AA, Lin H. Ultrasonography in community emergency departments in the United States: access to ultrasonography performed by consultants and status of emergency physician-performed ultrasonography. *Annals of Emergency Medicine*. 2006;47(2):147–153.

Shen AY, Dalziel P, Liteplo AS, et al. Focused assessment with sonography in trauma and abdominal computed tomography utilization in adult trauma patients: trends over the last decade. *Emerg Med Int*. 2013:678380 2013.

CHAPTER 20

Sonographic Techniques in the Transplant Patient

Talisha M. Hunt

OBJECTIVES

On completion of this chapter, you should be able to:
- Understand the complexity of and criteria for receiving a transplant
- Gain knowledge of surgical techniques of liver, renal, and pancreatic transplants
- Identify the necessary imaging protocol needed for imaging the transplanted organ
- Recognize and define normal sonographic features of the transplant patient
- Recognize and define common and complex pathologies
- Know the importance of imaging in the immediate postoperative patient
- Identify and describe immediate complications after transplantation and those that occur within the months and years to follow
- Understand your role in donating life

OUTLINE

Who Needs a Transplant? 584
   History and Criteria for Liver Transplantation 584
   History and Criteria for Renal Transplantation 585
   History and Criteria for Pancreatic Transplantation 586
Liver Transplant 586
   Surgical Technique of the Liver Transplant 586
   Evaluation of the Liver Allograft 588
   Normal Sonographic Findings of the Liver Transplant 590
   Liver Allograft Imaging in the Immediate Postoperative Period 590

Liver Transplantation Complications in Routine Surveillance 590
Pathology of the Liver Transplant 593
Renal Transplant 608
   Surgical Technique of the Renal Transplant 608
   Evaluation of the Renal Allograft 610
   Normal Sonographic Findings of the Renal Transplant 612
   Renal Allograft Imaging in the Immediate Postoperative Period 613
   Renal Transplantation Complications in Routine Surveillance 615
   Pathology of the Renal Transplant 615

Pancreatic Transplant 624
   Surgical Technique of the Pancreatic Transplant 624
   Evaluation of the Pancreatic Allograft 627
   Normal Sonographic Findings of the Pancreatic Transplant 629
   Pancreatic Allograft Imaging in the Immediate Postoperative Period 630
   Pancreatic Transplantation Complications in Routine Surveillance 630
   Pathology of the Pancreatic Transplant 633
Your Role in Donating Life 638

KEY TERMS

Model for End-Stage Liver Disease (MELD)
Organ Procurement and Transplantation Network (OPTN)
Pediatric End-Stage Liver Disease (PELD)
Posttransplant lymphoproliferative disorder (PTLD)
Renal autotransplantation
Simultaneous pancreas-kidney transplant (SPK)
United Network for Organ Sharing (UNOS)

WHO NEEDS A TRANSPLANT?

According to the **Organ Procurement and Transplantation Network (OPTN)**, as of January 2021, there are more than 120,000 people in need of an organ transplant. Of these, 108,464 are actively waiting, and every 9 minutes a new candidate is added to the national transplant waiting list. The average wait time is 5 to 7 years. With this severe shortage of donor organs, 17 people die each day on average while waiting for their transplant. In 2020, 39,034 patients received a transplant, which was the 10th consecutive annual record, with 70% of these transplants coming from deceased donors. The number of living donor transplants were reduced due to the COVID-19 pandemic. Many transplant programs deferred living donor transplantation to reduce unnecessary exposure to the COVID-19 virus. The majority of transplant recipients were age 50 and older during the past 10 years, with the most common age range between 50 and 64 years.

To ensure a successful transplant, each patient needs to receive the best of care from the entire transplant team. The team consists of clinical transplant coordinators, transplant physicians and surgeons, financial coordinators, and social workers. The **United Network for Organ Sharing (UNOS)** celebrated 35 years in 2019. UNOS maintains a centralized computer networking system for all organ procurement organizations and transplant centers while seeking to be fair and effective in selecting transplant candidates. The UNOS database can be accessed 24 hours a day. Once a patient is referred to a transplant center, the patient will have a series of tests, and their mental and physical health will be evaluated by a physician. The social support available to the patient is also a consideration. If the center accepts the candidate, the medical information will be entered into the national organ transplantation waiting list. Once a deceased donor is located, a transplant coordinator from an organ procurement organization will access the UNOS database. Each patient on the waiting list is matched with the donor characteristics using the computer. The computer will then display the ranked list of the candidates according to the OPTN organ allocation process. Factors in receiving a transplant include tissue match, blood type, immune status, length of time on the waiting list, and the distance between the donor and recipient. The organ is offered to the transplant team and candidate that are on top of the list. The person at the top does not always receive the organ because they may be too unhealthy or laboratory results indicate an incompatible match and rejection would likely occur. Once the patient is selected, they would be contacted for the transplant surgery to be scheduled and performed.

History and Criteria for Liver Transplantation

Patients who have severe liver disease require a liver transplant for survival. Acute liver failure is sudden and most commonly caused from a drug-induced injury such as an acetaminophen overdose. Chronic liver failure or end-stage liver disease is progressive over a period of months and years. Scar tissue is formed within the liver and normal functioning liver tissue is reduced, creating cirrhosis. The most common reason for transplantation in the United States is cirrhosis due to chronic hepatitis C, followed by alcohol abuse (Fig. 20.1). Many other liver diseases can also cause the liver to fail resulting in the need for transplantation, including the following:

- Chronic hepatitis B and autoimmune hepatitis
- Nonalcoholic steatohepatitis, caused by fat and inflammation of the liver
- Hemochromatosis, due to iron overload within the liver
- Wilson disease, due to copper overload within the liver
- Budd-Chiari syndrome, caused by occlusion of the hepatic veins draining the liver
- Biliary diseases, including the following:
  - Biliary atresia, absent or blocked bile ducts and occurs only in infants
  - Alagille syndrome, blocked or malformed bile ducts and ductal paucity
  - Primary biliary cirrhosis, destruction of intrahepatic ducts
  - Primary sclerosing cholangitis (PSC), destruction of intrahepatic and extrahepatic ducts
  - Cancer originating in the liver such as hepatocellular carcinoma (HCC), hepatoblastoma, and cholangiocarcinoma

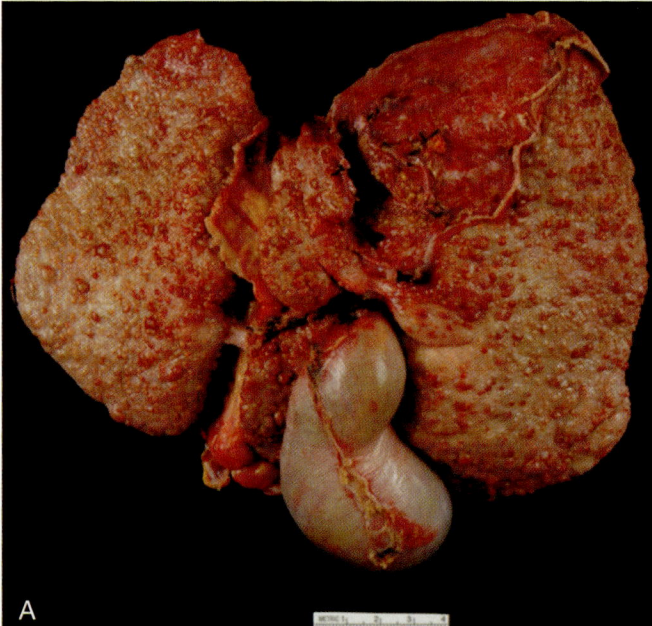
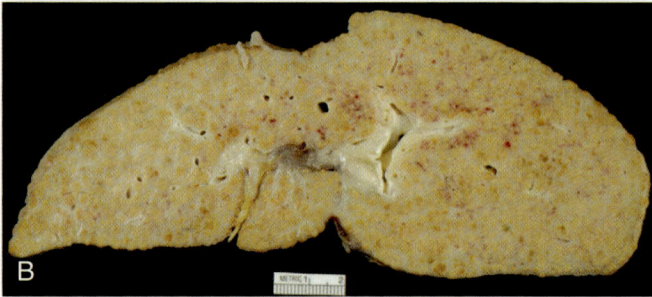

FIG. 20.1 Pathology liver specimen of cirrhosis due to alcoholic liver disease. (A) Surface nodularity is present. (B) Cross-sectional slice.

Symptoms of liver disease include jaundice, fatigue, weight loss, itching, abdominal ascites, bleeding in the stomach from varices, confusion, black stools, nausea, and loss of appetite. A patient may not be a liver transplant candidate if they present with severe irreversible illness, widespread cancer, human immunodeficiency virus/acquired immunodeficiency syndrome (HIV/AIDS), severe pulmonary hypertension, active infection, alcohol or drug abuse, or history of noncompliance.

Patients who are placed on the transplant waiting list receive a score that determines how urgently they need a new liver. Dr. Patrick Kamath originally developed the Mayo End-Stage Liver Disease Score at Mayo Clinic in 2001. With modification from UNOS, the **Model for End-Stage Liver Disease (MELD)** scale for adults and **Pediatric End-Stage Liver Disease (PELD)** for younger than 12 years are still actively used today. MELD was initially used to predict death within 3 months in patients who had a transjugular intrahepatic portosystemic shunt (TIPS) performed. This scale was also found to be beneficial in predicting prognosis and prioritizing liver transplant recipients. MELD scores range from 6 to 40 and PELD scores range from negative values to 99. The scores identify the likelihood of death within 3 months without receiving a transplant. Higher scores denote an increased need for a transplant. For example, a patient with a MELD score of 22 would have a 10% mortality risk at 3 months, whereas a patient with a score of 38 would have an 80% mortality risk. The MELD score is a mathematical calculation based on laboratory values of bilirubin (measurement of bile pigment), creatinine (kidney function), and international nationalized ratio (INR; blood clotting ability).

$$\text{MELD} = [0.957 \times \log(\text{creatinine}) + 0.378 \times \log(\text{bilirubin}) + 1.12 \times \log(\text{INR}) + 0.643] \times 10$$

In 2002 there was an immediate decrease by 12% of the time spent on the waiting list, which also led to a reduction of almost 15% mortality. The mean waiting time in the MELD era went from 656 to 416 days. The reduction in mortality went from 2046 deaths in 2001 to 1364 by 2005.[1] The average wait time in the United States based on the MELD scores is 21 months for a MELD of 11 to 18, 4 months for a MELD of 19 to 24, and 20 days for a MELD greater than 25.[2]

The Milan criteria also play a role in liver transplantation. If a cirrhotic patient has HCC, the patient may be considered for a transplant if they have one HCC smaller than 5 cm, or up to three lesions smaller than 3 cm without vascular invasion or extrahepatic involvement. HCC is the most common primary malignant tumor in the liver and is the fifth most common cancer. There is a 10% to 50% chance of recurrence at 2 years and 70% at 5 years with liver resection. Transplantation and radiofrequency ablation (RFA) are potentially curative options.[3]

Dr. Thomas Starzl performed the first liver transplant on March 1, 1963. The 3-year-old patient with biliary atresia died due to uncontrolled bleeding. The first five transplant recipients died within 23 days. In 1967 the first successful liver transplant performed by Dr. Starzl in Denver survived 1 year. The patient died of recurrent HCC.[2] With the help of Sir Roy Caine, cyclosporine was introduced in 1979, improving survival rates significantly. In 1989 Starzl and colleagues reported that 1179 patients survived between 1 and 5 years after transplantation. Since the first transplant, more than 10,000,000 liver transplants have been performed worldwide with an 80% to 90% survival rate within the first year.[4] There are currently more than 125 transplant programs performing approximately 5000 to 6000 transplants each year.[2] As of June 15, 2012, 16,773 patients were awaiting a deceased liver transplant.[5]

In 2020 the average cost of receiving a liver transplant was $878,400. If a patient received a combined liver and kidney transplant, the cost was $1,355,100. These costs include 30 days pretransplant, procurement, hospital transplant admission, transplant physician, 180 days posttransplant discharge, and immunosuppressants.

History and Criteria for Renal Transplantation

The most common cause for needing a renal transplant is chronic end-stage renal disease or renal failure. Acute renal failure may also occur, requiring transplantation, but this is significantly uncommon. Symptoms of renal failure begin when the kidney only has 10% functioning tissue. Some signs and symptoms are decreased urine output, edema in the legs or feet, shortness of breath, fatigue, confusion, nausea, chest pain, heart arrhythmias, difficulty sleeping, itching, hypertension, loss of appetite, muscle cramps, and seizures or coma in severe cases. Depending on the cause of renal impairment, it may be treatable, yet some may show irreversible damage. Renal function is evaluated using blood laboratory values of blood urea nitrogen, creatinine, and glomerular filtration rate. With progressive loss of kidney function, patients will ultimately require dialysis to filter waste and remove excess fluid from the blood. Dialysis is the only means of survival until a renal transplant becomes available. Patients may not receive a transplant if they have widespread cancer, active infection, HIV/AIDS, liver or heart disease, history of noncompliance, or alcohol or drug abuse. The following are causes that can lead to renal failure and a need for transplantation:

- Hypertension and renal artery stenosis or renal vein thrombosis
- Diabetes mellitus: high blood glucose can damage the filtering system (diabetic nephropathy)
- Urinary tract obstruction such as renal stones or certain cancers
- Inherited kidney disease such as polycystic kidney disease
- Glomerulonephritis: inflammation of small filters, glomeruli
- Interstitial nephritis: inflammation of kidney tubules
- Hemolytic uremic syndrome: premature destruction of red blood cells
- Systemic lupus erythematosus: immune system attacks kidney as foreign object
- Scleroderma: hardening and tightening of the skin and connective tissue
- Vasculitis: inflammation of blood vessels

- Toxins such as alcohol, cocaine, or heavy metals
- Recurrent kidney infection
- Medication therapy used for other diseases
- Severe dehydration

On December 23, 1954, Dr. Joseph Murray performed the first successful kidney transplant at Peter Bent Brigham Hospital in Boston. The surgery involved identical twins, Richard and Ronald Herrick, eliminating possible rejection.[6] In 1990 Dr. Murray won the Nobel Prize in Physiology of Medicine. Between 1954 and 1973, about 10,000 renal transplants were performed. More than 99,000 people were on the deceased kidney donor list as of June 15, 2012. Due to shortage of kidneys, the system of expanded criteria donors (ECDs) was introduced in 2002. This includes the kidneys that once were considered not suitable. ECD kidneys are any donors older than 60 years or ages 50 to 59 years with two of the following conditions: hypertension, serum creatinine greater than 1.5 mg/dL, or cause of death from a cerebrovascular accident.[5]

In 2020 the average cost of receiving a renal transplant was $442,500. If a patient received a combined kidney and liver transplant, the cost was $1,355,100. The cost of a combined kidney and pancreas transplant was $713,800. These costs include 30 days pretransplant, procurement, hospital transplant admission, transplant physician, 180 days posttransplant discharge, and immunosuppressants.

History and Criteria for Pancreatic Transplantation

More than 15 million people in the United States have diabetes mellitus, with 798,000 new patients diagnosed each year.[7] Patients receive a pancreas transplant in hopes to cure type 1 diabetes. In these patients, the pancreatic islet cells cannot produce enough insulin, resulting in dangerously elevated blood glucose. Insulin provides movement of the glucose in the blood into the muscles and fat to provide energy for the body. Initially, patients routinely receive insulin injections or take medications to help control blood glucose. Transplantation may be a consideration if glucose levels are poorly managed, if glucose levels show frequent insulin reactions, or if severe kidney damage occurs. It is common for a patient to receive a combined pancreas and renal transplant to ensure healthy organs are unlikely to be affected by the damage that comes from diabetes. High blood glucose can lead to many complications such as amputations, heart disease, stroke, vascular disease, blindness, nerve damage, or kidney damage.

Type 2 diabetes patients are not a consideration for pancreas transplant. In these patients, insulin is produced from the pancreas, but the body develops insulin resistance and a new pancreas will not be a cure in this case. Transplantation usually is not performed on a patient with cancer, active infection, HIV/AIDS, lung disease, obesity, severe heart disease, or an ongoing history of alcohol or drug abuse.

Dr. William Kelly and Dr. Richard Lillehei performed the first successful pancreas transplant combined with a kidney transplant on December 17, 1966, at the University of Minnesota.[7] The surgery was considered experimental until about 1990. There are about 1200 pancreas transplants performed each year in the United States, with 75% of cases being a **simultaneous pancreas-kidney transplant (SPK)**. There have been more than 23,000 pancreas transplants reported to the International Transplant Registry.[8]

In the United States there were 3202 patients that were listed for a pancreas transplant as of February 2014. During the years of 2012 and 2013, there were 16,410 deceased donors with only 2826 pancreas allografts procured. This shortage of organs is due to lack of procurement or the pancreas being deemed unsuitable. The ideal donor is between 10 and 40 years of age with a body mass index (BMI) less than 27.5 kg/m^2, and with a cause of death not from cerebrovascular disease.[9] Recent studies have suggested organs from extended criteria donors can receive similar graft survival as the "ideal" donor. The accumulation of risk factors and extended cold ischemic time should be avoided when possible to ensure a healthy allograft.[10]

In 2020 the average cost of receiving a pancreas transplant was $408,800. The cost of a combined pancreas and kidney transplant was $713,800. These costs include 30 days pretransplant, procurement, hospital transplant admission, transplant physician, 180 days posttransplant discharge, and immunosuppressants.

LIVER TRANSPLANT

Surgical Technique of the Liver Transplant

The liver can be preserved between 8 and 12 hours on ice and using a special preservation solution. The shorter the ischemic time, the better the allograft function once transplanted. For every liver transplant, the donor and recipient are rechecked to verify a match. The blood type and compatibility need to be confirmed and the UNOS database per protocol as well. Before coming into the operating room, the team will discuss the risks, benefits, and alternatives with the patient and obtain consent. All institutions have certain protocols and techniques that they follow. The following will discuss the basic current practices at my institution.

Cadaveric Liver Donation. The patient is brought into the operating room confirming patient identification and procedure to be performed. Following general anesthesia and line placement, a Foley catheter is placed into the bladder. The abdomen is prepped and draped sterilely. Bilateral subcostal skin incisions are made and extended to the midline up to the xiphoid process. The scar resembles a "Mercedes sign." The diseased liver is mobilized, vessels clamped and ligated, and dissected free from the body cavity becoming "anhepatic." This diseased liver is sent for pathologic examination.

The procured liver is prepared on the "back table" for any reconstruction to occur and submerged into a saline slush solution. Patients present with variant anatomy and that needs to be taken into consideration. Some may have normal anatomic variants such as additional veins or arteries to anastomose or vessels need to be trimmed down to size. Some may have short veins or arteries that are not long enough and require an interposition graft in which a deceased donor iliac artery or vein may be used. The iliac vein can act as a conduit between the recipient superior mesenteric vein and the donor portal vein. The iliac artery can be used as a conduit between the recipient infrarenal aorta and the donor hepatic artery.

Once the donor liver has been prepared, it is placed within the recipient's abdominal cavity and covered with laparotomy pads containing saline slush. Vent tubing is placed in the infrahepatic cava to prepare the suprahepatic cava for anastomosis. The upper caval anastomosis is sewn end to side with running sutures. The recipient portal vein is occluded with a clamp and flushed with glycine irrigant, and then an end-to-end portal vein anastomosis is sewn with sutures. The recipient common hepatic artery is flushed with heparinized saline, and occluded with a clamp. The donor and recipient common hepatic arteries are then sewn end-to-end using running sutures to create the arterial anastomosis. The arterial and portal venous clamps are removed and the liver flushed with blood to begin reperfusion. The surgeon examines all the anastomoses to ensure they are dry and do not have a leak and makes sure the patient is hemodynamically stable. At this point, a cholecystectomy is performed on the donor liver. A choledochodochostomy is sewn between donor and recipient common bile ducts using running sutures. The anastomosis is sewn over a polyurethane biliary stent or tube, which is brought out through the cystic duct stump. The catheter is then secured to the stump with a suture. Another option would be an end-to-side choledochojejunostomy using a suture over the jejunal biliary tube. In patients with PSC or retransplantation, a roux-en-Y limb is created for reconstruction (Fig. 20.2). The patient is rechecked for any significant bleeding. Drains are placed within the right and left subhepatic spaces and secured to the skin with stitches. Sponge, needle, and instrument counts are conducted before closure. If indicated, the patient will receive units of blood, platelets, or fresh frozen plasma. The incision is closed in two layers with a running layer suture on the midline and posterior fascia and then anterior fascia is closed. The skin is closed with staples. The wound is dressed with a dry sterile dressing and the patient is transported to the intensive care unit (ICU) when stable.

Living Donor Liver Donation. There is a shortage of organs available for donation. Living donor organ donation offers the alternative for ones waiting for a transplant and also increases the existing organ supply. A friend or family member may consider being a donor for their loved one. If the donor is not a match, there is a paired exchange program. The donor's organ would go to someone else for a better match rather than directly going to their friend or family member. The one needing the transplant will receive their organ in the exchange that meets their match.

The first adult living liver donor donation was performed in 1989; more than 4000 have been performed in the United States. The 1-, 3-, and 5-year survival rates are 90%, 83%, and 78%, respectively.[2] Ultimately, a donor liver will regenerate to more than 85% of its original volume. Living donor transplantation has many ethical issues and has been a source of some controversy. Donors may experience a psychological

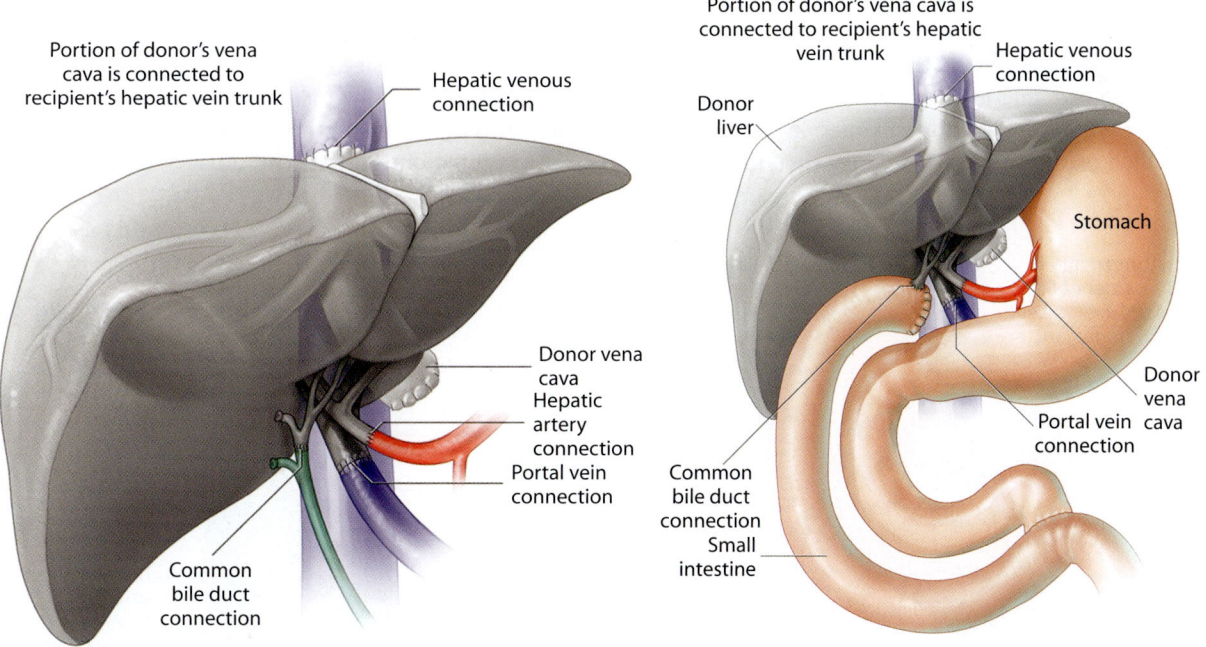

FIG. 20.2 Anastomosis sites of cadaveric liver transplant. (A) Duct-duct procedure. (B) Roux-en-Y procedure. (Courtesy Mayo Foundation for Medical Education and Research.)

syndrome due to the stress of surgery. Gokce and colleagues showed that 21% of donors feel anxious about the complications and quality of life after surgery. The donor complication rate is 40% with incision infection, biliary leak, or stricture being the most common. Some donors develop complications that lead them to suicide or drug overdose.[11] Living donor liver transplants are optimal in urgent situations; however, 27.1% of living donors demonstrated one or more complications in the postoperative period.[12]

The surgical technique is very similar compared with a cadaveric liver. The allograft may demonstrate better function more quickly due to the decreased preservation time in a living donor. The recipient will receive part of a liver rather than a full organ, usually the right hepatic lobe. The patient is brought into the operating room confirming patient identification and procedure to be performed. Following general anesthesia and line placement, a Foley catheter is placed into the bladder. The abdomen is prepped and draped sterilely. Bilateral subcostal skin incisions are made and extended to the midline up to the xiphoid process. The scar resembles a Mercedes sign. The diseased liver is mobilized, vessels clamped and ligated, and dissected free from the body cavity becoming anhepatic. This liver is sent off for pathologic examination.

The procured liver is prepared on the back table for any reconstruction to occur and submerged into a saline slush solution. Patients present with variant anatomy and that needs to be taken into consideration. Some may have additional veins or arteries to anastomose or vessels need to be trimmed down to size, or some may have short vessels and require an interposition graft. Once the donor liver is prepared, it is placed within the recipient's abdominal cavity and covered with laparotomy pads containing saline slush. The recipient's left middle hepatic vein trunk is stapled and the right hepatic vein is occluded using a clamp. The donor right hepatic vein opening is extended inferiorly on the vena cava, and two sutures are placed on the superior and inferior venotomy. The sutures are then placed through the donor right hepatic vein.

An end-to-end anastomosis is performed between the donor and recipient right hepatic vein and vena cava using running sutures. The recipient portal vein is flushed free of clot, and an end-to-end portal vein anastomosis is created using running sutures. Reperfusion of the liver is accomplished by releasing the venous and portal vein clamps. Following reperfusion, the perihepatic area is carefully inspected for hemostasis. If bleeding is noticed, the surgeon will control using additional sutures. The donor right hepatic artery is flushed with heparinized saline and occluded with a clamp. The recipient gastroduodenal artery is ligated and divided. The common hepatic artery is occluded with a clamp and divided in its distal portion. An end-to-end anastomosis is performed between the donor right hepatic artery and the recipient common hepatic artery using running sutures. Once arterial reperfusion is achieved, the perihepatic area is again carefully inspected for hemostasis. An end-to-end duct anastomosis is created. In patients with PSC or retransplantation, a roux-en-Y limb is created for reconstruction. An end-to-side hepaticojejunostomy is performed using a running suture on the posterior layer and an interrupted suture on the anterior layer (Fig. 20.3). Hemostasis is again ensured. Two drains are placed posterior to the liver and inferior to the incision. Sponge, needle, and instrument counts are conducted before closure. If indicated, the patient will receive units of blood, platelets, or fresh frozen plasma. The incision is closed with a running suture in the anterior and posterior layers and in the midline. Staples are used for skin closure. The wound is dressed with a dry sterile dressing and the patient is transported to the ICU when stable.

Evaluation of the Liver Allograft

As a sonographer, evaluate the liver transplant as a native liver. Assess the size, echotexture, contour, biliary tree, and vasculature, and look for any masses, fluid collections, or ascites. Institutions instill their own routine protocols on timing of examinations and specific images that are required. The

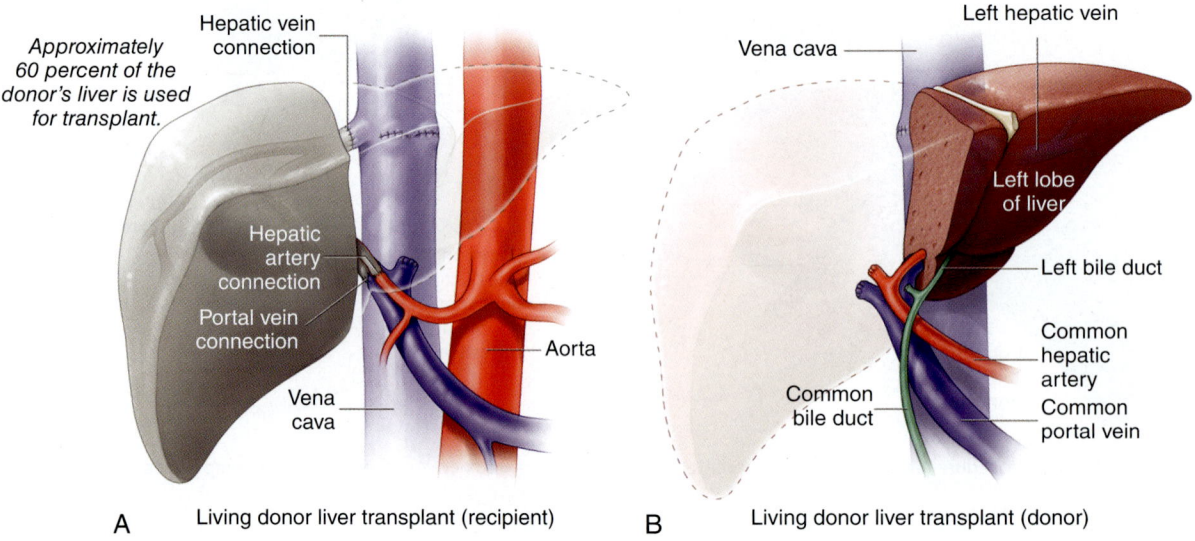

FIG. 20.3 **Anastomosis sites of living donor liver transplant.** (A) Liver transplant (recipient). (B) Native liver (donor). (Courtesy Mayo Foundation for Medical Education and Research.)

following is the basis of what my institution practices. Once the patient has arrived at the ICU from the surgical suite, the sonographer will go remotely to perform the "day 0" examination. Typically the patient will receive an ultrasound examination on postoperative day 1 and day 7 as well. The patient's liver function is closely monitored and if any issues arise, the transplant physicians will tailor their imaging requests. The patient usually has a follow-up ultrasound every 6 months to 1 year if there are no complications.

It is best to image using a 2.5- to 5.0-MHz curvilinear transducer and have the patient fasting 4 to 6 hours. Obese patients and livers with fatty infiltration will likely require lower frequencies. It is helpful to ask the patient to take a breath in and hold it if they are able to do so. This will give better visualization of the liver and reduce respiratory motion. Rolling the patient left lateral decubitus will also help aid visualizing the right lobe more clearly.

The sonographer should scan completely through the liver before taking any images using subcostal and intercostal approaches while adjusting the frequency, depth, gain, time-gain compensation (TGC), and focal zones as they go. Once the liver is fully accessed, the examination needs to include gray-scale longitudinal and transverse images of the left and right hepatic lobes including the caudate lobe and vascular landmarks of the inferior vena cava (IVC), hepatic veins (HVs), and portal veins (PVs). The right lobe of the liver should be compared with the right kidney to evaluate the echogenicity. Document any pathology in two planes with and without measurements and include color Doppler flow. Knowing the type of transplant the patient received (i.e., living or cadaveric) is helpful before scanning because in living donor transplanted patients only the right lobe will be present. The donor liver receives a cholecystectomy during the surgical process and, as a result, no gallbladder images will be acquired. The biliary tree needs to be evaluated for intrahepatic and extrahepatic ductal dilation, wall thickening, biliary leaks, and stones or sludge. It is common for biliary stents to be present. Quadrant images need to be obtained checking for free fluid or signs of bleeding.

The Doppler portion is crucial for the transplanted liver. Venous and arterial color and spectral Doppler needs to be obtained looking for any signs of thrombus or stenosis. Ultrasound is commonly the first method of imaging in these patients, and the sonographer can help the physicians diagnose the patient and treatment will be administered quickly. The hepatic arteries (HAs) are not routinely included in the native liver examination, but they are very important to image in your transplanted patient. It is critical to angle correct in the left, right, and main HAs with pulsed-wave Doppler to accurately assess for stenosis. The sonographer will need to measure the peak systolic and end diastolic velocities to obtain the resistive index (RI) measurement. This is a common indirect Doppler technique to evaluate the HA. A low RI can be a strong indicator of a proximal stenosis the sonographer may not be able to otherwise identify or a presence of an arteriovenous fistula (AVF). A high RI may indicate rejection or hepatic venous congestion. These vessels are small in size, and the sonographer may choose to use the zoom feature on the ultrasound machine for better visualization. Although sometimes it may be difficult to identify the anastomosis, attempt to evaluate the HA as proximally as possible. If a stenosis is present, the anastomotic site is the most common location. Color flow aliasing in the PVs, HVs, or IVC, should be further evaluated with spectral Doppler to help identify a narrowing. For all spectral Doppler, the angle should be parallel with the vessel that is being sampled and less than 60 degrees to avoid falsely elevated velocities. To increase diagnostic accuracy, all of the spectral waveforms should fill the spectral window while eliminating spectral aliasing.

When very slow flow is present in a vessel, a Doppler signal can be difficult to obtain and either the Doppler scale will need to be decreased or the color gain will need to be increased. Some ultrasound machines may have special settings to detect slow flow. These can often be found in other settings besides the abdominal settings such as those for detecting low flow in a lower extremity vein or the iliac vein. If these are not available, the renal artery setting can be helpful filling in the vessels as well. Sometimes the wall filter needs to be decreased if the very slow frequencies are rejected as "cluttered noise" (Fig. 20.4). For obese patients, decreasing

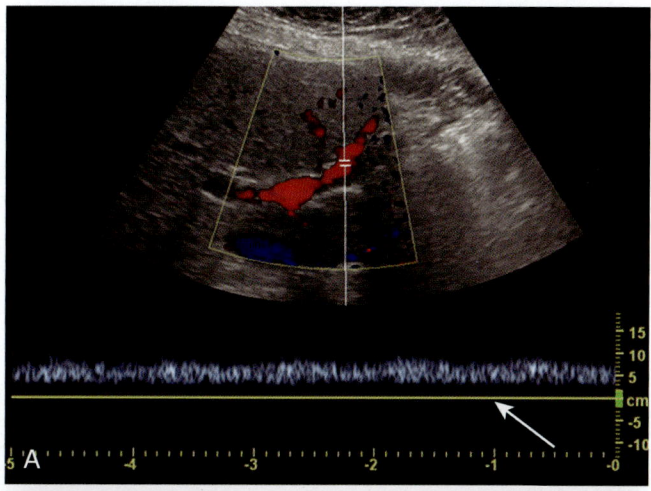
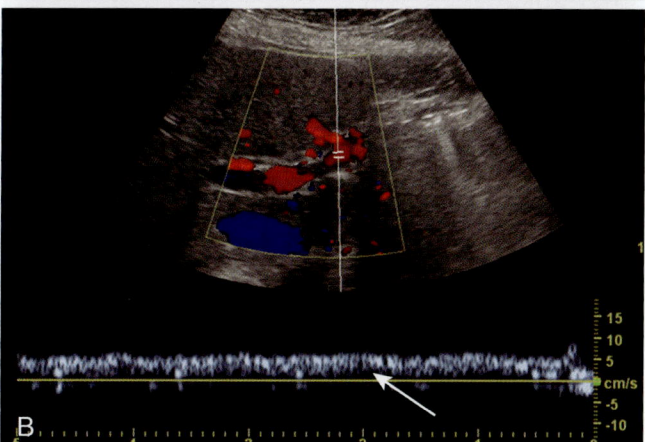

FIG. 20.4 Wall filter settings. (A) High wall filter is used and more noise is filtered on the spectral Doppler ultrasound. (B) Low wall filter is used and can pick up more noise on the spectral Doppler ultrasound.

the gray scale, color, and spectral Doppler frequencies will enable deeper penetration.

Normal Sonographic Findings of the Liver Transplant

On gray-scale imaging, the liver parenchyma should appear smooth and homogeneous being isoechoic relative to the right renal cortex. All vessels and biliary ducts should be anechoic. The HVs and IVC lack a distinct wall whereas the PVs, HAs, and ducts demonstrate echogenic walls running parallel from the liver hilum and branching within the liver. A normal common hepatic duct (CHD) ranges in diameter from 3 to 7 mm, and the common bile duct (CBD) can range from 5 to 9 mm. See Chapter 9 for a more detailed explanation of normal liver anatomy.

The Doppler portion of the transplanted liver examination is crucial to perform. Some vascular complications can only be diagnosed using color and spectral Doppler. The HA will be red on color imaging and the spectral waveform demonstrates a rapid systolic upstroke with continuous diastolic flow above baseline demonstrating a low-resistance waveform. The velocities should be below 200 cm/sec. A normal RI in the HA is in the range of 0.50 to 0.70. The PV flow should be toward the liver showing flow above the baseline with a red color. The spectral waveform of the PV has continuous flow with minimal respiratory changes. The IVC and HVs should be primarily blue in color with a phasic bidirectional spectral Doppler waveform representing changes in the cardiac cycle. The LHV can appear more pulsatile because you are in closer proximity to the heart (Fig. 20.5). When measuring velocities using spectral Doppler imaging, turbulence or any velocity doubling or tripling in the vessel from one location to the next should not be seen.

Liver Allograft Imaging in the Immediate Postoperative Period

It is imperative to image the newly transplanted liver in the immediate postoperative period. Ultrasound is the initial modality of choice. There is no ionizing radiation, and the cost is relatively inexpensive compared with computed tomography (CT) or magnetic resonance imaging (MRI). A skilled sonographer provides early detection of transplant complications and prevents misdiagnosis.

On day 0 of ultrasound examination, the patient will be in the ICU and intubated. As a result, these patients will not be able to roll onto their side or help assist with their breathing. It is very helpful to image the patient without bandages on, if possible. This helps attain the best imaging windows possible and prevents missing pathology. Although this is not a sterile scanning environment, using sterile gel while the patient's incisions are healing can potentially reduce the risk of infection. It is common and helpful to have a member of the transplant team or surgeon present for this examination. They want to ensure that the allograft has adequate arterial and venous flow and look for signs of hemorrhage.

If there is an urgent complication noted, the surgeon can transfer the patient back to the operating room to correct the issue immediately. Not all complications are considered urgent, and a follow-up ultrasound will often be recommended within 24 hours to ensure stability or determine whether the issue has resolved or is getting worse. Urgent findings include, but are not limited to, HA thrombosis, PV, HV or IVC thrombus or occlusion, or active bleeding. It is very common to see postoperative fluid collections, and these usually resolve on their own. Fluid collections will be monitored on serial ultrasound examinations making sure they are not enlarging and causing liver function problems. Another common finding involves the vasculature. Postoperative edema can create elevated blood flow velocities within the HAs or venous system. In this situation, the HAs can have an elevated RI and may demonstrate little or no diastolic flow. It may be common to see reversal of flow within the LPV due to the high flow volume state. Once the edema decreases, the vessels should return to their normal state (Fig. 20.6). Once the ultrasound examination has been completed, the incision should be redressed to help prevent infection. If no complications arise during recovery in the transplant unit, the liver transplant patient is typically discharged from the hospital around postoperative day 5.

Liver Transplantation Complications in Routine Surveillance

Once patients receive their liver transplant, they are closely monitored with routine follow-up examinations and procedures. Blood levels to monitor hepatic function and coagulation studies are checked frequently: daily for 1 week, then 3 times a week, then 2 times a week, then once weekly for 4 months, then monthly. Ultrasound examinations are routinely performed on days 0, 1, and 7. If the transplant team is concerned with complications, the patient will often have more frequent follow-up ultrasounds. Long term, the liver transplant patient typically is followed with a yearly ultrasound.

It is common to perform a routine parenchymal biopsy around day 7 after transplantation, and some patients may require a biopsy yearly to ensure no disease recurrence and rule out rejection. If the patient is symptomatic with pain, fever, or elevated liver function tests (LFTs), a biopsy may be ordered if the ultrasound does not help provide a diagnosis (Fig. 20.7).

Complications may arise while performing these biopsies. The most common complication is bleeding. The patient's INR and platelet counts are checked before the procedure. To reduce the risk of bleeding, patients are asked to stop taking anticoagulants 3 to 5 days before the procedure. Another risk of bleeding is elevated blood pressure or hypertension. Some patients may have known hypertension and be placed on an antihypertensive medication, and this should be taken as usual. Anxiety can significantly worsen hypertension as well in the acute setting. Blood pressures should not exceed 160/90 mm Hg. The radiologist or physician performing the biopsy may administer mild to moderate sedation to help

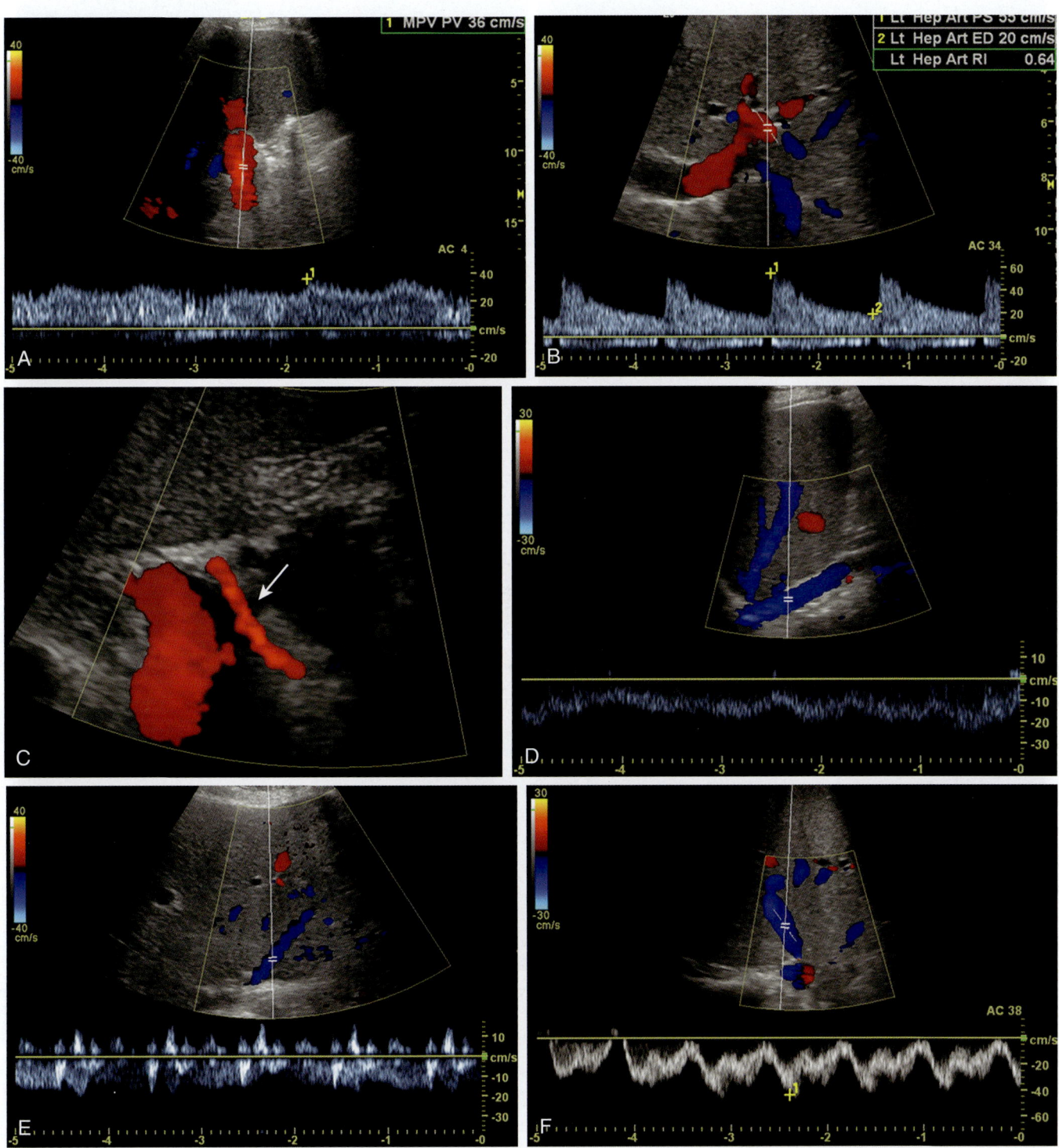

FIG. 20.5 **Normal liver Doppler.** (A) Main portal vein spectral waveform using ultrasound shows a normal velocity with continuous hepatopetal flow. (B) Left hepatic artery spectral waveform using ultrasound shows a normal velocity and resistive index (RI) with a sharp systolic upstroke and continuous diastolic flow. (C) Main hepatic artery color Doppler ultrasound shows no signs of aliasing or narrowing and is widely patent. (D) Inferior vena cava spectral waveform using ultrasound shows phasic flow. (E) Left hepatic vein spectral waveform using ultrasound appears more pulsatile in relation to the heart. (F) Right hepatic vein spectral waveform using ultrasound shows phasic flow.

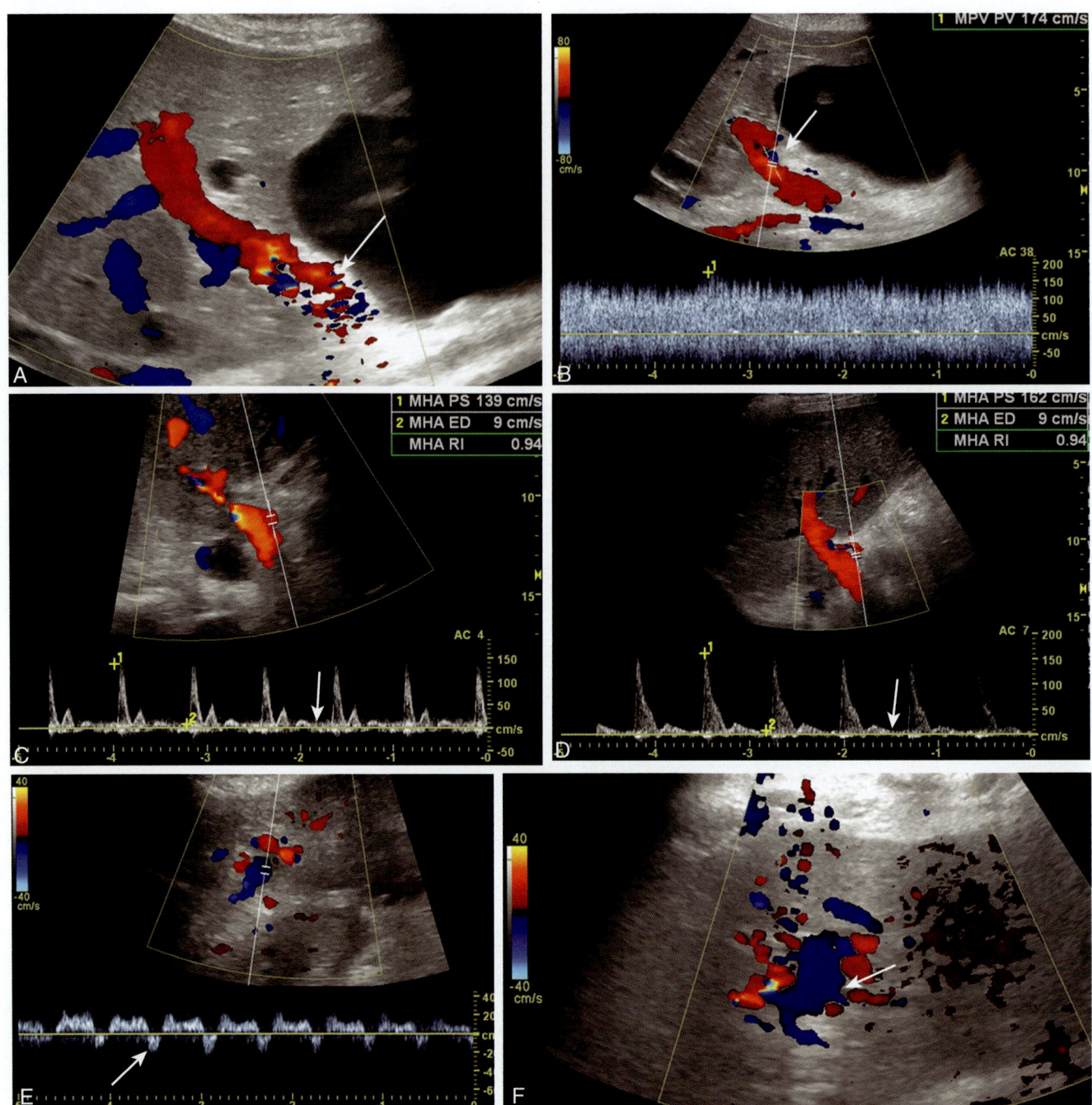

FIG. 20.6 Common temporary postoperative edema findings. (A) Main portal vein color Doppler ultrasound shows aliasing. (B) Main portal vein spectral Doppler ultrasound shows turbulence and elevated velocities. (C–D) Main hepatic artery spectral Doppler ultrasound shows high resistance with little diastolic flow. (E) Left portal vein spectral waveform using ultrasound shows to-and-fro flow. (F) Left portal vein color Doppler ultrasound shows hepatofugal flow.

calm the patient, reducing these pressures. Even after preventive measures, bleeding may still occur. Following the biopsy, the physician should image the site assessing for a bleed. Arterial flow along the biopsy tract outside of the liver parenchyma may be visualized on ultrasound. Color and spectral Doppler should be used to document the bleed. At times, a large collection of lidocaine may collect mimicking a subcapsular bleed. This area should be noted before the procedure so it is not confused with a postprocedural hematoma. The bleeding may be painful if it is associated with the liver capsule or painless. Most bleeds will stop on their own after applying moderate pressure over the biopsy tract. If the bleeding is severe, the patient may become vasovagal and blood pressure may drop. Fluids should be given, and the head should be lowered. If there is active bleeding that cannot be controlled, the patient may be transferred to the interventional radiology department for further imaging and possible embolization.

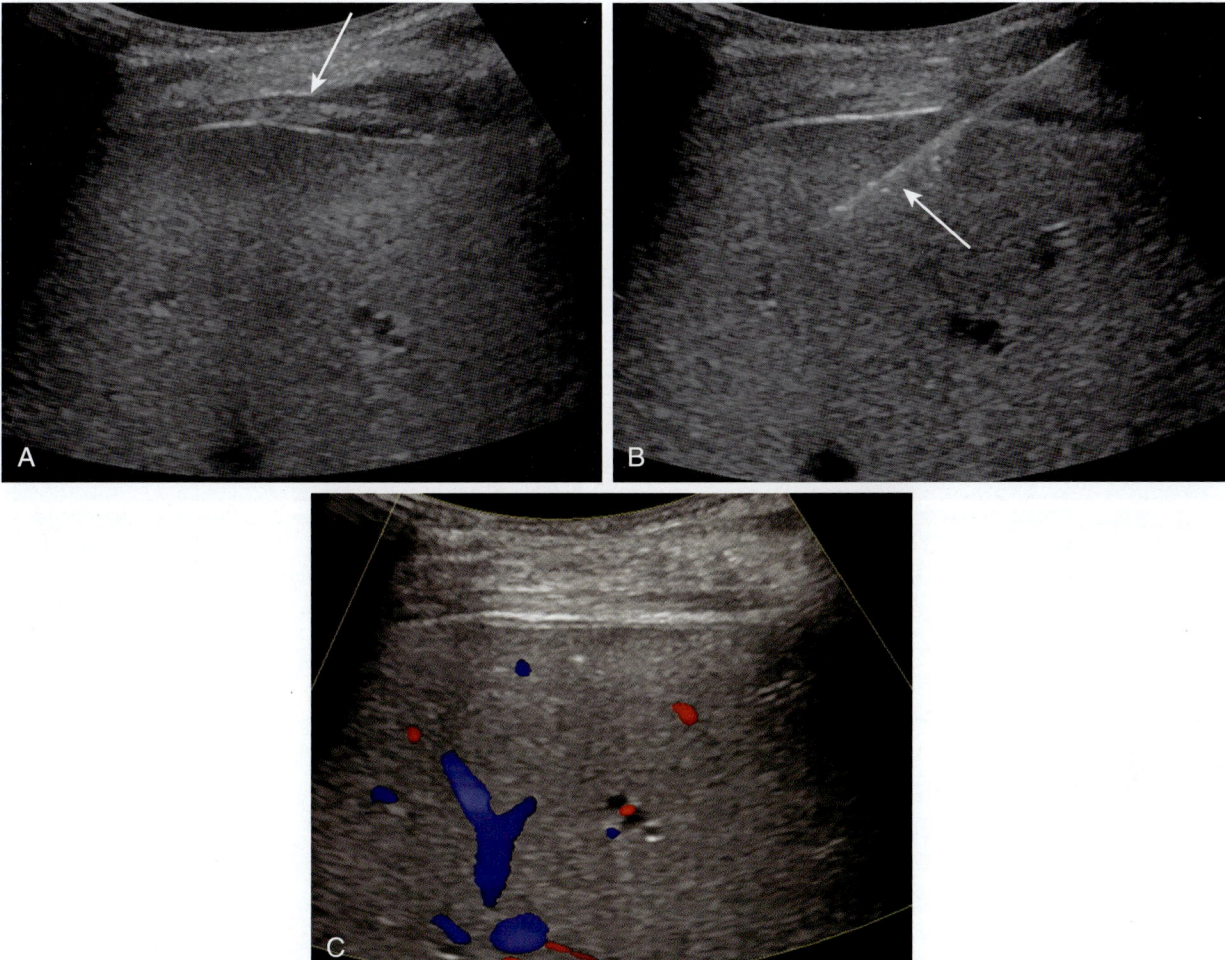

FIG. 20.7 **Normal routine liver biopsy.** (A) A prebiopsy lidocaine wheel outside the liver capsule visualized on ultrasound. (B) Ultrasound-guided needle biopsy pass remaining away from large vessels. (C) Ultrasound after biopsy shows no sign of bleeding on color imaging.

The biopsy needle is ultrasound guided to avoid major blood vessels and biliary ducts. At times, the needle path may cross small vessels for a potential risk creating an AVF or small intrahepatic ducts causing a bile leak forming a biloma (Fig. 20.8). Another rare complication after biopsy is creating a hepatic artery pseudoaneurysm. You can visualize the to-and-fro waveform on spectral Doppler imaging. These findings are usually clinically insignificant and will likely just be followed on serial ultrasound examinations. The radiologist can reduce these risks by avoiding the liver hilum.

Pathology of the Liver Transplant

Rejection. The most common cause for liver transplant failure is rejection. Acute rejection occurs within the first 10 days of transplantation. Some signs and symptoms include right upper quadrant pain, fever, tachycardia, hepatomegaly, and ascites. Liver function tests may be elevated and the patient may develop encephalopathy. Chronic rejection evolves over an extended period of time slowly deteriorating the liver graft, causing fibrosis. The ultrasound findings of rejection are often nonspecific and can include an elevated RI or periportal edema, most often requiring a liver biopsy for diagnosis.[13]

Infection and Abscesses. Intrahepatic abscesses are localized fluid collections of necrotic inflammatory tissue that contains purulent material and an infectious organism. Common signs and symptoms are fever, right upper quadrant pain, and jaundice. These abscesses are often seen secondary to a liver infarction. Patients who are on immunosuppressive medications who present with biliary stricture or arterial insufficiency are at increased risk for developing an infection. Infection is likely to spread to the chest and lungs in the immunocompromised patient.[14] On ultrasound imaging, an abscess will typically have thick walls and be hypoechoic and complex in appearance with an air-fluid level with poorly defined borders. Gas bubbles may be present within the abscess and will appear as a "dirty" shadow. Abscesses can have varied appearances though and may have internal septations or some may even appear solid mimicking a mass. The treatment of choice is usually a percutaneous drainage catheter using CT or ultrasound guidance and antibiotics (Fig. 20.9).

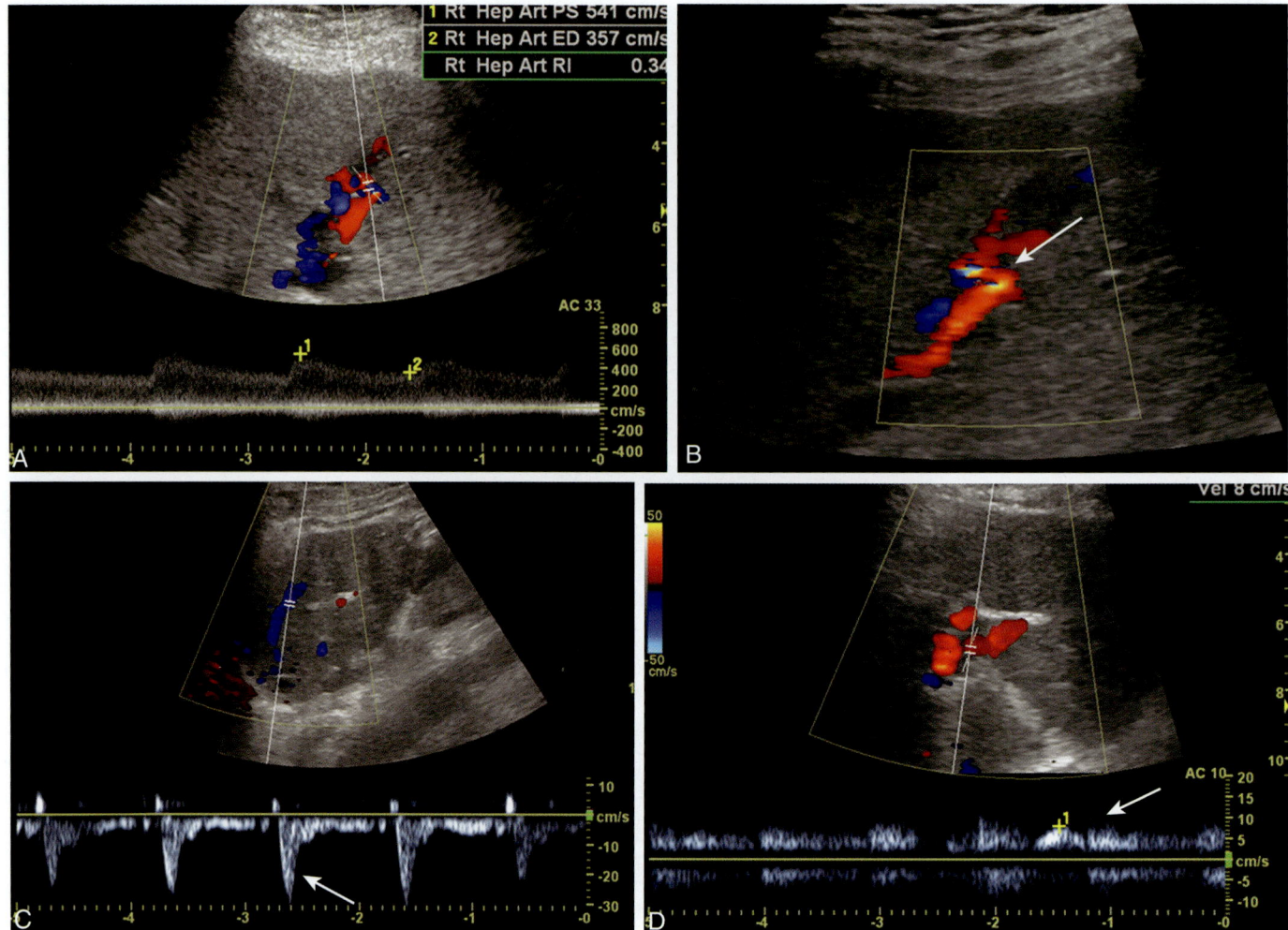

FIG. 20.8 **Liver biopsy complications.** (A) Spectral Doppler ultrasound shows an arteriovenous fistula (AVF) between the right hepatic artery (RHA) and right portal vein (RPV) with an elevated velocity and low resistive waveform. (B) Color Doppler ultrasound shows the connection of the right hepatic artery and RPV. (C) Left hepatic vein spectral Doppler ultrasound shows very pulsatile flow typically seen in an AVF. (D) Very slow flow of the left portal vein on spectral Doppler ultrasound is also highly suggestive of an AVF.

Vascular Compromise

Hepatic Vein and Inferior Vena Cava Thrombosis and Stenosis. There is less than a 1% complication rate involving the IVC and HVs after transplantation. Thrombosis and stenosis most commonly occur at the anastomosis sites due to size discrepancy between the native and transplant vessels or suprahepatic caval kinking. Chronic IVC stenosis is more common in retransplanted or pediatric patients.[13] The IVC can be narrowed from extrinsic compression from postoperative edema or a large hematoma creating a stenosis. Color Doppler aliasing and tripling of the spectral Doppler waveform velocities demonstrating turbulence may be visualized. Hepatic vein dilation with a dampened monophasic waveform may also be visualized. Angioplasty with stent placement is the treatment of choice (Fig. 20.10). Stenosis of the HV mostly occurs in living donor transplants. A focal narrowing along with aliasing on color Doppler and a monophasic, turbulent waveform demonstrating elevated velocities on spectral Doppler imaging will be seen. IVC and HV thrombosis is caused from a hypercoagulable state and surgical factors. Intraluminal thrombus is identified filling the vessel with no color Doppler flow. There may be imaging features of Budd-Chiari syndrome (Fig. 20.11). If the ultrasound examination is inconclusive, CT or MRI may be considered to confirm diagnosis.[13,14] These patients are typically treated with anticoagulants.

Portal Vein Thrombus and Stenosis. Portal vein stenosis occurs in about 1% of patients after transplantation. Stenosis is usually found at the anastomosis site and may occur when there is a size discrepancy of the vessels.[13] On ultrasound imaging, the PV will demonstrate color and spectral Doppler aliasing, typically with a 3:1 ratio. Patients may undergo balloon angioplasty, stent placement, or resection. Thrombosis of the PV occurs in about 3% of liver transplants.[14] This commonly results from mismatched caliber differences in the vessels, stretching of the PV near the anastomotic site, slow portal inflow, or hypercoagulable states. Fresh thrombus appears echogenic and can be either occlusive or nonocclusive. Occlusive thrombus will demonstrate no flow with color or spectral Doppler (Fig. 20.12). With nonocclusive

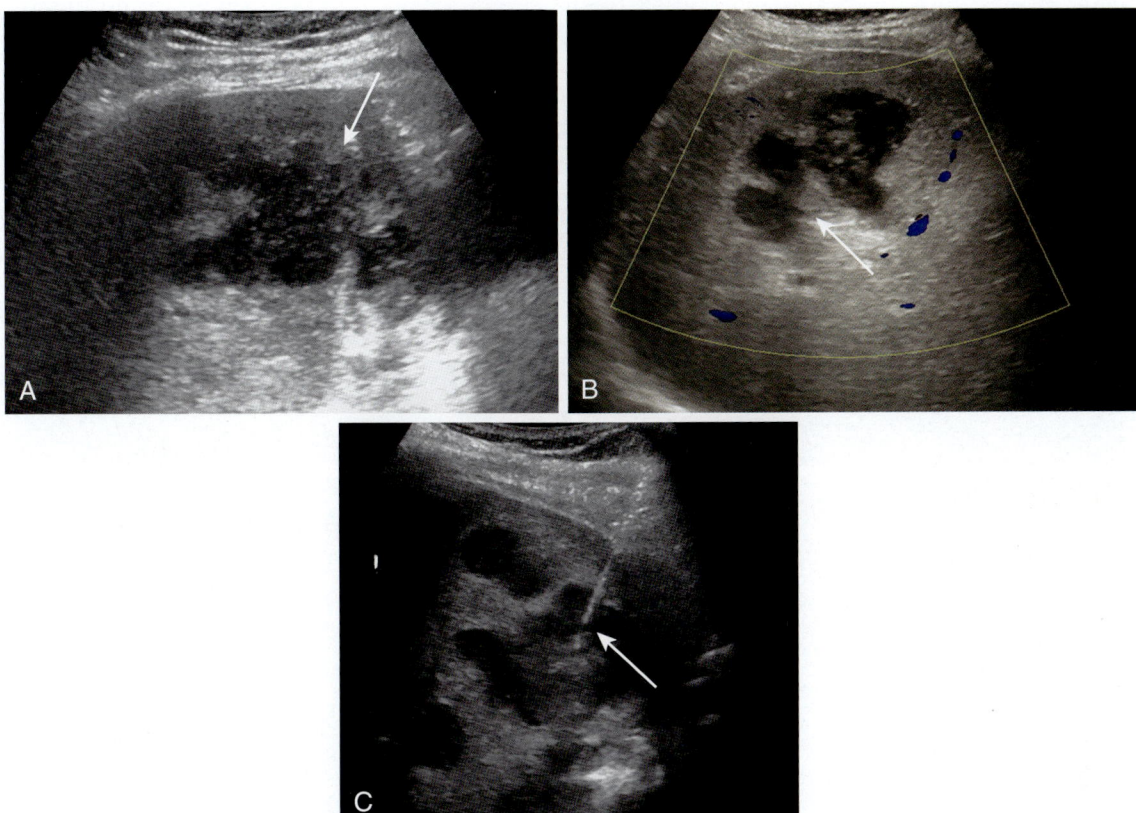

FIG. 20.9 **Intrahepatic liver abscess.** (A) Gray-scale ultrasound of the collection shows irregular, poorly defined borders with debris. (B) Color Doppler ultrasound shows no flow within the complex collection. (C) Ultrasound-guided percutaneous drain placement within the abscess.

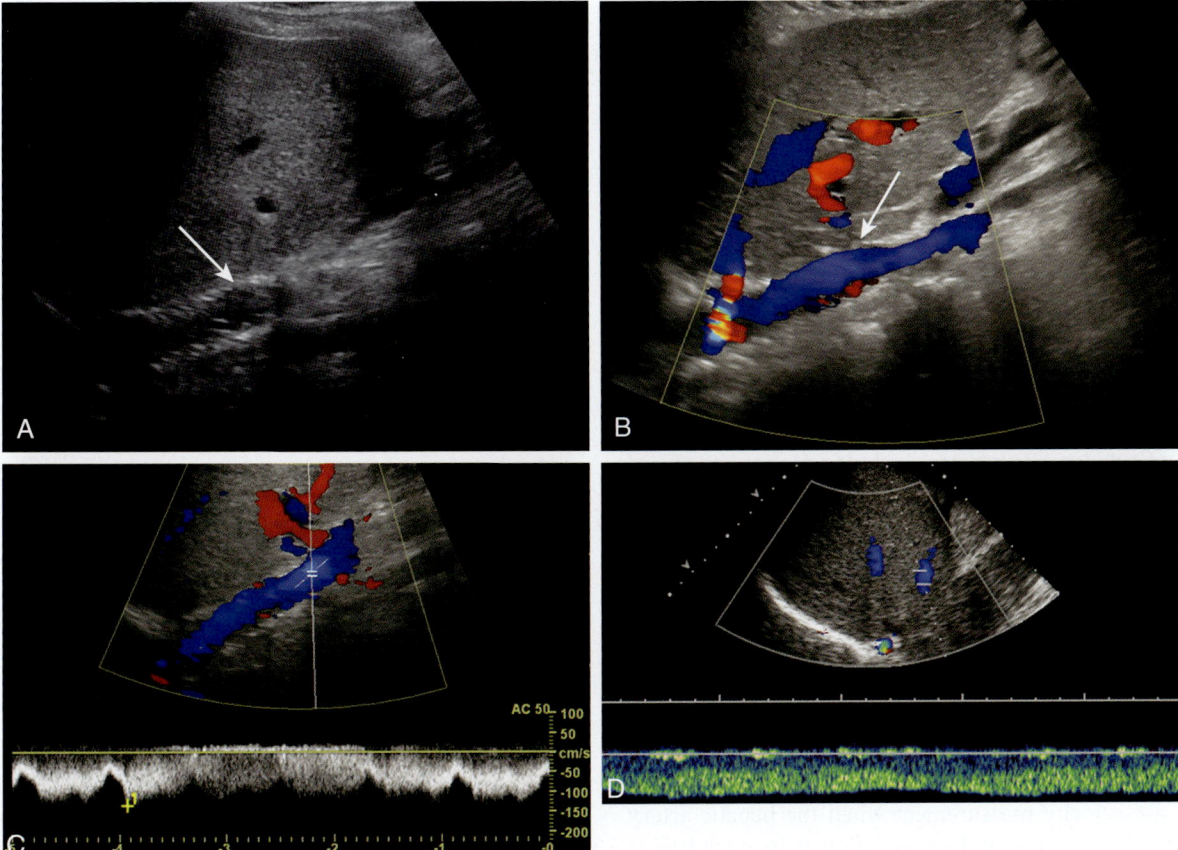

FIG. 20.10 **Inferior vena cava (IVC) stenosis and stent placement.** (A) Longitudinal gray-scale ultrasound shows a stent within the IVC. (B) Color Doppler ultrasound within the stent shows no signs of aliasing or narrowing. (C) IVC spectral Doppler ultrasound shows normal velocities within the stent. (D) Spectral Doppler ultrasound of a hepatic vein shows a flat monophasic waveform suggestive of IVC stenosis.

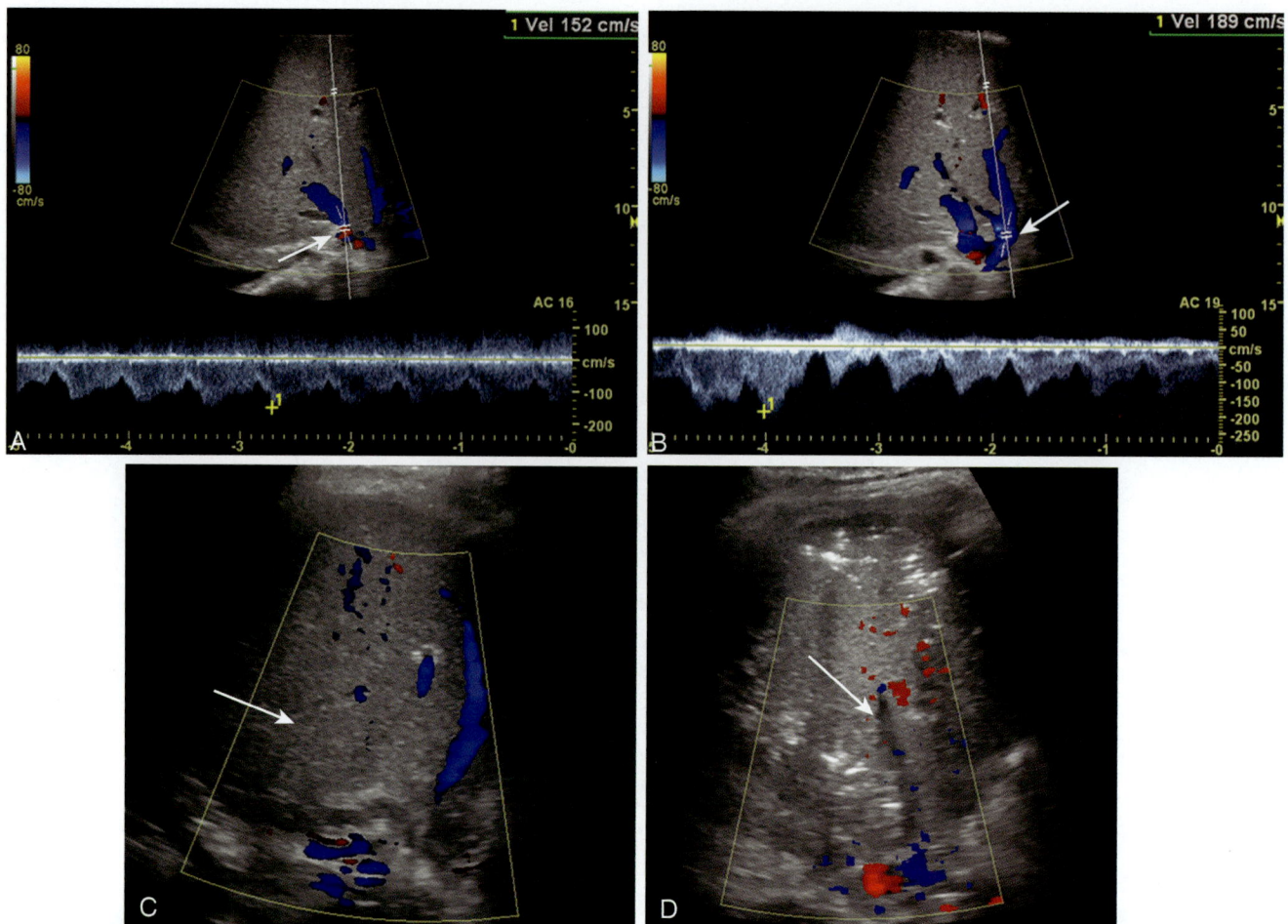

FIG. 20.11 Hepatic vein stenosis and thrombosis. (A–B) Spectral Doppler ultrasound of the right hepatic vein (RHV) and middle hepatic vein (MHV) shows turbulence with elevated velocities near the anastomosis sites. (C–D) Color Doppler ultrasound shows no flow within the RHV and MHV suggestive of complete thrombosis.

thrombus, some flow will be visualized around the thrombus. As a thrombus ages, it typically becomes more anechoic. In the symptomatic patient, thrombectomy, thrombolysis, stent placement, or a venous graft may be necessary[13] (Fig. 20.13). With chronic PV thrombosis, cavernous transformation can occur with the hepatic artery.

Hepatic Artery Stenosis. Hepatic artery stenosis occurs in 2% to 11% of liver transplant patients with a median time to diagnosis of 100 days. Risk factors include rejection, poor surgical technique, or clamp injury. The sonographer will notice color and spectral Doppler aliasing with turbulent flow. Pulsed-wave Doppler will demonstrate a low RI (less than 0.50) with a velocity greater than 200 cm/sec and a tardus parvus waveform. In the early postoperative period, less than 72 hours of transplantation, the RI can be elevated greater than 0.80, but usually will return to normal within a few days. The most common cause for this is postoperative edema. The increased hepatic artery resistance can be associated with an older donor age and an extended period of ischemic time. It is common to get an elevated false velocity measurement when the hepatic artery is tortuous. If the ultrasound examination is inconclusive, a CT angiography (CTA) or MR angiography (MRA) should be considered. Treatment may include balloon angioplasty with stent placement or surgical revision[14] (Fig. 20.14). If the stenosis is left untreated, it may lead to HA thrombosis, liver ischemia, biliary stricture, sepsis, and allograft loss. Early detection is critical to avoid the need for retransplantation.[13]

Hepatic Artery Thrombosis. The most common vascular complication of liver transplantation is HA thrombosis.[14] Thrombosis occurs in 4% to 12% of adults and 42% of children between postoperative days 15 and 132.[13,14] Risk factors include rejection, short warm ischemic time, end-to-end anastomosis, and pediatric transplantation. HA thrombosis and stenosis can lead to biliary ischemia because the HA is the only vascular supply to the biliary ducts. There will be absence of color and no flow on spectral Doppler imaging. On gray scale, echogenic thrombus filling the HA lumen may be visualized. When there is slow flow present due to low cardiac output or arterial spasm, ultrasound may not detect flow leading to a false-positive diagnosis when the hepatic artery is patent. If the ultrasound is inconclusive, a CTA may ultimately be required. CT may demonstrate areas of infarction as well. Treatment includes an emergent thrombectomy, but many cases ultimately require retransplantation[14] (Fig. 20.15).

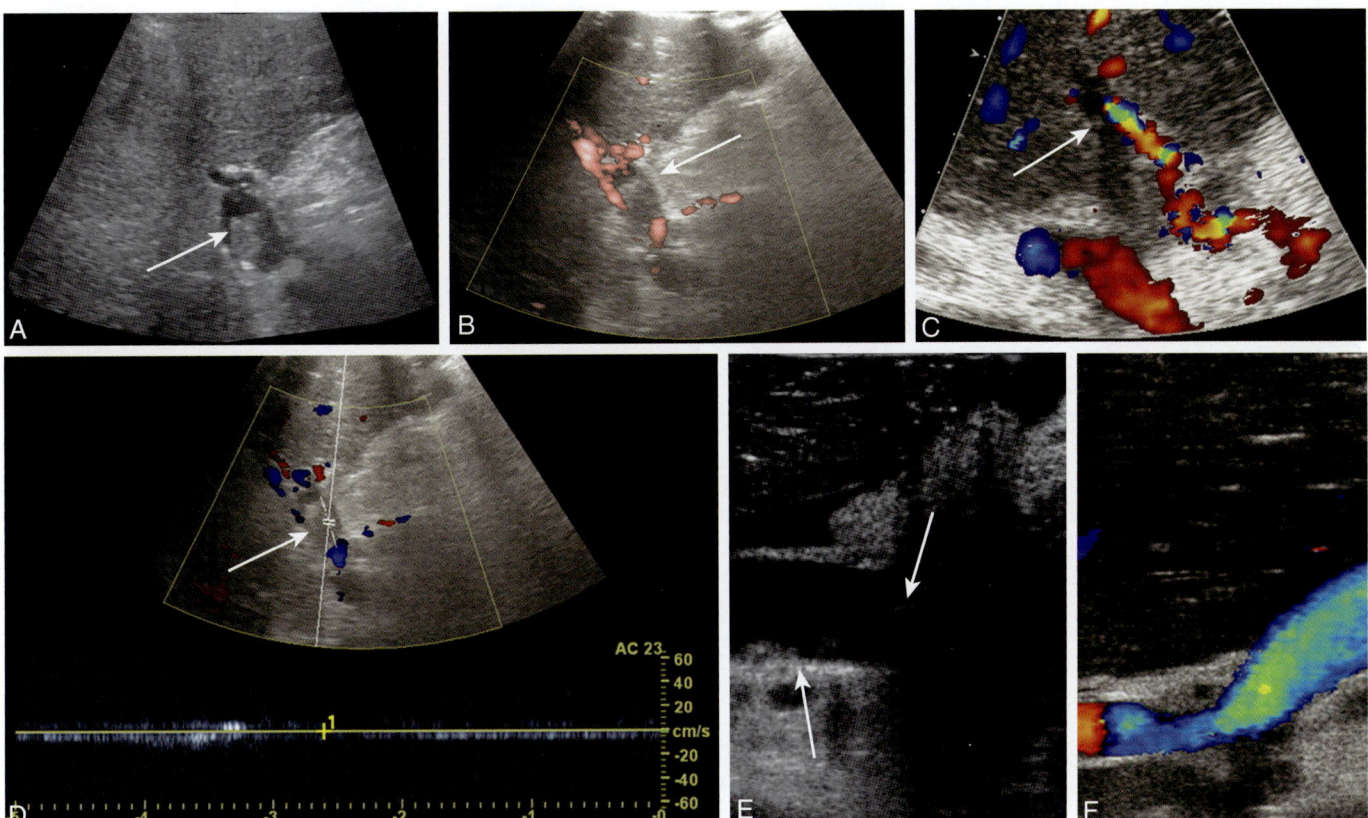

FIG. 20.12 **Immediate postoperative acute portal vein occlusive thrombus.** (A) Gray-scale ultrasound of main portal vein (MPV) shows acute thrombus within the vessel. (B) Power Doppler ultrasound shows no flow within the MPV. (C) MPV shows no flow on color Doppler ultrasound. (D) Spectral Doppler ultrasound shows no flow within the MPV. (E) Intraoperative MPV gray-scale ultrasound shows a small amount of residual thrombus following a thrombectomy. (F) Intraoperative color Doppler ultrasound shows the MPV widely patent following a thrombectomy.

Infarction and Necrosis. In a native liver, it is rare for an infarction to take place. If the HA were to occlude, collateral vessels would take over to give collateral flow to the liver. Within a transplant, development of collateral vessels is not usually possible as most of the collateral vessels are ligated during the surgical process. In 85% of cases, hepatic infarction is associated with HA complications with portal vein occlusion being less likely. Ischemic areas within the liver can liquefy over time and may become infected and calcifications may be present.[13] Infarction usually appears hypoechoic and wedge shaped located along the periphery. Infarcts can be difficult to distinguish from focal abscesses and an aspiration or biopsy may be needed for confirmation (Fig. 20.16).

Hepatic Artery Pseudoaneurysms. Hepatic artery pseudoaneurysms are relatively uncommon and usually located at the anastomosis site or occur due to angioplasty complications. These may also be intrahepatic secondary to a liver biopsy, biliary procedures, or infection. Patients are most often asymptomatic. If the pseudoaneurysm ruptures, however, the patient may go into acute shock and a portal or biliary fistula can develop. Treatments for extrahepatic pseudoaneurysms include resection, coil embolization, or stent placement. The treatment option of choice for an intrahepatic pseudoaneurysm is coil embolization. On ultrasound imaging, a pseudoaneurysm appears as an anechoic structure often containing nonocclusive thrombus along the walls, and located along the course of the HA. On Doppler imaging, it fills with color and there is a disorganized, bidirectional flow pattern. A characteristic "yin-yang" pattern of flow on Doppler imaging has been described.[13,14] Pseudoaneurysms can be visualized using CTA or MRA. These appear as round masses at the anastomotic site and enhance avidly during the arterial phase. If slow flow is present, enhancement may only be noted during the portal or delayed venous phases[15] (Fig. 20.17).

Biliary Complications. In about 5% to 15% of liver transplant patients, biliary complications occur. These typically occur within the first 3 months after transplantation.[14] Complications include biliary ductal obstruction, stenosis or stricture at the anastomosis, stone formation, biliary necrosis, sphincter of Oddi dysfunction, and recurrent biliary disease. Bile leaks and bilomas are also complications that are discussed later in this chapter. Biliary complications taken as a whole are the second most common cause of allograft dysfunction following rejection.[13]

Obstruction is the most common biliary complication usually caused from a stricture at the anastomosis but may also be secondary to choledocholithiasis.[13,14] The donor CBD will demonstrate postobstructive dilation in patients with choledocholithiasis. It is important to note that some patients may present with nonobstructive ductal dilation secondary

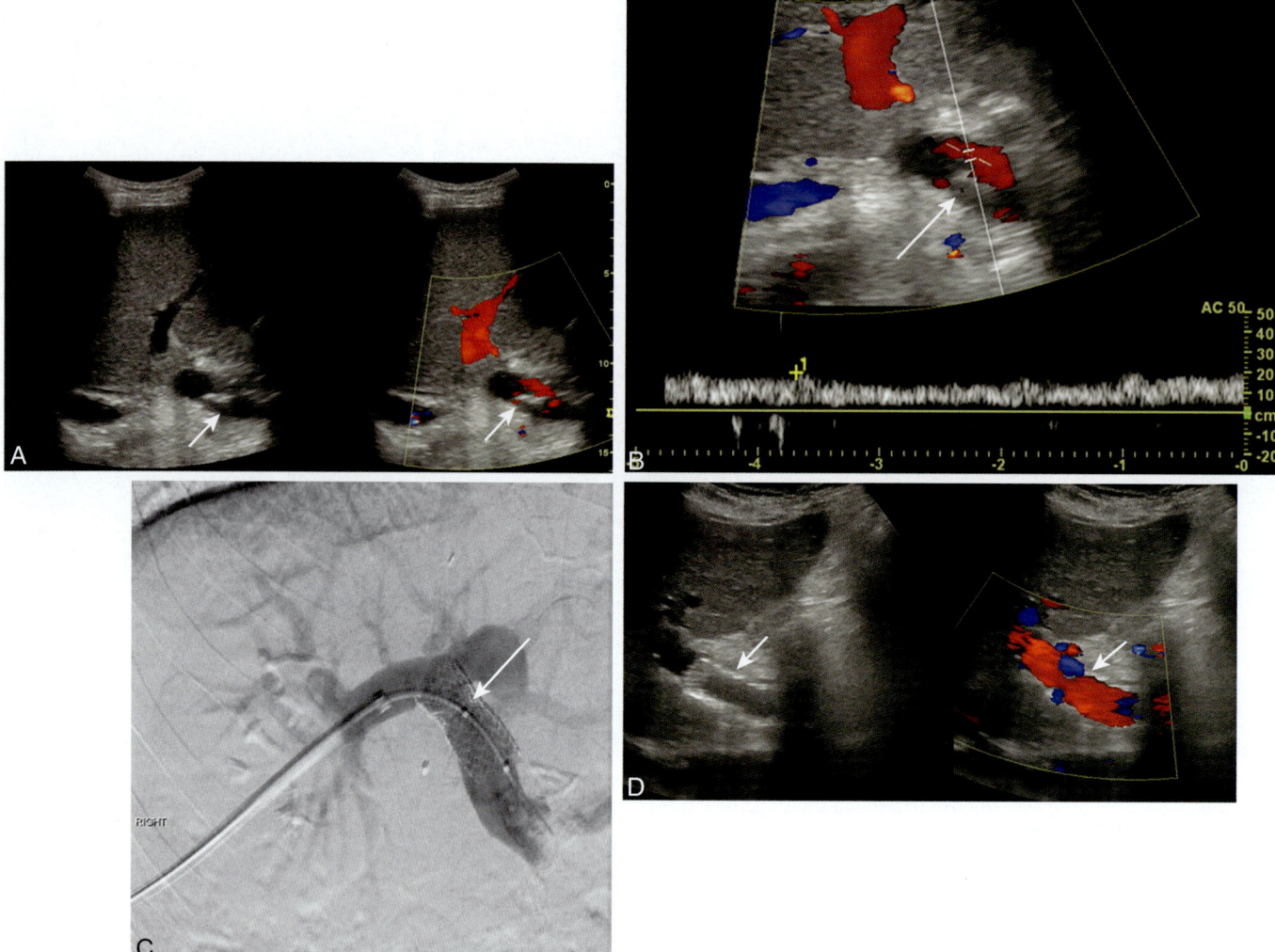

FIG. 20.13 Portal vein nonocclusive thrombus. (A) Gray-scale and color Doppler ultrasound show thrombus along the wall with some flow within main portal vein (MPV). (B) Spectral Doppler ultrasound of the MPV shows a patent segment flowing around the thrombus. (C) Interventional radiology stent placement within the MPV. (D) Gray-scale and color Doppler ultrasound show no signs of a filling defect within the stent.

to papillary dyskinesia and may be clinically insignificant. Imaging findings should be correlated with clinical findings and symptoms. Ultrasound is less reliable when mild ductal obstruction is present. As a result, MRI cholangiopancreatography is useful in detecting biliary obstruction. Most strictures are extrahepatic and near the anastomosis caused from fibrotic tissue scarring. These are usually treated with angioplasty with or without stent placement. As opposed to extrahepatic strictures, intrahepatic strictures are due to ischemia or cholangitis and treatment includes percutaneous biliary drain placement (Fig. 20.18). Stones, sludge, and debris can be found in 5.7% of liver transplants. Altering the bile composition could be a predisposing factor for stone and sludge formation. Choledocholithiasis is usually treated with an endoscopic sphincterotomy and stone retrieval[14] (Figs. 20.19 and 20.20). Biliary ductal ischemia is secondary to HA thrombosis or stenosis as the ducts are dependent on the HA for their only blood supply. Biliary necrosis occurs and biliary stenosis, bile leaks, and bilomas may follow. If angioplasty of the stenotic duct is not successful, retransplantation is often necessary.[13]

Fluid Collections

Bleeding and Hematomas. Hematomas are collections of blood and usually occur within the first 2 weeks postoperatively, and most are present and can be visualized on day 0 ultrasound examination. Hematomas are most common along the perihepatic spaces and near the vascular and biliary anastomoses sites. Most hematomas will resolve spontaneously with no intervention needed. At rare times, there may be an underlying infection within a hematoma and a percutaneous drainage catheter may need to be placed.[13,14] Hematomas can have variable appearances as they age. They typically have irregular walls, are ovoid in shape, and decrease in size over time. Fresh hematomas have more internal echoes and can appear echogenic. As they age, they liquefy and become more anechoic and may contain septations[15] (Fig. 20.21).

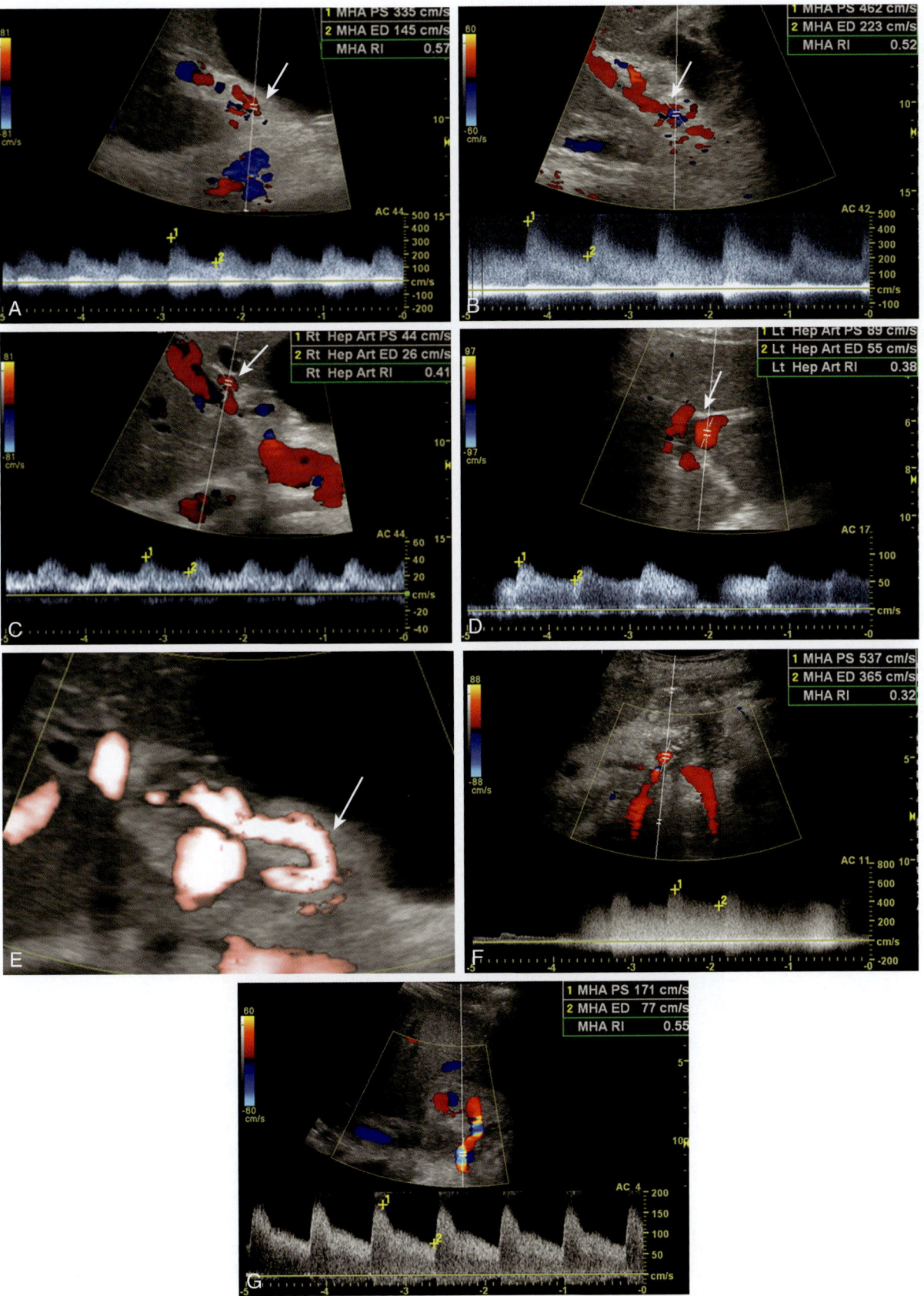

FIG. 20.14 **Hepatic artery stenosis.** (A–B) Spectral Doppler ultrasound of the main hepatic artery (MHA) shows turbulence and elevated velocities. (C–D) Spectral Doppler ultrasound of the right hepatic artery and left hepatic artery shows a low resistive index (RI) concerning for a proximal stenosis. (E) Power Doppler ultrasound of the MHA shows tortuosity in which elevated velocities may be present. (F) Spectral Doppler ultrasound of a severe MHA stenosis at 537 cm/sec. (G) Spectral Doppler ultrasound following a hepatic artery anastomosis reconstruction shows improvement.

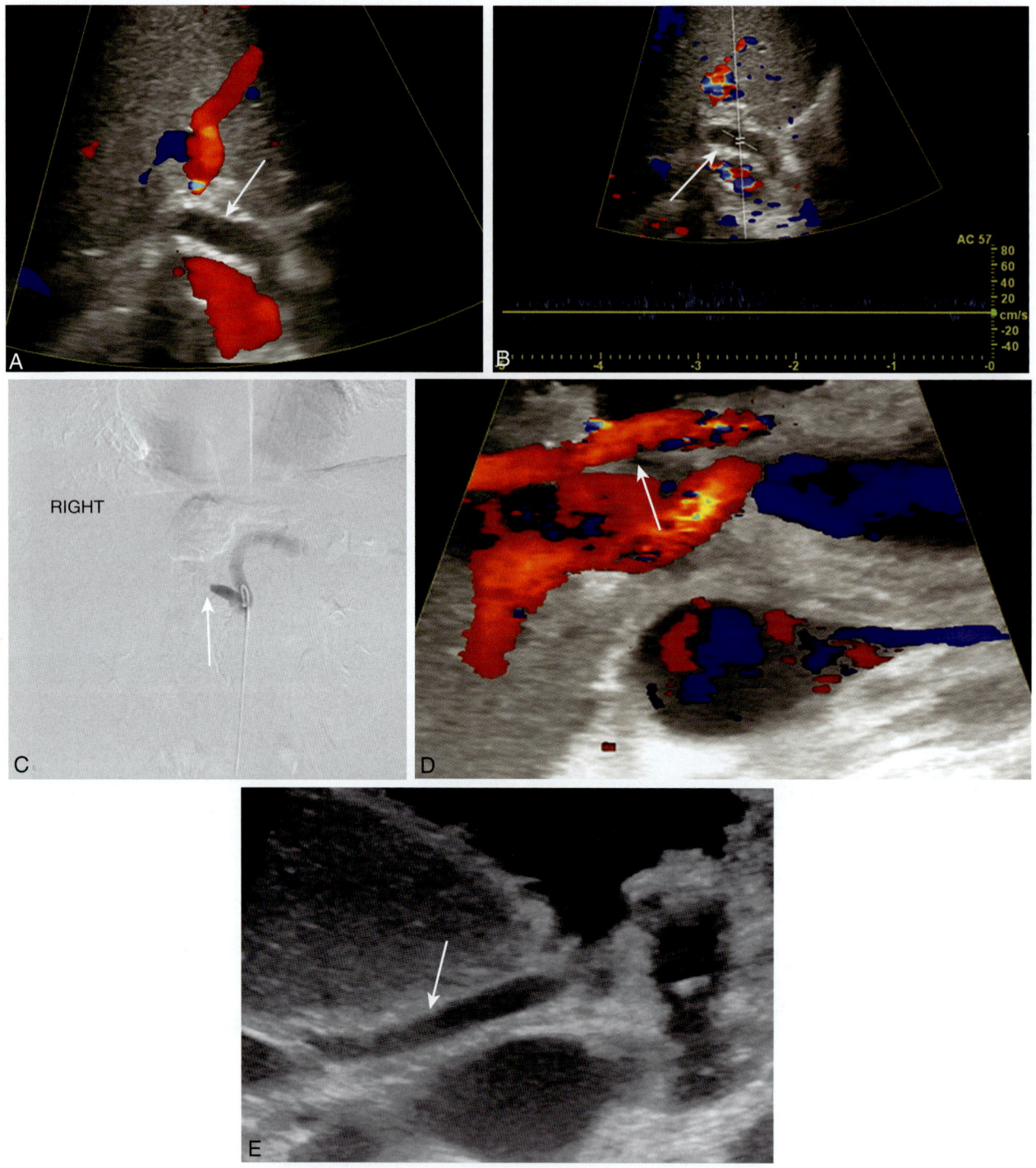

FIG. 20.15 **Acute hepatic artery thrombosis.** (A) Color Doppler ultrasound of the main hepatic artery (MHA) shows no flow within the vessel. (B) Spectral Doppler ultrasound of the MHA shows no flow within the vessel. (C) Interventional angiogram shows no flow within the MHA. (D–E) Intraoperative color Doppler and longitudinal gray-scale ultrasound shows no sign of thrombus and is widely patent following a thrombectomy.

Seromas. Seromas are clear, serous fluid collections that are usually found within the first few days after transplantation. They are most common along the perihepatic spaces and near the vascular and biliary anastomoses sites. Most seromas will resolve spontaneously within a few weeks. On ultrasound, a seroma is a round, localized, anechoic, thin-walled fluid collection, which may contain debris or septations. Ultrasound is very sensitive to diagnose a fluid collection but not specific of contents. Unfortunately, blood, pus, lymph, bile, and serosanguineous fluid can have similar appearances on ultrasound, and ultimately CT or MRI is helpful in differentiating the collections. If there is concern the fluid collection is infected or creating mass effect on the vasculature, an aspiration may be performed[13] (Fig. 20.22).

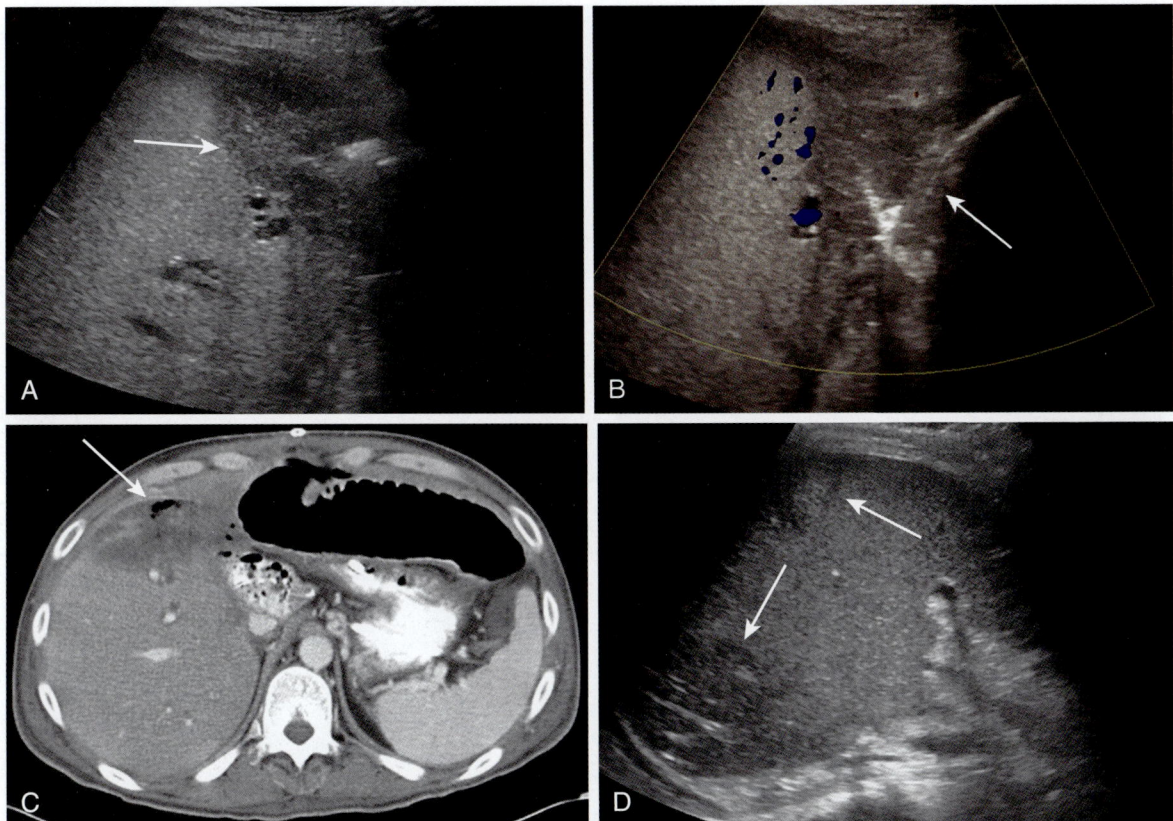

FIG. 20.16 **Hepatic infarction caused from previous hepatic artery thrombosis.** (A) Gray-scale ultrasound shows a hypoechoic wedge-shaped area along the periphery. (B) Color Doppler ultrasound shows no flow within the infarcted segment. (C) Computed tomography shows the peripheral infarction with a small amount of gas. (D) Transverse gray-scale ultrasound of other infarcted areas within the liver.

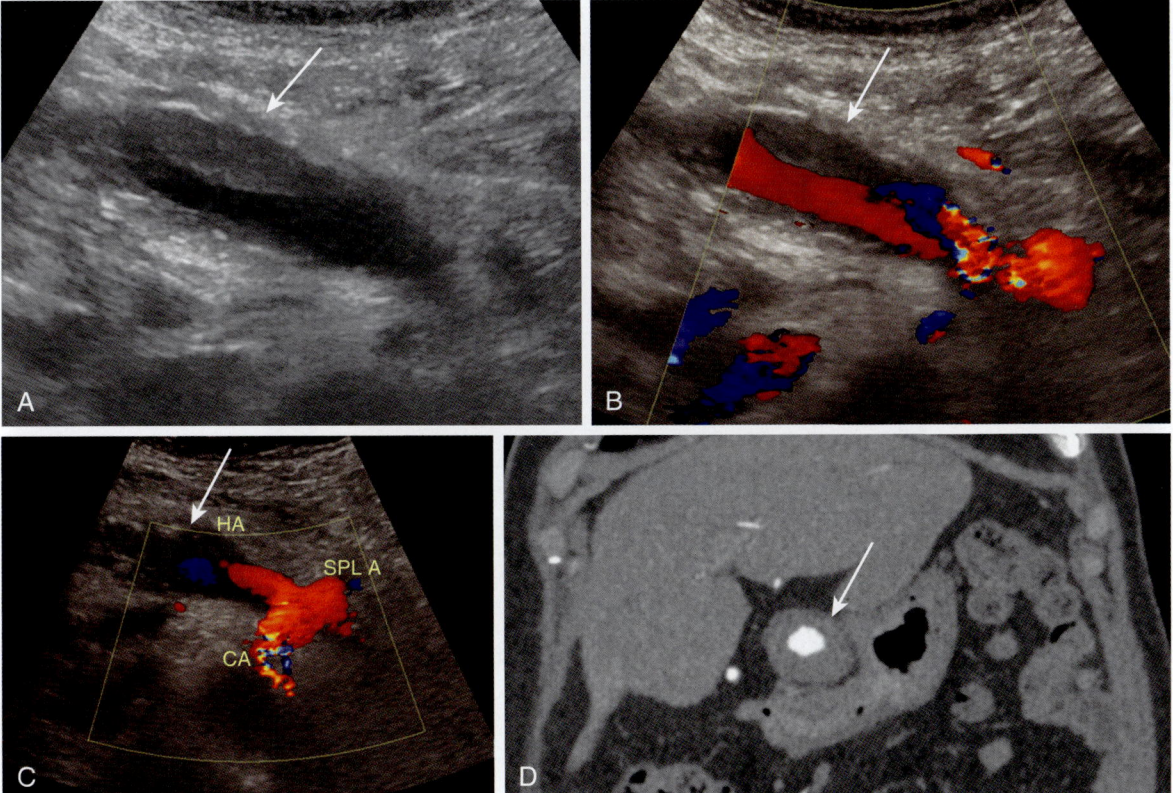

FIG. 20.17 **Hepatic artery pseudoaneurysm.** (A) Longitudinal gray-scale ultrasound of a pseudoaneurysm measured at 3 cm. (B) Color Doppler ultrasound shows thrombus along the arterial wall. (C) Color Doppler ultrasound shows the relation between the splenic artery and celiac artery. (D) Computed tomography shows a cross-sectional image of the main hepatic artery pseudoaneurysm with thrombus lining the arterial wall.

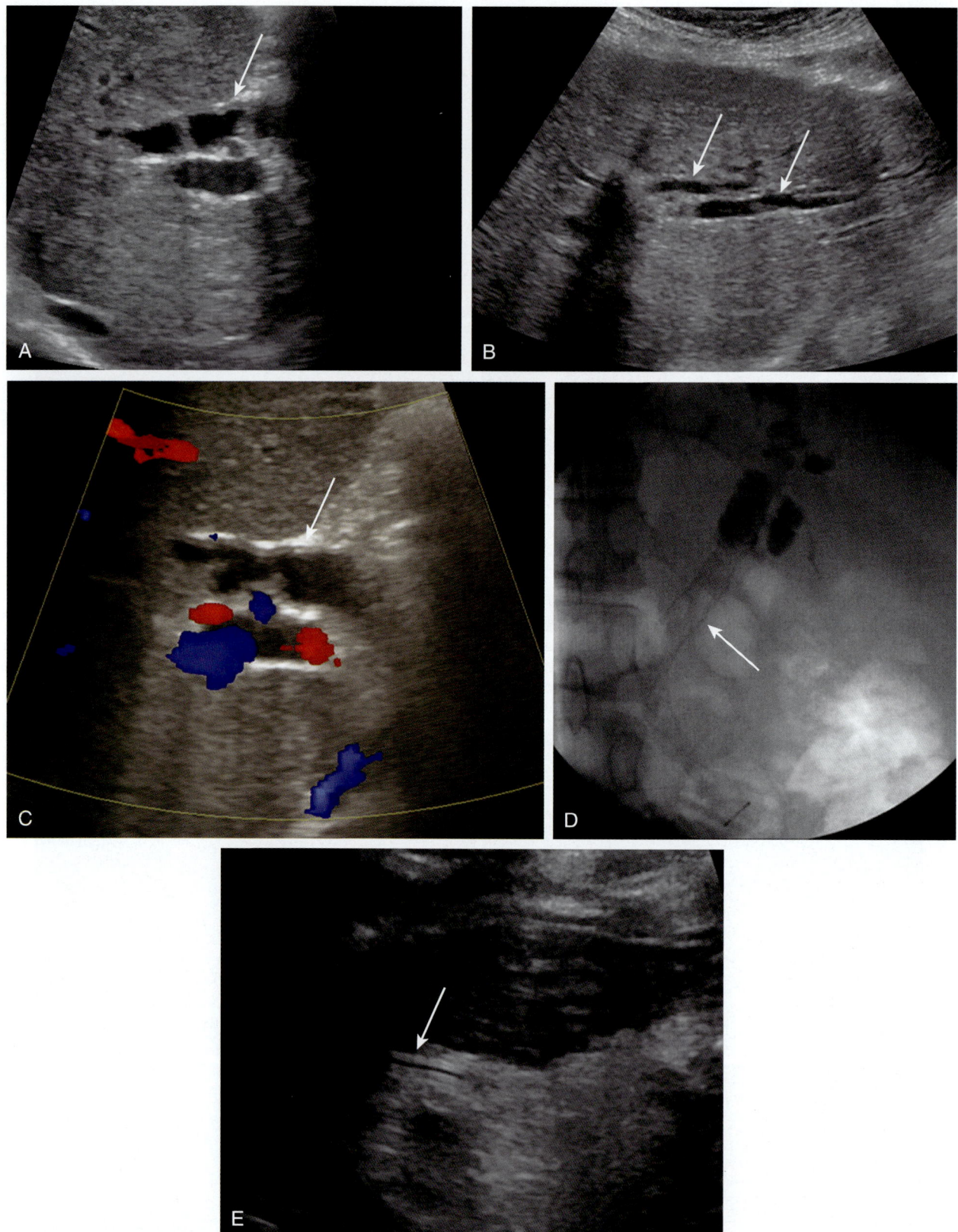

FIG. 20.18 Chronic cholangiopathy. (A–B) Gray-scale ultrasound of dilated ducts shows thickened walls and debris. (C) Color Doppler ultrasound shows no flow. (D) Endoscopic retrograde cholangiopancreatography shows changes of cholangitis and the stricture was balloon dilated and stent placement followed. (E) Longitudinal gray-scale ultrasound of a biliary stent.

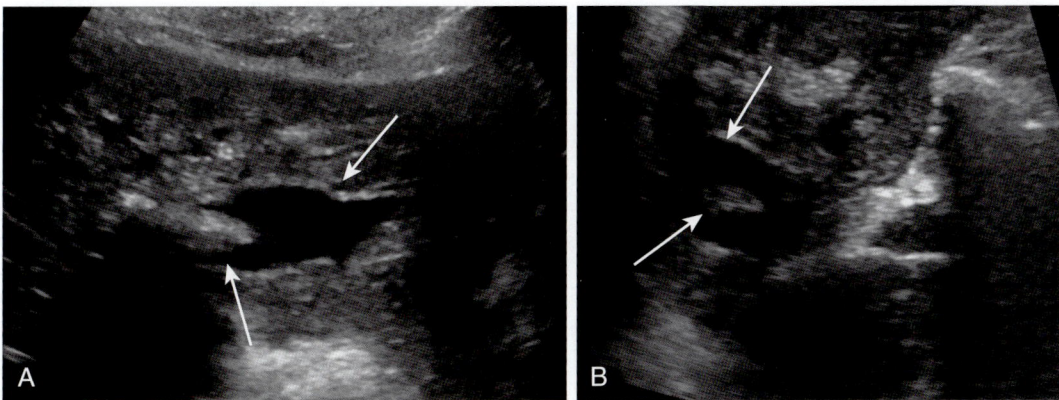

FIG. 20.19 **Intrahepatic ductal dilation with stones.** (A) Transverse gray-scale ultrasound shows shadowing from the stones. (B) Longitudinal gray-scale ultrasound.

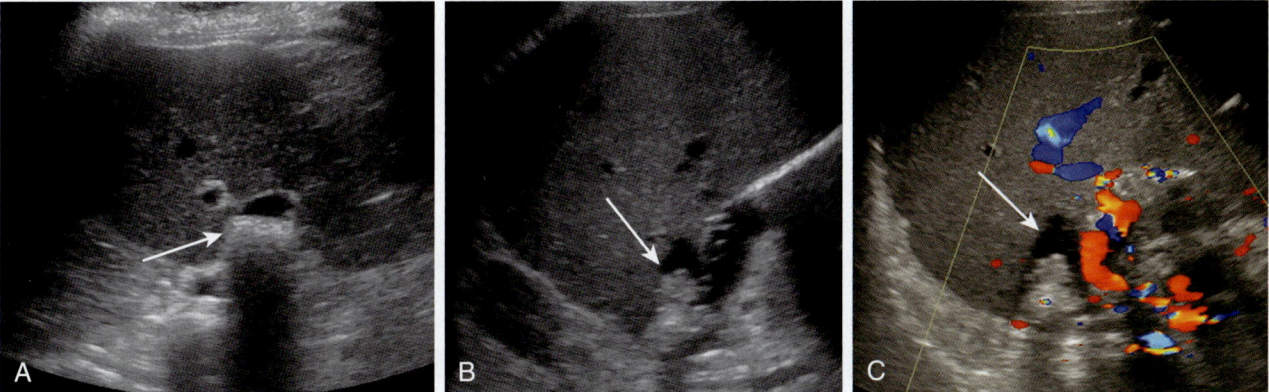

FIG. 20.20 **Cystic duct remnant with stones and debris.** (A) Transverse gray-scale ultrasound shows shadowing from the stones. (B) Longitudinal gray-scale ultrasound. (C) Color Doppler ultrasound shows "twinkle" artifact from stones.

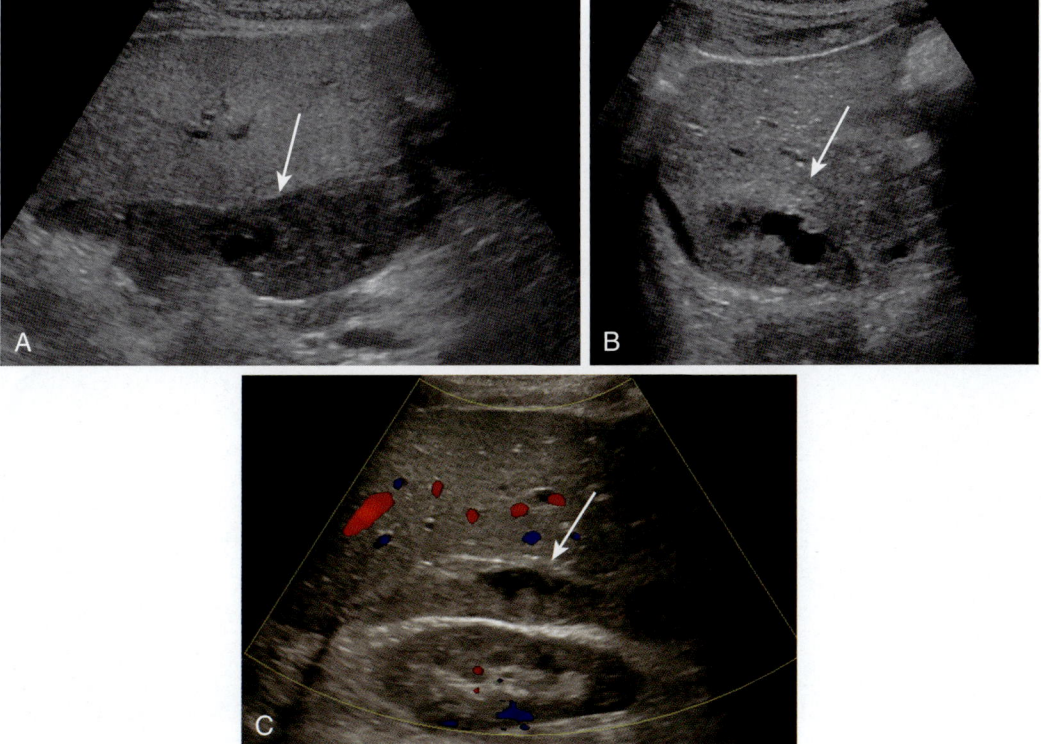

FIG. 20.21 **Postoperative hematoma.** (A) Longitudinal gray-scale ultrasound shows hypoechoic internal echoes consistent with a resolving hematoma. (B) Transverse gray-scale ultrasound shows some liquefying components. (C) Recurrent fresh echogenic hematoma following evacuation; color Doppler ultrasound shows no active bleed.

Lymphoceles. A surgical disruption of lymphatic channels causes lymph fluid leakage into the soft tissue space creating a lymphocele. These are typically found in the groin or retroperitoneal space. On ultrasound imaging, debris or septations within the fluid collection may be seen. Ultrasound is very sensitive to diagnose a fluid collection, although the contents are difficult to distinguish. CT or MRI is very helpful in differentiating among lymph, blood, bile, pus, or serosanguineous fluid.[13] The most common complication of venovenous bypass during liver transplantation is a lymphocele, which can be seen between 10% and 30%. Spontaneous resolution is rare. Treatment includes percutaneous drain placement used in conjunction with sclerotherapy. Surgical repair is the optimal choice of treatment. Methylene blue dye injected through the lymphatic system makes it possible to identify the leak source during an open repair. This complication fortunately is now only rarely seen, as the venovenous bypass is no longer routinely used for liver transplantation surgery.[16]

Bile Leak and Bilomas. Bile leaks occur in about 5% of liver transplant patients. These typically present in the early postoperative period with more than 70% within the first month of transplantation. Leaks are most often located at the biliary tube site with rare occurrences at the anastomotic site. Bile seeps into the peritoneal cavity and may form a contained perihepatic collection, or biloma. Treatment includes stent placement over the biliary leak and possibly placement of a percutaneous drainage catheter.[13] On ultrasound imaging, a biloma is a discrete, round, hypoechoic or anechoic fluid collection demonstrating no vascular flow. Ultrasound may have a difficult time differentiating biliary leaks from other fluid collections such as hematomas, abscesses, seromas, or ascites. Cholangiography and cholescintigraphy are sensitive and specific modalities that are helpful in biliary leakage evaluation[14] (Fig. 20.23).

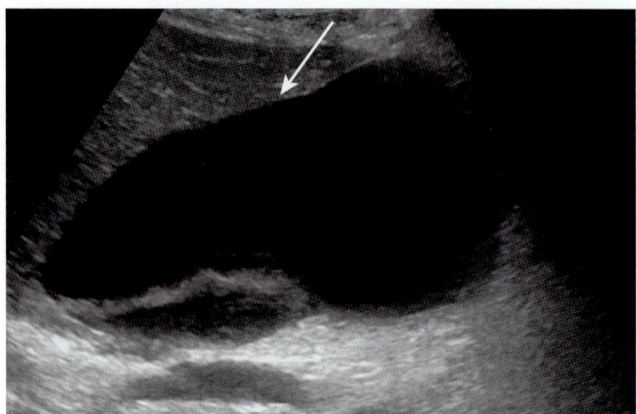

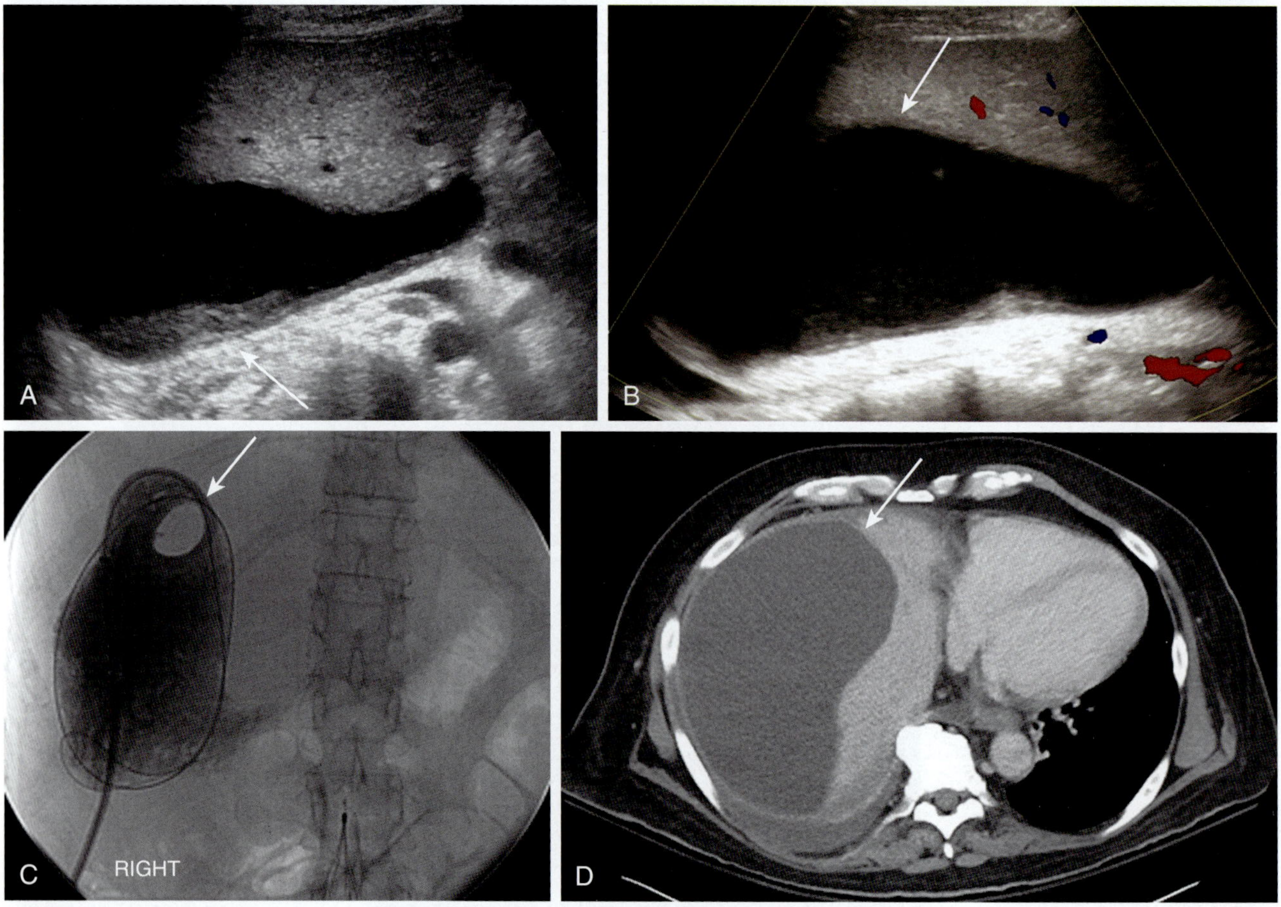

FIG. 20.22 **Seroma**. Longitudinal gray-scale ultrasound shows a simple fluid collection.

FIG. 20.23 **Biloma**. (A) Longitudinal gray-scale ultrasound shows a fluid collection with debris and posterior acoustic enhancement. (B) Color Doppler ultrasound shows no flow within the collection. (C) Interventional radiology sinogram shows a drain within the infected biloma. (D) Computed tomography shows a large biloma caused by a biopsy complication.

Free Fluid. Ascites is usually present in small amounts in the early postoperative period. It may contain debris or blood products. The ascites commonly resolves in 7 to 10 days following transplantation. If the patient is having pain and remains uncomfortable with a large amount of free fluid, a therapeutic paracentesis can be performed[15] (Fig. 20.24).

Hepatocellular Carcinoma and Metastatic Disease. Patients who initially present with small HCC lesions with no extrahepatic involvement typically have a reasonable long-term survival following liver transplantation. Recurrence of HCC is seen in about 40% of patients after their transplant, however. This may occur when chronic cirrhosis is present or microscopic extrahepatic lesions are not identified at the time of transplantation. This may create distant metastasis in other organs.[17] The most common site of HCC recurrence is the lung followed by the liver.[13]

Ultrasound can be quite sensitive for detecting HCC, but the experience and skill of the sonographer are critical for localizing these smaller tumors. Their appearance is typically hypoechoic with variability in size. Some tumors may appear hyperechoic and can be misdiagnosed as a benign hemangioma. Ultrasound imaging is useful in evaluating presence of flow and detecting vascular invasion. A dedicated contrast CT or MRI is helpful in identifying a benign versus a malignant process (Fig. 20.25).

The most common malignancies after liver transplantation are skin cancer (excluding melanoma), Kaposi sarcoma, and non-Hodgkin lymphoma. Long-term immunosuppression, a previous viral infection, chronic use of alcohol before transplantation, and acute rejection are risk factors contributing to malignant disease. Lymphoma may be seen intrahepatic or extrahepatic demonstrating a hypoechoic soft tissue mass or multiple liver lesions. The mass may encase the hilum affecting the vasculature or biliary tree.[13] Other metastasis from a different primary source may also be visualized (Fig. 20.26).

Hepatitis Recurrence. Hepatitis C virus (HCV) reinfection occurs in nearly all patients who receive a liver transplant for HCV cirrhosis.[15] An infected liver will have a heterogeneous

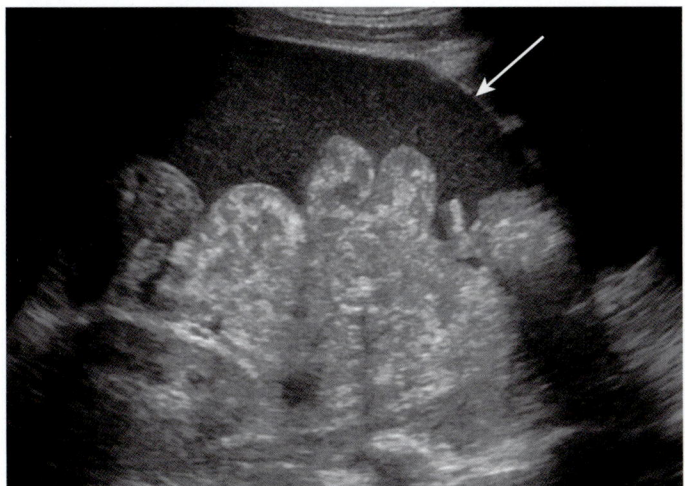

FIG. 20.24 Debris-filled ascites due to hemorrhage on gray-scale ultrasound.

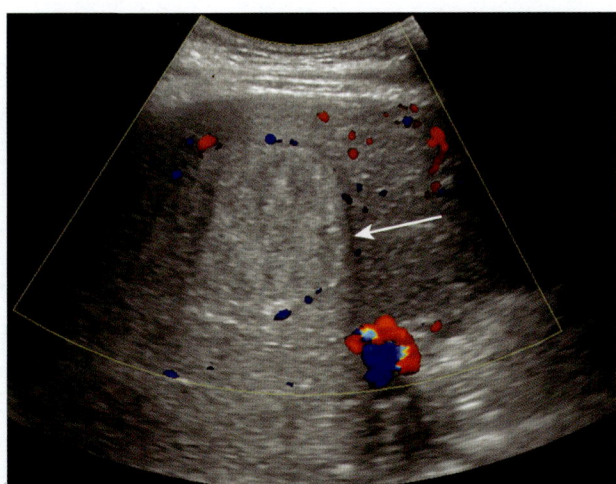

FIG. 20.25 Primary hepatocellular carcinoma in recurrent hepatitis C. Color Doppler ultrasound shows no flow within but along the periphery of the mass.

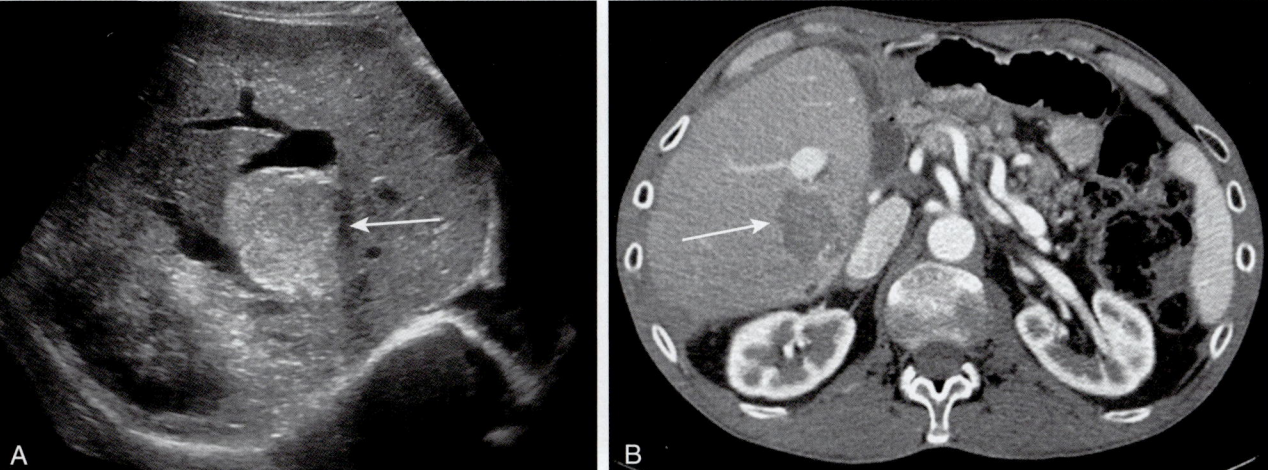

FIG. 20.26 **Islet cell metastasis.** (A) Transverse gray-scale ultrasound shows a hyperechoic mass within the right lobe of the liver. (B) Computed tomography shows a mass with irregular borders within the right lobe of the liver.

and coarsened echotexture on ultrasound imaging (Fig. 20.27). Risk factors for recurrence include donor age, immunosuppression, cytomegalovirus infection, metabolic syndrome, and IL28B genotype. Donor age over 40 years old has a significant impact on HCV infection and graft loss. Ideally, patients awaiting a liver transplant with HCV are placed on antiviral medication to eradicate the viral process before transplantation. Recurrence following transplant is immediate and universal in patients who are viremic at the time of surgery. Viral levels 1 year after surgery are 10 to 20 times greater than pretransplant. Recurrence is often associated with rapid fibrosis leading to higher mortality and allograft loss rates. About 20% of these patients will develop cirrhosis within 5 years of transplantation. Retransplantation remains controversial in these patients compared with other reasons for transplant loss such as primary nonfunction or hepatic arterial thrombosis.[18] Patients with coinfection of HIV and HCV are also debated in regard to receiving a liver transplant. The argument for transplantation in these patients is that HCV is more aggressive after liver transplantation in a patient with HIV and HCV, and is the major source of graft loss and death. In patients in whom HCV infection resolves, there is an 80% survival rate.[19]

Portal Venous Gas and Bowel Ischemia. Portal venous gas is a common finding on ultrasound during the early postoperative period following transplantation.[15,20] Beyond the early postoperative state, air visualized within the portal and mesenteric veins is associated with a poor prognosis. Some underlying causes of the portal venous gas are intestinal ischemia and necrosis (75% of patients), followed by ulcerative colitis (8%) and intraabdominal abscess (6%).[21] Bowel ischemia is an unfortunately common and dangerous condition, especially in the elderly. There is a high mortality rate of 75% to 90% of cases. Damage to the mucosal intestinal layer leads to overdistention of bowel loops and gas moves from the intestinal lumen to the mesenteric veins, through the portal veins, and into the liver parenchyma. Portal venous gas can be diagnosed on x-ray, CT, or ultrasound. Prompt treatment results in reducing the mortality rates. The prognosis is ultimately dependent on the underlying condition.[20] Using ultrasound, portal venous gas should be easily detectable on

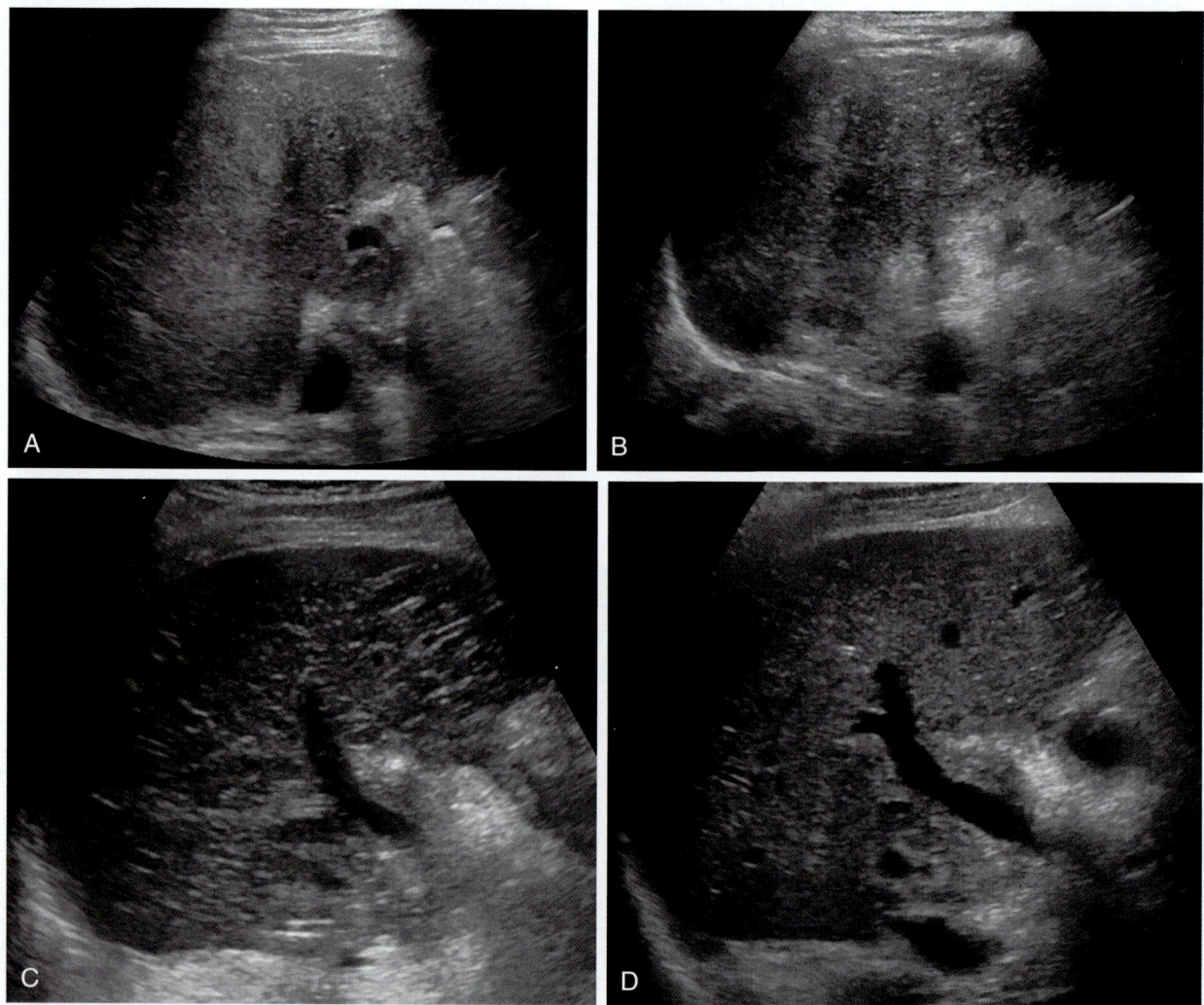

FIG. 20.27 **Hepatitis C recurrence.** (A) Longitudinal gray-scale ultrasound shows a coarsened liver parenchyma. (B) Transverse gray-scale ultrasound of a heterogeneous liver. (C) Immediate postoperative edema can have the appearance of chronic liver disease on gray-scale ultrasound. (D) Longitudinal gray-scale ultrasound of the liver parenchyma returns to a normal appearance 1 day later.

real-time imaging and should appear as echogenic foci flowing through the vein on gray scale. Clip stores can help aid in this diagnosis. On spectral Doppler, the turbulent flow can often be heard and sharp spikes can be seen on the venous waveform. In severe cases, echogenic foci can fill the entire liver parenchyma (Fig. 20.28).

Posttransplant Lymphoproliferative Disorder. Posttransplant lymphoproliferative disorder (PTLD) is one of the most severe complications found in solid organ as well as stem cell transplantation. PTLD occurs in 1% to 20% of patients who receive a transplant. In one study, PTLD was found to occur in 0.8% of liver transplant patients.[22] Chronic use of

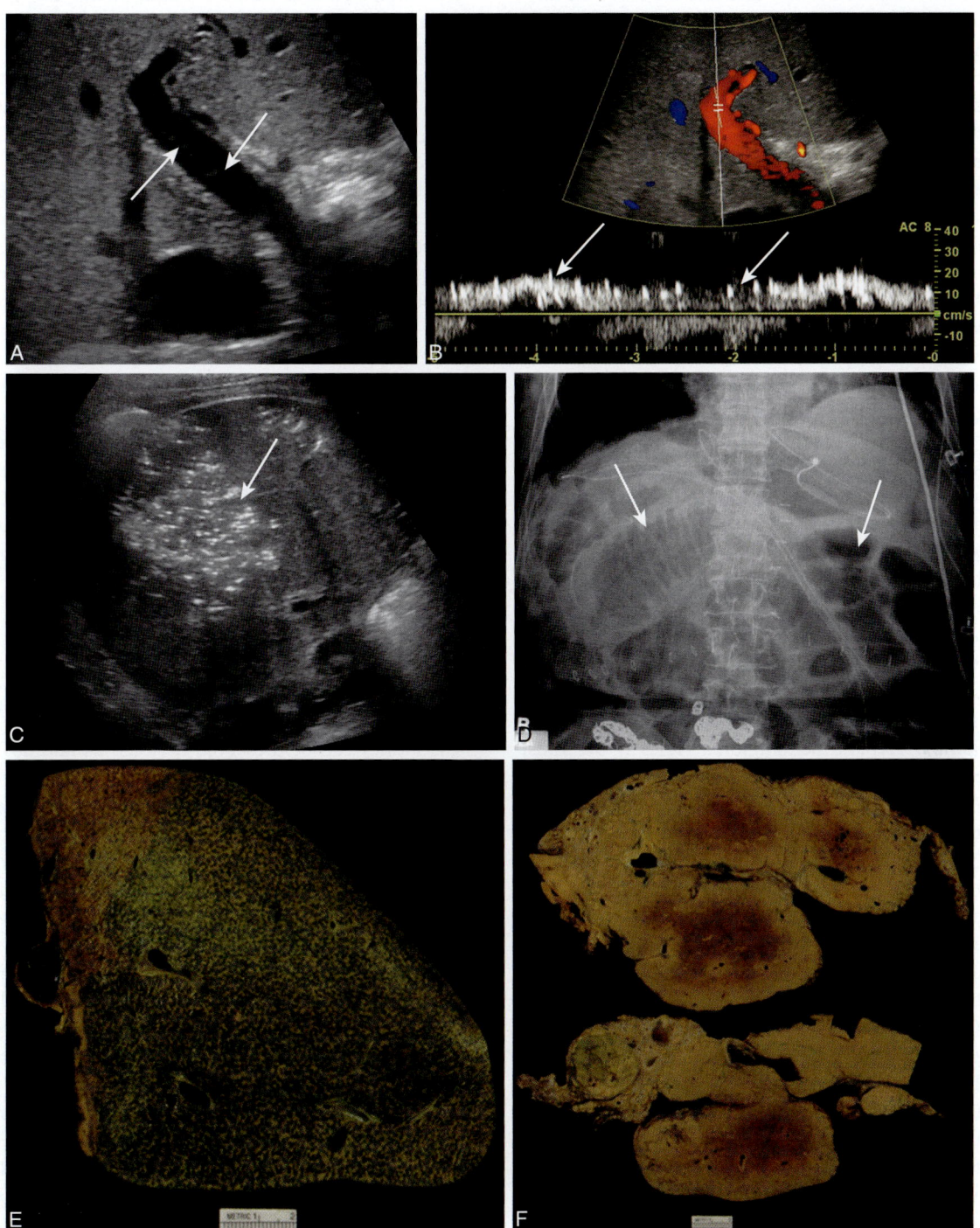

FIG. 20.28 Portal vein gas. (A) Longitudinal gray-scale ultrasound of the main portal vein (MPV) shows gas bubbles flowing within the vessel. (B) Spectral Doppler ultrasound of the MPV shows sharp spikes within the venous waveform. (C) Severe portal vein gas on gray-scale ultrasound shows echogenic foci throughout the liver parenchyma. (D) Radiograph of thickened and dilated loops of bowel is suggestive of bowel ischemia. (E–F) Pathology specimen of a necrotic liver.

immunosuppressant medication increases the risk of malignancies 2 to 5 times more than the general population. PTLD can range from benign reactive hyperplasia of tissue to malignant lymphoma. Most polymorphic masses are caused from the Epstein-Barr virus (EBV), occurring 60% to 80% and within 1 year of transplantation. Most of the monomorphic masses are found to be non-Hodgkin lymphoma and have a B-cell origin. Treatment for EBV-induced PTLD includes reducing the dosages of immunosuppressant drugs to allow the natural immune system to help fight the disorder. Dose reduction has been found to be effective in 23% to 50% of cases. In patients who do not respond to reduction of immunosuppression, immunotherapy with monoclonal antibodies such as rituximab may be given. Success using this treatment is seen in 40% to 68% of cases.[22] If left untreated, mortality with PTLD can be as high as 71%. The location of PTLD can be focal or diffuse and more commonly is extrahepatic. On ultrasound imaging, PTLD usually appears as a hypoechoic soft tissue mass and may encase the hepatic hilum.[15]

Common Benign Findings. Initially, the liver transplant is evaluated by the sonographer just as the native organ would be. Document any pathology visualized. The following are common findings that may be encountered within the liver and are not specific to transplantation.

Cysts. Simple hepatic cysts are benign liver lesions. They are common, occurring in 2% to 7% of the general population,[23,24] and can be diagnosed using CT, MRI, or ultrasound. Cysts can be focal or multiple, vary in size, and usually are found incidentally with most patients remaining asymptomatic. True cysts contain serous fluid with a thin wall.[23] On ultrasound evaluation, cysts appear round and anechoic with no color flow. The wall is thin with a well-defined border, and posterior acoustic enhancement can be visualized. Septations or debris may also be present.

Hemangiomas. Hepatic hemangioma (HH) is the most common benign liver tumor. It is hypervascular and supplied from the HA. Most are found incidentally and asymptomatic. HH can range from a few millimeters up to 40 cm, do not increase in size, and are found 0.4% to 20% within the general population. Symptoms are most common with large HH. Less than half of patients presenting with HH have significant symptoms, which include right upper quadrant pain, nausea, vomiting, loss of appetite, or fullness. HH can be diagnosed using ultrasound, CT, MRI, angiography, or nuclear medicine scans. On ultrasound, HH is a well-defined hyperechoic lesion demonstrating posterior acoustic enhancement with little or no Doppler flow. In patients with a hyperechoic fatty liver, HH may appear hypoechoic and can mimic a metastasis. Not all hyperechoic lesions are benign HH. Some of these lesions may represent hepatic metastasis or HCC and correlation with clinical history and other imaging modalities may be necessary. Typically there is no treatment necessary. Surgical resection of HH, RFA, or arterial embolization can be performed in rare circumstances when the clinical situation dictates.[25]

Pneumobilia. Pneumobilia is air within the biliary tree and suggests an abnormal connection of the intestinal tract with the biliary system or, less likely, infection from gas-forming bacteria. It is important to distinguish this relatively benign finding from the more ominous finding of portal venous gas. The most common causes of pneumobilia are recent biliary procedures such as an endoscopic retrograde cholangiopancreatography (ERCP), incompetent sphincter of Oddi, biliary-enteric surgical anastomosis, or a spontaneous biliary-enteric fistula.[26] Pneumobilia can be diagnosed on radiography, CT, or ultrasound. Ultrasound is sensitive in detection, and echogenic foci movement within the biliary tree on real-time imaging on gray scale can be seen. These foci can produce a shadowing or reverberation artifact (Fig. 20.29).

Fatty Liver and Focal Sparing. Fatty liver is a common condition affecting 20% to 30% of adults and 70% in diabetic patients. If left untreated, a fatty liver can lead to long-term illness and cirrhosis. Liver steatosis can be diffuse, focal, geographic, subcapsular, multifocal, or perivascular. Diagnosis can be made on CT, MRI, or ultrasound. Ultrasound is the first choice of imaging in chronic liver disease. Diffuse fatty liver is the most prevalent form involving the entire liver accumulated with fat. On ultrasound, the liver is hyperechoic or echogenic compared with the right kidney. It can be difficult to penetrate and a lower-frequency transducer is recommended. Focal fatty sparing is the geographic absence of fat within an otherwise diffusely fatty liver. This has a hypoechoic appearance and can mimic a mass. It tends to have a wedge-shaped margin with no mass effect on the vasculature or biliary tree.[27]

RENAL TRANSPLANT

Surgical Technique of the Renal Transplant

The kidney can be preserved between 24 and 36 hours on ice and using a special preservation solution. The shorter the ischemic time, the better the allograft function. For every transplant, the donor and recipient are rechecked to verify a match. The blood type and compatibility need to be confirmed as well as the UNOS database per protocol. Before coming into the operating room, the team will discuss the risks, benefits, and alternatives with the patient and obtain consent. All institutions have defined and specific protocols and techniques they follow. Every patient is unique, however, and individual surgeons will have different techniques they prefer.

Cadaveric Renal Donation. The 5-year survival rate for cadaveric transplantation from 1991 to 1995 was found to be 60%.[28] The patient is brought into the operating room confirming patient identification and procedure to be performed. Following general anesthesia and line placement, a Foley catheter is placed into the bladder. The abdomen is prepped and draped sterilely. The kidney back bench preparation includes removal of excess perinephric fat, the renal artery and vein are freed from surrounding structures, the ureter is dissected, and the tributary vessels are ligated. The kidney is flushed with HTK solution, packed, and placed on ice until transplantation is ready to occur. A nephrectomy is not routinely performed

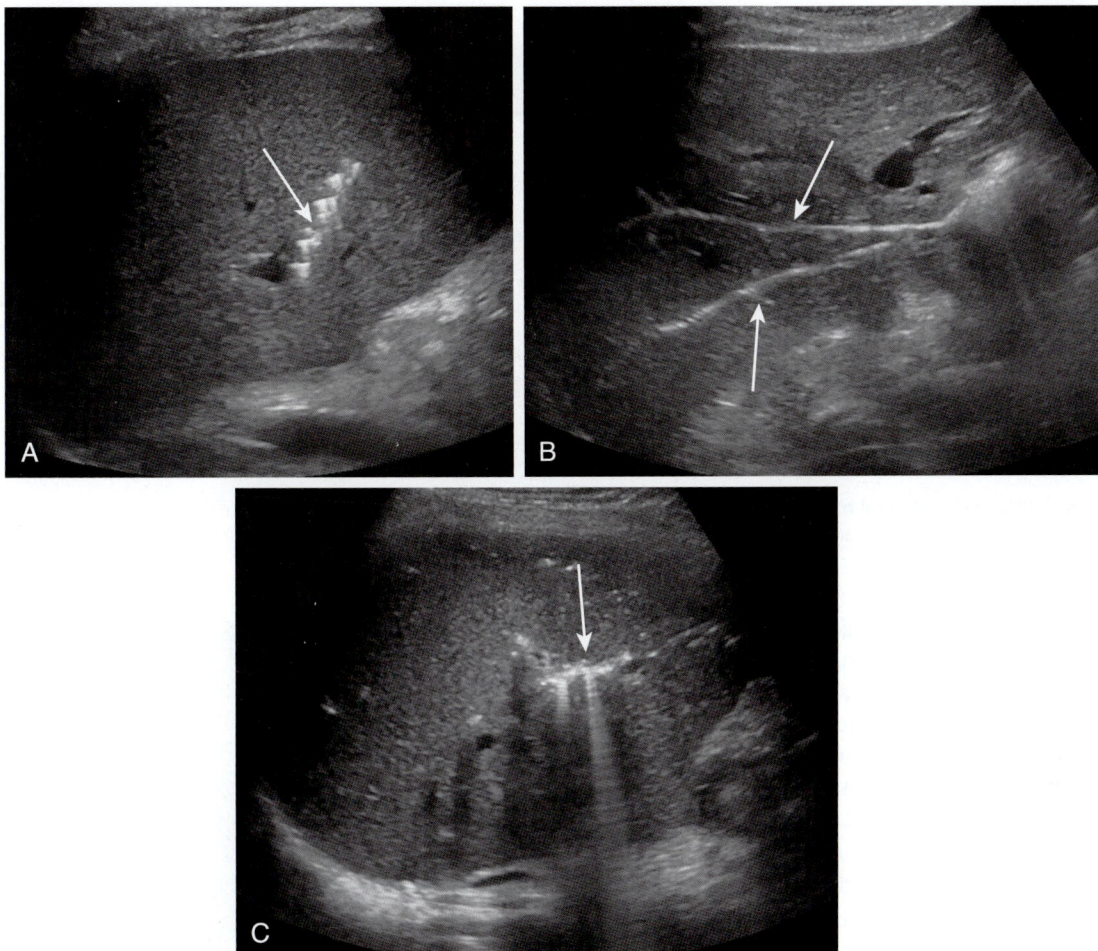

FIG. 20.29 **Pneumobilia.** (A) Longitudinal gray-scale ultrasound shows echogenic foci within the biliary tree. (B) Transverse gray-scale ultrasound shows the echogenic air within the biliary tree of the right hepatic lobe. (C) Transverse gray-scale ultrasound shows the reverberation artifact.

and native kidneys remain in the retroperitoneum. Commonly, the renal transplant will be placed into the right iliac fossa. If combined renal and pancreas transplants are to be performed, the incision will be midline from about 5 cm above the umbilicus down to the pubis. The kidney typically will be placed in the left iliac fossa and the pancreas will be placed in the right iliac fossa. If the patient has a previous renal transplant, the surgeon will typically choose the opposite side for placement if there are no vascular contraindications.

A lower quadrant incision is made, and a retractor is placed. Colon is mobilized exposing the external iliac artery and vein. The vein and artery are clamped, and the renal vein is anastomosed end-to-side to the external iliac vein with a suture. Similarly, an end-to-side anastomosis is performed between the renal artery and external iliac artery using running sutures. Clamps are removed and the kidney is reperfused. The surgeon carefully looks for any bleeding points. After obtaining hemostasis, the ureter is spatulated and anastomosed to the anterior bladder wall using a running suture. This is done over a double-J stent, which is secured to the tip of the Foley catheter (Fig. 20.30). A drain may be placed before closure and secured to the skin with sutures. The abdomen is closed in two layers. Sponge, needle, and instrument counts are conducted before closure. If indicated, the patient will receive units of blood, platelets, or fresh frozen plasma. The wound is dressed with a dry sterile dressing and the patient is extubated and transferred to the recovery room and later moved into the ICU when stable.

Living Donor Renal Donation. The 5-year survival rate of living donor transplantation from 1991 to 1995 was found to be 75%.[28] Living donation provides better allograft survival compared with the deceased donation, especially in patients who have not begun dialysis yet. In 2004 living kidney donation celebrated 50 years using a kidney from an identical twin. Living donation has become the predominant form of renal transplantation with the annual number of living donors surpassing the number of deceased donors in 2001.[29]

The surgical technique and back bench table preparation are nearly exact compared with a cadaveric kidney. The allograft may demonstrate better function more quickly due to the decreased preservation time in a living donor. With the shortage of organs available for donation, living donor organ donation offers the alternative for those waiting for a transplant and also increases the existing organ supply. A friend or family member may consider being a donor for their loved one. If the donor is not a match, there is a paired exchange

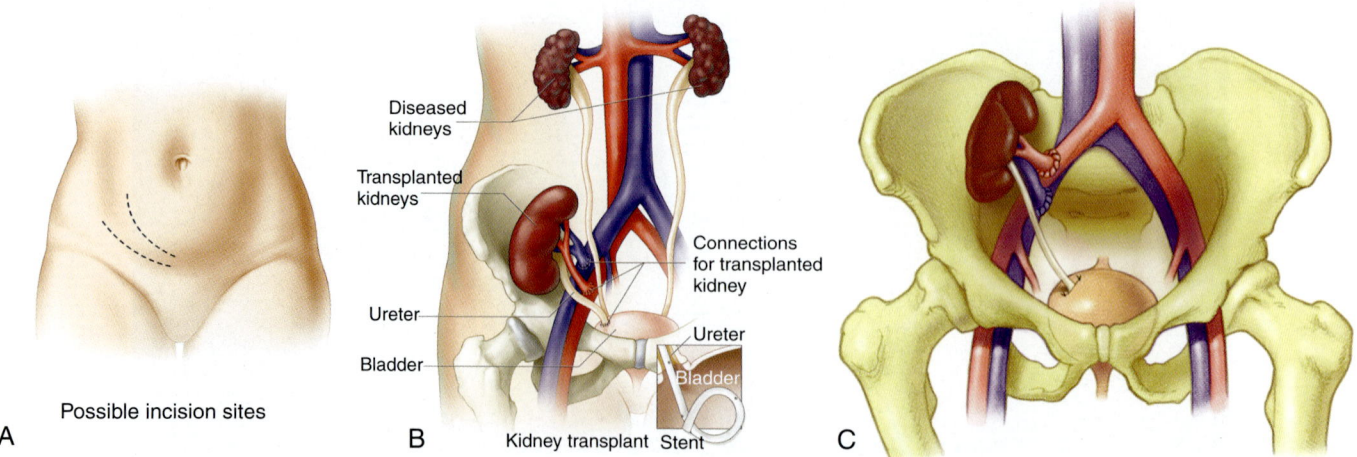

FIG. 20.30 **Surgical technique of renal transplantation.** (A) Possible incision sites. (B) Renal transplant in relation to the diseased native kidneys showing anastomotic sites. (C) Right lower quadrant renal transplant shows the anastomoses. (Courtesy Mayo Foundation for Medical Education and Research.)

program. The donor's organ would go to someone else for a better match rather than directly going to their friend or family member. The one needing the transplant will receive their organ in the exchange for one that meets their need.

Autotransplantation. Renal autotransplantation was first performed in 1963 by James Hardy to repair a high ureteral injury during an aortic surgery. The patient's own kidney is removed from the retroperitoneum and reimplanted into the iliac fossa. The autotransplant is performed to help treat or manage ureteral injuries or stenosis due to retroperitoneal fibrosis, renovascular disease such as renal artery stenosis or aneurysms, renal cell carcinoma (RCC), ureteral cancer, severe cases of nephrolithiasis, and severe loin pain–hematuria syndrome when all other conventional methods have failed.[30] The surgical technique and back bench table preparation are similar compared with a cadaveric or living donor kidney.

Evaluation of the Renal Allograft

The renal transplant is evaluated by the sonographer as a native kidney and renal artery examination would be, assessing the size, echotexture, and vasculature and looking for hydronephrosis, masses, fluid collections, or ascites. Institutions instill their own routine protocols on timing of examinations and certain images that are required. The following is the basis of what my institution practices. Once the patient has arrived at the recovery room from the surgical suite, the sonographer will go portably to perform the immediate postoperative examination. The patient's creatinine and urine output are closely monitored and if any issues arise, the transplant physicians will tailor their imaging requests. The blood values are evaluated weekly for the first 2 months, then every other week for 4 months, then monthly for 1 year, then every 3 months. The patient usually has a follow-up ultrasound every 4 to 6 months and then annually if there are no complications.

It is best to image using a 2.5- to 5.0-MHz curvilinear transducer and have the patient fasting 4 to 6 hours. Obese patients will require lower frequencies. The renal transplant is

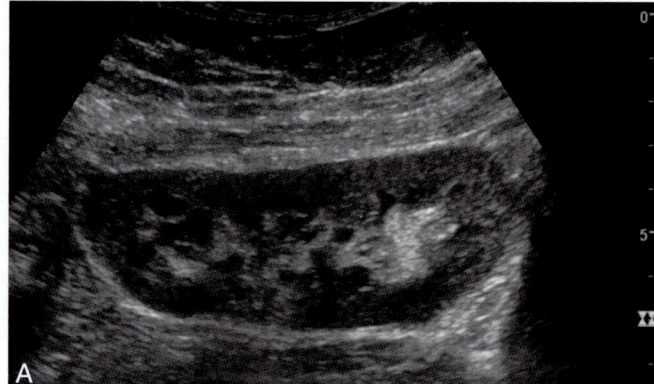

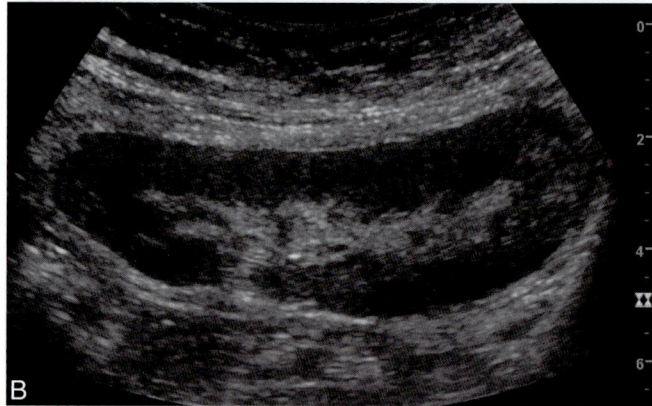

FIG. 20.31 **Renal transplant imaging using different patient positions.** (A) Longitudinal gray-scale ultrasound while the patient is supine. (B) Longitudinal gray-scale ultrasound with the patient rolled onto the side brings the kidney more superficial.

typically located in either the right or left lower quadrant and usually superficial. As a result, higher-frequency transducers are most commonly used. Breath holding is usually not necessary as respiratory motion of the pelvic structures is minimal. Depending on location, rolling the patient left lateral decubitus or right lateral decubitus may help move overlying bowel or bring the kidney to a more superficial position in the obese patient (Fig. 20.31).

The sonographer should scan completely through the kidney before taking any images while adjusting the frequency, depth, gain, TGCs, and focal zones as they go. Once the renal transplant has been fully evaluated, the examination needs to include a length measurement along with medial and lateral gray-scale longitudinal images. Gray-scale transverse images of the upper, mid, and lower poles also need to be obtained. Document any pathology in two planes with and without measurements and include color Doppler flow. Longitudinal and transverse gray-scale images should be taken of the bladder assessing for masses, bladder distention, or signs of infection. Most patients will typically have a urinary catheter in place immediately after surgery; this should not be confused with a bladder mass. Quadrant images need to be obtained checking for free fluid or signs of bleeding.

The Doppler portion is crucial for the transplanted kidney. Venous and arterial color and spectral Doppler need to be obtained looking for any signs of thrombus or stenosis. Ultrasound is commonly the first method of imaging in these patients, critical in helping the physicians diagnose the patient and ensure treatment will be administered quickly. Color Doppler and power Doppler should be used to judge adequate perfusion throughout the kidney (Fig. 20.32). The arcuate arteries within the parenchyma are evaluated in the upper, mid, and lower poles to obtain an RI measurement using the peak systolic and end-diastolic velocities. This is a common indirect Doppler technique to evaluate the arterial and venous flow. Angle correction is not necessary when obtaining an RI. The sweep speed can be increased, which will help spread the waveform over a period of 2 to 3 seconds. This helps magnify a particular part of the waveform for better interrogation and a more accurate measurement. A low RI can be a strong indicator of a proximal stenosis that may not be able to be otherwise identified. A high RI may indicate rejection, renal venous congestion, or chronic small vessel disease. These vessels are small in size and magnifying the image may help with visualization. Color images of the renal artery (RA) and renal vein (RV) should be included. Adjusting the color scale appropriately is important so areas of aliasing can be identified in the areas of the highest velocities. When evaluating the RA, it is critical to angle correct with pulsed-wave Doppler to accurately assess for stenosis or else a falsely elevated velocity may be obtained. The sonographer should document the transplanted renal artery similar to a native renal artery, including spectral Doppler with velocity measurements in the distal, mid, and proximal RA and at the anastomosis between the iliac artery and RA. The iliac artery and vein at the anastomosis and proximal to it should be evaluated and documented with spectral Doppler as well. If a stenosis is present, the anastomotic sites are the most common location. Some patients may have peripheral vascular disease, and an inflow stenosis may be identified affecting flow into the kidney allograft. A stenosis may undergo a balloon angioplasty with possible stent placement (Fig. 20.33). For all spectral Doppler, the angle should be parallel with the vessel that is sampled and less than 60 degrees to ensure accurate velocity measurements. The common femoral artery (CFA)

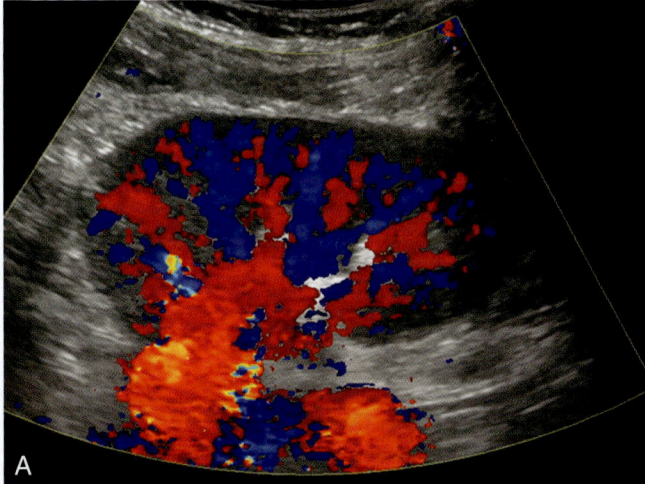
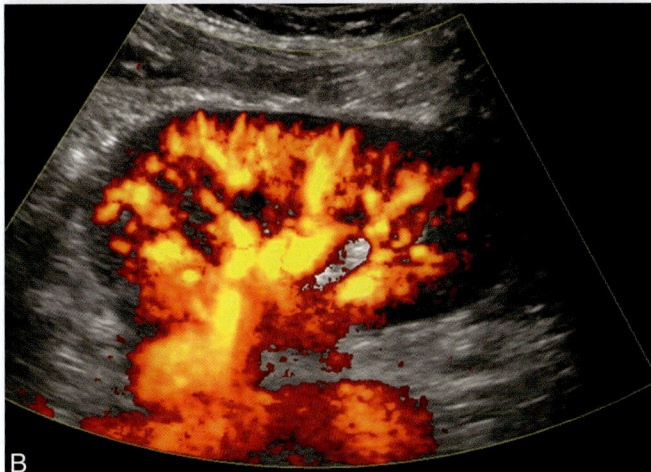

FIG. 20.32 Renal transplant perfusion. (A) Color Doppler ultrasound shows normal perfusion throughout the renal parenchyma. (B) Power Doppler ultrasound shows normal perfusion throughout the renal parenchyma without direction of flow identification.

should be documented to ensure adequate flow to the leg. All of the spectral waveforms should fill the spectral window while eliminating aliasing. There is a risk of arterial injury including complete occlusion or dissection. Dissection of the external iliac artery is rare, which can cause allograft loss and limit blood flow to the leg. The most common cause is traumatic handling. Treatment includes immediate intimal repair by means of stenting or artificial bypass grafting (Fig. 20.34). If the arterial segment occludes, emergent thrombectomy is required to try to salvage the graft[31] (Fig. 20.35).

Sometimes there may be difficulty obtaining a Doppler signal when there is very slow flow present within the vessels. Decreasing the color Doppler scale and increasing the color gain may help identify this slow flow. Some ultrasound machines enable slow flow settings such as lower extremity vein or iliac vein settings. A renal artery setting can also be helpful filling in the vessels as well. If the very slow frequencies are rejected as "cluttered noise," the wall filter should be decreased. If the patient is obese, the sonographer may also need to decrease the gray scale, color, and spectral Doppler frequencies enabling deeper penetration.

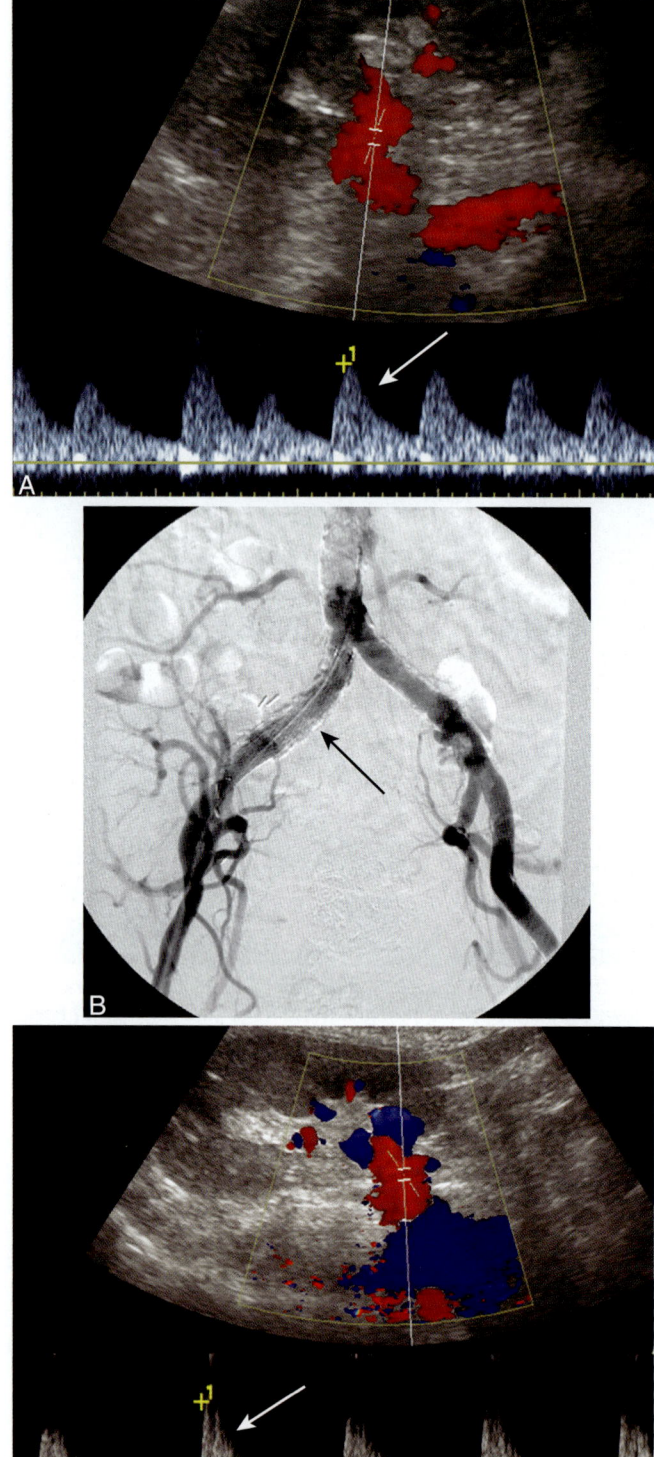

FIG. 20.33 **Inflow stenosis affecting renal function.** (A) Spectral Doppler ultrasound of the renal artery (RA) shows a monophasic waveform suggestive of an upstream stenosis. (B) Catheter angiography shows stent placement to treat a multifocal right common iliac artery stenosis. (C) Spectral Doppler ultrasound of the RA shows a normalized waveform following stent placement.

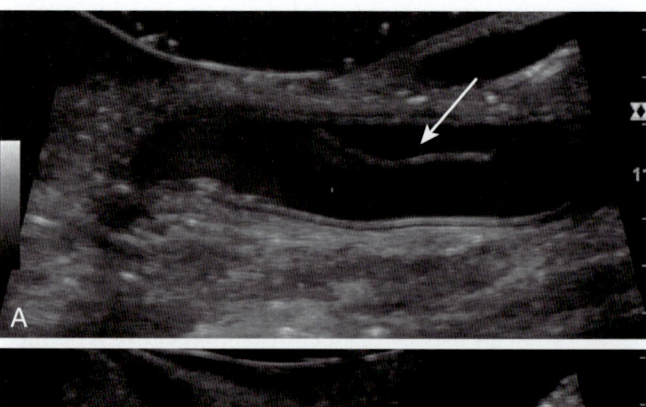
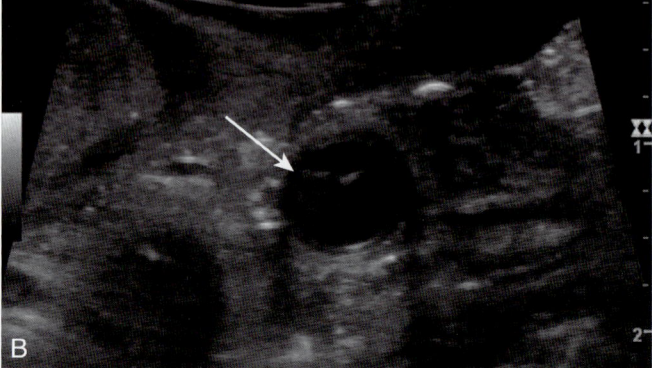
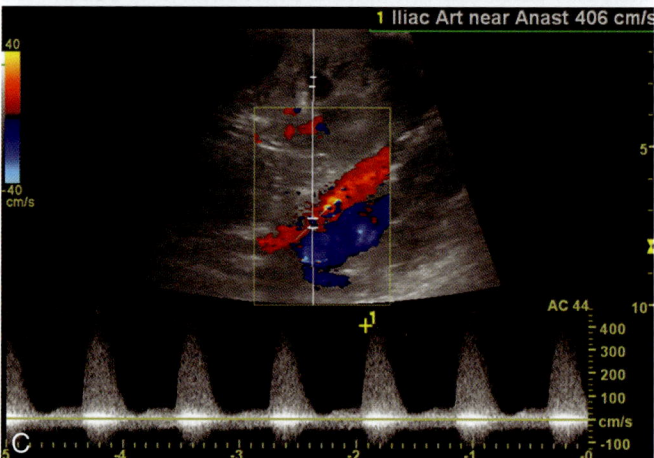

FIG. 20.34 **External iliac artery (EIA) injury.** (A) Intraoperative ultrasound shows longitudinal gray scale of the EIA with a dissection. (B) Intraoperative transverse gray-scale ultrasound of the EIA shows a dissection. (C) Spectral Doppler ultrasound shows elevated velocities associated with the EIA flap.

Normal Sonographic Findings of the Renal Transplant

On gray-scale imaging, the renal parenchyma should appear hypoechoic relative to the liver with the sinus fat being echogenic. Normal pyramids may be noted if using higher-frequency transducers due to the transplant being more superficial than native kidneys. The kidney has a reniform shape with a normal length of 9 to 13 cm. Renal length will vary depending on age and size of the donor. The collecting

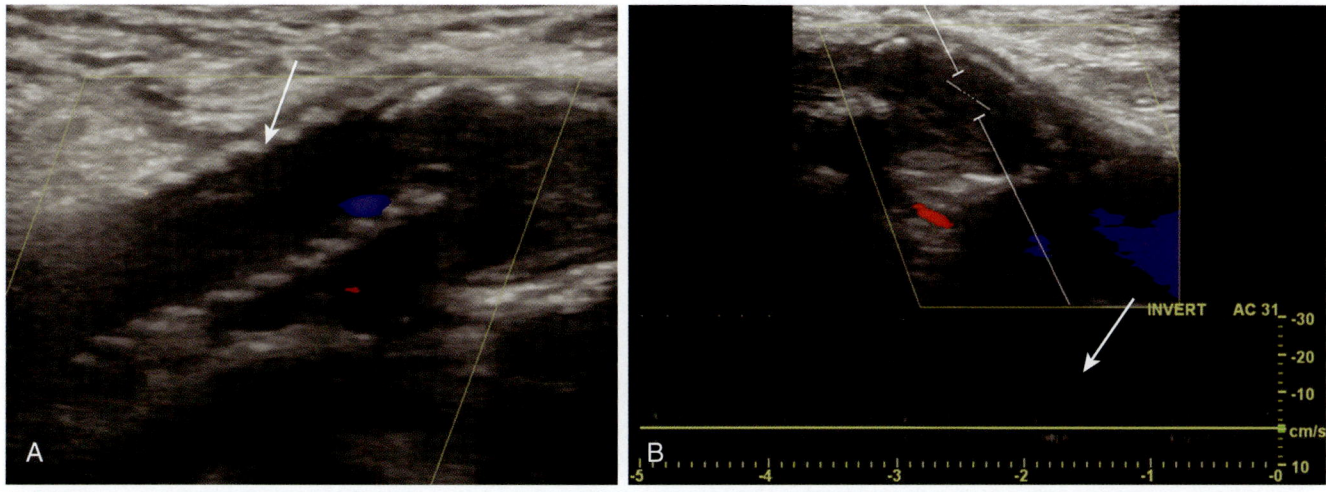

FIG. 20.35 **Arterial occlusion from clamp injury.** (A) Color Doppler ultrasound shows no flow within the aortic graft limb distally. (B) Spectral Doppler ultrasound shows no flow detected within the common femoral artery.

system should be free of fluid or debris. It is common to see a mildly dilated pelvis or extrarenal pelvis in these patients due to high urinary output through a single functioning kidney. In the immediate postoperative period, the urinary stents that are temporarily placed may be able to be visualized. When evaluating the bladder, it should have thin walls when distended and be free of debris (Fig. 20.36). In some patients, the Foley catheter may be visualized if they have one in place. See Chapter 15 for a more detailed explanation of the normal urinary tract and renal anatomy.

The Doppler portion of the transplanted kidney examination is crucial to perform. Some vascular complications can only be diagnosed using color and spectral Doppler. The RA will be red on color imaging bringing flow into the kidney and the spectral waveform demonstrates a rapid systolic upstroke with continuous diastolic flow above baseline demonstrating a low-resistance waveform. The velocities should be below 250 cm/sec with a renal to iliac artery ratio less than 3.0. A normal RI in the arcuate artery is in the range of 0.60 to 0.70 with borderline values between 0.70 and 0.80. The RV drains the kidney showing flow below the baseline with a blue color. The spectral waveform of the RV and iliac vein has continuous monophasic flow with minimal respiratory changes. The iliac artery and CFA should demonstrate a triphasic waveform with spectral Doppler imaging (Fig. 20.37). When measuring velocities using spectral Doppler imaging, turbulence or any doubling or tripling of velocities in the vessel from one location to the next should not be seen.

Renal Allograft Imaging in the Immediate Postoperative Period

It is imperative to image the newly transplanted kidney in the immediate postoperative period. Ultrasound is routinely used for this initial examination. The cost of sonography imaging is relatively low compared with CT or MRI and without the use of ionizing radiation. A skilled sonographer can provide

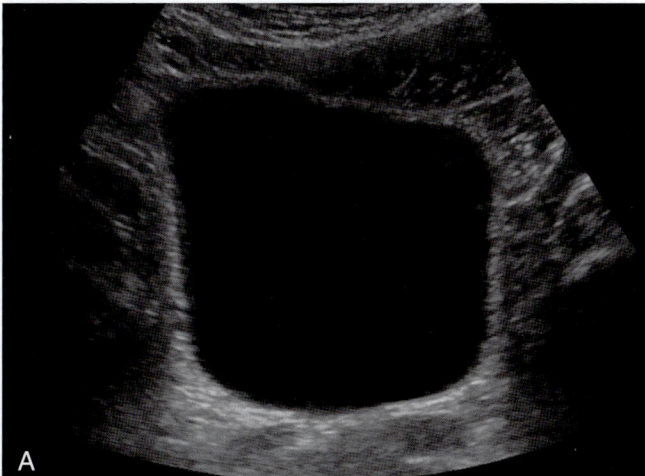
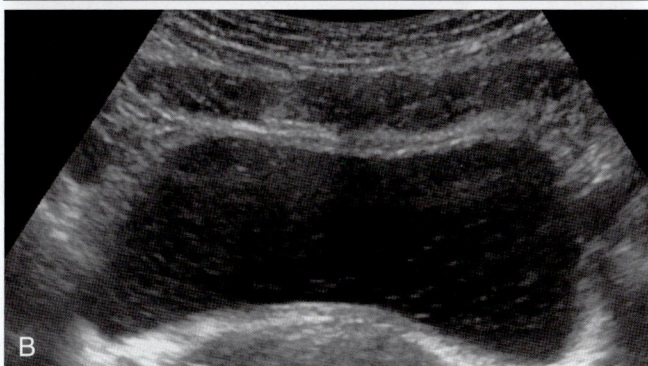

FIG. 20.36 **Bladder findings.** (A) Transverse gray-scale ultrasound shows a normal bladder with thin walls and free of debris. (B) Transverse gray-scale ultrasound shows a bladder with debris present consistent with a urinary tract infection.

pertinent images to the physician to help aid in diagnosis and transplant complications. Emergent findings can be treated quickly when the patient is routinely monitored with imaging.

During the postoperative ultrasound examination, the patient will be in the recovery unit while the general anesthesia

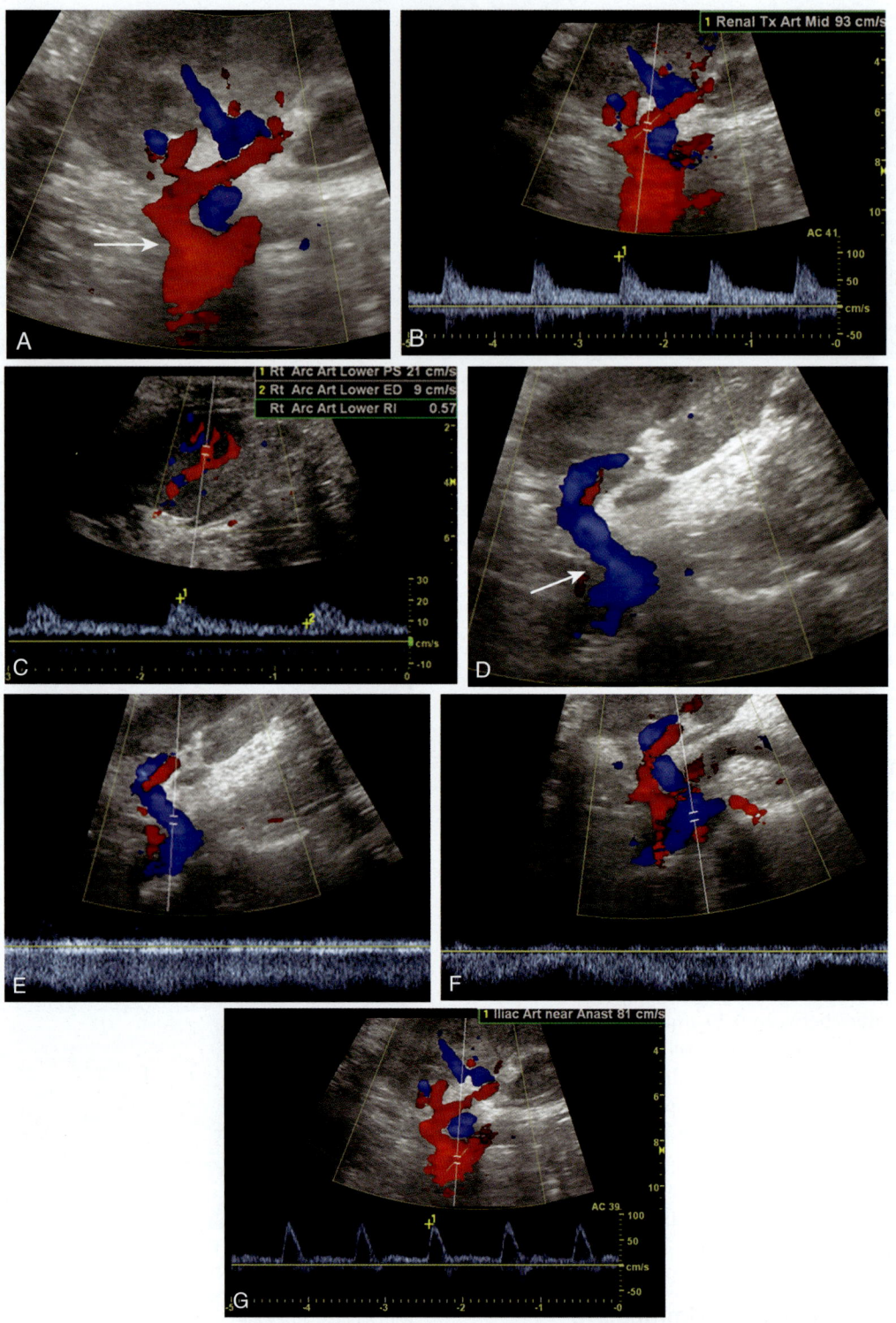

FIG. 20.37 **Normal renal Doppler.** (A) Color Doppler ultrasound shows a widely patent renal artery (RA) and anastomosis site without evidence of narrowing or focal stenosis. (B) Spectral Doppler ultrasound shows a normal RA waveform with a sharp systolic upstroke and continuous diastolic flow without elevated velocities. (C) Spectral Doppler ultrasound of the renal lower pole arcuate artery shows a normal resistive index (RI) with a sharp systolic upstroke and continuous diastolic flow. (D) Color Doppler ultrasound shows a widely patent renal vein (RV) and anastomosis site draining the kidney without evidence of narrowing or focal stenosis. (E) Spectral Doppler ultrasound of the RV near the anastomosis shows continuous monophasic flow. (F) Spectral Doppler ultrasound of the iliac vein shows continuous monophasic flow. (G) Iliac artery on spectral Doppler ultrasound shows a triphasic waveform without elevated velocities.

is wearing off. As a result, these patients will not be able to roll onto their side or help assist with their breathing. Sometimes the patient may become combative or confused. Reassure the patient that surgery is over and they are recovering. One of the common statements from patients is that they need to urinate. Again, reassure these patients that they are okay and that they have a catheter in place to help them. The nurses can give a medication to relieve this sensation as well. It is very helpful to have the patient's bandages taken off. This helps obtain the best imaging windows possible and prevents missing pathology. Although this is not a sterile scanning environment, using sterile gel while the patient's incisions are healing can potentially reduce the risk of infection. It is common to have a member of the transplant team or surgeon present for this examination. The physician wants to ensure the allograft has adequate arterial and venous flow and look for signs of hemorrhage. If there is an urgent complication noted, the surgeon could transfer the patient back to the operating room to correct the concerning issue immediately. Not all complications are considered urgent, and the radiologist likely will recommend a follow-up ultrasound within 24 hours to ensure stability or determine whether the issue has resolved or is getting worse. Urgent findings include the following: (1) RA severe stenosis or kinking of vessel affecting the flow within the renal parenchyma; (2) RA, RV, CFA, iliac artery or vein thrombus, or occlusion; or (3) an identified source of active bleeding. It is very common to see postoperative fluid collections, and these usually are self-limited and resolve on their own. Fluid collections will be monitored in serial ultrasound examinations making sure they are not enlarging or causing renal function problems. Another common finding involves the vasculature. Postoperative edema can create elevated blood flow velocities within the RA or RV and the arcuate arteries can have an elevated RI as well, demonstrating little or no diastolic flow. Once the edema decreases, the vessels usually return to a normal appearance. Once the ultrasound examination has been completed, remember to redress the incision with clean bandages or ask the patient's nurse to help assist. If the patient is stable and no complications arise during the recovery in the transplant unit, the patient is typically discharged from the hospital on postoperative day 3.

Renal Transplantation Complications in Routine Surveillance

It is common to perform routine protocol parenchymal biopsies around 4 months after transplantation followed by 1 year, 5 years, and 10 years. If the patient is symptomatic with pain, fever, or elevated creatinine, a biopsy may be ordered sooner. If a virus or rejection is discovered from the pathology results, the patient will be treated with medication for 1 month and then another biopsy will take place to evaluate the treatment plan (Fig. 20.38).

Biopsy complications may occur, with bleeding being the most common. The patient's INR and platelet counts are checked immediately before the biopsy. Patients are asked to stop taking anticoagulants 3 to 5 days before the procedure. Elevated blood pressure or hypertension is also a risk

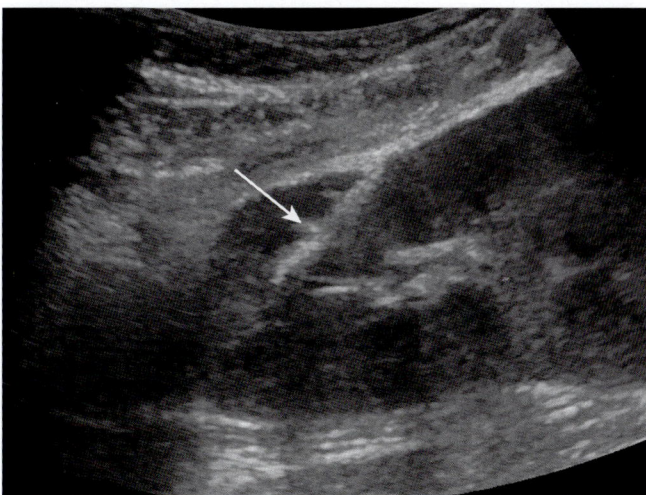

FIG. 20.38 Normal routine renal biopsy. Ultrasound-guided needle biopsy is aimed in the lateral renal cortex of the upper pole.

factor for bleeding. Some patients with known hypertension should take their antihypertensive medication as usual. Patients may come to the department showing anxiety. This may elevate the blood pressure as well. Pressures should not exceed 160/90 mm Hg. The radiologist or physician performing the biopsy may administer mild to moderate sedation to help relax the patient, reducing the blood pressure. Even after preventive measures, bleeding may still occur. A hematoma can form outside of the kidney capsule, and the patient may or may not develop pain (Fig. 20.39). Most bleeds will stop on their own after applying moderate pressure over the biopsy tract. If the bleeding is severe, the patient may become vasovagal and the blood pressure may drop. The patient's head should be lowered and saline fluids given. If there is active bleeding that cannot be controlled, the patient may be transferred to the interventional radiology department for further imaging and possible coil embolization (Fig. 20.40).

The biopsy needle is ultrasound guided to avoid major blood vessels and the collecting system. At times, the needle path may cross small vessels for a potential risk of creating an AVF. Inadvertent damage to the collecting system or ureter can also create a urine leak forming a urinoma. The radiologist will typically aim as lateral as possible within the cortex to retrieve enough glomeruli for the pathologist to evaluate while staying away from the renal hilum. Creating an AVF occurs in about 10% of patients. Depending on size and renal function, the AVF may be routinely followed or may be treated with embolization. Spectral Doppler will demonstrate a high velocity with a low resistive waveform. The renal vein will typically show arterialization near the fistula site[32] (Fig. 20.41).

Pathology of the Renal Transplant

Rejection and Acute Tubular Necrosis. Causes of graft dysfunction include rejection, acute tubular necrosis (ATN), and drug nephrotoxicity. Chronic parenchymal disease and chronic rejection will eventually lead to renal failure. The most common complications immediately postoperative and within the

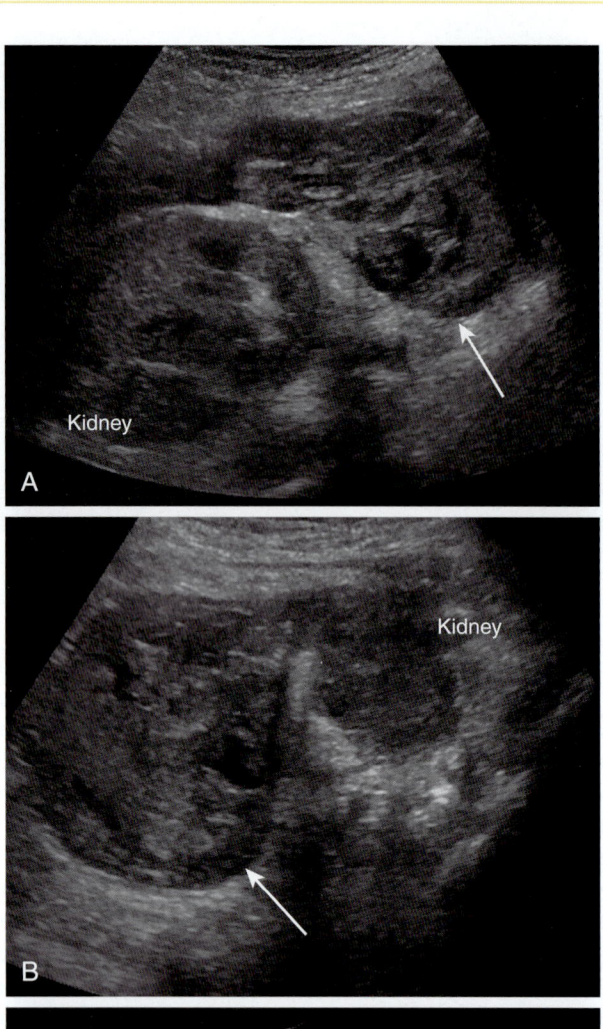

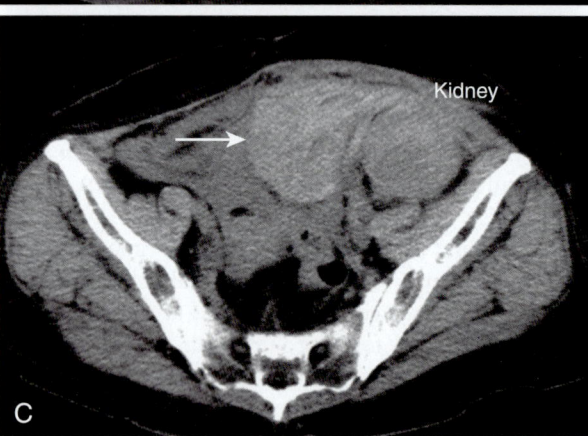

FIG. 20.39 **Renal biopsy hematoma complication.** Longitudinal (A) and transverse (B) gray-scale ultrasounds show a large hematoma that occurred after a renal biopsy. (C) Computed tomography imaging shows a large hematoma following a renal biopsy.

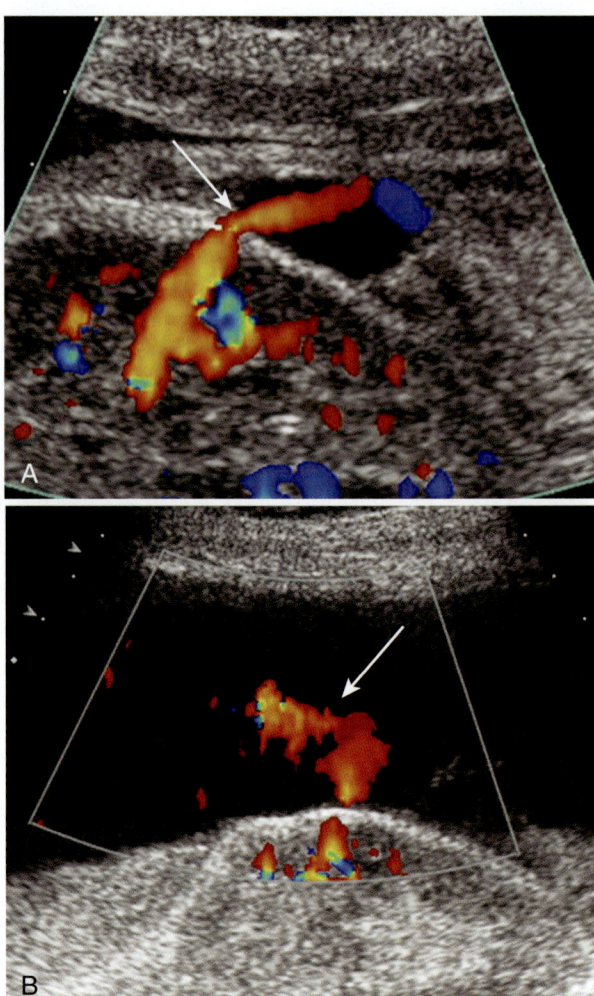

FIG. 20.40 **Renal biopsy active bleeding complication.** (A) Color Doppler ultrasound shows an active bleeding site along the biopsy tract into the abdomen. (B) Color Doppler ultrasound shows an active site of bleeding in a patient with ascites that could not be controlled by applying pressure to the biopsy site.

Infection and Abscesses. More than 80% of renal transplant recipients develop at least one infection within the first year. These can include pneumonia, wound infections, or urinary tract infections. Patients may present with fever or pain over the allograft. Peritransplant abscesses are uncommon and usually occur within the first few weeks after transplantation. These may be treated with percutaneous drain placement along with antibiotics. Any peritransplant fluid collection should be considered infected in the symptomatic patient. Acute pyelonephritis can also mimic acute rejection. Focal pyelonephritis can be an isolated area of increased or decreased echogenicity with nonspecific findings. Emphysematous pyelonephritis contains gas within the collecting system. The gas produces shadowing or reverberation artifacts. Fungus balls may also be seen within the collecting system. These masses appear echogenic with weak shadowing. Debris or low-level echoes within a dilated collecting system suggests pyonephrosis in a patient who presents with fever[33] (Fig. 20.43).

Urinary Obstruction and Stones. Urinary obstruction is seen in about 2% of renal transplant recipients and almost always

first year of transplantation are acute rejection and ATN. The kidney will usually be enlarged and edematous. A nonspecific finding of elevated RIs between 0.80 and 0.90 can be an indicator of dysfunction. A biopsy is required for diagnosis and differentiation of other pathologies. In the early stages following transplantation, acute rejection is the most common cause of hypertension. About 50% of patients will develop hypertension after receiving their kidney transplant[32] (Fig. 20.42).

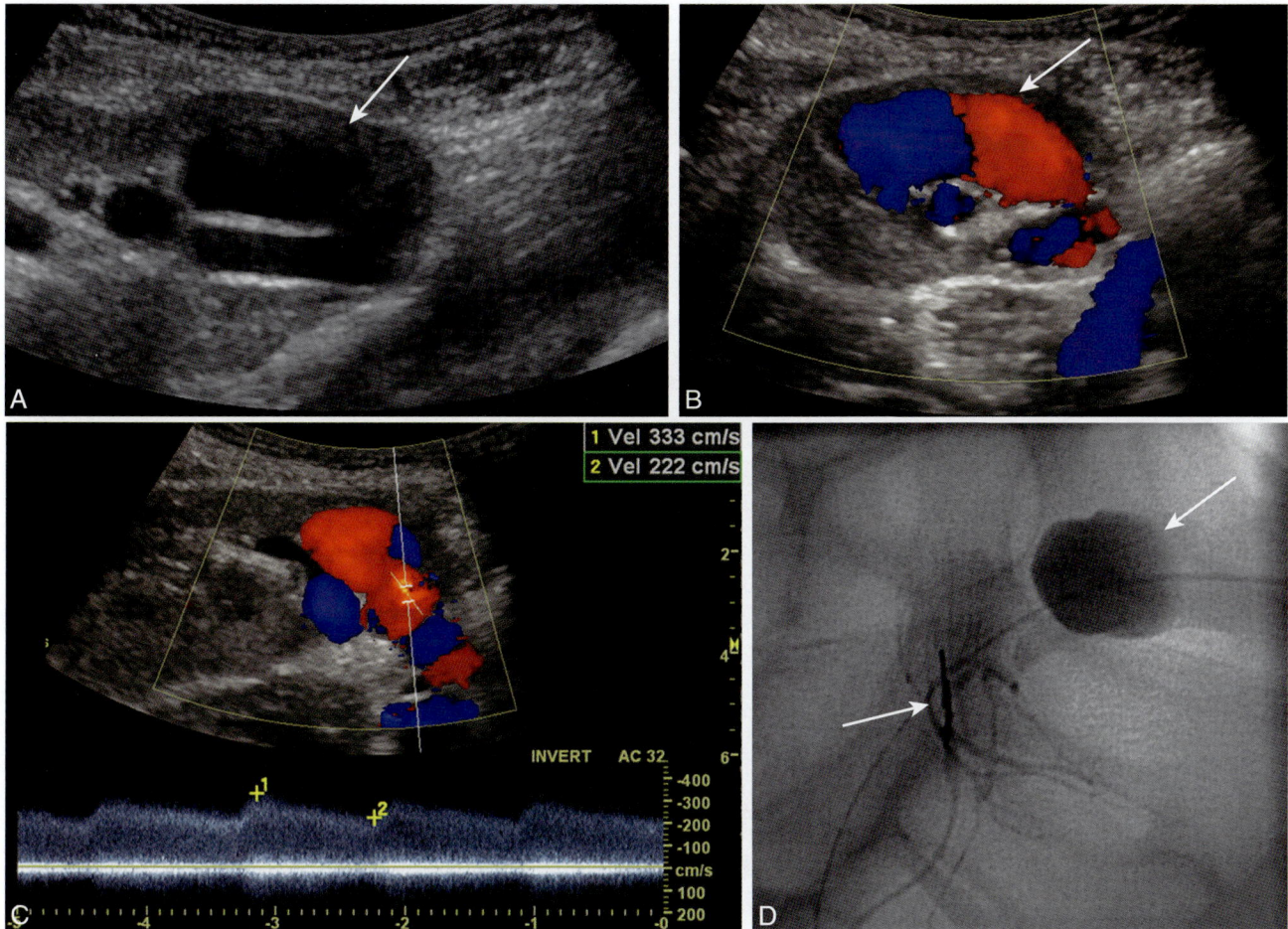

FIG. 20.41 **Renal biopsy arteriovenous fistula (AVF) complication.** (A) Longitudinal gray-scale ultrasound shows a large AVF of the lower renal pole caused from a biopsy site. (B) Transverse color Doppler ultrasound shows the flow within the AVF. (C) Spectral Doppler ultrasound shows a low resistive waveform and the elevated velocity within the AVF. (D) Interventional radiology shows a large AVF using coil embolization as treatment.

within the first 6 months after transplantation. The most common site of obstruction is at the site of ureteral implantation into the bladder. Ureteral stenoses are found in the distal third in more than 90% of these patients. Narrowing distally may be due to scarring caused from ischemia or rejection, surgical technique, or kinking. Other causes of obstruction include pelvic fibrosis, stones, papillary necrosis, fungus balls, clots, or extrinsic compression from a mass or fluid collection. Clinically the patient will have elevated creatinine levels making it difficult to distinguish from chronic rejection. Ultrasound is very sensitive for detecting hydronephrosis, the dilation of the urinary collecting system (Fig. 20.44). A percutaneous nephrostomy tube helps relieve the obstruction allowing for balloon dilation and stent placement. Dilation is successful in 90% of cases and may prevent the need for long-term stent placement, which can increase the risk of infection in the immunocompromised patient. Stents are usually removed after 10 days.[32,33]

Renal transplant recipients are at a higher risk for developing urinary calculi. If the patient's renal function is quickly declining, renal stones are considered. About 1% to 2% of patients develop a significant stone and require treatment. Percutaneous nephrostolithotomy or electrohydraulic lithotripsy may be used.[33] Stones and calculi can usually be visualized on ultrasound if large enough. You will visualize echogenic foci within the collecting system, ureter, or bladder, which may demonstrate shadowing or "twinkle" artifact on color Doppler imaging (Fig. 20.45).

Vascular Compromise

Renal Vein Stenosis and Thrombosis. Renal vein thrombosis is a rare complication that usually occurs within the first week of transplantation and is seen in less than 5% of patients. Clinical concerns include low urinary output and pain or swelling over the renal allograft. Slow flow, extrinsic compression, or a narrowing at the anastomosis may be a precursor to develop thrombus. On gray-scale imaging, the kidney may be edematous from venous congestion, and thrombus may be visualized within the vein lumen. On color and spectral Doppler, there will be absence of flow within the vein. There will often be increased resistance within the arterial system and demonstrate reversal of diastolic flow on spectral Doppler. Nonocclusive thrombus may also be observed with little venous flow along with a monophasic waveform (Fig. 20.46). CT or MRI may be helpful in diagnosis if

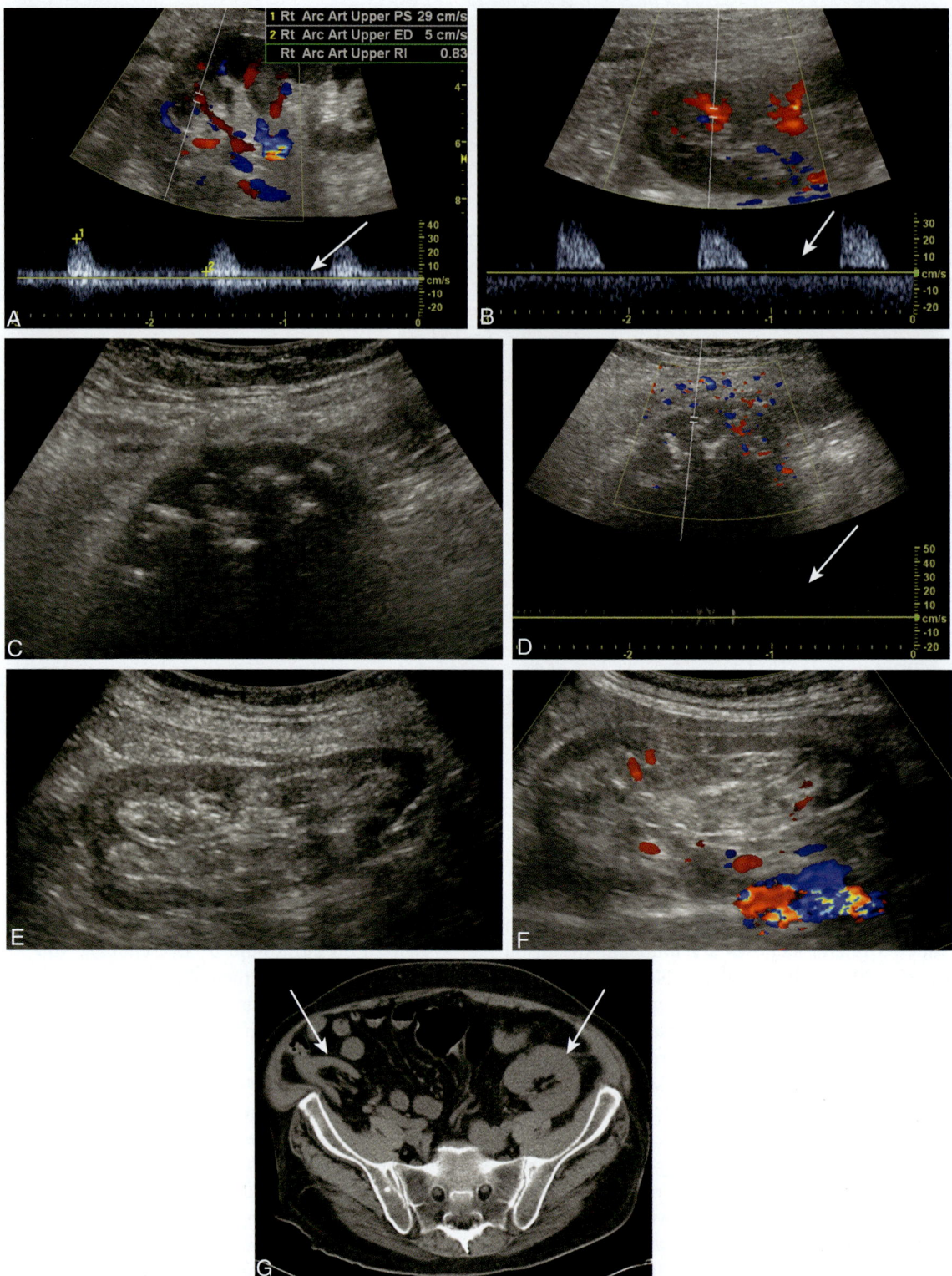

FIG. 20.42 Rejection and graft failure. (A) Spectral Doppler ultrasound shows an elevated resistive index (RI) within the upper arcuate artery with little diastolic flow and biopsy proven as acute rejection. (B) Spectral Doppler ultrasound shows the absence of diastolic flow within the upper arcuate artery demonstrating chronic parenchymal disease. (C) Longitudinal gray-scale ultrasound shows a calcified failed renal transplant. (D) Spectral Doppler ultrasound shows absence of flow within the renal parenchyma. (E) Longitudinal gray-scale ultrasound shows an atrophic kidney with a thinned cortex demonstrating renal transplant failure. (F) Color Doppler ultrasound shows minimal flow within the failed renal transplant. (G) Noncontrast computed tomographic imaging shows an atrophic right lower quadrant renal transplant compared with the normal left lower quadrant renal transplant.

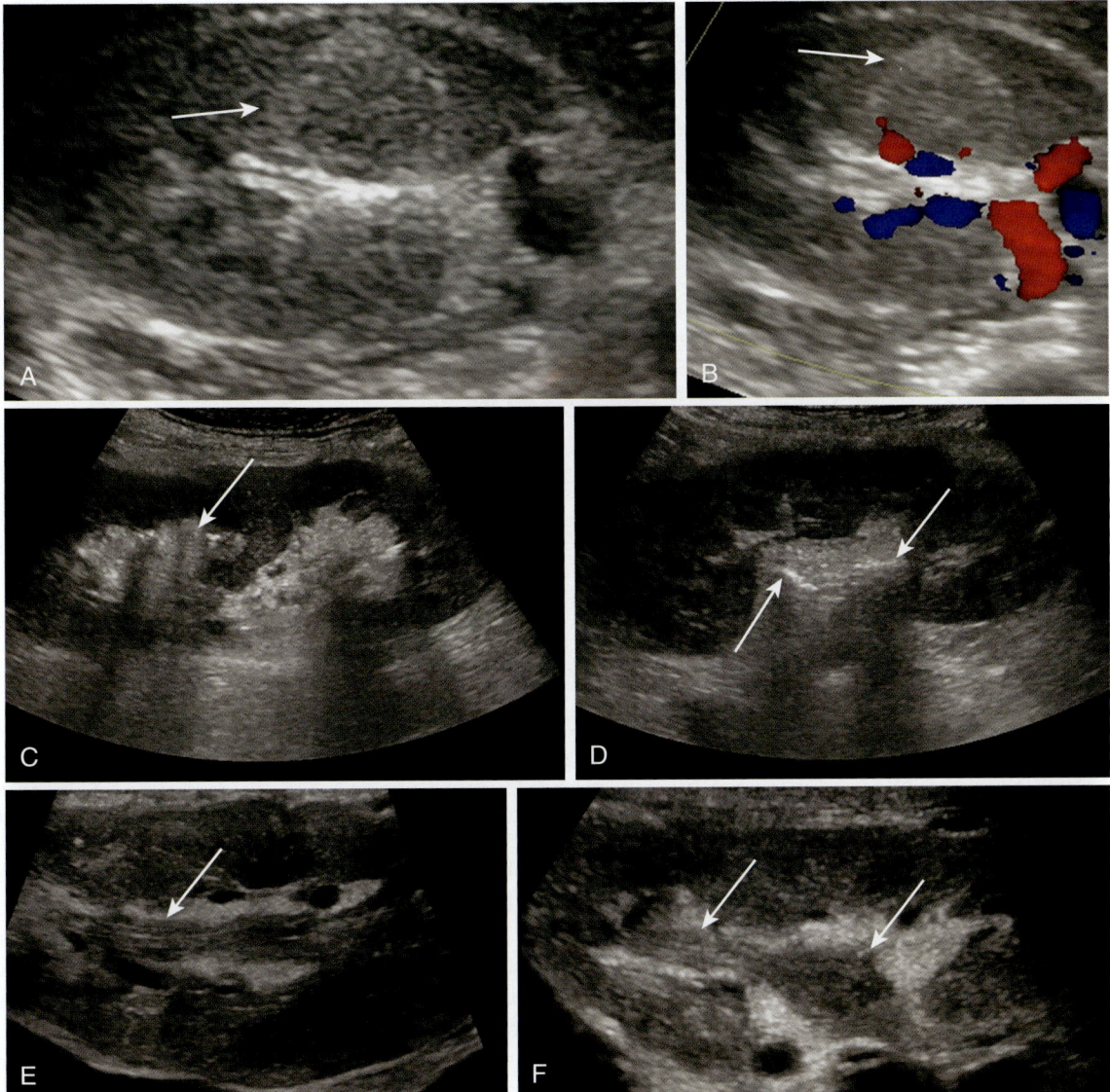

FIG. 20.43 **Renal infection.** (A) Transverse gray-scale ultrasound shows an echogenic area demonstrating focal pyelonephritis that can mimic a mass. (B) Color Doppler ultrasound shows no flow within the focally infected area. (C-D) Longitudinal gray-scale ultrasound shows gas within the collecting system creating shadowing and demonstrating emphysematous pyelonephritis. (E-F) Longitudinal gray-scale ultrasound shows thick debris and pus within the collecting system demonstrating pyonephrosis in the febrile patient.

thrombus is not directly visualized. Acute renal vein thrombosis is an urgent finding and the patient should undergo thrombectomy to avoid allograft loss. Infarction may occur due to late diagnosis and a nephrectomy may ultimately be required to prevent subsequent infection.[32,33] Renal vein stenosis usually occurs near the anastomosis site. The sonographer should look for color aliasing and doubling velocities within the vein on spectral Doppler. This should be routinely monitored to ensure stability or resolution. Commonly this is visualized in the immediate postoperative state due to surrounding soft tissue edema (Fig. 20.47).

Renal Artery Stenosis and Thrombosis. Renal artery stenosis is one of the most common vascular complications and usually occurs within the first year following transplantation. The stenosis may be related to the surgical technique and occur at the anastomosis or may be caused from atherosclerosis in the donor artery. The artery may also have a kink due to positioning. About 80% of end-stage renal disease patients develop hypertension. After transplantation, nearly two-thirds have improvement in their hypertension.[33] Patients who have multiple renal arteries have a slight increased risk of stenosis.[32] On ultrasound imaging, color flow will demonstrate aliasing in the area of stenosis. Blood flow velocities exceeding 250 cm/sec and an RA to iliac artery ratio above 3.0 strongly suggest stenosis. Tardus-parvus arcuate artery waveforms are indicative of a proximal stenosis as well. Within the immediate postoperative period, it is common to visualize elevated blood flow velocities due to soft tissue edema, but this usually resolves within a few days and does not usually affect renal function. This should be routinely monitored to ensure stability or resolution. Treatment of choice when needed is percutaneous transluminal angioplasty with or without stent

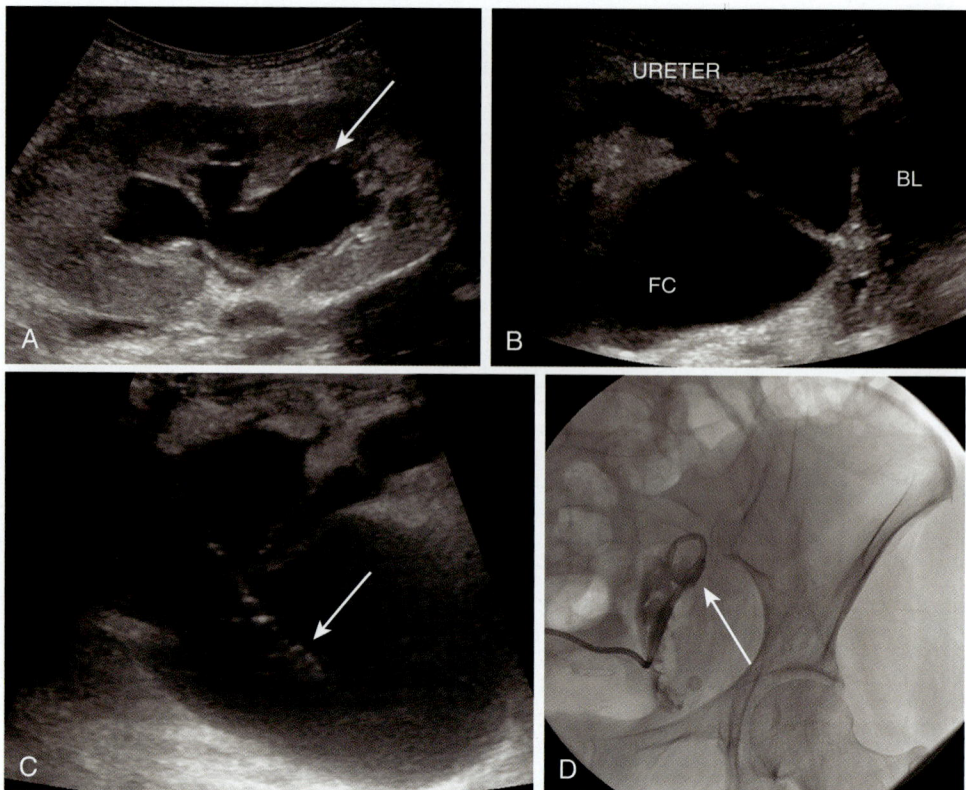

FIG. 20.44 **Urinary obstruction.** (A) Longitudinal gray-scale ultrasound shows moderate hydronephrosis. (B) Gray-scale ultrasound shows a pelvic fluid collection (FC) compressing the ureter. (C) Ultrasound-guided drain placement into the fluid collection. (D) Sonogram performed to check drain placement. *BL*, Bladder.

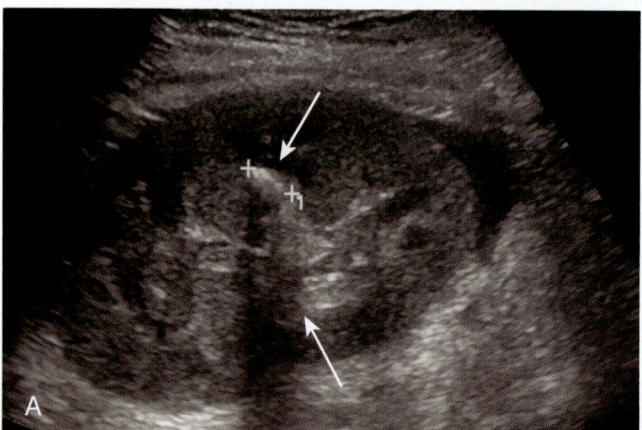

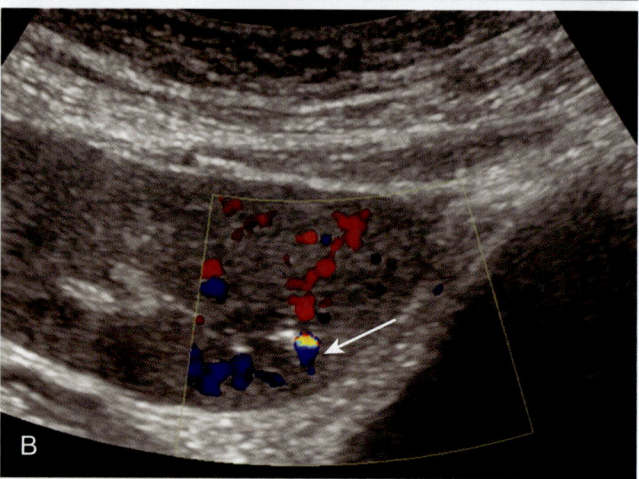

FIG. 20.45 **Renal stones.** (A) Longitudinal gray-scale ultrasound shows a stone with posterior shadowing. (B) Color Doppler ultrasound shows "twinkle" artifact associated with the renal stone.

placement. Success rates have been seen in 73% of patients. This typically reduces blood pressure and creatinine levels in 1 day[33] (Fig. 20.48). Arterial thrombus and thrombosis is a rare but very severe complication that usually leads to renal allograft loss. Early detection within 24 hours can salvage the transplant using fibrinolysis treatment.[34]

Infarction and Necrosis. Segmental infarction within the transplant is a result of vascular thrombosis, hyperacute rejection, kinking of the artery, dissection, or anastomotic occlusion (Fig. 20.49). Patients present with no urinary output and may have swelling or pain over the allograft. Infarcts may be diffuse or focal and have a hypoechoic wedge-shaped appearance on ultrasound. No color flow is visualized within the infarcted area. Power Doppler is useful in detecting slow flow. With complete vascular obstruction, there will be no arterial or venous flow identified within the renal transplant. Early detection is crucial to salvage the allograft by means of interventional or surgical techniques.[32,33]

Pseudoaneurysms. A pseudoaneurysm is a focal disruption of the artery with no direct communication with a vein and can occur in any vessel. On ultrasound, a pseudoaneurysm appears as a round cystic structure and demonstrates disorganized "yin-yang" color flow within. On spectral Doppler imaging, a to-and-fro waveform may be noted. A pseudoaneurysm can be due to surgical technique, trauma, or infection. Depending on size and location, these can be observed over time or treated surgically.[32]

Fluid Collections

Bleeding and Hematomas. It is common for patients to develop a hematoma, a collection of blood, in the immediate postoperative period with an overall incidence of 4% to 8%.

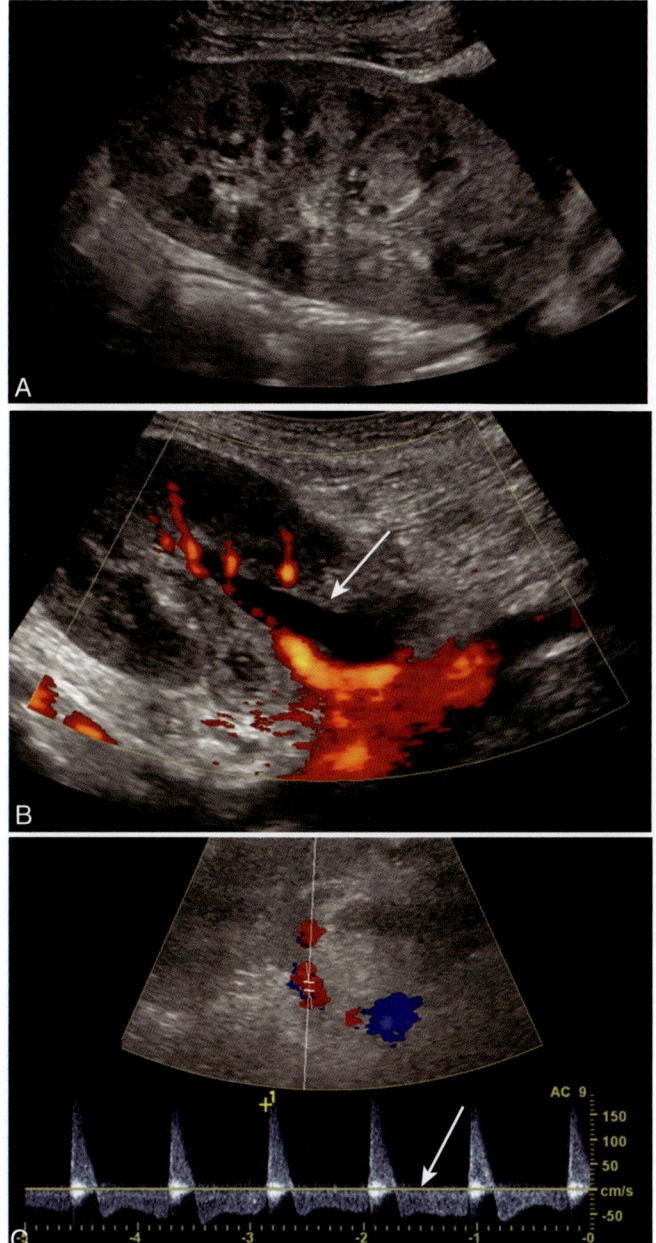

FIG. 20.46 Renal vein (RV) thrombosis. (A) Longitudinal gray-scale ultrasound shows an echogenic edematous kidney demonstrating venous congestion. (B) Power Doppler ultrasound shows absence of flow within the RV. (C) Spectral Doppler ultrasound within the renal artery shows reversal of diastolic flow consistent with RV thrombosis.

Hematomas may also be caused from trauma or at a biopsy site and usually resolve on their own.[35] Subcapsular hematomas may compress the parenchyma and affect renal function[32] (Fig. 20.50). Large hematomas may displace the kidney or cause compression of the ureter, and hydronephrosis may develop. On ultrasound, hematomas appear as a complex fluid collection and may have debris or septations. Fresh blood has an echogenic appearance whereas old hematomas become anechoic. If an infectious source is suspected, an aspiration can be obtained. If there is no infection present, drain placement is typically not recommended, as there is an increased risk of infection.[33]

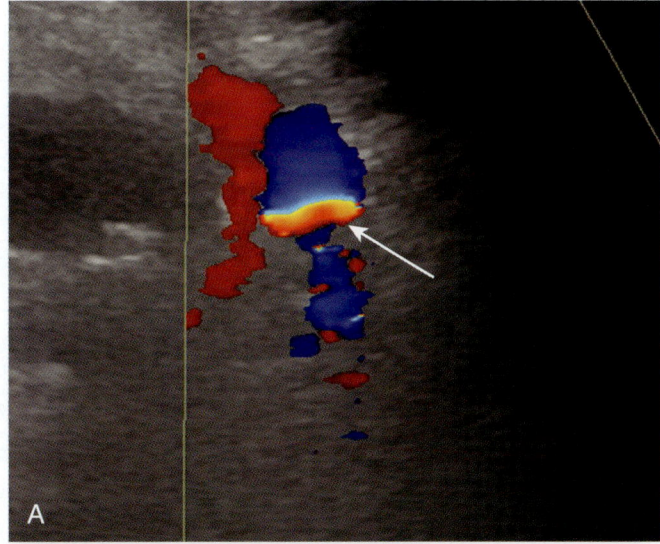

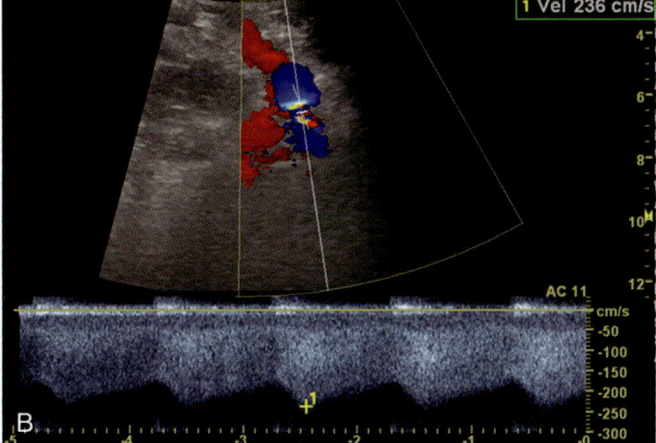

FIG. 20.47 Renal vein (RV) stenosis. (A) Color Doppler ultrasound shows aliasing within the RV near the anastomosis. (B) Elevated velocities are visualized indicating a narrowing within the RV on spectral Doppler ultrasound.

Seromas. Seromas are clear, serous fluid collections that are typically found within the early postoperative period and are most common along the vascular anastomoses sites. A seroma will usually resolve on its own with no treatment. If there is concern that the fluid collection is infected or if it is creating a mass effect on the vasculature or the ureter, an aspiration may be performed. A seroma is a round, localized, anechoic, thin-walled fluid collection, which may contain debris or septations on ultrasound imaging. Ultrasound is very sensitive to diagnose a fluid collection, but it remains difficult to determine the contents. CT or MRI may be helpful in differentiating the collections[13] (Fig. 20.51).

Lymphoceles. The most common peritransplant fluid collection is a lymphocele occurring in 0.5% to 20% of cases. These are usually an early complication seen within the first 2 months following transplantation but can also develop years later. A surgical disruption of lymphatic channels causes lymph fluid leakage into the soft tissue space, creating a lymphocele. These are typically found medial to the transplant and are the most common fluid collection that causes

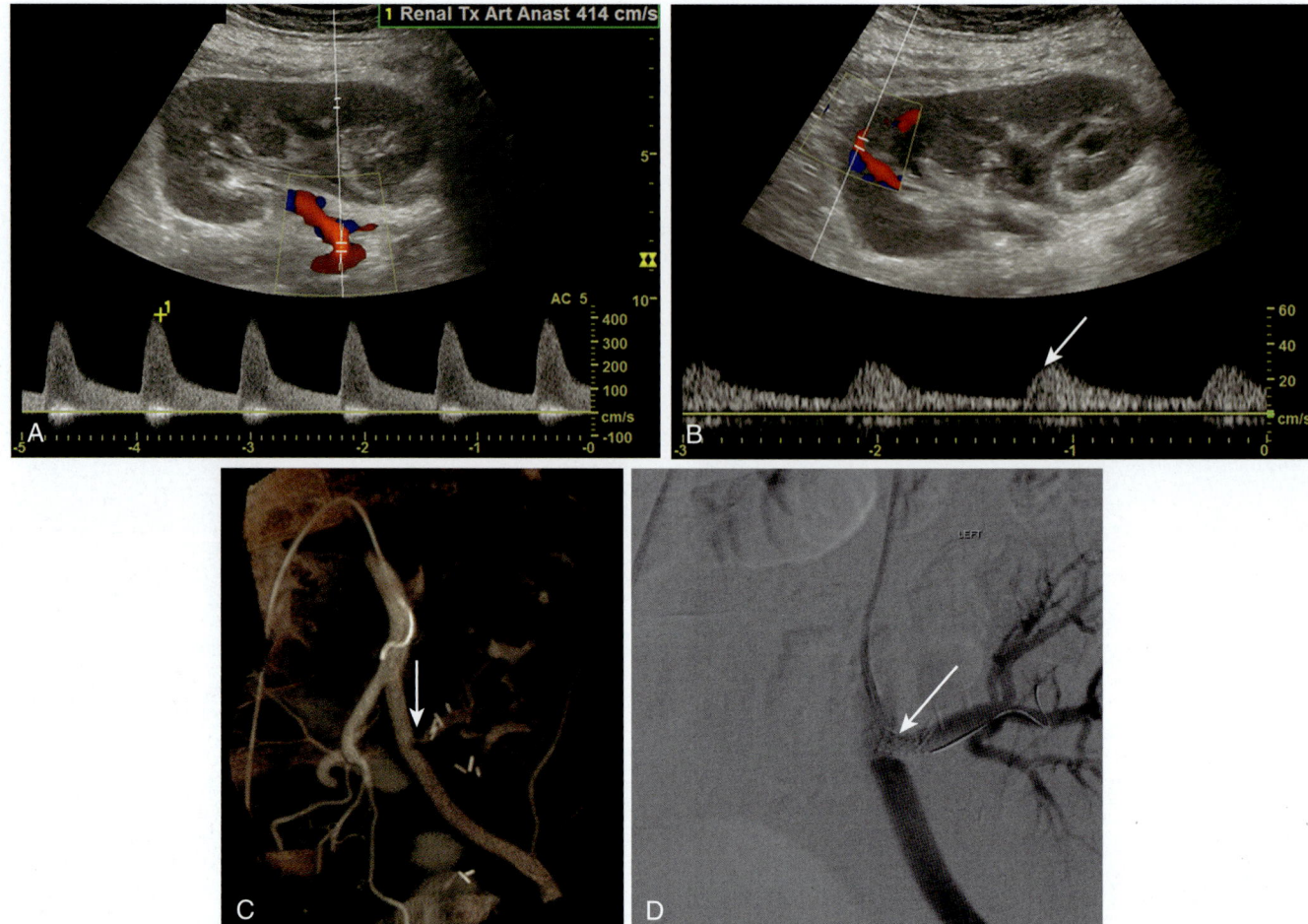

FIG. 20.48 **Renal artery (RA) stenosis.** (A) Elevated velocities near the RA anastomotic site are seen on spectral Doppler ultrasound. (B) The upper arcuate artery shows a tardus-parvus waveform with a dampened systolic upstroke on spectral Doppler ultrasound. (C) Three-dimensional angiography shows a severe RA stenosis near the anastomosis. (D) Interventional radiology successfully placed an RA stent for treatment.

hydronephrosis. Lymphoceles may also compress the iliac or femoral vein, causing leg edema.[33] On ultrasound imaging, you may see debris or septations within the fluid collection. Ultrasound is very sensitive to diagnose a fluid collection but as with other fluid collections is not specific for the contents.[13] Spontaneous resolution is rare. Treatment includes percutaneous drain placement in conjunction with sclerotherapy with a 97% success rate. Frequent aspirations increase the risk of infection and may require a drain placement along with antibiotic medications. Lymphoceles commonly recur after simple aspiration and ultimately may need surgical repair[33] (Fig. 20.52).

Urine Leak and Urinomas. Urine leaks and urinomas are rare complications and usually found within the first 2 weeks after transplantation. Urine may leak from the renal pelvis, ureter, or ureteroneocystostomy site due to ureteral necrosis. Urine seeps into the peritoneal cavity forming a contained fluid collection, a urinoma. Urinomas can vary in size and are typically visualized between the kidney and bladder. On ultrasound, a urinoma appears as an anechoic, well-defined fluid collection with no septations, and rapidly increases in size (Fig. 20.53). The patient may present with little or no urine output and have fullness or pain over the allograft. Large urinomas may rupture, creating urinary abdominal ascites and increasing the risk for infection and abscess formation. Early detection and treatment reduces the patient mortality rate. Treatment includes ultrasound-guided aspiration and percutaneous nephrostomy tube and stent placement. Stents should remain in place for 6 to 8 weeks to allow complete healing of the ureter. If the ureter fails to heal, ureteral reimplantation may be necessary.[33]

Renal Cell Carcinoma. Renal cell carcinoma (RCC) is rare within a renal transplant. Renal transplant tumors may be transmitted from donors, metastasis from the native kidneys, or new carcinomas arising after transplantation. A study reported 4.6% of posttransplant cancers were found to be renal carcinomas with 10% within the allograft itself.[36] Long-term immunosuppression increases the risk 100 times the normal risk for developing a malignancy and occurs in about 6% of patients. The most common malignancies are skin cancers and lymphoma. Patients with glomerulopathy and recurrent glomerulonephritis cause microhematuria and increase the risk of developing neoplasms. Ultrasound imaging of renal cell carcinomas typically demonstrates a solid

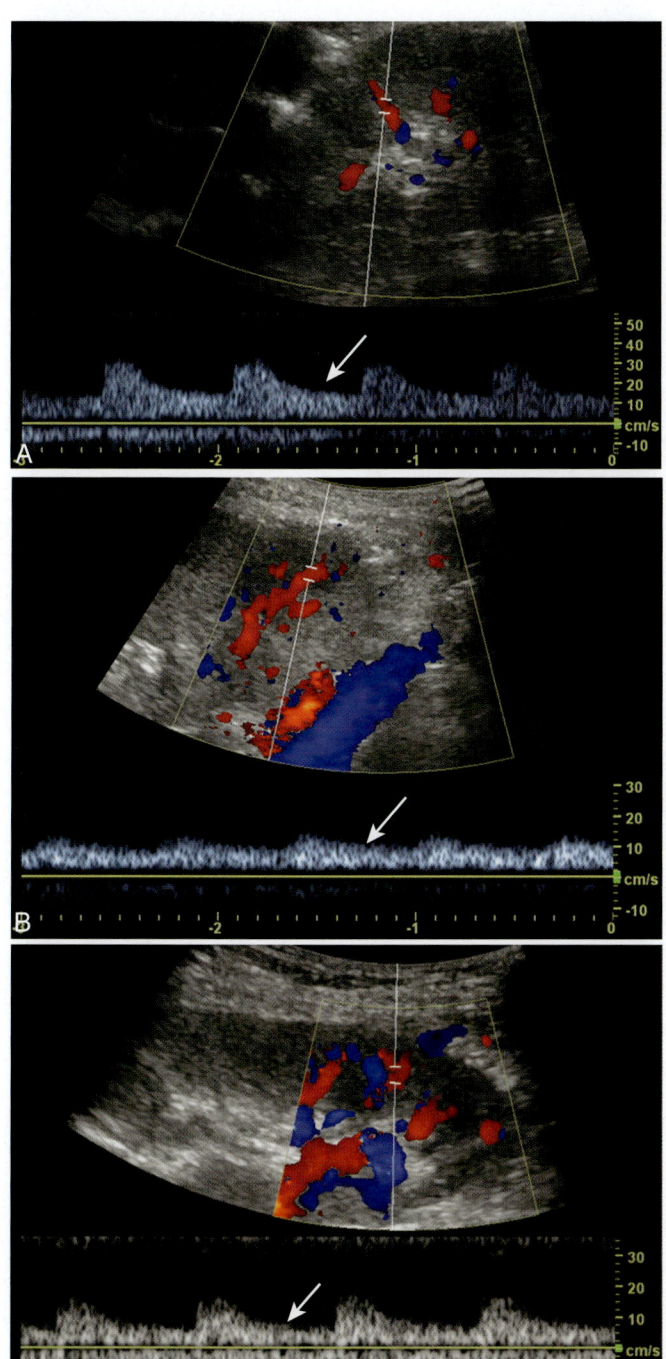

FIG. 20.49 Surgical ligation of an accessory renal artery. (A) Spectral Doppler ultrasound of a normal upper arcuate artery. (B) Spectral Doppler ultrasound of the lower pole arcuate artery shows a low resistive index with high diastolic flow. (C) Spectral Doppler ultrasound of the lower pole arcuate artery on a follow-up examination appears to return to normal as collateral flow helped establish more flow.

heterogeneous mass with a well-defined border that may contain cystic components in some cases. CT or MRI may be helpful in diagnosis. It is recommended that the native kidney be evaluated when an RCC is suspected. A final diagnosis can be made performing a mass biopsy. Treatment includes removal of the renal allograft or percutaneous ablation[33] (Fig. 20.54).

Transitional Cell Carcinoma. Transitional cell carcinoma (TCC) of the urinary tract occurs more often in the transplanted patient compared with the general population and is seen in about 0.07% to 1.9% of patients. TCC is rare within the transplanted patient and only a few cases have been published. The BK virus and human papillomavirus (HPV) have been shown to carry an increased risk of TCC. Most of these tumors are found within the bladder but can occur anywhere along the urinary tract. TCC within the transplanted patient tend to be more aggressive, rapidly progressive, poorly differentiated, and more fatal in comparison with the general population. Ultrasound may note an irregular mass within the bladder demonstrating vascular flow (Fig. 20.55). Final diagnosis is typically made with cystoscopy and biopsy. Treatments may include a radical cystectomy or nephroureterectomy in cases that involve the native upper tract. If TCC is present within the transplant, a complete allograft nephrectomy needs to be performed.[37]

Posttransplant Lymphoproliferative Disorder. PTLD occurs in 1% to 20% of patients who receive a transplant. In one study, PTLD was found to occur in 0.8% of renal transplant patients.[22] PTLD is the most severe complication found in solid organ and stem cell transplantation. Patients who are taking immunosuppressant medication increase the risk of malignancies 2 to 5 times more than the general population. PTLD can present as benign reactive hyperplasia of tissue to fulminant lymphoma. Most polymorphic masses are caused by the EBV, occurring 60% to 80% and within 1 year of transplantation. Most of the monomorphic masses are found to be non-Hodgkin lymphoma and have B-cell origin. Reducing immunosuppressant drugs is a recommended treatment in those patients with EBV-induced PTLD, effective in 23% to 50% of cases. Some patients may not positively respond to the reduction of immunosuppression; therefore immunotherapy with monoclonal antibodies such as rituximab is given. From 40% to 68% of cases have shown success using this treatment.[22] PTLD can occur in any solid organ or viscera.[32] The most common sites of involvement are the lymph nodes followed by the liver, brain, and lung. If the small intestine is involved, the patient presents with a generalized disease.[33] On ultrasound imaging, PTLD usually appears as a hypoechoic soft tissue mass and may be found near the renal hilum[32] (Fig. 20.56).

Common Benign Findings. The renal transplant is evaluated by the sonographer in a similar fashion as the native organ. The following are common findings that may be encountered within the kidney and are not specific to transplantation.

Cysts. Renal cysts are a common benign finding. They have well-defined margins, thin walls, and are anechoic with posterior acoustic enhancement on ultrasound examination. Some may have thin septations or demonstrate debris representing a hemorrhagic cyst. If a thick irregular wall or internal vascularity is noted, the possibility of an RCC should be raised and further evaluated with other imaging modalities or biopsy. Cysts typically remain asymptomatic and are incidental findings. Renal cysts increase with age and occur in 40% of the population who have a CT scan.[38] One study reported

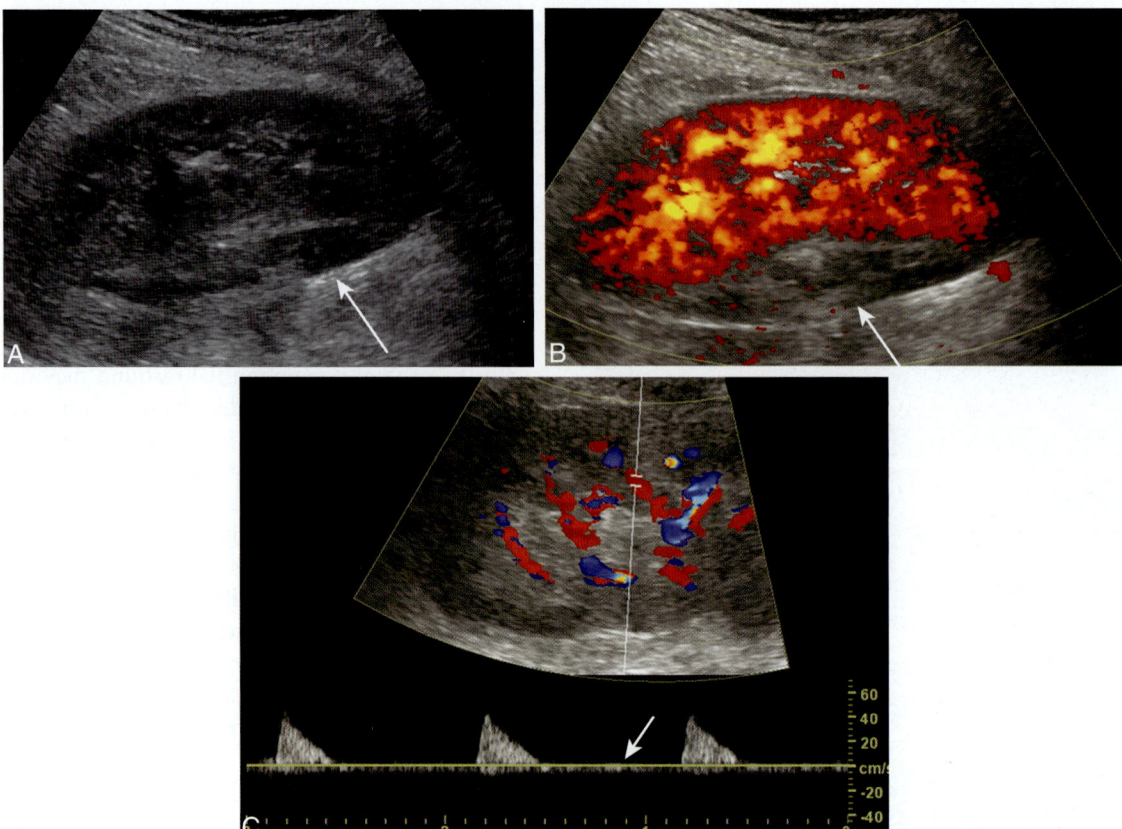

FIG. 20.50 **Hematoma.** (A) Longitudinal gray-scale ultrasound shows a subcapsular hematoma posteriorly. (B) Longitudinal power Doppler ultrasound shows mass effect on the renal parenchyma. (C) Spectral Doppler ultrasound of the mid arcuate artery shows no diastolic flow consistent with impaired renal function.

that cystic lesions found within the transplant did not cause dysfunction or related complications. An ultrasound or CT scan is commonly recommended for routine follow-up.[39]

Angiomyolipomas. Angiomyolipoma (AML) is the most common benign kidney lesion. It is composed of adipose tissue, smooth muscle, and vessels occurring in 0.1% to 0.22% of patients. AMLs are usually sporadic but can be associated with tuberous sclerosis, an autosomal dominant genetic disorder with other systemic findings. AMLs tend to be asymptomatic and incidental findings. AML is the second most common cause of retroperitoneal hemorrhage due to the potential risk of rupture, especially when larger than 4 cm. On ultrasound examination, AML is highly echogenic and may produce posterior shadowing. Treatment is usually not necessary unless the lesion is large enough for potential rupture or to cause renal failure. Embolization is the treatment of choice. An AML should not be a contraindication as a renal transplant donor.[40]

PANCREATIC TRANSPLANT

Surgical Technique of the Pancreatic Transplant

The pancreas can be preserved between 12 and 18 hours on ice and using a special preservation solution (e.g., UW, HTK, or Celsior). Shorter ischemic time leads to better allograft function. For every transplant, the donor and recipient are rechecked to verify a match. The blood type and compatibility need to be confirmed, as well as the UNOS database per protocol. Before coming into the operating room, the team will discuss the risks, benefits, and alternatives with the patient and obtain consent. All institutions have certain protocols and techniques they follow. Every patient has a unique situation, and the surgeons have different techniques they prefer.

Cadaveric Pancreatic Donation. The patient is brought into the operating room confirming patient identification and procedure to be performed. Following general anesthesia and line placement, a Foley catheter is placed into the bladder. The abdomen is prepped and draped sterilely. A primary midline incision is made. The subcutaneous tissues and rectus fascia are divided to enter the peritoneum, and the colon is mobilized to the hepatic flexure. The surgeon may choose a right lower quadrant or a left lower quadrant location. The right lower quadrant is typically the preferred choice. The distal IVC and common iliac artery and vein are dissected free from surrounding tissues.

The back bench table preparation includes performing a splenectomy, oversewing the stapled ends of the duodenum and the root of the mesentery using running sutures. The portal vein, superior mesenteric artery (SMA), and splenic artery (SA) are dissected free from surrounding tissues. A donor iliac artery bifurcation (Y graft) is anastomosed to the SMA and SA using continuous sutures. Once prepared,

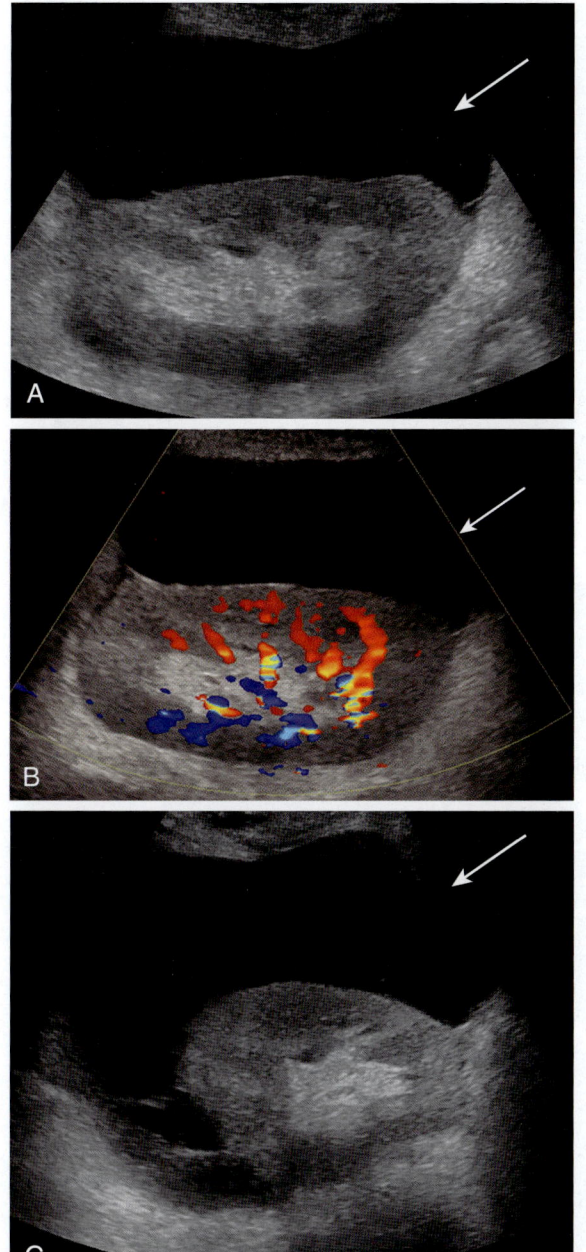

FIG. 20.51 Seroma. (A) Longitudinal gray-scale ultrasound shows a simple fluid collection anterior to an echogenic kidney. (B) Color Doppler ultrasound shows absence of flow within the collection. (C) Transverse gray-scale ultrasound demonstrates a mostly simple seroma with some debris.

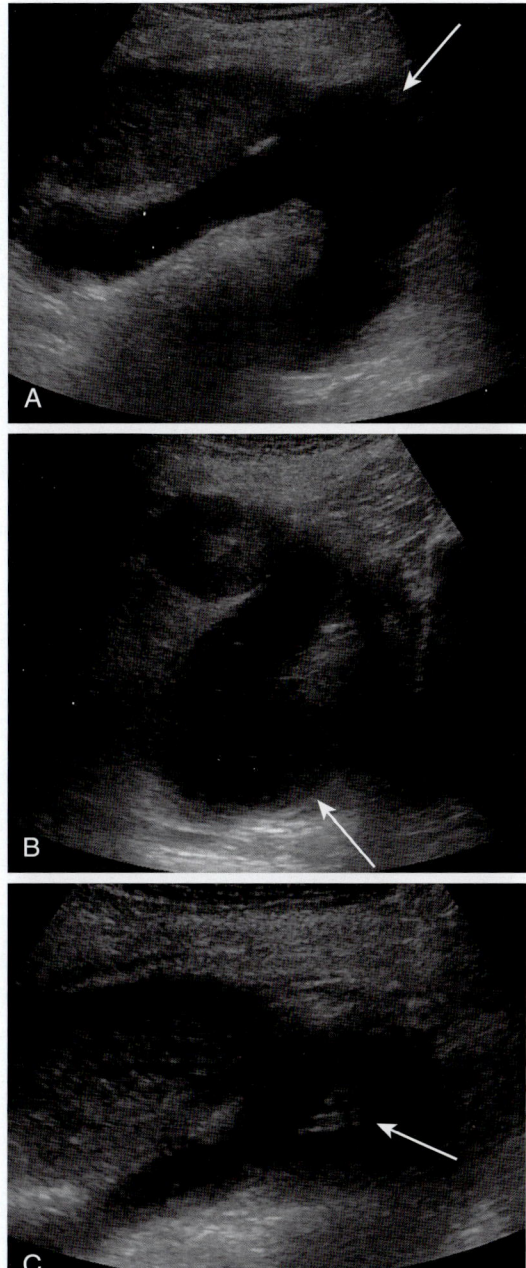

FIG. 20.52 Lymphocele. (A) Longitudinal gray-scale ultrasound shows a fluid collection with minimal debris. (B) Transverse gray-scale ultrasound shows a fluid collection with minimal debris. (C) Ultrasound-guided drain placement within the recurrent lymphocele.

the pancreas is repacked and placed on ice containing UW solution while awaiting transplantation.

Before vascular clamps are placed, the patient receives intravenous heparin. An end-to-side anastomosis is created between the donor portal vein and the recipient common iliac vein and IVC confluence. An end-to-side anastomosis is created between the common channel of the iliac Y graft and the common iliac artery of the recipient using continuous sutures. The clamps are released and the pancreas is reperfused. The surgeon will carefully look at the anastomosis sites and check for bleeding. If bleeding points are identified, they are controlled using sutures. The pancreas is then laid underneath the colon. A side-to-side anastomosis is fashioned between the terminal ileum and the allograft duodenum using sutures for the outer and inner layers. If needed, a drain may be placed near the pancreas bed. Once hemostasis has been achieved, the muscular fascia is closed with running sutures, and the skin is closed using staples (Fig. 20.57). Sponge, needle, and instrument counts are conducted before closure. If indicated, the patient will receive units of blood, platelets, or fresh frozen plasma. The wound is dressed with a dry sterile dressing, and the patient is extubated and transferred to the recovery room and later moved into the ICU when stable.

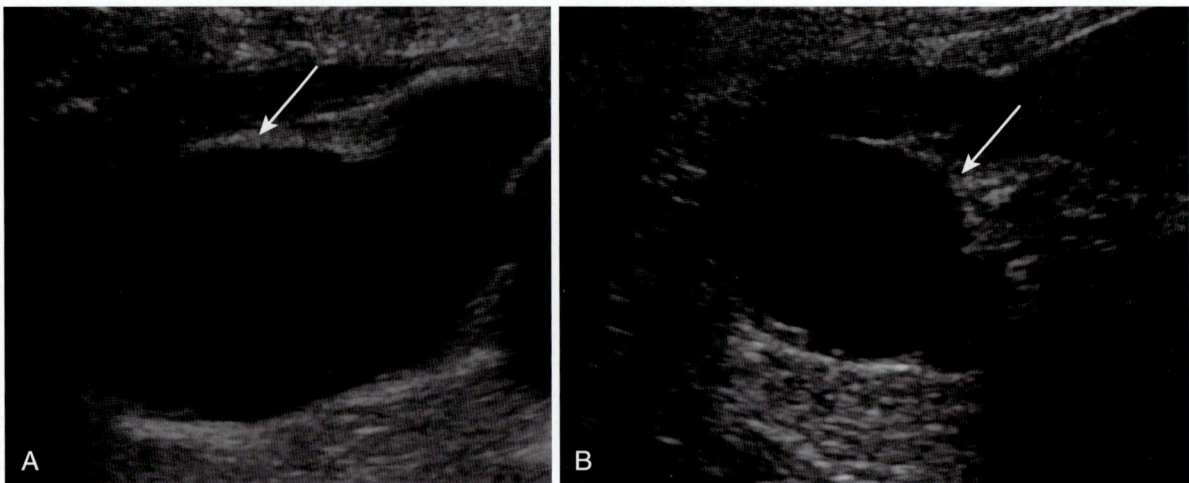

FIG. 20.53 Urinoma. (A) Longitudinal gray-scale ultrasound shows a simple fluid collection with no debris or septations. (B) Transverse gray-scale ultrasound shows a simple fluid collection medial to the transplant.

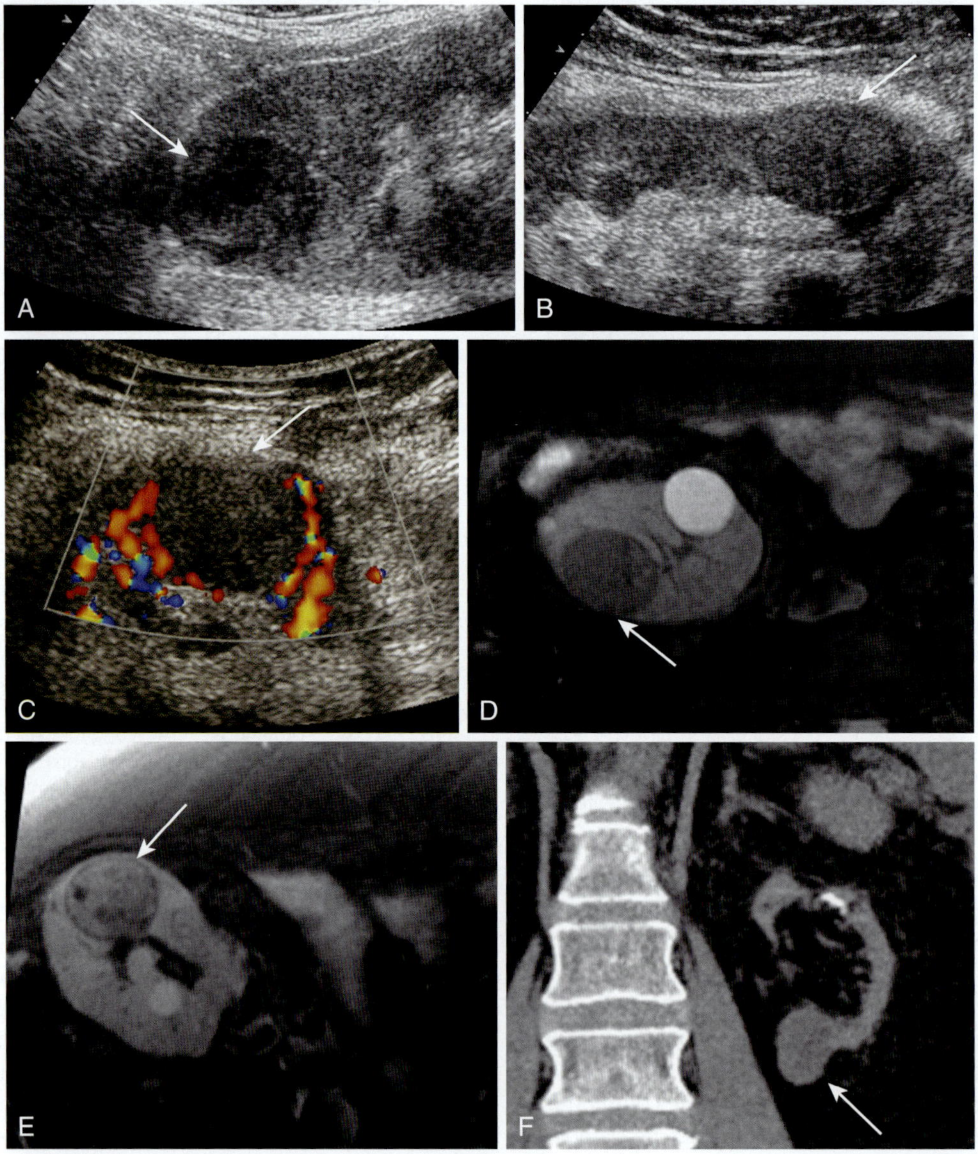

FIG. 20.54 Renal cell carcinoma. (A) Longitudinal gray-scale ultrasound shows an upper pole solid hypoechoic mass. (B) A lower pole solid mass is also seen on longitudinal gray-scale ultrasound. (C) Color Doppler ultrasound shows splaying of vascularity around one of the masses. (D) Magnetic resonance imaging (MRI) shows the upper pole mass. (E) The lower pole mass is visualized on MRI. (F) After metastatic renal cell carcinoma was found in the renal transplant, computed tomography showed a suspicious solid mass within the left native kidney on the lower pole.

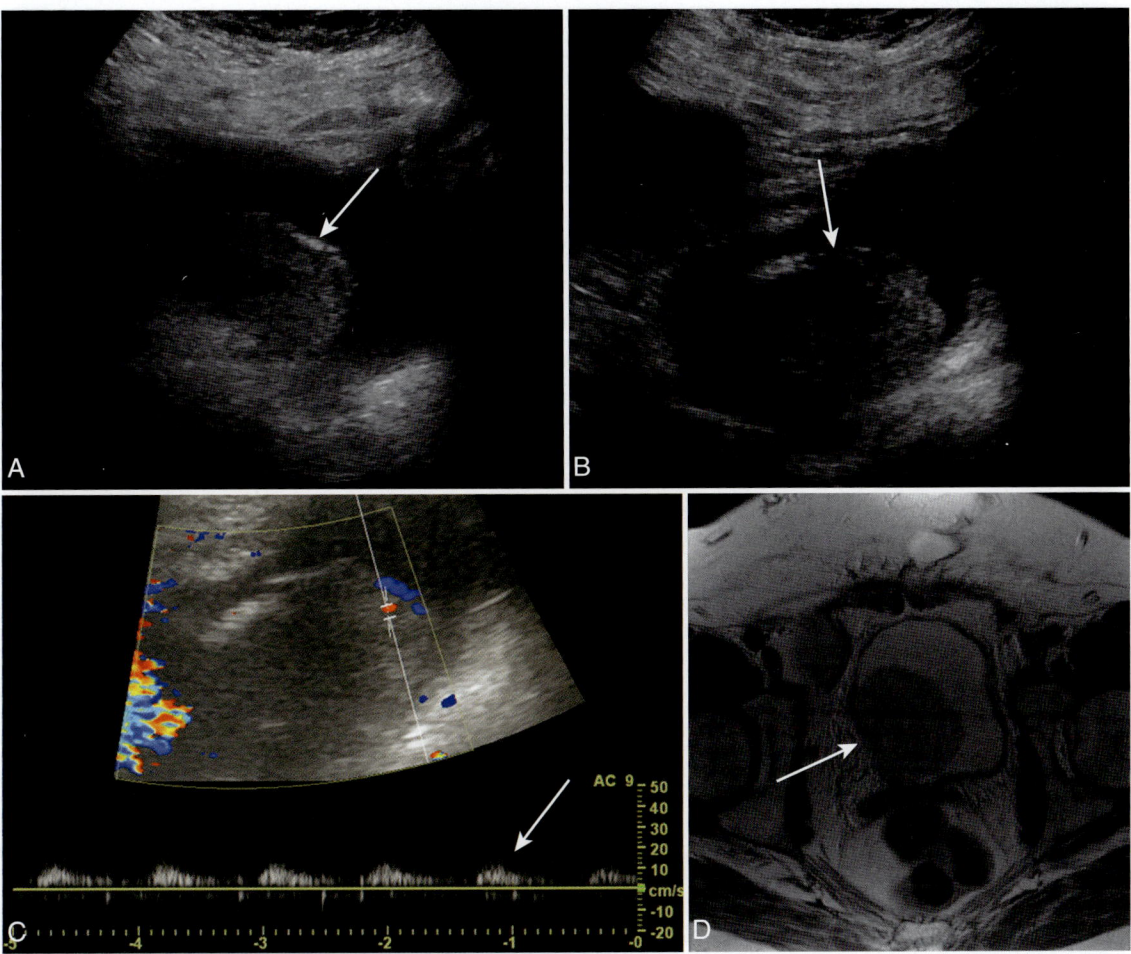

FIG. 20.55 Transitional cell carcinoma. (A) Transverse gray-scale ultrasound shows a solid hypoechoic mass with irregular borders within the bladder. (B) Longitudinal gray-scale ultrasound of the solid bladder mass. (C) Spectral Doppler ultrasound shows arterial vascular flow within the mass. (D) Magnetic resonance imaging shows a large mass adhering to the bladder wall.

Pancreatic Islet Cell Transplantation. Islet cells can be transplanted using minimally invasive techniques versus a full pancreatic organ transplant, allowing lower morbidity rates. Clinical trials have demonstrated restoration of the beta islet cell function and subsequent insulin production to regulate the blood glucose. For an autotransplant, islet cells are retrieved from the patient and a pancreatectomy is performed due to chronic pain such as pancreatitis or, rarely, trauma. For an allotransplant, the islet cells come from a donor. These cells are isolated and purified and then the islet cell clusters are infused into the hepatic sinusoids using a catheter in the portal vein. There is risk of portal vein thrombosis during this procedure. Posttransplant limitations include not being able to image these patients to determine function. These patients are monitored by checking blood glucose level, renal function, lipid levels, and liver function.[41] There were 471 patients who received islet cell transplants from 1999 to 2004.[42]

Evaluation of the Pancreatic Allograft

The pancreas transplant is evaluated by the sonographer as a native pancreas would be, but with some additional Doppler imaging. Assessing the echotexture and vasculature and looking for any masses, fluid collections, or ascites are important. Institutions have their own routine protocols on timing of examinations and specific images that are required.

Once the patient has arrived at the recovery room from the surgical suite, the sonographer will go portably to perform the immediate postoperative examination. The patient's amylase, lipase, and glucose are closely monitored and if any issues arise, the transplant physicians will tailor their imaging requests. These blood values are evaluated weekly for the first 2 months, then every other week for 4 months, then monthly for 1 year, then every 3 months. The patient usually only has a follow-up ultrasound if the patient is symptomatic or develops surgical complications.

It is best to image using a 2.5- to 5.0-MHz curvilinear transducer and have the patient fasting 4 to 6 hours. Obese patients will require lower frequencies. The pancreatic transplant is placed in either the right or left lower quadrant and typically superficial. As a result, higher-frequency transducers are most commonly used. Breath holding is usually not necessary as respiratory motion is limited. Depending on location, rolling the patient left lateral decubitus or right lateral decubitus will help move overlying bowel or bring the pancreas to a more superficial position in the obese patient.

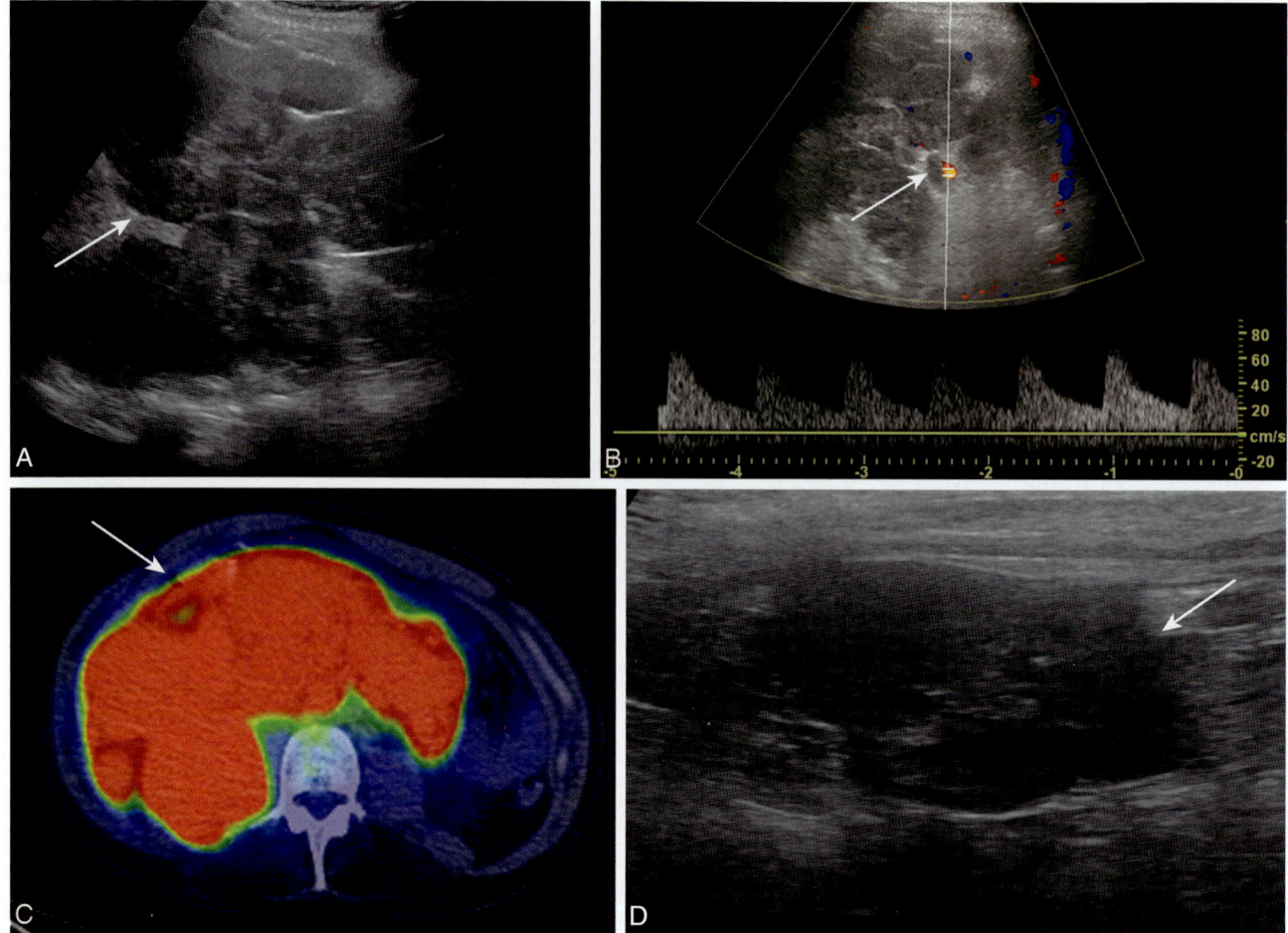

FIG. 20.56 **Posttransplant lymphoproliferative disease.** (A) Transverse gray-scale ultrasound shows a large solid mass with irregular margins in the right lower quadrant. (B) Spectral Doppler ultrasound shows arterial blood flow within the mass. (C) Positron emission tomography/computed tomography shows a large mass with fluorodeoxyglucose-avid uptake in the right lower quadrant. (D) Longitudinal gray-scale ultrasound shows an overall decreased size of the mass after chemotherapy treatment.

Most of these patients are very thin due to type 1 diabetes and obesity is less likely to be a problem.

The sonographer should scan completely through the pancreas before taking any images while adjusting the frequency, depth, gain, TGCs, and focal zones. Once the pancreatic transplant has been fully accessed, the examination needs to include a few representative gray-scale longitudinal images. Gray-scale transverse images of the upper, middle, and lower thirds also need to be obtained. Document any pathology in two planes with and without measurements and include color Doppler flow. Quadrant images need to be obtained checking for free fluid or signs of bleeding.

The Doppler portion is crucial for the transplanted pancreas. Venous and arterial color and spectral Doppler needs to be obtained looking for any signs of thrombus or stenosis. Ultrasound is commonly the first method of imaging in these patients, and the skilled sonographer can help the physicians diagnose the patient and treatment will be administered quickly. Color Doppler and power Doppler should be used to ensure adequate perfusion throughout the pancreatic tissue (Fig. 20.58). The intraparenchymal arteries and veins within the pancreas are evaluated in the upper, middle, and lower thirds. The sonographer should obtain an RI measurement using the peak systolic and end-diastolic velocities on these arterial waveforms. This is a common indirect Doppler technique to evaluate the arterial and venous flow. Angle correction is not necessary while obtaining the RI. Adjusting the sweep speed will spread the waveform over a period of 2 to 3 seconds, which will help magnify a particular part of your waveform for better interrogation and a more accurate measurement. A low RI is a strong indicator of a proximal stenosis that might not otherwise be able to be identified. A high RI may indicate rejection or venous congestion. Color images of the pancreatic artery and pancreatic vein should be included. Adjusting the color scale appropriately will help identify the highest velocities. When evaluating the pancreatic artery, it is critical to angle correct with pulsed-wave Doppler to accurately assess for stenosis. Spectral Doppler with velocity measurements in the distal, mid, proximal pancreatic artery and at the anastomosis between the iliac artery and pancreatic artery should also be included. The iliac artery and vein at the anastomosis and proximal to it should be evaluated and documented with spectral Doppler as well. If color flow aliasing in the pancreatic vein or iliac vein is visualized, angle correcting

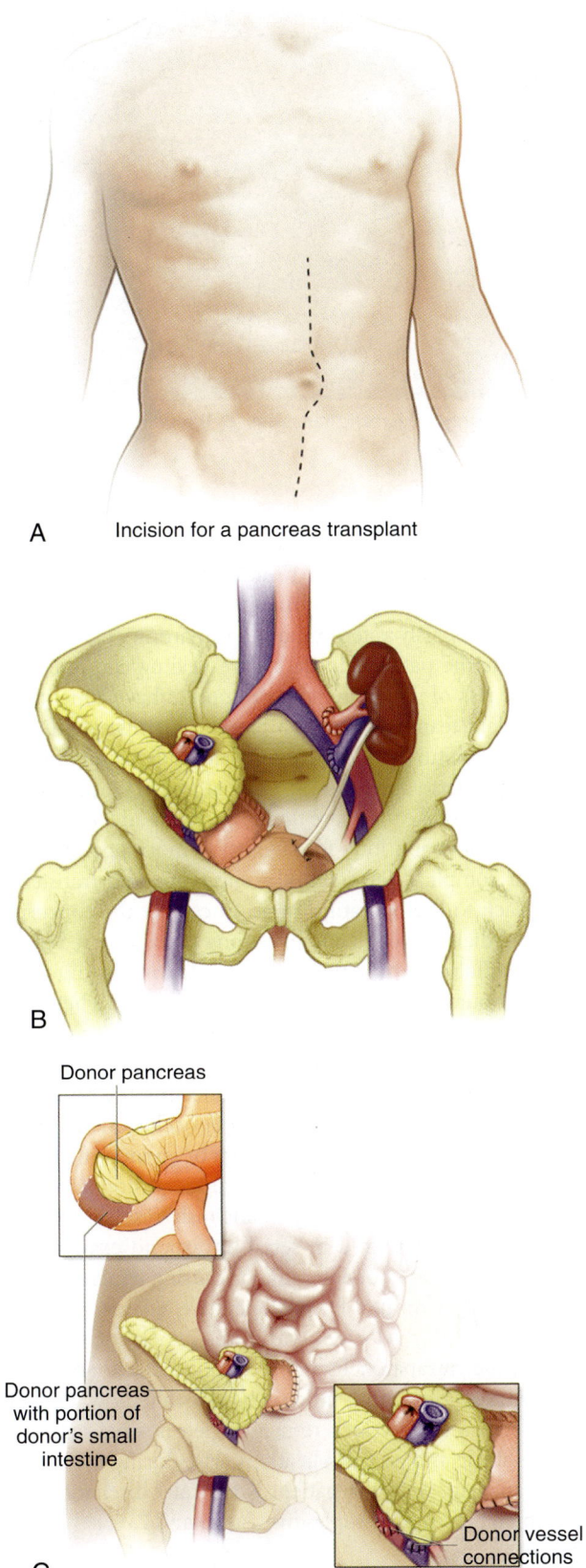

FIG. 20.57 **Surgical technique of pancreatic transplantation.** (A) Incision site. (B) The pancreas transplant is shown in relation to a possible combined renal transplant demonstrating the anastomoses sites. (C) The pancreas transplant anastomoses are demonstrated. (Courtesy Mayo Foundation for Medical Education and Research.)

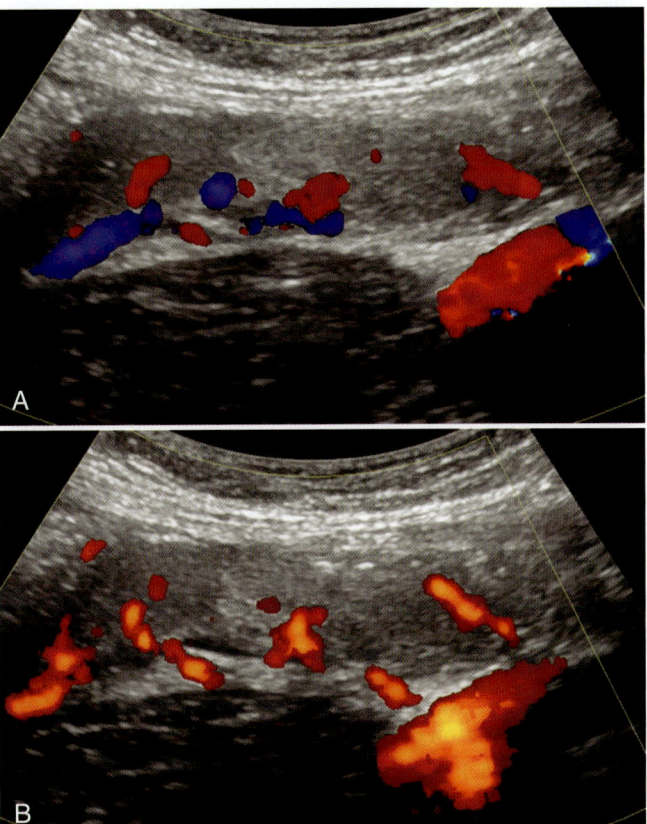

FIG. 20.58 **Pancreatic parenchymal perfusion.** (A) Normal perfusion using color Doppler ultrasound. (B) Power Doppler ultrasound shows adequate perfusion.

during your spectral Doppler images is important and will be helpful in identifying a focal narrowing. For all spectral Doppler, the angle should be parallel to the vessel that is being sampled and less than 60 degrees to ensure an accurate velocity measurement. The CFA should be documented to ensure adequate flow to the leg. All of the waveforms should fill the spectral window while eliminating aliasing.

Slow flow may be present within the vessels, and this can make it difficult to obtain a Doppler signal at times. The sonographer should try decreasing the color Doppler scale, and increasing the color gain. Using a slow flow setting such as a lower extremity vein or iliac vein model can be very useful if available on the ultrasound machine. The renal artery setting can also be helpful filling in the vessels as well. If the very slow frequencies are rejected as "cluttered noise," the wall filter needs to be decreased. If the patient is obese, decreasing the gray scale, color, and spectral Doppler frequencies will enable deeper penetration.

Normal Sonographic Findings of the Pancreatic Transplant

On gray-scale imaging, the pancreas parenchyma should appear homogeneous and hypoechoic relative to the mesenteric fat. The pancreas will appear different from the native organ and typically has a "blob" appearance, and the borders

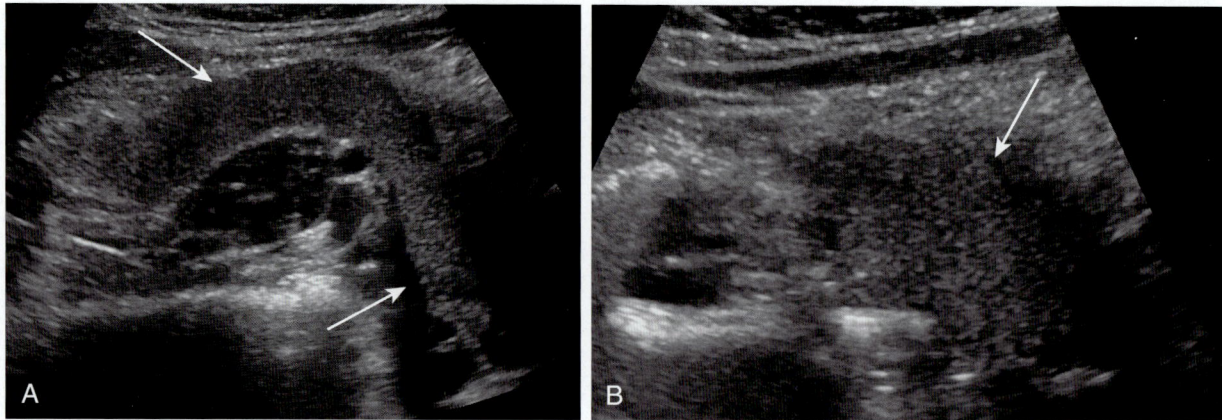

FIG. 20.59 **Normal pancreas.** (A) Longitudinal gray-scale ultrasound shows a normal-appearing pancreatic transplant. (B) Transverse gray-scale ultrasound shows normal pancreatic tissue separate from the neighboring bowel loops.

can be difficult to visualize at times. The bowel can be confused with the transplant at times and looking for peristalsis can help differentiate (Fig. 20.59). The pancreatic duct is usually not visualized unless it is abnormally dilated. The duct should measure less than 3 mm. See Chapter 12 for a more detailed explanation of the normal pancreatic anatomy.

The Doppler portion of the transplanted pancreas examination is crucial to perform. Some vascular complications can only be diagnosed using color and spectral Doppler. The pancreatic artery (Y graft of SMA and splenic artery) will be red on color imaging bringing flow into the pancreas, and the spectral waveform demonstrates a rapid systolic upstroke with continuous diastolic flow above baseline demonstrating a low-resistance waveform. The velocities should be below 200 cm/sec. A normal RI in the intraparenchymal artery should be below 0.80. The pancreatic vein drains the pancreas showing flow below the baseline with a blue color. The spectral waveforms of the intraparenchymal, pancreatic, and iliac veins have continuous monophasic flow with minimal respiratory changes. The iliac artery and CFA should demonstrate a classic triphasic waveform with spectral Doppler imaging. When measuring velocities using spectral Doppler imaging, turbulent flow or doubling or tripling of velocities in a vessel should not be seen as it indicates potential focal stenosis (Fig. 20.60).

Pancreatic Allograft Imaging in the Immediate Postoperative Period

It is imperative to image the newly transplanted pancreas in the immediate postoperative period. Ultrasound is the initial modality of choice. There is no ionizing radiation and the cost is relatively inexpensive compared with CT or MRI. These patients will be closely monitored and scanned routinely so there will be no delay in treatment if needed. A skilled sonographer provides early detection of transplant complications and prevents misdiagnosis.

The patient will be in the recovery unit while the general anesthesia is wearing off during the initial ultrasound examination. These patients will not be able to roll onto their side or help assist with breathing techniques if needed. Sometimes the patient may be confused or combative. Reassure your patient that surgery is over and the patient is recovering. The patient's dressings should be removed to help attain the best imaging windows possible and prevent missing pathology. Even though this is not necessarily a sterile scanning environment, using sterile gel while the patient's incisions are healing can potentially reduce the risk of infection. It is common to have a member of the transplant team or a surgeon present for this examination. This is very helpful to the sonographer to understand the surgical technique performed and variant anatomy of the patient. The physician would like to ensure the allograft has adequate arterial and venous flow and look for signs of hemorrhage. If there is an urgent complication noted, the surgeon could transfer the patient back to the operating room to correct the concerning issue immediately. Not all complications are considered urgent, and the radiologist may recommend a follow-up ultrasound within 24 hours to ensure stability or determine whether the issue has resolved or is getting worse. Urgent findings include, but are not limited to, the following: severe stenosis of the pancreatic artery or kinking of the vessel affecting the flow within the pancreatic parenchyma; thrombus or occlusion of the CFA, iliac artery, or pancreatic artery or vein; or an identified source of active bleeding. It is very common to see postoperative fluid collections and these usually spontaneously resolve. Fluid collections will be monitored in serial ultrasound examinations, making sure they are not enlarging or causing pancreatic function problems. Commonly, postoperative edema can create elevated blood flow velocities within the pancreatic artery and vein, and the intraparenchymal arteries can have an elevated RI as well, demonstrating little or no diastolic flow. Once the edema decreases, the vessels return to their normal state. If the patient is stable and no complications arise during the recovery in the transplant unit, the patient is typically discharged from the hospital between postoperative days 5 and 7.

Pancreatic Transplantation Complications in Routine Surveillance

It is common to perform routine protocol parenchymal biopsies around 4 months after transplantation followed by 1 year, 5 years, and 10 years. If the patient is symptomatic with pain and fever or has elevated amylase, lipase, or glucose, a biopsy

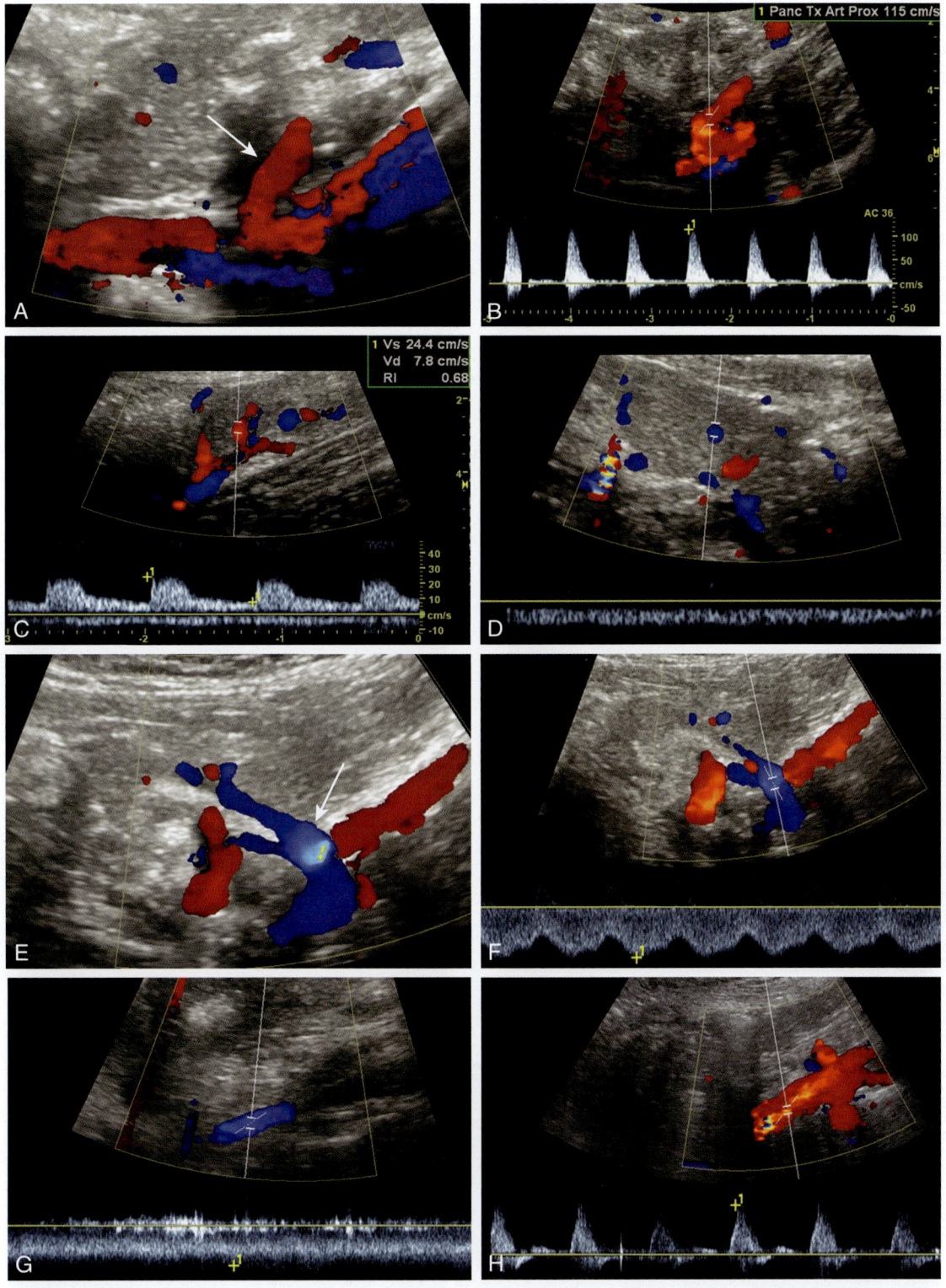

FIG. 20.60 Normal pancreas Doppler. (A) A widely patent pancreatic artery is identified without areas of aliasing or narrowing using color Doppler ultrasound. (B) Spectral Doppler ultrasound shows a normal high resistive waveform within the pancreatic artery without presence of an elevated velocity. (C) Spectral Doppler ultrasound of a normal waveform and resistive index (RI) within an intraparenchymal artery. (D) Spectral Doppler ultrasound of a normal monophasic waveform within an intraparenchymal vein. (E) Color Doppler ultrasound shows a normal pancreatic vein and anastomosis without evidence of aliasing or narrowing. (F) Spectral Doppler ultrasound shows a normal monophasic venous waveform within the pancreatic vein near the anastomosis. (G) The iliac vein seen on spectral Doppler ultrasound has a normal monophasic venous waveform. (H) The common femoral artery visualized on spectral Doppler ultrasound has a classic triphasic waveform.

may be ordered. If rejection is discovered from the pathology results, the patient will be treated with medication for 1 month and then another biopsy will take place to evaluate the treatment plan. If the patient clinically has pancreatitis, the biopsy will not be performed, as this could potentially aggravate the pancreatic tissue more (Fig. 20.61).

While performing these biopsies, there are potential risks of complications. Bleeding is the most common complication observed. The patient's INR and platelet counts are checked before the procedure and patients are asked to stop taking anticoagulants 3 to 5 days before the procedure. Elevated blood pressure or hypertension is an associated risk factor for bleeding. If the patient currently takes antihypertensive medication routinely, this should be taken as usual. Patients may become anxious about the procedure, thereby elevating the blood pressure. Pressures should not exceed 160/90 mm Hg. The radiologist or physician performing the biopsy may choose to administer mild to moderate sedation to help relax the patient, reducing these pressures. Bleeding may still occur after preventive measures are taken. You may see a hematoma form outside of the pancreatic tissue, and the patient may or may not develop pain. Usually bleeding will cease on its own after applying moderate pressure over the biopsy tract. If the bleeding is severe, the patient may become vasovagal and the blood pressure may drop. It is helpful to lower the head of the patient and give IV fluids as necessary. If there is an active bleed that cannot be controlled, the patient could be transferred to the interventional radiology department for further imaging and possible coil placement.

The biopsy needle is ultrasound guided to avoid major blood vessels and the pancreatic duct, although this can be difficult to visualize. At times the needle path may cross small vessels for a potential risk of creating an AVF, or damage to the duct can create a pancreatic leak forming a pseudocyst. The radiologist will aim away from the hilum of the pancreas and stay clear of the nearby bowel. If overlying bowel seems to be a problem, obtaining a biopsy using ultrasound guidance or CT may be beneficial to use for guidance by accurately visualizing the bowel (Fig. 20.62).

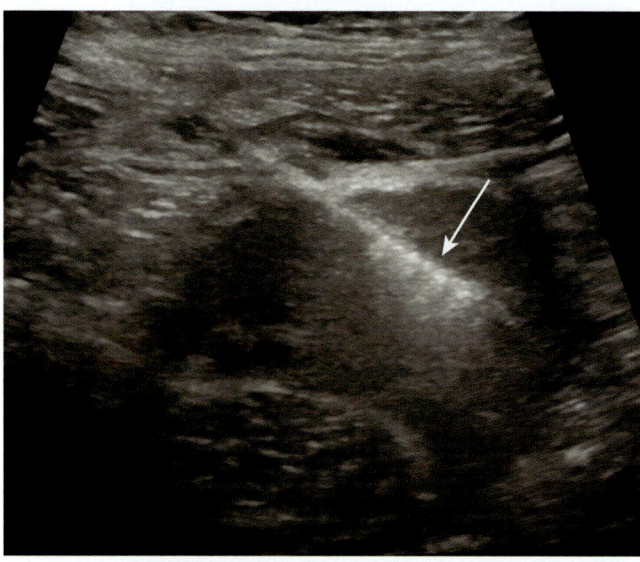

FIG. 20.61 **Routine pancreatic biopsy**. Ultrasound-guided needle biopsy staying clear of nearby bowel and pancreatic hilum.

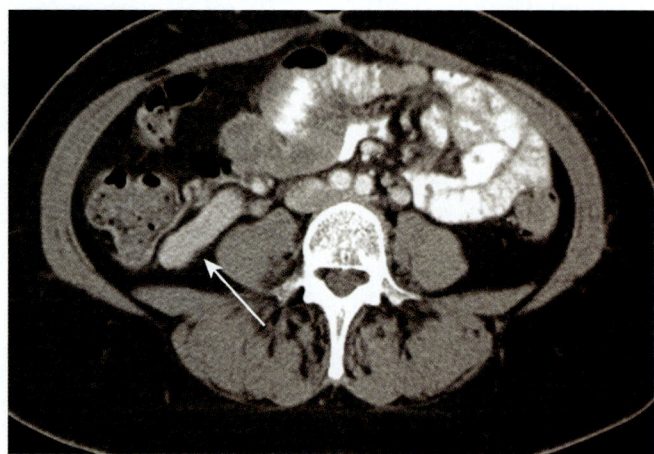

FIG. 20.62 Computed tomography (CT) imaging of the pancreas transplant covered by overlying bowel.

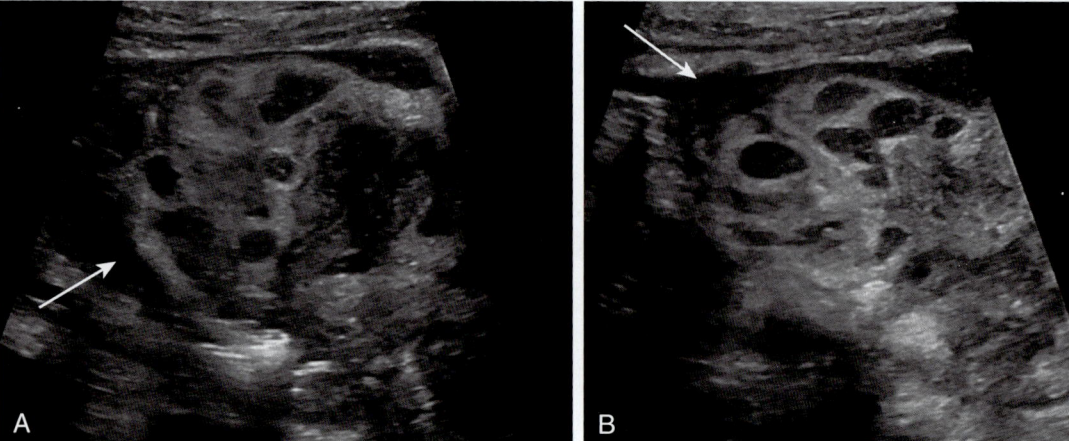

FIG. 20.63 **Acute rejection**. Transverse (A) and longitudinal (B) gray-scale ultrasound shows an enlarged pancreas with heterogeneous echotexture.

Pathology of the Pancreatic Transplant

Rejection. Rejection is the primary cause of allograft loss, occurring between 5% and 25% of the time. Hyperacute rejection is rare and occurs immediately postoperative and causes thrombosis and graft loss. Acute rejection usually occurs 1 to 3 weeks following transplantation. If left untreated, infarction may occur resulting from an autoimmune vasculitis. Chronic rejection is the major long-term cause of graft failure after the first 6 months, occurring in 4% to 10% of patients. It may be due to multiple episodes or partially treated acute rejection, resulting in fibrosis and atrophy of the pancreas. An elevation of serum glucose, amylase, and lipase poorly correlates with the severity of rejection. Ultrasound findings are nonspecific and may demonstrate pancreatic enlargement and a heterogeneous echotexture in the acute stages (Fig. 20.63). With chronic rejection, the pancreas is markedly atrophied and may not be visualized on ultrasound (Fig. 20.64). Percutaneous biopsy is required for diagnosis and grading either with ultrasound or CT guidance.[43]

Pancreatitis. Pancreatitis is the second most common complication following transplantation.[44] Within the first 4 weeks of transplantation, mild pancreatitis is present in about 35% of patients. This is usually caused from reperfusion injury. The patient may develop pain over the allograft, and elevated serum amylase and lipase are usually noted. Nonspecific ultrasound findings include pancreatic enlargement and heterogeneous echotexture. Ultrasound may visualize a pseudocyst, free fluid, infarction, or necrosis[43] (Fig. 20.65).

Infection and Abscesses. Infection at the surgical site occurs in 50% of patients. Superficial infections are more common and can be treated with antibiotics. Deep infections are associated with greater morbidity, mortality, and allograft loss. Percutaneous drain placement is the treatment of choice for localized abscesses. An infected collection may be filled with debris or presence of gas on ultrasound creating a "dirty" shadow.[43] Abscesses typically demonstrate thicker, irregular walls, and are associated with adjacent inflammatory tissue. At times, abscess formation may be associated with enteric leakage. Hyperemia may be present within the abscess wall or surrounding soft tissue using color Doppler.[45] It is sometimes difficult to determine the contents, and aspiration is beneficial for diagnosis and treatment. CT or MRI may also be helpful aiding in diagnosis[43] (Fig. 20.66).

Vascular Compromise

Pancreatic Venous and Arterial Thrombosis. Acute pancreatic transplant thrombosis occurs in 2% to 10% of patients and is more common on the venous side but can be visualized within the arterial system as well. Venous thrombosis is the second most common cause of allograft failure and is typically seen within the first 6 weeks following transplantation. Patients may present with elevated glucose and amylase, and note pain and swelling over the allograft. If detected early, the patient may be sent to the operating

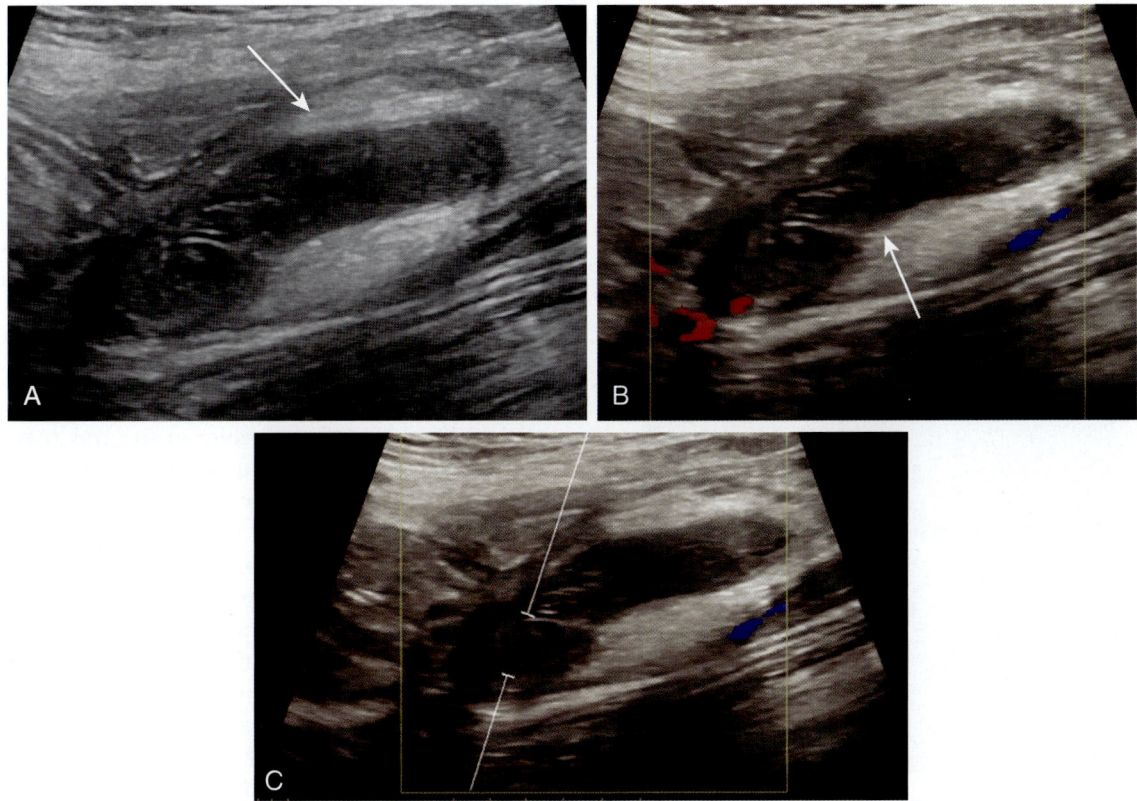

FIG. 20.64 Chronic rejection and failure. (A) Longitudinal gray-scale ultrasound shows an atrophic echogenic pancreas. (B) Color Doppler ultrasound shows no flow within the dilated pancreatic vein. (C) Absence of pancreatic venous flow is seen on spectral Doppler ultrasound.

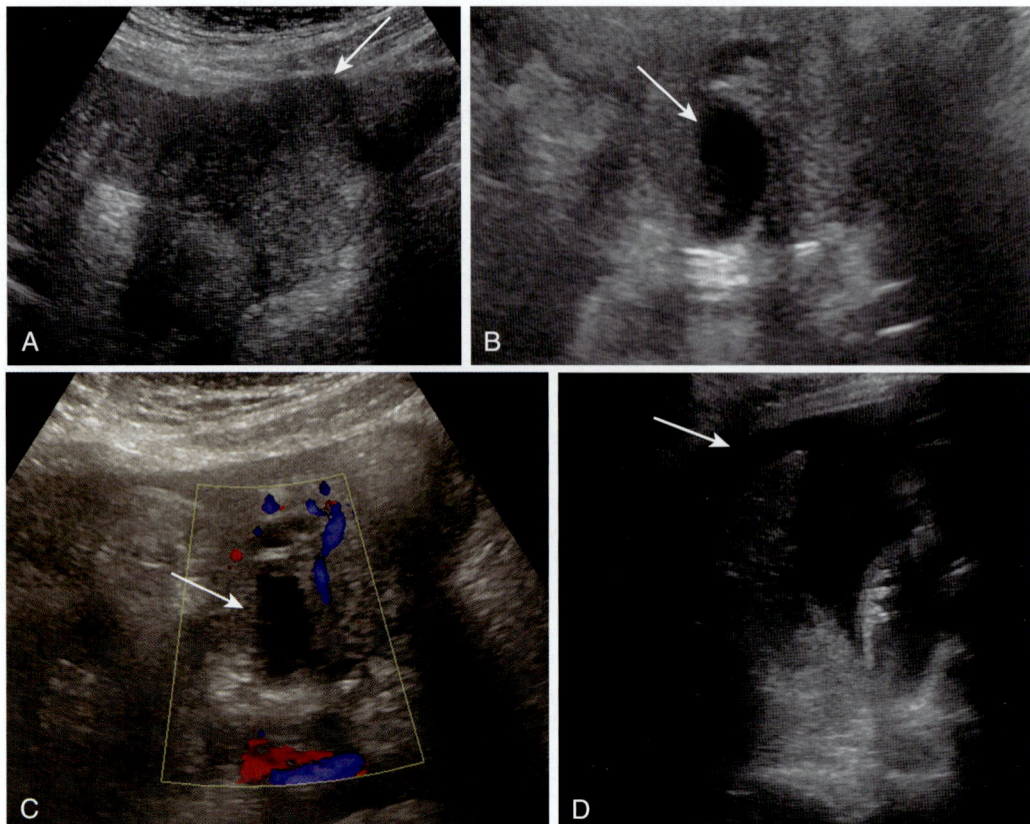

FIG. 20.65 **Pancreatitis with elevated amylase and lipase levels.** Longitudinal gray-scale ultrasound shows mild enlargement of the inhomogeneous pancreas (A) and a small fluid collection representing a pseudocyst (B). (C) Color Doppler ultrasound shows no vascular flow within the collection. (D) Gray-scale ultrasound shows new abdominal ascites.

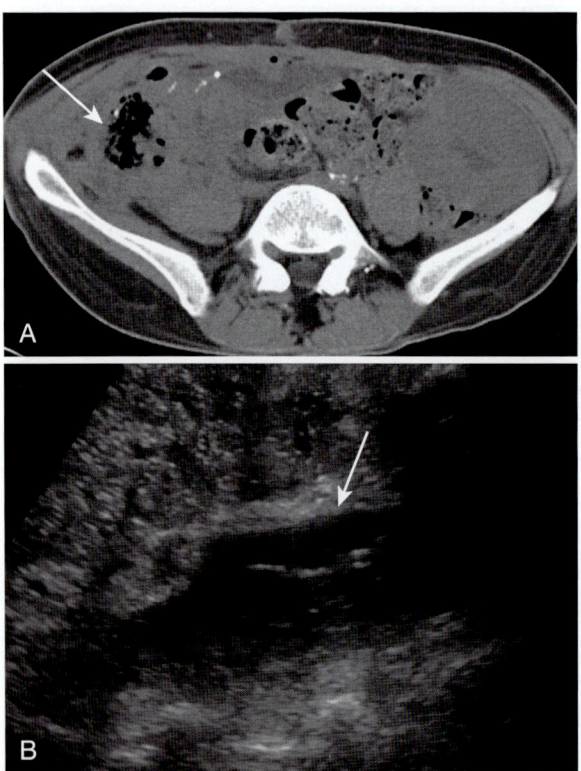

FIG. 20.66 **Abscess.** (A) Computed tomographic imaging shows an infected collection near the pancreas transplant. (B) Gray-scale ultrasound shows the drainage catheter within the abscess.

room to attempt to salvage the pancreas. Thrombectomy and thrombolysis are limited treatment options to short segments of thrombosis without developing necrosis. Some risk factors of thrombosis include severe pancreatitis, arterial wall injury, or superior mesenteric and splenic arterial and venous stump thrombus. Stump thrombus may be incidental and usually does not interfere with pancreatic function. If treatment is not successful or the thrombosis is found too late in the disease process, extensive thrombosis can lead to necrosis requiring an emergent pancreatectomy to reduce the risk of infection and mortality. With an arterial occlusion, collateral vessels may develop, preserving the tissue and function. Echogenic thrombus filling the vessel lumen with no flow identified on color or spectral imaging is demonstrated using ultrasound. With the presence of venous thrombosis, the arterial waveforms usually demonstrate high resistance with reversal in diastole (Figs. 20.67 and 20.68). If necrosis and infarction develop, the pancreas will be enlarged and hypoechoic with lack of blood flow. The pancreas may become atrophic and echogenic with chronic thrombosis and may be difficult to visualize on ultrasound. CTA or MRA may be beneficial aiding in diagnosis when the ultrasound remains inconclusive.[43]

Pancreatic Arterial and Venous Stenosis. Stenosis may uncommonly develop at the pancreatic arterial or venous anastomoses sites. Many patients are found to have peripheral vascular disease. As a result, inflow may be compromised

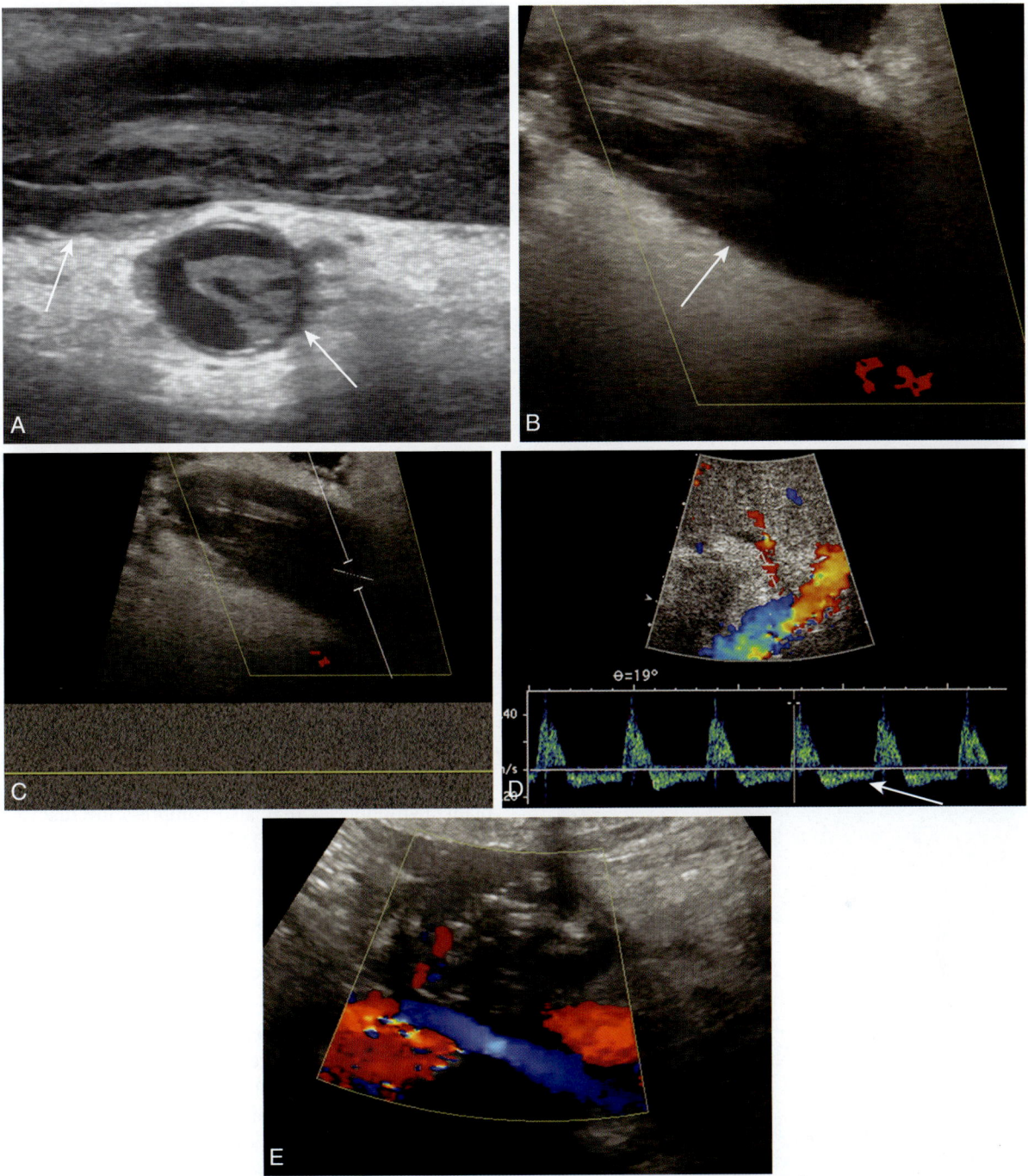

FIG. 20.67 Pancreatic venous and arterial thrombus. (A) Intraoperative gray-scale ultrasound shows thrombus within the longitudinal vein and transverse of the artery. (B) Intraoperative color Doppler shows absence of flow within the pancreatic vein. (C) Intraoperative spectral Doppler shows no venous flow present. (D) Spectral Doppler ultrasound of the pancreatic artery shows reversal of diastolic flow consistent with pancreatic vein thrombus or occlusion. (E) Color Doppler ultrasound could not identify a pancreatic vein.

due to a proximal stenosis. If a stenosis is identified, balloon angioplasty and stenting may be performed. The artery or vein may kink or twist on itself. As with other transplants, it is common to see elevated velocities in the immediate postoperative examination due to edema. On ultrasound, assess for color flow aliasing and turbulence with velocity measurement doubling on spectral Doppler[43] (Fig. 20.69).

Pseudoaneurysms. A pseudoaneurysm is a focal disruption of the artery with no direct communication with a vein and can occur in any vessel. On ultrasound, it appears as a round cystic structure and demonstrates disorganized "yin-yang" color flow within. On spectral Doppler imaging, a to-and-fro waveform is typically seen. These complications are rare and can be due to surgical technique, infection, pancreatitis, or biopsy. A pseudoaneurysm is typically asymptomatic but may be associated with a high risk of bleeding and allograft loss. Treatment depends on size and location and most can usually be followed

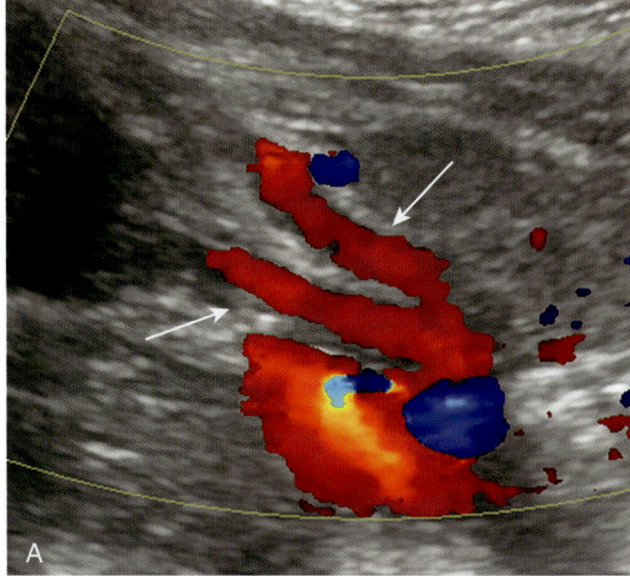
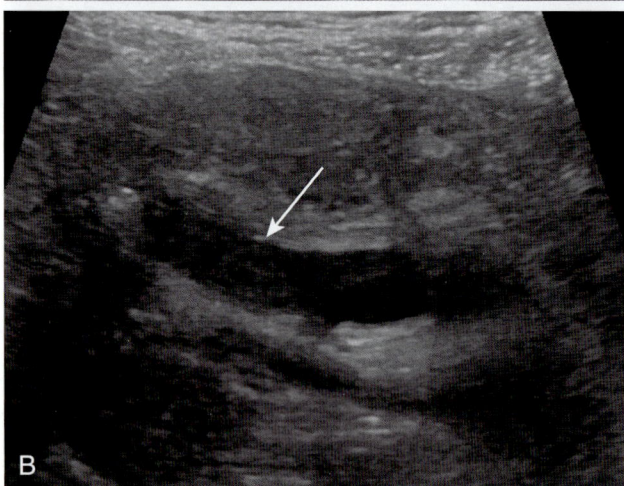
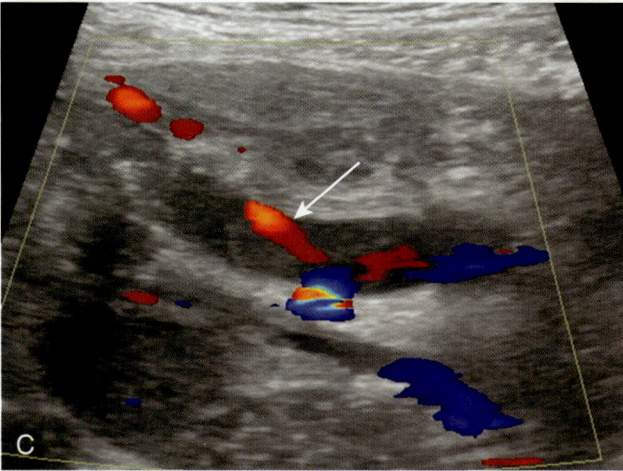

FIG. 20.68 **Pancreatic artery stump thrombus.** (A) Color Doppler ultrasound shows the normal branches, superior mesenteric artery (SMA), and splenic artery of the Y graft. (B) Gray-scale ultrasound shows arterial thrombus in the blind end of the SMA or splenic artery. (C) Color Doppler ultrasound shows the incomplete filling of blood flow within the stump of the branch.

conservatively. Some cases may require surgical or interventional treatments.[32,43]

Fluid Collections

Bleeding and Hematomas. Fluid collections are the most common complication following pancreatic transplantation, with the most common being a hematoma. Fresh hematomas usually appear echogenic with well-defined borders and absence of blood flow. Over a period of time, the hematoma may develop debris and septations and then liquefy, becoming anechoic. Hematomas typically spontaneously resolve without treatment. Percutaneous drain placement may only be needed when the collection is proven infectious by obtaining a diagnostic aspiration. CT or MRI may also be helpful aiding in diagnosis.[45]

Seromas. Seromas are clear, serous fluid collections that are usually found within the first few days of transplantation, being most common along the vascular anastomoses sites. Usually seromas will resolve spontaneously within a few weeks. If there is concern that it is part of an infectious process or creating a mass effect and compressing vasculature, an aspiration may be performed. A seroma is described as a round, localized, anechoic, thin-walled fluid collection, which may contain debris or septations found on ultrasound imaging. Fluid collections are easily identified on ultrasound, but not specific determining the contents. CT or MRI can be very helpful in differentiating the collections.[13,45]

Lymphoceles. A surgical disruption of lymphatic channels causes lymph fluid leakage into the soft tissue space, creating a lymphocele. These are typically found medial to the transplant. Lymphoceles may also compress the iliac or femoral vein causing leg edema.[33] Debris or septations within the fluid collection may be visualized on ultrasound. Ultrasound is very sensitive to diagnose a fluid collection but not specific of the contents because blood, pus, lymph, and serosanguineous fluid appear very similar. CT or MRI is helpful in differentiating the collections.[13,45] Spontaneous resolution is rare, and treatment is required. Percutaneous drain placement along with sclerotherapy has been shown to have a 97% success rate. The risk of infection increases with each aspiration and may require a drain placement along with antibiotic medications. Lymphoceles commonly recur after a simple aspiration and ultimately may need surgical repair.[33]

Pancreatic Fistulas and Pseudocysts. Following pancreatic transplantation, fistulas or leakage has been reported in as many as 30.8% of cases. This may be related to ischemia-reperfusion injury and usually does not significantly impair allograft function or survival.[46] A pseudocyst may ultimately develop. Pseudocysts may be caused from multiple episodes of pancreatitis and are usually found within the pancreatic parenchyma or surrounding tissues. Abscess formation may be a complication related to the pseudocyst, but usually has a simple appearance. On ultrasound, pseudocysts appear anechoic, with well-defined borders and thin walls with occasionally layering debris[13,45] (Fig. 20.70).

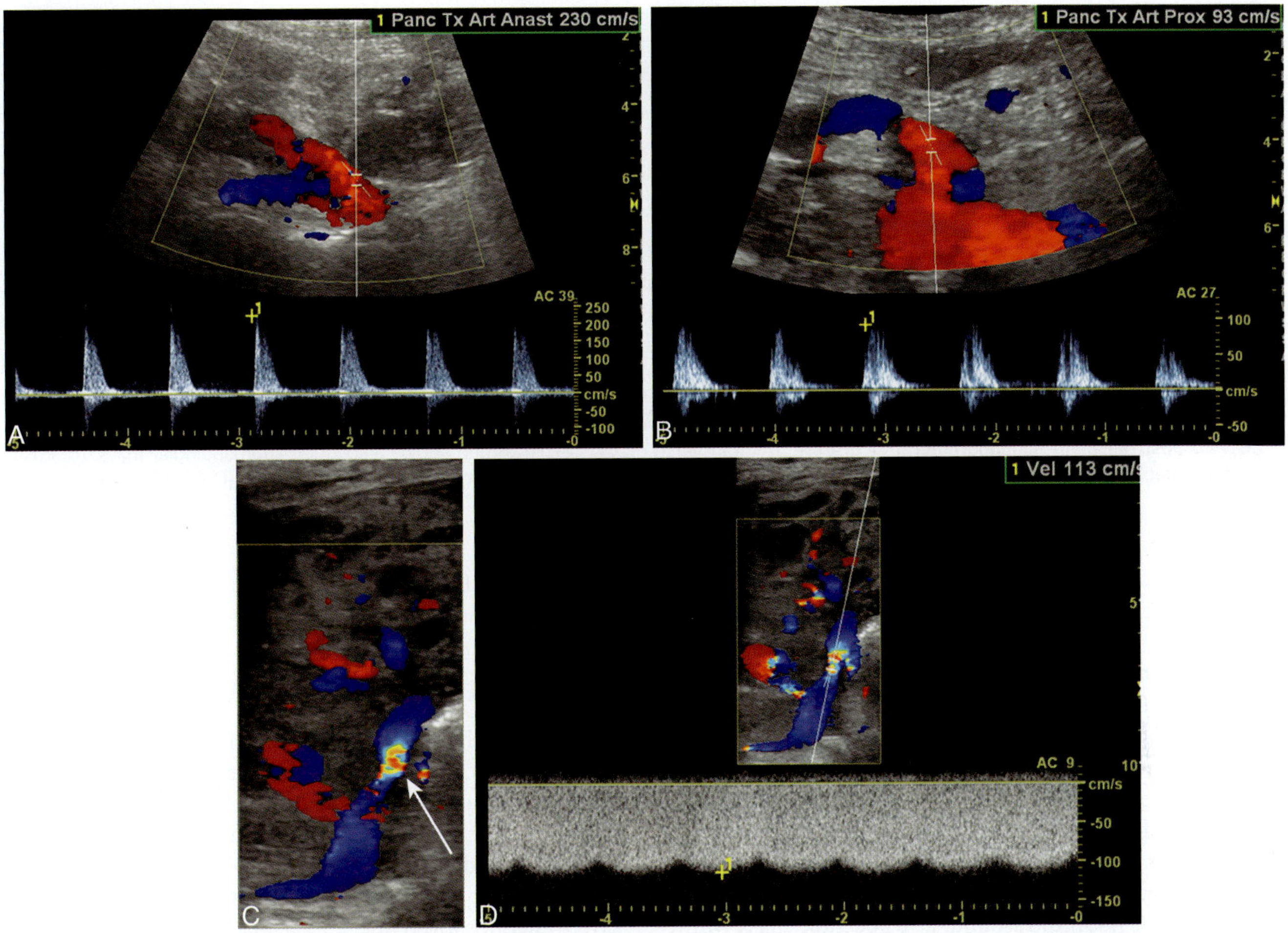

FIG. 20.69 **Pancreatic artery and vein stenosis**. (A) Spectral Doppler ultrasound shows elevated velocities near the anastomosis likely due to postoperative edema. (B) Spectral Doppler follow-up ultrasound shows the velocities decreased over a period of time. (C) Color Doppler ultrasound shows aliasing identifying a narrowing within the pancreatic vein. (D) Elevated velocities are documented near the anastomosis site of the pancreatic vein on spectral Doppler ultrasound.

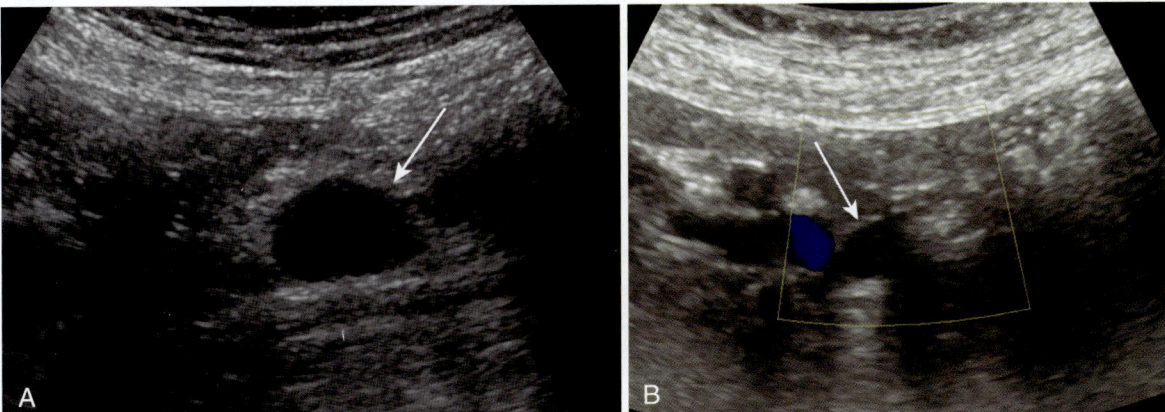

FIG. 20.70 **Pseudocyst**. (A) Transverse gray-scale ultrasound shows an anechoic cystic area with some debris within and posterior acoustic enhancement. (B) Color Doppler ultrasound shows absence of flow within the pseudocyst.

Cysts. As technology advancements continue to improve, pancreatic cystic neoplasms are now found more frequently. A subset of pancreatic cystic neoplasms has been shown to have malignant potential. Studies that have used CT and MRI to identify these cysts have reported that 2.5% of the population have them and are asymptomatic and incidentally noted. Ten percent of people 70 years or older have a pancreatic cyst. Some cysts may be observed over time to ensure stability, or some patients may undergo fine-needle aspiration and/or surgical resection. Most cysts are anechoic and thin walled, with well-defined borders and posterior acoustic enhancement with some containing debris and no vascular flow

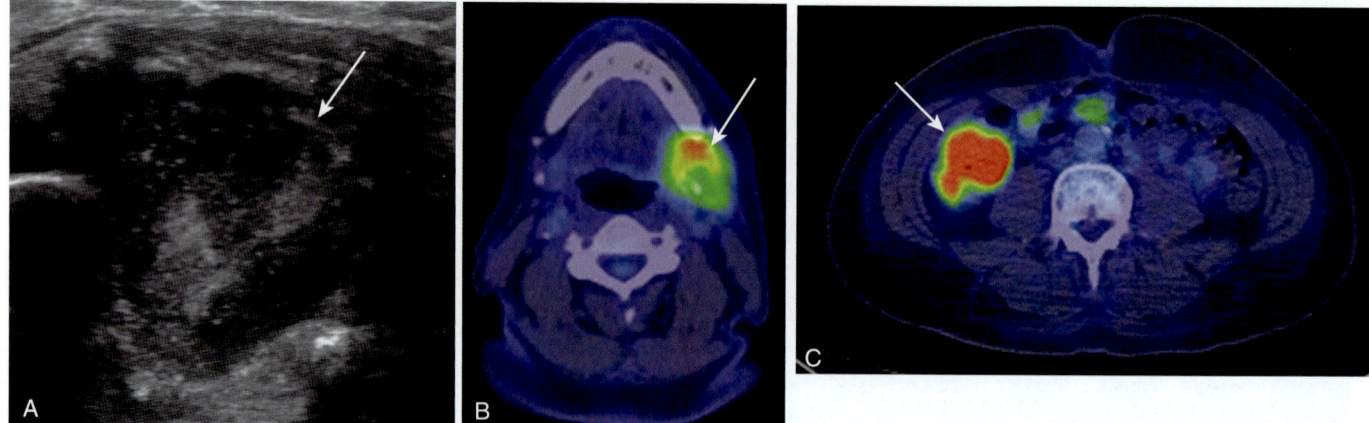

FIG. 20.71 **Posttransplant lymphoproliferative disease.** (A) Transverse gray-scale ultrasound shows a solid left submandibular mass. (B) Positron emission tomography/computed tomography (PET/CT) demonstrates a left submandibular fluorodeoxyglucose-avid mass. (C) PET/CT also shows colon involvement.

within on ultrasound imaging. A concerning cystic lesion would contain mural nodules or solid components with vascularity noted.[47]

Pancreatic Adenocarcinoma. Pancreatic adenocarcinoma is the fourth most common cause of cancer-related deaths with only 5% of patients surviving 5 years. The only treatment is complete resection of the tumor with less than 20% having a possible cure on new diagnosis. Unfortunately, many patients do not develop symptoms until the later stages of disease when metastases are already present. Early detection is essential with various imaging modalities, including ultrasound, MRI, or CT. On ultrasound, a hypoechoic mass with pancreatic ductal dilation is very suspicious for pancreatic adenocarcinoma. Unfortunately, ultrasound has a low sensitivity (50% to 90%) for detecting these lesions in the native pancreas.[48]

Posttransplant Lymphoproliferative Disorder. PTLD occurs in 1% to 20% of patients who receive a transplant.[22] In one study, PTLD was found to occur in 6.1% of pancreas transplant patients diagnosed between 1.3 months and 6.1 years.[49] PTLD is the most severe complication found in solid organ and stem cell transplantation. Patients who are on long-term use of immunosuppressant medication have an increased risk of malignancies 2 to 5 times more than the general population. PTLD can be in the form of benign tissue hyperplasia or present as malignant lymphoma. Most polymorphic masses are caused from the EBV, occurring 60% to 80% and within 1 year of transplantation. Most of the monomorphic masses are found to be non-Hodgkin lymphoma and have B-cell origin. In 23% to 50% of cases, treatment has been shown to be successful in the EBV patients by reducing the immunosuppressants. Patients have better outcomes when diagnosed in the early stages of PTLD. Immunotherapy with monoclonal antibodies such as rituximab may be given to patients as another treatment option with a 40% to 68% success rate.[22] PTLD can occur in any solid organ or viscera.[32] In 39% to 40% of cases, PTLD involves the lymph nodes and liver, followed by the gastrointestinal tract in 33%, and it is considered rare to involve the pancreas itself (10%). On ultrasound imaging, PTLD usually appears as a hypoechoic soft tissue mass and demonstrates lymphadenopathy[43] (Fig. 20.71).

YOUR ROLE IN DONATING LIFE

This chapter should provide new insight into what receiving a transplant is like. It is a very long and challenging struggle with a failing organ in the hope you can live to see the next day. If you are interested in more information about becoming an organ donor or would like to share with others, visit donatelife.net. Please consider the gift of life and how you can save someone's loved one.

> **Key Pearls**
>
> - Transplant ultrasound requires specialized knowledge of transplant anatomy in order to detect pathology and monitor transplant viability.
> - A standardized protocol for how and when to image transplants is important for each institution to develop in collaboration with the transplant surgeons.
> - With the shortage of transplants, specialized imaging, of which ultrasound is the prime modality, is critical to maintaining healthy and viable transplants.

REFERENCES

1. Kamath PS, Kim WR. The model for end-stage liver disease (MELD). *Hepatology*. 2007;45(3):797–805.
2. Bachir NM, Larson AM. Adult liver transplantation in the United States. *Am J Med Sci*. 2012;343(6):462–469.
3. Kornberg A. Liver transplantation for hepatocellular carcinoma beyond Milan criteria: multidisciplinary approach to improve outcome. *ISRN Hepatol*. 2014;2014:25.
4. Meirelles Jr RF, Salvalaggio P, Rezende MB, et al. Liver transplantation: history, outcomes and perspectives. *Einstein (Sao Paulo)*. 2015;13(1):149–152.
5. Smith JM, Biggins SW, Haselby DG, et al. Kidney, pancreas and liver allocation and distribution in the United States. *Am J Transplant*. 2012;12(12):3191–3212.

6. Leeson S, Desai SP. Medical and ethical challenges during the first successful human kidney transplantation in 1954 at Peter Bent Brigham Hospital, Boston. *Anesth Analg.* 2015;120(1):239–245.
7. Han DJ, Sutherland DE. Pancreas transplantation. *Gut Liver.* 2010;4(4):450–465.
8. Hampson FA, Freeman SJ, Ertner J, et al. Pancreatic transplantation: surgical technique, normal radiological appearances and complications. *Insights Imaging.* 2010;1(5-6):339–347.
9. Fridell JA, Powelson JA, Kubal CA, et al. Retrieval of the pancreas allograft for whole-organ transplantation. *Clin Transplant.* 2014;28(12):1313–1330.
10. Maglione M, Ploeg RJ, Friend PJ. Donor risk factors, retrieval technique, preservation and ischemia/reperfusion injury in pancreas transplantation. *Curr Opin Organ Transplant.* 2013;18(1):83–88.
11. Yang X, Gong J. The value of living donor liver transplantation. *Ann Transplant.* 2012;17(4):120–124.
12. Cheng YF, Ou HY, Yu CY, et al. Interventional radiology in living donor liver transplant. *World J Gastroenterol.* 2014;20(20):6221–6225.
13. Caiado AH, Blasbalg R, Marcelino AS, et al. Complications of liver transplantation: multimodality imaging approach. *Radiographics.* 2007;27(5):1401–1417.
14. Singh AK, Nachiappan AC, Verma HA, et al. Postoperative imaging in liver transplantation: what radiologists should know. *Radiographics.* 2010;30(2):339–351.
15. Zamboni GA, Pedrosa I, Kruskal JB, Raptopoulos V. Multimodality postoperative imaging of liver transplantation. *Eur Radiol.* 2008;18(5):882–891.
16. Rao AR, Chui AK, Shi LW, et al. Technique for repair of lymphocele after liver transplantation using patent blue dye. *Transplant Proc.* 2000;32(7):2221–2222.
17. Zimmerman MA, Ghobrial RM, Tong MJ, et al. Recurrence of hepatocellular carcinoma following liver transplantation: a review of preoperative and postoperative prognostic indicators. *Arch Surg.* 2008;143(2):182–188.
18. deLemos AS, Schmeltzer PA, Russo MW. Recurrent hepatitis C after liver transplant. *World J Gastroenterol.* 2014;20(31):10668–10681.
19. Miro JM, Stock P, Teicher E, et al. Outcome and management of HCV/HIV coinfection pre- and post-liver transplantation. A 2015 update. *J Hepatol.* 2015;62(3):701–711.
20. Abboud B, El Hachem J, Yazbeck T, Doumit C. Hepatic portal venous gas: physiopathology, etiology, prognosis and treatment. *World J Gastroenterol.* 2009;15(29):3585–3590.
21. Sivrioglu AK, Incedayi M, Saglam M, Sonmez G. Portomesenteric venous gas and pneumatosis intestinalis due to intestinal ischaemia. *BMJ Case Rep.* 2013; bcr2013009214.
22. Petrara MR, Giunco S, Serraino D, et al. Post-transplant lymphoproliferative disorders: from epidemiology to pathogenesis-driven treatment. *Cancer Lett.* 2015;369(1):37–44.
23. Mortele KJ, Ros PR. Cystic focal liver lesions in the adult: differential CT and MR imaging features. *Radiographics.* 2001;21(4):895–910.
24. Horton KM, Bluemke DA, Hruban RH, et al. CT and MR imaging of benign hepatic and biliary tumors. *Radiographics.* 1999;19(2):431–451.
25. Bajenaru N, Balaban V, Savulescu F, et al. Hepatic hemangioma—review. *J Med Life.* 2015;8(Spec Issue):4–11.
26. Sherman SC, Tran H. Pneumobilia: benign or life-threatening. *J Emerg Med.* 2006;30(2):147–153.
27. Decarie PO, Lepanto L, Billiard JS, et al. Fatty liver deposition and sparing: a pictorial review. *Insights Imaging.* 2011;2(5):533–538.
28. Cecka JM. The UNOS Scientific Renal Transplant Registry. *Clin Transpl.* 1996:1–14.
29. Davis CL, Delmonico FL. Living-donor kidney transplantation: a review of the current practices for the live donor. *J Am Soc Nephrol.* 2005;16(7):2098–2110.
30. Azhar B, Patel S, Chadha P, Hakim N. Indications for renal autotransplant: an overview. *Exp Clin Transplant.* 2015;13(2):109–114.
31. Chen CH, Hsieh SR, Shu KH, Ho HC. Salvage of external iliac artery dissection immediately after renal transplant. *Exp Clin Transplant.* 2013;11(3):274–277.
32. Weber TM, Lockhart ME. Renal transplant complications. *Abdom Imaging.* 2013;38(5):1144–1154.
33. Akbar SA, Jafri SZ, Amendola MA, et al. Complications of renal transplantation. *Radiographics.* 2005;25(5):1335–1356.
34. Rouviere O, Berger P, Beziat C, et al. Acute thrombosis of renal transplant artery: graft salvage by means of intra-arterial fibrinolysis. *Transplantation.* 2002;73(3):403–409.
35. Sharfuddin A. Renal relevant radiology: imaging in kidney transplantation. *Clin J Am Soc Nephrol.* 2014;9(2):416–429.
36. Banshodani M, Kawanishi H, Marubayashi S, et al. De novo renal cell carcinoma in a kidney allograft 20 years after transplant. *Case Rep Transplant.* 2015;2015:679262.
37. Hevia V, Gomez V, Alvarez S, et al. Transitional cell carcinoma of the kidney graft: an extremely uncommon presentation of tumor in renal transplant recipients. *Case Rep Transplant.* 2013;2013:196528.
38. Carrim ZI, Murchison JT. The prevalence of simple renal and hepatic cysts detected by spiral computed tomography. *Clin Radiol.* 2003;58(8):626–629.
39. Grotemeyer D, Voiculescu A, Iskandar F, et al. Renal cysts in living donor kidney transplantation: long-term follow-up in 25 patients. *Transplant Proc.* 2009;41(10):4047–4051.
40. Abboudi H, Chandak P, Kessaris N, Fronek J. A successful live donor kidney transplantation after large angiomyolipoma excision. *Int J Surg Case Rep.* 2012;3(12):594–596.
41. Pileggi A.: Islet transplantation. In De Groot LJ, Beck-Peccoz P, Chrousos G, et al., editors: Endotext, South Dartmouth, MA, 2000.
42. Shapiro AM, Lakey JR, Paty BW, et al. Strategic opportunities in clinical islet transplantation. *Transplantation.* 2005;79(10):1304–1307.
43. Vandermeer FQ, Manning MA, Frazier AA, et al. Imaging of whole-organ pancreas transplants. *Radiographics.* 2012;32(2):411–435.
44. Nadalin S, Girotti P, Konigsrainer A. Risk factors for and management of graft pancreatitis. *Curr Opin Organ Transplant.* 2013;18(1):89–96.
45. Heller MT, Bhargava P. Imaging in pancreatic transplants. *Indian J Radiol Imaging.* 2014;24(4):339–349.
46. Woeste G, Moench C, Hauser IA, et al. Incidence and treatment of pancreatic fistula after simultaneous pancreas kidney transplantation. *Transplant Proc.* 2010;42(10):4206–4208.
47. Farrell JJ. Prevalence, diagnosis and management of pancreatic cystic neoplasms: current status and future directions. *Gut Liver.* 2015;9(5):571–589.
48. Lee ES, Lee JM. Imaging diagnosis of pancreatic cancer: a state-of-the-art review. *World J Gastroenterol.* 2014;20(24):7864–7877.
49. Issa N, Amer H, Dean PG, et al. Posttransplant lymphoproliferative disorder following pancreas transplantation. *Am J Transplant.* 2009;9(8):1894–1902.

PART III

Superficial Structures

Chapter 21 Breast
Chapter 22 The Thyroid and Parathyroid Glands
Chapter 23 Scrotum
Chapter 24 Musculoskeletal System

CHAPTER 21

Breast

Kathryn Gill

OBJECTIVES

On completion of this chapter, you should be able to:
- Describe breast anatomy and sonographic layers
- Understand breast physiology
- Explain the difference between breast screening and breast imaging
- Summarize the indications for the use of ultrasound in breast imaging
- Describe the correct sonographic technique for imaging the breast
- Know how to use standard methods of identifying and labeling breast anatomy and masses
- Identify the sonographic characteristics associated with benign and malignant breast masses
- Identify the mammographic characteristics associated with malignant breast masses
- Understand ultrasound-guided interventional procedures

OUTLINE

Physiology of the Breast 644
Anatomy of the Breast 645
    Normal Anatomy and Sonographic Appearance 645
    Vascular Supply 649
    Lymphatic System 651
    The Male Breast 651
Breast Evaluation Overview 652
    Breast Screening 652
    Screening Mammography 653
    Breast Evaluation 654
    Diagnostic Breast Interrogation 654
    Interventional Breast Procedures 654
    Targeted Versus Whole Breast Scan 654
    Sonographic Evaluation of the Breast 654
    American College of Radiology Sonography Descriptive Form 658
Pathology of the Breast 658
    Clinical Evaluation 658
    Benign Breast Conditions 659

Fibrocystic Dysplasia/Fibrocystic Changes 660
Benign Fibroadenoma of the Breast 661
Pregnant and/or Lactating Patient 662
Other Breast Problems 663
Mastitis 663
Breast Abscess 664
Fat Necrosis 664
Breast Hematoma 664
Seroma/Lymphocele 665
Lipoma 665
Intraductal Papilloma 665
Diabetic Mastopathy 666
Breast Augmentation and Implant Complications 666
    Sonographic Characteristics of Malignant Breast Masses 669
Malignant Pathology of the Breast 671
    Ductal Carcinoma In Situ 671
    Invasive Ductal Carcinoma 672
    Comedocarcinoma 672

Papillary Carcinoma 672
Paget Disease 673
Inflammatory Carcinoma 673
Lobular Carcinoma in Situ/Lobular Neoplasia 673
Invasive Lobular Carcinoma 673
Medullary Carcinoma 673
Tubular Carcinoma 674
Scirrhous Carcinoma 674
Colloid/Mucinous Carcinoma 675
Cystosarcoma Phyllodes 675
Lymphoma 676
Metastatic Disease 676
Ultrasound-Guided Interventional Procedures 676
Other Imaging Modalities 676
    Ductography/Galactography 676
    Magnetic Resonance Imaging 676
Single Photon Emssion Computed Tomography 677
    Sentinel Node Procedure/Lymphoscintigraphy 678
    Emerging Sonographic Technologies 678

KEY TERMS

123-ABC method
Acini
ACR FORM breast disease
Adenosis
Antiradial plane
Apocrine metaplasia
Areola
Axilla
Breast
Breast cancer
Breast cancer screening
Breast Imaging Reporting and Data System (BI-RADS)
Breast self-examination (BSE)
Carcinoma
Clinical breast examination (CBE)
Clock face method
Cooper's ligaments
Diagnostic breast interrogation
Digital mammography
Fibroadenoma

Focal fibrosis
Granulomatous mastitis
Gynecomastia
Infiltrating (invasive) ductal carcinoma
Interventional breast procedures
Invasive carcinoma
Mammary Layer
Mastodynia
Microcalcifications
Noninvasive carcinoma
Paget disease
Peau d'orange
Periductal mastitis
Radial plane
Retromammary layer
Rotter's node
Sarcoma
Sentinel node
Side/quadrant method
Spiculation
Subcutaneous layer
Targeted scan
Tail of Spence
Terminal ductal lobar units (TDLUs)

One out of eight American women will develop **breast cancer**. It is the most common type of cancer among women in the United States and is the second leading cause of cancer death among women between the ages of 40 and 59 years. It is estimated that the lifetime risk of breast cancer development is approximately 12%. Early detection of breast cancer is vital because cancer can be difficult to eradicate once it has spread. Ultrasound evaluation of the breast plays a significant role in the early detection and characterization of breast masses and provides real-time guidance during interventional breast procedures. This chapter presents an overview of breast anatomy, physiology, sonographic evaluation techniques, and breast pathology with emphasis on breast cancer diagnosis and staging.

Although mammography is still considered by most the gold standard for breast imaging, improvements in sonographic technology and technique are making significant headway in breast imaging. This is especially true for younger women and those with dense breast tissue. As an adjunct to the breast exam on a patient with a palpable lump or a mammogram with worrisome findings, sonography can often provide a more definitive diagnosis. Performing a sonographic examination of the breast requires collection of pertinent clinical information including the patient's age, the location and clinical impression of any breast lumps, history of trauma to the breast, or previous breast surgery. Risk factors for breast cancer, if the patient has any, should also be noted (Box 21.1). The referring physician should provide clinical information including the size and location of a lump, when it was noticed, and its relation to the menstrual cycle. The referring physician's clinical impression (e.g., suspicion of cancer, probable fibrocystic condition, possible abscess) can help focus the sonographer's examination.

Common indications for the use of breast sonography include the following:

1. Evaluate a palpable mass in women younger than 30 years or women who are pregnant or lactating
2. Evaluate questionable findings on a mammogram
3. Evaluate breast implants and associated problems
4. Evaluate the radiographically dense breast
5. Serial monitoring of a benign mass
6. Evaluate axillary lymph nodes
7. Provide localization and guidance during interventional procedures
8. Assist with treatment planning for radiation therapy
9. Evaluate the male breast
10. Evaluate the breast when mammography is compromised or contraindicated

> **BOX 21.1 Risk Factors for Breast Cancer**
>
> - Female sex
> - Increasing age
> - Family history of breast cancer
> - Personal history of breast cancer
>   - First-degree relative (mother, sister, daughter)
>   - Premenopausal breast cancer
>   - Multiple affected first- and second-degree relatives
>   - Associated cancers (ovarian, colon, prostate)
> - Biopsy-proven atypical proliferative lesions
>   - Lobular neoplasia (lobular carcinoma in situ)
>   - Atypical epithelial hyperplasia
> - Prolonged estrogen effect
>   - Early menarche
> - Late menopause
> - Nulliparity
> - Late first pregnancy

PHYSIOLOGY OF THE BREAST

The primary function of the female breast is to produce milk for nutrition of the infant and baby through lactation. Milk is produced within the acini and is carried to the nipple by the ducts. During lactation, the transport of milk depends on the action of the two epithelial cells that make up the ductal network: luminal cells, which secrete the milk components into the ductal lumen, and myoepithelial cells, which contract to aid in the ejection of milk.

The breast includes fat, ligaments, glandular tissue, and a ductal system that work together to provide fluid transport. This ductal system is critical in the transport of fluids within the breast and is also where many pathologic conditions originate. The female breast is remarkably affected by changing hormonal levels during each menstrual cycle and is further affected by both pregnancy and lactation (breastfeeding). Breast development begins before menarche and continues until the female is approximately 16 years old. During this time, the ductal system proliferates under the influence of estrogen. During pregnancy, acinar development is accelerated to enable milk production by estrogen, progesterone, and prolactin. Prolactin is a hormone produced by the pituitary gland that stimulates the acini to produce and excrete milk. Prolactin levels usually rise during the latter part of pregnancy, but milk production is suppressed by high levels of progesterone. Expulsion of the placenta after the birth of a baby causes a drop in circulating progesterone, initiating milk production within the breasts. The physical stimulation of suckling by the baby initiates the release of oxytocin (produced by the hypothalamus and released by the pituitary gland), which further incites prolactin secretion, stimulating additional milk production. Full maturation of the acini occurs during lactation and is thought to be mildly protective against the development of breast cancer. At the end of lactation, the breast tissue parenchyma involutes. Aside from milk production, the **breast** is a modified sweat gland located in the superficial fascia of the anterior chest wall.

Breast evaluation by mammography can be difficult in a dense, lactating breast; therefore mammographic screening of the breast usually is not performed until at least 6 months after cessation of lactation.

ANATOMY OF THE BREAST

Normal Anatomy and Sonographic Appearance

The major portion of the breast tissue is situated between the second and third rib superiorly, the sixth and seventh costal cartilage inferiorly, the anterior axillary line laterally, and the sternal border medially. In many women, the breast extends deep toward the lateral upper margin of the chest and into the **axilla**. This extension is referred to as the axillary tail of the breast, or the **tail of Spence**.

The surface of the breast is dominated by the nipple and the surrounding **areola**. A few women may have ectopic breast tissue or accessory (supernumerary) nipples. Ectopic breast tissue and accessory nipples are usually located along the mammary milk line, which extends superiorly from the axilla downward and medially in an oblique line to the symphysis pubis of the pelvis (Fig. 21.1).

Sonographically, the breast is divided into three layers located between the skin and the pectoralis major muscle on the anterior chest wall. These layers are the **subcutaneous layer**, the **mammary (glandular) layer**, and the **retromammary layer** (Fig. 21.2). The subcutaneous and retromammary layers are usually quite thin and consist of fat surrounded by connective tissue septa. Although fat is often highly echogenic in other parts of the body, it is the least echogenic tissue within the breast. The fatty tissue appears hypoechoic, and the ducts, glands, and supporting ligaments appear echogenic (Fig. 21.3).

The mammary/glandular layer includes the functional portion of the breast and the surrounding supportive (stromal) tissue. The functional portion of the breast is made up of 15 to 20 lobes, which contain the milk-producing glands, and the ductal system, which carries the milk to the nipple. The lobes emanate from the nipple in a pattern resembling the spokes of a wheel. The upper outer quadrant of the breast contains the highest concentration of lobes. This concentration of lobes in the upper outer quadrant of the breast is the reason why most tumors are found here, as most tumors originate from

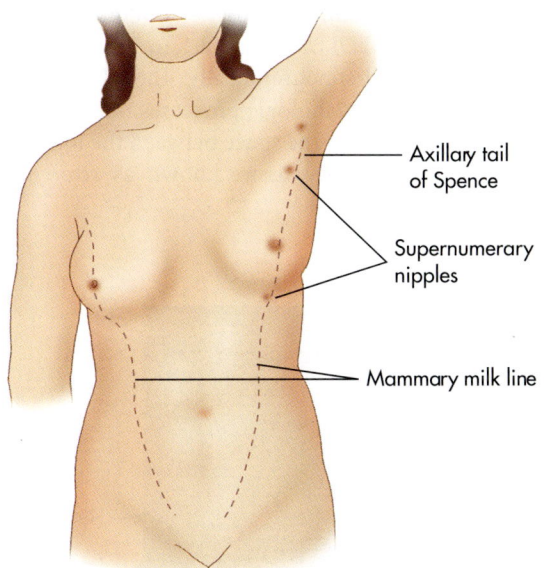

FIG. 21.1 The mammary milk line is the anatomic line along which breast tissue can be found in some women. The axillary tail of Spence is an extension of breast tissue into the axilla that is present in some women.

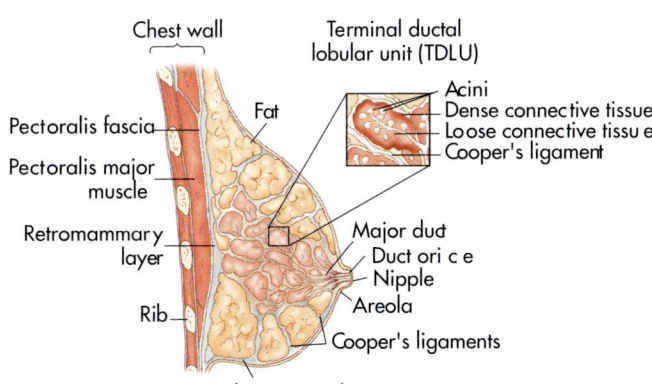

FIG. 21.2 Breast anatomy. Fifteen major ductal systems are present within the breast. Each gives rise to many separate terminal ductal lobular units (TDLUs) containing the terminal ducts, at least one lobule, and the separate acinar units (milk-producing glands) within each lobule. Each TDLU is surrounded by varying amounts of loose and dense connective tissue. The TDLU represents the site of origin of nearly all pathologic processes of the breast. Cooper's ligaments surround and suspend each of the TDLUs within the surrounding fatty tissue. The ligaments extend to the subcutaneous layer of the skin and the deep retromammary layer next to the pectoralis fascia overlying the chest wall.

within the ducts. The lobes of the breast resemble a grapevine branch; the major duct branches into smaller branches called lobules. Each lobule contains **acini** (milk-producing glands; singular *acinus*), which are clustered on the terminal ends of the ducts like grapes on a vine. Literally hundreds of acini are present within each breast. The terminal ends of the duct and the acini form small lobular units referred to as **terminal ductal lobular units (TDLUs)**, each of which is surrounded by both loose and dense connective tissue. The TDLUs are invested within the connective tissue skeleton of the breast (Fig. 21.4). Normal TDLUs measure 1 to 2 mm and usually are not differentiated sonographically. The TDLU is significant in that nearly all pathologic processes that occur within the breast originate here. The space between the lobes is filled with connective and fatty tissue known as *stroma*. These stromal elements are located both between and within the lobes and consist of dense connective tissue, loose connective tissue, and fat. The connective tissue septa within the breasts form a fibrous "skeleton," which is responsible for maintaining the shape and structure of the breast. These connective tissue septa are collectively termed **Cooper's ligaments**; they connect to the fascia around the ducts and glands and extend out to the skin (Fig. 21.5).

The boundaries of the breast are the skin line, nipple, and retromammary layer (Fig. 21.6A). These generally give strong, bright echo reflections. The areolar area may be recognized by its slightly lower echo reflection compared with the nipple and the skin. The internal nipple may show low to bright reflections with posterior shadowing, and it has a variable appearance (see Fig. 21.6B).

Subcutaneous fat generally appears hypoechoic, whereas Cooper's ligaments and other connective tissue appear echogenic and are dispersed in a linear pattern (Fig. 21.7). Cooper's ligaments are best identified when the beam strikes them at a perpendicular angle; compression of the breast often enhances the ability to visualize them.

The mammary/glandular layer lies between the subcutaneous fatty layer anteriorly and the retromammary layer posteriorly (Fig. 21.8). The fatty tissue interspersed throughout the mammary/glandular layer dictates the amount of intensity reflected from the breast parenchyma. If little fat is present, a uniform architecture with a strong echogenic pattern

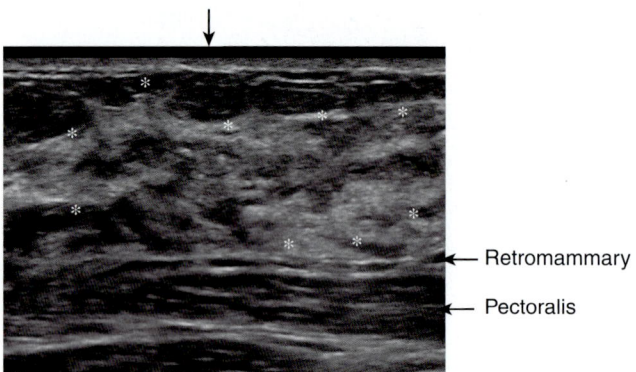

FIG. 21.3 Sonographic layers of breast tissue. The three layers of breast tissue are bordered by the skin and chest wall muscles *(arrows)*. The subcutaneous fat layer and the retromammary fat layer are usually very thin. The mammary layer *(asterisks)* varies remarkably in thickness and in echogenicity, depending on location within the breast (most glandular tissue is located in the upper outer quadrant) and the patient's age, hormonal status (e.g., pubertal, mature, gravid, lactating, postmenopausal), and inherited breast parenchymal pattern.

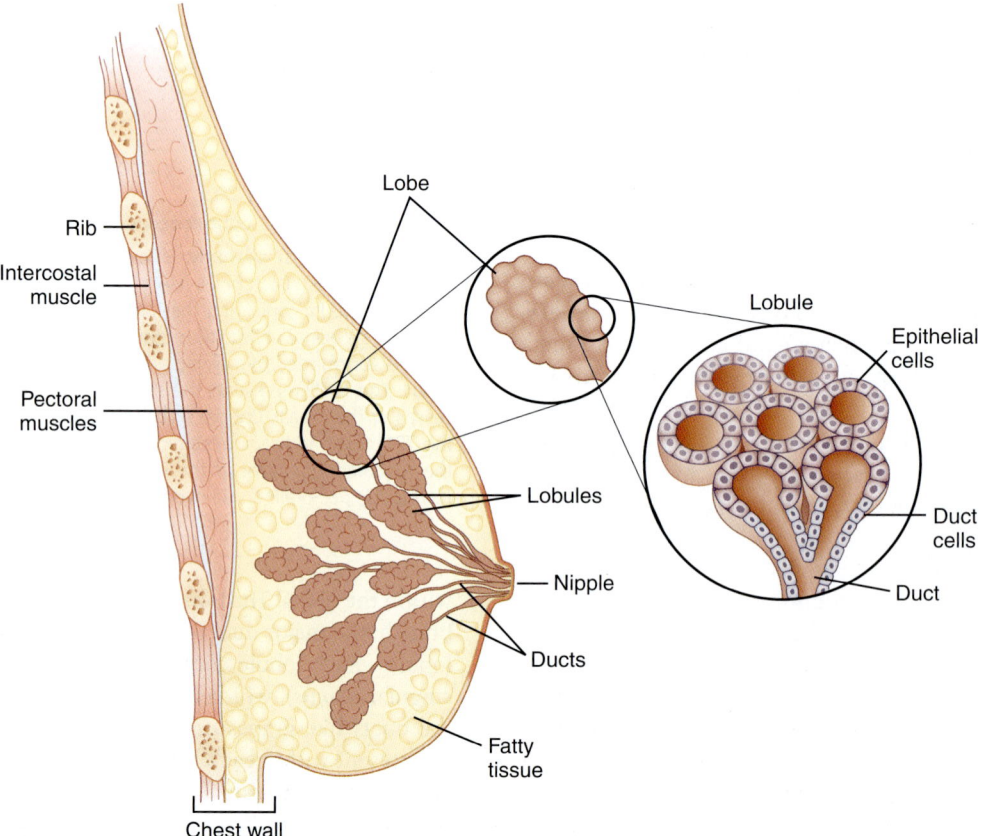

FIG. 21.4 The terminal ends of the duct and the acini form small lobular units referred to as terminal ductal lobular units, each of which is surrounded by both loose and dense connective tissue.

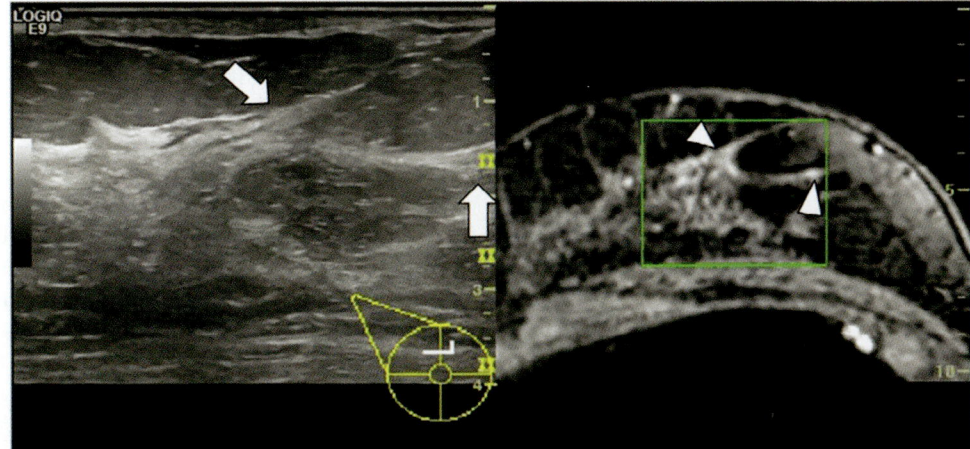

FIG. 21.5 The connective tissue septa within the breasts form a fibrous "skeleton" that is responsible for maintaining the shape and structure of the breast. These connective tissue septa are collectively termed Cooper's ligaments; they connect to the fascia around the ducts and glands and extend out to the skin.

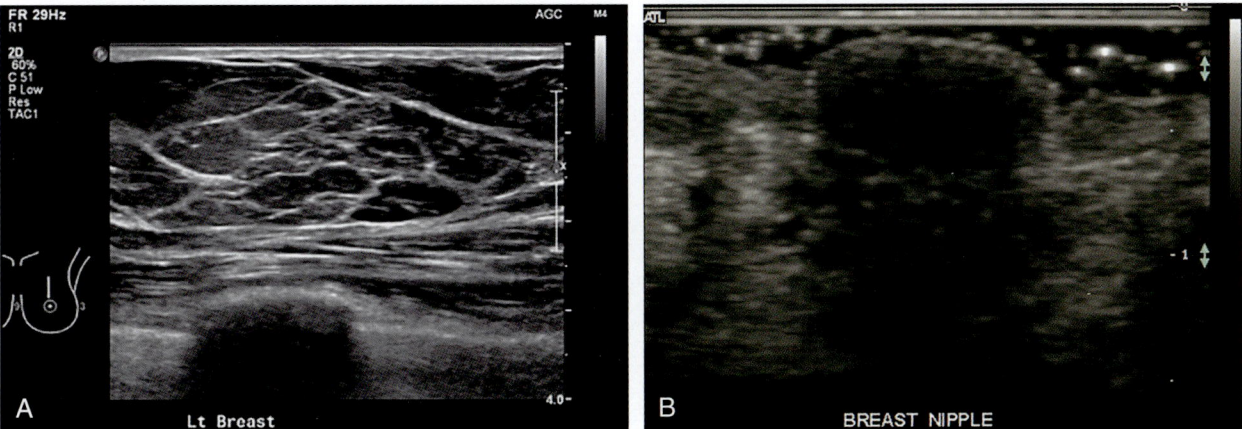

FIG. 21.6 (A) The boundaries of the breast are the skin line, nipple, and retromammary layer. (B) The internal nipple may show low to bright reflections with posterior shadowing with a variable echo appearance.

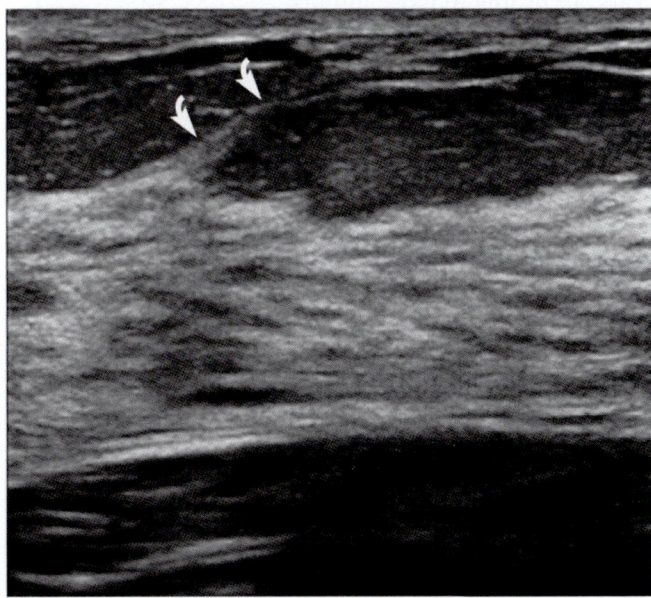

FIG. 21.7 The subcutaneous fat is hypoechoic, whereas Cooper's ligaments appear echogenic within the subcutaneous layer *(arrows)*.

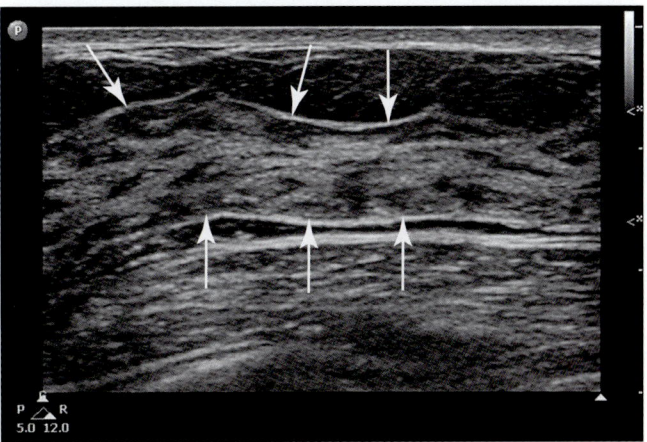

FIG. 21.8 The mammary/glandular layer lies between the subcutaneous fatty layer and the retromammary layer posteriorly *(arrows)*.

(because of collagen and fibrotic tissue) is seen throughout the mammary/glandular layer. When fatty tissue is present, areas of low-level echoes become intertwined with areas of strong echoes from the active breast tissue. Analysis of this pattern becomes critical to the final diagnosis, and one must be able to separate lobules of fat from a marginated lesion.

The retromammary layer is similar in echogenicity and echotexture to the subcutaneous layer, although the boundary echoes resemble skin reflections (Fig. 21.9A). The pectoral muscles appear as low-level echo areas posterior to the retromammary layer. The ribs appear sonographically as rounded structures with dense posterior shadowing (see Fig. 21.9B–C). They are easily identified by their occurrence at regular intervals along the chest wall. Between each rib one can see the intercostal muscles. The thin echogenic line seen posterior to the ribs is produced by the pleura and aerated lung.

Imaging of the breast must include the area past the glandular tissue to the pectoralis muscle. This verifies one has completely evaluated all tissues of the breast. As with most muscle tissue, the pectoralis muscle will be striated and hypoechoic. The pectoralis major muscle lies posterior to the retromammary layer. It originates at the anterior surface of the medial half of the clavicle and anterolateral surface of the sternum and inserts into the intertubercular groove on the anteromedial surface of the humerus. The lower border of the pectoralis major muscle forms the anterior margin of the axilla. The pectoralis minor muscle lies superolateral and posterior to the pectoralis major. The pectoralis minor courses from its origin near the costal cartilages of the third, fourth, and fifth ribs to where it inserts into the medial and superior surface of the coracoid process of the scapula. These muscles sonographically appear as a hypoechoic interface between the retromammary layer of the breast and the ribs. Although most lesions are found within the glandular tissue of the breast, it is important to evaluate tissue all the way to the chest wall.

Parenchymal Patterns. The size and shape of the breasts vary remarkably from woman to woman and may vary over time because of changes that occur during the menstrual cycle, with pregnancy and breastfeeding, and during menopause. Generally, in a young woman, fibrous tissue elements predominate, and the resulting appearance on mammography and ultrasound is a dense echogenic pattern of tissue. A common cause of breast lumps in young girls is the developing breast bud immediately behind the nipple (which should not be mistaken for an abnormal mass and surgically removed). Ultrasound is the primary tool in breast imaging for all women younger than 30 years, according to most authors.

The involutional changes that occur in the breast throughout life affect the appearance and pattern of the breast parenchyma. Most women in their reproductive years will show distinct mammary layers due to the prominent glandular tissue. Young patients with dense breasts are a challenge even for mammography, and the modality is not usually indicated for patients younger than 20 to 25 years. Sonography, therefore, is typically used (Fig. 21.10).

Involution is hallmarked in breast imaging by the remodeling process that causes glandular tissue to be slowly replaced by fatty tissue. This accounts for differences in the size, shape, and architecture of breast tissue. As a woman ages, the glandular breast tissue undergoes cell death and is remodeled by the infiltration of fatty tissue. The tissue is progressively replaced by fat and, with the onset of menopause, the ducts atrophy, resulting in a mammographic and sonographic pattern with less fibrous tissue elements (Fig. 21.11). This fatty breast is most difficult to image by sonography, as all three layers of the breast appear hypoechoic, with less distinction between the layers. Although sonography of the

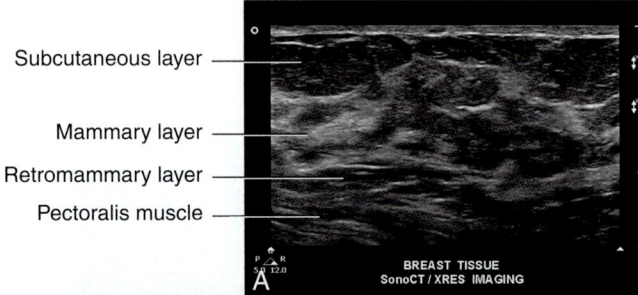
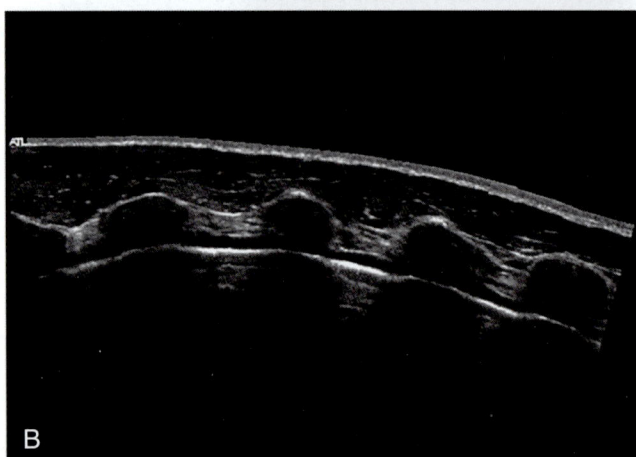
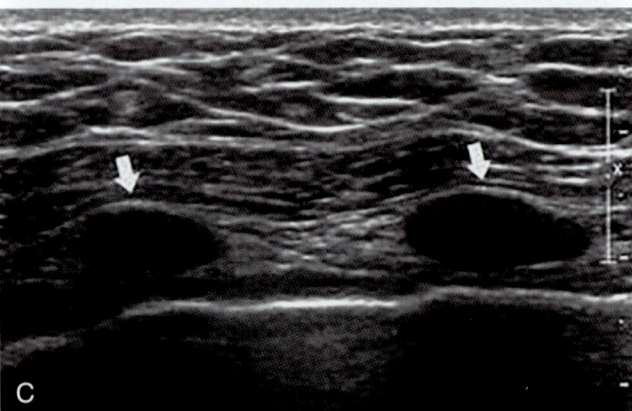

FIG. 21.9 (A) The retromammary layer is similar in echogenicity and echo texture to the subcutaneous layer. (B–C) The ribs appear sonographically as rounded structures with dense posterior shadowing. Between each rib lie the intercostal muscles. The thin echogenic line posterior to the ribs is produced by the pleura and aerated lung.

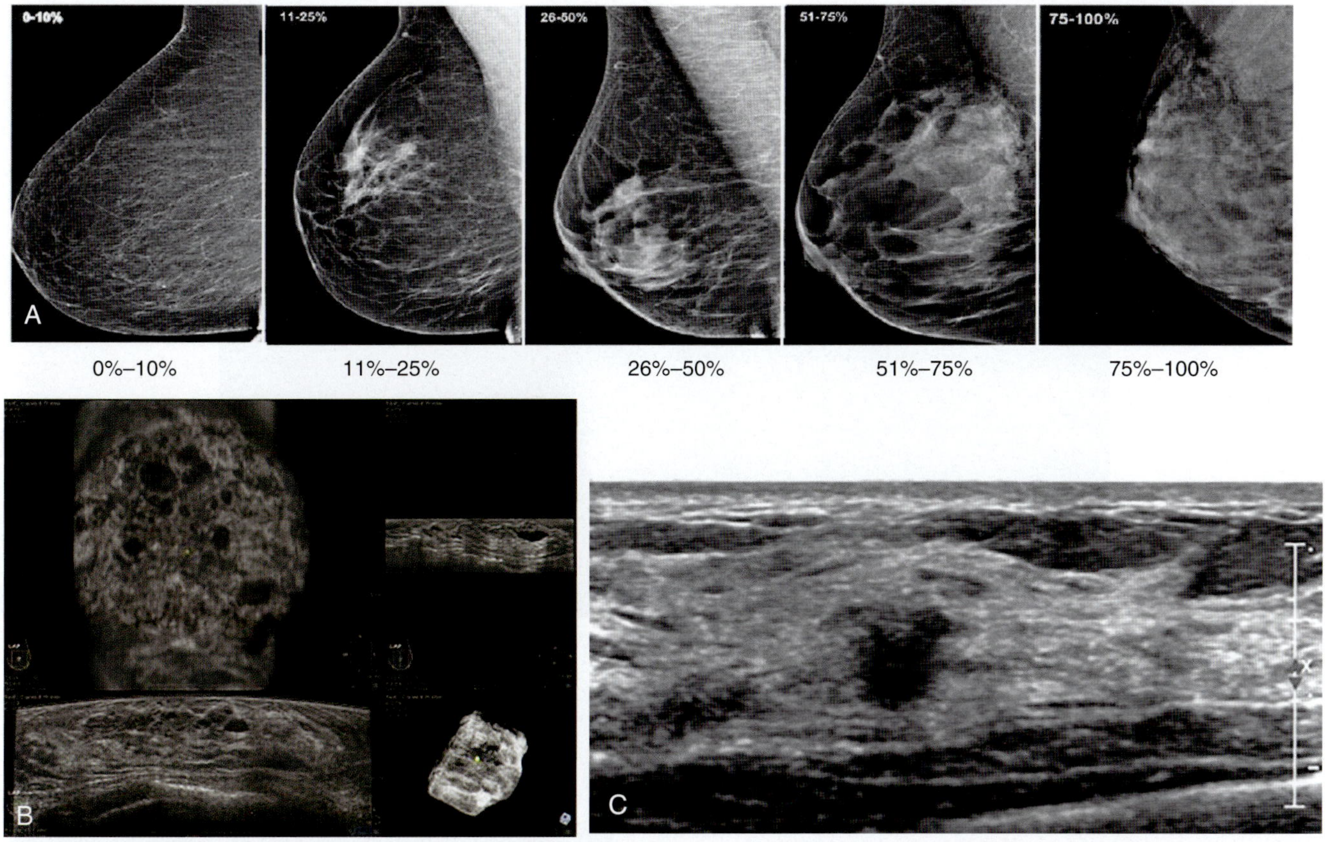

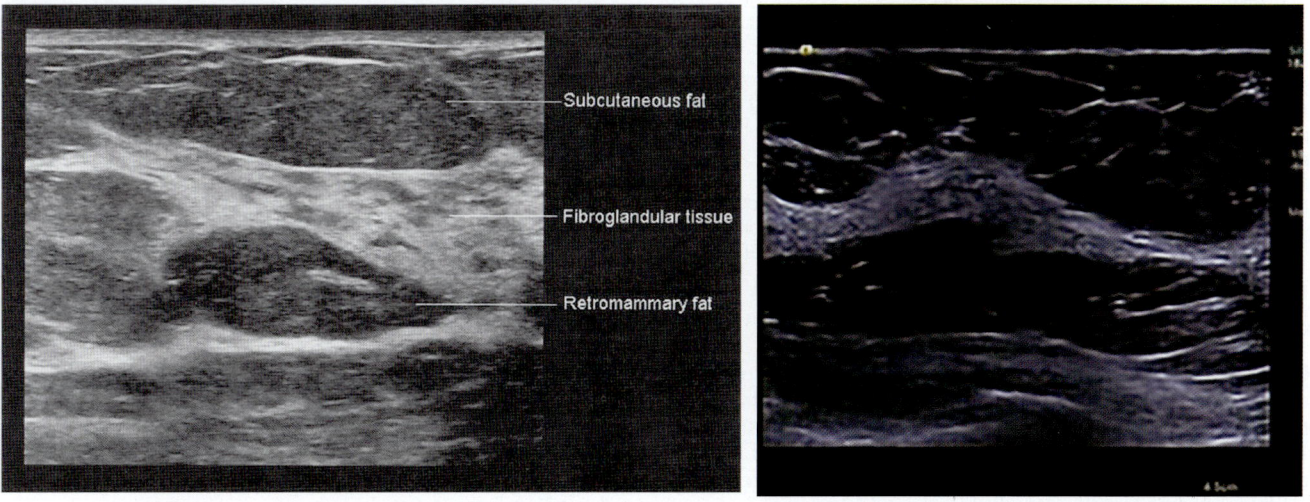

FIG. 21.10 (A) Classification of breast density using a 4-level density scale. (B) Automated ultrasound images of the dense breast pattern. (C) Traditional ultrasound images of the heterogeneous dense breast.

FIG. 21.11 Involution is hallmarked in breast imaging by the remodeling process that causes glandular tissue to be slowly replaced by fatty tissue.

fatty breast is difficult, mammography images this type of breast very well.

Pregnant or Lactating Patient. Sonography is the primary tool for breast imaging in a pregnant patient. In a pregnant or lactating woman, the glandular portions of the breast proliferate remarkably in both density and volume, creating interfaces that are less echogenic (Fig. 21.12).

Vascular Supply

The main arterial supply to the breast comes from the internal mammary and the lateral thoracic arteries (Fig. 21.13). More than half of the breast—mainly the central and medial portions—is supplied by the anterior perforating branches of the internal mammary artery. The remaining portion—the

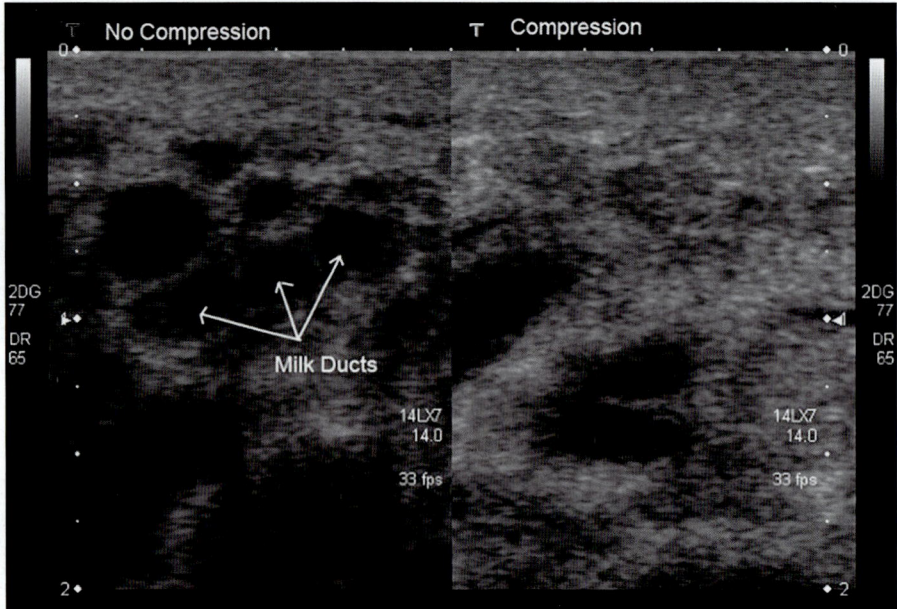

FIG. 21.12 Ultrasound of the dilated milk ducts with and without compression.

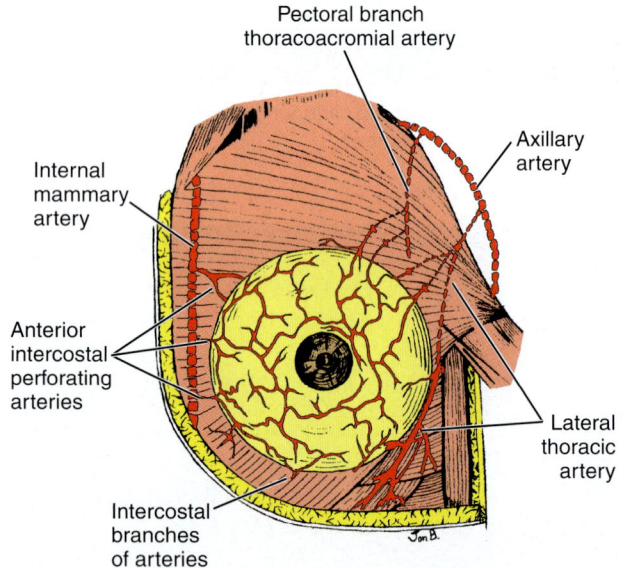

FIG. 21.13 The main arterial supply to the breast comes from the internal mammary and the lateral thoracic arteries. The central and medial portion is supplied by the anterior perforating branches of the internal mammary artery. The upper outer quadrant is supplied by the lateral thoracic artery. The intercostal, subcapsular, and thoracodorsal arteries contribute in lesser ways to the blood supply.

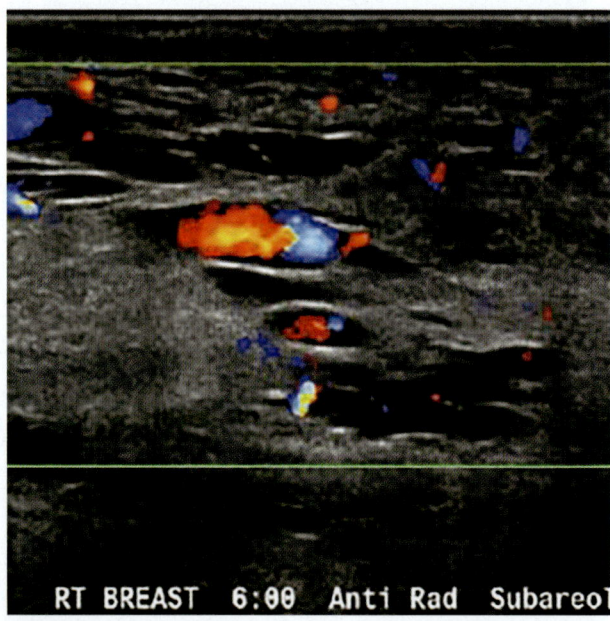

FIG. 21.14 Color Doppler will help separate vascular structures from dilated ducts in the breast.

upper outer quadrant—is supplied by the lateral thoracic artery. The intercostal, subcapsular, and thoracodorsal arteries contribute in lesser ways to the blood supply.

Venous anatomy largely parallels the arterial anatomy in the deep breast. However, venous drainage is mainly provided by unpaired superficial veins that can be seen sonographically just under the skin. These surface veins are often enlarged with superior vena cava syndrome or chronic venous thrombosis of the subclavian vein, as well as when arteriovenous shunts are placed in patients with chronic renal insufficiency. Fig. 21.14 shows an example of a grossly dilated surface vein in the breast. When there is doubt concerning the vascular nature of a long tubular anechoic structure on breast ultrasound, such as the distinction between a dilated duct and a vessel, color flow vascular imaging or Doppler ultrasound techniques can easily resolve this situation.

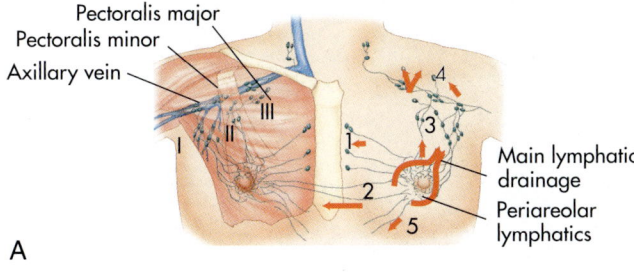

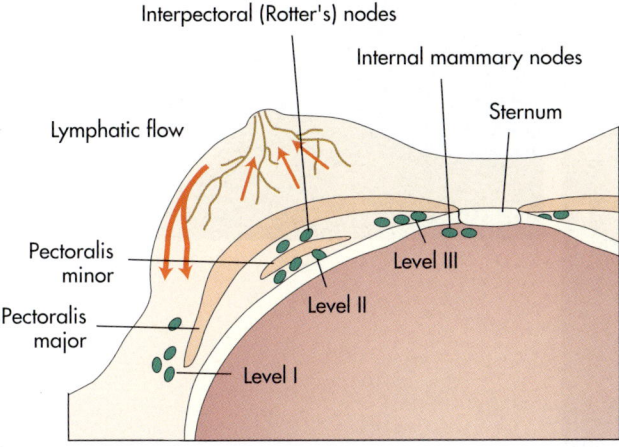

FIG. 21.15 **Lymphatic drainage of the breast.** (A) General position of the major axillary lymphatic groups I, II, and III in relation to the pectoralis major and minor muscles of the chest wall. On the right side of the figure, the major lymphatic flow from the periareolar plexus toward the axilla is shown. Alternative routes of lymphatic flow include retromammary nodes (1), contralateral flow to the opposite breast (2), interpectoral (Rotter's) nodes located between the pectoralis major and minor muscles (3), supraclavicular nodes (4), and diaphragmatic nodes (5). (B) Same information in cross section.

Lymphatic System

Lymphatic drainage from all parts of the breast generally flows to the axillary lymph nodes. The flow of lymph is promoted by valveless lymphatic vessels that allow the fluid to mingle and proceed unidirectionally from superficial to deep nodes of the breast. The flow of lymph moves from the intramammary nodes and deep nodes centrifugally toward the axillary and internal lymph node chains (Fig. 21.15). It has been estimated that only about 3% of lymph is eliminated by the internal chain, whereas 97% of lymph is removed by the axillary chain. Although most tumors can infiltrate and spread via the axillary lymph nodes, they may begin their infiltration by using alternative lymph channels, such as the internal mammary chain within the chest, across the midline to the contralateral breast, deep into the interpectoral (Rotter's) nodes, or into the supraclavicular nodes (Fig. 21.16).

The Male Breast

In males, the nipple and the areola remain relatively small. The male breast normally retains some ductal elements beneath

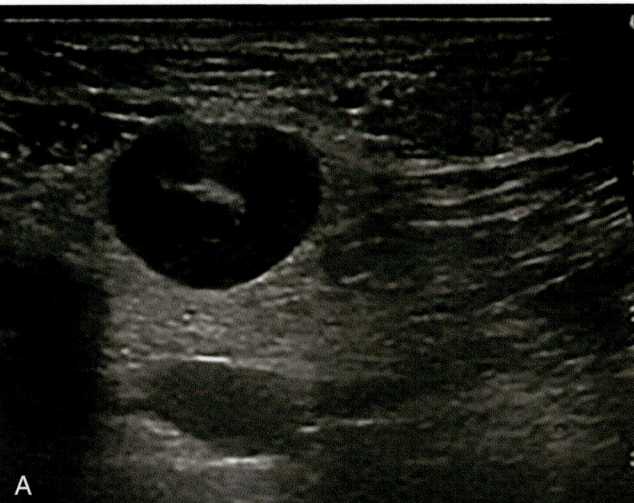

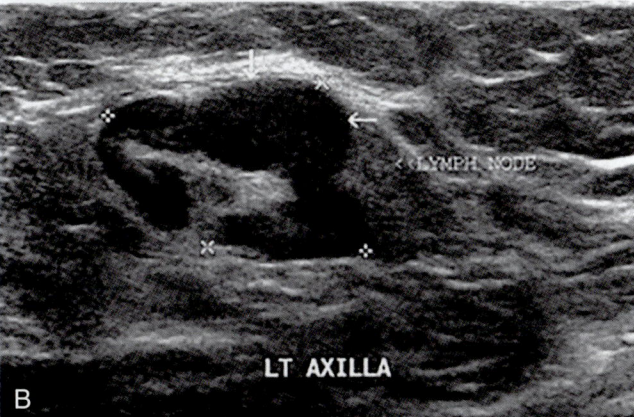

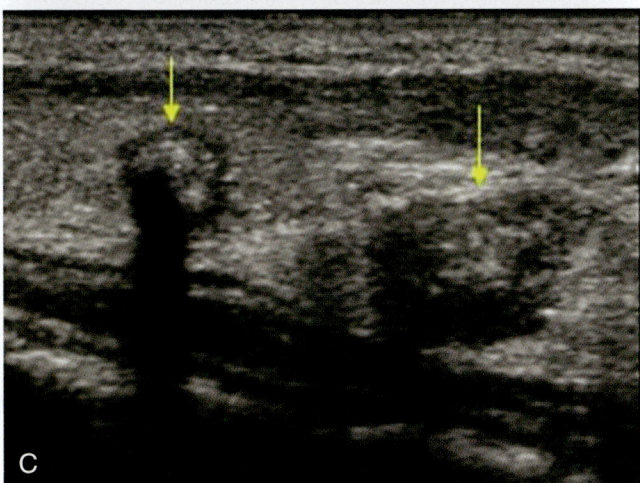

FIG. 21.16 Images of the abnormal lymph nodes within the breast (A) and axilla (B). The nodes may calcify, causing the shadow artifact beyond (C).

the nipple, but it does not develop the milk-producing lobular and acinar tissue. The ductal elements usually remain small but can hypertrophy during puberty and later in life under the influence of hormonal fluctuations, disease processes, or medications. This condition, in which the ductal elements hypertrophy, is called benign **gynecomastia** (Fig. 21.17). Imaging with mammography and ultrasound is often requested to exclude breast cancer as a cause. Although breast cancer is uncommon

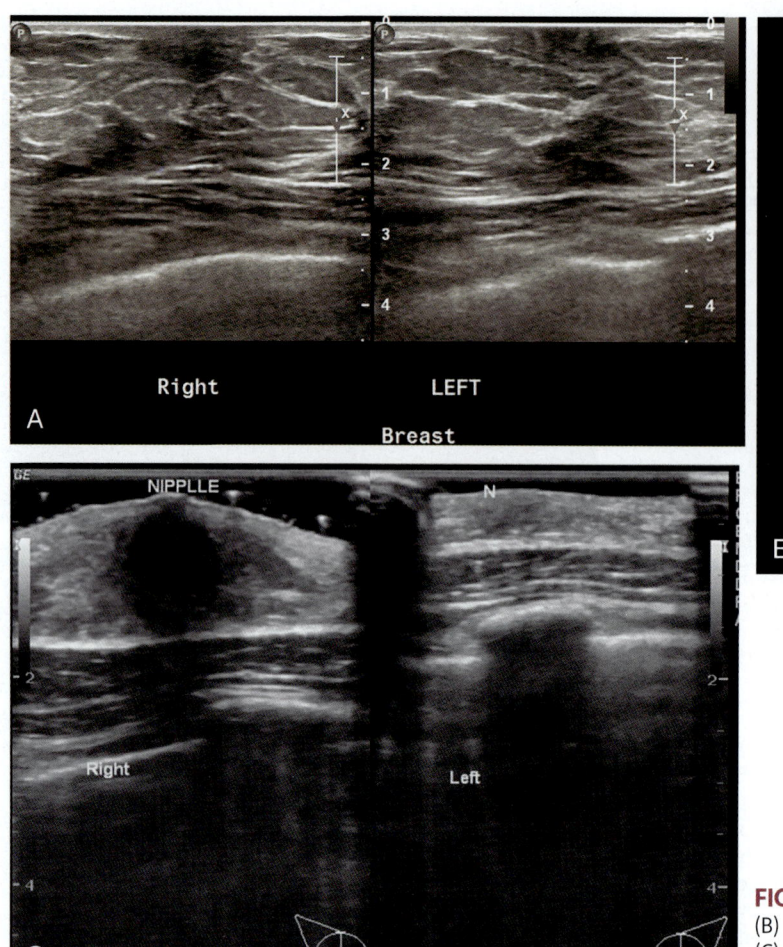
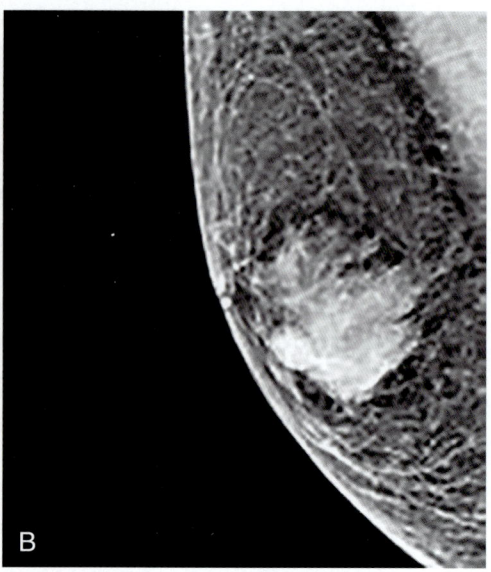

FIG. 21.17 (A) Bilateral gynecomastia in a male patient. (B) Mammogram on a male patient with a breast mass. (C) Bilateral breast ultrasound demonstrates the mass in the right breast.

BOX 21.2	Male Patients at Increased Risk for Breast Cancer

Klinefelter syndrome
Male-to-female transgender
History of prior chest wall irradiation (especially for Hodgkin lymphoma)
History of orchitis or testicular tumor
Liver disease
Genetic predisposition (*BRCA2* gene mutation, breast cancer in female relatives, p53 mutation)

in males, it does occur. Approximately 1300 new cases are diagnosed each year within the United Sates. The occurrence approximates 1% of the incidence in women. Box 21.2 lists male patients who have an increased risk for breast cancer.

BREAST EVALUATION OVERVIEW

Three general categories of diagnostic breast imaging are available, two of which involve breast ultrasound. These three categories include **breast cancer screening** (generally performed by physical breast evaluation with mammography), diagnostic interrogation (consultation, problem solving, workup), and **interventional breast procedures** (histologic diagnosis and/or localization). Mammography, sonography, and magnetic resonance imaging (MRI) are the primary imaging tools used for diagnostic breast evaluation.

Breast Screening

In recent years, we have seen an increase in breast cancer incidence worldwide, and it has surpassed lung cancer as the most common cause of cancer deaths among women. Therefore, the primary purpose of breast screening is the detection and diagnosis of breast cancer in its earliest and most curable stage. Accurate identification of benign breast lesions during cancer screening is also important for good care because it can save the patient from unnecessary surgical procedures and resultant tissue scarring.

According to the American Cancer Society, breast cancer screening involves monthly **breast self-examination (BSE)** and regular **clinical breast examination (CBE)** by a physician or other health care provider. Monthly BSE is best performed at the end of menses and should begin at age 20. Seventy percent of cancers are found as lumps felt during BSE and CBE. BSE and CBE may also identify other signs or symptoms of possible breast cancer that require further evaluation by diagnostic breast imaging (Box 21.3).

BOX 21.3	Breast Cancer Screening

Breast Self-Examination
- Monthly beginning at age 20 years

Clinical Breast Examination by a Health Care Provider
- Ages 20–39: every 3 years
- Ages ≥40: yearly

Screening Mammography
- Ages 40–44: yearly if desired by patient
- Ages 45–54: yearly
- Ages ≥55: every 2 years

Exceptions: Personal history of breast cancer, first-degree relative (mother or sister) with premenopausal breast cancer, atypical hyperplasia or lobular carcinoma in situ on prior breast biopsy, and known breast cancer gene mutation (*BRCA1* or *BRCA2*).

Screening Mammography

It is recommended that screening mammography begin yearly starting at age 40 years. Mammography, still the gold standard for breast cancer screening, provides a sensitive method of two-dimensional imaging for breast cancer. Analog mammography has been replaced with **digital mammography**, which provides images with more contrast, allows image manipulation, and archives films. There is no limitation on breast size, and cancer cells can be detected earlier than with analog imaging.

A relatively new technology is digital breast tomosynthesis or 3D mammography. This system allows for improved detection and characterization of breast masses, especially in younger patients, or those with less fatty and denser breast tissue. When a breast lesion is identified by mammography, it is normally described using guidelines contained within the Breast Imaging Reporting and Data System (BI-RADS). BI-RADS was developed by the American College of Radiology (ACR). A key component of this system is an overall outcome assessment category that indicates the suspicion of malignancy (Table 21.1). The mammographic signs of breast cancer listed in Box 21.4 present mammographic and sonographic examples of various BI-RADS category masses.

Diagnostic breast interrogation (i.e., consultation, workup, problem solving) is performed on all patients who present with any clinical signs of possible breast cancer found on CBE or BSE and on patients who are recalled for additional evaluation because of an abnormal screening mammogram. Diagnostic mammography involves specialized detailed views to analyze specific areas of the breast in question. In at least one-third of cases, adjunctive ultrasound of the breast is used to further evaluate questionable mammographic or clinical findings.

Patient With a Difficult or Compromised Mammogram. For some patients, breast imaging by mammography is limited in its sensitivity (as in the case of very dense breast tissue) or in its ability to visualize the breast tissue (as in the case of retroglandular breast implants).

Distinguishing between scar tissue and breast cancer is difficult with mammography. With more women having breast reduction surgeries, these reduction scars, along with previous open biopsy scars, form tissue that is distorted and is difficult to distinguish from breast cancer distortion of normal tissue.

For other patients, examination of breast tissue is compromised because of postsurgical or post-radiation changes. This is a common situation in the patient who has had breast-conserving therapy for early-stage breast cancer located close to the chest wall or in the axillary tail near the armpit. As technologic advances in ultrasound continue to improve its

TABLE 21.1	ACR BI-RADS Assessment Categories for Mammographic Masses
Category/Recommended Action	**Description**
1. Negative	Nothing to comment on. Breasts are symmetric; no masses, architectural distortion, or suspicious calcifications.
2. Benign finding(s)	Involuting, calcified fibroadenomas, multiple secretory calcifications, fat-containing lesions.
3. Probable benign finding(s)/initial short-term follow-up	Noncalcified circumscribed solid mass; focal asymmetry; cluster of round (punctate) calcifications. Less than 2% chance of malignancy.
4. Suspicious abnormality/consider biopsy	Findings do not have classic appearance of malignancy but have wide range of probability of malignancy greater than those in Category 3.
5. Highly suggestive of malignancy/appropriate action needed	Classic breast cancers with a 95% or greater likelihood for malignancy.

ACR, American College of Radiology; *BI-RADS*, Breast Imaging and Reporting Data System.
Courtesy American College of Radiology.

BOX 21.4	Signs of Breast Cancer on Mammography

Primary Signs
Common
Irregular (spiculated), high-density mass
Clustered pleomorphic microcalcifications
Focal distortion (with no history of prior biopsy, infection, or trauma)

Less common
Focal asymmetric density (with associated palpable lump or solid sonographic mass)
Developing density

Secondary Signs
Common
Nipple or skin retraction
Skin thickening
Lymphedema pattern
Increased vascularity

> **BOX 21.5 Breast Ultrasound Applications**
>
> Further characterization of mammographic masses
> Evaluation of a palpable breast lump
> Young patient with dense breasts
> Pregnant or lactating patient
> Patient with breast augmentation
> Difficult or compromised mammogram
> Image-guided procedures

sensitivity and specificity, the routine use of adjunctive breast ultrasound and mammography in certain high-risk or complicated patients is being advocated (Box 21.5). Although sonography is an invaluable aid to breast imaging, it should not be used as a substitute for mammography because microcalcifications and focal distortion, which are two of the three principal signs of breast cancer seen by mammography, are often difficult to visualize with ultrasound.

Tissue Diagnosis. Tissue diagnosis is suggested in high-risk patients or patients with larger masses. The size cut-off for tissue diagnosis versus follow-up varies. In a high-risk patient or in a patient who is not comfortable waiting on follow-up for an answer, tissue diagnosis can be pursued more aggressively. Options include fine-needle aspiration cytology, large-core needle biopsy, vacuum-assisted biopsy, and surgical excisional biopsy.

Breast Evaluation

The overall goal of breast evaluation is the proper classification of a breast lesion according to the level of suspicion for breast cancer. Thorough evaluation takes into account the results of both the breast imaging assessment and the clinical assessment. The appropriate next step in patient management is dictated by the level of suspicion for cancer in any breast lesion and takes into account the age and individual risk factors for each particular patient.

Clinical Assessment. It is important to recognize clinical signs or symptoms of possible breast cancer. Patients with clinical indications of breast cancer generally undergo diagnostic breast interrogation. Diagnostic imaging of the breast is tailored to the patient's age and specific clinical problem. Clinical history and examination of the patient with a breast problem help determine the next diagnostic step. In the patient with no signs or symptoms of possible breast cancer, screening mammography is typically the first diagnostic test performed.

Diagnostic Breast Interrogation

Diagnostic breast interrogation (consultation, workup, problem solving) is performed on all patients who present with any clinical signs of possible breast cancer found on CBE or BSE and on patients who are recalled for additional evaluation because of an abnormal screening mammogram. Diagnostic mammography involves specialized detailed views to analyze specific areas of the breast in question. In at least one-third of cases, adjunctive ultrasound of the breast is used to further evaluate questionable mammographic or clinical findings (see later discussion).

Interventional Breast Procedures

In some breast lesions, interventional procedures are necessary for definitive diagnosis. A common example is a smooth, benign-appearing mass identified by mammography that correlates with a hypoechoic sonographic lesion but does not meet the criteria for interpretation as a simple cyst. Cyst aspiration can be performed to determine whether the lesion is a complex cyst or truly a solid mass. Under real-time sonographic guidance, a needle is guided into the lesion in an attempt to aspirate fluid. Successful fluid aspiration is diagnostic of a complex cyst. The same approach can be used to guide fine-needle aspiration for cytology, core-needle biopsies for histology, and preoperative needle wire localization of masses for surgery, and for the injection of radioactive tracers for sentinel node identification and mapping.

In some cases, a patient has a clinical sign or symptom of possible breast cancer, and yet diagnostic breast imaging shows no abnormality. The most common clinical scenario is the patient with a breast lump and negative breast imaging. If no imaging correlation can be identified to explain the patient's breast lump, the patient must be managed clinically, which means that she is examined sequentially through at least one menstrual cycle. In the overwhelming majority of cases, the breast lump will improve or resolve completely, confirming the diagnosis of clinical fibrocystic condition. If the breast lump does not improve or continues to grow, surgical biopsy is performed.

Targeted Versus Whole Breast Scan

When examining for a palpable mass or for correlation with an abnormal mammogram, some centers scan only the area of interest. This is referred to as a **targeted scan**. For example, if a mass in the upper inner quadrant of the right breast is seen on the mammogram, then only the upper inner quadrant of the right breast will be scanned by ultrasound. The targeted scan is a more specific approach to lesion evaluation, results in fewer cases of false-positive sonographic findings, and is more cost effective than scanning the entire breast. Although some imaging centers routinely scan the entire breast, this technique is best performed with a real-time automated breast scanner.

Sonographic Evaluation of the Breast

The sonographer must have basic clinical information regarding any patient who is referred for breast ultrasound. Pertinent clinical information includes the patient's age, risk factors for breast cancer, symptoms, as well as the location and clinical impression of any breast lumps. Any history of trauma to the breast or previous breast surgery is also helpful. Inspection of the breast during the ultrasound examination often reveals pertinent findings. For example, the examiner should make note of any surface nipple erosion (possible Paget disease), nipple or skin retraction, skin thickening (edema, scarring, or peau d'orange), scars, signs of inflammation (induration and erythema), or contusion. Sonography is normally used as an adjunct to mammography but may be the initial method of imaging when a breast lump is palpable; it may also be used in a young patient with dense breasts, in a pregnant or lactating patient, in a patient with breast augmentation, or in a patient with a difficult or compromised mammogram.

Before the breast ultrasound examination begins, the sonographer must review the request to determine the scope of the exam requested (targeted/whole breast) and the clinical indication. When possible, imaging tests such as a mammogram or previous sonogram should also be reviewed. Imaging results may also be obtained from the patient's medical record. Clinical information should be obtained from the patient to include visual assessment of the patient's breasts to look for asymmetry, scars, moles, dermatologic conditions, contour changes, dimpling, skin thickening, discolorations, nipple retraction, and flattening or discharge. If the patient presents with a palpable mass, the sonographer should ask the patient to palpate the mass and then feel it for oneself. Any of these findings should be marked on an anatomical drawing to assist the sonologist with interpretation of the sonographic exam. Image optimization is achieved by using the highest-frequency transducer available that will allow visualization of all levels of the breast from skin line to the deeper echogenic chest wall. Adjustment of electronic focusing, overall gain, and time-gain compensation should be made to balance the detail within the breast tissue.

Patient Positioning. Position the patient in a supine position with the arm of the side being examined extended over her head (Fig. 21.18). Next, ask the patient to roll in a posterior oblique fashion so that the side to be evaluated is elevated slightly. This will allow the breast tissues to be evenly distributed over the chest wall with the nipple being centrally located. This position flattens the breast tissue and allows us to scan more perpendicularly to the chest wall. The straight supine position may help in evaluating the medial portion of the breast. For the lateral margin of the breast, the patient can be rolled slightly toward the opposite side (approximately 30 to 45 degrees) and stabilized with a cushion under her shoulder and hips. In some instances, a palpable mass may only be palpated in another position including upright. Other positions should be employed if they better facilitate identification and scanning of the tissues in question. For example, if a lesion identified on a mammogram cannot be located sonographically, the sonographer might try positioning the breast in the same positions used to obtain the mammogram. This allows easier localization and a similar frame of reference.

Scan Technique. The transducer orientation should remain the same as with conventional ultrasound examinations (i.e., the patient's right side is oriented to the left of the screen on transverse images, and the notch of the transducer is directed cephalad on longitudinal images). If a breast mass is identified, it should be thoroughly scanned in orthogonal planes (90 degrees apart) for evaluation of the lesion in three dimensions. This can be recorded using sagittal and transverse images or using radial/antiradial transducer positions (Fig. 21.19). Use of radial/antiradial positions is unique

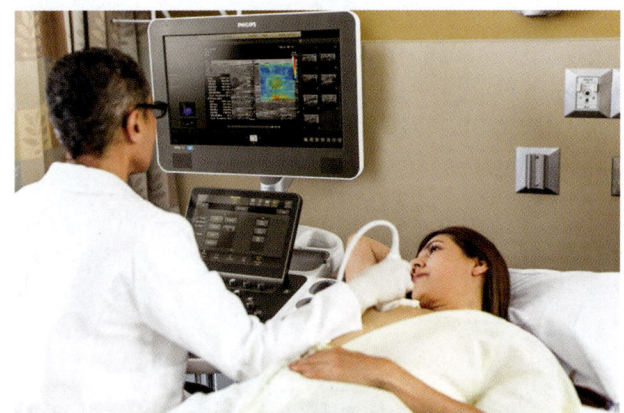

FIG. 21.18 Place the patient in a supine position with the arm of the side being examined extended over her head.

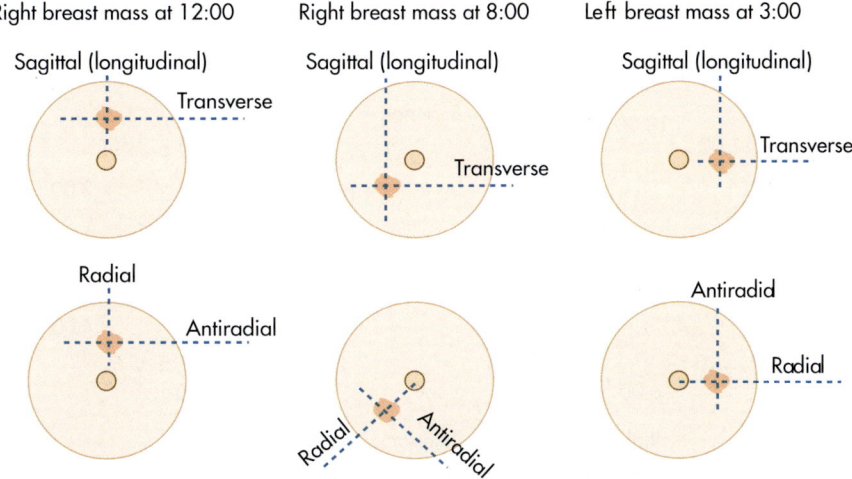

FIG. 21.19 Sagittal and transverse, plus radial and antiradial, transducer positions.

to the breast and can often pick up subtle abnormalities extending toward the nipple along the ductal system from the mass. All dominant solid masses are generally recorded with 3D measurements (length, width, and height) to facilitate management decisions and future follow-up.

Finally, your examination should include the areola, nipple, and skin line. Following the ducts to the nipple requires some special maneuvering and imaging the nipple can be accomplished two different ways. The **rolled nipple technique** is where you place one finger alongside the nipple and, with the pressure from the transducer, you roll the nipple over the finger so you are scanning parallel to the duct (Fig. 21.20A).

The skin line and superficial structures may be difficult to evaluate without the use of an acoustic stand-off pad. There are several commercially available pads or one can use a large dollop of gel (see Fig. 21.20B). The standoff thickness, however, should not exceed 1 cm due to the elevation plane focus which is fixed.

Annotation. There are several different methods of annotating breast images including the clock face method, the quadrant method, and the 123-ABC method. The **clock face method** involves viewing each breast as if it were the face of a clock. The scan plane is performed radially in the same direction as hands of a clock or spokes of a wheel. The specific location of a mass would be described according to the position on the clock. Directly above the nipple on either breast is 12 o'clock. Right medial breast and left lateral breast are 3 o'clock. Directly below the nipple bilaterally is 6 o'clock, and right lateral breast and left medial breast are 9 o'clock, respectively (Fig. 21.21).

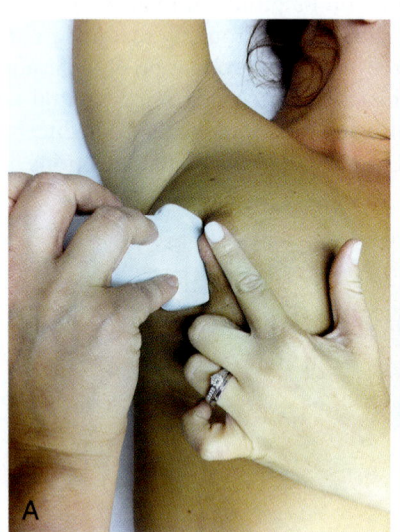
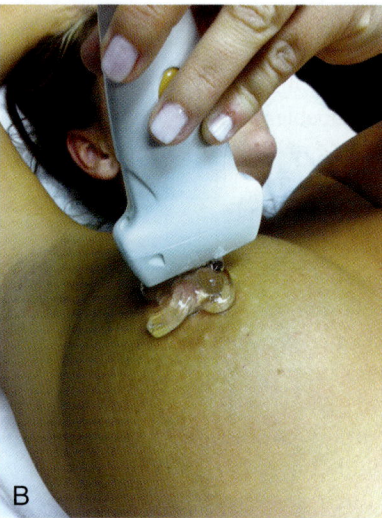

FIG. 21.20 Nipple roll. (A) The rolled nipple technique for evaluating the duct within the nipple. (B) Use of a thick dollop of gel as a stand-off material to better visualize the nipple and skin line.

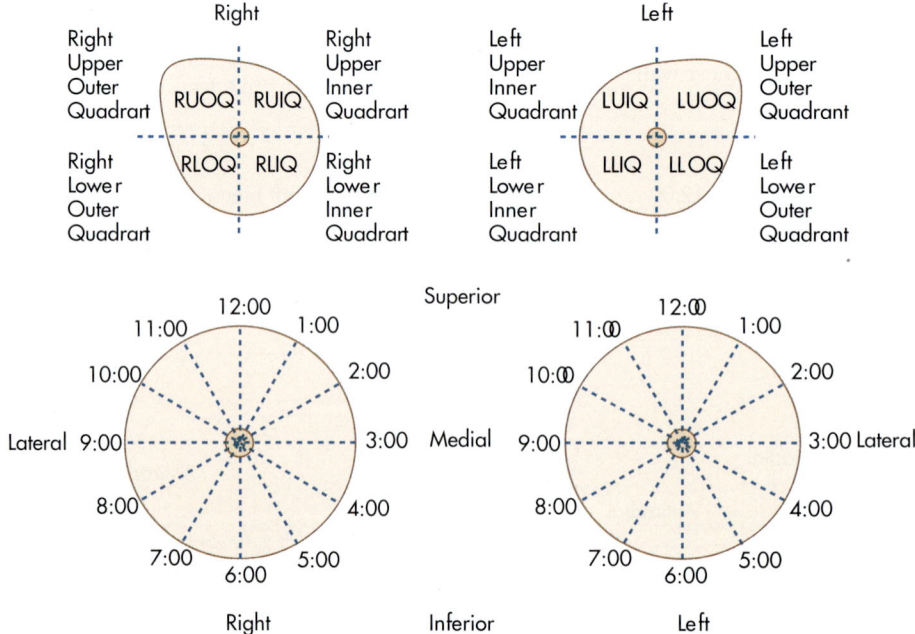

FIG. 21.21 Breast anatomy is described by two methods: the quadrant method (right/left, upper/lower, and inner/outer quadrants) and the clock face method.

The **side/quadrant method** divides the breast into four quadrants which are labeled as indicated in Box 21.6. The sonographer can choose either longitudinal/transverse planes or radial/antiradial planes using this method.

The **123-ABC method** is the most specific way of describing mass location when combined with either the clock face or side/quadrant methods. 123 refers to the approximate distance from the nipple. Three equal-width imaginary rings encircle the breast. 1 is the area closest to the nipple and 3 is the most peripheral aspect of the breast (Fig. 21.22). ABC indicates how deep a mass is located. A would be in the subcutaneous layer, B in the mammary zone, and C is the retromammary zone. A mass labeled as Lt. 2:00 3 C would indicate a mass in the left breast at the 2:00 o'clock position deep near the chest wall and peripheral outer quadrant.

If the abbreviations RAD or AR are included, the scan planes utilized were radial (RAD) or antiradial (AR). It is important to document the orientation of the mass, in addition to its location. The orientation of a lesion is determined by aligning the transducer with the longest axis of a lesion and identifying whether the long axis is oriented in a **radial or antiradial plane**. This is important because malignancies tend to grow within the ducts and often follow the ductal system in a radial plane toward the convergence at the nipple.

High-quality sonographic imaging of a solid breast mass is accurate in characterizing a lesion as probably benign or probably malignant in a majority of cases (Table 21.2). It is important, however, to realize that there is significant overlap in the appearance of benign and malignant lesions; ultrasound cannot be used as a substitute for tissue diagnosis when sonographic findings are indeterminate or when a biopsy is

BOX 21.6	ANNOTATION: Side/Quadrant Method

RUOQ: right upper outer quadrant
RUIQ: right upper inner quadrant
RLOQ: right lower outer quadrant
RLIQ: right lower inner quadrant
LUOQ: left upper outer quadrant
LUIQ: left upper inner quadrant
LLOQ: left lower outer quadrant
LLIQ: left lower inner quadrant
SA: subareolar
AX: axilla

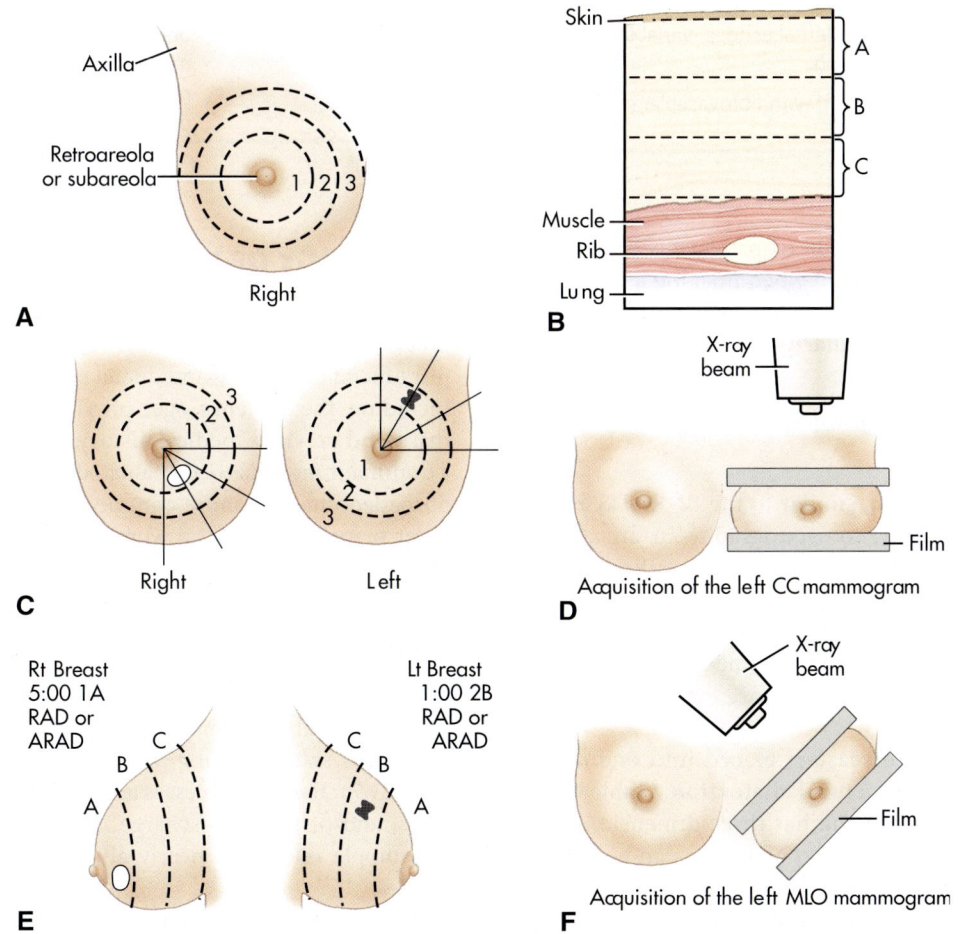

FIG. 21.22 (A) Zones of the breast. (B) Documentation of depth of tissue. (C) Localization of mass in the right breast. (D) Anterior and posterior mammogram of the breast. (E) Longitudinal view of the breast mass. (F) Medial to lateral mammogram acquisition. *ARAD*, Antiradial; *CC*, craniocaudal; *MLO*, mediolateral; *RAD*, radial.

TABLE 21.2	Sonographic Characteristics of Common Lesions
Mass	**Characteristics**
Simple cyst	Oval or round, anechoic, imperceptible capsule, posterior acoustic enhancement, edge refraction shadowing, often compressible.
Fibrocystic changes	Multiple cysts, well circumscribed, thin walls, increased fibrous stroma.
Complex cyst	Irregular or thickened wall, mural nodule, fluid levels, debris, particulate echoes, variable degrees of shadowing.
Benign fibroadenoma	Oval or gently lobular, hypoechoic, uniform echogenicity, smooth, distinct margins, wider than tall, posterior acoustic enhancement, edge refraction shadow.
Lipoma	May be large, smooth walls, hypoechoic (isoechoic with fat), posterior acoustic enhancement, easily compressible.
Fat necrosis	Irregular, complex mass with low-level echoes; may have posterior acoustic shadow, separate from breast parenchyma.
Abscess	Hypoechoic, complex lesion, posterior enhancement, thick walls, fluid levels.
Cystosarcoma phyllodes	Large, hypoechoic tumor, well-defined margins, decreased through-transmission, fine or coarse internal echoes, variable amounts of shadowing.
Intraductal papilloma	Intracystic lesion with fibrovascular stalk.

TABLE 21.3	American College of Radiology Descriptive Form for Breast Evaluation: Ultrasound Lexicon	
Breast composition	a. Homogeneous—fat b. Homogeneous—fibroglandular c. Heterogeneous	
Mass	Shape:	Oval, round, irregular
	Margin:	Circumscribed or not circumscribed: indistinct, angular, microlobulated, spiculated
	Orientation:	Parallel, not parallel
	Echo pattern:	Anechoic, hyperechoic, complex cystic/solid hypoechoic, isoechoic, heterogeneous
	Posterior features:	No features, enhancement, shadowing, combined pattern
Calcifications	In mass, outside mass, intraductal	
Associated features	Architectural distortion, duct changes, skin thickening, skin retraction, edema, vascularity (absent, internal, rim), elasticity	
Special cases (cases with a unique diagnosis)	Simple cyst, clustered microcysts, complicated cyst, mass in or on skin, foreign body (including implants), intramammary lymph node, arteriovenous malformation, Mondor disease, postsurgical fluid collection, fat necrosis	

indicated by clinical examination or patient history. Several characteristics must be observed when imaging a solid mass including **margins, shape, orientation, echo pattern, mobility, compressibility**, and **vascularity**.

American College of Radiology Sonography Descriptive Form

ACR has published a form, similar to the BI-RADS assessment for mammography, for sonography in an attempt to standardize descriptive terms and classifications of breast masses seen with sonography. BI-RADS stands for BI-RADS and the categories are defined in Table 21.1. It is important that everyone use the same terms to describe masses in order to accurately diagnose breast disease and specific lesions.

ACR FORM breast disease is placed into one of two groups: **mass** and **architectural distortion** (Table 21.3). A mass is space occupying and has three dimensions. The form and structure *(morphology)* of a mass can be characterized under primary and secondary features as shown in Table 21.3. Dynamic maneuvers should be performed to determine mobility and compressibility. When available, color Doppler should be used to detect the presence or absence of blood flow.

PATHOLOGY OF THE BREAST

The most common benign pathologic lesions of the female breast include cysts, fibrocystic dysplasia, fibroadenoma, intraductal papilloma, and ductal ectasia. Several parameters, including the patient's age, physical characteristics of the mass, and previous medical history, must be considered when a dominant mass has been palpated. Fibrocystic dysplasia and fibroadenomas are more common in younger women while older or postmenopausal women are more likely to present with intraductal papilloma and ductal ectasia.

Clinical Evaluation

Clinical symptoms of breast disease include pain with or without a palpable mass, spontaneous or induced nipple discharge, skin dimpling, ulceration, and nipple retraction (Box 21.7). Benign processes are usually associated with pain, mass, and/or nipple discharge. Skin dimpling or ulceration and nipple retraction nearly always appear with malignant masses.

Benign tumors are rubbery, mobile, and well defined (as seen in a fibroadenoma), whereas malignant tumors are often stone hard and irregular with a gritty feel. Soft tumors usually represent a lipoma (fatty tissue). Cystic masses are like a

> **BOX 21.7 Clinical Evaluation of the Patient With a Breast Problem**
>
> **History**
> Patient age
> Risk factors for breast cancer
> Onset and duration of mass
> Relation to menstrual cycle
>
> **Breast Examination (for Palpable Mass)**
> **Location of Mass**
> Clock face or quadrant
>
> **Characteristics of Mass**
> Size
> Shape (round, oval, lobular, irregular)
> Surface contour (smooth, irregular)
> Consistency (soft, rubbery, firm, hard, gritty)
> Mobility (movable, fixed)

> **BOX 21.8 Sonographic Characteristics of Breast Lesions**
>
> **Simple Cyst**
> - Smooth walls
> - Anechoic
> - Posterior enhancement
>
> **Complicated Cyst**
> - Wall thickening or irregularities
> - Septations
> - Internal echoes
>
> **Solid Mass**
> Margins
> - Benign: smooth, rounded
> - Malignant: indistinct, fuzzy, spiculated
>
> Disruption of breast architecture
> - Benign: grow within tissue, causing compression of the tissue adjacent to the mass
> - Malignant: grow through tissue without compressing adjacent tissue and may cause retraction of the nipple or dimpling of the skin
>
> Shape
> - Benign: rounded or oval, large lobulations (<3)
> - Malignant: sharp, angular microlobulations (≥3)
>
> Orientation
> - Malignant: taller than wide highly suspicious; radial growth suspicious for intraductal lesions
>
> Internal echo pattern
> - Benign: isoechoic, hyperechoic
> - Malignant: hypoechoic, weak internal echoes, clustered microcalcifications
>
> Attenuation effects
> - Benign: posterior enhancement
> - Malignant: strongly attenuating
>
> Mobility
> - Benign: some mobility
> - Malignant: firmly fixed
>
> Compressibility
> - Benign: fatty tumors are usually compressible
> - Malignant: rigid, noncompressible
>
> Vascularity
> - Malignant: hypervascular; feeder vessel may be identified

balloon of water, well-delineated, but not as mobile as fibroadenomas because they form part of the breast parenchyma, whereas a fibroadenoma has a capsule (Box 21.8).

Benign solid masses have relatively smooth margins or may be mildly lobulated. Lobulations associated with benign fibroadenomas are usually large, rounded lobulations and do not exceed three in number. The normal tissue planes of the breast are horizontally oriented. Benign lesions tend to grow within the normal tissue planes, and their long axis lies parallel to the chest wall. These lesions are noted to be "wider than tall."

Benign Breast Conditions

Breast Cysts. Cysts of the breast are commonly seen in women age 35 to 55 years and particularly in women who are perimenopausal. Symptoms include history of palpable lump(s) that change in size with the menstrual cycle, pain (especially when the cyst is growing rapidly), and tenderness. Cysts are basically dilated ducts caused by accumulated secretions caused by either an intrinsic or extrinsic process. Cysts commonly resolve after menopause although certain factors may predispose a woman to develop cysts such as hormone replacement therapy, the use of blood pressure medications, steroids, or digitalis. All have been linked to the formation of breast cysts in the postmenopausal patient. Small cysts may not regress completely and may persist from one cycle to the next. Most cysts will resolve after menopause unless the patient uses hormone replacement therapy.

Simple cysts meet all the criteria of a simple cyst anywhere else in the body. Cysts may be singular, clustered, simple, or complex. Complex cysts include those containing cholesterol crystals, hemorrhagic, infected debris, internal septations, and wall irregularities. A complex cyst is one that cannot be categorized as solid but does not meet all criteria for a cyst and aspiration is generally performed to confirm a benign etiology. A septated cyst with thin septae is usually treated as a simple cyst. Cysts will compress upon applying transducer pressure and are slightly moveable upon physical exam. Cysts are frequently round or oval (long axis toward nipple), smooth, and soft. Some cysts under tension can be firm and are often tender. The usual approach to a small, smooth, round, or oval benign-appearing solid mass in low-risk patients favors close interval follow-up breast imaging.

Sonographic Evaluation of a Cyst. Evaluation of a breast lesion normally begins with determination of whether a lesion is cystic or solid. The distinction between a cyst and a solid mass is extremely important for management purposes.

Simple Cyst. A cyst that meets the requirements of a simple cyst on ultrasound is universally considered benign. To be considered a simple cyst, a lesion must meet the following criteria on ultrasound: (1) the cyst must be devoid of internal echoes (anechoic), (2) show smooth inner margins with a defined, well-circumscribed capsule, and (3) demonstrate posterior acoustic enhancement (Fig. 21.23). In the case of simple cysts, usually, no further work up is required.

Complex Cyst. If the cyst has internal echoes, wall irregularity, mural nodularity or septations, shadowing, nonuniform internal echoes, or any other feature not associated with a simple cyst it is by definition a complex cyst (Fig. 21.24). Complex cysts are usually benign but may appear solid unless one can identify layering or floating crystals. Features that might suggest an **inflammatory reaction** would include internal fluid-debris levels that are gravity dependent, isoechoic wall thickening, and Color Doppler flow seen within the wall due to hyperemia. If a complex cyst is found, aspiration and/or biopsy should be considered.

Complex cysts are often indistinguishable from homogeneous solid sonographic masses because of their thick proteinaceous fluid content. Other complex cysts have thick or irregular capsules, a possible intracystic mass, or dependent debris. Cysts with layering calcifications or floating crystals are benign, although careful ultrasound evaluation is required to distinguish these cysts from those requiring further evaluation.

Subcutaneous cysts, such as epidermal, sebaceous, and epidermal inclusion cysts, are often complex containing keratin or sebum. They occur just under the skin from an obstructed sebaceous gland or hair follicle. They may also originate secondary to trauma.

Fibrocystic Dysplasia/Fibrocystic Changes

Fibrocystic dysplasia is the most common cause of breast masses in premenopausal patients. Fibrocystic changes produce histologic alterations in the terminal ducts and lobules of the breast in both epithelial and connective tissues and, although it may be asymptomatic, most cases are accompanied by pain or tenderness representing normal physiologic processes of breast tissue that fluctuate under the influence of female hormonal cycles. Other symptoms can include discomfort under the arms, breasts that feel swollen and heavy, and a dark brown or green discharge from the nipple. In most cases, both breasts are equally involved.

Imaging signs of fibrocystic dysplasia may be visible on the mammogram or breast ultrasound. On a mammogram, fibrocystic dysplasia may cause diffuse benign microcalcifications and multiple round masses. Sonographically, the breast may include scattered calcifications and cystic changes, such as simple cysts, complicated cysts, clustered cysts, and clustered microcysts (Fig. 21.25).

The first stage of fibrocystic changes is breast pain referred to as **mastodynia**, seen in younger women. Patients complain of painful breasts in the premenstrual period. This stage may regress with time, medications, or pregnancy. The second stage is called adenosis, predominantly seen in women aged 25 to 40 years. This stage can be accompanied by painful, lumpy breasts and nipple discharge. Postmenopausal women experience less severe pain. Sonographically, the fibrous glandular tissue appears hyperechoic and numerous small cysts may be seen scattered throughout along with some larger cysts. Late-stage cystic disease seen in women 35 to 55 years of age will present with more large cysts (macrocystic), increased pain, and defined palpable lump(s).

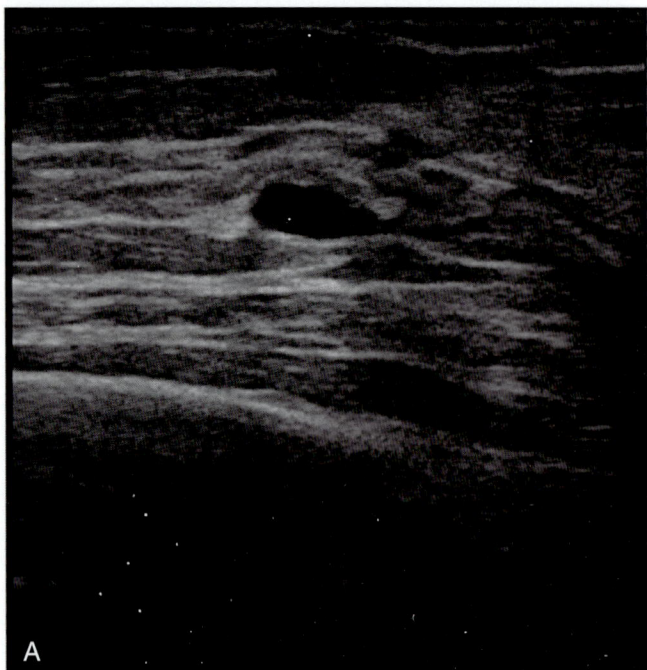
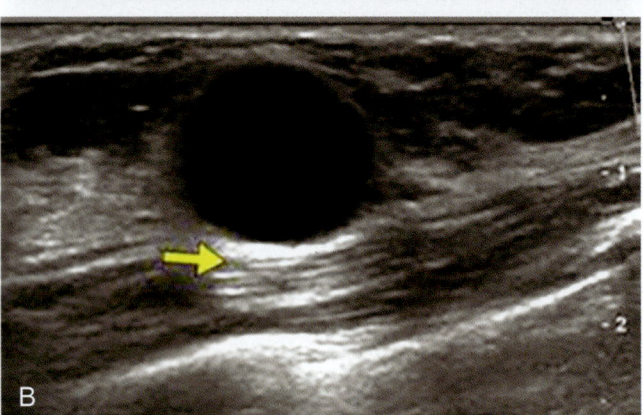
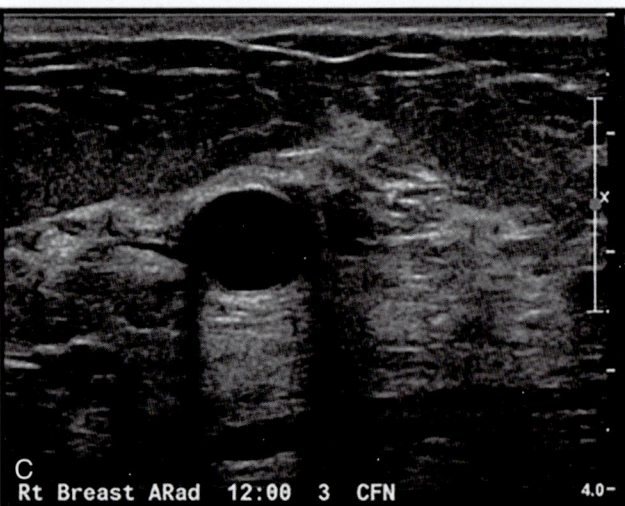

FIG. 21.23 To be considered a simple cyst, a lesion must meet the following criteria on ultrasound: (A) the cyst must be devoid of internal echoes (anechoic; A), show smooth inner margins with a defined, well-circumscribed capsule (B), and demonstrate posterior acoustic enhancement (C).

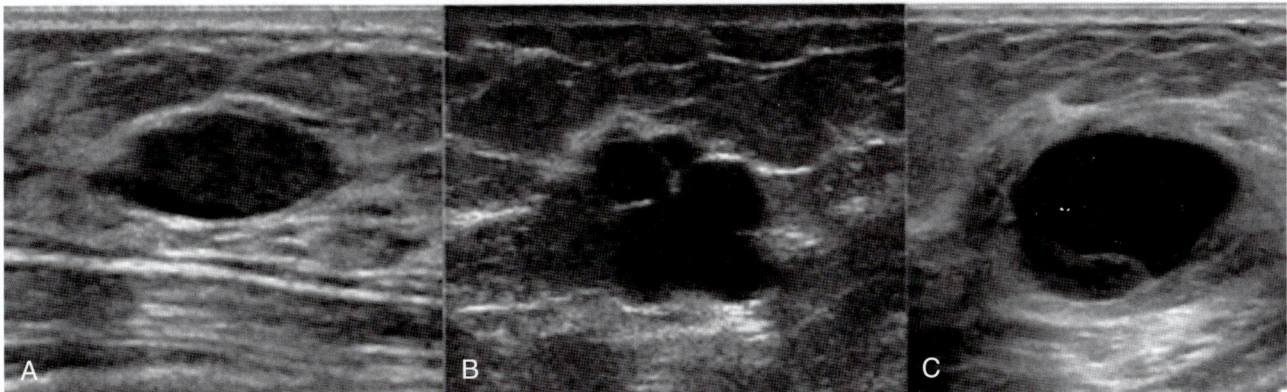

FIG. 21.24 A complex mass in the breast may appear with a variety of patterns: low level echoes (A), "strains" within the complex cyst (B), or a combination of loculated low level echoes within the smooth cystic mass (C).

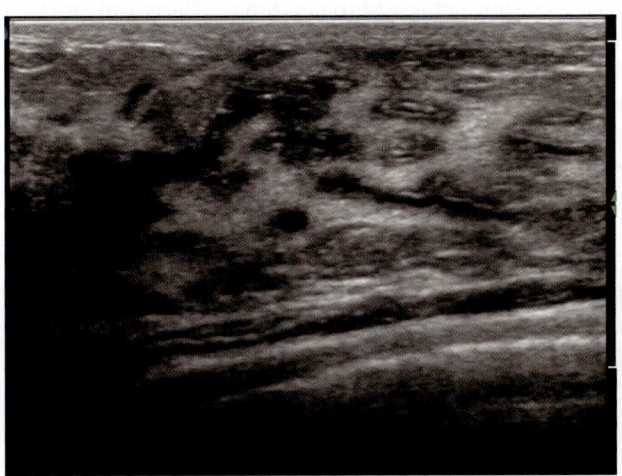
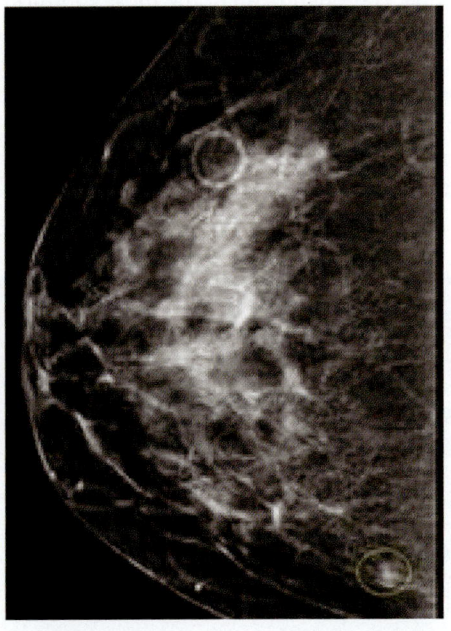

FIG. 21.25 Fibrocystic dysplasia on ultrasound and mammography demonstrated scattered calcifications and cystic changes.

Many separate tissue processes of fibrocystic dysplasia are recognized by the pathologist in reviewing breast tissue under a microscope, including **apocrine metaplasia**, fibrosis, epithelial ductal hyperplasia, and sclerosing adenosis. In correlating the pathologic results of a breast biopsy with the indication for biopsy (i.e., palpable breast lump, suspicious mammographic or sonographic mass, or clustered microcalcifications), it is very important for the physician to document that the pathologic results are concordant with the targeted lesion. If a breast biopsy was performed because of suspicious microcalcifications, for example, the pathology report should state that microcalcifications were seen. If no microcalcifications were seen on pathology slides, then this is a discordant result, and further investigation will be required.

Sonographic Findings of Fibrocystic Disease. Patients with fibrocystic disease of the breast may present with multiple well-circumscribed cystic lesions with thin walls and increased fibrous stroma

Benign Fibroadenoma of the Breast

The most common benign breast tumor is the fibroadenoma, and it occurs primarily in young women with an age range of 15 to 40 years. Fibroadenomas may be found in one or both breasts. The growth of a fibroadenoma is stimulated by estrogen. Under normal circumstances, hormonal influences on the breast (estrogen) result in the proliferation of epithelial cells in lactiferous ducts and in stromal tissue during the first half of the menstrual cycle. During the second half of the cycle, this condition regresses, thus allowing breast tissue to return to its normal resting state. In certain disturbances of this hormonal mechanism, regression fails to occur, resulting in the development of fibrous and epithelial nodules, separate from the ductal system, that become fibroadenomas, fibromas, or adenomas, depending on the predominant cell type. They may also be related to pregnancy and lactation.

Clinically, a fibroadenoma is firm, rubbery, freely mobile, and is clearly delineated from the surrounding breast tissue. It is round or ovoid, and smooth or lobulated, and usually does not cause loss of contour of the breast unless it develops to a large size. It rarely causes mastodynia, and it does not change size during the menstrual cycle. Fibroadenomas tend to grow very slowly. A sudden increase in size with acute pain may be the result of hemorrhage within the tumor. However, a growth greater than 20% within 6 months may suggest a phyllodes tumor, which warrants further investigation. Calcification may follow hemorrhage or infarction; thus the tumor may have calcifications and may mimic the appearance of a carcinoma on mammography.

There is a variant of the fibroadenoma which is seen in adolescent females (ages 10 to 20 years), called the giant (juvenile) fibroadenoma. These tumors can grow quite large and may contain dilated veins. Although benign, the most common treatment approach is needle biopsy followed by surgical excision.

Sonographic Findings of Fibroadenoma. Sonographically, fibroadenomas have benign characteristics with smooth, rounded margins and low-level homogeneous internal echoes. The fibroadenoma may demonstrate intermediate posterior enhancement. Fibroadenomas are normally hypoechoic, but occasionally are hyperechoic to the fat within the breast. Echo patterns vary from homogenous to heterogeneous (Fig. 21.26). Lesions that appear isoechoic with the breast parenchyma or have echoes equivalent to or brighter than that of fat are most often benign. Larger benign lesions often cause compression of tissue adjacent to the mass, implying that the mass is pushing against adjacent breast tissue, as opposed to infiltrating it. Poor enhancement behind a lesion is normally caused by a weakly attenuating structure; it usually indicates that the lesion is made up of fluid and is a characteristic associated with benign lesions. Note that most solid lesions, with the exception of a fibroadenoma, will not enhance.

Pregnant and/or Lactating Patient

Most masses that present in a pregnant or lactating patient are benign fibroadenomas. These can often enlarge rapidly because of the marked increase in circulating hormone levels during pregnancy and lactation. The increase in circulating hormones, however, can have a similar effect on breast cancers. In patients who develop breast cancer during pregnancy, cancers are often diagnosed at a later stage than in the nonpregnant patient.

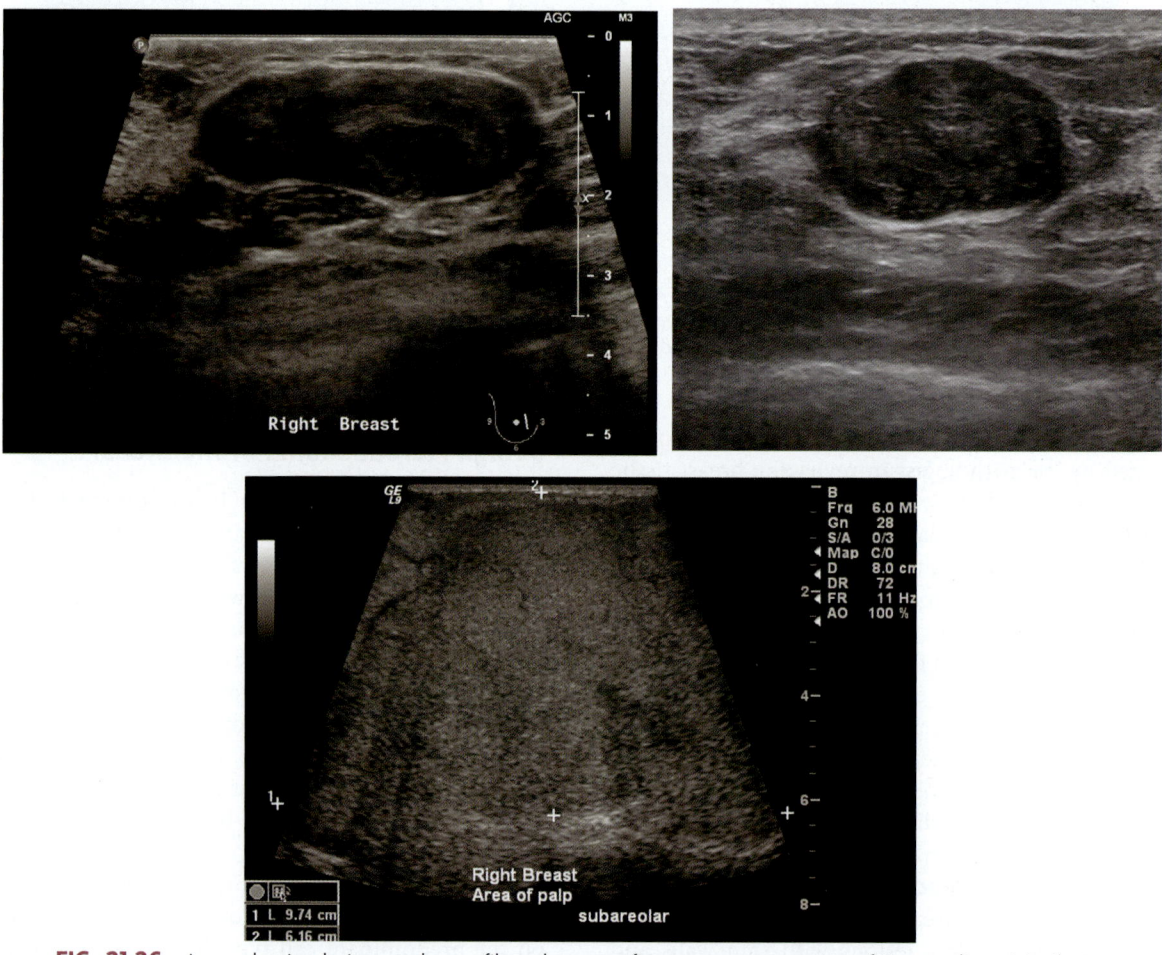

FIG. 21.26 Larger benign lesions such as a fibroadenoma often cause compression of tissue adjacent to the mass, implying that the mass is pushing against adjacent breast tissue, as opposed to infiltrating it. Poor enhancement behind a lesion is normally caused by a weakly attenuating structure.

Other Breast Problems

Other breast problems that may arise during pregnancy or lactation include mastitis, abscesses, cysts, or galactoceles (cysts containing milk). In the case of a galactocele, a fat-fluid level may be visible both by mammography and by ultrasound, but more commonly, this lesion appears as a complex cyst. Galactoceles or cysts can be aspirated easily under ultrasound guidance (Fig. 21.27).

Mastitis

Mastitis is categorized as **puerperal, periductal,** and **granulomatous**. Of the three, puerperal is the most common acute type occurring during lactation. **Periductal mastitis** is a noninfectious form of mastitis seen in perimenopausal and menopausal women. **Granulomatous mastitis** results from a traumatic injury, foreign body (silicone-sutures/clips-scar-sponge-pacemaker) or fungal infection (histoplasmosis), parasitic disease (hydatid-schistosomiasis), and autoimmune disorders (polyarteritis).

Acute Mastitis. Acute mastitis may result from infection, trauma, mechanical obstruction in the breast ducts caused by milk or mucus, or other conditions. It most often occurs during lactation, beginning in the lactiferous ducts (localized) and spreading via the lymphatic or blood (diffuse). Clinically, acute mastitis causes an enlarged, reddened, tender breast, and is often confined to one area of the breast. The galactocele, associated with lactation, is a milk-filled cyst which can develop within the TDLU (peripheral location) or within the lactiferous sinus of a main duct (central location). If the galactocele becomes infected, it can lead to mastitis and abscess formation while a persistent galactocele may turn into a lipid or oil cyst (Fig. 21.28). Diffuse mastitis results when infection

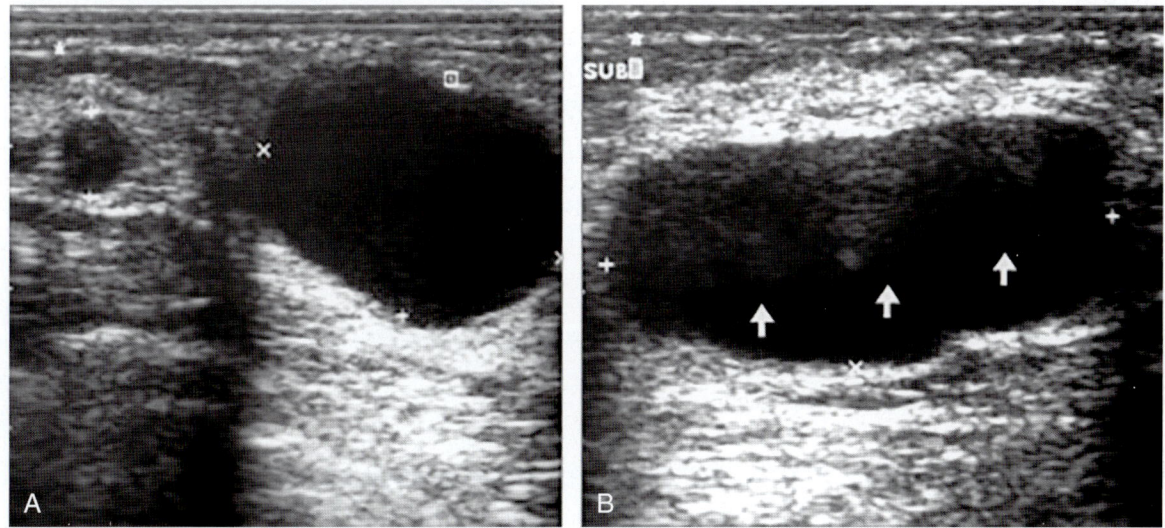

FIG. 21.27 Breast ultrasound in this postpartum patient reveals a large galactocele with low-level internal echoes.

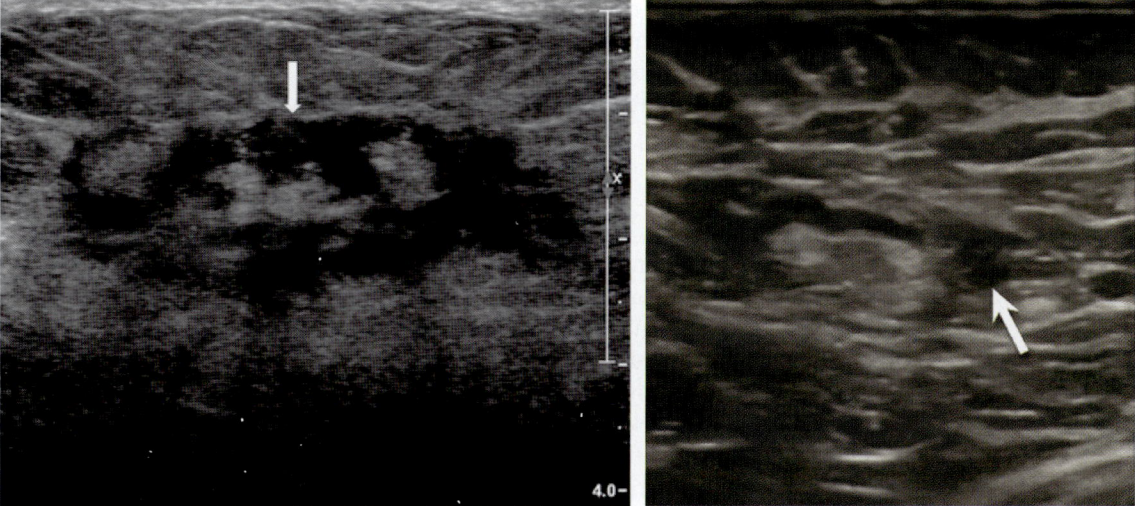

FIG. 21.28 Acute mastitis most often occurs during lactation, beginning in the lactiferous ducts (localized) and spreading via the lymphatic or blood (diffuse).

is carried via the blood or breast lymphatics and thus affects the entire breast. Patients are treated initially with antibiotics and are referred for breast imaging when acute inflammatory symptoms are sufficiently reduced to allow good-quality mammography and breast ultrasound to rule out inflammatory breast cancer as a cause.

Chronic Mastitis. An inflammation of the glandular tissue is considered to be chronic mastitis. This is very difficult to differentiate by ultrasound; the echo pattern is mixed and diffuse with sound absorption. The condition is usually found in elderly women. Thickening of the connective tissue results in narrowing of the lumina of the milk ducts. The cause is inspissated intraductal secretions, which are forced into the periductal connective tissue. Clinically, the patient usually has a nipple discharge; frequently, the nipple has retracted over a period of years. Palpation reveals some subareolar thickening, but no dominant mass.

Breast Abscess

Because obstructed ducts are prone to infection, acute mastitis can develop into an abscess. Abscesses are relatively rare, occurring in only a small percentage of patients, and may be single or multiple. Abscesses develop from bacteria entering through a cracked nipple or skin wound and are most often found in the subareolar area. However, they can form virtually in any part of the breast. Acute abscesses have a poorly defined border, whereas mature abscesses are well encapsulated with sharp borders. A definite diagnosis cannot be made from a mammogram alone, and either an aspiration or core needle biopsy is necessary to determine a diagnosis. An aspiration or biopsy is necessary to determine a diagnosis, but clinical findings help diagnose breast abscesses. Patients may present with pain, swelling, and reddening of the overlying skin. The patient may be febrile, and swollen painful axillary nodes may be present.

▸ **Sonographic Findings.** Ultrasound may show a diffuse, mottled appearance of the breast, irregular margins, posterior enhancement, and low-level internal echoes (Fig. 21.29). If associated with mastitis, skin thickening is almost always present, and edema leads to diffusely increased echogenicity of the breast tissue. Color or power Doppler of the breast may be helpful to document hyperemia associated with increased vascularity, which may tip the scales toward abscess rather than hematoma.

Fat Necrosis

Injury to breast fat may cause a common benign inflammatory process known as fat necrosis. Injuries include trauma to the breast, surgery, radiation treatments, or plasma cell mastitis or may be related to an involutional process or other disease present in the breast, such as cancer. It is more frequently found in older women. Clinical palpation reveals a spherical nodule that is generally superficial under a layer of calcified necrosis. A deep-lying focus of necrosis may cause scarring with skin retraction and thus may mimic carcinoma. Benign lesions normally demonstrate a limited degree of mobility or

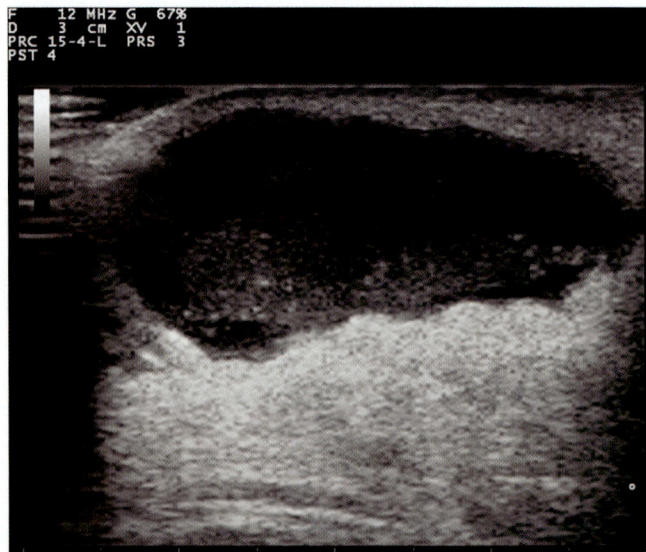
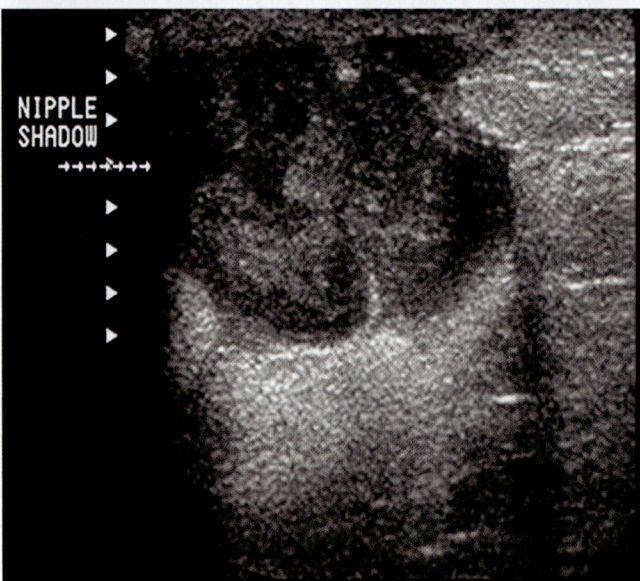

FIG. 21.29 Breast abscess on ultrasound appears as a complex mass without increased enhancement.

may roll away as they are palpated. If pressure applied by the transducer causes the lesion to compress or change shape, the lesion is probably benign and most likely represents a fat lobule.

▸ **Sonographic Findings.** Sonographically, fat necrosis may appear a number of ways. It may appear as a solid lesion, as a complex mass with mural nodules or echogenic bands, as an anechoic mass with either posterior acoustic enhancement or with shadowing, or without a visible mass. This variability may mimic a malignant lesion; however, it is separate and distinct from the rest of the breast parenchyma (Fig. 21.30).

Breast Hematoma

Breast hematomas may develop as a result of trauma or occur spontaneously in patients who take prescribed anticoagulants (coumadin/heparin) or in patients afflicted with a bleeding

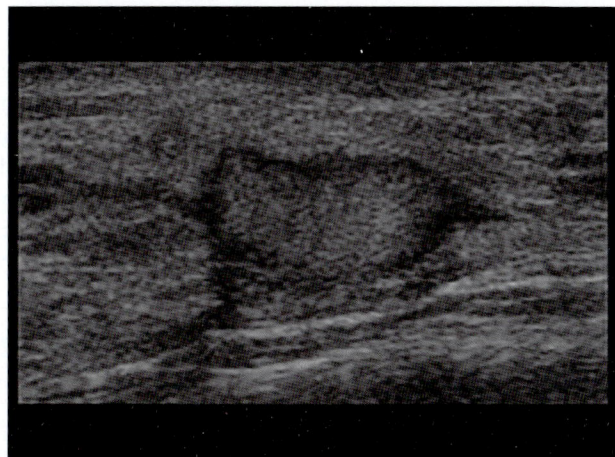

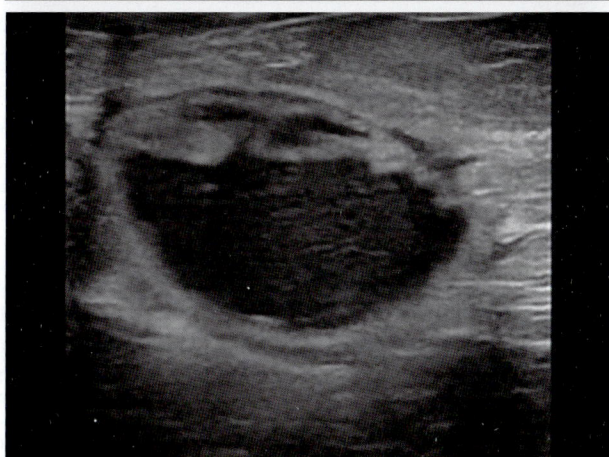

FIG. 21.30 Fat necrosis may appear as a solid lesion, as a complex mass with mural nodules or echogenic bands, as an anechoic mass with either posterior acoustic enhancement or with shadowing, or without a visible mass.

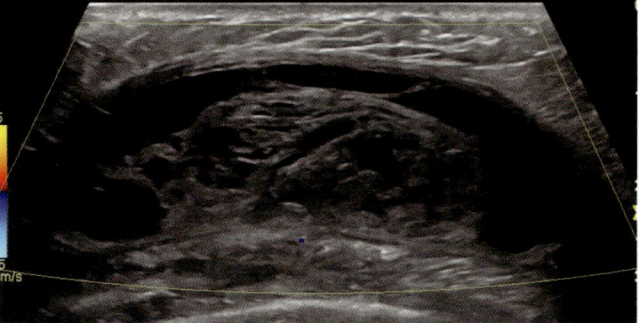

FIG. 21.31 Seroma of the breast following a surgical procedure.

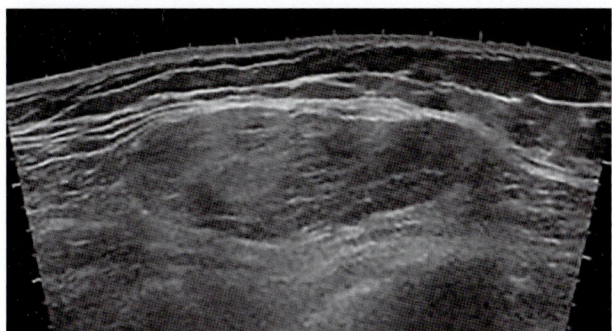

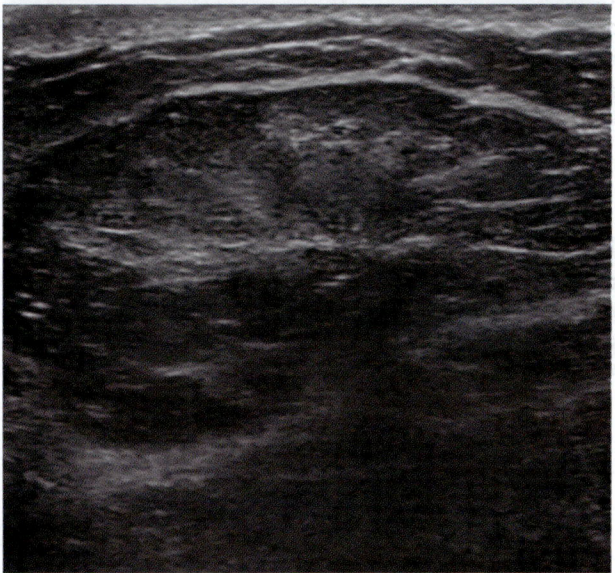

FIG. 21.32 Lipoma of the breast is very difficult to separate from fatty breast tissue.

disorder such as leukemia, thrombocytopenia, or hemophilia. Breast trauma can occur from the seat belt or air bag in an automobile accident or from an invasive procedure such as biopsy, cyst aspiration, or surgery.

Seroma/Lymphocele

A seroma is a collection of clear serous fluid consisting of the watery portion of blood, while a lymphocele is clear lymph fluid. Of the two, the seroma is the most common (Fig. 21.31). Such fluid collections may develop after a surgical procedure and cannot be differentiated sonographically.

Lipoma

A pure lipoma consists entirely of fatty tissue. Other forms of lipoma consist of fat with fibrous and glandular elements interspersed (fibroadenolipoma). A lipoma may grow to a large size before it is clinically detected. It is usually found in middle-aged or menopausal women. Clinically, on palpation, a large, soft, poorly demarcated mass is felt that cannot be clearly separated from the surrounding parenchyma. No thinning or fixation of the overlying skin is noted.

Sonographic Findings. Sonographically, it may be difficult or impossible to distinguish a lipoma in a fatty breast. Lipomas typically have smooth walls, are hypoechoic, and appear similar to fat. They often demonstrate posterior enhancement and are soft and easily compressible (Fig. 21.32).

Intraductal Papilloma

An intraductal papilloma is a small, benign tumor that grows within the acini of the breast. It occurs most frequently in women age 35 to 55 years. The predominant symptom is spontaneous nipple discharge arising from a single duct. When the discharge is copious, it is usually preceded by a sensation of fullness or pain in the areola or nipple area that is relieved as the fluid is expelled. It has a raspberry-like" configuration on the mammogram and in this way helps to promote correlation between the mammogram and the sonogram.

Sonographic Findings. Papillomas are usually small, multiple, and multicentric. They consist of simple proliferations of duct epithelium projecting outward into a dilated lumen from one or more focal points, each supported by a vascular stalk from which it receives the blood supply. Trauma may rupture the stalk, filling the duct with blood or serum. Papillomas may grow to a large size and thus become palpable lesions. They are somewhat linear, resembling the terminal duct, and are usually benign (Fig. 21.33).

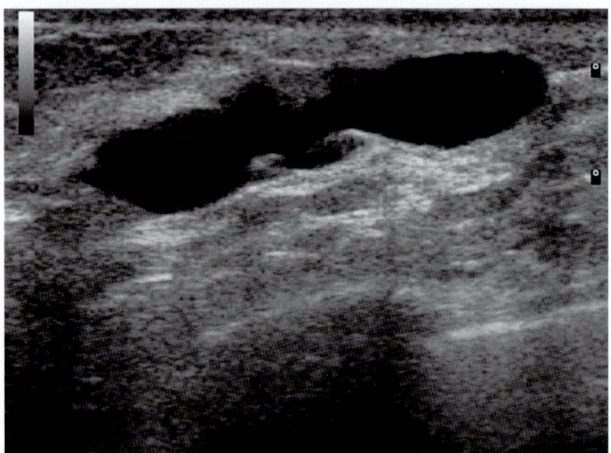

FIG. 21.33 Papillomas are usually small, multiple, and multicentric. They consist of simple proliferations of duct epithelium projecting outward into a dilated lumen from one or more focal points, each supported by a vascular stalk from which it receives the blood supply.

Diabetic Mastopathy

A feature associated with diabetes is disorders of collagen metabolism and the premenopausal Type I diabetic woman is at risk for developing benign breast fibrosis. **Focal fibrosis** usually appears in the upper outer quadrants as a highly echogenic mass that is well circumscribed but does not have a capsule. Diabetic mastopathy can simulate breast cancer on clinical examination as well as on various imaging techniques.

BREAST AUGMENTATION AND IMPLANT COMPLICATIONS

Sonographic evaluation of the breast in a patient who has had breast augmentation or reconstruction with silicone implants has been shown to be of benefit. Mammography is often limited in its ability to image beyond the implant, whereas ultrasound has the ability to evaluate the tissue surrounding the implant, search for the presence of defects in the membrane, and look for leakage into the breast parenchyma.

Although the primary indication for breast implants is cosmetic, implants may also be sought for congenital amastia, severe hypoplasia, breast asymmetry or tissue defects, and post-mastectomy reconstruction. Location for implants include subglandular, subpectoral, subcutaneous, or intramammary (Fig. 21.34).

The most common types of implants include saline- and/or silicone gel-filled, single or double lumen, with smooth or textured surface. Texturing is thought to reduce fibrous scarring around the implant which is typically seen. Some saline implants are expandable and will have ports or valves that can be identified sonographically.

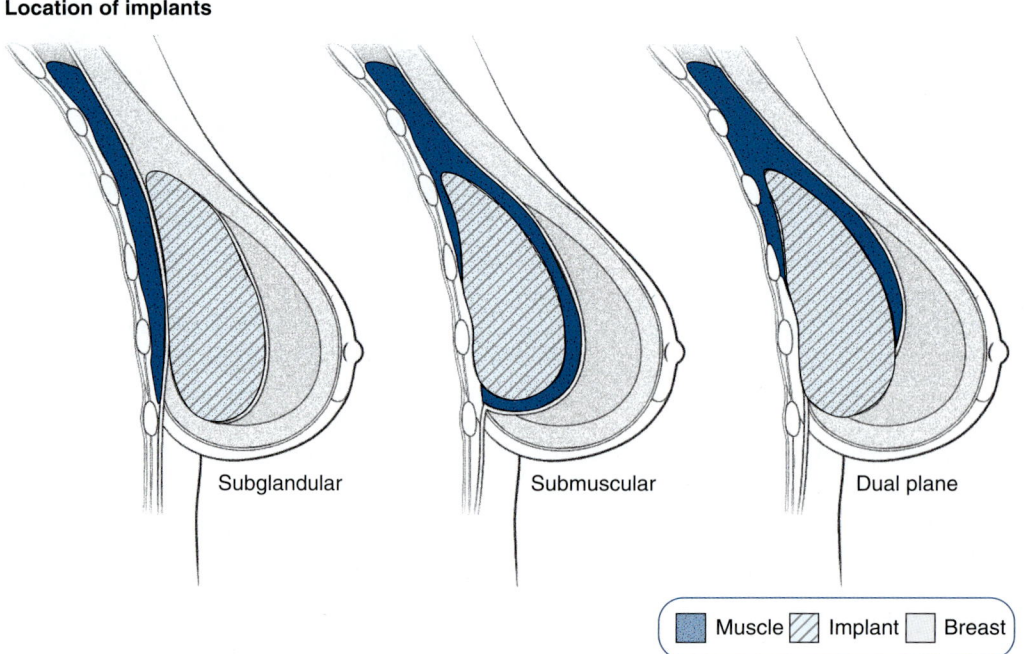

FIG. 21.34 Location for implants include subglandular, subpectoral, subcutaneous, or intramammary.

Sonographic Findings. The normal implant should have a well-defined outline and along the interface between the implant and patient's tissue, one should see two to three closely spaced linear echoes (Fig. 21.35). These will correspond to the anterior and posterior surface of the shell (two lines) and the fibrous capsule (third line). Whether one sees two or three lines will depend on equipment resolution. Saline implants and tissue expanders usually show a port or valve along the anterior surface and are often located beneath the subareolar area and may be palpable. Another common and normal finding is the peripheral or radial fold which extends from the wall of the implant.

Implant Complications. Implant complications can be classified as acute or chronic and may occur shortly after implantation or years later. Acute complications include pain/tenderness, loss of sensation of the nipple, hematoma, abscess, and seroma. Chronic complications are more likely to present in the sonography lab. They include capsular fibrosis/contracture, herniation, migration, rupture, silicone granuloma, and chronic infection.

The development of the fibrous capsule is one of the more common complications where a thin rim of scar tissue forms around the implant usually within weeks of implantation. This scar is the body's normal reaction to a foreign substance.

Capsular contracture occurs as the fibrous capsule gets harder and begins to tighten progressively around the implant. This tightening effect will cause the implant to become too rounded causing asymmetry between the breasts. More commonly seen with smooth shelled subglandular implants, capsular contracture is associated with a fibrous capsule that measures more than 1.5 mm. In some cases, capsular calcifications may develop over time. If there is a localized tear in the fibrous capsule, the intact implant can be seen to herniate through the opening (Fig. 21.36). This herniation may be palpable and easily identified on sonography and MRI.

Nonenhanced MRI is considered the best imaging modality for evaluating breast implant integrity and is particularly good at identifying failure of double-lumen implants.

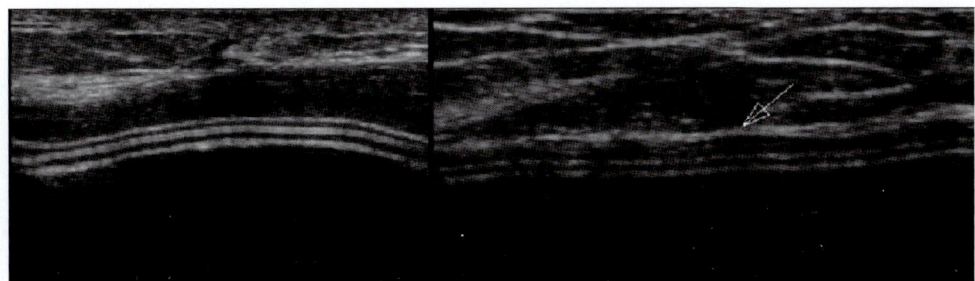

FIG. 21.35 The normal implant should have a well-defined outline and along the interface between the implant and patient's tissue; one should see two to three closely spaced linear echoes.

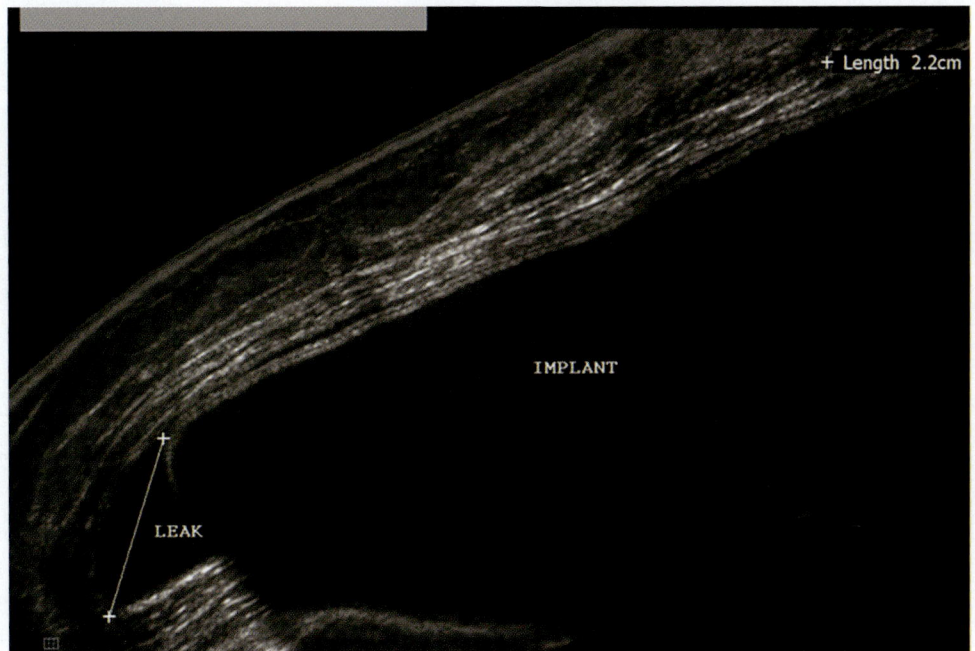

FIG. 21.36 If there is a localized tear in the fibrous capsule, the intact implant can be seen to herniate through the opening.

Common features of an **intracapsular** silicone rupture include the **"linguine"/wavy-line sign** and the **teardrop/noose sign** (Fig. 21.37).

The "linguine" sign shows the collapsed elastomer shell suspended within the silicone which is contained within a fibrous capsule while the teardrop sign is the result of an uncollapsed rupture within silicone gel that is trapped inside a peripheral fold. Extracapsular ruptures will show silicone granulomas outside the fibrous capsule and MRI can identify the presence, amount, and location of the extravasated silicone even within adjacent lymph nodes. These granulomas will appear hypointense on T1-weighted images with silicone suppression and hyperintense with T2-weighted images with water suppression.

Implant Rupture. Implant rupture is considered the second most common complication. Rupture can be intracapsular or extracapsular. Trauma and implant age are common risk factors. Silicone implants are more likely to rupture with age between 11 and 15 years. Silicone rupture into the tissue of the body can result in granuloma formation and inflammatory reactions including the development of autoimmune disorders. Saline implant rupture simply causes deflation of the implant causing obvious breast asymmetry but is absorbed by the body without consequence.

Sonographic Findings for Intracapsular Rupture. Most silicone implant ruptures are intracapsular where gel leaks outside the implant but is still contained by the fibrous capsule. It is best diagnosed sonographically when there is significant collapse of the implant. As the implant infolds on itself, it will produce the classic *stepladder* or *parallel-line sign* (Fig. 21.38). Although not as reliable as the stepladder sign, a secondary finding is when the silicone gel becomes more echogenic due to the silicone mixing with bodily fluids, proteins, and salts. The echoes may be diffuse, focal, or globular. One must keep in mind, however, that substances injected into the silicone gel at the time of implantation may also cause it to appear more echogenic or heterogeneous than normal. Saline, antibiotics, steroids, and povidone-iodine are used to help combat infection and fibrous encapsulation.

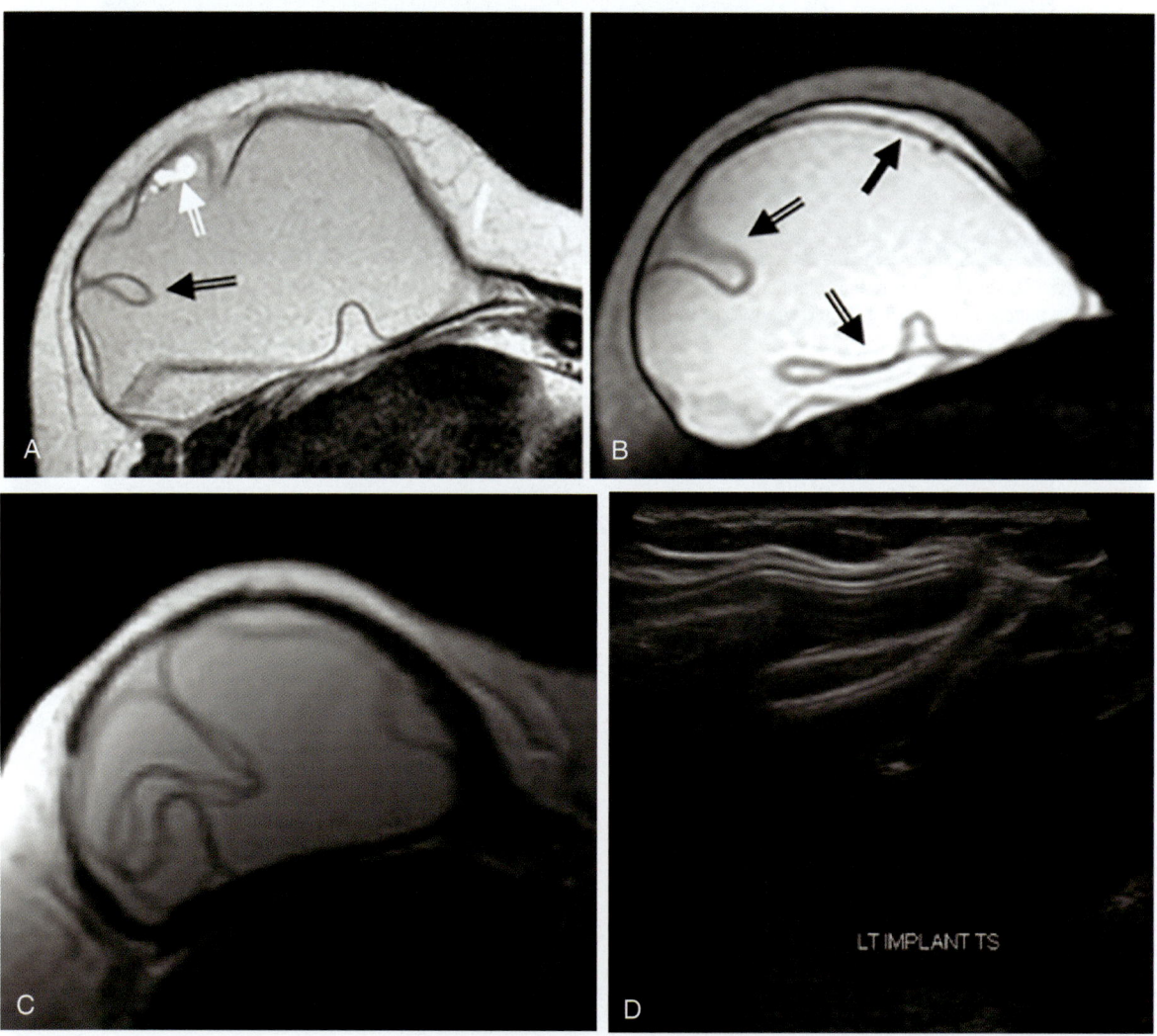

FIG. 21.37 Magnetic resonance images of the teardrop/noose sign (A–B) and the "linguine"/wavy-line sign (C). (D) Ultrasound image of the linguine sign.

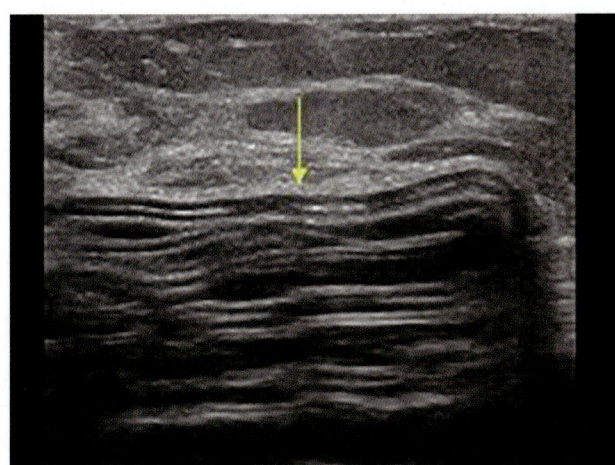

FIG. 21.38 **Ruptured breast implant.** As the implant unfolds on itself, it will produce the classic stepladder or parallel-line sign.

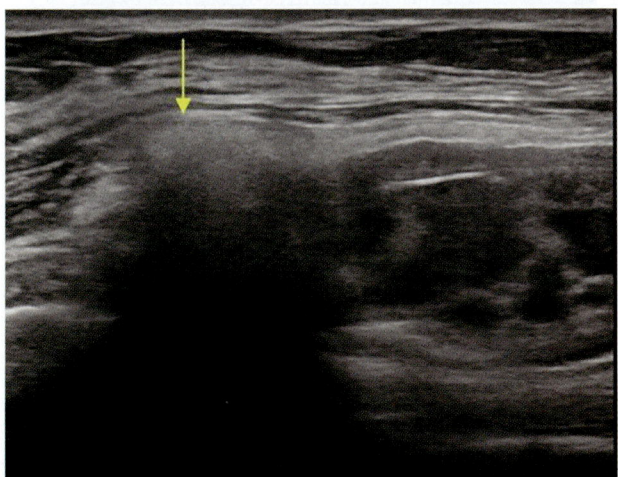

FIG. 21.39 An extracapsular rupture is when there is a break in the implant shell and fibrous capsule allowing silicone to seep into the tissues of the breast, along the chest wall and axilla. Infiltrated tissues will be hyperechoic and exhibit dirty shadowing.

Sonographic Findings for Extracapsular Rupture. An extracapsular rupture is when there is a break in the implant shell and fibrous capsule allowing silicone to seep into the tissues of the breast, along the chest wall and axilla. The most classic sonographic appearance is the "snowstorm" sign, or echogenic noise. Infiltrated tissues will be hyperechoic and exhibit dirty shadowing (Fig. 21.39).

Sonographic Characteristics of Malignant Breast Masses

Margins. Malignant masses usually have irregular or ill-defined margins. A technique called *fremitus* can be used to identify and confirm the margins of a mass. Fremitus is a palpable tremor or vibration of the chest wall. Using power Doppler, have the patient hum. The vibrations of the chest wall will carry through to the breast tissue, creating a power Doppler signal. The lesion is normally void of signal, making it easier to identify its margins. This technique can be useful in confirming the presence of a mass when in doubt, identifying multifocal masses, differentiating diffuse masses, and locating palpable masses that are isoechoic with the breast parenchyma.

Malignant tumors are aggressive and tend to grow through tissue via finger-like extensions termed **spiculation**. Spiculated margins are highly suspicious for malignancy and correlate with mammographic spiculation. Sonographic spiculations appear as small lines that radiate outward from the surface of a mass (Fig. 21.40A). They are typically alternating hypoechoic and hyperechoic lines. Ductal extensions project radially from the tumor and are oriented toward the nipple. Small extensions may not be visible sonographically, making the margins of a lesion appear indistinct. As malignant masses enlarge, they may cause retraction of the nipple or dimpling of the skin as the spiculations pull on Cooper's ligaments.

Shape. Sharp angular margins are associated with malignancy as are microlobulations (very small 1- to 2-mm lobulations) (see Fig. 21.40B). Microlobulations associated with malignancy are usually much smaller than lobulation seen with fibroadenomas, sharper, and more numerous.

Orientation. Malignant lesions are able to grow through the connective tissue and may have a vertical orientation when the breast is imaged from anterior to posterior. If a mass measures longer in the anteroposterior dimension (height) than in the transverse or sagittal plane (width), it has a vertical orientation, is usually described as "taller than wide," and is highly suspicious for malignancy (see Fig. 21.40C).

Internal Echo Pattern. A solid lesion that is markedly hypoechoic relative to the normal breast parenchyma is more suspicious for malignancy (see Fig. 21.40D). Malignant lesions tend to be extremely hypoechoic relative to fat and usually have weak internal echoes. They are often associated with dense posterior shadowing, making the lesion difficult to penetrate.

Attenuation Effects. Shadowing behind a solid breast mass is another suspicious sonographic sign for malignancy because malignant tumors tend to be highly attenuating (see Fig. 21.40A). Posterior shadowing should not be confused with edge or refraction shadowing, in which shadowing occurs at the curved edge of a smooth, benign mass.

Microcalcifications within a solid mass are associated with a breast malignancy. Ultrasound is less sensitive than mammography in the detection of microcalcifications due to the heterogeneous appearance of normal breast tissue. Microcalcifications seen with ultrasound are typically very small echogenic foci that do not create shadows because of their small size. Although calcifications are not visualized frequently by sonography, their detection in a hypoechoic mass is suspicious for malignancy.

Mobility. Because of the spiculations associated with malignancy, malignant lesions are normally very fixed or rigid in their position.

Compressibility. Malignant lesions normally are very hard and noncompressible.

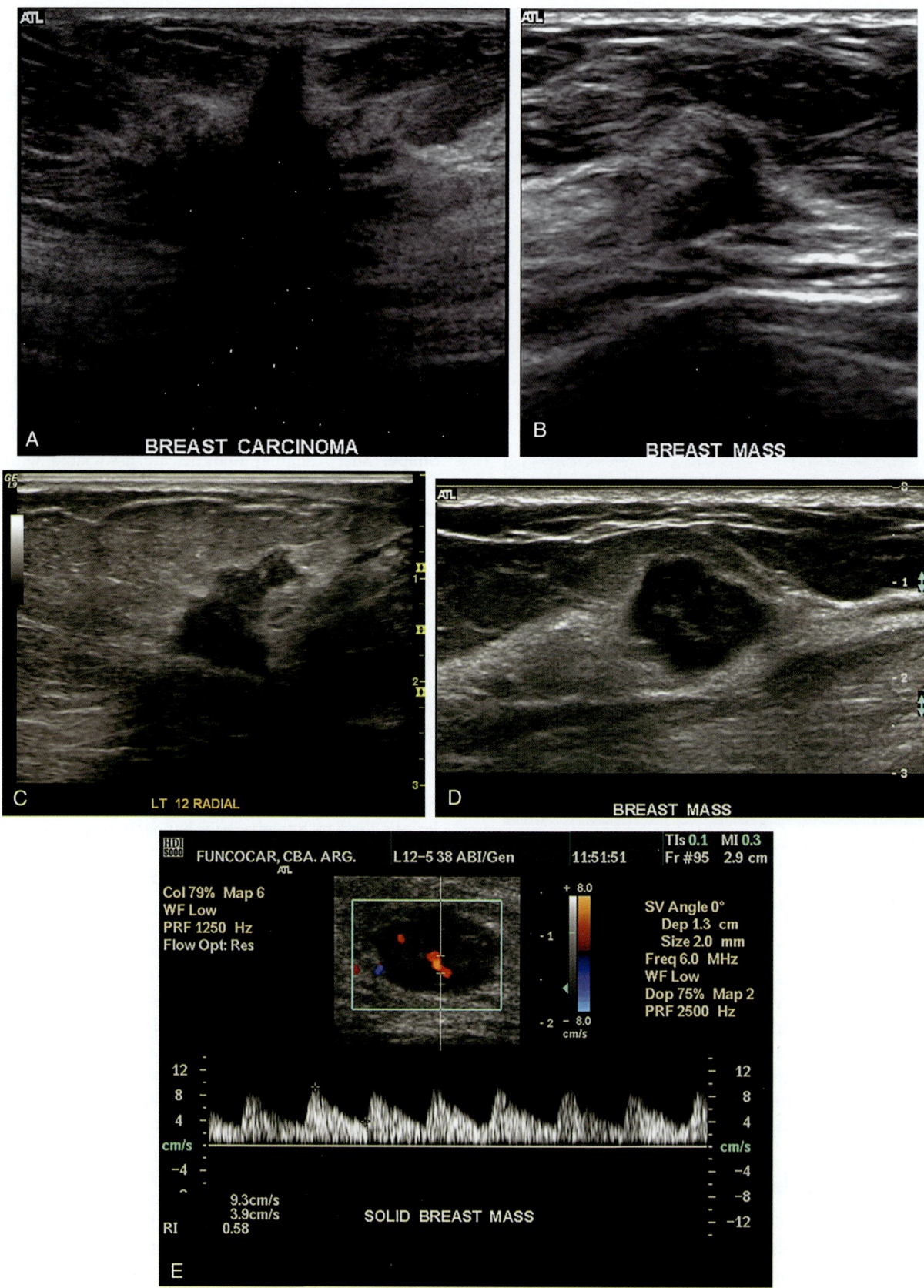

FIG. 21.40 (A) Spiculated margins are finger-like extensions that grow through tissue in malignant tumors. (B) Sharp, angular margins are associated with malignancy. (C) Malignant lesions are able to grow through the connective tissue and may have a vertical orientation when the breast is imaged from anterior to posterior. (D) Malignant lesions tend to be hypoechoic relative to fat and may have weak internal echoes. (E) Malignant tumors demonstrate increased vascularity within the lesion and often have a feeder vessel.

Vascularity. Doppler interrogation of a breast lesion is an essential element of the study. Although breast lesions are not associated with consistent resistance patterns on Doppler ultrasound, malignant masses often demonstrate increased vascularity within the lesion and often have a feeder vessel, which can be identified on careful evaluation (see Fig. 21.40E). Vessels that penetrate a mass are highly suspect for malignancy and should be checked using color or power Doppler to ascertain the number and to look for intratumoral vessels.

MALIGNANT PATHOLOGY OF THE BREAST

Breast cancer, by contrast, will generally be painless (although some cancers are associated with focal pain), lobular or irregular in shape, uneven in surface contour (sometimes gritty in texture), and fixed or poorly movable (see Box 21.8). Some will present with a palpable mass, spontaneous or induced nipple discharge, skin dimpling, ulceration, and nipple retraction. Skin dimpling or ulceration and nipple retraction nearly always result from cancer.

Breast cancers are classified as either **invasive** (85%) or **noninvasive carcinomas**. Of these, most arise from the ducts or lobules of the breast. Tumors usually originate within the **extralobular terminal duct (ELTD)** of the **TDLU** close to the junction with the lobule. This allows cells to disseminate into the main duct as well as the smaller ones. Since the breast lobules are concentrated in the upper outer quadrant of the breast, it is not surprising that a majority of breast cancers (50%) are found there.

Carcinoma refers to breast tumors that arise from the epithelium, in the ductal and from systemic neoplasms, such as leukemia or lymphoma. Breast carcinomas are generally categorized by two factors: where the cancer cells originate (ductal or lobular) and whether the cancer is prone to spreading (noninvasive or invasive). Most breast carcinomas begin within the ducts of the breast and are called ductal or intraductal carcinomas. Breast cancers that form in the lobules are called lobular carcinomas.

Sarcoma refers to breast tumors that arise from supportive or connective tissues. Sarcomas tend to grow rapidly and invade fibrous tissue. The term noninvasive or **in situ** means the tumor is localized to its site of origin. These tumors are confined to the duct and have not grown past the basement membrane and therefore, they are not likely to have metastasized. Invasive or **infiltrating** carcinomas grow past the site of origin and can gain access to the blood vessels and lymphatic channels near the duct resulting in metastases, increasing patient morbidity and mortality.

Multifocality is defined as the presence of additional tumors within one breast quadrant or ductal system. **Multicentricity** is the presence of multiple tumors in different quadrants or tumors separated by a distance of 5 cm or more. Multicentricity is less common and may present as the same or different histologic types. Both multicentric and multifocal tumors are more likely to recur, and therefore carry a poorer prognosis.

Ductal Carcinoma In Situ

Ductal carcinoma in situ (DCIS) is also known as intraductal carcinoma and is the most common noninvasive breast malignancy. DCIS is characterized by excessive growth of abnormal epithelial cells within the duct. These abnormal cells have not yet spread through the walls of the ducts into the fatty tissue of the breast, hence the term in situ. Calcifications and ductal enlargement with extension within the ducts are common (Fig. 21.41).

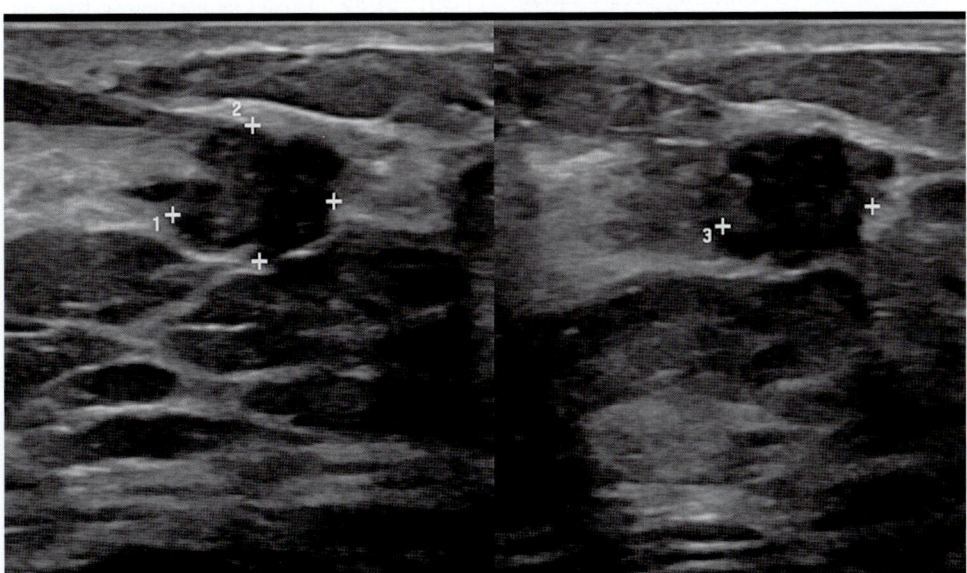

FIG. 21.41 Ductal carcinoma in situ, also known as intraductal carcinoma, is characterized by excessive growth of abnormal epithelial cells within the duct. These abnormal cells have not yet spread through the walls of the ducts into the fatty tissue of the breast, hence the term in situ. Calcifications and ductal enlargement with extension within the ducts are common.

Invasive Ductal Carcinoma

Invasive ductal carcinoma not otherwise specified is the most common breast cancer, accounting for nearly 85% of breast cancers. Similar to DCIS, these cancers begin in the ducts, but in contrast to DCIS, they invade the fatty tissue of the breast and have the potential to metastasize via the bloodstream or the lymphatic system. It is important to get a definitive diagnosis and begin treatment before cancer spreads to other organs.

The grading system for DCIS is classified as *low nuclear grade/non-comedo type, intermediate grade, and high nuclear grade/comedo type*. **Non-comedo** lesions have a better prognosis than those of higher grades. Atypical ductal hyperplasia is thought to be a precursor. The **comedo type** is a more aggressive tumor that is poorly differentiated. It can quickly become invasive and recurs more often and faster. Usually, the ducts are enlarged and filled with a plug of cottage cheese–like material containing many calcifications referred to as *comedocarcinoma*.

Comedocarcinoma

Intraductal solid carcinoma in which the lactiferous ducts are filled with a yellow paste-like material that looks like small plugs (comedones) when sectioned is called comedocarcinoma. Histologically, the ducts are filled with plugs of an epithelial tumor that have a central necrosis, giving rise to the paste-like material. Both invasive and noninvasive forms exist.

Noninvasive forms may lack any clinical or palpatory findings. If a nipple discharge occurs, it is more frequently clear than bloody (unlike papillary carcinoma, in which bloody discharge is typical). The patient may complain of pain or the sensation of insects crawling on the breast. With early invasion, minimal thickening of the surrounding breast tissue may be palpated. In the advanced stage, clinical signs include nipple retraction, dominant mass, and fixation.

Microcalcifications are commonly seen on mammography and may be picked up sonographically. Intraductal carcinomas have malignant characteristics, including irregular margins, a diffuse internal echo pattern, and attenuation with shadowing (Fig. 21.42). Other forms of DCIS include **intracystic papillary carcinoma** and **Paget disease** of the nipple.

Papillary Carcinoma

Papillary carcinoma is a tumor that initially arises as an intraductal mass. It may also take the form of an intracystic tumor, which is rare. The early stage of papillary carcinoma is noninvasive. The tumor occasionally arises from a benign ductal papilloma. It is associated with little fibrotic reaction. The earliest clinical sign of intraductal papillary carcinoma is bloody nipple discharge. Occasionally, a mass can be palpated as a small, firm, well-circumscribed area and may be mistaken for a fibroadenoma (Fig. 21.43). Nodules of blue or red discoloration may be found under the skin with central ulceration.

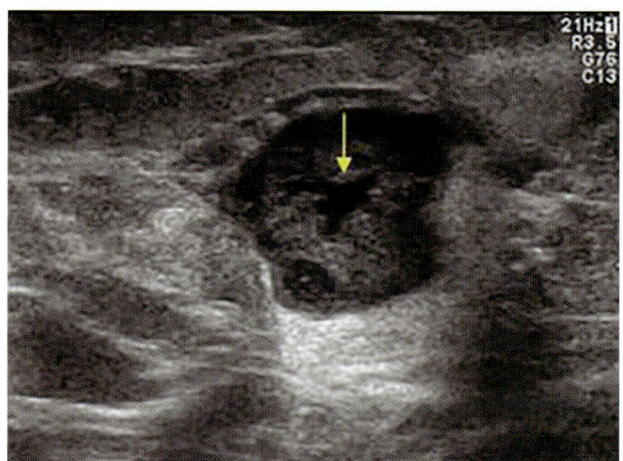

FIG. 21.42 Intraductal carcinomas have malignant characteristics, including irregular margins, a diffuse internal echo pattern, and attenuation with shadowing.

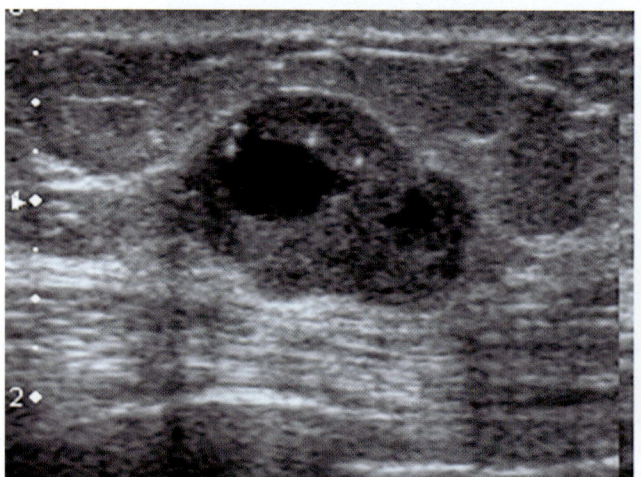 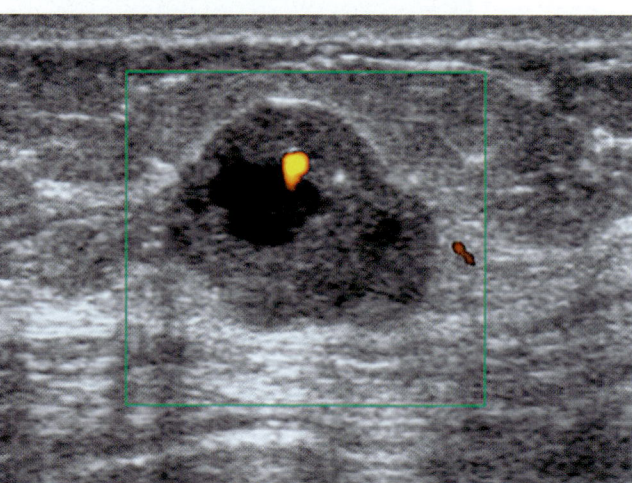

FIG. 21.43 Papillary carcinoma is a tumor that initially arises as an intraductal mass. Occasionally, a mass can be palpated as a small, firm, well-circumscribed area and may be mistaken for a fibroadenoma.

A diffusely nodular appearance overlying the skin is a special variant of multiple intraductal papillary carcinoma. Intracystic papillary carcinoma is clinically indistinguishable in its early stages from a cyst or fibroadenoma. When the tumor has invaded through the cyst wall, it is palpable as a poorly circumscribed mass. Malignant lesions, when compared to benign papillomas, usually expand and extend further into a duct (>1.5 cm) and other branching ducts. On mammogram, one can see microcalcifications and clustered nodules within a single quadrant of the breast. Papillary carcinoma typically has a more favorable prognosis than other types of carcinoma.

Paget Disease

Paget disease arises in the retroareolar ducts and grows in the direction of the nipple, spreading into the intraepidermal region of the nipple and areola, and has a rash-like appearance that may be confused with a melanoma. Any ulceration, enlargement, or deformity of the nipple and areola should suggest Paget disease. This is a relatively rare tumor and it typically occurs in women over 50 years of age. Differential diagnosis includes benign inflammatory eczematous condition of the nipple as palpatory findings frequently are not present. The primary ductal cancer may be quite deep or embedded in fibrotic tissue. Sonographically, Paget disease will present as a retroareolar mass with irregular margins, heterogeneous internal echoes, and attenuation with posterior shadowing (Fig. 21.44).

Inflammatory Carcinoma

Inflammatory carcinoma is where a highly malignant cancer invades and blocks the lymphatic channels of the skin. Edematous skin changes are caused by tumor clots within the dermal lymphatic system. This may occur with other primary tumors that are either multifocal or multicentric as well. Inflammatory carcinoma is rare, but metastases is rapid and diffuse which results in a poor prognosis. Clinically, the breast will be red and swollen with one-third of cases presenting the classic peau d'orange, or orange-peel appearance. The skin is feverish, breast is hard to palpation, and axillary lymph nodes are enlarged. On sonography, the skin is thick with increased echogenicity of the fat and dilation of the superficial veins and lymphatic channels (Fig. 21.45). It can look very similar to mastitis.

Lobular Carcinoma in Situ/Lobular Neoplasia

Lobular carcinoma in situ (LCIS) is not considered a cancer because it has a low malignant potential. LCIS is often referred to as *lobular neoplasia* and is classified as a precancerous growth that begins in the lobule. LCIS is confined to the gland and does not penetrate through the wall of the lobule. This process can be difficult to identify with mammography and sonography as it does not usually form a distinct mass. Women with LCIS are at higher risk of developing invasive breast cancer later on.

Invasive Lobular Carcinoma

Invasive lobular carcinoma (ILC) begins in the lobule, where it extends into the fatty tissue of the breast. Similar to invasive ductal carcinoma, ILC has the potential to metastasize and spread to other parts of the body. ILC is the second most common type of invasive tumor, accounting for 10% to 15% of all breast cancers. ILC is often bilateral, multicentric, or multifocal (Fig. 21.46). Compared with invasive ductal carcinoma, ILC carries a poorer prognosis.

The more favorable cancers remain localized to the breast longer, and treated patients have a 75% survival rate after 10 years. They represent only 10% to 12% of all breast cancers. This group includes medullary, intracystic papillary, papillary, colloid, and tubular carcinomas.

Medullary Carcinoma

Medullary carcinoma is a densely cellular tumor that contains large, round, or oval tumor cells. It usually is a well-circumscribed mass, with the center frequently necrotic and/or hemorrhagic. Medullary carcinomas are relatively rare, accounting for less than 5% of breast cancers. The age of occurrence is slightly lower than for the average breast cancer, with a majority of cases occurring in women younger than 50 years. Medullary carcinomas are usually well circumscribed, are often large, often smoothly lobulated, are mobile, nontender masses that show mild compressibility (Fig. 21.47). The tumor may resemble a **fibroadenoma** but tends to grow rapidly but carries a good prognosis as the incidence of lymph node involvement is usually low. Discoloration of the overlying skin may be seen as a clinical finding, and bilateral occurrence is more frequent with medullary carcinoma than with other cancers.

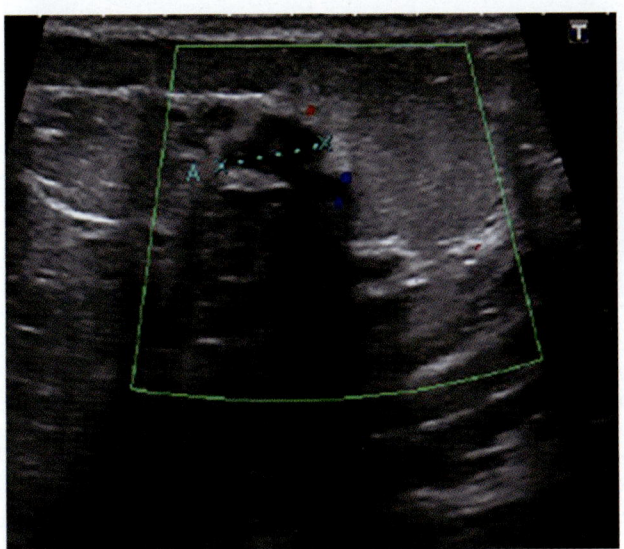

FIG. 21.44 Sonographically, Paget disease will present as a retroareolar mass with irregular margins, heterogeneous internal echoes, and attenuation with posterior shadowing, mistaken for a fibroadenoma.

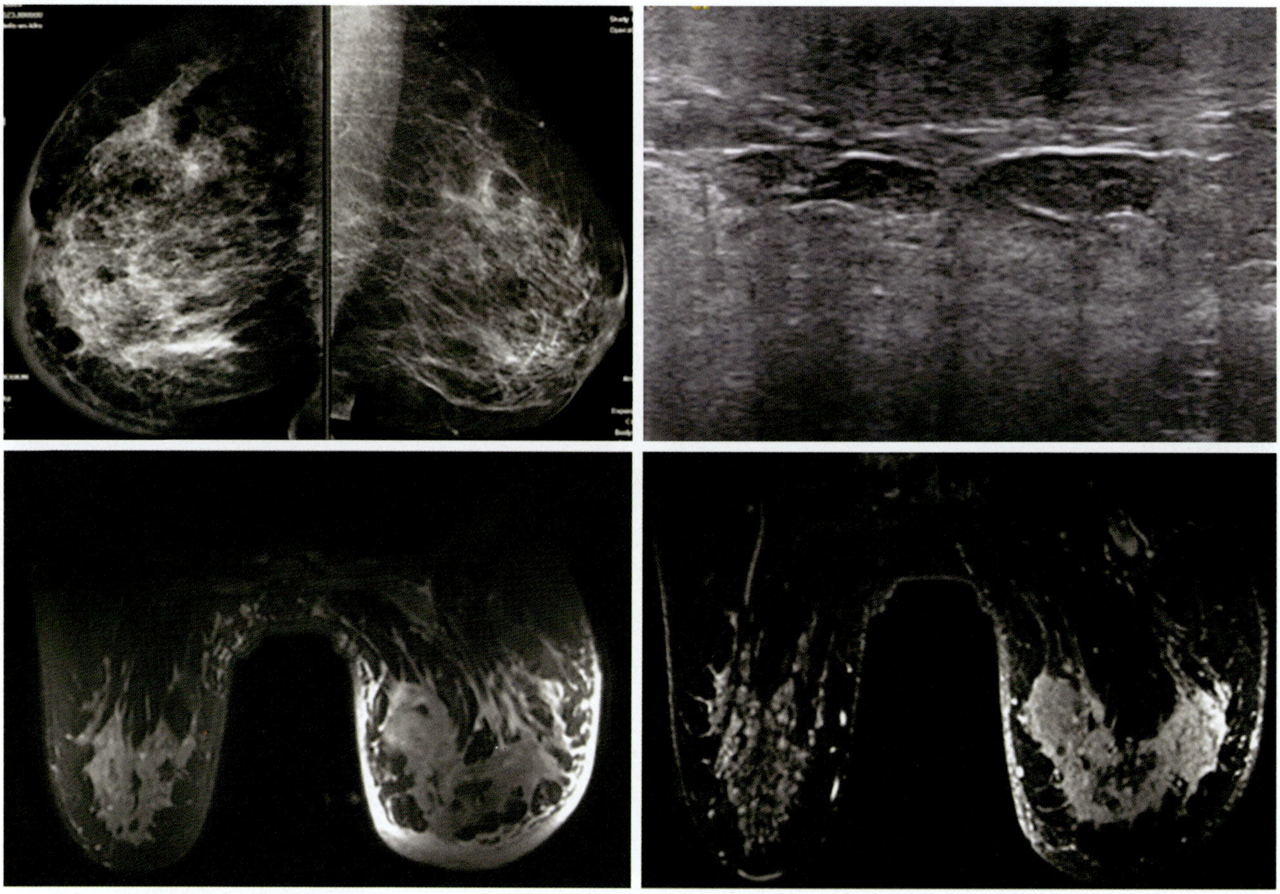

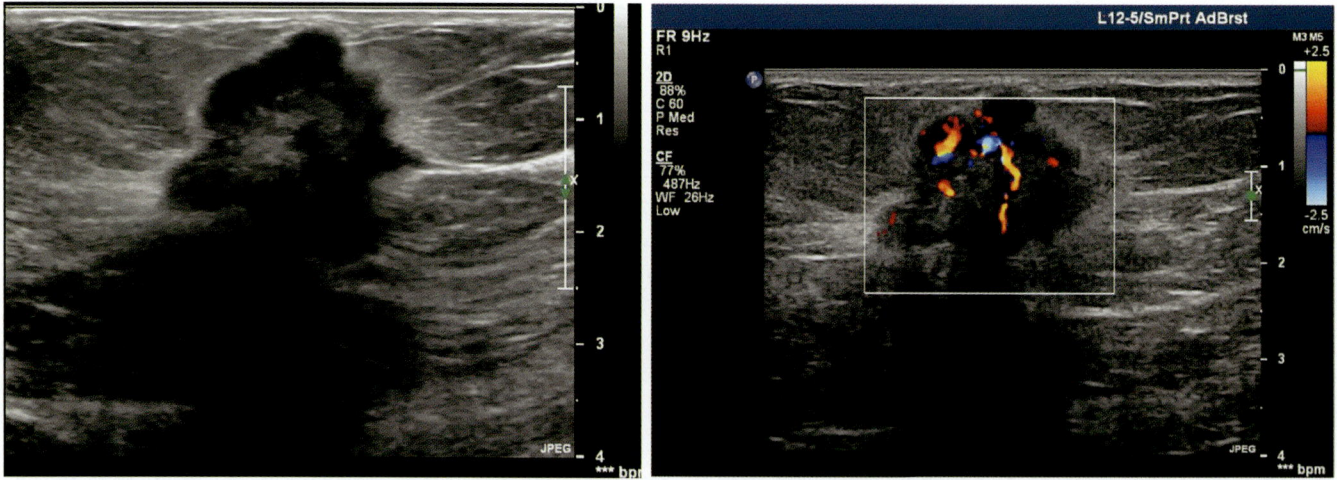

FIG. 21.45 **Inflammatory carcinoma.** On sonography, the skin is thick with increased echogenicity of the fat and dilation of the superficial veins and lymphatic channels. It can look very similar to mastitis.

FIG. 21.46 Invasive lobular carcinoma begins in the lobule, where it extends into the fatty tissue of the breast.

Tubular Carcinoma

Tubular carcinoma represents an uncommon, extremely well-differentiated form of infiltrating (invasive) ductal carcinoma usually less than 2 cm in dimension. Tubular carcinoma occurs in women with an average age of 50 years and has a favorable prognosis with a low rate of recurrence or metastasis. Death is rare. Tubular carcinoma typically has poorly circumscribed margins and a hard consistency.

Scirrhous Carcinoma

Scirrhous carcinoma is a type of intraductal tumor with extensive fibrous tissue proliferation (very dense fibrosis). Focal calcification may also be present. Scirrhous carcinoma is the pathological subtype of invasive ductal carcinoma and often has no specific histologic findings or patterns; therefore it is often classified as ductal carcinoma that is not otherwise specified. The classic clinical signs include a very firm

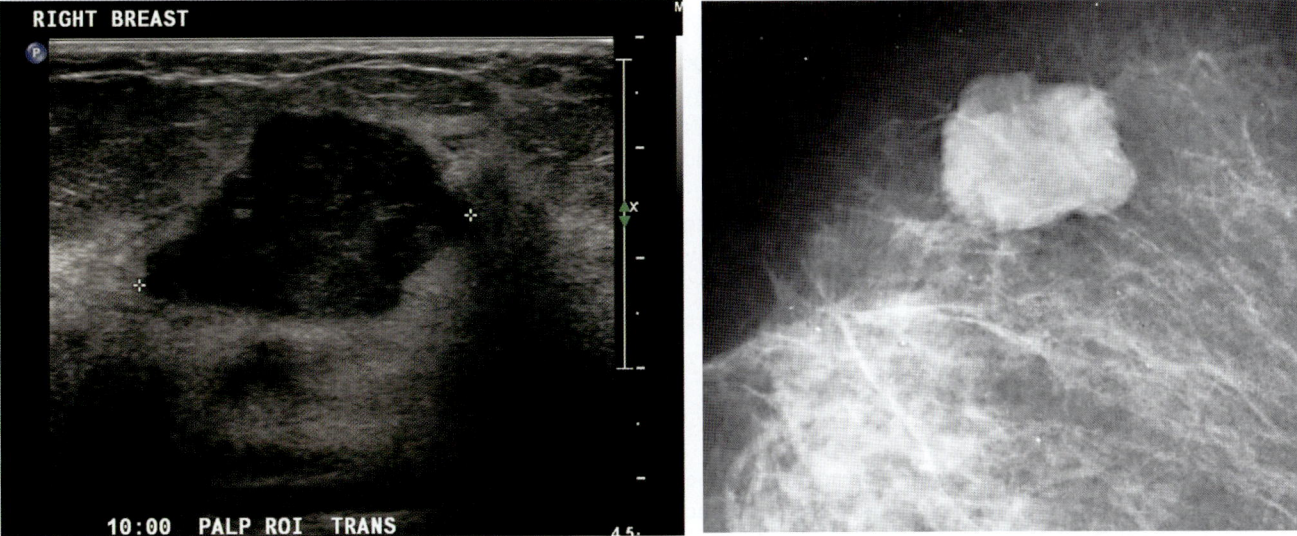

FIG. 21.47 Medullary carcinoma is a densely cellular tumor that contains large, round, or oval tumor cells. It usually is a well-circumscribed mass, with the center frequently necrotic and/or hemorrhagic.

nodular, frequently nonmovable mass, often with fixation and flattening of overlying skin and nipple retraction. The retraction is a result of an infiltrative shortening of Cooper's ligaments caused by productive fibrosis. Fixation and retraction of the nipple may be the result of a subareolar carcinoma but may also be caused by benign fibrosis of the breast. It is important to note that some patients normally have inverted nipples. The size of the cancer may vary from a few millimeters to involvement of nearly the entire breast. The deep-lying scirrhous carcinoma may grow into and become fixed to the thoracic wall. A bloody discharge is rare with this tumor.

Colloid/Mucinous Carcinoma

Colloid carcinoma (mucinous) is a relatively rare type of ductal carcinoma mostly seen in patients older than 75 years. The cells of the tumor produce gelatinous material that fill lactiferous ducts or stromal tissues in which the tumor cells are invading making the mass feel soft. The sonographic appearance is often similar to a fibroadenoma with smooth margins and posterior enhancement. The echotexture has been described as having a "salt and pepper" appearance.

Cystosarcoma Phyllodes

Other malignant tumors that have a better than average prognosis after treatment include malignant cystosarcoma phyllodes and stromal sarcomas, because they rarely metastasize to regional nodes. Cystosarcoma phyllodes is a rare, predominantly benign breast neoplasm that has malignant potential. It accounts for less than 1% of all breast neoplasms, yet it is the most frequent sarcoma of the breast, considered the malignant counterpart to the fibroadenoma. The larger the tumor, the more likely it is to be malignant. It is more commonly found in women 45 to 50 years of age and usually is unilateral. Many patients may notice that a small breast mass that has been present for a long time suddenly begins to

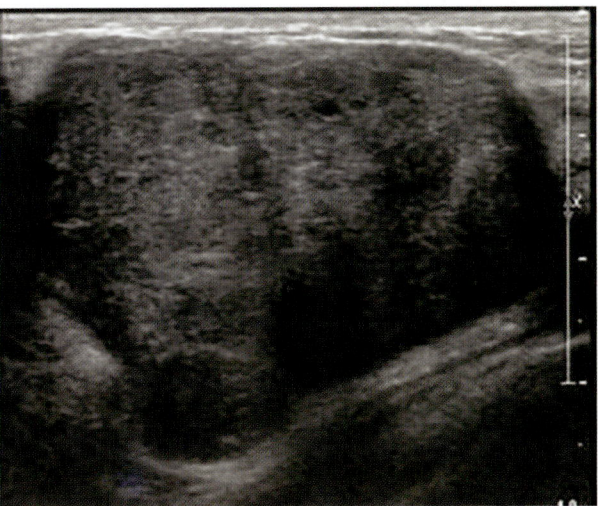

FIG. 21.48 Sonographic findings of cystosarcoma phyllodes include a large, hypoechoic tumor with well-defined margins and decreased through-transmission. Internal echoes may be fine or coarse with variable amounts of shadowing.

grow rapidly. Although it is considered a benign lesion, 27% of these tumors are malignant, and 12% metastasize.

When the tumor is small, it is well delineated, firm, and mobile, much like a fibroadenoma. As it enlarges, the surface may become irregular and lobulated. Skin changes can develop from increasing pressure. Edema may produce a skin change. Increasing pressure causes trophic changes and eventual skin ulcerations. Infection and abscess formation may be a secondary complication. The tumor never adheres to adjacent soft tissue or underlying pectoral muscle; therefore dimpling of the skin or fixation of the tumor is not observed. Sonographic findings include a large, hypoechoic tumor with well-defined margins and decreased through-transmission. Internal echoes may be fine or coarse with variable amounts of shadowing (Fig. 21.48).

Lymphoma

Lymphoma to the breast is rarely a primary process, but rather lymphomatous invasion from non-Hodgkin lymphoma. Usually, the patient will present with enlarged nodes within the breast and axillary region or show hypoechoic round or oval masses that are homogenous and show posterior enhancement. With diffuse infiltration, the appearance may be similar to inflammatory carcinoma. Biopsy is the only way to differentiate between inflammatory carcinoma, lymphomatous or leukemic infiltration, or other nodular masses of the breast.

Metastatic Disease

Primary breast cancer is most likely to spread first to the lymph nodes and then to bone, lung, brain, and liver. Bone metastases are considered the most common distant site.

Metastatic lesions in the breast are rare. The most common would develop from the contralateral breast. Extramammary primaries would include melanoma, lung, ovary, sarcoma, and the gastrointestinal tract. Of these, melanoma is the most common primary to metastasize to the breast in women. The most common hematologic primaries are lymphoma and leukemia.

Ultrasound-Guided Interventional Procedures

Preoperative Needle Wire Localization. Ultrasound offers a quick method for placement of a percutaneous needle wire assembly for preoperative localization of a nonpalpable breast lesion for surgical excision (Fig. 21.49) and offers a significant advantage in complicated cases, such as localization of a lesion adjacent to a breast implant, a lesion close to the chest wall, or a lesion in other areas not easily approached under mammographic guidance.

Large-Core Needle Biopsy. Ultrasound offers a fast and easy method for guiding large-core needle biopsy of solid masses. Patient comfort is enhanced, procedure time is often shorter, and ultrasound guidance is more cost effective in general than prone stereotactic procedures. It should be noted, however, that stereotactic guidance is still the preferred method for evaluation of clustered pleomorphic microcalcifications, which are difficult to see by ultrasound.

OTHER IMAGING MODALITIES

Ductography/Galactography

A ductogram may be indicated in the nonpregnant/nonlactating patient who presents with a worrisome nipple discharge. The procedure involves the retrograde injection of a contrast agent, using a 30-g sialography needle, into the orifice of secreting lactiferous duct. Once the contrast is injected, multiple mammographic or fluoroscopic images are taken to look for a filling defect within the ductal system. The benign papilloma is the most common cause of such a nipple discharge which can be clear, bloody, brown, yellow, or black. Ductography would be contraindicated in patients with mastitis or abscess and those who are pregnant or lactating (Fig. 21.50A and B).

Magnetic Resonance Imaging

MRI may be used to provide additional characterization and further interrogation of breast lesions that are not well visualized by mammography. MRI allows for improved discrimination between malignant and benign breast lesions by way of multiparametric assessment of the lesion. It has the highest sensitivity for breast cancer detection when compared with other imaging modalities. The technique is also helpful in preoperative staging and monitoring treatment response.

MRI uses a large and powerful magnet to cause hydrogen atoms within the tissues of the body to give off radio frequency waves. These waves received from the breast tissues are manipulated by a computer to produce an image of the breast and the internal architecture. The image provides a landscape view of the breast from any plane or direction and provides and offers improved contrast resolution in soft tissue lesions and in the extent of the disease process.

With MRI imaging, a paramagnetic contrast agent such as Gadolinium is injected through an IV. Malignant tumors, because of their vascularity, will show moderate to marked contrast enhancement rather quickly and then wash out. Lesions that show rim enhancement are very suggestive of malignancy. Contrast enhanced MRI is considered the most sensitive supplemental imaging technique for detecting breast cancer, both primary, nodal, multifocality, and multicentricity (Fig. 21.51).

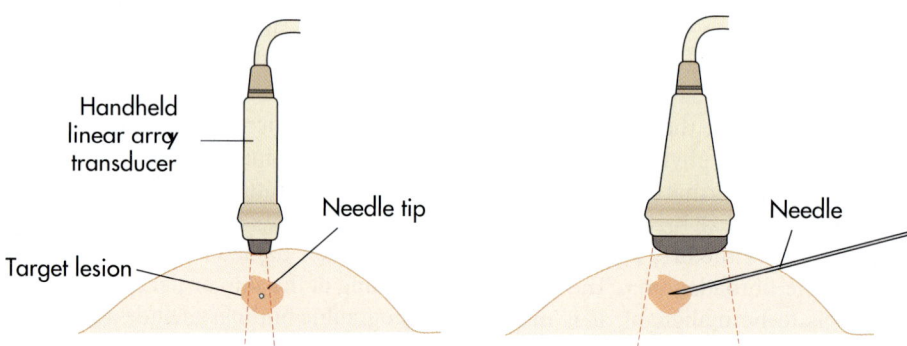

FIG. 21.49 Placement of the needle tip is facilitated by keeping it in the field of vision and as parallel as possible to the transducer surface.

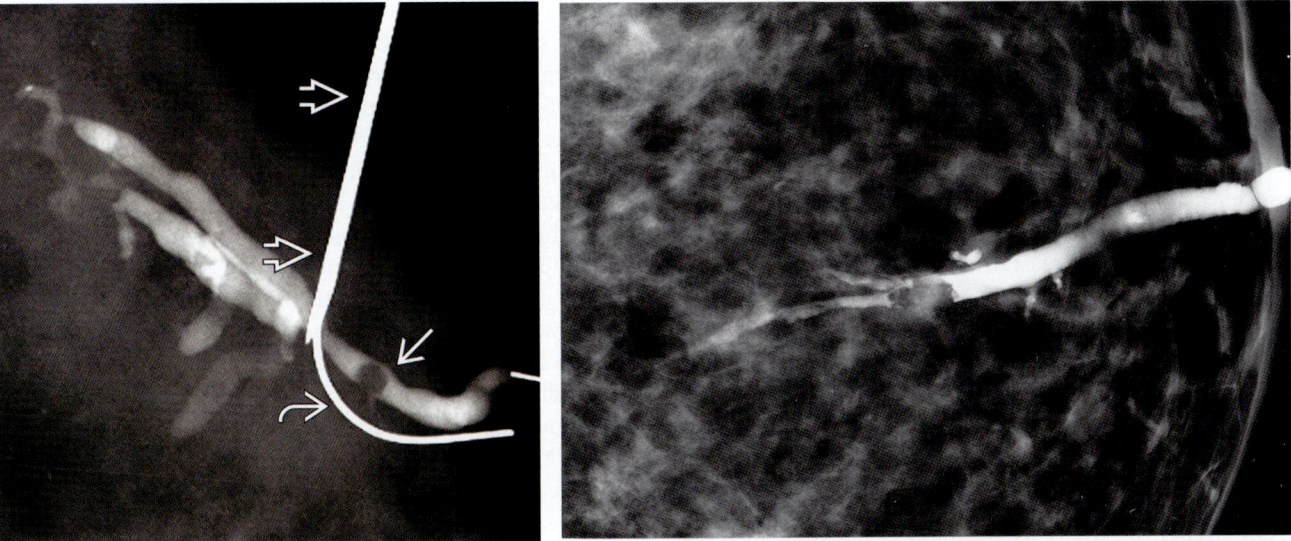

FIG. 21.50 A ductogram may be indicated in the nonpregnant/nonlactating patient who presents with a worrisome nipple discharge.

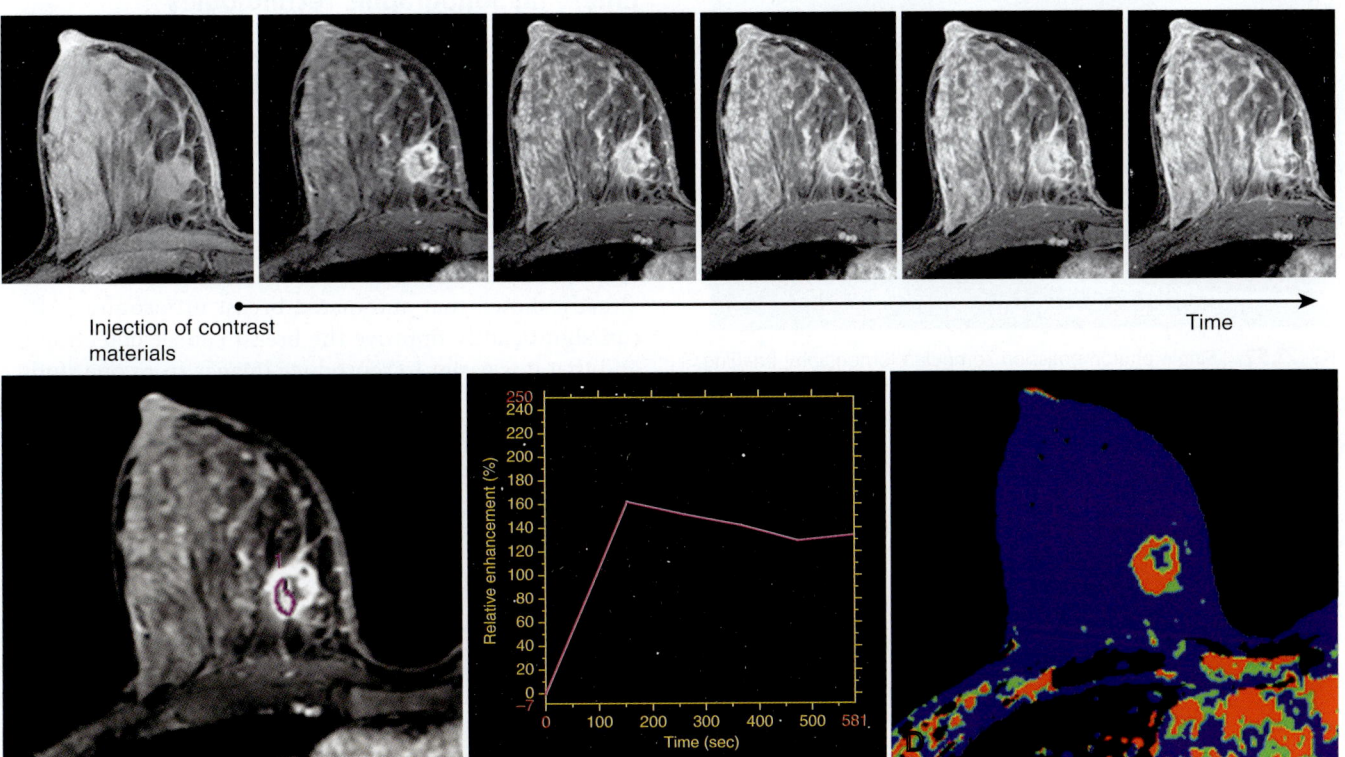

FIG. 21.51 Breast imaging with magnetic resonance imaging (MRI). With MRI imaging, a paramagnetic contrast agent such as gadolinium is administered intravenously. Malignant tumors, because of their vascularity, will show moderate to marked contrast enhancement rather quickly and then wash out.

Unfortunately, MRI breast imaging is not available in some areas and can be cost prohibitive for screening purposes. Another contraindication would be that MRI images are produced by two large, very strong magnets therefore not all patients are good candidates for the modality (e.g., patients with pacemakers or metal artificial joints). Finally, patients who suffer from uncontrolled claustrophobia are also not good candidates for MRI.

SINGLE PHOTON EMSSION COMPUTED TOMOGRAPHY

Single photon emission computed tomography (SPECT) imaging requires the injection of a small amount of radioactive material into the patient. The distribution of the radioactivity can be traced to locate cancer cells and track blood flow (Fig. 21.52). It has also proven to be more sensitive in detecting sentinel nodes in obese and overweight patients when compared with planar imaging.

Sentinel Node Procedure/Lymphoscintigraphy

The first node to receive lymph drainage from a primary breast cancer is called the sentinel node and is the node most at risk for metastasis. This node is typically an axillary node as 75% of lymph from the breast drains to this area. The sentinel node procedure involves injecting a blue dye and/or radioisotope, such as technetium-99m labeled as filtered sulfur colloid mixed with saline. The injection is made in front of the breast tumor and/or in the periareolar area. These mapping agents will flow through the lymphatic system and concentrate in the sentinel node creating a "hot spot" on the nuclear medicine image identifying the sentinel node. The surgeon will then use a scintillation counter or gamma probe to locate the radioactive node for removal and biopsy. The blue dye will have also collected within the node (Fig. 21.53).

This procedure, when the node is negative, has a 95% to 100% success rate for determining a clear axillary nodal basin indicating no metastasis. Many have chosen to rely on the sentinel node procedure as opposed to performing the complete axillary lymph node dissection (ALND) due to the high incidence of complications associated with the procedure such as arm lymph edema and the loss of the use of one's arm and shoulder due to nerve damage.

Emerging Sonographic Technologies

Automated Breast Ultrasound. Automated whole breast ultrasound is not a new idea but has re-emerged in order to standardize breast sonography and improve diagnostic quality by decreasing operator dependency. By evaluating the whole breast, there is less chance of missing small cancers and a better chance of catching them earlier. The application has also proven to be quite helpful in evaluating those patients with dense breast tissue. Several studies have already shown that automated breast ultrasound (ABUS) can significantly improve the breast cancer detection rate and that it is easier to reproduce images from one study to the next. ABUS is a volumetric sonographic technique that provides multiplanar reconstruction of the breast giving

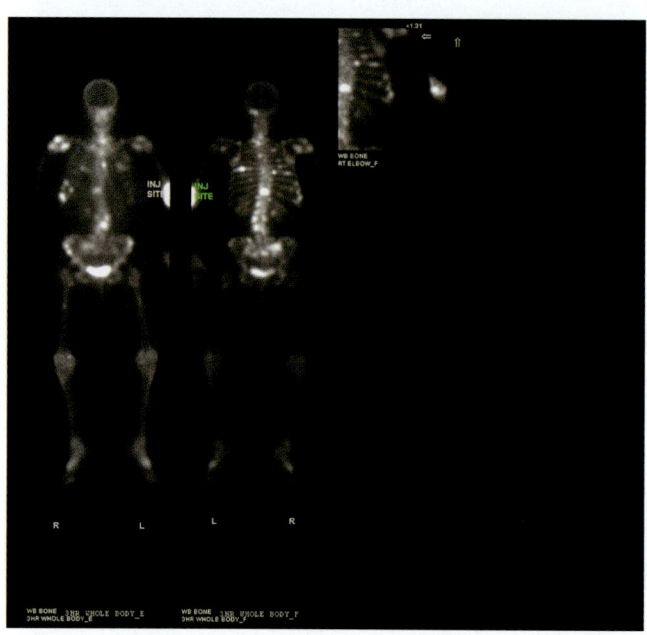

FIG. 21.52 Single photon emission computed tomography imaging requires the injection of a small amount of radioactive material into the patient. The distribution of the radioactivity can be traced to locate cancer cells and track blood flow.

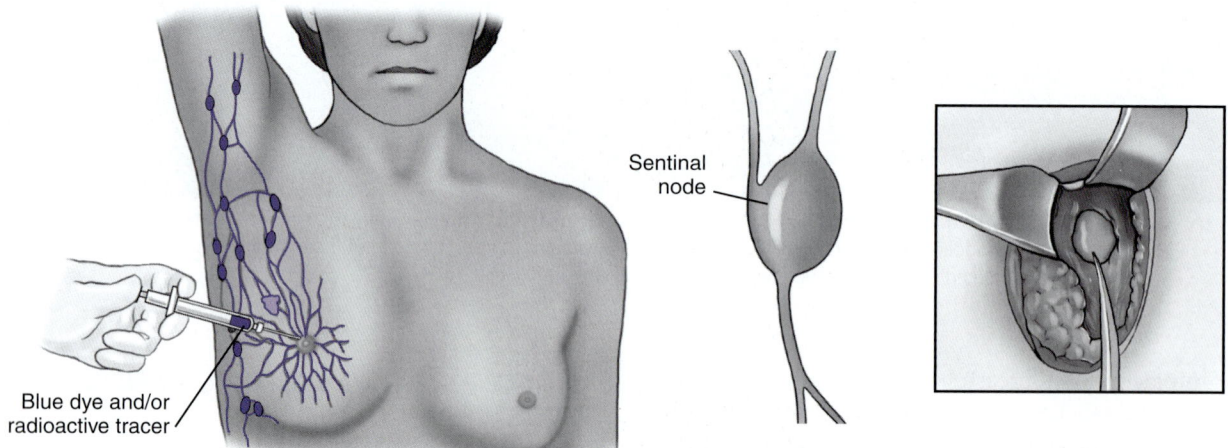

FIG. 21.53 The sentinel node procedure involves injecting a blue dye and/or radioisotope, such as technetium-99m labeled as filtered sulfur colloid mixed with saline. The injection is made in front of the breast tumor and/or in the periareolar area. These mapping agents will flow through the lymphatic system and concentrate in the sentinel node, creating a "hot spot" on the nuclear medicine image. The surgeon then uses a scintillation counter or gamma probe to locate the radioactive node for removal and biopsy. The blue dye also collects within the node.

a 3D view of the anatomy. A water path system is placed over the breast allowing for compression which provides for better visualization of the mammary tissues. Images are obtained by the automated transducer and the B-mode data is correlated by the system and combined in a series of gray-scale cine images forming the whole breast image (Fig. 21.54).

Breast Elastography. Ultrasound elastography is a noninvasive technique that provides information about the stiffness of a lesion. It can increase the specificity of conventional B-mode sonography by providing a more precise characterization of breast masses. Several studies have shown that breast elastography can increase the sensitivity, specificity, and overall diagnostic accuracy in differentiating benign from malignant solid breast masses (Fig. 21.55). There are two important characteristics of real-time ultrasound elastography and those are size and stiffness of the mass. Malignant breast masses tend to be harder or stiffer than benign masses. Relative to size, malignant masses tend to measure larger on elastography when compared to the conventional B-mode ultrasound image. This is thought to be due to the desmoplastic response of the tissue surrounding the tumor. Color coding allows for easy recognition of tissues that are hard versus soft (Fig. 21.56).

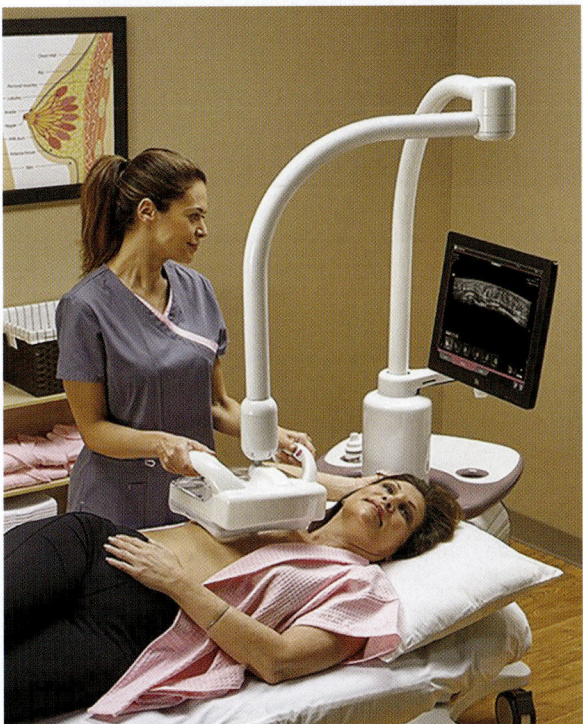

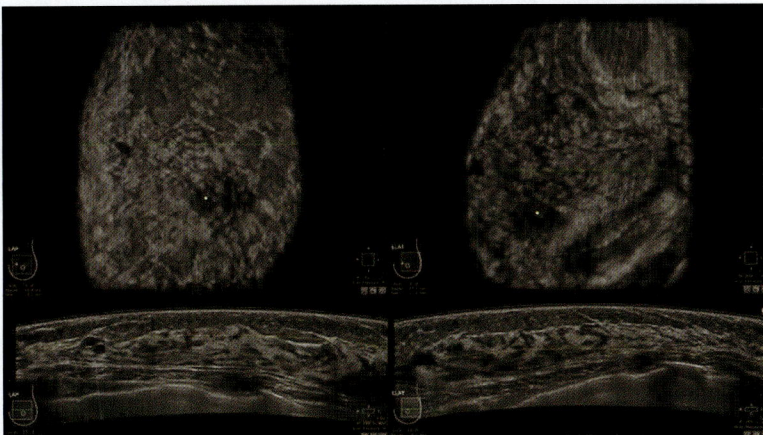

FIG. 21.54 An automated water path system is placed over the breast allowing for compression, which provides for better visualization of the mammary tissues. Images are obtained by the automated transducer, and the B-mode data is correlated by the system and combined in a series of gray-scale cine images forming the whole breast image.

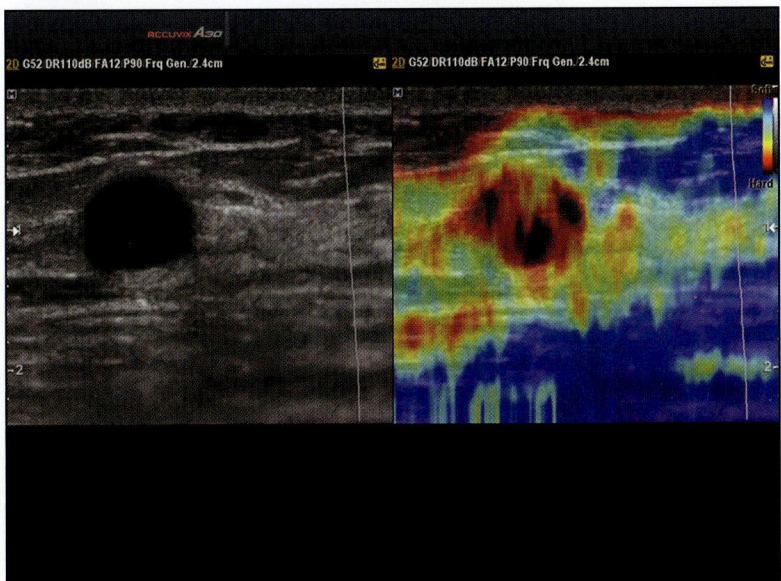

FIG. 21.55 Breast elastography can increase the specificity of conventional B-mode sonography by providing a more precise characterization of breast masses. Several studies have shown that breast elastography can increase the sensitivity, specificity, and overall diagnostic accuracy in differentiating benign from malignant solid breast masses.

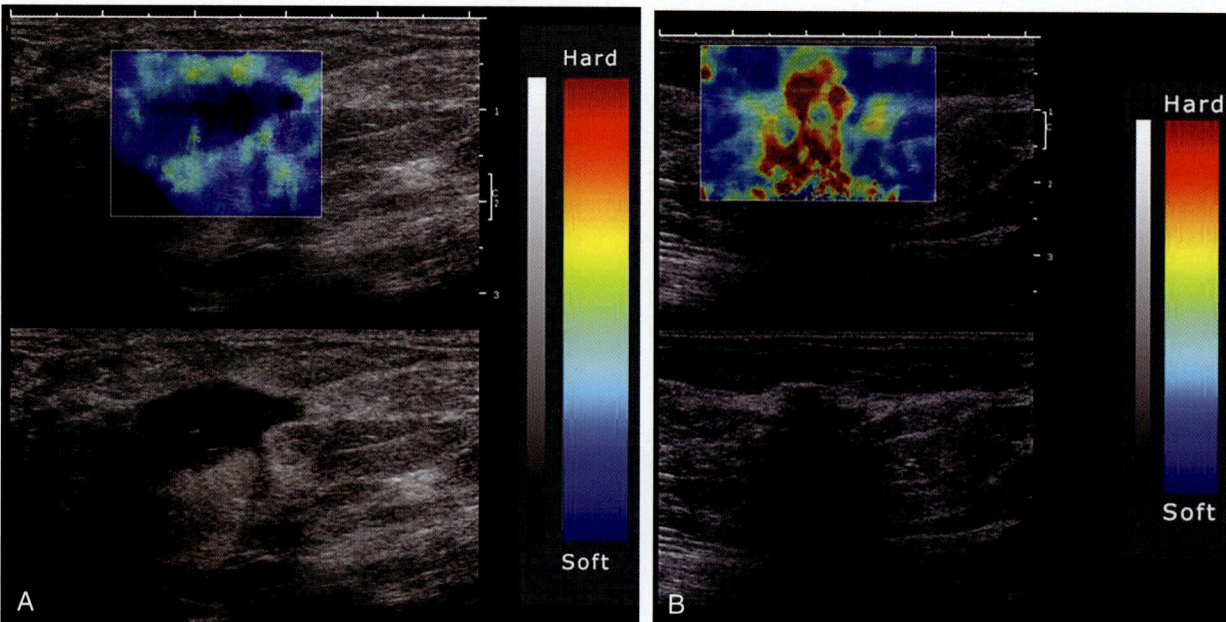

FIG. 21.56 (A) Lobular carcinoma of the breast. Malignant breast masses tend to be harder or stiffer than benign masses. (B) Mastitis abscess. Breast elastography can increase the sensitivity, specificity, and overall diagnostic accuracy in differentiating benign from malignant solid breast masses.

Key Pearls

- Sonographically, the breast is divided into three layers located between the skin and the pectoralis major muscle on the anterior of the chest wall. These layers are the subcutaneous layer, the mammary (glandular) layer, and the retromammary layer.
- The fatty tissue appears hypoechoic, and the ducts, glands, and supporting ligaments appear echogenic.
- The terminal ends of the duct and the acini form small lobular units referred to as TDLUs, each of which is surrounded by both loose and dense connective tissue.
- These connective tissue septa are collectively called Cooper's ligaments; they connect to the fascia around the ducts and glands and extend out to the skin.
- Lymphatic drainage from all parts of the breast generally flows to the axillary lymph nodes.
- The primary function of the breast is fluid transport.
- Three general categories of diagnostic breast imaging are available, two of which involve breast ultrasound. These three categories are breast cancer screening (generally performed by physical breast evaluation with mammography), diagnostic interrogation (consultation, problem solving, workup), and interventional breast procedures (histologic diagnosis and/or localization).
- The overall goal of breast evaluation is the proper classification of a breast lesion according to the level of suspicion for breast cancer.
- Most breast masses that arise during the teen years are fibroadenomas.
- Breast problems that may arise during pregnancy or lactation include mastitis, abscesses, cysts, or galactoceles (cysts containing milk).
- Sonographic evaluation of a breast lesion normally begins with determination of whether a lesion is cystic or solid.
- Cysts within the breast can be multilocular with thin internal septations.
- If the cyst has internal echoes, wall irregularity, mural nodularity or septation, shadowing, nonuniform internal echoes, or any other feature not associated with a simple cyst, it is by definition a complex cyst, and aspiration and/or biopsy should be considered.
- Benign lesions usually have smooth, rounded margins.
- Malignant tumors are aggressive and tend to grow through tissue via finger-like extensions called spiculation. As malignant masses enlarge, they may cause retraction of the nipple or dimpling of the skin as the spiculations pull on Cooper's ligaments.
- A rounded or oval shape is usually associated with benign lesions; sharp, angular margins are associated with malignancy.
- The normal tissue planes of the breast are horizontally oriented. Benign lesions tend to grow within the normal tissue planes, and their long axis lies parallel to the chest wall. These lesions are noted to be "wider than tall."
- Malignant lesions are able to grow through the connective tissue and may have a vertical orientation when the breast is imaged from anterior to posterior.
- Lesions that appear isoechoic with the breast parenchyma or have echoes equivalent to or brighter than that of fat are most often benign.
- A solid lesion that is hypoechoic relative to the normal breast parenchyma is more suspicious for malignancy.
- Microcalcifications within a solid mass are associated with a breast malignancy.
- Most solid lesions, with the exception of a fibroadenoma, will not enhance.

- Benign lesions normally demonstrate a limited degree of mobility or may roll away as they are palpated.
- If pressure applied by the transducer causes the lesion to compress or change shape, the lesion is probably benign and most likely represents a fat lobule. Malignant lesions normally are very hard and noncompressible.
- Vessels that penetrate a mass are highly suspect for malignancy and should be checked using color or power Doppler to ascertain the number and to look for intratumoral vessels.
- Symptoms of breast masses include pain, a palpable mass, spontaneous or induced nipple discharge, skin dimpling, ulceration, and nipple retraction.
- Skin dimpling or ulceration and nipple retraction nearly always result from cancer.
- Benign tumors are rubbery, mobile, and well defined (as seen in a fibroadenoma), whereas malignant tumors are often stone hard and irregular with a gritty feel.

BIBLIOGRAPHY

American Cancer Society: Breast Cancer Statistics. https://www.cancer.org/breast-cancer/about-howcommon-is-breast-cancer.html

American College of Radiology (ACR) *Breast imaging reporting and data system (BI-RADS) atlas.* ed 4 Reston: American College of Radiology; 2003.

Booi RC, Carson PL, O'Donnell M, et al. Diagnosing cysts with correlation coefficient images from 2-dimensional freehand elastography. *J Ultrasound Med.* 2007;26:1201–1207.

Cho SH, Park SH. Mimickers of breast malignancy on breast sonography. *J Ultrasound Med.* 2013;32:2029–2036.

Handel ER, Jackson VP. Other sonographically guided interventional procedures. In: Bassett LW, Jackson VP, Fu KL, Fu YS, eds. *Diagnosis of diseases of the breast.* ed 2 Philadelphia: Elsevier; 2005.

Hashimoto BE. New sonographic breast technologies. *Semin Roentgenol.* 2011;46(4):292–301.

Ikeda D. *Breast imaging: the requisites.* St Louis: Mosby; 2005.

Iorfida M, Maiorano E, Orvieto E, et al. Invasive lobular breast cancer: subtypes and outcome. *Breast Cancer Res Treat.* 2012;133:713–723.

Jesinger RA. Breast anatomy for the interventionalist. *Tech Vasc Interv Radiol.* 2014;17(1):3–9.

Kim SJ, Park YM, Jung SJ, et al. Sonographic appearances of juvenile fibroadenoma of the breast. *J Ultrasound Med.* 2014;33:1879–1884.

Norton K, Wininger M, Bhanot G, et al. A 2D mechanistic model of breast ductal carcinoma in situ (DCIS) morphology and progression. *J Theor Biol.* 2010;263:393–406.

Nwariaku FE. Sentinel lymph node biopsy, an alternative to elective axillary dissection for breast cancer. *Am J Surg.* 1998;176:529.

Romrell LJ, Bland KI. Anatomy of the breast, axilla, chest wall, and related metastatic sites. In: Bland KI, Copeland EM, eds. *The breast: comprehensive management of benign and malignant diseases.* ed 4 Philadelphia: Elsevier; 2010.

Schwartz T, Cyr A, Margenthaler J. Screening breast magnetic resonance imaging in women with atypia or lobular carcinoma in situ. *J Surg Res.* 2015;193:519–522.

Seymour MT, Moskovic EC, Walsh G, et al. Ultrasound assessment of residual abnormalities following primary chemotherapy for breast cancer. *Br J Cancer.* 1997;76:371.

Veronesi U, Paganelli G, Viale G, et al. Sentinel lymph node biopsy and axillary dissection in breast cancer: results in a large series. *J Natl Cancer Inst.* 1999;91:368.

Wilhelm MC, Langenburg SE, Wanebo HJ. Cancer of the male breast. In: Bland KI, Copeland EM, eds. *The breast: comprehensive management of benign and malignant diseases.* ed 4 Philadelphia: Elsevier; 2010.

Wilson M, Remlinger R, Wilson A. Critical thinking for sonographic breast imaging. *J Diagn Med Sonogr.* 2010;26(5):226–237.

CHAPTER 22

The Thyroid and Parathyroid Glands

Sandra L. Hagen-Ansert

OBJECTIVES

On completion of this chapter, you should be able to:
- Discuss the embryology of the thyroid and parathyroid glands
- Describe the normal anatomy and physiology of the thyroid and parathyroid glands
- Define the relational anatomy of the thyroid and parathyroid glands
- Discuss the laboratory values and clinical findings of the thyroid and parathyroid glands
- Describe the sonographic examination of the thyroid and parathyroid glands
- Differentiate the sonographic features of pathologic conditions found in the thyroid and parathyroid glands

OUTLINE

Embryology of the Thyroid Gland 683
Anatomy of the Thyroid Gland 683
   Size 683
   Relational Anatomy 683
   Vascular Supply 684
Thyroid Physiology and Laboratory Data 684
   Euthyroid, Hypothyroidism, and Hyperthyroidism 685
   Tests of Thyroid Function 685
Sonographic Evaluation of the Thyroid Gland 686

Congenital Abnormalities of the Thyroid Gland 690
Pathology of the Thyroid Gland 690
   Nodular Thyroid Disease 690
   Benign Lesions 691
   Malignant Lesions 693
   Diffuse Thyroid Disease 698
Embryology of the Parathyroid Gland 700
Anatomy of the Parathyroid Gland 700

Parathyroid Physiology and Laboratory Data 700
   Nuclear Medicine Scintigraphy 701
Sonographic Evaluation of the Parathyroid Gland 701
Pathology of the Parathyroid Gland 702
   Primary Hyperparathyroidism 702
   Secondary Hyperparathyroidism 704
Miscellaneous Neck Masses 704
   Developmental Cysts 704

KEY TERMS

Abscess
Adenoma
Branchial cleft cyst
Calcitonin
Endemic goiter
Euthyroid
Follicular adenoma
Follicular carcinoma
Graves disease
Goiter
Hashimoto thyroiditis
Hyperthyroidism
Hypothyroidism
Isthmus
Longus colli muscle
Medullary carcinoma
Multinodular goiter (MNG)
Nontoxic (simple) goiter
Papillary carcinoma
Parathyroid hormone (PTH)
Parathyroid hyperplasia
Primary hyperparathyroidism
Pyramidal lobe
Secondary hyperparathyroidism
Sternocleidomastoid muscles
Strap muscles
Subacute (de Quervain) thyroiditis
Thyroglossal duct cyst
Thyroid-stimulating hormone (TSH)
Thyrotoxicosis
Thyrotropin-releasing hormone (TRH)
Thyroxine (T_4)
Toxic goiter
Triiodothyronine T_3

The thyroid gland is an organ of the endocrine system that maintains body metabolism, growth, and development through the synthesis, storage, and secretion of thyroid hormones. A hormone triggers a reaction in a specific, targeted cell. Thyroid hormones include triiodothyronine (T_3), thyroxine (T_4), and calcitonin. The primary hormones, **triiodothyronine (T_3)** and **thyroxine (T_4)**, stimulate cell metabolism, which is the body's ability to break down food and convert it to energy. The third hormone, **calcitonin**, plays a minor role to regulate blood calcium levels. Disorders of the thyroid may result from thyroid gland dysfunction, which is regulated by the pituitary and hypothalamus glands (located in the brain).

The thyroid is located on the anterior lower neck on either side of the midline and is not easily palpated by physical examination. General enlargement of the thyroid gland is called a **goiter**. A localized enlargement is a *nodular goiter*, and multiple thyroid nodules are described as a **multinodular goiter (MNG)**. Both insufficient and excessive secretion of thyroid hormones may cause thyroid gland enlargement.

Because the thyroid gland is superficial, high-resolution sonography is used to evaluate the gland. The examination is easy to perform and is well tolerated by patients. Sonography of the thyroid is used to evaluate gland size, shape, and echogenicity and determine the sonographic appearance of a palpable lesion (i.e., solid or cystic, complex or calcified) and whether the lesion is single or multiple. The nodule size and location and the evaluation of the adjacent anatomy (i.e., lymph node adenopathy) may be imaged. Color Doppler, power Doppler, and pulsed wave Doppler are used to determine vascularity. Thyroid sonography will not determine the physiology of the thyroid gland. The functional state is better determined by nuclear medicine scintigraphy and laboratory measurements of the thyroid hormones present in the blood. Interventional procedures under sonographic guidance, including fine-needle aspiration (FNA) biopsy, are important applications of sonography. Sonographic evaluation of the parathyroid gland and other lesions of the neck will also be presented in this chapter.

EMBRYOLOGY OF THE THYROID GLAND

The thyroid gland is the first endocrine gland to develop in the human embryo. It develops at the floor of the primitive pharynx at the same location of the base of the tongue. The developing thyroid gland will migrate inferiorly along the anterior neck region to the lower neck anteriorly to the trachea. The migration may leave behind embryonic remnants or ectopic thyroid tissue that should atrophy but may form developmental cysts.

ANATOMY OF THE THYROID GLAND

The thyroid gland is located inferior to the thyroid cartilage (Adam's apple) in the anteroinferior neck. The gland has an "H" or a "U" configuration and consists of right and left lobes that consist of upper, middle, and lower poles that are connected across the midline by a thin bridge of thyroid tissue called the **isthmus**. The isthmus straddles the trachea anteriorly, whereas the paired lobes extend on either side of the trachea, bounded laterally by the common carotid arteries and internal jugular veins. When present, the **pyramidal lobe** arises from the isthmus and tapers superiorly just anterior to the thyroid cartilage and may be seen in 15% to 30% of patients (Fig. 22.1A). The pyramidal lobe is most commonly visualized in pediatric patients and usually atrophies with age. A fascia surrounds the thyroid, trachea, esophagus, and parathyroid glands (see Fig. 22.1B).

The thyroid gland is made up of two types of cells: follicular and parafollicular cells. Follicular cells make up the majority of thyroid tissue and secrete the main thyroid hormones T_3 and T_4. The follicular cells require an adequate supply of iodine to produce the correct amount of thyroid hormones. The parafollicular cells (also called C cells) secrete calcitonin.

Size

The size and shape of the thyroid gland vary with gender, age, and body surface area, with females having a slightly larger gland than males (Table 22.1). In tall individuals, the lateral lobes of the thyroid have a longitudinally elongated shape on sagittal scans, whereas in shorter individuals, the gland is more oval shaped. As a result, the normal dimensions of the gland have a wide range of variability. The lobes are normally equal in size. At age 1 year, the mean length is 25 mm, anteroposterior (AP) diameter is 12 to 15 mm, and width is 10 to 15 mm. In the normal adult, the thyroid gland measures 40 to 60 mm in length, 20 to 30 mm in AP diameter, and 15 to 20 mm in width. The isthmus is the smallest portion of the gland, with an AP diameter of 4 to 6 mm. The gland is considered enlarged when the thyroid lobe AP diameter measures greater than 20 mm and when the isthmus measures 10 mm or greater.

Due to shape variations, the thyroid volume is more useful to determine gland enlargement. The method commonly used to calculate thyroid volume is based on the ellipsoid formula with a correction factor (length × width × thickness × 0.523 for each lobe). The normal mean thyroid volume is 10 to 12 ± 3 mL. The volume in men is slightly more than in women. Volume measurement can be used to assess the need for surgery, calculate iodine-131 dosage for treatment of **thyrotoxicosis** (a toxic condition resulting from excessive amounts of thyroid hormones occurring in extreme hyperthyroidism), or evaluate the response to suppression treatments.

Relational Anatomy

Anterior. Along the anterior surface of the thyroid gland lie three **strap muscles**, including the sternohyoid, sternothyroid, and omohyoid, with the anterolateral **sternocleidomastoid muscles** (see Fig. 22.1).
Lateral. Directly lateral to each thyroid lobe are the common carotid artery, internal jugular vein, and vagus nerve within the carotid sheath.
Posterior. Along the posterior border adjacent to thyroid tissue lie the superior and inferior parathyroid glands along with the anastomosis between the superior and inferior thyroid arteries. The **longus colli muscle** is posterior and lateral to each thyroid lobe along the anterior surface of the cervical vertebrae (see Fig. 22.1).

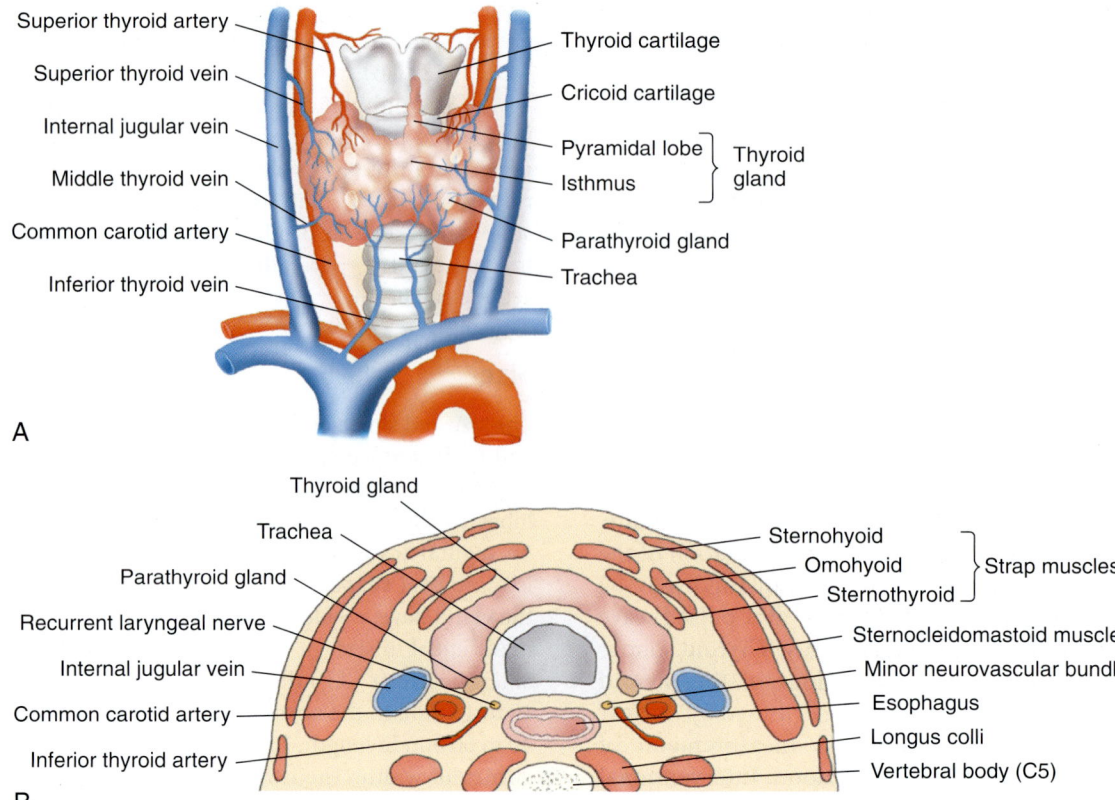

FIG. 22.1 (A) Anterior view of the thyroid and parathyroid glands. (B) Cross section of the thyroid region showing the thyroid gland and the vascular and muscular relationships to one another.

TABLE 22.1	Size of the Thyroid	
Dimension	Adults	Children
Length	40–60 mm	20–30 mm
Anteroposterior	20–30 mm	12–15 mm
Width	15–20 mm	10–15 mm
Volume	10–12 ± 3 mL	

Medial. Medial anatomy consists of the larynx, the trachea, and the inferior constrictor muscle of the pharynx. The esophagus is considered an anatomically midline structure but is usually found sonographically to the left of midline lateral to the trachea (see Fig. 22.1). It is identified by the target appearance in the transverse plane and confirmed during real time evaluation by its peristaltic movements when the patient swallows.

Vascular Supply

The thyroid gland is supplied by four arteries and considered highly vascular. Two superior thyroid arteries branch from the external carotid arteries and descend to the upper poles of the thyroid. Two inferior thyroid arteries arise from the thyrocervical trunk of the subclavian arteries and ascend to the lower poles of the thyroid. Corresponding superior thyroid veins drain into the internal jugular veins, and the inferior thyroid veins drain into the brachiocephalic veins (see Fig. 22.1).

THYROID PHYSIOLOGY AND LABORATORY DATA

The role of the thyroid is to maintain normal body metabolism, physical and mental growth, and development by the synthesis, storage, and secretion of thyroid hormones. Every cell in the body depends on thyroid hormones for regulation of its metabolism. The mechanism for producing thyroid hormones is through iodine metabolism. The thyroid follicular cells are the only cells in the body that can absorb iodine. Through a series of chemical reactions, the thyroid produces T_3 and T_4. Most endocrine glands do not store their hormones, but thyroid hormones are stored in the colloid material of the gland to be secreted when needed into the blood. In terms of amount of hormone secretion, T_4 is more abundant at 80%, whereas T_3 is 20% of secretion; however, T_3 is more potent.

When thyroid hormones are needed in the body, they are released into the bloodstream by the action of thyrotropin, or **thyroid-stimulating hormone (TSH)**, which is produced by the pituitary gland. The secretion of TSH is regulated by **thyrotropin-releasing hormone (TRH)**, which is produced by the hypothalamus. The level of TRH is controlled by the basal metabolic rate in a negative feedback system. Low concentration of thyroid hormones causes a decrease in the basal metabolic rate, which results in an increase in TRH. This causes an increased secretion of TSH and a subsequent increase in the release of thyroid hormones. When the blood level of thyroid hormones is returned to normal, the basal metabolic rate returns to normal and TSH secretion stops. In summary, the hypothalamus signals the pituitary gland to tell the thyroid gland to produce more or less thyroid hormones.

Calcitonin decreases the concentration of calcium in the blood by first acting on bone to inhibit its breakdown of calcium. When less calcium is being resorbed into the blood, less calcium moves out of the bone into the blood with a decrease in blood calcium levels. Calcitonin secretion will increase after any concentration of blood calcium increases.

Euthyroid, Hypothyroidism, and Hyperthyroidism

Euthyroid. When the thyroid is producing the correct amount of thyroid hormones, it is considered to be normal or **euthyroid**.

Abnormal thyroid hormone secretion is classified as either primary, if caused by inherent dysfunction of thyroid gland, or secondary, if there is failure of the pituitary or hypothalamus glands to correctly stimulate the thyroid gland to release hormones or possibly a pituitary mass.

Hypothyroidism. Undersecretion of thyroid hormones is called **hypothyroidism** and is the most common thyroid disorder. In the adult, it can be referred to as *myxedema*. Hypothyroidism can occur spontaneously from inability of the thyroid to produce the proper amount of thyroid hormones or a problem with the pituitary gland. Most commonly (75%), hypothyroidism is caused by a chronic thyroid inflammatory process called Hashimoto thyroiditis. The inflammatory process can also be the result of an autoimmune response that damages a large percentage of thyroid cells, and the thyroid is inadequate to produce sufficient hormones. Other causes include medications or radiation exposure to the head or neck. Radiation treatments to the neck and upper chest are associated with certain types of lymphoma. Box 22.1 lists the common disorders associated with hypothyroidism.

Clinical signs and symptoms of hypothyroidism include weight gain, hair loss, increased subcutaneous tissue around the eyes, lethargy, intellectual and motor slowing, cold intolerance, constipation, and a deep husky voice. Medical treatment with synthetic thyroid hormone can successfully treat, manage, and reverse the condition. A rare, more severe complication of hypothyroidism could lead to a life-threatening coma.

Hyperthyroidism. The oversecretion of thyroid hormones is called **hyperthyroidism**. This occurs when the entire gland is not functioning properly, usually from diffuse enlargement or localized nodule or **adenoma** causing overproduction of thyroid hormones, called **Graves disease**. Box 22.2 lists the common disorders associated with hyperthyroidism.

Clinical signs and symptoms of hyperthyroidism include weight loss, increased appetite, high degree of nervous energy, irritable, tremor, excessive sweating, heat intolerance, palpitations, impaired fertility, and exophthalmos (protruding eyes). An extreme form of hyperthyroidism is thyrotoxicosis.

Tests of Thyroid Function

Laboratory Tests. The most common laboratory test to evaluate thyroid function is serum T_4. This test reflects the amount of T_4 in the blood and is considered a good screening test of thyroid function. Serum T_3 reflects the amount of T_3 in the blood. Measurements of both thyroid hormones may be used to give a more accurate picture of thyroid function. The TSH (serum thyrotropin) laboratory test will also indicate thyroid function and may be the first to elevate as an indication of hypothyroidism. Often the TSH level is opposite the T_4 and T_3 levels with thyroid dysfunction (i.e., low TSH with elevated T_4 and T_3 indicates hyperthyroidism). If the TSH, T_3, and T_4 levels are all low, this could indicate pituitary dysfunction or pituitary mass from secondary hypothyroidism. The laboratory findings associated with common thyroid disorders are listed in Table 22.2.

Calcitonin helps to maintain homeostasis of blood calcium levels and helps to prevent increased amounts of

---

BOX 22.1	Disorders Associated With Hypothyroidism

Common
Chronic inflammatory process (most common Hashimoto thyroiditis)
Endemic iodine deficiency
Uncommon
Hyperfunctioning thyroid cancer
Thyroid-stimulating hormone–secreting pituitary adenoma
Neonatal thyrotoxicosis associated with maternal Graves disease

---

BOX 22.2	Disorders Associated With Hyperthyroidism

Common (account for 99% of cases)
Diffuse toxic hyperplasia (most common Graves disease)
Toxic multinodular goiter
Toxic adenoma
Uncommon
Acute or subacute thyroiditis
Hyperfunctioning thyroid cancer
Choriocarcinoma or hydatidiform mole
Thyroid-stimulating hormone–secreting pituitary adenoma
Neonatal thyrotoxicosis associated with maternal Graves disease

calcium in the blood (hypercalcemia). In addition, calcitonin is not a common indicator of thyroid function but can be a laboratory test for medullary carcinoma with elevated calcitonin used as a tumor marker.

Nuclear Medicine or Scintigraphy. Scintigraphy can be used to determine the thyroid function with two tests that can be performed together: iodine uptake scan and thyroid scan. For an iodine uptake scan, a capsule containing a small amount of radioactive iodine (called a radiotracer) is ingested by mouth. The amount of radioactivity accumulated in the thyroid gland is measured at multiple time points for up to 24 hours by a gamma camera. In comparison with normal thyroid uptake, patients with hyperthyroidism have a higher percentage of radioactivity in the thyroid gland; a lower percentage of radioactivity is present with hypothyroidism.

The thyroid scan will detect the amount of radioactive tracer to image the thyroid gland and demonstrate the thyroid size, shape, and position. In addition, if the thyroid has a concentrated amount of radioactivity, this will be imaged as a "hot" (hyperfunctioning) nodule (see Fig. 22.2A). An area of the thyroid with lower concentration of the radioactive tracer will demonstrate absence of uptake as a "cold" (nonfunctioning) nodule (see Fig. 22.2B). The majority (80% to 85%) of nodules in a thyroid scan are demonstrated as a cold nodule, with the remaining (15% to 20%) seen as a hot nodule. Hot nodules are considered to be benign. Cold nodules have the potential to be malignant, but only 10% to 15% of cold nodules are shown to be malignant with FNA biopsy.

Other imaging modalities for thyroid include computed tomography (CT) and magnetic resonance imaging (MRI) to determine thyroid size, shape, position, and imaging characteristics of masses within the gland and neck area.

SONOGRAPHIC EVALUATION OF THE THYROID GLAND

No patient preparation is required for thyroid sonography. The sonographer should review the examination indication and the available imaging results (i.e., previous thyroid sonography, scintigraphy, CT, or MRI). A thorough patient clinical history should be obtained before the sonographic examination. Pertinent information includes results of the physician's physical examination (e.g., palpable nodule or goiter), pain/duration, history of hyperthyroidism, hypothyroidism, thyroiditis and symptoms related to thyroid disorders, thyroid medications, or surgery. If the patient has a previous history of cancer, along with prior history of radiation or surgery to the neck and upper chest, this should be noted in the examination record. If the patient has a palpable mass, ask the patient to indicate the location or obtain a description of the palpable area from the ordering physician.

The examination procedure should always be explained to the patient before scanning. The patient is placed in the supine position with a pillow or pad under both shoulders to provide moderate hyperextension of the neck with chin elevated to place the thyroid more horizontal and bring the inferior portion of the gland more superior for visualization (Fig. 22.3). If the lower pole of the thyroid is still difficult to view, having the patient swallow will move the entire gland superiorly. Having the patient elevate the chin superiorly and turn to the opposite side will enable better visualizing of each lobe. It is important to be conscious of elderly patients or those who may experience dizziness or neck strain and make positioning adjustments as needed.

A high-frequency (7 to 15 MHz) linear array transducer should be used, selecting the highest frequency to penetrate

TABLE 22.2	Laboratory Findings With Common Thyroid Disorders			
Laboratory Test	Normal Thyroid (Euthyroid)	Hyperthyroidism	Primary Hypothyroidism	Secondary Hypothyroidism (Possible Pituitary Dysfunction or Mass)
T_4, T_3	Normal	High	Low	Low
TSH	Normal	Low	High	Low

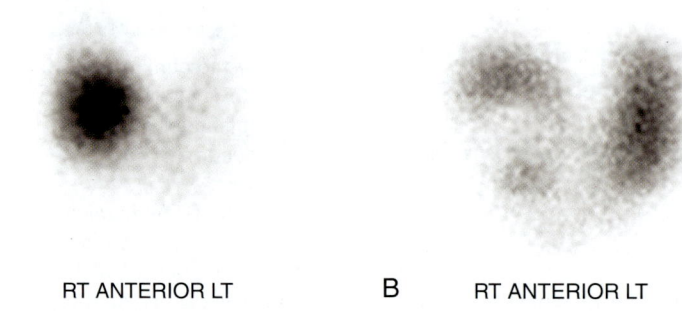

FIG. 22.2 (A) Scintigraphy of the thyroid gland demonstrating a "hot" nodule. (B) Scintigraphy of the thyroid demonstrating a "cold" nodule.

the entire thyroid and surrounding musculature. Each lobe and isthmus should be carefully surveyed in transverse and longitudinal planes. The survey should also extend superior, inferior, and lateral of the thyroid gland to identify and document any enlarged cervical lymph nodes (Fig. 22.4). The transverse survey is completed scanning from above to below the thyroid to note gland symmetry. Multiple transverse images of the superior, mid, and inferior levels of each lobe are imaged and labeled accordingly (Fig. 22.5). Virtual convex, split screen, or panoramic features may provide imaging of larger glands (Fig. 22.6).

Transverse and longitudinal survey of the isthmus is completed with images recorded and labeled. Transverse imaging landmarks include the trachea, common carotid artery, and internal jugular vein. The trachea is noted in the midline posterior to the isthmus with posterior shadowing. The common carotid artery is a circular, pulsatile structure directly lateral and adjacent to the gland. The oval-shaped internal jugular vein lies lateral to the common carotid artery (Fig. 22.7).

To locate the longitudinal scan plane of the thyroid gland, it is helpful to align the longitudinal axis of the common carotid artery and slide medially. Longitudinal survey is completed by scanning from the lateral to internal jugular vein to the midline isthmus. Multiple longitudinal images of the lateral, mid, and medial portions of each lobe are imaged individually and labeled accordingly (see Fig. 22.4). On longitudinal scans, landmarks include the recurrent laryngeal nerve and inferior thyroid artery, which may be seen between the thyroid lobe and esophagus on the left and between the thyroid lobe and longus colli muscle on the right.

During the examination, obtain three measurements of each lobe for volume calculations at maximum length, AP, and width of gland. The AP measurement of isthmus should be imaged in the transverse plane (Fig. 22.8). Examination protocol should

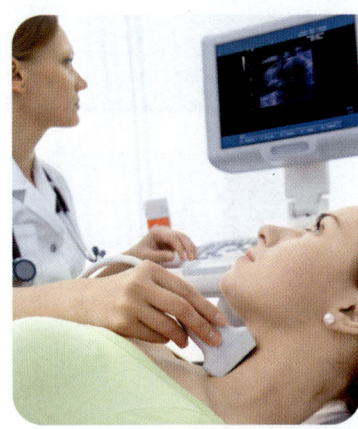

FIG. 22.3 The patient is placed in the supine position with a pillow or pad under both shoulders to provide moderate hyperextension of the neck and with the chin elevated to place the thyroid more horizontal and bring the inferior portion of the gland more superior for visualization.

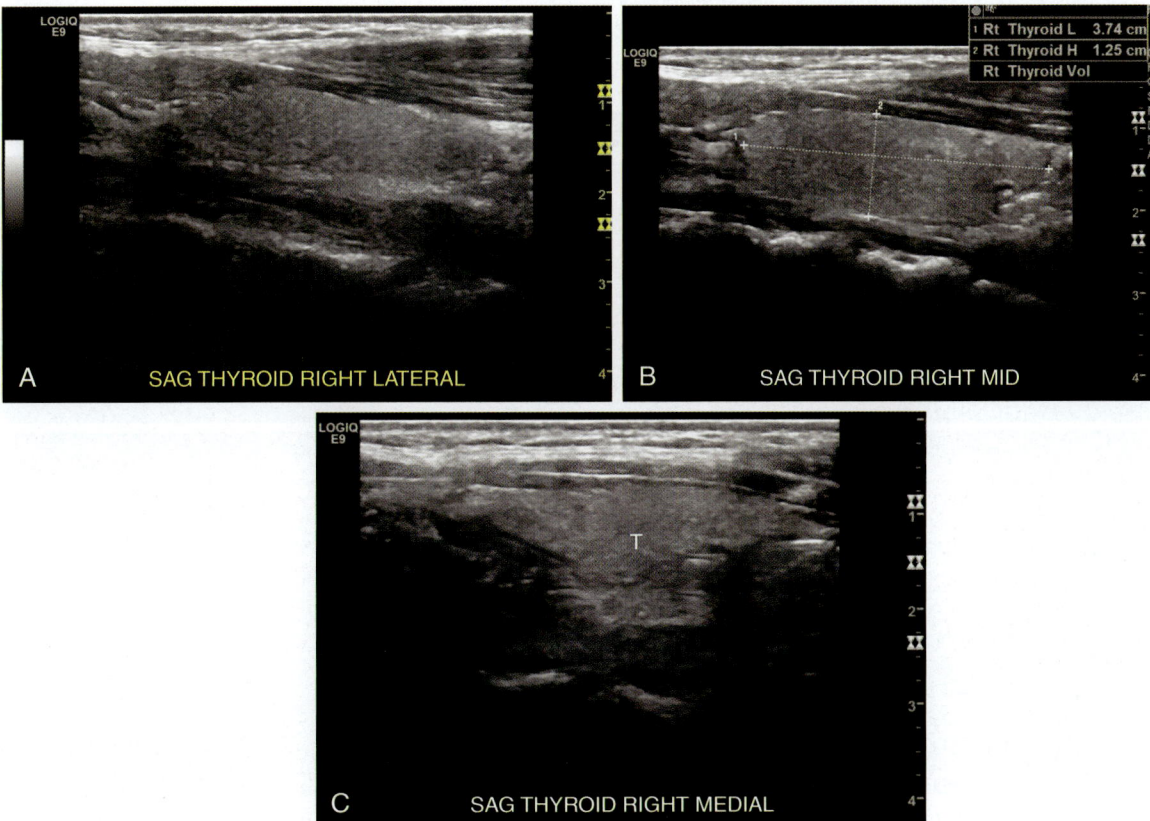

FIG. 22.4 Longitudinal images of the normal thyroid gland. (A) Long, lateral. (B) Long, mid. Measurement of the length and anteroposterior dimension of the gland. (C) Long, medial. *T*, Thyroid.

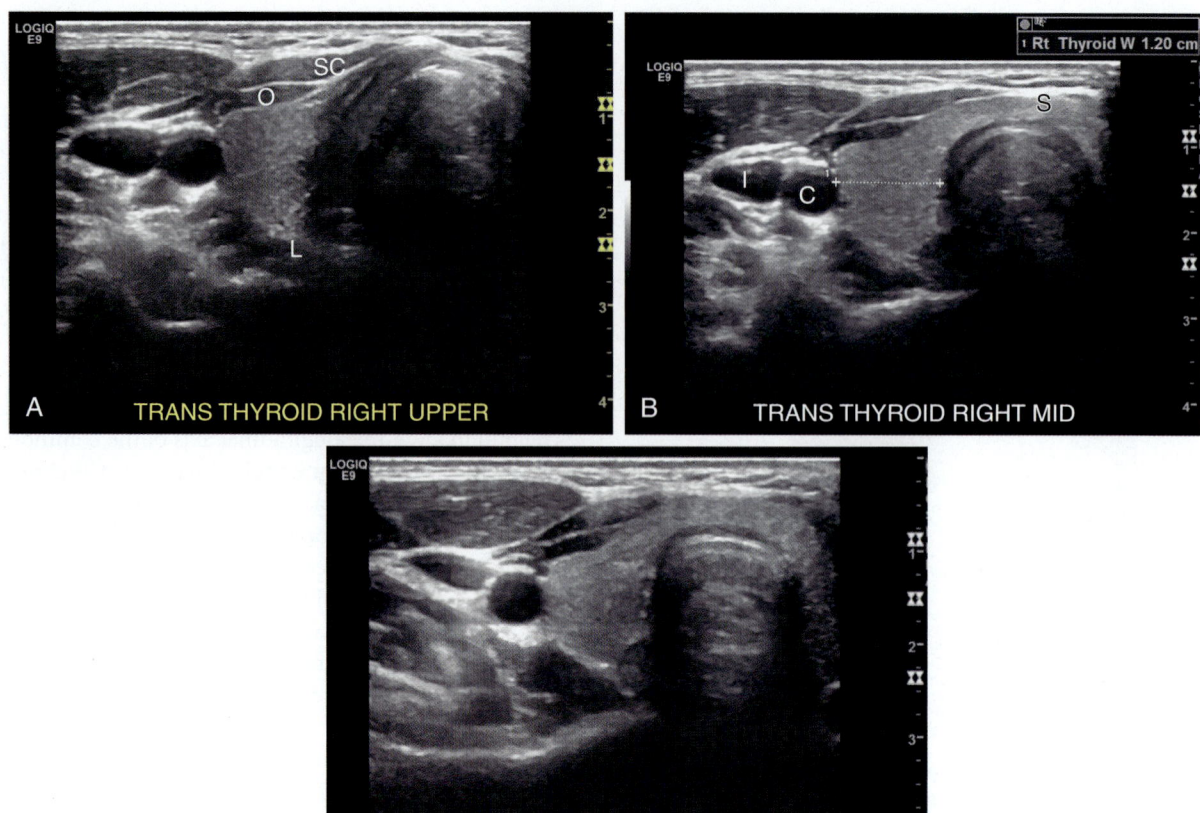

FIG. 22.5 Transverse images of the normal thyroid gland. (A) Trans, superior. (B) Trans, mid. Measurement of the width of the gland. (C) Trans, inferior. *C,* Carotid artery; *I,* internal jugular vein; *L,* longus colli muscle; *O,* omohyoid muscle; *S,* sternohyoid muscle; *SC,* sternocleidomastoid.

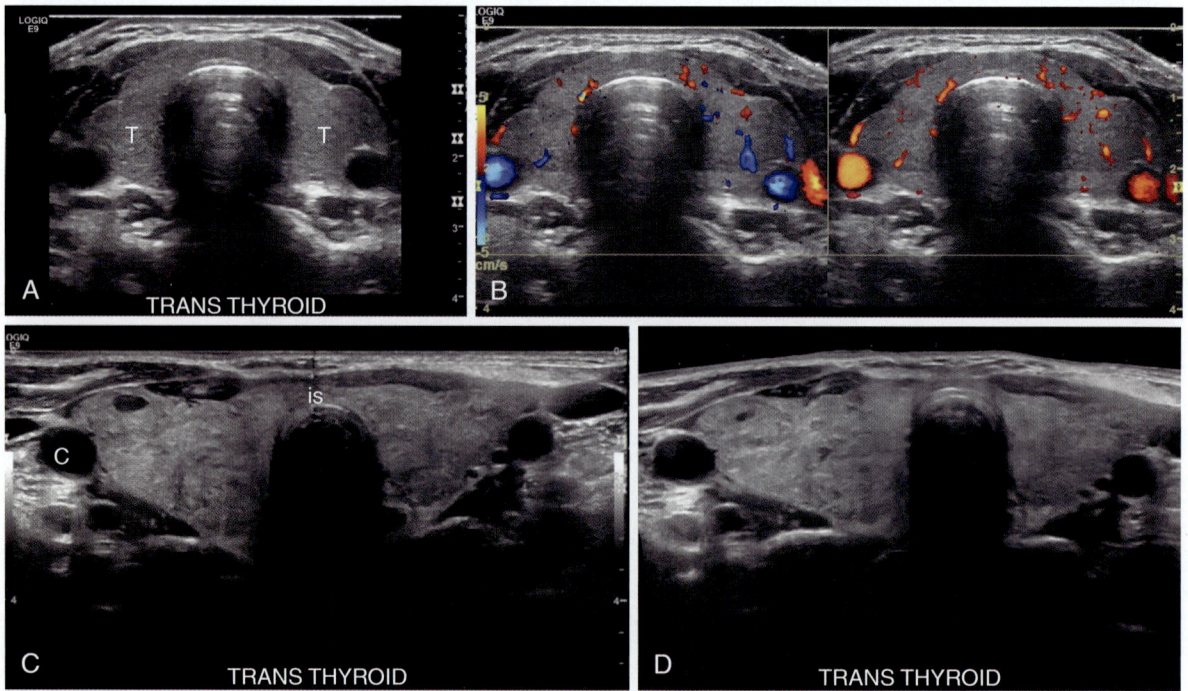

FIG. 22.6 (A) Transverse image of both lobes of the thyroid to show the comparable homogeneity of each lobe. (B) Color and power Doppler of both lobes. (C) Split-screen transverse image of both lobes. (D) Panoramic image of both lobes. *C,* Carotid; *is,* isthmus; *T,* thyroid.

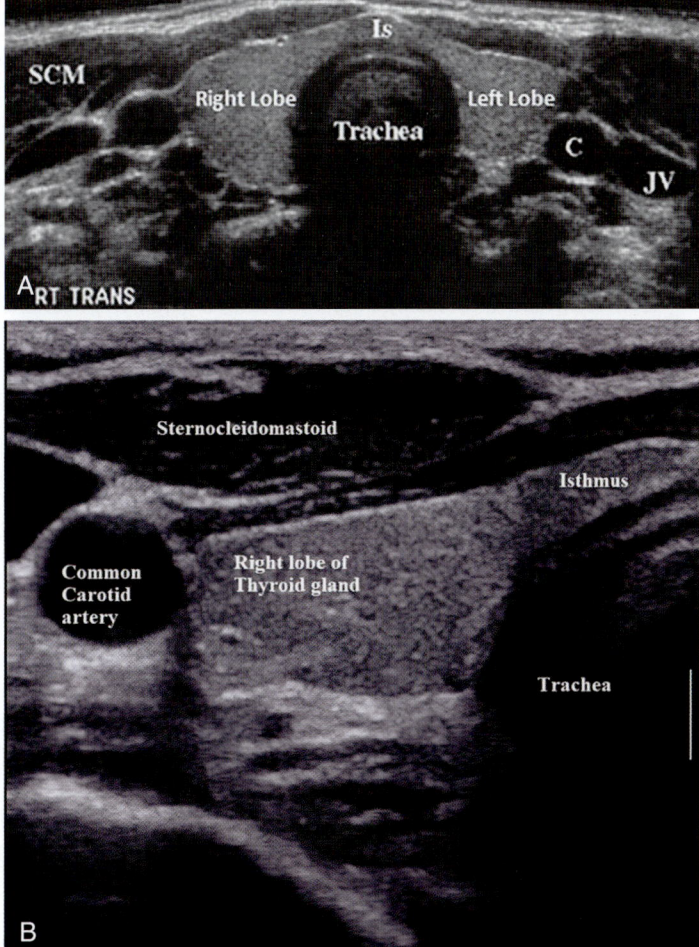
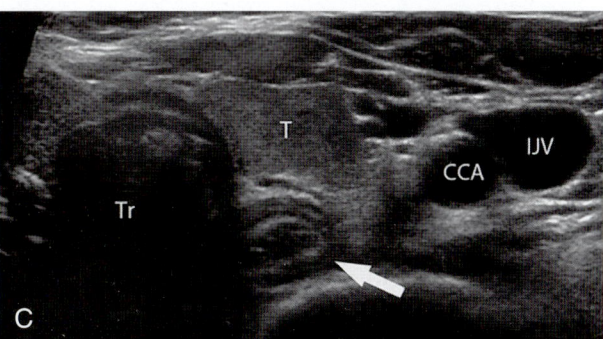

FIG. 22.7 Transverse and longitudinal survey of the isthmus is completed with images recorded and labeled. Transverse imaging landmarks include the trachea (Tr), common carotid artery (CCA), and internal jugular vein (IJV). The trachea is noted in the midline posterior to the isthmus (Is) with posterior shadowing. The common carotid artery is a circular, pulsatile structure directly lateral and adjacent to the gland. The oval-shaped internal jugular vein lies lateral to the common carotid artery. *C*, Carotid; *JV*, jugular vein.

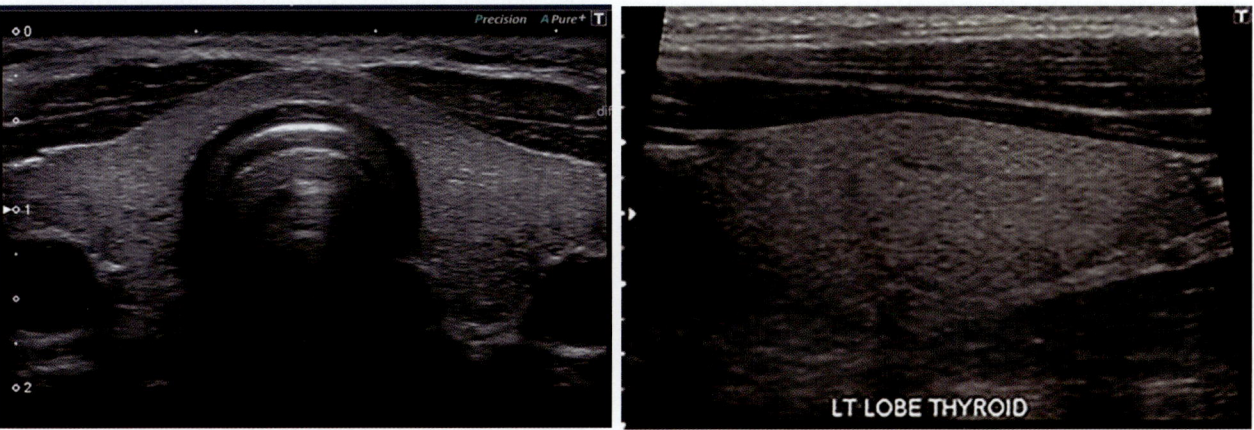

FIG. 22.8 Obtain three measurements of each lobe for volume calculations at maximum length, anteroposterior, and width of gland.

also include color Doppler images of both transverse and longitudinal planes of the middle portion of the thyroid demonstrating gland vascularity (see Fig. 22.6B). A low pulse repetition frequency is chosen for the color Doppler scale to distinguish all vascular structures. Power Doppler or pulsed wave Doppler may also contribute information on vascular hemodynamics and should be obtained as needed.

Normal sonographic appearance of the thyroid gland is fine homogeneous echotexture that is slightly more echogenic than the surrounding musculature. The thyroid capsule is imaged as a thin, hyperechoic line that outlines the gland from surrounding relational anatomy. The air-filled trachea is demonstrated as a curvilinear structure with acoustic shadowing. Multiple, tiny vascular structures may be seen as tubular anechoic structures more apparent at the periphery and upper and lower poles within the gland representing the superior and inferior thyroid arteries and veins. Normal pulsed Doppler spectrum will demonstrate peak systole velocities of 20 to 40 cm/sec in the major thyroid arteries and 15 to 30 cm/sec in intraparenchymal arteries.

The surrounding musculature of the thyroid gland is hypoechoic compared with the normal thyroid parenchyma. The strap muscles are anterior to the gland with the larger sternocleidomastoid muscle imaged more anterolateral to the gland. The hypoechoic longus colli muscle is found posterior to each lobe of the thyroid (see Fig. 22.5). The recurrent laryngeal nerve and the inferior thyroid artery pass in the angle between the trachea, esophagus, and thyroid lobe. The esophagus is adjacent to the trachea, with a hypoechoic rim surrounding an echogenic center more commonly visualized slightly to the left of the midline, next to the trachea, with peristalsis noted in real time with patient swallowing (Fig. 22.9).

CONGENITAL ABNORMALITIES OF THE THYROID GLAND

Congenital abnormalities of the thyroid gland include aplasia, hypoplasia, and ectopic locations of the thyroid gland. Aplasia is congenital absence of gland and may affect one lobe, the isthmus, or the entire gland. Complete absence of the thyroid gland has a severe impact on physical and mental development. Hypoplasia refers to underdevelopment of any part of the gland and may be associated with congenital hypothyroidism.

Ectopic locations may be present along the path of embryonic descent if the thyroid migrates too little or too far. Most commonly, ectopic tissue may be present posterior to the tongue (sublingual or lingual thyroid). Other ectopic locations include larynx (prelaryngeal thyroid) or mediastinum (substernal thyroid). Scintigraphy is best for visualization of ectopic thyroid tissue.

PATHOLOGY OF THE THYROID GLAND

Pathology identified in the thyroid and adjacent neck structures should always be documented in both longitudinal and transverse scan planes. The gland measurements and volume should be obtained and parenchyma defined as homogeneous or heterogeneous. If a nodule is visualized, the location should be noted in relationship to gland (e.g., right thyroid transverse upper; left thyroid long lateral) and also measured in three dimensions. The sonographic appearance should be demonstrated and echogenicity described (e.g., hypoechoic, hyperechoic, and whether cystic, complex cystic, solid, and/or presence and type of calcifications). In addition, the nodule borders should be described as ill defined or well defined and whether a hypoechoic halo is surrounding the nodule. It is not uncommon for sonography to demonstrate multiple nodules (MNG) in a gland. Vascularity should also be demonstrated with color or power Doppler and possibly pulsed wave Doppler.

Nodular Thyroid Disease

Nodular Hyperplasia, Multinodular Goiter, and Adenomatous Hyperplasia. Approximately 80% of nodular thyroid disease is due to hyperplasia or compensatory hypertrophy forming micronodules and macronodules of the gland. This can lead to overall enlargement (goiter) or MNG that may be unilateral or bilateral; it is seen more commonly in women with increasing age. When evaluated microscopically, most benign nodules are classified as hyperplastic, adenomatous, and colloid type nodules.

The most common cause of thyroid disorders worldwide is iodine deficiency, which leads to nodule and goiter formation. Often the gland is able to keep up with the demand and provide normal release of thyroid hormones. However, in some cases, the gland lags behind the demand and the patient develops hypothyroidism. In the first stage, hyperplasia occurs; in the second stage, colloid involution occurs. Progression of this process leads to an asymmetric and multinodular gland with areas of hemorrhage and calcification (Fig. 22.10).

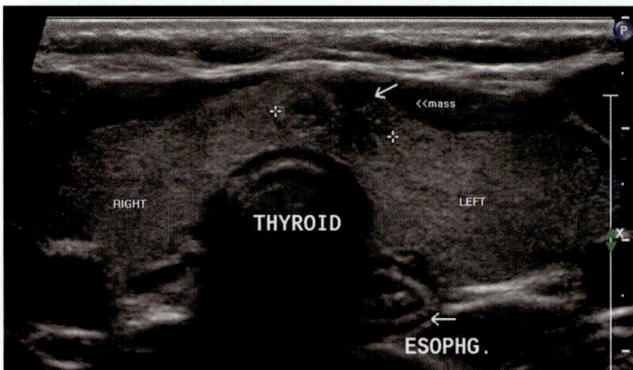

FIG. 22.9 The esophagus is adjacent to the trachea with a hypoechoic rim surrounding an echogenic center more commonly visualized slightly to the left of the midline, next to the trachea with peristalsis noted in real time with patient swallowing.

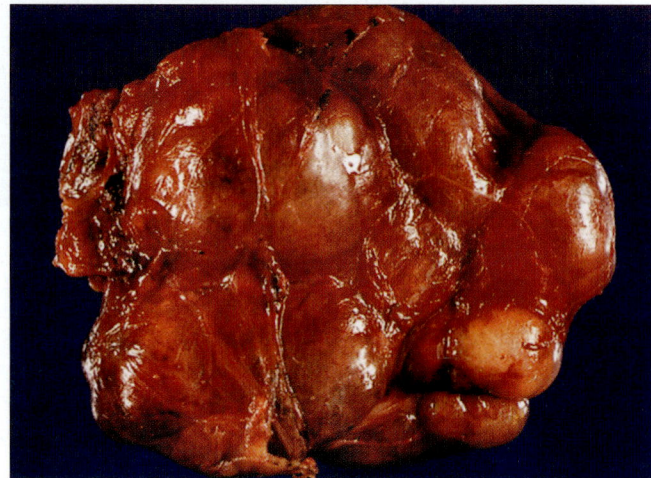

FIG. 22.10 Gross pathology of a nodular goiter. The thyroid is enlarged with nodules that vary in size and shape.

An **endemic goiter** may affect large groups of people in a specific geographic area where iodine levels in the soil, food, and water are low (e.g., mountainous areas or the Great Lakes region). Certain types of food (cabbage, turnips, and other related vegetables) when ingested in large quantities may increase blood synthesis of T_3 and T_4 but increase TSH secretion from the pituitary gland. This dietary deficiency can cause hyperplasia and hypertrophy and can promote goiter formation in the thyroid gland. Iodized salt as a dietary supplement usually corrects the iodine deficiency. In areas not deficient in iodine, autoimmune processes (Graves disease or Hashimoto thyroiditis) are believed to be the basis for most cases of thyroid disease.

A **toxic goiter** is a condition in which nodular enlargement causes hyperactivity of the thyroid gland and hyperthyroidism. **Nontoxic (simple) goiter** occurs when nodular enlargement is not associated with thyroid dysfunction (hypothyroidism or hyperthyroidism).

Clinical Findings. A goiter may first present visibly as an anterior protrusion on the neck on thin patients. The clinician may palpate an enlarged thyroid during a physical examination. A goiter may become very large, compressing the esophagus with difficulty swallowing (dysphagia), pressure on the trachea (inspiratory stridor) or neck veins (venous distention), or laryngeal nerve (hoarseness). Patients may also present with clinical symptoms of hypothyroidism or hyperthyroidism. Table 22.3 lists the common findings, sonographic appearances, and differential considerations for nodule thyroid disease.

Sonographic Findings. Sonographic appearance of nodular thyroid disease will vary. There can be diffuse symmetric gland enlargement (Fig. 22.11) or localized discrete nodule(s). Enlargement can involve both lobes and isthmus with several nodules, described as an MNG (Fig. 22.12), or one lobe. Nodules can also vary in echogenicity (i.e., isoechoic, hyperechoic, and complex cystic) due to fibrosis, colloid, focal scarring, ischemia, cystic degeneration, or calcification formation. Nodules may present as poorly circumscribed or well defined and encapsulated by a thin, peripheral hypoechoic halo due to surrounding compressed tissue and should be documented (Fig. 22.13). Hyperfunctioning nodules usually demonstrate increased perinodular and intranodular vascularity on color or power Doppler as seen in Fig. 22.12B.

Benign Lesions

A discrete, palpable nodule of the thyroid gland is the most common indication for a thyroid sonography. Nodular thyroid disease is frequently encountered in the adult population, with up to 7% found to have benign nodule, with women affected more frequently than men. Sonography is useful to locate the palpable nodule and describe sonographic appearance.

Cyst. A true epithelial-lined cyst within the thyroid is uncommon and considered benign. Most represent cystic degeneration of a follicular adenoma. Cystic component may represent serous fluid, colloid fluid, or hemorrhage and may contain blood or debris within the nodule.

TABLE 22.3 Thyroid Findings: Nodular Thyroid Disease

Clinical Findings	Sonographic Appearances	Differential Considerations
Nontoxic Simple Goiter		
Thyroid enlargement	Sometimes smooth, sometimes nodular; possible compression of surrounding structures	Thyroiditis Hypothyroidism Neoplasm
Toxic Multinodular Goiter		
Thyroid enlargement	Enlarged inhomogeneous gland; can have focal scarring, focal ischemia, necrosis, and cyst formation	Neoplasm Cyst
Graves Disease		
Diffuse toxic goiter	Diffusely homogeneous and enlarged	Neoplasm Ophthalmopathy Cutaneous manifestations Hyperthyroidism
Thyroiditis		
Swelling and tenderness of the thyroid; later, hypothyroidism	Homogeneous enlargement with nodularity; later, inhomogeneous	Neoplasm
Benign Lesions		
Cysts		
Solitary nodules or multiple nodules	Anechoic areas, echogenic fluid, or moving fluid levels	Toxic multinodular goiter
Adenoma		
Usually euthyroid or hyperthyroidism	Compression of adjacent structures; fibrous encapsulation; ranges from anechoic to hyperechoic; may have halo	Graves disease

Sonographic Findings. A true thyroid cyst demonstrates the sonographic appearance of a simple cyst as round, anechoic, and well defined, with thin echogenic walls and distal acoustic enhancement (Fig. 22.14A). Colloid cyst will demonstrate a cyst with a tiny echogenic focus (see Fig. 22.14B) and often demonstrates a comet tail artifact. Hemorrhage cyst may demonstrate low-level echoes with possible fluid and debris level with possible wall irregularities and internal septation(s) (see Fig. 22.14C). Vascularity should always be obtained on all thyroid masses with color

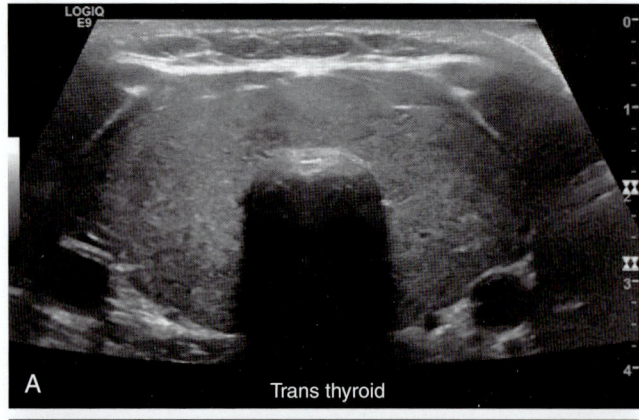
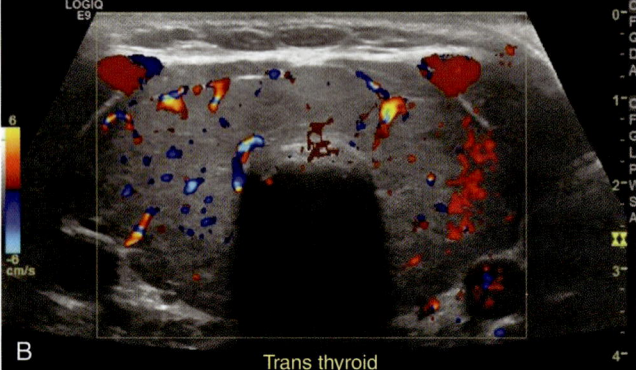

FIG. 22.11 (A) A patient with a goiter demonstrating diffusely enlarged thyroid gland. (B) Vascularity of the diffusely enlarged thyroid gland.

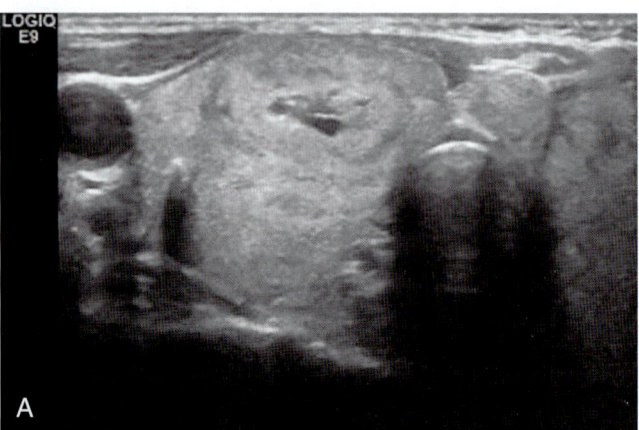
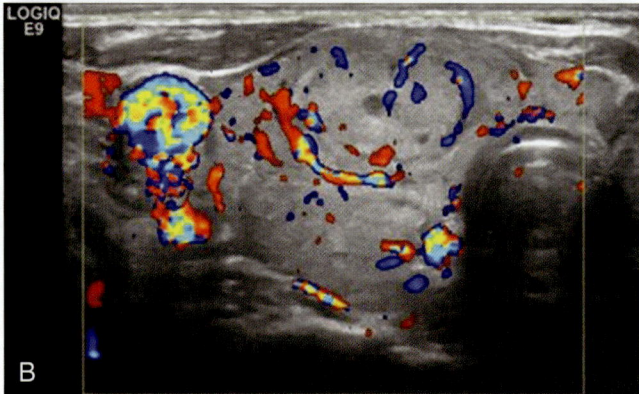

FIG. 22.12 (A) Multinodular goiter is seen as an inhomogeneous enlarged tissue mass within the thyroid gland. (B) Increased vascularity is shown in a patient with a multinodular goiter.

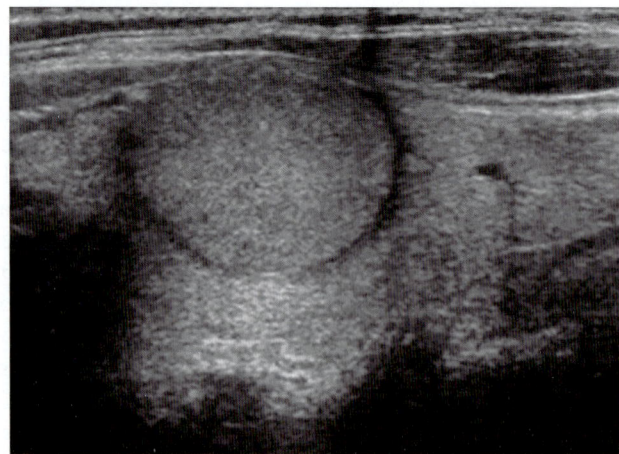

FIG. 22.13 Nodules may present as poorly circumscribed or well defined and encapsulated by a thin, peripheral hypoechoic halo due to surrounding compressed tissue and should be documented.

Doppler images. Thyroid carcinoma could present as complex cystic nodule, so FNA biopsy would be necessary to evaluate any suspicious cystic masses.

Adenoma. A **follicular adenoma** is a benign thyroid neoplasm that represents 5% to 10% of all nodular diseases of the thyroid. It is seven times more common in women than in men (Fig. 22.15). Other rarer subtypes of follicular adenomas that are distinguished histologically include fetal adenoma, embryonal adenoma, and Hürthle cell adenoma. A Hürthle cell adenoma should be further evaluated when found after FNA because 15% to 25% will have malignant cells found within the adenoma after excision.

The adenoma is often solitary and slow growing unless hemorrhage occurs that could cause sudden and painful enlargement. Most patients with a thyroid adenoma do not have thyroid dysfunction (euthyroid), and less than 10% develop hyperthyroidism (toxic nodule). Rarely, a toxic nodule may cause extreme hyperthyroidism or thyrotoxicosis and would require immediate treatment. Sonography cannot distinguish between a toxic and nontoxic adenoma.

Sonographic Findings. Adenomas have a broad spectrum of sonographic appearances. They are most often solitary, homogeneous, and variable in size and range in echogenicity from anechoic, hypoechoic, or isoechoic to hyperechoic. The presence of a thin hypoechoic rim or halo due to compressed tissue surrounding the adenoma is a relatively consistent finding with a benign adenoma (Fig. 22.16). However, it is not always present or may be seen less commonly (10% to 24%) with malignancy. Adenomas may contain anechoic areas from hemorrhage or cystic degeneration and may be irregular in outline. Calcification along the rim with an "eggshell" appearance with shadowing can also be demonstrated with an adenoma. Rim calcification with shadowing may obscure visualization. Color or power Doppler will demonstrate enhanced blood flow patterns along the peripheral borders or within the lesion but not specific to separate a benign from malignant process.

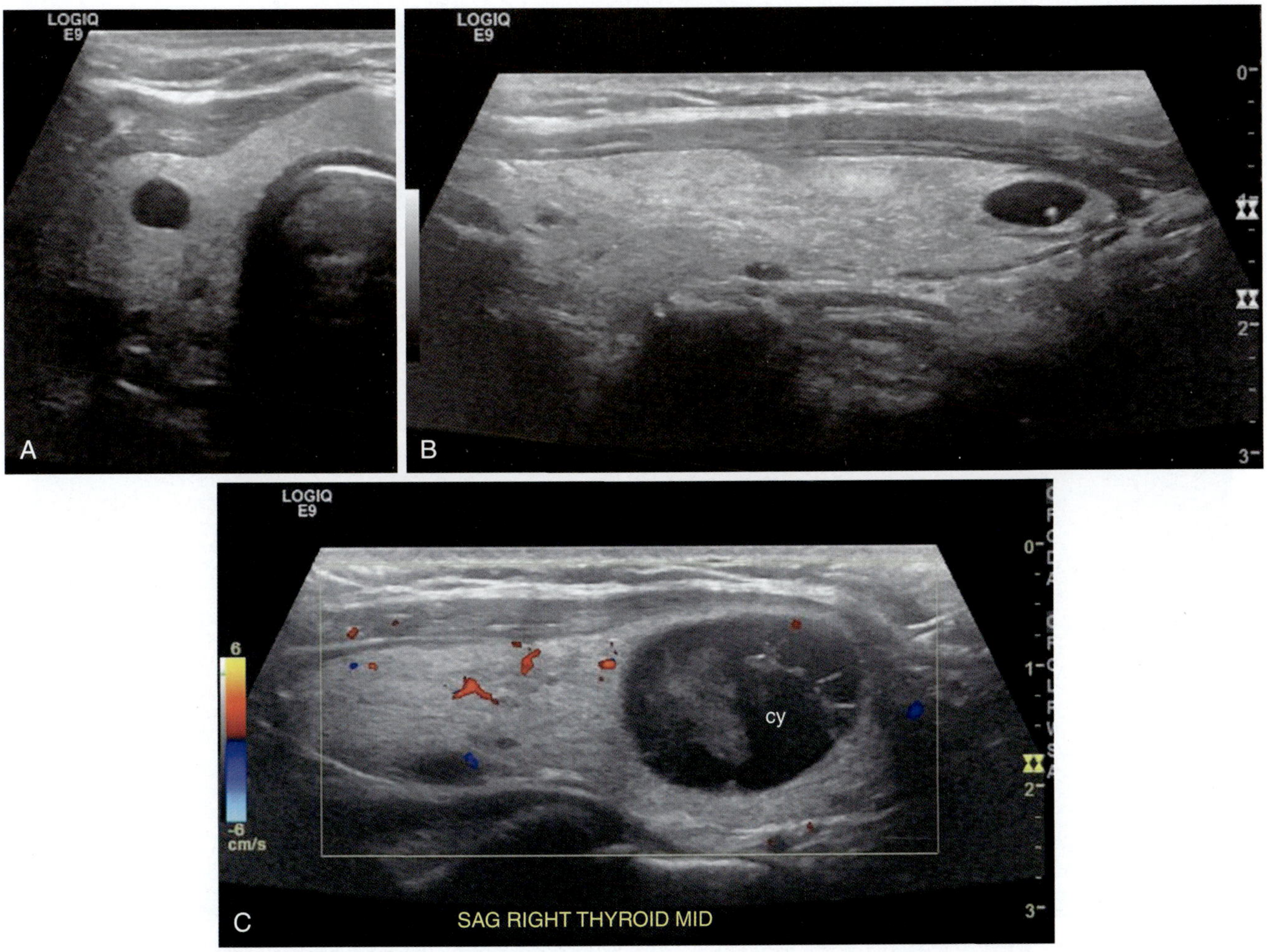

FIG. 22.14 (A) An anechoic cyst (cy) is seen within the normal thyroid gland. (B) Colloid cyst with echogenic focus. (C) Hemorrhagic cyst with color Doppler.

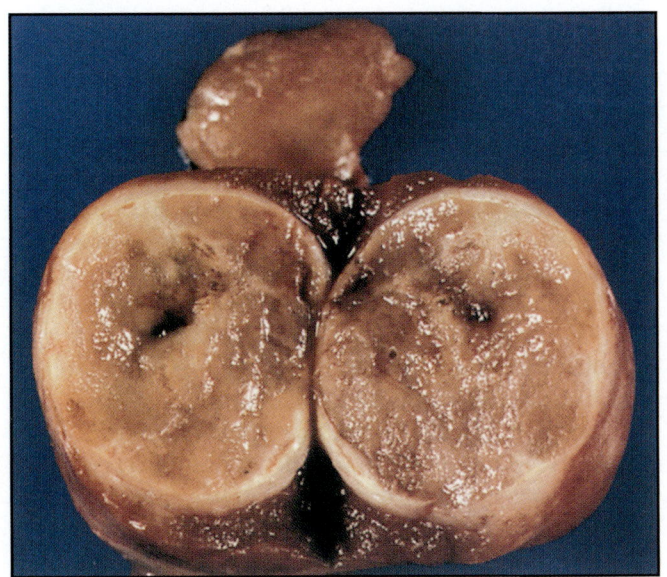

FIG. 22.15 Gross pathology of follicular adenoma. The nodule is well circumscribed with a fibrous capsule separating it from the normal parenchyma.

Malignant Lesions

Carcinoma of the thyroid is rare. A solitary nodule may be malignant in a small percentage of cases, but the risk of malignancy decreases with the presence of MNG. A solitary markedly hypoechoic thyroid nodule with the presence of cervical lymphadenopathy on the same side suggests malignancy. A prior history of neck or upper chest radiation is associated with the most common type of thyroid malignancy.

Clinical Findings. Thyroid malignancy is associated with the presence of a painless, palpable, hard, firm solitary nodule. If more advanced, the patient may present with compression of adjacent structures with hoarseness, cough, dysphagia, or dyspnea.

Sonographic Findings. Sonographic appearance of thyroid cancer is highly variable, making the distinction between benign and malignant nodules by sonography alone difficult. As stated previously, a malignant lesion is most often single but could be multiple; it may be variable in size, solid, partially cystic, or a largely cystic mass. In

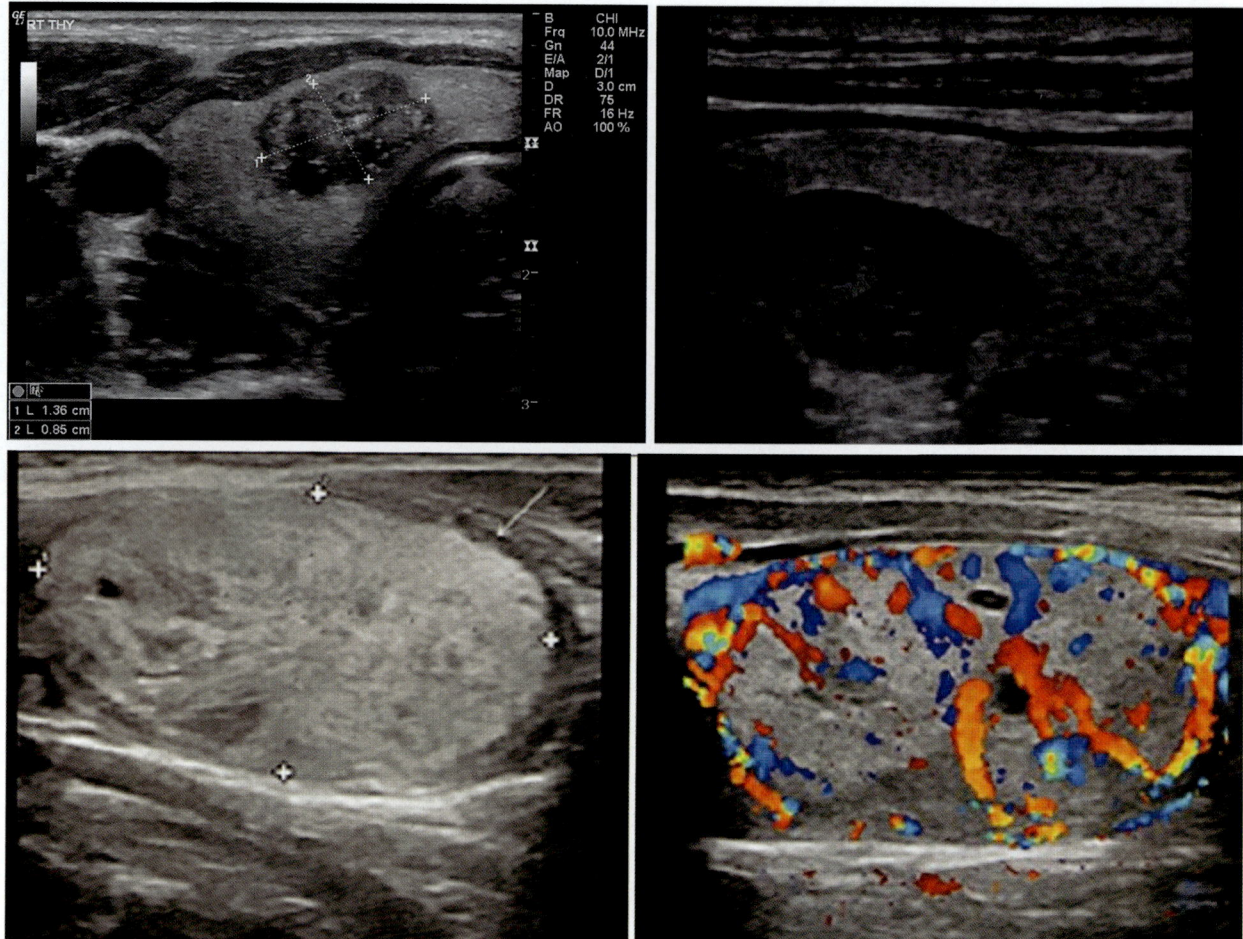

FIG. 22.16 Adenomas have a broad spectrum of sonographic appearances. They are most often solitary, homogeneous, and variable in size and range in echogenicity from anechoic, hypoechoic, isoechoic, to hyperechoic. The presence of a thin hypoechoic rim or halo due to compressed tissue surrounding the adenoma is a relatively consistent finding with a benign adenoma.

general, the sonographic characteristic that suggests malignancy is a solitary, solid mass that is markedly hypoechoic compared with strap muscles, with irregular or microlobulated margins that may be taller than wide. In addition, there are often small, punctate internal microcalcifications (<2 mm). Microcalcifications are present in 50% to 80% of thyroid carcinoma. Increased vascularity may be noted with color Doppler, with a more disorganized internal flow pattern (Fig. 22.17). Definitive diagnosis would need to be determined by FNA biopsy.

Papillary Carcinoma. The most common of the thyroid malignancies is **papillary carcinoma**, which comprises approximately 70% of all thyroid cancers. It is considered the least aggressive type of tumor, with excellent prognosis if found early and a 20-year survival rate greater than 90%. Females are affected three times more often than males and usually seen between the ages of 20 and 40 years. There is a higher incidence with clinical history of neck or upper chest radiation. The major route of spread of papillary carcinoma is through the lymphatic system to the nearby cervical lymph nodes, with metastatic cervical adenopathy seen in approximately 20% to 50% of patients when diagnosed.

Sonographic Findings. Sonographic characteristics of papillary carcinoma include solid texture with marked hypoechogenicity when compared with strap muscles (reported in 90% of cases). Incomplete halo or ill-defined borders surrounding the nodule, "taller than wide," internal microcalcifications that appear as tiny, punctate hyperechoic foci (less than 2 mm with or without acoustic shadowing), and increased vascularity with color or power Doppler are seen in 90% of cases (Fig. 22.18). Papillary carcinoma may also present as complex cystic in appearance. Ipsilateral cervical lymph node metastasis seen in approximately 20% to 50% of cases (see Fig. 22.16).

Follicular Carcinoma. Follicular carcinoma is the second most common type (10% to 20%) of well-differentiated thyroid cancer. It affects females three times more often than males, is seen between the ages of 40 and 60 years, and is not associated with prior neck and upper chest radiation. There are two types of follicular carcinoma: minimally invasive and widely invasive. The minimally invasive type is well encapsulated, which is best differentiated histologically from benign follicular adenoma by the demonstration of focal invasion of capsular blood vessels of the fibrous

CHAPTER 22 The Thyroid and Parathyroid Glands

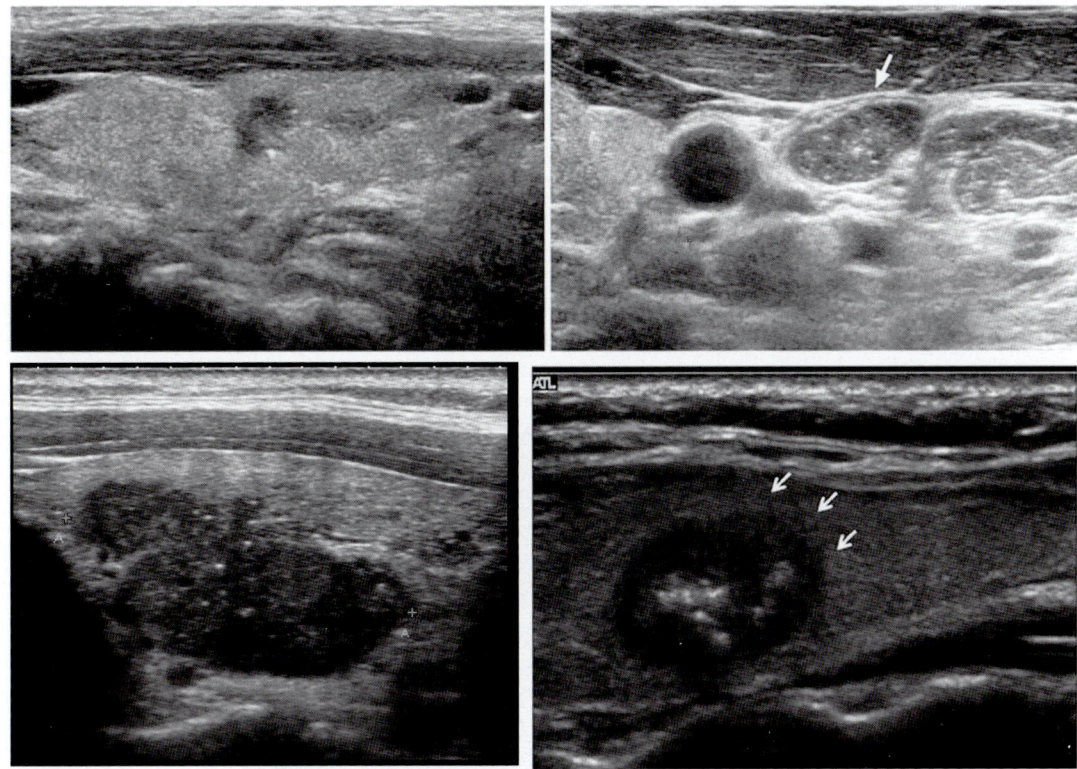

FIG. 22.17 In general, the sonographic characteristic that suggests malignancy is a solitary, solid mass that is markedly hypoechoic compared with strap muscles, with irregular or microlobulated margins that may be taller than wide. In addition, there are often small, punctate internal microcalcifications (<2 mm).

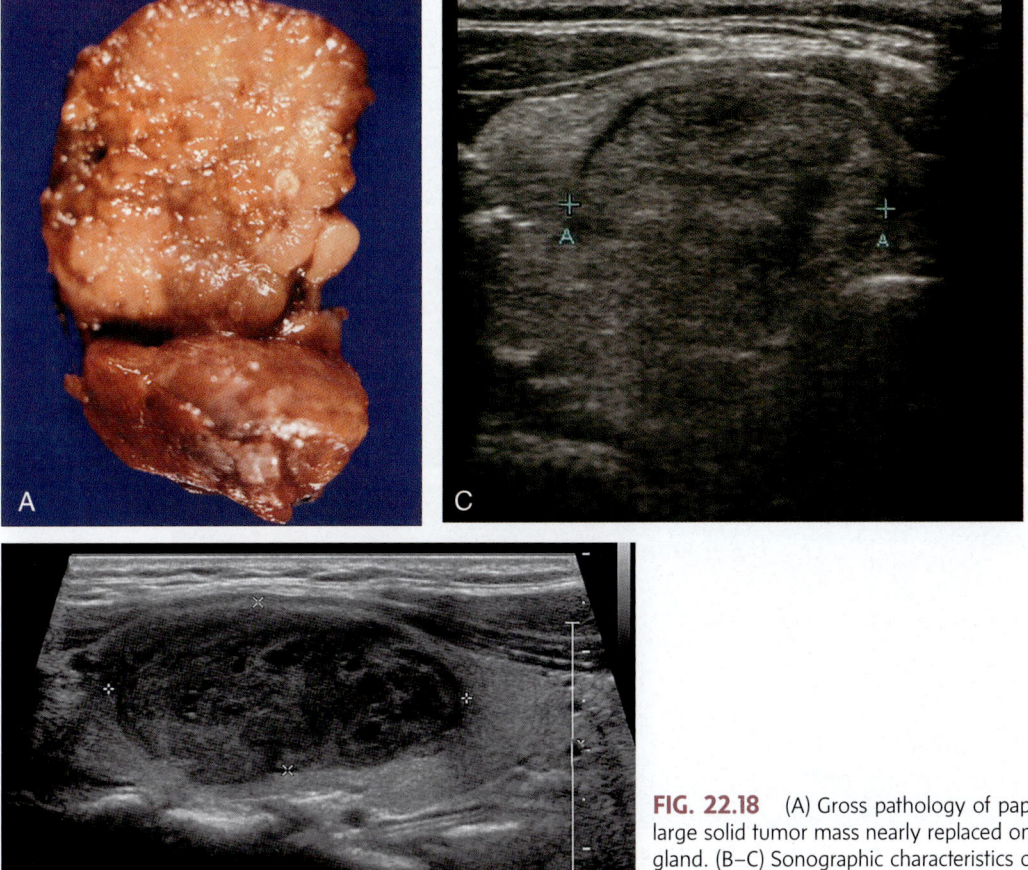

FIG. 22.18 (A) Gross pathology of papillary carcinoma. The large solid tumor mass nearly replaced one lobe of the thyroid gland. (B–C) Sonographic characteristics of papillary carcinoma include solid texture with marked hypoechogenicity when compared with strap muscles.

capsule. The widely invasive type is not encapsulated and will demonstrate invasion of the tumor blood vessels into adjacent thyroid tissue. Follicular carcinoma spreads through the bloodstream rather than by the lymphatic system with metastases to bone, lung, brain, and liver. Lymph node involvement is less common (10%). Follicular carcinoma usually presents as a solitary thyroid mass and may not be differentiated pathologically with FNA biopsy and may require surgical removal of the entire gland to confirm diagnose. It is more aggressive than papillary cancer, with a 20-year mortality rate of approximately 20%.

Sonographic Findings. Sonographic features are similar to benign follicular adenoma, but malignancy should be suspected with presence of thick irregular halo and tortuous internal blood vessels with increased vascularity with color or power Doppler. These findings along with cervical lymphadenopathy are characteristics but not specific for follicular carcinoma (Fig. 22.19).

Medullary Carcinoma. **Medullary carcinoma** accounts for 5% of thyroid cancers. This cancer derives from the parafollicular or C cells of the thyroid that secrete calcitonin. Calcitonin will be elevated and used as a laboratory tumor

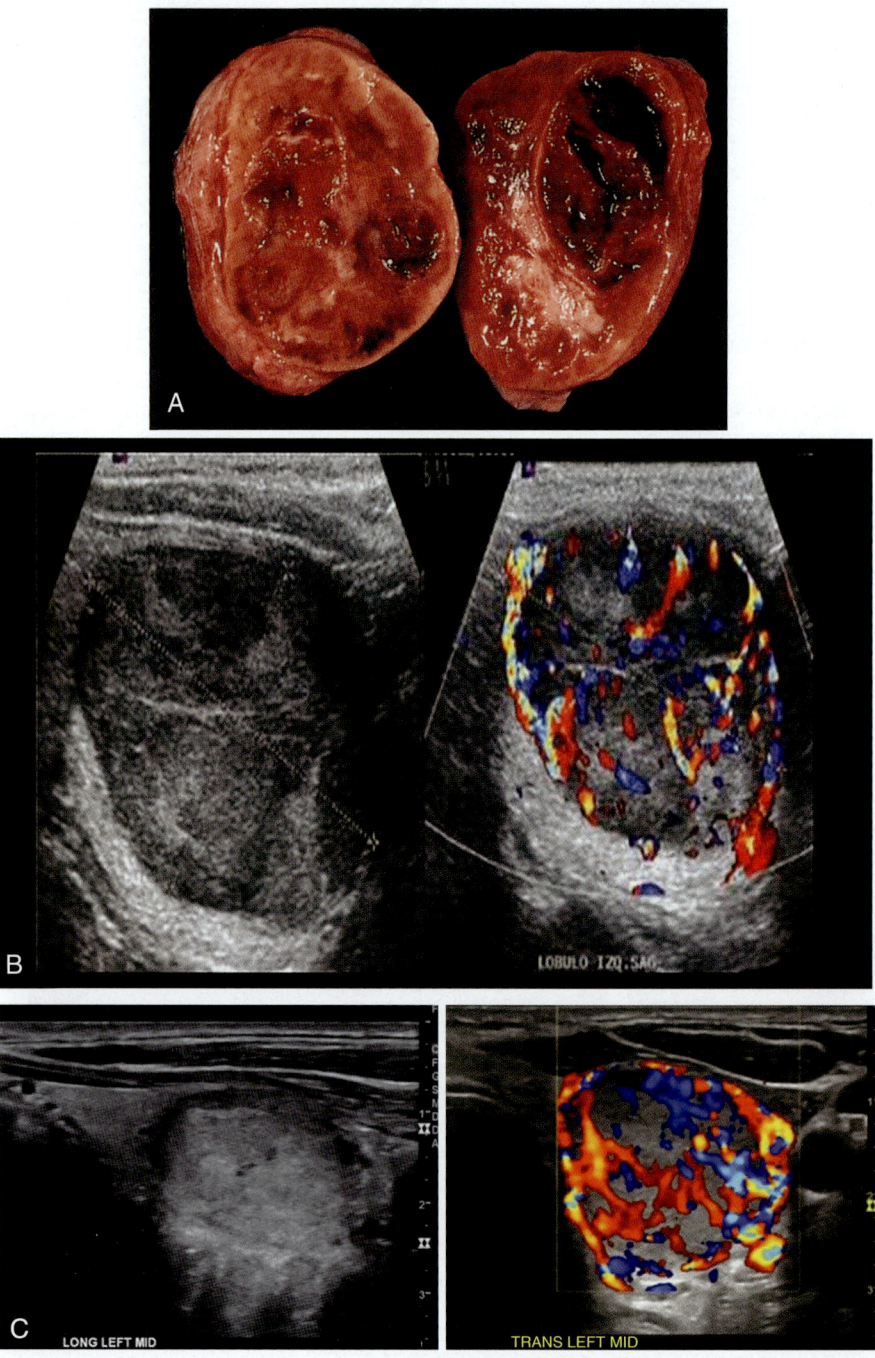

FIG. 22.19 (A) Gross pathology of a follicular carcinoma shows a well-circumscribed tumor. (B–C) Sonographic features are similar to benign follicular adenoma, but malignancy should be suspected with presence of thick irregular halo and tortuous internal blood vessels with increased vascularity with color or power Doppler.

marker. This has only a slightly higher female-to-male ratio of 3:2 and is not associated with prior neck or upper chest radiation exposure.

It may also be familial (20%) and associated with other disorders such as multiple endocrine neoplasia type 2 (MEN 2) syndrome and subtypes. MEN 2 syndrome is a hereditary condition associated with three primary types of endocrine tumors: medullary thyroid cancer, parathyroid tumors, and adrenal medullary tumors. A higher incidence of metastatic involvement of the cervical lymph nodes (80%) and liver metastasis has been reported, yielding a worse prognosis.

Sonographic Findings. Medullary carcinoma will appear sonographically similar to papillary carcinoma as a solid mass that is marked by hypoechogenicity and calcifications (Fig. 22.20). Hypervascularity may also be noted. Careful evaluation of the liver and entire neck area for cervical lymph node metastasis should be completed.

Anaplastic Carcinoma. Anaplastic carcinoma (*anaplastic* means undifferentiated) is rare, accounts for less than 2% of thyroid cancers, and is considered most deadly. It is considered undifferentiated because it may be associated with papillary or follicular carcinomas. It is twice as common in men and usually occurs after age 60 years. It may be seen many years after radiation exposure to the neck or upper chest, with lung metastasis seen in 50% of patients along with 90% cervical lymph node involvement. It is usually diagnosed at stage IV when found, and the 5-year mortality rate is 90% to 95%.

Clinically, the patient presents with a rapidly enlarging, hard, fixed mass and commonly dyspnea, dysphagia, hoarseness, and cough. It grows quickly with local invasion of the surrounding neck structures and widespread metastasis. It usually causes death by compression and asphyxiation due to invasion into the trachea.

Sonographic Findings. Anaplastic thyroid carcinoma presents as a large, hypoechoic mass with encasement and invasion of surrounding structures and vasculature of the neck. Careful evaluation of the liver and entire neck area for cervical lymph node metastasis should be completed (Fig. 22.21). CT and MRI may be more accurate to demonstrate the entire extent of the mass.

Lymphoma. Lymphoma within the thyroid is primarily non-Hodgkin type and accounts for 4% of all thyroid malignancies. It affects older females four times more often

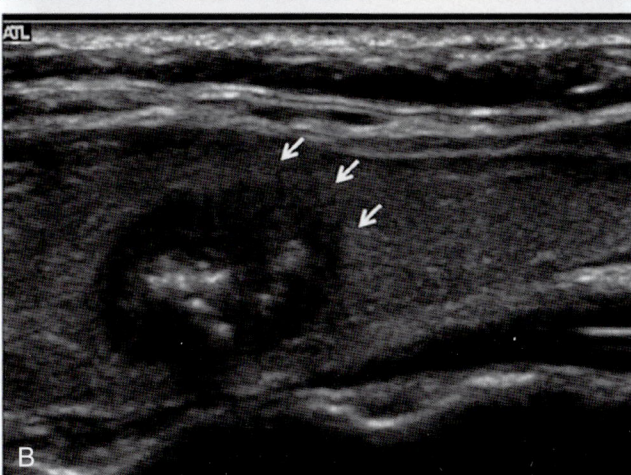

FIG. 22.20 (A) Gross pathology of medullary carcinoma is shown as a well-defined mass in the thyroid gland. (B) Medullary carcinoma will appear sonographically similar to papillary carcinoma as a solid mass that is marked by hypoechogenicity and calcifications.

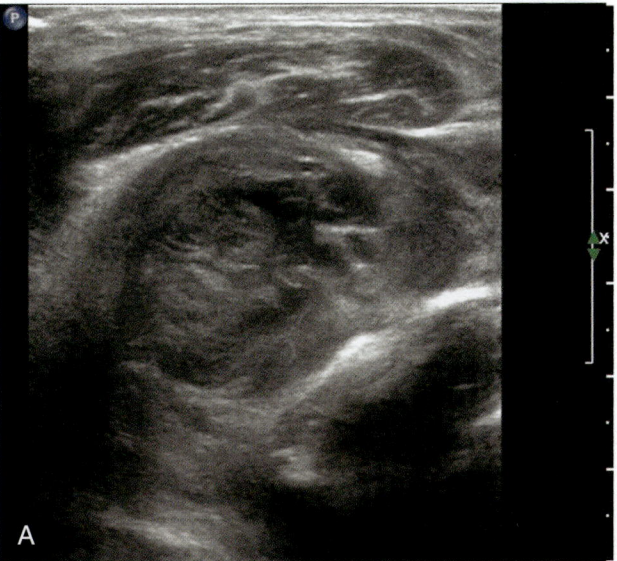
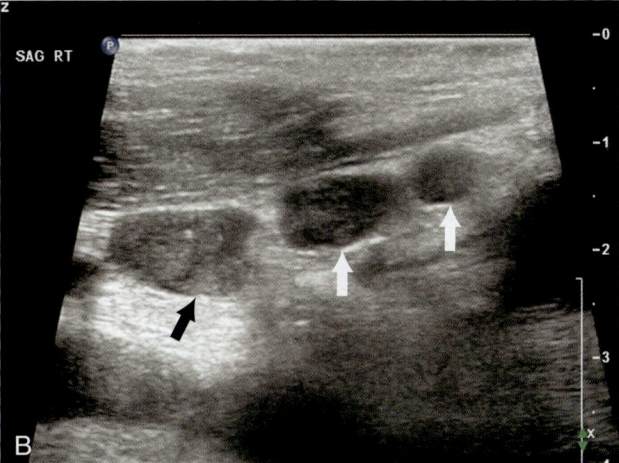

FIG. 22.21 (A) Large solitary lesion representing an anaplastic carcinoma causing enlargement of the thyroid gland. (B) Several enlarged cervical lymph nodes noted with anaplastic carcinoma *(arrows)*.

than men. In many cases, the patient has a preexisting chronic lymphocytic thyroiditis (Hashimoto disease) with subclinical or overt hypothyroidism. Clinically the patient has a rapidly growing neck mass, possibly with partial airway obstruction (dyspnea). Prognosis is good if found in early stages but poor if found in a more advanced stage.

▶ **Sonographic Findings.** Lymphoma is characterized by a large, nonvascular, hypoechoic, and lobulated solid mass (Fig. 22.22). There may be large areas of cystic necrosis within the tumor, along with encasement of adjacent neck vessels. The adjacent thyroid parenchyma may be heterogeneous secondary to associated chronic thyroiditis.

Thyroid Metastasis. The thyroid gland is not a common site for metastasis and usually occurs later in spread of the neoplasm. When found, it is usually from melanoma, breast, or renal cell carcinoma.

▶ **Sonographic Findings.** Metastasis can present as a solitary, well-defined hypoechoic nodule or diffuse gland involvement. There are no distinctive sonographic features, but it should be questioned if there is a known primary carcinoma and a new thyroid mass is sonographically demonstrated.

Elastography. A new sonographic application, elastography, is used to evaluate the tissue stiffness. There are several methods to evaluate the stiffness of normal tissue and solid thyroid lesions, such as strain elastography, acoustic radiation force impulse, and shear wave elastography. Medical studies are being used to investigate and validate whether elastography methods can be used to manage thyroid nodules and limit the number of FNAs. Fig. 22.23 shows elastography images demonstrating soft areas as blue and hard areas as red within the thyroid gland.

Diffuse Thyroid Disease

Several diseases of the thyroid are characterized by diffuse involvement of the gland causing enlargement (goiter) without palpable nodules. Conditions that produce diffuse enlargement of the gland include Graves disease, thyroiditis, and colloid or adenomatous goiter. Specific diagnosis is made on the basis of clinical and laboratory findings and possibly FNA biopsy. Sonography is usually not indicated with a diffusely enlarged gland; however, it may be indicated if a suspected thyroid mass is present.

Graves Disease. Graves disease is an autoimmune disorder and the most common (85%) cause of hyperthyroidism. With Graves disease, the immune system attacks the thyroid gland and causes it to produce thyroid hormones. It occurs five to eight times more frequently in women than men and usually is seen after 30 years of age. Graves disease is characterized by a triad of clinical findings: hypermetabolism, diffuse toxic goiter,

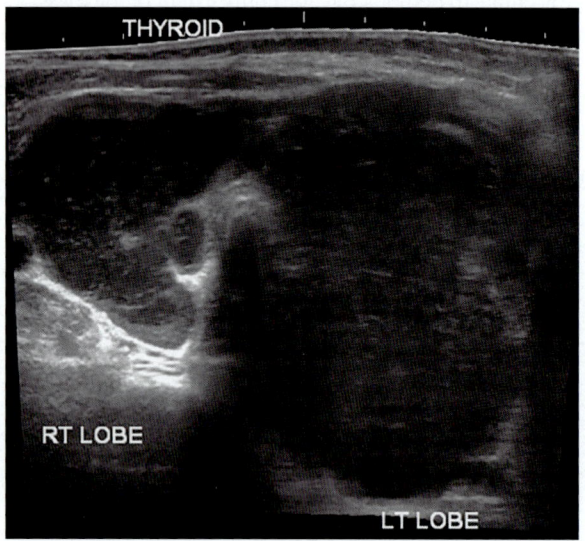

FIG. 22.22 Lymphoma is characterized by a large, nonvascular, hypoechoic, and lobulated solid mass.

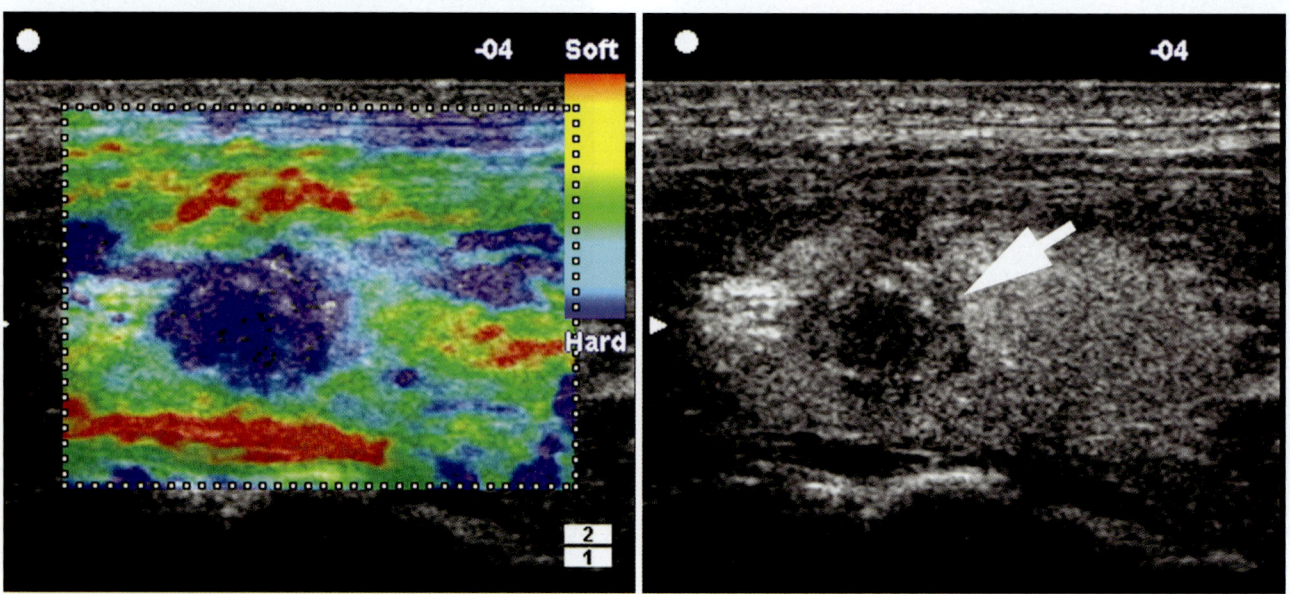

FIG. 22.23 Elastography images that demonstrate soft areas of blue and hard areas of red of nodules within the thyroid gland.

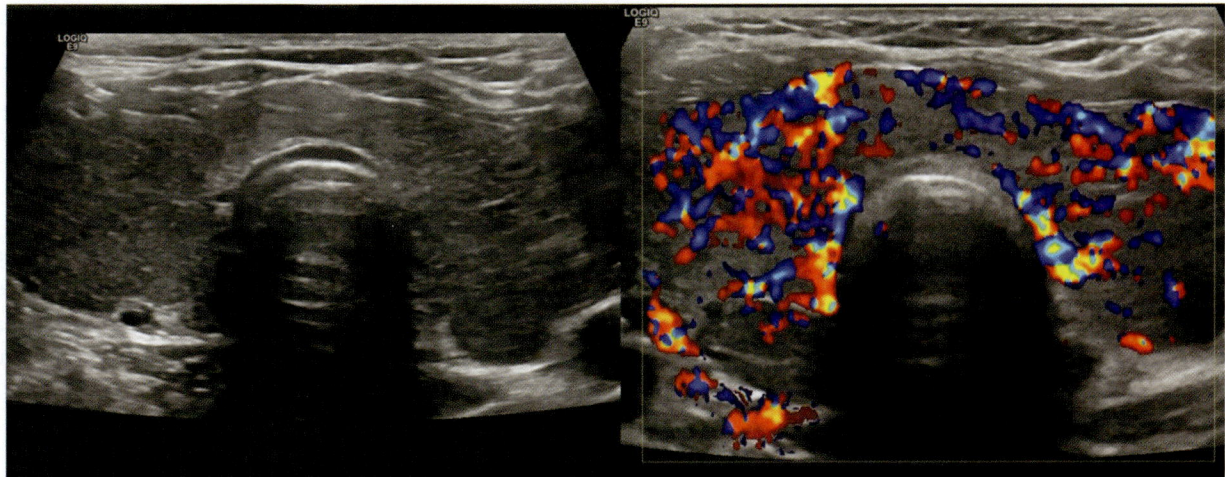

FIG. 22.24 The overactivity of Graves disease often demonstrates increased vascularity on color Doppler imaging, leading to the term *thyroid inferno*.

and exophthalmos (bulging eyes due to inflammatory infiltration of the tissue surrounding the orbit). Exophthalmos is also clinically characterized by the presence of protruding, staring eyes with decreased movement. The patient also presents with an enlarged thyroid associated with diffuse hyperplastic goiter. There may also be thickening of the dermis of the legs (pretibial areas) and dorsum of the feet. Laboratory tests will demonstrate elevated serum T_3 and T_4 but very low TSH.

Uncontrolled acute hyperthyroidism may cause a severe complication of Graves disease called thyrotoxicosis, thyrotoxic crisis, or thyroid storm. It usually occurs after recent infection or surgery and may be life threatening due to resulting hyperthermia, tachycardia, heart failure, and delirium.

Sonographic Findings. Graves disease can demonstrate a normal thyroid gland appearance or present as an enlarged and inhomogeneous gland because of large intraparenchymal vessels. In young patients, the gland may be hypoechoic secondary to extensive lymphocytic infiltration or predominant cellular parenchyma that is devoid of colloid substance. The overactivity of Graves disease often demonstrates increased vascularity on color Doppler imaging, leading to the term *thyroid inferno* (Fig. 22.24). Spectral Doppler may show low resistive flow with peak systolic velocities greater than 70 cm/sec.

Thyroiditis. Thyroiditis is a group of disorders that include inflammation of the thyroid gland with several causes, such as bacteria or viral infections, postpartum, post–radiation ablation technique, drug induced, or related to autoimmune abnormalities. All usually result in hypothyroidism. Types of thyroiditis include acute suppurative thyroiditis, subacute granulomatous thyroiditis (de Quervain disease), and chronic lymphocytic thyroiditis (Hashimoto disease). Clinical findings may vary from mild to severe swelling and tenderness of the thyroid followed later by symptoms of hypothyroidism.

Sonographic Findings. The appearance can change with acute to chronic disease progression. With acute disease the thyroid is hypoechoic, is enlarged, and may have increased color flow visualized. Sonography can be used to determine whether

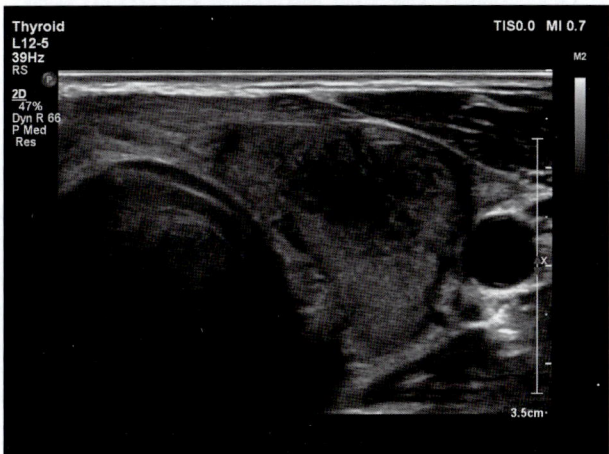

FIG. 22.25 Subacute thyroiditis may demonstrate an enlarged and hypoechoic thyroid with normal or decreased vascularity secondary to diffuse edema of the gland. The process could also present as focal hypoechoic regions within the thyroid gland.

an abscess is present and location. An abscess usually appears as an irregular, ill-defined, hypoechoic, heterogeneous mass with internal debris and possible septation(s) and could have gas present with shadowing. Chronically, the thyroid will become more inhomogeneous and fibrotic with nodular borders.

Subacute (de Quervain) Thyroiditis. Subacute (de Quervain) **thyroiditis** is probably caused by a viral infection of the thyroid, which results in diffuse inflammation of the thyroid with dysphagia, fever, pain, tenderness, enlargement, and malaise. The disease has a gradual or fairly abrupt onset, and the pain may be severe. de Quervain thyroiditis may cause transient hyperthyroidism, but in a period of weeks or a few months, the swelling and pain subside with the gland returning to normal function.

Sonographic Findings. These findings may demonstrate an enlarged and hypoechoic thyroid with normal or decreased vascularity secondary to diffuse edema of the gland. The process could also present as focal hypoechoic regions within the thyroid gland (Fig. 22.25).

Hashimoto thyroiditis. Hashimoto thyroiditis is the most common form of thyroiditis. It is associated with a destructive autoimmune disorder, which leads to chronic inflammation of the thyroid. The outstanding clinical feature is a painless, diffusely enlarged gland seen most often in young or middle-aged women. The entire gland may be involved, with an inflammatory reaction with enlargement that is not necessarily symmetric. Eventually, the gland becomes severely compromised with resultant hypothyroidism. Laboratory tests will demonstrate low serum T_3 and T_4 but elevated TSH levels.

Sonographic Findings. Sonographic findings demonstrate heterogeneous gland enlargement with micronodulation with ill-defined hypoechoic areas (pseudolobules) (Fig. 22.26). Color Doppler shows normal to decreased flow velocity, although occasionally the "thyroid inferno" with high peak systolic velocity is seen when hypothyroidism develops. Adjacent cervical lymphadenopathy may also be demonstrated.

EMBRYOLOGY OF THE PARATHYROID GLAND

The parathyroid glands are derived from endoderm germ cell tissue in the embryo. The parathyroid glands begin as separate paired glands. The superior parathyroid glands develop in the primitive pharyngeal region and migrate inferiorly to the dorsal aspect of the upper to middle portion of the thyroid gland. The paired inferior parathyroid glands develop in the area of the thymus gland and also migrate, but during migration the parathyroid glands should normally lose their connection with the thymus gland and rest at the inferior dorsal aspect of thyroid gland. Normal migration occurs in 60% of patients, with the remaining having ectopic location of parathyroid glands that can extend from the submandibular to the mediastinal region. Other ectopic locations are retrotracheal, intrathyroid, and along the carotid sheath.

ANATOMY OF THE PARATHYROID GLAND

The parathyroid glands are endocrine organs normally located on the posterior surface of the thyroid gland (Fig. 22.27). Most people have four parathyroid glands, but some individuals could have three or five parathyroid glands. The four parathyroid glands are paired and embedded within the fascia surrounding the thyroid gland. Two lie posterior to each superior pole of the thyroid, and the other two lie posterior to the inferior pole.

Normal parathyroid glands are small, flat, and disc shaped with normal size up to $5 \times 3 \times 1$ mm. Due to their small size and position, normal parathyroid glands are commonly not demonstrated sonographically.

PARATHYROID PHYSIOLOGY AND LABORATORY DATA

The parathyroid glands are considered the calcium-sensing organs of the body. Total body calcium is stored in bone in the form of phosphate, with only a smaller portion of calcium in the blood. The parathyroid glands produce **parathyroid hormone (PTH)** to control the serum calcium concentration using a feedback mechanism. When the serum calcium level decreases, the parathyroid glands are stimulated to release PTH. When the serum calcium level increases, the PTH level decreases. Abnormalities are initially suspected clinically when routine laboratory screening demonstrates an elevated serum calcium level (hypercalcemia), elevated urine calcium level (hypercalciuria), and low serum phosphorus levels (hypophosphatemia). It is important to note that elevated serum calcium levels may be associated clinically with other conditions including chronic renal failure and vitamin D deficiency that would also elevate serum calcium (secondary hyperparathyroidism).

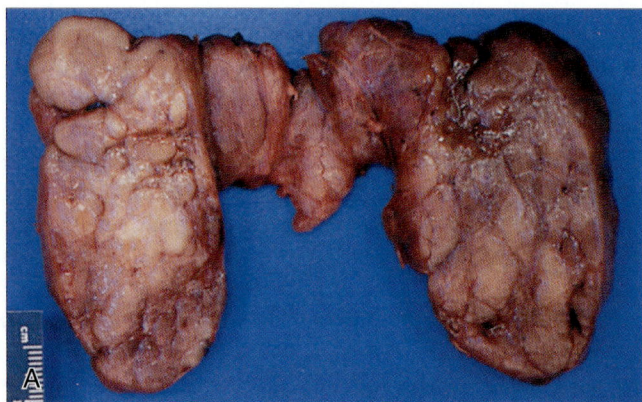
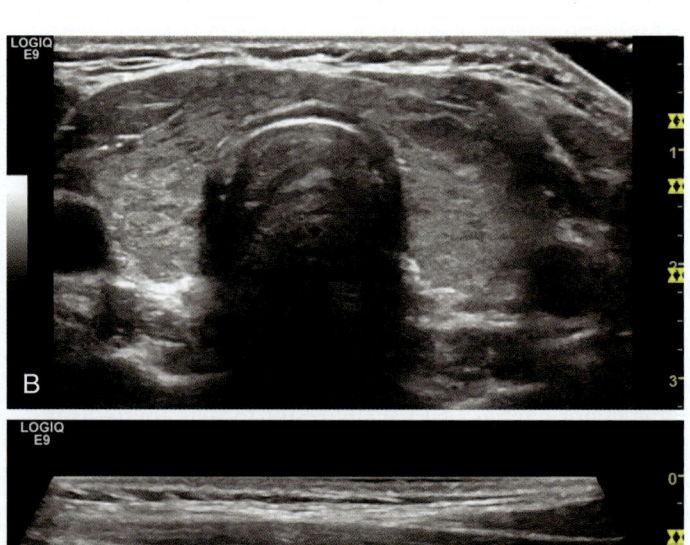

FIG. 22.26 (A) Gross pathology of a patient with Hashimoto thyroiditis. The enlarged gland is multinodular with multiple lymphoid infiltrates. (B) Image of heterogeneous, irregular thyroid gland seen in a patient with Hashimoto thyroiditis. (C) Sagittal image of prominent lymph nodes noted posterior and inferior to the thyroid gland seen with Hashimoto thyroiditis.

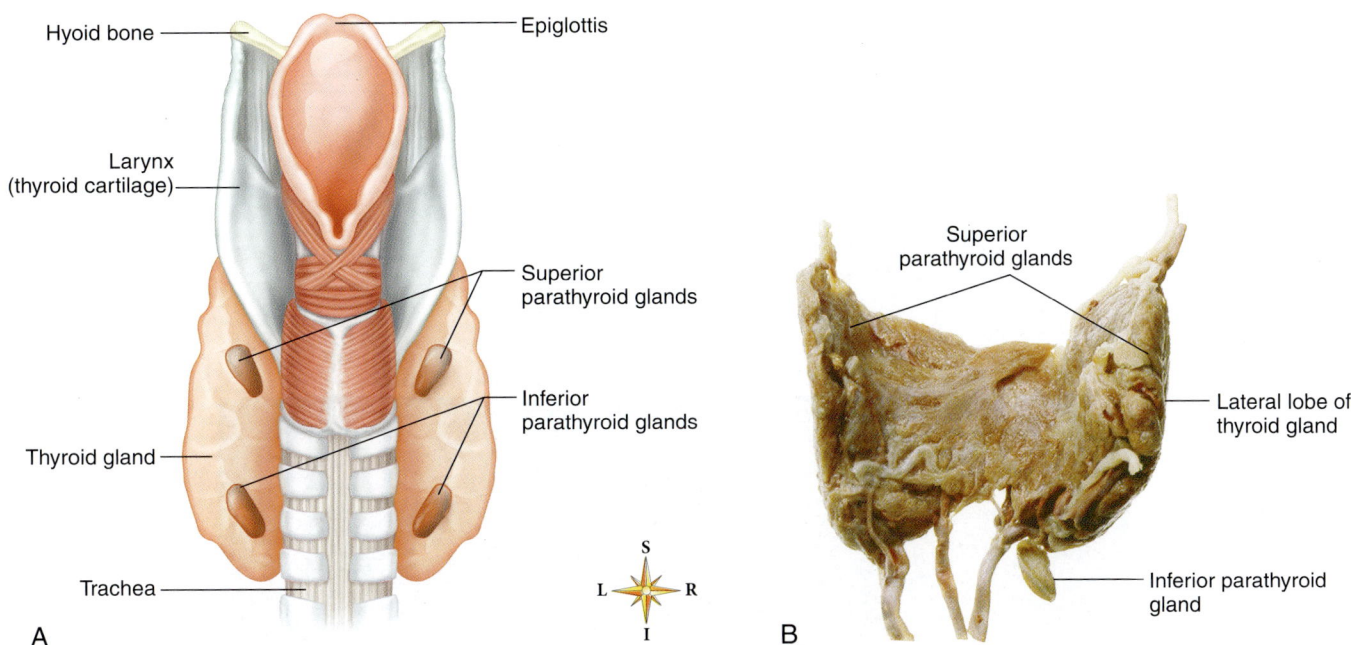

FIG. 22.27 Variations of parathyroid gland locations.

PTH acts on several target organs (skeletal system, kidneys, and intestines) to increase calcium absorption into the blood. The elevated serum calcium levels could be asymptomatic or lead to abdominal and/or musculoskeletal pain. It could also lead to the formation of renal stones (nephrolithiasis), ulcers, pancreatitis, or bone pain related to loss of bone calcium (osteopenia or osteoporosis). There can also be a clinical manifestation that is neurologic with increased depression, nervousness, confusion, and headaches. The primary physician may order a PTH laboratory test to look for abnormal PTH elevation that, along with elevated serum calcium levels, could indicate primary hyperparathyroidism.

Nuclear Medicine Scintigraphy

A nuclear medicine test called a *sestamibi parathyroid scan* is often completed to try to locate abnormally functioning parathyroid gland(s). The patient is given a radiopharmaceutical (Tc-99m sestamibi) and then imaged along with delay scan to note any increased uptake to the parathyroid gland(s). If available, sestamibi parathyroid scan results should be evaluated and correlated with sonography examination findings (Fig. 22.28). One of the advantages of a nuclear medicine examination is to locate increased activity from an ectopic parathyroid gland that cannot be imaged by sonography, especially if it is within the mediastinum.

SONOGRAPHIC EVALUATION OF THE PARATHYROID GLAND

Correct sonographic imaging of parathyroid abnormalities requires use of a high-resolution (7- to 15-MHz) linear array transducer. A thorough clinical history is obtained that includes previous diagnosis of parathyroid disease, kidney stones, ulcer, pancreatitis, and/or osteoporosis. It is also important to determine whether the patient has chronic renal failure or is receiving renal dialysis that could explain abnormal laboratory data (secondary hyperparathyroidism). The referring physician should also provide recent laboratory values on serum calcium and PTH levels. On clinical examination, enlarged parathyroid glands are usually soft and not palpable and have no association with dysphagia.

The examination should always be explained to the patient. The patient is then placed supine with a pillow or pad placed under the shoulders to hyperextend the neck. To investigate all locations for enlarged parathyroid glands and possible ectopic glands, the entire anterior and lateral neck should be surveyed. This should extend superiorly from the submandibular region to inferiorly to the sternal notch in transverse and longitudinal planes and laterally to the internal jugular veins with representative images recorded. Attention should be focused on the areas adjacent to the superior and inferior poles of both thyroid glands. To detect the inferior parathyroid glands, the patient should be asked to swallow to elevate the thyroid gland superiorly during real time scanning. It is important to note that the parathyroid glands will move with the thyroid gland when swallowing because they are located within the same fascia. Due to their small and flat shape and their close proximity to the thyroid, normal parathyroid gland(s) can be a challenge to visualize.

In transverse images, a prominent longus colli muscle located posteriorly to the thyroid may be confused with an enlarged parathyroid gland and should be evaluated with the opposite side for muscle symmetry. In addition,

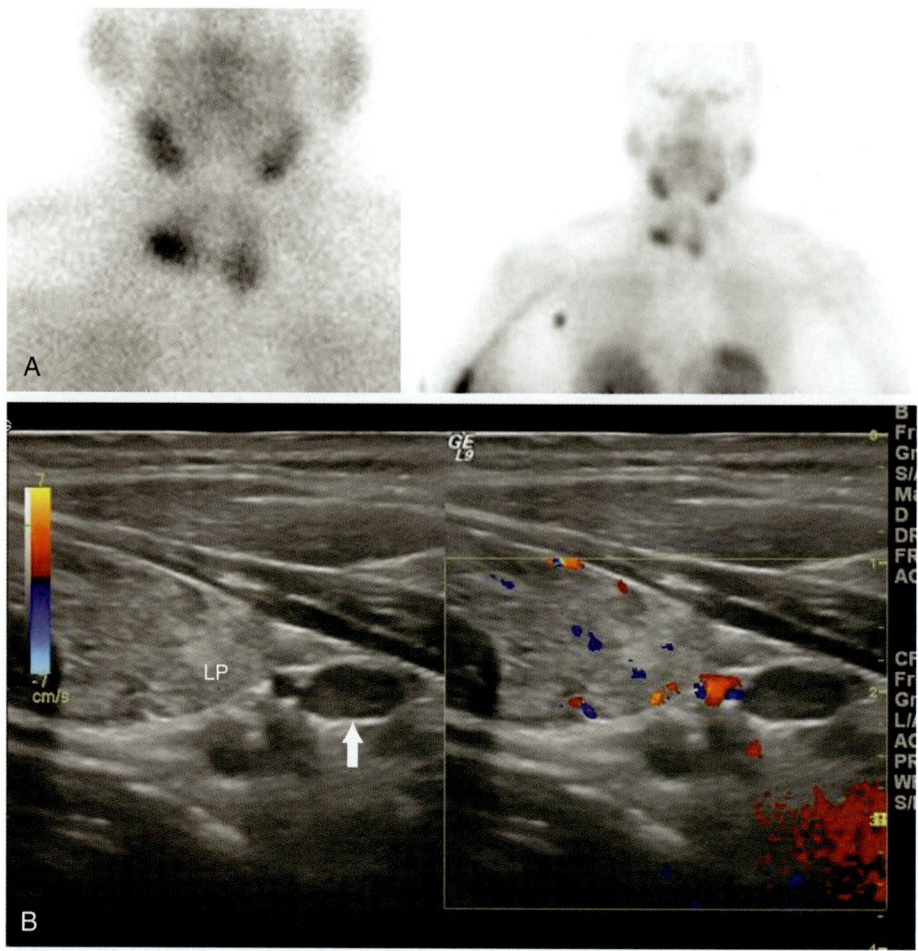

FIG. 22.28 (A) Scintigraphy demonstrating increased uptake associated with parathyroid adenoma. (B) Longitudinal image of a typical parathyroid adenoma with two-dimensional and color Doppler. Parathyroid adenoma *(arrow)*. *LP,* Lower pole of thyroid gland.

longitudinal images will be differentiated when the muscle elongates into the linear muscle appearance. If present, cervical lymph nodes that are located near the thyroid borders can be confused for an enlarged parathyroid gland. This can be differentiated by the demonstration of the echogenic hilum and central flow that is present in the sonographic appearance of normal lymph nodes. In addition, the minor neurovascular bundle, consisting of the inferior thyroid artery and recurrent laryngeal nerve, may be confused for the parathyroid glands. Longitudinal images can often eliminate this confusion by identifying the bundle's tubular appearance along with color or power Doppler demonstration of vascular flow.

PATHOLOGY OF THE PARATHYROID GLAND

Primary Hyperparathyroidism

Primary hyperparathyroidism is an endocrine disorder caused by the increased function of the parathyroid gland. It is more commonly seen after age 40, affecting women two to three times more than men. Primary hyperparathyroidism is characterized by abnormal secretion of PTH, which then signals more calcium to be released into the blood. Laboratory findings include hypercalcemia, hypercalciuria, and elevated PTH levels with hypophosphatemia. Most patients are asymptomatic without manifestation of primary hyperparathyroidism, such as nephrolithiasis, abdominal or musculoskeletal pain, or osteopenia. The role of sonography is to determine whether primary hyperparathyroidism is caused by a parathyroid adenoma (PTA), parathyroid hyperplasia, or, rarely, carcinoma of the parathyroid gland.

Adenoma. A PTA is a benign, solid mass and the most common (80% to 85%) cause of primary hyperparathyroidism. The exact cause is unknown. PTAs are usually oval and solitary but could involve one or more of four parathyroid glands causing enlargement. Because surgical removal is the only definitive treatment, location of an enlarged parathyroid gland within the complex anatomy of the neck will significantly aid the surgeon by indicating the affected side and whether the PTA is demonstrated superior or inferior to thyroid gland.

Sonographic Findings. PTAs are oval, hypoechoic, homogeneous, and usually solid (Fig. 22.29). They can often

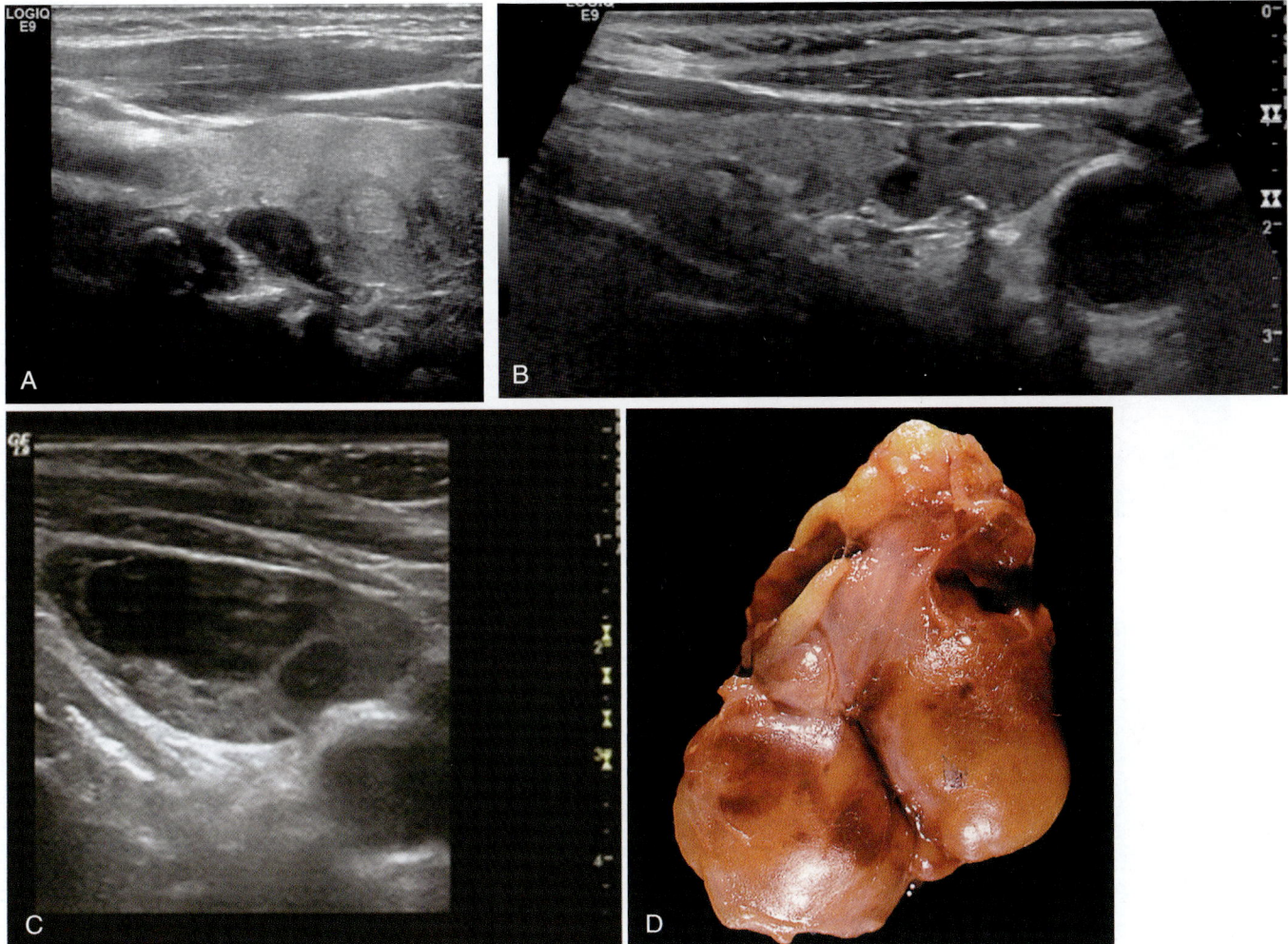

FIG. 22.29 Sonographic variations of parathyroid adenomas. (A) Parathyroid adenoma located along the posterior border of the upper pole of the thyroid. (B) Irregular parathyroid adenoma with calcification and shadowing. (C) Complex cystic parathyroid adenoma inferior to the thyroid gland. (D) Gross pathology of parathyroid adenoma. The gland is enlarged and nodular.

become more oblong, tubelike, or bilobar in shape. Smaller adenomas are usually less than 3 cm in size, with larger adenomas measuring 5 cm or greater in length. Superior PTAs are usually located adjacent to the posterior aspect of the superior to midportion of the thyroid, but inferior PTAs are more variable and could extend inferiorly from the lower pole of the thyroid to the sternal notch. Color and power Doppler may show vascularity to the gland that is usually more peripheral or a peripheral vascular arc pattern. This will help to differentiate from central hilum flow seen in hyperplastic regional lymph nodes. Less commonly, a PTA may have cystic components or calcifications. Pitfalls to be aware of in diagnosing parathyroid enlargement include recognition of normal cervical structures, longus colli muscle, esophagus, and vasculature, which could result in false-positive findings. An inferior PTA may be visualized by having the patient swallow and will demonstrate movement with the thyroid gland to help confirm identification. The parathyroid gland may also be ectopic, making it difficult to locate by sonography. Common locations are mediastinal, retrotracheal, intrathyroidal, and carotid sheath/undescended.

Parathyroid Hyperplasia. Approximately 10% to 15% of patients with primary hyperparathyroidism have parathyroid hyperplasia. **Parathyroid hyperplasia** is defined as enlargement and hyperfunction of the parathyroid gland with no apparent cause. Only one gland may be significantly enlarged, with the remaining glands only mildly affected, or all glands may be enlarged (Fig. 22.30).

Sonographic Findings. Noting enlargement of several glands will help differentiate hyperplasia from multiple PTAs (Fig. 22.31). If adjacent glands become enlarged, it becomes more difficult to separate the enlarged glands with sonography.

Parathyroid Carcinoma. Only 1% of patients with primary hyperparathyroidism have a parathyroid carcinoma. The histologic differentiation of adenoma and carcinoma is very difficult. Metastasis to regional lymph nodes or distant organs or local occurrence must be present for cancer to be diagnosed. Clinically, most parathyroid cancers are small and irregular but, as they enlarge, will become firm or hard masses and adhere to or invade surrounding structures.

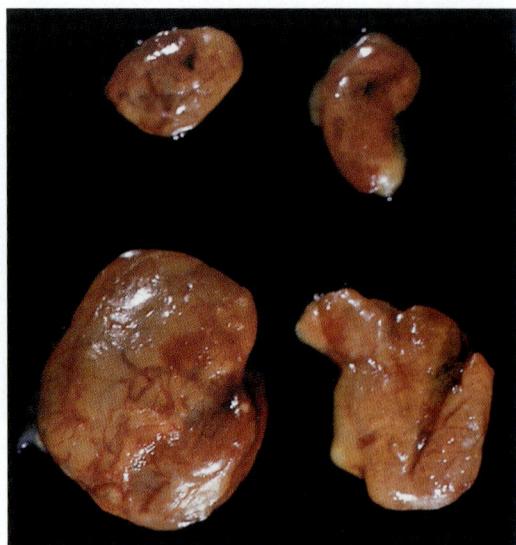

FIG. 22.30 Gross pathology of parathyroid hyperplasia with enlargement of all four parathyroid glands.

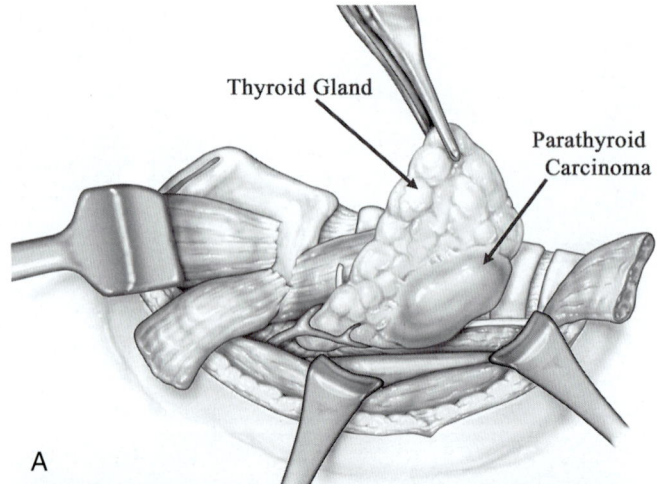

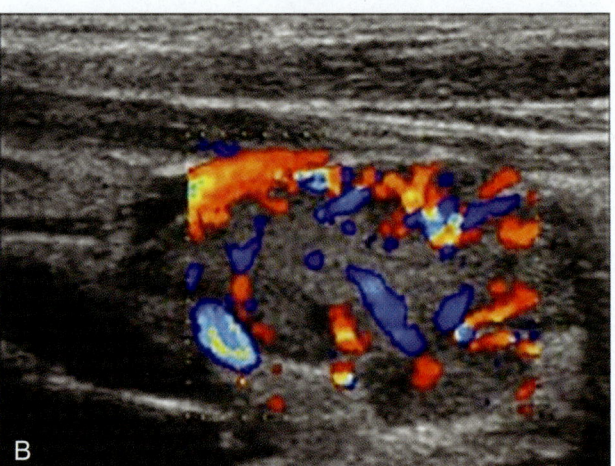

FIG. 22.32 (A) The sonographic appearance of parathyroid cancer is usually larger, more irregular in shape, or with a lobulated contour. (B) Note the prominent internal vascularity of the carcinoma.

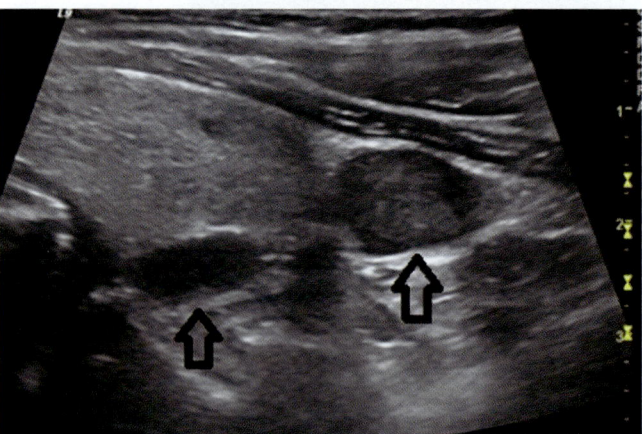

FIG. 22.31 Sonographic images that demonstrate enlargement of two parathyroid glands *(arrows)* in the lower pole of the thyroid.

It is seen equally in males and females. Laboratory findings of parathyroid cancer will usually demonstrate very high serum calcium levels.

Sonographic Findings. The sonographic appearance of parathyroid cancer is usually larger, more irregular in shape, or with a lobulated contour (Fig. 22.32). Gland orientation may be taller than wide, more heterogeneous, with increased vascularity or internal cystic components. Because a large adenoma may have some of these same sonographic findings, the diagnosis of malignancy may not be made until surgical removal. Metastases to regional nodes or distant organs, capsular invasion, and local recurrence are more reliable to diagnose parathyroid cancer by sonography.

Secondary Hyperparathyroidism

Secondary hyperparathyroidism occurs when the serum PTH level is increased due to chronic hypocalcemia. Increased PTH level is not caused by a dysfunction of the parathyroid gland but is stimulated by a compensatory reaction by the hypocalcemia usually from chronic renal failure, vitamin D deficiency or rickets, or intestinal malabsorption syndromes. Laboratory findings will demonstrate elevated PTH levels with low calcium levels. Secondary hyperparathyroidism may demonstrate enlargement of all four parathyroid glands.

MISCELLANEOUS NECK MASSES

When a palpable neck mass is present, the role of sonography is to determine the origin of the mass by demonstration of the location, sonographic characteristics, and vascularity of the mass.

Developmental Cysts

Thyroglossal Duct Cyst. The most common congenital cystic anomaly is **thyroglossal duct cyst**, which is usually located (70%) in the midline of the neck anterior to the trachea or within 2 cm of the midline. During embryology, a narrow, hollow tract connects the thyroid lobes to the flow of the pharynx between the base of the tongue, at or below the level of the hyoid bone. This tract should atrophy with age. If the tract persists, it creates a potential space for fluid to collect into a cystic mass anywhere along the tract from above to below the level of the hyoid bone. It is usually seen in the pediatric population, with 90% found before age 10 years.

Sonographic Findings. The thyroglossal duct cyst may have the same sonographic characteristics of a cyst, often oval or spherical in shape and located in the midline. The cyst may often be more complex in appearance and rarely larger than 2 or 3 cm (Fig. 22.33).

Branchial Cleft Cyst. Branchial cleft cyst is a congenital cystic mass that is located in the lateral portion of the neck. It may vary in location but usually is found laterally in the submandibular region. During embryonic development, the branchial cleft is a slender tract extending from the pharyngeal cavity to an opening near the auricle or into the neck. A diverticulum may extend laterally from the pharynx or medially from the neck and fill with fluid causing a cyst formation. It is usually single, but 2% to 3% are bilateral, and it is found more often in older children or young adults.

Sonographic Findings. The branchial cleft cyst appearance can vary; although primarily cystic, it may present as complex or solid components with low-level echoes, particularly if it has become infected (Fig. 22.34).

Abscess. An **abscess** can arise in any location of the neck and can have acute onset and progress quickly. Common clinical presentation of neck abscess is pain, erythema, edema, and fever, with a palpable mass. Sonography is also used to discern the nature of the palpable mass and involvement of adjacent anatomy. Sonography may also be used to guide for percutaneous needle aspiration and imaging after surgical or medical treatment.

Sonographic Findings. An abscess can range in its sonographic appearance from primarily fluid filled to completely echogenic. Most commonly, an abscess will appear as a complex cystic mass with low-level echogenicity and irregular walls (Fig. 22.35). Presence of air within and

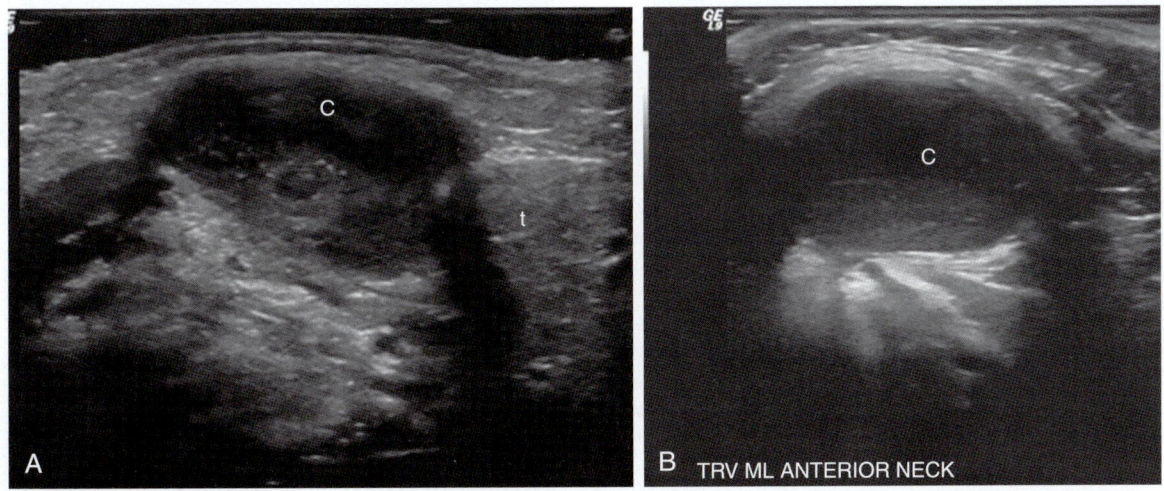

FIG. 22.33 (A) Sagittal image of a thyroglossal duct cyst (C) located in the midline superior to the thyroid gland (t). (B) Transverse image superior to the thyroid gland demonstrating a thyroglossal duct cyst in the midline.

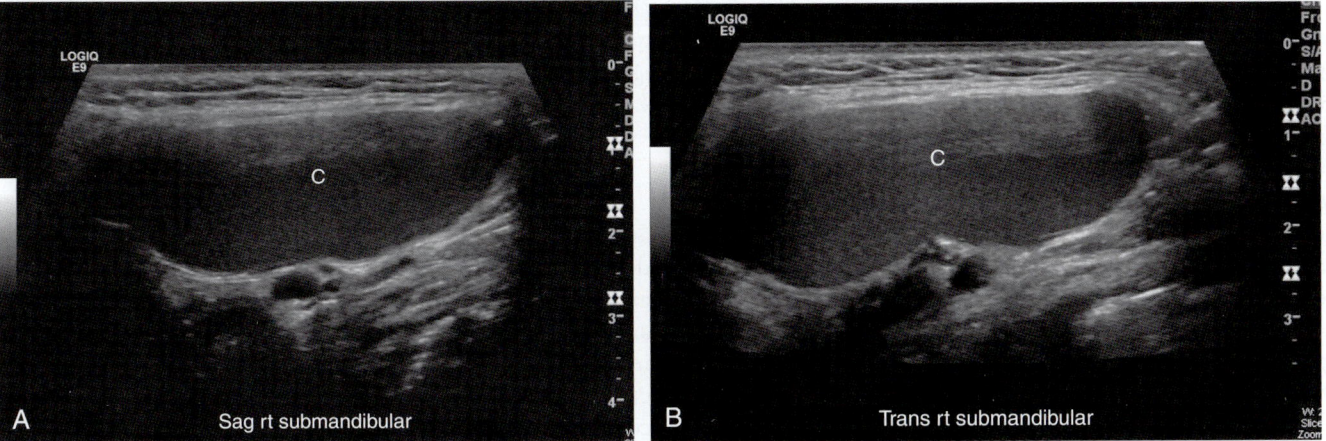

FIG. 22.34 (A) Longitudinal image at the angle of the mandible demonstrating a branchial cleft cyst (C) located inferior to the angle of the mandible. (B) Transverse image of the branchial cleft cyst.

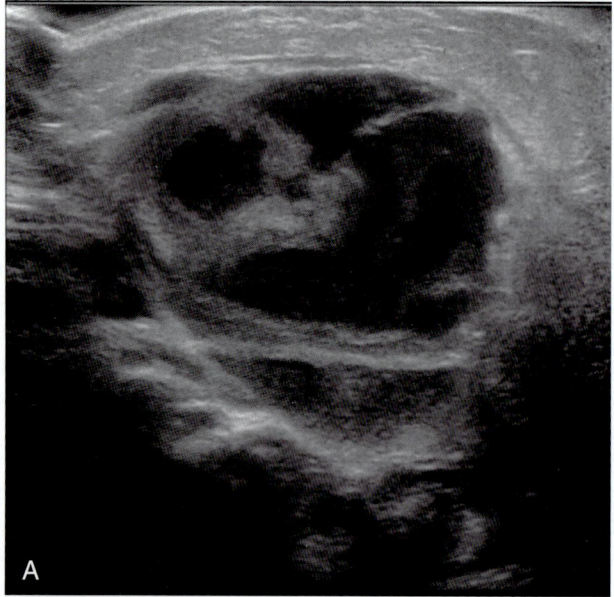
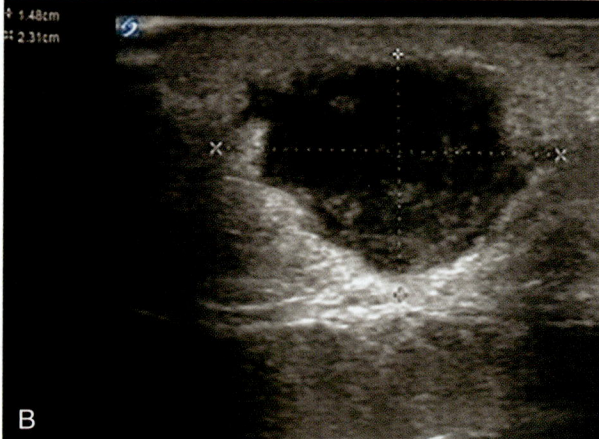

FIG. 22.35 An abscess can range in its sonographic appearance from primarily fluid filled to completely echogenic. Most commonly, an abscess will appear as a complex cystic mass with low-level echogenicity and irregular walls.

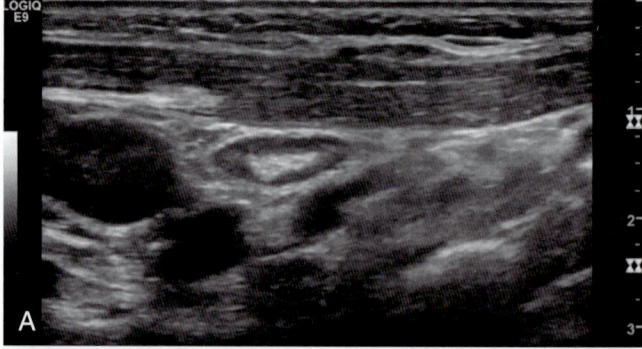
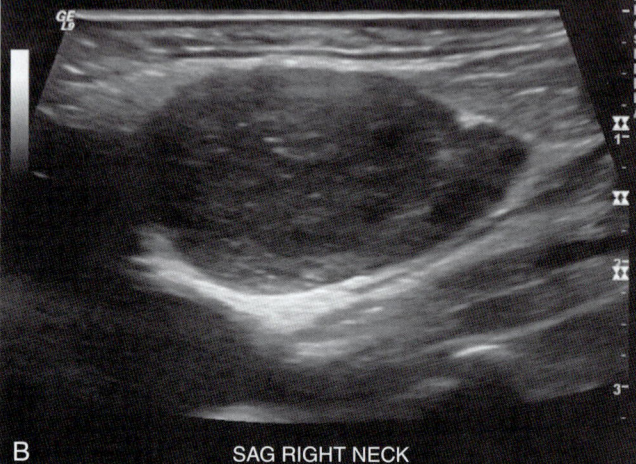
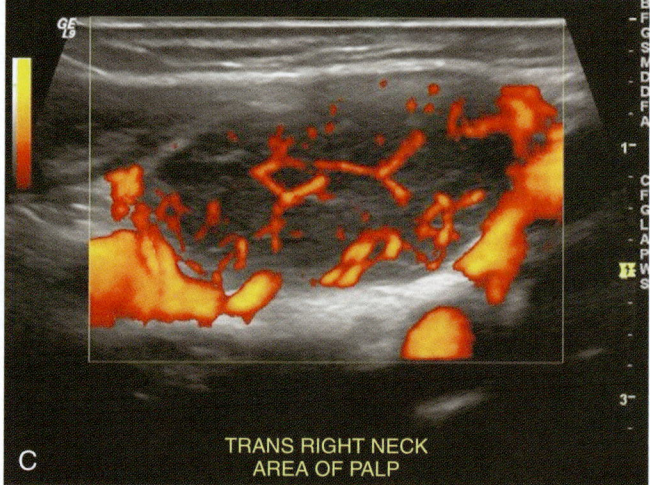

FIG. 22.36 (A) Normal cervical lymph node with echogenic hilum. (B) Enlarged, hypoechoic, lobulated abnormal lymph node. (C) Increased vascularity noted within an enlarged lymph node with power Doppler.

ring-down artifact or shadowing will confirm the suspected etiology of the mass as an abscess. Chronic abscesses may be particularly difficult to demonstrate because there are usually indistinct margins and they are more isoechoic with the surrounding neck anatomy.

Cervical Lymphadenopathy. *Lymphadenopathy* is a localized or generalized enlargement of the lymph nodes. A lymph node can become prominent due to reactive hyperplasia but could be enlarged due to neoplasm, metastasis, or an inflammatory process. Sonography can be an important imaging modality to assist tumor staging and careful evaluation of the neck regions for cervical lymphadenopathy with postthyroidectomy patients.

Sonographic Findings (Normal Lymph Node). Sonographic appearance of a normal lymph node is oval in shape with a symmetric, homogeneous, thin outer cortex, and an echogenic central hilum. Size typically does not exceed 1 cm (Fig. 22.36A). Color or power Doppler settings should be lowered to demonstrate flow entering the hilum.

Sonographic Findings (Lymphadenopathy). Appearance may vary, but cervical lymphadenopathy will usually demonstrate a more rounded shape or more lobulated shape and loss of the echogenic hilum. The cortex may be thickened and symmetric or show localized asymmetry with lobulated or irregular boarders. Color may also demonstrate increased vascularity or avascularity to lymph node (see Fig. 22.36B–C). Less commonly, lymphadenopathy may present with calcification(s) and a more complex cystic appearance from necrosis. Presence of multiple enlarged nodes is abnormal. Differentiation between inflammation, neoplasm, or metastatic processes is confirmed with FNA biopsy.

Postthyroidectomy Neck Sonography. Sonography plays an important role in the evaluation and management of patients after total thyroidectomy for thyroid cancer. A detailed scanning technique is being requested more often by endocrinologists and surgeons to detect potential regional recurrences or metastases. The sonographer will carefully evaluate and image the neck region to map the level and compartment of any enlarged lymph nodes. Sonography can also be invaluable as guidance for FNA of suspicious lymph nodes.

ACKNOWLEDGMENT

I acknowledge Janette Wybo for her contribution to this chapter in the previous edition.

Key Pearls

- Sonography is an excellent modality when clinically indicated for high-resolution evaluation of the thyroid gland for gland size, shape, location, and parenchyma echogenicity.
- Sonography can visualize the nature of palpable nodules as simple cyst, complex cystic, or solid and document associated calcifications.
- Thyroid pathology that includes inflammatory processes and benign and malignant conditions can be demonstrated by sonography but cannot be reliably differentiated.
- Sonographic characteristics that are suspicious for malignant thyroid nodule are a solid mass that is markedly hypoechoic with irregular margins that may be taller than wide. Visualization of microcalcifications and increased vascularity may be noted with color Doppler with a more disorganized internal flow pattern.
- Interventional procedures often use sonographic guidance for FNA of thyroid nodules.
- The parathyroid gland is often not visualized by high-resolution sonography unless enlarged, most often due to the presence of parathyroid adenoma, hyperplasia, or carcinoma of gland.
- Sonography can play an important role for the surgeon to locate enlarged parathyroid gland(s) before surgical removal of the abnormal gland(s).

BIBLIOGRAPHY

Barreda R, Kaude JV, Fagein M, et al. Hypervascularity of non-toxic goiter as shown by color-coded Doppler sonography. *Am J Roentgenol.* 1991;156:199.

Brant W, Helms C. *Fundamentals of diagnostic radiology.* 4th ed. Philadelphia: Lippincott Williams & Wilkins; 2012.

Brkljacic B, Cuk V, Tomic-Brzak H, et al. Ultrasonic evaluation of benign and malignant nodules in echographically multinodular thyroids. *J Clin Ultrasound.* 1994;22:71.

Chang DG, Yang PC, Yu CJ, et al. Differentiation of benign and malignant cervical lymph nodes with color Doppler sonography. *Am J Roentgenol.* 1994;162:956–960.

Clark KJ, Cronan JJ, Scola FH. Color Doppler sonography: anatomic and physiologic assessment of the thyroid. *J Clin Ultrasound.* 1995;23:215–223.

Esseig G, Meyers A: Parathyroid physiology. http://emedicine.medscape.com/article/874690.

Gladziwa U, Ittel TH, Dakshinamurty KV, et al. Secondary hyperparathyroidism and sonographic evaluation of parathyroid gland hyperplasia in dialysis patients. *Clin Nephrol.* 1992;38:162.

Goldberg B, McGahan J. *Atlas of ultrasound measurements.* 2nd ed. St. Louis: Elsevier; 2006.

Hennemann G. Non-Toxic Goiter. *Clin Endocrinol Metab.* 1999;8:167.

Holmes EC, Morton DL, Ketcham AS. Parathyroid carcinoma: a collective review. *Ann Surg.* 1999;169:631.

Kerr L. High-resolution thyroid ultrasound: the value of color Doppler. *Ultrasound Q.* 1994;12:21.

Kohri K, Ishikawa Y, Kodama M, et al. Comparison of imaging methods for localization of parathyroid tumors. *Am J Surg.* 1992;164:140–145.

Kuntz KM. Neck mass. In: Henningsen C, ed. *Clinical guide to ultrasonography.* St. Louis: Mosby; 2004.

Meola M, Barsotti M, Lenti C, et al. Color-Doppler in the imaging work-up of primary hyperparathyroidism. *J Nephrol.* 1999;12:270.

Montazemi M. There is a mass in the neck (presentation). Society of Diagnostic Medical Sonography, 2012.

Rosai J. *Rosai and Ackerman's surgical pathology.* 9th ed. St. Louis: Mosby; 2004.

Rumack C, Wilson S, Charboneua JW, et al. *Diagnostic ultrasound.* 4th ed. Elsevier; 2011.

Sargis R: Thyroid gland overview: a major player in regulating your metabolism. Available at www.endocrineweb.com.

Takashima S, Morimoto S, Ikezoe J, et al. Primary thyroid lymphoma: comparison of CT and US assessment. *Radiology.* 1995;171:439.

Thibodeau G, Patton K. *Structure and function of the body.* 14th ed. St. Louis: Elsevier; 2012.

CHAPTER 23

Scrotum

Cindy A. Owen

OBJECTIVES

On completion of this chapter, you should be able to:
- Identify the normal anatomy of the scrotum
- Explain the vascular supply to the scrotal contents
- Describe patient positioning, scanning protocol, and technical considerations for an ultrasound examination of the scrotum
- Discuss the role of color and spectral Doppler in scrotal imaging
- Describe the ultrasound characteristics of scrotal pathology

OUTLINE

Anatomy of the Scrotum 709
   Vascular Supply 710
   Patient Positioning and Scanning Protocol 712
Technical Considerations 713
Scrotal Pathology 717
   Acute Scrotum 717
   Extratesticular Masses 722
   Varicocele 722
   Scrotal Hernia 723
   Hydrocele, Pyocele, and Hematocele 725
   Sperm Granuloma 726
   Benign Testicular Masses 726
   Malignant Testicular Masses 728
   Lymphoma and Leukemia 730
   Congenital Anomalies 730

KEY TERMS

Centripetal arteries
Cremasteric artery
Cremasteric muscle
Cryptorchidism
Deferential artery
Ejaculatory duct
Epididymal cysts
Epididymis
Epididymitis
Hematocele
Hydrocele
Mediastinum testis
Pampiniform plexus
Pudendal artery
Pyocele
Recurrent rami
Rete testis
Scrotum
Seminal vesicles
Septa testis
Spermatic cord
Spermatoceles
Testicle
Testicular arteries
Testicular vein
Tunica albuginea
Tunica vaginalis
Urethra
Varicocele
Vas deferens
Verumontanum

Ultrasound is the imaging modality of choice for evaluating the scrotum. High-frequency ultrasound imaging, combined with color and spectral Doppler, quickly and reliably provides valuable information in the assessment of scrotal pain or mass. In particular, color Doppler has a central role in the evaluation of suspected testicular torsion because it can demonstrate absence of flow in the affected testis. Color Doppler also plays a key role in the evaluation of testicular infection by demonstrating hyperemic flow on the affected side. Ultrasound imaging accurately differentiates intratesticular from extratesticular masses and cystic from solid masses. Advances in the development of ultrasound equipment have provided improved spatial and contrast resolution, reduced speckle artifact, and increased sensitivity to the display of scrotal perfusion. The steady progress in ultrasound image quality has enhanced our ability to clearly define the scrotal anatomy and to depict and differentiate abnormalities more accurately. This chapter covers the pertinent anatomy of the scrotum and its contents, including the vascular supply. The ultrasound scanning protocol is discussed, along with tips on scanning techniques and potential pitfalls. A review of the disease processes affecting the scrotum is provided, including a description of sonographic findings.

ANATOMY OF THE SCROTUM

The testes are symmetric, oval-shaped glands residing in the **scrotum**. In adults, the testis measures approximately 3 to 5 cm in length, 2 to 4 cm in width, and approximately 3 cm in height. Each testis is divided into more than 250 to 400 conical lobules containing the seminiferous tubules. These tubules converge at the apex of each lobule and anastomose to form the **rete testis** in the mediastinum. The rete testis drains into the head of the epididymis through the efferent ductules (Fig. 23.1). Sonographically, the testes appear as smooth, medium-gray structures with a fine echotexture.

The epididymis is a 6- to 7-cm tubular structure beginning superiorly and then coursing posterolateral to the testis. It is divided into head, body, and tail. The head is the largest part of the epididymis, measuring 6 to 15 mm in width. It is located superior to the upper pole of the testis (Fig. 23.2). It contains 10 to 15 efferent ductules from the rete testis, which converge to form a single duct in the body and tail. This duct is known as the ductus epididymis. It becomes the vas deferens and continues in the spermatic cord. The body of the epididymis is much smaller than the head. It is difficult to see with ultrasound on normal individuals. It follows the posterolateral aspect of the testis from the upper to the lower pole. The tail of the epididymis is slightly larger and is positioned posterior to the lower pole of the testis. The appendix of the epididymis is a small protuberance from the head of the epididymis. Postmortem studies have shown the appendix epididymis in 34% of testes unilaterally and 12% of testes bilaterally. The normal epididymis usually appears as isoechoic or hypoechoic compared with the testis, although the echotexture is coarser.

At the upper pole of the testis, the appendix testis is attached. It is located between the testis and the epididymis. Postmortem studies have shown the appendix testis to be present in 92% of testes unilaterally and 69% bilaterally (Fig. 23.3).

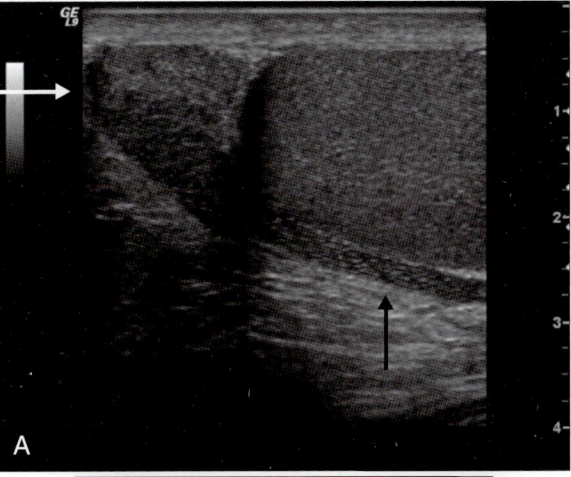

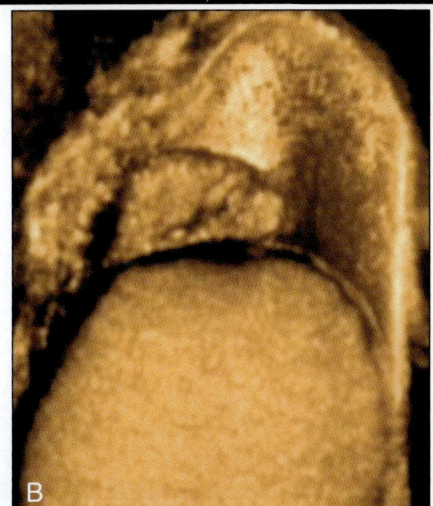

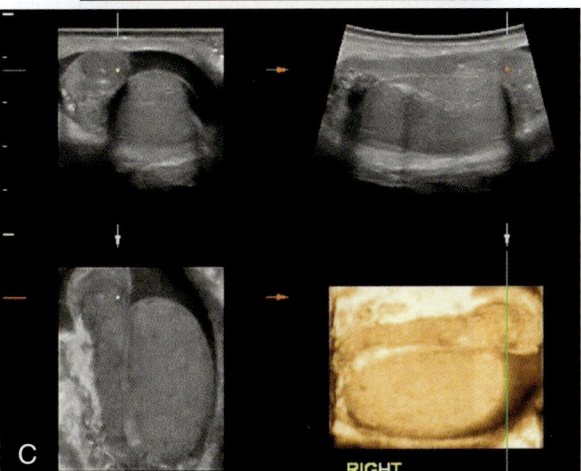

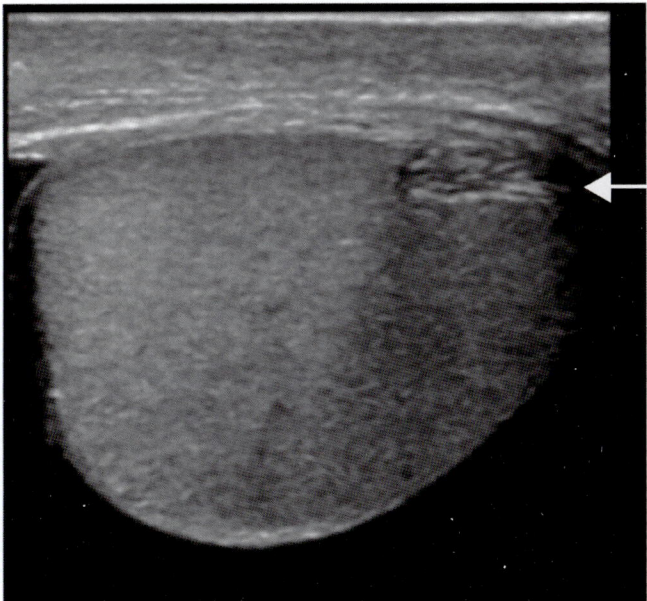

FIG. 23.1 **Transverse ultrasound scan of the normal rete testis.** With the use of high-resolution imaging and transducer frequencies of 10 MHz or greater, the normal rete testis can sometimes be depicted with ultrasound. It appears as tiny tubules adjacent to the epididymal head and the testis mediastinum *(arrow)*.

FIG. 23.2 (A) Sagittal ultrasound scan of a normal epididymis and testis. The head of the epididymis is seen superior to the upper pole of the testis *(white arrow)*. The body of the epididymis is seen posterior to the testis *(black arrow)*. Note the coarse echotexture of the epididymis compared with the fine texture of the testis. (B) Three-dimensional (3D) view rendered in the coronal plane demonstrates the relationship of the normal epididymal head to the superior pole of the testis. (C) 3D view shows orthogonal planes of enlarged epididymis in patients with epididymitis. An axis point *(small white dot)* is placed on the epididymal head to demonstrate the same point in three orthogonal views. The 3D data set allows manipulation of the volume in an infinite number of imaging planes. This allows the sonographer to adjust the display so that the entire length of the epididymis can be demonstrated.

The testis is completely covered by a dense, fibrous tissue termed the **tunica albuginea**. The posterior aspect of the tunica albuginea reflects into the testis to form a vertical septum known as the **mediastinum testis**. Multiple septa (**septa testis**) are formed from the tunica albuginea at the mediastinum. They course through the testis and separate it into lobules. The mediastinum supports the vessels and ducts coursing within the testis. The mediastinum is often seen on ultrasound as a bright hyperechoic line coursing craniocaudal within the testis (Fig. 23.4). The **tunica vaginalis** lines the inner walls of the scrotum, covering each testis and epididymis. It consists of two layers: parietal and visceral. The parietal layer is the inner lining of the scrotal wall. The visceral layer surrounds the testis and epididymis. A small bare area is posterior. At this site, the testicle is against the scrotal wall, preventing torsion.

Blood vessels, lymphatics, nerves, and spermatic ducts travel through the area (see Fig. 23.1). The space between the layers of the tunica vaginalis is where hydroceles form. It is normal to see a small amount of fluid in this space.

The **vas deferens** is a continuation of the ductus epididymis. It is thicker and less convoluted. The vas deferens dilates at the terminal portion near the **seminal vesicles**. This portion is termed the *ampulla* of the deferens. The vas deferens joins the duct of the seminal vesicles to form the **ejaculatory duct**, which, in turn, empties into the **urethra**. The junction of the ejaculatory ducts with the urethra is termed the **verumontanum**. The urethra courses from the bladder to the end of the penis. In men, the urethra transports both urine and semen outside the body.

The vas deferens, testicular arteries, venous pampiniform plexus, lymphatics, autonomic nerves, and fiber of the cremaster form the **spermatic cord**. The cord extends from the scrotum through the inguinal canal and internal inguinal rings to the pelvis. The spermatic cord suspends the testis in the scrotum.

Vascular Supply

Right and left **testicular arteries** arise from the abdominal aorta just below the level of the renal arteries. They are the primary source of blood flow to the testis. The testicular arteries descend in the retroperitoneum and enter the spermatic cord in the deep inguinal ring. Then they course along the posterior surface of each testis and pierce the tunica albuginea, forming the capsular arteries, which branch over the surface of the testis. With high-frequency ultrasound imaging, the capsular artery is sometimes seen as a hypoechoic linear structure on the surface of the testis. Color Doppler can be used to confirm its identity (Fig. 23.5). The capsular arteries give rise to **centripetal arteries**, which course from the testicular surface toward the mediastinum along the septa. Before

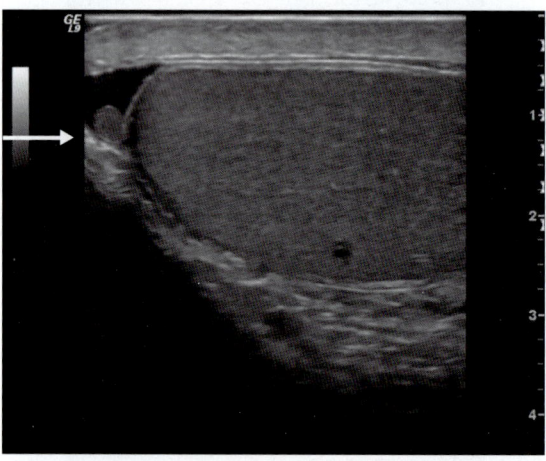

FIG. 23.3 Sagittal ultrasound scan of the normal testis demonstrates the appendix testis as a small structure superior to the testis *(arrow)*. The appendix testis is isoechoic to the testis. A small hydrocele improves the visibility of the appendix testis.

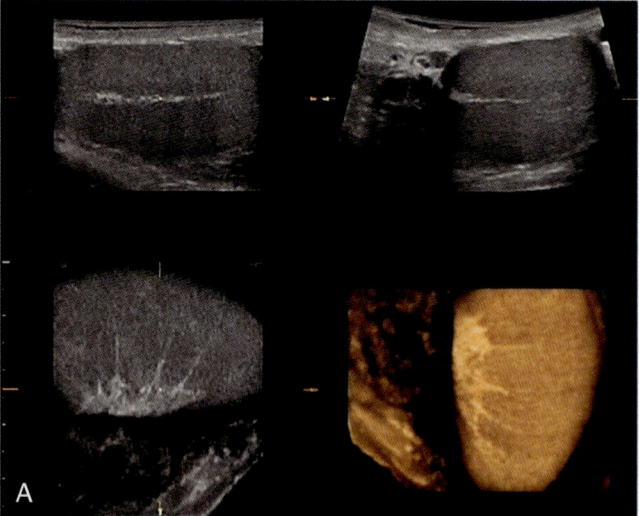 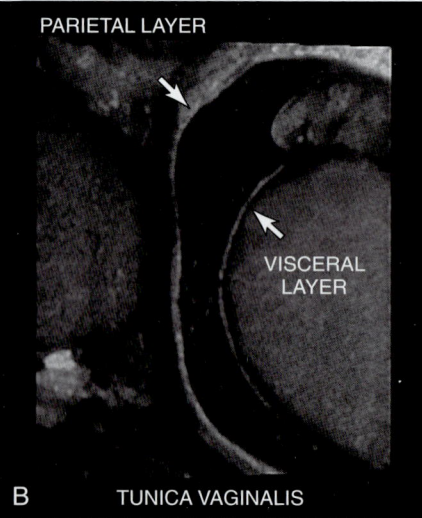

FIG. 23.4 (A) Three-dimensional (3D) view showing the mediastinum testis in orthogonal planes with the septa. This image was obtained with a 3D transducer sweeping in the sagittal plane *(upper left)*. The transverse image is derived from the 3D volume and is displayed upper right. 3D view allows visualization of the coronal plane *(lower left)*. The coronal plane is rarely imaged with traditional 2D imaging. A rendered view of the testis is seen in the lower right. (B) 3D coronal view demonstrating the layers of the tunica vaginalis *(arrows)*. This is well demonstrated because of the presence of a hydrocele. Hydroceles form between the parietal and visceral layers of the tunica vaginalis.

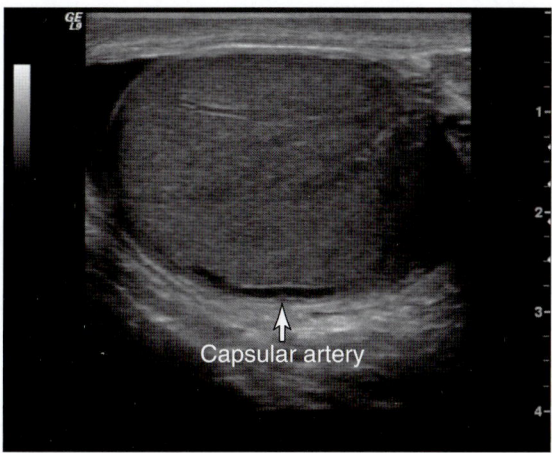

FIG. 23.5 Transverse ultrasound view of the testis depicting the capsular artery in a patient with orchitis. The capsular artery is seen as an anechoic structure coursing along the surface of the testis *(arrow)*.

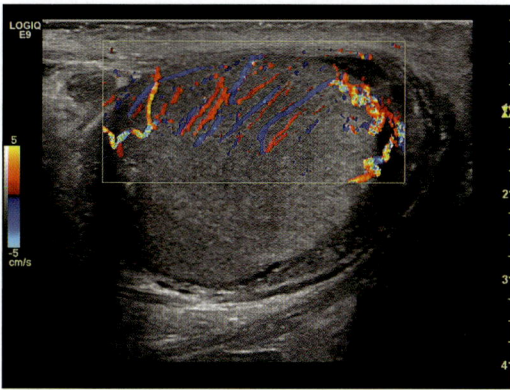

FIG. 23.7 Color Doppler image of the testis depicting the recurrent rami. A centripetal artery is seen coursing from the testicular capsule. Before reaching the mediastinum, it turns backward in a candy cane pattern, forming the recurrent rami.

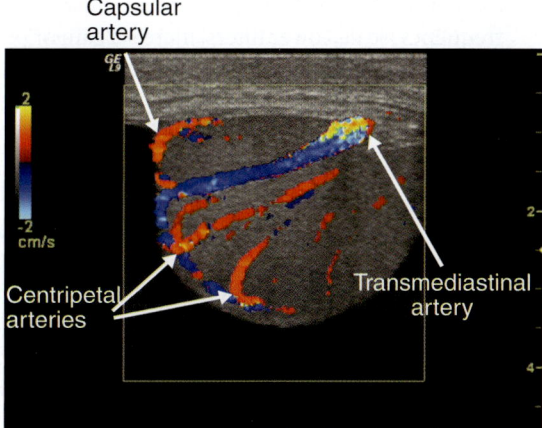

FIG. 23.6 Color Doppler image of the testis depicting the capsular artery giving rise to centripetal arteries. A transmediastinal artery is seen coursing from the mediastinum to the testicular surface. It then branches across the top of the testis as capsular arteries. The flow direction in the transmediastinal artery *(blue)* is opposite to that in the centripetal arteries *(red)*. The centripetal arteries rise from the capsular arteries with a flow direction through the testis toward the mediastinum, whereas the blood flow in the transmediastinal artery courses from the mediastinum to the testicular capsule.

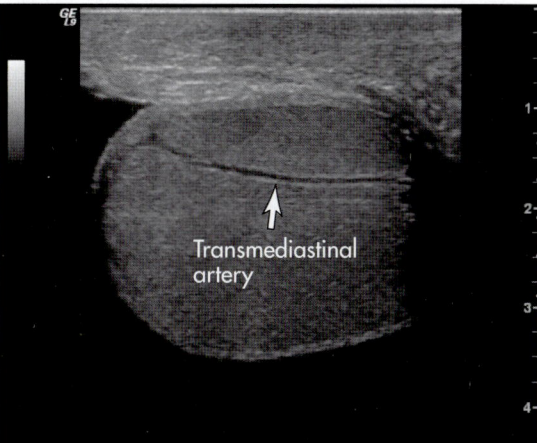

FIG. 23.8 Transverse ultrasound image shows a normal transmediastinal artery coursing from the mediastinum to the testicular capsule. It appears as an anechoic or hypoechoic tube. Transmediastinal arteries are seen in approximately 50% of testes.

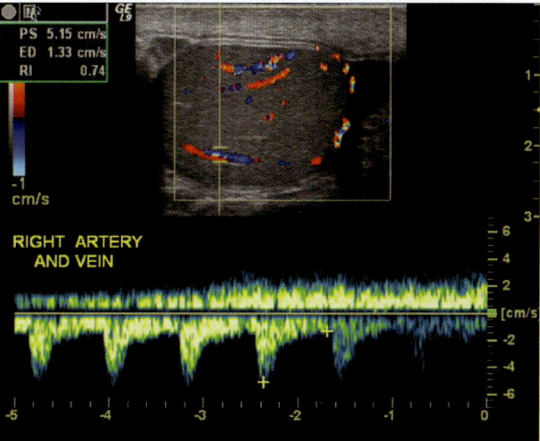

FIG. 23.9 Spectral Doppler image showing the normal low-resistance waveform pattern of the intratesticular arteries. A low-resistance waveform demonstrates forward flow during both systole and diastole. In this image, the Doppler sample volume includes both a transmediastinal artery and its accompanying vein. The venous and arterial flow signals are on opposite sides of the Doppler baseline, as their flow is in opposite directions.

reaching the mediastinum, they curve backward, forming the **recurrent rami** (centrifugal arteries) (Fig. 23.6). These centrifugal arteries branch farther into arterioles and capillaries. With sensitive color Doppler settings, the recurrent rami may be seen giving a candy cane appearance (Fig. 23.7).

In approximately one-half of normal testes, a transmediastinal (or transtesticular) artery is visualized coursing through the mediastinum toward the testicular capsule. A large vein is often identified adjacent to the artery (Fig. 23.8). On color Doppler, the transmediastinal artery will have a different color than the centripetal arteries because its flow is directed away from the mediastinum and toward the capsule. On reaching the testicular surface opposite the mediastinum, the transmediastinal artery courses along the capsule as capsular arteries. Spectral Doppler waveforms obtained from the capsular, centripetal, or transmediastinal arteries show a low-resistance waveform pattern in normal individuals (Fig. 23.9). Box 23.1 diagrams arterial branching in the testicles.

BOX 23.1	Testicular Arterial Branching

Testicular artery
↓
Capsular artery
↓
Centripetal artery
↓
Recurrent rami

BOX 23.2	Sonographer Tips

- Explain procedure and preparation to patient, and then allow the patient to get ready in private.
- Be sure to take an image of right and left testicles together for comparison in both gray-scale and color Doppler.
- Perform Valsalva maneuver when a varicocele is suspected.
- Sensitize color Doppler for slow flow when evaluating torsion.
- Torsion is a surgical emergency; perform the examination in a timely manner.

The **cremasteric artery** and **deferential artery** accompany the testicular artery within the spermatic cord to supply the extratesticular structures. They also have anastomoses with the testicular artery and may provide some flow to the testis. The cremasteric artery branches from the inferior epigastric artery (a branch of the external iliac artery). It provides flow to the **cremasteric muscle** and peritesticular tissue. The deferential artery arises from the vesicle artery (a branch of the internal iliac artery). It mainly supplies the epididymis and vas deferens. The scrotal wall is also supplied by branches of the **pudendal artery**.

Venous drainage of the scrotum occurs through the veins of the **pampiniform plexus**. The pampiniform plexus exits from the mediastinum testis and courses in the spermatic cord. It converges into three sets of anastomotic veins: testicular, deferential, and cremasteric. The right **testicular vein** drains into the inferior vena cava, and the left testicular vein joins the left renal vein. The deferential vein drains into the pelvic veins, and the cremasteric vein drains into tributaries of the epigastric and deep pudendal veins.

Patient Positioning and Scanning Protocol

Scrotal Protocol. High-resolution ultrasound imaging is the primary screening modality for most testicular pathology. Applications include inflammatory processes of the testes and epididymis, tumors, trauma, torsion, hydrocele, varicocele, hernias, spermatoceles, and undescended testes.
1. Patient preparation: none.
2. Transducer selection: 8- to 12-MHz linear array.
3. Patient position: supine (Valsalva maneuver or upright position to check for varicocele).
4. Images and observations should include the following:
   - Gray scale.
   - Long testicle (include medial, mid, and lateral).
   - Long epididymis.
   - Anteroposterior (AP) and long measurements of above anatomy.
   - Transverse scan of each testis (upper, mid, lower).
   - Transverse scan of head of epididymis.
   - Include AP and transverse measurements of the middle pole of the testicles.
   - If possible, a split-screen image should be obtained to compare the echogenicity of each testis.
   - Images of the extratesticular area should be obtained to determine the presence of hydrocele, hernia, or other conditions.
- Doppler flow analysis of the scrotal area:
  - When indicated, color and pulsed Doppler analysis of intratesticular flow with resistance measurements should be obtained.
  - The scanning instrument should be optimized for slow flow detection (e.g., decrease pulse repetition frequency/scale, lower filters, increase gain or power).

Ultrasound examination of the scrotum is performed with the patient in the supine position. The penis is positioned on the abdomen and covered with a towel. The patient is asked to place his legs close together to provide support for the scrotum. Alternatively, a rolled towel placed between the thighs can support the scrotum. It is often unnecessary to place a towel for support if the legs are positioned close together. This may be more comfortable for the patient in pain.

A generous amount of warmed gel is applied to the scrotum to ensure adequate probe contact and eliminate air between the probe and the skin surface. Rarely, a stand-off pad may be necessary to improve imaging of very superficial structures such as a tunica albuginea cyst. However, with the use of high-frequency probes (10 to 14 MHz), this is usually not necessary. Instead of a stand-off pad, an extra-thick mound of gel may be adequate to improve near-field imaging.

Before beginning the scrotal ultrasound, it is necessary to determine clinical findings. Was this patient referred because of a palpable mass, scrotal pain, swollen scrotum, or other reasons? It is important to ask the patient to describe his symptoms, including history, location, and duration of pain. Can he feel a mass? If so, ask the patient to find the lump. Then place the probe exactly over this location to examine the site. Did the patient experience trauma? When did the trauma occur? Ask him to describe what happened. Has he had a vasectomy? When? Not only is this information helpful in guiding the examination, but it is important to the interpreting physician and gives confidence to the patient regarding the quality of the ultrasound study. Box 23.2 lists important tips when performing an ultrasound examination of the scrotum.

Scrotal ultrasound is always a bilateral examination, with the asymptomatic side used as a comparison for the symptomatic side. To begin, it is best to perform a brief survey scan to determine what abnormalities, if any, are present. Each testis is scanned from superior to inferior and is carefully examined to determine whether abnormal findings are present.

The size, echogenicity, and structure of each testis are evaluated. The testicular parenchyma should be uniform with equal echogenicity between sides. Think of these questions as you scan: Is the parenchyma homogeneous or heterogeneous? Is there a mass? If so, is it cystic or solid? Is it intratesticular or extratesticular? Is one testis much larger than the other? Which side is swollen, or is one side shrunken? All testes should appear similar in size and shape. Is the epididymis normal? Is the skin thickened? Turn on color Doppler to assess the flow. Is there an absence of flow in the testis, or is it hyperemic? How does the color Doppler compare between sides? Testes should show about the same amount of flow when the same color Doppler setup is used. Check the flow in each epididymis. Again, compare between sides. They should be similar. After the survey scan, images are obtained that demonstrate the findings.

Representative images are obtained in at least two planes—transverse and sagittal—with additional imaging planes scanned as needed to demonstrate the findings. In transverse, images are taken that show the superior, mid, and inferior portions of each testis. The width of the testis is measured in the midtransverse view. A transverse view of the head of the epididymis is included. Superior to the epididymal head, an image is obtained to demonstrate the area of the spermatic cord. In the sagittal plane, images are taken to show the medial, mid, and lateral portions. A long axis measurement of testicular length is obtained in the midsagittal image. Again, additional images may be taken to demonstrate abnormal areas. An image is obtained of the epididymal head superior to the **testicle**. The body and tail of the epididymis can be demonstrated coursing posteriorly on each side. Scrotal skin thickness is evaluated and compared from side to side. At least one image is taken to show both testes at the same time, so the interpreting physician can compare size and echogenicity (Fig. 23.10). Additional views may be taken in patients with suspected varicocele. These include upright positioning and the Valsalva maneuver. Color and spectral Doppler are used in all examinations, with representative images taken to demonstrate both arterial and venous flow in each testis. Table 23.1 lists the scanning protocols for scrotal ultrasound.

TECHNICAL CONSIDERATIONS

High-frequency linear-array transducers are preferred for scrotal imaging because they provide the best spatial resolution. However, the field of view is limited with linear arrays. Occasionally, a larger field of view is required to measure anatomy or display anatomic relationships. Ultrasound systems provide numerous methods to meet this need, including virtual convex imaging, panoramic imaging, stitching images together, and using a curved-array transducer.

Real-time imaging of the scrotum is performed with a high-frequency linear-array probe of at least 7.5 MHz. Because high-frequency transducers have better spatial and contrast resolution compared with lower-frequency transducers, they are preferred for scrotal imaging. Probes with frequencies of 10 to 15 MHz are usually best. Because there is a tradeoff between frequency and penetration, the highest frequency providing adequate penetration should be used. In patients with considerable wall edema and thickening, frequencies as low as 5 to 7.5 MHz may be necessary to adequately penetrate the testis.

Many ultrasound systems have a trapezoid or virtual convex feature that can be selected with the linear-array probe. This is very helpful for measuring the long axis of the testis or when an abnormal area cannot be entirely imaged with the standard linear format (Fig. 23.11A). It is best to use this feature selectively instead of routinely because steering the beam to create the wider format has a negative impact on image quality; steering widens the distance between scan lines and degrades lateral resolution.

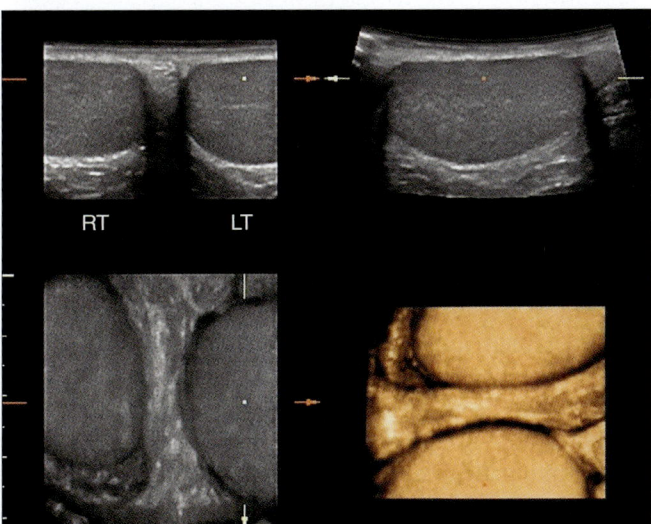

FIG. 23.10 Transverse three-dimensional sweep obtained at the midline in a normal patient demonstrating both testes. The size, echogenicity, and texture are similar between sides. It is advisable to obtain an image like this in all cases to allow comparison between the testes.

TABLE 23.1	Ultrasound Scrotal Scan Protocol
Transverse Image	Sagittal Image
Spermatic cord area	Spermatic cord area
Epididymal head	Epididymal head with superior testis
Superior testis	Long axis mid-testis with measurement
Mid testis with measurement	Medial long axis
Inferior testis	Lateral long axis
Transverse view showing both testes	Color Doppler of epididymal head
	Color Doppler of mid-testis
	Spectral Doppler of artery
	Spectral Doppler of vein

In patients with suspected varicocele, additional views include upright view of spermatic cord with and without Valsalva maneuver.

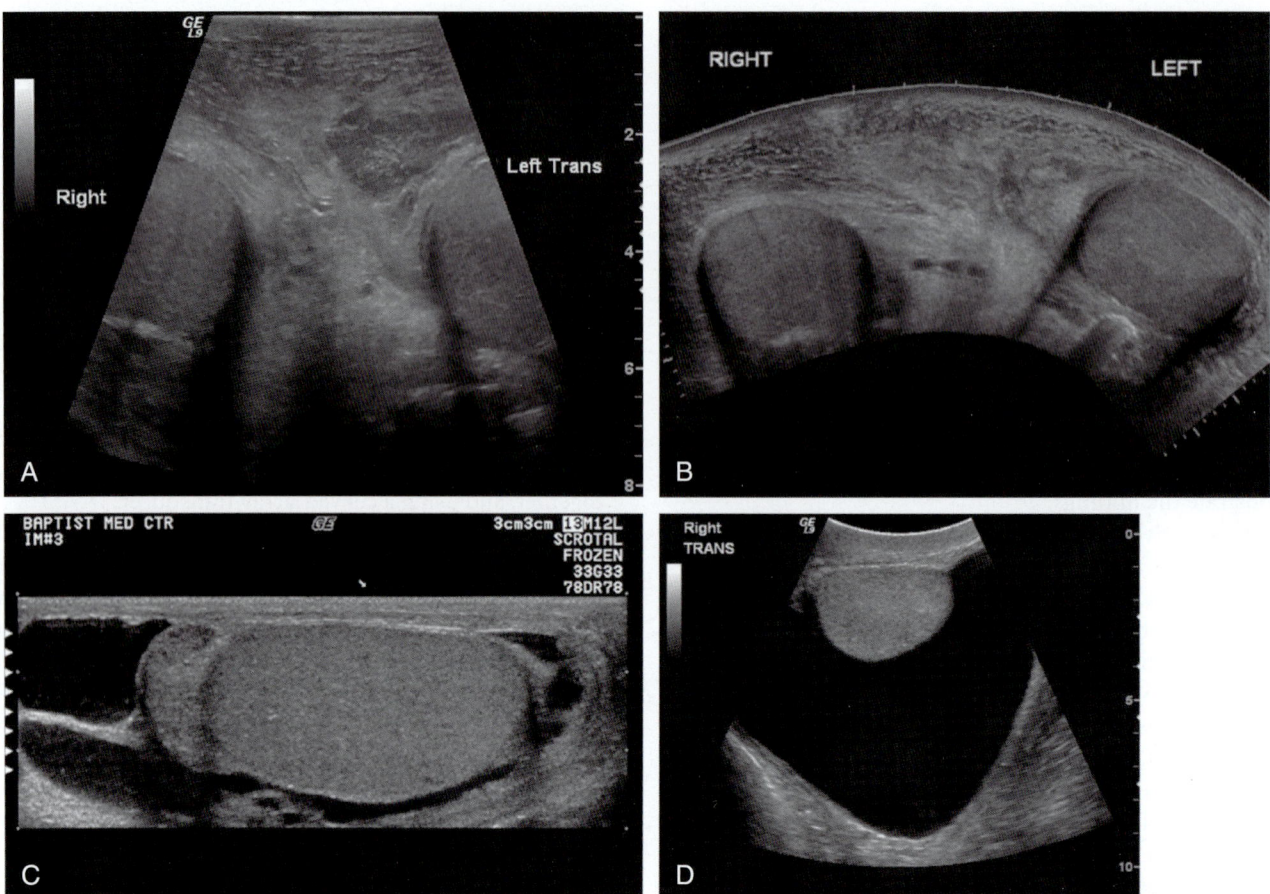

FIG. 23.11 (A) Transverse ultrasound scan of a scrotal hematoma using a virtual convex to create a sector or trapezoidal format using a linear-array probe. The field of view is enlarged to allow better depiction of the size and location of the hematoma compared with the testes. This feature is useful for measuring testicular length and showing abnormal areas that are too large to view with the standard linear format. However, because the scan lines are steered to create this image, lateral resolution is decreased compared with the standard format. (B) Transverse ultrasound view of the same scrotal hematoma using a panoramic setting. This feature allows the image to build as the transducer is moved across the anatomy. It is very useful for showing large masses and anatomic relationships. (C) Sagittal ultrasound image in a patient with epididymitis and hydrocele. The image was obtained by stitching together two images in a combined mode. This is another useful tool when a larger field of view is necessary to demonstrate anatomy. (D) Sagittal ultrasound image of the testis surrounded posteriorly by a large hydrocele. The linear-array format could not display the entire hydrocele, so a 7-MHz curved-array transducer was used to better demonstrate a pathologic condition.

In cases of large hydroceles, hematomas, or swelling, an even larger field of view may be required. In these cases, a panoramic tool may be useful. This tool allows the image to build as the probe is moved over the skin surface. A very long image can be obtained that shows anatomic relationships (see Fig. 23.11B). Images may also be stitched together in a combined mode. The first image is obtained in one window; then the probe is moved, and another image is obtained by attempting to match the boundaries of the first image (see Fig. 23.11C). Another way to obtain a larger field of view is to use a 5- to 7.5-MHz curved-array transducer for a portion of the examination to demonstrate the entire scrotal contents. Again, this should be done selectively to obtain the necessary images and should be followed by a return to the high-frequency linear-array probe for further evaluation of each testis (see Fig. 23.11D).

Most modern ultrasound scanners offer additional features that enhance the quality of the ultrasound image. These features include, but are not limited to, compound imaging, harmonics, extended field-of-view imaging, virtual convex, speckle reduction algorithms, and use of multiple focal zones (Table 23.2). All these controls may be adjusted to improve image quality.

Color and spectral Doppler play an important role in scrotal ultrasound. The typical color/spectral Doppler frequencies used for scrotal ultrasound are between 4 and 8 MHz. The upper-frequency range is used to improve sensitivity to slow flow. This is important in evaluation of testicular torsion or tumor vascularity. Penetration is decreased with higher frequencies, so it is important to make sure that the color penetrates to the depth of interest. Color and spectral Doppler findings on the symptomatic side are always compared with the asymptomatic side.

Power Doppler is often used to quickly get to a sensitive setting that will demonstrate slow flow. Power Doppler shows the amplitude or power of the moving signal, whereas color Doppler shows the frequency shift. Power Doppler does not demonstrate flow direction or aliasing and, to some, offers a

TABLE 23.2	Scanning Features		
Feature	What Is It?	Advantage	Disadvantage
Harmonics	Selective reception of penetration (uses frequencies generated within tissue)	Improved contrast resolution Improved visibility of low-level echoes Reduction of artifacts	Less harmonic penetration (uses higher frequency)
Compound imaging	Uses multiple-angled firings to create one image	Improved border definition Reduced speckle Less angle dependence	Slowed frame rate Loss of some beneficial artifacts (i.e., shadowing, refraction, and enhancement)
Speckle reduction algorithms	Sophisticated algorithms applied to the image to reduce speckle (salt and pepper appearance of ultrasound image)	Improved contrast resolution Improved conspicuity of masses	None
Extended field of view imaging	Image builds up as probe is moved across anatomy	Improved ability to show anatomic relationships of structures too large to fit in linear-array format	May be difficult to perform on uncooperative patient or over sharply curving interface
Trapezoid or virtual convex imaging	Steering of linear-array probe to create sector format	Larger field of view with linear-array probes	Reduced lateral resolution
Multizone focus	Use of multiple focal zones to create an extended area of focus on one image	Improved lateral resolution	Slowed frame rate

TABLE 23.3	Color/Power Doppler Parameters	
Parameter	What Is It?	How to Adjust
Gain	Amplification of selected frequency shift signal	Turn up until noise is present and then decrease until noise goes away
Pulse repetition frequency (PRF)	PRF is the number of pulses transmitted per second; sets the Nyquist limit; main control affecting sensitivity to flow	Adjust on the asymptomatic side so that flow is visible without too much flash or motion artifact; decrease to improve sensitivity to slow flow; increase to reduce aliasing
Wall filter	Color signals received below the wall filter setting do not appear on the image	Decrease to improve sensitivity and to reduce flash/motion artifact
Line density	Density of scan lines contained within the color box	Turn up to improve lateral resolution of vessels; turn down to increase frame rate
Threshold	Level of gray-scale brightness that is allowable to be overwritten by color when both gray-scale and color information are obtained for the same pixel location within the image	Turn up so that color information is prioritized compared with gray-scale information; if the threshold (also known as color/write priority) is set too low, small intratesticular vessels will not be filled with color
Packet size	Number of pulses on each color scan line	Turn up to improve signal-to-noise ratio and turn down to improve frame rate sensitivity
Color box size	Region of interest that is color encoded within the image	Set just over the area of interest; increasing color box size or depth will slow frame rate

more straightforward display of blood flow. Presets for power Doppler are often set at a lower pulse repetition frequency (PRF) than color Doppler because aliasing is not an issue, so pushing the power Doppler button may show more flow with fewer adjustments to the controls. This often provides a quick way to get to a more sensitive flow setting. Persistence is usually much greater with power Doppler, requiring a steady hand and slower movement of the probe. To further enhance power Doppler, the same parameters are adjusted as for color Doppler.

Familiarity with color Doppler controls is very important when performing scrotal ultrasounds. The sonographer may need to adjust some of the following color Doppler parameters throughout the study to enhance the visibility of scrotal perfusion (Table 23.3):

- *Gain*—The color gain control is used to amplify the reflected color Doppler signal. Whenever the expected amount of color is not visible in the image, the color gain should be increased until noise is present. Once color noise is visible, the gain can be decreased until it just disappears. At this point, the color gain setting is optimized.
- *Scale/PRF*—The PRF is the number of pulses transmitted in 1 second. This important color parameter affects the sensitivity of the system in displaying slow flow. It also sets

the point at which color aliasing occurs (Nyquist limit). The control has different names depending on the ultrasound equipment being used. It is variably named scale, PRF, or flow rate. The PRF is reduced to improve sensitivity to slow flow. This is critical when ruling out testicular torsion. If the PRF is set too high, slow flow may not be visible. When the PRF is set too low, excessive color aliasing occurs, which makes it impossible to determine flow direction or to assess flow quality. Neither of these factors is significant in scrotal ultrasound, so it is common to use low PRF settings. However, flash artifact from patient motion is more apparent with very low PRFs and may make scanning difficult. It is recommended to adjust the PRF so that the asymptomatic testicular flow is well demonstrated without excessive flash artifact. Then compare the same settings on the contralateral side (Fig. 23.12).

- *Wall filter*—The wall filter acts as an electronic eraser. Color echoes that fall below the filter cutoff do not appear on the image display. The wall filter is adjusted downward to enhance flow sensitivity. It is turned up to reduce flash artifact. On most ultrasound systems, the wall filter is automatically adjusted with the PRF. But in some instances, it may be beneficial to make further adjustments.
- *Line density*—The line density is the number or density of scan lines contained within the color box. It affects the lateral resolution of the color display. As line density is increased, lateral resolution is improved. The size of the intratesticular arteries is displayed more accurately when line density is high. Frame rate becomes slower as line density is increased because more transmitted pulses are required to create each image frame. If the frame rate becomes too slow, the line density can be decreased. The user must choose the tradeoff between resolution and frame rate (Fig. 23.13).
- *Threshold or color/tissue priority*—The B/color threshold is used to determine whether a gray scale or a color pixel is displayed in any given location on the image. Color and power Doppler images are color overlays on top of an

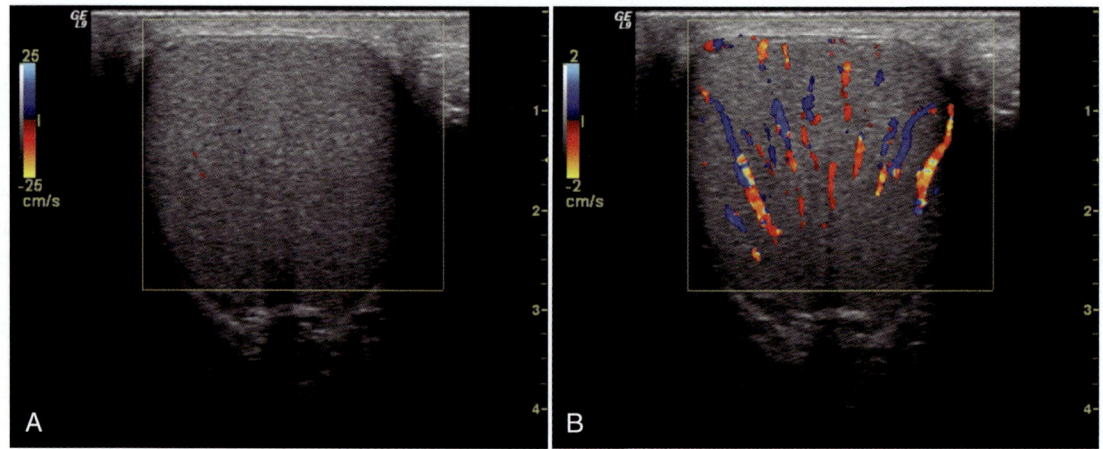

FIG. 23.12 (A) Transverse color Doppler image of a normal testis. Almost no color signal is apparent in the testis because of the high pulse repetition frequency (PRF) setting. The velocity scale values adjacent to the color bar show a velocity sensitivity of 25 cm/sec. (B) Image of the same testis, using a much lower PRF setting. The velocity scale shows a flow sensitivity of 2 cm/sec. Many intratesticular vessels can now be seen with color Doppler.

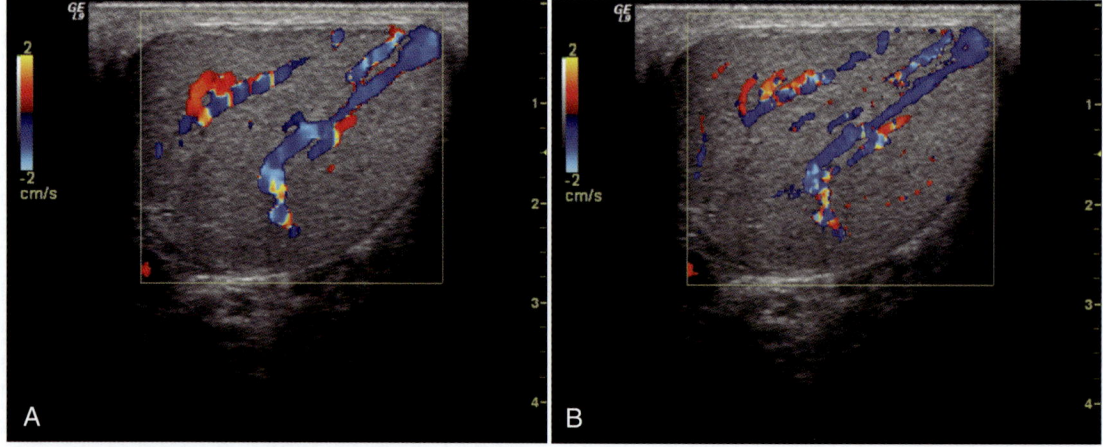

FIG. 23.13 (A) This image was obtained at a low line density setting. The vessels appear wider than expected (poor lateral resolution). (B) When the line density is increased, the vessel size is more accurately displayed. Frame rate is slower because more scan lines are present within the same-sized color box.

existing gray-scale image. A problem arises when gray-scale and color information are received for the same pixel location. The threshold control allows the user to prioritize either gray scale or color. For ultrasound of most small parts, including scrotal imaging, it is best to set the threshold so that color is prioritized. Based on the setting, when color and gray-scale information is received for an identical pixel location, the one displayed is determined by the brightness (amplitude) of the gray-scale dot and the frequency shift and/or power level of the color signal. This feature is not as important when looking at large vessels, such as the common carotid artery, because the vessel lumen typically does not contain gray-scale information, and color can be freely displayed in those pixels. However, in small parts imaging, most vessels are so small that the lumen is not visible or may contain gray-scale echoes caused by volume averaging. In these instances, color will not be displayed unless the threshold control is set to a level that prioritizes color.

- *Packet size*—The packet size is the number of sound pulses transmitted on each scan line within the color box. The packet size is usually set between 8 and 20 pulses for each scan line. The packet size affects the signal-to-noise ratio, improving color sensitivity when more pulses are used. The frame rate gets slower as the number of packets (pulses) is increased on each scan line. The packet size can be reduced to raise the frame rate when necessary or increased to improve color sensitivity. The key factor affecting color sensitivity, however, is the PRF.
- *Color box/region of interest*—The color box or region of interest is the area within the gray-scale image where flow is color encoded. The width of the color box affects the frame rate. If the color box is very wide, more scan lines are required to complete each image frame. This means that a greater number of pulses must be transmitted. This takes more time, so the frame rate is reduced. Color box depth also affects frame rate. When the color box is placed deep in the image, the round-trip time for the sound is increased. This slows down the frame rate.

An understanding of the factors affecting color frame rate, sensitivity, and resolution allows the sonographer to optimize the color parameters for each clinical situation. Most systems have specific presets for each ultrasound application. Selection of the scrotal preset will set the color parameters near an optimal setting for a typical normal examination. However, the user must further adjust the controls to enhance the visibility of scrotal perfusion in abnormal states.

SCROTAL PATHOLOGY

Table 23.4 lists the pathology and sonographic appearance associated with scrotal trauma, infection, and fluid collection. Although the sonographer is not responsible for the interpretation of ultrasound images, an understanding of the various differential considerations is useful to fully evaluate the lesion. Table 23.5 lists many of the common and uncommon masses or fluid collections found within or surrounding the testes.

TABLE 23.4 Scrotal Infection, Trauma, and Fluid Collections

Pathology	Sonographic Appearance
Infection	
Epididymitis	Enlarged epididymis Heterogeneous texture Hypoechoic, may contain hyperechoic areas Blood flow in the epididymis
Focal orchitis	Hypoechoic area within testis Blood flow in the testis
Diffuse orchitis	Enlarged, hypoechoic testis Echogenicity of the whole testis
Trauma	
Rupture	Irregular contour Focal alteration in echogenicity
Hematoma	Heterogeneous area Becomes hyperechoic as the blood clot ages Avascular
Torsion	Gray-scale image of testis normal when duration <4 h Testis enlarged and hypoechoic 4–12 h Testis heterogeneous after 24 h Absence of testicular flow
Fluid Collections	
Hydrocele	May be anechoic, but often contains low-level echoes Surrounds anterolateral aspect of testis
Spermatocele	Located in head of epididymis May contain internal echoes and/or septations Smooth walls Posterior acoustic enhancement
Epididymal cyst	May be located anywhere in epididymis Usually small, anechoic Ultrasound cannot differentiate between spermatocele and epididymal cyst Posterior acoustic enhancement
Varicocele	Tortuous, dilated veins Increased size with Valsalva maneuver or patient standing Dilated veins fill with color on Valsalva maneuver Spectral Doppler confirms venous flow
Hematocele	Contains low-level echoes May contain septations and loculations

Acute Scrotum

Scrotal Trauma. Scrotal trauma presents a challenge to the sonographer because the scrotum is often painful and swollen. Trauma may be the result of motor vehicle accident, athletic injury, direct blow to the scrotum, or straddle injury. The most important goal of the ultrasound examination in testicular trauma is to determine whether a rupture has occurred.

TABLE 23.5	Differential Considerations: Extratesticular Fluid Collections or Masses	
Scrotal Masses		
Common		Hydrocele
		Varicocele
		Ascites
		Hematocele
		Spermatocele
		Epididymitis
Uncommon		Cysts
		Pyoceles
		Herniated bowel
		Metastasis
		Polyorchidism
		Extratesticular Seminoma
Extratesticular Cystic Mass		
Common		Hematocele
		Spermatocele
Uncommon		Pyocele
		Epididymal cyst
		Herniated bowel
Hypoechoic Lesion		
Common		Seminoma
		Embryonal cell carcinoma
		Choriocarcinoma
		Mixed cell tumor
		Lymphoma
		Leukemia
Uncommon		Teratoma
		Torsion
		Metastasis
		Epididymal tumor
		Abscess
Enlarged Testicle		
Common		Tumor
		Edematous testis caused by trauma
		Torsion
Uncommon		Myeloma of testicle
		Idiopathic macro-orchidism
Enlarged Epididymis		
Common		Epididymitis
		Sperm granuloma
Uncommon		Polyorchidism
		Lipoma
Hypoechoic Band in Testis		
Common		Normal mediastinum testis
		Normal vessels

Rupture of the testis is a surgical emergency that requires prompt diagnosis. If surgery is performed within 72 hours following injury, up to 90% of testes can be saved, but only 45% can be saved after 72 hours. Hydrocele and hematocele are both complications of trauma. However, neither is specific to trauma. Hematoceles contain blood and are also found in advanced cases of epididymitis or orchitis.

Sonographic Findings. The sonographic findings associated with scrotal rupture include focal alteration of the testicular parenchymal pattern, interruption of the tunica albuginea, irregular testicular contour, scrotal wall thickening, and **hematocele**. These findings may also be associated with abscess, tumor, or other clinical conditions. When combined with a history of trauma, they suggest rupture.

The sonographic appearance of hematoceles varies with age. An acute hematocele is echogenic with numerous, highly visible echoes that can be seen to float or move in real-time. Over time, hematoceles show low-level echoes and develop fluid-filled levels or septations. The presence of a hematocele does not confirm rupture. Hematoceles result from bleeding of the pampiniform plexus or other extratesticular structures.

Hematomas associated with trauma may be large and may cause displacement of the associated testis. Hematomas appear as heterogeneous areas within the scrotum. They tend to become more complex over time, developing cystic components. Hematomas may involve the testis or epididymis, or they can be contained within the scrotal wall. Because hematomas are avascular, color Doppler is helpful in identifying them as areas with no flow (Fig. 23.14).

Other uses of color Doppler in testicular trauma include identification of blood flow disruption across the surface of the testis. This is an indication of rupture. Color Doppler can aid in separating a normally vascularized testis from one that is disrupted by hematoma. Epididymitis may result from trauma, and color Doppler imaging can be used to identify the associated increased vascularity in the **epididymis**. Torsion may also be associated with trauma. Color Doppler is used to confirm the absence of flow in the testis with torsion.

Epididymo-orchitis. Epididymo-orchitis is infection of the epididymis and testis. It most commonly results from the spread of a lower urinary tract infection via the spermatic cord. Less common causes include mumps, syphilis, tuberculosis,

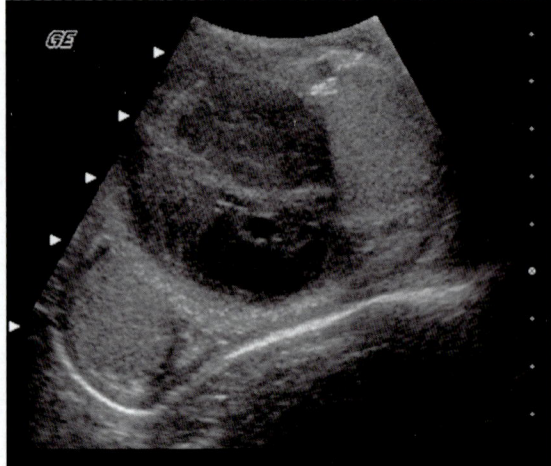

FIG. 23.14 Complex hematoma in a patient with hemophilia following scrotal trauma. Transverse ultrasound scan of both testes shows a large heterogeneous mass adjacent to the left testis. Color Doppler (not shown) demonstrated the mass to be avascular.

viruses, trauma, and chemical causes. Epididymo-orchitis represents the most common cause of acute scrotal pain in adults. The epididymis is the organ primarily involved with infection, which spreads to the testis in about 20% to 40% of cases. Orchitis almost always occurs secondary to epididymitis. Patients typically have increasing scrotal pain over 1 or 2 days. The pain may be mild or severe. Symptoms may also include fever and urethral discharge.

Sonographic Findings. Epididymitis appears as an enlarged, hypoechoic gland. If secondary hemorrhage has occurred, the epididymis may contain focal hyperechoic areas. Hyperemic flow is confirmed with color Doppler (Fig. 23.15). The normal epididymis shows little flow with color Doppler. The amount of color flow signal should be compared between sides. The affected side shows significantly more flow than the asymptomatic epididymis. It is important to use the same color Doppler settings when comparing the amount of flow between sides.

With epididymitis, Doppler waveforms demonstrate increased velocities in both systole and diastole. A low-resistance waveform pattern is present (see Fig. 23.15). If the infection is isolated to the epididymis, the testis will appear normal. When orchitis has developed, ultrasound imaging will show an enlarged testis. The infection may be focal or diffuse, and affected areas may appear hypoechoic compared with the surrounding tissue. Focal areas of infection within the testis will result in a heterogeneous appearance on ultrasound. A diffusely infected testis will appear enlarged and homogeneous with a hypoechoic echogenicity (Fig. 23.16). Up to 20% of cases will have a normal-appearing epididymis and testis on ultrasound. Ultrasound gray-scale findings associated with epididymo-orchitis are not specific and may also be seen with torsion or tumor. Color and spectral Doppler are key tools in differentiating between epididymo-orchitis and torsion in the patient with acute scrotal pain.

Epididymo-orchitis causes hyperemic flow with a significantly greater number of visible vessels on color Doppler compared with the asymptomatic side. Hyperemic flow is seen in the epididymis and testis when both are involved but is isolated to the epididymis when the testis is normal. Documentation of findings on ultrasound must include an image showing both testes, so the size and echogenicity can be compared.

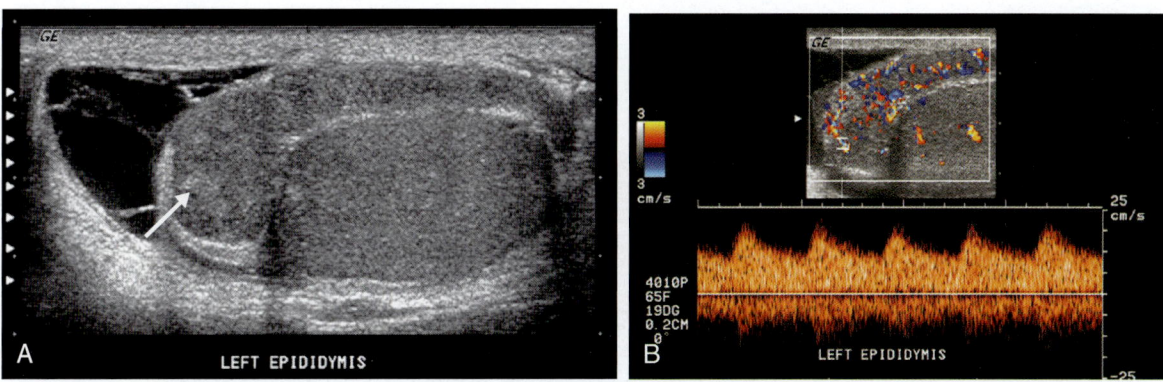

FIG. 23.15 (A) Sagittal ultrasound image in a patient with severe epididymitis shows an enlarged epididymis with a heterogeneous echotexture. Focal hyperechoic areas *(arrow)* within the epididymis may represent hemorrhage. A complex hydrocele with numerous septations is shown near the epididymal head. (B) Color Doppler shows hyperemic flow within the epididymis. A Doppler waveform obtained from the epididymal head shows increased diastolic flow associated with inflammation.

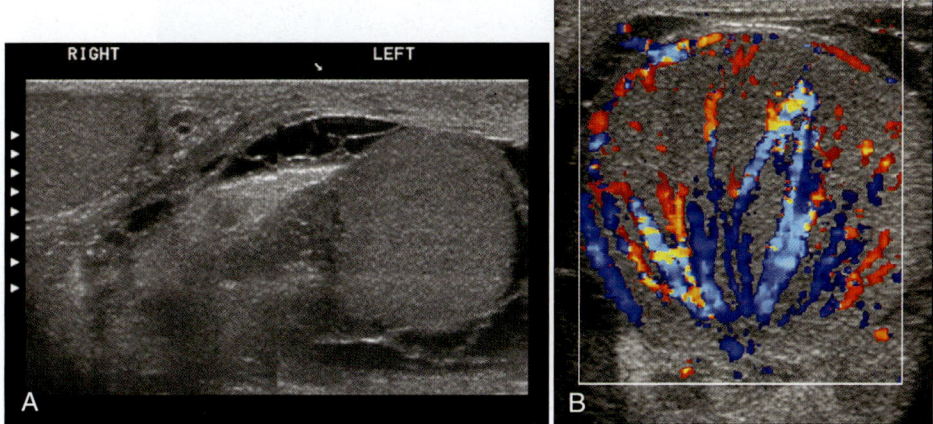

FIG. 23.16 (A) Orchitis in a patient presenting with severe scrotal pain and swelling. Transverse stitched ultrasound scan shows an enlarged left testis and a normal right testis. A complex hydrocele surrounds the left testis. Marked skin thickening is present on the left side compared with the normal right side. (B) Color Doppler shows hyperemic flow.

It is also recommended to obtain an image with the color box opened wide enough to show portions of both testes so that the amount of flow between sides can be easily compared.

Other findings associated with epididymitis and epididymo-orchitis include scrotal wall thickening and **hydrocele**. Hydroceles are found around the anterolateral aspect of the testis. They may appear anechoic or may contain low-level echoes. Complex hydroceles may be associated with severe epididymitis and orchitis. These have thick septations and contain low-level echoes. In severe cases, a pyocele may be present. A **pyocele** occurs when pus fills the space between the layers of the tunica vaginalis. It usually contains internal septations, loculations, and debris. This same appearance may be noted following trauma or surgery.

In severe cases of orchitis, testicular infarction may occur. The swollen testis is confined within a rigid tunica albuginea. Excessive swelling can cause obstruction to the testicular blood supply. Color Doppler will show decreased or absent flow compared with the contralateral testis. With decreased flow, spectral Doppler waveforms will have high resistance with little or no diastolic flow. A Doppler waveform demonstrating reversed diastolic flow is a serious finding, indicating threatened testicular infarction (Fig. 23.17). Infarction can affect the entire testis or may be confined to a focal area. With focal infarction, the color will show perfusion only in portions of the testis that have an absence of color signals in the affected areas. Gray-scale imaging will depict a heterogeneous pattern. Areas of infarction tend to appear hypoechoic compared with the surrounding testicular parenchyma. If the entire testis becomes infarcted, findings cannot be differentiated from testicular torsion.

Torsion. Torsion of the spermatic cord occurs as a result of abnormal mobility of the testis within the scrotum. An anomaly termed the *bell clapper deformity* is the most common cause of this condition. Normally, the testis and epididymis are surrounded by the tunica vaginalis, except at the bare area where they are attached to the posterior scrotal wall. The bell clapper anomaly occurs when the tunica vaginalis completely surrounds the testis, epididymis, and distal spermatic cord, allowing them to move and rotate freely within the scrotum. This movement is similar to that of a clapper inside a bell, hence the name. Torsion results when the testis and epididymis twist within the scrotum, cutting off the vascular supply within the spermatic cord. Up to 60% of patients with torsion will have an anatomic anomaly on both sides. Undescended testes are 10 times more likely to be affected by torsion than normal testes. Torsion compromises blood flow to the testis, the epididymis, and the intrascrotal portion of the spermatic cord. Venous flow is affected first, with occluded veins causing swelling of the scrotal structures on the affected side. If torsion continues, the arterial flow is obstructed, and testicular ischemia follows.

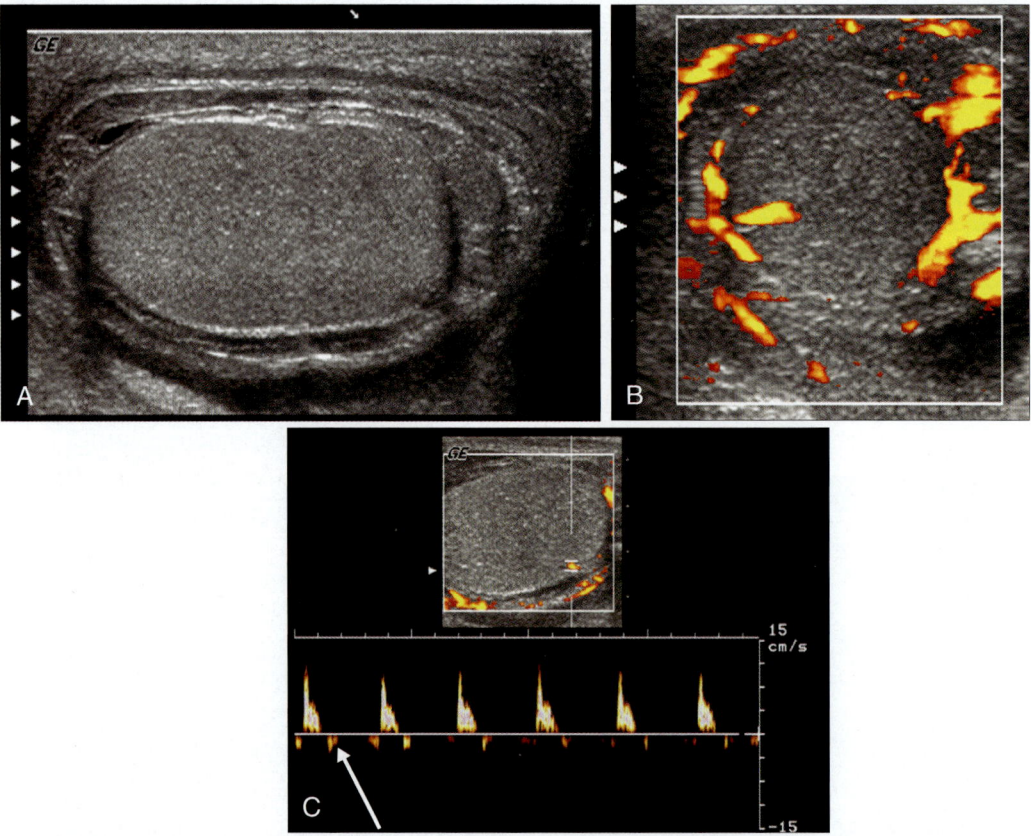

FIG. 23.17 (A) Severe epididymo-orchitis in patient with scrotal pain, swelling, and edema. The testis is swollen against a rigid tunica albuginea. Scrotal skin thickening is evident. (B) Power Doppler shows hyperemic perfusion surrounding the testis but little intratesticular flow, despite the use of sensitive Doppler settings. (C) Spectral Doppler waveform of an intratesticular artery demonstrates a high-resistance waveform. Reversed flow is seen in diastole *(arrow)*. This is a serious finding, indicating threatened infarction.

Torsion of the spermatic cord is a surgical emergency. It is important to obtain diagnostic images as quickly as possible because the salvage rate of the testis depends on the elapsed time since torsion. If surgery is performed within 5 to 6 hours of the onset of pain, 80% to 100% of testes can be salvaged. Between 6 and 12 hours, the salvage rate is 70%, but after 12 hours, only 20% will be saved. The degree of torsion (or the number of twists) also affects testicular salvage.

Torsion is the most common cause of acute scrotal pain in adolescents. Although it is more common in young adults and adolescents, torsion can occur at any age, with peak incidence at age 14. Patients with torsion most often present with sudden onset of scrotal pain accompanied by swelling on the affected side. The severe pain causes nausea and vomiting in many patients. Patients with torsion frequently report previous episodes of scrotal pain. The clinical differentiation between torsion and epididymo-orchitis is difficult in that patients have similar symptoms. Ultrasound plays a key role in helping to differentiate these entities.

Sonographic Findings. Gray-scale findings on ultrasound depend on how much time has passed since the torsion occurred. In the early stages, scrotal contents may have a normal sonographic appearance. After 4 to 6 hours, the testis becomes swollen and hypoechoic (Fig. 23.18). The lobes within the testis are usually well identified during this time as a result of interstitial and septal edema. After 24 hours, the testis becomes heterogeneous as a result of hemorrhage, infarction, necrosis, and vascular congestion (Fig. 23.19).

The epididymal head appears enlarged and may have decreased echogenicity or may become heterogeneous. In some cases, the twisted spermatic cord knot may be seen as a round or oval extratesticular mass that can be traced back to normal spermatic cord. Other findings may include scrotal skin thickening and reactive hydrocele.

Because ultrasound gray-scale findings are similar to those noted with epididymo-orchitis, Doppler evaluation in testicular torsion is very important. Color Doppler imaging is used to make diagnostic images of torsion. The absence of perfusion in the symptomatic testis with normal perfusion on the asymptomatic side is diagnostic of torsion. Color or power Doppler parameters must be adjusted for optimal detection of slow flow. The PRF and wall filter should be set at a low level. Flow around the ischemic testis will appear normal or decreased.

Spontaneous detorsion can produce a very confusing picture both clinically and by ultrasound. Depending on how long the testis was torsed and how long it has been since relief was attained, the intratesticular flow may be minimal or hyperemic. Extratesticular flow is usually increased. This is very difficult to differentiate from epididymo-orchitis.

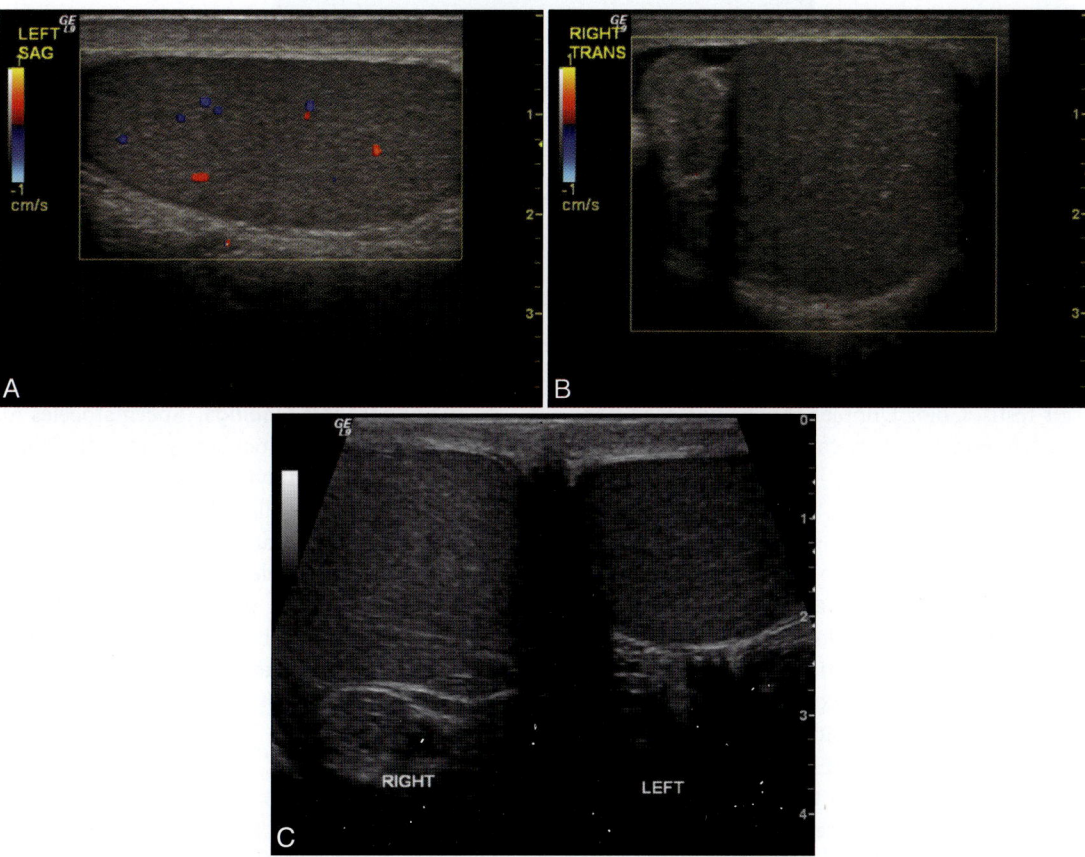

FIG. 23.18 Testicular torsion in an adolescent patient with sudden onset of right testicular pain, accompanied by nausea and vomiting. (A) Color Doppler shows normal flow within the parenchyma of the left testis. (B) The right testis and epididymis are avascular with color Doppler imaging, with the same settings used to show flow on the asymptomatic side. (C) Transverse ultrasound image showing both testes in right testicular torsion. The right testis is swollen and hyperechoic compared with the normal left testis.

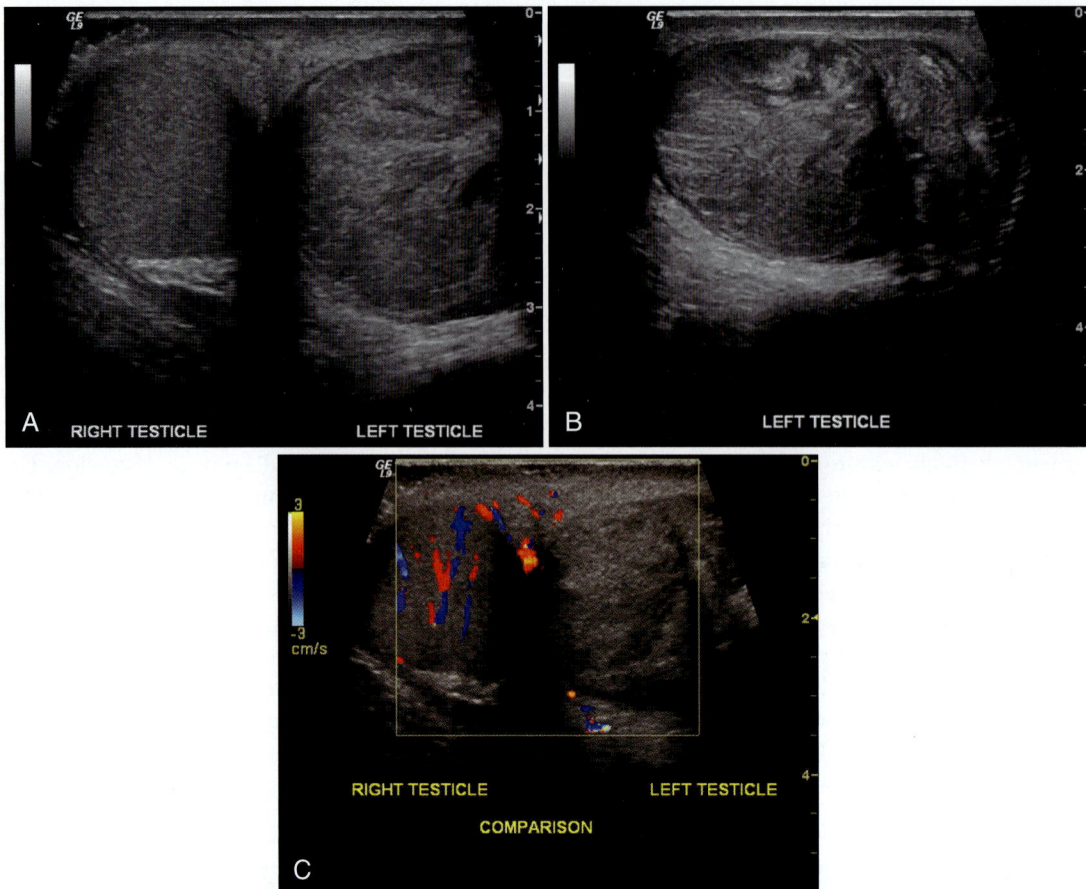

FIG. 23.19 Left spermatic cord torsion in adolescent with a history of scrotal pain of duration greater than 24 hours. (A) Transverse ultrasound image showing both testes. The left testis is enlarged and heterogeneous. (B) Sagittal ultrasound image of the left testis. The infarcted testis has a mixed echo pattern caused by the hemorrhage, necrosis, and vascular congestion associated with spermatic cord torsion exceeding 24 hours. (C) Transverse color Doppler image showing normal perfusion to the right testis with absence of detectable signal on the left side. Paratesticular blood flow is increased around the abnormal testis.

Torsion of the appendix epididymis and the appendix testis also occurs and further complicates the clinical picture. The clinical presentation is similar to that of testicular torsion and epididymo-orchitis. Ultrasound may show a small, hypoechoic mass located between the head of the epididymis and the superior testis. Color Doppler shows increased flow around the mass. Hemorrhage may cause the mass to appear hyperechoic.

Extratesticular Masses

Epididymal Cysts, Spermatoceles, and Tunica Albuginea Cysts. Cysts are benign fluid collections that may be located within the testis or in the extratesticular structures. Most scrotal cysts are extratesticular. Extratesticular cysts are found in the tunica albuginea or epididymis. These include spermatoceles, epididymal cysts, and tunica albuginea cysts. **Spermatoceles** are cystic dilations of the efferent ductules of the epididymis. They are always located in the epididymal head. Spermatoceles contain proteinaceous fluid and spermatozoa. They may be seen more often following vasectomy.

Epididymal cysts are small, clear cysts that contain serous fluid (Fig. 23.20). They can be found anywhere within the epididymis. Small cysts are sometimes found between the layers of the tunica vaginalis or between the tunica vaginalis and the tunica albuginea. All three entities are generally asymptomatic, although they may be palpable and may cause the patient to be concerned.

Sonographic Findings. Spermatoceles may be seen as simple cysts or multilocular cystic collections that contain internal echoes. Epididymal cysts appear as simple fluid-filled structures with thin walls and posterior acoustic enhancement. Ultrasound imaging cannot reliably differentiate epididymal cysts from spermatoceles. Tunica albuginea cysts are usually small and appear as anechoic, thin-walled structures on ultrasound. They can become large and cause displacement and distortion of the testis. This helps to differentiate them from hydroceles, which do not distort the testis.

Varicocele

A **varicocele** is an abnormal dilation of the veins of the pampiniform plexus (located within the spermatic cord). Varicoceles are usually caused by incompetent venous valves within the spermatic vein. These are called primary varicoceles. They are more common on the left. This is probably due

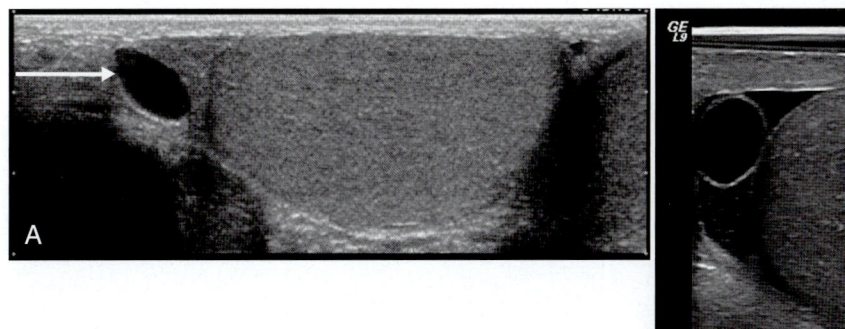
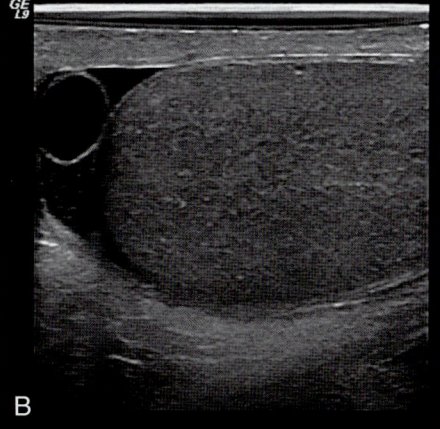
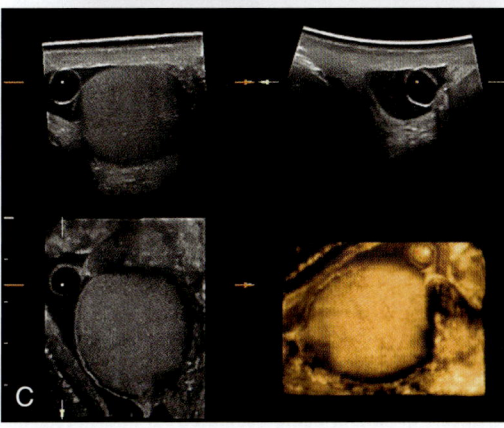

FIG. 23.20 (A) Sagittal image of a patient with a palpable scrotal mass. This image was obtained by scanning directly over the palpable area. It shows a fluid-filled mass with posterior acoustic enhancement located in the head of the epididymis *(arrow)*. This finding is consistent with both spermatocele and epididymal cyst. (B) Conventional two-dimensional sagittal image demonstrated a cystic mass slightly superior and lateral to the right testis. (C) Three-dimensional volume from the same patient showing orthogonal planes and surface rendering *(lower right)* demonstrated smooth walls and confirmed the extratesticular location of the cyst near the epididymal head. The coronal plane image *(lower left)* demonstrated a stalk connecting the cyst to the epididymal head, confirming the diagnosis of a pedunculated cystic appendix epididymis.

to the mechanics pertaining to the left spermatic vein and the left renal vein. The spermatic vein empties into the left renal vein at a steep angle, which may inhibit blood flow return. The left renal vein can become compressed between the aorta and the superior mesenteric artery. Secondary varicoceles are caused by increased pressure on the spermatic vein. This may be the result of renal hydronephrosis, an abdominal mass, or liver cirrhosis. An abdominal malignancy invading the left renal vein may cause a varicocele with noncompressible veins. Any noncompressible varicocele in a man older than 40 years of age should prompt a search for a retroperitoneal mass.

Varicoceles have a relationship with impaired fertility. They are more common in infertile men. Treatment of the varicocele has been shown to improve sperm count in up to 53% of cases, but controversy surrounds the treatment of varicoceles for infertility. Uncommonly, varicoceles may extend within the testis. These will be located near the mediastinum. Intratesticular varicoceles have unknown clinical significance, but it is possible that they will affect male fertility by the same mechanism as extratesticular varicoceles.

Sonographic Findings. Ultrasound imaging of a varicocele shows numerous tortuous tubes of varying sizes within the spermatic cord near the epididymal head. The tubes may contain echoes that move with real-time imaging. This represents slow venous flow (Fig. 23.21). Varicoceles measure more than 2 mm in diameter. They tend to increase diameter in response to the Valsalva maneuver. Scanning with the patient in an upright position will enhance the visibility of a varicocele because the veins will become more distended. Some authors advocate using a standing position routinely; others believe that supine scanning with the Valsalva maneuver and color Doppler imaging is adequate. With either protocol, color and spectral Doppler are used to confirm the presence of venous flow and to demonstrate retrograde filling with the Valsalva maneuver (see Fig. 23.21C). Color Doppler settings must be sensitized for slow flow to detect the venous signal in varicoceles. Flash artifact may be a problem with color Doppler imaging during a Valsalva maneuver. It is helpful to instruct the patient to hold as still as possible during the maneuver and to carefully adjust the color settings so that the PRF and wall filter are sensitized but not so low that flash artifact fills the screen with a small movement.

Intratesticular varicocele has the sonographic appearance of straight or serpiginous channels coursing from the mediastinum into the testicular tissue. Color and spectral Doppler are used to identify these channels as dilated veins. On grayscale imaging, the appearance can mimic that of tubular ectasia of the rete testis. Color Doppler will differentiate between intratesticular varicocele and tubular ectasia of the rete testis, as the latter shows no flow (Fig. 23.22).

Scrotal Hernia

Hernias occur when bowel, omentum, or other structures herniate into the scrotum. Clinical diagnosis is usually sufficient, but ultrasound imaging is helpful when findings are

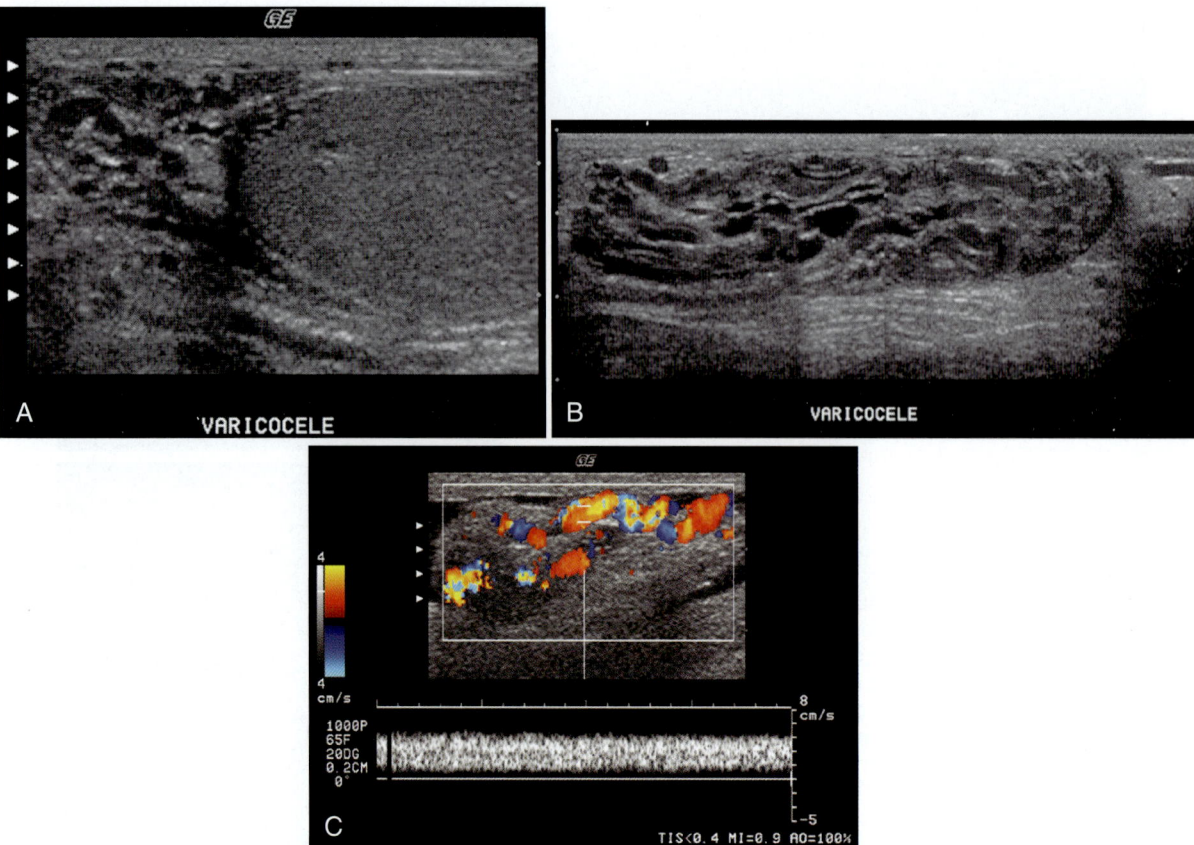

FIG. 23.21 **Varicocele in patient being evaluated for infertility.** (A) Sagittal view of the testis shows dilated tubular structures superiorly. (B) Stitched ultrasound image shows prominent serpiginous venous channels forming a large varicocele on the left. (C) Doppler ultrasound with Valsalva maneuver shows venous flow within the dilated vascular channels, confirming the diagnosis of varicocele.

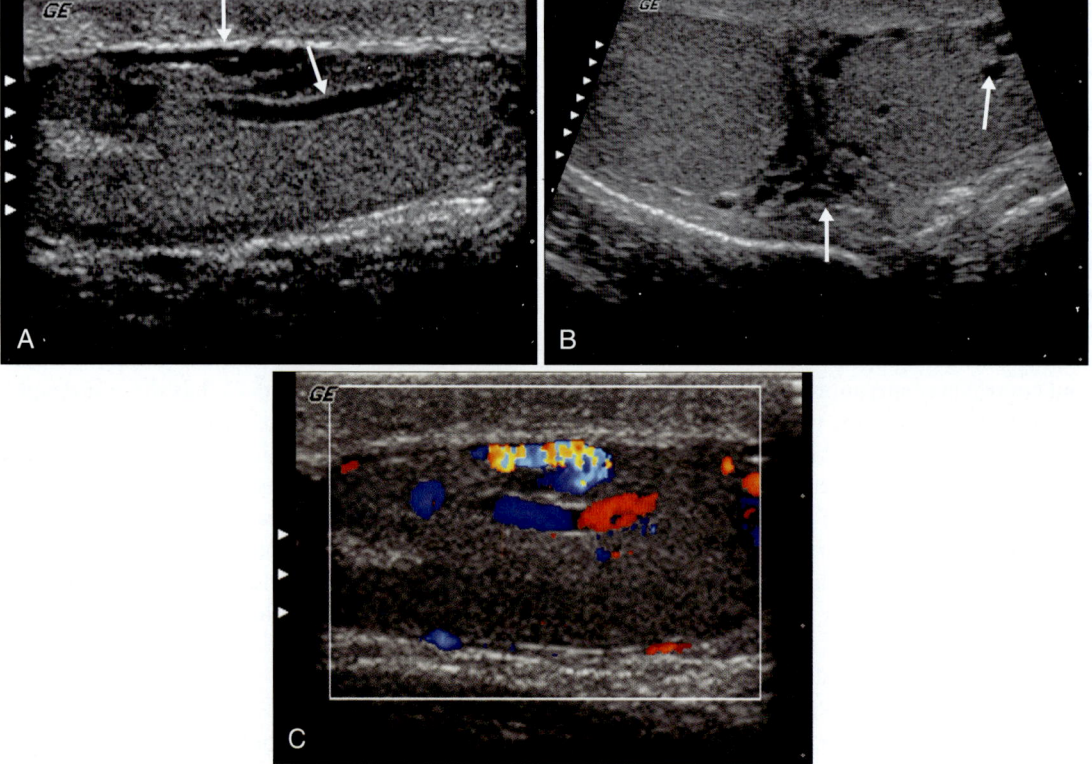

FIG. 23.22 **Intratesticular varicocele.** (A) Sagittal ultrasound image shows prominent connecting tubes with the testis *(arrows)*. (B) Transverse ultrasound image of both testes shows an intratesticular and extratesticular varicocele on the left side *(arrows)*. (C) Color Doppler is used to detect flow within the dilated intratesticular veins during Valsalva maneuver.

equivocal. The bowel is the most commonly herniated structure, followed by the omentum.

Sonographic Findings. Peristalsis of the bowel, seen on real-time imaging, confirms the diagnosis of a scrotal hernia (Fig. 23.23). This can be captured on videotape or as a cine clip for the interpreting physician to review. Unfortunately, peristalsis may not always be visible. Fluid-filled bowel loops are easily recognizable by ultrasound. Air-filled loops and loops that contain solid stool are more difficult to recognize. On ultrasound, air appears as bright echoes with a dirty acoustic shadow or ring artifact. Omental hernias appear brightly echogenic because of the omental fat (Fig. 23.24).

Hydrocele, Pyocele, and Hematocele

A potential space exists between the visceral and parietal layers of the tunica vaginalis. This space is the place where a hydrocele, pyocele, or hematocele will develop. Normally, a small amount of fluid is present in this cavity, and this should not be confused with the presence of a hydrocele. A hydrocele contains serous fluid and is the most common cause of painless scrotal swelling. Hydroceles may have an unknown cause (idiopathic) but are commonly associated with epididymo-orchitis and torsion. They may also be found in patients following trauma or development of a neoplasm. Hydroceles associated with neoplasms tend to be smaller than those associated with other causes. Pyoceles and hematoceles are much less common than hydroceles.

A pyocele is a collection of pus. Pyoceles occur with untreated infection or when an abscess ruptures into the space between the layers of the tunica vaginalis. Hematoceles are associated with trauma, surgery, neoplasms, or torsion. They are collections of blood.

Sonographic Findings. A hydrocele displays a fluid-filled collection located outside the anterolateral aspect of the testis. Hydroceles may be anechoic but most often contain some low-level echoes as a result of cellular debris (Fig. 23.25). The display of low-level echoes is enhanced by high-frequency transducers and harmonic imaging. Hydroceles are more likely

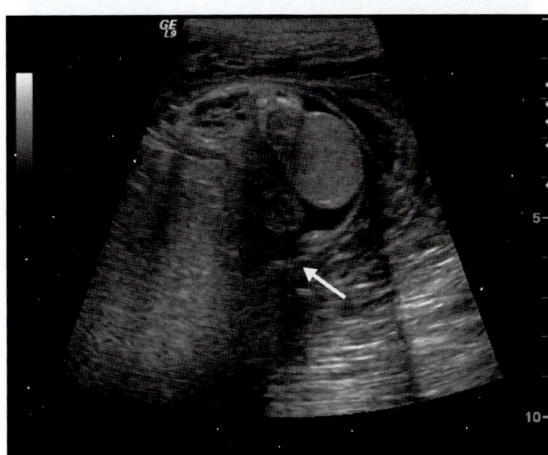

FIG. 23.24 Scrotal hernia. Sagittal ultrasound image in a patient with chronic heart failure and scrotal edema. A large amount of edema is seen in the tissue surrounding the normal testis. A small hydrocele is present. A large hernia is seen protruding into the scrotum and displacing the testis inferiorly (arrow). The hyperechoic appearance of the hernia suggests omental fat content.

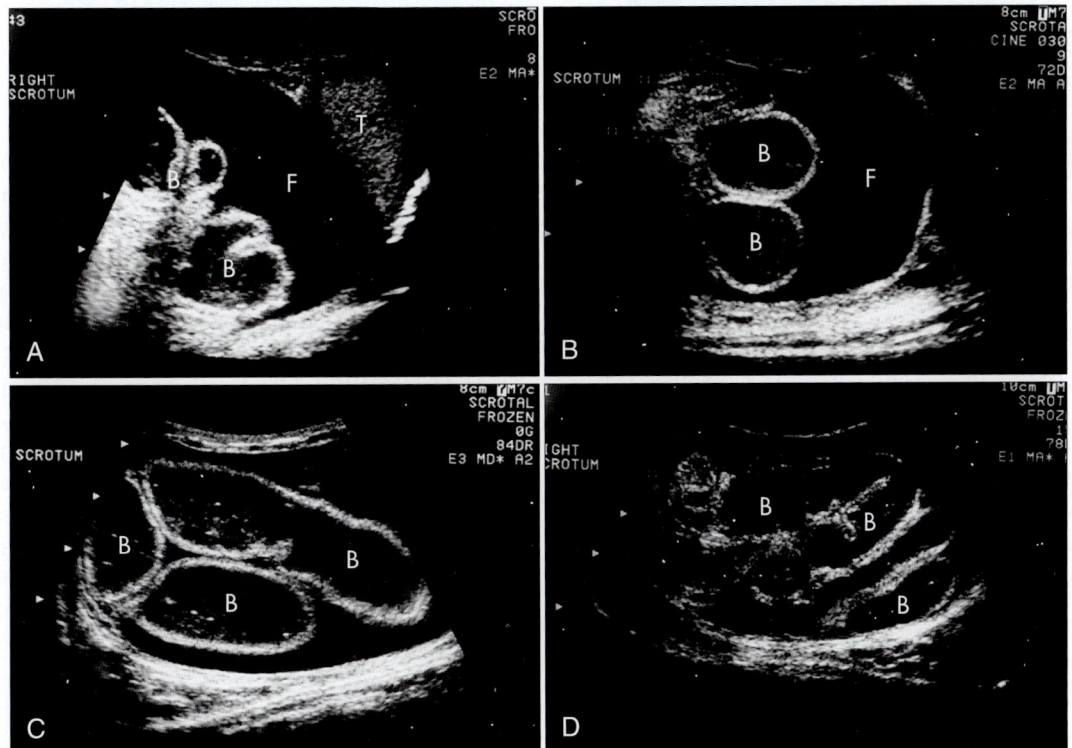

FIG. 23.23 (A–D) Small bowel herniated into the scrotum, representing scrotal hernia. Peristalsis was noted on real-time imaging. *B*, Bowel; *F*, fluid; *T*, testicle.

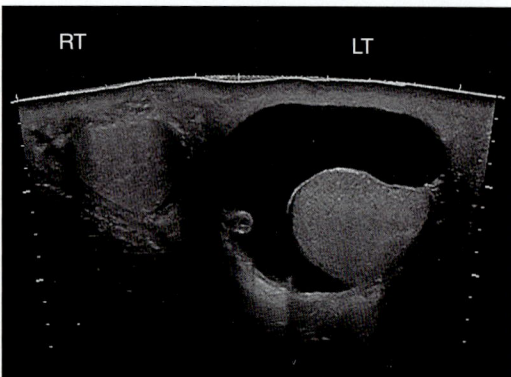

FIG. 23.25 Idiopathic hydrocele formation in patient with scrotal swelling and tenderness. Panoramic view shows the normal right testis. The left testis is compressed because of the large hydrocele.

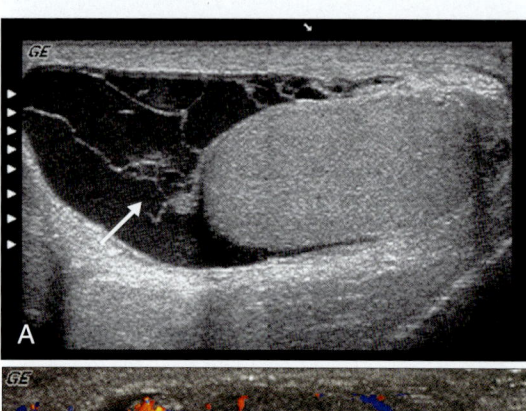

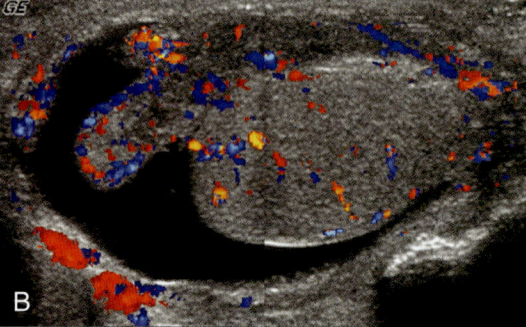

FIG. 23.26 Pyocele formation in patient with severe, untreated epididymo-orchitis. (A) Sagittal ultrasound image shows the multiseptated fluid collection containing internal debris *(arrow)*. (B) Color Doppler image shows increased perfusion in the epididymis, testis, and surrounding tissue.

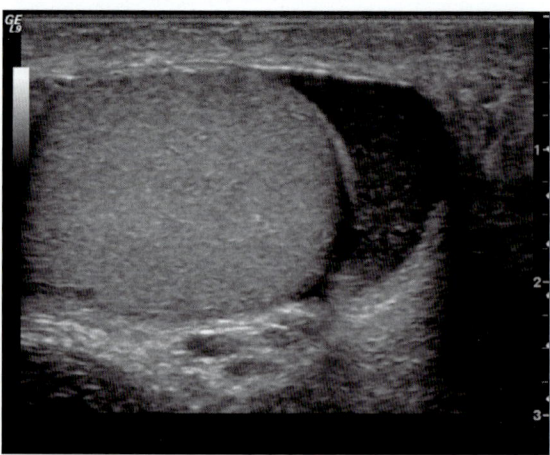

FIG. 23.27 **Hematocele in patient from the emergency department with scrotal trauma.** Sagittal ultrasound image shows a small fluid collection with numerous bright echoes.

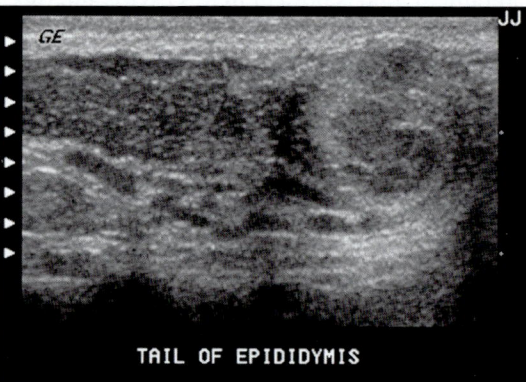

FIG. 23.28 **Painful epididymal mass in patient with history of vasectomy.** Sagittal ultrasound image of epididymis shows a small, heterogeneous mass in the tail of the epididymis, possibly representing a sperm granuloma.

to appear anechoic with transducer frequencies below 7 MHz or when low dynamic range settings are used. Hydroceles associated with infection show more internal echoes and septations. Sonographically, pyoceles and hematoceles are indistinguishable. They both contain internal echoes, thickened septations, and loculations (Figs. 23.26 and 23.27). Ultrasound depiction of air within the space indicates an abscess, although an abscess may occur without the presence of air.

Sperm Granuloma

Sperm granulomas occur as a chronic inflammatory reaction to extravasation of spermatozoa. They are most frequently seen in patients with a history of vasectomy. A sperm granuloma may be located anywhere within the epididymis or the vas deferens. The main role of ultrasound imaging is to determine whether the mass is intratesticular or extratesticular. Extratesticular masses have a much lower rate of malignancy compared with intratesticular masses. Sperm granulomas cannot be reliably differentiated from epididymal tumors by ultrasound imaging. However, a clinical history of vasectomy will help to target the differential diagnosis. Additionally, sperm granulomas are often painful. This aids in their differentiation from epididymal tumors, which are usually painless.

Sonographic Findings. Sonographic imaging shows a well-defined solid mass that may appear hypoechoic or isoechoic to the epididymis. These masses are often heterogeneous (Fig. 23.28). Calcifications are not commonly present. Increased flow may be seen with color Doppler when inflammation is present.

Benign Testicular Masses

Tubular Ectasia of the Rete Testis. The rete testis is located at the hilum of the testis, where the mediastinum resides.

Tubular ectasia of the rete testis is an uncommon, benign condition. It is associated with the presence of a spermatocele, an epididymal or testicular cyst, or other epididymal obstruction on the same side as the dilated tubules. It is more commonly seen in patients 45 years of age or older.

Sonographic Findings. The normal rete testis may not be clearly depicted with ultrasound imaging. High-resolution imaging sometimes allows visualization of the normal rete testis as very tiny tubular structures near the mediastinum. Tubular ectasia appears as prominent hypoechoic channels near the echogenic mediastinum testis (Fig. 23.29). Color Doppler can confirm the avascular nature of the tubules. Tubular ectasia has a similar sonographic appearance to intratesticular varicocele. These conditions can be differentiated using Doppler interrogation because the varicocele will demonstrate slow venous flow. To demonstrate slow flow, the color Doppler must be sensitized by using a low PRF and wall filter setting. The Valsalva maneuver should be used to enhance flow if a varicocele is present. If these and other adjustments are not made to the color controls, flow within a varicocele may not be detected, and results may be misinterpreted.

Cyst. Intratesticular cysts were once thought to be uncommon but are seen more often with more frequent use of ultrasound imaging. Cysts are common in men older than 40 years of age and have an association with extratesticular spermatoceles. They are located near the mediastinum. They may be single or multiple and of variable size. Cysts are incidental findings on sonography and do not require treatment.

Sonographic Findings. The sonographic appearance of cysts is the same throughout the body. Simple cysts are anechoic with posterior acoustic enhancement and a smooth border (Fig. 23.30).

Microlithiasis. Microlithiasis is an uncommon condition characterized by tiny calcifications within the testis. These microcalcifications are smaller than 3 mm. Microlithiasis is usually a bilateral condition. It has been reported to have an

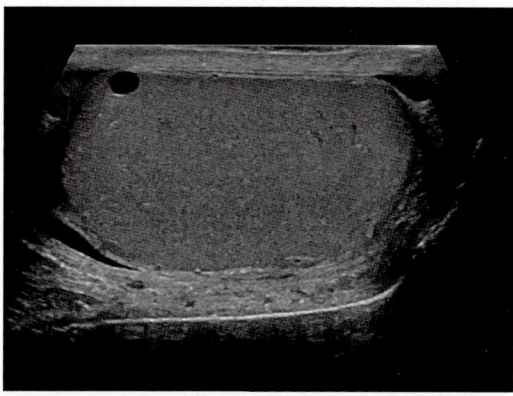

FIG. 23.30 Simple testicular cyst. Sagittal ultrasound image was obtained using virtual convex to obtain a wide field of view. A small, simple cyst is shown in the superior pole of the testis. Note the smooth borders and the posterior acoustic enhancement.

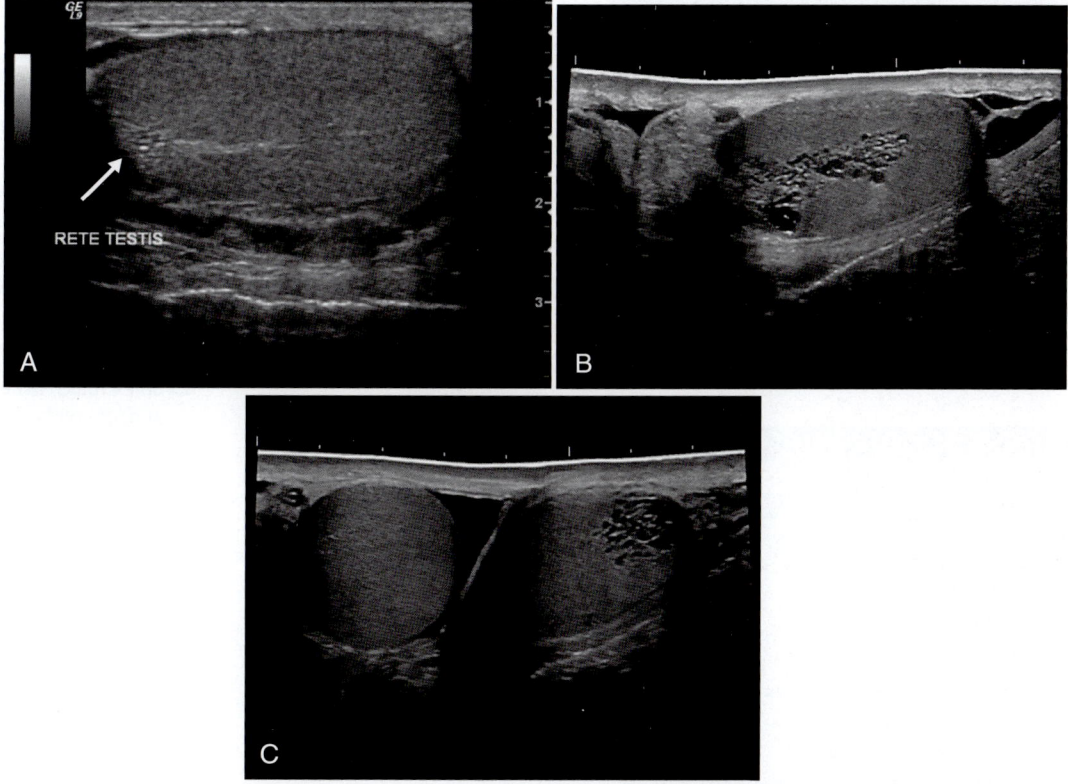

FIG. 23.29 (A) Mild dilation of the rete testis in patient with spermatocele. Sagittal ultrasound image shows enlarged tubular structures located near the mediastinum testis. (B) Sagittal panoramic view on the same patient demonstrates the dilated tubules of the rete testis in the area of the testicular mediastinum. (C) Panoramic transverse image through the right and left testis shows dilation of the rete testis on the left in a patient with a large spermatocele (not shown).

association with testicular malignancy, but the exact nature of this is unknown. Annual follow-up of patients with testicular microlithiasis is recommended by some to exclude the development of neoplasm. Microlithiasis has also been associated with cryptorchidism, Klinefelter syndrome, infertility, varicoceles, testicular atrophy, and male pseudohermaphroditism.

Sonographic Findings. The sonographic appearance of testicular microlithiasis is of multiple bright, nonshadowing foci scattered throughout the testis (Fig. 23.31). The microliths may be numerous or few but are not considered to be abnormal unless more than five appear on any single image (Fig. 23.32).

Malignant Testicular Masses

Table 23.6 lists the sonographic findings for solid malignant masses.

Germ Cell Tumors. Testicular cancer is not common, accounting for only 1% of cancers in men, but it is the most common malignancy in men between 15 and 35 years of age. Fortunately, testicular cancer is one of the most curable forms of cancer. It is more common in white men than black men. Testicular cancer occurs most frequently between ages 20 and 34 years. Undescended testes are 2.5 to 8 times more likely to develop cancer.

Most patients have no other symptoms except a painless lump, testicular enlargement, or vague discomfort in the scrotum. The primary goal of the ultrasound examination in testicular tumors is to determine the mass location and differentiate between cystic and solid composition. Extratesticular masses are usually benign, whereas intratesticular masses are more likely to be malignant. Intratesticular cysts are benign masses, but care must be taken to ensure that a cyst is simple because some testicular cancers contain cystic components. Some benign conditions may mimic malignancy. These include hematoma, orchitis (especially when focal), abscess, infarction, and sperm granuloma. Obtaining a thorough patient history is very important because it will help to differentiate among these conditions.

In general, testicular tumors are divided into germ cell and non–germ cell tumors. Germ cell tumors are associated with elevated levels of human chorionic gonadotropin and alpha-fetoprotein. Approximately 95% of all testicular tumors are of germ cell type and are highly malignant. Non–germ cell tumors are generally benign. The most common type of germ cell tumor is seminoma, followed by mixed embryonal cell tumors and teratocarcinomas. Other less common germ cell tumors include yolk sacs, choriocarcinomas, teratomas, and other combinations of these cell types. The sonographer

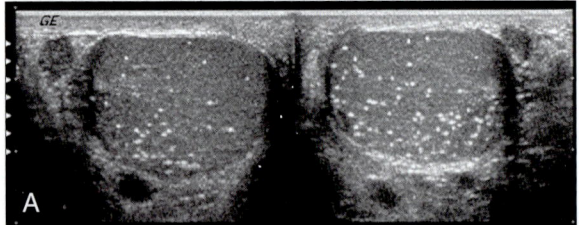
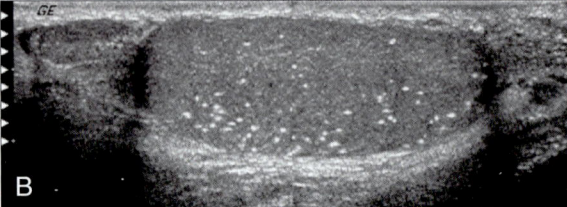

FIG. 23.31 Testicular microlithiasis. (A) Stitched transverse ultrasound image showing both testes with numerous brightly echogenic foci throughout. (B) Sagittal ultrasound image showing testis with fewer microliths.

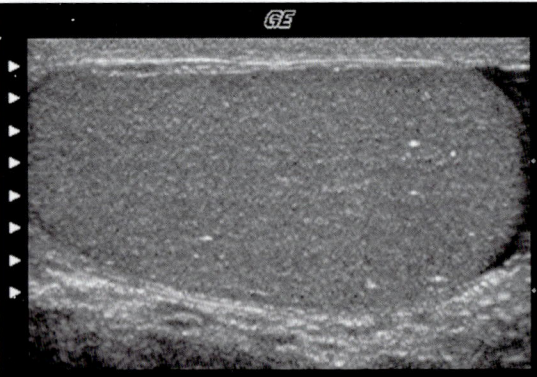

FIG. 23.32 Sagittal ultrasound image showing testis with fewer microliths. More than five microcalcifications per image are considered abnormal. Note the absence of shadowing.

TABLE 23.6	Solid Malignant Masses
Tumor	Sonographic Findings
Seminoma	Hypoechoic lesion Smooth, well-defined borders
Embryonal cell carcinoma	Small hypoechoic mass Areas of increased echogenicity due to calcification Irregular borders May contain cystic areas
Teratoma	Complex mass, usually cystic and/or solid Well-defined borders Acoustic shadowing
Choriocarcinoma	Irregular borders Complex lesion Metastasis usually seen
Metastasis	Solid hypoechoic lesion (uncommonly may appear as hyperechoic or mixed echogenicity)
Lymphoma and leukemia	Enlarged testis Diffuse or focal areas of decreased echogenicity
Chronic lymphocytic leukemia	Well circumscribed Anechoic Through-transmission

must remember that although testicular masses can be clearly described and differentiated using ultrasound, the examination cannot confirm the histology of the neoplasm. However, the sonographic features of a mass may suggest a certain type of tumor.

Sonographic Findings. Ultrasound is nearly 100% sensitive for detecting tumors. Sonographically, most tumors appear as focal, hypoechoic masses (see Table 23.6). Seminomas tend to be homogeneous, hypoechoic masses with a smooth border (see Figs. 23.27, 23.33, and 23.34). They often do not contain calcification or cystic components. In comparison, embryonal cell carcinoma is heterogeneous and is less well circumscribed. It may contain areas of increased echogenicity resulting from calcification, hemorrhage, or

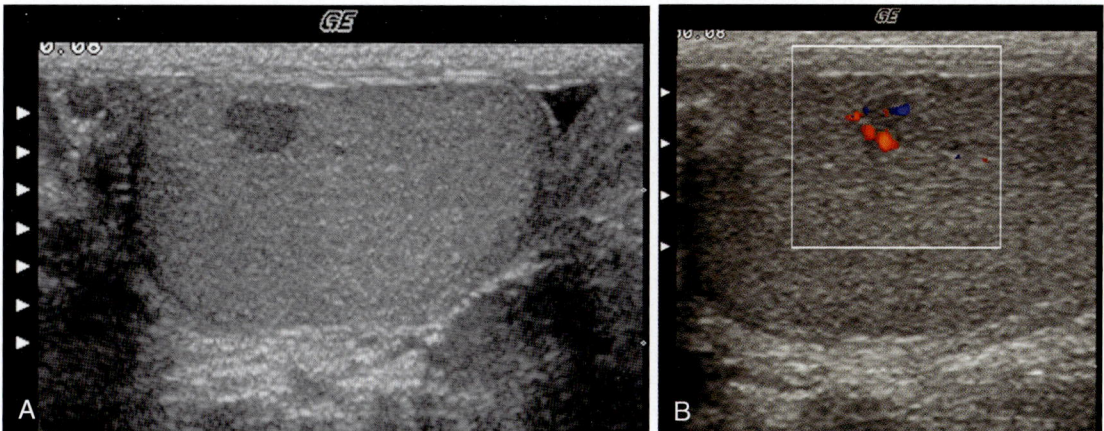

FIG. 23.33 **Small seminoma.** (A) Sagittal ultrasound image shows a small, hypoechoic mass within the testis. Note the presence of a small hydrocele. (B) Color Doppler shows increased vascularity to the mass.

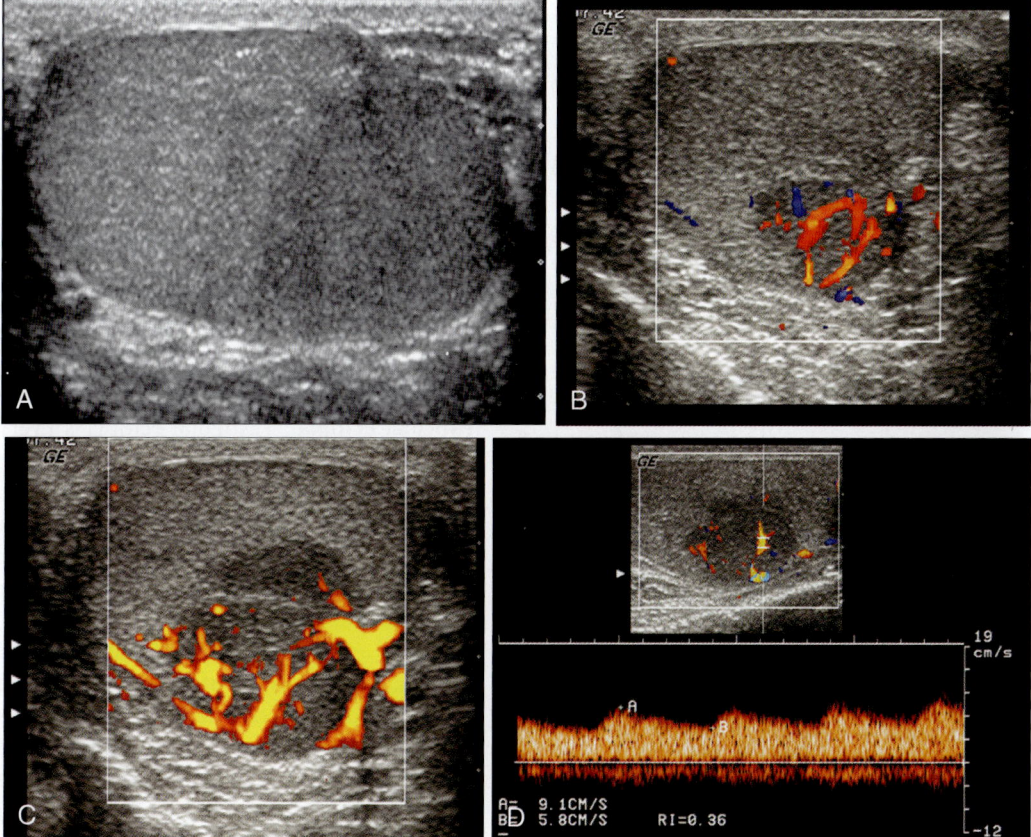

FIG. 23.34 **Germ cell testicular tumor.** (A) Transverse ultrasound image shows heterogeneous echotexture throughout the testis. The tumor is primarily hypoechoic. (B) Color Doppler shows distortion of the normal vessel architecture within the testis. Increased flow is seen within the mass. (C) Power Doppler clearly shows the distorted vasculature of the testis within the mass. (D) Spectral Doppler waveforms obtained within the mass show low resistance with prominent end-diastolic velocities characteristic of tumor flow. Doppler waveforms have not been shown to reliably differentiate between benign and malignant flow patterns.

fibrosis (see Fig. 23.28). Cystic components are found in up to one-third of embryonal cell carcinomas (Fig. 23.35). Embryonal cell tumors are more aggressive than seminomas, often invading the tunica albuginea and distorting the testicular contour. Teratomas may show dense foci that produce acoustic shadowing. They are normally heterogeneous but have well-defined borders. Teratomas are usually benign in children but malignant in adults. Choriocarcinoma has a varied sonographic appearance because of mixed cell types. Its appearance is determined by the dominant cell type, but it typically has irregular borders (see Fig. 23.29). Ultrasound imaging cannot differentiate malignant from benign masses. Neither color Doppler nor Doppler waveforms can reliably distinguish between flow patterns of benign and malignant tumors.

Metastasis. Metastasis to the testicle is rare, normally occurring later in life. The primary tumor may originate from the prostate or kidneys; less common sites include lung, pancreas, bladder, colon, thyroid, and melanoma. Metastasis to the testicle is bilateral, with multiple lesions found.

▸ *Sonographic Findings.* Sonographically, metastasis appears as a solid hypoechoic mass, although it has been reported as hyperechoic or a mixture of both (see Table 23.6).

Lymphoma and Leukemia

Malignant lymphoma makes up 1% to 7% of all testicular tumors and is the most common bilateral secondary testicular neoplasm affecting men older than 60 years.

Leukemic involvement of the testicle is the next most common secondary testicular neoplasm, most often found in children. Of children with leukemia, 8% have been reported to have testicular involvement.

Clinically, patients may experience weight loss, anorexia, and weakness. The testicle may become enlarged, and the tumor may be bilateral or unilateral.

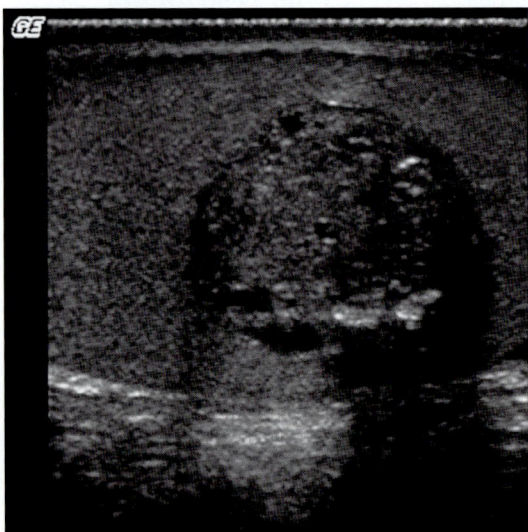

FIG. 23.35 Heterogeneous testicular tumor. Sagittal ultrasound image of a testicular tumor containing calcium and cystic components. Although this pattern is not specific, it is typical of embryonal cell tumor.

▸ *Sonographic Findings.* Sonographically, lymphoma and leukemia appear similar. The testes may appear homogeneously hypoechoic or may contain multiple focal areas of decreased echogenicity (see Table 23.6). Chronic lymphocytic leukemia may appear as a focal, well-circumscribed, anechoic mass with through-transmission. Increased vascularity is seen with color Doppler imaging.

Congenital Anomalies

Cryptorchidism (Undescended Testicle). During fetal growth, the testes first appear in the retroperitoneum near the kidneys. They descend into the scrotum from the inguinal canal shortly before birth or early in the neonatal period. The terms *undescended testis* and **cryptorchidism** describe a condition in which the testis has not descended into the scrotum and cannot be brought into the scrotum with external manipulation. The undescended testis may be in the abdomen, inguinal canal, or other ectopic location. In most cases (up to 80%), the testis is found in the inguinal canal and is usually palpable. Because the testes do not descend until late in pregnancy, this condition is more common in premature babies. Cryptorchidism is bilateral in 10% to 25% of cases.

Surgical treatment of an undescended testicle by freeing it from the structures and implanting it into the scrotum is known as *orchiopexy*. If orchiopexy is not performed at an early age, multiple complications can occur. Exposure of the testis to higher temperatures than that found in the scrotum can prohibit spermatogenesis and result in infertility. Undescended testes are much more likely to develop testicular cancer. The risk of cancer is not reduced by orchiopexy, but it does allow the testis to be more easily palpated so that a lump may be detected and treated earlier. Testicular torsion is also more common with undescended testes.

▸ *Sonographic Findings.* On ultrasound, the undescended testis is smaller and less echogenic than the normal testis. It is usually oval with a homogeneous texture (Fig. 23.36). Rarely, the mediastinum is seen.

Testicular Ectopia. Testicular ectopia is a very rare condition. Unlike an undescended testicle, an ectopic testicle cannot be manipulated into the correct path of descent. The most common site for the ectopic testicle to rest is the superficial inguinal pouch. Other sites include the perineum, femoral canal, suprapubic area, penis, diaphragm, and the other scrotal compartment.

Anorchia. Anorchia is rare. Unilateral anorchia, or monorchidism, is found in 4% of patients with a nonpalpable testis. It is more common on the left side, and definitive diagnosis depends on surgical diagnosis. Causes include intrauterine testicular torsion and other forms of decreased vascular supply to the testicle in utero. Bilateral anorchia is found in only 0.6% to 1.0% of patients with a nonpalpable testis. Patients have a male XY genotype. On physical examination, the scrotum is an empty, hypoplastic sac with a micropenis. These patients also have delayed onset of puberty, usually caused by an imbalance of hormones.

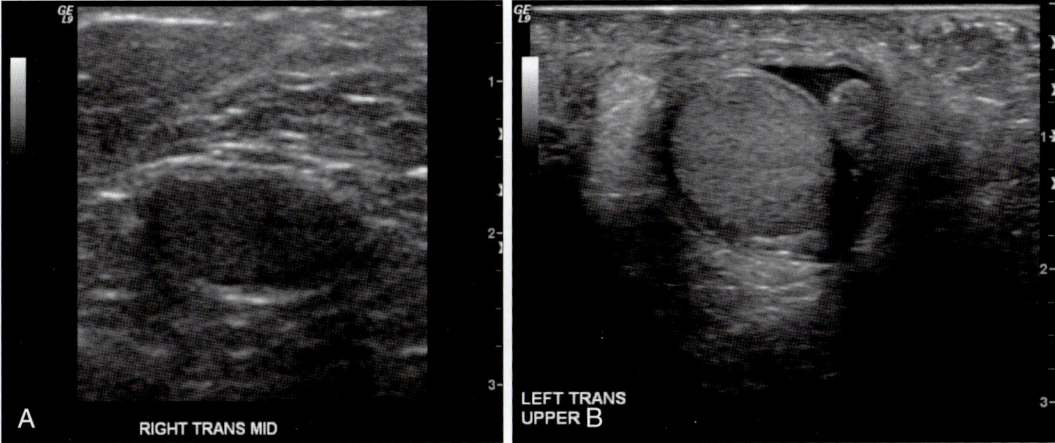

FIG. 23.36 Undescended right testicle (A) with normal left testicle (B). The undescended testis is smaller and hypoechoic compared with the normal left testis. The right testicle was located within the right inguinal canal.

Polyorchidism (Testicular Duplication). Polyorchidism is a very rare disorder, with only 80 cases reported. It is more common on the left side (75%) and is bilateral in 5% of cases. Testicular duplication is usually found in the scrotum but has also been found in the inguinal canal or retroperitoneum. The incidence of malignancy, cryptorchidism, inguinal hernia, and torsion is increased with polyorchidism. The duplicated testis is usually small, and its efferent spermatic system is completely absent.

Key Pearls

- The testes are symmetric, oval-shaped glands residing in the scrotum.
- Sonographically, the testes appear as smooth, medium-gray structures with a fine echotexture.
- The epididymis is a 6- to 7-cm tubular structure beginning superiorly and then coursing posterolateral to the testis.
- Right and left testicular arteries arise from the abdominal aorta just below the level of the renal arteries.
- Venous drainage of the scrotum occurs through the veins of the pampiniform plexus.
- The sonographic findings associated with scrotal rupture include focal alteration of the testicular parenchymal pattern, interruption of the tunica albuginea, irregular testicular contour, scrotal wall thickening, and hematocele.
- Epididymo-orchitis is infection of the epididymis and testis and most commonly results from the spread of a lower urinary tract infection via the spermatic cord.
- Torsion of the spermatic cord occurs as a result of abnormal mobility of the testis within the scrotum. An anomaly termed the *bell clapper deformity* is the most common cause of this condition.
- Cysts are benign fluid collections that may be located within the testis or in the extratesticular structures. Most scrotal cysts are extratesticular.
- A varicocele is an abnormal dilation of the veins of the pampiniform plexus (located within the spermatic cord). Varicoceles are usually caused by incompetent venous valves within the spermatic vein.
- Hernias occur when bowel, omentum, or other structures herniate into the scrotum.
- A potential space exists between the visceral and parietal layers of the tunica vaginalis. This space is the place where a hydrocele, pyocele, or hematocele will develop.
- A hydrocele contains serous fluid and is the most common cause of painless scrotal swelling. Hydroceles may have an unknown cause (idiopathic) but are commonly associated with epididymo-orchitis and torsion.
- A pyocele is a collection of pus. Pyoceles occur with untreated infection or when an abscess ruptures into the space between the layers of the tunica vaginalis.
- Sperm granulomas occur as a chronic inflammatory reaction to extravasation of spermatozoa. They are most frequently seen in patients with a history of vasectomy.
- The rete testis is located at the hilum of the testis, where the mediastinum resides. Tubular ectasia of the rete testis is an uncommon, benign condition. It is associated with the presence of a spermatocele, an epididymal or testicular cyst, or other epididymal obstruction on the same side as the dilated tubules.
- The sonographic appearance of testicular microlithiasis is of multiple bright, nonshadowing foci scattered throughout the testis.
- Extratesticular masses are usually benign, whereas intratesticular masses are more likely to be malignant.
- In general, testicular tumors are divided into germ cell and non–germ cell tumors.
- Germ cell tumors are associated with elevated levels of human chorionic gonadotropin and alpha-fetoprotein.
- Seminomas tend to be homogeneous, hypoechoic masses with a smooth border.
- Embryonal cell carcinoma is heterogeneous and is less well circumscribed. It may contain areas of increased echogenicity resulting from calcification, hemorrhage, or fibrosis; it may also have cystic components.
- Teratomas may show dense foci that produce acoustic shadowing. They are normally heterogeneous but have well-defined borders.

- Malignant lymphoma makes up 1% to 7% of all testicular tumors and is the most common bilateral secondary testicular neoplasm affecting men older than 60 years.
- The terms *undescended testis* and *cryptorchidism* describe a condition in which the testis has not descended into the scrotum and cannot be brought into the scrotum with external manipulation.
- Surgical treatment of an undescended testicle by freeing it from the structures and implanting it into the scrotum is known as *orchiopexy*.

BIBLIOGRAPHY

American College of Radiology: *ACR standard for performance of scrotal ultrasound examination*, 2001. http://www.acr.org.

Berman JM, Beidle TR, Kunberger LE, et al. Sonographic evaluation of acute intrascrotal pathology. *Am J Roentgenol.* 1996;166:857–861.

Black JAR, Patel A. Sonography of the abnormal extratesticular space. *Am J Roentgenol.* 1996;167:507–511.

Bree RL, Hoang DT. Scrotal ultrasound. *Radiol Clin North Am.* 1996;34:1183.

Dambro TJ, Stewart RR, Carroll BA. The scrotum. In: Rumack CM, Wilson SR, Willi J, eds. *Diagnostic Ultrasound.* ed 2, St Louis: Mosby; 1998.

Dogra VS, Gottlieb RH, Oka M, et al. Sonography of the scrotum. *Radiology.* 2003;227:18–36.

Feole JB, Lee FT. Jr: Doppler sonography in testicular and scrotal imaging. *Curr Opin Urol.* 1998;8:87.

Figler TJ, Olson MC, Kinzler GJ. Polyorchidism and rete testis adenoma: ultrasound and MR findings. *Abdom Imaging.* 1996;21:470.

Horstmann WG, Middleton WD, Melson GL. Scrotal inflammatory disease: color Doppler sonographic findings. *Radiology.* 1991;179:55.

Morse MJ, Whitmere WF. Neoplasm of the testis. In: Walsh P, ed. *Campbell's urology.* ed 7 Philadelphia: Saunders; 1998.

Oh C, Nisenbaum HL, Langer J, et al. Sonographic demonstration, including color Doppler imaging of recurrent sperm granulomas. *J Ultrasound Med.* 2000;19:333–335.

Older RA, Watson LR. Tubular ectasia of the rete testis: a benign condition with a sonographic appearance that may be misinterpreted as malignant. *J Urol.* 1994;152:477–478.

Prando D. Torsion of the spermatic cord. *Ultrasound Q.* 2002;18:41–57.

Ragheb D, Higgins JL. Ultrasonography of the scrotum, technique, anatomy, and pathologic entities. *J Ultrasound Med.* 2002;21:171–185.

Weiss AJ, Kellman GM, Middleton WD, et al. Intratesticular varicocele: sonographic findings in two patients. *Am J Roentgenol.* 1992;158:1061–1063.

CHAPTER 24

Musculoskeletal System

Kevin R. Volz

OBJECTIVES

On completion of this chapter, you should be able to:
- Identify the normal anatomic location and function of the tendon, ligament, muscle, nerve, and bursa
- Know the advantages and disadvantages of sonographic artifacts in musculoskeletal imaging
- Summarize the basic sonographic examinations of the shoulder, wrist/hand, and ankle
- Distinguish normal anatomy from common pathologic conditions of the musculoskeletal system

OUTLINE

Anatomy of the Musculoskeletal System 734
- Skeletal Muscle 734
- Tendons 736
- Ligaments 737
- Bursa 738
- Nerves 739

Musculoskeletal Sonography Artifacts 740
- Anisotropy 741
- Reverberation 742
- Refractile Shadowing 742
- Speed Error Artifacts 743

Sonographic Evaluation of the Musculoskeletal System 743
- Shoulder 744
- Wrist/Hand 747
- Ankle 749

Pathology of the Musculoskeletal System 751
- Shoulder Biceps Tendon Subluxation/Dislocation 751
- Rotator Cuff Tears 751
- Tendinitis 753
- Muscle Tears 754
- Carpal Tunnel Syndrome 755

KEY TERMS

Achilles tendon
Acromioclavicular (AC) joint
Anisotropy
Aponeuroses
Biceps tendon
Bursa
Carpal tunnel
Cartilage interface sign
"Clapper in the bell" sign
Comet-tail artifact
Dorsiflexion
Epineurium
Fasciculi

Guyon canal
Infraspinatus tendon
Ligaments
Muscle
Myelin
Naked tuberosity sign
Nerves
Pennate
Perineurium
Phalen sign
Plantar flexion
Refractile shadowing (edge artifact)
Reverberation

Rotator cuff
Seroma
Speed error artifact
Subscapularis tendon
Synovial sheath
Tendinitis
Tendon
Teres minor tendon
Thompson's test
Tinel sign
Volar

The use of ultrasound imaging to evaluate anatomy and disorders of the musculoskeletal system first began in the 1970s to evaluate Baker cysts and calf inflammation. Since this initial application, musculoskeletal ultrasound imaging has come a long way and has seen a particularly rapid increase both in use and its variety of applications over the last decade. This can be attributed to technological refinements of the ultrasound modality, which have elevated image resolution, tissue contrast, and signal-to-noise ratios pathing the way for significant advancements in soft tissue imaging. For example, the 5- or 7-MHz transducer commonly used in the 1990s is no longer acceptable for imaging superficial structures. Current transducers image clinically using insonating frequencies as high as 17 MHz and exist above 50 MHz, although these only exist for imaging research purposes.

Musculoskeletal ultrasound imaging has been widely used in Europe; furthermore, it is now beginning to reach similar levels of popularity in the United States. Magnetic resonance imaging (MRI) is still considered the gold standard for musculoskeletal imaging; however, ultrasound has demonstrated the ability to serve as a trusted initial diagnostic imaging technique while remaining much more cost-effective than other imaging modalities. Recent literature reported in 2016 that musculoskeletal disorders accounted for $380 billion in US healthcare dollar spending, which was the highest of any other examined health condition.

Other characteristics of ultrasound imaging that make it a great modality to perform imaging of the musculoskeletal system are that it is portable, which enables point of care (POC) imaging in the field or workplace where musculoskeletal injuries are more likely to occur, it provides dynamic imaging capabilities so joints and other musculoskeletal structures can be evaluated while in motion, and of course, is noninvasive and does not require the use of ionizing radiation.

This chapter is intended to provide a foundation for a basic musculoskeletal ultrasound. Imaging of the muscular system is not limited only to muscles but also associated structures such as the tendons, nerves, ligaments, and bursa. Typically, musculoskeletal ultrasound examinations are characterized by the joint or structure in need of evaluation. The most common are the shoulder, elbow, wrist/hand, knee, and ankle/foot. Beyond these joints, musculoskeletal ultrasound is used to image superficial structures in other areas in the presence of pain or inflammation following trauma while attempting to detect foreign bodies and evaluate disease processes. These might include pathologies of the musculoskeletal structures mentioned above but is also commonly used in pediatric imaging, as a guidance tool during interventional procedures, and postoperatively to assess healing.

While musculoskeletal ultrasound has many applications and will undoubtedly continue to grow in popularity, it is technically difficult. Musculoskeletal ultrasound can be overwhelming due to the similar appearance of many different muscles, ligaments, tendons, and nerves. All joints contain similar anatomic structures, and in general, tendons, ligaments, and nerves have a similar sonographic imaging appearance to the untrained eye, regardless of the joint. Further, muscle attachments also appear similar on ultrasound imaging. As such, musculoskeletal ultrasound requires an incredibly strong knowledge of musculoskeletal anatomy coupled with a deep understanding of ultrasound technical settings to detect and accurately evaluate structures and pathology. The first step in sonographic imaging of any musculoskeletal structure is knowing the details of its anatomy and function, followed by its sonographic appearance.

ANATOMY OF THE MUSCULOSKELETAL SYSTEM

Skeletal Muscle

Skeletal muscle is muscle that attaches to bone and is composed of long organized muscle cells, also referred to as *muscle fibers*. The characteristic long muscle fibers are under voluntary control for **muscle** contraction and subsequent joint movement. Groups of muscle fibers are encapsulated by a thin connective tissue layer called the perimysium. These groupings of muscle fibers are referred to as muscle bundles. Several muscle bundles exist within each muscle and can be thought of as muscle fibers compartments that exist parallel to one another. The fibrous tissue of the perimysium appears echogenic sonographically compared to the surrounding hypoechoic muscle fiber tissue, giving muscles a distinct spotted appearance in the short axis, helping to differentiate from other superficial structures.

Also located among and parallel to the muscle bundles are blood vessels, structures of the lymphatic system, and nerve fibers. These are held in place by an outer layer of fibrous connective tissue known as the epimysium that encases the entire muscle, encapsulating all the muscle bundles along with any other anatomical structures. Similar to the perimysium, the fibrous epimysium causes muscles to have an echogenic border and likewise aids in their visualization.

When referring to the anatomical locations of skeletal muscle, the terms origin and insertion are used to describe the locations of muscle attachment to bone. The portion of the muscle that attaches to the mobile bone for which that muscle action controls is designated as the insertion, while the part of the muscle attached to the stationary (or immobile) bone is referred to as the origin. It is a common misconception that the origin refers to the more proximal attachment sites. While this is often happening to align with the proper designation, it is not always the case. Finally, some muscles may have two or more heads and can have more than one origin in more than one location on the bone.

Muscles have fibers that run parallel to the bone, have a fan shape, or form a **pennate** pattern. These feather-like patterns run oblique to the long axis of the muscle and are unipennate, bipennate, multipennate, or circumpennate. Using the feather as a metaphor, feather fibers originate from a central section and spread outward. This is much like the appearance of muscle patterns. Half of a feather is unipennate, whereas the entire feather is bipennate. A multipennate muscle is a division of several feather-like sections in one muscle, and the circumpennate is the convergence of fibers to a central tendon (Fig. 24.1A). The deltoid muscle itself is an example of a unipennate muscle, although it has unipennate, bipennate, multipennate muscle attachments (see Fig. 24.1B). The gastrocnemius muscle in the posterior calf is a bipennate muscle in which the muscle fibers have a central origin (see Fig. 24.1C). The large, flat muscles of the external oblique or the trapezius attach with a large, flat aponeurosis (see Fig. 24.1D).

To begin learning the normal sonographic appearance of muscles, it is easy to use the large quadriceps muscle located in the anterior thigh or the calf muscles of the posterior lower leg. Skeletal muscle imaged in a longitudinal plane appears homogeneous with multiple, fine parallel echoes. Fig. 24.2 provides an example of this as seen on the bipennate gastrocnemius muscle of the calf. The connective tissue epimysium surrounding the muscle fiber bundles produces these echogenic bands. The main portions of the muscle fibers are hypoechoic and radiate toward a central tendon

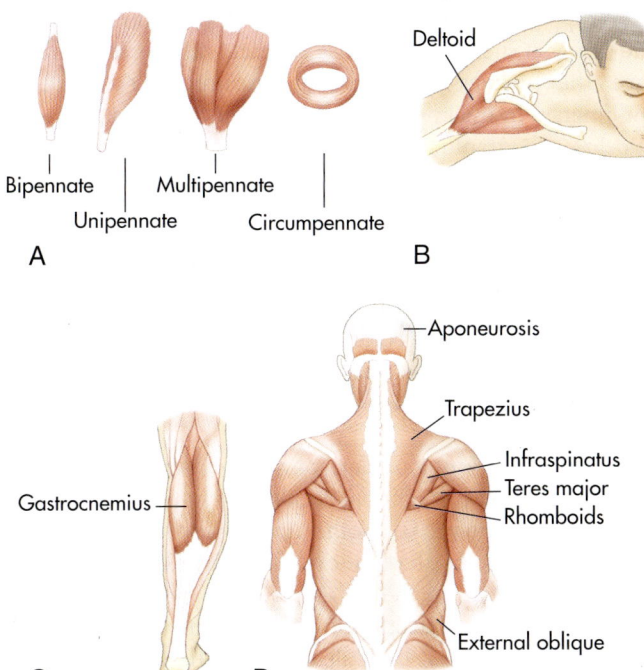

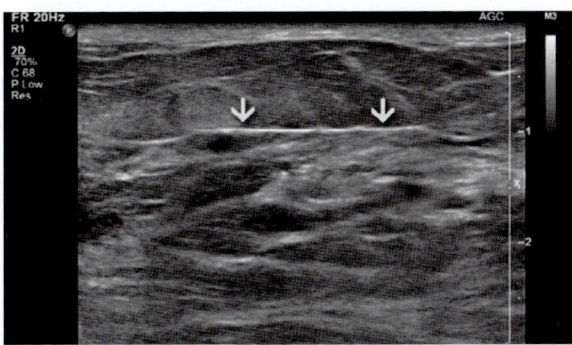

FIG. 24.1 Different muscle types. (A) Unipennate, bipennate, multipennate, and circumpennate muscle patterns. (B) The deltoid muscle is an example of a unipennate muscle and has feather-like fascicles with a unipennate, bipennate, or multipennate attachment. (C) The gastrocnemius muscle in the calf is a bipennate muscle whose fibers have a central origin. (D) The large, flat muscles of the external oblique or the trapezius attach with a large, flat aponeurosis.

FIG. 24.3 Longitudinal gray-scale image showing the dense aponeurosis tissue that connects the muscle to bone. The aponeurosis tissue appears as an echogenic linear structure *(arrows)*.

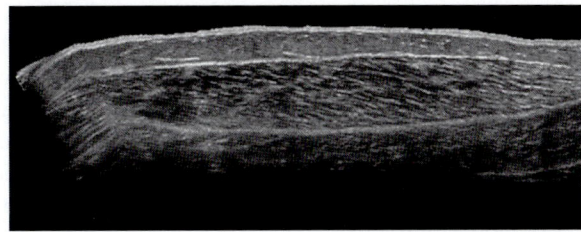

FIG. 24.4 Panoramic gray-scale imaging allows global study of this normal gastrocnemius muscle in the transverse plane.

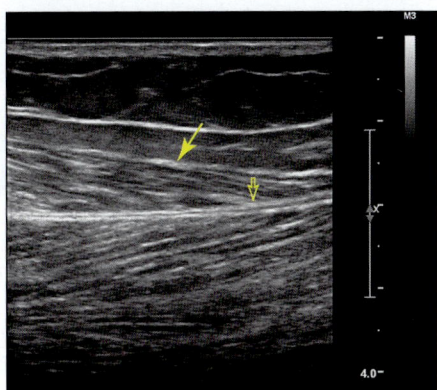

FIG. 24.2 Gray-scale image of the bipennate gastrocnemius muscle in the longitudinal plane demonstrating echogenic obliquely oriented connective tissue *(solid arrow)* between the muscle bundles. A small central tendon *(open arrow)* serves as the anchor for these bundles.

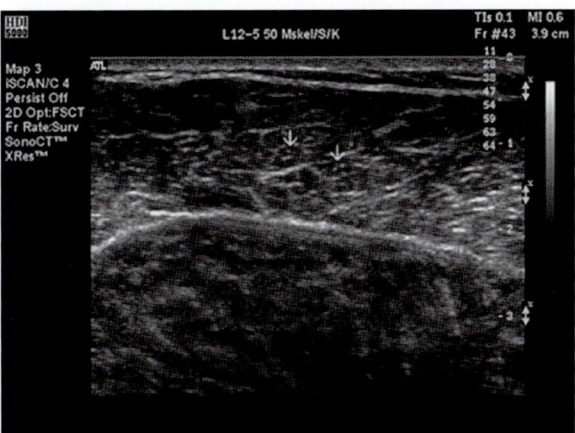

FIG. 24.5 Small punctate echogenicities *(arrows)* image on the transverse muscle.

or aponeurosis (Fig. 24.3). The transverse plane shows a less organized pattern of fine punctate echoes scattered through the muscle bundle. As mentioned previously, the fibrous perimysium fascia tissue that encases the muscle fibers cause these sporadic echogenic areas (Figs. 24.4 and 24.5). Although perimysium fascia appear more echogenic than the sheathed muscle fibers, both are less echogenic than bordering subcutaneous fat or nearby tendons in the extremities.

Several different types of muscles exist in the human body and vary in sonographic appearance based on their type and location. Differing muscle appearance can be deceiving in some areas, such as the hand, in which normal musculature appears similar in echogenicity to a mass or tenosynovitis. Careful scanning and transducer rotation help image the pennate structure of the muscle, aiding in its identification. Normal muscle dynamics are easily imaged in real-time using ultrasound. As muscle contraction occurs, the muscle increases in both thickness and hypoechogenicity. In addition, echogenic connective tissue bands increase in obliquity. Sustained contraction of the muscle has the same sonographic appearance as muscle bundles found in the athletic patient. This reduced muscle echogenicity is a result of hypertrophy and is a normal finding in this patient population.

The operator can also influence muscle echogenicity. Excess external compression from the transducer causes muscle tissue to condense, resulting in increased echogenicity. This can also be influenced by transducer orientation. An oblique orientation will result in falsely increased muscle echogenicity. Ensuring a longitudinal and transverse plane relative to the muscle being imaged with appropriate contact pressure reduces the likelihood of introducing artifactual information. Scanning the contralateral normal side is helpful to ensure scanning technique or the presence of normal anatomical variants do not result in a misinterpretation of images or a misdiagnosis.

Tendons

Attachment of the muscle occurs at the proximal and distal portions of the bundle. This attachment, which is a collection of tough collagenous fibers, is known as a **tendon**. Tendons may be cordlike or flat sheets called **aponeuroses**. This type of attachment occurs in flat muscles, such as the rectus abdominis in the abdomen. Tendons consist of elastic collagen fibers which enable them to stretch and flex around other structures. Tendons are avascular, meaning they are minimally perfused. They heal slowly following injury, which is why tendon injuries are often incapacitating.

Tendons exist with or without a surrounding tubular sac called the **synovial sheath**. The synovial sheath has two layers separated by fluid (synovial membrane). They are found in the tendons of the shoulder, hand, wrist, and ankle. This sheath plays an important role while imaging with ultrasound, as the surrounding sheath causes the tendon to appear with an echogenic border (Fig. 24.6). Knowing this feature can assist in the identification of these tendons and delineation of their borders. The biceps tendon of the shoulder is another example of a tendon with a synovial sheath (Fig. 24.7). Other tendons, such as the Achilles and patellar, do not have this sheath and instead are surrounded by a layer of lipids or loose connective tissue, causing them to be more difficult to visualize sonographically.

Wrapped around the tendon, the smooth inner layer of the synovial sheath lies in close contact with the tendon surface. The thickness of this sheath measures only a couple of millimeters in thickness; however, because it is fluid filled, it appears sonographically as a hypoechoic halo surrounding the tendon. Inflammation of synovial sheath (often including tendon involvement) can occur but is often easily recognized with ultrasound imaging as an increase in the size of the hypoechoic halo from the increased amount of fluid present in the synovium in the acute phase. Hyperemia may also be seen if imaged with color Doppler imaging. Areas of high stress in the hand, wrist, and ankle also contain tendons with sheaths and will be discussed in further detail throughout this chapter.

Paratenon, a loose areolar connective tissue, fills the fascial compartment of tendons lacking a synovial sheath. The dense epitendineum is another layer of connective tissue that closely adjoins the tendon. The epitendineum appears slightly echogenic to the adjacent tendon with ultrasound. Unfortunately, the densities of the epitendineum and tendon are similar, making it difficult to differentiate the interfaces of these two structures. Fortunately, tendons without a synovial sheath tend to be large in size and can be imaged without

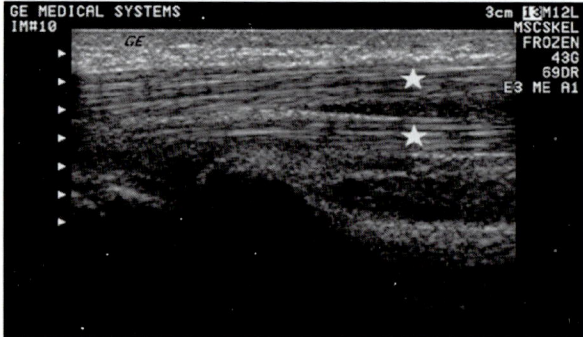

FIG. 24.6 Superficial and deep flexor tendons *(stars)* have a surrounding synovial sheath that allows smooth motion of the pulley system within the hand. Tendon movement can be seen in real-time with movement of the digits.

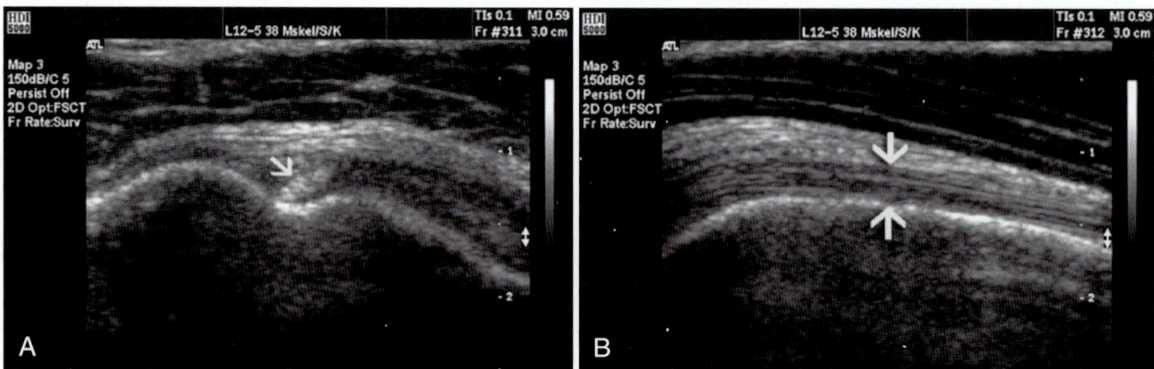

FIG. 24.7 (A) Gray-scale image of the rounded biceps tendon in the transverse plane. The tendon is seen as a hyperechoic structure sitting within the bicipital groove of the humerus *(arrow)*. (B) The longitudinal view has the characteristic pattern seen in tendons encased within a synovial sheath *(arrows)*.

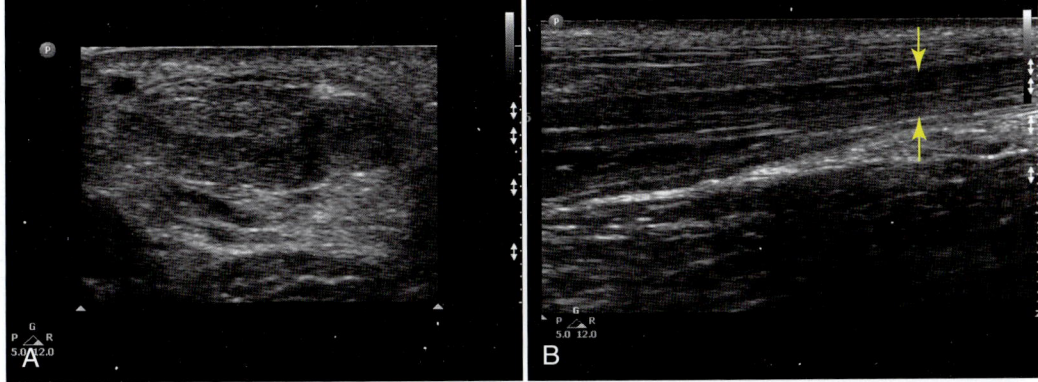

FIG. 24.8 (A) Gray-scale image of the distal Achilles tendon in the transverse plane demonstrates a characteristic oval appearance. With decreased use, the tendon changes shape, becoming round in the sedentary individual. (B) The lack of synovial sheath is evident in the longitudinal view of the tendon. The slight increase in echogenicity *(arrows)* on each side of the tendon is the epitendineum.

much difficulty. Examples of tendons without a synovial sheath include the Achilles, patellar, proximal gastrocnemius, and semimembranosus tendons (Fig. 24.8).

Tendons are high density due to their composition of interwoven and interconnected collagen fibers that run in a parallel path, giving tendons their tubular structure. The numerous interfaces of collagen fascicles provide a strong linear reflector that images well with ultrasound. With increasing transducer insonating frequency, these fibers can be visualized with higher resolution for a more thorough inspection of their quality and a more accurate representation of tendon health. This underscores the need to utilize a transducer capable of imaging at operating frequencies greater than 7 MHz. The ability to depict normal fibrillar hypoechoic pattern in detail is a key component of diagnosing several associated abnormalities.

Care must be taken when imaging tendons because just a slight rotation off axis can produce an image that incorrectly suggests tendinitis. Both transverse and longitudinal planes help image the tendon, along with side-by-side (dual) comparison views with the contralateral side.

The tendon insertion site has its own sonographic characteristics. The joining of the tendon to the bone (enthesis) occurs via a narrow band of fibrocartilage. This avascular structure is approximately 1 cm long and images as a triangular hypoechoic area in the longitudinal plane at the distal end of the tendon. Familiarity with the normal sonographic appearance is important because injury to the tendon in this area results in thickening of the insertion site (Fig. 24.9).

As with all musculoskeletal structures, MRI has been the modality of choice as of late for physicians in the United States when radiologically evaluating suspected musculoskeletal pathology. However, in the context of evaluating tendinous structures, the advent of high-resolution ultrasound has challenged the superiority of MRI, especially when performed by a skilled sonographer using high-quality equipment. Ultrasound's ability to image in real-time and visualize dynamic movement enables clinicians to fully evaluate tendon range of motion to better inform patient management decisions. The high resolution made possible by modern

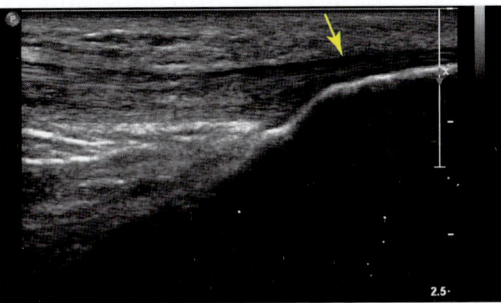

FIG. 24.9 Gray-scale image of the normal Achilles tendon insertion *(arrow)* insertion on the calcaneus and mimics cartilage found in other parts of the body.

high-frequency transducers also allows visualization of the fine tendon fibers compared to normal (healthy) tendons using dual imaging display techniques.

Ligaments

Joint support and strength are largely due to associated **ligaments**, short bands of tough fibrous connective tissue that connect bones to other bones. Ligaments are especially important in the knees, ankles, and shoulders, which are subjected to significant stress from continual and often rapid movements. Like tendons, ligaments are elastic and allow joint flexibility; however, they also limit movement to protect joints from hyperextension or hyperflexion beyond the normal range of motion. As such, ligaments provide support to the joints and are why in situations of ligament injury, stability of the associated joint is compromised.

Compared with other structures in the musculoskeletal system, ligaments are thin and therefore often difficult to image. They typically measure between 2 and 3 mm in thickness (AP). Ligaments are also located outside and superficial to the joint during imaging, so a higher-frequency transducer—10 MHz or greater—and possibly a stand-off pad to aid in visualization should be used during sonographic evaluation. For accurate identification of ligaments, it is critical to adjust ultrasound technical settings throughout the imaging examination. Inappropriately elevated gain settings (from either increased overall gain or time gain compensation [TGC] settings) result in loss of detail due to strong bone reflections. Unlike imaging in other areas of the body, longitudinal imaging of the ligament is the only plane used to visualize injuries. Transverse views are of little help when imaging ligaments as they blend in with surrounding fat of similar echogenicity. As with tendons, dual imaging or side-by-side imaging can help visualize ligaments, especially when compared with the contralateral side.

The composition of ligaments is similar to that of tendons; however, ligaments have less collagen content. This causes them to be less echoic than tendons, but they have the same parallel fascicular echogenic appearance (Fig. 24.10).

The medial collateral ligament (MCL) or tibial collateral ligament connects the medial femoral condyle to the medial proximal tibia and deviates from the usual ligament appearance. This wide, smooth ligament is about 9 cm long and has deep as well as superficial portions. The external superficial portion consists of connective tissue appearing as a dense band connecting the medial femoral condyle to the proximal tibia. The deep layer connects the medial meniscus to the femur and tibia. Sonographic imaging of the MCL reveals a three-layer structure. The superficial and deep layers have a hypoechoic-separating layer. Loose connective tissue forms the middle layer, which provides a potential space for bursae in some individuals (Fig. 24.11).

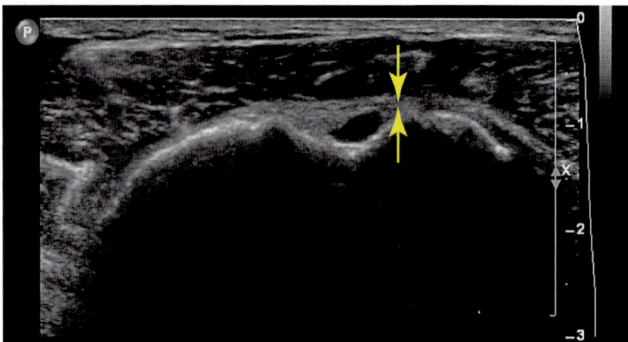

FIG. 24.10 Gray-scale image of the coracohumeral ligament *(between arrows)*. The coracohumeral ligament helps maintain proper location of the long biceps tendon within the bicipital groove. In this image, the biceps tendon demonstrates tenosynovitis with inflammation of the tendon and sheath, resulting in a hypoechoic appearance.

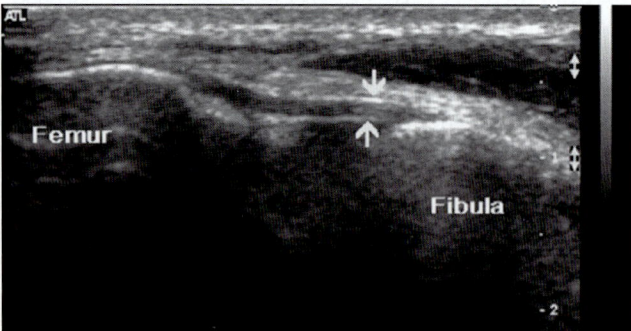

FIG. 24.11 The fibular collateral ligament has a hypoechoic linear structure *(arrows)* as it passes over the lateral meniscus at a slightly oblique course to connect the fibula to the lateral side of the femur.

Bursa

Bursae (**bursa** in the singular form) are saclike structures surrounding muscles, tendons, and ligaments. Bursae contain viscous synovial fluid and are located between bone and soft tissue to reduce friction between bones and other structures of the musculoskeletal system during movement, particularly over bony projections (Figs. 24.12 and 24.13). A synovial membrane encapsulates the bursa, which is the source of synovial fluid production for the bursa. There are over 140 bursae throughout the body. The knee joint has nine bursae—three located anterior and six on the popliteal side of the joint. The major bursa of the body is the subacromial-subdeltoid bursa, found in the shoulder, covering the deep surface of the deltoid muscle.

Two types of bursae are found in the body: communicating and noncommunicating. This categorization describes the relationship of the bursa to the joint space. As the name suggests, the synovial membrane of communicating bursae interacts with the joint space. Bursa-containing joints are referred to as synovial joints.

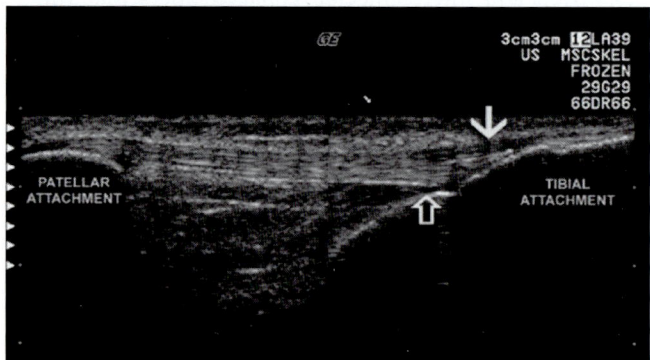

FIG. 24.12 Gray-scale panoramic image of a normal infrapatellar tendon which has multiple bursae, which typically blend in with surrounding tissue. One bursa is seen between the skin and fascia anterior to the tibial tuberosity *(arrow)*, and a second deep bursa is seen between the patellar ligament and the tibial tuberosity *(open arrow)*.

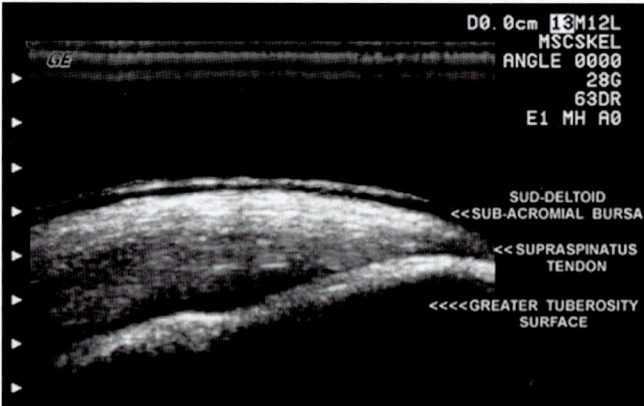

FIG. 24.13 Reconstructed three-dimensional gray-scale image of the subdeltoid-subacromial bursa, which clearly demonstrates the external synovial layer with hypoechoic lubricating fluid. New sonographic technologies, such as three-dimensional imaging, have the ability to remove surrounding tissue signals from the acquired ultrasound data set, making it ideal for bursa imaging.

Because bursae are fluid-filled structures, they are hypoechoic on ultrasound imaging, but in the normal patient are often difficult to image due to their small size. As part of the inflammatory process, fluid accumulation will cause bursae to increase in size and become more echogenic, taking on an appearance similar to that of a complex cyst. Any bursa larger than 2 mm in any dimension is considered abnormal and should be compared with the normal contralateral side. In the presence of enlarged bursae, color Doppler can assist with differentiation from vasculature. A color Doppler finding of hyperemia in the surrounding area to the bursa can also contribute evidence in support of an inflammatory response finding.

One finding related to a communicating bursa often encountered by sonographers is the Baker cyst, located in the medial popliteal fossa. A Baker cyst has a connecting neck between the semimembranosus and medial gastrocnemius tendons to a bursa contained within the knee joint. However, it is more common during musculoskeletal ultrasound imaging to image bursae that do not communicate with the joint space. An example of a superficial noncommunicating type of bursa is the prepatellar bursa.

Nerves

Nerves conduct electrical impulses that transmit motor and sensory signals between the central nervous system and the periphery. Efferent motor nerves originate from the central nervous system and extend into the extremities, among other locations, ending at neuromuscular junctions, also called motor endplates, within skeletal muscles. These nerves innervate skeletal muscles to control movement.

Elements of the peripheral nerve include the nerve fibers, arranged into bundles (**fasciculi**), each encapsulated by dense insulating sheaths of **myelin** (Schwann cells) and connective tissue. The **perineurium** layer surrounds nerve fiber bundles to create compartments of bundles throughout the nerve. These run parallel within the nerve, along with nerve microvasculature in a space called the interfascicular epineurium. The interfascicular epineurium and all its containing structures are surrounded by the outer layer of the nerve—the **epineurium**.

The normal nerve has a mixed echogenic appearance. Nerves appear hyperechoic compared with muscle tissue but are hypoechoic compared with tendons. The echogenicity can be dependent on its location and the surrounding anatomy. However, in general, in the longitudinal plane, peripheral nerves appear hypoechoic from the interfascicular epineurium with a fibrillar pattern of parallel hyperechoic inner linear echoes similar to the tendon. These linear echoes are the hyperechoic perineurium. The outer edge also appears hyperechoic from the collagenous epineurium (Fig. 24.14). In the transverse plane, the nerve fibers and perineurium appear as sporadic hyperechoic echoes within the hypoechoic interfascicular epineurial space (Fig. 24.15). The circular border of the epineurium again appears echogenic.

Differentiating nerves from tendons is a simple task when contrasting the two structures. Dynamic imaging shows

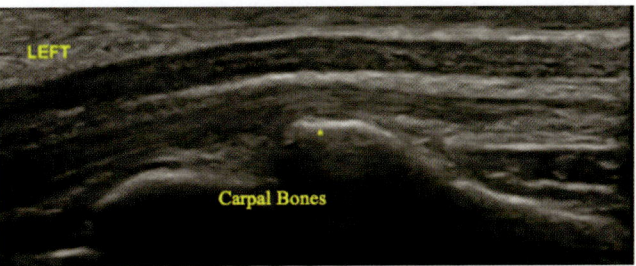

FIG. 24.14 Longitudinal gray-scale image of the median nerve on the ventral side of the forearm and wrist. Deep to the nerve, the carpal bones are seen, more specifically, the lunate *(left)* and the distal radius *(asterisk)*.

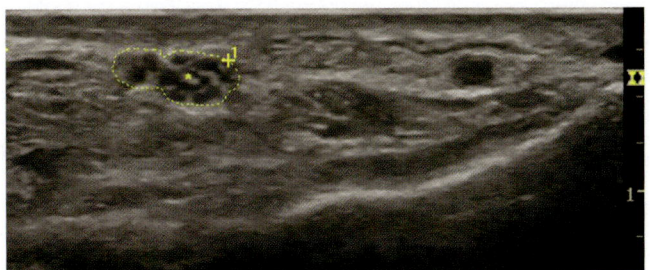

FIG. 24.15 Transverse gray-scale image of the median nerve. The nerve is seen outlined in yellow, within the hyperechoic nerve fibers, and can be appreciated in the hypoechoic nerve.

TABLE 24.1	Nerves Commonly Evaluated With Sonography
	Location
Lower Limb	
Sciatic	Posterior thigh lateral to the hamstring muscle
Popliteal	Popliteal fossa superficial to the popliteal artery and vein
Upper Limb	
Suprascapular	Deep to the trapezius to the infraspinatus fossa
Median	Medial to the biceps tendon and brachial artery, elbow, proximal to and within the carpal tunnel
Radial	Between the brachioradialis and brachialis muscles
Ulnar	Median epicondyle of the elbow, medial to the ulnar artery in Guyon canal

tendons that move when the corresponding joint or muscle contracts. The nerve structure will remain stable within the muscle tissue during movement, but within, excursion of the nerve fibers is seen during associated joint movement. Finally, sonographic artifacts, such as anisotropy (described in the next section of this chapter), are more evident in the tendon than the nerve. Nerves are best imaged with operating frequencies of 10 MHz or greater. Power Doppler is especially helpful in nerve identification, as nerve microvasculature within the interfascicular epineurial space can be detected. Table 24.1 lists nerves commonly evaluated with sonography.

Table 24.2 summarizes the normal sonographic appearance of tendons, ligaments, nerves, muscles, and bursae.

TABLE 24.2	Normal Sonographic Appearance		
Anatomy	General	Longitudinal	Transverse
Muscle	Muscular bundles: hypoechoic Perimysium, epimysium, fascia, fat plane: hyperechoic	Parallel echogenic linear striations within hypoechoic muscle tissue; pennate pattern	Punctate echogenic areas within the hypoechoic muscle
Tendon	Hyperechoic fibrillar linear structure Dynamic with movement of corresponding joint/muscle	Cordlike	Hyperechoic; oval, round, or cuboid
Ligament	Thin, hypoechoic, weakly hyperechoic striations	Striated structures connecting bone to bone	Difficult to image on the transverse plane, similar echogenicity to surrounding soft tissue
Nerve	Mixed echogenic appearance (hypoechoic with hyperechoic linear echoes) Echogenic outer border Hypoechoic to tendons, hyperechoic to muscle May or may not be dynamic with movement of corresponding joint/muscle	Cordlike tubular structure	Hypoechoic with sporadic echogenic fascicles
Bursa	Thin, hypoechoic	Thin linear hypoechoic structure adjacent to a tendon	—

MUSCULOSKELETAL SONOGRAPHY

The musculoskeletal ultrasound examination uses high frequency (>7 MHz) ultrasonic imaging to evaluate superficial structures of the musculoskeletal system and associated pathology. Unlike other areas of sonographic imaging, MSK relies heavily on the dynamic evaluation of structures imaged. Movement of the joint during imaging reveals the full extent of the joint, often enabling visualization of pathology that would not otherwise be seen. Specific movements are part of the examination procedure and should be standardized when developing various joint image acquisition protocols. This is an added layer of complexity compared with other ultrasound imaging areas and requires a thorough understanding of musculoskeletal anatomy. Patient movements also increase the technical difficulty of scanning protocols. The sonographer must maintain consistent imaging while instructing and often assisting the patient in performing the required positional movement. The sonographer must also know to identify abnormalities while scanning, as additional imaging to further evaluate pathologies should be performed whenever it is identified.

Common joints imaged with musculoskeletal ultrasound follow the shoulder, wrist/hands, and ankle/foot. Each of these examinations is described in this section, along with a description of associated anatomy, common pathology, imaging considerations, and recommended views for a standardized examination protocol. In addition, the musculoskeletal sonographer should also be able to image areas outside of these joints. Musculoskeletal ultrasound is commonly used to evaluate trauma or evaluate potential foreign bodies, either of which can occur at any location in the body. Additionally, musculoskeletal interventional procedures are routinely performed under ultrasound guidance, so it is important that the musculoskeletal sonographer be familiar with the general appearance of various musculoskeletal structures and abnormalities to apply this knowledge to any area of the body imaged. Along these lines, sonographers must understand the artifacts specific to the musculoskeletal system so as not to misinterpret them as pathology.

ARTIFACTS

Sonographers and sonologists have the daily challenge of separating artifacts from useful image information. All ultrasound equipment includes algorithms to convert received acoustic soundwaves into an ultrasound image viewable by the operator. Some basic assumptions within these algorithms are a constant speed of sound through soft tissue densities assumed to be 1540 m/sec, the area imaged is within the central beam, and that incident and reflected soundwaves travel in a straight line. Artifacts occur when these basic principles are not met, causing distortion or obstruction of the image. Often these appear as objects not present in the patient but can also present as a structure being erroneously positioned, displaying improper brightness, or completely absent from the image. With ongoing advancements in ultrasound technology, the frequency and severity of artifacts are continuously being reduced; however, it is still critical that anyone performing ultrasound imaging is well aware of the appearance and circumstances that create artifacts. The inability to recognize image artifacts as such can result in image misinterpretation leading to mismanagement of the patient.

Musculoskeletal imaging is plagued with many of the same artifacts seen in other areas of the body; however, this chapter will focus on those common or unique to musculoskeletal imaging. More specifically, those that are a result of musculoskeletal structures which are superficial, linear in shape, and/or are highly reflective. Artifacts that appear anterior to highly reflective bone can be particularly problematic, while others can assist in identifying pathologic conditions and structures; further still, others disguise and even mimic disease.

Several artifact types—anisotropy, reverberation, speed error, and refractile shadowing (edge artifact)—are important in musculoskeletal ultrasound. Understanding how artifacts occur and how to correct images when they appear increases both diagnostic confidence and image accuracy.

Anisotropy

The anisotropic phenomenon is one that occurs not only in sonography but also in other professions, such as astronomy, geology, and chemistry. **Anisotropy** occurs when the incident angle of insonating frequencies from the transducer is not perpendicular to the structure being imaged. The angle and direction of the reflected soundwave depend on the angle of incidence, as well as the shape of the reflector. This causes soundwave reflections away from the transducer instead of directly back at 90 degrees. This commonly occurs when imaging linear structures such as tendons, ligaments, and nerves, particularly when not situated in a straight line, as curvature accentuates this problem (Fig. 24.16). Anisotropy is also frequently seen when imaging muscles, although not as common as the other musculoskeletal structures just mentioned.

The reflection coefficient is a function of the incident angle and is susceptible to anisotropic alterations when the reflected soundwave does not return to the transducer at a 90-degree angle or misses the transducer receiver altogether. As mentioned, this is accentuated in nonperpendicular tissue interfaces and results in differing image properties depending on the angle of incidence and shape of the reflector. In general, anisotropy will appear as an anechoic area or area of reduced echoes due to the reduced amount or amplitude of the signal received (Fig. 24.17), the degree of which depends on the amount of reflected signal loss, with greater signal loss occurring as the angle of incidence departs from 90 degrees.

Although not nearly as common outside of musculoskeletal imaging, anisotropy is evident during renal ultrasound imaging by the loss of definition of the curved upper pole of the right kidney. Muscles, ligaments, tendons, and nerves all image as anisotropic reflectors because of the plane they occupy, with tendons having the most pronounced anisotropy of the structures seen during musculoskeletal imaging. To correct or reduce anisotropy artifact, the transducer can be repositioned to achieve perpendicular insonation of the target structure. The heel-to-toe transducer rocking technique can be helpful to create the optimal 90-degree angle (Fig. 24.18).

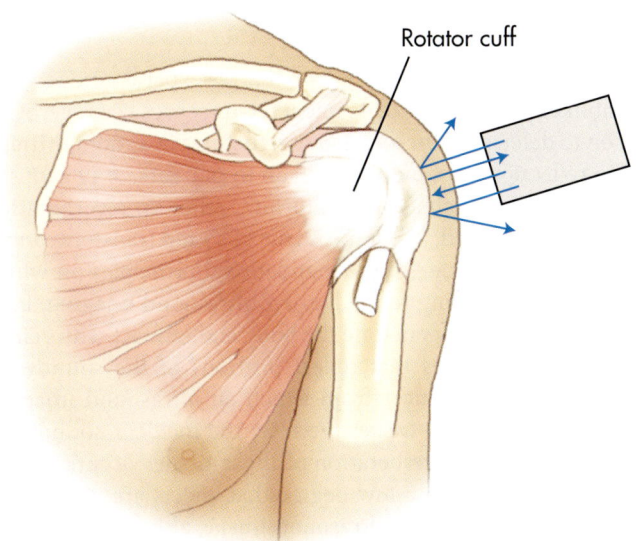

FIG. 24.16 Physics that result in anisotropy artifact. Perpendicular or 90-degree angle of soundwave insonation with the reflecting structure results in the greatest amount of reflection and optimal images. At nonperpendicular insonation, part of the incident soundwave misses the transducer, resulting in an anechoic area on the associated image.

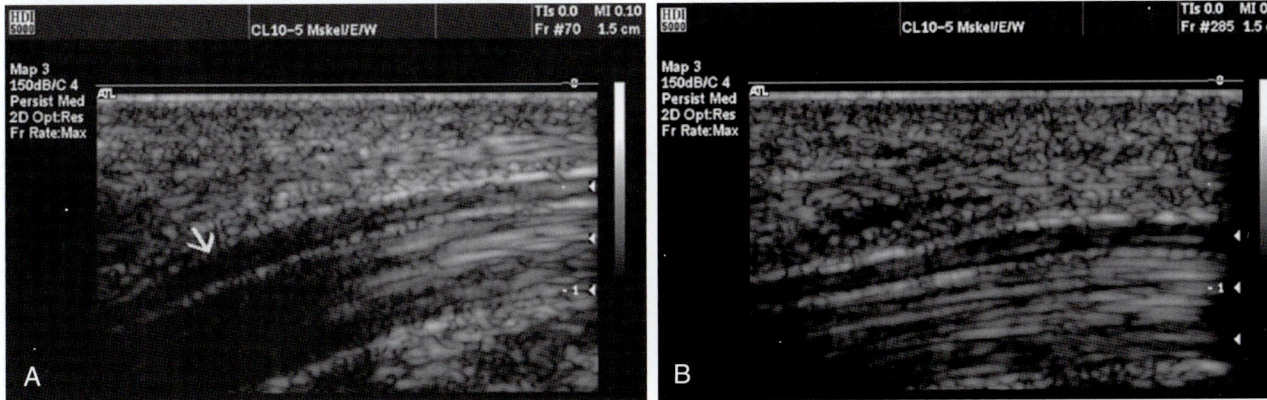

FIG. 24.17 Gray-scale image of the (A) median nerve demonstrating a large anisotropy artifact due to the angle of insonation that is not 90 degrees, resulting in a hypoechoic appearance of the tendon and nerve *(arrow)*; and (B) deep flexor tendon that is of similar shape and location of the median nerve, but without anisotropy artifact as a result of repositioning the transducer to achieve an angle of incidence with the tendon near 90 degrees, thereby eliminating the artifact.

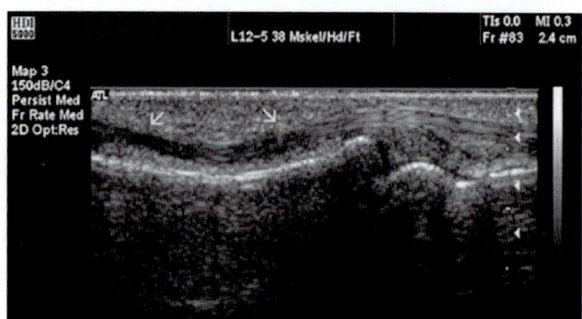

FIG. 24.18 Longitudinal gray-scale image of the digital flexor tendon. Changes in direction of the tendon due to its curvature cause multiple areas of anisotropy *(arrows)* due to changes in the angle of soundwave reflection.

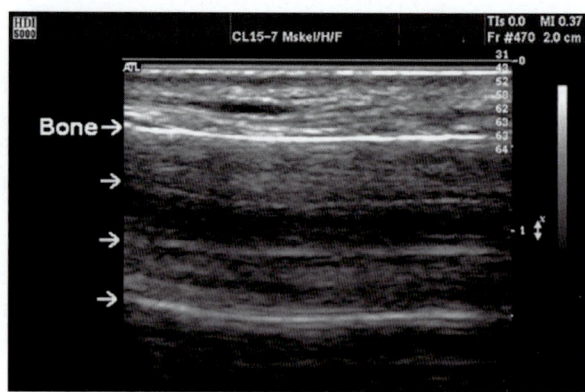

FIG. 24.19 Reverberation artifact resulting from soundwaves interacting with bone, which is a strong linear reflector.

Reverberation

Reverberation is a phenomenon that we experience every day but likely do not realize its impact. Our senses use reverberation to determine the location of structures in a room through the reflection of soundwaves back to our ears. Any acoustic environment, such as an auditorium, relies on reverberation to transmit sound. The same is true of sound transmitted into the body and is one of the foundational principles on which ultrasound imaging relies. During ultrasound imaging, incident soundwaves penetrate the body and interact with reflective tissue surfaces that reflect portions of the soundwave back to the transducer from which an ultrasound image is generated. At each tissue interface, the incident soundwave encounters, the reverberation of those tissues occurs. Often, this occurs at such a low degree that effects are not able to be appreciated on the ultrasound image, although occasionally, and frequent to certain musculoskeletal structures such as bone, the effect of reverberation can be seen on ultrasound and may be beneficial or detrimental to image quality. Multiple delayed reflections from strong tissue boundaries, such as bone, result in a linear artifact that *decreases* in intensity with depth. This collection of reflected sound is superimposed over the primary signal, adding phantom information to the image (Fig. 24.19).

As mentioned, reverberation is not always detrimental. One type of reverberation artifact, comet tail, results from the reverberation of metal, such as clips, sutures, staples, or foreign objects. The **comet-tail artifact** is a function of sound reflecting between two closely placed reflectors. In the case of a pin surgically placed within a bone, the anterior and posterior borders of the hardware are both strong reflecting surfaces. The reverberation occurs within the metal object. Each time sound returns to the anterior border, some of the sound escapes. The resultant artifact resembles a comet tail, hence its name (Fig. 24.20).

Refractile Shadowing

When the incident soundwave interacts with a curved surface, causing the soundwave to redirect in an oblique path,

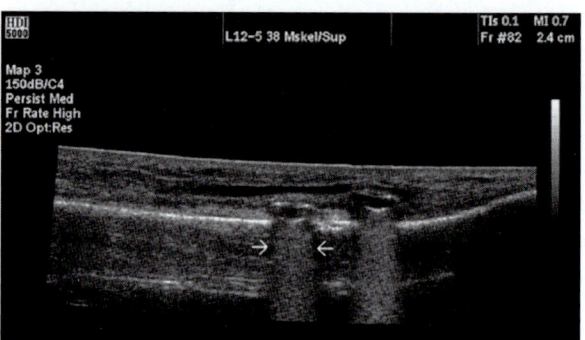

FIG. 24.20 Comet-tail artifact *(arrows)* seen posterior to tibial pins placed to stabilize a tibial fracture. Note the widening of the posterior reverberation, which is due to reverberation within the metal pins. This widening is common with metal placed within musculoskeletal structures and is still a comet-tail artifact even though it does not narrow in the distal area.

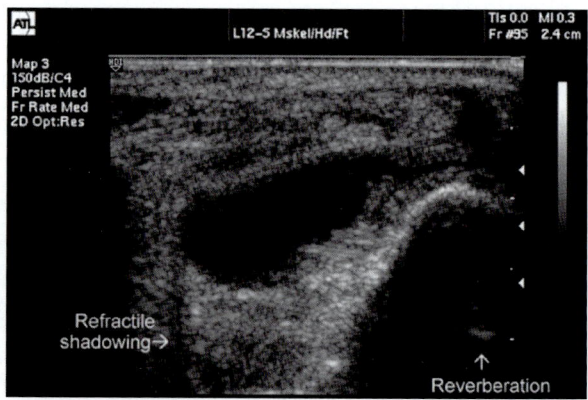

FIG. 24.21 Ganglion cyst located in the ankle demonstrating refractile shadowing.

it is referred to as **refractile shadowing (edge artifact)** on the sonographic image. This change in direction causes a hypoechoic band posterior to the target structure. Another cause of refractile shadowing is a tissue impedance mismatch greatly differing from the average assumed speed of sound within soft tissue (1540 m/sec). This is seen at the edge of round or oval ligaments (Fig. 24.21) or in instances

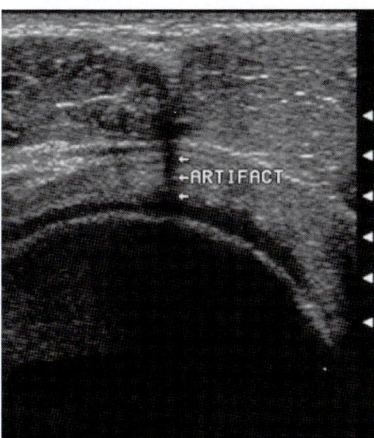

FIG. 24.22 Refractile shadowing from a normal structure anterior to the area of interest (supraspinatus tendon).

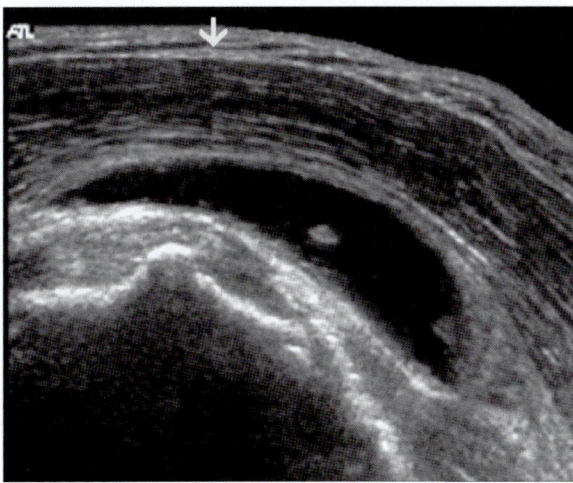

FIG. 24.23 Panoramic gray-scale image of a rotator cuff tear demonstrates very subtle speed error artifact.

of traumatic tear of a musculoskeletal structure (Fig. 24.22). Most commonly seen with a complete tendon tear, the angles formed from the retracted tendon cause refractile shadowing. This shadowing is often used to determine the distance between ligaments by measuring from one artifact edge to the other.

Speed Error Artifacts

Several speed error artifacts are associated with the deviations from the assumption that incident and returning soundwaves travel at a constant speed of 1540 m/sec within soft tissue. These are also referred to as time-of-flight or speed-of-sound artifacts. Of course, not all soft tissue of the human body is homogeneous in density, making errors associated with the speed of sound in the body inevitable. However, when differences in tissue density exist that significantly stray from the assumed speed of 1540 m/sec, speed error effects can be seen on the ultrasound image as associated artifacts.

More specifically, these occur when returning soundwaves interact with two tissue interfaces with markedly different densities, causing markedly different soundwave reflection speeds. The **speed error artifact** displaces the associated structures in the anteroposterior (axial) plane of the image. If the speed of sound is less than the assumed 1540 m/sec, the artifactual effect results in the structure appearing farther away from the transducer in the image. On the contrary, in highly dense tissue, the speed of soundwave travel is greater than 1540 m/sec and results in the structure appearing artifactually closer to the transducer on the image. The creation of this type of artifactual information occurs most commonly during musculoskeletal ultrasound of obese patients at muscle-fat interfaces (Fig. 24.23).

Encountering speed error artifacts coupled with refraction artifacts is not uncommon in musculoskeletal imaging to. This results in structures displayed at incorrect locations and in incorrect shapes.

Table 24.3 lists the techniques for correcting the artifacts discussed previously.

TABLE 24.3	Correction Techniques for Artifacts
Artifact	**Technique**
Anisotropy	Reposition transducer for a perpendicular angle of incidence with the target structure; Heel-to-toe rocking of the transducer
Reverberation	Anterior reverberation can be minimized with the use of a stand-off pad or by changing the angle of incidence.
Refractile	Use of newer technologies, such as compound shadowing imaging or tissue harmonics, helps reduce or eliminate. Changing the angle of incidence may move the artifact out of the region of interest.
Speed error	May not be able to eliminate as a result of tissue artifact sound properties. Change the angle of incidence to demonstrate surrounding tissue.

SONOGRAPHIC EVALUATION OF THE MUSCULOSKELETAL SYSTEM

Sonographic imaging of the joints begins with the proper choice of transducers. Superficially located joints and structures image well with high-frequency transducers capable of imaging at frequencies 7 MHz or greater. The tradeoff between image resolution and image depth must be understood when making transducer selection to ensure imaging is performed using the highest possible frequency considering the depth of the structures needing evaluation.

Positioning of the patient (and joint of interest) is also an important part of the examination. The patient should be placed in a comfortable position that allows the sonographer to maintain ergonomically correct positions to prevent the development of musculoskeletal injuries. A final consideration is the dynamic portion of the examination. Moving the joint to fully evaluate all its components is often required, so space must be left to allow joint movement during imaging at its full range of motion.

Shoulder

The American Institute for Ultrasound Medicine (AIUM) recommends middle frequencies of 7 and 10 MHz for imaging shoulder structures; however, deeper rotator cuff structures may require as low as 5 MHz. Shoulder anatomy is complex, with numerous bursae, muscles, and tendons surrounding the joint. The **rotator cuff** is the focus of a basic shoulder sonographic examination. Box 24.1 lists the minimum recommended 11 shoulder views for rotator cuff evaluation. As with any examination, documentation includes both longitudinal and transverse views of the anatomy. Comparison with the contralateral normal shoulder is also recommended as a comparator and can be helpful to determine absence or presence of disease. To perform a shoulder examination, the patient is placed in an erect position seated on a rotating chair with a back. The rotation of the chair allows easy repositioning of the shoulder during imaging.

Biceps Tendon. The shoulder examination begins by locating the biceps tendon. The **biceps tendon** is one of the easiest structures to image in the adult shoulder, making it a good anatomical landmark to serve as a starting point while performing shoulder musculoskeletal imaging. To view the biceps tendon, place the patient with a slight internal rotation of the shoulder by placing the arm in the lap with the fingers facing the opposite shoulder (Fig. 24.24). The sonographer is situated facing the patient to ensure correct transducer orientation while scanning. When the sonographer faces the patient and to image the right shoulder, the lateral anatomy displays on the left side of the image and the medial anatomy on the right. When the sonographer scans posterior shoulder structures, the image corresponds to the patient position.

The biceps tendon is 3- to 5-mm-thick and is easily located in the transverse plane, appearing as an echogenic oval structure within the bicipital groove of the humerus. The bicipital groove is an indentation on the humerus located between the greater and lesser tuberosities. The overlying transverse ligament encloses the open portion of the groove to house the biceps tendon. Once identified, images at several different levels help determine normalcy. A small amount of fluid (less than 1.5 mm) is normal. Care must be taken to use minimal transducer pressure because small amounts of fluid may be compressed out of the imaging plane (Fig. 24.25). A longitudinal image of the tendon requires some rocking of the transducer to obtain images with minimal anisotropic artifacts. When scanning the biceps tendon, take note of the fibrillar pattern of the normal tendon because disruptions indicate a possible pathologic condition (Fig. 24.26).

Subscapularis Tendon. Next, the **subscapularis tendon** is evaluated. Subscapularis imaging begins by identifying the biceps tendon in the transverse plane at the level of the humeral head. Using the biceps tendon as a landmark, the transducer is angled anteromedially to view the subscapularis. The transverse view displays the tendon as a soft oval tissue structure (Fig. 24.27). Note the transverse view of the tendon requires a longitudinal transducer orientation. External rotation of the arm while scanning aids in visualization of the tendon and determination of normal movement. The subscapularis tendon inserts into the lesser tuberosity at an angle requiring slight rotation of the transducer to obtain its longitudinal view (transverse transducer position).

Supraspinatus Tendon. Imaging proceeds with the supraspinatus tendon, a 3- to 7-mm tendon located lateral and posterior to the biceps tendon. This bandlike tendon has a medium-level echo texture and originates from the greater tuberosity of the humerus. The acromion limits the field of view, requiring careful transducer and patient positioning. A portion of the tendon called the critical zone is the most likely location for injury. The critical zone is located 1 cm posterolateral to the biceps tendon. Care must be taken here because improper scanning results in false-positive or false-negative findings. The dual- or split-screen function allows for normal versus abnormal/injured shoulder comparisons, which help identify small tears.

Initial transverse and longitudinal views begin with the patient's arm in a neutral position; however, after localization of the tendon, the arm is repositioned into the Bouffard or Crass position (Fig. 24.28). Whether the shoulder can be externally rotated into these positions depends on the patient's ability to place the arm behind the back or on the hip. This stresses the tendons of the rotator cuff to emphasize any abnormalities. Another benefit of this position is that it causes the supraspinatus to move anterior and out from under the

---

BOX 24.1 Minimum Shoulder Views of the Rotator Cuff

Views 1 and 2: biceps tendon longitudinal and transverse
Views 3 and 4: subscapularis tendon longitudinal and transverse
Views 5 through 8: supraspinatus tendon in neutral and internal rotation
View 9: infraspinatus tendon
View 10: posterior glenoid labrum
View: 11: teres minor tendon

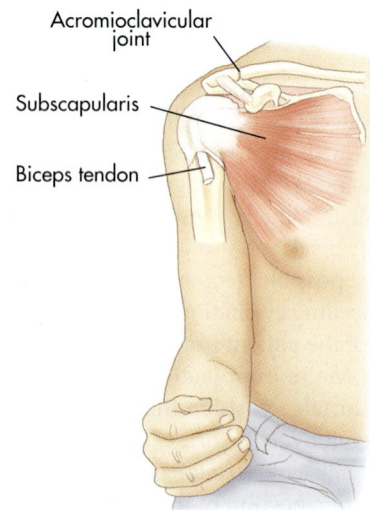

FIG. 24.24 Anatomical diagram of the subscapularis, biceps tendon, and acromioclavicular joint. These structures image easily from an anterior approach. This is considered a neutral position for the shoulder.

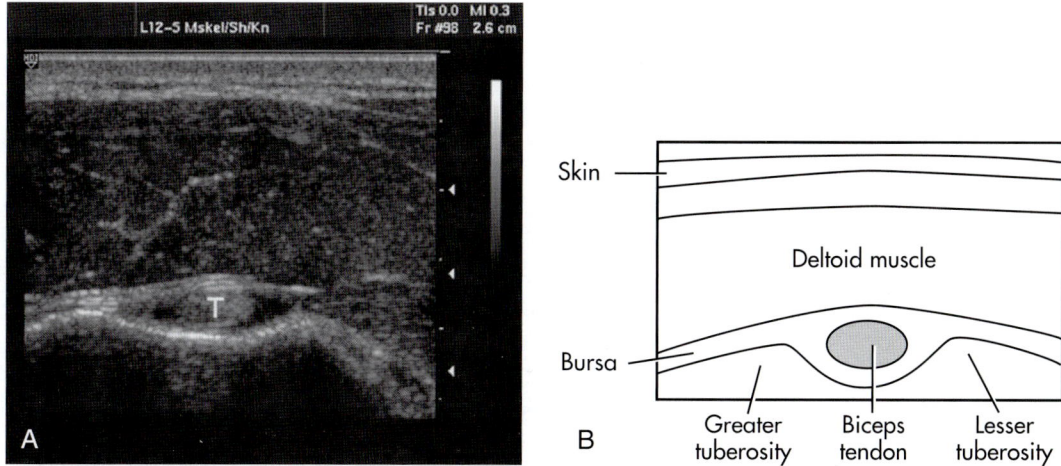

FIG. 24.25 (A) Transverse gray-scale image of the normal echogenic biceps tendon (T) within the bicipital groove. The anechoic effusion of tenosynovitis surrounding the tendon aids in visualization. (B) Diagram of associated anatomy.

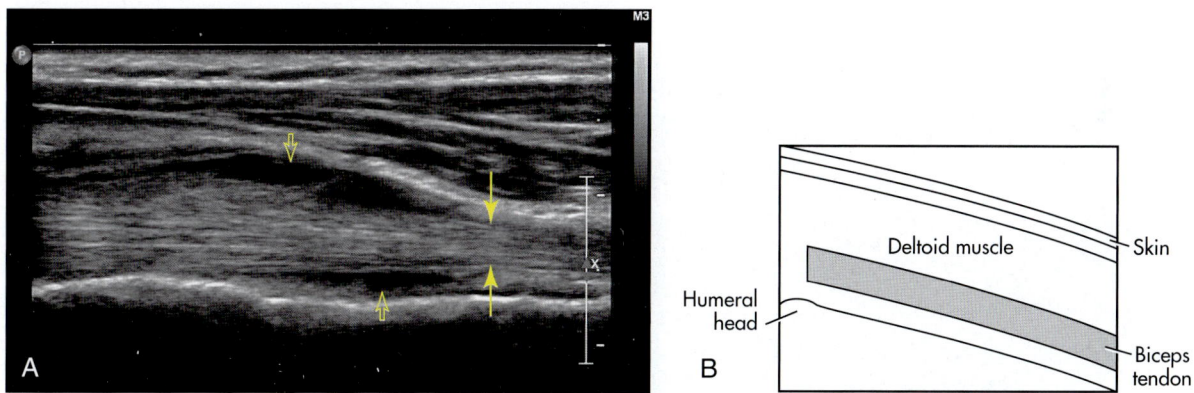

FIG. 24.26 (A) Longitudinal gray-scale image of the biceps tendon *(solid arrows)* demonstrating a fibrillar pattern characteristic of tendons. A small amount of effusion *(open arrows)* is seen posterior to the tendon indicating mild tenosynovitis. (B) Associated anatomy.

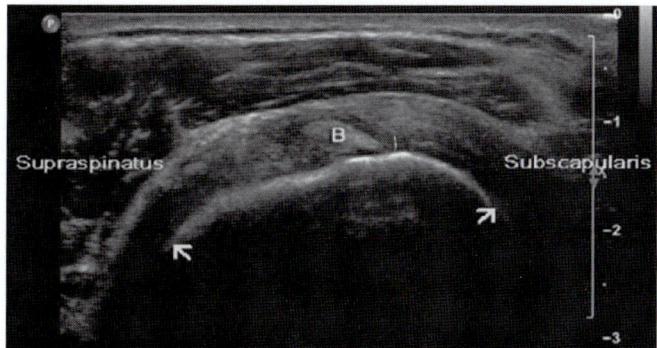

FIG. 24.27 Gray-scale image of the biceps tendon (B) in the transverse plane between the anteromedially located subscapularis tendon and the posterolateral supraspinatus. The biceps tendon is a recommended landmark while locating the subscapularis and supraspinatus tendons. Note anisotropy artifact *(arrows)* seen as the tendons curve with the surface of humeral head.

acromion, allowing better visualization and a more thorough assessment of the tendon (Figs. 24.29 through 24.32).

Infraspinatus Tendon. The infraspinatus tendon is the next structure imaged; two methods are available to localize the tendon. The first involves rotating the patient to gain access to the posterior shoulder and positioning the hand on the patient's opposite shoulder. The posterior glenoid labrum is a good landmark to help find the anteriorly located infraspinatus tendon (Fig. 24.33). A second method has the patient's arm in the same position used while imaging the biceps tendon, locating the supraspinatus tendon, moving posterior and parallel to the scapular spine, and locating the infraspinatus tendon at its attachment to the posterior greater tuberosity of the humerus. Fluid imaged superficial to the infraspinatus tendon indicates bursal fluid, whereas posterior fluid indicates joint effusion. Take note of the humeral head contours because irregularities indicate a pathologic condition.

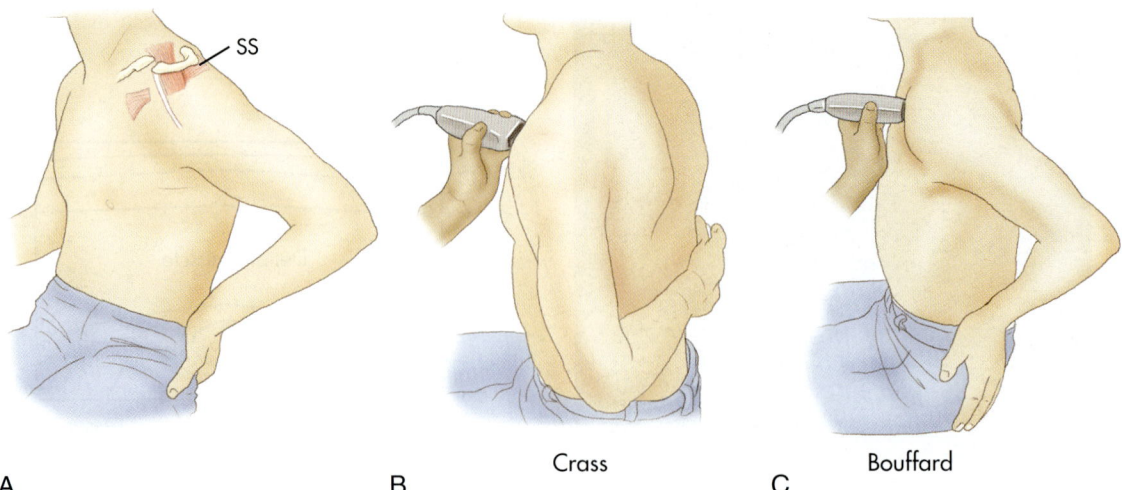

FIG. 24.28 (A) Supraspinatus (SS) in the neutral position of the shoulder. Shoulder imaging using the Crass (B) and Bouffard (C) positions.

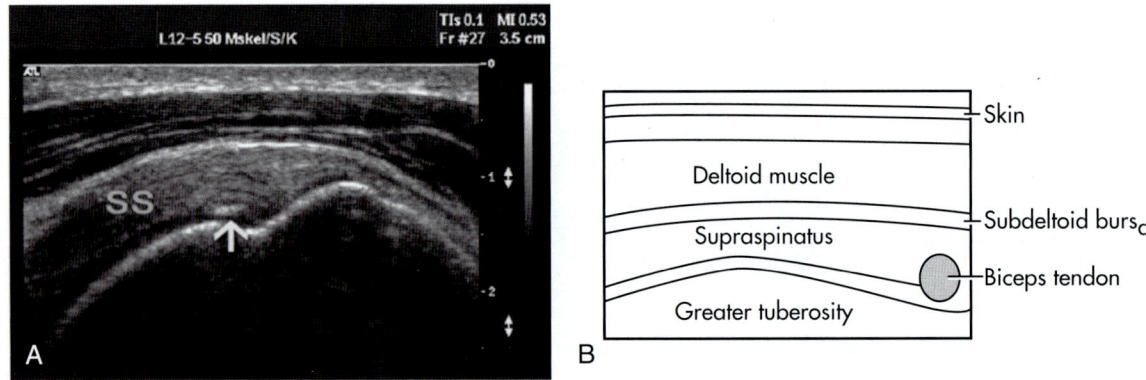

FIG. 24.29 (A) Gray-scale image of the medially located biceps tendon *(arrow)* helps locate the supraspinatus (SS) located anteriorly. The biceps tendon is imaged from the acromion to the greater tuberosity to detect any changes in echogenicity or the presence of fluid. (B) Associated anatomy.

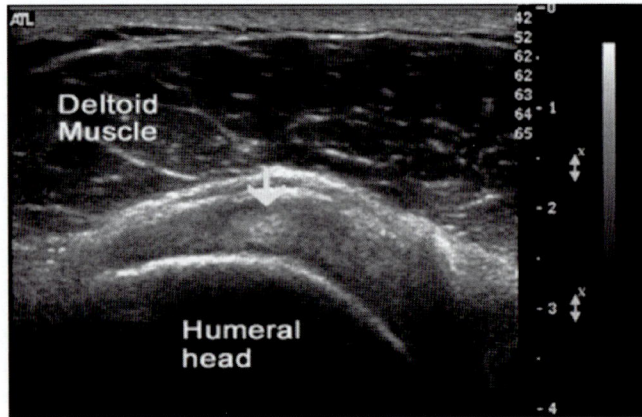

FIG. 24.30 Gray-scale transverse image of the supraspinatus tendon *(arrow)* demonstrating mild hyperechogenicity.

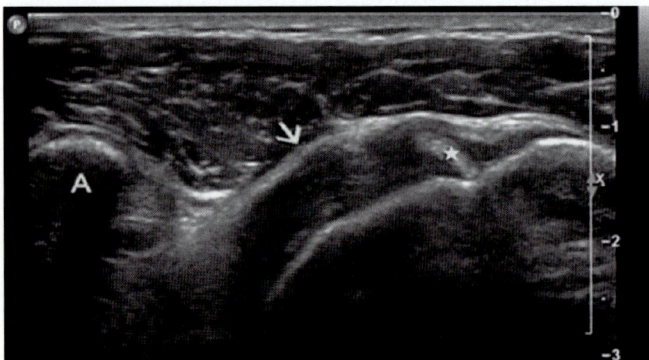

FIG. 24.31 Gray-scale image of the shoulder in a neutral position. To locate the supraspinatus, use the biceps tendon *(star)* as a landmark, then rotate the transducer until the acromion (A) comes into view. The supraspinatus tendon *(arrow)* is located between these two structures. Note the anisotropy artifact that partially hinders visualization of the tendon.

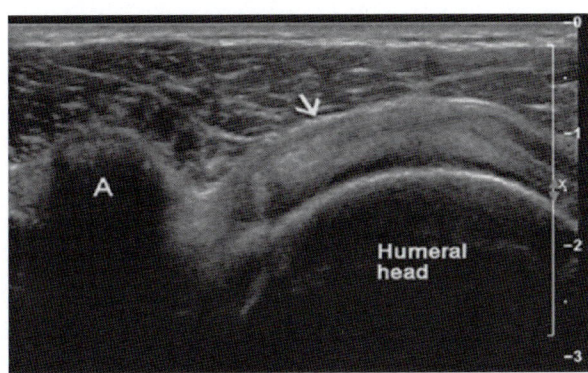

FIG. 24.32 Gray-scale image of the shoulder internally rotated into the Bouffard position. The supraspinatus tendon *(arrow)* is seen extending to the acromion (A). Note that most of the anisotropic artifact is no longer present because the tendon is closer to perpendicular with the transducer.

Teres Minor Tendon. Although injury to the teres minor tendon is uncommon, imaging ensures complete visualization of the infraspinatus tendon because of their proximity. The **teres minor tendon** lies parallel to the scapular spine and inferior to the infraspinatus tendon. To differentiate the infraspinatus tendon from the teres minor, pay close attention to the plane of the tendon fibers. Horizontal fibers indicate the infraspinatus, whereas the teres minor is on an oblique plane. The teres minor tendon appears as a trapezoidal structure inferior to the infraspinatus tendon.

During examination of rotator cuff structures, it is important to note any bursal thickening, tendon calcifications, bony irregularities, loose bodies, or fluid collections. Many other non–rotator cuff structures can also be imaged, such as the **acromioclavicular (AC) joint**. Because of the superficial location of the AC joint, separations are easily imaged and are especially evident when compared with a normal contralateral joint. As with any other portion of the body, soft tissue masses and injury, foreign bodies, and fluid collections are easily identified (Figs. 24.34 and 24.35).

Box 24.2 lists common indications for shoulder sonography.

Wrist/Hand

The wrist joint is easily examined because of its accessibility, size, and lack of overlying bony structures. This ease of imaging implies that the wrist is an uncomplicated joint to image; however, familiarity with wrist anatomy reveals a very complex set of structures. The complexity of the wrist is underscored by the fact that some orthopedic surgeons specialize in just this one joint. Eight small carpal bones make up the wrist joint between the proximal ulna and radius and the distal metacarpal bones of the hand. The eight carpal bones are organized into a proximal row (scaphoid, lunate, triquetrum, pisiform) and distal row (trapezium, trapezoid, capitate, hamate), which articulate to allow wrist flexion and extension. Distal to the carpal bones are the five metacarpals

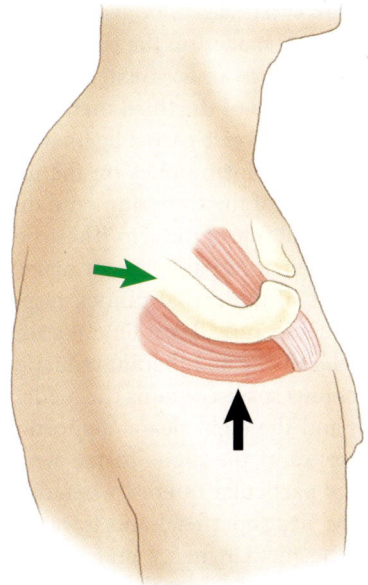

FIG. 24.33 The infraspinatus tendon *(black arrow)* lies lateral and inferior to the scapular spine *(green arrow)*.

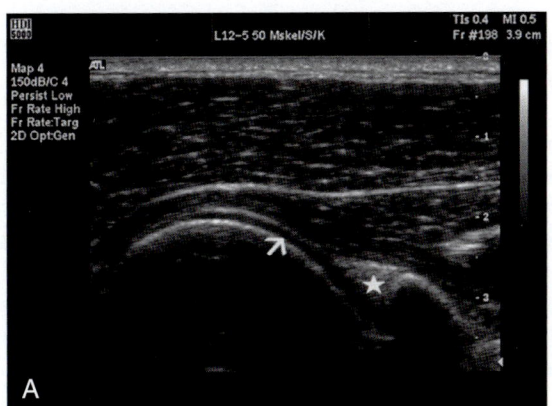

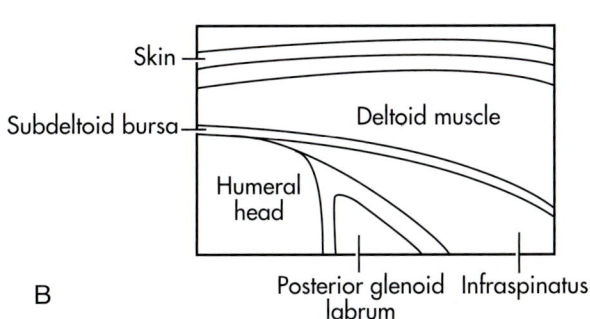

FIG. 24.34 (A) Gray-scale image of the posterior glenoid labrum *(star)*, which appears as a triangular hyperechoic structure deep to the infraspinatus tendon. The thin hypoechoic layer of cartilage superficial to the bony surface of the humeral head can also be appreciated *(arrow)*. (B) Associated anatomy.

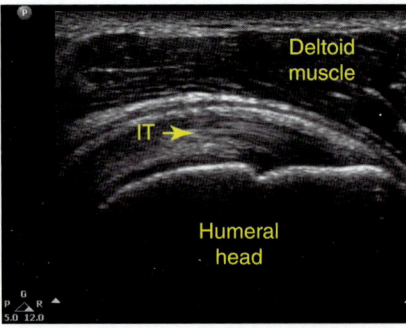

FIG. 24.35 Gray-scale image of the infraspinatus tendon (IT) appearing as a triangular structure at its posterior attachment with the greater tuberosity. This image helps determine its echogenic consistency when coupled with external and internal rotation maneuvers.

BOX 24.2	Common Indications for Shoulder Sonography

- Pain or swelling
- Pain with joint rotation
- Weakness with arm elevation
- Trauma
- Decreased range of motion
- Evaluation of soft tissue masses

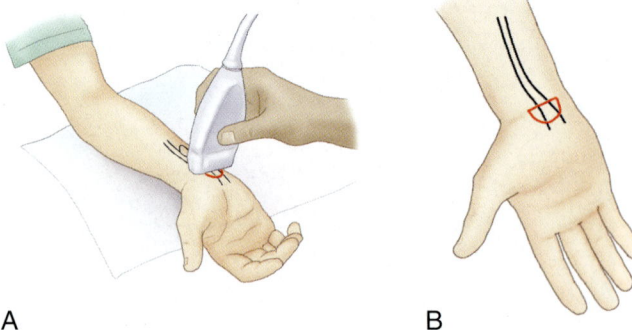

FIG. 24.36 (A) Patient positioning (wrist on a pillow on the patient's lap) for imaging wrist structures with a volar approach. (B) The retinaculum *(red)*, a strong fibrous tendinous structure that attaches to the pisiform on the lateral side and the hook of the hamate medially.

bones that comprise the hand. Distal to the metacarpal bones are the phalanges that articulate at the metacarpophalangeal joints. Phalanges are the bones of the digits. There are 14 phalanges on each hand, two in the thumb and three in the rest of the digits, separated by interphalangeal joints.

To perform a sonographic wrist examination, the patient is positioned with the arm at a 90-degree angle, and the palm pronated or supinated on the lap of the patient (Fig. 24.36). Placing a small rolled-up towel under the wrist when examining the palmar (**volar**) portion of the wrist places the joint in a neutral position. The towel also helps dorsal imaging of the wrist when the hand is palm down. These positions allow imaging of carpal tunnel structures, ganglion and synovial cysts, tears of the triangular fibrocartilage, tenosynovitis, and any other tumors. This positioning also allows easy imaging of the contralateral wrist for comparisons.

Another benefit of sonographic wrist imaging is its ability to demonstrate the dynamics of the wrist and associated masses with finger movement. The smaller wrist joint requires a higher-frequency transducer in the 10- to 20-MHz range. Manufacturers also offer transducers with smaller footprints, which allow easier scanning than some of the larger linear transducers. "Hockey stick" probes are typically the transducer of choice when imaging the wrist, hand, and fingers. An excess amount of gel or stand-off pad should be used to optimize very superficial wrist structures. Clinically, sonographic evaluations of the wrist typically consist of focused imaging at the symptomatic area; however, symptoms associated with median nerve pain or carpal tunnel syndrome are the most common indications for this type of imaging.

The **carpal tunnel** is located between the carpal bones and the overlying flexor retinaculum on the palmar side of the wrist. The flexor retinaculum, also known as the transverse carpal ligament, makes up the superficial border of the carpal tunnel and covers an area extending from the distal radius to the metaphysis of the third metacarpal. The attachment points of the transverse carpal ligament are the hook of the hamate and the pisiform bones on the ulnar side of the arm, and the tubercle of the trapezium and distal pole of the scaphoid on the radial side of the arm. These bony attachment points of the transverse carpal ligament make up the medial and lateral borders of the carpal tunnel, respectively. Along with the median nerve, nine flexor tendons also pass through the carpal tunnel, causing an inherent reduction

This fibro-osseous space contains the median nerve, flexor pollicis longus, and the eight flexor digitorum tendons that connect the muscles of the digits to the wrist. The median nerve, which is of particular interest when diagnosing carpal tunnel syndrome, lies superficial and toward the radial side of the tunnel. The median nerve and its branches provide sensory innervation of the lateral portion of the hand, the palmar surface of the thumb index, middle finger, and lateral half of the ring finger. The median nerve provides motor innervation to the abductor pollicis brevis, opponens pollicis, superficial head of the flexor pollicis brevis, and the first and second lumbrical muscles. As a result, loss of sensory or motor function to any of those aforementioned areas suggests carpal tunnel syndrome and are common symptoms for the basis of the wrist sonogram. **Guyon canal** is a tunnel on the ulnar side of the wrist formed by the hook of the hamate and pisiform bones, through which the ulnar nerve passes. The ulnar nerve can become the victim of a compression disorder due to Guyon canal (referred to as ulnar tunnel syndrome), just as the median nerve within the carpal tunnel. Ulnar tunnel syndrome frequently occurs in long-distance cyclists, following wrist trauma or as a result of repetitive wrist actions.

To investigate the contents of the carpal tunnel, imaging in the transverse plane is the easiest approach to begin the examination. Locating the ulnar artery at the wrist crease helps orientation and subsequent identification of wrist structures. Care must be taken to maintain a perpendicular scan plane to reduce anisotropic effects. The flexor digitorum tendons are hypoechoic structures just posterior to the median nerve. Fibrillary hyperechoic tendon patterns help differentiate from the hypoechoic median nerve. The median nerve also has a distinct hyperechoic border. The rounded or oval median nerve flattens as it continues through the carpal tunnel (Figs. 24.37 and 24.38).

The median nerve imaged in a longitudinal plane appears as a parallel structure superficial to the flexor digitorum tendons. The nerve sheath appears as a continuous hyperechoic structure on the anterior and posterior borders of the nerve. Tendons located posterior to the median nerve have the characteristic hyperechoic fibrillar pattern seen with tendons in other areas of the body (Fig. 24.39).

Digit ultrasound examinations are primarily performed to assess the digital flexor tendons of the hand and associated annular digital pulleys. Flexor tendons appear similar to other tendons of the body, as echogenic, fibrillar structures parallel and superficial to the bones. Annular pulleys appear as anechoic anisotropic bands covering the flexor tendons. Imaging is performed from the volar aspect of the digits in both the longitudinal and transverse planes.

Similar to wrist imaging, the imaging protocol of the digits is driven by symptom location. The painful area should be imaged in both the longitudinal and transverse planes.

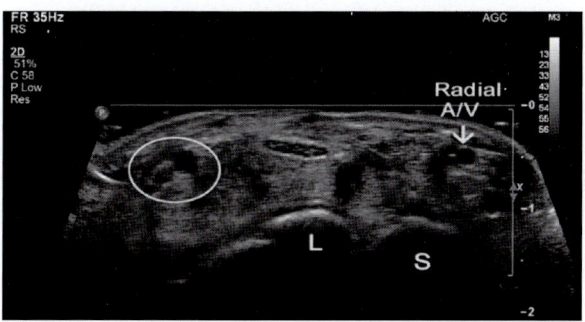

FIG. 24.37 Transverse gray-scale image acquired from the volar side of the wrist at the crease demonstrates the complicated wrist anatomy from this approach. Large amounts of gel allow for imaging with minimal artifact on the lateral curved edges. Guyon canal *(circle)* contains the ulnar vein and vessels demarcating the medial carpal tunnel border. The lunate (L) and scaphoid bone (S) mark the posterior boundaries of the carpal tunnel. The median nerve is slightly flattened at this level, which is a normal finding.

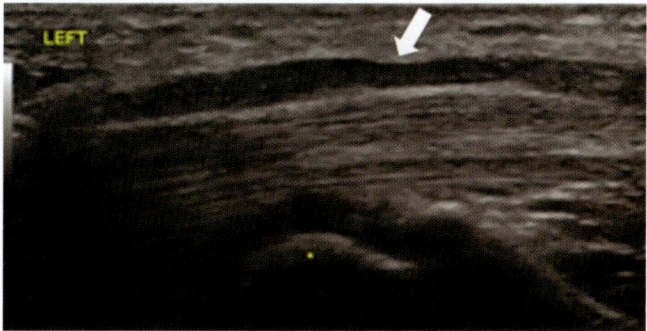

FIG. 24.38 Gray-scale longitudinal image of a median nerve with flattening *(arrow)* at the level of the distal radius.

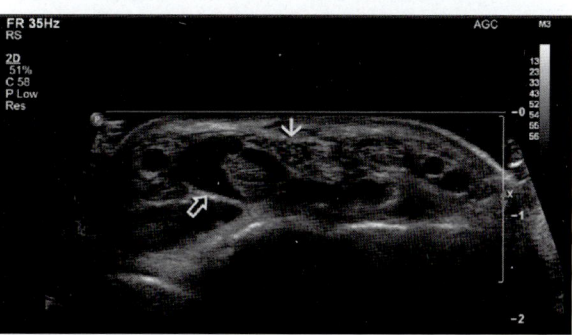

FIG. 24.39 Gray-scale transverse image acquired proximal to Fig. 24.37 demonstrates a more oval, less flattened median nerve *(solid arrow)*. The flexor pollicis longus tendon and the beginning of the muscle *(open arrow)* appear as a hypoechoic structure.

BOX 24.3	Indications for Wrist/Hand Sonography

- Palpable mass
- Loss or decrease of digital mobility
- Pain and swelling
- Trauma
- Foreign body location
- Numbness of the middle and index fingers
- Weakness or clumsiness of the hand
- Tingling with nerve percussion (Tinel sign)
- Pain with wrist flexion when sustained for a minute or longer (Phalen sign)

Color and power Doppler imaging should also be employed to detect areas of hyperemia, which can be an indicator for pathologic processes such as rheumatoid arthritis. Common indications for digit imaging, along with wrist and hand imaging, are included in Box 24.3.

Ankle

Like the wrist, the ankle joint is very superficial and is easily visualized with ultrasound imaging. Structures of the ankle and their associated views are detailed in Table 24.4. The sonographic evaluation of the ankle is often driven by symptomatology, so familiarity with the various musculoskeletal structures of the ankle and how they are imaged is important.

One of the most common MSK structures of the ankle evaluated using ultrasound imaging is the **Achilles tendon**. Named after the Greek mythology figure Achilles, this large, strong fibrous tendon connects the gastrocnemius and soleus muscles to the calcaneus. Although the Achilles tendon (as with any tendon) has many variations, it originates from the gastrocnemius muscle in about two-thirds of the population and from the soleus muscle in the other third. The Achilles tendon enables plantar flexion and flexion of the knee from the muscles of the calf and heel. This allows moving the foot downward to push off when walking and to rise up on the toes. Achilles tendon injuries can significantly impede walking and often result in permanent painful gait.

TABLE 24.4	Musculoskeletal Structures of the Ankle Identifiable With Sonography
Approach	**Structure**
Anterior	Extensor tendons: tibialis anterior, extensor hallucis longus, extensor digitorum longus
	Tibialis anterior tendon
	Anterior recess of the tibiotalar joint
	Anterior talofibular ligament
	Anterior tibiofibular ligament
	Calcaneofibular ligament
	Dorsal midtarsal ligaments
Lateral	Peroneal tendons
Medial	Tibialis posterior
	Flexor digitorum longus tendons
	Tarsal tunnel and tibial nerve
	Flexor hallucis longus tendon (transverse)
	Deltoid ligament
Posterior	Flexor hallucis longus tendon (longitudinal)
	Posterior joint recess
	Achilles tendon

Tendinitis of the Achilles tendon is not uncommon in active patients and athletes. Any activity that involves rapid, high-intensity ankle movements such as jumping and sudden stopping and starting stresses the tendon. Overstretching of the Achilles can result in a partial or complete tear, with the most common site of occurrence being the distal portion of the tendon near the insertion to the calcaneus. Unfortunately, this is also the location of the tendon with the most limited blood supply. The longitudinal arteries that run the length of the gastrocnemius and soleus muscles perfuse the Achilles tendon, although overall perfusion of the tendon is low compared with other structures. A limited blood supply to the Achilles tendon slows the healing process after injury and results in an increased risk of chronic and more severe outcomes. Chances of rupture and inflammation increase with age as the result of a diminishing blood supply.

The Achilles tendon is relatively easy to image sonographically as it is the largest tendon in the body, is conveniently located superficially at the posterior ankle, and has distinct echo characteristics. A connective tissue sheath called the paratenon surrounds the Achilles tendon that promotes tendon gliding of 2 to 3 cm during movement. The lack of a true synovial sheath results in a less echogenic border between the tendon and the surrounding tissue.

To begin the examination, position the patient prone with the foot hanging over the edge of the cart or bed. The foot may also be supported on a pillow or sponge for easier scanning and patient comfort. Patients unable to lie prone may be scanned while on their side if the injured Achilles tendon is accessible.

The size of the Achilles allows imaging at frequencies as low as 5 MHz, although higher frequencies should be used as long as the image quality of the tendon is maintained. The tendon is followed from its origin at the gastrocnemius and soleus muscles to the insertion on the calcaneus. A complete scan includes transverse and sagittal views, with anteroposterior (AP) measurements obtained in the transverse view. The AP diameter of the normal tendon is approximately 5 to 6 mm, varying with patient gender and body habitus. AP measurements should always be performed in the transverse plane, as diameters in the longitudinal plane tend to overestimate distance because of the oblique course of the tendon. **Dorsiflexion** and **plantar flexion** of the foot, best imaged on the sagittal plane, increase the ability to detect an Achilles tendon tear. The **Thompson's test** (plantar flexion with squeezing of the calf) may be used to evaluate the integrity of the Achilles tendon. The patient kneels on the examination table with the feet hanging off the edge; the examiner squeezes the calf while observing for plantar flexion. The result is positive if no movement of the foot is noted; this indicates Achilles tendon rupture.

When scanning the patient in the prone position, special attention must be given to the hypoechoic Kager's fat pad or pre-Achilles fat pad located deep in the Achilles tendon. Displacement of this triangular fat pad is one radiographic marker for the Achilles tendon and can serve as a landmark during the sonographic examination. Scanning the contralateral side also aids in determining tendon normalcy (Figs. 24.40 and 24.41).

Box 24.4 lists the indications for Achilles tendon sonography.

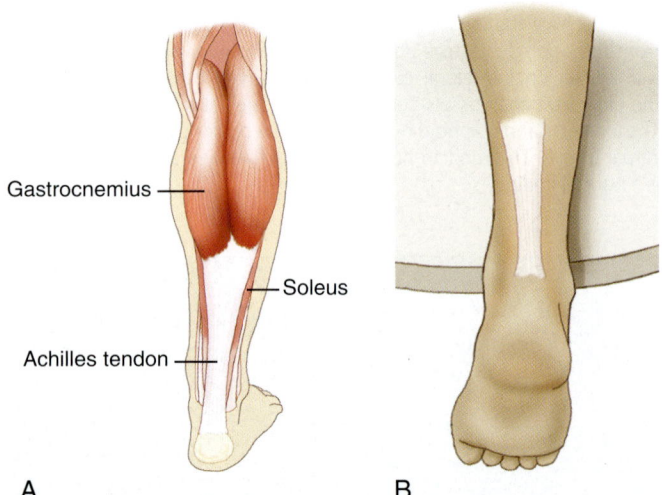

FIG. 24.40 (A) Anatomy of the posterior calf. The Achilles tendon extends from the origin at the gastrocnemius and soleus muscles to the insertion on the calcaneus. (B) Placing the patient prone with the foot over the cart edge allows easy access to the tendon and dorsal and plantar flexion of the foot.

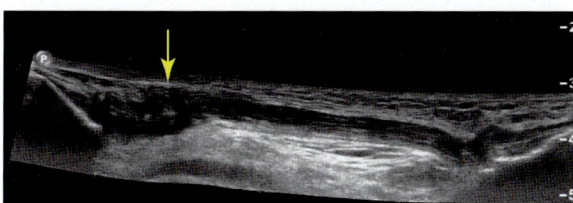

FIG. 24.41 Panoramic or extended field of view gray-scale imaging allows imaging of a greater length of the Achilles tendon. This enables comparison of echogenicity in different areas of the tendon. Kager's fat pad *(arrow)* images as a hypoechoic structure.

BOX 24.4	Indications for Achilles Tendon Sonography

- Abnormal Thompson's test (toes point toward the plantar surface of the foot when the calf is squeezed)
- Trauma
- Displacement of Kager's fat pad on a radiograph
- Knot or bulge over the proximal tendon
- Audible pop or snap followed by a sharp pain
- Inability to stand on toes
- Swelling
- Heel pain for longer than 4 weeks
- Decreased strength or mobility
- Postoperative monitoring

PATHOLOGY OF THE MUSCULOSKELETAL SYSTEM

Familiarity with the sonographic appearance of injury, inflammation, and chronic pathology enables a more thorough and accurate musculoskeletal ultrasound examination to be performed. Some pathology occurs more frequently in some joints than others; however, the sonographic appearance of the various pathologies is similar in the muscles, tendons, and ligaments, regardless of location.

Shoulder Biceps Tendon Subluxation/Dislocation

Dislocation (also called *subluxation*) of the biceps tendon from the bicipital groove may be caused by abnormalities with the transverse humeral ligament, abnormal development of the bicipital groove or supraspinatus, and/or subscapularis tears. The most common dislocation site is deep to the subscapularis anterior to the glenohumeral joint capsule. This medial dislocation results in an empty groove that may fill with granulation and fibrous tissue. Rotating the arm from a neutral to external position allows real-time imaging of tendon dislocation (Figs. 24.42 and 24.43).

Rotator Cuff Tears

Tears of the rotator cuff can be classified as partial-thickness or full-thickness tears (Fig. 24.44). The two types are differentiated by abnormal communication with the glenohumeral joint and the subacromial bursa. Full-thickness tears have this communication, while partial-thickness tears do not.

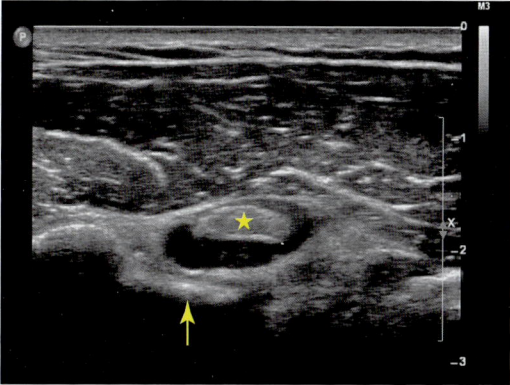

FIG. 24.42 Gray-scale image demonstrating subluxation and complete or incomplete dislocation of the biceps tendon *(star)* out of the bicipital groove *(arrow)* of the humerus.

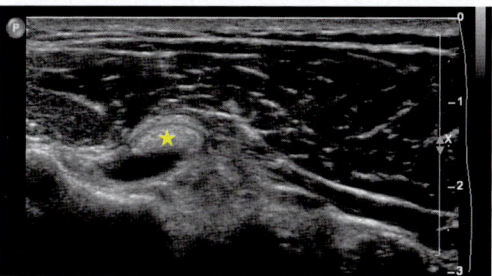

FIG. 24.43 Gray-scale image demonstrating complete dislocation of the biceps tendon *(star)* outside of the biceps groove of the humerus.

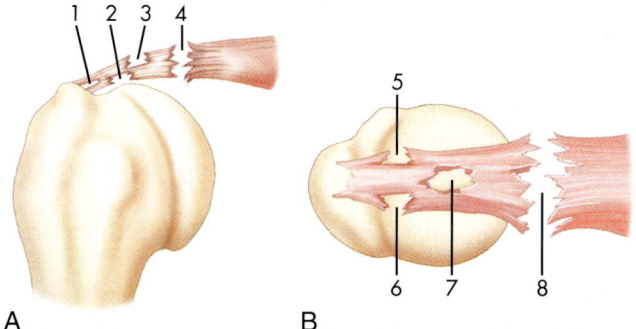

FIG. 24.44 The shoulder, as seen from the coronal view (A) and from above (B), showing tears of the supraspinatus tendon. Tears can occur anywhere along the supraspinatus tendon and range from an intrasubstance tear (1) to a complete full-thickness, full-width tear (8). The range includes partial-thickness humeral surface tear (2), partial-thickness bursal surface tear (3), full-thickness tear (4), full-thickness tear posteriorly (partial width; 5), full-thickness tear posteriorly (partial width; 6), and full-thickness tear centrally (partial width; 7).

Rotator cuff pathology may occur as an acute or chronic processes. Biceps tendon ruptures, trauma, and shoulder dislocations are a few common causes of acute rotator cuff tears. A chronic process occurs as a cumulative progression of injury from activities that involve moving the arms over the head, such as placing items on high shelves, playing tennis, swimming, or rock climbing. Impingement between the humeral head and the acromion causes tendon microtrauma during movement and results in cuff degeneration and eventual tear. Rotator cuff tears are divided into three stages: stage I, swelling and mild pain; stage II, inflammation and scarring; and stage III, partial or complete tears of the rotator cuff.

The supraspinatus, similar to all tendons of the shoulder, is a straplike tendon with three dimensions. Tears in width, length, and thickness occur, and a complete examination includes documentation of the tear in all planes. A tear located on the sagittal plane appears as a disruption on the thickness or AP dimension of the tendon. This only partially depicts the tear, however, as an orthogonal view will provide the location and extent of the tear on the width of the tendon.

It is important to remember the shape of tendons when assessing them for possible tears. Their curved shape causes them to have an increased likelihood of producing anisotropic artifact, which appears similar to a tear. Internally rotating or extending the arm will alter the imaging plane and help to reduce the artifact but also accentuate the appearance of any tears present.

Partial-Thickness Tear. Partial-thickness tears may involve the bursal or articular cuff surface or the intrasubstance material, although instances of intrasubstance tears are rare. Tears begin in the critical zone of the anterolateral supraspinatus tendon and image as focal disruptions of the tendon fibers. This zone is located 1 cm from the insertion into the greater tuberosity. When injured, the acute tendon tear appears as an anechoic defect in the rotator cuff. As tears become chronic, they will appear with greater levels of echogenicity caused by the mixing of blood and bursal granulation tissue in the frayed tendon area. Diffuse thinning of the tendon is another indication of a chronic partial-thickness tear.

The most common type of tear is the articular cuff surface defect. The following criteria help to establish the presence of a partial-thickness tear:
1. Critical zone focus of mixed hyperechoic and hypoechoic echogenicity (focal discontinuity).
2. Bursal or articular extension of any hypoechoic areas imaged in two orthogonal planes.
3. Irregularity of the anterior greater tuberosity (occurs in ~75% of partial-thickness tears), such as bone cortex defects, fragmentation, and/or spurring.
4. Decreased tendon thickness.

Fluid seen within the biceps tendon indicates possible articular surface tear. Large amounts of fluid in the subacromial-subdeltoid bursa decrease the ability to visualize a full-thickness tear.

Hypoechoic concave bursal surface tears are the second most common type of partial rotator cuff tears (Fig. 24.45).

Box 24.5 lists the sonographic criteria for partial-thickness tears.

Full-Thickness Tear. Tears that involve the full thickness and width of a rotator cuff tendon is considered a full-thickness tear. Retraction of multiple tendons occurs with separation between 2 and 4 cm from the torn tendon ends. The frequency of tendon tearing in descending order occurs in the supraspinatus, infraspinatus, and subscapularis, and, very rarely, the teres minor.

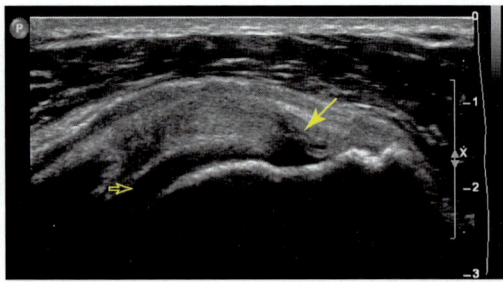

FIG. 24.45 Gray-scale image demonstrating a bursal side partial-thickness tear *(solid arrow)*, with a hypoechoic appearance compared with the surrounding rotator cuff. Fluid, blood, and debris collect in the bursa, producing an anechoic structure *(open arrow)*.

BOX 24.5	Sonographic Criteria for Partial-Thickness Tears

- Critical zone of the supraspinatus imaging with a hypoechoic or hyperechoic focus
- Articular or bursal extension of a hypoechoic lesion on two orthogonal planes
- Hypoechoic or echogenic line within the cuff substance
- Anterior greater tuberosity regional irregularities
- Effusions of the biceps tendon sheath
- Concave subdeltoid bursal surface

Images of the tear on sagittal and transverse planes not only confirm the full-thickness nature of the tear but also allow measurements between the torn tendon edges (Figs. 24.46 through 24.48). The largest obtained measure is used to classify the tear. The **cartilage interface sign** is the echogenic line on the anterior surface of the cartilage surrounding the humeral head. The four classifications of rotator cuff vary in the literature; however, the criteria below reflect a composite of published categorizations:
1. Partial-thickness tear
2. Small full-thickness tear 1 to 2 cm in AP dimension over the greater tuberosity
3. Large full-thickness tear 2 to 4 cm
4. Complete tears greater than 4 cm

During the real-time ultrasound imaging, perform a simple compression test over the area being examined. The normal tendon cannot be compressed; however, the injured tendon flattens as the torn edges move apart. Long-standing cuff injuries may also result in atrophy or nonvisualization of muscle. Rupture of the subscapularis tendon results in retraction of muscle between the scapula and the chest wall. Fatty infiltration of the supraspinatus and infraspinatus fossae changes this area's echogenic appearance, giving a false appearance of normalcy and underscoring the importance of scanning the contralateral side for a healthy comparator. The **naked tuberosity sign** is defined as the deltoid muscle on the humeral head; it is seen with full-thickness tears of the rotator cuff.

Joint effusion around the biceps tendon combined with subacromial-subdeltoid (SASD) bursitis create the double

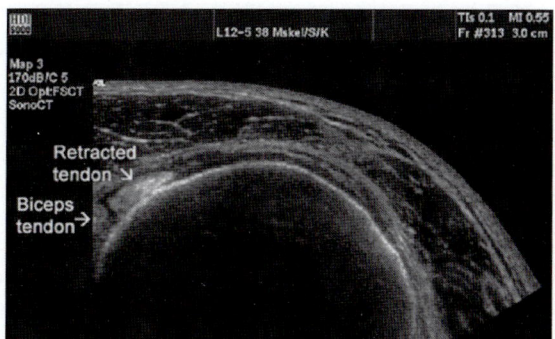

FIG. 24.46 Gray-scale panoramic image demonstrating a complete full-thickness tear (complete rupture) shows the biceps tendon retraction at the far left. The deltoid muscle is located anterior to the greater tuberosity.

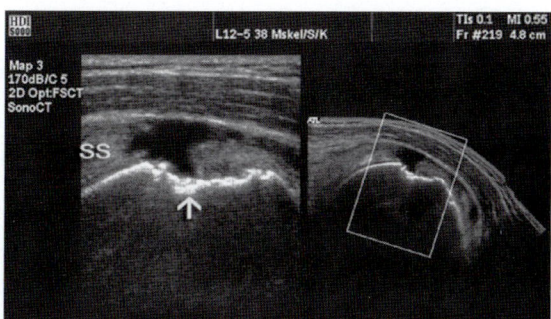

FIG. 24.47 Dual gray-scale panoramic image *(right)* and its magnification *(left)* show a complex subdeltoid bursa with hemorrhage after a rotator cuff tear. The retracted supraspinatus (SS) leaves a space for fluid and blood to collect. Note the irregularity of the biceps groove *(arrow)*.

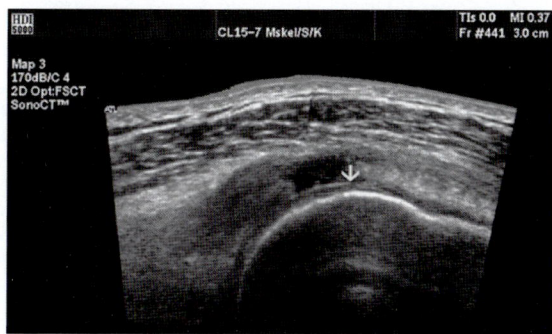

FIG. 24.48 Gray-scale image of the humeral head. The cartilage of the humeral head interface *(arrow)* is seen as the echogenic anterior border surrounding the humeral head. This is seen through the anechoic or hypoechoic complete rotator cuff tear.

> **BOX 24.6** **Primary and Secondary Sonographic Signs of a Full-Thickness Tear**
>
> **Primary Signs**
> - Naked tuberosity sign
> - Tendon edge atrophy in a chronic tear
> - Retracted tendons
> - Fiber discontinuity with interposed fluid
> - A cleft in the cuff of hypoechoic or anechoic echotexture
> - Distended SASD bursa in direct communication with the joint
> - Compressed tendon
> - Absence of the rotator cuff
> - Deltoid muscle or SASD bursa herniation into the rotator cuff
>
> **Secondary Signs**
> - Long head biceps tendon effusion
> - Double effusion sign
> - Erosion of the greater tuberosity of the humerus
> - Cartilage interface sign
> - Glenohumeral joint effusion

SASD, Subacromial-subdeltoid.

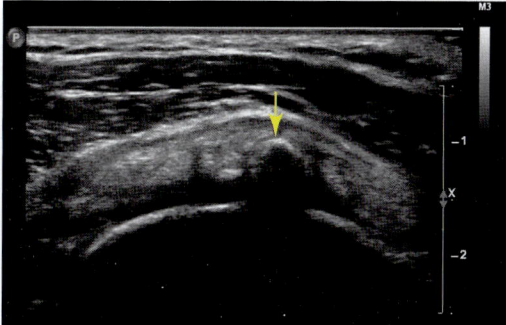

FIG. 24.49 Gray-scale image of the rotator cuff with intratendinous calcifications *(arrow)*. This is a common finding in chronic tendinitis.

Box 24.6 lists the primary and secondary sonographic signs of a full-thickness tear.

Tendinitis

One of the most common tendon abnormalities is inflammation due to age-related elasticity loss, diseases such as rheumatoid arthritis, overuse, or acute trauma. **Tendinitis** can occur in any tendon but is most commonly seen in the shoulder, wrist, heel, and elbow. This inflammatory condition has the following characteristic clinical symptoms: pain at the tendinous insertion into the bone, palpable mass in the area of pain, and decreased range of movement. Treatment is important to correct tendinitis in the acute stage, as chronic tendinitis may lead to a weakening of the tendon and rupture (Fig. 24.49).

Ultrasound images tendinitis well because of inflammatory changes in surrounding tissues (Fig. 24.50). Acute tendinitis (also called *tenosynovitis*) involves not only the tendon but also the surrounding synovial sheath. Ultrasound imaging demonstrates a fluid increase within

effusion sign sonographically. This is a sign specific to rotator cuff tears and has been reported to have a diagnostic positive predictive value as high as 95%. Arm extension and internal rotation help image lateral greater tuberosity bursal fluid. Light transducer pressure is important so as not to compress the fluid into other nonimaged areas of the joint. This indirect sign is important enough to warrant complementary imaging, typically arthroscopy or MRI.

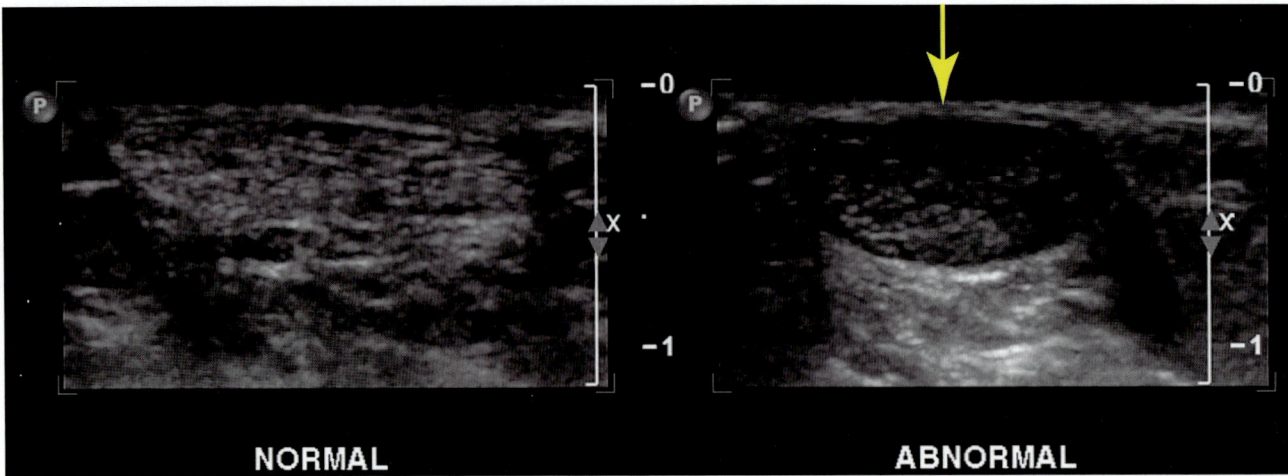

FIG. 24.50 Dual gray-scale image comparing the normal *(left)* with the injured tendon *(right)*. The abnormal tendon reveals a focal area of inflammation *(arrowhead)*.

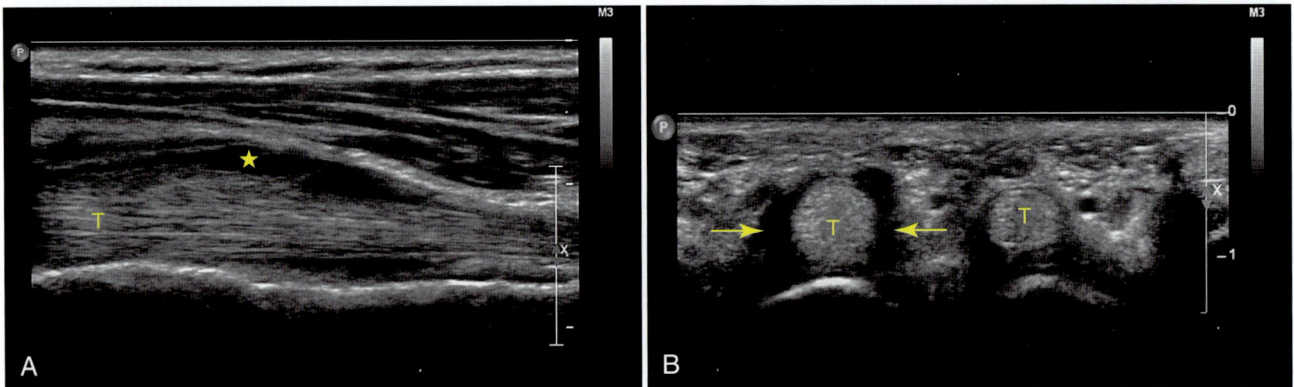

FIG. 24.51 (A) Gray-scale image of the extensor tendons in the hand of a patient with tenosynovitis displays the characteristic anechoic fluid *(star)* surrounding the tendon (T). (B) The fluid within the tendon sheath creates a halo effect *(arrows)* around the tendon on the transverse image.

the synovial sheath, which appears as a halo effect in the transverse plane (Fig. 24.51). The normal synovial sheath appears as a hypoechoic halo around the tendon. Fluid surrounding the tendon may be anechoic or complex if debris-containing.

A focal or diffuse decrease in echogenicity within tendon fibers is a sonographic sign of tendinitis. An increase in blood flow on color or power Doppler imaging in the periphery detects hyperemia. Any discrepancy in thickness measurements greater than 1.5 mm is also highly suspicious of a focal lesion. Areas of injury may be subtle; comparing the abnormal side with the contralateral healthy side helps confirm the diagnosis (see Fig. 24.50).

De Quervain tendinitis is a form of tendinitis with which many sonographers and sonologists may be inherently familiar. This type of tendon inflammation results in pain on the lateral side of the wrist and may result in an audible creaking called *crepitus* during movement. Continuous use of the hand and thumb in a twisting, pinching, or grasping fashion increases the chances of developing swelling in this area. During the acute phase, sonographic imaging of the large abductor pollicis longus and small extensor pollicis brevis

> **BOX 24.7** **Sonographic Features of Tendinitis**
>
> - Focal or diffuse hypoechogenicity
> - Enlargement of the tendon in a focal or diffuse pattern
> - Echogenic tendon fibrils within the area of inflammation
> - Calcifications with chronic tendinitis
> - Increased color or power Doppler signals in the periphery
> - Coexisting bursitis
> - Excess synovial sheath fluid

tendon reveals hypoechoic tendons and synovium. As the process becomes chronic, fibrosis forms, increasing echogenicity. Fibrosis results in restriction of the tendons through the dorsal compartment of the hand, leading to decreased thumb mobility, more specifically the ability to move the thumb away from the hand or straighten after grasping.

Box 24.7 lists the sonographic features of tendinitis.

Muscle Tears

Ultrasound's ability to reveal subtle changes in internal muscle structure allows accurate identification of traumatic muscle injury. Tears are the most common pathologic condition of muscles in the limbs. A muscle strain from overexertion does not cause visual changes in muscle visualized with ultrasound; however, this is a common indication for musculoskeletal imaging examinations as ultrasound is able to correct a strain diagnosis if a tear is observed. Two types of muscle tears can occur: distraction (indirect) and compression (direct). Abrupt stretching of the muscle beyond its maximum length results in distraction tears. These are usually due to sudden interruption of a movement, such as kicking or improper body alignment. External force resulting in a crush injury is considered a compression tear. This type of trauma causes the muscle to crush against underlying bone and results in symptoms ranging from a bruise to a large hematoma. Hematomas associated with muscle injury have variable sonographic appearances. The characteristics of hematoma secondary to muscle injury help determine the extent of underlying damage. The hematoma mass structure pushes apart muscle fibers and often appear diffuse and ill-defined. Acute hematomas initially appear anechoic; however, they become heterogeneous in echogenicity within the muscle fibers as coagulation occurs. Within a few days, the hematoma becomes more well-defined; this often increases detection (Fig. 24.52). As the hematoma ages, it liquefies into a hypoechoic to anechoic mass, and a **seroma** (accumulation of serous fluid within tissue) forms within the muscle defect. This typically occurs within a few weeks. Once healed, a hyperechoic fibrous scar or calcifications within the muscle after reabsorption of the serous material can be visualized. The hematoma that conforms to the fibrous layers may mimic deep vein thrombosis within the calf or arm muscles.

The sonographic appearance of a muscle tear varies with the type of injury. A full-thickness muscle tear images with the torn muscle end outlined by fluid. The muscle belly appears thick with a whorled circular pattern compared with the healthy contralateral side (Fig. 24.53). As the hematoma resolves, it becomes smaller, and echogenicity increases.

A complete muscle tear has a straightforward appearance of a retracted hyperechoic muscle surrounded by a hematoma (**"clapper in the bell" sign**). The partial tear may be as subtle

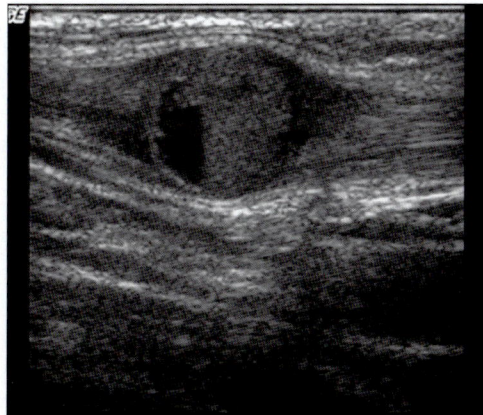

FIG. 24.52 Gray-scale image of an intramuscular hematoma appears as an organized heterogeneous thrombus.

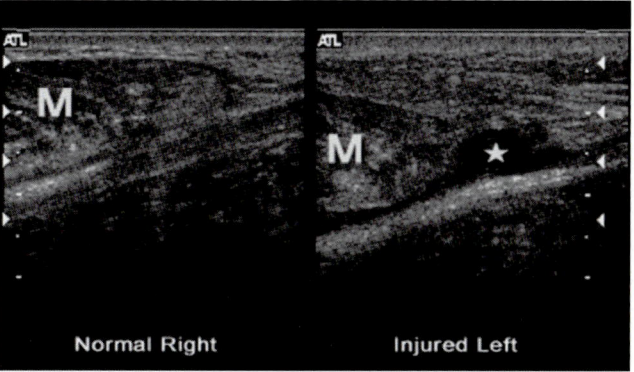

FIG. 24.53 Dual gray-scale image of a normal *(left)* and torn *(right)* gastrocnemius muscle (M) results in a hematoma *(star)* at the area of the injury. Comparison of the normal and injured sides confirms the muscle tear, which is more commonly seen in athletes participating in jumping activities.

TABLE 24.5	Sonographic Appearance of Muscle Tear Grades
Grade	Appearance
I (elongation injury)	Normal, flame-shaped focal fiber discontinuity, small hematoma (<1 cm)
II (partial rupture)	<⅓ of muscle fibers disrupted, hematoma <3 cm, interfascial hematoma, hypoechoic gap within the muscle that changes position with transducer pressure
III (complete rupture)	>⅓ rupture of muscle resembling a soft tissue mass, hematoma >3 cm, large interfascial hematoma

as a discontinuity of the muscle fibers and septa or as obvious as a hematoma with echoic debris. This type of tear may be difficult to separate from the earlier mentioned edge artifact because of similarities in appearance. The true torn muscle with irregular margins will have the same sonographic appearance at varying angles of incidence, whereas the edge artifact will occur only at a 90-degree angle. Examination of the injured muscle includes images with the muscle contracted and at rest in both longitudinal and transverse planes. An area of rupture may also image with a hyperechoic halo surrounding the jagged rupture margins. As the muscle heals, the edges of the tear increase in echogenicity and thickness. The normal muscle architecture becomes evident with healing. The hyperechoic linear, stellate, or nodular scar or an intramuscular cyst provides evidence of an abnormal healing process.

Table 24.5 lists the sonographic appearance of muscle tears by grade.

Carpal Tunnel Syndrome

Carpal tunnel syndrome (CTS) is an entrapment syndrome of the median nerve characterized by median nerve compression and neuropathy. Continued use of the same muscle group results in hypertrophied muscles, and repeated trauma

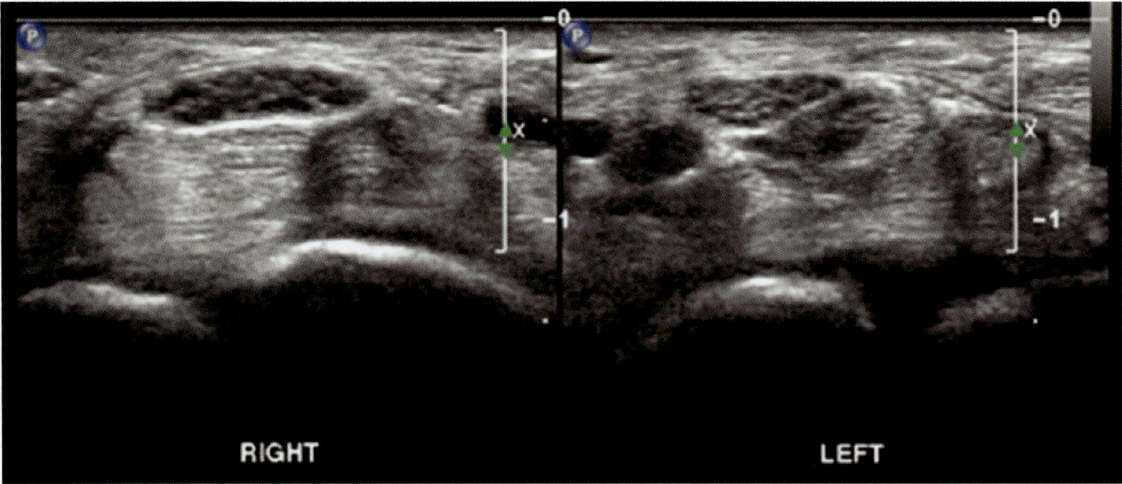

FIG. 24.54 Dual gray-scale image of the right median nerve demonstrates notable flattening in this symptomatic patient. The left median nerve *(right side of image)* is also mildly flattened.

to the tendon sheath may cause tendon (traumatic synovitis) and muscle enlargement, resulting in tunnel narrowing (Fig. 24.54). Repetitive wrist movements cause excursion of the median nerve through the already crowded carpal tunnel. Continued friction within the tunnel causes microtrauma to the epineurium of the median nerve, resulting in inflammation. Increase in median nerve size from inflammation further contributes to limiting the space inside the carpal tunnel.

Occupations that require repetitive wrist movements cause repetitive stress on the median nerve, resulting in the pain and paresthesias characteristic of this CTS. The sonography profession is one that is highly susceptible to CTS from repetitive scanning motions, forceful exertion in obese patients, and fine movements of the ultrasound transducer. In addition to repetitive movements, CTS can also occur secondary to pregnancy, chronic renal failure, diabetes mellitus, rheumatoid arthritis, amyloidosis, and tenosynovitis. Extrinsic causes include accessory muscles, soft tissue masses, and ganglions.

The patient suffering from CTS typically presents with numbness of the middle and index fingers, weakness or clumsiness of the hand, and pain. The clinical examination is positive for **Tinel sign** or **Phalen sign**, and weakness is seen in the affected hand in chronic stages.

The normal median nerve is elliptical proximal to the wrist and flattens distally as the nerve passes under the flexor retinaculum and through the carpal tunnel. The transverse median nerve in a patient with CTS reveals a nerve that severely flattens and often disfigures within the carpal tunnel, with bowing of the flexor retinaculum.

Increased nerve size can also be appreciated from inflammation; however, normal variations in nerve area occur throughout the course of the median nerve. Cross-sectional area (CSA) calculations are helpful to detect an increase in median nerve size and are calculated using an ellipsoid formula of Area = $\pi(D1 \times D2)/4$. Because normal variations in nerve size occur, several area thresholds have been proposed; however, it is generally accepted that nerve CSA greater than 15 mm² at the level of the proximal tunnel is considered enlarged. As with assessments of other musculoskeletal structures, comparison with the healthy contralateral side is helpful to assist in detection of abnormalities.

Box 24.8 describes the sonographic appearance of median nerve compression.

BOX 24.8	Sonographic Appearance of Median Nerve Compression

- Focal or diffuse enlargement proximal to the carpal tunnel
- Increased cross-sectional area (>15 mm²)
- Deformation of oval shape in transverse view at the level of the distal radius (within the carpal tunnel)
- Tenosynovitis with >4mm dorsal bowing of the flexor retinaculum

Key Pearls

- Skeletal muscle contains long organized skeletal muscle cells, also called muscle fibers, organized into muscle bundles.
- Muscles fibers may run parallel to the bone, have a fan shape, or form a pennate pattern.
- Pennate pattern muscle fibers appear feather-like and run oblique to the long axis of the muscle and can be unipennate, bipennate, multipennate, or circumpennate.
- Attachment of the muscle occurs at the proximal and distal portions of the muscle bundles
- Tendons are tough collagenous fibers that attach muscles to bones.
- Tendons may be cordlike or flat sheets called aponeuroses. Aponeuroses attachments occur in flat muscles, such as the rectus abdominis in the abdomen. Tendons may or may not have a synovial sheath outer covering.
- The synovial sheath is a tubular sac that surrounds a tendon. They have two layers and consist of synovial fluid.

- The support and strength of joints are due in part to ligaments. Ligaments are short bands of tough fibers that connect bones to other bones.
- Bursae are fluid-filled saclike structures that surround joints and tendons. Bursae contain synovial fluid that reduces friction between musculoskeletal structures during movement.
- Nerves conduct electrical impulses that carry sensory and motor information to and from the central nervous system muscles, respectively.
- Anisotropy is an artifact that occurs commonly in musculoskeletal imaging. It occurs when imaging a structure while not perpendicular, which results in soundwave reflections not returning to the transducer. This also commonly occurs when imaging curved structures. The angle and direction of the reflected soundwave depend on the angle of incidence.
- A comet-tail artifact is seen when soundwaves reflect multiple times between two closely placed reflectors. In the case of a pin surgically placed within a bone, the reflecting surfaces are the anterior and posterior borders of the hardware.
- Redirection of the incident soundwave to an oblique path occurs often and is seen as an edge artifact (refractile shadowing) on the sonographic image. This change in direction of the soundwave results in a hypoechoic band posterior to the structure.
- Speed error artifact, also referred to as time-of-flight or speed-of-sound error, occurs when the returning soundwave passes through tissues with markedly different densities, deviating from the assumed speed of sound in soft tissue of 1540 m/sec.
- The Achilles tendon is a large, strong fibrous tendon that connects the gastrocnemius and soleus muscles to the calcaneus. This tendon helps move your foot downward, push off when walking, and rise up on your toes. Injury to this tendon can make it impossible to walk without pain.
- Thompson's test (plantar flexion with squeezing of the calf) may be used to evaluate the integrity of the Achilles tendon.
- Dislocation (also called *subluxation*) of the biceps tendon from the bicipital groove may be caused by abnormalities with the transverse humeral ligament, abnormal development of the bicipital groove or supraspinatus, and/or subscapularis tears.
- Rotator cuff pathology may occur as acute or chronic processes. Biceps tendon ruptures, trauma, and shoulder dislocations are a few common causes of acute rotator cuff tears.
- One of the most common tendon abnormalities is inflammation due to age-related elasticity loss, diseases such as rheumatoid arthritis, overuse, or trauma. Tendinitis can occur in any tendon but is often seen in the shoulder, wrist, heel, and elbow.
- A complete muscle tear has a straightforward appearance of a retracted hyperechoic muscle surrounded by a hematoma ("clapper in the bell" sign).
- The carpal tunnel is formed by the carpal bones and overlying flexor retinaculum on the palmar side of the wrist. Carpal tunnel syndrome is an entrapment disorder causing compression and neuropathy of the median nerve.

BIBLIOGRAPHY

American Institute of Ultrasound in Medicine: AIUM practice guidelines for the performance of a shoulder ultrasound examination, Laurel, MD, 2007, AIUM.

Azar FM, Beaty JH, Canale TS, eds. *Campbell's Operative Orthopaedics*, vol 1, 13th ed. Philadelphia: Elsevier; 2017.

Bianchi S, et al. Ultrasound of the digital flexor system: normal and pathological findings. *J ultrasound*. 2007;10(2):85–92.

Bianchi S. Ultrasound of the peripheral nerves. *Jt Bone Spine*. 2008;75:643–649.

Bradley M, O'Donnell P. *Atlas of musculoskeletal ultrasound anatomy*. Cambridge: Greenwich Medical Media Limited; 2007.

Dieleman Joseph L, et al. US health care spending by payer and health condition, 1996-2016. *Jama*. 2020;323(9):863–884.

Dondelinger R, ed. *Peripheral musculoskeletal ultrasound atlas: a CD-ROM atlas*. New York: Thieme; 2001.

Elangovan Sakktivel, Tan York Kiat. The role of musculoskeletal ultrasound imaging in rheumatoid arthritis. *Ultrasound Med & Biol*. 2020

Fessell D, Jacobson J. Ultrasound of the hindfoot and midfoot. *Radiol Clin North Am*. 2008;46:1027–1043.

Finlay K, Friedman L. Ultrasonography of the lower extremity. *Orthop Clin North Am*. 2006;37:245–275.

Grainger A. Internal impingement syndromes of the shoulder. *Semin Musculoskelet Radiol*. 2008;12:127–135.

Harvey C, Hart J, Lloyd C, Barbar S. Musculoskeletal ultrasound in adults. *Br J Hosp Med*. 2008;69:M100–M103.

Hirji Z, Jaspal S, Hema N. Imaging of the bursae. *J Clin imaging Sci*. 2011;1

Hodgson RJ, O'Connor P, Grainger A. Tendon and ligament imaging. *Br J radiology*. 2012;85(1016):1157–1172.

Jacobson J. *Fundamentals of musculoskeletal ultrasound*. ed 2 Philadelphia: Elsevier; 2013.

Jamadar D, Jacobson J, Caoili E, et al. Musculoskeletal sonography technique: focused versus comprehensive evaluation. *Am J Roentgenol*. 2008;190:5–9.

Kremkau F. *Diagnostic ultrasound: principles and instruments, ed 7*. Philadelphia. : Saunders; 2006.

Lew H, Chen C, Wang T, Chew K. Introduction to musculoskeletal diagnostic ultrasound: examination of the upper limb. *Am J Phys Med Rehabil*. 2007;86:310–321.

Lin J, Fessell D, Jacobson J, et al. An illustrated tutorial of musculoskeletal sonography: part 3, lower extremity. *Am J Roentgenol*. 2000;175:1313–1321.

Ly J, Bui-Mansfield L. Anatomy of and abnormalities associated with Kager's fat pad. *Am J Roentgenol*. 2004;182:147–154.

McDonald DG, Leopold GR. Ultrasound B-scanning in the differentiation of Baker's cyst and thrombophlebitis. *Br J Radiol*. 1972;45:729–732.

Martinoli Carlo. Musculoskeletal ultrasound: technical guidelines. *Insights into imaging*. 2010;1(3):99–141.

Moore K, Dalley A, Agur A, eds. *Clinically oriented anatomy*. ed 6 Philadelphia: Lippincott Williams & Wilkins; 2010.

O'Neill J, ed. *Musculoskeletal ultrasound: anatomy and technique*. New York: Springer; 2008.

Peetrons P. Ultrasound of muscles. *Eur Radiol*. 2002;12:35–43.

Schmidt W, Backhaus M. What the practicing rheumatologist needs to know about the technical fundamentals of ultrasonography. *Best Pract Res Clin Rheumatol*. 2008;22:981–999.

Tagliafico A, Rubino M, Autuori A, et al. Wrist and hand ultrasound. *Semin Musculoskelet Radiol*. 2007;11:95–104.

Torriani M, Kattapuram S. Dynamic sonography of the forefoot: the sonographic Mulder sign. *Am J Roentgenol*. 2002;180:1121.

van Holsbeeck M, Introcaso J. *Musculoskeletal ultrasound*. ed 2 St Louis: Mosby; 2001.

Walker F, Cartwright M, Wiesler E, et al. Ultrasound of nerve and muscle. *Clin Neurophysiol.* 2004;115:495–507.

Wiesler E, Chloros G, Cartwright M, et al. The use of diagnostic ultrasound in carpal tunnel syndrome. *J Hand Surg Am.* 2006;31:726–732.

Winter T, Teefey S, Middleton W. Musculoskeletal ultrasound: an update. *Radiol Clin North Am.* 2004;39:465–483.

Wu Wei-Ting, et al. Artifacts in musculoskeletal ultrasonography: from physics to clinics. *Diagnostics.* 2020;10(9):645.

Zagzebski J. *Essentials of ultrasound physics.* St Louis: Mosby; 1997.

PART IV

Pediatrics

Chapter 25 Neonatal and Pediatric Abdomen
Chapter 26 Neonatal and Pediatric Adrenal and Urinary System
Chapter 27 Neonatal and Infant Head
Chapter 28 Infant and Pediatric Hip
Chapter 29 Neonatal and Infant Spine

CHAPTER 25

Neonatal and Pediatric Abdomen

Kathryn E. Zale

OBJECTIVES

On completion of this chapter, you should be able to:
- Understand the different pediatric stages/ages and how to increase patient cooperation
- List the more common hepatobiliary, pancreatic, and splenic reasons for acute abdominal pain in the pediatric population
- List the more common acquired and hereditary diseases and how pediatric sonography can monitor the associated chronic or malignant processes
- List the causes of jaundice in the neonate and pediatric patient
- Distinguish obstructive from nonobstructive jaundice
- List the common primary hepatic tumors in children
- List the most common gastrointestinal surgical conditions in the pediatric population
- Describe the sonographic appearance of the pathologic conditions discussed in this chapter

OUTLINE

Examination Preparation 762
Normal Anatomy and Sonographic Findings 764
Hepatobiliary, Pancreatic, and Splenic Pathology 766
  Common Presenting Diseases 767
  Abdominal Tumors 772
Gastrointestinal Pathology 775
  Common Surgical Conditions 775
  Other Surgical Conditions 787

KEY TERMS

Acholic (stools)
Appendectomy
Appendicitis
Appendicolith
Atretic
Beckwith-Wiedemann syndrome
Biliary atresia
Choledochal cyst
Extracorporeal membrane oxygenation (ECMO)
Hemihypertrophy
Hypertrophic pyloric stenosis (HPS)
Hypomotility
Inspissated
Intussusception
Kasai portoenterostomy
McBurney's point
Midgut malrotation
Mucosa
Neonatal intensive care unit (NICU)
Neuroblastoma
Nonalcoholic steatohepatitis
Pancreatic lipomatosis
Projectile vomiting
Pyloric canal
Pyloromyotomy
Scintigraphy
Short bowel syndrome
Target sign ("cinnamon bun" sign)
Ultrasound-first approach
Umbilical vein catheter
Ventriculoperitoneal shunt
Wilms' tumor (nephroblastoma)

Sonography is often the first imaging procedure used to evaluate the neonatal and pediatric abdomen. Pediatric sonography is a powerful imaging specialty, providing excellent visualization of the anatomy in an infant or a child. Furthermore, it does not subject them to ionizing radiation, iodized contrast material, or anesthesia. It is portable, inexpensive, relatively painless, and generally well tolerated. It is important to relay that children often have different diseases than adults with their own features; therefore, this chapter focuses on the more common, as well as critical, abdominal diagnoses specific to the pediatric population. Abdominal conditions discussed here are primarily focused on hepatobiliary (along with some pancreatic and splenic diseases) and common surgical gastrointestinal conditions, such as appendicitis, intussusception, and hypertrophic pyloric stenosis (HPS).

Many of these diagnoses will require surgical treatment, and using the **ultrasound-first approach** may, in some cases, obviate the need for more testing or imaging. Finally, although this section focuses on diseases specific to the neonate and child, pediatric sonographers must also have an in-depth comprehension of adult pathology. The increase in childhood obesity, for example, may accompany an earlier onset of adult disease processes, such as nonalcoholic fatty liver disease (NAFLD). Additionally, some pediatric hospitals may follow patients affected by chronic congenital or childhood diseases for life (e.g., cystic fibrosis [CF] and myelomeningoceles).

EXAMINATION PREPARATION

Special attention is always required with pediatric patients, and it is imperative to remember that children are not just small adults. Gaining the trust of the patient and the patient's family to facilitate the examination is best captured in the famous quote by the late pediatric radiologist, Dr. Armand Brodeur, "To stand tall in pediatrics, you have to get down on your knees." Getting down to the child's level requires patience, preparation, and sometimes, creativity. Being mindful of the patient's developmental stage (mentally, physically, and emotionally) and having a basic understanding of their normal age group are important. The pediatric stages and scanning tips provided in Table 25.1 aim to help minimize patient discomfort and optimize image quality. Moreover, our society has seen a rise in pediatric conditions, such as attention deficit–hyperactivity disorder, autism, Down

TABLE 25.1 Pediatric Stages, Ages, and Scanning Tips

Stage/Age	Considerations
Preterm infant: <37 weeks of gestation	• Use 9–12 MHz curved array or linear transducer • Extra infection control measures are critical in this delicate population; use gel packets if possible, to decrease contamination risks • Susceptible to hypothermia; always use warm gel, but be sure it is not too hot • Remove gel as soon as possible; it gets cold quickly • Keep preemie securely wrapped in a blanket when not scanning • Observe and note all monitors in the **neonatal intensive care unit (NICU)**; always obtain the nurse's permission before starting any examination • Scan through the portholes of an isolette to maintain body temperature

Neonate: first 28 days of life
Infant: first year of life after the first 28 days
	• Use 7.5–10 MHz curved array or linear transducer
	• Use warm gel and be sure it is not too hot
	• Wrap blankets around infant as needed
	• Use good infection control techniques
	• Let mother hold child until calm
	• Neonates and infants up to 6 months old:
	  • Use pacifier, cuddling, or changing diaper when necessary to keep comfortable
	  • Feeding okay if not contraindicated or after biliary evaluation and pancreas completed in full abdominal study
	  • Glycogen and water bottles should be handy (dip binky into sugar solution; may repeat while scanning until able to give milk/formula)
	  • Palpate abdomen when muscles are relaxed
	  • Have plenty of distractions ready (e.g., noisy bright-colored toys, keys, singing)
	• Infants >6 months old (in addition to above infant information)
	  • Separation and stranger anxiety developing, keep parents near, examine on parent's lap if necessary
	  • Smile and talk to infant throughout the examination

Toddler: between 1 and 3 years **Preschooler:** between 3 and 5 years	• Use 6–9 MHz linear, curved array, or sector • Tell the child what you are doing at each step • Provide positive feedback when cooperating • Give them choices when possible; they may prefer the cold gel • Let the child touch the gel beforehand • Offer to scan favorite doll/teddy first to reduce anxiety • Have plenty of distractions ready (e.g., stickers, televisions, mobiles, or ultrasound itself ["watch the movie"]). • If toddler becomes too stressed, give the child a rest • Allow child to lie next to parent or caregiver on table if feasible
School-age: between 6 and 12 years	• Use 5–7.5 MHz curved array or sector • Usually understand and cooperative at this age; explain what you are doing and why • Distract with questions about favorite color, pets, classes, etc • Provide positive feedback when cooperating • Develop modesty at this age, so be sure to explain procedure before child undresses
Teenager/adolescent: between 12 and 18 years	• Use 2–5 MHz curved array or sector • Provide privacy for undressing if required • Provide chaperone when parent or accompanying adult is unavailable • Adolescents have a lot of concerns about their developing bodies; provide reassurance when appropriate

TABLE 25.2	Pediatric Considerations
Condition/Issue	Considerations
Attention deficit–hyperactivity disorder (ADHD)	One of the most common childhood disorders; median age of onset is 6 years; affects nearly 9% of children ages 13–18, with boys diagnosed 3× more often than girls. Children with ADHD experience inattentiveness, hyperactivity, and impulsivity. Be clear and consistent, focus on the positive, and provide praise/rewards when following the rules.
Autism spectrum disorder (ASD)	Occurs in 1 of 54 children in the United States, affecting boys 4× more than girls. Inhibits a child's ability to interact socially; usually plays alone or shows little eye contact. Often appears within the first 2 years of life, although may be diagnosed later. ASD is a spectrum and is different from child to child; it is important to carefully observe parent-child interaction for guidance on approach. Be very clear in directions and sensitive to sensory issues (e.g., touch), which are common.
Family dynamics and structures	Many different family dynamics/structures exist. Never assume the person with the child is the parent/grandparent, etc., and be mindful and respectful of all family types.
Child abuse	May take on the form of sexual abuse, physical abuse, or neglect. Physical abuse and neglect by caregivers have not declined in recent years, although some trends show overall child abuse is down. Health care workers are obligated under law to report ANY suspicion of abuse.
Food allergies	Allergies are on the rise, with roughly 30%–35% of all children affected. As health care workers with direct contact with children, it is especially important to wash hands after handling potential allergens and keep clothes clean of them; even a small amount of peanut dust may send a child who is very allergic to peanuts into anaphylactic shock.
Childhood obesity	Rates have doubled in children and quadrupled in adolescents in the past 30 years; 1 in 5 children or adolescents is affected in the United States. There is an increased risk for cardiovascular disease and greater risk for bone and joint problems, sleep apnea, and social and psychological issues stemming from stigmatization and poor self-esteem.
Critically ill and dying infant/child	Perhaps the most difficult part of scanning children is dealing with the critically ill or dying patient. In these cases, it becomes increasingly important to have a child-centered approach and respect for the family, keeping in mind they are dealing with an immense amount of grief and stress, however expressed. It is also equally important to acknowledge one's own feelings to perform examinations without emotions interfering in providing quality patient care.

syndrome, cerebral palsy, and childhood obesity, among others. Table 25.2 provides more information on some of these issues to consider carefully when dealing with children.

The sonographer should first allow sufficient time to calmly explain the examination to the parents and the child who is old enough to comprehend the proceedings. Recruiting the parent(s) is an invaluable resource and can help reassure and quiet the patient. Therefore, parents are highly encouraged to be present during the examination. Talking to the patient in age-appropriate terms and speaking with a soft voice will also facilitate cooperation. It is always best to make eye contact on the child's level, keeping the eye contact steady and concentrating on the child. Towering over a child and wearing white coats can be intimidating. It is also best to start the examination in a well-lit room, as not to scare the child. Sedation and immobilization techniques are generally not required or recommended. A pacifier may serve well when examining infants. Toys, books, keys, televisions, mobiles, and various other distracting devices can help quiet the frightened young child. A good attitude and a dose of fun can go a long way, too.

Patient preparation will depend on the type of abdominal examination being performed and emergent status. Formula feeding is generally not recommended and contraindicated if they are a surgical candidate. Some laboratories may offer glucose "sugar" water or Pedialyte feedings when examining a neonate for pyloric stenosis, but it is always best to ask the radiologist and emergency department before offering. When imaging the biliary system feedings should be withheld for a short time according to the patient's age (Box 25.1).

> **BOX 25.1 Pediatric Ultrasound Examination Prep**
>
> **Abdominal Ultrasound[a]**
> Age-specific guidelines of nothing by mouth (NPO) prior to study:
> - Infants: NPO 2–3 h
> - 1–4 years: NPO 3–4 h
> - 5–10 years: NPO 5–6 h
> - 11+ years: NPO 8 h
>
> **Pelvic Ultrasound**
> Age-specific guidelines of pushing fluids (noncarbonated, preferably water) to obtain a full urinary bladder:
> - Infants–2 years: feed fluids 1 hour prior to study. Recommend bringing extra bottle or juice for use during study.
> - 3–5 years: drink 8 oz of fluid 30–60 minutes prior to study, and do not void.
> - 6–10 years: drink 16–24 oz of fluid 45–60 minutes prior to study, and do not void.
> - 11+ years: drink 32 oz of fluid 1 hour prior to study, and do not void.
>
> [a]Whenever possible, patients should not void for 1 hour prior to study.

Adequate distention of the urinary bladder is also desirable when examining the pelvis (see Box 25.1). This not only allows assessment of the bladder itself but also facilitates the identification of dilated distal ureters, free peritoneal fluid, the pelvic reproductive organs, and pelvic masses. A urine-filled bladder may, in some cases, help localize gastrointestinal abnormalities, such as appendicitis and intussusception. In females, pelvic structures are examined with a well-filled but not overly distended bladder.

Pediatric scanning will require some technical changes as well. Because imaging infants and children involves countless different body habitus, utilizing a wide array of probe frequencies and footprints is not unusual. The information provided on transducer selection is merely a guideline, and the highest-frequency transducer and smallest footprint for the imaged area are best. Avoid "shooting the table" or including nondiagnostic information posterior to the spine; a 5 MHz just utilized for an adolescent will provide poor diagnostic images on an infant. However, if the optimal frequency is unavailable, use sequential focusing and zoom for better resolution instead of decreasing depth. Optimization to improve image quality should always be performed while keeping the aggregate ultrasound exposure as low as reasonably achievable.

Maintaining body temperature in the neonate is very important because small infants can quickly lose a potentially dangerous amount of body heat. Whenever possible, scanning through the portholes of an Isolette provides an optimal environment for the premature or otherwise fragile neonate. When the examination is performed outside of the Isolette, body heat loss can be minimized using heat lamps and by exposing only the area of the body being interrogated.

It will also be necessary to learn how to acquire images quickly when imaging infants and young children, and cine clips can serve well in depicting difficult anatomy or pathology in the unruly child. It may also be best to put the gel on the probe instead of directly on the patient to improve child cooperation. Careful consideration is necessary to determine a child's patience and/or ability to withstand an examination, as in the case of a critically ill preemie or uncooperative child. Therefore, modifying protocols to tailor to these individuals may be necessary. Finally, before beginning any pediatric examination, a review of the medical record and any previous imaging (paying close attention to ultrasound transducer selection and settings) will aid in providing a more thorough and time-efficient study.

NORMAL ANATOMY AND SONOGRAPHIC FINDINGS

A full abdominal ultrasound examination is required when evaluating the neonatal or pediatric abdomen. Limited abdominal studies are only relegated for follow-ups or the emergent, acute abdomen for gastrointestinal conditions. Ultrasound is the modality of choice to document organ size and other abnormalities in the pediatric abdomen. Therefore, it is important to be well acquainted with the normal pediatric abdomen and document organ growth and properly utilize size charts.

In the upper abdomen, the pancreas should be examined for normal size and echotexture, without evidence of peripancreatic fluid, adenopathy, dilation of the distal common bile duct or pancreatic duct, which should not exceed 2 mm in diameter. The size of the pancreas should increase with the child's age (Table 25.3). The normal texture is homogenous and may appear slightly hyperechoic, or even isoechoic, compared with the normal liver texture, as little fatty tissue has yet invaded the islets of Langerhans (Fig. 25.1).

TABLE 25.3	Normal Dimensions of the Pancreas as a Function of Age		
	Maximum AP Dimension in cm (SD)		
Patient Age	Head	Body	Tail
Neonate	1.0 (0.4)	0.6 (0.2)	1.0 (0.4)
1 month–1 year	1.5 (0.5)	0.8 (0.3)	1.2 (0.4)
1–5 years	1.7 (0.3)	1.0 (0.2)	1.8 (0.4)
5–10 years	1.6 (0.4)	1.0 (0.3)	1.8 (0.4)
10–19 years	2.0 (0.5)	1.1 (0.3)	2.0 (0.4)

AP, Anteroposterior; *SD*, standard deviation.
Data from Siegel MJ, Martin KW, Worthington JL. Normal and abnormal pancreas in children: US studies. *Radiology*. 1987;165:15–18.

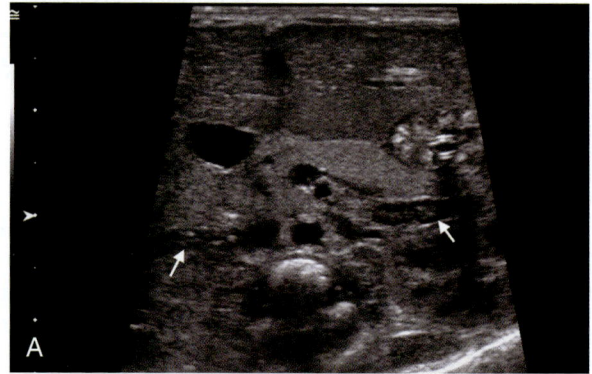

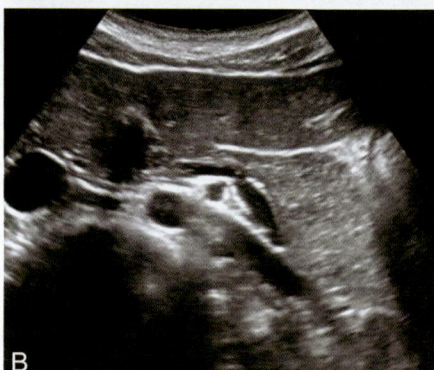

FIG. 25.1 Normal neonatal and pediatric pancreas. Evaluation of the pancreas is unremarkable without evidence of focal mass. Uncinate process, head, and body of pancreas are well visualized. Tail of the pancreas seen in its entirety. (A) Neonatal pancreas imaged with a linear transducer. Bilateral adrenal glands are also visualized *(arrows)*. (B) Adolescent pancreas. (A, Courtesy Chester County Hospital, West Chester, PA. B, Courtesy Nationwide Children's Hospital, Columbus, OH.)

The size and texture of the liver should be evaluated (Fig. 25.2). The right hepatic lobe should not extend more than 1 cm below the costal margin in a young infant without pulmonary hyperaeration and should not extend below the right costal margin in older infants and children. The echogenicity is normally low to medium homogeneity with clear definition of the portal venous vasculature. Documentation with a linear transducer over the capsule is recommended. The right hemidiaphragm and pleural space should be evaluated as well.

The portal vein diameter helps determine the presence of portal hypertension (Fig. 25.3) and increases in size with age and weight (Box 25.2). Color and pulsed wave Doppler should be used to determine flow direction and patency.

Careful evaluation of the biliary system should be made to exclude ductal dilation. The common bile duct should measure less than 1 mm in neonates, less than 2 mm in infants up to 1 year, less than 4 mm in older children, and less than 6 mm in adolescents and adults (see Box 25.2).

The gallbladder size and wall thickness should be assessed. In infants under one year of age, the gallbladder length is 1.5 to 3 cm, and in older children, it is 3 to 7 cm. The length of the

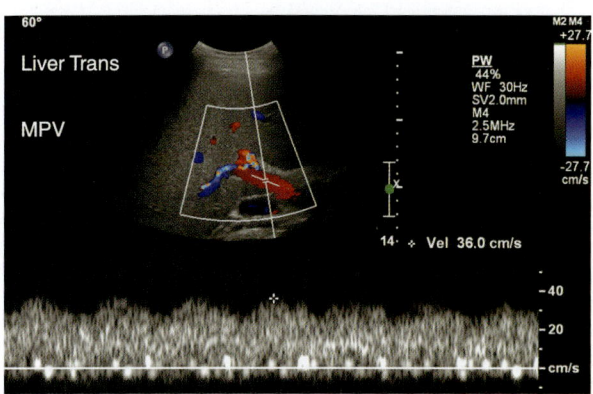

FIG. 25.3 Normal pediatric main portal vein. The portal vein is normal in size with hepatopetal phasic flow patterns shown with color Doppler and angle-corrected pulsed Doppler. (Courtesy Nationwide Children's Hospital, Columbus, OH.)

BOX 25.2 Normal Sonographic Measurements

Pancreas[a]
- Head: 1.0–2.5 cm
- Body: 0.6–1.4 cm
- Tail: 1.0–2.4 cm
- Duct: <2 mm

Liver
- Infants: right lobe should not extend >1 cm below costal margin
- Older infants and children: right lobe should not extend below right costal margin

Portal Vein Diameter (Upper Limits)
- Neonates: 3–5 mm
- Children <10 years: 8.5 mm
- Children >10 years: 10 mm
- Adolescents ≤20 years: 7–13 mm

Biliary Ducts
- Neonates: CBD <1 mm
- Infants (≤1 year): CBD <2 mm
- Older children (1–10 years): CBD <4 mm
- Adolescents: CBD <6 mm

Gallbladder Length
- Infants (<1 year): 1.5–3 cm
- Children >1 year: 3–7 cm

Spleen Length (Upper Limits)
- Small-for-date neonates: 3.0 cm (average size)
- Infants
  - 0–3 months: ≤6 cm
  - 3–6 months: ≤6.5 cm
  - 6–12 months: ≤7 cm
- Toddlers/preschoolers
  - 1–2 years: ≤8 cm
  - 2–4 years: ≤9 cm
- Children
  - 4–6 years: ≤9.5 cm
  - 6–8 years: ≤10 cm
  - 8–10 years: ≤11 cm
  - 10–12 years: ≤11.5 cm
- Older children
  - 12–15 years: ≤12 cm
  - 15–20 years: ≤12 cm (female)
  - 15–20 years: ≤13 cm (male)

[a]Size increases with age; see Table 25.3 for specific age criteria.
CBD, Common bile duct.

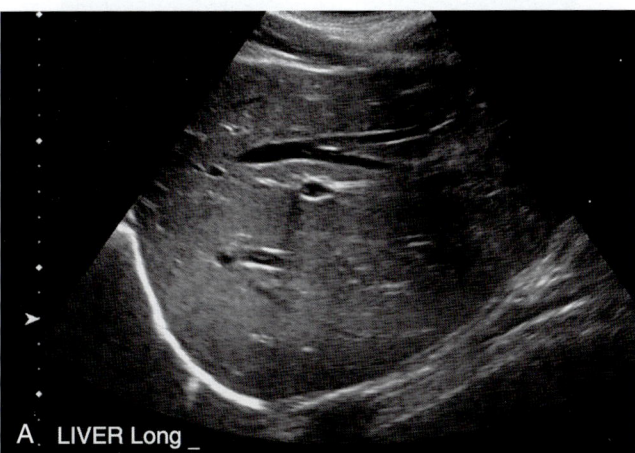
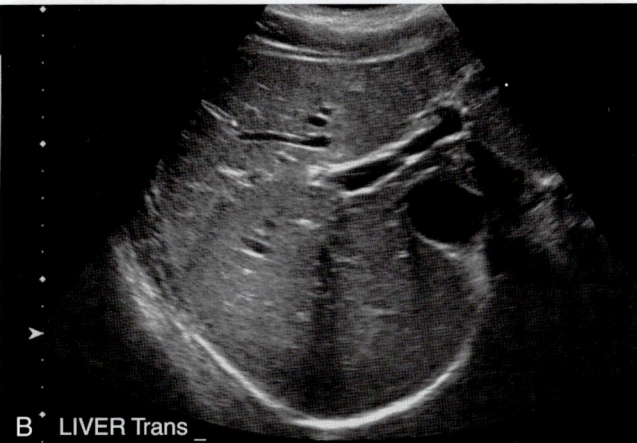

FIG. 25.2 Normal pediatric liver. The liver is normal in size and contour without focal mass or marginal irregularity. (A) Longitudinal right lobe of the liver showing normal hepatic veins. (B) Transverse right lobe of the liver showing right and left portal vein split, and gallbladder in transverse. (Courtesy Nationwide Children's Hospital, Columbus, OH.)

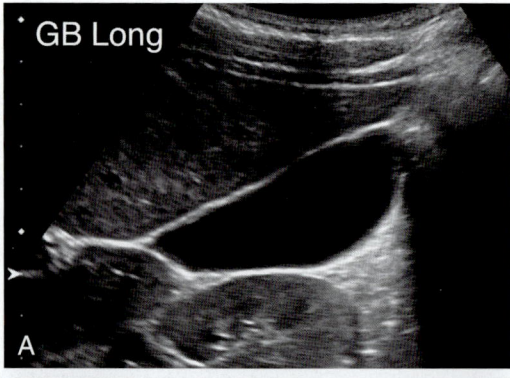
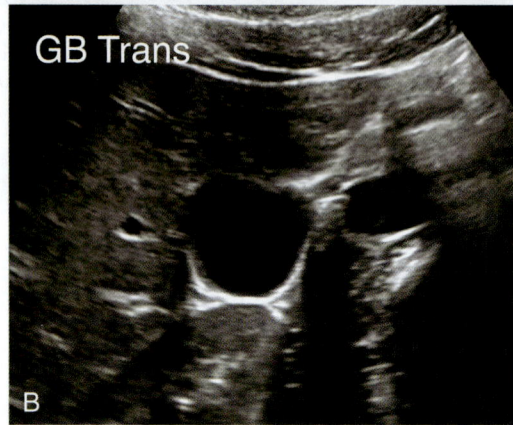
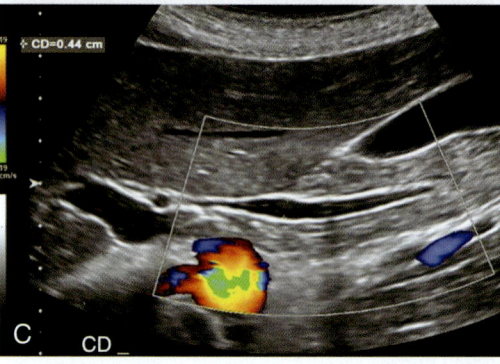

FIG. 25.4 Normal pediatric gallbladder and common bile duct. Gallbladder is unremarkable without wall thickening, pericholecystic fluid, or cholelithiasis. No ductal dilation is seen. (A) Longitudinal gallbladder. (B) Transverse gallbladder. (C) Common bile duct measurement is within normal limits for this adolescent patient. (Courtesy Nationwide Children's Hospital, Columbus, OH.)

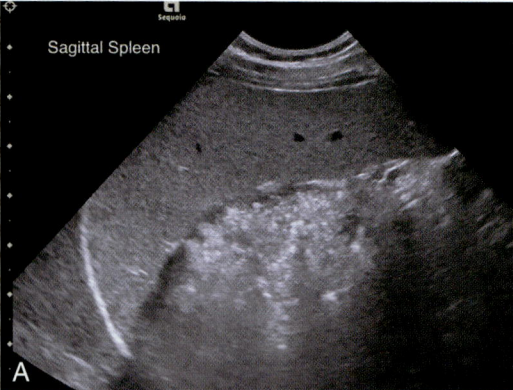
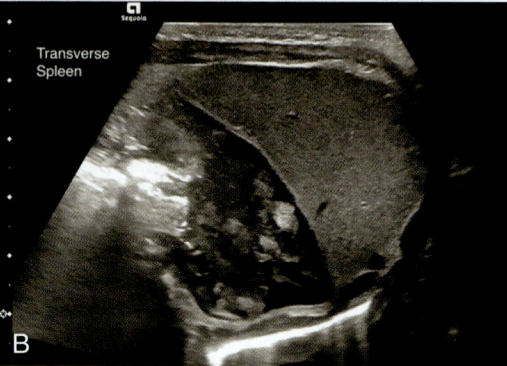

FIG. 25.5 Normal pediatric and neonatal spleen. (A) Pediatric sagittal spleen. The spleen is normal in size, contour, and echogenicity. No focal masses are seen. (B) Transverse neonatal spleen. Stomach posteriorly is full and mostly fluid-filled. (Courtesy of Siemens Healthineers USA, Inc.)

gallbladder should not exceed the length of the kidney. The normal gallbladder should show a smooth-walled anechoic structure without internal echoes (Fig. 25.4). Pericholecystic fluid should not be present.

The splenic size and texture should be evaluated. Often, the stomach contents can be visualized posteriorly (Fig. 25.5). The upper limits of normal splenic length range from 6.0 cm in infants less than 3 months old to 12 cm in children older than 12 years. Polysplenia, as with any anatomic anomaly, should be ruled out. The left hemidiaphragm and pleural space should be evaluated when viewing the spleen as well.

Finally, the retroperitoneal area should be closely evaluated throughout the abdominal sonographic evaluation as most malignant abdominal masses arise from the retroperitoneum in both infants and children. The inferior vena cava (IVC) and aorta vessels are documented. Proper positioning and relationship should be established to rule out situs inversus, and both vessels should be free of any thrombus. This is a critical finding. Lymph nodes are not normally visualized and abnormal when detected. They can be indicated in lymphomas, as well as malignant abdominal and pelvic masses.

Normal bowel peristalsis should be observed in the lower abdomen, and the bowel should not appear thickened. When distended, the bowel wall should measure less than 3 mm in the large bowel, and less than 2.5 mm in the small bowel. It may be up to 4 to 6 mm when collapsed. When unobstructed by gas, the normal five bowel layers, from outer serosa to inner mucosa, also called the *gut signature*, should be observed (Fig. 25.6).

The lower abdomen should be free of any pelvic mass or free fluid. Free fluid is often abnormal, except for a little free fluid in the menstruating female or a patient with a **ventriculoperitoneal shunt**. If a shunt is present, the tip should be documented to rule out the development of an abdominal cerebrospinal fluid pseudocyst.

HEPATOBILIARY, PANCREATIC, AND SPLENIC PATHOLOGY

A wide variety of pathologies may be seen within the pediatric abdomen, and it is important to remember the cause may

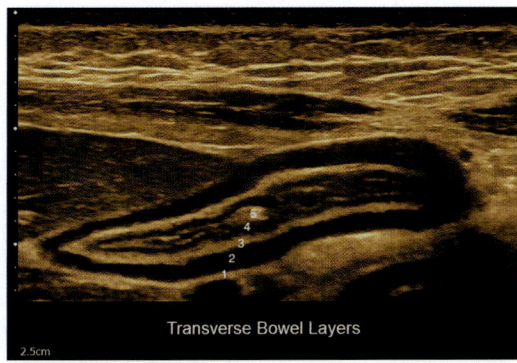

FIG. 25.6 **Normal bowel wall layers.** All five layers are well visualized in the collapsed large transverse colon. From outer to inner layer, they include: *1*, echogenic outer serosa; *2*, hypoechoic muscularis; *3*, echogenic submucosa, which is often indicated in gastrointestinal inflammation; *4*, hypoechoic muscularis mucosa; *5*, and echogenic inner mucosa. (Courtesy Siemens Healthineers USA, Inc.)

arise from any of the body's systems. So, ruling out disease can be as important as ruling it in. Given the wide range of ages and developmental stages within the pediatric population, it is vital to be cognizant of the general disease processes as well as the sonographic appearance of the presenting pathology. Nonneoplastic disease entities of the neonatal/pediatric abdomen may be acute, chronic, congenital, or acquired.

Common Presenting Diseases

Acute Abdominal Pain. Acute abdominal pain is one of the most common complaints among children. Many underlying surgical and nonsurgical conditions vary according to age, associated symptoms, and pain location. The most common nonsurgical condition is gastroenteritis, and the most common surgical condition is appendicitis. Gastrointestinal conditions (see Gastrointestinal Pathology later in this chapter) are often the underlying cause, but other reasons for acute abdominal pain in the child include trauma, pancreatitis, splenic sequestration, and choledocholithiasis.

Trauma. Accidents (unintentional injuries) are the leading cause of mortality for children in all age groups. At ages 1 to 9 years this is followed by congenital malformations, chromosomal abnormalities, and cancer, while at ages 10 to 14 years, suicide and cancer prevail. Blunt abdominal trauma (caused by motor vehicle accidents, falling, and child abuse) may cause laceration of abdominal organs, bowel perforation, ischemia of organs due to vascular injury, and intramural hematoma. In neonates, traumatic delivery or resuscitation efforts may cause liver or splenic injury. Children have incomplete rib ossification, making the liver the most commonly injured abdominal organ versus the spleen in adults. In half of the liver cases, other abdominal organs are affected, too, especially the spleen. The pancreas (Fig. 25.7) and duodenum may also be injured.

Ultrasound is often used for follow-up imaging of trauma in children. Hepatic subcapsular hematomas may be observed, as well as parenchymal hematomas, lacerations, and fractures. Liver lacerations will usually appear slightly echogenic in the acute stage and become more hypoechoic or cystic in the following days. Pseudoaneurysms and bilomas may also develop as later complications. A complex appearance and gas due to tissue necrosis and calcifications may be depicted sonographically in an aging liver hematoma.

Pancreatitis. Acute and chronic pancreatitis in childhood can cause significant morbidity and mortality. Often, acute inflammation is due to trauma or structural abnormalities, multisystemic disease, or drugs and toxins, but in nearly a quarter of children, the cause is idiopathic. Ultrasound is the imaging modality of choice in the setting of acute pancreatitis. It allows for the exclusion of extrapancreatic diseases, such as gallstones or choledocholithiasis. The most useful diagnostic finding is an enlarged pancreatic duct, which should measure less than 2 mm. Pancreatic enlargement or swelling is present in up to half of patients with acute pancreatitis. Peripancreatic fluid and fluid collections (pseudocysts), as well as peripancreatic fatty infiltration, may be present.

Chronic inflammation of the pancreas is more often caused by CF (see Acquired and Hereditary Diseases later in this chapter), fibrosing pancreatitis, hereditary chronic pancreatitis, or inborn errors of metabolism. In chronic pancreatitis, the pancreas may appear echogenic with calcifications, both shadowing and nonshadowing.

Splenic Sequestration Syndrome. Splenic sequestration syndrome presents with rapid splenic enlargement and an acute fall in hematocrit. It causes extreme pain and, if left untreated, can be fatal. Often, it occurs in children younger than 2 years with sickle cell disease, but it can occur in older children with blood disorders or neonates/infants on **extracorporeal membrane oxygenation (ECMO)**. Ultrasound will reveal a grossly enlarged spleen with peripheral low echogenicity foci (corresponding to hemorrhage on magnetic resonance imaging), but internal blood flow will be preserved.

Chole(docho)lithiasis. The incidence of gallstones in children, though still uncommon, has been increasing over the past few decades. The widespread use of ultrasound in detecting asymptomatic cholelithiasis and increasing childhood obesity are key reasons for this trend. In neonates and infants, causes of cholelithiasis or choledocholithiasis include sepsis, total parenteral nutrition, and diuretics. Fetal gallstones, however, will often resolve spontaneously within the first year of life. In older children, causes include hemolytic anemia (such as sickle cell disease), CF, and small bowel diseases. Echogenic foci may be detected within the lumen of the gallbladder or anywhere along the biliary tract. Distal ductal dilation may be present as well. Documenting gallstone mobility is encouraged. Since up to half of pediatric biliary stones are calcified, especially among those with hemolytic disease, color Doppler may aid in producing a "twinkle" artifact in a nonmobile focus. This artifact is best produced by increasing the color Doppler scale and the color gain.

Acquired and Hereditary Diseases. Acquired and hereditary diseases need to be carefully monitored and screened in the pediatric population. Some hereditary diseases may predispose an infant or child to develop certain cancers

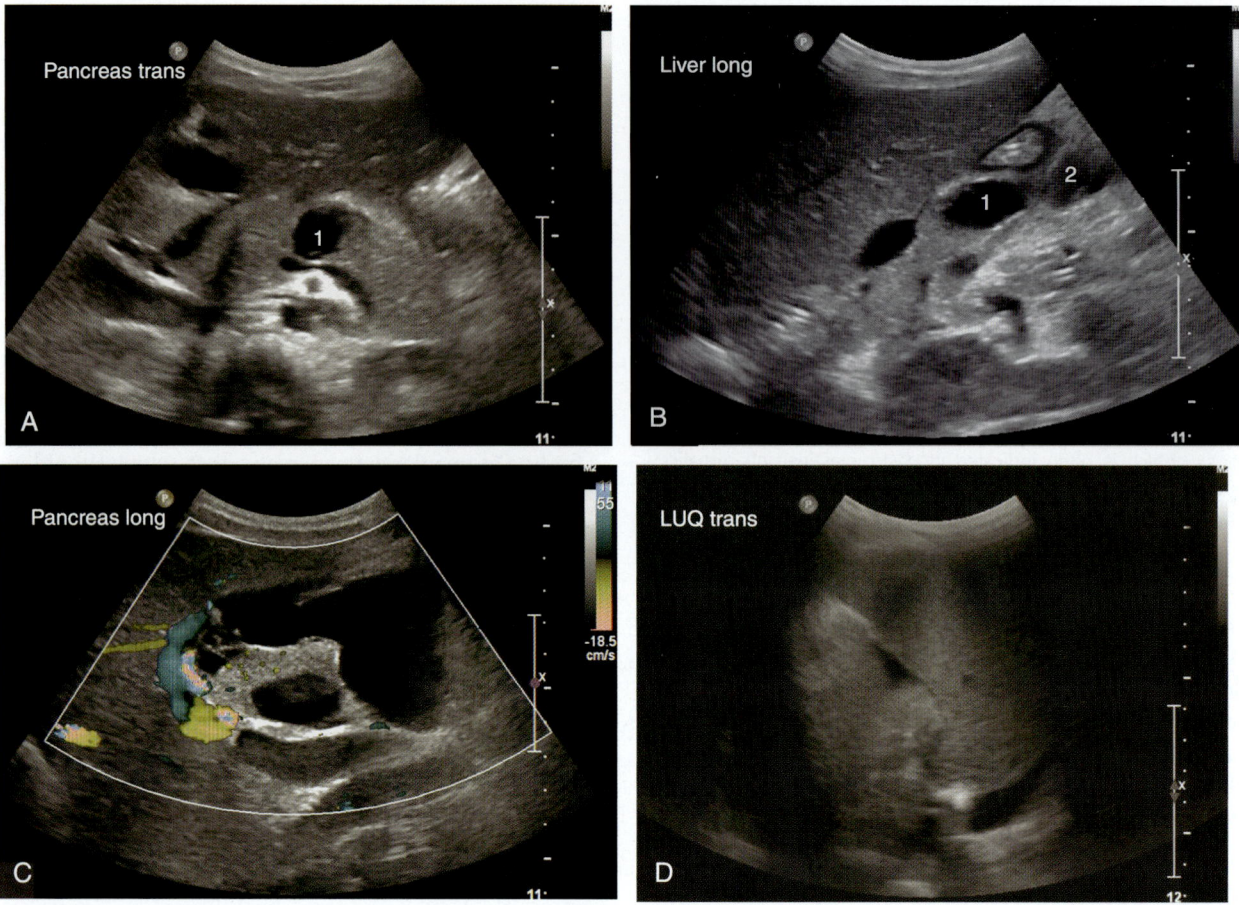

FIG. 25.7 Transected pancreas from trauma. An 11-year-old had increased abdominal pain that did not subside with medication several days after blunt trauma to the abdomen from handlebars on her bike. (A) In the transverse plane, a fluid collection is seen within the body of the pancreas (1). (B) Longitudinal view color Doppler reveals two fluid collections within the pancreas (1 and 2). (C) Large (7.5 × 4.7 cm) peripancreatic fluid collection is seen in the inferior longitudinal view. (D) Perisplenic fluid was also detected. (Courtesy Nationwide Children's Hospital, Columbus, OH.)

(e.g., Beckwith-Wiedemann syndrome's increased risk of hepatoblastoma) and/or chronic conditions (e.g., CF's high association with chronic pancreatitis). These abdominal disorders, common in children, are described here.

Hepatobiliary Disease.

Fatty Liver. Once only seen in adults, NAFLD is now considered one of the most prevalent chronic liver diseases in children, with an estimated 3% to 10% of the pediatric population affected (mostly adolescents). This increase is directly linked to increased obesity among children and resulting fatty deposition within the liver. It may lead to **nonalcoholic steatohepatitis**. Sonographically, the same four general categories of fatty liver classification (absent, mild, moderate, and severe) are used in children, as with adults.

Cirrhosis. Although less common than in their adult counterparts, cirrhosis and portal hypertension are found in the pediatric population. The cause of cirrhosis in children is often divided into four categories: (1) biliary (biliary atresia, Alagille syndrome, alpha-1 antitrypsin deficiency, and CF); (2) metabolic (errors resulting in excessive copper buildup with Wilson disease, or excessive iron buildup with hemochromatosis); (3) postnecrotic cirrhosis (neonatal, postviral, or autoimmune hepatitis); and (4) unknown causes. Sonographically, cirrhosis displays the same adult characteristics, such as abnormal liver surface, with increased echogenicity and nodular changes of the parenchyma being the most specific.

Elastography Assessment. In pediatrics, elastography is becoming routinely utilized, in conjunction with the standard liver sonogram, to assess liver tissue stiffness. It can aid in selecting children who should undergo a liver biopsy, which is the gold standard to definitively diagnose and determine both cirrhosis and NAFLD extent (Fig. 25.8).

Portal Hypertension. If portal hypertension is suspected, it is imperative to use Doppler imaging with angle correction, not only on the main portal vein but also on the right and left intrahepatic veins, as hepatofugal flow may only be involved with one of these. Pulsatility of the portal vein is highly sensitive for identifying portal hypertension, showing a to-and-fro pattern. A hepatofugal flow pattern may emerge, as well. Portal hypertension may also be suspected when portal flow peak systolic velocities are low (dropping below 20 cm/sec). Elevated peak systolic velocities in the hepatic artery with velocities greater than three times the portal vein flow may also indicate portal hypertension in the pediatric patient.

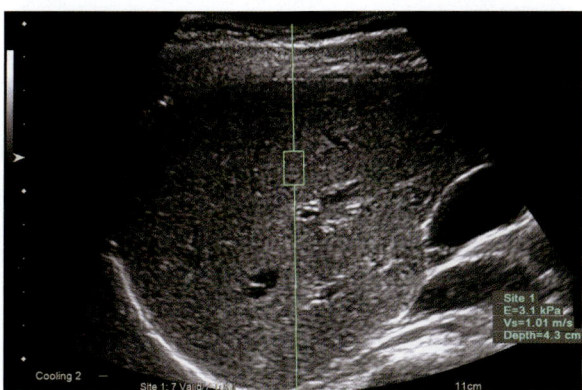

FIG. 25.8 **Elastography liver stiffness in hereditary hemochromatosis.** Shear wave elastography of the liver demonstrates increased liver stiffness in a teenager with hemochromatosis, a hereditary metabolic disease. The average of 10 samples obtained for this patient was 3.0 m/sec. The normal range for this population is 1.16 ± 0.14 m/sec. This indicates the presence of liver fibrosis, the first stage of cirrhosis. (Courtesy Chester County Hospital, West Chester, PA.)

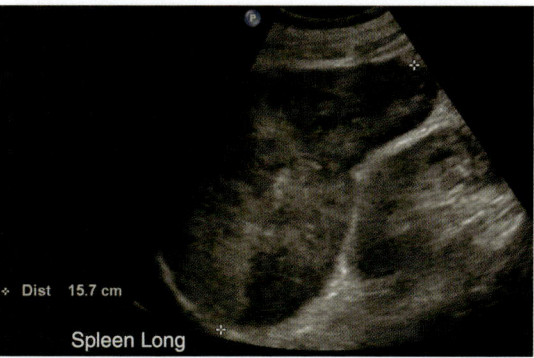

FIG. 25.9 **Splenomegaly in 17-year-old male with leukemia.** The patient had acute lymphoblastic or lymphocytic leukemia, the most common childhood leukemia, which presents with portal hypertension and splenomegaly; the spleen measures 15.7 cm in longitudinal dimension. The diseased spleen is enlarged and grossly inhomogeneous. (Courtesy Nationwide Children's Hospital, Columbus, OH.)

Cholangitis. Infection of the biliary tract can occur in children and is often associated with congenital or immune-related biliary abnormalities and immunodeficiency states. It may also result from surgery, such as correction of biliary atresia (Kasai procedure) or liver transplantation. Often the cause is bacterial, but it may be parasitic, viral, or fungal in an immune-suppressed child. Ultrasound is the modality of choice, and it is used to identify underlying structural bile duct abnormalities or identify causes of bile flow obstruction.

Primary sclerosing cholangitis, a distinct type, is increasingly being found in children. It is a chronic condition with unknown causes, although 70% to 80% of those afflicted also have inflammatory bowel disease. This progressive cholestatic disease may result in cirrhosis, portal hypertension, and ultimately liver failure. Intrahepatic or extrahepatic duct dilation may be present on ultrasound, along with cirrhotic liver changes and splenomegaly.

Pancreatic Disease. Pancreatic pathology in children may be associated with Beckwith-Wiedemann syndrome, von Hippel–Lindau disease, autosomal dominant polycystic kidney disease, CF, and Shwachman-Diamond syndrome. The last two often present with **pancreatic lipomatosis** and resulting pancreatic insufficiency. Beckwith-Wiedemann syndrome is associated with pancreaticoblastoma (a solid malignant tumor), whereas von Hippel–Lindau and polycystic kidney disease present with associated cysts or lesions within the pancreas.

Cystic Fibrosis. CF is an autosomal recessive disease involving abnormal chloride metabolism, which often affects exocrine glands (i.e., sweat glands, pancreatic exocrine glands), leading to increased viscosity. As with many inherited disorders, many different organs and systems can be involved. CF frequently affects the biliary epithelium resulting in end-stage liver cirrhosis and pancreatic atrophy. Serious liver disease affects 13% to 25% of children with CF; however, pancreatic disease is more prevalent in children, affecting 85% to 90% of CF pediatric patients. As normal pancreatic tissue is replaced by fatty tissue due to blocked ducts, ultrasound often reveals increased echogenicity. Cyst formation, calcifications, and atrophy of the pancreas may also be seen.

Splenic Disease. The spleen is implemented in many acquired and hereditary childhood diseases, as it is part of the body's immune response and blood formation. Furthermore, the spleen is often involved with leukemias and lymphomas, the most prevalent cancers among children. Hepatosplenomegaly is a common presentation for newly diagnosed leukemia. The most common childhood cancer, specifically, is acute lymphoblastic (lymphocytic) leukemia. Palpation alone is not accurate enough to diagnose an enlarged liver or spleen, highlighting why the spleen is often included in the pediatric abdominal evaluation.

Splenomegaly may be seen in children affected by diseases such as mononucleosis, hemolytic anemias (sickle cell disease), leukemias (Fig. 25.9), lymphomas, liver cirrhosis, and other diseases, both viral and bacterial.

Cat-Scratch Disease. Cat-scratch disease is one such disease that may cause splenomegaly. The gram-negative bacterium is spread by a cat and accompanying fleas when a child is scratched or bitten. It often appears within 1 to 2 weeks following the incident. A thorough history is important to rule out other more serious etiologies, such as malignancies (lymphoma or metastasis) or granulomatous disease (tuberculosis, sarcoidosis). Previous contact with a cat or kitten is vital to the diagnosis. Although relatively rare, it occurs most commonly in children 5 to 9 years of age, in the southern regions, and during winter months. It presents with fever (also referred to as *cat-scratch fever*) and lymphadenopathy and is often self-limiting.

Abdominal reactive lymph nodes may be seen with ultrasound. Both splenic and hepatic round, hypoechoic, well-defined nodules are often visualized (Fig. 25.10). Histologically, the lesions may be vascular proliferative lesions (peliosis) or necrotizing granulomatous lesions. It may take a month or two for them to resolve radiographically. Contrast-enhanced ultrasound may help better define such lesions.

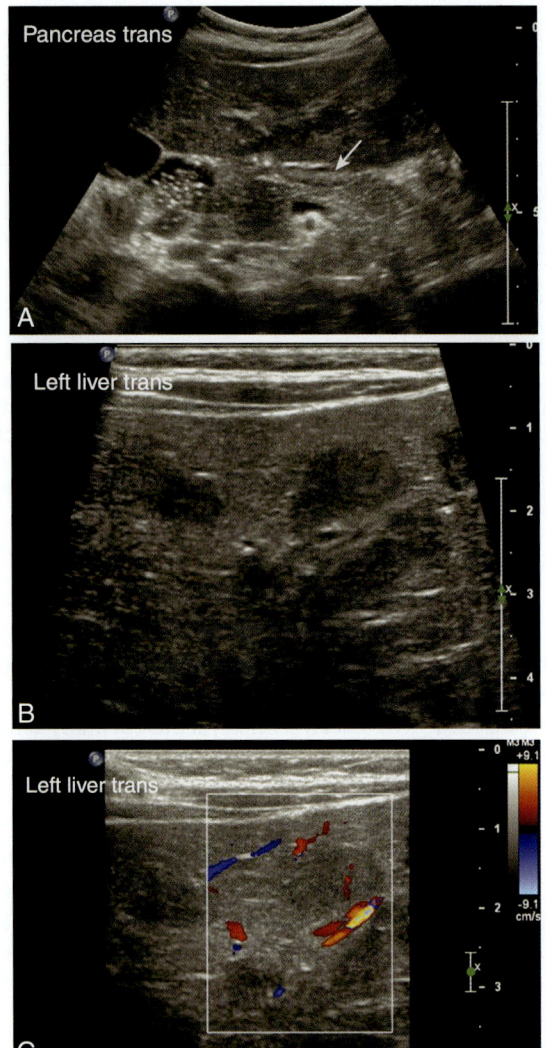

FIG. 25.10 Cat-scratch disease. (A) Reactive lymph node anterior to the pancreas *(arrow)* in a 2-year-old patient with cat-scratch disease. (B) Multiple round, hypoechoic nodules are seen throughout the liver, shown here with a high-frequency transducer. (C) Color Doppler of a liver lesion. (Courtesy Nationwide Children's Hospital, Columbus, OH.)

Neonatal Jaundice. During the first few weeks of life, many neonates, especially preemies, experience transient jaundice due to an excess of bilirubin at birth and a liver not quite ready for the task of conjugating it. Unconjugated hyperbilirubinemia occurs in approximately 60% of normal term infants and 80% of preterm infants. However, persistent jaundice beyond the 2-week postdelivery date is abnormal. In the case of bile obstruction, biliary atresia, or metabolic disease, it is important the neonate is treated early before cirrhosis occurs, and a diagnosis must be made soon after delivery.

Neonatal jaundice may be difficult to define because clinical and laboratory features may be similar in *hepatocellular jaundice* (treated medically) and *obstructive jaundice* (often necessitates surgery).

Obstructive Jaundice. Jaundice may be caused by either *extrahepatic* or *intrahepatic* obstruction to bile flow. The extrahepatic obstruction in the neonate includes conditions such as choledochal cyst, biliary atresia, or spontaneous perforation of the bile ducts. The intrahepatic causes of neonatal jaundice include hepatitis and metabolic disease. Systemic diseases that cause *cholestasis* include heart failure, shock, sepsis, neonatal lupus, histiocytosis, and severe hemolytic disease.

Nonobstructive Jaundice. Nonobstructive jaundice may be caused by hepatitis or hemolytic disease, which occurs due to the excessive breakdown of red blood cells, increasing bilirubin production.

Differentials in Neonatal Jaundice. Jaundice in infants and children may be due to cirrhosis, benign strictures, and neoplastic processes. Sonographic evaluation is used to help differentiate between obstructive versus nonobstructive jaundice. Ultrasound is useful in demonstrating the gallbladder with **inspissated** bile and biliary duct stones. It may also reveal a coarse and echogenic liver on ultrasound; however, various other conditions, including hepatic inflammatory, obstructive, and metabolic processes, have a similar sonographic appearance. Therefore, other studies, such as hepatic **scintigraphy** or liver biopsy, may be necessary to further narrow the differential considerations.

Since several differentials for persistent neonatal jaundice are possible, both a clinical and a laboratory workup is necessary to identify the underlying infectious, metabolic, or structural causes. Laboratory workup may include liver function tests, evaluation for hepatitis B antigen, sepsis, metabolic screening, sweat test, and TORCH infections (toxoplasmosis, other [syphilis, varicella-zoster, parvovirus B19], rubella, cytomegalovirus [CMV], and herpes) to rule out fetomaternal disease.

Causes and Diagnosis of Neonatal Jaundice. The three most common causes of jaundice in the neonatal period are hepatitis, biliary atresia, and choledochal cyst. See Table 25.4 for clinical findings, sonographic findings, and differential considerations for the diseases and conditions discussed here.

Neonatal Hepatitis. Neonatal hepatitis is an infection of the liver that occurs within the first 3 months after birth. There are several causes of neonatal hepatitis, including infections, metabolic disorders, recurrent familial cholestasis, or idiopathic causes. The infection may reach the liver through the placenta (via the vagina from infected maternal secretions) or through catheters or blood transfusions. Transplacental infection occurs most readily during the third trimester of pregnancy via TORCH infections. Bacterial hepatitis is most commonly acquired secondary to an upward spread of organisms from the vagina, infecting the endometrium, placenta, and amniotic fluid. During delivery, direct contact with the herpes virus, CMV, human immunodeficiency virus (HIV), and *Listeria* may lead to hepatitis. Blood transfusions may contain the hepatitis virus, Epstein-Barr virus, or HIV. In addition, bacterial hepatitis or abscess formation may be obtained from an **umbilical vein catheter** after delivery.

Sonographic Findings. The liver may be normal-sized or enlarged. The parenchyma pattern is hyperechoic and coarse, with decreased visualization of the peripheral portal venous

TABLE 25.4	Most Common Causes of Neonatal Jaundice	
Clinical Findings	Sonographic Findings	Differential Considerations
Neonatal Hepatitis		
Hepatomegaly	Liver normal or enlarged	Biliary atresia
Jaundice when obstruction is present	Liver parenchyma echogenic with decreased vascularization of peripheral portal venous structures	
	When severe, gallbladder may be small in size	
Biliary Atresia		
Persistent jaundice	Liver may be enlarged	Neonatal hepatitis
Acholic (colorless) stools	Echogenicity of liver parenchyma may be normal or increased with slight decrease in visualization of portal structures	
Dark urine		
Distended abdomen		
	Intrahepatic ducts not dilated	
	Polysplenia may be present	
Choledochal Cyst		
Jaundice	Fusiform dilation of the common bile duct	Duplicated gallbladder
Pain		Liver cyst
Palpable mass may be present	Associated intrahepatic ductal dilation	Fluid in duodenum

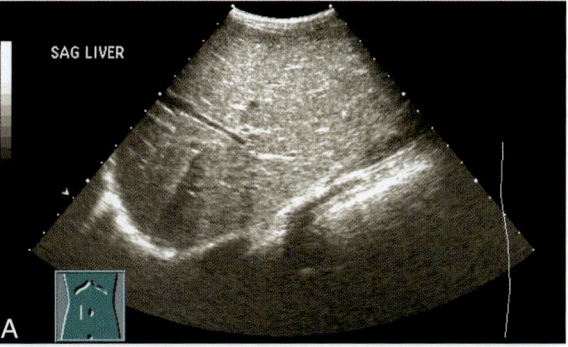

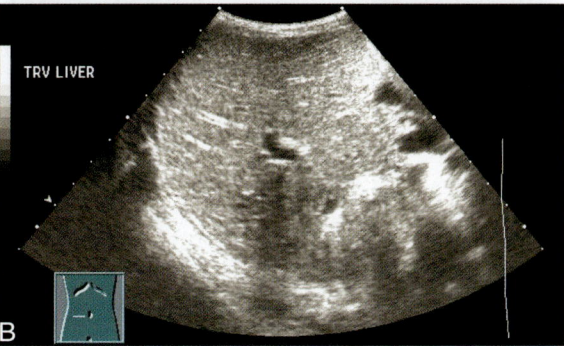

FIG. 25.11 Hepatitis. Liver size and texture should be evaluated in a patient with hepatitis. The liver may appear normal or enlarged, often with a coarser and more echogenic echotexture. (A) Sagittal liver. (B) Transverse liver.

structures (Fig. 25.11). The biliary ducts and gallbladder are not enlarged. If the hepatocellular dysfunction is severe, the gallbladder may be small due to the decreased bile production. The differential of neonatal hepatitis and biliary atresia may be difficult when the gallbladder is small; therefore, nuclear scintigraphy will allow visualization of the biliary function.

Biliary Atresia. **Biliary atresia** is the narrowing or underdevelopment of the biliary ductal system. This serious disease is seen more commonly in males and may be congenital or result from inflammation of the hepatobiliary system. Biliary atresia may affect the intrahepatic or extrahepatic ducts and may or may not involve the gallbladder, although the latter is the most common form with the absence of the gallbladder. However, sonographers should recognize the pseudo-gallbladder, or abnormally shaped gallbladder, sometimes seen in neonates with biliary atresia. The clinical features of biliary atresia in the neonate include persistent jaundice, acholic stools (colorless), dark urine, and distended abdomen from hepatomegaly. Early surgical intervention (**Kasai portoenterostomy** to repair biliary atresia) is often necessary to prevent serious complications, including cirrhosis, liver failure, and subsequent death. Biliary atresia remains the leading cause of liver transplants in children.

Sonographic Findings. Sonographic findings in a neonate with biliary atresia may vary depending on the disease type and severity. The liver size may be normal or enlarged. The echogenicity of the liver parenchyma may be normal or increased with a slight decrease in the visualization of the peripheral portal venous vasculature (indicative of fibrosis). The intrahepatic ducts are not dilated, although a remnant duct may be identified with some types of atresia. A small hyperechoic focal triangular area often referred to as the "triangular cord" sign may be seen anterior to the portal vein bifurcation on an oblique transverse view, a hypoplastic fibrotic remnant of the biliary structure.

A normal-sized gallbladder may be seen when the **atretic** common bile duct is distal to the insertion of the cystic duct. However, if a gallbladder is present with biliary atresia, it is often the small pseudo-gallbladder, which appears as a fluid-filled structure less than 15 mm in length within the interlobar fissure region, often without a normal gallbladder wall (Fig. 25.12). However, as mentioned earlier, a small gallbladder is nonspecific and may be seen with either hepatitis or biliary atresia. However, a decrease in the gallbladder size after a milk feeding suggests normal patency of the common hepatic and common bile ducts and would suggest neonatal hepatitis.

The abdomen should be closely evaluated for the presence of polysplenia if there is suspicion for biliary atresia because

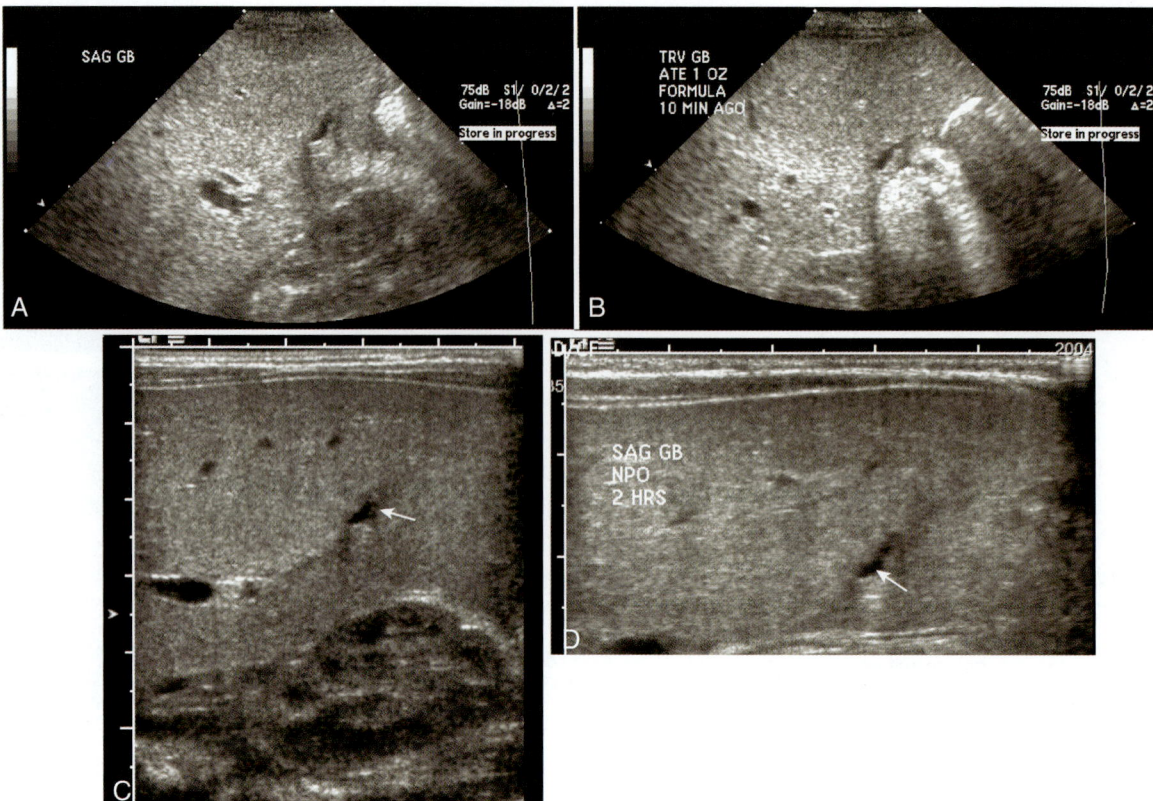

FIG. 25.12 Biliary atresia. A 5-day-old infant presented with direct hyperbilirubinemia of unknown origin with liver congestion, inflammation, and ductal blockage. The liver is enlarged with a homogeneous appearance. The neonate had eaten just before the study and the gallbladder was contracted and measured less than 1 cm. The patient was scanned after 2 hours, and the gallbladder did not change in appearance, as normally expected. The common bile duct was not identified. (A) Sagittal gallbladder. (B) Transverse gallbladder after patient had 1 oz of formula. (C) Sagittal gallbladder *(arrow)* utilizing higher-frequency linear transducer. (D) Sagittal gallbladder *(arrow).* No change was seen after the patient was NPO for 2 hours.

there is a high association of this abnormality. There are also known associations of situs inversus, interrupted IVC, or enlarged hepatic artery. Signs of end-stage liver disease (e.g., ascites, hepatofugal flow, and collateral venous channels) should also be documented. Ultrasound has a very high accuracy differentiating biliary atresia from other causes of increased conjugated hyperbilirubinemia if all these sonographic features are carefully evaluated.

Choledochal Cyst. A **choledochal cyst** is an abnormal cystic dilation of the biliary tree, frequently affecting the common bile duct. There are five types of choledochal cysts, with type I being the most common (80% to 90% of cases). The basic choledochal cysts are summarized here:

Type I—fusiform dilation of the common bile duct (CBD)
Type II—one or more diverticula of the CBD
Type III—dilation of the intraduodenal portion of the CBD (choledochocele)
Type IV—dilation of the intrahepatic and extrahepatic ducts
Type V—Caroli disease (see Chapter 10) with dilation of intrahepatic ducts

The neonate clinically presents with jaundice and pain. A palpable mass may be felt in the right upper quadrant. Sonography is used to identify dilation of the ductal system and the presence or absence of a gallbladder or mass (Fig. 25.13). There is usually fusiform dilation of the common bile duct with associated intrahepatic ductal dilation when a choledochal cyst is present.

Causes of Pediatric Jaundice. In the older pediatric patient, jaundice may be caused by several processes, including hepatocellular disease, cholelithiasis, choledocholithiasis, and cirrhosis. Hepatic neoplasms may also be a cause of both pediatric and infant jaundice.

Abdominal Tumors

Pediatric abdominal masses are often differentiated based on a patient's age (neonate/young infant versus older infant and child) and symptoms (symptomatic versus asymptomatic). Usually, but certainly not always (as in the case of ovarian torsion), abdominal masses of the gastrointestinal tract are symptomatic and others asymptomatic. In all age groups, most neoplasms arise from the retroperitoneum, particularly the kidneys.

Less often, masses may arise from the adrenals, reproductive organs (ovarian cysts, teratomas, hydrocolpos,

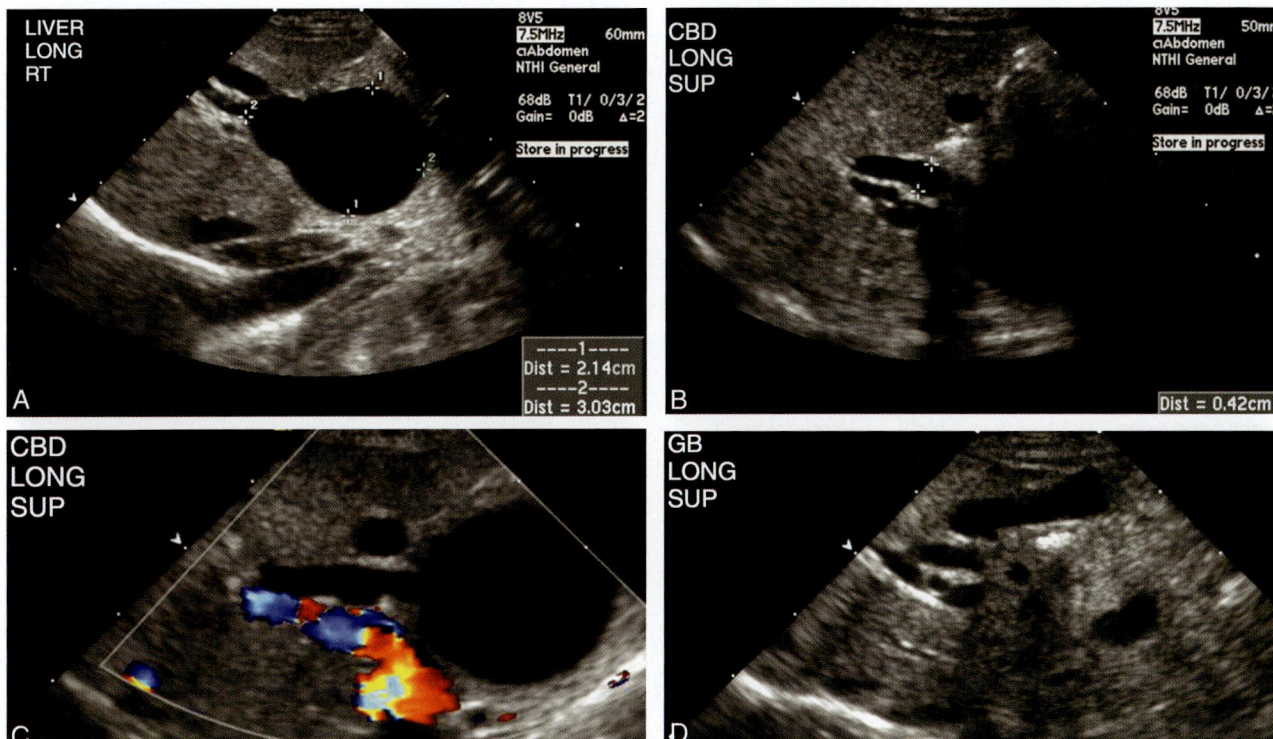

FIG. 25.13 Choledochal cyst in a 5-day-old infant. Follow-up to an abdominal polycystic mass on prenatal ultrasound. The gallbladder is seen without evidence of gallstones or wall thickening. A thin-walled fluid collection is seen in the right upper quadrant (RUQ) measuring 2 × 3 × 2.2 cm. The cystic mass is separate from the gallbladder and does not demonstrate flow. The RUQ cyst is connected to the common bile duct (CBD), consistent with a choledochal cyst type II. (A) Sagittal right liver showing large cystic area (with measurements) near the CBD. (B) Dilated CBD measuring 4 mm. (C) Supine position showing CBD connection to cyst, while color Doppler shows CBD separate from vascular structures. (D) Sagittal gallbladder. (Courtesy Nationwide Children's Hospital, Columbus, OH.)

hydrometrocolpos), gastrointestinal tract (lymphoma), liver, and biliary tract (choledochal cysts). Pancreatic masses are rare, but if seen in infants and young children, the pancreatic blastoma may be suspected, which presents as a large, hypoechoic, solitary mass. The often-large, solid, and pseudopapillary epithelial neoplasm (SPEN) may be indicated in adolescent girls and young women.

Liver Tumors. Although more common in children, primary liver tumors only account for 5% to 6% of all intraabdominal masses and 1% to 4% of all solid tumors in the pediatric population. However, nearly two-thirds of all childhood hepatic tumors are malignant. Sonography plays an important role in their detection and in defining the origin, size, number, Doppler flow characteristics, IVC involvement, location for potential resection, and response to therapy. The two most common neoplasms (Table 25.5) in the pediatric population often present as an asymptomatic mass: hepatoblastoma and infantile hepatic hemangiomas (IHHs).

Malignant Liver Tumors. The distinction between benign and malignant mass with sonography is impossible; only histologic diagnosis is definitive. However, the clinical history, laboratory results, and sonographic findings may provide a differential for the clinician. The two most common malignant tumors in childhood are hepatoblastoma and hepatocellular carcinoma. The undifferentiated sarcoma and biliary rhabdomyosarcoma are rare. Metastases to the liver may arise from neuroblastoma, Wilms tumor, leukemia, or lymphoma.

Hepatoblastoma. Hepatoblastoma is the most common primary malignant disease of the liver and occurs most frequently in children under 4 years of age, with the majority occurring in children under 1 year of age. It is the third most common pediatric abdominal malignancy after **Wilms tumor (nephroblastoma)** and **neuroblastoma** (see Chapter 26). It is sometimes considered the infantile form of hepatocellular carcinoma. The tumor may be familial. Hepatoblastoma has been associated with **Beckwith-Wiedemann syndrome, hemihypertrophy,** familial adenomatous polyposis, precocious puberty, congenital anomalies, fetal alcohol syndrome, and very low birth weight (generally defined as less than 1500 g).

Pathologically, the tumor is single, solid, large, or mixed echogenicity and poorly marginated, with small cysts and rounded or irregularly shaped calcium deposits. The tumor may show areas of necrosis, hemorrhage, and calcification (Fig. 25.14). It usually does not show diffuse infiltration; the remaining liver may be normal. The intrahepatic vessels are displaced or amputated by the mass.

Clinical findings include a palpable abdominal mass and a highly elevated serum alpha-fetoprotein level. Patients may be symptomatic with fever, pain, anorexia, and subsequent weight loss. The prognosis is dependent on the resectability of the mass.

TABLE 25.5	Most Common Hepatic Neoplasms	
Clinical Findings	Sonographic Findings	Differential Considerations
Hepatoblastoma		
Most common malignant tumor of the liver	Hepatomegaly	Hepatocellular carcinoma
Less than 4 years of age	Calcification may occur	Adenoma
	Solitary heterogeneous mass	Focal nodular hyperplasia
Palpable abdominal mass	Portal vein thrombosis	Cirrhosis—regenerating nodules
Elevated serum alpha-fetoprotein levels in 90% of patients	Area around mass is hyperechoic	Hemangioendothelioma
	Doppler shows high-velocity, low-resistance flow	Biliary rhabdoma/sarcoma
Fever		Lymphoma
Pain		Metastasis
Infantile Hepatic Hemangiomas (Infantile Hemangioendotheliomas)		
First 6 months of life	Multiple hypoechoic lesions or solitary mass in liver	Adenoma
Rapid growing benign tumors		Focal nodular hyperplasia
Hepatomegaly	Hepatomegaly	Cirrhosis—regenerating nodules
Congestive heart failure	Tumor is heterogeneous or isoechoic with cystic components	Hepatoblastoma
Cutaneous hemangiomas		Biliary rhabdoma/sarcoma
Serum alpha-fetoprotein level rarely elevated	Calcification may be present	Lymphoma
	Well circumscribed to poorly marginated	Metastasis
	Doppler may show arteriovenous shunt	

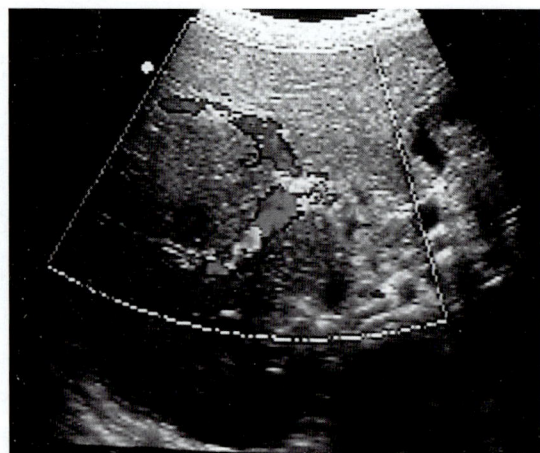

FIG. 25.15 Hepatoblastoma. The portal veins are displaced by the large mass.

may be hypoechoic areas with necrosis or hemorrhage. The fleshy areas around the mass are often mildly hyperechoic. It becomes important to identify the hepatic vessels, as hepatic and portal venous thrombosis may be present. Color Doppler is useful to detect flow in the malignant neovasculature, while pulsed Doppler shows a high-velocity, low-resistance flow pattern.

Hepatocellular Carcinoma. Hepatocellular carcinoma, also known as hepatoma, is the second most common malignant liver tumor in childhood, after hepatoblastoma. It usually affects children older than 3 years, and half will have preexisting liver disease, such as hepatitis or type I glycogen storage disease. This liver tumor is often a multicentric solid mass involving the whole liver, usually without calcification and variable echogenicity on sonography. Color Doppler should be used to evaluate the portal venous and hepatic structures to look for thrombus or tumor invasion, as patients often present with sudden liver failure due to invasion of these vessels.

Benign Liver Tumors. IHHs are the most common benign liver tumor and account for 12% of childhood hepatic neoplasms. Mesenchymal hamartoma, adenoma, and focal nodular hyperplasia together make up roughly half of all benign liver tumors.

Infantile Hepatic Hemangiomas. Perhaps the most perplexing hepatic tumors in infancy are the IHHs, previously well-known as the infantile hemangioendothelioma, and may also be referred to as a hepatic vascular tumor. This tumor has recently been divided histologically into hepatic infantile hemangioma (type I) and congenital hepatic vascular malformation (type II). It has been suggested that type I is the hepatic counterpart to the common cutaneous hemangioma, which also has positive immunoreactivity to erythrocyte-type glucose transporter protein 1 (GLUT-1), whereas type II may represent a vascular malformation and does not show GLUT-1 reactivity. However, type II tumor histology reports are differing and have been reported as vascular malformations with capillary proliferation and as vascular hepatic lesions that do involute. Likely, these type II tumors represent a heterogeneous type of lesion.

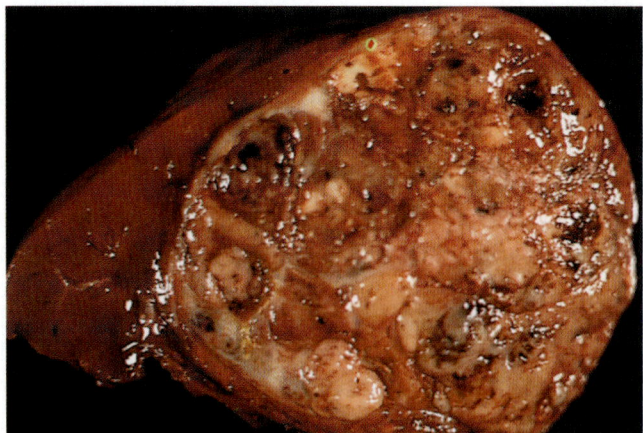

FIG. 25.14 Hepatoblastoma specimen. Lobular tumor with areas of necrosis.

Sonographic Findings. The sonographic appearance of the hepatoblastoma shows hepatomegaly with a large solitary mass (Fig. 25.15). Calcifications are common. The heterogeneous mass is predominantly solid; however, there

TABLE 25.6	Infantile Hepatic Hemangiomas by Type and Histologic Findings
Clinical Findings	**Sonographic Findings**
Type I: Infantile Hepatic Hemangioma	
High association with cutaneous hemangiomas Glucose transporter protein 1 (GLUT-1) positive Proliferation, usually third of fourth month, followed by involution Often asymptomatic, but some may have congestive heart failure (CHF)	Multifocal masses Small with no central necrosis on pathology, homogeneous in appearance
Type II: Congenital Hepatic Vascular Malformation (With Associated Capillary Proliferation or Vascular Hepatic Lesions That Involute)	
Rarely associated with cutaneous hemangiomas GLUT-1 negative Manifests in perinatal period Involute by 12–14 months of age Patient is usually symptomatic and may present with CHF	Large solitary mass with central hemorrhage, necrosis or fibrosis on pathology, calcifications and mixed heterogeneity

Not surprisingly, there is an ongoing debate over the nomenclature of this pathology that has been previously classified by the clinical appearance of multifocal, focal, or diffuse. It is unclear which histologic type the diffuse type belongs; however, the uniform appearance and low association with congestive heart failure (CHF) may indicate type I or a combination (Table 25.6).

Regardless, IHHs make up the most common benign vascular liver tumors of early childhood, with a peak diagnosis at 6 months of life, with one-third diagnosed in the first month of life. They grow rapidly after birth, causing abdominal distention. Fewer than 5% are diagnosed after the first year.

The clinical presentation for infants with IHH is hepatomegaly, which may be accompanied by CHF and/or cutaneous hemangioma. CHF and high cardiac output are seen in 50% to 60% of patients due to increased blood volume and output needed to maintain vascular bed perfusion. A biopsy is not recommended due to an increased risk of bleeding in these high-flow lesions. The serum alpha-fetoprotein level may be elevated. These benign tumors usually spontaneously regress by 12 to 18 months of age.

Sonographic Findings. The most common sonographic appearance of IHH is hepatomegaly, with half presenting as multiple hypoechoic lesions (hemangiomatosis) and the other half as a solitary mass. The tumor may be isoechoic or heterogeneous and may contain cystic components from the vascular-stroma structure (Fig. 25.16). Speckled areas of calcification may be seen within the mass. Interestingly, infantile hemangiomas do not show calcifications or arteriovenous shunting, whereas congenital vascular malformations may. The tumor may be well-circumscribed or poorly marginated.

Color Doppler shows high flow in the dilated vascular spaces and may be used to show the arteriovenous shunting that accompanies this lesion. When arteriovenous shunting is severe, the celiac axis, hepatic artery, and veins are dilated, and the infraceliac aorta is tapered. Doppler characteristics may overlap with malignancies, showing higher diastolic flow. It is suspected this is likely associated with type II, which may be more aggressive. Evaluation with contrast-enhanced ultrasound is helping to provide more diagnostic criteria to identify these tumors.

Hepatic Hemangiomas. Hepatic hemangiomas may be infantile or juvenile. The juvenile appearance is similar to that of the adult hepatic hemangioma. The hepatic hemangioma is characterized by active endothelial growth. The vessel growth slows down as the tumor matures, but the existing vessels may form "lakes" within the lesion with little blood flow. The sonographic pattern (hyperechoic) is similar to that found in the adult.

Sometimes, infants with common cutaneous hemangiomas (vascular lesions of proliferative endothelium present on the superficial skin) will have a screening ultrasound of the liver, spleen, and brain for concomitant visceral lesions. Risk factors for cutaneous hemangiomas include prematurity, female sex (3:1 to 4:1), and fair skin. The hepatic hemangioma is the most common extracutaneous hemangioma, also with a female prevalence, and is more likely to occur in those patients presenting with five to six cutaneous lesions, with one over 5 cm, or with a miliary or disseminated form.

Mesenchymal Hamartoma. This is a rare tumor in the asymptomatic infant younger than 2 years. The tumor has multiseptate cystic masses derived from periportal mesenchyma.

Adenoma. This tumor is not commonly seen in the infant unless liver disease is present (i.e., glycogen storage disease). Laboratory values will show normal serum alpha-fetoprotein levels. The sonographic appearance ranges from hyperechoic to hypoechoic and is nonspecific.

GASTROINTESTINAL PATHOLOGY

Sonography is routinely used to triage and diagnose common surgical conditions in infants and children. The sonographic evaluation of the gastrointestinal system has been increasing, owing to efforts to reduce ionizing radiation exposure among children. Although considered an inferior imaging modality to computed tomography for gastrointestinal pathology, the increased reliance on ultrasound for appendicitis in pediatric institutions, for example, has resulted in a stable frequency of appendiceal perforations and emergency department revisits, while negative appendectomy rates have slightly decreased.

Common Surgical Conditions

Pediatric patients commonly present to the emergency department with gastrointestinal symptoms, including abdominal pain and vomiting. Sonography is critical in differentiating common and self-limiting processes, such as viral gastroenteritis, from life-threatening surgical emergencies. Three common pediatric surgical conditions evaluated

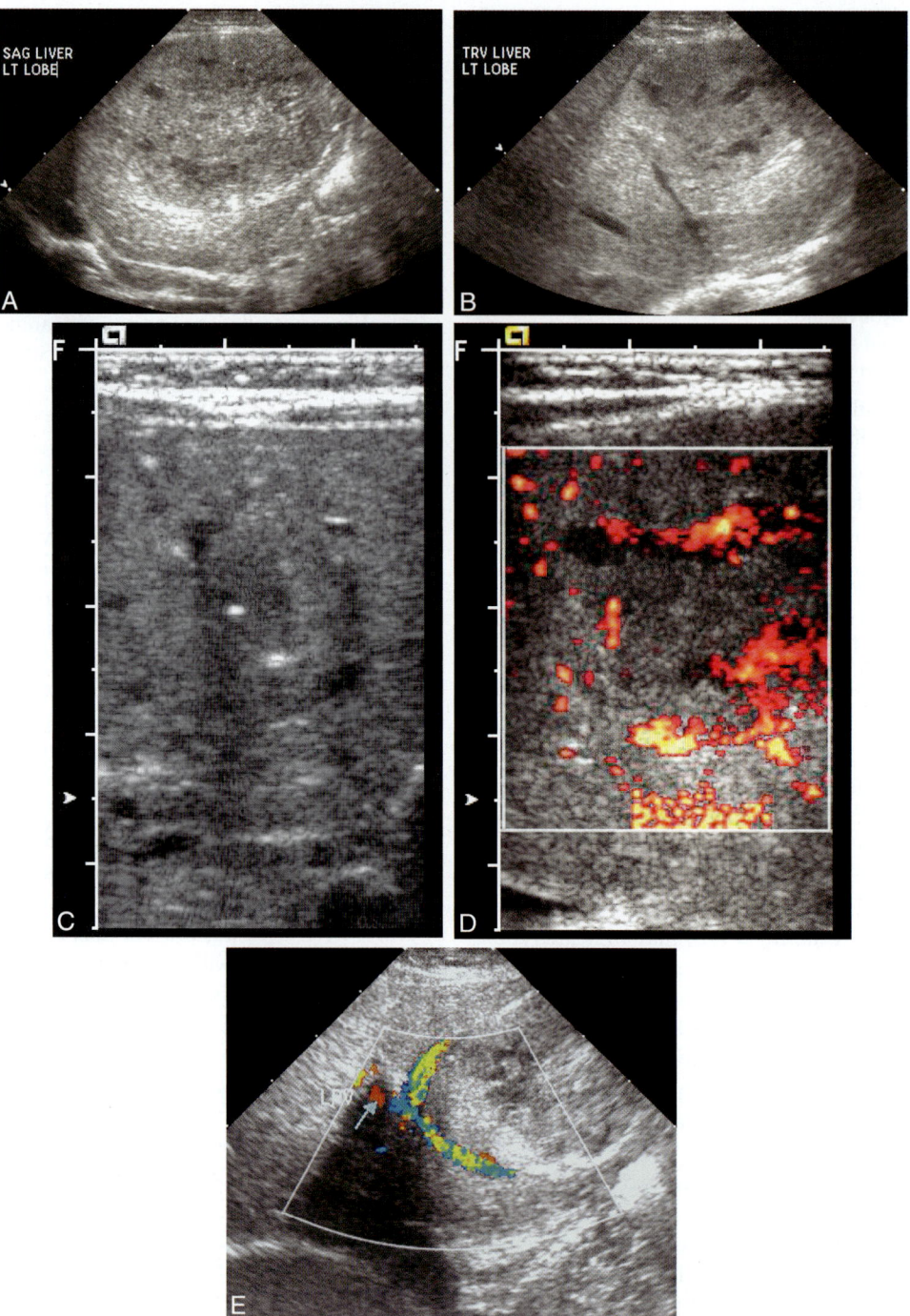

FIG. 25.16 Infantile hepatic hemangioma. A 2-month-old infant with a liver vascular tumor (likely infantile hemangioendothelioma type II) shows a well-circumscribed heterogeneous mass with focal areas of calcium in the left lobe of the liver. There is predominant flow around the mass. There were normal waveforms in both the main portal vein and the left hepatic artery. (A) Sagittal left lobe liver with large heterogeneous mass and right pleural effusion superior to diaphragm. (B) Transverse left lobe of liver with mass. (C) Sagittal views of mass showing areas of calcification that appear echogenic on sonography. (D) Power Doppler shows increased vascularity within the mass (shown), while color Doppler helps to define the vascularity of the mass and the relationships of the portal and hepatic veins to the mass lesion. (E) Color flow in portal veins displaced around the mass.

by ultrasound are appendicitis, intussusception, and HPS (Table 25.7).

Appendicitis. **Appendicitis** is the most common cause of emergent surgical abdominal pain in children. It mostly occurs in patients ages 5 to 15 years but may occur as young as 3 months (although rare under age 2) and has a male (1.7:1) prevalence. Appendicitis occurs when the appendiceal lumen becomes obstructed and subsequently infected and inflamed (Fig. 25.17).

In infants and young children, the progression of acute appendicitis to perforation is more rapid than in older children and adults, sometimes occurring within 6 to 12 hours. Perforation of the appendix is a serious complication of appendicitis, along with peritonitis, abscess formation, and

TABLE 25.7	Most Common Gastrointestinal Surgical Conditions	
Clinical Findings	**(+) Sonographic Findings**	**(−) Differential Considerations**
Appendicitis		
Right lower quadrant pain Nausea, vomiting Increased white blood cell count Fever	Noncompressible appendix Maximum outer diameter >6 mm Rebound pain	Mesenteric lymphadenitis Gastroenteritis Meckel diverticulum Pelvic mass Distal Ileitis
Intussusception		
Colicky abdominal pain Vomiting Bloody stools Abdominal mass	Alternating hypoechoic and hyperechoic rings surrounding an echogenic center (target sign or "cinnamon bun" sign) Free peritoneal fluid	Colic Intestinal wall thickening Inflammatory bowel Colitis Perforated appendix Viral disease Lymphoma Benign tumors
Hypertrophic Pyloric Stenosis (HPS)		
Male infants Projectile vomiting Dehydration and weight loss	Distended stomach Pyloric wall muscle ≥3 mm Hypertrophied pyloric muscle with a canal >15–16 mm	Pseudoechogenic muscle secondary to beam angulation Antropyloric (pyloric antrum) canal posteriorly oriented Pylorospasm with minimal muscular hypertrophy Prostaglandin-induced HPS

sepsis. Classic physical and laboratory findings may be absent or confusing in children, making the diagnosis difficult.

Right lower quadrant pain and vomiting are common clinical presentations. Pain may originate in the umbilicus area and migrate to **McBurney's point** (Fig. 25.18). In addition to appendicitis, diagnostic considerations include mesenteric lymphadenitis, lymphoma, inflammatory bowel disease, and enteritis or small bowel inflammation (Fig. 25.19).

The differentials broaden to include gynecologic processes in girls, such as ovarian cysts or neoplasms and ovarian torsion. It is important to note that females (and those presenting after hours) may have a significant delay in having an **appendectomy**. Although unusual in the first 12 hours in older children, perforation of the appendix is directly proportional to delayed diagnosis thereafter.

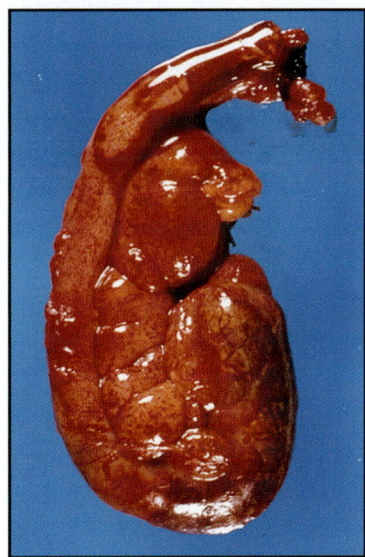

FIG. 25.17 Gross pathology of appendicitis. Gross pathology of acute appendicitis demonstrates inflammation extending to the serosa, which appears hyperemic.

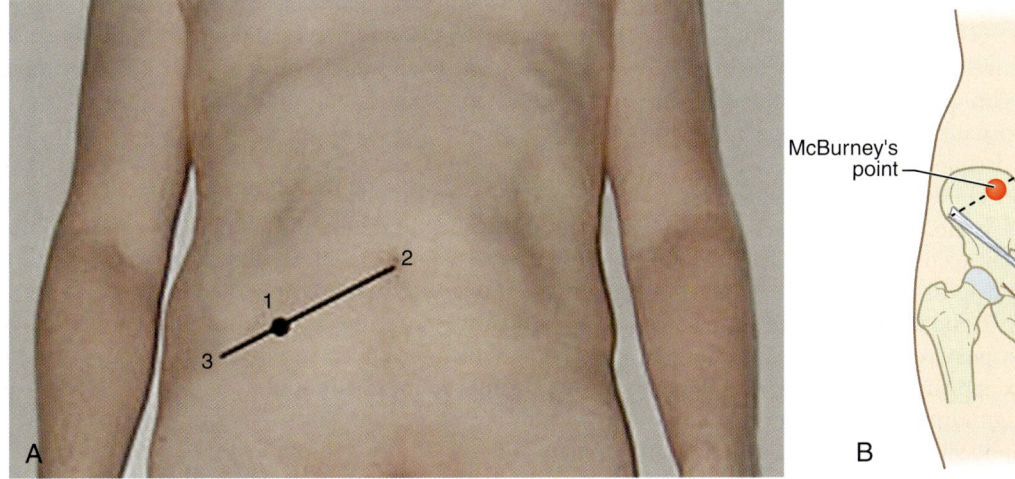
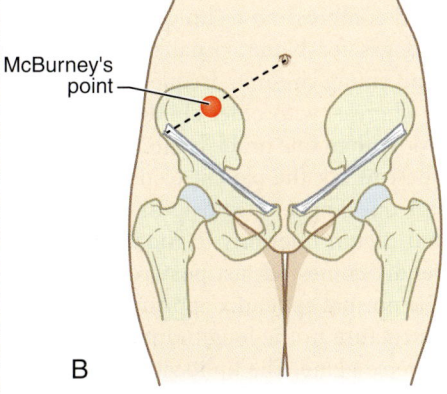

FIG. 25.18 McBurney's point. This common area of the appendiceal attachment to the cecum is found one-third the distance between the right anterior superior iliac spine and the umbilicus. (A) McBurney's point is shown with a black dot (1) on a child. (B) Exact anatomic location.

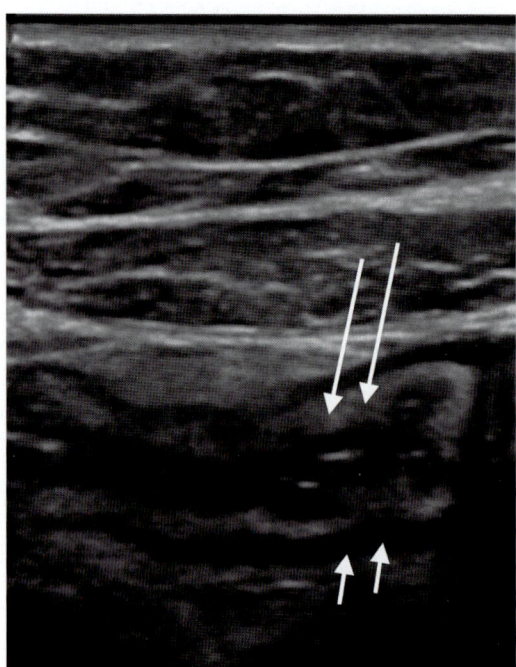

FIG. 25.19 **Enteritis.** The small bowel is slightly thickened in an adolescent with right lower quadrant pain and a normal appendix. There is a loss of the bowel wall signature. In gastrointestinal inflammation, increased thickness often appears in the hyperechoic submucosal layer *(long arrows)*, surrounded by the muscularis halo *(arrows)*. (Courtesy Nationwide Children's Hospital, Columbus, OH.)

Examination Technique. Sonography has proven to be very accurate in confirming appendicitis. The patient begins in a supine position, and a survey of the abdomen is first performed using a curved-array transducer, suitable to the age and body habitus. Specifically, the cul-de-sac posterior to the bladder and Morison's pouch is evaluated for the presence of free fluid. To view deeper structures, and in girls, the adnexal areas should be examined with a distended urinary bladder. However, bladder-filling techniques will vary depending on clinical presentation.

Be sure to explain to the patient what you will do before beginning the compression portion of the examination. Pain is a limiting factor in effectively performing this technique. The graded compression technique displaces adjacent bowel loops and gas for better visualization of the appendix. In infants and young children, frequencies of 12 to 17 MHz may be used, whereas, with older children, 5 to 9 MHz will often suffice. More than one probe is often necessary.

It is best to ask the patient to point to the place of most pain with one finger. It is helpful to follow the ascending colon and cecum inferiorly to the ileocecal junction, where the appendix comes off just posteromedial (inferior) to this valve. The normal appendix appears as a blind-ending, long, tubular structure in the longitudinal plane and a bullseye in the transverse plane. The tip location is variable but must be seen to rule out focal appendiceal tip appendicitis or appendicolith. A cine clip of the transverse appendix leading to the blind-ending is very helpful to the reading radiologist.

Maneuvers to Help Visualize the Appendix. The appendix must be visualized for the examination to be deemed diagnostic. Nonvisualization of the appendix (or equivocal examination) may occur for multiple reasons and is not a definite indication of a normal appendix. Appendiceal nonvisualization may result from any of the following: (1) being obscured by overlying bowel, (2) retrocecal position or deep pelvic position of the appendix, (3) overdistention or nondistention of the urinary bladder, which alters the position of the appendix and overlying bowel, or (4) lack of sonographer experience.

If the appendix cannot be identified, the following maneuvers may be helpful to locate it more readily. The child in pain may be moving, and the normal appendix moves quite a bit, so changing pressure too fast may move the appendix out of view. Changing the patient's position and emptying or filling the urinary bladder may facilitate visualization of both the normal and the abnormal appendix. Finally, scanning all over is helpful, as the appendiceal tip may be located as superior as the right kidney.

Upward Graded Compression. Starting over the area of the appendix in the right lower quadrant, position the linear array transducer in the transverse plane. Next, angle up toward the liver and slowly begin a gradual graded compression upward. The appendix is usually seen anteromedial to the psoas muscle and anterolateral to the iliac vessels.

Left Lateral Decubitus Compression. The patient lies in a left lateral decubitus (LLD) position while imaging both with and without compression. This technique, along with the upward graded compression maneuver, is best for identifying appendices in a retrocecal location.

Posterior Bimanual Compression. This technique is most helpful when imaging muscular or obese patients. It is performed by placing the left hand underneath the patient (on the back) and pressing upward toward the transducer, simultaneously gently pushing toward the patient's back with the transducer in the right scanning hand. A variation of this technique may also be performed with the patient in a LLD position (LLD bimanual compression).

Sonographic Findings. Peristalsis is not seen in the appendix, allowing differentiation of the normal appendix and adjacent small bowel, which is similar in appearance. The appendix may be tortuous and therefore difficult to visualize in its entirety. The walls are not thickened, and the maximal mural thickness normally measures less than 1.7 mm (range, 1.1 to 2.7 mm). Yet, in children under 6 years of age, a maximum mural thickness less than 3 mm may be considered normal. The normal appendix compresses easily, and the lumen may be empty or filled with gas or fecal material (Fig. 25.20).

Sonographically, the acutely inflamed appendix is noncompressible. The appendix is measured from outer-to-outer wall, using the maximum outer diameter (MOD), with and without compression. Measurements are best made in the plane with the most well-defined wall, as acute appendicitis may present with a less defined or ragged wall or loss of the normal gut signature. MOD of 7 mm or greater with compression is consistent with appendicitis in both children and

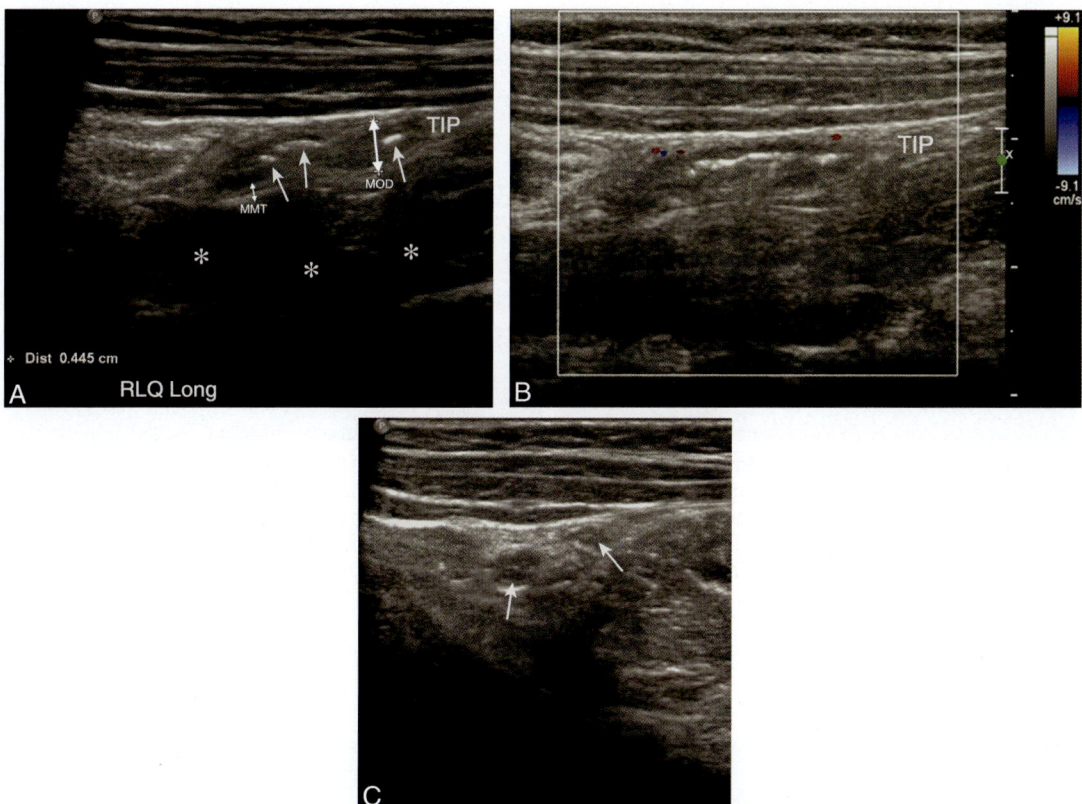

FIG. 25.20 **Normal appendix.** Compressible appendix is visualized with no secondary signs of appendicitis. (A) Normal appearing distal appendix in the longitudinal plane measuring 4.5 mm in the maximum outer diameter (MOD) is within the normal limits of <6 mm. *Double arrows* show MOD and maximal mural wall thickness (MMT). It is helpful to label the tip, as it can be faint and difficult to see in a static image. *Arrows* point to air in the appendix, and *asterisks* show the psoas muscle. (B) No hyperemia detected with color Doppler. (C) Transverse view of the same normal appendix; two sections of this tortuous proximal appendix are visualized *(arrows)*. (Courtesy Nationwide Children's Hospital, Columbus, OH.)

adults. MOD of 6 mm or less indicates a normal appendix, while a MOD between 6 and 7 mm is indeterminate and often established by each institution based on their outcomes. In this case, secondary signs of appendicitis may be helpful (Fig. 25.21). Furthermore, the wall of the appendix will become thickened with acute appendicitis. Institutional criteria may vary on a cutoff maximal mural thickness; however, a measurement over 1.7 mm is above the average. Often there is thickening within the submucosal layer of the appendiceal (same as the bowel) wall layers.

The only statistically significant secondary sign for predicting acute appendicitis is increased peri-appendiceal echogenic fat. This increased echogenicity may be seen in the surrounding mesentery secondary to inflammation, and subsequent **hypomotility** of bowel peristalsis may be present. Rebound pain and localized pain produced by overlying transducer pressure is an additional clinical finding consistent with appendicitis. Color Doppler is useful to document increased blood flow (hyperemia) of the appendiceal wall (Fig. 25.22). Beware, however, a gangrenous appendix may not show signs of hyperemic blood flow. Other findings in appendicitis may include free peritoneal fluid or a loculated fluid collection in the lower abdomen. Mesenteric lymph nodes are another nonspecific secondary finding, and sonographers should report size, number, location, and hyperemia.

Confirmation of an appendicolith in a symptomatic patient is virtually diagnostic (Fig. 25.23). An **appendicolith** is hyperechoic, produces a classic acoustic shadow, may be single or multiple, and may be intraluminal or surrounded by a periappendiceal phlegmon or abscess. The right kidney may at times become dilated due to ureteral inflammation.

The perforated appendix may or may not be visualized. If decompressed, an abnormally thick bowel wall may be apparent. A localized, well-defined right lower quadrant phlegmon or abscess with or without an appendicolith may be present. Free peritoneal fluid may be the lone abnormal sonographic finding. An abscess far from the right lower quadrant is another potential intraabdominal complication of an appendiceal perforation (Fig. 25.24).

Enlarged reactive lymph nodes may accompany appendicitis (Fig. 25.25), and they may also be a pitfall in mimicking appendicitis. The single most common differential diagnosis for appendicitis is mesenteric lymphadenitis, which presents with prominent lymph nodes (generally defined as three or more lymph nodes, oval, greater than 5 mm in the short axis) and flulike symptoms previous to illness. Color Doppler imaging may help the sonographer to determine increased blood flow in the inflamed appendix from the enlarged lymph node.

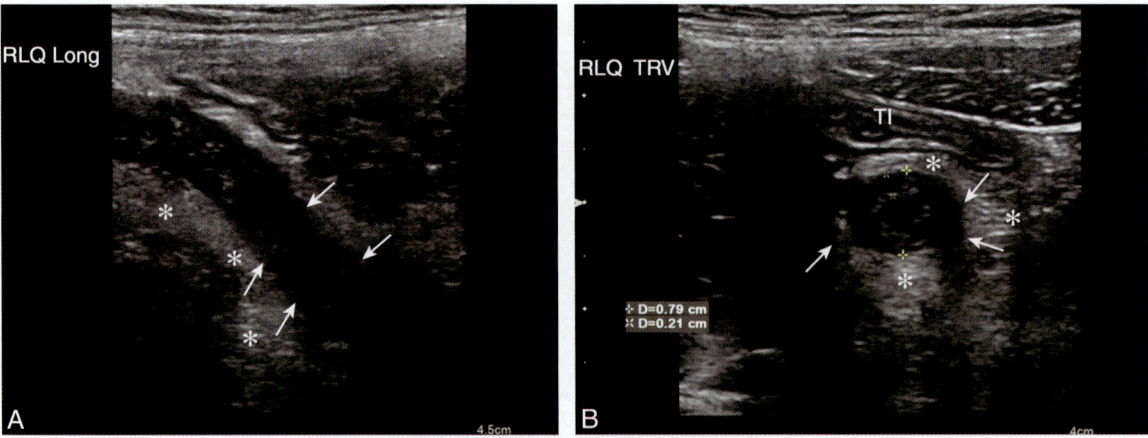

FIG. 25.21 Acute appendicitis. Noncompressible appendix measuring nearly 8 mm in the maximum outer diameter (MOD) and wall measuring >2 mm, indicating appendicitis. Notice the increased echogenicity of the periappendiceal fat *(asterisks)* and loss of wall delineation *(arrows)*. Terminal ilium (TI) is seen superior to appendix in transverse image. (A) Longitudinal view of inflamed appendix, seen diving posterior. (B) Transverse or axial view of appendicitis with MOD wall thickness measurements. (Courtesy Nationwide Children's Hospital, Columbus, OH.)

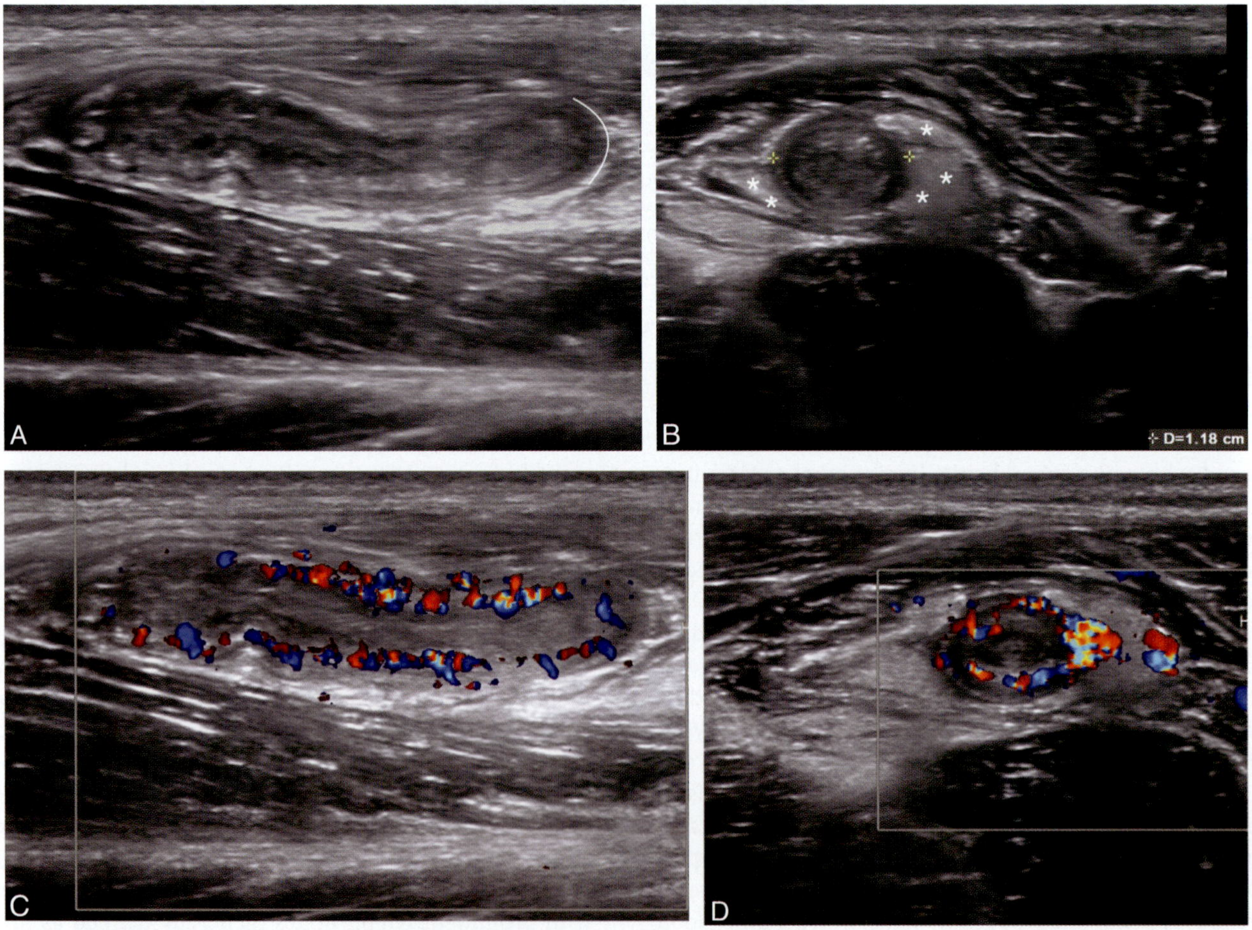

FIG. 25.22 Acute appendicitis. (A) Sagittal view of appendicitis with the tip outlined by the *curved line*. (B) Transverse anteroposterior measurement of the appendiceal tip, measuring nearly 1.2 cm. Increased echogenic fat *(asterisks)* surrounds the inflamed appendix. Color Doppler demonstrating hyperemia of the appendiceal wall in the sagittal (C) and transverse (D) views. (Courtesy Chester County Hospital, West Chester, PA.)

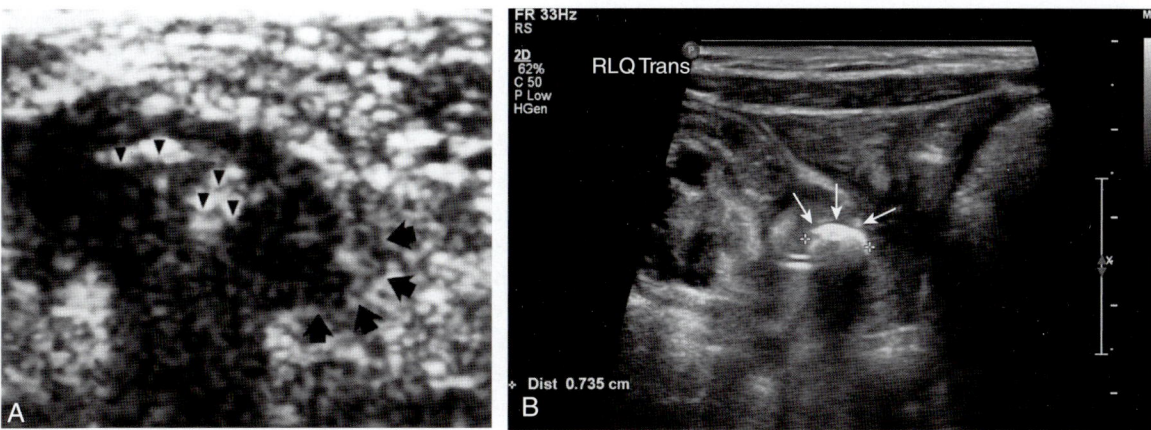

FIG. 25.23 Appendicolith(s). (A) Longitudinal image of an inflamed appendix containing multiple echogenic foci *(arrowheads)* consistent with appendicoliths, which cast acoustic shadows. The blind-ending tip *(arrows)* confirms the echogenic foci are within the appendix and are not gas moving through the small bowel. (B) Transverse image of an inflamed appendix in a different patient. There is a solitary appendicolith *(arrows)* measuring 7 mm. (B, Courtesy Nationwide Children's Hospital, Columbus, OH.)

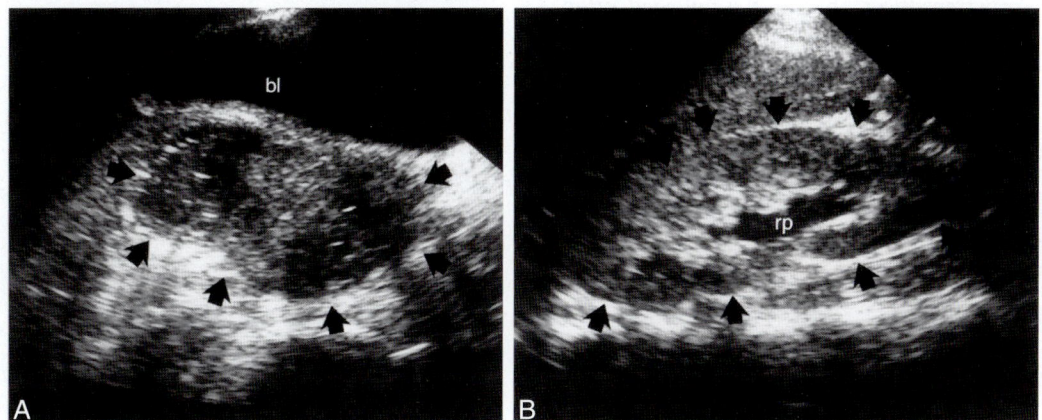

FIG. 25.24 Appendiceal abscess. (A) Midline sagittal image in a boy with an appendiceal abscess *(arrows)* posterior to the urinary bladder (bl). The appendiceal abscess appears heterogeneous in echogenicity and is well demarcated from the surrounding bowel, which was actively peristaltic on real-time examination. (B) Longitudinal image of the right kidney *(arrows)* in the same patient shows moderate urinary tract dilation because of distal ureteral inflammation from the abscess. A fluid-filled right renal pelvis (rp) may be a secondary sign of a right lower quadrant or pelvic process.

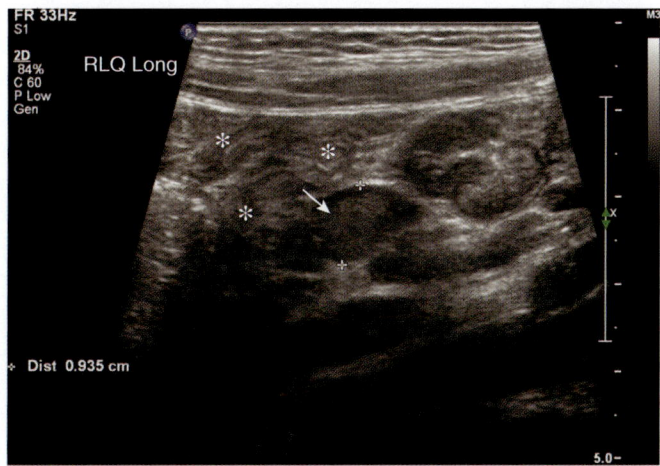

FIG. 25.25 Reactive lymph nodes. Patient positive for appendicitis has an accompanying reactive mesenteric lymph node *(arrow)* seen within the small bowel *(asterisks)*. Short-axis measurement demonstrates an anteroposterior dimension of 9 mm. (Courtesy Nationwide Children's Hospital, Columbus, OH.)

Intussusception. **Intussusception** is the most common acute abdominal disorder in early childhood. This condition occurs when the bowel prolapses into a more distal bowel and is propelled in an antegrade fashion. Telescoping of the bowel in this manner causes obstruction. The ileum may invaginate into more distal ileum, causing an ileoileal intussusception, which often resolves on its own. However, if there is further progression through the ileocecal valve, an ileocolic intussusception results (Fig. 25.26).

Traditionally, intussusception in 90% of cases includes the prolapse of the ileum into the cecum or beyond, producing an ileocolic intussusception. Ileocolic intussusception is usually seen in children between the ages of 6 months and 2 years. Older children with Henoch-Schönlein purpura are also at risk. A higher incidence has been reported in males (2:1), along with a cold/flu seasonal prevalence. Frequently, there is a history of an antecedent upper respiratory tract infection. Associated inflammation of lymphoid tissue in the ileocolic region may act as a lead point for the telescoping phenomenon.

Children may present with colicky abdominal pain, vomiting, and bloody (currant jelly) stools. Abdominal distention or a mass may also be palpable in up to 50% of patients with intussusception. In patients with this classic clinical presentation, sonography has established itself as the imaging modality of choice, with sensitivity and specificity of nearly 98% and a negative predictive value at nearly 100%. Therapeutic reduction is almost entirely undergone by fluoroscopic means (often an air enema), although sonographically guided saline enemas may also reduce intussusceptions. Failure to reduce an intussusception mandates immediate surgical intervention. Likewise, surgical intervention is indicated in patients with a classic clinical presentation of intussusception who have developed fever and peritoneal signs.

Examination Technique. The patient is examined in the supine position. A brief survey of the entire abdomen is performed, dividing the abdomen into four quadrants, followed by an examination focusing on the bowel using a 5 to 12 MHz linear or curved array transducer. The bowel is followed, often starting at the cecum in the right lower quadrant.

Sonographic Findings. The sonographic appearance of intussusception is of alternating hypoechoic and hyperechoic rings surrounding an echogenic center, as seen in a short-axis view of the involved area. This is known as the **target** (or **"cinnamon bun"**) sign (Fig. 25.27). Often the ileoileal intussusception will measure less than 3 cm in the transverse plane, whereas the pathologic ileocolic intussusception will measure greater than 3 cm.

In the long-axis view, hypoechoic layers on each side of the echogenic center result in a pseudo-kidney or "sandwich" sign appearance (Fig. 25.28). The sonolucent ring represents the edematous infolded loop of the intussusceptum, whereas the echogenic central area represents its compressed **mucosa**. Other concentric rings are present, resulting

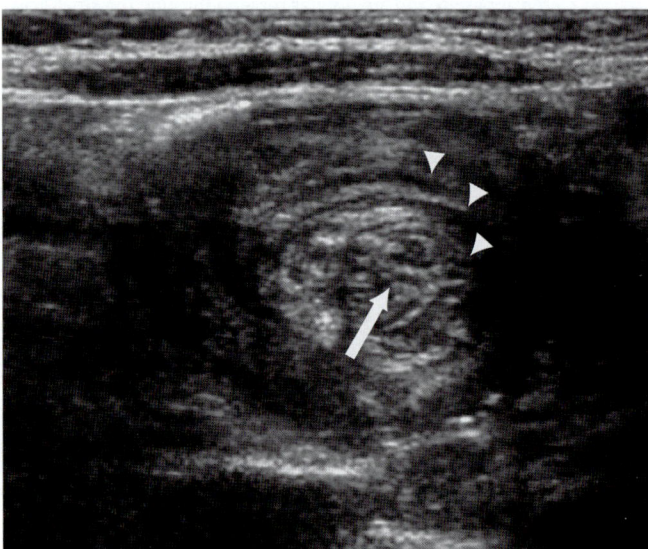

FIG. 25.27 **Intussusception target or "cinnamon bun" sign.** Transverse image of an intussusception showing a target or cinnamon bun sign. There are several circumferential layers of increased and decreased echogenicity *(arrowheads)* because of the telescoping bowel. The lumen *(arrow)* may contain fluid or lymph node(s). (Courtesy Nationwide Children's Hospital, Columbus, OH.)

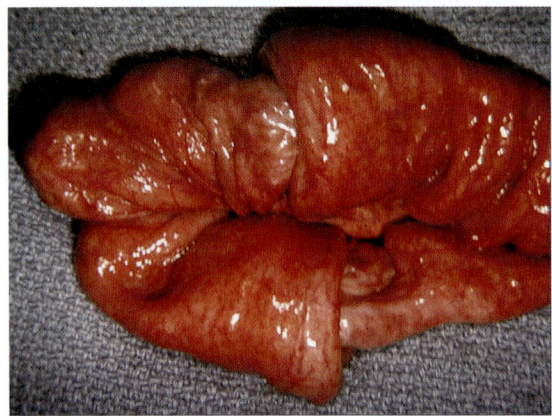

FIG. 25.26 **Gross pathology of intussusception.** Specimen shows the loops of bowel invaginating into each other.

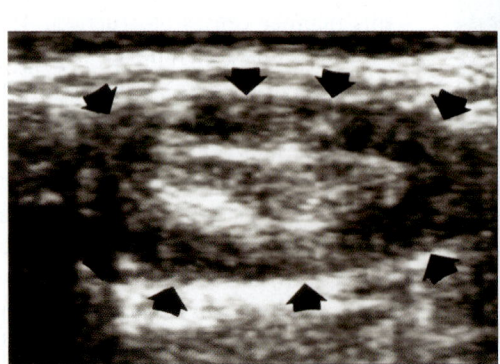
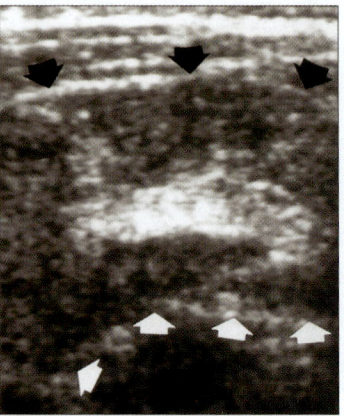

FIG. 25.28 **Intussusception pseudo-kidney or "sandwich" sign.** *Left:* Longitudinal image of the intussusception in the right lower quadrant demonstrates a *pseudokidney* appearance *(arrows)*. A normal kidney was documented in each renal fossa, so this is not a pelvic kidney. *Right:* Longitudinal image of an intussusception *(arrows)* in the right lower quadrant in a different patient shows a sandwich appearance.

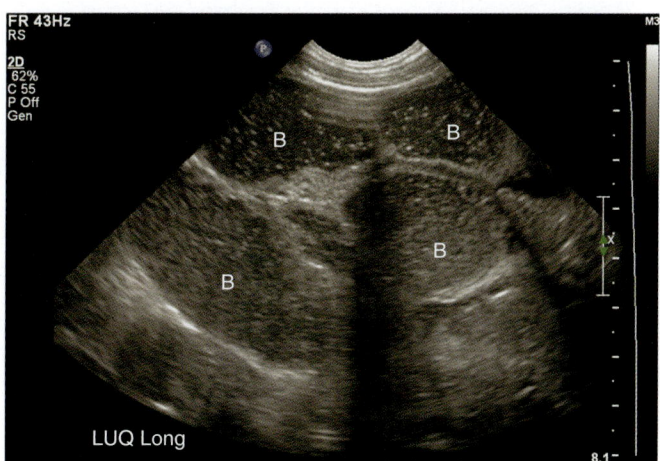

FIG. 25.29 Dilated fluid-filled bowel loops. Dilated bowel (B) located proximal to an intussusception. Multiple, dilated fluid-filled bowel loops are seen within the left upper quadrant. (Courtesy Nationwide Children's Hospital, Columbus, OH.)

from visualization of additional bowel wall layers within the intussusception. Dilated loops of obstructed proximal bowel may also be seen (Fig. 25.29). Free peritoneal fluid is not an uncommon finding with uncomplicated intussusception. Color Doppler (Fig. 25.30) may help determine the success of an air reduction enema; if there is good color flow to all areas of the telescoping bowel, the chances are better for a reduction. Poor color Doppler may indicate ischemia to the area of the affected bowel and is likely irreducible with air or hydrostatic enema, necessitating surgery.

When an intussusception is documented sonographically, an associated mass or cause, though relatively uncommon (5% to 10%), should be sought. A *double target sign* has been reported as being diagnostic of intussuscepted Meckel diverticulum. Other causes, such as a small bowel tumor, polyp, or duplication cyst, may likewise be identified.

After reduction, an edematous ileocecal valve may be seen on fluoroscopy that may mimic a residual intussusception. Sonography helps distinguish between persistent intussusception and an edematous ileocecal valve. The edematous valve appears as a small sonolucent rim with an echogenic center. It is distinguishable from intussusception because its cross-sectional diameter is smaller than that of an intussusception, and it lacks the diagnostic concentric rings.

In addition to intussusception, conditions that can produce a target-like sonographic appearance include primary bowel tumors, such as lymphoma, and thickened bowel wall in post–stem-cell transplant or bone marrow transplant patients and patients with inflammatory bowel disease.

Hypertrophic Pyloric Stenosis. The **pyloric canal** is located between the stomach and duodenum. In some infants, the pyloric muscle can become hypertrophied, resulting in gastric obstruction. Hypertrophy of the circular muscle of the pylorus is an acquired condition that narrows the pyloric canal (Fig. 25.31). The pyloric canal itself is not intrinsically stenotic or narrowed, but it functions as if it were due to the abnormally thickened surrounding muscle.

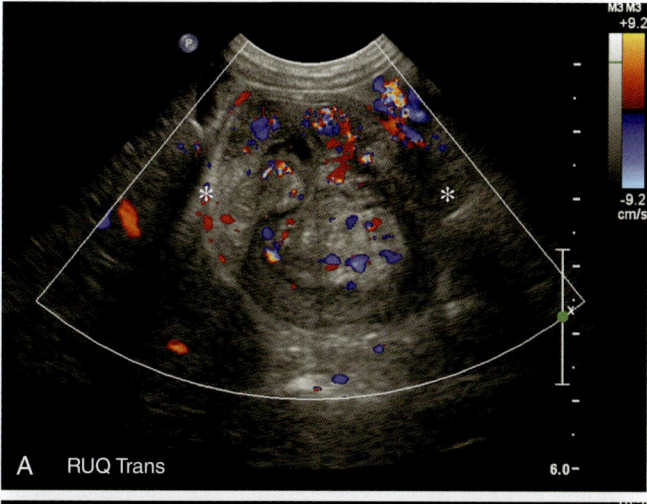

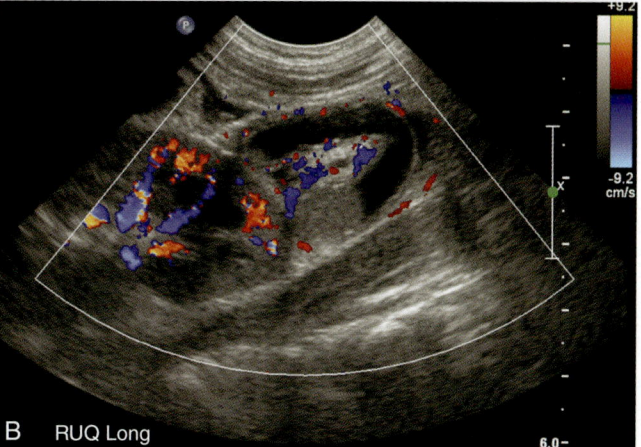

FIG. 25.30 Ileocolic intussusception. A 1-year-old with a positive ileocolic intussusception successfully underwent a single air enema for resolution. (A) Transverse view showing good color Doppler flow measured *(asterisks)* over 3 cm, indicating an ileocolic intussusception. (B) Longitudinal view with color Doppler flow. (Courtesy Nationwide Children's Hospital, Columbus, OH.)

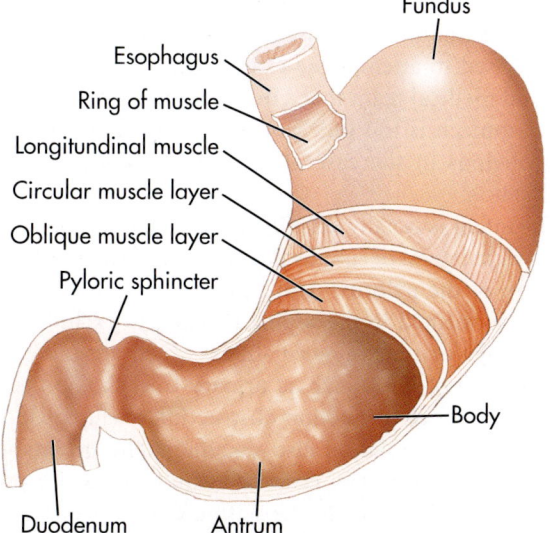

FIG. 25.31 Stomach and pyloric canal. The pylorus muscle (sphincter) connects the antrum of the stomach with the duodenum of the small intestine.

Hypertrophic pyloric stenosis (HPS) appears most commonly in male infants (4:1) with 95% of cases occurring between 3 and 12 weeks of age, often peaking at 4 weeks. Rarely, it becomes apparent at birth or as late as 5 months of age. The incidence of HPS is approximately 3 in 1000 neonates. Bile-free vomiting in an otherwise healthy infant is the most frequent clinical sign. As the pyloric muscle thickens and elongates, the stomach outlet obstruction increases and vomiting is more constant and projectile. Dehydration and weight loss may ensue.

Often acute-onset patients will present very colicky, whereas those who show signs of dehydration and weight loss are often lethargic and too sick to cry and struggle. Peristaltic waves and reverse peristaltic waves crossing the upper abdomen may be observed during or after feeding as the stomach attempts to force its contents through the abnormal canal, often resulting in **projectile vomiting**. In these infants, palpation of an olive-shaped mass at the epigastrium is diagnostic and is treated by surgical **pyloromyotomy**. In infants with a suggestive history or an equivocal physical examination, diagnostic imaging is required to directly visualize the pyloric muscle.

The neonate with projectile vomiting is frequently sent directly from the physician's office or the hospital emergency department. In pediatric imaging departments and in other ultrasound departments where there is appropriate expertise, sonography is the imaging method of choice to establish the diagnosis of HPS. If HPS is not a primary diagnostic consideration, or if the sonogram is not diagnostic, conventional contrast radiography of the upper gastrointestinal tract is necessary to assess other potential causes of vomiting. The differential considerations include pylorospasm, gastrointestinal reflux, antral web, hiatal hernia, and duodenal obstruction caused by stenosis or midgut malrotation with bands or volvulus.

Examination Technique. Ideally, the infant will be on a nothing by mouth (NPO, nil per os) status for a couple of hours before scanning, as too much fluid or no fluid in the stomach is undesirable. However, this is rarely the case, and it is advised to attempt the examination, warning the parents and medical team that a delay period may be necessary if the stomach is too full. However, it is often sonographically obvious in the case of a positive HPS, regardless of NPO status.

The infant is usually examined first in the supine and then in the right lateral decubitus position, which aids in the visualization of the pylorus. A preliminary survey of the abdomen is performed in the supine position to exclude adrenal hemorrhage or renal abnormalities, which are increased in the presence of HPS, such as urinary tract dilation secondary to ureteropelvic junction obstruction or duplex kidneys. The sonographer should also document the orientation of the superior mesenteric artery and vein to assess for **midgut malrotation**, especially in the setting of negative findings of HPS (Fig. 25.32). A positive finding of midgut malrotation may appear with an inability to show the normal relationship or a "whirlpool sign" of these vessels.

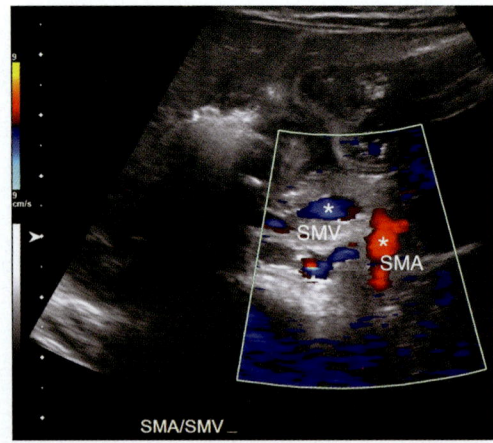

FIG. 25.32 **Normal superior mesenteric artery/superior mesenteric vein relationship.** Transverse plane of the abdomen at the level of the pancreas showing the normal superior mesenteric artery/superior mesenteric vein relationship, ruling out midgut malrotation abnormalities. (Courtesy Chester County Hospital, West Chester, PA.)

Real-time imaging is then performed using a high-frequency linear array or small curved array transducer (5 to 12 MHz). Before administering fluid, preliminary imaging of the pylorus is first performed to assess the amount of gastric fluid in the antrum of the stomach, and radiologist discretion is advised.

The associated pitfalls of having an improper amount of gastric fluid are as follows: (1) *No fluid in the antrum of the stomach.* Inadequate gastric fluid will not accurately distinguish the normally collapsed antrum from the pylorus (Fig. 25.33). (2) *Having an overly distended stomach.* This can displace the pyloric muscle posteriorly, making sonographic delineation much more difficult to obtain accurate measurements, or render it impossible (Fig. 25.34). In this instance, scanning from a prone approach may do the trick. If not, and the patient is positive for HPS, he or she may vomit the contents out. Occasionally, aspiration of gastric contents via a nasogastric tube is required. If the pyloric muscle is normal, the gastric contents will pass through the canal of their own volition.

If there are adequate amounts of fluid in the antrum, the longitudinal images of the pyloric muscle are obtained by placing the transducer transversely across the right upper quadrant, just below the level of the xiphoid process. The head of the pancreas and gallbladder may be initially identified, and the transducer is then rotated obliquely until the pyloric muscle is visualized in its long axis. Transverse short-axis images of the pyloric muscle are often obtained from the right coronal plane angled medially when the pylorus is abnormal (Fig. 25.35).

If there is not enough residual gastric fluid present and a positive diagnosis has not been established, the patient is often administered a small amount, 30 to 90 mL (1 to 3 oz), of glucose water with a bottle or syringe. The infant is placed in the right lateral decubitus position for feeding, and the transducer is again placed transversely in the right upper quadrant, allowing for maximum long-axis visualization of the

CHAPTER 25 Neonatal and Pediatric Abdomen

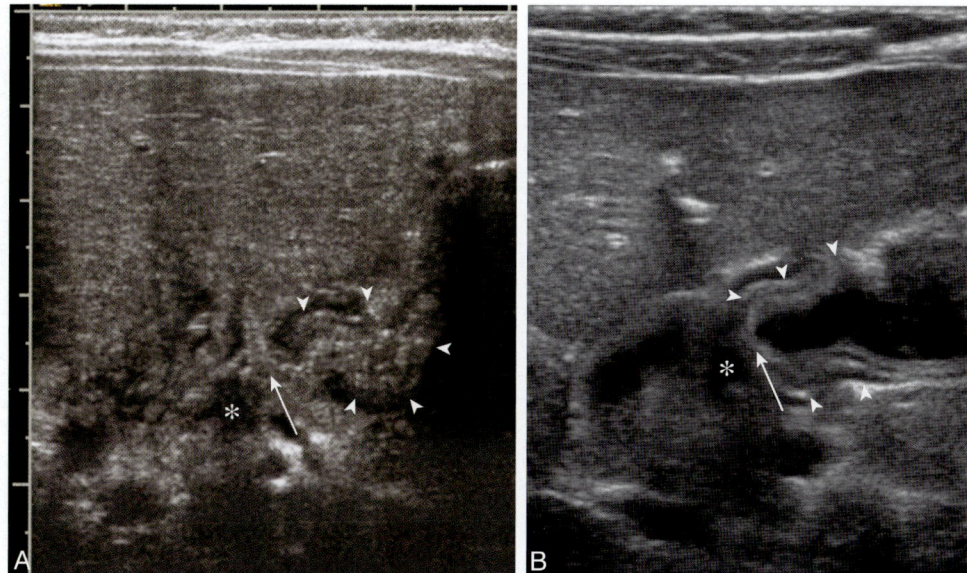

FIG. 25.33 **Pitfalls of an empty stomach (and collapsed antrum).** (A) Long-axis view of an empty gastric antrum in a normal pyloric muscle *(arrow)*. The antrum is seen anterior and lateral to the muscle *(arrowheads)*. Fluid in the duodenum *(asterisk)* is often triangular and is seen inferior and medial to the muscle. (B) Long-axis view of a properly filled antrum in a normal pylorus. A clearer delineation of the pyloric muscle *(arrow)*, gastric antrum *(arrowheads)*, and duodenum *(asterisk)* is seen. (Courtesy Nationwide Children's Hospital, Columbus, OH.)

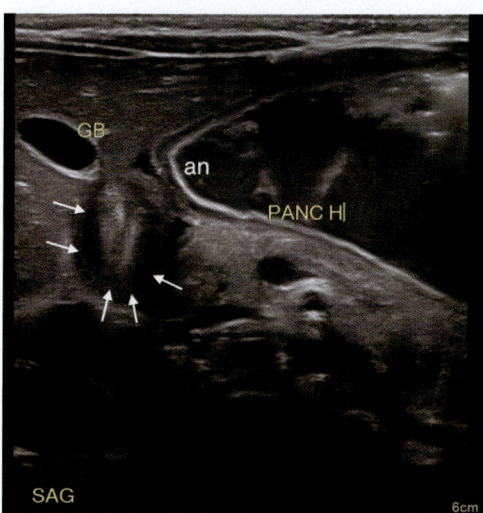

FIG. 25.34 **Pitfalls of an overdistended stomach.** Transverse view of the right upper quadrant in a neonate with hypertrophic pyloric stenosis. The fluid-distended antrum (an) has pushed the elongated pyloric muscle *(arrows)* posteriorly, precluding accurate measurement of the length of the pyloric canal. The pylorus sits between the gallbladder (GB) and pancreatic head (PANC H). (Courtesy Chester County Hospital, West Chester, PA.)

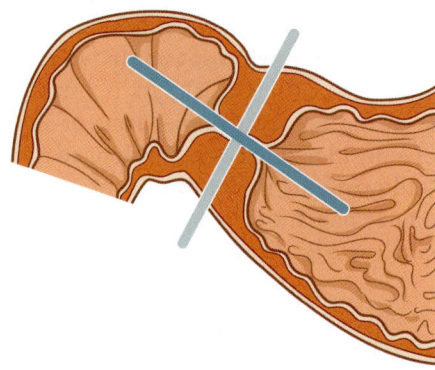

FIG. 25.35 **Pylorus transducer angles.** Long-axis angle *(dark blue line)* and short-axis angle *(light blue line)* of the transducer placement in evaluating pylorus.

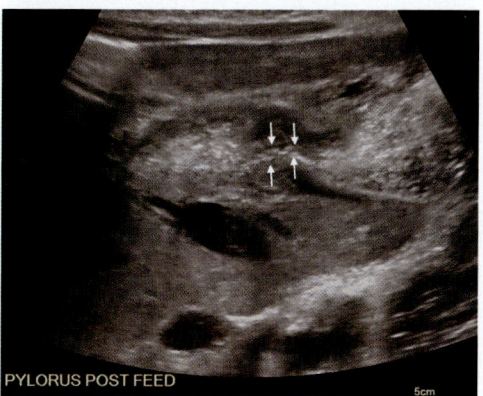

FIG. 25.36 **Normal pylorus after feeding.** After feeding the infant, the echogenic contents of the stomach are seen moving freely through the normal pylorus *(arrows)*. (Courtesy Chester County Hospital, West Chester, PA.)

stomach and pyloric canal, and is most advantageous for documenting the transit of gastric contents into the duodenum (Fig. 25.36). Often, no more than 30 mL is required. Pedialyte (and often breast milk) will have a similar appearance as water; however, the formula will appear more echogenic, occluding a good view, and is not advised. Sometimes gastrointestinal reflux may be seen as well. This documentation of fluid passing through the canal is important, and a cine clip will garner better appreciation.

Sonographic Findings. Sonographic measurement of the pyloric muscle thickness enables the diagnosis of HPS. Pyloric muscle measurements can be made in both the long- and short-axis planes. If the image is oblique, measurements will be overestimated. Muscle thickness greater than or equal to 3 mm is the most diagnostic measurement. The thickness is measured from the periphery of the hypoechoic muscle to its junction with the echogenic central canal.

An elongated channel length greater than 15 to 16 mm (often established by institutions) on the long-axis view is also a reliable indicator of HPS. Pyloric channel length is measured from the proximal to the distal extremes of the echogenic central canal (Fig. 25.37).

Transverse views will also allow for the measurement of the pylorus muscle wall thickness. A "bagel" or "donut" appearance of a hypertrophied pyloric muscle and the echogenic central canal is seen. The pyloric muscle frequently has a nonuniform echo pattern, with the near and far fields appearing more echogenic (Fig. 25.38).

In addition to these sonographic findings and measurements, another significant finding is the presence of active antegrade and reverse gastric peristalsis. With positive HPS, fluid will often not pass through the canal on fluid-aided real-time sonography. However, fluid may occasionally pass through the crevices of the compressed echogenic mucosa, which appears as the double-track sign. This sign may also be seen with pylorospasm, in which the canal is elongated, but the muscle thickness is often within normal limits. In the case of pylorospasm (or if there is any question of a positive diagnosis), prolonged observation is necessary, allowing the infant to rest for 10 minutes without scanning or palpation, and will often show the pyloric channel opening (Fig. 25.39).

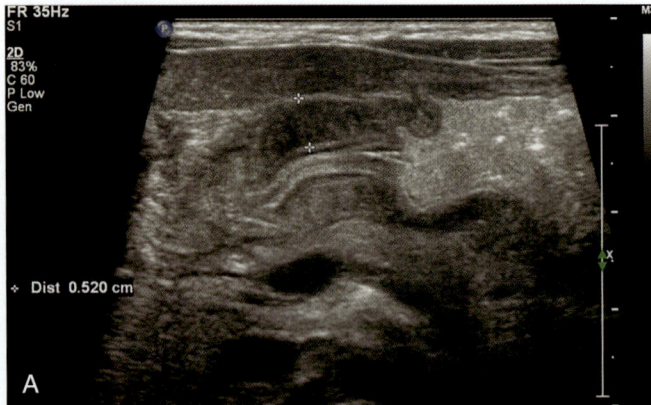
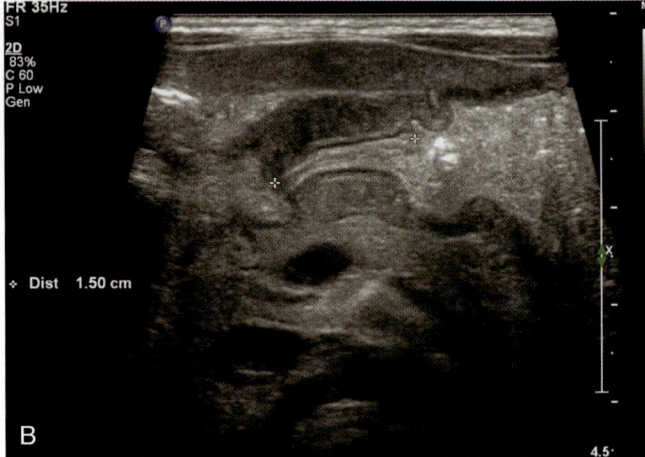

FIG. 25.37 **Positive hypertrophic pyloric stenosis.** Positive hypertrophic pyloric stenosis seen in 26-day-old neonate with vomiting. Patient had a positive upper gastrointestinal fluoroscopy study previously (and unnecessarily) at an outside hospital. (A) Long-axis pyloric muscle thickness measurement (anteroposterior) is abnormal at >5 mm. Pancreas is seen directly posterior to enlarged pylorus. (B) Pyloric channel length measurement is 15 mm. (Courtesy Nationwide Children's Hospital, Columbus, OH.)

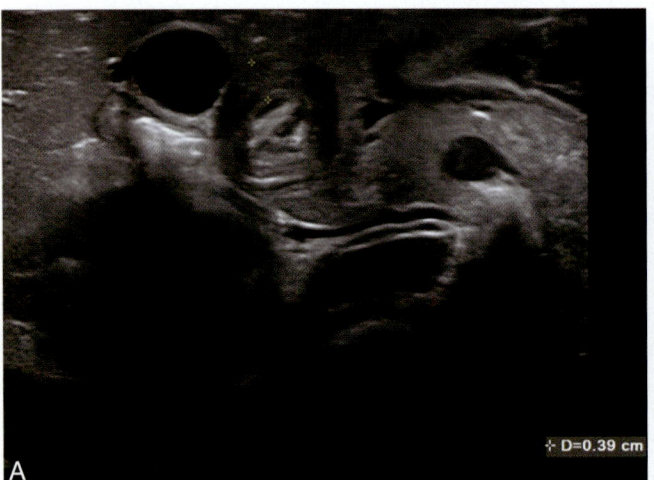
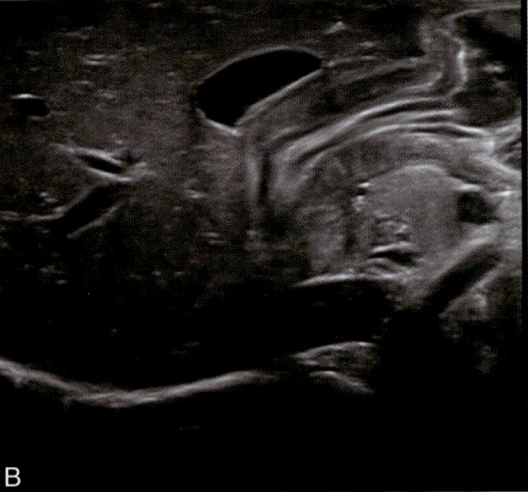

FIG. 25.38 **Positive hypertrophic pyloric stenosis "bagel" or "donut" sign.** (A) Short-axis view of the hypertrophied pyloric muscle measuring 3.9 mm demonstrating the bagel or donut sign. The muscle thickness is measured from the outer border to the mucosal-muscle interface. (B) Long-axis view in the same 3-week-old neonate. (Courtesy Chester County Hospital, West Chester, PA.)

Other Surgical Conditions

Other conditions that may lead to surgical correction may be seen less frequently through the ultrasound department in the neonate. These conditions include midgut malrotation (Fig. 25.40), mesenteric or omental cysts (often large), bowel duplication cysts, duodenal atresia, and meconium peritonitis. Older infants and children may present with Meckel diverticulum, incarcerated hernia, duplication cysts of the bowel, and hematomas of the bowel resulting from trauma.

Necrotizing Enterocolitis. Necrotizing enterocolitis (NEC) is a serious condition seen in premature infants, causing high morbidity and mortality. In NEC, the bowel undergoes necrosis and must be surgically removed, resulting in **short bowel syndrome**. Once developed, one out of four extremely preterm infants will die from this condition. It is the second leading cause of death in preemies after respiratory distress. Whereas other causes of mortality in this age group have declined, NEC mortality has been increasing.

Plain abdominal radiography is the imaging modality of choice, yet sonography can help depict intraabdominal fluid and/or abscess formation before and after surgery in the neonate with abdominal distention or other clinical symptoms. Ultrasound is also helpful in showing bowel wall thickness. However, the most useful sonographic sign is intramural gas, which appears as small, punctate, hyperechoic foci *within* the intestinal wall, with an associated loss of the normal hypoechoic muscularis halo. Intraluminal gas, on the other hand, will be seen floating within normal intraluminal fluid. Portal venous gas and free intraperitoneal gas may also be detected sonographically.

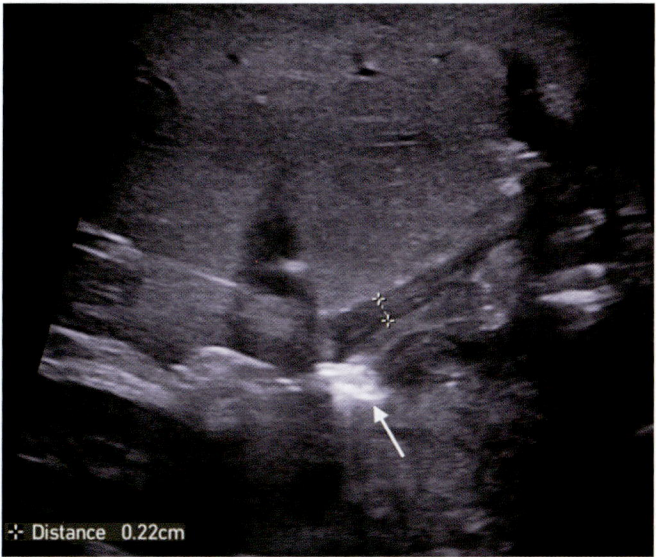

FIG. 25.39 Pylorospasm. Imaging transverse across the right upper quadrant using the liver as an acoustic window, the long axis of the pylorus, shown here, appears at first to be positive for hypertrophic pyloric stenosis. While the channel length varied from 11 to 15 mm, the thickened muscle, at 2.2 mm, did not meet the cut-off criteria of 3 mm. The contents of the stomach passed through to the duodenum *(arrow)* with feeding. However, due to the patient's clinical presentation and ultrasound findings, the neonate was transferred to surgical care to be observed and reevaluated. (Courtesy Chester County Hospital, West Chester, PA.)

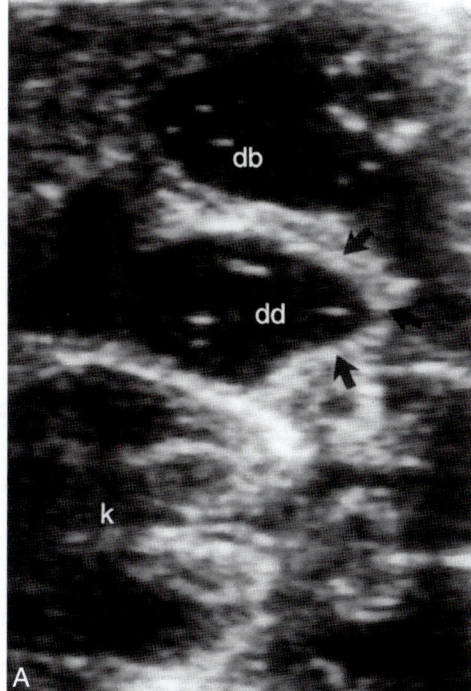
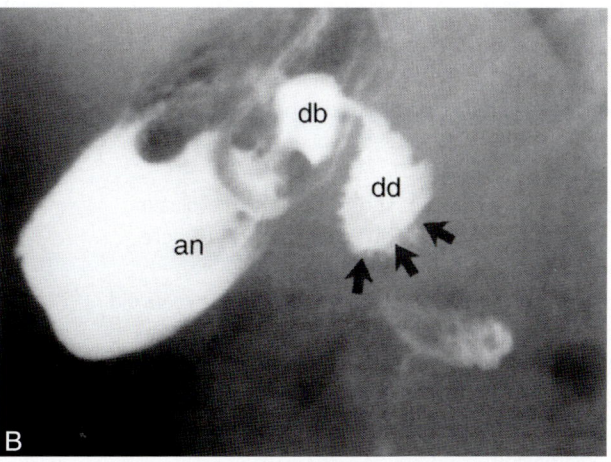

FIG. 25.40 Midgut malrotation. (A) Transverse image of a 4-week-old infant with projectile vomiting. There was to-and-fro peristalsis in the fluid-filled duodenal bulb (db) and descending duodenum (dd). The descending duodenum tapered abruptly *(arrows)* and could not be traced distally. The right kidney (k) is posterior to the descending duodenum. A hypertrophied pyloric muscle was not identified. (B) Right lateral view from a barium examination in the same patient shows the stomach, antrum (an), duodenal bulb (db), and descending duodenum (dd). The descending duodenum tapers abruptly *(arrows)* and then spirals inferiorly. The barium examination delineates the surgically emergent malrotation, which could not be identified on the sonogram.

Key Pearls

- Sonography is the imaging modality of choice to evaluate the neonatal and pediatric abdomen, as it provides excellent visualization of the abdominal organs and structures without ionizing radiation.
- Knowledge of a pediatric patient's developmental stage can greatly aid a sonographer in obtaining high-quality diagnostic images.
- Scanning techniques, probe frequencies, and footprints will vary widely across age groups, and continual probe changes and optimization are in order.
- Knowledge of normal organ sizes and reference charts are necessary for the normal pediatric abdominal examination.
- Retroperitoneal and vascular structures should be closely evaluated to rule out malignant processes in the pediatric patient.
- Pancreatitis, trauma, and choledocholithiasis are common reasons for acute upper abdominal pain.
- Childhood obesity is on the rise and is associated with an increased risk of gallstones and nonalcoholic fatty liver disease.
- Acquired and hereditary diseases need to be carefully monitored in children, as there may be increased associated risks of both chronic and malignant processes.
- Most pediatric patients with cystic fibrosis will develop pancreatitis.
- The spleen plays a role in many childhood diseases, as it plays a role in the body's immune response and blood formation.
- Sonography is used to differentiate obstructive from nonobstructive neonatal jaundice in neonates.
- Neonatal hepatitis, biliary atresia, and choledochal cyst are the most common causes of neonatal jaundice.
- Abdominal tumors must be carefully evaluated to determine their organ of origin, blood flow patterns, and morphology and to see any associated lymph nodes or vessel thrombus.
- Two-thirds of all pediatric liver masses are malignant.
- Most malignant pediatric masses are asymptomatic, whereas symptomatic ones tend to be of a gastrointestinal origin.
- The most common surgical conditions diagnosed with sonography are appendicitis, intussusception, and hypertrophic pyloric stenosis.
- Multiple sonographic techniques should be used in evaluating the appendix to overcome an equivocal examination where the appendix is not visualized.
- Intussusception commonly occurs in children under 2 years old and may obstruct the bowel if in an ileocolic location.
- Hypertrophic pyloric stenosis (HPS) is more commonly seen in males (4:1) and peaks at 1 month of life.
- Too much fluid and too little fluid in the stomach are both pitfalls of HPS imaging.
- Ultrasound may detect other gastrointestinal surgical conditions. Although it may not diagnose them all, ultrasound may be the first imaging procedure in children, so it is good to be aware of these differential diagnoses.

BIBLIOGRAPHY

American Institute of Ultrasound in Medicine: AIUM practice parameter for the performance of an ultrasound examination of the abdomen and/or retroperitoneum, 2017. https://www.aium.org/resources/guidelines/abdominal.pdf

Amodio J, Fefferman N. Ultrasound of pediatric abdominal and scrotal emergencies. *Appl Radiol*. 2007;36(12):22–29.

Askew N. An overview of infantile hypertrophic pyloric stenosis. *Paediatr Nurs*. 2010;22(8):27–30.

Aziz S, Wild Y, Rosenthal P, Golstein RB. Pseudo gallbladder sign in biliary atresia—an imaging pitfall. *Pediatr Radiol*. 2011;41(5):620–626.

Babcock DS. Sonography of the acute abdomen in the pediatric patient. *J Ultrasound Med*. 2002;21:887–899.

Bachur RG, Dayan PS, Bajaj L, et al. The effect of abdominal pain duration on the accuracy of diagnostic imaging for pediatric appendicitis. *Ann Emerg Med*. 2012;60(5):582–590.

Bachur RG, Levy JA, Callahan MJ, et al. Effect of reduction in the use of computed tomography on clinical outcomes of appendicitis. *JAMA Pediatr*. 2015;169(8):755–760.

Baker ME, Nelson RC, Rosen MP, et al. *Expert Panel on Gastrointestinal Imaging: ACR Appropriateness Criteria: acute pancreatitis*. Reston, VA: American College of Radiology; 2013.

Balachandran B, Singhi S, Lal S. Emergency management of acute abdomen in children. *Indian J Pediatr*. 2013;80(3):226–234.

Bhisitkul DM, Listernick R, Shkolnik A, et al. Clinical application of ultrasonography in the diagnosis of intussusception. *J Pediatr*. 1992;121:182.

Butler M, Servaes S, Srinivasan A, et al. US depiction of the appendix: role of abdominal wall thickness and appendiceal location. *Emerg Radiol*. 2011;18(6):525–531.

Centers for Disease Control and Prevention. Autism spectrum disorder. https://www.cdc.gov/ncbddd/autism/data.html

Centers for Disease Control and Prevention, National Center for Health Statistics Underlying Cause of Death 1999–2019 on CDC WONDER Online Database, released in 2020. http://wonder.cdc.gov/ucd-icd10.html. http://wonder.cdc.gov/ucd-icd10.html.

Centers for Disease Control and Prevention: Childhood obesity facts. https://www.cdc.gov/nchs/fastats/child-health.htm.

Chiorean L, et al. Benign liver tumors in pediatric patients—review with emphasis on imaging features. *World J Gastroenterol*. 2015;21(28):8541–8561.

Chung EM, Cube R, Lewis RB, Conran RM. From the archives of the AFIP: pediatric liver masses: radiologic-pathologic correlation part 2. Malignant tumors. *Radiographics*. 2011;31(2):483–507.

Coley BD. Pediatric applications of abdominal vascular Doppler imaging: part I. *Pediatr Radiol*. 2004;34(10):757–771.

Cogley J, O'Connor S, Houshyar R, Dulaimy K. Emergent pediatric US: what every radiologist should know. *Radiographics*. 2012;32(3):651–665.

Cyr J, Johnston DL. Accuracy of physical examination versus ultrasound in the detection of hepatosplenomegaly at diagnosis of pediatric leukemia. *J Hematol Malign*. 2013;3(1):24.

Danon O, et al. Hepatic and splenic involvement in cat-scratch disease: imaging features. *Abdom Imaging*. 2000;25(2):182–183.

Dias SC, Swinson S, Torrão H, et al. Hypertrophic pyloric stenosis: tips and tricks for ultrasound diagnosis. *Insights Imaging*. 2012;3(3):247–250.

Epelman M, et al. Necrotizing enterocolitis: review of state-of-the-art imaging findings with pathologic correlation. *Radiographics*. 2007;27(2):285–305.

Finkelhor D, Turner H, Ormrod R, Hamby S. Trends in childhood violence and abuse exposure: evidence from 2 national surveys. *Arch Pediatr Adolesc Med*. 2010;164(3):238–242.

Fordham LA. Approach to the pediatric patient. *Ultrasound Clin*. 2009;4:439–443.

Goldberg BB, McGahan JP. *Atlas of ultrasound measurements*. ed 2 St Louis: Elsevier; 2006.

Goldin AB, Khanna P, Thapa M, et al. Revised ultrasound criteria for appendicitis in children improve diagnostic accuracy. *Pediatr Radiol.* 2011;41(8):993–999.

Gongidi P, Bellah RD. Ultrasound of the pediatric appendix. *Pediatr Radiol.* 2017;47(9):1091–1100. 4.

Haller JO, Slovis TL, Babcock DS, Teele RL. Early history of pediatric ultrasound. *J Ultrasound Med.* 2004;23:323–329.

Heller ME, Veach LM. Evaluation and care of the pediatric patient. In: Heller ME, Veach LM, eds. *Clinical medical assisting: a professional, field smart approach to the workplace.* ed 1 New York: Cengage; 2009:426–435.

Herman TE, Siegel MJ. Infantile hepatic hemangioendothelioma. *J Perinatol.* 2000;20:447–449.

Hernanz-Schulman M, Ambrosino MM, Freeman PC, Quinn CB. Common bile duct in children: sonographic dimensions. *Radiology.* 1995;195(1):193–195.

Hilmes MA, Strouse PJ. The pediatric spleen. *Semin Ultrasound CT MRI.* 2007;28(1):3–11.

Humphrey TM, Stringer MD. Biliary atresia: US diagnosis 1. *Radiology.* 2007;244(3):845–851.

Hwang M, Piskunowicz M, Darge K. Advanced Ultrasound Techniques for Pediatric Imaging. *Pediatrics.* 2019;143(3):e20182609.

Ikeda S, Sera Y, Ohshiro H. Gallbladder contraction in biliary atresia: a pitfall of ultrasound diagnosis. *Pediatr Radiol.* 1998;28:451–453.

Ingram JD, Yerushalmi B, Connell J, et al. Hepatoblastoma in a neonate: a hypervascular presentation mimicking hemangioendothelioma. *Pediatr Radiol.* 2000;30:794–797.

Itagaki A, Uchida M, Ueki K. Double targets sign in ultrasonic diagnosis of intussuscepted Meckel diverticulum. *Pediatr Radiol.* 1991;21:148.

Karlapudi A, Gunderman RB. To stand tall in pediatric radiology, you have to get down on your knees: Dr. Armand Brodeur. *Pediatr Radiol.* 2021;51(9):1559–1561.

Kendrick A, Phua K, Ooi B, et al. Making the diagnosis of biliary atresia using the triangular cord sign and gallbladder length. *Pediatr Radiol.* 2000;30:69–73.

Kim EH, et al. Clinical features of infantile hepatic hemangioendothelioma. *Korean J Pediatr.* 2011;54(6):260–266.

Kim JS. Acute abdominal pain in children. *Pediatr Gastroenterol Hepatol Nutr.* 2013;16(4):219–224.

Kotagal M, et al. Improving ultrasound quality to reduce computed tomography use in pediatric appendicitis: the Safe and Sound campaign. *Am J Surg.* 2015;209(5):896–900.

Le J, et al. Do clinical outcomes suffer during transition to an ultrasound-first paradigm for the evaluation of acute appendicitis in children? *AJR Am J Roentgenol.* 2013;201(6):1348.

Lee HC, et al. Dilation of the biliary tree in children: sonographic diagnosis and its clinical significance. *J Ultrasound Med.* 2000;19:177–182.

London M, Ladewig P, Ball J, Binler R. Pediatric assessment. In: London M, Ladewig P, Ball J, Binler R, eds. *Maternal and child nursing care.* ed 2 London: Pearson; 2007:961–1022.

Loomba R, Sirlin CB, Schwimmer JB, Lavine JE. Advances in pediatric nonalcoholic fatty liver disease. *Hepatology.* 2009;50(4):1282–1293.

Martin AE, Vollman D, Adler B, Caniano DA. CT scans may not reduce the negative appendectomy rate in children. *J Pediatr Surg.* 2004;39(6):886–890.

Martin-Hirsel A, Cantrell CJ, Hulka F. Antenatal diagnosis of a choledochal cyst and annular pancreas. *J Ultrasound Med.* 2004;23:315–318.

Matz S, Connell M, Sinha M, et al. Clinical outcomes of pediatric patients with acute abdominal pain and incidental findings of free intraperitoneal fluid on diagnostic imaging. *J Ultrasound Med.* 2013;32(9):1547–1553.

Megremis SD, Vlachonikolis JG, Tsilimigaki AM. Spleen length in childhood with US: normal values based on age, sex, and somatometric parameters. *Radiology.* 2004;231(1):129–134.

Milla SS, Lee EY, Buonomo C, Bramson RT. Ultrasound evaluation of pediatric abdominal masses. *Ultrasound Clin.* 2007;2(3):541–559.

National Institute of Mental Health: Attention deficit/ hyperactivity disorder. https://www.nimh.nih.gov/health/statistics/attention-deficit-hyperactivity-disorder-adhd.shtml.

Nelson CA, Saha S, Mead PS. Cat-Scratch Disease in the United States, 2005-2013. *Emerg Infect Dis.* 2016;22(10):1741–1746.

Nielsen JW, et al. Reducing computed tomography scans for appendicitis by introduction of a standardized and validated ultrasonography report template. *J Pediatr Surg.* 2015;50(1):144–148.

Nievelstein RAJ, Robben SJF, Blickman JG. Hepatobiliary and pancreatic imaging in children—techniques and an overview of non-neoplastic disease entities. *Pediatr Radiol.* 2011;41:55–75.

Park NH, Park CS, Lee EJ, et al. Ultrasonographic findings identifying the faecal-impacted appendix: differential findings with acute appendicitis. *Br J Radiol.* 2007;80(959):872–877.

Patel RM, Kandefer S, Walsh MC, et al. Causes and timing of death in extremely premature infants from 2000 through 2011. *N Engl J Med.* 2015;372(4):331–340.

Pepper VK, Stanfill AB, Pearl RH. Diagnosis and management of pediatric appendicitis, intussusception, and Meckel diverticulum. *Surg Clin North Am.* 2012;92(3):505–526.

Redmon S. Pediatric sonography: funography for kids. *J Diagn Med Sonogr.* 2007;23:110–111.

Restrepo R, Palani R, Cervantes LF, et al. Hemangiomas revisited: the useful, the unusual and the new. Part 1: overview and clinical and imaging characteristics. *Pediatr Radiol.* 2011;41(7):895–904.

Restrepo R, Palani R, Cervantes LF, et al. Hemangiomas revisited: the useful, the unusual and the new. Part 2: endangering hemangiomas and treatment. *Pediatr Radiol.* 2011;41(7):905–915.

Rioux M. Sonographic detection of the normal and abnormal appendix. *Am J Roentgenol.* 1992;158:773.

Saigal G, Therrien JR, Kuo F. Ultrasound in pediatric emergencies. *Appl Radiol.* Aug 2014:6–16. Available at. http://appliedradiology.com/articles/ultrasound-in-pediatric-emergencies.

Sato M. Liver tumors in children and young patients: sonographic and color Doppler findings. *Abdom Imaging.* 2000;25:596–601.

Siegel MJ. Pediatric abdominal masses. In: Sanders RC, Winter T, eds. *Clinical sonography: a practical guide.* ed 4 Baltimore, MD: Lippincott Williams & Wilkins; 2007:321–340.

Siegel MJ. *Pediatric sonography.* Philadelphia, PA: Lippincott Williams & Wilkins; 2010.

Siegel MJ, Martin KW, Worthington JL. Normal and abnormal pancreas in children: US studies. *Radiology.* 1987;165:15–18.

Sivit CJ. Diagnosis of acute appendicitis in children: spectrum of sonographic findings. *Am J Roentgenol.* 1993;161:147.

Sivit CJ, Newman KD, Boenning DA, et al. Appendicitis: usefulness of US in diagnosis in a pediatric population. *Radiology.* 1992;185:549.

Roos JE, Piffner R, Stallmach T, et al. Infantile hemangioendothelioma. *Radiographics.* 2003;23(6):1649–1655.

Rosenberg HK, et al. Normal splenic sizes in infants and children: sonographic measurements. *AJR Am J Roentgenol.* 1991;157:119–121.

Samuel M. Pediatric appendicitis score. *J Pediatr Surg.* 2002;37:877–881.

Sanchez TRS, Potnick A, Graf JL, et al. Sonographically guided enema for intussusception reduction a safer alternative to fluoroscopy. *J Ultrasound Med.* 2012;31(10):1505–1508.

Sargar KM, Siegel MJ. Sonography of acute appendicitis and its mimics in children. *Indian J Radiol Imaging.* 2014;24(2):163.

Sepulveda A, Buchanan EP. Vascular tumors. *Semin Plast Surg.* 2014;28:49–57.

Spector LJ, Birch J. The epidemiology of hepatoblastoma. *Pediatr Blood Cancer.* 2012;59(5):776–779.

Stringer MD, Capps SNJ, Pablot SM. Sonographic detection of the lead point in intussusception. *Arch Dis Child.* 1992;67:529.

Swischuk LE, Stansberry SD. Ultrasonographic detection of free peritoneal fluid in uncomplicated intussusception. *Pediatr Radiol.* 1991;21:350.

Trout AT, Sanchez R, Ladino-Torres MF, et al. A critical evaluation of US for the diagnosis of pediatric acute appendicitis in a real-life setting: how can we improve the diagnostic value of sonography? *Pediatr Radiol.* 2012;42(7):813–823.

Trout AT, Sanchez R, Ladino-torres MF. Reevaluating the sonographic criteria for acute appendicitis in children: a review of the literature and a retrospective analysis of 246 cases. *Acad Radiol.* 2012;19(11):1382–1394.

van Rijn RR, Nievelstein RAJ. Paediatric ultrasonography of the liver, hepatobiliary tract and pancreas. *Eur J Radiol.* 2014;83(9):1570–1581.

Varich L. Ultrasound of pediatric liver masses. *Ultrasound Clin.* 2010;5(1):137–152.

Verschelden P, Filiatrault D, Garel L, et al. Intussusception in children: reliability of US in diagnosis—a prospective study. *Radiology.* 1992;184:741.

Vignault F, Filiatrault D, Brandt ML, et al. Acute appendicitis in children: evaluation with US. *Radiology.* 1990;176:501.

Wiersma F, Srámek A, Holscher HC. US features of the normal appendix and surrounding area in children. *Radiology.* 2005;235(3):1018–1022.

Wilkinson A. The role of ultrasound in the diagnosis and treatment of intussusception in children. *Ultrasound.* 2007;15(2):86–92.

Wilson BG. Chapter 11: Patient Interactions. In: Adler AM, Carlton RR, eds. *Introduction to radiologic and imaging sciences and patient care.* 6th ed: Elsevier; 2016:139.

Zavras N, Dimopoulou A, Machairas N, et al. Infantile hepatic hemangioma: current state of the art, controversies, and perspectives. *Eur J Pediatr.* 2020;179:1–8.

Zave C. Allergies in children. *Paediatr Child Health.* 2001;6(8):555.

CHAPTER 26

Neonatal and Pediatric Adrenal and Urinary System

Kathryn E. Zale

OBJECTIVES

On completion of this chapter, you should be able to:
- Discuss the sonographic approach to imaging neonatal/pediatric kidneys and adrenal glands
- Distinguish normal anatomy and sonographic findings from abnormal findings
- List and discuss the pathologic conditions covered in this chapter

OUTLINE

Examination Preparation 792
Normal Anatomy and Sonographic Findings 792
    Kidneys 792
    Adrenal Glands 794
    Urinary Bladder 794
Contrast Evaluation of the Urinary System 795
Renal, Adrenal, and Bladder Pathology 796
    Congenital Urinary Tract Anomalies 798
Hereditary Renal Cystic Disease 804
Acquired Pathology 805
Malignant Tumors 807

KEY TERMS

Adrenal hemorrhage
Angiomyolipomas
Arcuate artery
Autosomal dominant polycystic kidney disease (ADPKD)
Autosomal recessive polycystic kidney disease (ARPKD)
Congenital mesoblastic nephroma
Cortex
Corticomedullary differentiation

Ectasia
Ectopic ureterocele
Medullary pyramids
Multicystic dysplastic kidney (MCDK)
Nephroblastomatosis
Neuroblastoma
Patent urachus
Polycystic renal disease
Posterior urethral valves (PUVs)
Potter facies

Prune-belly syndrome
Pulmonary hypoplasia
Pyelonephritis
Renal vein thrombosis
Ureteropelvic junction obstruction (UPJ)
Urinary tract dilation (UTD)
VACTERL
Vesicoureteral reflux (VUR)
Wilms tumor (nephroblastoma)

Sonography is the diagnostic imaging method of choice when a renal or an adrenal abnormality is suspected in the neonate or pediatric patient. While there are numerous indications for this examination during the newborn period, an abnormality detected during prenatal sonography (such as **urinary tract dilation [UTD]** or a two-vessel umbilical cord) is common. Other conditions or findings in the newborn associated with renal abnormalities are anuria, oliguria, hematuria, urinary tract infection (UTI) or sepsis, ambiguous external genitalia, and prune-belly syndrome. Skin tags found near the ear and associated cardiac anomalies may also be an indicator. Additionally, a palpable flank mass or abdominal distention may be concerning. Renal masses make up about 70% of abdominal masses in neonates, and nearly all are asymptomatic. Flank masses in neonates may also arise from the adrenal glands, although less often. These conditions usually indicate the renal study is for screening the kidneys with no particular renal symptoms present.

In the older infant and child, indications often include screening for known congenital anomalies or acquired conditions presenting with symptoms, such as flank pain and hematuria.

EXAMINATION PREPARATION

The urinary bladder is considered an important part of the renal sonographic examination, and therefore any child who has bladder control should come to the examination with a full bladder. Full bladder preparation recommendations, along with general aspects of scanning the neonate and pediatric patient, are described in Chapter 25. Keep in mind that maintaining the body temperature is important in the preemie and neonate.

A 10-MHz curved array (slightly more curved than an adult footprint) is ideal for scanning neonates and infants, whereas a 7.5-MHz transducer with a similar footprint can provide excellent visualization in a young or thin child. A 3- to 6-MHz curved array is typical for an older child or adolescent. Additionally, a 9- to 12-MHz linear array will provide better detail resolution when imaging premature infants, scanning from the prone position, or when pathology is suspected.

Scanning is gently initiated over the suprapubic region due to the infant's tendency to urinate spontaneously and a young child's inability to hold the bladder for extended periods. If the urinary bladder is not distended at the time, or if voiding occurs before adequate detail can be obtained, the pelvis can be reexamined after imaging the kidneys and retroperitoneum, documenting the aorta, inferior vena cava, and adrenal glands or area superior to the kidneys. Filling of the urinary bladder is relatively rapid if the infant is fed or parenteral fluids are being administered. A pre-void bladder volume and bladder wall thickness measurement should be obtained with a full bladder.

Next, longitudinal and transverse views of the kidneys are documented in the supine or decubitus position. Renal measurements and volumes should be obtained, as well as documentation of the renal echogenicity compared with the liver and spleen. In the infant and young child (or when feasible), dedicated renal views are obtained by scanning the patient's back from the prone position with a linear transducer. It should be noted the renal length may be slightly shorter from this position, and prone-dependent renal dilation may occur.

In the toilet-trained or older child, the patient is then instructed to urinate fully. The bladder is reexamined in longitudinal and transverse views, including a post-void bladder volume and bladder wall measurement.

In the setting of urinary tract dilation (UTD), an anterior-posterior measurement of any dilated renal pelvis or ureter should be obtained. Furthermore, supine renal scanning before and after the infant or child voids can provide useful information. When imaging an infant or a child who needs to urinate before instructed to do so, it is ideal to document the kidneys while the bladder is still full. One sagittal and one mid-pole transverse image will often suffice to detect fluid in the kidneys. Likewise, similar post-void images of the kidneys should be obtained in an older child if any UTD was seen throughout the examination.

NORMAL ANATOMY AND SONOGRAPHIC FINDINGS

Kidneys

The sonographic appearance of the kidneys varies, depending on the age of the child. This is especially apparent in the young infant. Keep in mind, premature infants are adjusted to their gestational age until they are 2 years old. (For example, a 5-month-old, born 2 months early, would be evaluated as a 3-month-old.) In the second trimester, the kidneys grow from small renunculi that are composed of a central large pyramid, with a thin peripheral rim of the cortex. As these renunculi fuse progressively, their adjoining cortices form the columns of Bertin. The former renunculi are then called *lobes*. Remnants of these lobes, with somewhat incomplete fusion, are termed *fetal* or *renal lobulation* and should not be confused with renal abnormalities or scars. Renal lobulation is most prominent at birth and in the neonatal period, often disappearing completely by 6 years of age. Even after birth, the pyramids remain large compared to the thin rim of the cortex that surrounds them. The glomerular filtration rate is low right after birth but increases rapidly thereafter. The cortex continues to grow throughout childhood, whereas the pyramids become smaller. The sinus fat often seen in adults is not present in the neonate and is rarely observed in the pediatric patient.

The normal kidney in the neonate and infant is characterized by a distinct demarcation of the cortex and medullary pyramids, or **corticomedullary differentiation**, owing to a larger medullary volume. The **medullary pyramids** are prominent and hypoechoic and should not be mistaken for dilated calyces or cysts. They are typically less prominent by 1 year of age. The surrounding **cortex** is quite thin at birth, and echogenicity varies by age.

Premature infants tend to have more echogenic kidneys, owing to underdevelopment of the renal structures. Echogenicity in the full-term neonate may be similar to, or slightly greater than, the normal liver and splenic parenchyma. This increased cortical echogenicity is only seen in the neonatal period, up to 1 month of age (Fig. 26.1). Renal cortical echogenicity normally decreases to less than the liver parenchyma by 4 to 6 months.

The increased cortical echogenicity may result from the glomeruli occupying a larger proportion of cortical volume and the location of the loops of Henle within the cortex (20% versus 9% in adults) as opposed to within the medulla. Due to a paucity of fat in the renal sinus of the neonate and infant, this area is generally hypoechoic and therefore indistinct.

The sonographic renal anatomy in children and adolescents is similar to an adult. The normal cortex is thick and produces low-level, back-scattered echoes. The medullary pyramids are relatively hypoechoic and arranged around the central, echo-producing renal sinus (Fig. 26.2).

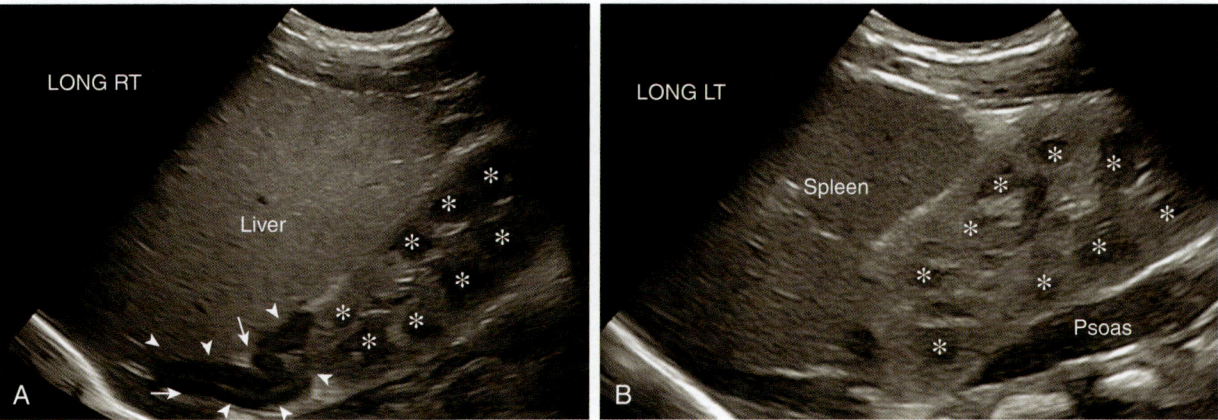

FIG. 26.1 **Normal kidneys in a full-term neonate.** The medullary pyramids *(asterisks)* appear as triangular hypoechoic areas. (A) Longitudinal supine view of the normal right kidney (isoechoic compared with the liver parenchyma). Normal adrenal gland is also visualized *(arrows)*. (B) Longitudinal supine view of the normal left kidney (hyperechoic compared to the spleen). Adrenal gland is not visualized. (Courtesy Nationwide Children's Hospital, Columbus, OH.)

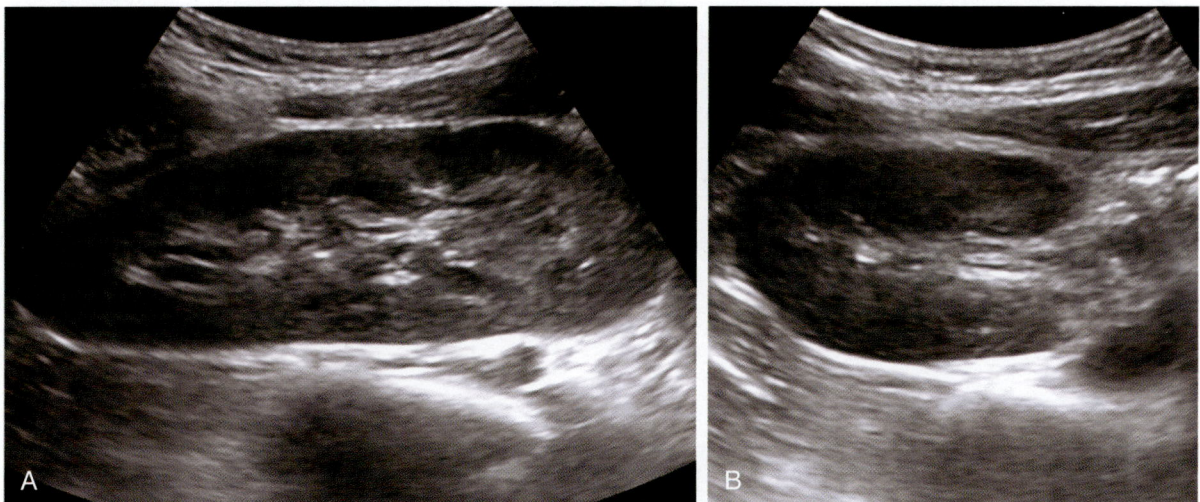

FIG. 26.2 **Normal kidney in an adolescent.** (A) Mid-longitudinal view of a normal right kidney in a 15-year-old. The sonographic renal anatomy is similar to an adult with a thick cortex. The medullary pyramids are relatively hypoechoic, arranged around the central, echogenic renal sinus. (B) Mid-transverse view of the same right kidney. (Images courtesy Chester County Hospital, West Chester, PA.)

The **arcuate artery** vessels may be seen as intense specular echoes at the corticomedullary junction. Color Doppler is often used to document the renal artery and vein in the pediatric renal examination and is best taken in a mid-transverse view. This also aids in differentiating a prominent vein from dilation in the renal pelvis.

Pulsed Doppler can detect cases of renal vein thrombosis, hypertension, or other suspected vascular diseases. A dedicated renal duplex examination reports the direct methods of the peak systolic velocities of the renal artery and aorta. The peak systolic velocity of the renal artery should be less than 180 cm/sec, and the RAR (renal artery and abdominal aorta ratio) less than 3.5:1. Indirect methods include sampling the segmental, or arcuate arteries, and measuring the resistive index (RI) and acceleration time (same criteria as in adults, less than 70 msec) in the superior, mid, and inferior poles. The normal RI value varies greatly within the first year: preterm infant, up to 0.9; neonate, 0.6 to 0.8; and by the end of the first year show values similar to those found in adults, 0.5 to 0.7. It is important to keep in mind that cardiac disease, coarctation of the aorta, and patent ductus arteriosus may also affect the RI.

The normal renal length varies with the age of the neonate or pediatric patient (Fig. 26.3). Accurate and consistent measurements are important to document normal growth and to help detect abnormalities. Although the left kidney is often somewhat longer, a kidney measurement greater than 1 cm side to side should be monitored closely; and may indicate infection, scarring, or congenital abnormalities, such as hypotrophy or a duplex collecting system.

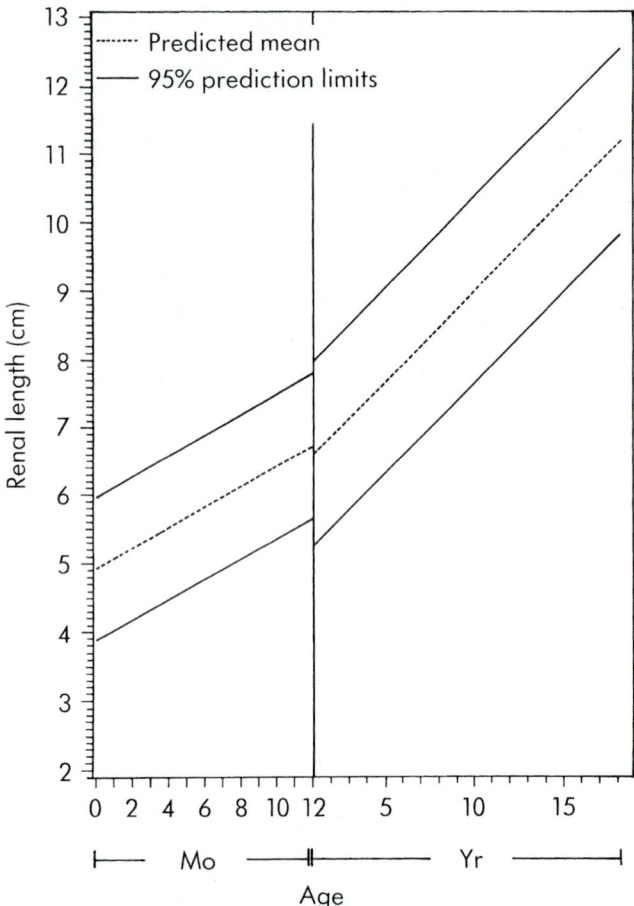

FIG. 26.3 Normal renal length versus age.

Adrenal Glands

The normal adrenal glands are larger and more easily identified in the neonate than in the older infant or young child. In fact, the prominent size of the adrenal gland at birth will normally decrease rapidly within the first 10 days and then slowly atrophy over the next few weeks. At 1 year of age, it takes on the appearance of an adult adrenal gland. Each gland lies immediately superior to the upper pole of the kidney. The left adrenal gland extends slightly more medial than the right. The gland has an inverted V or Y shape in the longitudinal plane (Fig. 26.4). In the transverse plane, the portion of the gland delineated has a linear or curvilinear outline. When the kidney is absent or ectopic, the ipsilateral adrenal gland remains in the renal fossa, but as a result, it may have an altered elongated "lying down" configuration. Sonographically, the central adrenal medulla in the neonate is relatively thin, appearing as a distinctly echogenic stripe, surrounded by the more prominent and less echogenic adrenal cortex (Fig. 26.5).

Urinary Bladder

The normal urinary bladder is thin-walled in the distended state and should measure less than 3 mm (mean, 1.5 mm) in the anterior-posterior (AP) dimension. When empty, the wall thickness increases but remains less than 5 mm. In pediatrics, the anterior bladder wall may be difficult to accurately measure due to excessive ring-down artifact and the prominent urachal remnant sometimes seen in children. Therefore, the posterior

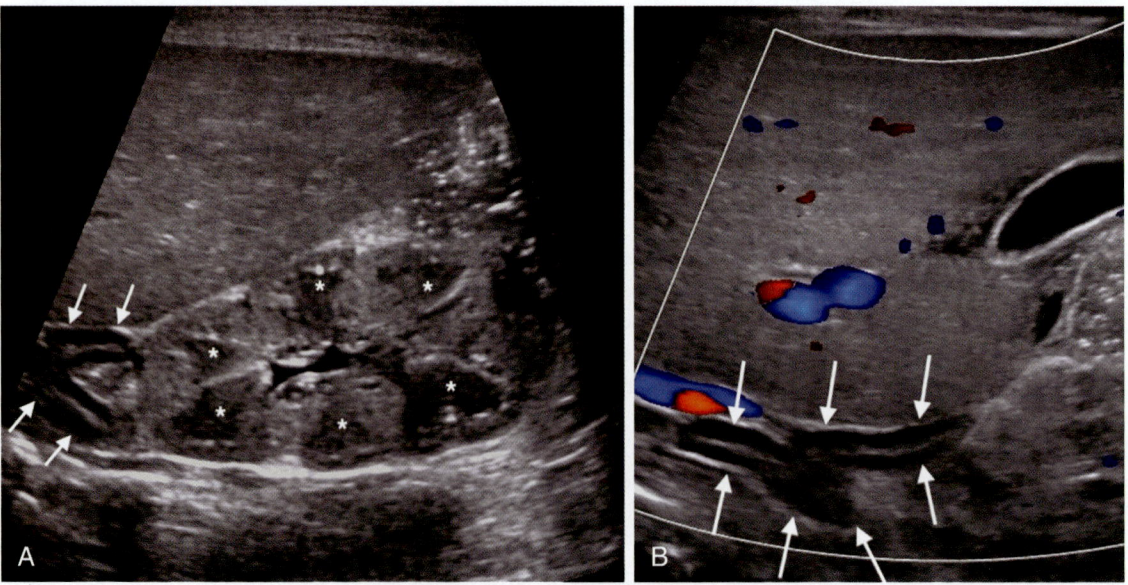

FIG. 26.4 Normal sagittal neonatal adrenal gland and kidney. (A) Sagittal view of a normal adrenal gland *(arrows)* and kidney in a 1-day-old infant. The adrenal gland has an inverted-V configuration at the level of the kidney. Kidney has fetal lobulation appearance with hypoechoic renal pyramids *(asterisks)*. (B) Sagittal view of the same normal adrenal gland *(arrows)* taken at the level above the kidney and appears as an inverted-Y. Color Doppler reveals no detectable flow within the normal adrenal gland. (Courtesy Chester County Hospital, West Chester, PA.)

bladder wall is measured, and the posterolateral wall has been suggested to avoid the thickened posterior region of the trigone, which has different characteristics than the detrusor muscle. The bladder should normally empty completely or at least 90% of the bladder capacity. An exception is made for infants, as they often retain urine in their bladder (Fig. 26.6). Visualization of the bladder also includes the assessment for distal ureteral dilation. Color Doppler aids in depicting the normal distal ureteral jets as they enter the posterior wall of the bladder.

Contrast Evaluation of the Urinary System

The use of contrast in the pediatric population has elevated the role of sonography from a screening examination to a critical tool in disease diagnosis and monitoring. *Contrast-enhanced ultrasound* (CEUS) detects blood perfusion abnormalities in real-time with the use of intravascular microbubble agents. Due to different vascularization patterns of benign and malignant lesions, tumors may be evaluated with CEUS to exclude malignancy, with immediate results. This obviates the need for further testing and reduces stress for both parents and children alike. Furthermore, if a biopsy is found to be necessary, CEUS can detect areas of viable tumor versus areas of necrosis, reducing false-negative results.

Contrast-enhanced voiding urosonography (ceVUS) administers these same microbubble agents via a urinary catheter to sonographically evaluate for vesicoureteral reflux. The higher

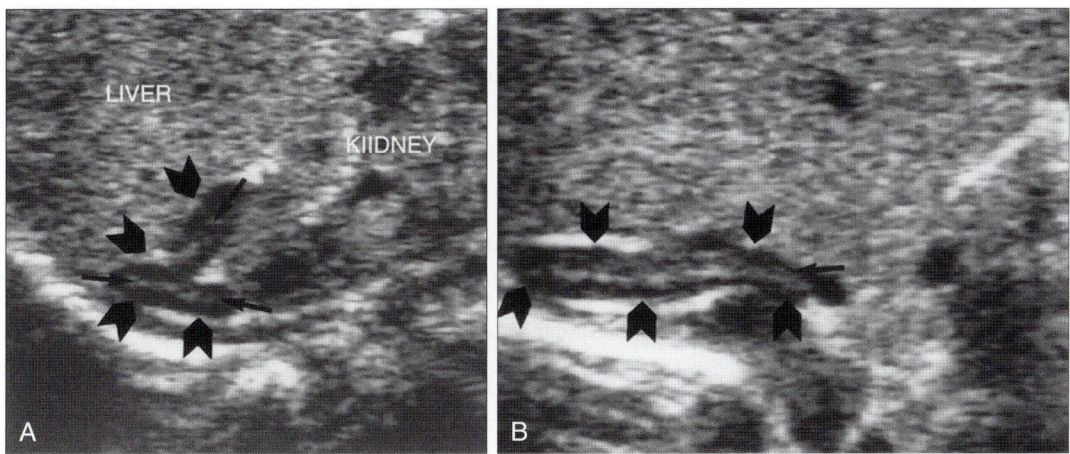

FIG. 26.5 Normal adrenal gland. (A) Longitudinal view of a normal adrenal gland *(arrowheads)* in a 1-day-old infant with ambiguous genitalia. The adrenal medulla *(arrows)* appears as a central echogenic stripe, surrounded by the hypoechoic cortex. The adrenal gland has an inverted-Y configuration. (B) Transverse view through a portion of a normal adrenal gland *(arrowheads)* demonstrating the curvilinear shape in this plane.

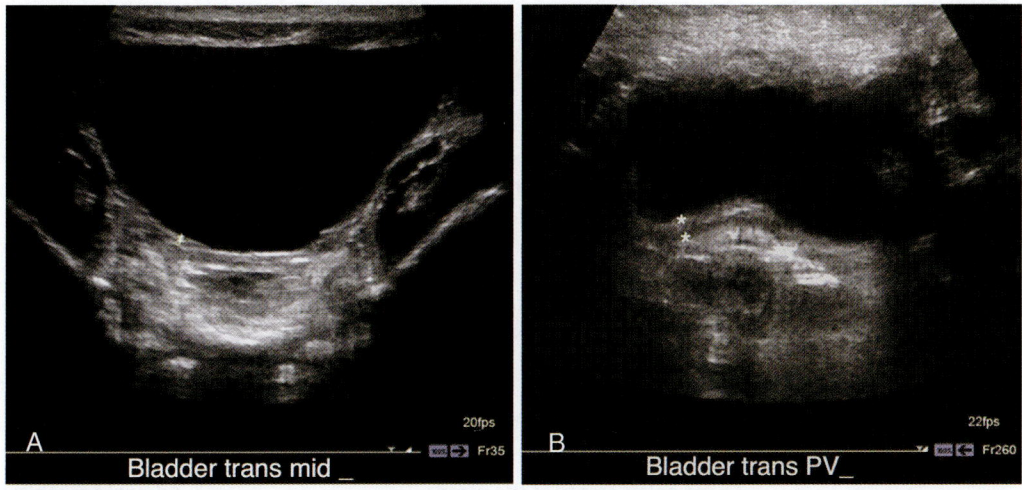

FIG. 26.6 Normal bladder. (A) Normal mid-transverse view of the bladder in a 1-day-old infant. Pre-void bladder wall measurement *(asterisks* posteriorly) was 0.7 mm. The urinary bladder is well distended, appearing anechoic with a thin bladder wall. (B) Post-void bladder wall measurement *(asterisks)* is also normal at 2.2 mm. Post-void fluid retention in the bladder is typical during the neonatal period. (Courtesy Nationwide Children's Hospital, Columbus, OH.)

sensitivity of ceVUS, coupled with a detailed evaluation of the urethra, provides a safe and radiation-free alternative to the voiding cystourethrogram (Fig. 26.7).

RENAL, ADRENAL, AND BLADDER PATHOLOGY

Congenital anomalies, hereditary renal cystic disease, acquired pathologies, and malignant tumors of the neonatal and pediatric urinary tract and adrenals are presented here. Although discussed separately, it should be understood congenital or genetic abnormalities might contribute to an increased risk of acquired or malignant processes.

The pathologies discussed, underlying benign renal and adrenal enlargement, are summarized in Table 26.1, while malignant tumor findings are provided in Table 26.2. Furthermore, abnormalities in the urinary tract can often be related to abnormalities of the reproductive system, hence the genitourinary system. When renal abnormalities are detected, a pelvic ultrasound exam may be subsequently ordered, and keeping the bladder full may be prudent (Fig. 26.8).

TABLE 26.1 Most Common Benign Retroperitoneal Findings

Clinical Findings	Sonographic Findings	Differential Considerations
UTD (Hydronephrosis)		
Flank pain	Dilation of the renal pelvis Dilation of the central calyces (and possibly with the peripheral calyces) Ureter is dilated when vesicoureteral reflux or primary megaureter is present	Parapelvic cyst Extrarenal sinus Congenital megacystis Multiple renal cysts Multicystic renal disease Functional dilation Duplex collecting system
Duplex Collecting System (With Ectopic Ureterocele)		
Recurrent urinary tract infection	Enlarged kidney unilaterally (often left side) Fluid within the superior pole of the kidney Dilated ureter Ballooning or pouch of the ureterocele in bladder inferior to normal ureter	Renal cyst in superior pole with vesicoureteral obstruction due to a ureterocele
Posterior Urethral Valves		
Decreased urine output	Enlarged bladder with a thickened bladder wall May see thickened valves in the urethra Bilateral UTD Dilated ureters	Pelvic mass or tumor Bilateral megaureters
Multicystic Dysplastic Kidney		
	Unilateral multicystic mass in kidney Contralateral ureteropelvic junction	UTD
Autosomal Recessive Polycystic Renal Disease		
Pulmonary hypoplasia Potter facies	Enlarged kidneys Echogenic kidneys	
Prune-Belly Syndrome		
Absence of abdominal muscle Undescended testes Dilated bladder, ureter, prostatic urethra	Kidney is normal, dilated, or dysplastic Dysplastic enlarged kidneys Dilated ureters Dilated bladder	Posterior urethral valves
Congenital Mesoblastic Nephroma		
Found in children <1 year of age	Hyperechoic or hypoechoic or mixed	Adrenal tumor Neuroblastoma Benign renal tumor Abscess
Adrenal Hemorrhage		
Abdominal mass Jaundice Anemia	Ovoid enlargement of the gland Anechoic to hyperechoic No detection of blood flow within the mass using color or power Doppler	Adrenal neuroblastoma Adrenal cyst Adrenal neoplasm

UTD, Urinary tract dilation.

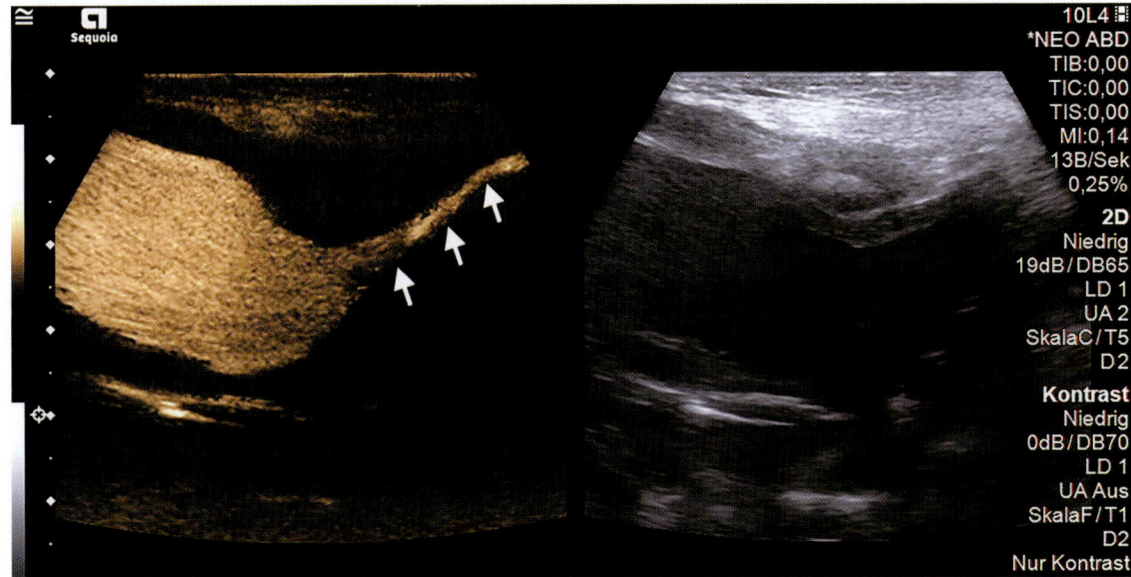

FIG. 26.7 Contrast-enhanced voiding urosonography. Evaluation with contrast-enhanced voiding urosonography depicting a normal neonatal urethra *(arrows)*, captured while the infant voided. Dual-screen image simultaneously captures microbubble contrast agents filling urinary tract *(left)* and standard grayscale sonogram *(right)*. (Courtesy Siemens Healthineers USA, Inc.)

TABLE 26.2	Most Common Malignant Retroperitoneal Findings	
Clinical Findings	**Sonographic Findings**	**Differential Considerations**
Neuroblastoma		
Nystagmus Unsteady gait	Mass usually in the adrenal gland Echogenic Calcification Look for metastasis to the liver	Adrenal hemorrhage Benign renal tumor Abscess
Wilms Tumor		
Hypertension Palpable abdominal or flank mass Weight loss, fever, anemia, pain	Complex mass in the kidney Well-circumscribed mass Isoechoic to echogenic May have calcification Look for tumor extension into the renal vein or inferior vena cava	Mesoblastic nephroma Renal cell carcinoma Retroperitoneal sarcoma Adrenal cortical carcinoma Multicystic renal hamartoma

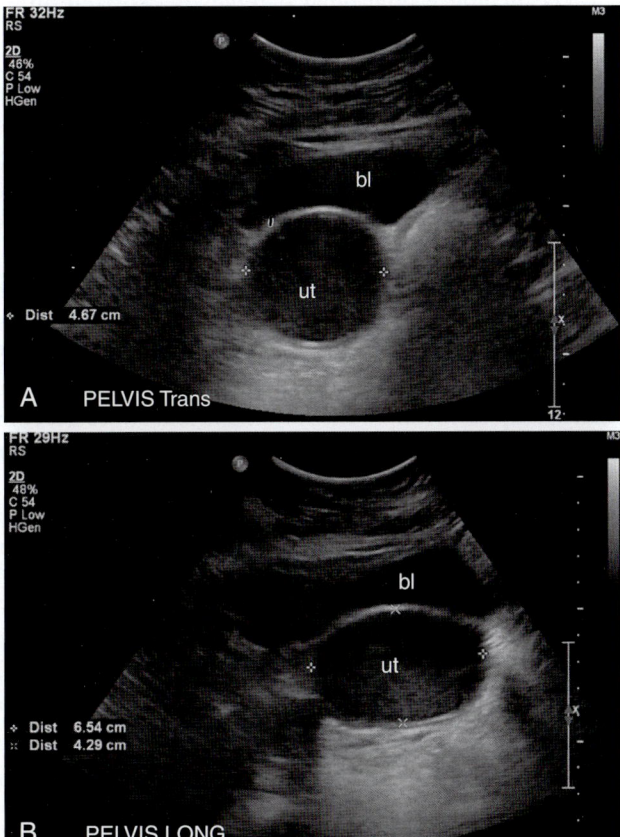

FIG. 26.8 Genitourinary pathology. A 12-year-old girl with a history of caudal regression, neurogenic bladder, and left solitary kidney. Renal sonography incidentally detected uterine hematocolpos/hydrocolpos (likely hematocolpos). This was confirmed with magnetic resonance imaging, which showed duplicated uteri with fluid in the right uterus filled with blood/fluid. (A) Transverse image of the pelvis shows the urinary bladder (bl) and right uterus (ut) posterior. (B) Longitudinal view. (Courtesy Nationwide Children's Hospital, Columbus, OH.)

Congenital Urinary Tract Anomalies

Pediatric sonography plays a vital role in the detection of congenital urinary tract anomalies, which account for half of all congenital anomalies and occur in 3% to 11% of the general population. These anomalies may be isolated, exist in tandem, or occur as part of the **VACTERL** association (vertebral defects, anal atresia, cardiac defects, tracheoesophageal fistula, renal anomalies, and limb abnormalities). Abnormalities of the collecting system are the most common and are the primary focus of this section. The multicystic dysplastic kidney, crossed-fused renal ectopia, and patent urachus are presented here. The reader is referred to Chapter 15 for further discussion on other anomalies that may be encountered, such as abnormal renal number (renal agenesis and supernumerary kidney) and anomalies related to renal position (ectopic kidney) and renal form (horseshoe kidney).

Urinary Tract Dilation. Dilation of the urinary tract has many causes, and sonography allows for the detection and differentiation of the many possible underlying conditions. UTD, also known as hydronephrosis, describes the dilation of the urinary collecting system. It is also the most common cause of a palpable mass in the neonate, accounting for 50% of congenital malformations. The most common causes of UTD are obstruction, reflux, or abnormal muscle development. Since the urine is made in the kidneys, dilation will occur proximal to any obstruction. Sonography is sensitive in detecting small amounts of fluid in the renal pelvis. The sonographer is able to determine the severity of the UTD, whether the condition is unilateral or bilateral, if the ureters and bladder are dilated, and the status of the renal parenchyma.

Sonographic Findings. Sonographic features found in UTD include visible renal parenchyma surrounding a central cystic component, small peripheral cysts (dilated calyces) budding off a large central cyst (renal pelvis), and visualization of a dilated ureter. Renal dilation must be distinguished from the noncommunicating cysts of multicystic dysplastic kidneys.

Urinary Tract Dilation Classification. Commonly referred to as hydronephrosis, the degree of dilation within the urinary tract has not been uniformly classified over the years. Classification systems include the Society for Fetal Urology grading system (SFU grades I-IV), the radiology grading system (RAD I-V), as well as the updated Onen system (ONEN grades I-IV). In each of these systems, a renal pelvis dilation is normal up to 10 mm in the AP dimension. However, common terminology and classification were needed to define abnormal dilation.

Recently, a multidisciplinary consensus on terminology and classification for UTD was created to unify the prenatal and postnatal language around urinary tract findings. Previously, various terms for UTD were nonspecific and had only implied meanings; common terms relating to UTD include *hydronephrosis, pyelectasis, pelviectasis,* and *pelvic fullness*. Additionally, calyceal descriptors, such as the term *major calyces* to describe the centrally located calyces and the term *minor calyces* used to describe the peripherally located calyces, should also be avoided. The use of these more confusing terms is discouraged, and UTD is preferred. However, while the UTD terminology is being adopted, the use of the term *urinary tract dilation* (UTD) is used in place of the word *hydronephrosis* throughout this text.

Unified language around this prevalent pathology will allow for clearer communication among clinicians and improve research outcomes. The full postnatal UTD classification system is provided in Table 26.3. The system uses six ultrasound findings to classify and describe both antenatal and postnatal UTD. Both prenatal and antenatal classifications include *normal, UTD 1, UTD 2,* and *UTD 3*. The postnatal findings would be termed *UTD P1*, whereas the antenatal equivalent would be termed *UTD A1*. The antenatal findings are used after 16 weeks gestation, while the first postnatal evaluation should occur 48 hours after birth. The diagnosis is more severe as the number increases, with UTD 3 being the most critical. The UTD classification system is based on the following criteria:

1. Measurement of the greatest AP distention within the dilated renal pelvis (intrarenal) in the transverse view. It is recommended this measurement be taken with the patient in the *prone position*. It is called the AP renal pelvic diameter (Fig. 26.9)
2. Involvement of calyceal dilation (the distinction between central and peripheral calyces is only made postnatally)
3. Renal parenchyma thickness
4. Appearance of the renal parenchyma
5. Abnormalities of the bladder
6. Abnormalities of the ureter

Although this system has slowly been adopted, the extent of this adoption remains unclear. However, in a small survey via the SFU, roughly 70% of pediatric urologists were still using the SFU grading system and 19% were now using the UTD system.

TABLE 26.3	Urinary Tract Dilation Postnatal Classification System[a]			
	Normal	UTD P1	UTD P2	UTD P3
APRPD (anterior-posterior renal pelvic diameter)	<10 mm	≥10–15 mm	≥15 mm	≥10 mm
Dilation of the calyces	None	Central only	Peripheral	N/A
Parenchymal thickness	N	N	N	A
Parenchymal appearance	N	N	N	A
Ureters	N	N	A	N/A
Bladder	N	N	N	A

[a]Valid 48 hours after birth.
A, Abnormal; *N,* normal; *N/A,* not applicable (or irrelevant due to the severe loss of papillary impressions and parenchymal disease already present); *P,* postnatal; *UTD,* urinary tract dilation.
Modified from Chow JS, Koning JL, Back SJ, et al. Classification of pediatric urinary tract dilation: the new language. *Pediatr Radiol.* 2017;47(9):1109–1115.

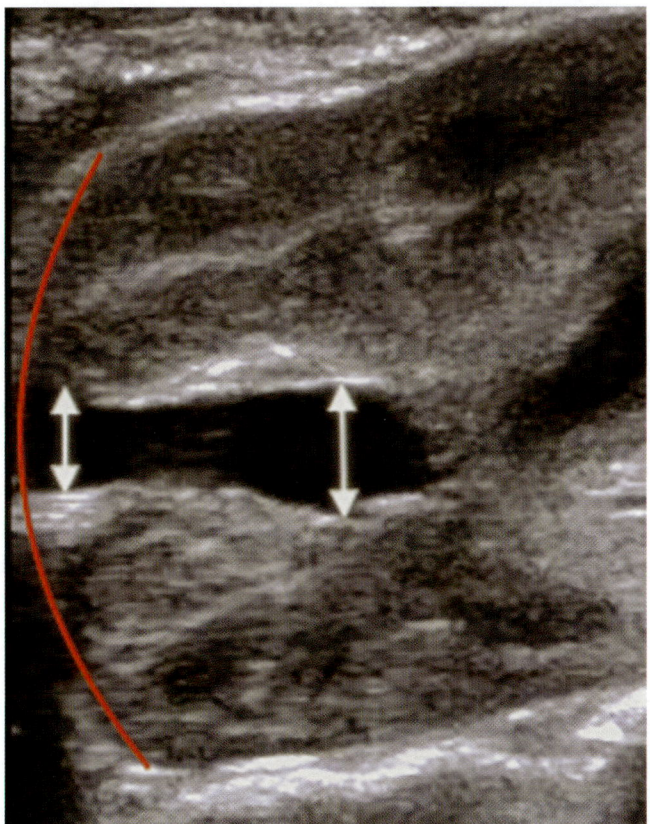

FIG. 26.9 **Anterior-posterior renal pelvic diameter.** Transverse view of the kidney provides two examples *(arrows)* of ways to properly measure the renal pelvis for dilation. The larger measurement should be recorded (here it is the longer *double arrow at right*) and may be taken anywhere within the pelvis but should not extend outside the kidney where there is no surrounding parenchyma. The *red line* outlines the renal parenchyma, and measurements should not be obtained beyond it. (Courtesy Chester County Hospital, West Chester, PA.)

However, 54% of the respondents stated they preferred the SFU system for a unified classification, while 34% favored the UTD system. It is unknown how much these preferences extend to pediatric radiology, whose societies proposed the UTD classification. Furthermore, inter-rater reliability was substantial with the UTD system and moderate with the SFU system. Another small study to compare the fetal renal dilation between the SFU and UTD studies also found a higher inter-rater reliability among the UTD classification system.

More research and validity of the UTD system will likely be necessary for furthering its adoption. Regardless of the system utilized, the features presented in this classification are reported and may be used to describe UTD and the various causes listed below.

Vesicoureteral Reflux. **Vesicoureteral reflux (VUR)** is a common nonobstructive cause of UTD and is indicated in up to 33% of prenatally diagnosed UTD. VUR is the abnormal refluxing of urine from the urinary bladder through the ureters back into the kidney.

It is often treated conservatively because it is nonobstructive. In severe cases, a shunt from the kidney to the bladder may need to be placed. Many cases, often males, and an appreciable number of moderate UTDs, resolve on their own within the first 2 years of life. Unilateral or bilateral UTD may occur, and different sides may have different reflux levels (i.e., severity of UTD). Although ultrasound can often detect the higher levels of VUR, it may be helpful to detect lower grades by using both pre-void and post-void renal imaging. Additionally, waiting 48 hours to perform a postnatal ultrasound is recommended, as low urine output is typical at birth. It is definitively diagnosed by a voiding cystourethrogram or ceVUS.

Sonographic Findings. Sonographic findings for VUR are often nonspecific and may or may not include UTD, renal pelvic or ureteral wall thickening (also termed urothelial or uroepithelial thickening, which is due to irritation of the epithelial lining), intermittent dilation of the collecting system, or displaced ureteral jet in the bladder.

Ureteral Dilation (Megaureter). Dilation of the ureter may be seen in vesicoureteral reflux and may also be caused by nonobstructive primary megaureter or obstruction (causing megaureter). Nonobstructive primary megaureter implies a congenitally expanded or widened ureter, which does not function normally, resulting in reflux from the bladder back into the affected ureter.

In obstructive primary megaureter, the ureter may be congenitally constricted anywhere along its course or, most commonly, at the ureterovesical junction causing renal dilation. In secondary megaureter, the ureter is obstructed in the more distal urinary tract, bladder, or urethra. Also, a secondary process such as abscess, previous surgery (e.g., for appendicitis), lymphoma, and urolithiasis may cause obstruction to the ureter. Ureteral atresia or an ectopic ureter may be the underlying cause as well.

Sonographic Findings. With megaureter, sonography shows UTD involving the ureters and the kidneys. A small segment of the distal ureter is seen behind the bladder. The best way to demonstrate the dilated ureters at the vesicoureteral (bladder/ureter) junction is in the longitudinal scan plane (Fig. 26.10).

The increased peristalsis in the ureter distal to the obstruction may be seen with sonography as the probe is held over the dilated ureter, and the sonographer watches for the peristaltic movement. M-mode may enable a semi-quantified assessment of this ureteral peristalsis. A diminished ureteral inflow jet may be seen at the lower margin of the bladder with color Doppler on the side of the obstruction.

Ureteropelvic Junction Obstruction. **Ureteropelvic junction (UPJ) obstruction** is the most common type of obstruction causing UTD of the upper urinary tract and occurs in 1 in 2000 children with a male prevalence (3:1), accounting for about 10% of prenatally diagnosed UTD. It most often results from intrinsic narrowing or extrinsic vascular compression at the level of the ureteropelvic junction. The obstruction produces proximal dilation of the collecting system, and the distal ureter is often normal in size. There is an increased incidence of abnormalities of the contralateral kidney, such as multicystic dysplastic kidney or vesicoureteral reflux.

Sonographic Findings. Sonographically, there is pelvocaliectasis (dilation of both the renal pelvis and calyces). When the obstruction is pronounced, the dilated renal pelvis extends inferiorly and medially outside the renal parenchyma, forming an extrarenal pelvis. Normally, it presents without ureteral dilation (Fig. 26.11). However, in the setting of vesicoureteral reflux or primary megaureter, the ureter may also be dilated.

Duplex Collecting System (With Ectopic Ureterocele). The duplex collecting system may frequently be encountered, as it is the most common congenital ureteral anomaly. It may be also be referred to as a duplex or "double" kidney. It occurs more often in girls and is common enough in children to be considered a normal variant. The kidney of one side, more commonly the left, has a duplicated collecting system. If completely duplicated, two ureters are present on one side, and the duplicated ureter that drains the upper pole of the kidney inserts into the bladder ectopically. As a result, the upper moiety of a completely duplicated renal collecting system often shows a little dilation of fluid. This fluid in the superior pole often diminishes with urination.

Usually, the duplex collecting system does not cause any issues; however, it may have a role in recurrent urinary tract infections (UTIs) due to urinary tract dilation and vesicoureteral reflux from the ectopic ureter. It may also present with a cystic dilation of the distal ureter, called an ectopic ureterocele. This ballooning into the bladder may cause too much fluid to be backed up into the kidney, and surgery is often required. A duplex collecting system is one of the most common causes of a ureterocele in children (Fig. 26.12).

Sonographic Findings. The first indication of a duplicated collecting system may simply be that it measures more than 1 cm longer than the contralateral kidney. Fluid is often detected in the superior pole of the longer kidney. The ectopic ureterocele is seen as a fluid mass within the urinary bladder, often located inferomedial to the ureteral insertion of the normal lower pole ureter. Low-level echoes may be seen in the ureter and ureterocele, representing debris. Postoperatively, following the incision of the ureterocele, the structure may be seen in a collapsed state. The sonographic delineation of an upper pole fluid mass, in continuity with a dilated ureter and the aforementioned ureterocele, is diagnostic of this entity. Distention and effacement or contraction of the ureterocele may be evident during the real-time study (Fig. 26.13).

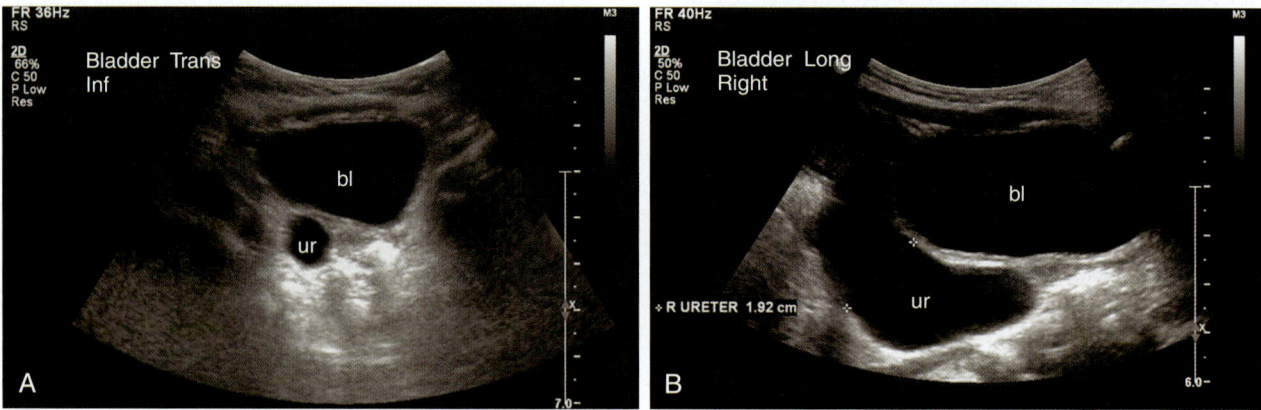

FIG. 26.10 Dilation of the ureter (megaureter). (A) Transverse image of the pelvis in a 28-day-old infant with severe diffuse right dilated ureter with primary refluxing megaureter suspected. The urinary bladder (bl) is well distended. Dilation of the distal right ureter (ur) is seen posterior to the bladder in cross-section. (B) Longitudinal view shows the distal ureter measuring nearly 2 cm. (Courtesy Nationwide Children's Hospital, Columbus, OH.)

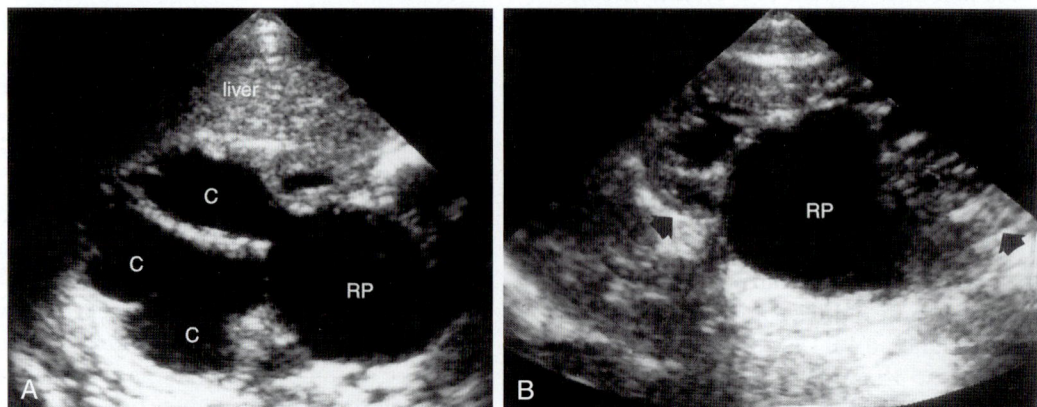

FIG. 26.11 Ureteropelvic junction obstruction. (A) Ureteropelvic junction obstruction in a 2-week-old girl with an abnormal prenatal ultrasound. Marked dilation of the renal pelvis (RP) and calyces (C) is present on this transverse view. Parenchymal loss is also noted. The distal ureter was not identified. Radionuclide imaging confirmed the diagnosis. (B) Uteropelvic junction obstruction in a 1-day-old infant. Longitudinal image of the kidney (arrows) identifies marked dilation of the renal pelvis (RP).

CHAPTER 26 Neonatal and Pediatric Adrenal and Urinary System

Posterior Urethral Valves. Bilateral UTD may be caused by bilateral vesicoureteral reflux but is frequently caused by obstruction at the level of the bladder or bladder outlet. The bladder may be obstructed by a neurogenic bladder, a pelvic mass, or a congenital anomaly. A pelvic mass or tumor may also cause the bladder to be distended with a thickened wall.

Congenital anomalies causing bladder outlet obstructions include posterior urethral valves and prune-belly syndrome. **Posterior urethral valves (PUVs)** are the most common congenital cause of bladder outlet obstruction in the male neonate and are due to excessive flaps of tissue in the posterior urethra only found in males. On the other hand, **prune-belly syndrome** (or abdominal muscle deficiency syndrome) is a rare congenital anomaly of unknown etiology, affecting males in 96% of cases, with severe cases resulting in early infant death from pulmonary hypoplasia (due to related oligohydramnios in utero). It includes a triad of hypoplasia or deficiency of the abdominal musculature, cryptorchidism, and urinary tract anomalies. This anomaly includes congenital absence or deficiency of the abdominal musculature, large hypotonic dilated tortuous ureters, a large bladder, a patent urachus, bilateral cryptorchidism, and a dilated prostatic urethra. Eighty-five

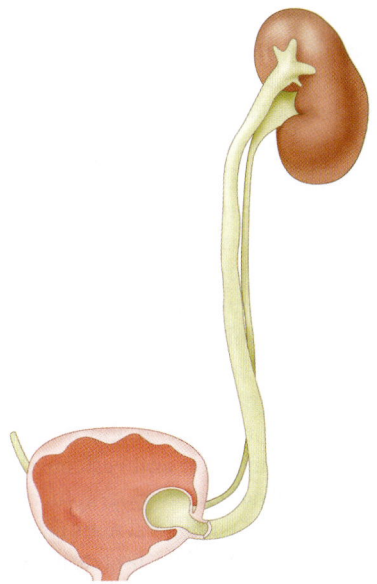

FIG. 26.12 **Duplex collecting system with ectopic ureterocele.** The obstructed ureter, associated with the superior pelvis of the duplicated collecting system, inserts ectopically into a ureterocele, resulting in dilation of the superior pole.

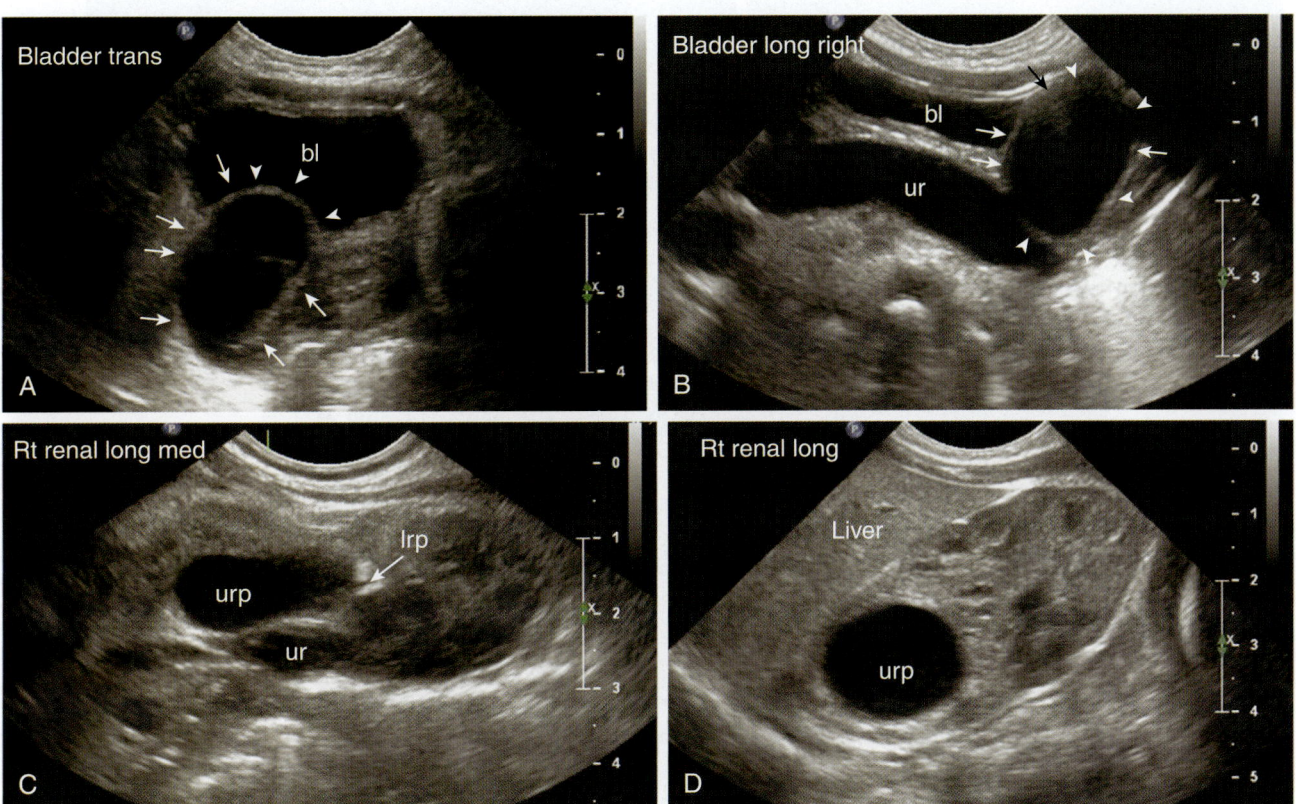

FIG. 26.13 **Duplex collecting system with ectopic ureterocele in a neonate.** A 13-day-old girl with possible right-sided renal urinary tract dilation on prenatal sonogram was referred for a renal ultrasound. A complete duplication of the right collecting system with a dilated upper pole and ureter (measuring 1 cm) was seen along the entire course to an inferior ectopic insertion into the bladder terminating in a ureterocele. Bladder wall thickness and left kidney were normal. (A) Transverse image of the urinary bladder (bl). A large, thin-walled ureterocele *(arrows)* is seen in the right posterior aspect of the bladder. (B) Longitudinal view of the bladder shows the dilated ureter (ur) and ureterocele *(arrows)*. (C) Longitudinal prone view of the medial aspect of the kidney demonstrates a duplex collecting system with notable dilation of the upper renal pelvis (urp) and no dilation of the lower renal pelvis (lrp). The ureter from the upper pole segment (ur) is seen posterior to the kidney. (D) Dilated upper renal pole (urp) and isoechoic renal parenchyma compared with the liver, as seen from a right supine longitudinal view. (Courtesy Nationwide Children's Hospital, Columbus, OH.)

percent of patients with prune-belly syndrome will have associated VUR. Physically, the wrinkled, prune-like abdomen aids in the clinical diagnosis.

Sonographic Findings. The wall of the urinary bladder appears thickened and trabeculated with PUVs. Midline sagittal imaging with caudal angulation through the bladder may allow visualization of the distended posterior urethra. Alternatively, the posterior urethra can be imaged directly from a perineal approach. The resultant UTD of the kidneys and ureters is usually bilateral. Urinary ascites or a perirenal urinoma can result from high-pressure VUR, rupturing a calyceal fornix, or tearing the renal parenchyma. The perirenal urinoma is usually anechoic, but septations may be noted (Fig. 26.14). Other potential causes of perirenal urine extravasation include trauma, ureteropelvic junction obstruction, ureterovesical junction obstruction, and pelvic masses that obstruct the bladder or ureter.

Multicystic Dysplastic Kidney. Multicystic dysplastic kidney (MCDK) is the most common cause of renal cystic disease in the neonate, with an incidence of 1 in 4300 live births. When UTD is excluded, it is the most common cause of an abdominal mass in the newborn. The MCDK is a congenital, usually sporadic, renal dysplasia, which is thought to be secondary to severe, generalized interference with ureteral bud function during the first trimester. The malformation results from ureteral obstruction. High ureteral atresia and pelvicocalyceal occlusion are almost always present.

In utero, the obstruction interferes with ureteral bud division and inhibits the maturation of nephrons in the kidney. Thus, the collecting tubules enlarge, becoming cystic and grossly distorting the shape of the kidney. The remaining renal parenchyma becomes virtually nonfunctioning. Nearly half of the cases have contralateral abnormalities (e.g., ureteropelvic junction obstruction and vesicoureteral reflux).

Sonographic Findings. Sonographically, the classic appearance of MCDK is of a unilateral mass resembling a cluster of grapes, which represents multiple discrete noncommunicating

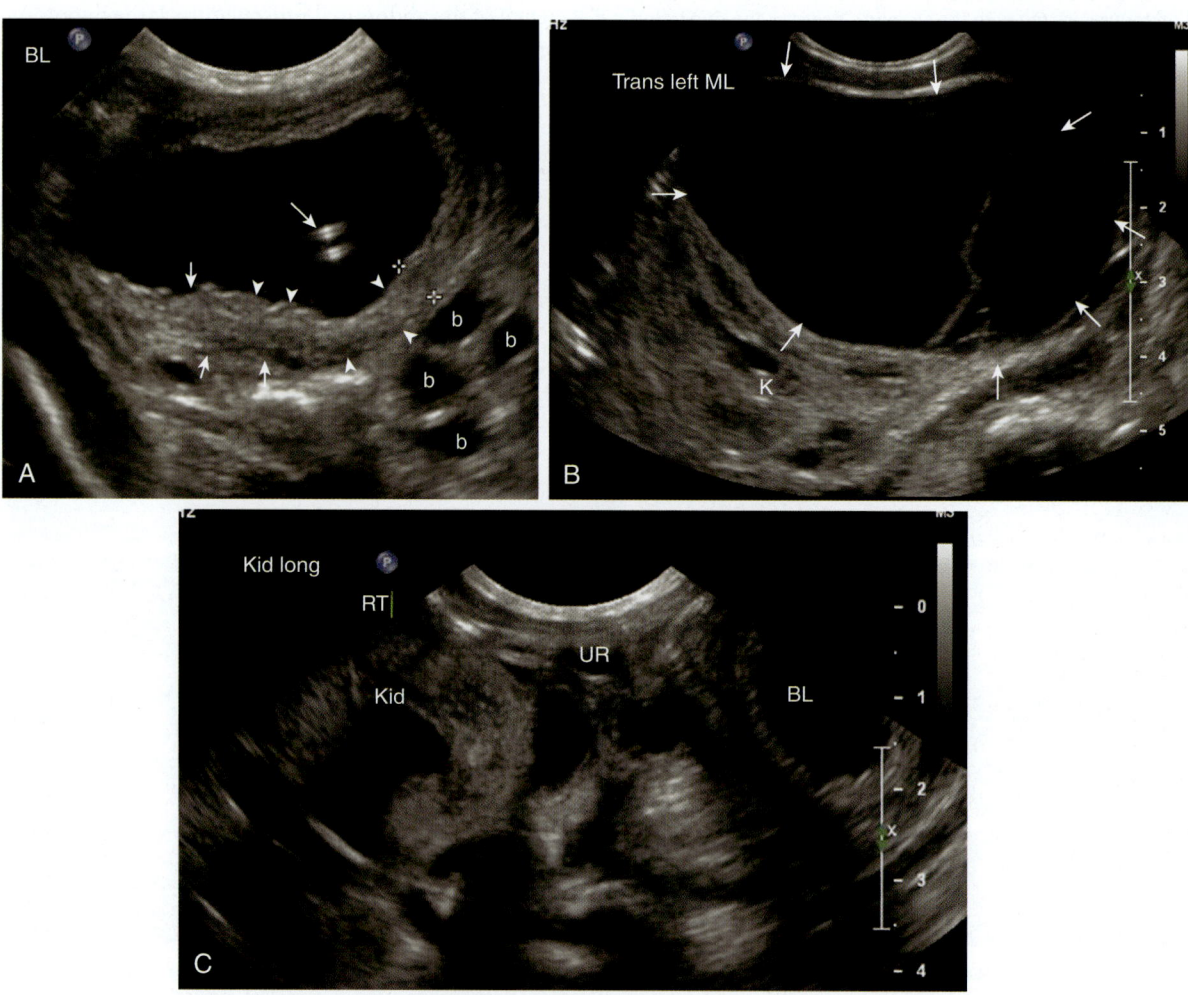

FIG. 26.14 Posterior urethral valves with urinoma. Posterior urethral valves in an 11-day-old boy. Patient had a bladder catheter placed and a large urinoma drained; however, this follow-up scan showed a distended bladder, and the urinoma had reaccumulated. (A) Transverse view of the urinary bladder shows the thickened bladder wall *(short arrows, arrowheads)* and catheter *(long arrow).* Dilated distal ureters were identified in this patient but are not shown here. Posteriorly, normal fluid-filled bowel (b) could be seen peristalsing on real-time imaging. (B) Longitudinal view of the same patient's left kidney shows a large left perinephric urinoma *(arrows)* measuring 8 cm in its greatest dimension, compressing the kidney (k) posteriorly. (C) Right longitudinal image shows the relationship between the kidney (Kid) with urinary tract dilation of the kidney, dilated ureter (UR), and thickened bladder. (Courtesy Nationwide Children's Hospital, Columbus, OH.)

cysts, the largest of which are peripheral. These cysts may be variable in size. There is no identifiable renal pelvis (Fig. 26.15).

A less common and dilating form of MCDK has been described in which a renal pelvis is identified. The association with contralateral ureteropelvic junction obstruction has been noted. Bilateral MCDK may be fatal in the absence of dialysis or renal transplant.

At times, sonographic differentiation of MCDK from severe ureteropelvic junction obstruction may be difficult. In such instances, radionuclide documentation of renal function usually indicates severe UTD. The use of ultrasound has led to conservative management of MCDK. These abnormal kidneys most often involute and disappear completely or result in a small dysplastic kidney. If there is evidence of growth, resection is usually undertaken.

Crossed-Fused Renal Ectopia. While rare, crossed-fused renal ectopia, or crossed renal ectopia with fusion, is the second most frequent fusion abnormality after horseshoe kidney. It occurs when a kidney crosses to the opposite side, and the two kidneys are located on the same side. The left kidney crosses to the right more frequently, and in most cases they fuse at the parenchyma. (It is referred to as simply crossed renal ectopia when unfused, a positional anomaly.) The ureter of the crossed kidney inserts normally, which is now situated contralateral from the kidney. There is a male predominance, and the most common associated anomaly is anorectal malformation. There may be associated ureteropelvic junction obstruction, ureterovesical junction obstruction, and vesicoureteral reflux.

Sonographic Findings. At least one kidney will be absent from the renal fossa, revealing an abnormally shaped adrenal gland. The kidney is discovered on the opposite side of the body. Two renal pelvises with two distinct renal cortexes will be present. Both kidneys may be in the pelvis (more frequently) or in a normal location on one side. In a majority of cases, the two kidneys are fused. There are a variety of ways the kidneys may be fused together: at the superior poles, at midline, and so forth. The kidneys may demonstrate excess fluid if obstruction or reflux is present (Fig. 26.16).

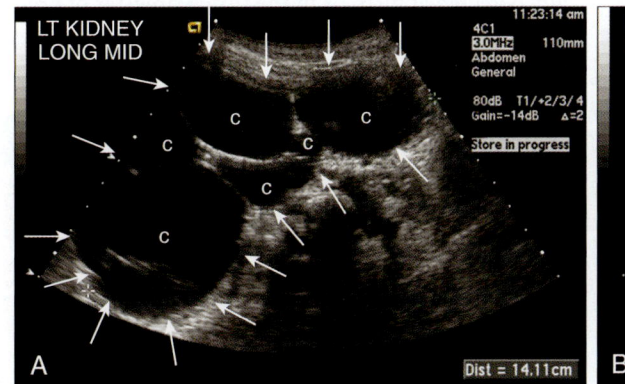
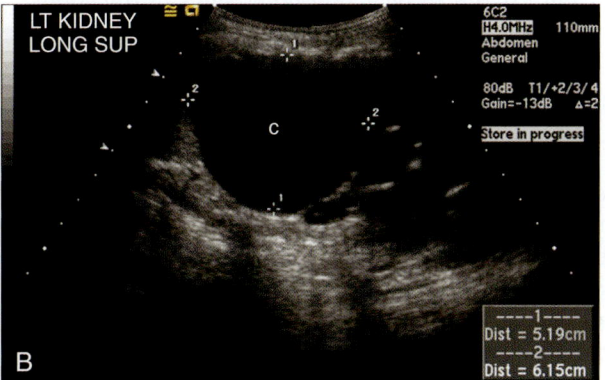

FIG. 26.15 **Multicystic dysplastic kidney (MCDK) (arrows) in a 4-year-old boy.** There was no apparent left renal pelvis, and follow-up imaging a year later showed most of the cysts had involuted. (A) Sagittal view of the left flank demonstrates multiple noncommunicating cysts (c) of varying sizes, distinguishing it from urinary tract dilation. Left MCDK measuring >14 cm. (B) The largest cyst located in the superior pole measured 6 × 5 cm in the sagittal view. (Courtesy Nationwide Children's Hospital, Columbus, OH.)

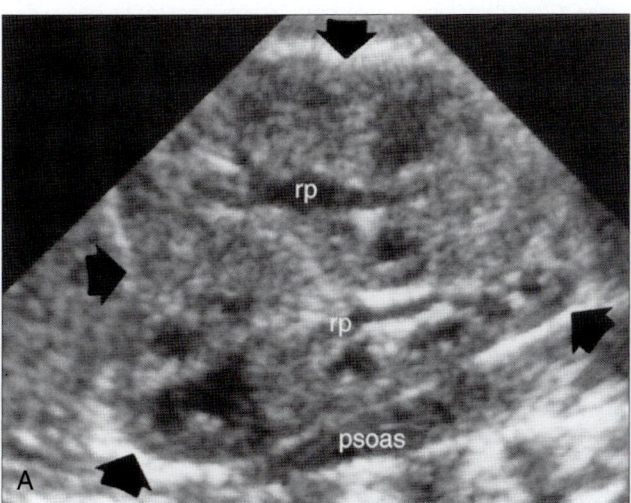
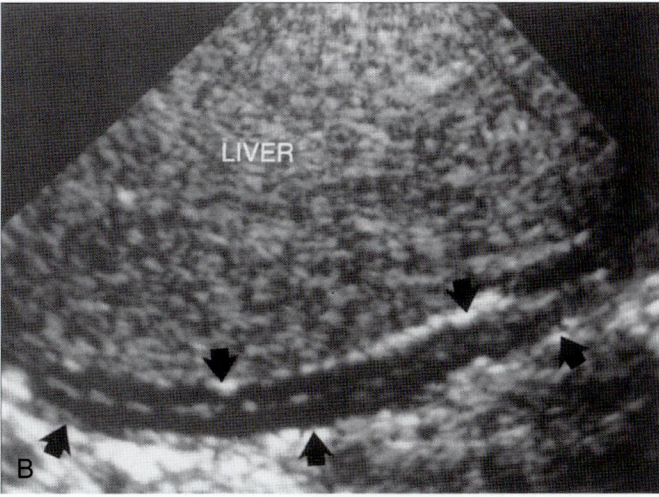

FIG. 26.16 **Crossed-fused renal ectopia.** (A) Crossed-fused renal ectopia (arrows) in a 1-day-old boy with imperforate anus. Sonogram through the left flank demonstrates the renal pelvis (rp) of each kidney. (B) Longitudinal image through the right flank demonstrates an elongated "lying down" adrenal gland (arrows) resulting from the absence of a kidney in this renal fossa.

Patent Urachus. The urachus is a long, tubular structure, which connects the dome of the bladder to the umbilicus. Normally, it closes during the fourth and fifth months of gestation and is often completely fibrotic at birth, or at least sealed off in the neonatal period. Sometimes, however, the urachus remains patent, either from the bladder end or the umbilical end and at times from both sides. Sonography plays a role in detecting suspected **patent urachus**, which may present as a cystic mass under the umbilicus at birth or drainage of fluid from the umbilicus, but often the patent urachus presents with symptoms of infection. This is also called an infected umbilical remnant.

Sonographic Findings. High-resolution sonography over the superior bladder will reveal a hypoechoic tract tracing to the umbilicus. Fluid may be present on either end. In the case where the urachal remnant is patent at the bladder end and closed at the umbilicus, a cyst will form, appearing as a hypoechoic mass seen just posterior to the umbilicus. In case of infection, surrounding edema may also be present (Fig. 26.17). Color or power Doppler and compression can aid in detecting other signs of infection, such as hyperemia and fluid.

Hereditary Renal Cystic Disease

Renal cystic disease is often found as part of the initial workup for renal failure, a prenatal ultrasound, or known family history. Prenatal or incidental sonographic findings may also detect these diseases. Hereditary renal cystic diseases, which may present in the neonate or pediatric patient, include **autosomal recessive polycystic kidney disease (ARPKD),** autosomal dominant polycystic kidney disease, tuberous sclerosis, and von Hippel–Lindau disease.

These diseases should not be confused with nonhereditary and incidental multiple renal cysts. Just as in adults, incidental simple cysts may occur in children as well or be associated with a more serious underlying hereditary disease. Furthermore, there may be a high association of cortical renal cysts and bilateral Wilms tumor development. Therefore, monitoring is important, in conjunction with laboratory testing, family history, and associated symptoms or findings.

Autosomal Recessive Polycystic Kidney Disease. Polycystic renal disease identified in the neonatal period is most often ARPKD, previously known as *infantile polycystic disease.* This disease is not common, occurring in 1 in 6000 to 14,000 births, with a female predominance (2:1). As the name suggests, it is transmitted by autosomal recessive inheritance. The typical pathologic presentation is diffuse enlargement, sacculations, and cystic diverticula of the medullary portions of the kidneys (Fig. 26.18).

The degree of renal cystic disease determines the severity of renal dysplasia, which can lead to renal failure and eventual hepatic fibrosis and liver failure. ARPKD is also associated with biliary **ectasia**, which is proportional to the degree of renal involvement. The most severe form is seen in the neonatal stage, and the least severe form is seen in the infantile to juvenile stage.

The perinatal form, in which the dilated kidneys occupy nearly the entire abdomen and cause the abdomen to protrude, is the most common. This diagnosis may be made in utero as early as 16 to 18 weeks of gestation; however, it is usually detected at birth or in the third trimester of pregnancy in the presence of severe oligohydramnios and nonvisualization

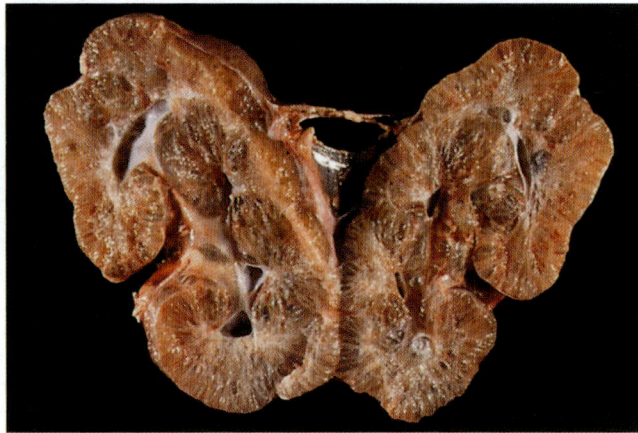

FIG. 26.18 Autosomal recessive polycystic kidney disease specimen. Gross pathology of autosomal recessive polycystic kidney disease demonstrates bilateral renal enlargement with diffuse cysts replacing the tubules and collecting ducts.

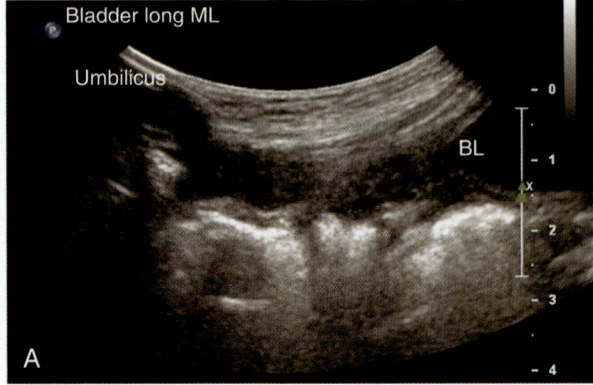 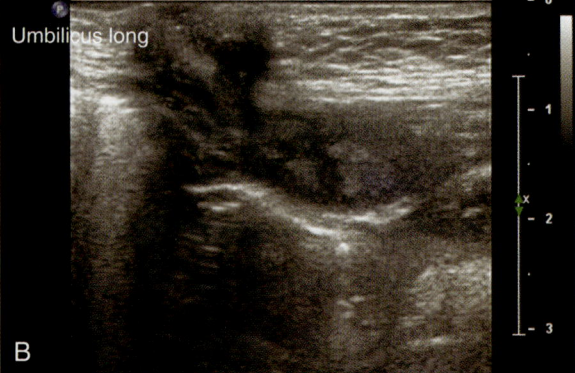

FIG. 26.17 Infected patent urachus in a 4-month-old. The patient presented with purulent drainage from the umbilicus. (A) Sagittal image shows a mostly hypoechoic tract extending from the dome of the bladder to the umbilicus. (B) Closer sagittal view over the umbilicus reveals an inhomogeneous mass extending toward the bladder (BL) inferiorly. (Courtesy Nationwide Children's Hospital, Columbus, OH.)

of the bladder. These manifestations, due to low urine output, may result in **pulmonary hypoplasia** with respiratory distress and **Potter facies**. Over a quarter of affected neonates will die from resulting respiratory insufficiency.

In the juvenile form of ARPKD, symptoms can occur later in childhood. The renal tubular ectasia and the resultant renal symptomatology are overshadowed by hepatic fibrosis leading to portal hypertension and gastrointestinal bleeding. In this condition, the dilated renal collecting tubules produce an accentuated medullary echogenicity, and the renal cortex has an essentially normal appearance. Increased liver echogenicity reflects hepatic fibrosis.

Sonographic Findings. The most striking feature is bilateral renal enlargement with diffuse increased echogenicity and loss of definition throughout the renal sinus, medulla, and cortex. The macroscopic cyst-like appearance throughout both kidneys actually reflects dilated renal tubules that are generally less than 2 mm in diameter. The innumerable acoustic interfaces that present due to this morphologic abnormality result in notable echogenicity, obscuring corticomedullary differentiation. A thin, peripheral, hypoechoic renal rim may be demonstrated, representing the renal cortex compressed by the expanded pyramids, which appear as elongated thin-walled cystic spaces (Fig. 26.19). Less severe cases may show hepatosplenomegaly and portal hypertension, with the renal parenchyma normal to echogenic. Additionally, associated mild hepatic fibrosis and ductal hyperplasia can produce a heterogeneous increase in echogenicity of liver parenchyma.

Autosomal Dominant Polycystic Kidney Disease. More than 90% of patients with **autosomal dominant polycystic kidney disease (ADPKD)** have a gene locus on the short arm of chromosome 16 and was previously referred to as *adult polycystic disease*. There is wide variation in the severity of the disease. The adult dominant form of polycystic kidney disease usually appears during middle age. On rare occasions, however, it has been reported in a young infant. Sonography of parents and siblings of patients with ADPKD has proven helpful in identifying this abnormality in afflicted persons who are asymptomatic. More typically, the disease becomes manifest during the fourth decade of adulthood, with hypertension, hematuria, and enlarged kidneys.

Sonographic Findings. Sonographic findings include well-defined bilateral cysts of various sizes as the tubular and ductal cells become engorged. Cysts are macroscopic and of varying size and can also form in the liver, spleen, and pancreas. There is an increased incidence of renal cell carcinoma in patients with ADPKD. Cerebral berry aneurysms are also known to occur in 10% to 15% of patients with ADPKD.

Tuberous Sclerosis and von Hippel–Lindau Disease. Just as in the adult patient, renal cysts may appear in the kidney and may be found associated with various multisystemic syndromes such as tuberous sclerosis and von Hippel–Lindau disease. Both tuberous sclerosis and von Hippel–Lindau disease are associated with an increased incidence of renal cell carcinoma.

Sonographic Findings. Patients with the autosomal disease of tuberous sclerosis have a 40% incidence of having renal cysts, which may resemble polycystic renal disease. Multiple **angiomyolipomas** may be present, and their echogenicity is determined by the amount of fatty tissue within the lesion.

In patients with von Hippel–Lindau disease, multiple bilateral cysts are often present. Cysts may also be found in the pancreas and liver.

Acquired Pathology

Children, like adults, may acquire both acute and chronic pathology of the urinary tract. Often, acquired pathology of the kidney and bladder is associated with congenital

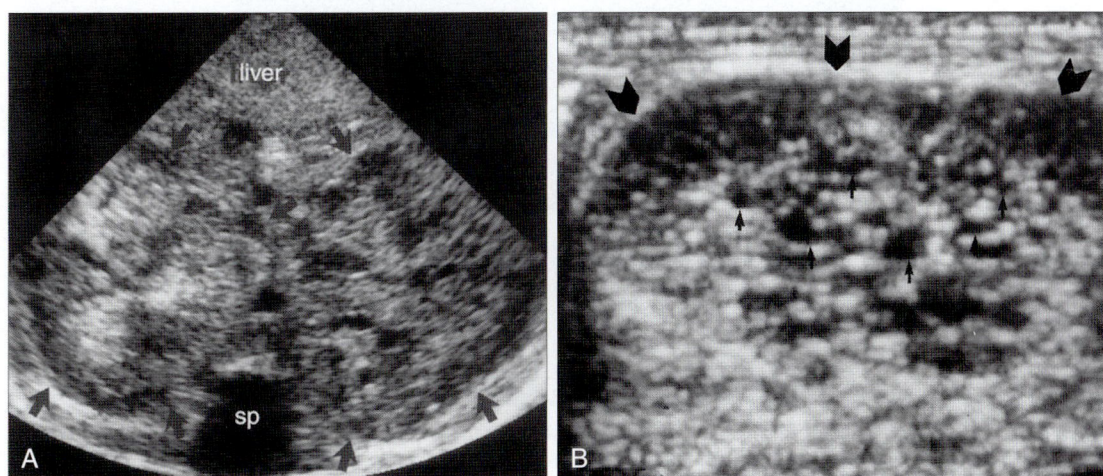

FIG. 26.19 **Autosomal recessive polycystic kidney disease (ARPKD) in a 1-day-old boy with abdominal distention.** (A) Transverse image of the upper abdomen using the liver as an acoustic window shows the kidneys are enlarged and echogenic with a hypoechoic peripheral rim *(arrows)*. This appearance is typical for ARPKD. (B) Higher-resolution 7-MHz linear image of the kidney *(arrowheads)* in the same patient reveals multiple small cysts *(arrows)*. *sp*, Spine.

anomalies, medications, or even prematurity. For example, children with congenital UTD are at risk for UTIs.

Infection of the Urinary Tract. UTI is the most common bacterial infection among children. Children younger than 5 years with a UTI are often referred for renal sonography to rule out congenital anomalies. UTI is the first sign of an anomaly in 30% of children with a urinary tract abnormality. It is important for the clinician to rule out the presence of kidney abnormalities that may lead to renal infection and subsequent scarring.

Acute Pyelonephritis. Clinical symptoms of acute **pyelonephritis** include sudden fever, flank pain, and tenderness. The infection usually begins in the bladder and ascends the ureter into the renal pelvis.

Sonographic Findings. On sonography, the renal size may be slightly enlarged with an altered renal parenchymal echogenicity secondary to edema. As the infection spreads into the renal pyramids, there may be increased echogenicity in this triangular area. The renal pelvis and ureter may show urothelial thickening secondary to inflammation. The infection may be diffuse or localized. Power Doppler may be used in detecting and better defining pyelonephritis, with the area of infection showing decreased or absent flow.

As the infection begins to wall itself into an abscess formation, a mixed echogenic pattern is demonstrated within the renal parenchyma. Sonography may be useful to demonstrate retraction of the lesion in a patient receiving antibiotic therapy (Fig. 26.20).

Chronic Pyelonephritis. This results when repeated episodes of acute pyelonephritis cause the kidney to become scarred, leading to an overall decrease in renal size.

Sonographic Findings. The outline of the kidney may be irregular as the parenchyma becomes scarred. The renal cortex becomes increasingly more echogenic than the liver

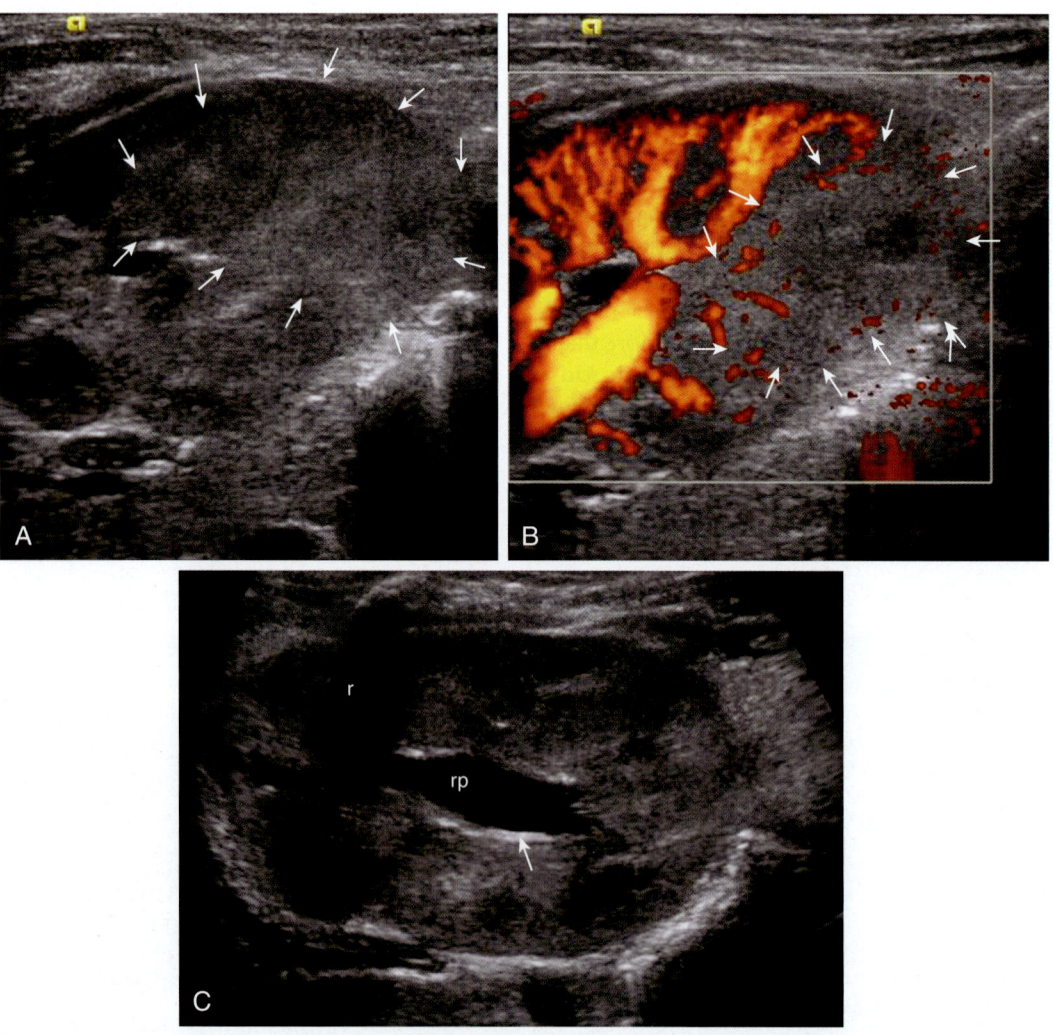

FIG. 26.20 Acute pyelonephritis in a 22-day-old boy with *Escherichia coli* urinary tract infection and bacteremia. The right kidney shows focal increased echogenicity in the upper pole. There was associated mild pelvic dilation and uroepithelial thickening. (A) Upper pole lacks normal corticomedullary differentiation *(arrows)*, and the increased echogenicity within it suggests pyelonephritis based on the patient's history. (B) Upper pole view, using power Doppler to define the area, showing a lack of color Doppler fill in the suspected area. (C) Sagittal mid-view showing dilation in the right renal pelvis (rp) and associated uroepithelial lining *(arrow)* thickening. Rib shadow (r) seen due to the prone position. (Courtesy Nationwide Children's Hospital, Columbus, OH.)

parenchyma. The renal pyramids become difficult to separate from the renal parenchyma.

Medullary Nephrocalcinosis. Once known as Albright calcinosis, nephrocalcinosis is another possible acquired renal pathology. It is the calcification of the renal parenchyma, often in the pyramid and rarely in the cortex. Nephrocalcinosis may be encountered in the premature infant, with a wide range reported from 6 to 41%, with the strongest factor associated with very low birth weight. It has many underlying causes, often associated with hypercalcemia, including infants receiving vitamin D therapy, long-term furosemide for lung or heart disease, among other medications, and medullary sponge kidney (Cacchi-Ricci disease), or Bartter syndrome.

▸ *Sonographic Findings.* Nephrocalcinosis appears sonographically with echogenic renal pyramids and a remaining normal hypoechoic cortex. While the renal pyramids normally appear hypoechoic in infancy, the echogenic pyramids are the first sonographic sign (Fig. 26.21). While echogenic, it does not usually cause shadowing, although kidney stones or nephrolithiasis may be present in the adjacent calyces.

Renal Vein Thrombosis. **Renal vein thrombosis** is most likely to occur in the dehydrated or septic infant and is more prevalent in infants of diabetic mothers. It may occur in infants with shock, glomerulonephritis, or nephrotic syndrome. It may also be indicated when malignancy is present, so a full workup is critical. One or both kidneys may be involved. There is renal enlargement, hematuria, proteinuria, and a low platelet count.

▸ *Sonographic Findings.* Thrombosis occurs initially in the small intrarenal venous branches, and at this stage, the enlarged kidney has a nonspecific disordered heterogeneous internal echogenicity corresponding to the extent and severity of the process (Fig. 26.22). If the thrombus reaches the renal vein or inferior vena cava, it may be directly visualized within these vascular structures. There may be coexistent adrenal hemorrhage, particularly on the left side, where the adrenal vein drains directly into the renal vein. Calcification within the involved veins may eventually result. The use of color and pulsed Doppler helps the sonographer to identify whether the flow is present, reversed, or obstructed.

Adrenal Hemorrhage. Difficult delivery, large size, infants of diabetic mothers, stress and hypoxia at delivery, septicemia, and shock all predispose the neonate to the development of an adrenal hemorrhage. The newborn with **adrenal hemorrhage**, however, may have none of these associated factors and still presents with abdominal mass, jaundice, and anemia. Usually, the hemorrhage is found secondary to other complications, such as uncontrolled bleeding, jaundice, intestinal obstruction, hypertension, adrenal abscess, or impaired renal function.

▸ *Sonographic Findings.* Sonographically, adrenal hemorrhage results in ovoid enlargement of the gland or a portion of the gland. The appearance of the hemorrhagic gland can range from anechoic to hyperechoic or may be a mixture of echogenicities, depending on the extent, age, and severity of the process (Fig. 26.23).

When enlargement is significant, a characteristic blunting of the superior pole of the underlying kidney is produced, along with inferior displacement of the kidney. The initial appearance of adrenal hemorrhage may render it indistinguishable from an adrenal neuroblastoma. Follow-up sonography can differentiate these two entities. Unlike a neoplasm, a hemorrhagic adrenal gland does not enlarge but rather decreases in size. Generally, within 4 to 6 weeks, the lesion becomes appreciably smaller, and subsequent calcification may be identified on a sonogram or a radiograph.

Malignant Tumors

Most malignant tumors of the abdomen in children arise from the kidneys. Although malignant tumors of the retroperitoneum are far less common than UTD or multicystic renal dysplasia for palpable mass in the infant or child, they must be considered. When the child presents in the ultrasound department, it is the responsibility of the sonographer to determine the origin of the mass (whether it is part of the liver, kidney, reproductive system, etc.), the internal pattern

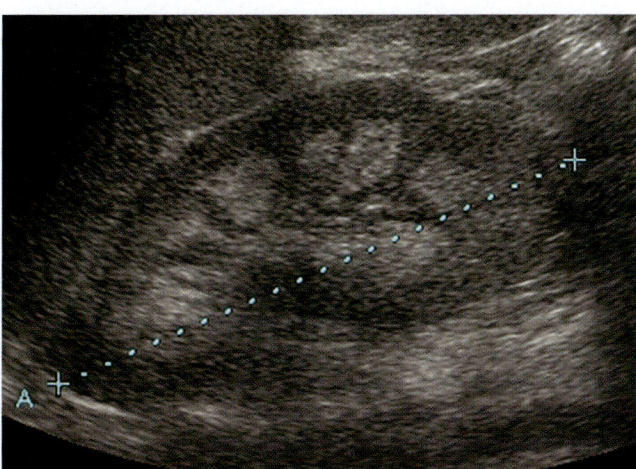

FIG. 26.21 **Medullary nephrocalcinosis.** Sagittal view of the mid-kidney demonstrates the classic appearance of medullary nephrocalcinosis with echogenic pyramids while the outer cortex remains hypoechoic.

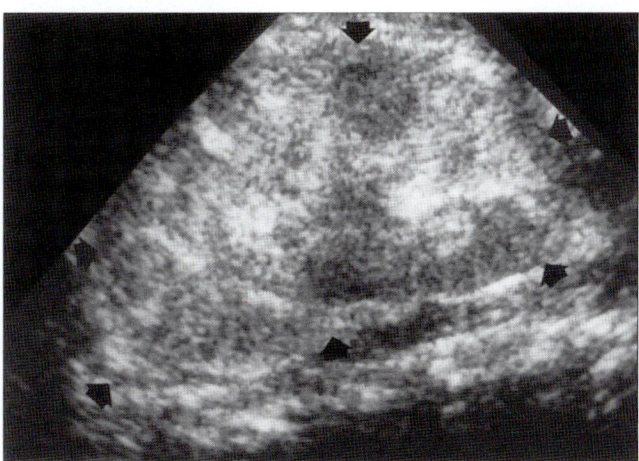

FIG. 26.22 **Renal vein thrombosis in a 3-day-old term newborn with hematuria.** Sagittal sonogram of the left flank demonstrates an enlarged kidney *(arrows)* with patchy areas of increased echogenicity.

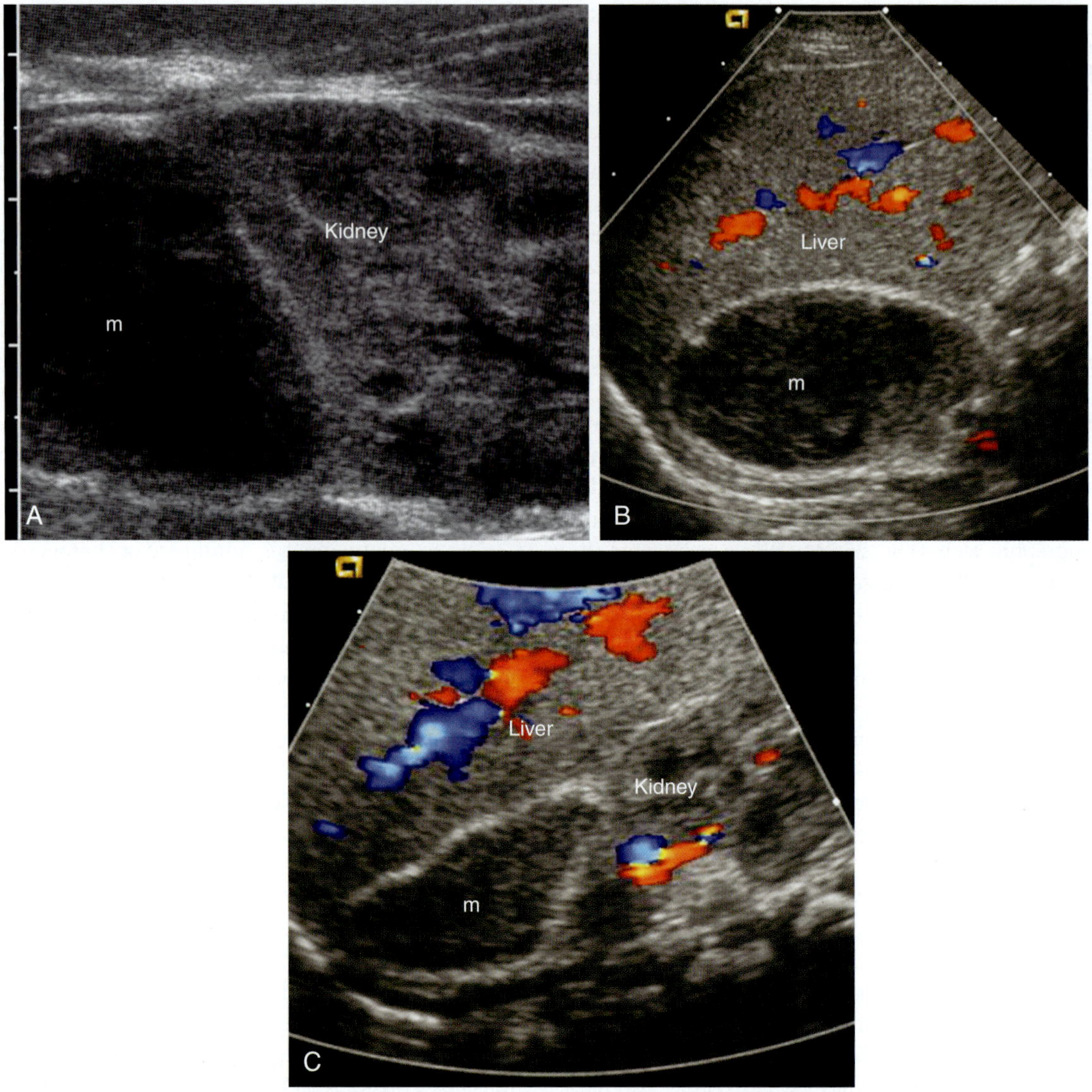

FIG. 26.23 Adrenal hemorrhage. An 8-day-old boy had a history of traumatic delivery and jaundice. (A) Magnified sagittal sonogram demonstrates a suprarenal hypoechoic mass (m) just superior to the right kidney. (B) Sagittal image of the mass through the liver appears ovoid without evidence of vascularity. The adrenal hemorrhage measured 4 × 3.8 × 2.2 cm. A normal adrenal gland was not identified. (C) The same patient 2 weeks later shows the mass has decreased in size (2.6 × 3.1 × 1.7 cm), and there is still no evidence of vascularity, confirming the diagnosis. (Courtesy Nationwide Children's Hospital, Columbus, OH.)

(cystic, solid, or mixed), and whether the mass has vascular flow. The most common urinary tract and adrenal malignant tumors of childhood are presented here.

Nephroblastoma (Wilms Tumor). Wilms tumor (nephroblastoma) is the most common intraabdominal malignant renal tumor in young children. The incidence of this tumor peaks between 2 and 5 years of age. This tumor is usually unilateral, although in a small percentage, it may occur bilaterally. Wilms tumor is bulky and expands within the renal parenchyma, resulting in distortion and displacement of the collecting system and capsule (Fig. 26.24). Many pediatric laboratories will sonographically monitor both those predisposed to the tumor and those with a history or a family history of Wilms tumor, including patients with either proven or potential **nephroblastomatosis** or Beckwith-Wiedemann syndrome. It is important to note that Wilms tumor may also occur spontaneously. Additionally,

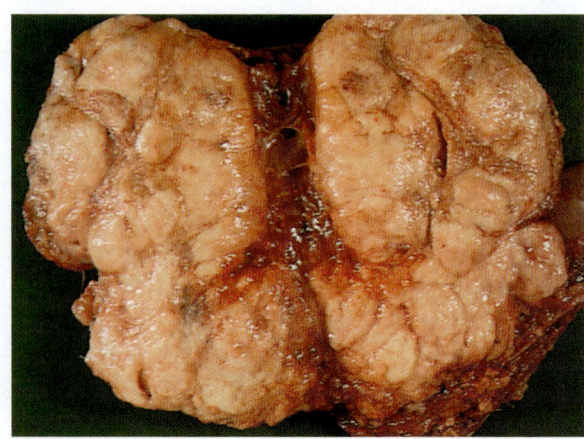

FIG. 26.24 Wilms tumor specimen. Gross pathology demonstrates the multinodular tumor replacing a large portion of the renal parenchyma.

sonography may be used to monitor the size of the tumor while a patient is treated with chemotherapy drugs to shrink the tumor. Therefore, the size of the tumor is documented, and the appropriate time for surgery is chosen. Early surgical removal and treatment yield a favorable prognosis.

Significant differentials for Wilms tumor in children younger than 1 year include the neuroblastoma and **congenital mesoblastic nephroma** (also known as *fetal renal hamartoma* or *congenital Wilms tumor*). Though rare (8 in 1 million births), the mesoblastic nephroma is the most common solid renal tumor of the neonate. This tumor is benign but is indistinguishable from a Wilms tumor by any method of imaging. Because the tumor may invade adjacent structures, nephrectomy is indicated.

Sonographic Findings. The sonographic appearance of a Wilms tumor is variable (Fig. 26.25), extending from a homogeneous to a complex texture. The mass usually has areas of echogenicity and may have calcifications within. The liquefaction may represent necrosis and hemorrhage. The borders are sharply marginated and well-defined but bulky, with a hypoechoic to hyperechoic rim surrounding the mass. The adjacent renal tissue becomes compressed with the growth of the mass. The large solid mass generally is seen to completely distort the renal sinus, pyramids, cortex, and contour of the kidney. The mass may be so large as to protrude into the hepatic capsule (Fig. 26.26). Resultant UTD may be present.

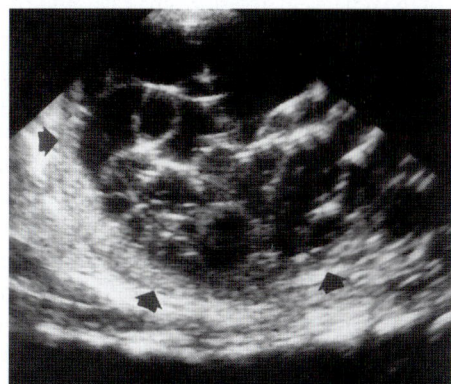

FIG. 26.25 Wilms tumor in an infant. A 7-month-old presented with an abdominal mass. The sonogram revealed a large mass with multiple cystic areas occupying the renal fossa *(arrows)*. This represents an unusual presentation of a Wilms tumor; more frequently, a large solid component is present in these masses.

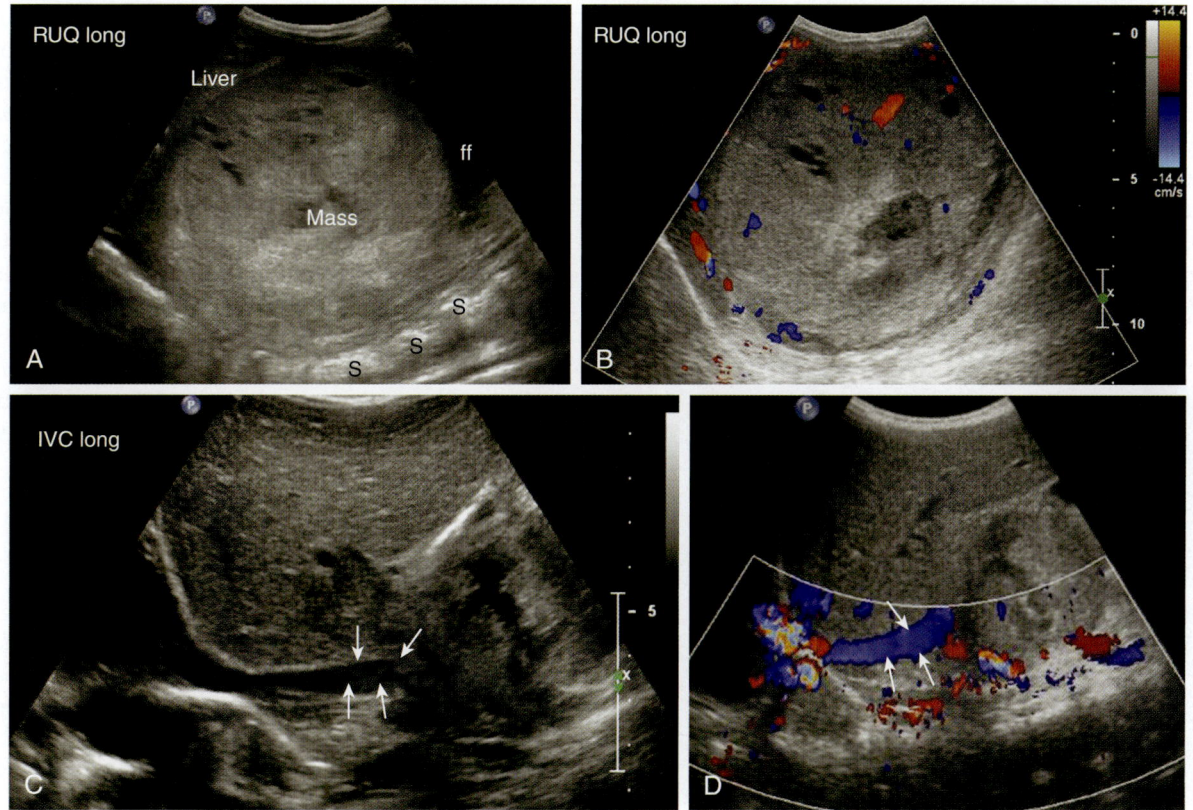

FIG. 26.26 Wilms tumor in a 1-year-old boy. The child presented with an enlarged liver and spleen. (A) Sagittal view of the right renal fossa demonstrates a large (10 × 10 cm) complex mass displacing the liver anteriorly. Free fluid (ff) is seen inferior to the mass, and the mass can be seen pushing against the spine (S). (B) Longitudinal evaluation of the mass with color Doppler. (C) Careful evaluation of the inferior vena cava (IVC) showed no extension of the tumor into the IVC, and no metastases were seen. Proximal IVC *(arrows)* appears to be disrupted by the large tumor. (D) Color Doppler (shown) in the proximal portion of the IVC, along with pulsed Doppler, was used for the vessel's entire length to demonstrate patency. IVC and other midline structures, such as the pancreas, were displaced to the left. (Courtesy Nationwide Children's Hospital, Columbus, OH.)

Sonography is valuable in detecting the extension of a Wilms tumor into the renal vein, inferior vena cava, right atrium, and contralateral kidney. The tumor spreads through direct extension into the renal sinus and peri-pelvic soft tissues, the lymph nodes in the renal hilum, and the para-aortic areas. Careful evaluation of the renal vein, inferior vena cava, and right atrium of the heart is important to document the possible extension of the tumor. Documentation of tumor extension can have a significant bearing on the surgical approach to the patient. When the tumor extends into the right atrium, cardiopulmonary bypass may be necessary to resect the tumor completely.

Neuroblastoma. Neuroblastoma is the most common malignancy in children less than 1 year of age, with an incidence rate twice that of leukemia. It arises in the sympathetic chain ganglia and adrenal medulla and may be detected on prenatal sonography or at birth. This is the second most common abdominal tumor of childhood, occurring between the ages of 2 months and 2 years. About half of these tumors arise in the medulla of the adrenal gland, although tumors have also been found in the neck, mediastinum, retroperitoneum, and pelvis.

Clinical findings depend on the location of the tumor. Tumors that arise within the adrenal gland show an abdominal mass, hypertension, diarrhea, and bone pain if metastasis is involved. If the tumor is detected in infants under 1 year of age, the prognosis is often good, whereas aggressive treatment methods are often needed in older children. Overall, they carry a worse prognosis than a Wilms tumor.

Sonographic Findings. Neuroblastoma is usually highly echogenic. Intrinsic calcification may be identified. The smaller tumors may appear homogeneous and hyperechoic, whereas the large tumors are more complex in appearance. A cystic form of neuroblastoma has also been described. The adjacent kidney is displaced inferiorly and at times laterally (Fig. 26.27). Doppler evaluation may help to differentiate the tumor from an adrenal hemorrhage because there is increased vascularity within the neoplastic growth.

The tumor spreads early and wide, with the majority of patients presenting with metastases. Careful sonographic evaluation of the liver should be made for evidence of metastatic disease. The mass also spreads around the aorta, celiac, and superior mesenteric arteries. The spread of this tumor helps to distinguish a neuroblastoma from a Wilms tumor. The neuroblastoma is poorly defined and heterogeneous, with irregular hyperechoic areas caused by calcifications. Intraspinal extension is reported to occur in as many as 15% of patients. Since ultrasonography can successfully define the spinal canal in young infants, a neonatal spine evaluation may be considered to evaluate an infant with suspected neuroblastoma.

Other Malignant Retroperitoneal Tumors. Renal cell carcinoma infrequently occurs in childhood, accounting for 1.8% to 6.3% of all malignant renal tumors in childhood. It appears as an isoechoic to slightly hypoechoic mass within the kidney.

The rhabdomyosarcoma is the fourth most common solid malignancy of childhood, behind central nervous system neoplasms, neuroblastoma, and Wilms tumor. It often arises from the head and neck, but also the genitourinary system, including the bladder. The average age of presentation for this tumor is 7 years old. It may arise posterior to the bladder causing urethral obstruction. The sonographer should always allow for adequate visualization posterior to the bladder, and in the case of extreme distention, catheterization may be required.

Though rare, adrenal malignant tumors include the pheochromocytoma, an adrenal neuroendocrine tumor of childhood. Patients present with headache, palpitations, and sweating. Roughly half will present with a palpable abdominal mass and may also have hypertension. Adrenocortical carcinomas are another malignant adrenal tumor, with most cases occurring before 3 years of age. However, any adrenal tumor or hyperplasia may be indicated in precocious puberty, defined as sexual maturation in boys younger than 9 years old or girls younger than 8 years old.

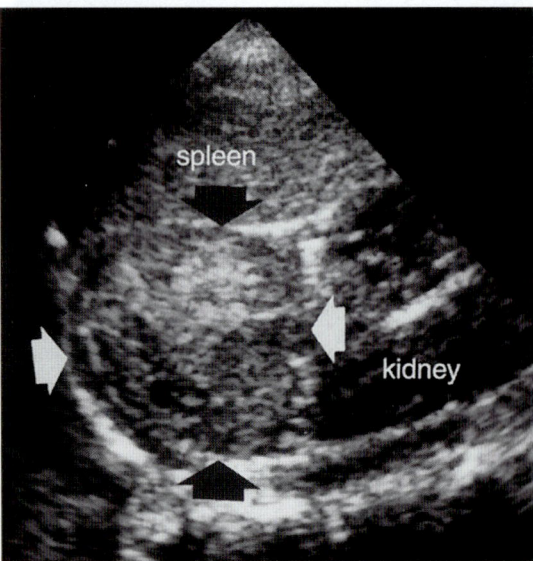

FIG. 26.27 Adrenal neuroblastoma in a neonate. A 1-week-old girl with a history of a left kidney mass seen on a fetal sonogram. Sagittal image through the left flank reveals a large heterogeneous mass *(arrows)* displacing the left kidney inferiorly.

Key Pearls

- Neonatal kidneys may appear hyperechoic or isoechoic compared with the liver parenchyma, which is normal up to 1 month. However, they should be less echogenic than the liver and spleen parenchyma by 4–6 months of age.
- The medullary pyramids are hypoechoic and prominent up to the first year and should not be mistaken for urinary tract dilation (UTD) or cysts.
- Renal length varies by age, with the left kidney being a bit longer. A measurement greater than 1 cm from side to side may indicate a congenital anomaly or possible pathology.
- Accurate and consistent renal measurements are important and allow for the documentation of normal growth and accurate follow-up studies.

- Congenital urinary tract anomalies are common and account for half of all congenital anomalies.
- It is important to visualize the bladder, often imaged first, and should be properly prepped in those old enough to hold a full urinary bladder.
- Infants are likely to retain urine in the bladder after voiding and is a normal finding.
- Allow for adequate posterior viewing of the bladder to identify dilated ureters, pathology of the uterus, and masses.
- Adrenals may easily be seen in neonates, often prominent at birth and rapidly decrease in size in the first 10 days of life.
- It is critical to differentiate communicating cysts (UTD) from noncommunicating cysts of multicystic dysplastic kidney disease.
- UTD is the most common cause of a palpable mass in the neonate.
- There are many causes of UTD, including vesicoureteral reflux, ureteropelvic junction obstruction, ectopic ureterocele associated with a duplex collecting system, and bladder outlet obstruction (posterior urethral valves and prune-belly syndrome).
- Ureteropelvic junction obstruction is the most common type of obstruction in UTD.
- Multicystic dysplastic kidney disease is the most common renal cystic diagnosis in a neonate.
- Hereditary renal cystic disease is often found prenatally, incidentally, or as part of a workup for renal failure.
- Multiple simple cysts may be benign or part of a serious hereditary disease; therefore a workup and history are important.
- Multisystemic diseases, such as tuberous sclerosis and von Hippel–Lindau disease, increase a patient's risk for developing renal cell carcinoma.
- Urinary tract infection is the most common bacterial infection in children, and sonography is used to rule out any underlying congenital anomalies.
- Medullary nephrocalcinosis is often associated with very low birth weight and preterm birth.
- Adrenal hemorrhage is often ovoid and will not show any color Doppler flow; follow-up is necessary to confirm the diagnosis.
- Wilms tumor (nephroblastoma) is the most common intraabdominal malignant tumor in young children, whereas the neuroblastoma is the most common tumor in infants under 1 year of age, although it may present between 2 months and 2 years of age.
- Wilms tumor peaks at 2–5 years of age and has a better prognosis than neuroblastoma, which often presents with metastases.
- Careful evaluation of the inferior vena cava and renal veins is important to exclude vascular extension of any abdominal tumor.

BIBLIOGRAPHY

Abdellah A, Selma K, Elamin M, et al. Renal cell carcinoma in children: case report and literature review. *Pan Afr Med J*. 2015;20:84.

Aderotimi TS, Kraft JK. Ultrasound of the adrenal gland in children. *Ultrasound*. 2021 Feb;29(1):48–56.

American Institute of Ultrasound in Medicine: AIUM practice guideline for the performance of an ultrasound examination in the practice of urology, 2011. http://www.aium.org/resources/guidelines/urology.pdf.

Becker A, Baum M. Obstructive uropathy. *Early Hum Dev*. 2006;82(1):15–22.

Belarmino JM, Kogan BA. Management of neonatal hydronephrosis. *Early Hum Dev*. 2006;82(1):9–14.

Bhansali A, Rajput R, Behra A, et al. Childhood sporadic pheochromocytoma: clinical profile and outcome in 19 patients. *J Pediatr Endocrinol Metab*. 2006;19(5):749–756.

Blane CE, Ritchey M, DiPietro M. Single system ectopic ureters and ureteroceles associated with dysplastic kidney. *Pediatr Radiol*. 1992;22:217.

Chalmers DJ, Meyers ML, Brodie KE, Palmer C, Campbell JB. Interrater reliability of the APD, SFU and UTD grading systems in fetal sonography and MRI. *J Pediatr Urol*. 2016;12(5):305.e1–305.e5.

Chen JJ, Pugach J, Patel M, et al. The renal length nomogram: multivariable approach. *J Urol*. 2002;168(5):2149–2152.

Chow JS, Koning JL, Back SJ, Nguyen HT, Phelps A, Darge K. Classification of pediatric urinary tract dilation: the new language. *Pediatr Radiol*. 2017;47(9):1109–1115.

Cohan RH, Ellis JH. Renal masses: imaging evaluation. *Radiol Clin North Am*. 2015;53(5):985–1003.

Coley BD. Pediatric applications of abdominal vascular Doppler: part II. *Pediatr Radiol*. 2004;34(10):772–786.

Creel S, Anderson J, Michael K, Pinkerman B. Evaluation of pediatric renal size by sonography. *J Diagn Med Sonogr*. 1999;15(1):1–6.

Fang SB, Lee H, Sheu J. Prenatal sonographic detection of adrenal hemorrhage confirmed by postnatal surgery. *J Clin Ultrasound*. 1999;27:206–209.

Fenichel G. *Clinical pediatric neurology*. ed 6 Philadelphia: Saunders; 2009.

Fisher JP, Tweddle DA. Neonatal neuroblastoma. *Semin Fetal Neonatal Med*. 2012;17(4):207–215.

Garel L. Renal cystic disease. *Ultrasound Clin*. 2010;5(1):15–59.

Gray MC, Zillioux JM, Varda B, et al. Assessment of urinary tract dilation grading amongst pediatric urologists. *J Pediatr Urol*. 2020;16(4):457.e1–457.e6.

Heikkilä J, Taskinen S, Rintala R. Urinomas associated with posterior urethral valves. *J Urol*. 2008;180(4):1476–1478.

Houat AP, Guimarães CT, Takahashi MS, et al. Congenital anomalies of the upper urinary tract: a comprehensive review. *RadioGraphics*. 2021;2:462–486.

Hwang M, Piskunowicz M, Darge K. Advanced ultrasound techniques for pediatric imaging. *Pediatrics*. 2019;143(3):e20182609.

Jakubowska A, Grajewska-Ferens M, Brzewski M, Sopylo B. Usefulness of imaging techniques in the diagnostics of precocious puberty in boys. *Pol J Radiol*. 2011;76(4):21–27.

Jequier S, Rousseau O. Sonographic measurements of the normal bladder wall in children. *AJR Am J Roentgenol*. 1987;149(3):563–566.

Kasap B, Soylu A, Türkmen M, Kavukcu S. Relationship of increased renal cortical echogenicity with clinical and laboratory findings in pediatric renal disease. *J Clin Ultrasound*. 2006;34(7):339–342.

Lawande A. Ultrasonography in pediatric renal masses. *Ultrasound Clin*. 2010;5(4):433–441.

Lee HS, Sung IK, Kim SJ, et al. Risk factors associated with nephrocalcinosis in preterm infants. *Am J Perinatol*. 2014;31(4):279–286.

Lee W, Comstock CH, Jurcak-Zaleski S. Prenatal diagnosis of adrenal hemorrhage by ultrasonography. *J Ultrasound Med*. 1992;11:369.

Letourneau K, Harrington C, Reed M, et al. Tuberous sclerosis complex: typical and atypical sonographic findings. *J Diagn Med Sonogr*. 2015;21:491–496.

Leung VY, Chu WC, Yeung CK, et al. Nomograms of total renal volume, urinary bladder volume and bladder wall thickness index in 3,376 children with a normal urinary tract. *Pediatr Radiol*. 2007;37(2):181–188.

Lin CC, Tsai JD, Sheu JC, et al. Segmental multicystic dysplastic kidney in children: clinical presentation, imaging finding, management, and outcome. *J Pediatr Surg*. 2010;45(9):1856–1862.

Loganathan AK, Bal HS. Crossed fused renal ectopia in children: a review of clinical profile, surgical challenges, and outcome. *J Pediatr Urol*. 2019;15(4):315–321.

Luckens JN. Neuroblastoma in the neonate. *Semin Perinatol*. 1999;23:263–273.

Margraf LR. Diagnosis and discussion: autosomal recessive polycystic kidney disease. *Am J Dis Child*. 1993;147:77.

Matos F, Carneiro L, Oeiras L. Retroperitoneal masses in children—beyond neuroblastoma and Wilms tumor. *Eur Congr Radiol*. 2011;1970:1–20.

Mchugh K. Renal and adrenal tumours in children. *Cancer Imaging*. 2007;7:41–51.

Nadler EP, Barksdale Jr EM. Adrenal masses in the newborn. *Semin Pediatr Surg*. 2000;9:156–164.

Nguyen HT, Benson CB, Bromley B, et al. Multidisciplinary consensus on the classification of prenatal and postnatal urinary tract dilation (UTD classification system). *J Pediatr Urol*. 2014;10(6):982–998.

Orazi C, Fariello G, Malena S: Renal vein thrombosis and adrenal hemorrhage in the newborn: ultrasound evaluation of 4 cases. *J Clin Ultrasound*. 1993;21(3):163–9.

Resontoc LP, Yap HK. Renal vascular thrombosis in the newborn. *Pediatr Nephrol*. 2016;31(6):907–915.

Riccabona M. Urinary tract imaging in infancy. *Pediatr Radiol*. 2009;39(Suppl 3):436–445.

Riccabona M. Obstructive diseases of the urinary tract in children: lessons from the last 15 years. *Pediatr Radiol*. 2010;40(6):947–955.

Robert A, Leroy V, Riquet A, et al. Renal involvement in tuberous sclerosis complex with emphasis on cystic lesions. *Radiol Med*. 2016;121(5):402–408.

Rumack CM, Wilson SR, Charboneau JW, Johnson J. *Diagnostic ultrasound*. vol 2. St. Louis: Elsevier; 2010.

Samal SK, Rathod S. Prune belly syndrome: a rare case report. *J Natl Sci Biol Med*. 2015;6(1):255–257.

Scott EM, Thomas A, Mcgarrigle HH, Lachelin GC. Serial adrenal ultrasonography in normal neonates. *J Ultrasound Med*. 1990;9(5):279–283.

Siegel MJ. Pediatric abdominal masses. In: Sanders RC, Winter T, eds. *Clinical sonography: a practical guide*. ed 4 Baltimore, MD: Lippincott Williams & Wilkins; 2007:321–340.

Siegel MJ. *Pediatric sonography*. Philadelphia, PA: Lippincott Williams & Wilkins; 2010.

Simanovsky N, Revel-Vilk S, Weintraub M, Hiller N. Association between renal cystic lesions and bilateral Wilms' tumours. *Eur Radiol*. 2016;26(6):1665–1669.

Simõese Silva AC, Oliveira EA. Update on the approach of urinary tract infection in childhood. *J Pediatr (Rio J)*. 2015;91(6 Suppl 1):S2–S10.

Sivit CJ. Sonography of pediatric urinary tract emergencies. *Ultrasound Clin*. 2006;1(1):67–75.

Soundappan SV, Lam AH, Cass DT. Traumatic adrenal haemorrhage in children. *Aust N Z J Surg*. 2006;76(8):729–731.

Stark JE, Weinberger E. Ultrasonography of the neonatal genitourinary tract. *Appl Radiol*. 1993;22:50.

Strife JL, et al. Multicystic dysplastic kidney in children: US follow-up. *Radiology*. 1993;186:785.

Sweeney WE, Avner ED. Diagnosis and management of childhood polycystic kidney disease. *Pediatr Nephrol*. 2011;26(5):675–692.

Swenson DW, Darge K, Ziniel SI, Chow JS. Characterizing upper urinary tract dilation on ultrasound: a survey of North American pediatric radiologists's practices. *Pediatr Radiol*. 2015;45(5):686–694.

Teele RL, Share JC. Evaluating an abdominal mass. In: Teele RL, Share JC, eds. *Ultrasonography of infants and children*. Philadelphia: Saunders; 1991.

Valdespino RS. The importance of sonography in the evaluation of neonatal adrenal hemorrhage. *J Diagn Med Sonogr*. 2009;25(4):221–225.

Yeung CK, Sreedhar B, Leung YF, Sit KY. Correlation between ultrasonographic bladder measurements and urodynamic findings in children with recurrent urinary tract infection. *BJU Int*. 2007;99(3):651–655.

Zerin JM, Blane CE. Sonographic assessment of renal length in children: a reappraisal. *Pediatr Radiol*. 1994;24(2):101–106.

CHAPTER 27

Neonatal and Infant Head

Kathryn E. Zale

OBJECTIVES

On completion of this chapter, you should be able to:
- Recognize normal neuroanatomy as it pertains to the ultrasound examination of the preterm and term neonate
- Describe the coronal, sagittal, and mastoid view studies
- Discuss the sonographic findings in neonatal brain pathology

OUTLINE

Normal Anatomy And Sonographic Findings 814
- Fontanels (Fontanelles) 814
- Meninges 815
- Ventricular System 815
- Cerebrum 817
- Basal Ganglia 818
- Brainstem 818
- Cerebellum 819
- Cerebrovascular System 819

Examination Preparation 819

Neonatal Head Examination 821
- Overview of the Standard Evaluation 821
- Additional/Modified Evaluation 821
- Advanced Techniques in Neurosonography 821
- Coronal Study 824
- Sagittal Study 827
- Posterior Fossa Study 828

Hydrocephalus (Ventriculomegaly) 829

Acquired Brain Lesions 832
- Intracranial Hemorrhage 832
- Hypoxic-Ischemic Injury Lesions 836

Congenital Brain Malformations 838
- Disorders of Neural Tube Closure 838
- Disorders of Diverticulation and Cleavage 842
- Destructive Lesions 843
- Cystic Lesions 844

Brain Infections 846
- Congenital Infections 846
- Ventriculitis 847
- Ependymitis 847

KEY TERMS

Aqueductal stenosis
Asphyxia
Atrium (trigone) of the lateral ventricle
Brainstem
Caudothalamic groove or notch
Cerebellum
Cerebrum
Chiari malformations
Choroid plexus

Dandy-Walker malformation
Ependyma
Extracorporeal membrane oxygenation (ECMO)
Falx cerebri
Fontanels
Germinal matrix
Holoprosencephaly
Hydrocephalus
Hypoxia

Increased intracranial pressure (ICP)
Intraventricular hemorrhage (IVH)
Mega cisterna magna
Meninges
Periventricular leukomalacia (PVL)
Sulcus
Tentorium cerebelli
Ventriculoperitoneal shunt

Neurosonography is the primary imaging modality for high-risk and unstable premature infants because it is portable, nonionizing, noninvasive, and can be tolerated by the sickest infants, even immediately after birth. Furthermore, it is safe when adhering to the ALARA (as low as reasonably achievable) principle and is without contraindications, thus allowing for serial imaging of brain maturation and lesion evolution. In the hands of a skilled sonographer or physician, it is a reliable tool for the detection of most hemorrhage cystic and ischemic brain lesions, structural brain anomalies, calcifications, and cerebral infections. Although some conditions are not treatable, neurosonography allows for the assessment of neurologic prognosis, which aids parental counseling, as well as decisions on the continuation of neonatal intensive care. Furthermore, it helps to optimize treatment of the infant and provides support to the family, both during and after the neonatal period.

Neurologic impairment is one of the primary health concerns for premature infants. Prematurity is defined as a birth occurring before term, or 37 weeks of gestation. Most infants in the late-preterm category (34 to 36 weeks' gestation) are often spared neurologic impairment, but the risk increases the more premature an infant is at birth (Table 27.1 for prematurity categories). Intraventricular and subependymal hemorrhages (SEHs) occur in 40% to 70% of premature neonates under 34 weeks of gestation. Multifocal necrosis of the white matter, referred to as periventricular leukomalacia (PVL), may develop in 12% to 20% of infants weighing less than 2000 g (5 lb, 5 oz). Additionally, any neonate who suffered a difficult delivery associated with **hypoxia** or **asphyxia** may be examined for PVL. These lesions are associated with increased mortality and abnormal neurologic outcomes.

This chapter provides an introduction to the neonatal head examination, and therefore the focus is on normal cranial anatomy, along with sonographic findings and protocols. Pathology in this chapter includes hydrocephalus, intracranial hemorrhage (ICH), hypoxic-ischemic lesions, congenital malformations, and infection in the neonate.

NORMAL ANATOMY AND SONOGRAPHIC FINDINGS

Knowledge of the normal cranial anatomy is essential to perform the neonatal head examination confidently. The cranial cavity contains the brain and its surrounding meninges and portions of the cranial nerves, arteries, veins, and venous sinuses. The following neonatal head structures and sonographic findings are provided to aid in performing neurosonography.

Fontanels

The **fontanels** are unossified spaces between the bones of the infant skull, allowing for compression at birth and rapid brain growth thereafter. Colloquially termed "soft spots," they provide the sonographer with acoustic windows, where the transducer is carefully placed to visualize and record brain structures (Fig. 27.1). It is important to note their closure, which heavily hampers or completely impairs sonographic imaging. Generally, an acoustic window becomes limited at the beginning of the respective fontanel closure timeframe. Furthermore, these timeframes are relative to a term neonate, and preterm infants will be adjusted according to their gestational age at birth (Box 27.1).

Neurosonography primarily utilizes the anterior and mastoid fontanels. The anterior fontanel is the largest at birth and provides an optimal sonographic view of the brain until 9 to 12 months of age, when it begins to close. This fontanel may remain open longer than the normal range in cases of prematurity, hydrocephalus, hypothyroidism, and some bone disorders and chromosomal abnormalities, such as trisomy 13, 18, and 21. If **hydrocephalus** is present, it is felt to be bulging. Compressed or overlapping fontanelles, on the other hand, due to oligohydramnios or a difficult delivery, may be difficult to palpate and provide a limited acoustic window to adequately image the structures of the brain.

TABLE 27.1	Preterm Infants, Gestational Age, and Preterm Birth Weight Categories	
Preterm Definition	**Gestational Age at Birth**	**Birth Weight Categories and Corresponding Median Gestational Ages**
Late preterm (or near-term)	34 to <37 weeks	• Most premature births occur during this stage and carry the lowest risk among preterm infants for morbidity and mortality. • LBW is defined as weighing <2500 g (5 lb, 8 oz) at birth. • Median GA weight of 2500 g at birth: 　• Male (35 weeks) 　• Female (35.5 weeks)
Moderately preterm	32 to <34 weeks	• Most births during this GA are below the LBW category, around 2000 g (5 lb, 5 oz). • Median GA weight of 2000 g at birth: 　• Male (33 weeks) 　• Female (33.5 weeks)
Very preterm	28 to <32 weeks	• VLBW is defined as weighing <1500 g (3 lb, 5 oz) at birth. • Median GA weight of 1500 g at birth: 　• Male (30.5 weeks) 　• Female (31 weeks)
Extremely preterm	<28 weeks	• ELBW is defined as weighing <1000 g (2 lb, 3 oz) at birth. • Median GA weight of 1000 g at birth: 　• Male (27.5 weeks) 　• Female (28 weeks)

Birth weights are representative of 50th percentile for gestational age.
ELBW, Extremely low birth weight; *GA*, gestational age; *LBW*, low birth weight; *VLBW*, very low birth weight.

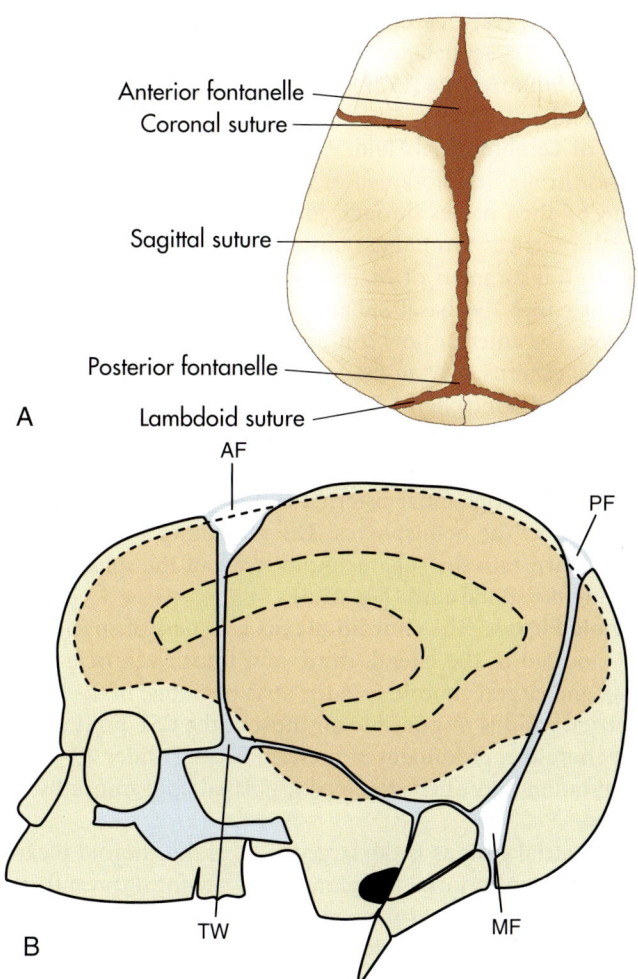

FIG. 27.1 Acoustic windows. (A) Top view of the neonatal skull showing the sutures and open anterior and posterior fontanel. (B) Sagittal view of the neonatal skull, showing the anterior fontanel (AF), posterior fontanel (PF), temporal window (TW) (or sphenoidal fontanel), and mastoid fontanel (MF).

BOX 27.1　Normal Fontanel Closure Timeframes

Anterior: 9–15 months (median, 13.8 months)
Mastoid: 6 and 18 months
Sphenoidal (temporal window): 6 months
Posterior: 8–12 weeks; some may be closed at birth

Meninges

There are three membranes called **meninges** that surround and form a protective covering for the brain: the dura mater, arachnoid mater, and pia mater. The pia mater, or "soft mother," lies against the delicate brain parenchyma; the arachnoid membrane is in the middle; and the dura mater, or "tough mother," is a double-layered outer membrane that forms the strongest barrier (Fig. 27.2).

Lying between the delicate pia mater and arachnoid mater, the subarachnoid space contains cerebrospinal fluid (CSF) and branches of the arteries and veins of the brain. The intercommunication between these vascular channels and the CSF plays an important role in the blood-brain barrier. It connects to the pia matter via the arachnoid trabeculae, and to the dura matter, via arachnoid granulations.

The **falx cerebri** is a fibrous structure composed of a double fold of dura mater, separating the right and left cerebral hemispheres. The **tentorium cerebelli** is an extension of the falx cerebri and separates the cerebrum from the cerebellum. Structures superior to this inverted echogenic V-shaped structure are supratentorial, and structures below it, infratentorial. The infratentorial structures of the brain are collectively referred to as the *posterior fossa*.

Ventricular System

The ventricular system is filled with CSF, which surrounds and protects the brain and spinal cord from physical impact. It also acts as a communication route for hormones and transmitters between areas of the central nervous system (CNS). The CSF-filled ventricular system includes the ventricles, their connecting foramina, and subarachnoid space, which are all contiguous with the central spinal column through the foramen magnum.
Lateral Ventricles. The lateral ventricles, located on either side of the brain, are the largest of the CSF-filled cavities located within the cerebral hemispheres and appear anechoic sonographically. The lateral ventricles are divided into four segments and are generally named after the lobe of the brain into which they project: the frontal horns, central body, temporal horns, and occipital horns. The body is the central section, just posterior to the frontal horn. The **atrium (or trigone) of the lateral ventricle** is the site where the body, occipital, and temporal horns join (Fig. 27.3).
Third and Fourth Ventricles. The lateral ventricles communicate with the third ventricle through paired foramina, individually referred to as the intraventricular foramen, or foramen of Monro. The third ventricle is a narrow, irregularly shaped opening, which sits inferior and midline between the lateral ventricles. The roof is formed by the corpus callosum. Often, the third ventricle is not visualized beyond 32 weeks of gestation. The cerebral aqueduct, or aqueduct of Sylvius, connects the third and fourth ventricles and is the narrowest passage. It is also the most common site for intraventricular blockage of CSF in the neonate.

The fourth ventricle is diamond-shaped and sits within the pons, or upper portion of the brain stem, between the cerebellar peduncles. Anteriorly, the lower floor surface is formed by the medulla oblongata. The roof is formed by the cerebellar vermis posteriorly. Three apertures allow the CSF to leave the fourth ventricle, one centrally and two laterally, into the subarachnoid cisterns. The lateral angles of the fourth ventricle form the foramina of Luschka, which drain into the lateral cerebellopontine cisterns. The inferior angle, the middle foramen of Magendie, drains into the cerebellomedullary cistern,

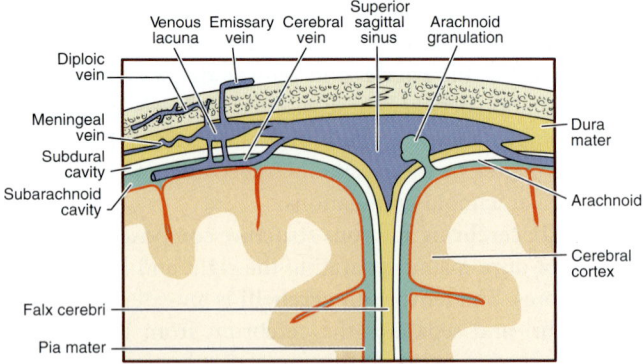

FIG. 27.2 Meningeal membranes. Coronal diagram showing the three meningeal layers (dura, arachnoid, and pia mater) and their cavities.

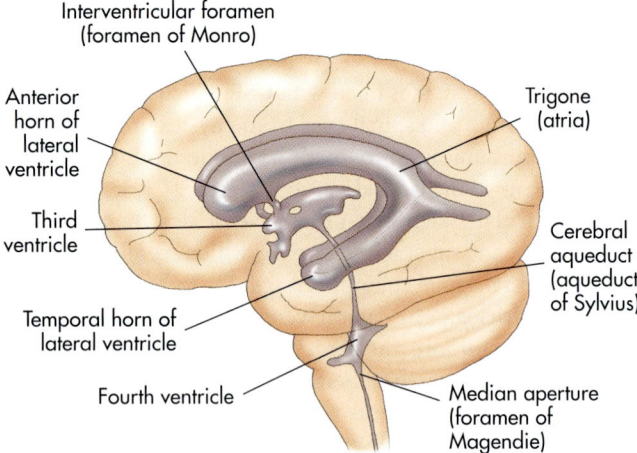

FIG. 27.3 Sagittal view of the ventricular system. Note the atria of the lateral ventricles angle out laterally from than the more medial frontal horns.

which is continuous with the cisterna magna and central canal of the spinal cord.

Subarachnoid Space and Cisterns. Like the ventricles, the subarachnoid space and cisterns also play a role in the flow of CSF. The narrow subarachnoid space surrounding the brain and spinal cord contains a small amount of CSF. The subarachnoid cisterns are the spaces at the base of the brain where the arachnoid becomes widely separated from the pia, giving rise to large cavities. The cisterna magna is one of the largest of these subarachnoid cisterns and is consistently seen with ultrasound, appearing anechoic; it is in the posterior fossa between the medulla oblongata, cerebellar hemispheres, and occipital bone.

Ventricular Size and Variants. The sonographer should be aware that ventricular size varies with gestational age, and the premature infant will normally have larger-appearing ventricles than the term infant. Also, dilation of the lateral ventricles often begins in the occipital horns. Minor asymmetry of the lateral ventricles is not uncommon, occurring in 20% to 40% of infants. The left side is often larger than the right. Another rarer variant is coarctation of the ventricle (Fig. 27.4), which will appear as a cyst in coronal view at the superior and lateral ventricle, often at the level of the intraventricular foramen. In both variant cases, care should be taken to make certain the cause is not a sequela, or sequential result, of an **intraventricular hemorrhage (IVH)**, such as ventricular dilation or a subependymal cyst.

Flow of Cerebrospinal Fluid. CSF from the lateral ventricles passes through the foramen of Monro to the third ventricle. The CSF then passes through the aqueduct of Sylvius to the fourth ventricle. From that point, the CSF may leave through the central foramen of Magendie or the lateral foramen of Luschka into the basal subarachnoid cisterns and cisterna magna. The anterior flow continues upward through the chiasmatic cisterns, sylvian fissure, and the pericallosal cisterns up over the hemispheres, where it is reabsorbed by the arachnoid granulations in the sagittal sinus. Posteriorly the CSF flow moves around the cerebelli, through the tentorial incisure, the quadrigeminal cistern, the posterior callosal cistern, and up over the hemispheres. The remaining small amount flows down into the subarachnoid space of the spinal canal, bathing the spinal cord (Fig. 27.5).

Choroid Plexus. The **choroid plexus** is a mass of specialized cells located in the lateral, third, and fourth ventricles. The main and largest choroid is in the atria (atriums) of the lateral ventricles and is responsible for most of the CSF production. The choroid is prominent in preterm infants under 25 weeks of gestation and often develops a normal appearance by 30 weeks.

The atrial glomus is the largest part of the choroid plexus and tapers posteriorly. The glomus is a site for intraventricular bleeding in the term neonate compared with the much more common intraventricular hemorrhage in the caudothalamic groove in premature infants. The periventricular blush, or white matter, is the area of parenchyma surrounding the lateral ventricle containing the glomus. It is a major site for hypoxic-ischemic injury. The choroid plexus should always appear more echogenic than the surrounding brain tissue (Fig. 27.6).

Other structures that produce CSF in the ventricular system include the intracranial and spinal subarachnoid lining. Additionally, the ventricles are lined with specialized **ependyma** that also produce CSF. These cells, along with the choroid plexus, regulate the normal intraventricular pressure by both secreting and absorbing CSF. However, in the setting of pathology, CSF production does not appreciably change, and absorption does not keep up, which may result in the ventricles enlarging, putting increased pressure on the brain parenchyma (intracranial pressure).

Cavum Septum Pellucidum (and Vergae). The cavum septum pellucidum (CSP) is a thin triangular space filled with CSF and lies between the anterior horn of the lateral ventricles and forms the floor of the corpus callosum. Thus, the CSP is inferior to the corpus callosum. The CSP is present at birth in 50% to 61% of normal neonates and often closes within the first 3 to 6 months of life. However, it may persist for life in some individuals. The cavum vergae is a posterior extension of the CSP and is often closed in term neonates. However, it may be seen in some preterm infants, as it normally closes around 6 months gestation.

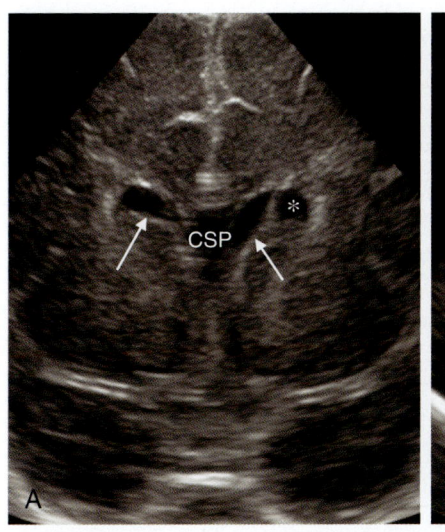
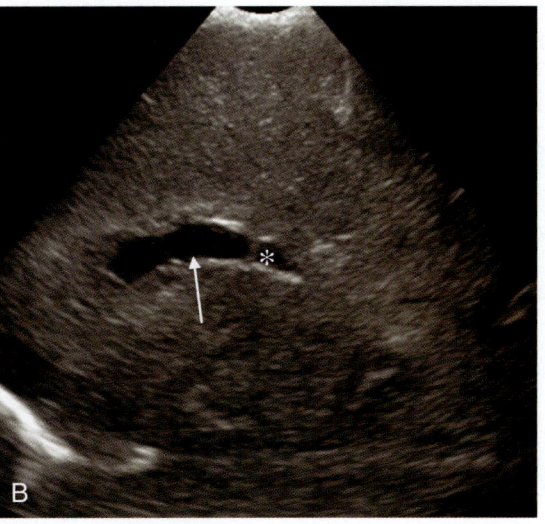

FIG. 27.4 Coarctation of the lateral ventricles. Seen at the level of the left intraventricular foramen. (A) Coronal view shows a cyst *(asterisk)* at the superolateral aspect of the left ventricle. *Arrows* point to the lateral ventricles. (B) Parasagittal view of the same ventricle demonstrates a large septation-like divide within the cavity posteriorly. *CSP,* Cavum septum pellucidum. (Courtesy Nationwide Children's Hospital, Columbus, OH.)

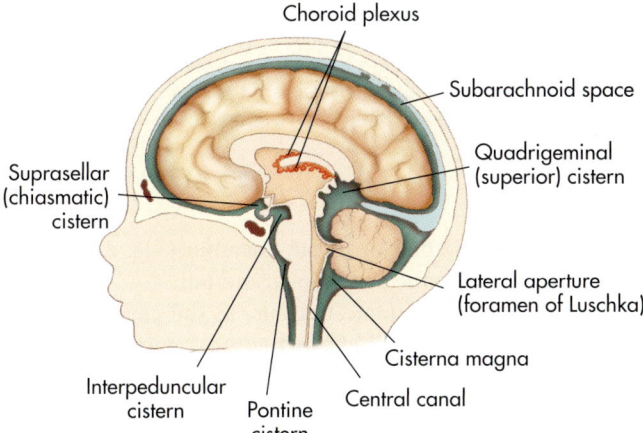

FIG. 27.5 Sagittal view outlining the subarachnoid space/cisterns. The subarachnoid cisterns of the ventricular system and the choroid plexus are shown.

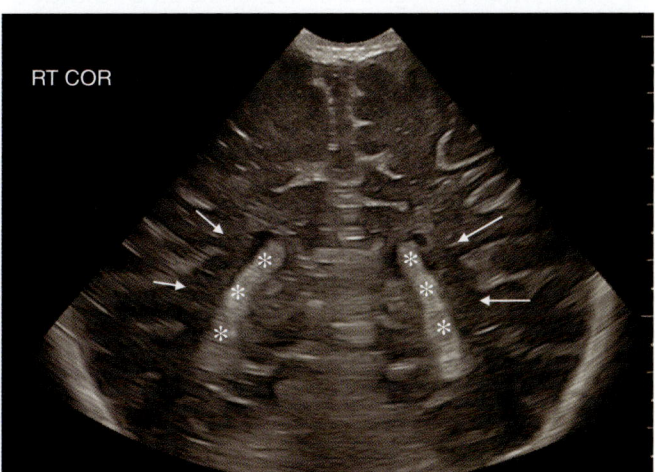

FIG. 27.6 Normal glomus of the choroid plexus. The choroid plexus glomi *(asterisks)* are prominent, seen here in a term 2-week-old on a posterior coronal sonogram. Note, the choroid is normally more echogenic in relation to the surrounding brain parenchyma or periventricular white matter *(arrows).* (Courtesy Nationwide Children's Hospital, Columbus, OH.)

Cerebrum

Cerebral Hemispheres. There are two cerebral hemispheres connected by the corpus callosum. They extend from the frontal to the occipital bones above the anterior and middle cranial fossae. Posteriorly, they extend above the tentorium cerebelli. They are separated by a longitudinal fissure into which the falx cerebri projects. The cerebrum consists of the gray and white matter. The outermost portion of the cerebrum is the cerebral cortex (composed of gray matter). White matter is located at the innermost portion of the cerebrum. The largest and densest bundle of white matter is the corpus callosum.

Lobes of the Brain. The cortex is divided into four sections or lobes. These lobes correspond to the cerebral cortex located under the cranial bone of the same name and include the frontal, parietal, occipital, and temporal lobes (Fig. 27.7).

Sulci and Gyri. The gyri are convolutions on the surface of the brain caused by infolding of the cortex. The **sulcus** is a groove or depression on the surface of the brain separating the gyri. The sulci further divide the hemispheres into frontal, parietal, occipital, and temporal lobes. Sulci and gyri development is heavily dependent on the age of an infant. Sulci develop first around 22 weeks of gestation, with most formed by 28 weeks. However, sulci are not detected sonographically until around 26 weeks, and extremely premature brains have a smooth appearance. The midline cingulate sulcus forms fully between 28 and 31 weeks of gestation. Gyral development occurs after sulci development, and even at 32 weeks, this may be seen as asymmetric, with the right side more advanced.

Fissures. The interhemispheric fissure is the area in which the falx cerebri sits and separates the two cerebral hemispheres. The sylvian fissure is located along the lateral-most aspect of the brain and is the area through which the middle cerebral artery courses (Fig. 27.8). The quadrigeminal fissure is located posterior and inferior to the cavum vergae. The vein of Galen is also posterior, so the sonographer must be aware that Doppler should be utilized to make sure it is a

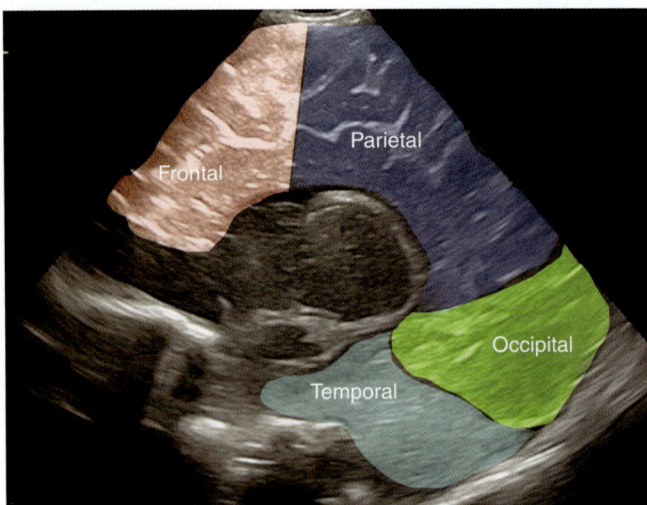

FIG. 27.7 Normal parasagittal view of the cerebrum. Parasagittal view showing the four lobes of the normal neonatal cerebrum. (Courtesy Nationwide Children's Hospital, Columbus, OH.)

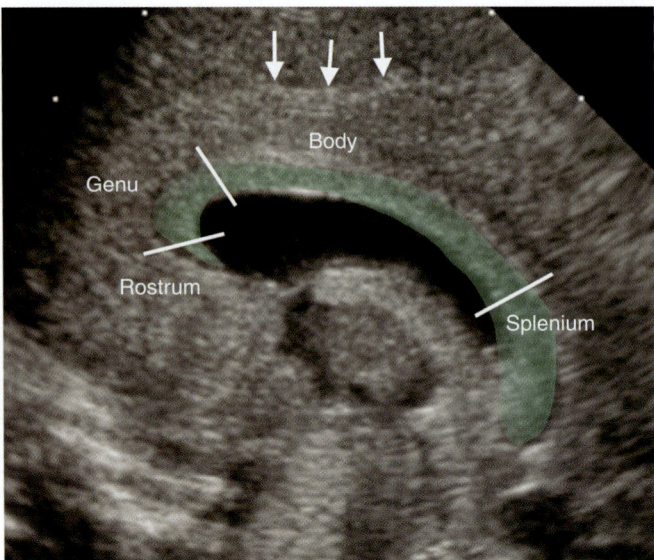

FIG. 27.9 Corpus callosum. Midsagittal image of the corpus callosum in an extremely premature infant. Note that it sits superior to the cavum septum pellucidum and posterior cavum vergae. The rostrum, genu, body, and splenium are identified. *Arrows* point to the underdeveloped cingulate sulcus. There is also a lack of gyri development in the brain parenchyma. (Courtesy Nationwide Children's Hospital, Columbus, OH.)

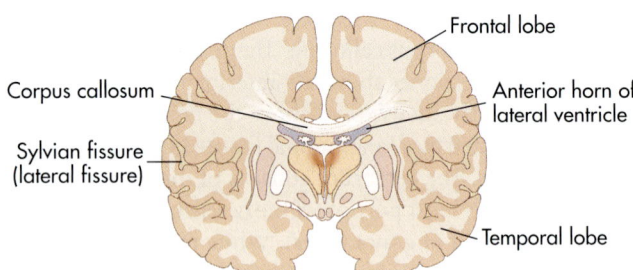

FIG. 27.8 Coronal cerebrum diagram. Coronal view of cerebral lobes, corpus callosum, anterior horns of the lateral ventricle, and sylvian fissures.

fissure, when prominent, and not a malformation of the vein of Galen.

Corpus Callosum. The corpus callosum forms broad bands of connecting fibers between the cerebral hemispheres. This structure forms the roof of the lateral ventricles. The corpus callosum sits superior to the CSP (Fig. 27.9). The development of the corpus callosum occurs between the 8th and 18th week of gestation, beginning ventrally and extending dorsally. The genu of the corpus callosum develops first, followed by the body and splenium (the posterior element). The rostrum develops last. If a uterine insult occurs, development may be partially arrested, or complete agenesis may occur. If partial, the genu will be preserved, whereas those portions that develop later will be absent. This is known as agenesis or dysgenesis of the corpus callosum, respectively.

Basal Ganglia

The basal ganglia are a collection of gray matter that includes the caudate nucleus, lentiform nucleus, claustrum, and thalamus. The caudate nucleus is the portion of the brain that forms the lateral borders of the frontal horns of the lateral ventricles and lies anterior to the thalamus (Fig. 27.10). It is further divided into the head, body, and tail.

The head of the caudate nucleus, at the **caudothalamic groove or notch** (Fig. 27.11), is the most common site for hemorrhage. The caudate nucleus and lentiform nucleus are the largest basal ganglia. They serve as relay stations between the thalamus and the cerebral cortex.

The thalamus consists of two ovoid, egg-shaped brain structures situated on either side of the third ventricle, superior to the brainstem. The thalamus borders the third ventricle and connects through the middle of the third ventricle by the massa intermedia, which is composed of gray matter and exists in most neonatal brains. The hypothalamus forms the floor of the third ventricle. The pituitary gland is connected to the hypothalamus by the infundibulum.

The **germinal matrix** includes periventricular tissue and the caudate nucleus. It is located 1 cm above the caudate nucleus in the floor of the lateral ventricle, at the caudothalamic groove. It sweeps from the frontal horn posteriorly into the temporal horn. It is indicated in 90% of premature brain bleeds and is made up of a highly vascular bed of delicate blood vessels, especially in infants under 34 weeks of gestation.

Brainstem

The **brainstem** is the part of the brain connecting the forebrain (cerebral hemispheres, thalamus, and hypothalamus) and the spinal cord. It consists of the midbrain, pons, and medulla oblongata.

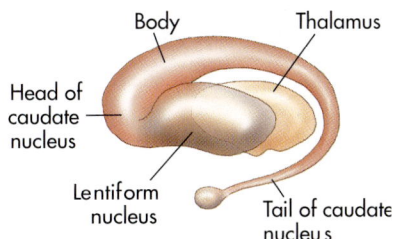

FIG. 27.10 Basal ganglia. Lateral view of the basal ganglia with the caudate nucleus.

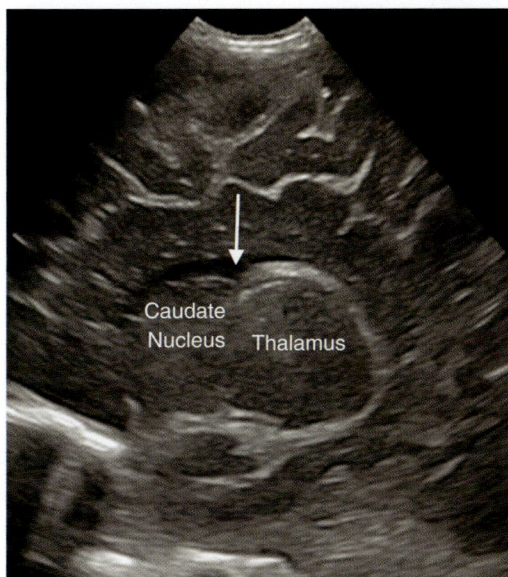

FIG. 27.11 Caudothalamic groove. Normal caudothalamic groove *(arrow)*, where the germinal matrix lies, which is a common site of hemorrhage in the premature infant. (Courtesy Nationwide Children's Hospital, Columbus, OH.)

Midbrain. The midbrain portion of the brain is narrow and connects the forebrain to the hindbrain. It consists of two halves called the cerebral peduncles, the cerebral aqueduct, the tectum, and the tegmentum.

Pons and Medulla Oblongata. The pons and medulla oblongata are part of the brainstem and hindbrain. The pons is found on the anterior surface of the cerebellum below the midbrain and above the medulla oblongata.

The medulla oblongata extends from the pons to the foramen magnum, where it continues as the spinal cord. This structure contains the fiber tracts between the brain and the spinal cord and the vital centers that regulate important internal activities of the body (heart rate, respiration, and blood pressure).

Cerebellum

The **cerebellum**, part of the hindbrain, is composed of two hemispheres that have a cauliflower-like appearance. The central cerebellar white matter is referred to as the *arbor vitae* ("tree of life") due to its appearance and function of bringing motor and sensory information to and from the cerebellum. The cerebellum lies in the posterior cranial fossa under the tentorium cerebelli. The two hemispheres are connected by the vermis.

Fig. 27.12 summarizes the major anatomy of the midline sagittal plane. Fig. 27.13 summarizes the major sonographic anatomy of the midsagittal view for both a term infant and an extremely premature infant. (Notice the development of the gyri and cingulate sulcus and lack of a cavum vergae pellucidum in the term neonate. Also, the structures are better visualized in the premature infant due to a wider anterior fontanel and more prominent ventricular system.)

Cerebrovascular System

The cerebrovascular system consists of the internal cerebral arteries, vertebral arteries, the circle of Willis, and its major branches. The anterior cerebral artery (ACA) is one such major branch of the circle of Willis and can be visualized in a midsagittal plane. Branches of the ACA are routinely evaluated and include the pericallosal artery and callosomarginal artery. The pericallosal artery is frequently used to evaluate blood flow to the infant brain, and, as the name suggests, it flows up and around the corpus callosum. The cerebrovascular system is discussed in more detail in Chapter 38.

EXAMINATION PREPARATION

For the premature or sick infant, most neurosonography examinations are performed portably in the neonatal intensive care unit. Only well, term, or older infants may be examined in the ultrasound laboratory, either on the examination table, in a car seat, or on the parent's lap. For inpatients, the sonographer must be aware of the infant's condition before the examination, and therefore should never begin an examination before first contacting the infant's nurse.

Two key concerns are keeping the premature infant both safe and warm. They can lose a potentially dangerous amount of body heat quickly, so a small amount of warm gel (ideally from an individual packet) should be used while scanning through the isolette portholes. If a large amount of cold gel is applied to the fontanel, or if the isolette is open for an extended period, the infant's temperature may drop, which will often set off the infant's thermal regulation (and alarms). Likewise, applying too much pressure while performing the examination may bring about bradycardia (and more alarms). Additionally, the sonographer should be acutely aware of any lifesaving wires, tubes (e.g., endotracheal tubes) and monitors, limit head and neck movement, and practice good infection control techniques to minimize the spread of disease in this vulnerable population.

Neurosonology is performed primarily through the anterior fontanel or easily felt "soft spot" on top of the head. If a good view is not readily obtained in the general area, palpating a fontanel beforehand may be helpful. Additionally, when possible, it is best to rest the hand to keep steady, even if just a single finger atop the infant's head is achievable. Performing the exam requires staying stationary over the scanning window, using only very small movements.

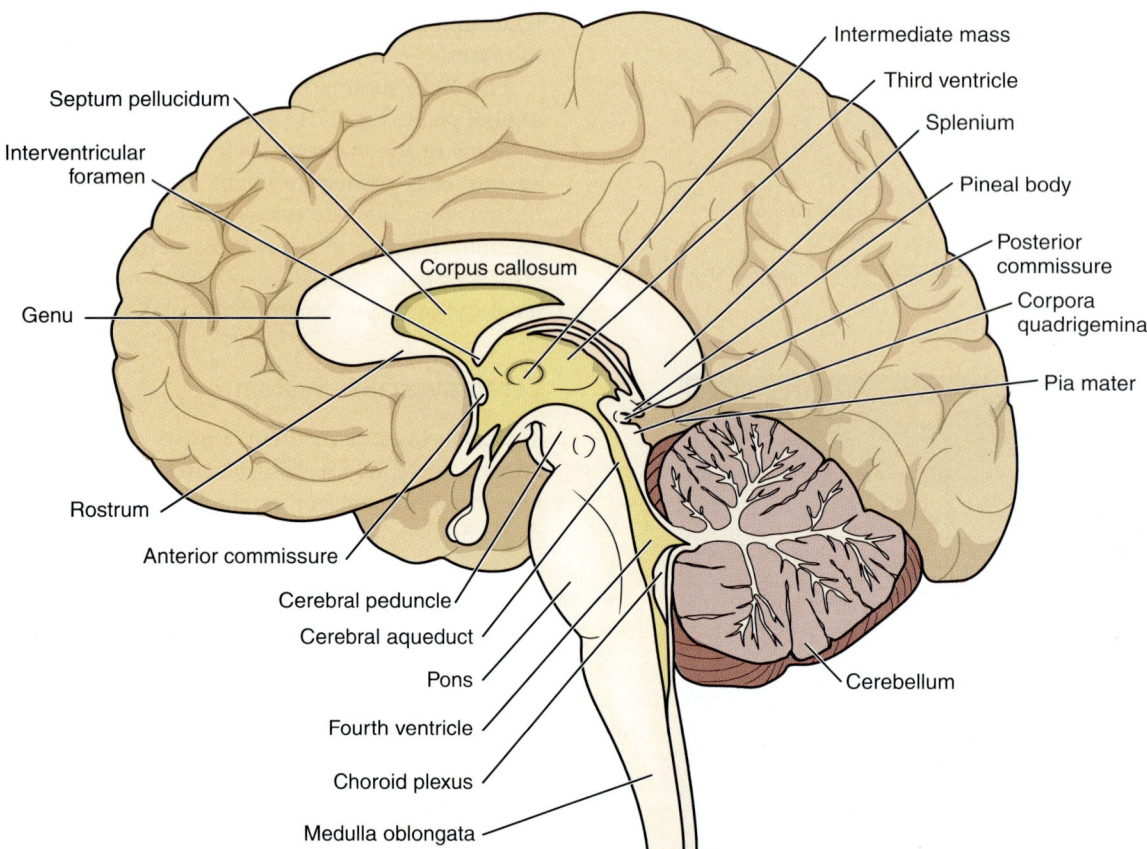

FIG. 27.12 Midsagittal brain anatomy. Midline sagittal view of the midline structures in the brain.

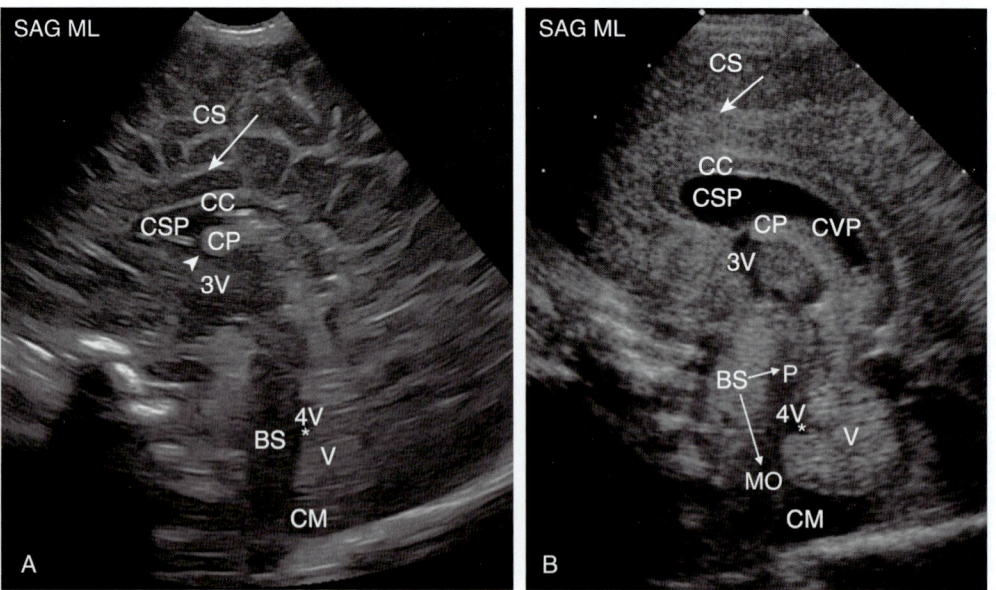

FIG. 27.13 Normal midsagittal brain anatomy in a term infant and extremely premature infant. View of the midline structures in both a term neonate (A) and an extremely premature infant (B). *Supratentorial structures:* cingulate sulcus (CS, *arrow*), corpus callosum (CC), cavum septum pellucidum (CSP), cavum vergae pellucidum (CVP), choroid plexus (CP), and third ventricle (3V, *arrowhead* in term infant). *Infratentorial structures:* brainstem (BS) (with *arrows* to the pons (P) and medulla oblongata (MO) in the premature infant), cerebellar vermis (V), cisterna magna (CM), and fourth ventricle (4V). (Courtesy Nationwide Children's Hospital, Columbus, OH.)

A curved-array or sector high-frequency transducer of 7 to 10 MHz is best for imaging most preterm infants and neonates, whereas lower frequencies of 5 to 7 MHz may be needed for older infants with closing fontanels or infants with thick hair. A 3- to 5-MHz transducer may also be necessary to visualize deeper structures.

More than one transducer is often necessary and recommended. First, a dedicated neonatal head probe will provide the much-desired small footprint and 110- to 130-degree angle needed to obtain excellent contact and brain visualization. Second, a small linear array, high-frequency transducer (10 to 15 MHz), with or without a standoff pad, may be used to image the extra-axial fluid space and any abnormalities in the near-field. Specialized settings with low grayscale contrast and multiple focal zones throughout the depth of the image help to optimize the lateral resolution of brain parenchyma to detect any subtle changes.

NEONATAL HEAD EXAMINATION

Overview of the Standard Evaluation

Sonography of the neonatal brain is initiated through the anterior fontanel in coronal and sagittal views to study the supratentorial and infratentorial compartments (Box 27.2). Since the structures in the infratentorial compartment are located relatively far from the transducer, the alteration of a deep focal placement and lowering the transducer frequency are recommended. In older infants, two transducers may be needed, one for the supratentorial structures and another for the infratentorial structures. The posterior cranial bones should always be present in the standard images to ensure the entire brain is being visualized.

The mastoid fontanel is used to better visualize the cerebellum and infratentorial compartment, or posterior fossa, in younger infants. Cine clips should be used when possible to show the coronal and sagittal sweeps through the neonatal head. Additional magnified views are also encouraged to provide better resolution of any abnormal or high-risk areas (e.g., the caudothalamic groove in a preterm infant). Color Doppler evaluation (and pulsed wave Doppler, when indicated) of the pericallosal artery in the midsagittal view is also encouraged.

Knowing the gestational age of the premature infant when performing a neonatal sonogram of the head is essential. Table 27.2 summarizes the general sonographic findings in the term versus preterm neonate.

Additional/Modified Evaluation

While the posterior fontanel is often not useful beyond the neonatal period, or first four 4 weeks of life, it can provide more up-close sagittal and coronal views of the occipital horns, periventricular blush, and cerebellum in premature infants and neonates. It may be used routinely in this population or when pathology is suspected. It may also be used if imaging is restricted due to overlapping bones in the area of the anterior fontanel. The posterior fontanel approach is most helpful for any critical neonate on **extracorporeal membrane oxygenation (ECMO)**, where the mastoid view may be unattainable.

Pathology should always be evaluated in multiple planes and with color and/or power and spectral Doppler. Additional views of pathology may be obtained from the posterior or mastoid fontanel, the foramen magnum, or thin areas over the temporal and parietal bones. Clot in the occipital horns is best evaluated from a posterior approach (mastoid or posterior fontanel), and the foramen magnum is useful to evaluate the proximal end of the spinal canal, often in the setting of known or suspected Chiari malformation (type I or II). Additionally, any open suture, burr hole, or craniotomy defect can also serve as an acoustic window.

High-frequency linear array transducers used in the near-field can identify superior sagittal sinus thrombosis, cerebral edema, and subdural hematomas or subdural abscess secondary to meningitis. It is also used in evaluating for possible craniosynostosis, holding it perpendicular to the anticipated course of the coronal, sagittal, lambdoid, and metopic sutures.

Finally, although standard protocols are provided, additional oblique or axial views are very helpful and encouraged. This is particularly true in patients with ventricular shunt tubes, in which oblique angles help to identify the shunt and tip. When clinically indicated, the circle of Willis and its major branches are evaluated with pulsed wave and color Doppler ultrasound from a transtemporal approach in determining cerebral blood flow patterns.

Advanced Techniques in Neurosonography

Three-dimensional (3D) sonography is showing promise as an emerging method in imaging the neonatal head. This technique can reduce inter-operator variability and significantly reduce the time required to perform a neurosonology examination (about 15 minutes down to 1 to 2 minutes.) Research shows this is achievable without compromising diagnostic quality in comparison to the standard two-dimensional approach. It also allows for later 3D reconstructions and may be useful in better evaluating brain anomalies. The 3D assessment of fluid volume in the setting of ventriculomegaly may be more accurate.

Additionally, ultrafast Doppler is a newer Doppler technique capable of quickly mapping cerebral vascular resistivity in neonates. It has superior temporal resolution, surpassing functional magnetic resonance imaging (MRI), sending out greater than 100,000 frames per second. For comparison, conventional color Doppler sends out around 50 frames per second. It has been called ultrasound angiography. It offers the evaluation of blood flow speed at a subcardiac cycle time scale, which other angiographic modalities are unable to assess. This may be useful for monitoring hypoxic-ischemic injuries (HIIs) in the future, as well as opening up knowledge about cerebrovascular regulation in infants in general.

BOX 27.2 Supratentorial and Infratentorial Structures

Supratentorial
Cerebral hemispheres
Basal ganglia
Lateral and third ventricles
Interhemispheric fissure
Subarachnoid space around the hemispheres

Infratentorial
Cerebellum
Brainstem
Fourth ventricle
Basal cisterns

TABLE 27.2	Term vs. Preterm Neonate Normal Sonographic Findings	
	Term (> 37 Weeks)	**Preterm (<37 Weeks)**
Sulci and gyri	• Well developed.	• Still developing or may be nearly absent in extremely preterm infants; also called the "smooth" brain appearance.
Ventricles	• Slit-like ventricles or width increasing from 2 mm AP at frontal horns to 3–6 mm AP maximum at trigone on coronal study. • Height of the bodies of the lateral ventricles is normally >7 mm AP at the level of mid-thalamus on a parasagittal study.	• Preterm infants, in general, will have larger appearing ventricles.
Third ventricle	• Not usually seen on the coronal study and may only be visualized as an echogenic formation immediately below the septum pellucidum.	• Prominent and easily seen in premature infants <32 weeks.
CSP	• Seen in 50%–61% of term neonates.	• Nearly always visualized in preterm infants.
Cavum vergae	• Not visualized.	• May be present in very preterm infants; seen as a posterior extention of the CSP.
Choroid plexus	• Between 30–40 weeks. • About 2–3 mm at the body of the lateral ventricles and 4–5 mm at the atria (or glomus).[a]	• Very large in extremely preterm infants (≤25 weeks); should not be mistaken for intraventricular hemorrhages. • Appearance similar to term neonate after 30 weeks.
Caudate nuclei	• Show isoechoic or low areas of echogenicity compared with surrounding brain parenchyma.	• Basal ganglia and thalami[b] may have a higher echogenicity than the surrounding brain parenchyma in preterm infants <32 weeks.
Periventricular white matter	• Has a low echogenicity, with thin echogenic streaks corresponding to small vessels. • Should be less echogenic than the choroid.	• Area[c] may show a slight increased echogenicity due to anisotropy in preterm infants. • Scanning from the posterior fontanel, this "blush" or "halo" should disappear.

[a]The glomus is a common site for intraventricular bleeding in the full-term neonate.
[b]Not to be confused with the caudothalamic groove, which is the most common site for intracranial hemorrhage, often in preterm infants <34 weeks.
[c]The periventricular area is where most white matter necrosis or periventricular leukomalacia occurs in the preterm infant.
AP, Anterior-posterior; *CSP*, cavum septum pellucidum.

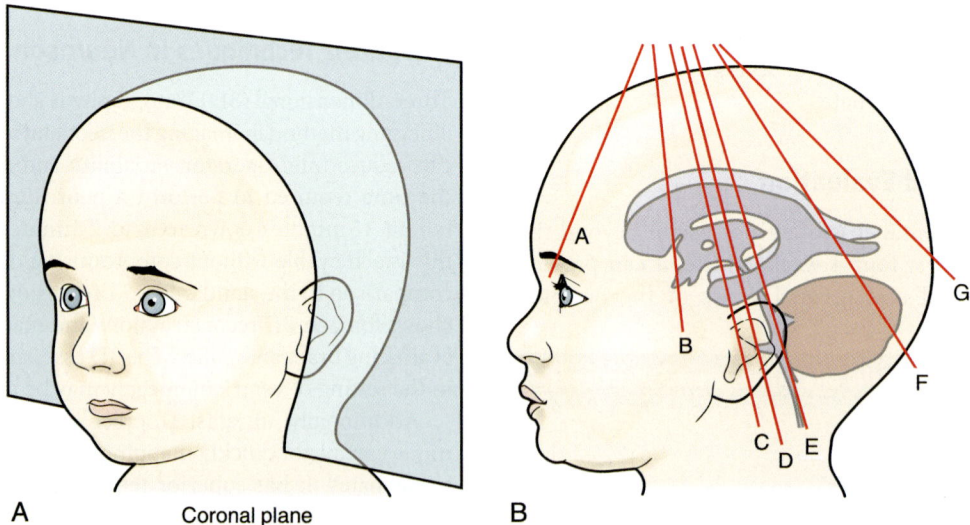

FIG. 27.14 Coronal scanning planes. (A) The transducer is placed on the anterior fontanel, perpendicular to the neonatal head, with the notch to the infant's right. (B) The transducer is angled from the anterior to the posterior skull as described in the text. A through G indicate the different coronal scanning planes. A is the most anterior, and G is the most posterior.

Contrast-enhanced ultrasound allows for detailed perfusion studies of the infant head in the setting of post-cardiac arrest. Finally, shear-wave and strain elastography are also emerging in providing more information about hypoxic-ischemic events and the periventricular gray-white matter softening that can follow. All the above techniques provide clinicians a portable, relatively low-cost, and quick evaluation without sedation, providing valuable

CHAPTER 27 Neonatal and Infant Head   823

TABLE 27.3 Coronal Study Protocol With Anatomy

Coronal Protocol (Corresponds to Images A–I in Fig. 27.15)	Labeled Anatomic Structures (**Bold Numbers** Also Correspond to Sagittal Image Structures)	
A. Level of the Orbits		
• Orbits are deep in the skull base, showing the frontal lobes and anterior interhemispheric fissure.	1. Interhemispheric fissure 2. Frontal lobe	3. Orbits 4. Skull
B. Level of the Frontal Horns and CSP		
• Frontal horns of the lateral ventricles and interhemispheric fissure. • The corpus callosum is seen just anterior to the fluid-filled CSP, which is between the two frontal horns. The head of the caudate nucleus is also seen.	1. Interhemispheric fissure 2. Frontal lobe 5. Frontal horn of lateral ventricle 6. Caudate nucleus (area of caudothalamic groove, *arrows* on image)	7. Thalamus 8. Sylvian fissure 9. Temporal lobe 10. CSP 11. Corpus callosum
C. Level of the Third Ventricle		
• Third ventricle is just below the echogenic anterior choroid plexus. Intraventricular foramen (of Monro) is also seen at the point where the lateral ventricles and third ventricle communicate. • Temporal lobes are visualized posteriorly.	1. Interhemispheric fissure 2. Frontal lobe 5. Frontal horn of lateral ventricle 6. Caudate nucleus 8. Sylvian fissure	9. Temporal lobe 12. Intraventricular foramen (of Monro) 13. Third ventricle 14. Cingulate sulcus 15. Anterior choroid plexus in the roof of the third ventricle *(asterisk)*
D. Level of the Third Ventricle (Angled Posteriorly)		
• Echogenic anterior choroid plexus seen in the roof of the third ventricle. Third ventricle may not be directly visualized in a full-term infant. • Brainstem is visualized posteriorly.	1. Interhemispheric fissure 2. Frontal lobe 5. Frontal horn of lateral ventricle 6. Caudate nucleus 8. Sylvian fissure 9. Temporal lobe	14. Cingulate sulcus 15. Anterior choroid plexus *(asterisk)* 16. Thalamus 18. Hippocampal fissure 19. Mesencephalic aqueduct 21. Pons 22. Medulla oblongata
E. Level of the Cerebellum		
• Thalami seen anterior to the quadrigeminal cistern (echogenic star shape). • Tentorium is visualized, with echogenic vermis and cerebellum underneath. Cisterna magna is anechoic.	1. Interhemispheric fissure 7. Thalamus 8. Sylvian fissure 9. Temporal lobe 15. Choroid plexus 17. Body of lateral ventricle	20. Parietal lobe 23. Tentorium *(arrows)* 24. Cerebellar vermis 25. Cerebellar hemispheres 26. Cisterna magna 27. Quadrigeminal cistern
F. Level of the Choroid Plexus		
• Choroid plexus glomi within the trigones of the lateral ventricles and periventricular white matter.	1. Interhemispheric fissure 9. Temporal lobe 15. Choroid plexus	20. Parietal lobe 28. Trigone of the lateral ventricle 29. Periventricular white matter
G. Level of the Occipital Lobes		
• Periventricular white matter (periventricular blush), gyri and sulci of occipital lobe, and posterior interhemispheric fissure.	1. Interhemispheric fissure 20. Parietal lobe	29. Periventricular white matter 30. Occipital lobe
H. Off-Axis Views of Cerebral Hemispheres/Pathology		
• Extra views, especially in the setting of pathology. • Tilted views from side to side. Image as much of the superficial peripheral surface of the cerebral hemispheres as possible.	1. Interhemispheric fissure 6. Caudate nucleus (*arrows* point to a bleed within the caudate, seen as echogenic as the choroid)	15. Choroid plexus (*long arrow* to small cyst within the choroid) 20. Parietal lobe
I. Magnification View of Extra-axial Spaces		
• Evaluate the extra-axial fluid spaces using a high-frequency linear transducer at the level of the frontal horns, separated by the CSP. • Include peripheral structures, such as the superior sagittal sinus. • Measure fluid as shown: (1) craniocortical distance, (2) sinocortical distance, and (3) width of the interhemispheric fissure (see Box 27.3).	1. Interhemispheric fissure 5. Frontal horn of lateral ventricle 10. CSP 31. Sagittal sinus (transverse view of the vein; *asterisk*)	

CSP, Cavum septum pellucidum.

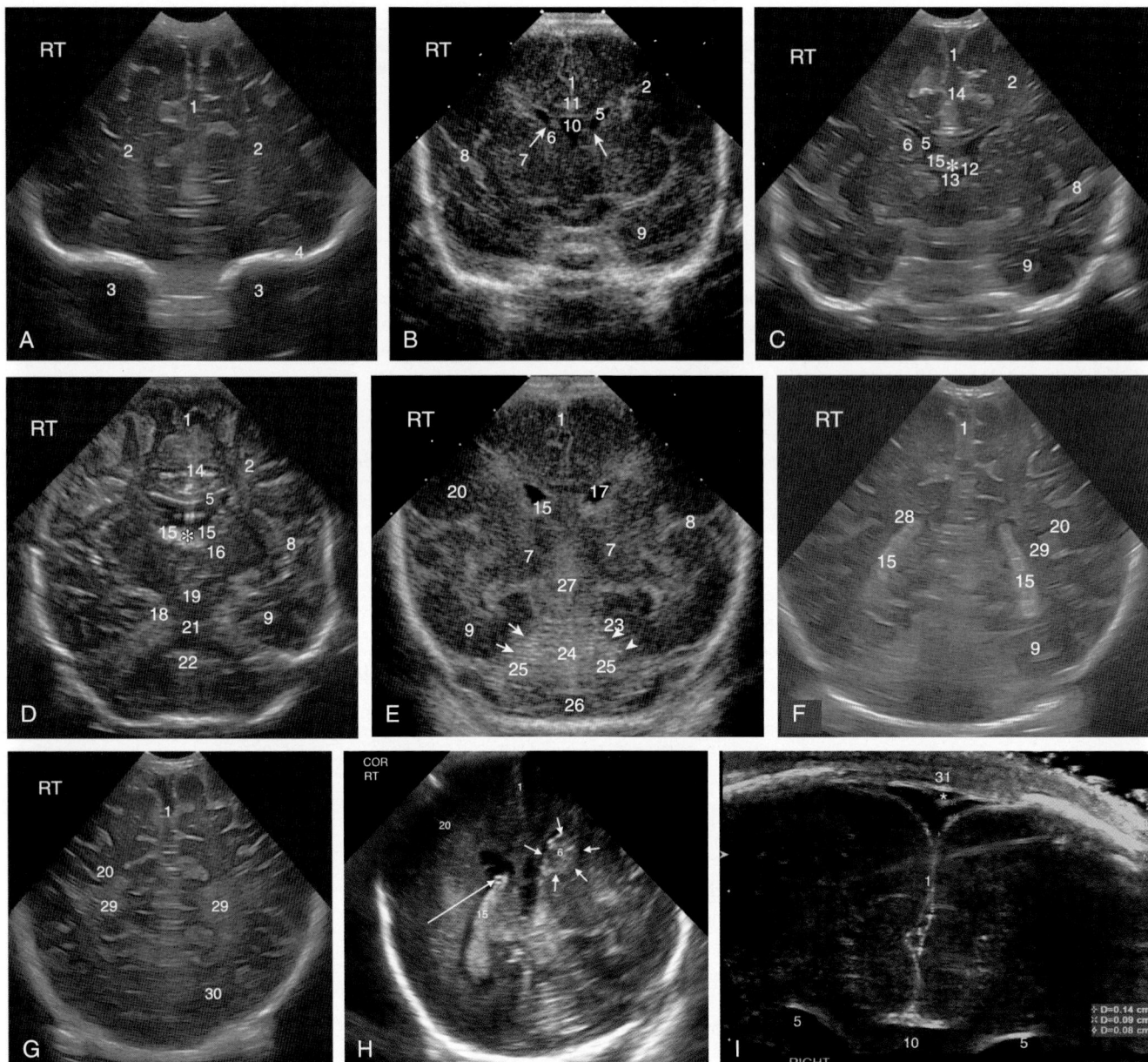

FIG. 27.15 Coronal protocol images. Normal protocol for coronal images beginning with the transducer angled toward the anterior skull (orbits) and fanning posteriorly. Images A–I correspond to Table 27.3, and structures correspond to the numbers labeled here. Images B and E are from a premature infant, and the remainder are from a term neonate. Image H shows an off-axis view to better evaluate pathology (*arrows*) in an extremely premature neonate. Image I was taken with a high-frequency linear array transducer. (A–G, Courtesy Nationwide Children's Hospital, Columbus, OH. H–I, Courtesy Chester County Hospital, West Chester, PA.)

information, which may be used in serial monitoring of pathology.

Coronal Study

To obtain the coronal views, the transducer is placed with the notch to the infant's right side on the anterior fontanel with the scanning plane following the coronal suture. When looking at the coronal sections, the vertex of the skull is at the top, and the left side of the brain is to the right of the image and should be annotated as such. The middle of the transducer must be centered in the coronal suture to reduce bone interference and to procure the most extensive image of the brain.

Symmetric images must be obtained; this is accomplished by using the skull bones and the middle cerebral arteries at the sylvian fissure as landmarks. The skull bones and the arteries should be the same size bilaterally. In the coronal plane, the transducer is angled from the anterior to the posterior skull to completely visualize the lateral and third ventricles, the deep subcortical white matter, the basal ganglia, as well as the peripheral brain parenchyma. The coronal view orientation and angles are summarized in Fig. 27.14, with corresponding protocol images and annotations found in Fig. 27.15 and Table 27.3, respectively.

Evaluation of the Lateral Ventricles. When the transducer is angled anteriorly, the frontal horns of the lateral

TABLE 27.4	Sagittal Study Protocol With Anatomy[a]	
Sagittal Protocol (Corresponds to Images A–F in Fig. 27.17)	**Labeled Anatomic Structures (Bold Numbers Also Correspond to Coronal Image Structures)**	
A. Midline Sagittal View • Midline structures include the corpus callosum, cavum septum pellucidum, third and fourth ventricles, cerebral aqueduct, and cingulate sulcus. • Inferiorly, includes the brainstem, cerebellar vermis (tentorium), and cisterna magna.	1. Massa intermedia 2. Frontal lobe 4. Skull 10. CSP 11. Corpus callosum 13. Third ventricle 14. Cingulate sulcus	19. Mesencephalic aqueduct 21. Pons 22. Medulla 23. Fourth ventricle 24. Cerebellar vermis 26. Cisterna magna 27. Quadrigeminal cistern 30. Occipital lobe
A. Midline Sagittal View With Color Doppler • Color Doppler images demonstrate the branches of the anterior cerebral artery. • Pulsed Doppler may be taken at this level, as indicated, often in the setting of suspected hypoxia-ischemia.	See Fig. 27.18	
B. Level of the Caudothalamic Groove • Parasagittal view of the caudothalamic groove (notch). • Preterm infants as a hypoechoic structure inferior to middle choroid.	2. Frontal lobe 5. Frontal horn of lateral ventricle 6. Caudate nucleus (area of caudothalamic groove, *arrow*)	7. Thalamus 15. Choroid plexus 17. Body of lateral ventricle 20. Parietal lobe 30. Occipital lobe
C. Level of Lateral Ventricles and Choroid Plexus • Parasagittal view of choroid plexus through the body of the lateral ventricle. The periventricular white matter should also be demonstrated.	7. Thalamus 9. Temporal lobe 15. Choroid plexus 17. Body of lateral ventricle 18. Hippocampal fissure	25. Cerebellar hemispheres 28. Trigone of the lateral ventricle 29. Periventricular white matter 30. Occipital lobe
D. Level of the Sylvian Fissure and Insula • Lateral-most required parasagittal angle shows brain parenchyma lateral to the ventricles; should include sylvian fissure and pulsations from the middle cerebral artery. • Shows periventricular regions (deep white matter).	2. Frontal lobe 3. Insula 8. Sylvian fissure 9. Temporal lobe	20. Parietal lobe 29. Periventricular white matter 30. Occipital lobe
E. Level of the Lateral-Most Brain Parenchyma • A common extra parasagittal view, past the sylvian fissure, demonstrating gyri development in the neonatal brain.		
F. Magnification View of Extra-axial Spaces • View with a high-frequency linear transducer. Document color flow within the superior sagittal sinus, as needed. • Note any color fill defects and report any clot; this is a critical finding.	31. Sagittal sinus (sagittal view of the vein, *arrows*)	
Additional Views if Necessary • Any additional parasagittal views necessary to include all parts of the lateral ventricles.		

[a]Performed on both the right and the left sides.
CSP, Cavum septum pellucidum.

ventricles appear as slit-like hypoechoic or cystic formations. As the transducer is angled posteriorly, the ventricles acquire a comma-like shape, and their width increases from the frontal horns to the atria or trigone. The choroid plexus is an echogenic structure inside the ventricular cavities surrounding the thalamic nuclei. It lies along the floor of the lateral ventricles, extending from the temporal horn into the atrium and body of the lateral ventricles. It should not appear extending anterior into the frontal horns or posterior into the occipital horns. Increased hyperechoic areas in the floor of the ventricles, anterior to the third ventricle, would indicate hemorrhage at the caudothalamic groove.

Evaluation of the Third Ventricle and Choroids. At the intraventricular foramen, the choroid plexus enters the third ventricle. The choroid plexus becomes enlarged at the level of the atria (glomus of the choroid plexus) and can almost entirely fill the ventricular cavity.

The third ventricle is not well visualized in the normal coronal study in the term neonate. An off-axis approach and high-frequency transducer may be helpful to identify

826 CHAPTER 27 Neonatal and Infant Head

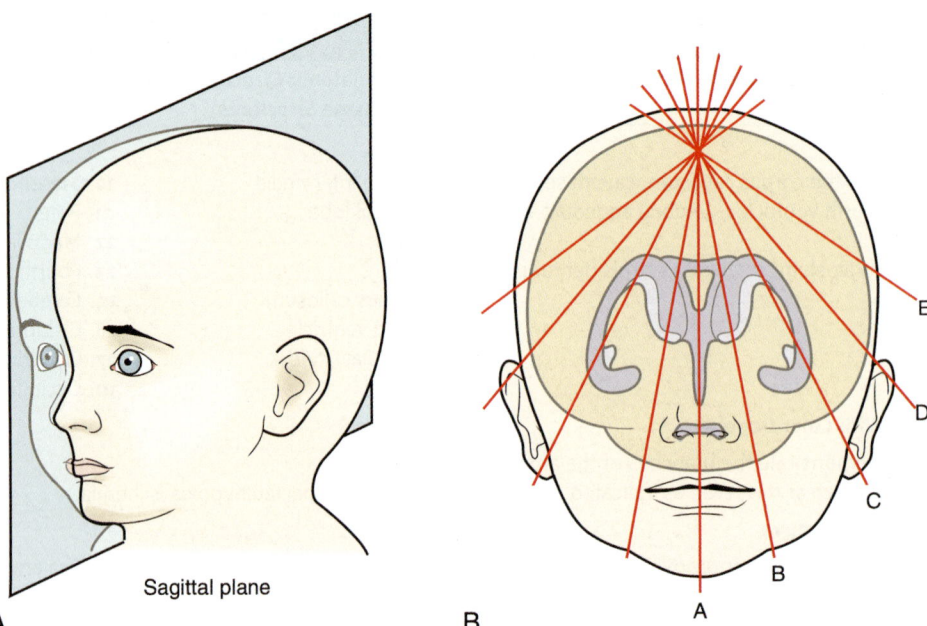

FIG. 27.16 Sagittal scanning planes. (A) The transducer is placed on the anterior fontanel, perpendicular to the skull, and rotated 90 degrees from the coronal plane to the sagittal plane, with the notch to the infant's nose. The transducer uses the midsagittal plane as the primary landmark; slight angulation of the transducer away from the midline will show the parasagittal planes. (B) Line *A* indicates the midline sagittal plane, and the other lines indicate the lateral sagittal or parasagittal planes.

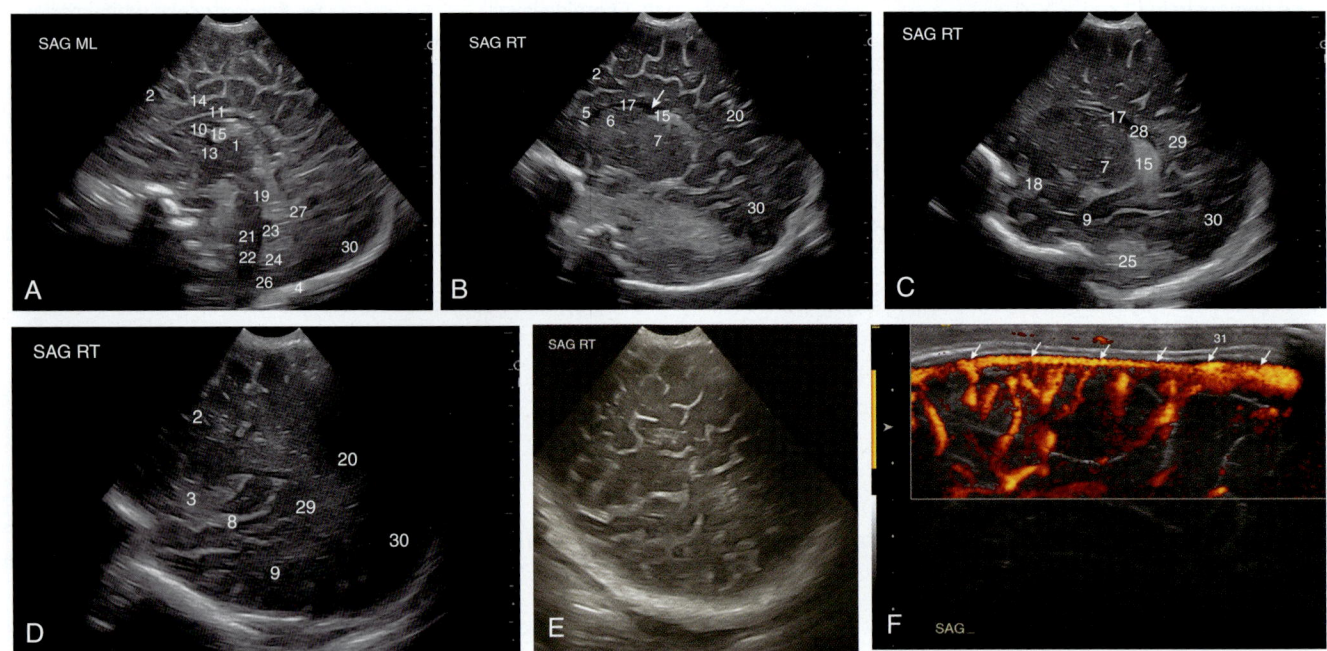

FIG. 27.17 Sagittal protocol images. Normal protocol for sagittal images beginning with the transducer midline parallel to the skull and then angling obliquely to one side and then the other (only the right side is shown). Images A–F correspond to Table 27.4, and structures correspond to numbers labeled here on a term neonate. Image F was taken with a high-frequency linear array transducer with power Doppler. (A–E, Courtesy Nationwide Children's Hospital, Columbus, OH. F, Courtesy Chester County Hospital, West Chester, PA.)

it. Occasionally, a thin and very echogenic formation can be seen in the midline immediately below the septum pellucidum. This echogenic image corresponds to the choroid plexus extending into the roof of the third ventricle.

Evaluation of the Cavum Septum Pellucidum. The septum pellucidum appears as a midline hypoechoic cystic structure separating the bodies and frontal horns of the lateral ventricles. The CSP appears inferior to the corpus callosum. In extremely premature infants, it may be visualized with the extension of the posterior cavum vergae. In some term and older infants, the CSP may be completely absent.

Evaluation of the Deep White Matter. Coronal and modified coronal views also visualize the basal ganglia and the white matter. The white matter has low echogenicity with thin echogenic streaks that correspond to small vessels. In premature infants this area is known as a *watershed zone*, or terminal ends of the vessel bed, and may be used to describe the periventricular white matter or periventricular blush. This area should be evaluated carefully. The echogenicity should never be greater than that of the choroid plexus; if it is, hemorrhage or infarction should be suspected, and follow-up studies are required.

Evaluation of the Cerebellum. The cerebellar vermis is a very echogenic structure, seen deep in the midline. The fourth ventricle appears in the midline as a small anechoic space located anteriorly to the vermis and is not always seen in the coronal view. The cerebellar hemispheres are contiguous with the vermis. The cisterna magna corresponds to the anechoic space between the vermis, the cerebellar hemispheres, and the occipital bone. The mastoid study provides better resolution in evaluating these structures.

Sagittal Study

The sagittal study is made by rotating the coronal plane approximately 90 degrees, positioned over the anterior fontanel, and aligning with the sagittal suture. These sections are viewed with the anterior brain to the left and the occipital portion of the brain to the right. Sagittal studies provide the most extensive visualization of the brain.

The straight sagittal view should be obtained first and may be used as a guide to stay in axis and determine whether a parasagittal study corresponds to the right or left side. The sonographer must always be careful to properly annotate the images right, left, and midline. Protocol for the sagittal view is often dependent on sonographer or physician preference. One may start midline and scan out to the right, back to center, and then out to the left; or one may start laterally, often the right side, and fan sequentially through to the lateral-most left side. If obtaining a cine clip sweep; the latter may be faster. The sagittal view orientation and angles are summarized in Fig. 27.16, with corresponding protocol images found in Figs. 27.17 and 27.18, with anatomical annotations in Table 27.4.

Midline Sagittal View. The straight midsagittal view is critical and can rule out many midline anomalies. The study shows the midline structures in the supratentorial and infratentorial compartments. Supratentorially, the corpus callosum appears as two thin hyperechoic parallel lines separated by a thin hypoechoic space. The cingulate sulcus is found anterior and parallel to the corpus callosum. It may be less defined in the preterm infant. The septum pellucidum appears as an anechoic (cystic) structure immediately below the corpus callosum. The third ventricle is normally anechoic and is located inferiorly to the CSP anteriorly. The echogenic choroid plexus appears to enter the top of the third ventricle through the foramen of Monro.

Infratentorially, in the straight or midline sagittal plane, the vermis of the cerebellum appears as a very echo dense

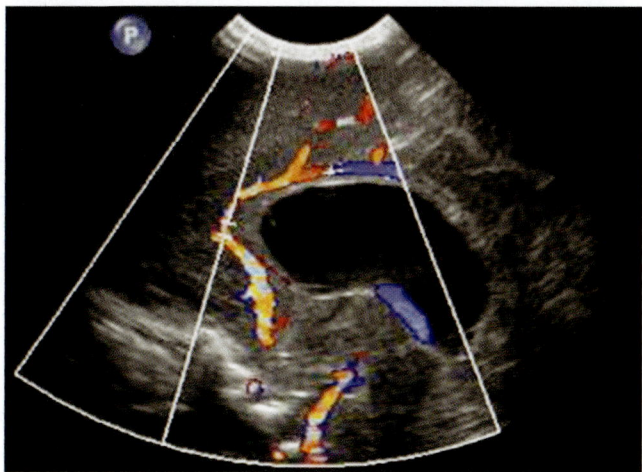

FIG. 27.18 Midsagittal color Doppler. Color Doppler of the anterior cerebral artery and pericallosal artery branch in the midline sagittal view seen coursing over the corpus callosum. Spectral Doppler gate placement is also shown. This 12-day-old extremely preterm neonate demonstrates a large cavum septum and cavum vergae pellucidum. (Courtesy Nationwide Children's Hospital, Columbus, OH.)

formation, separated from the occipital bone by an anechoic space corresponding to the cisterna magna. The other cisterns also are anechoic spaces located above and behind the cerebellar vermis. The fourth ventricle appears as a small sideways "V" with the vertex oriented posteriorly inside the echogenic vermis. The fourth ventricle is limited anteriorly by the brainstem. The brainstem has low echogenicity, with an echodense anterior border demarcated by the basilar artery.

Finally, the pericallosal artery, a branch of the ACA, may be seen with color Doppler, shown in Fig. 27.18 with spectral Doppler gate placement.

Parasagittal Views. After having studied the midline, the sonographer obtains parasagittal by angling the transducer to the right or left side of the skull. Four parasagittal studies should be performed at minimum, and often more are taken at the caudothalamic groove and at the very lateral brain parenchyma. The first parasagittal image should be close to the midline to visualize the caudate nuclei in detail because SEHs begin in the germinal matrix that is located at the caudothalamic groove. These views image the frontal horn and body of the lateral ventricles, the thalamus, the head of the caudate nucleus, and the choroid plexus. The frontal horns of the lateral ventricles appear as narrow sonolucent cavities. The choroid plexus ends at the caudothalamic groove and appears as an echogenic structure (2 to 3 mm high) lying against the thalamus.

The second parasagittal image is made slightly lateral to the first image and includes the entire ventricular cavity. Because the ventricular cavity is not entirely parallel to the midline (i.e., the posterior horns are more lateral or external than the anterior horns), the transducer must be rotated slightly to form an acute angle with the sagittal suture anteriorly. These views show the entire ventricular horns; the choroid plexus, including the glomus; the thalami; the caudate nuclei; and the white matter superior and posterior to the lateral ventricles.

The third parasagittal view images the white matter located lateral (externally) to the lateral ventricles. This view is useful for studying intraparenchymal hemorrhages (IPHs), porencephaly, and PVL. It will also demonstrate the sylvian fissure, middle cerebral artery, and insula. The insula is considered by some to be the fifth brain lobe, and it remains open until 24 to 26 weeks of gestation.

The fourth parasagittal view depicts the very lateral brain parenchyma. However, more views are often required to fully evaluate the lateral ventricles completely, and more are taken showing the caudothalamic grove, including magnified images, which is always encouraged.

Posterior Fossa Study

The integration of the mastoid view of the posterior fossa (infratentorial compartment) in the routine neonatal head examination increases the detection of congenital anomalies relating to the third and fourth ventricles, as well as the cerebellum. Furthermore, the detection of cerebellar hemorrhages is very limited from the anterior fontanel approach, and this view better visualizes and defines these bleeds.

The transducer is placed just behind the ear after gently bending the auricle forward. If the transducer notch is pointing upward in a vertical position, this will correspond to a coronal plane, whereas if the notch is turned to the right in a horizontal position, it will correspond to a transverse or axial plane.

The side of the head being examined should be clearly annotated, and often one side will clearly visualize both cerebellar hemispheres. However, in the case of difficult visualization of the opposite cerebellar hemisphere, both mastoid fontanels may need to be examined. In the coronal view, the fourth ventricle should not be larger than half the size of the vermis (Fig. 27.19). As with any interrogation, the sonographer should make sure to sweep through the entire viewable area.

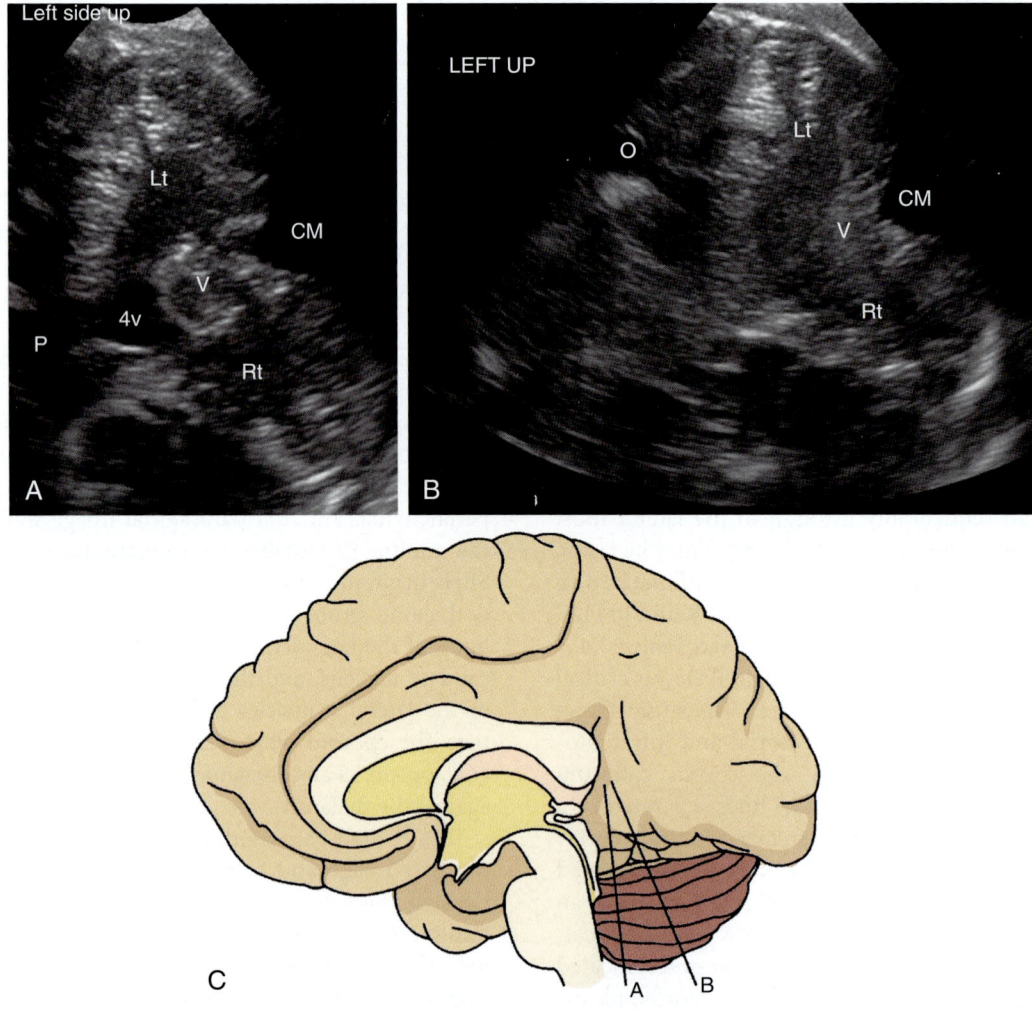

FIG. 27.19 Posterior fossa study. Evaluation from the mastoid fontanel shows the normal cauliflower-like appearance of the cerebellum. Annotation indicates this image was taken from the left mastoid fontanel. Vermis (V), right (Rt) and left (Lt) cerebellar hemispheres, and pons (P). (A) View at the level of the fourth ventricle (4v) and cisterna magna (CM). (B) A more posterior view can also show the occipital horns (O) of the lateral ventricles. (C) Diagram of the coronal views (A and B) from the mastoid fontanel. (A–B, Courtesy Nationwide Children's Hospital, Columbus, OH.)

HYDROCEPHALUS (VENTRICULOMEGALY)

Ventriculomegaly is the most common disorder of the neonatal brain and is marked by the dilation of the ventricular system. Ventricular enlargement may be caused by a variety of conditions leading to the obstruction, overproduction, or decreased absorption of CSF. Often, regarding the neonatal brain, the terms *ventriculomegaly* and *hydrocephalus* are used interchangeably. Differing definitions of hydrocephalus have emerged, and it may be defined as ventricular enlargement caused by obstruction or when increased intracranial pressure (ICP) is present. Nevertheless, hydrocephalus puts neonates at high risk for brain parenchyma loss and subsequent neurodevelopmental impairment.

Neonates may be diagnosed with ventriculomegaly or hydrocephalus in utero or may present clinically with a bulging anterior fontanel and/or macrocephaly. However, initial ventricular dilation occurs without changes in the head circumference, and hydrocephalus may be silent because the white matter of newborn infants is very compliant and easily compressed as the ventricles widen. The head circumference starts to enlarge only after significant compression of the white matter has developed. Therefore, screening and sequential neonatal head sonography for infants at risk play an important role in diagnosing ventricular dilation in the silent phase, as well as determining underlying etiology.

Hydrocephalus may be acquired or congenital. Acquired hydrocephalus may result from CSF obstruction from an ICH, also known as posthemorrhagic hydrocephalus (PHH), when severe dilation occurs or after the loss of deep white matter in PVL. Ex vacuo hydrocephalus describes the dilation of ventricles due to parenchymal loss and can be caused by either ICH or PVL. Congenital hydrocephalus occurs before birth and may be due to structural malformations or congenital brain infections. In general, the earlier that hydrocephalus occurs in utero, the greater the enlargement of the neonatal head.

Hydrocephalus is divided into communicating and noncommunicating forms. The latter is also referred to as obstructive hydrocephalus and is characterized by blockage of the CSF anywhere within the ventricular system itself, causing subsequent enlargement of the ventricular cavities *proximal to the obstruction*. The most common cause of both acquired and congenital hydrocephalus is **aqueductal stenosis**. The aqueduct of Sylvius, situated in the midbrain, is narrowed or replaced by multiple small channels with blind ends. Occasionally, aqueductal stenosis may be caused by extrinsic lesions posterior to the brainstem, such as congenital aneurysm of the vein of Galen or brain tumors. Congenital brain tumors (which have been defined from birth to 12 months) are quite rare of all pediatric brain tumors, with neuroblastomas making up the largest majority at 26%.

In communicating hydrocephalus, the CSF pathways are open within the ventricular system, but there is either decreased absorption via occluded arachnoid granulations or overproduction of CSF. Hydrocephalus is infrequently caused by overproduction of fluid. Excessive fluid production may occur in infants with papilloma of the choroid plexus, a tumor that actively secretes CSF.

Sonographic Findings. The sonographer should look for the blunting of the outer angles of the lateral ventricles (Fig. 27.20). In the setting of aqueductal stenosis, there is a widening of the lateral and third ventricles, with a normal-size fourth ventricle. If the hydrocephalus is very large, the posterior fossa is smaller than usual, and the cerebellum is displaced toward the occipital bone with the disappearance of the cisterna magna. However, the cerebellum is not dislodged into the foramen magnum, thus differentiating aqueductal stenosis from the Arnold-Chiari and Dandy-Walker malformations.

Ultrasound is very useful both during and after **ventriculoperitoneal shunt** placements to access tip placement and monitor the drainage of the dilated ventricle. These shunts are placed in the ventricles, routed through the body, and typically drain in the lower abdomen. Shunts are often seen as echogenic bright parallel lines in a long-axis view and echogenic foci in the short-axis view. In a decompressed ventricle, they will have a distal shadow.

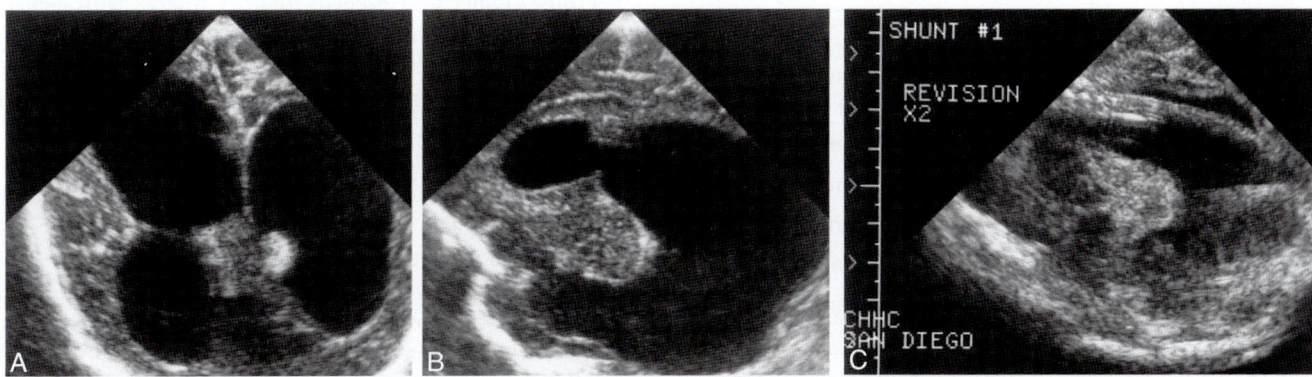

FIG. 27.20 Severe hydrocephalus with ventriculoperitoneal shunt. A 4-month-old infant with hydrocephalus shows gross dilation of the lateral ventricles. (A) Coronal view. (B) Sagittal view. (C) Follow-up study after ventriculoperitoneal shunt placement shows shunt tubing in place for drainage of the cerebrospinal fluid. This sagittal view shows the start of some decompression of the lateral ventricle.

Increased Intracranial Pressure. Of particular concern in the neonate with hydrocephalus is the development of **increased intracranial pressure (ICP)**, which is the cause of, or result of, brain injury. Increased ICP restricts cerebral blood flow and is a serious medical condition. Increased ICP, bradycardia, and apnea may follow days or weeks after the onset of ventricular dilation. The drainage of CSF via a ventricular shunt or reservoir plays a central role in treatment. Serial sonography aids in this therapeutic decision using both ventricular measurements and spectral Doppler assessment.

Ventricular Measurements. The four most reproducible ventricular biometric measurements are the ventricular index (VI), anterior horn width (AHW), frontal temporal horn ratio (FTHR), and thalamo-occipital distance (TOD).

1. *The ventricular index* measurements are taken at the level of the third ventricle in a coronal view, with VI measured at the widest point to the falx (Fig. 27.21). The VI is the most commonly used metric and shows a considerable increase with maturation (Table 27.5). These absolute VI measurements alone are very useful in determining the degree of ventricular dilation present.

2. *Anterior horn width* is also measured from the same coronal view as the VI. The AHW is measured across the widest point of the ventricle at a diagonal (Fig. 27.22A). AHW, regardless of gestational age, over 4 mm may indicate dilation.

3. Additionally, from this same coronal view at the level of the third ventricle, the *frontal temporal horn ratio* may be calculated = bilateral frontal horn dimension + biooccipital horn dimension/2 × biparietal calvarial dimension. The bifrontal horn dimension is measured at the greatest width across both frontal horns, the biparietal calvarium is measured from the greatest width of one side of the calvarium to the other, and the biparietal occipital horn is measured at the greatest transverse dimension of the occipital horn anterior to the brainstem (see Fig. 27.22B).

   The FTHR value has been shown to have excellent interrater reliability and concordance with MRI of the same ratio and is a reliable index to follow ventriculomegaly.

4. Finally, the *thalamo-occipital distance* (TOD) is taken from a parasagittal view and is measured from the outermost part of the occipital horn to the junction of the choroid with the outermost part of the thalamus (Fig. 27.23). Some will also measure the midbody height at the level of the thalamus from a parasagittal view or the AHW, which is the anterior-posterior measurement in a coronal view. Preterm infants with a TOD measurement over 19 mm and term infants with a TOD over 21 mm may indicate ventricular dilation.

Measurements beyond the normative 95th percentile represent ventricular dilation. Sonographers should be aware that head position within 3 hours of a positioning change could affect measurements. These measurements help to define ventricular enlargement in the premature and term neonate, but it is unclear at what degree ventricular dilation is associated with ICP, although a VI measurement 4 mm above the 97th percentile for gestational age may be a strong indicator for therapeutic intervention. Additional measurements at the third and fourth ventricle, as well as Doppler assessment, are helpful.

Spectral Doppler Measurements. Hemodynamic changes showing increased blood flow resistance may be recorded by spectral Doppler and used to identify infants with elevated ICP. A tracing from the pericallosal artery, the most distal portion of the anterior cerebral artery (ACA), is obtained from the anterior fontanel. If a reversal of flow already exists, this is an indication of elevated ICP, and fontanel pressure is not recommended. If no reversal is detected, light pressure is applied to the anterior fontanel. A reversal of flow in diastole with pressure is also an indication, and no resistive index (RI) measurement is needed (Fig. 27.24).

Often, though, the RI is measured at a state with and without pressure, annotated for clarity. An RI change greater than 0.1 above the baseline is indicated in elevated ICP.

While performing this technique, prolonged pressure (greater than 3 to 5 seconds) is not recommended and may cause bradycardia. Also, any change in thermal regulation or

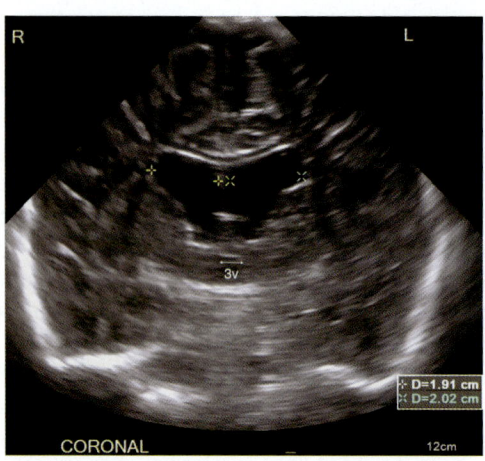

FIG. 27.21 Ventricular index. A 4-month-old with macrocephaly showed mildly dilated lateral ventricles and mild dilation *(double arrow)* within the third ventricle (3v), which should appear slit-like at this age. Coronal image at the level of the third ventricle shows the ventricular index measurement being taken bilaterally from the widest point of the frontal horn to the falx. The head ultrasound also revealed increased extra-axial fluid. (Courtesy Chester County Hospital, West Chester, PA.)

TABLE 27.5	Ventricular Index for Select Gestational Ages	
Gestational Age	Mean[a] (0–6 Days)	97.5th Percentile[b] (0–6 Days)
26 weeks	8.5–8.7 mm	10.1–10.3 mm
30 weeks	9.5–9.7 mm	11.2–11.4 mm
34 weeks	10.4–10.6 mm	12.3–12.5 mm
38 weeks	11.3–11.4 mm	13.3–13.5 mm
42 weeks	11.7–11.8 mm	13.8–14.0 mm

[a]Mean calculation = $0.550280 + (0.359138 \times GA) + (-0.002034 \times GA^2)$
[b]97.5th percentile calculation = $0.642056 + (0.424486 \times GA) + (-0.002409 \times GA^2)$
Data from Brouwer MJ, De Vries LS, Groenendaal F, et al. New reference values for the neonatal cerebral ventricles. *Radiology.* 2012;262(1):224–233.

desaturation in the neonate during normal compression is a signal to remove pressure immediately, and this should be reported, as it is likely an indication of elevated ICP.

Extra-axial Spaces. The extra-axial spaces are evaluated routinely for increased extra-axial fluid. Color Doppler is utilized to show the normal cortical vasculature within the subarachnoid space, crossing through the CSF.

Previously referred to as "benign" extra-axial fluid or benign external hydrocephalus, evidence is emerging in linking increased extra-axial fluid to autism spectrum disorder

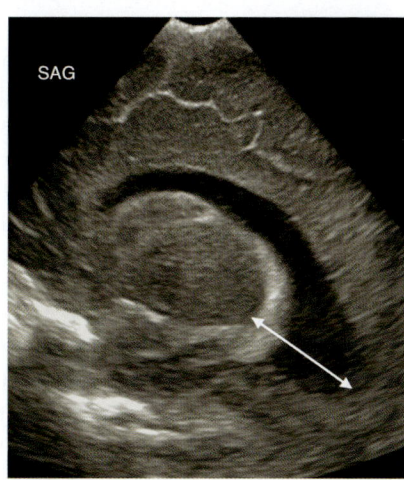

FIG. 27.23 **Parasagittal view demonstrates thalamo-occipital distance.** Measurement shown by the *arrow*. (Courtesy Nationwide Children's Hospital, Columbus, OH.)

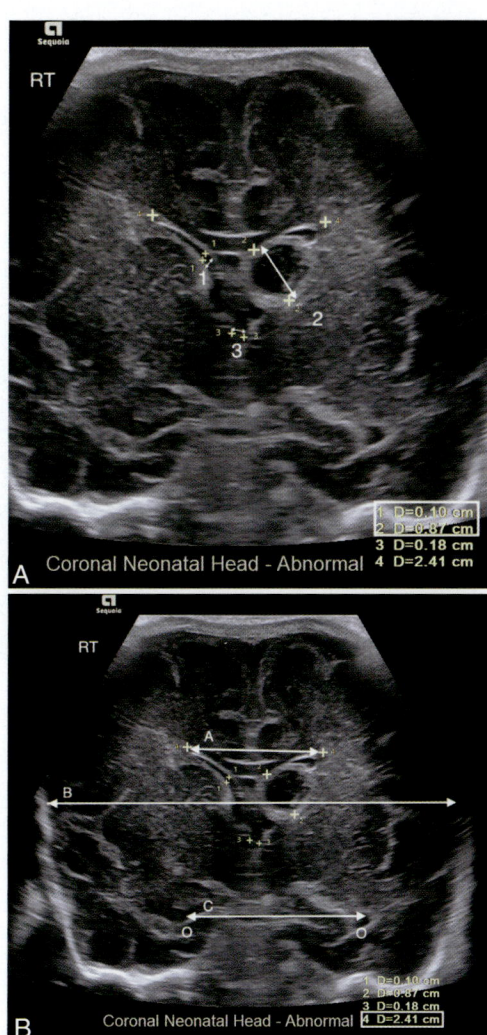

FIG. 27.22 **Anterior horn width and frontal temporal horn ratio.** Coronal view at the level of the third ventricle in a premature infant shows a resolving left bleed and subsequent dilation of the affected frontal horn of the lateral ventricle. (A) Anterior horn width (AHW) is measured bilaterally. The right side AHW *(arrow 1)* is very small and normal, while the left side AHW *(arrow 2)* is mildly dilated at almost 9 mm (normal, <4 mm). The third ventricle is also shown here measured side to side *(arrow 3)*. Often this measurement is used for follow-up studies. (B) The frontal temporal horn ratio is derived from three measurements across the ventricles and brain in the coronal view. The bifrontal horn dimension is shown with *arrow A* and measures 2.4 cm. The biparietal calvarium is indicated by *arrow B*, and the biparietal occipital horn is *arrow C*. The occipital horns in this infant are not distended and marked (O) just below them. (Courtesy Siemens Healthineers USA, Inc.)

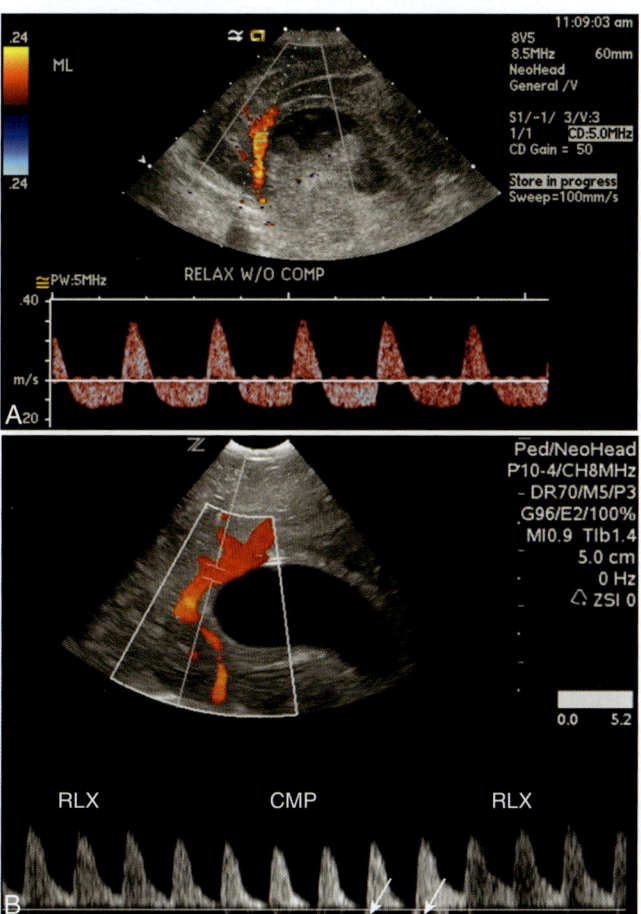

FIG. 27.24 **Spectral Doppler to evaluate for increased intracranial pressure.** Spectral Doppler of the pericallosal artery in the presence of hydrocephaly to evaluate for intracranial pressure (ICP). (A) Neonate with bilateral grade IV hemorrhage and a diffusely echogenic and swollen brain demonstrates reversal of diastolic flow without compression, indicating elevated ICP. (B) Premature infant with bilateral periventricular leukomalacia shows an absence of diastolic flow with compression on the anterior fontanel. The small bit of reversal of flow shown with *arrows* indicates ICP is increasing. *CMP*, With transducer compression; *RLX*, with relaxation. (Courtesy Nationwide Children's Hospital, Columbus, OH.)

(ASD). Furthermore, as fluid volume increases, there is a correlating decrease in the thickness of the cortical surface. It is hypothesized that immature arachnoid granulations in infancy may cause CSF to accumulate in the subarachnoid space. The arachnoid granulations only form at birth and develop until 18 months. Before birth, lymphatic pathways are utilized; this drainage also continues throughout the neonatal period. Twenty percent more extra-axial fluid may be detected in infants with ASD over normal infants at 6 to 9 months, 33% greater fluid at 12 to 15 months, and 22% greater fluid at 18 to 24 months. Infants and toddlers who have the longest persistent extra-axial fluid are at the greatest risk. Sonographically, a transcranial approach has been used to show increased extra-axial spaces in children with ASD.

The extra-axial space may also be evaluated for critical results after a brain injury or meningitis, resulting in thrombosis in the superior sagittal sinus, cerebral edema, and subdural hematoma. Furthermore, a subdural abscess may form secondary to meningitis. While uncommon, all these findings can be life threatening.

Sonographic Findings. In the setting of increased extra-axial fluid, the craniocortical distance, sinocortical distance, and interhemispheric fissure width measurements will all increase (Box 27.3 and Fig. 27.25A). If cortical vessels are seen passing through the superficial fluid, also known as the cerebral cortical vein sign, it suggests a subarachnoid fluid collection (see Fig. 27.25B).

An acutely threatening subdural collection, on the other hand, would show vessels along the periphery. This is not definitive; care must be taken to evaluate for debris or compressed vessels posteriorly, which may suggest a subdural bleed, even in the presence of the cortical vein sign. Furthermore, the superior sagittal sinus should demonstrate blood flow and be free from clot. A sagittal view is best to further investigate this vessel for venous thrombus. Power Doppler may be helpful to detect the low blood flow in the area (see Fig. 27.17F).

ACQUIRED BRAIN LESIONS

Sonography is ideal for timing the onset and sequentially following the evolution of brain lesions that may develop in the premature infant.

BOX 27.3 Extra-Axial Fluid Measurements

Craniocortical distance: measured in the straight AP dimension from the cranium to the edge of the cerebral cortex
Sinocortical distance: measured from the outer edge of the sagittal sinus in an oblique AP angle to the edge of the cerebral cortex
Interhemispheric fissure width: measured across (width) at the widest gap in the interhemispheric fissure. All measurements are taken at the level of the frontal horns and cavum septum pellucidum.

AP, Anterior-posterior.

Intracranial Hemorrhage

The premature neonate is at the greatest risk for ICH, and it is a major cause of mortality and morbidity (cerebral palsy) in this population. The *germinal matrix–intraventricular hemorrhage* (GM-IVH) is the most common hemorrhagic lesion in preterm neonates. They are also known as subependymal hemorrhages (SEHs). They affect 40% to 70% of infants less than 34 weeks of gestation, with an increased risk in infants less than 32 weeks of gestation or weighing less than 1500 g at birth. ICH is rare beyond the first week of life, with most bleeds occurring within the first 3 days.

ICH is a developmental disease that originates in the subependymal germinal matrix and can spread throughout the ventricular system in the worst case, into the parenchyma. The four grades of ICH are described in Box 27.4. Sonography is the most reliable technique to diagnose and follow changes in intraventricular clots and ventricle size. ICHs may resolve

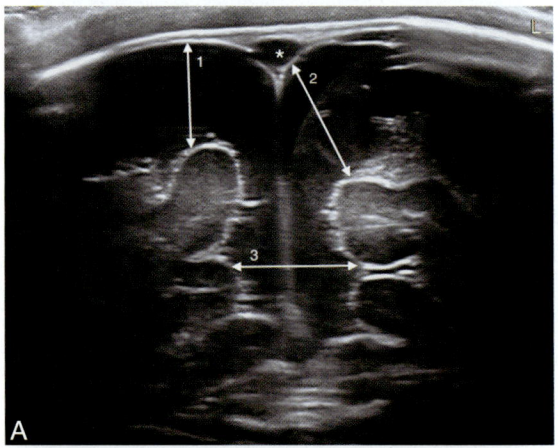
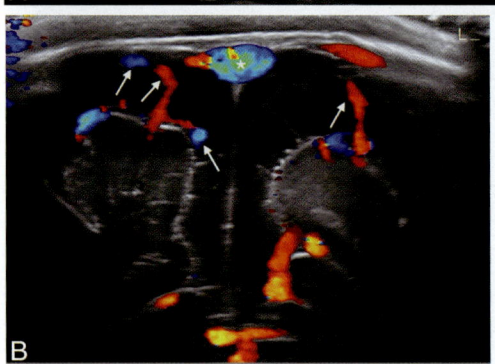

FIG. 27.25 Extra-axial fluid measurements and cerebral cortical vein sign. Coronal image with a high-resolution linear transducer demonstrates increased extra-axial fluid in an infant with macrocephaly. (A) Fluid is seen enlarging the space between the cerebral cortex and the cranium. The interhemispheric fissure also widens as it fills with extra-axial cerebrospinal fluid. Measurements show the craniocortical distance *(arrow 1)*, sinocortical distance *(arrow 2)*, and width of the interhemispheric fissure *(arrow 3)*. Note that subarachnoid and subdural fluid collections cannot be differentiated with gray-scale imaging alone. The superior sagittal sinus *(asterisk)* is seen anteriorly. (B) Cortical vessels *(arrows)* are seen coursing through the fluid on color Doppler, demonstrating the cerebral cortical vein sign. The superior sagittal sinus is shown here in cross-section *(asterisk)* and should also be evaluated for patency. It will not fill with color Doppler in the presence of thrombus. (Courtesy Chester County Hospital, West Chester, PA.)

in several days or weeks, depending on the size of the bleed and on the individual patient.

ICH changes in appearance over time, and in the acute stage, it will have an echogenicity equal to or greater than the choroid plexus. These ICHs are easily detected with ultrasound as echogenic structures because fluid and clotted blood have higher acoustic impedance than the brain parenchyma and the CSF. As the clot lyses, it will become hypoechoic or cystic centrally, with the periphery still echogenic. Therefore the degree of echogenicity will depend on the acute-chronic process of the hemorrhage.

Grade I: Germinal Matrix/Subependymal Hemorrhages. SEHs are caused by capillary bleeding in the germinal matrix. The germinal matrix is the tissue where neurons and glial cells develop before migrating from the subventricular (subependymal) region to the cortex. The germinal matrix is highly cellular, has poor connective supporting tissue, and is richly vascularized with very thin, fragile capillaries, which explains the high frequency of these hemorrhages in tiny infants. By 24 weeks of gestation, most of the neuronal and glial migration has occurred; however, pockets of germinal matrix remain until 40 weeks of gestation in the subependymal area at the head of the caudate nuclei. The most frequent location is at the caudothalamic groove. These lesions are not associated with any morbidity or mortality.

Sonographic Findings. A germinal matrix hemorrhage is usually seen at the caudothalamic notch as a very echogenic lesion pushing up the floor and external wall of the lateral ventricle with partial obliteration of the ventricular cavity. An untrained eye may miss small germinal matrix bleeds (Fig. 27.26).

Subependymal Cysts. These are most commonly the result of the sequelae of germinal matrix hemorrhage in premature infants. These present as discrete cysts in the lining of the ventricles and are seen as a smooth-walled spherical cyst in the lateral ventricle at the caudothalamic groove where there was a previous clot.

Grades II and III: Intraventricular Hemorrhage. The germinal matrix or subependymal hemorrhage can extend by continuous bleeding and perforate the ventricular wall with partial or total flooding of the ventricular system (Fig. 27.27), known as a grade II IVH. Depending on the amount of blood, the ventricle can become full and dilated. If dilation occurs, it is said to be a grade III IVH. Subsequently, the IVH may obstruct the circulation and absorption of the CSF, causing the ventricles to dilate further with CSF and ultimately resulting in post-hemorrhagic hydrocephalus, where intervention is required. This complication occurs in approximately 35% of infants with large hemorrhages. Mild to moderate ventricular dilation usually resolves spontaneously.

BOX 27.4 Intracranial Ventricular Hemorrhage Classification

Grade I: GM/subependymal hemorrhage only
Grade II: IVH without ventricular enlargement
Grade III: IVH with ventricular enlargement
Grade IV: IVH with intraparenchymal hemorrhage (with or without ventricular enlargement)

ªGrade I may also be referred to as a GM hemorrhage.
GM, Germinal matrix; *IVH*, intraventricular hemorrhage.

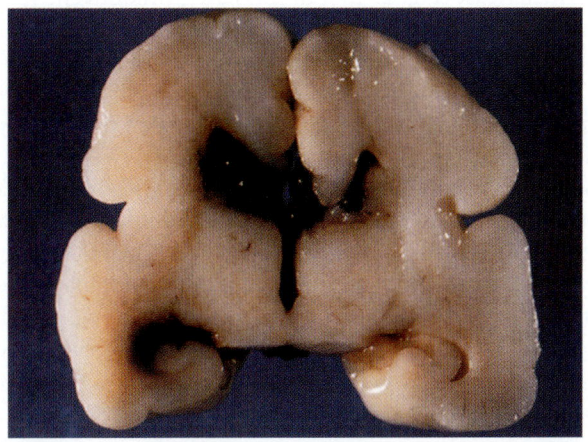

FIG. 27.27 **Intraventricular hemorrhage** specimen. Subependymal hemorrhage extending into the ventricles, containing coagulated blood.

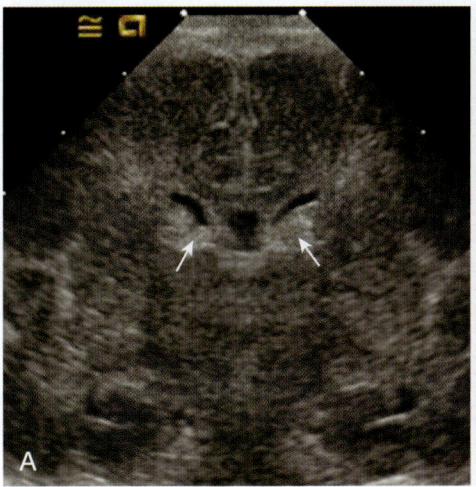
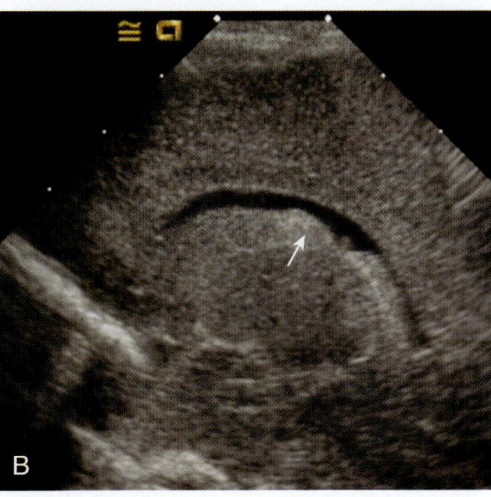

FIG. 27.26 Grade I germinal matrix hemorrhage seen bilaterally in a 1-day-old, 28-week preterm infant. (A) Coronal image showing two small germinal matrix bleeds *(arrows)*. (B) Sagittal image of the left germinal matrix hemorrhage *(arrow)*. (Courtesy Nationwide Children's Hospital, Columbus, OH.)

IVHs are not a sudden event; they usually expand slowly. Typically, when a small GM-IVH progresses to a large IVH (usually during the first 4 postpartum days), the IVH is asymptomatic. Because approximately 70% of hemorrhages are asymptomatic, it is necessary to have a technique, such as ultrasound, to routinely scan all the infants at risk for these lesions.

However, in some infants, the GM hemorrhage expands very rapidly to a more severe IVH; the sudden flooding and distention of the ventricles by hemorrhage is associated with the clinical symptoms of shock, seizures, hypoxemia, and a sudden decrease in hematocrit.

Sonographic Findings. IVHs appear as echogenic structures inside the anechoic ventricular cavities. Blood may fill just a small portion of the ventricle or the entire cavity. Care should be taken for small IVHs because studies from the anterior fontanel may not detect them, as blood tends to "settle out" in the posterior horns (Fig. 27.28). These small IVHs can be diagnosed when the occipital horns are visualized in the axial plane from the mastoid or posterior fontanels. Furthermore, even small IVHs may occlude the foramen of Monro or the aqueduct of Sylvius and thereby produce moderate to large dilation of the lateral ventricles by CSF.

When blood fills the entire ventricle, it is referred to as a ventricular cast (Fig. 27.29). In this case, without ventricular dilation, the ventricle may become isoechoic with the other structures in the brain, making definition of the borders of the ventricular wall difficult. Large cystic IVH may cause persistent ventricular dilation despite drainage of the CSF by a ventriculoperitoneal shunt.

Grade IV: Intraparenchymal Hemorrhages. IPHs complicate GM-IVHs in approximately 15% to 25% of infants. IPHs are a severe complication because they indicate the brain parenchyma has been destroyed. Although IPHs originally were considered an extension of GM-IVHs, evidence suggests this lesion is an infarction of the periventricular and subcortical white matter with destruction of the lateral wall of the ventricle, occurring secondary to obstruction of the terminal veins by the GM bleed. When the necrotic tissue liquefies, the IVH extends into the necrotic areas.

Sonographic Findings. IPHs appear as very echogenic zones in the white matter adjacent to the lateral ventricles. Echogenic areas in the white matter may correspond to IPHs or to hemorrhagic infarctions or extensive PVL. In the classic grade IV IPH, there is a clot extending from the white matter into the ventricular cavity (Fig. 27.30).

Intraparenchymal clots follow the same evolution as intraventricular clots. A few days after the acute bleeding, the clots become cystic and are reabsorbed completely in 3 or 4 weeks, leaving a cavity communicating with the lateral ventricle (porencephalic cyst).

When GM-IVHs associated with IPH evolve to PHH, the increased intraventricular pressure is transmitted to the porencephalic cyst. Hydrocephalus after hemorrhage associated with porencephaly is an indication for early ventriculoperitoneal shunt placement to minimize the deleterious effects of progressive compression and ischemia of the brain parenchyma.

Intracerebellar Hemorrhages. In premature neonates, there are areas of germinal matrix located around the fourth ventricle in the cerebellar hemispheres. The cerebellar germinal matrix has the same vulnerability to hemorrhage in the telencephalic germinal matrix. Intracerebellar hemorrhages have been reported in approximately 5% to 10% of postmortem studies of neonatal populations. The incidence in live infants is significantly lower.

Sonographic Findings. These hemorrhages appear as very echogenic structures inside the less echogenic cerebellar parenchyma (Fig. 27.31). Coronal views through the mastoid fontanel may be essential to differentiate intracerebellar hemorrhages from large subarachnoid hemorrhages in the cisterna magna, the supracerebellar cistern, or both.

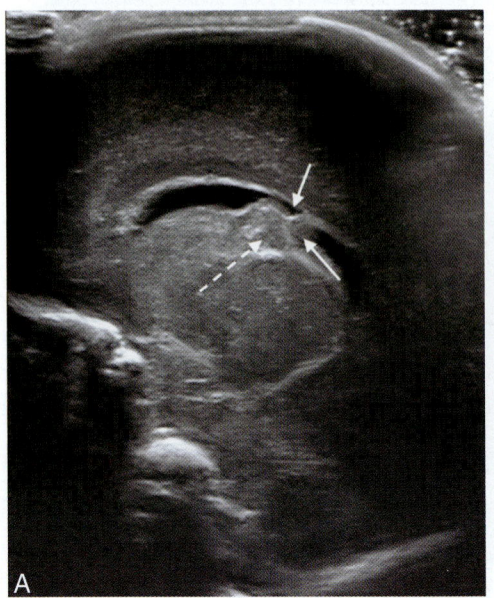
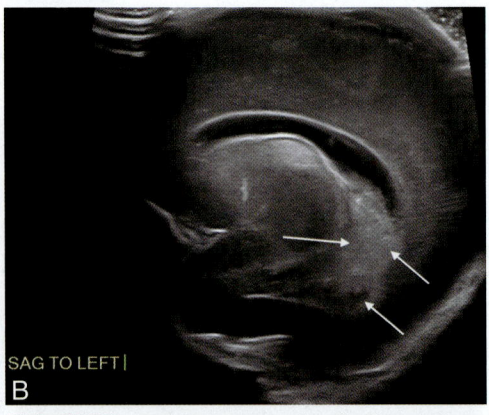

FIG. 27.28 Grade II intraventricular hemorrhage in an extremely premature 4-week-old. (A) Magnified sagittal view, just past midline in the area of the caudothalamic groove *(dashed arrow)*, helps to delineate that the hemorrhage is out of the germinal matrix and in the ventricle *(solid arrows)*. (B) A more lateral parasagittal view shows the echogenic blood has coagulated in the posterior portions of the ventricles *(arrows)*, making the choroid plexus appear bulky. The blood was not found to be outside the ventricles, and the ventricle size was not enlarged for this premature infant. (Courtesy Chester County Hospital, West Chester, PA.)

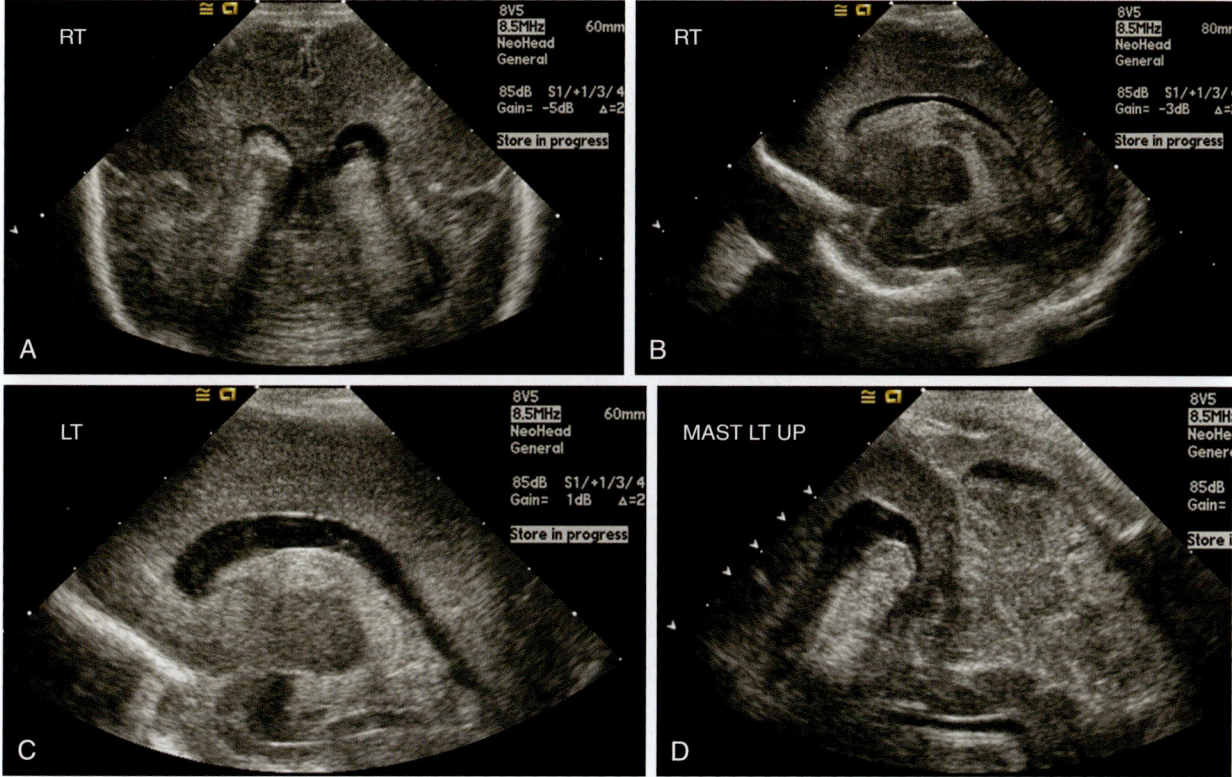

FIG. 27.29 **Grade III intraventricular hemorrhage.** Expansion of a germinal matrix bleed seen in the same 1-day-old 28-week preterm infant shown in Fig. 27.26 who had the grade I subependymal bleed bilaterally. Patient had pulmonary hemorrhage on day 2 of life followed by grade III intraventricular hemorrhage seen on a follow-up study on day 3. (A) Coronal view. (B) Right parasagittal image. (C) Left parasagittal image. (D) Mastoid view depicting the dilated, blood-filled occipital horns more clearly. (Courtesy Nationwide Children's Hospital, Columbus, OH.)

Intracerebellar hemorrhages become cystic with time, leaving cavitary lesions in the cerebellar hemispheres. These characteristic sequential changes are useful in making a positive diagnosis of intracerebellar hemorrhages.

Epidural Hemorrhages and Subdural Collections. Epidural hemorrhages and subdural fluid collections are better diagnosed by MRI or computed tomography; because these lesions are located peripherally along the surface of the brain, they are often not adequately visualized by ultrasound. However, if superficial fluid is seen, care should be taken to better detail it with color Doppler and proper gray-scale settings to differentiate it from subarachnoid fluid.

Sonographic Findings. Epidural hemorrhages are seen as echogenic formations located immediately underneath the calvarium. Subdural collections appear as nonechogenic spaces between the echogenic calvarium and the cortex. Also, color Doppler may be helpful to distinguish a subdural hemorrhage from a subarachnoid hemorrhage. Both will produce widening of the interhemispheric fissure, but only a subarachnoid one will cause widening of the sylvian fissures. Additionally, any break in the bone of the calvarium can appear with a step-off or step-down effect and may be incidentally found imaging the convexities of the brain. In the absence of birth trauma, this may indicate nonaccidental abuse if a subdural bleed is detected.

Extracorporeal Membrane Oxygenation. Neonatal ultrasound is primarily used to monitor hemorrhage in the brain tissue of infants on ECMO. ECMO is used for pulmonary and circulatory support in many neonatal conditions to allow additional time for the lungs to develop. Infants born with diaphragmatic hernia, persistent pulmonary hypertension, meconium aspiration, and congenital heart disease may be recommended for ECMO to give the infant's lungs a chance to mature. The ECMO cannula is often inserted into the right internal jugular vein and carotid artery (the vessels are ligated above their insertion site). Therefore the ECMO pump procedure can cause a notable change in cerebral circulation. After the vessel ligation, there is a 50% abrupt decrease in intracranial blood flow with a return of peak systolic velocities to nearly pre-ECMO levels within 3 to 5 minutes. The end-diastolic velocity is increased, and Doppler is used to monitor for hypoxic-ischemic encephalopathy.

Hemorrhage and ischemia are common in children on ECMO, both from the effects of ECMO itself and from the conditions leading to the use of ECMO. Preexisting hypoxic-ischemic encephalopathy with an abnormal RI has been shown to lead to ICH in a high percentage of infants. Bleeding may occur in the parenchyma, ventricle, or posterior fossa, but the cerebellum is also a common site. Increased extra-axial fluid is a common finding in infants on ECMO as well.

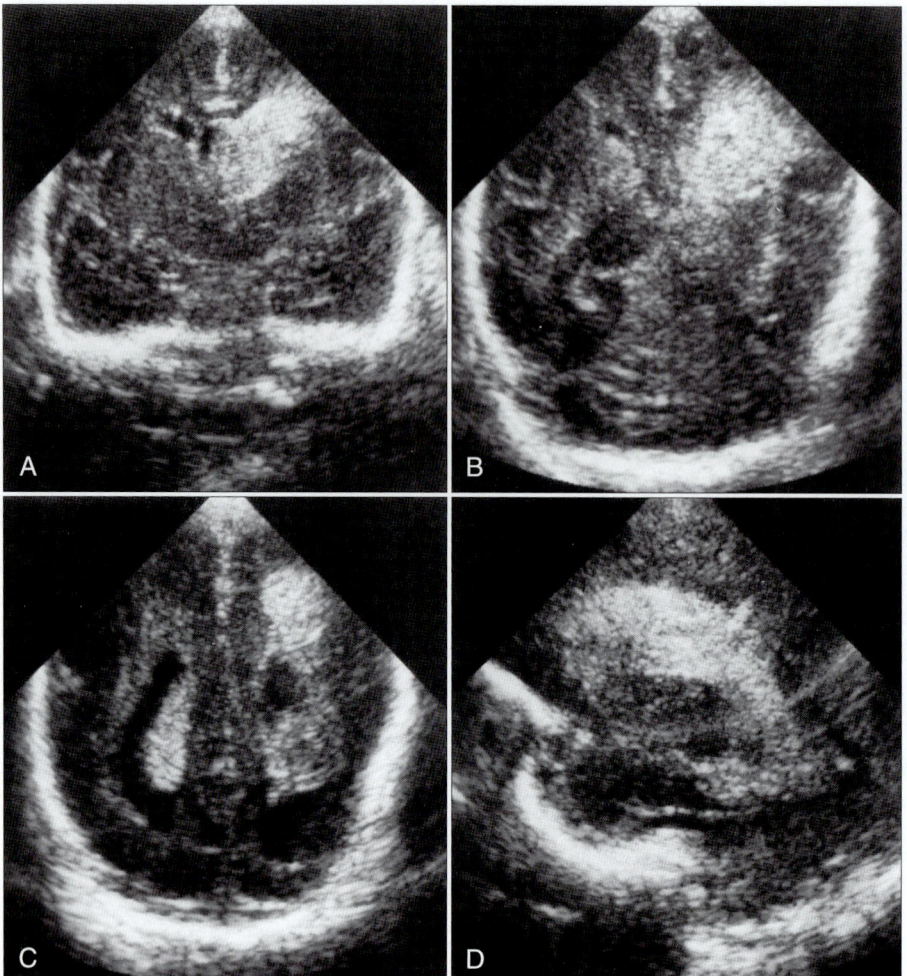

FIG. 27.30 **Grade III intraventricular hemorrhage and grade IV intraparenchymal hemorrhage.** A 3-day-old premature infant had a grade III bleed on the right and grade IV bleed on the left with extension into the brain parenchyma. (A) Coronal view at the frontal horns of the lateral ventricles shows hyperechoic hemorrhage extending into brain parenchyma on the left side. (B) Coronal view just posterior, at the body of the lateral ventricles, shows clot in the right ventricle as well as a left intraparenchymal bleed. (C) Coronal view showing dilation of the right and left posterior horn with bleed anterior to the left ventricle and attachmen to the glomus, distorting its normal shape. (D) Left parasagittal view showing intraparenchymal bleed.

Hypoxic-Ischemic Injury Lesions

HII is a frequent complication of sick newborn infants. The premature neonate is physiologically delicate at birth and, as a result, is subject to many stresses that, in turn, can cause hemorrhage and brain injury. Hypoxia is the lack of adequate oxygen to the brain, whereas ischemia is the lack of adequate blood flow to the brain. These occurrences can result from a variety of insults, including respiratory failure, congenital heart disease, and sepsis.

In the term neonate, HII tends to occur in watershed regions between the vascular territories of the major cerebral vessels, located at the cerebral cortex and subcortical white matter. With severe insults, the basal ganglia and thalami may also be involved. The cortex is usually preserved in the preterm infant as a result of anastomotic communicating vessels from the meningeal circulation that serve to preserve cortical blood flow. The preterm infant suffers injury primarily at their watershed zone located at the periventricular white matter, occurring most commonly near the atria of the lateral ventricles posteriorly and near the foramen of Monro, but can occur anywhere within the corona radiata and even the corpus callosum. White matter ischemia leads to white matter volume loss or PVL (**periventricular leukomalacia**). These lesions in the brain are usually associated with abnormal neurologic outcomes.

Five major types of neonatal hypoxic-ischemic brain injury have been described in the neonatal brain, and MRI is the modality of choice to diagnose them. The initial gray-scale sonographic evaluation for HII is often normal; however, it can be very useful in following multifocal white matter necrosis (PVL) and focal ischemic lesion development.

Doppler sonography can be very useful in the earlier detection of neonates with hypoxia/ischemia and may be the only sonographic indication that HII has occurred. To increase cerebral perfusion, end-diastolic flow rises, leading to a lower RI. The ACA should normally have an RI of 0.70. A low RI (less than 0.6), fluctuating RI, and hyperemia are

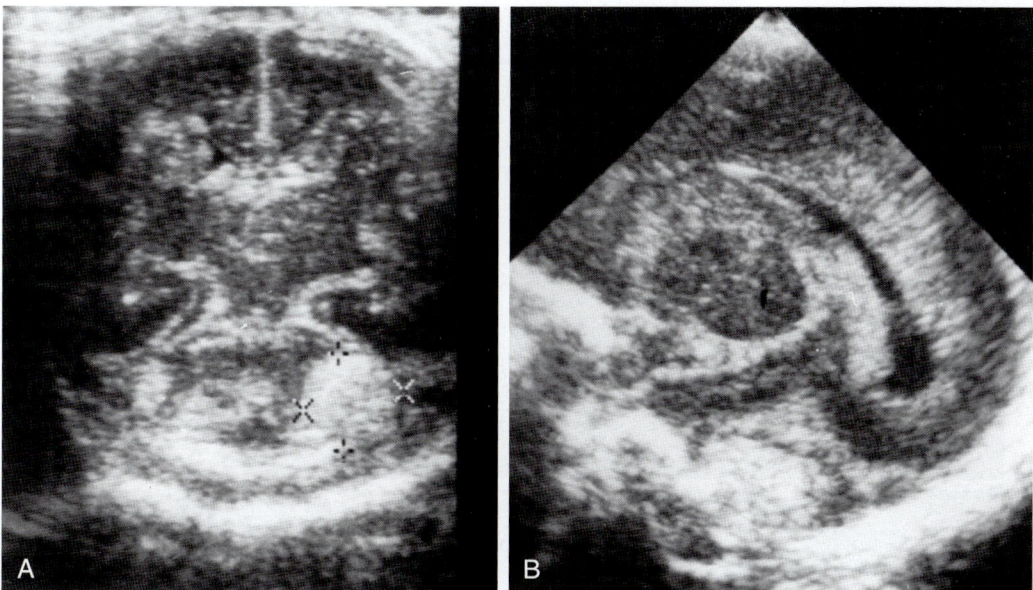

FIG. 27.31 Cerebellar hemorrhage in a premature infant born after 27 weeks of gestation. In 5 days, the bleed had progressed throughout the cerebellar compartment. (A) Coronal view with largest measurement within a portion of the bleed. (B) Parasagittal view.

useful Doppler findings in infants who have suffered HII. Fluctuations in RI likely reflect the loss of cerebrovascular autoregulation.

Periventricular Leukomalacia. Multifocal white matter necrosis, or PVL, is the most frequent ischemic lesion in the immature brain. This lesion is associated with anomalous myelination of the immature brain and abnormal neurologic development, including cerebral palsy. PVL is probably the most important cause of abnormal neurodevelopmental sequelae in preterm infants.

PVL is found in 20% to 80% of neonatal autopsies. Pathologists describe an acute phase characterized by multiple foci or coagulation necrosis in deep and periventricular white matter and a chronic phase depicted by cavitation and scarring appearing 1 or more weeks after cerebral insult. Early in the chronic stage, multiple cavities develop in the necrotic white matter adjacent to the lateral walls of the frontal horns, body, atria, and occipital horns of the lateral ventricles. These lesions are frequently located in the lateral wall of the atria and occipital horns, causing damage to the optic radiations. Eventually, the cavities resolve, leaving gliotic scars and diffuse cerebral atrophy. Necrotic lesions with only microscopic cavities may also lead to cerebral atrophy.

Sonographic Findings. PVL may be detected by sonography only 1 to 2 days after the HII. This "acute" stage of PVL is characterized by highly echogenic areas in the cerebral white matter superior and lateral to the frontal horns, bodies, atria, and occipital horns of the lateral ventricles (Fig. 27.32). In preterm infants, echogenic areas, or a periventricular blush, are present during the first week after delivery. However, they usually resolve in the following weeks, suggesting the echogenicities may be associated only with congestion and microhemorrhages without necrosis. If necrosis is present in the echogenic areas, cavitary lesions appear 2 or more weeks after the ischemic insult. Therefore careful follow-up studies are required. The chronic stage and definitive diagnosis of PVL with sonography are when echolucencies develop in the echogenic white matter (Fig. 27.33).

Keep in mind that cystic lesions in white matter may be microscopic or smaller than the resolution of the ultrasound scanners. Consequently, PVL may exist in the absence of cavitary lesions on ultrasound. Both neuropathologic and MRI studies have shown that a period of 1 to 6 weeks ensues between the acute stage of PVL and the development of cystic lesions. Echogenic areas and cysts decrease in size and eventually disappear 2 to 5 months after the diagnosis of acute necrosis. If the necrosis was extensive, brain atrophy may be the only indication that PVL occurred during the perinatal period. Sonography is also useful to diagnose the chronic atrophic stage of PVL. Brain atrophy is identified by an enlarged subarachnoid space, widened interhemispheric fissure, and persistent ventricular dilation in an infant with a normal or small head circumference.

Focal Brain Necrosis. These necrotic lesions occur within the distribution of large arteries. This complication is present in term and preterm infants, but it is infrequent under 30 weeks of gestation. Vascular maldevelopment, asphyxia or hypoxia, embolism from the placenta, infectious diseases, thromboembolism secondary to disseminated intravascular coagulation, and polycythemia have been implicated as causal factors in this condition. These insults may occur prenatally or early in postnatal life, leading subsequently to the dissolution of the cerebral tissues and formation of cavitary lesions. The term *porencephaly* is used to describe a single cavity, *multicystic encephalomalacia* for multiple cavities, and *hydranencephaly* for a large single cavity with the entire disappearance of the cerebral hemispheres.

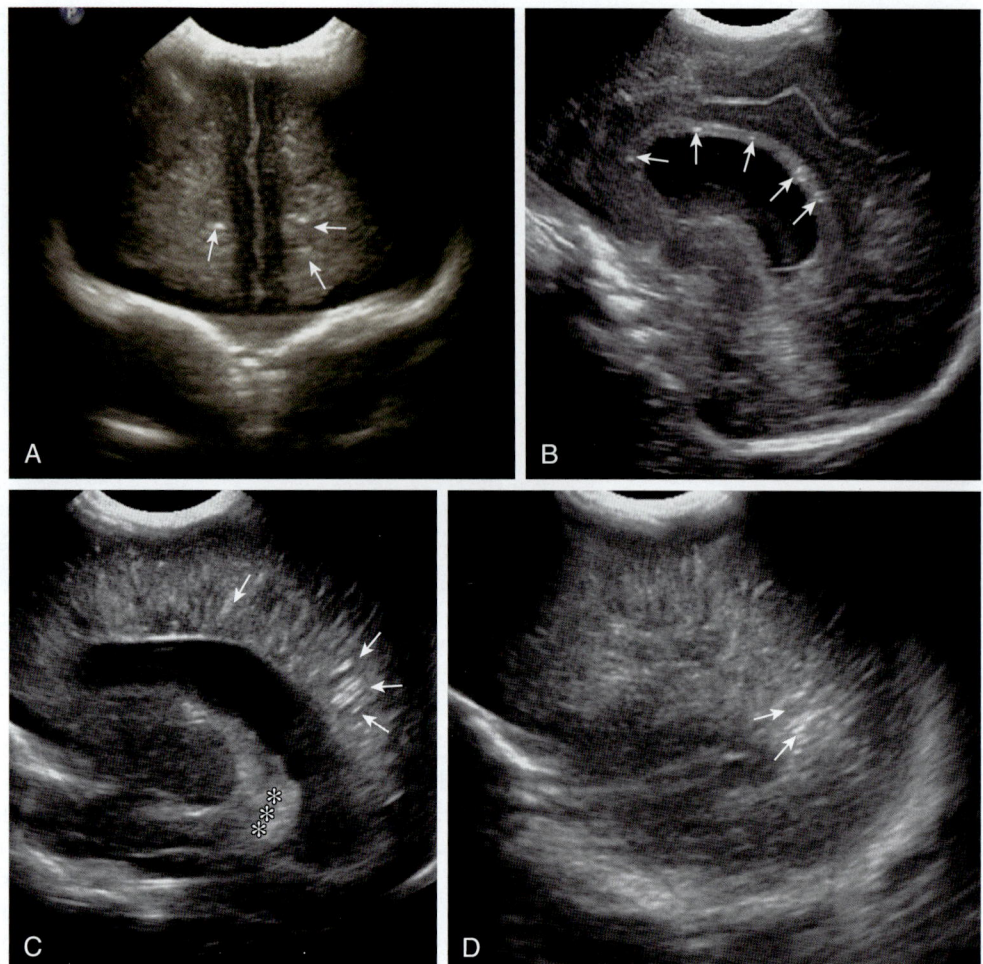

FIG. 27.32 Acute periventricular leukomalacia. An 8-day-old extremely premature infant with an acute drop in hematocrit was referred for a head ultrasound to evaluate for intracranial hemorrhage. Bilateral subependymal bleeds were seen, but the major concern was the increased echogenicity of the bilateral periventricular white matter and hyperechoic foci within the corpus callosum. (A) Coronal view of the anterior periventricular area; *arrows* show increased echogenicity. (B) Midline sagittal view demonstrating echogenic foci within the corpus callosum *(arrows)*. (C) Left parasagittal view showing increased periventricular white matter *(arrows)*, seen more echogenic than the choroid plexus *(asterisks)*. (D) Right parasagittal view showing increased echogenicity of the periventricular white matter *(arrows)*. (Courtesy Nationwide Children's Hospital, Columbus, OH.)

Sonographic Findings. Ultrasound images of these injuries show very echogenic localized lesions within the distribution of the major vessels. The echodense lesions are considered to correspond to cerebral infarctions. After several days, sonolucencies appear within the echogenic areas. Subsequently, the infarcted regions are replaced by cavities that may or may not communicate with the ventricle.

Lenticulostriate Vasculopathy. Lenticulostriate vasculopathy (LSV) lesions may be seen in neonates with HII. Hemodynamics in the premature brain is indicated in their pathogenesis. LSV has also been associated with congenital anomalies, chromosomal anomalies, prematurity, perinatal insult, and congenital infection. Isolated findings of LSV have a good prognosis; however, 18.9% to 55% are shown to have neurodevelopmental delay, but this is likely associated with underlying abnormalities and brain insult.

Sonographic Findings. LSV is characterized by linear echogenic foci branching within the basal ganglia and thalamus.

CONGENITAL BRAIN MALFORMATIONS

A number of different malformations may occur in fetal brain development and may be related to neural tube closure, diverticulation, vessel formation, neural tissue migration, or sulcation (sulci development). Congenital brain anomalies are rare and occur in only 3% to 8% of all births, including stillbirths. It is important to keep in mind that brain malformations are often accompanied by characteristic clinical observations, hydrocephalus, and other cerebral malformations. Furthermore, in some cases, "the face reflects the brain," meaning they present with distinct facial features. If the anterior fontanel is open, sonography can reliably diagnose these malformations; however, more extensive diagnostics can be achieved through a cranial MRI.

Disorders of Neural Tube Closure

The more commonly encountered neural tube defects encountered in neonatal head sonography are discussed here.

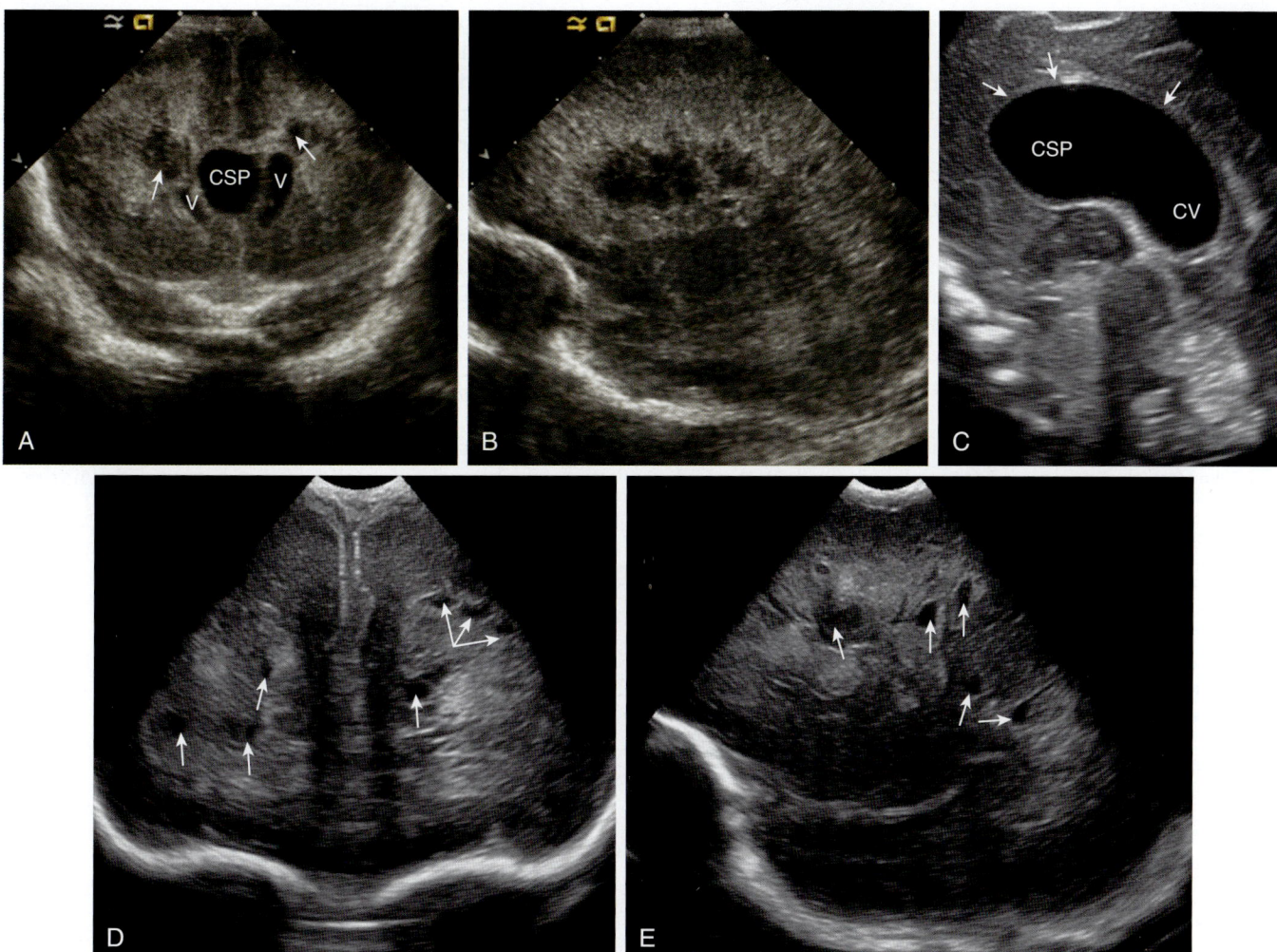

FIG. 27.33 **Chronic periventricular leukomalacia.** Cavitations or cystic formation within the increased periventricular white matter within 2 weeks of hypoxic-ischemic injury in the same extremely premature infant shown in Fig. 27.32 with bilateral grade I (germinal matrix) bleeds who also subsequently developed posthemorrhagic hydrocephalus. (A) At 4-day follow-up, the coronal view of the anterior horns of the lateral ventricles shows increased echogenicity, and adjacent hypoechoic areas *(arrows)* are indicative of brain liquefaction. (B) Right parasagittal view showing same parenchymal pattern lateral to the ventricles. (C) At 2-week follow-up, there is thinning of the corpus callosum *(arrow)*. (D) Coronal view of anterior periventricular white matter confirms an increased number of small cystic spaces *(arrows)* of liquefaction, developing porencephaly. (E) Right parasagittal view of periventricular white matter with same cysts *(arrows)*. *CSP*, Cavum septum pellucidum; *CV*, cavum vergae; *V*, ventricle. (Courtesy Nationwide Children's Hospital, Columbus, OH.)

Information on anomalies, such as anencephaly, myelomeningocele, meningocele, and encephalocele, are discussed in more detail in Chapter 60.

Arnold-Chiari Malformation. Chiari malformations are some of the most common brain anomalies encountered, comprising 50% of all cerebral malformations. There are three types, of which type I and type III are rare. Type I is not usually diagnosed until adulthood, and type III is associated with encephaloceles. The most common is type II, also called Arnold-Chiari malformation, and is of the greatest clinical importance in the setting of the neonatal brain because of its association with myelomeningoceles and myeloceles. In the early development of the brain, abnormal neural tube closure may result in a spinal defect, such as a myelomeningocele. About 80% to 90% of infants with myelomeningocele have Chiari malformations.

In Arnold-Chiari malformation, the cerebellum and brainstem are pulled downward (often from an open neural tube defect, such as myelomeningocele) toward the spinal cord through the foramen magna obstructing CSF flow, and secondary hydrocephalus develops. Aqueductal stenosis is present in 40% to 75% of infants with Chiari malformations. Hydrocephalus may also be caused by obstruction at the fourth ventricle or posterior fossa. Arnold-Chiari often leads to underdevelopment of the posterior fossa bony structures with a resulting small posterior fossa.

Sonographic Findings. Sagittal studies from the anterior fontanel show a small and dysplastic cerebellum, absence of the cisterna magna, low position of the fourth ventricle, and displacement of the cerebellum through the foramen magnum. The cavum septum pellucidum may be partially or completely absent.

With compression of the cerebellum, the cerebellar tonsils and vermis are herniated into the spinal canal through an enlarged foramen magnum, and the cisterna magna is not visualized due to this caudal displacement. The pons and medulla are inferiorly displaced, and the fourth ventricle becomes elongated. In addition, enlargement of the massa intermedia may be noted on the coronal and midline sagittal images.

Hydrocephalus is present in 90% of cases and to varying degrees but is often not symmetrically dilated as in the case of PHH. The third ventricle may be slightly dilated and is often dysplastic. Rarely with Arnold-Chiari are the temporal horns dilated. The frontal horns are often small with a batlike configuration, whereas the posterior horns of the ventricles are quite enlarged (Fig. 27.34). Often ventricular enlargement worsens after the myelomeningocele is repaired, as the CSF cannot enter the spinal defect. Commonly, it necessitates treatment with a life-long ventriculoperitoneal shunt.

Agenesis of the Corpus Callosum. The corpus callosum (or great commissure) is a white matter structure that connects both cerebral hemispheres. The presence of the corpus callosum is important in coordinating information and exchanging sensorial stimuli between the two hemispheres. Development of the corpus callosum occurs between the 8th and 12th weeks of gestation, beginning ventrally and extending dorsally. Depending on the timing of the intrauterine insult, the development of the corpus callosum can be partially arrested, or complete agenesis can occur. Absence of the corpus callosum may also be induced by ischemic lesions in the midline or by intrauterine encephalomalacia.

Agenesis of the corpus callosum has been associated with over 80 chromosomal, genetic, and sporadic syndromes,

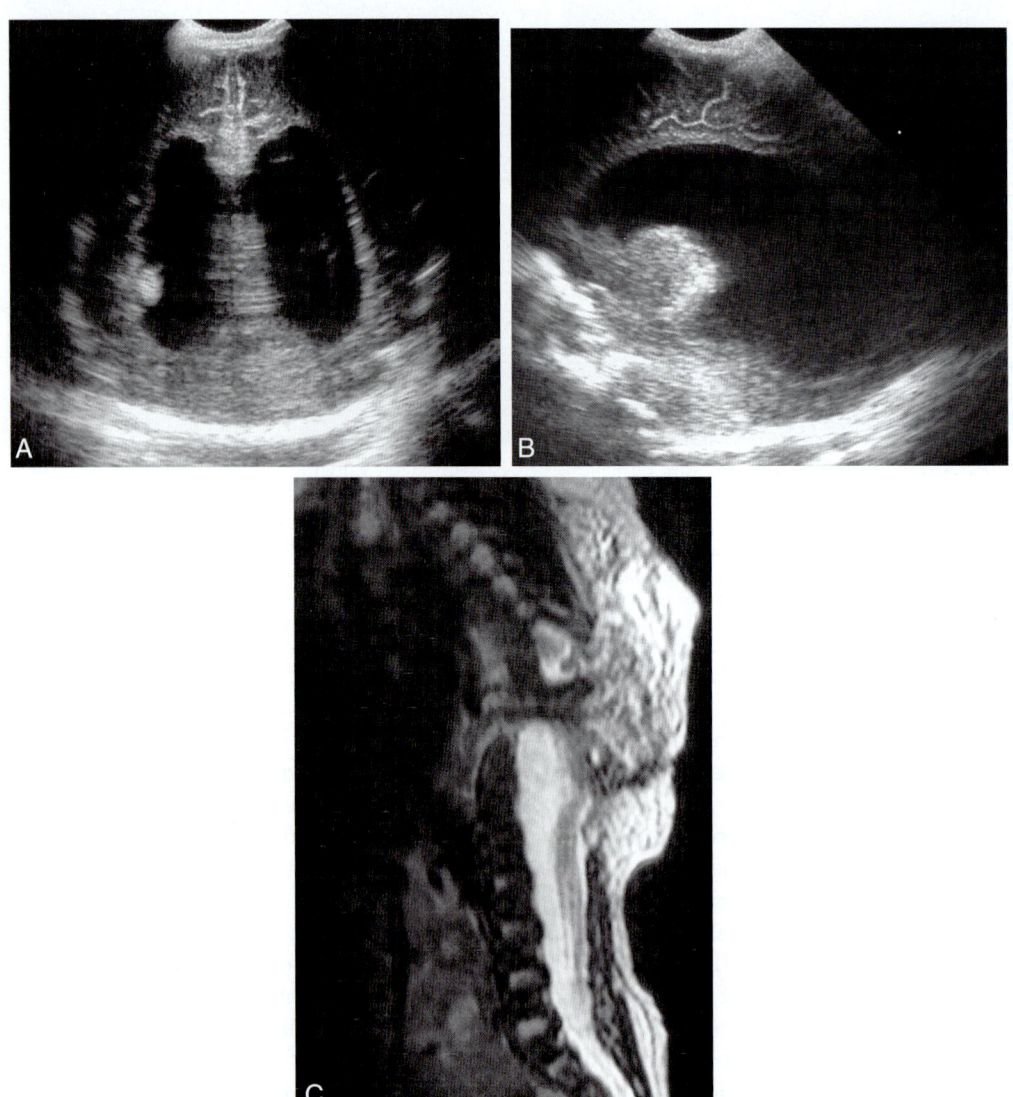

FIG. 27.34 **Chiari malformation type II.** The infant was delivered by cesarean section at 39 weeks of gestation for thoracic spina bifida. Chiari malformation type II was identified. Enlarged ventricles can be seen in both views of the head. (A) Posterior coronal view. (B) Midsagittal view showing obliteration of the cisterna magna, downward displacement of the midline structures, and a prominent massa intermedia. (C) Magnetic resonance imaging shows the spinal defect.

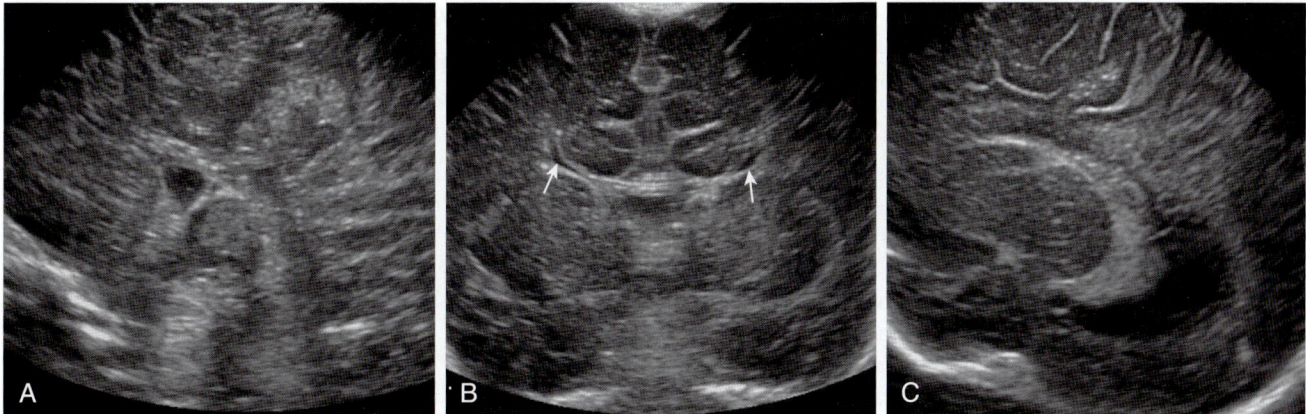

FIG. 27.35 **Agenesis of the corpus callosum.** Agenesis of the corpus callosum seen in an 11-day-old term infant. (A) Although randomizing of the cingulate sulcus is not as obvious in this infant, absence of the corpus callosum is easily noted. (B) Coronal view at the frontal horns shows a winglike or "bat-wing" appearance *(arrows)*. (C) Colpocephaly, or enlargement of the occipital horns, seen from a coronal view. (Courtesy Nationwide Children's Hospital, Columbus, OH.)

including Arnold-Chiari malformation. Agenesis of the corpus callosum is highly associated with Dandy-Walker malformation, affecting one-third of those diagnosed. It is often combined with migrational disorders, such as heterotopias and polymicrogyria. Other defects associated with this anomaly are porencephaly, hydrocephalus, microgyria, and fusion of the hemispheres. The corpus callosum is absent in severe holoprosencephaly. In neonates with this anomaly, the cerebral hemispheres have ventricles with pointed upper corners (bat-wing appearance). Correspondingly, the eyes in these neonates tend to be very wide apart.

Sonographic Findings. In neonates with this anomaly, the corpus callosum will be absent. The cingulate sulcus is randomized or spiraled because of the midline defect, and the pericallosal artery may have an abnormal course or be absent. The third ventricle may appear to be "high riding" between the ventricles where the CSP normally sits. The CSP is absent when due to developmental destruction and should not be confused for the third ventricle. The cerebral hemispheres have ventricles with pointed upper corners (bat-wing appearance), and colpocephaly is present. Colpocephaly refers to teardrop-like enlarged occipital horns (Fig. 27.35). Midline cysts may also be present and may or may not communicate with the lateral ventricles. Partial agenesis of the corpus callosum occurs when the genu, the splenium, and the rostrum are absent.

Dandy-Walker Malformation. Dandy-Walker syndrome is a group of congenital brain anomalies involving the disruption in development of the cerebellar vermis and roof of the fourth ventricle. There are several manifestations of this developmental differentiation just after the neural tube closes, which include both the Dandy-Walker malformation and Dandy-Walker variant. *Dandy-Walker complex* is a newer terminology for Dandy-Walker syndrome and includes **mega cisterna magna** and arachnoid cysts of the posterior cranial fossa.

Dandy-Walker malformation is the most serious of this complex, in which a huge fourth ventricle cyst (Fig. 27.36) occupies the area where the cerebellum usually lies, with secondary dilation of the third and lateral ventricles. The vermis

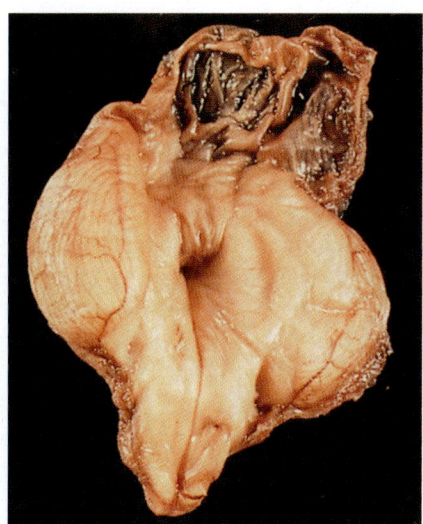

FIG. 27.36 **Dandy-Walker malformation specimen.** Hypoplastic vermis and cyst are reflected to expose a dilated fourth ventricle.

is hypoplastic or, roughly 25% of the time, absent. The fourth ventricle is enlarged. The posterior fossa is enlarged with the elevation of the tentorium cerebelli, straight sinus, and torcular herophili at the venous sinus confluence. The brainstem may be compressed anteriorly or become hypoplastic. Obstructive hydrocephalus occurs in 70% to 80% of patients and is not often pronounced at birth but develops within the first 3 months of life.

Dandy-Walker malformation may be associated with other CNS anomalies, which include hydrocephalus, partial or complete agenesis of the corpus callosum, encephalocele, holoprosencephaly, microcephaly, infundibular hamartomas, or brainstem lipomas.

Sonographic Findings. The typical Dandy-Walker malformation is characterized by absence or hypoplasia of the cerebellar vermis, enlarged fourth ventricle connecting to the development of a large cyst in the posterior fossa (Dandy-Walker cyst), hypoplastic cerebellar hemispheres that are often not connected, displaced laterally by the fourth ventricle, and a small brainstem. A large posterior fossa is present with an elevated tentorium. Ventricular dilation is symmetric. In many cases, the corpus callosum may be absent as well (Fig. 27.37).

Dandy-Walker Variant. In the Dandy-Walker variant, the posterior fossa is not enlarged, and the cerebellar hemispheres are normally developed. Ventricular dilation is rare. The fourth ventricle is only slightly dilated but communicates with the cyst.

Mega Cisterna Magna. The cistern magna is enlarged without cerebellar involvement and is considered a normal variant. No mass effect is found and no association with the development of hydrocephalus. There is a normal cerebellar vermis, fourth ventricle, and cerebellar hemisphere.

A posterior fossa arachnoid cyst can be differentiated from Dandy-Walker malformation or variant by the lack of communication of the cyst with the fourth ventricle. The arachnoid cyst displaces the normal fourth ventricle, vermis, and cerebellum.

Disorders of Diverticulation and Cleavage

Holoprosencephaly. Holoprosencephaly is a complex development abnormality of the brain arising from failure of cleavage of the prosencephalon or forebrain. This failure occurs early in gestation. It is characterized by a grossly abnormal brain in which there is a common large central ventricle (Fig. 27.38). The neuropathologic features include a single cerebrum with a single ventricular cavity, absence of the corpus callosum and frontal horns, and a thin membrane arising from the roof of the third ventricle, which may extend posteriorly, forming a supratentorial cyst. In addition, anomalies of the face also accompany this condition.

Holoprosencephaly represents a spectrum of malformations that form a continuum from most severe, with no separation of the telencephalon (alobar), to least severe, with partial separation of the dorsal aspects of the brain (lobar). A third classification of intermediate severity between alobar and lobar is semilobar holoprosencephaly. The mildest form

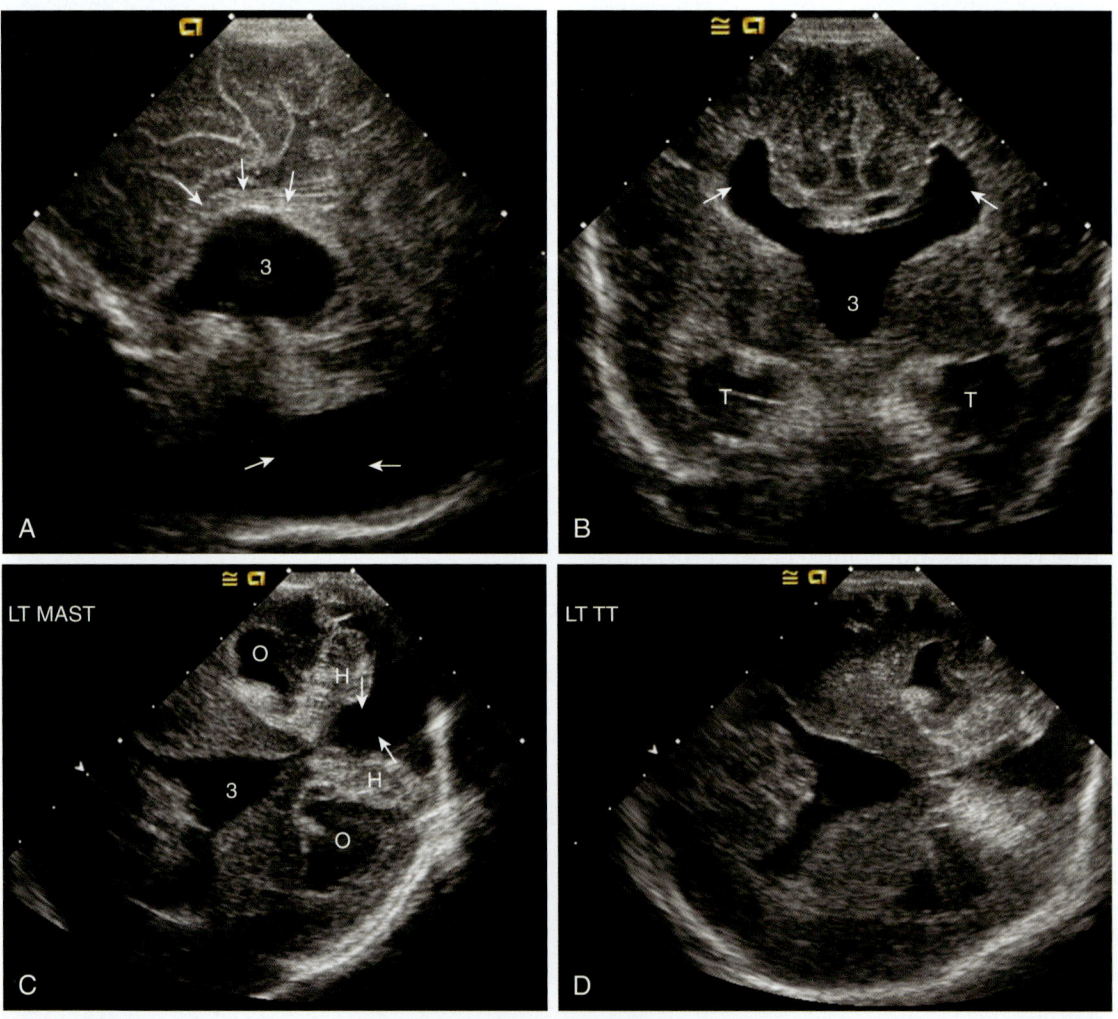

FIG. 27.37 Dandy-Walker malformation with agenesis of the corpus callosum. (A) Midline sagittal view in a term neonate shows an absence of both the cerebellar vermis and corpus callosum *(arrows)* and a very enlarged and superiorly positioned third ventricle (3). (B) Coronal view shows grossly enlarged lateral ventricles *(arrows)* with a bat-wing configuration communicating with the third ventricle (3). The temporal horns (T) are also seen dilated in this view. (C) Mastoid view of the cerebellum shows an absent vermis *(arrows)*, the space now occupied with cerebrospinal fluid, and hypoplastic cerebellar hemispheres (H). The occipital horns (O) are also enlarged. (D) A transtemporal approach demonstrating the entire anomaly. (Courtesy Nationwide Children's Hospital, Columbus, OH.)

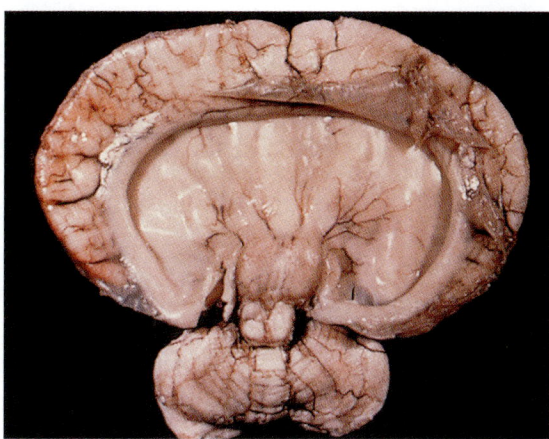

FIG. 27.38 Holoprosencephaly specimen. This posterior coronal view shows the reflected cyst wall communicating with a univentricle.

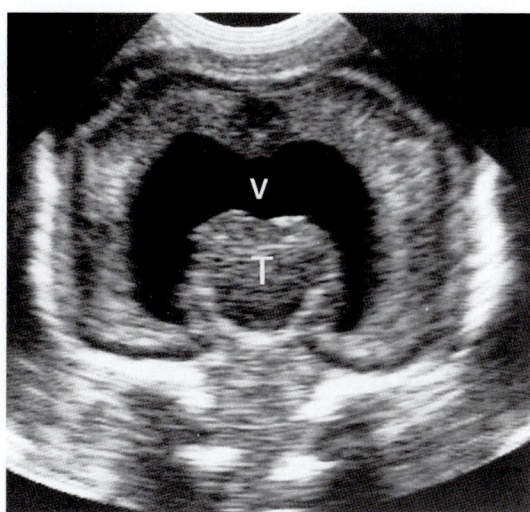

FIG. 27.39 Alobar holoprosencephaly demonstrating a single ventricle (V) and thalamus (T). The falx cerebri is absent.

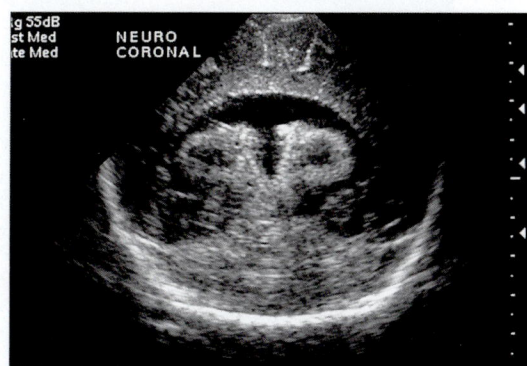

FIG. 27.40 Semilobar holoprosencephaly. Variable fusion is identified in semilobar holoprosencephaly, shown here with a split thalamus and univentricle.

of lobar prosencephaly is septo-optic dysplasia, known as De Morsier syndrome, in which there is absence of the cavum septum pellucidum and optic nerve hypoplasia. Generally, the eyes are close set in those with holoprosencephaly, and the degree varies based on the type.

Alobar Holoprosencephaly. This is the most severe form of holoprosencephaly. Multiple facial anomalies (i.e., cebocephaly, cyclopia, and ethmocephaly) are present. The brain surrounds a single midline crescent-shaped ventricle with a thin, primitive cerebral cortex surrounding the large ventricle. The thalami and hemispheres are fused; therefore the falx, corpus callosum, and interhemispheric fissure are not present. The fused thalami are seen anterior to the fused hyperechogenic choroid plexus (Fig. 27.39). The third ventricle is absent, causing the dilated single ventricle to communicate directly with the aqueduct of Sylvius. A large dorsal cyst may also be present.

Semilobar Holoprosencephaly. A single ventricle is evident; however, more brain parenchyma is present. A small portion of the falx and interhemispheric fissure develops in the occipital cortex posteriorly. There may be separate occipital and temporal horns. The splenium and genu of the corpus callosum are often formed and may be seen on midline sagittal images. The thalami are partially separated, and the third ventricle is rudimentary (Fig. 27.40). Mild facial anomalies (i.e., hypotelorism and cleft lip) may be present.

Lobar Holoprosencephaly. This is the least severe form of holoprosencephaly. There is nearly complete separation of hemispheres with the development of a falx and interhemispheric fissure. There may be fusion of the frontal lobes. The septum pellucidum is absent. The anterior horns of the lateral ventricles are fused; however, the occipital horns are separated (Fig. 27.41). The third ventricle is present and separates the thalami. The splenium and body of the corpus callosum are present with the absence of the genu and rostrum. Facial anomalies are mild.

▸ ***Sonographic Findings.*** When holoprosencephaly is suspected, it is important to obtain coronal studies of the whole frontal lobes to determine whether one frontal horn or thalamus is present and to document if the falx is absent or partial.

Destructive Lesions

Hydranencephaly. Hydranencephaly is an ischemic lesion believed to be the result of bilateral occlusion of the internal carotid arteries during fetal development between the third and sixth months of pregnancy, but it may result from any number of intracranial destructive processes. Brain tissue is destroyed, and the cerebrum is replaced by CSF. Because the posterior communicating arteries are preserved, the midbrain and cerebellum are present. The basal ganglia, choroid plexus, and thalamus may also be spared. It has a similar appearance to alobar holoprosencephaly. As in holoprosencephaly, there is a single ventricular cavity and absence of the corpus callosum. However, the presence of midline structures, such as the falx and two frontal horns or thalami, helps differentiate these malformations caused by ischemic lesions from true holoprosencephaly.

▸ ***Sonographic Findings.*** There is absence of normal brain tissue with almost complete replacement by CSF (Fig. 27.42).

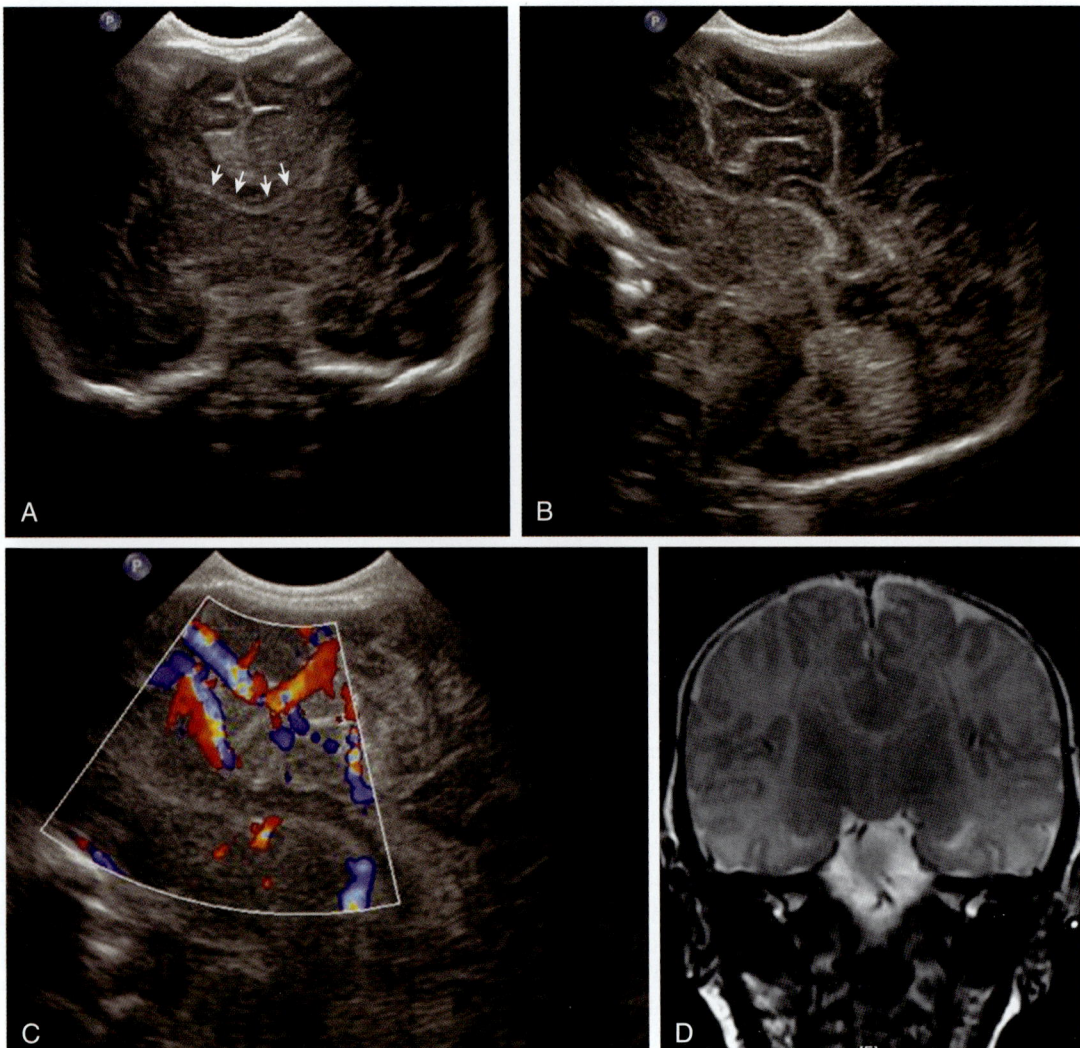

FIG. 27.41 **Lobar holoprosencephaly.** This brain anomaly was seen in a 2-day-old with a cranial deformity. (A) Coronal view demonstrates fusion of the anterior lateral ventricles *(arrows).* The ventricular system is completely decompressed, making visualization of the structures more difficult. (B) Sagittal midline view does not demonstrate a corpus callosum or cavum septum pellucidum. (C) Sagittal midline view with color Doppler demonstrates an abnormal pericallosal artery. (D) Coronal T2-weighted magnetic resonance imaging shows same fused anterior horns of the lateral ventricles and confirmed the patient had lobar holoprosencephaly with partial agenesis of the corpus callosum. (Courtesy Nationwide Children's Hospital, Columbus, OH.)

Unlike alobar holoprosencephaly, the midline structures, such as the interhemispheric fissure, falx cerebri, and third ventricle, may be preserved. A high-frequency linear transducer may help to visualize the superficial falx. Two thalami and two frontal horns may be identified. The midbrain, basal ganglia, and cerebellum are seen. Macrocephaly may be present. Doppler flow in the carotid arteries is absent.

Porencephalic Cyst. A porencephalic cyst, also known as porencephaly, is a cyst filled with CSF that communicates with the ventricular system or subarachnoid space. These cysts may result from hemorrhage, infarction, delivery trauma, or inflammatory changes in the nervous system. The affected brain parenchyma undergoes necrosis, brain tissue is reabsorbed and, as CSF fills in the space, a cystic lesion remains.

Sonographic Findings. A cyst is seen within the brain parenchyma without a mass effect. There may be communication of the cyst with the ventricle or subarachnoid space. A reduction in the size of the affected hemisphere may cause a midline shift and contralateral ventricular enlargement.

Cystic Lesions

Choroid Plexus Cysts. Choroid plexus cysts are common and may be seen in early development, as well as after delivery. The cysts tend to be singular and present as an isolated finding, not associated with other CNS or chromosomal abnormalities. However, when the cysts are greater than 10 mm and multiple, these may be associated with chromosomal abnormalities, particularly trisomy 18.

Sonographic Findings. On sonography, the choroid plexus cyst appears as a well-defined anechoic mass within the dorsal choroid plexus. They range in size from 4 to 7 mm and are usually unilateral, with the left larger than the right.

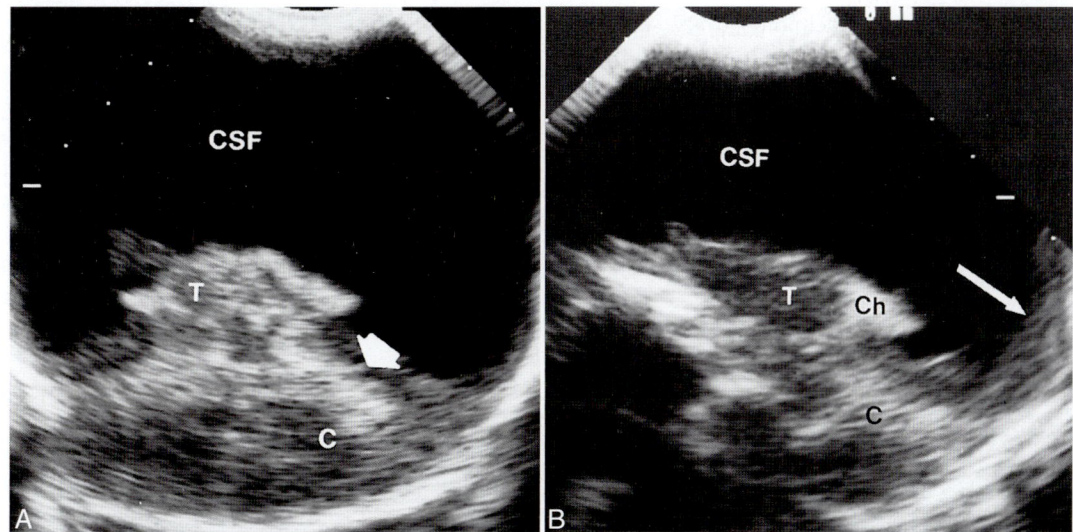

FIG. 27.42 **Hydranencephaly.** Coronal (A) and sagittal (B) midline views. Tentorium cerebelli *(thick arrow)*; thin remnant of cerebral cortex *(thin arrow)*; *C*, Cerebellum; *Ch*, choroid plexus; *CSF*, cerebrospinal fluid; *T*, thalamus.

They should be differentiated from subependymal cysts formed within the ventricular cavity (see Fig. 27.43).

Galenic Venous Malformation. The galenic venous malformation represents dilation of the vein of Galen within the quadrigeminal cistern caused by a vascular malformation that is fed by large arteries off the anterior or posterior cerebral artery circulation. Infants with this condition usually present with congestive heart failure.

Sonographic Findings. This malformation appears as an anechoic, cystic mass between the lateral ventricles. It lies posterior to the foramen of Monro, superior to the third ventricle, and primarily in the midline. The large feeding vessels help to differentiate this lesion from other cystic masses (Fig. 27.44). Hydrocephalus may or may not be present, and calcification may occur if there is thrombosis in the malformation.

Arachnoid Cysts. Arachnoid cysts are lined by arachnoid tissue and contain CSF and may arise within any of the three meninges. There are three major causes postulated to explain the formation of these cysts: (1) localized entrapment of fluid during embryogenesis, (2) residual subdural hematoma, and (3) fluid extravasation secondary to leptomeningeal tear or ventricular rupture.

The cysts may be in the infratentorial or supratentorial compartments. Arachnoid cysts in the posterior fossa are associated with a normal vermis and a normal fourth ventricle, which differentiates arachnoid cysts from the Dandy-Walker malformation. In a supratentorial compartment, these cysts usually arise from the suprasellar or quadrigeminal plate cisterns. The most frequent locations are the interhemispheric fissure, the suprasellar region, and the cerebral convexities. These cysts may be symptomatic secondary to cerebral compression or hydrocephalus, or they may be totally asymptomatic.

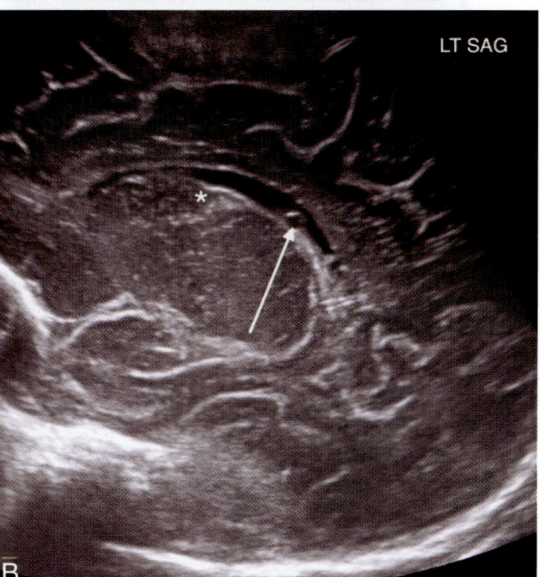

FIG. 27.43 **Choroid plexus cyst.** (A) Coronal view of a left choroid plexus cyst *(arrow)* in a 36-week-old neonate. (B) Parasagittal view of the choroid plexus cyst *(arrow)*. Note the location is more posterior than the caudothalamic groove *(asterisk)* indicated in germinal matrix bleeds. (Courtesy Chester County Hospital, West Chester, PA.)

▶ **Sonographic Findings.** Arachnoid cysts usually appear on sonography as a sonolucent structure arising from the quadrigeminal plate cistern or the suprasellar region (Fig. 27.45). Sagittal studies are useful to determine the location and size of these cysts. Sequential studies should be obtained in infants with this complication, as the cysts may have progressive growth and may need to be drained by ventriculoperitoneal shunts. Color Doppler may be used to verify that these are not venous malformations.

BRAIN INFECTIONS

Congenital Infections

Congenital infections of the brain can have serious consequences for the neonate, including death, intellectual disability, or developmental delay. The most frequent congenital infections are commonly referred to by the acronym TORCH (*Toxoplasma gondii*, other infections that cross the placenta during pregnancy, Rubella virus, cytomegalovirus, and

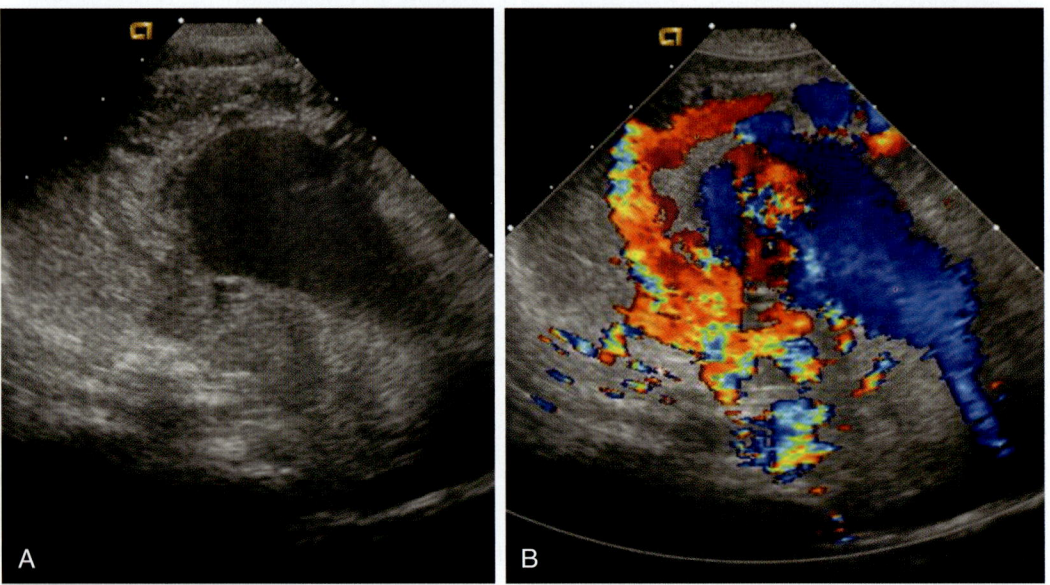

FIG. 27.44 **Vein of Galen malformation.** (A) Large cyst is visualized on a sagittal view. (B) Color Doppler shows blood flow within the cyst, confirming the diagnosis. (Courtesy Nationwide Children's Hospital, Columbus, OH.)

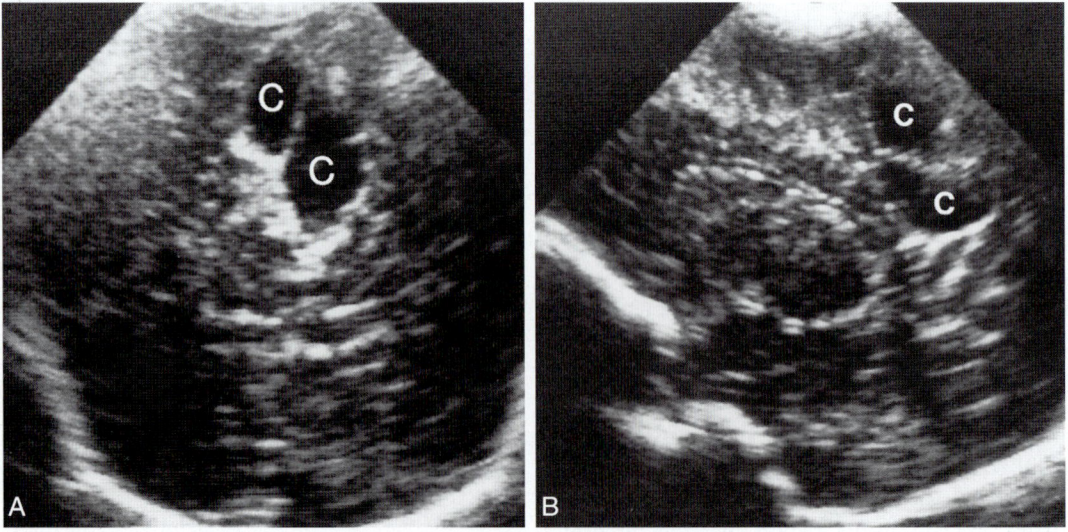

FIG. 27.45 **Midline arachnoid cyst.** Coronal (A) and sagittal (B) scans show two arachnoid cysts (C), one in the interhemispheric fissure and the other just at left; both are above the lateral ventricle.

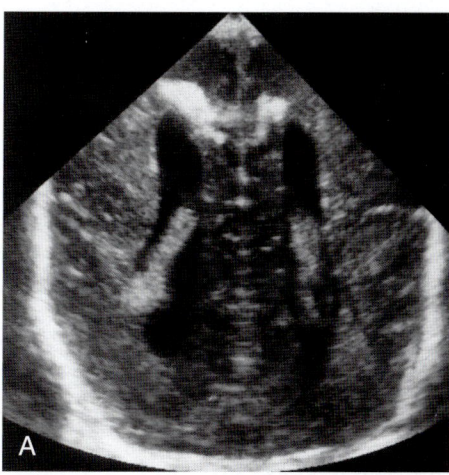 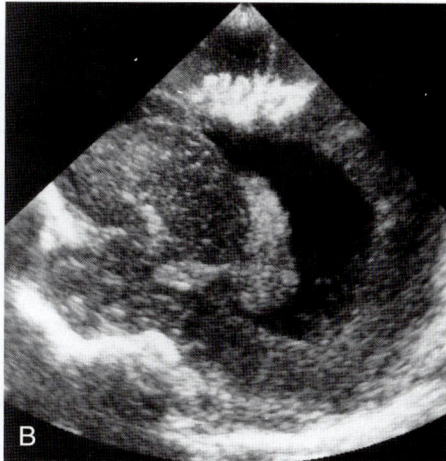

FIG. 27.46 **Calcifications due to a congenital cytomegalovirus infection.** A 1-month-old infant with bright calcifications seen bilaterally secondary to a cytomegalovirus congenital infection. (A) Coronal image. (B) Right parasagittal image.

herpes simplex virus). Other agents, such as syphilis, may cause acute meningitis. The most common of these vertically transmitted diseases is cytomegalovirus, and toxoplasmosis is the second most common.

Sonographic Findings. Sonography may detect parenchymal calcifications (Fig. 27.46) and LSV. LSV is highly associated with neonatal brain infections. Other complications that may arise include hydrocephalus, abscess, white matter softening or loss (encephalomalacia), and infarctions.

Ventriculitis

Ventriculitis is a common complication of purulent meningitis in newborn infants. Ventriculitis probably is caused by the hematogenous spread of the infection to the choroid plexus. The presence of a foreign body in the ventricular cavity, such as a catheter from a ventriculoperitoneal shunt, may provide a nidus for persistent infection of the ventricular cavities.

Sonographic Findings. Ventriculitis leads to compartmentalization of the ventricular cavities by inflammatory adhesions extending from wall to wall. The first stage of ventriculitis is seen in ultrasound as thin septations extending from the walls of the lateral ventricles. The septa become thicker and lead to multilocular hydrocephalus and extensive disorganization of the brain anatomy. Sequential studies in patients with meningitis or with ventriculoperitoneal shunts can provide an early diagnosis of this severe complication.

Ependymitis

Ependymitis occurs when the ependymal lining of the ventricles becomes inflamed as a result of irritation from hemorrhage within the ventricle.

Sonographic Findings. The ependymal lining will appear thickened and hyperechoic. This is more common and occurs earlier than ventriculitis, which can also develop from intraventricular hemorrhage.

Key Pearls

- Sonography plays a very important role in the diagnosis and follow-up of intracranial problems in the neonate.
- Care must be taken to keep the infant warm and safe (good disinfectant techniques, minimize movement, etc.).
- Knowing the approximate gestational age of the premature infant and the associated sonographic findings is critical.
- Fontanel closure, around 9 months, makes sonographic imaging difficult after this time.
- The midline sagittal view is critical to rule out many congenital anomalies.
- Sagittal and coronal views are used to image the supratentorial and infratentorial structures.
- A mastoid view is very helpful in better depicting the deep infratentorial structures in most infants under 6 months of age when the fontanel typically closes.
- Use multiple acoustic windows in the presence of pathology, if possible.
- Ventriculomegaly is very common, and ventricular measurements and Doppler of the pericallosal artery can help track enlargement and increased intracranial pressure (ICP).
- Increased ICP is of great clinical concern and is treated with the placement of a ventricular shunt.
- Any superficial fluid should be investigated with color or power Doppler to determine whether it is extra-axial or subdural in location.
- The caudothalamic groove is a common source of subependymal bleeds in infants less than 34 weeks, with increased risk under 32 weeks and under 1500 g.
- In term infants, bleeds often occur in the glomus of the choroid plexus.
- Intracranial hemorrhages (ICHs) may be classified as grades I through IV depending on the location of the bleed, ventricular dilation, or parenchymal involvement.
- An ICH starts in the germinal matrix or caudothalamic groove and is a progressive disease.

- The periventricular white matter should never appear more hyperechoic than the choroid plexus and is a common place for white matter necrosis (periventricular leukomalacia [PVL]) to occur in the premature infant.
- PVL initially appears echogenic, and over the course of weeks, cystic areas develop as a result of necrosis.
- LSV may also occur in patients who have undergone a hypoxic-ischemic injury.
- Agenesis of the corpus callosum is indicated in many congenital anomalies, and the associated cingulate gyri and sulci will have a sunburst appearance.
- Dandy-Walker complex includes an array of anomalies, the most severe of which is the Dandy-Walker malformation, which presents with a large cystic area under the cerebelli tentorium due to a missing cerebellar vermis. Cerebellar hemispheres may be absent or hypoplastic.
- Chiari malformations involve the hindbrain and type II, called Arnold-Chiari malformation, is nearly always associated with spina bifida.
- Holoprosencephaly is a spectrum of malformations due to abnormal diverticulation in utero. This disorder may be divided into the alobar, semilobar, and lobar types.
- Congenital infections, most commonly the TORCH complex, may present with calcification or lenticulostriate vasculopathy (LSV).

BIBLIOGRAPHY

AIUM Practice Parameter for the Performance of Neurosonography in Neonates and Infants. *J Ultrasound Med*. 2020;39(5):E57-E61.

Amodio J, Spektor V, Pramanik B, et al. Spontaneous development of bilateral subdural hematomas in an infant with benign infantile hydrocephalus: color Doppler assessment of vessels traversing extra-axial spaces. *Pediatr Radiol*. 2005;35(11):1113-1117.

Bacani M. The neonatal brain. In *Diagnostic medical sonography: abdomen and superficial structures*. ed 3, Philadelphia: Lippincott Williams & Wilkins; 2012:735-747.

Bhat V. Neonatal neurosonography: a pictorial essay. *Indian J Radiol Imaging*. 2014;24(4):389-400.

Bradstreet JJ, Pacini S, Ruggiero M. A new methodology of viewing extra-axial fluid and cortical abnormalities in children with autism via transcranial ultrasonography. *Front Hum Neurosci*. 2014;7:934.

Brouwer MJ, De Vries LS, Pistorius L, et al. Ultrasound measurements of the lateral ventricles in neonates: why, how and when? A systematic review. *Acta Paediatr*. 2010;99(9):1298-1306.

Brouwer MJ, De Vries LS, Groenendaal F, et al. New reference values for the neonatal cerebral ventricles. *Radiology*. 2012;262(1):224-233.

Brown PD, Davies SL, Speake T, Millar ID. Molecular mechanisms of cerebrospinal fluid production. *Neuroscience*. 2004;129(4):957-970.

Chapman T, Mahalingam S, Ishak GE, et al. Diagnostic imaging of posterior fossa anomalies in the fetus and neonate: part 2. Posterior fossa disorders. *Clin Imaging*. 2015;39(2):167-175.

Cinalli G, Spennato P, Nastro A, et al. Hydrocephalus in aqueductal stenosis. *Childs Nerv Syst*. 2011;27(10):1621-1642.

Coley BD, Rusin JA, Boue DR. Importance of hypoxic/ischemic conditions in the development of cerebral lenticulostriate vasculopathy. *Pediatr Radiol*. 2000;30(12):846-855.

Correa FF, Lara C, Bellver J, et al. Potential pitfalls in fetal neurosonography. *Prenat Diagn*. 2006;26(1):52-56.

Daneman A, Epelman M. Neurosonography: in pursuit of an optimized examination. *Pediatr Radiol*. 2015;45(Suppl 3):406-412.

Daneman A, Epelman M, Blaser S, Jarrin JR. Imaging of the brain in full-term neonates: does sonography still play a role? *Pediatr Radiol*. 2006;36(7):636-646.

Deeg KH, Gassner I. Sonographic diagnosis of cerebral malformations in infancy. Part 1: Chiari and Dandy-Walker malformations. *Ultraschall Med*. 2010;31(5):446-462.

Deeg KH, Gassner I. Sonographic diagnosis of brain malformations, part 2: holoprosencephaly—hydranencephaly—agenesis of septum pellicidum—schizencephaly—septo-optical dysplasia. *Ultraschall Med*. 2010;31(6):548-560.

Demené C, Pernot M, Biran V, et al. Ultrafast Doppler reveals the mapping of cerebral vascular resistivity in neonates. *J Cereb Blood Flow Metab*. 2014;34(6):1009-1017.

Duan Y, Sun FQ, Li YQ, et al. Prognosis of psychomotor and mental development in premature infants by early cranial ultrasound. *Ital J Pediatr*. 2015;41:30.

Ecker JL, Shipp TD, Bromley B, et al. The sonographic diagnosis of Dandy-Walker and Dandy-Walker variant: associated findings and outcomes. *Prental Diagn*. 2000;20:328-332.

Engle WA. A recommendation for the definition of "late preterm" (near-term) and the birth weight-gestational age classification system. *Semin Perinatol*. 2006;30(1):2-7.

Evans DH. Doppler ultrasound and the neonatal cerebral circulation: methodology and pitfalls. *Biol Neonate*. 1992;62:271.

Fenton AC, Shortland DB, Papathoma E, et al. Normal range for blood flow velocity in cerebral arteries of newly born term infants. *Early Hum Dev*. 1990;22:73.

Fenton AC, Papathoma E, Evans DH, et al. Neonatal cerebral venous flow velocity measurement using a color flow Doppler system. *J Clin Ultrasound*. 1991;19:69.

Fenton TR, Tanis R, Kim JH. A systematic review and meta-analysis to revise the Fenton growth chart for preterm infants. *BMC Pediatr*. 2013;13(1):59.

Fox TB. Sonography of the neonatal brain. *J Diagn Med Sonogr*. 2009;25(6):331-348.

Fox LM, Choo P, Rogerson SR, et al. The relationship between ventricular size at 1 month and outcome at 2 years in infants less than 30 weeks' gestation. *Arch Dis Child Fetal Neonatal Ed*. 2014;99(3):F209-F214.

Frankel DA, Fessell DP, Wolfson WP. High resolution sonographic determination of the normal dimensions of the intracranial extraaxial compartment in the newborn infant. *J Ultrasound Med*. 1998;17(7):411-415.

Fritz J, Polansky SM, O'Connor SC. Neonatal neurosonography. *Semin Ultrasound CT MRI*. 2014;35(4):349-364.

Govaert P, De Vries LS. *An atlas of neonatal brain sonography*. ed 2, Cornwall, UK: Mac Keith Press; 2010.

Hamrick SE, Miller SP, Leonard C, et al. Trends in severe brain injury and neurodevelopmental outcome in premature newborn infants: the role of cystic periventricular leukomalacia. *J Pediatr*. 2004;145(5):593-599.

Hervey-Jumper SL, Cohen-Gadol AA, Maher CO. Neurosurgical management of congenital malformations of the brain. *Neuroimaging Clin North Am*. 2011;21(3):705-717.

Hong SY, Yang JJ, Li SY, Lee IC. Lenticulostriate vasculopathy in brain ultrasonography is associated with cytomegalovirus infection in newborns. *Pediatr Neonatol*. 2015;56(6):1-7. http://www.ncbi.nlm.nih.gov/pubmed/26073370.

Horbar JD, Leahy KA, Lucey JF. Ultrasound identification of lateral ventricular asymmetry in the human neonate. *J Clin Ultrasound*. 1983;11(2):67-69.

Hwang SW, Su JM, Jea A. Diagnosis and management of brain and spinal cord tumors in the neonate. *Semin Fetal Neonatal Med*. 2012;17(4):202-206.

Hwang M, Piskunowicz M, Darge K. Advanced Ultrasound Techniques for Pediatric Imaging. *Pediatrics*. 2019;143(3):e20182609.

International Society for Pediatric Neurosurgery: Ultrasound of ventricles in the brains of infants, 2010. https://www.ispn.guide/hydrocephalus-and-other-anomalies-of-csf-circulation-in-children/hydrocephalus-after-intraventricular-hemorrhage-in-infants-homepage/.

Kliegman RM, et al. *Nelson textbook of pediatrics*. ed 19, Philadelphia: Elsevier; 2011.

Lowe LH, Bailey Z. State-of-the-art cranial sonography: part 2, pitfalls and variants. *AJR Am J Roentgenol*. 2011;196(5):1034–1039.

Makhoul IR, Eisenstein I, Sujov P, et al. Neonatal lenticulostriate vasculopathy: further characterisation. *Arch Dis Child Fetal Neonatal Ed*. 2003;88(5):F410–F414.

Mandiwanza T, Saidlear C, Caird J, Crimmins D. The open fontanelle: a window to less radiation. *Childs Nerv Syst*. 2013;29(7):1177–1181.

Mondal P, Mukhopadhyay J, Sural S, et al. A robust method for ventriculomegaly detection from neonatal brain ultrasound images. *J Med Syst*. 2012;36(5):2817–2828.

Monteagudo A. Fetal neurosonography: should it be routine? Should it be detailed? *Ultrasound Obstet Gynecol*. 1998;12(1):1–5.

Orman G, Benson JE, Kweldam CF, et al. Neonatal head ultrasonography today: a powerful imaging tool! *J Neuroimaging*. 2015;25(1):31–55.

Perlman JM. White matter injury in the preterm infant: an important determination of abnormal neuro development outcome. *Early Hum Dev*. 1998;53:99–120.

Rabiner JE, Friedman LM, Khine H, et al. Accuracy of point-of-care ultrasound for diagnosis of skull fractures in children. *Pediatrics*. 2013;131(6):e1757–e1764.

Radhakrishnan R, Brown BP, Kralik SF, et al. Frontal occipital and frontal temporal horn ratios: comparison and validation of head ultrasound-derived indexes with MRI and ventricular volumes in infantile ventriculomegaly. *AJR Am J Roentgenol*. 2019;213(4):925–931.

Riccabona M. Neonatal neurosonography. *Eur J Radiol*. 2014;83(9):1495–1506.

Romero JM, Madan N, Betancur I, et al. Time efficiency and diagnostic agreement of 2-D versus 3-D ultrasound acquisition of the neonatal brain. *Ultrasound Med Biol*. 2014;40(8):1804–1809.

Rosenberg HK, et al. Normal splenic sizes in infants and children: sonographic measurements. *AJR Am J Roentgenol*. 1991;157:119–121.

Rumack CM, ed. *Diagnostic ultrasound*. ed 3, St Louis: Elsevier; 2005.

Rumack C, Drose J. Neonatal and infant brain imaging. In *Diagnostic ultrasound*, vol 2, ed 4, St. Louis: Elsevier; 2011:1623–1695.

Seibert JJ, Avva R, Hronas TN, et al. Use of power Doppler in pediatric neurosonography: a pictorial essay. *Radiographics*. 1998;18(4):879–890.

Shekdar K. Posterior fossa malformations. *Semin Ultrasound CT MRI*. 2011;32(3):228–241.

Shen EY, Weng SM, Kuo YT, et al. Serial sonographic findings of lenticulostriate vasculopathy. *Acta Paediatr Taiwan*. 2005;46(2):77–81.

Shen MD, Nordahl CW, Young GS, et al. Early brain enlargement and elevated extra-axial fluid in infants who develop autism spectrum disorder. *Brain*. 2013;136(Pt 9):2825–2835.

Siegel MJ. Neonatal intracranial problems. In: Sanders RC, Winter T, eds. *Clinical sonography: a practical guide*. ed 4 Baltimore: Lippincott Williams & Wilkins; 2007:341–364.

Siegel MJ. *Pediatric sonography*. Philadelphia: Lippincott Williams & Wilkins; 2010.

Taylor GA, Madsen JR. Neonatal hydrocephalus: hemodynamic response to fontanel compression—correlation with intracranial pressure and need for shunt placement. *Radiology*. 1996;201(3):685–689.

van de Bor M, Walther FJ, Sims ME. Acceleration time in cerebral arteries of preterm and term infants. *J Clin Ultrasound*. 1990;18:167.

van Wezel-Meijler G. *Neonatal cranial ultrasonography*. Berlin: Springer; 2007.

van Wezel-Meijler GV, De Vries LS. Cranial ultrasound—optimizing utility in the NICU. *Curr Pediatr Rev*. 2014;10(1):16–27.

Volpe JJ. Brain injury in the premature infant: overview of clinical aspects, neuropathology, and pathogenesis. *Semin Pediatr Neurol*. 1998;5:135–151.

Winter TC, Kennedy AM, Byrne J, Woodward PJ. The cavum septi pellucidi: why is it important? *J Ultrasound Med*. 2010;29(3):427–444.

Whitelaw A. Intraventricular hemorrhage and post-hemorrhagic hydrocephalus: pathogenesis, prevention and future interventions. *Semin Neonatol*. 2001;6:135–146.

CHAPTER 28

Infant and Pediatric Hip

Kathryn E. Zale

OBJECTIVES

On completion of this chapter, you should be able to:
- Discuss anatomy of the neonatal hip
- Describe normal movements of the hip
- Describe sonographic evaluation of the neonatal hip, including technique and protocol
- Describe the normal sonographic appearance of the neonatal hip
- Describe the sonographic evaluation of the neonatal hip for developmental displacement of the hip
- Define the Barlow and Ortolani maneuvers
- Differentiate between subluxation of the hip and dislocation of the hip

OUTLINE

Normal Anatomy and Sonographic Findings 851
    Bony Pelvic Girdle ("Socket") 851
    Femoral Head ("Ball") 851
    Hip Joint ("Ball-and-Socket") 851
    Supporting Ligaments and Muscles 853
    Movements of the Hip 853
Sonographic Examination 854
    Sonographic Examination Overview 854
    Examination Preparation 854
    Sonographic Protocol 855
Developmental Displacement of the Hip 857
    Hip Dislocation 857
    Hip Dislocation and Subluxation 857
    Physical Examination 858
    Abnormal Sonographic Findings 859
    Sonographic Technique/Assessment 860
    Treatment and Sonographic Follow-up 866
    Etiology 866
Joint Effusions of the Hip 867
    Sonographic Technique 867
Other Hip Conditions (Incidental Findings) 868

KEY TERMS

Abduction
Adduction
Barlow maneuver
Developmental displacement of the hip (DDH)
Extension
Flexion
Frank dislocation
Galeazzi sign
Hip joint
Labrum
Medial and lateral rotation
Ortolani maneuver
Pelvic girdle

Sonographic evaluation of the neonatal hip allows for a dynamic view of the soft tissues and cartilaginous structures, with the added advantages of being low cost and free from ionizing radiation, contrast media, and sedation. It plays an important role in the diagnosis and management of developmental displacement of the hip (DDH) in the infant, which is among one of the most common causes of disability in children. Sonography can also easily detect fluid within the joint space, providing clinicians a quick way to assess for joint effusions or septic arthritis in the child with a painful hip.

Until the femoral head ossifies around 4 to 6 months of age, sonography is optimal for evaluating DDH in the neonatal/infant hip compared with other imaging modalities. Although magnetic imaging can provide excellent anatomic detail of the hip anatomy in the young infant, it does not capture live movement of the hip joint, requires a long scanning period, is expensive, and requires sedation. Computed tomography is also non-dynamic and requires gonadal ionizing radiation and sedation but may be helpful in infants confined to a cast. Radiography, although it was originally used to diagnose DDH in young infants, is not reliable in detecting the soft cartilaginous structures of the hip, not yet ossified in this population.

This chapter provides the necessary anatomy, sonographic findings, and techniques to better assess the hip conditions for which sonography offers advantages over other imaging modalities: (1) developmental dislocation or dysplasia of the hip, which is seen in the first 6 months of life, and (2) hip pain, which is seen in the young child and may be caused by inflammatory or traumatic conditions.

NORMAL ANATOMY AND SONOGRAPHIC FINDINGS

The anatomy assessed in the pediatric hip consists of the bony pelvic girdle, superior portions of the femur, hip joint (including the acetabulum and acetabular labrum), and supporting ligaments and muscles.

Bony Pelvic Girdle ("Socket")

The bony pelvis is a ring-like bony structure composed of two hipbones (or pelvic bones), the sacrum, and the coccyx. The sacroiliac joints unite these two hipbones with the sacral part of the vertebral column. The pubic symphysis is where these two hipbones unite with each other anteriorly. The two hipbones (also referred to as the **pelvic girdles** or hip girdles) serve as attachment sites, one for each side of the lower limbs, to the axial skeleton. Each pelvic girdle is made up of a single hip (or coxal) bone and, collectively, may be referred to as the innominate bones or os coxae. The pelvic girdle is ossified at birth and consists of three joined bones, individually identified as the ilium, ischium, and pubis.

Within the pelvic girdle, these bones join and form the bony acetabulum. The acetabulum makes up the hip socket and is normally a deep, cup-shaped structure. In childhood, the *triradiate cartilage* connects these three bones and is made of three distinct growth plates, or physes, that do not ossify until around puberty. The cartilage, once ossified, becomes part of the adult bony acetabulum, or hip socket (Fig. 28.1).

Femoral Head ("Ball")

The bone of the upper thigh is the femur, which is surrounded by muscles, ligaments, and tendons. The upper part of the femur, the head, articulates with the hipbone to make the hip joint (Fig. 28.2). The shaft (or diaphysis) of the femur is ossified at birth and sonographically appears hyperechoic, casting an acoustic shadow.

The greater and lesser trochanters, as well as the neck and head of the femur, are cartilaginous at birth and seen well with sonography. The greater trochanter sits superolateral, whereas the lesser trochanter projects from the posteromedial proximal femoral shaft. The neck of the femur tapers medial, superior, and anterior toward the femoral head.

The *femoral head* appears as a large hypoechoic circle and typically ossifies between 3 and 8 months of age. Ossification begins centrally (which may be seen as early as 2 to 4 weeks of age), with girls often showing earlier ossification than boys. The sonographic value in evaluating the hip greatly decreases as the femoral head ossifies. Ossification as the infant ages, combined with structures located deeper in the body, equates

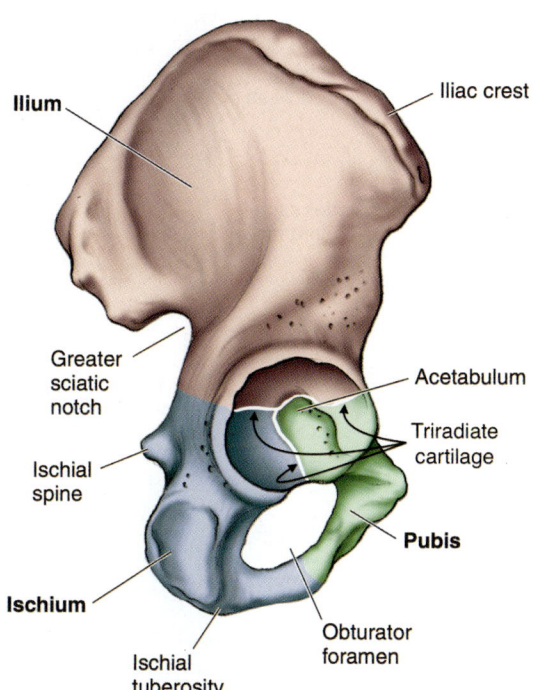

FIG. 28.1 **Bony pelvic girdle.** Lateroposterior view of the right pelvic girdle made up of the ilium, ischium, and pubis. These bones join together at the acetabulum, making up the bony hip socket. The triradiate cartilage seen in childhood *(arrows)* within the acetabulum is outlined in white.

to a substantial diminishment in image quality around 4 to 6 months of age. Once the femoral head is completely ossified, it is difficult to obtain adequate sonographic images because of the beam artifact interference (Fig. 28.3). Radiography is the preferred modality after 4 to 6 months of age unless the acetabulum and triradiate cartilage can be adequately identified with ultrasound.

Hip Joint ("Ball-and-Socket")

The rounded femoral head and the cup-shaped bony acetabulum form the freely movable "ball-and-socket" **hip joint**. The hip joint is not directly palpable because it is surrounded and protected by muscles of the upper thigh. The greater trochanter of the femur forms a palpable knob at the side of the region.

Within the hip joint, the bony acetabulum has a smaller articular surface than the femur's articular surface and is often referred to as the *bony acetabular roof*. The acetabulum is made deeper by a rim of cartilage that surrounds it, called the acetabular **labrum**. The labrum is mostly composed of hyaline cartilage and is hypoechoic, except at the lateral marginal tip, where it changes to fibrocartilage and appears echogenic and triangular. Furthermore, this lateral margin forms an extension of the acetabular roof (often referred to as the *cartilaginous roof*). The acetabular labrum narrows the acetabulum and increases its depth, functioning to stabilize and support the femoral head articulation within the acetabulum.

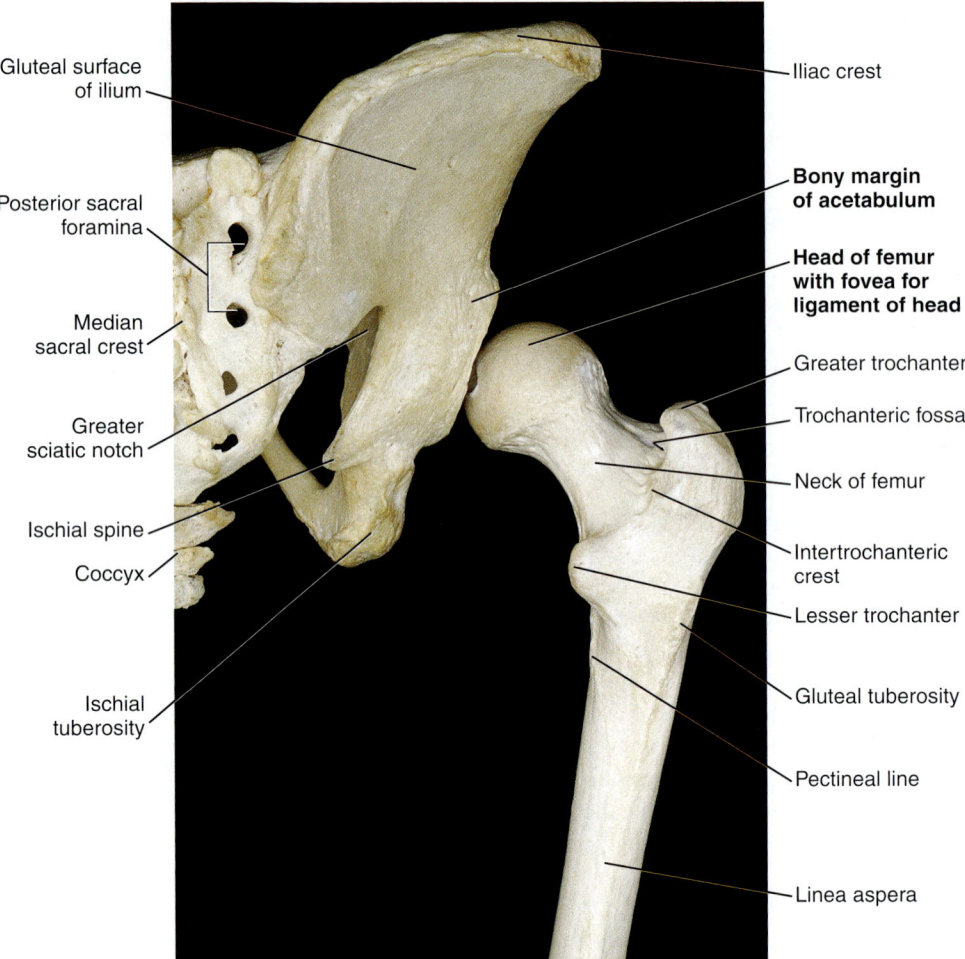

FIG. 28.2 **Hip joint: posterior osteology.** Posterior view of the right hip joint. The femur has been partly dislocated so that its posterior surface can be completely visualized.

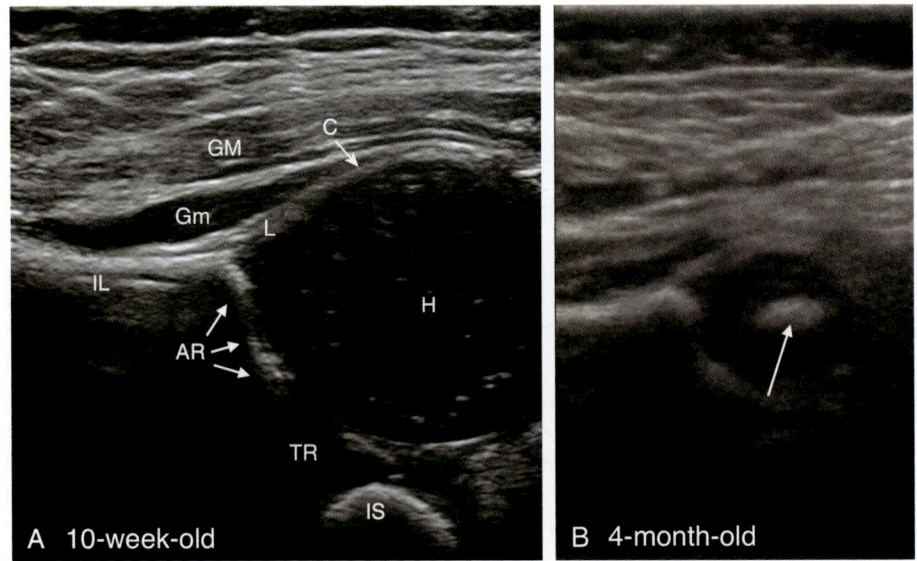

FIG. 28.3 **Normal anatomy and femoral head development.** A normal coronal flexion view of the hip joint is seen in both images. (A) A 10-week-old infant has a cartilaginous and hypoechoic femoral head with smooth borders and fine-stippled echoes dispersed throughout. (B) The femoral head shows central ossification *(arrow)* in this 4-month-old infant. *AR*, Bony acetabular roof; *C*, capsule; *GM*, gluteus medius; *Gm*, gluteus minimus; *H*, head of femur; *IL*, ilium; *IS*, ischium; *L*, labrum; *TR*, triradiate cartilage. (Courtesy Nationwide Children's Hospital, Columbus, OH.)

Normally, the labrum, or cartilaginous acetabulum, covers two-thirds of the femoral head. Sonographically, the labrum is best depicted from a coronal view and appears superolateral to the femoral head, adjacent to the ilium. Both the bony and cartilaginous roofs are evaluated and may be measured.

The *acetabular notch* is a bony deficiency at the inferior portion of the central acetabular depression and is covered by a band of fibrous tissue called the transverse acetabular ligament. The ligamentum teres of the femur runs from this acetabular notch through a foramen to the pit or *fovea* in the head of the femur, through which nerves and blood vessels pass. In the younger child, this ligament contains the *branch of the obturator artery* to supply the femoral head. The artery usually disintegrates by 7 years of age (Fig. 28.4).

Within the hip joint evaluation, the triradiate cartilage is a useful landmark, lying posterior to the femoral head, and appears hypoechoic in the neonate. The posterior rim of the acetabulum, part of the triradiate cartilage in the immature skeleton, is often referred to as the *posterior lip*.

Supporting Ligaments and Muscles

The hip joint is surrounded by a tough *capsule*, which attaches to the intertrochanteric line of the femur and is reinforced by outside ligaments and muscles. This fibrous capsule covers the labrum and appears sonographically to extend from it inferiorly. The psoas tendon crosses the center of the hip joint just inferior to the inguinal ligament. The iliacus muscle sits lateral to the psoas tendon and, along with the psoas muscle, flexes the hip.

The most important hip ligament is the iliofemoral ligament, which passes from the anterior inferior iliac spine to each end of the intertrochanteric line. It is one of the strongest ligaments in the body and is very important for standing and maintaining correct upright balance.

The large gluteus maximus muscle overlies other muscles superior and posterior to the hip joint. The gluteus maximus is a powerful extensor of the hip. The *gluteus minimus* muscle is the immediate cover for the upper part of the hip joint. The *gluteus medius* and gluteus minimus pass from the outer surface of the hipbone to the greater trochanter. Together they act as abductors of the hip joint. Their most important function is to prevent adduction and to keep the pelvis level while walking.

Movements of the Hip

The movements of the hip are somewhat limited in range because of the tight fit between the femur and acetabulum and because the hipbone is immobile. The following are the hip movements and their actions. Note that sonographic evaluation is primarily concerned with the abduction and adduction motions.
- Flexion—bending forward
- Extension—bending backward
- Abduction—moving sideways outward
- Adduction—moving sideways inward
- Medial rotation
- Lateral rotation

Flexion (bending forward) and **extension** (bending backward): The primary flexors of the hip are the psoas major, iliacus, and rectus femoris. Extension is limited to 20 degrees and is brought about by the hamstrings and gluteus maximus.

Adduction (moving sideways inward) and **abduction** (moving sideways outward): An example of hip adduction is crossing your legs when in a seated position, an action performed by the adductor group of muscles. In abduction, the gluteus medius and minimus muscles open the limbs. The more important function of these muscles, however, is to prevent adduction, which is the function they perform when walking (Fig. 28.5).

Medial and lateral rotation is related to the angle at which rotation occurs at the head of the femur, which is about 120 degrees angle to the shaft of the femur. When the trochanter moves forward, the femur rotates medially, and when the trochanter moves backward, the femur rotates laterally. Thus, the medial rotators are the anterior fibers of the gluteus medius and minimus. The lateral rotators are the small muscles at the back of the joint: piriformis, obturator internus, and quadratus femoris, with assistance from the gluteus maximus.

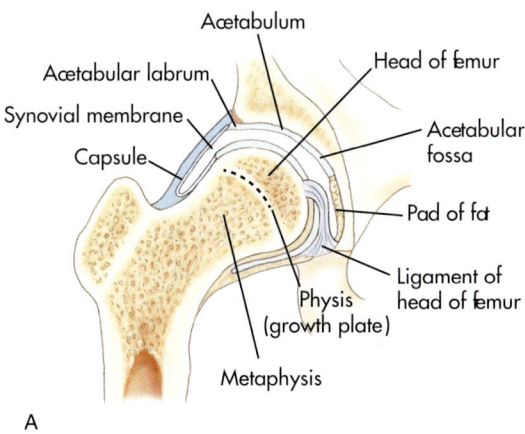
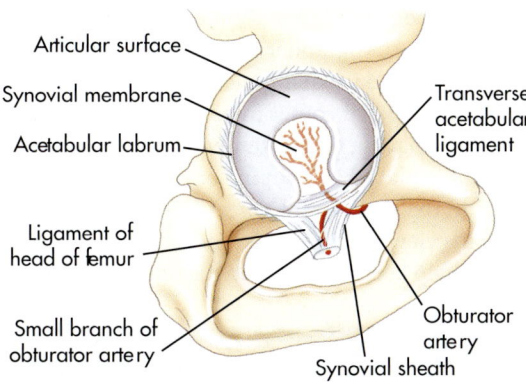

FIG. 28.4 (A) Coronal section of the right hip joint. (B) Lateroposterior view of the articular surface of the right hip joint and arterial supply of the femoral head.

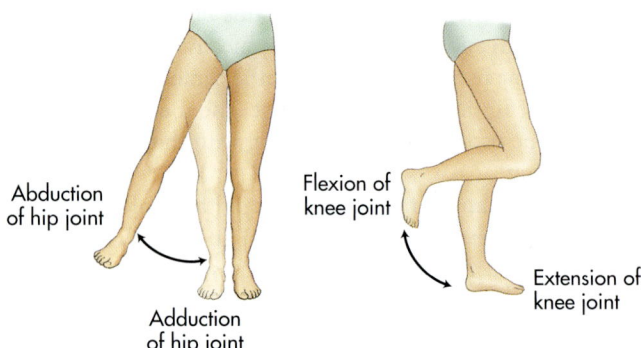

FIG. 28.5 Anatomic terms used in relation to the movement of the hip.

SONOGRAPHIC EXAMINATION

Sonography is the preferred imaging modality in the detection of DDH in infants. It is more sensitive than the physical examination and has been shown to change the diagnosis in over half of cases. Furthermore, it has changed the management plan in one-third of cases in infants presenting to pediatric orthopedist surgeons for suspected DDH. Given its ability to detect this condition, universal screening sonography has been recommended and implemented in some places. Unfortunately, screening has not been shown to decrease the rate of late diagnoses.

The most important factor influencing the outcome is the age at which the diagnosis is made and treatment initiated. Treatment should begin before the patient walks, and an early diagnosis is vital so that treatment can be instituted as early as possible. Currently, selective screening sonography is indicated in infancy after the neonatal period; if the physical examination is abnormal or unequivocal, risk factors, associated congenital anomalies, or neuromuscular conditions are present; or if there is a need to evaluate the response to treatment, often a Pavlik harness. Risk factors include female sex, breech presentation, oligohydramnios, or a family history of DDH.

The ultrasound examination may be repeated as often as necessary to follow the progression of treatment. However, if the patient is in a harness, do not remove the harness unless instructed to do so by the ordering physician or orthopedic doctor. Infants are often examined in the harness, and the stress maneuvers are not performed.

Sonography for DDH is practical for most infants from 4 to 6 weeks up 4 to 6 months of age. Exceptions may include older infants if the femoral head is not yet ossified. Neonates are not typically evaluated, and infants should be at least 44 gestational weeks of age, adjusted for prematurity. Typically, after 4 to 6 months of age, radiography is the preferred imaging modality.

Sonographic Examination Overview

The sonographic examination for DDH moves through a series of images in the coronal and transverse planes, taken at rest and with stress, allowing the sonographer to assess the position and stability of the femoral head in the hip joint.

Stability. Stability of the hip is determined through the guided motion and application of gentle stress. These gentle "push-pull" stress movements are the imaging counterparts of the Barlow (adduction) and Ortolani (abduction) physical screening maneuvers. Stability testing is reported as normal, lax, subluxable, dislocatable, and reducible or irreducible.

Femoral Head Coverage. Position of the hip is determined by the degree to which the femoral head is covered by the labrum, as well as the position of the femoral head in the acetabulum. The sonographic appearance of the femoral head location is described as normal, subluxed, or dislocated.

Bony and Cartilaginous Acetabulum. Additionally, the development of the bony and cartilaginous acetabulum is sonographically described as normal, immature, or dysplastic.

Measurements. Ideally, validation of the femoral head position is achieved through measurements quantifying the amount of femoral head coverage. Likewise, the acetabular morphology is assessed with drawn angles, which correspond to the degree of the bony acetabulum (alpha angle) and the labrum or cartilaginous acetabulum (beta angle).

Examination Preparation

To achieve a satisfactory examination, the infant should be relaxed and as comfortable as possible. Parental assistance is helpful to keep the infant calm. Having them stand on the opposite side of the bed allows the parent to be near the infant's head. Feeding before or during the examination helps to soothe the infant. Make sure the room is warm, and keep blankets close for warmth. Toys and other distractions help to quiet the infant so that the examination may be performed.

Sonography of the neonatal hip is performed with a high-frequency linear-array transducer, often a 10 to 12 MHz (Box 28.1). Sector or curved-array transducers will distort anatomy and are not recommended. This examination is always performed on both hips. Because ambidextrous scanning (commonly with the aid of a foot pedal) is a requisite, the sonographer often requires a good amount of experience before feeling fully competent. Scanning with the dominant hand first may be helpful. The right hip is examined with the transducer in the sonographer's left hand and vice versa. The opposite hand is used for manipulation of the hip being examined, while a foot pedal comes in handy to freeze and capture images without having to constantly reposition the infant.

The infant is placed in a supine or decubitus position perpendicular to the table with the feet toward the sonographer. In a decubitus view, rolled towels, bolsters, or even specialized cradles may help keep the child on his or her side. It is wise to

BOX 28.1	Linear-Array Transducer Recommendations

Premature infants: 12–15 MHz
Average-sized infant ≤3 months: 9–12 MHz
Infants 3–7 months: 6–9 MHz

leave the diaper on through the examination and expose only the side of the hip being examined.

Sonographic Protocol

The basic hip anatomy may be imaged in four different views. A two-word combination labels the view by both the plane of the body (coronal or transverse) and hip position (neutral or with flexion). While institutions may vary on which ones are performed, they include (1) coronal/neutral, (2) coronal/flexion, (3) transverse/neutral, and (4) transverse/flexion. Next, dynamic stress maneuvers from the flexed transverse position are then often performed. A coronal posterior lip view with stress may also be obtained. In the setting of pathology, a 3D acquisition of the coronal views is possible. Finally, measurements for a quantifiable evaluation are obtained from the coronal view(s) and may be performed by either the sonographer or radiologist, preferably by the latter.

Hip Views Positioning. All views are performed with the infant in the supine or lateral decubitus position with the transducer placed on the posterolateral aspect of the hip joint. The hand performing manipulation holds the infant's leg, often at the level of the low thigh or knee, and should stabilize it gently and steadily so the infant does not move too much and feels secure. In the neutral view, the infant's leg is straightened to a physiologic neutral position, or 15 to 20 degrees of flexion. The flexed view involves moving the knee upward toward the infant's chest so the hip is at 90 degrees of flexion.

Angling the probe in both the flexed and neutral positions should be strictly avoided. It is difficult to make the abnormal hip appear normal; however, one can make the normal hip appear abnormal—this has to do with probe angulation, which results in misalignment. Instead, the entire transducer should be moved to align properly with the anatomic structures to avoid tilting and oblique planes. When first learning, it may help to check the probe placement on the infant. Correct positioning is so important that Graf, whose series of lines and angle measurements are utilized to assess the acetabulum, recommends the use of a specialized cradle and probe guide system to reduce any such operator errors.

Coronal/Neutral View. The coronal view is crucial for assessing acetabular development. It is obtained by aligning the probe along the lateral shaft of the femur, demonstrating a straight iliac line to the inferior tip of the os ilium (iliac bone) at the midportion of the acetabulum (Fig. 28.6). The hypoechoic cartilage of the acetabular roof extends lateral to the acetabular lip. The echogenic tip of the labrum should also be visualized. The femoral head is resting against the bony acetabulum. The acetabular roof should have a concave configuration and cover over half of the femoral head. According to Graf, the coronal/neutral plane must meet certain checklist criteria to be considered diagnostic (Fig. 28.7 and Box 28.2).

Coronal/Flexion View. The coronal/flexion view is also made at the midacetabulum with similar sonographic features to the coronal/neutral view. First, the head of the femur is a bit more difficult to find in the flexed position but scanning in a posterior direction along the femoral shaft is helpful. However, unlike its neutral counterpart, the echogenic femoral metaphysis is not visualized in the coronal/flexion

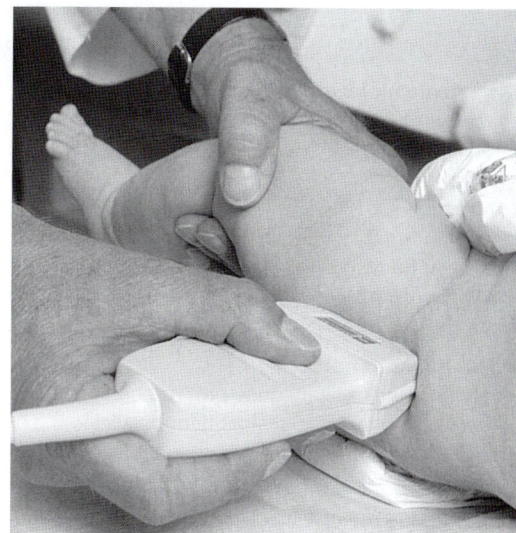

FIG. 28.6 Coronal/neutral positioning. The transducer is coronal with respect to the hip joint, aligned along the iliac bone. The femur is in a physiologic neutral position for the infant (slight hip flexion).

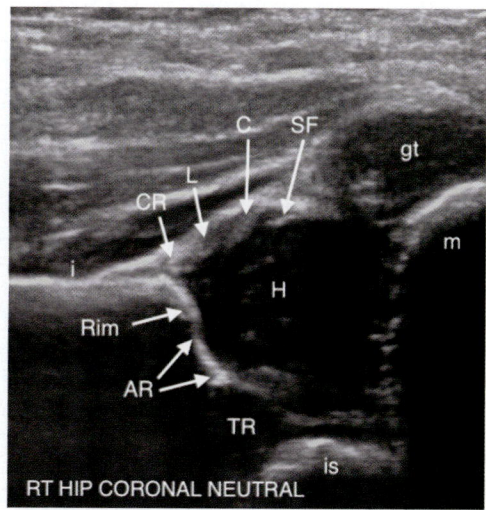

FIG. 28.7 Normal coronal/neutral view. This view demonstrates Graf's checklist (Box 28.2) and shows the fibrocartilaginous tip of labrum (L), triradiate cartilage (TR), ilium (i), femoral head (H), metaphysis (m) of the femoral neck, synovial fold (SF), joint capsule (C), cartilaginous roof (CR), bony acetabular roof (AR), and bony rim (Rim). Also shown is the ischium (is) and greater trochanter (gt). (Courtesy Chester County Hospital, West Chester, PA.)

position. Also, the coronal/flexion view provides more of a "ball on a spoon" appearance. The gluteus minimus muscle is another landmark of this view and is seen as a hypoechoic structure superolateral to the labrum (Fig. 28.8).

Transverse/Flexion View. In the transverse view, the transducer is rotated 90 degrees and moved posteriorly into a posterolateral position over the hip joint (Fig. 28.9). The transverse/flexion study is normally performed with the hip flexed 90 degrees. One static transverse/flexion view is normally imaged, along with one adduction stress, including a cine clip, and one abduction image (see Dynamic Harcke Technique, later in this chapter). Keep in mind that the hip is naturally already in an adducted position in the normal transverse/flexion view.

BOX 28.2 Graf Checklist for Coronal/Neutral View

Checklist 1: Anatomic identification
M—Metaphysis or osteochondral border
H—Femoral head
SF—Synovial fold
C—Joint capsule
CR—Cartilaginous roof
AR—Acetabular Bony roof
Rim—Bony rim (normally concave)
L—Labrum

Checklist 2: Usability Check
1—Lower limb of the os ilium (bony rim) is seen
2—Os ilium (iliac bone) contour straight or parallel to the probe
3—Tilting and oblique planes are avoided[a]

[a]Graf recommends the use of a specialized cradle and probe guide system to reduce error.

The bony shaft of the femur gives off brightly reflected echoes anteriorly, adjacent to the femoral head. The echoes from the bony acetabulum appear posteriorly to the femoral head, and in the normal hip, a U configuration is produced (Fig. 28.10A).

The relationship of the femoral head to the acetabulum is observed during flexion of the hip from adduction to abduction. In adduction, the femoral head moves little while adding stress, whereas the femoral shaft moves upwards to become straight across and the femoral head forms a deep U configuration with maximum abduction (see Fig. 28.10B). Ensure that the transducer is posterior enough to image the medial bony acetabulum, or the hip may appear falsely displaced. The hip is stressed with a gentle posterior push, downwards toward the transducer, in adduction (Barlow maneuver). In the normal hip, the femoral head will remain deep within the acetabulum in contact with the ischium with stress (see Fig. 28.10C). The normal hip flexion images are summarized in Fig. 28.11.

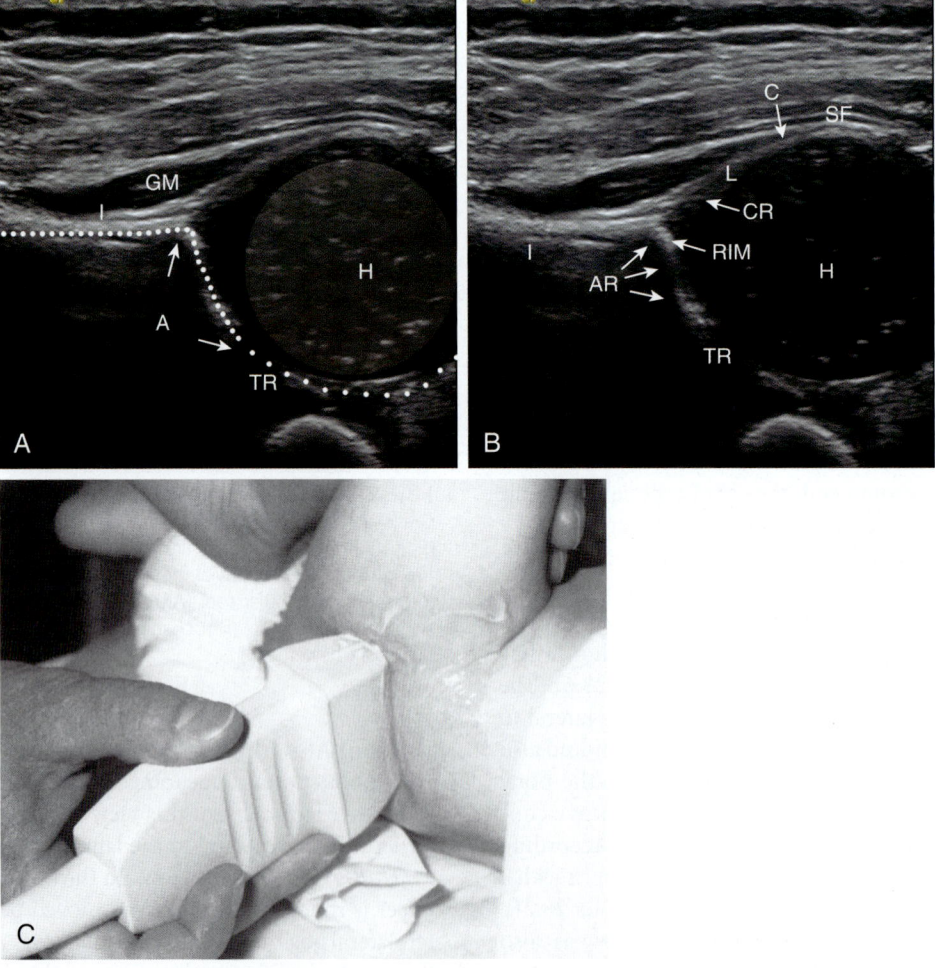

FIG. 28.8 Normal coronal/flexion view and positioning. (A) Normal "ball on a spoon" appearance of the coronal/flexion view. The femoral head (H) is the ball, the acetabulum (A) forms the spoon, and the iliac (I) line is the handle. The triradiate cartilage (TR) and gluteus minimus muscle (GM) are also seen. (B) Corresponding anatomic anatomy with coronal/neutral position (notice metaphysis is missing). (C) Normal coronal/flexion view with the hips now drawn up. *AR*, Bony acetabular roof; *C*, joint capsule; *CR*, cartilaginous roof; *H*, femoral head; *I*, ilium; *L*, labrum; *Rim*, bony rim; *SF*, synovial fold; *TR*, triradiate cartilage. (Courtesy Nationwide Children's Hospital, Columbus, OH.)

Transverse/Neutral View. From the transverse/flexion view, the leg is brought down into a neutral position. The transducer is now horizontal to the acetabulum from the lateral aspect of the hip. The plane passes through the femoral head into the acetabulum at the center of the triradiate cartilage. The exam is begun caudally over the bony shaft of the femur. Moving cephalad, the transition from bone to cartilage in the proximal femur becomes apparent, and the circular cross section of the spherical femoral head is identified.

In the normal hip, the sonolucent femoral head is positioned against the bony acetabulum over the triradiate cartilage. The images of the sonogram represent the parts of a flower. The femoral head is the flower; the bright echoes from the ischium posteriorly and pubis anteriorly represent the leaves at its base. The stem is formed by echoes that pass through the triradiate cartilage into the area of acoustic shadowing created by the osseous structures.

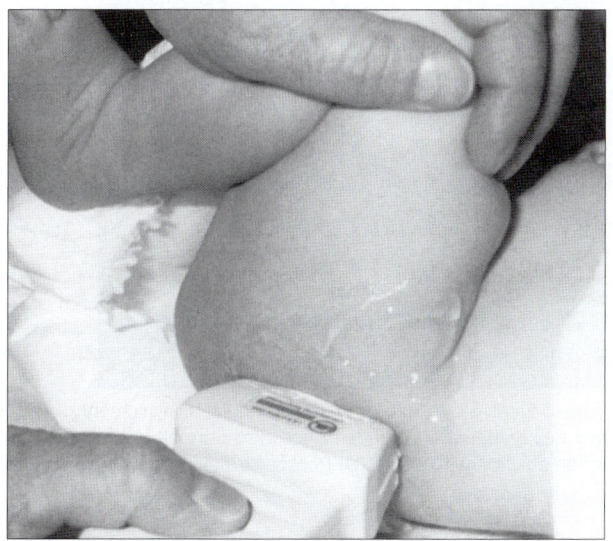

FIG. 28.9 **Transverse/flexion positioning**. The transducer is in the axial plane posterolateral over the hip joint with the hip flexed.

DEVELOPMENTAL DISPLACEMENT OF THE HIP

Developmental dysplasia/dislocation of the hip has been described as far back as Hippocrates. Formerly known as congenital hip dislocation, this misleading term referred to a spectrum of pathology that usually develops after birth. Therefore, the term **developmental displacement of the hip (DDH)**, or developmental dysplasia of the hip, is now used. DDH encompasses a broad spectrum of pathologies from the mildly subluxated hip to the fully dislocated hip.

Hip Dislocation

Neonatal hip dislocation is often not present at birth and may be acquired, teratogenic, or developmental. Acquired causes of hip dislocation can be traumatic or nontraumatic (i.e., neuromuscular diseases). Teratogenic dislocations occur in utero and are associated with neuromuscular disorders.

Hip Dislocation and Subluxation

In the newborn period, the femoral head may dislocate in a lateral and posterosuperior position relative to the acetabulum. The femoral head is found completely separated from the joint in dislocated hips. However, if the femoral head is only partially dislocated out of the joint, the hip is said to be subluxated (Fig. 28.12). When a hip joint is lax, or the femoral head is seated too shallow in the acetabulum, the hip may be manipulated (via the Barlow maneuver) and easily dislocated. Such hips are described as being dislocatable. When dislocation does occur, the femoral head can usually be reduced (via the Ortolani maneuver) without deformity to the joint. When the femoral head cannot be reduced back into the bony socket, the hip is described as dislocated.

When dislocation is not recognized early, the muscles tighten and limit movement over time, which causes the acetabulum to become dysplastic because it lacks the stimulus of

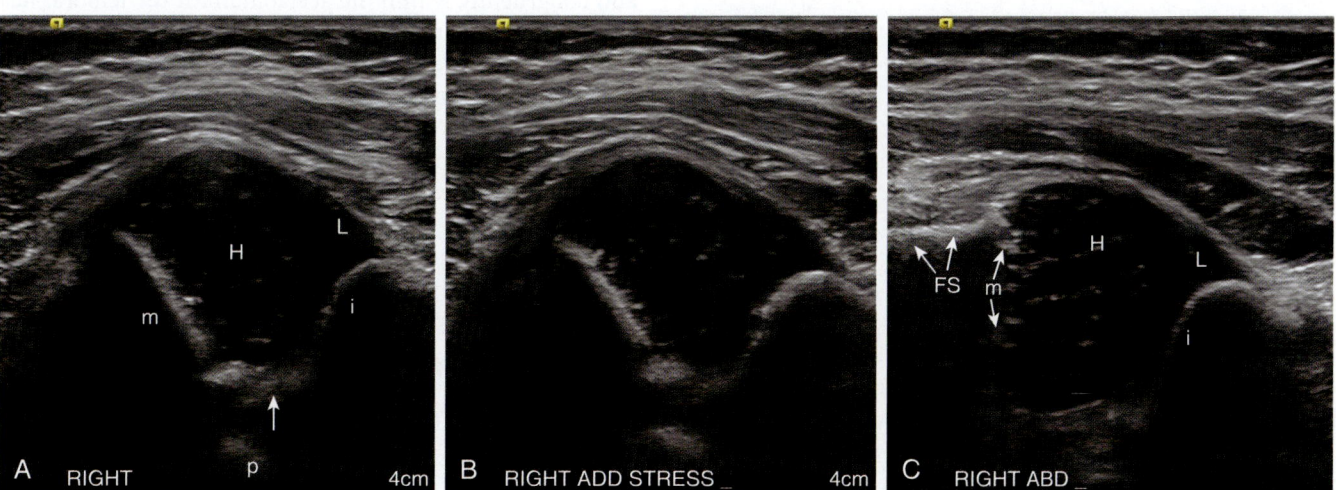

FIG. 28.10 **Normal transverse/flexion view with and without stress**. Normal sonographic appearance of the transverse/flexion study. (A) Transverse flexion image (adduction position)—normal U shape. (B) Transverse image with added stress from the same adduction (ADD) position— very little to no change is normal. (C) Transverse image showing the abduction (ABD) position—the femoral shaft is now straight across with the femoral head appearing deeper. *Arrow* points to area of triradiate cartilage. *FS*, Femoral shaft; *H*, head; *I*, ischium; *l*, labrum; *m*, metaphysis; *p*, pubis. (Courtesy Nationwide Children's Hospital, Columbus, OH.)

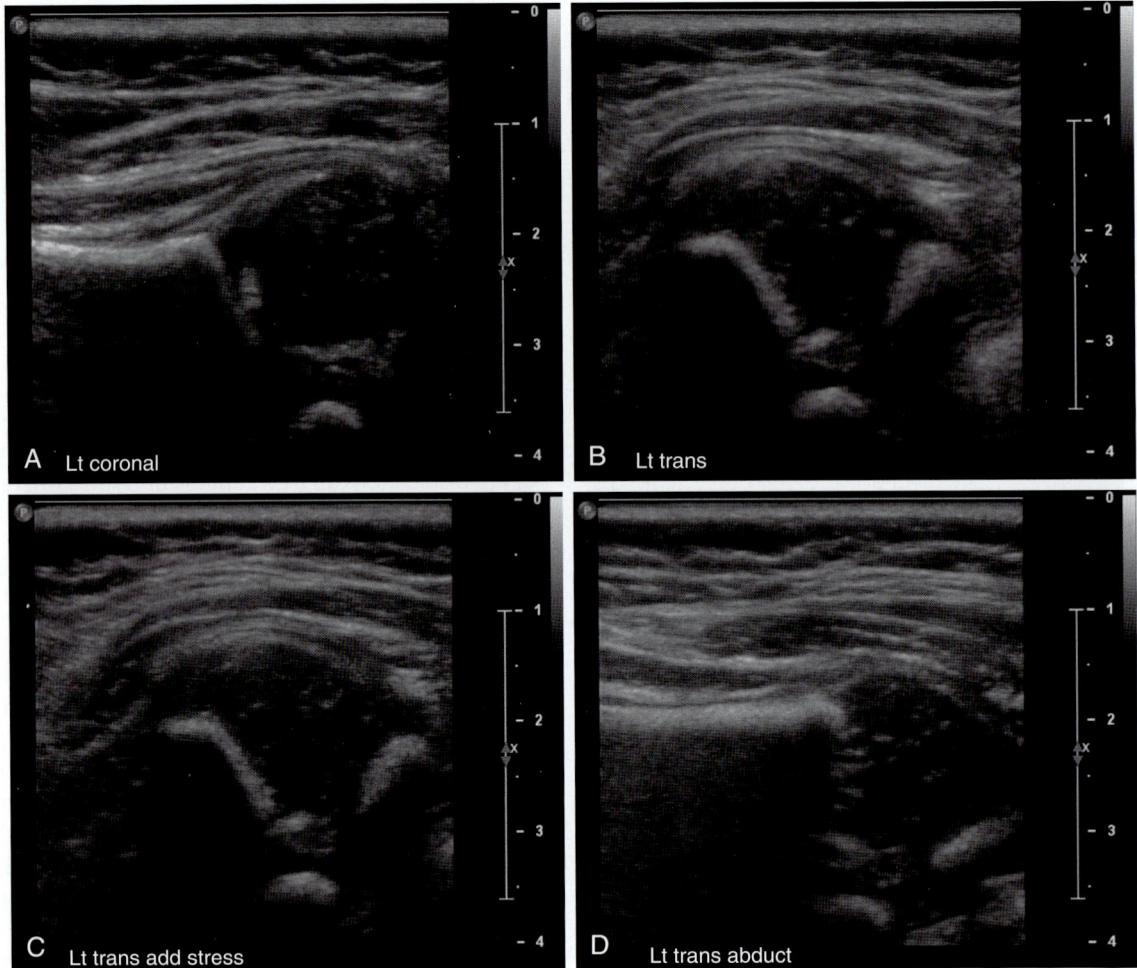

FIG. 28.11 **Infant hip flexion views.** Normal sonographic study of the left hip of a 10-week-old to rule out developmental displacement of the hip. Remember that this is a bilateral examination; in this case, the right hip images were nearly identical to the left ones, also normal. (A) Coronal/flexion view. (B) Transverse/flexion (adduction) view. (C) Transverse/flexion view in an adduction position with stress. (D) Transverse/flexion view in an abduction position. (Courtesy Nationwide Children's Hospital, Columbus, OH.)

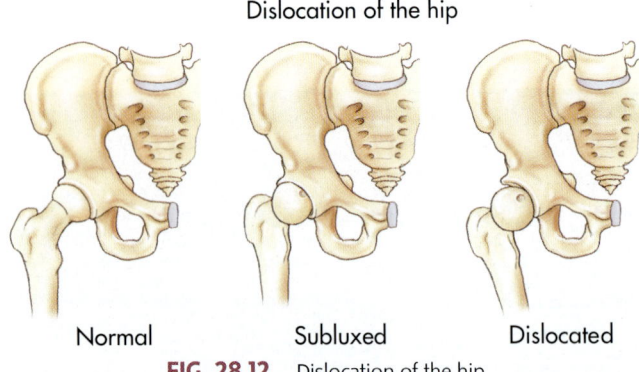

FIG. 28.12 Dislocation of the hip.

the femoral head for proper growth. In turn, the ligamentous structures stretch, and fibrofatty tissue fills in the acetabular void, making it impossible to return the femoral head into the acetabulum. This *fibrofatty pulvinar* may also develop in subluxation.

Abnormal Hip Development (Developmental Displacement of the Hip). Most frequently, pathology in the neonatal and infant hip is developmental. Development of the neonatal hip requires both sides of the femoral head to be seated normally and congruently within the acetabulum. If the femoral head and acetabulum are not in their normal position, both sides of the hip will develop abnormally. A displacement of the hip is a relatively common abnormality, and when diagnosed in the neonatal period (up to 4 to 6 weeks of age), it is often attributed to normal laxity of the hips. Whereas 90% of mild cases diagnosed with sonography may resolve, more severe cases of DDH can cause impaired function and degenerative joint disease. Diagnosis should be made early, and treatment instituted promptly.

Physical Examination

The sonographer should be acquainted with the physical examination to screen for DDH. The same maneuvers are employed for the stress portion of the examination, and it provides more context when abnormal findings are the reason for the sonographic study.

A careful physical examination remains the universal screening for DDH and is therefore critical to the diagnosis.

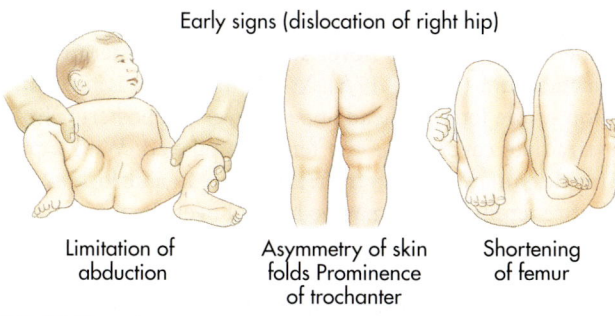

FIG. 28.13 Physical signs of developmental displacement of the hip.

DDH detection, however, may vary widely between novice clinicians and experienced pediatric orthopedists. On visual inspection, the dislocated hip shows asymmetric skin folds and shortening of the affected thigh. The knee is lower in position on the affected side when the patient is supine and the knees are flexed, known as the **Galeazzi sign** (Fig. 28.13).

Hip instability may resolve after 4 to 6 weeks due to waning maternal hormones. Therefore, neonates with a slightly positive or inconclusive physical examination, and newborns with a risk factor for DDH, should be examined with sonography after this period to reduce false-positive results. Neonates with a grossly positive physical examination result or dislocation, however, may be scanned earlier.

The two following basic maneuvers are helpful in the diagnosis of DDH. The Barlow maneuver determines whether the hip can be dislocated, and the Ortolani maneuver determines whether the dislocated femoral head can be reduced back into the acetabulum.

Barlow Maneuver. In the Barlow maneuver (Fig. 28.14), the patient lies in the supine position with the hip flexed 90 degrees and adducted. Downward and outward pressure is then applied. If the hip can be dislocated, the examiner will feel the femoral head move out of the acetabulum with his or her fingers.

Ortolani Maneuver. In the **Ortolani maneuver** (Fig. 28.15), the patient lies in the supine position. The examiner's hand is placed around the hip to be examined, with the fingers over the femoral head. The examiner's middle finger lies over the greater trochanter, and the thumb is over the lesser trochanter. The hip is flexed 90 degrees, and the thigh is abducted. Movement in the normal hip should feel smooth. In cases of DDH, a "clunk" is appreciated as the femoral head returns into the acetabulum. A "click" does not necessarily imply DDH. Each hip should be examined individually.

Abnormal Sonographic Findings

Abnormal Coronal/Neutral View. In the coronal view, when a hip becomes subluxed or dislocated, the femoral head gradually migrates laterally and superiorly with progressively decreased coverage of the femoral head. Echogenic soft tissue (fibrofatty pulvinar) may be interposed between the femoral head and the bony acetabulum. In hip dysplasia, the bony acetabular roof is irregular and rounded, and the

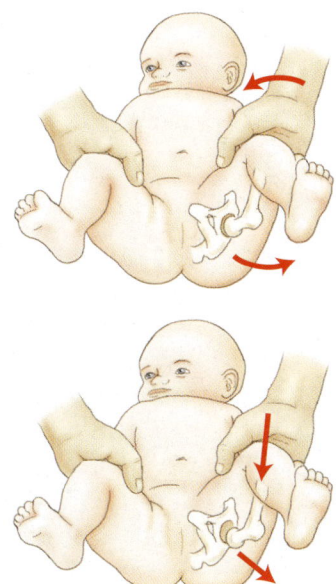

FIG. 28.14 Dynamic hip evaluation with the Barlow maneuver. Examiner is evaluating if the hip is abnormal and can easily be dislocated.

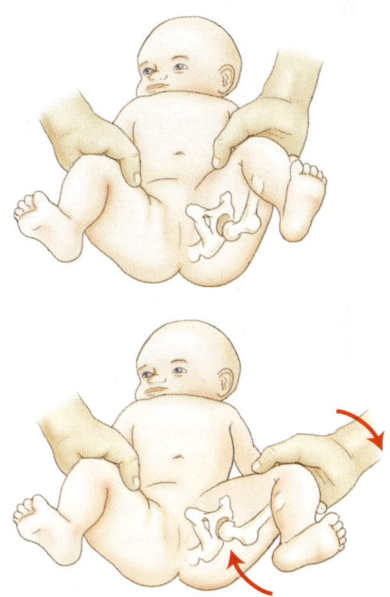

FIG. 28.15 Dynamic hip evaluation with the Ortolani maneuver. Examiner is evaluating if a dislocated hip can be reduced (bringing the femoral head back into the acetabulum.)

labrum is defected superiorly and becomes echogenic and thickened. When the hip is frankly dislocated, the labrum may be deformed, which will contribute to irreducibility (Fig. 28.16).

Abnormal Coronal/Flexion View With Stress (Posterior Lip View). From the coronal/flexion view, the transducer is moved posteriorly; the scan plane is over the posterior margin of the acetabulum showing the posterior lip of the triradiate cartilage.

In subluxation, the femoral head is displaced laterally, posteriorly, or both with respect to the acetabulum. Between the

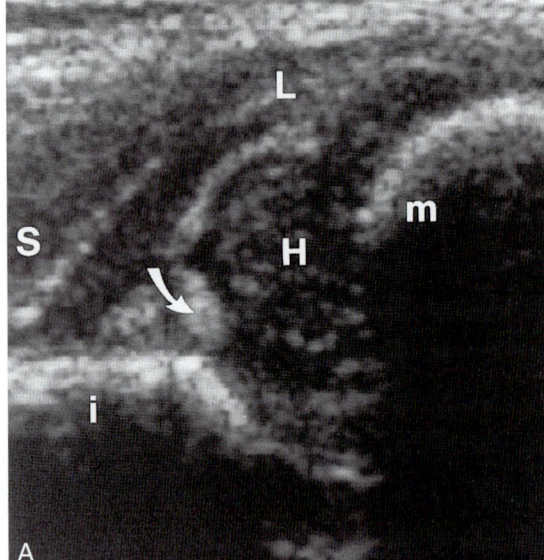

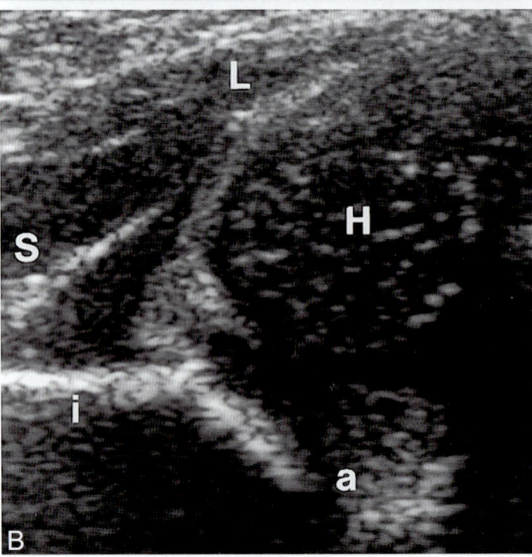

FIG. 28.16 Abnormal coronal views. (A) Coronal/neutral view of a dislocated hip shows displacement of the femoral head laterally with deformity of the labrum *(arrow)*. (B) Coronal/flexion view of a dislocated hip has similar findings to image A and shows soft tissue echoes in the acetabulum (fibrofatty pulvinar) that may prevent the hip from being reduced without surgical intervention. *a*, Acetabulum; *H*, femoral head; *i*, iliac line; *L*, lateral; *m*, femoral metaphysis; *S*, superior.

femoral head and the bony reflections, soft tissue echoes from the medial acetabulum are seen. In dislocation, the femoral head is completely out of the acetabulum. With superior dislocations, the femoral head may rest against the iliac bone. In posterior dislocations, the femoral head is seen lateral to the posterior lip of the triradiate cartilage. The acetabulum may not be visualized in a dislocation because the bony shaft of the femur blocks the view.

This view involves a dynamic "push-pull" maneuver. In many clinical sites, the pediatric orthopedist, the radiologist, or the experienced pediatric sonographer performs this examination. The **Barlow maneuver** is performed with adduction and gentle pushing against the knee. In the normal hip, the femoral head is never seen over the posterior lip of the acetabulum (Fig. 28.17A). When instability is present, a portion of the femoral head appears over the posterior lip of the triradiate cartilage as the femur is pushed. With a pull, the head again disappears from the plane. In a dislocated hip, the entire femoral head may be located over the posterior lip and may or may not move out of the plane with traction (Fig. 28.17B).

Abnormal Transverse/Flexion View. In the transverse view, if subluxation is present, the hip will be normally positioned or mildly displaced at rest, and there will be further lateral displacement from the medial acetabulum with stress, but the femoral head will remain in contact with a portion of the ischium. If the femoral head dislocates laterally, the central femoral head does not align with the iliac wing. A line drawn through the iliac wing will pass through the medial aspect of the femoral head. If the femoral head dislocates posteriorly, only an echogenic arc (representing one side of the head) is seen. With **frank dislocation**, however, the hip will be laterally and posteriorly displaced to the extent that the femoral head has no contact with the acetabulum, and the normal U configuration cannot be obtained (Fig. 28.18). With abduction (Ortolani maneuver), the dislocated hip may be reduced, returning it to the acetabulum.

Abnormal Transverse/Neutral View. In this view, malpositioned hips show soft tissue echoes between the femoral head and acetabulum. The width and configuration of the gap depend on the nature of the displacement. With subluxation, the femoral head usually moves posteriorly and remains in contact with the posterior aspect of the acetabulum. In more severe cases, the lateral displacement accompanies posterior migration. Most dislocations are lateral, posterior, and superior.

Sonographic Technique/Assessment

Two general sonographic techniques are used in the assessment for DDH: the static (morphologic) Graf technique and the dynamic Harcke technique. A combination of these and their modifications may be performed across institutions, and the techniques are not mutually exclusive. However, regardless of the Graf method or modification used at an institution, the assessment of hip stability and morphology appears feasible and accurate given a well-organized, high-quality service.

Static Graf and Modified Graf Technique. The standard Graf sonographic image is acquired in the coronal plane at the midacetabular level from the lateral aspect of the hip in a neutral position. This image includes the femoral head, acetabulum, labrum, and iliac bone as it meets the triradiate cartilage. The inclusion of these structures ensures a proper image from which the radiologist or physician can measure the alpha and/or beta Graf angles (Fig. 28.19). It is from these angles (Box 28.3) that the neonatal hip is assessed quantitatively. The alpha angle is normally greater than 60 degrees, and the beta angle is usually less than 55 degrees. Software is

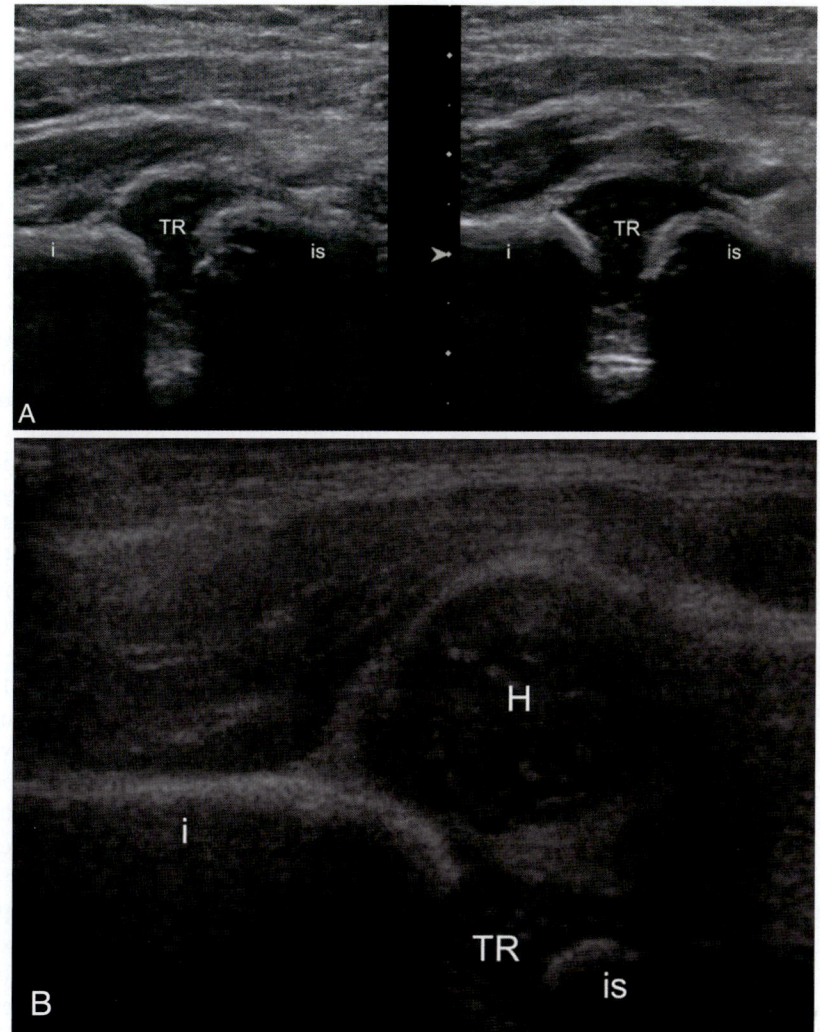

FIG. 28.17 Normal and dislocated hip in the posterior lip view. (A) A normal hip shows the triradiate cartilage (TR) of the posterior acetabular lip between the ilium (i) and ischium (is). The image on the *right* shows there is no change with the push stress portion of the "push-pull" maneuver. (B) A fully dislocated hip abnormally shows the femoral head over the triradiate cartilage of the posterior lip of the acetabulum. If irreducible, the femoral head would not disappear from this view upon the pull movement. (Courtesy Chester County Hospital, West Chester, PA.)

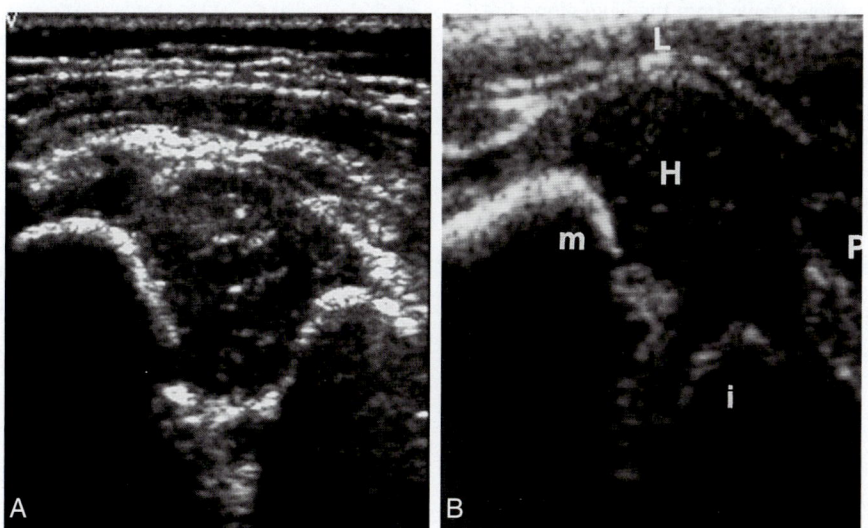

FIG. 28.18 Normal and dislocated hip in the transverse/flexion view. (A) Normal hip sonogram shows echolucent femoral head surrounded by metaphysis (anterior) and ischium (posterior), forming a U shape around the femoral head. (B) Dislocated hip sonogram shows sonolucent femoral head displaced posterolaterally. The U configuration of normal metaphysis and ischium is not seen. *H*, Femoral head *i*, ischium; *L*, lateral; *m*, metaphysis; *P*, posterior.

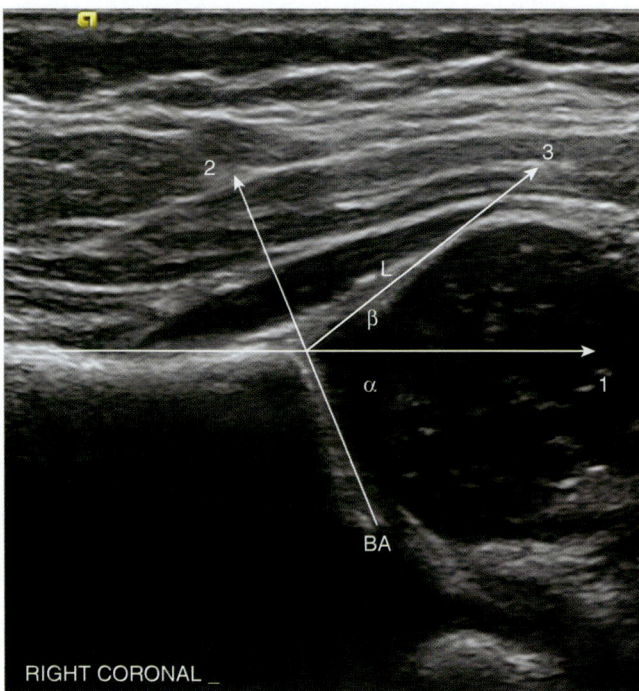

FIG. 28.19 Normal Graf angle assessment. Normal hip and coronal view measuring alpha and beta angles. Alpha angle (α) is between lines 1 and 2. Beta angle (β) is between lines 1 and 3. *BA*, Edge of the bony acetabulum (deepest point); *L*, center of the labrum. (Courtesy Nationwide Children's Hospital, Columbus, OH.)

BOX 28.3   Graf's Alpha and Beta Angles

Graf used a series of lines and angle measurements to evaluate the morphology of the acetabulum (Fig. 28.19):

Line 1: Baseline, drawn along the ilium, extending through the head of the femur

Line 2: Provides the alpha angle, drawn from bony edge of acetabulum at the triradiate cartilage to the lowest point of the ilium.

Line 3: Provides the beta angle drawn from the ilium along the labrum.

Alpha Angle (α)
- Measures the acetabular depth
- The alpha angle reflects changes in the osseous portion of the acetabulum, which occur gradually
- Normally ≥60 degrees

Beta Angle (β)
- The beta angle reflects changes in the cartilaginous acetabulum (labrum), which occur more quickly than do changes in the osseous acetabulum
- Normally ≤55 degrees

---

also available on ultrasound systems, making it possible for sonographers to measure these angles from the machine.

Modifications to the original Graf technique have allowed the inclusion of hip shape and stability to be examined. The Rosendahl, or modified Graf, method involves measuring only the alpha angle of the bony acetabulum in a coronal/flexion view. Meanwhile, Graf encourages using the beta angle, as it reflects changes to the cartilaginous acetabulum, which occur more quickly than do changes in the osseous acetabulum and may be more sensitive than the alpha angle. However, studies have found both techniques to be comparable in their findings. The modified Graf method may include a separate dynamic assessment of the hip joint for stability. The usual practice for this modification is having the femur flexed at 90 degrees, allowing for consistency with any possible follow-up examinations when the infant is in a harness.

The four types of neonatal hip displacements are described in Table 28.1, showing the Graf and modified Graf (Rosendahl) criteria. Normal hips (type I) require no further evaluation. Immature hips (types IIa and IIb) must be monitored, and follow-up studies are required. Mild hip dysplasia (types IIc and IId) is monitored and may or may not require treatment. Severe hip dysplasia (types III and IV) must be treated.

Additional subjective sonographic signs of DDH are also assessed, which include delayed ossification of the femoral head and acetabular abnormalities (see Table 28.2). Fibrofatty pulvinar may also be present.

The osteochondral plate sign (Fig. 28.20) may be added for obtaining the standard Graf image in the neutral coronal position. The sign should show a perpendicular angle of the osteochondral border, or metaphysis, to the transducer. It may aid in providing better reproducibility of Graf measurements, especially among borderline alpha angle values.

A normal sonogram does not absolutely exclude DDH, although the sensitivity and specificity of sonography approach 100%. The accuracy and specificity of this technique increase with age and are highest at 3 months of age and lowest before 4 weeks of age. Furthermore, a learning curve to obtain experience with normal and abnormal hips is important to the reproducibility and accuracy of the sonographic evaluation. Harcke has suggested that at least 100 infant hip examinations should be performed to acquire sufficient experience. Fig. 28.21 demonstrates all the different modified Graf hip types, defined by alpha angle and appearance.

Static Femoral Head Coverage Measurement. Another widely used measurement is the femoral head coverage, which can be used in adjunct to the Graf measurements, although it is not required. Simply, the height of the femoral head is measured and compared with the height of the bony acetabular coverage within the femoral head in a coronal/flexion view (Fig. 28.22). Normally, the mean femoral head coverage is between 54% and 56% (in females and males, respectively), with a lower limit of 45%. Fifty percent is considered the limit between normal and potentially abnormal. Subluxation is reached when femoral head coverage is less than 39% and dislocation less than 10%.

Dynamic Harcke Technique. Harcke formulated basic standards for dynamic hip sonography, which are currently used in most clinical settings today. In the flexed position, the hip may be stressed and evaluated in the transverse or coronal plane. If evaluated in the coronal view, the tip of the labrum must be included in the image. Often, though, the transverse plane is more widely used. It is important to label

CHAPTER 28 Infant and Pediatric Hip

TABLE 28.1 Classification of Neonatal Hips and Angle Measurements

Modified (Rosendahl) Graf Classification		Graf Hip Classification			
Description	Modified Graf Angle Measurements[a]	Classification	Description	Graf Angle Measurements[b]	Age
Normal	α ≥ 60°	Type I	Normal	α >60° β <55°	Any
Immature	α 50–60°	Type IIa	Physiologically immature	α 50–60° β 55–77°	<3 months
		Type IIb	Immature	α 50–59° β 55–77°	>3 months
Mild dysplasia	α 43–50°	Type IIc	Acetabular deficiency	α 43–49° β >77°	Any
		Type IId	Everted labrum with subluxation	α 43–49° β >77°	Any
Severe dysplasia	α < 43°	Type III	Everted labrum with dislocation	α <43° β >77°	Any
		Type IV	Dislocation	α <43° β >77°	Any

[a]Modified Graf measurements taken from a flexed coronal position.
[b]Graf measurements taken from a neutral coronal position.
α, Alpha angle; β, beta angle.

TABLE 28.2 Description of Acetabulum by Graf Type

Hip Graf Classification Type	Bony Roof Development	Ossific Rim Shape	Cartilaginous Rim (Labrum) Appearance
Type I	Good	Sharp or angular	Extends over femoral head and is narrow
Type II	Deficient or severely deficient	Rounded or rounded/flat	Covers femoral head and may be thinned and compressed
Type III	Poor	Flat	Displaced upward and may be echo-poor or more reflective than femoral head, may be thinned or rounded
Type IV	Poor	Flat	Inverted into the acetabulum

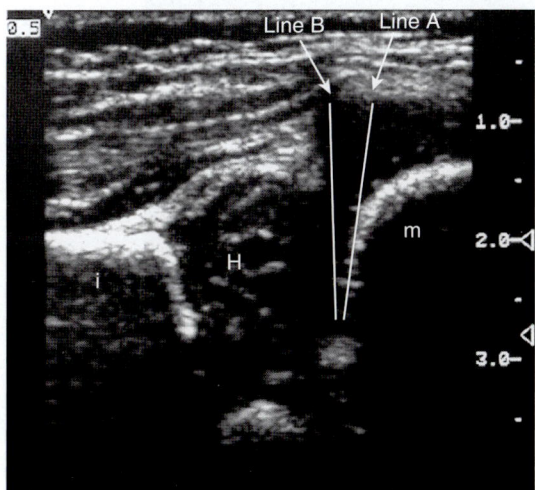

FIG. 28.20 Osteochondral plate sign shown in a normal hip in the coronal/neutral view. *Line A* is drawn along the osteochondral border, or metaphysis (m). For increased reproducibility, this osteochondral border line should be angled so it is near parallel with the transducer scan lines *(line B)*.

the appropriate view and stress maneuver used (abduction/adduction).

The thigh of the hip being examined is slightly adducted and abducted while simultaneously exerting a downward force, while imaging is performed with the opposite hand. This is known as the "push-pull" method or "piston" maneuver. Images are obtained at rest and at maximum pressure, showing any movement of the femoral head. Cine clips are very useful, too. With added stress in adduction, the femoral head should normally remain resting against the osseous acetabulum. If the hip is unstable, the femoral head will be identified posterior (superior and lateral) to the acetabulum (Fig. 28.23). The sonographer will often feel the hip displace out of the joint, and any instability felt in the hip is noted. If the hip does become subluxed or dislocated, the Ortolani maneuver is performed to assess if the hip can be reduced (this is the abduction view). The often accompanying "click" or "clunk" sounds are reported; a "click" sound is not definitive for hip displacement, but a "clunk" diagnoses it.

Hips are classified according to their behavior under stress as normal, unstable, or dislocated. The femoral head should be stable within the acetabulum with stress after 4 weeks of age. Unstable hips are divided into subluxable and dislocatable. A subluxable hip, or an immature hip due to physiologic laxity, is one in which the proximal femur moves (more than 6 mm on the left and 4 mm on the right) within the acetabulum, but it cannot be displaced out of it. A dislocatable hip is one in which the proximal femur can be displaced out of the acetabulum, but it can be reduced. A dislocated hip is one in which the femoral head is displaced out of the acetabulum and cannot be reduced.

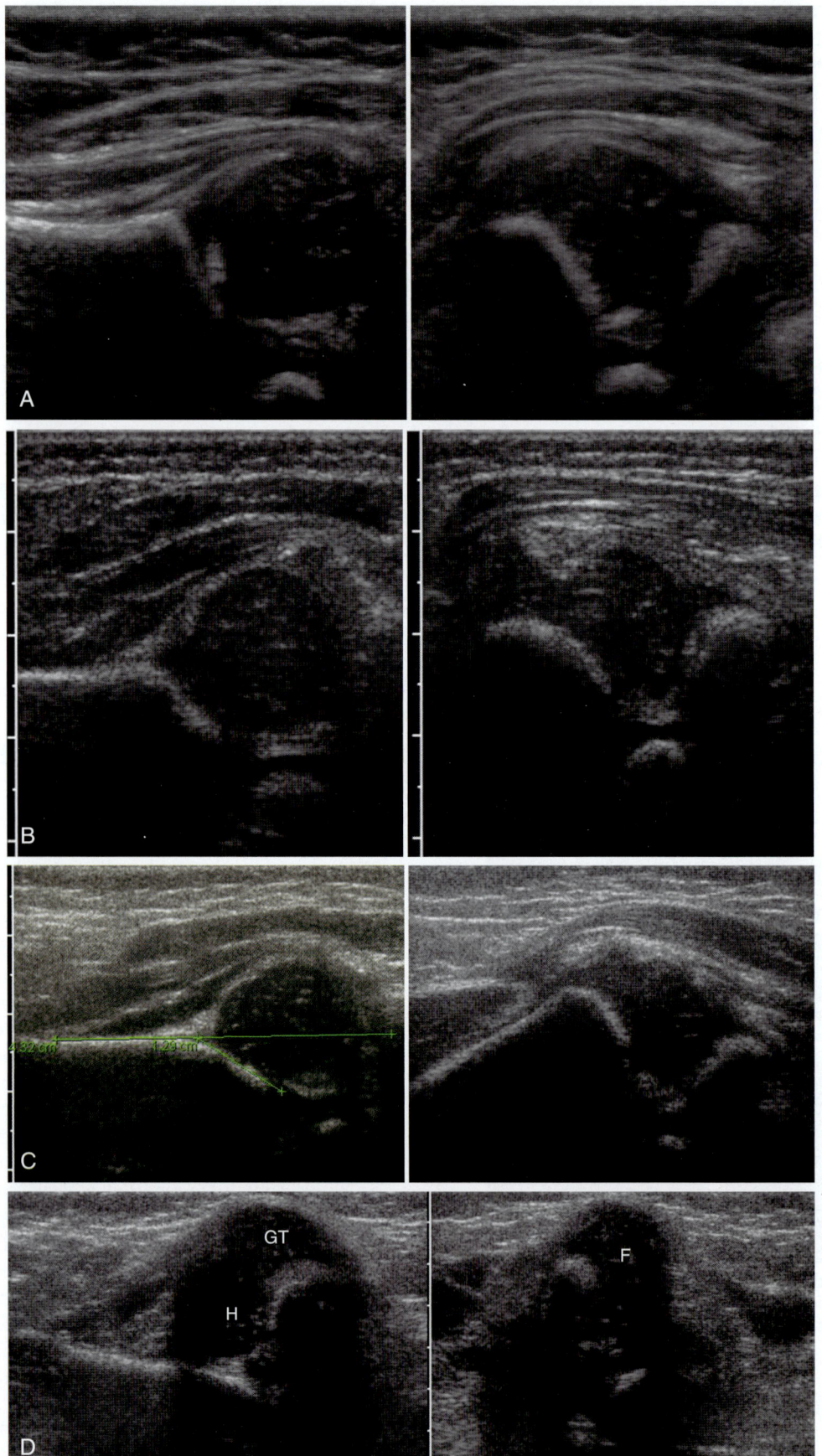

FIG. 28.21 Flexed coronal and transverse views of the different modified Graf types. Images on the *left* show a coronal/flexion view and images on the *right* show a static transverse/flexion view. (A) Normal hips. (B) Immature hips. (C) Mild hip dysplasia. Hip click was heard in this patient. (D) Severe hip dysplasia with frank dislocation and associated severe acetabular dysplasia. *GT*, Greater trochanter; *H*, femoral head. (Courtesy Nationwide Children's Hospital, Columbus, OH.)

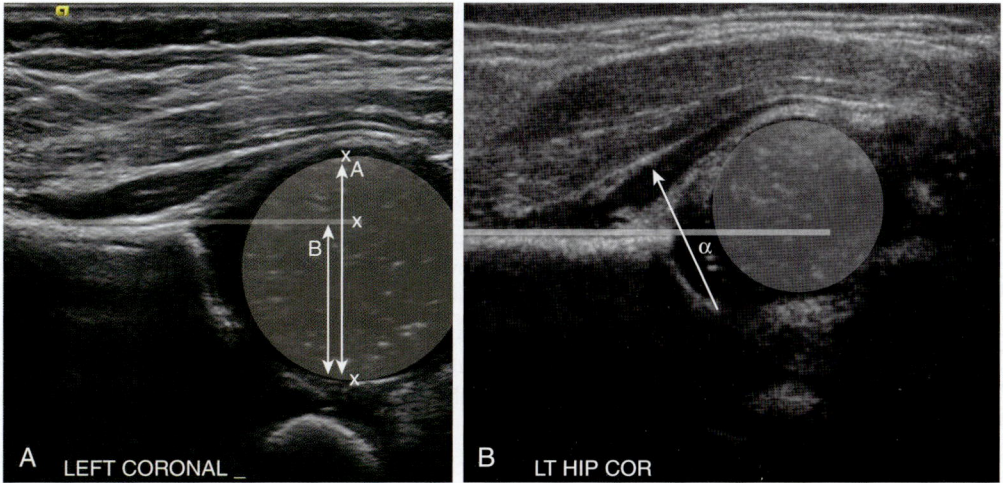

FIG. 28.22 Femoral head coverage measurement. (A) Normal hip in a coronal/flexion view demonstrating the caliper placements (x) and line measurements *(arrows)* for the femoral head coverage technique. Femoral head coverage % = B/A × 100%. (B) Abnormal hip in a 2-week-old girl with risk factors and abnormal physical examination. Coronal image shows bony roof covering less than 50% of the femoral head. Alpha angle was between 53 and 57 degrees. Acetabular morphology was of concern, with the labrum slightly more horizontal than normal, while the superior bony rim was a bit more rounded on both sides. Although no hip instability was noted on stress movements, due to acetabular morphology, consideration for treatment and a follow-up were strongly suggested. (Courtesy Nationwide Children's Hospital, Columbus, OH.)

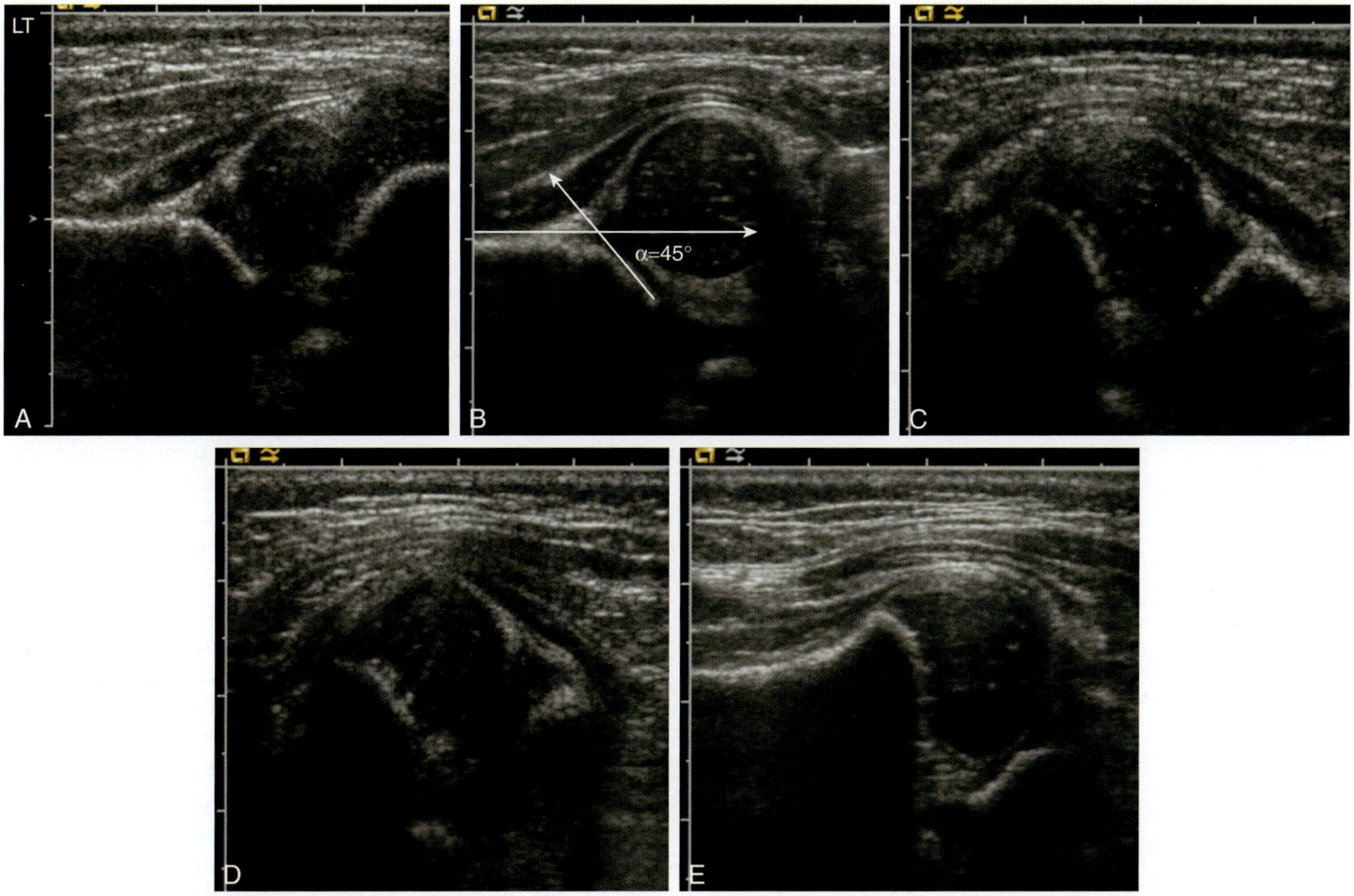

FIG. 28.23 Dynamic technique shown in a mildly dysplastic hip. The sonographer reported a lax unstable hip. (A) Coronal/neutral position. (B) Coronal/flexion position with the modified Graf angle measuring 45 degrees. (C) Transverse/flexion. (D) Transverse/flexion with adduction stress. Hip appears to move away from the acetabulum, slightly lateral and superior. (E) Transverse/flexion with abduction, showing abnormal bony rim morphology. (Courtesy Nationwide Children's Hospital, Columbus, OH.)

Treatment and Sonographic Follow-up

The most important factor influencing the outcome of DDH is the age at which the diagnosis is made and treatment initiated. Treatment should begin before the patient walks and ideally long beforehand. Delayed diagnosis often requires more complex treatment and with worse outcomes. The principle of treatment is that a subluxed hip in the neutral or rest position will seat itself with continuous flexion and abduction. The initial treatment of uncomplicated DDH is closed reduction. This may be accomplished either by placing two diapers on the neonate or by using a spica cast, brace, or Pavlik harness (Fig. 28.24). The hip should be positioned in flexion, with abduction and external rotation.

The position of the femoral head relative to the acetabulum can be determined with follow-up sonography. If the patient has a cast, a "window" must be cut into the cast so the transducer can be placed directly on the skin. Fortunately, the Pavlik harness is more commonly used, allowing easy access to demonstrate the hip joint's response to treatment (Fig. 28.25). Within 6 to 8 weeks of treatment, the hip joint often stabilizes.

Causes of failure of closed reduction include inversion of the labrum or capsule and invagination of the iliopsoas muscle, which can be imaged most efficiently by sonography and magnetic resonance imaging. If closed reduction fails or the dislocation is teratogenic, the patient usually requires open reduction or surgical means.

Etiology

Incidence of Developmental Displacement of the Hip. The incidence of hip dislocation is difficult to define as there is no gold standard test, but it is estimated to be between 1.5 and 20 cases per 1000 live births. Milder forms of displacement, such as subluxation, are more common and when the diagnosis is based on diagnostic sonographic findings, the rate may be as high as 40 to 60 cases per 1000 infants. However, epidemiologic and demographic data vary widely, ranging from 0.06 per 1000 live births among Africans in Africa to 76.1 per 1000 among some Native Americans.

Multiple risk factors may contribute to the condition. Approximately 12% to 16% of all newborns have one or more of these factors and are at a higher risk of developing DDH. The most salient factors include breech presentation in both pregnancy and delivery, which increases the risk nearly four times over the general population. Females are affected 4 to 6 times more frequently than males. The left hip is affected 64% of the time owing to the common left occiput anterior position in utero; likewise, DDH occurs unilaterally 64% of the time. It is also more common among firstborn children and those with a family history of DDH.

The condition also affects certain races, such as Caucasians and certain North American tribes, more than those of African or Asian descent. Some suspect these differences may be due to swaddling practices. Improper swaddling, where the hips cannot move freely, has been strongly associated with DDH, which has a higher prevalence of being diagnosed in winter months as well. Other risk factors may include maternal hypertension, fetal growth restriction, oligohydramnios, premature rupture of membranes, prolonged gestation, increased birth weight, Potter syndrome, and neonatal intensive care. Congenital muscular torticollis and congenital foot deformities are also associated factors. Prematurity, however, is not a predisposing risk factor for DDH.

Causes of Developmental Displacement of the Hip. Although the exact etiology of DDH is unknown, the primary root is thought to be increased laxity within the joint capsule, causing a gradual migration of the femoral head away from the acetabulum. Hormonal, mechanical, and genetic factors are thought to play a role.

Hormonal Factors. The hormonal theory suggests that the sex hormones act on the laxity of the connective hip joint tissue. The maternal hormonal effect of estrogen, which increases muscle laxity late in pregnancy (aiding childbirth), is thought to account for increased risk among female neonates, as this effect is reduced by the male sex hormones. Other sex hormones affecting laxity include progesterone and estrogen. Progesterone increases the collagen content in the joint capsule, likely facilitating hip dislocation, whereas estrogen has the opposite effects.

Mechanical Factors. As for the mechanical causes of DDH, swaddling, oligohydramnios, breech presentation, and the primigravid uterus are considered risk factors because each limits the mobility of the hip in its own way. Improper swaddling may keep the hips in an adducted position if swaddled too tight and straight; instead, the legs should be able to bend up and out of the hips. Oligohydramnios limits mobility because less than a normal amount of amniotic fluid is present for the fetus to move freely within the amniotic sac. In breech presentation, the fetal hip rests against the maternal sacrum and is usually flexed, limiting movement. This usually affects the left hip. The frank breech presentation of the fetus is the highest risk because the hips are maximally flexed, and the knees are extended. The primigravid uterus is smaller

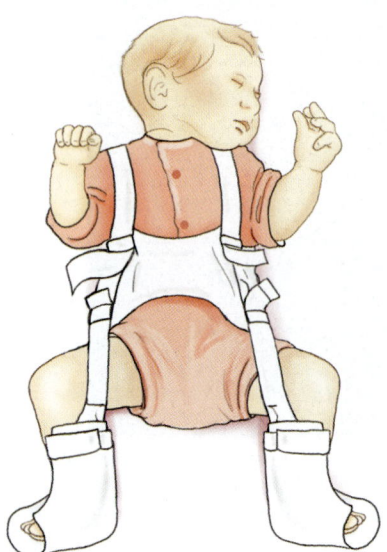

FIG. 28.24 The Pavlik harness may be used in the treatment of hip dysplasia.

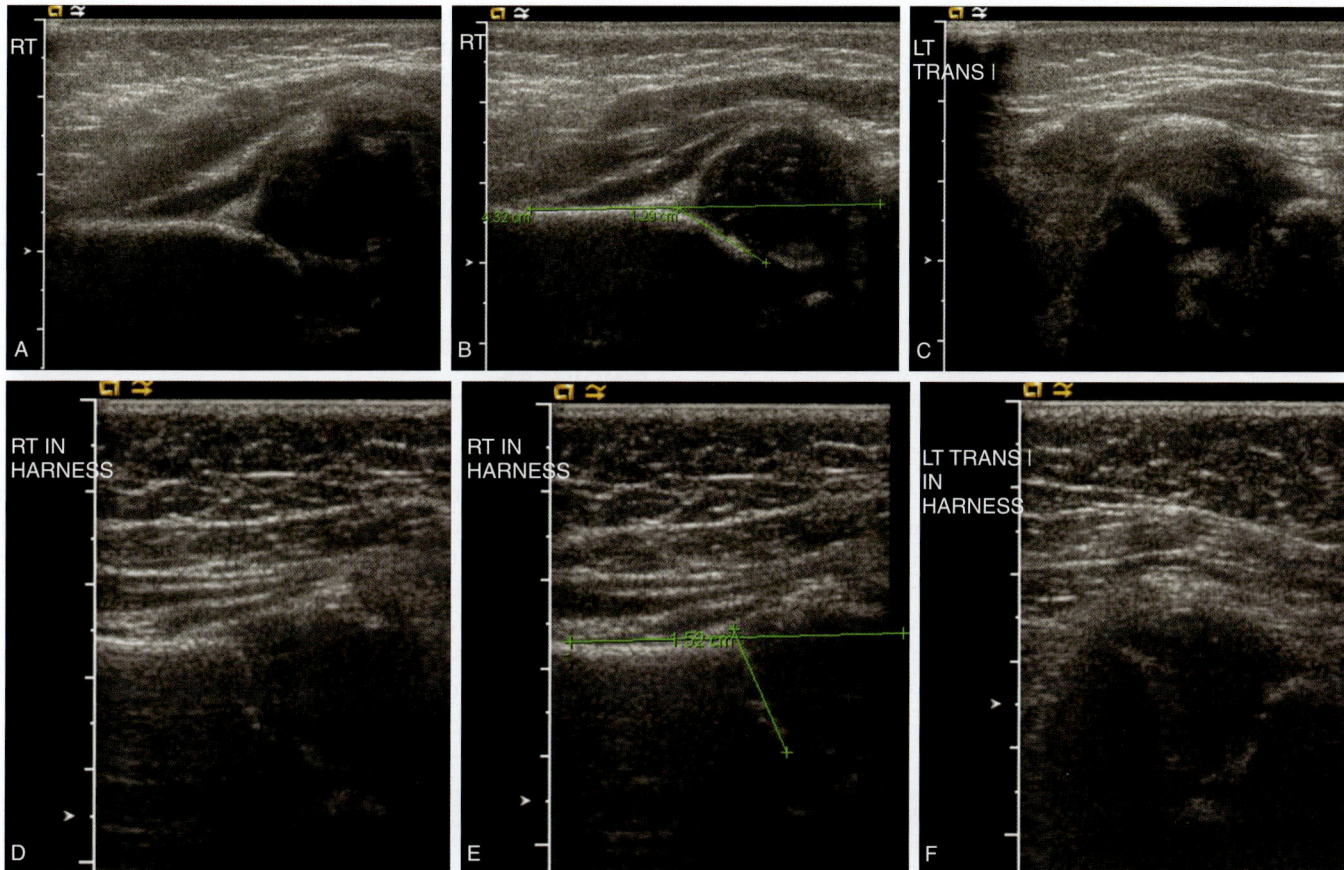

FIG. 28.25 Pavlik harness follow-up. Pretreatment and posttreatment images of a patient wearing a Pavlik harness for follow-up assessment of developmental displacement of the hip. Patient presented with mild dysplasia bilaterally, and both normalized with harness treatment. In the harness, stress maneuvers are not performed. (A) Pre–right hip coronal/flexion view at 4 weeks of age. (B) Pre–right hip modified Graf alpha angle measured 45 degrees, consistent with mild dysplasia. (C) Pre–transverse sonogram of left hip, also mildly dysplastic. (D) Post–right hip coronal/flexion view at 3.5 months of age. (E) Post–right hip modified Graf alpha angle measured over 60 degrees on follow-up, consistent with a normal hip. (F) Post–left hip transverse image shows the femoral head seated normally within the acetabulum. (Courtesy Nationwide Children's Hospital, Columbus, OH.)

than the multigravida uterus and is more confining, limiting mobility.

Genetic Factors. Genetic factors are currently being investigated in DDH, and findings from family and twin heritability suggest a strong genetic predisposition at onset (although less so with regard to progression or severity). Evidence shows that there is a 5% chance that a child will be affected if a sibling has DDH and a 36% chance if one sibling and one parent are affected. There is a 12% chance that an affected individual will have a child with DDH.

JOINT EFFUSIONS OF THE HIP

Joint effusions occur when synovial fluid builds up in the hip capsule—it may be transient or suggest septic arthritis. Transient synovitis is the most common cause of hip pain in children ages 3 to 10 years old. It is more common in males and is thought to be caused by an inflammatory response due to viral infection. Young children often present clinically to the emergency department with localized pain, refusal to bear weight, limping, limited movement of the affected hip, or fever. Additionally, the child may have had a viral infection 1 to 2 weeks earlier.

Sonography offers a rapid and sensitive technique to detect joint effusions of the hip. If a joint effusion is present, the synovial fluid needs to be aspirated (arthrocentesis); this is often performed under sonographic guidance. The fluid is then evaluated in the laboratory to determine whether it is transient synovitis versus septic arthritis. Fluid analysis is the definitive diagnosis, although laboratory values may show increased leukocytosis, among others. Transient synovitis can often bring relief with just the removal of the fluid, whereas septic arthritis is a true emergency and is more serious, requiring intravenous antibiotic treatment, orthopedic consultation, and admission. Delayed treatment can result in severe damage to the hip joint and may even necessitate a hip replacement.

Sonographic Technique

A high-frequency linear transducer is used to view the longitudinal anterior femoral neck, where synovial fluid may accumulate in the anterior recess of the joint space. Frequencies will range from 5 to 12 MHz, depending on age and body habitus. The patient is placed in a supine position with the legs extended straight in a neutral position. Pain may limit the patient's ability to reach a fully neutral position; in this case, using a small roll under the knee may help the patient relax enough to get a good view. The femoral head and neck are located, and the transducer is aligned with the hip capsule and overlying iliopsoas muscle—often at a slight oblique-sagittal plane with the notched end of the footprint more medial. The sonographer should be careful to keep pressure to a minimum so as not to displace the fluid. Two longitudinal images of each hip are taken, along with anterior-posterior measurements of the hip capsule or fluid, as necessary, and power Doppler to detect any soft tissue swelling. Finally, a comparison of the bilateral longitudinal views is taken.

Sonographic Findings. As with any musculoskeletal pathology, comparing the symptomatic side with the asymptomatic side is important. The normal hip capsule is 2 to 5 mm in thickness and should appear concave and symmetric. Capsular thickness greater than 5 mm or more than 2 mm in difference side to side is indicative of a hip effusion. If a hip effusion is detected, fluid within the synovium will be present, and the anterior-posterior diameter is measured. The overlying muscles often appear to bulge toward the transducer as a result of the convex appearance of the abnormal joint capsule (Fig. 28.26). Debris in the synovial fluid and power Doppler detection of hyperemia likely suggest a septic hip. However, if these are not present, the condition cannot be ruled out, and it may be too early in the course for these findings to show up sonographically.

OTHER HIP CONDITIONS (INCIDENTAL FINDINGS)

Other conditions of the infant and pediatric hip are often found incidentally on the sonographic evaluation for DDH or painful hip and may be further evaluated in conjunction with other imaging modalities. Although sonographers are focused on a particular disease process while scanning the hip, they should also be cognizant of the surrounding areas and differential diagnoses.

There is always the potential for neoplasm in the pediatric patient. Rhabdomyosarcoma is the most common malignant

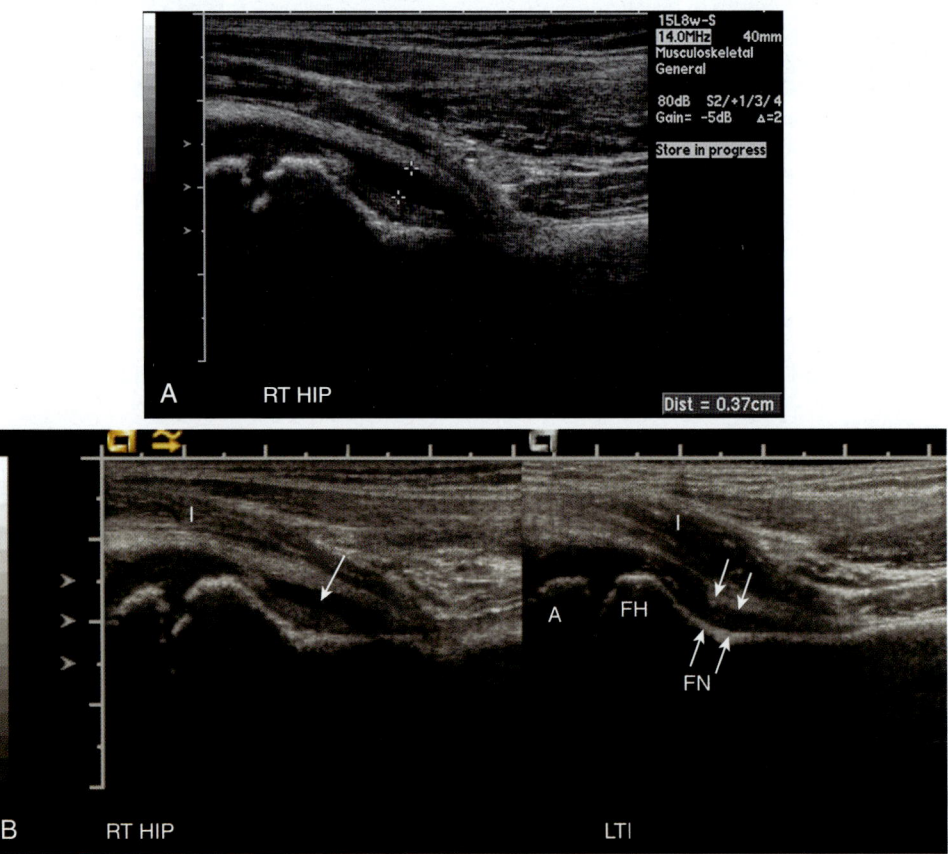

FIG. 28.26 **Hip effusion.** Sonographic hip evaluation for joint effusion in a young child who presented with hip pain and limping. (A) Image shows anterior-posterior measurement of nearly 4 mm of fluid found within the symptomatic right hip. (B) Sonogram shows a side-by-side comparison of the abnormal right hip capsule with an effusion *(left)* and normal left hip capsule *(right)*. Arrow on the *left* points to the fluid and shows an approximate path for fluid aspiration. *Down arrows* on the *right* point to the collapsed normal hip capsule of the left hip. Notice the concavity of the normal hip capsule compared with the one distended with fluid. The acetabulum (A), femoral head (FH), and femoral neck (FN, *up arrows*) are useful landmarks. The iliopsoas muscle (I) sits just above the joint capsule. In this case, the left iliopsoas appears a bit more distressed and hypertrophied compared with the right, likely attributed to overuse of the asymptomatic limb. (Courtesy Nationwide Children's Hospital, Columbus, OH.)

soft tissue tumor in children and often occurs in the head, neck, gastrointestinal tract, and extremities. Two thirds of these tumors are found in children under 6 years old. This malignancy, among others, may be detected from associated psoas irritation, and scanning the psoas up into the pelvis is advised. Osteomyelitis and myositis remain as differential diagnoses in the child with a painful hip as well. Deep soft tissue swelling is present, and periosteal fluid or cortical erosion may be seen along the bone. Cellulitis and abscess are additional possibilities.

Finally, in evaluating for DDH, proximal focal femoral deficiency may be identified. Although a rare congenital anomaly, there is a wide range of severity from decreased ossification of the femoral head to the complete absence of the hip joint. Half of these patients have concomitant limb anomalies, such as coxa vera, which is often accompanied by a shortened bowed femur on the affected side. Radiographs are helpful when available and should be reviewed by the sonographer. Although ultrasound cannot provide an unequivocal diagnosis, recognizing the normal hip structures may help differentiate it from type IV dysplasia.

Key Pearls

- The infant hip can often be evaluated up to 4 to 6 months of age for developmental displacement of the hip (DDH). Thereafter, radiography is used due to bone ossification.
- Sonographic assessment for DDH is often performed after 4–6 weeks of age (at least 44 weeks of gestation) to decrease false-positive results due to physiologic laxity and immaturity in the neonatal hip joint.
- Risk factors for DDH include breech position, female gender, positive family history, and improper swaddling.
- The Barlow and Ortolani tests are part of the clinical examination and correspond to adduction and abduction, respectively, in the dynamic sonographic techniques.
- Static coronal images and dynamic transverse imaging are standard for the DDH bilateral sonographic evaluation.
- Angulation and misalignment should be avoided, and care should be taken to obtain a precise midacetabular coronal image.
- The coronal view may be evaluated in a neutral or flexed position, corresponding to the Graf or modified Graf technique used.
- There are four types of hip joint classifications, which are based on criteria developed by Graf.
- Sonography is a quick and sensitive way to detect hip joint effusions, and aspiration of fluid is necessary to evaluate for septic arthritis.
- Knowledge of normal anatomy and differential diagnoses can greatly aid in providing patients with the best patient care to get appropriate prompt treatment.

BIBLIOGRAPHY

Abrahams PH, Spratt J, Loukas M, VanSchoor A. *Abrahams' and McMinn's Clinical Atlas of Human Anatomy*. ed 8. St Louis: Elsevier; 2018.

Adhikari S, Blaivas M. Utility of bedside sonography to distinguish soft tissue abnormalities from joint effusions in the emergency department. *J Ultrasound Med*. 2010;29(4):519–526.

AIUM-ACR-SPR-SRU Practice Parameter for the performance of an ultrasound examination for detection and assessment of developmental dysplasia of the hip. *J Ultrasound Med*. 2018;37(11): E1–E5.

Arti H, Mehdinasab SA, Arti S. Comparing results of clinical versus ultrasonographic examination in developmental dysplasia of hip. *J Res Med Sci*. 2013;18(12):1051–1055.

Ashby E, Roposch A. Diagnostic yield of sonography in infants with suspected hip dysplasia: diagnostic thinking efficiency and therapeutic efficiency. *AJR Am J Roentgenol*. 2015;204(1):177–181.

Barrera CA, Cohen SA, Sankar WN, et al. Imaging of developmental dysplasia of the hip: ultrasound, radiography and magnetic resonance imaging. *Pediatr Radiol*. 2019;49:1652–1668.

Committee on Quality Improvement Subcommittee on Developmental Dysplasia of the Hip: Clinical practice guideline: early detection of developmental dysplasia of the hip. *Pediatrics*. 2000;105(4 Pt 1): 896–905.

Cook MA. Developmental displacement of the neonatal hip. In: Haller JO, ed. *Textbook of neonatal ultrasound*. New York: Parthenon Publishing Group; 1998.

Coskun G, et al. Proximal femoral focal deficiency. *Eur J Radiol*. 2010;76(3):e99–e101.

Di Pietro MA: Sonography of the pediatric spine and hip, 2015. http://www.sonoworld.com.

Dogruel H, Atalar H, Yavuz OY, Sayli U. Clinical examination versus ultrasonography in detecting developmental dysplasia of the hip. *Int Orthop*. 2008;32(3):415–419.

Falliner A, Schwinzer D, Hahne HJ, et al. Comparing ultrasound measurements of neonatal hips using the methods of Graf and Terjesen. *J Bone Joint Surg Br*. 2006;88(1):104–106.

Filly AL, Robnett-filly B, Filly RA. Syndromes with focal femoral deficiency: strengths and weaknesses of prenatal sonography. *J Ultrasound Med*. 2004;23(11):1511–1516.

Gardiner HM, Dunn PM. Controlled trial of immediate splinting versus ultrasonographic surveillance in congenitally dislocatable hips. *Lancet*. 1990;336(8730):1553–1556.

Gerscovich EO. Infant hip in developmental dysplasia: facts to consider for a successful diagnostic ultrasound examination. *Appl Radiol*. 1999;28(3):18–25.

Graf R. Fundamentals of sonographic diagnosis of infant hip dysplasia. *J Pediatr Orthop*. 1984;4:735–740.

Graf R, Mohajer M, Plattner F. Hip sonography update. Quality-management, catastrophes—tips and tricks. *Med Ultrason*. 2013;15(4):299–303.

Grissom LE, Harcke HT. The pediatric hip and musculoskeletal ultrasound. In: Rumack C, Levine D, eds. *Diagnostic ultrasound*. ed 5. St Louis: Elsevier; 2017.

Gunay C, Atalar H, Dogruel H, et al. Correlation of femoral head coverage and Graf alpha angle in infants being screened for developmental dysplasia of the hip. *Int Orthop*. 2009;33(3):761–764.

Harcke HT. Screening newborns for developmental displacement of the hip: the role of sonography. *Am J Roentgenol*. 1994;152:395–397.

Harcke HT, Grissom LE. Performing dynamic sonography of the infant hip. *Am J Roentgenol*. 1990;155:837–844.

Harcke HT, Grissom LE. Infant hip sonography: current concepts. *Semin Ultrasound CT MRI*. 1994;15(4):256–263.

Henningsen C. *Clinical guide to ultrasonography*. St Louis: Elsevier; 2004.

Henningsen C. *The infant hip joint. Diagnostic medical sonography: abdomen and superficial structures.* ed 3. Philadelphia: Lippincott Williams & Wilkins; 2012:749–748.

Holroyd B, Wedge J. Developmental dysplasia of the hip. *Orthop Trauma.* 2009;23(3):162–168.

Jacobson JA. *Fundamentals of musculoskeletal ultrasound.* ed 2. Philadelphia: Elsevier; 2013.

Jain N, Sah M, Chakraverty J, et al. Radiological approach to a child with hip pain. *Clin Radiol.* 2013;68(11):1167–1178.

Karnik A. Hip ultrasonography in infants and children. *Indian J Radiol Imaging.* 2007;17(4):280.

Kayser R, Mahlfeld K, Grasshoff H, Merk HR. Proximal focal femoral deficiency—a rare entity in the sonographic differential diagnosis of developmental dysplasia of the hip. *Ultraschall Med.* 2005;26(5):379–384.

Kolb A, Schweiger N, Mailath-Pokorny M, et al. Low incidence of early developmental dysplasia of the hip in universal ultrasonographic screening of newborns: analysis and evaluation of risk factors. *Int Orthop.* 2016;40(1):123–127.

Loder RT, Skopelja EN. The epidemiology and demographics of hip dysplasia. *ISRN Orthop.* 2011;2011:238607.

MacPherson L, Brockley C. Developmental dysplasia of the infant hip. In: Sanders RC, Hall-Terracciano B, eds. *Clinical Sonography: A Practical Guide.* ed 5. Baltimore, MD: Wolters Kluwer; 2015.

Mahan ST, Katz JN, Kim YJ. To screen or not to screen? A decision analysis of the utility of screening for developmental dysplasia of the hip. *J Bone Joint Surg Am.* 2009;91(7):1705–1719.

Marks DS, Clegg J, al-Chalabi AN. Routine ultrasound screening for neonatal hip instability. *Can it abolish late-presenting congenital dislocation of the hip? J Bone Joint Surg Br.* 1994;76(4):534–538.

Moraleda L, Albiñana J, Salcedo M, Gonzalez-Moran G. [Dysplasia in the development of the hip]. *Rev Esp Cir Ortop Traumatol.* 2013;57(1):67–77.

Neriman D, Basit R, Howlett DC. Imaging of the symptomatic pediatric hip. *Foundation Years.* 2009;5(2):84–87.

Orak MM, Onay T, Gümüştaş SA, et al. Is prematurity a risk factor for developmental dysplasia of the hip? A prospective study. *Bone Joint J.* 2015;97-B(5):716–720.

Ortiz-Neira CL, Paolucci EO, Donnon T. A meta-analysis of common risk factors associated with the diagnosis of developmental dysplasia of the hip in newborns. *Eur J Radiol.* 2012;81(3):e344–e351.

Pillai A, Joseph J, Mcauley A, Bramley D. Diagnostic accuracy of static Graf technique of ultrasound evaluation of infant hips for developmental dysplasia. *Arch Orthop Trauma Surg.* 2011;131(1):53–58.

Rosendahl K, Aslaksen A, Lie RT, Markestad T. Reliability of ultrasound in the early diagnosis of developmental dysplasia of the hip. *Pediatr Radiol.* 1995;25(3):219–224.

Rosendahl K, Toma P. Ultrasound in the diagnosis of developmental dysplasia of the hip in newborns. The European approach. A review of methods, accuracy and clinical validity. *Eur Radiol.* 2007;17(8):1960–1967.

Shipman SA, Helfand M, Moyer VA, Yawn BP. Screening for developmental dysplasia of the hip: a systematic literature review for the US Preventive Services Task Force. *Pediatrics.* 2006;117(3):e557–e576.

Sewell MD, Rosendahl K, Eastwood DM. Developmental dysplasia of the hip. *BMJ.* 2009;339:b44–b54.

Terjesen T, Holen KJ, Tegnander A. Hip abnormalities detected by ultrasound in clinically normal newborn infants. *J Bone Joint Surg Br.* 1996;78(4):636–640.

Vasilescu D, Cosma D, Vasilescu DE, et al. A new sign in the standard hip ultrasound image of the Graf method. *Med Ultrason.* 2015;17(2):206–210.

Weintroub S, Grill F. Ultrasonography in developmental dysplasia of the hip. *J Bone Joint Surg.* 2000;82A:1004–1018.

CHAPTER 29

Neonatal and Infant Spine

Kathryn E. Zale

OBJECTIVES

On completion of this chapter, you should be able to:
- Describe the sonographic technique to image the neonatal and infant spinal column
- Describe the sonographic appearance of normal anatomy of the spinal cord, the dura, the nerve roots, and the cauda equina
- Describe how to determine the level of the lumbar vertebrae in the sonographic examination
- Describe the different clinical presentations associated with a tethered cord
- List the common pathologic conditions of the spinal cord and their sonographic appearances

OUTLINE

Embryogenesis 871
Normal Anatomy and Sonographic Appearance 872
    Normal Anatomy of the Spine 872
    Normal Sonographic Appearance of the Spine 875
Sonographic Evaluation of the Neonatal and Infant Spine 876
    Scanning Technique 876
    Important Features Used in the Sonographic Evaluation 878
Pathology of the Neonatal and Infant Spine 880
    Closed Spinal Dysraphism 880
    Lipomas 882
    Diastematomyelia 883
    Hydromyelia 883
    Sinus Tracts (Pseudosinus Versus Dorsal Dermal Sinus) 883
Other Indications 883
    Open Spinal Dysraphism 883
    Spinal Cord Injury 886

KEY TERMS

Cauda equina
Conus medullaris
Diastematomyelia
Dysraphism
Filum terminale
Hydromyelia
Lipoma
Meningocele
Myelocele
Myelomeningocele
Myeloschisis
Spina bifida aperta
Spina bifida occulta
Tethered spinal cord
Vertebral arch
Vertebral foramen

The spinal canal and its contents can be demonstrated sonographically with great clarity in the neonatal and early infant periods. Thus, high-resolution sonography of the spine has emerged as a widely used first-line clinical tool to detect certain congenital conditions, such as a **tethered spinal cord**.

Sonography is used to determine the relationship of abnormal clinical findings to deformities in the spinal canal. The infant may present with a sacral dimple or defect anywhere along the posterior surface of the body adjacent to the spinal canal. Although it is not uncommon for the buttocks to contain a shallow dimple near the anus, at times, the dimple appears unusually deep or asymmetric. This may suggest the possibility of an underlying maldevelopment of the spinal column. If these abnormalities are not recognized early, the patient may have difficulty walking or experience other neurologic problems in infancy and childhood.

Advantages of sonography include performing the procedure easily, dynamically, and at the bedside without ionizing radiation. The availability of high-frequency transducers now leaves operator inexperience as the main reason for unsuccessful neonatal spinal sonography. The sonographer may observe the spinal cord as it pulsates normally within the spinal canal, and the vascular supply to the canal may be evaluated with color Doppler. The development of fluid collections, cysts, or fatty tumors (lipomas) may be seen. Malformations of the spinal cord may be imaged and will be presented in this chapter.

EMBRYOGENESIS

The fetal central nervous system begins developing in the first 3 to 4 weeks of the embryonic period. The ectoderm, or outer layer of the trilaminar embryonic disk, gives rise to the neural tube and subsequent spinal cord and brain. During *neurulation* or neural tube development, the ectoderm differentiates into the neuroectoderm, forming the neural plate posteriorly. The neural plate then wraps in on itself and fuses at the dorsal midline forming the neural tube. Simultaneously, the neural tube separates from the outer ectoderm and sinks below the mesoderm, or middle embryonic layer. The mesoderm, which forms the bony spine, meninges, and muscle, comes to lie between the neural tube and the outer cutaneous ectoderm.

Defects of the spinal canal may occur at any time during these first 8.5 weeks of development. Failure of the neural tube to fold and fuse in the midline results in neural tube defects, such as spina bifida. Failure of the neural tube to completely separate from the outer ectoderm may result in cord tethering, diastematomyelia, or a dorsal dermal sinus. Finally, if the cutaneous ectoderm prematurely separates from the neural tube, it may result in the formation of abnormal mesenchymal or primary mesodermal elements, such as lipomas, between the neural tube and skin.

NORMAL ANATOMY AND SONOGRAPHIC APPEARANCE

Normal Anatomy of the Spine

The vertebral column extends from the base of the skull to the tip of the coccyx along the posterior surface of the body and serves as its central bony stabilizer. Within the vertebral cavity lie the spinal cord, the roots of the spinal nerves, and the covering meninges, all bathed in cerebrospinal fluid (CSF). The meninges and CSF protect the vertebral column. The vertebral column consists of 33 vertebrae: 7 cervical, 12 thoracic, 5 lumbar, 5 sacral (fused to form the sacrum), and 4 coccygeal (fused to form the tailbone) (Fig. 29.1). The pads of fibrocartilage, called intervertebral disks, are found between each vertebra and allow flexibility in the spine.

Vertebrae. Each vertebra consists of a rounded body anteriorly and a vertebral arch posteriorly (Fig. 29.2). These enclose a space called the **vertebral foramen**, through which the spinal cord and its coverings run. The **vertebral arch** consists of a pair of cylindrical pedicles, which form the sides of the arch, and a pair of flattened laminae, which complete the arch posteriorly. The vertebral arch gives rise to seven processes: one spinous, two transverse, and four articular. The two superior articular processes of one vertebral arch articulate with the two inferior articular processes of the arch above, forming two synovial joints.

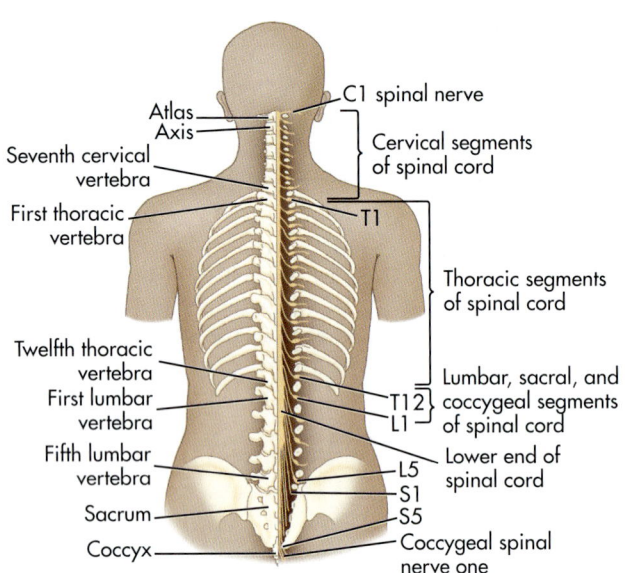

FIG. 29.1 Vertebral column. Posterior view of the vertebral column, indicating the vertebral levels. On the right, the laminae have been removed to expose the right half of the spinal cord and nerve roots.

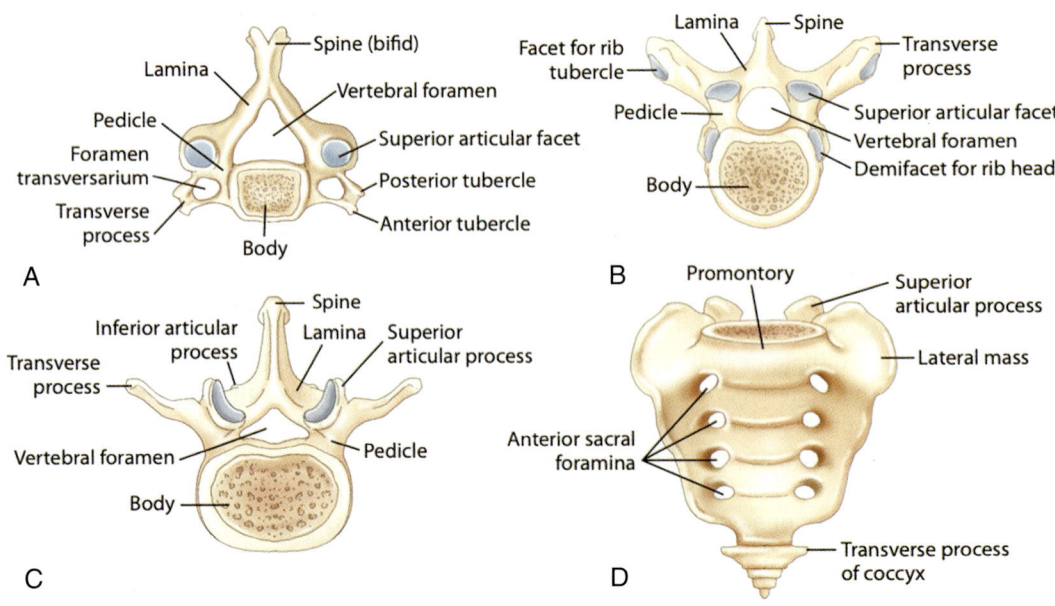

FIG. 29.2 Basic vertebrae features. (A) Cervical vertebrae. (B) Thoracic vertebrae. (C) Lumbar vertebrae. (D) Fused sacral vertebrae and coccyx.

The pedicles are notched on their upper and lower borders, forming the superior and inferior vertebral notches. On each side, the superior notch of one vertebra and the inferior notch of an adjacent vertebra together form the intervertebral foramen. These foramina transmit the spinal nerves and blood vessels.

In the neonate, problems typically occur in the lower back near the area of the lumbar vertebrae and the sacrum. Characteristics of the lumbar vertebrae include a large and oval body, strong pedicles directed posterior, and thick laminae with a triangular vertebral foramen. Additionally, the transverse processes are short, flat, and project backward.

Sacrum. The sacrum consists of five bones fused together. The upper border articulates with the fifth lumbar vertebra. The narrow inferior border articulates with the coccyx. Laterally, the sacrum articulates with the two iliac bones to form the sacroiliac joints. The anterior and upper margin of the first sacral vertebra bulges forward as the posterior margin of the pelvic inlet and is known as the sacral promontory.

The vertebral foramina are present and form the sacral canal. The laminae of the fifth sacral vertebra (and occasionally the fourth) do not fuse at the midline, forming the sacral hiatus. The sacral canal contains the anterior and posterior roots of the sacral and coccygeal spinal nerves, the **filum terminale**, and fibrofatty material. It also contains the lower part of the subarachnoid space, where the dural or thecal sac ends at the second sacral vertebra (Fig. 29.3).

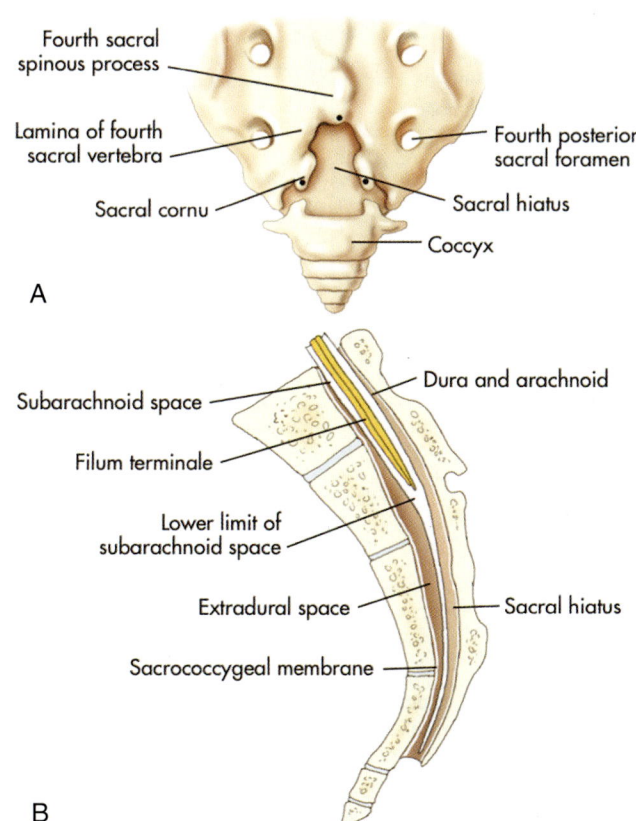

FIG. 29.3 Sacrum. (A) Coronal plane of the sacral hiatus, with black dots indicating the bony landmarks. (B) Longitudinal plane of the sacrum.

Intervertebral Disks. The intervertebral disks make up one-fourth of the length of the vertebral column. They are thickest in the cervical and lumbar regions, where the movements of the vertebral column are greatest. Each disk consists of a peripheral part, the annulus fibrosus, and a central part, the nucleus pulposus (Fig. 29.4). The annulus fibrosus consists of fibrocartilage. The nucleus pulposus is an ovoid mass of gelatinous material containing a large amount of water, a small number of collagen fibers, and a few cartilage cells.

Ligaments and Nerves. The anterior and posterior longitudinal ligaments run as continuous bands down the anterior and posterior surfaces of the vertebral column from the skull to the sacrum. Transverse dentate ligaments extend laterally from the spinal cord. The small meningeal branches of each spinal nerve innervate the joints between the vertebral bodies.

Spinal Cord. The spinal cord is a cylindrical, grayish-white structure that begins superiorly at the foramen magnum, where it is continuous with the medulla oblongata of the brain. The cord has a deep longitudinal fissure in the midline anteriorly. The size and shape of the spinal cord vary along its length. Its diameter is narrowest in the midthoracic and thoracolumbar junctions. Inferiorly, the cord tapers off into the **conus medullaris**, where it ends at its tip.

In the adult, the tip of the conus medullaris terminates below the level of the lower border of the first lumbar (L1) vertebra. At birth, the conus tip may end between the L2 and L3 vertebra, but often it does not extend beyond the second lumbar vertebra. The conus may end even lower, between L2 and L4, in the preterm infant. By 3 months of age, the tip of the conus is at the L1 to L2 level. From its apex, the filum terminale, a thin fibrous cord, descends to be attached to the back of the coccyx to provide stability to the spinal cord (Fig. 29.5).

Roots of the Spinal Nerves. Along the length of the spinal cord are attached 31 pairs of spinal nerves. Each spinal nerve root connects to the central spinal nerve by one dorsal root (carrying sensory fibers to the cord) and one ventral rootlet (carrying sensory fibers away from the cord). The lower nerve roots typically project from the segments lower than L1 to L5 and collectively are called the **cauda equina** (Latin for "horse's tail") (see Fig. 29.5).

Meninges of the Spinal Cord. The spinal cord is surrounded by three meninges: the dura mater, the arachnoid mater, and the pia mater. The dura mater is the most external membrane and is a dense, strong, fibrous sheet that encloses the spinal cord and cauda equina. Collectively, the lowest portion containing CSF is called the thecal sac, or dural sheath, located inferiorly as the lower border of the second sacral vertebra. Superiorly, it is continuous through the foramen magnum with the meningeal layer of dura covering the brain. The arachnoid mater is a delicate impermeable membrane covering the spinal cord and lies between the pia mater internally and the dura mater externally. It is separated from the dura by the subdural space, which contains a thin film of tissue fluid. The arachnoid is separated from the pia mater

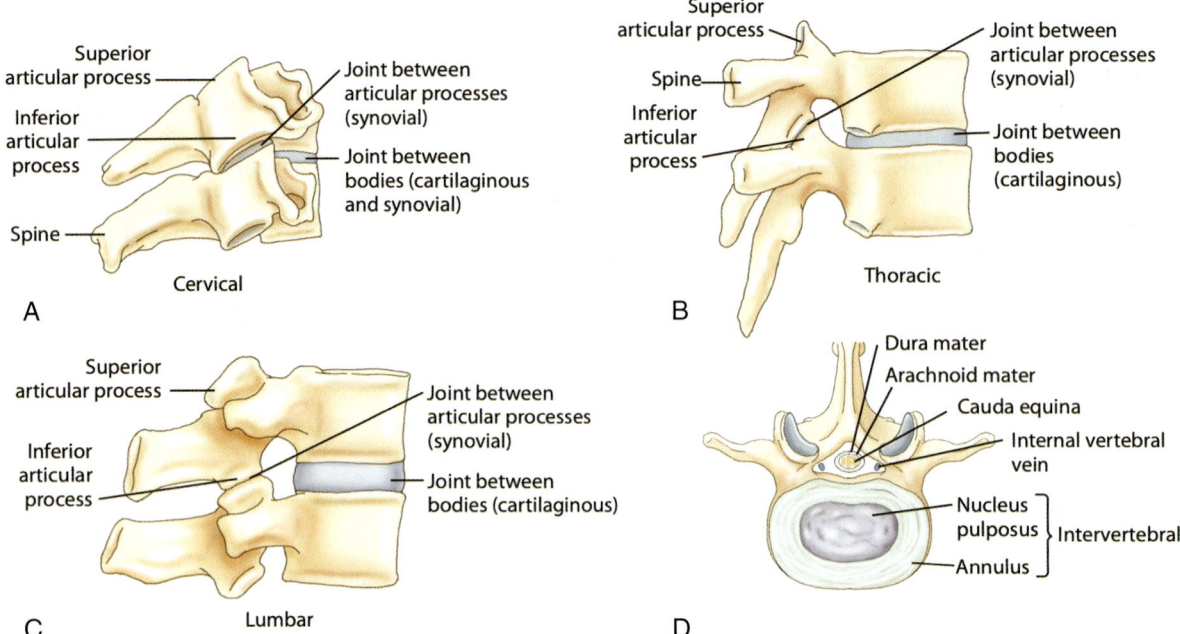

FIG. 29.4 Disk joints of the vertebral column. (A) Cervical region. (B) Thoracic region. (C) Lumbar region. (D) Third lumbar vertebra, seen from above, showing the relationship between intervertebral disk and cauda equina.

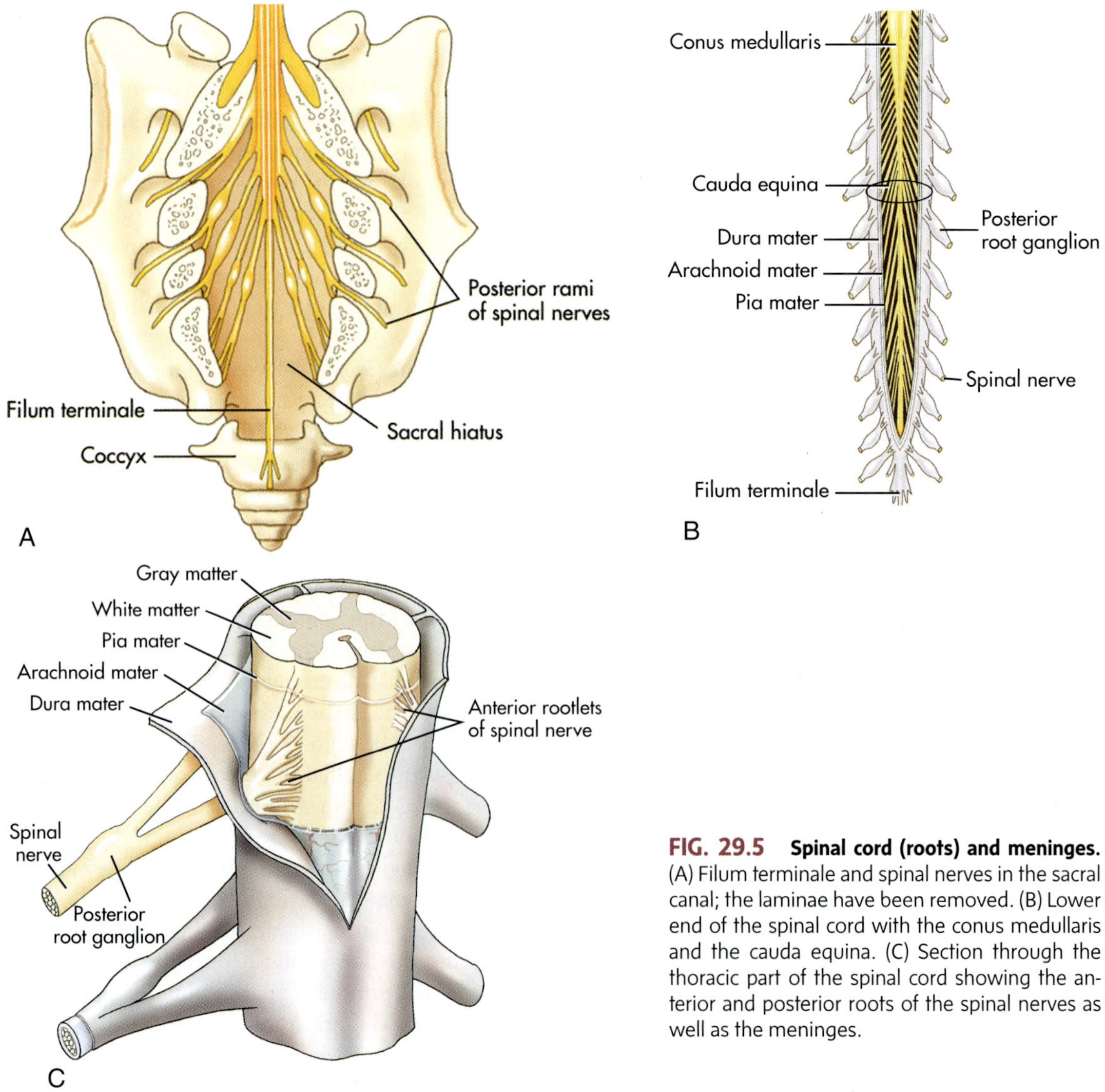

FIG. 29.5 Spinal cord (roots) and meninges. (A) Filum terminale and spinal nerves in the sacral canal; the laminae have been removed. (B) Lower end of the spinal cord with the conus medullaris and the cauda equina. (C) Section through the thoracic part of the spinal cord showing the anterior and posterior roots of the spinal nerves as well as the meninges.

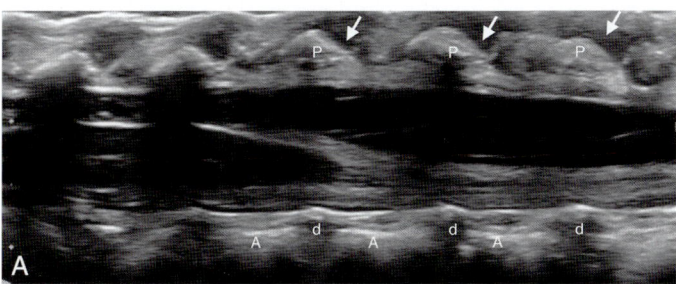 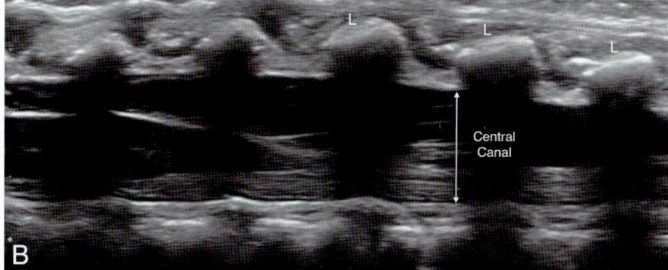

FIG. 29.6 Sagittal view of the normal thoracic/lumbar spine. (A) Approach should be directly over the echogenic inverted U-shaped posterior spinal processes allowing for good visualization. Posterior spinous processes (P), anterior vertebral bodies (A), intervertebral disks (d), and *short arrows* point toward the cartilaginous tips of the hypoechoic spinous processes. (B) When the approach is slightly off midline, over the flat posterior arch laminae (L), shadowing is increased within the central canal. (Courtesy Nationwide Children's Hospital, Columbus, OH.).

by a wide space, the subarachnoid space, which contains cerebrospinal fluid. The pia mater is a vascular membrane that closely covers the spinal cord. It is continuous above the neck, through the foramen magnum, with the pia covering the brain. Inferiorly, the pia mater fuses with the filum terminale (see Fig. 29.5).

Normal Sonographic Appearance of the Spine

Vertebrae. With sonography, the hypoechoic spinal canal is demarcated by the posterior elements anteriorly and the echogenic anterior vertebral bodies posteriorly. In the sagittal plane, scanning directly over the incompletely ossified posterior spinous processes, they will look, individually, like an echogenic upside down U. It should be noted, the tips of the posterior spinous processes are cartilaginous, being a secondary ossification center, and appear hypoechoic in infancy (Fig. 29.6A). Laminae are seen when scanning slightly off midline and appear more flat, similar to overlapping roof tiles (see Fig. 29.6B). In the transverse plane, scanning over the unossified cartilaginous midline tips of the posterior spinous process allows for better visualization (Fig. 29.7).

Spinal Cord. The spinal cord is surrounded by cerebrospinal fluid and appears hypoechoic with slightly echogenic borders and an echogenic line extending longitudinally along its midline. This central echo complex represents the cord's central canal (Fig. 29.8A). The cord's anterior longitudinal midline fissure may be seen on a transverse image. The spinal cord should taper at its end, called the conus medullaris.

A slight anechoic prominence or widening of the central canal at the caudal end of the cord is a common finding in neonates. This normal variant is often called ventriculus terminalis, also referred to as the *fifth ventricle*, and it typically disappears within the first few weeks of life (Fig. 29.8B). In neonates, this widening is no more than 2 to 4 mm in a transverse diameter and extends longitudinally for 8 to 10 mm. It should be closely investigated to rule out an abnormal cavity, or syrinx, within the canal.

Cauda Equina. Nerve roots that surround the spinal cord are echogenic and form the cauda equina. They are especially noticeable at and below the conus medullaris. Dorsal and

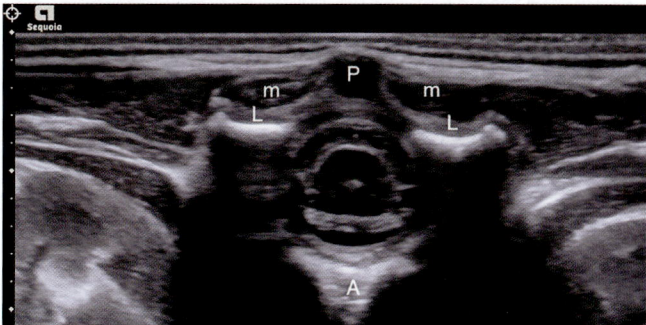

FIG. 29.7 Transverse view of the normal thoracic spine. Approach is over the unossified tips of the posterior spinous process (P). Laminae of vertebral arches (L) and muscle (m) in the epidural space anterior to the spinal canal. Anterior vertebral body (A) is shown posterior to the spinal canal. (Courtesy Siemens Healthineers USA, Inc.)

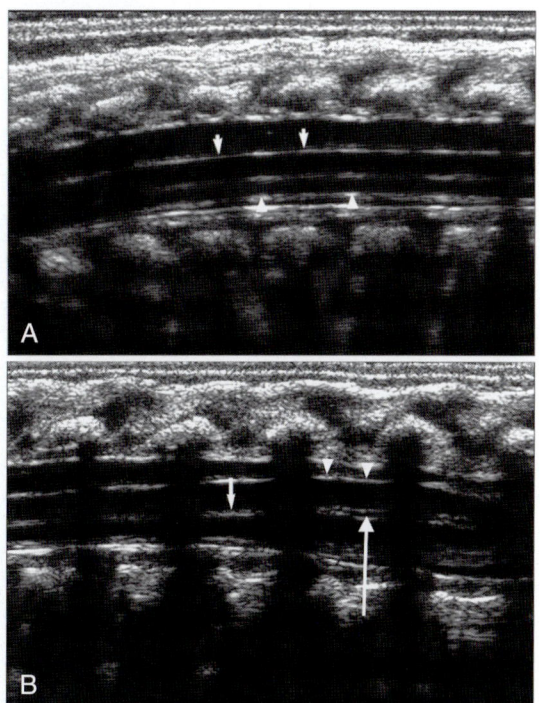

FIG. 29.8 Sagittal view of the normal thoracic spinal cord and ventriculus terminalis variant. (A) Sagittal view shows the posterior *(arrows)* and the anterior aspects of the thoracic spinal cord *(arrowheads)*. (B) Normal variant, ventriculus terminalis, causes a slight widening of the spinal cord *(arrowheads)*. The normal central echo complex *(short arrow)* is shown cranially, in contrast to the anechoic central canal prominence *(long arrow)* caudally.

ventral nerve roots can have a spider-like configuration at the tip of the conus in the transverse view (Fig. 29.9). They may also appear as an echogenic clump in the middle of the spinal canal or as bilateral clusters, sometimes in an upside-down V configuration.

Filum Terminale. The filum terminale, or filum, appears as a thin, cord-like, echogenic structure stretching from the tip of the conus medullaris to the end of the spinal canal. A magnified view of the filum terminale demonstrates an echogenic outer linear interface with a hypoechoic central potion. A normal variant to be aware of is the filar cyst. These small cysts in the filum terminale might be remnants of a terminal ventricle or an arachnoid pseudocyst and have no known clinical significance (Fig. 29.10).

Coccyx and Meninges. In the infant, the coccyx is unossified and appears hypoechoic. The C1 segment may be ossified but will appear rounder, differentiating it from the squarer sacral vertebrae (Fig. 29.11).

Finally, the dura mater and the pia mater appear echogenic at their interface. CSF fills the subarachnoid space around the hypoechoic spinal cord, appearing anechoic (Fig. 29.12).

SONOGRAPHIC EVALUATION OF THE NEONATAL AND INFANT SPINE

Scanning Technique

Imaging of the spine is ideally performed in the neonatal period, up to 3 to 4 months of age, before there is too much ossification of the posterior spinal elements. It is not possible after 6 months of age. Feeding prior to the examination is encouraged to calm the infant.

A posterior approach is used with the patient in a prone or lateral decubitus position. When prone, this is accomplished by having the baby lie over a small pillow or a rolled towel. Slight elevation of the upper part of the body will better distend the caudal aspect of the thecal sac. Likewise, a sitting position, bending forward, will also help separate the interlaminar spaces with the accumulation of CSF.

Since movement makes this examination extremely tricky, it may be necessary to have the parent hold the baby over their shoulder in a "burping" position. It is crucial to have the spine flexed or rounded enough to separate the posterior spinal elements. Care must be taken that flexion is not so extreme as

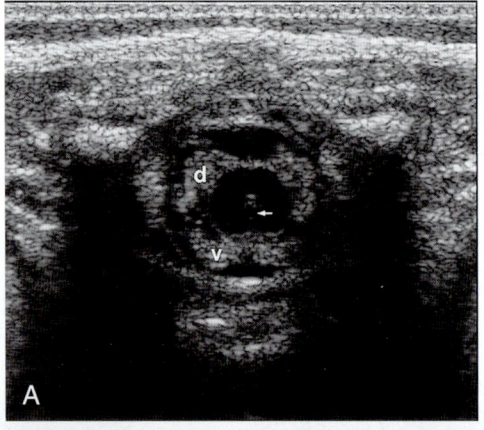

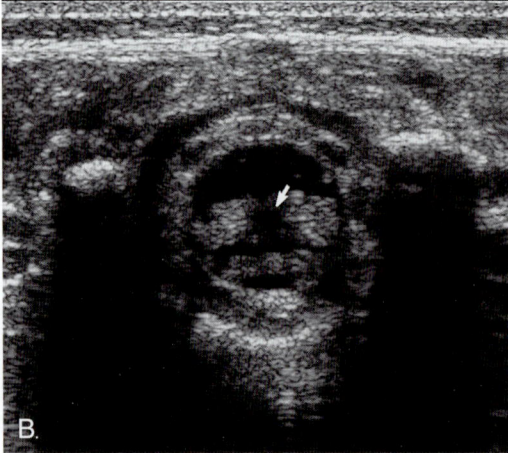
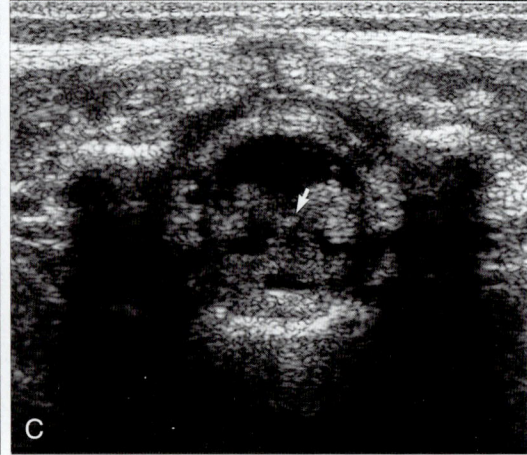

FIG. 29.9 Normal lumbar spinal cord and nerve roots. (A) Transverse view of the lumbar spinal cord, dorsal (d) and ventral (v) nerve roots, as well as the anterior median fissure, are visible *(arrow)*. (B) Transverse view near the tip of the conus medullaris demonstrates the relatively hypoechoic substance of the cord *(arrow)* in the center of the more echogenic nerve roots making up the caudate equina. (C) The beginning of the filum terminale is seen as a central, slightly echogenic focus *(arrow)* in the transverse plane.

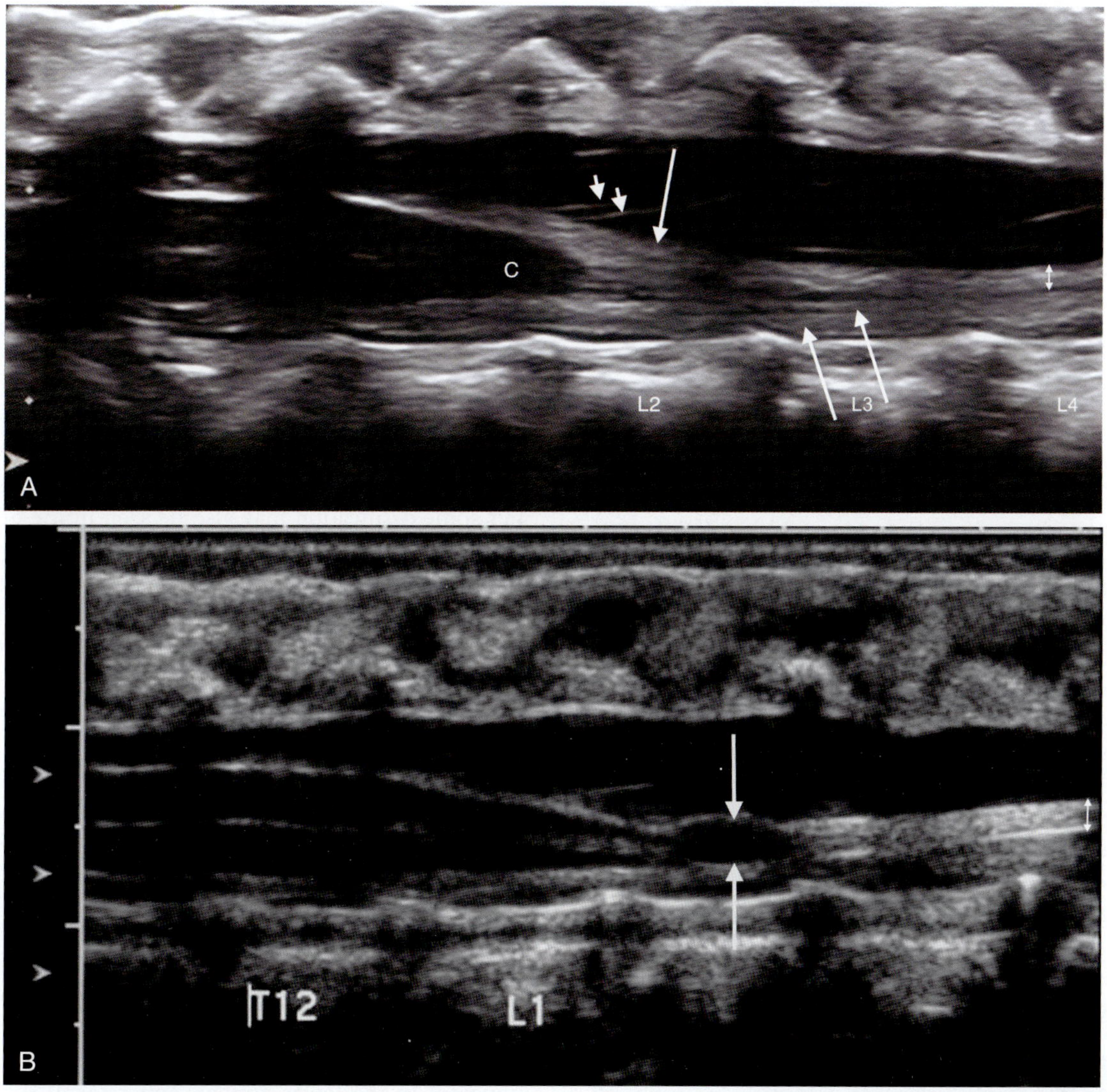

FIG. 29.10 Normal filum terminale and filar cyst variant. (A) Tip of the conus medullaris (c) should taper gradually. Filum terminale *(double arrow)* is best defined more distal from the conus around the L4–L5 level, where it is not in the thick of the cauda equina *(long arrows)*. Individual dorsal nerve roots are also visible *(short arrows)*. (B) Normal filar cyst variant *(arrows)* appears as a small anechoic fluid collection seen in the filum *(double arrow)*, among the nerve roots of the cauda equina, just below the tip of the conus medullaris. (Courtesy Nationwide Children's Hospital, Columbus, OH.)

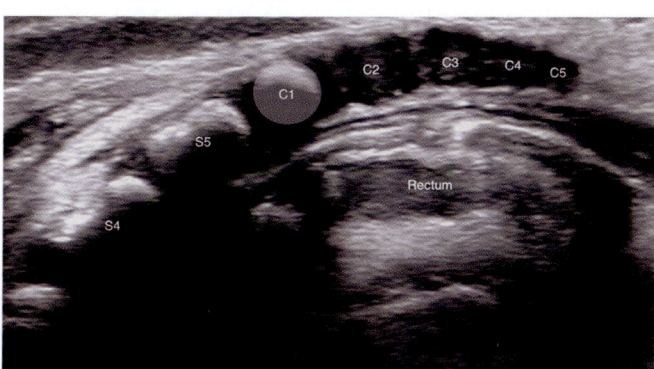

FIG. 29.11 Normal coccyx. Sagittal view over the hypoechoic coccyx. The first coccyx (C1) vertebra in this neonate is partially ossified and has a rounded appearance, differentiated from the squarer sacral (S) vertebrae. Rectum appears posterior and is anatomically anterior. (Courtesy Nationwide Children's Hospital, Columbus, OH.)

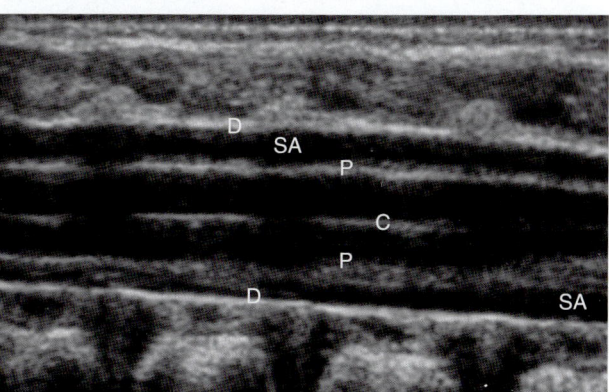

FIG. 29.12 Normal meningeal layers. Normal ultrasound of the neonatal spinal canal showing the thick, fibrous dura mater (D), or dural sac, enclosing the spinal cord. The subarachnoid space (SA) filled with cerebro spinal fluid separates the arachnoid mater (dural side) and pia mater (spinal cord side). The pia mater (P) surrounds the posterior and anterior margins of the spinal cord. The echogenic central canal (or central echo complex) of the spinal cord (C) is seen in the middle. (Courtesy Nationwide Children's Hospital, Columbus, OH.)

to compromise the infant's breathing. This consideration is amplified if the baby has been sedated. The infant usually falls asleep during the procedure once the warm coupling gel is applied and the transducer is gently rubbed along the spine.

The sonographer should use the highest frequency transducer available to obtain the greatest soft tissue detail; a 12 MHz is often utilized. Small neonates will require higher frequencies (15 MHz), whereas chunky or older babies will require lower frequencies (7 MHz). The linear array transducer works the best to completely scan along the spinal canal. Sector transducers may be used in older infants with a limited acoustic window.

Scanning is performed in the midline sagittal (longitudinal) and axial (transverse) planes, and probe orientation is the same as conventional abdominal imaging. The longitudinal images are obtained directly over the spine and optimized with panoramic sonography (Fig. 29.13A). If the infant is older and ossification obscures this view, a parasagittal approach is best. Transverse images are taken mainly between the more ossified portions of the spinous processes over the cartilaginous midline.

The spinal canal is usually easily identified, and the depth of the image is adjusted so the vertebral bodies are at the bottom of the image. It is helpful to scan the sacral region first, where the canal is easily identified by the stepwise ascent of the sacral vertebral elements (Fig. 29.13B), and then follow the spinal canal in a cranial direction. A standoff pad may be used to examine the soft tissue dorsal to the spine when looking for a sinus tract.

The integrity of the entire spinal canal is examined, with the lumbar spinal canal receiving the most attention. While protocols may vary, imaging often includes the mid to lower portions of the thoracic spine to the tip of the coccyx.

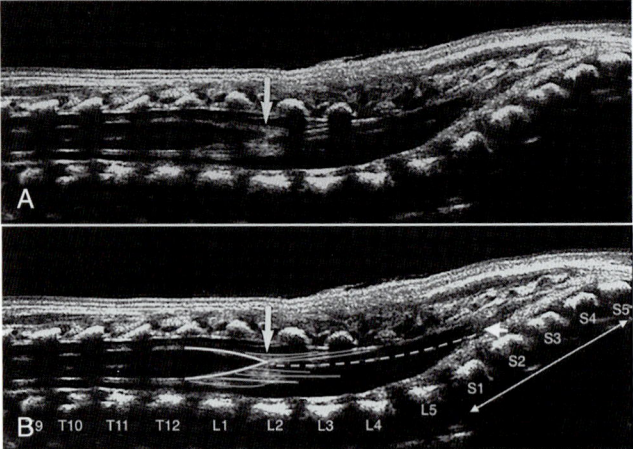

FIG. 29.13 Panoramic view of the spine. (A) Lumbosacral spine. Extended field of view image reveals detailed anatomy of the course and contour of the neonatal lumbosacral spine. The tip of the conus medullaris *(arrow)* is clearly visible. (B) The tapered conus medullaris is outlined, and the tip is seen *(arrow)*. Filum terminale extends from the tip of the conus to the end of the thecal sac *(dashed line)*. The thecal sac ends at the S2 vertebra *(short arrow)*. Caudate equina nerve roots are accentuated *(thin lines around filum)*. Stepwise ascent of the sacral vertebral elements is shown *(double arrow)*. Thoracic (T), lumbar (L), and sacral (S) vertebrae are labeled.

Important Sonographic Features to Evaluate

Level of the Conus Medullaris.
The single most important determination is the level of the tip of the tapered conus medullaris, since most examinations are performed to exclude an occult tethered spinal cord. In the infant, it is normally found above the superior endplate of L3, with most cords ending at the mid-L2 level. Since the conus medullaris tip moves upward with age, some variations in the normal lumbar vertebral level exist.

The lumbar vertebral level may be determined in several different ways and, ideally, more than one method is used to confirm the level of the conus tip. This is often achieved by counting cranially in a longitudinal orientation from the caudal end. There are several different approaches: (1) *Use the last ossification center*. This is often the last sacral vertebra (S5), but some ossification may also be seen in the first coccygeal level (C1). Shape helps differentiate the squarer S5 from the more circular C1. (2) *Use the lumbosacral junction* or normal curvature of the spine seen between the last lumbar and first sacral vertebra (L5/S1). (3) *Use the caudal end of the thecal, or dural, sac*, normally at the S2 level, and at times the S1 level. Panoramic imaging is especially helpful for these methods (Fig. 29.14).

The transverse orientation can also be utilized to determine the relationship of the vertebral level to normal anatomic structures. (1) *Use the psoas muscle*, which runs longitudinally along much of the lower spine, with the top of this muscle correlating to the L1 level. In the transverse view, the psoas muscle can be visualized directly anterolateral to the spine and medial to the kidneys. The psoas is best identified slightly off-axis from the midline or over the semi-ossified posterior spinous processes, where the canal is shadowed out (and not normally imaged). Furthermore, the psoas is more apparent in the lower lumbar, upper sacral regions, so it is best to start caudally to identify it and then travel superiorly to where it ends, correlating with the L1 vertebra (Fig. 29.15). (2) *The renal hilum correlates to the L1 to L2 level*. (3) *Iliac crest correlates to the L5 level*. A transverse projection is followed across the midline from the palpated apex of the iliac crest to the L5 vertebra. (4) *Use the ribs*. Finally, the ribs may be used in two ways to determine vertebral level. First, a projection followed from the lowest palpable rib end is often the L2 vertebral level.

Second, the lowest rib on the back can be identified with ultrasound. Then, moving directly medial in the transverse projection, scanning over each kidney, brings the transducer to a corresponding vertebral body. This vertebral level can be assigned as T12. Turning sagittal then provides the relationship to the conus (Fig. 29.16). These methods to determine the tip of the conus medullaris are summarized in Box 29.1.

The ribs could be off by a level if the patient has an anatomic variant of 11 or 13 pairs of ribs. If the conus tip is mid-lumbar, its exact level might need to be determined by a correlative radiograph. The conus tip is carefully noted in both longitudinal and transverse sonographic projections,

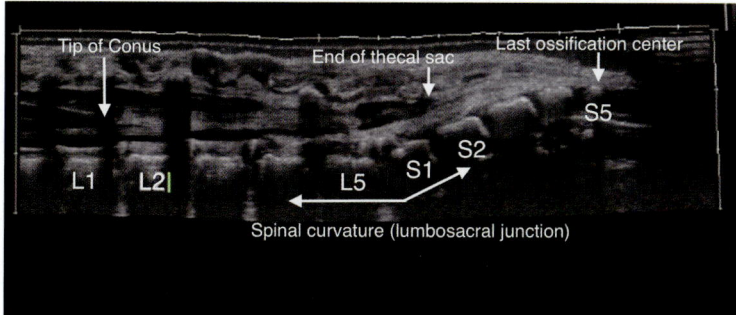

FIG. 29.14 Vertebral level by counting vertebrae. Utilizing the panoramic function, counting may begin with S5, the last ossified bone before the coccyx; the end of the thecal sac at S2; or the lumbosacral junction (L5–S1) shown with *double arrow*. This conus medullaris ends between L1 and L2. (Courtesy Nationwide Children's Hospital, Columbus, OH.)

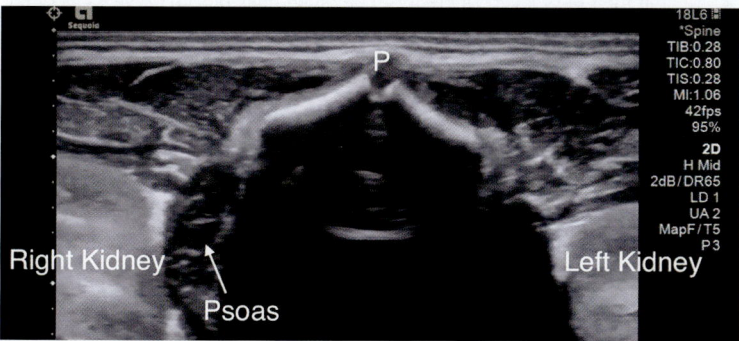

FIG. 29.15 Vertebral level using the psoas muscle. The psoas is well visualized adjacent to the anterolateral spine at the level of the kidneys. Following it to the origin corresponds to the L1 level. It is most obvious below this level, as shown; it is slightly off-axis and over the more ossified portion of the posterior spinous process (P), causing shadowing in the canal. (Courtesy Siemens Healthineers USA, Inc.)

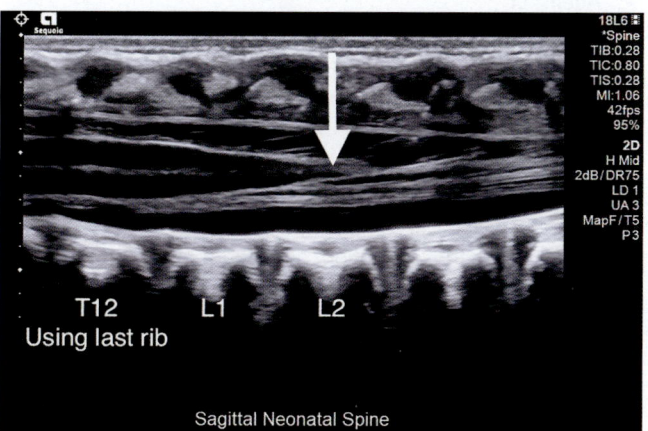

FIG. 29.16 Vertebral level using the last rib. The last rib-bearing vertebral segment is the T12 vertebra, which corresponds to and is followed from the lowest rib over each kidney in the back. This conus medullaris (*arrow*) therefore ends at the typical mid-L2 vertebra. (Courtesy Siemens Healthineers USA, Inc.)

BOX 29.1 Methods to Determine Vertebral Level of the Conus Medullaris

Sagittal View Using Panoramic Function
Last ossification center:
- Squarer shaped (S5)
- Circular shaped (C1)

Caudal end of the dural sac (S2)
Curvature of the spine (L5–S1)

Transverse View Using Anatomic Projections
Top of psoas muscle (L1)
Renal hilum (L1–L2)
Iliac crest (L5)
Ribs
- Lowest palpated rib (L2)
- Lowest rib seen with ultrasound from the back (T12)

---

and this position is marked on the skin by a radiopaque marker, such as a nipple B-B marker. Most tethered cords, however, are unquestionably low, and correlative radiographs are usually not necessary.

Anterior Position of the Spinal Cord. The spinal cord should lie one-third to halfway toward the anterior (ventral) vertebrae in the spinal canal when the infant is lying in the prone position. This indicates that the cord's position is gravity dependent and free flowing.

Normal Pulsatile Movement of the Cauda Equina. The spinal cord and roots of the cauda equina are normally observed to move freely and may be documented with M-mode or a cine clip over the tip of the conus medullaris or just beyond it (Fig. 29.17). This is best observed when the image persistence or frame averaging is minimized. Dorsoventral oscillations occur at the frequency of the heartbeat, and there is also a superimposed motion, which occurs with respirations. These movements are variably present in neonates but are almost always seen after 1 or 2 months of age. In one study, the average M-mode oscillation amplitude of the cauda equina was 0.52 mm at the L5–S1 level. Motion may indicate cord tethering if the oscillation amplitude is less than 0.3 mm.

Clusters of the normal nerve roots of the cauda equina might be mistaken for an echogenic intracanalicular mass. However, as mentioned, nerves will be observed to move and change configuration as one scans along the canal in real

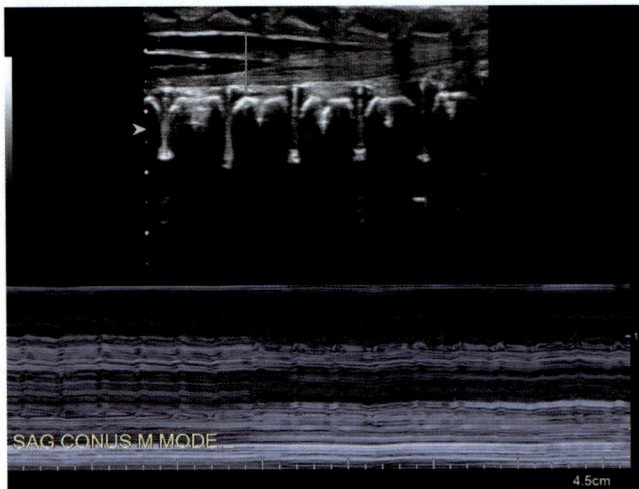

FIG. 29.17 **M-Mode capturing normal cauda equina movement.** The nerve roots of the cauda equina should move freely, in a pulsatile fashion, and are demonstrated using a cine clip or M-mode. Normal movement is shown in a neonate, captured at the level of the conus medullaris. (Courtesy Chester County Hospital, West Chester, PA.)

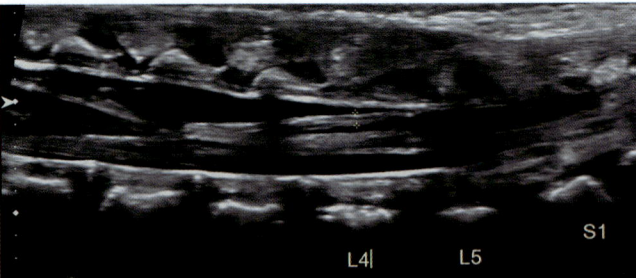

FIG. 29.18 **Measuring the filum terminale.** Normal filum terminale is shown measuring 1.2 mm. It should measure <2 mm and is best viewed at the L4–L5 level, where it can be differentiated from nerve roots of the cauda equina. (Courtesy Chester County Hospital, West Chester, PA.)

time. Another potential false-positive finding is the bilateral dorsal and ventral roots at the tip of the conus that can superficially mimic a split cord (**diastematomyelia**). Although they appear similar on the sonographic image, they are readily distinguished during real-time scanning in both projections, above and below the area of concern.

Finally, it is important to note that the normal, brisk oscillation of the cord is not as apparent in normal neonates as it is in older infants; therefore, looking for dampened or absent oscillations in neonates with tethered cords may have limited usefulness (false positives). Most nonoscillating cords in neonates are normal and are not due to tethering. Furthermore, these oscillations usually diminish as the child grows out of infancy, presumably because the cord is anchored and is being stretched.

Thickness of the Filum Terminale. Although the filum is normally larger than the cauda equina nerves, it should measure less than 2 mm in the anterior to posterior (AP) dimension. Use real-time imaging to be sure to capture just this structure and not a clump of nerve roots, as this is a potential pitfall. This is best performed at the lower lumbar spine (L4/L5), with less nerve root clumping (Fig. 29.18). These four important sonographic features are summarized in Box 29.2.

PATHOLOGY OF THE NEONATAL AND INFANT SPINE

Closed Spinal Dysraphism

Spinal sonography is performed primarily to evaluate the spinal canal for closed dysraphic conditions, which are often associated with midline cutaneous abnormalities over the lower back. Spinal **dysraphism** includes a wide range of developmental anomalies of the spinal canal and is broadly divided into open and closed types. Neural tube defects are a type of spinal dysraphism involving the absent or incomplete closure of the neural tube. The severity of the defect ranges from mild **spina bifida occulta** to severe **spina bifida aperta**. Open (aperta) spinal dysraphisms have a skin defect with the neural tissue exposed to the environment and spinal sonography is contraindicated when the skin is thin or no longer intact; therefore, occult conditions are the primary focus of the sonographic infant spine evaluation.

Closed Dysraphic Associations. Midline dimples over the lower back occur in approximately 2% to 4.3% of newborns, and most are low sacral or coccygeal pits without an associated tethered cord. However, the dimple may be suspicious if it is more than 25 mm above the anus, larger than 5 mm, or associated with other spinal lesions. Cutaneous back masses and midline deformities called lumbosacral stigmata (Box 29.3) are known to be highly associated with spinal dysraphism and tethered cord.

BOX 29.2 Summary of Important Sonographic Features to Evaluate

Level of the Conus Medullaris
Determine the conus tip is at the appropriate level and not too low. Normal vertebral locations of the conus medullaris:
- Preterm neonates: L2–L4
- Term neonates: L2–L3, usually mid-L2 level
- ≥1 Month: L1–L2, above L2 level
- Adults: L1

Anterior Position of the Spinal Cord
- Spinal cord lies one-third to halfway toward the anterior spinal canal (infant lying in a prone position)
- Gravity dependent and free flowing

Normal Pulsatile Movement of the Cauda Equina
- Dorsoventral movement at the frequency of a heartbeat
- M-mode or cine-clips for documentation
- Normal M-mode oscillation amplitude ≥0.3 mm (average ~0.5 mm)
- Best observed over conus, or just beyond it

Thickness of the Filum Terminale
- Normal <2 mm (anterior-posterior dimension)
- Best measured at L4–L5 level

Closed dysraphism of the spine is also associated with other congenital anomalies, such as anorectal malformations, including imperforate anus and patients with VACTERL syndrome, caudal regression syndrome, cloacal exstrophy, and developmental and motor delays, as well as neurogenic bladder. However, MRI is the imaging modality of choice to depict the more complex conditions associated with anal and urogenital malformations.

Closed dysraphisms presented in this chapter include tethered spinal cord, along with lipomas, hydromyelia, diastematomyelia, and sinus tracts. Other conditions touched upon include open dysraphisms and the sequelae of spinal cord injuries. However, since open spinal anomalies are best diagnosed during obstetric sonographic evaluation; more extensive information is covered on this topic in Chapter 60. Table 29.1 lists the clinical findings, sonographic findings, and differential considerations for neonatal and infant spinal anomalies.

Tethered Spinal Cord. The most common request for the sonographic spine study is to search for an occult tethered cord in the setting of a suspicious lumbosacral dimple or mark (see Box 29.3). This may be a primary closed dysraphic condition, known as tight filum terminale syndrome, or it may be associated with other dysraphic anomalies, oftentimes a fibrolipoma.

The tethered spinal cord is a pathologic fixation of the spinal cord in an abnormal caudal location so that the cord, and surrounding nerve roots, suffer mechanical stretching, distortion, and ischemia with daily activities and development. As the child grows, the spinal cord is not able to freely move with normal growth, stretching, or bending, resulting in terrible consequences if not treated. Surgical release is the corrective course for this condition. Untreated, children may have pain or lose function of their legs, bowel, or bladder. Onset of symptoms is often seen around 3 years of age.

TABLE 29.1 Summary of Neonatal and Infant Spinal Anomalies

Abnormality	Definition/Clinical Findings	Sonographic Findings
Tethered spinal cord	• Tethered cord is a group of complicated developmental malformations of the spinal cord • Benign; terrible consequences if not treated; children may have pain or lose function of legs, bowel, or bladder • As children grow, the spinal cord is not able to grow because of the abnormal structures holding onto the cord • Fatty mass may be present on mid to lower back • Increased areas of pigmentation • Dimples on back • Large collections of hair on back	• Low-lying conus medullaris below L2–L3 level in an infant • Cord fixed centrally within spinal canal • Decreased cord oscillations • Thick, echogenic filum terminale
Lipomas	• Fatty lump on lower back	• Echogenic small to large mass • May be inside the spinal canal or outside of it • May be associated with a myelocele or myelomeningocele
Diastematomyelia	• A congenital fissure or splitting of the spinal cord, frequently associated with spina bifida cystica (meningocele)	• Cord split at one or more sites by osseous cartilaginous or fibrous septum • Vertebral column is always abnormal
Hydromyelia	• Increased fluid in the central canal of the spinal cord	• Prominence of central canal at caudal end of cord • Focal hydromyelia present cephalad to site of tethered cord
Dorsal dermal sinus	• Open tract from skin to the spinal canal • Increased risk for meningitis • Present as deep pits • May leak CSF • May be associated with a tethered cord or diastematomyelia	• Tract from suspected sinus through the dermal layer into the spinal cord • Often appear anechoic and disrupt the echogenic dural line • May be filled with CSF
Pseudosinus tract	• Often has an associated sacral dimple • Normal common variant of a fibrous cord that extends from coccyx to a sacral dimple • Mimics true dermal tract but is not associated with a tethered cord or diastematomyelia	• Hypoechoic tract from tip of the coccyx to the sacral dimple • Does not extend into the dural sheath
Myelomeningocele	• Spina bifida with a portion of the spinal cord and meninges protruding	• Flat nontubulated cord with nerve roots extending into the defect
Meningocele	• Congenital hernia in which the meninges protrude through a defect in the skull or spinal column	• Shows only fluid within the sac • May have fine, lacelike strands into the sac • Cord may be eccentric or tethered

CSF, Cerebrospinal fluid.

Sonographic Findings. Tethered cord is often not a subtle pathology. The diagnosis corresponds to abnormalities of the four primary evaluative sonographic features (see Box 29.2). Positive signs are (1) a low-lying conus medullaris beyond the L2–L3, or appropriate level, (2) a caudal or posterior position of the spinal cord, (3) absent or dampened pulsations of the spinal cord and nerve roots (Fig. 29.19), and (4) thickened filum terminale (>2 mm) (Fig. 29.20). Additionally, the cord is often accompanied by a filar lipoma or cyst (Fig. 29.21).

Lipomas

A lipoma is a benign tumor composed of fat cells. Spinal lipomas are fatty masses that have a connection with the spinal cord. These lipomas may be further divided into four categories of *intradural lipomas, lipomyelocele, lipomyelomeningocele,* and *fibrolipomas* of the filum terminale. Intradural lipomas are situated in a subpial position in a dorsal cleft of the open spinal cord. The lipomyelocele is analogous to the open myelocele, but there is a covering of attached lipoma and intact skin. In patients with lipomyelomeningocele, there is expansion of the subarachnoid space ventral to the placode (Fig. 29.22).

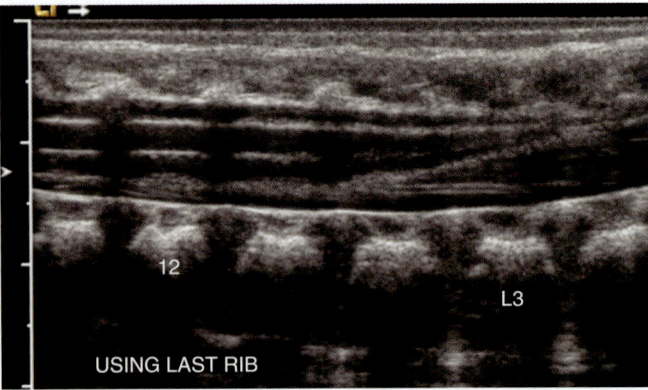

FIG. 29.19 Tethered cord. A 2-week-old neonate positive for tethered cord. Sagittal image shows the tip of the conus is extending beyond the L3 level. Poor motion of the cauda equina was noted in real time with a cine clip. Furthermore, the cord is seen abnormally located against the posterior portion of the spinal canal. (Courtesy Nationwide Children's Hospital, Columbus, OH.)

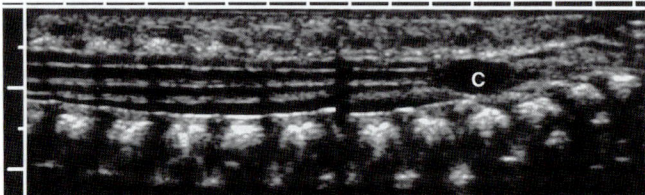

FIG. 29.21 Tethered cord with filar cyst. A newborn with a low-lying tethered cord and filar cyst (C).

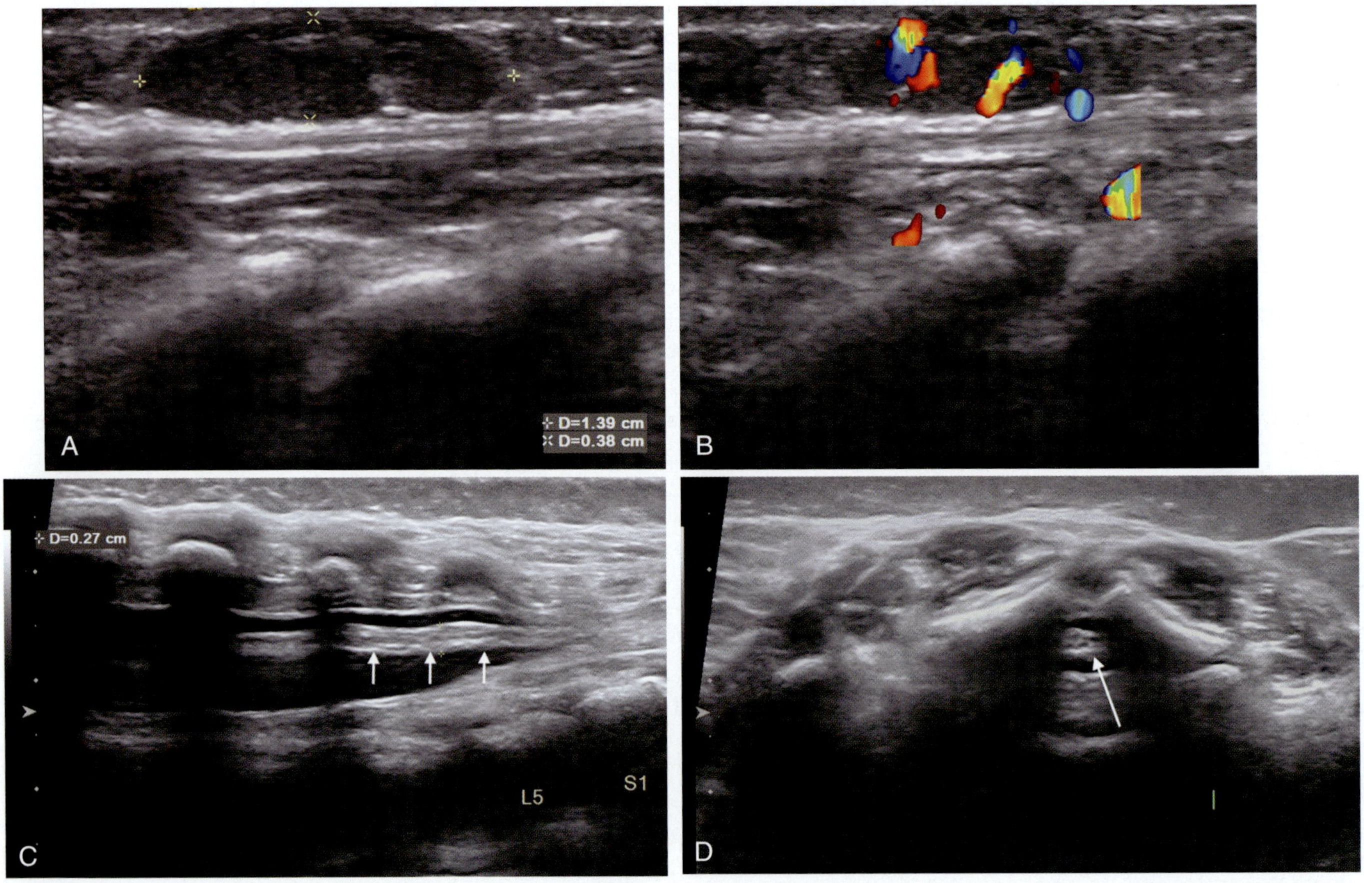

FIG. 29.20 Suspected tethered cord and thickened filum terminale. A 2-month-old presented with a cutaneous hemangioma on the lower back at the T12 level and a low positioning of the conus at the L2–L3 level with a thickened filum. Magnetic resonance imaging was recommended to further evaluate for a suspected tethered cord. (A) Sagittal view over the superficial hemangioma, measuring 1.4 × 0.4 cm. (B) Color Doppler demonstrating blood flow in the lesion. (C) Thickened echogenic filum terminale *(arrows)* measures 2.9 mm in a sagittal view. (D) Transverse view of filum terminale *(arrow)*. (Courtesy Chester County Hospital, West Chester, PA.)

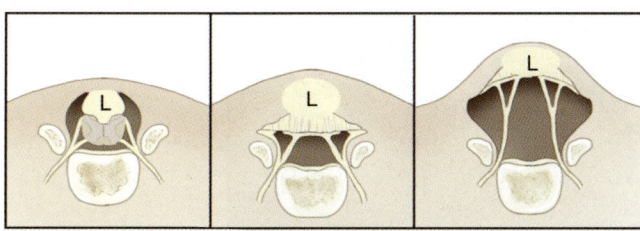

Intradural lipoma   Lipomyelocele   Lipomyelomeningocele

FIG. 29.22 Diagram of closed dysraphisms with lipomas. Diagrams are shown with the dorsal side up, the position used when scanning the spine of an infant. Intradural lipoma is situated within the dura or spinal canal. Lipomyelocele is similar to a myelocele, but the defect is not open and instead is covered by the fatty tumor. Lipomyelomeningocele has a lipoma sitting atop a myelomeningocele, which projects the nerves outward, into and along with the subarachnoid space.

Fibrolipomas of the filum terminale are a unique form of lipoma that may represent a variant of normal development. It is often associated with a tethered cord and comprises 20% to 50% of spinal dysplasias.

■ *Sonographic Findings.* On sonography, lipomas are usually echogenic and may present as a small or large mass. Fibrolipomas are seen as a thickened, echogenic filum terminale, sometimes with an undulating contour (Fig. 29.23). Lipomas can be isolated to the filum terminale or extend to and infiltrate the spinal cord and conus medullaris to varying degrees, such as the intradural juxtamedullary lipoma. (Fig. 29.24). The mass often has lipomatous elements and can be continuous with the subcutaneous tissues and present as a fatty lump on the lower back, constituting a lipomyelocele or lipomyelomeningocele (Fig. 29.25).

Diastematomyelia

Diastematomyelia is a condition in which there is sagittal division of the cord into two hemicords, each containing a central canal, a single dorsal horn, and a single ventral horn. The cord is split at one or more sites by an osseous, cartilaginous, or fibrous septum. The vertebral column is virtually always abnormal on plain radiography in patients with diastematomyelia.

Hydromyelia

Hydromyelia is an abnormal widening of the central canal that can put pressure on the spinal cord. It is also referred to as a syrinx. The cavity is filled with CSF. Remember, a slight prominence of the central canal at the caudal end of the cord is a common finding in neonates. Focal hydromyelia is often present just cephalad to the site of tethering in dysraphic conditions such as myelomeningocele or lipomyelomeningocele. Hydromyelia is present in about 50% of cases of diastematomyelia in one or both cords.

■ *Sonographic Findings.* The two segments of the cord in diastematomyelia can be seen most clearly on transverse views. They might rejoin caudal to the cleft. Hydromyelia often accompanies diastematomyelia and is another sonographically observable abnormality of the spinal cord that can be seen in variable degrees (Fig. 29.26)

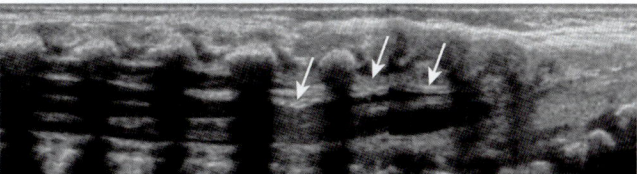

FIG. 29.23 Tethered cord with thickened filum and suspected fibrolipoma. Sagittal view of a prominent echogenic filum *(arrows)* with a "stuck" posterior appearance and undulating contour, reported as a subtle lipomatous collection. This 2-week-old male had a subcutaneous hemangioma overlying the sacrum. Magnetic resonance imaging was recommended. (Courtesy Nationwide Children's Hospital, Columbus, OH.)

Sinus Tracts (Pseudosinus Versus Dorsal Dermal Sinus)

A true sinus tract of the spine is the dorsal dermal sinus. It is a thin, epithelial-lined passage extending from the skin surface to the spinal canal by various lengths. Although they may occur anywhere along the spine, they are most common in the lumbosacral region, followed by the occipital region. Patients are at risk for meningitis due to this tract opening directly into the spinal canal. It may be associated with a tethered cord, intrathecal mass, or diastematomyelia. They often present clinically as deep midline pits and may leak cerebrospinal fluid.

A pseudosinus, on the other hand, is a common variant and is a normal fibrous cord that extends from a sacral dimple to the sacral or coccygeal fascia. Importantly, it is not connected to the spinal canal and never extends intraspinally, nor is it associated with a tethered cord.

■ *Sonographic Findings.* It is important to differentiate a true dorsal dermal sinus from a pseudosinus. Dural penetration may be difficult to ascertain or exclude on sonography, which is why care should be taken and settings optimized. If a dorsal dermal sinus is suspected, sterile gel is advised to minimize the risk of infection. A dorsal dermal sinus tract will often appear anechoic in the subcutaneous tissues and disrupt the echogenic dural line with extension into the subarachnoid space. It may be filled with cerebrospinal fluid.

A pseudosinus tract will not extend into the spinal canal and can be seen by following the tract from the sacral dimple to the coccyx (Fig. 29.27). The neonatal coccyx is usually of very low echogenicity and should not be mistaken for a cyst or fluid collection in these cases.

OTHER INDICATIONS

Sonography of the spine may also be used to assess open spina bifida and spinal cord injury. It can also evaluate for cord retethering postoperatively or visualize the spinal fluid for characteristics of blood products in patients with intracranial hemorrhage.

Open Spinal Dysraphism

Spina bifida aperta is a type of open spinal dysraphism, and the different types are classified according to what structures herniate through the open vertebral defect.

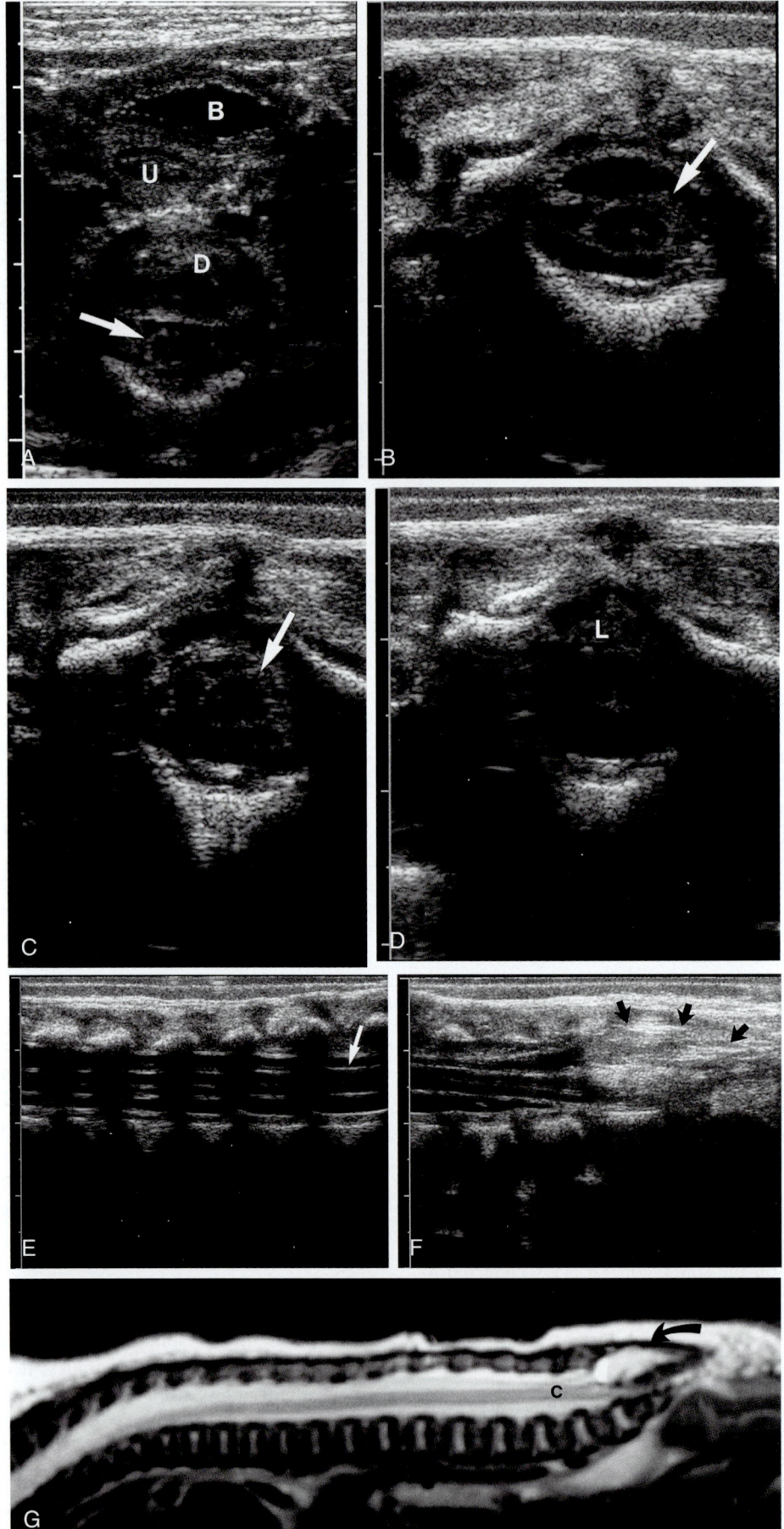

FIG. 29.24 Intradural juxtamedullary lipoma in a 2-week-old female neonate. (A) The conus medullaris of the spinal cord *(arrow)* is situated too low and is visible from an anterior approach. Transverse view of the pelvis shows the partially full urinary bladder (B), the newborn uterus (U), and an abnormal intervertebral disk space of the sacrum (D). (B–D) Traditional posterior transverse views of the spine scanning progressively inferior reveal the rightward skew of the abnormally low spinal cord *(arrow)* that is also pulled into an abnormal dorsal position by the lipoma (L). (E–F) Sagittal views of the low cord *(white arrow)* with the clearly visible tethering lipoma *(black arrows)*. (G) The correlative sagittal T2-weighted magnetic resonance image, oriented to match the sonogram, reveals the abnormally low cord (C) and the lipoma *(arrow)*.

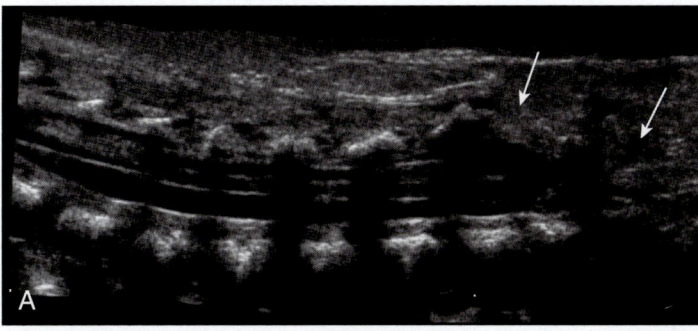
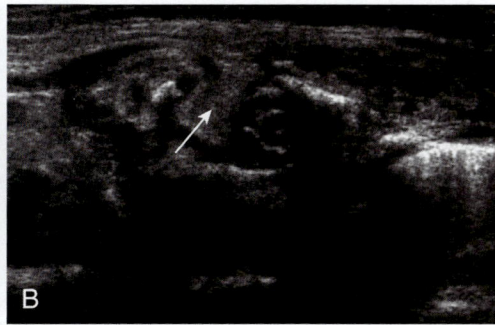

FIG. 29.25 **Lipomyelomeningocele in a 1-day-old neonate with an associated back mass (lipoma).** (A) Longitudinal image shows a large lobulated, slightly echogenic mass *(arrows)* tethering the cord inferiorly. (B) Transverse image shows the mass *(arrow)* against the superolateral aspect of the spinal canal. (Courtesy Nationwide Children's Hospital, Columbus, OH.)

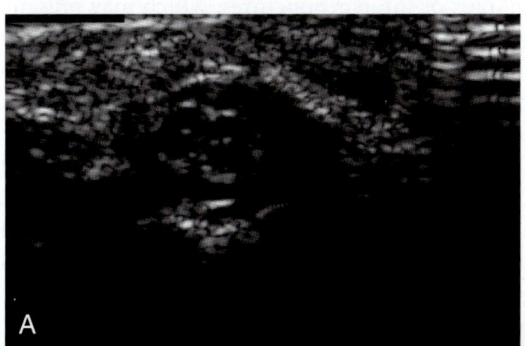

FIG. 29.26 **Diastematomyelia with hydromyelia.** (A) Transverse scan of the lumbar spinal canal shows left and right hemicords. Each hemicord has an eccentric central canal. (B) Panoramic image reveals acute kyphosis (flexion) of the spine at the thoracolumbar junction and a dilated central canal *(arrow)*. (C) Longitudinal image at the level of the thoracolumbar junction. (Courtesy Nationwide Children's Hospital, Columbus, OH.)

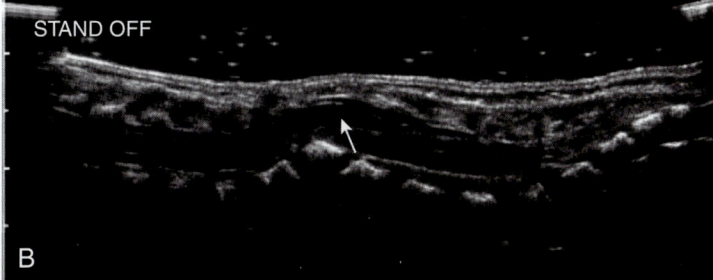
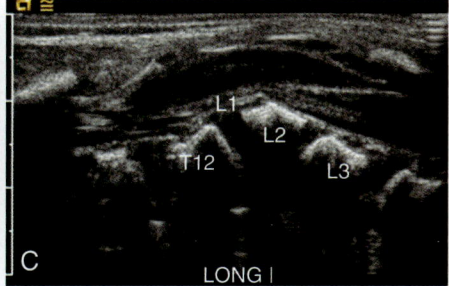

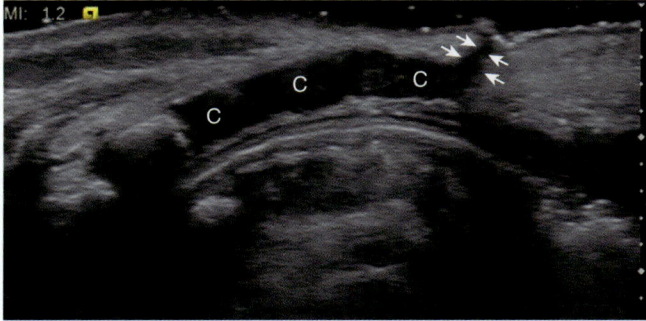

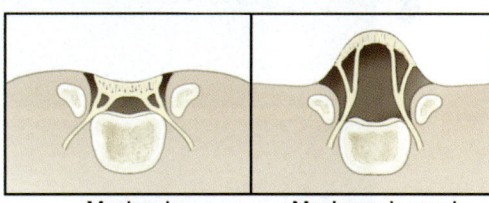

FIG. 29.28 **Open dysraphisms.** Dorsal side-up view of the open neural tube defects myelocele and myelomeningocele.

FIG. 29.27 **Pseudosinus tract.** Newborn with a sacral dimple was referred to sonography because the physician was unclear whether the dimple was open or closed. Fibrous tract *(arrows)* seen extending to the very tip of the coccyx (C), demonstrating a pseudosinus tract. There was no evidence of the tract extending into the spinal canal or cord tethering. (Courtesy Nationwide Children's Hospital, Columbus, OH.)

Myelomeningoceles are the most common open spinal defects, occurring 98% of the time, whereas **myeloceles** comprise about 2% of open dysraphisms. Myelomeningoceles are a herniation of both the meninges (meningo-) and nerves (myelo- or "marrow" of the spinal cord). Myelocele, also referred to as **myeloschisis**, occurs if the defect is uncovered, exposing the nerves, and is the most severe form (Fig. 29.28). **Meningocele** is the least common form of open spina bifida and contains the herniated meninges and cerebrospinal fluid without neural involvement; it is often referred to as spina bifida cystica (Fig. 29.29).

The primary reason for studying the spinal cord in cases of clinically obvious open dysraphism is to exclude additional cord pathology, such as diastematomyelia, which in conjunction with the myelomeningoceles and myeloceles are called hemimyelomeningocele and hemimyelocele, respectively.

Sonographic Findings. Intraoperative sonography has been successfully used to detect the margin of an open neural defect. The curved array may be helpful to scan at this margin.

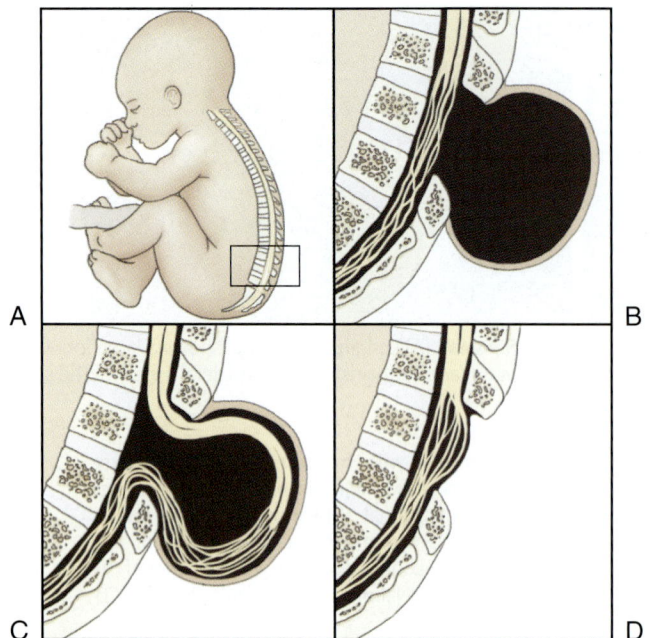

FIG. 29.29 **Spina bifida classifications.** (A) Sagittal view of lumbosacral spine, the most common area of herniation. (B) Meningoceles only contain meninges and fluid. (C) Myelomeningoceles include neural elements. (D) The defect is uncovered in myeloschisis, exposing the neural elements.

Additionally, the anatomy of the cord, adhesion of the cord to the dorsal aspect of the spinal canal cephalad to the defect, and the appearance of the neural placode and nerve roots in the defect can all be seen on a sonogram.

Spinal Cord Injury

Spinal sonography may also follow sequelae in spinal cord injury. Injury may occur as a result of birth trauma or a failed lumbar puncture. Although MRI evaluates most cases of birth trauma, in the case of a rare cord transection, sonography provides a useful, quick, and portable examination.

More commonly, ultrasound is used to evaluate failed spinal taps or lumbar punctures, which may present with an associated epidural hematoma. Sonography is useful in determining whether the cerebrospinal fluid has leaked and/or reaccumulated to avoid another failed puncture.

Sonographic Findings. After a failed or traumatic lumbar puncture, the epidural space will accumulate blood products. The cauda equina may have a thickened cord appearance from congealed blood. The presence or absence of the anechoic cerebrospinal fluid is an important determination (Fig. 29.30). Additionally, sonographic guidance for lumbar puncture can be beneficial to ensure success.

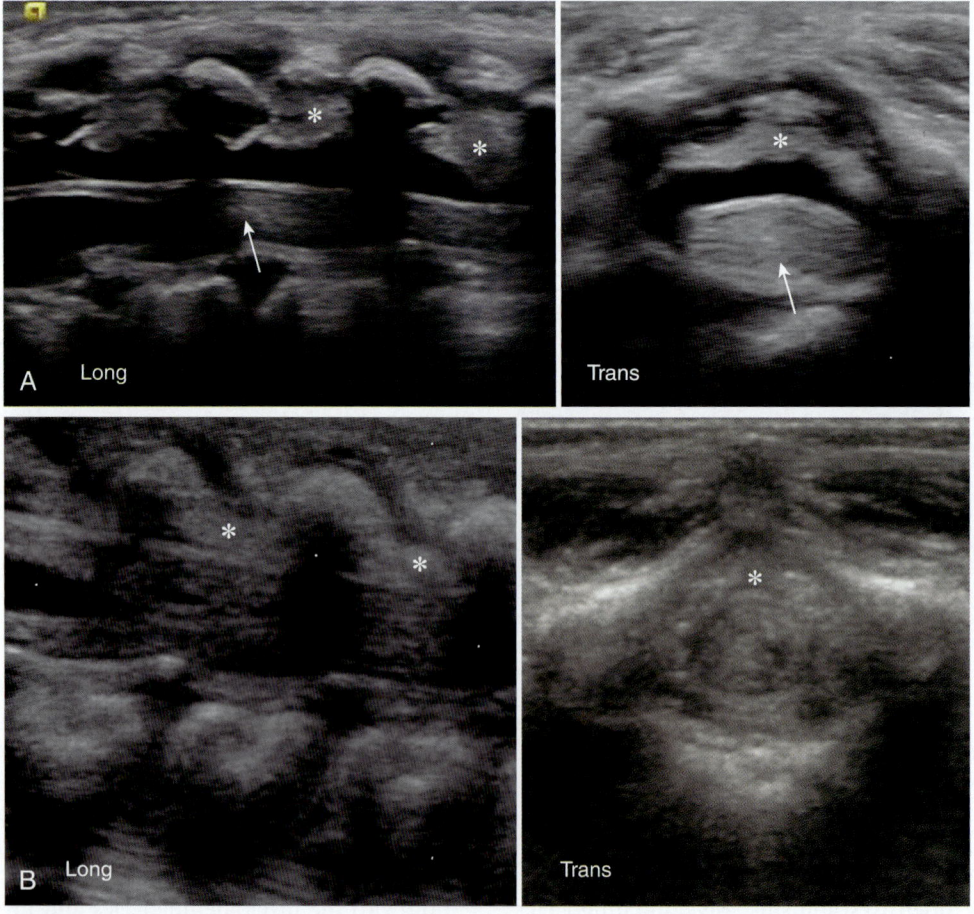

FIG. 29.30 **Failed lumbar puncture.** (A) Failed lumbar puncture attempt in a 2-month-old infant reveals an epidural hematoma *(asterisks)*; cauda equina has a thickened cord appearance from congealed blood *(arrows)*, although still in a normal anterior position. (B) Follow-up 2 days later shows the cerebrospinal fluid (CSF) has completely leaked out and the hematoma has slightly decreased in size *(asterisks)*. Another lumbar puncture is not indicated until the CSF reaccumulates. (Courtesy Nationwide Children's Hospital, Columbus, OH.)

> **BOX 29.3 Lumbosacral Stigmata Associated With Closed Spinal Dysraphism**
>
> - Dimples 25 mm above the anus or >5 mm
> - Midline or paramedian masses
> - Hair tufts
> - Skin tags or discolorations
> - Large, pigmented nevi (moles)
> - Hemangiomas
> - Pinpoint midline dimples
> - Paramedian deep dimples
> - Tail-like projection

Key Pearls

- Spinal sonography is usually diagnostic until 3–4 months of age and is performed with a 7- to 15-MHz linear-array transducer.
- The most common indication is a midline cutaneous abnormality to look for occult dysraphic conditions, such as tethered cord.
- An extended field of view is optimal and helpful in counting vertebrae.
- A tethered cord may be indicated when a dimple is more than 25 mm above the anus, larger than 5 mm, and when associated with other spinal lesions.
- Sonographically, tethering may present with a low-lying conus medullaris, posterior position of the spinal canal, thickened and echogenic filum terminale, and decreased pulsations and movement of the nerve roots within the spinal canal.
- Most defects occur in the lower lumbosacral spine, but they may occur anywhere.
- A dorsal dermal sinus should be differentiated from a pseudosinus tract, as the latter is not associated with a tethered cord, but a dorsal dermal sinus often is and is open to the skin surface. Sterile gel is recommended.
- Diastematomyelia is the split of the cord into two complete hemicords.
- Myelomeningocele and myelocele are open dysraphic abnormalities without intact skin, a contraindication to perform a spinal sonographic examination.
- Sonography may be indicated for evaluation of spinal cord injury, such as birth trauma or a failed lumbar puncture.

BIBLIOGRAPHY

AIUM Practice Parameter for the Performance of an Ultrasound Examination of the Neonatal and Infant Spine. *J Ultrasound Med.* 2016;35(9):1–11.

Beek FJA, Bax KMA. Mali WFTM: Sonography of the coccyx in newborns and infants. *J Ultrasound Med.* 1994;13:629–634.

Castro-Aragon I et al. The pediatric spinal canal. In: Rumack CM, Levine D, eds. Diagnostic ultrasound, ed 5. St Louis: Elsevier; 2018.

Chern JJ, Kirkma JL, Shannon CN, et al. Use of lumbar ultrasonography to detect occult spinal dysraphism: clinical article. *J Neurosurg Pediatr.* 2012;9(3):274–279.

Dick EA, Patel K, Owens CM. Spinal ultrasound in infants. *Br J Radiol.* 2002;75:384–392.

DiPietro MA. The conus medullaris: normal US findings throughout childhood. *Radiology.* 1993;188:149–153.

DiPietro MA: Sonography of the pediatric spine and hip [lecture], 2015. http://www.sonoworld.com.

Glasier CM, Chadduck WM, Leithiser Jr RE, et al. Screening spinal ultrasound in newborns with neural tube defects. *J Ultrasound Med.* 1990;9:339–343.

Hung PC, Wang HS, Lui TN, Wong AMC. Sonographic findings in a neonate with diastematomyelia and a tethered spinal cord. *J Ultrasound Med.* 2010;29(9):1357–1360.

Irani N, Goud AR, Lowe LH. Isolated filar cyst on lumbar spine sonography in infants: a case-control study. *Pediatr Radiol.* 2006;36(12):1283–1288.

Kriss VM, Desai NS. Occult spinal dysraphism in neonates: assessment of high-risk cutaneous stigmata on sonography. *Am J Roentgenol.* 1998;171(4):1687–1692.

Kriss VM, Kriss TC, Babcock DS. The ventriculus terminalis of the spinal cord in the neonate: a normal variant on sonography. *Am J Radiol.* 1995;165:1491–1493.

Nair N, Sreenivas M, Gupta AK, Kandasamy D, Jana M. Neonatal and infantile spinal sonography: A useful investigation often underutilized. *Indian J Radiol Imaging.* 2016;26(4):493–501.

Meyers AB, Chandra T, Epelman M. Sonographic spinal imaging of normal anatomy, pathology and magnetic growing rods in children. *Pediatr Radiol.* 2017;47(9):1046–1057.

McGovern M, et al. Ultrasound investigation of sacral dimples and other stigmata of spinal dysraphism. *Arch Dis Child.* 2013;98(10):784–786.

Rypens F, Avni EF, Matos C, et al. Atypical and equivocal sonographic features of the spinal cord in neonates. *Pediatr Radiol.* 1995;25:429–432.

Rufener S, Ibrahim M, Parmar HA. Imaging of congenital spine and spinal cord malformations. *Neuroimag Clin North Am.* 2011;21(3):659–676.

Schenk JP, Herweh C, Günther P, et al. Imaging of congenital anomalies and variations of the caudal spine and back in neonates and small infants. *Eur J Radiol.* 2006;58(1):3–14.

Scottoni F, Iacobelli BD, Zaccara AM, et al. Spinal ultrasound in patients with anorectal malformations: is this the end of an era? *Pediatr Surg Int.* 2014;30(8):829–831.

Siegel MJ. *Pediatric sonography.* Philadelphia, PA: Lippincott Williams & Wilkins; 2010.

Simanovsky N, Stepensky P, Hiller N. The use of ultrasound for the diagnosis of spinal hemorrhage in a newborn. *Pediatr Neurol.* 2004;31(4):295–297.

Unsinn KM, Geley T, Freund MC, et al. US of the spinal cord in newborns: spectrum of normal findings, variants, congenital abnormalities, and acquired diseases. *Radiographics.* 2000;20(4):923–938.

GLOSSARY FOR VOLUME 1

abdominal aortic aneurysm   localized dilation of an artery, with an increase in diameter of 1.5 times its normal diameter

abduction   to move away from the body

abscess   localized collection of pus surrounded by inflamed tissue

absorption   process of nutrient molecules passing through wall of intestine into blood or lymph system

accessory spleen   results from the failure of fusion of separate splenic masses forming on the dorsal mesogastrium; most commonly found in the splenic hilum or along the splenic vessels of associated ligaments

acholic (stools)   describes absence or deficiency of bile secretion or failure of bile to enter the alimentary tract (secondary to obstruction); stools are claylike and colorless

acini   glandular component of the breast lobule; the breast contains hundreds of lobules, each containing several small glands or acini

acini cells   cells that perform exocrine function

acoustic emission   occurs when an appropriate level of acoustic energy is applied to the tissue, the microbubbles first oscillate and then rupture; the rupture of the microbubbles in random Doppler shifts appearing as a transient mosaic of colors on a color Doppler display

acoustic impedance   measure of a material's resistance to the propagation of sound; expressed as the product of acoustic velocity of the medium and the density of the medium

acromioclavicular joint (AC)   the joint found in the shoulder that connects the clavicle to the acromion process of the scapula

Addison disease   condition caused by hyposecretion of hormones from the adrenal cortex

adduction   to move toward the body

adenoma   benign neoplasm characterized by complete fibrous encapsulation

adenomyomatosis   small polypoid projections arising from the gallbladder wall

adenopathy   multiple, enlarged lymph nodes

adenosis   overgrowth of the acini within the terminal ductal lobular unit of the breast

adrenal hemorrhage   occurs when the fetus is stressed during a difficult delivery or a hypoxic insult

adrenocorticotropic hormone (ACTH)   hormone secreted by the pituitary gland

afferent arteriole   carries blood into the glomerulus of the nephron

alanine aminotransferase (ALT)   enzyme of the liver

aliasing   indicates improper representation of information that has been sampled insufficiently; usually occurs in pulsed Doppler imaging in which a high-frequency Doppler shift is interpreted as a lower frequency

alimentary tract   also known as the digestive tract; includes the mouth, pharynx, esophagus, stomach, duodenum, small and large intestine

alkaline phosphatase   enzyme of the liver

alpha fetoprotein (AFP)   a laboratory test that measures levels of alpha fetoprotein in blood serum; an elevated level could indicate a liver lesion

amplitude   strength of the ultrasound wave measured in decibels

ampulla of Vater   small opening in the duodenum in which the pancreatic and common bile duct enter to release secretions

amylase   enzyme secreted by the pancreas to aid in the digestion of carbohydrates

amyloidosis   metabolic disorder marked by amyloid deposits in organs and tissue

anastomosis   communication between two blood vessels without any intervening capillary network

anatomic position   individual is standing erect, arms are by the sides with the palms facing forward, face and eyes are directed forward, and heels are together, with the feet pointed forward

angiomyolipomas   most common benign tumor of the kidney; appears as a hyperechoic mass composed of blood vessels, muscle cells, and fat cells; strongly associated with tuberous sclerosis, often bilaterally

angle of incidence   angle at which the sound beam strikes the interface

angle of reflection   angle at which the beam of the sound is reflected from an interface; the angle of reflection equals the angle of incidence

anisotropy   the quality of comprising varying values of a given property when measured in different directions

anterior (ventral)   toward the front of the body or in front of another structure

anti-radial   plane of imaging on ultrasound that is perpendicular to the radial plane of imaging

aorta   largest arterial structure in the body

apnea   spontaneous breathing that stops for any reason

apocrine metaplasia   form of fibrocystic change in which the epithelial cells of the acini undergo alteration

aponeurosis   band-like flat tendons connecting muscle to the bone

appendicolith   a fecalith or calcification located in the appendix

aqueductal stenosis   blockage of the duct connecting the third and fourth ventricles, which causes their dilation

arcuate artery   small arteries that lie at the bases of the renal pyramids and appear as echogenic structures

areola   the pigmented skin surrounding the breast nipple

arrhythmia   any irregular heartbeat; also called dysrhythmia

arteries   vascular structures that carry blood away from the heart

arteriosclerosis   a disease of the arterial vessels marked by thickening, hardening, and loss of elasticity in the arterial walls

arteriovenous fistula   communication between an artery and vein

ascites   free fluid in the abdominal cavity

aspartase aminotransferase (AST)   enzyme of the liver

asphyxia   severe hypoxia, or inadequate oxygenation

atherosclerosis   condition in which the aortic wall becomes irregular from plaque build-up

atretic   describes the congenital absence or closure of a normal body opening or tubular structure

atrium (trigone) of the lateral ventricle   junction of the anterior, occipital, and temporal horns of the lateral ventricles

attenuation reduction in the amplitude and intensity of a sound wave as it propagates through a medium; attenuation coefficient increases with increasing frequency

atypical hyperplasia abnormal proliferation of cells with atypical features involving the terminal ductal lobular unit

autoimmune hemolytic anemia anemia caused by antibodies produced by the patient's own immune system

autosomal dominant polycystic renal disease (ADPKD) hereditary polycystic disease that usually presents in middle age

autosomal recessive polycystic renal disease (ARPKD) rare, hereditary polycystic disease (infantile polycystic disease)

axial resolution refers to the minimum distance between two structures positioned along the axis of the beam where both structures can be visualized as separate objects

axilla the axilla contains lymph nodes that drain the majority of breast tissue

bare area area superior to the liver that is not covered by peritoneum so that the inferior vena cava may enter the thoracic cavity

Barlow maneuver the patient lies in the supine position with the hip flexed 90 degrees and adducted; downward and outward pressure is applied; if the hip is dislocated, the examiner will feel the femoral head move out of the acetabulum

Beckwith-Wiedemann syndrome hereditary disorder transmitted as an autosomal recessive trait; clinical manifestations include umbilical hernia (exomphalos), macroglossia, and gigantism. Often accompanied by visceromegaly and dysplasia of the renal medulla; also called exophthalmos-macroglossia-gigantism (EMG) syndrome

biliary atresia closure or absence of some or all of the major bile ducts

bilirubin yellow pigment in bile formed by the breakdown of red blood cells; excreted by the liver and stored in the gallbladder

blood urea nitrogen (BUN) measures amount of nitrogenous waste (along with creatinine); waste products accumulate in the blood when kidneys malfunction

blunt abdominal trauma (BAT) injury to the abdomen caused by a blunt (not penetrating) object or surface

body mechanics theory and practice of using the correct muscles to complete a task safely, efficiently, and without undue strain on any joints or muscles

body of the pancreas lies in the mid-epigastrium anterior to the superior mesenteric artery and vein, aorta, and inferior vena cava

Bowman's capsule part of the filtration process; contains water, salts, glucose, urea, and amino acids

bradycardia a heart rate of less than 60 beats/min

brainstem part of the brain connecting the forebrain and the spinal cord; consists of the midbrain, pons, and medulla oblongata

branchial cleft cyst remnant of embryonic development that appears as a cyst in the neck

Budd-Chiari syndrome thrombosis of the hepatic veins

Bulk modulus amount of pressure required to compress a small volume of material a small amount

bull's eye (target) lesion hypoechoic mass with an echogenic central core (abscess, metastases)

bursa a saclike structure containing thick fluid that surrounds areas subject to friction, such as the interface between bone and tendon

bursitis inflammation of a bursa

calcitonin a thyroid hormone that is important for maintaining a dense, strong bone matrix and regulating the blood calcium level

calyx part of the collecting system adjacent to the pyramid that collects urine and is connected to the major calyx

capillaries minute vessels that connect the arterial and venous systems

cardiac orifice entrance of the esophagus into the stomach

carpal tunnel the canal in the wrist bounded by osteofibrous material through which the flexor tendons and the median nerve pass

cartilage interface sign echogenic line on the anterior surface of the cartilage surrounding the humeral head

cauda equina bundle of nerve roots from the lumbar, sacral, and coccygeal spinal nerves that descend nearly vertically from the spinal cord until they reach respective openings in the vertebral column

caudal pancreatic artery branch of the splenic artery that supplies the tail of the pancreas

caudal toward the feet

caudate lobe small lobe of the liver situated on the posterosuperior surface of the left lobe; the ligamentum venosum is the anterior border

caudothalamic groove or notch the region at which the caudate nucleus and thalamus join; the most common location of germinal matrix hemorrhage

cavernous transformation of the portal vein periportal collateral channels in patients with chronic portal vein obstruction

centripetal artery terminal intratesticular arteries arising from the capsular arteries

cerebellum area of the brain that lies posterior to the brainstem below the tentorium

cerebrum largest part of the brain consisting of two equal hemispheres

Chiari malformations congenital defect in which the cerebellum and brainstem are pulled toward the spinal cord ("banana sign" seen with sonography); frontal bossing or a lemon-shaped neonatal head can be observed

cholangitis inflammation of the bile ducts

cholecystectomy removal of the gallbladder

cholecystitis inflammation of the gallbladder; may be acute or chronic

cholecystokinin hormone secreted into the blood by the mucosa of the upper small intestine; stimulates contraction of the gallbladder and pancreatic secretion of enzymes

choledochal cyst cystic growth on the common bile duct that may cause obstruction

choledocholithiasis stones in the bile duct

cholelithiasis gallstones in the gallbladder

cholesterosis variant of adenomyomatosis; cholesterol polyps

choroid plexus echogenic cluster of cells important in the production of cerebrospinal fluid that lie along the atrium of the lateral ventricles

clapper-in-the-bell sign hypoechoic hematoma found at the end of a completely retracted muscle fragment

C-loop of the duodenum forms the lateral border of the head of the pancreas

coagulopathy a defect in blood-clotting mechanisms

collateral circulation develops when normal venous channels become obstructed

color flow Doppler velocity in each direction is quantified by allocating a pixel to each area

columns of Bertin bands of cortical tissue that separate the renal pyramids; a prominent column of Bertin may mimic a renal mass on sonography

common bile duct extends from the point where the common hepatic duct meets the cystic duct; drains into the duodenum after it joins with the main pancreatic duct

common hepatic artery arises from the celiac trunk to supply the liver; forms the right superior border of the body and head of the pancreas and gives rise to the gastroduodenal artery

common hepatic duct bile duct drains from the liver to the hepatic duct, which joins the cystic duct to form the common bile duct

common iliac arteries the abdominal aorta bifurcates at the level of the umbilicus into common iliac arteries to supply blood to the lower extremities

compression region of increased particle density

congenital mesoblastic nephroma most common benign renal tumor of the neonate and infant

continuous wave Doppler (CW) one transducer continuously transmits sound while one transducer continuously receives sound; used in high-velocity flow patterns

contrast-enhanced sonography (CES) agent used to reduce or eliminate some of the current limitations of ultrasound imaging and Doppler blood flow detection color flow imaging

conus medullaris caudal end of the spinal cord; it should taper

converse piezoelectric effect property of piezoelectric materials whereby an electric stimulus causes the dipolar material to expand and contract, producing a sound wave

Cooper's ligaments connective tissue septa that connect perpendicularly to the breast lobules and extend out to the skin

coronal lengthwise plane running from side to side, dividing the body into anterior and posterior portions

cortex (adrenal) outer parenchyma of the adrenal gland that secretes steroid hormones, commonly called corticoids

cortex (kidney) outer parenchyma of an organ; in the kidney, it contains the renal corpuscle and proximal and distal convoluted tubules of the nephron

corticomedullary differentiation the distinct separation and normal sonographic appearance of the cortex and medulla within the pediatric kidney; when poor, it may be indicative of renal pathology

Courvoisier's gallbladder enlargement of the gallbladder caused by a slow progressive obstruction of the distal common bile duct from an external mass

cranial toward the head

creatinine (Cr) one of the laboratory tests used to measure the ability of the kidney to get rid of waste; waste products accumulate in the blood when the kidneys are malfunctioning

cremasteric artery small artery arising from the inferior epigastric artery (a branch of the external iliac artery), which supplies the peritesticular tissue, including the cremasteric muscle

cremasteric muscle an extension of the internal oblique muscle that descends to the testis with the spermatic cord; contraction of the cremasteric muscle shortens the spermatic cord and elevates the testis

Crohn disease inflammation of the bowel, accompanied by abscess and bowel wall thickening

cryptorchidism (undescended testes) testicles remain within the abdomen or groin and fail to descend into the scrotal sac

culling process by which the spleen removes abnormal red blood cells as they pass through

curved array probe large footprint that allows good near field and far field visualization with limited intercostal access

Cushing syndrome condition caused by hypersecretion of hormones from the adrenal cortex

cyanosis bluish discoloration of the skin and mucous membranes caused by lack of oxygen in the blood

cycle a sequence of events occurring at regular intervals; a wavelength cycle is that of a particle density that varies from maximum in the compression zone to a minimum in the reflection zone and back to maximum in the successive compression zone to complete one cycle

cystic duct connects the gallbladder to the common hepatic duct

cystic medial necrosis weakening of the arterial wall

Dandy-Walker malformation abnormal development of the fourth ventricle, often accompanied by hydrocephalus

dartos layer of muscle underneath the scrotal skin

decibel (dB) unit used to quantitatively express the ratio of two amplitudes or intensities

deferential artery arises from the vesicle artery (a branch of the internal iliac artery) and supplies the vas deferens and epididymis

developmental displacement of the hip (DDH) abnormal condition of the hip that results in congenital hip dysplasia; includes dysplastic, subluxated, dislocatable, and dislocated hips

diagnostic peritoneal lavage (DPT) procedure to determine the presence of free-floating fluid in the abdominal cavity

diastematomyelia a congenital fissure of the spinal cord, frequently associated with spina bifida cystica

diffuse hepatocellular disease affects hepatocytes and interferes with liver function

dissecting aneurysm tear in the intima and/or media of the abdominal aorta

distal away from the point of origin or away from the body

diverticulum a pouch-like herniation through the muscular wall of a tubular organ that occurs in the stomach, small intestine, or colon

Doppler angle the angle the reflector path makes with the ultrasound beam; the most accurate velocity is when the beam is parallel to flow

Doppler gate the sample site from which the signal is obtained with pulsed wave Doppler

Doppler shift change in frequency of a reflected wave; caused by motion between the reflector and the transducer's beam

dorsal pancreatic artery branch of the splenic artery that supplies the body of the pancreas

dorsiflexion upward movement of the hand or foot

dromedary hump normal variant that occurs on the left kidney as a bulge on the lateral border

duct of Santorini small accessory duct found in the head of the pancreas

duct of Wirsung largest duct that drains the tail, body, and head of the pancreas; it joins the common bile duct to enter the duodenum through the ampulla of Vater

duodenal bulb first part of the duodenum

dynamic range ratio of the largest to smallest signals that an instrument or component of an instrument can respond to without distortion

dyspnea a shortness of breath or the feeling of not getting enough air, which may leave a person gasping

dysraphism abnormalities associated with incomplete embryologic development of the dorsal aspect of an embryo; abnormalities of the spine and spinal cord

ectasia dilation of any tubular vessel

ectopic kidney located outside of the normal position, most often in the pelvic cavity

ectopic ureterocele ectopic insertion and cystic dilation of the distal ureter of a duplicated renal collecting system (duplex kidney); occurs more commonly in females and on the left side

efferent arteriole blood from this structure supplies the peritubular capillaries, which also supply the convoluted tubules

ejaculatory ducts connect the seminal vesicle and the vas deferens to the urethra at the verumontanum

endocrine production of the hormone insulin

enhancement strengthening of echoes from reflectors that lie behind a weakly attenuating structure

ependyma the inside lining of the cerebral ventricles and central canal of the spinal cord

epicondylitis (lateral and medial) inflammation of the humerus and surrounding tissues

epididymis anatomic structure formed by the network of ducts leaving the mediastinum testis that combine into a single, convoluted epidiymal tubule; located on the posterolateral aspect of the testis; the epididymis consists of the head, the body, and the tail; spermatozoa mature and accumulate within the epididymis

epididymal cyst mass filled with clear, serous fluid located in the epididymis

epididymitis inflammation of the epididymis

epigastrium area between the right and left hypochondrium that contains part of the liver, duodenum, and pancreas

epineurium the covering of a nerve that consists of connective tissue

ergonomics the science concerned with fitting a job to a person's anatomical, physiological, and psychological characteristics in a way that enhances human efficiency and well-being

erythrocyte red blood cell

euthyroid refers to a normal functioning thyroid gland

exocrine production and digestion of pancreatic juice

external outside

extracorporeal membrane oxygenation (ECMO) intensive treatment for infants with severe respiratory failure who have not responded to maximal conventional ventilator support

extrahepatic outside the liver

falciform ligament extends from the umbilicus to the diaphragm in a sagittal plane and contains the ligamentum teres

false pelvis portion of the pelvic cavity that is above the pelvic brim

falx cerebri echogenic fibrous structure (portion of the dura mater) that descends through the interhemispheric fissure, separating the cerebral hemispheres

fan micro movement when the probe is minutely angled, pivoting on a point of interest

far field (Fraunhofer zone) the field farthest from the transducer during the formation of the sound beam

fasciculi term describing a small bundle of muscles, nerves, and tendons

fecalith calculus that may form around fecal material; associated with appendicitis

fibroadenoma most common benign solid tumor of the breast

filum terminale slender tapering terminal section of the spinal cord, contiguous with the pia mater

fine needle aspiration (FNA) the use of a fine-gauge needle to obtain cells from a mass

first-generation contrast agents agents containing room air (i.e., Albunex)

focal zone the region over which the effective width of the sound beam is within some measure of its width at the focal distance

focused assessment with sonography for trauma (FAST) exam limited survey of the chest, abdomen, and pelvis to evaluate for free fluid or pericardial fluid

follicular carcinoma a malignant thyroid neoplasm showing follicular cell differentiation but lacking the diagnostic features of papillary carcinoma

fontanels soft space between the bones; usually large enough to accommodate the ultrasound transducer until 9–12 months of age

frame rate rate at which images are updated on the display; dependent on frequency of the transducer and depth selection

frank dislocation lateral and posterior displacement of the hip to the extent that the femoral head has no contact with the acetabulum and the normal "U" configuration in the transverse view cannot be obtained on ultrasound

frequency number of cycles per second that a periodic event or function undergoes per unit of time

fusiform aneurysm circumferential enlargement of a vessel with tapering at both ends

gain measure of the strength of the ultrasound signal expressed in decibels

Galeazzi sign on physical examination, the knee is lower in position on the affected side of the neonate with developmental displacement of the hip (DDH) when the patient is supine and the knees are flexed

gallbladder storage pouch for bile

gastrin endocrine hormone released from the stomach that stimulates secretion of gastric acid

gastroduodenal artery branch of the common hepatic artery to supply to stomach and duodenum

gastrosplenic ligament ligament between the greater curvature of the stomach and spleen that helps hold the spleen in place

Gaucher disease storage disease in which fat and proteins are deposited abnormally in the body

germinal matrix fragile periventricular tissue (includes the caudate nucleus) that easily bleeds in the premature infant

Gerota's fascia another term for the renal fascia; the kidney is covered by the renal capsule, perirenal fat, Gerota's fascia, and pararenal fat

glomerulus part of the filtration process in the kidney

glucagon stimulates the liver to convert glycogen to glucose

goiter enlargement of the thyroid gland that can be focal or diffuse; multiple nodules may be present

grating lobes additional beams emitted from an array transducer that are stronger than the side lobes of individual elements

Graves disease autoimmune disorder of diffuse toxic goiter characterized by bulging eyes (exophthalmos)

gray scale B-mode technique that permits the brightness of the B-mode dots to be displayed in various shades of gray to represent different echo amplitudes

gray scale harmonic imaging allows detection of contrast-enhanced blood flow and organs with grayscale ultrasound;

in the harmonic-imaging mode, the echoes from the oscillating microbubbles have a higher signal-to-noise ration than found in conventional ultrasound; regions with microbubbles (e.g., blood vessels and organ parenchyma) are better visualized

greater omentum   known as the "fatty apron" double fold of the peritoneum attached to the duodenum, stomach, and large intestine; helps support the great curve of the stomach

Guyon's canal or tunnel   fibrous tunnel that contains the ulnar artery and vein, ulnar nerve, and some fatty tissue

gynecomastia   hypertrophy of residual elements that persist behind the nipple in the male

harmonic imaging (HI)   mode in which the ultrasound system is configured to receive only echoes at the second harmonic frequency, which is twice the transmit frequency

Hartmann's pouch   small outpouching of the gallbladder fundus that lies near the cystic duct that may collect gallstones

Hashimoto thyroiditis   chronic inflammation of the thyroid gland caused by the formation of antibodies against normal thyroid tissue

haustra   normal segmentation of the wall of the colon

head of the pancreas   lies in the C-loop of the duodenum; the gastroduodenal artery is the anterolateral border and the common bile duct is the posterior border

Heimlich maneuver   emergency treatment to clear an upper airway obstruction that is preventing normal breathing

Heister's valve   tiny valves found within the cystic duct

hematocele   blood located between the visceral and parietal layers of the tunica vaginalis

hematopoiesis   blood cell production

hemihypertrophy   excessive development of one side or one half of the body or an organ

hemoglobin   oxygen-binding protein found in red blood cells

hemolytic anemia   anemia resulting from hemolysis of red blood cells

hemoperitoneum   collection of bloody fluid in the abdomen or pelvis secondary to trauma or surgical procedure

hemorrhage   collection of blood

hepatic flexure   ascending colon rises from the right lower quadrant to bend at this point to form the transverse colon

hepatic veins   three large veins that drain the liver and empty into the inferior vena cava at the level of the diaphragm

hepatocellular disease   refers to liver cells or hepatocytes as primary problem

hepatocyte   a parenchymal liver cell that performs all functions ascribed to the liver

hepatofugal   flow away from the liver

hepatopedal   flow toward the liver

hertz (Hz)   unit for frequency, equal to 1 cycle per second

hilus   area of kidney where vessels, ureter, and lymphatics enter and exit

hip joint   formed by the articulation of the head of the femur within the acetabulum of the hip bone

Hodgkin disease   malignant disease that involves lymphoid tissue

holoprosencephaly   congenital defect caused by an extra chromosome and characterized by abnormal single ventricular cavity with some form of thalami fusion; the prosencephalon fails to divide into hemispheres during embryonic development

homeostasis   maintenance of normal body physiology

horseshoe kidney   congenital malformation in which both kidneys are joined together by an isthmus, most commonly at the lower poles

hydrocele   fluid formed between the visceral and parietal layers of the tunica vaginalis

hydrocephalus   ventriculomegaly in the neonate; abnormal accumulation of cerebrospinal fluid within the cerebral ventricles resulting in compression and frequently destruction of brain tissue

hydromyelia   dilation of the central canal of the spinal cord

hydronephrosis   dilation of the renal collecting system

hydrops   massive enlargement of the gallbladder

hypercalcemia   elevated levels of calcium in the blood

hyperglycemia   uncontrolled increase in glucose

hyperlipidemia   congenital condition in which elevated fat levels cause pancreatitis

hyperparathyroidism   disorder associated with elevated serum calcium level, usually caused by a benign parathyroid adenoma

hyperplasia   enlargement

hypertension   blood pressure higher than 130/90 mm Hg

hyperthyroidism   oversecretion of thyroid hormones

hypoglycemia   deficiency of glucose

hypomotility   abnormally decreased motility or movement of the bowel; can be associated with appendicitis, constipation, and other gastrointestinal conditions

hypophosphatasia   low phosphatase level; sometimes seen with hyperparathyroidism

hypotension   blood pressure lower than 115/75 mm Hg; decreased systolic and diastolic blood pressure below normal; may occur with shock, hemorrhaging, infection, fever, cancer, anemia, neurasthenia, and Addison disease

hypothyroidism   underactive thyroid hormones

hypoxia   decreased oxygen in the body

incarcerated hernia   imprisonment or confinement of a part of the bowel in which the visceral contents cannot be reduced

increased intracranial pressure (ICP)   increased pressure inside the skull compressing the brain and restricting blood flow; in the neonate it is often caused by hydrocephalus, but may be due to brain edema

induced acoustic emission   after the injection of the tissue-specific contrast agent, the reflectivity of the contrast-containing tissue increases; when the right level of acoustic energy is applied to tissue, the contrast microbubbles eventually rupture, resulting in random Doppler shifts, which appear as a transient mosaic of colors on the color Doppler display; masses that have destroyed or replaced normal Kupffer cells will be displayed as color-free areas

infarction   interruption in the blood supply to an area that may lead to necrosis of that area

inferior   below

inferior mesenteric artery   arises from the anterior aortic wall at the level of the third or fourth lumbar vertebra to supply the left transverse colon, descending colon, sigmoid colon, and rectum

inferior mesenteric vein   drains the left third of the colon and upper colon and joins the splenic vein

inferior vena cava   largest venous abdominal vessel that conveys blood from the body below the diaphragm to the right atrium of the heart

infiltrating ductal carcinoma   cancer of the ductal epithelium

infiltrating (invasive) lobular carcinoma cancer of the lobular epithelium of the breast

inspissated thickened by absorption, evaporation, or dehydration

insulin hormone that causes glycogen formation from glucose in the liver and allows cells within insulin receptors to take up glucose to decrease blood sugar

intensity power per unit area

interface surface forming the boundary between media having different properties

internal inside

international normalized ratio (INR) method developed to standardize prothrombin time (PT) results among laboratories by accounting for the different thromboplastin reagents used to determine PT

intrahepatic within the liver

intraperitoneal within the peritoneal cavity

intravenous (IV) therapy administration of liquid substances directly into a vein

intraventricular hemorrhage (IVH) hemorrhage that has burst through the germinal matrix or subependymal bleed and lies within the ventricular cavity; depending on severity and location, it may cause ventricular enlargement

intussusception when bowel prolapses into distal bowel (telescoping) and is propelled in an antegrade fashion, causing bowel obstruction

islets of Langerhans small cells that comprise the endocrine portion of the pancreas for the production of insulin, glucagon, and somatostatin

isolated systolic hypertension condition that occurs when systolic pressure is above 140 mm Hg but diastolic pressure remains below 90 mm Hg

isthmus small piece of thyroid tissue connecting the right and left lobes of the gland

jaundice excessive bilirubin accumulation causing yellow pigmentation of the skin

junctional fold small septum within the gallbladder, usually arising from the posterior wall

kilohertz (kHz) 1000 Hz

Klatskin tumor cancer at the bifurcation of the hepatic ducts; may cause asymmetric obstruction of the biliary tree

labrum fibrocartilage (rubbery tissue) that attaches the rim of a socket to keep the ball joint in place; in the hip, the acetabular labrum has a fibrous echogenic tip and increases the ball (femoral head) depth in the socket

laminar normal pattern of vessel flow; flow in the center of the vessel is faster than at the edges

lateral farther from the midline or to the side of the body

lateral resolution the minimal distance between two objects where they can still be displayed as separate objects

left gastric artery arises from the celiac axis to supply the stomach and lower third of the esophagus

left hepatic artery small branch the supplies the caudate and left lobes of the liver

left hypochondrium left upper quadrant of the abdomen that contains the left lobe of the liver, spleen, and stomach

left lobe of the liver lies in the epigastrium and left hypochondrium

left portal vein supplies the left lobe of the liver

left renal artery arises from the posterolateral wall of the aorta directly into the hilus of the kidney

left renal vein leaves the renal hilum, travelling anterior to the aorta and posterior to the superior mesenteric artery to enter the lateral wall of the inferior vena cava

lesser omentum suspends the stomach and duodenum from the liver; helps support the lesser curvature of the stomach

leukocytolysis destruction of leukocytes

leukopenia abnormal decrease of white blood corpuscles

lienorenal ligament ligament between the spleen and kidney that helps support the great curvature of the stomach

ligament fibrous band of tissue connecting bone or cartilage to bone that aids in stabilizing a joint

ligamentum teres along with falciform ligament, divides medial and lateral segments of the left lobe of the liver; appears as a bright echogenic foci on transverse images

ligamentum venosum separates left lobe from caudate lobe; shown as echogenic line on transverse and sagittal images

lipase pancreatic enzyme that breaks down fats; is elevated in pancreatitis and remains increased longer than amylase

lipoma common benign tumor composed of fat cells

liver function tests specific laboratory tests that look at liver function (aspartase or alanine aminotransferase, lactic acid dehydrogenase, alkaline phosphatase, and bilirubin)

longitudinal plane that is parallel to the long axis of the body or part

longus colli muscle wedge-shaped muscle posterior to the thyroid lobes

loop of Henle portion of a renal tubule lying between the proximal and distal convoluted portions; reabsorption of fluid, sodium, and chloride occurs here

lymph an alkaline fluid found in the lymphatic vessels

lymphoma malignancy that primarily affects the lymph nodes, spleen, or liver

macro movement movement of the probe used with the sweep and slight motion in which the probe is moved greater than 1 centimeter

main lobar fissure boundary between the right and left lobes of the liver; seen as hyperechoic line on the sagittal image extending from the portal vein to the neck of the gallbladder

main portal vein enters the liver at the porta hepatis

major calyces (also known as the infundibulum) receives urine from the minor calyces to convey to the loop of Henle

mammary layer middle layer of the breast tissue between the skin and the chest wall that contains the ductal, glandular, and stromal portions of the breast

Marfan syndrome hereditary disorder of connective tissue, bones, muscles, ligaments, and skeletal structures

McBurney's point site of maximal tenderness in the right lower quadrant; usually with appendicitis; located by drawing a line from the right anterosuperior iliac spine to the umbilicus; at approximately the midpoint of this line lies the root of the appendix

mechanical index (MI) an index that defines the low acoustic output power that can be used to minimize the destruction of microbubbles by energy in the acoustic field; when the microbubbles in microbubble-based ultrasound contrast agents are destroyed, contrast enhancement is lost

Meckel's diverticulum congenital sac or blind pouch found in the lower portion of the ileum

medial nearer to or toward the midline

median plane vertical plane that bisects the body into right and left halves

mediastinum testis central linear structure formed by the convergence of multiple thin septations within the testicle; the septations are invaginations of the tunica albuginea

medulla (aderenal) central tissue of the adrenal gland that secretes epinephrine and norepinephrine

medulla (renal—also known as the pyramid) refers to the inner portion of the renal parenchyma that contains the loop of Henle

medullary carcinoma neoplastic growth that accounts for 10% of thyroid malignancies

medullary pyramids large and hypoechoic in the neonate should not be mistaken for hydronephrosis. Triangular in shape, they consist mainly of tubules, which transport urine from the cortex to the calyces

mega cisterna magna normal variant without associated neurological impairment, in which there is an enlarged cisterna magna without a mass effect

megahertz (MHz) 1,000,000 Hz

meninges three membranes enclosing the brain and spinal cord

meningocele open defect in which the spinal cord, not the nerve roots, just fluid is exposed

mesentery projects from the parietal peritoneum and attaches to the small intestine, anchoring it to the posterior abdominal wall

mesothelium fifth layer of bowel

metastatic disease most common form of neoplasm of the liver; primary sites are colon, breast, and lung

micro movement movement of the probe used with the sweep and slight motion in which the probe is moved less than 1 centimeter

midgut malrotation congenital anomaly in which the bowel did not properly rotate during embryogenesis, with sonography may show an inversion of the normal SMA and SMV positioning

minor calyces receives urine from the renal pyramids; forms the border of the renal sinus

mirror image shows structures that exist on one side of a strong reflector as being present on the other side as well

Model for End-Stage Liver Disease (MELD) mathematical calculation based on lab values of bilirubin (measurement of bile pigment), creatinine (kidney function), and International Nationalized Ratio (INR) (blood clotting ability); used to predict death within 3 months in patients with a transjugular intrahepatic portosystemic shunt (TIPS)

molecular contrast imaging agents agents include Optison, Definity, Imagent, Levovist, SonoVue

mononucleosis acute infection caused by the Epstein-Barr virus that most commonly affects teenagers and young adults; symptoms include fever, sore throat, enlarged lymph nodes, abnormal lymphocysts, and hepatosplenomegaly

Morison's pouch right posterior subhepatic space located anterior to the kidney and inferior to the liver where fluid may accumulate

mucosa innermost layer of the bowel wall, or lining of the gastrointestinal tract, often appearing hyperechoic with sonography (first layer of bowel)

multicystic dysplastic kidney disease (MCDK) multiple cysts replace normal renal tissue throughout the kidney; usually causes renal obstruction; most common cause of renal cystic disease in the neonate; may have contralateral ureteral pelvic junction (UPJ) obstruction

multinodular goiter (MNG) nodular enlargement of the thyroid associated with hyperthyroidism

Murphy's sign positive sign implies exquisite tenderness over the area of the gallbladder upon palpation

muscle a type of tissue consisting of contractile cells or fibers that affects movement of an organ or part of the body

muscularis third layer of bowel

myelin a substance forming the sheath of Schwann cells

myelomeningocele defect in which the spinal cord and nerve roots are exposed, often adhering to the fine membrane that overlies them

myeloschisis cleft spinal cord resulting from failure of the neural tube to close

naked tuberosity sign notes when the deltoid muscle is on the humeral head; seen with a full-thickness tear of the rotator cuff

nasal cannula device for delivering oxygen through two small tubes inserted into the nostrils

nasal catheter piece of tubing longer than a cannula that is inserted through the nostril and into the back of the patient's mouth to provide continuous oxygen

near field (Fresnel zone) the field closest to the transducer during the formation of the sound beam

neck of the pancreas small area of the pancreas between the head and the body

neonatal intensive care unit (NICU) ICU for newborns requiring specialized medical treatment; includes a diverse team of clinicians, social workers and respiratory therapists, etc.; requires three levels of accreditation, with level 3 providing the highest level of care for the smallest infants, often <30 weeks gestational age

neoplasm any new growth (benign or malignant)

nephroblastomatosis lesion often found in the cortex or along the columns of Bertin; may replace parenchyma and appear hypoechoic and focal, multifocal, or diffuse

nephron functional unit of the kidney; includes a renal corpuscle and a renal tubule

neuroblastoma malignant, often adrenal, tumor that is seen in pediatric patients; hemorrhagic tumor principally consisting of cells resembling neuroblasts

neuroectodermal tissue early embryonic tissue that will eventually develop into the brain and spinal cord

nodular hyperplasia degenerative nodules within the thyroid

noise internally generated electronic distortion when Doppler gain is set too high

non-alcoholic steatohepatitis the most extreme form of non-alcoholic fatty liver disease, causing histologic damage to the liver; signs of hypertension and cirrhosis may be among the first manifestations

non-Hodgkin lymphoma a malignant disease of lymphoid tissue

non-resistive vessels that have high diastolic component and supply organs that need constant perfusion (i.e., internal carotid artery, hepatic artery, and renal arteries)

non-toxic (simple) goiter or nodule a compensatory enlargement of the thyroid gland due to thyroid hormone deficiency

nosocomial infections hospital-acquired infection

Nyquist limit maximum frequency shift that can be measured in pulsed wave Doppler without aliasing

obstructive disease bile excretion blocked within the liver or biliary system

omentum double fold of peritoneum attached to the stomach and connecting it with certain abdominal viscera

Organ Procurement and Transplantation Network (OPTN) United States organ allocation organization

Ortolani maneuver with the patient supine, the examiner's hand is placed around the hip to be examined with the fingers over the femoral head; the hip is flexed 90 degrees and the thigh is abducted

ostomy surgical procedure in which an opening is made to allow the passage of urine from the bladder or intestinal contents from the bowel to a surgically created opening, or stoma, in the wall of the abdomen

oximetry noninvasive method of monitoring blood oxygen levels

Paget disease (of the breast) surface erosion of the nipple resulting from direct invasion of the skin from underlying breast cancer

pampiniform plexus plexus of veins in the spermatic cord that drain into the right and left testicular veins; when a varicocele is present, dilation and tortuosity may develop

pancreatic ascites occurs when a pancreatic pseudocyst ruptures into the abdomen; free-floating pancreatic enzymes are very dangerous to surrounding structures

pancreatic duct travels horizontally through the pancreas to join the common bile duct at the ampulla of Vater

pancreatic lipomatosis the fatty replacement of normal pancreatic tissue

pancreatic pseudocyst "sterile abscess" collection of pancreatic enzymes that accumulated in the available space in the abdomen, usually near the pancreas

pancreatitis inflammation of the pancreas

papillary carcinoma cancer that forms in follicular cells in the thyroid and grows in small finger-like shapes

paralytic ileus dilated, fluid-filled bowel loops without peristalsis

parathyroid hormone (PTH) hormone secreted by the parathyroid glands, which regulate serum calcium levels

parathyroid hyperplasia enlargement of multiple parathyroid glands

partial thromboplastin time (PTT) laboratory test that can be used to evaluate the effects of heparin, aspirin, and antihistamines on the blood clotting process; detects clotting abnormalities of the intrinsic and common pathways

patent urachus the urachal remnant (or tube) extending from the superior bladder to the belly button; does not properly close (fibrotic by birth); can be open on either ends or both ends; may be a source of infection

patient-focused care (PFC) national movement to recapture the respect and goodwill of the American public and to ensure that every patient receives the best possible medical care

peau d'orange descriptive term for skin thickening of one breast that resembles an orange

pediatric end-stage liver disease (PELD) disease severity scoring system for children younger than 12 years

pelvic girdle formation of the hip bones by the ilium, ischium, and pubis

pelviectasis dilation of the renal pelvis only; pelvicaliectasis or pyelocaliectasis would include dilation of the renal pelvis and calyces; also called pyelectasis

pennate feather-like pattern of muscle growth

perineurium surrounding connective tissue of muscle

period (ultrasound physics) time it takes for one cycle to occur; decreases as frequency increases

peritoneal lavage invasive procedure used to sample the intraperitoneal space for evidence of damage to viscera and blood vessels

peritonitis inflammation of the peritoneum

periventricular leukomalacia (PVL) echogenic white matter necrosis best seen posterior to the brain or adjacent to the ventricular system

phagocytosis process by which the red pulp destroys the degenerating red blood cells

Phalen's sign (test, maneuver, or position) increase in wrist compression due to hyperflexion of the wrist for 60 seconds; test is done with the patient holding the forearms upright and pressing the ventral side of the hands together

pheochromocytoma benign adrenal tumor that secretes hormones that produce hypertension

phrenocolic ligament ligament between the spleen and the colon

Phrygian cap gallbladder variant in which part of the fundus is bent back on itself

piezoelectric effect generation of electric signals as a result of an incident sound beam on a material that has piezoelectric properties

pitting process by which the spleen removes nuclei from blood cells without destroying the erythrocytes

plantar flexion pointing of the toes toward the plantar surface of the foot

pneumothorax a collection of air or gas in the pleural cavity

polycystic renal disease poorly functioning enlarged kidneys

polycythemia excess of red blood cells

polycythemia vera chronic, life-shortening condition of unknown cause involving bone marrow elements; characterized by an increase in red blood cell mass and hemoglobin concentration

polyp small, well-defined soft tissue projection from the gallbladder wall; a small tumor-like growth that projects from a mucous membrane surface

polysplenia condition in which there is more than one spleen

porcelain gallbladder calcification of the gallbladder wall

porta hepatis central area of the liver where the portal vein, common duct, and hepatic artery enter

portal vein formed by the union of the superior mesenteric vein and splenic vein near the porta hepatis of the liver

portal venous hypertension may result from intrinsic liver disease or obstruction of the portal veins, hepatic veins, inferior vena cava, or prolonged congestive heart failure

posterior (dorsal) toward the back of the body or in back of another structure

posterior urethral valve (PUV) the presence of a valve in the posterior urethra; occurs only in male fetuses; most common cause of bladder outlet syndrome

Post-transplant lymphoproliferative disorder (PTLF) Rare immune complication of solid organ or stem cell transplantation

potter facies distinct facial features in infants with severe oligohydramnios in utero, which causes deformation through restraint; characterized by infraorbital folds, micrognathia, abnormal ear lobulation, and flattened nasal tip

power rate of energy flow over the entire beam of sound; measured in watts (W) or milliwatts (mW)

prehypertension blood pressure readings associated with prehypertension are 120 to 139 mm Hg systolic pressure, and 80 to 89 mm Hg diastolic pressure

primary hyperparathyroidism oversecretion of parathyroid hormone, usually from a parathyroid adenoma

projectile vomiting condition found in pyloric stenosis in the neonatal period; after drinking, the infant often experiences violent (across the room) vomiting secondary to obstruction

prone lying face down

prostate specific antigen (PSA) protein made by the prostate gland; elevated levels could indicate prostate cancer

prothrombin time (PT) time it takes for a blood sample to coagulate after thromboplastin and calcium are added; detects clotting abnormalities of the extrinsic pathway

protocol standardization of specific anatomical structures that should be imaged in a complete or focused sonographic examination

proximal closer to the point of origin or closer to the body

prune-belly syndrome dilation of the fetal abdomen secondary to severe hydronephrosis and fetal ascites; fetus also has oligohydramnios and pulmonary hypoplasia

pseudoaneurysm pulsatile hematoma that results from leakage of blood into soft tissues abutting the punctured artery with fibrous encapsulation and failure of the vessel wall to heal

pseudodissection condition seen in a patient with aortic dissection; there is no intimal flap seen, only hypoechoic thrombus near the outer margin of the aorta with echogenic laminated clot

pudendal artery internal and external pudendal arteries partially supply the scrotal wall and epididymis and occasionally the lower pole of the testis

pulmonary hypoplasia small, underdeveloped lungs with resultant reduction in lung volume; secondary to prolonged oligohydramnios or as a consequence of a small thoracic cavity

pulse a way to measure heart rate; recorded as beats/min

pulse duration time interval required for generating the transmitted pulse; the pulse duration is calculated by multiplying the number of cycles in the pulse by the period

pulse pressure difference between the systolic and diastolic blood pressures

pulse repetition frequency (PRF) number of times the system is pulsed each second

pulsed wave (PW) Doppler sound transmitted and received intermittently with one transducer

pyelonephritis infection of the kidneys; often the result of infection spread from the bladder through the ureters

pyloric canal canal located between the stomach and proximal duodenum; surrounded by the pyloric sphincter muscle

pyloromyotomy Surgical procedure used in treating hypertrophic pyloric stenosis in which the pyloric muscle is split longitudinally not to violate the mucosa; pyloric muscle will appear abnormally large for up to 12 weeks post-surgery

pyocele pus located between the visceral and parietal layers of the tunica vaginalis

pyogenic producing pus

pyogenic abscess pus-forming collection of fluid

pyramidal lobe present in small percentage of patients; extends superiorly from the isthmus pyramidal lobe

pyramids convey urine to the minor calyces

range ambiguity misplacement of an interface when the assumption that each echo is derived from the most recent pulse is violated

real-time ultrasound instrumentation allowing the image to be displayed multiple times per second to achieve a "real-time" image of movement

recurrent rami terminal ends of the centripetal (intratesticular) arteries that curve backward toward the capsule

red pulp consists of reticular cells and fibers (cords of Billroth); surrounds the splenic sinuses

reducible hernia capable of being replaced in a normal position, and the visceral contents can be returned to normal intraabdominal location

refractile shadowing (edge artifact) bending of the sound beam at the edge of a circular structure resulting in the absence of posterior echoes

refraction change in the direction of propagation of a sound wave transmitted across an interface where the speed of sound varies

renal agenesis interruption in the normal development of the kidney resulting in absence of the kidney; may be unilateral or bilateral

renal autotransplantation patient's own kidney is removed from the retroperitoneum and reimplanted into the iliac fossa

renal capsule first layer adjacent to the kidney that forms a tough, fibrous covering

renal corpuscle part of the nephron that consists of Bowman's capsule and the glomerulus

renal hilum area in the midportion of the kidney where the renal vessels and ureter enter and exit

renal pelvis area in the midportion of the kidney that collects urine before entering the ureter

renal sinus central area of the kidney that includes the calyces, renal pelvis, renal vessels, fat, nerves, and lymphatics

renal vein thrombosis obstruction of the renal vein resulting in an enlarged and edematous kidney

resistance passive force in opposition to another active force; occurs when tissue exerts pressure against the flow

resistive vessels that have little or reversed flow in diastole and supply organs that do not need a constant blood supply (i.e., external carotid artery and brachial arteries)

resolution ability of the transducer to distinguish between two structures adjacent to one another

respiration process of inhaling and exhaling air

rete testis network of channels formed by the convergence of the straight seminiferous tubules in the mediastinum testis; these channels drain into the head of the epididymis

reticuloendothelial cells phagocytic cells found in the liver and spleen comprising the reticuloendothelial system; play a role in the synthesis of blood proteins and hemopoiesis

retromammary layer deepest of the three layers of the breast

retroperitoneum space behind the peritoneal lining of the abdominal cavity

reverberation Multiple reflections that occur between the transducer and a strong reflector; multiple echoes may be sufficiently strong to be detected by the instrument and to cause confusion on the display (additional echoes that do not represent additional structures); results in the display of additional reflectors that are not real

right gastric artery supplies the stomach

right hepatic artery supplies the gallbladder via the cystic artery

right hepatic vein supplies the right lobe of the liver; branches into anterior and posterior segments

right hypochondrium right upper quadrant of the abdomen that contains the liver and gallbladder

right renal artery arises from the lateral wall of the aorta, travels posterior to the inferior vena cava to enter the medial segment of the right kidney

right renal vein leaves the medal renal hilum to enter the lateral wall of the inferior vena cava

rock slowly angling the probe back and forth in one place to image the area completely or to follow the anatomical structure

rotate motion used to navigate between the ribs or to change from transverse to longitudinal planes

rugae inner folds of the stomach wall

saccular aneurysm localized dilation of the vessel

sagittal lengthwise plane running from front to back; divides the body or any of its parts into right and left sides, or two equal halves (known as the midsagittal plane)

scan window areas in the body that allow the sound beam to penetrate without obstruction

scintigraphy nuclear medicine diagnostic test of photographing the scintillations emitted by radioactive substances injected into the body to determine the outline and function of structures in which the radioactive substance collects or is secreted

scrotum sac containing the testes and epididymis

second generation contrast agents agents containing heavy gases (e.g., Optison)

secondary hyperparathyroidism enlargement of parathyroid glands in patients with renal failure or vitamin D deficiency

secretin released from small bowel as antacid; stimulates secretion of bicarbonate

section thickness beam width perpendicular to the scan plane resulting in section-thickness artifacts

sector array probe small face transducer that allows adequate intercostal visualization although the near field is reduced

seminal vesicles reservoirs for sperm located posterior to the bladder

sentinel node represents the first lymph node along the axillary node chain

sepsis the spread of an infection from its initial site to the bloodstream, initiating a systemic response that adversely affects blood flow to vital organs

septa testis multiple septa formed from the tunica albuginea that course toward the mediastinum testis and separate the testicle into lobules

septicemia presence of pathogenic microorganisms in the blood

seroma accumulation of serous fluid within tissue

serosa fourth layer of bowel

serum amylase pancreatic enzyme that is elevated during pancreatitis

shadowing reduction in echo amplitude from reflectors that lie behind a strongly reflecting or attenuating structure

short bowel syndrome malabsorption disorder often resulting from the surgical removal of the small intestine; also called short gut syndrome

sickle cell anemia inherited disorder transmitted as an autosomal recessive trait that causes an abnormality of the globin genes in hemoglobin

sickle cell crisis condition in sickle cell anemia in which the sickled cells interfere with oxygen transport, obstruct capillary blood flow, and cause fever and severe pain in the joints and abdomen

slice thickness thickness of the section in the patient that contributes to echo signals on any one image

slide this motion is used when the probe is physically moved along the area of interest

sludge low-level echoes found along the posterior margin of the gallbladder

spatial pulse length product of a number of cycles in the pulse and wavelength of the pulse

specific gravity lab tests that measure how much dissolved material is present in the urine

speckle interference pattern incident on a transducer produced by echoes that have undergone multipath scattering; the signal does not exhibit a 1:1 correspondence with the scatters

spectral analysis analysis of the entire frequency spectrum

spectral broadening "fill-in" of the spectral window that is proportional to the severity of the high flow patterns or increased gain

speed error propagation speed error occurs when the assumed value for propagation speed (1.54 mm/microsecond, leading to the 13 microsecond/cm round-trip travel-time rule) is incorrect

spermatic cord structure made up of vas deferens, testicular artery, cremasteric artery, and pampiniform plexus that suspends the testis in the scrotum

spherocytosis hereditary condition in which erythrocytes assume a spheroid shape

sphincter of Oddi small muscle that guards the ampulla of Vater

spiculation finger-like extension of a malignant tumor

spina bifida aperta open (non-skin-covered) neural tube defects, such as myelomeningocele and meningocele

spina bifida occulta closed (skin-covered) neural tube defects, such as spinal lipoma and tethered cord

SPK simultaneous pancreas-kidney transplant

splaying widening

splenic agenesis complete absence of the spleen

splenic artery branch of the celiac axis; arises from the celiac trunk to supply the spleen

splenic flexure point where the transverse colon bends to form the descending colon

splenic hilum site in the center of the spleen where the vessels and lymph nodes enter and exit

splenic vein drains the spleen and travels horizontally across the abdomen, posterior to the pancreas, to join the superior mesenteric vein to form the portal vein

splenomegaly enlargement of the spleen

standard precautions basic infection control guidelines used to reduce the risks of infection spread through the three transmission modes: airborne, droplet, and contact

strangulated hernia incarcerated hernia with vascular compromise

strap muscles group of three muscles (sternothyroid, sternohyoid, and omohyoid) that lie anterior to the thyroid

subacute (de Quervain) thyroiditis viral infection of the thyroid that causes inflammation

subcutaneous layer most superficial of the three layers of the breast

subhepatic below the liver

submucosa second layer of bowel

subphrenic below the spleen

sulcus groove on the surface of the brain that separates the gyri

superior above

superior mesenteric artery arises inferior to the celiac axis to supply the proximal half of the colon and small intestine

superior mesenteric vein drains the proximal half of the colon and small intestine and travels vertically, slightly anterior to the inferior vena cava, to join the splenic vein to form the portal vein

supine lying face up

sweep movement in which a large wrist motion, with the probe perpendicular to the skin surface, is swept across the area of interest

synovial sheath membrane surrounding a joint, tendon, or bursa that secretes a viscous fluid called synovia

tachycardia heart rate more than 100 beats/min

tadpole sign narrow bands of acoustic shadowing posterior to the margins of the cyst along the lateral borders of enhancement

tail of Spence normal extension of breast tissue into the axillary or arm pit region

tail of the pancreas tapered end of the pancreas that lies in the left hypochondrium near the hilus of the spleen and upper pole of the left kidney

target (donut) sign characteristic of gastrointestinal wall thickening seen on cross-sectional imaging, consisting of an echogenic center and hypoechoic rim

temporal resolution ability of the system to accurately depict motion

tendinitis (tendinopathy, tendinosis, or tenosynovitis) inflammation of a tendon

tendon fibrous tissue connecting muscle to bone

tendonitis inflammation of a tendon

tenosynovitis inflammation of a tendon sheath

tentorium cerebelli echogenic V-shaped "tent" structure in the posterior fossa that separates the cerebellum from the cerebrum

terminal ductal lobar units (TDLU) smallest functional portion of the breast involving the terminal duct and its associated lobule containing at least one acinus

testicle male gonad that produces hormones that induce masculine features and spermatozoa

testicular artery artery arising from the aorta just distal to each renal artery; divides into two major branches supplying the testis medially and laterally

testicular vein pampiniform plexus forms each testicular vein; the right testicular vein drains directly into the inferior vena cava, and the left testicular vein drains into the left renal vein

tethered spinal cord fixed spinal cord that is positioned in an abnormal way

thalassemia group of hereditary anemias occurring in Asian and Mediterranean populations

thoracentesis surgical puncture of the chest wall for removal of fluids; usually done with a large-bore needle

thoracic outlet syndrome complex symptom caused by conditions in which nerves or vessels are compressed in the neck or axilla

thyroglossal duct cysts congenital anomalies that present in the midline of the neck anterior to the trachea

thyrotoxicosis toxic condition caused by hyperactivity of the thyroid gland

thyroxine one of the main hormones secreted by the thyroid that increases the use of all food types for energy production and increases the rate of protein synthesis in most tissues

time gain compensation (TGC) a setting applied in diagnostic ultrasound imaging to account for tissue attenuation

Tinel's sign (Hoffmann-Tinel sign, Tinel's symptom, or Tinel-Hoffmann sign) pins-and-needles tingling felt distally to a percussion site

tissue-specific ultrasound contrast agent contrast agent whose microbubbles are removed from the blood and are taken up by specific tissues in the body (e.g., Sonazoid)

transducer in ultrasound, a piezoelectric crystal that converts an electrical stimulus into an ultrasound pulse and the returning echo into an electrical signal

transjugular intrahepatic portosystemic shunt (TIPS) radiology procedure in which a tubular device is inserted in the middle of the liver to redirect blood flow

transverse plane horizontal to the body

trigger finger state in which flexion or extension of a digit is temporarily arrested, then completed with a jerking motion

tunica adventitia outer layer of the vascular system

tunica albuginea inner fibrous membrane surrounding the testicle

tunica intima inner layer of the vascular system

tunica media middle layer of the vascular system; veins have thinner tunica media than arteries

tunica vaginalis membrane consisting of a visceral layer (adherent to the testis) and a parietal layer (adherent to the scrotum) lining the inner wall of the scrotum; a potential space between these layers is where hydroceles may develop

ultrasound contrast agents (UCAs) agents that can be administered intravenously to evaluate blood vessels, blood flow, and solid organs

umbilical vein catheter passes through the umbilicus, umbilical vein (which is still patent in neonates), left portal vein, ductus venosus, middle or left hepatic vein, and into the inferior vena cava; used for vascular access in infants (more commonly premature neonates)

uncinate process small, curved tip of the pancreatic head that lies posterior to the superior mesenteric vein

United Network for Organ Sharing (UNOS) Organization that maintains a centralized computer networking system for all organ procurement organizations and transplant centers while seeking to be fair and effective in selecting transplant candidates

ureteropelvic junction (UPJ) obstruction most common neonatal obstruction of the urinary tract, causing hydronephrosis; results from intrinsic narrowing or extrinsic vascular compression

ureters retroperitoneal structures that exit the kidney to carry urine to the urinary bladder

urethra small membranous canal that excretes urine from the urinary bladder; tubular structure that extends from the bladder to the end of the penis

urinary bladder muscular retroperitoneal organ that serves as a reservoir for urine

urinoma cyst containing urine

urolithiasis stone within the urinary system

VACTERL (VATER) vertebral abnormalities, anal atresia, cardiac abnormalities, tracheoesophageal fistula, renal and limb abnormalities; VATER excludes cardiac and limb anomalies

valvulae conniventes normal segmentation of the small bowel

varicocele dilated veins in the pampiniform plexus

vas deferens tube that connects the epididymis to the seminal vesicle

vasa vasorum tiny arteries and veins that supply the walls of blood vessels

vascular ultrasound contrast agents contrast agent whose microbubbles are contained in the body's vascular spaces (e.g., Optison, Definity, Imagent, Levovist, SonoVue)

vasovagal relating to or denoting a temporary fall in blood pressure, with pallor, fainting, sweating, and nausea, caused by overactivity of the vagus nerve, especially as a result of stress

veins collapsible vascular structures that carry blood back to the heart

velocity rate and direction at which sound propagates through a medium; the average velocity of sound in soft tissues is 1540 m/sec

ventriculoperitoneal (VP) shunt tube placed by a neurosurgeon to relieve intracranial pressure due to increased cerebral spinal fluid (hydrocephalus); extends from the ventricles in the brain to the lower abdominal (peritoneal) cavity

vertebral arch part of the vertebral bones, which make up the vertebral opening or foramen

vertebral foramen opening in the vertebral bones through which the spinal cord runs

verumontanum junction of the ejaculatory ducts with the urethra

vesicoureteral reflux (VUR) abnormal reflux of urine from the bladder through the ureters and, at times, back into the renal pelvis and calyces

villi inner folds of the small intestine

vital signs medical measurements used to ascertain how the body is functioning

volar relating to the palm of the hand or sole of the foot

wall echo shadow (WES) sign sonographic pattern found when the gallbladder is packed with stones

"wandering" spleen spleen that has migrated from its normal location in the left upper quadrant

wave propagation of energy that moves back and forth or vibrates at a steady rate

wavelength length of space over which one cycle occurs; decreases as frequency increases

white blood cells cells that defend the body by destroying invading microorganisms and their toxins

white pulp consists of lymphatic tissue and lymphatic follicles

Wilms tumor (nephroblastoma) most common malignant renal tumor in the neonate and infant; an embryonal tumor arising in the kidneys, which is often unilateral, though may be bilateral

INDEX

Note: Page numbers followed by b indicate boxed material; those followed by f indicate figures; those followed by t indicate tables.

A

Abdomen
- FAST scan of, 563f
- fetal, 1572, 1590b–1591b
  - cystic masses of, 1590–1591
  - ultrasound, 1408t
- pain in, 84, 85t
- pseudopulsatile masses of, 195
- quadrants of, 88f
- regions of, 99f
- trauma to, 561–563
- ultrasound protocols for, 134–141, 134f
- viscera of, 88–89, 89f

Abdominal abscesses, 420–421, 423f

Abdominal aorta, 172, 173f, 174f, 178t
- branches of, 179–180
  - anterior, 179–180
    - celiac trunk, 179–180, 179f
    - inferior mesenteric artery, 184, 184f
    - superior mesenteric artery, 180–182, 183f
  - dorsal, 187
  - lateral, 185–187
- coronal plane of, 173, 176f
- Doppler flow patterns in, 212–214, 212b, 213f
- longitudinal plane of, 172–178, 175f, 176f
- longitudinal scans of, 130f, 131f, 140–141
- measurement of, 174–178, 177f
- size of, 176–178
- sonographic evaluation of, 172, 174b
- subcostal view of, 911f
- transverse plane of, 174, 177f
- transverse scans, 135–140, 136f, 137f, 138f, 139f

Abdominal aortic aneurysms, 188–193, 189f, 190f
- classification of, 190–191, 191f
- descriptive terms for, 191–192, 192f
- epigastric pain and, 569–570, 569f, 570f
- features of, 189b
- graft repair of, 194–195, 196f
- growth rate of, 190t
- risk factors for, 188, 190b
- symptoms of, 188–190, 190t

Abdominal cavity, 88–92
- abdominal muscles, 90–92, 90f
- abdominal wall, 89–90, 90f
- diaphragm, 88–89
- sonographic evaluation of, 1576–1580
  - gastrointestinal system, 1576–1579
  - hepatobiliary system, 1579–1580
- visceral organs of, 88–89

Abdominal circumference, 1291, 1577, 1577f

Abdominal cysts, 426, 427f

Abdominal hernias, 432, 432f

Abdominal muscles, 90–92, 90f

Abdominal pain
- acute, 767–775, 768f
- in children, 767–775, 768f
- description of, 84, 85t

Abdominal planes, 104–105, 104f
- body sections, 105, 105b, 105f

Abdominal quadrants, 104–105, 104f

Abdominal regions, 104–105, 104f

Abdominal scanning
- abnormalities in, 131
- clinical considerations before
  - documentation, 125
  - general abdominal examination, 125
  - patient positions, 125, 125f
  - scanning techniques, 125
  - transducer positions, 126–128, 129f
  - transducer selection, 125–126, 126f, 127f
  - written order for examination, 125
- criteria for adequate scan in, 134, 135f
- Doppler evaluation, 141–146, 209–217
- fasting before, 125
- labeling scans, 124
- patient breathing technique tip in, 124
- sectional anatomy and, 102, 105–122, 122b
  - in longitudinal plane, 104, 108–122
    - at aorta and superior mesenteric artery level, 109, 121f
    - at inferior vena cava, left lobe of the liver, and pancreas level, 109, 120f
    - at liver, caudate lobe, and psoas muscle, 109, 119f
    - at liver, duodenum, and pancreas level, 109, 120f
    - at liver, gallbladder, and right kidney level, 108–109, 118f
    - at liver, inferior vena cava, pancreas, and gastroduodenal artery level, 109, 120f
    - at liver and gallbladder level, 108–109, 118f
    - at right lobe of the liver level, 108, 117f
  - in transverse plane, 104–108
    - at bifurcation of aorta level, 108, 112f
    - caudate lobe and celiac axis, 106–107, 108f
    - at caudate lobe level, 106, 107f
    - at dome of the liver level, 106–108, 106f
    - at external iliac arteries level, 108, 113f
    - at external iliac veins level, 108, 113f
    - at female pelvis level, 108, 116f
    - at gallbladder and right kidney level, 107, 110f
    - at liver, gallbladder, and right kidney level, 107, 111f
    - at male pelvis level, 108, 114f
    - at right lobe of the liver level, 107, 112f
    - at superior mesenteric artery and pancreas level, 107, 109f

Abdominal sonography, 129

Abdominal wall, 89–90, 90f, 434b
- anatomy of, 413–419, 414f–415f, 416f, 1161
- embryology of, 1560–1562, 1561f, 1562f, 1563f
- fetal, 1562
- hernia of, 432–434, 432f, 433f
- masses of, 428
- neoplasms of, 432
- pathology of, 428–434
- regions of, 105f
- sonographic evaluation of, 413–419, 414f–415f, 416f

Abdominal wall defects, 1338–1339, 1339f

Abdominopelvic cavity, 88–102

Abdominopelvic membranes and ligaments, 95–98, 96f

Abduction
- of hip joint, 853
- of scanning arm, 74f, 76

ABI. *see* Ankle-brachial index

Abortion
- complete, 1322
- incomplete spontaneous, 1322, 1322f
- threatened, 1320

Abruptio placentae, 1285, 1455

Abscesses
- abdominal, 420–421, 423f
- amebic, 264t, 266–267, 269f
- biloma, 425, 425f
- breast, 658t, 664, 664f
- definition of, 420
- gas-containing, 421–422, 423f
- lesser-sac, 423, 424f
- in liver transplantation patients, 593, 595f
- neck, 705–706, 706f
- pancreatic, 369t, 375–377
- in pancreatic transplantation patients, 633, 634f
- pelvic, 425–426, 425b, 426f
- pyogenic, 264t, 265–266, 267f
- in renal transplantation patients, 616, 619f
- splenic, 342–344, 345f, 346f
- subphrenic, 423–424, 424f
- tubo-ovarian, 1261b, 1263–1264
- ultrasound-guided draining and collection of, 534–535, 559

Absent cardiac activity, 1327, 1327f

Absorption, 12, 393

ACA. *see* Anterior cerebral artery

Acalculous cholecystitis, 294t–295t, 297, 300f

Acardiac anomaly, 1423, 1423f

Acceptance, illness and, 60

Accessory fissures, 239

Accessory spleen, 329, 331f

Acetabular notch, 853

Acetabulum, 851
- bony and cartilaginous, 854

Achilles tendon, 736, 749, 750f, 751b

Achondrogenesis, 1623t, 1626, 1626f, 1627f

Achondroplasia, 1623t, 1626

Acidic solution, 83

Acidosis, 83

Acini, 645–646

Acini cells, 360–361

ACKD. *see* Acquired cystic kidney disease

Acoustic emission, 514–515, 515f

Acoustic impedance, 11t, 12, 13f

Acoustics, 10–14, 11f, 11t

Acquired cystic disease of dialysis, 454t–458t

Acquired cystic kidney disease (ACKD), 460–461

Acquired immunodeficiency syndrome (AIDS)
- sonographic findings in, 471, 471f, 472f
- spleen in, 344

ACR FORM breast disease, 658

Acrania, 1335, 1336f, 1336t, 1524
- sonographic findings in, 1524, 1526f

Acromioclavicular joint, 744f

I-1

ACTH. *see* Adrenocorticotropic hormone
Acute appendicitis, 403–405, 404*t*, 406*f*
Acute cholecystitis, 293, 297*f*
 complications of, 296–297, 299*f*
 right upper quadrant pain in, 567–568, 568*f*
 sonographic findings in, 296, 298*f*, 299*f*
Acute glomerulonephritis, 454*t*–458*t*, 470
Acute hepatitis, 243*t*, 246, 246*f*
Acute interstitial nephritis, 470–471, 471*f*
Acute liver failure, 584–585
Acute mastitis, 663–664, 663*f*
Acute pancreatitis, 369–371, 369*t*, 370*f*
 extrapancreatic fluid collections and edema, 371–372, 372*f*
 sonographic findings in, 370–371, 371*f*
Acute pelvic pain, 578–579
Acute pyelonephritis, 806
Acute renal failure, 454*t*–458*t*, 473
Acute tubular necrosis (ATN), 473
 in renal transplantation patients, 615–616, 618*f*
 sonographic findings in, 473–474, 474*f*
Addison disease, 497, 499–500, 502*t*
Adduction, of hip joint, 853
Adenocarcinoma
 macrocystic, 380
 pancreatic, 638
 pancreatic ductal, 381, 384*f*, 385*f*
Adenoma, 775
 adrenal, 503–504, 504*f*
 cortical, 500–501
 follicular, 692, 693*f*
 gallbladder, 294*t*–295*t*, 305, 308*f*
 hepatic, 250*f*, 269–270, 273*f*
 liver cell, 271*t*
 parathyroid, 702–703
 renal, 454*t*–458*t*
 thyroid, 692, 694*f*
Adenomatoid malformation, congenital cystic, 1552–1554, 1553*f*
 sonographic findings in, 1554, 1554*b*
 type I, 1553–1554, 1553*f*
 type II, 1553–1554
 type III, 1553–1554, 1554*f*
Adenomatous tumors, renal, 468, 470*f*
Adenomyomas, 1212–1214
Adenomyomatosis of gallbladder, 294*t*–295*t*, 304, 307*f*
Adenomyosis, 1212–1216, 1260
 sonographic findings in, 1214
 transvaginal scanning of, 1212–1216
ADHD. *see* Attention-deficit/hyperactivity disorder
Adhesions
 female infertility and, 1277
 fluid collections in, 1240, 1241*f*
Administrative controls, 73–74
Adnexa
 interventional ultrasound of, 1270, 1270*f*
 pathology of, 1260, 1271*b*
  endometriosis and endometriomas, 1267–1270, 1268*f*, 1269*f*
  endometritis, 1266–1267, 1267*f*
  pelvic inflammatory disease, 1260–1266, 1261*b*, 1261*f*
  peritonitis, 1264–1266, 1266*f*
  salpingitis, hydrosalpinx, and pyosalpinx, 1261–1263, 1262*f*, 1262*t*, 1263*f*, 1264*f*
 postoperative ultrasound for, 1271
 tubo-ovarian abscesses, 1261*b*, 1263–1264
 ultrasound examination of, 1178*b*

Adnexal cysts, 1415, 1416*f*
Adnexal masses
 with ectopic pregnancy, 1330–1332, 1331*f*
 resistive index and, 1236
Adolescents
 benign ovarian cysts in, 1240
 special needs of, 58
ADPKD. *see* Autosomal dominant polycystic kidney disease
Adrenal cortex, 497
Adrenal cysts, 502–503, 502*f*, 503*f*
Adrenal glands, 88
 anatomy of, 494, 494*f*
 fetal ultrasound, 1408*t*
 neonatal/pediatric, 494
  adrenal hemorrhages, 796*t*
  anatomy of, 794, 794*f*
  hydronephrosis, 796*t*
  pathology of enlargement of, 796*t*
   adrenal hemorrhages, 796*t*, 807, 808*f*
   hydronephrosis, 796*t*
   prune belly syndrome, 796*t*, 801–802
   renal cystic disease, 804–805, 804*f*
   renal vein thrombosis, 807, 807*f*
 sonographic evaluation of, 497–498, 498*f*, 499*f*, 791
 vascular supply of, 496–497
Adrenal hemorrhage
 description of, 503, 503*f*
 neonatal/pediatric, 796*t*, 807, 808*f*
Adrenal medulla, 497
 neonatal, 795*f*
 tumors, 505–506
Adrenal neuroblastoma, 505–506, 506*f*, 810*f*
Adrenal tumors, 503–505
 malignant, 504, 504*f*
Adrenocorticotropic hormone (ACTH), 497
Adrenogenital syndrome, 500, 502*t*
Advanced maternal age (AMA), 1407
AED. *see* Automated external defibrillation
AFC. *see* Antral follicle count
Afferent arterioles, 437
AFP. *see* Alpha-fetoprotein
Afterload, 903–904, 910
Agenesis
 corpus callosum, 840–841, 841*f*, 1523*t*, 1535–1536
  sonographic findings in, 1536, 1536*f*
 liver, 239
 pancreatic, 359
 splenic, 327–329
Aging, 57
Agnathia, 1500–1501
AHW. *see* Anterior horn width
AI. *see* Aortic insufficiency
AIDS. *see* Acquired immunodeficiency syndrome
Airborne precautions, 54
Airborne transmission, of infections, 50
AIUM. *see* American Institute of Ultrasound in Medicine
Alanine aminotransferase (ALT), 228, 228*t*, 230
ALARA principle, 1288
Albumin, 228, 231
Alcoholic cirrhosis, 247*f*
Aliasing, 24
 color Doppler, 160, 161*f*, 162*f*
 definition of, 156
 elimination of, 159*b*
 range-ambiguity artifact values and, 157*t*
 reduction of, 159*b*
 spectral Doppler, 156

Alimentary tract, 389–390, 390*f*
Alkaline phosphatase, 228, 228*t*, 231
Alkaline solution, 83
Alkalosis, 83
Allantoic ducts, 1460–1461
Alloimmune thrombocytopenia, 1411
Alobar holoprosencephaly, 843, 843*f*, 1532–1533, 1532*f*
Alpha angle, Graf's, 860–866, 862*b*, 862*f*
Alpha cells, 361
Alpha-fetoprotein (AFP), 531–532
 prenatal diagnosis of congenital anomalies, 1427–1429, 1427*b*, 1427*f*, 1428*b*
ALT. *see* Alanine aminotransferase
AMA. *see* Advanced maternal age
Amaurosis fugax, 1072
Ambiguous genitalia, 1617–1618, 1618*f*
Amebic abscess, 264*t*, 266–267, 269*f*
Amenorrhea, 1174
American College of Radiology (ACR), Standard for the Performance of Ultrasound Examination of the Female Pelvis, 1177
American College of Radiology Sonography Descriptive Form, 658, 658*t*
American Institute of Ultrasound in Medicine (AIUM), 6
 pelvic ultrasound standards, 1177
 shoulder imaging recommendations, 744
American Registry for Diagnostic Medical Sonography (ARDMS), 4, 6
American Society of Echocardiography (ASE), 6
Ammonium, 229
Amniocentesis, 1285
 prenatal diagnosis of congenital anomalies, 1430–1431, 1430*f*, 1431*f*
Amnion, 1289–1290, 1443*f*, 1462*f*
 embryonic development of, 1327
 evaluation of, 1327
 sonographic findings of, in abnormal intrauterine pregnancies, 1324*b*
Amniotic band syndrome, 1564, 1566, 1568*f*
 amniotic fluid and, 1483–1485
 fetal membranes and, 1483–1485, 1485*f*, 1486*f*
Amniotic cavity, 1308–1310, 1474
Amniotic fluid, 1374, 1375*f*, 1599
 abnormal volumes, 1479–1481
  oligohydramnios, 1480–1481, 1480*b*, 1481*f*
  polyhydramnios, 1479–1480, 1480*b*, 1480*f*
 amniotic band syndrome, 1483–1485
 amniotic fluid index, 1477–1478, 1477*f*
 assessment of, 1475–1477
  quantitative, 1476–1477
  subjective, 1476, 1476*f*, 1477*f*
 characteristics of, 1475, 1475*b*, 1475*f*, 1476*f*
 derivation, 1474–1475
 fetal membranes and, 1474, 1489*b*–1490*b*
 single pocket assessment, 1478, 1478*f*
 twin pregnancies, assessment in, 1478–1479, 1478*f*, 1479*f*
 two-diameter pocket assessment, 1478, 1478*f*
 volume, abnormal, 1600, 1600*b*
Amniotic sac, 1443*f*, 1462*f*
Amniotic sludge, 1475
A-mode transducers, 528, 529*f*
Amplitude, 11–12
Amplitude modulation (A-mode), 17, 18*f*
Ampulla of Vater, 282
Amputation, 1118

Amylase, 360–361, 361t
　diseases that affect, 361t, 362, 362t
　urine, 362
Amyloid cardiomyopathy, 992, 994f
Amyloidosis, 339–340, 339f
Anaplastic carcinoma, 697, 697f
Anasarca, 1407
Anastomosis, 206
　stenosis at, 1124f
Anatomic directions, 132–134, 135f
Anatomy, 80, 101b
Androgen, 1234
Anechoic, 130, 133f
Anembryonic pregnancy, 1320, 1323, 1323f, 1324b
Anemia
　autoimmune hemolytic, 341
　hemolytic, 341
　sickle cell
　　description of, 340
　　illustration of, 340f
　　stroke in, 1102, 1103f
Anencephaly, 1292, 1335, 1336f, 1336t, 1523–1524
　differential considerations for, 1524t
　sonographic findings in, 1524, 1525f
Aneuploidies, 1285, 1287–1288
Aneurysms
　arterial duplex imaging of, 1124–1126, 1125f
　cervical carotid system, 1078
　definition of, 971
　false, 190–191, 191f, 974t
　fusiform, 191, 192f
　graft repair complications, 194–195, 196f
　iliac, 195
　inflammatory aortic, 192
　mycotic, 192
　popliteal artery, 1125f
　saccular, 191, 192f
　sinus of Valsalva, 974, 976f
　sonographic findings of, 192, 193b, 193f
　splanchnic, 185–187, 185f, 195
　thoracic, 195
　true, 190–191, 191f, 974t
　vein of Galen, 1537
Angiogram, ultrasound, 516f
Angiolipomas, 454t–458t, 469f
Angiomyolipoma, renal, 467, 469f, 624
Angle of incidence, 6
Angle of reflection, 6
Anisotropy, 741, 741f, 743t
Ankle, 749–750, 750t
Ankle-brachial index (ABI), 1115, 1115t
Annotation, 656–658, 656f, 657b, 657f, 658t
Annular pancreas, 360, 361f
Anophthalmia, 1501
Anophthalmos, 1392
Anorectal atresia, 1585, 1588
Anotia, 1500, 1501f
Anteflexion, 1166f, 1207f
Anterior, 132
Anterior abdominal wall
　abnormalities of, 1562–1571, 1564b, 1564t
　　amniotic band syndrome, 1566, 1568f
　　Beckwith-Wiedemann syndrome, 1566–1567, 1568f
　　bladder and cloacal exstrophy, 1567–1568, 1568f, 1569f
　　limb-body wall complex, 1570–1571, 1570f
　　pentalogy of Cantrell, ectopia cordis, and cleft sternum, 1568–1570, 1569f

Anterior abdominal wall (Continued)
　fetal, 1560, 1570b–1571b
　muscles of, 1161f
Anterior cerebral artery (ACA), 1089–1090
Anterior communicating artery (ACoA), 1090
Anterior horn width (AHW), 830, 831f
Anterior pararenal space, 92, 492, 492b, 493f
Anterior/posterior direction, 132
Anterior tibial artery, 1112
Anterior tibial veins (ATVs), 1130f, 1131
Anterior urethral valves, 1612–1614, 1614f
Anteversion, 1162–1163, 1166f, 1207f
Antiradial plane, 657
Antral follicle count (AFC), 1277
Aorta
　abdominal, 172, 173f, 174f, 178t
　　dorsal branches of, 187
　　lateral branches of, 185–187
　abdominal scanning of, at bifurcation level, 108, 112f
　abnormalities, 971–979, 973f
　anatomy of, 971
　ascending, 172
　atherosclerosis of, 974, 977f
　descending, 172
　Doppler flow patterns in, 145, 212–214, 212b, 213f
　fetal circulation, 1446f
　pathology of, 187–195, 187f
　　tumors, 978–979, 978f
　retroperitoneum and, 494f, 496
　root of, 171, 172f
　sections of, 171–172
　sections/segments of, 971
　sonographic evaluation of, 179–180, 179f
Aortic aneurysms, 971–974
　abdominal, 188–193, 189f, 190f
　　classification of, 190–191, 191f
　　descriptive terms for, 191–192, 192f
　　epigastric pain and, 569–570, 569f, 570f
　　features of, 189b
　　graft repair of, 194–195, 196f
　　growth rate of, 190t
　　risk factors for, 188, 190b
　　symptoms of, 188–190, 190t
　aortic ectasia versus, 187
　causes of, 971–974
　diagnosis of, 972–973
　fusiform, 191, 192f
　rupture of, 192–193, 192f
　sonographic findings of, 192, 193b, 193f
Aortic arches, 901, 901f, 1008–1009, 1009b, 1009f
　Doppler measurements, 1014t
　extracranial cerebrovascular imaging, 1070
　fetal circulation, 1446f
　interrupted, 1056–1057
　oblique long axis view of, 1026–1029, 1027f, 1028f
Aortic branches, 901, 901f
Aortic dissection, 193–194, 194f, 195f, 572–573, 572f
　causes of, 572, 572b
　classification of, 974
　clinical findings for, 572–573, 573t
　complications of, 974
　DeBakey and Stanford classification of, 974, 974f
　imaging of, 973
　sonographic findings of, 573, 574f
　type I, 974, 974f, 975f
　type II, 974, 974f, 975f
　type III, 974, 974f, 976f

Aortic ectasia, 187
Aortic insufficiency (AI), 956, 963–966, 963t
Aortic regurgitation, 963, 963t, 964f, 965f, 966f
Aortic root motion, 989, 991f
Aortic sclerosis, 967
　types of, 966
Aortic stenosis, 964t, 966–970, 966f, 967f, 969b, 969f, 970b, 970f, 972t, 1050–1052
　critical, 1050, 1051f
　subvalvular/supravalvular, 1050–1052, 1051f, 1052f
Aortic ulcer, penetrating, 977, 977f
Aortic valve, 901, 901f
　atherosclerosis of, 968f
　bicuspid, 966–967, 968f
　Doppler measurements, 1014t
　M-mode imaging of, 935f, 945–946, 946f, 950f
　unicuspid, 967f
Aortic valve area (AVA), 967
Aphasia, 1072
Apical transducer location, 918, 919f
Apical views
　two-chamber, 933, 938b, 940f, 941f, 944f
　four-chamber, 572f, 911, 911f, 912f, 921f, 922b, 922f, 941f, 943f
　right heart, 938b
　five-chamber, 922b, 932–938, 936f, 937f, 938b
　for color flow mapping, 932–938, 944f
　long-axis, 938b
　for pericardial effusion, 1036f
　two-dimensional, 932–938, 936f, 937f, 938b
Apical window, 924b
Apocrine metaplasia, 661
Aponeuroses, 736
Aponeurosis tissue, 735f
Appendectomy, 777
Appendiceal abscess, 781f
Appendicitis
　acute, 403–405, 404t, 406f
　pediatric, 776–781, 777f, 780f, 781f
　retrocecal, 404
　right lower quadrant pain in, 573t, 574–575, 576f
Appendicoliths, 404, 779, 781f
Appendix
　abnormalities of, mucocele, 404t, 405–408, 408f
　normal, 779f
　sonographic evaluation of, 398, 404–405, 407f
Appendix testis, 710f
Aqueductal stenosis, 829, 1536, 1537f
Arachnoid cysts, 845–846, 846f, 1523t, 1540f
Arachnoid mater, 873–875
Architectural distortion, 658
Arcuate arteries, 436
　calcifications of, 1192–1193
　neonatal, 793
　in renal allograft, 611
Arcuate vessels, 1192–1193, 1193f
ARDMS. see American Registry for Diagnostic Medical Sonography
Areola, 645
Arhinia, 1505
Arnold-Chiari malformation, 839–840, 840f
　type II, 1392–1393
Arrhenoblastoma, 1256
Arrhythmia
　causes of, 35
　definition of, 35
　fetal, 1012–1013

ART. *see* Assisted reproductive technology
Arterial duplex imaging, 1118–1126
　interpretation of, 1120–1122, 1120*b*, 1121*f*, 1122*b*, 1122*f*
　　aneurysms and pseudoaneurysms, 1124–1126, 1125*f*
　　bypass graft surveillance, 1122–1123, 1122*f*, 1123*f*
　　dialysis access grafts, 1123–1124, 1123*f*, 1124*f*
　lower extremity, 1119–1120, 1119*f*, 1120*f*
　upper extremity, 1120, 1120*f*
Arterial occlusive disease, 1117, 1117*f*
Arterial stress testing, 1116
Arterial system, 1134
Arterial testing, indirect, 1114–1118
Arterial thrombosis, 633–634, 635*f*, 636*f*
Arteries, 171
　anatomy of, 1111
　femoral, 178*t*
　layers of, 171, 171*f*
　lower extremity, 1111–1112, 1111*f*
　upper extremity, 1112, 1112*f*
　veins *versus*, 1134
Arterioles, 437
Arteriosclerosis, 187–188, 188*f*
Arteriovenous fistulas (AVFs), 482–483, 484*f*, 589, 617*f*
Arteriovenous malformations (AVMs), 1216, 1217*f*
Arthrogryposis multiplex congenita, 1632–1633, 1632*f*
Artifacts, 147, 165*b*
　attenuation, 153–156
　　enhancement and, 156, 156*f*, 157*f*
　　shadowing and, 153–156, 155*f*
　color Doppler, 160–163
　　aliasing and, 160, 161*f*, 162*f*
　　mirror image, shadowing, clutter, and noise and, 160–163, 162*f*, 163*f*
　definition of, 147
　musculoskeletal imaging, 740–743, 741*f*, 742*f*, 743*t*
　propagation of, 147–153
　　grating lobes and, 151, 153*f*
　　mirror image and, 149, 151*f*
　　range ambiguity and, 151–152, 154*f*
　　refraction and, 149, 152*f*
　　reverberation and, 148–149, 149*f*, 150*f*, 151*f*
　　section thickness and, 148, 148*f*
　　speckle and, 148, 149*f*
　　speed error and, 151, 154*f*
　reverberation, 129, 132*f*, 149*f*
　spectral Doppler, 156–160
　　aliasing and, 156, 159*b*
　　mirror image and, 160, 160*f*
　　noise and, 160, 160*f*
　　Nyquist limit and, 156–159, 157*f*, 158*f*, 159*b*, 159*f*
　　range ambiguity and, 157*f*, 159–160
　speed error, 743, 743*t*
　types of, 129
As low as reasonably achievable (ALARA) principle, 1091
Ascariasis, 318, 319*f*
Ascending aorta, 172

Ascites, 96, 408
　after liver transplantation, 605, 605*f*
　fetal, 1589*f*, 1590
　hydrops and, 1486–1487
　inflammatory, 420, 422*f*
　malignant, 420, 422*f*
　pancreatic, 374–375
　peritoneal, 419–420, 421*f*, 422*f*
　ultrasound-guided draining of, 559
ASD. *see* Autism spectrum disorder
ASE. *see* American Society of Echocardiography
Aspartate aminotransferase (AST), 228, 228*t*, 230
Asphyxia, neonatal, 814
Asphyxiating thoracic dystrophy, 1546
Aspiration, of renal masses, 449–450, 452*t*
Asplenia, 1581
Assisted reproductive technology (ART), 1278–1279, 1279*f*
AST. *see* Aspartate aminotransferase
Ataxia, 1072
Atherosclerosis
　aortic, 974, 977*f*
　description of, 187, 188*f*, 480
Atherosclerotic disease, 1076–1077, 1077*f*, 1078*f*
ATN. *see* Acute tubular necrosis
Atoms, 81
Atresia
　laryngeal, 1554–1555
　tracheal, 1554–1555, 1555*f*
Atretic common bile duct, 771
Atrial septal defect, 1036–1038, 1037*f*
　ostium primum, 1037–1038, 1037*f*, 1038*f*
　ostium secundum, 1037, 1037*f*
　sinus venosus septal defect, 1037*f*, 1038, 1038*f*
Atrial systole, 901*b*
Atrialized chamber, 1043
Atrioventricular block, 1064–1066, 1064*f*
Atrioventricular canal
　division of, 1009
　partitioning of, 1010*f*
Atrioventricular node, 1010
Atrioventricular septal defect (AVSD), 1041–1043, 1041*f*
Atrioventricular valves, 902
Atrium
　of lateral ventricles, 815, 816*f*
　primitive, 1010*f*
Atrophy
　renal, 454*t*–458*t*, 472
　splenic, 336
Attention-deficit/hyperactivity disorder (ADHD), 763*t*
Attenuation
　artifacts associated with, 153–156
　　enhancement and, 156, 156*f*, 157*f*
　　shadowing and, 153–156, 155*f*
　description of, 12*t*, 14, 14*f*
Attenuation effects, 669
ATVs. *see* Anterior tibial veins
Audio signals, 920–923
Augmentation, 1140*f*
　lower extremity, 1140–1141
　upper extremity, 1140
Autism spectrum disorder (ASD), 763*t*, 831–832
Autoimmune hemolytic anemia, 341
Automated external defibrillation (AED), 66, 66*f*
Automated whole breast ultrasound, 678–681, 679*f*

Autonomy, 1296–1297
Autosomal dominant polycystic disease, 377
Autosomal dominant polycystic kidney disease (ADPKD), 378*t*, 461, 1607–1608, 1608*f*, 1609*f*
　neonatal/pediatric, 805
　sonographic findings in, 461–462, 462*f*
Autosomal recessive polycystic kidney disease (ARPKD), 461
　neonatal/pediatric, 804*f*, 805*f*
AVA. *see* Aortic valve area
AVFs. *see* Arteriovenous fistulas
AVMs. *see* Arteriovenous malformations
AVSD. *see* Atrioventricular septal defect
Axial imaging, 1177–1178
Axial resolution, 13–14, 13*f*
Axilla, 645, 645*f*
Axillary artery, 1112, 1120, 1120*f*
Axillary vein, 1133
Azimuthal resolution, 13–14

B

BA. *see* Basilar artery
Back muscles, 91
Bacteremia, 332–333
Bacterial cholangitis, 315, 318*f*
Baker, Donald, 8–10, 10*f*
Baker cyst, 579, 580*f*, 739, 1147, 1147*f*
Ballantyne syndrome, 1487
Banana sign, 1351, 1392–1393, 1530*f*
Banding, 157*f*
Bandwidth, 13
Barber, Frank, 8–10
Bare area, 219, 220*f*, 417
Barlow maneuver, 859, 859*f*
Barrier devices, 54
Basal ganglia, neonatal, 818, 819*f*
Basal plate, 1443, 1443*b*
Baseline, 26
Baseline shift, 156–160
Basic ultrasound imaging, 123, 146*b*
Basilar artery (BA), 1089
Basilic vein, 1140
"Basket sign," 464, 464*f*
Battledore placenta, 1444–1445
B-cell tumor, 381, 384*f*
Beckwith-Wiedemann syndrome, 1510, 1511*f*, 1566–1567, 1568*f*
　pediatric, 773, 807–808
　sonographic findings of, 1564*t*
Bed rest, 48–49
Bedpans, 48–49, 48*f*
Beemer-Langer dysplasia, 1630
Bell clapper deformity, 720
Beneficence, 1296
Benign conditions, breast, 659–660
Benign lesions, thyroid gland, 691–693, 693*f*
Benign ovarian cysts
　in adolescents, 1240
　paraovarian cysts, 1240, 1240*b*, 1241*f*
　peritoneal inclusion cysts, 1239–1242, 1240*f*
　simple cysts in postmenopausal women, 1240–1242
Benign testicular masses, 726–728, 727*f*
Benign tumors
　hepatic, 268–269
　liver, pediatric, 773–775
　renal, 467, 469*f*, 488–490

Benign tumors *(Continued)*
    adenomatous tumors, 468, 470*f*
    angiomyolipoma, 467, 469*f*
    lipomas, 454*t*–458*t*, 468, 470*f*
    oncocytoma, 468, 470*f*
    splenic, 349, 350*f*
Bernoulli equation, 913–914, 914*f*
Beside ultrasound, 63–64, 63*f*, 64*f*
Beta angle, Graf's, 860–866, 862*b*, 862*f*
Beta cells, 361
Bezoars, gastric, 399–400, 400*t*, 401*f*
Biceps tendon, 736, 736*f*
    sonographic evaluation of, 744, 744*f*, 745*f*
    subluxation/dislocation of, 751, 751*f*
Bicornuate uterus, 1208*f*, 1273*f*
Bicuspid aortic valve, 966–967, 968*f*, 973, 1033, 1050, 1050*f*
Bifid renal pelvis, 436–437, 446
Bilateral pararectal space, 496, 496*f*
Bilateral venous duplex imaging, 1148
Bile, 83, 230, 230*f*
Bile ducts, 282, 282*f*
    cholangitis and, 315–318
    sonographic evaluation of, 289, 292*f*, 293*f*
Bile leaks, 604, 604*f*
Bile pigments, 230
Biliary atresia, neonatal, 771, 771*t*, 772*f*
Biliary cirrhosis, 247*f*
Biliary dilation, 568, 569*f*
Biliary ductal ischemia, 597–598
Biliary neoplasms, intrahepatic, 318
Biliary obstructions, 312, 313*f*
    distal, 259, 261*t*, 262*f*
    extrahepatic, 312–313, 313*f*
    proximal, 258–259, 261*f*, 261*t*, 262*f*
Biliary system, 281, 322*b*–323*b*
    anatomy of, 281–285, 282*f*
    laboratory data regarding, 285
    pathology of, 289–308, 294*t*–295*t*
        cholelithiasis, 294*t*–295*t*, 300, 301*f*, 302*f*, 303*f*, 304*f*
        gallbladder carcinoma, 306–308, 309*f*, 310*f*
        gallbladder disease, 290–293
        gallbladder torsion, 299–300
        gallbladder wall thickening, 293, 296*b*, 296*f*
        sludge, 290–293, 294*t*–295*t*, 295*f*
    pediatric, 765, 765*b*, 766*f*
    physiology of, 285
    sonographic evaluation of, 285–289, 290*b*
        bile ducts, 289, 292*f*, 293*f*
        gallbladder, 284*f*, 286*f*, 287–289, 290*f*, 291*f*, 292*f*
        protocol, 285–287, 289*f*, 290*f*
    transverse scans of, 134
    ultrasound protocol for, 289*t*
    vascular supply of, 285
Biliary tree pathology, 308–321
    ascariasis, 318, 319*f*
    Caroli disease, 310, 311*f*
    cholangiocarcinoma, 318–321, 319*f*, 320*f*
    cholangitis, 315–318
    dilated biliary ducts, 311–312, 312*f*
    hemobilia, 315, 317*f*
    intrahepatic biliary neoplasms, 318
    metastases, 321
    pneumobilia, 315, 317*f*

Bilirubin, 285
    definition of, 225
    detoxification of, 229
    direct-acting, 229, 229*t*
    indirect-acting, 229, 229*t*
    liver function tests, 231
Biloma, 425, 593, 594*f*, 604, 604*f*
Biometry, fetal ultrasound, 1408*t*
Biophysical profile (BPP), 1399–1401, 1399*b*
    amniotic fluid volume, 1401, 1401*f*
    fetal body and trunk gross movements, 1400*f*, 1401
    fetal breathing movements, 1399, 1400*f*
    fetal tone, 1401, 1401*f*
Biopsy, 543–548, 543*f*, 544*f*, 545*f*, 546*f*, 547*f*, 548*f*
    after renal transplants, 555, 555*f*
    breast, large-core needle, 676
    complications of, 539–540, 539*f*
    contraindications for, 531, 531*f*
    core, 533, 533*f*, 534*f*
    indication for, 530–531, 531*f*
    kidney, 554–555, 555*f*
    liver, 552–553, 552*f*, 553*f*, 554*f*
    lung, 556–557, 556*f*
    musculoskeletal, 557–558, 557*f*, 558*f*
    neck nodes and masses, 557
    pancreatic, 553–554
    pelvic mass, 558
    prostate, 558, 558*f*, 559*f*
    renal, 548*f*, 555*f*, 615*f*, 616*f*, 617*f*
    retroperitoneal lymph nodes, 555–556, 556*f*
    thyroid, 557, 557*f*
Biopsy gun, 533
Biparietal diameter (BPD), 1291, 1383, 1384*b*, 1384*f*, 1384*t*, 1385*f*
BI-RADS. *see* Breast Imaging Reporting and Data System
Bladder, 89
    as acoustic window, 1189, 1189*f*
    anatomy of, 86, 437, 1161–1162, 1162*b*, 1163*f*
    development of, 1595
    distended, 1178, 1266*f*
    exstrophy of, 1564*t*, 1567–1568, 1568*f*, 1569*f*
    extrophy of, 1603–1604, 1604*f*
    fetal
        not seen, 1600
        sonographic evaluation of, 1596
    neonatal/pediatric
        anatomy of, 794–795, 795*f*
        sonographic evaluation of preparation for, 792
    sonographic evaluation of, 451–453, 1177, 1179*f*, 1182*f*
    tumors of, 486–487, 488*f*
Bladder diverticulum, 485, 488*f*
Bladder-flap hematoma, 430
Bladder outlet obstruction, neonatal/pediatric, 801–802, 802*f*
Bleeding, first-trimester, 1320–1326
    abnormal sac criteria, 1322–1323
    absent intrauterine sac, 1320–1322, 1321*t*, 1322*f*
    anembryonic pregnancy, 1323, 1323*f*, 1324*b*
    gestational sac without embryo or yolk sac, 1322
    gestational trophoblastic disease, 1323–1326, 1324*f*, 1325*f*, 1326*f*
    placental hematomas, 1320
    subchorionic hemorrhage, 1320, 1321*f*
Blighted ovum, 1320

Bliss, William Roderic, 7, 8*f*
Blood
    composition of, 81, 82*f*
    functions of, 81–83
    in urine, 437–438
Blood-borne precautions, 55
Blood flow
    direction of, in transcranial color Doppler imaging, 1096
    physiology of, 908
    principles of, 905–907, 905*f*
    velocity of, 910, 910*f*
Blood flow analysis, 209–210
Blood glucose, 361*t*, 362
Blood pressure
    definition of, 36
    in gastrointestinal assessment, 84
    measurement of, 36, 36*f*, 37*b*, 37*f*
Blood pressure cuff, 36, 37*f*
Blood urea nitrogen (BUN), 229, 439
Blood vessels, 1008, 1008*f*
Blunt trauma
    abdomen, 767
    FAST scan in, 563–567, 563*b*, 563*f*, 564*b*, 564*f*, 565*f*
    sonographic findings of, 564–566, 566*f*
    splenic, 345–348, 350*f*
B-mode transducers, 528, 529*f*
Bochdalek, foramen of, 1555, 1556*f*
Body cavities, 88, 88*f*
Body fluids, sonographer exposure to, 67
Body mechanics
    definition of, 38
    patient transfer and, 38–39
Body systems, 81–88, 82*t*
Bones
    hip, 851, 851*f*
    nasal, 1317–1318, 1317*f*
Bony pelvis, 1159–1160, 1159*f*, 1189
Bosniak classification, of cysts, 449, 452*t*, 458–459
Bouffard position, 747*f*
Bowel, 1174–1175
    fetal
        abnormalities of, 1586–1590
        sonographic evaluation of, 1578–1579, 1579*f*
    herniation of, 1561–1562, 1565–1566, 1567*f*
    hyperechoic, 1589, 1589*b*
    layers of, 394, 394*b*
    physiologic herniation of, 1313, 1314*f*
    sonographic evaluation of, 1198–1199, 1198*f*
Bowel herniation, 1338, 1339*f*
Bowel ischemia, 606–607, 607*f*
Bowel omphaloceles, 1563, 1566*f*
Bowman capsule, 437
Boyle, Robert, 6
BPD. *see* Biparietal diameter
BPP. *see* Biophysical profile
Brachial artery, 1112
Brachial pressures, 1115
Brachial veins, 1133
Brachiocephalic artery, 901
Bradycardia
    definition of, 35
    embryonic, 1327
    fetal, 1012
Brain death, 1103
Brainstem, neonatal, 818–819
Branchial apparatus, 1493

Branchial cleft cysts, 705, 705f, 1512
Breast, 643, 680b–681b
   abscesses of, 658t, 664, 664f
   anatomy of, 645–652
      clock face method, 656f
      lymphatic drainage of, 651, 651f
      male, 651–652, 652b, 652f
      normal, 645–648, 645f, 646f, 647f, 648f
      quadrant method, 656f
      vascular supply, 649–650, 650f
   augmentation of, 666–671, 666f, 667f
   biopsy of, large-core needle, 676
   clinical evaluation of patient with problem, 659b
   dense, 648, 649f
   evaluation of, 652–658
      clinical assessment, 654
      diagnostic breast interrogation, 654
      interventional breast procedures, 654
      screening, 652, 653b
      targeted *versus* whole breast scan, 654
   fatty, 648–649, 649f
   interventional procedures, 654
   lumps in, 654
   parenchymal patterns, 648–649, 649f
   pathology of, 658–666
      abscesses, 658t, 664, 664f
      acute mastitis, 663–664, 663f
      chronic mastitis, 664
      cystosarcoma phyllodes, 658t, 675, 675f
      diabetic mastopathy, 666
      fat necrosis, 658t, 664, 665f
      fibroadenoma, 658t, 661–662, 662f
      fibrocystic changes, 658t
      fibrocystic dysplasia/fibrocystic changes, 660–661, 661f
      hematoma, 664–665
      intraductal papilloma, 658t, 665–666, 666f
      lipomas, 658t, 665, 665f
      lymphoma, 676
      metastatic disease, 676
      pregnant and/or lactating patient, 662
      seroma/lymphocele, 665, 665f
   physiology of, 644–645
   sonographic evaluation of, 654–658
      automated whole breast ultrasound, 678–681, 679f
      elastography, 679–681, 679f, 680f
      patient positioning for, 655, 655f
      technique for, 655–656, 655f, 656f
      ultrasound-guided interventional procedures in, 676
      large-core needle biopsy, 676
      preoperative needle wire localization, 676, 676f
   zones of, 657f
Breast cancer, 644, 671
   in males, 651–652, 652b, 652f
   mammographic findings in, 653–654, 653b, 653t, 654b
   risk factors for, 644b
   screening for, 652, 653b
   signs and symptoms of, 653b
   types of
      colloid/mucinous carcinoma, 675
      comedocarcinoma, 672, 672f
      ductal carcinoma in situ, 671, 671f
      inflammatory carcinoma, 673, 674f

Breast cancer *(Continued)*
      invasive ductal carcinoma, 672
      invasive lobular carcinoma, 673, 674f
      medullary carcinoma, 673, 675f
      Paget disease, 654–655, 673, 673f
      papillary carcinoma, 672–673, 672f
      scirrhous carcinoma, 674–675
      tubular carcinoma, 674
Breast cysts
   description of, 659
   sonographic evaluation of, 659–660
Breast hematoma, 664–665
Breast Imaging Reporting and Data System (BI-RADS), 653
   categories of mammographic masses, 653t
Breast implants
   complications of, 667–668, 667f
   extracapsular, 669, 669f
   intracapsular, 668, 669f
   ruptured, 668–669, 669f
Breast masses
   in males, 652f
   sonographic characteristics of, 669–671
      attenuation effects, 669
      compressibility, 669
      internal echo pattern, 669
      margins, 669, 670f
      mobility, 669
      orientation, 669
      shape, 669
      vascularity, 671
   vascularity, 657–658
Breast self-examination (BSE), 652, 653b
Breathing, by patient
   in abdominal scanning, 124
   extreme shortness of breath, 570–572
Breech, 1346–1347, 1347f
Brescia-Cimino graft, 1124f
Brightness modulation (B-mode), 17–18, 18f
Broad ligaments, 1165, 1166f
Bronchial atresia, congenital, 1554
Bronchogenic cysts, 1550, 1551f
Brown, Tom, 7
Bruit, 1072
B-scanners, 7–8
BSE. *see* Breast self-examination
Budd, George, 256–257
Budd-Chiari syndrome, 258
   liver findings in, 258t
   sonographic findings in, 258, 259f
Buffers, 83
Bulbus cordis, 1009
Bull's eye (target) lesion, 266
Bull's eye sign, 406f
BUN. *see* Blood urea nitrogen
Bundle of His, 903
Bursa, 738–739, 738f, 740t
Bursitis, 72
Bypass graft surveillance, 1122–1123, 1122f, 1123f

C

CA. *see* Celiac axis
CA 125 test, 1244–1245
"Cake" kidney, 1601f
Calcifications
   arcuate arteries, 1192–1193
   dermoid tumors, 1253f
   intratendinous, 753f

Calcifications *(Continued)*
   periventricular, 1541f
   urinary tract, 479, 480f
   uterine, 1210–1212, 1213f
Calcitonin, 682–683
Calcium, serum, 700–701
Calf vein imaging, 1149
   duplex imaging, 1149
   evaluation of, 1149
Calyx, 436–437
Camptomelic dysplasia, 1623t, 1629, 1630f
Candidiasis
   hepatic, 264t, 266, 267f
   hepatosplenic, 344
Capillaries, 171
Capsular arteries, 710–711, 711f
Carbohydrates, 227
Carbon dioxide reactivity, 1097
Carcinoma, 671
   anaplastic, 697, 697f
   cervical, 1204, 1206b, 1206f
   cholangiocarcinoma, 318–321, 319f, 320f
   colloid, 675
   colorectal, 520f
   endometrial, 1223–1224, 1224b, 1224f
   fallopian tube, 1257
   follicular, 694–696, 696f
   gallbladder, 306–308, 309f, 310f
   gastric, 400t, 401–402, 402f
   ovarian, 1244–1246, 1246f, 1247f
   parathyroid, 703–704
   transitional cell, 454t–458t, 464–466
Cardiac abnormalities, 1058–1062
   cardiosplenic syndromes, 1060–1062
   congenital vena cava to left atrial communication, 1059–1060
   cor triatriatum, 1059, 1059f
   ectopia cordis, 1062, 1062f
   single ventricle, 1058–1059, 1058f, 1059f
   total anomalous pulmonary venous return, 899, 1060, 1060f, 1061f
Cardiac anomalies, 1334
Cardiac arrest, 66
Cardiac axis, 1018f
Cardiac cycle, 901–903, 902f, 909–910, 909f
Cardiac enlargement, 1034–1036
Cardiac malposition, 1033, 1035f
Cardiac masses, 1005b
   definition of, 995
   normal variants *versus*, 995, 998b
   subacute bacterial endocarditis, 1000–1006, 1004f, 1005f
   thrombus, 998–1000, 1003f
   vegetations, 1000–1006, 1004f, 1005f
Cardiac nerves, 903
Cardiac orifice, 390
Cardiac output (CO), 910, 914, 990b, 1097, 1097b
Cardiac structures, M-mode imaging of, 920, 943–952, 950b
   aortic valve, 935f, 945–946, 946f, 950f
   interventricular septum, 946, 951f
   left atrium, 945–946, 950f
   left ventricle, 946, 951f
   mitral valve, 943–944, 950f
   normal measurements, 950t
   pulmonary valve, 950–952, 951f
   tricuspid valve, 946
Cardiac tamponade, 982–983, 984f, 985b, 985f

Cardiac tumors, 1058
　categories of, 995–998, 999f
　lipomatous hypertrophy, 998, 1001f
　malignant primary, 998, 1002f
　myxomas, 998, 999f
　papillary fibroelastoma, 998, 1000f
　rhabdomyoma, 998, 1001f
Cardinal ligaments, 1165, 1165f
Cardiomyopathy, 1005b, 1034–1036, 1036f
　amyloid, 992, 994f
　categories of, 985–986
　definition of, 985–986
　dilated, 986–993, 988b, 988f, 989f, 990b, 990f, 991f, 992b
　eosinophilic, 992, 993f
　hypertrophic, 993–995, 996f, 997b, 997f
　idiopathic restrictive, 992
　infiltrative, 990–992, 992b
　ischemic, 989
　nonischemic, 989
　predictors of, 992b
　prognosis of, 990
　restrictive, 990–992, 992b
　Takotsubo, 993
Cardiopulmonary resuscitation (CPR), 66–67, 66f
Cardiosplenic syndromes, 1060–1062
Cardiovascular system, embryology of, 1008–1010
Caroli disease, 310, 311f
Carotid artery disease, 1082–1083
Carotid artery stenting, 1083–1084, 1084f
Carotid body tumors, 1078, 1079f
Carotid duplex imaging, 1070f
　after stent placement or endarterectomy, 1083–1084, 1084f
　aneurysms, 1078
　atherosclerotic disease, 1076–1077, 1077f, 1078f
　carotid body tumors, 1078, 1079f
　dissection, 1078, 1079f
　fibromuscular dysplasia, 1078–1079
　interpretation of, 1079–1082, 1080t, 1081f, 1082b
　intraoperative use of, 1083
　normal findings of, 1074–1076, 1074f, 1075f
　procedure, 1073–1074, 1073f
　pseudoaneurysms, 1078
　technical aspects of, 1072–1079
　three-dimensional, 1084–1085, 1085f
Carotid intima-media thickness, 1081
Carotid pulse, 35, 36f
Carotid sheath, 1070
Carotid siphon, 1088, 1094
Carpal tunnel
　definition of, 72
　sonographic evaluation of, 748, 749f
Carpal tunnel syndrome (CTS), 755–757, 756b, 756f
Carpenter syndrome, 1633f
Cartilage interface sign, 752
Catheters, urinary, 43–44, 44f
Cat-scratch disease, 769, 770f
Cauda equina, 873, 874f, 875–876, 876f
　normal pulsatile movement of, 879–880, 880f
Caudal direction, 132–134
Caudal pancreatic artery, 180, 359
Caudal regression syndrome (CRS), 1414, 1631–1632, 1631f, 1632f

Caudate lobe
　abdominal scanning of, 106–107, 108f
　at celiac axis level, 106–107, 108f
　description of, 221
　at liver and psoas muscle level, 106, 107f
Caudate nucleus, 818, 819f
Caudothalamic groove, 818, 819f, 827
Caudothalamic notch, 818
Cavernous hemangioma
　contrast-enhanced imaging of, 518, 520f
　hepatic, 268, 271t, 272f
Cavernous transformation, of portal vein, 214, 260t
Cavum septum pellucidum, 816, 826
Cavum vergae, 816
CBD. *see* Common bile duct
CBE. *see* Clinical breast examination
CCA. *see* Common carotid artery
CCAM. *see* Congenital cystic adenomatoid malformation
CDH. *see* Congenital diaphragmatic hernia
Cebocephaly, 1503, 1534–1535, 1535f
Celiac axis (CA)
　abdominal transverse scanning of, at level of caudate lobe, 106–107, 108f
　Doppler flow patterns in, 212–214, 212b, 213f
　pancreas and, 358f, 359
Celiac trunk, 179–180, 179f
Cell-free DNA testing, prenatal diagnosis of congenital anomalies, 1429
Cells, 81
Centesis catheter, 534, 534f
Central nervous system anomalies, in fetus, embryology of, 1522
Centripetal arteries, 711, 711f
Cephalic direction, 132–134
Cephalic index, 1385, 1386f
Cephalic vein, 1124f, 1133–1134
Cephalocele, 1336, 1336t, 1337f, 1503, 1523t, 1525–1526, 1527f
　differential considerations for, 1524t
　sonographic findings in, 1526, 1527f, 1528f
Cerclage placement, 1285
Cerebellum, 1351
　fetal, 1392, 1393b, 1393f
　neonatal, 819, 820f
Cerebral circulatory arrest, 1103–1104
Cerebral hemispheres, neonatal, 817
Cerebral vasospasm, 1099
Cerebrospinal fluid (CSF), neonatal, 816, 817f
Cerebrovascular accident
　costs associated with, 1069
　risk factors for, 1070
　warning signs and symptoms of, 1071–1072, 1072b
Cerebrovascular evaluation
　extracranial, 1069, 1085b
　　anatomy for imaging in, 1070–1071
　intracranial, 1087, 1107b
　　anatomy for imaging in, 1088–1090, 1088f
　　physiology in, 1090
Cerebrovascular system, neonatal, 819
Cerebrum
　hemispheres of, 817
　neonatal, 817–818, 818f
Certification, in ultrasound, 6
Cervical canal, 1443f
Cervical carcinoma, 1204, 1206b, 1206f

Cervical carotid system aneurysms, 1078
Cervical leiomyoma, 1204, 1205f
Cervical polyps, 1204
Cervical pregnancy, 1332–1333
Cervical stenosis, 1204, 1205f
Cervix, 1162, 1165b, 1375, 1375b
　coronal view of, 1163f
　female infertility and, 1272–1273
　lateral view of, 1162f
　pathology of, 1203–1207
　　benign conditions, 1203–1204, 1203f, 1204b
　　cervical carcinoma, 1204, 1206b, 1206f
　transvaginal scanning of, 1187f, 1193f
CEUS. *see* Contrast-enhanced ultrasound imaging
ceVUS. *see* Contrast-enhanced voiding urosonography
CFM. *see* Color flow mapping
CFV. *see* Common femoral vein
Chest, fetal ultrasound, 1408t
CHF. *see* Congestive heart failure
CHI. *see* Contrast harmonic imaging
Chiari, Hans, 256–257
Chiari malformations, 821, 839
Children
　abuse of, 763t
　acute abdominal pain in, 767
　cat-scratch disease in, 769, 770f
　cholangitis in, 769
　choledocholithiasis in, 767
　cirrhosis in, 768–769
　critically ill, 763t
　cystic fibrosis in, 769
　fatty liver in, 768–769
　food allergies in, 763t
　obesity in, 763t
　pancreatic disease in, 769
　pancreatitis in, 767
　portal hypertension in, 768–769
　special needs of, 58–59
　splenic disease in, 769
　splenic sequestration syndrome in, 767
　splenomegaly in, 769f
　trauma in, 767
Chlamydia trachomatis, 1261
Choking, 65–66, 65b, 65f
Cholangiocarcinoma, 318–321, 319f, 320f
Cholangiopathy, 602f
Cholangitis, 315–318, 769
Cholecystectomy, 285
Cholecystitis, 293–299, 297b
　acalculous, 294t–295t, 297, 300f
　chronic, 294t–295t, 300
　clinical findings for, 573t
　emphysematous, 294t–295t, 296–297
　gangrenous, 294t–295t, 297, 300f
　hyperplastic, 303–306, 306f, 307f
Cholecystokinin, 289, 393
Choledochal cysts, 308–311
　fetal, 1582, 1584b
　pediatric, 771t, 772, 773f
　sonographic findings in, 294t–295t, 308, 310f, 311f
Choledocholithiasis
　in children, 767
　description of, 294t–295t, 313, 316f, 597–598
Cholelithiasis, 294t–295t, 300, 301f, 302f, 303f, 304f
　fetal, 1582, 1584f
　right upper quadrant pain in, 567–568, 568f
　sonographic findings in, 300–303, 302f, 304f, 305f

Cholesterolosis, 303–304, 306f
Chorioamnionitis, 1483
Chorioangioma, placental tumors, 1457, 1457f
Choriocarcinoma, 728t, 1326
Chorion, 1289–1290
Chorion frondosum, 1443, 1443b, 1443f
Chorion laeve, 1443b, 1443f
Chorionic cavity, 1308–1309, 1462f
Chorionic or gestational sac, 1379
Chorionic plate, 1443, 1443b
Chorionic sac, 1462f
Chorionic villi, 1443, 1443f
Chorionic villus sampling (CVS), 1300–1301
 prenatal diagnosis of congenital anomalies, 1429–1430, 1429f, 1430f
Choroid plexus, neonatal, 816, 817f, 825–826
Choroid plexus cysts, 844–845, 845f, 1537–1538, 1537f
 subependymal cysts *versus*, 845
Chromosomal abnormalities, congenital heart disease and, 1032, 1032t
Chromosomal disorder, 1433
Chronic cholecystitis, 294t–295t, 300
Chronic granulomatous disease, 264t, 266, 268f
Chronic hepatitis, 243t, 246, 247f
Chronic kidney disease (CKD), 474
Chronic liver failure, 584–585
Chronic lymphocytic leukemia, 728t
Chronic pancreatitis, 369t, 372–373, 373f
Chronic pyelonephritis, 806–807
Chronic renal failure, 454t–458t
Circle of Willis, 1088f, 1089, 1351f
 transtemporal approach to, 1092–1093, 1092f
Circulation
 coronary, 906–907
 fetal
  description of, 1010–1012
  illustration of, 1011f
  neonatal, 1012f
Circulatory system, 81–83, 170–171
Circumvallate/circummarginate placenta, 1454, 1455f
Cirrhosis, 246–248, 247f
 in children, 768–769
 intrahepatic portal hypertension and, 251
 liver transplantation for, 584–585, 584f
 pathology of, 584f
 sonographic findings in, 243t, 246–248, 248f
Cisterna magna, 816, 1351
Cisterns, neonatal, 816
CKD. *see* Chronic kidney disease
"Clapper-in-the-bell" sign, 755–756
Claudication, 1114
Clear cell tumors, 1249–1250
Cleft lip/palate, 1506, 1507f, 1508f, 1509f, 1510b, 1510f, 1511f, 1512f
Cleft sternum, 1568–1570, 1569f
Clicks, 905
Clinical breast examination (CBE), 652, 653b
Clinical laboratory orientation, 124–125
Clinical sonography, foundations of, 3, 27b
Cloacal exstrophy, 1564t, 1567–1568, 1568f, 1569f, 1603–1604
Clock face method, 656, 656f
C-loop of duodenum, 356–358, 358f
Closed dysraphic associations, 880–881, 881t
Closed spinal dysraphism, 880–881
Cloverleaf skull, 1498–1499, 1499f

Clubfoot, 1633–1635, 1635f
Clutter, 160–163, 162f, 163f
CO. *see* Cardiac output
Coagulopathy, 532
Coarctation of aorta, 1032t, 1048, 1055–1056, 1057f
Coccygeus muscles, 94f, 1160, 1160f
Coccyx, 876, 877f
Code of Ethics for the Profession of Diagnostic Medical Sonography, 1295
Colitis, 410f
Collateral circulation, 252–253, 252f, 254f, 255t, 256t
Collateral pathways, 1071, 1100–1101
Colloid carcinoma, 675
Colon
 sonographic evaluation of, 398–399, 399f
 tumors of, 409–412
"Color blooming" artifacts, 515–516
Color box size, 715t
Color Doppler imaging, 24–25, 26f, 211–212
 of acoustic emission, 514–515, 515f
 of arteriovenous malformations, 1216
 artifacts of, 160–163
  aliasing and, 160, 161f, 162f
  mirror image, shadowing, clutter, and noise and, 160–163, 162f, 163f
 carotid duplex
  procedure, 1073
  of tortuous arteries, 1075–1076, 1076b, 1076f
  of vertebral arteries, 1081
 of collateral circulation, 252–253, 254f, 255t, 256t
 color flow, 912, 912f
 contrast-enhanced
  of renal artery flow, 512f
  of renal artery stenosis, 521, 521f
  of right renal artery, 512f
 of ovaries, 1236, 1236f
 of pancreatic mass, 553–554
 of pelvic vascularity, 1190
 principles of, 912, 912f, 913f
 of renal transplantation complications, 555, 555f
 of scrotum, 715t, 718
  epididymo-orchitis, 718
  hematoceles, 726f
  torsion, 710f, 722f
  tubular ectasia of the rete testis, 726–728
  varicoceles, 722–723, 724f
 of spleen, 335–336, 336f
 of testes, 716f
 transorbital approach, 1094, 1094f
 venous, 1147f
Color flow Doppler, 24, 1015, 1015f
Color flow imaging
 of renal artery flow, 512f
 of single ventricle, 1059f
Color flow mapping (CFM)
 apical view for, 933–936, 944f
 examination, 919–920, 922b, 922f
 M-mode, 920, 943–952, 950b
 parasternal views
  long-axis, 920f, 922b, 925–928, 927f
  short-axis, 922b, 929–931, 931f, 932f, 933f, 934f
 right parasternal window for, 928, 930f
 subcostal view for, 938, 948b
 suprasternal view for, 939–943

Colostomies, 47
Colpocephaly, 840–841
Columns of Bertin, 444, 446f
Comedocarcinoma, 672, 672f
Comet tail artifacts, 148–149, 150f, 742, 742f
Common atria, 1042
Common bile duct (CBD), 282, 282f
 atretic, 771
 pancreas and, 358f, 359
 pediatric, 765, 765b, 766f
 right upper quadrant pain and, 568, 569f
 sonographic evaluation of, 289, 292f, 293f
 stones of, 313
 stricture of, 259
Common carotid artery (CCA), 1070, 1070f
Common femoral artery, 178t, 611, 1111–1112, 1143f
Common femoral vein (CFV), 1131
 venous duplex imaging of, 1147f
Common hepatic artery, 179–180, 180f
 color Doppler technique for, 255t
 pancreas and, 359
Common hepatic duct, 282, 282f
Common iliac arteries, 178–179, 178f, 178t
Common iliac vein, 1131
Communicating hydrocephalus, 829, 1540, 1540f
Communication, sonographers and, 5b, 550
Compartments
 intraperitoneal, 417–418, 418f, 419f
 lower abdominal, 418–419, 419f
 pelvic, 418–419, 419f
 perihepatic, 417–418
 psoas, 495, 495f
 upper abdominal, 417–418, 418f
Complete atrioventricular septal defect, 1041–1043, 1042f
Complete blood count, 83
Complete duplication, 447, 450f, 451f
Complex cysts
 breast, 658t, 659b, 660, 661f
 renal, 458, 459b, 459f, 460f
Complex lung masses, 1554–1555
Complicated cyst, in breast, 659b
Compound imaging, 540, 715t
Compression, 10
Compression therapy, 1125–1126
Computed tomography (CT), 103–104, 103t
 abdominal trauma on, 562
 of calcified dermoid tumor, 1253f
 fusion technology and, 540, 540f, 541f
 noncontrast, 439
Conceptional age, 1378
Conduction system, of heart
 development of, 1010
 electrical, 903, 903f
 mechanical, 903–904
Confidentiality, of findings, 1298
Confluence of splenic and portal veins, 107
Congenital anomalies
 of face, 1492
 prenatal diagnosis of, 1426, 1441b
  chromosomal abnormalities, 1433–1441
   nuchal translucency, 1433, 1433f
   triploidy, 1438
   trisomy 13, 1437–1438, 1438f, 1439f, 1440f
   trisomy 18, 1436–1437, 1436f, 1437f, 1438f
   trisomy 21, 1433–1436, 1434f, 1435f, 1436f
   Turner syndrome, 1438–1441, 1440f

Congenital anomalies *(Continued)*
   chromosomal disorders, 1426–1427
   diagnostic screening tests, 1429–1432
     amniocentesis, 1430–1431, 1430f, 1431f
     chorionic villus sampling, 1429–1430, 1429f, 1430f
     cordocentesis, 1432
     genetic amniocentesis, 1431–1432, 1431f, 1432f
     multiple gestations, genetic amniocentesis and, 1432
   first trimester screening, 1432–1433
     human chorionic gonadotropin, 1432–1433
     pregnancy-associated plasma protein A, 1432
   genetic screening tests, 1427–1429
     alpha-fetoprotein, 1427–1429, 1427b, 1427f, 1428b
     cell-free DNA testing, 1429
     quadruple screen, 1429
   medical genetics, 1433
   scrotal, 728t, 730–732
   splenic, 327–329, 331f
   uterus, 1273–1274, 1273f, 1274f
Congenital bronchial atresia, 1554
Congenital cystic adenomatoid malformation (CCAM), 1552–1554, 1553f
   sonographic findings in, 1554, 1554b
   type I, 1553–1554, 1553f
   type II, 1553–1554
   type III, 1553–1554, 1554f
Congenital diaphragmatic hernia (CDH), 1555–1558, 1556b
Congenital heart disease, 1065b–1066b
   atrioventricular septal defect, 1041–1043, 1041f
   cardiac abnormalities, 1058–1062
     single ventricle, 1058–1059, 1058f, 1059f
   cardiac enlargement, 1034–1036
   cardiac malposition terms, 1033, 1035f
   cardiac tumors, 1058
   cardiosplenic syndromes, 1060–1062
   chromosomal abnormalities and, 1032, 1032t
   congenital vena cava to left atrial communication, 1059–1060
   cor triatriatum, 1059, 1059f
   ectopia cordis, 1062, 1062f
   familial risks of, 1033
   fetal echocardiography of, 1008
   four-chamber view of, 1033, 1034f
   great vessel abnormalities, 1054–1058
     coarctation of the aorta, 1055–1056, 1057f
     ductal constriction, 1057
     interrupted aortic arch, 1056–1057
     transposition of the great arteries, 1054, 1054f, 1055f
     truncus arteriosus, 1054–1055, 1055f, 1056f
   incidence of, 1007, 1033
   left ventricular inflow disturbance, 1048–1050
   left ventricular outflow tract disturbance, 1050–1054
     aortic stenosis, 1050–1052
     bicuspid aortic valve, 1033, 1050, 1050f
     hypoplastic left heart syndrome, 1052–1054, 1052f, 1053f
   mitral regurgitation, 1050
   prenatal evaluation of, 1033
   right ventricular inflow disturbance, 1043–1045
   right ventricular outflow disturbance, 1045–1048
   single ventricle, 1058–1059, 1058f, 1059f

Congenital heart disease *(Continued)*
   total anomalous pulmonary venous return, 1060, 1060f, 1061f
Congenital hepatic cysts, 264
Congenital hydrocephalus, 829
Congenital hypophosphatasia, 1628
Congenital lobar emphysema, 1554
Congenital mesoblastic nephroma, 796t
Congenital mitral stenosis, 1048–1050, 1048f, 1049f
Congenital spherocytosis, 340, 341f
Congenital vena cava to left atrial communication, 1059–1060
Congestive heart failure (CHF), 1076, 1077f, 1142f
Congestive splenomegaly, 338b, 339
Conjoined twins, 1419–1420, 1421f, 1423
Conn syndrome, 500–501, 502t
Consent
   form, 33f, 543
   patient, 32, 33f
   verbal, 32
   written, 32
Constrictive pericarditis, 983–985, 986b, 986f, 987f
Contact precautions, 54
Continuity equation
   aortic stenosis assessments using, 971b
   description of, 915, 915f
   mitral stenosis assessments using, 960–961, 961f
Continuity principle, 915
Continuous murmur, 905
Continuous wave (CW) Doppler, 23, 25f
   aortic regurgitation, 963–964
   description of, 913, 913f
   echocardiography, 923, 923f
   hypertrophic cardiomyopathy evaluations, 995, 997f
   mitral regurgitation, 956, 957f
   transducers for, 913f
Continuous wave probe, 923, 924f
Contrast-enhanced ultrasound imaging (CEUS), 511
   focal nodular hyperplasia, 518, 520f
   harmonic imaging for, 515–516
   hepatic blood flow, 517
   hepatic tumors, 517f, 518, 518f, 519f, 520f, 521f
   intermittent imaging and, 516
   liver metastases, 520f
   organ transplants and, 523–524
   pancreatic applications of, 523
   renal masses, 522, 522f
   splenic applications of, 522–523
Contrast-enhanced voiding urosonography (ceVUS), 795–796, 797f
Contrast harmonic imaging (CHI), 515–516
Conus medullaris, 873, 874f, 878–879, 879b, 879f
Cooper's ligaments, 645–646, 647f
Copper 7, 1227–1228
Cor triatriatum, 1059, 1059f
Coracohumeral ligament, 738f
Cordis, ectopia, 1564t
Cordocentesis, 1410–1411, 1411f
   prenatal diagnosis of congenital anomalies, 1432
Core biopsy, needles for, 533, 533f, 534f
Coronal imaging, transvaginal, 1186, 1186b, 1187f
Coronal plane
   abdominal, 104–105
   neonatal head examination, 822f, 823t, 824–827, 824f
Coronary circulation, 906–907

Corpus callosum
   agenesis of, 840–841, 841f, 1523t, 1535–1536
     sonographic findings in, 1536, 1536f
   neonatal, 818, 818f
Corpus luteum, 1168, 1198
Corpus luteum cysts, 1236–1237, 1237b, 1237f, 1329t, 1340, 1341f
   hemorrhagic, 1237, 1238f
   sonographic findings in, 1237, 1237f
Cortex, 792
   adrenal, 497
   renal, 436, 444
Corticomedullary differentiation, 792
Corticosteroid therapy, 1483
Costal margin, 891–892
Costophrenic sinus, 892
Couinaud's system, of hepatic nomenclature, 219–220, 220b, 221f
Courvoisier sign, 289, 292f
CPR. *see* Cardiopulmonary resuscitation
Craig, Marveen, 69
Cranial cavity, 88
Cranial direction, 132–134
Cranial meningocele, 1525–1526
Craniostenosis, 1523t
Craniosynostosis, 1496, 1624
Cranium
   embryonic
     anomalies of, 1334–1338, 1335f, 1336t
     sonographic findings of, 1310–1313, 1311f, 1312f
   fetal, 1348–1352, 1348f, 1349f, 1350f, 1351f, 1352f
Cranium bifidum, 1527f
Crass position, 746f
Creatinine (Cr), 438–439
Creatinine clearance, 439
Cremasteric artery, 712
Cremasteric muscle, 712
Crepitus, 754
Crisscross view, 1021, 1022b, 1022f
Critical aortic stenosis, 1050, 1051f
CRL. *see* Crown-rump length
Crohn's disease, 404t, 409, 409f
Crossed-fused renal ectopia, 448–449, 451f, 452f, 800, 803f
Cross-talk, 160
Crown-rump length (CRL), 1301, 1304f, 1315, 1315f, 1316f, 1381–1382, 1381b, 1381f, 1382f, 1382t
CRS. *see* Caudal regression syndrome
Crus of diaphragm, 106, 107f
Crying patients, 57
Cryptorchidism, 1617
   neonatal/pediatric, 730–732, 731f
Crystals, piezoelectric, 12–13, 13f
CSF. *see* Cerebrospinal fluid
CT. *see* Computed tomography
CTS. *see* Carpal tunnel syndrome
Cubital tunnel, 72
Cuffs, blood pressure, 36, 37f
Cul-de-sac
   fluid, 1198f
   sonographic evaluation of, 578
   ultrasound examination of, 1178b
Culling, 332
Curie, Paul-Jacques, 6
Curie, Pierre, 6

Curved array transducer, 16–17, 125, 127f, 128f
Cushing syndrome, 502, 502t
Cushions, 78
Cushman, Richard, 7
CVS. see Chorionic villus sampling
Cyanosis, 38
Cyclopia, 1503, 1504f, 1534–1535, 1535f
Cyst(s)
  abdominal, 426, 427f
  adrenal, 502–503, 502f, 503f
  arachnoid, 845–846, 846f, 1523t, 1540f
  Baker, 579, 580f, 1147, 1147f
  Bosniak classification of, 449, 452t, 458–459
  branchial cleft, 705, 705f, 1512
  bronchogenic, 1550, 1551f
  choledochal, 308–311
    fetal, 1582, 1584b
    pediatric, 771t, 772, 773f
    sonographic findings in, 294t–295t, 308, 310f
  choroid plexus, 844–845, 845f, 1537–1538, 1537f
    subependymal cysts versus, 845
  complex, renal, 458, 459b, 459f, 460f
  corpus luteum, 1236–1237, 1237b, 1237f, 1329t, 1340, 1341f
    hemorrhagic, 1237, 1238f
    sonographic findings in, 1237, 1237f
  developmental, of neck, 704–707
  duplication, 399, 400f, 400t
  echinococcal, 264t, 267–268, 270f
  epididymal, 717t, 722, 723f
  follicular, 1198, 1231–1233, 1233f
  Gartner duct, 1203, 1203f
  glioependymal, 1523t
  hepatic, 260–262, 264t
  intratesticular, 727, 727f
  kissing, 459, 460f
  masses within, 468–470, 470f
  medullary, 454t–458t
  mesenteric, 426, 427f
  nabothian, 1193, 1193f, 1204, 1204b, 1204f, 1205f
  pancreatic, 1583
  paraovarian, 1240, 1240b, 1241f
  peribiliary, 264, 265f
  peritoneal, 426
  peritoneal inclusion, 1239–1242, 1240f
  renal
    simple, 453, 459f
      sonographic findings in, 453–458
    sinus parapelvic, 454t–458t, 459–460
  simple, hepatic, 262–264, 264t, 265f
  splenic, 337t, 348–349, 349f, 1583–1584
  subependymal, 845
  sublingual, 1512f
  theca-lutein, 1237, 1238b, 1239f
  thyroglossal duct, 704–705, 705f
  tunica albuginea, 718
  urachal, 427, 427f
  von Hippel-Lindau, 454t–458t, 460
Cystadenocarcinomas
  mucinous, 1247, 1248b, 1249f
  ovarian, 1247
  serous, 1248–1249, 1249b, 1250f, 1251f
Cystadenomas
  mucinous, 382f, 1247, 1248b, 1249f
  ovarian, 1235
  serous, 1249b, 1250f, 1252f

Cystic adenomatoid malformation
  AFP and, 1428
  congenital, 1552–1554, 1553f
    sonographic findings in, 1554, 1554b
    type I, 1553–1554, 1553f
    type II, 1553–1554
    type III, 1553–1554, 1554f
Cystic degeneration of myomas, 1210
Cystic duct, 282f, 283
Cystic fibrosis
  in children, 769
  meconium ileus and, 1587
  pancreatic lesions, 377, 379f
Cystic hygroma
  AFP and, 1428
  cephaloceles versus, 1527
  fetal, 1513–1514, 1513f, 1514f, 1515f, 1516f
  first-trimester, 1339–1340, 1339f
  Turner syndrome, 1440, 1440f
Cystic lesions
  hepatic, 262–265, 264t
  neonatal, 844–846
  pancreatic, 377, 378t
Cystic masses
  abdomen, fetal, 1590–1591
  left upper quadrant, 396
  lung, 1549–1550, 1551b
  ovarian, 1234, 1234b, 1234f, 1235f
Cystic medial necrosis, 193–194
Cystic pancreatic neoplasms, 377–381
Cystic rhombencephalon, 1335f
Cystitis, 485–486
Cystosarcoma phyllodes, 658t, 675, 675f
Cytopathology, 538–539

D
da Vinci, Leonardo, 6
Dacryocystoceles, 1501
Dandy-Walker malformation, 841–842, 841f, 1336, 1336t, 1338f, 1523t, 1531
  differential considerations for, 1524t
  sonographic findings in, 1531, 1532f
  sonographic findings of, 841, 842f
"Dangling choroid" sign, 1541
DCIS. see Ductal carcinoma in situ
DDH. see Developmental displacement of the hip
De Quervain disease, 72
De Quervain tendinitis, 754
De Quervain thyroiditis, 699
DeBakey model, 194, 194f
Decibel (dB) unit, 11–12, 12t
Decidua basalis, 1307, 1443b, 1443f
Decidua capsularis, 1307, 1443, 1443b, 1443f
Decidua vera (parietalis), 1443b, 1443f
Decidual septum, 1443f
Deciduas basalis, 1443
Dedication, 5b
Deep flexor tendon, 736f
Deep structures, 134
Deep vein thrombosis (DVT), 1130, 1134–1136, 1147f
  bilateral symptoms, 1148–1149
  complications of, 1130
  diagnostic approach to, 1145
  risk factors for, 1135b
  signs and symptoms of, 1130, 1135b
Deep veins
  lower extremity, 1130–1131, 1130f
  upper extremity, 1133–1134, 1133f

Deferential artery, 712
Deformation sequence, 1496
Delta cells, 361
Denial, illness and, 60
Depth gain compensation (DGC), 21–22
Dermal sinus, 883, 885f
Dermoid cyst, 1416f
Dermoid tumors, 1250–1251, 1252b, 1252f, 1253f
Descending aorta, 172, 1111
Desmoid tumor, 432, 432f
Detailed fetal anatomic survey ultrasound, 1407
Detoxification
  bilirubin, 229
  drug, 230
  hormone, 230
  liver, 229–230, 229t
Developmental cysts, of neck, 704–707, 705f
Developmental displacement of the hip (DDH), 857–867
  abnormal, 858
  Barlow maneuver for, 859, 859f
  causes of, 866–867
  genetic factors, 867
  hormonal factors, 866
  incidence of, 866
  mechanical factors, 866–867
  Ortolani maneuver for, 859, 859f
  physical examination for, 858–859, 859f
  signs of, 859f
  sonographic findings of
    coronal/flexion view, 855, 856f, 859–860, 861f
    coronal/neutral view, 855, 855f, 856b, 859, 860f
    dynamic Harcke technique, 862–863, 865f
    follow-up, 866, 866f, 867f
    Graf checklist, 856b
    linear-array transducer for, 854, 854b
    modified Graf technique, 860–866, 862b, 862f, 863f, 863t, 864f
    overview of, 854
    positioning for, 855
    preparation for, 854–855
    static femoral head coverage measurement with, 862, 865f
    static Graf technique, 860–866, 862b, 862f, 863f, 863t, 864f
    techniques used in, 860–866
    transverse/flexion view, 855–856, 857f, 858f, 860, 861f
    transverse/neutral view, 857, 860
  treatment of, 866, 866f, 867f
Dextrocardia, 1033, 1035f
Dextroposition, 1033, 1035f
Dextroversion, 1035f
DGC. see Depth gain compensation
Diabetes, 1413–1415
  type 1, pancreatic transplantation for, 586
Diabetic mastopathy, 666
Diagnostic breast interrogation, 653–654
Diagnostic medical ultrasonography, 4
Diagnostic peritoneal lavage (DPL), 562, 562f
Dialysis, description of, 585–586
Dialysis access grafts, 1123–1124, 1123f, 1124f
Diaphragm, 88–89, 90f
  abnormalities of, 1555–1558, 1555f
  anatomy of, 88
  longitudinal scans of, 141, 141f
  thoracic vessels and, fetal, 1360–1362, 1361f, 1362f, 1363f

Diaphragmatic crura, 172
  anatomy of, 444, 445f, 494, 494f
  sonographic evaluation of, 498, 500f
Diaphragmatic hernia
  right-side, 1556
  sonographic criteria of, 1556b
Diarrhea, 84–86, 85t
Diastematomyelia, 872, 879–880, 883, 885f
Diastole, 909, 926–928
Diastolic measurement, 36
Diastolic murmur, 905
Diastrophic dysplasia, 1628–1629, 1629f
Diffuse disease, 340–342
  autoimmune hemolytic anemia, 341
  cirrhosis, 243t, 246–248, 247f
  congenital spherocytosis, 340, 341f
  fatty infiltration, 243–244, 244b
  glycogen storage disease, 243t, 248–249, 250f
  granulocytopoietic abnormalities, 342
  Hand-Schüller-Christian disease, 342
  hemochromatosis, 243t, 249, 250f
  hemolytic anemia, 341
  hepatitis, 244–246
    acute, 243t, 246, 246f
    chronic, 243t, 246, 247f
  hepatocellular, 243
  Letterer-Siwe disease, 342
  myeloproliferative disorders, 342, 343f
  polycythemia vera, 341
  reticuloendotheliosis, 342
  sickle cell anemia, 340
  thalassemia, 341–342, 343f
  thyroid gland, 698–700, 699f, 700f
Diffuse orchitis, 717t
Digestive system, 84f
  embryology of, 1572–1576, 1573f, 1574f
Digital subtraction angiography, 1083
Dilated biliary ducts, 311–312, 312f
Dilated posterior urethra, 1600
Dilation, lower gastrointestinal, 403, 404t, 405f
Diplopia, 1072
Direct-acting bilirubin, 229, 229t
Disbelief, illness and, 60
Discriminatory level, 1323
Disinfection technique, 1187–1189
Dislocation
  neonatal hip, 857, 858f
  shoulder biceps tendon, 751, 751f
Disruption sequence, 1496
Dissecting aneurysm, 194, 194f
Dissection, carotid artery, 1078, 1079f
Distal cholangiocarcinoma, 321, 322f
Distal direction, 132–134
Distal femoral and proximal tibial epiphyseal ossification centers, 1390
Disturbed flow, 905
Diverticulum, 408–409
Dolichocephaly, 1424
Dome of liver, 106–108, 106f
Dominant disorder, 1433
Donald, Ian, 7
Doppler, Christian Johann, 6
Doppler angle, 23
Doppler effect, 6, 22–23, 22f, 23f, 910–911, 911f
Doppler flow patterns
  in abdominal vessels, 212–214, 212b
  aorta, 212–214, 212b, 213f
  cardiac, 920, 922f

Doppler flow patterns (Continued)
  celiac axis, 212–214, 212b, 213f
  hepatic artery, 212–214, 212b, 213f
  inferior vena cava and hepatic veins, 214, 214b, 215f
  portal vein, 214, 214b, 215f
  renal artery, 212b, 214, 214f
  renal vein, 214, 214b, 215f
  splenic artery, 212–214, 212b, 213f
  superior mesenteric artery, 212b, 213f, 214
Doppler frequency shift, 910–911, 910f, 911f
Doppler interrogation, 253
Doppler quantitation, 924, 924t
Doppler sample volume, 210
Doppler shift, 23, 1091
Doppler sonography, fetal growth assessment, 1402–1404, 1402f
  quantitative and qualitative measurements, 1403, 1403b, 1403f, 1404f
Doppler spectral analysis
  of intracranial carotid arterial system, 1090–1091
  venous reflux imaging, 1145–1146, 1145f
Doppler ultrasound, 22–28
  abdominal
    scanning techniques, 145–146, 145f
    techniques, 209–217
      blood flow analysis, 209–210
  artifacts in, 147, 165b
  cirrhosis, 248, 249f
  color flow, 24
  for echocardiography, 920
    audio signals and spectral display of Doppler signals, 920–923
    continuous-wave Doppler, 923, 923f
    Doppler examination, 924, 924b
    Doppler quantitation, 924, 924t
    normal cardiac Doppler flow patterns, 920, 922f
    pulsed wave Doppler, 923, 923f
  endometrial carcinoma, 1224, 1224f
  examination, 925–943, 925f, 926f, 927b
  left parasternal window for, 928, 930f
  lower extremity veins, 1140
  methods of, 211–212, 212f
  optimization of, 25–28
  ovaries, 1236, 1236f, 1245–1246
  parasternal short-axis window for, 922–923, 928, 932f, 935f
  pitfalls in, 970–971, 971f, 972f
  portal hypertension, 252, 253b
  right parasternal window for, 928, 930f
  segmental pressures, 1114–1116, 1115t
  spectral, 945b
  subcostal window for, 924b, 938–939
  suprasternal window for, 941–943, 949f
  technical considerations, 970–971, 971f, 972f
  venous, 1142f
Doppler waveform analysis, abdominal techniques, 210
Dorsal aortic branches, 187
Dorsal cavity, 88, 88f
Dorsal direction, 132
Dorsal pancreatic artery, 359
Dorsalis pedis artery, 1112
Dorsiflexion, 750
Double bubble sign, 1585, 1586b, 1586f
Double decidual sac sign, 1307, 1379, 1379f

Double-layer thickness, 1277–1278
Double-outlet right ventricle, 1032t, 1046
Douglas, pouch of, 564, 566f, 1174
Down syndrome, 1032, 1042
  absent nasal bone in, 1505, 1507f
  midface hypoplasia and, 1506, 1508f
DPL. see Diagnostic peritoneal lavage
Drainage
  of abscess, 534–535, 559
  of ascites, 559
Drains, 46–47
Dressings, 46–47
Dromedary hump, 444, 446t
Droplet precautions, 54
Droplet transmission, of infections, 50
Drug detoxification, 230
Duct of Santorini, 358–359
Duct of Wirsung, 358–359, 358f
Ductal arch view, 1026–1029, 1027f, 1028f
Ductal carcinoma in situ (DCIS), 671, 671f
Ductal constriction, 1057
Ductography, of breast, 676, 677f
Ductus arteriosus, 1010
  fetal circulation, 1446f
Ductus venosus, 1288, 1446, 1461
  fetal circulation, 1446f
Duke University, 10
Duodenal atresia, 1574, 1585
Duodenal bulb, 390
Duodenal stenosis, 1574
Duodenum
  abdominal scanning of, at level of liver and pancreas, 109, 120f
  abnormalities of, 1584–1586
  C-loop of, 356–358, 358f
  embryology of, 1574
  segments of, 390, 392f
  sonographic evaluation of, 396–397, 397f
Duplex collecting, 446t
Duplication cysts, 399, 400f, 400t
Dura mater, 873–875
Dussik, Karl, 7, 7f
DVT. see Deep vein thrombosis
Dynamic range, 22
Dysarthria, 1072
Dysgerminoma, 1252, 1254f
Dysmenorrhea, 1174, 1204
Dysphagia, 1072
Dysplasia
  frontonasal, 1503, 1505f, 1510
  thanatophoric, 1499f
Dyspnea, 38
Dysrhythmias
  atrioventricular block, 1064–1066, 1064f
  ectopy, 1062–1063
  fetal, 1062–1066, 1062t, 1063f
  supraventricular tachyarrhythmias, 1063–1064, 1064f
Dysuria, 86, 87t

E
Ear
  abnormalities of, 1500–1501, 1501f
  development of, 1494–1495
Early proliferative phase, 1195
Ebstein anomaly, 1043–1045, 1044f
EBV. see Epstein-Barr virus
ECA. see External carotid artery

Echinococcal cyst, 264t, 267–268, 270f
Echinococcus, 348–349
Echocardiography, 920, 952b
  cardiac protocol for, 927b
  constrictive pericarditis, 983–985, 986b, 986f, 987f
  definition of, 4
  Doppler applications and technique, 920–925
    audio signals and spectral display of Doppler signals, 920–923
    cardiac Doppler flow patterns, 920, 922f
    continuous-wave Doppler, 923, 923f
    Doppler examination, 924, 924b
    Doppler quantitation, 924, 924t
    pulsed wave Doppler, 942f
  examination for, 925–943, 925f, 926f, 927b
  pericardial disease, 980–985
  pericardial effusion, 981–982, 981f, 981t, 982f, 983f
  positioning for, 927b
  subcostal views, 938–939, 948b
  techniques, 916
  transducers for, 918–919, 919f
  two-dimensional, 917–919, 917f, 918f
Echogenic, 130, 133f
Echogenic intracardiac focus (EIF), 1359–1360
Echogenic kidneys, enlarged, 1600
Eclampsia, 1415
ECMO. *see* Extracorporeal membrane oxygenation
Ectasia
  aortic, 187
  neonatal/pediatric, 804–805
Ectocervix, 1204
Ectopia
  renal, 448–449, 451f, 452f, 800, 803f
  testicular, 730
Ectopia cordis, 1062, 1062f, 1564t, 1568–1570, 1569f
Ectopic kidneys, 448–449, 451f, 452f
Ectopic pancreatic tissue, 359
Ectopic pregnancy, 1257, 1327–1333, 1328f
  adnexal mass with, 1330–1332, 1331f
  human chorionic gonadotrophin levels in, 1303
  sonographic findings in, 1328–1330, 1328f, 1329f, 1329t, 1330f, 1331f
Ectopic ureterocele, 450
  neonatal/pediatric, 797–798, 801f
  sonographic findings, 450–453
Ectopy, 1062–1063
Ectrodactyly, 1633f
Edler, Inge, 7, 8f
Edwards syndrome. *see* Trisomy 18
Efferent arteriole, 437
EFW. *see* Estimated fetal weight
EHR. *see* Embryonic heart rate
EIF. *see* Echogenic intracardiac focus
Ejaculatory ducts, 710
EJV. *see* External jugular vein
Elastography, 679–681, 679f, 680f
  assessment, in children, 768–769, 769f
  thyroid gland applications of, 698, 698f
Elderly, special needs of, 57–58
Electrical conduction system, 903, 903f
Electrocardiography, 904, 904f
Ellis-van Creveld syndrome, 1631

Embryo, 1289–1290, 1301
  aortic arches in, 1009f
  gestational sac without, 1322
  sonographic findings of
    at 6 to 10 weeks of gestational age, 1310–1313, 1310t
      embryonic cranium and spine, 1310–1313, 1311f, 1312f
      embryonic heart, 1313, 1314f, 1314t
      limb development, 1313, 1313f
      physiologic herniation of bowel, 1313, 1314f
      skeletal ossification, 1313, 1313f
    in abnormal intrauterine pregnancies, 1324b
    during fetal period, 1308–1310, 1309f, 1310f
Embryo in amniotic sac, 1443f
Embryo transfer, 1278
Embryogenesis, spine and, 871–872
Embryologic age, 1301
Embryology
  abdominal wall, 1560–1562, 1561f, 1562f, 1563f
  cardiovascular system, 1008–1010
  definition of, 80
  digestive system, 1572–1576, 1573f
  of face, 1493–1495, 1493f
  of neural axis, 1522–1523
  thoracic cavity, 1545
Embryonal cell carcinoma, 728t
Embryonic abnormalities, 1333–1340
  abdominal wall defects, 1338–1339, 1339f
  cardiac anomalies, 1334
  cranial anomalies, 1334–1338, 1335f, 1336t
  cystic hygroma, 1339–1340, 1339f
  first-trimester umbilical cord cysts, 1340, 1340f
  nuchal translucency, 1333–1334, 1334f
  obstructive uropathy, 1339
Embryonic bradycardia, 1327
Embryonic demise, 1320
Embryonic development, 1304t, 1311f
Embryonic heart, 1313, 1314f, 1314t
Embryonic heart rate (EHR), 1382, 1383b, 1383f
Embryonic oligohydramnios, 1327
Embryonic period, 1310
Embryonic tachycardia, 1327
Emergency medical situations, 65–67
  cardiopulmonary resuscitation, 66–67, 66f
  choking, 65–66, 65b, 65f
Emergent ultrasound procedures, 561, 581b
  abdominal trauma assessment, 561–563
  in acute pelvic pain, 578–579
  in appendicitis, 573–575, 574f, 576f
  in epigastric pain, 568–570
  in extremity swelling and pain, 579–581, 580f
  in flank pain caused by urolithiasis, 573–574, 573t
  in paraumbilical hernia, 573t, 575–578, 576f, 577f
  in pericardial effusion, 570–571, 571f, 572f
  in right upper quadrant pain, 567–568
  in scrotal trauma and torsion, 579, 579f, 580f
Emesis basins, 49, 49f
Emotional stability, 5b
Emphysematous cholecystitis, 294t–295t, 296–297
Emphysematous pyelonephritis, 478, 479f
Employment, 5–6
Encephalocele, 1497, 1498f, 1504f, 1525–1526, 1527f, 1568
  Meckel-Gruber syndrome and, 1528f
  occipital, 1527f

Endarterectomy, 1083–1084, 1084f
End-diastolic velocity, 1112–1113
Endemic goiter, 691
Endocardial cushion, 1048
Endocardium, 896
Endocrine, 360
Endodermal sinus tumors, 1252
Endometrial canal, 1185f, 1195, 1196f
Endometrial carcinoma, 1223–1224, 1224b, 1224f
Endometrial fluid, 1223f, 1224–1225
Endometrial fluid collections
  large, 1225, 1225f
  small, 1224–1225, 1225f
Endometrial hyperplasia, 1220, 1220b, 1221f
Endometrial polyps
  description of, 1220–1221
  sonographic findings in, 1221, 1222f
Endometriomas, 1243, 1243f, 1267–1270, 1268f, 1269f
Endometriosis, 1242–1243, 1242f, 1260, 1267–1270, 1268f, 1268t, 1269f
  female infertility and, 1277
  pelvic sites of, 1268f
  sonographic findings in, 1242, 1242f, 1243f, 1268t, 1269–1270
Endometritis, 1221–1222, 1222b, 1260, 1261b, 1261f, 1266–1267, 1267f
Endometrium, 1165
  blood supply to, 1169
  changes in, 1172–1174, 1172f, 1173f
  female infertility and
    evaluation of, 1274–1275, 1274f, 1275f
    monitoring of, 1277–1278
  measurement of, 1186, 1218, 1218t
  pathology of, 1217–1225
    carcinoma, 1223–1224, 1224b, 1224f
    endometritis, 1221–1222, 1222b
    hyperplasia, 1220, 1220b, 1221f
    intrauterine synechiae, 1222–1223, 1223f
    large endometrial fluid collections, 1225, 1225f
    small endometrial fluid collections, 1224–1225, 1225f
    polyps, 1220–1221, 1222f
  sonographic evaluation of, 1195–1196, 1195f
  sonohysterography of, 1218–1220, 1219f
  thickness of, 1218t
  transabdominal pelvic ultrasound of, 1181
Endovascular aneurysm repair, 523f, 524
Endovascular graft, 196f
End-to-side hepaticojejunostomy, 588
Enhancement, 156, 156f, 157f
  definition of, 156
  increased through-transmission, 130, 133f
Enteric isolation, 55
Environment cleanliness, 57
Environmental control, 47–48, 47f, 48f
Enzymes, hepatic, 228–229, 228t
Eosinophilic cardiomyopathy, 992, 993f
Ependymitis, 847–848
Epicardium, 896
Epicondylitis, 72, 72f
Epididymal cysts, 717t, 722
Epididymis
  description of, 709
  enlarge, 718t
  sonographic evaluation of, 709f
Epididymitis, 579f, 717t, 719, 719f

Epididymo-orchitis, 718
Epidural hemorrhages, 835
Epigastric hernias, 433
Epigastric pain, 568–570, 573t
Epigastrium, 219, 564
Epignathus, 1512, 1512f
Epineurium, 739
Epiploic foramen, 98, 99f
Epispadias, 1603
Epithelial ovarian tumors
    mucinous cystadenocarcinoma, 1247, 1248b, 1249f
    mucinous cystadenoma, 1247, 1248b, 1249f
    serous cystadenocarcinomas, 1248–1249, 1249b, 1250b, 1251f
    serous cystadenomas, 1249b, 1249f, 1250f, 1252f
Epstein-Barr virus (EBV), 623
Ergonomic exam tables, 78
Ergonomics
    definition of, 68
    economics of, 77–78
    history of, 68–70
    industry awareness/changes and, 72–74
    work practice changes and, 74–77, 76f, 77f
    work-related musculoskeletal disorders (WRMSDs), 70, 71f
    workstation setup, 78–79, 79f
EROA. see Estimated regurgitant orifice area
Erythrocytes, 83, 332
Erythropoiesis, 83
Esophageal stenosis, 1573
Esophagus
    anatomy of, 390, 390f
    atresia of, 1584–1585, 1585f
    fetal
        abnormalities of, 1584–1586, 1585f
        embryology of, 1573
        sonographic evaluation of, 1577, 1577f
    vascular anatomy of, 392, 394f
Estimated fetal weight (EFW), 1397
Estimated regurgitant orifice area (EROA), 955–956
Estrogen, 497, 1168, 1220b, 1234
ESWL. see Extracorporeal shockwave lithotripsy
Ethics, for obstetric sonography, 1294, 1299b
    confidentiality of findings, 1298
    defined, 1294–1295
    medical
        history of, 1295
        principles, 1295–1298
Ethmocephaly, 1503, 1504f, 1534–1535, 1535f
Euthyroid, 685
Ex utero intrapartum treatment (EXIT) procedure, 1512
Exam tables, ergonomic, 78
Excitation contraction coupling, 904
Excretion, urinary, 438
Exencephaly, 1568
Exercise, 77, 77f
Exocoelomic cavity, 1443f
Exocrine, 360
Exophthalmia, 1502
Exophthalmos, 698–699
Explicit permission, 1298
Exstrophy, bladder, 1564t, 1567–1568, 1568f, 1569f
Extension, 853
External carotid artery (ECA), 1070–1071, 1075

External genitalia
    development of, 1595, 1595f, 1596f
    female, 1159, 1159f, 1595
    male, 1595
External iliac arteries, 108, 113f, 612f, 1169, 1170f
External iliac veins, 108, 113f, 1131
External jugular vein (EJV), 1133
External oblique muscle, 90, 90f
Extracorporeal liver, 1564t
Extracorporeal membrane oxygenation (ECMO)
    description of, 767, 821
    in neonates, 835
Extracorporeal shockwave lithotripsy (ESWL), 483–485
Extracranial carotid system, 1070f
Extracranial cerebrovascular evaluation, 1069, 1085b
    anatomy, 1070–1071
Extrahepatic biliary atresia, 1574
Extrahepatic biliary obstructions, 312–313, 313f
Extrahepatic mass, 259, 261t, 263f
Extrapancreatic fluid collections, 371–372, 372f
Extraperitoneal hematomas, 430, 431f
Extrarenal pelvis, 444–445, 446f, 448f
Extratesticular cystic mass, 718t
Extratesticular masses, 718t, 722
Extreme shortness of breath, 570–572
Extremities
    fetal ultrasound, 1408t
    swelling of, 579–581, 580f
Eye, protection for, 56

F

Face, fetal, 1352–1355, 1492, 1518b. see also Facial profile, fetal
    abnormalities of, 1496–1518
    congenital anomalies of, 1492
    coronal facial view, anatomic landmarks of, 1354, 1354f
        fetal ears, 1355, 1355f
        fetal lips, 1354–1355, 1354f
        fetal tongue, 1354
    embryology of, 1493–1495, 1493f
    facial profile, 1352–1354, 1353f
    fetal eye orbits, 1352, 1353f
    nasal bone, 1354
    sonographic evaluation of, 1495–1496, 1495f, 1496b
        additional imaging, 1517–1518, 1517f
        three-dimensional, 1516–1517, 1517f
    ultrasound, 1408t
Face shield, 56
Facial clefting, 1508f, 1509–1510, 1511f
Facial profile, fetal
    abnormalities of, 1496–1518, 1496b
        ear, 1500–1501, 1501f
        face, 1506–1509
        forehead, 1496–1498, 1497f, 1498f, 1499f
        larynx, 1511–1512, 1512f
        lip, 1506–1509, 1508f, 1509f
        mandible, 1499–1500, 1500b, 1500f
        mid-face, 1503–1510, 1506f, 1507f
        neck, 1512–1516
        nose, 1505–1506, 1507f
        orbits, 1501–1503, 1502f, 1503f
        palate, 1506–1509, 1508f, 1509f, 1510f
        skull, 1498–1499, 1499f
        tongue, 1510–1511, 1511f, 1512f
        trachea, 1511–1512, 1512f
    sonography of, 1496b

Falciform ligament (FL), 98, 106, 221–223, 222f
Fallopian tubes, 93f, 1167, 1167b, 1167f
    carcinoma of, 1257
    female infertility and, 1275–1276, 1275f
    sonographic evaluation of, 579, 1196–1197, 1197f
    ultrasound examination of, 1178b
False aneurysm, 190–191, 191f, 974t
False lumen, 1078
False-negative hydronephrosis, 477–478
False pelvis, 93f, 94, 94f, 495, 1159–1160, 1159f
    anatomy of, 492
    muscles of, 1160f, 1161
False-positive hydronephrosis, 477, 478b
Falx cerebri, 815
Fan, 126
Fasciculi, 739
FAST. see Focused assessment with sonography for trauma
Fat necrosis, 658t, 664, 665f
Fats, 227–228
    retroperitoneal, 506
    subcutaneous, 646, 647f
Fatty breast, 648–649, 649f
Fatty infiltration, 243–244, 244b
    causes of, 244b
    focal, 244, 245f
    sonographic findings in, 244, 244f, 245f
Fatty liver, 243–244, 244b
    in children, 768–769
    description of, 227–228, 608
Fear, illness and, 60
Fecalith, 404
Female infertility
    evaluation of, 1272, 1279b
        cervix, 1272–1273
        endometrium, 1274–1275, 1274f, 1275f
        fallopian tubes, 1275–1276, 1275f
        ovaries, 1276–1277, 1276f, 1277f
        uterus, 1273, 1273f
    peritoneal factors in, 1277
    treatment options for, 1277–1278
        endometrial monitoring, 1277–1278, 1278f
        intrauterine insemination, 1278
        ovulation induction therapy, 1277, 1277f
        in vitro fertilization and embryo transfer, 1278
Female pelvis, 92, 1157, 1175b, 1201b
    abdominal scanning at level of, 108, 116f
    bladder, 1161–1162, 1162b, 1163f
    blood supply to, 1191–1192
    bowel, 1174–1175, 1174b
    endometrial changes and, 1172–1174, 1172f, 1173f
    follicular development and ovulation and, 1170–1172, 1171f
    landmarks of, 1158f, 1159–1160
        bony pelvis, 1159–1160, 1159f
        external, 1159, 1159f
        pelvic cavity and perineum, 1160, 1160b, 1160f
    muscles of, 1160–1161, 1160b
    recesses, 1174–1175
    ureters, 1161–1162, 1162b, 1163f
    vasculature of, 1168b, 1169, 1169f, 1170f
Female pseudohermaphrodites, 1618
Femoral arteries, 178t, 1111–1112
    Doppler image of, 1121f
    narrowing of, 1121f
    stenosis in, 1121f

Femoral head, 851, 852f
  coverage of, 854
Femoral veins, 1130f, 1131, 1142f
Femur length (FL), 1389, 1389b, 1389f, 1389t
Fetal age, 1378
Fetal capillaries in villi, 1443f
Fetal circulation, 1010–1012, 1011f, 1012f, 1446f
Fetal death, 1417, 1417f
Fetal echocardiography, 1008, 1030b
  color flow Doppler, 1015, 1015f
  ductal and aortic arch views, 1026–1029, 1027f, 1028f
  evaluation, 1017–1030
  four-chamber view, 1017–1021, 1018b, 1019f, 1020f, 1021f
  instrumentation, 1013
  landmarks, 1016–1017, 1016f, 1017f, 1018f
  left and right ventricular outflow tracts
    crisscross view, 1021, 1022b, 1022f
    five-chamber view, 1021, 1021b, 1022f
    long-axis view, 1022–1023, 1023b, 1023f, 1024f, 1025f, 1026f
    short-axis view, 1023–1026, 1026b, 1026f, 1027f
  motion mode imaging, 1013, 1014f, 1014t
  pulsed Doppler, 1014, 1014f, 1014t
  risk factors indicating, 1012–1013
  three-dimensional imaging, 1015, 1015f
  three-vessel view, 1029–1030, 1029f
  transducer requirements, 1013, 1013f
Fetal growth assessment, by sonography, 1395, 1405b
  diagnostic criteria, 1396b, 1397–1399
    abdominal circumference, 1397
    biparietal diameter, 1397
    estimated fetal weight, 1398
    head circumference to abdominal circumference ratio, 1397–1398, 1398f
  fetal well-being, tests of, 1399–1404, 1399f
    biophysical profile, 1399–1401, 1399b
    Doppler sonography, 1402–1404, 1402f
    nonstress test, 1401–1402, 1402f
  intrauterine growth restriction, 1395–1397, 1396b
  macrosomia and large for gestational age, 1404–1405
Fetal heart rate, 1012
Fetal lobulation, 444–445, 446t, 447f
Fetal measurements, 1382–1388
  biparietal diameter, 1383, 1384b, 1384f, 1384t, 1385f
    growth-adjusted sonar age, 1384–1385
  cephalic index, 1385
  coronal view, vertical cranial diameter, and 3D biparietal diameter correction, 1387, 1387b, 1387f
  head circumference, 1384b, 1385, 1385f, 1386b, 1386t
Fetal membranes, 1481–1486, 1482f
  amniotic band syndrome, 1483–1485, 1485f, 1486f
  amniotic fluid and, 1474, 1489b–1490b
  amniotic sheets, 1485–1486, 1486f
  ruptured, 1482–1483, 1484f
Fetal period (weeks 9-14), 1306–1313
  embryo during, 1308–1310, 1309f, 1310f
  gestational sac during, 1307–1310, 1307f, 1307t
  yolk sac during, 1307–1308, 1307f, 1308f

Fetal presentation, sonography of second and third trimesters, 1345–1348, 1345f, 1346f
  breech, 1346–1347, 1347f
  situs, 1347
  transverse, 1347, 1348f
  vertex, 1345–1346, 1346f
Fetal thoracic circumference measurements, 1550t
Fetor hepaticus, 229
Fetus, 1301
  abdominal wall of, 1562
  diaphragm of, abnormalities of, 1555–1558, 1555f
  heart of
    crisscross view of, 1021, 1022b, 1022f
    five-chamber view of, 1021, 1021b, 1022f
    four-chamber view of, 1017–1021, 1018b, 1019f, 1020f, 1021f
Fetus papyraceous, 1421, 1422f
Fibrinogen, 81
Fibroadenoma, 658t, 661–662, 662f
Fibrocystic dysplasia/fibrocystic changes, 660–661, 661f
Fibroelastoma, papillary, 998, 1000f
Fibroids, 1340, 1341f
  submucosal, 1275f
  uterine, 1273f, 1274–1275
    various locations, 1210f
Fibrolipomas, 883, 883f, 884f, 885f
Fibromas, 1254–1255, 1256f
Fibromuscular dysplasia (FMD), 480–481, 1078–1079
Fibrosarcomas, 507
Fibrosis, retroperitoneal, 509–510, 509f
Fibrous pericardium, 980, 981f
Fibula, fetal measurement, 1390, 1390b, 1390f
Field of view, 22
Filum terminale, 873, 876, 877f, 880, 880b, 880f
Fimbriae, 1167
Fine-needle aspiration (FNA), 532–533
  needles for, 532–533, 533f
First-degree heart block, 1065
First trimester pregnancy
  complications during, 1316, 1319, 1342b
    abnormal or absent cardiac activity, 1326–1327, 1326t
    bleeding, 1320–1326
      abnormal sac criteria, 1322–1323
      absent intrauterine sac, 1320–1322, 1321t, 1322f
      anembryonic pregnancy, 1323, 1323f, 1324b
      gestational sac without embryo or yolk sac, 1322
      gestational trophoblastic disease, 1323–1326, 1324f, 1325f, 1326f
      placental hematomas, 1320
      subchorionic hemorrhage, 1320, 1321f
    embryonic abnormalities, 1333–1340
      abdominal wall defects, 1338–1339, 1339f
      cardiac anomalies, 1334
      cranial anomalies, 1334–1338, 1335f, 1336f
      cystic hygroma, 1339–1340, 1339f
      nuchal translucency, 1333–1334, 1334f
      obstructive uropathy, 1339
      umbilical cord cysts, 1340, 1340f
    embryonic development of yolk sac and amnion, 1327
    pelvic masses, 1329t, 1340
    positive hCG with intrauterine fluid collection without yolk sac or embryo, 1316

First trimester pregnancy *(Continued)*
    positive hCG without intrauterine fluid collection or adnexal mass, 1316
  early embryonic stage, 1300, 1317b
  embryology of, 1305–1306, 1306b, 1306f
  gestational age assessment, 1379–1382
    crown-rump length, 1381–1382, 1381b, 1381f, 1382f, 1382t
    embryonic heart rate, 1382, 1383b, 1383f
    gestational sac diameter, 1379–1381, 1379b, 1379f, 1380f, 1380t, 1381b, 1381f
  gestational age determination, 1313–1316
  overview of, 1301–1303
  risk assessment, 1316–1318
  sonography during, indications for, 1284b, 1289–1290
  transvaginal sonographic technique and evaluation during, 1305–1306, 1305f
  at 6 to 10 weeks of gestational age, 1310–1313, 1310t
    embryonic cranium and spine, 1310–1313, 1311f, 1312f
    embryonic heart, 1313, 1314f, 1314t
    limb development, 1313, 1313f
    physiologic herniation of bowel, 1313, 1314f
    skeletal ossification, 1313, 1313f
  fetal period (weeks 9-14), 1306–1313
    embryo during, 1308–1310, 1309f, 1310f
    gestational sac during, 1307–1310, 1307f, 1307t
    yolk sac during, 1307–1308, 1307f, 1308f
Fissures
  liver, 221–223, 222f, 239
  neonatal, 817–818, 818f
Fistula
  arteriovenous, 482–483, 484f, 589, 617f
  dialysis, 1123f
  pancreatic, 636, 637f
Five-chamber view
  apical, 922b, 932–938, 936f, 937f, 938b
  of left and right ventricular outflow tracts, 1021, 1021b, 1022f
  of ventricular septal aneurysm, 1040f
FL. *see* Falciform ligament
Flank pain, 573–574, 573t
Flat flow velocity profile, 905–906
Flexion, 853
"Floating gallstones," 303, 305f
Flow cytometry, 538–539
Fluid collections
  in adhesions, 1240, 1241f
  endometrial
    large, 1225, 1225f
    small, 1224–1225, 1225f
  pleural, 559
  retroperitoneal, 508–509
  scrotal, 718t
  ultrasound-guided, 534–535
Fluid-fluid level, 130
FMD. *see* Fibromuscular dysplasia
FNA. *see* Fine-needle aspiration
FNH. *see* Focal nodular hyperplasia
Focal banding, 156, 157f
Focal brain necrosis, 837–838
Focal enhancement, 156, 157f
Focal fatty infiltration, 244, 245f
Focal fatty sparing, 244, 245f

Focal hepatic disease, 260–265, 264t
Focal nodular hyperplasia (FNH), 268–269, 272f
   contrast-enhanced ultrasound imaging of, 518, 520f
   liver findings, 271t
Focal orchitis, 717t
Focal pyelonephritis, 806f
Focal sparing, 608
Focal zone, 13–14, 22, 22f
Focused assessment with sonography for trauma (FAST), 563f
   in blunt trauma, 563–567, 563b, 563f, 564b, 564f, 565f
   in parenchymal injury, 566–567, 567f
Foley catheter, 43–44
Follicle-stimulating hormone (FSH), 1171, 1231–1233
Follicular adenomas, 692
Follicular carcinoma, 694–696
Follicular cysts
   description of, 1231–1233, 1233f
   ovarian, 1231–1233, 1233f
Follicular development, 1170–1172, 1171f
Fontanels, 814, 815b, 815f
   anterior, 822f, 824, 824f
Food allergies, 763t
Foot, ulcers of, 1118
Foramen of Bochdalek, 1555, 1556f
Foramen of Monro, 816
Foramen of Morgagni, 1555–1556, 1556f
Foramen ovale, 1014t
   fetal circulation, 1446f
Foramen secundum, 1009, 1010f
Ford Motor Company, 69
Foregut, 1573–1574, 1574f
Forehead, abnormalities of, 1496–1498, 1497f, 1498f, 1499f
Formed elements, 81
Fornices, 1162, 1164f
Fossa ovale, 1010
Fossa ovalis, 1037
Four-chamber view
   apical, 572f, 921f, 922b, 922f, 941f, 943f
      right heart, 938b
   of congenital heart disease, 1033, 1034f
   of cor triatriatum, 1059f
   of critical aortic stenosis, 1051f
   of Ebstein anomaly, 1043–1045, 1044f
   of fetal heart, 1017–1021, 1018b, 1019f, 1020f, 1021f
   of fetus, 1017–1021, 1018b, 1019f, 1020f, 1021f
   of hypoplastic left heart, 1053f
   of membranous septal defect, 1040f
   of mitral and tricuspid valves, 1014f
   of ostium primum atrial septal defect, 1038f
   of rhabdomyomas, 1058f
   of single ventricle, 1058–1059, 1058f, 1059f
   subcostal, 939f, 947f
   of total anomalous pulmonary venous return, 1060f
   of transposition of the great arteries, 1054f
Four-chambered heart, 1009, 1010f
Four-dimensional ultrasound, 20–21, 20f
Fourth ventricle, neonatal, 827
Fracture bedpan, 48, 48f
Frame rate, 18
Frank dislocation, 860
Frank-Starling law of the heart, 903

Free-hand techniques, 535–536
   one-person, 536f
   two-person, 535f
Frequency, 12, 12t
Frequency shift, 22
Fresnel, Augustin, 6
Frontal bossing, 1352–1354, 1497, 1497f
Frontonasal dysplasia, 1503, 1505f, 1510
Fry, William, 7
FSH. see Follicle-stimulating hormone
Full-thickness rotator cuff tears, 752, 753b, 753f
Functional cysts, 1236
   corpus luteum cysts, 1236–1237, 1237b, 1237f
   follicular cysts, 1236, 1237b
   hemorrhagic cysts, 1237, 1238f
   theca-lutein cysts, 1237, 1238b, 1239f
Fundus
   description of, 390, 1162–1163
   illustration of, 1166f
   transvaginal scanning of, 1186, 1186f, 1193
Fused crossed renal ectopia, 448
Fusiform aneurysm, 191, 192f
Fusion technology, 540–542, 540f, 541f, 542f

G

Gain, 21–22, 21f, 26, 715–716, 715t
Galactoceles, 663, 663f
Galactography, of breast, 676, 677f
Galeazzi sign, 858–859, 859f
Galenic venous malformation, 845, 846f
Galilei, Galileo, 6
Gallbladder, 88, 89f
   abdominal scanning of
      at level of liver, 108–109, 118f
      at level of liver and right kidney transverse, 107, 111f
      at level of liver and right kidney longitudinal, 107, 111f
      at level of right kidney, 107, 111f
   anatomy of, 282f, 283
      variations in, 283f, 285, 287f
   double, 288f
   fetal
      abnormalities of, 1582–1583
      sonographic evaluation of, 1579
   laboratory data of, 285
   longitudinal scans of, 141
   pathology of, 289–308, 294t–295t
      carcinoma, 306–308, 309f, 310f
      cholelithiasis, 294t–295t, 300, 301f, 302f, 303f, 304f
      gallbladder disease, 290–293
      porcelain gallbladder, 294t–295t, 303, 305f
      sludge, 290–293, 294t–295t, 295f
      torsion, 299–300
      wall thickening, 293, 296b, 296f
   pediatric, 765–766, 765b, 765f
   physiology of, 285
   removal of, 285
   septations of, 288f
   sonographic evaluation of, 284f, 286f, 287–289, 290f, 291f, 292f
Gallbladder wall, thickening of, 293, 296b, 296f
Gallstones
   in children, 767
   fetal, 1582, 1584f
   floating, 303, 305f
   in hepatic duct, 262f

Gallstones (Continued)
   pancreatitis and, 370
   sonographic findings of, 296, 298f, 299f
Galton, Sir Francis, 6
Gangrenous cholecystitis, 294t–295t, 297, 300f
Garrett, William, 7–8
Gartner duct cyst, 1203, 1203f
GASA. see Growth-adjusted sonar age
Gas-containing abscesses, 421–422, 423f
Gastric bezoars, 399–400, 400t, 401f
Gastric carcinoma, 400t, 401–402, 402f
Gastric tumors, 400–401
Gastrin, 393
Gastrinoma, 381, 384f
Gastrocnemius muscle, 735f, 755f
Gastrocnemius veins, 1139
Gastroduodenal artery (GDA), 179–180, 180f
   abdominal scanning of
      at gallbladder and right kidney level, 107, 110f
      at level of liver, inferior vena cava, and pancreas, 109, 120f
   pancreas and, 359
Gastroesophageal junction, 395, 396f
Gastrohepatic ligament, 390
Gastrointestinal (GI) system, 83–86
   assessment of, 84
   diseases and disorders of, 84–86, 85t
   fetal, 1365–1366, 1365f, 1576–1579
   normal findings for, 84
Gastrointestinal (GI) tract
   anatomy of, 389–393, 390f, 411b–412b
   fetal, abnormalities of, 1584–1590, 1584b
      bowel, 1586–1590
      esophagus, stomach, duodenum, 1584–1586, 1585f
   pathology of, 399–412, 400t
      acute appendicitis, 403–405, 404t, 406f
      Crohn's disease, 404t, 409, 409f
      duplication cysts, 399, 400f, 400t
      gastric bezoars, 399–400, 400t, 401f
      gastric carcinoma, 400t, 401–402, 402f
      leiomyomas, 400, 400t, 401f
      leiomyosarcoma, 400t, 402, 403f, 404t
      lymphoma, 400t, 402, 402f, 404t
      Meckel's diverticulitis, 404t, 408–409
      metastatic disease, 400t, 402, 403f
      mucocele, 404t, 405–408, 408f
      obstruction and dilation, 403, 404t, 405f
      polyps, 400, 400t, 401f
   physiology and laboratory data of, 393–394
   sonographic evaluation of, 394–399, 396f
      appendix, 398
      colon, 398–399, 399f
      duodenum, 396–397, 397f
      layers of bowel and, 394, 394b
      small bowel, 397–398, 398f
      stomach, 395–396, 396f
   vascular anatomy of, 392–393, 394f
Gastrophrenic ligament, 390
Gastroschisis, 1338, 1466–1467, 1466f, 1562, 1564t, 1565–1566, 1566f, 1575–1576, 1575f
   left-side, 1567f
   omphalocele versus, 1562, 1564b
   sonographic findings in, 1565, 1567f
Gastrosplenic ligament, 326, 328f, 390, 418, 418f
Gate, 23–24
Gaucher disease, 332, 340

G-cell tumors, 381, 384f
GDA. see Gastroduodenal artery
Gender pronouns, 62t
Genetic amniocentesis, prenatal diagnosis of congenital anomalies, 1431–1432, 1431f, 1432f
Genital ridge, 1593
Genitalia
　external female, 1159, 1159f
　fetal, 1368–1369, 1368f, 1369f
　　ultrasound, 1408t
　sonographic evaluation of, 1596–1598, 1598f
Genitourinary pathology, 797f
Genitourinary system, 86–88
Germ cell tumors, 507–508, 728, 1250–1252
　dysgerminoma, 1252, 1254f
　endodermal sinus tumors, 1252
　sonographic findings in, 728–730, 729f
　teratomas
　　dermoid tumors, 1250–1251, 1252b, 1252f, 1253f
　　immature and mature, 1251–1252, 1253f
Germinal epithelium, 1168
Germinal matrix, 818, 832
Germinal matrix-intraventricular hemorrhages (GM-IVHs), 832, 833b
Gerota fascia, 92, 436, 492
Gestational age, 814t, 1284–1285, 1301, 1378
　determination of, first trimester, 1313–1316
　　crown-rump length, 1301, 1304f, 1315, 1315f, 1316f
　　mean gestational sac size, 1314, 1314f, 1315f
Gestational sac, 1289–1290
　abnormal
　　absent intrauterine sac, 1320–1322, 1321t, 1322f
　　criteria, 1322–1323
　　sonographic findings associated with, 1324b
　　without embryo or yolk sac, 1322
　　sonographic findings of, during fetal period, 1307–1310, 1307f, 1307t
Gestational sac diameter (GSD), 1379–1381, 1379b, 1379f, 1380f, 1380t, 1381b, 1381f
Gestational trophoblastic disease, 1323–1326, 1324f, 1325f, 1326f, 1456–1457, 1457f
Gilbreth, Frank, 69
Gilbreth, Lillian, 69
Glioependymal cyst, 1523t
Glisson's capsule, 221–223
Globulins, 81, 231
Glomerulus, 437
Gloves
　removing, 52
　standard precautions and, 56, 56f
Glucagon, 361, 361t
Glucocorticoids, 497
Glucose, 362
Gluteus maximus, 115f, 853
Gluteus medius, 853
Gluteus minimus, 853
Glycogen storage disease, 243t, 248–249, 250f
GM-IVHs. see Germinal matrix-intraventricular hemorrhages
Goiters, 683
　endemic, 691
　fetal, 1514–1515, 1516f
　nontoxic simple, 691, 691t
Gonadal artery, 186
Gonadal veins, 203–204

Gonadotropin-releasing hormones (GnRHs), 1171
Gowns
　donning, 54
　standard precautions and, 57
Graafian follicles, 1171–1172
Graf's alpha angle, 860–866, 862b, 862f
Graf's beta angle, 860–866, 862b, 862f
Graft, aortic, 194–195, 196f
Granulocytes, 83
Granulocytopoietic abnormalities, 342
Granulomas, sperm, 726, 726f
Granulomatous disease, chronic, 264t, 266, 268f
Granulomatous mastitis, 663
Granulosas, 1255, 1256f
Grating lobes, 151, 153f
Graves disease, 698–699
　hyperthyroidism caused by, 685, 685b
　sonographic findings in, 699, 699f
Gravidity, 1286
Gray scale, 17–18
Gray-scale harmonic imaging (GSHI), 516f, 1137–1140
Great pancreatic artery, 180
Great vessels
　abnormalities of, 1054–1058
　　coarctation of the aorta, 1055–1056, 1057f
　　ductal constriction, 1057
　　interrupted aortic arch, 1056–1057
　　transposition of the great arteries, 1054, 1054f, 1055f
　　truncus arteriosus, 1054–1055, 1055f, 1056f
　anatomy of, 894–901, 895f, 896f
Greater omentum, 97, 97f, 390, 413–414, 416f
Greater sac, 97, 98f, 414, 416f
Greater saphenous vein (GSV), 1132
Greater trochanter, 851
Grey Turner sign, 188, 375
Griffith, James, 8
Gross anatomy, 80
Growth-adjusted sonar age (GASA), 1384–1385
Growth restriction, 1327
GSD. see Gestational sac diameter
GSHI. see Gray-scale harmonic imaging
GSV. see Greater saphenous vein
Gutters, 99–100, 414
Guyon canal, 748, 749f
Gynecomastia, 651–652, 652f
Gyrus, 817

H

Hamartoma
　mesenchymal, 775
　of spleen, 349–351
"Hamburger" sign, 1598, 1598f
Hammurabi, Prince, 1295
Hand, 747–749
　anomalies, 1633, 1633f, 1634f
Hand sanitizers, 53, 53b
Hand-Schüller-Christian disease, 342
Hand washing, 52–53, 53b
Harmonic imaging (HI), 18–20, 19f, 515–516, 540
　gray-scale, 516f
　intermittent imaging and, 516
Hartmann pouch, 285
Hashimoto thyroiditis, 700, 700f
Haustra, 390–391
Haustral folds, 1578, 1579f

HCC. see Hepatocellular carcinoma
hCG. see Human chorionic gonadotropin
Head and neck, fetal ultrasound, 1408t
Health Insurance Portability and Accountability Act (HIPAA), 32, 62–63, 1298
Heart
　aortic arch and branches, 901, 901f
　aortic valve, 901, 901f, 935f, 945–946, 946f, 950f
　apical views of, 919f, 922b
　auscultation of valves of, 904–905, 905f
　cardiac cycle, 901–903, 901b, 902f
　development of, 1009–1010, 1009f, 1010f
　electrical activity of, 904, 904f
　electrical conduction system, 903, 903f
　embryonic, 1313, 1314f, 1314t
　FAST scan of chambers of, 564, 564f
　fetal, 1359–1360, 1360f, 1361f
　　crisscross view of, 1021, 1022b, 1022f
　　five-chamber view of, 1021, 1021b, 1022f
　　four-chamber view of, 1017–1021, 1018b, 1019f, 1020f, 1021f
　Frank-Starling law of, 903
　great vessels of, 894–901, 895f, 896f
　heart wall linings, 896–897, 897f
　interatrial septum, 897, 897f
　interventricular septum, 900, 900f, 946, 951f
　intracardiac pressures and volumes, 909–910, 909f
　left atrium, 894, 899, 899f, 945–946, 950f
　left ventricle, 946, 951f
　mechanical conduction system, 903–904
　mitral valve, 899, 899f, 900f, 943–944, 950f
　M-mode imaging of, 920, 943–952, 950b
　pericardial sac, 895f, 896
　pulmonary trunk, 898, 898f
　pulmonary valve, 898, 898f
　right atrium, 897, 897f
　subcostal view of, 564f
　thorax and, fetal ultrasound, 1408t
　tricuspid valve, 897, 897f
Heart failure, AFP and, 1428
Heart rate
　fetal, 1012
　intracranial arterial velocities and, 1097, 1097b
Heart sounds, 904–905
Height-adjustable stools, 78
Heimlich maneuver
　definition of, 65
　techniques of, 65
Heister valve, 285
Hemangioblastoma, 377
Hemangioendothelioma, infantile, 774–775, 775t
Hemangiomas, 1497–1498, 1498f, 1499f
　cavernous
　　contrast-enhanced imaging of, 518, 520f
　　hepatic, 268, 271t, 272f
　of cord, 1467, 1467f
　hepatic, 608
　liver, 519f
Hemangiosarcoma, splenic, 352
Hematoceles, 579, 717t, 725–726
Hematochezia, 85t, 86
Hematocrit, 83, 332–333, 438, 1097
Hematomas
　bladder-flap, 430
　of cord, 1467
　extraperitoneal, 430, 431f
　intramural, 977, 977f
　intramuscular, 580f, 738f

Hematomas (Continued)
  in liver transplantation patients, 598, 603f
  in Morison's pouch, 539f
  in pancreatic transplantation patients, 636
  placental, 1320
  in renal transplantation patients, 620–621, 624f
  scrotal, 714f, 717t
  splenic, 347–348, 348f, 349f, 566f
  subfascial, 430
Hematometrocolpos, 1205f, 1225
Hematopoiesis, 326, 337b, 1307
Hematuria, 438
Hemianopsia, 1072
Hemifacial microsomia, 1500–1501
Hemihypertrophy, 773
Hemiparesis, 1072
Hemobilia, 315, 317f
Hemochromatosis, 243t, 249, 250f
Hemodynamics, 915ba
  Bernoulli equation, 913–914, 914f
  cardiac cycle, 909–910, 909f
  cardiac output, 910, 1097
  in cardiac tamponade, 985b
  color Doppler imaging, 912, 912f, 913f
  continuity principle, 915
  continuous wave Doppler, 913, 913f
  definition of, 908
  Doppler effect, 910–911, 911f
  Doppler frequency shift, 910–911, 910f, 911f
  extracranial arterial, 1071
  pulsed wave Doppler, 911–912, 911f
  right atrial pressure, 914, 914f
  stroke volume, 910, 914
  terminology associated with, 908
Hemoglobin, 83, 332, 438
Hemolysis, 1409
Hemolytic anemia, 341
Hemoperitoneum, 563
Hemopoiesis, 1574
Hemorrhage, 399, 426
  adrenal
    description of, 503, 503f
    illustration of, 503f
    neonatal/pediatric, 796t, 807, 808f
  epidural, 835
  intracerebellar, 834–835, 837f
  intracranial, 832–836, 833b, 1523t
  intraparenchymal, 566, 834, 836f
  intraventricular, 816, 833–834, 833f, 834f, 835f
  retroperitoneal, 508, 508f
  subchorionic, 1320, 1321f
Hemorrhagic corpus luteum cysts, 1237, 1238f
Hemorrhagic cysts, 1237, 1238f
Hemorrhagic pancreatitis, 369t, 375, 376f
Hemosiderin, 332
Henry, Walter, 8
Hepatic adenoma, 250f, 269–270, 273f
Hepatic arteries, 223, 225f
  anomalies in, 242–243
  Doppler observations of, 256t
  sonographic findings of, 260t
Hepatic artery
  Doppler flow patterns in, 212–214, 212b, 213f
  pseudoaneurysms of, 597, 601f
  stenosis of, after liver transplantation, 596, 599f
  thrombosis of, after liver transplantation, 596, 600f
Hepatic blood flow, 517
Hepatic candidiasis, 264t, 266, 267f

Hepatic congestion, passive, 259–260, 261t, 263f
Hepatic cyst, 260–262, 264t, 608
Hepatic duct, 262f, 282, 282f
Hepatic flexure, 390–391
Hepatic hemangiomas, 775
Hepatic tumors, 268–280, 271t
  benign, 268–269
  contrast-enhanced evaluation of, 517f, 518, 518f, 519f, 520f, 521f
  malignant, 270–280
    hepatocellular carcinoma, 270–271, 271t, 274f, 275f
    lymphoma, 271t, 274–280, 277f
    metastatic disease, 271–274, 271t, 276f
Hepatic vasculature technique, 255t
Hepatic veins (HV), 204–206, 205f, 223, 226f
  abdominal scanning of
    at level of caudate lobe, 106, 107f
    at level of inferior vena cava, pancreas, and superior mesenteric vein, 106f
  characteristics of, 223–225, 227f
  Doppler flow patterns in, 145, 146f, 214, 214b, 215f
  sonographic findings of, 198, 205f, 206f
  stenosis and thrombosis of, after liver transplantation, 594, 595f, 596f
Hepatitis, 244–246
  A, 245–246
  acute, 243t, 246, 246f
  B, 245–246
  C, 245–246, 605–606
  chronic, 243t, 246, 247f
  neonatal, 770, 771f, 771t
Hepatobiliary system
  abnormalities of, 1580–1584
  embryology of, 1574
  physiology and laboratory data of, 225–231
  sonographic evaluation of, 1579–1580
  upper abdomen and, fetal, 1363–1365, 1364f, 1365f
Hepatoblastoma, 773, 774f
Hepatocellular carcinoma (HCC), 270–271, 271t, 274f, 275f
  after liver transplantation, 605, 605f
  contrast-enhanced ultrasound imaging of, 518, 519f
  pediatric, 774
Hepatocellular disease, 228t
  definition of, 225–226
  obstructive disease versus, 225–226
Hepatocytes, 229
Hepatofugal flow, 209, 231
Hepatopetal flow, 209, 231
Hepatorenal recess, 420, 422f
Hepatosplenic candidiasis, 344
Hermaphroditism, true, 1618
Hernia
  abdominal, 432–434, 432f, 433f
  bowel, 1561–1562, 1565–1566, 1567f
  congenital diaphragmatic, 1555–1558, 1556b
  epigastric, 433
  incarcerated, 575
  inguinal, 577f
  left congenital, 1557b
  paraumbilical, 573t, 575–578, 576f, 577f
  reducible, 575
  scrotal, 723–725, 725f
  spigelian, 433
  strangulated, 575
  umbilical, 1563

Hertz, Hellmuth, 7, 8f
Hertz (Hz), 10, 12t
Heterogeneous, 130, 133f
Heterogeneous testicular tumor, 730f
Heterotopic pregnancy, 1279, 1279f, 1332, 1332t
Heterozygous achondroplasia, 1626
HI. see Harmonic imaging
HIFU. see High-intensity focused ultrasound
High-intensity focused ultrasound (HIFU), 1210
High-risk pregnancy
  sonography and, 1406, 1424b–1425b
  fetal factors, 1417–1418
    fetal death, 1417, 1417f
    large for gestational age, 1417
    small for gestational age, 1417–1418, 1418f
  maternal diseases of pregnancy, 1413–1416
    adnexal cysts, 1415
    diabetes, 1413–1415, 1414b, 1414f
    hyperemesis, 1415
    hypertension, 1415
    obesity, 1416
    systemic lupus erythematosus, 1415
    urinary tract disease, 1415
    uterine fibroids, 1416
  maternal factors, 1407–1413
    advanced maternal age, 1407
    alloimmune thrombocytopenia, 1411
    immune and nonimmune hydrops, 1407–1412
    nonimmune hydrops, 1411
    vaginal bleeding, 1412–1413, 1412f, 1413f
  multiple gestation pregnancy, 1418–1424, 1418b
  screening tests, 1406–1407, 1408t
  ultrasound in labor and delivery, 1416–1417
  systemic lupus erythematosus, 1064f
Hilar cholangiocarcinoma, 318
Hilus, 436
Hindgut, 1574f, 1576
Hip
  anatomy of, 851–854
  bones of, 851, 851f
  ligaments of, 853
  movements of, 853, 854f
  muscles of, 853
  stability of, 854
HIPAA. see Health Insurance Portability and Accountability Act
Hippocrates, 1295
Hirschsprung disease, 1588, 1589f
His, bundle of, 903
Histology, 80
History, 1177
Hodgkin lymphoma, 274–280, 351
Holmes, Joseph, 7
Holoprosencephaly, 842–843, 1336, 1336t, 1337f, 1502, 1503f, 1504f, 1523t, 1531–1533, 1532f, 1533f
  alobar, 843, 843f
  definition of, 842
  lobar, 843, 844f
  semilobar, 843, 843f, 1542f
  sonographic findings in, 1533, 1533f, 1534f, 1535f
Homeostasis, 81, 438
Homogeneous, 130, 133f
Homozygous achondroplasia, 1626
Hormone detoxification, 230

Hormone replacement therapy (HRT), 1172–1174
　description of, 1205f
　in menopausal women, 1220b
Horseshoe kidney, 446t, 448–449, 452f, 1601f, 1602–1603
Howry, Douglass, 7, 8f
HPS. *see* Hypertrophic pyloric stenosis
HRT. *see* Hormone replacement therapy
HSG. *see* Hysterosalpingography
Human chorionic gonadotropin (hCG), 1277, 1301
　in ectopic pregnancy, 1303
　prenatal diagnosis of congenital anomalies, 1432–1433
Humerus, fetal measurement, 1390, 1390b, 1391f
HV. *see* Hepatic veins
Hyaloid artery, 1502f
Hydatidiform mole, 1285, 1323–1324, 1324f, 1325f
Hydranencephaly, 837, 843–844, 1538–1539
　differential considerations for, 1524t
　sonographic findings in, 843–844, 845f, 1539, 1539f
Hydrocele, 579f, 710f, 714f, 720, 1617
　idiopathic, 726f
　sonographic appearance of, 717t
Hydrocephalus, 829–832, 1540–1542. *see also* Ventriculomegaly
　acquired, 829
　communicating, 829, 1540, 1540f
　congenital, 829
　definition of, 829
　description of, 814
　Doppler measurements in, 830–831, 831f
　extra-axial spaces in, 831–832, 832b, 832f
　increased intracranial pressure and, 830
　neonatal, 829–832
　noncommunicating, 1540, 1540f
　pericallosal artery in, 831f
　posthemorrhagic, 829
　ventricular measurements, 830
　ventriculoperitoneal shunt for, 829, 829f
Hydrocephaly, 1540f
Hydrometra, 1224
Hydrometrocolpos, 1618
Hydromyelia, 883, 885f
Hydronephrosis, 474–475
　causes of, 475b
　false-negative, 477–478
　false-positive, 477, 478b
　fetal, 1609–1610
　　clinical findings in, 1609–1610, 1610b, 1610f
　　etiology of, 1609
　　in one pole of kidney, 1599–1600
　　prognosis, 1609–1610
　　sonographic findings in, 1610, 1611f
　neonatal/pediatric, 796t
　nonobstructive, 477
　obstructive, 454t–458t, 475–476, 477f
　urinary tract obstruction, 474, 475f, 476f
Hydrops, 1486–1489, 1486f, 1487f
　immune, 1487–1488, 1488f
　nonimmune, 1488–1489, 1489f
Hydrops fetalis, 292f, 1407
Hydrosalpinx, 1261–1263, 1262f, 1262t, 1263f, 1264f
　infertility and, 1275–1276, 1275f
Hydrothorax, 1550–1551
Hydroureters, 1600

Hypercalcemia, 372
Hypercapnia, 1097
Hyperechoic bowel, 1366, 1589, 1589b
Hyperemesis gravidarum, 1415
Hyperglycemia, 227
Hyperlipidemia, 372
Hyperparathyroidism
　primary, 702–704, 703f
　secondary, 704
Hyperplasia
　adrenal, 497
　endometrial, 1220, 1220b, 1221f
　nodular, 690–691, 692f
Hyperplastic cholecystosis, 303–306, 306f, 307f
Hypertelorism, 1392, 1503, 1504f, 1505f
Hypertension, 84, 1415
　dissection caused by, 1079f
Hypertensive nephropathy, 454t–458t, 471
Hyperthyroidism, 685, 685b
Hypertrophic cardiomyopathy, 993–995, 996f, 997b, 997f
Hypertrophic pyloric stenosis (HPS), 777t, 783–787, 783f, 784f, 785f, 786f, 787f
Hypoalbuminemia, 228
Hypocapnia, 1097
Hypoechoic, 130, 133f
Hypoechoic lesion, 718t
Hypoechoic masses, differential considerations for, 728t
Hypoglycemia, 227
Hypomotility, 779
Hypophosphatasia
　congenital, 1628
　sonographic findings in, 1623t
Hypoplasia
　midface, 1505–1506, 1507f, 1508f
　renal, 445–446
Hypoplastic left heart syndrome, 1052–1054, 1052f, 1053f
Hypoplastic right heart syndrome, 1045, 1045f
Hypospadias, 1601
Hypotelorism, 1392, 1502–1503, 1503f, 1534–1535, 1535f
Hypotension, 84
Hypothalamus, neonatal, 818
Hypothyroidism, 685
Hypoxia, neonatal, 814
Hypoxic-ischemic injury lesions, 836–838
Hysterosalpingography (HSG), 1272–1273

I

IA. *see* Iliac arteries
IAE. *see* Induced acoustic emission
ICA. *see* Internal carotid artery
IHF. *see* Immune hydrops fetalis
IJV. *see* Internal jugular vein
ILC. *see* Invasive lobular carcinoma
Ileostomies, 47
Iliac aneurysm, 195
Iliac arteries (IA), 108, 113f, 172, 173f, 174f, 178t, 1169, 1170f
Iliac fossa, 492b, 495
Iliac veins, 108
Iliacus muscle, 94, 495f, 1161
Iliofemoral ligament, 853
Iliopectineal line, 1159–1160, 1159f
Iliopsoas muscle, 94, 94f, 495f, 1160f, 1190–1192, 1191f

Illness, patient reactions to, 60–61
IMA. *see* Inferior mesenteric artery
Image resolution, 13–14
Immune and nonimmune hydrops, 1407–1412
Immune hydrops, 1407, 1409f
　cordocentesis, 1410–1411, 1411f
　sonographic surveillance, 1409–1410, 1409f, 1410f
Immune hydrops fetalis (IHF), 1487–1488, 1488f
Imperforate anus, 803f
In vitro fertilization, 1278
Incarcerated hernia, 575
Inclusion cysts, peritoneal, 1239–1242, 1240f
Incompetent cervix, 1285
Incomplete atrioventricular septal defect, 1041, 1042f
Incomplete duplication, 446
Increased intracranial pressure, 830
Independence, 5b
Indirect-acting bilirubin, 229, 229t
Indirect arterial testing, 1114–1118
Induced acoustic emission (IAE), 514–515, 515f
Infant head, 813, 847b–848b
Infant hip, 850, 869b
Infantile hemangioendothelioma, 774–775, 775t
Infantile polycystic kidney disease (IPKD), 1605–1606, 1606f
Infarction
　renal, 454t–458t, 481–482
　splenic, 337t, 344–345, 347f
Infection
　after liver transplantation, 593, 595f
　after pancreatic transplantation, 633, 634f
　after renal transplantation, 616, 619f
　neural axis, 1523t
　nosocomial, 50
　renal, 478, 479f, 616, 619f
　splenic, 344, 344f, 347f
　urinary tract, neonatal/pediatric, 806–807
Infection prevention, 49–53, 50f, 51f
　nosocomial infection and, 50
　standard precautions and, 49–53, 50f, 51f
Infectious disease, of liver, 265–268
Inferior direction, 132–134
Inferior mediastinum, 892, 893b
　illustration of, 892
Inferior mesenteric artery (IMA), 184, 184f
　abdominal scanning of, at liver, gallbladder, and right kidney level, 107, 111f
　sonographic evaluation of, 184–195
Inferior mesenteric vein, 209
　sonographic findings of, 198
Inferior vena cava (IVC), 195–206, 197f, 198f, 199f
　abdominal scanning of
　　at level of caudate lobe, 106, 107f
　　at level of hepatic vein, pancreas and superior mesenteric vein, 109, 121f
　　at level of left lobe of the liver and pancreas, 109, 120f
　　at level of liver, pancreas, and gastroduodenal artery, 109, 120f
　abnormalities, 198–199
　anatomy of, 92, 195–197
　anterior tributaries to, 204–206
　color Doppler technique for, 255t
　congenital left atrial communication with, 1059, 1060f
　diagnostic criteria for, 260t

Inferior vena cava (IVC) *(Continued)*
   dilation or compression of, 198–199, 201*f*
   Doppler flow patterns in, 214, 214*b*, 215*f*
   Doppler ultrasound of, 146, 256*t*
   fetal circulation and, 1010, 1446*f*
   hepatic portion of, 198
   lateral tributaries to, 199–204
   longitudinal scans of, 141, 198
   pancreatic portion of, 198
   renal vein obstruction, 202–203
   retroperitoneum and, 496
   small bowel (lower) segment of, 198
   sonographic findings of, 198–204, 200*f*, 201*f*, 202*f*
   stenosis of, after liver transplantation, 594, 595*f*, 596*f*
   thrombosis of, 199–204
   tributaries of, 197
   tumors of, 198
Inferior vena cava filters, 199–204, 203*f*
Infertility
   female. *see* Female infertility
   male, 724*f*
Infiltrating, 131, 133*f*
Infiltrating carcinomas, 671
Infiltrative cardiomyopathy, 990–992, 992*b*
Inflammatory aortic aneurysm, 192
Inflammatory ascites, 420, 422*f*
Inflammatory carcinoma, 673, 674*f*
Inflammatory reaction, 660
Informed consent, 1295–1296
Infracristal defects, 1038–1039
Infrapatellar tendon bursa, 738*f*
Infrasound, 11*t*
Infraspinatus tendon, 745, 747*f*
Infundibulum, 1167, 1167*f*
Inguinal canal, 100–101, 100*f*
Inguinal hernia, 577*f*
Inguinal ligament, 90–91
Initiative, 5*b*
Injuries
   parenchymal, 566–567, 567*f*
   in sonography, 70–72, 71*f*, 71*t*
Innominate artery, 1070, 1112
Innominate veins, 1133
INR. *see* International normalized ratio
Inspissated bile, 770
Instrumentation
   fetal echocardiography, 1013
   pulse-echo, 21–22, 21*f*
   transcranial color Doppler imaging, 1091
Insulin, 361*t*
Insulinoma, 381, 383*f*, 384*f*
Integrity, 1297–1298
Intellectual curiosity, 5*b*
Intensity, 11–12
Interatrial septum, 897
Interface, 12
Intermittent imaging, 516
Internal carotid artery (ICA), 1070, 1071*f*, 1088, 1088*f*
   diagnostic criteria for, 1080, 1080*t*
   hemodynamics of, 1071
   occlusion of, 1077, 1078*f*, 1080–1081
   stenosis of, 1080, 1081*f*
Internal iliac arteries, 1169
Internal iliac vein, 1131
Internal jugular vein (IJV), 1133

Internal oblique muscle, 90, 90*f*
Internal os, 1191
International normalized ratio (INR), 532
Interrupted aortic arch, 1056–1057
Interstitial nephritis, acute, 454*t*–458*t*, 470–471
Interstitial pregnancy, 1332, 1333*f*
Intertubercular plane, 105
Interventional ultrasound, of adnexa, 1270*f*
Interventricular septum, 900, 900*f*
   description of, 1023
   M-mode imaging of, 946, 951*f*
Intervertebral disks, 873, 874*f*
Intervillous space, 1443*f*
Intervillous thrombosis, 1456, 1456*f*
Intestinal obstructions, 1586–1587, 1587*f*
Intestine, 1462*f*
Intima-media thickness, 1081
Intracerebellar hemorrhage, 834–835, 837*f*
Intracorporeal liver, 1564*t*
Intracranial arteries
   anatomy of, 1088–1090, 1088*f*
   identification of, 1096*t*
   occlusion of, 1100
   stenosis of, 1100
   velocities
      normal, 1096*t*, 1097–1099, 1098*f*
      physiologic factors, 1096–1097
Intracranial cerebrovascular evaluation, 1087, 1107*b*
   anatomy for imaging in, 1088–1090, 1088*f*
   physiology in, 1090
Intracranial hemorrhage, 1523*t*
Intracranial venous evaluation, 1104
Intraductal papillary mucinous neoplasms, 379–380, 382*f*
Intraductal papilloma, 658*t*, 665–666, 666*f*
Intrahepatic biliary neoplasms, 318
Intrahepatic cholangiocarcinoma, 319–320, 321*f*
Intrahepatic ducts, 136
Intrahepatic masses, 260–262
Intrahepatic vessels and ducts, 223–225
Intraluminal transducer, 17, 17*f*
Intramural benign gastric tumors, 400–401
Intramural hematoma, 977, 977*f*
Intramural leiomyomas, 1209, 1209*b*
Intrapancreatic obstruction, 312, 314*f*
Intraparenchymal hemorrhage, 566, 834, 836*f*
Intraperitoneal compartments, 417–418, 418*f*, 419*f*
Intraperitoneal organ, 326
Intratesticular cysts, 727, 727*f*
Intratesticular varicocele, 724*f*
Intrauterine contraceptive devices (IUCDs), 1225–1228, 1226*f*–1227*f*
Intrauterine growth restriction (IUGR), 1284–1285, 1388, 1395–1397, 1396*b*
   asymetric, 1397
   small for gestational age, 1397
   symmetric, 1397
Intrauterine insemination, 1278
Intrauterine pregnancy (IUP), 1306
   abnormal
      cardiac activity and, 1326
      sonographic findings associated with, 1324*b*
   assisted reproductive technology and, 1279, 1279*f*
Intrauterine sac, absent, 1320–1322, 1321*t*, 1322*f*
Intrauterine synechiae, 1222–1223, 1223*f*
Intravenous (IV) injection, 513

Intravenous (IV) therapy
   definition of, 41–42
   patient care and, 41–43, 41*f*, 42*f*, 43*f*
Intravenous urography (IVU), 573
Intraventricular hemorrhage (IVH), 816, 833–834, 833*f*, 834*f*, 835*f*
Intrinsic factor, 83
Intussusception, 777*t*, 781–783, 782*f*, 783*f*
Invasive ductal carcinoma, 672
Invasive lobular carcinoma (ILC), 673, 674*f*
IPKD. *see* Infantile polycystic kidney disease
Irregular borders, 131, 133*f*
Ischemic cardiomyopathy, 989
Ischemic rest pain, 1114
Islet cell tumors, nonfunctioning, 381, 384*f*
Islet cells
   metastasis of, 605*f*
   transplantation of, 627
Islets of Langerhans, 359, 361
Isoechoic, 131
Isolation precautions, 53–55, 53*b*
Isovolumetric contraction, 901*b*
Isovolumic contraction, 909
Isthmus
   of fallopian tubes, 1167*f*
   thyroid, 683, 684*f*
IUCDs. *see* Intrauterine contraceptive devices
IUGR. *see* Intrauterine growth restriction
IUP. *see* Intrauterine pregnancy
IVC. *see* Inferior vena cava
IVH. *see* Intraventricular hemorrhage
IVU. *see* Intravenous urography
Izumi, Kato, 8–10
Izumi, T., 8–10

J

Jastrzebowski, Wojciech, 68
Jaundice, 83
   bilirubin elevations in, 229
   gallbladder disease and, 290–293
   neonatal, 770
   nonobstructive, 770
   obstructive, 770
Jaw index, 1499, 1500*b*
Jejunoileal atresia, 1586
Jeune syndrome, 1631
Joint, hip, 851–853, 853*f*
Joint effusions, of hip, 867–868, 868*f*
Joint Review Committee on Education in Cardiovascular Technology (JRC-CVT), 6
Joint Review Committee on Education in Diagnostic Medical Sonography (JRC-DMS), 6
JRC-CVT. *see* Joint Review Committee on Education in Cardiovascular Technology
JRC-DMS. *see* Joint Review Committee on Education in Diagnostic Medical Sonography
Junctional fold, 287–289
Junctional parenchymal defects, 444, 446*f*, 447*f*
Justice, 1298
Juxtamedullary lipoma, 884*f*

K

Kager's fat pad, 751*f*
Kasai, Chihiro, 8–10
Kasai portoenterostomy, 771–772

KDOQI. see Kidney Disease Outcomes Quality
    Initiative
Key bladder sign, 1600
Kidney(s), 88
    agenesis of, 445–446, 449f
    anatomy of, 86, 435–437, 436f
    ectopic, 448–449, 451f, 452f
    fetal
        congenital malformations of, 1601–1605
        development of, 1593–1594, 1593f, 1594f
        not seen, 1600
        sonographic evaluation of, 1595–1599, 1597f,
            1597t, 1598f
    function of, 438
    medullary sponge, 454t–458t, 462, 479, 480f
    neonatal/pediatric
        anatomy of, 792–793, 793f, 810b–811b
        hydronephrosis, 796t
        pathology of enlargement of, 796, 796t, 797t
            adrenal hemorrhages, 796t, 807, 808f
            hydronephrosis, 796t
            prune belly syndrome, 796t, 801–802
            renal cystic disease, 804–805, 804f
            renal vein thrombosis, 807
        sonographic evaluation of, 792–793,
            793f, 794f
    physiology of, 438–439
    secondary malignancies of, 466, 468f, 469f
    sonographic evaluation of, 439–444, 766f
        patient position and technique in, 439, 440f,
            441f, 442f
        renal medulla, 444
        renal parenchyma, 440–441, 442f, 443f
        renal vessels, 441–444, 443f, 444f, 445f
    transverse scans of, 141, 144f
    ultrasound-guided biopsy of, 554–555, 555f
    variants of, 444, 446f
        columns of Bertin, 444, 446f
        extrarenal pelvis, 444–445, 446t, 448f
        fetal lobulation, 444–445, 446t, 447f
        junctional parenchymal defects, 444,
            446f, 447f
        sinus lipomatosis, 444, 447f
Kidney disease, chronic, 474
Kidney Disease Outcomes Quality Initiative
    (KDOQI), 1123–1124
Kilohertz (kHz), 10
Kissing cysts, 459, 460f
Klatskin tumor, 320–321, 322f
Kleeblattschädel, 1498–1499, 1499f
Knobology, 126
Kossoff, George, 7–8
Krause, Walter, 8
Krukenberg tumors, 1256–1257, 1257f

L

Labeling scans, 124
Labia majora, 1159, 1159f
Labia minora, 1159, 1159f
Labor and delivery
    preterm labor, 1416–1417
    ultrasound in, 1416–1417
Laboratory orientation, 124–125
Laboratory tests
    pancreatic, 361, 362t
    renal disease, 438–439
    thyroid function, 685–686, 686t
    ultrasound-guided, 531–532

Labrum, acetabular, 851–853
Lactating patient, breast imaging in, 649, 650f, 662
Lactic acid dehydrogenase, 230–231
Lacunae, 1301
Laminar flow, 23, 905
Langevin, Paul, 6
Large for gestational age (LGA), 1404, 1417
Large intestine, 89, 93f. see also Bowel
    anatomy of, 392, 395f
    vascular anatomy of, 390–391, 393f, 395f
Large-core needle biopsy, ultrasound-guided, 676
Larynx, abnormalities of, 1511–1512, 1512f
Last menstrual period (LMP), 1378
Late proliferative phase, 1195
Lateral arcuate ligament, 89
Lateral direction, 132
Lateral resolution, 13–14
Lateral rotation, 853
Lateral ventricles
    atrium (trigone) of, 815, 816f
    neonatal, 816f, 824–825
Lateroconal fascia, 492–493, 493f
LCIS. see Lobular carcinoma in situ
Left atrial appendage, 1000
Left atrium, 894, 899, 899f
    congenital vena cava communication,
        1059–1060
    development of, 1009
    fetal circulation, 1446f
    M-mode imaging of, 945–946, 950f
Left congenital hernia, 1557b
Left crus of diaphragm, 89, 89f
Left gastric artery, 180
Left hepatic artery, 180, 255t
Left hepatic vein, 223, 255t
Left hypochondrium, 219
Left kidney, abdominal scanning at level of spleen
    and, 109, 122f
Left lateral decubitus compression, 778
Left lateral decubitus position, 239
Left lobe of liver, 219f, 221
    abdominal scanning at level of inferior vena
        cava, pancreas, and, 109, 120f
    transverse scanning of, 143f
Left lower quadrant (LLQ), 88, 88f
Left parasternal window for Doppler, 928, 930f
Left portal vein, 206, 208f, 223, 224f, 255t
Left renal artery (LRA), 185, 441, 444f
Left renal vein (LRV), 200–202, 204f, 441, 445f
Left subclavian artery, 901
Left upper quadrant (LUQ), 88, 88f, 396
Left ventricle, 894, 900
    dilation of, 988f
    formation of, 1009
    M-mode imaging of, 946, 951f
Left ventricular inflow disturbance, 1048–1050
Left ventricular outflow tract disturbance, 1050–1054
    aortic stenosis, 1050–1052
    bicuspid aortic valve, 1033, 1050, 1050f
    in hypertrophic cardiomyopathy, 993–995, 997b
    hypoplastic left heart syndrome, 1052–1054,
        1052f, 1053f
Left ventricular outflow tracts, 914
    crisscross view, 1021, 1022b, 1022f
    five-chamber view of, 1021, 1021b, 1022f
    long-axis view of, 1022–1023, 1023b, 1023f,
        1024f, 1025f, 1026f
    short-axis view of, 1023–1026, 1026b, 1026f, 1027f

Left ventricular thrombus, 988, 989f
Left ventricular volumes, 990b
Left-sided valvular heart disease, 953,
    978b–979b
    aortic atherosclerosis, 974, 977f
    aortic dissection, 973–974
    aortic insufficiency, 956, 963–966, 963t
    aortic regurgitation, 963, 963t, 964f,
        965f, 966f
    aortic stenosis, 964t, 966–970, 966f, 967f, 969b,
        969f, 970b, 970f
    aortic tumors, 978–979, 978f
    intramural hematoma, 977, 977f
    mitral regurgitation, 953–957, 954f, 955b, 955f,
        956f, 957f, 958f
    mitral stenosis. see Mitral stenosis
    penetrating aortic ulcer, 977, 977f
    pseudoaneurysm, 973
    sinus of Valsalva, 974, 976f
Lehman, Stauffer, 7, 9f
Leiomyoma, 1207–1210, 1209f
    cervical, 1204, 1205f
    characteristics of, 1209b
    gastrointestinal, 400, 400t, 401f
    intramural, 1209, 1209b, 1210f
    submucosal, 1209, 1209b
    subserosal, 1209, 1209b, 1210f
    uterine, 1209, 1209b
        first-trimester, 1329t
        locations of, 1209, 1209b, 1210f
        sonographic findings in, 1210, 1211f,
            1212f, 1213f
        treatment of, 1210
Leiomyosarcoma
    colon, 409–412, 411f
    gastrointestinal
        upper, 400t, 402, 403f, 404t
        primary retroperitoneal tumor and,
            507, 507f
    uterine, 1216–1217, 1217b
Lemon sign, 1392–1393, 1530
Lenticulostriate vasculopathy, 838
Lesser omental bursa, 418
Lesser omentum, 97, 390, 414
    pancreas and, 358f, 359
Lesser sac
    abscesses of, 423, 424f
    description of, 97, 414
    illustration of, 416f
Lesser saphenous vein, 1132, 1132f
Lesser trochanter, 851
Lethal multiple pterygium syndrome, 1632
Letterer-Siwe disease, 342
Leukemia
    lymphatic, 83
    myelogenous, 83
    testicular, 730
Leukocytes, 83, 438
Leukocytosis, 333, 420
Leukopenia, 333
Leukopoiesis, 83
Levator ani muscles, 1160, 1160f, 1190, 1190f
Levocardia, 1033, 1035f
Levoposition, 1033
Levoversion, 1035f
LGA. see Large for gestational age
Lienorenal ligament, 328f, 390
Lifting, 38

Ligaments
  hip joint, 853
  liver, 221–223, 222f
  peritoneal, 98, 99f
  sonographic appearance of, 737–738, 738f, 740t
  vertebral column, 873
Ligamentum arteriosum, 898
Ligamentum teres, 98, 221–223
Ligamentum venosum, 106, 107f, 221–223, 222f, 1446
Likelihood ratios, 1375
Limb abnormalities, 1633–1635, 1633f, 1634f, 1635f
Limb development, 1313, 1313f
Limb-body wall complex, 1564t, 1570–1571, 1570f
Lindegaard ratio, 1100
Line density parameters, 715t, 716, 716f
Linea alba, 90f, 91
Linea semilunaris, 90, 419
Linear-array transducers, 16, 17f, 854, 854b, 1146
Linens, 50
"Linguine" sign, 667–668, 668f
Lip, abnormalities of, 1506–1509, 1508f, 1509f
Lipases, 361t, 362
Lipoma
  breast, 658t, 665, 665f
  juxtamedullary, 884f
  renal, 454t–458t, 468, 470f
  spinal, 882, 883f
Lipomatous hypertrophy, 998, 1001f
Lipomyelomeningocele, 885f
Lipoproteins, 227–228
Lips, development of, 1493–1494, 1493f
Lissencephaly, 1523t
Lister, Joseph, 49
Liver, 88, 89f, 218, 277b–280b
  abdominal scanning of
    at level of caudate lobe and psoas muscle, 107, 119f
    at level of duodenum and pancreas, 109, 120f
    at level of gallbladder, 108–109, 118f
    at level of gallbladder, right kidney, and longitudinal, 107, 111f
    at level of inferior vena cava, pancreas, and gastroduodenal artery, 109, 120f
  anatomy of, 219–225, 219f, 220f
    ligaments and fissures, 221–223, 222f
    lobes of, 219–223
    vascular supply, 221, 222f, 223–225
  bile and, 230, 230f
  biopsy of, ultrasound-guided, 552–553, 552f, 553f, 554f
  detoxification functions of, 229–230, 229t
  dome of, 106–108, 106f
  extracorporeal, 1564t
  FAST scan of, 564, 565f
  fatty, 243–244, 244b, 608
  fetal
    abnormalities of, 1580–1581, 1581f
    embryology of, 1574
    sonographic evaluation of, 1579, 1580f
  hepatic versus obstructive disease, 225–226
  intracorporeal, 1564t
  metabolic functions of, 227–229
  metastases to, 520f
  pathology of, 239–280
    developmental anomalies, 239–243
    diffuse parenchymal abnormalities, 258–260, 261t

Liver (Continued)
  focal hepatic disease, 260–265, 264t
  infectious disease, 265–268
  vascular flow abnormalities
    Budd-Chiari syndrome. see Budd-Chiari syndrome
    diagnostic criteria for imaging, 260t
    portal hypertension. see Portal hypertension
  pediatric, 765, 765b, 765f
  physiology of, 225, 227b
  segmental anatomy of, 220b, 221f
  sonographic evaluation of, 231–239, 232f, 233f, 234f
    anatomy and texture in, 234–235
    assessment criteria in, 233, 235f
    diagnostic criteria for, 260t
    in lateral decubitus plane, 239
    in sagittal plane, 235–239, 236f–237f, 238f
    in transverse plane, 239, 240f–241f, 242f
  ultrasound protocol for, 233–234, 235t
  vascular supply, 221, 222f, 223–225
Liver calcifications, in pregnancy affected by cytomegalovirus, 1418f
Liver cell adenoma, 271t
Liver disease, 585
  AFP and, 1428
Liver function tests, 230–231
Liver hemangioma, 519f
Liver Imaging Reporting & Data Systems (LI-RADS) system, 518
Liver omphaloceles, 1566f
Liver parenchyma
  diffuse abnormalities of, 258–260, 261t
  longitudinal scans of, 141
  sonographic findings, 590
Liver transplantation
  allograft
    Doppler evaluation of, 589
    evaluation of, 588–590, 589f
    postoperative imaging of, 590, 592f
    rejection of, 593
  biopsy after, 590, 593f, 594f
  cadaveric liver donation for, 586–587, 587f
  for cirrhosis, 584–585, 584f
  complications of
    abscesses, 593, 595f
    ascites, 605
    bile leaks, 604, 604f
    biliary, 597–598, 602f, 603f
    biloma, 604, 604f
    bleeding, 598, 603f
    bowel ischemia, 606–607, 607f
    cholangiopathy, 602f
    fatty liver, 608
    hematomas, 598, 603f
    hepatic artery pseudoaneurysms, 597, 601f
    hepatic artery stenosis, 596, 599f
    hepatic artery thrombosis, 596, 600f
    hepatic cysts, 608
    hepatic hemangioma, 608
    hepatic vein stenosis and thrombosis, 594, 595f, 596f
    hepatitis C recurrence, 605–606, 606f
    hepatocellular carcinoma, 605, 605f
    infarction and necrosis, 597, 601f
    infection, 593, 595f
    inferior vena cava stenosis, 594, 595f, 596f

Liver transplantation (Continued)
    intrahepatic abscesses, 593, 595f
    intrahepatic ductal dilation with stones, 603f
    islet cell metastasis, 605f
    lymphoceles, 604
    metastatic disease, 605, 605f
    pneumobilia, 608, 609f
    portal vein thrombus and stenosis, 594–596, 597f, 598f
    portal venous gas, 606–607, 607f
    rejection, 593
    seromas, 600, 604f
    surveillance for, 590–593, 593f, 594f
  cost of, 585–586
  criteria for, 584–585
  Doppler imaging of, 589–590
  expanded criteria donors for, 586
  history of, 584–585
  living donor for, 587–588, 588f
  Milan criteria for, 585
  Model for End-stage Liver Disease scale for, 585
  parenchymal biopsy after, 590, 593f, 594f
  Pediatric End-Stage Liver Disease scale for, 585
  rejection of, 593
  sonographic findings in, 590, 591f
  surgical technique of, 586–588
  waiting list for, 585
Liver tumors, pediatric, benign, 774–775, 775t, 776f
Living donor liver transplantation, 587–588, 588f
LLQ. see Left lower quadrant
Lobar dysmorphism, 444–445, 446t
Lobar holoprosencephaly, 843, 844f
Lobular carcinoma in situ (LCIS), 673
Lobular neoplasia, 673
Loculated mass, 131, 133f
Loeffler endocarditis, 992, 993f
Long-axis view
  apical, 938b
  of atrioventricular septal defect, 1041f
  ductal and aortic arch, 1026–1029, 1027f, 1028f
  of left ventricular outflow tracts, 1022–1023, 1023b, 1023f, 1024f, 1025f, 1026f
  parasternal
    of aortic stenosis, 1051f
    for color flow mapping, 922b, 925–928, 927f
    of congenital mitral stenosis, 1048f
    two-dimensional, 926–928, 927f
Longitudinal plane, abdominal, 104
Longitudinal scanning
  abdominal, 108–122, 128–129, 130f, 131f
  protocols for, 140–141
  transabdominal pelvic, 1178–1181
Longus colli muscle, 683, 684f
Loop of Henle, 437
Lower abdominal compartments, 418–419, 419f
Lower abdominal pain, 573t
Lower extremity
  arterial duplex imaging of, 1119–1120, 1119f, 1120f
  deep veins of, 1130–1131, 1130f
  fetal, 1369–1371, 1369f, 1370f, 1371f, 1372f
  superficial veins of, 1132–1133, 1132f
  venous duplex imaging of
    examination, 1146
    tips for, 1141t

Lower gastrointestinal tract
    acute appendicitis, 403–405, 404t, 406f
    Crohn's disease, 404t, 409, 409f
    Meckel's diverticulitis, 404t, 408–409
    mucocele, 404t, 405–408, 408f
    obstruction and dilation, 403, 404t, 405f
Lower urinary tract, 450, 453b, 453f
Lower uterine segment (LUS), 1448
Ludwig, George, 7
Lumason, 514
Lumbar artery, 187
Lumbar myelomeningocele, 1531f
Lumbar puncture, failed, 886f
Lumbosacral spine, neonatal, 878f
Lung
    anatomy of, 892–894, 893f, 894f, 895f
    fetal
        abnormalities of, 1548–1555, 1549f, 1550t
            cystic lung masses, 1549–1550, 1551b
            pleural effusions. see Pleural effusions
            pulmonary hypoplasia, 1549, 1550b, 1551f
            solid masses, 1551–1554
                congenital bronchial atresia, 1554
                congenital cystic adenomatoid malformation, 1552–1554, 1553f, 1554f
                pulmonary sequestration, 1552, 1552b, 1552f
    ultrasound-guided biopsy of, 556–557, 556f
Lung masses
    complex, 1554–1555
    solid, 1551–1554
        congenital bronchial atresia, 1554
        congenital cystic adenomatoid malformation, 1552–1554, 1553f, 1554f
        pulmonary sequestration, 1552, 1552b, 1552f
Lupus nephritis, 454t–458t, 471
LUQ. see Left upper quadrant
LUS. see Lower uterine segment
Luteal phase deficiency (LPD), 1274
Luteinization, 1172
Luteinizing hormone (LH), 1171–1172, 1231–1233
Lymph nodes
    abnormal, 651f
    normal, 651f
    para-aortic, 494–495, 494f, 498–499, 500f, 501f
    retroperitoneal
        ultrasound-guided biopsy of, 555–556, 556f
        visualization of, 550f
Lymph vessels, 326
Lymphadenopathy, 498, 706–707, 706f
    cervical, 706–707
Lymphangiectasia, 1551
Lymphangioma, 351, 351f
Lymphatic leukemia, 83
Lymphatic system
    of breast, 651, 651f
    in fetus, 1513, 1513f
Lymphoceles, 428–430, 430f, 604, 621–622, 625f, 636, 665, 665f
Lymphocytes, 83
Lymphoma, 676
    colon, 409, 410f
    gastrointestinal
        lower, 402–412, 404t, 406f
        upper, 400t, 402, 402f
    hepatic, 271t, 274–280, 277f
    mesentery, 428, 429f

Lymphoma (Continued)
    omentum, 428, 429f
    renal, 454t–458t, 466, 467f
    retroperitoneal, 506–507, 507f
    splenic, 351, 352f
    testicular, 730
    thyroid gland, 697–698, 698f
Lymphoscintigraphy, of breasts, 677–681, 678f

M

Macro movement, 126
Macrocephaly, 1531
Macroglossia, 1510
Macronodular cirrhosis, 246, 247f
Macrosomia, 1284–1285, 1404, 1413–1414
"Magic triangle," 78–79, 79f
Magnetic resonance angiography (MRA), 1083
Magnetic resonance imaging (MRI), 103t, 104
    of breasts, 652, 676–677, 677f
    fusion technology and, 540, 540f, 541f
    of kidneys, 439
    of tendons, 733–734
Main lobar fissure, 221–223, 290f
Main portal vein, 223, 224f, 255t
Main pulmonary artery, 1010
Majewski syndrome, 1630
Major calyces, 436–437
Male infertility, 724f
Male pelvic cavity, 94–95
Male pelvis, 108, 115f
Male pseudohermaphrodites, 1618
Male urethral discharge, 87
Male urinary hesitancy, 87
Malformation sequence, 1496
Malignant ascites, 420, 422f
Malignant primary cardiac tumors, 998, 1002f
Malignant tumors. see also Carcinoma
    adrenal, 504, 504f
    gastrointestinal, 401–402
    hepatic, 270–280
        hepatocellular carcinoma, 270–271, 271t, 274f, 275f
        lymphoma, 271t, 274–280, 277f
        metastatic disease, 271–274, 271t, 276f
    parapancreatic, 386–388, 386f
    pediatric, 773–774
    renal
        renal cell carcinoma. see Renal cell carcinoma
        squamous cell carcinoma, 454t–458t, 466, 467f
        transitional cell carcinoma, 454t–458t, 464–466
    spleen, 351–354
    testicular, 728–730, 728t
    thyroid gland, 693–698, 695f
Malpighian corpuscles, 330
Mammary layer, 645, 645f, 646f
Mammography
    benign gynecomastia on, 651–652, 652f
    BI-RADS categories of masses on, 653t
    breast cancer on
        males, 651–652, 652b, 652f
        signs of, 653b
    dense breast on, 648, 649f
    difficult or compromised, 653–654, 654b
    fatty tissue on, 648–649, 649f
    screening, 653–654, 653b, 653t, 654b
Mandible, abnormalities of, 1499–1500, 1500b, 1500f

Marfan syndrome, 193–194, 974
Marginal abruption, 1456, 1456f
Marginal insertion, placenta, 1444–1445
Marginal lake, 1443f
Masks
    oxygen, 45–46, 46f
    standard precautions and, 56
Mass(es)
    abdominal wall, 428
    adnexal
        with ectopic pregnancy, 1330–1332, 1331f
        resistive index and, 1236
    breast. see Breast masses
    cystic. see Cystic masses
    extrahepatic, 259, 261t, 263f
    extratesticular, 718t, 722
    liver, 552–553, 554f
    mesenteric, 426t
    neck
        developmental, 704–707
        ultrasound-guided biopsy of, 557
    omental, 426, 426t
    ovarian
        complex, 1234–1235, 1235b, 1235f
        first-trimester, 1340, 1341f
        simple cystic, 1234, 1234b, 1234f, 1235f
    pancreatic, 553–554
    pelvic, 1257–1258
        biopsy, 558
        first-trimester, 1329t, 1340
    peritoneal, 426t
    pseudopulsatile abdominal, 195
    retroperitoneal, 555–556
    scrotal, 718t, 723f
    testicular
        benign, 726–728, 727f
        malignant, 728–730, 728t
    uterine, 1340
Mastitis
    acute, 663–664, 663f
    chronic, 664
Mastodynia, 660
Mastoid fontanel, 821
Maternal anatomy, fetal ultrasound, 1408t
Maternal diseases of pregnancy, 1413–1416
    adnexal cysts, 1415
    diabetes, 1413–1415, 1414b, 1414f
    hyperemesis, 1415
    hypertension, 1415
    obesity, 1416
    systemic lupus erythematosus, 1064f, 1415
    urinary tract disease, 1415
    uterine fibroids, 1416
Maternal serum alpha-fetoprotein (MSAFP), 1285
    multiple gestation pregnancy and, 1418
Maternal serum quad screen, 1407
Maxillary prominences, 1493–1494
Maximum vertical pocket, 1478
MCA. see Middle cerebral artery
McBurney's point, 398, 398f, 777f, 778f
McBurney's sign, 403
MCDK. see Multicystic dysplastic kidney
MCL. see Medial collateral ligament
Mean flow velocity, 1097
Mean gestational sac size, 1314, 1314f, 1315f
Mean pressure gradient, 959
Mechanical conduction system, 903–904
Mechanical index (MI), 516

Mechanical macrosomia, 1405
Meckel-Gruber syndrome, 1528f
Meckel's diverticulitis, 404t, 408–409
Meckel's diverticulum, 408–409, 408f, 1576, 1576f
Meconium ileus, 1587, 1588b, 1588f
Meconium peritonitis, 1589
Medial arcuate ligament, 89
Medial collateral ligament (MCL), 738, 738f
Medial rotation, 853
Medial/lateral direction, 132
Median nerve, 739t
   compression of, 756–757, 756b
   illustration of, 739f
Mediastinum, 892
   inferior, 892, 893b
   superior, 893b
Mediastinum testis, 710, 710f
Medical ethics
   history of, 1295
   principles, 1295–1298
Medulla, 436, 497
Medulla oblongata, neonatal, 819
Medulla tumor, 502t
Medullary carcinoma
   of breast, 673, 675f
   of thyroid gland, 696–697, 697f
Medullary cystic disease, 454t–458t, 462–463
   nephronophthisis and, 463, 463f
Medullary nephrocalcinosis, neonatal/pediatric, 807f
Medullary pyramids
   description of, 440, 443f
   neonatal/pediatric, 792, 793f
Medullary sponge kidney, 454t–458t, 479
Mega cisterna magna, 842
Megacolon, 1588
Megacystis, 1608–1609
Megahertz (MHz), 10
Megaureter, 1610–1611
Meigs' syndrome, 1254
Melanoma, metastatic disease from, 555f
Membranes, fetal, 1374–1375
Membranous septal defect, 1038–1040, 1040f
Menarche, 1170, 1177
Meninges
   neonatal, 815, 816f
   spinal cord, 873–876, 874f, 877f
Meningocele, 883–885, 1528
Meningomyelocele, 1528, 1529f, 1530f
Menopause, 1170
   definition of, 1177
   hormonal regimens for women in, 1220b
Menorrhagia, 1174
Menses, endometrium and, 1164, 1172
Menstrual age, 1378. see also Gestational age
Menstrual cycle, 1170, 1171b, 1171f
   abnormal, 1174
   endometrial changes during, 1172
   endometrial thickness related to phases of, 1218t
Menstruation, 1170, 1171b, 1195, 1196f. see also Menstrual cycle
Mesenchymal hamartoma, 775
Mesenteric cysts, 426, 427f
Mesentery, 96–97, 97f, 390, 414
   lymphoma, 428, 429f
   pathology of, 426–428, 426t
Mesoblastic nephroma, 1615, 1616f
   congenital, 796t, 809

Mesocardia, 1033, 1035f
Mesocaval shunt, 256–257, 257f
Mesonephroi, 1593
Mesosalpinx, 1165
Mesothelium, 95
Mesovarium, 1165, 1166f
Metabolic macrosomia, 1405
Metabolism, 81, 227–229
Metastatic disease, 676
   adrenal glands, 504–505, 505f
   biliary tree, 321
   gastrointestinal, 400t, 402, 403f
   hepatic, 271–274, 271t, 276f, 520f
   from melanoma, 555f
   pancreas, 386
   peritoneal, 427–428, 429f
   splenic, 352–354, 353f
   testicular, 730
Methicillin-resistant *Staphylococcus aureus* (MRSA), 52
Metrorrhea, 1214
Meyers, Russell, 7
"Mickey Mouse" sign, 289
Micro movement, 126
Microcalcifications, 669, 693–694
Microcephaly, 1502, 1523t, 1542–1543
   sonographic findings in, 1542–1543, 1542f
Microemboli detection, 1102, 1102f
Micrognathia, 1352–1354, 1499–1500, 1500f
Microlithiasis, testicular, 727–728, 728f
Micronodular cirrhosis, 246, 247f
Microphthalmia, 1501
Microphthalmos, 1392
Microsomia
   craniofacial, 1498–1499
   hemifacial, 1500–1501
Microtia, 1496
Midaxillary line, 891–892
Midbrain, 819
Middle cerebral artery (MCA), 1089, 1093
   Doppler spectral waveform from, 1098f
   right, 1093f
Middle hepatic vein, 223, 255t
Mid-face, abnormalities of, 1503–1510, 1506f, 1507f
Midface hypoplasia, 1505–1506, 1507f, 1508f
Midgut, 1574f
   development and rotation of, 1563f
   embryology of, 1574–1575, 1575f
   malformations of, 1575–1576
Midgut malrotation, 784
Midsternal line, 891–892
Mineralocorticoids, 497
Minor calyces, 436–437
Mirizzi syndrome, 312, 314f
Mirror image artifacts
   color Doppler, 160–163, 162f, 163f
   description of, 149, 151f
   spectral Doppler, 160, 160f
Mirror syndrome, 1487
Mirror-image artifacts
   description of, 129
   illustration of, 132f
Mitral annular calcification, 957–958
Mitral atresia, 1049–1050, 1049f
Mitral regurgitation, 930f, 995, 1050

Mitral stenosis
   causes of, 957–963
   congenital, 1048–1050, 1048f, 1049f
   degenerative, 957–958
   echocardiographic evaluation of, 959
   hemodynamic measurements of, 959
   management of, 963
   pathophysiology of, 958–963, 958f, 959f
   percutaneous mitral balloon valvuloplasty for, 963
   rheumatic, 957–959, 958f
   severity assessments, 954, 955b, 959
   severity of, 960t
   treatment of, 963t
Mitral valve, 899, 899f, 900f
   fetal circulation and, 1010–1011
   M-mode imaging of, 943–944, 950f
   normal Doppler measurements, 1014t
   "parachute," 1048
   regurgitation of. see Mitral regurgitation
   stenosis of. see Mitral stenosis
Mitral valve area, 954f, 960, 961b, 961f
Mitral valve disease
   anatomy of, 953–963, 954f
   mitral regurgitation, 953–957, 954f, 955b, 955f, 956f, 957f, 958f
Mittelschmerz, 1172
M-mode imaging, 18, 19f
   of cardiac structures, 920, 943–952, 950b
      aortic valve and left atrium, 935f, 945–946, 950f
      interventricular septum, 946, 951f
      left ventricle, 946, 951f
      mitral valve, 943–944, 950f
      normal measurements, 950t
      pulmonary valve, 950–952, 951f
      tricuspid valve, 946
   color flow mapping, 920, 943–952, 950b
   fetal, 1013, 1014f, 1014t
   of hypertrophic cardiomyopathy, 997b
   of hypoplastic left heart syndrome, 1053
   of mitral stenosis, 959, 960f
Model for End-stage Liver Disease (MELD) scale, 585
Modified coronal plane, 827
Molar pregnancy, 1456–1457
Molecular imaging agents, 514
Molecules, 81
Monckeberg's arteriosclerosis, 1210–1212
Monocytes, 83
Mononucleosis, 341
Morality, 1294–1295
Morbidly adherent placenta, 1452–1454, 1453f, 1454f
Morgagni, foramen of, 1555–1556, 1556f
Morison's pouch, 98, 108–109, 417, 418f, 436
   FAST scan of, 563f, 564, 565f, 566f
   hematoma in, 539f
Mosaicism, 1433
Mouth, development of, 1494, 1494f
MPV. see Main portal vein
MRI. see Magnetic resonance imaging
MRSA. see Methicillin-resistant *Staphylococcus aureus*
MSAFP. see Maternal serum alpha-fetoprotein
Mucinous cystadenocarcinoma, 1247, 1248b, 1249f
Mucinous cystadenoma, 382f

Mucinous cystadenomas, 1247, 1248b, 1249f
Mucinous cystic neoplasms, 377–379
Mucocele, 404t, 405–408, 408f
Mucosa, 390, 782–783
Multicentricity, 671
Multicultural patients, 59
Multicystic dysplastic kidney disease (MDKD), 1606–1607, 1606f, 1607f
   neonatal/pediatric, 796t, 802–803, 803f
   sonographic findings in, 454t–458t, 461f, 462
Multicystic encephalomalacia, 837
Multielement transducer, 16, 16f
Multifactorial condition, 1433
Multifocality, 671
Multinodular goiter (MNG), 683, 690–691, 691t, 692f
Multiple gestation pregnancy, 1418–1424, 1418b, 1419f, 1420f
   anomalies specific to twin pregnancies, 1422–1423
   dizygotic twins, 1419, 1420f
   genetic amniocentesis and, prenatal diagnosis of congenital anomalies, 1432
   monozygotic twins, 1419–1421, 1420f, 1421f, 1422f
   placental tumors, 1457–1459, 1458b, 1458f
   scanning, 1408t, 1423–1424, 1424f
Murmurs, 905
Murphy sign, 296
Muscle(s)
   abdominal, 90–92, 90f
   back, 91
   false pelvis, 1160f, 1161
   hip, 853
   pelvis, 1160–1161, 1160b, 1189–1192, 1190f
   sonographic appearance of, 740t
   transvaginal scanning of endometrium during, 1195f
   types of, 735, 735f
Muscle tears, 754–755, 755f
Muscularis propria, 408–409
Musculoskeletal system, 733
   anatomy of, 734–740, 735f, 756b–757b
   artifacts, 740–743, 741f, 742f, 743t
   pathology of, 751–757
     carpal tunnel syndrome, 755–757, 756b, 756f
     muscle tears, 754–755, 755f
     shoulder biceps tendon subluxation/dislocation, 751, 751f
     tendinitis, 753–754, 753f, 754b, 754f
   sonographic appearance and evaluation, 740, 743–751
     Achilles tendon, 736, 749, 750f, 751b
     bursa, 738–739, 738f
     carpal tunnel, 748, 749f
     ligaments, 737–738, 738f, 740t
     muscles, 735, 735f, 740t
     nerves, 739, 739f, 739t, 740t
     rotator cuff, 744, 744b
        biceps tendon, 744, 744f, 745f
        indications for, 749b
        infraspinatus tendon, 745, 747f
        subscapularis tendon, 744, 745f
        supraspinatus tendon, 744–745, 746f
     tendons, 736–737, 736f, 737f, 740t
   work-related disorders of. see Work-related musculoskeletal disorders
Mycotic aneurysm, 192

Myelin, 739
Myeloceles, 883–885
Myelogenous leukemia, 83
Myelomeningocele, 1531f
Myeloproliferative disorders, 342, 343f
Myeloschisis, 883–885, 1528, 1528f
Myocarditis, 1034–1036
Myocardium, 896
Myoma, calcifications within, 1214f
Myometritis, 1260
Myometrium, 1181, 1192f, 1443f
Myxedema, 685
Myxomas, 998, 999f

N

Nabothian cysts, 1193, 1193f, 1204, 1204b, 1204f, 1205f
Nägele's rule, 1287, 1287b
Naked tuberosity sign, 752
Namekawa, Koroku, 8–10
Nasal bone, 1317–1318, 1317f
Nasal cannula, 45
Nasal pits, 1494, 1494f
Nasogastric (NG) tubes, 43, 44f
National Certification Examination for Ultrasound, 6
National patient safety standards, 544
Naumoff syndrome, 1630
Nausea, 85t, 86
NCCT. see Noncontrast computed tomography
Neck
   fetal, 1492, 1518b
     abnormalities of, 1496–1518
     embryology of, 1493–1495, 1493f
   twisting of, 75–76
Neck masses
   developmental cysts, 704–707, 705f
   fetal, 1512, 1516b
   miscellaneous, 704–707, 705f
   ultrasound-guided biopsy of, 557
Neck nodes, 557
Necrosis
   acute tubular. see Acute tubular necrosis
   focal brain, 837–838
   papillary, 454t–458t, 471–472
Necrotizing enterocolitis (NEC), 787–788, 787f
Needle biopsy, large-core, 676
Needle tips, finding, 550–551, 551f
Needles
   attached to transducer, 536–538, 536f
   for core biopsy, 533, 533f, 534f
   deviation of, 551–552, 551f, 552f
   for fine-needle aspiration, 532–533, 533f
Neonatal abdomen, 788b
   examination of, preparation for, 762–764, 762t, 763b
   pathology of
     liver tumors, 774, 775t, 776f
        benign, 773
        malignant, 773–774
     neonatal jaundice, 770
   sonographic evaluation of, 766
     biliary system, 765, 765b, 766f
     liver, 765, 765b, 765f
     normal measurements, 765b
     pancreas, 764, 764f, 764t
     portal vein, 765b, 765f
     spleen, 765b, 766f, 767f

Neonatal abdomen (Continued)
   surgical conditions, 775–787
     appendicitis, 776–781, 777f, 780f, 781f
     hypertrophic pyloric stenosis, 777t, 783–787, 783f, 784f, 785f, 786f, 787f
     intussusception. see Intussusception
Neonatal brain
   acquired lesions of
     epidural hemorrhages, 835
     extracorporeal membrane oxygenation for, 835
     focal brain necrosis, 837–838
     germinal matrix/subependymal hemorrhages, 833, 833f
     hypoxic-ischemic injury lesions, 836–838
     intracerebellar hemorrhage, 834–835, 837f
     intracranial hemorrhage, 832–836, 833b
     intraparenchymal hemorrhage, 834, 836f
     intraventricular hemorrhage, 833–834, 833f, 834f, 835f
     lenticulostriate vasculopathy, 838
     periventricular leukomalacia, 837, 838f, 839f
     subependymal cysts, 833
   anatomy of, 814–819
     basal ganglia, 818, 819f
     brainstem, 818–819
     cerebellum, 819, 820f
     cerebrovascular system, 819
     cerebrum, 817–818, 818f
     cisterns, 816
     fontanels, 814, 815b, 815f
     meninges, 815, 816f
     ventricular system, 815–817, 817f
   congenital malformations of
     cystic lesions, 844–846
     destructive lesions, 843–844
     neural tube defects, 838–842
        agenesis of corpus callosum, 840–841, 841f
        Arnold-Chiari malformation, 839–840, 840f
        Dandy-Walker malformation, 841–842, 841f
        disorders of diverticulation and cleavage, 842–843
   examination preparation of, 819–821
   focal necrosis of, 837–838
   infections of, 846–848
     congenital, 846–847, 847f
Neonatal head, 813, 847b–848b
Neonatal head examination, 821–829, 821b, 822t
   coronal plane, 822f, 823t, 824–827, 824f
   modified coronal plane, 827
   parasagittal views of, 825t, 827–828
   posterior fossa study, 828, 828f
   sagittal plane, 825t, 826f, 827–828, 827f
   three-dimensional neurosonography for, 821–824
Neonatal hepatitis, 770, 771f, 771t
Neonatal hip
   anatomy of, 851–854
   classification of, 863t
   movements of, 853, 854f
   pathology of
     developmental displacement of the hip. see Developmental displacement of the hip
     dislocation and subluxation of, 857–858, 858f
   sonographic findings of, 851–854
Neonatal intensive care unit (NICU), 762t

Neonatal jaundice, 770, 771t
Neonatal spine, 871, 887b
   anatomy of, 872, 872f
   embryogenesis and, 871–872
   pathology of, 880–883
      diastematomyelia and hydromyelia, 883, 885f
      lipoma, 882, 883f
      myelomeningoceles, 883–885, 885f
      tethered spinal cord, 881–883, 882f
   sonographic evaluation of, 871, 875–880, 878f
Neoplasia, lobular, 673
Neoplasms. see also Adenocarcinoma; Carcinoma
   endocrine pancreatic, 381–386, 383f
   parapancreatic, 386–388, 386f
Nephritis
   acute interstitial, 454t–458t, 470–471
   lupus, 454t–458t, 471
Nephroblastoma, 467. see also Wilms tumor
Nephroblastomatosis, 807–808
Nephrocalcinosis, medullary, 463f, 479, 481f
Nephroma
   congenital mesoblastic, 809
   mesoblastic, 1615, 1616f
Nephronophthisis, 463, 463f
Nephrons, 436–437
Nephropathy
   hypertensive, 454t–458t, 471
   sickle cell, 454t–458t, 471
Nerve(s), 739, 739f, 739t, 740t
   cardiac, 903
   sciatic, 739t
   sonographic appearance, 739, 739f, 739t, 740t
   vertebral column, 872f, 873
Nerve roots, spinal, 873
Neural axis, fetal, 1522, 1543b
Neural tube defects, 838–842
   agenesis of corpus callosum, 840–841, 841f
   Arnold-Chiari malformation, 839–840, 840f
   Dandy-Walker malformation, 841–842, 841f
Neuroblastoma, 773
   adrenal, 505–506, 506f, 807–808, 808f, 809f, 810f
   neonatal/pediatric, 808f, 809–810, 809f, 810f
   pediatric, 274–280
Neuroectodermal tissue, 505
Newton, Isaac, 6
Niemann-Pick disease, 340
Nightingale, Florence, 30
NIH. see Nonimmune hydrops
Nimura, Yasuhara, 8–10
Nodular hyperplasia, 268–269, 271t, 272f, 690–691
Nodular thyroid disease, 690–691, 690f, 691t, 692f
Noise
   as artifact, 156, 157f
   color Doppler, 160–163, 162f, 163f
   spectral Doppler, 160, 160f
Nomograms, fetal eye orbits, 1352
Nonalcoholic steatohepatitis, 768–769
Noncommunicating hydrocephalus, 1540, 1540f
Noncontrast computed tomography (NCCT), 439
Non-Hodgkin lymphoma, 351
Nonimmune hydrops (NIH), 1411, 1411b
   sonographic findings, 1412, 1412f
Nonimmune hydrops fetalis (NIHF), 1488–1489, 1489f
Nonischemic cardiomyopathy, 989
Nonmaleficence, 1295–1296
Nonobstructive hydronephrosis, 477

Nonobstructive jaundice, 770
Nonresistive vessels, 210
Nonstress test (NST), 1401–1402, 1402f
Nontoxic (simple) goiter, 691, 691t
Nose
   abnormalities of, 1505–1506, 1507f
   development of, 1494, 1494f
Nosocomial infection, 50
Nuchal translucency, 1286, 1433, 1433f
   embryonic abnormalities and, 1333–1334, 1334f
   first trimester, measurement, 1317, 1317b, 1317f
Nuclear medicine scintigraphy, 701, 702f
Nucleus, 81
Nyquist limit
   color Doppler artifacts and, 160, 161f
   definition of, 156–159, 715–716
   pulsed wave Doppler and, 911–912
   spectral Doppler artifacts and, 156–159, 157t, 158f, 159b, 159f
Nyquist sampling limit, 24

O

Obesity, 1416
   childhood, 763t
Obstetric measurements and gestational age, 1378, 1379b, 1393b–1394b
   gestational age assessment
      first trimester, 1379–1382
      second and third trimester, 1382–1394
Obstetric sonography
   classification of, 1285–1286, 1286b
   clinical ethics for, 1294, 1299b
      confidentiality of findings, 1298
      defined, 1294–1295
      history of, 1295
      principles, 1295–1298
   diagnostic and screening aspects of, 1292–1293
   Doppler for, 1288–1289
   examination guidelines, 1289–1292
      documentation in, 1289
      equipment specifications, 1289
      first-trimester protocol, 1284b, 1289–1290
      quality control, 1289
      second- and third-trimester protocol, 1284b, 1290–1292, 1292b
   indications for, 1284–1285, 1284b
   patient history, 1286–1288
      clinical dates, 1287
      gravidity and parity, 1286
      maternal risk factors, 1287–1288
      Nägele's rule, 1287, 1287b
   role of, 1283, 1292b–1293b
   safety of, 1288
Obstructions
   biliary. see Biliary obstructions
   bladder outlet, neonatal/pediatric, 801–802, 802f
   intestinal, 1586–1587, 1587f
   lower gastrointestinal, 403, 404t, 405f
   ureteral, 802
   ureteropelvic junction, neonatal/pediatric, 799, 800f, 802
   urinary tract. see Obstructive urinary tract abnormalities
Obstructive cystic dysplasia, 1608, 1609f
Obstructive disease
   definition of, 225–226
   hepatic disease versus, 225–226

Obstructive hydronephrosis, 454t–458t, 475–476, 477f
Obstructive jaundice, 770
Obstructive urinary tract abnormalities, 1608–1615
   anterior urethral valves, 1612–1614, 1614f
   hydronephrosis. see Hydronephrosis
   posterior urethral valve (PUV) obstruction, 1611–1612, 1612f, 1613f, 1614f
   prune belly syndrome, 796t, 801–802
   ureteropelvic junction (UPJ) obstruction, 1610, 1611f, 1612f
   ureterovesical junction (UVJ) obstruction, 1610–1611, 1612f
Obstructive uropathy, 1339
Obturator internus muscles, 1161, 1161f, 1189–1190, 1190f
Occipital encephalocele, 1527f
Occlusion
   internal carotid artery, 1077, 1078f, 1080–1081
   intracranial arteries, 1100
Occupational Safety and Health Act (OSHA), 69
OHS. see Ovarian hyperstimulation syndrome
Oligohydramnios, 1285, 1422, 1480–1481, 1480b, 1481f
   embryonic, 1327
Oligomenorrhea, 1174
Omental cysts, 426–427, 427f
Omentum, 97
   lymphoma, 428, 429f
   pathology of, 426–428, 426t
   tumors of, 428, 430f
Omoto, Ryozo, 8–10
Omphaloceles, 1338, 1428, 1466, 1466f, 1562–1565, 1565f, 1566f, 1575–1576, 1575f
   bowel, 1563, 1566f
   gastroschisis versus, 1562, 1564b
   liver, 1566f
   sonographic findings in, 1563–1565, 1564t, 1566f
Omphalomesenteric cyst, 1467, 1467f
Oncocytoma, 468, 470f
123-ABC method, 657
Oocyte, 1170–1171
Oophoritis, 1260
Open spinal dysraphism, 883–886, 885f, 886f
Ophthalmic artery, 1088, 1094, 1094f
Optison, 513
Oral cavity, abnormalities of, 1510–1512
Orbits
   abnormalities of, 1501–1503, 1502f, 1503f
   fetal, 1392, 1392b, 1393f
Orchiopexy, 730
Orchitis, 717t
Organ Procurement and Transplantation Network (OPTN), 584–585
Organ transplants, 523–524
Organelles, 81
Organism, from atom to, 81
Organomegaly, 1510
Ortolani maneuver, 859, 859f
OSHA. see Occupational Safety and Health Act
Ossification, skeletal, 1313, 1313f
Osteochondral plate sign, 862, 863f
Osteochondrodysplasia, 1623t
Osteogenesis imperfecta, 1623t, 1626–1628, 1627f, 1628f
Ostium primum atrial septal defect, 1037–1038, 1037f, 1038f

Ostium secundum atrial septal defect, 1037, 1037f
Ostomy, 47
Otocephaly, 1499
Ovarian carcinoma, 1244–1246, 1246f, 1247f
Ovarian cysts
　benign, 1239–1242
　　in adolescents, 1240
　　paraovarian cysts, 1240, 1240b, 1241f
　　peritoneal inclusion, 1239–1242, 1240f
　　simple cysts in postmenopausal women, 1240–1242
　complex, 1234–1235, 1235b, 1235f
　fetal, 1618–1619, 1619f
　functional, 1236
　　corpus luteum cysts, 1236–1237, 1237b, 1237f
　　follicular cysts, 1236, 1237b
　　hemorrhagic cysts, 1237, 1238f
　　theca-lutein cysts, 1237, 1238b, 1239f
　hemorrhagic, 1237, 1238f
Ovarian follicles, multiple, 1277f
Ovarian hyperstimulation syndrome (OHSS), 1237–1239, 1239f, 1278, 1279f
Ovarian ligaments, 1168f, 1169
Ovarian masses
　complex, 1234–1235, 1235b, 1235f
　first-trimester, 1340, 1341f
　simple cystic, 1234, 1234b, 1234f, 1235f
Ovarian neoplasms, 1244
Ovarian pregnancy, 1333
Ovarian remnant syndrome, 1239
Ovarian tumors
　epithelial, 1246–1250, 1248f
　　mucinous cystadenocarcinoma, 1247, 1248b, 1249f
　　mucinous cystadenoma, 1247, 1248b, 1249f
　　serous cystadenocarcinomas, 1248–1249, 1249b, 1250b, 1251f
　　serous cystadenomas, 1249b, 1250f, 1252f
　solid, 1235–1236, 1236b
Ovaries
　anatomy of, 1168, 1169f, 1231–1234, 1231f
　blood supply to, 1191–1192
　cyclic changes of, 1172f, 1232f
　Doppler ultrasound of, 1236, 1236f
　female infertility and, 1276–1277, 1276f, 1277f
　ligaments of, 1168f, 1169
　pathology of, 1230, 1258b
　　endometriosis, 1242–1243, 1242f
　　epithelial tumors. see Epithelial ovarian tumors
　　fluid collections in adhesions, 1240, 1241f
　　functional cysts. see Functional cysts
　　germ cell tumors. see Germ cell tumors
　　ovarian carcinoma, 1244–1246, 1246f, 1247f
　　ovarian hyperstimulation syndrome, 1237–1239, 1239f
　　ovarian remnant syndrome, 1239
　　paraovarian cysts, 1240, 1240b, 1241f
　　polycystic ovarian syndrome, 1238–1239, 1239b, 1240f
　　simple cysts in postmenopausal women, 1240–1242
　　stromal tumors, 1252–1257, 1255f
　peritoneal inclusion cysts, 1239–1242, 1240f
　position and size of, 1167–1168, 1167b, 1167t, 1168b, 1168f
　sonographic evaluation of, 578, 1191f, 1197–1198, 1197f, 1231–1233, 1232f, 1233f

Ovaries (Continued)
　complex masses, 1234–1235, 1235b, 1235f
　ovarian neoplasms, 1244
　simple cystic masses, 1234, 1234b, 1234f, 1235f
　solid tumors, 1235–1236, 1236b
　transvaginal, 1186b, 1197–1198, 1197f, 1198f
　volume measurements, 1233
　torsion, 1243–1244, 1243b, 1244f
　ultrasound examination of, 1178b
Ovulation, 1170–1172, 1171f, 1231–1233
Ovulation induction therapy, 1277, 1277f
Ovum, 1168
Oximetry, 36–37, 38f
Oxygen masks, 45–46, 46f
Oxygen therapy, 45–46, 45f, 46f

P

P wave, 904, 904f
Packet size, 715t, 717
PACS. see Premature atrial contractions
Paget disease, 654–655, 673, 673f
Pain
　abdominal
　　acute, 767–775, 768f
　　in children, 767–775, 768f
　　description of, 84, 85t
　defined, 1296
　epigastric, 568–570, 573t
　flank, 573–574, 573t
　gallbladder disease and, 290–293
　lower abdominal, 573t
　pelvic, acute, 578–579
　right lower quadrant, 573t, 574–575
　right upper quadrant, 567–568, 573t
　scrotal, 720f
　thoracic, 573t
Palate
　abnormalities of, 1506–1509, 1508f, 1509f, 1510f. see also Cleft lip/palate
　development of, 1494, 1495f
Pampiniform plexus, 712
Pan Scanner, 8f
Pancreas, 88, 89f, 355, 387b
　abdominal scanning of
　　at level of liver, inferior vena cava, and gastroduodenal artery, 109, 120f
　　at level of liver and duodenum, 109, 120f
　　at level of superior mesenteric artery, 107, 109f
　abscesses, 369t, 375–377
　adenocarcinoma of, 381, 384f, 385f
　anatomy of, 356–360, 356f, 357f
　annular, 360, 361f
　biopsy of, 553–554
　body of, 358, 358f
　congenital anomalies, 359–360
　Doppler imaging of, 631f
　ectopic tissue, 359
　endocrine function of, 361, 361t
　exocrine function of, 360–361, 361t
　fetal
　　abnormalities of, 1583
　　embryology of, 1574
　　sonographic evaluation of, 1580, 1580f
　head of, 356–358, 356f, 357f, 360
　　pancreatic landmark, 363–364, 364b
　size of, 359

Pancreas (Continued)
　inflammation of, 371f, 767
　laboratory tests, 361, 362t
　masses of, 553–554
　neck of, 356f, 358
　　pancreatic landmark, 363–364, 364b
　neoplasms of, 381–386, 383f
　　endocrine pancreatic, 381–386
　pancreatitis. see Pancreatitis
　parenchyma of, 629–630
　pathology of, 368–388
　　cystic lesions, 377, 378t
　　metastatic disease, 386
　　neoplasms, 377–381, 379t
　　　parapancreatic, 386–388, 386f
　physiology of, 360–361, 361t
　size of, 359
　sonographic evaluation of, 362–368, 362t
　　contrast-enhanced, 523
　　normal characteristics of, 363, 363b, 363f
　　pancreatic duct, 367, 368f
　　pediatric, 764, 764f, 764t
　　in sagittal plane, 366–367, 367f, 368f
　　technique for, 363–368, 363f, 364f
　　in transverse plane, 364–366, 366f
　　windows for visualization, 364, 365f
　tail of, 358, 358f
　　pancreatic landmark, 363–364, 364b
　transplantation of. see Pancreatic transplantation
　transverse scans of, 136–138, 143f
　ultrasound-guided biopsy of, 553–554
　vascular and ductal landmarks, 359
　vascular supply of, 358f, 359
　walled-off fluid collections, 373–374
Pancreas divisum, 359, 360f
Pancreatic ascites, 374–375
Pancreatic cyst(s), 1583
　after pancreatic transplantation, 637–638
　in autosomal dominant polycystic kidney disease, 378t
Pancreatic disease
　laboratory values for, 361, 362t
　metastatic, 386
Pancreatic duct, 282, 358–359, 358f
　acute pancreatitis and, 369–371, 369t, 370f
　as pancreatic landmark, 364b, 367, 368f
　sonographic evaluation of, 367, 368f
Pancreatic ductal adenocarcinoma (PDAC), 523
Pancreatic lipomatosis, 769
Pancreatic neuroendocrine tumor, 377
Pancreatic pseudocysts, 374, 375f, 376f
　after pancreatic transplantation, 636, 637f
　locations of, 374
　sonographic findings in, 377, 377f
Pancreatic transplantation
　allograft for
　　computed tomography of, 632f
　　Doppler imaging of, 628–629
　　evaluation of, 627–629, 629f
　　perfusion of, 629f
　　postoperative imaging of, 630
　　rejection of, 632f, 633, 633f
　biopsy of, 630–632, 632f
　cadaveric pancreas for, 624–625, 629f
　complications of
　　abscesses, 633, 634f
　　adenocarcinoma, 638

Pancreatic transplantation (Continued)
    arterial thrombosis, 633–634, 635f, 636f
    biopsy-related, 630–632
    cysts, 637–638
    fistula, 636, 637f
    hematomas, 636
    infection, 633, 634f
    lymphoceles, 636
    pancreatic artery stenosis, 634–635, 637f
    pancreatic vein stenosis, 634–635, 637f
    pancreatitis, 633, 634f
    posttransplant lymphoproliferative disorder, 638, 638f
    pseudoaneurysm, 635–636
    pseudocysts, 636, 637f
    rejection, 632f, 633, 633f
    seromas, 636
    surveillance for, 630–632, 632f
    venous thrombosis, 633–634, 635f, 636f
  cost of, 586
  criteria for, 586
  history of, 586
  islet cells, 627
  kidney transplantation with, 586
  rejection of, 632f, 633, 633f
  simultaneous pancreas-kidney transplant with, 586
  sonographic findings of, 629–630, 630f, 631f
  surgical technique of, 624–627
  for type 1 diabetes, 586
Pancreaticoduodenal arteries, 358f, 359
Pancreatitis, 368–373
  acute. see Acute pancreatitis
  after pancreatic transplantation, 633, 634f
  in children, 767
  complications of, 373
    chronic pancreatitis, 369t, 372–373, 373f
    pancreatic abscesses, 369t, 375–377
    walled-off pancreatic fluid collections associated with, 373–374, 374f
  definition of, 368–373
  epigastric pain with, 568–569, 569f, 573t
  hemorrhagic, 369t, 375, 376f
  phlegmonous, 369t, 375, 376f
Papillary carcinoma
  of breast, 672–673, 672f
  of thyroid gland, 694, 695f
Papillary fibroelastoma, 998, 1000f
Papillary necrosis, 454t–458t, 471–472
Para-aortic lymph nodes
  anatomy of, 494–495, 494f
  sonographic evaluation of, 498–499, 500f, 501f
Parabolic flow velocity profile, 905–906
Paracolic gutters, 99–100, 100f
Paralytic ileus, 403
Parametritis, 1260
Paraovarian cysts, 1240, 1240b, 1241f
Parapancreatic neoplasms, 386–388, 386f
Parapelvic cysts, 454t–458t, 459–460
Pararectal space, bilateral, 496, 496f
Parasternal transducer location, 919f
Parasternal views
  Doppler ultrasound, 928
    two-dimensional, 929–931, 935f
  long-axis
    of aortic stenosis, 1051f
    for color flow mapping, 922b, 926–928, 927f
    of congenital mitral stenosis, 1048f

Parasternal views (Continued)
    Doppler window, 920f, 924, 927b
    with patient in left lateral decubitus position, 936–937, 936f, 945b, 945f
    two-dimensional, 925–926, 927b, 928b, 928f, 929f
  of pulmonary stenosis, 1047f
  right, for Doppler, 927b, 928
  short-axis
    for color flow mapping, 922b, 929–931, 931f, 932f, 933f, 934f
    Doppler ultrasound, 928, 932f, 935f
Paratenon, 736–737
Parathyroid adenomas, 703f
Parathyroid carcinoma, 703–704
Parathyroid glands, 682, 707b
  anatomy of, 684f, 700, 701f
  embryology of, 700
  nuclear medicine of, 686
  pathology of, 702–704, 703f
  physiology and laboratory data of, 700–701
  scintigraphy of, 686, 686f
  sonographic evaluation of, 701–702
Parathyroid hormone (PTH), 700–701
Parathyroid hyperplasia, 703, 704f
Paraumbilical hernia, 573t, 575–578, 576f, 577f
Parenchyma
  injuries to, 566–567, 567f
  liver
    diffuse abnormalities of, 258–260, 261t
    longitudinal scans of, 141
    sonographic findings, 590
  renal
    angiomyolipoma and, 480f
    biopsy, 555
    junctional defects, 444, 446f, 446t, 447f
    sonographic evaluation of, 440–441, 442f, 443f
Parenchymal patterns, 648–649, 649f
Parietal epicardium, 980, 981f
Parietal peritoneum, 95, 562, 1174
Parity, 1286
Partial anomalous pulmonary venous return, 1036
Partial situs inversus, 1581, 1583f
Partial thromboplastin time (PTT), 532
Partial-thickness rotator cuff tears, 752, 752b, 752f
Parvus-tardus, 483f
Passive hepatic congestion, 259–260, 261t, 263f
Patau syndrome. see Trisomy 13
Patent ductus arteriosus, 1011–1012
Patent urachus, 804, 804f, 1604
Pathology
  in abdominal scanning, identifying, 131
  definition of, 80
Patient(s)
  breathing by
    in abdominal scanning, 124
    extreme shortness of breath, 570–572
  transfer techniques for, 38–40
    in assisting patients from the scanning stretcher into the wheelchair, 40, 41f
    body mechanics and, 38–39
    in moving patients toward the head of a stretcher, 39–40
    in moving patients up in bed, 39, 40f
    in stretcher transfer, 39, 39f
    in turning patients, 40
    in wheelchair transfer, 39, 39f

Patient breathing technique tip, 124
Patient care. see also Patient-focused care
  emergency medical situations. see Emergency medical situations
  equipment for, 57
  evaluating patient reactions to illness, 60–61
  infection prevention, 49–53, 50f, 51f
  for patients with tubes and tubing, 40–47, 41f
    catheters, 43–44, 44f
    colostomies and ileostomies, 47
    intravenous therapy, 41–43, 41f, 42f, 43f
    nasogastric tubes, 43, 44f
    ostomy, 47
    oxygen therapy, 45–46, 45f, 46f
    wounds, drains, and dressings, 46–47
  professionalism and, 61
  for special needs patients, 57–60
  during strict bed rest, 48–49
  for terminal patients, 60–61
  transfer techniques for, 38–40
Patient care partnership, 61
Patient consent, 32, 33f
Patient privacy, 32
Patient refusal, 32, 33f
Patient-centered care, 30–35
Patient-focused care, 61
Patients' Bill of Rights, 61
PCAs. see Posterior cerebral arteries
PCoA. see Posterior communicating artery
PCOS. see Polycystic ovarian syndrome
Peak systolic velocity, 1112–1113
Peau d'orange, 654–655
Pectoralis muscle, 645f, 648
Pediatric abdomen, 788b
  conditions that affect, 775–787
    appendicitis, 776–781, 777f, 780f, 781f
    hypertrophic pyloric stenosis, 777t, 783–787, 783f, 784f, 785f, 786f, 787f
  examination of, preparation for, 762–764, 762t, 763b
  pathology of
    liver tumors, 773–775
      benign, 773
    neonatal jaundice, 770, 771t
  sonographic evaluation of, 765b
    biliary system, 765, 765b, 766f
    liver, 765, 765b, 765f
    normal measurements, 765b
Pediatric End-Stage Liver Disease (PELD) scale, 585
Pediatric hip, 850, 869b
Pediatric patients. see also Adolescents; Children
  special needs of, 58–59
Pedicles, 873
Peliosis, 769
Pelvic abscesses, 425–426, 425b, 426f
Pelvic cavity, 92–95, 92f, 1160, 1161f
  blood supply to, 1170f
  FAST scan of, 564, 565f
  sonographic evaluation of, 1197f
Pelvic cyst, 154f
Pelvic floor muscles, 1190, 1190f
Pelvic fluid, 567
Pelvic girdle, 851, 851f
Pelvic inflammatory disease (PID), 1260–1266, 1261b, 1261f
  peritonitis, 1264–1266, 1266f
  salpingitis, hydrosalpinx, and pyosalpinx, 1261–1263, 1262f, 1262t, 1263f, 1264f

Pelvic inflammatory disease (PID) *(Continued)*
   sonographic findings in, 1261*b*, 1262
   tubo-ovarian abscesses, 1261*b*, 1263–1264
Pelvic kidney, 1594, 1601*f*
Pelvic landmarks, 1158*f*, 1159–1160
   bony pelvis, 1159–1160, 1159*f*
   external, 1159, 1159*f*
   pelvic cavity and perineum, 1160, 1160*b*, 1160*f*
Pelvic mass, 1618–1619
   anechoic tortuous, 1600
Pelvic masses, 1257–1258
   biopsy, 558
   first-trimester, 1329*t*, 1340
Pelvic muscles, 1160–1161, 1160*b*, 1189–1192, 1189*f*
Pelvic pain, acute, 578–579
Pelvic recesses, 1174–1175, 1174*b*
Pelvic retroperitoneum, 495–496, 496*f*
Pelvic ultrasound, 1158
   of bony pelvis, 1189, 1189*f*
   of bowel and rectouterine recess, 1198–1199, 1198*f*
   of fallopian tubes, 1178*b*
   of ovaries, 1197–1198, 1197*f*
   patient preparation and history for, 1177
   of pelvic muscles, 1189–1192, 1189*f*
   performance standards for, 1177
   three-dimensional, 1199–1201, 1200*f*
Pelvis
   acute pain in, 578–579
   false. *see* False pelvis
   female. *see* Female pelvis
   male, 108, 115*f*
   muscles of, 1160–1161, 1160*b*
   neonatal/pediatric, 763*b*
   sonographic evaluation of. *see* Pelvic ultrasound
   ultrasound-guided biopsy of, 558
   vasculature of, 1168*b*, 1169, 1169*f*, 1170*f*
Pena-Shokeir syndrome, 1632–1633
Penetrating aortic ulcer, 977, 977*f*
Pennate patterns, 734
Pentalogy of Cantrell, 1568–1570, 1569*f*
   fetus with, 1062*f*
   sonographic findings in, 1564, 1564*t*, 1570
Percival, Thomas, 1295
Percutaneous mitral balloon valvuloplasty, 963
Perforating veins, 1132–1133
Peribiliary cysts, 264, 265*f*
Pericardial disease, 980–985, 1005*b*
   cardiac tamponade, 571, 982–983, 984*f*, 985*b*, 985*f*
   constrictive pericarditis, 983–985, 986*b*, 986*f*, 987*f*
   pericardial effusion. *see* Pericardial effusion
Pericardial effusion, 1036, 1036*f*
   echocardiography of, 981–982, 981*f*, 981*t*, 982*f*, 983*f*
   extreme shortness of breath and, 570–571, 571*f*, 572*f*
   fluid estimations for, 981–982, 981*t*
   hydrops and, 1487
   size of, 981*t*, 982*f*
   with supraventricular tachyarrhythmias, 1064*f*
   transthoracic echocardiography of, 981, 981*f*
Pericardial sac, 88, 563, 895*f*, 896
Pericarditis, constrictive, 983–985, 986*b*, 986*f*, 987*f*
Pericardium, 896
   fibrous, 980, 981*f*
   serous, 980, 981*f*

Periductal mastitis, 663
Perihepatic compartments, 417–418
Perimetrium, 1164
Perineum, 94, 1160
Perineurium, 739
Periovarian inflammation, 1260
Peripheral arterial disease (PAD)
   pathophysiology of, 1113–1114
   physiology of, 1112–1113
   risk factors for, 1113–1114
   symptoms of, 1110–1111, 1113–1114
   treatment of, 1113
Peripheral arterial evaluation, 1110, 1127*b*
   anatomy associated with
     lower extremity, 1111–1112, 1111*f*
     upper extremity, 1112, 1112*f*
   guidelines for, 1126–1127, 1126*b*, 1126*t*
   indirect testing, 1114–1118
   purpose of, 1111*b*
Peripheral venous evaluation, 1129, 1150*b*–1151*b*
Perirenal space, 92, 491–493, 492*b*, 492*f*, 493*f*
Peristalsis, 393, 1578
Peritoneal cavity, 96, 1174, 1174*f*
   anatomy of, 413–414, 414*f*–415*f*, 416*f*, 434*b*
     intraperitoneal compartments, 417–418, 418*f*, 419*f*
     intraperitoneal location, 414–417, 417*f*, 418*f*
     lower abdominal and pelvic compartments, 418–419, 419*f*
   pathology of, 419–426
     abscess formation and pockets in abdomen and pelvis, 420–421, 423*f*
     ascites, 419–420, 421*f*, 422*f*
   sonographic evaluation of, 413–419, 414*f*–415*f*, 416*f*
Peritoneal cysts, 426
   inclusion cysts, 1239–1242, 1240*f*
Peritoneal lavage, 562, 562*f*
Peritoneal ligaments, 98, 99*f*
Peritoneal pseudocyst, 1264*f*
Peritoneal recesses, 99
Peritoneum, 95–96, 95*f*, 96*f*, 1166*f*
   definition of, 413–414
   metastases to, 427–428
   pathology of, 426–428, 426*t*
   tumors of, 428, 430*f*
Peritonitis, 422–423, 1264–1266, 1266*f*
Periventricular calcifications, 1541*f*
Periventricular leukomalacia (PVL), 837, 838*f*, 839*f*
Peroneal artery, 1112
Peroneal veins, 1131, 1139*f*
Perseverance, 5*b*
Persistent intrahepatic right umbilical vein, 1472–1473, 1472*f*
Persistent trophoblastic disease, 1325–1326
Personal protective equipment (PPE), 55–57, 73–74, 75*f*
pH, urine, 438
Phagocytosis, 332
Phalen sign, 756
Phenylketonuria (PKU), 1502
Pheochromocytoma, 502*t*, 505, 505*f*
Phlegmasia alba dolens, 1135
Phlegmasia cerulea dolens, 1135
Phlegmonous pancreatitis, 369*t*, 375, 376*f*
Photoplethysmography, 1117
Phrenic arteries, 185

Phrenocolic ligament, 326, 328*f*
Phrygian cap, 285, 288*f*
PHT. *see* Portal hypertension
Physiology, 80
Pia mater, 873–875
PID. *see* Pelvic inflammatory disease
Pierre Robin syndrome, 1500
Piezoelectricity, 6
Piriformis muscle, 94*f*, 1161
Pitting, 332
Placenta, 1373–1374, 1373*f*, 1374*f*, 1442, 1459*b*. *see also* Embryogenesis
   abnormalities of, 1450–1455, 1451*t*
     circumvallate/circummarginate placenta, 1454, 1455*f*
     morbidly adherent placenta, 1452–1454, 1453*t*, 1454*f*
     placenta previa, 1451–1452, 1451*f*, 1452*b*, 1452*f*, 1453*f*
     placental hemorrhage, 1455
     placentomegaly, 1451, 1451*b*
     succenturiate placenta, 1454, 1454*f*, 1455*f*
     vasa previa, 1452, 1453*f*
   amniotic sac and amniotic fluid, 1445
   Doppler evaluation of, 1449–1450, 1450*f*
   embryogenesis, 1443–1445, 1443*b*, 1443*f*
     cordal attachments, 1444–1445, 1444*f*, 1445*f*
     fetal-placental-uterine circulation, 1444
     membranes, 1445
     placental implantation, 1445
   evaluation after delivery, 1450
     fibrin deposition, 1450
   fetal circulation, 1446
   fetal ultrasound, 1408*t*
   functions of, 1444*b*
   hematomas, 1320
   normal, sonographic evaluation of, 1446–1449, 1447*f*, 1448*f*
     placental position, 1448–1449, 1448*f*, 1449*f*
   placental abruption, 1455–1456, 1455*f*
     intervillous thrombosis, 1456, 1456*f*
     marginal abruption, 1456, 1456*f*
     placental infarct, 1456
     retroplacental abruption, 1456, 1456*f*
   placental tumors, 1456–1459
     chorioangioma, 1457, 1457*f*
     gestational trophoblastic disease, 1456–1457, 1457*f*
     multiple gestation, 1457–1459, 1458*b*, 1458*f*
   umbilical cord, 1445–1446
     sonographic evaluation of, 1446, 1446*f*
Placenta accreta, 1413*f*, 1452–1453, 1453*t*
Placenta increta, 1452–1453, 1453*t*
Placenta percreta, 1452–1453, 1453*t*
Placenta previa, 1285, 1445, 1451–1452, 1451*f*, 1452*b*, 1452*f*, 1453*f*
Placental abruption, 1412–1413
Placental calcifications, 1418*f*
Placental edema, hydrops and, 1487
Placental hemorrhage, 1455
Placental infarct, 1418*f*, 1456
Placental insufficiency, 1481
Placental lesions, AFP and, 1428
Placental sonolucencies, 1447
Placentomegaly, 1447*f*, 1451, 1451*b*
Planimetry, for mitral valve area evaluations, 961
Plantar flexion, 750
Plaque, common carotid artery, 1077*f*

Plasma, 81
Plethysmography, 1117
Pleural effusions, 1409f, 1550–1551
    hydrops and, 1486–1487
    sonographic findings in, 1551, 1552f
Pleural fluid, 559
Plug flow, 210
Pneumobilia, 315, 317f, 608, 609f
Pneumocystis carinii, 268, 270f
Pneumothorax, 529
Polycystic kidney disease, 454t–458t, 461
    AFP and, 1428
    autosomal dominant. *see* Autosomal dominant polycystic kidney disease
    autosomal recessive. *see* Autosomal recessive polycystic kidney disease
    infantile, 454t–458t
Polycystic liver disease, 264–265, 264t, 266f
Polycystic ovarian syndrome (PCOS), 1238–1239, 1239b, 1240f, 1276, 1277f
Polycystic renal disease, autosomal recessive, 796t, 804–805
Polycythemia, 341
Polycythemia vera, 341
Polydactyly, 1630, 1631f, 1633f, 1634f
Polyhydramnios, 1285, 1410f, 1414, 1422, 1479–1480, 1480b, 1480f
    anencephaly and, 1524
    cephaloceles and, 1527
Polyhydramnios-oligohydramnios (poly-oli) sequence, 1422–1423, 1422f
Polymenorrhea, 1174
Polyorchidism, 731–732
Polyps, 400, 400t, 401f
    cervical, 1204
    endometrial, 1220–1221, 1274–1275, 1275f
        sonographic findings in, 1221, 1222f
    gallbladder, 304
Polysplenia, 327–329, 1581
Polysyndactyly, 1633f
Pons, neonatal, 819
Popliteal artery
    aneurysms of, 1125f
    description of, 1111–1112
    illustration of, 158f
Popliteal nerve, 739t
Popliteal vein, 1131, 1132f
    evaluation of, 1138
Porcelain gallbladder, 294t–295t, 303, 305f
Porencephalic cyst, 844
    sonographic findings in, 844
Porencephalic cysts, 1538
Porencephaly, 837, 1523t
    differential considerations for, 1524t
Porta hepatis
    description of, 282
    illustration of, 283f
    obstruction of, 312, 315f, 316f
    ultrasound protocol for, 233–234, 235t
Portal caval shunts, 254–257, 257f
Portal hypertension (PHT), 249–258
    in children, 768–769
    indications for, 251b
    portal caval shunts and, 254–257, 257f
    secondary to portal vein thrombosis, 253–258, 256f
    sonographic evaluation of
        collateral circulation, 252–253, 254f, 255t, 256f

Portal hypertension (PHT) *(Continued)*
    diagnostic criteria for, 260t
    Doppler interrogation, 253
    Doppler technique in, 252, 253b, 336f
    patient preparation and positioning for, 251–252, 252b
    vascular ultrasound contrast agents and, 517
    venous, 250–251, 251b, 252f, 252t
Portal sinus, fetal circulation, 1446f
Portal triad, 223f, 289, 292f
Portal vein, 206, 207f, 223, 223f
    characteristics of, 223–225, 227f
    Doppler flow patterns in, 214–217, 214b, 215f
    fetal circulation, 1446f
    pancreas and, 356–359, 357f
    pediatric, 765b, 765f
    sonographic findings of, 206, 208f, 209f, 260t
    stenosis, after liver transplantation, 594–596, 597f, 598f
    thrombosis of, 253–258, 256f, 594–596, 597f, 598f
Portal venous gas, 606–607, 607f
Portal venous hypertension, 209
Portal venous system
    anomalies in, 242–243
    Doppler ultrasound of, 146, 146f
    inferior mesenteric vein, 209
    splenic vein, 206–207
    superior mesenteric vein, 207–209
Portal-splenic confluence, 356–358
Posakony, Gerald J., 7, 8f
Positioning
    for abdominal scanning, 125, 125f
    Bouffard position, 747f
    for breast evaluation, 655, 655f
    for carotid duplex imaging, 1072
    Crass position, 746f
    for echocardiography, 927b
    for kidney evaluation, 439, 440f, 441f, 442f
    for portal hypertension, 251–252, 252b
    for scrotum evaluation, 712–713, 712b
    for spleen evaluation, 334–336
    for venous duplex imaging, lower extremity, 1137
Posterior arch vein, 1132
Posterior bimanual compression, 778–779
Posterior cerebral arteries (PCAs), 1090
Posterior communicating artery (PCoA), 1090, 1094, 1094f
Posterior direction, 132
Posterior fossa, studies of, 828, 828f
Posterior pararenal space, 92, 492b, 492f, 495
Posterior tibial artery, 1112
Posterior tibial veins, 1131, 1136f, 1139f
Posterior triangle, 94
Posterior urethral valve, 1600
    illustration of, 802f
    neonatal/pediatric
        bladder outlet obstruction and, 801–802
        sonographic findings in, 796t
    obstruction, 1611–1612, 1612f, 1613f, 1614f
Posthemorrhagic hydrocephalus, 829
Postoperative ultrasound, 1271
Postthyroidectomy neck sonography, 707
Posttransplant lymphoproliferative disorder (PTLD), 607–608
    in pancreatic transplantation patients, 638, 638f
    in renal transplantation patients, 623, 628f

Posttrauma brain injury, 1103
Postural anomalies, 1632
Potter facies, 804–805
Potter sequence, 1605
Potter syndrome, 1601
Pouch of Douglas, 564, 566f, 1162f, 1174, 1198–1199, 1198f, 1203, 1204f
Pourcelot resistive index, 1191
Power, 11–12, 12t, 26–27
Power Doppler imaging, 25, 27f
    vascular ultrasound contrast agents with, 513f
Power output, 21
PPE. *see* Personal protective equipment
P-R interval, 904
Precocious puberty, 810–811
Preeclampsia, 1415
    multiple gestation pregnancy, 1418
Pregnancy. *see also* Obstetric sonography
    anembryonic, 1320, 1323, 1323f, 1324b
    breast imaging in, 649, 650f, 662
    cervical, 1332–1333
    early, maternal serum analysis in, 1303–1305, 1304t
    ectopic, 1257, 1327–1333, 1328f
        adnexal mass with, 1330–1332, 1331f
        human chorionic gonadotrophin levels in, 1303
        sonographic findings in, 1328–1330, 1328f, 1329f, 1329t, 1330f, 1331f
    failed, 1320, 1327
    first-trimester. *see* First trimester pregnancy
    heterotopic, 1279, 1279f, 1332, 1332t
    interstitial, 1332, 1333f
    intrauterine. *see* Intrauterine pregnancy
    maternal diseases of, 1413–1416
        adnexal cysts, 1415
        diabetes, 1413–1415, 1414b, 1414f
        hyperemesis, 1415
        hypertension, 1415
        obesity, 1416
        systemic lupus erythematosus, 1064f, 1415
        urinary tract disease, 1415
        uterine fibroids, 1416
    molar, 1324
    multiple gestation. *see* Multiple gestation pregnancy
    normal progression, 1301–1303, 1301f, 1302f, 1303f, 1304f, 1304t
    second trimester. *see* Second trimester pregnancy
    third trimester. *see* Third trimester pregnancy
Pregnancy-associated plasma protein-A (PAPP-A), 1305
    prenatal diagnosis of congenital anomalies, 1432
Pregnancy-induced hypertension (PIH), 1415
Preload, 910
Premature atrial contractions (PACs), 1062–1063
Premature rupture of membranes (PROM), 1414, 1482
Premature ventricular contractions (PVCs), 1062–1063
Premenarche, 1170, 1177
Premenopause, 1177
Preoperative needle wire localization, 676, 676f
Presacral space, 496
Pressure, 908
Pressure amplitude, 12t

Pressure half-time (PHT), 960–961, 961f, 962f
Preterm infants, 814t
Preterm labor, 1416–1417, 1416b
    premature rupture of membranes, 1416–1417
    sonographic findings, 1408t, 1416, 1416f
Preterm premature rupture of the membranes (PPROM), 1482
Prevesical space, 495
PRF. see Pulse repetition frequency
Primary hyperparathyroidism, 702–704, 703f
Primary yolk sac, 1301
Primitive atrium, 1009, 1010f
Primitive ventricle, 1010f
Privacy, patient, 32
Proboscis, 1503f, 1504f, 1534f
Professionalism, 61
Profunda femoris artery, 1111–1112
Profunda femoris vein, 1131
Progesterone, 1168, 1220b
Projectile vomiting, 784
Proliferative phase, 1171b, 1172, 1195, 1196f
PROM. see Preterm premature rupture of the membranes
Pronephros, 1593
Propagation artifacts, 147–153
    grating lobes and, 151, 153f
    mirror image and, 149, 151f
    range ambiguity and, 151–152, 154f
    refraction and, 149, 152f
    reverberation and, 148–149, 149f, 150f, 151f
    section thickness and, 148, 148f
    speckle and, 148, 149f
    speed error and, 151, 154f
Prostate gland, 558, 558f, 559f
Prostate-specific antigen (PSA), 531–532
Proteins
    liver production of, 228
    urinary, 438
Prothrombin time (PT), 231, 532
Proximal isovelocity surface area (PISA), 954, 957f
    in mitral stenosis, 954, 957f
Proximal/distal direction, 132–134
Prune-belly syndrome, 796t, 801–802, 1614–1615, 1615b
Pseudoaneurysms, 482–483, 484f
    arterial duplex imaging of, 1124–1126, 1125f
    carotid duplex imaging of, 1078
    computed tomography of, 973, 973f, 974f
    definition of, 597, 635–636, 973
    description of, 190–191, 191f
    Doppler imaging of, 145
    hepatic artery, 597, 601f
    in pancreatic transplantation patients, 635–636
    in renal transplantation patients, 620
Pseudoascites, 1581–1582, 1583f
Pseudocysts. see also Cyst(s)
    pancreatic. see Pancreatic pseudocysts
    peritoneal, 1264f
    uriniferous, 427
Pseudodissection, 573
Pseudogestational sac, 1329, 1329f
Pseudomyxoma peritonei, 405, 407–408
Pseudopulsatile abdominal masses, 195
Pseudotoxemia, 1487
Psoas compartment, 495, 495f
Psoas muscles, 94, 495, 495f
    psoas major, 107, 109f, 495f, 1160f, 1161
PT. see Prothrombin time

PTH. see Parathyroid hormone
PTT. see Partial thromboplastin time
Pudendal artery, 712
Pudendum, 1159
Puerperal mastitis, 663
Pulmonary capillary wedge, 909
Pulmonary embolism (PE), 1134–1135, 1135b, 1149–1150
Pulmonary hypertension, 988–989
Pulmonary hypoplasia, 1549, 1550b, 1551f
Pulmonary sequestration, 1552, 1552b, 1552f
Pulmonary stenosis, 1032, 1046–1047, 1047f
    sonographic findings of, 1046–1047, 1047f
    supravalvular, 1048, 1048f
Pulmonary trunk, 898
    fetal circulation, 1446f
Pulmonary valve, 898, 898f, 950–952, 951f
Pulmonary veins
    fetal circulation, 1446f
Pulmonic valve, 1014t
Pulsatility, 1141
Pulsatility index (PI), 1098, 1191, 1403
    definition of, 1236
    ovaries and, 1236
Pulse, 84
    measurement of, 35, 35f, 36f
Pulse duration, 13
Pulse oximetry, 36–37, 38f
Pulse repetition frequency (PRF), 27, 151–152, 253b, 923
    Nyquist limit and, 156–159, 158f, 911–912
    parameters for scrotum evaluation, 715t
Pulse volume recordings, 1117, 1117f
Pulsed wave Doppler, 23–24, 1014, 1014f, 1014t, 1402–1403
    apical four-chamber view with, 911, 911f
    description of, 145, 911–912
    echocardiography, 923, 923f
    hypertrophic cardiomyopathy evaluations, 995, 997f
    illustration, 1014f
    Nyquist limit and, 911–912
    transducers used in, 911, 911f
Pulsed wave transducer, 923
Pulse-echo display modes, 17–18
Pulse-echo instrumentation, 21–22, 21f
PVCs. see Premature ventricular contractions
PVL. see Periventricular leukomalacia
Pyelectasis, 1366, 1610
Pyelonephritis
    acute, 806
    chronic, 806–807
    emphysematous, 478, 479f
    xanthogranulomatous, 454t–458t, 478–479, 480f
Pyloric canal, 390, 783
Pyloromyotomy, 784
Pylorus, description of, 390, 392f
Pyocele, 720, 726f
Pyogenic abscess, 264t, 265–266, 267f
Pyogenic infection, 430–432
Pyometra, 1225
Pyonephrosis, 454t–458t, 478, 479f
Pyosalpinx, 1261–1263, 1262f, 1262t, 1263f, 1264f
Pyramidal lobe, 683
Pyramids, medullary, 440, 443f
Pythagoras, 6
Pyuria, 438

Q

QRS complex, 904
Quad screen, 1285
Quadrant method, 656f, 657
Quadratus lumborum muscle, 492–493, 495f
Quadruple screen, prenatal diagnosis of congenital anomalies, 1429

R

Rachischisis, 1528, 1528f
Radial artery, 1112
Radial nerve, 739t
Radial plane, 657
Radial pulse, 35, 35f
Radial ray defects, 1633, 1634f
Radial veins, 1133
Radiography, 104
Radius, fetal measurement, 1390, 1391b, 1391f
Railway sign, 1355
Ramazzini, Bernardino, 68
Range ambiguity
    propagation, 151–152, 154f
    spectral Doppler, 157t, 159–160
Rarefaction, 10
RAS. see Renal artery stenosis
Raynaud phenomenon, 1118
RBCs. see Red blood cells
RCC. see Renal cell carcinoma
Reaching, 77
Reactive lymph nodes, 779, 781f
Real-time imaging, 18
Recessive disorder, 1433
Recovery, illness and, 60
Rectouterine pouch, 94
Rectouterine recess, 1174, 1198–1199, 1198f, 1203, 1203f, 1204f
Rectovesical spaces, 495
Rectus abdominis muscles, 90, 91f, 419, 420f, 1189, 1189f
Rectus sheath, anatomy of, 90, 1189, 1189f
Recurrent rami, 710–711, 711f
Red blood cells (RBCs), 83
Red pulp, of spleen, 330, 332f
Reducible hernia, 575
Reflection, 12, 12f
Refractile shadowing, 742–743, 742f, 743f
Refraction, 12, 149, 152f
Refusal, 30
    patient, 32, 33f
Reid, John, 8–10
Reidel lobe, 234–235
Rejection, 22
    liver transplantation, 593
    pancreatic transplantation, 632f, 633, 633f
    renal transplantation, 615–616, 618f
Renal adenomatous tumors, 468, 470f
Renal agenesis, 445–446, 449f, 1601–1602, 1602f, 1603b
Renal angiomyolipoma, 467, 469f
Renal anomalies, 445–447, 448f, 797–798
    horseshoe kidney, 448–449, 452f
    renal agenesis, 445–446, 449f
    renal ectopia, 448–449, 451f, 452f
Renal arteries, 185–187, 185f
    accessory, 623f
    Doppler flow patterns in, 212b, 214, 214f
    occlusion, 214
    sonographic findings of, 186, 186f, 187f

Renal arteriography, 481–482, 481f, 482f, 483f
Renal artery stenosis (RAS), 195, 197f, 480–481
   after renal transplantation, 622f
   contrast-enhanced evaluation of, 521, 521f
   sonographic findings in, 481–482, 481b, 481f, 482f, 483f
Renal atrophy, 454t–458t, 472
   sonographic findings in, 472–473, 473f
Renal biopsy, 548f, 555f
Renal capsule, 466–467
Renal cell carcinoma (RCC), 454t–458t, 464
   in children, 810–811
   in renal transplantation patients, 622–623, 626f
   sonographic findings in, 464–466, 464f, 465f, 466b, 466f
Renal corpuscle, 437
Renal cortex, 436–437, 444
Renal cystic disease, 453, 454t–458t, 458b, 1605–1608, 1605b, 1605t
   autosomal dominant polycystic kidney disease. see Autosomal dominant polycystic kidney disease
   autosomal recessive polycystic kidney disease. see Autosomal recessive polycystic kidney disease
   medullary cystic disease, 454t–458t, 462–463
   multicystic dysplastic kidney. see Multicystic dysplastic kidney
   polycystic kidney disease. see Polycystic kidney disease
   renal cysts associated with renal tumors, 460–461
   simple, 453, 459f
   sinus parapelvic, 454t–458t, 459–460
Renal cysts, 1600
   artifactual range-ambiguity echoes within, 154f
   complex, 458, 459b, 459f, 460f
   in renal transplantation patients, 624
   simple, 453, 459f
Renal disease, 468–470
   acquired immunodeficiency syndrome and, 454t–458t, 471, 471f, 472f
   acute interstitial nephritis, 470–471
   cystic. see Renal cystic disease
   hypertensive nephropathy, 454t–458t, 471
   laboratory tests for, 438–439
   lupus nephritis, 454t–458t, 471
   papillary necrosis, 454t–458t, 471–472
   renal atrophy, 454t–458t, 472
   sickle cell nephropathy, 454t–458t, 471
Renal ectopia, 448–449, 451f, 452f, 800, 803f, 1603, 1603f
Renal failure, 473
   acute, 454t–458t, 473, 585–586
   causes of, 473b
   chronic, 454t–458t, 473
   dialysis for, 585–586
   renal transplantation for, 585–586
   signs and symptoms of, 585–586
Renal hilum, 436
Renal hypoplasia, 445–446
Renal infarction, 454t–458t, 481–482
Renal infection, 478, 479f
Renal lymphoma, 454t–458t, 466, 467f
Renal masses
   aspiration of, 449–450, 452t
   complex, 458, 459b, 459f, 460f
   evaluation of, 449
   sonographic evaluation of, 522, 522f
   ultrasound-guided biopsy of, 554, 555f

Renal medulla, 444
Renal neoplasms, 463–464
Renal parenchyma
   angiomyolipoma and, 480f
   biopsy, 555
   junctional defects, 444, 446f, 446t, 447f
   sonographic evaluation of, 440–441, 442f, 443f
Renal pelvis, 436–437
Renal pyramids, 436
Renal sinus, 436–437
Renal sinus lipomatosis, 454t–458t
Renal stones. see Urolithiasis
Renal transplantation
   allograft for
     evaluation of, 610–611, 610f, 611f, 612f, 613f
     perfusion of, 611f
     postoperative imaging of, 613–615
     rejection of, 615–616, 618f
   autotransplantation, 610
   biopsy after, 615, 615f, 616f, 617f
   cadaveric kidney for, 608–609, 610f
   complications of
     abscesses, 616, 619f
     acute tubular necrosis, 615–616, 618f
     angiomyolipoma, 624
     biopsy-related, 615, 615f, 616f, 617f
     hematomas, 620–621, 624f
     infarction, 620, 623f
     infection, 616, 619f
     lymphoceles, 621–622, 625f
     necrosis, 620, 623f
     posttransplant lymphoproliferative disorder, 623, 628f
     pseudoaneurysms, 620
     rejection, 615–616, 618f
     renal artery stenosis and thrombosis, 619–620, 622f
     renal cell carcinoma, 622–623, 626f
     renal cysts, 623–624
     renal vein stenosis and thrombosis, 617–619, 621f
     seromas, 621, 625f
     transitional cell carcinoma, 623, 627f
     urinary obstruction, 616–617, 620f
     urinary stones, 616–617, 620f
     urine leak, 622, 626f
     urinomas, 622, 626f
   criteria for, 585–586
   history of, 585–586
   living donor kidney for, 609–610
   pancreas transplantation with, 586
   reasons for needing, 585–586
   rejection of, 615–616, 618f
   for renal failure, 585–586
   simultaneous pancreas-kidney transplant with, 586
   sonographic findings of, 612–613, 613f, 614f
   surgical technique of, 608–610
   ultrasound contrast agents and, 523–524
   ultrasound-guided biopsy after, 555, 555f
Renal tumors
   benign, 467, 469f, 488–490
     adenomatous tumors, 468, 470f
     angiomyolipoma, 467, 469f
     lipoma, 454t–458t, 468, 470f
     oncocytoma, 468, 470f
   fetal, 1615–1616, 1616f, 1617b, 1617f
   lymphoma, 454t–458t, 466, 467f
   renal cell carcinoma. see Renal cell carcinoma

Renal tumors (Continued)
   renal cysts associated with, 460–461
   squamous cell carcinoma, 454t–458t, 466, 466f, 467f
   Wilms tumor. see Wilms tumor
Renal variants
   columns of Bertin, 444, 446f
   dromedary hump, 444, 446t
   extrarenal pelvis, 444–445, 446t, 448f
   fetal lobulation, 444–445, 446t, 447f
   sinus lipomatosis, 444, 447f
Renal vein thrombosis, 807, 807f
Renal veins, 199–203, 203f, 438
   Doppler flow patterns in, 214, 214b, 215f
   left, 200–202, 204f
   obstruction of, 202–203
   renal transplantation complications of, 617–619, 621f
   right, 202–203, 204f
   stenosis of, 617–619, 621f
   thrombosis of, 202–203, 204f, 617–619, 621f, 807
Renunculi, 444, 446f, 447f, 792
Resistance, 12
Resistive index (RI), 210, 589, 1098, 1403
   definition of, 1236
   ovaries and, 1236
   urinary tract obstruction and, 476–478
Resistive vessels, 210
Resolution
   axial, 13–14
   azimuthal, 13–14
   lateral, 13–14
Resonance, 148–149
Resource organizations, 6
Respect for persons, 1296
Respiration, 84
   assessment of, 37–38
   definition of, 37–38
Respiratory phasicity, 1140
Restrictive cardiomyopathy, 990–992, 992b
Rete testis, 709, 709f
Reticuloendothelial system (RES), 326, 330, 514
Reticuloendotheliosis, 342
Retrocecal appendicitis, 404
Retrofascial space, 492b, 495, 495f
Retroflexion, 1166f, 1207f
Retromammary layer, 645, 645f, 646f
Retroperitoneal abscess, 508–509, 509f
Retroperitoneal fat, 506
Retroperitoneal fibrosis, 509–510, 509f
   with aneurysms, 192
Retroperitoneal fluid collections, 508–509
Retroperitoneal lymph nodes
   ultrasound-guided biopsy of, 555–556, 556f
   visualization of, 550f
Retroperitoneal spaces, 91f, 92, 492f
Retroperitoneal tumor
   primary, 506–508, 507f
   secondary, 508
Retroperitoneum, 435–437, 491, 510b
   anatomy of, 491–497, 492b, 492f, 493f
     adrenal glands, 494, 494f
     anterior pararenal space, 492, 492b, 493f
     diaphragmatic crura, 494, 494f
     iliac fossa, 492b, 495
     para-aortic lymph nodes, 494–495, 494f
     pelvic retroperitoneum, 495–496, 496f
     perirenal space, 491–493, 492b, 492f, 493f

Retroperitoneum (Continued)
    posterior pararenal space, 492b, 492f, 495
    retrofascial space, 492b, 495, 495f
    pathology of, 499-510
        adrenal cortical syndromes, 499-502, 502t
        adrenal cysts, 502-503, 502f, 503f
        adrenal hemorrhage, 503, 503f
        adrenal medulla tumors, 505-506
        adrenal tumors, 503-505
        primary retroperitoneal tumor, 506-508, 507f
        retroperitoneal fat, 506
        retroperitoneal fibrosis, 509-510, 509f
        retroperitoneal fluid collections, 508-509
        secondary retroperitoneal tumor, 508
    physiology and laboratory data of, 497
    sonographic evaluation of, 497-499
        adrenal glands, 497-498, 498f, 499f
        diaphragmatic crura, 498, 500f
        para-aortic lymph nodes, 498-499, 500f, 501f
        pitfalls in, 498
    vascular supply for, 496-497
Retroplacental abruption, 1456, 1456f
Retropubic space, 1174
Retroversion, 1166f, 1207f
Retrovesical space, 418-419
Reverberation, 742, 742f
Reverberation artifacts, 129, 132f, 148-149, 149f, 150f, 151f
Reverse isolation, 55
Reversible ischemic neurologic deficit (RIND), 1072
Rhabdomyoma, 998, 1001f, 1058, 1058f
Rhabdomyosarcomas, 507
Rheumatic fever, 957
Rheumatic heart disease
    aortic stenosis caused by, 967, 968f
    mitral stenosis caused by, 958-959, 958f
Rhombencephalon, 1522
Right atrial pressure, 914
Right atrium, 897, 897f, 1009, 1010f
    fetal circulation, 1446f
Right crus of diaphragm, 89, 89f
Right gastric artery, 179-180
Right hepatic artery, 180, 255t
Right hepatic vein, 223, 255t
Right hypochondrium, 88, 219
Right kidney
    abdominal scanning of
        at level of gallbladder, 107, 111f
        at level of liver and gallbladder longitudinal, 107-109, 111f, 118f
        power Doppler imaging with vascular UCA of, 513f
        transverse scanning of, 140f
Right lobe of liver, 219f, 220-221
    longitudinal scanning of, 108, 117f
    transverse scanning of, 107, 112f, 142f
Right lower quadrant (RLQ)
    description of, 88f
    pain in, 573t, 574-575
Right middle cerebral artery, 1093f
Right parasternal window, 927b, 928, 948b
Right portal vein (RPV), 206, 208f, 223, 224f
    color Doppler technique for, 255t
Right renal artery (RRA), 185
    color Doppler imaging with vascular ultrasound contrast agents of, 512f
    sonographic findings in, 186, 186f, 443f

Right renal vein (RRV), 202-203, 204f, 441-444, 444f
Right upper quadrant (RUQ), 88, 88f, 567-568, 573t
Right ventricle, 898, 898f
    anterior view of, 892f
    fetal circulation and, 1010
Right ventricular inflow disturbance, 1043-1045
Right ventricular outflow disturbance, 1045-1048
Right ventricular outflow tracts
    crisscross view, 1021, 1022b, 1022f
    five-chamber view of, 1021, 1021b, 1022f
    long-axis view of, 1022-1023, 1023b, 1023f, 1024f, 1025f, 1026f
    short-axis view of, 1023-1026, 1026b, 1026f, 1027f
Right-side diaphragmatic hernia, 1556
RIND. see Reversible ischemic neurologic deficit
Ring-down artifacts, 148-149, 151f
Roberts syndrome, 1500-1501, 1629-1630
Robinson, David, 7-8
Rock, 127-128
Rolled nipple technique, 656
Root, aortic, 171, 172f
Rotate motion, 128
Rotator cuff
    injuries to, 72
    minimum shoulder views of, 744b
    sonographic evaluation of, 744, 744b
        biceps tendon, 744, 744f, 745f
        indications for, 748b
        infraspinatus tendon, 745, 747f
        subscapularis tendon, 744, 745f
        supraspinatus tendon, 744-745, 746f
    tears of, 751-753, 751f
        full-thickness, 752, 753b, 753f
        partial-thickness, 752, 752b, 752f
Round ligaments, 1165-1166
Roux-en-Y procedure, 587f
RPV. see Right portal vein
RRA. see Right renal artery
RRV. see Right renal vein
Rubin's test, 1276
Rugae, 390
RUQ. see Right upper quadrant
Rushmer, Robert, 8-10

S

Saccular aneurysm, 191, 192f
Sacral hiatus, 873f
Sacrococcygeal teratomas
    AFP and, 1427-1428
Sacrum, 873, 873f
Safety, national patient standards for, 544
Sagittal imaging
    of female pelvis, 1184
    of hepatic structures, 235-239, 236f-237f, 238f
    in neonatal head examination, 825t, 826f, 827-828, 827f
    of pancreas, 366-367, 367f, 368f
    transabdominal, 1178-1180, 1179f, 1180f
    transvaginal, 1186, 1186b, 1186f, 1193f
Sagittal plane, abdominal, 104
Saldino-Noonan syndrome, 1630
Salpingitis, 1260-1263, 1262f, 1262t, 1263f, 1264f
Sample volume, 920, 1096
"Sandwich sign," 428
Sarcoma, 671

Satomura, Shigeo, 8-10
Scale, 26
Scalp edema, 1409f
Scan window, 125
Scanning, 124
    criteria for adequate scans, 134, 135f
Scattering, 12, 13f
Schizencephaly, 1523t, 1538, 1539f
Sciatic nerve, 739t
Scintigraphy, 770
Scirrhous carcinoma, 674-675
Sclerosing cholangitis, 315, 318f
Sclerotherapy, 1136-1137
Scoliosis, 1563-1564
Screening
    breast, 652, 653b
    mammography, 653-654, 653b, 653t, 654b
Scrotal cavity, 87t, 94-95
Scrotum
    anatomy of, 709-713, 709f, 710f, 731b-732b
    pathology of, 717-732
        congenital anomalies, 728t, 730-732
        epididymo-orchitis, 718
        extratesticular masses, 718t, 722
        hematomas, 714, 714f
        hernias, 723-725, 725f
        hydroceles, pyoceles, and hematoceles, 725-726, 726f
        lymphoma and leukemia, 728t, 730
        masses, 718t
        sperm granulomas, 726, 726f
        torsion, 710f, 720, 722f
        trauma, 717-722, 718f
        varicoceles, 717t, 722-723
    sonographic evaluation of
        patient positioning and scanning protocol, 712-713, 712b, 713f, 713t
        technical considerations for, 713-717, 714f, 715t
    swollen, 87t
    technical considerations for, 713-717, 714f
    testicular masses
        benign, 726-728, 727f
        malignant, 728-730, 728t
    torsion, 579, 579f, 580f
    trauma, 579, 579f, 580f
    vascular supply of, 710-712, 711f, 712b
SDMS. see Society of Diagnostic Medical Sonography
Second trimester pregnancy
    gestational age assessment, 1382-1394
        abdominal circumference, 1388-1389, 1388b, 1388f
        bone lengths, 1389-1390
        fetal measurements, 1382-1388
        fetal weight estimation, 1391-1392, 1392t
        multiple parameters, 1390-1391
        parameters, 1392-1394
    indications for, 1284b, 1290-1292, 1292b
    sonography of, 1343
Secondary hyperparathyroidism, 704
Secondary retroperitoneal tumor, 508
Secondary yolk sac, 1301, 1302f
Second-degree heart block, 1065-1066
Secretin, 393
Secretory phase
    description of, 1171b, 1172
    endometrium during, 1195, 1196f

Section thickness artifacts, 148, 148f
Sectional anatomy, 102
Sector array transducer, 134–135
Sector phased-array transducer, 16, 17f
Segmental Doppler pressures, 1114–1116, 1115t
Semilobar holoprosencephaly, 843, 843f, 1532–1533, 1532f, 1542f
Semilunar valves, 902–903
Seminoma, 728–729, 728t, 729f
Sensitization, 1407–1409
Sentinel node procedure, of breasts, 677–681, 678f
Sepsis, generalized, 420
Septa testis, 710
Septal defects
　atrial, 1036–1038, 1037f
　　ostium primum, 1037–1038, 1037f, 1038f
　　ostium secundum, 1037, 1037f
　　sinus venosus septal defect, 1037f, 1038, 1038f
　atrioventricular, 1041–1043, 1041f
　ventricular, 1038–1041, 1038f, 1039f
　　incidence of, 1032t, 1033
　　membranous septal defect, 1038–1040, 1040f
　　muscular defect, 1040–1041
Septicemia, 430–432
Septum primum, 1009, 1010f
Septum secundum, 1009, 1010f
Seroma
　after liver transplantation, 600, 604f
　after pancreatic transplantation, 636
　after renal transplantation, 621, 625f
　breast, 665, 665f
　definition of, 600
　muscle, 754
Serosa, 398
Serous cystadenocarcinomas, 1248–1249, 1249b, 1250b, 1251f
Serous cystadenoma, 1249b, 1249f, 1250f, 1252f
Serous cystic tumors, 377, 380f, 381f
Serous pericardium, 980, 981f
Sertoli-Leydig cell tumors, 1255–1256, 1256f
Serum albumin, 81, 228t
Serum amylase, 362
Serum calcium, 700–701
Serum creatinine, 439
Sestamibi parathyroid scan, 701
Sex hormones, 497
SGA. see Small for gestational age
Shadowing
　attenuation, 153–156, 155f
　causes of, 314–315
　color Doppler, 160–163, 162f, 163f
　definition of, 129, 153–156
　endometrial, 1208b
　example of, 131, 133f
　refractile, 742–743, 742f, 743f
　sonographic findings in, 314–315, 317f
Shone complex, 1048, 1049f
Short bowel syndrome, 787–788
Short-axis view
　of left and right ventricular outflow tracts, 1023–1026, 1026b, 1026f, 1027f
　parasternal
　　for color flow mapping, 922b, 929–931, 931f, 932f, 933f, 934f
　　Doppler window, 922–923, 931b, 931f, 932f, 933f, 934f
　　of pulmonary stenosis, 1047f

Short-rib polydactyly syndrome, 1623t, 1630–1631, 1631f
Shoulder biceps tendon, 751, 751f
Shoulder dystocia, 1413–1414
Sickle cell anemia
　description of, 340
　illustration of, 340f
　stroke in, 1102–1103, 1103f
Sickle cell crisis, 340
Sickle cell nephropathy, 454t–458t, 471
Side lobes, 129, 132f, 151
Silicone breast implants
　low propagation speed in, 154f
　ruptured, 668, 669f
Simple call button, 34, 34f
Simple cysts
　in breast, 658t, 659, 659b, 660f
　hepatic, 262–264, 264t, 265f, 608
　ovarian
　　in postmenopausal women, 1240–1242
　　sonographic evaluation of, 1234, 1234b, 1234f, 1235f
　renal, 454t–458t
Simultaneous pancreas-kidney transplant (SPK), 586
Single photon emission computed tomography (SPECT), of breasts, 677–681, 678f
Single umbilical artery, 1470–1472, 1471f
Single ventricle, 1058–1059, 1058f, 1059f
Sinoatrial node, 1010
Sinus lipomatosis, 444, 447f
Sinus of Valsalva aneurysm, 974, 976f
Sinus venosus septal defect, 1037f, 1038, 1038f
Sinuses of Valsalva, 903, 974
Sirenomelia, 1631–1632, 1631f, 1632f
Situs ambiguous, 327–329
Situs inversus, 327–329, 1035f, 1577, 1581, 1582f
　partial, 1581, 1583f
　sonographic findings in, 1581
Situs solitus, 327–329, 1035f, 1582f
Skeletal dysplasia, 1622–1623, 1635b–1636b
　achondrogenesis, 1623t, 1626, 1626f, 1627f
　achondroplasia, 1623t, 1626
　arthrogryposis multiplex congenita, 1632–1633, 1632f
　camptomelic dysplasia, 1623t, 1629, 1630f
　caudal regression syndrome, 1631–1632, 1631f, 1632f
　congenital hypophosphatasia, 1628
　diastrophic dysplasia, 1628–1629, 1629f
　Ellis-van Creveld syndrome, 1631
　Jeune syndrome, 1631
　limb abnormalities, 1633–1635, 1633f, 1634f, 1635f
　osteogenesis imperfecta, 1623t, 1626–1628, 1627f, 1628f
　Roberts syndrome, 1629–1630
　short-rib polydactyly syndrome, 1623t, 1630–1631, 1631f
　sonographic evaluation of, 1623–1624, 1624t, 1625f
　thanatophoric dysplasia, 1623t, 1624–1626, 1625f
Skeleton, fetal, 1622, 1635b–1636b
　abnormalities of, 1622–1633. see also Skeletal dysplasia
　embryology of, 1622
Skin edema, hydrops and, 1486–1487

Skull. see also Cranium
　fetal, abnormalities of, 1498–1499, 1499f
　neonatal, 815f
Slice thickness, 13–14
Slide motion, 127
Sludge, 290–293, 294t–295t, 295f
Small for gestational age (SGA), 1390, 1397, 1417–1418, 1418f
Small intestine, 89, 89f. see also Bowel
　anatomy of, 390, 392f, 393f
　sonographic evaluation of, 399f
　vascular anatomy of, 392, 395f
Small saphenous vein (SSV), 1132
Society for Vascular Ultrasound (SVU), 6
Society of Diagnostic Medical Sonography (SDMS), 6
　sonographer's shoulder complaints received by, 69
Soldner, Richard, 8
Soleal sinuses, 1131
Solid lung masses, 1551–1554
　congenital bronchial atresia, 1554
　congenital cystic adenomatoid malformation, 1552–1554, 1553f, 1554f
　pulmonary sequestration, 1552, 1552b, 1552f
Somer, Jan, 8
Sonar, 7
Sonazoid, 514–515
Sonographers, 4
　commitments of, 30–35
　essentials of patient care for, 29, 67b
　in interventional procedures, 548–550, 549f, 550f
　physical health of, 5b
　qualities of, 5b
　resource organizations for, 6
　role of, 4–6
　training of, 129
Sonography
　career in, 5–6
　definition of, 4
　of second and third trimesters, 1343, 1376b
　　diaphragm and thoracic vessels, 1360–1362, 1361f, 1362f, 1363f
　　equipment and practices, 1344
　　extrafetal obstetric overview, 1371–1375
　　　amniotic fluid, 1374, 1375f
　　　cervix, 1375, 1375b
　　　membranes, 1374–1375
　　　placenta, 1373–1374, 1373f, 1374f
　　　umbilical cord, 1372–1373, 1372f, 1373f
　　fetal anatomy, 1348–1371
　　　cranium, 1348–1352, 1348f, 1349f, 1350f, 1351f, 1352f
　　　face, 1352–1355
　　fetal circulation, 1362–1363, 1363f, 1364f
　　fetal presentation, 1345–1348, 1345f, 1346f
　　gastrointestinal system, 1365–1366, 1365f
　　genetic sonogram, 1375–1376
　　genitalia, 1368–1369, 1368f, 1369f
　　heart, 1359–1360, 1360f, 1361f
　　hepatobiliary system and upper abdomen, 1363–1365, 1364f, 1365f
　　initial steps and examination overview, 1344–1348
　　suggested protocol, 1344, 1344b
　　thorax, 1357–1359, 1358f, 1359f

Sonography *(Continued)*
    upper and lower extremities, 1369–1371, 1369f, 1370f, 1371f, 1372f
    urinary system, 1366–1368, 1366f, 1367f
    vertebral column, 1355–1357, 1356f, 1357f
Sonohysterography, 1199, 1200f
    of endometrium, 1218–1220, 1219f
Sonolucent, 130
SonoVue, 514, 517
Sound
    measurement of, 11–12
    propagation through tissue, 12
    velocity of, 10
Sound frequency ranges, 11t
Sound theory, 6–10
Space of Retzius, 1174
Spalding sign, 1417
Spallanzani, Lazzaro, 6
Spaulding's classification system, 51–52, 51t, 52f
Special needs patients, 57–60
    adolescent patients, 58
    crying/upset patients, 57
    elderly patients, 57–58
    multicultural patients, 59
    pediatric patients, 58–59
Specific gravity, 438
Speckle
    algorithms for reduction of, 715t
    description of, 148, 149f
Spectral analysis, 23, 24f, 922–923, 923f
Spectral analysis waveform, 922–923
Spectral broadening, 23, 212, 1098–1099
Spectral Doppler analysis
    of renal artery flow, 512f
    scrotal, 713
Spectral Doppler artifacts, 156–160
    aliasing and, 156, 159b
    mirror image and, 160, 160f
    noise and, 160, 160f
    Nyquist limit and, 156–159, 157t, 158f, 159b, 159f
    range ambiguity and, 157f, 159–160
Speed error artifacts, 743, 743t
Speed error propagation, 151, 154f
Sperm granulomas, 726, 726f
Spermatic cord
    description of, 710
    torsion of, 579, 720, 721f, 722f
Spermatoceles, 717t, 722
Spherocytosis, congenital, 340, 341f
Sphincter of Oddi, 283
Spiculation, 669, 670f
Spigelian fascia, 419
Spigelian hernia, 433
Spina bifida, 1337–1338, 1338f, 1392–1393, 1523t, 1527–1529, 1528f
    sonographic findings in, 1529, 1529f, 1530f, 1531f
Spina bifida aperta, 880, 1528
Spina bifida cystica, 1528f
Spina bifida occulta, 880, 1528, 1528f
Spinal canal, 88, 871, 875, 875f
Spinal cord
    anatomy of, 873, 874f
    anterior position of, 879
    injury, 886–887, 886f
    meninges of, 873–875, 874f
    primitive, 1523

Spinal cord *(Continued)*
    sonographic appearance of, 875, 875f
    tethered, 871, 881–883, 882f
Spinal degeneration, 72
Spinal dysraphism, lumbosacral stigmata associated with, 887b
Spinal nerve roots, 873
Spine. *see also* Vertebral column
    embryonic, 1310–1313, 1311f, 1312f
    fetal ultrasound, 1408t
    neonatal. *see* Neonatal spine
Spiral arteries, 1443f
Splanchnic aneurysm, 185–187, 185f, 195
Spleen, 88, 325, 333b, 335f, 353b
    abdominal scanning of, at level of left kidney, 109, 122f
    abscesses of, 337t, 342–344, 346f
    accessory, 329, 331f
    agenesis, 327–329
    anatomy of, 326–327
        normal, 326, 327f, 328f
        relational, 326, 331f
        size, 326, 329f
        vascular supply, 326, 330f
    atrophy, 336
    congenital anomalies of, 327–329, 331f
    diffuse disease, 340–342, 340f, 341f
    displacement of, 326–327
    fetal
        abnormalities of, 1583–1584
        embryology of, 1574
        sonographic evaluation of, 1580, 1580f
    functions of, 332, 332b
    hematoma, 566f
    infarction, 337t, 344–345, 347f
    infection, 344, 344f, 347f
    laboratory data of, 332–333
    longitudinal scans of, 141
    nonvisualization of, 336
    pathology of, 336
        acquired immunodeficiency syndrome, 344
        benign primary tumors, 349–351, 350f
        congestion, 337b, 337t
        cysts, 337t, 348–349, 349f
        diffuse disease, 340, 341f
        hamartoma, 349, 351f
        hematoma, 347–348, 348f, 349f
        infarction, 337t, 344–345
        malignant primary tumors, 351–354
        storage disease, 339–340, 339f
        trauma, 337t, 345–348, 347f, 350f
    pediatric, 765b, 766f, 767f
    physiology of, 329–333
    pulp of, 329
    sonographic evaluation of, 333–336
        normal texture and patterns in, 333–334, 334f
        patient position and technique in, 334–336, 335f
        size in, 333, 333f, 337t
    transverse scanning of, 139, 139f, 141
    wandering, 327
Splenic artery, 106, 106f, 109, 180, 326
    Doppler flow patterns in, 212, 212b, 213f
    pancreas and, 358f, 359
    sonographic evaluation of, 181f, 182f
Splenic flexure, 390–391
Splenic hilum, 326, 330f
Splenic sequestration syndrome, 767–775

Splenic vein, 106–108, 106f, 206–207
    anatomy of, 326, 330f
    color Doppler technique for, 255t
    pancreas and, 358, 358f
    sonographic findings of, 206, 210f
Splenomegaly, 326, 336–338, 336f, 337t, 338b, 338f, 338t, 339f, 342f
    in adolescents, 769f
    congestive, 338b, 339
    patterns, 339f
    sonographic evaluation of, 337t, 499, 501f
Splenorenal ligament, 326, 328f, 418, 418f
Split-hand deformity, 1633f
Sponge kidney, medullary, 454t–458t, 462, 479, 480f
Spontaneous abortion, 1322, 1322f
Spontaneous flow, 1140–1141
Spontaneous rupture of the membranes (SPROM), 1482
Squamous cell carcinoma
    cervical, 1204–1206, 1206f
    renal, 454t–458t, 466, 466f, 467f
Standard evaluation, fetal ultrasound, 1408t
Standard precautions, 49–53, 50f, 51f
Starzl, Thomas, 585
Static Graf technique, 860–866, 862b, 862f, 863f, 863t, 864f
Stein-Leventhal syndrome, 1238–1239
Stepladder sign, 668, 669f
Sternal angle, 891–892
Sternocleidomastoid muscles, 683, 684f
Sternum, absent, 1564t
Stoma, 47
Stomach, 88, 89f, 219, 220f
    anatomy of
        normal, 390, 391f
        vascular, 392, 394f
    antrum of, 367, 368f
    fetal
        abnormalities of, 1584–1586
        embryology of, 1573–1574
        sonographic evaluation of, 1576–1577, 1577f
    sonographic evaluation of, 395–396, 397f
Stools, height-adjustable, 78
Storage disease, 339–340, 339f
Strabismus, 1502
Strangulated hernia, 575
Strap muscles, 683, 684f
Stress testing, arterial, 1116
Stressors, 81
Stretches, 77f
Striations, 1160–1161
Strict isolation, 55
Strictures, ureteral, 450
Stroke volume, 910, 914, 990b
Stroma ovarii, 1250–1251
Stromal tumors, 1252–1257, 1255f
Strutt, John William, 6
Stuck twin. *see* Polyhydramnios-oligohydramnios (poly-oli) sequence
Subacute bacterial endocarditis, 1000–1006, 1004f, 1005f
Subacute (de Quervain) thyroiditis, 699–700
Subarachnoid space, 816
Subcapsular collections, 424–425, 425f
Subchorionic hemorrhage, 1320, 1321f, 1456
Subclavian artery, 162f, 1112
Subclavian steal syndrome, 1081f, 1101, 1101f

Subclavian vein, 1133
Subcostal plane, 105
Subcostal transducer location, 918, 919f
Subcostal view
　for color flow mapping, 938, 948b
　for Doppler, 924b, 938–939
　transducer position, 938–939, 948b
　two-dimensional, 938, 938b, 948f
Subcostal window, 924b, 938–939
Subcutaneous fat, 646, 647f
Subcutaneous layer, 645, 645f, 646f
Subependyma, cysts of, 833, 845
Subfascial hematoma, 430
Subfertility, 1272–1273
Subhepatic lesion, 414
Subhepatic spaces, 99f
Sublingual cysts, 1512f
Subluxation
　of neonatal hip, 857–858, 858f
　of shoulder biceps tendon, 751, 751f
Submandibular window
　intracranial arterial identification criteria, 1096t
　for transcranial color Doppler imaging, 1095–1096
Submucosa, 390
Submucosal leiomyomas, 1209, 1209b
Suboccipital window, 1095, 1095f
Subphrenic abscesses, 423–424, 424f
Subphrenic space, 98, 99f, 219
Subpulmonic stenosis, 1047–1048, 1047f
Subscapularis tendon, 744, 745f
Subserosal leiomyomas, 1209, 1209b, 1210f
Subvalvular aortic stenosis, 966, 967f, 1050–1052, 1051f, 1052f
Subvalvular pulmonary stenosis, 1047f
Succenturiate lobes, 1454
Succenturiate placenta, 1449, 1454, 1454f, 1455f
Suffering, 1296
Sulcus, 817
Superficial flexor tendon, 736f
Superficial inguinal ring, 90
Superficial structures, 134
Superficial veins
　lower extremity, 1132–1133, 1132f
　mapping of, 1146
　upper extremity, 1134f
Superficial venous thrombosis, 1136
Superior mesenteric artery (SMA), 180–182, 183f
　abdominal scanning of
　　at level of aorta, 109, 121f
　　at level of pancreas, 107, 109f
　Doppler flow patterns in, 212b, 213f, 214
　longitudinal scans of, 141
　pancreas and, 358f, 359
　sonographic evaluation of, 182–184, 183f
Superior mesenteric vein (SMV), 207–209
　pancreas and, 356, 357f, 358, 365f
　sonographic findings of, 198, 211f
Superior vena cava
　congenital left atrial communication with, 1059–1060, 1060f
　fetal circulation, 1446f
　fetal circulation and, 1010
Superior vesical arteries, 1461
Superior/inferior direction, 132–134
Supine, 132
Support cushions, 78
Supracolic compartment, 99f

Supracristal defects, 1038–1039
Suprapancreatic obstruction, 312, 314f
Suprarenal veins, 204–206
Suprascapular nerve, 739t
Supraspinatus tendon
　sonographic evaluation of, 746f
　tears of, 752
Suprasternal notch, 891–892, 948b
Suprasternal notch view, 924b, 949f
Suprasternal transducer location, 918, 919f
Suprasternal views
　for color flow mapping, 940–941, 949f
　for Doppler, 941–943, 949f
　transducer position, 949f
　two-dimensional, 939–940, 948b, 948f
Supravalvular aortic stenosis, 966, 966f, 1050–1052, 1051f, 1052f
Supravalvular pulmonary stenosis, 1048, 1048f
Supraventricular tachyarrhythmias, 1063–1064, 1064f
Supravesical space, 418–419
Surgery, for hypertrophic pyloric stenosis, 787–788, 787f
Suspensory ligament, 1169
Sweep motion, 127
Swelling
　extremity, 579–581, 580f
　scrotum, 87t
Swyer syndrome, 1630f
Sylvian fissure, 818f
Syncope, 1072
Synechiae
　intrauterine, 1222–1223, 1223f
　uterine, 1275f
Synovial sheath, 736, 736f
Systemic lupus erythematosus (SLE), 1064f, 1415, 1415f
Systole, 909, 926–928
Systolic measurement, 36
Systolic murmur, 905
Systolic to diastolic (S/D) ratio, 1191, 1403

T
T wave, 904
T_3. see Triiodothyronine
T4. see Thyroxine
Tachyarrhythmias, supraventricular, 1063–1064, 1064f
Tachycardia, 84
　definition of, 35
　embryonic, 1327
　fetal, 1012
Tail of Spence, 645
Takotsubo cardiomyopathy, 993
Talipes. see Clubfoot
Tamoxifen, 1224
Tardus-parvus, 481, 483f
Target sign, 404
　double, 783
Tatum T, 1227–1228
Taylor, Frederick Winslow, 68
TCC. see Transitional cell carcinoma
Teardrop/noose sign, 667–668, 668f
Technical aptitude, 5b
TEE. see Transesophageal echocardiography
Temporal resolution, 18
Tendinitis, 72, 753–754, 753f, 754b, 754f
　acute, 753–754
　de Quervain, 754
　sonographic features of, 755t

Tendons, 736–737, 736f, 737f
Tenosynovitis, 72, 753–754, 754f
Tentorium cerebelli, 815
Teratogens, 1533
Teratoma, 508
　dermoid tumors, 1250–1251, 1252b, 1252f, 1253f
　fetal neck, 1515, 1516b, 1516f
　immature and mature, 1251–1252, 1253f
Teres minor tendon, 747, 747f, 748f
Terminal ductal lobular units (TDLUs), 645–646, 646f
Terminal patients, 60–61
Testes, 709
　enlarged, 718t
　hypoechoic band in, 718t
　undescended. see Cryptorchidism
Testicular arteries, 710–711, 712b
Testicular duplication, 731–732
Testicular ectopia, 730
Testicular masses, benign, 726–728, 727f
　malignant, 728–730, 728t
Testicular microlithiasis, 728, 728f
Testicular vein, 712
Tethered spinal cord, 871, 881–883, 882f
Tetralogy of Fallot, 1045–1046, 1046f
TGC. see Time gain compensation
Thalamo-occipital distance (TOD), 830, 831f
Thalamus, neonatal, 818, 819f
Thalassemia, 341–342, 343f
Thanatophoric dysplasia, 1499f, 1623t, 1624–1626, 1625f
Theca-lutein cysts, 1237, 1238b, 1239f, 1325, 1326f
Thecomas, 1254–1255, 1255f
Thermal index (TI), 1288
Third trimester pregnancy
　gestational age assessment, 1382–1394
　　abdominal circumference, 1388–1389, 1388b, 1388f
　　bone lengths, 1389–1390
　　fetal measurements, 1382–1388
　　fetal weight estimation, 1391–1392, 1392t
　　multiple parameters, 1390–1391
　　parameters, 1392–1394
　indications for, 1284b, 1290–1292, 1292b
　sonography of, 1343
Third ventricle, neonatal, 815–816, 825–826
Third-degree heart block, 1065–1066
Thompson's test, 750
Thoracentesis, 543
Thoracic aneurysms, 195
Thoracic cavity, 88, 88f
　abnormalities of, 1548–1558
　　diaphragm, 1555–1558, 1555f
　　lung, 1548–1555, 1549f, 1550t
　anatomy of, 891–892, 892f, 893b, 906b–907b
　embryology of, 1545
Thoracic circumference measurements, fetal, 1550t
Thoracic outlet syndrome (TOS), 72, 1117–1118
Thoracic pain, 573t
Thorax, 891–892, 892f
　fetal, 1357–1359, 1358f, 1359f, 1545, 1558b.
　　see also Thoracic cavity
　sonographic characteristics of, 1545–1548, 1546b
　　position, 1546–1547, 1548f
　　respiration, 1547–1548, 1548f
　　size, 1546, 1546f, 1547f
　　texture, 1547, 1548f

Threatened abortion, 1320
Three-dimensional (3D) imaging
  echocardiography, 916–917
  of female pelvis, 1199–1201, 1200f
  fetal echocardiography, 1015, 1015f
  gray-scale harmonic imaging with vascular UCA, 516, 516f
  for lost intrauterine contraceptive devices, 1225–1228, 1226f–1227f, 1228f
  of ovaries, 1233
  of scrotum, 710f, 713f
Three-dimensional ultrasound (3DU), 20–21, 20f
Threshold level, 1323
Threshold parameters for scrotum evaluation, 715t
Thrombocytes, 83
Thrombocytopenia, 333
Thrombolytic therapy, 1135
Thrombosis
  after pancreatic transplantation, 633–634, 635f, 636f
  inferior vena cava, 199–204, 260t
  renal veins, 202–203, 204f, 617–619, 621f, 805–806
  of umbilical vessels, 1467, 1468f
Thrombus, cardiac, 998–1000, 1003f
Thyroglossal duct cysts, 705, 705f
Thyroid gland, 682, 707b
  anatomy of, 683–684, 684f
    relational, 683–684, 684f
    size, 683, 684t
  aplasia, 690
  blood supply of, 684
  congenital abnormalities of, 690
  ectopic, 690
  elastography of, 698, 698f
  embryology of, 683
  pathology of, 690–700
    benign lesions, 691–693, 693f
    diffuse thyroid disease, 698–700
    malignant lesions, 693–698, 695f
    nodular thyroid disease, 690–691, 690f, 692f
  physiology and laboratory data of, 684–686, 685b
  sonographic evaluation of, 686–690, 687f, 688f, 689f, 690f
  ultrasound-guided biopsy of, 557, 557f
Thyroid inferno, 699
Thyroid metastasis, 698
Thyroiditis, 699
  de Quervain, 699
  Hashimoto, 700, 700f
Thyroid-stimulating hormone (TSH), 684–685
Thyromegaly, 1514, 1516f
Thyrotoxic crisis, 699
Thyrotoxicosis, 683
Thyroxine (T_4), 682–683
TIA. see Transient ischemic attack
Tibia, fetal measurement, 1390, 1390b, 1390f
Tibial-peroneal trunk, 1112
Ticlopidine, 1135
Time gain compensation (TGC), 21–22, 124, 231–232, 439
Time-of-flight artifacts, 743, 743f
Tinel sign, 756
"Tip of the iceberg," 1251
TIPS. see Transjugular intrahepatic portosystemic shunt
Tissue
  definition of, 81
  propagation of sound through, 12

Tissue characterization, 209
Tissue Doppler imaging, 995
Tissue plasminogen activators (tPAs), 1135
Tissue-specific ultrasound contrast agents, 514–515, 515f
TOAs. see Tubo-ovarian abscesses
Toe pressures, 1115
Toe-brachial index (TBI), 1116–1117
Tongue, abnormalities of, 1510–1511, 1511f, 1512f
TORCH, 770
Torsion
  gallbladder, 299–300
  ovarian, 1243–1244, 1243b, 1244f
  scrotal, 579, 579f, 580f, 717t, 720, 722f
Tortuous arteries, 1075–1076, 1076b, 1076f
Tortuous pelvic mass, anechoic, 1600
TOS. see Thoracic outlet syndrome
Total anomalous pulmonary venous return (TAPVR), 899, 1060, 1060f, 1061f
Toxemia, 1415
Toxic goiter, 691, 691t
Trachea, abnormalities of, 1511–1512, 1512f
Tracheoesophageal septum, 1573
Transabdominal (TA) ultrasonography, 1158, 1178–1181, 1181b
  levator ani muscles, 1190, 1190f
  longitudinal, 1178–1181, 1194, 1194f
  obturator internus muscles, 1189–1190, 1190f
  of ovaries, 1231–1234
  patient preparation and history for, 1178–1181
  pelvic vascularity, 1181f, 1190, 1192f
  protocol for, 1181b, 1185
  sagittal imaging, 1178–1180, 1179f, 1180f
    of distended bladder, 1179f, 1180f
  transverse, 1179f, 1180f
  of tubo-ovarian abscess, 1263–1264, 1265f, 1266f
  of uterus
    longitudinal, 1178–1181
    sagittal, 1181f, 1182f
    transverse, 1183f
Transcranial Doppler (TCD) imaging, 1087–1088
  advantages of, 1104–1107
  applications of, 1087–1088, 1088b, 1099–1104
  of brain death, 1103
  of collateral pathways, 1100–1101
  diagnostic pitfalls of, 1105–1107, 1107f
  guidelines for, 1105b
  interpretation of, 1096–1099
  intracranial disease diagnosed using, 1100–1103
  intracranial venous evaluation by, 1104
  intraoperative use of, 1104
  limitations of, 1104–1107, 1104b
  sickle cell disease examination, 1102–1103, 1103f
  technical aspects of, 1090–1096
    hints on, 1106t
    instrumentation, 1091
    technique, 1091–1096, 1092f
      submandibular window, 1095–1096
      suboccipital window, 1095, 1095f
      transorbital window, 1094, 1094f
      transtemporal window, 1092–1094, 1092f, 1093f, 1094f
  vasospasm diagnosis using, 1099–1100
Transducer(s)
  cable management, 76–77
  continuous-wave Doppler, 913f

Transducer(s) (Continued)
  curved-array, 16–17
  definition of, 14–15
  Doppler frequency shift and, 25
  for echocardiography, 918–919, 919f
  gripping pressure, 74–75
  intraluminal, 17, 17f
  linear-array, 16, 17f, 854, 854b
  multielement, 16, 16f
  needles attached to, 536–538, 536f
  for neonatal head examination, 820
  placement for transcranial color Doppler, 1092
  positions of
    in abdominal scanning, 126–128, 129f
    cardiac protocol and, 927b
    in echocardiography, 918–919, 919f
    radial/antiradial, 657
  prepping, 544–546, 545f, 546f
  pulsed wave Doppler, 911, 911f, 923, 923f
  requirements for fetal echocardiography, 1013
  sector phased-array, 16, 17f
  selection of, 14–17, 14f, 15f
    in abdominal scanning, 125–126, 126f, 127f
  transvaginal, 1180–1181, 1305
  types of, 14
Transducer angle, 1096
Transesophageal echocardiography (TEE), 916–917
Transfer, of patient, 38–40
  in assisting patients from the scanning stretcher into the wheelchair, 40, 41f
  body mechanics and, 38–39
  in moving patients toward the head of a stretcher, 39–40
  in moving patients up in bed, 39, 40f
  in stretcher transfer, 39, 39f
  in turning patients, 40
  in wheelchair transfer, 39, 39f
Transient ischemic attack (TIA), 1071
Transitional cell carcinoma (TCC), 454t–458t, 464–466, 623, 627f
Transitional cell tumors, 1249–1250, 1252f
Transjugular intrahepatic portosystemic shunt (TIPS), 257, 257f, 517
Translabial sonography, 1187, 1206–1207
Transmediastinal artery, 711, 711f
Transmission, abnormal structures affecting, 134b
Transorbital approach, 1094, 1094f, 1096t
Transorbital window, 1094, 1094f
Transperineal approach, 1177
Transperineal sonography, 1187, 1206–1207
Transplant patient, sonographic techniques in, 583, 638b
Transplantation, 523–524
  liver. see Liver transplantation
  pancreatic. see Pancreatic transplantation
  renal. see Renal transplantation
  team-based approach to, 584
  waiting list for, 584
Transposition of the great arteries, 1054, 1054f, 1055f
  corrected, 1054
  sonographic findings in, 1054, 1055f
Transpyloric plane, 88, 105
Transtemporal approach
  bony landmarks from, 1092–1093, 1092f, 1093f
  intracranial arterial identification criteria, 1096t
  for transcranial Doppler, 1092–1094, 1092f, 1093f, 1094f

Transtemporal window, 1092-1094, 1092f, 1093f, 1094f
Transtesticular artery, 711
Transvaginal transducers, 126, 128f, 1305
Transvaginal (TV) ultrasonography, 1158, 1183-1189
  of adenomyosis, 1212-1216
  of cervix
    benign conditions, 1203-1204, 1203f, 1204b
    cervical carcinoma and, 1204, 1206b, 1206f
  disinfection technique, 1187-1189
  endometrial hyperplasia, 1220, 1220b, 1221f
  of endometriomas, 1267-1270, 1268f, 1269f
  of endometrium, 1195-1196, 1195f, 1196f
    carcinoma, 1223-1224, 1224b, 1224f
    endometritis, 1221-1222, 1222b
  examination technique, 1183-1184
  of fallopian tubes, 1196-1197, 1197f
  first trimester, 1305-1306, 1305f
    at 6 to 10 weeks of gestational age, 1310-1313, 1310t
      embryonic cranium and spine, 1310-1313, 1311f, 1312f
      embryonic heart, 1313, 1314f, 1314t
      limb development, 1313, 1313f
      physiologic herniation of bowel, 1313, 1314f
      skeletal ossification, 1313, 1313f
    fetal period (weeks 9-14), 1306-1313
      embryo during, 1308-1310, 1309f, 1310f
      gestational sac during, 1307-1310, 1307f, 1307t
      yolk sac during, 1307-1308, 1307f, 1308f
  of ovaries, 1186b, 1197-1198, 1197f
    dermoid tumors, 1250-1251, 1252b, 1252f, 1253f
    hemorrhagic corpus luteum cysts, 1237, 1238f
    hemorrhagic cysts, 1237, 1238f
    ovarian hyperstimulation syndrome, 1237-1239, 1239f
    simple cystic masses, 1234, 1234b, 1234f, 1235f
    torsion, 1243-1244, 1243b, 1244f
  paraovarian cysts, 1240, 1240b, 1241f
  patient instructions for, 1183
  of pelvic inflammatory disease, salpingitis, hydrosalpinx, and pyosalpinx, 1261-1263, 1262f, 1262t, 1263f, 1264f
  pelvic vascularity, 1181f, 1190, 1192f
  of peritonitis, 1264-1266, 1266f
  polyps, 1220-1221, 1222f
  probe preparation for, 1183, 1184f
  protocol, 1186b
  scan orientation, 1184, 1185f
  scanning planes, 1184
  scanning techniques, 1184-1185
  small endometrial fluid collections, 1224-1225, 1225f
  technique, 1187-1189, 1188f
  of uterine leiomyosarcoma, 1216-1217, 1217f
  of uterus
    coronal, 1186, 1186b, 1187f
    with hypoechoic myoma, 1206f
    sagittal, 1186, 1186b, 1186f, 1193f, 1197f
Transverse fetal lie, 1345, 1345f
Transverse pancreatic artery, 180
Transverse plane, 88
  abdominal, 104, 106-108
  of abdominal aorta, 174, 177f

Transverse scanning
  abdominal, 128. see also Abdominal scanning
  of abdominal aorta, 138-139, 138f
  of biliary system, 134
  of gallbladder, 141, 144f
  of hepatic structures, 239, 240f-241f, 242f
  of pancreas, 136-138, 364-366, 366f
  protocols for, 135-140, 136f, 137f
  of spleen, 139, 139f, 141
  suprasternal notch view, 949f
Transversus muscle, 90, 90f
Trauma
  abdominal, 561-563
  blunt. see Blunt trauma
  scrotal, 579, 579f, 580f, 717-722, 718f
  splenic, 337t, 345-348, 347f, 350f
Treacher Collins syndrome, 1500
Tricuspid annular plane systolic excursion (TAPSE), 988-989, 990f
Tricuspid regurgitation, 988-989, 990f, 1045f
Tricuspid valve, 897, 897f
  atresia of, 1043, 1043f
  Ebstein anomaly of, 1043-1045, 1044f
  fetal circulation and, 1010
  M-mode imaging of, 946
  normal Doppler measurements, 1014t
Trigger finger, 72
Trigonocephaly, 1498-1499
Triiodothyronine (T_3), 682-683
Trimesters, 1287
Triploidy, 1438
Trisomy 13, 1032, 1437-1438, 1438f, 1439f, 1440f
  sonographic findings in, 1535f
Trisomy 18, 1032, 1436-1437, 1436f, 1437f, 1438f
Trisomy 21, 1433-1436, 1434f, 1435f, 1436f
Trophoblastic layer, 1443f
Trophoblastic reaction, 1324b
True aneurysm, 190-191, 191f
True hermaphroditism, 1618
True pelvis
  description of, 1159-1160
  illustration of, 94, 1161f
  muscles of, 1161, 1161f
Truncus arteriosus, 1054-1055, 1055f
  partitioning of, 1009
  sonographic findings in, 1055, 1056f
Trunk twisting, 75f, 77
Tuberous sclerosis, 454t-458t, 460, 805
Tubes and tubing, 40-47, 41f
  catheters, 43-44, 44f
  colostomies and ileostomies, 47
  drains, 46-47
  dressings, 46-47
  intravenous therapy, 41-43, 41f, 42f, 43f
  nasogastric tubes, 43, 44f
  ostomy, 47
  oxygen therapy, 45-46, 45f, 46f
  wounds, 46-47
Tubo-ovarian abscesses (TOAs), 1261b, 1263-1264
Tubo-ovarian complex, 1221, 1260
Tubular carcinoma, 674
Tumor(s). see also Carcinoma; Neoplasms
  abdominal, 772-775
  adrenal, 503-505
    neonatal/pediatric, 807-811
  adrenal medulla, 505-506
  bladder, 486-487, 488f

Tumor(s) (Continued)
  cardiac. see Cardiac tumors
  carotid body, 1078, 1079f
  dermoid, 1250-1251, 1252b, 1252f, 1253f
  endodermal sinus, 1252
  epithelial ovarian, 1246-1250, 1248f
  gastrointestinal, 401-402
  intrahepatic biliary, 318
  Krukenberg, 1256-1257, 1257f
  liver, 773-775, 774t
    benign, 773
    malignant, 773-774
  medulla, 502t
  mesentery, 428, 430f
  omentum, 428, 430f
  ovarian
    solid, 1235-1236, 1236b
    sonographic evaluation of, 1244
  peritoneal, 428, 430f
  retroperitoneal
    primary, 506-508, 507f
    secondary, 508
  Sertoli-Leydig cell, 1255-1256, 1256f
  splenic, 337t
    benign, 349-351
    malignant, 351-354
  uterine, 1207-1208
Tunica adventitia, 171, 171f, 1111
Tunica albuginea
  cysts of, 722
  description of, 710
Tunica intima, 171, 171f, 1111
Tunica media, 171, 171f, 1111
Tunica vaginalis, 710, 710f
Turbulent flow, 23
Turner syndrome, 1032, 1339, 1438-1441, 1440f, 1513, 1514f
Twin anemia-polycythemia syndrome (TAPS), 1420-1421, 1423
Twin pregnancy, intrauterine, 1279, 1279f
"Twinkling" artifact, 160-163, 163f
Twinkling sign, 485, 485f
Twin-to-twin transfusion syndrome (TTTS), 1412f, 1422, 1422f
Two-dimensional imaging
  ability to conceptualize, 5b
  apical views, 932-938, 936f, 937f, 938b
  echocardiography, 917-919, 917f, 918f
  parasternal long-axis views, 925-926, 927b, 928b, 928f, 929f
  subcostal views, 938, 938b, 948f
  suprasternal views, 939-940, 948b, 948f

U

UCAs. see Ultrasound contrast agents
Ulcerative colitis, 410f
Ulna, fetal measurement, 1390, 1391b, 1391f
Ulnar artery, 1112
Ulnar nerve, 739t
Ulnar veins, 1133
Ultrasonic Institute, 7-8, 9f
Ultrasound, 14, 103, 103t
  annotation of images, 128-129
  certification for, 6
  criteria for identifying abnormal structures, 134b
  definition of, 4, 10
  efficiency in patient care, 34-35

Ultrasound *(Continued)*
  explanation of, 31–32
  historical overview of sound theory and, 6–10
  postoperative uses of, 1271
  principles of, 10–28
    acoustics, 10–14, 11*f*, 11*t*
    harmonic imaging, 18–20, 19*f*
    pulse-echo display modes, 17–18
    system controls for image optimization, 21–22
    three-dimensional and four-dimensional ultrasound, 20–21, 20*f*
    transducer selection, 14–17, 14*f*, 15*f*
  protocols used in
    abdominal survey, 134–135, 134*f*
    biliary system, 289*t*
    liver, 233–234, 235*t*
    longitudinal scans, 140–141
    porta hepatis, 233–234, 235*t*
    transverse scans, 135–140, 136*f*, 137*f*, 138*f*, 139*f*
  resource organizations for, 6
  systems
    ergonomic, 73, 73*f*
    illustration of, 130*f*
  terminology, 129–131, 130*f*
Ultrasound angiogram, 516*f*
Ultrasound contrast agents (UCAs), 511
  abdominal applications of, 511, 524*b*
  clinical applications of, 517–524
    hepatic applications, 517–521
    organ transplants, 523–524
    pancreatic applications of, 523
    renal applications, 521–522
    splenic applications, 522–523
  modes of, 515–516, 516*f*
  types of, 511–515
    tissue-specific, 514–515, 515*f*
    vascular, 511–514, 512*f*, 513*f*, 513*t*, 514*t*
Ultrasound first, 761–762
Ultrasound-guided procedures, 529–530, 529*f*, 530*f*, 531*f*, 559*b*
  abscess drainage and fluid collection, 534–535, 559
  advantage of, 529, 530*f*
  ascites drainage, 559
  in breast, 676
    large-core needle biopsy, 676
      preoperative needle wire localization, 676, 676*f*
  deviation of needles, 551–552, 551*f*, 552*f*
  equipment and techniques of, 532–535, 533*f*, 534*f*, 535*f*
  finding the needle tips, 550–551, 551*f*
  fusion technology and, 540–542, 540*f*, 541*f*, 542*f*
  growth in, 528–529
  laboratory tests, 531–532
  limitations of, 529–530, 530*f*
  methods for, 535–538, 535*f*, 536*f*, 537*f*, 538*f*
    free-hand techniques, 535–536, 535*f*, 536*f*
    needles attached to transducer, 536–538, 536*f*
  new applications of, 559–560
  pleural fluid collections, 559
  sonographer's role in, 548–550, 549*f*, 550*f*
Umbilical arteries, 1443*f*
  fetal circulation, 1446*f*
Umbilical cord, 1291, 1372–1373, 1372*f*, 1373*f*, 1443*f*, 1460, 1472*b*–1473*b*

Umbilical cord *(Continued)*
  abnormal dimensions, 1462–1464, 1464*f*, 1465*f*
  development and anatomy of, 1460–1462
    embryologic development, 1460–1461, 1461*f*
    normal anatomy, 1461, 1462*f*
    sonographic evaluation, 1461, 1462*f*, 1463*f*, 1464*f*
  insertion, 1577–1578, 1578*f*
  insertion abnormalities, 1468–1470
    marginal insertion of the cord (Battledore placenta), 1468, 1469*f*
    membranous or velamentous insertion of the cord, 1469–1470, 1470*f*
  knots, 1467–1468
    false, 1468, 1468*f*
    nuchal cord, 1468, 1469*f*
    true, 1467–1468, 1468*f*
  masses, 1464–1467
    gastroschisis, 1466–1467, 1466*f*
    hemangioma of the cord, 1467, 1467*f*
    hematoma of the cord, 1467
    omphalocele, 1466, 1466*f*
    omphalomesenteric cyst, 1467, 1467*f*
    thrombosis of the umbilical vessels, 1467, 1468*f*
    umbilical herniation, 1467, 1467*f*
  persistent intrahepatic right umbilical vein, 1472–1473, 1472*f*
  prolapse of, 1470, 1470*f*
    cord presentation with prolapse, 1470
    multiple pregnancy, 1470
    obstetric procedures, 1470
    prematurity, 1470
  single umbilical artery, 1470–1472, 1471*f*
  varix of umbilical vein, 1471*f*, 1472
  vasa previa and prolapse of the cord, 1470, 1470*f*
    cord presentation with prolapse, 1470
    multiple pregnancy, 1470
    obstetric procedures, 1470
    prematurity, 1470
Umbilical cord cysts, first-trimester, 1340, 1340*f*
Umbilical cord Doppler, 1424
Umbilical hernia, 1563, 1576, 1576*f*
Umbilical herniation, 1467, 1467*f*
Umbilical vein, fetal circulation, 1446*f*
Umbilical vein catheter, 770
Umbilical vesicle, 1462*f*
Uncinate process, 356–358, 356*f*
Undescended testis, 1617
Unilateral venous duplex imaging, 1140
United Network for Organ Sharing (UNOS), 584
Upper abdominal compartments, 417–418, 418*f*
Upper extremity
  arterial duplex imaging of, 1120, 1120*f*
  arteries of, 1112, 1112*f*
  fetal, 1369–1371, 1369*f*, 1370*f*, 1371*f*, 1372*f*
  venous duplex imaging of, tips for, 1141*t*
Upper gastrointestinal tract, 399–402, 400*t*
  duplication cysts, 399, 400*f*, 400*t*
  gastric bezoars, 399–400, 400*t*, 401*f*
  gastric carcinoma, 400*t*, 401–402, 402*f*
  leiomyomas, 400, 400*t*, 401*f*
  lymphoma, 400*t*, 402, 402*f*
  metastatic disease, 400*t*, 402, 403*f*
  polyps, 400, 400*t*, 401*f*
Upward graded compression, 778
Urachal abnormalities, 1604–1605, 1604*f*

Urachal cysts, 427, 427*f*, 1604
Ureter(s), 450, 453*b*, 453*f*, 1161–1162, 1162*b*, 1163*f*
  anatomy and physiology of, 86, 437
  narrowing of, 450, 453*b*
  sonographic evaluation of, 1596
  strictures of, 450, 453*b*
Ureteral jet phenomenon, 476–478, 477*f*, 478*f*, 574, 575*f*
Ureterocele, 450, 453*f*, 1599–1600, 1615, 1615*f*, 1616*f*
  ectopic, 450
    neonatal/pediatric, 797–798, 801*f*
    sonographic findings, 450–453
Ureteropelvic junction (UPJ), 1599, 1608–1609
  obstructions, 1610, 1611*f*, 1612*f*
    neonatal/pediatric, 799–800
    sonographic findings in, 799–800
Ureterovesical junction (UVJ), 1599, 1608–1609
  obstruction, 1610–1611, 1612*f*
Urethra
  anatomy of, 86, 437, 710
  sonographic evaluation of, 1596
Urethral atresia, 1608
Urethral discharge, 87, 87*t*
Urinals, 48–49, 48*f*
Urinalysis, 438, 573–574
Urinary anomalies, 1615–1616
Urinary bladder. *see* Bladder
Urinary hesitancy, 87*t*
Urinary incontinence, 86, 87*t*
Urinary obstruction, 616–617, 620*f*
Urinary stones, 616–617, 620*f*
Urinary system, 435, 488*b*–490*b*. *see also* Bladder; Genitourinary system; Kidney(s); Urinary tract
  anatomy of, 86, 86*f*, 435–438, 436*f*
  contrast evaluation of, 795–796
  dysfunction of, 86–88
  fetal, 1366–1368, 1366*f*, 1367*f*
  laboratory data of, 438–439
  lower urinary tract, 450, 453*b*, 453*f*
  pathology of, 453, 453*b*
    arteriovenous fistulas and pseudoaneurysms, 482–483, 484*f*
    bladder diverticulum, 485, 488*f*
    bladder tumors, 486–487, 488*f*
    cystitis, 485–486
    renal infarction, 454*t*–458*t*, 481–482
    renal infection, 478, 479*f*
  physiology of, 438–439
  sonographic evaluation of, 439–444
    normal texture and patterns, 439, 439*f*, 440*f*, 441*f*, 442*f*
    renal anomalies, 445–447, 448*f*
    in renal variants, 444, 446*f*
      columns of Bertin, 444, 446*f*
      dromedary hump, 444, 446*t*
      extrarenal pelvis, 444–445, 446*t*, 448*f*
      fetal lobulation, 444–445, 446*t*, 447*f*
      junctional parenchymal defects, 444, 446*f*, 447*f*
      sinus lipomatosis, 444, 447*f*
  urinary tract calcifications, 479, 480*f*
  vascular supply for, 437–438, 437*f*
Urinary tract
  abnormalities of, 1601, 1601*f*
  calcifications, 479, 480*f*
  dilation of, 1599, 1599*f*

Urinary tract dilation (UTD), 791, 798–799, 798t, 799f, 800f
  classification, 798–802
Urinary tract disease, 1415
Urinary tract obstruction (UTO), 474, 475f, 476f
  AFP and, 1428
Urine amylase, 362
Urine leak, 622, 626f
Urine pH, 438
Uriniferous pseudocysts, 427
Urinoma, 427, 428f, 508, 622, 626f, 802f
Urogenital fetal malformations, 1593t
Urogenital ridge, 1593
Urogenital system, fetal, 1592, 1619b–1620b
  abnormalities of, 1599–1601
  development of, 1593–1595
  embryology of, 1593
  sonographic evaluation of, 1595–1599, 1596b
Urolithiasis, 483–485, 573–574
  clinical findings for, 573–574, 573t
  sonographic findings in, 485, 485f, 486f, 487f, 574, 575f
Uterine artery, 1169, 1170f
Uterine artery embolization, 1210
Uterine cavity, 1225, 1443f
Uterine fibroids, 1416, 1416f
Uterine leiomyoma, 1209
  characteristics of, 1209b, 1210
  first-trimester, 1329t
  locations of, 1209b
Uterine masses, 1340
Uterine supply
Uterine synechiae, 1275f
Uterosacral ligaments, 1165–1166
Uterus, 89, 93f
  anatomy of, 1162–1164, 1164b, 1164t, 1165b, 1165f
    layers of, 1164, 1165b
    size of, 1162, 1164b, 1165f
  bicornuate, 1207, 1208f, 1273f
  blood supply to, 1169, 1191–1192
  calcifications, 1210–1212, 1213f
  congenital anomalies, 1273–1274, 1273f, 1274f
  coronal view of, 1163f
  leiomyomas, 1207–1208
    characteristics of, 1209b, 1210
    locations of, 1209b
    treatment of, 1210
  leiomyosarcoma, 1216–1217, 1218f
  ligaments of, 1165–1166, 1165b, 1165f, 1166f
  measurement of, 1212f
  pathology of, 1207–1217, 1207f, 1208b, 1228b–1229b
    adenomyosis, 1212–1216, 1215f, 1216f
    arteriovenous malformations, 1216, 1217f
    differential considerations for, 1207
    enlarged uterus, 1207
    uterine leiomyosarcoma, 1216–1217, 1218f
  positions of, 1166–1167, 1166b, 1166f, 1207f
  sonographic evaluation of, 578, 578f, 1177–1189, 1178b
  three-dimensional ultrasound, 1199–1201, 1200f
  transabdominal, 1195f
    longitudinal, 1178–1180, 1195f
    sagittal, 1181f, 1182f
    transverse, 1183f
  transvaginal, 1186, 1187f, 1192–1195, 1194f
    coronal, 1186, 1186b, 1187f

Uterus (Continued)
  with hypoechoic myoma, 1206f
  sagittal, 1186, 1186b, 1186f, 1193f
  tumors, 1207–1208
  variations of, 1207, 1207f
  width of, 1186, 1187f, 1194f

V

VACTERL association, 1572, 1632
VACTERL syndrome, 881
VACTERL-H syndrome, 1632
Vagina, 1159, 1162, 1163b, 1163f, 1164f
  blood supply to, 1170f, 1191, 1192f
  coronal view of, 1163f
  pathology of, 1203, 1203f
Vaginal artery, 1170f
Vaginal bleeding, 1412–1413, 1412f, 1413f
Vaginal cuff, 1203
Valves, venous, 1130
Valvulae conniventes, 390
Valvular aortic stenosis, 966–967
Vanishing twin, 1421
Varicoceles, 717t, 722–723, 724f
Varicose veins, 1136
Varix of umbilical vein, 1471f, 1472
Vas deferens, 710
Vasa previa, 1412, 1444–1445, 1452, 1453f, 1470, 1470f
Vasa vasorum, 171
Vascular malformations, 1523t
Vascular supply
  for biliary system, 285
  for breast, 649–650, 650f
  for liver, 223–225
  of pancreas, 358f, 359
  for retroperitoneum, 496–497
  for scrotum, 710–712, 711f, 712b
  for spleen, 326, 330f
  for urinary system, 437–438, 437f
Vascular system, 169, 170f, 215b–217b
  inferior mesenteric vein, 209
  splenic vein, 206–207
  superior mesenteric vein, 207–209
Vascular ultrasound contrast agents, 511–514, 512f, 513f, 513t, 514t
  hepatic blood flow and, 517
  3D gray-scale harmonic imaging and, 516f
Vasospasm, 1099–1100
Vegetations, cardiac, 1000–1006, 1004f, 1005f
Vein(s), 171
  deep
    lower extremity, 1130–1131, 1130f
    upper extremity, 1133–1134, 1133f
  functions of, 1134
  physiology of, 1134
Vein mapping, 1146–1147
Vein of Galen aneurysm, 1537
  differential considerations for, 1524t
  sonographic findings in, 1537
Velamentous insertion, placenta, 1444–1445, 1445f
Velocity
  definition of, 908
  of propagation, 10
  of sound, 10–11
Vena contracta, 957b, 957f, 958f
Venous disease
  risk factors for, 1135, 1135b
  symptoms of, 1135b

Venous duplex imaging, 1130–1134
  anatomy for, 1130–1134
    lower extremity, 1130–1133, 1130f
    upper extremity, 1133–1134, 1133f
  controversies of, 1147–1150
    bilateral symptoms, 1148–1149
    calf vein imaging, 1149
    complete versus limited examination, 1147–1148
    emergent venous duplex imaging, 1149
    pulmonary embolism assessments, 1149–1150
    unilateral versus bilateral, 1148
  guidelines for, 1150–1151, 1150b
  interpretation of, 1140–1144, 1141t, 1142f, 1143f, 1144f, 1145f
    criteria for, 1140, 1141t
    technical adjustments for, 1144t
    tips for, 1141t
  technical aspects of, 1137–1140
    lower extremity, 1137b, 1138f
Venous insufficiency, 1136–1137
Venous reflux, 1136–1137
Venous reflux imaging, 1145–1146, 1145f
Venous sinuses, 1443f
Venous thromboembolism (VTE), 1134–1135
Venous thrombosis, 633–634, 635f, 636f
Venous valves, 1130
Ventral, 132
Ventral cavity, 88
Ventral direction, 132
Ventricles. see also Lateral ventricles; Left ventricle; Right ventricle
  formation of, 1009, 1010f
Ventricular diastole, 901b
Ventricular ejection, 906
Ventricular index, 830, 830f, 830t
Ventricular septal defects, 1038–1041, 1038f, 1039f
  incidence of, 1032t, 1033
  membranous septal defect, 1038–1040, 1040f
  muscular defect, 1040–1041
Ventricular system, neonatal, 815–817, 817f
Ventriculitis, 847
Ventriculomegaly, 1336, 1336t, 1337f, 1540–1542. see also Hydrocephalus
  anomalies associated with, 1523t
  definition of, 829
  meningomyelocele and, 1530f
  myelomeningocele and, 1530f
  sonographic findings in, 1541f, 1542, 1542f
Ventriculoperitoneal shunt, 766, 829, 829f
Venturi mask, 45–46
Veracity, 1297–1298
Verbal consent, 32
Vernix caseosa, 1475
Vertebrae, 872–873, 872f, 875, 875f
Vertebral arch, 872
Vertebral arteries, 1071, 1075f
Vertebral column
  anatomy of, 872, 872f
  fetal, 1355–1357, 1356f, 1357f
Vertebral foramen, 872, 872f
Vertebrobasilar system, 1089
Vertigo, 1072
Verumontanum, 710
Vesicoallantoic cyst, 1604
Vesicoureteral reflux, 799
Vesicouterine pouch, 94, 1174b

Vidoscan, 8
Villi, 390
Virchow, Rudolph, 1135
Virchow triad, 1135
Virtual beam-forming artifacts, 163, 164b, 164f, 164t
Viscera, abdominal, 88
Visceral peritoneum, 95–96, 413–414
Vital signs, 35–38, 63
  definition of, 35
  homeostasis and, 81
Vitamin K, 81, 228
Volar, 748
Volume, 908
Vomiting, 85t, 86
  basins for, 49
  projectile, 784
von Gierke disease, 248
Von Hippel-Lindau cysts, 454t–458t, 460
Von Hippel-Lindau disease, 805
Von Hippel-Lindau syndrome, 377–381, 378f
Vulva, 1159

W

Wall echo shadow (WES) sign, 300, 301f
Wall filter, 27–28, 589–590, 589f, 715t
Walled-off pancreatic fluid collections, 373–374, 374f
Wandering spleen, 327
Waterhouse-Friderichsen syndrome, 502, 502t
Wave, 10
Wavelength, 12, 12f
Wavy-line sign, 667–668, 668f
WBCs. see White blood cells
WES sign. see Wall echo shadow (WES) sign
Wharton jelly, 1445, 1461
Wheelchair transfer, 39, 39f
Whirlpool sign, 1243–1244
White blood cells (WBCs), 83
White coat hypertension, 36
White pulp, of spleen, 330, 332f
Wild, John, 7
Williams syndrome, 966, 1051
Wilms tumor, 199–204, 274–280, 773
  neonatal/pediatric, 467, 773, 807–808
  sonographic findings in, 454t–458t, 468f, 469f
Work-related musculoskeletal disorders (WRMSDs)
  definition of, 70, 78b
  economics of, 77–78
  history of, 69
  incidence of, 69
  industry awareness/changes and, 72–74
  mechanisms of injury in, 70–72, 71f, 72f
  OSHA and, 69–70
  risk factors for, 70, 71f
  surveys of, 70, 71t
  types of, 72, 72f
  work practice changes and, 74–77, 76f, 77f
  workstation setup, 78–79, 79f
Workstation setup, 78–79, 79f
World Health Organization (WHO), 532
Wounds, patient care and, 46–47
Wrists, 747–749
  carpal tunnel and, 748, 749f
  flexion and extension, 75
Written consent, 32
WRMSDs. see Work-related musculoskeletal disorders

X

Xanthogranulomatous pyelonephritis, 478–479, 480f
Xiphisternal joint, 891–892
X-linked disorders, 1433

Y

Yolk sac, 1289–1290, 1443f
  embryonic development of, 1327
  embryonic evaluation, 1327
  gestational sac without, 1322
  sonographic findings of
    in abnormal intrauterine pregnancies, 1324b
    during fetal period, 1307–1308, 1307f, 1308f
  tumors of. see Endodermal sinus tumors
Yolk stalk, 1309–1310, 1460–1461

Z

Zygote, 1290, 1301

TEXTBOOK OF DIAGNOSTIC SONOGRAPHY

TEXTBOOK OF DIAGNOSTIC SONOGRAPHY

9TH EDITION

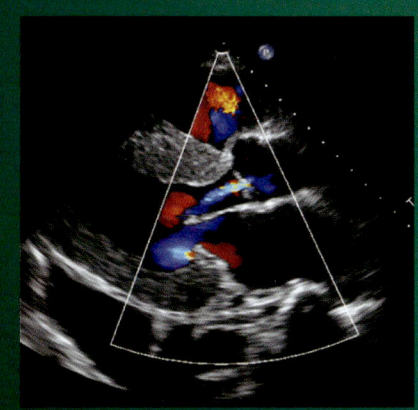
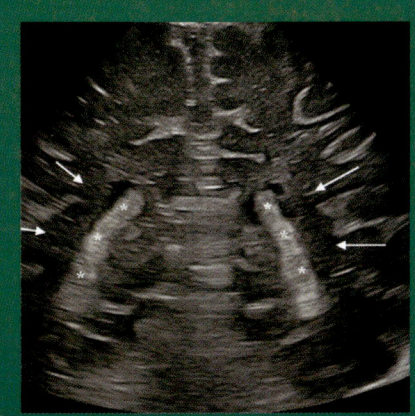
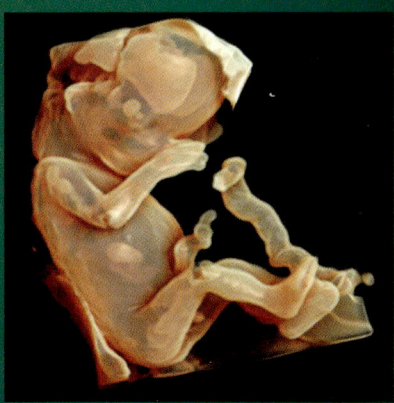

SANDRA L. HAGEN-ANSERT,
MS, RDMS, RDCS, FASE, FSDMS (RETIRED)

Cardiology Department Manager, Echo Labs
Scripps Clinic & Hospitals—La Jolla, California

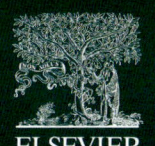

ELSEVIER

ELSEVIER
3251 Riverport Lane
St Louis, Missouri 63043

TEXTBOOK OF DIAGNOSTIC SONOGRAPHY, NINTH EDITION
ISBN: 978-0-323-82646-4
Volume 1 ISBN: 978-0-323-82761-4
Volume 2 ISBN: 978-0-323-82762-1

Copyright © 2023 by Elsevier Inc. All rights reserved.
No part of this publication may be reproduced or transmitted in any form or by any means, electronic or mechanical, including photocopying, recording, or any information storage and retrieval system, without permission in writing from the publisher. Details on how to seek permission, further information about the Publisher's permissions policies and our arrangements with organizations such as the Copyright Clearance Center and the Copyright Licensing Agency, can be found at our website: www.elsevier.com/permissions.

This book and the individual contributions contained in it are protected under copyright by the Publisher (other than as may be noted herein).

Notices

Knowledge and best practice in this field are constantly changing. As new research and experience broaden our understanding, changes in research methods, professional practices, or medical treatment may become necessary.

Practitioners and researchers must always rely on their own experience and knowledge in evaluating and using any information, methods, compounds, or experiments described herein. In using such information or methods they should be mindful of their own safety and the safety of others, including parties for whom they have a professional responsibility.

With respect to any drug or pharmaceutical products identified, readers are advised to check the most current information provided (i) on procedures featured or (ii) by the manufacturer of each product to be administered, to verify the recommended dose or formula, the method and duration of administration, and contraindications. It is the responsibility of practitioners, relying on their own experience and knowledge of their patients, to make diagnoses, to determine dosages and the best treatment for each individual patient, and to take all appropriate safety precautions.

To the fullest extent of the law, neither the Publisher nor the authors, contributors, or editors, assume any liability for any injury and/or damage to persons or property as a matter of products liability, negligence or otherwise, or from any use or operation of any methods, products, instructions, or ideas contained in the material herein.

Previous editions copyrighted 2018, 2012, 2006, 2001, 1995, 1989, 1983, and 1978.

Executive Content Strategist: Meg Benson
Content Development Manager: Danielle Frazier
Publishing Services Manager: Catherine Jackson
Senior Project Manager/Specialist: Carrie Stetz
Design Direction: Amy Buxton

Printed in India
Last digit is the print number: 9 8 7 6 5 4 3 2 1

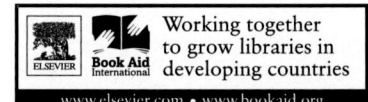

To my family,
Art, Aly, Kati, Becca and Eric, Adeline and Osborne,
who mean the world to me

CONTRIBUTORS

Alicia Armour, MA, ACS, RDCS, FASE
Health Center Administrator
Duke Triangle Heart Associates
Duke University Health System
Durham, North Carolina

Joan P. Baker, MSR, RDMS, FSDMS
President, Sound Ergonomics, LLC
Kenmore, Washington

Carolyn T. Coffin, MPH, RDMS, RVT, RDCS
CEO and Consultant
Sound Ergonomics LLC
Kenmore, Washington

M. Robert DeJong, RDMS, RDCS, RVT, FSDMS, FAIUM
Bob DeJong, LLC
Ultrasound Educational Services
Rosedale, Maryland;
Former Radiology Technical
 Manager–Ultrasound
Russell H. Morgan Department
 of Radiology and Radiological
 Science
Johns Hopkins Hospital
Baltimore, Maryland

Kelsey Doyle, MEd, RDMS, RVT
Education and Outreach
 Coordinator
Center for Perinatal Care
UnityPoint Health-Meriter/University
 of Wisconsin–Madison
Madison, Wisconsin

John Eisenbrey, PhD
Associate Professor of Radiology
Department of Radiology
Thomas Jefferson University
Philadelphia, Pennsylvania

Kathryn Gill, MS, RDMS, RVT, FSDMS
Sonographer
Program Director
Institute of Ultrasound Diagnostics &
 Medscan Clinic
Spanish Fort, Alabama

Joy Guthrie, PhD, ACS, RDMS, RDCS, RVT, FSDMS, RCS, RCCS, RVS
Advanced Practice Sonographer
Program Director, Diagnostic Medical
 Sonography
Researcher, Community Regional
 Medical Center
Fresno, California

Sandra L. Hagen-Ansert, MS, RDMS, RDCS, FASE, FSDMS (Retired)
Cardiology Department Manager,
 Echo Labs
Scripps Clinic & Hospitals
La Jolla, California

Talisha M. Hunt, BSRT, RDMS, RDCS, RVT
Lead Sonographer
Assistant Professor of Radiology
Mayo Clinic
Rochester, Minnesota

Mariana Kozirovsky, MS, RDMS, RDCS
Assistant Professor
Long Island University
Brooklyn, New York;
Research Scientist
NYU Grossman School of Medicine
New York, New York

Frederick W. Kremkau, PhD, RACR, RAIMBE, FAIUM, FASA
Professor of Radiologic Sciences
Director, Program for Medical
 Ultrasound
Center for Experiential and Applied
 Learning
Wake Forest University School of
 Medicine
Winston Salem, North Carolina

Dan Lebovic, MD
Professor
Department of Obstetrics and
 Gynecology
Washington University in St. Louis
St. Louis, Missouri

Daniel Merton, BS, RDMS, FSDMS, FAIUM
Diagnostic Ultrasound Specialist and
 Principal Project Officer
Health Devices Group
ECRI Institute
Plymouth Meeting, Pennsylvania

Carol Mitchell, PhD, ACS, RDMS, RDCS, RVT, RT(R), FASE, FSDMS
Associate Professor
Department of Medicine
School of Medicine and Public Health
University of Wisconsin–Madison
Madison, Wisconsin

Tanya Nolan, EdD, RDMS, RT(R)(ARRT)
Associate Professor
Director, Diagnostic Medical Sonography
Director, MSRS Innovation and
 Improvement
School of Radiologic Sciences
Weber State University
Ogden, Utah

Cindy A. Owen, RDMS, RVT, RT, FSDMS
Former Director, Clinical Insights and
 Development
GE Healthcare, Point of Care Ultrasound
Milwaukee, Wisconsin

Mitzi Roberts, EdD, RDMS, RDCS, FSDMS, RT(R)
Associate Professor
Baptist Health Sciences University;
Clinical Sonographer
Mid-South Maternal-Fetal Medicine
Memphis, Tennessee

Jean Lea Spitz, MPH, RDMS
Executive Director
Perinatal Quality Foundation
Oklahoma City, Oklahoma

Christina Taff, BS, RDMS
Lead Clinical Coordinator
Mid-South Maternal Fetal Medicine
Memphis, Tennessee

Shpetim Telegrafi, MD
Research Professor
Director of Diagnostic Ultrasound
Department of Urology
NYU Grossman School of Medicine
New York, New York

Barbara Trampe, BA, RN, RDMS
Education and Outreach
 Coordinator
Maternal-Fetal Medicine
University of Wisconsin/UnityPoint
 Health Meriter
Madison, Wisconsin

Kevin R. Volz, PhD, RVT
Research Lab Manager
Laboratory for Investigative Imaging
Former Instructor/Vascular Technology
 Clinical Coordinator
School of Health and Rehabilitation
 Sciences
Division of Radiologic Sciences and
 Therapy
The Ohio State University College of
 Medicine
Columbus, Ohio

Kelsi Weakley, MS, RDMS
Clinical Coordinator
Maternal-Fetal Medicine
Regional One Health
Memphis, Tennessee

**Kerry Weinberg, PhD, MPA, MA,
 RDMS, RDCS, RT(T), FSDMS**
Associate Professor and Program
 Director
Diagnostic Medical Sonography
Long Island University
Brooklyn, New York

**Michelle Wilson, EdD, RDMS, RDCS,
 FSDMS**
Former Clinical Sonographer and
 Educator
Kaiser Permanente Medical Center and
 Kaiser School of Allied Health
Napa, California;
Adjunct Associate Professor
DMS Program
University of Southern Indiana
Evansville, Indiana

Kathryn Zale, MS, RDMS, RVT
Faculty Instructor
Diagnostic Medical Sonography
Pennsylvania College of Health
 Sciences
Lancaster, Pennsylvania;
Sonographer
Department of Radiology
Children's Hospital of Philadelphia
King of Prussia, Pennsylvania

PREFACE

INTRODUCING THE NINTH EDITION

The ninth edition of *Textbook of Diagnostic Sonography* continues the tradition of excellence that began when the first edition was published in 1978. Like other medical imaging fields, diagnostic sonography has seen dramatic changes and innovations since its first clinical experimental days. Phenomenal strides in transducer design, instrumentation, three-dimensional (3D) and four-dimensional (4D) imaging, image processing, tissue harmonics, elastoraphy, and contrast agents continue to improve image resolution and the diagnostic clinical value of sonography. The ninth edition has kept abreast of advancements in the field by inviting new contributors currently working in different areas of medical sonography throughout the country. The critiques and suggestions from multiple reviewers have helped ensure that this edition includes the most complete and up-to-date information needed to meet the requirements of the modern student of sonography.

Distinctive Approach

This textbook can serve as an in-depth resource both for students of sonography and for practitioners in any number of clinical settings, including hospitals, clinics, and private practices. Care has been taken to cultivate readers' understanding of the patient's total clinical picture even as they study sonographic examination protocol and technique. To this end, each chapter covers the following:
- Key terminology
- Normal anatomy (including cross-sectional anatomy)
- Normal physiology
- Laboratory data and values
- Pathology
- Sonographic evaluation of an organ
- Sonographic findings
- Pitfalls in sonography
- Clinical findings
- Differential considerations
- "Key Pearls"

The full-color art program is of great value to the student of anatomy and pathology for sonography. Detailed line drawings illustrate the anatomic information a sonographer must know to successfully perform specific sonographic examinations. Multiple color photographs of gross pathology help the reader visualize some of the pathology presented, with 3D and color Doppler illustrations included where relevant.

To make important information easy to find, key points are pulled out into numerous boxes; tables throughout the chapters summarize the pathology under discussion and break down the information into Clinical Findings, Sonographic Findings, and Differential Considerations.

Sonographic findings for particular pathologic conditions are always preceded in the text by the following special heading:

Sonographic Findings

This icon makes it very easy for students and practicing sonographers to locate this clinical information quickly.

Study and Review Opportunities

Study and review are also essential to gaining a solid grasp of the concepts and information presented in this textbook. Learning objectives, chapter outlines, "Key Pearls" that summarize the chapter highlights, comprehensive glossaries of key terms, and full references for cited material all help students learn the material in an organized and thorough manner.

Scope and Organization of Topics

The *Textbook of Diagnostic Sonography* is divided into eight parts:

Part I introduces the reader to the foundations of sonography and patient care and includes the following:
- Foundations of sonography, which include the basic principles of ultrasound physics and medical sonography
- Terminology frequently encountered by the sonographer
- Patient care for the sonographer
- Ergonomics and musculoskeletal issues for practitioners
- Anatomic and physiologic relationships within the abdominopelvic cavity
- Comparative sectional anatomy of the abdominopelvic cavity
- Imaging and Doppler artifacts

Part II presents the abdomen in depth. The following topics are discussed:
- Anatomic relationships and physiology
- Abdominal scanning techniques and protocols
- Abdominal applications of ultrasound contrast agents
- Ultrasound-guided interventional techniques
- Emergent abdominal ultrasound procedures
- Sonographic techniques in the transplant patient
- Separate chapters for the vascular system, liver, gallbladder and biliary system, spleen, pancreas, gastrointestinal tract, urinary system, retroperitoneum, peritoneal cavity, and abdominal wall

Part III focuses on the superficial structures of the body, including the breast, thyroid and parathyroid glands, scrotum, and musculoskeletal system.

Part IV is completely updated and explores sonographic examination of the neonate and pediatric patient, including abdomen, adrenal and urinary system, neonatal head, neonatal hip, and neonatal spine.

Part V focuses on the thoracic cavity and includes the following topics:
- Anatomic and physiologic relationships within the thoracic cavity
- Hemodynamics
- Echocardiographic evaluation and techniques
- Introduction to clinical echocardiography
- Fetal echocardiography
- Congenital heart disease

Part VI is composed of four updated chapters on extracranial and intracranial cerebrovascular imaging and peripheral arterial and venous sonographic evaluation.

Part VII is devoted to gynecology and includes the following topics:
- Normal anatomy and physiology of the female pelvis
- Sonographic and Doppler evaluation of the female pelvis
- Separate chapters on the pathologic conditions of the uterus, ovaries, and adnexa
- Updated chapter on the role of sonography in evaluating female infertility

Part VIII takes a thorough look at obstetric sonography. The following topics are discussed:
- The role of sonography in obstetrics
- Clinical ethics for obstetric sonography
- Normal first-trimester findings and first-trimester complications
- Sonography of the second and third trimesters
- Obstetric measurements and gestational age and fetal growth assessment
- Sonography in the high-risk pregnancy
- Prenatal diagnosis of congenital anomalies
- Chapters are devoted to the placenta, umbilical cord, amniotic fluid and fetal membranes, fetal face and neck, neural axis, thorax, anterior abdominal wall, abdomen, urogenital system, and skeleton

New to This Edition

Eight new contributors joined the ninth edition to update and expand existing content, bringing with them a fresh perspective and an impressive knowledge base. They also helped contribute the more than 1000 images new to this edition, including color Doppler, 3D and 4D, and contrast-enhanced images. More than 30 new line drawings complement the new chapters found in the ninth edition.

As the reader proceeds through each chapter, terminology is introduced to lay the foundation for the reader as they study the specific chapters. Information that may seem repetitive to the experienced sonographer is reinforcement for student sonographers as they build their understanding of the many concepts that must be mastered for their clinical experience.

Foundations of Ultrasound (Chapter 1) introduces the reader to the field of sonography, including the role of the sonographer, historical overview of the development of ultrasound, as well as an introduction to basic ultrasound principles and terminology.

Essentials of Patient Care for the Sonographer (Chapter 2) covers all aspects of patient care the sonographer may encounter, including obtaining and understanding vital signs, handling patients on strict bed rest, patients with tubes and oxygen, patient transfer techniques, infection control, isolation techniques, emergency medical situations, assisting patients with special needs, and patient rights.

Ergonomics and Musculoskeletal Issues in Sonography (Chapter 3) outlines the importance of proper technique and positioning throughout the sonographic examination as a way to avoid long-term disability problems that may be acquired with repetitive scanning.

Anatomic and Physiologic Relationships Within the Abdominopelvic Cavity (Chapter 4) introduces the reader to body systems and anatomic relationships, which include membranes and ligaments and potential spaces in the body.

Comparative Sectional Anatomy of the Abdominopelvic Cavity (Chapter 5) is an introduction to sectional anatomy incorporating gross anatomy with comparative ultrasound and computed tomography sectional images. This chapter provides the groundwork for understanding sectional anatomy.

Basic Ultrasound Imaging: Techniques, Terminology, and Tips (Chapter 6) describes scanning techniques, terminology, abdominal ultrasound protocol, and abdominal Doppler technique.

Imaging and Doppler Artifacts (Chapter 7) is an outstanding review of all the artifacts commonly encountered by sonographers. There are numerous examples of the various artifacts and detailed explanations of how these artifacts are produced and how to avoid them.

The abdominal chapters (Chapter 8-19) have all been updated with new images that include ultrasound, CT, and MRI.

Sonographic Techniques in the Transplant Patient (Chapter 20) has been updated to focus on criteria required for organ transplantation, including liver transplant, renal transplant, and pancreatic transplant.

The Breast (Chapter 21) has been updated by a new contributor with new techniques and images.

The Musculoskeletal System (Chapter 24) has been updated by a new contributor with beautiful illustrations and a comprehensive bibliography.

The entire pediatrics section (Chapters 25 to 29) has been fully updated with exquisite new illustrations for each chapter.

Understanding Hemodynamics (Chapter 31) introduces the student to blood flow dynamics, intracardiac pressures and volumes, Doppler basics, and quantification of intracardiac pressures by ultrasound.

Introduction to Clinical Echocardiography: Left-Sided Valvular Heart Disease (Chapter 33) and *Introduction to Clinical Echocardiography: Pericardial Disease, Cardiomyopathies, and Tumors* (Chapter 34) have been included in this edition to provide a basic understanding of significant cardiac findings that may be encountered by the general sonographer or clinician. The fetal echocardiography chapters (Chapters 35 and 36) have been updated to include current protocol and image acquisition.

The entire cerebrovascular section (Chapters 37 to 40) has been updated with new images and current techniques for the sonographer.

Several new contributors have provided their expertise in the obstetrics section (Chapters 47 to 65). *Sonography of the Second and Third Trimesters, Prenatal Diagnosis of Congenital Anomalies, The Placenta, Fetal Face and Neck, Fetal Neural Axis,* and *Fetal Skeleton* chapters have all been updated with new images and references.

Student Resources

Workbook. Available for separate purchase, the *Workbook for the Textbook of Diagnostic Sonography* has also been completely updated. This resource gives the learner ample opportunity to practice and apply the information presented in the textbook.
- Each workbook chapter covers all the material presented in the textbook.
- Each chapter includes exercises on image identification, anatomy identification, key term definitions, and sonographic technique.
- Case studies using images from the textbook invite students to test their skills at identifying key anatomy and pathology and describing and interpreting sonographic findings.
- Students can also test their knowledge with the hundreds of multiple-choice questions found in the four examinations covering different content areas: General Sonography, Pediatric, Cardiovascular Anatomy, and Obstetrics and Gynecology.

Evolve. On the Evolve site, students will find review questions for each chapter.

Instructor Resources

Resources for instructors are also provided on the Evolve site to assist in the preparation of classroom lectures and activities.
- Extensive PowerPoint lectures for each chapter that include illustrations
- Test bank of 1500 multiple-choice questions in Exam View and Word
- Electronic image collection that includes all the images from the textbook both in PowerPoint and in .jpeg format

Evolve Online Course Management. Evolve is an interactive learning environment designed to work in coordination with the *Textbook of Diagnostic Sonography*. Instructors may use Evolve to include an Internet-based course component that reinforces and expands on the concepts delivered in class. Evolve may be used to do all of the following:
- Publish the class syllabus, outlines, and lecture notes
- Set up virtual office hours and email communication
- Share important dates and information on the online class calendar
- Encourage student participation with chat rooms and discussion boards
- Post examinations and manage grade books
- For more information, visit http://www.evolve.elsevier.com/HagenAnsert/diagnostic/ or contact an Elsevier sales representative.

ACKNOWLEDGMENTS

I would like to express my gratitude and appreciation to a number of individuals who have served as mentors and guides throughout my years in sonography. It all began with Dr. George Leopold at UCSD Medical Center. His quest for knowledge and his perseverance for excellence have been the mainstay of my career in sonography. I would also like to recognize Drs. Dolores Pretorius, Nancy Budorick, Wanda Miller-Hance, and David Sahn for their encouragement throughout the years at the UCSD Medical Center in both Radiology and Pediatric Cardiology.

I would also like to acknowledge Dr. Barry Goldberg for the opportunity he gave me to develop countless numbers of educational programs in sonography in an independent fashion and for his encouragement to pursue advancement. I would also like to thank Dr. Daniel Yellon for his early-hour anatomy dissection and instruction; Dr. Carson Schneck, for his excellent instruction in gross anatomy and sections of "Geraldine"; and Dr. Jacob Zutuchni, for his enthusiasm for the field of cardiology.

I am grateful to Dr. Harry Rakowski for his continued support in teaching fellows and students while I was at the Toronto General Hospital. Dr. William Zwiebel encouraged me to continue writing and teaching while I was at the University of Wisconsin Medical Center, and I appreciate his knowledge, which found its way into the liver physiology section of this textbook.

My good fortune in learning about and understanding the total patient must be attributed to a very dedicated cardiologist, James Glenn, with whom I had the pleasure of working while I was at MUSC in Charleston, South Carolina. It was through his compassion and knowledge that I grew to appreciate the total patient beyond the transducer, and for this I am grateful.

For their continual support, feedback, and challenges, I would like to thank and recognize all the students I have taught in the various diagnostic medical sonography programs: Episcopal Hospital, Thomas Jefferson University Medical Center, University of Wisconsin-Madison Medical Center, UCSD Medical Center, and Baptist College of Health Science. These students continually work toward the development of quality sonography techniques and protocols and have given back to the sonography community tenfold.

The continual push towards excellence has been encouraged on a daily basis by our Scripps Clinic Medical Director of the Echo Lab, Dr. David Rubenson, and outstanding staff of Scripps Clinic Cardiologists.

The Cardiac Sonographers at Scripps Clinic Anderson Medical Pavillion have been invaluable in their excellent image acquisition. Special thanks to Kristen Billick for her excellent echocardiographic images. The general sonographers at Scripps Clinic have been invaluable in providing the outstanding images for the obstetrics and gynecology chapters.

I would like to thank the very supportive and capable staff at Elsevier who have guided me though yet another edition of this textbook. Danielle Frazier, Carrie Stetz, and the staff at Elsevier are to be commended on their perseverance to make this an outstanding textbook.

I would like to thank my family, Art, Becca, Aly, and Kati, for their patience and understanding, as I thought this edition would never come to an end. My recent retirement and the pandemic lockdown provided an excellent opportunity for total undivided dedication to this edition.

I think that you will find the 9th Edition of the *Textbook of Diagnostic Sonography* reflects the contribution of so many individuals with attention to detail and a dedication to excellence. I hope you will find this educational experience in sonography as rewarding as I have throughout the past 50 years.

Sandra L. Hagen-Ansert,
MS, RDMS, RDCS, FASE, FSDMS (Retired)

CONTENTS

VOLUME ONE

PART I Foundations of Sonography

1. Foundations of Clinical Sonography, 3
2. Essentials of Patient Care for the Sonographer, 29
3. Ergonomics and Musculoskeletal Issues in Sonography, 68
4. Anatomic and Physiologic Relationships Within the Abdominopelvic Cavity, 80
5. Comparative Sectional Anatomy of the Abdominopelvic Cavity, 102
6. Basic Ultrasound Imaging: Techniques, Terminology, and Tips, 123
7. Imaging and Doppler Artifacts, 147

PART II Abdomen

8. Vascular System, 169
9. The Liver, 218
10. The Gallbladder and the Biliary System, 281
11. The Spleen, 325
12. The Pancreas, 355
13. The Gastrointestinal Tract, 389
14. The Peritoneal Cavity and Abdominal Wall, 413
15. Urinary System, 435
16. The Retroperitoneum, 491
17. Abdominal Applications of Ultrasound Contrast Agents, 511
18. Ultrasound-Guided Interventional Techniques, 528
19. Emergent Ultrasound Procedures, 561
20. Sonographic Techniques in the Transplant Patient, 583

PART III Superficial Structures

21 Breast, 643

22 The Thyroid and Parathyroid Glands, 682

23 Scrotum, 708

24 Musculoskeletal System, 733

PART IV Pediatrics

25 Neonatal and Pediatric Abdomen, 761

26 Neonatal and Pediatric Adrenal and Urinary System, 791

27 Neonatal and Infant Head, 813

28 Infant and Pediatric Hip, 850

29 Neonatal and Infant Spine, 871

Glossary, G-1 to G-12

VOLUME TWO

PART V The Thoracic Cavity

30 Anatomic and Physiologic Relationships Within the Thoracic Cavity, 891

31 Understanding Hemodynamics, 908

32 Introduction to Echocardiographic Techniques, Terminology, and Tips, 916

33 Introduction to Clinical Echocardiography: Left-Sided Valvular Heart Disease, 953

34 Introduction to Clinical Echocardiography: Pericardial Disease, Cardiomyopathies, and Tumors, 980

35 Fetal Echocardiography: Beyond the Four Chambers, 1007

36 Fetal Echocardiography: Congenital Heart Disease, 1031

PART VI Cerebrovascular

37 Extracranial Cerebrovascular Evaluation, 1069

38 Intracranial Cerebrovascular Evaluation, 1087

39 Peripheral Arterial Evaluation, 1110

40 Peripheral Venous Evaluation, 1129

PART VII Gynecology

41 Normal Anatomy and Physiology of the Female Pelvis, 1157

42 Sonographic and Doppler Evaluation of the Female Pelvis, 1176

43 Pathology of the Uterus, 1202

44 Pathology of the Ovaries, 1230

45 Pathology of the Adnexa, 1260

46 Role of Ultrasound in Evaluating Female Infertility, 1272

PART VIII Obstetrics

47 The Role of Sonography in Obstetrics, 1283

48 Clinical Ethics for Obstetric Sonography, 1294

49 The Early Embryonic Stage of the First Trimester, 1300

50 First-Trimester Complications, 1319

51 Sonography of the Second and Third Trimesters, 1343

52 Obstetric Measurements and Gestational Age, 1378

53 Fetal Growth Assessment by Sonography, 1395

54 Sonography and High-Risk Pregnancy, 1406

55 Prenatal Diagnosis of Congenital Anomalies, 1426

56 Placenta, 1442

57 The Umbilical Cord, 1460

58 Amniotic Fluid and Fetal Membranes, 1474

59 Fetal Face and Neck, 1492

60 Fetal Neural Axis, 1522

61 The Fetal Thorax, 1545

62 The Fetal Anterior Abdominal Wall, 1560

63 The Fetal Abdomen, 1572

64 Fetal Urogenital System, 1592

65 Fetal Skeleton, 1622

Glossary, G-13 to G-24

Illustration Credits, C-1 to C-10

Index, I-1 to I-40

PART V

The Thoracic Cavity

Chapter 30 Anatomic and Physiologic Relationships Within the Thoracic Cavity
Chapter 31 Understanding Hemodynamics
Chapter 32 Introduction to Echocardiographic Techniques, Terminology, and Tips
Chapter 33 Introduction To Clinical Echocardiography: Left-Sided Valvular Heart Disease
Chapter 34 Introduction To Clinical Echocardiography: Pericardial Disease, Cardiomyopathies, and Tumors
Chapter 35 Fetal Echocardiography: Beyond the Four Chambers
Chapter 36 Fetal Echocardiography: Congenital Heart Disease

CHAPTER 30

Anatomic and Physiologic Relationships Within the Thoracic Cavity

Sandra L. Hagen-Ansert

OBJECTIVES

On completion of this chapter, you should be able to:
- Describe the landmarks of the thoracic cavity
- Define the relational landmarks of the heart
- Discuss the function of the pericardial sac
- Differentiate the three layers of the heart wall
- Describe the anatomic landmarks of the cardiac chambers, valves, and interventricular septum

OUTLINE

The Thorax and the Thoracic Cavity 891
The Lungs 892
The Heart and Great Vessels 894
   Pericardial Sac 896
   Linings of the Heart Wall 896
   Right Atrium and Interatrial Septum 897
   Tricuspid Valve 897
   Right Ventricle 898
   Pulmonary Valve and Trunk 898
   Left Atrium 899

Mitral Valve 899
Left Ventricle 900
Interventricular Septum 900
Aortic Valve 901
Aortic Arch and Branches 901
The Cardiac Cycle 901
The Electrical Conduction System 903
   Bundle of His 903
   Cardiac Nerves 903
The Mechanical Conduction System 903

Electrocardiography 904
   P Wave 904
   QRS Complex 904
   P-R Interval 904
   T Wave 904
Auscultation of the Heart Valves 904
Principles of Blood Flow 905
   Ventricular Ejection 906
   Coronary Circulation 906

KEY TERMS

Atrioventricular valves
Continuous murmur
Costal margin
Depolarization
Diastolic murmur
Electrocardiography
Endocardium
Epicardium

Frequency
Heart murmurs
Intensity
Midaxillary line
Midclavicular line
Murmur
Myocardium
Pathologic murmur

Pericardium
Repolarization
Semilunar valves
Sternal angle
Suprasternal notch
Systolic murmur
Xiphisternal joint
Xiphoid

The cardiovascular system delivers oxygenated blood to tissues in the body and removes waste products from these tissues. The heart pumps blood to all the organs and tissues of the body. The autonomic nervous system controls how the heart pumps, and the vascular network (arteries and veins) carries blood throughout the body, keeps the heart filled with blood, and maintains blood pressure.

THE THORAX AND THE THORACIC CAVITY

The thorax constitutes the upper part of the body between the neck and the diaphragm. There are eight external landmarks of the thorax (Fig. 30.1). The **costal margin** is the lower boundary of the thorax; it is formed by the cartilages of the seventh through tenth ribs and the ends of the eleventh and twelfth

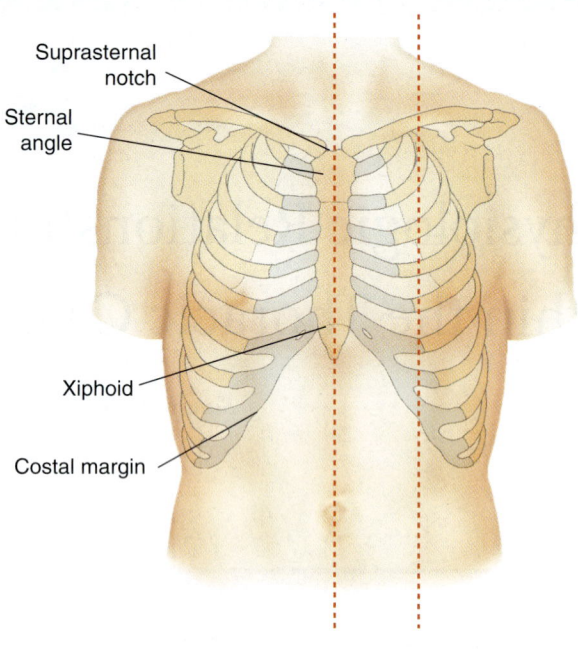

FIG. 30.1 External landmarks of the thorax. The thorax constitutes the upper part of the body between the neck and the diaphragm.

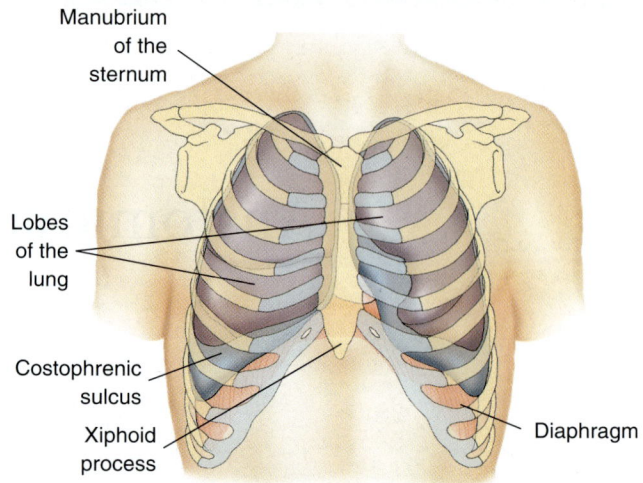

FIG. 30.2 Anterior view of the thorax. The thoracic cavity lies within the thorax and is separated from the abdominal cavity by the diaphragm.

cartilages. The **midaxillary line** runs vertically from a point midway between the anterior and posterior axillary folds. The **midclavicular line** is a vertical line from the midpoint of the clavicle. The *midsternal line* lies in the median plane over the sternum. The **sternal angle** is the angle between the manubrium and the body of the sternum; it is also known as the angle of Louis. The **suprasternal notch** is the superior margin of the manubrium sterni, lying opposite the lower border of the body of the second thoracic vertebra. The **xiphisternal joint** is the junction between the xiphoid and the sternum. The final external landmark of the thorax is the **xiphoid**, the lowest point of the sternum.

The thoracic cavity lies within the thorax and is separated from the abdominal cavity by the diaphragm (Fig. 30.2). The diaphragm reaches upward as high as the midaxillary level of the seventh rib. The mediastinum is the medial portion of the thorax, and the pleurae and lungs are the lateral components.

Superiorly, the upper thoracic cavity gives access to the root of the neck. It is bounded by the upper part of the sternum, the first ribs, and the body of the first thoracic vertebra.

Anteriorly, the sternum consists of the manubrium, the corpus sterni (body), and the xiphoid process. The junction between the manubrium and the body of the sternum is a prominent ridge; together they form the angle of Louis. This palpable landmark is important in locating the superior mediastinum or the second rib cartilages, which articulate with the sternum at this point.

The greater part of the thoracic cavity is occupied by the two lungs, which are enclosed by the pleural sac. To understand the pleural sac, imagine a deflated plastic bag covering your fist. Your fist should be enveloped by both sides of the bag to simulate the pleural sac. The internal layer, or visceral pleura, is adherent to each lobe of the lung. The external layer, or parietal pleura, is adherent to the inner surface of the chest wall (costal pleura), diaphragm (diaphragmatic pleura), and mediastinum (mediastinal pleura). The two layers become continuous with each other by a "cuff" of pleura that surrounds the structures at the hilum of the lung.

The costophrenic sinus is the pleural reflection between the costal and diaphragmatic portions of the parietal pleura. This space lies lower than the edge of the lung and, in most cases, is never occupied by the lung. When pleural fluid accumulates, its most common location is in the costophrenic sinus. On a radiographic examination, the costophrenic angle is blunted by the presence of pleural effusion.

The mediastinum is the median partition of the thoracic cavity. The mediastinum is a movable, thick structure and extends superiorly to the thoracic inlet and the root of the neck and inferiorly to the diaphragm. It extends anteriorly to the sternum and posteriorly to the twelfth thoracic vertebra. Within the mediastinum are found the remains of the thymus, the heart and great vessels, the trachea and esophagus, the thoracic duct and lymph nodes, the vagus and phrenic nerves, and the sympathetic trunks.

The mediastinum may be divided into a superior and inferior mediastinum by an imaginary plane from the sternal angle to the lower body of the fourth thoracic vertebra (Box 30.1). The inferior mediastinum is subdivided into three parts: (1) middle, which contains the pericardium and the heart; (2) anterior, which is a space between the pericardium and sternum; and (3) posterior, which lies between the pericardium and vertebral column.

THE LUNGS

The evaluation of the lungs with ultrasound is primarily based on the interpretation of artifacts produced at the pleural surface. Most of these artifacts relate to the interaction of ultrasound and air. Although ultrasound can be used to interpret

CHAPTER 30 Anatomic and Physiologic Relationships Within the Thoracic Cavity

> **BOX 30.1 Major Mediastinal Structures From Anterior to Posterior**
>
> **Superior Mediastinum**
> - Thymus
> - Great veins
> - Great arteries
> - Trachea
> - Esophagus and thoracic duct
> - Sympathetic trunks
>
> **Inferior Mediastinum**
> - Thymus
> - Heart within the pericardium with the phrenic nerves on either side
> - Esophagus and thoracic duct
> - Descending aorta
> - Sympathetic trunks

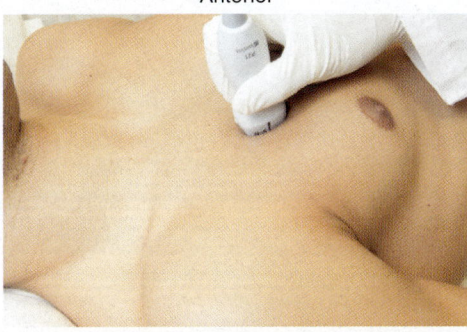
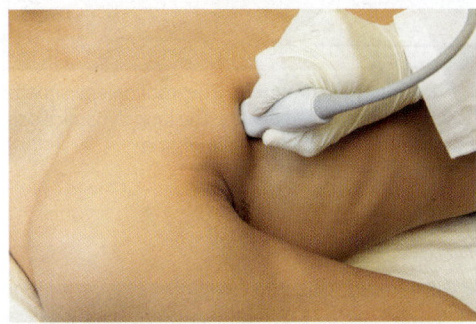
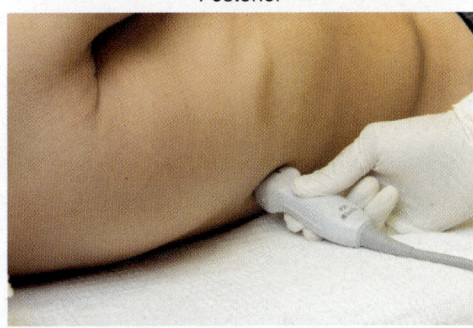

FIG. 30.3 The probes utilized to evaluate the lungs include the curvilinear (for good penetration with low frequency), the linear (for pleural surface detail with high frequency, shown here), or the phased array transducer (for visualization of the pleural surface and the pleural fluid).

the characteristics of the surface of an air interface, it cannot penetrate gas; therefore, pathology lying deep to air cannot be visualized with ultrasound. With the exception of the mediastinal reflections, ultrasound can be used to explore most of the pleural surface of the lungs. There is frequently an overlap in the sonographic appearance of differing conditions, and integration with the clinical picture is important.

In trauma cases the patient is supine, which is convenient for the detection of a pneumothorax where free pleural air gathers at the most apical point of the thoracic cavity. The detection of a hemothorax—which is more dependent—is challenging, with a posterolateral approach required using the liver or spleen as an acoustic window. Intubated patients are generally supine for the anterior, lateral, and posterior approach—with the patient rolled to one side or other. The conscious patients in acute respiratory distress usually sit up to optimize their ventilators. Access to the entire chest wall is possible with this approach. If the patient is not acutely distressed and is sitting on a chair or stool, maximal chest wall accessibility is possible. Ask the patient to hug themselves or put their arms out forward to move the scapula around the chest wall to help access the upper posterior lung.

The probes utilized to evaluate the lungs include the curvilinear (for good penetration with low frequency), the linear (for pleural surface detail with high frequency; Fig. 30.3), or the phased array transducer (for visualization of the pleural surface and the pleural fluid).

Ultrasound evaluation of the pleural line to look for lung sliding (Fig. 30.4) or lung pulse is done by looking for movement at the pleural line. Vertical artifacts below the pleural lining may represent comet tails or B-lines (Fig. 30.5). Horizontal artifacts below the pleural line may be seen when the pleural line is perpendicular to the line of interrogation of the ultrasound beam (Fig. 30.6).

Lung that is normally aerated has a characteristic pattern of air artifact designated as A-lines (Fig. 30.7). These A-lines indicate air, whether physiologic of pathologic. A-lines are

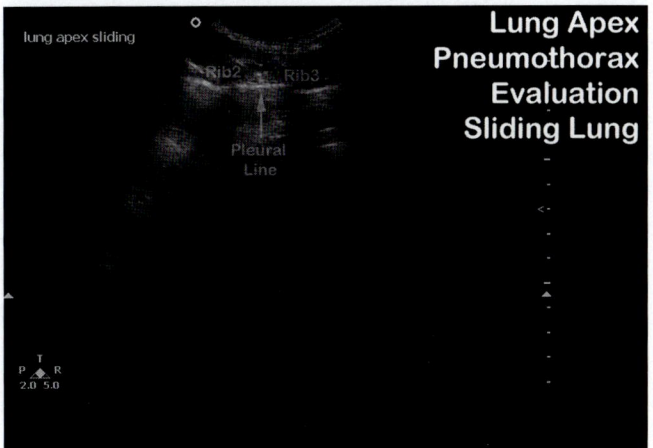

FIG. 30.4 Ultrasound evaluation of the pleural line to look for lung sliding or lung pulse is done by looking for movement at the pleural line. (Courtesy fpnotebook.com.)

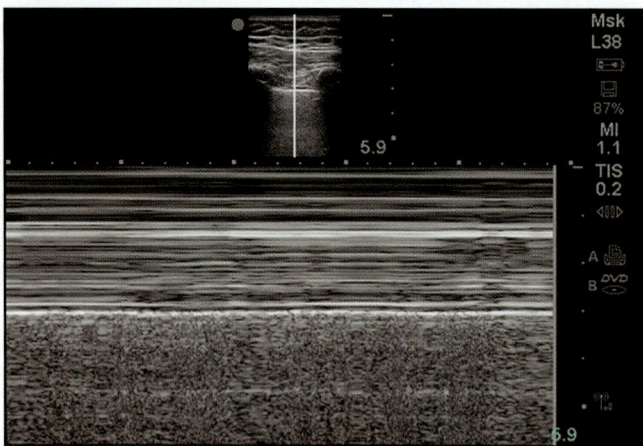

FIG. 30.5 **Normal lung/M-mode.** The motionless superficial layers generate horizontal lines, called *B-lines*. The lung dynamics generate lung sliding (sandy pattern), called the *seashore sign*.

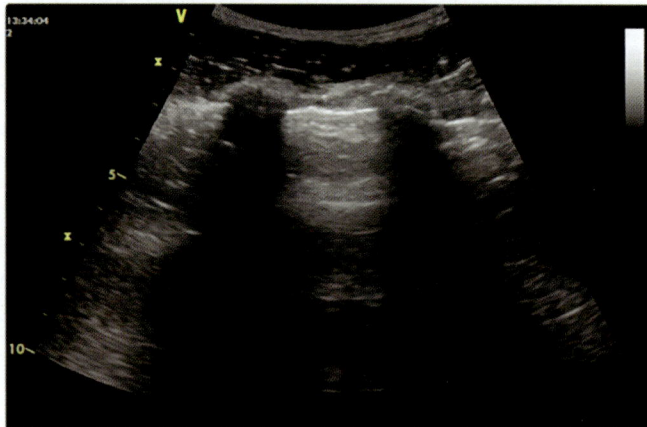

FIG. 30.6 Horizontal artifacts, or B-lines, below the pleural line may be seen when the pleural line is perpendicular to the line of interrogation of the ultrasound beam.

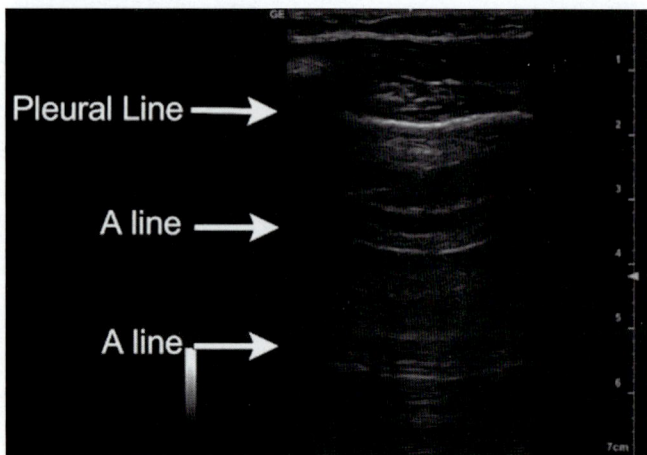

FIG. 30.7 Lung that is normally aerated has a characteristic pattern of air artifact designated as A-lines. These A-lines indicate air, whether physiologic of or pathologic. A-lines are horizontally oriented hyperechoic lines seen deep to the pleural line.

horizontally oriented hyperechoic lines seen deep to the pleural line. They represent reverberation artifacts from the ultrasound reflection between the pleural surface and the outer surface of the chest wall. Therefore, their depth is a multiplicative of the distance between the skin surface and the pleural line.

In the presence of a pleural effusion, the costophrenic angle is filled with fluid that allows the ultrasound to reach the spine (Fig. 30.8). A loculated effusion may not involve the costophrenic angle and requires scanning multiple zones (Fig. 30.9).

THE HEART AND GREAT VESSELS

The heart lies obliquely in the chest, posterior to the sternum, with the greater portion of its muscular mass lying slightly to the left of midline. The heart is protected within the chest by the sternum and rib cage anteriorly and the vertebral column and rib cage posteriorly. The other structures within the thoracic cavity in close approximation to the heart are the lungs, esophagus, and descending thoracic aorta.

Contrary to most simplified anatomic illustrations, the heart is not situated with its right chambers lying to the right and its left chambers to the left. It may be better considered as an anteroposterior structure, with its right-side chambers located more anterior than its left-side chambers. As we look at the embryologic development, the heart forms as a tubular right-to-left structure. However, as development continues, the right side becomes more ventral and the left side remains dorsal.

In addition, another change in axis causes the apex (or the inferior surface of the heart) to tilt anteriorly. The final development of the heart presents the right atrium anterior to the left atrium and to the right of the sternum, whereas the right ventricle presents anterior to the left ventricle and slightly to the left of the sternum. The left atrium becomes the most posterior chamber to the left of the sternum, whereas the left ventricle swings its posterior axis slightly toward the anterior chest wall.

The heart has three surfaces: sternocostal (anterior), diaphragmatic (inferior or apex), and base (posterior) (Fig. 30.10). The right atrium forms the right border of the heart to the right of the sternum. The vertical atrioventricular groove separates these two structures.

The left border is formed by the left ventricle and left atrial appendage. The right and left ventricles are separated by the anterior interventricular groove (Fig. 30.11). The diaphragmatic surface of the heart is formed principally by the right and left ventricles, separated by the posterior interventricular groove. A small part of the inferior surface of the right atrium also forms this surface.

The base of the heart is formed by the left atrium, into which the four pulmonary veins enter from the lungs. The right atrium contributes a small part to this posterior surface (Fig. 30.12). The left ventricle forms the apex of the heart, which can be palpated at the level of the fifth intercostal space, about 9 cm from the midline.

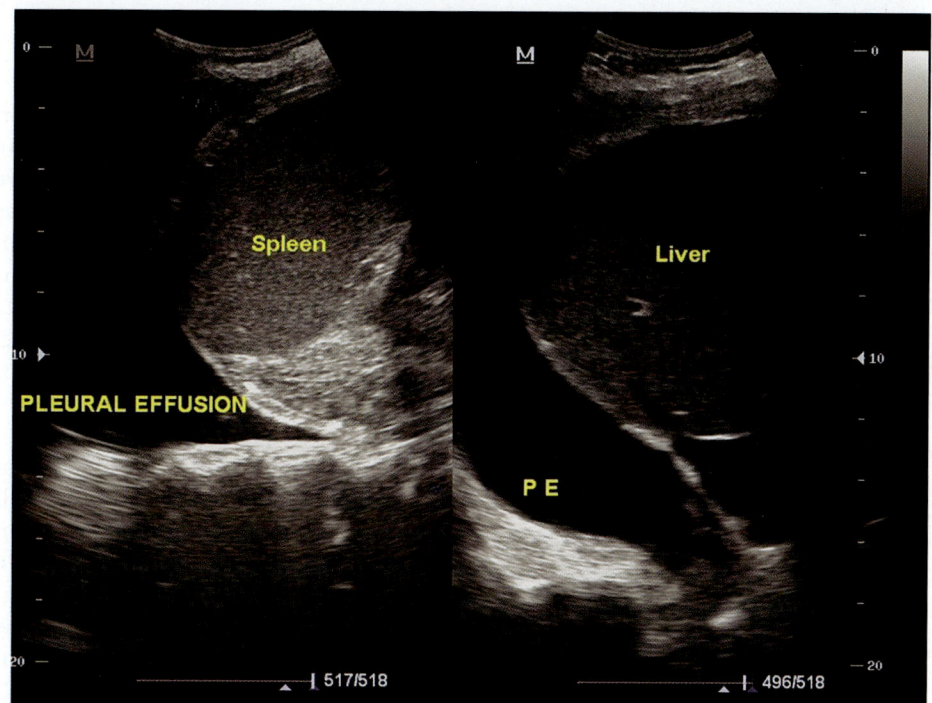

FIG. 30.8 In the presence of a pleural effusion, the costophrenic angle is filled with fluid that allows the ultrasound to reach the spine.

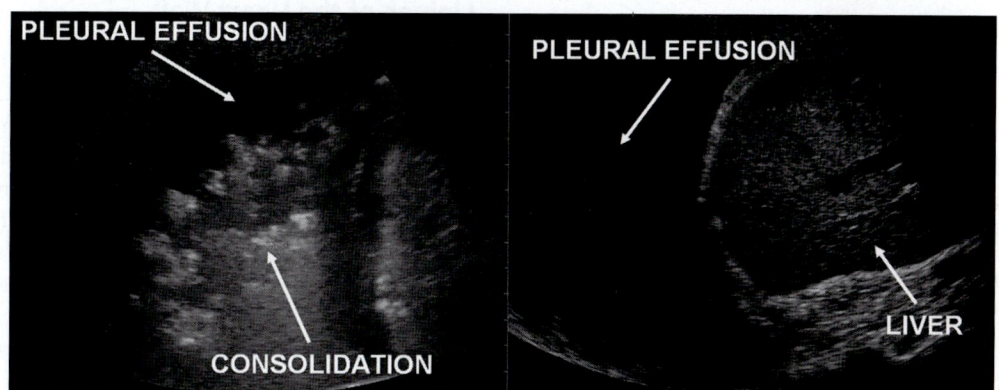

FIG. 30.9 **Consolidation/pleural effusion.** A loculated effusion may not involve the costophrenic angle and requires scanning multiple zones.

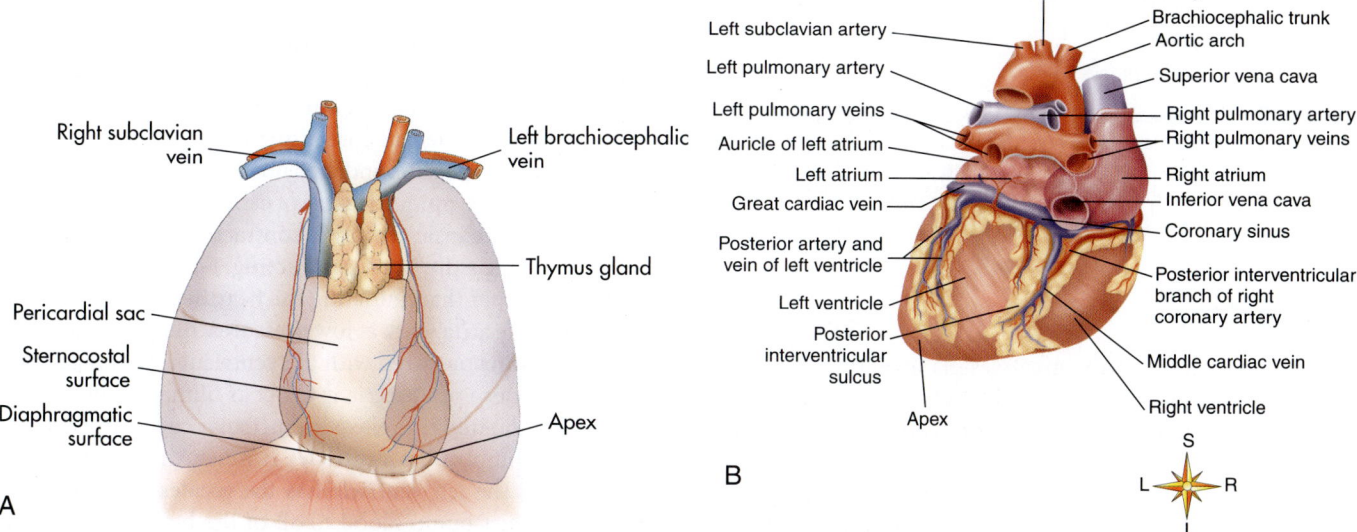

FIG. 30.10 (A) Anterior view of the heart and great vessels. The heart has three surfaces: sternocostal (anterior), diaphragmatic (inferior or apex), and base (posterior). (B) Posterior view of the cardiac structures.

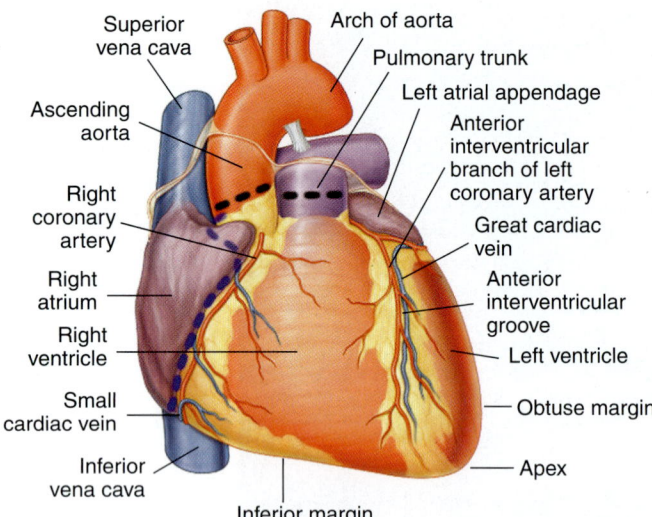

FIG. 30.11 The left border is formed by the left ventricle and left atrial appendage. The right and left ventricles are separated by the anterior interventricular groove.

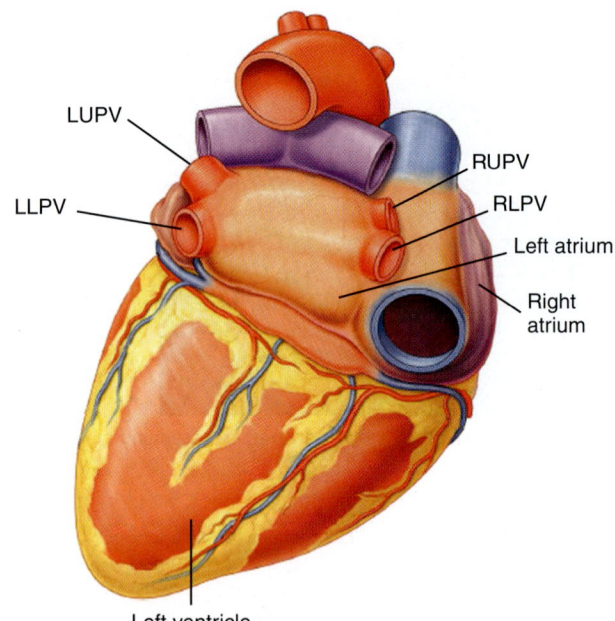

FIG. 30.12 The base of the heart is formed by the left atrium, into which the four pulmonary veins enter from the lungs. The right atrium contributes a small part to this posterior surface. *LLPV,* Left lower pulmonary vein; *LUPV,* left upper pulmonary vein; *RLPV,* right lower pulmonary vein; *RUPV,* right upper pulmonary vein.

Pericardial Sac

The heart and roots of the great vessels lie within the pericardial sac (see Fig. 30.10). Like the pleura of the lungs, the **pericardium** is a double sac. The fibrous pericardium limits the movement of the heart by attaching to the central tendon of the diaphragm below and the outer coat of the great vessels above. The sternopericardial ligaments attach to it in the front. The serous pericardium is divided into parietal and visceral layers. The parietal layer lines the fibrous pericardium and is reflected around the roots of the great vessels to become continuous with the visceral layer of serous pericardium. The visceral layer is closely applied to the heart and is often called the epicardium. The slit between the parietal and visceral layers is the pericardial cavity. This cavity normally contains a small amount of fluid that lubricates the heart as it moves.

The pericardial sac protects the heart against friction. If the serous pericardium becomes inflamed, pericarditis will develop, or if too much pericardial fluid, fibrin, or pus develops in the pericardial space, the visceral and parietal layers may adhere to one another.

The pericardial sac does not totally encompass the heart. On the posterior left atrial surface of the heart, the reflection of serous pericardium around the pulmonary veins forms the recess of the oblique sinus. This may be an important landmark in the echocardiographic separation of pericardial effusion from pleural effusion. The transverse sinus lies between the reflection of serous pericardium around the aorta and pulmonary arteries and between the reflections around the pulmonary veins.

Linings of the Heart Wall

The chambers of the heart are lined by the endocardium, myocardium, and epicardium. (Fig. 30.13) The **endocardium** is the intimal lining of the heart and is continuous with the intima of the vessels connecting to it. The endocardium is similar to the intima of blood vessels. It also forms the valves that lie between the filling (atria) and pumping (ventricle) chambers of the heart and along each base of the two great arterial trunks leaving the heart (the aorta and pulmonary artery).

The muscular part of the heart, the **myocardium**, is a special type of muscle found only in the heart and great vessels. This cardiac muscle is equivalent to the media of a blood vessel. The cardiac muscle is complex compared with other muscular fibers. Although it is striated like voluntary muscle, the fibers of the cardiac muscle branch and anastomose so that it is impossible to determine the limits of a fiber. The myocardium of both ventricles is one continuous muscle mass, as is the myocardium of both atria. Because of this continuity, an impulse for contraction originating in the atrium can spread throughout the atrial musculature; similarly, an impulse originating in a ventricle can spread throughout the ventricular musculature. A special bundle of fibers connects the atria to the ventricles. The unique feature of cardiac muscle is the ability to possess intrinsic rhythmic contractility. It is this rhythmicity that keeps the heart contracting, with nerve impulses modifying rather than initiating the heartbeat.

Because the atria work at low pressures, the musculature of the atria is thin compared with the ventricular wall mass. The primary purpose of the atria is to act as filling chambers that drive the blood into the relaxed ventricular cavity. In contrast, the myocardium of the ventricles is much thicker than that of the atria. The left ventricle has the greatest muscle mass, because it must pump blood to all of the body, whereas the right ventricle needs only enough pressure to pump the blood to the lungs.

The outside layer of the heart is the **epicardium**, or the visceral layer of the serous pericardium. The outer surface of the epicardium is a single layer of mesothelial cells continuous with the serous (inner) surface of the pericardium.

Right Atrium and Interatrial Septum

The right atrium forms the right border of the heart (Fig. 30.14). The superior vena cava enters the upper posterior border, and the inferior vena cava enters the lower posterolateral border. The posterior wall of the right atrium is directly related to the pulmonary veins (which flow from the lungs to empty into the left atrium). The medial wall of the right atrium is formed by the interatrial septum. The septum angles slightly posterior and to the patient's right, so the atrium lies in front and to the right of the left atrium. The central ovale portion of the septum is thin and fibrous. Just superior and in front of the opening of the inferior vena cava lies a shallow depression, the fossa ovalis. Its borders are the limbus fossae ovalis and the primitive septum primum. The foramen ovale lies under the most superior part of the limbus fossae. The limbus fossae ovalis is the remainder of the atrial septum and forms a ridge around the fossa ovalis.

The atrioventricular part of the membranous septum separates the right atrium and left ventricle. Atrial septal defects can occur in this area, causing blood to flow from the high-pressured left ventricle into the right atrial cavity.

The anterior and lateral walls of the right atrium are ridged by the pectinate muscles. The superior portion of the right atrium, the right atrial appendage, contains the most prominent pectinate muscles. The posterior and medial walls are smooth, probably because of the continual flow of blood from the inferior and superior venae cavae and coronary sinus.

The inferior vena cava is guarded by a fold of tissue called the eustachian valve, and the coronary sinus is guarded by the thebesian valve.

The coronary sinus drains the blood supply from the heart wall. It is bordered by the fossa ovalis and the tricuspid valve.

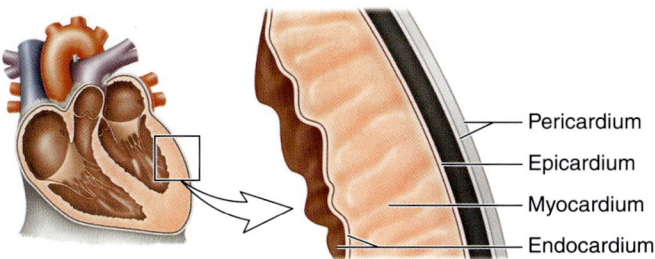

FIG. 30.13 The chambers of the heart are lined by the endocardium, myocardium, and epicardium.

Tricuspid Valve

The tricuspid valve separates the right atrium from the right ventricle. It has three leaflets: anterior, septal, and inferior (or mural) (Fig. 30.15). The septal leaflet may be underdeveloped in association with such conditions as ostium primum defect or ventricular septal defect. The leaflets are attached by their base to the fibrous atrioventricular ring. The chordae tendineae attach the leaflets to the papillary muscles. As these muscles contract with ventricular contraction, the leaflets are pulled together to prevent their being pulled into the atrial cavity. The septal and anterior leaflets are connected to the same papillary muscle, which helps in this process.

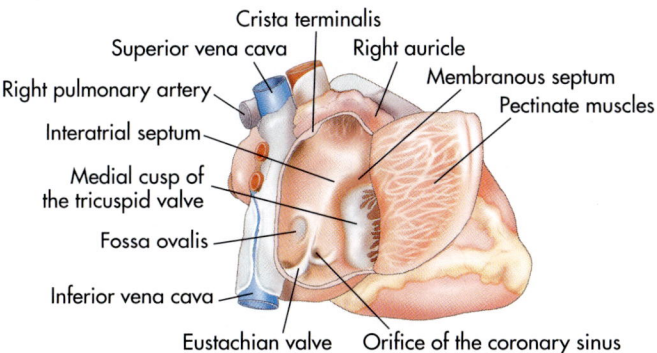

FIG. 30.14 The right atrium forms the right border of the heart.

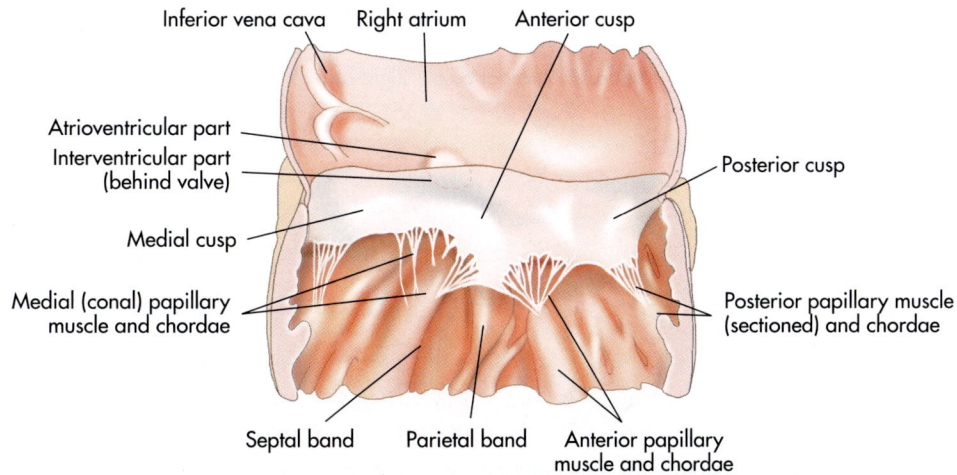

FIG. 30.15 The tricuspid valve has three leaflets: anterior, septal, and inferior (or mural).

Right Ventricle

The base of the right ventricle lies on the diaphragm, and the roof is occupied by the crista supraventricularis, which lies between the tricuspid and pulmonary orifices (Fig. 30.16). The right ventricle is essentially divided into two parts: the posteroinferior inflow portion (containing the tricuspid valve) and the anterosuperior outflow portion (containing the origin of the pulmonary trunk). The demarcation between these two parts is several prominent bands: the parietal band, supraventricular crest, septal band, and moderator band (see Fig. 30.16). Together, these bands form an almost circular orifice that normally is wide and forms no impediment to flow.

The inflow tract of the right ventricle is short and heavily trabeculated. It extends from the tricuspid valve and merges into the trabecular zone. This zone is the body of the right ventricle. The trabeculae carneae enclose an elongated ovoid opening. The inflow tract unites with the outflow tract, which extends to the pulmonary valve. The outflow portion of the right ventricle, or infundibulum, is smooth walled and contains few trabeculae.

The right ventricle has two walls: an anterior wall (corresponding to the sternocostal surface) and a posterior wall (formed by the ventricular septum).

Pulmonary Valve and Trunk

The pulmonary valve lies at the upper anterior aspect of the right ventricle. It has three cusps: anterior, right, and left (Fig. 30.17). The wall of the pulmonary artery bulges out adjacent to each cusp to form pockets known as the pulmonary sinuses of Valsalva.

The pulmonary trunk passes posterior and slightly upward from the right ventricle. It bifurcates into the right and left pulmonary arteries just after leaving the pericardial cavity. The ligamentum arteriosum connects the upper aspect of the bifurcation to the anterior surface of the aortic arch. (The ligamentum arteriosum is a remnant of the fetal ductus arteriosus.)

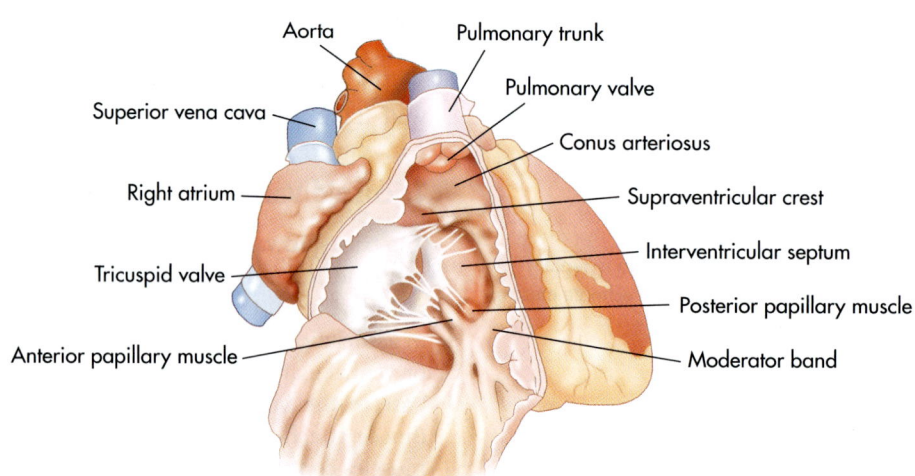

FIG. 30.16 The base of the right ventricle lies on the diaphragm, and the roof is occupied by the crista supraventricularis, which lies between the tricuspid and pulmonary orifices.

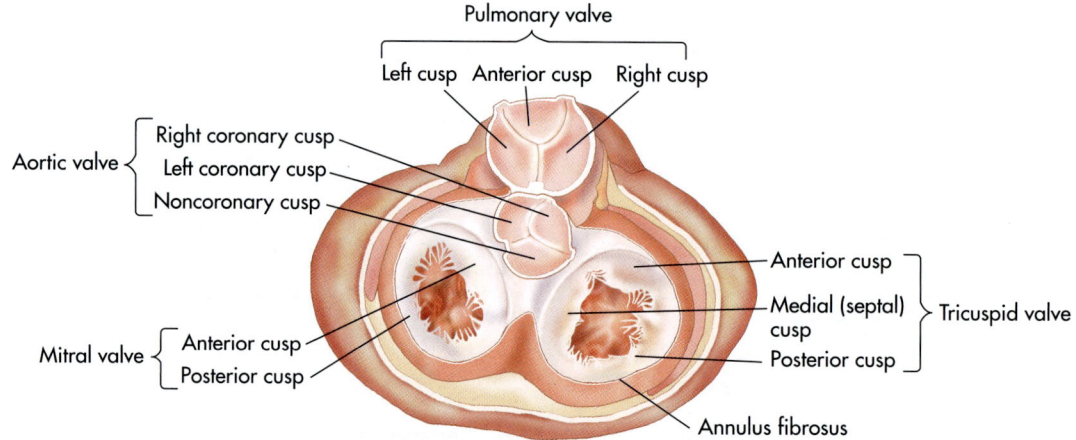

FIG. 30.17 Heart viewed from the base with the atria removed. The pulmonary valve lies at the upper anterior aspect of the right ventricle. It has three cusps: anterior, right, and left.

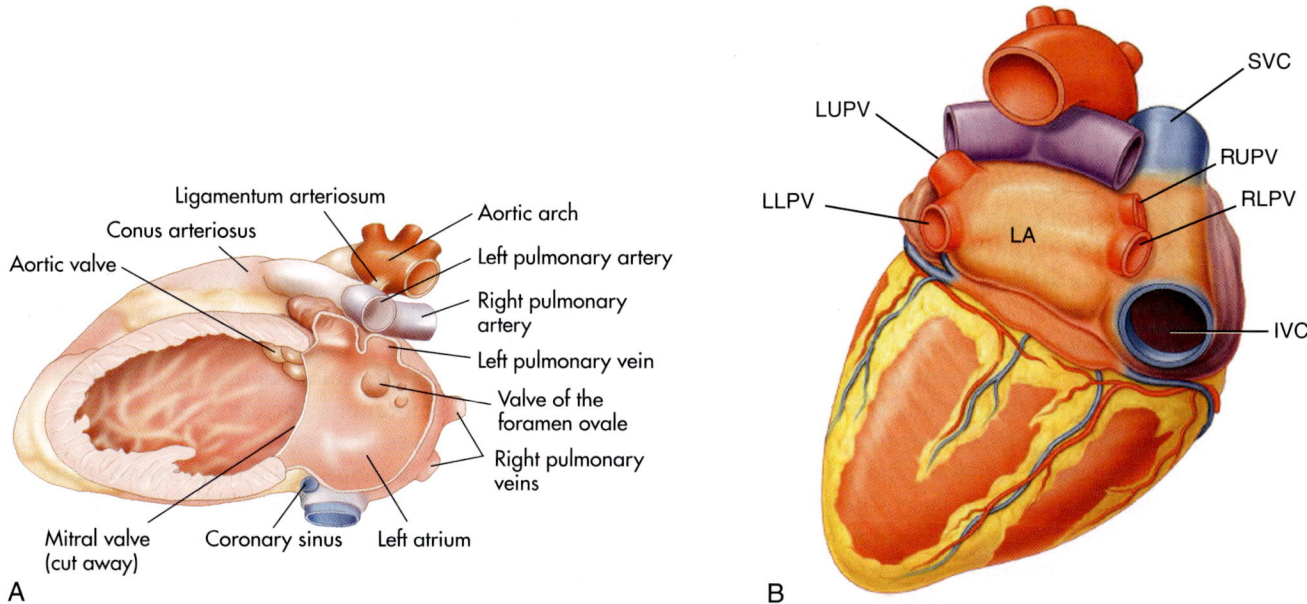

FIG. 30.18 (A) The left atrium is a smooth-walled, circular sac that lies posterior in the base of the heart. (B) Four pulmonary veins enter posteriorly on either side of the cavity. *LA*, Left atrium; *IVC*, inferior vena cava; *LLPV*, left lower pulmonary vein; *LUPV*, left upper pulmonary vein; *RLPV*, right lower pulmonary vein; *RUPV*, right upper pulmonary vein; *SVC*, superior vena cava.

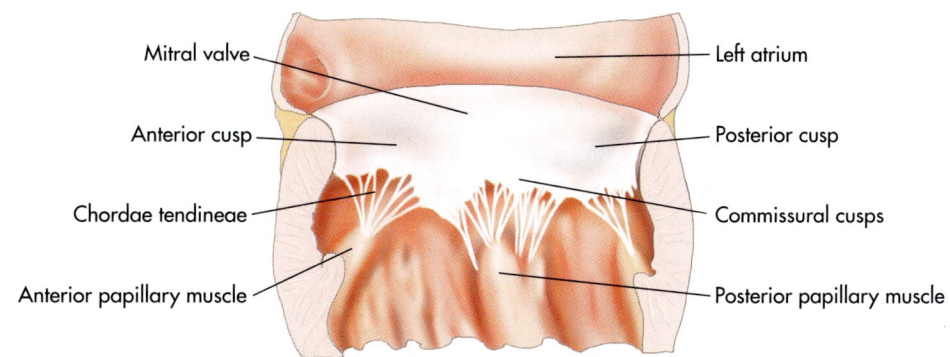

FIG. 30.19 The mitral valve separates the left atrium from the left ventricle. It consists of two large principal leaflets (anterior and posterior) and two small commissural cusps (which usually merge with the posterior leaflet).

Left Atrium

The left atrium is a smooth-walled, circular sac that lies posterior in the base of the heart. Four pulmonary veins enter posteriorly on either side of the cavity (Fig. 30.18). The four pulmonary veins are named according to their anatomic placement: right upper, right lower, left upper, and left lower. Occasionally, these veins unite before entering the atrium, and sometimes there are more than two veins on either side. The veins may also be congenitally defective and enter the right atrium or other areas in the thoracic cavity. This absence of pulmonary veins entering the left atrial cavity is known as *total anomalous pulmonary venous return*.

The septal surface of the atrium is fairly smooth. A somewhat irregular area indicates the position of the fetal valve of the foramen ovale. The left auricle, or left atrial appendage, is a continuation of the left upper anterior part of the left atrium. Small pectinate muscles are located within its lumen.

Mitral Valve

The mitral valve separates the left atrium from the left ventricle. It consists of two large principal leaflets (anterior and posterior) and two small commissural cusps, which usually merge with the posterior leaflet. The anterior leaflet is much longer and larger than the posterior leaflet. It projects downward into the left ventricular cavity. The leaflets are thick membranes that are trapezoidal with fine irregular edges (Figs. 30.19 and 30.20). They originate from the annulus fibrosus and are attached to the papillary muscles by chordae tendineae. The functions of the chordae tendineae are to prevent the opposing borders of the leaflets from inverting into the atrial cavity, to act as mainstays of the valves, and to form bands or fold-like structures that may contain muscle.

Left Ventricle

The left ventricle is conical or egg shaped. The smaller end of the ventricle represents the apex of the heart, and the larger end—near the orifice of the mitral valve—is near the base of the heart (see Fig. 30.20). The left ventricle has a short inflow tract from the mitral valve to the trabecular zone that merges with the outflow tract extending to the aortic valve. Unlike the right side of the heart, where there is no continuity between the tricuspid and pulmonary valves, the anterior leaflet of the mitral valve is continuous with the posterior aortic wall, and the left side of the interventricular septum is continuous with the anterior aortic wall.

The left ventricle has several wall segments that can be recognized in relation to their surrounding structures. The medial wall is formed by the ventricular septum. The lateral wall, posterior wall, posterior-basal wall, and apex are all formed by their relative locations in the heart. The lateral wall is covered with trabeculae, which are finer and more numerous than those found in the right ventricle.

As mentioned previously, the wall of the ventricle consists of the endocardium, the myocardium, and the epicardium. This wall thickness is two to three times thicker than the right ventricular wall because it must handle the increased pressures in the left ventricular cavity.

Interventricular Septum

The septum is somewhat triangular in shape, with its apex corresponding to the apex of the heart and its base fusing posteriorly and superiorly with the atrial septum. The ventricular septum is formed of membranous, inflow, trabecular, and infundibular parts (see Fig. 30.20). These parts arise from the endocardial cushions, the primitive ventricle, and the bulbus cordis. The membranous septum varies in size and shape. It merges into the tissue at the aortic root and infundibular septum but is sharply demarcated from the muscular portion of the septum.

Most of the interventricular septum is muscular and thicker than the membranous portion of the septum. The muscular septum makes up about two-thirds of the septal length, with the membranous septum located just inferior to the aortic root in the area of the left ventricular outflow tract. Most interventricular septal defects occur in this thin, membranous part of the septum. The muscular septum consists of two layers: a thin layer on the right side and a thicker layer on the left side. The major septal arteries run between these layers. The muscular portion of the septum has approximately the same thickness as the left ventricular wall.

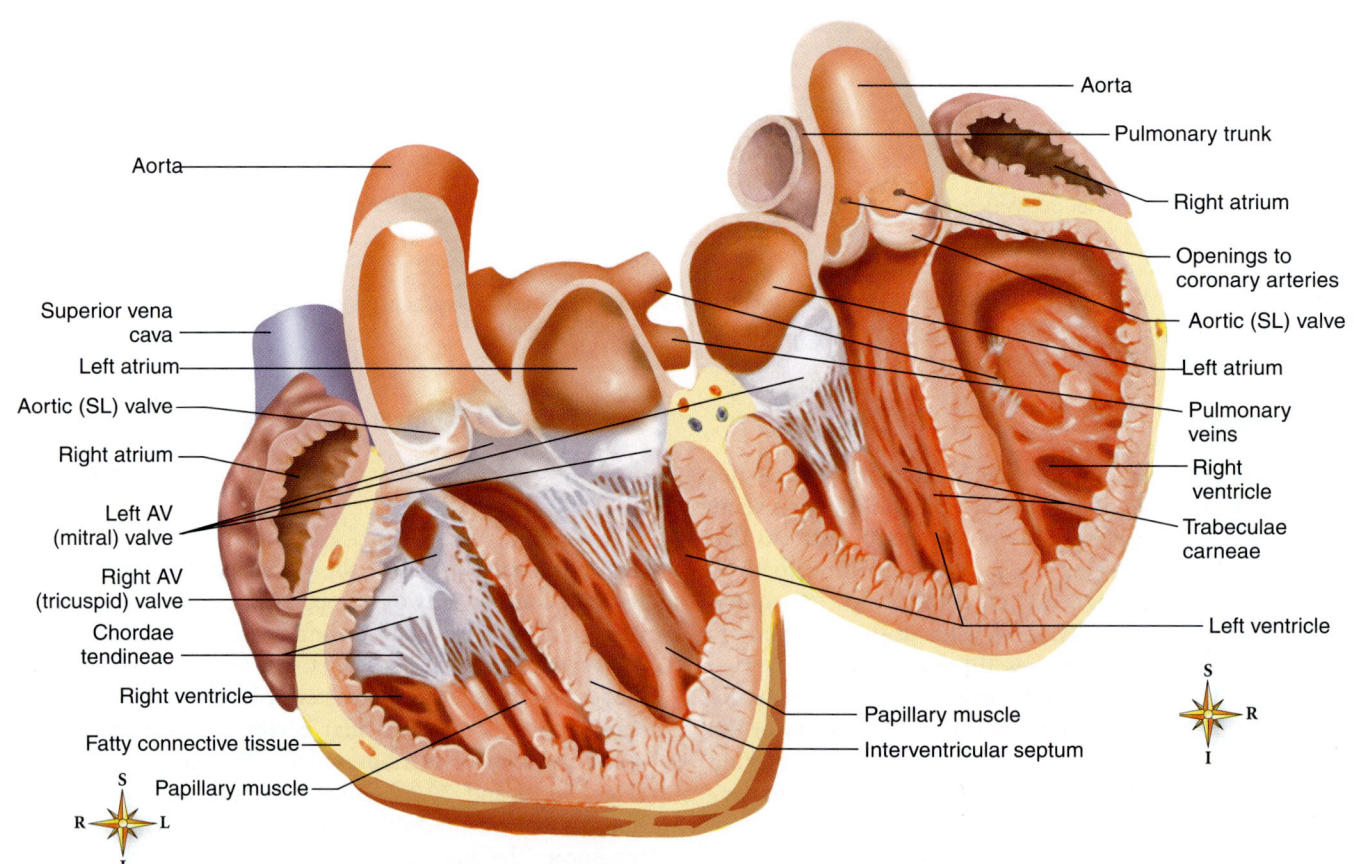

FIG. 30.20 (A) The left ventricle is conical or egg shaped. The smaller end of the ventricle represents the apex of the heart, and the larger end, near the orifice of the mitral valve, is near the base of the heart. (B) The left ventricle has a short inflow tract from the mitral valve to the trabecular zone that merges with the outflow tract extending to the aortic valve.

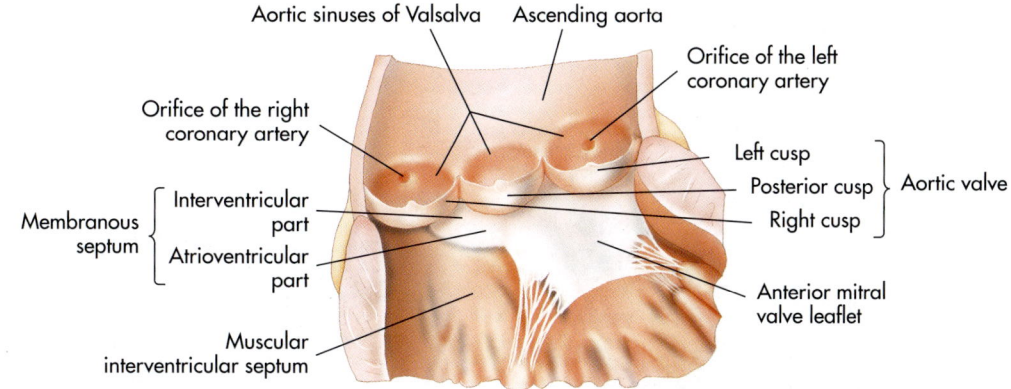

FIG. 30.21 The aortic valve lies at the root of the aorta and has right, left, and posterior (or noncoronary) cusps.

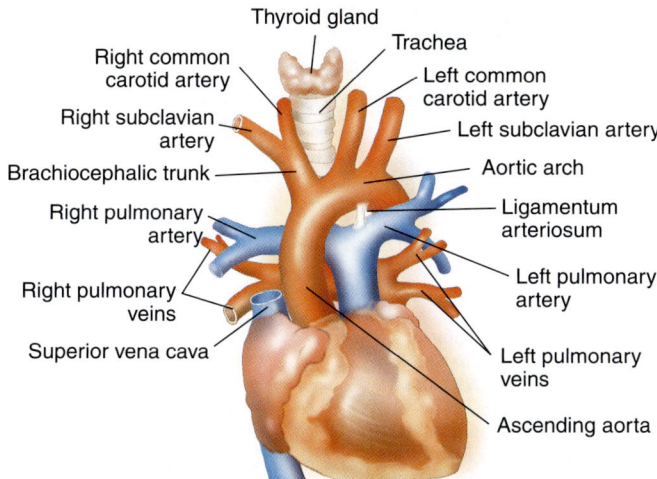

FIG. 30.22 The aortic arch is a continuation of the ascending aorta with three major branches: left subclavian, left common carotid, and the brachiocephalic trunk that further branches into the right subclavian and right common carotid artery.

Aortic Valve

The aortic valve lies at the root of the aorta and has right, left, and posterior (or noncoronary) cusps (Fig. 30.21). The wall of the aorta bulges slightly at each cusp to form the sinus of Valsalva. The main coronary arteries arise from the right and left coronary cusps. At the center of each cusp is a small fibrous nodule, Arantius nodule, which aids in preventing leakage of blood from the left ventricle when the aortic cusps are closed. Often it becomes the site of calcification in patients in whom arteriosclerosis develops.

Aortic Arch and Branches

The aortic arch is a continuation of the ascending aorta (Fig. 30.22). The arch lies behind the manubrium sterni and runs upward, backward, and to the left in front of the trachea. It then passes downward to the left of the trachea to become continuous with the descending aorta at the sternal angle.

The brachiocephalic artery arises from the convex surface of the arch. It passes upward and to the right of the trachea and divides into the right subclavian and common carotid

> **BOX 30.2** **Phases of the Cardiac Cycle (Electromechanical Events)**
>
> 1. **Passive Filling Phase (Ventricular Diastole)**
>   Early diastole, blood enters ventricles through atrioventricular valves
>   Venous blood continues to enter atria during this phase
>   Ventricles expand and pressure slowly rises as ventricular volume increases
>   Inflow volume diminishes in mid-diastole
> 2. **Atrial Systole (P Wave on Electrocardiogram, Late Diastole)**
>   Active contraction of atria stops venous inflow
>   Rapid push of blood into ventricles
>   Causes pressure rise in both atria and ventricles (a wave)
> 3. **Isovolumetric Contraction**
>   Part of pre-ejection period from onset of QRS complex to onset of ventricular ejection
>   Occurs from closure of atrioventricular valves to onset of ventricular ejection (opening of semilunar valves)
> 4. **Ventricles Contract Isovolumetrically**
>   - Pressure rises in ventricles until pressure reaches that of the corresponding great vessel
>   - Pulling down of mitral/tricuspid valve ring causes fall in atrial pressure
>   - Rate of change in left ventricular pressure during isometric ventricular contraction is known as dp/dt (change in pressure over change in time).

arteries. The left common carotid artery arises from the aortic arch on the left side of the brachiocephalic artery. It runs upward and to the left of the trachea and enters the neck behind the left sternoclavicular joint.

The left subclavian artery arises from the arch behind the left common carotid artery. It runs upward along the right side of the trachea and the esophagus to enter the root of the neck.

THE CARDIAC CYCLE

The heart is a muscular pump that propels blood to all parts of the body. It is able to act in definite strokes, or beats, and beats in sinus rhythm at 70 times per minute in the normal adult usually. The cardiac cycle is the series of changes that the heart undergoes as it fills with blood and empties (Box 30.2).

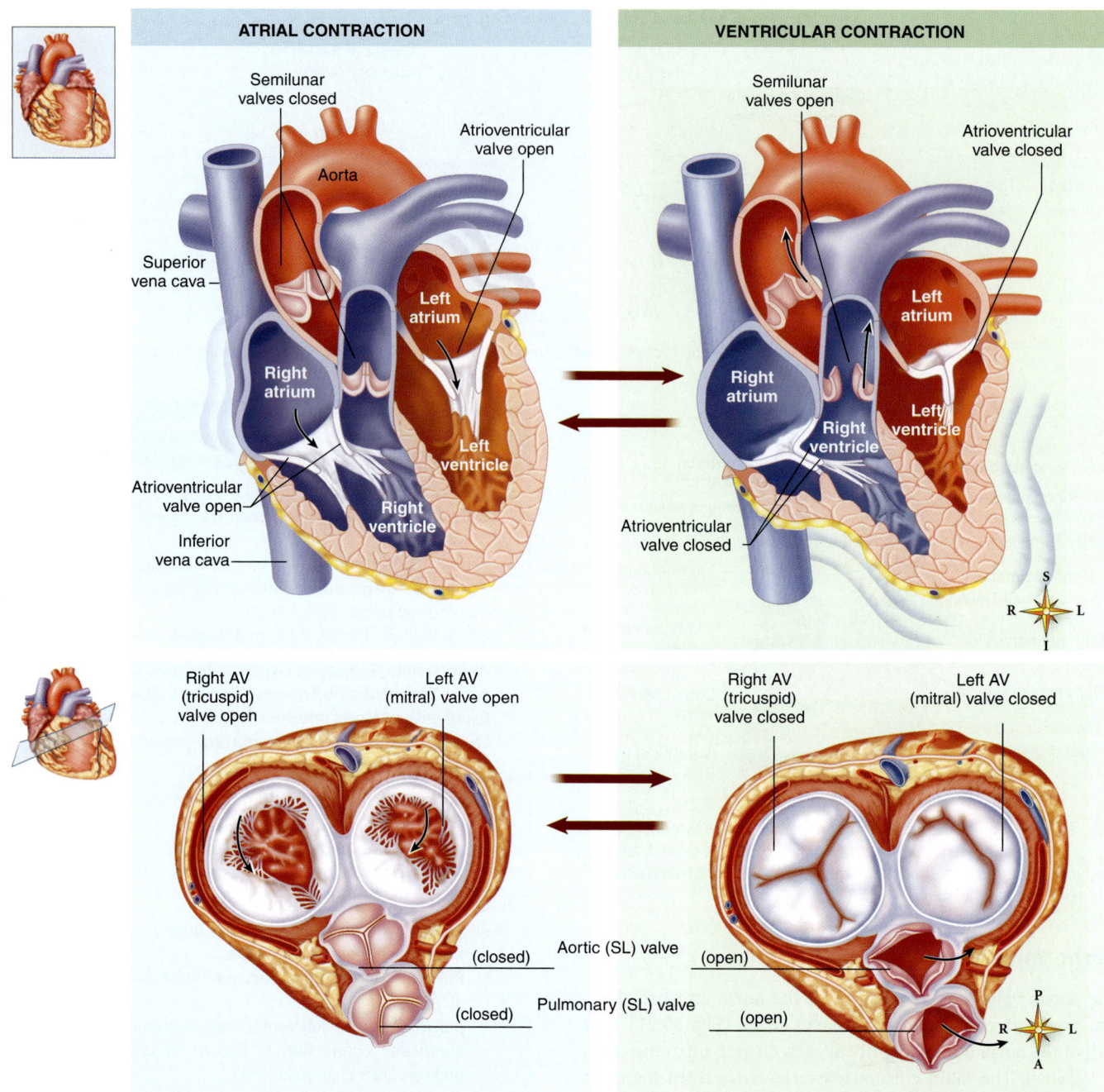

FIG. 30.23 The forceful contraction of the cardiac chambers is *systole*, and the relaxed phase of the cycle is *diastole*. Atrial contraction (atrial systole) corresponds to ventricular diastole; the atrioventricular valves (tricuspid and mitral) between the atria and ventricles are open so that the blood may flow from the atria into the ventricles. Ventricular contraction (atrial diastole) corresponds to ventricular systole. The rising pressure in the ventricular cavity closes the atrioventricular (AV) valves. As the pressure increases in the ventricles, the semilunar (SL) valves (pulmonary and aortic) open so that blood can be forced into the lungs and body, respectively.

Rhythmic contraction of the heart causes blood to be pumped through the chambers of the heart and out through the great vessels. The forceful contraction of the cardiac chambers is *systole*, and the relaxed phase of the cycle is *diastole* (Fig. 30.23).

During diastole the venous blood enters the right atrium from the superior and inferior venae cavae. At the same time, the oxygenated blood returns from the lungs through the pulmonary veins to enter the left atrium. At this point, the **atrioventricular valves** (tricuspid and mitral) between the atria and ventricles are open so that the blood may flow from the atria into the ventricles. The next phase allows atrial contraction to squeeze the remaining blood from the atria into the ventricles. The combination of atrial contraction and increased pressure of the full atrial cavities ultimately drains the atrial blood into the ventricles.

Shortly after this phase, the ventricles contract (ventricular systole). The rising pressure in the ventricular cavity closes the atrioventricular valves. As the pressure increases in the ventricles, the **semilunar valves** (pulmonary and aortic) open so that blood can be forced into the lungs and body, respectively.

The ventricles relax when contraction is completed (ventricular diastole). The blood in the aorta is under very high pressure, and the decreased pressure in the ventricles would cause it to flow backward into the ventricle. However, the semilunar valves prevent this reverse flow. The blood fills the sinuses of Valsalva and forces the valves to close. During ventricular contraction, the atria relax and the venous blood starts to fill them again. When the ventricles are completely relaxed, the atrioventricular valves open and blood flows into the ventricles to begin the next cardiac cycle.

THE ELECTRICAL CONDUCTION SYSTEM

The heart consists of a syncytium of striated muscle cells held together with fibrous tissue. The specialized muscle cells with a high degree of inherent rhythmicity are present in conduction tissue in the areas concerned with the generation and propagation of excitatory electrical activity.

The electrical conduction system of the heart consists of specialized cardiac muscle in the sinoatrial node, atrioventricular node, atrioventricular bundle and its right and left terminal branches, and subendocardial plexus of Purkinje fibers (Fig. 30.24). The sinoatrial node initiates the normal cardiac impulse and is often called the pacemaker of the heart. It is situated on the lateral wall of the right atrium, at the upper part of the sulcus terminalis just to the right of the opening of the superior vena cava. Once activated, the cardiac impulse spreads through the atrial myocardium to reach the atrioventricular node. The atrioventricular node is located in the right posterior portion of the interatrial septum. It lies subendocardially in the medial wall of the right atrium to the left of the ostium of the coronary sinus and immediately posterior to the basal attachment of the septal cusp of the tricuspid valve.

Bundle of His

The atrioventricular node is continuous with the bundle of His, which forms the common bundle that passes along the posterior edge of the membranous septum. The bundle branches include the common bundle and the right and left branches. The common bundle divides into the right and left bundle branch and extends subendocardially along both septal surfaces. The left branch divides into anterior and posterior branches that run along the left interventricular septal surface into the Purkinje fibers, which spread to all parts of the ventricular myocardium.

Cardiac Nerves

The heart is innervated by cholinergic fibers from the vagus nerve and by adrenergic fibers arising from the thoracolumbar sympathetic system and passing through the superior, middle, and inferior cervical ganglions.

THE MECHANICAL CONDUCTION SYSTEM

The Frank-Starling law of the heart states that the output of the heart increases in proportion to the degree of diastolic stretch of the muscle fibers. When a sarcomere is maximally shortened, the actin filaments overlap in the middle, covering up and eliminating from cross-linkage a number of active sites. As the sarcomere is stretched, more sites are uncovered and made available for cross-linkage, increasing the force that is developed. The longer the initial resting length of the cardiac muscle (preload), the greater the strength of contraction of the following beat. A further stretch beyond the normal range cuts the amount of overlap and the force of contraction by reducing the number of cross-bridges.

The shortening velocity of cardiac muscle is inversely related to *afterload*, or the force opposing ventricular ejection. The long interval between beats increases the strength

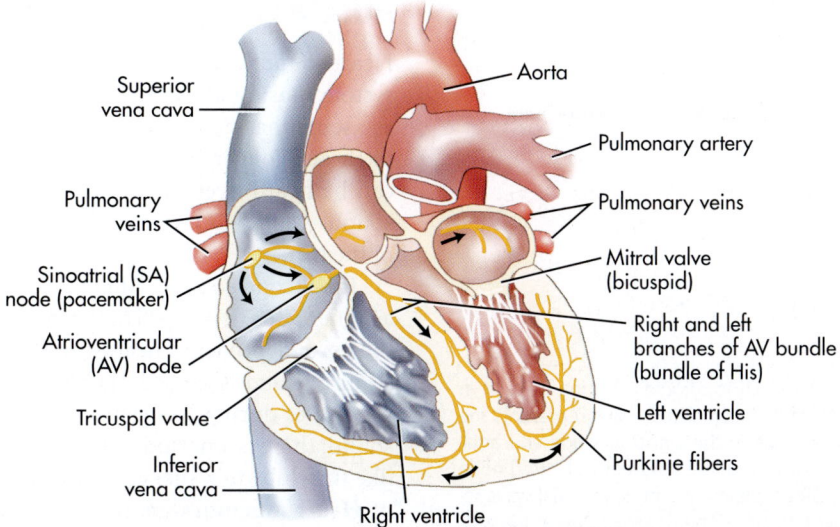

FIG. 30.24 The electrical conduction system of the heart consists of specialized cardiac muscle in the sinoatrial node, atrioventricular node, atrioventricular bundle and its right and left terminal branches, and subendocardial plexus of Purkinje fibers.

of the next cardiac contraction. Tachycardia causes increased strength of contraction. The intracellular calcium ion concentration is probably involved in cellular mechanism.

ELECTROCARDIOGRAPHY

Electrocardiography is a method of recording the heart's electrical activity. It is used to assess cardiac function and disorders of the heart. The contraction of the heart muscle is accompanied by electrical changes, which can be detected by electrodes placed on the skin's surface, and they can be recorded as an electrocardiogram (ECG) on a sheet of graphic paper. On stimulation of a muscle or nerve, the cell membranes are **depolarized**. On recovery, they are **repolarized**. These electrical events are spread throughout the body and can be detected with suitable instruments applied to the skin's surface at considerable distances from the sites of origin. There are various standard positions on the front of the chest on which the electrodes are placed to obtain an adequate electrical signal.

The heart's electrical activity is propagated in the following manner (Fig. 30.25):
- It starts with firing of the sinoatrial (SA) node.
- Electrical events precede mechanical events: atrial contraction follows the P wave on ECG and generates the atrial systolic activity (a wave). Activation proceeds in an orderly, repetitive fashion as the impulse spreads by several internodal pathways through both atria.
- When the impulse reaches the atrioventricular (AV) node near the tricuspid valve, the cells of the bundle of His are activated and the impulse passes via the right and left bundle branches, the latter splitting into the anterior and posterior divisions.
- The impulse spreads via the Purkinje fibers to activate the ventricles, generating the Q, R, and S waves of the ECG (ventricular depolarization).
- After the ventricles depolarize, they begin to repolarize; this repolarization is demarcated by the T wave on the ECG.

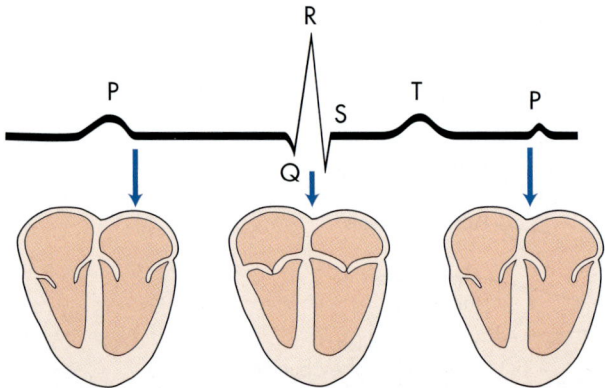

FIG. 30.25 Components of the electrocardiogram tracing as seen in conjunction with the conduction of the heart. The P wave represents the depolarization of cardiac muscle tissue in the sinoatrial node and atrial walls. Before the QRS complex is observed, the atrioventricular (AV) node and AV bundle depolarize. The QRS complex occurs as the atrial walls repolarize and the ventricular walls depolarize. The T wave occurs as the ventricular walls repolarize. Depolarization triggers contraction in the affected muscle tissue. Cardiac muscle contraction occurs after depolarization.

In echocardiography examinations, three ECG lead wires are used for the ECG tracing. Two ECG leads are placed on the patient's right and left shoulders and a ground lead on the right hip. The ECG has three components: P, QRS, and T waves.

P Wave

The impulse is initiated by the SA node and spreads over the atria. The P wave represents the electrical activity associated with the spread of the impulse over the atria (i.e., the wave of depolarization or activity of the atria).

QRS Complex

The wave of depolarization spreads from the SA node over the bundle branches (bundle of His) and Purkinje system to activate both ventricles simultaneously. The QRS complex is the result of all electrical activity occurring in the ventricles.

P-R Interval

The P-R interval is measured from the beginning of the P wave to the beginning of the QRS complex. It indicates the time that elapses between activation of the SA node and activation of the AV node.

T Wave

The T wave represents ventricular repolarization. The echocardiographic examination is always performed with an ECG. This allows the cardiac sonographer to assess cardiac events as they occur in systole and diastole.

Excitation Contraction Coupling. The cardiac muscle is a type of striated muscle tissue. The cells are joined by intercalated disks. The calcium ions are stored and released in response to electrical activity.

AUSCULTATION OF THE HEART VALVES

Heart sounds are associated with the initiation of ventricular systole, closing of the atrioventricular valves, and opening of the semilunar valves (Fig. 30.26). The first sound is lower in pitch and longer in duration than the second. Both sounds can be heard over the entire area of the heart, but the first sound—"lub"—is heard most clearly in the region of the apex of the heart.

The second sound—"dub"—is sharper and shorter and has a higher pitch. It is heard best over the second right rib because the aorta approaches nearest to the surface at this point. The second sound is caused mainly by the closing of the semilunar valves during ventricular diastole. Following the second sound, there is a period of silence. Thus, the sequence sounds like this: lub, dub, silence; lub, dub, silence; and so on.

Heart murmurs are heart sounds produced when blood flows across one of the heart valves that is loud enough to be heard with a stethoscope. There are basically two types of

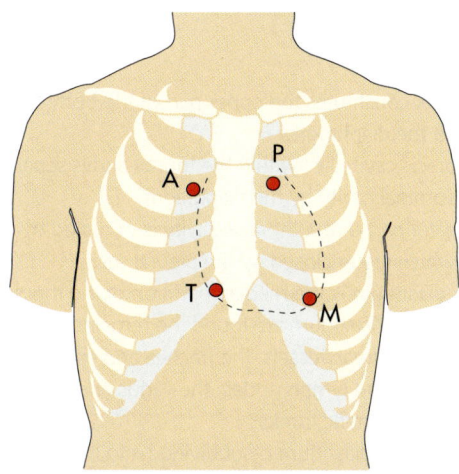

FIG. 30.26 The valve opening and closing sounds may be heard best with the least interference at the location of the circles. *A*, Aortic valve; *M*, mitral valve; *P*, pulmonic valve; *T*, tricuspid valve.

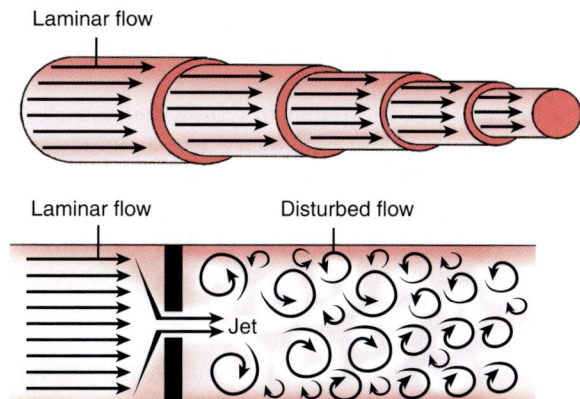

FIG. 30.27 Blood flow may be described in terms of laminar flow or disturbed flow. *Laminar flow* means that blood moves in smooth layers that slide against each other. The blood cells move with similar velocities and directions in an organized manner. *Disturbed flow* means that blood cells move in different directions with varying velocities (disorganized flow). The turbulence denotes the presence of random vortices (flow eddies).

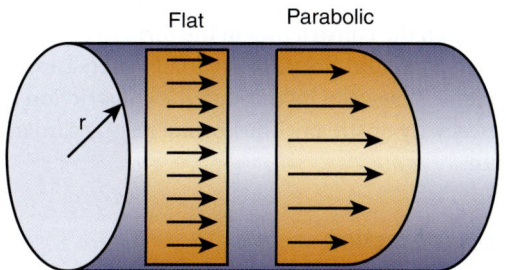

Flow = CSA × velocity
CSA = π × r^2

FIG. 30.28 The velocity profile indicates two pathways: parabolic flow or flat flow. The *parabolic flow velocity profile* is such that as fluid moves through a tube, fluid layers in the center have a higher velocity than those on outer surfaces. The *flat flow velocity profile* states that as flow accelerates and converges, more fluid travels at velocities closer to peak velocity as layers in the center. This is characteristic of high-velocity flow and at the inlets of the great vessels. *CSA,* Curved surface area; *r*, radius.

murmurs: functional or pathologic. A functional murmur, or *physiologic murmur*, is a heart murmur that is primarily due to physiologic conditions outside the heart. Other types of murmurs are due to structural defects in the heart itself. Functional murmurs are benign and often referred to as an "innocent murmur." Murmurs may also be the result of various problems, such as narrowing or leaking of valves, or the presence of abnormal passages through which blood flows in or near the heart. Such murmurs are considered as **pathologic murmur** and usually are further characterized by a specialist.

Heart murmurs are most frequently categorized by timing, into systolic heart murmurs and diastolic heart murmurs, differing in the part of the heartbeat on which they can be heard. Sometimes, a murmur is heard through both systolic and diastolic and is known as a "continuous murmur."

Defects in the valves can cause excessive turbulence or regurgitation of the blood. As described, these are extra abnormal sounds and are called **murmurs** or clicks. If the valves fail to close tightly and blood leaks back, a hissing murmur is heard in the area of the affected valve; thus, if the mitral valve is affected, it will be heard in the first sound. Another condition giving rise to an abnormal sound is stenosis or stiffening of a valve orifice. In this case, a rumble is heard in the area of the affected valve. A **diastolic murmur** begins with or after the time of the second heart sound and ends at or before the time of the first heart sound. A **systolic murmur** begins with or after the time of the first heart sound and ends at or before the time of the second heart sound. A **continuous murmur** begins in systole and continues without interruption through the time of the second heart sound into all or part of diastole. Murmurs are graded according to **frequency** and **intensity**.

It is beyond the scope of this text to present an in-depth approach to auscultation, and the reader is referred to the Bibliography for additional reading on this subject. An understanding of auscultation will help in understanding cardiac physiology and echocardiographic differential considerations.

PRINCIPLES OF BLOOD FLOW

Blood flow may be described in terms of laminar flow or disturbed flow (Fig. 30.27). *Laminar flow* means that blood moves in smooth layers that slide against each other. The blood cells move with similar velocities and directions in an organized manner. *Disturbed flow* means that blood cells move in different directions with varying velocities (disorganized flow). The turbulence denotes the presence of random vortices (flow eddies).

The flow dynamics depend on the fluid viscosity and the momentum of molecules in the fluid. The velocity profile indicates two pathways: parabolic flow or flat flow. The parabolic flow velocity profile is such that as fluid moves through a tube, fluid layers in the center have a higher velocity than those on outer surfaces (Fig. 30.28). The flat flow velocity profile states that as flow accelerates and converges, more fluid travels at velocities closer to peak velocity as layers in the center. This is characteristic of high-velocity flow and at the inlets of the great vessels.

The heart is a pulsatile pump. In systole, the ventricles eject blood into the aorta and pulmonary artery. In diastole, the ventricles fill with blood from the atria and flow to the body organs. The damping effect is achieved because of the elasticity of great vessels as they absorb high-flow pulsatility of the heart and smooth it out before sending it to the blood downstream. The blood vessels stretch in response to an increase in pressure (compliance). The increase in fluid pressure during systole causes the aorta and pulmonary artery to expand and store some of the ejected blood. Blood is prevented from reentering the ventricles by the closure of the valves. Stored blood is pushed downstream into circulation when the aorta and pulmonary artery begin to return to normal dimensions in diastole. The hardening of the arteries results in loss of vessel compliance. The circulatory impedance occurs because of resistance to flow downstream in small vessels and capillaries. Flow is produced when a pressure gradient exists. The blood flow through a constriction creates a high fluid pressure upstream from constriction. The high fluid pressure forces blood through the constriction in the form of a laminar high-velocity jet. The fluid pressure gradually decreases as it goes downstream. Flow velocity through the constriction is higher than the velocity upstream. The normal resting cardiac output is 5 L/min.

Ventricular Ejection

Both ventricles eject the same proportion of contents with systole. The normal left ventricular ejection fraction is 67%. The normal stroke volume is 45 ± 13 mL/m^2. The amount of filling (preload) influences the pressure developed during the next systole via the Frank Starling mechanism. The output of the ventricle depends on resistance encountered by the contracting ventricle when the aortic valve opens during systole (afterload). The most important indicator of cardiac work is the metabolic cost of cardiac activity, which is given by the oxygen consumption of the myocardium.

Coronary Circulation

The coronary flow is essential to myocardial performance. The right and left coronary arteries arise from the base of the ascending aorta. The left coronary artery flow is mainly diastolic. The right coronary artery flow is more evenly spread through systole and diastole. The flow goes from the epicardium to the endocardium. The diastolic aortic pressure is a major factor in coronary perfusion. Myocardial ischemia may occur in situations in which blood pressure is acutely lowered. The arteries and arterioles anastomose with one another and the small collateral channels increase in number when vessels are occluded.

Key Pearls

- The thorax constitutes the upper part of the body between the neck and the diaphragm.
- The thoracic cavity lies within the thorax and is separated from the abdominal cavity by the diaphragm.
- The greater part of the thoracic cavity is occupied by the two lungs, which are enclosed by the pleural sac.
- The mediastinum is the median partition of the thoracic cavity. Within the mediastinum are found the remains of the thymus, the heart and great vessels, the trachea and esophagus, the thoracic duct and lymph nodes, the vagus and phrenic nerves, and the sympathetic trunks.
- The inferior mediastinum is subdivided into three parts: (1) middle, which contains the pericardium and the heart; (2) anterior, which is a space between the pericardium and sternum; and (3) posterior, which lies between the pericardium and vertebral column.
- The heart lies obliquely in the chest, posterior to the sternum, with the greater portion of its muscular mass lying slightly to the left of midline.
- The heart may be better considered as an anteroposterior structure, with its right-side chambers located more anterior than its left-side chambers.
- The heart has three surfaces: sternocostal (anterior), diaphragmatic (inferior or apex), and base (posterior).
- The right atrium forms the right border of the heart to the right of the sternum. The vertical atrioventricular groove separates these two structures.
- The left border is formed by the left ventricle and left atrial appendage. The right and left ventricles are separated by the anterior interventricular groove.
- The base of the heart is formed by the left atrium, into which the four pulmonary veins enter from the lungs. The right atrium contributes a small part to this posterior surface.
- The heart and roots of the great vessels lie within the pericardial sac.
- The serous pericardium is divided into parietal and visceral layers. The slit between the parietal and visceral layers is the pericardial cavity.
- On the posterior left atrial surface of the heart, the reflection of serous pericardium around the pulmonary veins forms the recess of the oblique sinus.
- The transverse sinus lies between the reflection of serous pericardium around the aorta and pulmonary arteries and between the reflections around the pulmonary veins.
- The chambers of the heart are lined by the endocardium, myocardium, and epicardium.
- The musculature of the atria is thin compared with the ventricular wall mass.
- The left ventricle has the greatest muscle mass because it must pump blood to all of the body, whereas the right ventricle needs only enough pressure to pump the blood to the lungs.
- The right atrium forms the right border of the heart. The superior vena cava enters the upper posterior border, and the inferior vena cava enters the lower posterolateral border.

- The inferior vena cava is guarded by a fold of tissue called the eustachian valve, and the coronary sinus is guarded by the thebesian valve.
- The coronary sinus drains the blood supply from the heart wall. It is bordered by the fossa ovalis and the tricuspid valve.
- The tricuspid valve separates the right atrium from the right ventricle. It has three leaflets: anterior, septal, and inferior.
- The right ventricle is essentially divided into two parts: the posteroinferior inflow portion (containing the tricuspid valve) and the anterosuperior outflow portion (containing the origin of the pulmonary trunk).
- The pulmonary valve lies at the upper anterior aspect of the right ventricle. It has three cusps: anterior, right, and left.
- The pulmonary trunk passes posterior and slightly upward from the right ventricle. It bifurcates into the right and left pulmonary arteries just after leaving the pericardial cavity.
- The left atrium is a smooth-walled, circular sac that lies posterior in the base of the heart. Four pulmonary veins enter posteriorly on either side of the cavity.
- The mitral valve separates the left atrium from the left ventricle. It consists of two large principal leaflets (anterior and posterior) and two small commissural cusps, which usually merge with the posterior leaflet.
- The left ventricle is conical or egg shaped. The smaller end of the ventricle represents the apex of the heart, and the larger end—near the orifice of the mitral valve—is near the base of the heart.
- The left ventricle has a short inflow tract from the mitral valve to the trabecular zone that merges with the outflow tract extending to the aortic valve.
- The ventricular septum is formed of membranous, inflow, trabecular, and infundibular parts.
- The muscular septum makes up about two-thirds of the septal length, with the membranous septum located just inferior to the aortic root in the area of the left ventricular outflow tract. The aortic valve lies at the root of the aorta and has right, left, and posterior (or noncoronary) cusps.
- The wall of the aorta bulges slightly at each cusp to form the sinus of Valsalva. The main coronary arteries arise from the right and left coronary cusps.
- The aortic arch is a continuation of the ascending aorta. The arch lies behind the manubrium sterni and runs upward, backward, and to the left in front of the trachea. It then passes downward to the left of the trachea to become continuous with the descending aorta at the sternal angle.
- The cardiac cycle is the series of changes that the heart undergoes as it fills with blood and empties.
- The forceful contraction of the cardiac chambers is systole, and the relaxed phase of the cycle is diastole.
- The electrical conduction system of the heart consists of specialized cardiac muscle in the sinoatrial node, atrioventricular node, atrioventricular bundle and its right and left terminal branches, and subendocardial plexus of Purkinje fibers.
- Electrocardiography is a method of recording the heart's electrical activity. It is used to assess cardiac function and disorders of the heart.
- On stimulation of a muscle or nerve, the cell membranes are depolarized. On recovery, they are repolarized.
- Heart sounds are associated with the initiation of ventricular systole, closing of the atrioventricular valves, and opening of the semilunar valves.
- Heart murmurs are heart sounds produced when blood flows across one of the heart valves that is loud enough to be heard with a stethoscope.
- Pathologic murmurs may be the result of various problems, such as narrowing or leaking of valves, or the presence of abnormal passages through which blood flows in or near the heart.
- Blood flow may be described in terms of laminar flow or disturbed flow.

BIBLIOGRAPHY

Abrahams PH, Boon J, Spratt JD. *McMinn's clinical atlas of human anatomy*. ed 6. St Louis: Mosby; 2008.

Dubin D. *Rapid interpretation of EKGs*. ed 6. Tampa, FL: Cover Publishing Company; 2004.

McMinn RMH, Gaddum-Rosse P, Hutchings RT, Logan BM. *McMinn's Functional & Clinical Anatomy*. St. Louis: Mosby; 1995.

Oh JK, Seward JB, Tajik AJ. *The echo manual*. ed 4. Mayo Foundation for Medical Education and Research; 2018.

Snell RS. *Clinical anatomy*. ed 7. Philadelphia: Lippincott Williams & Wilkins; 2004.

Sokolow M, McIlroy MB. *Clinical Cardiology*. San Francisco: Lange Medical Publications; 1977.

Tilkian AG, Conover MB. *Understanding heart sounds and murmurs with an introduction to lung sounds*. ed 4. Philadelphia: Saunders; 2001.

CHAPTER 31

Understanding Hemodynamics

Alicia Armour

OBJECTIVES

On completion of this chapter, you should be able to:
- Understand the fundamental concepts of hemodynamics as applied to ultrasound
- State basic knowledge of the cardiac cycle, normal intracardiac pressures and volumes, cardiac output, stroke volume, and its mechanisms
- Describe the principles of blood flow velocity profiles, how they are displayed, and how they are evaluated by Doppler ultrasound
- Demonstrate knowledge of how to apply Doppler ultrasound to calculate pressures, velocities, and output

OUTLINE

The Cardiac Cycle 909
   Normal Intracardiac Pressures and Volumes 909
   Cardiac Output, Stroke Volume, and Its Mechanisms 910
   Blood Flow Velocity Profiles 910
Doppler Basics 910
   Doppler Effect and Frequency Shift 910
Pulsed Wave Doppler 911
Color Doppler 912
Continuous Wave Doppler 913
Quantification of Intracardiac Pressures With Ultrasound 913
   Pressure-Velocity Relationship: Bernoulli Equation 913
   Right Atrial Pressure 914
Cardiac Output and Stroke Volume Measured by Ultrasound 914
Continuity Principle and Equation: Valve Area 915

KEY TERMS

Afterload
Bernoulli equation
Blood flow velocity
Cardiac output
Color Doppler
Continuity principle

Continuous wave Doppler
Doppler effect
Doppler frequency shift
Hemodynamics
Preload
Pressure

Pulsed wave Doppler
Stroke volume
Velocity
Volume

Hemodynamics is the study of the forces involved with blood flow and circulation. This chapter focuses on blood flow and circulation as it moves through the body. It is important to understand hemodynamics because the forces involved with blood flow and circulation allow us to answer important questions regarding a patient's condition, such as cardiac output, right ventricular systolic pressure (RVSP), and degree of valvular stenosis or regurgitation. Doppler principles can be applied using ultrasound to indirectly measure such information.

Some basic terms that are used frequently throughout this chapter include pressure, volume, and velocity. **Pressure** is defined as the exertion of force on a surface by an object or a fluid it is in contact with, or the force per unit area. Pressure will be used in the context of the force of fluid per unit area. **Volume** is the amount of space occupied by a three-dimensional object as measured in cubic units such as cubic centimeters (cm) or milliliters (mL). **Velocity** is the speed with which something moves in a given direction.

Before discussing basic principles of blood flow, one must review how blood moves through the heart. Blood flow enters the heart through the vena cava (superior and inferior) into the right atrium, through the tricuspid valve, and into the right ventricle (RV). From the RV, blood travels to the pulmonary circuit through the pulmonary valve and pulmonary artery (PA). The PA bifurcates, and blood flows through to the pulmonary capillaries and circuit, eventually back to the pulmonary veins. The pulmonary veins bring blood into the left atrium (LA), through the mitral valve, and into the left ventricle (LV). Blood leaves the heart through the aortic valve and aorta to the systemic circulatory system.

THE CARDIAC CYCLE

The cardiac cycle can be best described by the Wiggers diagram (Fig. 31.1). This diagram shows the interaction of pressure and volume changes with electrical and mechanical systole and diastole. The two major components of the cardiac cycle are systole and diastole. Within these two major components, there are six minor components of the cardiac cycle; systole can be divided into isovolumic contraction and ejection, and diastole consists of isovolumic relaxation, rapid inflow, diastasis, and atrial systole. During systole, the volume in the ventricles decreases as the ventricular and aortic pressure rises. Throughout diastole, the pressures in the ventricles stabilize while the ventricular volume gradually increases.

Normal Intracardiac Pressures and Volumes

As shown in Fig. 31.1, the pressures in the cardiac chambers are constantly changing throughout the cardiac cycle. Fig. 31.2 shows normal pressures in the various cardiac chambers. It is important to remember that there are ranges of pressures, both normal and abnormal, but these are typical. In both the right and LVs, the pressure in early diastole drops to 0 mm Hg (middle number) and then slowly rises. Note that the right and left atrial pressures are a mean or average over the cardiac cycle. Pulmonary capillary wedge is a substitute for left atrial pressure. Pulmonary capillary wedge is obtained using a Swan-Ganz catheter primarily in intensive care settings.

The average pressures in each cardiac chamber, which can be measured directly through cardiac catheterization or indirectly through Doppler ultrasound, are as follows:

Right atrium: 1–5 mm Hg	Left atrium: 2–12 mm Hg
Right ventricle: 15–30 mm Hg in systole 1–7 mm Hg in diastole	**Left ventricle:** 90–140 in systole 5–12 mm Hg in diastole
Pulmonary artery: 15–30 mm Hg in systole 4–12 in diastole	**Aorta:** 90–140 mm Hg in systole 60–90 mm Hg in diastole

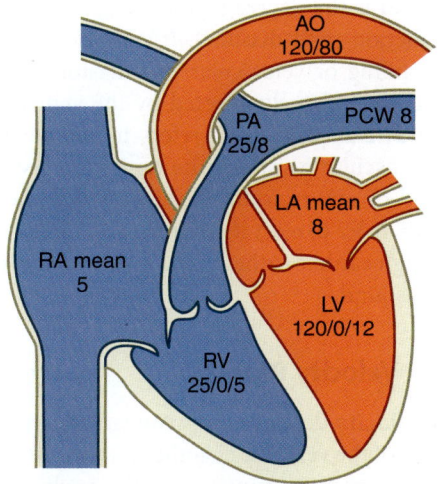

FIG. 31.2 Normal pressures in the cardiac chambers and great vessels. See text for ranges. *AO*, Aorta; *LA*, left atrium; *LV*, left ventricle; *PA*, pulmonary artery; *PCW*, pulmonary capillary wedge; *RA*, right atrium; *RV*, right ventricle.

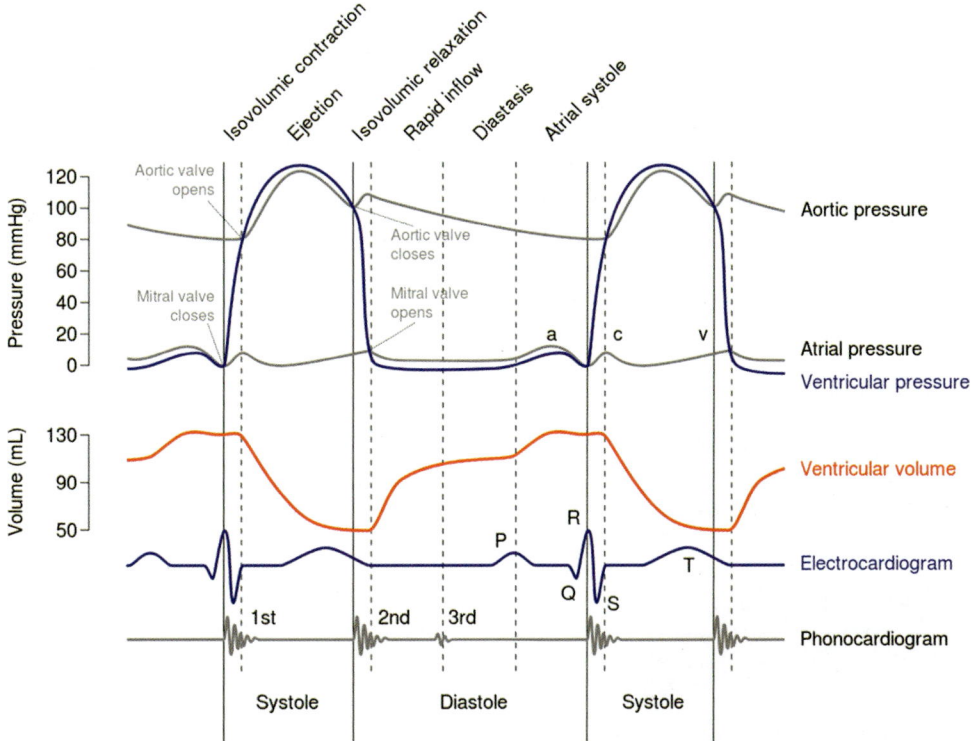

FIG. 31.1 The Wiggers diagram shows the normal relationships between the chamber pressures, volumes, and heart sounds timed with the electrocardiogram for the left side of the heart.

Cardiac Output, Stroke Volume, and Its Mechanisms

Some basic aspects of blood flow as it relates to the heart include cardiac output, stroke volume (SV), preload, and afterload. **Cardiac output** (CO) refers to the amount of blood pumped by each ventricle in 1 minute. It is the product of SV and heart rate (HR). The average CO for adults is 4 to 8 L/min. Cardiac output has a direct effect on blood pressure; as the cardiac output increases, so does the blood pressure. **Stroke volume** is the volume of blood ejected by the ventricles with each contraction. Any effect on SV or HR affects the cardiac output. **Preload** is the degree that the muscle fiber stretches before contraction (end-diastole). It can also be considered the diastolic filling or ventricular end-diastolic volume and pressure. Preload is largely affected by the ventricle's ability to stretch and relax. **Afterload** refers to the aortic arterial pressure and vascular resistance the ventricle must overcome to eject blood or any resistance against which the ventricle must pump in order to eject its volume. CO can be measured directly through cardiac catheterization or indirectly through Doppler ultrasound.

Blood Flow Velocity Profiles

Blood flow velocity depends on many factors, including the shape and size of the vessel or chamber it is traveling through, wall characteristics, the timing within the cardiac cycle, flow rate, and the viscosity of the blood. Flow starts uniformly with similar velocity flow profiles giving a "flat," laminar appearance (Fig. 31.3, *top*). Most of the flow is traveling at the same velocity as laminar flow. As the shape of the surface blood travels through changes, so does the flow velocity profile. As this change in shape or additional forces continue, the flow will vary so that it appears more parabolic with varying flow velocities. The flow velocities will be highest toward the middle of the vessel or area and slowest along the walls or edges of the surface it travels through. Flow can become turbulent when it travels through an area of obstruction or smaller surface area (Fig. 31.3, *bottom*). The flow velocities vary significantly when turbulent with high velocity and multidirectional flow. These blood flow velocities can be interrogated by Doppler with ultrasound, which will be discussed further within this chapter.

DOPPLER BASICS

Doppler provides clinical information about blood flow, including the direction and velocity as well as the timing during the cardiac cycle. Qualitative (color flow) and quantitative (pulsed and continuous wave) Doppler aids in the evaluation of stenosis, insufficiency, and shunt lesions. It can also provide estimates of cardiac function, such as CO.

Doppler Effect and Frequency Shift

The **Doppler effect** refers to a change in the frequency of waves (through sound, light, etc.) that occurs as the source and observer change in motion relative to each other (away or toward). The Doppler effect will be discussed relative to the frequency of sound waves for the purposes of this chapter. With sound, the frequency will increase as the source and observer move toward each other and decrease as they move apart, as demonstrated in Fig. 31.4.

Blood flow velocities, as mentioned previously, are interrogated by Doppler in ultrasound. The change or shift in the received sound waves allows for the calculation of the blood flow velocity. **Doppler frequency shift** refers to the change or shift in received sound waves from the initial transmitted sound waves or pulse. Because the Doppler frequency shift is evaluating blood flow velocities, these shifts can be positive or negative. When the flow is moving away from the transducer or source, the velocity will be negative, displaying a negative shift with lower frequencies. As flow moves toward the transducer or source, the velocity is positive, displaying a positive shift. If flow is perpendicular to the transducer, it will exhibit no change in frequency, giving no frequency shift.

It is important to keep in mind that the Doppler shift is relative to the position of the transducer. Blood flow moving away from the transducer has a lower frequency and is negative because of the movement away from the transducer, whereas blood flow moving toward the transducer has a higher frequency and is positive because the flow is moving

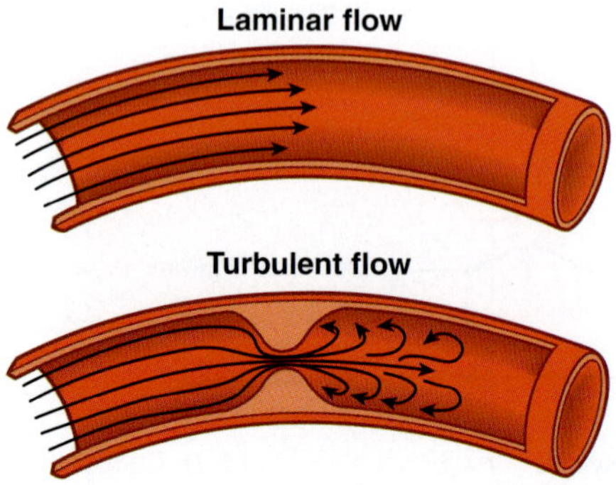

FIG. 31.3 Examples of normal (laminar) flow in a blood vessel versus abnormal (turbulent) flow as might be seen in valvular stenosis or regurgitation.

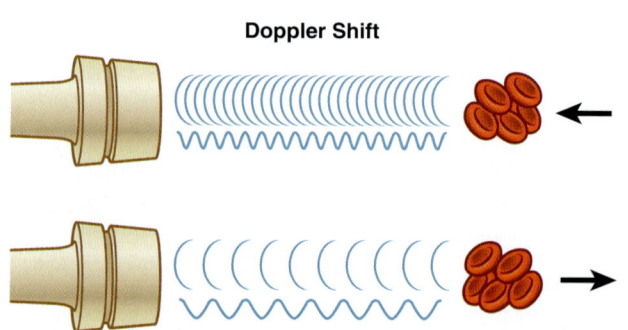

FIG. 31.4 The Doppler shift showing higher returning frequencies when encountering blood flow toward the transducer *(top)* compared with lower returning frequencies when flow is away from the transducer *(bottom)*.

toward the transducer. This is clearly seen in Fig. 31.5, where flow toward the transducer is shown above the baseline in the Doppler spectral display and flow away from the transducer is below the baseline. The Doppler spectral display is used in both pulsed and continuous wave Doppler to show the timing, direction, and velocity of blood flow.

Pulsed Wave Doppler

Pulsed wave Doppler transducers send and receive ultrasound pulses at timed intervals so that the location of where the sample volume is positioned can be known. This allows the detection of flow in specific areas of vessels and organs. Pulsed wave Doppler is usually combined with an imaging transducer so that accurate placement can be accomplished. Fig. 31.6 is a schematic showing how an ultrasound machine can calculate the distance the sample volume is positioned since the transit time is known for the speed of an ultrasound pulse in tissue.

Fig. 31.7 is an apical four-chamber view with a pulsed Doppler sample volume positioned at the tips of the mitral valve leaflets. Doppler controls allow the operator to position the sample volume anywhere within the image. The resultant spectral trace shows the typical mitral inflow pattern with early diastolic filling followed by late diastolic flow from atrial contraction. Fig. 31.8 is another example from the subcostal view of the abdominal aorta containing a pulsed wave Doppler sample volume recording systolic flow. The spectral Doppler displays normal velocity flow above the baseline due to the angle of the aorta with the flow moving toward the transducer.

One of the limitations of pulsed wave Doppler is that higher velocities will exceed the Nyquist limit, and aliasing of the spectral trace will occur. The Nyquist limit equals the pulse repetition frequency (PRF) divided by 2 (one-half the PRF). The PRF is changed based on the depth of the sample volume as a longer distance from the transducer to the

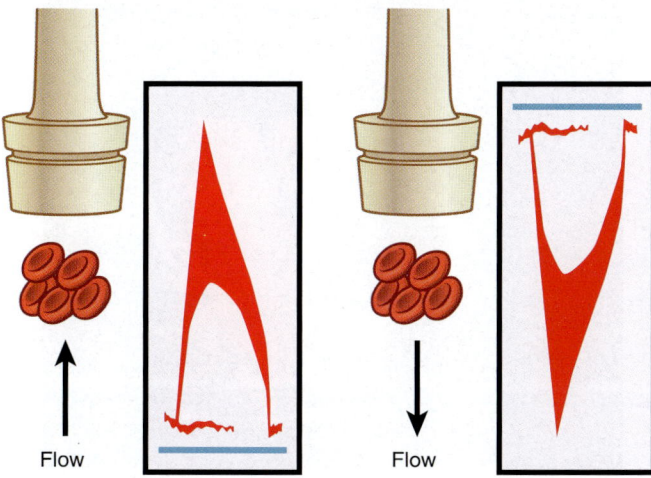

FIG. 31.5 Doppler display showing spectral trace of velocities above the baseline by convention when encountering blood flow toward the transducer *(left)*. Spectral direction is below the baseline when flow is away from the transducer *(right)*.

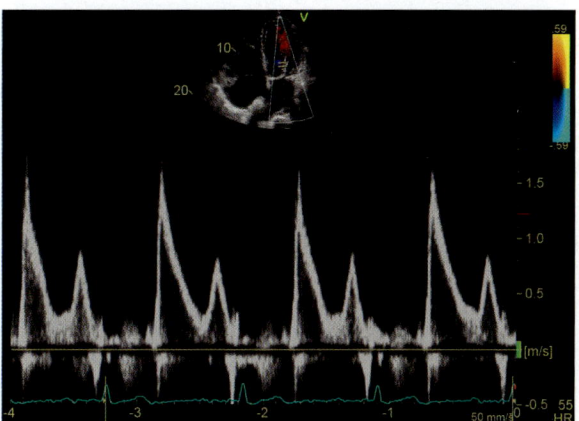

FIG. 31.7 Apical four-chamber view with a pulsed Doppler sample volume positioned at the tips of the mitral valve leaflets. The resultant spectral trace shows the typical mitral inflow pattern with early diastolic filling followed by late diastolic flow from atrial contraction.

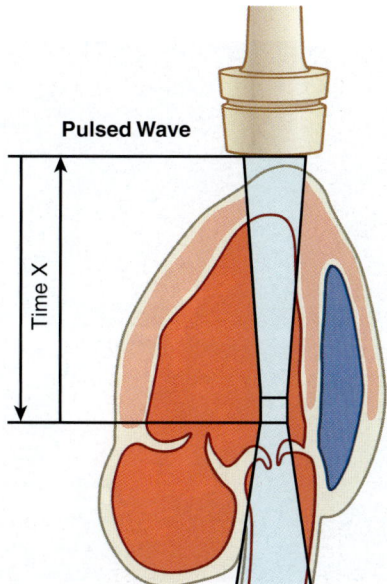

FIG. 31.6 Pulsed wave Doppler transducers send and receive ultrasound pulses at timed intervals so that the location of where the sample volume is positioned can be known. This allows the detection of flow in specific areas of vessels and organs.

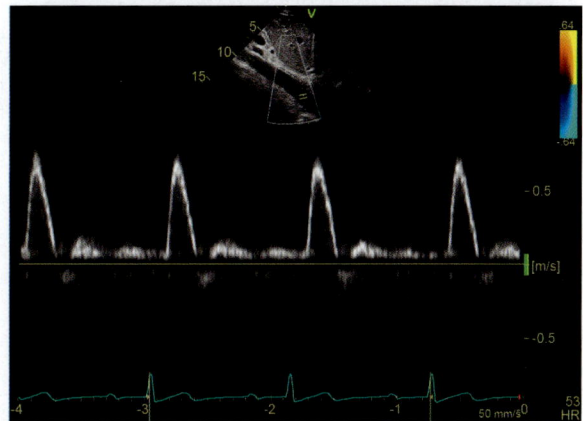

FIG. 31.8 Subcostal view of the abdominal aorta containing a pulsed wave Doppler sample volume recording systolic flow. The spectral Doppler displays normal velocity flow above the baseline due to the angle of the aorta because the flow is toward the transducer.

sample site requires more time for the pulses to be transmitted and received. An example of aliasing is seen in Fig. 31.9, where tricuspid regurgitation (TR) was interrogated in a patient with pulmonary hypertension. With the sample volume positioned on the right atrial side of the tricuspid valve, the true velocity of the systolic regurgitation cannot be measured.

Color Doppler

The addition of color Doppler to ultrasound images helped tremendously in the assessment of flow dynamics. Especially in echocardiography, the ability to semiquantitate the degree of regurgitation or follow blood flow across shunts has decreased the time it used to take for finding abnormal flows. Fig. 31.10 is a diagram showing how color flow Doppler is a pulsed wave technique with multiple gates for averaging flow velocities and then assigning a color. Fig. 31.11 demonstrates color Doppler diastolic flow in a normal apical four-chamber view. Flow can be seen coming from the pulmonary veins at the bottom of this image, traveling across the LA and entering the LV. As the flow accelerates through the mitral valve, the increase in normal velocity changes from red to yellow, as

indicated on the color map in the upper right corner. An apical four-chamber view showing color Doppler systolic flow is seen in Fig. 31.12. As the blood flows through the aortic valve (out of plane in this image), there is blue seen in the LV. During ventricular systole, there is normal flow from the pulmonary veins into the LA so that flow is colored red because it is toward the transducer. In Fig. 31.13, systolic mitral regurgitation is seen in an apical four-chamber view with color Doppler. The regurgitant jet is colored green to denote turbulent flow, as seen in the color flow map in the upper right corner of this image.

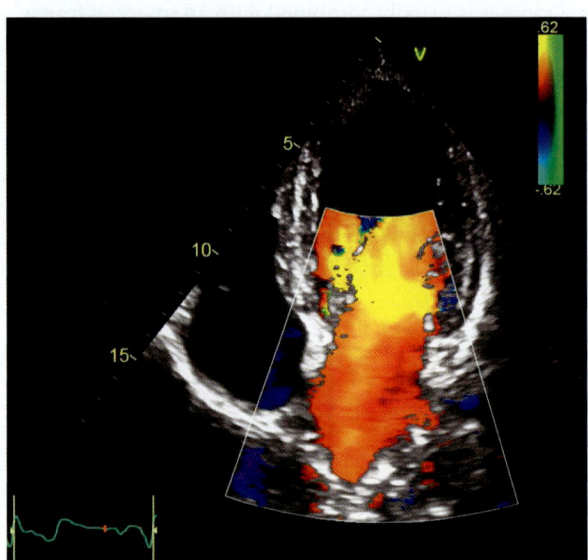

FIG. 31.11 **Apical four-chamber view showing color Doppler diastolic flow.** As the flow accelerates through the mitral valve, the increase in normal velocity changes from red to yellow, as indicated on the color map in the upper right corner.

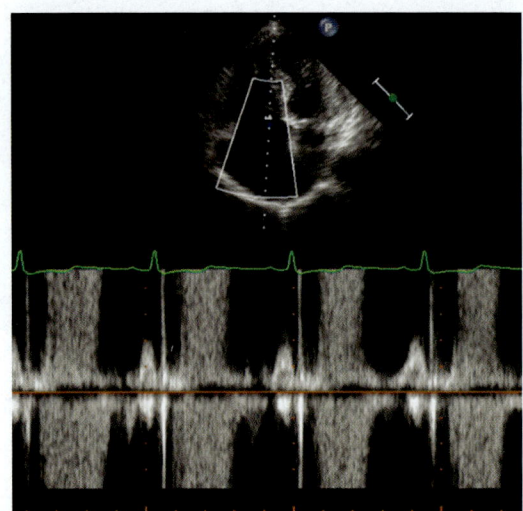

FIG. 31.9 Apical four-chamber view in a patient with an enlarged right side and pulmonary hypertension. The pulsed wave Doppler sample volume is positioned on the atrial side of the tricuspid valve and records the systolic regurgitation flow. The spectral display has aliased due to the high velocity, and the true velocity is not known.

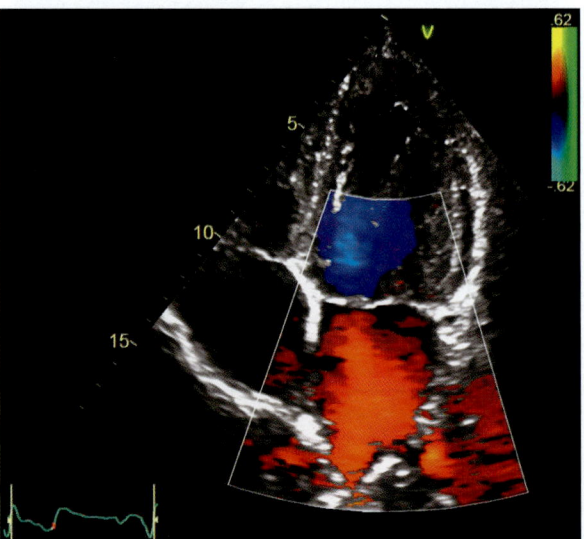

FIG. 31.12 **Apical four-chamber view showing color Doppler systolic flow.** As the blood flows through the aortic valve (not seen in this view), there is blue seen in the left ventricle. During systole, there is normal flow from the pulmonary veins into the left atrium so that flow is colored red because it is toward the transducer.

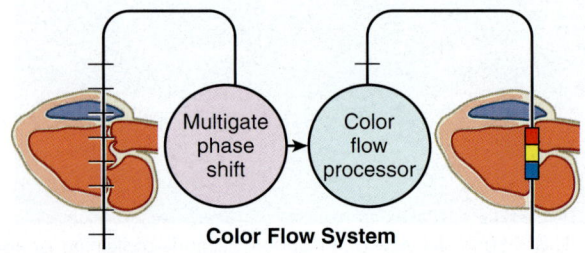

FIG. 31.10 A diagram showing how color flow Doppler is a pulsed wave technique with multiple gates for averaging flow velocities and then assigning a color.

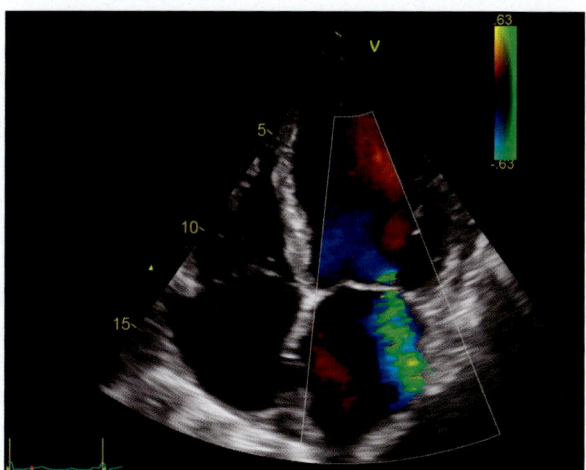

FIG. 31.13 **Apical four-chamber view with color Doppler showing mitral regurgitation during systole.** The regurgitant jet is colored green to denote turbulent flow.

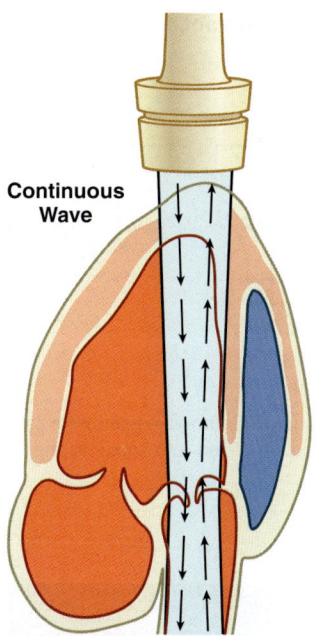

FIG. 31.14 **Continuous wave Doppler transducers continuously send and receive ultrasound pulses.** Continuous wave is best used for high-velocity flows as the spectral display will not alias.

Continuous Wave Doppler

Continuous wave Doppler delivers continuous pulses out and back; it constantly transmits and receives, with no specific pulse duration or sample volume area (Fig. 31.14). These low-amplitude pulses sample along the cursor as seen, obtaining peak velocity Doppler information. This information is not specific to a region but along the whole line of transmit and receive from the Doppler crystals. Although continuous wave Doppler has the ability to assess peak information, beam angle still plays an important role. The Doppler equation is seen in Fig. 31.15, solved for velocity (V). One important component of the Doppler equation is the cosine of the angle between the ultrasound beam and the blood flow vector. Fig. 31.16 shows the impact on Doppler angle to flow on the velocities recorded when the true velocity is 2.0 m/sec. An angle of 60 degrees would result in a displayed velocity of half the actual one. In echocardiography, every attempt is made to align the Doppler beam as parallel to flow by using multiple windows on the chest, especially in patients with aortic stenosis.

QUANTIFICATION OF INTRACARDIAC PRESSURES WITH ULTRASOUND

Pressure-Velocity Relationship: Bernoulli Equation

The original **Bernoulli equation** (Fig. 31.17) for calculating a peak pressure gradient can be simplified into squaring the Doppler velocity and multiplying by 4 ($4V^2$). Anytime there is a spectral display of Doppler velocities, using this simplified calculation can turn velocities into pressure gradients. Fig. 31.18 is a schematic of continuous wave Doppler obtained from the suprasternal notch in a patient with valvular aortic stenosis. The spectral trace shows a high-velocity profile of approximately 5 m/sec, indicating a peak gradient of 100 mm Hg between the LV and aorta. The noninvasive Doppler gradients are often compared with those obtained invasively in

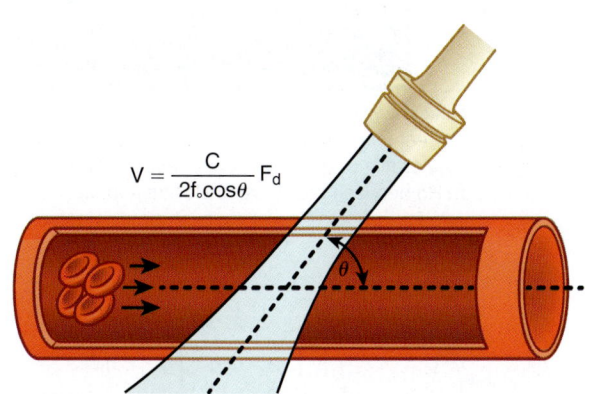

FIG. 31.15 The Doppler equation for calculating velocity (V) is highly dependent on the angle between the Doppler beam and the direction of blood flow.

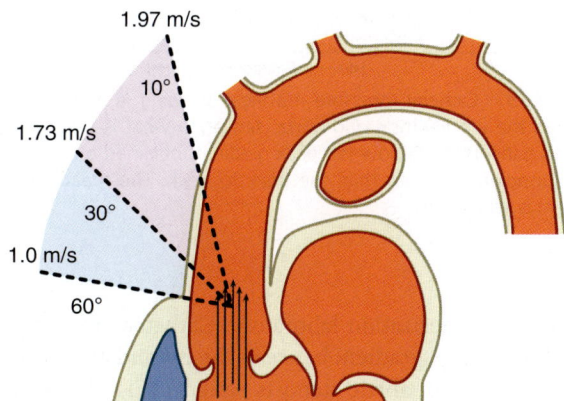

FIG. 31.16 An example of the impact on Doppler angle to flow on the velocities recorded when the true velocity is 2.0 m/sec. An angle of 60 degrees would result in a displayed velocity of half the true one.

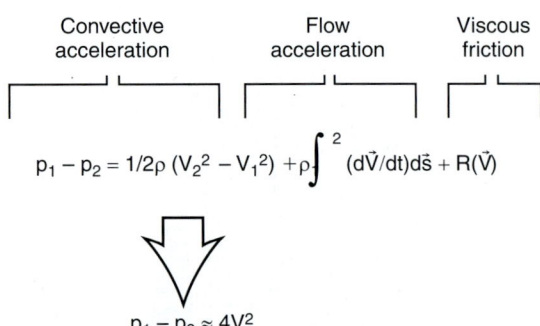

FIG. 31.17 The original Bernoulli equation for calculating a peak pressure gradient can be simplified into squaring the Doppler velocity and multiplying by 4.

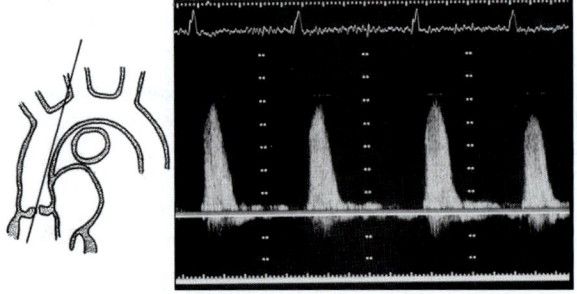

FIG. 31.18 Continuous wave Doppler with the probe in the suprasternal notch in a patient with valvular aortic stenosis. The spectral trace shows a high-velocity profile of approximately 5 m/sec, indicating a peak gradient of 100 mm Hg between the left ventricle and aorta.

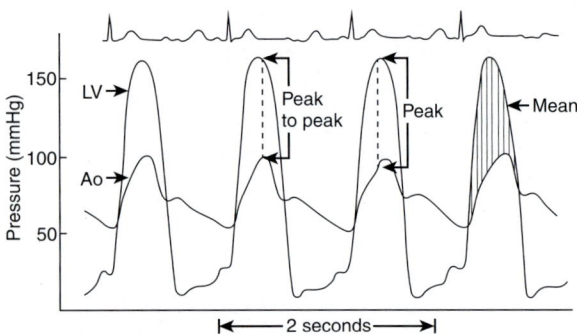

FIG. 31.19 Catheter pressure tracings showing a large gradient between the left ventricle and aorta, similar to what is seen in aortic stenosis patients. Note how the peak gradient, obtained by continuous wave Doppler, is higher than the peak to peak. The mean LV–aorta gradient is also shown.

the heart catheterization laboratory. Catheter pressure tracings show a large gradient between the LV and aorta, similar to what is seen in aortic stenosis patients (Fig. 31.19). Note how the peak gradient, obtained by continuous wave Doppler, is higher than the peak to peak. The mean LV-aorta gradient is also shown on the far right.

Right Atrial Pressure

The right atrial pressure (RAP) is estimated by ultrasound from the size and collapsibility of the inferior vena cava (IVC). If the IVC is normally sized (≤ 2.1 cm) and collapses with respiration, generally, the RAP is estimated at 3 mm Hg (based on the American Society of Echocardiography guidelines). If the IVC is dilated (>2.1 cm) and does not collapse with respiration, the RAP is generally estimated at 15 mm Hg. Anywhere in between these two would give an RAP estimate of 8 mm Hg. RVSP is four times the peak velocity of the TR squared plus the estimated RAP. Fig. 31.20 is an apical four-chamber view in the same patient seen in Fig. 31.9 when the TR velocity by pulsed Doppler aliased. The continuous wave Doppler records the systolic regurgitation flow, and the spectral display has not aliased, so the true velocity is known and approximates 4 m/sec. Using the simplified Bernoulli equation ($4V^2$), the gradient between the RV and atrium would be 64 mm Hg. If, for example, you estimated the RAP to be 8 mm Hg, adding these two together would give you an RVSP of approximately 72 mm Hg. With no significant gradient between the RV and PA, RVSP is equal to systolic pulmonary pressure.

Cardiac Output and Stroke Volume Measured by Ultrasound

To calculate this by ultrasound, two images will be required. One image is the radius of the outflow tract (generally a zoomed two-dimensional image of the left ventricular outflow tract [LVOT]). The other is a pulsed wave spectral Doppler image in the LVOT. Given that CO = SV × HR, one needs to know how to calculate SV ultrasound (SV = VTI_{LVOT} × CSA_{LVOT}). SV is the product of the velocity time integral (VTI) of the LVOT and the cross-sectional area (CSA) of the LVOT. The CSA is the radius of the LVOT in centimeters, squared and multiplied by pi (CSA = πr^2).

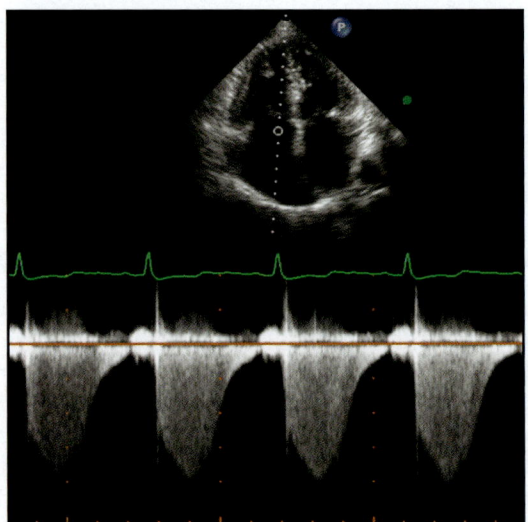

FIG. 31.20 Apical four-chamber view in a patient with an enlarged right side and pulmonary hypertension. The continuous wave Doppler records the systolic regurgitation flow. The spectral display has not aliased so the true velocity is known and approximates 4 m/sec.

Continuity Principle and Equation: Valve Area

The **continuity principle** and equation are derived from one of the fundamental laws of physics, the conservation of energy, which states that energy cannot be created or destroyed, only transferred from one form to another. This principle can be applied to fluid dynamics. Fig. 31.21 displays flow moving from one area to another where the flows are equal. Fluid flow, or volume flow, is expressed in volume per unit of time (mL/sec, L/min, etc.). The continuity equation breaks down fluid flow, which is the area multiplied by the velocity of the flow (see Fig. 31.21). One can break down the equation to find the area the flow travels through to get from one side to the next. This equation can also be used to find the velocity on one side if the other variables (A_1, V_1, and A_2) are known.

An example of the continuity equation can best be described when one is looking for the degree of aortic stenosis. To find the aortic valve area, the radius of the LVOT, velocity through the LVOT, and peak velocity through the aortic valve will be needed. As seen in Fig. 31.21, the LVOT diameter, velocity from the pulsed wave of the LVOT, and peak velocity from the continuous wave Doppler of the aortic valve are entered into the equation to solve the aortic valve area.

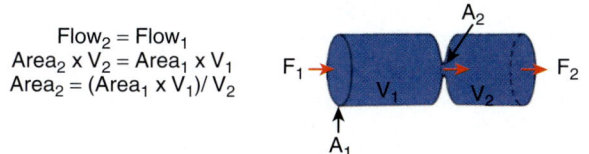

Continuity equation

$Flow_2 = Flow_1$
$Area_2 \times V_2 = Area_1 \times V_1$
$Area_2 = (Area_1 \times V_1)/V_2$

FIG. 31.21 The continuity equation can be rearranged to calculate the aortic valve area in stenosis patients.

By the continuity equation, we know that the $Area_2 = [Area_1(2\pi r^2) \times V_1] \div V_2$, where r = LVOT diameter, V_1 is the pulsed wave Doppler velocity through the LVOT, and V_2 is the peak velocity (continuous wave) through the aortic valve.

 Key Pearls

- Doppler echocardiography provides clinical information about blood flow, including the direction and velocity as well as the timing during the cardiac cycle.
- Doppler velocities can turn velocities into pressure gradients by using the simplified Bernoulli equation ($4V^2$).
- With pulsed wave Doppler, higher velocities will exceed the Nyquist limit (one-half the pulse repetition frequency), and aliasing of the spectral trace will occur.
- Continuous wave Doppler can accurately record high velocities as long as the angle between the ultrasound beam, and the blood flow vector is 10 degrees or less.

BIBLIOGRAPHY

Des Jardins T. *Cardiopulmonary anatomy and physiology*. ed 4. Albany, NY: Delmar; 2002.

Kisslo J, Adams D, Mark D. *Basic Doppler echocardiography*. New York: Churchill Livingstone; 1986.

Lang RM, Badano LP, Mor-Avi V, et al. Recommendations for Cardiac Chamber Quantification by Echocardiography in adults: an update from the American Society of Echocardiography and the European Association of Cardiovascular Imaging. *J Am Soc Echocardiogr*. 2015;28:1–39.

Martini FH, Bartholomew EF. *Essentials of anatomy and physiology*. Glenview, IL: Pearson Education; 2007. ed 4.

O'Toole MT., ed. *Miller-Keane encyclopedia and dictionary of medicine, nursing, and allied health*. ed 7. St. Louis: Elsevier; 2003.

CHAPTER 32

Introduction to Echocardiographic Techniques, Terminology, and Tips

Sandra L. Hagen-Ansert

OBJECTIVES

On completion of this chapter, you should be able to:
- Explain the transducer selection and patient position for a cardiac examination
- Describe the imaging planes used in echocardiography
- Define *suprasternal, subcostal, apical,* and *parasternal*
- Describe a normal cardiac examination using two-dimensional, color flow, Doppler, and M-mode imaging modes
- List and discuss the applications of color flow Doppler in the echocardiographic examination

OUTLINE

Two-Dimensional Echocardiography 917
  Equipment Setup and Patient Examination Techniques 917
  Transducers 918
Cardiac Color Flow Examination 919
Doppler Applications and Technique 920
  Normal Cardiac Doppler Flow Patterns 920

Audio Signals and Spectral Display of Doppler Signals 920
Pulsed Wave and Continuous Wave Doppler 923
Continuous Wave Doppler 923
Doppler Quantitation 924
Doppler Examination 924
The Echocardiographic Examination 925
  Parasternal Views 925
  Apical Views 932

Subcostal Views 938
Suprasternal Views 939
M-Mode Imaging of the Cardiac Structures 943
  Mitral Valve 943
  Aortic Valve and Left Atrium 945
  Interventricular Septum 946
  Left Ventricle 946
  Tricuspid Valve 946
  Pulmonary Valve 950

KEY TERMS

Color flow mapping (CFM)
Continuous wave probe

Diastole
Pulsed wave transducer

Spectral analysis waveform
Systole

The widespread clinical acceptance of echocardiography has tremendously aided the diagnostic results of the cardiac examination. Improved transducer design, resolution capabilities, focus parameters, gray-scale differentiation, gain control factors, cine loop functions, and other software capabilities have enabled the cardiac sonographer to record consistent, high-quality images from the multiple scan planes necessary to obtain a dynamic composite image of the cardiac structures. Color flow Doppler allows the cardiac sonographer to obtain additional velocity information in detecting intracardiac shunt flow, mapping regurgitant jets, and determining obstructive flow pathways.

The evaluation of cardiac structures by echocardiography is regarded as an essential diagnostic tool in clinical cardiology. The reason for its widespread use in the evaluation of cardiac disease is its noninvasive, reproducible, and accurate assessment of cardiac structures. Echocardiography further exploded when three- or four-dimensional (3D/4D) echocardiography was developed, which allowed the cardiac structures to be anatomically and dynamically visualized in real-time. Thus the echocardiographer can assess the four chambers of the heart, the cardiac valves, the intracardiac anatomy, and the intracardiac lesions; observe contractility; determine valvular function; and assess hemodynamics. The combination of 2D/3D/4D, Doppler, tissue Doppler imaging, strain, and color flow mapping provides an extremely accurate means to evaluate wall or valve thickness, valvular orifice and chamber size, and contractility of the cardiac structures. Transesophageal echocardiography and 3D echocardiography has enabled exquisite visualization of the heart while the transducer is guided through the mouth and into the esophagus to closely image the cardiac anatomy and guide intracardiac interventional procedures.

Contrast injected through an intravenous line into the bloodstream has provided an additional pathway to enhance cardiac endocardial borders and clearly demonstrate cardiac thrombus and mass lesions. Saline bubble injections have been a clinical aid to determine the presence and direction of interatrial septal shunt flow.

Exercise stress echocardiography, supine bike stress echocardiography, and dobutamine stress echocardiography have provided additional information about the contractility, hemodynamics, and performance of the left ventricle in a simulated stress situation.

To perform an echocardiographic examination of good diagnostic quality, the sonographer must understand the anatomic, hemodynamic, and pathophysiologic parameters of the heart and be able to incorporate the physical principles of sonography into the routine examination. This chapter introduces the reader to the basic technical components of echocardiography through 2D, M-mode, Doppler, and color Doppler imaging. Emphasis will be on common findings the general sonographer may encounter "above the diaphragm" in the subsequent Clinical Echocardiography chapters.

TWO-DIMENSIONAL ECHOCARDIOGRAPHY

Equipment Setup and Patient Examination Techniques

Most echocardiographic examinations are performed with the sonographer's left hand. The ultrasound equipment is placed on the right side of the echo bed by the head of the patient. The ergonomic echo chair and echo bed (Fig. 32.1) are essential to avoid future musculoskeletal problems. The echo bed should have at least a thick 3-inch cushion, a large drop-down component for the apical views, a backrest to support the patient when lying in a decubitus position, and adequate space for the patient's shoulder and head. The bed should be able to raise and lower to allow the sonographer to be on the same plane as the patient, as the sonographer may rest their elbow on the echo bed when performing the parasternal views.

The patient is examined while in the left lateral decubitus position. This position allows the heart to move away from the sternum and closer to the chest wall, thus allowing a better cardiac window. The *cardiac window* may be considered the area on the anterior chest where the heart is just beneath the skin surface and free of lung interference; it is usually found between the third and fifth intercostal spaces, slightly to the left of the sternal border.

The cardiac sonographer must keep in mind that different body shapes require variations in transducer position. An obese patient may have a horizontal transverse heart, and thus a slight lateral movement from the sternal border may be needed to record cardiac structures (Fig. 32.2). A thin patient may have a long and slender heart, requiring a lower, more

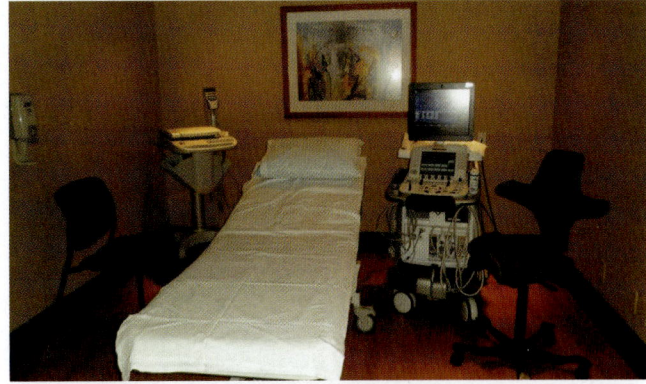

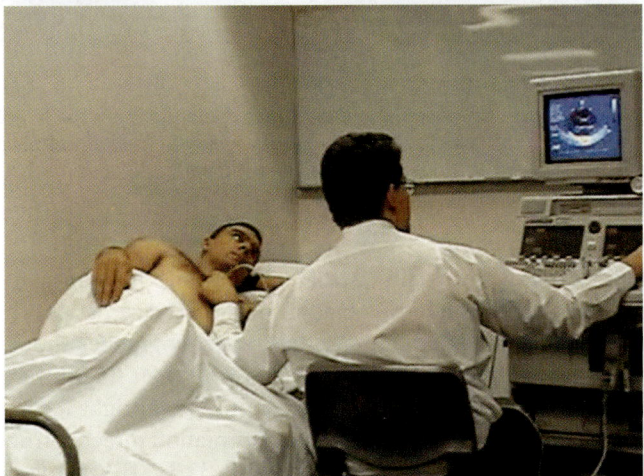

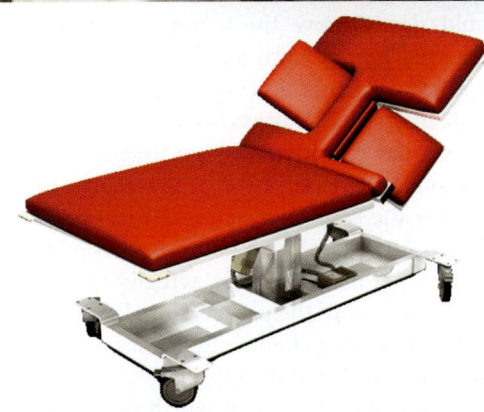

FIG. 32.1 Most echocardiographic examinations are performed with the sonographer's left hand. The ultrasound equipment is placed on the right side of the bed by the head of the patient. The ergonomic chair and bed are essential to avoid future musculoskeletal problems. The bed should have at least a 3-inch-thick cushion, a large drop-down component for the apical views, a back rest to support the patient when lying in a decubitus position, and adequate space for the patient's shoulder and head. The bed should be able to raise and lower to allow the sonographer to be on the same plane as the patient, as the sonographer may rest their elbow on the echo bed when performing the parasternal views.

medial transducer position. Barrel-chested patients may have echocardiographic difficulties because of the lung absorption interference, and it may be necessary to turn these patients completely on their left side. Sometimes in these patients, the upright or slightly forward-bent position is useful in forcing the heart closer to the anterior chest wall.

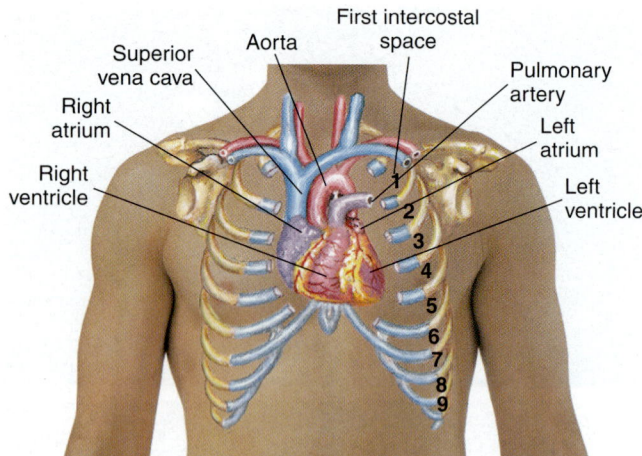

FIG. 32.2 The heart lies obliquely in the chest, posterior to the sternum, with the greater part of muscular mass lying slightly to the left of midline in the normal patient. An obese patient may have a horizontal transverse heart, and thus a slight lateral movement from the sternal border may be needed to record cardiac structures.

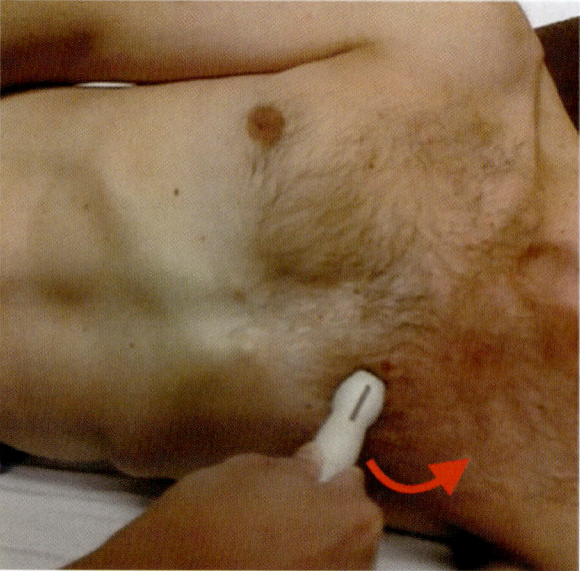

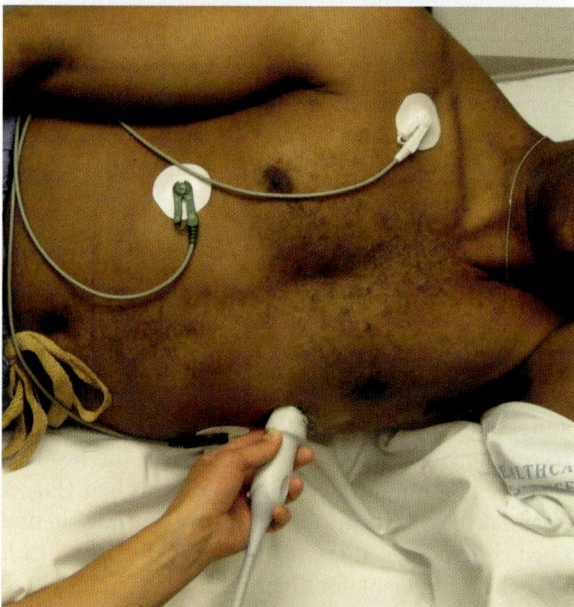

FIG. 32.3 In the initial echocardiographic study, the sonographer should hold the transducer in their left hand with their fingers near the base of the probe. The notch should be upright for the parasternal long-axis view with slight rotation directed from the right shoulder to the left hip.

The following techniques are beginning guidelines for the echocardiographic evaluation of the average patient. In the initial echocardiographic study, the sonographer should hold the transducer in their left hand with their fingers near the base of the probe. The notch should be upright for the parasternal long-axis view with slight rotation directed from the right shoulder to the left hip (Fig. 32.3). The sonographer should slowly move the transducer freely along the mid–left sternal border until all the cardiac structures are easily identified is a better practice than restricting the transducer to one interspace. Stay as close to the sternal border as possible; if cardiac pulsations are not imaged, move slightly lateral, but angle the base of the probe medial towards the sternum to see the cardiac structures. This procedure saves time and gives the examiner a better understanding of cardiac relationships. If the heart is actually medial, the best study is performed with the patient completely on his or her left side. Observing the patient's respiratory pattern may help the sonographer identify if the lungs overshadow the cardiac structures. Controlled breathing will help to obtain good-quality images. If the lung interference clouds the cardiac structures, the patient should breathe in and then exhale for as long as possible to move the lungs away from the field of view. This usually gives the examiner adequate time to record valid information.

Transducers

Several types of transducers are available for echocardiographic techniques. Most adult cardiac sonographers use multifocal transducers that range from 1.5 to 4.5 MHz with either a manually controlled or an automatic focus. A pediatric patient generally requires a multifocal higher-frequency transducer for improved resolution and near-field definition.

Transducer Location and Imaging Planes. The Committee on Nomenclature and Standards in Two-Dimensional Echocardiography of the American Society of Echocardiography recommends the following nomenclature and image orientation standards for transducer locations (Fig. 32.4):

- *Suprasternal:* Patient is supine; transducer placed in the suprasternal notch.
- *Subcostal:* Patient is supine; transducer located near the body midline and beneath the costal margin.
- *Apical:* Patient is in left lateral decubitus position; transducer located over the cardiac apex (at the point of maximal impulse).
- *Parasternal:* Patient is in left lateral decubitus position; transducer placed over the area bounded superiorly by the left clavicle, medially by the sternum, and inferiorly by the apical region.

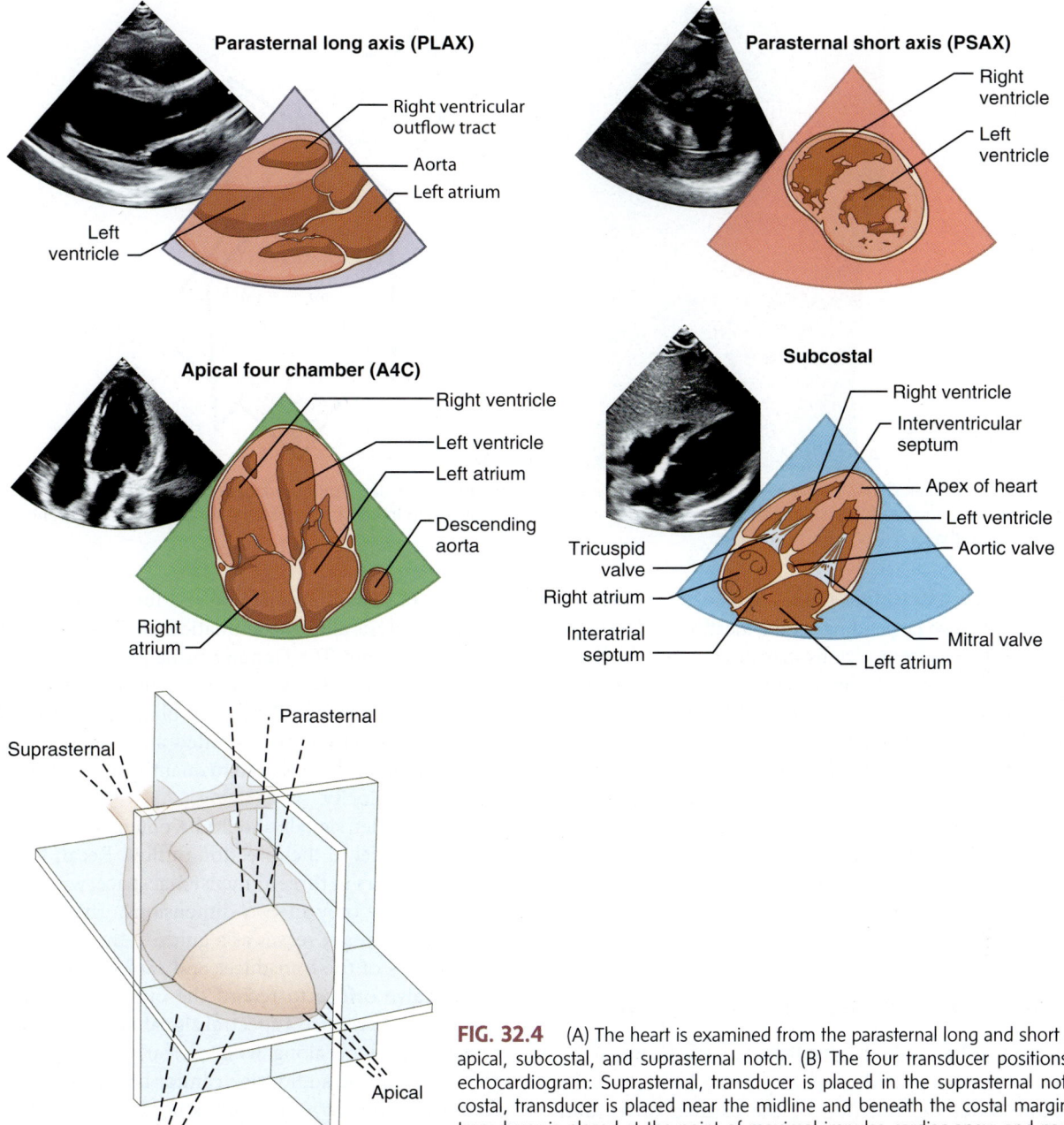

FIG. 32.4 (A) The heart is examined from the parasternal long and short axis, the apical, subcostal, and suprasternal notch. (B) The four transducer positions for the echocardiogram: Suprasternal, transducer is placed in the suprasternal notch; subcostal, transducer is placed near the midline and beneath the costal margin; apical, transducer is placed at the point of maximal impulse cardiac apex; and parasternal, transducer is placed just left of the sternum about the fourth intercostal space.

The imaging planes are described by the manner in which the 2D transducer transects the heart:
- *PLAX (parasternal long axis):* Transects the heart perpendicular to the dorsal and ventral surfaces of the body and parallel with the long axis of the heart (Fig. 32.5).
- *PSAX (parasternal short axis):* Transects the heart perpendicular to the dorsal and ventral surfaces of the body and perpendicular to the long axis of the heart (see Fig. 32.5).
- *APICAL four chamber:* Transects the heart approximately parallel with the dorsal and ventral surfaces of the body (Fig. 32.6).

CARDIAC COLOR FLOW EXAMINATION

The **color flow mapping (CFM)** examination is generally performed along with the conventional 2D examination. The advantage of CFM is its ability to rapidly investigate flow direction and movement within the cardiac chambers (Box 32.1). Flow toward the transducer is recorded in red, and flow away from the transducer is blue (Fig. 32.7). This is denoted on the color bar on the right upper side of the image. As the velocities increase, the flow pattern in the variance mode turns from red to various shades of red, orange, and yellow before it aliases. Likewise, flow away from the transducer is recorded in

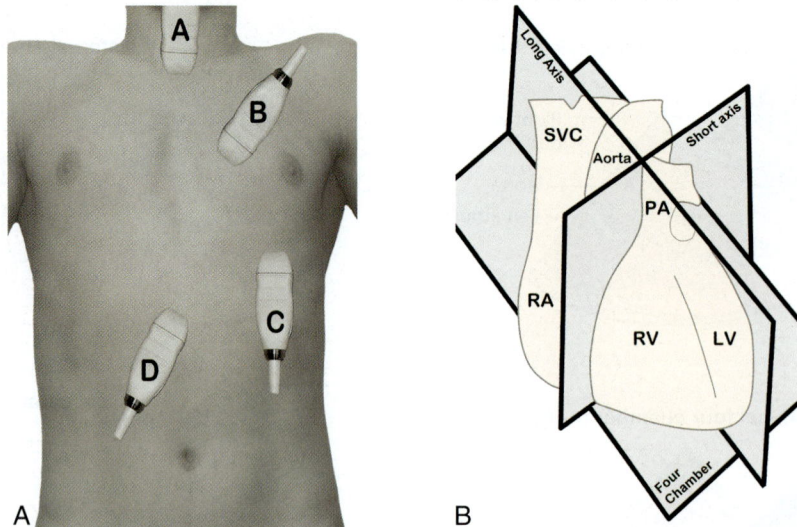

FIG. 32.5 (A) Parasternal long axis transects the heart perpendicular to the dorsal and ventral surfaces of the body and parallel with the long axis of the heart. Parasternal short axis transects the heart perpendicular to the dorsal and ventral surfaces of the body and perpendicular to the long axis of the heart.

blue; this color turns to various shades of blue, turquoise, and green before it aliases. Depending on the location of the transducer, the flow signals from various structures within the heart appear as different colors. An understanding of cardiac hemodynamics helps the examiner understand the flow patterns.

Although normal cardiac flows are difficult to accurately time during the CFM examination because of its slow frame rate, the use of color M-mode (with a faster frame rate) allows one to precisely determine specific cardiac events in correlation with the ECG. The color M-mode is made in the same manner as a conventional M-mode study (Fig. 32.8). The cursor is placed through the area of interest, and the flow is evaluated using an autocorrelation technique.

DOPPLER APPLICATIONS AND TECHNIQUE

Doppler echocardiography is established as a valuable, noninvasive tool in clinical cardiology to provide hemodynamic information about the function of the cardiac valves and chambers of the heart. When combined with conventional 2D echo, Doppler techniques may be focused to provide specific information on the velocity flow patterns of a particular area within the heart. The ability to provide qualitative and quantitative information in evaluating valvular function, intracardiac shunts, dysfunction of a native or prosthetic valve, or the obstruction of a surgically inserted shunt has contributed to the clinical care of the cardiac patient. Understanding cardiac physiology and hemodynamics is critical to the interpretation of the Doppler information. In addition, the sonographer must clearly understand Doppler principles, artifacts, and pitfalls in order to produce a quality study.

Normal Cardiac Doppler Flow Patterns

Understanding the relationship between the 2D echo and the Doppler flow study is important. The 2D echo allows assessment of cardiac anatomy and function; Doppler velocity flow analysis allows examination of blood flow rather than cardiac anatomy. The Doppler principle on which this technique is based involves the backscatter of transmitted ultrasonic waves from circulating red blood cells. The difference in frequency between transmitted and backscattered sound waves (Doppler shift) is used to quantify forward or backward blood flow velocity.

The Doppler signals should be obtained with the sample volume parallel to the direction of flow. Recall that the flow of blood occurs in three-dimensional space, whereas the real-time image is only in two dimensions. Therefore the two-dimensional image serves as a guide to the operator as small adjustments of the transducer and sample volume are made in the valve orifice to record the optimal Doppler signals. The key is to produce a spectral signal to show a well-defined velocity envelope along with a clearly defined audio tone. The clarity of the audio tone cannot be emphasized enough. Frequently the clarity of tone is used to guide the Doppler cursor into the correct plane to record the maximum velocity.

Blood flow toward the transducer is displayed by a time velocity waveform above the baseline at point zero or a positive deflection (Fig. 32.9). Flow away from the Doppler signal is displayed below the baseline or as a negative deflection. A simultaneous ECG should be displayed to help time the cardiac cycle.

Audio Signals and Spectral Display of Doppler Signals

The best Doppler signals are obtained when the ultrasound beam is parallel or nearly parallel to the flow of blood; therefore the best windows used to record the 2D images may not be the best windows to record Doppler flow patterns. This section discusses the technique for recording quality Doppler signals from the inflow and outflow tracts through the cardiac valves.

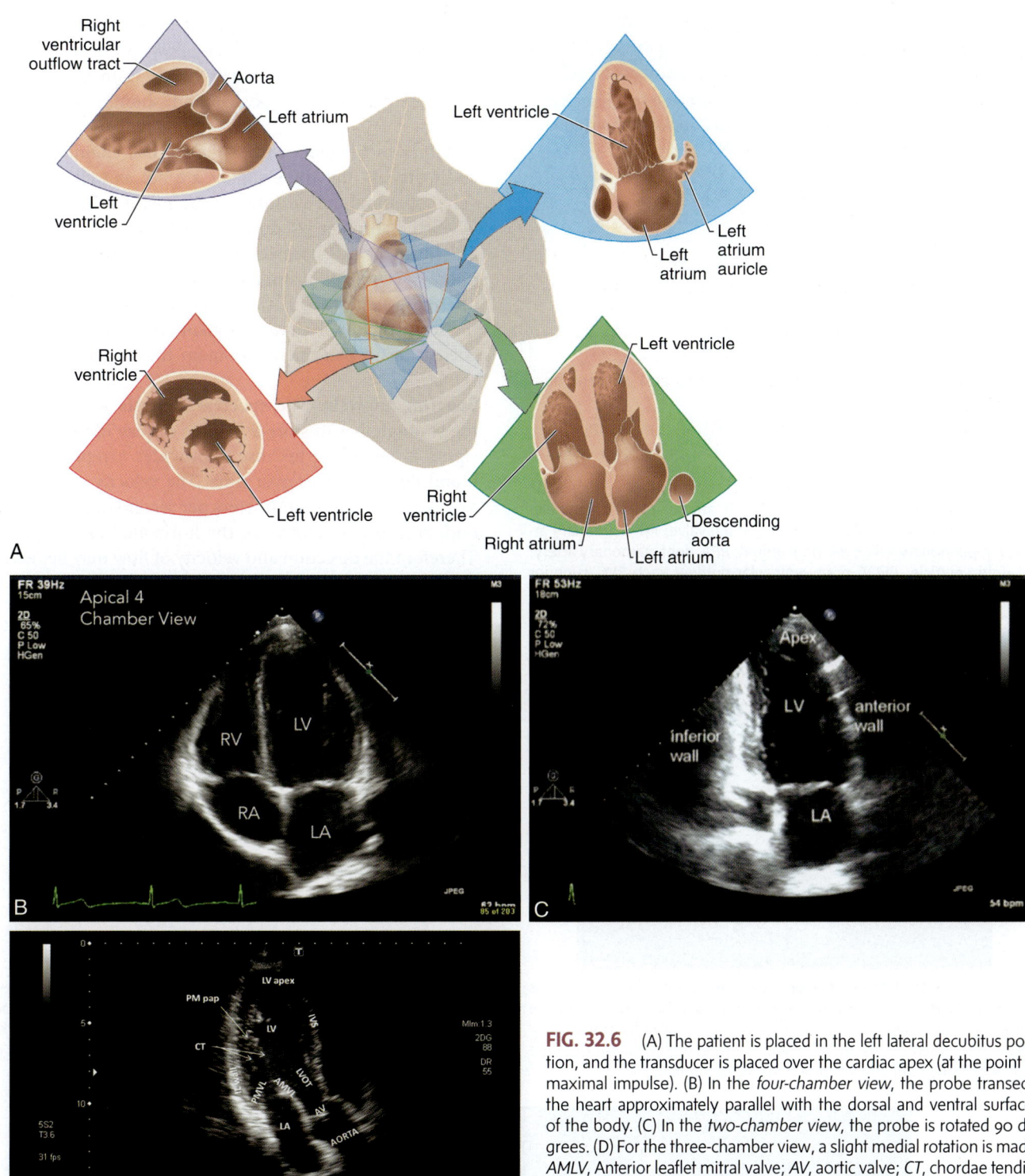

FIG. 32.6 (A) The patient is placed in the left lateral decubitus position, and the transducer is placed over the cardiac apex (at the point of maximal impulse). (B) In the *four-chamber view*, the probe transects the heart approximately parallel with the dorsal and ventral surfaces of the body. (C) In the *two-chamber view*, the probe is rotated 90 degrees. (D) For the three-chamber view, a slight medial rotation is made. *AMLV*, Anterior leaflet mitral valve; *AV*, aortic valve; *CT*, chordae tendineae; *IVS*, interventricular septum; *LA*, left atrium; *LVOT*, left ventricular outflow tract; *LV*, left ventricle; *PLMV*, posterior leaflet mitral valve; *PM pap*, posterior papillary muscle; *RA*, right atrium; *RV*, right ventricle.

Audio Signals. Doppler produces an audible sound which helps guide the sonographer to obtain the highest velocity signal. The signal from the arterial flow is very different from that of the venous flow; likewise, mitral and tricuspid patterns differ from the aortic and pulmonary valve patterns. The blood flow velocity determines the pitch or frequency of the audio signal. As the velocity becomes higher, the pitch becomes higher; as the velocity decreases, so does the pitch.

Normal blood flow across the cardiac valves demonstrates a narrow range of velocity with a smooth and even Doppler audio signal. When the flow becomes disturbed, as occurs

> **BOX 32.1** **Normal Color Flow Mapping Examination and Techniques**
>
> - The color flow mapping examination is generally performed in the same planes used for conventional Doppler examination.
> - Parasternal long-axis view: MV, TV, AO
> - Parasternal short-axis view: AO, PA, RVOT, IAS, TV
> - Parasternal short-axis view: MV, TV, AO, PV
> - Apical four-chamber plane: MV, TV
> - Apical five-chamber plane: LVOT, AV
> - Apical long-axis, two-chamber view: LV, MV, LA
> - Subcostal four-chamber view: IAS, IVS, RV, LV, RA, LA
> - Subcostal view: IVC, hepatic veins
> - Subcostal five-chamber view: AO, LVOT
> - Subcostal short-axis view: AO, PA, RVOT
> - Suprasternal view (long axis): ascending and descending aorta, SVC
> - Suprasternal view (short axis): arch, RPA, LA, SVC, pulmonary veins

AO, Aorta; *AV*, aortic valve; *IAS*, interatrial septum; *IVC*, inferior vena cava; *IVS*, interventricular septum; *LA*, left atrium; *LV*, left ventricle; *LVOT*, left ventricular outflow tract; *MV*, mitral valve; *PA*, pulmonary artery; *PV*, pulmonary valve; *RA*, right atrium; *RPA*, right pulmonary artery; *RV*, right ventricle; *RVOT*, right ventricular outflow tract; *SVC*, superior vena cava; *TV*, tricuspid valve.

distal to an obstruction or regurgitation of the valve, the tone becomes harsh. The high-velocity flows produce a very high-frequency signal with a sharp whistling-hissing tone. This signal may be found in obstruction, shunts, and regurgitant lesions.

Other movements within the cardiac chambers produce audio signals, but these signals are not as well defined. The valve opening and closure can be heard as a discrete click when the Doppler window is located too close to the valve. The normal cardiac function causes the valve to move in and out of the Doppler beam, producing a lower-frequency signal. Therefore careful angulation along with the audio signal helps the sonographer observe the dynamics of the cardiac cycle for correct beam placement to obtain the best-quality Doppler signal.

Spectral Analysis. The **spectral analysis waveform** allows the sonographer to store a graphic display of what the audio signal is recording because it provides a representation of blood flow velocities over time. The velocity on the vertical axis is measured in centimeters per second or meters per second, and time is shown on the horizontal axis (Fig. 32.10). Therefore the direction and velocity of flow may be measured very accurately when the beam is parallel to the flow.

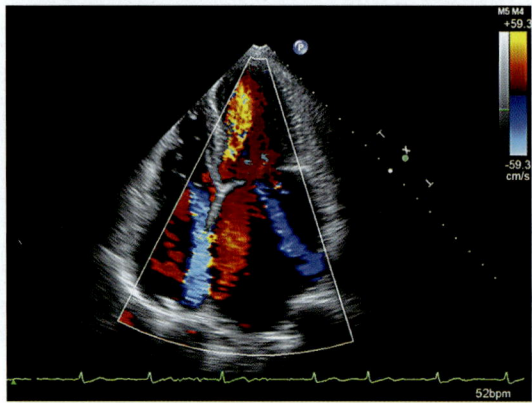

FIG. 32.7 Apical four-chamber view with color. The color bar is shown along the right margin; yellow and red indicate flow toward the transducer, and blue and turquoise indicate flow away from the transducer. This patient has both mitral and tricuspid regurgitation. Note the blue flow in the right and left atria from the regurgitant jet.

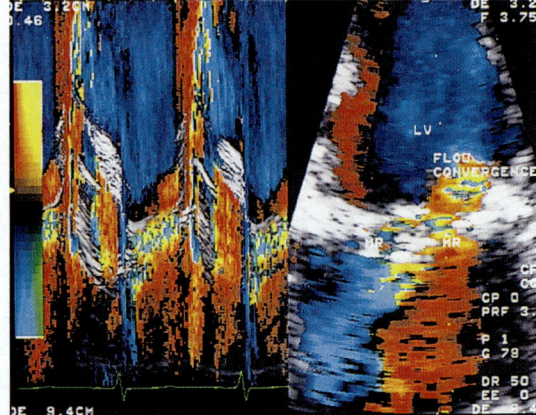

FIG. 32.8 Flow convergence as imaged in the four-chamber view and M-mode/color flow mapping image. The red inflow is from the pulmonary veins into the left atrium, the blue is swirling flow within the left atrium, and the multicolored flow at the level of the mitral valve is regurgitant flow. *LV*, Left ventricle; *MR*, mitral regurgitation.

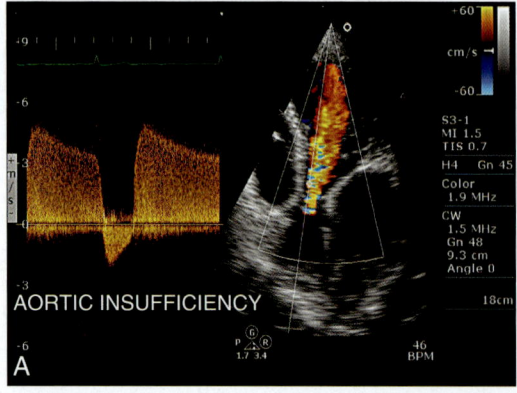
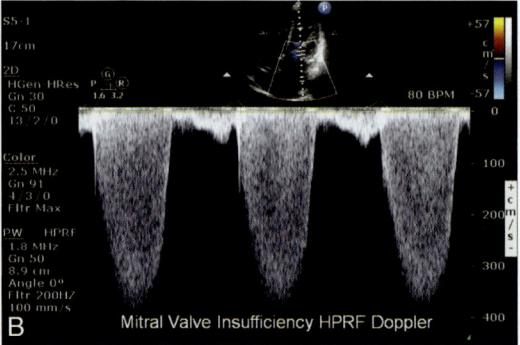

FIG. 32.9 (A) Flow above the baseline represents forward flow, as seen in this patient with aortic insufficiency. (B) Flow below the baseline represents flow moving away from the transducer, as seen in this patient with mitral regurgitation.

A normal spectral display pattern has a typical appearance. In normal blood flow, the cells generally have a uniform direction with similar velocities. The spectral tracing appears as a smooth mitral velocity pattern bordered by a narrow band of velocities. As the velocity increases, so does the turbulence within the border of the narrow-band velocities, producing a filling of the velocity curve. As the cardiac structure moves in and out of the beam, the Doppler frequency shift is recorded as tall artifact spikes.

Pulsed Wave and Continuous Wave Doppler

There are two types of Doppler signals that are utilized in echocardiography: pulsed wave and continuous wave (Fig. 32.11).

A **pulsed wave transducer** is constructed with a single crystal that sends bursts of ultrasound at a rate called the *pulse repetition frequency* (PRF). The transducer receives sound waves backscattered from moving red blood cells during a limited time between transmitted pulses. A time gating device is then used to select the precise depth from which the returning signal has originated because the signals return from the heart at different times.

The particular area of interest undergoing Doppler evaluation is referred to as the sample volume. The sample volume and directional line placement of the beam are moved by use of the trackball. The exact size and location of the sample volume can be adjusted at the area of interest. Some instruments have a fixed sample volume size. Others allow the operator to select the size appropriate for the particular study.

Velocities less than 2 m/sec are recorded without an alias pattern. However, pulsed Doppler is limited in its ability to record high-velocity patterns. The maximum frequency shift that can be measured by a pulsed Doppler system is called the Nyquist limit and is one-half the PRF. Velocities that exceed this limit are known to produce an aliasing pattern (Fig. 32.12). Normal cardiac structures do not exceed the Nyquist limit and are easily measured with the pulsed Doppler system.

Continuous Wave Doppler

The **continuous wave probe** differs from the pulsed wave probe in that it is able to both send and receive sound (see Fig. 32.11). One crystal continuously emits sound; the other receives sound as it is backscattered to the transducer. This probe may be part of a phased or annular array imaging probe or may be a stand-alone independent probe. If it is part of a 2D imaging transducer, the sample direction can be steered by use of the trackball.

The Pedof continuous wave (nonimaging) probe is smaller than the 2D imaging probe and thus has advantages

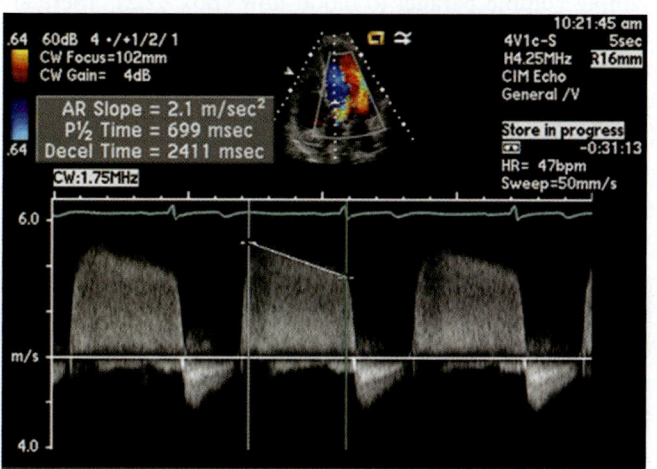

FIG. 32.10 The spectral analysis waveform allows the sonographer to store a graphic display of what the audio signal is recording because it provides a representation of blood flow velocities over time. The velocity on the vertical axis is measured in centimeters per second or meters per second, and time is shown on the horizontal axis.

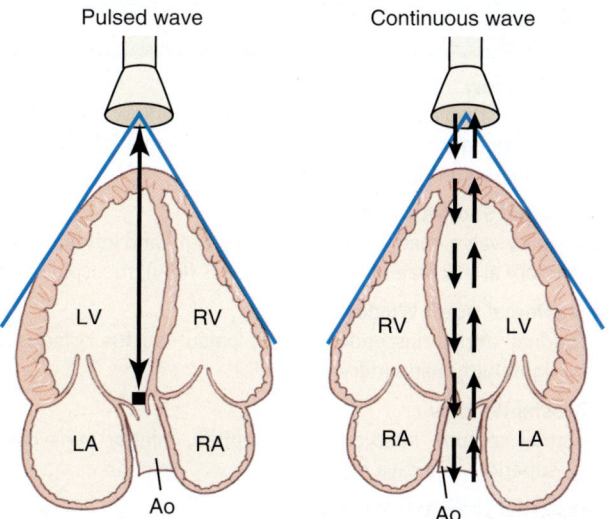

FIG. 32.11 Pulsed wave and continuous wave Doppler echocardiography with the transducer placed in the point of maximal impulse at the apex of the heart. *Ao*, Aorta; *LA*, left atrium; *LV*, left ventricle; *RA*, right atrium; *RV*, right ventricle.

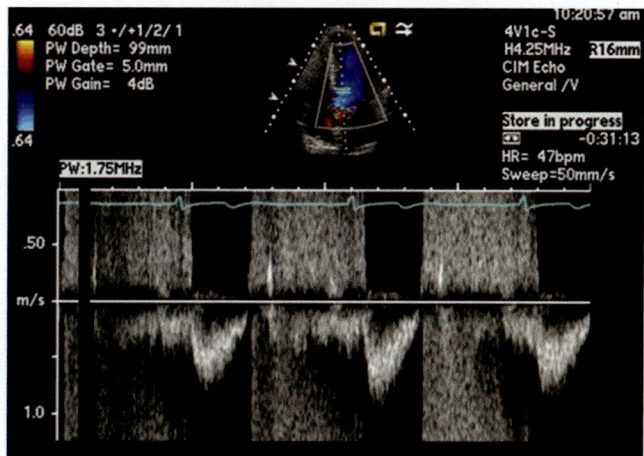

FIG. 32.12 Example of the high-velocity flow produced from aortic insufficiency, which shows an alias pattern *(arrow)*. The maximum frequency shift that can be measured by a pulsed Doppler system is called the *Nyquist limit* and is one-half the pulse repetition frequency. Velocities that exceed this limit are known to produce an aliasing pattern.

in obtaining a good Doppler study (Fig. 32.13). This small diameter allows greater flexibility to angle between small rib interspaces or obtain signals from the suprasternal notch or right parasternal border. The audio portion of the Doppler examination becomes a critical factor in this study because 2D is not available to guide the transducer location.

Often both 2D–continuous wave and Pedof probes are used within the echocardiographic study. Once the proper transducer position is found with the imaging transducer, the angulation and window are marked for proper placement of the Pedof probe. The audio sound and spectral wave pattern are then used to guide the correction angulation of the beam for maximum-velocity recordings. Because there is not a particular sample volume site within the continuous wave beam, velocities are recorded from several points along the linear beam. This technique has the ability to record maximum velocities without alias patterns and is especially useful for very high-velocity patterns, as seen in regurgitant lesions or stenotic valves.

Doppler Quantitation

Quantitation of the Doppler signal to obtain hemodynamic information is derived from the measurement of blood flow velocity (Table 32.1). As explained previously, it is critical that the angle of the Doppler signal be as parallel to flow as possible. The Doppler equation is based on the principle that the velocity of blood flow is directly proportional to the Doppler frequency shift and the speed of sound in tissue, and it is inversely related to twice the frequency of transmitted ultrasound and the cosine of the angle of incidence between the ultrasound beam and the direction of blood flow. Therefore the relationship between the angle and its cosine becomes significant and can be a source of error if ignored. If the angle is less than 20 degrees, the cosine is close to 1 and can be ignored. If the angle increases beyond 20 degrees, the cosine becomes less than 1 and may produce an underestimation of velocity.

Doppler Examination

The Doppler examination is performed along with the 2D study of the cardiac structures. During this conventional study, the sonographer notes structures that may need special attention during the Doppler examination (e.g., a redundant mitral valve leaflet may indicate the need to search for mitral regurgitation). Throughout the Doppler study, various patient positions and transducer rotations are necessary to place the sample volume parallel to blood flow (Box 32.2). There are basically five transducer positions used to record quality Doppler flow patterns: the apical four chamber, the left parasternal, subcostal, suprasternal, and the right parasternal. The patient should be forewarned about the audio sounds produced by the Doppler signal because some find the sound alarming if the volume is set too high.

TABLE 32.1	Maximal Velocities Recorded With Doppler in Normal Individuals	
	Children (cm/sec)	Adults (cm/sec)
Mitral flow	80–130	60–130
Tricuspid flow	50–80	30–70
Pulmonary artery	70–110	60–90
Left ventricle	70–120	70–110
Aorta	120–180	100–170

BOX 32.2	Doppler and Color Doppler Windows

Apical Window
Mitral valve, tricuspid valve, left ventricular outflow tract, aortic valve, pulmonary vein inflow, superior vena cava inflow, interventricular septum, interatrial septum

Parasternal Short-Axis Window
Pulmonary valve, main pulmonary artery, right and left branches pulmonary artery (patent ductus arteriosus flow), tricuspid valve

Suprasternal Notch Window
Ascending aorta, descending aorta, patent ductus arteriosus flow, right pulmonary artery

Subcostal Window
Interatrial septum, interventricular septum, inferior vena cava flow, superior vena cava flow

Parasternal Long-Axis Window
Mitral regurgitation, tricuspid regurgitation, aortic regurgitation

Right Parasternal Window
Ascending aorta

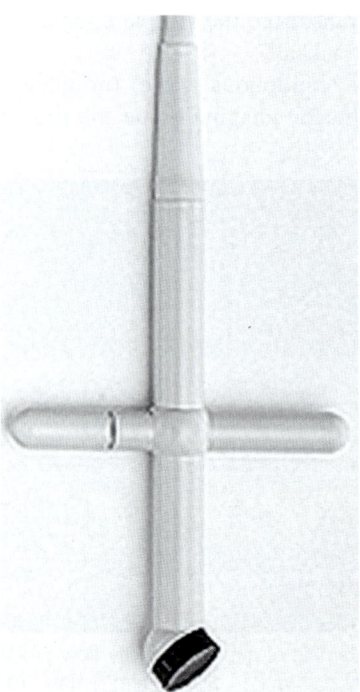

FIG. 32.13 The small pencil-like Pedof non-imaging probe allows continuous wave imaging of the flow dynamics.

THE ECHOCARDIOGRAPHIC EXAMINATION

The cardiac sonographer is responsible for acquiring the blood pressure, height, and weight (to calibrate the body surface area) of each patient. The sonographer should know the reason for the echo examination and review the available previous echo images prior to the exam. The sonographer should note clinical information regarding the specific cardiac symptoms and heart conditions. The patient is positioned on the echo bed with their left arm tucked under their head (Fig. 32.14). The bed should be raised to the level of the sonographer so the elbow may rest on the edge of the bed for stability in acquiring the images.

Ideally, the sonographer should digitally acquire the cine loop of one or more cardiac cycles as needed for quantification and analysis. If an irregular rhythm is present (i.e., atrial fibrillation, flutter, or frequent ectopy), the sonographer should acquire 3 to 5 consecutive cardiac cycles for 2D; Doppler will need 4 to 10 consecutive beats averaged. If two or more myocardial segments of the left ventricle are not well visualized, the use of an approved injectable contrast agent, such as Definity, should be considered if no contraindications are present. The sonographer should always compare the echocardiographic images to the previous study when preparing the preliminary report.

The protocol for the evaluation of cardiac structures begins with the parasternal long- and short-axis views, followed by the apical four-chamber, two-chamber, and three-chamber views (Fig. 32.15). The subcostal and suprasternal views complete the study. The sonographer should acquire the respective cine loop(s) for 2D and color flow Doppler and acquire the representative still frames for M-modes and pulsed wave/continuous wave Doppler. The color Doppler *sector* should be long, spanning the entire cardiac image from top to bottom. This sector should be narrow enough to obtain the frame rate greater than or equal to 17 Hz (Box 32.3).

The following protocol is a *minimum* standard to be performed for all complete 2D/M-mode, color flow Doppler, and spectral Doppler examinations. Additional views are often required and are based on the presence of disease and clinical indications. The order of acquisition is important and should always follow this sequence: (1) 2D image, then (2) full-screen color flow Doppler of the same image, followed by (3) spectral Doppler of the same view. The intent is to show anatomy first (zoom as needed), then color flow of that anatomy (zoom as needed), then spectral. Labeling views or structures is strongly recommended whenever there is an interruption in the 2D/color flow Doppler/spectral format or if nonstandard images are used. Either mode may not increase frame rate depending on harmonic frequency selection. Digitally acquire the following views in the order listed below.

Parasternal Views

Parasternal Long-Axis Two-Dimensional View. The parasternal long-axis view (PLAX) is the initial image in the complete echocardiographic examination. An attempt should be made to record as many of the cardiac structures as possible, from the base of the heart to the apex. Generally, this is accomplished by placing the long axis of the transducer (with the "dot" of the probe towards the head) slightly to the left of the sternum in about the fourth intercostal space. When the bright echo reflection of the pericardium is noted, the transducer is gradually rotated until a long-axis view of the heart is obtained. This view will demonstrate the right ventricle, aorta/ascending aorta, left atrium, mitral leaflets, interventricular septum, and left ventricle (Fig. 32.16). If it is not possible to record the entire long axis on a single scan, the transducer should be gently rocked cephalad to caudad in an "ice pick" fashion to record all the information from the base to the apex of the heart (Boxes 32.4 and 32.5 for protocols).

With slight medial angulation of the probe in the PLAX view, the tricuspid valve, right ventricle, and right atrium will be demonstrated (Fig. 32.17).

The cardiac sonographer should observe the following structures and functions in the PLAX:

1. Composite size of the cardiac chambers
2. Contractility of the right and left ventricles
3. Thickness of the right ventricular wall
4. Continuity of the interventricular septum with the anterior wall of the aorta
5. Pliability of the atrioventricular and semilunar valves
6. Coaptation of the atrioventricular valves
7. Presence of increased echoes on the atrioventricular and semilunar valves (increased echoes may represent calcification, fibroelastoma, vegetations, or other abnormality)
8. Systolic clearance of the aortic cusps (aortic leaflets should open fully in systole)
9. Presence of abnormal echo collections in the chambers or attached to the valve orifice (thrombus may occur if there are wall motion abnormalities)
10. Presence and movement of chordal-papillary muscle structure
11. Thickness of the septum and posterior wall of the left ventricle
12. Uniform texture of the endocardium and myocardium
13. Size of the aortic root and left atrium

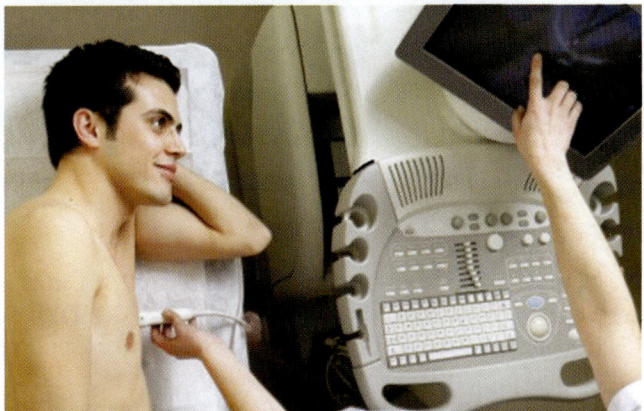

FIG. 32.14 The patient is positioned on the bed with their left arm tucked under the head.

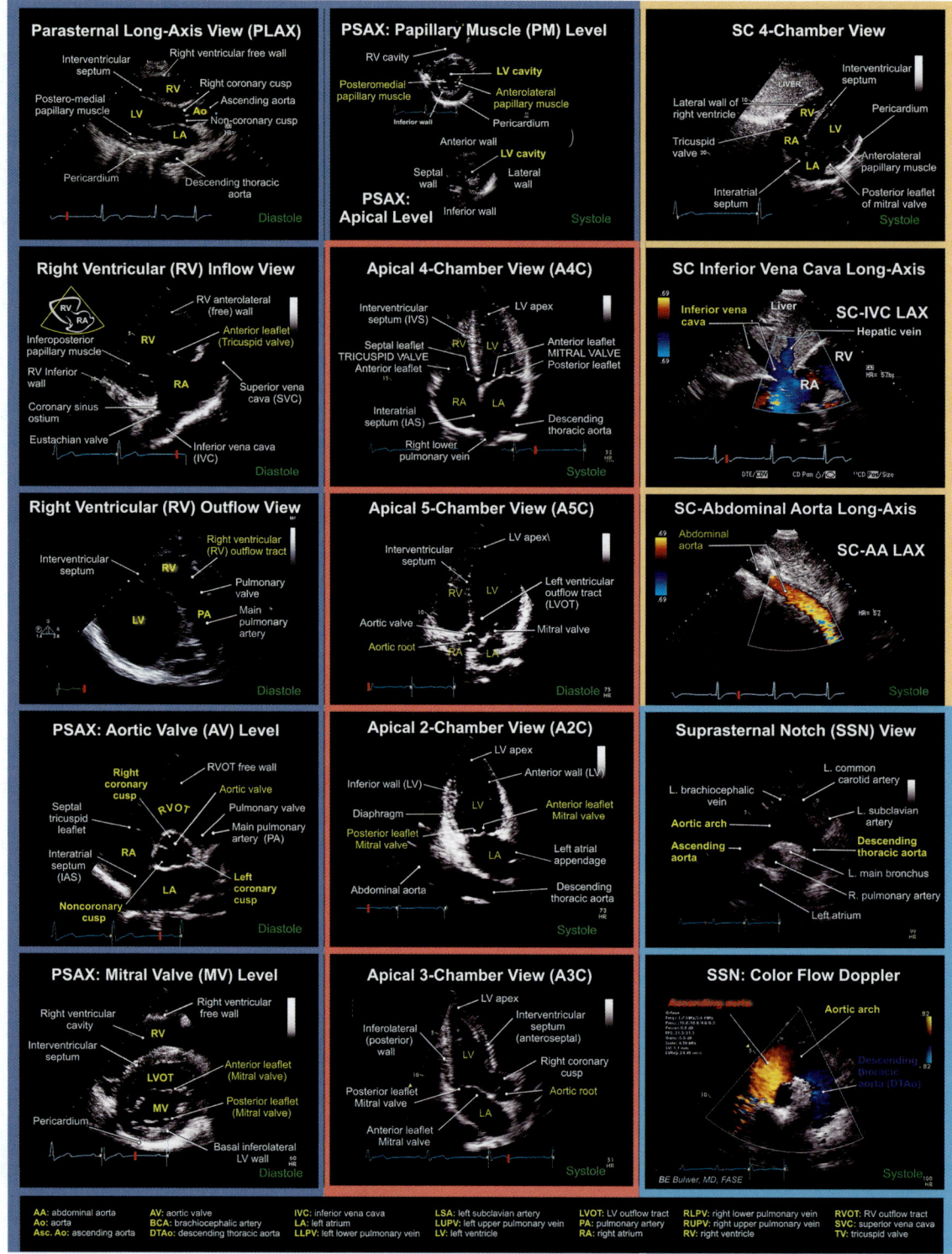

FIG. 32.15 The protocol for the evaluation of cardiac structures begins with the parasternal long- and short-axis views, followed by the apical four-chamber, two-chamber, and three-chamber views. The subcostal and suprasternal views complete the study.

14. M-mode of the aortic root/left atrium (Fig. 32.18), mitral leaflets (Fig. 32.13C), and left ventricle (Fig. 32.13D)
15. Evaluation of the aortic root, aortic sinus, and ascending aorta (Fig. 32.19)

Parasternal Long-Axis View for Color Flow Mapping. In **diastole**, the PLAX shows the left atrium filled with various shades of red as the pulmonary venous flow enters the atrial cavity from the right and left branches. While the blood is pushed toward the mitral leaflets, some turbulence is shown when the flow enters the left ventricle.

During ventricular **systole**, the mitral leaflets close, and the ventricle contracts to push the blood through the left ventricular outflow tract through the open aortic cusps. The blood is now flowing toward the transducer and is shown as a

CHAPTER 32 Introduction to Echocardiographic Techniques, Terminology, and Tips

BOX 32.3	Transducer Position and Cardiac Protocol (See Fig. 32.10)

Parasternal
Long-axis view
Short-axis view

Apical
Four-chamber view
Five-chamber view (including aorta)
Two-chamber view

Subcostal Window
Inferior vena cava, hepatic veins
RV and LV inflow
LV, aorta
RV outflow

Suprasternal Notch Window
Ascending aorta
Descending aorta
Right pulmonary artery
Left atrium

Right Parasternal Window
Ascending aorta

LV, Left ventricle; *RV,* right ventricle.

BOX 32.4	Parasternal Long-Axis View (PLAX)

1. Record deep PLAX (regardless of presence of effusion); typical depths are 20–24 cm; far field should not be dark unless there is effusion; adjust TGC gain accordingly.
2. PLAX full screen (not zoomed).
3. Color Doppler full screen of aortic, mitral valve, LVOT, and include RVOT in color Doppler.
4. PLAX 2D zoom as needed to show anatomy/pathology better and then zoom of same image with color.
5. PLAX color IVS to rule out shunt.
6. M-mode cursor through the minor axis of the aorta and left atrium.
7. M-mode cursor through mitral valve leaflet tips.
8. M-mode cursor through minor axis of LV just superior to papillary muscle.
9. High PLAX window to assess ascending aorta; color flow Doppler as needed to differentiate between artifact and a dissection; also high PSAX 2D and with color flow Doppler if needed to help differentiate between an artifact and a dissection.

2D, Two-dimensional; *IVS,* interventricular septum; *LV,* left ventricle; *LVOT,* left ventricular outflow tract; *PSAX,* parasternal short-axis view; *RVOT,* right ventricular outflow tract; *TGC,* time gain compensation.

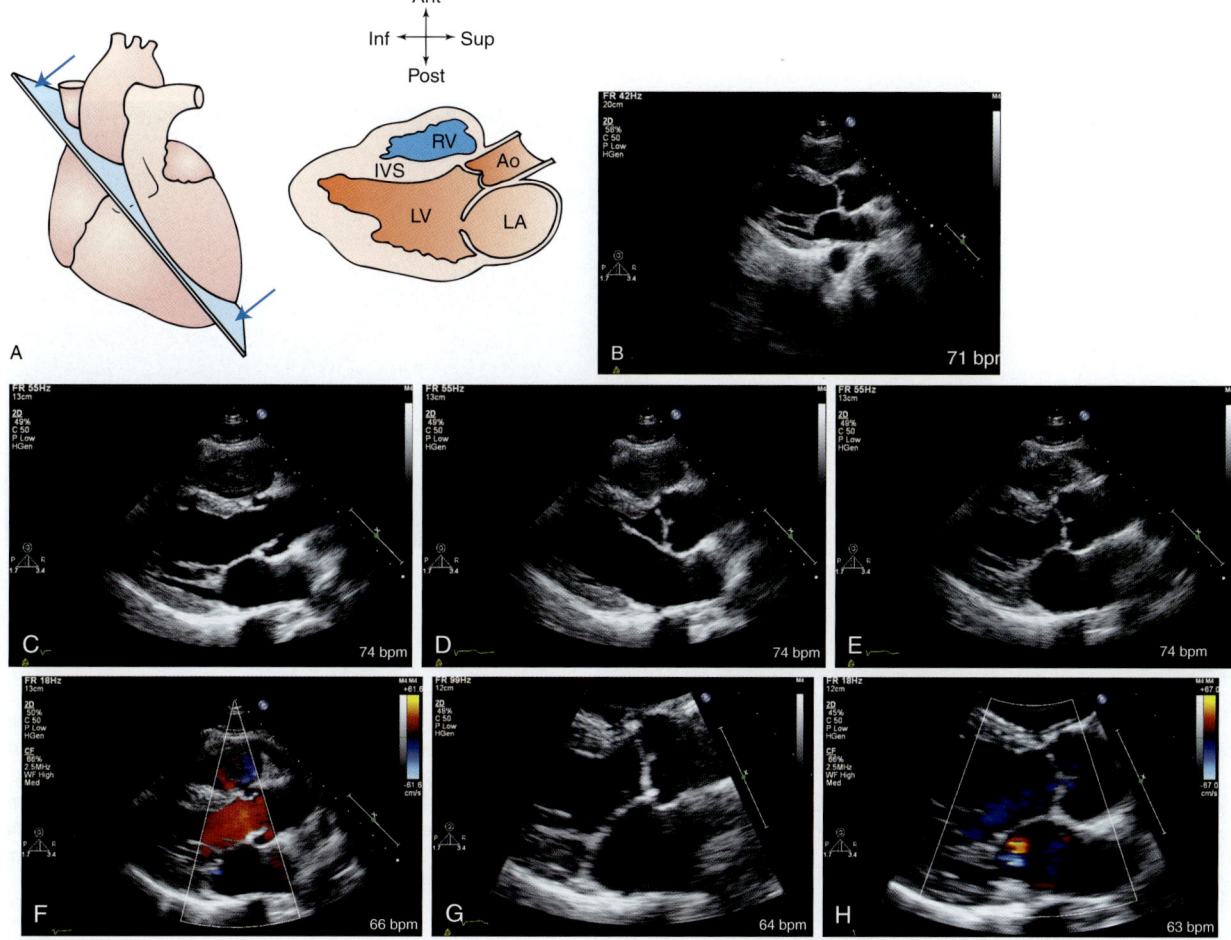

FIG. 32.16 (A) The two-dimensional parasternal long-axis view of the heart with reduced field of view to see beyond the pericardium. (B) End systole; note aortic valve closure and mitral valve closure (C). Early systole shows the mitral leaflets closed, aortic valve is open (D), and end diastole (E) shows mitral leaflets closed. The thickness of the anterior leaflet of the mitral valve is measured. Color Doppler (F) shows the mitral valve closed (systole) with red flowing from the left ventricle into the aorta. (G) Zoom of the mitral valve. (H) Color Doppler of the mitral valve and aortic root. *Ao,* Aortic root; *IVS,* interventricular septum; *LA,* left atrium; *LV,* left ventricle; *RV,* right ventricle.

shade of red with some yellow highlights as it approaches the aortic root (see Fig. 32.16F). No color flow is seen to cross at the level of the membranous septum in the normal patient.

Left Parasternal Window for Doppler. The PLAX with the patient rolled in a left lateral decubitus position has limited applications with Doppler. The transducer is more perpendicular to the cardiac structures than parallel, so the maximum velocity is difficult to record. However, disturbances in flow, especially mitral, aortic, and tricuspid (with the transducer angled medially) regurgitation, may be recorded in some patients with this view. Thickened cusps may direct the regurgitant flow in a pathway not typically seen as well on the apical view as on the PLAX (Fig. 32.20). A ventricular septal defect may be visualized in this view because the flow of blood is more parallel to the beam. Both muscular and membranous defects may be imaged from this view, along with the apical and subcostal views.

Right Parasternal View for Color Flow Mapping. The right parasternal view is performed after the patient has been rolled into a steep right decubitus position. The transducer is placed along the right sternal border in the second intercostal space. This view may be useful for visualization of the entrance of the superior vena cava into the right atrium (Fig. 32.21). The caval flow appears red as it enters the right atrium. This view also provides another window to image the entrance of the pulmonary veins into the left atrium. Flow patterns from the veins may be seen, whereas the actual veins are difficult to image on the 2D study.

Right Parasternal Window for Doppler. The right parasternal position is most useful in the difficult-to-image adult or older pediatric patient after surgery who has a jet of aortic stenosis directed more to the right. The patient is rolled into a steep right decubitus position and the transducer placed in the first, second, or third intercostal space to the right of the sternum. Often the Pedof probe is easier to position in this patient, with the audible sound as the guide to the maximal velocity jet.

BOX 32.5 Right Ventricular Inflow View

1. RA/RV, full screen.
2. Color Doppler of RA/RV.
3. Whether or not tricuspid regurgitation is seen, attempt continuous wave Doppler for peak tricuspid regurgitation velocity and record.

RA, Right atrium; *RV*, right ventricle.

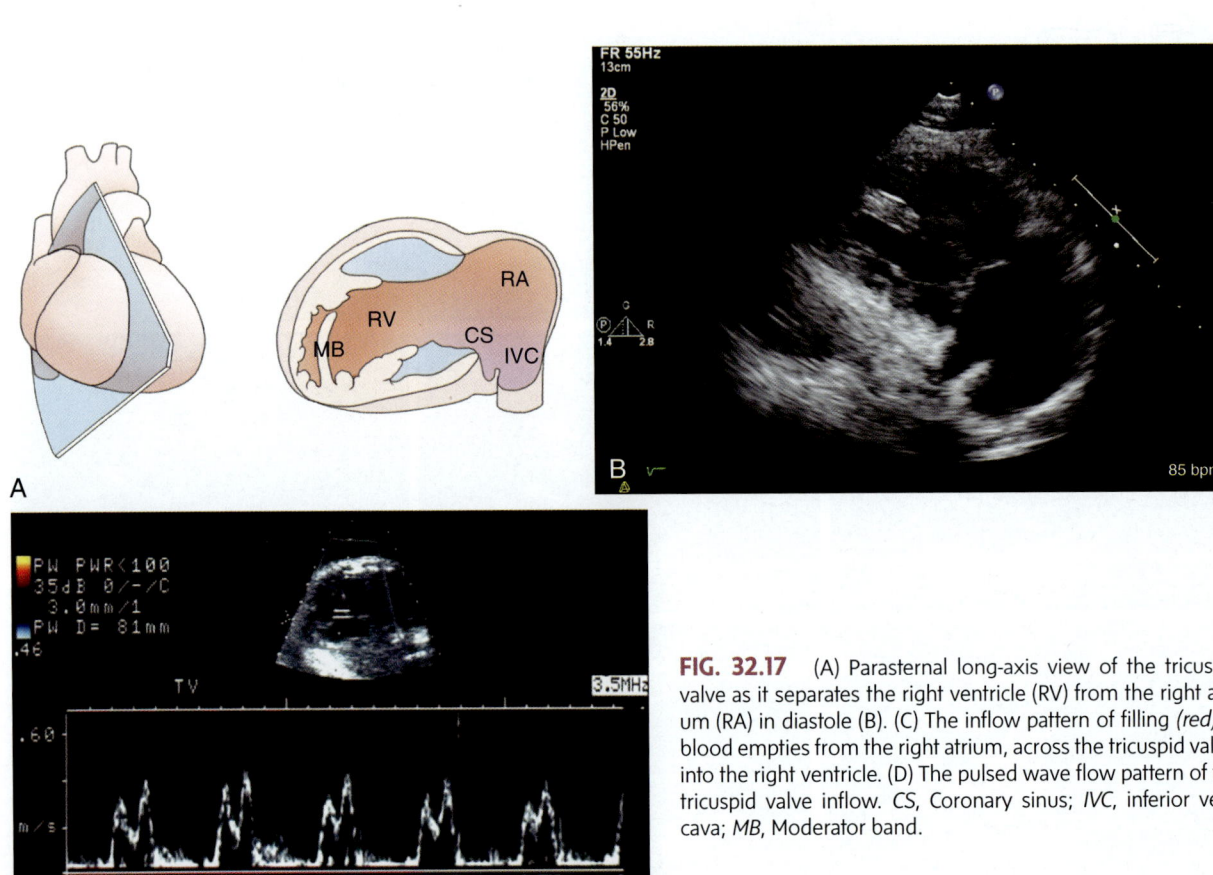

FIG. 32.17 (A) Parasternal long-axis view of the tricuspid valve as it separates the right ventricle (RV) from the right atrium (RA) in diastole (B). (C) The inflow pattern of filling *(red)* as blood empties from the right atrium, across the tricuspid valve, into the right ventricle. (D) The pulsed wave flow pattern of the tricuspid valve inflow. *CS*, Coronary sinus; *IVC*, inferior vena cava; *MB*, Moderator band.

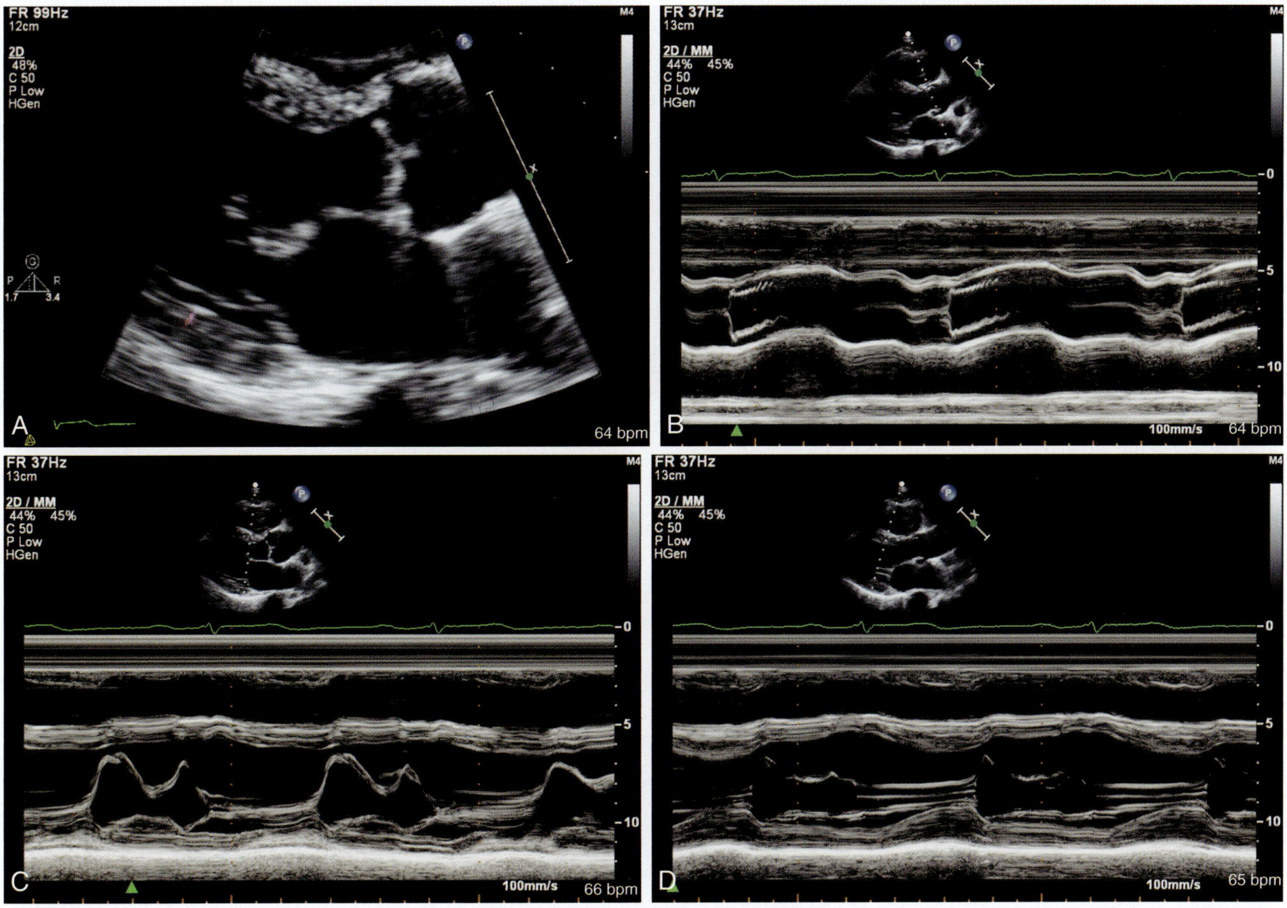

FIG. 32.18 (A) Parasternal long-axis view is used to record M-mode tracings through the aortic leaflets (B), mitral leaflets (C), and left ventricle (D).

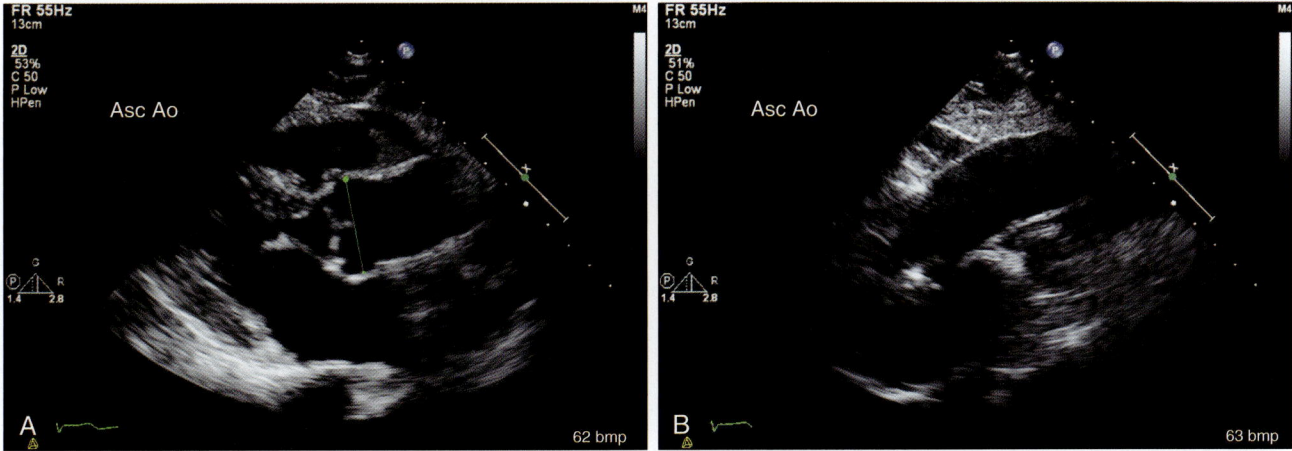

FIG. 32.19 (A) Parasternal long-axis view of the ascending aorta. (B) The sonographer should follow the root of the aorta and slowly move the transducer up an interspace to see the ascending aorta (Asc Ao).

Parasternal Short-Axis Two-Dimensional View. The transducer should be rotated 90 degrees from the PLAX to obtain multiple transverse short-axis views of the heart, particularly at the following four levels. See Box 32.6 for the protocol.

1. The low parasternal short-axis view should demonstrate the right ventricle, left ventricle, and papillary muscles (chordal echoes may also be seen) (Fig. 32.22):
   a. Contractility of the septum and posterior wall of the left ventricle
   b. Thickness of the septum and posterior wall
   c. Size of the left ventricle
   d. Presence or absence of mural thrombus or other mass
   e. Presence or absence of pericardial fluid, constriction, or restriction
   f. Presence of increased echo density in posterior wall
   g. Number of papillary muscles and their location within the left ventricular cavity

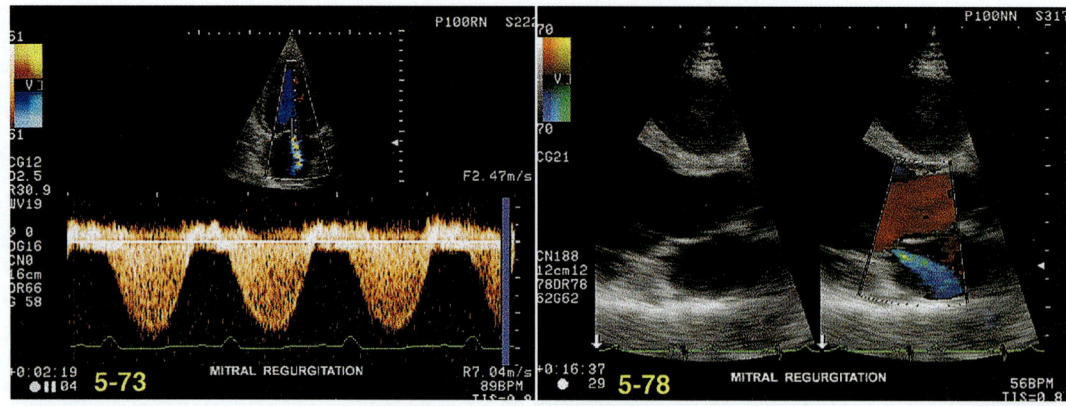

FIG. 32.20 Parasternal long-axis view in a patient with mitral regurgitation (blue flow in the left atrium). The continuous wave flow is recorded in the apical position to measure 5 m/sec.

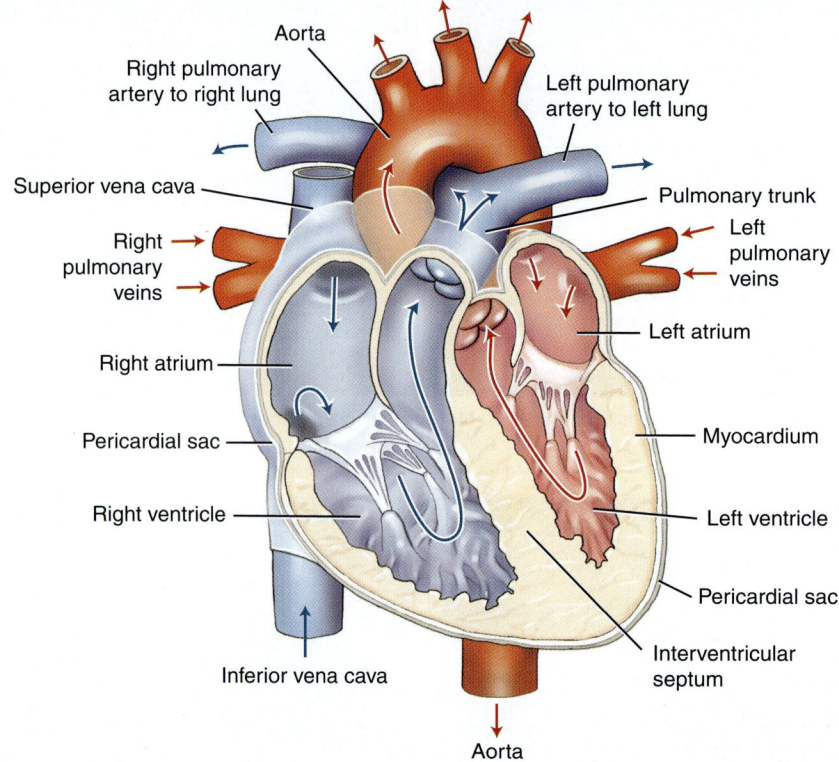

FIG. 32.21 The superior vena cava drains into the medial superior wall of the right atrium.

2. The midparasternal short-axis view should demonstrate the right ventricle, left ventricular outflow tract, and anterior and posterior leaflets of the mitral valve (Fig. 32.23):
   a. Size of the septum and posterior wall
   b. Presence of mass lesions in left or right ventricle
   c. Mobility and thickness of the mitral valve
   d. Presence of a flutter on the septum or anterior leaflet of the mitral valve or both
   e. Systolic apposition of mitral valve leaflets
   f. Contractility of septum and posterior wall
3. The moderate to high parasternal short-axis view should demonstrate the right ventricular outflow tract, main pulmonary artery, tricuspid valve, aortic cusps, coronary arteries, right and left atria, and interatrial septum (Fig. 32.24):
   a. Size of right ventricle and left atrium
   b. Presence of mass lesions in right or left atrium
   c. Mobility and thickness of tricuspid and aortic valves
   d. Continuity of interatrial septum
   e. Right ventricular wall thickness
   f. Presence of trileaflet aortic valve
4. The high parasternal short-axis view should demonstrate the pulmonary valve, right ventricular outflow tract, and aorta (Fig. 32.25):
   a. Typical sausage-shaped right ventricular outflow tract and pulmonary artery draped anterior to circular aorta
   b. Semilunar cusp thickness and mobility
   c. Presence of calcification, extraneous echoes, or both in right ventricle or valve areas
   d. Pulmonary valve mobility and thickness

CHAPTER 32 Introduction to Echocardiographic Techniques, Terminology, and Tips

> **BOX 32.6 Parasternal Short-Axis View (PSAX)**
>
> 1. PSAX at level of papillary muscles, full screen.
> 2. PSAX at level of left ventricular apex, full screen.
> 3. PSAX at level of mitral leaflet tips, full screen.
> 4. PSAX color flow Doppler of MV; include entire annulus, and if MVR, include entire ring to assess for paravalvular leak.
> 5. PSAX at level of aortic valve and LA, full screen.
> 6. Zoom of aortic valve and then with color flow Doppler if AI present.
> 7. Often, PA, TV, and RV are not well visualized from PSAX AO/LA; take additional loops separately emphasizing PA, RV, and TV by 2D.
> 8. PSAX of PA to bifurcation (without color Doppler).
> 9. PSAX with long color flow Doppler sector of the RVOT and PA, including the bifurcation.
> 10. PW Doppler of RVOT at the level of the pulmonic annulus with closing click seen for PVR application.
> 11. CW Doppler through PA as needed to assess for PS or if PS not ruled out by color Doppler screen; also CW Doppler of PI signal.
> 12. PSAX of TV, RA, and RV.
> 13. PSAX color flow Doppler of TV, RA, RV, and interatrial septum.
> 14. Whether or not tricuspid regurgitation is seen, attempt CW Doppler for peak tricuspid regurgitation velocity and record.

2D, Two-dimensional; *CW*, continuous wave; *AI*, aortic insufficiency; *AO*, aorta; *CW*, continuous wave; *LA*, left atrium; *MV*, mitral valve; *MVR*, mitral valve replacement; *PA*, pulmonary artery; *PI*, pulmonary insufficiency; *PS*, pulmonary stenosis; *PVR*, pulmonary vascular resistance; *PW*, pulsed wave; *RA*, right atrium; *RV*, right ventricle; *RVOT*, right ventricular outflow tract; *TV*, tricuspid valve.

5. The high parasternal short-axis view is also good to demonstrate the right ventricular outflow tract, tricuspid leaflets, and right atrium. The transducer should be angled medially from the pulmonary artery to image the tricuspid leaflets (Fig. 32.26).

Parasternal Short-Axis View for Color Flow Mapping. At the level of the aortic valve, the blood flow appears as a blue signal moving from the right ventricular outflow tract into the main pulmonary artery (Fig. 32.27). Flow into the coronary arteries is sometimes seen in the right coronary, left main coronary, and circumflex and proximal left anterior descending arteries. Depending on the orientation of the coronary arteries, the blood flow appears yellow-red or bluish.

With slight angulation of the transducer, flow from the inferior vena cava can be seen while it flows into the right atrium. This flow appears red. When atrial systole occurs, blue signals can be seen moving from the right atrium into the inferior vena cava. Blue signals can also be seen as blood leaves the right ventricular outflow tract to enter the pulmonary valve and main pulmonary artery in systole. While the transducer is angled slightly, the flow from the main pulmonary artery is seen to move into the bifurcation of the right and left pulmonary arteries. This flow is still primarily blue while it moves away from the transducer.

A short-axis view at the level of the mitral valve in diastole may show flow signals in the mitral orifice and the right

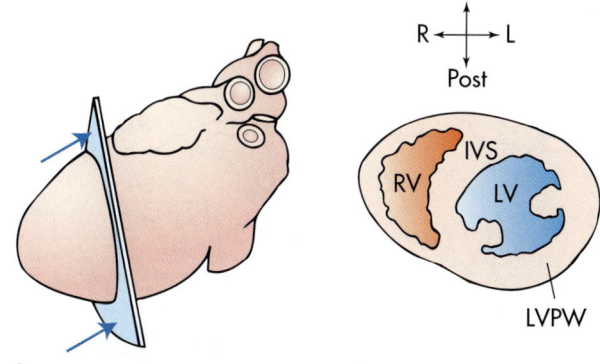

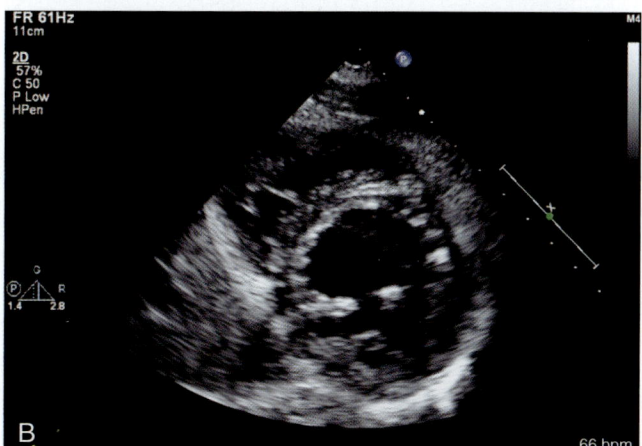

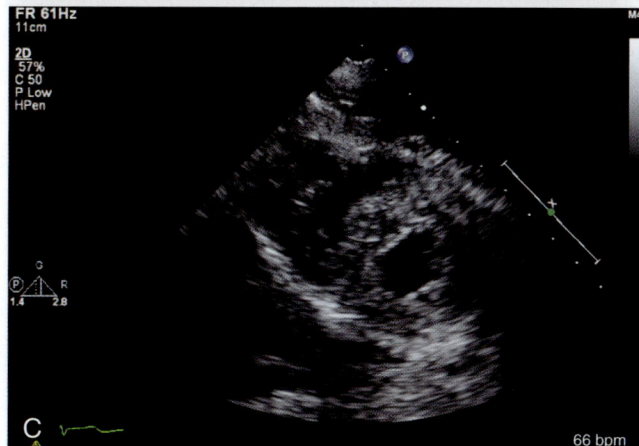

FIG. 32.22 (A) Parasternal short-axis view of the left ventricle. (B) Low parasternal short-axis view of the right ventricle (RV), left ventricle (LV), and posterior papillary muscle *(arrows)* in end diastole. (C) End-systolic squeeze of the left ventricle (LV). *IVS*, Interventricular septum; *LVPW*, left ventricular posterior wall.

ventricle. When the transducer is angled medially, the right ventricular inflow plane may show flow signals while they arise from the coronary sinus into the right heart during diastole.

Parasternal Short-Axis Window for Doppler. The parasternal short-axis view is very useful for recording flow from the right ventricular outflow tract and pulmonary artery. The sample volume should be placed distal to the pulmonary cusps to record flow in the main pulmonary artery (see Fig. 32.26).

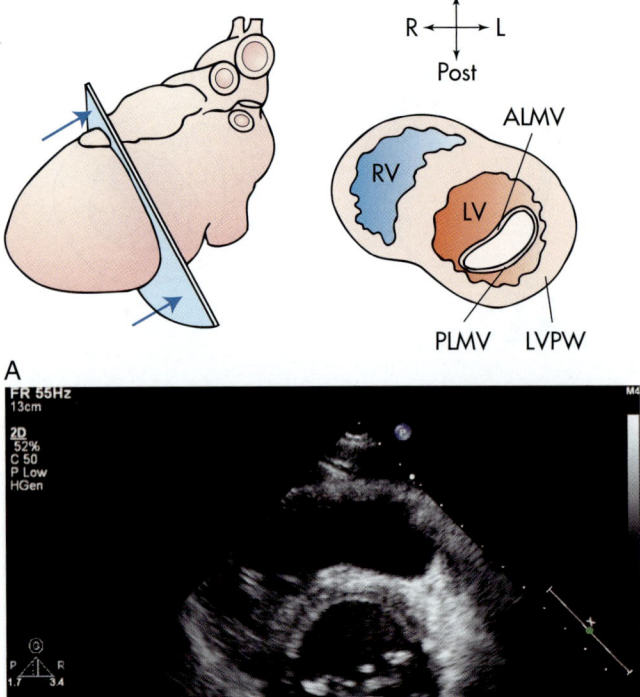

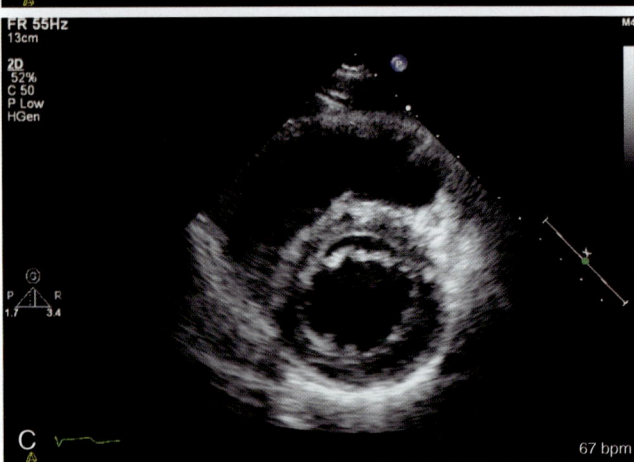

FIG. 32.23 (A) Parasternal short-axis view. (B) Midparasternal short-axis view of the right ventricle, interventricular septum, anterior leaflet mitral valve, posterior leaflet mitral valve, and left ventricle in systole and diastole (C). *ALMV*, Anterior leaflet mitral valve; *LV*, left ventricle; *LVPW*, left ventricular posterior wall; *PLMV*, posterior leaflet mitral valve; *RV*, right ventricle.

The flow pattern is similar to that obtained from the aortic flow when the transducer is placed in the apical position but with a slightly slower upstroke. The spectral display shows a velocity curve below the baseline with a narrow band of frequencies. Normal pulmonary flow velocities range from 60 to 90 cm/sec in adults and 70 to 110 cm/sec in children. This view is useful for recording pulmonary regurgitation and stenosis, as well as abnormal patent ductus arteriosus flow that may be present in the neonate or child.

As the sample volume is positioned closer to the bifurcation of the pulmonary artery, the flow velocity increases slightly. To record velocities in the right ventricular outflow tract, the sample volume is placed just proximal to the pulmonary valve. The flow pattern is similar to the pulmonary outflow but has a slightly lower velocity. This view is especially useful for detecting a left-to-right shunt at the membranous ventricular septum, a coronary artery fistula, or a muscle bundle in the right ventricular outflow tract.

Apical Views

Three apical views are very useful: the four-chamber view, the two-chamber view, and the apical long-axis view. The cardiac sonographer should palpate the patient's chest to detect the point of maximal impulse (PMI) (Fig. 32.28A). The transducer should then be directed in a transverse plane at the PMI and angled sharply cephalad to record the four chambers of the heart. If there is too much lung interference, the proper cardiac window has not been found, and care should be taken to adjust the patient's position or the transducer position to adequately see all four chambers of the heart. Many laboratories have found it useful to use the special echocardiographic bed in which a dropout enables the sonographer to readily access the cardiac apex. This allows the transducer more flexibility for recording the apical views.

The apical views are excellent for assessing cardiac contractility, size of cardiac chambers, presence of mass lesions, alignment of atrioventricular valves, coaptation of atrioventricular valves, septal or posterior wall hypertrophy, chordal attachments, and the presence of pericardial effusion (Fig. 32.29). The student will find more difficulty in obtaining an adequate image from the apical view than from the parasternal views. This is because the ribs may interfere with the probe access to image the cardiac structures without artifacts or lungs interfering with the sound beam transmission. Once the perfect cardiac window has been located, the sonographer should carefully sweep the probe slightly anterior to posterior to be sure the ventricles are not foreshortened. The effort is made to elongate the ventricular cavity to show the thin apical segment. If the ventricle appears "roundish," the probe should be directed more posterior to "open up" the ventricular cavity. Breathing the patient helps with these views in the apex. The goal is to watch what happens to the lungs when the patient takes in a breath and then lets the breath out. Practicing breathing techniques on every patient will help your images become stellar.

The four-chamber view does not provide a good window to evaluate the presence of an atrial septal defect because the beam is parallel to the thin foramen ovale, and the septum commonly appears as an artifactual defect in this view. The subcostal four-chamber view is much better for evaluating the presence of such a defect. See Boxes 32.7 through 32.11 for apical protocols.

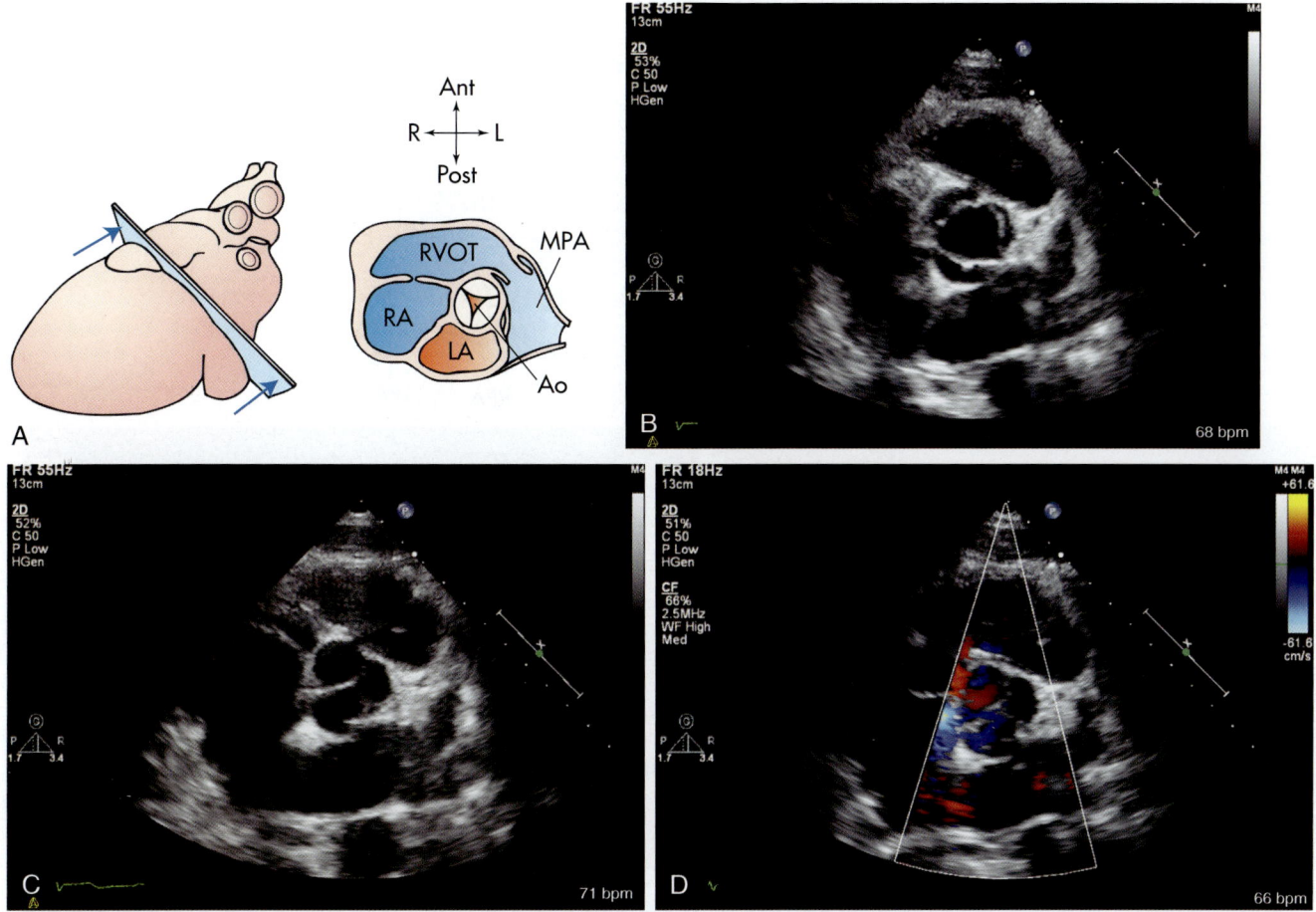

FIG. 32.24 (A) Parasternal short-axis view. (B) High mid-parasternal short-axis view of the right ventricular outflow tract, tricuspid valve, right atrium, aortic cusp (open in systole), and left atrium. (C) Aortic cusps are closed in diastole. (D) Color Doppler of the end-diastolic phase. *Ao,* Aorta; *LA,* left atrium; *MPA,* main pulmonary artery; *RA,* right atrium; *RVOT,* right ventricular outflow tract.

The cardiac sonographer should observe the following structures:

1. Size of the cardiac chambers
2. Contractility of right and left ventricles
3. Septal and posterior wall thickness, contractility, and continuity
4. Coaptation of atrioventricular valves
5. Alignment of atrioventricular valves
6. Presence of increased echoes on valve apparatus
7. Presence of mass or thrombus in cardiac chambers
8. Entrance of pulmonary veins into left atrial cavity
9. Size of left ventricular outflow tract, signs of obstruction, mobility of aortic cusps, absence of subaortic membrane
10. Entrance of inferior and superior vena cava into the right atrium

From the four-chamber view, the probe is slightly angled anterior to obtain the five-chamber view (Fig. 32.30). This view outlines the left ventricular outflow tract, aortic root and leaflets, and the ascending aorta.

To obtain the apical two-chamber view, the transducer is rotated 90 degrees from the apical four-chamber view to visualize the left ventricle, left atrium, and mitral valve. The anterior and posterior walls of the left ventricle are well seen (Fig. 32.31).

The apical long-axis view is very useful for evaluation of the left ventricular cavity and aortic outflow tract (Fig. 32.32). From the two-chamber view, the transducer is angled slightly anterior to see the left ventricular outflow tract and ascending aorta. This view permits the cardiac sonographer to evaluate the wall motion of the posterior basal segment of the left ventricle, the septal wall, and the apex of the left ventricle. It also permits another view of the left ventricular outflow tract, which may be useful in determining aortic cusp motion or the presence of a subvalvular membrane.

The apical four-chamber view allows good visualization of the left atrial cavity and pulmonary venous inflow (Fig. 32.33). It also provides excellent visualization of the mitral valve inflow patterns at rest and with Valsalva to assess diastology (Fig. 32.34). Doppler tissue imaging is useful to quantify diastolic parameters. Pulmonary venous inflow is also recorded from this view. Analysis of the right side of the heart and tricuspid valve is made in the apical four-chamber view (Fig. 32.35).

Apical View for Color Flow Mapping. The apical four-chamber view is one of the most useful views in color flow mapping. In the typical four-chamber view, the operator can follow blood flow as it enters the atrial cavities and flows through the atrioventricular valves in diastole to enter the ventricular

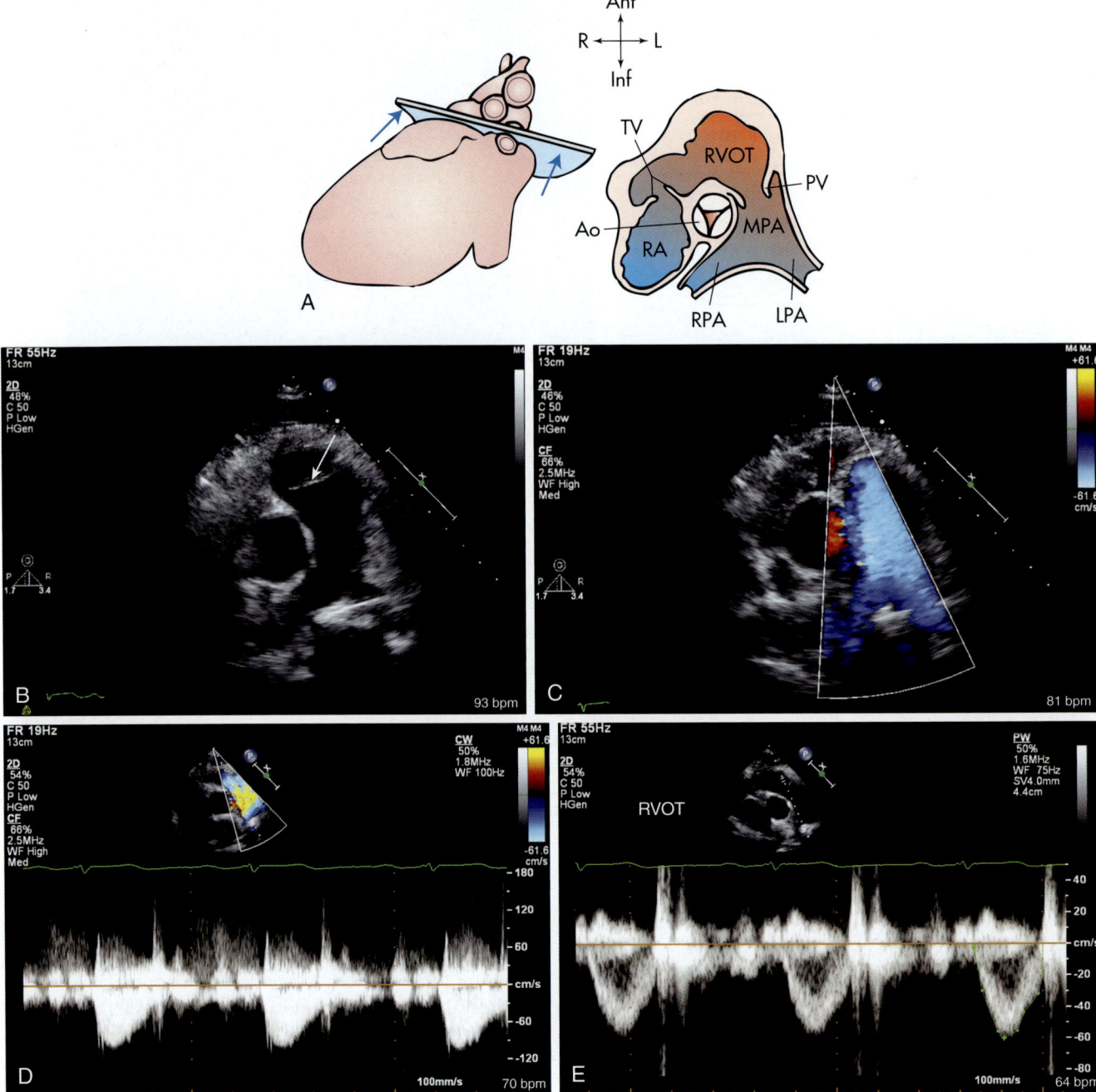

FIG. 32.25 (A) Parasternal short-axis view. (B) High parasternal short-axis view of the aorta pulmonary cusp *(arrow)*, main pulmonary artery, right pulmonary artery, and left pulmonary artery. (C) Color *(blue)* shows the flow leaving the right ventricle through the pulmonary valve into the main pulmonary artery. Continuous wave (D) and pulsed wave (E) Doppler taken at the level of the right ventricular outflow tract. *Ao*, Aorta; *LPA*, left pulmonary artery; *MPA*, main pulmonary artery; *PV*, pulmonary valve; *RA*, right atrium; *RPA*, right pulmonary artery; *RVOT*, right ventricular outflow tract; *TV*, tricuspid valve.

chambers before it exits through the great arteries. The flow towards the transducer is laminar (depicted in red). As the velocity increases, the flow becomes turbulent and turns yellow. In contrast, the laminar flow away from the transducer is "blue" while the turbulent flow becomes "greenish" (Fig. 32.36).

The right-side events appear slightly earlier as the tricuspid valve opens before the mitral valve. When blood fills the atrial cavities, it appears red as it flows toward the transducer (Fig. 32.37B). Pulmonary venous inflow to the left atrial cavity may be seen in this four-chamber view (see Fig. 32.37C). Flow from the right and left upper veins appears reddish with some yellow, whereas flow from the lower left pulmonary vein appears blue as it moves away from the transducer. Although the transducer is angled more posterior and medial, inflow from the superior vena cava is red when it enters the medial aspect of the right atrium along the border of the interatrial septum.

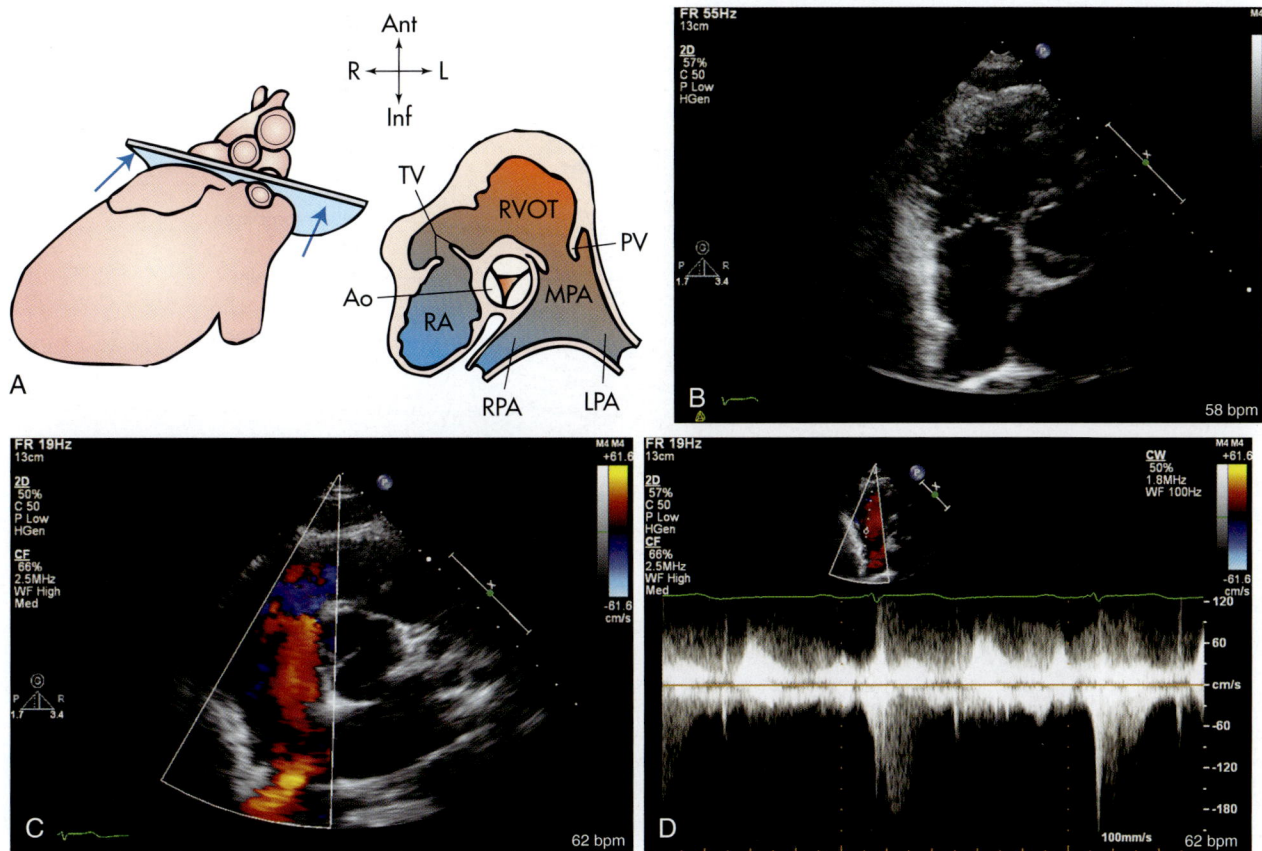

FIG. 32.26 (A) Parasternal short-axis view. (B) The transducer is angled slightly medial to show the right atrium (RA), tricuspid valve (TV), and right ventricle. (C) Color Doppler shows the red inflow from the superior vena cava into the right atrial cavity. (D) Continuous wave Doppler through the tricuspid leaflets demonstrates trace tricuspid insufficiency below the baseline. *Ao*, Aorta; *LPA*, left pulmonary artery; *MPA*, main pulmonary artery; *PV*, pulmonary valve; *RPA*, right pulmonary artery; *RVOT*, right ventricular outflow tract.

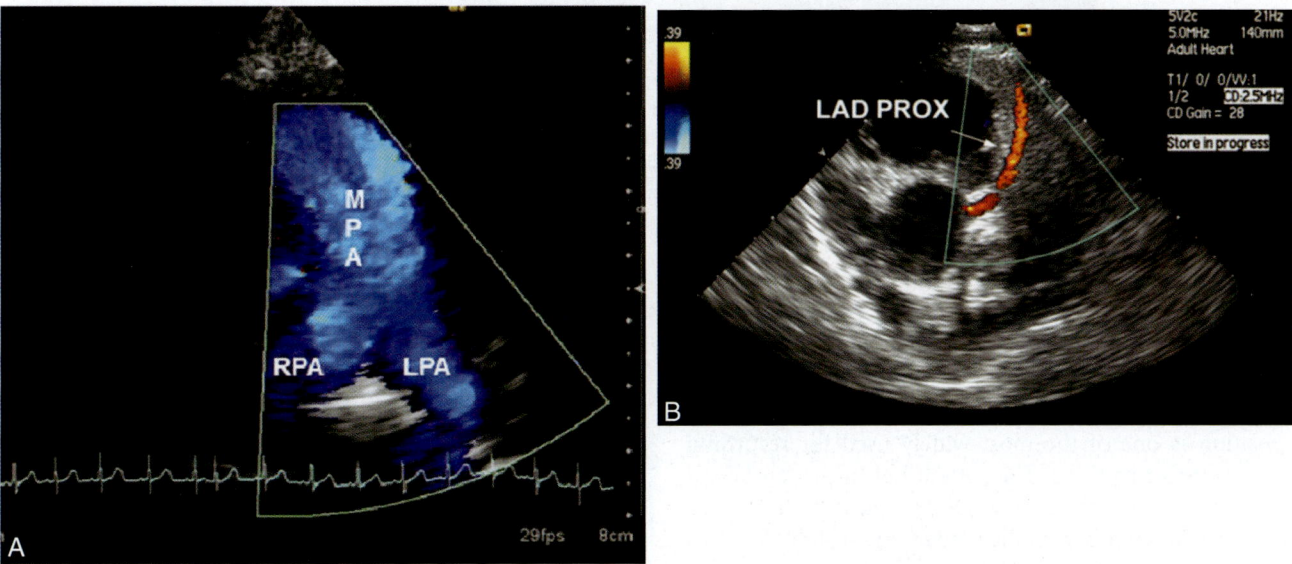

FIG. 32.27 (A) At the level of the aortic valve, the blood flow appears as a blue signal moving from the right ventricular outflow tract into the main pulmonary artery to bifurcate into the right and left pulmonary arteries. (B) The left anterior descending (LAD) arterial flow appears yellow-red.

Diastolic flow through the atrioventricular orifice occurs at a slightly higher velocity, giving rise to changes in colors from red to yellow (see Fig. 32.37D). The flow returns to red as the inflow chamber of the ventricles fills. When the flow reaches the apex, it begins to swirl toward the ventricular outflow tract, and the color changes to blue. Again, the velocity increases as the flow moves toward the leaflets of the aorta in systole, changing the color into more intense blue

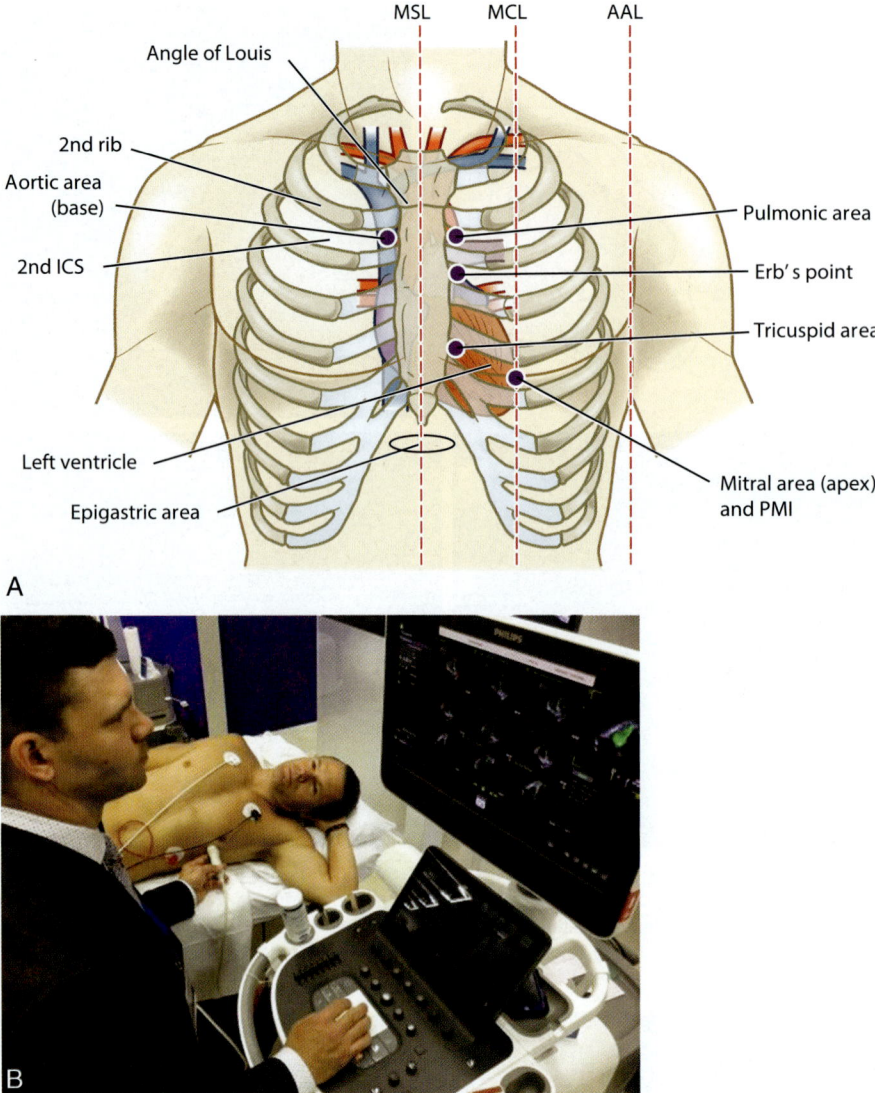

FIG. 32.28 (A) The cardiac sonographer should palpate the patient's chest to detect the point of maximal impulse (PMI). (B) The transducer should then be directed in a transverse plane at the PMI and angled sharply cephalad to record the four chambers of the heart. *AAL*, Anterior axillary line; *ICS*, intercostal space; *MCL*, midclavicular line; *MSL*, midsternal line.

shades. Flow in the ascending aorta should be a uniform blue. Regurgitant flow into the left atrium from the incompetent mitral or tricuspid valve will appear as a blue-green mixed pattern.

Apical Window for Spectral Doppler. The apical four-chamber position is one of the most widely used for recording multiple Doppler patterns. The patient lies in the left lateral decubitus position with the transducer placed at the apical impulse and directed toward the patient's right shoulder. This position allows sampling of flow through the mitral, tricuspid, and aortic valves at nearly parallel angles to the beam. See Boxes 32.12 and 32.13 for protocols.

Inflow through the mitral valve leaflets may be recorded by placing the Doppler signal at the level of the tips of the leaflets. The pulsed sample volume may be moved from the tips of the leaflets to the level of the mitral annulus to obtain a clean recording. The normal mitral flow velocity tracing is similar to that found on an M-mode recording. The vertical markings are in cm/sec, while the horizontal markings denote the time.

The initial peak occurs during the rapid-filling phase of diastole (see Fig. 32.37). The smaller second peak occurs late in diastole (with atrial contraction). In patients with decreased left ventricular compliance, the first peak may be lower and the second peak higher. Normal flow velocity across the mitral valve ranges from 60 to 130 cm/sec in adults and similar velocities in children.

The tricuspid valve flow may be recorded in the apical position while the transducer is angled slightly to the right. With the transducer position at the level of the leaflets, a pattern similar to mitral valve flow is recorded with two peaks during diastole. The first occurs during ventricular filling and the second with the onset of atrial contraction. The velocity pattern is much lower in the tricuspid valve, with significant

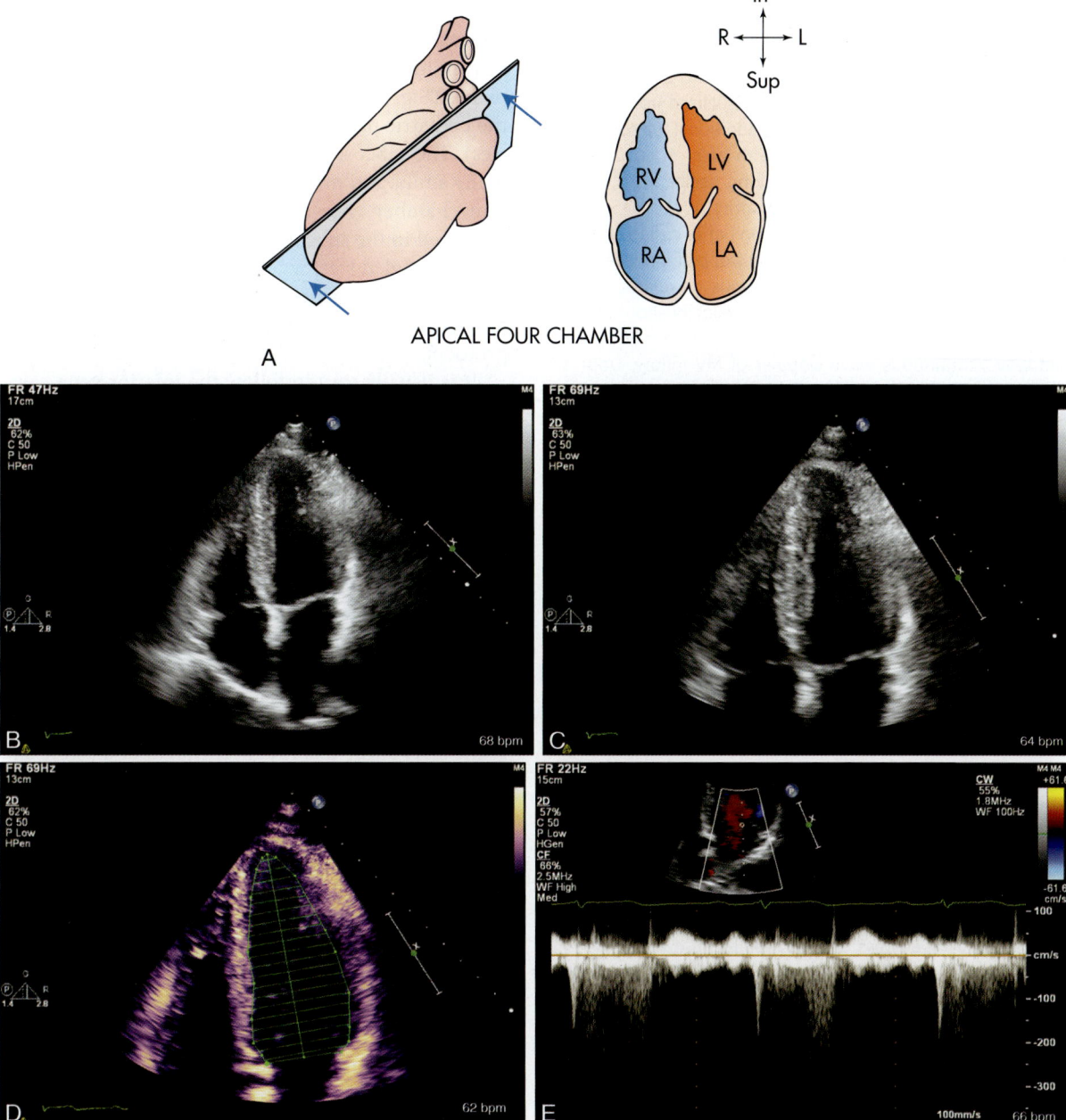

FIG. 32.29 (A–B) Apical four-chamber view. The transducer is placed at the posterior maximum impulse (near the midcoronal plane) and angled steeply toward the right shoulder. The patient should be rolled completely on their side for this examination. (C) Zoom image of the left ventricular cavity. (D) The image is frozen at end diastole to trace the endocardial border. (E) The image is then scrolled to end systole to again trace the endocardial border to determine the ejection fraction of the left ventricle (LV). (F) Color and spectral Doppler shows the high-velocity flow as blood empties from the left atrium (LA) into the left ventricular cavity. *RA*, Right atrium; *RV*, right ventricle.

respiratory changes that increase during inspiration and decrease during expiration (Fig. 32.38). The normal velocity range is 30 to 70 cm/sec for adults and is similar for children (see Table 32.1).

In the apical position, the transducer may be angled slightly anterior or rotated into a long-axis view to record blood flow from the left ventricular outflow tract as it enters the aortic root and ascending aorta. With the pulsed wave sample volume placed just proximal to the aortic root (in the left ventricular outflow tract), the flow is away from the transducer during systole. The spectral display shows a narrow band of frequencies below the baseline (Fig. 32.39).

The normal velocity pattern in the left ventricular outflow tract in the adult is 70 to 110 cm/sec, and it is similar in children. As the sample volume is moved across the aortic valve, flow can be recorded within the ascending aorta. This velocity pattern is slightly higher and peaks earlier. Normal velocities range from 100 to 170 cm/sec in adults and 120 to 180 cm/sec in children.

| BOX 32.7 | Apical Four-Chamber View (Ap4C) |

1. Ap4C showing all four chambers and atrioventricular valves, full screen.
2. If right heart and left heart are not well visualized from one Ap4C view, take left heart images now; additional full screen Ap4C loops of the right heart will be taken later.
3. Ap4C color flow Doppler of the MV (long sector from the apex through the MV and the entire left atrium).
4. Zoom on left heart structures as needed to better define anatomy/pathology, then zoomed color flow Doppler if needed.
5. If mitral regurgitation is present, continuous wave Doppler of mitral regurgitation for dp/dt and peak velocity should be taken.
6. Pulsed wave/continuous wave Doppler of MV inflow, Doppler tissue imaging lateral and septal MV annulus, and right pulmonary vein and, if needed, MV Valsalva.

dp/dt, Change in pressure over change in time; *MV*, mitral valve.

| BOX 32.8 | Apical Five-Chamber View (Ap5C) |

1. Ap5C full screen then zoom AoV as needed to show anatomy/pathology better.
2. Ap5C color flow Doppler of the aortic valve with color sector box from apex through aortic valve and aorta; if there is aortic insufficiency, record continuous wave Doppler signal.
3. If there is LVOT obstruction, show pulsed wave before obstruction and then continuous wave through obstruction; also, pulsed wave/continuous wave Doppler of LVOT and then AoV.

AoV, Aortic valve; *LVOT*, left ventricular outflow tract.

| BOX 32.9 | Apical Four-Chamber View (Ap4C): Right Heart |

1. Ap4C emphasizing RV, TV, and RA (do not use narrow sector).
2. Perform and measure TAPSE and TA Doppler tissue imaging.
3. Ap4C color flow Doppler of TV from RV apex through TV and entire RA; include interatrial septal interrogation or perform separately.
4. Whether or not tricuspid regurgitation is seen, attempt continuous wave Doppler for peak tricuspid regurgitation velocity and record.
5. Coronal RV view is not routinely mandatory, but if performed should be done if there is concern for pathology in the RV or tricuspid valve.

RA, Right atrium; *RV*, right ventricle; *TV*, tricuspid valve; *TA*, tricuspid annulus; *TAPSE*, tricuspid annular plane systolic excursion.

| BOX 32.10 | Apical Two-Chamber View (Ap2C) |

1. Ap2C, full screen.
2. Ap2C color flow Doppler of the mitral valve from the apex through the mitral valve and entire left atrium.

| BOX 32.11 | Apical Long-Axis View (Ap LAX) |

1. Ap LAX, full screen.
2. Ap LAX color flow Doppler of mitral and aortic valves from apex through valves and beyond.

Subcostal Views

Subcostal Two-Dimensional View. The subcostal view also has multiple windows in the four-chamber and short-axis planes (Fig. 32.40A). Many of the views are only available in the pediatric patient (because of the flexible abdominal muscles). The subcostal four-chamber view is generally useful in many adults and may serve as an alternative view if the apical four-chamber view is unobtainable. The transducer should be placed in the subcostal space and, with moderate pressure applied, angled steeply toward the patient's left shoulder. The plane of the transducer is transverse for visualization of the four chambers of the heart. See Box 32.14 for the subcostal protocol.

It is usually easy to follow the inferior vena cava into the right atrium of the heart. With careful angulation, the interatrial septum may be visualized between the anterior right atrial chamber and the posterior left atrial chamber (Fig. 32.41B–G). It is usually more difficult to open the right ventricular cavity in this view; therefore, no size assessment should be made. This view is usually very good for assessing the presence of pericardial effusion, especially because it surrounds the anterior segment of the right side of the heart.

Subcostal View for Color Flow Mapping. The subcostal long-axis view shows the inferior vena cava inflow pattern as it enters the right atrial cavity. The flow from the hepatic veins appears blue when blood enters the inferior vena cava at the level of the diaphragm throughout diastole and systole. During atrial systole, some retrograde flow is seen as it moves from the right atrium into the inferior vena cava and hepatic veins (see Fig. 32.41). With the transducer angled slightly to the left, pulsatile flow signals through the descending and abdominal aorta may be seen in systole.

In the subcostal short-axis view, the right ventricular outflow tract and pulmonary artery may be demonstrated. The right ventricular outflow tract appears blue as it leaves the right ventricle to enter through the pulmonary cusps. The velocity increases slightly, causing some color change from blue to turquoise and green before returning to blue when it enters the main pulmonary artery. Some aliasing may be experienced as the flow bounces off the tricuspid leaflets and right ventricular walls. Red and yellow flow can be seen arising from the coronary artery along the posterior wall of the right ventricle. Superior vena cava inflow appears as red and orange flow as it enters the right atrium.

Subcostal Window for Spectral Doppler. The subcostal four-chamber view is especially useful in the neonatal and pediatric population because the transducer is placed in the subcostal region, and, with gentle pressure applied, the transducer is angled superiorly to record the four chambers of the heart. In adults with pulmonary obstructive disease, this view is useful because the increased size of the lungs pushes the heart into the view of the transducer without too much pressure on the diaphragm.

In this position, the interatrial and interventricular septa are perpendicular to the transducer, so the presence of a left-to-right defect shows positive high-velocity flow from the

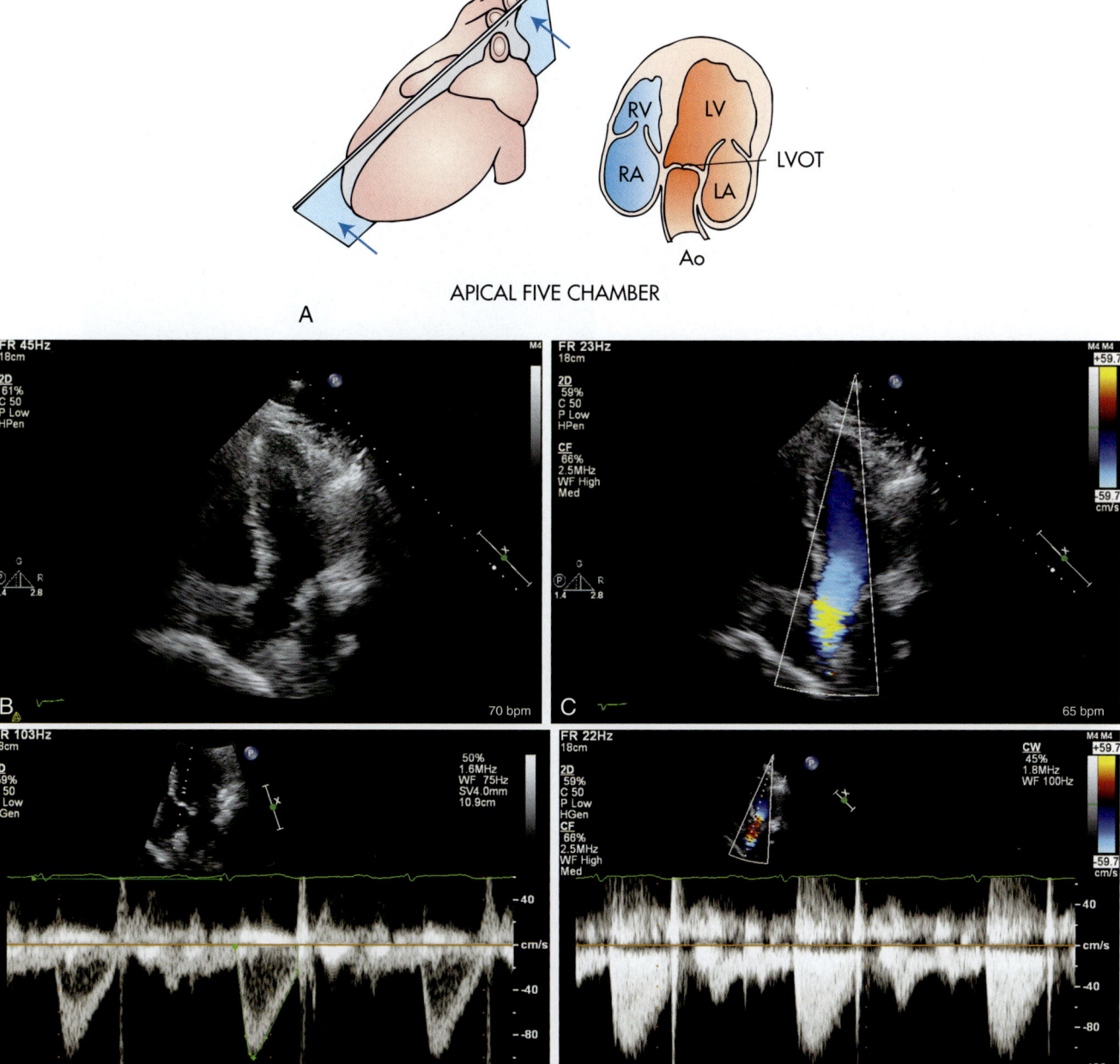

FIG. 32.30 (A) Apical five-chamber view. Anterior angulation from the four-chamber view will demonstrate the left ventricular outflow tract (LVOT) and the ascending aorta (Ao). (B) Midsystolic frame of the LVOT with the aortic cusps open. (C) Color Doppler shows the blue flow leaving the left ventricle (LV) into the ascending aorta. (D) Pulsed wave Doppler taken at the level of the LVOT. (E) Continuous wave Doppler is taken in the ascending aorta. *LA*, Left atrium; *RA*, right atrium; *RV*, right ventricle.

baseline on the spectral display, and the flow is parallel to the beam. A right-to-left flow shows as a negative deflection on the spectral display. This view may also be useful for recording the flow pattern from the pulmonary veins (upper right and left and lower left) when they enter the left atrium.

The superior vena cava flow is shown as a high-pitched, low-velocity, positive deflection from the baseline on the spectral display. The inferior vena cava flow may be recorded as a negative display on the spectral display. A better view of the inferior vena cava flow is made in the subcostal long-axis view through the right lobe of the liver. The inferior vena cava may be well seen as it moves slightly anterior to pierce the diaphragm before it enters the right atrial cavity. This display would project as a low-velocity positive reflection from the baseline.

Suprasternal Views

Suprasternal Two-Dimensional View. In the suprasternal view, the transducer is directed transversely in the patient's

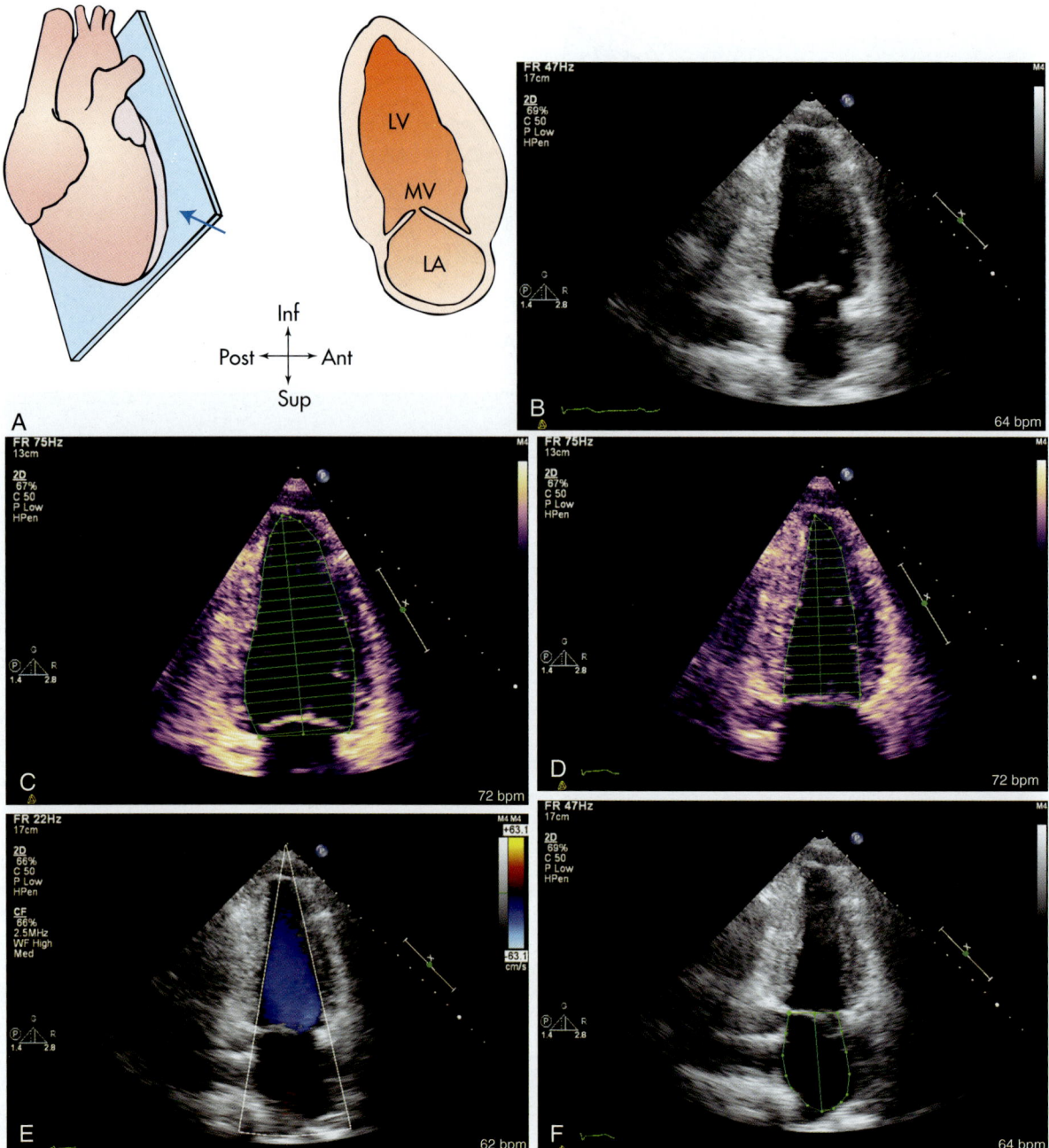

FIG. 32.31 (A–B) Apical two-chamber view. The transducer is rotated 90 degrees from the apical four-chamber view to show only the left ventricle (LV), mitral valve (MV), and left atrium (LA). (C) End-diastolic frame with tracing along the endocardial border. (D) End-systolic frame with tracing along the endocardial border to determine the ejection fraction by method of discs. (E) Color Doppler at end systole shows the blue flow as it leaves the left ventricle into the ascending aorta. (F) tracing of the left atrial diameter.

suprasternal notch and angled steeply toward the arch of the aorta (Fig. 32.42). This view is only useful if the transducer is small enough to fit well into the suprasternal notch. The patient is best prepared if several towels or a pillow is placed under the shoulders. In this position, the patient's neck should flex, avoiding interference with the neck of the transducer and cable. The patient's head should be turned to the right, again to avoid interference with the cable. With careful angulation, the cardiac structures visualized are the aortic arch, brachiocephalic vessels, right pulmonary artery, left atrium, and left main bronchus. This view is especially useful in determining supravalvular enlargement of the aorta, coarctation of the aorta, or dissection of the aorta. See Boxes 32.15 and 32.16 for the suprasternal notch and right parasternal border protocols.

Suprasternal View for Color Flow Mapping. In the suprasternal long-axis plane of the ascending aorta, arch, and descending aorta, flow signals begin as red in the ascending

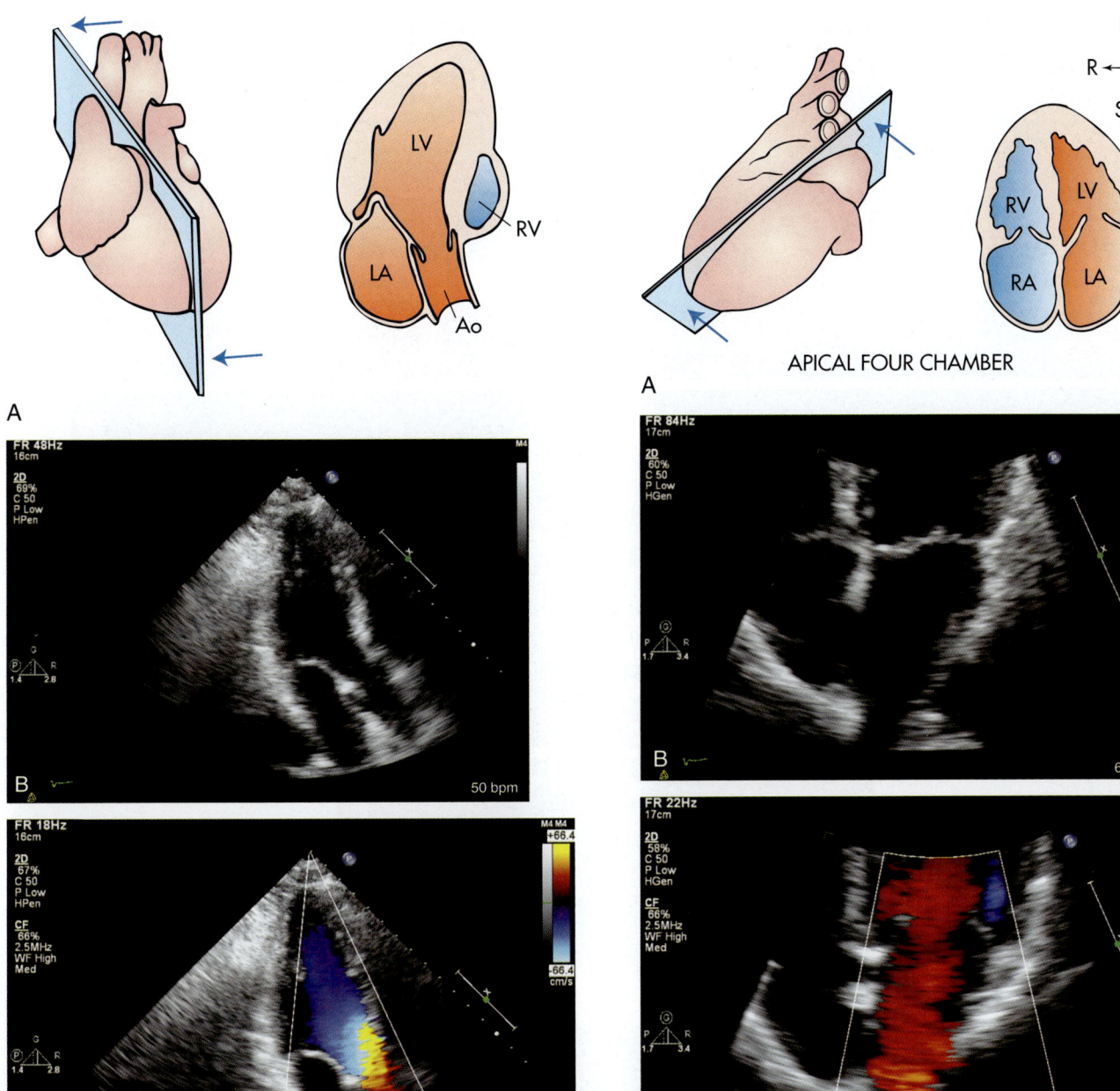

FIG. 32.32 (A) Medial angulation from the two-chamber view will show the left ventricular outflow tract and aorta (Ao). (B) Three-chamber view. The parasternal short-axis and apical two-chamber views are used to show abnormal motion in the posterobasal segment of the left ventricular wall. (C) Color Doppler shows the yellow-red outflow through the aortic leaflets. *LA*, Left atrium; *LV*, left ventricle; *RV*, right ventricle.

FIG. 32.33 (A) Apical four-chamber view. (B) Focus on the left atrium and mitral valve inflow. (C) The pulmonary venous inflow appears as red. *LA*, Left atrium; *LV*, left ventricle; *RA*, right atrium; *RV*, right ventricle.

aorta and turn to blue when flow moves into the arch (some aliasing and reversal of color are seen along this point as the flow bounces off the walls in the arch). When the flow enters the descending aorta, a bright blue color is seen (Fig. 32.43). The atrial and ventricular septa are well seen on this view, and adequate visualization of a possible defect may be made in this imaging plane.

In the short-axis plane, the superior vena cava flow is blue when it enters the right atrium. Flow within the aortic arch and right pulmonary artery is also seen. In some patients, pulmonary venous inflow may be seen in the suprasternal view.

Suprasternal Window for Spectral Doppler. The suprasternal position is used to record velocities in the ascending and descending aorta, right pulmonary artery, superior vena cava inflow, and pulmonary venous return into the left atrium. Initially, the patient's shoulders are elevated by a pillow, the neck is extended, and the transducer is placed in the suprasternal notch with an inferior angulation of the beam.

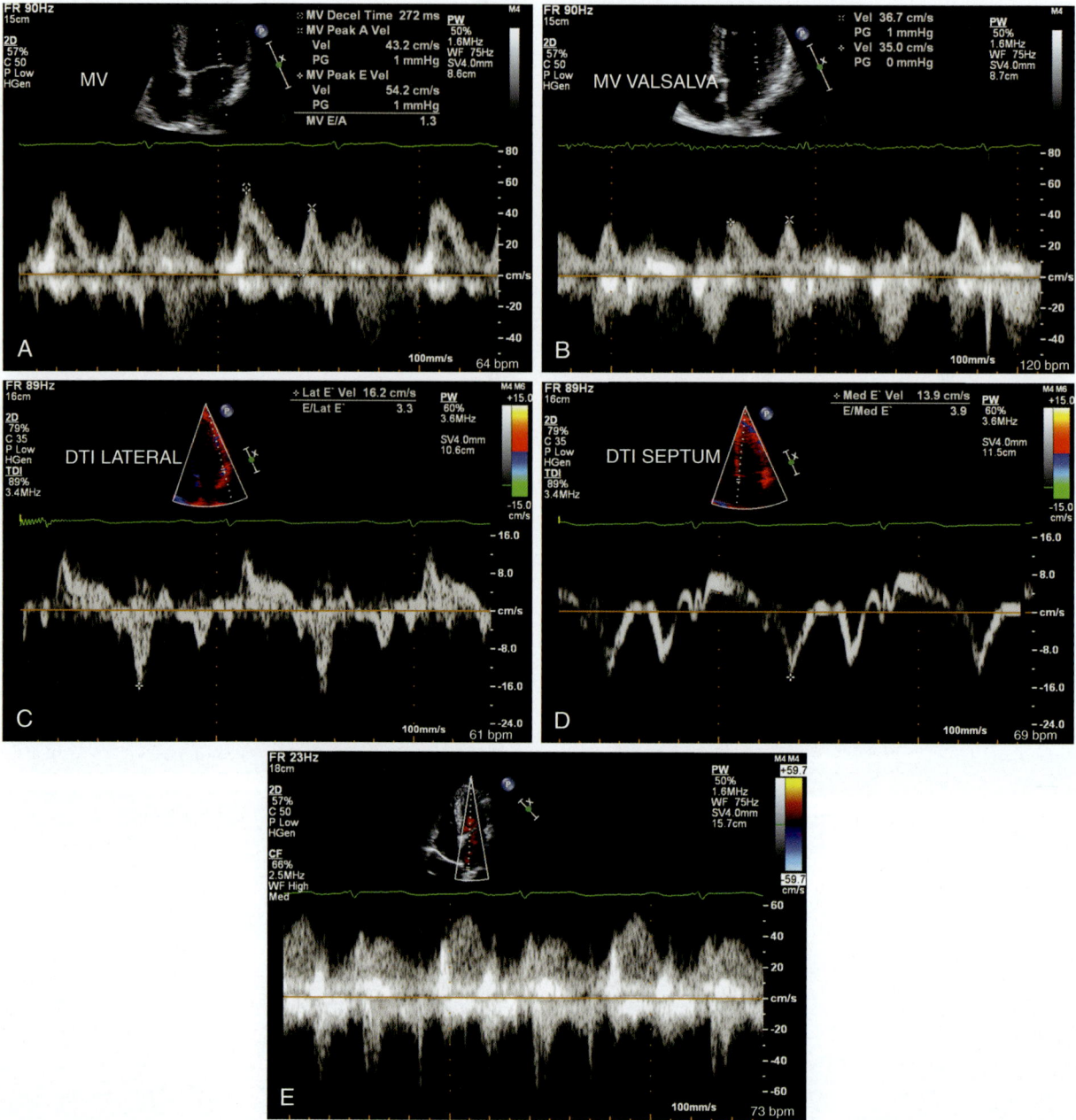

FIG. 32.34 (A) Pulsed wave Doppler of the mitral valve inflow. The initial peak occurs during the rapid-filling phase of diastole. The smaller second peak occurs late in diastole with atrial contraction. (B) The patient should perform a Valsalva maneuver to see if there are changes in the mitral valve inflow pattern. (C–D) Pulsed wave Doppler tissue imaging is recorded from the lateral and septal mitral annulus. The septal velocity (B) is slightly smaller than the lateral wall velocity. (E) Pulsed wave Doppler at the level of the pulmonary veins is taken with the sample volume placed 1 cm into the pulmonary vein. The systolic, diastolic, and aortic regurgitation flow is observed.

The transducer sample volume is placed in the ascending aorta when the walls of the aorta are as nearly perpendicular to the beam as possible. The flow is then parallel to the pulsed Doppler cursor, and a positive deflection with a narrow band of frequencies is shown above the baseline. Careful sweeping back and forth allows the operator to determine the highest velocity possible. The audio sound helps direct the probe to the maximal jet flow. If high velocities are suspected, the continuous wave probe is used.

The spectral tracing from this probe contains a wider range of frequencies with the same peak velocity measurements as the pulsed wave. As the transducer is angled to the left and posterior, velocity from the descending aorta is recorded. Generally, with the pulsed Doppler, the sample volume is placed near the level of the left subclavian artery to record the maximum flow away from the transducer as it flows down the descending aorta to the abdominal aorta (Fig. 32.44E).

The flow pattern of the superior vena cava may be recorded from the suprasternal position while the transducer is directed inferiorly and to the right (medial) of the ascending aorta. Flow away from the transducer is recorded with

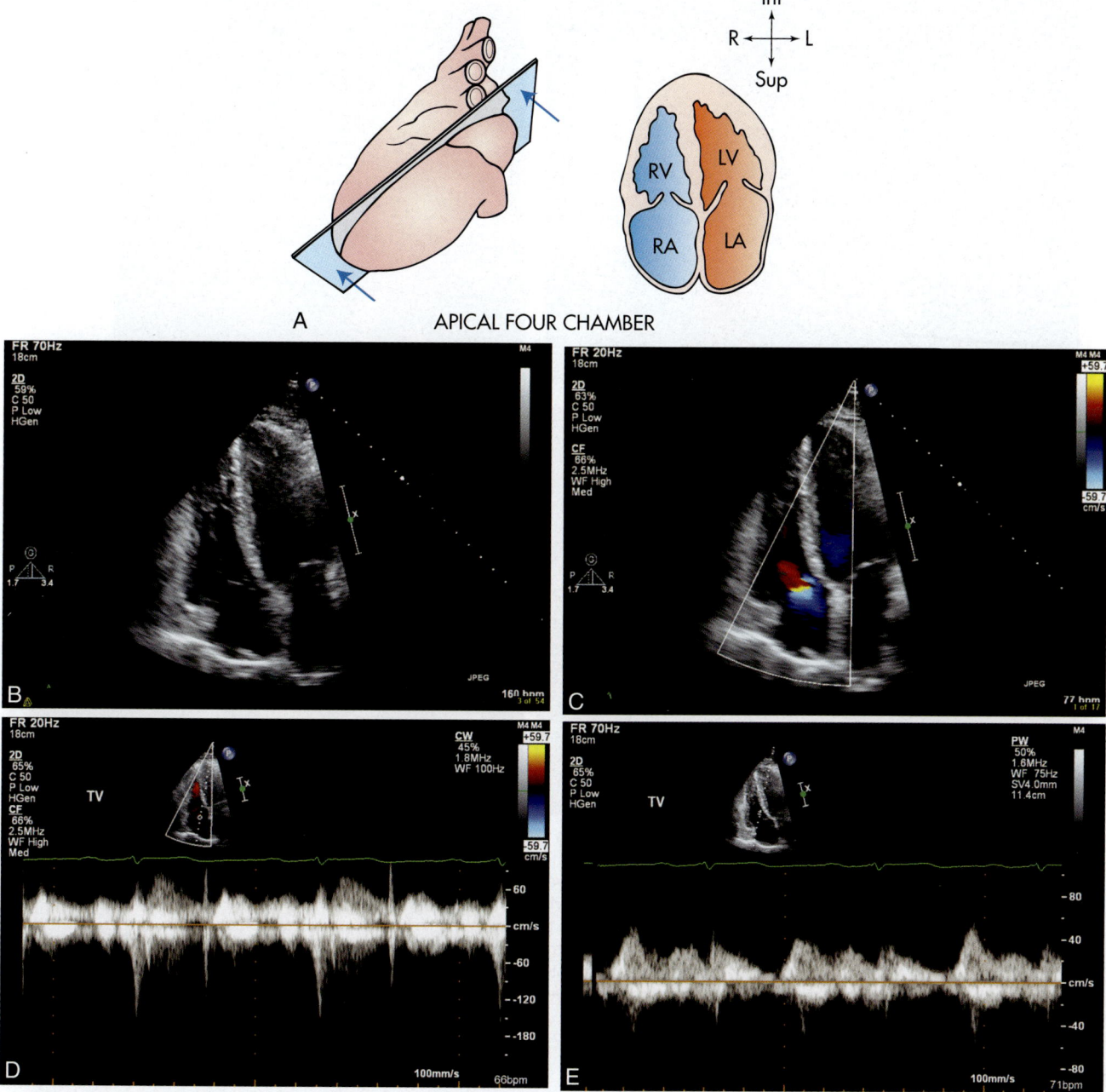

FIG. 32.35 (A) Apical four-chamber view of the right ventricle (RV) and right atrium (RA) at end systole. (B) The transducer is angled medial from the traditional four-chamber view to image the free wall of the right ventricle. (C) Color Doppler at end systole shows a small yellow flow representing trace tricuspid regurgitation. (D) Continuous wave through the tricuspid regurgitation. (E) Pulsed wave through the tricuspid inflow. *LA,* Left atrium; *LV,* left ventricle.

two low-velocity peaks in systole and diastole, which may increase in height during inspiration. This view is useful for recording flow patterns that may be obstructed in the area of the superior vena cava.

The demonstration of the pulmonary veins from the suprasternal notch is more difficult to obtain. With the transducer aligned with the ascending aorta, the beam is angled more posterior to record the dorsal aspect of the left atrial cavity (see Fig. 32.44). The right and left upper pulmonary veins appear as a negative flow away from the baseline, whereas the right and left lower veins appear as a positive flow from the baseline. The velocity is low, with changes in respiration and cardiac motion.

M-MODE IMAGING OF THE CARDIAC STRUCTURES

Table 32.2 and Box 32.17 list normal M-mode measurements for cardiac structures and left ventricular ejection fraction.

Mitral Valve

Echographically, the mitral valve is one of the easiest cardiac structures to recognize. With M-mode, the mitral valve has the greatest amplitude and excursion and can be unquestionably recognized by its "double," or biphasic, kick. This

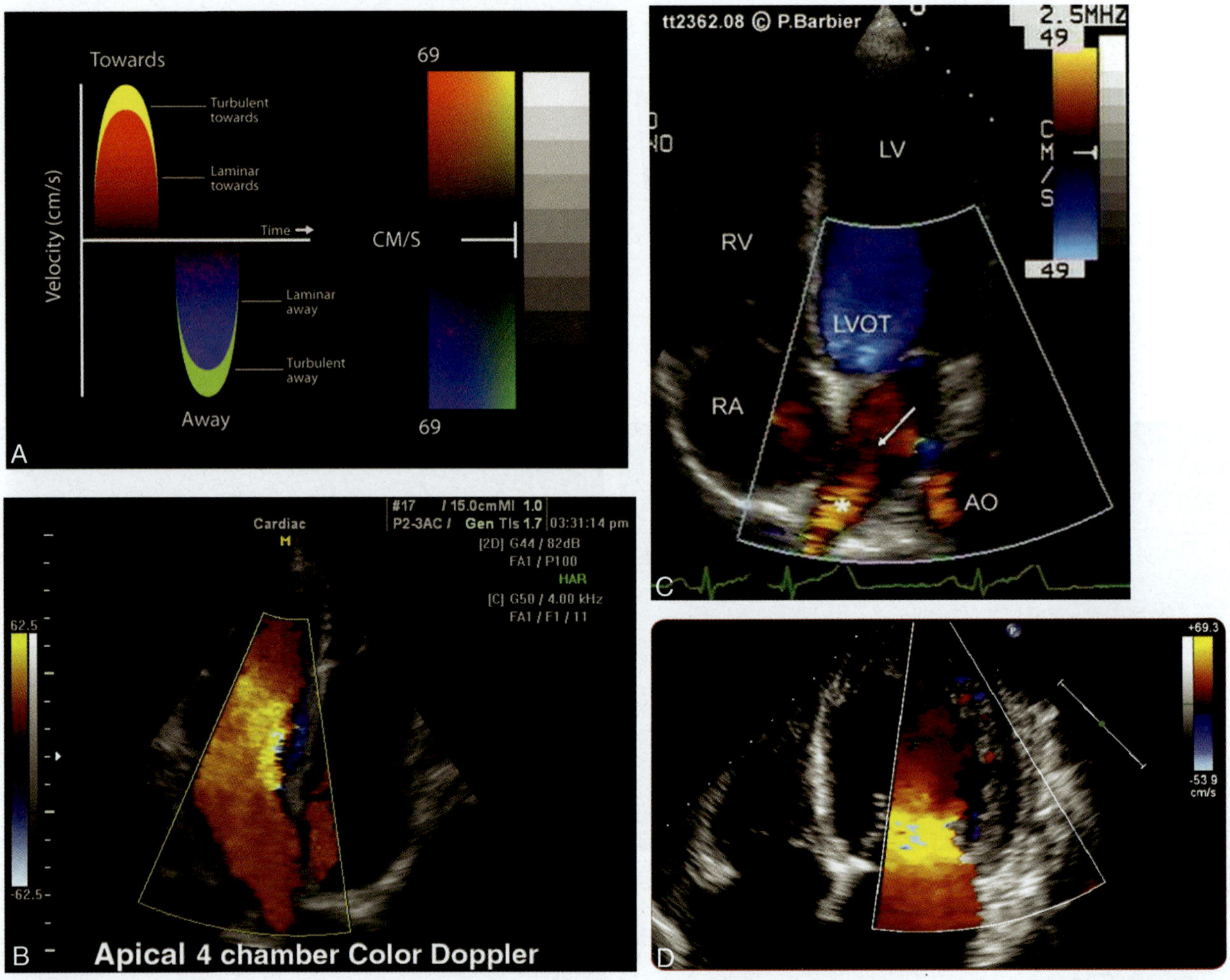

FIG. 32.36 (A) The flow towards the transducer is laminar (red). As the velocity increases, the flow becomes turbulent and turns yellow. In contrast, the laminar flow away from the transducer is blue, while the turbulent flow becomes greenish. (B) The right-side events appear slightly earlier as the tricuspid valve opens before the mitral valve. When blood fills the atrial cavities, it appears red as it flows toward the transducer. (C) Pulmonary venous inflow to the left atrial cavity may be seen in this four-chamber view. Flow from the right and left upper veins appears reddish with some yellow, whereas flow from the lower left pulmonary vein appears blue as it moves away from the transducer. Although the transducer is angled more posterior and medial, inflow from the superior vena cava is red when it enters the medial aspect of the right atrium along the border of the interatrial septum. (D) Diastolic flow through the atrioventricular orifice occurs at a slightly higher velocity, giving rise to changes in colors from red to yellow.

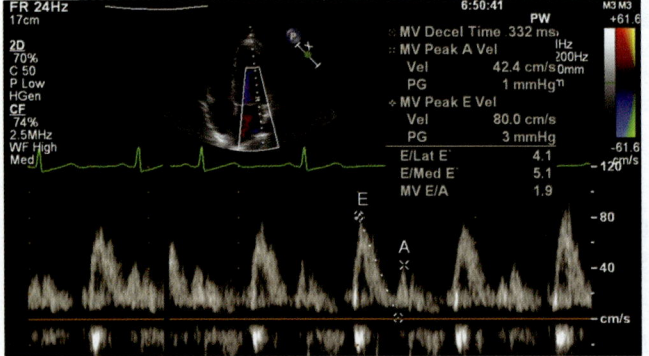

FIG. 32.37 Inflow through the mitral valve leaflets may be recorded by placing the Doppler signal at the level of the tips of the leaflets. The pulsed sample volume may be moved from the tips of the leaflets to the level of the mitral annulus to obtain a clean recording. The normal mitral flow velocity tracing is similar to that found on an M-mode recording. The initial peak occurs during the rapid-filling phase of diastole (E point). The smaller second peak occurs late in diastole, at A (with atrial contraction).

kick is caused by the initial opening of the valve in ventricular diastole and the atrial contraction at end diastole (Fig. 32.45).

As shown in Fig. 32.45, when diastole begins, the anterior mitral leaflet executes a rapid anterior motion, coming to a peak at point E. While the ventricle fills rapidly with blood from the left atrium, the valve drifts closed at point F. The rate at which this movement takes place represents the rate of left atrial emptying and serves as an important indicator of altered mitral function. As the left atrium contracts, the mitral valve opens in a shorter anterior excursion and terminates at point A, which occurs just after the P wave on the electrocardiogram. This motion is followed by a rapid posterior movement from point B to point C, which coincides with the QRS systolic component on the electrocardiogram produced by the left ventricular contractility closing the valve.

BOX 32.12 Spectral Doppler

Every effort should be made to avoid measuring post–ectopic beats. Average 3–10 consecutive beats if frequent ectopy (i.e., bigeminy) or atrial fibrillation/flutter is present. Every effort should be made to align Doppler parallel to flow. Doppler should be recorded at 100 mm/sec sweep speed except when needing to average consecutive beats or when documenting for respiratory variations. Acquire spectral signal at end-expiration or during quiet breathing. All signals should be set with minimal "wall filter" to show signal intersecting with baseline to allow for more accurate time measurements. PW Doppler should be recorded with gains/reject set to show clear envelope. Sample volume size should be between 2 and 5 mm.

1. PW Doppler transmitral flow recording with sample volume at the leaflet; tips during opening; sample volume beyond leaflet tips and into left ventricle makes signal less crisp; MV sample volume at annulus for regurgitant fraction calculations and to better see the "A" kick on the mitral leaflet for the *A duration* measurement.
2. PW Doppler tissue imaging is recorded from lateral and septal mitral annulus; septal velocity should be slightly smaller; use clinical eye if big discrepancy exists.
3. PW Doppler of pulmonary veins with sample volume >1 cm in the pulmonary vein for cleanest signal; signal should be free of MR jet signal and truly reflect pulmonary vein in systole and diastole and aortic regurgitation flow.
4. CW Doppler between MV and LVOT for IVRT; avoid AI and MR signals (PW may be necessary).
5. PW Doppler of MV with Valsalva as needed for differentiation between stage 3 and 4 diastolic dysfunction and stage 2 from normal.
6. PW Doppler of LVOT about 0.5–1.0 cm below AoV; if LVOT obstruction present, show pre-obstruction and post-obstruction Doppler signals.
7. CW Doppler through AoV.

AI, Aortic insufficiency; *AoV*, aortic valve; *CW*, continuous wave; *IVRT*, isovolumic relaxation time; *LVOT*, left ventricular outflow tract; *MR*, mitral regurgitation; *MV*, mitral valve; *PW*, pulsed wave.

BOX 32.13 2D and Doppler Measurements and Calculations

1. LV diastolic and systolic volumes from Ap4C and Ap2C for biplane-MOD EF%. May substitute Ap LAX for Ap2C if Ap2C is technically inadequate. May use Definity to trace volumes. Keep in mind apex does not move inward toward annulus; rather, annulus moves toward apex. This will provide a more accurate LAX length for biplane-MOD. Begin trace at MV annulus and not in LV cavity.
2. LA biplane-MOD volume from Ap4C and Ap2C. May need to optimize a separate image to visualize LA. Exclude LAA, pulmonary vein ostium, and atrial septal anomalies (i.e., aneurysm) from trace. Stop trace at MV annulus (i.e., do not include area under leaflet tips). Correct LAX dimension.
3. RVSP = TR gradient + CVP where CVP equals:
   5 mm Hg if IVC is normal size and collapses ≥ 50% with inspiration
   10 mm Hg if IVC is large and collapses ≤ 50% with inspiration
   15 mm Hg if IVC is large, shows no collapse, and presence of significant TR and RA enlargement
4. Normal RVd2 measurement per ASE poster mandatory for all RV cases. IVC size is <2.2 cm, although athletic individuals are an exception.
5. For all aortic stenosis and prosthetic AoV cases report the following in AoV section of echocardiography report: AoV area by continuity, AoV peak/mean pressure gradient, and dimensionless index. Use the previous echocardiogram's LVOT diameter when present. For prosthetic valves, use preprosthetic valve LVOT diameter when present. Otherwise, LVOT diameters are generally between 1.9 and 2.3 cm. For serial echo comparisons, compare only AoV area changes in interpretation summary section of report.
6. Measure and label MV deceleration time.
7. Measure and label MV E and A waves.

2D, Two-dimensional; *AoV*, aortic valve; *Ap2C*, apical two-chamber view; *Ap4C*, apical four-chamber view; *Ap LAX*, apical long-axis view; *ASE*, American Society of Electrocardiography; *AVA*, aortic valve area; *CVP*, central venous pressure; *EF%*, ejection fraction; *IVC*, inferior vena cava; *LA*, left atrium; *LAA*, left atrial appendage; *LAX*, long-axis view; *LV*, left ventricle; *LVOT*, left ventricular outflow tract; *MOD*, method of discs; *MV*, mitral valve; *RA*, right atrium; *RV*, right ventricle; *RVd2*, right ventricle in diastole; *RVSP*, right ventricular systolic pressure; *TR*, tricuspid regurgitation.

Aortic Valve and Left Atrium

The echoes recorded from the aortic root on M-mode should be parallel, moving anteriorly in systole and posteriorly in diastole. When the transducer is angled slightly medial, two of the three semilunar cusps can be visualized. The right coronary cusp is shown anterior and the noncoronary cusp posterior (Fig. 32.46). When seen, the left coronary cusp is shown in the midline between the other two cusps. The onset of systole causes the cusps to open to the full extent of the aortic root. The extreme force of blood through this opening causes a fine flutter to occur during systole. As the pressure relents in the ventricle, the cusps begin to drift to a closed position until they are fully closed in diastole.

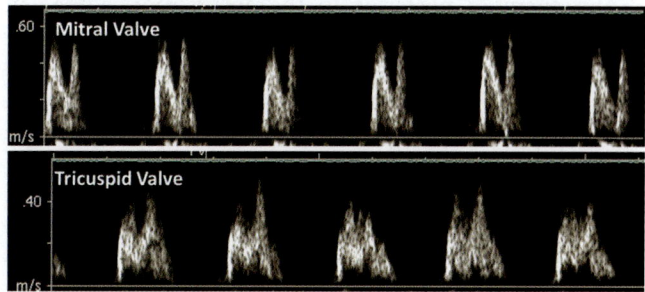

FIG. 32.38 With the transducer position at the level of the leaflets, a pattern similar to mitral valve flow is recorded with two peaks during diastole. The first occurs during ventricular filling and the second with the onset of atrial contraction. The velocity pattern is much lower in the tricuspid valve, with significant respiratory changes that increase during inspiration and decrease during expiration.

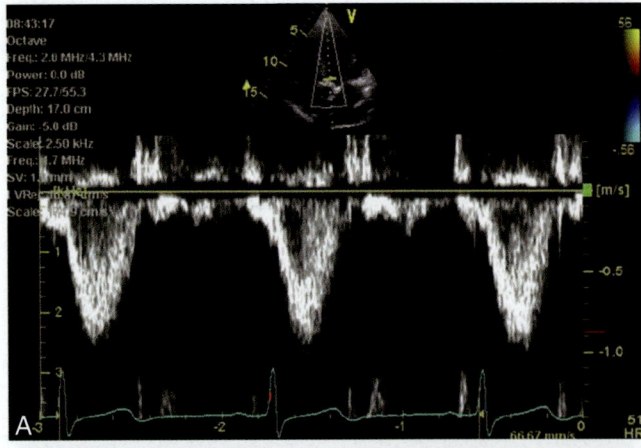

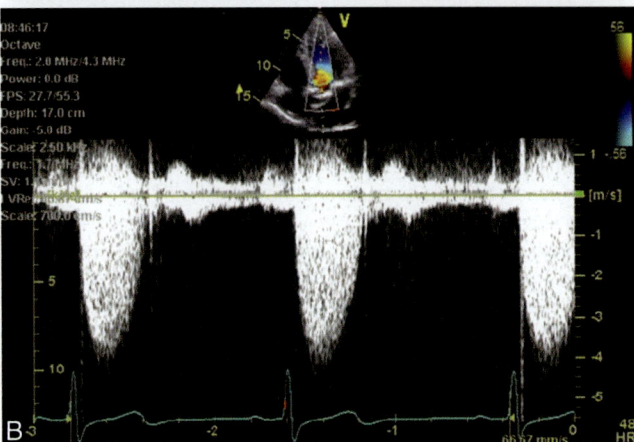

FIG. 32.39 **Spectral Doppler pulsed wave of the aortic valve.** In the apical position, the transducer may be angled slightly anterior or rotated into a long-axis view to record blood flow from the left ventricular outflow tract as it enters the aortic root and ascending aorta. With the pulsed wave sample volume placed just proximal to the aortic root (in the left ventricular outflow tract), the flow is away from the transducer during systole. (A) The spectral pulsed wave display shows a narrow band of frequencies below the baseline. (B) Continuous wave Doppler of the aortic valve is used when velocities exceed 2 m/sec.

The chamber posterior to the aortic root is the left atrium, which can be recognized by its immobile posterior wall. As one sweeps from the mitral apparatus medially and superiorly, the left ventricular wall blends into the atrioventricular groove and finally into the left atrial wall. Thus the sweep demonstrates good contractility in the left ventricle, with anterior wall motion in systole to the atrioventricular area, where the posterior wall starts to move posteriorly in systole, and then to the left atrium, where there is no movement.

Other structures posterior to the left atrial cavity that may lead to confusion in the identification of the left atrial wall are the left atrial appendage and descending aorta. The left atrial appendage may appear prominent posterior to the left atrial wall if there is severe enlargement of the left atrial cavity (especially seen in patients with severe mitral valve disease). The 2D evaluation with the transducer in the apical four-chamber position clarifies the atrial appendage as a separate structure. The descending aorta may also be recognized as a parallel, pulsating, tubular structure posterior to the left atrial cavity. The aorta is not continuous with the left ventricular wall, as is the left atrial wall. Thus the cardiac sonographer should be able to distinguish this echo reflection as normal anatomy.

Interventricular Septum

The septum thickens in systole at the midportion of the ventricular cavity (Fig. 32.47). The measurement and evaluation of septal thickness and motion should be made at the onset of systole at the QRS on the ECG. Normal septal thickness should match that of the posterior left ventricular wall and not exceed 1.2 cm.

Left Ventricle

Correct identification of the left ventricle may be made when both sides of the septum are seen to contract with the posterior heart wall. If the septum is not well defined or does not appear to move well, a more medial placement of the transducer along the sternal border with a lateral angulation may permit better visualization of this structure.

The three layers of the posterior heart wall—the endocardium (inner layer), myocardium (middle layer), and epicardium (outer layer)—should be identified separately from the pericardium (Fig. 32.48). Sometimes it is difficult to separate the epicardium from the pericardium until the gain is reduced. The myocardium usually has a fine scattering of echoes throughout its muscular layer. The endocardium may be a more difficult structure to record because it reflects a weak echo pattern. The chordae are much denser structures than the endocardium. They generally are shown in the systolic segment along the anterior surface of the endocardium. As the ventricle contracts, the endocardial velocity is greater than the chordae tendineae velocity.

Tricuspid Valve

When the transducer has recorded the mitral apparatus, the beam should be angled slightly medially under the sternum to record the tricuspid valve. The normal pattern of the tricuspid valve is very similar to that of the mitral leaflet. It is fairly easy to identify the whipping motion of the anterior valve in systole and early diastole. However, the complete diastolic period reveals the pathologic changes of stenosis and regurgitation; careful angulation may allow this phase to be recorded.

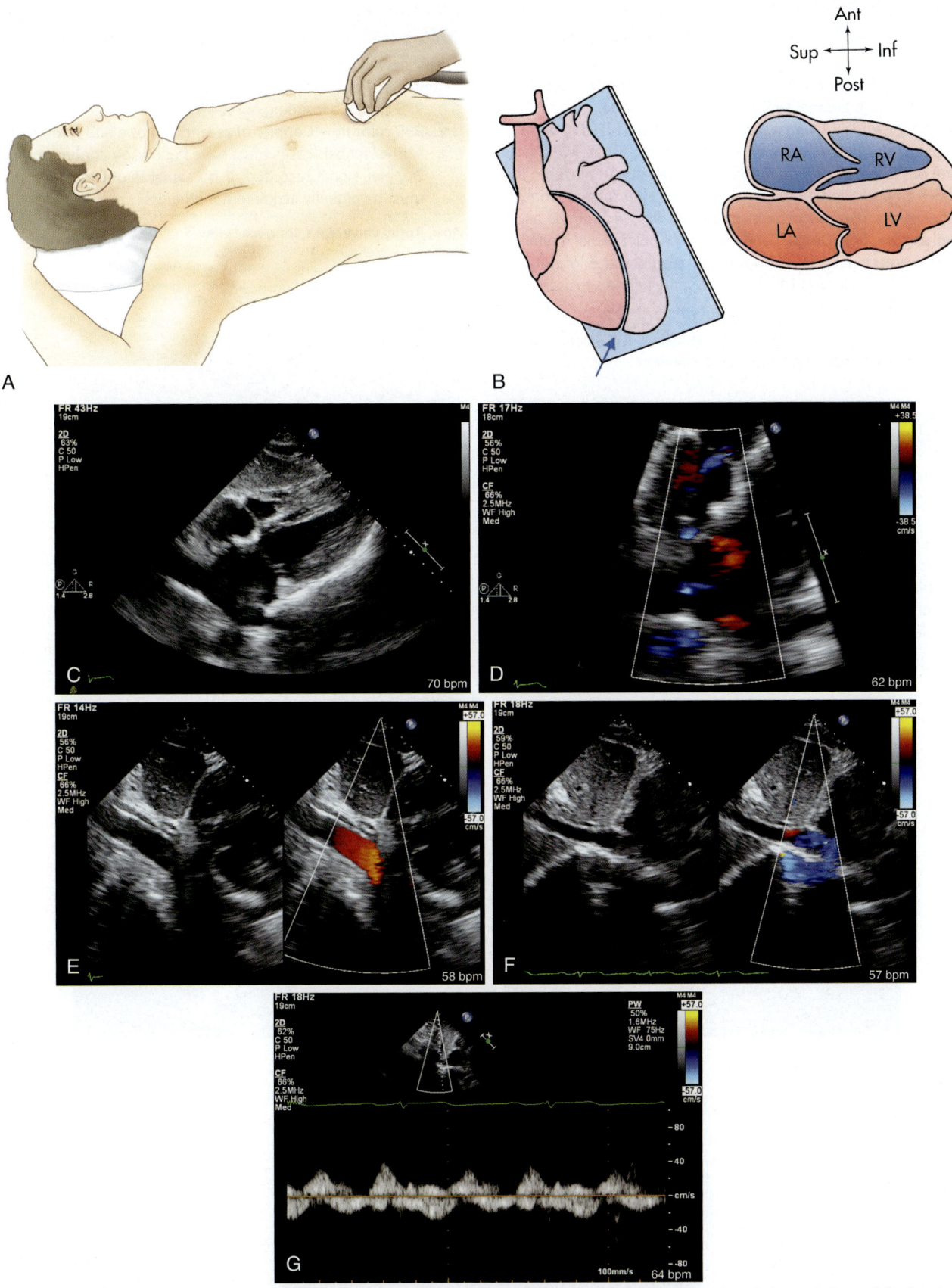

FIG. 32.40 (A) Subcostal four-chamber view. The transducer is placed below the costal margin and angled steeply toward the head. (B) Subcostal view shows the four chambers of the heart and the interatrial and interventricular septa. (C) Subcostal four-chamber view. (D) Color Doppler with low pulse repetition frequency is taken in the subcostal view of the atrial cavities to look for the presence of intra-atrial shunt flow. (E) Subcostal image of the aorta is made with the transducer angled slightly to the left of midline. (F) Subcostal image of the inferior vena cava is made with the transducer midline or slightly angled to the right. (G) Pulsed wave of the hepatic veins. *LA*, Left atrium; *LV*, left ventricle; *RA*, right atrium; *RV*, right ventricle.

BOX 32.14 Subcostal Four-Chamber View (SC4C)

1. SC4C, full screen.
2. SC4C color flow Doppler of interatrial septum; may be necessary to zoom interatrial septum to keep frame rate ≥17 Hz.
3. SC SAX showing IVC and hepatic veins; demonstrate IVC with inspiration or sniff maneuver; hepatic vein interrogation if unsure of TR grade (TDS) or if moderate or greater TR present.
4. Show any additional structures not well interrogated from other views because of poor image quality; include 2D as well as color flow Doppler and spectral Doppler (usual digital format order); deep SC4C toward right pleural space for right pleural effusion for all CHF cardiomyopathy patients to assess for decompensation.

2D, Two-dimensional; *CHF*, congestive heart failure; *IVC*, inferior vena cava; *SAX*, short-axis view; *TR*, tricuspid regurgitation.

BOX 32.15 Suprasternal Notch (SSN)

This view is mandatory for aortic disease, stroke, and patent ductus arteriosus.
1. SSN LAX of aortic arch and descending aorta.
2. SSN LAX color flow Doppler.
3. Aortic stenosis cases must have Pedof AoV continuous wave Doppler signal recorded.

If no signal is obtainable, attempt must be digitally acquired nonetheless.

AoV, Aortic valve; *LAX*, long-axis view.

BOX 32.16 Right Parasternal Border (RPS)

This view is mandatory for aortic stenosis. Patient should be in right lateral decubitus position.
1. RPS LAX of ascending aorta.
2. RPS color flow Doppler of ascending aorta and through AoV.
3. Aortic stenosis cases must have Pedof AoV continuous wave Doppler signal recorded; if no signal is obtainable, attempt must be digitally acquired nonetheless.

AoV, Aortic valve; *LAX*, long-axis view.

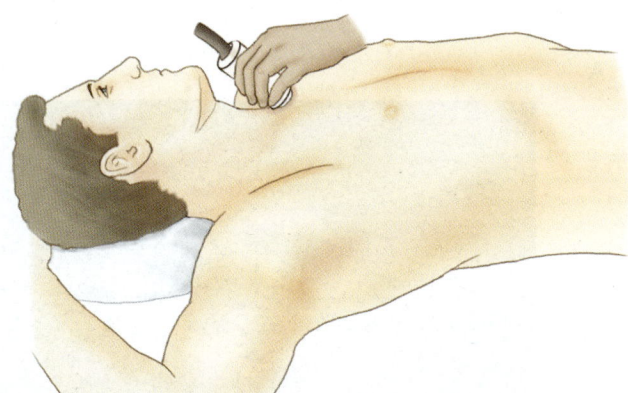

FIG. 32.42 **Suprasternal view.** The transducer is placed in the suprasternal notch and angled steeply toward the arch of the aorta.

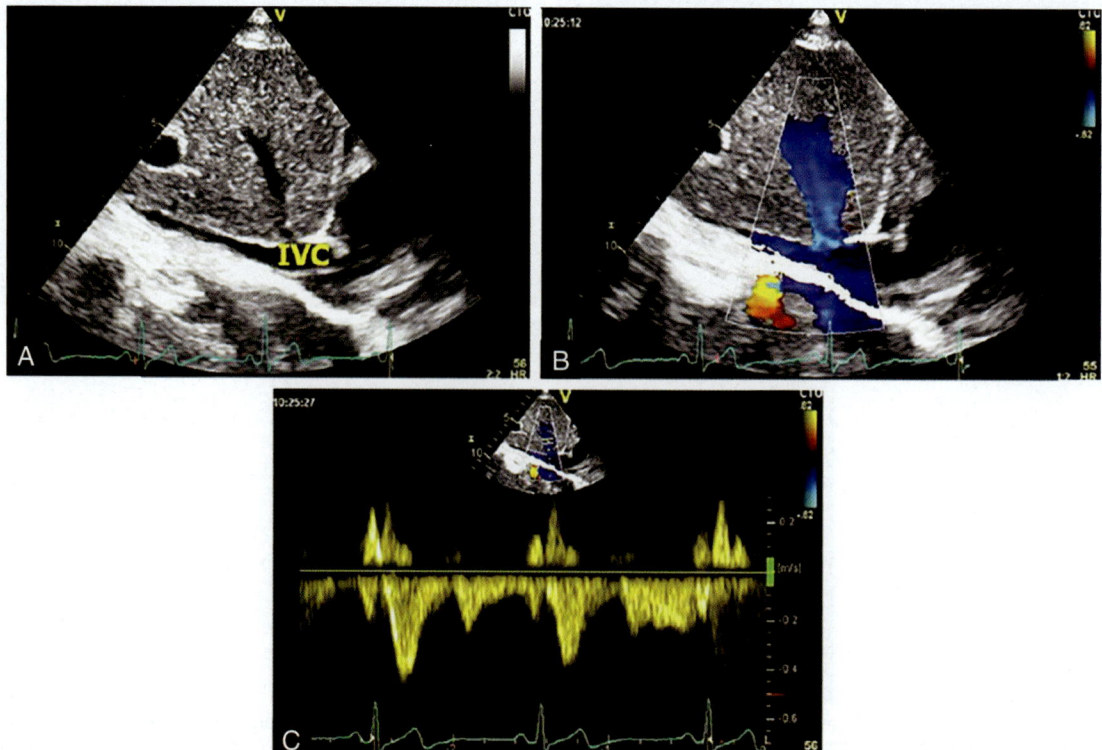

FIG. 32.41 (A) The subcostal long-axis view shows the inferior vena cava inflow pattern as it enters the right atrial cavity. (B) The flow from the hepatic veins appears blue when blood enters the inferior vena cava at the level of the diaphragm throughout diastole and systole. (C) During atrial systole, some retrograde flow is seen as it moves from the right atrium into the inferior vena cava and hepatic veins.

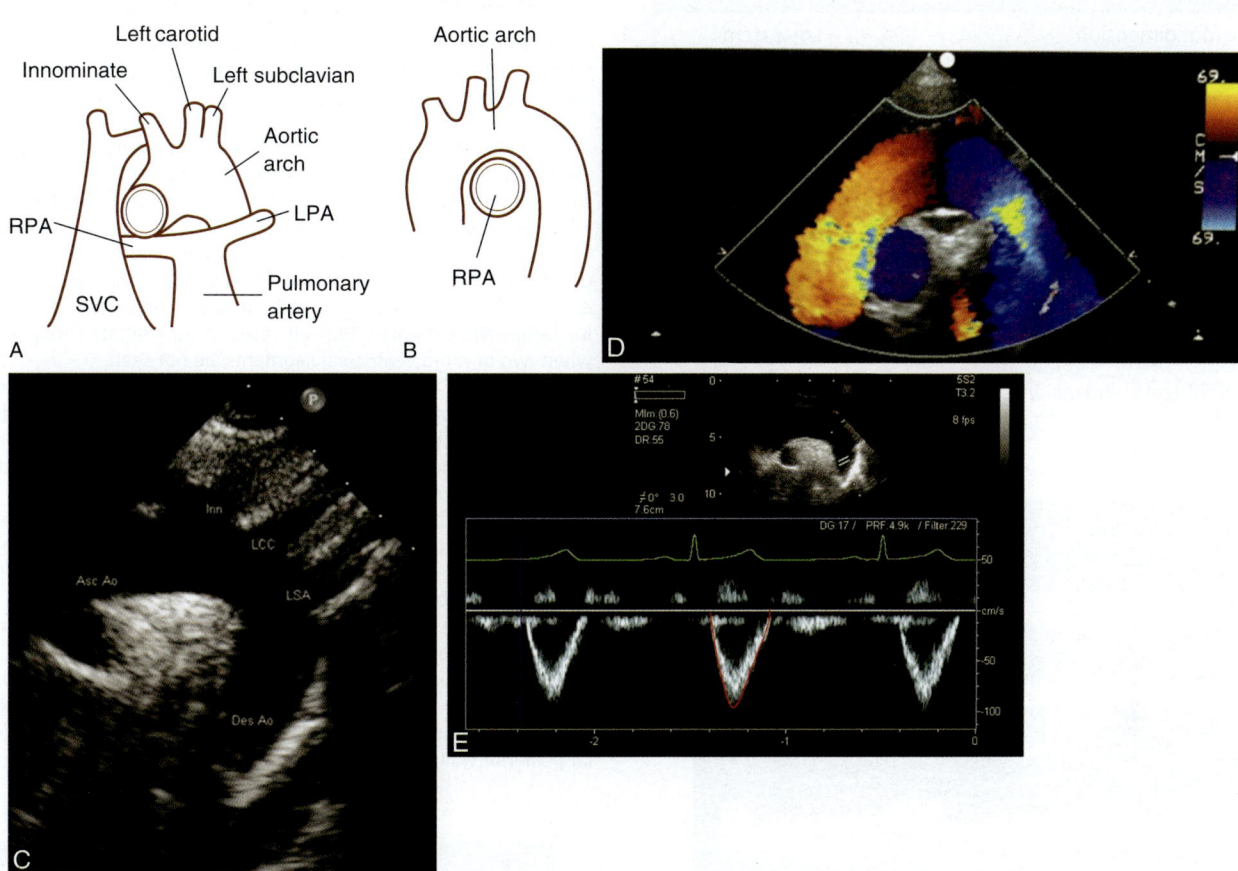

FIG. 32.43 (A) Transverse suprasternal notch view of the superior vena cava (SVC) as it lies to the right of the arch of the aorta. The right pulmonary artery (RPA) is posterior to the arch of the aorta. (B) Longitudinal suprasternal notch view of the ascending aorta and right pulmonary artery. (C) Suprasternal long view of the ascending arch (Asc Ao) and descending aorta (Des Ao). (D) Color Doppler at the level of the arch shows the flow in red in the ascending aorta/arch and blue in the arch/descending aorta. (E) Pulsed wave Doppler of the normal flow in the descending aorta. *Inn*, Innominate; *LCC*, left common carotid; *LPA*, left pulmonary artery; *LSA*, left subclavian artery.

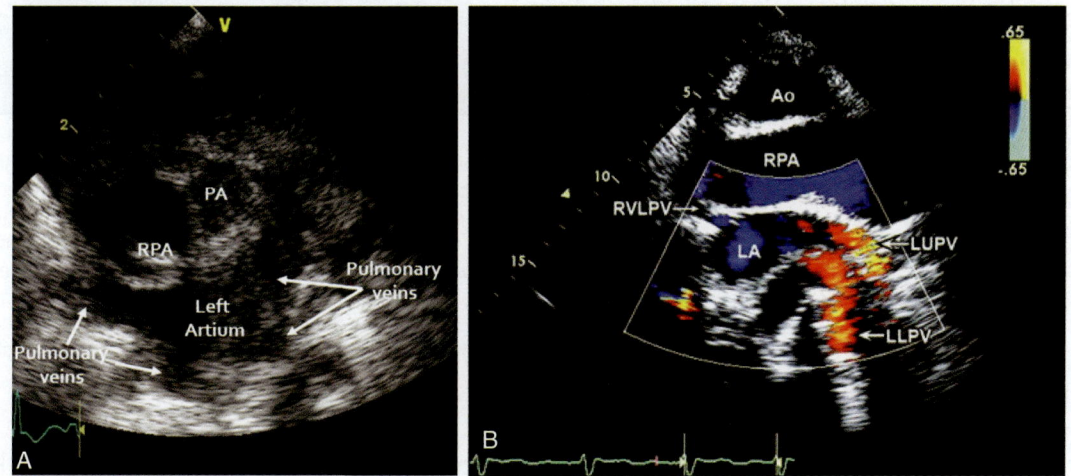

FIG. 32.44 The demonstration of the pulmonary veins from the suprasternal notch is more difficult to obtain. With the transducer aligned with the ascending aorta (Ao), the beam is angled more posterior to record the dorsal aspect of the left atrial cavity. The right and left upper pulmonary veins (RUPV, LUPV) appear as a negative flow away from the baseline, whereas the right and left lower veins (LLPV) appear as a positive flow from the baseline. The velocity is low, with changes in respiration and cardiac motion. *PA*, Pulmonary artery; *RPA*, right pulmonary artery.

TABLE 32.2	Normal M-Mode Measurements
Aortic root dimension	1.9–4.0 cm
Aortic cusp separation	1.5–2.6 cm
Left atrial dimension	1.9–4.0 cm
Mitral valve excursion	1.6–3.0 cm
Left ventricular end-diastolic dimension	3.5–5.7 cm
Left ventricular end-systolic dimension	2.5–4.0 cm
Left ventricular ejection fraction	>55%
Interventricular septal thickness	0.6–1.2 cm
Posterior left ventricular thickness	0.6–1.2 cm
Right ventricular dimension	0.7–2.7 cm

> **BOX 32.17 M-Mode/2D Measurements and Calculations**
>
> If M-mode angles are oblique, measurements should be made using 2D with 2D calipers placed along minor axis. Even if oblique, include M-mode in study for motion of structures.

LVIDd, LVIDs: Measure LVIDs for all patients with moderate or greater aortic insufficiency but do not label; use dropdown in left ventricle size/shape section to report. Include only one EF% on the report. Multiple EF% values on a report are confusing to clinicians. Calculate EF% by biplane-MOD. It is okay to give EF% as range for atrial fibrillation/flutter or frequent ectopy, but range should agree with calculated EF%. Visual estimation of EF% is not recommended and is only used as a last resort for technically extremely difficult cases; echo contrast should be used when two or more ventricular segments are not seen.

IVS, LVPW: The IVS and LVPW should be measured in the parasternal long axis view at end-systole. IVSd measurements may be made from apical four-chamber view when not clearly seen in parasternal long-axis view. It is okay to measure (but do not label) discrete septal thickening separately so as not to misrepresent left ventricle mass.

LA, AVD: The left atrium is measured in the parasternal long axis view at end-systole. Aortic root measurement is performed at sinus of Valsalva. Omit left atrium single plain dimension from report if it does not agree with left atrium biplane volume.

Ascending Aorta: Ascending aorta measurement is done at largest minor axis seen (not necessarily at sinotubular junction).

2D, Two-dimensional; *EF%*, ejection fraction; *IVSd*, interventricular septum in diastole; *LVIDd*, left ventricular internal dimension in diastole; *LVIDs*, left ventricular internal dimension in systole; *LVPW*, left ventricular posterior wall; *MOD*, method of discs.

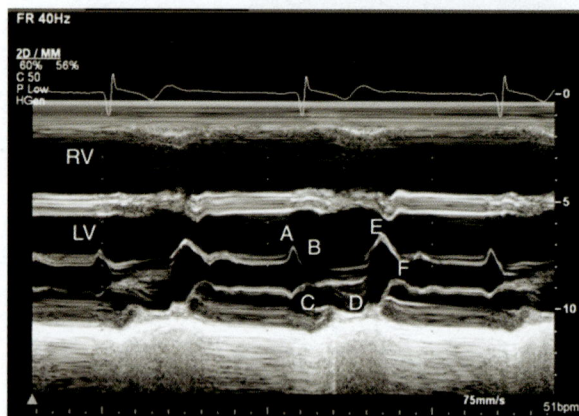

FIG. 32.45 With M-mode, the mitral valve has the greatest amplitude and excursion and can be unquestionably recognized by its "double," or biphasic, kick. This kick is caused by the initial opening of the valve in ventricular diastole and the atrial contraction at end diastole. When diastole begins, the anterior mitral leaflet executes a rapid anterior motion, coming to a peak at point E. While the ventricle fills rapidly with blood from the left atrium, the valve drifts closed at point F. The rate at which this movement takes place represents the rate of left atrial emptying and serves as an important indicator of altered mitral function. As the left atrium contracts, the mitral valve opens in a shorter anterior excursion and terminates at point A, which occurs just after the P wave on the electrocardiogram. This motion is followed by a rapid posterior movement from point B to point C, which coincides with the QRS systolic component on the electrocardiogram produced by the left ventricular contractility closing the valve. *LV*, Left ventricle; *RV*, right ventricle.

Pulmonary Valve

The anterior aortic root forms the posterior boundary of the pulmonary valve area. The appearance of the pulmonic cusp is similar to the aortic cusp and requires very slight angulations of the beam to demonstrate fully. With 2D capabilities, the optimal view is generally a high-parasternal short-axis view with a slight angulation of the beam toward the left shoulder.

At the beginning of diastole, the pulmonary valve is displaced downward and is represented anteriorly on the ultrasound recording. The low transducer position with upward

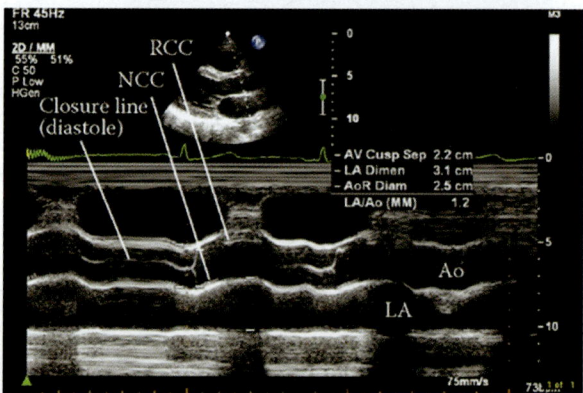

FIG. 32.46 The echoes recorded from the aortic root on M-mode (parasternal long-axis view) should be parallel, moving anteriorly in systole and posteriorly in diastole. When the transducer is angled slightly medial, two of the three semilunar cusps can be visualized. The right coronary cusp is shown anterior and the noncoronary cusp posterior. The onset of systole causes the cusps to open to the full extent of the aortic root. The extreme force of blood through this opening causes a fine flutter to occur during systole. As the pressure relents in the ventricle, the cusps begin to drift to a closed position until they are fully closed in diastole.

beam angulation, together with the vertical inclination of the pulmonary ring, results in the examination of the valve from below. All elevations of the pulmonary valve in the stream of flow are represented as posterior movements on the echo. Likewise, downward movements are represented by anterior cusp positions on the trace.

CHAPTER 32 Introduction to Echocardiographic Techniques, Terminology, and Tips

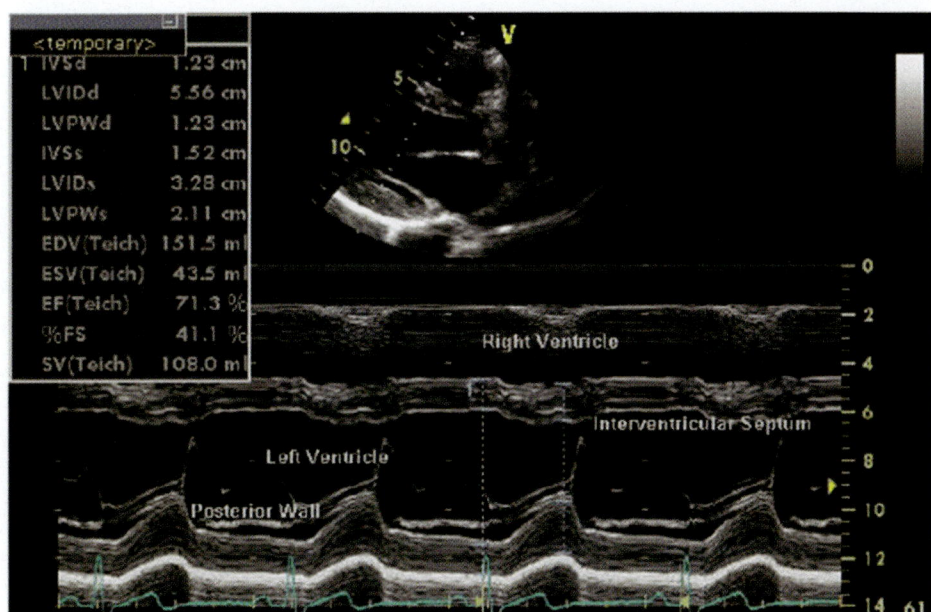

FIG. 32.47 *The septum thickens in systole at the midportion of the ventricular cavity.* The measurement and evaluation of septal thickness and motion should be made at the onset of systole (at the QRS).

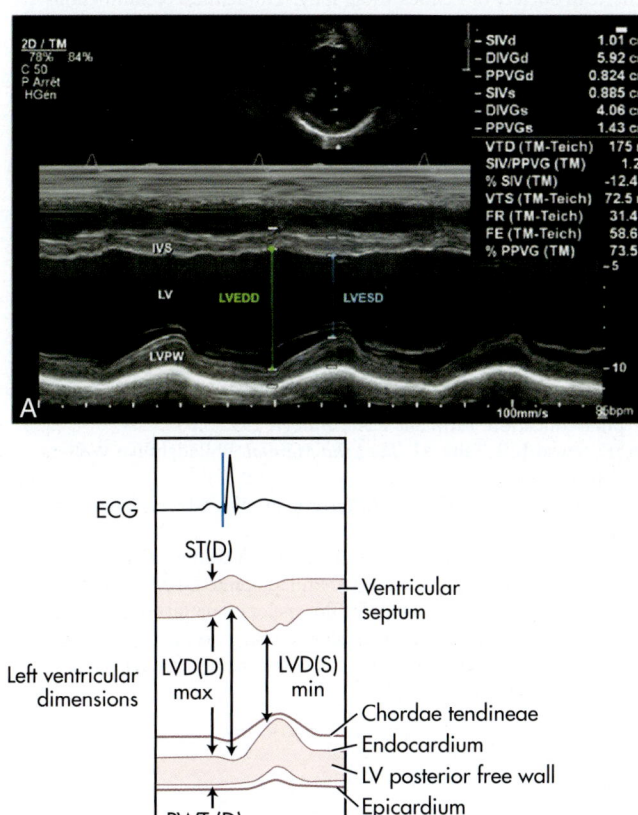

FIG. 32.48 Measurements of the interventricular septum (IVS), left ventricle (LV) in diastole (LVDD) and systole (LVDS), and the posterior wall (LVPW) are made. M-mode recording in the left ventricular cavity demonstrates the layers of the posterior heart wall: endocardium, myocardium, epicardium, pericardium, and chordae tendineae. The distinction between the endocardium and chordal structures may be made by assessing the velocity of the two structures. The normal endocardial velocity is always much greater than the chordal velocity. *LVEDD,* lLeft ventricular end diastolic diameter; *LVESD,* left ventricular end systolic diameter.

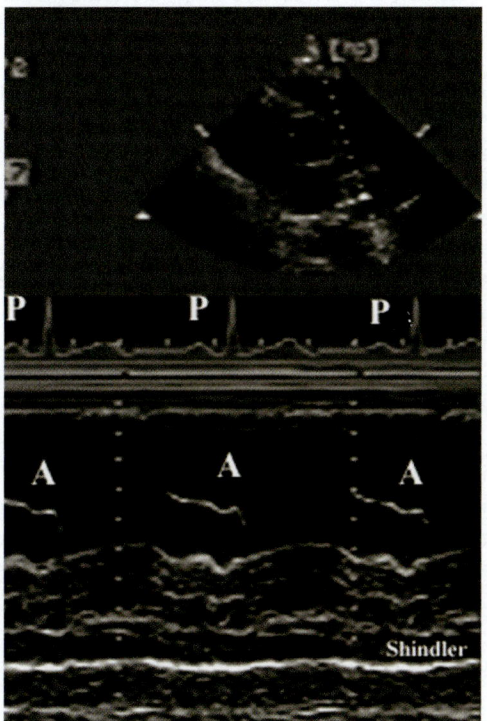

FIG. 32.49 *M-mode recording of the posterior cusp of the pulmonary valve.* The cusp opens in systole and closes in diastole. *A,* A wave of the pulmonic cusp; *P,* P wave of electrocardiogram; *PLPV,* posterior leaflet of the pulmonary valve.

The pulmonary valve begins to move posteriorly (points e to f) in a gradual manner as the right ventricle fills in diastole (Fig. 32.49). Atrial systole elevates the valve and produces a 3- to 7-mm posterior movement a (dip). The valve completes the opening (points *b* and *c*), and, at the *c* to *d* point, the valve moves upward with ventricular systole.

Key Pearls

- Review American Society of Echocardiography guidelines and for direction on protocol development for your laboratory.
- The "cardiac window" may be considered that area on the anterior chest where the heart is just beneath the skin surface, free of lung interference, and is usually found between the third and fifth intercostal spaces, slightly to the left of the sternal border.
- The color flow mapping (CFM) examination is performed with the conventional 2D examination. The advantage of CFM is its ability to rapidly investigate flow direction and movement within the cardiac chambers. Flow toward the transducer is recorded in red, and flow away from the transducer is blue; this is denoted on the color bar on the right upper side of the image. As the velocities increase, the flow pattern in the variance mode turns from red to various shades of red, orange, and yellow; or from blue to blue-green before it aliases.
- Doppler echocardiography is established as a valuable noninvasive tool in clinical cardiology to provide hemodynamic information about the function of the cardiac valves and chambers of the heart.
- A pulsed wave transducer is constructed with a single crystal that sends bursts of ultrasound at a rate called the pulsed repetition frequency. The transducer receives sound waves backscattered from moving red blood cells during a limited time between transmitted pulses.
- The continuous wave probe differs from the pulsed wave probe in that it is able to both send and receive sound. One crystal continuously emits sound; the other receives sound as it is backscattered to the transducer.
- The best Doppler signals are obtained when the ultrasound beam is parallel or nearly parallel to the flow of blood.
- The Pedof continuous wave (non-imaging) probe is smaller than the 2D imaging probe and thus has advantages in obtaining a good Doppler study. This small diameter allows greater flexibility to angle between small rib interspaces or obtain signals from the suprasternal notch or right parasternal border.
- The spectral analysis waveform allows the sonographer to store a graphic display of what the audio signal is recording because it provides a representation of blood flow velocities over time. The velocity on the vertical axis is measured in centimeters per second or meters per second, whereas time is shown on the horizontal axis.
- The protocol for the evaluation of cardiac structures begins with the parasternal long- and short-axis views, followed by the apical four-chamber, long-axis, and two-chamber views. The subcostal and suprasternal views complete the study. The sonographer should acquire the respective cine loop(s) for 2D and color flow Doppler and acquire the representative still frames for M-modes and PW/CW Doppler. The color Doppler sector should be long, spanning the entire cardiac image from top to bottom. This sector should be narrow enough to obtain the frame rate (FR) ≥ 17 Hz.
- M-mode recording should be obtained for the mitral valve, aortic valve, and the left ventricle.

REFERENCES

American Society of Echocardiography: Guidelines: recommendations for cardiac chamber quantification by echocardiography in adults: an update from the American Society of Echocardiography and the European Association of Cardiovascular Imaging. *JASE*. 2015;28:1–39.

American Society of Echocardiography: Guidelines for the echocardiographic assessment of the right heart in adults. *JASE*. 2010;23: 685–713.

American Society of Echocardiography: Guidelines: recommendations for quantification of Doppler echocardiography. *JASE*. 2002;15: 167–184.

American Society of Echocardiography: Guidelines: current and evolving echocardiographic techniques for the quantitative evaluation of cardiac mechanics: ASE/EAE consensus statement on methodology and indications. *JASE*. 2011;24:277–313.

Garner CJ, Brown S, Hagen-Ansert S. Guidelines for cardiac sonographer education. *J Am Soc Echocardiogr*. 1992;5:635.

Oh JK, Seward JB, Tajik AJ. *The Echo Manual*. Philadelphia: Wolters Kluwer; 2018.

Otto CM. *Textbook of Clinical Echocardiography*. ed 6 Philadelphia: Elsevier; 2018.

Otto CM, Bonow R. *Valvular Heart Disease: A Companion to Braunwald's Heart Disease*. ed 5. Philadelphia: Elsevier; 2020.

Reynolds T, Appleton CP. Doppler flow velocity patterns of the superior vena cava, inferior vena cava, hepatic vein, coronary sinus, and atrial septal defect: a guide for the echocardiographer. *J Am Soc Echocardiogr*. 1991;4:503.

CHAPTER 33

Introduction to Clinical Echocardiography: Left-Sided Valvular Heart Disease

Sandra L. Hagen-Ansert

OBJECTIVES

On completion of this chapter, you should be able to:
- Define the characteristics and causes of mitral regurgitation
- Know how to calculate the proximal isovelocity surface area method
- Describe the common causes of mitral stenosis
- Explain the causes of aortic regurgitation
- List the echocardiographic features of acute versus chronic aortic regurgitation
- State the three types of aortic stenosis and their echocardiographic features
- Explain how to calculate the aortic valve area
- Define *aortic aneurysm*
- State the difference between a true aneurysm and a pseudoaneurysm
- Describe the echocardiographic findings in aortic dissection

OUTLINE

Left-Sided Valvular Heart Disease 953
Mitral Valve Disease 953
   Mitral Regurgitation 953
   Mitral Stenosis 957
Aortic Valve Disease 963

Aortic Insufficiency 963
Aortic Stenosis 966
Technical Considerations and Pitfalls in Doppler Measurements 970
Aortic Abnormalities 971

Aortic Aneurysm 971
Aortic Atherosclerosis 974
Penetrating Aortic Ulcer 977
Intramural Hematoma 977
Aortic Tumors 978

KEY TERMS

Aortic insufficiency/regurgitation
Aortic stenosis
Aortic valve area (ARA)
Bicuspid aortic valve
Deceleration time (DT)
Dissection
Estimated regurgitant orifice area (EROA)

Mitral regurgitation
Mitral stenosis
Mitral valve area (MVA)
Percutaneous mitral balloon valvuloplasty (PBV)
Pressure half-time (PHT)
Proximal isovelocity surface area (PISA) method

Pseudoaneurysm
Transvalvular aortic valve replacement (TAVR)
Velocity-time interval (VTI)
Vena contracta

LEFT-SIDED VALVULAR HEART DISEASE

This chapter focuses on left-sided valvular heart disease, namely mitral regurgitation, mitral stenosis, aortic valve insufficiency, and aortic stenosis, as well as a brief discussion of aortic abnormalities. The normal anatomy of the valves has been presented in Chapter 32.

MITRAL VALVE DISEASE

Recall that the mitral apparatus consists of two leaflets (anterior and posterior), the annulus, chordae tendineae, and papillary muscles (Fig. 33.1). The anterior and posterior leaflets are pliable, with chordae tendineae attached to the tips of the leaflets. The chordae tendineae are attached to the anterior and posterior papillary muscles that are attached to the left ventricular myocardium. The mitral leaflets open in diastole and close in systole. The thickness of the leaflets should measure less than 4 mm. The anterior and posterior leaflets are further classified according to their scallop location (Fig. 33.2).

Mitral Regurgitation

Mitral regurgitation is defined as the systolic retrograde flow from the left ventricle into the left atrium. This occurs when there is dysfunction or altered anatomy of the mitral annulus,

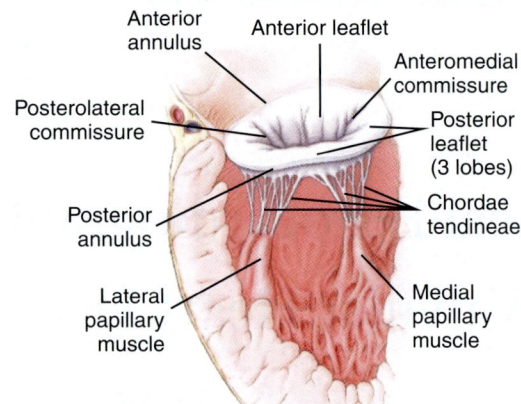

FIG. 33.1 The mitral apparatus is comprised of two leaflets (anterior and posterior), anterior and posterior annulus, posterolateral and anteromedial commissure, chordae tendineae, and lateral and medial papillary muscles.

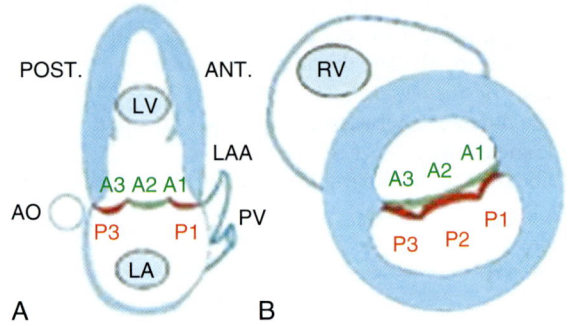

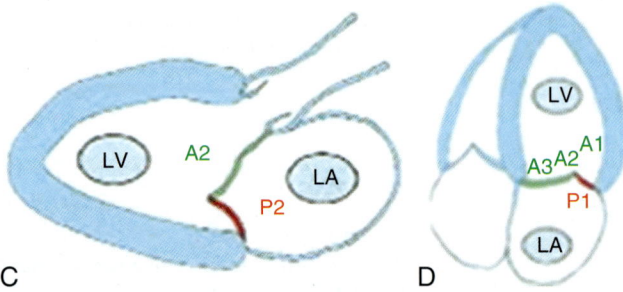

FIG. 33.2 The anterior and posterior leaflets are further classified according to their scallop location. The anterior leaflets are classified as A1 (lateral), A2 (mid), and A3 (medial). The posterior leaflets are classified as P1 (lateral), P2 (mid), and P3 (medial). (A–B) Two-chamber view. (C) Parasternal long-axis view. (D) Four-chamber view. *AO,* Aorta; *LA,* left atrium; *LAA,* left atrial appendage; *LV,* left ventricle; *PV,* pulmonary veins; *RV,* right ventricle.

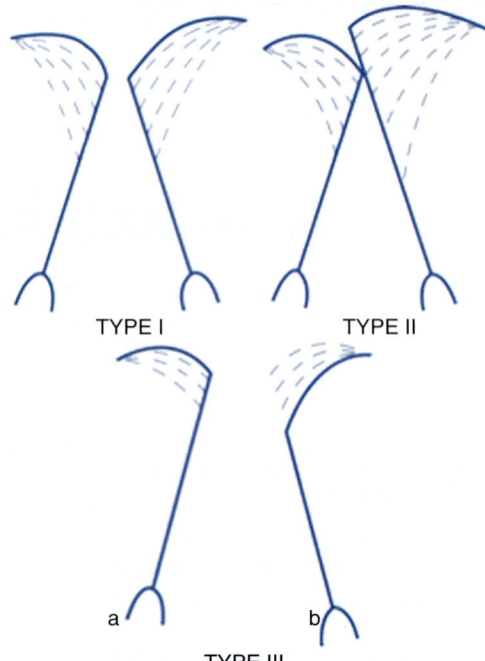

FIG. 33.3 The functional classification of mitral regurgitation is known as Carpentier's classification with three specific types. Type I shows normal leaflet motion with the mitral regurgitation due to annular dilation, perforation, or cleft; type II shows excessive leaflet motion due to mitral valve prolapse or chordal rupture; and type III shows restricted leaflet motion (two forms, *a* and *b*) due to rheumatic heart disease or dilated cardiomyopathy.

the mitral leaflets, the chordae, the papillary muscles, or the left ventricular myocardium. Mitral regurgitation occurs secondary to the reduction or elimination of the normal systolic coaptation between the anterior and posterior mitral leaflets. If the left atrium or ventricle is dilated, annular dilation may occur, which may result in poor mitral leaflet coaptation. Calcification of the mitral annulus also may cause mitral regurgitation.

Various diseases that may affect the mitral leaflets, such as myxomatous disease, rheumatic disease, endocarditis, Marfan syndrome, infiltrative diseases, and systemic inflammatory disorders, may also alter the normal coaptation of the mitral leaflets, which results in regurgitation.

The functional classification of mitral regurgitation is known as Carpentier's classification with three specific types: type I shows normal leaflet motion with the mitral regurgitation due to annular dilation, perforation, or cleft; type II shows excessive leaflet motion due to mitral valve prolapse or chordal rupture; and type III shows restricted leaflet motion due to rheumatic heart disease or dilated cardiomyopathy (Fig. 33.3).

Causes of mitral regurgitation include leaflet and annulus disorders, defective tensor apparatus, and alterations of left ventricular and left atrial size and/or function. The severity of mitral regurgitation is variable, ranging from tenting of the leaflets with left ventricular dilation and dysfunction to mitral valve prolapse or flail leaflet (Fig. 33.4). When the chordal structure is disrupted, a flail leaflet is displaced into the left atrial cavity with mitral regurgitation (Box 33.1).

The determination of the severity of mitral regurgitation requires a combination of both two-dimensional (2D) echocardiography and Doppler evaluation. The sonographer should assess the structural appearance of the valve, the size of the left atrium and ventricle, and the function of the left ventricle and quantify the flow velocity of the regurgitant jet and pulmonary vein with pulsed wave (PW) and continuous wave (CW) Doppler (Fig. 33.5). Color flow Doppler is useful to determine the direction of the jet, the number of jets present, the width of the vena contracta, and the **proximal isovelocity surface area (PISA) method** to calculate the effective regurgitant orifice area to determine regurgitant volume and fraction (Fig. 33.6).

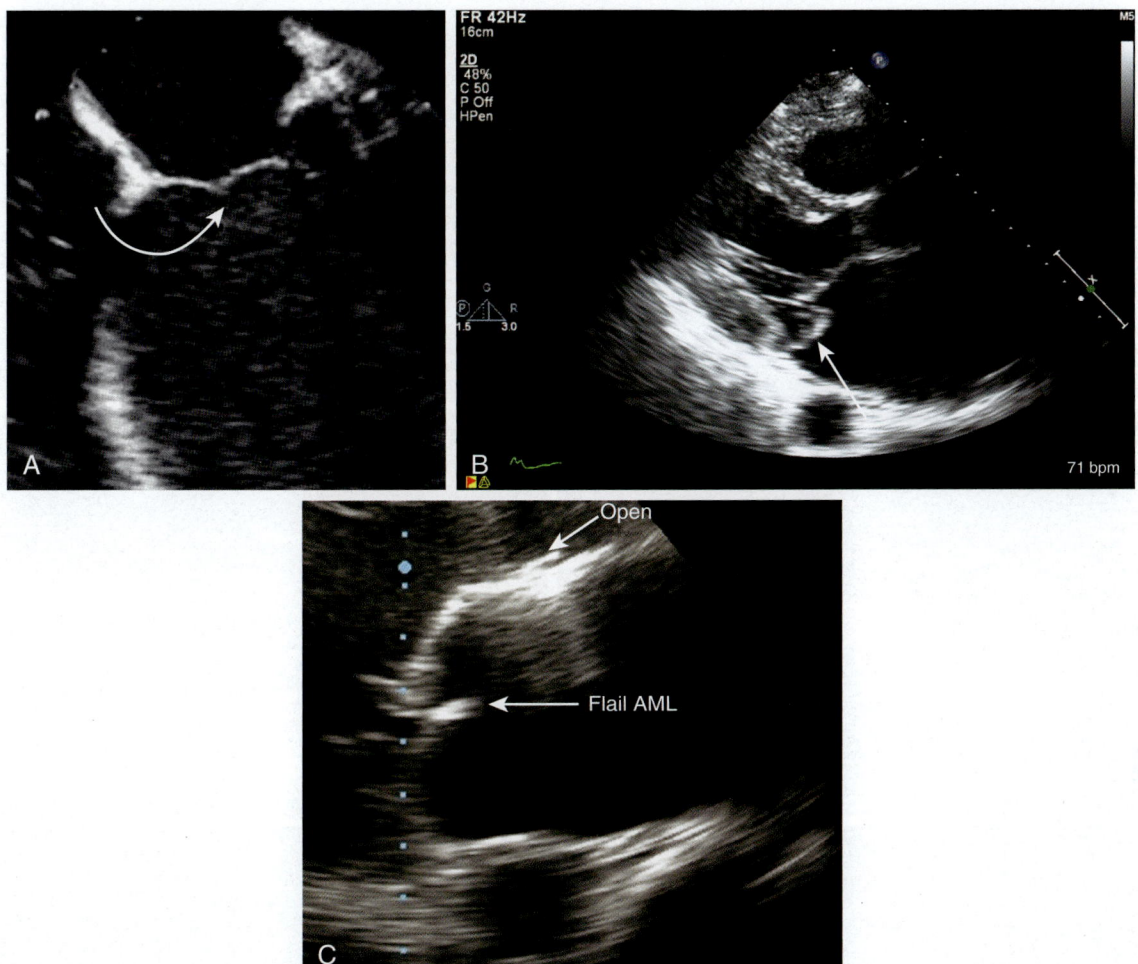

FIG. 33.4 (A) Tenting of the mitral leaflets *(arrow)*. (B) Mitral valve prolapse of the posterior leaflet *(arrow)*. (C) Flail anterior leaflet of the mitral valve (AML).

BOX 33.1 Causes of Mitral Regurgitation

Leaflet and Annulus Disorders
Myxomatous degeneration (mitral valve prolapse)
Flail leaflet
Mitral annulus calcification
Infective endocarditis
Rheumatic heart disease
Congenital abnormalities (cleft, double orifice)
Rare causes: tumor, lupus, connective tissue disease, endomyocardial fibrosis

Defective Tensor Apparatus
Ruptured chordae tendineae
Papillary muscle abnormalities

Alterations of LV and LA Size and/or Function
LA enlargement
Dilated LV
Hypertrophic cardiomyopathy

LA, Left atrium; *LV*, left ventricle.

The **vena contracta** width (Fig. 33.7) should be measured in the parasternal long-axis view at the narrowest portion of the regurgitant jet, just after the orifice. This correlates with the width of the regurgitant orifice and the severity of mitral regurgitation (Box 33.2).

The PISA or flow convergence method to calculate regurgitant orifice area is based on the continuity equation and properties of flow dynamics. Flow accelerates proximal to a narrowed orifice and forms concentric shells of increasing velocity and decreasing hemispheres. As the velocity exceeds the Nyquist limit (aliasing velocity), there is an abrupt change in color. This is seen as a distinct colored hemisphere with color flow Doppler. Per the continuity equation, blood flow at the surface of this hemisphere is the same as the flow through the regurgitant orifice.

To measure the **estimated regurgitant orifice area (EROA)** by the PISA method, these steps are recommended:

1. Center the mitral valve and apply color flow Doppler. Use the apical four-chamber view that shows the convergence zone optimally.
2. Zoom in on the flow convergence area on the ventricular side of the mitral valve, and adjust the Nyquist limit to obtain a hemispheric flow convergence area.

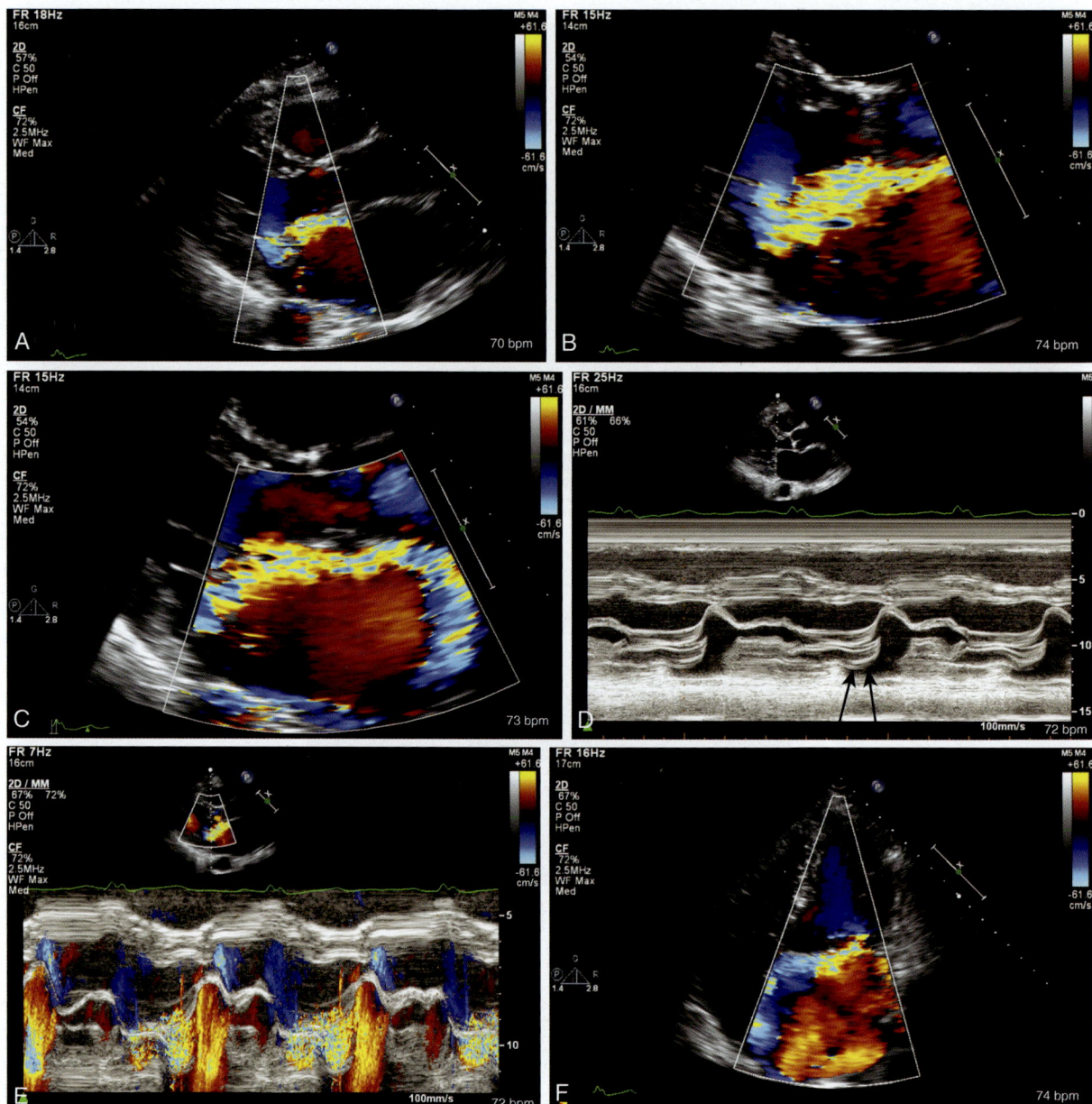

FIG. 33.5 (A) Parasternal long-axis view (PLAX) shows the anterior direction of the mitral regurgitation. (B) Zoom PLAX of the mitral regurgitation. (C) The regurgitant jet flows to the base of the atria. (D) M-mode demonstrating the midsystolic prolapse of the posterior leaflet mitral valve *(arrow)*. (E) M-color Doppler of the regurgitant jet. (F) Four-chamber view of the posterior-directed jet.

3. Measure the distance between the edge of the hemisphere where color flow Doppler abruptly changes colors to the valve orifice; this is the radius of the hemisphere (r).
4. Obtain CW signal of mitral regurgitation jet and measure the peak velocity; this is the mitral regurgitation peak velocity.
5. Calculate EROA using the following formula:

$$\text{EROA} = 2\pi r^2 \times (\text{Alias velocity} / \text{Mitral regurgitation peak velocity})$$

The limitations of the PISA method are that it is inaccurate when the orifice is nonspherical, the flow convergence zone is nonhemispheric due to eccentric jets, and when multiple jets or regurgitant orifices are present.

The regurgitant volume and fraction can be measured using the continuity equation at the mitral inflow and left ventricular outflow tract. The mitral inflow equals the left ventricular outflow unless there is mitral regurgitation or **aortic insufficiency (AI)**. The regurgitant volume equals the mitral inflow minus left ventricular outflow. In patients with severe mitral regurgitation, the regurgitant volume is greater than 60 mL, and the regurgitant fraction is greater than 50%.

Quantification of mitral regurgitation by CW Doppler will display severe regurgitation to produce higher intensity Doppler envelopes with high flow velocities. On the other hand, PW Doppler of the mitral valve inflow will show a dominant E wave peak velocity with a short **deceleration time (DT)** due to the elevated left atrial pressure. If the E point is less than the A point, the mitral regurgitation is probably not severe. This cannot be used if mitral stenosis is present.

Analysis of the pulmonary vein flow into the left atrium with PW Doppler may show systolic flow blunting or reversal

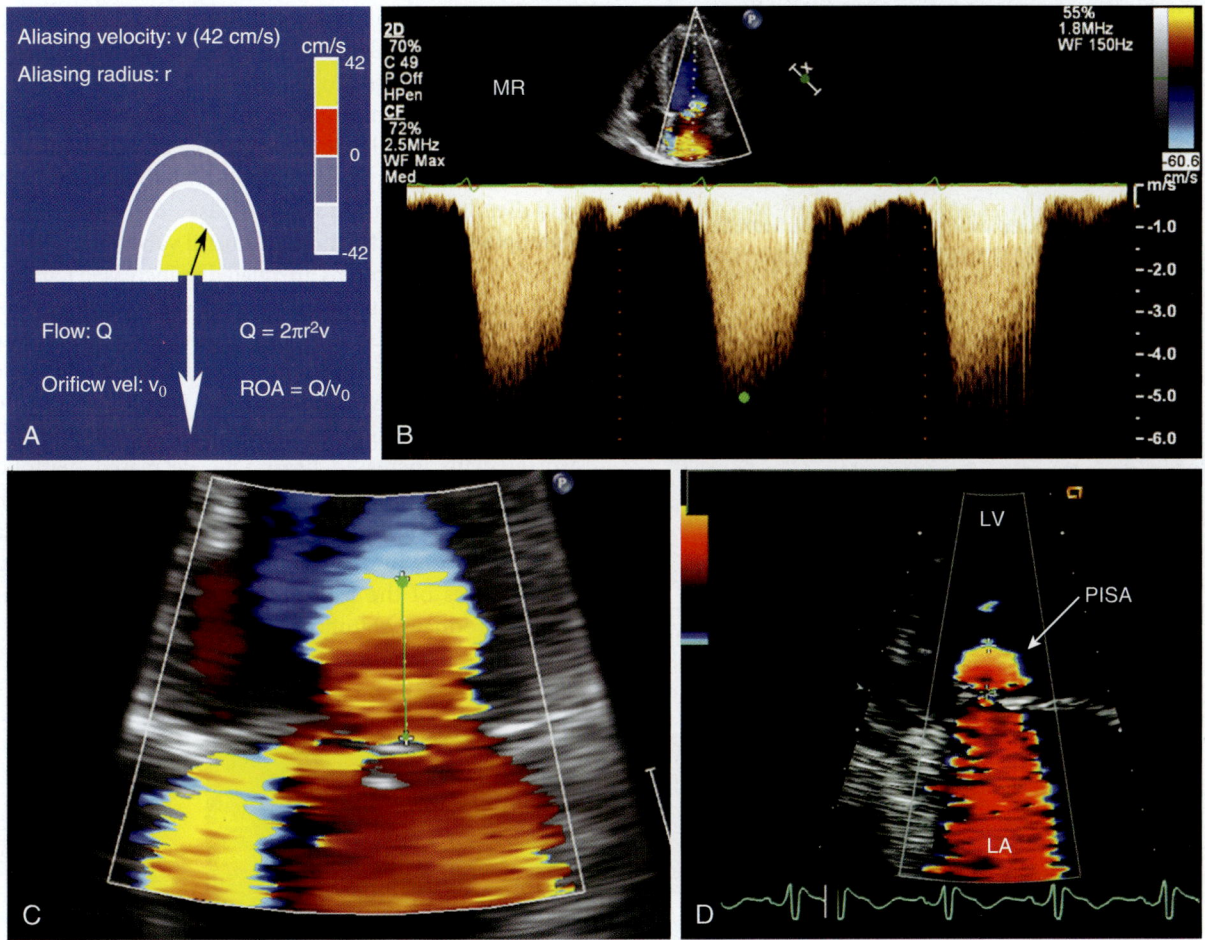

FIG. 33.6 (A) Proximal isovelocity surface area (PISA) method: flow at the surface of the hemisphere equals flow through the regurgitant orifice. (B) Measurement of the mitral regurgitant jet with continuous wave Doppler. (C–D) Measure the hemisphere of the PISA. *LV*, Left ventricle; *MV*, mitral valve.

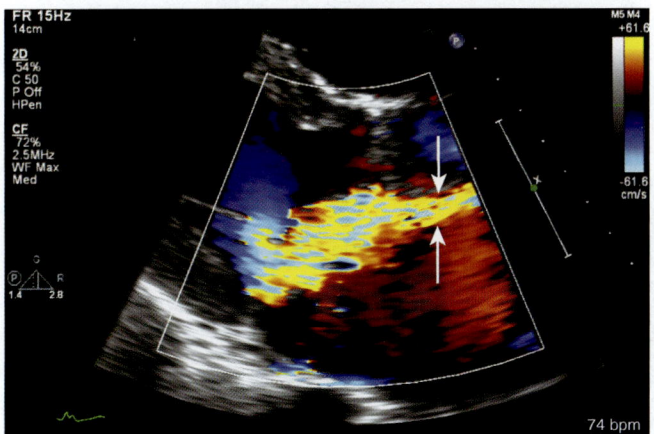

FIG. 33.7 The vena contracta should be measured in the parasternal long-axis view at the narrowest portion of the regurgitant jet, just after the orifice *(arrows)*.

BOX 33.2	Vena Contracta Width

Mild mitral regurgitation: <0.3 cm
Moderate mitral regurgitation: 0.30–0.69 cm
Severe mitral regurgitation: >0.7 cm

due to the mitral regurgitation jet and elevated LA pressure. The blunting of the systolic component of the pulmonary venous inflow indicates moderate mitral regurgitation. The systolic flow reversal indicates severe mitral regurgitation. It is useful to map the regurgitant jet with color Doppler to see if it travels into the pulmonary vein (Fig. 33.8).

Mitral Stenosis

The two common causes of mitral stenosis are rheumatic fever and degenerative **mitral stenosis**. The most frequent valvular complication of rheumatic fever is the development of mitral stenosis. The inflammation from rheumatic fever causes the valves to thicken and eventually calcify, thus causing restriction of blood flow through the mitral leaflets. There is commissural fusion, chordal shortening and fusion, and thickening of the mitral leaflets at the tips; these conditions lead to restriction of leaflet motion. The development of mitral stenosis usually has a slow, stable course in the early years, followed by progressive acceleration later in life. Once the patient develops symptoms, it can take up to a decade before the symptoms become disabling.

Degenerative mitral stenosis is secondary to mitral annular calcification, which is associated with advanced age,

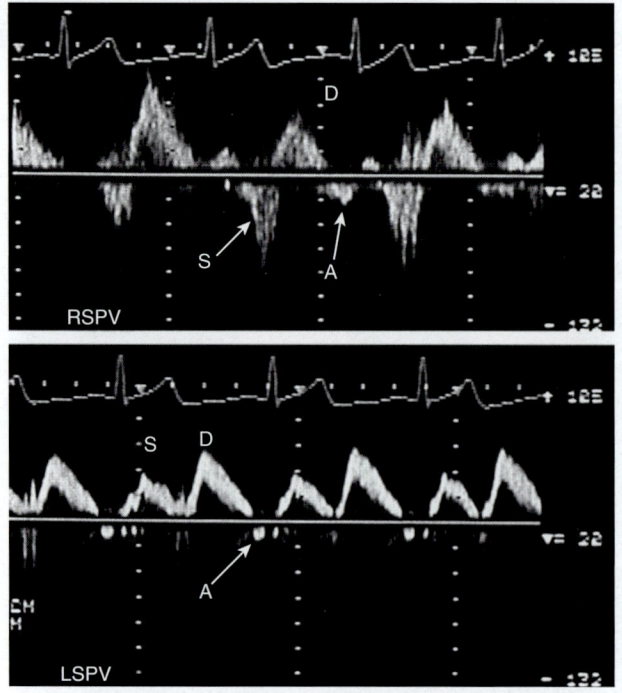

FIG. 33.8 The blunting of the systolic component of the pulmonary venous inflow indicates moderate mitral regurgitation. The systolic flow reversal indicates severe mitral regurgitation. *LSPV*, Left superior pulmonary vein; *RSPV*, right superior pulmonary vein.

hypertension, atherosclerosis, and renal disease/dialysis. In degenerative mitral stenosis, the sonographer may find annular calcification, valve thickening, and calcification at the base of the leaflets leading to restriction of leaflet mobility.

Other uncommon causes include congenital malformation of the mitral leaflets, infiltrative diseases, inflammatory conditions (e.g., systemic lupus and rheumatoid arthritis), and diet drug–induced valve disease.

Pathophysiology. The normal **mitral valve area (MVA)** is 4 to 6 cm². Patient symptoms are related to increased left atrial pressure and dyspnea and usually occur when the MVA is less than 1.5 cm². This reduced valve area leads to decreased diastolic flow into the left ventricle, causing elevation of the left atrial pressure and pulmonary venous pressure, which leads to pulmonary edema and right-sided heart failure. The patient's symptoms worsen with increased heart rate, decreased diastolic filling time, and loss of atrial contraction, known as atrial fibrillation.

Rheumatic heart disease is the most common cause of mitral stenosis and results in leaflet thickening beginning at the edges of the leaflets and fusion of the commissures, which produces significant narrowing of the mitral orifice (Fig. 33.9). In addition, there may be subvalvular involvement with calcification and thickening of the chordal apparatus. In

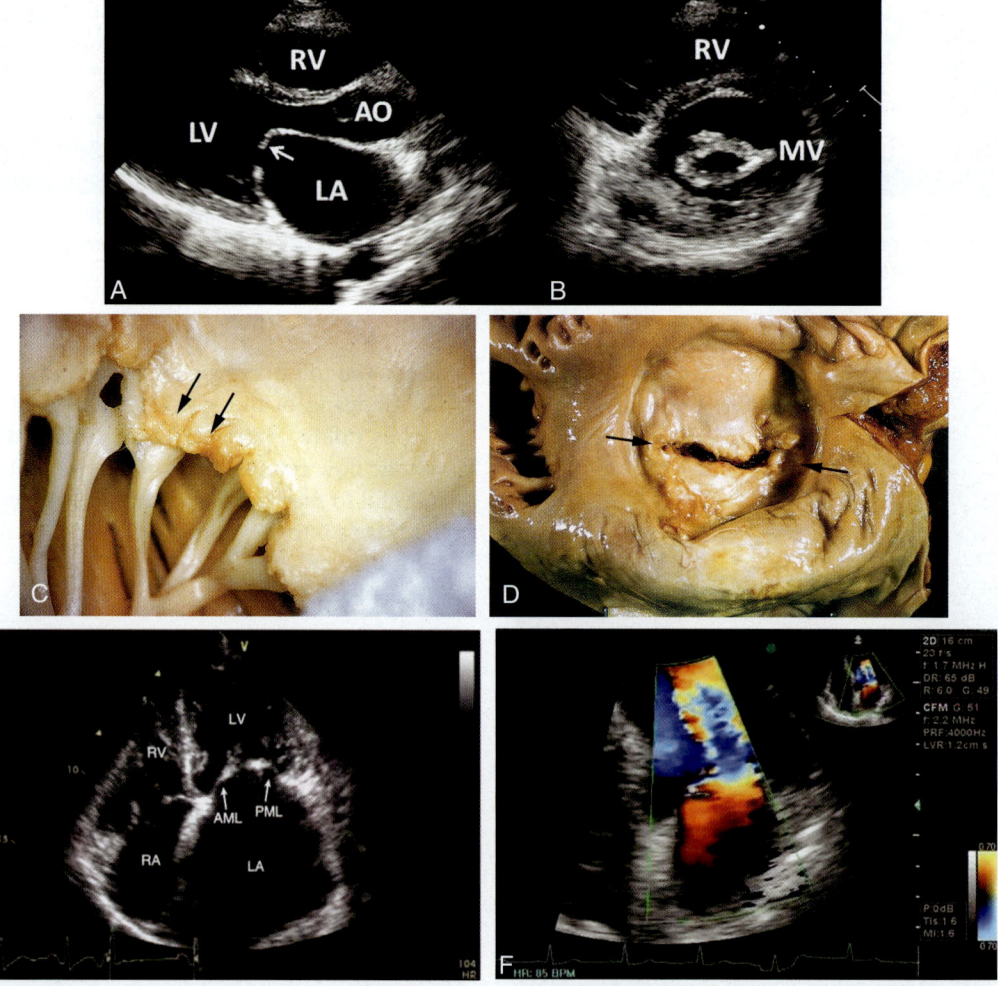

FIG. 33.9 Rheumatic heart disease is the most common cause of mitral stenosis that results in leaflet thickening beginning at the edges of the leaflets and fusion of the commissures, which produces significant narrowing of the mitral orifice. (A), "Hockey stick" appearance of the restricted mitral apparatus. (B) Short-axis image of the mitral valve orifice (MV) shows restricted opening. (C–D) Gross specimens of the mitral leaflet; note the nodular thickening along the tips of the leaflet. (E) Apical four-chamber view of the thickened mitral apparatus and enlarged left atrium. (F) Color Doppler shows increased flow across the stenotic mitral valve.

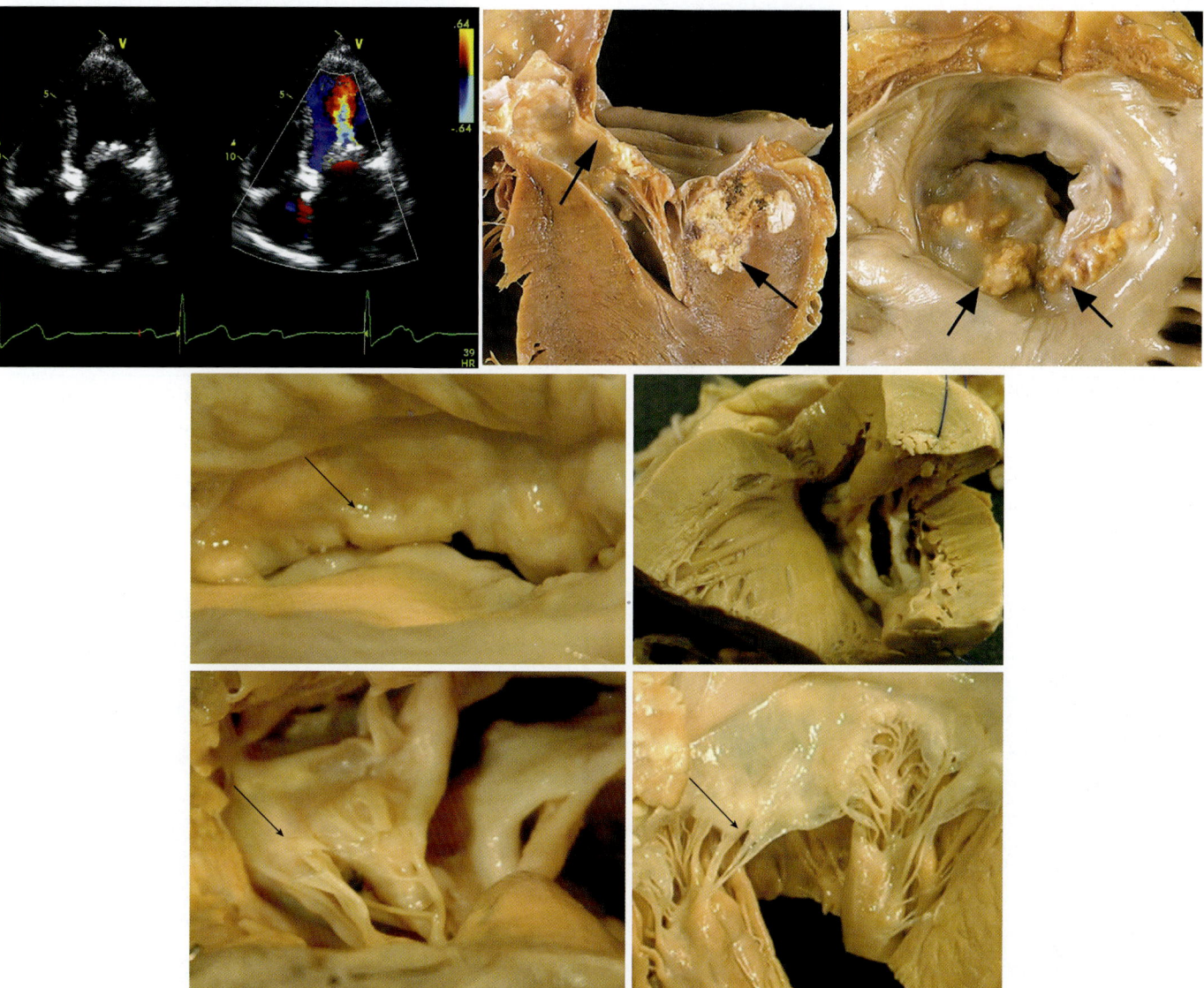

FIG. 33.10 Mitral stenosis may have subvalvular involvement with calcification and thickening of the chordal apparatus.

nonrheumatic mitral stenosis, the annular calcification may extend down the leaflets to cause the restricted mobility of the leaflets (Fig. 33.10).

The goals of echocardiographic evaluation of the patient with suspected mitral stenosis are to establish an equivocal diagnosis and to identify the valve anatomy and involvement of the subchordal structures to determine the success of a possible valvuloplasty. Hemodynamic measurements are made to acquire the mitral valve gradients, determine the valve area, and calculate the pulmonary artery systolic pressure. The supine bike stress echo or the treadmill stress echo may be used to determine the hemodynamic response to exercise in patients with symptoms out of proportion to their valve indices.

On 2D and M-mode echocardiography, there are distinct features of mitral stenosis (Fig. 33.11): (1) thickened and calcified mitral leaflets and subvalvular apparatus, (2) decreased E-F slope on M-mode, (3) "hockey stick" appearance of the anterior leaflet in diastole on the parasternal long-axis view, (4) immobility of the posterior leaflet (often the posterior leaflet moves anterior with the anterior leaflet, instead of the normal mirror movement), (5) "fish mouth" orifice of the mitral valve in the parasternal short-axis view, and (6) increased left atrial size.

In patients with rheumatic mitral stenosis, there is thickening and fusion of the mitral valve commissural edges and chordae that result in the reduction of the orifice and conversion of the normal tubular channel into a funnel-shaped orifice. Over time, progressive fibrosis at the fusion sites and chordae results in stiffening and calcification. Thus, on echocardiography the thickening is demonstrated at the leaflet tips, which causes the valve to "dome" in diastole due to the commissural fusion. This is known as the "hockey stick" abnormality of the anterior leaflet of the mitral valve (ALMV).

In patients with calcific mitral stenosis, the annular calcification extends down the leaflets, often into the chordal apparatus, which causes reduced mobility and restriction of the mitral opening in diastole (see Fig. 33.10).

To assess the severity of mitral stenosis (Table 33.1), there are several indices that may be used in echocardiography: mean pressure gradient, MVA by planimetry, pressure half time, MVA by PISA, and the continuity equation (Gorlin formula):

1. The *mean pressure gradient* is the diastolic pressure gradient $\Delta P = 4V^2$. The use of CW Doppler is preferred to ensure the maximum velocities are recorded (Fig. 33.12). The mean pressure gradient is greater than 10 mm Hg for severe mitral stenosis. The pressure gradient will vary based on several factors, including the mitral orifice area, transvalvular flow, diastolic filling time, cardiac output, and heart rate.

2. *Mitral valve area* may be obtained by planimetry, pressure half time, and continuity equation (Box 33.3). The planimetry method is the direct tracing of the mitral orifice in the parasternal short-axis view at the tip of the leaflets in mid-diastole. This requires a good acoustic window and clear visualization of the mitral leaflets (Fig. 33.13). Pitfalls in obtaining MVA by planimetry include the following: optimal view of the valve orifice may be "off axis" to short-axis of the ventricle; heavy calcification may cause underestimation of the MVA; and severe subchordal involvement may produce a tunnel rather than a single level of obstruction.

3. The **pressure half-time (PHT)** method is the time in milliseconds for the transmitral pressure gradient to decrease by half of its original peak value. This calculation may also be calculated from the deceleration slope. It is affected by

TABLE 33.1	Mitral Stenosis Severity		
Method	Mild	Moderate	Severe
MVA (cm²)	<2.0	1.0–1.5	<1.0
PAP (mm Hg)	<30	30–50	>50
Mean ΔP (mm Hg)	<5	5–10	>10

MVA, Mitral valve area; *PAP*, pulmonary artery pressure.

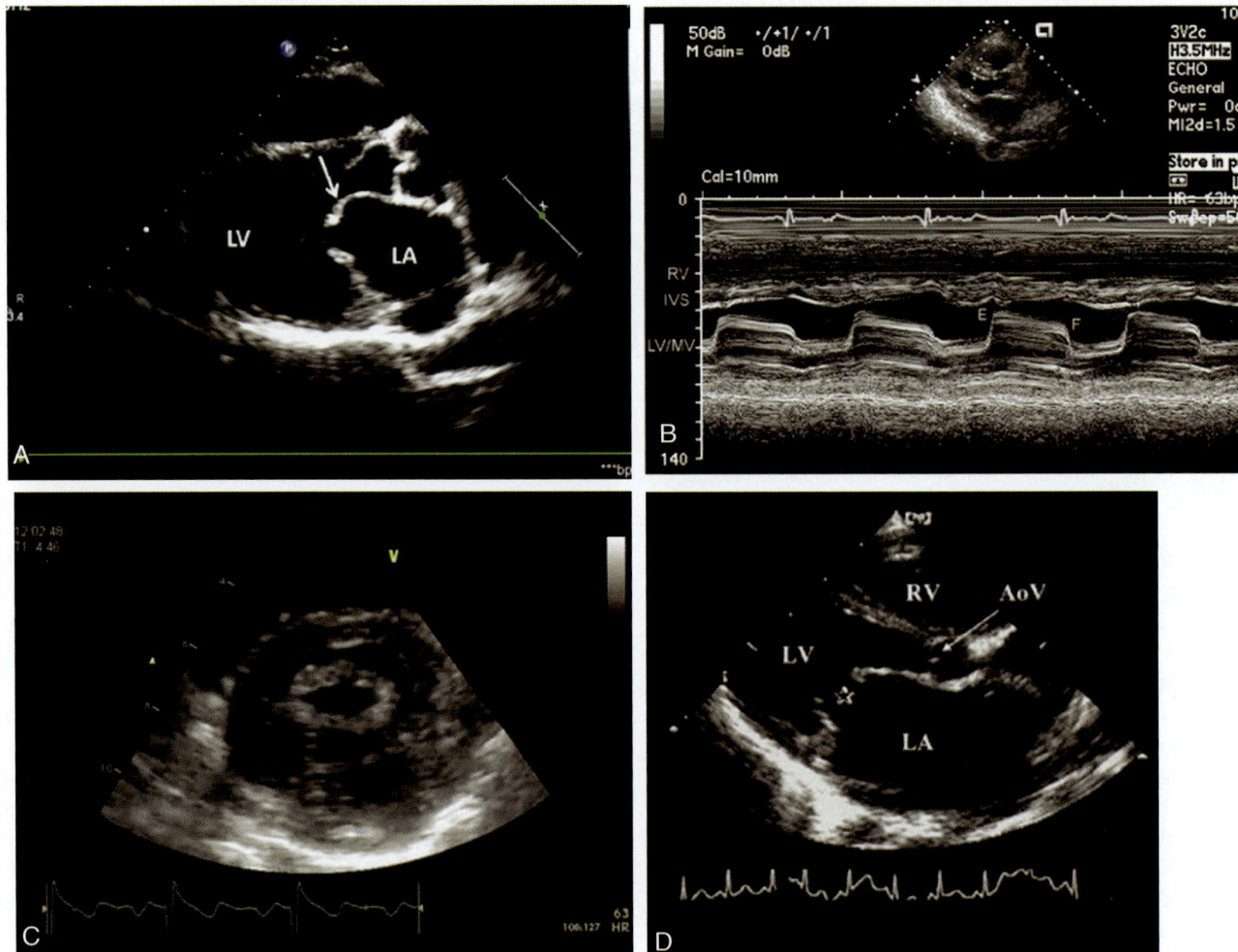

FIG. 33.11 Two-dimensional and M-mode echocardiography reveal distinct features of mitral stenosis. (A) Thickened and calcified mitral leaflets and subvalvular apparatus with "hockey stick" appearance of the anterior leaflet in diastole on the parasternal long-axis view *(arrow)*. (B) Decreased E-F slope on M-mode with immobility of the posterior leaflet (often the posterior leaflet moves anterior with the anterior leaflet, instead of the normal mirror movement). (C) "Fish mouth" orifice of the mitral valve in the parasternal short-axis view. (D) Increased left atrial size. *LA*, Left atrium; *LV*, left ventricle.

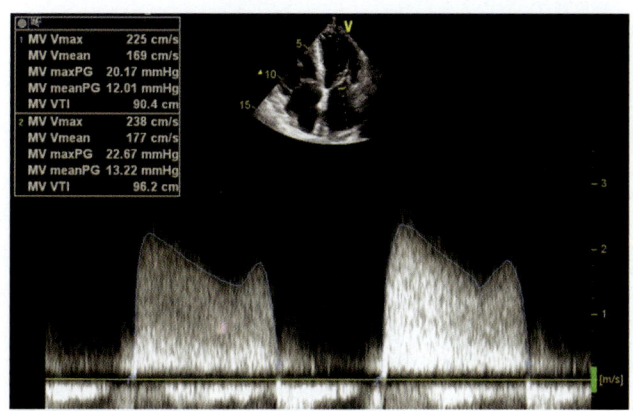

FIG. 33.12 The mean pressure gradient is the diastolic pressure gradient $\Delta P = 4V^2$. This patient has a mitral valve maximal gradient of 22.67 mm Hg.

left atrial compliance, left ventricle compliance, and the presence of AI or atrial septal defect. By using the formula MVA − 220/PHT, the PHT may be computed. In Fig. 33.14, the MVA is 220/178, which calculates the MVA as 1.2 cm². Limitations of this method include the following: an abnormal myocardial relaxation can lead to increased PHT and overestimate mitral stenosis severity, and a rapid increase in left ventricular diastolic pressure (as in aortic regurgitation) can shorten the PHT and underestimate the severity of the stenosis.

4. MVA by PISA (Fig. 33.15) measures the MVA as 1.1 cm².
5. The *continuity equation* (Fig. 33.16) may be used in the absence of valvular regurgitation with the premise that mitral valve inflow equals left ventricular or aortic valve outflow. This formula may be used:

$$MVA = LVOT \times D^2 \times 0.785 \times (VTI\ LVOT/VTI\ MV)$$

where LVOT is left ventricular outflow tract, D is diameter, and VTI is **velocity-time interval**. The presence of mitral regurgitation will overestimate the severity of mitral stenosis. If AI is present, the severity of mitral stenosis will be underestimated. The continuity equation is useful to determine MVA when there is a discrepancy between the severity with pressure half time and mitral gradients.

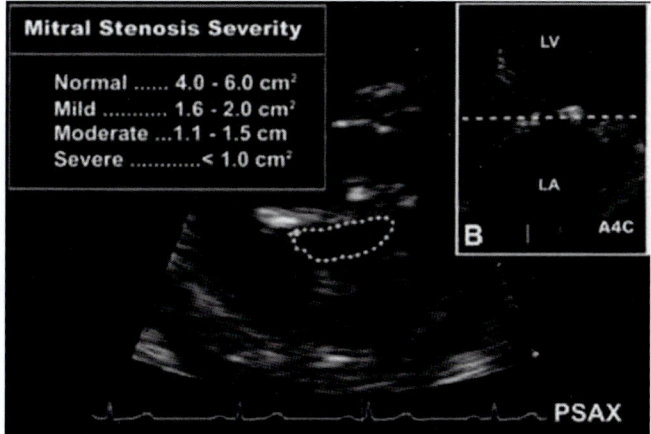

FIG. 33.13 One method to assess mitral stenosis is the direct tracing of the mitral orifice in the parasternal short-axis view (PSAX) at the tip of the leaflets in mid-diastole. This requires a good acoustic window and clear visualization of the mitral leaflets. *A4C*, Apical four-chamber view; *LA*, left atrium; *LV*, left ventricle.

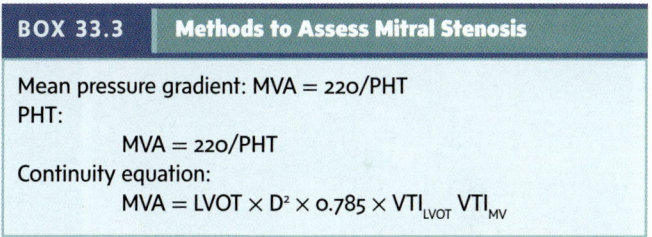

BOX 33.3 Methods to Assess Mitral Stenosis

Mean pressure gradient: MVA = 220/PHT
PHT:
    MVA = 220/PHT
Continuity equation:
    MVA = LVOT × D² × 0.785 × VTI$_{LVOT}$ VTI$_{MV}$

D, Diameter; *LVOT*, left ventricular outflow tract; *MV*, mitral valve; *MVA*, mitral valve area; *PHT*, pressure half-time; *VTI*, velocity-time interval.

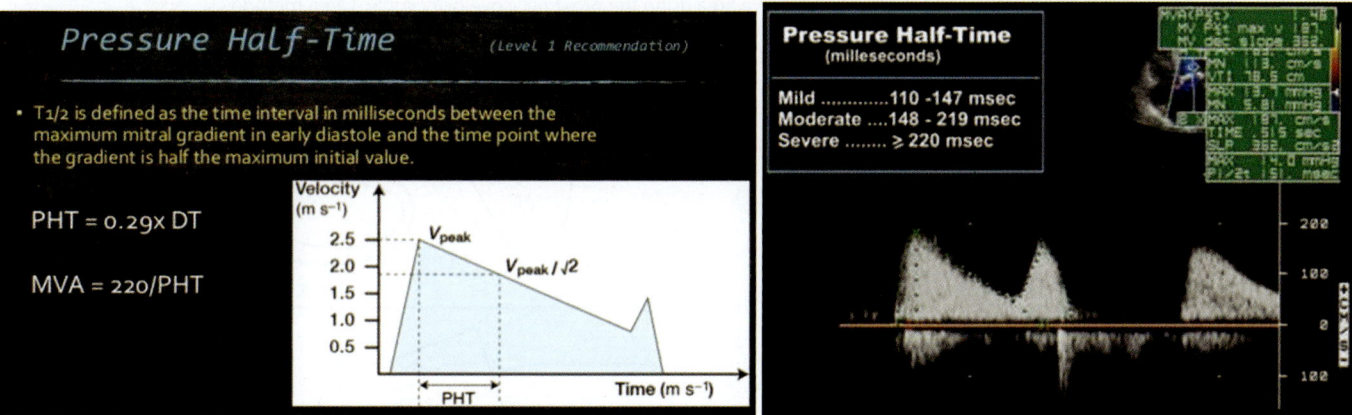

FIG. 33.14 The pressure half-time method is the time in milliseconds for the transmitral pressure gradient to decrease by half of its original peak value. *DT*, Deceleration time; *MVA*, mitral valve area; *PHT*, pressure half-time.

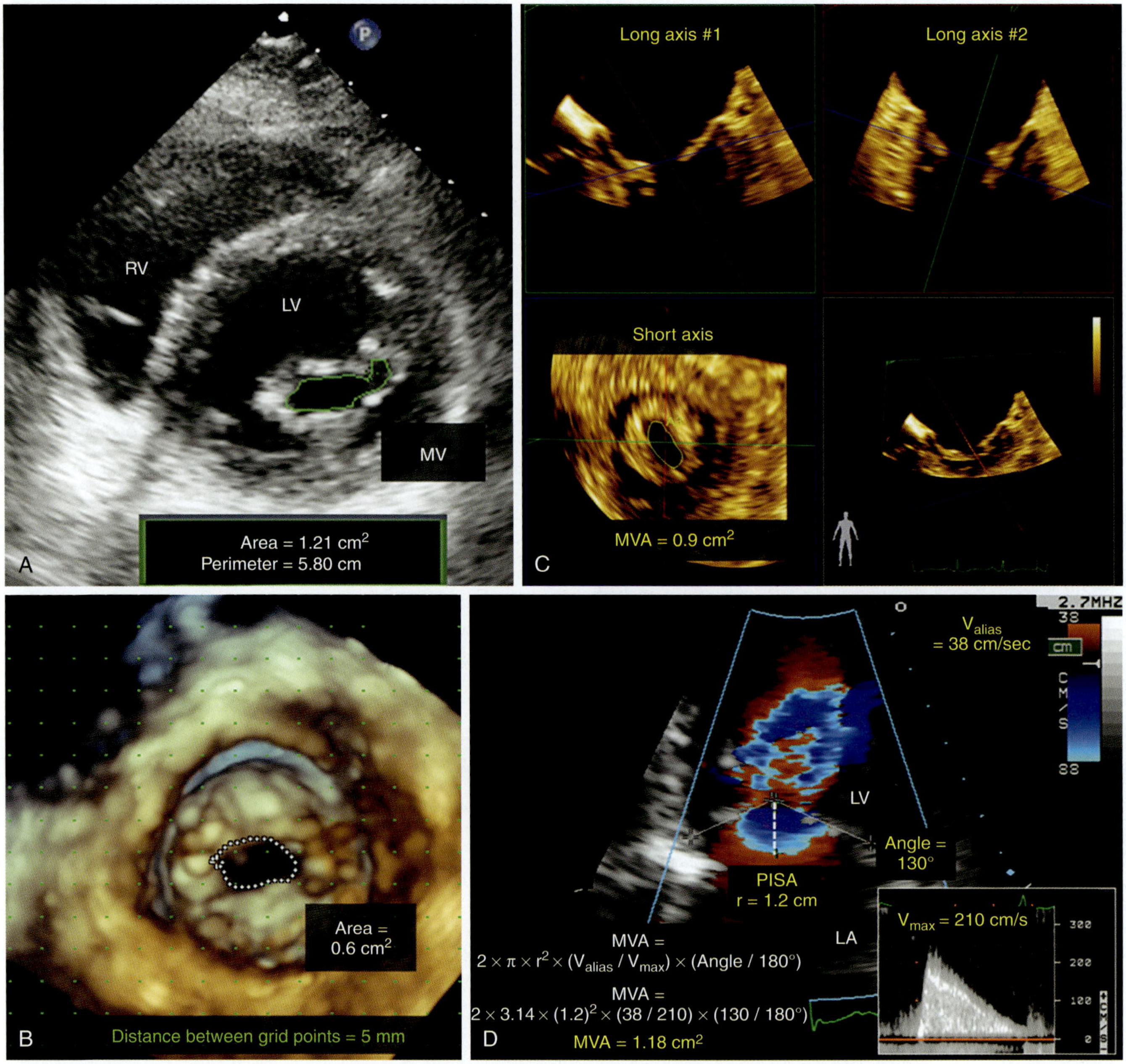

FIG. 33.15 Calculation of the mitral valve area using the proximal isovelocity surface area method.

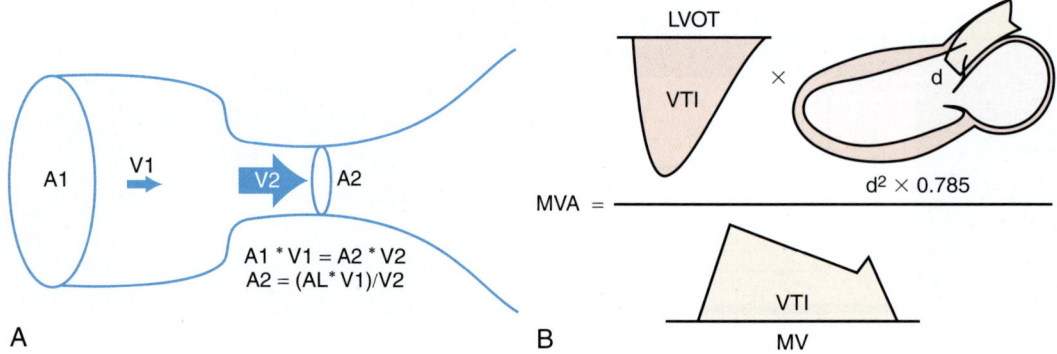

FIG. 33.16 The continuity equation may be used in the absence of valvular regurgitation with the premise that mitral valve inflow equals left ventricular or aortic valve outflow. *d*, Diameter; *LVOT*, left ventricular outflow tract; *MV*, mitral valve; *MVA*, mitral valve area; *VTI*, velocity-time interval.

Other echocardiographic findings may include left atrial enlargement, pulmonary hypertension, pulmonary artery dilation, right ventricular enlargement and hypertrophy, and left atrial appendage thrombus.

Transesophageal echocardiography (TEE) may be useful in defining further findings in the patient with mitral stenosis to outline medical versus surgical treatment. TEE will clearly define the anatomy of the mitral apparatus to determine whether the valve is suitable for **percutaneous mitral balloon valvuloplasty (PBV)**. It will define the presence of a thrombus in the left atrial appendage, left atrium, or left ventricle. In addition, TEE will detect any concomitant aortic or tricuspid valve disease that may be present.

Management of Mitral Stenosis. The definitive treatment is PBV or surgery. The medical therapy is directed toward slowing the heart rate to increase diastolic filling time, managing atrial fibrillation, reducing pulmonary edema, and lowering the risk of embolic episodes.

The PBV is considered the gold standard for patients who meet the criteria. The mitral valve anatomy may be assessed for severity and treatment options to see if the patient is a candidate for balloon valvuloplasty using the Wilkins score (Table 33.2). The Wilkins score ranges from 1 for mild up to 4 for severe to judge the valve in four categories: (1) leaflet mobility, (2) leaflet calcification, (3) leaflet thickening, and (4) subvalvular involvement. A Wilkins score of less than 8 and minimal mitral regurgitation is associated with a more favorable result from mitral balloon valvuloplasty. Severe subvalvular involvement and significant mitral regurgitation are definite contraindications. A score of greater than 8 does not preclude the option of valvuloplasty.

Surgical repair of the mitral valve may be performed with a closed or open commissurotomy or complete mitral valve replacement with a bioprosthetic valve.

AORTIC VALVE DISEASE

Aortic Insufficiency/Regurgitation

The development of aortic regurgitation may be the result of multiple causes: congenital malformation of the aortic valve, rheumatic disease, dilated aortic root, Marfan syndrome, endocarditis, aortic dissection, prosthetic valve dysfunction, or degenerative or calcified aortic valve.

Aortic regurgitation may be acute or chronic. With acute aortic regurgitation, there is a sudden large regurgitant volume on the left ventricle, causing early closure of the mitral valve. This may be secondary to aortic dissection, infective endocarditis, or postsurgical prosthetic valve implantation. There is an abrupt increase in the left ventricle end-diastolic volume with a decrease in the forward stroke volume leading to compensatory tachycardia, pulmonary edema, or cardiogenic shock. Myocardial ischemia may occur secondary to decreased perfusion pressure in the subendocardium (Table 33.3).

Patients with chronic aortic regurgitation are monitored by echocardiography by carefully following the left ventricular size. They may show an increase in the left ventricular end-diastolic volume, an increase in chamber compliance, eccentric and concentric hypertrophy, and pressure overload of the left ventricle. Once the left ventricle is dilated, the patients should have follow-up echocardiograms every 6 to 12 months.

Indirect echocardiographic signs of aortic regurgitation are reflected on the ALMV. There may be increased E point septal separation as the AI impinges on the ALMV, causing impaired opening. It is common to see high-frequency fluttering of the anterior mitral valve leaflet on both 2D and M-mode (Fig. 33.17). Severe insufficiency may cause reverse doming of the ALMV.

Multiple echocardiographic modalities are used to assess aortic regurgitation: 2D, M-mode, PW/CW Doppler, and color flow Doppler (Table 33.4). The comprehensive echocardiographic examination for AI includes evaluation of the vena contracta; jet width of AI compared with LVOT; flow reversal in the abdominal aorta; CW Doppler for PHT and DT; PW Doppler for regurgitant volume, regurgitant fraction, and

TABLE 33.3	Left Ventricle Response to Aortic Regurgitation[a]	
Parameter	Acute	Chronic[o]
LV size	Normal	Dilated
LVEDP	Elevated	Normal
Pulse pressure	Narrow	Wide
CW Doppler slope	Steep	Flat

[a]Acute aortic insufficiency has a short interval from onset to volume overload.
CW, Continuous wave; *LV*, left ventricle; *LVEDP*, left ventricular end-diastolic pressure.

TABLE 33.2	Wilkins Score to Assess Treatment Options			
Grade	Mobility	Subvalvular Thickening	Valvular Thickening	Calcification
1	Highly mobile valve with only leaflet tips restricted	Minimal thickening just below the mitral leaflets	Leaflets nearly normal in thickness (4–5 mm)	Single area of increased echo brightness
2	Leaflet mid and basal portions normally mobile	Thickening of chordal structures extending up to one-third of chordal length	Mid leaflets normal, considerable thickening of margins (5–8 mm)	Scattered areas of brightness confined to leaflet margins
3	Valve continues to move forward in diastole, mainly from base	Thickening extending to the distal third of chords	Thickening extending through the entire leaflet (5–8 mm)	Brightness extending into midportion of the leaflets
4	No or minimal forward movement of the leaflets in diastole	Extensive thickening and shortening of all chordal structures extending down to papillary muscles	Considerable thickening of all leaflet tissue (>8–10 mm)	Extensive brightness throughout much of the leaflet tissue

effective regurgitant orifice area; and measurement of the left ventricular size and shape and aortic dimension.

Echocardiographic parameters used to assess aortic regurgitation include measurement of the vena contracta in the parasternal long-axis view (mild is <0.3 cm, severe is >0.6 cm). The vena contracta is measured in the parasternal long-axis view with the beam perpendicular to the jet of regurgitation at the smallest neck of the flow region at the level of the aortic valve immediately below the flow convergence region (Fig. 33.18). This assessment cannot be used when there are multiple or eccentric jets. If eccentric jets are present, the diameter is measured perpendicular to the long axis of the jet, not the long axis of the outflow tract.

The jet width may be assessed in the left ventricular outflow tract; severe is greater than 60%, and mild is less than 25%. The jet area and length may provide additional information, although the jet length has been found to be unreliable in assessing severity. The jet width is assessed immediately below or within 1 cm of the aortic valve and its ratio to the left ventricular outflow tract in the parasternal long-axis view (Fig. 33.19). Eccentric jets tend to underestimate the severity of regurgitation, whereas central jets tend to expand fully in the outflow tract and may be overestimated.

Other useful assessments include the PHT and rate of deceleration and diastolic flow reversal in the descending

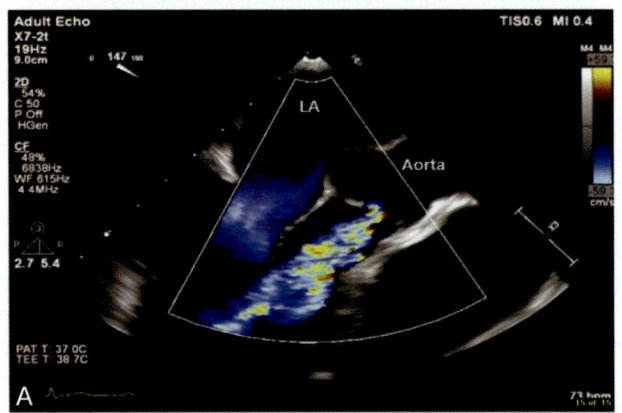
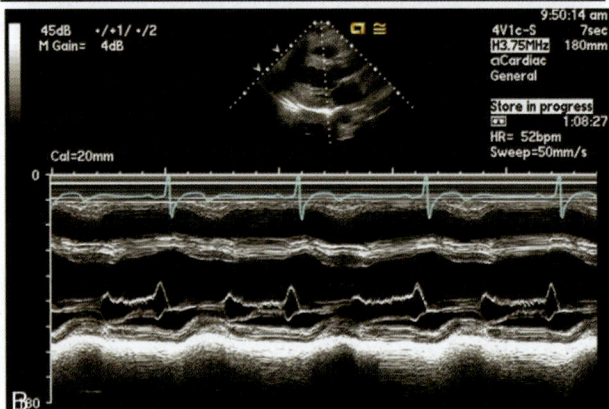

FIG. 33.17 Indirect echocardiographic signs of aortic regurgitation are reflected on the anterior leaflet of the mitral valve. (A) There may be increased E-point septal separation as the aortic insufficiency impinges on the anterior mitral valve leaflet, causing impaired opening. (B) It is common to see high-frequency fluttering of the anterior mitral valve leaflet on both two-dimensional and M-mode echocardiography. *LA,* Left atrium.

TABLE 33.4	Aortic Regurgitation	
	Severe	Mild
LV diastolic dimension	7.5 cm	5.5 cm
Regurgitant jet width/ LVOT diameter ratio	≥60%	30%
Vena contracta width	6 mm	3 mm
Regurgitant jet area/ LVOT area ratio	60%	30%
Aortic regurgitant PHT	<250 msec	>500 msec
	Restrictive mitral flow pattern; flutter ALMV	No change on ALMV
Low reversal in descending aorta	Holodiastolic	Mild early diastolic flow reversal
CW Doppler	Dense	Faint

ALMV, Anterior leaflet of the mitral valve; *CW,* continuous wave; *LV,* left ventricle; *LVOT,* left ventricular outflow tract; *PHT,* pressure half-time.

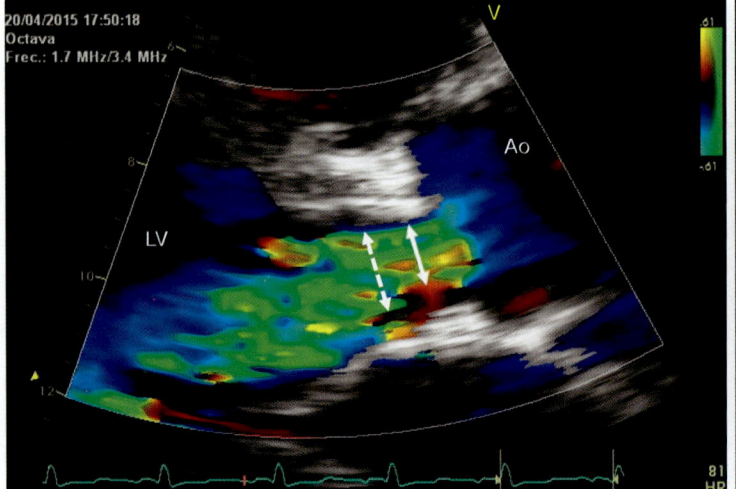
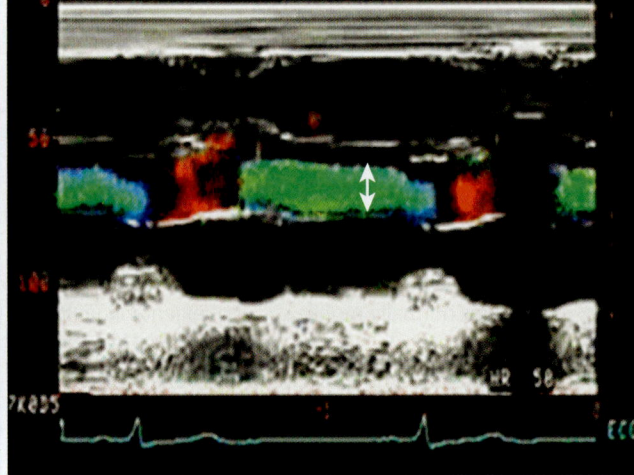

FIG. 33.18 The vena contracta is measured in the parasternal long-axis view with the beam perpendicular to the jet of regurgitation at the smallest neck of the flow region at the level of the aortic valve immediately below the flow convergence region.

aorta. The aortic regurgitant jet DT and PHT reflect the rate of equalization of aortic and left ventricular diastolic pressure. PHT is the time required for the pressure to fall to half of the peak value (velocity). In patients with increasing aortic regurgitant severity, the PHT becomes shorter and steeper in its DT. The formula is PHT = 0.29 × DT; a PHT of greater than 500 msec is mild regurgitation, and when the PHT is less than 200 msec, it is severe regurgitation. In patients with chronic severe AI, there is an increased pulse pressure with a low end-diastolic pressure. Thus the sonographer will note a rapid rate of decline in the aortic pressure on the CW Doppler tracing with a steep diastolic deceleration slope. The flat slope with a long pressure half-time, less than 500 msec, indicates mild AI; the steep slope with a short pressure half-time, less than 200 msec, indicates severe AI (Fig. 33.20).

Flow reversal in the descending aorta is imaged from the suprasternal notch view (Fig. 33.21). The distal descending

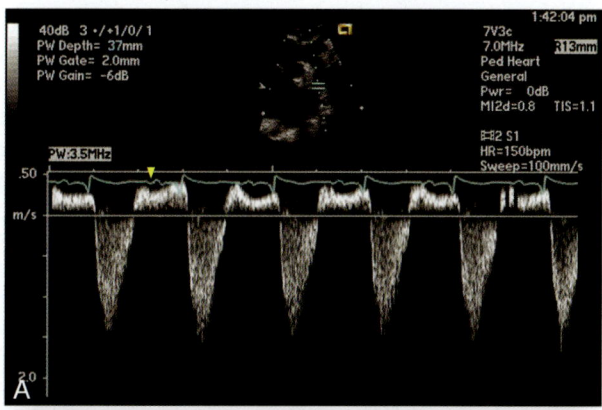

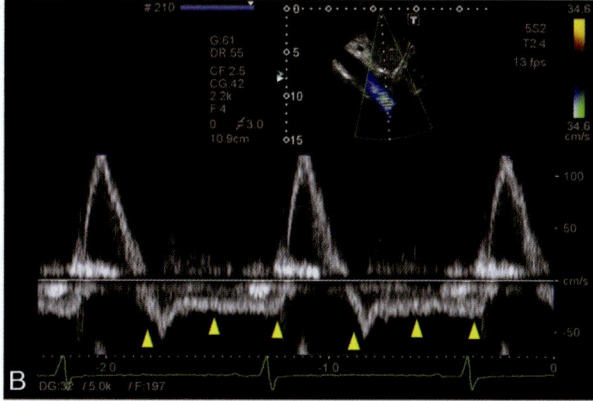

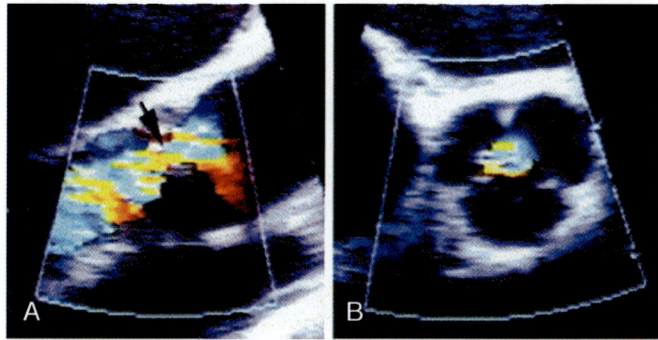

FIG. 33.19 The jet width is assessed immediately below or within 1 cm of the aortic valve and its ratio to the left ventricular outflow tract in the parasternal long-axis view. The diameter is assessed in the short-axis view.

FIG. 33.21 (A) Flow reversal in the descending aorta is imaged from the suprasternal notch view *(arrow)*. (B) From the subcostal window, the long axis of the abdominal aorta may be evaluated with color and spectral Doppler to search for flow reversal. The holodiastolic reversal is seen in patients with at least moderate aortic regurgitation. The distal descending aorta flow reversal may be imaged from the apical long-axis view *(arrows)*.

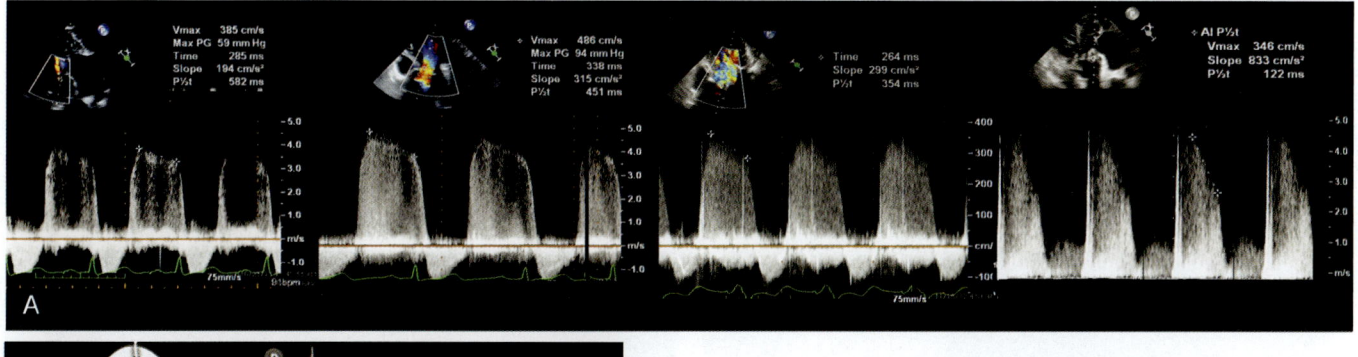

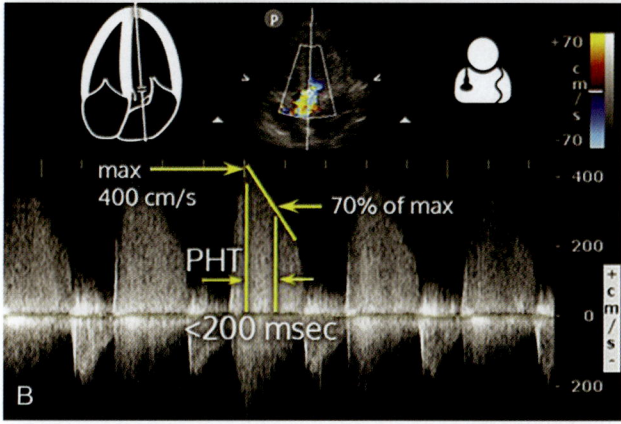

FIG. 33.20 The flat slope with a long pressure half-time (<500 msec) indicates mild aortic insufficiency (A), while the steep slope with a short pressure half-time (<200 msec) indicates severe aortic insufficiency (B).

aorta flow reversal may be imaged from the apical long-axis view. From the subcostal window, the long axis of the abdominal aorta may be evaluated with color and spectral Doppler to search for flow reversal. The holodiastolic reversal is seen in patients with at least moderate aortic regurgitation. Keep in mind that a false-positive flow reversal may be seen in patients with a patent ductus arteriosus. The proximal diastolic flow reversal seen in the descending aorta is less specific and can be seen with moderate AI.

CW Doppler is best recorded from the apical five-chamber view, as seen in Fig. 33.22. The Doppler signal has its onset at the closure of the aortic valve. There is a gradual decline in velocity during diastole. The flow reversal is easily recorded in moderate to severe AI, and the shape of the CW VTI curve can reflect the chronicity and severity of insufficiency.

Aortic Stenosis

There are three types of **aortic stenosis**: supravalvular, subvalvular, and valvular. A supravalvular aortic stenosis is uncommon and is seen more in the pediatric population (Fig. 33.23). This involves a narrowing of the proximal aortic root just above the sinotubular junction and is most often associated with Williams syndrome. The subvalvular stenosis occurs inferior to the aortic leaflets in the left ventricular outflow tract (Fig. 33.24). This membrane is best seen in the parasternal long-axis view. The membrane is separate from the aortic leaflets and causes increased velocity in the left ventricular outflow tract and aorta.

The most common lesion is valvular aortic stenosis, which will be discussed in this chapter. Valvular stenosis

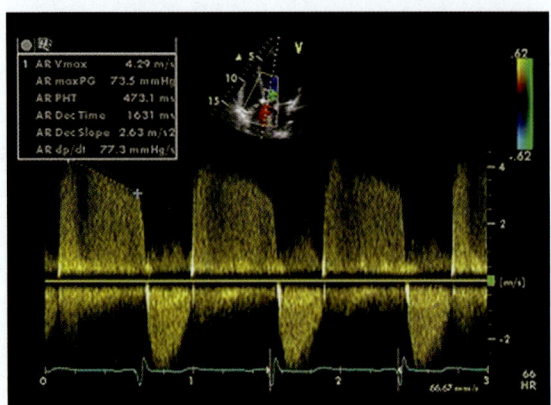

FIG. 33.22 The continuous wave Doppler is best recorded from the apical five-chamber view. The Doppler signal has its onset at the closure of the aortic valve. There is a gradual decline in velocity during diastole. The flow reversal is easily recorded in moderate to severe aortic insufficiency, and the shape of the continuous wave velocity-time interval curve can reflect the chronicity and severity of insufficiency.

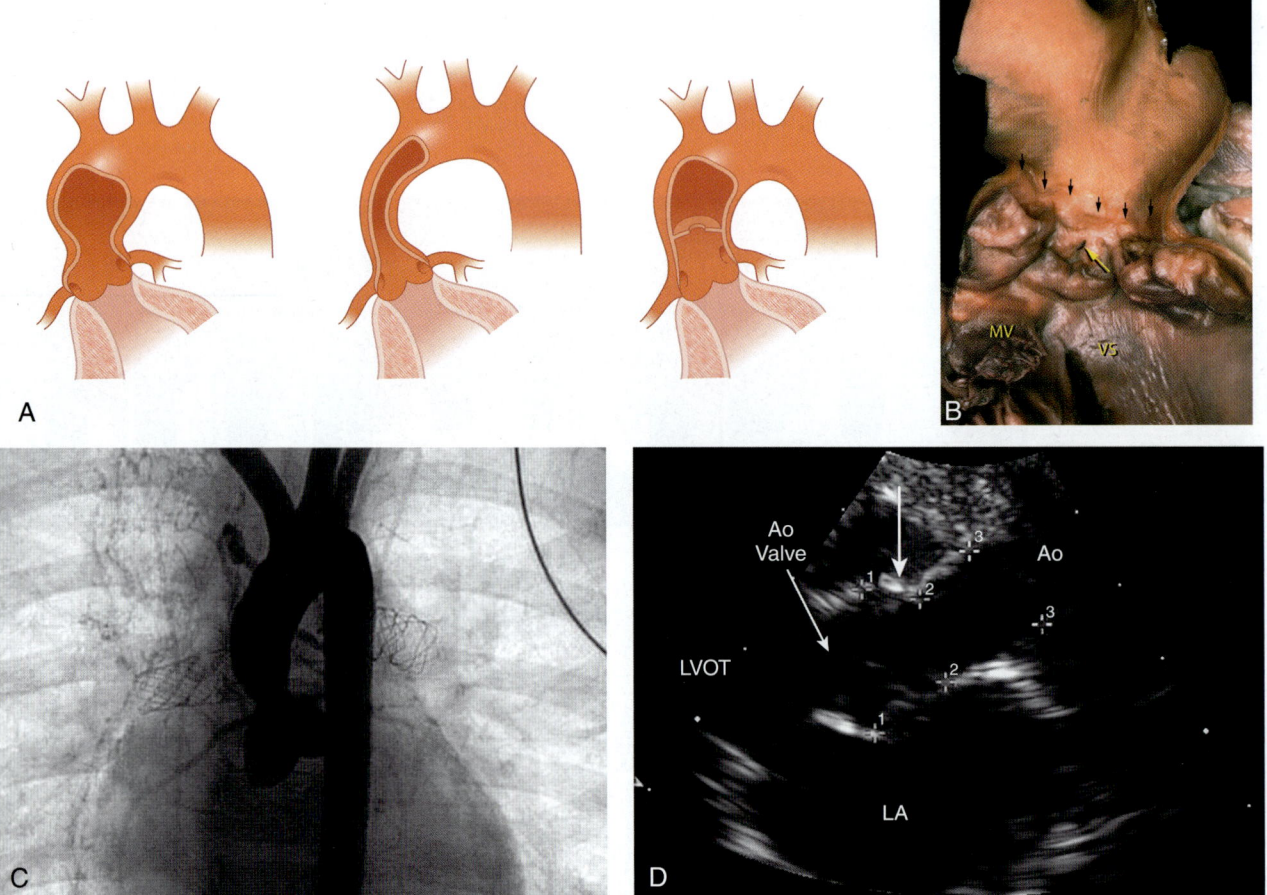

FIG. 33.23 (A–B) Supravalvular aortic stenosis involves a narrowing of the proximal aortic root just above the sinotubular junction and is most often associated with Williams syndrome. (C–D) Radiograph of the supravalvular aortic stenosis with corresponding echo.

may be caused by a congenital malformation of the leaflets, as shown in Fig. 33.25: unicuspid or bicuspid leaflet. Of the congenital variety, the most common abnormality is the **bicuspid aortic valve**, which occurs in 1% to 2% of the population. The bicuspid valve usually has a fused raphe between two of the leaflets that may develop calcification and reduced mobility with age.

Rheumatic heart disease may affect the heart valves, causing thickening and fibrosis that leads to aortic stenosis (Fig. 33.26). This is characterized by commissural fusion and thickening of the leaflet edges that are sometimes associated with leaflet retraction, aortic regurgitation, and mitral leaflet involvement.

The most common cause of aortic stenosis is calcific and senile or degenerative disease. Aortic sclerosis is found in 25% of the North American population, and 1 in 6 of these affected people will proceed to develop aortic stenosis (Fig. 33.27). Furthermore, 4% of the North American population older than 75 years has aortic stenosis; 50% of those with mild to moderate aortic stenosis will proceed to hemodynamically significant aortic stenosis; however, only 33% to 50% of patients with severe stenosis are symptomatic. Once the stenosis becomes moderate, the average rate of progression is as follows:

- Aortic jet velocity increases by about 0.3 m/sec per year.
- Mean transvalvular gradient increases at 7 mm Hg/year.
- **Aortic valve area (AVA)** is reduced by 0.1 cm^2/year.

There is an average survival of 2 to 3 years after the onset of symptoms. The predictors of survival include the transaortic gradient, the left ventricular systolic function, and the patient's age and gender. There is a risk of sudden death in patients with aortic stenosis if left untreated. The risk stratification selects those patients who are likely to benefit from early elective valve replacement once symptoms appear. Patients are now

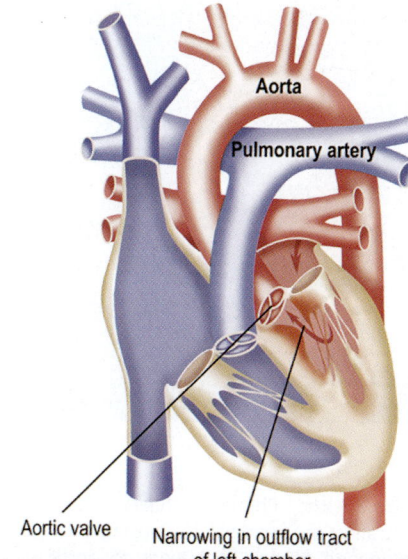
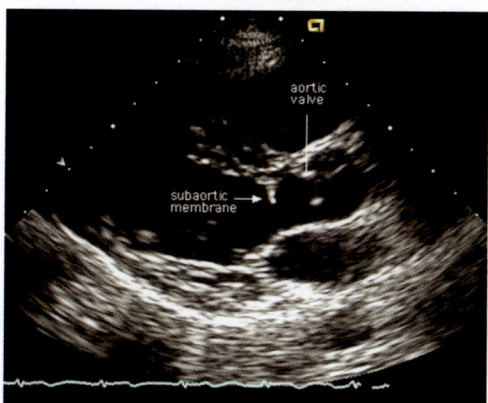

FIG. 33.24 **Subvalvular stenosis occurs inferior to the aortic leaflets in the left ventricular outflow tract.** This membrane is best seen in the parasternal long-axis view. The membrane is separate from the aortic leaflets and causes increased velocity in the left ventricular outflow tract and aorta.

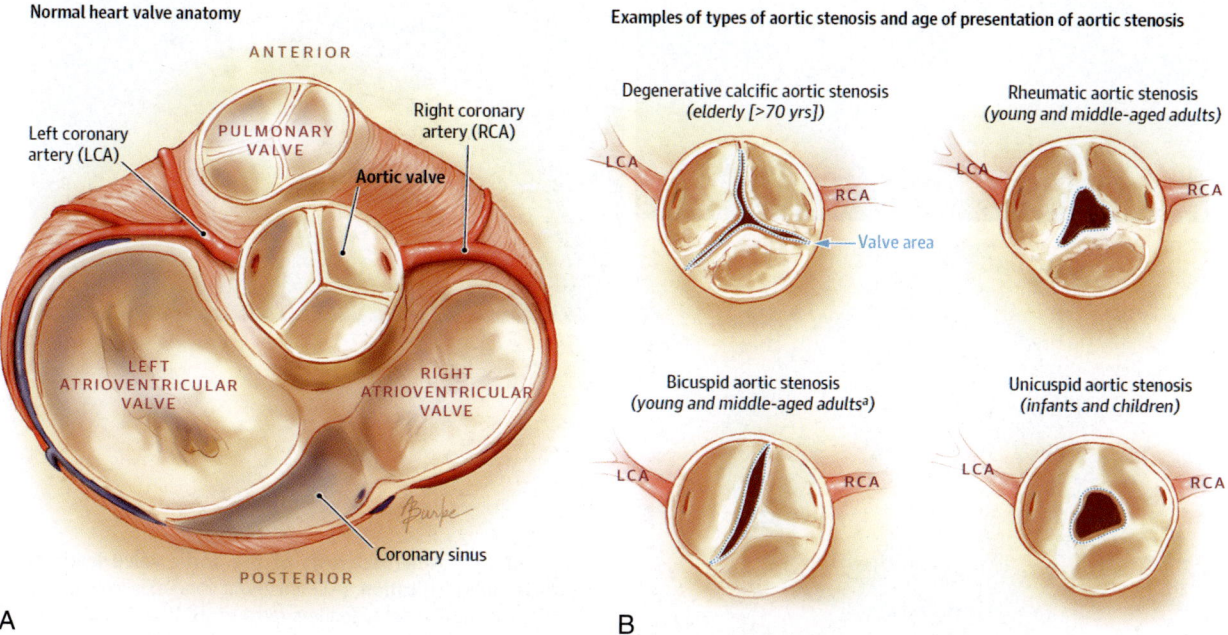

FIG. 33.25 **Valvular stenosis may be caused by a congenital malformation of the leaflets.** The bicuspid aortic valve occurs more commonly than does the unicuspid valve.

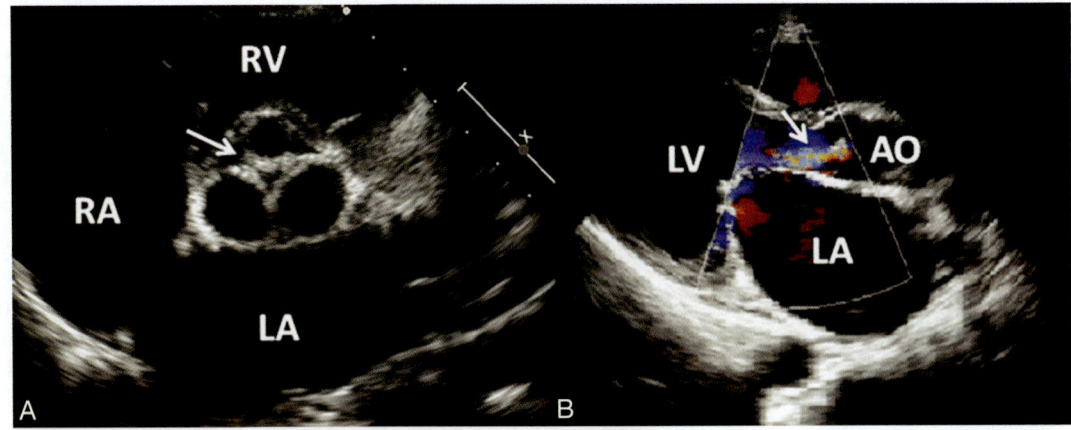

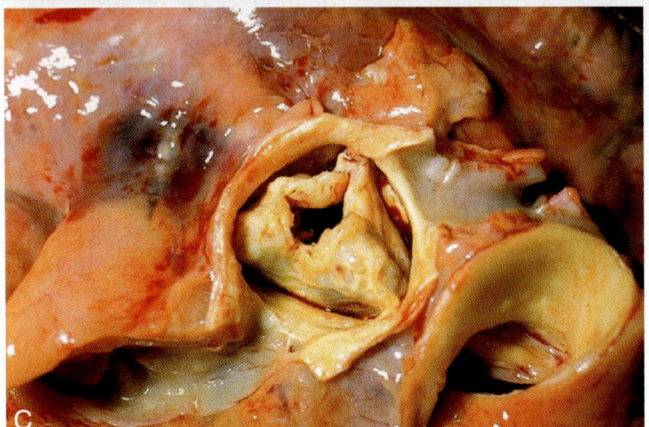

FIG. 33.26 Rheumatic heart disease may affect the heart valves, causing thickening and fibrosis that leads to aortic stenosis. This is characterized by commissural fusion and thickening of the leaflet edges that is sometimes associated with leaflet retraction, aortic regurgitation, and mitral leaflet involvement. (A) Parasternal short-axis view of the thickened aortic leaflets *(arrow)*. (B) Parasternal long-axis view of the thickened aortic leaflets failure to close completely, causing aortic regurgitation *(arrow)*. (C) Gross specimen of the restricted aortic leaflets.

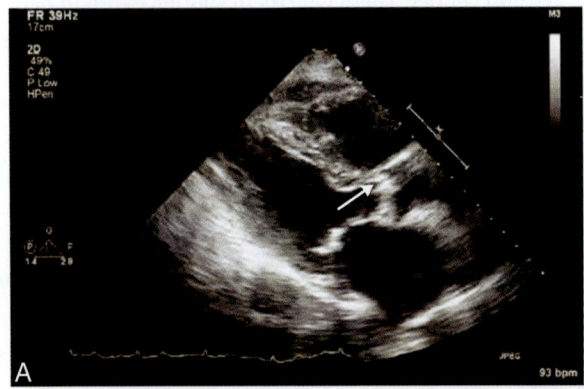

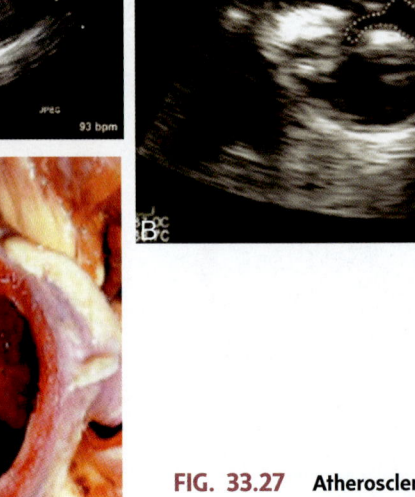

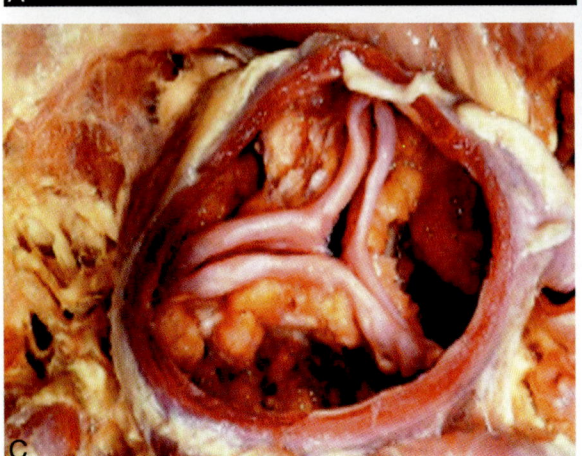

FIG. 33.27 Atherosclerosis of the aortic valve leads to fibrosis and calcification. (A) Parasternal long-axis view of the calcified immobile aortic leaflets *(arrow)*. (B) Parasternal short-axis tracing of the thickened and fibrotic aortic valve area. (C) Gross specimen of the atherosclerotic aortic valve.

given an opportunity to have a **percutaneous transvalvular aortic valve replacement (TAVR)** implanted if they met certain criteria versus the surgical replacement of the aortic valve.

The evaluation of the patient to assess the severity of aortic stenosis is made by echocardiography on an annual or biannual basis, depending on the patient's symptoms. The echocardiogram parameters will assess the left ventricular wall thickness, size, and function, as well as assess the gradients across the aortic valve (Fig. 33.28). The chronic pressure overload leads to impaired early diastolic relaxation, causing reduced early diastolic filling velocity (reduced mitral valve inflow). The diastolic dysfunction varies in aortic stenosis, but as the patient becomes more symptomatic, the dysfunction becomes more pronounced.

The echocardiographic assessment of hemodynamic severity of aortic stenosis includes the peak aortic flow velocity, mean pressure gradient, effective orifice area, and left ventricular outflow tract velocity time interval proximal to and through the aortic valve (Box 33.4).

There are several important Doppler measurements that are useful in determining the severity of aortic stenosis:

BOX 33.4 Aortic Stenosis: Assessment of Hemodynamic Severity

Peak aortic flow velocity (velocity in cm/sec; VTI in cm)
Mean pressure gradient (mm Hg)
Effective orifice area (AoV area, in cm^2)
LVOT/VTI$_{AoV}$ velocity proximal to, and through, the AoV
Normal aortic valve area of 3–4 cm^2
Normal opening results in about 2 cm of leaflet separation

AoV, Aortic valve area; *LVOT*, left ventricular outflow tract; *VTI*, velocity-time interval.

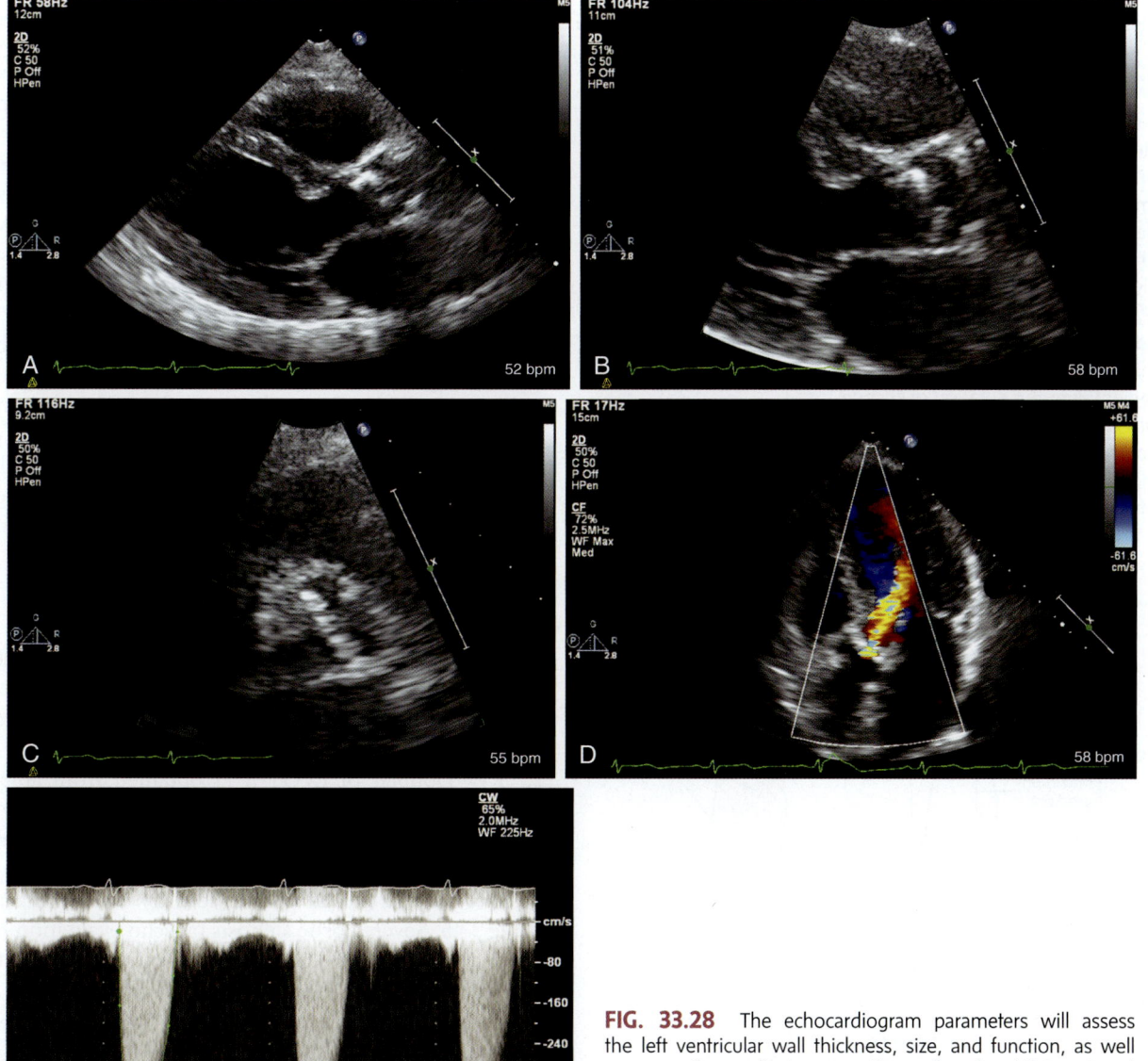

FIG. 33.28 The echocardiogram parameters will assess the left ventricular wall thickness, size, and function, as well as assess the gradients across the aortic valve. (A) Parasternal long-axis view shows the calcified aortic leaflets. (B) Zoom of the domed leaflets. (C) Parasternal short-axis view shows the bicuspid aortic valve. (D) There is both aortic stenosis and regurgitation. (E) The maximum gradient is 68 mm Hg.

transvalvular gradients include the peak transaortic pressure gradient and the mean pressure gradient. The peak transaortic pressure gradient is derived from velocities using the Bernoulli equation (Box 33.5). The mean pressure gradient is calculated by integrating the peak gradient over the duration of systole. With increasing severity of stenosis, the peak gradient occurs later during systole (see Box 33.4).

Doppler mean gradients and measured gradients in the catheterization laboratory represent the average pressure difference between the aorta and the left ventricle over the systolic ejection period (Fig. 33.29). The peak Doppler echo gradient corresponds to the maximal difference between the aortic and instantaneous LV pressure. The peak-to-peak gradient corresponds to the difference between peak aortic pressure and peak LV pressure; because they do not occur at the same time, it does not exist physiologically and cannot be measured by Doppler echocardiography.

> **BOX 33.5 Doppler Measurements: Transvalvular Gradients**
>
> - Peak transaortic pressure gradient is derived from velocities using the Bernoulli equation.
> - Conservation of energy in a closed system.
> - Simplified Bernoulli equation ignores viscous losses and the effects of flow acceleration: $\Delta P = 4v^2$.
> - In the presence of accelerated flow or less significant stenosis, valve gradient is better estimated by the following equation: $\Delta P = 4(v_2^2 - v_1^2)$ where v_2 and v_1 represent the transvalvular and the proximal flow velocities, respectively.
> - Mean pressure gradient is calculated by integrating the peak gradient over the duration of systole.
> - With increasing stenosis severity, the peak of the gradient occurs later during systole.
> - Linear relationship between peak and mean transaortic gradients is given by the following equations:
>
>   Mean ΔP = (Max ΔP/1.45) − 2.2 mm Hg
>
>   Mean $\Delta P = 2.4 (V_{max})^3$

TECHNICAL CONSIDERATIONS AND PITFALLS IN DOPPLER MEASUREMENTS

It is important to note that any misalignment of the transducer to the jet direction leads to underestimation. The probe must be aligned parallel to the jet flow. Multiple transducer positions must be used to obtain the maximum velocity flow signal: right parasternal, suprasternal and right sternal border, apical, and subcostal. Always document where the highest peak velocity is obtained so follow-up examinations will be able to follow jet progression accurately. If the aortic valve root is heavily calcified, consider another nonregurgitant orifice to calculate stroke volume (right ventricular outflow tract or mitral valve). For patients in atrial fibrillation or flutter, use an average of 5 to 10 cycles to determine the velocity-time interval (VTI), or velocity ratio. Be cautious to isolate the aortic jet from other systolic Doppler findings such as mitral regurgitation, LVOT obstruction, tricuspid regurgitation, or pulmonary stenosis. In patients with mitral regurgitation, the pressure crossover occurs earlier compared with the flow signal from aortic stenosis (Fig. 33.30). Also, the velocity is usually much higher in mitral regurgitation than in aortic stenosis.

Other pitfalls the sonographer should be aware of in patients with aortic stenosis involve high and low flow rates. High flow rate (hyperdynamic status secondary to AI) may lead to overestimation of the severity of aortic stenosis. Low flow rate (left ventricular dysfunction or mitral regurgitation) may lead to underestimation of the severity of aortic stenosis. Further evaluation with a dobutamine stress echo may help the cardiologist determine whether the ejection fraction improves enough to cause the aortic flow velocity to increase.

This measurement is obtained from the continuity equation as explained in Box 33.6. Therefore, calculating the AVA with the continuity equation requires (1) LVOT diameter, (2) LVOT VTI, and (3) aortic jet VTI. The simplified continuity equation is shown in Fig. 33.31:

$$AVA = (CSA_{LVOT} \times V_{LVOT})/V_{AS\text{-}jet}$$

where CSA is cross-sectional area and AS is aortic stenosis. Fig. 33.32 demonstrates the valve area calculation:

1. LVOT diameter is measured from the posterolateral long-axis view for CSA calculation.
2. PW Doppler of LVOT VTI obtained from apical five-chamber view.
3. CW Doppler of aortic stenosis jet VTI obtained from the window with the highest velocity signal.

The assessment of aortic severity is summarized in Table 33.5. Severe aortic stenosis by echo evaluation requires the peak aortic jet velocity to exceed 4 m/sec; the AVA to measure less than 1 cm²; the aortic mean gradient to be greater than 40 mm Hg; and the LVOT/VTI aortic ratio (dimensionless index) to calculate less than 0.25.

Aortic stenosis in the presence of left ventricular dysfunction should be carefully assessed. Severe left ventricular dysfunction leads to low cardiac output. The aortic stenosis may be underestimated with a false, low-pressure gradient, or the

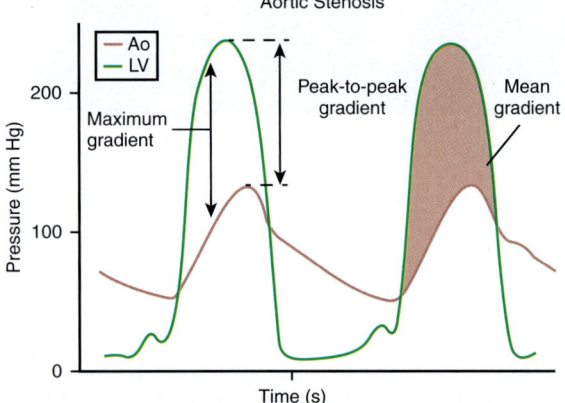

FIG. 33.29 Even though the peak measurements differ between echocardiogram and catheterization, there is a good correlation of the valve gradient by both; however, by catheterization, the peak-to-peak gradient is less than the peak instantaneous gradient by echocardiogram. *Ao*, Aorta; *LV*, left ventricle.

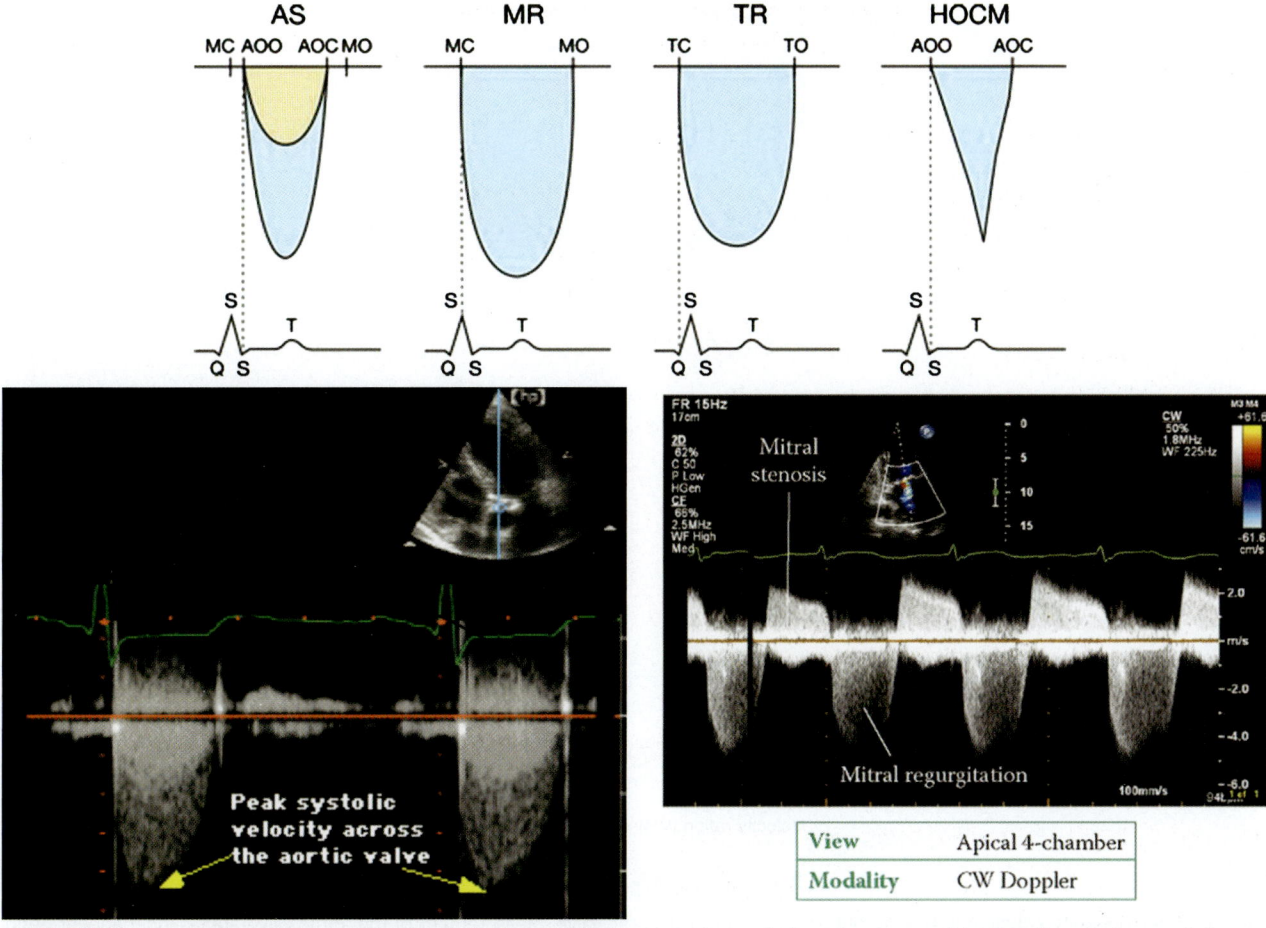

FIG. 33.30 **Comparison of the aortic and mitral valve velocity tracings.** The aortic flow signal occurs later than the mitral regurgitation flow. Be cautious to isolate the aortic jet from other systolic Doppler findings such as mitral regurgitation (MR), left ventricular outflow tract obstruction, tricuspid regurgitation (TR), or pulmonary stenosis. In patients with MR, the pressure crossover occurs earlier compared with the flow signal from aortic stenosis (AS). Also, the velocity is usually much higher in MR than in AS. *AOO,* Aortic opening; *AOC,* aortic closure; *HOCM,* hypertrophic obstructive cardiomyopathy; *MC,* mitral closure; *MO,* mitral opening.

BOX 33.6 Valve Area Calculation: Continuity Equation

Stroke volume just proximal to AoV (SV_{LVOT}) and that in the stenotic valve orifice (SV_{AO}) are equal:

$$SV_{LVOT} = SV_{AO}$$

If flow is laminar with a spatially flat velocity profile:
$SV = CSA \times VTI$

Because flow both proximal to and in the aortic jet itself is laminar with a reasonably flat velocity profile:

$$CSA_{LVOT} \times VTI_{LVOT} = CSA_{Ao} \times VTI_{Ao}$$

Rearranging the equation:

$$AVA = \frac{CSA_{LVOT} \times VTI_{LVOT}}{VTI_{Ao}}$$

AVA, Aortic valve area; *CSA,* cross-sectional area; *LVOT,* left ventricular outflow tract; *VTI,* velocity-time interval.

---

aortic stenosis may be overestimated if there is inadequate valve opening secondary to the low cardiac output. These patients may be referred for a dobutamine stress echocardiogram to see if their gradient increases significantly, indicating severe aortic stenosis, or if their gradient increases slightly along with an increase in the AVA to indicate the stenosis is not severe.

AORTIC ABNORMALITIES

The ascending aorta can be divided into four segments (Fig. 33.33), which may be imaged with multiple echocardiographic windows. The parasternal long-axis view will image the aortic sinuses of Valsalva, the sinotubular junction, and, with medial angulation, the right parasternal view shows the mid ascending aorta. The aortic arch is seen from the suprasternal notch, the descending thoracic aorta is imaged from the apical two-chamber view, and the subcostal long-axis view demonstrates the distal thoracic and proximal abdominal aorta.

Abnormalities of the aorta include aneurysm, dissection, sinus of Valsalva aneurysm, atherosclerosis, penetrating aortic ulcer, intramural hematoma, and aortic tumors. These abnormalities will be briefly presented.

Aortic Aneurysm

The definition of an aneurysm implies that there has been 50% expansion of all three layers of the vessel wall in diameter.

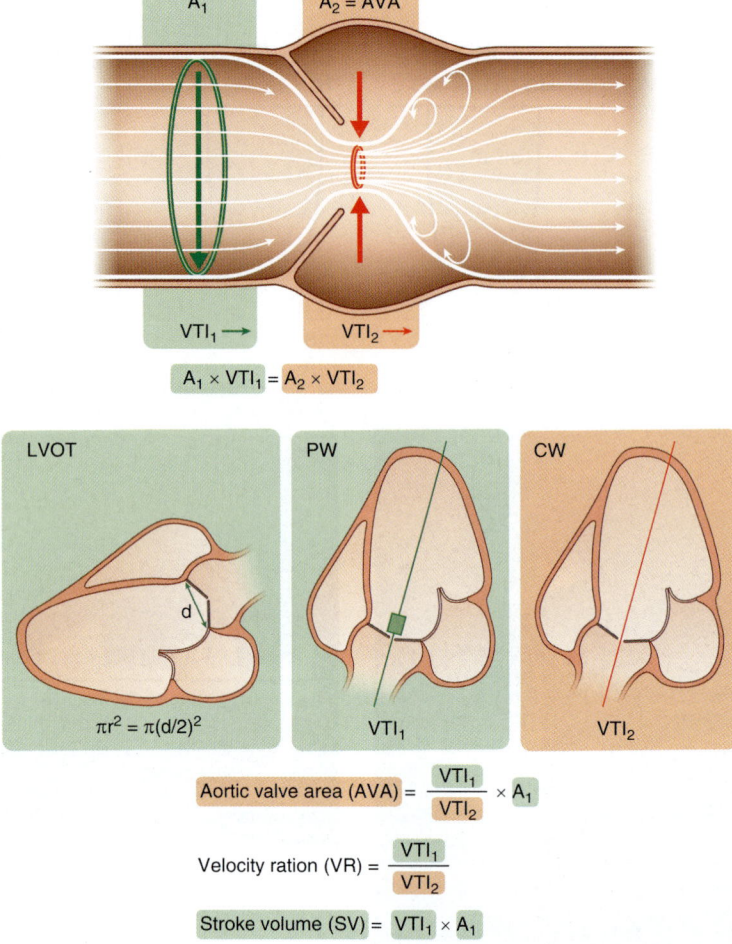

FIG. 33.31 The continuity equation is used to obtain the area of the aortic valve. Measurement of the aortic valve area is independent of flow rate influence. Calculation of the aortic valve area with the continuity equation requires (1) left ventricular outflow tract (LVOT) diameter, (2) LVOT velocity-time interval (VTI), and (3) aortic jet VTI.

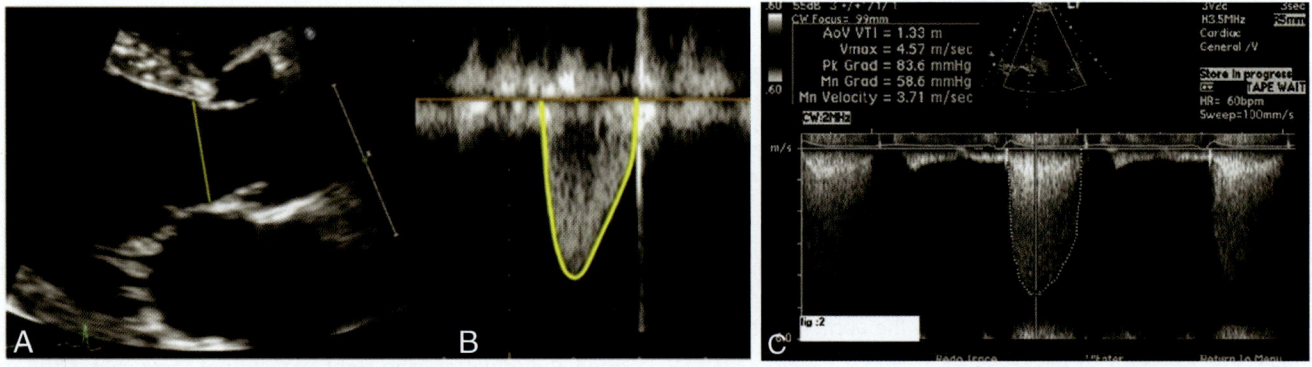

FIG. 33.32 (A) Left ventricular outflow tract (LVOT) diameter is measured from the parasternal long-axis view for cross-sectional calculation. (B) Pulsed wave Doppler of LVOT velocity-time interval (VTI) obtained from apical five-chamber view. (C) Continuous wave Doppler of aortic stenosis jet VTI obtained from the window with the highest velocity signal.

TABLE 33.5 Assessment of Severity of Aortic Stenosis

	Normal	Mild	Moderate	Severe
V_{max} (m/sec)	<2.6	2.6–2.9	3.0–4.0	>4.0
AVA (cm²)	4.0–3.0	2.0–1.6	1.5–1.0	<1.0
Mean ΔP (mm Hg)	<10	11–25	25–40	>40
Dimensionless index	1.0	<0.5	<0.33	<0.25

AVA, Aortic valve area.

The causes of aneurysm formation are multiple and include structural/congenital abnormalities (bicuspid aortic valve), connective tissue disease (Marfan, Loeys-Dietz), inflammatory (ankylosing spondylitis, Takayasu arteritis), infectious (tertiary syphilis), and trauma/iatrogenic.

Most patients are asymptomatic and are diagnosed incidentally by echocardiogram or other imaging modality. The mean rate of growth for the aneurysm is 0.1 to 0.6 cm/year, although this is higher in patients with Marfan syndrome.

The risk of rupture is greatest when the aneurysm exceeds 6.0 cm or if the aneurysm is rapidly expanding. Patients with Marfan and a bicuspid aortic valve with an aneurysm of greater than 5.0 cm may be considered sooner for cardiovascular surgery.

The bicuspid aortic valve occurs in 1% to 2% of the population; of these affected patients, 50% with a bicuspid aortic valve develop aortopathy. The bicuspid aortic valve is associated with other lesions in the heart in the form of aortic stenosis, endocarditis, coarctation, aortic dilation, or aortic dissection.

Pseudoaneurysm. A **pseudoaneurysm** is the loss of integrity of the aortic wall with a blood collection outside the aorta. Common causes may include post-surgery for aortic disease (blood from the graft lumen into an area contained by surrounding scar tissue or the native aorta) and endocarditis. On an echocardiogram, the pseudoaneurysm shows a pedunculated echolucency (Fig. 33.34). Color Doppler may demonstrate the communication flow pathway.

Aortic Dissection. The **dissection** is a tear in the aortic intima that leads to a false lumen with blood between the intima and media and/or adventitia. The patient may have a variety of symptoms: acute chest pain, acute heart failure, acute aortic regurgitation, tamponade, syncope, cerebrovascular event, sudden cardiac arrest, or death. Clinically the patient may have a pulse deficit or blood pressure differential. This condition may require medical or surgical management.

The diagnostic choice of imaging is driven by the patient's hemodynamic status. Computed tomography (CT) and magnetic resonance angiogram (MRA) are the first choices in critical situations; these imaging techniques demonstrate the entire aorta and may show the point and extent of the dissection. If the patient is clinically stable, transthoracic echocardiography (TTE) and/or TEE imaging is performed. The TTE will show the dilated aortic lumen. The sonographer should search for a linear echogenic structure with independent motion, which would represent the flap in the lumen; color Doppler is helpful to show the movement of blood flow into the false lumen. TEE is performed with the transducer placed orally into the esophagus of the patient. This technique provides excellent segmental visualization of the entire aortic root.

The differentiation between the true and false lumen is found in Table 33.6. The true lumen expands with systole and shows normal laminar flow with color Doppler. The false

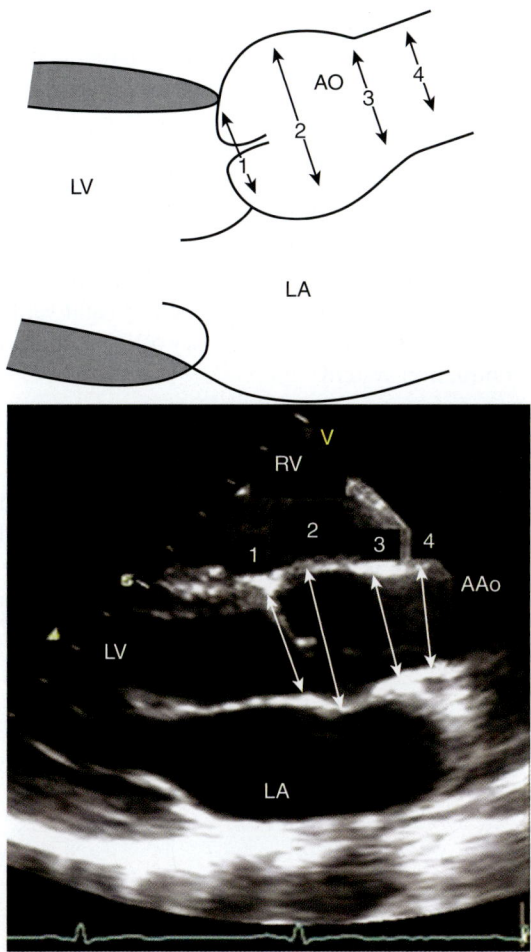

FIG. 33.33 Normal anatomy of the ascending aorta (AAo) with standard anatomic landmarks. *1*, Aortic annulus; *2*, sinuses of Valsalva; *3*, sinotubular junction; and *4*, proximal ascending aorta. *LA*, Left atrium; *LV*, left ventricle; *RV*, right ventricle.

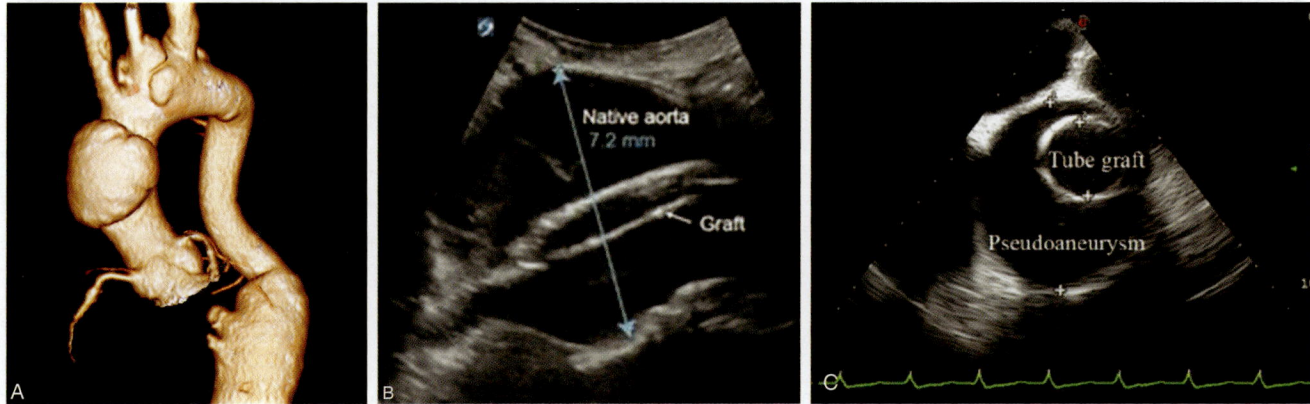

FIG. 33.34 (A) Three-dimensional computed tomography reconstruction of the aortic graft with a subsequent pseudoaneurysm at the root of the aorta. (B–C) On an echocardiogram, the pseudoaneurysm shows a pedunculated echolucency surrounding the graft.

lumen may be crescent-shaped, usually larger than the true lumen, with thrombosis within the lumen.

The classification of aortic dissection has been developed by DeBakey and Stanford (Fig. 33.35). Type I dissection originates in the ascending aorta and propagates distally to include at least the aortic arch and typically the descending aorta (Fig. 33.36); type II dissection originates in and is confined to the ascending aorta (Fig. 33.37); type III dissection originates in the descending aorta and propagates most often distally.

TABLE 33.6	Differentiation Between True and False Lumen	
	True Lumen	**False Lumen**
Size	True less than false	Usually false greater than true
Pulsation	Systolic expansion	Systolic compression
Flow direction	Systolic antegrade flow	Systolic antegrade flow reduced or absent, or retrograde flow
Communication flow	Extends from true to false lumen in systole	
Contrast echo flow	Early and fast	Delayed and slow

Type III is further divided into type IIIa, which is limited to the descending thoracic aorta, and type IIIb, which extends below the diaphragm (Fig. 33.38).

Complications of aortic dissection include compression of the true lumen (e.g., coronary ostial occlusion may lead to regional wall motion abnormalities or distal vessel obstruction may lead to stroke); thrombosis; acute aortic regurgitation; pericardial effusion and/or tamponade; acute aortic rupture with pleural effusion; and mediastinal hematoma.

Sinus of Valsalva Aneurysm. The aneurysm occurs at the base of the aorta in the area of the sinus of Valsalva (Fig. 33.39). The cause of this aneurysm may be congenital (Marfan syndrome, Ehler-Danlos syndrome, or bicuspid aortic valve); iatrogenic, secondary to surgery; or infectious (syphilis or infective endocarditis). Complications of this type of aneurysm may include obstruction of the left or right ventricular outflow tract, distortion of the coronary ostia, or compression of the conduction system.

Aortic Atherosclerosis

Atherosclerosis is easily imaged with both TTE and TEE modalities as the aortic walls become thickened and calcified (Fig. 33.40). There is a strong correlation between coronary artery disease and stroke risk, especially if there is a complex plaque (greater than 4 mm thick, mobile lesions, ulcers) seen in the descending aorta.

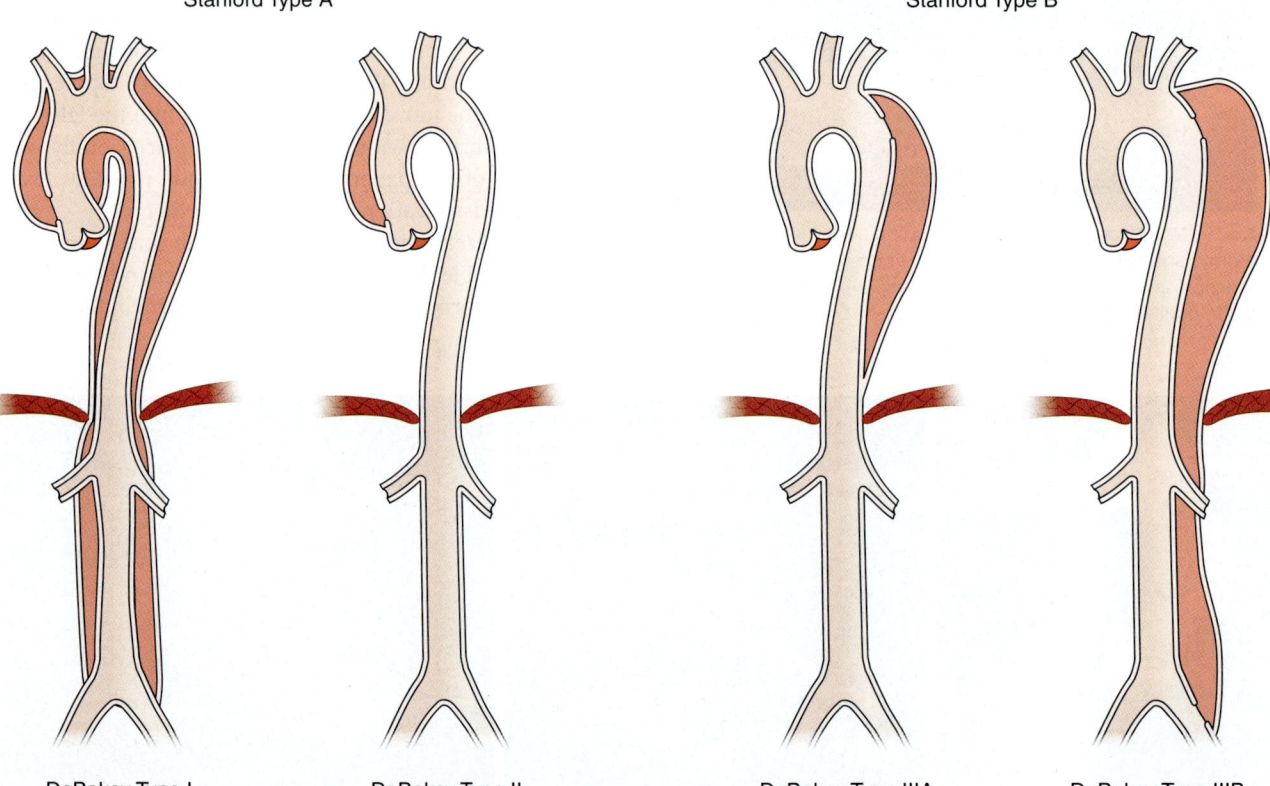

FIG. 33.35 **DeBakey and Stanford aortic dissection classification.** Type I dissection originates in the ascending aorta and propagates distally to include at least the aortic arch and typically the descending aorta; type II dissection originates in and is confined to the ascending aorta; type III dissection originates in the descending aorta and propagates most often distally. Type III is further divided into type IIIA, which is limited to the descending thoracic aorta, and type IIIB, which extends below the diaphragm.

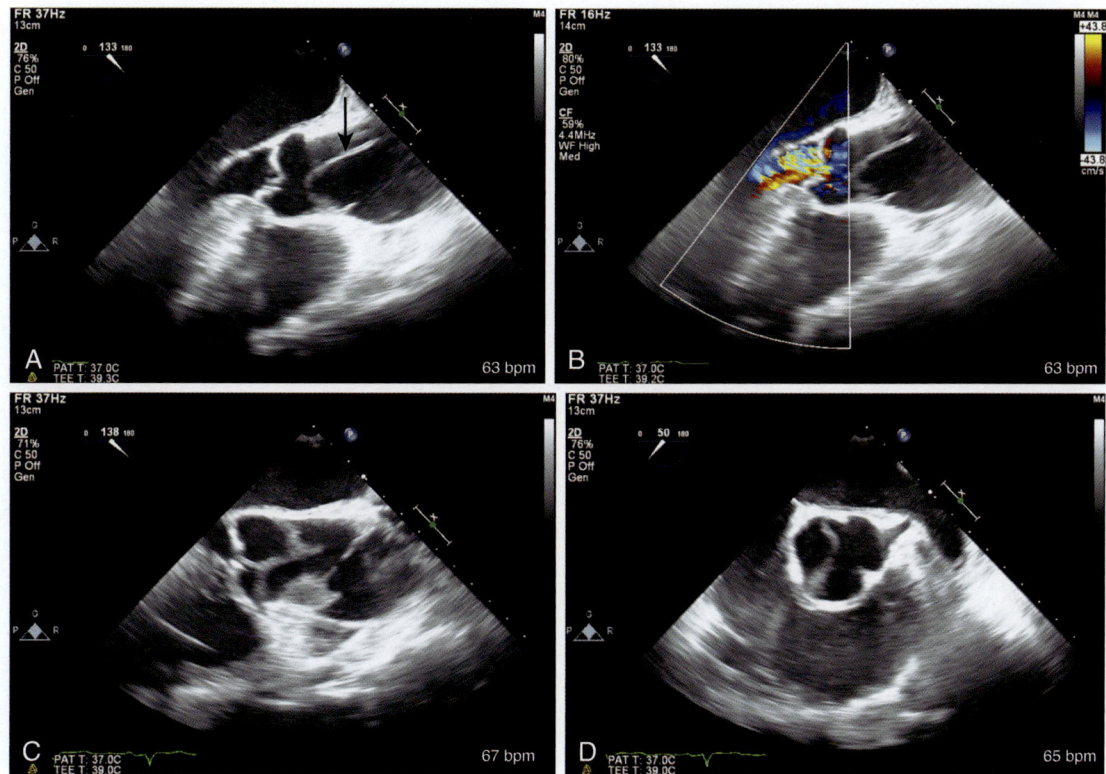

FIG. 33.36 Type I dissection originates in the ascending aorta and propagates distally to include at least the aortic arch and typically the descending aorta. (A–C) Transesophageal echocardiography images of the ascending aorta with the luminal flap *(arrow)*. (D) Short-axis view of the aortic root.

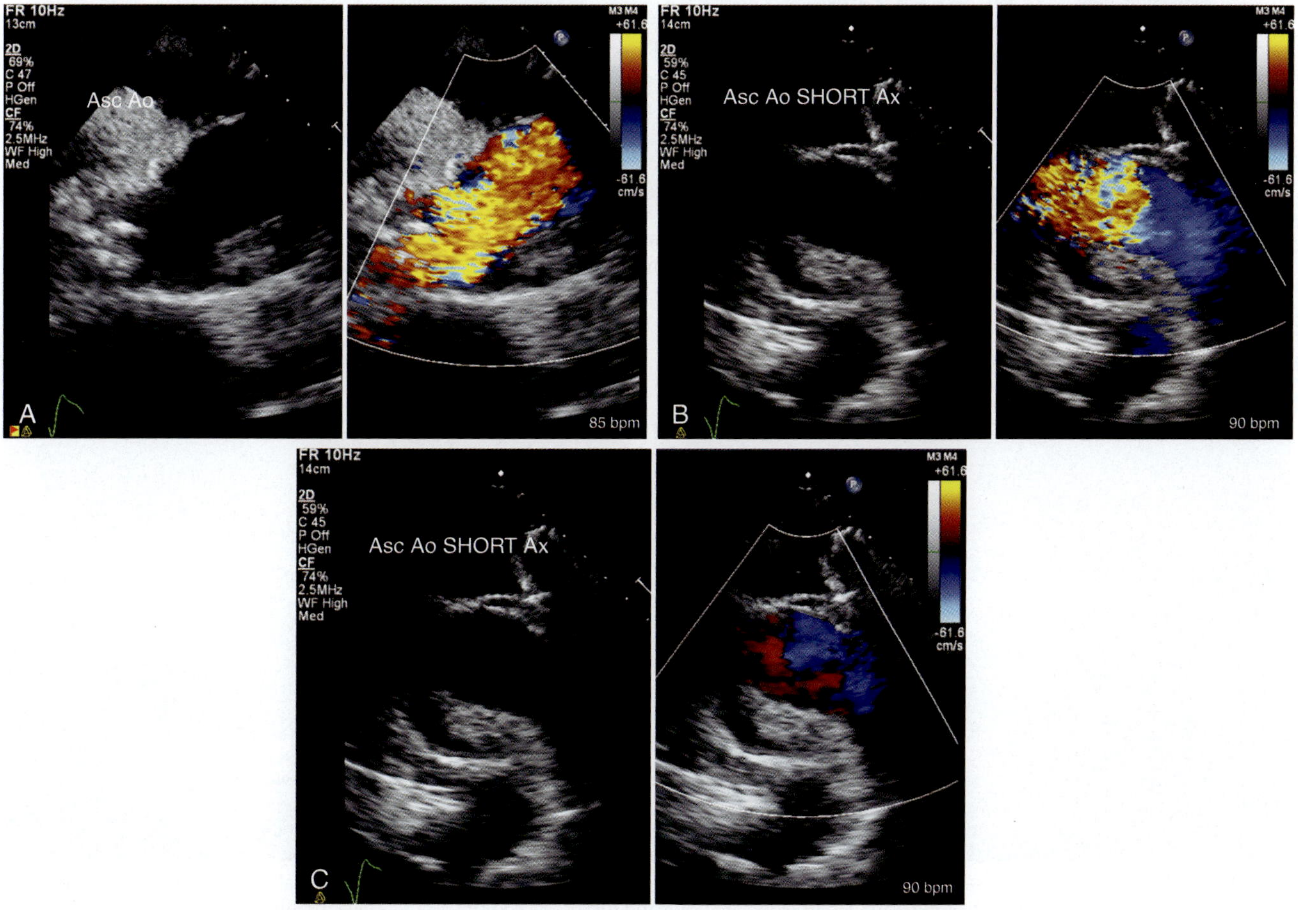

FIG. 33.37 Type II dissection originates in and is confined to the ascending aorta.

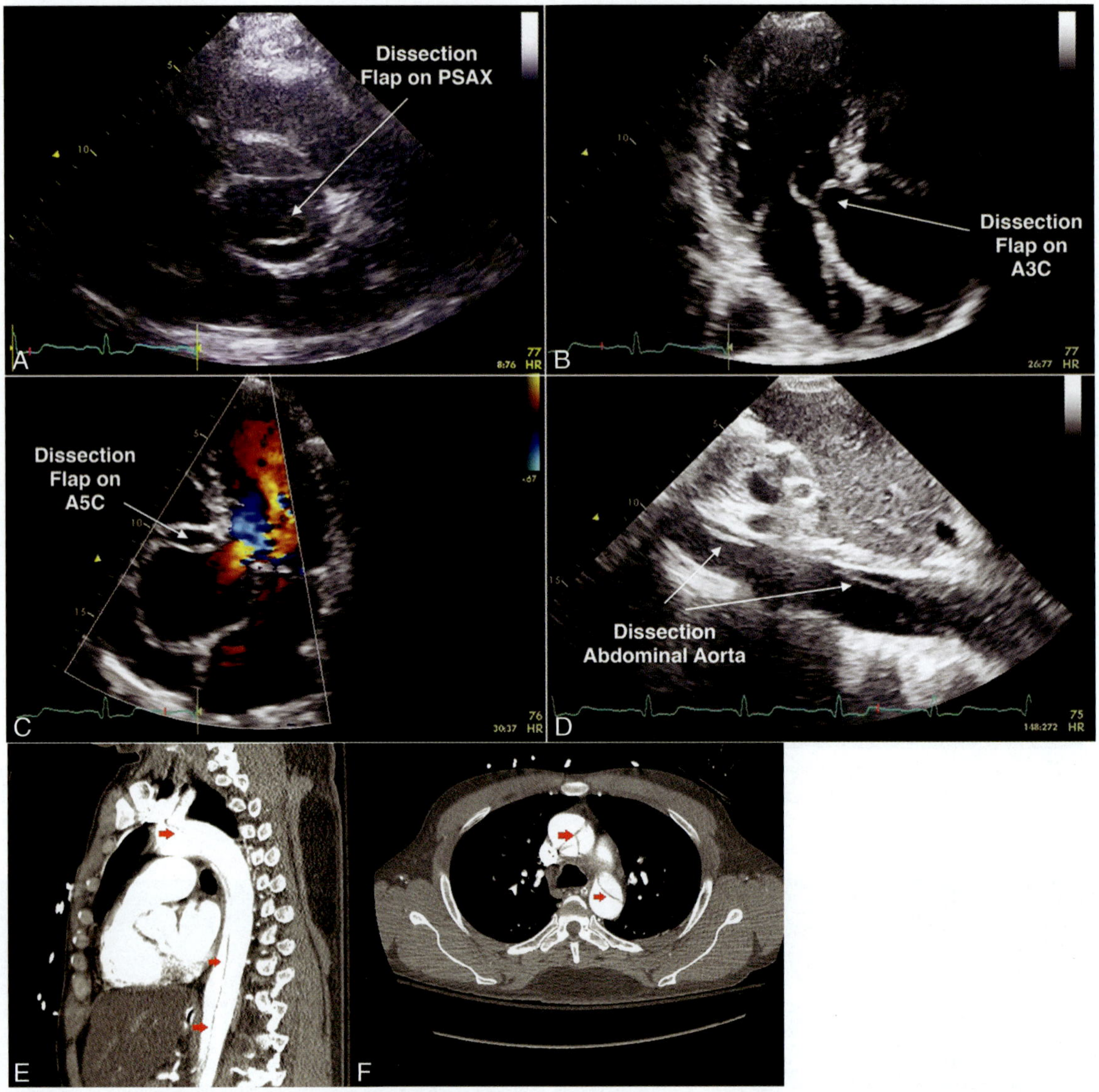

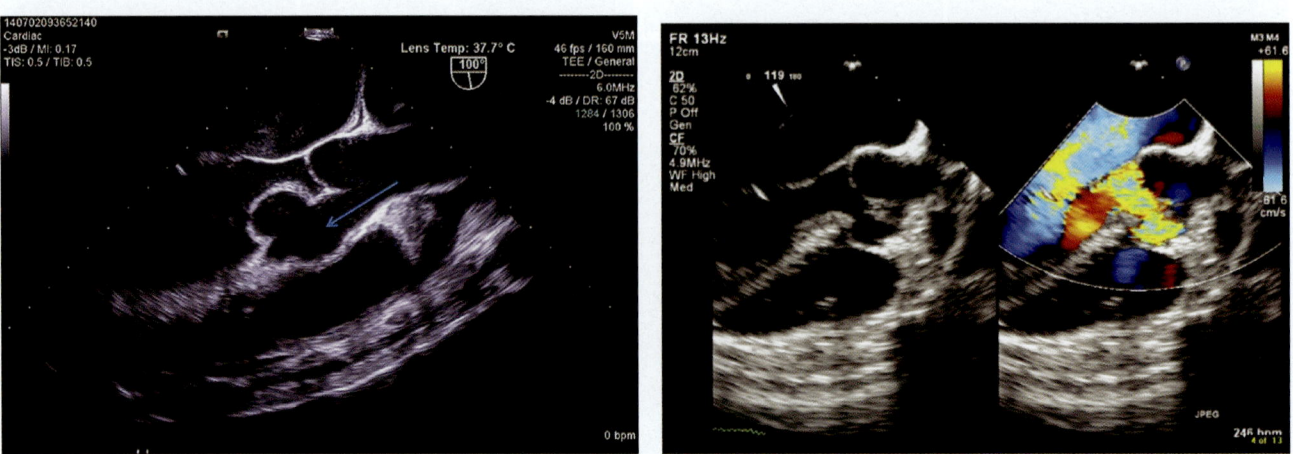

FIG. 33.38 Type III dissection originates in the descending aorta and propagates most often distally into the abdominal aorta, as demonstrated on the echocardiography (A–D) and contrast computed tomography (E–F) images. *A3C*, Apical three-chamber view; *A5C*, apical five-chamber view; *PSAX*, parasternal short-axis view.

FIG. 33.39 The sinus of Valsalva aneurysm occurs at the base of the aorta in the area of the sinus of Valsalva. These transesophageal images show the distorted base of the aorta. Color Doppler shows the rupture of the sinus of Valsalva into the right ventricular outflow tract.

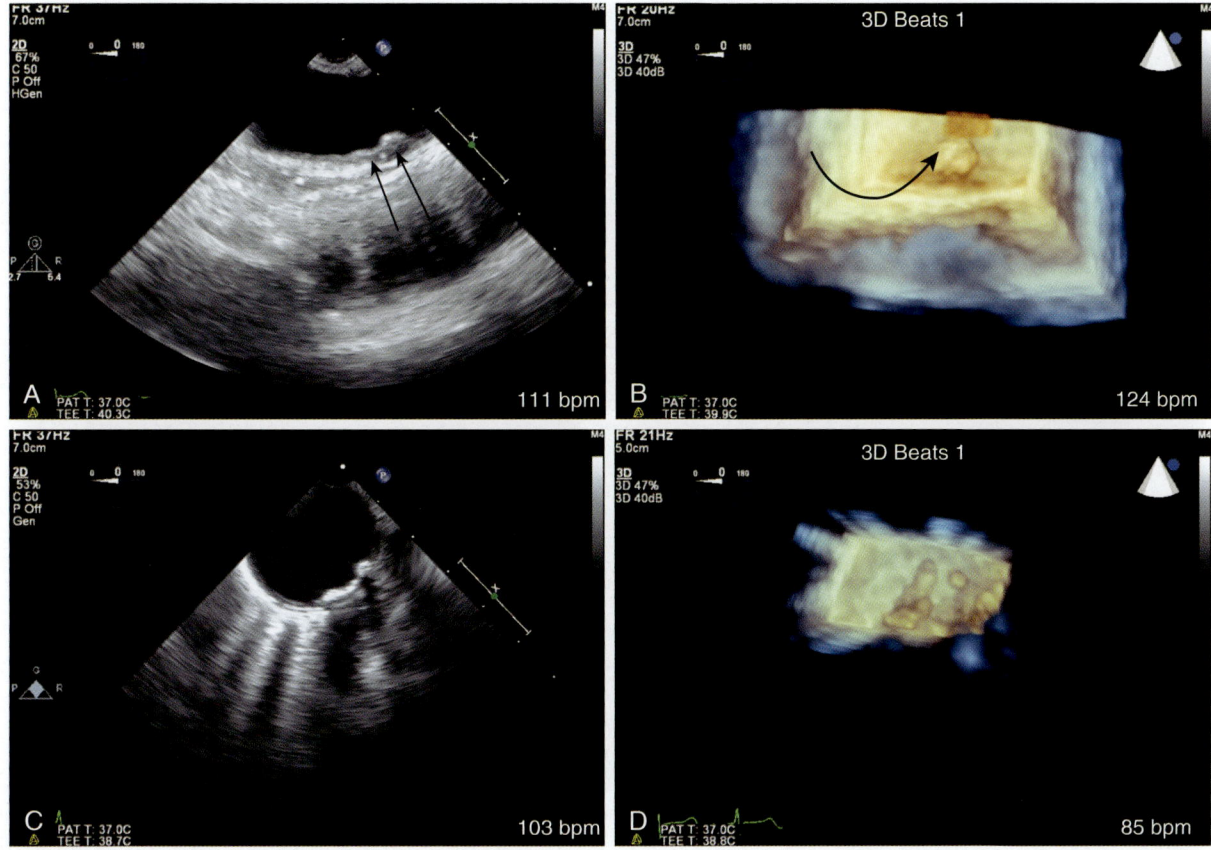

FIG. 33.40 Atherosclerosis is easily imaged with both transthoracic echocardiography and transesophageal echocardiography (TEE) modalities as the aortic walls become thickened and calcified. (A) TEE of the aortic arch shows the thickening along the posterior wall *(arrows)*. (B) Three-dimensional (3D) TEE demonstrates the extent of the plaque. (C) Irregular echo formation is seen on the posterior wall of the aortic arch in this TEE image. Note the shadowing posterior. (D) 3D TEE demonstrates several calcifications along the posterior wall not appreciated on the 2D TEE image.

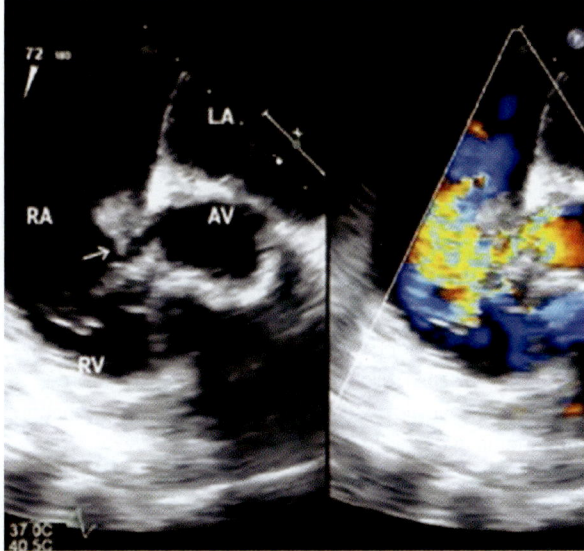

FIG. 33.41 Parasternal short-axis view of a penetrating aortic ulcer that has ruptured into the right ventricle.

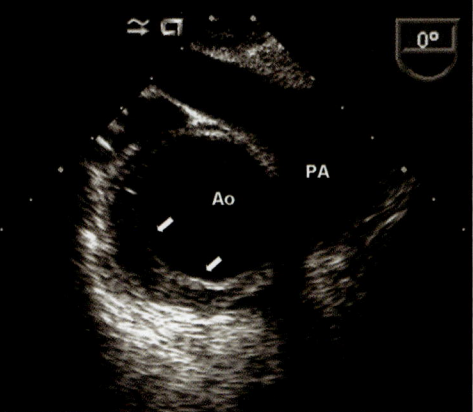

FIG. 33.42 An intramural hematoma is characterized by the absence of an intimal tear, layered thickening, crescent shape, and homogeneous appearance.

Penetrating Aortic Ulcer

This is an atheromatous plaque that ulcerates and disrupts the internal elastic lamina, burrowing deeply through the intima into the aortic media (Fig. 33.41). There may be involvement in the ascending aorta with true or pseudoaneurysm formation.

Intramural Hematoma

This hematoma occurs with the progression of a penetrating aortic ulcer. This may be found in hypertensive patients with spontaneous bleeding from the vasa vasorum into the media. The lesion is characterized by the absence of an intimal tear, layered thickening, crescent shape, and sonolucent to homogeneous appearance (Fig. 33.42).

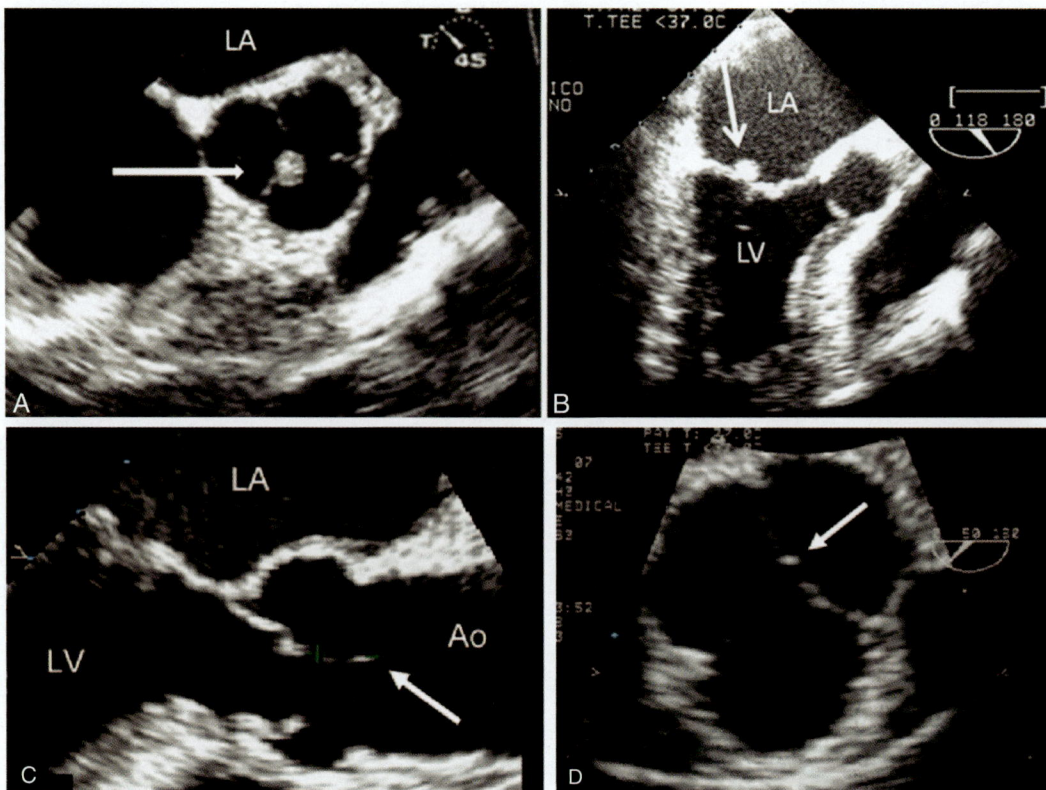

FIG. 33.43 Parasternal short-axis (A) and apical (B) views of a well-defined echogenic papillary fibroelastoma on the aorta and mitral valve *(arrow)*. (C–D) In contrast, the Lambl's excrescences are fine sail-like strings seen on the aortic leaflets. *Ao*, Aorta; *LA*, left atrium; *LV*, left ventricle.

Aortic Tumors

The most common benign tumor is a papillary fibroelastoma that is seen to arise on the valvular tissue. This presents as a small mass most commonly attached to the aortic or mitral leaflets that exhibit independent motion from the normal structures; less frequently, the fibroelastoma may also be seen attached to the tricuspid or pulmonary valves. The mass is most often found on the downstream side of the valve, closest to the ventricular cavity. The fibroelastoma may be similar to the smaller Lambl's excrescences, which are normally seen on the elderly valves (Fig. 33.43).

Primary tumors of the aorta are rare; sarcomas are found to be the majority of primary aortic tumors. The tumors classically arise in the intima and grow along the intimal surface into the aortic lumen. The morbidity and mortality are secondary to embolism.

Key Pearls

- Mitral regurgitation is defined as the systolic retrograde flow from the left ventricle into the left atrium.
- Causes of mitral regurgitation include leaflet and annulus disorders, defective tensor apparatus, and alterations of left ventricular and left atrial size and/or function.
- The two common causes of mitral stenosis are rheumatic fever and degenerative mitral stenosis.
- Differential diagnosis for mitral stenosis: cor triatriatum: subdivision of LA by a fenestrated membrane, atrial myxoma, or PV obstruction.
- Exercise hemodynamics should be performed in patients with symptoms out of proportion or discrepancies between valve area and gradients.
- Percutaneous balloon valvotomy should be the procedure of choice for those with mitral stenosis and a noncalcified, pliable valve.
- The development of aortic regurgitation may be the result of multiple causes: congenital malformation of the aortic valve, rheumatic disease, dilated aortic root, Marfan syndrome, endocarditis, aortic dissection, prosthetic valve dysfunction, or degenerative or calcified aortic valve.
- With acute aortic regurgitation, there is a sudden large regurgitant volume on the left ventricle, causing early closure of the mitral valve.
- There are three types of aortic stenosis: supravalvular, subvalvular, and valvular.
- The most common cause of aortic stenosis is calcific and senile or degenerative disease.
- The definition of an aneurysm implies that there has been 50% expansion of all three layers of the vessel wall in diameter.

- The mean rate of growth for the aneurysm is 0.1 to 0.6 cm/year, although this is higher in patients with Marfan syndrome. The risk of rupture is greatest when the aneurysm exceeds 6.0 cm or if the aneurysm is rapidly expanding.
- Bicuspid aortic valve is associated with other lesions in the heart in the form of aortic stenosis, endocarditis, coarctation, aortic dilation, or aortic dissection.
- The dissection is a tear in the aortic intima that leads to a false lumen with blood between the intima and media and/or adventitia.
- Complications of aortic dissection include compression of the true lumen (e.g., coronary ostial occlusion may lead to regional wall motion abnormalities or distal vessel obstruction may lead to stroke); thrombosis; acute aortic regurgitation; pericardial effusion and/or tamponade; acute aortic rupture with pleural effusion; and mediastinal hematoma.

BIBLIOGRAPHY

Baumgartner H, Hung J, Bermejo J, et al. EACVI/ASE clinical recommendations. Recommendations on the echocardiographic assessment of aortic valve stenosis: a focused update from the European Association of Cardiovascular Imaging and the American Society of Echocardiography. *J Am Soc of Echocardiogr.* 2017;30(4):373–390.

Oh JK, Kane GC, Seward JB, Tajik AJ, eds. *The echo manual.* ed 4. Philadelphia: Lippincott, Williams, Wilkins; 2018.

Otto CM. *The practice of clinical echocardiography.* Philadelphia. ed 6. Elsevier; 2023.

Zoghbi WA, Adams D, Bonow RO, et al. ASE guidelines and standards. Recommendations for noninvasive evaluation of native valvular regurgitation: a report from the American Society of Echocardiography Developed in collaboration with the Society for Cardiovascular Magnetic Resonance. *J Am Soc of Echocardiogr.* 2017;30(4):303–372.

CHAPTER 34

Introduction to Clinical Echocardiography: Pericardial Disease, Cardiomyopathies, and Tumors

Sandra L. Hagen-Ansert

OBJECTIVES

On completion of this chapter, you should be able to:
- Identify the echocardiographic distinction between pericardial effusion and pleural effusion
- Describe the echocardiographic findings in cardiac tamponade
- Describe the echocardiographic findings in dilated, restrictive, infiltrative, and hypertrophic cardiomyopathy
- Recognize the echocardiographic findings of tumors, thrombus, vegetations, and normal variants

OUTLINE

Pericardial Disease 980
    Pericardial Effusion 981
    Cardiac Tamponade 982
    Constrictive Pericarditis 983

Cardiomyopathies 985
    Dilated/Congestive Cardiomyopathy 986
    Takotsubo Cardiomyopathy 993
    Hypertrophic Cardiomyopathy 993

Cardiac Masses 995
    Cardiac Tumors 995
    Thrombus 998
    Subacute Bacterial Endocarditis/Vegetations 1000

KEY TERMS

Cardiac tamponade
Constrictive pericarditis
Dilated cardiomyopathy
Exudative
Fibrous pericardium
Hypertrophic cardiomyopathy
Lipomatous hypertrophy
Malignant primary cardiac tumors
Myxoma
Papillary fibroelastoma
Rhabdomyoma
Serous pericardium
Takotsubo cardiomyopathy
Transudative

In addition to valvular heart disease, the sonographer may encounter fluid within the pericardial sac secondary to pericardial disease; enlargement of the cardiac chambers with regurgitant valvular flow as a result of dilated cardiomyopathy; increased thickness of the myocardium secondary to infiltrative cardiomyopathy; abnormal thickness of the interventricular septum compared with the posterior wall as seen in hypertrophic cardiomyopathy; or abnormal lesions within the cardiac chambers that represent tumors, thrombus, or vegetations. Each of these areas will be presented briefly to provide a basic understanding and investigative pathway for the sonographer.

PERICARDIAL DISEASE

The normal pericardium has two layers: the outer sac is the **fibrous pericardium**, and the inner sac is the **serous pericardium**. The inner layer is further divided into the *visceral layer* (epicardium) that is continuous with the pericardial surface and covers the heart and proximal great vessels and the fibrous parietal layer (Fig. 34.1). The visceral layer is reflected to form the *parietal epicardium*. The visceral and parietal layers are separated by 15 to 50 mL of serous fluid. Their normal thickness is 1 to 2 mm and is abnormal if the thickness is greater than 4 mm.

CHAPTER 34 Introduction to Clinical Echocardiography: Pericardial Disease, Cardiomyopathies, and Tumors

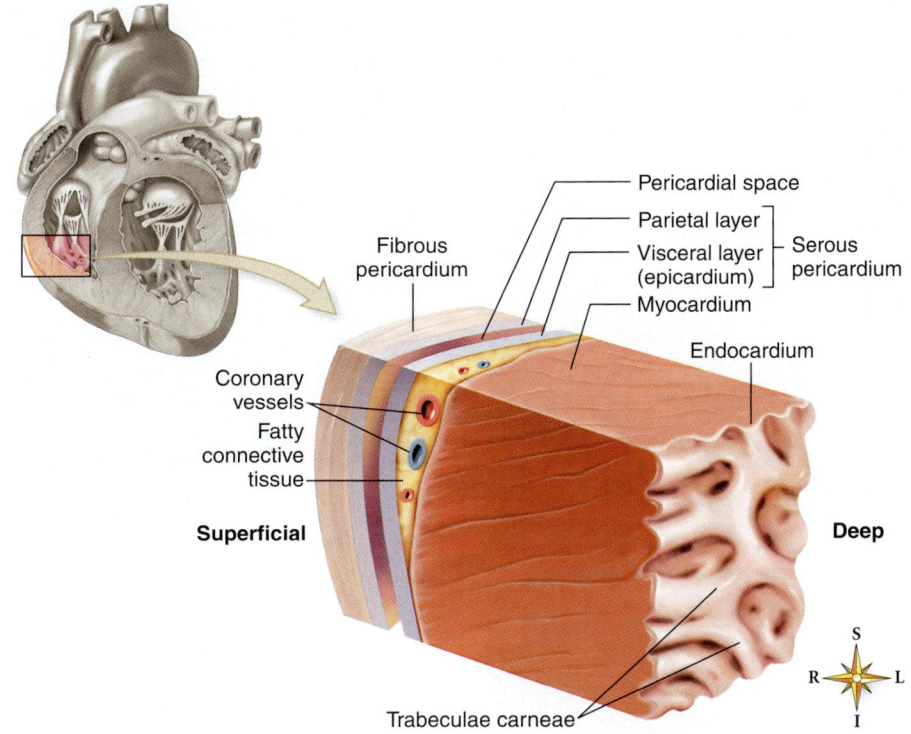

FIG. 34.1 The pericardium consists of two layers: the *fibrous outer layer* and the inner double-layered sac known as the *serous pericardium*.

The pericardium has many functions. It provides a mechanical protection to the heart, provides a barrier to infection, reduces friction, and hemodynamically limits acute distention. The pericardial sac also contributes to the diastolic coupling and ventricular interdependence.

Pericardial Effusion

The pericardial effusion is recognized as an echo-free space between the visceral and parietal pericardium. This fluid can be **transudative**, **exudative**, malignant, or hemorrhagic. The effusions first accumulate posterior to the heart and, as the size increases, extend laterally and then circumferentially.

Echocardiography is the primary method for the initial detection of pericardial effusion that occurs when fluid accumulates in the pericardial sac. This fluid usually accumulates posterior to the heart because this is the most dependent surface. As the effusion increases, it extends laterally and then may surround the apex and the anterior surface of the heart. It is important to distinguish the pericardial effusion from a possible pleural effusion. This is best imaged with transthoracic echocardiography (TTE) in the parasternal long-axis view with the deep image view. The round circle of the descending aorta may be seen posterior to the left atrium and serves as a landmark to distinguish pericardial from pleural effusion (Fig. 34.2). The pericardial effusion always is found anterior to the descending aorta, whereas the pleural effusion is posterior to the descending aorta. Recall that the pericardium reflects off the aorta at this junction.

The estimation of the amount of fluid around the heart may be made with echocardiographic evaluation (Table 34.1).

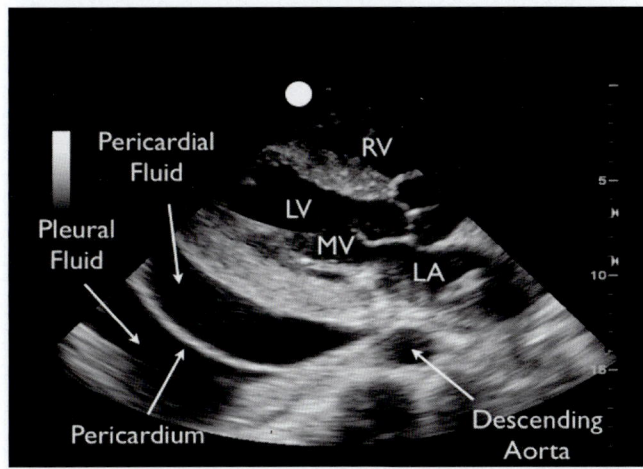

FIG. 34.2 The round circle of the descending aorta may be seen posterior to the left atrium and serves as a landmark to distinguish pericardial from pleural effusion. The pericardial effusion always is found anterior to the descending aorta, whereas the pleural effusion is posterior to the descending aorta. *LA,* Left atrium; *LV,* left ventricle; *MV,* mitral valve; *RV,* right ventricle.

TABLE 34.1	Size of Pericardial Effusion		
Size	Small	Medium	Large
Volume (mL)	<100	100–500	>500
Localization	Localized	Circumferential	Circumferential
Width (cm)	<1	1–2	>2

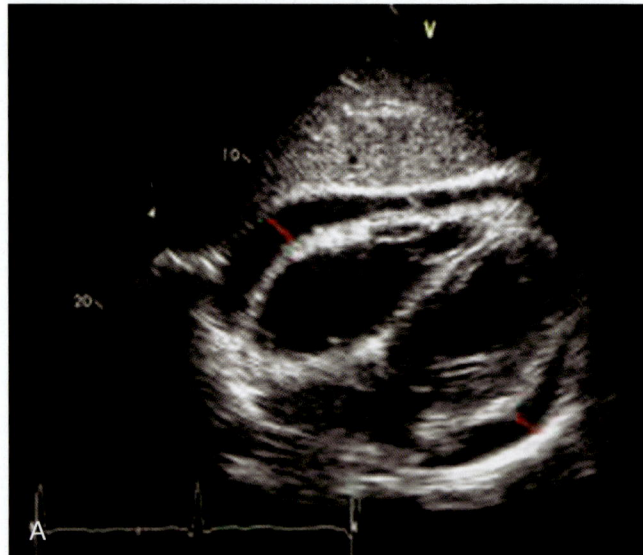

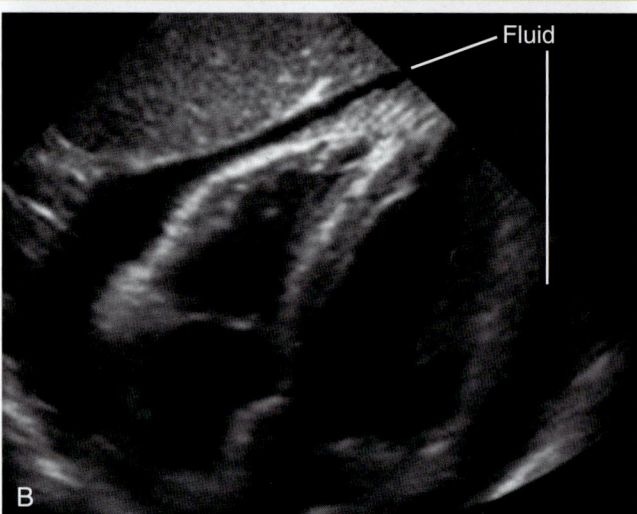

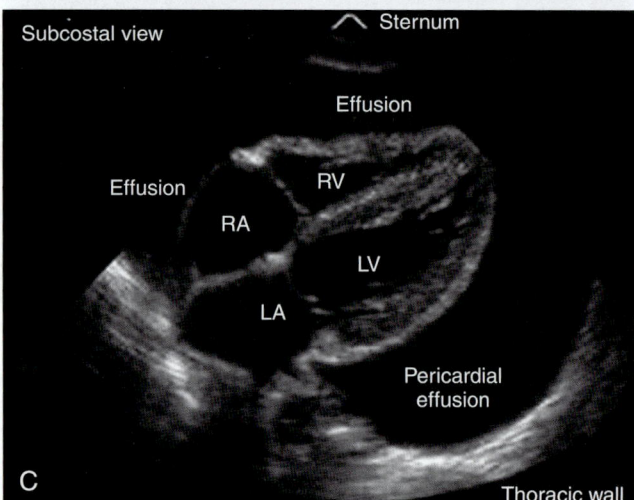

FIG. 34.3 A small pericardial effusion would measure <0.5 cm in systole (A); a moderate effusion would measure 0.5 to 2.0 cm (B); and a large effusion would be >2.0 cm (C). *LA*, Left atrium; *LV*, left ventricle; *RA*, right atrium; *RV*, right ventricle.

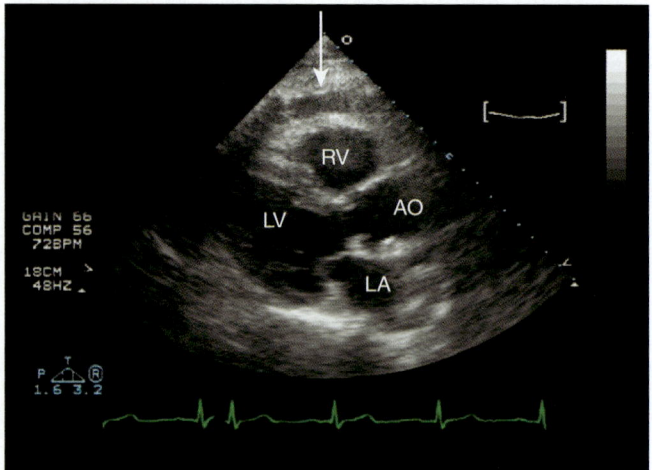

FIG. 34.4 If there is only an echo-free space anterior to the right ventricle, pericardial fat should be considered. *AO*, Aorta; *LA*, left atrium; *LV*, left ventricle; *RV*, right ventricle.

The small effusions are the most obvious during systole. If the effusion is greater than 25 mL, the echo-free space persists throughout the cardiac cycle. As the effusion increases in size, the parietal pericardium movement decreases. The small pericardial effusion would measure less than 0.5 cm in systole, a moderate effusion would measure 0.5 to 2.0 cm, and a large effusion would be greater than 2.0 cm (Fig. 34.3).

If there is only an echo-free space anterior to the right ventricle, the consideration of pericardial fat should be made (Fig. 34.4). If the patient has chronic effusions, fibrinous stranding within the fluid and on the epicardial surface of the heart may be noted. Pericardial effusion with hemorrhage or purulent fluid is more heterogeneous and echogenic; such hemorrhagic effusions are more common in patients with metastatic disease. Loculated effusions may be seen in postsurgical patients (Fig. 34.5).

Cardiac Tamponade

When a large volume of pericardial fluid accumulates rapidly, it becomes an emergent clinical problem. **Cardiac tamponade** occurs when the pressure in the pericardium exceeds the pressure in the cardiac chambers, which results in impaired cardiac filling. The intrapericardial pressure increases to the point of compromising systemic venous return to the right atrium. The pressure and volume relationship is much stiffer when fluid accumulates rapidly.

Clinically the patient will exhibit hypotension and tachycardia as manifested by symptoms of low cardiac output. The clinical finding of pulsus paradoxus is closely related to the echo findings of reciprocal respiratory changes in both the right and left ventricular filling and emptying.

Echocardiographic findings are quite specific for tamponade: moderate to large pericardial effusion, right atrial systolic

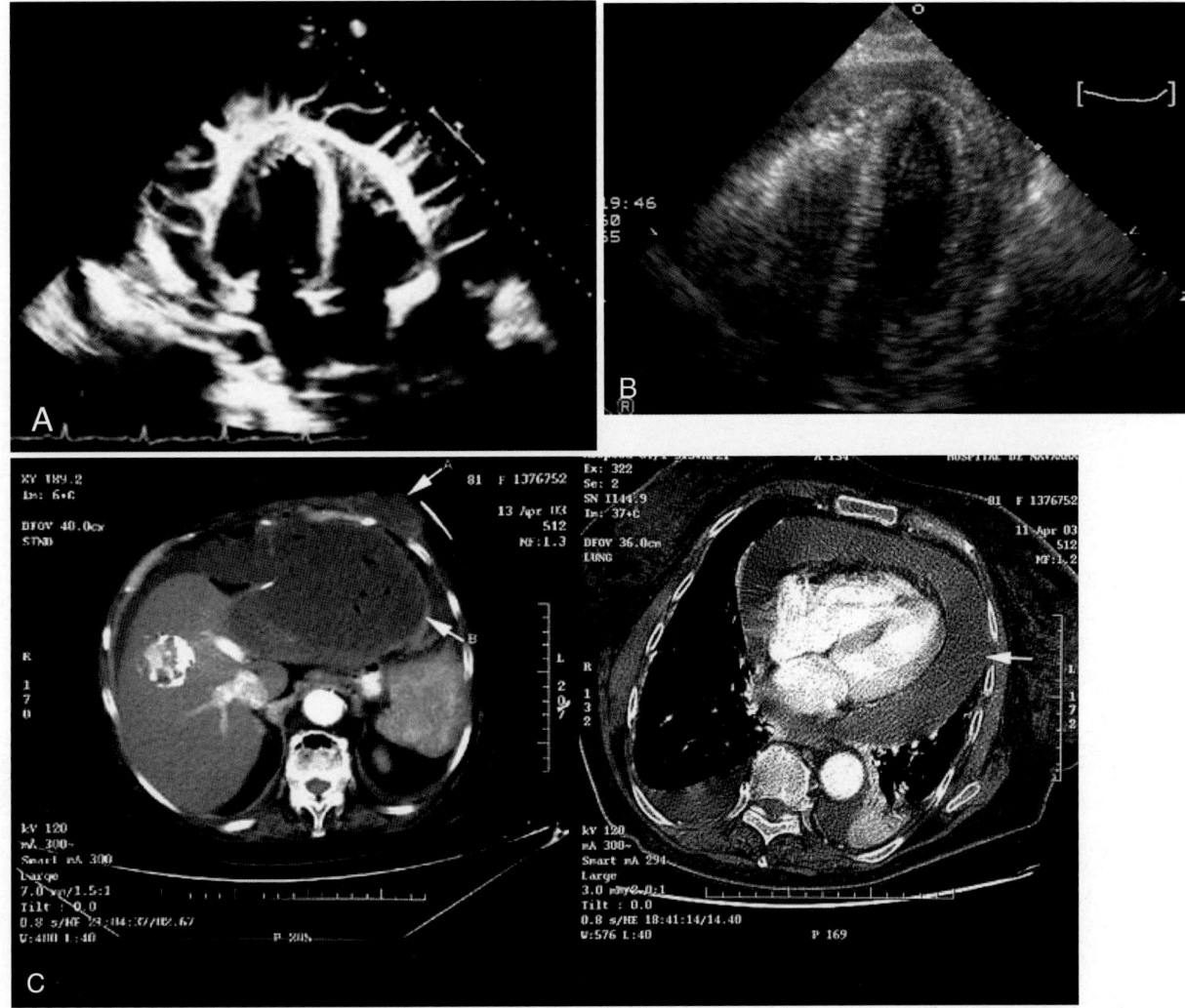

FIG. 34.5 (A) If the patient has chronic effusions, fibrinous stranding within the fluid and on the epicardial surface of the heart may be noted. (B) Pericardial effusion with hemorrhage or purulent fluid is more heterogeneous and echogenic. (C) Computed tomography image of the heterogeneous purulent fluid within the pericardial space.

collapse, right ventricle diastolic collapse, reciprocal respiratory changes in ventricular volumes, and a dilated inferior vena cava with lack of respiratory changes (Fig. 34.6). Doppler findings of the tricuspid and mitral inflow will show a respiratory variation in the right ventricular (greater than 40% variation) and left ventricular (greater than 25% variation) diastolic filling (Boxes 34.1 and 34.2). There is increased right ventricular filling on the first beat after inspiration and decreased left ventricular filling on the first beat after inspiration (Fig. 34.7).

Constrictive Pericarditis

In chronic pericardial disease the pericardium may become thickened and inelastic, which in turn limits the ventricular filling, leading to chronic biventricular diastolic dysfunction, right-sided heart failure, and low systemic output.

This condition is secondary to long-standing pericardial inflammation with pericardial scarring, thickening, fibrosis, and calcification. Causes of constriction include prior cardiac surgery, acute or chronic/recurrent pericarditis, mediastinal radiation, tuberculous pericarditis, trauma, or idiopathic.

On echocardiography there may be thickening of the pericardial layer with increased echogenicity (Fig. 34.8). There may be normal left ventricular size and systolic function. There is biatrial enlargement. The septum is quite abnormal: there may be an abrupt posterior motion of the ventricular septum in early diastole, a flat motion in middle diastole, an abrupt anterior motion following atrial contraction, or a septal "bounce" demonstrating an exaggerated interventricular dependence. The left ventricular posterior wall may be abnormal with a rapid movement during diastole, then flat during

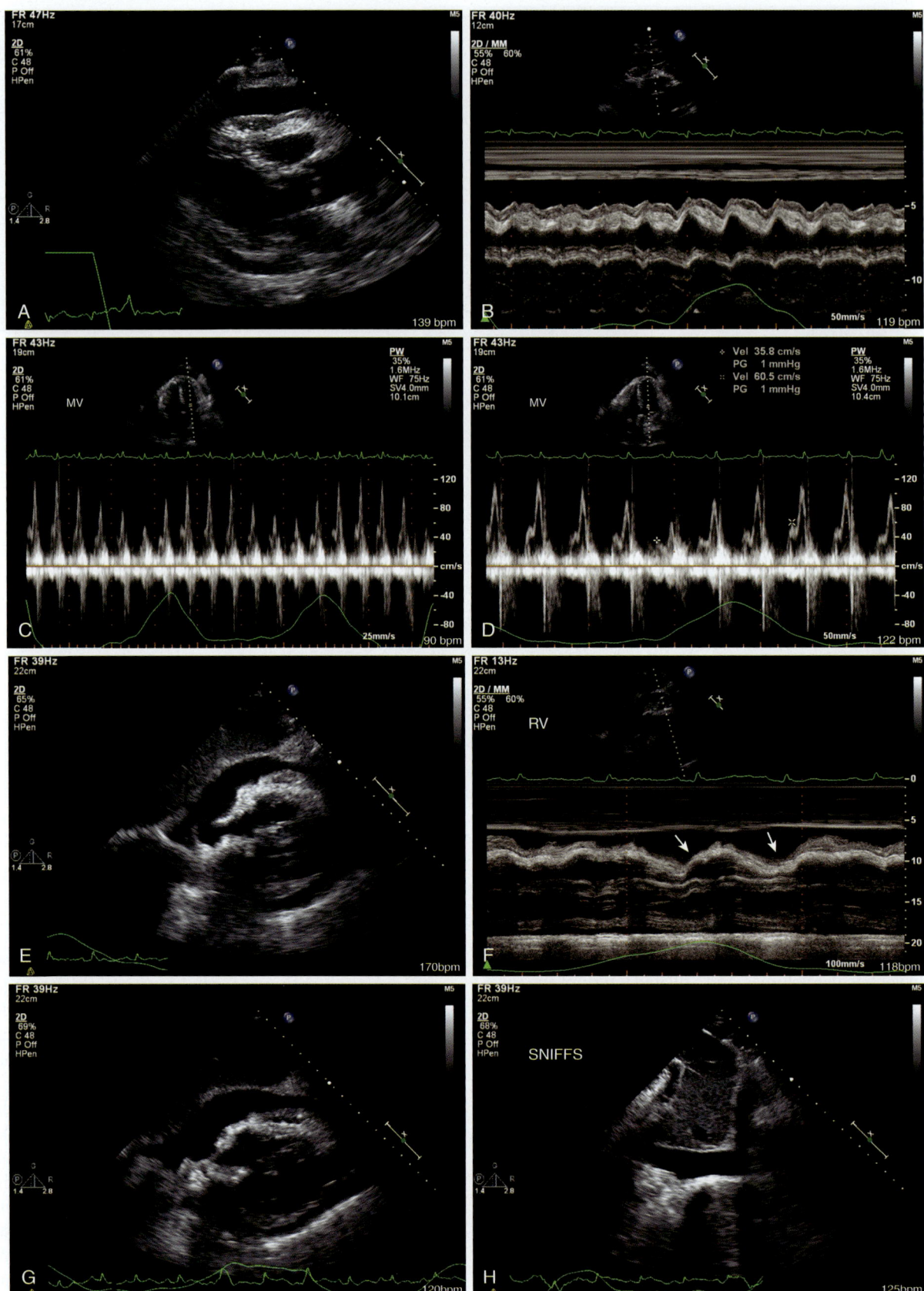

FIG. 34.6 (A) Parasternal long-axis view of a patient with an acute moderate size pericardial effusion causing right ventricular collapse. (B) M-mode tracing through the ventricles. (C–D) Doppler of the mitral valve inflow shows respiratory variation. (E) Subcostal image of the right heart diastolic collapse. (F) M-mode demonstrates the diastolic collapse of the right ventricle (arrows). (G) Subcostal view of the right atrial collapse. (H) The inferior vena cava remained dilated, even with "sniffs."

BOX 34.1	Cardiac Hemodynamics and Normal Respiratory Variation

With Inspiration
- Intrathoracic pressure decreases, transmitted to all cardiac chambers—intrapericardial and intracardiac pressures decrease.
- SVC and IVC are mostly extrathoracic, and pressure remains relatively constant.
- Pressure gradient between great veins and RA + RV increases, leading to increased right-sided heart filling. Tricuspid inflow varies by <25%.
- ↑ in RV volume causes small compensatory decrease in LV filling—"ventricular interdependence" (normal pulsus paradoxus <10 mm Hg).
- Pulmonary veins and LA + LV are entirely intrathoracic and have an almost equal decrease in pressures; hence overall pressure gradient between PV and LV remains constant with little change in LV filling through the respiratory cycle. Mitral inflow varies by <15%.

With Expiration
- Intrathoracic, intrapericardial, and intracardiac pressures increase, with a mild decrease in RV filling and a subsequent increase in LV filling.

IVC, Inferior vena cava; *LA*, left atrium; *LV*, left ventricle; *PV*, pulmonary vein; *RA*, right atrium; *RV*, right ventricle; *SVC*, superior vena cava.

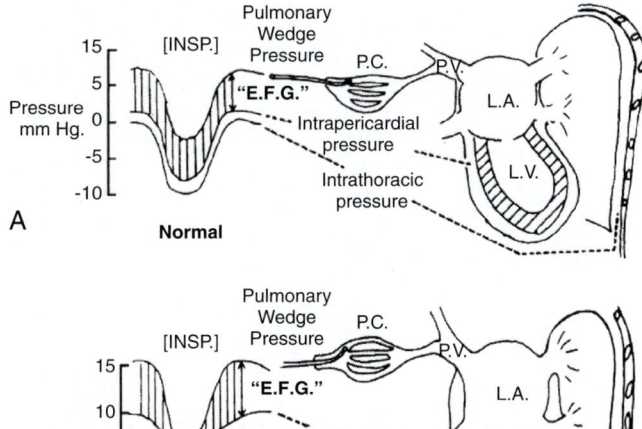

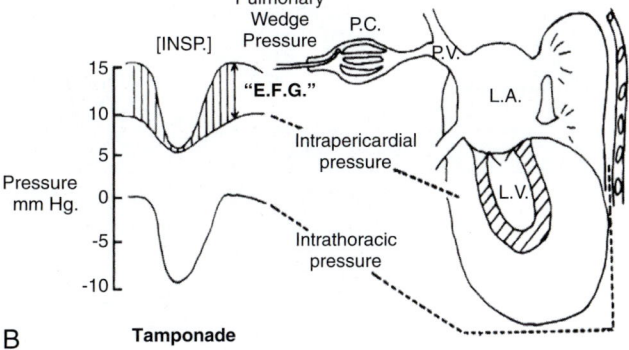

FIG. 34.7 (A) Left ventricle (LV) filling with inspiration (normal). Changes in intrathoracic pressure are transmitted equally to the pericardial sac and pulmonary veins (PV). The effective filling gradient (EFG) changes only slightly with respiration. (B) Left ventricle filling with inspiration (INSP) (tamponade). Changes in intrathoracic pressure are transmitted to the pulmonary veins but not to the pericardial sac; the EFG falls during inspiration. *P.C.*, pulmonary capillary.

BOX 34.2	Cardiac Hemodynamics and Respiratory Variation in Tamponade

With Inspiration
- On right side, decrease in intrathoracic pressure is transmitted to intrapericardial space and both pericardial and intracardiac pressures decrease relative to SVC/IVC pressures, leading to RV filling increases.
- Tricuspid inflow varies >25% with respiration.
- Ventricular interdependence makes septum bow toward LV to accommodate increased RV volume, leading to decreased LV filling.
- On left side, there is a decrease in intrathoracic and PV (PCWP) pressures but only a small decrease in intrapericardial and intracardiac pressures. Therefore LV filling gradient decreases, leading to decreased LV filling.
- Decreased LV filling allows for increased RV filling (ventricular interdependence).
- Mitral inflow varies >15%.

With Expiration
- RV filling is decreased slightly, and LV filling is restored.

IVC, Inferior vena cava; *LV*, left ventricle; *PCWP*, pulmonary capillary wedge pressure; *PV*, pulmonary vein; *RV*, right ventricle; *SVC*, superior vena cava.

mid to late diastole, with an abrupt termination of ventricular filling. The inferior vena cava is dilated with minimal respiratory variation.

Doppler findings in **constrictive pericarditis** reflect abnormal hemodynamics (Box 34.3 and Fig. 34.9). The mitral inflow pattern demonstrates increased early diastolic filling velocity followed by rapid deceleration, leading to a short filling time. There may be dynamic changes with respiration: early diastolic mitral inflow is reduced with the onset of inspiration, and the isovolumic relaxation time shortens and returns to normal with expiration. The pulmonary venous flow may show respiratory changes. The systolic wave and early diastolic wave velocities are increased during expiration and decreased during inspiration. The diastolic flow reversal is augmented in expiration in the hepatic vein flow. There may be a prominent y-descent on the hepatic vein or superior vena cava flow pattern.

CARDIOMYOPATHIES

Cardiomyopathy may be defined as a primary myocardial disorder that is not related to the effects of valvular heart disease, hypertension, or coronary artery disease. Traditionally

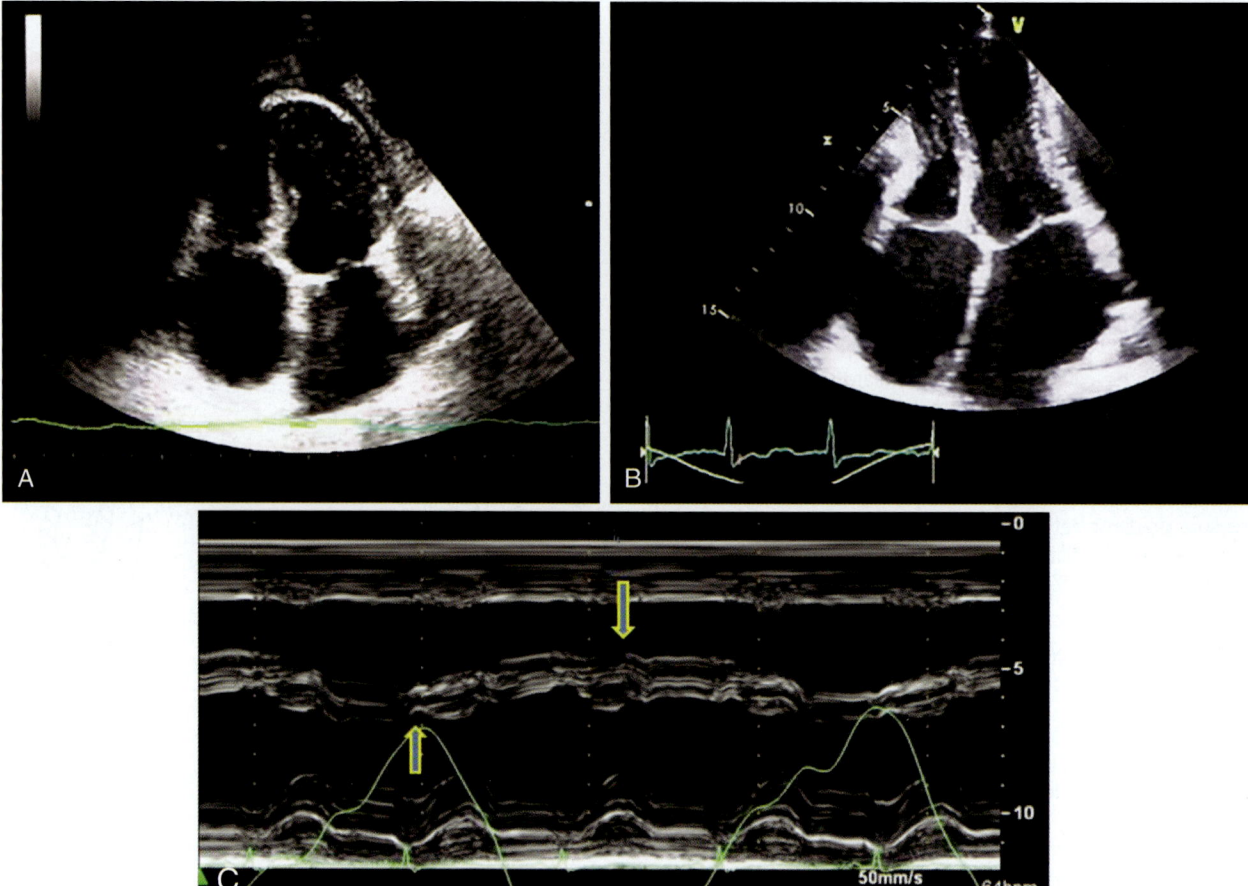

FIG. 34.8 (A) On echocardiography there may be thickening of the pericardial layer with increased echogenicity. There may be normal left ventricular size and systolic function. There is biatrial enlargement. (B–C) The septum is quite abnormal: there may be an abrupt posterior motion of the ventricular septum in early diastole, a flat motion in middle diastole, an abrupt anterior motion following atrial contraction, or a septal "bounce" demonstrating an exaggerated interventricular dependence *(arrow)*. The left ventricular posterior wall may be abnormal with a rapid movement during diastole, then flat during mid to late diastole, with an abrupt termination of ventricular filling. The inferior vena cava is dilated with minimal respiratory variation.

cardiomyopathies may be divided into these categories: dilated/congestive, restrictive/infiltrative, arrhythmogenic right ventricular dysplasia, hypertrophic, and unclassified (e.g., endomyocardial fibroelastosis). This section will focus on dilated, restrictive, and hypertrophic cardiomyopathies. Echocardiography plays a primary role in the assessment of the patient with congestive heart failure and suspected cardiomyopathy. The echocardiographic study not only provides prognostic information but also serves as a guide to the success of therapy.

BOX 34.3	Echocardiogram Findings in Constrictive Pericarditis

- Right atrial pressure: increased
- RV/LV filling pressures: increased RV, equivalent LV
- Pulmonary artery pressures: mild
- RV diastolic pressure plateau: greater than one-third peak RV pressure
- Diastolic filling: rapid, early, impaired late
- 2D echocardiography: pericardial thickening without effusion
- Doppler: E > a on LV inflow
- Prominent y-descent in hepatic vein
- Prominent a wave in pulmonary valve flow
- Respiratory variation in IVRT, E velocity
- Other diagnostic testing: CT or MRI for pericardial thickening

2D, Two-dimensional; *CT*, computed tomography; *IVRT*, isovolumic relaxation time; *LV*, left ventricle; *MRI*, magnetic resonance imaging; *RV*, right ventricle.

Dilated/Congestive Cardiomyopathy

Dilated cardiomyopathy is characterized by the dilation and reduced contractility of the left ventricle or both the left and right ventricles. There are multiple causes of dilated cardiomyopathy, as noted in Box 34.4. The abnormalities that may be seen with two-dimensional (2D) echocardiography include the following:
1. Left ventricular dilation (Fig. 34.10A).
2. Apical and lateral displacement of the papillary muscles with resultant functional mitral regurgitation (MR) due to the reduction in the length of the mitral valve apparatus in comparison with the annulus (Fig. 34.10B). The mitral valve leaflets may coapt only at the tips or not at all. In addition, there may be a shortened length of coaptation at the zona coapta.

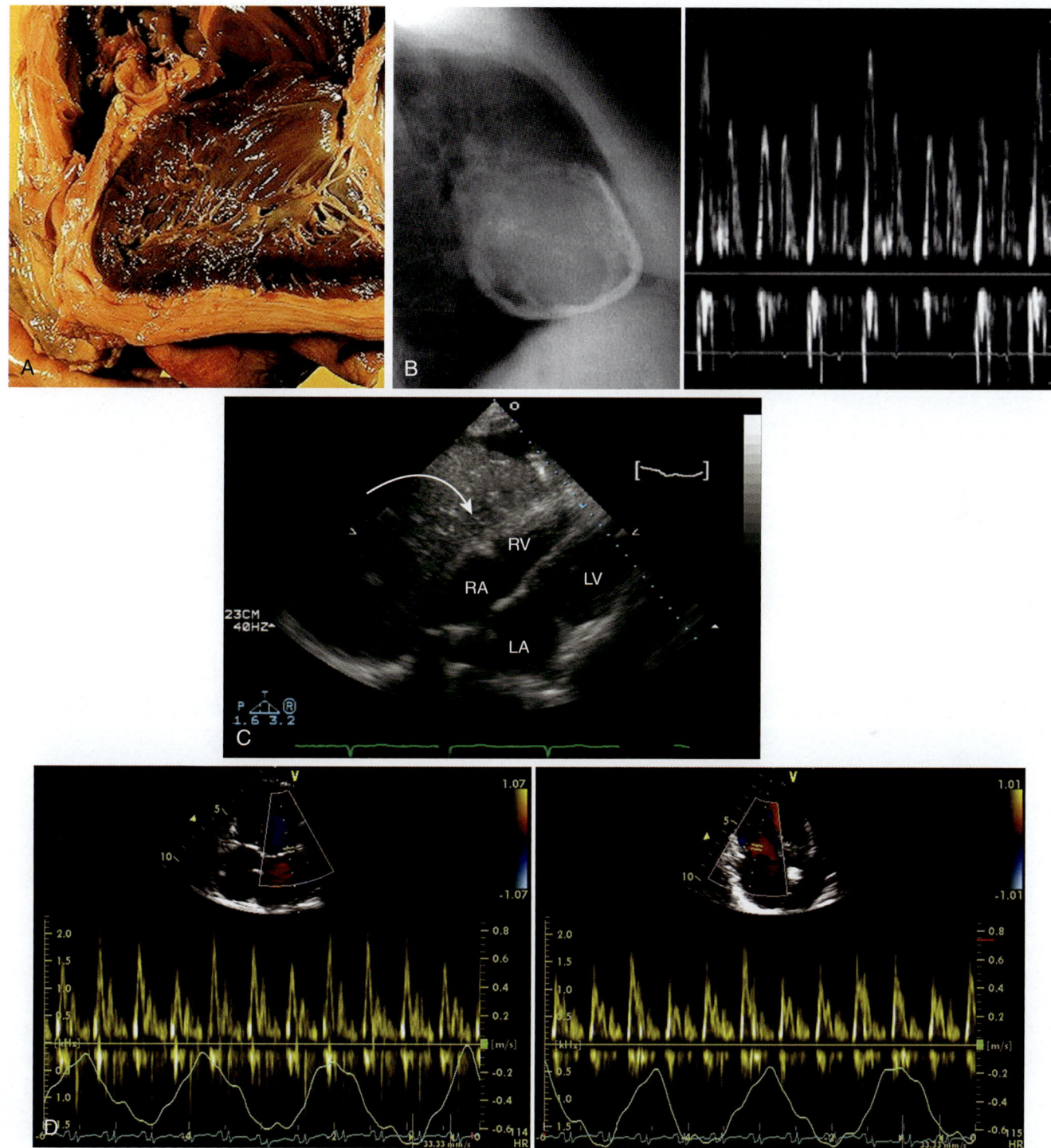

FIG. 34.9 (A) Gross specimen of the thickened pericardial layers as seen in pericardial constriction. (B) On radiography, the pericardium appears densely calcified. (C) Subcostal image demonstrates a thickened pericardial layer *(arrow)*. (D) Doppler evaluation of the mitral valve demonstrates increased early diastolic filling velocity followed by rapid deceleration, leading to a short filling time. *LA,* Left atrium; *LV,* left ventricle; *RA,* right atrium; *RV,* right ventricle.

BOX 34.4 Dilated Cardiomyopathy

Idiopathic
Familial
Noncompacted myocardium
Postpartum cardiomyopathy
Hemochromatosis
Infectious
- Postviral myocarditis
- Human immunodeficiency virus
- Legionella infection
- Gram-negative sepsis

Toxic cardiomyopathy
- Adriamycin/chemotherapy agents
- Alcohol
- Carbon monoxide poisoning

3. Increased distance between the interventricular septum and the E point of the anterior leaflet mitral valve (Fig. 34.10C).
4. "B" bump seen when there is a delayed closure of the mitral valve which correlates with an elevated end-diastolic pressure in dilated cardiomyopathy (Fig. 34.10D).
5. Left ventricular thrombus (Fig. 34.11). Contrast should be used if there are wall motion abnormalities and the endocardial layer is not clearly identified.
6. Normal to reduced wall thickness (Fig. 34.12).
7. Reduction of all of the systolic indices (see Fig. 34.12).

Additional echocardiographic findings may include the following changes. Left atrial dilation may be present; the degree of dilation is dependent on the duration of the cardiomyopathy. It also is a marker of more severe and long-standing ventricular dysfunction. Pulmonary hypertension may be

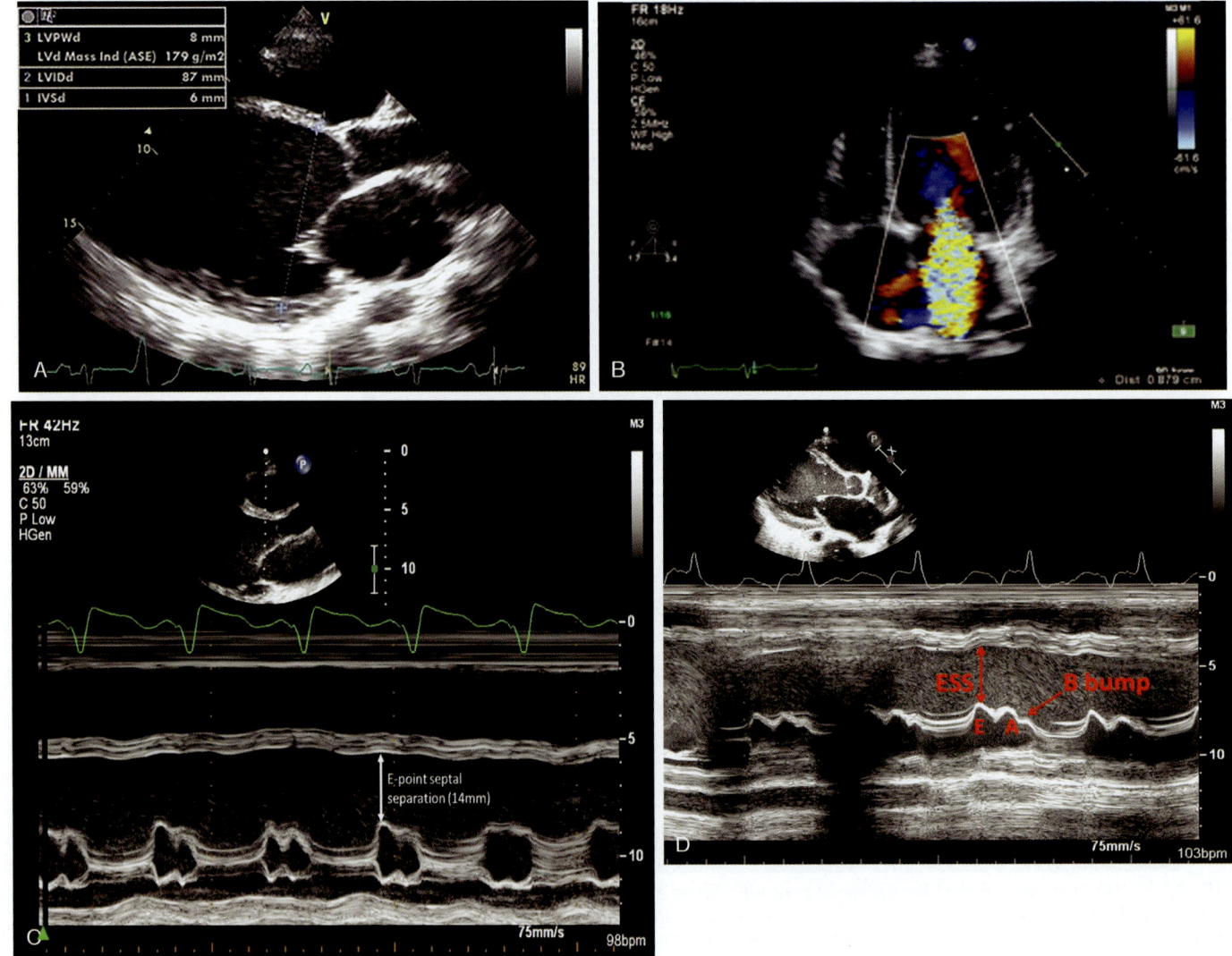

FIG. 34.10 (A) Left ventricular dilation. (B) Apical and lateral displacement of the papillary muscles with resultant functional mitral regurgitation due to the reduction in the length of the mitral valve apparatus in comparison to the annulus. (C) Increased distance between the interventricular septum and the E point of the anterior leaflet mitral valve. (D) "B" bump seen when there is a delayed closure of the mitral valve, which correlates with an elevated end-diastolic pressure in dilated cardiomyopathy.

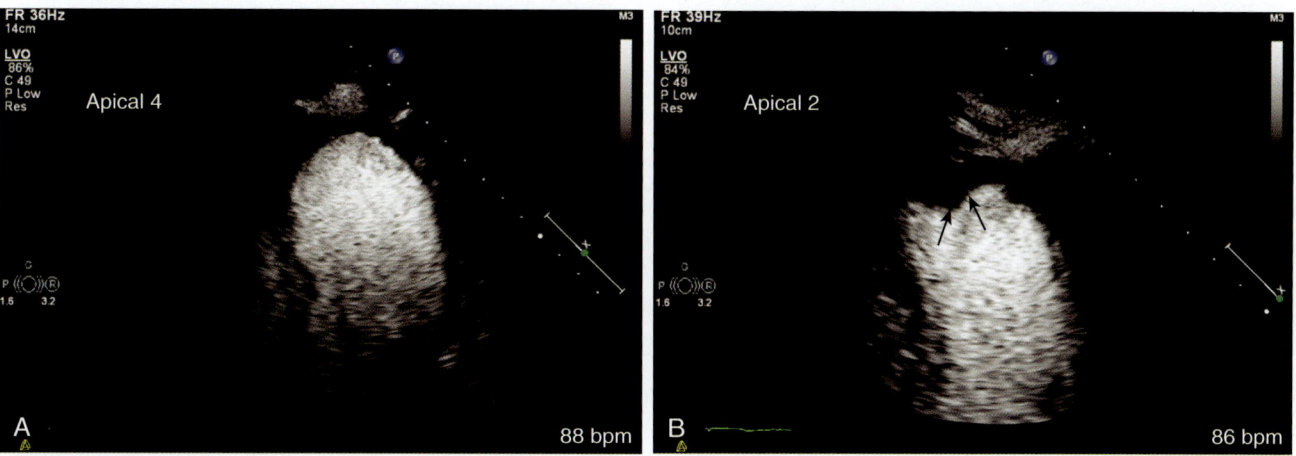

FIG. 34.11 (A) Contrast should be used if there are wall motion abnormalities and the endocardial layer is not clearly identified. (B) The apex of heart should be carefully evaluated with a slow sweep if wall motion abnormalities are identified to search for thrombus *(arrows)*.

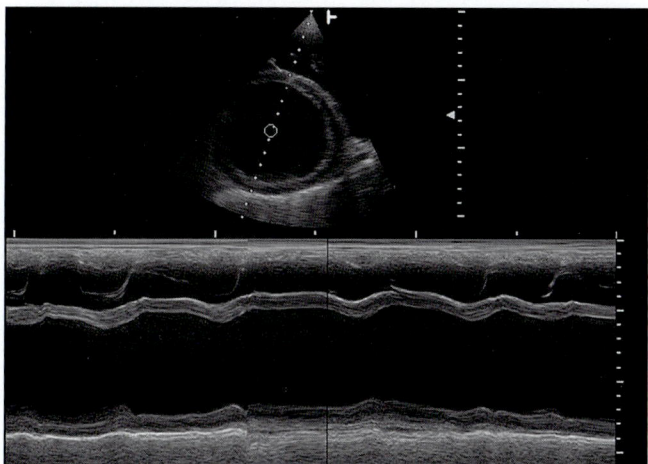

FIG. 34.12 M-mode of a patient with dilated cardiomyopathy. Note the reduced wall thickness and reduction of systolic indices.

present, as well as tricuspid regurgitation (Fig. 34.13). There may be dilation of the right ventricle with pulmonary hypertension, or there may be pathologic involvement of the right ventricle. The prognosis is worse when the right ventricle is involved. Measurement of tricuspid annular plane systolic excursion (TAPSE) of less than 15 mm indicates abnormal movement of the right ventricular free wall. This measurement is made with the M-mode cursor parallel to the base of the tricuspid annulus (Fig. 34.14).

It is challenging to distinguish with echo between ischemic and nonischemic cardiomyopathy. With end-stage ischemic disease, the sonographer will note regional wall motion abnormalities, calcification, and thin, bright, echogenic wall segments that may or may not have aneurysm formation. The left ventricular ejection fraction is moderately to severely depressed. The right ventricular systolic function is normal, whereas the pulmonary pressure is elevated. There is at least moderate MR.

Left ventricular volumes are useful to monitor clinical progress. Quantitative measurements should be obtained from all chambers with either 2D or three-dimensional (3D) imaging (Box 34.5). The end-diastolic volume index and end-systolic index should be calculated and related to body surface area. The M-mode analysis of the mitral valve tracing (Fig. 34.15) may demonstrate an increased distance between the E point of the anterior leaflet of the mitral valve and the corresponding (synchronous) interventricular septal endocardium. The normal E-point separation should be less than 6 mm; with ventricular enlargement, this distance increases. Also noted on this M-mode tracing is the "B bump," which signifies the delayed closure of the mitral leaflets between the leaflet coaptation points. This indicates increased left ventricular end-diastolic pressure (LVEDP), typically exceeding 20 mm Hg.

The aortic root motion may also indicate cardiac function. The systolic anterior motion (SAM) of the aortic root is proportional to the cardiac output (Fig. 34.16). The diastolic backward motion of the aortic root is determined by the emptying dynamics of the left atrium during left ventricular filling. This movement reflects the left ventricular diastolic filling pattern. The aortic root motion in low-cardiac-output state will demonstrate a reduced anterior systolic motion of the root. The aortic valve opening is also reduced and its duration is abbreviated with a slow closure at end systole.

If the patient has MR, the continuous wave (CW) Doppler velocity from the MR can be used as an index of global systolic function. The rate of rise of the Doppler velocity reflects the rate of rise of the left ventricular pressure. A dp/dt (change in pressure over change in time) less than 800 mm Hg/sec indicates severe dysfunction of the left ventricle (see Fig. 34.16C).

The Doppler evaluation of left ventricular function is outlined in Box 34.6. Forward flow and the diastolic properties of the right and left ventricles may be assessed. The assessment of forward flow is made through time velocity interval, stroke volume, and cardiac output (see Chapters 31 and 32). The diastolic properties of the left ventricle may be determined by the E/A ratio, dispersion of the E-wave velocity, color Doppler M-mode velocity of propagation, deceleration time, pulmonary vein flow, and annular Doppler tissue imaging. The diastolic properties of the right ventricle are determined by the

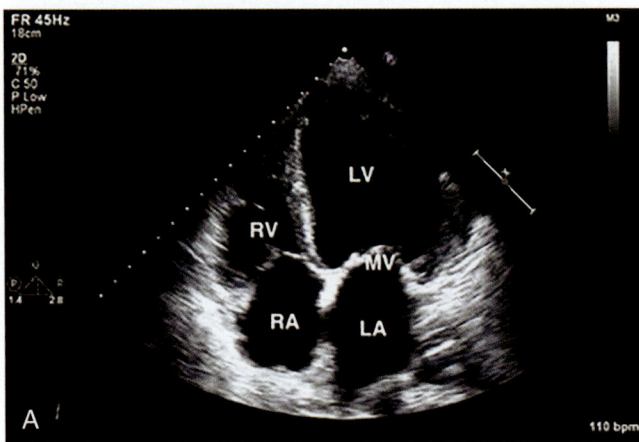
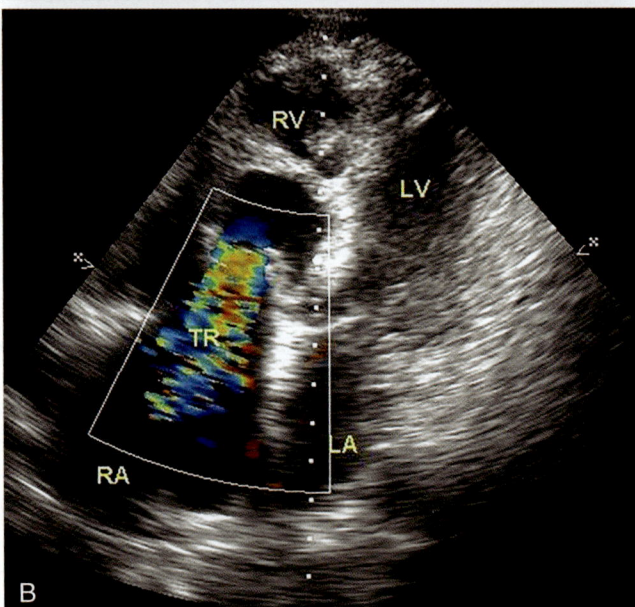
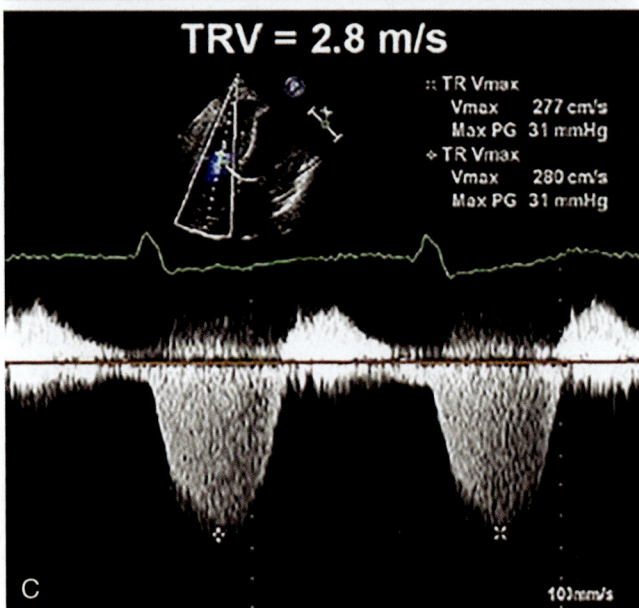

FIG. 34.13 Left atrial dilation may be present; the degree of dilation is dependent on the duration of the cardiomyopathy. It also is a marker of more severe and long-standing ventricular dysfunction. Pulmonary hypertension may be present, as well as tricuspid regurgitation. *LA*, Left atrium; *LV*, left ventricle; *RA*, right atrium; *RV*, right ventricle.

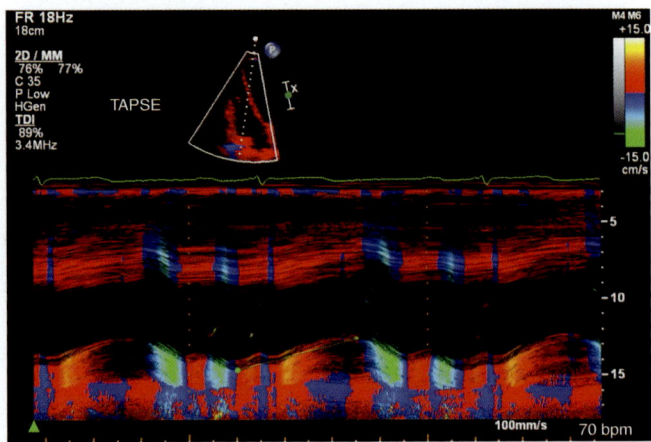

FIG. 34.14 Measurement of tricuspid annular plane systolic excursion <15 mm indicates abnormal movement of the right ventricular free wall. This measurement is made with the M-mode cursor parallel to the base of the tricuspid annulus.

BOX 34.5 Left Ventricle Volumes, Cardiac Output, and Stroke Volume

Quantitative measurements should be obtained from all chambers with 2D/3D imaging:
- End-diastolic volume index >100 mL/m²

Cardiac output calculations are frequently normal:
- EF usually between 20% and 40%
- Maintain high end-diastolic volumes and elevated heart rates

End-systolic volume index:
- Exceeds 30 mL/m² important indicator of global LV dysfunction
- ICM and global LV dysfunction with evidence of infarction, ESVI of 45 mL/m² identifies patients with a poor outcome

2D, Two-dimensional; *3D*, three-dimensional; *EF*, ejection fraction; *ESVI*, estimated stroke volume index; *ICM*, ischemic cardiomyopathy; *LV*, left ventricle.

Doppler flow in the hepatic veins and the Doppler flow in the superior vena cava.

The adverse prognosis of a patient with cardiomyopathy may be determined by the left ventricular size and function (Box 34.7) and the diastolic properties of the left ventricle.

Restrictive/Infiltrative Cardiomyopathy. There are many causes for restrictive/infiltrative cardiomyopathy (Box 34.8). The characteristics of restrictive cardiomyopathy include impaired ventricular filling due to increased stiffness of the myocardium, normal or reduced diastolic volume of either or both ventricles, and decreased ventricular compliance with an increase in LVEDP with respect to changes in left ventricular end-diastolic volume (LVEDV). This condition leads to increased biatrial enlargement. The valves may be thickened in infiltrative disorders. Apical obliteration with thrombus is a hallmark finding in endomyocardial fibrosis and hypereosinophilic heart disease. Pericardial effusion may be present. With the exception of infiltrative cardiomyopathy,

CHAPTER 34 Introduction to Clinical Echocardiography: Pericardial Disease, Cardiomyopathies, and Tumors

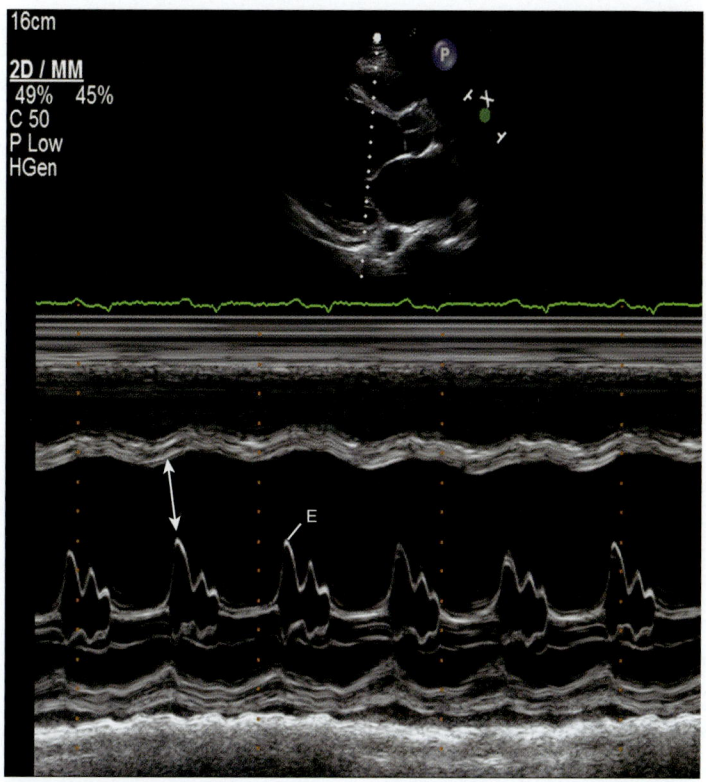

FIG. 34.15 M-mode tracing of the dilated left ventricle demonstrates an increased distance between the E point of the anterior leaflet of the mitral valve and the corresponding (synchronous) interventricular septal endocardium.

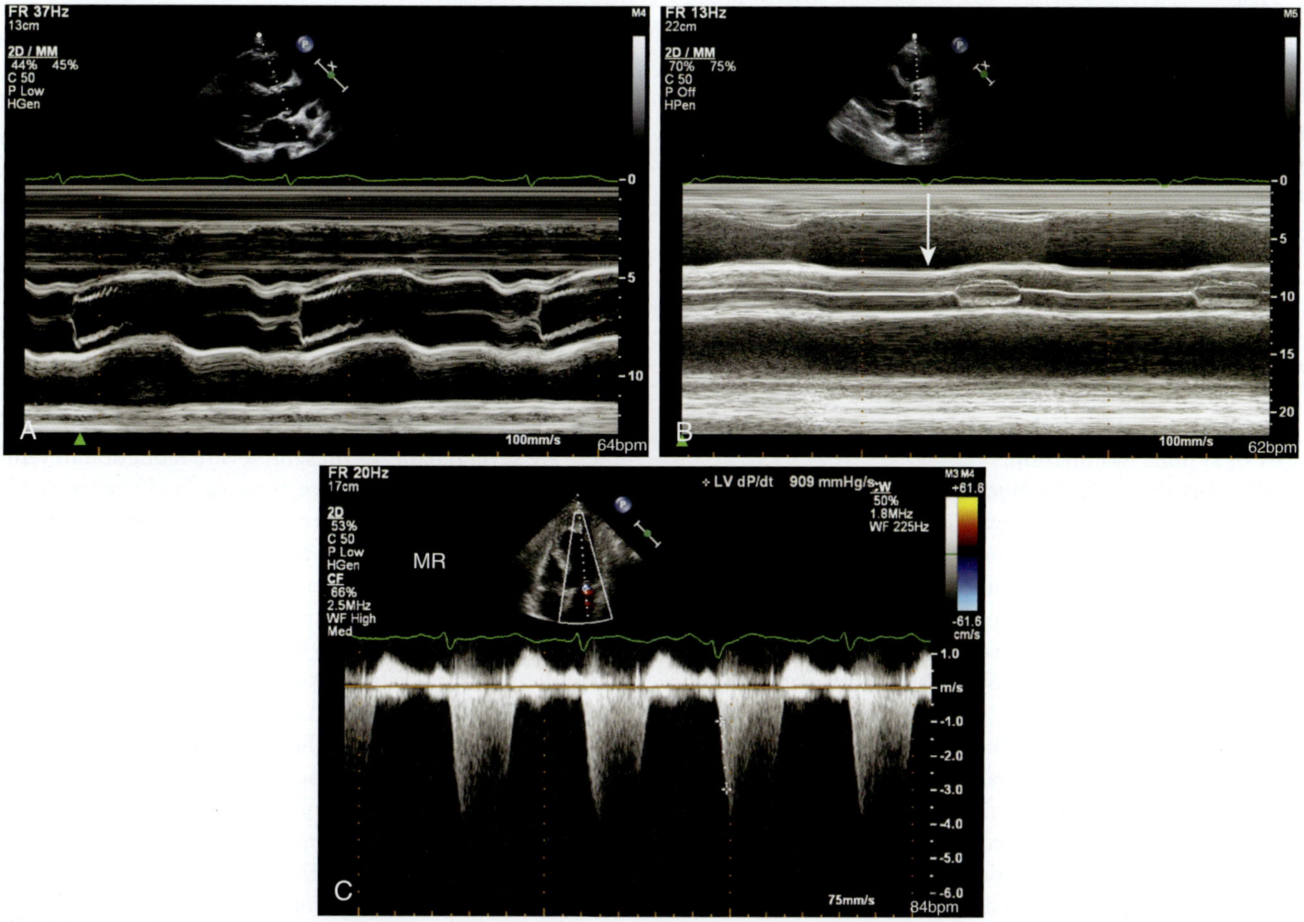

FIG. 34.16 The systolic anterior motion of the aortic root is proportional to the cardiac output. (A) Normal heart. (B) Heart with low cardiac output demonstrates reduced anterior systolic movement of the aortic root. (C) Doppler tracing of the patient with mitral regurgitation shows the left ventricular dp/dt of 909 mm Hg/sec. *MR*, Mitral regurgitation.

> **BOX 34.6 Doppler Evaluation**
>
> **Assessment of Forward Flow**
> Time-velocity interval
> Volume-based stroke volume
> Determine cardiac output
>
> **Diastolic Properties of the Left Ventricle**
> Mitral inflow pattern:
> - E/A ratio
> - Dispersion of E-wave velocity
> - Color Doppler M-mode velocity of propagation
> - Deceleration time
> - Isovolumic relaxation time
> - Pulmonary vein flow
>
> Annular Doppler tissue imaging
>
> **Diastolic Properties of the Right Ventricle**
> Doppler flow in hepatic veins
> Superior vena cava Doppler flow

> **BOX 34.7 Echocardiographic and Doppler Predictors of Adverse Prognosis in Cardiomyopathy**
>
> **LV Size and Function**
> LV internal dimension
> LV end-diastolic volume >75 mL/m^2
> LV end-systolic volume >55 mL/m^2
> EF <40%
> Sphericity index <1.5
> LV dp/dt <600 mm Hg/sec
> Myocardial performance index >0.4
>
> **Diastolic Properties of the LV**
> Restrictive mitral inflow pattern
> Pseudonormal mitral inflow pattern

dp/dt, Change in pressure over change in time; *EF*, ejection fraction; *LV*, left ventricle.

> **BOX 34.8 Classification of Restrictive/Infiltrative Cardiomyopathy**
>
> **Infiltrative**
> Amyloid heart disease (most common)
> Sarcoidosis
> Gaucher disease
> Hurler syndrome
> Fatty infiltration
>
> **Storage Diseases**
> Hemochromatosis
> Fabry disease
> Glycogen storage disease
>
> **Endomyocardial**
> Endomyocardial fibrosis
> Hypereosinophilic syndrome–Loeffler endocarditis
> Carcinoid heart disease
> X-ray therapy
> Metastatic cancers
> Anthracycline toxicity
>
> **Noninfiltrative**
> Idiopathic cardiomyopathy
> Familial cardiomyopathy
> Scleroderma
> Diabetic cardiomyopathy
> Hypertrophic cardiomyopathy

there may be normal or near-normal systolic function and wall thickness. Restrictive/infiltrative cardiomyopathy should be considered in a patient with heart failure without cardiomegaly or systolic dysfunction.

Idiopathic Restrictive Cardiomyopathy. This is a familial disorder that can be associated with distal skeletal myopathy. Echocardiographic findings include biatrial enlargement, appendageal thrombosis (common), normal left ventricle cavity size and thickness, and normal systolic function.

Eosinophilic Cardiomyopathy: Loeffler Endocarditis. This is a restrictive, obliterative cardiomyopathy with eosinophilic infiltration of the myocardium. There is direct damage from intracytoplasmic granules to the myocardium. The fibrosis can be localized, leading to valvular heart disease (regurgitation). On echocardiographic evaluation the following findings may be present: thickening of the inferior basal left ventricular wall, endocardial deposition of thrombus, and apical obliteration (best defined with contrast echocardiography) (Fig. 34.17).

Amyloid Cardiomyopathy. The heart is affected in nearly 90% of patients with amyloid cardiomyopathy; less than 5% have isolated cardiac involvement. The patient presents with diastolic heart failure with predominant right-sided symptoms. Classic echocardiographic features are commonly present in the later stages of disease (Fig. 34.18), which include the following: myocardial thickening with echogenic homogeneous granular sparkling appearance, thickening of the valve leaflets with resultant regurgitation, biatrial enlargement, normal left ventricle cavity size, gradual deterioration of ventricular systolic function, diastolic dysfunction, and pericardial effusion.

Restrictive Pattern With Severe Dysfunction. In this condition, the echocardiograph findings can be very useful because there are several patterns present: severe reduction in ventricular or pericardial compliance, increase in left ventricle filling pressures, increase in left atrial pressure, increase in transmitral gradient, increase in E-wave peak velocity, increased flow into a noncompliant ventricle leading to a rapid rise in LVEDP, shortened deceleration time of less than 150 msec, A wave reduced secondary to no atrial filling due to high LVEDP, and mitral valve E/A ratio greater than 1.5.

The patterns of abnormal pulmonary venous flow in restrictive cardiomyopathy show a marked decrease of relaxation and compliance that leads to elevation of left atrial pressure. There is reduced systolic antegrade flow and a small S wave on the pulmonary inflow. The antegrade flow shifts predominantly to diastole. The large E wave is present with abrupt cessation to flow. Small volume leads to an abrupt increase in LVEDP (Fig. 34.19).

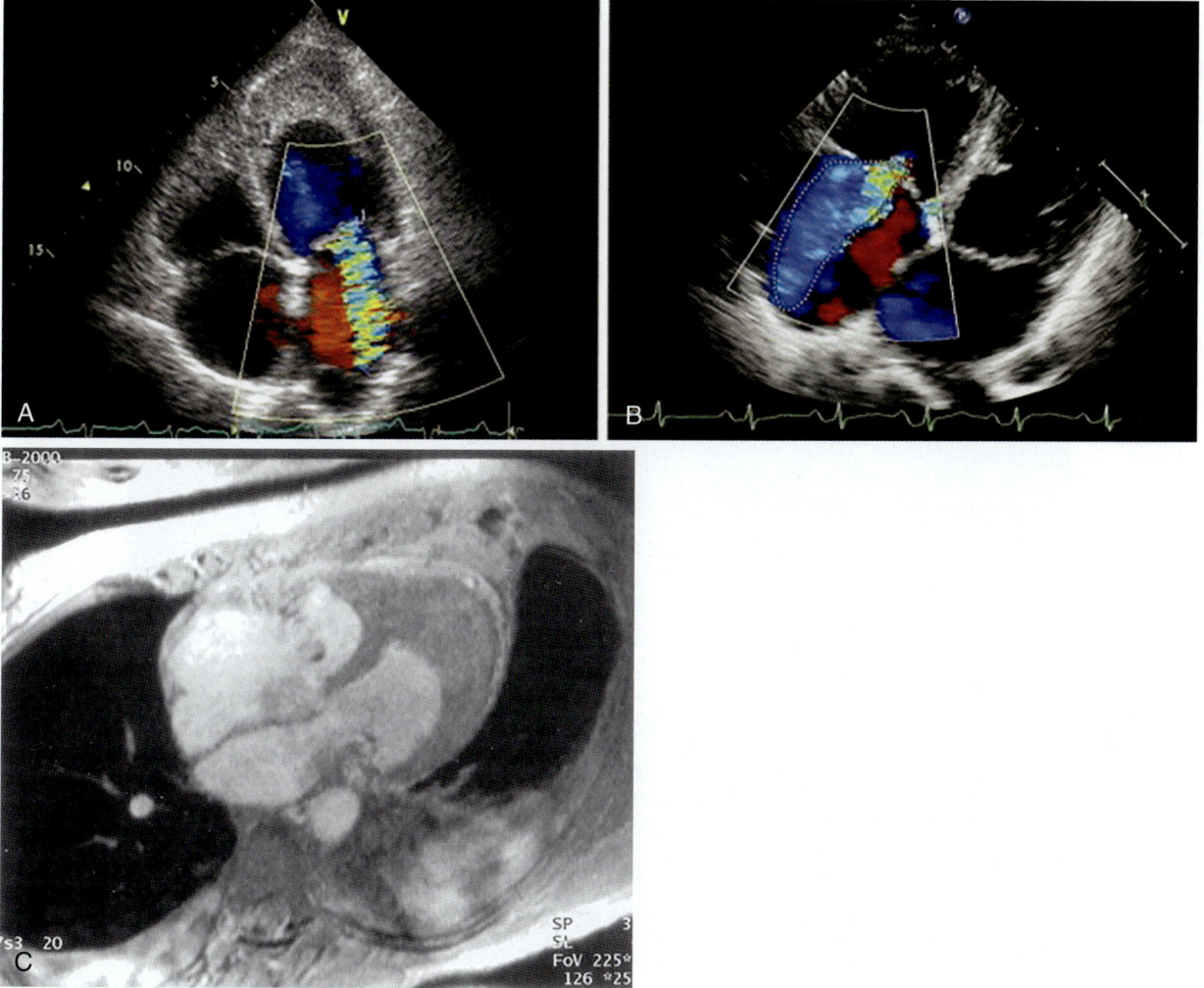

FIG. 34.17 Eosinophilic cardiomyopathy. (A–B) On echocardiographic evaluation the following findings may be present: thickening of the inferior basal left ventricular wall, endocardial deposition of thrombus, and apical obliteration (best defined with contrast echocardiography). (C) Magnetic resonance image demonstrates the endocardial deposition of thrombus with apical obliteration.

Takotsubo Cardiomyopathy

Takotsubo cardiomyopathy is an acute cardiac syndrome that is characterized by transient left ventricular regional wall motion abnormalities, chest pain and/or dyspnea, ST segment elevations, and minor elevations in cardiac enzymes. On echocardiography there is a marked reduction in left ventricular ejection fraction, apical hypokinesis in the setting of preserved basilar function, and apical ballooning. Subsequent follow-up echocardiograph evaluation will show the disappearance of these findings.

Hypertrophic Cardiomyopathy

The definition of **hypertrophic cardiomyopathy** is a hypertrophied, nondilated left ventricle in the absence of another cardiac or systemic disease capable of producing hypertrophy. The pathology of this condition denotes inappropriate hypertrophy, interstitial fibrosis, myofiber disarray, disorganized myocardial architecture, and impaired left ventricle performance. The differential diagnosis would include systemic hypertension, aortic stenosis, storage or infiltrative disorders, athletic heart, and elderly septal hypertrophy.

The predominant anatomic features of hypertrophic cardiomyopathy include a narrowed left ventricular outflow tract (LVOT) secondary to the asymmetric septal hypertrophy. The definition of asymmetric hypertrophy of the left ventricle is made when the septal/posterior left ventricular wall ratio is greater than 1.3 and with septal thickness greater than 15 mm. There is normal ventricular systolic function, impaired diastolic left ventricular function, and/or subaortic dynamic obstruction. An intrinsic abnormality of the mitral valve leaflets usually demonstrates the leaflets to be elongated with coaptation at the body rather than the tips. SAM of the mitral valve may be present, which further impedes flow in the LVOT. There may be anterior displacement of the mitral valve apparatus. The long mitral valve leaflets and anterior displacement of the papillary muscles lead to reduced chordal tension. The anterior leaflet, distal to the site of coaptation, is subject to Venturi (drag) forces resulting in anterior and superior angulation and contact with the septum in midsystole. This mitral leaflet-septal contact occurs

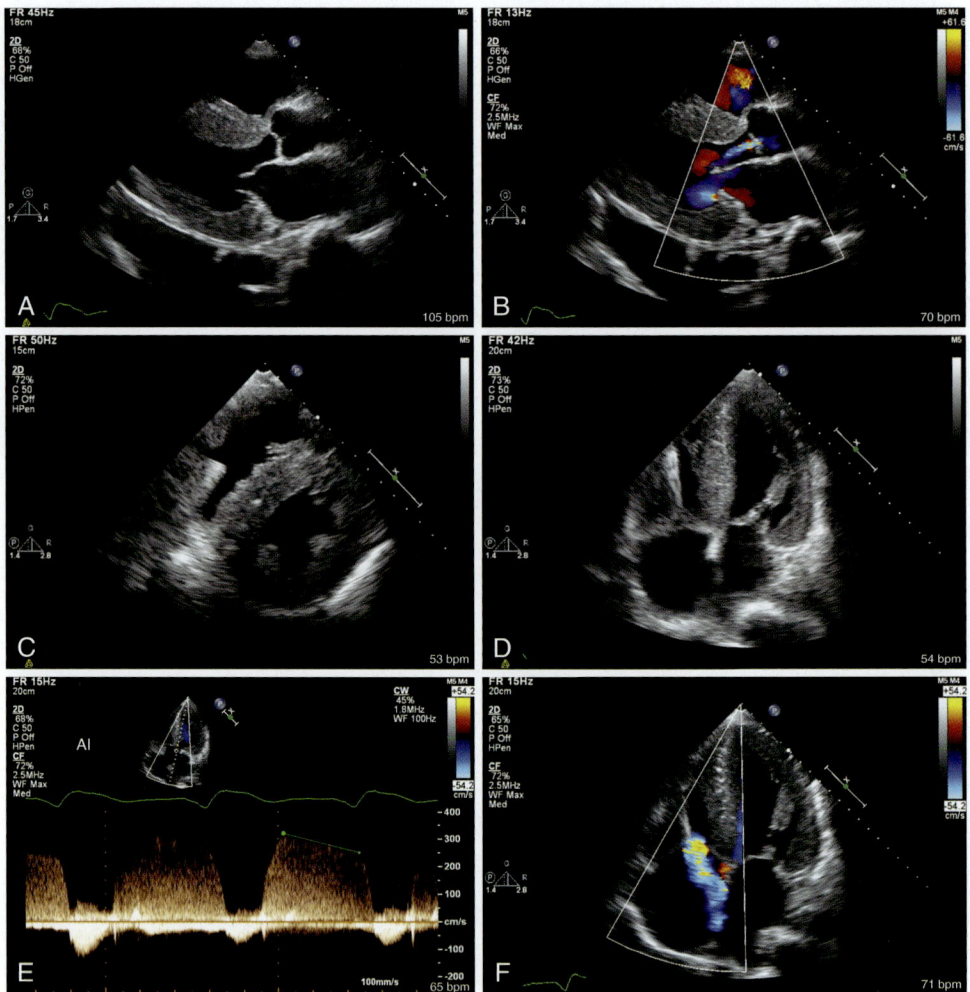

FIG. 34.18 Amyloid echocardiographic features. (A) Myocardial thickening with echogenic homogeneous granular sparkling appearance. (B) Thickening of the valve leaflets with resultant regurgitation. (C) Parasternal short-axis view of the thickened myocardium. (D) Apical four-chamber view shows normal ventricular size. (E) Continuous wave Doppler through the aortic valve demonstrates aortic regurgitation. (F) Apical four-chamber view shows tricuspid regurgitation.

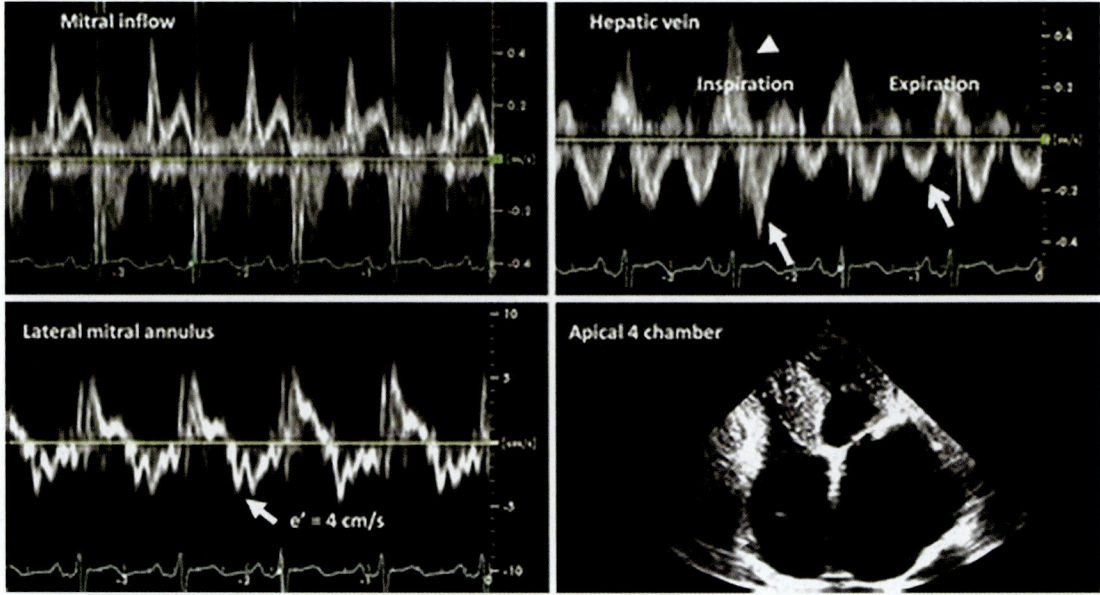

FIG. 34.19 In restrictive cardiomyopathy with left ventricular dysfunction there will be an increase in left ventricular filling pressures, an increase in left atrial pressure, an increase in transmitral gradient, an increase in E-wave peak velocity, increased flow into a noncompliant ventricle leading to a rapid rise in left ventricular end-diastolic pressure (LVEDP), shortened deceleration time of <150 msec, A wave reduced secondary to no atrial filling due to high LVEDP, and mitral valve E/A ratio >1.5.

almost simultaneously with the onset of the increased pressure gradient.

Hypertrophic cardiomyopathy may be nonobstructive or obstructive (hypertrophic obstructive cardiomyopathy). There are four patterns of left ventricular hypertrophy: type I, confined to anterior septal segment; type II, anterior/posterior septal segments; type III, basal segment of the posterior wall; and type IV, apical hypertrophy.

The echocardiographic analysis should include a complete echo evaluation, with 2D, M-mode, spectral, and color Doppler analysis. In the parasternal long-axis view, the evaluation of the thickness of the interventricular septum should be compared with the thickness of the posterior basal segment of the left ventricle (Fig. 34.20). The LVOT should be evaluated to see if the septal thickness causes obstruction to the LVOT. In addition, the presence of SAM of the mitral leaflet should be evaluated to see if further flow velocity is obstructed in the LVOT (Box 34.9). The dynamic outflow obstruction is determined by the amount of SAM present. The SAM may be restricted to redundant chordal SAM, which does not cause significant changes in flow velocity, or the SAM may touch the septum throughout systole, causing significant LVOT obstruction of flow and resultant mid-systolic closure of the aortic valve (Fig. 34.21). Keep in mind that there may be "normal" slight bulging of the septum into the LVOT in older patients. In addition, increased tortuosity of the aorta may lead to a more acute angle between the basal septum and the aortic root.

The sonographer should use both pulsed wave (PW) and CW Doppler to evaluate the flow velocity from the apical five-chamber view (Box 34.10). With PW Doppler, place the sample volume at the apex of the left ventricle to record the velocity; slowly move the sample volume to the mid-ventricle (annotate on the 2D image), and record the flow velocity. Then move the sample volume to the LVOT, still with PW Doppler to record the flow. With significant obstruction, you may reach the Nyquist limit of the PW probe; move the baseline up to record the maximum velocity. If you need to change to "high PRF," the sample volume is now made from multiple sites and averaged, and the LVOT flow will not be as accurate. Then use CW to record the flow velocity in the aorta. With obstruction, you will see a late-peaking "dagger" with CW Doppler (Fig. 34.22). You may also use the Valsalva maneuver to perform this Doppler interrogation to see the change in flow obstruction. Be certain to annotate your position in the ventricle as you move the sample volume and if you use the Valsalva maneuver.

Tissue Doppler imaging may help to differentiate between the variants of left ventricular hypertrophy such as hypertrophic cardiomyopathy, hypertensive left ventricular hypertrophy, and athlete's heart. The systolic and early diastolic mitral annular velocities (a measure of longitudinal systolic function) are attenuated in hypertrophic cardiomyopathy, even in nonhypertrophied segments. The tissue Doppler imaging–derived myocardial strain and strain rate imaging allow for accurate estimation of regional myocardial deformation.

Associated MR may be present in patients with hypertrophic cardiomyopathy. The abnormal SAM demonstrates a late systolic failure of coaptation of the mitral leaflet causing a posterior-directed mitral regurgitant jet. In these patients, the anterior leaflet is usually found to have a larger surface area and longer length. In a small percentage of patients there is an abnormal papillary muscle insertion that contributes to the regurgitant jet. If the mitral regurgitant jet is anteriorly directed, there may be intrinsic mitral leaflet disease independent of SAM (mitral prolapse, ruptured chordae, calcification, or leaflet trauma). The high-velocity systolic signal of LVOT obstruction may be contaminated by the jet of MR.

CARDIAC MASSES

The definition of a *cardiac mass* is an abnormal structure within or immediately adjacent to the heart. There are several types of cardiac masses, including tumor, thrombus, vegetation, iatrogenic material, normal variant, and extracardiac structures. The definitive diagnosis depends on several factors, including the visualization of the mass throughout the cardiac cycle in the same anatomic region using more than one acoustic window. The sonographer should ensure that the findings actually represent an actual mass and not the unusual appearance of a normal structure. The echocardiograph findings and clinical data should be integrated into the final interpretation; for example, if the patient has rheumatic mitral stenosis, left atrial enlargement, or atrial fibrillation, one should look for the presence of thrombus within the left atrium. The sonographer should ensure that the cardiac mass is not due to an ultrasound artifact caused by beam width, electrical inference, or side-lobe artifact. Normal anatomic variants that may appear as artifacts to the inexperienced eye are listed in Box 34.11. An example of anatomic normal variants is found on the aortic valve leaflets, called Lambl excrescences. These appear as slightly thicken strands attached to the aortic leaflets.

Cardiac Tumors

The detection of an intracardiac mass is an important clinical finding for the echocardiographer. Once a mass has been found, it is important to identify the mass as distinct because normal variants may appear mass-like without careful investigation. Once the mass has been identified on TTE, it is not uncommon to further classify the anatomic attachment of the mass with transesophageal echocardiography (TEE).

There are two categories of cardiac tumors (Fig. 34.23): primary, originating from the heart; and secondary, originating from metastases from other malignancies elsewhere in the body but most likely from the lung or breast. Metastases may arise from lymphoma, melanoma, leukemia, stomach, liver, and colon and may also spread to the heart. Adenocarcinoma of the kidney may travel through the renal vein into the inferior vena cava and into the right atrium. The secondary

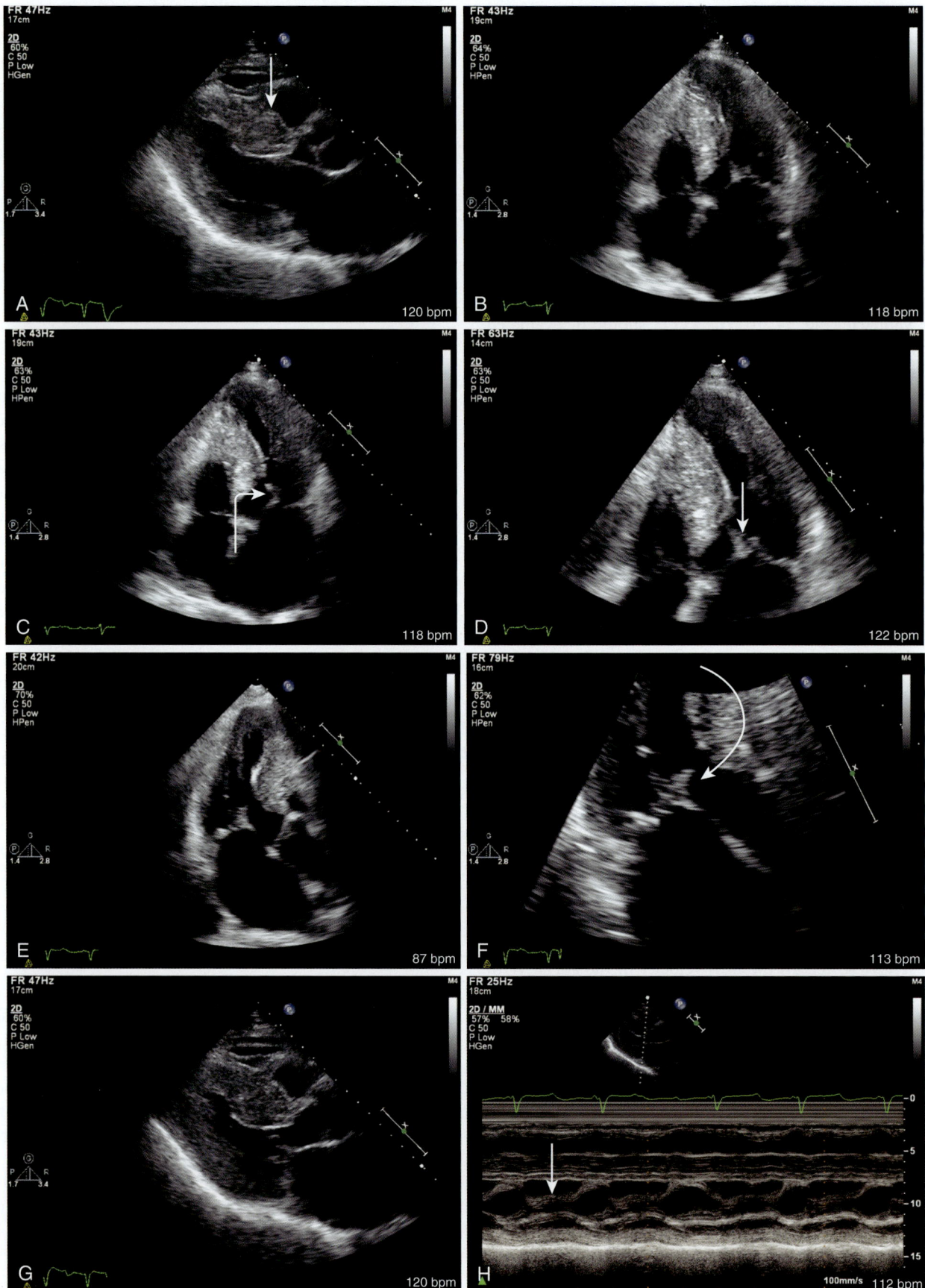

FIG. 34.20 **Hypertrophic obstructive cardiomyopathy.** (A) Parasternal long-axis (PLA) view shows the hypertrophied interventricular septum compared with the posterior wall left ventricle (PWLV). (B) Apical four-chamber view in the same patient demonstrates the enlarged left atrium and hypertrophied septum. (C–D) Apical four-chamber view shows the systolic anterior motion (SAM) *(arrow)* obstructing the left ventricular outflow tract. (E–F) Apical two-chamber view shows the hypertrophied septum and SAM. (G) PLA view shows the SAM obstructing the left ventricular outflow tract. (H) M-mode shows the anterior leaflet of the mitral valve touching the septum, and moderate SAM.

CHAPTER 34 Introduction to Clinical Echocardiography: Pericardial Disease, Cardiomyopathies, and Tumors

BOX 34.9	Evaluation by M-Mode

Narrowing of the LVOT
SAM
- Mild: SAM septal distance >10 mm
- Mod: SAM septal distance <10 mm (or brief mitral leaflet-septal contact)
- Severe: prolonged SAM septal contact, lasting >30% of systole

Midsystolic notching of AV

AV, Aortic valve; *LVOT*, left ventricular outflow tract; *SAM*, systolic anterior motion.

BOX 34.10	Left Ventricular Outflow Tract Obstruction

Dynamic
Defined as pressure gradient >30 mm Hg
Resting gradient >30 has prognostic significance and is a strong predictor of death and progression to heart failure
For those with resting gradient <30, provocation techniques include amyl nitrite, upright exercise, Valsalva maneuver, and dobutamine infusion

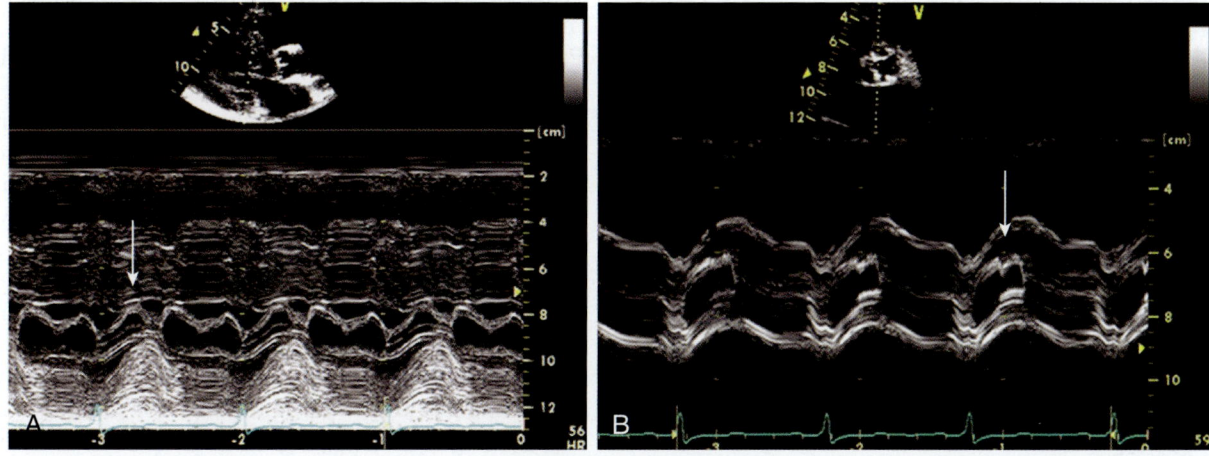

FIG. 34.21 (A) M-mode of the anterior leaflet of the mitral valve with severe systolic anterior motion touching the septum in systole. (B) The left ventricular outflow tract obstruction causes mid-systolic closure of the aortic leaflets *(arrows)*.

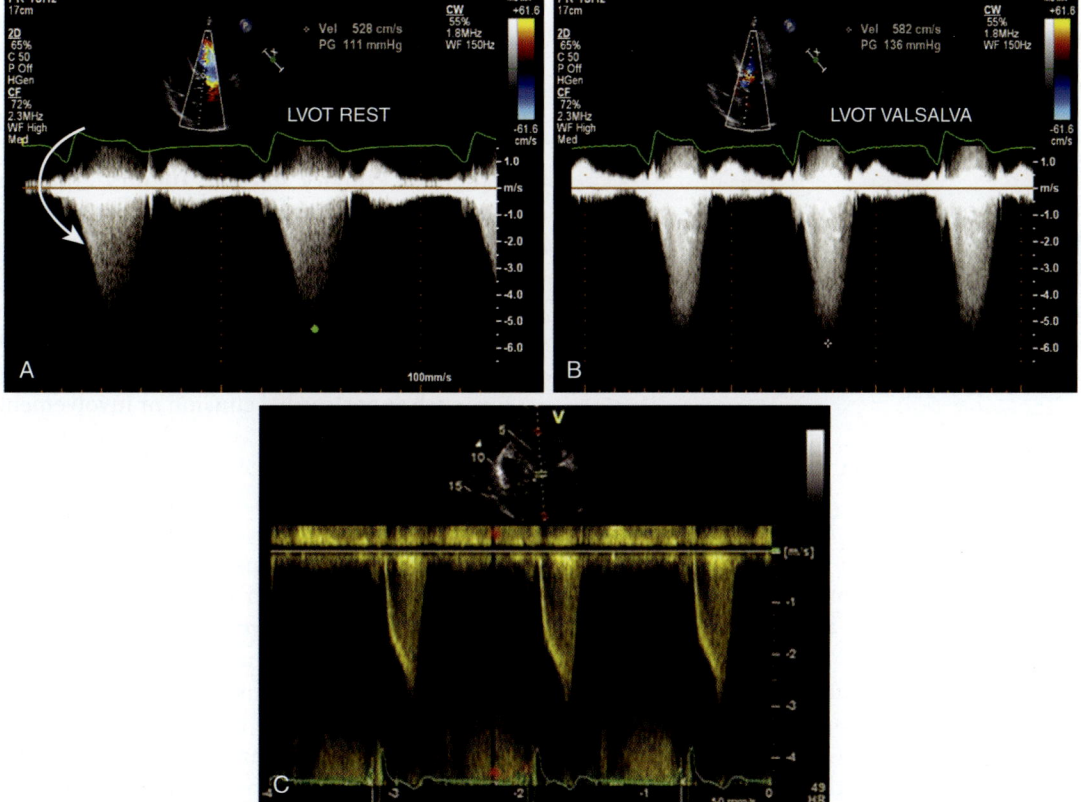

FIG. 34.22 (A) Continuous wave (CW) Doppler shows the late peaking "dagger" of the aortic outflow secondary to obstructive cardiomyopathy. (B) With Valsalva, the gradient increases from 111 to 136 mm Hg. (C) CW Doppler of another patient with severe obstructive cardiomyopathy and "dagger" aortic outflow velocity. *LVOT*, Left ventricular outflow tract.

BOX 34.11 Normal Variants

Left Ventricle
Papillary muscles
Left ventricle web (aberrant chordae)
Prominent apical trabeculations
Prominent MAC

Right Ventricle
Moderator band
Papillary muscles
Swan-Ganz/Pacer wire

Left Atrium
Dilated coronary sinus
Raphe between LSPV, LAA
Atrial suture line
Beam-width artifact from calcified aortic valve, prosthesis
IAS aneurysm

Right Atrium (Most Common Source)
Crista terminalis
Chiari network
Lipomatous hypertrophy of IAS
Trabeculation of RAA
Atrial suture
Pacer wire, Swan-Ganz, line
Eustachian valve
Fatty material surrounding tricuspid

Aortic Valve
Nodules of Arantius
Lambl excrescences
Base of leaflet en face

Mitral Valve
Redundant chordae
Myxomatous tissue
MAC

Pulmonary Artery
Left atrium appendage

Pericardium
Epicardial adipose tissue
Fibrinous debris in chronic organized pericardial effusion

IAS, Interatrial septum; *LAA,* left atrial appendage; *LSPV,* left superior pulmonary vein; *MAC,* mitral annular calcification; *RAA,* right atrial appendage.

---

tumors are 20 times more common than primary tumors of the heart.

The secondary cardiac malignancies may involve the pericardium, epicardium, myocardium (lymphoma and melanoma), and, rarely, the endocardium. Carcinoid malignancy affects the right side of the heart, causing severe tricuspid regurgitation.

Primary cardiac tumors may be divided into three categories: (1) benign (myxoma, lipoma, papillary fibroelastoma, hemangioma, and mesothelioma); (2) malignant (angiosarcoma, rhabdomyosarcoma, mesothelioma, fibrosarcoma, and malignant lymphoma); and (3) cysts (pericardial, bronchogenic). Keep in mind that most cardiac tumors are benign. Symptoms may include systemic symptomatology, arrhythmia, embolic events, chest pain, and congestive heart failure.

Myxomas. **Myxoma** is one of the more common benign tumors of the heart. The tumor is often single with an irregular shape or "cluster of grapes" appearance, with a stalk attached between the atrial wall and the tumor mass (Fig. 34.24). They can grow very large, causing the auscultation of tumor "plop" when the valve opens and the mass plops into the ventricular cavity. The tumor consistency is very inhomogeneous. The patient may present with embolic events as small pieces of the tumor break away. Tumors in the left atrial cavity may obstruct the LVOT, causing an outflow murmur.

Papillary Fibroelastoma. **Papillary fibroelastoma** arises on the aortic or mitral valve tissue and is usually quite small. This mass can usually be distinguished from the strand-like Lambl excrescences. The fibroelastoma has a stippled edge with a shimmer or vibration at the tumor-blood interface that is always found downstream of the flow (Fig. 34.25). Most of these lesions are singular, but a very small percentage appear as multiple lesions. The mass may mimic a small vegetation, and, if clinically indicated, a TEE examination may help to distinguish the lesion.

Lipomatous Hypertrophy. **Lipomatous hypertrophy** is a thickening that is seen along the superior/inferior interatrial septum (Fig. 34.26). The apical and subcostal four-chamber views best image this abnormality.

Rhabdomyoma. **Rhabdomyoma** is a benign cardiac tumor and is the most common tumor in children (often these children have tuberous sclerosis). These echogenic tumors are often multiple and seen within the right ventricle or right ventricular outflow tract (Fig. 34.27). They can be diagnosed before birth with fetal echo and may regress spontaneously after birth.

Malignant Primary Cardiac Tumors. The **malignant primary cardiac tumors** include angiosarcomas, rhabdomyosarcoma, mesothelioma, fibrosarcoma, and synovial fibrosarcoma (Fig. 34.28). The focus of the TTE examination is to identify the anatomic location and extent of the tumor involvement, the physiologic consequences (valve regurgitation, chamber obstruction), and associated findings such as pericardial effusion or involvement of the valves or conduction system.

Thrombus

Predisposing conditions for left ventricular thrombus include blood stasis with low-velocity flow, ventricular aneurysm, dilated cardiomyopathy with "swirling" blood flow, or pseudoaneurysm. If apical akinesis is present with a left ventricular aneurysm and a low ejection fraction less than 20%, caution should be made to clearly identify the apex of the heart to rule out thrombus. This requires the sonographer to carefully sweep anterior/posterior and medial/lateral through the apex to see if a thrombus is present. The thrombus is usually more echogenic than the underlying

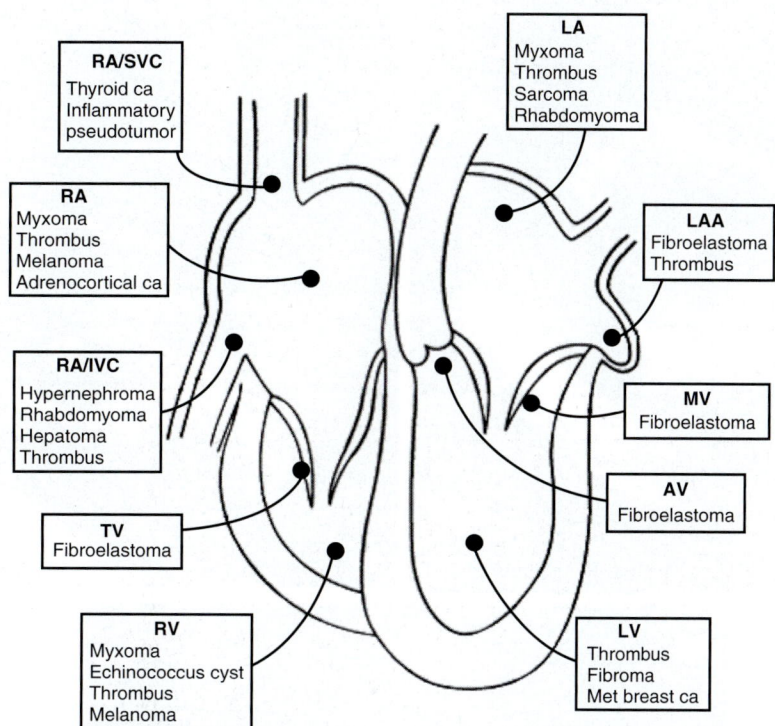

FIG. 34.23 There are two categories of cardiac tumors: primary, originating from the heart, and secondary, originating from metastases from other malignancies elsewhere in the body but most likely from the lung or breast. *AV,* Aortic valve; *ca,* cancer; *IVC,* inferior vena cava; *LA,* left atrium; *LAA,* left atrial appendage; *LV,* left ventricle; *Met,* metastatic; *MV,* mitral valve; *RA,* right atrium; *RV,* right ventricle; *SVC,* superior vena cava; *TV,* tricuspid valve.

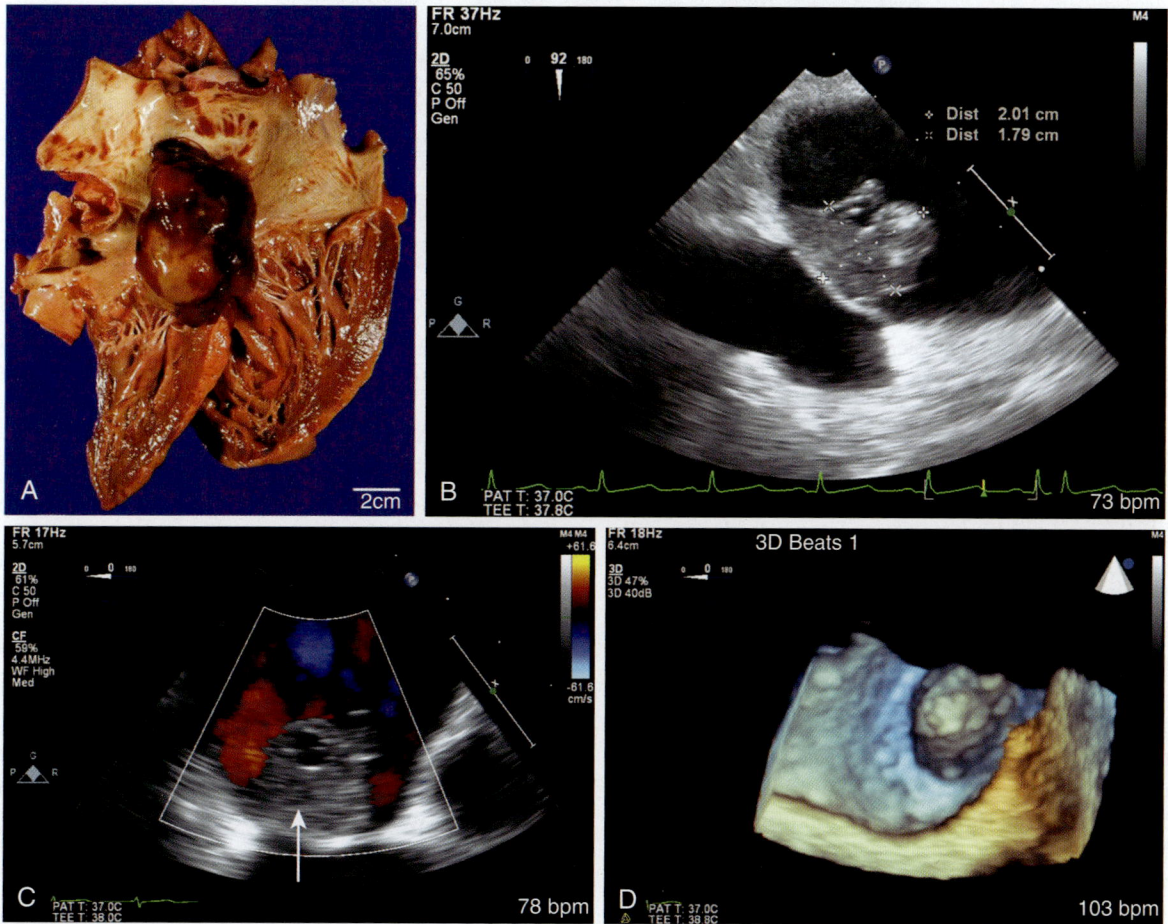

FIG. 34.24 (A) Gross anatomy of the atrial myxoma. (B) Transesophageal echocardiogram of a left atrial myxoma measuring 2.01 × 1.79 cm. (C) Color flow surrounds the myxoma. (D) Three-dimensional image of the myxoma.

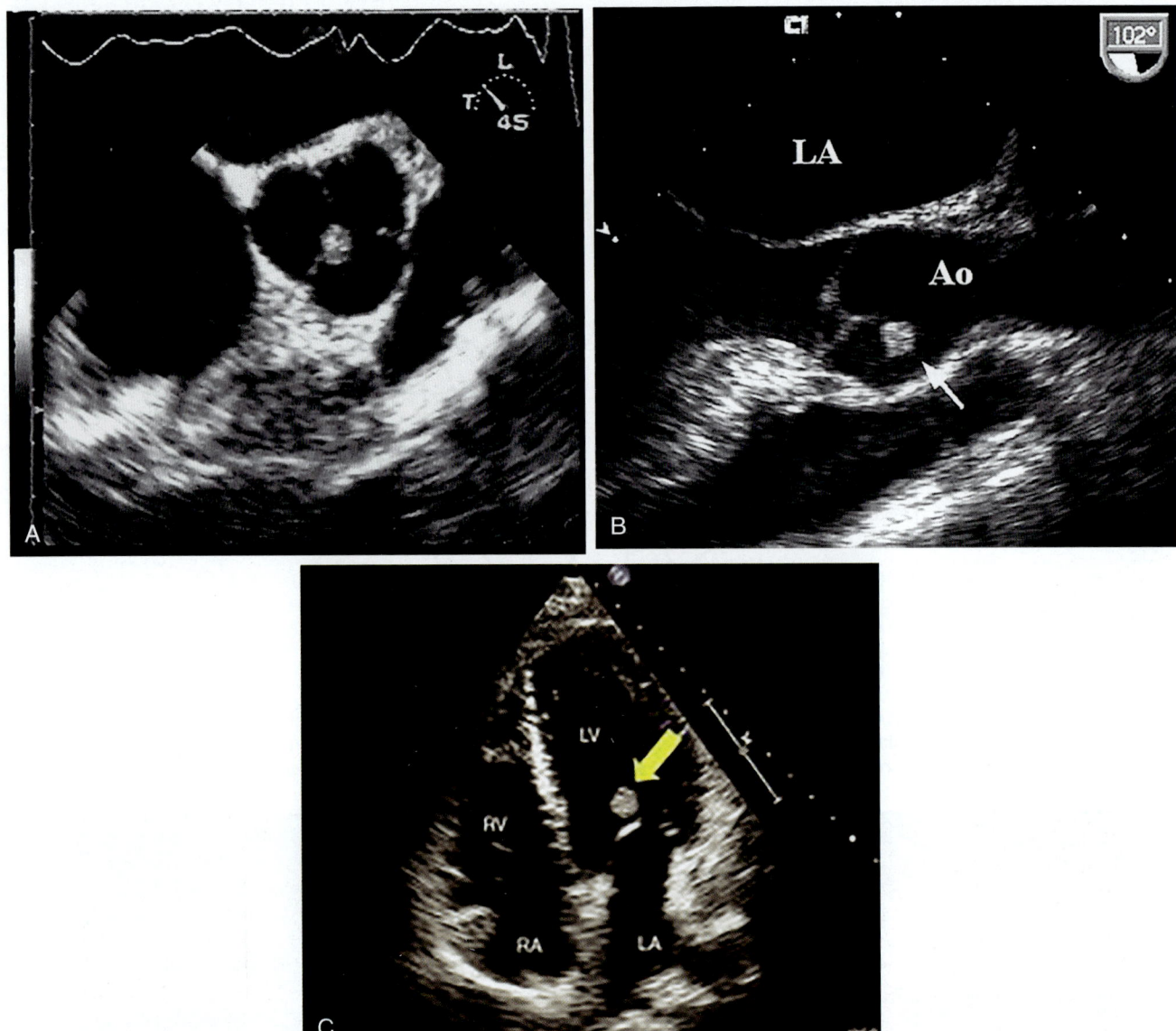

FIG. 34.25 Papillary fibroelastoma arises on the aortic or mitral valve tissue and is usually quite small. The fibroelastoma has a stippled edge with a shimmer or vibration at the tumor-blood interface that is always found downstream of the flow. (A–B) Transesophageal images of the short and long axis of the ascending aorta (Ao) shows the well-defined lesion of a fibroelastoma *(arrow)*. (C) Apical four-chamber view shows the fibroelastoma on the downstream of the mitral valve *(arrow)*. *LA*, Left atrium; *LV*, left ventricle; *RA*, right atrium; *RV*, right ventricle.

myocardium, whereas the laminated thrombus is more difficult to diagnose. Contrast injected into the heart will clearly demonstrate a dark anechoic area if thrombus is present (Fig. 34.29). The differential diagnosis would include hypereosinophilic cardiomyopathy where there is apical obliteration, deposits of thrombus, and eosinophils without impaired contractility.

Thrombus that occurs in the left atrial appendage is difficult to image with TTE but is always seen with TEE. Thrombus within the right atrial cavity is quite rare but may be seen in cases of severe right ventricle dilation and systolic dysfunction. A source of potential emboli may occur from indwelling catheters or pacer wires. Thrombus may also be seen to cross the patent foramen ovale as seen in Fig. 34.30.

Subacute Bacterial Endocarditis/Vegetations

Patients are usually very symptomatic with subacute bacterial endocarditis. They present with fever, chills, and perhaps a new cardiac murmur. Many of these patients have had a recent bacterial infection secondary to dental work. Vegetations on the cardiac valve leaflets may be seen on TTE

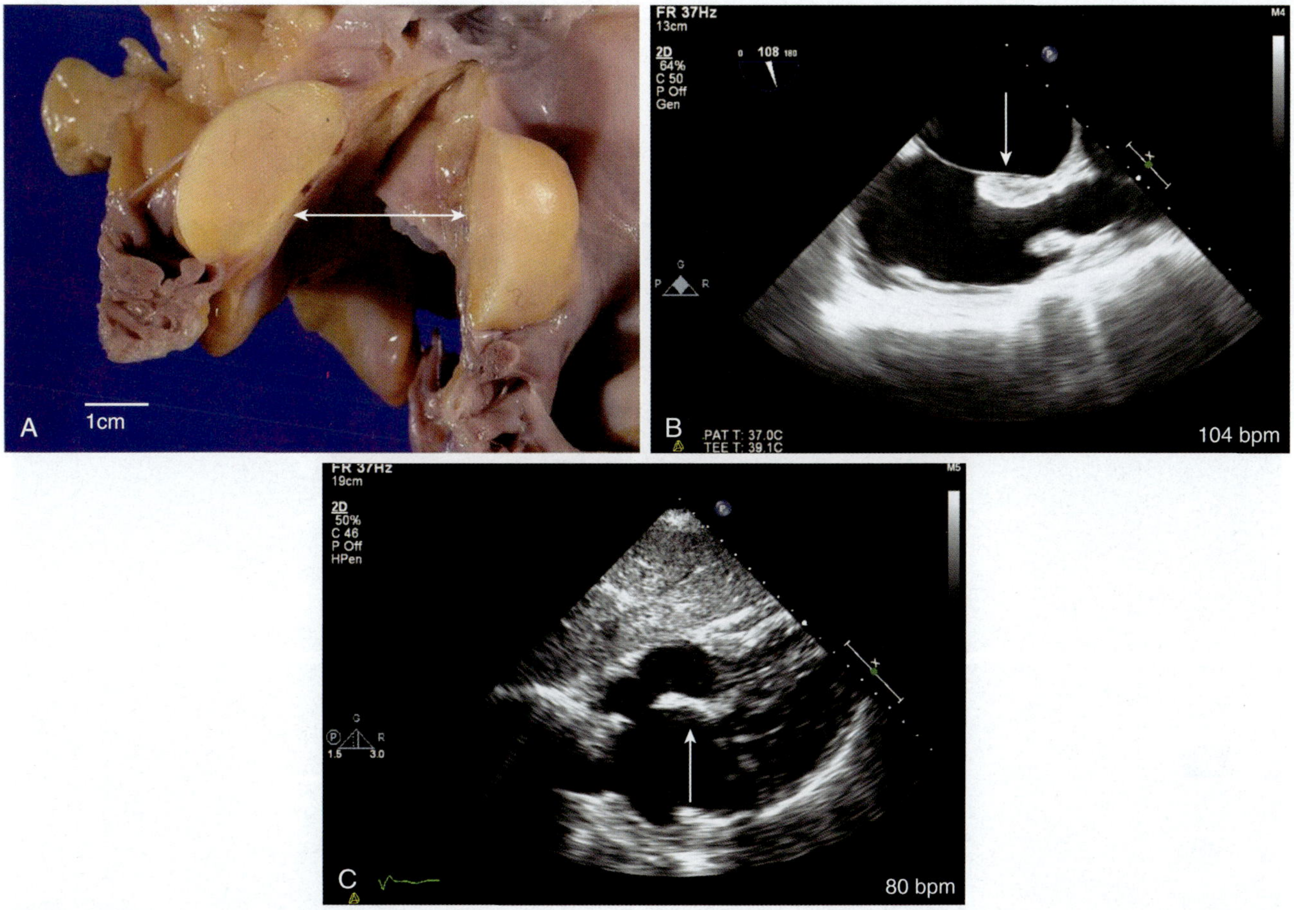

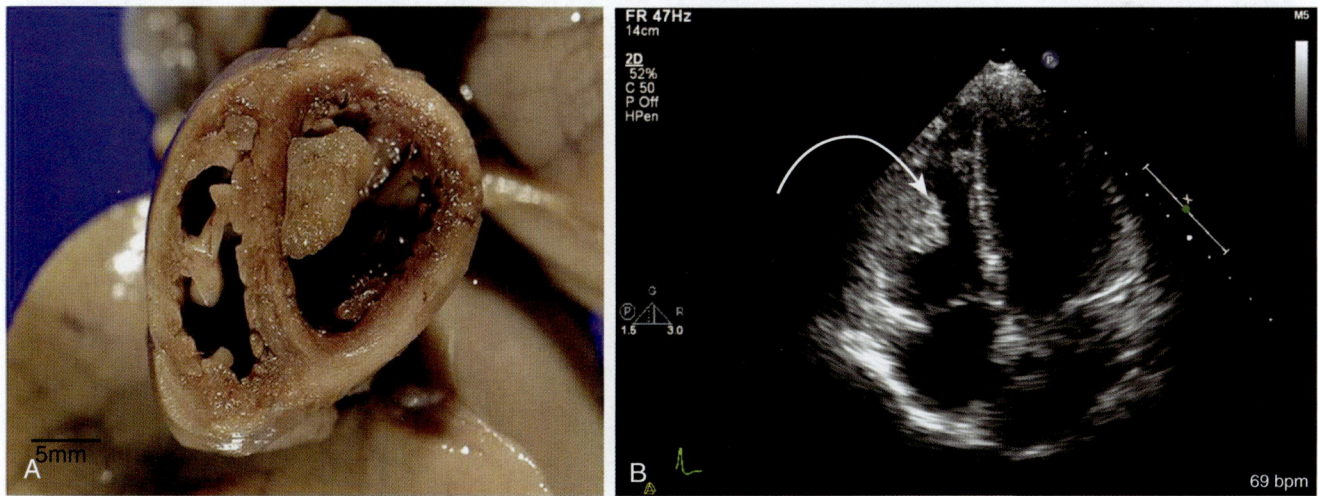

FIG. 34.26 (A) Gross anatomy of the lipomatous atrial septum. (B) Transesophageal echocardiogram of the lipomatous interatrial septum. (C) Subcostal image of the same patient with a lipomatous interatrial septum.

FIG. 34.27 (A) Gross anatomy of a rhabdomyoma. (B) Apical four-chamber view of the rhabdomyoma within the right ventricle.

examination if the vegetation is greater than 2 mm in size; however, TEE examination provides a better evaluation of the valve leaflets. These lesions are irregularly shaped and attached to the upstream side of the valve leaflet (Fig. 34.31). There is chaotic motion that differs from the leaflet motion.

There usually is valvular regurgitation and cardiac murmur. A paravalvular abscess may also be present, especially on the aortic valve in the area of the sinus of Valsalva. Vegetations may also be seen on pacemaker wires or other cardiac devices (Fig. 34.32).

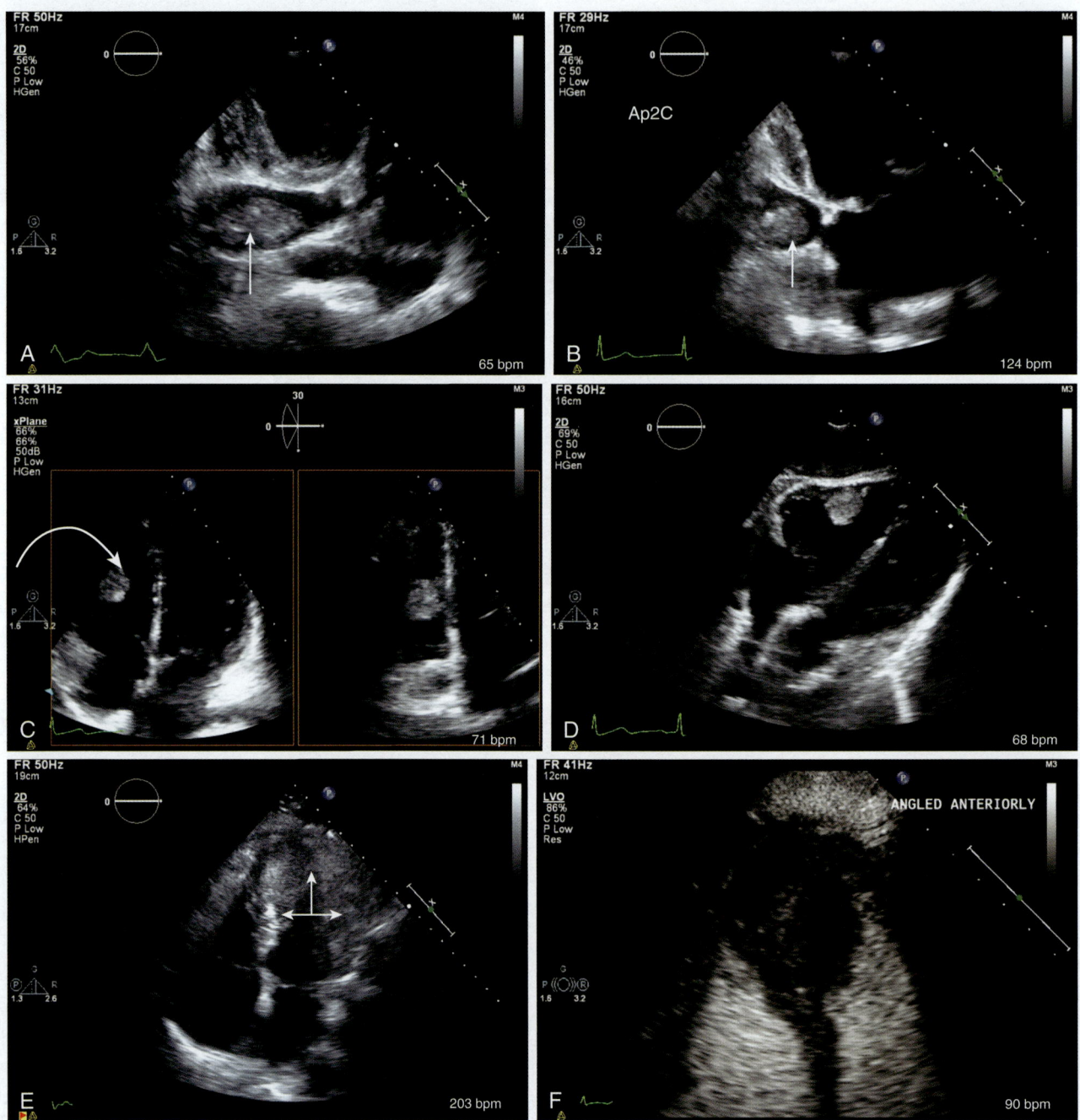

FIG. 34.28 Cardiac tumors. (A–B) Tumor within the coronary sinus *(arrows)*. (C–D) Tumor within the right ventricular cavity. (E–F) Eosinophilic tumor mass that infiltrated the myocardium.

CHAPTER 34 Introduction to Clinical Echocardiography: Pericardial Disease, Cardiomyopathies, and Tumors

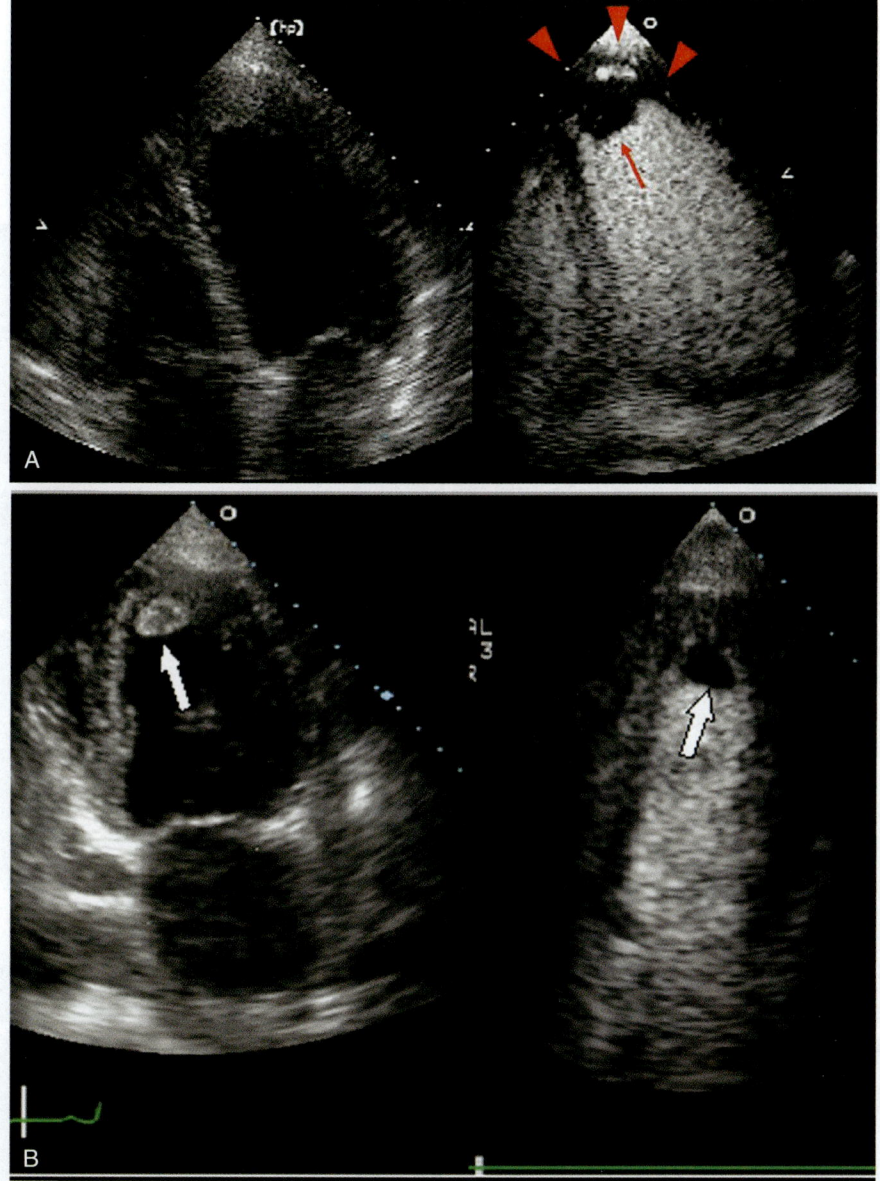

FIG. 34.29 Apical four-chamber view of apical akinesis. (A) The apex looks thickened and with contrast injection the thrombus clearly appears *(arrows)*. (B) The thrombus is more echogenic *(arrow)* and appears well defined at the apex of the two-chamber view with the injection of contrast.

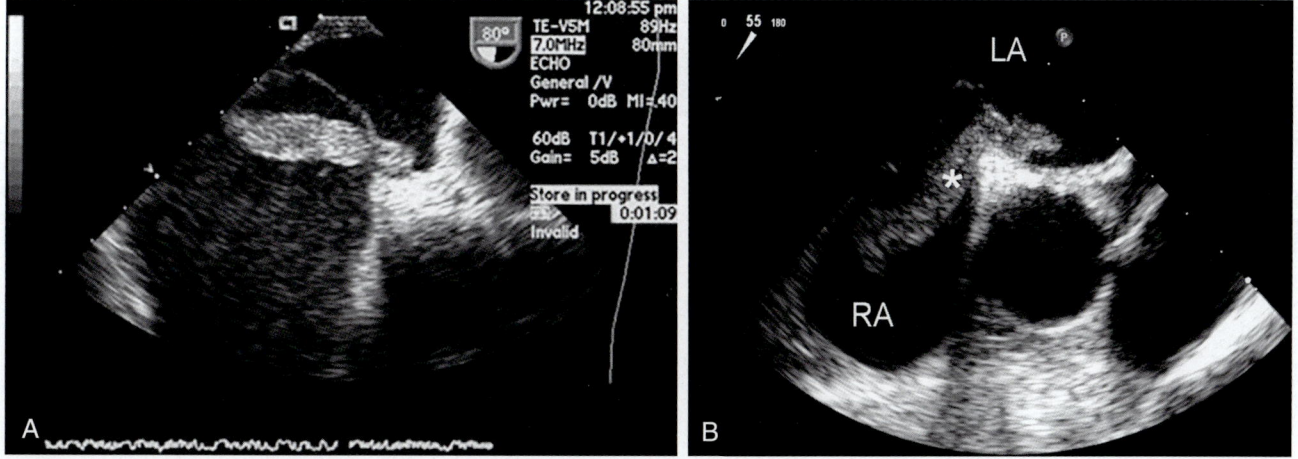

FIG. 34.30 An embolic event occurred in a patient with a patent foramen ovale. Transesophageal images demonstrated a large thrombus *(arrow)* across the patent foramen. *LA,* Left atrium; *RA,* right atrium.

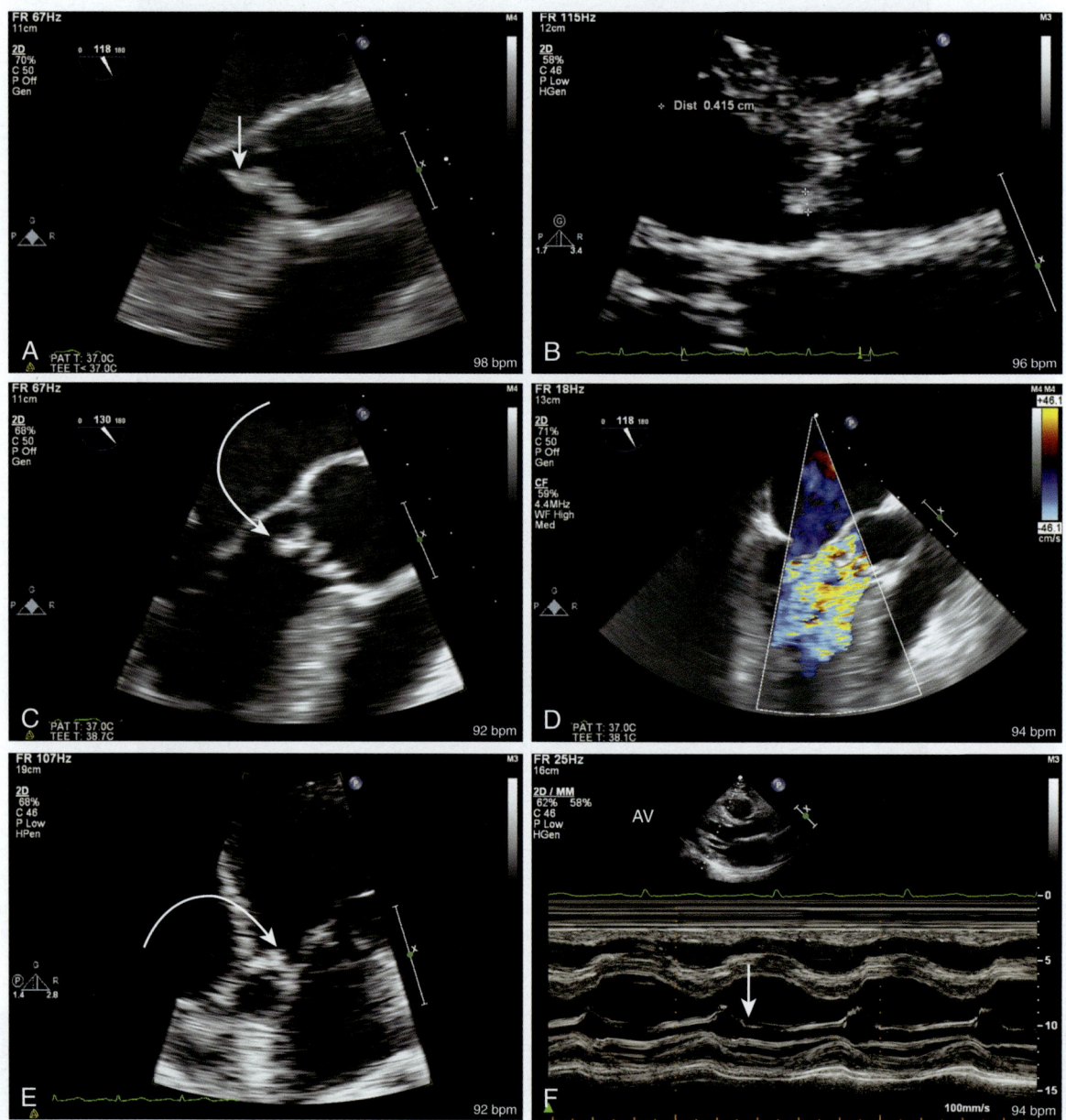

FIG. 34.31 Vegetations on the cardiac valve leaflets may be seen on transthoracic echocardiography (TTE) examination if the vegetation is >2mm in size; however, transesophageal echocardiography (TEE) examination provides a better evaluation of the valve leaflets. These lesions are irregularly shaped and attached to the upstream side of the valve leaflet. (A) TEE long axis of the aortic leaflets with a mobile mass *(arrow)* representing vegetations. (B) The vegetation measures 4mm. (C) TEE long axis shows the irregular mass on the aortic leaflets. (D) Severe aortic insufficiency is seen. (E) TTE five-chamber view of the aortic vegetation. (F) M-mode demonstrates early closure of the mitral valve secondary to acute aortic insufficiency.

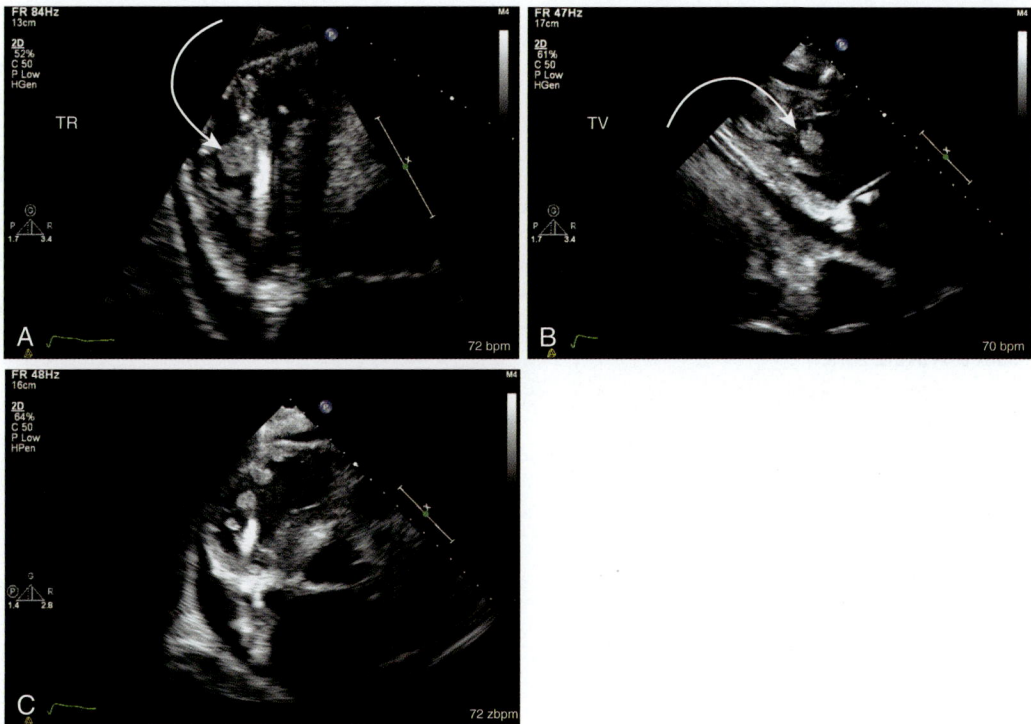

FIG. 34.32 Multiple vegetations are noted along the pacemaker wire *(arrow)* in this patient who presented with fever and chills for several weeks following dental surgery.

Key Pearls

- The normal pericardium has two layers: the outer sac is the fibrous pericardium and the inner sac is the serous pericardium.
- The pericardium has many functions. It provides a mechanical protection to the heart, provides a barrier to infection, reduces friction, hemodynamically limits acute distention, and contributes to the diastolic coupling and ventricular interdependence.
- The pericardial effusion is recognized as an echo-free space between the visceral and parietal pericardium.
- The effusions first accumulate posterior to the heart and as the size increases extend laterally and then circumferentially.
- The pericardial effusion always is found anterior to the descending aorta, whereas the pleural effusion is posterior to the descending aorta.
- Echocardiographic findings are quite specific for tamponade: moderate to large pericardial effusion, right atrial systolic collapse, right ventricle diastolic collapse, reciprocal respiratory changes in ventricular volumes, and a dilated inferior vena cava with lack of respiratory changes.
- In chronic pericardial disease the pericardium may become thickened and inelastic, which in turn limits the ventricular filling, leading to chronic biventricular diastolic dysfunction, right-sided heart failure, and low systemic output.
- Cardiomyopathy may be defined as a primary myocardial disorder that is not related to the effects of valvular heart disease, hypertension, or coronary artery disease.
- Cardiomyopathies may be divided into these categories: dilated/congestive, restrictive/infiltrative, arrhythmogenic right ventricular dysplasia, hypertrophic, and unclassified (e.g., endomyocardial fibroelastosis).
- The definition of a cardiac mass is an abnormal structure within or immediately adjacent to the heart.
- There are several types of cardiac masses, including tumor, thrombus, vegetation, iatrogenic material, normal variant, and extracardiac structures.
- There are two categories of cardiac tumors: primary, originating from the heart; and secondary, originating from metastases from other malignancies elsewhere in the body but most likely from the lung or breast.
- Myxoma is one of the more common benign tumors of the heart. The tumor is often single with an irregular shape or "cluster of grapes" appearance, with a stalk attached between the atrial wall and the tumor mass.
- The fibroelastoma arises on the aortic or mitral valve tissue and is usually quite small. This mass can usually be distinguished from the strand-like Lambl excrescences.
- The malignant primary cardiac tumors include angiosarcoma, rhabdomyosarcoma, mesothelioma, fibrosarcoma, and synovial fibrosarcoma.
- Predisposing conditions for left ventricular thrombus include blood stasis with low-velocity flow, ventricular aneurysm, dilated cardiomyopathy with "swirling" blood flow, or pseudoaneurysm.
- Vegetations on the cardiac valve leaflets may be seen on transthoracic echocardiography examination if the vegetation is greater than 2 mm in size; however, transesophageal echocardiography examination provides a better evaluation of the valve leaflets.

BIBLIOGRAPHY

Frischknecht BS, Jost CH, Occhslin EN, et al. Validation of noncompaction criteria in dilated cardiomyopathy, and valvular and hypertensive heart disease. *J Am Soc Echocardiogr*. 2005;18:865–872.

Kwan J, Shiota T, Agler DA, et al. Geometric differences of the mitral apparatus between ischemic and dilated cardiomyopathy with significant mitral regurgitation: Real-time three-dimensional echocardiographic study. *Circulation*. 2003;107:1135–1140.

Markiewicz W, Monakier I, Brik A, et al. Clinical-echocardiographic correlations in pericardial effusion. *Eur Heart J*. 1982;3:260–266.

Oh JK, Seward JB, Tajik AJ, eds. *The echo manual.* ed 4. New York: Lippincott Williams & Wilkins; 2018.

Otto CM. *The practice of clinical echocardiography.* ed 6. St. Louis: Elsevier; 2023.

Porter TR, Mulvagh SL, Abdelmoneium SS, et al. Clinical Applications of Ultrasonic Enhancing Agents in Echocardiography: 2018 American Society of Echocardiography Guidelines Update. *J Am Soc Echocardiogr*. 2018;31(3):241–275.

Reddy PS, Curtiss EL, Uretsky BF. Spectrum of hemodynamic changes in cardiac tamponade. *Am J Cardiol*. 1990;55:1487–1491.

Saric M, Armour AC, Arnaout MS, et al. Guidelines for the use of echocardiography in the evaluation of a cardiac source of embolism. *J Am Soc of Echocardiogr*. 2016;29(1):1–44.

Wann S, Passen E. Echocardiography in pericardial disease. *J Am Soc Echocardiogr*. 2008;21:7–13.

CHAPTER 35

Fetal Echocardiography: Beyond the Four Chambers

Sandra L. Hagen-Ansert and Joy Guthrie

OBJECTIVES

On completion of this chapter, you should be able to:
- Understand the embryologic development of the fetal heart
- Describe fetal circulation
- List the maternal risks factors that would require fetal echocardiography
- Explain how to sonographically evaluate the fetal heart with two-dimensional, M-mode, pulsed Doppler, and color flow Doppler imaging
- Locate fetal ultrasound landmarks
- Describe normal anatomy seen in the views discussed in this chapter

OUTLINE

Embryology of the Cardiovascular System 1008
   Development of Blood Vessels 1008
   Aortic Arches 1008
   Development of the Heart 1009
Fetal Circulation 1010
   Heart Rate 1012
Risk Factors Indicating Fetal Echocardiography 1012

Fetal Risk Factors 1012
Maternal Risk Factors 1013
Familial Risk Factors 1013
Beyond the Four-Chamber View 1013
   Transducer Requirements 1013
   Instrumentation 1013
   Motion Mode Evaluation 1013
   Pulsed Doppler Imaging 1014
   Color Flow Doppler Imaging 1015

Three-Dimensional Imaging 1015
Fetal Ultrasound Landmarks 1016
Echocardiographic Evaluation of the Fetus 1017
   Four-Chamber View 1017
   Left and Right Ventricular Outflow Tracts 1021
   Ductal and Aortic Arch Views: Oblique Long Axis 1026
   Three-Vessel View 1029

KEY TERMS

Atrioventricular node
Bicuspid aortic valve
Fossa ovale
Inferior vena cava

Left atrium
Left ventricle
Main pulmonary artery mitral valve
Patent ductus arteriosus

Pulmonary veins
Right atrium
Right ventricle
Tricuspid valve

The continued development and improvement of high-resolution, real-time sonography has enabled the sonographer to visualize fetal cardiac activity with transvaginal transducers early in the first trimester. Although the detailed visualization of all the anatomic structures of the fetal heart is best imaged in the second and third trimesters. This ability to visualize cardiac anatomy has aided in the prenatal diagnosis of congenital heart disease. The incidence of congenital heart disease is about 8%, or 30,000 infants per year in the United States. Sonographic visualization allows the sonographer and clinician to image the small cardiac structures and obtain hemodynamic information from the fetal heart.

Conditions such as small cardiac defects, abnormal size or location of cardiac structures, arrhythmias, or abnormal cardiac function may all be observed with fetal echocardiography. The information obtained from the sonogram regarding the congenital heart defect is then managed through a team effort of multiple clinicians—including the pediatric cardiologist, obstetrician, perinatologist, geneticist, cardiovascular surgeon, and imaging specialists—to allow the patient to make educated decisions regarding the opportunities and outcomes for her fetus with a congenital heart defect.

Improvement in high-resolution transducers has permitted good resolution and visualization of even the smallest structures within the fetal cardiac chambers. These transducers and dedicated cardiac instrumentation, complete with motion mode (M-mode), 2D, 3D, 4D, color and Doppler capabilities, enable the sonographer to perform a complete fetal echocardiogram on obstetric patients between their 16th week of pregnancy and the time of delivery. Although fetal heart motion may be seen within the gestational sac as early as 4 to 5 weeks, structural information may be seen with the transvaginal probe as early as 10 to 16 weeks of gestation, with even more detailed information available after 18 weeks of gestation. The optimum time to perform a complete anatomical fetal echocardiogram is 18 to 22 weeks.

Fetal echocardiography has been a tremendous clinical aid for the high-risk obstetric patient. The ability to map normal cardiac structures and ventricular function in a patient who has had a previous child with congenital heart disease helps relieve the pregnant patient of worry. Moreover, if a congenital heart condition is found, arrangements may be made to deliver the patient in a facility with the appropriate staff to manage such a neonate.

The addition of Doppler and color flow imaging has aided the diagnosis of congenital heart disease and has helped in the understanding of flow dynamics in the fetus. These two modalities, Doppler and color flow imaging, are used with discretion in the fetus with congenital heart disease. Three- and four-dimensional echocardiography has been introduced in fetal echocardiography to allow more intricate visualization of the cardiac structures. This technique still requires a good axis of the fetal heart to be obtained before adequate interpolation of the data is made.

EMBRYOLOGY OF THE CARDIOVASCULAR SYSTEM

A single major error in the genetic constitution is the basis of congenital malformations. Human teratogens produce or raise the incidence of congenital malformations; 7% are caused by environmental agents or teratogens. A spontaneous abortion usually occurs if the genetic malformation is severe.

The most sensitive period in the first trimester for cardiac development is between 3.5 and 6.5 weeks. The cardiovascular system is the first organ system to reach a functional state; by the end of the third week, circulation of blood has begun.

Development of Blood Vessels

The primitive heart is a tubular structure that forms like a large blood vessel from the mesenchymal cells in the cardiogenic area of the embryo. Paired endocardial heart tubes develop before the end of the third week and begin to fuse, thus forming the primitive heart.

The circulation of blood starts by the end of the third week as the tubular heart begins to beat. (Fig. 35.1). The embryo obtains sufficient nourishment during the second week of development by diffusion of nutrients from maternal blood flow. The vascular system begins during the third week in the wall of the yolk sac, the connecting stalk, and the chorion. The blood vessels begin to develop 2 days later. Blood islands are formed; cavities develop in the islands to form primitive blood cells and vessels. These primitive vessels form a vascular network in the wall of the yolk sac. Blood vessels form in the mesenchyme associated with the connecting stalk and chorion. Blood vessels also form in the embryo toward the end of the third week and join to form a continuous system of vessels on each side.

Blood vessels from the embryo join those on the yolk sac, connecting stalk, and chorion to form a primitive cardiovascular system (see Fig. 35.1). The cardinal veins return blood from the embryo, and the vitelline veins return blood from the yolk sac. The umbilical veins return oxygenated blood from the placenta (only one umbilical vein persists). Two dorsal aortas fuse in the caudal half of the embryo to form a single dorsal aorta. Blood formation in the embryo begins at the fifth week.

Aortic Arches

Each branchial arch is supplied by an aortic arch (Fig. 35.2). The arteries to the fifth pair are rudimentary or absent. The third pair of aortic arches becomes the common carotid artery and the proximal parts of the internal carotid arteries. The left fourth arch forms part of the arch of the aorta. The

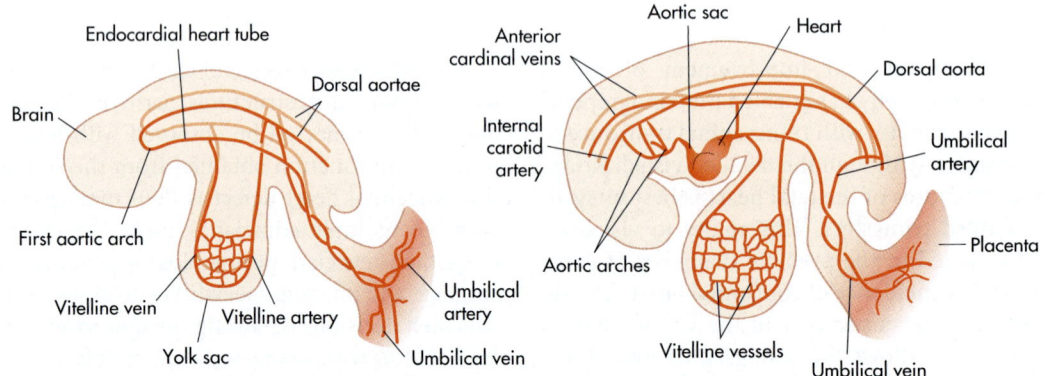

FIG. 35.1 Cardiovascular system in a 26-day-old embryo. The two endocardial heart tubes have fused to form a tubular heart ring. The umbilical vein carries oxygenated blood and nutrients to the embryo from the placenta.

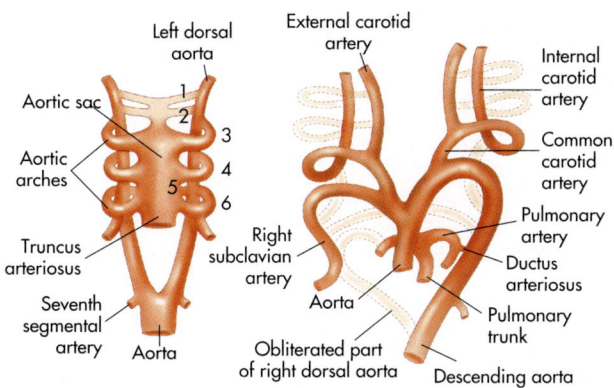

FIG. 35.2 Aortic arches in a 6-week embryo (*left*) and in an 8-week embryo (*right*).

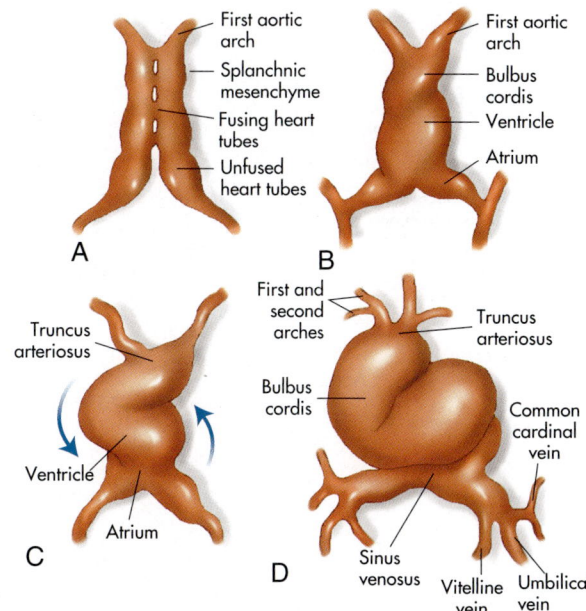

FIG. 35.3 **The heart during the fourth week of development.** The paired endocardial heart tubes (A) gradually fuse to form a single tubular heart (B). The fusion begins at the cranial end of the tubes and extends caudally until a single tubular heart is formed. As the heart elongates, it bends on itself (C–D).

BOX 35.1 Cardiac Development

- *Sinus venosus:* the caudal region of the primitive heart, which receives all blood returning to the heart from common cardinal veins, vitelline veins, and umbilical veins
- *Primitive atrium:* develops into the right and left atria
- *Primitive ventricle:* develops into the left ventricle
- *Bulbus cordis:* develops into the right ventricle
- *Truncus arteriosus:* dilates to form the aortic sac from which the aortic arches arise

---

right fourth arch forms the proximal part of the right subclavian artery. The right sixth aortic arch becomes the right pulmonary artery. The left sixth aortic arch forms the left pulmonary artery and the ductus arteriosus (Box 35.1).

Development of the Heart

The heart tube grows rapidly, bending on itself because it is fixed at its cranial and caudal ends. The bending forms a U-shaped bulboventricular loop. The sinus venosus is initially a separate chamber that opens into the **right atrium** (Fig. 35.3).

Right atrium. The left horn of the sinus becomes the coronary sinus. The right horn is incorporated into the wall of the right atrium (forms a smooth portion of the adult right atrial wall). The right half of the primitive atrium persists as the right auricle.

Left atrium. The **left atrium** is formed by incorporation of the primitive pulmonary vein. As the atrium grows, parts of this vein and its branches are absorbed. Four pulmonary veins eventually enter the left atrium from the lungs. The smooth wall of the left atrium is from the absorbed pulmonary vein. The left auricle is from the primitive heart.

Four-chambered heart. During the fourth and fifth weeks of fetal development, the division of the four chambers occurs (Fig. 34.4).

Division of the atrioventricular canal. Endocardial cushions develop in the atrioventricular region of the heart. The cushions grow toward each other and fuse to divide the atrioventricular canal into right and left canals.

Division of the primitive atrium. The **septum primum** grows from the dorsal wall of the primitive atrium and fuses with the endocardial cushions (see Fig. 35.4A–B). Before the fusion of the septum primum, a communication exists between the right and left halves of the primum atrium through the ostium primum or foramen primum. As the septum primum fuses with the endocardial cushions (obliterating the foramen primum), the superior part of the septum primum breaks down, creating an opening called the *foramen secundum* (see Fig. 35.4A–B). As this foramen develops, another membranous fold, the **septum secundum**, grows into the atrium to the right of the septum primum. The septum secundum overlaps the foramen secundum and the opening of the septum primum. There is also an opening between the free edge of the septum secundum and the dorsal wall of the atrium called the **foramen ovale** (see Fig. 35.4C).

Formation of the ventricles. The **left ventricle** is formed from the primitive vein. The right ventricle is formed from the **bulbus cordis**. The interventricular septum begins as a ridge in the floor of the primitive ventricle and slowly grows toward the endocardial cushions (see Fig. 35.4B–C). Until the seventh week, the right and left ventricles communicate through a large interventricular foramen. Closure of the interventricular foramen results in the formation of the membranous part of the interventricular septum.

Partitioning of bulbus cordis and truncus arteriosus. The division of this part of the heart results from the development and fusions of the truncal ridges and bulbar ridges (see Fig. 35.4D and E). Fused mesenchymal ridges form the aorticopulmonary septum, which divides the truncus arteriosus and bulbus cordis into the ascending aorta (AA) and pulmonary trunk.

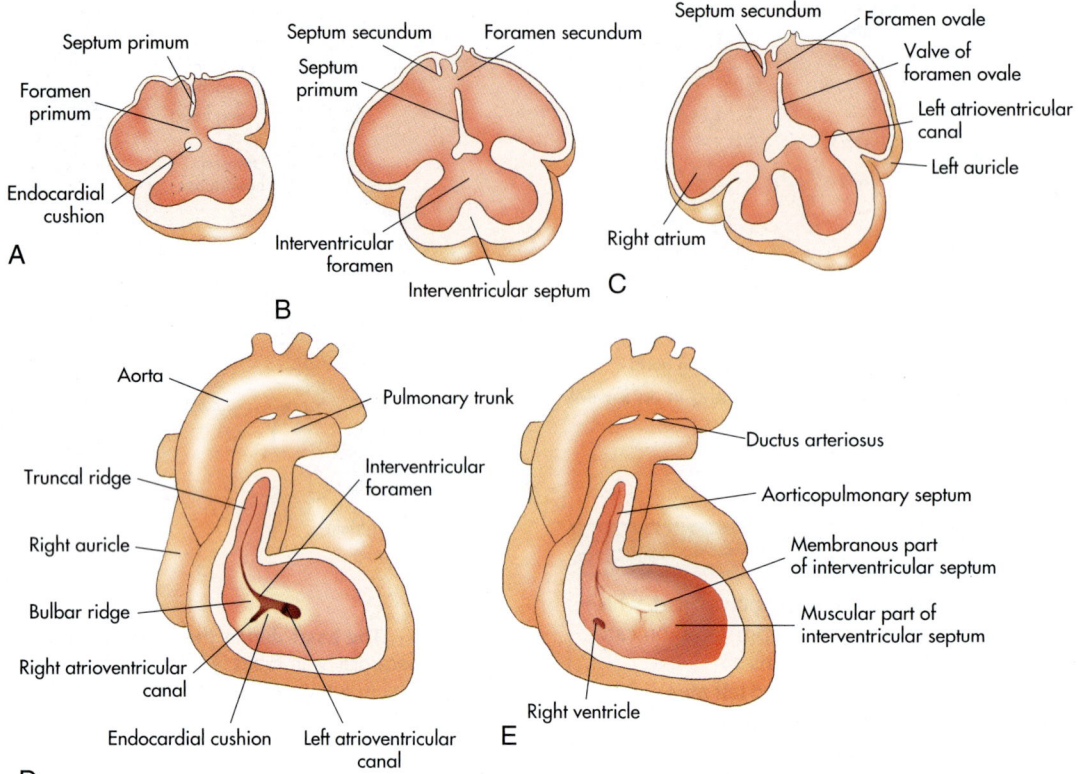

FIG. 35.4 **The partitioning of the primitive atrioventricular canal, atrium, and ventricle in the developing heart.** (A–C) Frontal sections of the embryonic heart during the fourth week. The heart at 5 weeks (D) and 7 weeks (E) shows closure of the interventricular foramen and formation of the interventricular septum. Note that the interventricular foramen is closed by tissues from three sources.

Development of the conduction system. The **sinoatrial node** forms in the wall of the sinus venosus near its opening into the right atrium; later it is incorporated into the right atrium with the right horn of the sinus venosus. The **atrioventricular node** and bundle are derived from cells in the walls of the sinus venosus and atrioventricular canal.

FETAL CIRCULATION

Blood flow in the fetus varies in two respects from the neonatal stage. Communication is open between the right and left sides of the fetal heart through the **fossa ovale** and between the aorta and the pulmonary artery via the **ductus arteriosus**. It is useful to know these important communications to appreciate the fetal physiology of the cardiac structures.

The primitive cardiovascular system is formed from the blood vessels in the embryo joining those on the yolk sac, connecting stalk, and chorion. The cardinal veins return blood from the embryo; vitelline veins return blood from the yolk sac; and umbilical veins return oxygenated blood from the placenta. Only one umbilical vein persists. Initially, there are two dorsal arteries, but these fuse together in the caudal half of the embryo to form a single dorsal aorta.

Before birth, the oxygenated blood is given to the fetus by way of the umbilical vein from the placenta to the heart. The design of the prenatal circulation is to ensure that the highly oxygenated blood from the umbilical vein quickly and efficiently flows into the heart. Approximately half of the blood passes through the hepatic sinusoids, whereas the remainder bypasses the liver to go through the ductus venosus into the inferior vena cava. Blood flows from the **inferior vena cava** and **superior vena cava** and enters into the right atrium (Fig. 35.5). Blood in the right atrium is less oxygenated than blood in the umbilical vein.

A small amount of oxygenated blood from the inferior vena cava is diverted by the crista dividens and remains in the right atrium to mix with deoxygenated blood from the superior vena cava and coronary sinus. The eustachian valve at the junction of the inferior vena cava and right atrium serves to direct the highly oxygenated umbilical venous flow toward the foramen ovale into the left atrium. Some of the blood from the inferior vena cava is directed by the lower border of the septum secundum (the crista dividens) through the foramen ovale into the left atrium.

The blood in the right atrium flows through the three-leaflet **tricuspid valve** into the **right ventricle** and leaves the right ventricle through the **main pulmonary artery** (MPA). This artery bifurcates into right and left pulmonary artery branches that lead to their respective lungs. However, most of this blood passes through the connection of the ductus arteriosus into the descending aorta; only a very small amount goes to the lungs.

The blood mixes with a small amount of deoxygenated blood as it returns from the lungs via the four **pulmonary veins** into the left atrium. The pulmonary veins enter the posterior of the left atrium. The four veins are named according to their locations: right upper, left upper, right lower, and left lower. The blood then flows from the left atrium into the

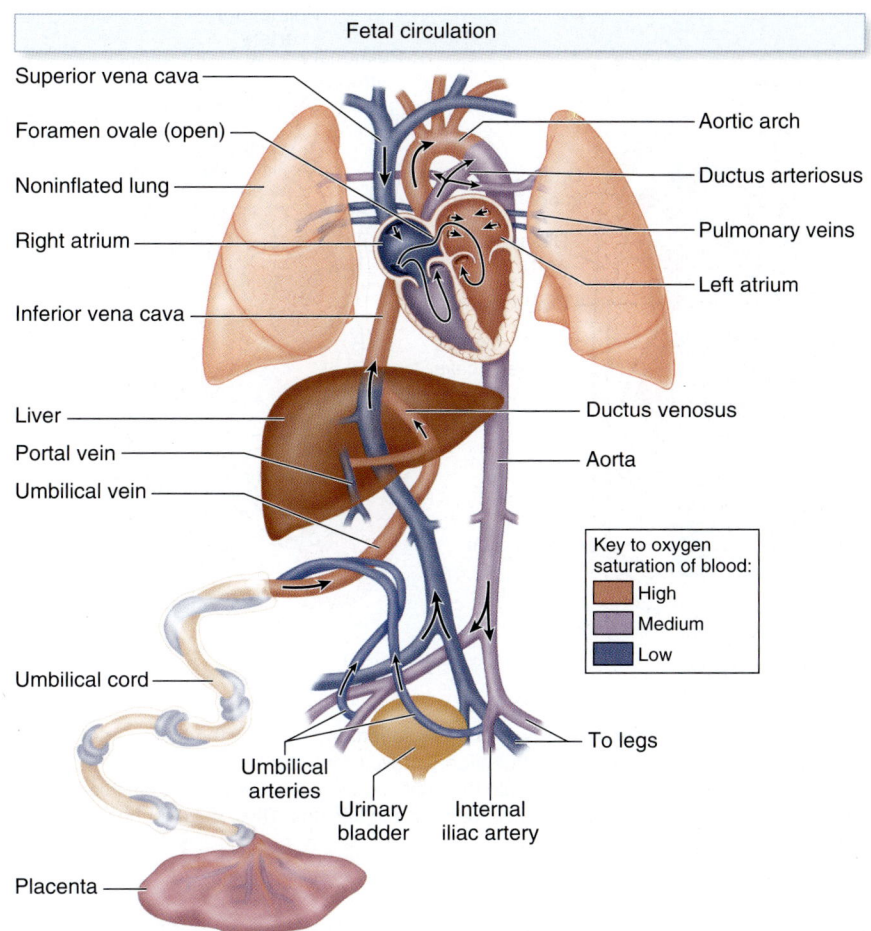

FIG. 35.5 Blood flows from the inferior vena cava and superior vena cava and enters into the right atrium. A small amount of oxygenated blood from the inferior vena cava is diverted by the crista dividens and remains in the right atrium to mix with deoxygenated blood from the superior vena cava and coronary sinus. The eustachian valve at the junction of the inferior vena cava and right atrium directs the oxygenated umbilical venous flow toward the foramen ovale into the left atrium. The blood in the right atrium flows through the tricuspid valve into the right ventricle and leaves the right ventricle through the main pulmonary artery that bifurcates into right and left pulmonary artery branches that lead to their respective lungs. However, most of this blood passes through the connection of the ductus arteriosus into the descending aorta; only a very small amount goes to the lungs. The blood mixes with a small amount of deoxygenated blood as it returns from the lungs via the four pulmonary veins into the left atrium. The pulmonary veins enter the posterior of the left atrium. The blood then flows from the left atrium into the left ventricle through the two-leaflet mitral valve and leaves the heart through the ascending aorta. The head, neck, and upper torso of the fetus are fed via the three branches arising from the aortic arch. The rest of the mixed blood in the descending aorta passes into the umbilical arteries and is returned to the placenta for reoxygenation.

left ventricle through the two-leaflet **mitral valve** and leaves the heart through the AA. The head, neck, and upper torso of the fetus are fed via the three branches arising from the aortic arch. These branches are the innominate, left carotid, and left subclavian arteries. The rest of the mixed blood in the descending aorta passes into the umbilical arteries and is returned to the placenta for reoxygenation. The remainder of the blood circulates through the lower part of the body.

At birth, the circulation of the fetal blood through the placenta ceases, the neonatal lungs begin to expand, and the blood flow to the lungs increases rapidly. The lungs are now able to provide oxygen and carbon dioxide exchange after the placenta has separated from the newborn infant. This expansion of the lungs causes several changes in the newborn. The fetal cardiac structures no longer necessary are the foramen ovale, ductus arteriosus, ductus venosus, and umbilical vessels (Fig. 35.6).

Omission of the placental circulation causes an immediate fall of blood pressure in the newborn's inferior vena cava and right atrium. As the lungs expand with air, there is a fall in the pulmonary vascular resistance. This causes an increase in pulmonary blood flow and a progressive thinning of the walls of the pulmonary arteries. Thus, the pressure in the left atrium becomes higher than that in the right atrium. This causes the foramen ovale to close. With time, complete closure of the foramen occurs from adhesion of the septum primum to the left margin of the septum secundum. The septum primum forms the floor of the fossa ovalis. The lower edge of the septum secundum forms the limbus fossae ovalis, which demarcates the former cranial boundary of the foramen ovale. If this foramen ovale does not close after birth, it is known as a patent foramen ovale.

The ductus arteriosus usually constricts shortly after birth (usually within 24 to 48 hours) once the left-sided pressures

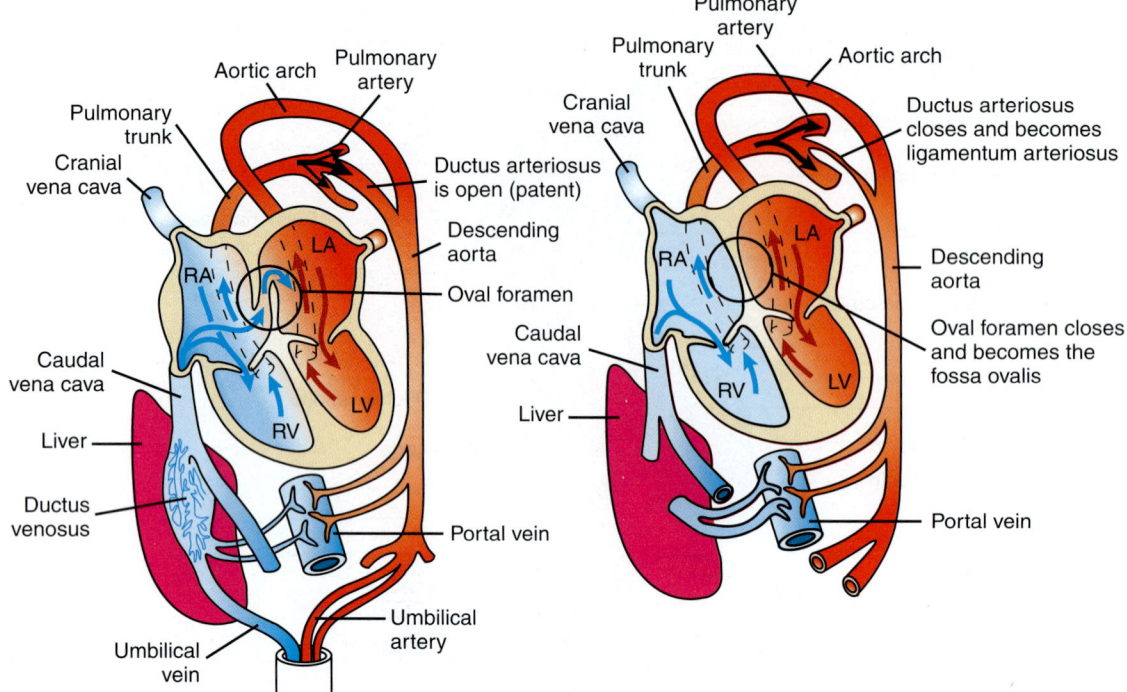

FIG. 35.6 **Comparison of the fetal circulation to the neonatal circulation.** In the fetus, the ductus arteriosus is open between the pulmonary artery and aorta; shortly after birth, this communication pathway should close, allowing the unoxygenated blood to leave the right ventricle via the pulmonary artery which bifurcate into the right and left pulmonary arteries that lead into the lungs. The other significant closure is the foramen ovale that is located between the right and left atria. Thus, the right heart carries unoxygenated blood and the left heart receives the oxygenated blood.

exceed the right-sided pressures. Often there is a small shunt of blood from the aorta to the pulmonary artery until these pressures adjust to neonatal life. Once the ductus closes, it is known as the ligamentum arteriosum in the neonate. If this communication persists, it is called a **patent ductus arteriosus**. This ligament passes from the left pulmonary artery to the arch of the aorta. The persistence of the ductus arteriosus may eventually cause an overload on the left heart; thus the goal is to close the patent ductus either medically or surgically.

The umbilical arteries also constrict after birth to prevent blood loss from the neonate. The umbilical vein may remain patent for some time after birth.

Heart Rate

The normal fetal heart rate is between 120 and 160 beats/min. In the first trimester of pregnancy, the heart rate begins around 90 beats/min and increases to 170 beats/min before returning to a normal rate and sinus rhythm. If the heart rate is too slow (less than 100 beats/min), it is called **bradycardia**; a heart rate more than 200 beats/min is termed **tachycardia**.

A slow fetal heart rate places the fetus at higher risk of associated heart disease; fetal echocardiography should be performed to rule out the presence of a structural heart defect. The association of complete heart block with structural cardiac defects appears to have a poor prognosis, presumably because of the adverse interaction and the atrioventricular valve regurgitation that commonly complicates the condition.

Connective tissue disorder (e.g., systemic lupus erythematosus) is associated with heart block and pericardial effusion.

RISK FACTORS INDICATING FETAL ECHOCARDIOGRAPHY

Specific risk factors indicate that the fetus is at a higher than normal risk for congenital heart disease and warrants a fetal echocardiogram. These may be divided into the following three categories: fetal risk factors, maternal risk factors, and familial risk factors.

Fetal Risk Factors

Fetal risk factors include the presence of intrauterine growth restriction, cardiac arrhythmias or abnormal heart rate, an abnormal amniocentesis result indicating a trisomy, abnormal amniotic fluid collections, thickened nuchal translucency, or other anomalies as detected by the sonogram, such as hydrops fetalis.

The presence of extracardiac abnormalities (e.g., renal anomalies, gastrointestinal anomalies, and single umbilical artery) in the fetus are frequently associated with congenital heart disease. If the abnormality is found in more than one organ system, the incidence of congenital heart disease increases further. Nonimmune hydrops may be cardiac related (heart failure) or associated with other problems in the fetus.

Cardiac arrhythmias in the fetus may be a common finding if they are simply *extra-systoles* (premature atrial beats secondary to the immature conducting system). A small percentage of arrhythmias are associated with significant heart disease. However, a fetus with congenital heart block is usually associated with structural abnormalities in about half of the cases, most commonly the atrioventricular septal defect as found in trisomy 21.

Maternal Risk Factors

Maternal risk factors include the previous occurrence of congenital heart disease in siblings or parents; a maternal disease known to affect the fetus, such as diabetes mellitus or connective tissue disease (e.g., lupus erythematosus); and maternal use of drugs, such as lithium, antidepressants, and alcohol.

The incidence of congenital heart disease in fetuses whose mothers have uncontrolled diabetes is much higher than when the diabetes is controlled. The most common anomalies are ventricular septal defect (VSD), transposition of the great arteries, and tetralogy of Fallot.

Excessive alcohol during pregnancy has known effects of fetal alcohol syndrome, which includes facial abnormalities, growth restriction, mental retardation, and cardiac abnormalities (VSD).

Indomethacin, a nonsteroidal antiinflammatory drug, has been used in the treatment of preterm labor. However, this drug has an effect on early closure of the patent ductus arteriosus. Evaluation of the fetus may be monitored with ultrasound to measure velocities across the patent ductus to detect if early closure is evident.

Familial Risk Factors

Familial risk factors include genetic syndromes or the presence of congenital heart disease in a previous sibling. The recurrence risk cited given a sibling with one of the most common cardiovascular abnormalities (VSD, atrial septal defect, patent ductus arteriosus, tetralogy of Fallot) varies from 2.5% to 3%. Similar data given one parent with a congenital heart defect suggest that for the common defects listed, the recurrence risk ranges from 2.5% (atrial septal defect) to 4% (VSD, patent ductus arteriosus, tetralogy of Fallot).

BEYOND THE FOUR-CHAMBER VIEW

Transducer Requirements

The ideal transducer for fetal echocardiography is a multifrequency transducer that can be quickly and easily changed from a low to a high frequency. This is especially useful when the fetus is located in a position far from the transducer face or when a lower-frequency Doppler signal is necessary to obtain a high-velocity flow profile.

The following guidelines may be used in selecting the proper multi-Hertz transducer for the fetal echocardiogram:
1. A 5.0-MHz transducer or higher with a medium focus is generally ideal for the typical pregnancy in a small to average-size patient in the second trimester.
2. A 3.5-MHz transducer with a medium-to-long focus may be used on patients of average to large build and on patients in the third trimester.
3. A 2.25-MHz transducer with medium-to-long focus is used for the obese patient in the second or third trimester.
4. The higher-frequency transvaginal probe is useful when the fetus is directed in a transverse lie. The small probe is placed on the mother's umbilicus with gentle pressure and angled toward the fetal heart.
5. The size of the transducer varies. The early second trimester fetus may be adequately imaged with a curved array transducer (Fig. 35.7); however, some laboratories prefer the small-sector, high-frequency probe.

Instrumentation

Other features useful on the ultrasound equipment include the following: cine-loop feature that allows imaging of the heart in frame-by-frame analysis, high-power resolution (write zoom) capability, simultaneous M-mode with range expansion (for cardiac arrhythmias), simultaneous Doppler capability with pulsed and continuous wave (to record high-velocity flow), color Doppler, and three-dimensional reconstruction when pathology is present.

Motion Mode Evaluation

M-mode is used to evaluate cardiac motion. Once the two-dimensional image is made, a single vertical line of information can be obtained from the face of the transducer through the fetal cardiac structures (Table 35.1). This image is electronically rotated 90 degrees so the depth of the image is along the vertical axis and the time display is shown along the horizontal axis (Fig. 35.8). Acquisition of heart wall motion, septal and valve movement, and cavity size may be easily obtained from this technique. Heart rate is generally calculated electronically on most units. However, it can also be measured by counting the number of beats that occur within a specific time frame, usually more than 1 second. If 2.5 beats were shown in a 1-second time period, the heart rate would be 2.5 beats × 60 seconds = 150 beats/min.

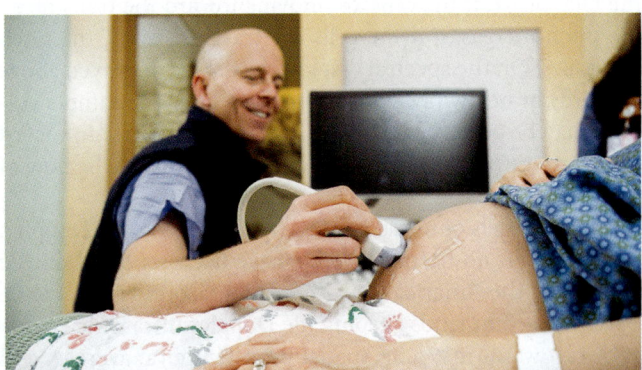

FIG. 35.7 The early second trimester fetus may be adequately imaged with a curved array transducer.

TABLE 35.1	Normal Fetal Motion Mode Cardiac Measurements (mm)			
	Cardiac Structure			
Weeks of Gestation	LV/RV	IVS	AO/PA	LA
20	6	1.5	4	5
22	8	1.7	4.8	6
24	9	2	5	6.5
28	10	2.3	6	8
32	12	3	7	10
36	14	3.5	8	11
40	16	3.8	9	12.5

AO, Aorta; *IVS*, interventricular septum; *LA*, left atrium; *LV*, left ventricle; *PA*, pulmonary artery; *RV*, right ventricle.

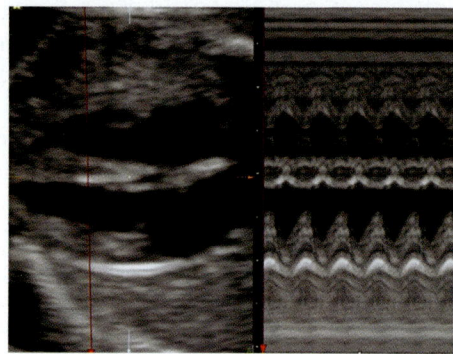

FIG. 35.8 Two-dimensional and M-mode of the ventricular cavities. On the motion mode, time is depicted along the horizontal axis *(dots along the top of the image)*. The distance between two dots represents 1 second. Distance is located along the vertical axis. The aorta is shown as the two parallel lines moving as a "unit" through systole (pumping) and diastole (resting).

Pulsed Doppler Imaging

Pulsed Doppler demonstrates the direction and characteristics of blood flow within the fetal heart and great vessels and allows the qualitative and quantitative definition of flow disturbances, such as those that occur with valvular stenotic or regurgitant lesions. Doppler uses the principle of the Doppler shift, or sound waves reflected from the red blood cells within the fetal heart: If the cells are moving toward the transducer, the pitch increases; if the cells are traveling away, the pitch decreases. On the spectral display, the flow is displayed above (toward) or below (away) from the baseline. The sample volume may be gated or moved to the area of interest to record the optimum signal as the transducer is parallel to the flow of blood (Fig. 35.9).

Higher levels of ultrasound energy are used with Doppler, and although no harmful effects have been reported on the fetal heart, the American Institute of Ultrasound in Medicine (AIUM) recommends keeping the Doppler ultrasonic energy at or below 100 mW/cm^2 spatial peak-temporal average, and Doppler interrogation should be limited to as short a time as possible (Table 35.2).

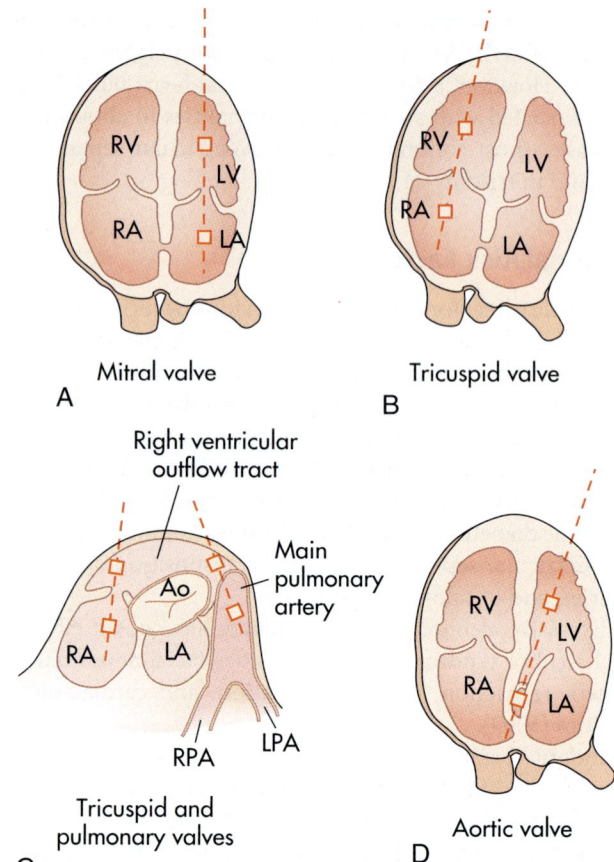

FIG. 35.9 Pulsed Doppler sample volume placement for fetal echo. (A–B) The four-chamber view is ideal to sample the velocity flow patterns of the mitral and tricuspid valves. The sample volume is initially placed at the annulus of the valve. To record regurgitation, the volume is moved into the atrial chamber; to record inflow of the valves, the sample volume is moved into the ventricular cavity. (C) The high short-axis view is best to obtain velocities from the tricuspid and pulmonary valves. The same procedure is used for the tricuspid valve as described in the four-chamber view. To record flow in the main pulmonary artery, the sample volume is placed at the level of the cusps and then moved back into the right ventricular outflow tract, then into the main pulmonary artery to look for abnormal flow patterns. (D) The five-chamber view is good to record velocity flow in the left ventricular outflow tract and the ascending aorta. The sample volume should be placed below the aortic leaflets in the left ventricular outflow tract and then slowly moved through the cusps into the ascending aorta to see flow velocities. *AO,* Aorta; *LA,* left atrium; *LPA,* left pulmonary artery; *LV,* left ventricle; *RA,* right atrium; *RPA,* right pulmonary artery; *RV,* right ventricle.

TABLE 35.2	Normal Doppler Measurements (Peak Systole)
Mitral valve	40–60–77 cm/sec
Tricuspid valve	47–65–83 cm/sec
Aortic valve	30–60–95 cm/sec
Pulmonic valve	25–55–80 cm/sec
Foramen ovale	20–30 cm/sec
Aortic arch, level of ductal insertion	120–150 cm/sec

Values at 20 weeks of gestation range from 25th to 50th to 95th percentiles.

Color Flow Doppler Imaging

Color flow Doppler may help detect flow disturbances and flow direction (to check whether vessels or chambers are patent) and should be integrated into the fetal echocardiogram. Color Doppler flow mapping is a multi-gated Doppler technique in which sampling along all of the scan lines and depths in the field occurs simultaneously. Color displays are usually oriented so that flow toward the transducer is projected in shades of red and orange, and flow away is projected in cool blue colors (Fig. 35.10). Disturbed flow is seen as a mixture of red, orange, and yellow or blues and greens. The color gain should be adjusted to each image to eliminate color "blooming."

Three-Dimensional Imaging

Clinical investigation of 3D echocardiography has been performed both with and without cardiac gating. The gated acquisition showed improved resolution of structures compared with the non-gated acquisition. Clarity of images is still the primary problem in this technique: the fetal heart is beating so quickly and the volume is too small to acquire enough data points to display an image better than the current real-time two-dimensional images (Fig. 35.11).

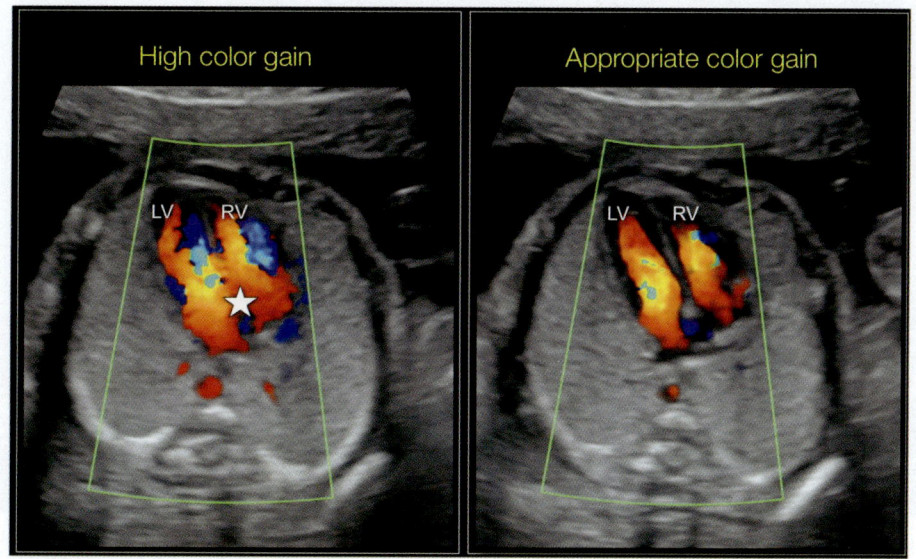

FIG. 35.10 Color displays are usually oriented so that flow toward the transducer is projected in shades of red and orange, and flow away is projected in cool blue colors. Disturbed flow is seen as a mixture of red, orange, and yellow or blues and greens. The color gain should be adjusted to each image to eliminate color "blooming." *LV*, Left ventricle; *RV*, right ventricle.

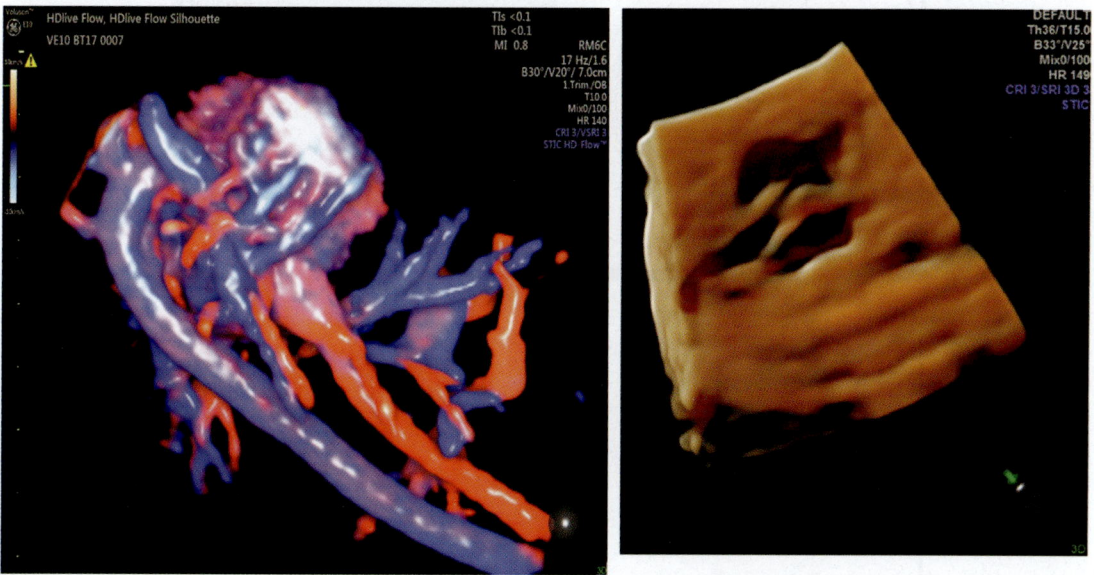

FIG. 35.11 Clinical investigation of three-dimensional echocardiography has been performed both with and without cardiac gating. The gated acquisition showed improved resolution of structures compared with the nongated acquisition. Clarity of images is still the primary problem in this technique: the fetal heart is beating so quickly and the volume is too small to acquire enough data points to display an image better than the current real-time two-dimensional images.

FETAL ULTRASOUND LANDMARKS

In most cases, the obstetric patient has had a previous baseline obstetrical ultrasound and is referred for a dedicated, or target, fetal echocardiographic examination. Generally, a dedicated fetal echocardiographic study may take 30 minutes to more than 1 hour, depending on the type of pathologic condition present. The cardiac sonographer must know certain characteristics that will help in the cardiac evaluation. (See Chapter 51 for illustrations of these normal structures.)

The fetal survey should demonstrate the following structures before focusing on the fetal heart:
1. The position of the fetus (vertex, breech, transverse).
2. The position of the fetal thorax (spine up or down; determine right side and left side).
3. The position of the fetal stomach; normal position is left of the fetal spine (Fig. 35.12).
4. The location of the apex of the heart (left, right, or midline) (Fig. 35.13).
5. The location of the fetal abdominal aorta and inferior vena cava (aorta left, close to spine, inferior vena cava right, and elevated from spine) (Fig. 35.14).
6. The position of the placenta is important to recognize as the anterior placenta may cause noise that interferes with visualization of the cardiac structures if the fetal thorax is adjacent to the placenta (Fig. 35.15).

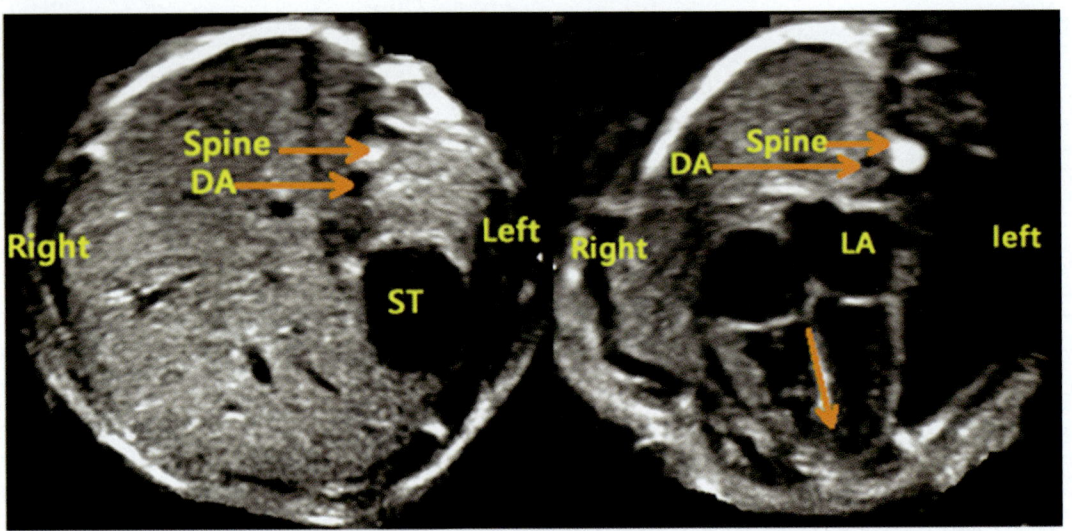

FIG. 35.12 The position of the fetal stomach; normal position is left of the fetal spine. *DA,* Descending aorta; *LA,* left atrium; *ST,* stomach.

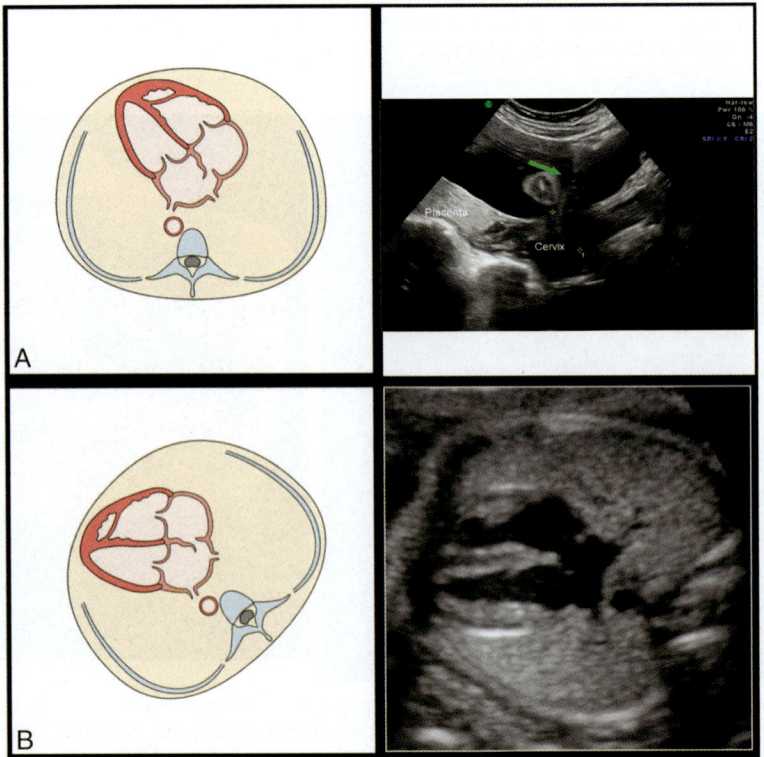

FIG. 35.13 The location of the apex of the heart should be noted. (A) Apex points to the left. (B) Apex is midline.

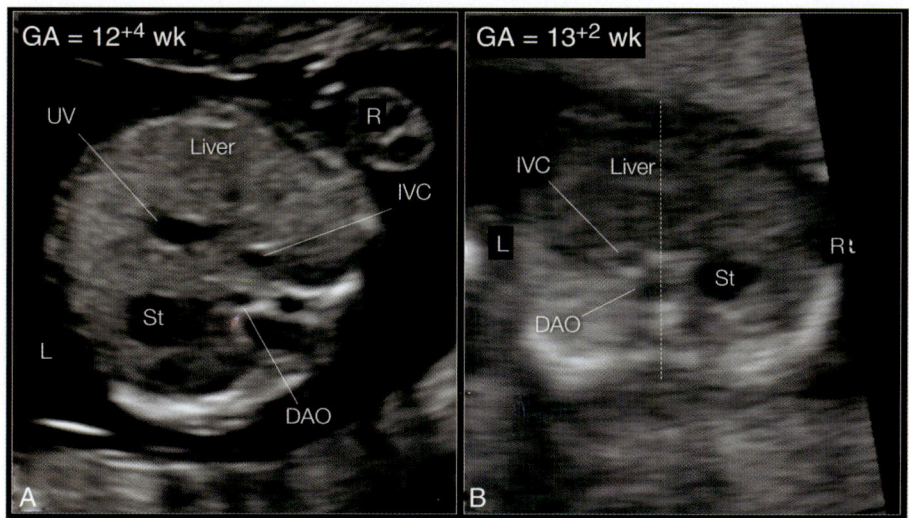

FIG. 35.14 The location of the fetal abdominal aorta and inferior vena cava should be noted; the abdominal aorta is left, close to spine, whereas the inferior vena cava lies to the right and is elevated from the spine. *DAO*, Descending aorta; *GA*, gestational age; *IVC*, inferior vena cava; *LV*, left ventricle; *St*, stomach.

(oligohydramnios), unusual fetal position (spine up, transverse, or low lie in the maternal pelvis), and maternal obesity. The diabetic mother is generally more difficult to scan; these patients are imaged best in the middle of the second trimester, between 24 and 26 weeks of gestation. Alterations of the maternal position sometimes helps encourage the fetus to move; the goal is to move the mother such that the fetal spine is down or away from the anterior maternal wall.

When the fetus is in a difficult-to-image position, the sonographer may ask the mother to get up, use the restroom, walk the hall for a few minutes, or perform toe touches or jumping jacks to encourage the fetus to change positions. This technique usually works.

ECHOCARDIOGRAPHIC EVALUATION OF THE FETUS

A normal cardiac study should include the following views: four-chamber, outflow tracts, and oblique long-axis view for the aortic arch and ductus arteriosus.

Four-Chamber View

The four-chamber view is probably one of the easiest views to demonstrate cardiac anatomy (Box 35.2). Recall that the fetal heart lies in a horizontal position within the thorax with the apex of the heart (the left ventricle) directed toward the left hip (Fig. 35.18). The transducer is angled in a cephalic direction through the fetal liver, which serves as a good window to visualize cardiac structures.

The sonographer should note the relative size and function of the atria and inflow ventricular cavities and the axis of the left ventricle. The right heart is slightly larger in utero than the left heart. The right and left sides may be identified by the opening flap of the patent foramen ovale: in utero, the foramen opens toward the left atrium as the pressure is slightly greater in the right atrium. After birth, the pressure in the left heart forces the foramen to close; failure for the foramen to close results in an atrial septal defect. The moderator band

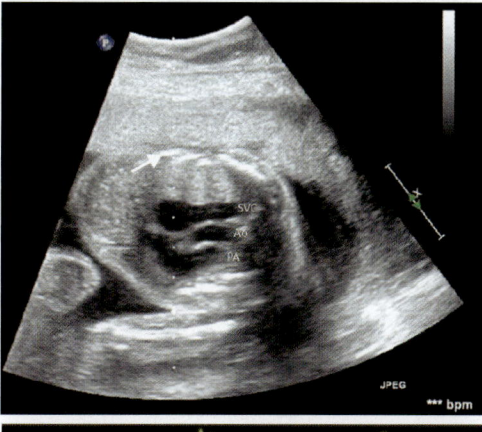

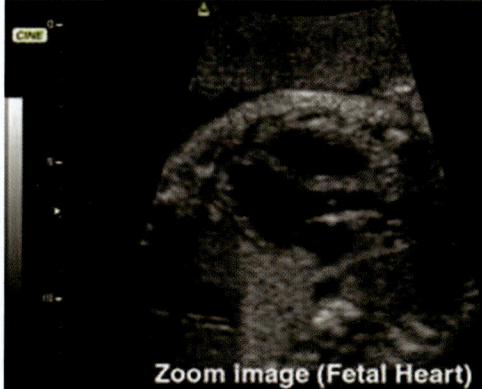

FIG. 35.15 The position of the placenta *(arrow)* is important as the anterior placenta may cause noise that interferes with visualization of the cardiac structures if the fetal thorax is adjacent to the placenta as noted on the lower image. *Ao*, Aorta; *PA*, pulmonary artery; *SVC*, superior vena cava.

7. The measurement of the biparietal diameter, abdominal circumference, and femur length is made to assess gestational age, see Chapter 52 (Fig. 35.16).
8. Measurement of the cardiothoracic circumference and/or area ratio and cardiac axis (Fig. 35.17).

The sonographer may encounter obstacles when performing a fetal echocardiogram. Such obstacles for obtaining an adequate image include decreased amniotic fluid

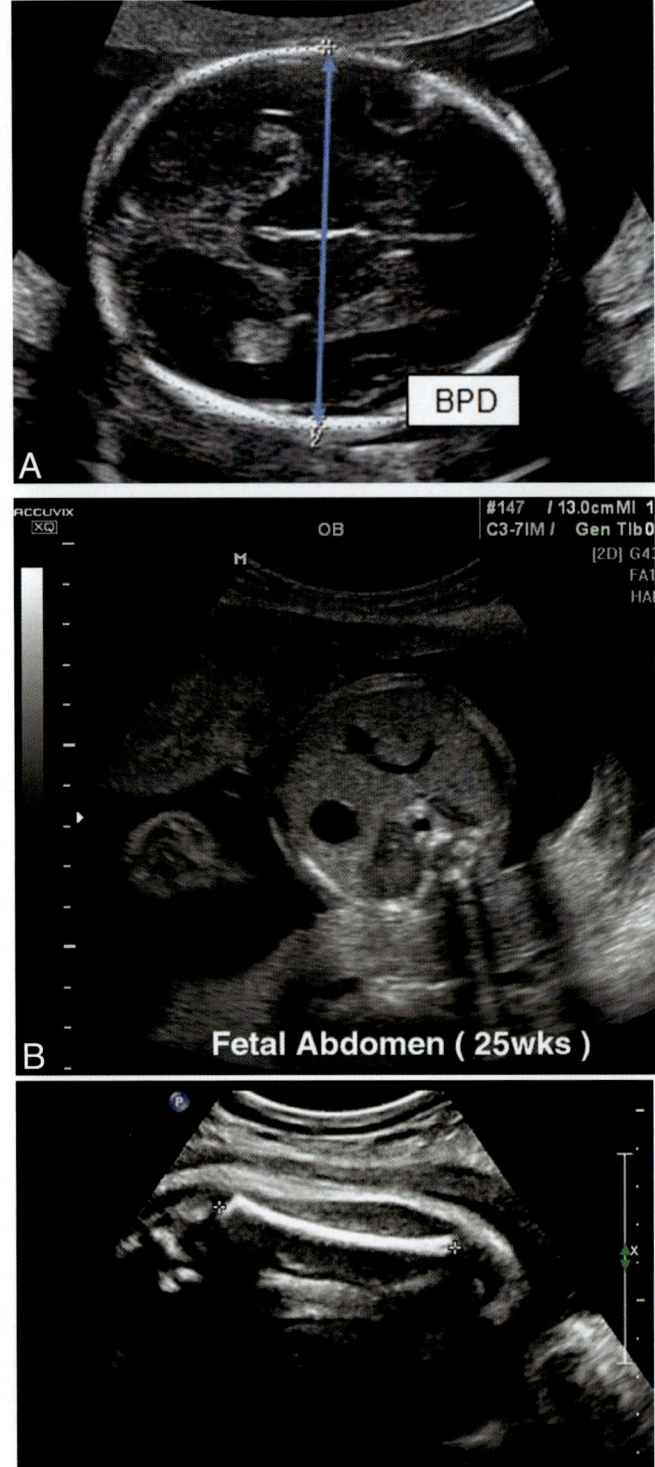

FIG. 35.16 Measurements of the biparietal diameter (BPD; A), abdominal circumference (B), and femur length (C) are made to assess gestational age.

can also be used to identify the right ventricle. It stretches horizontally across the right ventricle near the apex. The right ventricle is also more trabeculated than the left ventricle.

The position of the mitral and tricuspid leaflets (atrioventricular leaflets) should be assessed. Normally, the tricuspid valve is located just slightly inferior to the mitral valve.

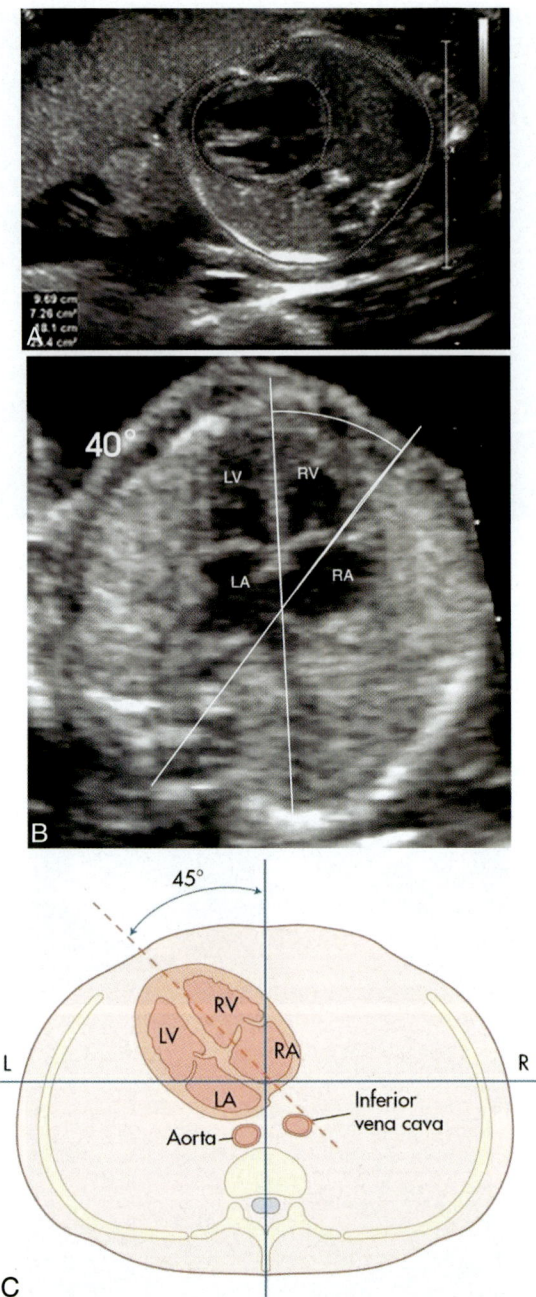

FIG. 35.17 Measurement of the cardiothoracic circumference and/or area ratio (A) and cardiac axis (B and C) from a four-chamber view of the fetal chest. The apex of the heart should not exceed a 45-degree angle from the line drawn perpendicular to the fetal spine. *LA*, Left atrium; *LV*, left ventricle; *RA*, right atrium; *RV*, right ventricle.

BOX 35.2	Four-Chamber View Anatomy

Right atrium and ventricle (with moderator band)
Tricuspid valve
Left atrium and ventricle
Mitral valve
Interventricular septum
Interatrial septum
Foramen ovale
Pulmonary veins as they enter the left atrium

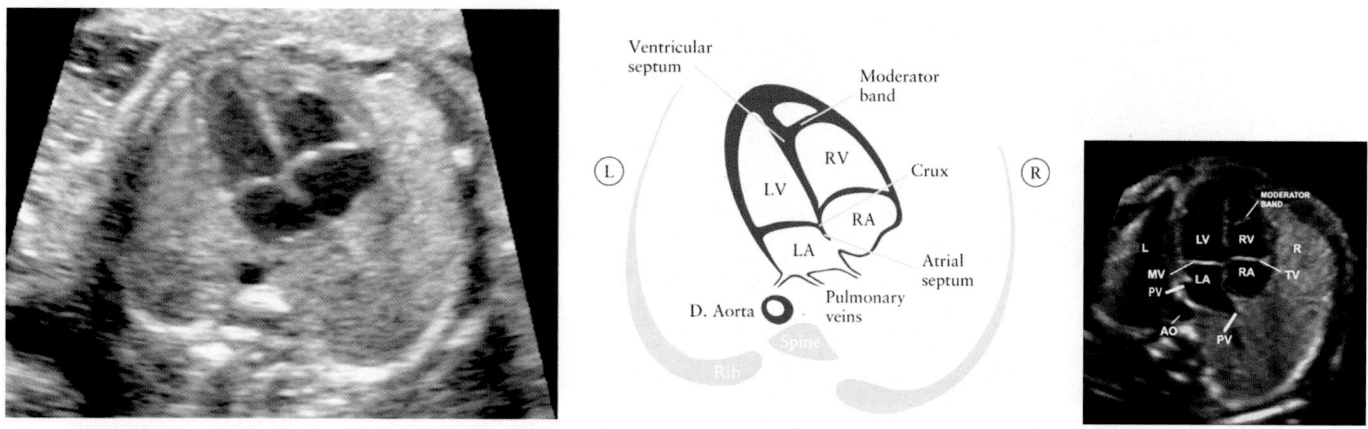

FIG. 35.18 The fetal heart lies in a horizontal position within the thorax with the apex of the heart directed toward the left hip. The right heart is slightly larger in utero than the left heart. The right and left sides may be identified by the opening flap of the patent foramen ovale *(small red arrow)*. The right and left atria and ventricles are separated respectfully by the tricuspid valve and mitral valve. *AO*, Aorta; *CS*, coronary sinus; *LA*, left atrium; *LV*, left ventricle; *MV*, mitral valve; *PV*, pulmonary vein; *RA*, right atrium; *RV*, right ventricle; *TV*, tricuspid valve.

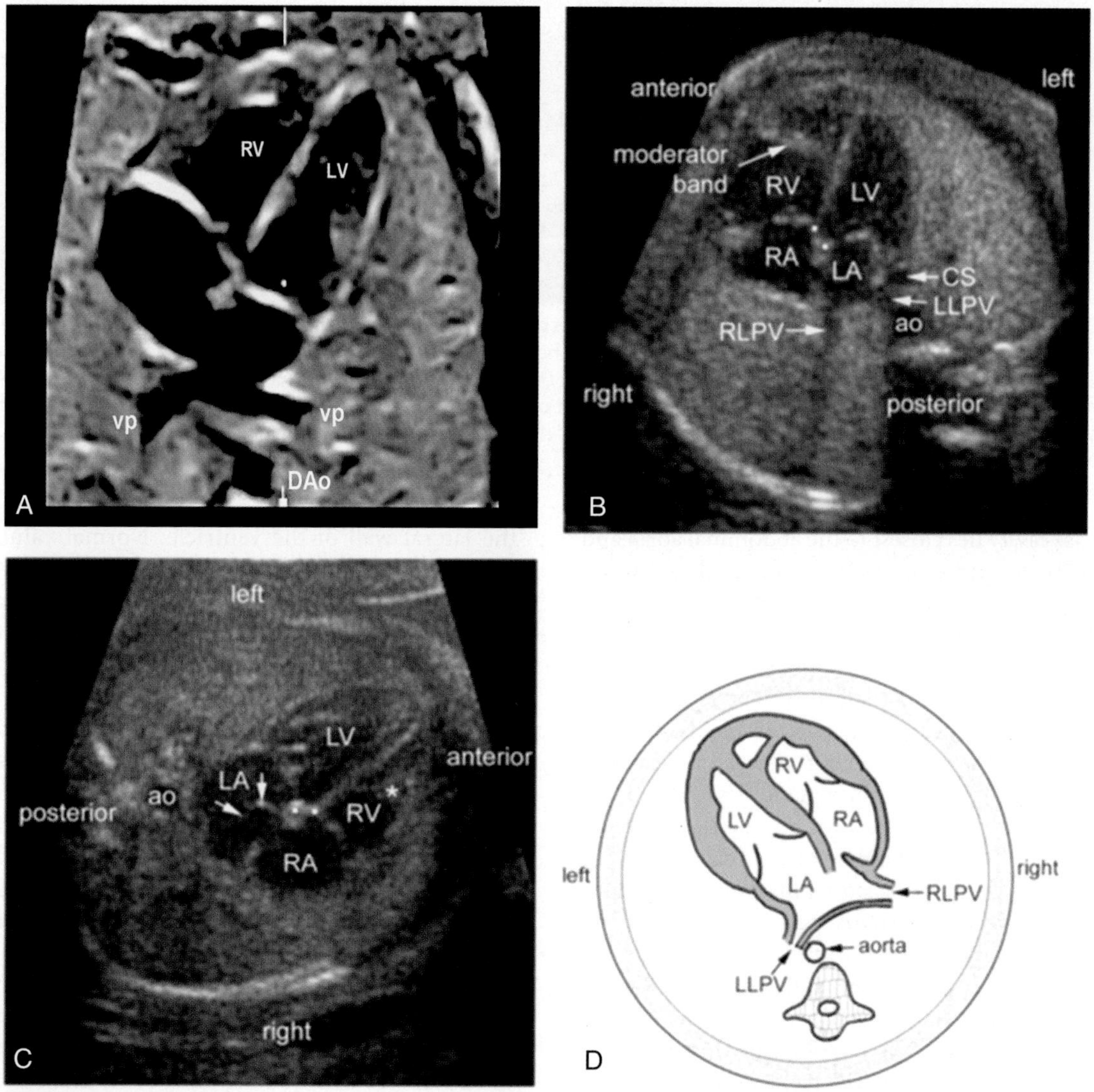

FIG. 35.19 The four pulmonic veins enter into the posterior wall of the left atrium. The right upper enters into the medial-posterosuperior wall; the left upper enters into the lateral-posterosuperior wall; the left lower enters the lateral inferior wall; and the right lower enters the medial inferior wall. *AO*, Aorta; *LA*, left atrium; *LLPV*, left lower pulmonary vein; *LV*, left ventricle; *RA*, right atrium; *RLPV*, right lower pulmonary vein; *RV*, right ventricle.

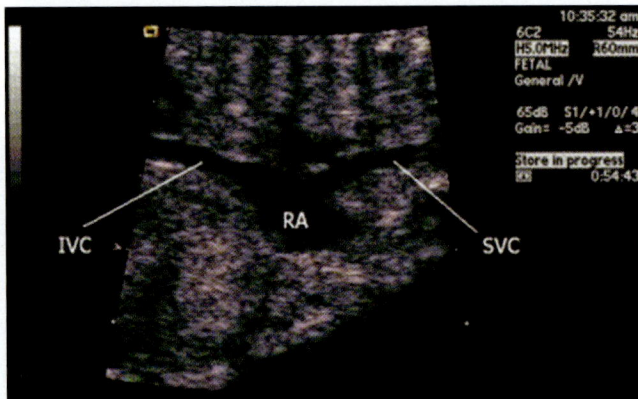 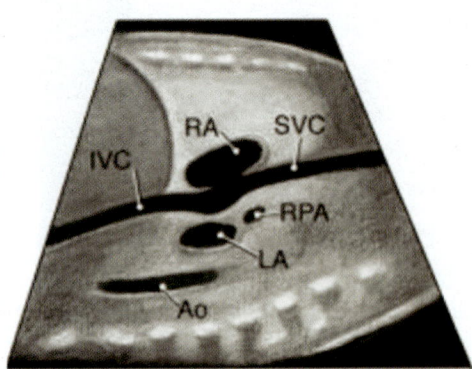

FIG. 35.20 The inferior and superior vena cava may be seen to enter the right atrium. The inferior vena cava (IVC) enters the posterior wall along the inferior lateral margin; the superior vena cava (SVC) enters the medial-posterosuperior wall. *Ao*, Aorta; *LA*, left atrium; *RA*, right atrium; *RPA*, right pulmonary artery.

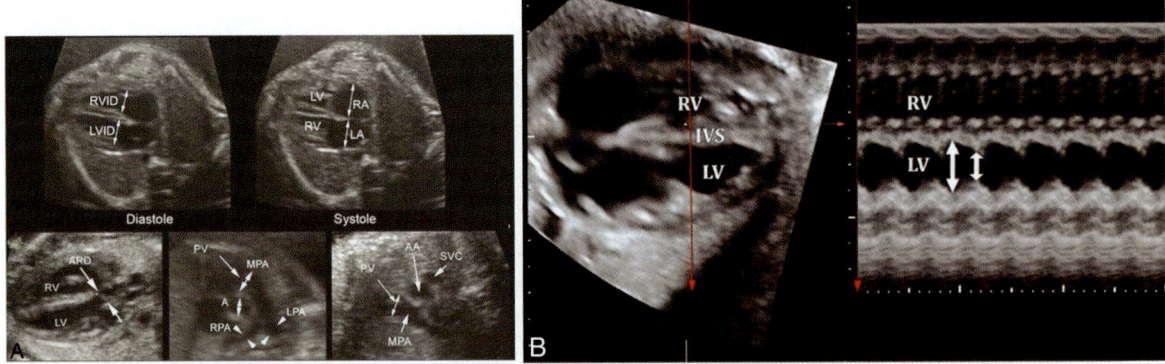

FIG. 35.21 (A) The right and left ventricular width measurements are performed in the four-chamber view at the level of the atrioventricular annulus in diastole. (B) M-mode measurement of the fetal heart. *A*, Aorta; *AA*, ascending aorta; *ARD*, aortic root diameter; *IVS*, interventricular septum; *LA*, left atrium; *LPA*, left pulmonary artery; *LV*, left ventricle; *LVID*, left ventricular internal dimension; *MPA*, main pulmonary artery; *PV*, pulmonary vein; *RA*, right atrium; *RPA*, right pulmonary artery; *RV*, right ventricle; *RVID*, right ventricular internal dimension; *SVC*, superior vena cava.

The left atrial cavity lies closest to the abdominal aorta and is generally about the same size as the right atrial cavity and is hypoechoic. The four pulmonic veins enter into the posterior wall of the left atrium. The right upper enters into the medial-posterosuperior wall; the left upper enters into the lateral-posterosuperior wall; the left lower enters the lateral inferior wall; and the right lower enters the medial inferior wall (Fig. 35.19). On the four-chamber view, all the pulmonary veins are imaged except for the right lower vein.

The inferior and superior vena cava may be seen to enter the right atrium (Fig. 35.20). The inferior vena cava enters the posterior wall along the inferior lateral margin; the superior vena cava enters the medial-posterosuperior wall.

The right and left ventricular width measurements are performed in the four-chamber view at the level of the atrioventricular annulus (Fig. 35.21). The sonographer should clean up the image as much as possible for this measurement by turning the gain down. The right ventricle is measured from the lateral wall, across the level of the tricuspid annulus, to the mid-portion of the septum. The left ventricle is measured from the mid-portion of the septum, across the level of the mitral annulus, to the endocardial surface of the lateral wall of the ventricle. Normal values have been established to correspond to appropriate gestational ages. At 18 weeks of gestation, the ventricles should each measure approximately 6 mm. M-mode tracings may be made with the transducer perpendicular to the ventricular cavity, see Fig. 35.21C.

If an abnormality exists in the atrioventricular valves or if the atria are enlarged, the four-chamber view is excellent to record Doppler tracings of blood flow (Fig. 35.22). The transducer should be parallel to the four-chamber view, with the cursor placed at the level of the annulus and slowly moved toward the apex, into the ventricular cavity to record atrioventricular inflow patterns. To record regurgitation of the atrioventricular valves, the cursor is slowly moved toward the base of the heart into the atrial cavity to map the flow pattern and assess flow dynamics. Normally there is no backward flow through the orifice. The sonographer can assess the atrial size as an additional determinant of the presence of regurgitation.

The atrioventricular valves have a "double peak" of blood flow on the Doppler tracing. The first peak, *e*, is termed the *passive filling phase*. (This increases with fetal breathing and

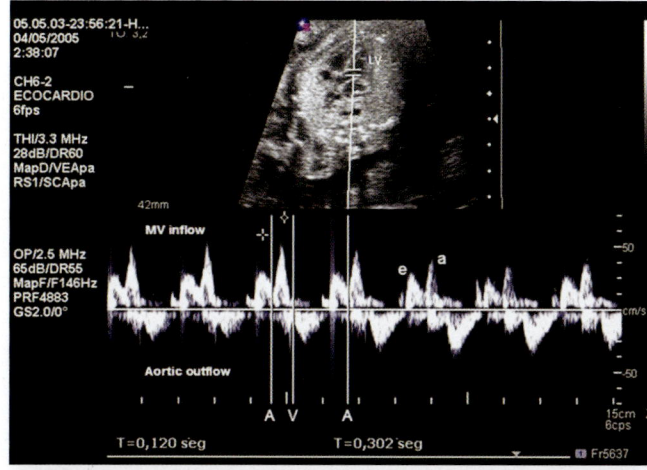

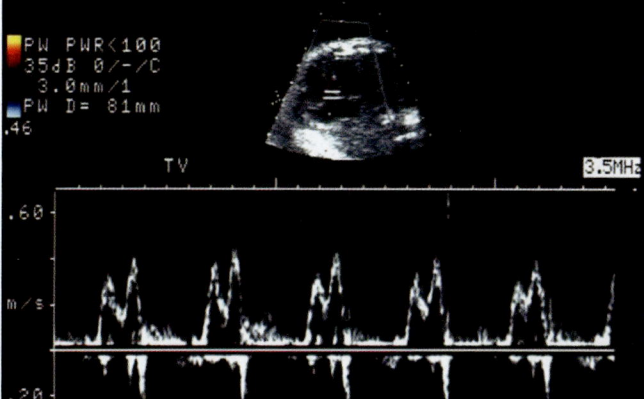

FIG. 35.22 The atrioventricular valves have a "double peak" of blood flow on the Doppler tracing. The first peak, *e*, is termed the *passive filling phase*. This peak is smaller than the second peak because the fetal heart is less compliant than the neonatal heart. The second, taller peak, *a*, is termed the *active atrial phase*. In later pregnancy, the *e* point equals or exceeds the *a* point on the Doppler tracing as the pressure on the left side exceeds the right-side pressure. The mean tricuspid valve velocity is 65 cm/sec; the mean mitral valve velocity is 60 cm/sec.

with gestational age.) This peak is smaller than the second peak because the fetal heart is less compliant than the neonatal heart. The second, taller peak, *a*, is termed the *active atrial phase*. In later pregnancy, the *e* point equals or exceeds the *a* point on the Doppler tracing as the pressure on the left side exceeds the right-side pressure. The mean tricuspid valve velocity is 65 cm/sec; the mean mitral valve velocity is 60 cm/sec^2.

Color flow Doppler (Fig. 35.23) may be useful in demonstrating the amount and path of regurgitation. A multicolored jet would be present in the atrial cavity posterior to the atrioventricular valve. Remember, the pressures in the fetal heart are different than after birth; therefore, the color and Doppler flow patterns will not be truly representative of the velocities obtained after birth.

Left and Right Ventricular Outflow Tracts

Five-Chamber View. Aortic flow may be recorded in the five-chamber view (Box 35.3); to obtain this view, the transducer should be angled slightly anterior from the four-chamber view to include the left ventricular and aortic outflow tract (Fig. 35.24). Doppler flow patterns of the aorta are recorded

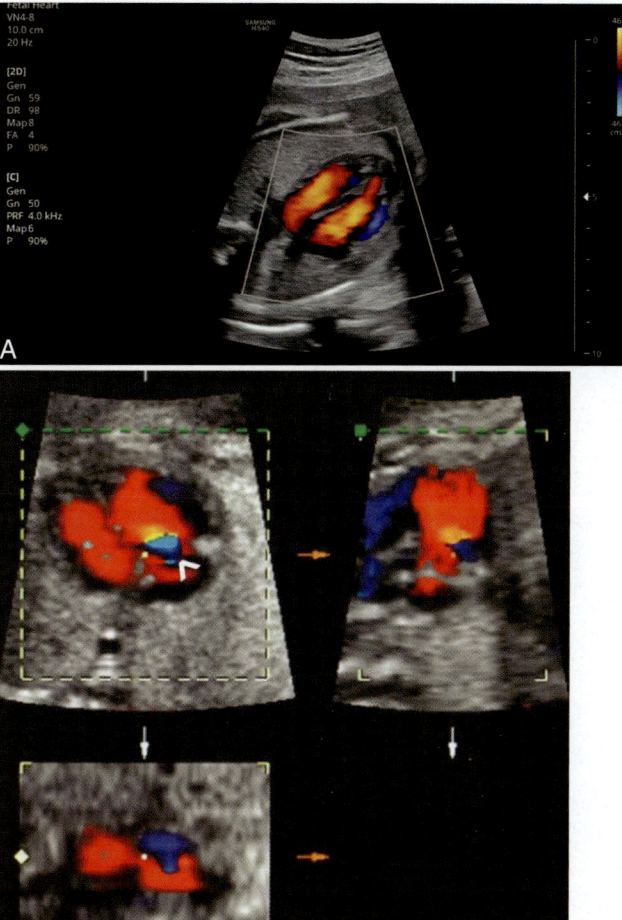

FIG. 35.23 Color flow Doppler may be useful in demonstrating the amount and path of regurgitation. A multicolored jet would be present in the atrial cavity posterior to the atrioventricular valve. (A) Normal color Doppler pattern. (B) *Arrowhead* points to the blue-yellow color Doppler of tricuspid regurgitation.

BOX 35.3	Five-Chamber View Anatomy
Left atrium	
Left ventricular outflow tract	
Aortic root	
Left ventricle	

with the transducer again parallel to flow and the cursor placed first at the level of the aortic cusps and then moved into the AA. The mean velocity in the aorta is 60 cm/sec.

Crisscross View. As the transducer is angled from the aorta slightly to the left, the pulmonary artery may be seen as it arises from the right ventricular outflow tract (Fig. 35.25). The pulmonary artery normally is anterior and to the left of the aorta. This sweep from the aorta to the pulmonary artery is called the *crisscross view* and allows the sonographer to see the normal relationship of the great arteries to one another (Box 35.4). Pulmonary flow patterns may be obtained in this view if the cursor is parallel with the flow. The cursor is moved into the MPA to record the flow patterns. The mean velocity in the pulmonary artery is 55 cm/sec.

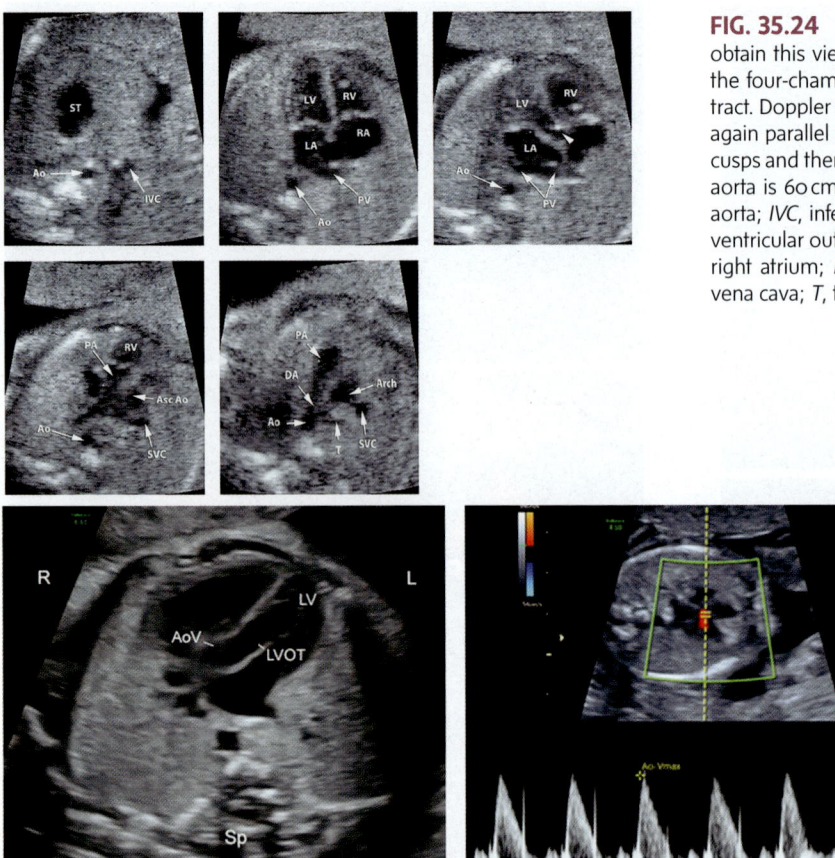

FIG. 35.24 Aortic flow may be recorded in the five-chamber view; to obtain this view, the transducer should be angled slightly anterior from the four-chamber view to include the left ventricular and aortic outflow tract. Doppler flow patterns of the aorta are recorded with the transducer again parallel to flow and the cursor placed first at the level of the aortic cusps and then moved into the ascending aorta. The mean velocity in the aorta is 60 cm/sec. *Ao*, Aorta; *AscAo*, ascending aorta; *DA*, descending aorta; *IVC*, inferior vena cava; *LA*, left atrium; *LV*, left ventricle; *LVOT*, left ventricular outflow tract; *PA*, pulmonary artery; *PV*, pulmonary veins; *RA*, right atrium; *RV*, right ventricle; *Sp*, spine; *ST*, stomach; *SVC*, superior vena cava; *T*, trachea.

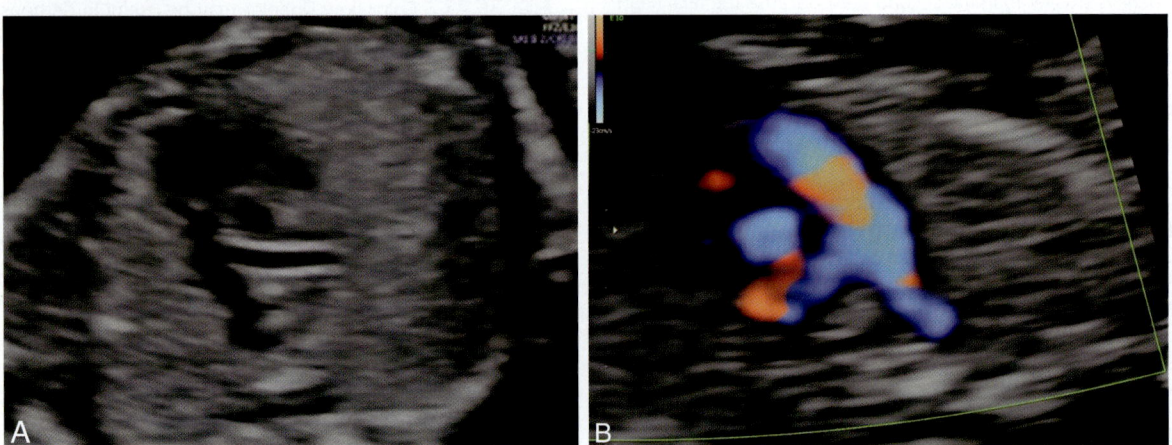

FIG. 35.25 As the transducer is angled from the aorta slightly to the left (A), the pulmonary artery may be seen as it arises from the right ventricular outflow tract (B). The pulmonary artery normally is anterior and to the left of the aorta. This "sweep" from the aorta to the pulmonary artery is called the crisscross view and allows the sonographer to see the normal relationship of the great arteries to one another.

BOX 35.4 Crisscross View of Great Arteries

Sweep from aorta (located posterior) to pulmonic vessel (located anterior and medial)
Left ventricular outflow tract
Right ventricular outflow tract

Long-Axis View. In the long-axis view (Fig. 35.26), the size of the right and left ventricles and the left atrial cavity should be assessed to obtain an overview of cardiac disease and contractility (Box 35.5). The left atrial cavity in this view is generally about the same size as the aorta and is hypoechoic. The crescent-shaped right ventricle is anterior to the left ventricle.

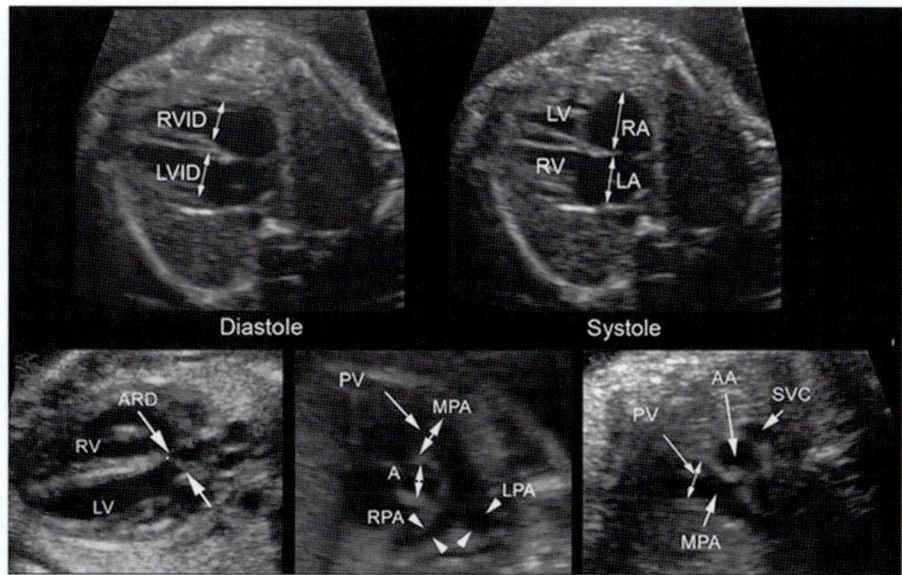

FIG. 35.26 In the long-axis view, the size of the right and left ventricles and the left atrial cavity should be assessed to obtain an overview of cardiac disease and contractility. The left atrial cavity in this view is generally about the same size as the aorta and is hypoechoic. *A*, Aorta; *AA*, ascending aorta; *ARD*, aortic root diameter; *LA*, left atrium; *LPA*, left pulmonary artery; *LV*, left ventricle; *LVID*, left ventricular internal diameter; *MPA*, main pulmonary artery; *PV*, pulmonary vein; *RA*, right atrium; *RPA*, right pulmonary artery; *RV*, right ventricle; *RVID*, right ventricular internal diameter; *SVC*, superior vena cava.

BOX 35.5	Long-Axis View

Right ventricle
Interventricular septum
Left ventricle
Mitral valve leaflets
Aorta with aortic cusps
Left atrium

The thickness of the interventricular septum may be assessed from the parasternal long-axis view when the transducer is perpendicular to the septum (Fig. 35.27). The septum is divided into membranous and muscular segments. The membranous portion is located just inferior to the aorta. This part of the septum is the last to develop and is very thin; it must be examined in several planes (apical, short axis, and subcostal) to evaluate its inflow and outflow sections. The inflow membranous septum is best seen on the apical four-chamber view with slight posterior angulation at the level of the atrioventricular valves, whereas the outflow may be seen on the long-axis view.

The septum thickens along its muscular component, which makes up the remaining two-thirds of the septum. The septum and the posterior left ventricular wall are generally the same thickness at the end of the ventricular systole. Normal septal thickness should correspond to the gestational age; a good rule of thumb is that the second-trimester septum should measure about 2 to 2.5 mm, and the third-trimester septum should measure less than 4 mm. If the septum measures over 5 mm, septal hypertrophy or concentric ventricular hypertrophy should be considered.

On the long-axis view (Fig. 35.28A), the continuity of the right side of the septum with the anterior wall of the aortic root is important to rule out the presence of a membranous VSD, conal truncal abnormality (such as truncus arteriosus), endocardial cushion defect, or tetralogy of Fallot. A very small VSD may not be visualized at this stage depending on the resolution of the equipment and quality visualization of the fetus. Generally, the septal defect must be at least half the size of the aortic diameter to be imaged by ultrasound. Multiple septal defects may be difficult to image in the second trimester.

As the transducer is angled slightly anterior and medial from the aortic root, the right ventricular outflow tract may be imaged (Fig. 35.28B). The pulmonary artery is slightly wider at its origin than the aorta and bifurcates into the right and left pulmonary arteries.

The size of the aorta should be assessed. A gestational age of 20 weeks would show a normal aortic measurement of 4 mm. The aortic cusp motion should be assessed on the long- and short-axis views. Normally, the three cusps open in systole to the full extent of the aortic root and close in a mid-position in diastole (Fig. 35.29). The cusps do not "flop" into the left ventricular outflow tract, as is sometimes seen to varying degrees with a bicuspid or unicuspid valve. The aortic root should be anechoic from its base throughout the arch and descending aorta. The presence of interluminal echoes with dilation may indicate some degree of aortic stenosis (with post-stenotic dilation). The presence of a membrane inferior to the aortic cusps may indicate subvalvular aortic obstruction.

Short-Axis View. Once the long-axis view has been obtained, the transducer is rotated 90 degrees to the transverse or short-axis view. Generally, the transducer is angled in a cephalic direction to make this a high parasternal short-axis view

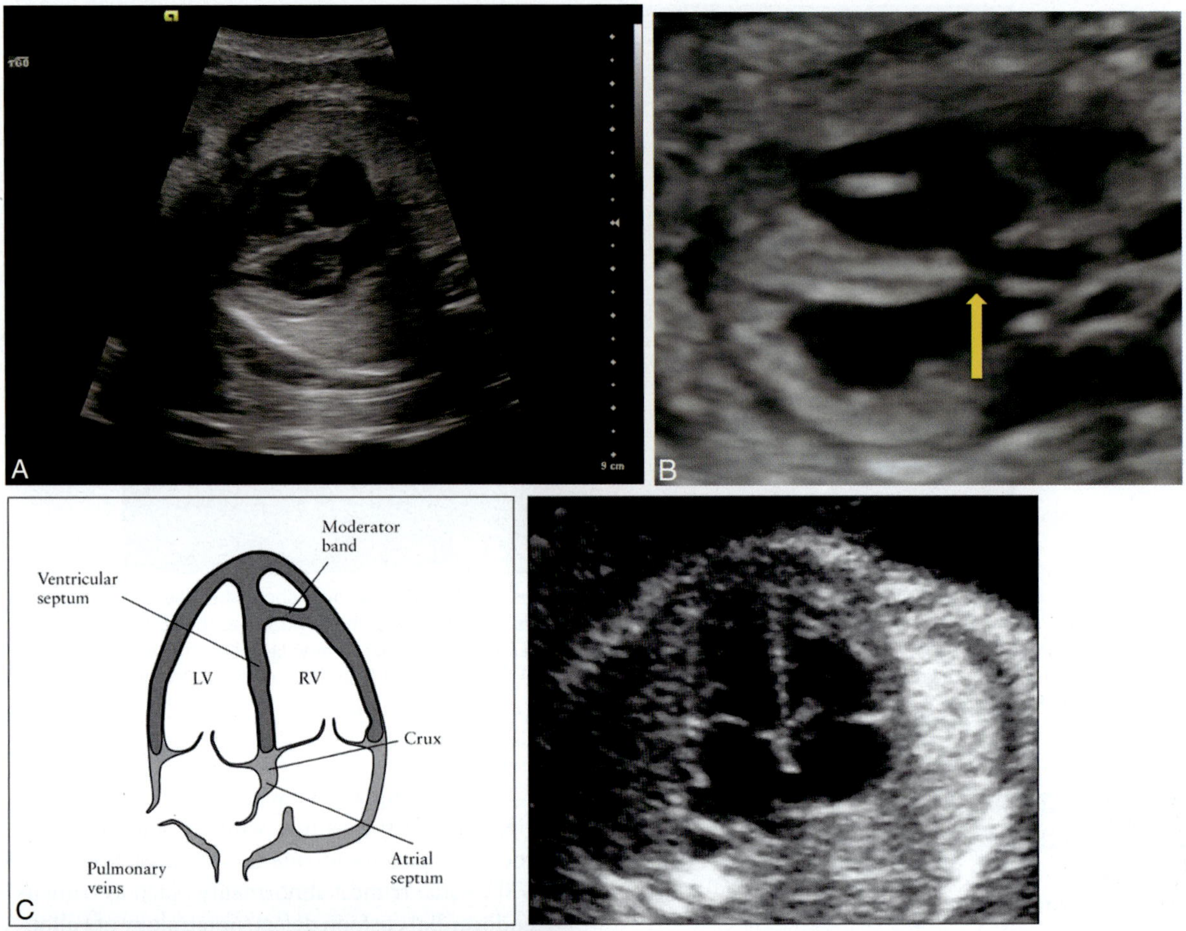

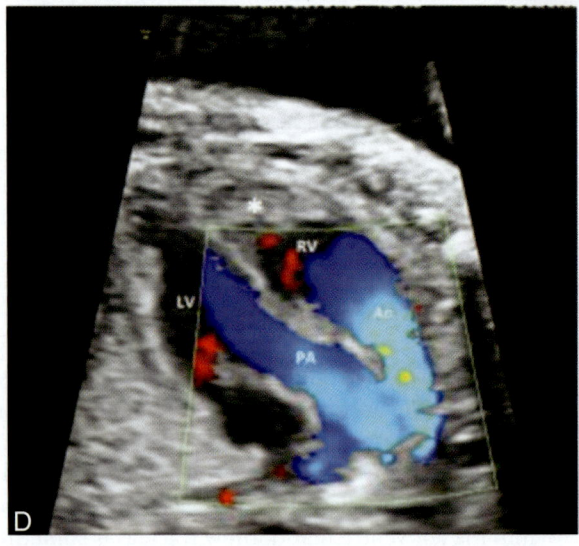

FIG. 35.27 (A) The thickness of the interventricular septum may be assessed from the parasternal long-axis view when the transducer is perpendicular to the septum. (B) The septum is divided into membranous and muscular segments. The membranous portion is located just inferior to the aorta. This part of the septum is the last to develop and is very thin; it must be examined in several planes (apical, short axis and subcostal) to evaluate its inflow and outflow sections. The inflow membranous septum is best seen on the apical four-chamber view with slight posterior angulation at the level of the atrioventricular valves, whereas the outflow may be seen on the long-axis view. (C) The membranous septum is not well defined when the apex is vertical to the transducer. (D) Normal color flow in the outflow tracts. *Ao*, Aorta; *LV*, left ventricle; *PA*, pulmonary artery; *RV*, right ventricle.

(see Fig. 35.29B). The structures listed in Box 35.6 should be visualized.

The high short-axis view is used to measure the diameter of the pulmonary artery and the aorta (see Fig. 35.29B). It is also important to visualize the bifurcation of the MPA into the right and left pulmonary arteries to demonstrate the normal relationship of the pulmonary artery as it lies anterior and to the right of the aorta. On the short-axis view, normally the right ventricular outflow tract and pulmonary artery "drape" anterior to the circular aorta. The great vessels are measured at the level of the semilunar cusps. At 20 weeks of gestation, both arteries should measure approximately 4 mm each.

The trileaflet aortic cusps may be visualized in this short-axis view. Abnormal development of the aortic cusps may lead to a two-leaflet or **bicuspid aortic valve** which appears as two cusps with or without eccentric closure, depending on the equal distribution of cusp tissue.

Pulmonic flow patterns are obtained parallel to flow in the high short-axis plane with the Doppler cursor at the level of the pulmonic cusps. The cursor is moved into the MPA to

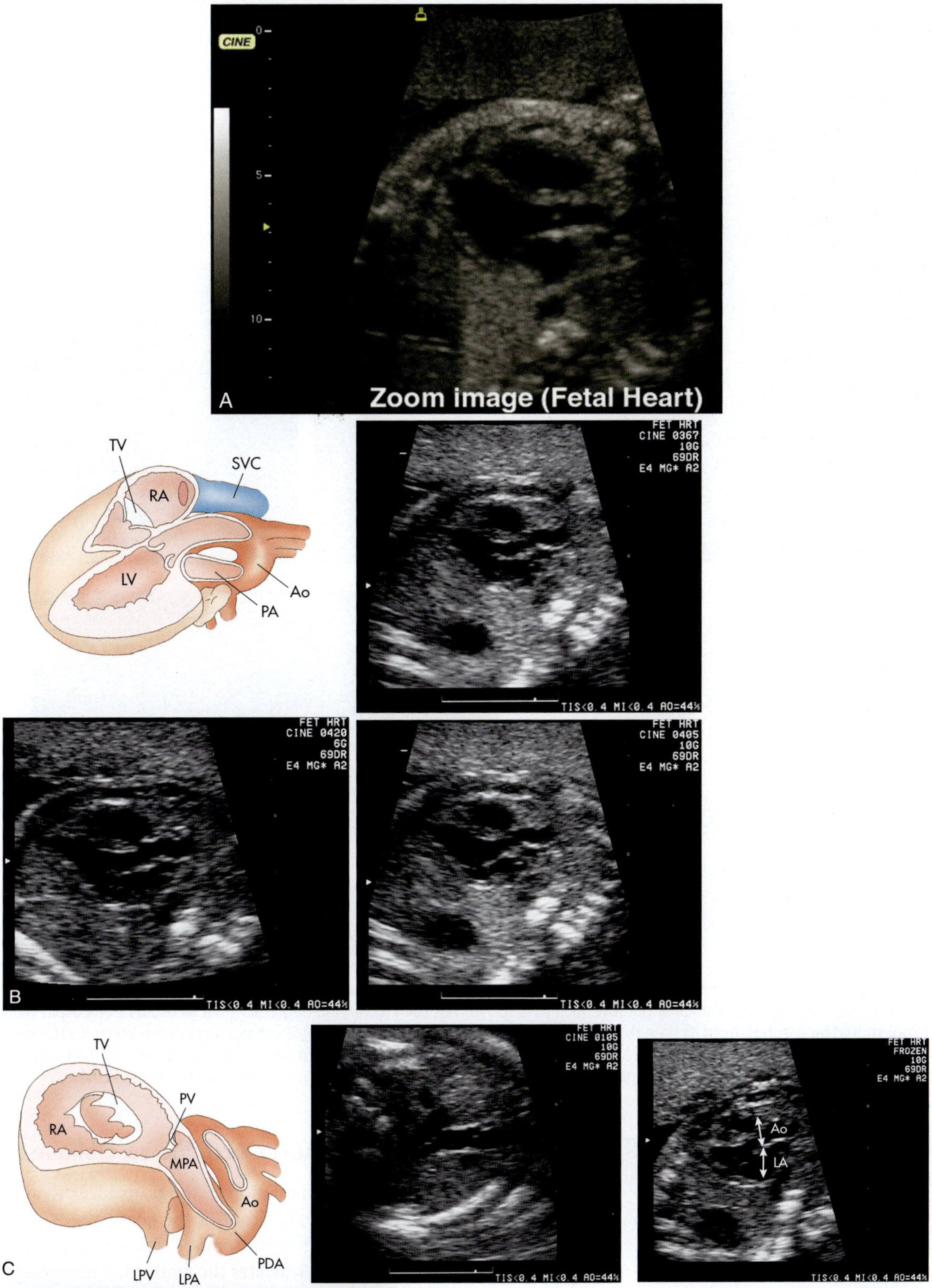

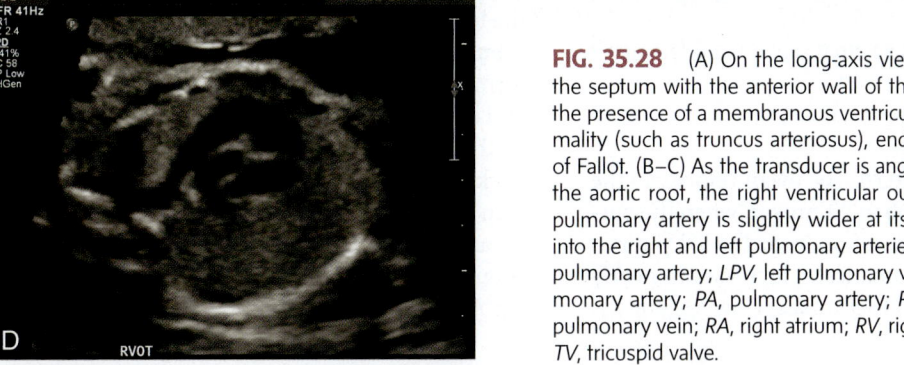

FIG. 35.28 (A) On the long-axis view, the continuity of the right side of the septum with the anterior wall of the aortic root is important to rule out the presence of a membranous ventricular septal defect, conal truncal abnormality (such as truncus arteriosus), endocardial cushion defect, or tetralogy of Fallot. (B–C) As the transducer is angled slightly anterior and medial from the aortic root, the right ventricular outflow tract may be imaged. (D) The pulmonary artery is slightly wider at its origin than the aorta and bifurcates into the right and left pulmonary arteries. *Ao*, Aorta; *LA*, left atrium; *LPA*, left pulmonary artery; *LPV*, left pulmonary vein; *LV*, Left ventricle; *MPA*, main pulmonary artery; *PA*, pulmonary artery; *PDA*, posterior descending artery; *PV*, pulmonary vein; *RA*, right atrium; *RV*, right ventricle; *SVC*, superior vena cava; *TV*, tricuspid valve.

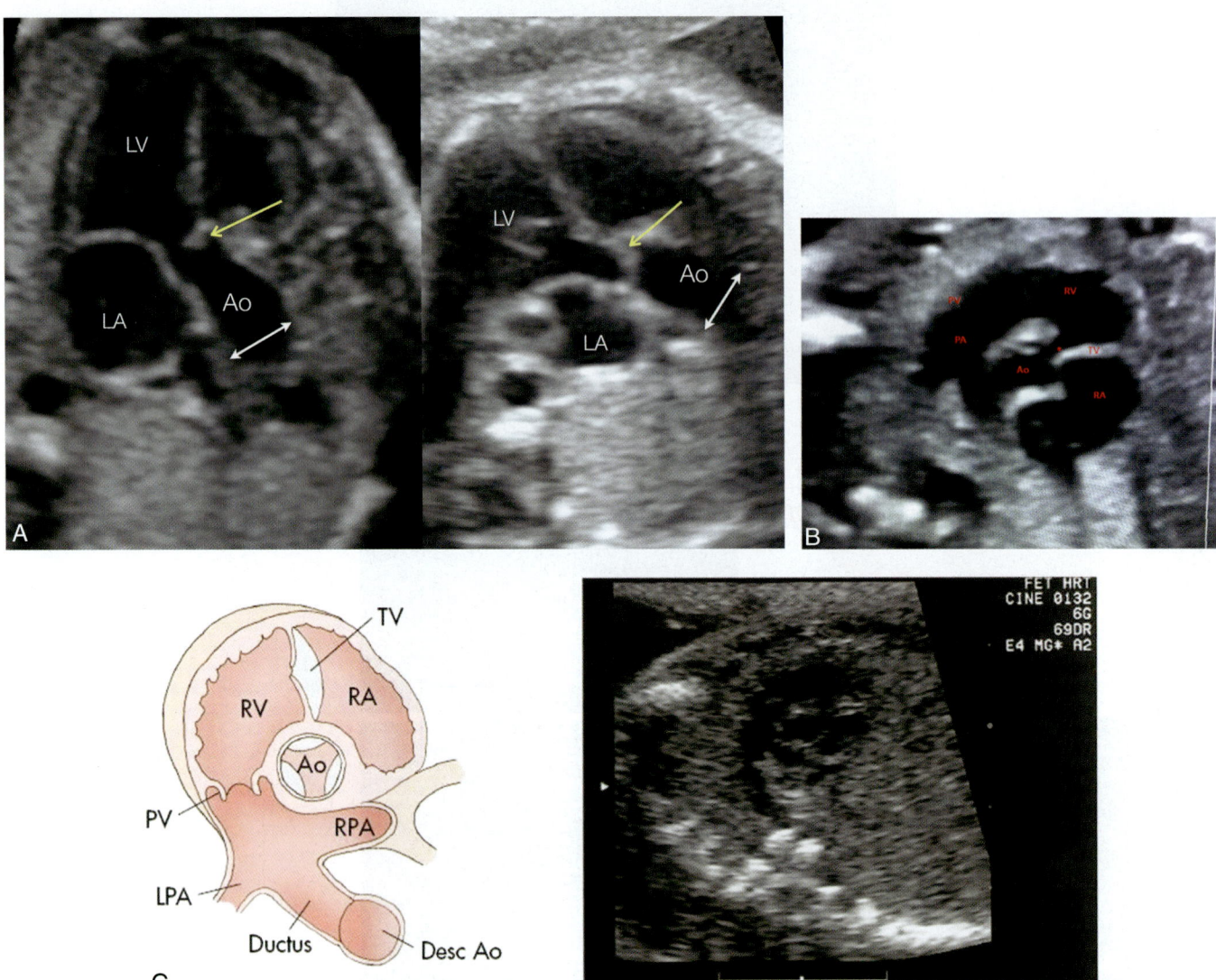

FIG. 35.29 (A) Normally the three cusps open in systole to the full extent of the aortic root and close in a mid-position in diastole. The cusps do not "flop" into the left ventricular outflow tract, as is sometimes seen to varying degrees with a bicuspid or unicuspid valve. The aortic root should be anechoic from its base throughout the arch and descending aorta. (B) Short-axis view of the aorta. (C) The three thin aortic leaflets are best seen in real time. *Ao,* Aorta; *Desc,* descending; *LA,* left atrium; *LPA,* left pulmonary artery; *LV,* Left ventricle; *PA,* pulmonary artery; *PV,* pulmonary vein; *RA,* right atrium; *RPA,* right pulmonary artery; *RV,* right ventricle; *TV,* tricuspid valve.

BOX 35.6	Short-Axis View

Right ventricular outflow tract
Tricuspid valve
Pulmonary cusps
Main pulmonary artery with bifurcation
Right and left pulmonary arteries
Aorta with cusps
Right and Left atrial cavity with interatrial septum and foramen ovale

map any changes in the flow pattern. The mean velocity in the pulmonary artery ranges from 60 to 80 cm/sec; when the cursor reaches the level of ductal insertion, near the left pulmonary branch artery, the flow dramatically increases to nearly double the velocity in the MPA (150 cm/sec) (Fig. 35.30).

Ductal and Aortic Arch Views: Oblique Long Axis

With careful angulation of the transducer to an oblique longitudinal plane, the root of the aorta, the AA, the arch, and the descending aorta may be assessed (Fig. 35.31A). Once the sonographer locates the fetal spine in the sagittal plane, if the spine is down, the probe is angled slightly inward toward the left chest to search for the descending aorta and arch. The tubular dimension of this vessel should be somewhat uniform as one follows the aorta from its base into the thorax and abdomen. As the sonographer carefully sweeps back and forth, the inner core should be anechoic. The three head and neck branch arteries (innominate, carotid, and left subclavian) may be seen to arise from the perfect curve of the aortic arch as they ascend into the fetal head. The sonographer should be able to demonstrate the "candy cane" appearance of the AA, arch, and descending aorta in one image plane.

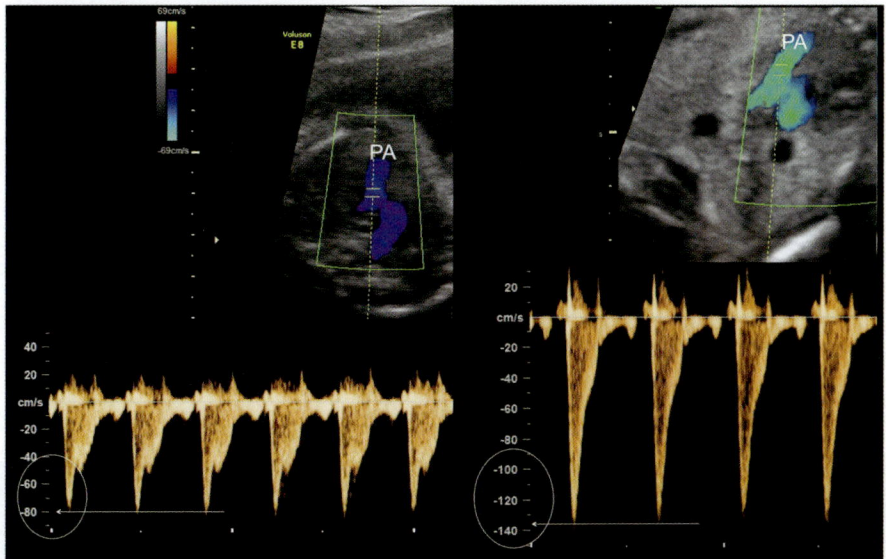

FIG. 35.30 Pulmonic flow patterns are obtained parallel to flow in the high short-axis plane with the Doppler cursor at the level of the pulmonic cusps. The cursor is moved into the main pulmonary artery to map any changes in the flow pattern. The mean velocity in the pulmonary artery ranges from 60 to 80 cm/sec. Note the high-velocity pulmonic flow on the right which could be from pulmonary stenosis. *PA*, Pulmonary artery.

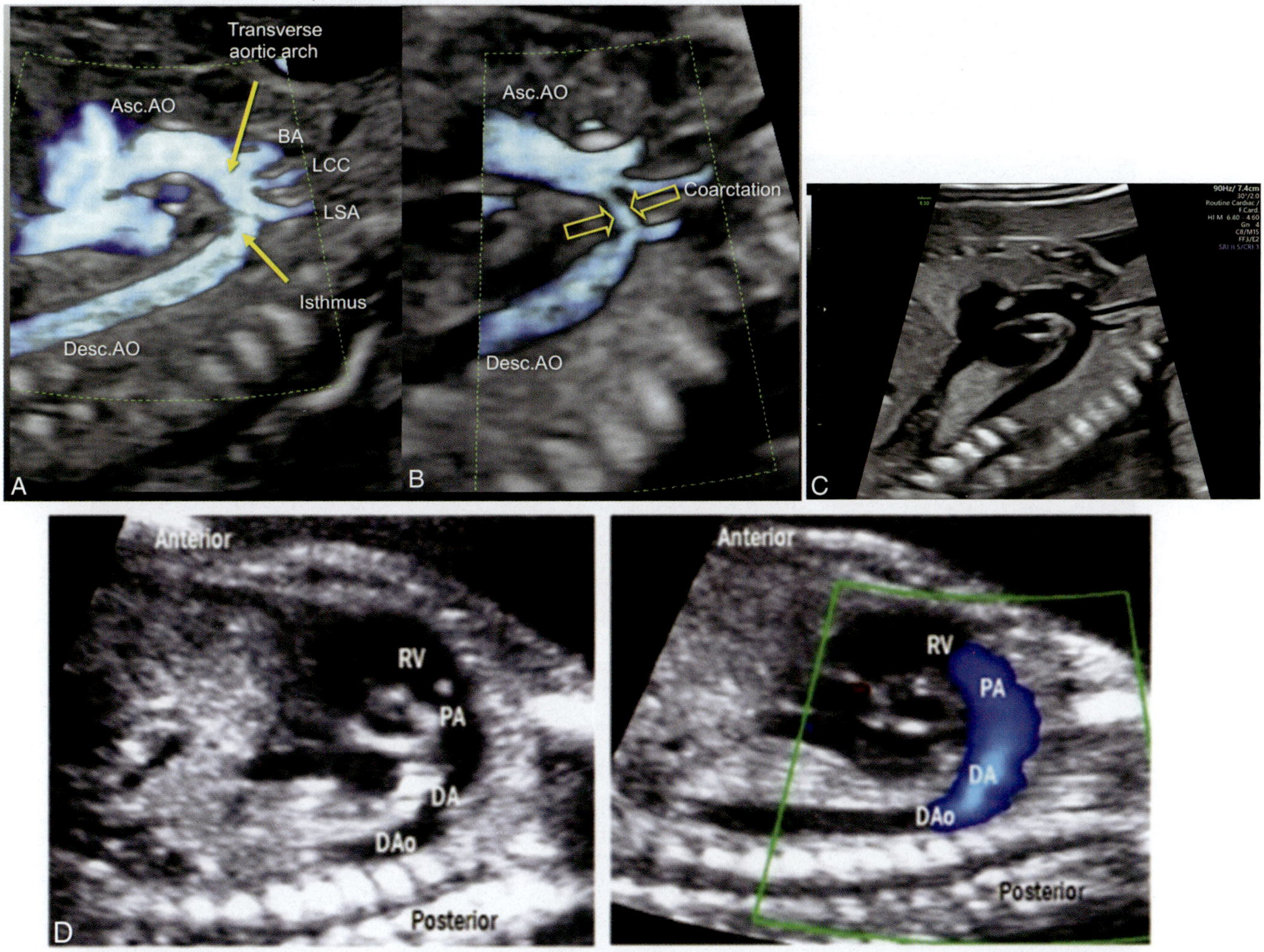

FIG. 35.31 (A–B) Once the sonographer locates the fetal spine in the sagittal plane, if the spine is down, the probe is angled slightly inward toward the left chest to search for the descending aorta and arch. The tubular dimension of this vessel should be somewhat uniform as one follows the aorta from its base into the thorax and abdomen. As the sonographer carefully sweeps back and forth, the inner core should be anechoic. The three head and neck branch arteries (innominate, carotid, and left subclavian) may be seen to arise from the perfect curve of the aortic arch as they ascend into the fetal head. Narrowing of the arch indicates coarctation of the aorta. (C–D) A second arch-type pattern (which appears as large as the aorta) is shown as the transducer is angled inferior from the aortic arch. This represents the patent ductus arteriosus, a communication between the pulmonary artery and the aorta that is patent during fetal life but closes shortly after birth. The ductus is slightly larger than the aortic arch and has a sharper angle ("hockey stick") as it drains into the descending aorta. The ductus does not have arterial structures arising from its wall as the aorta does. *Ao*, Aorta; *Asc*, ascending; *BA*, brachiocephalic artery; *DA*, ductus arteriosus; *DAo*, descending aorta; *LCC*, left common carotid; *LSA*, left subclavian artery; *PA*, pulmonary artery; *RV*, right ventricle.

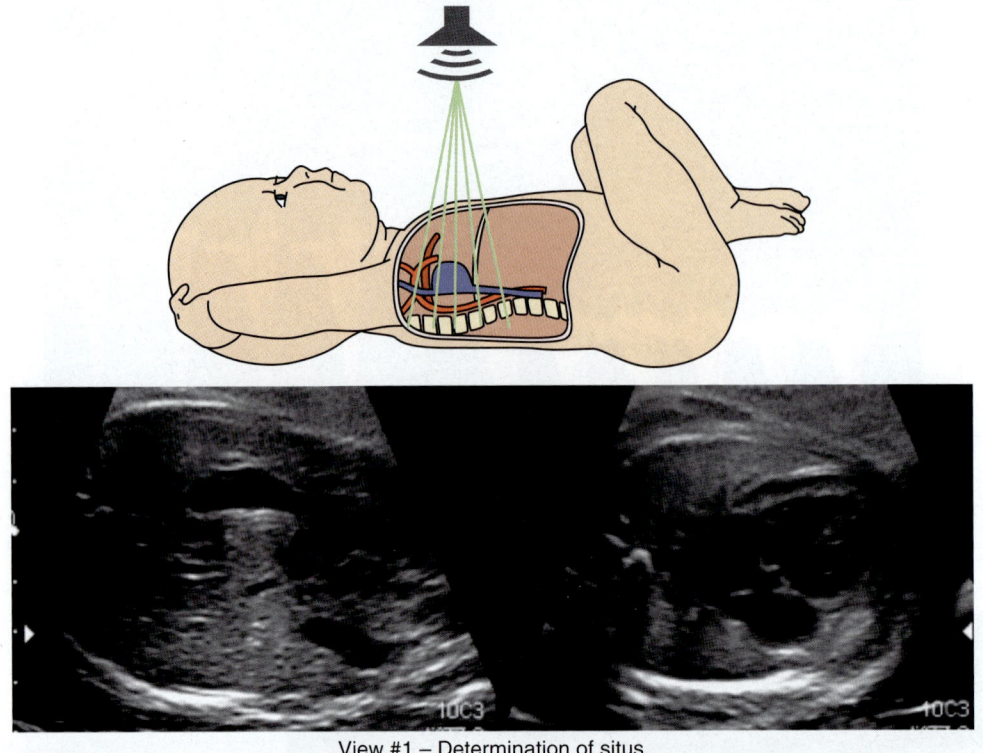
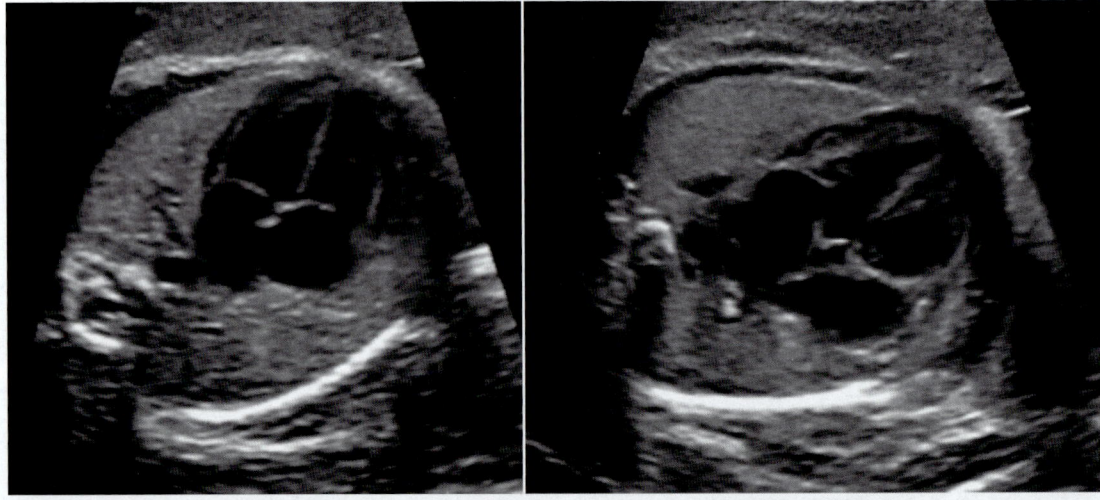
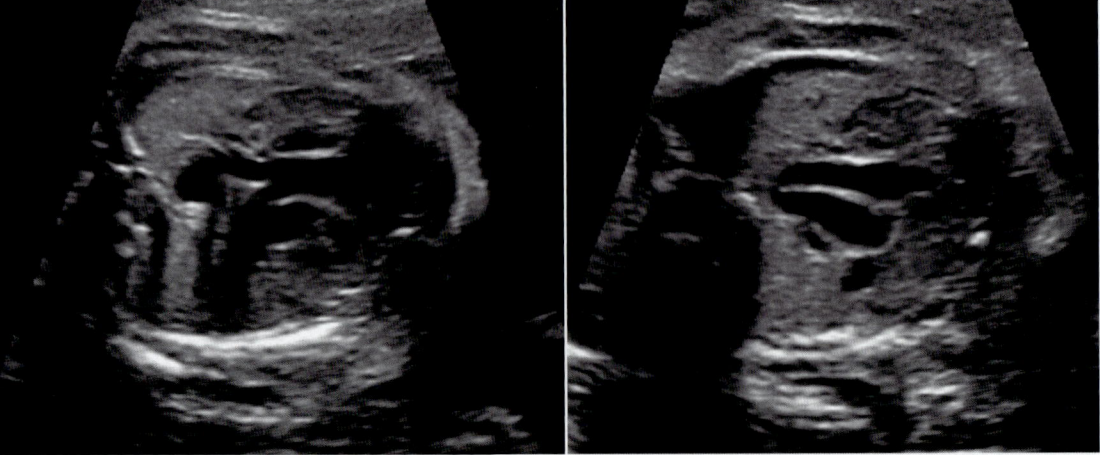

View #1 – Determination of situs

View #2 – Four-chamber view

View #3 – LVOT view

View #4 – RVOT view

View #5 – 3VT view

FIG. 35.32 Evaluation of the fetal heart should include the determination of situs, the four-chamber view, the left ventricular and right ventricle outflow views, and the three-vessel view. The three-vessel view is a transverse image of the fetal upper mediastinum that displays the main pulmonary artery, ascending aorta, and superior vena cava, obtained by angling the transducer cephalad from the four-chamber view.

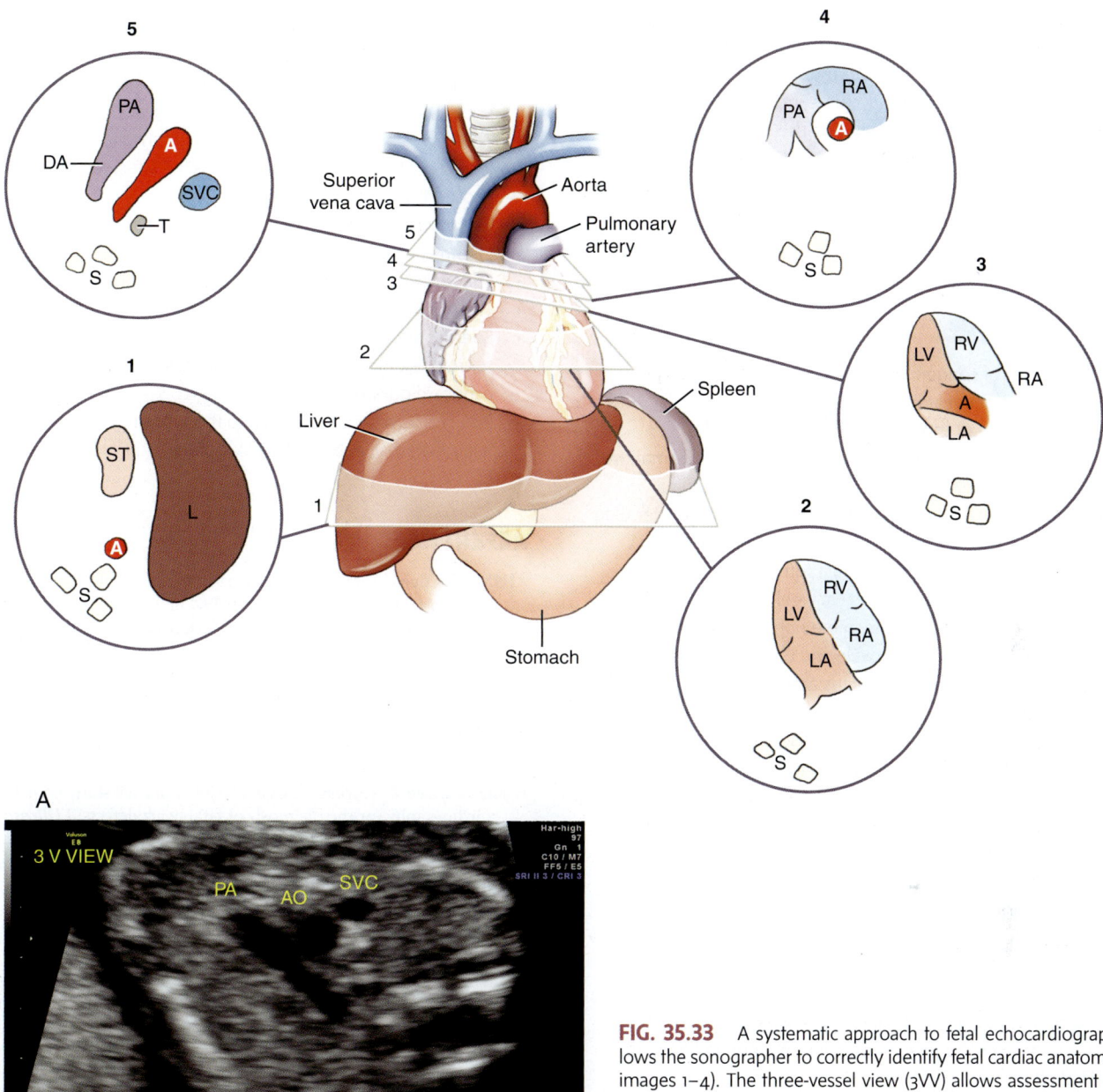

FIG. 35.33 A systematic approach to fetal echocardiography allows the sonographer to correctly identify fetal cardiac anatomy (see images 1–4). The three-vessel view (3VV) allows assessment of the superior vena cava *(yellow)*, ascending aorta (AA, *red*), and main pulmonary artery (MPA, *blue*). Screening fetal sonography showing a 3VV AA/MPA ratio of >1 suggests congenital heart disease and indicates the need for a detailed comprehensive fetal echocardiogram. *Ao*, Aorta; *PA*, pulmonary artery.

A second arch-type pattern (which appears as large as the aorta) is shown as the transducer is angled inferior from the aortic arch. This represents the patent ductus arteriosus, a communication between the pulmonary artery and the aorta that is patent during fetal life but closes shortly after birth. The ductus is slightly larger than the aortic arch and has a sharper angle ("hockey stick") as it drains into the descending aorta (Fig. 35.31D). The ductus does not have arterial structures arising from its wall as the aorta does.

Three-Vessel View

The three-vessel view (3VV) allows assessment of the superior vena cava, AA, and MPA (Fig. 35.32). Screening fetal sonography showing a 3VV AA/MPA ratio of greater than 1 suggests congenital heart disease and indicates the need for a detailed comprehensive fetal echocardiogram. Throughout gestation, the fetal MPA is normally equal to or slightly larger than the fetal AA. The exception occurs in the early second trimester, when the AA may be slightly larger than the

MPA. The size of the AA and MPA are preserved in growth-restricted fetuses. A larger than normal MPA suggests coarctation of the aorta, valvar pulmonary stenosis, an interrupted aortic arch, or hypoplastic left heart syndrome.

The 3VV is a transverse image of the fetal upper mediastinum that displays the MPA, AA, and superior vena cava, obtained by angling the transducer cephalad from the four-chamber view (Fig. 35.33).

Key Pearls

- The incidence of congenital heart disease is about 8%, or 30,000 infants per year in the United States.
- Although fetal heart motion may be seen within the gestational sac as early as 4 to 5 weeks, structural information is seen at 10–16 weeks of gestation with the transvaginal probe, with even more detailed information available after 18 to 22 weeks of gestation.
- The most sensitive period in the first trimester for cardiac development is between 3.5 and 6.5 weeks.
- Communication is open between the right and left sides of the fetal heart through the fossa ovale and between the aorta and the pulmonary artery via the ductus arteriosus.
- Before birth, the oxygenated blood is given to the fetus by way of the umbilical vein from the placenta to the heart.
- The blood enters the right atrium via the superior and inferior vena cava and flows through the three-leaflet tricuspid valve into the right ventricle and leaves the right ventricle through the main pulmonary artery.
- The main pulmonary artery bifurcates into right and left pulmonary artery branches that lead to their respective lungs; most of this blood passes through the connection of the ductus arteriosus into the descending aorta; only a very small amount goes to the lungs.
- The blood mixes with a small amount of deoxygenated blood as it returns from the lungs via the four pulmonary veins into the left atrium.
- The blood then flows from the left atrium into the left ventricle through the bicuspid mitral valve and leaves the heart through the ascending aorta.
- The rest of the mixed blood in the descending aorta passes into the umbilical arteries and is returned to the placenta for reoxygenation.
- After the fetus is born, omission of the placental circulation causes an immediate fall of blood pressure in the newborn's inferior vena cava and right atrium.
- As the lungs expand with air, there is a fall in the pulmonary vascular resistance.
- The pressure in the left atrium becomes higher than that in the right atrium which causes the foramen ovale to close.
- The ductus arteriosus usually constricts shortly after birth (usually within 24 to 48 hours) once the left-sided pressures exceed the right-sided pressures.
- The umbilical arteries also constrict after birth to prevent blood loss from the neonate.
- The umbilical vein may remain patent for some time after birth.
- The normal fetal heart rate is between 120 and 160 beats/min.
- Specific risk factors indicate that the fetus is at a higher than normal risk for congenital heart disease and warrants a fetal echocardiogram.
- Risk factors may be divided into the following three categories: fetal, maternal, and familial risk factors.

REFERENCES

AIUM Practice parameter for the performance of fetal echocardiography. *J of Ultrasound in Med*. 2019;39(1):E5–E16.

Allan LD, Cook AC, Huggon IC. *Fetal Echocardiography: A Practical Guide*. New York: Cambridge University Press; 2009.

Bronshtein M, Siegler E, Eshcoli Z, et al. Transvaginal ultrasound measurements of the fetal heart at 11 to 17 weeks of gestation. *Am J Perinatol*. 1992;9:38.

Callen PC. *Ultrasonography in Obstetrics and Gynecology*. ed 6. Philadelphia: Elsevier; 2016.

Espinoza J, Lee W, Cornstock C, et al. Collaborative study on 4-D echocardiography for the diagnosis of fetal heart defects. *J Ultrasound Med*. 2010;29(11):1573–1580.

Moore KL, Persaud TVN. *The Developing Human: Clinically Oriented Embryology*. ed 11. Philadelphia: Elsevier; 2019.

Rollins RB, Acherman RJ, Castillo WJ, et al. Aorta larger than pulmonary artery in the fetal 3-vessel view. *J Ultrasound Med*. 2009;28(1):9–12.

Rychik J, Ayres N, Cueno B, et al. American Society of Echocardiography guidelines and standards for performance of the fetal echocardiogram. *J Am Soc Echocardiogr*. 2004;17:803–810.

Sklansky M, Tang A, Levy D, et al. Maternal psychological impact of fetal echocardiography. *J Am Soc Echo*. 2002;15:159–166.

Smrcek JM, Berg C, Geipel A, et al. Early fetal echocardiography. *J Ultrasound Med*. 2006;25(2):173–182.

Starikov RS, Bsat FA, Knee AB, et al. Utility of fetal echocardiography after normal cardiac imaging findings on detailed fetal anatomic ultrasonography. *J Ultrasound Med*. 2009;28(5):603–608.

Wilson AD, Rao PS, Aeschlimann S. Normal fetal foramen flap and transatrial Doppler velocity pattern. *J Am Soc Echocardiogr*. 1990;3:491.

Wladimiroff JW. Normal fetal Doppler inferior vena cava, transtricuspid, and umbilical artery flow velocity waveforms between 11 and 16 weeks' gestation. *Am J Obstet Gynecol*. 1992;166:921.

CHAPTER 36

Fetal Echocardiography: Congenital Heart Disease

Joy Guthrie and Sandra L. Hagen-Ansert

OBJECTIVES

On completion of this chapter, you should be able to:
- List the three factors that contribute to congenital heart disease
- Describe why the four-chamber view cannot rule out all forms of congenital heart disease
- Discuss the pathologic conditions covered in this chapter
- Discuss the echocardiographic findings for septal defects, ventricular inflow and outflow tract disturbances, great vessel abnormalities, cardiac tumors, complex cardiac abnormalities, and dysrhythmias

OUTLINE

Relationship of Genetics to Congenital Heart Disease 1032
  Chromosomal Abnormalities 1032
  Familial Risks of Congenital Heart Disease 1033
Incidence of Congenital Heart Disease 1033
Prenatal Evaluation of Congenital Heart Disease 1033
  The Four-Chamber View 1033
Cardiac Malposition 1033
Cardiac Enlargement 1034
  Cardiomyopathy 1034
  Pericardial Effusion 1036
Septal Defects 1036
  Atrial Septal Defect 1036
  Ventricular Septal Defect 1038
  Atrioventricular Septal Defect 1041
Right Ventricular Inflow Disturbance 1043
  Tricuspid Atresia/Stenosis 1043
  Ebstein Anomaly of the Tricuspid Valve 1043

Right Ventricular Outflow Disturbance 1045
  Hypoplastic Right Heart 1045
  Tetralogy of Fallot 1045
  Pulmonic Stenosis 1046
  Subpulmonic Stenosis 1047
  Supravalvular Pulmonic Stenosis 1048
Left Ventricular Inflow Disturbance 1048
  Congenital Mitral Stenosis 1048
  Mitral Regurgitation 1050
Left Ventricular Outflow Tract Disturbance 1050
  Bicuspid Aortic Valve 1050
  Aortic Stenosis 1050
  Hypoplastic Left Heart Syndrome 1052
Great Vessel Abnormalities 1054
  Transposition of the Great Arteries 1054
  Truncus Arteriosus 1054
  Coarctation of the Aorta 1055

Interrupted Aortic Arch 1056
Ductal Constriction 1057
Cardiac Tumors 1058
  Rhabdomyomas 1058
Complex Cardiac Abnormalities 1058
  Single Ventricle 1058
  Cor Triatriatum 1059
  Congenital Vena Cava to Left Atrial Communication 1059
  Total Anomalous Pulmonary Venous Return 1060
  Cardiosplenic Syndromes 1060
  Ectopia Cordis 1062
Dysrhythmias 1062
  Ectopy 1062
  Supraventricular Tachyarrhythmia 1063
  Atrioventricular Block 1064

KEY TERMS

Aortic stenosis
Atrial septal defect
Atrioventricular block
Atrioventricular septal defect (AVSD)
Cardiomyopathy
Coarctation of the aorta
Corrected transposition of the great arteries
Cor triatriatum

Dextrocardia
Dextroposition
Ductal constriction
Ebstein anomaly of the tricuspid valve
Hypoplastic left heart syndrome
Hypoplastic right heart syndrome
Levocardia
Levoposition
Mesocardia

Mitral atresia
Mitral regurgitation
Myocarditis
Partial anomalous pulmonary venous return
Pericardial effusion
Premature atrial contractions (PACs)
Premature ventricular contractions (PVCs)

Pulmonary stenosis
Single ventricle
Subpulmonic stenosis
Supravalvular pulmonic stenosis
Supraventricular tachyarrhythmias
Tetralogy of Fallot
Total anomalous pulmonary venous return (TAPVR)
Transposition of the great arteries
Tricuspid atresia
Truncus arteriosus
Ventricular septal defect

This chapter presents the sonographer's approach to evaluating congenital heart disease with examples of the more common fetal heart abnormalities. As discussed in Chapter 35, the development of the fetal heart is completed by the eighth week of embryonic life. The presence of congenital heart disease is a result of an interrupted or abnormal cardiac development during this time period.

The most common types of congenital heart disease are the ventricular septal defect, atrial septal defects, bicuspid aortic valve, and **pulmonary stenosis**. The development of congenital heart disease is multifaceted. Environmental factors, chromosomal factors, and hereditary factors may influence the development of congenital heart disease in the fetus. Fetal echocardiography can help to establish the presence and severity of the cardiac abnormality. A simple acronym (CHRISTMAS) will assist the sonographer in prenatal detection of congenital heart disease:

C = Concordance and contractility
H = Hydrops
R = Risk factors and rhythm
I = Incorrect size (large or small for gestational age)
S = Symmetry
T = Tetralogy of Fallot, total anomalous pulmonary venous return, transposition, tricuspid atresia, truncus arteriosus
M = Masses and mobility
A = Aneuploidy
S = Situs

RELATIONSHIP OF GENETICS TO CONGENITAL HEART DISEASE

Chromosomal Abnormalities

The frequency of chromosomal abnormalities in infants with congenital heart disease is estimated as 5% to 10% from postnatal data. In a control study of 2100 live-born infants with cardiovascular malformations, chromosomal abnormalities were found in 13%.[1] In this study, Down syndrome occurred in more than 10% of the infants, with the other trisomies each constituting the remaining 3%.

The frequency of abnormal karyotypes in fetuses with cardiac defects has been commonly found at 30% to 40%. Of these fetuses, most have trisomy 21, followed by trisomy 13, trisomy 18, and Turner syndrome. The association of congenital heart defects and chromosomal abnormalities is lower in live-born infants than in fetuses because of the high in utero mortality of the fetus with trisomy 18, trisomy 13, and Turner syndrome (trisomy 45,X).

The occurrence of associated extracardiac abnormalities in fetuses with cardiac defects and chromosomal abnormalities is on the order of 50% to 70%. In the fetus with a single cardiac abnormality, the incidence of chromosomal abnormalities is still increased (15% to 30%). The most common single cardiac abnormality is the ventricular septal defect.

Certain cardiac abnormalities are more likely associated with chromosomal defects. In general, malformations of the right side of the heart are rarely associated with karyotypic abnormalities (e.g., pulmonic stenosis and tricuspid atresia). On the other hand, abnormalities such as atrioventricular septal defect (AVSD), perimembranous ventricular septal defect, tetralogy of Fallot, double-outlet right ventricle, coarctation of the aorta, and hypoplastic left heart are often associated with chromosomal abnormalities.

The incidence of cardiac defects in the fetus with trisomy is increased, with trisomy 21 showing the highest rate at 40% to 50%, Turner syndrome (45,X) showing 25% to 40%, and more than 90% having cardiac defects with trisomies 13 and 18 (see Table 36.1).

TABLE 36.1	Congenital Heart Disease and Chromosomal Abnormality		
Chromosomal Abnormality	Incidence at Live Birth	Associated Cardiac Abnormality	Common Cardiac Abnormalities
Trisomy 21	1:800	40%–50%	Atrioventricular septal defect
			Ventricular septal defect
			Cleft mitral valve
			Heart block
Trisomy 18	1:8,000	>90%	Ventricular septal defect
			Double-outlet right ventricle
Trisomy 13	1:20,000	>80%	Ventricular septal defect
			Atrial septal defect
Turner syndrome (trisomy 45,X)	1:10,000	25%–45%	Coarctation of the aorta
			Bicuspid aortic valve

Familial Risks of Congenital Heart Disease

Most congenital heart defects have more than one cause, with genetic and environmental factors both playing a role. Only about 10% to 15% of all congenital heart defects have been attributed to known chromosomal abnormalities, genetic syndromes, and teratogenic embryopathies.

The recurrence risk for an isolated congenital cardiovascular malformation is modified for each family based on the number of affected relatives and the severity of the abnormality. In general, a recurrence risk of 1% to 5% is estimated for the majority of congenital cardiac abnormalities.

Studies have shown that the contribution of genetic factors increases the risk of congenital heart disease significantly. For example, a mother who has had a child with an abnormality of the left side of the heart (mitral atresia or aortic atresia) has a significantly higher risk (13%) of delivering another child with a form of left-sided heart disease. This risk increases significantly with each pregnancy.

INCIDENCE OF CONGENITAL HEART DISEASE

Congenital heart disease is the most common severe congenital abnormality, with an incidence of 8% in live births. Approximately half of these defects are minor and may be corrected easily with surgery; the other half are responsible for more than 50% of the deaths from congenital abnormalities in childhood. Cardiac defects may account for as much as 4% of congenital heart disease in live births. Common cardiac defects include the bicuspid aortic valve, patent ductus arteriosus (common in premature infants), and ventricular septal defects. The incidence of the bicuspid aortic valve defect is 10 in 10,000 births; it may lead to aortic stenosis in adulthood.

PRENATAL EVALUATION OF CONGENITAL HEART DISEASE

The Four-Chamber View

All sonographers should be familiar with the routine four-chamber view that is part of the normal obstetric examination. This view is easily obtainable after 16 weeks of gestation, although the anatomy becomes more distinctly imaged with ultrasound between 18 and 22 weeks of gestation. The four-chamber view is normal when the following conditions are seen:

1. The fetal situs is normal. (The heart is in the left side of the chest and its apex points to the left, the stomach is to the left, the aorta is anterior and to the left of the spine, and the inferior vena cava is anterior and to the right of the spine; Fig. 36.1A).
2. The size of the heart in relation to the chest is normal (ratio of heart to thorax = 1:3) (see Fig. 36.1B).
3. The two atria are equal in size, and the flap of the foramen ovale is seen to move toward the left atrium. (The atria should constitute about one-third of the size of the heart; Fig. 36.1C).
4. The two ventricles are equal in size and contractility. (The ventricles should constitute about two-thirds of the size of the heart; Fig. 36.1D).
5. The interatrial and interventricular septa are completely formed and normal in thickness (see Fig. 36.1E).
6. The atrioventricular valves are normal in thickness, position, and opening (see Fig. 36.1F).

Several cardiac abnormalities may be recognized with the four-chamber view alone, such as a large ventricular septal defect, AVSD, hypoplastic left or right heart, mitral or tricuspid atresia, Ebstein anomaly, and total anomalous pulmonary venous return (TAPVR; discussed later in this chapter). However, many cardiac abnormalities may be missed with only the four-chamber view. Abnormalities of the cardiac structure (especially the great vessels) that are not located in the four-chamber plane may show a normal four-chamber view, but the specific abnormality will be missed if a complete fetal echocardiogram with multiple sweep cine loop images is not conducted (e.g., transposition of the great arteries, truncus arteriosus, coarctation of the aorta, small outlet ventricular septal defect, and tetralogy of Fallot). Chapter 35 covers the normal fetal echocardiographic examination.

CARDIAC MALPOSITION

When the heart is out of its normal position, several terms may be used to describe the exact position of the heart relative to location and position of the cardiac apex (Figs. 36.2 and 36.3). **Dextrocardia** means the heart is in the right side of the chest, with the apex pointed to the right of the thorax (Fig. 36.4A). Dextrocardia can be associated with a normal visceral situs, situs inversus, or situs ambiguous. **Dextroposition** of the heart refers to a condition in which the heart is located in the right side of the chest, and the cardiac apex points medially or to the left. This condition is usually found when extrinsic factors, such as a space-occupying large diaphragmatic hernia or hypoplasia of the right lung, are present (Fig. 36.4B–C).

Levocardia is the term used to denote the normal position of the heart in the left side of the chest (with the cardiac apex pointed to the left) and is often used when visceral situs abnormalities are present. Levocardia can be associated with normal situs, situs inversus (abdominal organs are located on the opposite side of normal), or situs ambiguous. **Levoposition** of the heart refers to the condition in which the heart is displaced further toward the left side of the chest, usually in association with a space-occupying lesion.

Mesocardia indicates an atypical location of the heart, with the cardiac apex pointing toward the midline of the chest. Usually, the heart is located more toward the midline. This may be found with the presence of an extracardiac mass or lung abnormalities (Fig. 36.4D).

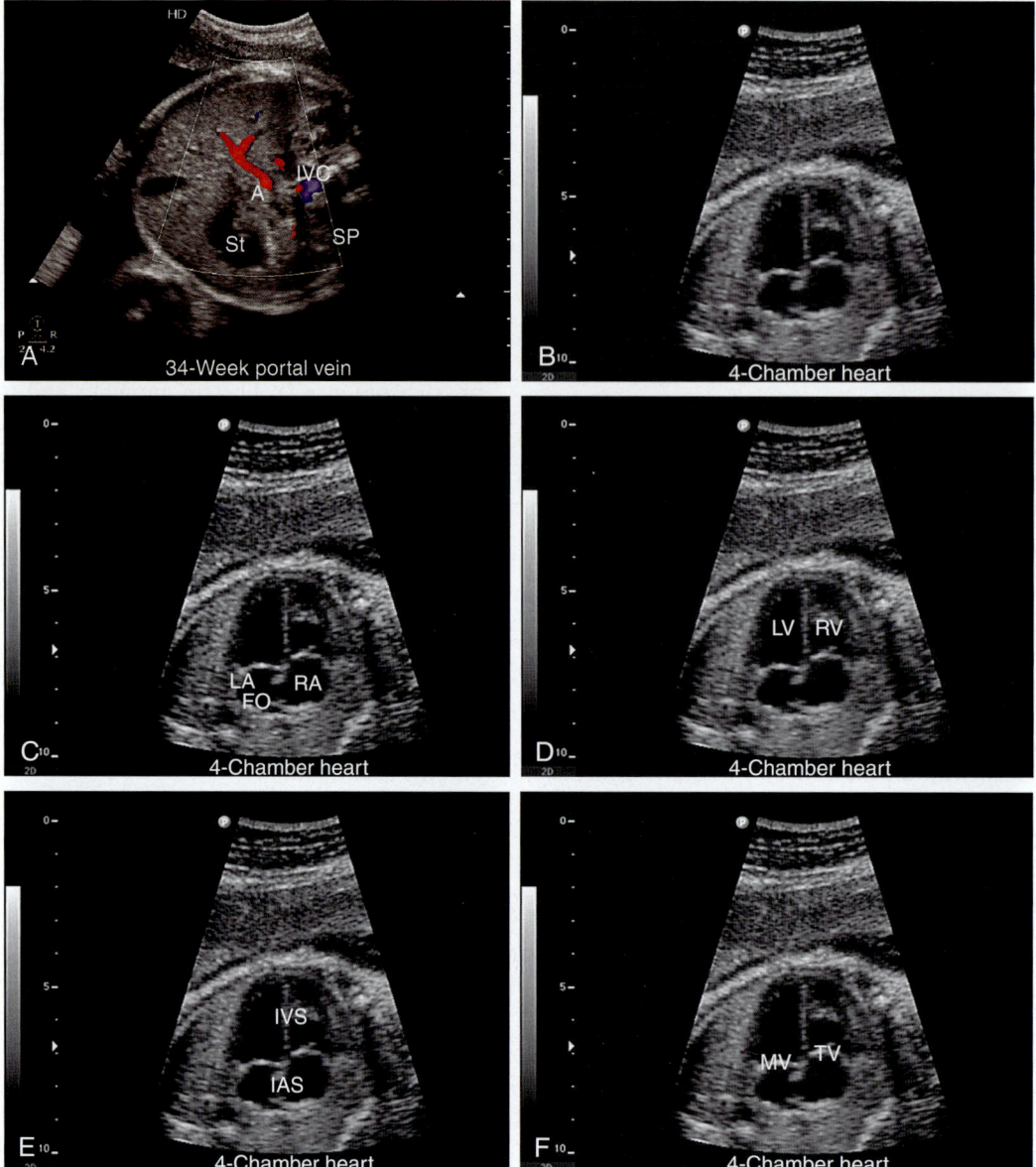

FIG. 36.1 (A) The fetal situs is normal. (Heart position is in the left chest and the apex of heart points to the left; stomach is to the left; aorta is anterior and to the left of the spine; and inferior vena cava is anterior and to the right of the spine.) (B) The size of the heart in relation to the chest is normal. (Ratio of heart to thorax = 1:3.) (C) The two atria are equal in size, and the flap of the foramen ovale is seen to move toward the left atrium. (The atrium should comprise about one-third the size of the heart.) (D) The two ventricles are equal in size and contractility. (The ventricles should comprise about two-thirds the size of the heart.) (E) The interatrial and interventricular septa are completely formed and normal in thickness. (F) The atrioventricular valves are normal in thickness, position, and opening. *A,* Aorta; *FO,* foramen ovale; *IAS,* interatrial septum; *IVC,* inferior vena cava; *IVS,* interventricular septum; *LA,* left atrium; *LV,* left ventricle; *MV,* mitral valve; *RA,* right atrium; *RV,* right ventricle; *St,* stomach; *TV,* tricuspid valve.

CARDIAC ENLARGEMENT

Cardiomyopathy

Cardiomyopathy is a condition of the myocardial tissue in the heart. This disease process may be caused by exposure to a virus (Coxsackie or mumps) or to bacteria, which leads to an infection that causes cardiomyopathy. Errors of metabolism may also cause cardiomyopathy. Endocardial fibroelastosis has also been associated with cardiomyopathies and hypoplastic left heart syndrome. Asymmetric septal hypertrophy (as seen in patients with hereditary idiopathic subaortic stenosis) and concentric hypertrophy (as seen in some uncontrolled diabetic mothers) have been reported.

Myocarditis is characterized by necrosis and destruction of myocardial cells and an inflammatory infiltrate. In a viral cardiomyopathy, all four chambers are dilated, with thinning of the myocardial walls. Gross valvular regurgitation may be present, resulting from the stretched mitral and tricuspid annulus

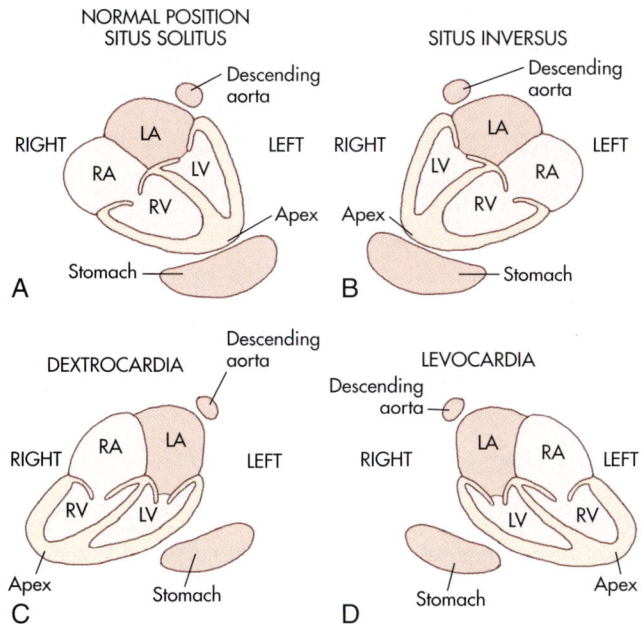

FIG. 36.2 The anatomic relationship of the descending aorta, left atrium, apex, and stomach in the four cardiac positions. (A) Normal position, situs solitus. (B) Situs inversus. (C) Dextrocardia. (D) Levocardia. *LA*, Left atrium; *LV*, left ventricle; *RA*, right atrium; *RV*, right ventricle.

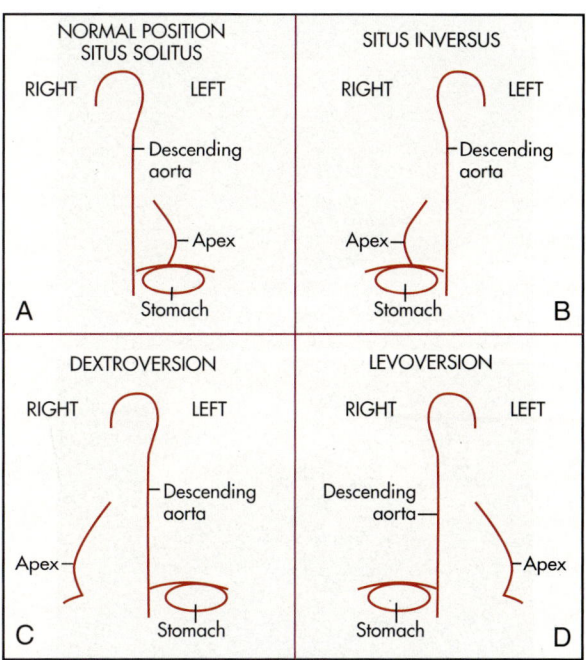

FIG. 36.3 The alignment of the descending aorta, apex, and stomach in the four basic cardiac positions from the frontal projection. (A) In situs solitus, the descending aorta, apex, and stomach are all on the left. (B) In situs inversus, the descending aorta, apex, and stomach are all on the right. (C) In dextroversion, the descending aorta and stomach are on the left, but the apex is on the right. (D) In levoversion, the descending aorta and stomach are on the right, but the apex is on the left.

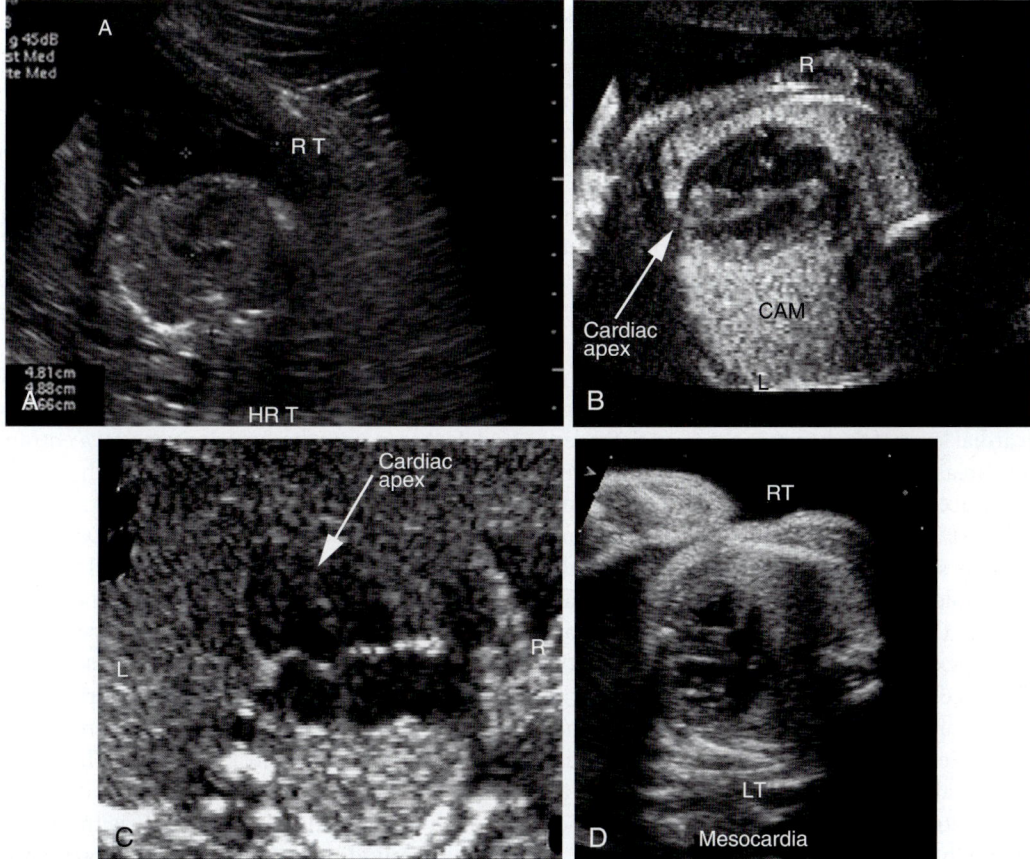

FIG. 36.4 Abnormal cardiac axis and position. (A) True dextrocardia. (B) Dextroposition secondary to a large left-sided cystic adenomatous malformation (CAM) that pushes the heart into the right chest. (C) Dextroposition caused by the presence of right lung hypoplasia. The heart shifts into the space lacking lung tissue but maintains a near-normal axis. (D) Mesocardia. *HRT*, Heart; *LT*, left; *RT*, right.

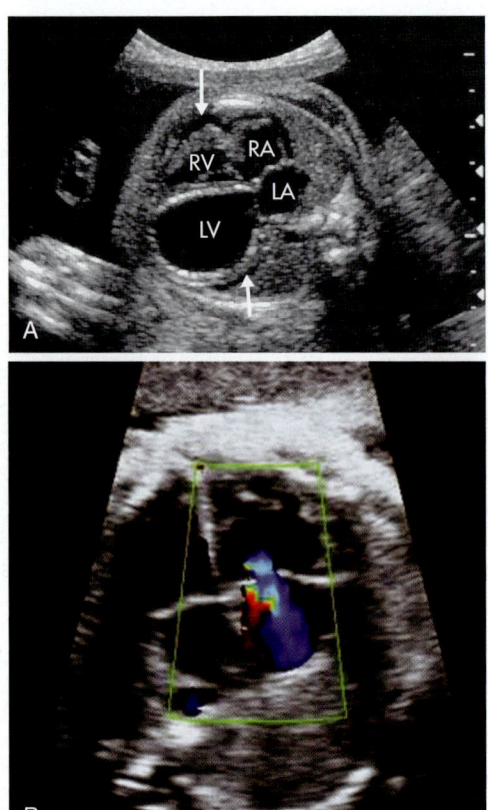

FIG. 36.5 (A) Four-chamber view of the heart shows dilation of all four chambers. (B) Regurgitation was present in the mitral and tricuspid valves. Pericardial effusion. *LA*, Left atrium; *LV*, left ventricle; *RA*, right atrium; *RV*, right ventricle.

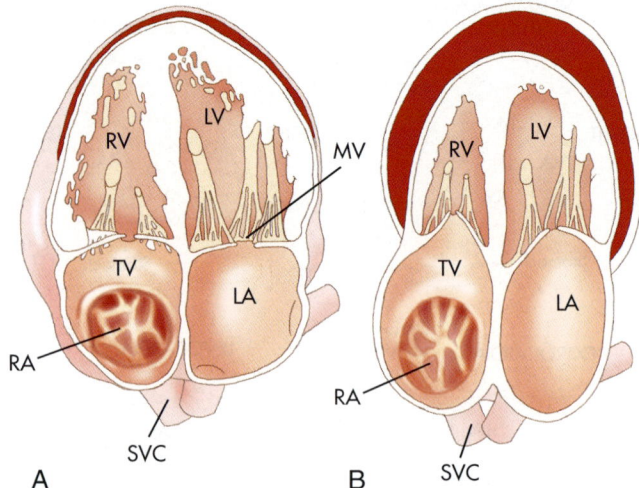

FIG. 36.6 (A) Apical view of a small pericardial effusion. (B) Apical view of a large pericardial effusion involving the right ventricle, apex, and left ventricle. *LA*, Left atrium; *LV*, left ventricle; *MV*, mitral valve; *RA* right atrium; *RV*, right ventricle; *SVC*, superior vena cava; *TV*, tricuspid valve.

(Fig. 36.5). Cardiac function is decreased severely, leading to congestive heart failure with pericardial effusion, bradycardia, and death. The general prognosis for a fetus with evidence for a cardiomyopathy is poor. Serial fetal echoes are performed to monitor chamber size, regurgitation, and contractility.

Pericardial Effusion

Pericardial effusion is an abnormal collection of fluid surrounding the epicardial layer of the heart. In the four-chamber view, a hypoechoic area in the peripheral part of the epicardial/pericardial interface of 2 mm or less is considered within normal limits and does not represent a pericardial effusion. The separation must be seen on the M-mode to separate both in systole and in diastole and be greater than 2 mm. A separation that surrounds the heart (from the atrioventricular junction around the apex of the heart) may be associated with hydrops fetalis (Fig. 36.6).

With a small pericardial effusion, the separation of the pericardium from the epicardium may localize toward the posterolateral and apical walls of the heart. The larger effusion will extend to the atrioventricular groove posteriorly and around the anterior right ventricular wall.

Pericardial effusion may be seen secondary to indomethacin therapy with premature closure of the patent ductus arteriosus.

Pericardial effusion has also been associated with coxsackievirus, cytomegalovirus, parvovirus, human immunodeficiency virus, intrauterine growth restriction, and aneuploidy.

SEPTAL DEFECTS

Atrial Septal Defect

An **atrial septal defect** allows communication between the left atrium and right atrium. The locations of three common atrial septal defects are shown in Fig. 36.7. There are three common forms of atrial septal defects: ostium secundum, ostium primum, and sinus venosus. The ostium secundum defect is the defect in the central atrial septum near the foramen ovale and is the most difficult to see in utero, as the flap of the foramen ovale is mobile at this period of development. The ostium primum defect is usually associated with the chromosomal abnormality of trisomy 21 and often will have a cleft mitral valve and abnormalities of the atrioventricular septum. The least common septal defect is the sinus venosus defect seen near the superior vena cava entrance into the right atrium. This may be associated with a **partial anomalous pulmonary venous return**.

The atrial septal defect is not always recognized during fetal life unless part of the intra-atrial septum is missing. The foramen ovale remains open in the fetal heart until after birth, and the pressures change between the right and left sides of the heart to force the foramen to close completely. Failure of the foramen to close may result in atrial septal defect, secundum type. An atrial septal defect provides communication between the right and left atrium. The defect must be quite large in the fetus to be identified by ultrasound.

The area of the foramen ovale is thinner in the fetus than the surrounding atrial tissue; therefore, with echocardiography, the area is prone to signal dropout, particularly in the apical four-chamber view when the transducer is parallel

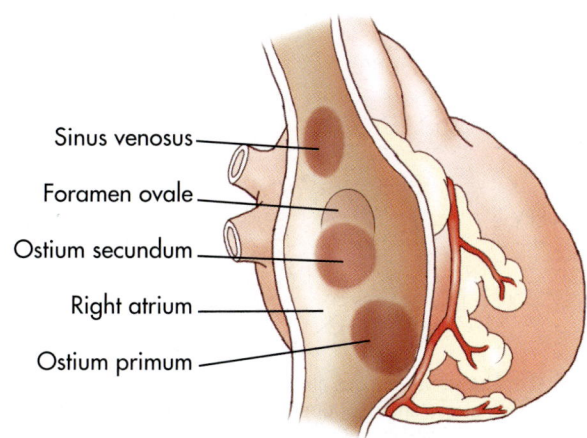

FIG. 36.7 Atrial septal defects: ostium secundum, ostium primum, and sinus venosus defects viewed from the right atrium.

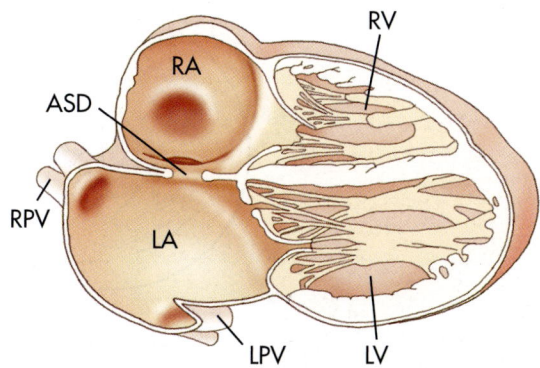

FIG. 36.8 Four-chamber view of the heart illustrating the absence of the flap of the foramen ovale. *ASD*, Atrial septal defect; *LA*, left atrium; *LPV*, left pulmonary vein; *LV*, left ventricle; *RA*, right atrium; *RPV*, right pulmonary vein; *RV*, right ventricle.

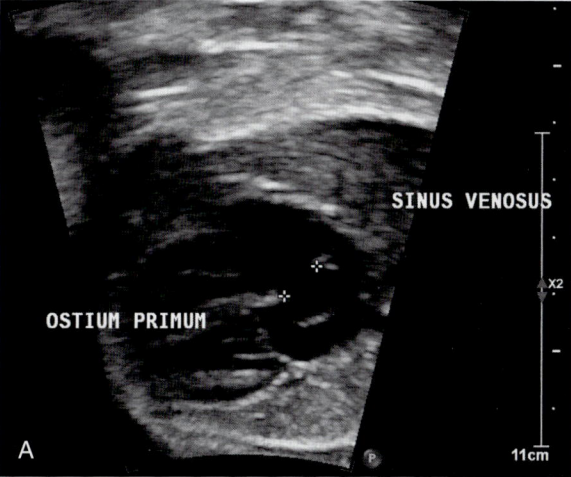

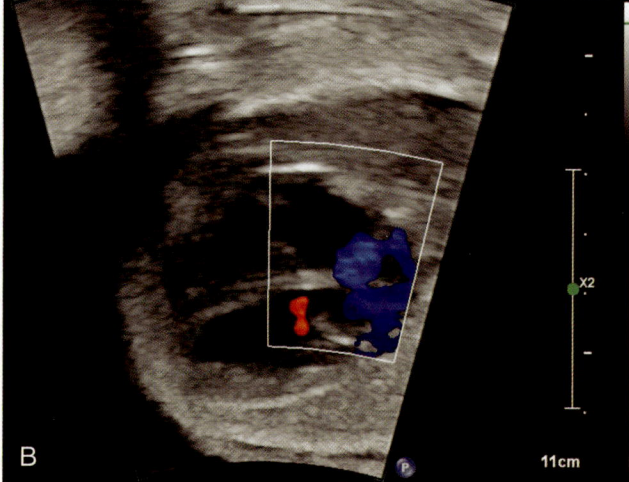

FIG. 36.9 (A) The most common type of atrial septal defects occurs in the area of the fossa ovalis, known as the secundum defect. (B) In the fetus, normal flow should occur at the level of the foramen ovale.

to the septum. Any break in the atrial septum in this view must be confirmed by the short-axis, or subcostal, view (the transducer is inferior to the heart and angled cephalad in a transverse or short-axis plane), in which the septum is more perpendicular to the transducer. Because of beam-width artifacts, the edges of the defect may be slightly blunted and appear brighter than the remaining septum.

In utero, the natural flow in the atrium is right to left across the foramen (as the pressures are slightly higher on the right). A small reversal flow may be present. The foramen should flap into the left atrial cavity. The flap should not be so large as to touch the lateral wall of the atrium; when this redundancy of the foramen occurs, the sinoatrial node may become agitated in the right atrium and cause fetal arrhythmias. The sonographer should be sure to sweep inferior to superior along the atrial septum to identify the three parts of the septum: the primum septum, fossa ovalis, and septum secundum.

Ostium Secundum Atrial Septal Defect. The most common atrial defect is the secundum atrial septal defect, which occurs in the area of the fossa ovalis (Fig. 36.8). Usually, an absence of the foramen ovale flap is noted, with the fossa ovalis opening larger than normal.

Sonographic Findings. Doppler tracings of the septal defect with the sample volume placed at the site of the defect show a right-to-left flow with a velocity of 20 to 30 cm/sec. Color flow Doppler is performed in the apical four-chamber and subcostal views and may be useful to outline the size and direction of flow as it crosses the foramen ovale (Fig. 36.9). The flow patterns of the mitral and tricuspid valves are slightly increased with the elevated shunt flow.

Ostium Primum Septal Defect. The primum septal defect is deficient in the lower (inferior) portion of the septum, near the crux of the heart (Fig. 36.10). It may be seen in AVSD malformation in which there is malalignment of the atrioventricular valves secondary to the defect. In addition, a cleft of the mitral valve is present, causing mitral regurgitation into the left atrial cavity.

Sonographic Findings. The primum septal defect is best imaged in the four-chamber plane that is parallel to the transducer beam. The gain should be reduced to clearly identify the atrial septum. Look for the flap of the foramen ovale. This defect may be part of an AVSD or a primary defect with or without a cleft mitral valve.

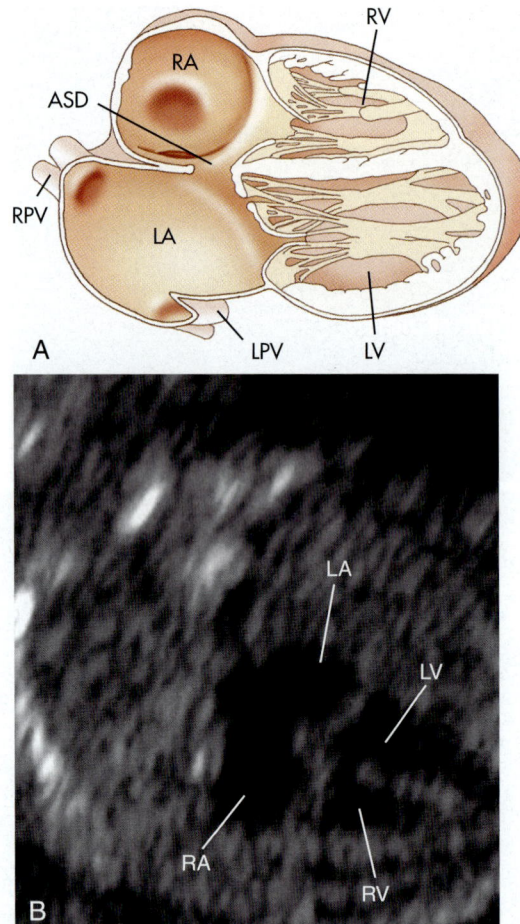

FIG. 36.10 (A) The ostium primum atrial septal defect in the four-chamber view. (B) Atrioventricular defect with a primum and membranous septal defect. *ASD*, Atrial septal defect; *LA*, left atrium; *LPV*, left pulmonary vein; *LV*, left ventricle; *RA*, right atrium; *RPV*, right pulmonary vein; *RV*, right ventricle.

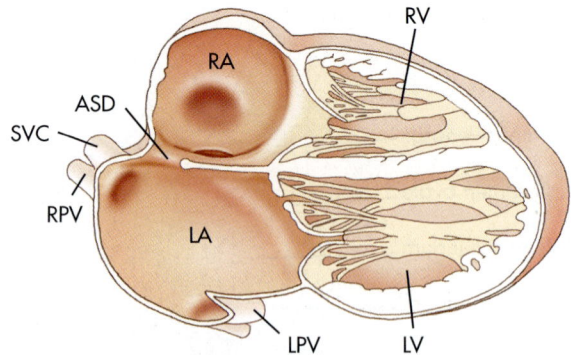

FIG. 36.11 The sinus venosus atrial septal defect near the entrance of the superior vena cava and right upper pulmonary vein (RPV). *ASD*, Atrial septal defect; *LA*, left atrium; *LPV*, left pulmonary vein; *LV*, left ventricle; *RA*, right atrium; *RPV*, right pulmonary vein; *RV*, right ventricle; *SVC*, superior vena cava.

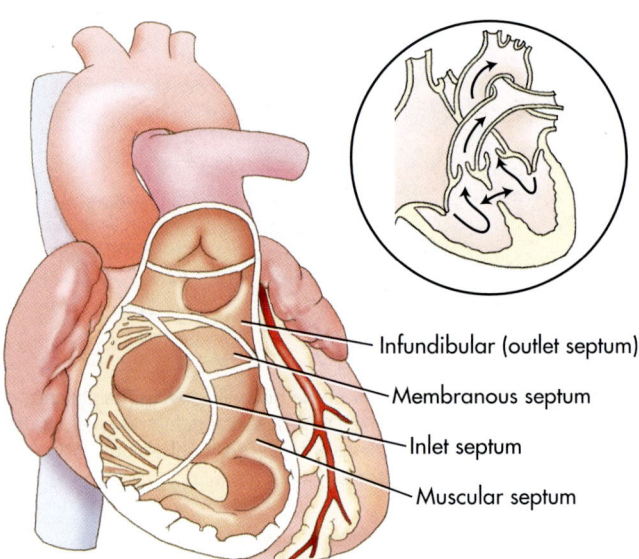

FIG. 36.12 Ventricular septal defect. Portions of the ventricular septum showing the infundibular (outlet septum), membranous septum, inlet septum, and muscular septa.

Sinus Venosus Septal Defect. The sinus venosus atrial septal defect is technically more difficult to visualize with echocardiography. This defect lies in the superior portion of the atrial septum, close to the inflow pattern of the superior vena cava (Fig. 36.11).

Sonographic Findings. Sinus venosus septal defects are best visualized with the subxiphoid four-chamber view. If signs of right ventricular volume overload are present, with no atrial septal defect obvious, care should be taken to study the septum in search of a sinus venosus type of defect. Partial anomalous pulmonary venous drainage of the right pulmonary vein is usually associated with this type of defect; thus it is important to identify the entry site of the pulmonary veins into the left atrial cavity. Color flow mapping is useful in this type of problem because it allows the sonographer to visualize the venous return to the left atrium and a flow pattern crossing into the right atrial cavity.

Ventricular Septal Defect

Ventricular septal defect is the most common congenital lesion of the heart, accounting for 30% of all structural heart defects. The septum is divided into two basic segments: the membranous and muscular areas (Fig. 36.12). The septum lies in a curvilinear plane and has different areas of thickness. There are several sites where ventricular septal defects may occur within the septum. Muscular defects occur more inferior in the septum, usually are very small, and may be multiple (Fig. 36.13). Often, smaller defects will close spontaneously shortly after birth. This type of muscular defect is more difficult to image with echocardiography.

Membranous Septal Defect. The (perimembranous) ventricular septal defect may be classified as membranous, aneurysmal, or supracristal (Fig. 36.14). The significant anatomic landmark is the crista supraventricularis ridge. The defect lies either above or below this ridge. Defects that lie above are called *supracristal*. Supracristal defects are located just beneath the pulmonary orifice so that the pulmonary valve forms part of the superior margin of the interventricular

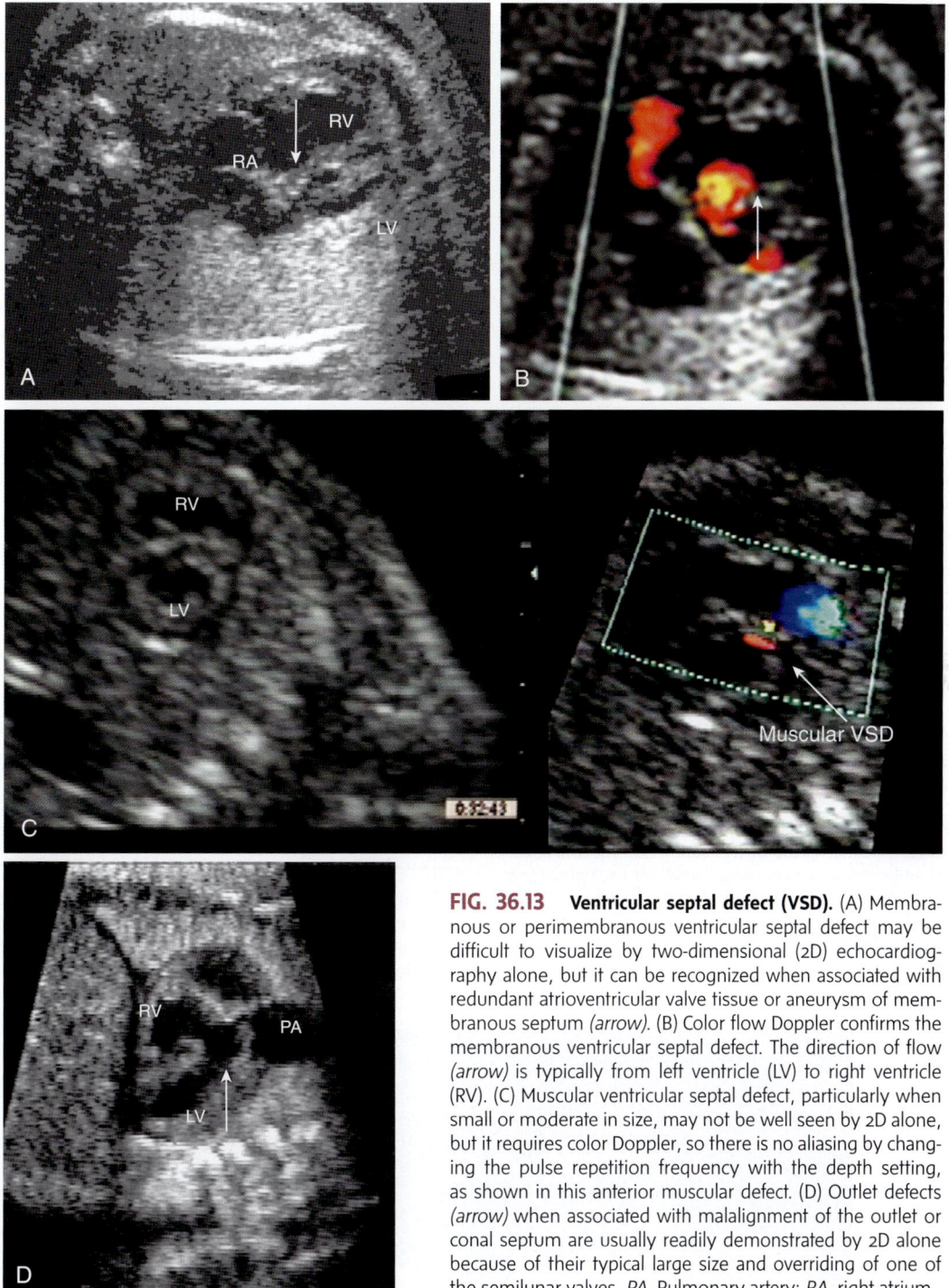

FIG. 36.13 Ventricular septal defect (VSD). (A) Membranous or perimembranous ventricular septal defect may be difficult to visualize by two-dimensional (2D) echocardiography alone, but it can be recognized when associated with redundant atrioventricular valve tissue or aneurysm of membranous septum *(arrow)*. (B) Color flow Doppler confirms the membranous ventricular septal defect. The direction of flow *(arrow)* is typically from left ventricle (LV) to right ventricle (RV). (C) Muscular ventricular septal defect, particularly when small or moderate in size, may not be well seen by 2D alone, but it requires color Doppler, so there is no aliasing by changing the pulse repetition frequency with the depth setting, as shown in this anterior muscular defect. (D) Outlet defects *(arrow)* when associated with malalignment of the outlet or conal septum are usually readily demonstrated by 2D alone because of their typical large size and overriding of one of the semilunar valves. *PA,* Pulmonary artery; *RA,* right atrium.

communication. Defects that lie below the crista are called *infracristal* and may be found in the membranous or muscular part of the septum. Infracristal defects are the most common.

Sonographic Findings. The lesion may be partially covered by the tricuspid septal leaflet, and the sonographer must carefully evaluate this area with Doppler and color flow tracings. The membranous defect is found just below the aortic leaflets; sometimes, the aortic leaflet is sucked into this defect (Fig. 36.15).

The presence of an isolated ventricular septal defect in utero usually does not change the hemodynamics of the fetus. Defects smaller than 2 mm are not detected by fetal echocardiography as these are beyond the limits of resolution. Care must be taken in the four-chamber view to carefully sweep the probe posterior to record the inlet part of the septum to anterior to record the outlet part of the septum.

Ventricular septal defects may close with the formation of aneurysm tissue, which is commonly found along the right side of the septal defect (Fig. 36.16). These aneurysms generally protrude into the right heart in one of the following three directions: (1) above the tricuspid valve and into the right atrium, (2) directly into the septal leaflet of the tricuspid valve, or (3) below the tricuspid leaflets and into the right ventricular cavity. Usually, these aneurysms are small, but obstruction may occur in the right ventricular outflow tract when they become large.

Muscular Defect. A less common infracristal defect is located in the muscular septum. These defects may be large or small, or they may be multiple fenestrated holes. The multiple defects are more difficult to repair, and their combination may have the same ventricular overload effect as a single large communication. Small muscular defects are usually found in the neonatal stage and often close spontaneously.

The prognosis is good for a patient with a single ventricular septal defect. However, the association with other cardiac anomalies, such as tetralogy of Fallot, single ventricle, transposition of the great arteries, and endocardial cushion defect, is increased when a ventricular septal defect is found.

Silverman and Schmidt[2] reported that 40% of ventricular septal defects are closed within 2 years of life and that 60% close by 5 years. The incidence of closure for membranous defects is 25% by 5 years and 65% for muscular defects by 5 years.

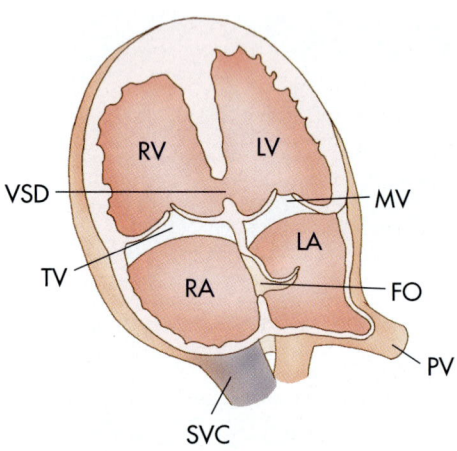

FIG. 36.14 The membranous septal defect is shown in this four-chamber view. This is located in the inflow of the ventricles. The muscular defect in this four-chamber view may be large, small, or multiple along the thicker part of the septum. *FO*, Foramen ovale; *LA*, left atrium; *LV*, left ventricle; *MV*, mitral valve; *PV*, pulmonary vein; *RA*, right atrium; *RV*, right ventricle; *SVC*, superior vena cava; *TV*, tricuspid valve; *VSD*, ventricular septal defect.

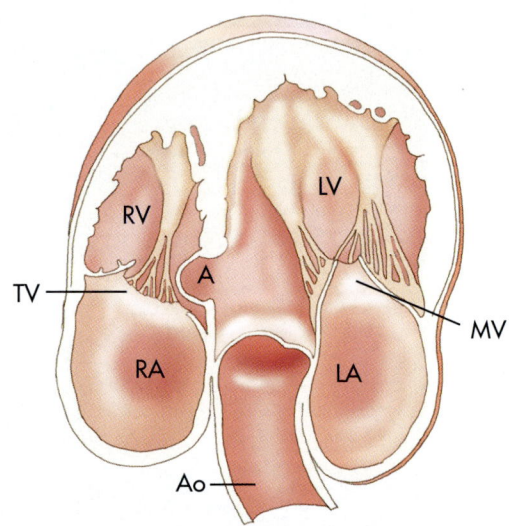

FIG. 36.16 Five-chamber view of the heart illustrating the presence of a ventricular septal aneurysm inferior to the aortic cusps near the septal leaflet of the tricuspid valve. *A*, Atrium; *Ao*, aorta; *LA*, left atrium; *LV*, left ventricle; *MV*, mitral valve; *RA*, right atrium; *RV*, right ventricle; *TV*, tricuspid valve.

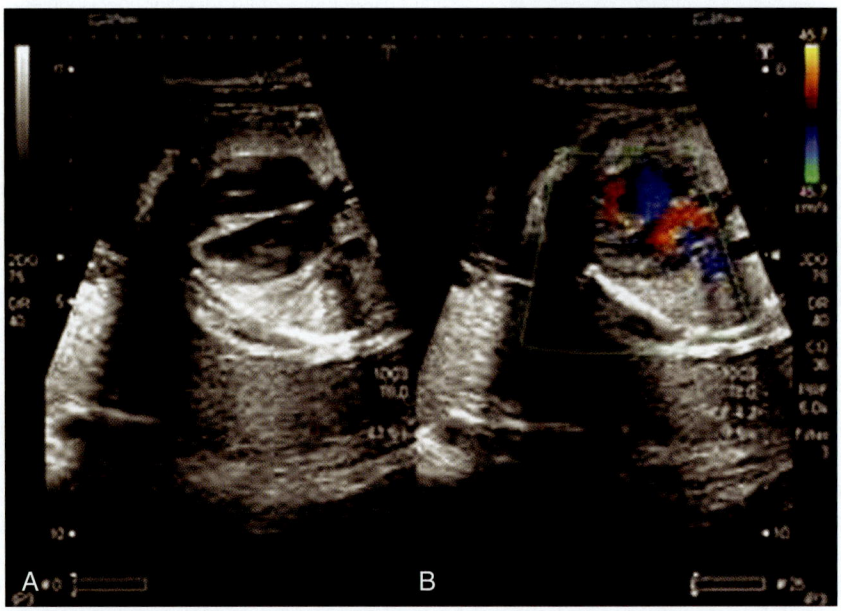

FIG. 36.15 **Ventricular septal defect.** (A) An isolated membranous septal defect shown in this four-chamber view. The edges of the defect are slightly brighter than the rest of the septum. (B) Color Doppler is helpful when the ventricular septal defect is large enough to allow crossover of flow from the higher-pressure right side of the heart into the left side of the heart.

▸ **Sonographic Findings.** The best echocardiographic views to image the septal defect in the outflow tract are the long-axis, short-axis, and five-chamber views. The septal defect in the inflow tract is best seen on the four-chamber view.

Evaluation of shunt flow and direction is made with color flow mapping. Remember that pressures between the right and left heart are almost the same in utero, so a small defect will probably not show a velocity change. If the defect is large, the sample volume should be placed directly in the defect to see the jet flow direction and velocity.

Atrioventricular Septal Defect

The endocardial cushion defect is also called *ostium primum atrial septal defect, atrioventricular canal malformation, endocardial cushion defect,* and **atrioventricular septal defect (AVSD)** (Fig. 36.17). These defects are subdivided into complete, incomplete, and partial forms.

Incomplete Atrioventricular Septal Defect. The failure of the endocardial cushion to fuse is termed an *incomplete atrioventricular septal defect.* This condition results in a membranous ventricular septal defect, abnormal tricuspid valve, primum atrial septal defect, and cleft mitral valve (Fig. 36.18). A cleft mitral valve means that the anterior part of the leaflet is divided into two parts (medial and lateral). When the leaflet closes, blood leaks through this hole into the left atrial cavity. The leaflet is usually somewhat malformed, further causing regurgitation into the atrium. In addition, there is a communication between the left ventricle and right atrium (left ventricular to right atrial shunt) because of the absent primum atrial septum and membranous interventricular septum. The ventricular septal defect occurs just below the mitral ring and is continuous with the primum atrial septal defect.

Complete Atrioventricular Septal Defect. The endocardial defect is characterized by the insertion of the chordae from the cleft mitral and tricuspid valve into the crest of the ventricular septum or a right ventricular papillary muscle (Fig. 36.19). The most primitive form is called a *complete atrioventricular septal defect.* This defect has a single, undivided, free-floating leaflet stretching across both ventricles. A two-dimensional (2D) sweep from the mitral to the aortic valves would show the anterior mitral leaflet swinging through the ventricular septal defect in continuity with the tricuspid valve. The tricuspid valve is said to *cap* the mitral valve. The anterior and posterior leaflets are on both sides of the interventricular septum, causing the valve to override or straddle the septum. This is a more complex abnormality to repair because the defect is larger, and the single atrioventricular valve is more difficult to manage clinically, depending on the amount of regurgitation present. The regurgitant jet may extend from the right ventricle to the left atrium, secondary

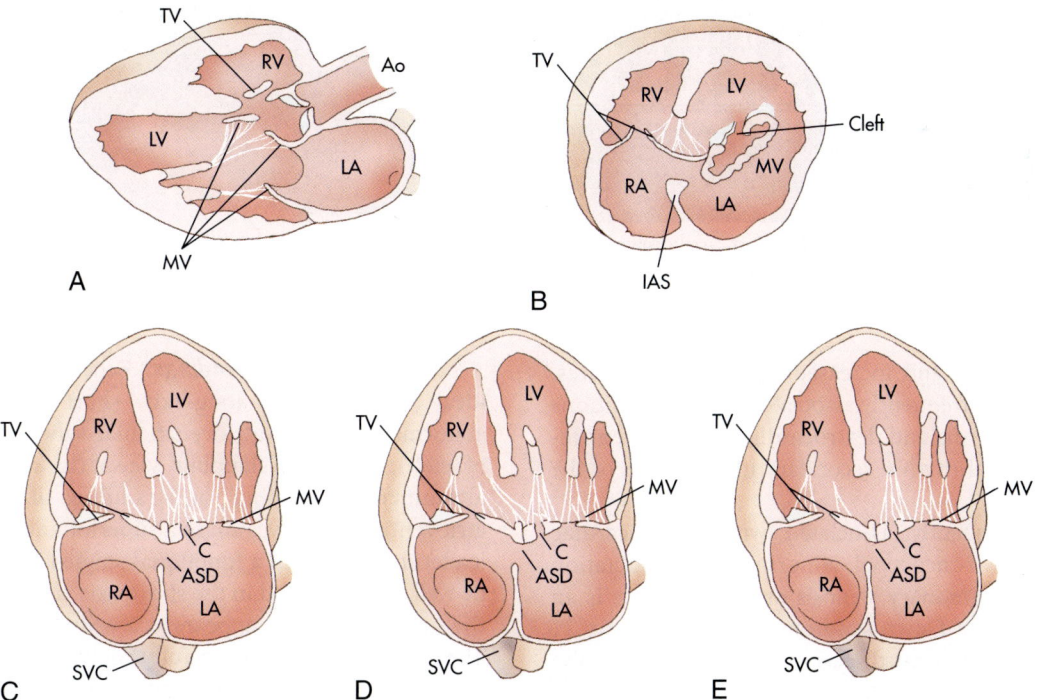

FIG. 36.17 Atrioventricular septal defect. (A) Long-axis view shows the discontinuity of the anterior leaflet of the mitral valve with the posterior wall of the aorta. The membranous septal defect is seen. (B) Short-axis view through the atrioventricular valves shows the cleft in the anterior leaflet of the mitral valve (MV). The primum septal defect is seen. (C) Four-chamber view showing the Rastelli type A large defect in the center (crux) of the heart. The membranous and primum septal defects are seen with the cleft mitral valve. There is a common leaflet from the anterior mitral leaflet to the septal tricuspid leaflet. (D) Rastelli type B defect shows the chordal attachments from the medial portion of the cleft mitral leaflet related to the papillary muscle on the right side of the septal defect. (E) Rastelli type C defect shows a free-floating common atrioventricular leaflet *(C). Ao,* Aorta; *ASD,* atrial septal defect; *IAS,* interarterial septum; *LA,* left atrium; *LV,* left ventricle; *RV,* right ventricle; *SVC,* superior vena cava; *TV,* tricuspid valve.

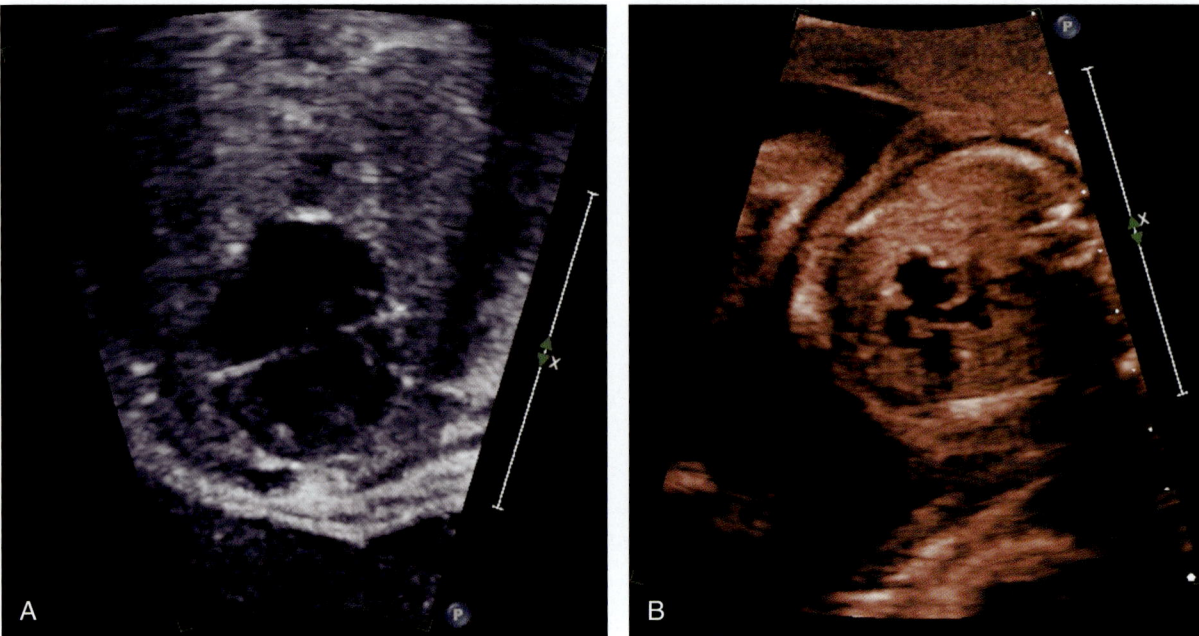

FIG. 36.18 Atrioventricular septal defect. (A) A patient with trisomy 21 had 2:1 heart block secondary to the complete atrioventricular septal defect, which included the membranous and atrial septa. (B) A patient with trisomy 21 had a huge atrioventricular defect. The membranous and part of the muscular septum is not present; the primum septum is also absent.

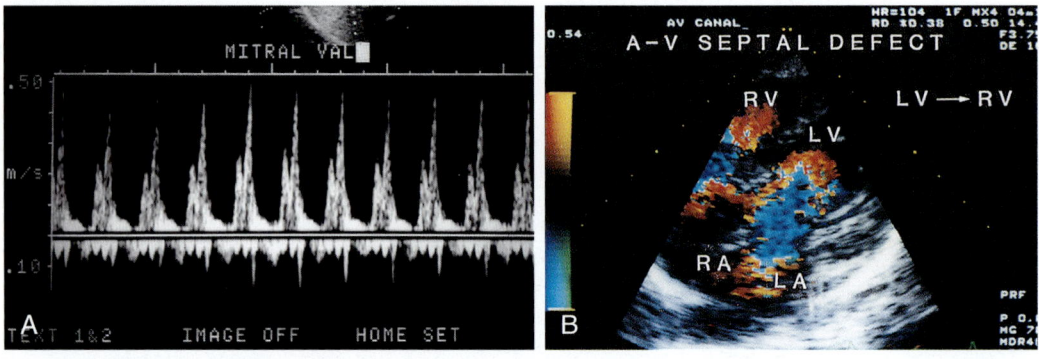

FIG. 36.19 Atrioventricular septal defect. (A) Prominent inflow velocities are seen across the mitral valve. There is a small regurgitant flow into the left atrium seen as flow reversal at the end of diastole below the baseline. (B) Color flow imaging is helpful to map the flow across the defect and to track regurgitation into the atria. *LA,* Left atrium; *LV,* left ventricle; *RA,* right atrium; *RV,* right ventricle.

to the valve deformity and increased right heart pressures. Complete AVSDs are frequently associated with malpositions of the heart (mesocardia and dextrocardia) and atrioventricular block (abnormal rhythm secondary to distortion of the conduction tissues).

AVSDs are frequently associated with other cardiac defects, including truncoconal abnormalities, coarctation of the aorta, and pulmonary stenosis or atresia. There is an increased incidence of Down syndrome (50% of trisomy 21 babies have congenital heart disease) and asplenia and polysplenia syndromes.

Occasionally, complete absence of the interatrial septum is noted in the fetal four-chamber view. With color flow, the entire atria are completely filled throughout systole and diastole. This is termed *common atria*.

With a partial AVSD, the fetus has only some of the previously described findings, usually an absent primum atrial septum and a cleft mitral valve.

Sonographic Findings. Echocardiographically, the ideal views are the long-axis, short-axis (to search for abnormalities in the atrioventricular valves, such as presence of cleft), and four-chamber views (to search for chordal attachment, overriding, or straddling of the valves). The atrioventricular valves share a superior and inferior bridging leaflet that results in a functional single large valve. This may be well demonstrated in the short-axis view of the ventricle as the single large valve appears as a wide circle *figure-of-8 sign*. The crux of the heart is carefully analyzed by slowly sweeping the transducer anterior (toward the aorta outlet) to posterior (toward the atrioventricular valve inlet) to record the outlet and inlet portions of the membranous septum.

Doppler and color flow techniques are extremely useful in determining the direction and degree of regurgitation present in the atrioventricular valves and the direction of shunt flow (increased right-sided heart pressure causes a right ventricular to left atrial shunt in the fetus).

RIGHT VENTRICULAR INFLOW DISTURBANCE

Abnormalities that primarily affect the right side of the heart are listed as inflow or outflow tract disturbances. Each lesion is presented, along with technical advice on how to obtain the ideal fetal cardiac image.

Tricuspid Atresia/Stenosis

Tricuspid atresia is the interruption of the growth of the tricuspid leaflet that begins early in cardiac embryology. This interruption involves the growth of the tricuspid apparatus, causing the valve to be hypoplastic or atretic.

In tricuspid atresia, the inflow portion of the right ventricle has failed to form, and a membrane or dimple in the floor of the right atrium represents the position where the tricuspid valve should have originated (Fig. 36.20). A ventricular septal defect may be present to help shunt blood into the hypertrophied right ventricle. The right ventricular outflow tract and pulmonary artery are generally diminished in size.

Sonographic Findings. Echocardiographically, the tricuspid valve is best visualized on the four-chamber view (Fig. 36.21). The findings in tricuspid atresia are a large dilated left ventricular cavity with a small, underdeveloped right ventricular cavity. The echogenic tricuspid annulus is seen with no valvular movement. The mitral valve is clearly the dominant atrioventricular valve. On the long- and short-axis views, the right ventricle is seen as a slit-like cavity just anterior to the interventricular septum.

Color flow imaging shows the incoming blood entering the right atrium and crossing the patent foramen ovale to enter the left side of the heart. If no blood flow passes the tricuspid orifice, pulmonary stenosis is present. However, if a ventricular septal defect is present, the blood flows from the high-pressure left ventricle across the defect into the hypertrophied right ventricle and out the pulmonary outflow tract.

Ebstein Anomaly of the Tricuspid Valve

Ebstein anomaly of the tricuspid valve is an abnormal displacement of the septal leaflet of the tricuspid valve toward the apex of the right ventricle (Fig. 36.22A). Tricuspid valvular tissue may adhere directly to the ventricular endocardium or may be closely attached to the ventricular wall by multiple, anomalous, short chordae tendineae. The portion of the right ventricle underlying the adherent tricuspid valvular tissue is quite thin and functions as a receiving chamber analogous to the right atrium. This is referred to as the *atrialized chamber* because it registers a right atrial pressure pulse.

The anterior leaflet of the tricuspid valve is the least affected of the three leaflets. The septal and posterior leaflets show the greatest deformity, and the posterior cusp may be rudimentary or entirely absent. The right atrium is usually massively

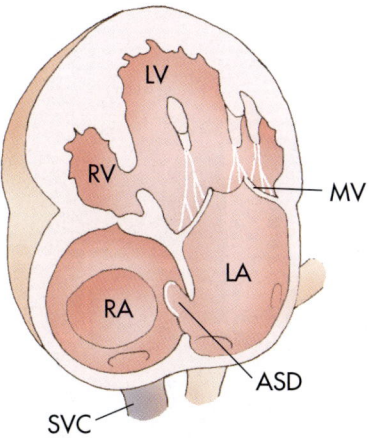

FIG. 36.20 The hypoplastic right ventricle and immobile echogenic tricuspid valve apparatus are key factors in the four-chamber view in the patient with tricuspid atresia. The right atrium (RA) is enlarged. *ASD,* Atrial septal defect; *LA,* left atrium; *LV,* left ventricle; *MV,* mitral valve; *RV,* right ventricle; *SVC,* superior vena cava.

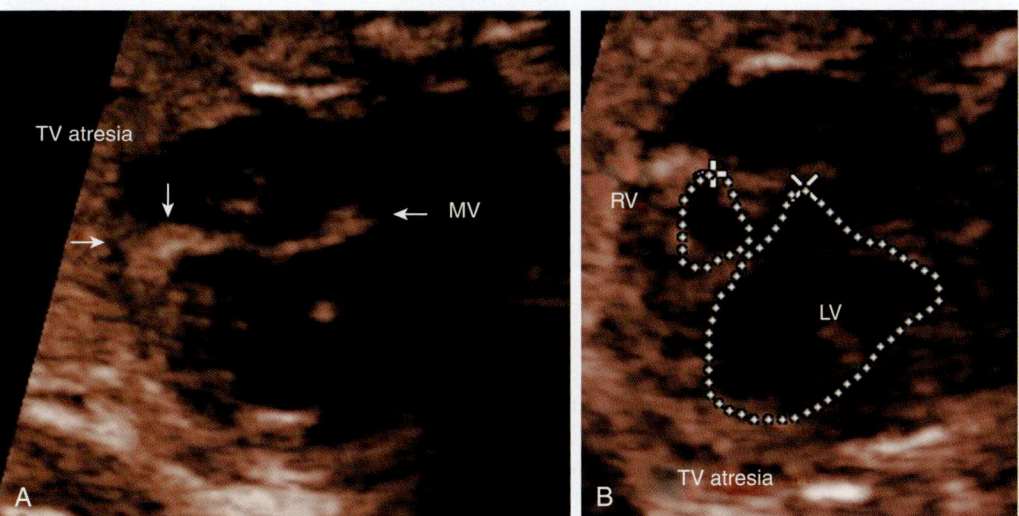

FIG. 36.21 **Tricuspid atresia.** (A) This patient presented in her 22nd week with the fetus demonstrating asymmetry of the ventricles. The annulus of the tricuspid valve (TV) was echogenic and immobile. The right ventricle was smaller than the left ventricle. The right atrium was enlarged. (B) Dramatic asymmetry of the right ventricle (RV) size compared with the left ventricle (LV) size. *MV,* Mitral valve.

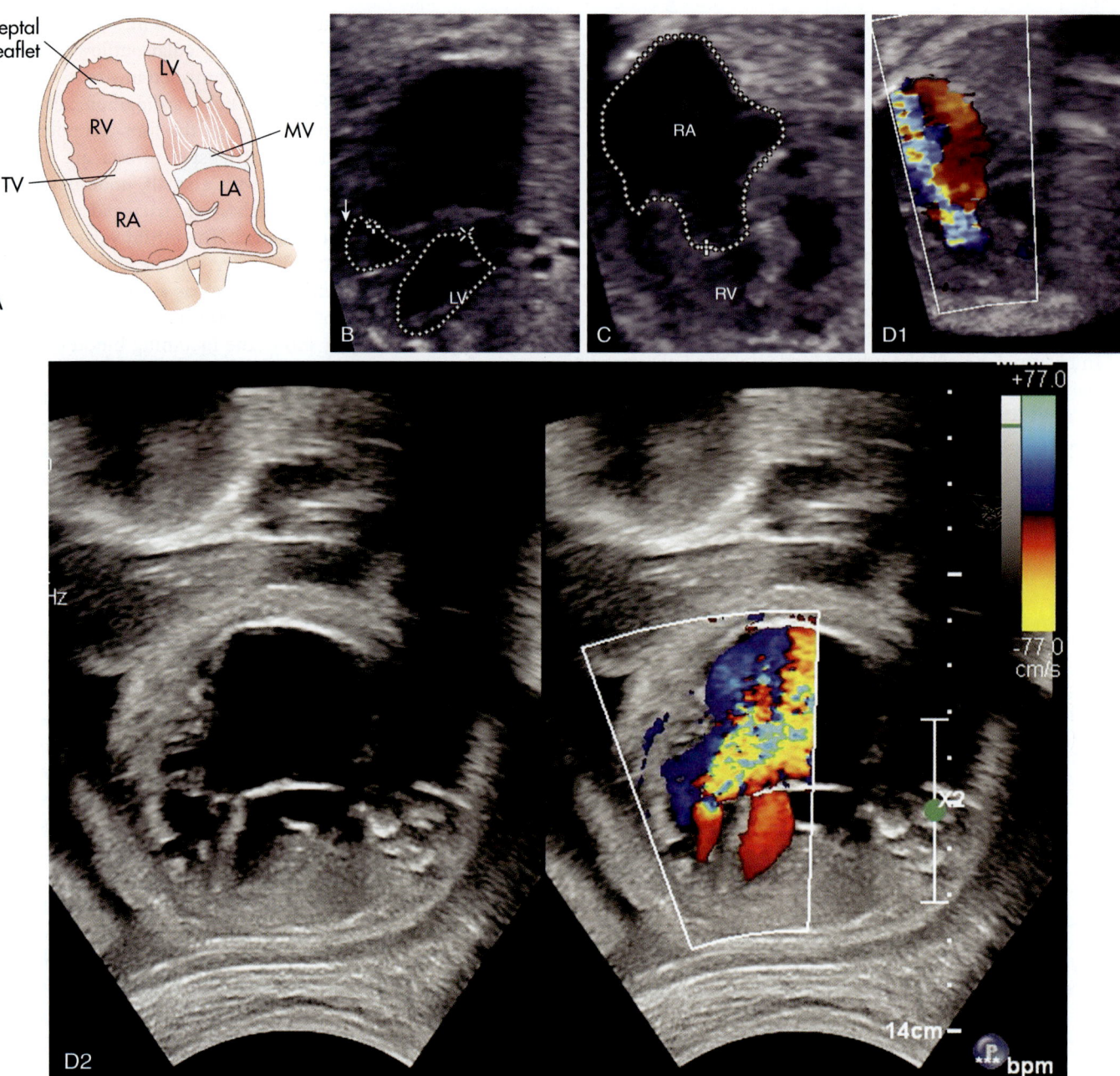

FIG. 36.22 (A) Four-chamber view of Ebstein anomaly shows the septal leaflet of the tricuspid valve (TV) inferiorly displaced from its normal insertion point. The right atrium (RA) is markedly enlarged. (B) Inferior displacement of the tricuspid valve into the apex of the right ventricle. (C) Huge right atrial enlargement with a dysplastic regurgitant valve (D1, D2). *LA*, Left atrium; *LV*, left ventricle; *MV*, mitral valve; *RV*, right ventricle.

dilated. Often these patients have an incompetent or fenestrated foramen ovale or a secundum atrial septal defect.

The abnormal function of the right side of the heart is related to the following three factors: (1) the malformed tricuspid valve, (2) the "atrialized" portion of the right ventricle, and (3) the reduced capacity of the pumping portion of the right ventricle.

Sonographic Findings. Echocardiographically, there is apical displacement of the septal leaflet of the tricuspid valve with resultant insufficiency (as seen on the apical four-chamber view) (see Fig. 36.22B–D). The atrialized right ventricle is well seen. Generally, right ventricular dysfunction is present, which results in an overload pattern of wall motion with paradoxic or anterior septal motion in systole. This right ventricular overload also shows flattening of the septum when viewed in the short-axis plane.

Doppler tracings are useful to record the amount of insufficiency present from the abnormal tricuspid valve. The sample volume should be placed at the annulus of the tricuspid valve and then mapped through the atrialized right ventricle into the right atrial cavity to record the maximum jet of insufficiency. One should note how far the regurgitant jet extends and the width of the jet to determine the degree of insufficiency.

RIGHT VENTRICULAR OUTFLOW DISTURBANCE

The normal pulmonic valve comprises three semilunar cusps that open in systole and close completely in diastole, just like the aortic cusps. These cusps are best imaged in the high short-axis plane or right long-axis plane of the right ventricular outflow tract.

Hypoplastic Right Heart

There are several forms of **hypoplastic right heart syndrome**: pulmonary atresia with an intact interventricular septum, pulmonary valve fusion with an intact interventricular septum and atrial septal defect, and pulmonary atresia with a normal aortic root diameter.

The right side of the heart is underdeveloped because of obstruction of the right ventricular outflow tract secondary to pulmonary stenosis. The tricuspid valve is small, and the pulmonary infundibulum is atretic (see Fig. 36.20).

Sonographic Findings. The sonographer must be careful not to call a hypoplastic right heart a hypoplastic left heart (which may be a lethal situation) (Fig. 36.23). Careful assessment of the situs of the fetus, great vessel relationships, and trabeculation pattern helps the sonographer determine right from left heart (the right heart is more trabeculated than the left). Care must also be taken to avoid mistaking the papillary muscle for the septum when a large membranous defect is present. In a fetus with a single ventricle (and essentially a hypoplastic right heart), it may be easy to confuse a large papillary muscle with the septum. In this case, it would be difficult to figure out the great vessel origin. A single ventricle usually has an associated transposition of the great arteries with a small pulmonary artery and large aorta.

Tetralogy of Fallot

Tetralogy of Fallot is the most common form of cyanotic heart disease in infants and children. The severity of the disease varies according to the degree of pulmonary stenosis present—the more stenosis, the greater the cyanosis. It is possible to have a mild form of pulmonary stenosis and not have any cyanosis after birth.

In tetralogy of Fallot, the outlet or conal septum is anteriorly and leftward deviated, resulting in impingement of flow through the pulmonary outflow tract. There is a large subaortic ventricular septal defect caused by the large aorta overriding the interventricular septum. This override of the aorta is best seen with a gradual sweep of the outflow tracts. If the pulmonary artery is stenotic, it may be hypoplastic and difficult to recognize as one sweeps from the large aorta to the area of the smaller pulmonary artery. The enlarged aorta is usually more anterior than in the normal heart. The hypoplasia of the pulmonary artery may extend into the branch pulmonary arteries with progressive pulmonary outflow tract obstruction. Color Doppler is often useful to demonstrate patency of flow in the outflow tracts, particularly if there is patency in the pulmonary outflow tract and the direction of flow through the main pulmonary artery. Patency of the ductus arteriosus is critical in planning postnatal management. If reversed flow is present in the ductus, severe pulmonary outflow obstruction may be present.

Tetralogy of Fallot has the following four characteristics (Fig. 36.24):
1. High, membranous ventricular septal defect
2. Large, anteriorly displaced aorta, which overrides the septal defect
3. Pulmonary stenosis
4. Right ventricular hypertrophy (not seen in fetal life; occurs after birth when pulmonary stenosis causes increased pressure in the right ventricle)

A large septal defect with mild to moderate pulmonary stenosis is classified as acyanotic disease, whereas a large septal defect with severe pulmonary stenosis is considered cyanotic disease ("blue baby" at birth).

In addition to the association of trisomy abnormalities (13, 18, and 21), other congenital cardiac malformations may occur in patients with pulmonic stenosis and ventricular septal defect, including the following:
- Right aortic arch
- Persistent left superior vena cava
- Anomalies of the pulmonary artery and its branches
- Absence of the pulmonary valve
- Incompetence of the aortic valve
- Variations in coronary arterial anatomy

The prognosis for a fetus with tetralogy of Fallot is good with surgical intervention. One of the first surgical approaches was developed to obviate the underperfusion of the lungs.

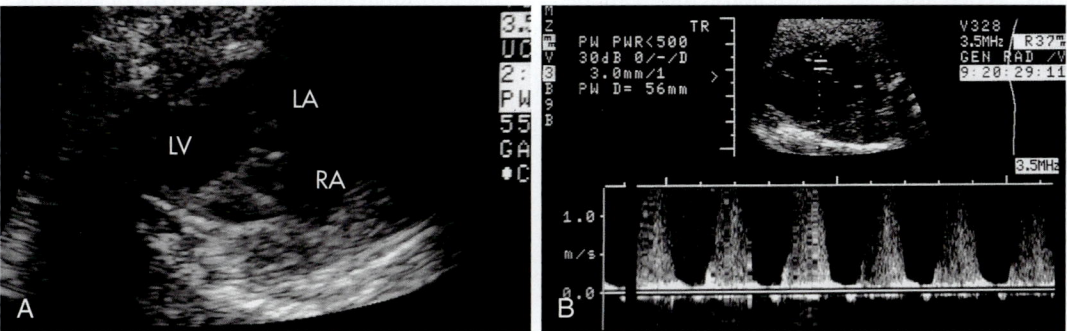

FIG. 36.23 Hypoplastic right heart. (A) Asymmetry of the ventricles with severe tricuspid regurgitation (B) into the right atrium (RA). *LA*, Left atrium; *LV*, left ventricle; *RV*, right ventricle.

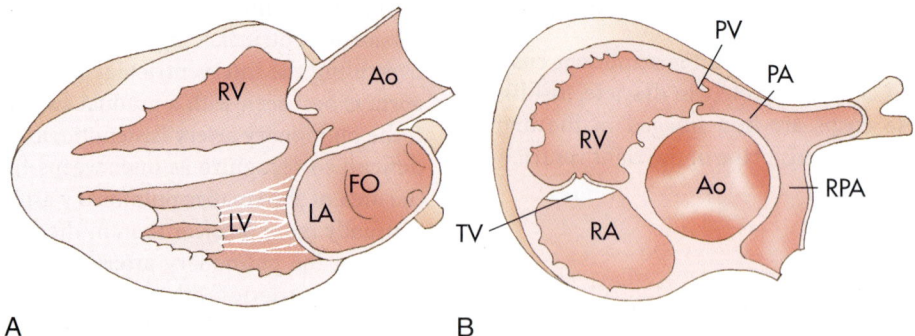

FIG. 36.24 Tetralogy of Fallot. (A) Long-axis view of the enlarged aorta (Ao) as it overrides the interventricular septum. The amount of aortic enlargement depends on the degree of pulmonary stenosis or atresia present. (B) Short-axis view of the small pulmonary artery (PA) displaced anteriorly by the enlarged aorta. *FO*, Foramen ovale; *LA*, left atrium; *LV*, left ventricle; *PV*, pulmonary valve; *RA*, right atrium; *RPA*, right pulmonary artery; *RV*, right ventricle; *TV*, tricuspid valve.

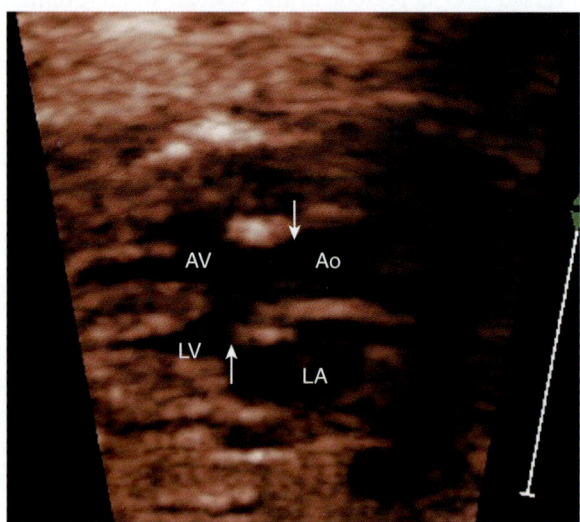

FIG. 36.25 Tetralogy of Fallot. Long-axis view of the heart shows the aorta as it overrides the septum and ventricular septal defect and enlarged overriding aorta (Ao). *AV*, Aortic valve; *LA*, left atrium; *LV*, left ventricle.

The Blalock-Taussig shunt was performed to anastomose the subclavian artery to the pulmonary artery.

The prognosis for tetralogy of Fallot with pulmonary atresia or an absent pulmonary valve is not as good. In the fetus shown in Fig. 36.25, a single large great vessel is identified (aorta) without a significant second great vessel. The aortic override is readily apparent on the long-axis view. The hypoplastic branch pulmonary arteries may be contiguous or discontinuous. When they are contiguous, they can be demonstrated as the "seagull sign." The lungs and pulmonary arteries receive their blood supply through a tortuous and small ductus arteriosus or collateral vessels that arise from the descending aorta or other systemic arteries. The absent pulmonary valve may cause congestive heart failure in the fetus. Aneurysmal dilation of the pulmonary artery and its branches may be a cause of pulmonary distress.

Sonographic Findings. Echocardiographically the demonstration of tetralogy of Fallot is distinguished on the parasternal long-axis view (see Fig. 36.25). The large aorta overrides the ventricular septum. If the override is greater than 50%, the condition is called a *double-outlet right ventricle*, meaning that both great vessels arise from the right side of the heart. A septal defect is present; the size may vary from small to large. The parasternal short-axis view shows the small, hypertrophied right ventricle (if significant pulmonary stenosis is present). The pulmonary artery is usually small, and the cusps may be thickened and domed or difficult to image well.

A sample volume should be made in the high parasternal short-axis view to determine the turbulence of the right ventricular outflow tract and pulmonary valve stenosis. Color flow is helpful in this condition to delineate the abnormal high-velocity pattern and to direct the sample volume into the proper jet flow. If the ventricular septal defect is large, increased flow is seen in the right side of the heart (increased tricuspid velocity, right ventricular outflow tract velocity, and increased pulmonic velocity). The best view for imaging the subvalvular portion of the right ventricular outflow tract is obtained with the subcostal short-axis plane. This view allows extensive visualization of the subpulmonary area so often affected in tetralogy of Fallot. In the fetus, the pulmonic obstructive flow patterns are not as pronounced as in the neonatal period.

Pulmonic Stenosis

The most common form of right ventricular outflow tract obstruction is pulmonary valve stenosis. In pulmonic stenosis, the abnormal pulmonic cusps become thickened and domed during diastole (Fig. 36.26A). The main pulmonary artery may be hypoplastic, or there may be poststenotic dilation of the pulmonary artery. Other forms of pulmonary stenosis may show subvalvular thickening just inferior to the cusp opening.

Sonographic Findings. The domed effect is not quite as noticeable on the fetal echocardiogram, but with careful evaluation, the thickness of the cusp may be compared with that of the aortic cusp. An M-mode image may be made through the area to further define cusp mobility and thickness. As with the aortic cusps, multiple degrees of stenosis and atresia may develop in the right ventricular outflow tract. The more atretic the cusp, the more hypoplastic the pulmonary artery becomes. Critical pulmonary atresia may be difficult to image in the early second-trimester fetus because the pulmonary outflow becomes so hypoplastic that it is difficult to recognize.

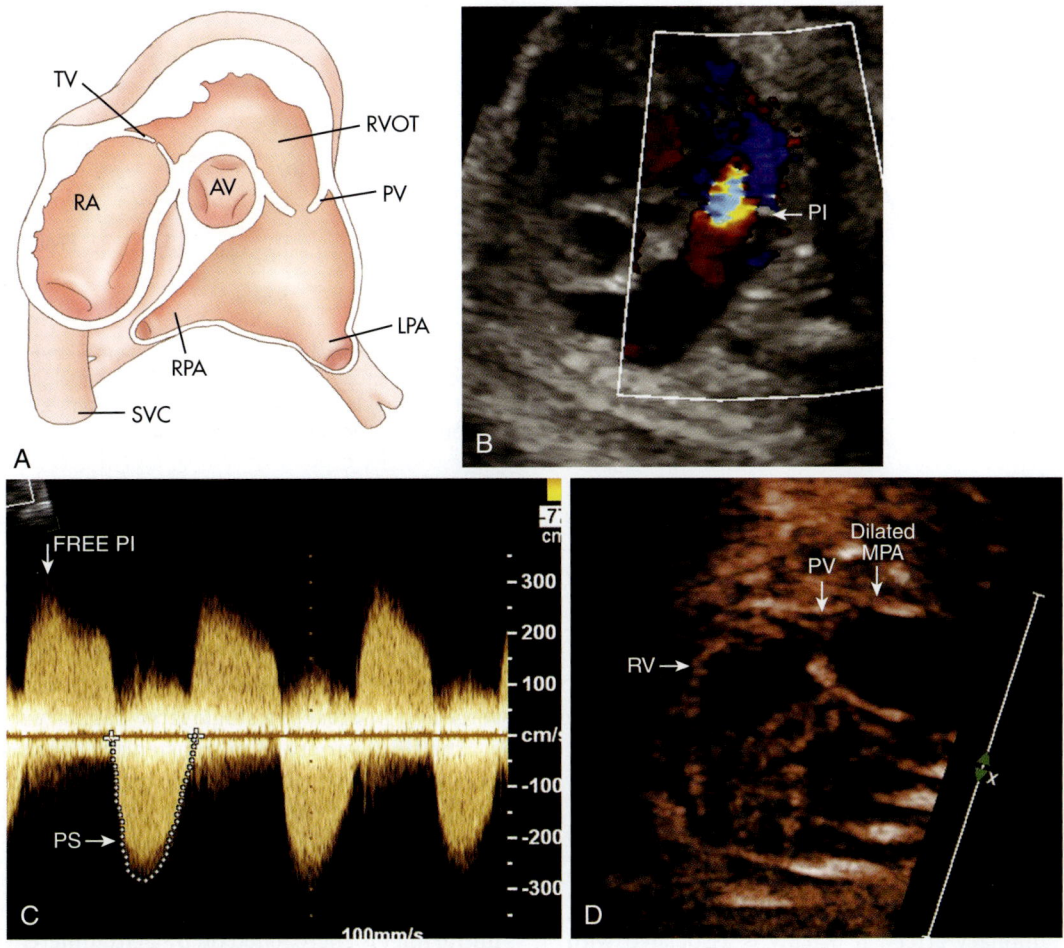

FIG. 36.26 Pulmonary stenosis. (A) Parasternal short-axis view of the domed pulmonary leaflets and some right ventricular hypertrophy. (B) Color Doppler of the RVOT at the level of the pulmonary valve shows high-velocity turbulence. (C) Continuous wave Doppler recorded at the level of the thickened pulmonary valve toward pulmonary insufficiency (PI; flow above the baseline) and increased velocities from pulmonary stenosis (PS; flow below the baseline). (D) Poststenotic dilation of the main pulmonary artery (MPA) secondary to severe pulmonic stenosis. *AV*, Aortic valve; *LPA*, left pulmonary artery; *PV*, pulmonary valve; *RA*, right atrium; *RPA*, right pulmonary artery; *RVOT*, right ventricular outflow tract; *SVC*, superior vena cava; *TV*, tricuspid valve.

It becomes even more difficult to diagnose when pulmonary stenosis is associated with another cardiac anomaly, such as transposition, double-outlet right ventricle, or tetralogy of Fallot. Secondary findings of dilation of the right ventricular cavity and right atrial cavity (secondary to tricuspid insufficiency) usually lead the investigator to the principal cause of the overload of the right side of the heart (pulmonic stenosis).

Color flow Doppler and spectral Doppler (Fig. 36.26B) evaluation is useful not only to assess the degree of obstruction but also to monitor the fetus in terms of following the course of disease.

Subpulmonic Stenosis

Subpulmonic stenosis occurs when a membrane or muscle bundle obstructs the outflow tract into the pulmonary artery (Fig. 36.27).

Sonographic Findings. If the right ventricular outflow tract can be imaged adequately, the actual obstruction may be imaged. The Doppler and color flow pattern shows a turbulent

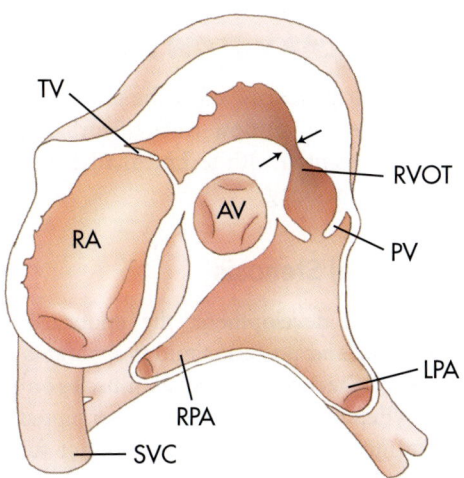

FIG. 36.27 Subvalvular pulmonary stenosis. The parasternal short-axis view shows the right ventricular hypertrophy *(arrows)* with thickening of the bands of the crista supraventricularis. *AV*, Aortic valve; *LPA*, left pulmonary artery; *PV*, pulmonary valve; *RA*, right atrium; *RPA*, right pulmonary artery; *RVOT*, right ventricular outflow tract; *SVC*, superior vena cava; *TV*, tricuspid valve.

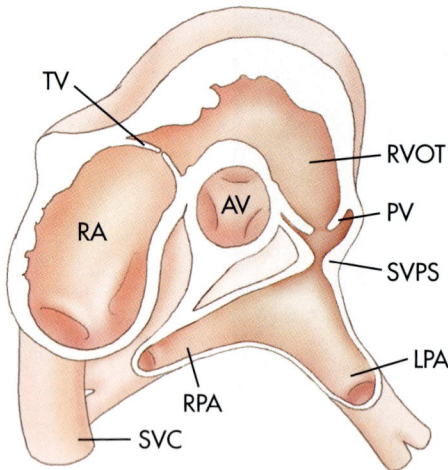

FIG. 36.28 **Supravalvular pulmonary stenosis (SVPS).** Domed pulmonary leaflets and a small pulmonary valve annulus compared with the normal-sized aortic root. There is poststenotic dilation in the main pulmonary artery. *AV,* Aortic valve; *LPA,* left pulmonary artery; *PV,* pulmonary valve; *RA,* right atrium; *RPA,* right pulmonary artery; *RVOT,* right ventricular outflow tract; *SVC,* superior vena cava; *TV,* tricuspid valve.

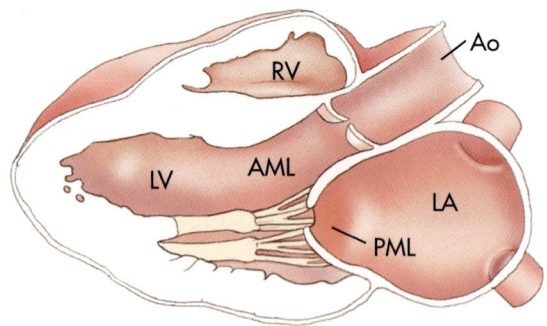

FIG. 36.29 **Mitral stenosis.** The parasternal long-axis view shows the thickened chordae and the doming of the mitral valve apparatus. *AML,* Anterior mitral leaflet; *Ao,* aorta; *LA,* left atrium; *LV,* left ventricle; *PML,* posterior mitral leaflet; *RV,* right ventricle.

obstructive pattern just before the pulmonary cusps. The velocity would not be as high as in the neonatal period but would measure at least 1.8 to 2 m/sec.

Supravalvular Pulmonic Stenosis

Supravalvular pulmonic stenosis is an abnormal narrowing in the main pulmonary artery. It usually is associated with Williams' syndrome and is hereditary (Fig. 36.28).

▶ **Sonographic Findings.** The parasternal short-axis view is best to image this condition. Prominent dilated right and left pulmonary branch arteries may be present. Again, color flow will show a turbulent high-velocity flow pattern across the narrowed vessel.

LEFT VENTRICULAR INFLOW DISTURBANCE

Abnormalities that primarily affect the left side of the heart are listed as inflow or outflow tract disturbances. Each of these lesions is presented with technical advice on obtaining the ideal fetal cardiac image.

Congenital Mitral Stenosis

In normal cardiac development, the endocardial cushion forms the anterior and posterior mitral apparatus with chordae tendineae attached to two papillary muscles on the left side of the heart. When this development is interrupted in the first trimester, the mitral valve apparatus may not fully develop, causing mitral atresia or stenosis (Fig. 36.29). Mitral valve stenosis and regurgitation rarely occur in isolation. They are usually associated with other forms of left-sided heart obstruction.

There are several anatomic varieties of congenital mitral stenosis. In one variety, the leaflets are thickened, nodular, and fibrotic; the commissures are rudimentary or absent; the chordae tendineae are shortened, thickened, and fused; and the papillary muscles are fibrosed. The mitral valve is a funnel-shaped, flat, or diaphragm-like structure.

The second variety consists of a "parachute" deformity of the valve. This occurs when the normal leaflets are drawn into close apposition by shortened chordae tendineae, which converge and insert into a single large papillary muscle.

The third variety of mitral stenosis consists of an anomalous arcade with obstructing papillary muscles that extend between the papillary muscles. The papillary muscles are so large that they encroach on the subvalvular area.

The last form of mitral stenosis occurs when the valve and its supporting structure are anatomically normal, but the mitral inlet is encroached on by a circumferential supravalvular ridge of connective tissue, which arises at the base of the atrial aspect of the mitral leaflets.

Shone complex is a rare congenital heart disease consisting of four defects (Fig. 36.30):
1. Coarctation of the aorta—a narrowing or constriction of the aorta, the large vessel that carries blood from the heart to the body tissues.
2. Valvular and subvalvular aortic stenosis—a narrowing of the valve and the channel below the aortic valve connecting the left ventricle to the aorta (additional forms of aortic stenosis may also be present).
3. "Parachute" mitral valve—a malformation of the mitral valve, the valve between the left atrium and left ventricle, in which the two valve leaflets are attached to one papillary muscle rather than two and remain close together. This results in a narrowing of the valve opening (mitral stenosis), obstructing blood flow and causing the valve to resemble a parachute in appearance.
4. Supravalvular mitral membrane, or mitral ring—an abnormal ridge or membrane of connective tissue around the circumference of the mitral valve on the atrial side that may protrude into the valve opening and/or adhere to the valve leaflets. Variable in size, this ring may obstruct blood flow through the mitral valve into the left ventricle.

These defects all affect the left side of the heart and interfere with the flow of blood into and out of the left ventricle, which pumps oxygen-rich blood through the aorta to the

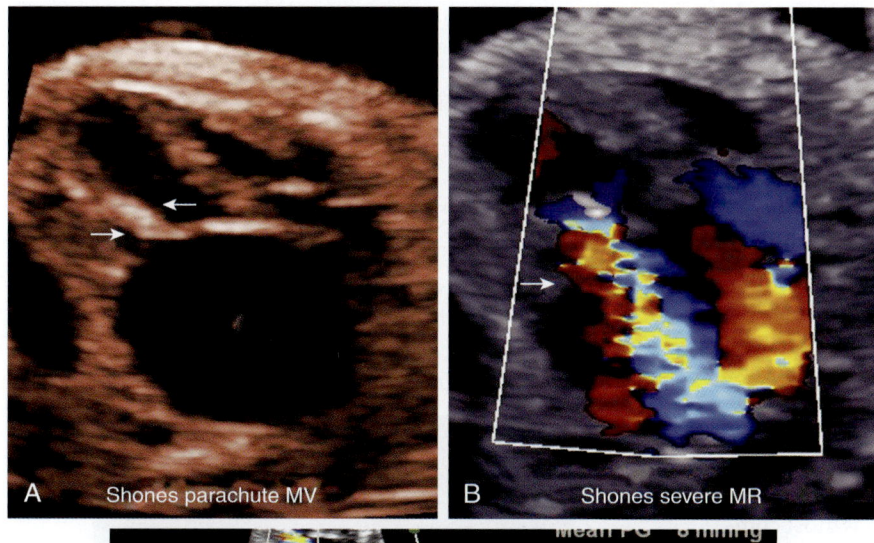

FIG. 36.30 **Shone complex.** (A) Four-chamber view shows a thickened, immobile mitral leaflet (parachute mitral valve) with a small left ventricular cavity. (B) Severe mitral regurgitation (MR) was present. (C) Doppler shows both mitral stenosis flow and mitral regurgitation. *MV*, Mitral valve.

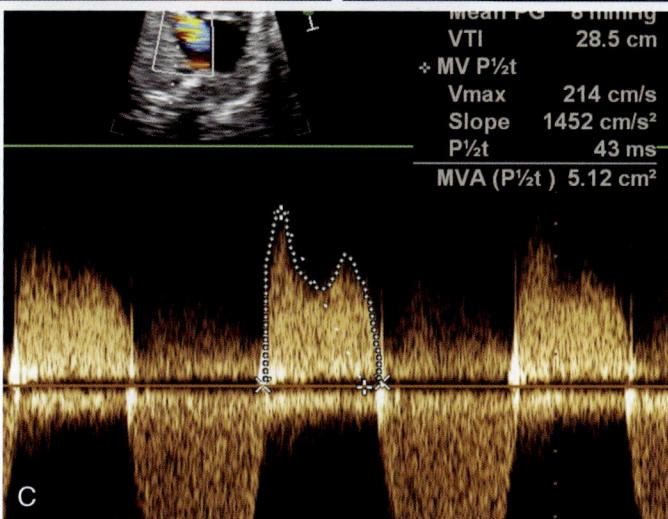

body. Shone complex has a broad spectrum of symptoms, treatments, and outcomes, depending on the severity and number of defects. There are also incomplete forms of the disease in which only two or three of these defects are present, and cases in which other congenital heart defects also occur (e.g., patent ductus arteriosus, interrupted aortic arch, bicuspid aortic valve, atrial septal defect, ventricular septal defect).

Sonographic Findings. The mitral valve should be evaluated from at least two cardiac windows: the long-axis and the four-chamber views. The long-axis view allows the examiner to evaluate the mobility of the anterior and posterior mitral valve leaflets as they open into the left ventricular cavity. The four-chamber view allows comparison of the mitral valve placement with the normal, slightly apical displacement of the tricuspid valve. It also allows observation of the pliability of the thin leaflets as they open in diastole and close in systole. The ideal Doppler waveform should be recorded from this apical position.

Mitral Atresia. In a fetus with **mitral atresia** or congenital mitral stenosis, the examiner sees a thickened mitral orifice with restriction of leaflet amplitude. The left ventricular cavity is reduced in volume because of decreased inflow (Fig. 36.31).

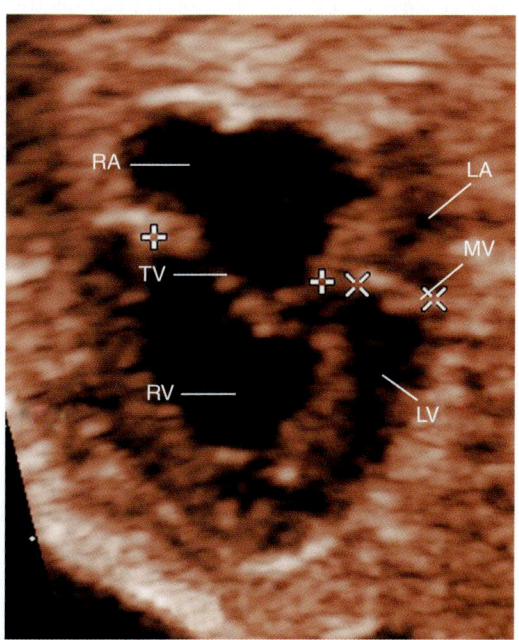

FIG. 36.31 **Mitral atresia.** The mitral valve is hypoplastic and atretic, causing the left ventricle to be underdeveloped. *LA*, Left atrium; *LV*, left ventricle; *MV*, mitral leaflet; *RA*, right atrium; *RV*, right ventricle; *TV*, tricuspid valve.

The myocardial thickness is increased (secondary to increased left ventricular pressure overload) if associated aortic atresia is present.

> **Sonographic Findings.** The mitral apparatus may appear thickened and dysplastic with shortened chordae and closely spaced papillary muscles or a single papillary muscle. The left ventricle is small relative to the right. Flow is usually redirected through the foramen; therefore the flow through the obstructed mitral valve is laminar. A left to right shunt through the fetal foramen ovale is consistent with mitral valve atresia. Color Doppler can be helpful to determine how much, if any, mitral inflow is present. The apical four-chamber view is again best to obtain this assessment.

Mitral Regurgitation

In fetal life, the presence of **mitral regurgitation** is most commonly secondary to a cleft mitral valve (endocardial cushion defect) or a congenital mitral stenosis. In the presence of mitral regurgitation, the left atrial cavity would become enlarged because of the leakage of blood from the defective mitral valve.

> **Sonographic Findings.** The color Doppler flow pattern of disturbed flow in the left atrial cavity would be seen on the apical four-chamber view and probably on the parasternal long-axis view.

LEFT VENTRICULAR OUTFLOW TRACT DISTURBANCE

The normal aortic valve comprises three semilunar cusps that open in systole and close completely in diastole. The cusps are best imaged in the long-axis and short-axis planes. The aortic root is measured in the short-axis plane as the transducer bisects the right ventricular outflow tract, the pulmonary artery, and the aortic root. Normal spectral Doppler flow is recorded in the aortic outflow tract (either from a five-chamber view or a modified long- or short-axis view).

Bicuspid Aortic Valve

If the development of the aortic valve is interrupted during the first trimester, the three aortic cusps may not fully separate. In this instance, the valve may be a *unicuspid* valve with a central opening and aortic stenosis or a *bicuspid* (two-leaflet) valve with asymmetric cusps (Fig. 36.32).

> **Sonographic Findings.** In this case, the raphe between the cusp tissue has not separated; thus the leaflet opens asymmetrically and may show doming on the parasternal long-axis view. In the fetus, a bicuspid valve may be difficult to image at 18 weeks, but it should be well visualized in the late second trimester at 27 weeks (Fig. 36.33).

Aortic Stenosis

Critical Aortic Stenosis. Aortic stenosis is an abnormal development of the cusps of the aortic valve that results in

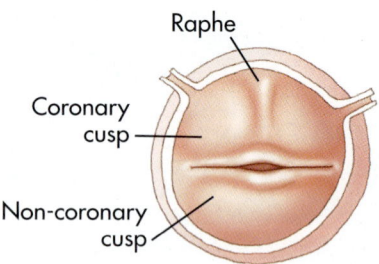

FIG. 36.32 Bicuspid aortic valve showing the noncoronary cusp and fused right and left coronary cusps with a raphe.

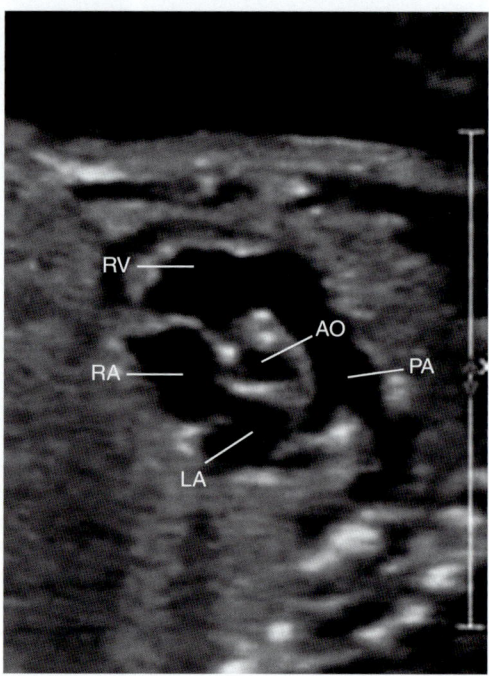

FIG. 36.33 Parasternal short-axis view is used to show the three separate aortic leaflets. *Ao*, Aorta; *LA*, left atrium; *PA*, pulmonary artery; *RA*, right atrium; *RV*, right ventricle; *TV*, tricuspid valve.

thickened and domed leaflets. Critical aortic stenosis signifies end-stage left ventricular dysfunction. At some point in the second or third trimester, an infection or other viral process has caused the aortic leaflet to thicken and close prematurely. The fetus shows a normal ascending and descending aorta with abnormal opening of the aortic cusps. The enlarged, dysfunctional left ventricle then "billows" from the increased pressure in the ventricle because the left ventricular outflow tract is blocked (Figs. 36.34 and 36.35A). The ventricular walls would be thin and bulge into the right ventricular cavity. The parasternal long-axis and apical four-chamber views are the most helpful to image this disease.

> **Sonographic Findings.** Color flow helps to assess the severity of the aortic stenosis to determine how much, if any, blood is flowing through the stenotic aortic leaflets (Fig. 36.35B).

Subvalvular or Supravalvular Aortic Stenosis. Subvalvular aortic stenosis occurs when a membrane covers the left

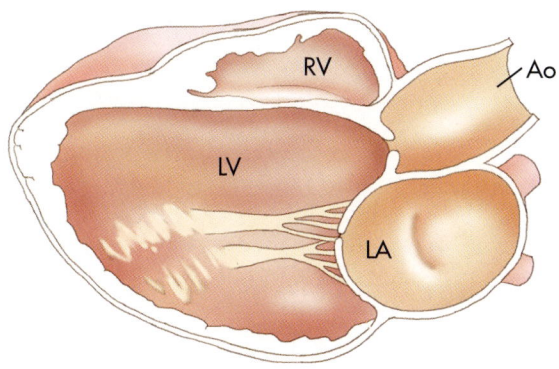

FIG. 36.34 Parasternal long-axis view of the domed aortic valve, dilated left ventricle, and poststenotic dilation of the ascending aorta. *Ao*, Aorta; *LA*, left atrium; *LV*, left ventricle; *RV*, right ventricle.

ventricular outflow tract (Fig. 36.36). Supravalvular aortic stenosis is a narrowing of the ascending aortic root.

Supravalvular aortic stenosis may be related to Williams syndrome (Fig. 36.37). Subaortic stenosis has been described in patients with Turner syndrome, Noonan syndrome, and congenital rubella.

Sonographic Findings. The left ventricular outflow tract should be carefully evaluated in the parasternal long-axis, apical five-chamber, and aortic arch views to image this thin membrane. The Doppler view shows increased velocity across the obstructive membrane, whereas color flow imaging shows increased turbulence at the area of narrowing.

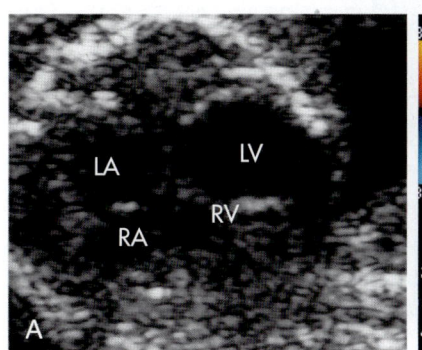
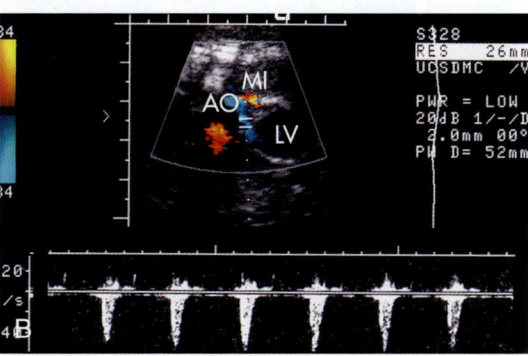

FIG. 36.35 **Critical aortic stenosis.** (A) Critical aortic stenosis appears in the second or third trimester. The four-chamber view shows a dilated left ventricular cavity (assumes the shape of a balloon). The ventricle is tense and quickly becomes noncompliant. (B) Color Doppler imaging shows aortic insufficiency *(blue)* and mitral insufficiency (MI, *red*). *AO*, Aorta; *LA*, left atrium; *LV*, left ventricle; *RA*, right atrium; *RV*, right ventricle.

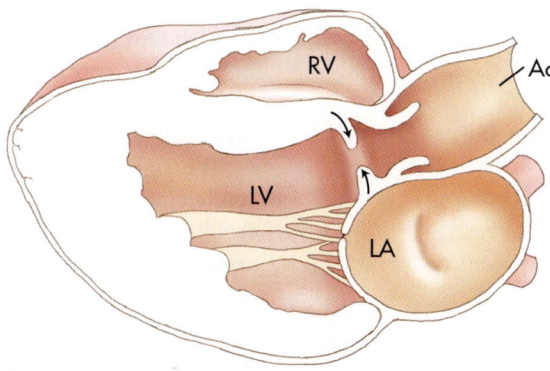

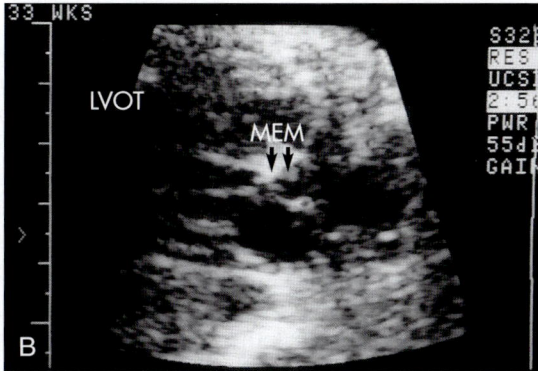
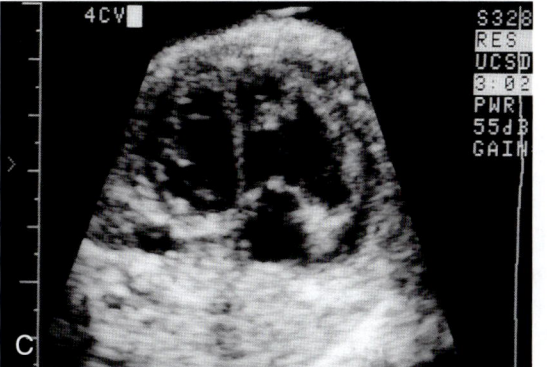

FIG. 36.36 **Submembranous aortic stenosis.** (A) A discrete membrane inferior to the aortic valve is shown in the parasternal long-axis view *(arrows)*. (B) Submembranous aortic obstruction. Long-axis view of the ascending aorta and left ventricle shows the thick membrane (MEM, *arrows*) located above the aortic cusps to cause obstruction to the left ventricular outflow tract (LVOT). (C) This outflow obstruction causes the left ventricle to enlarge, as seen on this four-chamber view, and go into failure. A small pericardial effusion is seen around the heart. *Ao*, Aorta; *LA*, left atrium; *LV*, left ventricle; *RV*, right ventricle.

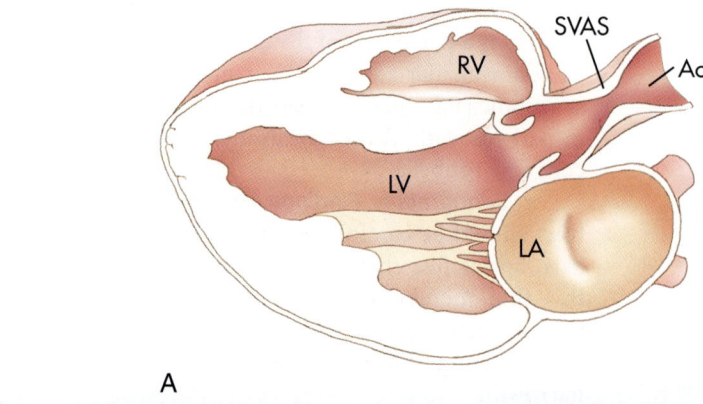

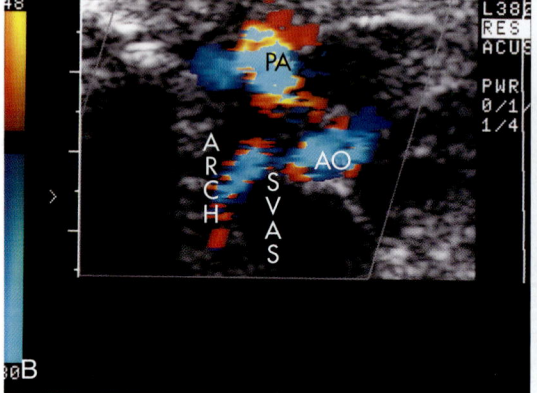
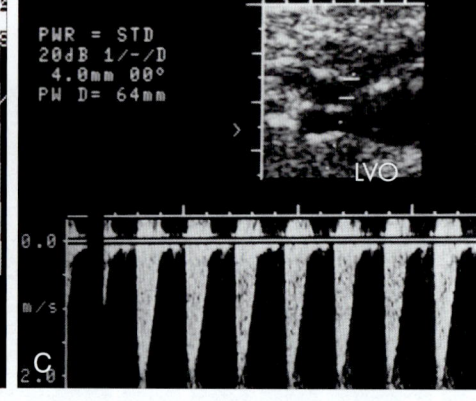

FIG. 36.37 **Supravalvular aortic stenosis (SVAS).** (A) The parasternal long-axis view shows the hourglass narrowing of the ascending aorta superior to the aortic valve. (B) Long-axis view of the ascending aorta (AO) and arch with the supravalvular narrowing. (C) Doppler velocities measure 200 cm/sec, well above the normal range. *LA*, Left atrium; *LV*, left ventricle; *PA*, pulmonary artery; *RV*, right ventricle.

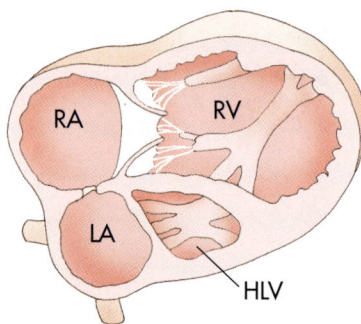

FIG. 36.38 Hypoplastic left heart syndrome is characterized by a small, hypertrophied left ventricle (HLV) with aortic and/or mitral atresia. *LA*, Left atrium; *RA*, right atrium; *RV*, right ventricle.

Hypoplastic Left Heart Syndrome

Hypoplastic left heart syndrome is characterized by a small, hypertrophied left ventricle with aortic or mitral dysplasia or atresia (Fig. 36.38). This syndrome is an autosomal recessive condition. If a couple has had one child with hypoplastic left heart syndrome, the recurrence is 4%; if two births have been affected, recurrence increases to 25%.

Although the cause of the hypoplastic left heart is unknown, it is thought to be decreased filling and perfusion of the left ventricle during embryologic development. It also may be associated with premature closure of the foramen ovale. When this closure occurs, the blood cannot cross the foramen to help the left ventricle grow. The real-time image shows a reduction in the size of the foramen ovale (the foramen should measure at least 0.6 multiplied by the diameter of the aortic root). Premature closure of the foramen would also show increased velocities across the interatrial septum (approximately 40 to 50 cm/sec).

The right ventricle supplies both the pulmonic and systemic circulations. The pulmonary venous return is diverted from the left atrium to the right atrium through interatrial communication. Through the pulmonary artery and ductus arteriosus, the right ventricle supplies the descending aorta and retrograde flow to the aortic arch and the ascending aorta. Overload on the right ventricle may lead to congestive heart failure in utero with the development of pericardial effusion and hydrops.

The ascending aorta is often hypoplastic and threadlike, with the distal arch having a slightly larger and more normal diameter. There is always retrograde flow in the distal aortic arch and left to right atrial flow across the foramen. The evaluation of the right ventricle should be made to ascertain normal function and competency of the tricuspid and pulmonic valve. If these valves are incompetent, cardiovascular compromise may occur. Flow across the atrial septum and pulmonary venous inflow should be assessed. If the foramen ovale flow is restricted, this could result in severe hypoxemia and respiratory distress after birth.

Sonographic Findings. A fetus with major disturbance to the development of the mitral valve or aortic valve shows dramatic changes in the development of the left ventricle. The amount of hypoplasia depends on when the left-sided atresia developed in the valvular area (Fig. 36.39). If the mitral atresia is the cause, the blood cannot fill the left ventricle to provide volume, and thus the aortic valve becomes atretic as well, with concentric hypertrophy of the small left ventricular cavity. If the cause is aortic stenosis, the myocardium shows extreme hypertrophy from the increased pressure overload (Fig. 36.40).

M-mode imaging may be used to further define the ventricular disproportion. The sonographer must be aware that even in normal fetuses, the M-mode and real-time measurements of the ventricles depend totally on the position of the fetus, position of the transducer, and angle of the cursor. Therefore it is important to make sure the transducer is directly perpendicular to the right and left ventricles before making an M-mode measurement. This measurement is always slightly smaller than the real-time direct measurement because the detail of the endocardium is better visualized on the M-mode than on the real-time image.

The prognosis for a fetus with a hypoplastic left heart has improved with cardiac transplantation. Norwood has developed a series of surgical repairs for the hypoplastic left heart patient. His repairs are based on the development of the aorta and aortic arch. Initial palliative procedures are done, including atrial balloon septostomy, banding of the pulmonary artery (to protect the potential volume overload to the lungs), and creation of an aortopulmonary shunt. The modified Fontan surgical procedure connects the left atrium to the tricuspid valve and the right atrium to the pulmonary artery. Norwood's challenge is to rebuild the hypoplastic aorta to improve blood flow into the left ventricle.

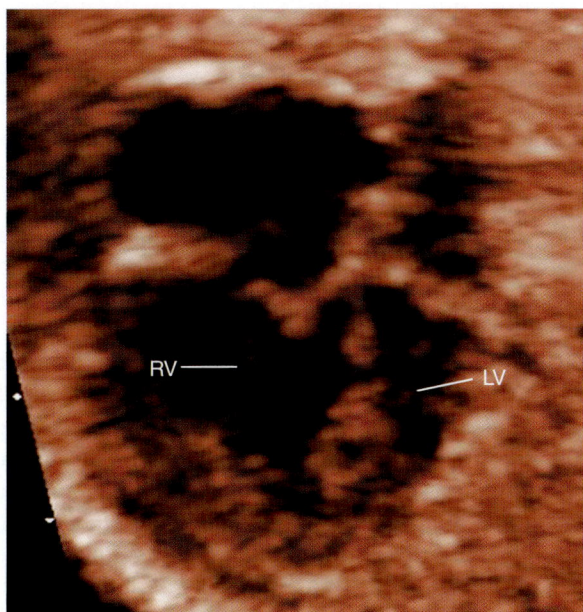

FIG. 36.39 Hypoplastic left heart. Four-chamber view shows asymmetry between the right ventricle (RV) and left ventricle (LV). The aorta and ascending aorta were also hypertrophied.

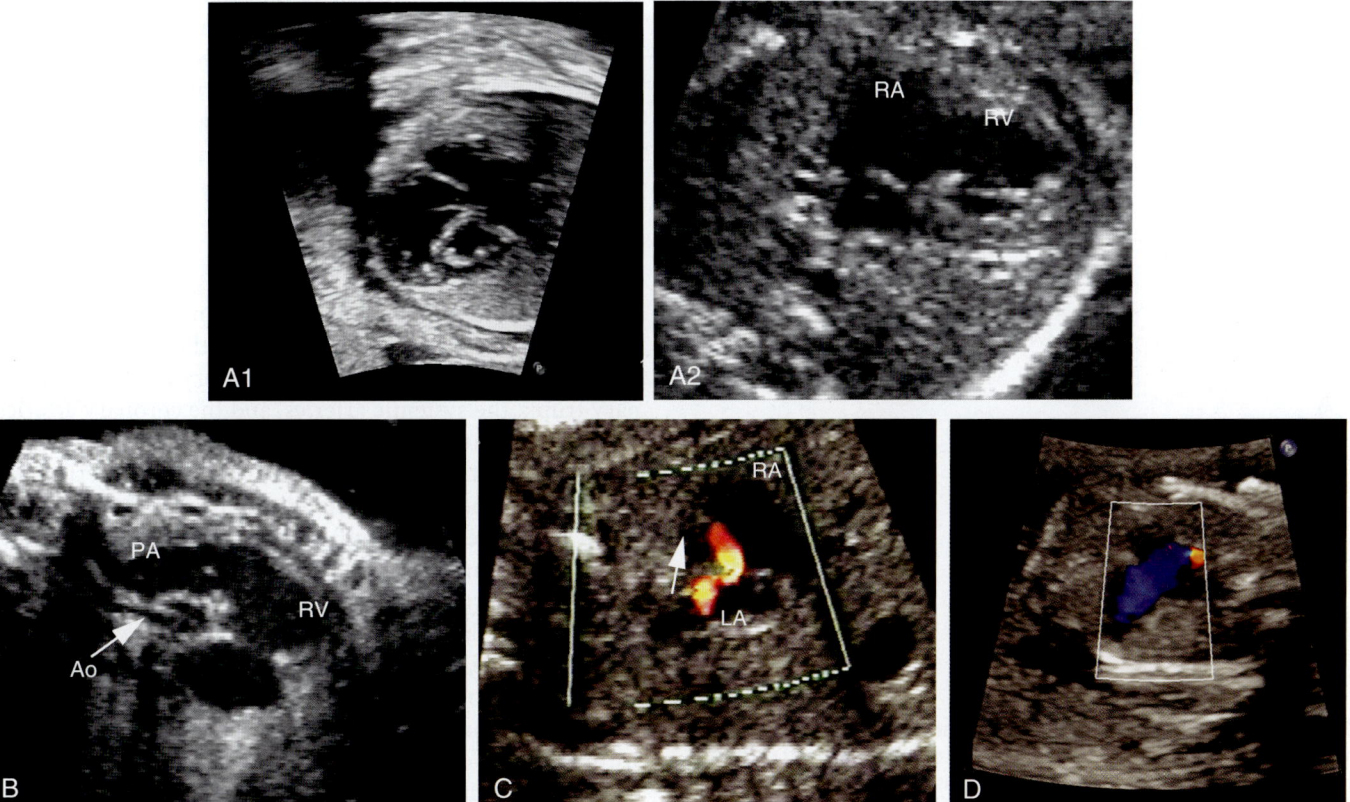

FIG. 36.40 Hypoplastic left heart syndrome. (A) Typical four-chamber view seen in this disease with a very small left atrium and left ventricle and prominent right atrium (RA) and right ventricle (RV). (B) Sagittal image demonstrates a large pulmonary artery (PA) arising from the right ventricle and a diminutive ascending aorta (Ao). (C) There is left (LA) to right atrial flow *(arrow)*, demonstrated by color Doppler.

GREAT VESSEL ABNORMALITIES

Great vessel abnormalities include interruption in the spiraling that occurs during early embryonic development. These anomalies also include complete transposition of the great arteries, corrected transposition of the great arteries, and truncus arteriosus.

Transposition of the Great Arteries

Transposition of the great arteries is an abnormal condition that exists when the aorta is connected to the right ventricle, and the pulmonary artery is connected to the left ventricle (Fig. 36.41). The atrioventricular valves are normally attached and related. This occurs because of an abnormal completion of the "loop" in embryology. The great vessels originate as a common truncus and undergo rotation and spiraling; if this development is interrupted, the great arteries do not complete their spiral, and thus transposition occurs. Usually, the aorta is anterior and to the right of the pulmonary artery. Less frequently, the two arteries are side by side, or the aorta is posterior.

In the fetal heart, no hemodynamic compromise is seen in the fetus when the great arteries are transposed. The problems occur in the neonatal period when there is inadequate mixing of oxygenated and unoxygenated blood.

The prognosis for a neonate with transposition of the great arteries is quite good with surgical intervention. The survival rate is 92% at 1 year with surgical correction. Survival depends on other cardiac anomalies that may also be present.

Other associated cardiac anomalies include atrial septal defects, anomalies of the atrioventricular valves, and underdevelopment of the right or left ventricles.

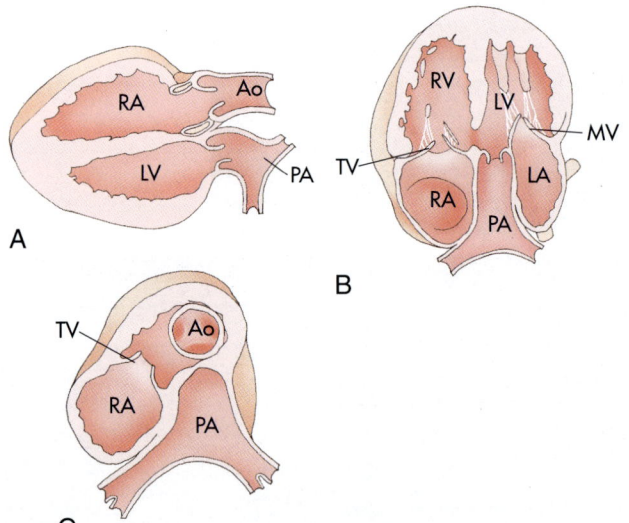

FIG. 36.41 Transposition of the great arteries. (A) Four-chamber view shows the aorta (Ao) anteriorly, arising from the right ventricle (RV), and the pulmonary artery (PA) posteriorly, arising from the left ventricle (LV). (B) Five-chamber view shows the PA arising from the LV; as the transducer follows the great artery, the bifurcation of the branch arteries is seen. (C) Short-axis view shows the aorta anterior to the PA. *LA*, Left atrium; *MV*, mitral valve; *RA*, right atrium; *TV*, tricuspid valve.

Sonographic Findings. The parasternal short-axis view is the key view to image the great arteries and their normal relationship (Fig. 36.42). In the parasternal short-axis view, the right ventricular outflow tract, pulmonary artery, and bifurcation should be seen anterior to the aorta. In transposition, this relationship is not present; it is impossible to demonstrate the bifurcation of the pulmonary artery because the aorta would be the anterior vessel. Sometimes the double circles of the great arteries can be seen in this view.

On the modified long-axis view, the normal crisscross pattern obtained from a normal fetal echocardiogram occurs when the transducer is swept from the left ventricular outflow tract anterior and medial into the right ventricular outflow tract. In a fetus with transposition, this crisscross sweep of the great arteries is not possible. The parallel great arteries are sometimes seen in this view as they both arise from the ventricles.

Corrected Transposition of the Great Arteries. Corrected transposition of the great arteries (now called L-transposition) is a cardiac condition in which the right atrium is connected to the morphologic left ventricle, and the left atrium is connected to the right ventricle (ventricular inversion). Although this is not a cyanotic lesion at birth, it can eventually cause right ventricular failure. The right ventricle is not designed at systemic pressure; therefore, surgical intervention (double-switch procedure) may be needed to restore normal hemodynamics.

Sonographic Findings. Corrected transposition is associated with malpositions of the heart and sometimes with situs inversus. A ventricular perimembranous septal defect may be present in half of the fetuses. The pulmonary artery may be seen to override the septal defect, with pulmonary stenosis in 50%. Abnormalities of the atrioventricular valves, such as an Ebstein type of malformation and straddling of the tricuspid valve, may be present. Atrioventricular heart block may also be recorded.

Truncus Arteriosus

Truncus arteriosus is a complex congenital heart lesion in which only one great artery arises from the base of the heart (Fig. 36.43). From this single great artery arise the pulmonary trunk, the systemic arteries, and the coronary arteries. This defect occurs in the early embryologic period when the conotruncus fails to separate into two great arteries. The conus corresponds to the middle third of the bulbus cordis. It gives rise to the outflow tract of both ventricles and to the muscular portion of the ventricles located between the atrioventricular and semilunar valves. The truncus is the distal part of the bulbus cordis. This structure rotates and divides into the two great semilunar valvular structures that represent the aortic and pulmonic leaflets. Failure of the bulbus to divide causes a single great artery with multiple cusps within.

Associated anomalies include mitral atresia, atrial septal defect, univentricular heart, and aortic arch abnormalities. In the neonatal stage, the prognosis is poor for truncus arteriosus.

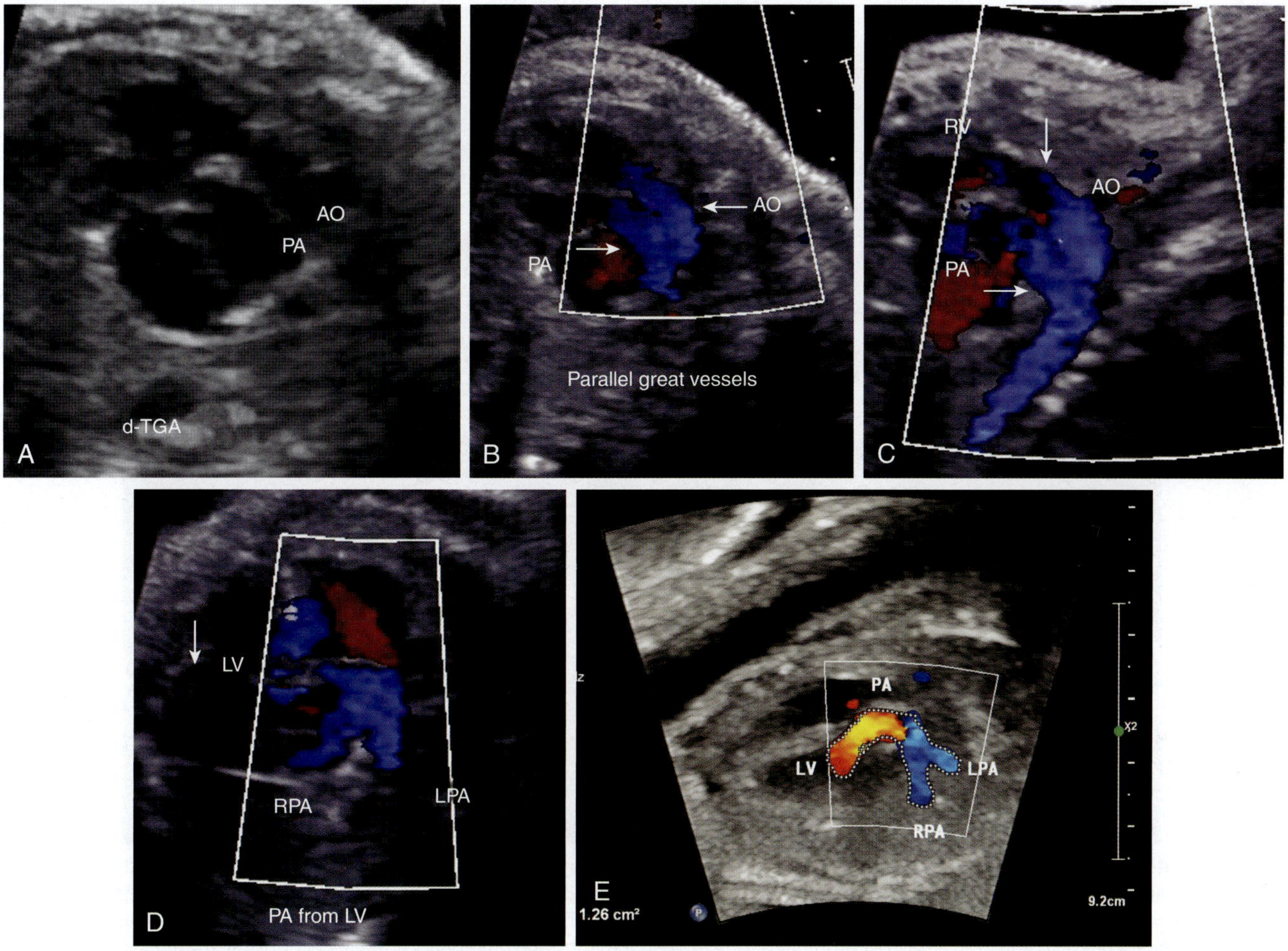

FIG. 36.42 **Transposition of the great arteries.** Arches can both be demonstrated in a single plane as a result of the parallel proximal origins of the great arteries. *Ao,* Aorta; *LPA,* left pulmonary artery; *LV,* left ventricle; *PA,* pulmonary artery; *RPA,* right pulmonary artery; *RV,* right ventricle.

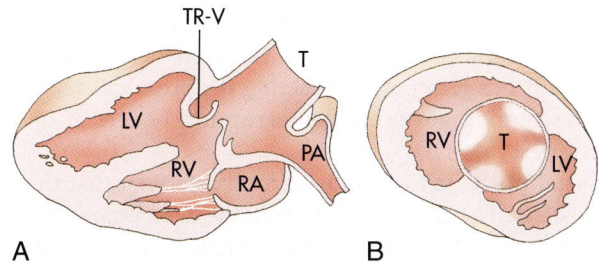

FIG. 36.43 Truncus arteriosus results when the aorta and pulmonary arteries (PA) fail to complete their rotations and divisions early in development. (A) A single large great artery is shown as it arises from the center of the heart on the long-axis view. (B) The short-axis view shows the single great artery with multiple cusps within. *LV,* Left ventricle; *RA,* right atrium; *RV,* right ventricle; *T,* truncus; *TR-V,* truncal valve.

Sonographic Findings. The fetal echocardiogram shows an abnormal, large, single great vessel arising from the ventricles (Figs. 36.44 and 36.45). Usually, an infundibular ventricular septal defect is present. Significant septal override is present. The truncal valve is usually dysplastic, thick, and domed. Multiple cusps are seen within the great artery. If truncal regurgitation is present, the prognosis is grim; the fetus usually develops congestive heart failure, pericardial effusion, and hydrops. Truncus arteriosus may be difficult to separate from a severe tetralogy of Fallot with pulmonary atresia (small pulmonary artery and large aorta overriding septal defect).

Coarctation of the Aorta

Coarctation of the aorta is a discrete shelflike lesion present in the isthmus of the arch or, more commonly, at the site of the ductal insertion near the left subclavian artery (Fig. 36.46). The coarctation may be discrete, long segment, or tubular.

Intracardiac-associated malformations are present in 90% of cases. These include aortic stenosis, aortic insufficiency, septal defects, transposition of the great arteries, truncus arteriosus, and double-outlet right ventricle. In Turner syndrome, coarctation of the aorta and ventricular septal defects are the most common cardiac defects found.

Sonographic Findings. If a bicuspid aortic valve is suspected, the aortic arch should be carefully searched for a narrowing or coarctation of the aorta. There is a 25% association of bicuspid aortic valves in fetuses with coarctation of the aorta. It is important to keep in mind that coarctation may be difficult to evaluate in the fetus because

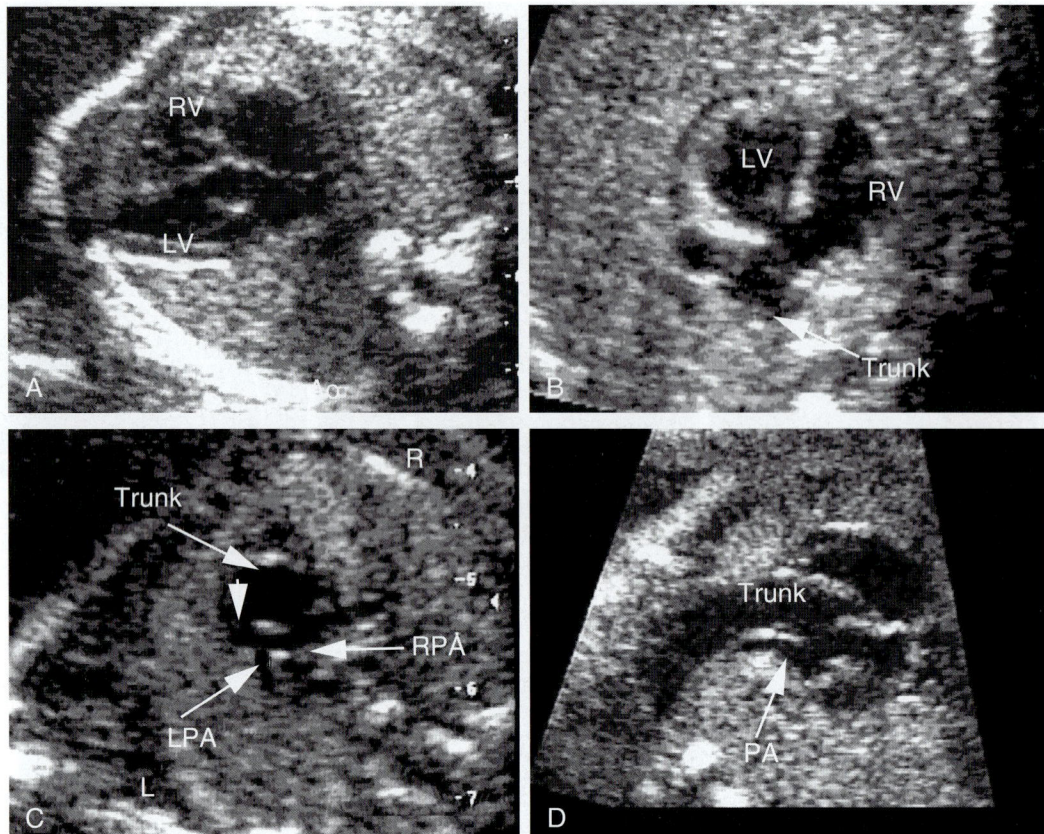

FIG. 36.44 **Truncus arteriosus.** (A) The four-chamber view may not be so abnormal in truncus arteriosus, other than the leftward axis. (B) Sweeping toward the outflow tract, only a single semilunar valve can be demonstrated, which overrides the ventricular septal defect. (C) Three-vessel view reveals one very large great artery, the trunk from which both brachiocephalic arteries and the main and branch pulmonary arteries (LPA and RPA) arise. (D) Communication between the trunk and pulmonary artery is demonstrated with an arrow. The pulmonary artery (PA) arises from the posterior or leftward aspect of the trunk.

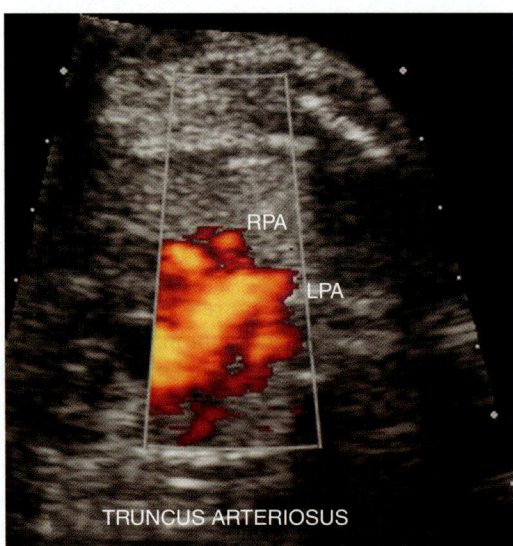

FIG. 36.45 Color Doppler of a fetal echocardiogram showing truncus arteriosus and the bifurcation of the pulmonary artery. *LPA*, Left pulmonary artery; *RPA*, right pulmonary artery.

the ductus arteriosus is patent, so some of the blood may flow into the arch during fetal life (see Fig. 36.46C). Once the fetus is delivered and the ductus closes, however, the narrowed portion of the arch becomes evident.

Interrupted Aortic Arch

Interruption of the aortic arch is characterized by complete anatomic interruption of the arch or, rarely, by an atretic fibrous remnant connecting the proximal arch with the descending aorta. The interruption occurs at one of three sites:

1. Distal to the left common carotid artery so that the left subclavian artery originates from the descending aorta
2. Just beyond the left subclavian so that all the brachiocephalic arteries arise from the arch and none from the descending aorta
3. Distal to the innominate artery so that the left common carotid and left subclavian arteries originate from the descending aorta

The descending aorta is really a continuation of the main pulmonary artery via the patent ductus. A ventricular septal defect is almost always present. After birth, these three items make a distinct congenital triad: interruption of the aortic arch, patent ductus arteriosus, and ventricular septal defect. In this condition, the conal septum is posteriorly deviated, thus restricting flow through the aortic outflow tract. A large, more subpulmonary ventricular septal defect, with or without true override of the main pulmonary artery, is the first clue to its diagnosis. A significant size discrepancy between

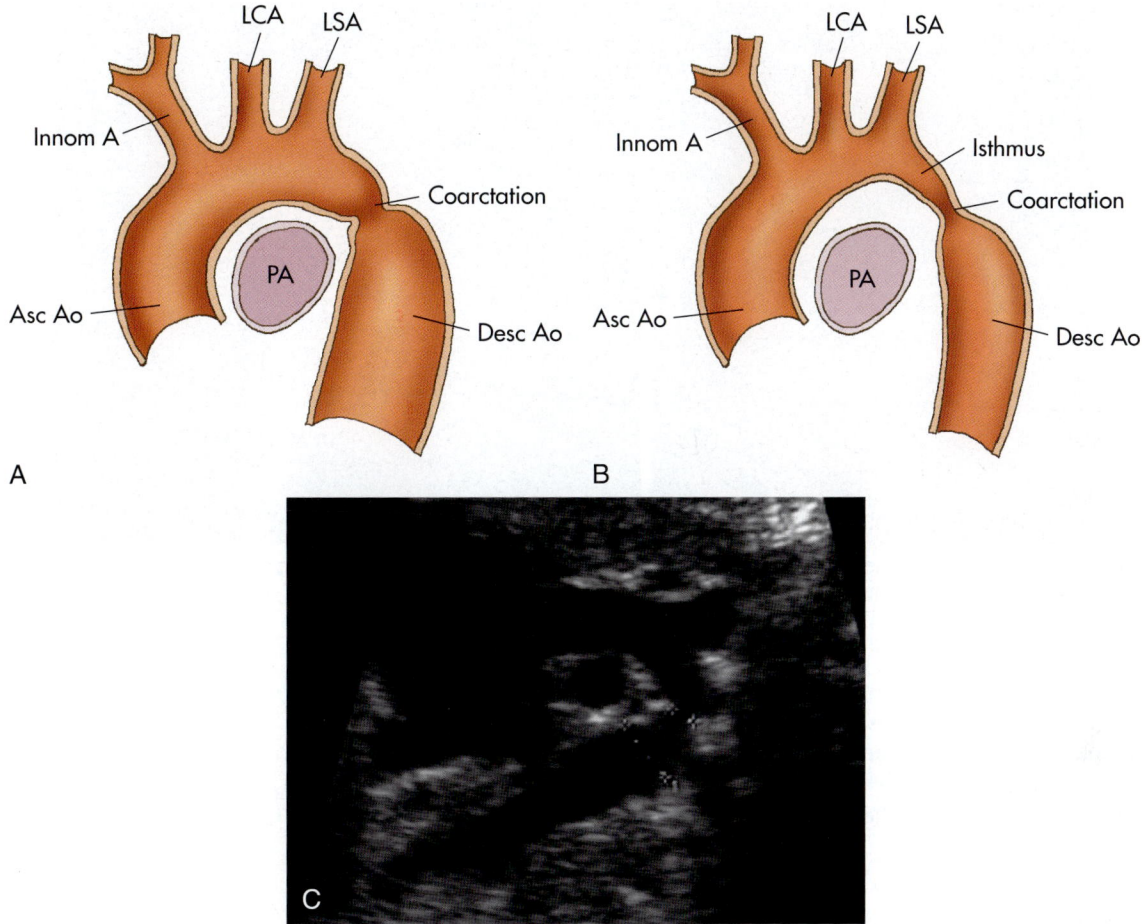

FIG. 36.46 Coarctation of the aorta occurs just inferior to the insertion of the left subclavian artery (LSA). (A) The coarctation may be discrete, with mild poststenotic dilation in the fetus. This narrowing usually is near the point of ductal insertion. (B) A long segment narrowing of the isthmus is more likely to be found by echocardiography. (C) A discrete narrowing was found in this 32-week fetus. Long-axis view of the aortic arch shows the narrowing at the level of the left subclavian artery. *Asc Ao*, Ascending aorta; *Innom A*, innominate artery; *LCA*, left carotid artery.

the greater arteries is apparent, with the main pulmonary artery appearing larger than the aorta.

The interruption of the aortic arch also tends to occur with a bicuspid or deformed aortic valve, subaortic stenosis, biventricular origin of the pulmonary trunk, or anomalous origin of the major branches of the ascending aorta.

Ductal Constriction

Ductal constriction occurs when flow is diverted from the ductus secondary to tricuspid or pulmonary atresia or secondary to maternal medications (indomethacin therapy) given to stop early contractions. In the normal fetus, the ductus arteriosus transmits about 55% to 60% of combined ventricular output from the pulmonary artery to the aorta. It joins the aorta at an obtuse inferior angle, presumably because flow is directed down to the descending aorta. If aortic atresia or aortic isthmus interruption were present, a much larger proportion of the output would have to flow through the ductus to maintain ventricular output; in fact, in aortic atresia, the total output—excluding pulmonary flow—would cross the ductus. Thus about 90% of combined ventricular output would be carried by the ductus, which could be considerably wider than normal (no change in Doppler velocities at the ductus).

In tricuspid or pulmonary atresia, no blood would be ejected from the right ventricle into the pulmonary artery. The flow through the ductus would occur from the aorta to the pulmonary arteries. Because this normally represents only about 10% of the combined ventricular output, the ductus may be quite narrow and underdeveloped (with high-velocity Doppler recordings at the level of the ductus). Furthermore, because flow is from the aorta to the pulmonary artery, the connection of the ductus with the aorta has an acute inferior angle.

The primary signs of ductal constriction include right atrial and ventricular dilation, right ventricular dysfunction, and pulmonary and tricuspid insufficiency. The Doppler flow pattern at the ductus increases in systolic and diastolic velocities. The diastolic velocity may reach peak velocities of greater than 30 cm/sec, and there is continuous flow in diastole rather than the more pulsatile flow as seen in the normal ductus arteriosus. Heart failure may develop if the ductal constriction is not reversed by discontinuing maternal oral therapy or through delivery of the infant. Ductal constriction can result in neonatal primary pulmonary hypertension.

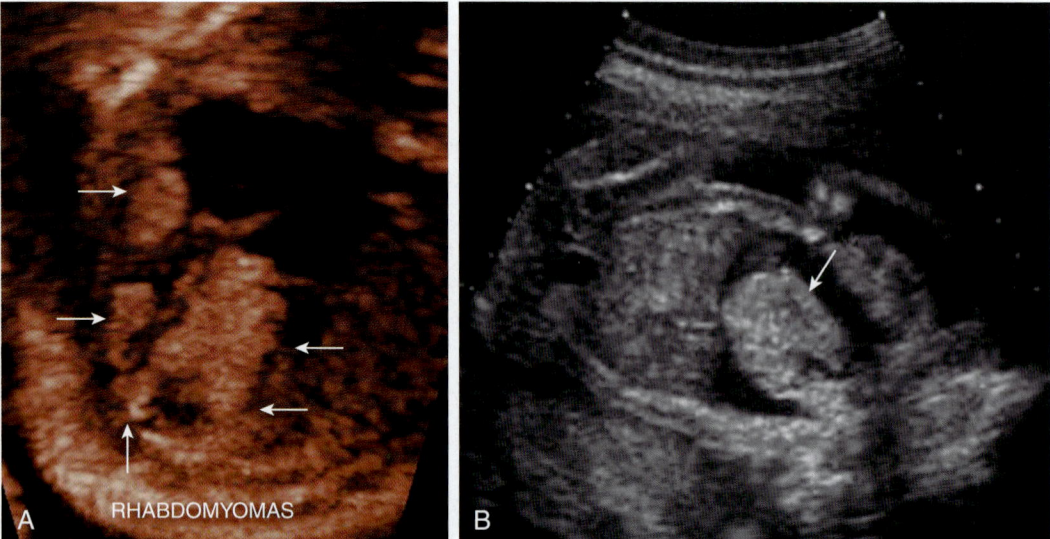

FIG. 36.47 (A) Four-chamber view of a fetus with a huge rhabdomyoma *(arrows)* completely filling the left ventricular cavity. (B) Long-axis view of the fetal heart with a huge teratoma *(arrow)*.

CARDIAC TUMORS

Cardiac tumors are very unusual. Most of these tumors are benign and isolated. The most common tumors are rhabdomyoma (58%) and teratoma (20%), followed by fibroma, myxoma, hemangioma, and mesothelioma. Less than 10% of cardiac tumors are malignant.

Rhabdomyomas

Rhabdomyomas tend to be multiple and involve the septum. This tumor is associated with tuberous sclerosis (50% to 86%). The fetus becomes symptomatic when the tumor is large and causes obstruction to the outflow tract, leading to congestive heart failure, pericardial effusion, hydrops, and death. The prognosis depends on the size of the tumor, its location, and its histologic type.

Sonographic Findings. If this mass is suspected, the sonographer should also look for associated tumor mass abnormalities in the kidneys and fetal head. The teratoma may be intrapericardial and extracardiac. The fibroma tumors account for 12% of all cardiac tumors in the neonate. This tumor is pedunculated and may calcify. The fetal echocardiogram shows the tumor best in the four-chamber view (Fig. 36.47). Close analysis should be made to search for regurgitation and obstruction. The right and left ventricular outflow tracts should be carefully studied with Doppler to record velocities in the subvalvular and supravalvular areas. Serial evaluation may be made with fetal echocardiography to follow the ventricular function and Doppler flow patterns.

COMPLEX CARDIAC ABNORMALITIES

Single Ventricle

Single ventricle is a congenital anomaly in which there are two atria but only one ventricular chamber, which receives

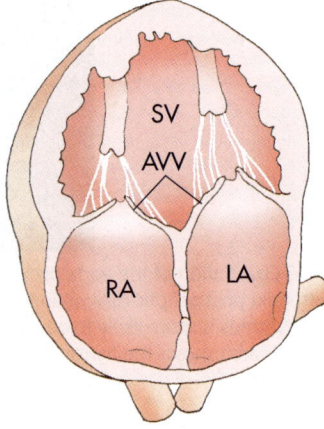

FIG. 36.48 Apical view shows a single inflow cavity (single ventricle [SV]). Two atrial cavities and atrioventricular valves (AVV) are present. *LA,* Left atrium; *RA,* right atrium.

both the mitral and tricuspid valves (Fig. 36.48). Both valves are patent, so mitral and tricuspid atresia can be excluded. (Occasionally, the mitral and tricuspid valves join to form a common atrioventricular valve.)

Sonographic Findings. The most common form of a single ventricle heart is a morphologic left ventricle with a small outlet chamber that represents the infundibular portion of the right ventricle. The right or left atrioventricular connection may be absent, and the great arteries may be transposed, with the aorta arising above the small outlet chamber. If transposition is present, the pulmonary artery lies posterior to the aorta. The infundibulum lies at the base of the ventricle, communicating with the aorta above and the single ventricle below. If the great vessels are normal, the infundibulum communicates with the pulmonary trunk. The outlet chambers may be left-side and anterior or right-side and anterior, but they commonly lie high on the cardiac silhouette. Pulmonary stenosis may or may not coexist.

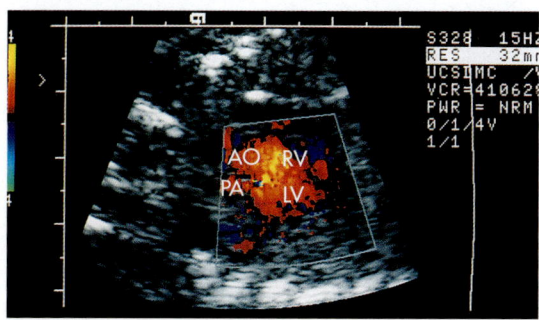

FIG. 36.49 Color flow image demonstrates complete filling of the essentially single ventricle in a patient with transposition of the great arteries and a huge ventricular septal defect. *AO*, Aorta; *LV*, left ventricle; *PA*, pulmonary artery; *RV*, right ventricle.

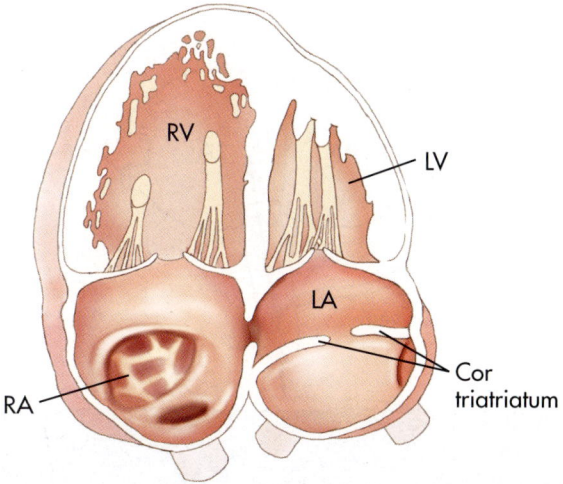

FIG. 36.50 **Cor triatriatum.** Four-chamber view of the heart shows the pulmonary veins draining into a segment of the left atrial cavity, separated from the mitral inflow by the subdividing membrane. The amount of obstruction into the left ventricle will depend on how tight the orifice of the cor triatriatum is.

If present, the pulmonary stenosis is usually valvular or subvalvular. The pulmonary trunk is usually slightly smaller than the aortic trunk.

The four-chamber view is the most useful window in delineating the cardiac anatomy (Fig. 36.49). The prominent papillary muscles should not be confused with the interventricular septum. In a single ventricle, the papillary muscles may be quite prominent. With careful transducer angulation, the chordal structures may be traced to these structures for correct delineation. The right ventricle may be just a slitlike cavity, as seen on the apical four-chamber view. The position of the great arteries should be assessed, and the aorta and pulmonary arteries should be delineated clearly. Regurgitant jets may be associated with abnormal chordal connections of the atrioventricular valves. Doppler evaluation of these valves is useful in depicting any regurgitation present. Color flow imaging is especially useful in outlining the direction of jet flow for proper Doppler evaluation.

Cor Triatriatum

Cor triatriatum occurs when the left atrial cavity is partitioned into two compartments. This anomaly is characterized by drainage of the pulmonary veins into an accessory left atrial chamber that lies proximal to the true left atrium (Fig. 36.50). The accessory chamber is believed to represent the dilated common pulmonary vein of the embryo. (This lesion has also been called stenosis of the common pulmonary vein.) The distal compartment communicates with the mitral valve and contains the left atrial appendage and usually the fossa ovalis. The fibrous or fibromuscular diaphragm that partitions the left atrium possesses one or more openings, and the size of these openings determines the degree of left atrial obstruction.

Congenital Vena Cava to Left Atrial Communication

Isolated connection of the superior or inferior vena cava to the left atrium is a rare congenital malformation. The left atrium occasionally receives other systemic veins, such as the coronary sinus, the azygous vein, or the hepatic vein.

Inferior Vena Cava. When the inferior vena cava communicates with the left atrium, the vessel usually has a normal abdominal course and penetrates the diaphragm at the expected site. An enlarged azygous vein may arise from the anomalous inferior cava and ultimately communicate with the right atrium (Fig. 36.51). Normally the azygous vein begins as a branch of the inferior vena cava, then proceeds upward through the aortic hiatus of the diaphragm, passes along the right side of the vertebral column, and finally arches forward to enter the superior vena cava. An enlarged azygous system can serve an important function as a conveyor of inferior vena caval blood to the right atrium even though the inferior cava itself communicates with the left atrium. Occasionally the inferior vena cava is absent, and infradiaphragmatic blood reaches the right atrium entirely via the azygous system.

Superior Vena Cava. Congenital abnormalities of the superior vena cava generally fall into two categories: anomalies of position and anomalies of drainage (Fig. 36.52). Anomalies of position, especially persistent left superior vena cava, are more frequent than those of drainage. A left superior vena cava itself causes no physiologic disturbance because it harmlessly drains into the right atrium via the coronary sinus. However, a persistent left superior vena cava assumes particular significance when it communicates with the left atrium. It also follows that when a superior vena cava drains into the left atrium, the anomalously draining vessel is likely to be a persistent left cava. A right superior vena cava usually coexists and enters the right atrium in normal fashion.

When two superior cavas are present, the right and left may be completely separate from each other or may be joined by means of an innominate vein. This innominate bridge can be widely patent, small, or atretic.

The intracardiac defects that may accompany caval drainage into the left atrium include atrial or ventricular septal defects, single atrium or ventricle, tetralogy of Fallot, transposition of the great vessels, and complex positional anomalies

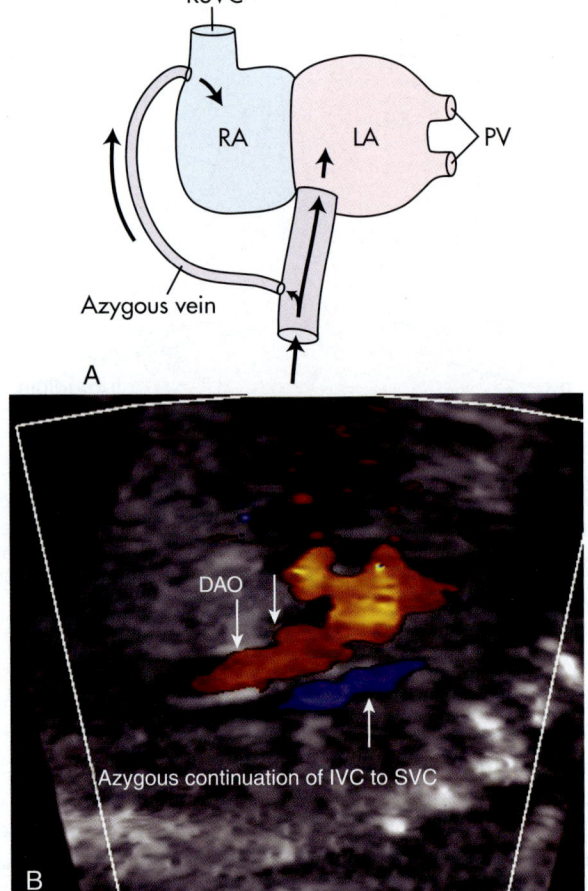

FIG. 36.51 (A) The inferior vena cava (IVC) communicates directly with the left atrium (LA). An enlarged azygous vein arises from the anomalous IVC and communicates with the right atrium (RA) via a normal right superior vena cava (RSVC). Inferior caval blood flows directly into the LA *(large arrow)*; a portion of the IVC blood is diverted through the azygous vein into the RSVC and right heart *(small arrow)*. (B) Sagittal view of the azygous continuation of the inferior vena cava (IVC) to the superior vena cava (SVC). *DAO*, Descending aorta; *PV*, pulmonary veins.

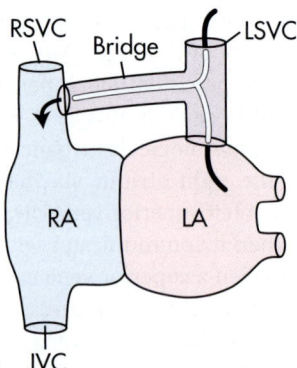

FIG. 36.52 Persistent left superior vena cava (LSVC) communicating with the left atrium (LA). The size of the bridge may vary; when very small, the LSVC blood flows entirely into the LA. *IVC*, Inferior vena cava; *RA*, right atrium; *RSVC*, right superior vena cava.

of the heart. The extracardiac anomalies that have been associated with this condition include coarctation of the aorta, pulmonary arteriovenous fistula, and inferior vena cava malformations.

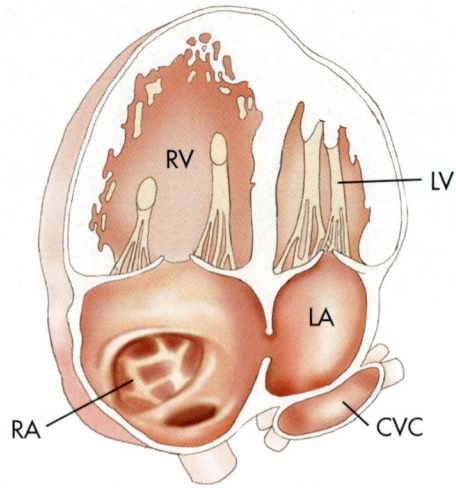

FIG. 36.53 Four-chamber view of the heart showing total anomalous pulmonary venous return. In this view, the veins are shown to enter the anomalous common venous chamber (CVC) superior to the left atrial cavity (LA). *LV*, Left ventricle; *RA*, right atrium; *RV*, right ventricle.

Total Anomalous Pulmonary Venous Return

The four pulmonary veins normally return blood into the left atrium from the lungs. When this fails to occur, the condition is termed **total anomalous pulmonary venous return (TAPVR)**. The venous return may be totally into the right atrium or into a "common chamber" posterior to the left atrium, into the superior or inferior vena cava, or into the left subclavian vein, azygous vein, or portal vein. The venous drainage may be total or partial (Fig. 36.53).

Sonographic Findings. In the fetus, TAPVR may not be evident unless the pulmonary veins are carefully recorded. The sonographer may image an enlarged right atrial cavity with the atrial septum bulging into the small left atrium. The normal pulmonary veins are seen on the four-chamber view (Fig. 36.54). The right upper vein is seen near the base of the heart at the level of the septum secundum, the left upper vein is seen at the lateral atrial wall near the base of the heart, and the left lower vein is seen just above the atrioventricular junction, along the lateral atrial wall. The right lower vein is not routinely imaged in a four-chamber view. Color Doppler imaging may help identify these venous structures.

TAPVR should be suspected in all cases of AVSDs and in asplenia and polysplenia syndromes. The prognosis is poor, with 75% dying within the first year after birth if no surgery is performed. Reconstruction of the pulmonary venous drainage into the left atrium has shown promising survival results.

Cardiosplenic Syndromes

Cardiosplenic syndromes are sporadic disorders characterized by a symmetric development of normally asymmetric organs or organ systems. The cardiosplenic syndromes are subdivided into asplenia and polysplenia syndromes. These two conditions are characterized by lack of the normal asymmetry of the visceral organs. The trunk tends to have

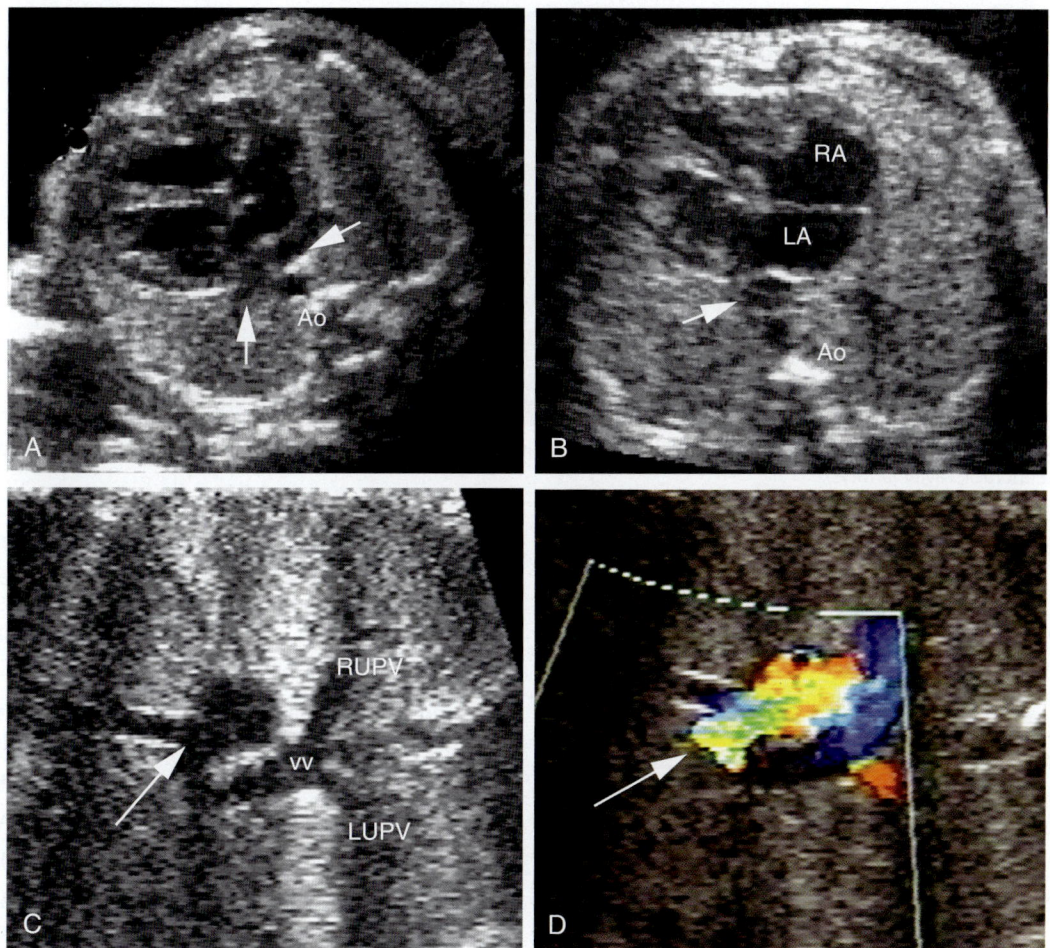

FIG. 36.54 **Total anomalous pulmonary venous return connection.** Anomalous pulmonary veins connected to a confluence, which joined a vertical vein, ultimately draining into the inferior vena cava near the ductus venosus. (A) Pulmonary vein connection *(arrows)* with the confluence that sits just in front of the descending aorta (Ao) behind the left atrium (LA) in part B clearly demonstrates the confluence, the presence of which results in a gap between the posterior wall of the left atrium and the descending aorta, which normally is minimal. (C) Pulmonary vein confluence then joins a vertical vein (vv) that ultimately connects below the diaphragm *(arrow)*. The left upper pulmonary vein (LUPV) and right upper pulmonary vein (RUPV) connection to the confluence can be seen. (D) Color Doppler confirms the direction of flow and presence of obstruction where the vertical vein connects with the inferior vena cava *(arrow)*.

two halves that are mirror images of one another. Generally speaking, asplenia is a condition of bilateral right-sidedness, and polysplenia is bilateral left-sidedness.

In a fetus with asplenia, the following anomalies have been seen: the spleen is absent; the lungs are bilaterally trilobed with morphologic right bronchi on both sides; the liver is central; the stomach may be right, left, or central; the gut is malrotated; the superior vena cava is bilateral; the inferior vena cava lies to the right or left of the spine; and the aorta and cava are seen on the same side of the spine (instead of the aorta on the left and the cava on the right). Asplenia syndrome is twice as common in males.

There is a high association between asplenia and congenital heart disease. TAPVR is seen in nearly all patients, AVSD in 85%, single ventricle in 51%, transposition of the great arteries in 58%, and pulmonary stenosis or atresia in 70%. In less than half of asplenic patients, dextrocardia is present.

Polysplenia syndrome is characterized by two or more spleens on both sides of the mesogastrium. Bilateral morphologic left lungs and bronchi are found in 68% of patients. The liver and stomach are on the right or left, malrotation of the bowel is found in 80%, bilateral superior vena cava is seen in half the fetuses, and the inferior vena cava is absent in 70% (blood is drained by the azygous vein, which may be on the right or left).

Cardiac malformations are frequent but not as common as with asplenia. The most common lesions found are TAPVR (70%), dextrocardia, atrial septal defect, AVSD, transposition of the great arteries, and double-outlet right ventricle.

The prognosis of this disease depends on the severity of the cardiac lesion. Surgical intervention has increased the survival rate.

Sonographic Findings. The recognition of the cardiosplenic syndrome relies on the demonstration of both the abnormal relationship between the abdominal organs and the associated cardiac deformities. The abdominal situs must be determined clearly—with the stomach on the left, heart apex on the left, aorta on the left, and inferior vena on the right—to rule out a cardiosplenic syndrome.

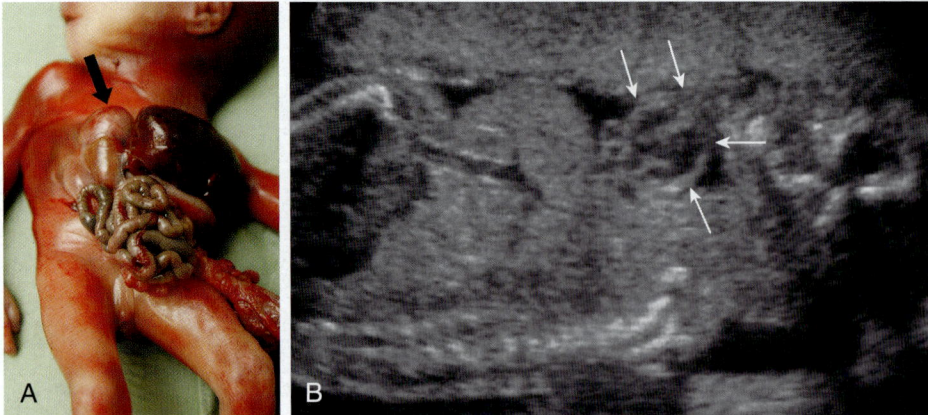

FIG. 36.55 (A) A fetus with pentalogy of Cantrell (multiple midline defects), including ectopia cordis. (B) The heart was completely outside the thoracic cavity *(arrows)*.

Ectopia Cordis

Ectopia cordis is a heart lesion that results from abnormal development of the primitive heart outside the embryonic disk in the early stage of development (Fig. 36.55).

Associated anomalies include facial and skeletal deformities, ventral wall defects, and central nervous system malformations (meningocele and cephalocele). Cardiac anomalies include tetralogy of Fallot and transposition of the great arteries. The prognosis is poor for this fetus.

DYSRHYTHMIAS

The fetal heart undergoes multiple changes during the embryologic stages. One of these stages is the progression of the cardiac electrical system, which matures to cause a normal sinus rhythm in the cardiac cycle. It is not uncommon during the course of a fetal echocardiogram to see the normal fetal heart rate decelerate from 150 beats/min to a bradycardia stage (under 55 beats/min), or even to pause for a few seconds. This may happen if the baby is lying on the umbilical cord or if the transducer pressure is too great. The fetus should be given a recovery time to bring the heart rate to a normal sinus rhythm. This is usually done by changing the position of the mother or releasing the pressure from the transducer.

Other changes in rhythm patterns seen during fetal development are listed in Table 36.2 and may result from premature atrial and ventricular contractions, supraventricular tachycardia, tachycardia, or atrioventricular block (Fig. 36.56).

Ectopy

Premature Atrial and Ventricular Contractions. Electrical impulses generated outside the cardiac pacemaker (sinus node) can cause **premature atrial contractions (PACs)** or **premature ventricular contractions (PVCs)**. The sinus node is located along the lateral right atrial wall. It is not clearly understood why some patients develop these ectopic premature contractions. Some investigators have tried to link them to increased amounts of caffeine, alcohol, or smoking, but none of our patients with PACs has these associations. An increased

TABLE 36.2	Sonographic Pitfalls for Arrhythmias	
Heart Rate (Beats/Min)	**Rhythm**	**Features: Atrial to Ventricular Association**
40–60	Complete heart block	A-V dissociation
60–90	Atrial bigeminy	Every other atrial impulse blocked
80–110	Sinus bradycardia	Normal A-V conduction
105–185	Normal sinus rhythm	Normal A-V conduction
180–210	Sinus tachycardia	Normal A-V conduction
150–220	Ventricular tachycardia	A-V dissociation or 1:1 V-A conduction
180	SVT (ectopic)	1:1 A-V conduction, incessant
220–260	SVT (reentrant)	A-V conduction with sudden onset and cessation
150–600	Atrial flutter	1:1 A-V conduction or 2:1, 3:1, 4:1 A-V block
Any rate	Ectopy or blocked atrial PVCs	Frequent or occasional PACs conducted

A-V, Atrioventricular; *PACs*, premature atrial contractions; *PVCs*, premature ventricular contractions; *SVT*, supraventricular tachycardia.

redundancy of the flap of the foramen ovale has been noted in these patients. The flap is larger than seen in the normal fetus and appears to swing with a great excursion from the left atrium into the right atrial cavity, touching the right atrial node.

The patient is usually referred for a fetal cardiac arrhythmia as heard on the routine obstetric examination by Doptone or auscultation. These techniques provide information about the ventricular rate only. To adequately assess the fetal rhythm, the ventricular and atrial rates must be analyzed simultaneously.

The atrium and ventricle may both experience extrasystoles and ectopic beats to give rise to complex echo patterns. The PACs may either be conducted to the ventricles or blocked, depending on the moment in which they occur in the cardiac cycle. Repeated PACs may lead to an increased or decreased

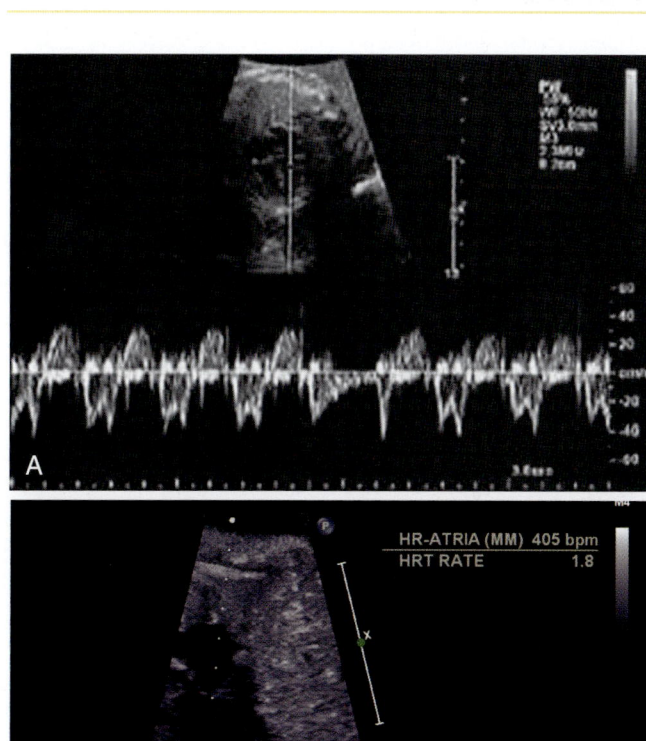

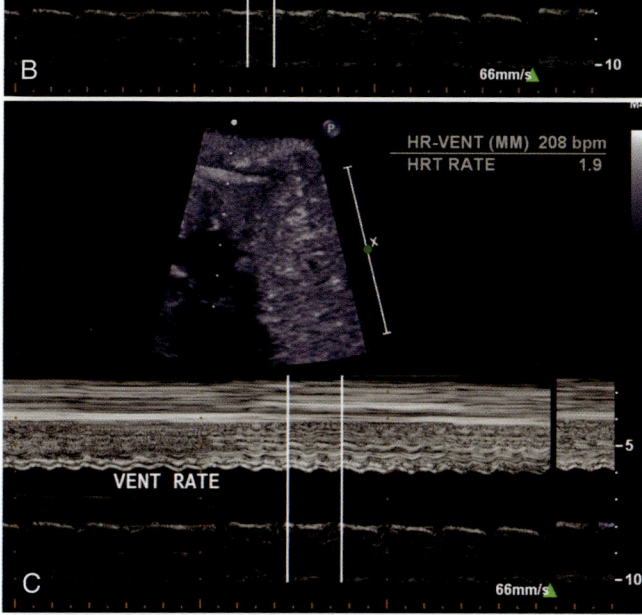

FIG. 36.56 **Fetus with premature atrial contractions.** The fetus had normal cardiac anatomy.

ventricular rate. A blocked PAC must be differentiated from an atrioventricular block. This distinction relies on the demonstration of an atrial contraction that appears prematurely. PVCs are characterized by a PVC that is not preceded by an atrial contraction.

Sonographic Findings. The sonographer can help sort out the rhythm with M-mode or Doppler. To record the atrial and ventricular rates simultaneously, the four-chamber heart must be perpendicular to the transducer (see Fig. 36.56A). The beam must dissect the ventricle and atria of the heart. It does not matter if the right or left side of the heart is more anterior. The best area to record atrial motion is usually just superior to the atrioventricular junction along the lateral wall of the atria. The atrial pattern appears to move with a box type of motion. The ventricular rate is best recorded at the level of the atrioventricular valve and is seen to move as a smooth, uniform, well-defined pattern.

The parasternal short-axis view may be used if the sonographer cannot obtain adequate images from the four-chamber view. The beam should be directed through the right atrial wall, aortic cusps, or the left atrial wall and aortic cusps. As the aorta moves in an anterior direction, the aortic cusps open in systole and close in diastole. Thus the aortic leaflets may signify the ventricular systolic event, whereas the atrial wall signifies the atrial event.

The M-mode should be expanded to its full extent to clearly see the movement of the atrial and ventricular walls. Changes in the atrioventricular valve patterns are also noted in patients with arrhythmias. Doppler imaging of the atrioventricular valves demonstrates whether regurgitation is present during the disturbance in rhythm.

Patients with PACs and PVCs are assured that this development is a normal, benign condition resulting from the immaturity of the heart's electrical conduction system. This pattern is not associated with other cardiac anomalies.

Supraventricular Tachyarrhythmia

Supraventricular tachyarrhythmias include abnormal rhythms above 200 beats/min, with a conduction rate of 1:1. These rhythm disturbances may be paroxysmal supraventricular tachycardia, paroxysmal atrial tachycardia, atrial flutter, or atrial fibrillation. The atrial rate is recorded at 300 to 460 beats/min in atrial flutter with a normal ventricular rate. Atrial fibrillation shows the atria to beat at more than 400 beats/min, with a ventricular rate of 120 to 200 beats/min.

Supraventricular tachycardia occurs by automaticity or reentry mechanisms. In cases of automatic induced tachyarrhythmias, an irritable ectopic focus discharges at a high frequency. The reentry mechanism consists of an electrical impulse reentering the atria, giving rise to repeated electrical activity. Reentry may occur at the level of the sinoatrial node, inside the atrium, at the atrioventricular node, and in the His-Purkinje system. Reentry may also occur along an anomalous atrioventricular connection, such as the Kent bundle in Wolff-Parkinson-White (WPW) syndrome.

Supraventricular tachycardia is the most frequent arrhythmia caused by atrioventricular nodal reentry, occurring in 1 in 25,000 births. Viral infections or hypoplasia of the sinoatrial tract may trigger supraventricular tachycardia.

Sonographic Findings. The finding of supraventricular tachycardia in a fetus is an emergency situation. The fetus should be scanned immediately to assess signs of heart rate, ventricular and atrial size, amount of regurgitation present, ventricular function, and presence of pericardial effusion and

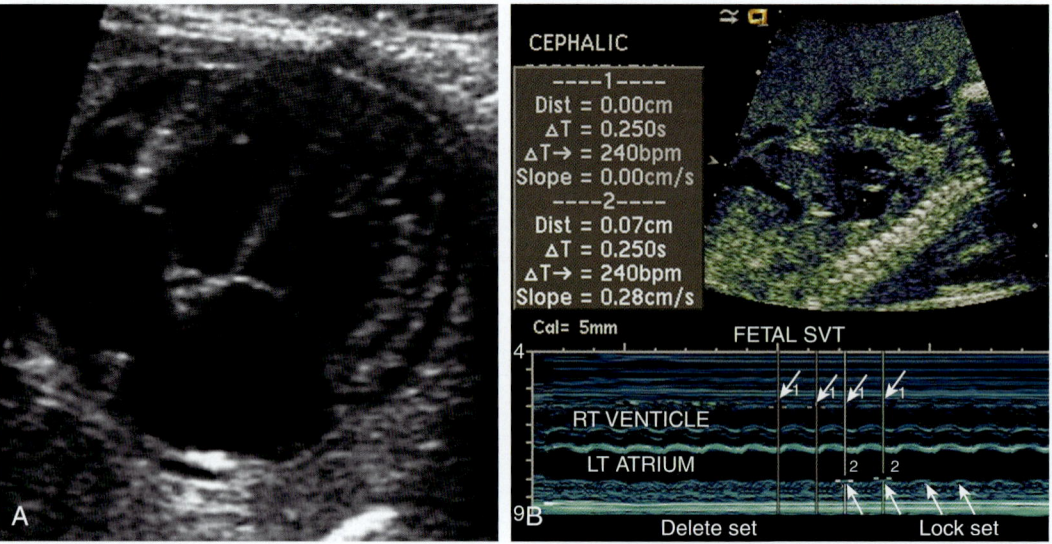

FIG. 36.57 (A) Pericardial effusion (pe) may be present if the arrhythmia is significant (i.e., supraventricular tachycardia). The fetus cannot withstand rapid changes in cardiac activity without developing signs of heart failure. (B) Fetus with supraventricular tachycardia showed normal conduction with a heart rate of more than 240 beats/min. SVT, Supraventricular tachycardia.

hydrops (Fig. 36.57). With supraventricular tachycardia, the fetus develops suboptimal filling of the ventricles, decreased cardiac output, and right ventricular volume overload leading to subsequent congestive heart failure.

Other cardiac anomalies associated with supraventricular tachycardia are atrial septal defects, mitral valve disease, cardiac tumors, and WPW syndrome.

Atrial flutter and fibrillation often alternate and are thought to result from a mechanism similar to that found in supraventricular tachycardia. Atrial flutter and fibrillation have been described in patients with WPW syndrome, cardiomyopathies, and thyrotoxicosis.

The fetus with this arrhythmia is usually admitted to the hospital and medically treated with antiarrhythmic drugs to control the ventricular rate, to convert the rate into normal sinus rhythm. Fetal echocardiography may be clinically useful in monitoring these patients' recovery.

Atrioventricular Block

When the electrical impulse transmission from the atria to the ventricles is blocked, the condition is called an **atrioventricular block**. Normally the atria fill in ventricular diastole and empty in ventricular systole. Just before ventricular systole occurs, the pressure in the atria is at its peak. (This corresponds to the P wave on the electrocardiogram.) The QRS complex signifies the onset of ventricular systole, causing the pressure from the atria to open the atrioventricular valves so the left ventricle may fill. If this electrical process is blocked, the blood remains in the atria and does not cause the atrioventricular valves to open so blood can fill the ventricular cavities. This condition may be attributed to immaturity of the conduction system, absence of connection to the atrioventricular node, or an abnormal anatomic position of the atrioventricular node. The fetus may have a first-, second-, or third-degree heart block.

The fetus with a third-degree atrioventricular block has been found to have associated structural anomalies, including

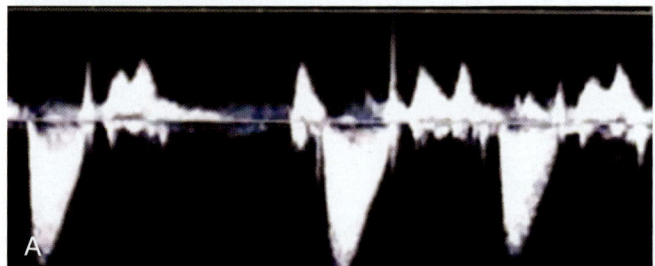
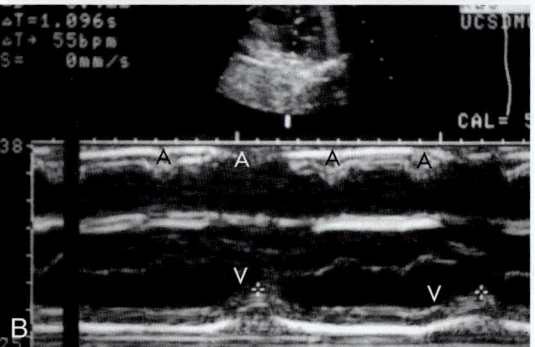

FIG. 36.58 (A) Doppler of the fetal heart rhythm demonstrates heart block. (B) Mother with systemic lupus erythematosus presented at 20 weeks of gestation because of a "slow heart rate." The fetus was in 2:1 heart block with the atria beating twice as fast as the ventricle; every other beat was conducted. A, Atrium; V, ventricle.

corrected transposition, univentricular heart, cardiac tumors, and cardiomyopathies. Patients with a connective tissue disorder, such as lupus erythematosus, have also been found to develop heart block.

First- and second-degree atrioventricular blocks are not associated with any significant hemodynamic disturbance. A complete heart block may result in bradycardia, leading to decreased cardiac output and congestive heart failure during fetal life.

Sonographic Findings. The fetal M-mode echocardiogram should be performed after the normal anatomic cardiac anatomy has been demonstrated (Fig. 36.58). As described in the supraventricular tachycardia section, the four-chamber and parasternal short-axis views are best used to record atrial and ventricular events simultaneously.

First-degree heart block is not seen in the fetus, as the heart rate and rhythm are normal. A normal atrial impulse blockage can be diagnosed by demonstrating a normally timed atrial contraction that is not followed by a ventricular contraction.

Second- and third-degree heart blocks are defined by observing the relationship between the atrial and ventricular rates. In second-degree Mobitz type I block, only a few atrial impulses are not conducted; in Mobitz type II block, a submultiple of atrial impulses is transmitted. In complete heart block, atrial and ventricular rates are independent of each other, with the atrial rate slower. The fetus becomes symptomatic when the cardiac output is decreased, and congestive heart failure develops.

Key Pearls

- The most common types of congenital heart disease are the ventricular septal defect, atrial septal defects, and pulmonary stenosis.
- A simple acronym (CHRISTMAS) will assist the sonographer in prenatal detection of congenital heart disease.
- The frequency of chromosomal abnormalities in infants with congenital heart disease is estimated as 5%–10% from postnatal data.
- The occurrence of associated extracardiac abnormalities in fetuses with cardiac defects and chromosomal abnormalities is on the order of 50% to 70%.
- In general, malformations of the right side of the heart are rarely associated with karyotypic abnormalities (e.g., pulmonic stenosis and tricuspid atresia).
- Abnormalities include atrioventricular septal defect, perimembranous ventricular septal defect, tetralogy of Fallot, double-outlet right ventricle, coarctation of the aorta, and hypoplastic left heart are often associated with chromosomal abnormalities.
- The incidence of cardiac defects in the fetus with trisomy is increased, with trisomy 21 showing the highest rate at 40% to 50%, Turner syndrome (trisomy 45,X) showing 25% to 40%, and more than 90% having cardiac defects with trisomies 13 and 18.
- Several cardiac abnormalities may be recognized with the four-chamber view alone, such as a large ventricular septal defect, atrioventricular septal defect, hypoplastic left or right heart, mitral or tricuspid atresia, Ebstein anomaly, and total anomalous pulmonary venous return.
- Anomalies of the great vessels and outlet lesions (transposition of the great arteries, truncus arteriosus, coarctation of the aorta, small outlet ventricular septal defect, and tetralogy of Fallot) need further investigation beyond the four-chamber view.
- When the heart is out of its normal position, several terms may be used to describe the exact position of the heart relative to location and position of the cardiac apex.
- The general prognosis for a fetus with evidence for a cardiomyopathy is poor. Serial fetal echoes are performed to monitor chamber size, regurgitation, and contractility.
- Pericardial effusion is an abnormal collection of fluid surrounding the epicardial layer of the heart.
- Atrial septal defects allow communication between the left atrium and right atrium.
- The perimembranous ventricular septal defect may be classified as membranous, aneurysmal, or supracristal.
- Ventricular septal defects may close with the formation of aneurysm tissue, which is commonly found along the right side of the septal defect.
- Small ventricular muscular defects are usually found in the neonatal stage and often close spontaneously.
- The failure of the endocardial cushion to fuse is termed an incomplete atrioventricular septal defect. This condition results in a membranous ventricular septal defect, abnormal tricuspid valve, primum atrial septal defect, and cleft mitral valve.
- A complete atrioventricular septal defect has a single, undivided, free-floating leaflet stretching across both ventricles.
- Atrioventricular septal defects are frequently associated with other cardiac defects, including truncoconal abnormalities, coarctation of the aorta, and pulmonary stenosis or atresia.
- Tricuspid atresia is the interruption of the growth of the tricuspid leaflet that begins early in cardiac embryology.
- Ebstein anomaly of the tricuspid valve is an abnormal displacement of the septal leaflet of the tricuspid valve toward the apex of the right ventricle.
- There are several forms of hypoplastic right heart syndrome: pulmonary atresia with an intact interventricular septum, pulmonary valve fusion with an intact interventricular septum and atrial septal defect, and pulmonary atresia with a normal aortic root diameter.
- Tetralogy of Fallot has four characteristics: (1) high, membranous ventricular septal defect; (2) large, anteriorly displaced aorta, which overrides the septal defect; (3) pulmonary stenosis; and (4) right ventricular hypertrophy.
- In pulmonic stenosis, the abnormal pulmonic cusps become thickened and domed during diastole.
- Mitral valve stenosis is usually associated with other forms of left-sided heart obstruction.
- In fetal life, the presence of mitral regurgitation is most commonly secondary to a cleft mitral valve (endocardial cushion defect) or a congenital mitral stenosis.
- If the development of the aortic valve is interrupted during the first trimester, the three aortic cusps may not fully separate, causing a unicusp or bicuspid leaflet.
- Aortic stenosis is an abnormal development of the cusps of the aortic valve that results in thickened and domed leaflets.
- Hypoplastic left heart syndrome is characterized by a small, hypertrophied left ventricle with aortic or mitral dysplasia or atresia.
- Transposition of the great arteries is an abnormal condition that exists when the aorta is connected to the right ventricle, and the pulmonary artery is connected to the left ventricle.

- Corrected transposition of the great arteries is a cardiac condition in which the right atrium and left atrium are connected to the morphologic left and right ventricle, respectively, and the great arteries are transposed.
- Truncus arteriosus is a complex congenital heart lesion in which only one great artery arises from the base of the heart.
- Coarctation of the aorta is a discrete shelflike lesion present in the isthmus of the arch or, more commonly, at the site of the ductal insertion near the left subclavian artery.
- Rhabdomyomas tend to be multiple and involve the septum and are associated with tuberous sclerosis.
- Single ventricle is a congenital anomaly in which there are two atria but only one ventricular chamber, which receives both the mitral and tricuspid valves.
- Cor triatriatum occurs when the left atrial cavity is partitioned into two compartments.
- Total anomalous pulmonary venous return may be totally into the right atrium or into a common chamber posterior to the left atrium, into the superior or inferior vena cava, or into the left subclavian vein, azygous vein, or portal vein.
- Ectopia cordis is a heart lesion that results from abnormal development of the primitive heart outside the embryonic disk in the early stage of development.
- Electrical impulses generated outside the cardiac pacemaker (sinus node) can cause premature atrial contractions or premature ventricular contractions.
- Supraventricular tachyarrhythmias include abnormal rhythms above 200 beats/min with a conduction rate of 1:1.
- When the electrical impulse transmission from the atria to the ventricles is blocked, the condition is called an atrioventricular block.

REFERENCES

1. Callen PC. *Ultrasonography in Obstetrics and Gynecology*. ed 4. Philadelphia: WB Saunders; 2000.
2. Silverman NH, Schmidt KG. Ventricular volume overload in the human fetus: observations from fetal echocardiography. *J Am Soc Echocardiogr*. 1990;3:20–29.

BIBLIOGRAPHY

Allen LD, Cook AC, Huggon IC. *Fetal Echocardiography: A Practical Guide*. New York: Cambridge University Press; 2009.

Beeby AR. Reproducibility of ultrasonic measurement of fetal cardiac haemodynamics. *Br J Obstet Gynaecol*. 1991;98:807.

Brand JM, Friedberg DZ. Spontaneous regression of a primary cardiac tumor presenting as fetal tachyarrhythmias. *J Perinatol*. 1992;12:48.

Callan NA, Maggio M, Steger S. Fetal echocardiography: indications for referral, prenatal diagnoses, and outcomes. *Am J Perinatol*. 1991;8:390.

Dolkart LA, Reimers FT. Transvaginal fetal echocardiography in early pregnancy: normative data. *Am J Obstet Gynecol*. 1991;165:688.

Feinstein JA, Benson DW, Dubin AM. Hypoplastic left heart syndrome: current considerations and expectations. *J Am Coll Cardiol*. 2012;59(1 suppl):S42.

Hornberg LK, Jaeggi ET, Trines J. The fetal heart. In: Rumack CW, Wilson SR, Charboneau JW, eds. *Diagnostic Ultrasound*. ed 3. St Louis: Elsevier; 2005.

Hornberger LK. Tricuspid valve disease with significant tricuspid insufficiency in the fetus: diagnosis and outcome. *J Am Coll Cardiol*. 1991;17:167.

Hornberger LK, Sanders SP, Rein AJ, et al. Left heart obstructive lesions and left ventricular growth in the midtrimester fetus: a longitudinal study. *Circulation*. 1995;92:1531–1538.

Kaltman J, Di H, Tian Z, et al. Impact of congenital heart disease on cerebrovascular blood flow dynamics in the fetus. *Ultrasound Obstet Gynecol*. 2005;25(1):32–36.

Moore KL, Persaud TVN. *The Developing Human: Clinically Oriented Embryology*. ed 8. Philadelphia: Elsevier; 2008.

Morris S, Ayres N, Espinoza J. *Sonographic evaluation of the fetal heart. Callen's Ultrasonography in Obstetrics and Gynecology*. ed 6. Philadelphia: Elsevier; 2017.

Perloff J. *The Clinical Recognition of Congenital Heart Disease*. ed 5. Philadelphia: Saunders; 2003.

Roberts DJ, Genest D. Cardiac histologic pathology characteristic of trisomies 13 and 21. *Hum Pathol*. 1992;23:1130.

Rychik J. Frontiers in fetal cardiovascular disease. *Pediatr Clin North Am*. 2004;51:6.

Rychik J, Tian T, Cohen MD, et al. Acute cardiovascular effects of fetal surgery in the human. *Circulation*. 2004;110:1549–1556.

van Velzen CL, Haak MC, Reijinders G. Prenatal detection of transposition of the great arteries reduces mortality and morbidity. *Ultrasound Obstet Gynecol*. 2015;45(3):320–325.

PART VI

Cerebrovascular

Chapter 37 Extracranial Cerebrovascular Evaluation
Chapter 38 Intracranial Cerebrovascular Evaluation
Chapter 39 Peripheral Arterial Evaluation
Chapter 40 Peripheral Venous Evaluation

CHAPTER 37

Extracranial Cerebrovascular Evaluation

Kevin R. Volz

OBJECTIVES

On completion of this chapter, you should be able to:
- List the risk factors, signs, and symptoms for stroke and carotid artery disease
- Distinguish normal from abnormal carotid anatomy
- Understand the physiology of the carotid arterial system
- Discuss the technical aspects of carotid duplex imaging
- Recognize pathology associated with the carotid anatomy
- Describe the sonographic findings associated with internal carotid artery disease, specifically stenosis and occlusion
- Discuss common errors associated with the interpretation of carotid duplex imaging examinations

OUTLINE

Anatomy for Extracranial Cerebrovascular Imaging 1070
  Aortic Arch 1070
  Common Carotid Artery 1070
  Internal Carotid Artery 1070
  External Carotid Artery 1070
  Vertebral Artery 1071
Extracranial Arterial Hemodynamics 1071
Carotid Disease and Stroke Risk Factors, Warning Signs, and Symptoms 1071

Technical Aspects of Carotid Duplex Imaging 1072
  Procedure 1073
  Normal Findings 1074
  Pathologic Findings 1076
Interpretation of Carotid Duplex Imaging 1079
Common Carotid Artery Disease Treatments 1082
Other Carotid Artery Imaging Modalities 1083

Other Carotid Duplex Imaging Applications and Emerging Techniques 1083
  Intraoperative Imaging 1083
  Carotid Duplex Imaging After Stent Placement or Endarterectomy 1083
  Three-Dimensional Carotid Duplex Imaging 1084

KEY TERMS

Amaurosis fugax
Aphasia
Ataxia
Bruit
Cerebrovascular accident (CVA)
Collateral pathway
Common carotid artery (CCA)

Diplopia
Dysarthria
Dysphagia
External carotid artery (ECA)
Hemianopsia
Hemiparesis
Innominate artery

Internal carotid artery (ICA)
Reversible ischemic neurologic deficit (RIND)
Syncope
Transient ischemic attack (TIA)
Vertebral artery
Vertigo

One of the most commonly ordered arterial vascular sonographic examinations is carotid duplex. Carotid duplex imaging is a noninvasive screening tool for atherosclerosis and prevention of stroke. A cerebrovascular accident, or stroke, is characterized by an interruption of blood flow to the brain (ischemic stroke) or by a ruptured intracranial blood vessel (intracranial hemorrhage). Approximately 85% of all strokes are ischemic; the remaining 15% are hemorrhagic. Stroke has an estimated prevalence of 2.5%, with 7 million reported in the United States, and often dramatically affects the life of an individual.[1] Stroke is a leading cause of serious long-term disability, and approximately 145,000 of the strokes that occur each year in the United States result in death.[1] The resulting financial burden is estimated to be $45.5 billion annually, comprised of direct costs (health care, rehabilitation, etc.) and indirect costs (missed work days, loss of productivity, etc.).[1]

Stroke is more prevalent among men, with risk increasing with age. Stroke is also almost twice as common in the black population than white, with the black, Hispanic, and native American populations all having an increased risk compared with the white population.[1] Because of the high prevalence and often fatal consequences, extracranial cerebrovascular ultrasound becomes an important imaging modality to identify disease that may be the potential cause of a stroke. Accurate and thorough imaging of the carotid artery is imperative, as prevention remains the best treatment for stroke.

ANATOMY FOR EXTRACRANIAL CEREBROVASCULAR IMAGING

Aortic Arch

The ascending aorta originates from the left ventricle of the heart. The transverse aortic arch lies in the superior mediastinum and is formed as the aorta ascends and curves posteroinferiorly from right to left, above the left mainstem bronchus. Three main arteries arise from the superior convexity of the arch in its normal configuration. The first branch is the innominate artery (brachiocephalic), the second is the left common carotid artery (CCA), followed by the left subclavian artery.

The **innominate artery** divides into the right CCA and the right subclavian artery, which gives rise to the right vertebral artery. The left CCA originates slightly to the left of the innominate artery, followed by the left subclavian artery, which likewise gives rise to the left vertebral artery.

Anatomic variants of the major arch vessels exist. The most common variant is the left CCA forming a common origin with or originating directly from the innominate artery, with an incidence of approximately 13%.[2] Less frequently, the left vertebral artery arises directly from the arch, the right subclavian artery originates from the arch distal to the left subclavian artery, the right CCA originates directly from the arch, and a left innominate artery may exist, from which the left common carotid and the left subclavian originate.[2]

Common Carotid Artery

The right and left **common carotid artery (CCA)** ascend through the superior mediastinum anterolaterally in the neck, located medial to the jugular vein (Fig. 37.1). The CCA usually measures between 6 and 8 mm in diameter. The left CCA is typically longer than the right, as it originates from the aortic arch. Bilaterally in the neck, the CCA, jugular vein, and vagus nerve are enclosed in a connective tissue called the *carotid sheath*. The vagus nerve lies between and dorsal to the artery and vein. The CCA typically does not have branches, but occasionally it is the origin of the superior thyroid artery. The CCA terminates at its bifurcation into the internal and external carotid arteries (ECAs). This occurs in the vicinity of the superior border of the thyroid cartilage at approximately C4; however, this level may be asymmetric and ranges from T2 to C1. At its bifurcation, the CCA has a slight dilation,

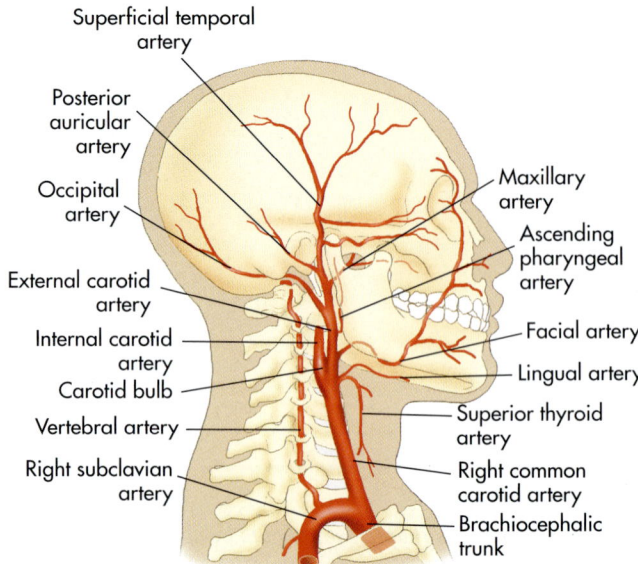

FIG. 37.1 The extracranial carotid system. During carotid duplex imaging, the area of focus is the common carotid bifurcation because of its propensity for atherosclerotic plaque formation.

known as the carotid bulb. The carotid bulb may include the distal CCA, the proximal internal, and the proximal ECAs.

Internal Carotid Artery

The **internal carotid artery (ICA)** originates at the CCA bifurcation and is usually the larger of the CCA terminal branches. It serves as the main conduit of perfusion to the brain. The ICA is divided into four main segments: cervical, petrous, cavernous, and cerebral. The cervical portion of the ICA is evaluated during carotid duplex imaging examinations. It begins at the CCA bifurcation (carotid bulb) and extends to the base of the skull. The ICA is located within the carotid sheath and travels deep to the sternocleidomastoid muscle. In the majority of individuals, the ICA is posterolateral to the ECA and courses medially as it ascends the neck. The cervical ICA usually does not have branches and measures between 5 and 6 mm in diameter. The first branch of the ICA is located in the cavernous portion, which cannot be visualized during an extracranial examination; however, it can be an important collateral in cases of cervical ICA obstruction. With advancing age and progressive disease, the cervical ICA may become tortuous, coiled, and/or kinked (Fig. 37.2). This may make visualization, vessel differentiation, and obtaining accurate Doppler signals difficult. Agenesis, or absence of the ICA, can occur, although it is rare. Agenesis of the ICA can be bilateral or unilateral, with a higher proportion of cases being unilateral.[3]

External Carotid Artery

The **external carotid artery (ECA)** originates at the CCA bifurcation. It is typically the smaller of the CCA terminal branches and perfuses the majority of the neck and face.

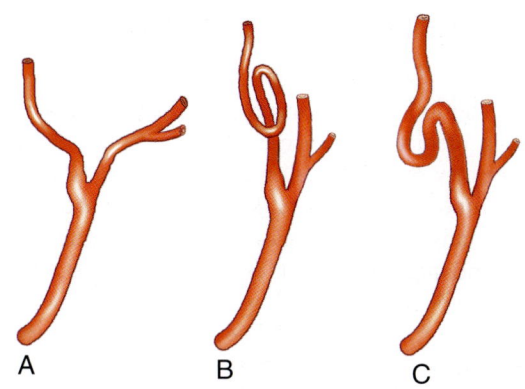

FIG. 37.2 Morphologic variations in the internal carotid artery. (A) Tortuosity: curving of the artery. (B) Coiling: a redundant curve. (C) Kinking: sharp and abrupt angulation.

It is located anteromedial to the ICA at its origin but courses posterolaterally as it ascends. In approximately 15% of the population, the ECA originates lateral to the ICA. This anatomic variation occurs three times more frequently on the right side. The normal ECA measures 3 to 4 mm in diameter.

There are eight named branches of the ECA (in ascending order): the superior thyroid, ascending pharyngeal, lingual, facial, occipital, posterior auricular, and terminal branches; the superficial temporal branch; and the internal maxillary branch. The first branch of the ECA, the superior thyroid artery is the most commonly visualized branch during carotid duplex imaging. The abundant number of anastomoses between the branches of the ECA and the intracranial circulation underscores the clinical significance of the ECA as a **collateral pathway** for cerebral perfusion when significant, flow-limiting disease is present in the ICA.

Vertebral Artery

The vertebral arteries are large branches of the subclavian arteries, with atherosclerotic changes usually occurring at their origin. Occasionally, the vertebral artery arises directly from the aortic arch (3% of cases on the left side and rarely on the right side).[2] The two vertebral arteries are asymmetric in size in about 75% of cases, with the left vertebral artery being the dominant artery. The **vertebral artery** can be divided into four segments: extravertebral, intervertebral, horizontal, and intracranial.

The extravertebral segment is evaluated during carotid duplex imaging. This segment courses superior and medial from its subclavicular origin and enters the transverse foramen of the sixth cervical vertebra. The proximal segment of the vertebral artery is approximately 4 to 5 cm in length and usually has no branches. The vertebral artery ascends within the transverse foramina of the upper cervical vertebrae (intervertebral segment), emerges from the transverse foramen of the atlas (horizontal segment), and becomes the intracranial portion as it pierces the spinal dura and arachnoid, just below the base of the skull at the foramen magnum. At this level, the right and left vertebral arteries combine to form the basilar artery.

EXTRACRANIAL ARTERIAL HEMODYNAMICS

The hemodynamics of arterial flow is governed by Poiseuille's law and is influenced by several factors, including vessel diameter, flow volume, vessel tortuosity, blood viscosity, and resistance. Resistance is determined by nature of the vascular bed arterial flow is perfusing. Arteries perfusing a dilated vascular bed (present on most organs) will have low resistive blood flow within them. Conversely, arteries supplying blood to a more constricted vascular bed, or arterioles, will maintain higher resistance.

The ICA and ECA are responsible for providing the majority of the head with oxygen- and nutrient-rich arterial blood. However, both have significantly different hemodynamic flow as a result of the different areas they perfuse. These hemodynamic characteristics must be understood to appropriately perform and interpret a carotid artery examination.

After originating from the CCA, the ICA typically travels deep toward the base of the skull. Once intracranial, the ICA branches form portions of the circle of Willis for neural perfusion. Because the brain requires a large amount of perfusion ~13% of systemic blood flow) the ICA tends to be larger than the ECA to account for the larger blood volume it transports. The ICA also maintains low-resistive arterial flow in the normal patient. This is in part due to its lack of extracranial branches, but more so a result of the low peripheral resistance placed upon it. Because of the brain's large blood volume requirement and its continual, adequate perfusion is critical, the vascular beds that perfuse it are of low resistance. This allows for constant perfusion throughout systole and diastole of the cardiac cycle. Similar to the ICA, the vertebral artery also contains low-resistive arterial flow, as it contributes a large portion of posterior neural circulation consisting of vascular beds applying minimal peripheral resistance.

Conversely, the ECA supplies blood to the majority of the neck, face, and scalp. These areas of the body require much less blood than an area such as the brain. Therefore, the capillary beds in these areas tend to be smaller and apply a higher amount of resistance. For this reason, coupled with its many extracranial branches, blood flow within the ECA is highly resistive, most evident by a reversal of flow component present during diastole.

CAROTID DISEASE AND STROKE RISK FACTORS, WARNING SIGNS, AND SYMPTOMS

Disease of the carotid arteries is caused by atherosclerotic plaque buildup along the vessel lumen. Continued plaque buildup causes vessel narrowing or occlusion in severe cases. When atherosclerotic plaque dislodges from the endothelium wall, it can propagate resulting in stroke, sudden vision loss, or a **transient ischemic attack (TIA)**. A TIA, often referred to as a *mini-stroke*, is an ischemic neurologic deficit lasting less than 24 hours.

Risk factors for carotid disease and stroke can be divided into two categories, those that are not modifiable and those that are modifiable. Nonmodifiable risk factors include age (risk of stroke dramatically increases with age), sex (incidence of stroke is higher in males), race (blacks have a higher stroke risk than other races), and family history of cerebrovascular disease. Modifiable, or controllable risk factors include hypertension, atrial fibrillation, and other cardiac diseases; diabetes mellitus; elevated cholesterol; smoking; and history of sedentary lifestyle and/or poor diet.

Patients may present either symptomatic or asymptomatic, but the majority of individuals with carotid disease will have no symptoms.[4] Asymptomatic patients are typically referred for carotid duplex imaging if they are at high risk for stroke or if a cervical bruit is detected. A cervical **bruit** located in the carotid artery is a noise that is audible while using a stethoscope. It is caused by high-velocity and/or turbulent blood flow, which in turn causes the auscultation of the vessel and vibration of surrounding tissues. Tissue vibration may also be visualized on the patient's neck in some cases. Symptomatic patients commonly present with symptoms including **aphasia**, dizziness, **dysphagia**, **diplopia**, and **hemianopsia**.

The five warning signs of stroke are listed in Box 37.1. Warning signs can also be remembered using the acronym FAST:
- Face
- Arm
- Speech
- Time

This stands for facial weakness, arm weakness, speech difficulties, and time to act if these symptoms are observed.[5] It is important to remember that symptoms of weakness or numbness of a leg or arm on one side of the body (**hemiparesis**) indicate disease in the contralateral carotid system. Ocular symptoms, however, suggest ipsilateral carotid disease. For example, transient blindness (**amaurosis fugax**) of the right eye is suggestive of right carotid system disease. Symptoms such as blurred vision, **dysarthria**, **ataxia**, **syncope**, **vertigo**, or overall weakness are nonspecific and can be confusing as to which vascular system is involved. Bilateral symptoms such as these may be related to the vertebral system, especially if disease is ruled out in the carotid system. The classification of cerebrovascular symptoms includes the following: *stroke*, or **cerebrovascular accident (CVA)**, defined as a permanent ischemic neurologic deficit; **reversible ischemic neurologic deficit (RIND)**, defined as a neurologic deficit that resolves between 24 and 72 hours; and TIA, defined as an ischemic neurologic deficit lasting less than 24 hours.

BOX 37.1 Classic Warning Signs of Stroke

Sudden numbness or weakness of face, arm, or leg, especially on one side of the body
Sudden confusion; trouble speaking or understanding
Sudden trouble seeing in one or both eyes
Sudden trouble walking or experiencing dizziness, loss of balance, or coordination
Sudden headache with no known cause

TECHNICAL ASPECTS OF CAROTID DUPLEX IMAGING

Before the carotid duplex imaging examination is performed, a thorough medical history must be taken from the patient. Medical history should focus on risk factors, signs, and symptoms of carotid disease and stroke. The patient should also be asked about any previous surgical interventions and any imaging he or she might have had, especially previous ultrasound studies. All information, including history, surgical history, and previous imaging studies, should be confirmed and augmented with a review of the patient's chart and any previous relevant imaging that is available for comparison. Once completed, the examination is explained and the patient is positioned supine, with the head resting on a pillow and turned slightly away from the side being scanned. The head of the bed can be raised slightly if the patient has trouble lying flat, but too much of a forward angle can hinder imaging and decrease examination quality.

Before duplex imaging begins, brachial pressures may be obtained. A difference of 20 mm Hg or greater between arms is suggestive of a proximal subclavian or innominate artery stenosis/occlusion, on the side with the lower pressure. Close examination of the neck should also be performed to check for presence of a cervical bruit. Not all stenoses in the carotid arteries will cause bruits, and on the contrary, a bruit may be identified in a normal artery. Furthermore, the bruit may also be transmitted (cardiac) from a distal location.

The carotid duplex imaging examination consists of grayscale (GS) images (used to identify vessels for Doppler interrogation, detect intimal thickening, evaluate location, extent, and characteristic of plaque, visualize other pathology); color Doppler (CD) imaging (provides a qualitative assessment of flow patterns, evaluates the amount of vessel filling [identifies area of stenosis]); and spectral Doppler (SD) imaging (obtains qualitative and quantitative information regarding flow characteristics).

Suggested technical parameters for carotid duplex imaging are as follows:
1. Use a high-frequency (7- to 12-MHz) linear-array transducer.
2. The image is oriented such that the head is to the left of the monitor.
3. Although CD is based on the direction of blood flow (toward or away) in relation to the transducer, red is typically assigned to arterial, and blue to venous blood flow. Follow your institution's guidelines.
4. Keep SD sample volume size (gate) small to acquire waveforms that accurately represent flow characteristics.
5. Use a 60-degree SD angle (or less) to the vessel wall. Make sure fine angle correction is parallel to the vessel walls. Any error can have a large effect on true velocity readings.
6. The CD and SD scale (pulse repetition frequency [PRF]) should be adjusted throughout the examination to evaluate changing velocity patterns.
7. The CD and SD wall filters are set low.
8. The CD region of interest size affects frame rate (number of image frames displayed per second), so CD display

should be kept as small as possible to maintain adequate frame rate.
9. The CD and SD gain should be adjusted throughout the examination as the signal strength changes.
10. Harmonics may be used during GS imaging to improve hypoechoic plaque visualization.
11. If available, compound imaging may increase the quality of GS imaging.
12. Beware of using time gain compensation controls to make vessels completely anechoic, as you may "erase" hypoechoic plaque or thrombus.

It is imperative that each institution develop a carotid imaging protocol that defines the standard examination. This protocol must include indications for a complete and/or limited examination, clinical applications, protocol and technique (arteries to be evaluated including the number and locations SD waveforms are obtained within each artery), interpretation criteria, quality assurance, and equipment maintenance. A standard complete examination usually includes GS, CD, and SD evaluation of the carotid and vertebral arterial systems, bilaterally.

Procedure

The transducer is placed above the clavicle on the neck. First, GS imaging is used to initially determine the locations of the arteries and CCA bifurcation, evaluate vessel tortuosity, and extent of atherosclerotic plaque. This may be performed in a transverse or longitudinal view, depending on the preference of the operator. Doing so provides global information regarding the anatomy and pathology, which will aid while imaging in a longitudinal plane.

Imaging longitudinally, the CCA is located and followed proximally as far as the clavicle will permit (Fig. 37.3). The CCA can be distinguished from the internal jugular vein, as the jugular will change shape with respiration and compresses with transducer pressure. Although the origin of the right CCA is often located as it arises from the innominate artery, the left CCA originates from the aortic arch and is not typically visualized using ultrasound imaging. The origin of the left CCA may be located in some cases by using a lower-frequency transducer with a smaller footprint angled inferiorly. The CCA is imaged superiorly to the level of the carotid bifurcation (carotid bulb). The CCA bifurcation is a common site for the development of atherosclerotic disease. At the bifurcation, the ultrasound transducer is moved slightly anterior and posterior to image the origin of the ICA and ECA. The ICA and ECA are individually followed distally to the angle of the mandible or as far as quality imaging is attainable.

The vertebral arteries are located by angling the transducer slightly lateral from a longitudinal view of the mid or proximal CCA. The vertebral artery lies deep to the CCA. Once correctly identified, it should be followed as far proximally as possible. Using CD will greatly assist in locating the vertebral artery and its origin, as well as determining the direction of vertebral artery blood flow. Decreasing the CD velocity scale (PRF) may be helpful while locating the vertebral artery. The more sensitive power Doppler may also prove helpful.

Multiple scanning approaches (anterior, lateral, and posterior to the sternocleidomastoid muscle) can be used to acquire carotid images. It is not uncommon for a carotid duplex to require the use of all four approaches to obtain high-quality longitudinal and transverse images to perform a complete assessment of the arteries of the neck due to vessel tortuosity and the eccentric shape and shadowing of atherosclerotic plaque. The lateral approach provides best visualization of the carotid system, while the distal ICA is typically best visualized from a posterior approach. The transverse plane provides a cross-sectional view of the artery; therefore, any measurement of vessel diameter or plaque should be performed in this plane.

The CD and SD interrogation of the carotid system is performed in the longitudinal plane using a 60-degree SD angle between the ultrasound beam and the vessel walls. Using constant and standard SD angle permits study reproducibility and proper comparison. SD angles greater than 60 degrees are not recommended, as they cause an increase in measurement error. The sample volume, or SD gate, should be placed in the center of the artery, and parallel to the vessel walls. Although SD images may only be obtained at certain areas within the carotid arteries, the SD gate should be moved slowly throughout the entire length of the artery while searching for the highest velocity. Spot Doppler checks at specified locations will result in errors, as areas of increased velocity and stenosis may be missed. The CD display will help guide proper placement of the SD gate and is useful in visually locating sites of increased velocity (aliasing). Although CD is helpful to locate areas of increased velocity and possible stenosis, care must be taken to evaluate that area to obtain its maximum velocity. This is done by slowly moving the SD gate in proximity of and throughout the color jet.

Commonly, SD waveforms are obtained in the proximal, mid, and distal CCA; the carotid bulb; the origin of the ECA; the proximal, mid, and distal ICA; the vertebral artery; and, in some institutions, the subclavian artery. This is most often done bilaterally, so a comparison between sides can be made. Additionally, if an area of stenosis is discovered, additional SD signals may be necessary in that area to further interrogate

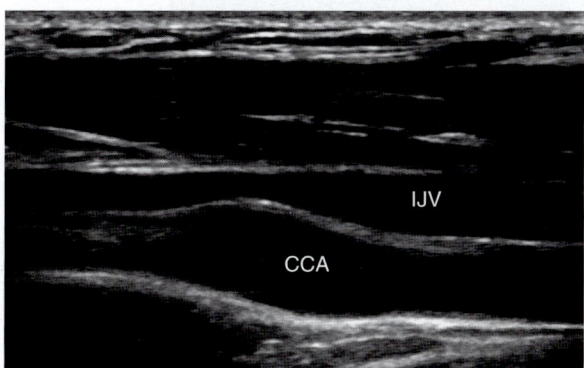

FIG. 37.3 Longitudinal gray-scale image of a normal common carotid artery (CCA) in which the internal jugular vein (IJV) can be seen anterior to the CCA.

the extent of disease. This can be done by obtaining SD signals just proximal to, within, and distal to the stenotic area. In these situations, additional GS images should also be obtained, both in the longitudinal plane (to evaluate plaque characteristics and extent) and in the transverse plane (to provide information regarding the severity of stenosis). This should be done in any vessel in which pathology is visualized. Manipulation of GSs via B-mode gain and time gain compensation is critical to obtain an accurate depiction of plaque that is present.

Common sources of technical errors that occur when performing carotid duplex imaging include the following: too high of insonating frequency for vessel depth, focal zone(s) inappropriately set, CD angle set too steep, CD gain set too low, and CD velocity scale (PRF) set too high. Cases of severe stenosis may not be detectable using CD; in these situations, power Doppler should be used to ensure the absence of flow before a determination of occlusion is made.

Normal Findings

In the normal patient, GS imaging should reveal smooth vessel walls with an anechoic lumen. No visual evidence of plaque formation or vessel wall deformities should be found.

Furthermore, all vessels can be fully visualized in both the longitudinal and transverse plane.

SD waveforms obtained within the CCA will demonstrate characteristics of both the low resistive ICA and the high resistive ECA (end diastole above baseline). The CCA SD waveforms will display a positive and continuous Doppler pattern throughout the cardiac cycle (Fig. 37.4A–B). At peak systole, the CD color map will fill the artery to the vessel walls and display an increased velocity (a lighter shade) in the center of the artery. These CD and SD waveform findings will be present in all locations of the CCA evaluated (proximal, midportion, and distal [just proximal to the bifurcation]). The CCA SD waveform is important because it can be an indicator of proximal or distal disease. However, investigators have shown that the peak systolic velocities (PSVs) recorded from the CCA change along its length and should not be considered a reliable marker for disease.[6-8] Instead, an ICA-to-CCA peak systolic ratio is recommended to compare the CCA and ICA within the individual. When selecting the SD waveform for use in the CCA/ICA ratio calculation, it is important the SD obtained is from the non-tortuous portion of the CCA. Most often this is the mid/distal CCA. Errors will occur if the SD waveform obtained from the proximal, tortuous CCA (increased velocity) or the distal CCA that may include the

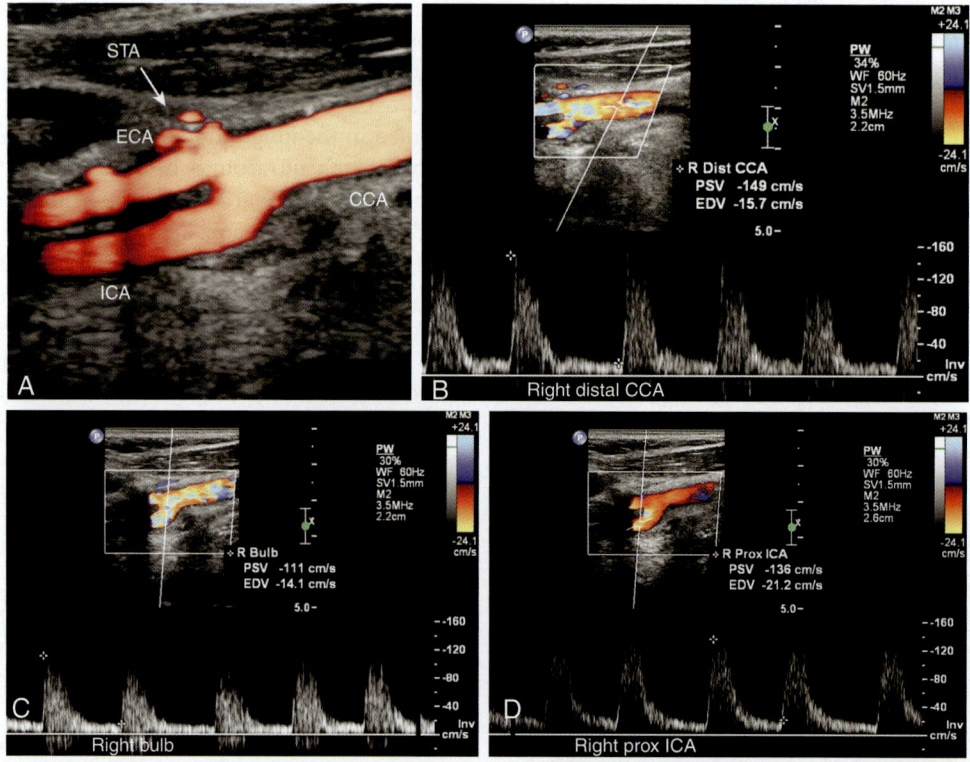

FIG. 37.4 (A) Power Doppler image of the carotid bifurcation in the longitudinal plane, as the common carotid artery (CCA) can be seen bifurcating into the internal (ICA) and external carotid artery (ECA). The superior thyroid artery (STA) is the first branch of the ECA and is also visualized in this image. (B) Spectral waveforms from the CCA demonstrating continuous antegrade flow, with characteristics of both the low resistive ICA and the high resistive ECA. (C) Spectral Doppler waveforms obtained at the level of the carotid bifurcation (carotid bulb), recognized by lower velocities and the presence of turbulence. (D) Spectral Doppler waveforms from the ICA demonstrate low resistance, evident by continuous antegrade flow and the absence of spectral broadening.

bulb (decreased velocity) is used. At the level of the CCA bifurcation, the carotid bulb can be visualized characterized by a slight dilation of the vessel. This increase in diameter causes a change in blood flow hemodynamics as compared with the CCA. Here, blood velocities are lower and flow is more turbulent (Fig. 37.4C). Boundary layer separation, which is a normal flow disturbance, may also be detected as a transient reversal of blood flow along the posterior wall of the bulb. Boundary layer separation may be visualized in the CD display and SD waveforms. Sample volumes for the ICA and ECA should start just distal to this area.

Proper identification of the ICA and ECA is not a problem in most patients, but it is essential for reporting accurate findings. The most reliable method to distinguish the ICA from the ECA is their hemodynamic characteristics demonstrated with the SD. The SD waveforms obtained in the ICA are low resistance with the absence of spectral broadening. The ICA also maintains continuous antegrade flow throughout the cardiac cycle, caused by the low peripheral resistance of the brain (Fig. 37.4D). This is demonstrated on SD by the waveforms remaining above the baseline and on CD by a continuous color pattern. Blood flow PSV may slightly decrease as evaluation progresses distally within the ICA, but SD waveform should remain consistent.

The ECA demonstrates a more pulsatile SD signal (high resistive, minimal diastolic flow) because it perfuses the skin and muscular bed of the scalp and face, which contain high resistant vascular beds (Fig. 37.5). On SD interrogation, the classic ECA waveform has a steep slope to peak systole and an end-diastolic velocity (EDV) that is very close to zero or absent. The normal color flow pattern of the ECA will also reflect the high resistance scalp and face vascular beds, decreasing during diastole. This may also disappear at end-diastole. Additionally, the ECA is smaller in diameter since it transports a lower blood volume, and typically originates anterior and medial at the carotid bifurcation. The ECA has extracranial (cervical) branches. The first branch of the ECA, the superior thyroid artery, is often visualized during a carotid duplex imaging examination. This can also aid in its identification. Lastly, a temporal tap maneuver can be used to confirm ECA and ICA differentiation. The temporal tap maneuver is performed by "tapping" on the superficial temporal artery while obtaining a SD waveform. Tapping will cause small deflections in the end-diastolic component of the ECA waveform, however, it will have no effect on an ICA waveform (see Fig. 37.5).

To reliably identify the vertebral artery, periodic shadowing over the artery is visualized as a result of the transverse vertebral processes (Fig. 37.6). Its identification can be further confirmed by obtaining SD waveforms, which are low resistive, similar to the CCA, but demonstrate lower PSVs (Fig. 37.7). Furthermore, they are also continuous and antegrade throughout the entire cardiac cycle in the absence of disease. Waveforms should be obtained near the origin of the vessel to identify any significant stenosis formation. Accordingly, continuous CD flow is seen throughout the cardiac cycle. Comparing the flow direction of the vertebral artery to the CCA will help confirm antegrade or retrograde flow.

Tortuous Arteries. During a carotid duplex imaging examination, encountering tortuous arteries is common (Fig. 37.8).

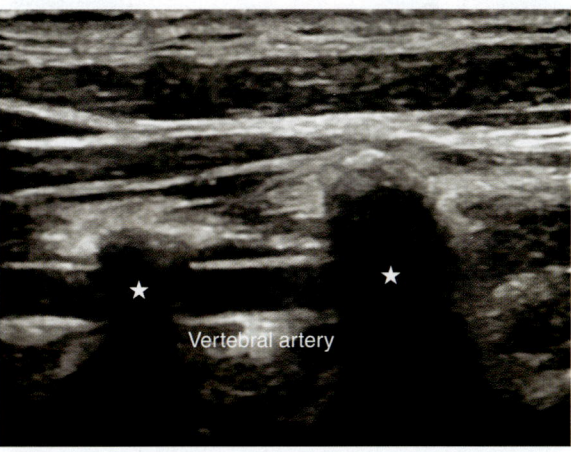

FIG. 37.6 Longitudinal gray-scale image of the vertebral artery, as it travels between the transverse processes *(stars)* of the cervical spine, as demonstrated by the areas of acoustic shadowing.

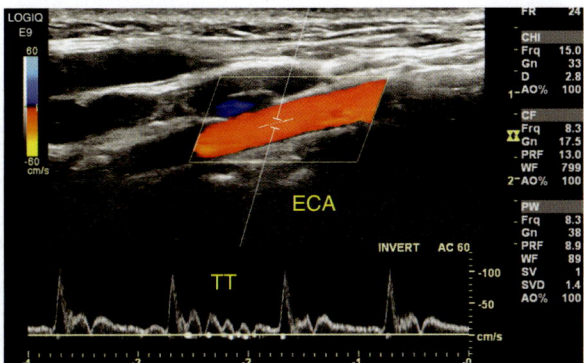

FIG. 37.5 Spectral Doppler waveforms from the external carotid artery (ECA) reflect a higher resistance flow pattern, evident by a rapid systolic acceleration, minimal diastolic flow. The second waveform in this ECA spectral Doppler signal also portrays deflections in the diastolic component caused by the temporal tap (TT) maneuver.

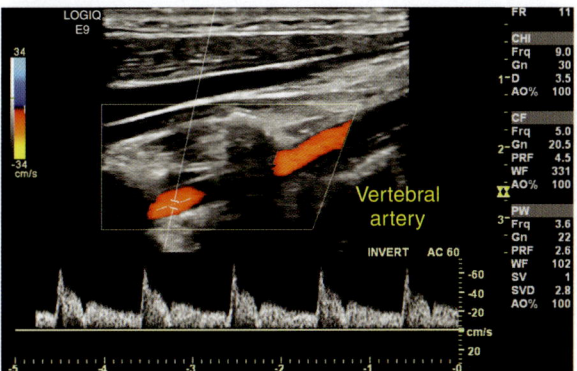

FIG. 37.7 Color and spectral Doppler image of a normal vertebral artery in a longitudinal view, as it travels between the bony transverse processes of the cervical spine. Note that the blood flow is in the correct direction (head is to the left on the image), and spectral Doppler waveforms are low resistive, continuous, and antegrade.

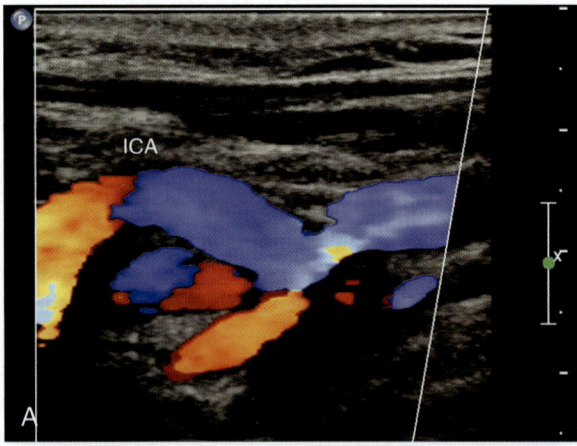
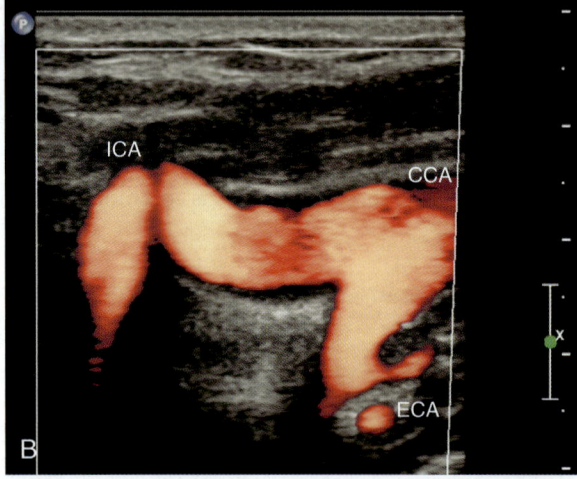

FIG. 37.8 (A) Color Doppler image of a tortuous internal carotid artery (ICA) at the level of the carotid bifurcation. (B) Power Doppler image of a tortuous ICA. Note that power Doppler imaging is helpful while imaging tortuous vessels, as it is not susceptible to Doppler signal loss at the location perpendicular to the insonating beam. The external carotid artery (ECA) and distal portion of the common carotid artery (CCA) are also seen.

Normal blood flow disturbances occur because of vessel tortuosity and typically result in an increase in PSV within tortuous portions of the artery. Correct placement of the SD gate and adjustment of the SD angle may be very difficult in some areas. In tortuous arteries, it is recommended that SD signals be obtained just distal to the curved portion of the vessel. Often, PSVs are found to be falsely elevated when obtained in the curve of an artery due to the acute Doppler angles relative to the changing blood flow direction. It is important for sonographers to understand this and be able to differentiate true increased PSV caused by stenosis from falsely elevated PSVs caused by an inaccurate SD angle. To ensure PSVs are truly increased as a result of disease, it is recommended that other evidence, such as post-stenotic turbulence on CD or GS images displaying a visual narrowing, be reported. Additionally, if SD angle other than 60 degrees is used, it should be documented to allow for the same angle to be used in follow-up examinations of that patient.

Currently, the best carotid duplex examinations will be achieved by proper attention to detail. Major areas of focus when performing carotid duplex imaging examinations are

> **BOX 37.2 Important Considerations for Carotid Duplex Examinations**
>
> Obtain a patient medical history focusing on risk factors, symptoms, history of stroke, vascular surgical interventions, and prior vascular imaging.
> Be familiar with cerebrovascular anatomy, physiology, and pathology.
> Optimize gray-scale images. Too much contrast can eliminate hypoechoic plaque and thrombus visualization.
> Understand how each color Doppler technical setting affects image quality.
> Use a small spectral Doppler sample volume (gate) and a 60-degree angle.
> Use color/power Doppler imaging as a guide to obtain spectral Doppler waveform information.
> Be aware of the spectral Doppler technical settings.
> Compare spectral Doppler waveforms obtained at each location with those of the contralateral side.
> Establish an institutional protocol that includes information regarding technique, diagnostic criteria, and quality assurance.

summarized in Box 37.2. Attention to these technical areas and interpretation details will ensure the accurate carotid duplex results.

Doppler Variations. Congestive heart failure can have a profound effect on the SD signal. Blood flow velocity in the carotid system decreases as congestive heart failure severity increases. This effect will be seen bilaterally. If it is seen unilaterally, large vessel obstruction should be considered as the reason for diminished flow velocities. Patients placed on balloon pumps following surgery also exhibit unique flow (Fig. 37.9). SD signal variations can also be seen with respiration. Typically, this does not occur, but some individuals who tend to take large breaths in and out can make obtaining SD waveforms difficult. One way to remedy this is to have the patient hold his/her breath while acquiring the SD signals.

Pathologic Findings

Atherosclerotic Disease. Plaque visualized at any time throughout a carotid imaging examination should be documented. Documentation should include location, extent, surface characteristics (smooth vs. irregular), and echogenicity (homogeneous, heterogeneous, calcified).[9] The extent of plaque may be measured in a longitudinal or transverse plane by tracing the plaque border using software measurement packages included with most imaging systems.

Plaque that is uniform in echogenicity and texture throughout its entirety is described as homogeneous. Plaque with mixed areas of echogenicity and textures are characterized as heterogeneous. Heterogeneity findings are important because they may represent degenerative changes in the plaque or hemorrhage, resulting in an increased risk of plaque embolization. Calcified plaque is very dense and is brightly echogenic that often shadow (Fig. 37.10). The characterization of plaque on GS imaging provides valuable information

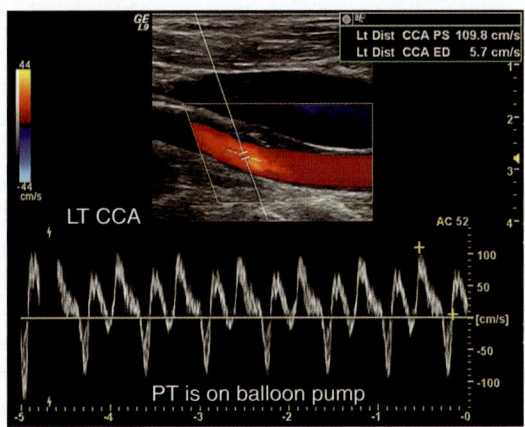

FIG. 37.9 Common carotid artery (CCA) waveform obtained from a patient on an intraaortic balloon pump.

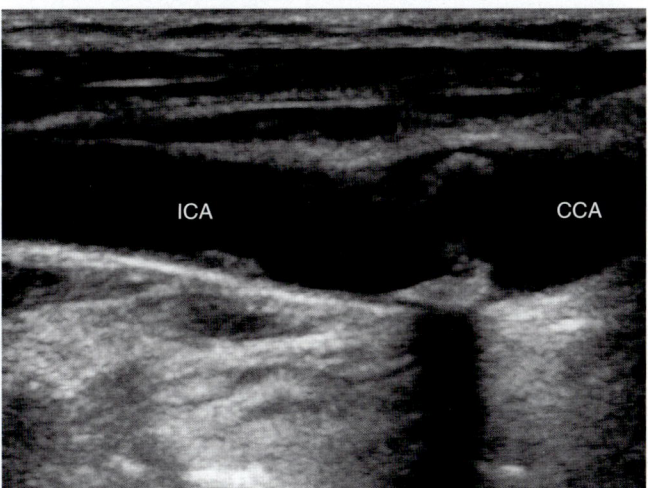

FIG. 37.10 Gray-scale image of calcified plaque near the origin of the internal carotid artery (ICA) at the level of the carotid bifurcation. Calcified plaque causes acoustic shadowing deep to their location. Shadowing artifact can affect the gray-scale and color Doppler display. The distal portion of the common carotid artery (CCA) is also visualized.

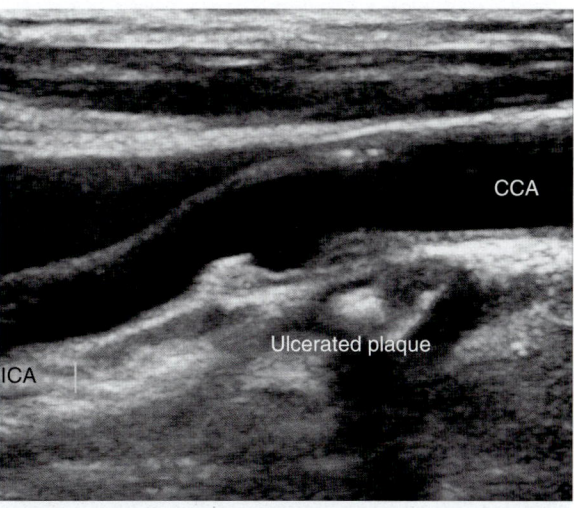

FIG. 37.11 A longitudinal gray-scale image of the internal carotid artery (ICA) containing irregular plaque. Another term for irregular plaque is *ulcerated plaque*. The distal portion of the common carotid artery (CCA) is also seen.

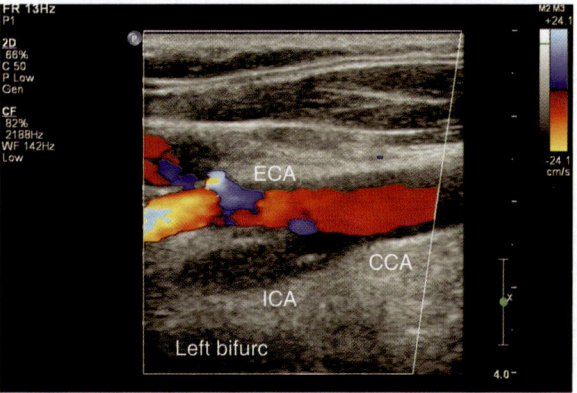

FIG. 37.12 Color Doppler image demonstrating an occlusion of the internal carotid artery (ICA); there is no color signal information. Blood flow is demonstrated in the external carotid artery (ECA) and common carotid artery (CCA).

regarding its morphology and composition.[9] Recent trends show a shift from the concept of linking stroke risk to degree of stenosis to focusing more on plaque morphology and composition.[10] It has been reported that the presence of vulnerable plaques, such as soft (anechoic) or irregular plaque (Fig. 37.11), significantly increases risk of TIA or stroke as compared with calcified plaque and are considered to be independent predictors of ischemic stroke.[11] Therefore, multiple scanning approaches should be used to obtain multiple views of an artery in the presence of plaque for its adequate visualization and characterization.

It is also very important for patient management to correctly differentiate between ICA high-grade stenosis and occlusion (Fig. 37.12). An occlusion of the ICA is not amenable to surgical intervention, whereas a stenosed ICA can typically be repaired. To characterize an ICA as occluded, the artery should be evaluated with SD, CD, and power Doppler imaging to rule out the presence of low-velocity trickle flow.

In doing so, the color and/or power Doppler PRF should be decreased to exclude the presence of any slow-moving blood flow, and the color and power Doppler gain should be increased to enhance any blood flow that may exist. The ICA should be sampled at multiple sites with SD. A large SD gate should be used in an attempt to identify any presence of blood flow. Secondary ultrasound characteristics of an ICA occlusion include echogenic material filling the lumen, lack of arterial pulsations, retrograde blood flow near the proximal origin of the occlusion, loss of diastolic blood flow in the ipsilateral CCA, elevated PSVs in the ipsilateral ECA, and elevated PSVs in the contralateral ICA. Occlusion of the ECA or CCA may also occur and should be documented during a carotid duplex imaging examination (Fig. 37.13). In some circumstances, the CCA may be occluded while the ICA and ECA remain patent, as retrograde ECA flow supplies the ICA. In this situation, it is important to document the blood flow direction and the velocity in the ECA and the ICA.

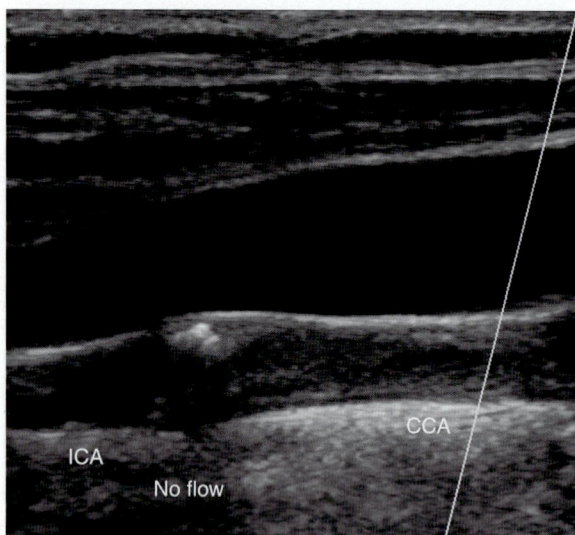

FIG. 37.13 A longitudinal image of an occluded common carotid artery (CCA). The occluded internal carotid artery (ICA) can also be seen.

Aneurysms. Aneurysms of the cervical carotid system are rare but can be associated with a higher risk of thromboembolic events.[12] Most patients present with a pulsatile mass of the neck, and a bruit is often observed.

Sonographic Findings. In cases of aneurysm, diameter of the afflicted artery will be significantly increased. An aneurysm finding can be considered if the diameter of the vessel is 50% larger than the diameter of the adjacent proximal segment. Abnormal blood flow patterns demonstrated within the aneurysm by CD and SD will depend on the size of the aneurysm; however, turbulent flow is the most common finding. Diameter measurements of the aneurysmal artery should be obtained on GS images in a transverse plane proximal to, within, and distal to the aneurysm. CD and SD images should also be obtained at these locations.

Pseudoaneurysms. Pseudoaneurysms—or false aneurysms—of the carotid arterial system can occur in the presence of trauma, iatrogenically, or in association with pathologies that weaken the arterial wall, such as dissection or arteritis. Patients will most commonly present with a pulsatile neck mass, and although rare, can be fatal if ruptured.[13]

Sonographic Findings. Pseudoaneurysms appear sonographically as round, mass-like lesions. The lesion may exhibit to-and-fro flow on CD and SD with a conduit connecting the pseudoaneurysm and the artery. This is known as a neck (tract) and should also be visualized. Sizes of the pseudoaneurysm and the neck connection can be variable depending on the cause and should be documented to help with patient management decisions. SD waveforms should be obtained within the pseudoaneurysm and its neck. Thrombosis may also be seen in cases of spontaneous occlusion.

Carotid Dissection. In the presence of an intimal tear, arterial blood can enter the wall of the artery, causing the separation of its layers and leading to a dissection.[14] A carotid artery dissection can occur between any layers of the arterial wall. Thin-walled dissections may represent a tear between the intimal and medial layers, whereas thick-walled dissections may represent medial and adventitial layer separation. Furthermore, dissections near the adventitial layer may result in a pseudoaneurysm. Flow between any of these walls is known as the false lumen. Dissections can be unilateral or bilateral. Evaluation of dissections is important because complete obstruction of carotid vessels can lead to ischemic stroke. Common causes of carotid artery dissection include blunt and penetrating trauma, acceleration or deceleration cervical injuries, and neck flexion.

Sonographic Findings. Different blood flow patterns in the two lumina is visualized and should be documented with CD imaging and SD waveforms. In some cases, the ICA has a gradual taper ending at the base of the skull, causing a decrease in PSV with a high resistance pattern. Vessel lumen narrowing without visualization of plaque is characteristic of dissection. GS images in the longitudinal and transverse planes should also be obtained for further investigation (Fig. 37.14).

Carotid Body Tumors. Carotid body tumors (CBTs) are slow-growing neoplasms of the carotid body.[15] The carotid body is a small (3 to 5 mm) chemoreceptor that lies within the adventitial layer on the posterior aspect of the carotid bifurcation. The carotid body assists in regulation of heart rate, blood pressure, and respiration. Findings of CBT are relatively rare, accounting for less than 0.03% of all neoplasms.[16-18] CBTs are further characterized as hypervascular structures typically located between the ICA and ECA. Blood is supplied to most CBTs via branches of the ECA.

Sonographic Findings. CBTs tend to be incidental findings on a carotid examination. They can be identified on GS imaging, as they typically cause displacement of the ICA and/or ECA. Their hypervascularity allows easy identification by CD imaging (Fig. 37.15). Along with CD images to document vascularity, GS images in the longitudinal and transverse planes should be acquired to obtain tumor measurements, as size will have a large influence on patient management decisions.

Fibromuscular Dysplasia. Fibromuscular dysplasia (FMD) is a nonatherosclerotic, noninflammatory disease that typically affects the media of the arterial wall in medium-sized vessels. FMD primarily affects women and is most commonly found in the renal, extracranial carotid, and vertebral arteries.[19,20] When found in the carotid or vertebral arteries, FMD may cause stroke, TIA, aneurysm, and carotid dissection.[21] Most patients present asymptomatic or with only minimal symptoms as a result of turbulent carotid or vertebral artery blood flow.[22] FMD has been visually described a "string of pearls" appearance on arteriography. This pattern causes multiple arterial dilations separated by concentric stenosis.

Sonographic Findings. Gross narrowing and thickened arterial walls may be visualized on GS imaging. CD imaging may reveal turbulent blood flow patterns adjacent to the arterial wall, along with the absence of atherosclerotic plaque in the proximal and distal segments of the artery. Turbulent flow characteristics will also be present in SD waveforms. Diagnosis of FMD is typically made in conjunction with

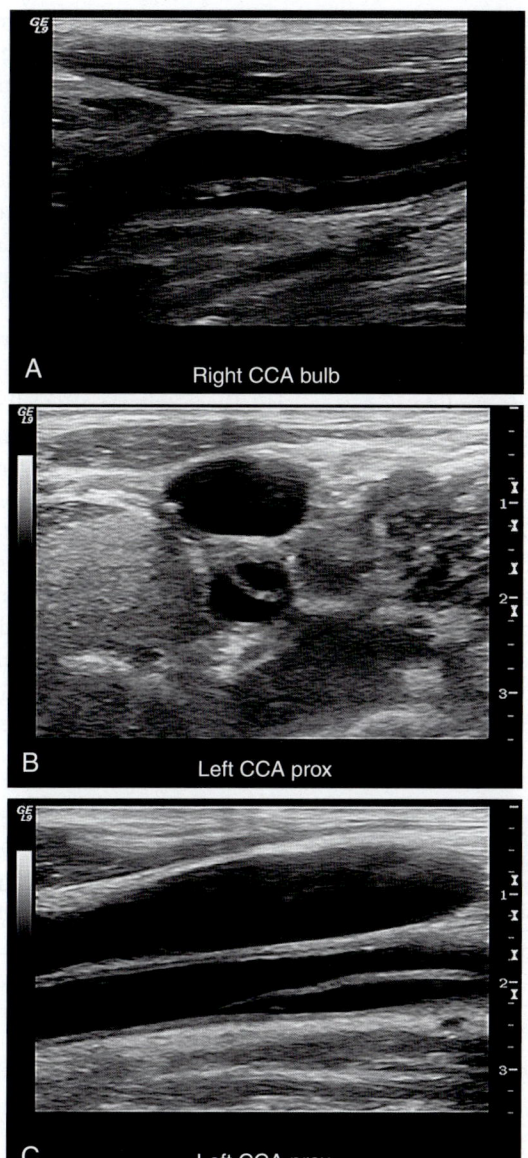

FIG. 37.14 A 39-year-old woman presented to the emergency department with stroke-like symptoms. Carotid gray-scale imaging revealed bilateral common carotid artery (CCA) dissections due to uncontrolled hypertension. (A) The right CCA and bulb demonstrating a thick dissection. (B) The left CCA imaged in a transverse plane; true and false lumina are seen. (C) Dissection is visualized in the proximal portion of the left CCA.

arteriography, computed tomography angiography (CTA), and/or magnetic resonance angiography (MRA) studies.

INTERPRETATION OF CAROTID DUPLEX IMAGING

Accurate interpretation of carotid duplex imaging depends on the quality, accuracy, and the thoroughness of the sonogram. This includes adapting to scanning challenges, such as patient body habitus or vessel tortuosity, optimizing GS and Doppler technical parameters to ensure optimal images obtained, and understanding differences in appearance between normal anatomy and pathology within the carotid

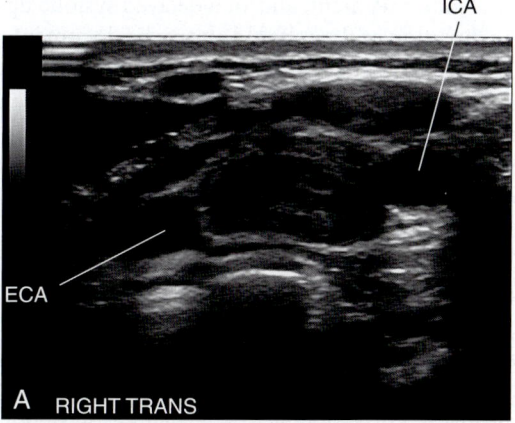
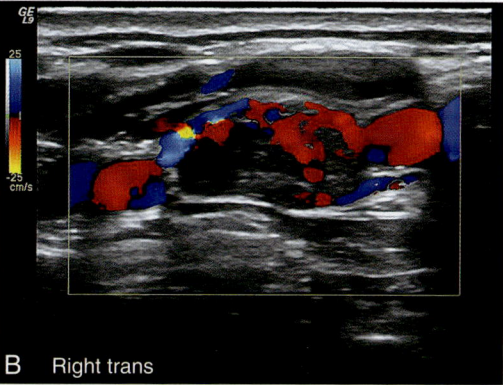

FIG. 37.15 (A) Transverse gray-scale image of a carotid body tumor. The internal carotid artery (ICA) and the external carotid artery (ECA) are seen being displaced on each side of the tumor. (B) Color flow visualized in the hypervascular carotid body tumor.

system. SD waveforms should be obtained throughout the carotid system bilaterally for a qualitative and quantitative assessment of the carotid system. This is done by comparing contralateral carotid spectral waveform morphology, direction of blood flow, PSV, and EDV. GS and CD images should also be obtained at multiple levels bilaterally to supplement the qualitative assessment of the carotid system, especially in areas of stenosis.

SD waveform morphology analysis provides information for qualitative evaluation of carotid system hemodynamics. The level of symmetry between spectral waveform morphology obtained at the same location on the contralateral side should be noted. Abnormal waveform morphology (increased or decreased pulsatility) may be an indicator of proximal (innominate, subclavian) or distal (intracranial) disease. The degree of spectral broadening within the SD waveform should also be assessed, as presence of spectral broadening is indicative of turbulent flow, often seen in the presence of a stenosis. CD imaging can also be used to detect blood flow turbulence within a stenosis, as demonstrated by aliasing and multidirectional flow. Post-stenotic disturbances located distal to the stenosed area will also demonstrate multidirectional turbulent blood flow patterns, which can be detected using CD. Spectral waveforms obtained distal to a stenotic region are characterized by turbulent flow, diminished PSV compared with the stenotic segment, and/or a delayed systolic upstroke. Last, the direction of flow should always be documented with both CD and SD. Retrograde flow is uncommon; however, it typically occurs in the vertebral artery in the presence of subclavian steal. Other causes of retrograde flow include aortic valve regurgitation, arrhythmias, dissections, and intraaortic balloon pumps.

A quantitative assessment of the carotid system is made using PSV and EDV values obtained from SD waveforms. Normal ICA PSVs range from 60 to 80 cm/sec in older individuals and 80 to 100 cm/sec in younger individuals. In the presence of stenosis, elevated PSVs are seen within the narrowed segment. The degree of PSV increase measured on SD waveforms corresponds to the degree of stenosis and is used to noninvasively evaluate disease severity. This is a widely used technique that demonstrates high levels of accuracy, sensitivity, and specificity.[23-25] Interpretation criteria of ICA velocities for degree of stenosis vary somewhat, so it is important that each institution develop its own stenosis criteria.[26] This can be done by comparing carotid duplex imaging results with other imaging modalities, most commonly CTA or surgical outcomes such as carotid endarterectomies.[27] The original carotid stenosis criteria was developed in 1987 at the University of Washington, which provided stenosis categories based on velocity ranges (as opposed to an absolute value or percentage of stenosis).[28] In 2002, the Society of Radiologists in Ultrasound convened a multidisciplinary panel of experts in the field of vascular sonography, which established consensus interpretation criteria for SD waveform velocities used in the diagnosis of carotid artery stenosis using measures of PSV and an estimate of plaque degree (lumen diameter reduction) (Table 37.1).[29] In 2020, these interpretation criteria were reiterated in a consensus statement from the Society for Vascular Medicine and the Society for Vascular Ultrasound.[30]

Another measure that can be used to aid in ICA stenosis grading is the ICA/CCA ratio. This measure is a ratio between velocities of the ICA and CCA and is used to control for technical or clinical factors that may cause falsely elevated or diminished PSV values.[29] It is also accepted that the ICA/CCA PSV ratio provides useful information while grading stenoses categorized as severe by PSV criteria (70% or more) to determine if surgical intervention (carotid endarterectomy [CEA]) is warranted.[31] This measure and SD waveform EDV values are considered by the 2002 Society of Radiologists in Ultrasound Consensus Panel to be secondary parameters that serve to aid in the determination of carotid stenosis severity (Table 37.2).[29] It is important to note that these stenosis criteria are specific to the ICA and cannot be appropriately applied to any other arteries of the carotid system. Criteria for stenosis within the CCA have been proposed but are not widely used.[32]

The criteria recommended in the 2002 consensus are currently thought to be the most commonly cited and clinically used for grading ICA stenosis.[9] These criteria are well documented and evidence based, as they were generated from data in the literature. They are a good starting point for any institution before establishing its own diagnostic criteria (Figs. 37.16 and 37.17).

When only one patent vessel can be identified distal to the carotid bifurcation, careful evaluation must occur to determine whether it is the ICA or the ECA that is occluded. In the presence of ICA occlusion, the contralateral ICA velocity may be elevated, causing the estimated level of stenosis in the patent ICA to be falsely elevated.[33] Therefore

TABLE 37.2	Diagnostic Criteria of the Secondary Parameters for Internal Carotid Artery Stenosis	
Classification	ICA/CCA PSV Ratio	ICA End-Diastolic Velocity
Normal	<2.0	<40 cm/sec
Mild	<2.0	<40 cm/sec
Moderate	2.0–4.0	40–100 cm/sec
Severe	>4.0	>100 cm/sec
Near occlusion	Variable	Variable
Total occlusion	N/A	N/A

CCA, Common carotid artery; *ICA*, internal carotid artery; *N/A*, not applicable; *PSV*, peak systolic velocity.
Data from Grant EG, Benson CB, Moneta GL, et al: Carotid artery stenosis: grayscale and Doppler ultrasound diagnosis—Society of Radiologists in Ultrasound Consensus Conference. *Radiology.* 2003;19(4):190–198.

TABLE 37.1	Diagnostic Criteria of the Primary Parameters for Internal Carotid Artery Stenosis		
Classification	Degree of Stenosis (%)	ICA Peak Systolic Velocity	Plaque Estimate (%)[a]
Normal	None	<125 cm/sec	None
Mild	<50	<125 cm/sec	<50
Moderate	50–69	125–230 cm/sec	≥50
Severe	≥70	>230 cm/sec	≥50
Near occlusion	N/A	High, low, or undetectable	Visible
Total occlusion	100	Undetectable	Visible, no detectable lumen

[a]Plaque estimates (diameter reduction) obtained using gray-scale and color Doppler ultrasound imaging.
ICA, Internal carotid artery; *N/A*, not applicable.
Data from Grant EG, Benson CB, Moneta GL, et al: Carotid artery stenosis: grayscale and Doppler ultrasound diagnosis—Society of Radiologists in Ultrasound Consensus Conference. *Radiology.* 2003;19(4):190–198.

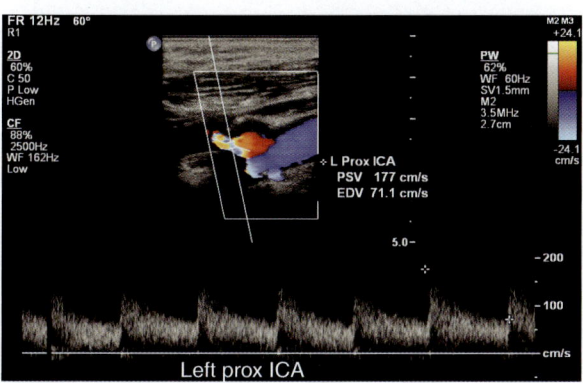

FIG. 37.16 An example of a 50% to 69% diameter reduction stenosis of the internal carotid artery (ICA). The peak systolic velocity (PSV) is approximately 175 cm/sec, and the end-diastolic velocity (EDV) is approximately 70 cm/sec. The color Doppler information was used as a guide to sweep the spectral Doppler gate through the area of suspected stenosis based on the color jet, represented by the aliasing artifact.

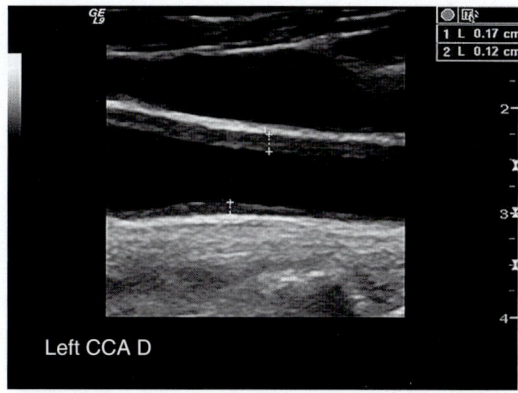

FIG. 37.18 Intima-media thickness measures being performed on a longitudinal gray-scale image of the distal common carotid artery (CCA). See the electronic distance measurement calipers on the anterior and posterior walls of the artery. Both of these demonstrate abnormal thickness.

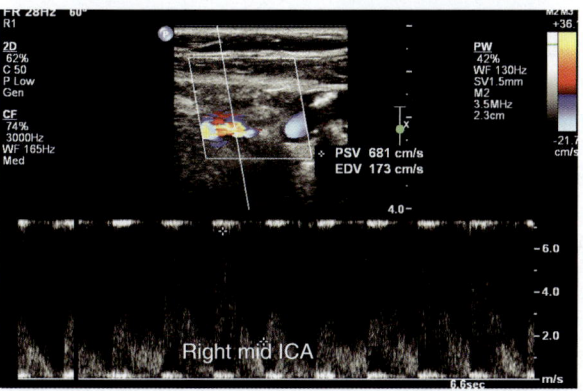

FIG. 37.17 An example of a greater than 70% diameter reduction stenosis of the internal carotid artery (ICA). The peak systolic velocity (PSV) is greater than 680 cm/sec, and the end-diastolic velocity (EDV) is greater than 170 cm/sec. Aliasing artifact can be seen on the color display and spectral waveforms, as the Nyquist limit is being exceeded.

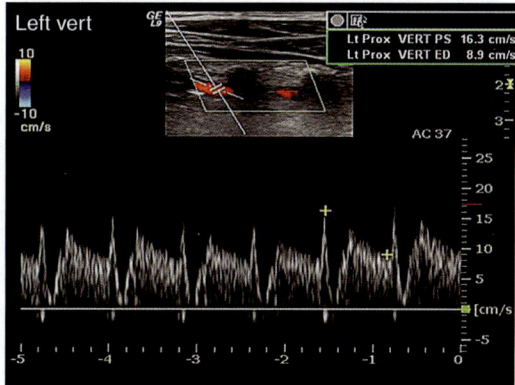

FIG. 37.19 A left vertebral artery exhibiting antegrade flow with a fast decline in flow velocity after the early systolic upstroke. This is what is known as the "bunny rabbit" sign. It represents an early indicator of subclavian steal syndrome.

in circumstances of unilateral ICA occlusion, ICA velocity stenosis criteria, which have been altered for this situation, should be used in the contralateral ICA.[33] This alternate criteria states ICA PSV 140 cm/sec or more (instead of 125 cm/sec or more) suggests stenosis with greater than 50% diameter reduction.[33]

Another parameter that provides quantitative information regarding carotid artery disease (CAD) progression is intima-media thickness (IMT). This measure provides an index of present or subclinical atherosclerotic plaque, which, if monitored consistently, can be used as a marker for the early detection of plaque progression or regression.[34,35] Obtained on a longitudinal GS image of the artery, measurements are made at the near or far wall of the vessel, including only the intima and media layers. This is the distance between the lumen-intima interface and the media-adventitia interface (Fig. 37.18). IMT measures can be performed in the CCA, bulb, and ICA, with a value of less than 1 mm considered normal.[36] To accurately measure carotid IMT, sonographers must be experienced, must be using modern equipment with a high-frequency transducer (greater than 7 MHz), and must acquire multiple samples.[36]

Normal vertebral arteries produce a wide variation in velocities, rendering absolute velocity values not useful for the diagnosis of vertebral artery stenosis. However, poststenotic disturbances demonstrated in the vertebral artery on CD and dampening of the SD waveform may suggest proximal obstruction. It is also important to evaluate direction of blood flow within the vertebral artery, as retrograde flow is indicative of a subclavian steal. A subclavian steal occurs secondary to significant obstruction proximal to the origin of the vertebral artery in the ipsilateral subclavian or innominate artery.[37] Early signs of subclavian steal include bidirectional SD signals in the vertebral artery (alternating pattern of antegrade and retrograde flow) or antegrade flow with a fast decline in flow velocity after the early systolic upstroke component (Fig. 37.19).

Information important to include in the interpretation of a carotid duplex examination is (1) location of stenosis, (2) extent of plaque and patency of the distal ICA, (3) presence of tortuous vessels, and (4) plaque characteristics (smooth

> **BOX 37.3 Essential Questions to Be Answered by Carotid Duplex Imaging**
>
> Is the ultrasound examination high quality and thorough?
> What level is the carotid bifurcation?
> Is disease present in the cervical carotid system?
> Where is the disease located?
> What is the percent diameter reduction of the stenosis?
> What is the extent (length of the plaque) of the disease?
> What are the characteristics of the plaque?
> Is the distal internal carotid artery (ICA) patent?
> Are the arteries tortuous?
> Are spectral Doppler waveforms bilaterally symmetric?
> Does the distal ICA spectral Doppler signal suggest distal (intracranial) disease?
> Is the proximal common carotid artery spectral Doppler signal normal or does it suggest proximal disease?
> What is the direction of blood flow in the vertebral arteries?
> Are any irregularities present along the walls of the carotid artery (e.g., dissection, fibromuscular dysplasia)?

> **BOX 37.4 Carotid Duplex Imaging Common Interpretation Errors**
>
> **Increased Velocity Without a Stenosis**
> Improper technique used to acquire images
> Internal carotid artery diagnostic criteria being applied to the common carotid, external carotid, or vertebral arteries
> Tortuous arteries
> Contralateral ICA high-grade stenosis or occlusion
> Distal arteriovenous malformation
> Cardiac function (affects signals bilaterally)
> Decreased hematocrit (affects Doppler signals bilaterally)
>
> **Normal Velocity With a Stenosis**
> Improper technique used to acquire images
> Velocity jet not identified
> Very high-grade stenosis (velocity decreases)
>
> **Absence of Blood Flow Velocity With Arterial Patency**
> Improper technique used to acquire images
> Improper technical settings
> Pseudo-occlusion because of low-volume flow
> Increased velocity missed
>
> **Blood Flow Velocity Recorded in Presence of Arterial Occlusion**
> Improper technique used to acquire images
> ECA and branches misidentified, thought to be the ICA
> Time interval between ultrasound evaluation and arteriography

ECA, External carotid artery; *ICA*, Internal carotid artery.

vs. irregular surface, calcification). Additionally, the report should include any variation from the standardized imaging protocol, quality of the examination, any findings of atypical SD waveforms, and any limitations of the examination. Common limitations of a carotid duplex examination include vessel tortuosity and heavy patient breathing causing inaccurate SD measures, shadowing artifact due to calcified vessels and patient body habitus leading to poor image quality, and vessel depth. Finally, if previous imaging studies are available, the report should include a comparison between the current and previous findings.

At many institutions, carotid duplex imaging may be the only diagnostic imaging modality performed before a patient undergoes CEA. Careful imaging technique and the appropriate interpretation of results are essential to address several important questions, as it may influence the physician's decision for surgical intervention. Questions that should be answered by a carotid duplex examination are listed in Box 37.3.

Consistency of protocol and findings on GS, CD, and SD imaging will limit errors in interpretation of carotid duplex examinations and decrease the likelihood of intraoperator and interoperator error. However, many pitfalls have been noted in the carotid duplex interpretation. Common examination interpretation errors are listed in Box 37.4. Proper technique is essential to perform accurate carotid duplex imaging and minimize errors in interpretation.

COMMON CAROTID ARTERY DISEASE TREATMENTS

The principal goal of CAD treatment methods is prevention of stroke. Depending on the degree and extent of carotid vessel narrowing and the characteristics and composition of the atherosclerotic plaque (smooth vs. irregular, homogeneous vs. calcified), a variety or combination of treatment types can be implemented. In less severe cases of stenosis, medical management is often elected, consisting of decreasing CAD risk factors through lifestyle modification, modified diet, and exercise. Pharmacologic agents can also be used, which aim to reduce the risk of stroke, as well as slow the progression of the CAD process. This is accomplished by targeting treatment to manage hypertension, maintaining appropriate glucose levels in the diabetic population, and treatment of hyperlipidemia, as well as anticoagulant and antithrombotic medications, which decrease platelet aggregation and thrombus formation.[38]

In more severe cases of carotid artery stenosis, endovascular or surgical intervention is often needed to reduce risk of stroke, prevent further vessel blockage, and reintroduce arterial flow through the carotid vessel. Using endovascular techniques, a percutaneous transluminal angioplasty procedure uses a balloon-tipped catheter, which is placed within the stenosis. The balloon is then inflated to compress present atherosclerotic plaque against the arterial wall and increase the size of the vessel lumen. Carotid stenting can also be performed as an endovascular intervention to promote arterial flow within the artery. This can be done using a variety of different stenting techniques. Although less invasive than surgical intervention, evidence suggests higher rates of infarct following carotid stenting compared with CEA procedures.[39]

Surgical intervention, in the form of a CEA, is the alternative to endovascular interventions in cases of severe CAD. This has historically been considered the gold standard of treatment in symptomatic and asymptomatic patients.[40] CEAs are performed by making an incision in the neck and carotid artery, at which point extracranial carotid plaque and thrombi are removed.[41,42]

Most commonly, a combination of medical management and surgical interventional methods for CAD are used to achieve optimal care and patient outcomes. As mentioned, treatment methods are dependent on CAD severity, plaque properties, and the overall health of the patient. Therefore, management of CAD often varies with each individual. It is important to understand the different interventions used to treat CAD, as this may affect the presentation and interpretation of carotid duplex examinations.

OTHER CAROTID ARTERY IMAGING MODALITIES

Although carotid ultrasound imaging is the initial modality of choice for the evaluation of CAD, multiple other imaging techniques are used to provide additional information. Carotid duplex findings of severe disease warrant additional imaging to confirm ultrasound imaging results and evaluate other areas for disease. Such other locations include the great vessels and the vessels of intracranial circulation and is most often done using CTA or MRA imaging.[11,16,43] CTA and MRA have reported similar high levels of sensitivity; however, CTA demonstrates higher levels of specificity than MRA.[43] While advantageously MRA does not require ionizing radiation, it is unable to visualize surrounding soft tissue structures causing a tendency to overestimate degree of carotid narrowing in the presence of disease.[44] Further, MR flow signals can be lost as a result of slow or turbulent flow found in atherosclerotic lesions. This causes inaccuracies in degree of stenosis measures, requiring contrast administration to resolve.[39,40] Similar to ultrasound imaging, MRA is able to visualize plaque, from which plaque morphology information can be obtained.

CTA imaging provides very high levels of spatial resolution for accurate evaluations of carotid stenosis.[43] As a result it has emerged as the noninvasive gold standard for detecting carotid disease, despite being historically reported as a less reliable technique to assess plaque morphology as compared with ultrasound and MRA.[45–48] However, more recent techniques are investigating quantitative assessments of plaque morphology, such as geometry and composition using semiautomated image analysis for reliable and standardized methods of assessing atherosclerotic lesions with CTA.[49] Unlike MRA and ultrasound, CTA imaging exposes the patient to ionizing radiation while acquiring images.

Digital subtraction angiography (DSA) is an invasive method of imaging that was previously considered to be the imaging gold standard for the assessment of CAD.[24] DSA maintains high levels of sensitivity (95%), specificity (99%), and accuracy (97%).[50] However, the femoral artery puncture required for intraarterial contrast administration leads to a higher rate of complications following DSA procedures compared with noninvasive imaging techniques. This, coupled with the technologic advancements and resultant increases in accuracy of noninvasive imaging methods (ultrasound, MRA, and CTA imaging), has led to the decreased use of DSA in the evaluation of CAD.

Maintaining an understanding of the different imaging modalities used for CAD evaluation, and the way in which a stenosis appears on imaging other than ultrasound, can provide valuable information regarding patient anatomy, as well as disease location, severity, and extent, before performing a carotid duplex examination. Using information obtained from previous imaging studies as a guide enables high-quality and accurate carotid duplex examinations to be performed in a timely and effective manner.

OTHER CAROTID DUPLEX IMAGING APPLICATIONS AND EMERGING TECHNIQUES

Intraoperative Imaging

Assessment of the carotid intervention site by duplex imaging for technical adequacy is an effective method to improve the results of the operation and reduce postoperative complications, including the need for reintervention. Intraoperative duplex imaging is done during CEA or stent-angioplasty procedures. It is used after ICA blood flow is restored but before skin closure, and a 10- to 15-MHz linear array transducer is used to evaluate the carotid system.[51] The transducer is placed over the artery within the incision, imaging from the distal CCA to the distal ICA. The ICA is assessed for anatomic abnormalities, such as dissection, residual plaque, thrombus, intimal flap, and suture stenosis. CD imaging is used to detect blood flow abnormalities and confirm vessel patency. SD waveforms are also obtained throughout the area imaged to ensure no marked increases in PSV are present. PSVs greater than 150 cm/sec are considered abnormal and may warrant additional imaging (angiography).[51] PSVs greater than 300 cm/sec indicate platelet aggregation and typically warrant reexploration.[51] End diastolic velocities greater than 50% of the PSV indicate hyperperfusion syndrome.[52] Although reported that only half of vascular surgeons use intraoperative carotid imaging following an endarterectomy procedure, it has been reported that its use decreases the likelihood of repair site thrombus to as low as 1% up to 3 months postoperative.[52,53]

Carotid Duplex Imaging After Stent Placement or Endarterectomy

Carotid duplex imaging is often used postoperatively to evaluate individuals who have undergone surgical intervention to restore carotid artery flow (carotid artery stenting or CEA). Carotid artery stenting is an alternative technique to the more invasive CEA surgical procedure, to restore blood flow through the carotid arteries. The GS image of a stent produces bright echoes (Fig. 37.20). The velocity criteria for detection of stenosis within a stent are not well established due to differences in stent and native vessel characteristics.[54] Stents tend to have smaller diameters than the native vascular lumen, also the lack of stent elasticity, both of which cause elevated PSVs, cause native carotid artery velocity criteria to be non-translatable to stent velocities. Velocity measures should still be obtained throughout the stent, however, to identify any marked increases in PSV between adjacent segments.[55] CD should also be used to interrogate blood flow within the stent for any hemodynamic disturbances. Last, a GS evaluation of the stent should be completed to assess any plaque formation and its morphology. Duplex imaging has been found useful in detecting carotid artery stent occlusion.

Follow-up duplex imaging should be performed 1 to 3 months after a CEA. The time interval for follow-up after the initial postoperative study depends on the status of the artery after the procedure and the amount of disease present in the contralateral ICA. If a carotid patch is used, imaging immediately after the endarterectomy is difficult because the synthetic material composing the patch retains air, making it not conducive to ultrasound imaging. As a result, images can only be obtained proximal and distal to the patch. Gas present in the synthetic material typically reabsorbs within a few days, at which point the carotid can be evaluated with duplex imaging. Typically, the carotid artery appears bulbous and enlarged at the bifurcation post-CEA, often extending into the proximal portion of the ICA (Fig. 37.21). PSVs are obtained throughout the carotid system just as in a routine carotid duplex examination. It is important to note that elevated PSVs may be found distal to the surgical site. If found, this area should be carefully interrogated to determine whether artery diameter reduction is due to plaque formation or surgical closure. The contralateral carotid artery should also be evaluated in CEA postoperative individuals, as its diameter reduction may increase the risk of carotid disease and may warrant more frequent follow-up imaging.[56]

Three-Dimensional Carotid Duplex Imaging

GS ultrasound imaging is widely used in the carotid duplex examination to evaluate plaque formation, extent, and morphology and to determine the residual area of the artery using IMT measures. This measure can be enhanced by using three-dimensional (3D) ultrasound technology, which can provide volumetric changes in blood flow throughout the vessel (Fig. 37.22). Although still not routinely implemented in many vascular labs, 3D ultrasound has demonstrated the ability to detect CAD and provide plaque volume measures at high levels of inter- and intra-reader repeatability; however, this has been debated in the literature and is a result of the difficulty in image acquisition.[55,57] Compared with 2D, 3D ultrasound has proven more reliable and sensitive in the evaluation of CAD.[55,58,59] As technology advances this area and 3D image acquisition techniques are refined and standardized, 3D ultrasound imaging is expected to become a promising tool in the evaluation of CAD.

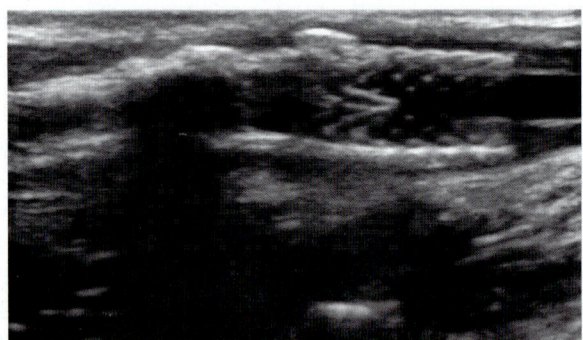

FIG. 37.20 Longitudinal gray-scale image of a carotid stent. The stent can be visualized as the bright echoes within the lumen. The stent is placed in the distal common carotid artery and extends into the bifurcation and the internal carotid artery.

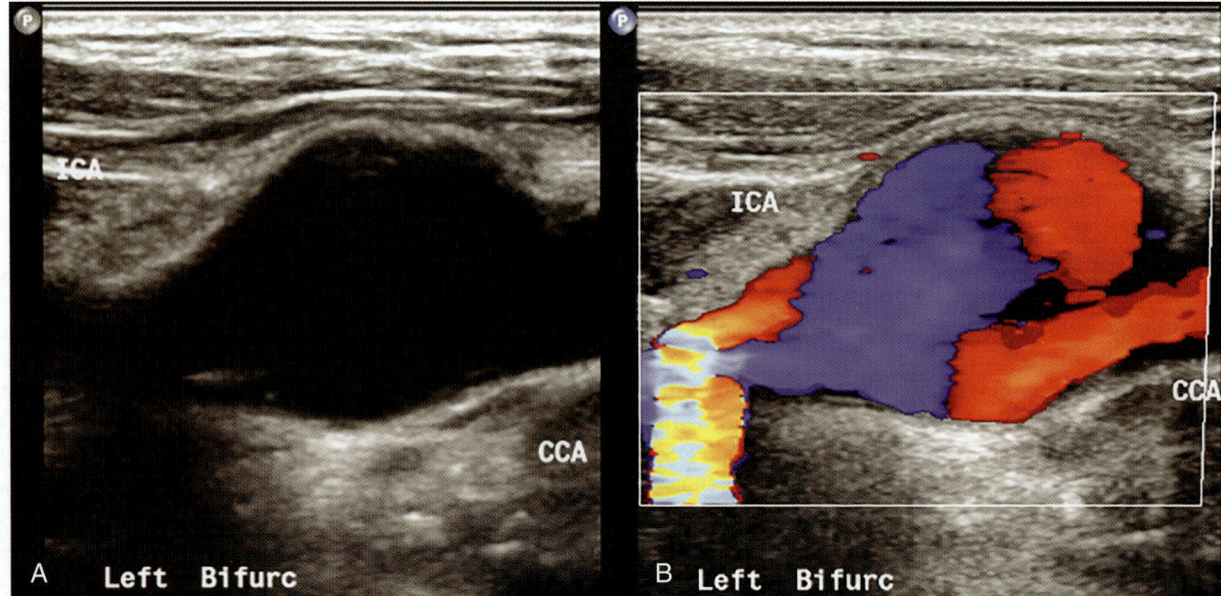

FIG. 37.21 Longitudinal gray-scale (A) and color Doppler (B) images of a dilated carotid artery at the level of the bifurcation post–carotid endarterectomy. *CCA,* Common carotid artery; *ICA,* Internal carotid artery.

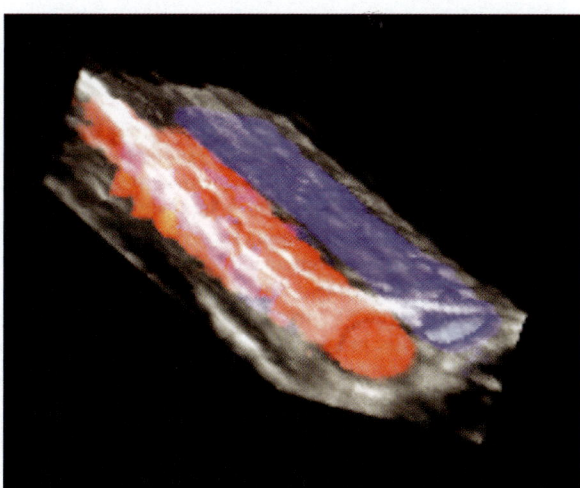

FIG. 37.22 Reconstructed three-dimensional ultrasound image of the internal carotid artery *(red)* and internal jugular vein *(blue)*.

Key Pearls

- A cerebrovascular accident, or stroke, is characterized by an interruption of blood flow to the brain (ischemic stroke) or by a ruptured intracranial blood vessel (intracranial hemorrhage).
- The hemodynamics of arterial flow can be influenced by a variety of factors, including vessel diameter, flow volume, vessel tortuosity, blood viscosity, and resistance.
- Because the brain requires a large amount of perfusion (~13% of systemic blood flow), the ICA tends to be larger than the ECA to account for the larger blood volume it transports.
- Disease of the carotid arteries is caused by atherosclerotic plaque buildup along the lumen of the vessels.
- If atherosclerotic plaque dislodges from the endothelium wall, it can propagate and cause a stroke, sudden vision loss, or a transient ischemic attack (TIA).
- Symptomatic patients commonly present with aphasia, dizziness, dysphagia, diplopia, and hemianopsia.
- Face, arm, speech, time (FAST) stands for facial weakness, arm weakness, speech difficulties, and time to act if these symptoms are observed.
- Spectral Doppler waveforms obtained within the CCA will demonstrate characteristics of both the low resistive ICA and the high resistive ECA.
- Plaque documentation should include its location, extent, surface characteristics (smooth vs. irregular), and echogenicity (homogeneous, heterogeneous, calcified).
- Pseudoaneurysms, or false aneurysms, of the carotid arterial system can occur in the presence of trauma, iatrogenically, or in association with pathologies that weaken the arterial wall, such as dissection or arteritis.
- A carotid artery dissection can occur between any layers of the arterial wall.
- Carotid body tumors are slow-growing neoplasms of the carotid body.
- Fibromuscular dysplasia is a nonatherosclerotic, noninflammatory disease that typically affects the media of the arterial wall in medium-sized arteries.

- Abnormal waveform morphology (increased or decreased pulsatility) may be an indicator of proximal (innominate, subclavian) or distal (intracranial) disease.
- Normal vertebral arteries produce a wide variation in velocities, rendering absolute velocity values not useful for vertebral artery stenosis diagnosis.
- Early signs of subclavian steal include bidirectional SD signals in the vertebral artery (alternating pattern of antegrade and retrograde flow) or antegrade flow with a fast decline in flow velocity after the early systolic upstroke component.
- Gray-scale ultrasound imaging is widely used in the carotid duplex examination to evaluate plaque formation, extent, and morphology and to determine the residual area of the artery using intima-media thickness measures.

REFERENCES

1. Bejamin EJ, et al. Heart disease and stroke statistics—2019 update: a report from the American Heart Association. *Circulation*. 2019;139(10):e56–e528.
2. Popieluszko P, et al. A systematic review and meta-analysis of variations in branching patterns of the adult aortic arch. *J Vasc Surg*. 2018;68(1):298–306.
3. Li S, et al. Internal carotid artery agenesis: A case report and review of literature. *The Neuroradiology J*. 2017;30(2):186–191.
4. Ratchford EV, Evans NS. Carotid artery disease. *Vasc Med*. 2014;19:512–515.
5. Kleindorfer DO, Miller R, Moomaw CJ, et al. Designing a message for public education regarding stroke: does FAST capture enough stroke? *Stroke*. 2007;38:2864–2868.
6. Slovut DP, Romero JM, Hannon KM, et al. Detection of common carotid artery stenosis using duplex ultrasonography: a validation study with computed tomographic angiography. *J Vasc Surg*. 2010;51:65–70.
7. Lee VS, Hertzberg BS, Workman MJ, et al. Variability of Doppler US measurements along the common carotid artery: effects on estimates of internal carotid arterial stenosis in patients with angiographically proved disease. *Radiology*. 2000;214:387–392.
8. Meyer JI, Khalil RM, Obuchowski NA, et al. Common carotid artery: variability of Doppler US velocity measurements. *Radiology*. 1997;204:339–341.
9. Huynh TT, Broadbent KC, Jacob AD, et al. Screening for carotid artery stenosis. *Semin Roentgenol*. 2015;50:127–138.
10. Saba L, et al. Vessel wall–imaging biomarkers of carotid plaque vulnerability in stroke prevention trials: a viewpoint from The Carotid Imaging Consensus group. *JACC Cardiovasc Imaging*. 2020:2445–2456.
11. Saba L, et al. Imaging biomarkers of vulnerable carotid plaques for stroke risk prediction and their potential clinical implications. *Lancet Neurol*. 2019;18(6):559–572.
12. Jiranukool J, Thiarawat P, Galassi W. Prevalence of intracranial aneurysms among acute ischemic stroke patients. *Surg Neurol Int*. 2020;11
13. Oh SH, Park JH, Choi SP. An unusual cause of epistaxis: rupture of a rapidly growing internal carotid artery pseudoaneurysm. *J Emerg Med*. 2013;45:e141–e143.
14. Urasyanandana K, et al. Treatment outcomes in cerebral artery dissection and literature review. *Interv Neuroradiol*. 2018;24(3):254–262.
15. Hoang VT, Trinh CT, et al. Carotid body tumor: a case report and literature review. *J Radiol Case Rep*. 2019;13(8):19.
16. Georgiadis GS, Lazarides MK, Tsalkidis Carotid body tumor in a 13-year-old child: case report and review of the literature. *J Vasc Surg*. 2008;47:874–880.
17. Patlola R, Ingraldi A, Walker C, et al. Carotid body tumor. *Int J Cardiol*. 2010;143:e7–e10.

18. Muduroglu A, Yuksel A. Carotid body tumors: A report of three cases and current literature review. *Vasc Dis Ther*. 2017;2:1–3.
19. Wake N, Marina I, Olin JW. Vascular function in fibromuscular dysplasia. *J Vasc Med Surg*. 2015;3:2.
20. Rana MN, Al-Kindi SG. Prevalence and manifestations of diagnosed fibromuscular dysplasia by sex and race: Analysis of >4500 FMD cases in the United States. *Heart Lung*. 2020;50(1):168–173.
21. Carrera JF, Southerland AM. Carotid artery fibromuscular dysplasia. *Carotid Artery Dis*. 2020:199–219.
22. Kerut CK, Sheahan C, Sheahan M. Carotid artery fibromuscular dysplasia: Ultrasound and CT imaging. *Echocardiography*. 2019;36(5):971–974.
23. Gorican K, et al. Diagnostic criteria for the determination of clinically significant internal carotid artery stenosis using duplex ultrasound. *Biomed Pap Med Fac Univ Palacky Olomouc Czech Repub*. 2020;164(3):255–260.
24. U-King-Im JM, Young V, Gillard JH. Carotid-artery imaging in the diagnosis and management of patients at risk of stroke. *Lancet Neurol*. 2009;8:569–580.
25. Dharmasaroja PA, et al. Accuracy of carotid duplex criteria in diagnosis of significant carotid stenosis in Asian patients. *J Stroke Cerebrovasc Dis*. 2018;27(3):778–782.
26. Columbo JA, et al. Variation in ultrasound diagnostic thresholds for carotid stenosis in the United States. *Circulation*. 2020;141(12):946–953.
27. Birmpili P, et al. Comparison of measurement and grading of carotid stenosis with computed tomography angiography and Doppler ultrasound. *Ann Vasc Surg*. 2018;51:217–224.
28. Taylor DC, Strandness DE. Carotid artery duplex scanning. *J Clin Ultrasound*. 1987;15:635–644.
29. Grant EG, Benson CB, Moneta GL, et al. Carotid artery stenosis: gray-scale and Doppler US diagnosis—Society of Radiologists in Ultrasound Consensus Conference 1. *Radiology*. 2003;229(2):340–346.
30. Kim ESH, et al. Interpretation of peripheral arterial and venous Doppler waveforms: a consensus statement from the Society for Vascular Medicine and Society for Vascular Ultrasound. *Vasc Med*. 2020;25(5):484–506.
31. Polak A, Joseph FP. Internal to common carotid artery peak systolic velocity ratios for predicting North American Symptomatic Carotid Endarterectomy Trial stenosis: derivation/validation study using a machine learning technique. *J Vasc Ultrasound*. 2019;43(4):182–185.
32. Oglat AA, et al. A review of medical doppler ultrasonography of blood flow in general and especially in common carotid artery. *J Med Ultrasound*. 2018;26(1):3.
33. Preiss JE, Itum DS, Reeves JG, et al. Carotid duplex criteria for patients with contralateral occlusion. *J Surg Res*. 2015;193:28–32.
34. O'Leary DH, Polak JF. Intima-media thickness: a tool for atherosclerosis imaging and event prediction. *Am J Cardiol*. 2002;90:L18–L21.
35. Baldassarre D, Amato M, Bondioli A, et al. Carotid artery intima-media thickness measured by ultrasonography in normal clinical practice correlates well with atherosclerosis risk factors. *Stroke*. 2000;31:2426–2430.
36. Tahmasebpour HR, Buckley AR, Cooperberg PL, et al. Sonographic examination of the carotid arteries 1. *Radiographics*. 2005;25:1561–1575.
37. Egan R. Anatomy and physiology of the cerebrovascular system. In: *Walsh and Hoyt's Clinical Neuro-Ophthalmology*. ed 6. Philadelphia: Lippincott Williams & Wilkins; 2005:1901–1966.
38. Naylor AR, et al. Editor's choice–management of atherosclerotic carotid and vertebral artery disease: 2017 clinical practice guidelines of the European Society for Vascular Surgery (ESVS). *Eur J Vasc Endovasc Surg*. 2018;55(1):3–81.
39. Jager HR, Moore EA, Bynevelt M, Coley S, Mounfeld P, Kitchen N, et al. Contrast-enhanced MR angiography in patients with carotid artery stenosis: comparison of two diferent techniques with an unenhanced 2D time-offight sequence. *Neuroradiology*. 2000;42(240–8):73.
40. Nederkoorn PJ, Van Der Graaf Y, Hunink MGM. Duplex ultrasound and magnetic resonance angiography compared with digital subtraction angiography in carotid artery stenosis: a systematic review. *Stroke*. 2003;34:1324–1331.
41. Batchelder AJ, Saratzis A, Naylor AR. Editor's choice–overview of primary and secondary analyses from 20 randomised controlled trials comparing carotid artery stenting with carotid endarterectomy. *Eur J Vasc Endovasc Surg*. 2019;58(4):479–493.
42. Yuan G, et al. Carotid artery stenting versus carotid endarterectomy for treatment of asymptomatic carotid artery stenosis: a meta-analysis study. *Int Heart J*. 2018;59(3):550–558.
43. Saxena A, Ng EYK, Lim ST. Imaging modalities to diagnose carotid artery stenosis: progress and prospect. *Biomed Eng online*. 2019;18(1):1–23.
44. Ricotta JJ, AbuRahma A, Ascher E, et al. Updated Society for Vascular Surgery guidelines for management of extracranial carotid disease. *J Vasc Surg*. 2011;54:e1–e31.
45. Budoff MJ, et al. Diagnostic performance of 64-multidetector row coronary computed tomographic angiography for evaluation of coronary artery stenosis in individuals without known coronary artery disease: results from the prospective multicenter ACCURACY (Assessment by Coronary Computed Tomographic Angiography of Individuals Undergoing Invasive Coronary Angiography) trial. *J Am Coll Cardiology*. 2008;52(21):1724–1732.
46. Meijboom WB, et al. Diagnostic accuracy of 64-slice computed tomography coronary angiography: a prospective, multicenter, multivendor study. *J Am Coll Cardiology*. 2008;52(25):2135–2144.
47. Miller JM, et al. Diagnostic performance of coronary angiography by 64-row CT. *N Engl J Med*. 2008;359(22):2324–2336.
48. Grønholdt MLM. B-mode ultrasound and spiral CT for the assessment of carotid atherosclerosis. *Neuroimaging Clin North Am*. 2002;12:421–435.
49. Chrencik MT, et al. Quantitative assessment of carotid plaque morphology (geometry and tissue composition) using computed tomography angiography. *J Vasc Surg*. 2019;70(3):858–868.
50. Chilcote WA, Modic MT, Pavlicek WA, Little JR, Furlan AJ, Duchesneau MP, et al. Digital subtraction angiography of the carotid arteries: a comparative study in 100 patients. *Radiology*. 1981;139:287–295.
51. Cyrek AE, et al. Assessment of intraoperative flow measurement as a quality control during carotid endarterectomy: a single-center analysis. *Scand J Surg*. 2020;1457496920971139.
52. Armstrong PA, Powell A, Bandyk DF. Intraoperative ultrasound assessment of carotid endarterectomy and stent angioplasty. In: AbuRahma AF, Bandyk DF, eds. *Noninvasive Vascular Diagnosis: A Practical Guide to Therapy*. New York: Springer; 2013:211–219.
53. Wallaert JB, Goodney PP, Vignati JJ, et al. Completion imaging after carotid endarterectomy in the Vascular Study Group of New England. *J Vasc Surg*. 2011;54:376–385.
54. Lal BK. Duplex ultrasound velocity criteria in carotid artery stenting patients. In: AbuRahma AF, Bandyk DF, eds. *Noninvasive Vascular Diagnosis: A Practical Guide to Therapy*. New York: Springer; 2013:183–188.
55. AlMuhanna K, Hossain MM, Zhao L, et al. Carotid plaque morphometric assessment with three-dimensional ultrasound imaging. *J Vasc Surg*. 2015;61:690–697.
56. AbuRahma AF, Srivastava M, AbuRahma Z, et al. The value and economic analysis of routine postoperative carotid duplex ultrasound surveillance after carotid endarterectomy. *J Vasc Surg*. 2015;62:378–384.
57. Landry A, Spence JD, Fenster A. Measurement of carotid plaque volume by 3-dimensional ultrasound. *Stroke*. 2004;35:864–869.
58. Schminke U, Motsch L, Hilker L, Kessler C. Three-dimensional ultrasound observation of carotid artery plaque ulceration. *Stroke*. 2000;31:1651–1655.
59. Heliopoulos J, Vadikolias K, Piperidou C, Mitsias P. Detection of carotid artery plaque ulceration using 3-dimensional ultrasound. *J Neuroimaging*. 2011;21:126–131.

CHAPTER 38

Intracranial Cerebrovascular Evaluation

Kevin R. Volz

OBJECTIVES

On completion of this chapter, you should be able to:
- Distinguish normal from abnormal intracranial arterial anatomy
- Understand the circle of Willis physiology and hemodynamics
- Outline the technical aspects and proper instrumentation and control settings used to perform high-quality transcranial Doppler imaging
- Describe the characteristics of spectral Doppler waveforms obtained from arteries evaluated during a transcranial Doppler examination
- List the clinical applications of transcranial Doppler imaging and describe associated expected findings and diagnostic criteria
- Discuss common errors associated with performing and interpreting transcranial Doppler imaging

OUTLINE

Intracranial Arterial Anatomy 1088
   Internal Carotid Artery 1088
   Ophthalmic Artery 1088
   Vertebral Arteries 1088
   Basilar Artery 1089
   Circle of Willis 1089
   Middle Cerebral Artery 1089
   Anterior Cerebral Artery 1089
   Anterior Communicating Artery 1090
   Posterior Cerebral Arteries 1090
   Posterior Communicating Artery 1090

Intracranial Arterial Physiology 1090
Technical Aspects of Transcranial Doppler Imaging 1090
   Instrumentation 1091
   Technique 1091
Interpretation of Transcranial Doppler Imaging 1096
   Physiologic Factors 1096
   Normal Intracranial Velocities 1097
Clinical Applications 1099
   Vasospasm 1099

Diagnosis of Intracranial Disease 1100
Cerebral Circulatory Arrest 1103
Intraoperative Use of Transcranial Doppler Technology 1104
Advantages and Limitations of Transcranial Doppler Imaging 1104
   Diagnostic Pitfalls 1105

KEY TERMS

Anterior cerebral artery (ACA)
Anterior communicating artery (ACoA)
Basilar artery (BA)
Cerebral vasospasm
Circle of Willis
Internal carotid artery (ICA)

Mean flow velocity (MFV)
Middle cerebral artery (MCA)
Ophthalmic artery
Posterior cerebral arteries (PCAs)
Posterior communicating artery (PCoA)
Pulsatility index (PI)

Resistive index (RI)
Subclavian steal syndrome
Submandibular window
Suboccipital window
Transorbital window
Transtemporal window
Vertebral arteries

As discussed in the previous chapter, noninvasive Doppler evaluation of the extracranial arterial vasculature has become a reliable and effective method for the detection and monitoring of arterial disease. However, the development of a noninvasive method to interrogate the intracranial arterial system has suffered in comparison because of the attention focused on surgically correctable lesions of the carotid bifurcation and the difficulty penetrating the skull using ultrasound technology.

Fortunately, technical sophistication has progressed, and experience has been gained in the area of transcranial Doppler (TCD) imaging since its inception into clinical use in 1982.[1]

TCD imaging was first used to detect cerebral arterial vasospasm after subarachnoid hemorrhage (SAH) but has since been used in a wide variety of clinical applications (Box 38.1). With its continued use and growing popularity as a noninvasive diagnostic tool, a better understanding of intracranial

BOX 38.1 Transcranial Color Doppler Imaging: Clinical Applications

- Assessment of intracranial collateral pathways
- Detection of cerebral emboli
- Detection of feeders of arteriovenous malformations
- Diagnosis and monitoring of intracranial vascular disease
- Documentation of the subclavian steal syndrome
- Evaluation of the hemodynamic effects of extracranial occlusive disease on intracranial blood flow
- Evaluation of the vertebrobasilar system
- Monitoring vasospasm in subarachnoid hemorrhage
- Monitoring evolution of cerebral circulatory arrest
- Monitoring during anticoagulative or fibrinolytic therapy
- Monitoring following traumatic brain injury
- Intraoperative monitoring
- Screening of children with sickle cell disease

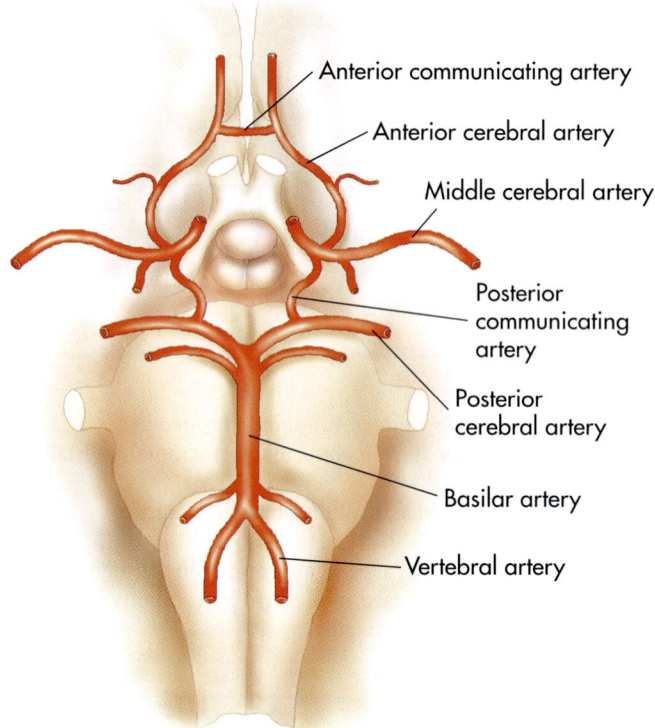

FIG. 38.1 Arteries comprising the circle of Willis.

arterial hemodynamics will be gained by using TCD in many different clinical settings. Although TCD imaging can provide valuable information regarding intracranial circulation, it is a technically difficult imaging modality to master; thorough knowledge of anatomy, physiology, and pathologies of the intracranial arterial system are required, in addition to technical skill. Furthermore, accurate TCD examination interpretation is not possible without knowledge of extracranial atherosclerotic disease location and extent. Carotid and vertebral duplex imaging should be performed before the TCD examination, as extensive extracranial disease may cause changes in the velocity profile or direction of blood flow in the intracranial arterial system.

INTRACRANIAL ARTERIAL ANATOMY

Blood supply to the brain is provided by the internal carotid (anteriorly) and vertebral (posteriorly) arteries, both of which originate extracranially and terminate intracranially. Familiarity with the anatomy of the large intracranial arteries and the arteries that compose the circle of Willis are prerequisites when it comes to performing accurate TCD imaging studies. Therefore this chapter will focus on the intracranial portions of the carotid and vertebral arteries, as well as the arteries that comprise the circle of Willis (Fig. 38.1). The extracranial portions of the internal carotid and vertebral arteries are discussed in Chapter 37.

Internal Carotid Artery

The **internal carotid artery (ICA)** is divided into four main segments: (1) the *cervical* ICA originates at the common carotid bifurcation (carotid bulb) and ends as it enters the carotid canal of the temporal bone at the base of the skull; (2) the *petrous* section of the ICA begins at the entrance of the carotid canal within the petrous portion of the bone and continues until it traverses the cranial portion of the foramen lacerum and passes into the cavernous sinus; (3) the *cavernous* segment extends from the foramen lacerum and cavernous sinus entrance to just medial of the anterior clinoid process; and (4) the *supraclinoid* portion of the ICA enters the intracranial space at the anterior clinoid and continues to its termination where it bifurcates into the middle cerebral and anterior cerebral arteries. During a TCD examination, the terminal portion of the ICA, just proximal to its bifurcation, and the more proximal carotid siphon are evaluated. The *carotid siphon* is an S-shaped curve in the ICA formed by a posterior and then anterior bend. This begins in the cavernous segment and continues to the ICA bifurcation. The internal carotid siphon is a common site of atherosclerotic disease in adults.[2-4]

Ophthalmic Artery

The **ophthalmic artery (OA)** originates as the first branch of the ICA just distal to the cavernous sinus. The OA travels anterolaterally and slightly deep through the optic foramen to perfuse the globe, orbit, and adjacent structures. This artery has three major groups of branches: (1) the ocular branches, (2) the orbital branches, and (3) the extraorbital branches. The branches of the OA often play an important role in collateral pathway formation as a result of internal or external carotid artery (ECA) disease. The OA is evaluated during a TCD examination.

Vertebral Arteries

The **vertebral arteries** are large branches of the subclavian arteries. The left vertebral artery is dominant in approximately

50% of individuals, the right in approximately 25%, and codominant in the remaining 25%; that is to say, vertebral artery size asymmetry is common.[5] The vertebral artery is divided into four segments: (1) extravertebral, (2) intervertebral, (3) horizontal, and (4) intracranial. The intracranial portion begins as it pierces the dura and arachnoid immediately below the base of the skull at the foramen magnum. It continues anterior and medial to the anterior surface of the medulla and unites with the contralateral vertebral artery to form the basilar artery. Several major branches arise from this segment of the vertebral artery, with the posterior inferior cerebral artery (PICA) being the largest and commonly arising approximately 1 to 2 cm proximal to the confluence of the two vertebral arteries forming the basilar artery. During TCD examinations, it is the intracranial segment of the vertebral arteries that is evaluated. The PICA, along with another branch of the vertebral artery, the anterior spinal artery, can occasionally be visualized on TCD imaging but are not routinely included as part of the examination.

Basilar Artery

The **basilar artery (BA)** is evaluated during TCD imaging and is formed by the union of the vertebral arteries at the lower border of the pons (pontomedullary junction). The basilar, when combined with the vertebral arteries, is often referred to as the *vertebrobasilar system*, which perfuses the posterior portion of the circle of Willis. From its origin, the BA extends anteriorly and superiorly and bifurcates into the paired posterior cerebral arteries. There are several branches of the BA, including the anterior inferior cerebellar arteries, the internal auditory (labyrinthine) arteries, the pontine branches, and the superior cerebellar arteries, just proximal to the posterior cerebral arteries. The BA is often variable in its path, size, and length; is typically tortuous; and may be duplicated or fenestrated.

Circle of Willis

The **circle of Willis** was first described in 1664 by Thomas Willis, characterized by the arterial anastomoses at the base of the brain.[6] The circle is composed of the A1 segments of the two anterior cerebral arteries, anterior communicating arteries (ACoAs), posterior communicating arteries (PCoAs), the terminal portions of the ICAs, and the P1 segments of the two posterior cerebral arteries. These intracranial arteries form a polygon vascular ring at the base of the brain that permits communication between the right and left cerebral hemispheres (via the ACoA) and the anterior and posterior systems (via the PCoA). These communications are important in the presence of significant disease or occlusion of a major cervical artery, as they serve as compensatory perfusion mechanisms. Variations in the circle of Willis are common, as it is estimated that an anatomically complete (classic) circle of Willis is present in only one-third of the population; however, a physiologically adequate circle of Willis exists in approximately two-thirds.[7] Significant hypoplasia and absence of the PCoA, the ACoA, the A1 segment of the anterior cerebral artery, and the P1 segment of the posterior cerebral artery are the most common variations.[8]

Middle Cerebral Artery

The **middle cerebral artery (MCA)** is the larger terminal branch of the ICA. From its origin, the MCA extends laterally and horizontally in the lateral cerebral fissure. The horizontal segment may course superficial or deep. The MCA either bifurcates or trifurcates before the limen insulae (a small gyrus), where the branches turn upward into the Sylvian fissure, forming its genu ("knee"). The vessels travel around the island of Reil, which is a triangular mound of cortex, and run posterosuperiorly within the Sylvian fissure. The terminal branches of the MCA anastomose with the terminal branches of the anterior cerebral and posterior cerebral arteries.

The MCA can be divided into four segments (M1 to M4). The main horizontal section of the MCA, from its origin to the limen insulae, is the M1 segment. The M1 segment gives rise to numerous small lenticulostriate branches. The M2 segment is composed of the branches overlying the insular surface in the deep Sylvian fissure. The M1 segment and the origin of the M2 segment are evaluated during TCD imaging. The initial MCA bifurcation is a common site for intracranial aneurysmal formation.[9] The MCA may also be the site of arterial stenosis and/or occlusion.

Anterior Cerebral Artery

The **anterior cerebral artery (ACA)** is the smaller of the two terminal branches of the ICA. From its origin, the ACA courses anteromedially over the optic chiasm and the optic nerve to the interhemispheric fissure (longitudinal cerebral fissure). The proximal horizontal portion of the ACA is known as the *A1 segment* and is connected to the contralateral A1 segment via the ACoA (see the following section). The A1 segment is evaluated during a TCD imaging examination and serves as a midline marker. The contour of the A1 segment may take a horizontal course, ascend, or slightly descend. The complete absence of the A1 segment is unusual. An anomalous origin of the ACA is rare, and asymmetry between the bilateral A1 segments is uncommon.[10] A direct inverse correlation tends to exist between the size of the A1 segment and the size of the ACoA. A small or hypoplastic A1 is typically found in conjunction with a large ACoA, as the contralateral A1 segment supplies most of the blood flow to both distal ACA territories.[11] It has been well documented that individuals with anomalies of the A1 segment have a higher incidence of ACoA aneurysms.[12-15] Stenosis or occlusion of the ACA may be found, but this has been found to be less common than in other intracranial vessels.

Distal to the ACoA, the ACA angles superiorly and travels in the interhemispheric fissure. The ACA curves anterosuperiorly around the genu of the corpus callosum. The segment of the ACA extending from the ACoA to the distal ACA bifurcation (callosomarginal artery and pericallosal artery) is termed the *A2 segment*. The proximal portion of the bilateral A2 segments may be visualized in some patients during TCD imaging and should be documented if possible. The distal A2 segments anastomose with branches of the posterior cerebral arteries. A large medial striate artery (recurrent artery of Heubner) is a major branch of the proximal A2 segment in approximately 20% of individuals, but this artery can also originate from the distal A1 segment (approximately 15%) or from the ACA/ACoA junction (approximately 60%).[16]

Anterior Communicating Artery

The **anterior communicating artery (ACoA)** is a short vessel that connects the A1 segments of the ACAs at the interhemispheric fissure. The ACoA is typically a single vessel but may be duplicated, absent, or a multichanneled system. The ACoA is typically short in length; however, this has been found to be variable. Longer ACoAs tend to be curved, tortuous, and/or kinked. The ACoA is often the location for congenital anomalies and is the most common site for intracranial aneurysm formation (25%), as well as the most common site for aneurysms associated with SAH.[11,12] A Doppler waveform of the ACoA may be captured at midline, but it cannot be visualized with TCD imaging.

Posterior Cerebral Arteries

At the approximate level of the pontomesencephalic junction, the basilar artery termination is its bifurcation into the bilateral **posterior cerebral arteries (PCAs)**. From their origin, each PCA travels anterolaterally to perfuse the posterior occipital lobe. The portion of the PCA extending from its origin to its junction with the PCoA can be referred to as the precommunicating portion but is more commonly termed the *P1 segment*. The P1 segment is evaluated during TCD imaging. Throughout this segment is the origin of many perforating branches that perfuse the brainstem and thalamus. The portion of the vessel extending posteriorly from the PCoA to the posterior aspect of the midbrain is the *P2 segment* of the PCA, which may be visualized with TCD imaging. The proximal portion of the PCA is typically asymmetric. In cases of "fetal" origin, the P1 segment is hypoplastic or smaller than the PCoA. It is uncommon for occlusive disease to be limited to the PCA, but if it does occur, the P2 segment is most commonly affected. The PCA is further divided into the P3 and P4 segments, but these cannot be visualized with TCD imaging.

Posterior Communicating Artery

The **posterior communicating artery (PCoA)** is a paired artery that travels posterior and medial to provide a connection between the ICA and PCA. The PCoA is highly variable in size and may angle upward or downward. Hypoplasia is a common PCoA anomaly, which occurs in an estimated 25% of individuals.[17] However, the PCoA can be enlarged in circumstances of a hypoplastic posterior cerebral artery, which occurs in 10% to 20% of cases.[18] This is termed a *fetal* origin of the posterior cerebral artery. The PCoA does not generally function as an important collateral pathway except in the presence of extensive bilateral extracranial occlusive disease or the absence of a patent ACA. The PCoA is typically evaluated during TCD imaging.

INTRACRANIAL ARTERIAL PHYSIOLOGY

The circle of Willis provides communication between the internal carotid, external carotid, and vertebrobasilar systems.[7] Upon its discovery, Thomas Willis stated its function to be a compensatory mechanism in the case of carotid or vertebral stenosis, a belief that is still largely accepted today.[6,19] In essence, the circle of Willis provides multiple communications between intracranial arteries and collateral pathways to ensure cerebral perfusion remains intact and the brain is adequately supplied with oxygenated blood, even in the presence of a flow-limiting lesion(s). Hemodynamic principles teach us that turbulent and low-velocity blood flow exists distal to significant stenosis. In cases of stenosis proximal to the intracranial arterial system, there is a risk of an inadequate amount of oxygenated blood reaching the area of the brain perfused by the stenosed artery. When this occurs, arteries composing the circle of Willis may shunt blood and be used as collateral pathways to provide arterial blood to the area in need. The same concept remains true during artery occlusion, in that collateral pathways are used to divert blood in an attempt to preserve adequate and entire brain perfusion.

An alternative and somewhat overlapping theory explains that the circle of Willis serves to dissipate areas of elevated pressure within the intracranial arterial system caused by significant distal stenoses.[6] As mentioned, a significant stenosis causes turbulent and low-velocity blood flow distal to the narrowed segment. This sudden deceleration of blood flow within a closed system causes the kinetic energy previously possessed by the blood to be transferred to the arterial walls, which propagates a shock wave toward the brain.[20] Therefore, the circle of Willis absorbs this shock wave by transferring pressure to another lower-pressure compartment in the intracranial arterial system.

TECHNICAL ASPECTS OF TRANSCRANIAL DOPPLER IMAGING

TCD imaging is used to investigate intracranial arterial circulation and has been referred to as one of the most complex and in-depth physiologic tests in vascular medicine, as it requires a thorough understanding of intracranial vascular anatomy, physiology, and pathology.[21] To consistently obtain reliable studies with TCD imaging, the operator must appreciate the importance of proper patient positioning, use available anatomic landmarks important for accurate identification of intracranial arteries, and be knowledgeable about the proper use of instrument controls. The accuracy of the examination will be elevated through the use of gray-scale (GS) image and color Doppler (CD) to guide the TCD evaluation. The outcome of a TCD examination is spectral Doppler

(SD) waveforms representing flow characteristics of the intracranial vasculature. The analysis of these waveforms provides information regarding hemodynamic properties and any fluctuations from normal physiologic flow.

Instrumentation

Instrument controls and technical settings vary depending on the manufacturer of the imaging system. Therefore it is important for the operator to be familiar with the particular imaging system being used. SD waveforms obtained are typically saved digitally and archived, but it may also prove beneficial to document the audio signal of waveforms being evaluated.

TCD imaging is performed using a low-frequency (4 MHz) phased-array imaging transducer, typically operating between 2 and 3.5 MHz.[7] High-quality TCD imaging depends on the proper adjustment of several instrument controls. This includes GS, CD, and SD imaging parameters. Deep knowledge of ultrasound physics is required to understand the effects adjusting various ultrasound settings will have on the image and how they will affect other settings. Improper settings may result in a false finding of the examination.

Instrument controls to consider when adjusting the GS image during TCD imaging are frequency, sector width, image depth, overall gain, time gain compensation, focal zone number and placement, frame rate, and dynamic range. Proper GS optimization is key as B-mode imaging plays an important role in performing an optimal TCD examination.

CD imaging is also very important when performing TCD, and its instrument controls should likewise be carefully optimized. Instrument controls to consider when adjusting the CD display during TCD include CD gain, scale (pulse repetition frequency [PRF]), wall filter, sensitivity (ensemble length), and persistence. As previously mentioned, CD imaging is integral to the TCD examination to visualize anatomic landmarks within the brain, as well as identify locations of certain intracranial vessels.[7] Conventional CD scale orientation for TCD examinations use the red portion of the scale to represent blood flow toward the transducer and the blue portion to indicate flow moving away from the transducer. Keeping this color assignment constant will allow intracranial blood flow direction in the arteries to be readily recognized. While imaging, the CD box, also known as the region of interest (ROI), is moved to the area being examined on the GS image. During TCD imaging, the entire circle of Willis can often be captured within a small color ROI. It is important to consider the size of the color ROI while scanning because its increasing size will negatively affect the imaging frame rate and hinder the performance of the examination. Therefore it is recommended that instead of a large color ROI, a small color ROI should be used, and the anterior and posterior circulations evaluated separately.

The third component of TCD imaging requires the use of SD imaging for real-time display of Doppler shift frequencies, represented by SD waveforms. Time is recorded along the horizontal axis and velocity (frequency shift) on the vertical axis. This allows velocity measurements of the SD waveforms to be recorded in centimeters per second. TCD imaging, like all ultrasound imaging, is based on the Doppler effect.[22] The ultrasound transducer emits a frequency of a known value and evaluates the value of the returned frequency to determine what is known as the *Doppler shift*.[23] A positive Doppler shift indicates blood flow toward the transducer and is displayed above the SD baseline, while a negative Doppler shift indicates blood flow away from the transducer and is displayed below the SD baseline. This means that information from SD waveforms depends on the direction of blood flow relative to the transducer; therefore, it is imperative that proper transducer placement and angle of insonation are practiced. Accurate recording of the intracranial SD waveform is critical, as this is the basis for interpretation of the TCD imaging examination. To this end, along with transducer placement, instrument controls to consider when obtaining SD waveforms are the SD gate (sample volume) size and position, SD gain, velocity (frequency shift) scale (PRF), baseline, wall filter, sweep speed, and output power. During TCD imaging, Doppler output power should be increased to ensure adequate penetration to enhance SD waveform quality. It is important to note, however, that output power increase should be done at the lowest level necessary and applied for the shortest duration possible while still obtaining accurate clinical information. This is in accordance with the as low as reasonably achievable (ALARA) principle, which should be applied during all TCD imaging examinations.[24–27]

TCD evaluation of the intracranial arteries is performed with a large sample volume (5 to 10 mm) to obtain a good signal-to-noise ratio. Furthermore, intracranial arterial SD waveforms are acquired without angle correction, as an assumption of a zero-degree angle is recommended.[7,28] This is due to a Doppler shift measurement error that occurs when the angle of insonation exceeds 30 degrees.[29] Several investigators have evaluated the potential use of angle-adjusted (corrected) velocities during TCD imaging which has resulted in somewhat of a controversy on the topic, stating that angle correction reduces the inaccuracy of velocity measures, allowing them to be compared with other arterial stenosis diagnostic criteria, all while maintaining acceptable levels of intrarater and interrater reproducibility.[30] This caused the release of a practice recommendation consensus statement in 2008, which states angle correction should only be performed in circumstances in which the SD sample volume can be positioned in a sufficiently long vessel segment and should be omitted in curved or tortuous vessels.[30] It is important to note that velocities obtained using angle correction tend to be elevated compared with those that have not.[31–34] To this end, follow-up TCD examinations for disease monitoring should not utilize angle correction techniques if this was not done in the previous study so appropriate comparisons can be made.[35,36]

Technique

Bone tissue comprising the skull heavily attenuates ultrasound waves, making insonation of the intracranial vasculature very difficult. Therefore thinner areas of the skull, or naturally occurring foramen or fissures, are instead used for insonation. These are known as acoustic windows. Four windows are commonly used during TCD imaging: the transtemporal, transorbital, suboccipital, and submandibular (Fig. 38.2). During every TCD examination, the operator should do the following:

1. Examine blood flow throughout the entire course of the circle of Willis and its major branches.
2. Identify, optimize, and acquire SD waveforms at a minimum of two locations in each artery.
3. Identify, optimize, and acquire any abnormal SD waveforms or CD signals.
4. Measure the highest velocity at each location in which SD waveforms are obtained.[28]

Transtemporal Window. The terminal ICA (t-ICA) or C1 segment of the ICA, MCA, ACA, PCA, and PCoA can be interrogated using the **transtemporal window** (Fig. 38.3).[37] This approach is performed with the patient in the supine position, with the patient's head aligned straight with the body. The transducer is placed on the temporal bone, cephalad to the zygomatic arch, and anterior to the ear. It is angled slightly upward and anterior to the contralateral ear.[7] This transducer orientation produces an imaging plane that is a transverse oblique view which in many patients provides simultaneous visualization of the anterior and posterior intracranial circulation. The ipsilateral hemisphere is at the top of the image and the contralateral hemisphere at the bottom. Accordingly, the left side of the image is anterior, and the right side of the monitor is posterior. Although the contralateral hemisphere is visualized in many patients, each hemisphere should be evaluated separately through the ipsilateral window to optimize artery-to-transducer angle. It is acceptable to evaluate the contralateral hemisphere in patients with only a unilateral transtemporal window.

A generous amount of acoustic gel is necessary to ensure good transducer-to-skin contact. Acoustic gel also allows the transducer to be angled at a higher degree in instances when it becomes necessary to lift the footprint from the skin surface in order to obtain optimal SD signals. Locating the transtemporal window can be difficult and, at times, frustrating, as it varies in size and location among patients, as well as bilaterally in the individual patient. Furthermore, transtemporal TCD imaging depends on ultrasound beam penetration through the temporal bone. Other windows used during the TCD examination tend to be less difficult to locate because they consist of the much less dense natural ostia, which is more favorable for intracranial penetration of the ultrasound beam. However, in situations of a dense and thick temporal bone, attenuation of the Doppler signal will be greater, resulting in less penetration of the ultrasound beam. It has been estimated that up to only 6% of the acoustic beam intensity reaches brain tissue while insonating through the cranial bones.[23] The ultrasound beam's ability to penetrate the temporal bone is also influenced by the age, sex, and race of the individual. Hyperostosis is the excessive growth of a bone and is the greatest obstacle for transtemporal TCD imaging. Hyperostosis increases in prevalence with age and also has a higher prevalence in females and those of African descent.[38,39] An estimated variation between 3% and 34% of individuals have inadequate or absent transtemporal acoustic windows.[38,40] One strategy to decrease the amount of time it takes to find the transtemporal window is to begin the TCD examination with maximum output power (100%), and once located, decrease the output power until an appropriate balance between image quality and patient safety is achieved.[28]

Once the transtemporal window is located, identifying bony landmarks ensures position at the correct level within the skull to locate the circle of Willis (Fig. 38.4).

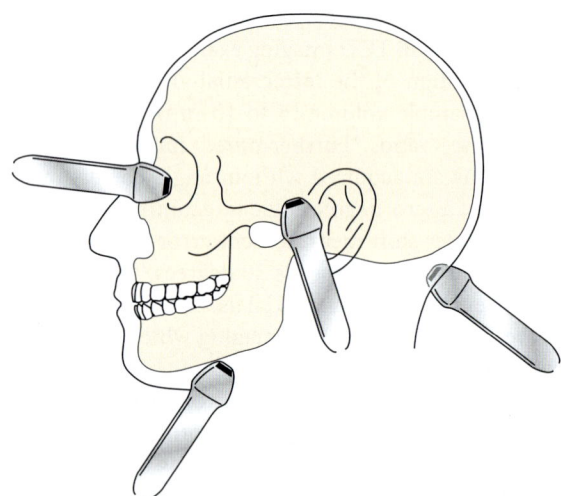

FIG. 38.2 Placement of the ultrasound transducer for the four transcranial Doppler acoustic windows: transtemporal, transorbital, suboccipital, and submandibular approaches.

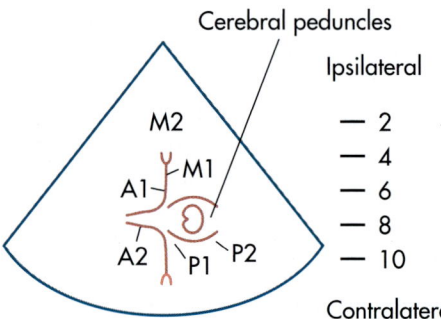

FIG. 38.3 Schematic of the arteries in the circle of Willis that can be visualized from the transtemporal approach.

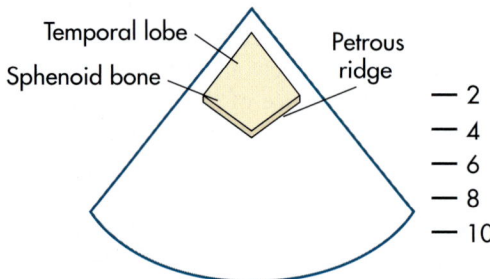

FIG. 38.4 Schematic of the bony landmarks visualized from the transtemporal approach.

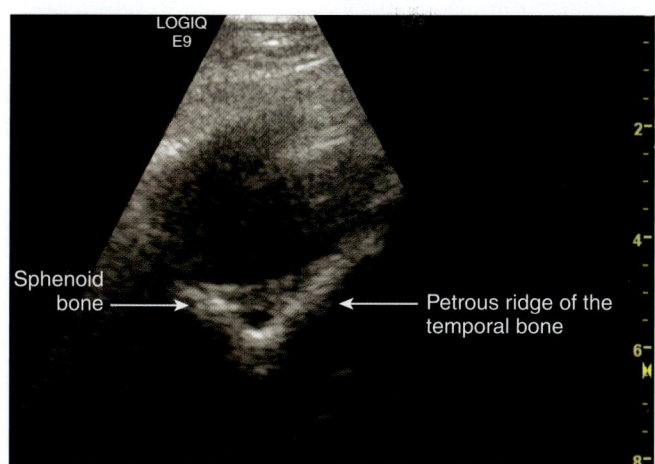

FIG. 38.5 Gray-scale image of the bony landmarks (lesser wing of the sphenoid bone and the petrous ridge of the temporal bone) from the transtemporal approach.

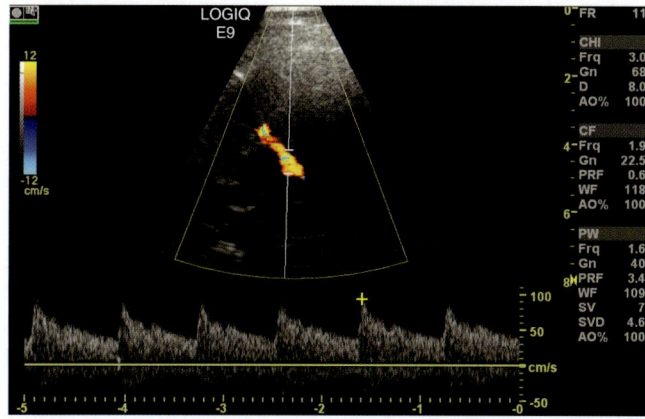

FIG. 38.7 Color and spectral Doppler image of the right middle cerebral artery. A zero-degree angle is used to obtain spectral Doppler waveforms. MCA blood flow is toward the transducer as represented in red on the color display and above the baseline on the spectral Doppler display.

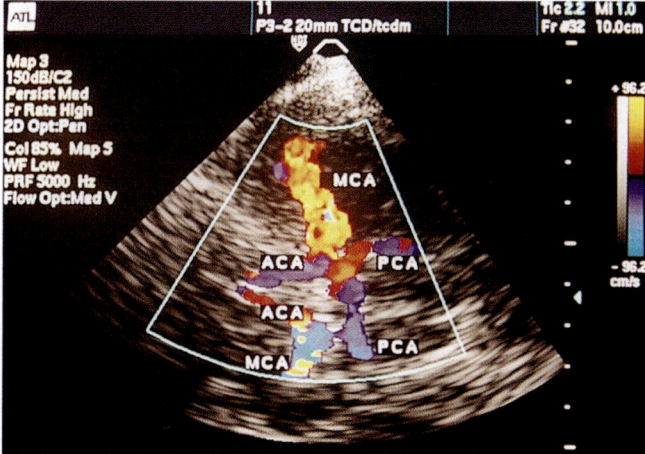

FIG. 38.6 Color Doppler image of the intracranial arteries from the transtemporal approach. The ipsilateral hemisphere is at the top of the image, and the contralateral hemisphere is at the bottom of the image. *ACA*, Anterior cerebral artery; *MCA*, middle cerebral artery; *PCA*, posterior cerebral artery.

In the transtemporal approach, these anatomic landmarks are the petrous ridge of the temporal bone, sphenoid bone, cerebral falx, suprasellar cistern, and cerebral peduncles. In this view, the highly reflective echoes of the lesser wing of the sphenoid bone can be seen extending anteriorly, and the petrous ridge of the temporal bone can be visualized extending posteriorly (Fig. 38.5). The ipsilateral temporal lobe is also typically seen at the top of the image in this view.

After bony landmarks have been identified, CD is activated to evaluate the intracranial vasculature via the transtemporal window (Fig. 38.6). First, visualization of the t-ICA is optimized by slightly angling the transducer inferior. Typically t-ICA blood flow direction is toward the transducer but depends on the artery's anatomic configuration. In the normal patient, t-ICA mean velocity is 39 ± 9 cm/sec. While imaging at this location, a mirror imaging artifact is present due to the adjacent bone.

Next, the transducer is angled slightly anterosuperior to image and evaluate the MCA and ACA. Using the aforementioned bony landmarks, the MCA is visualized traveling adjacent to the sphenoid wing. From this approach, blood flow in the main trunk of the MCA (M1 segment) should be traveling toward the transducer (Fig. 38.7). The normal mean velocity of the MCA is 62 ± 12 cm/sec. The M2 branches are also often visualized, typically traveling toward the transducer, but may appear to be traveling away due to curvature in their shape.

The A1 segment of the ACA is located just posterior to the MCA on the ultrasound image as it travels away from the transducer toward midline. It may be necessary to angle the transducer slightly anterior and superior to most optimally visualize the ACA. The normal ACA mean velocity is 50 ± 11 cm/sec. Here it may be necessary to decrease the CD PRF to enhance visualization of this artery due to its lower relative velocity and increased depth from the transtemporal window. The initial portion of the A2 segment is often visualized traveling away from the transducer in an anterior direction at midline.

The posterior circulation is imaged by angling the transducer slightly posterior and inferior, using the cerebral peduncles as an anatomic landmark. Typically, the two cerebral peduncles are identical in size and shape and are of intermediate echogenicity. Using this landmark, the P1 segment of the PCA can be visualized wrapping around the cerebral peduncle, traveling toward the transducer. For adequate interrogation of this artery, the CD PRF may need to be slightly decreased, as the PCA is characterized with a slower relative blood flow velocity (39 ± 10 cm/sec under normal circumstances). The ipsilateral and contralateral P1 segments can often be visualized at their origin at the bifurcation of the basilar artery. In this view, the ipsilateral P1 segment is traveling toward the transducer, and the contralateral P1 segment is traveling away. CD of the ipsilateral P2 segment may be displayed in red just distal to the origin of the PCoA but will be displayed in blue distally as it wraps around the cerebral peduncle and changes direction. The CD display of the P2 segment is variable due to the anatomic route and relative orientation to the transducer.

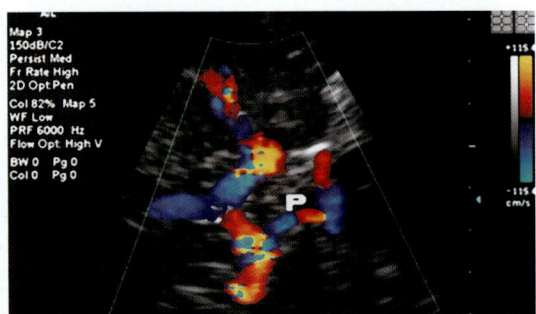

FIG. 38.8 Color Doppler image of the posterior communicating artery (P), visualized connecting the anterior and posterior intracranial arterial circulations.

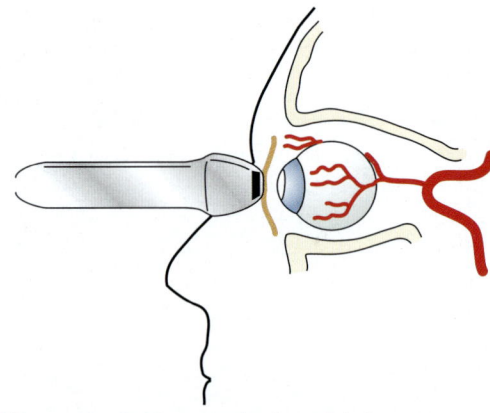

FIG. 38.9 **Transorbital approach.** The ophthalmic artery is a branch of the internal carotid artery that perfuses the orbit.

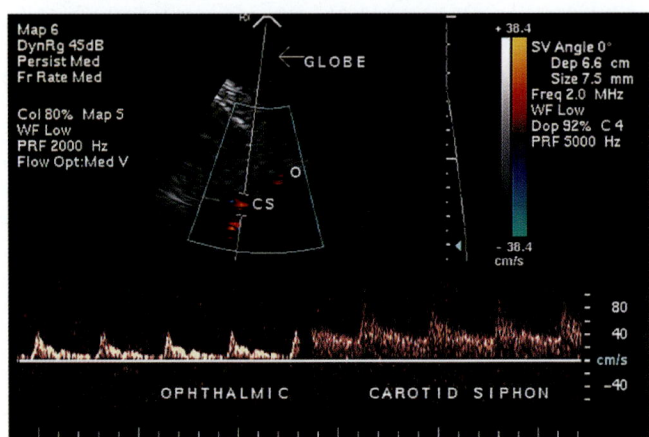

FIG. 38.10 **Color and spectral Doppler image from the transorbital approach.** The ophthalmic spectral Doppler waveform demonstrates a high resistance signal, and the carotid siphon (CS) demonstrates a low resistance signal. A mechanical index of 0.28 or less should be used when imaging via the transorbital approach. *O,* Ophthalmic artery.

The ACoA is not visualized with TCD imaging due to its short length. On the contrary, the longer PCoA can often be seen connecting the anterior and posterior circulations (ACA and PCA, respectively) (Fig. 38.8). The normal mean peak velocity in the PCoA is 36 ± 15 cm/sec, and the direction of blood flow may be toward or away from the transducer. Again, the CD PRF may need to be decreased to appropriately image the PCoA. Additionally, the use of power Doppler (PD) imaging may prove helpful while locating the PCoA, as PD imaging is not susceptible to a loss of information in the area of the vessel insonated at 90 degrees. This makes PD ideal for PCoA imaging, as it often courses parallel to the skin line.

It is important to note that although the anterior and posterior portions of the circle of Willis can often be simultaneously visualized on a single image, variations in anatomy among the population often require minor changes in transducer position on the surface of the skin or its angle of insonation, to permit individual evaluation of either portion.

Transorbital Window. The **transorbital window** allows for imaging and evaluation of the ophthalmic artery and the carotid siphon.[37] The US Food and Drug Administration has approved certain imaging transducers on various manufacturers' equipment for evaluation of the orbit. It is important for all operators to contact the appropriate ultrasound company to determine which transducer is approved for orbital imaging on their system. Furthermore, care should be taken to minimize the amount of acoustic energy exposed to the eye, as a traumatic subluxation of the crystalline lens can occur.[29] Therefore, the ultrasound output power should be significantly decreased and remain <10% for the entirety of transorbital window imaging.[28,29] In addition to acoustic energy concentration, the total time of insonation must also be minimized to prevent further soft tissue and ocular damage. Current maximum acoustic output levels (derated) for ophthalmic imaging allowable by the US Food and Drug Administration are a spatial peak temporal average intensity of 17 mW/cm² and a mechanical index of 0.28.

The transorbital window imaging portion of the TCD examination begins with the patient in the supine position, with the transducer gently placed on the closed eyelid. A liberal amount of acoustic gel is important to reduce the amount of transducer pressure needed. The ultrasound transducer is aligned in a transverse orientation, with the orientation marker pointing medial (while scanning on both the right and left sides). Thus, views from either eye show medial (nasal) on the left, lateral (temporal) on the right, and the globe at the top.

Once transorbital imaging has commenced, the transducer is pointed toward the optic canal to image the carotid siphon.[29] The carotid siphon is located in the medial portion of the transorbital window and is located at an approximate depth range of 58 to 65 mm. The direction of blood flow can be used to determine which portion of the carotid siphon (parasellar, genu, or supraclinoid) is seen (Fig. 38.9). Normal flow is toward the transducer in the parasellar portion, bidirectional in the genu, and away from the transducer in the supraclinoid portion. The mean velocity in the carotid siphon is 47 ± 14 cm/sec.

The ophthalmic artery is generally located adjacent to the optic nerve; therefore, the ultrasound beam should be directed slightly medial along the anteroposterior plane for its insonation. The CD PRF should be decreased to adequately visualize this vessel. Blood flow within the ophthalmic artery is toward the transducer under normal circumstances, with a mean velocity of 21 ± 5 cm/sec. Ophthalmic artery SD waveforms demonstrate higher resistivity than those from the carotid siphon, as the ophthalmic artery supplies blood to the globe and its structures (Fig. 38.10).

Suboccipital Window. Performing TCD imaging via the **suboccipital window** allows for evaluation of the vertebral and basilar arteries of the vertebrobasilar system (Fig. 38.11).[37] Before imaging, the patient should be lying on his or her side with the head bowed slightly toward the chest. This position increases the gap between the cranium and the atlas and has been found to create the best opportunity for TCD imaging. The orientation marker on the transducer is pointed to the patient's right side, while the transducer is placed on the posterior aspect of the neck, inferior to the nuchal crest. The best images from this approach are acquired with transducer placement slightly off midline and angled toward the bridge of the patient's nose.

On the GS image obtained through this acoustic window, the foramen magnum and the occipital bone can be used as the anatomic landmarks while locating the vertebrobasilar system. The foramen magnum will appear as a large, circular, anechoic area. The occipital bone is identified by its echogenic appearance. Under normal circumstances, blood flow within the vertebrobasilar system arteries will travel away from the transducer and can be visualized on CD imaging as a blue Y, which represents the confluence of the vertebral arteries to form the basilar artery (Fig. 38.12). Because of transducer orientation located on the posterior portion of the body, the right vertebral artery is displayed on the left side of the image, and the left vertebral is on the right. The basilar artery is located deep to the vertebral arteries. The mean velocity is 38 ± 10 cm/sec in the vertebral arteries and 41 ± 10 cm/sec in the basilar artery. Because the posterior circulation has lower velocities than the anterior circulation, the operator may need to decrease the CD PRF to visualize the arteries of the vertebrobasilar system.

Attention to the CD gain setting is critical when measuring the exact depth of the vertebral artery confluence. An inappropriately high setting could result in a falsely elevated measure. Appropriate CD settings will also aid in visualizing vertebral artery branches that can often be imaged with this approach. The most common branch visualized of the vertebral arteries is the PICA, which is seen curving as it transports blood away from the suboccipital window transducer location. Moving the transducer slightly inferior on the neck and angling superior provides optimal visualization of the distal portion of the basilar artery. The terminal portion of the basilar artery bifurcating into the PCAs cannot be visualized in this acoustic window.

Submandibular Window. Evaluation of the intracranial vasculature through the **submandibular window** is an approach that is a continuation of the TCD imaging examination, used to interrogate the distal portion of the ICA.[37] Before imaging, the patient is placed in the supine position, with the head tilted up slightly. The transducer is placed at the angle of the mandible and angled slightly medial and cephalad toward the carotid canal. The orientation marker on the transducer should be pointed superiorly. The distal ICA is typically found at a depth of 35 to 80 mm. Normal blood flow in the distal ICA travels away from the transducer. Careful Doppler evaluation is important to distinguish the ICA's low resistance signal from the higher resistance signal of the ECA. The mean velocity in the retromandibular portion of the ICA is normally 37 ± 9 cm/sec.

Intracranial image quality depends on proper ultrasound instrumentation adjustment and continual optimization throughout the examination. Initially, anatomic landmarks are identified using GS imaging to aid in locating various intracranial vessels. Therefore GS parameters such as frequency, sector width, image depth, overall gain, TGC, focal zone number and placement, frame rate, and dynamic range must be appropriately optimized. To obtain quality CD images, the color gain is increased to the appropriate level while maintaining a small sector width and color ROI to preserve frame rate. In addition, color PRF is adjusted depending on the vessel evaluated and the patient's individual hemodynamics. The operator should also remain aware of color sensitivity and persistence settings. Just as the GS image aids in locating intracranial arteries, the CD image aids in determining proper SD gate placement for SD waveform acquisition. The TCD examination is interpreted based on the information obtained from SD waveforms. Therefore SD signals are obtained along the path of the arteries using the color display as a road map. At each depth setting, it is important to adjust the SD gate and angle the transducer to optimize the

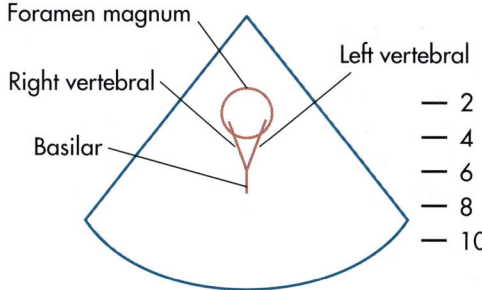

FIG. 38.11 The suboccipital approach used in transcranial Doppler imaging, where the vertebrobasilar system can be visualized.

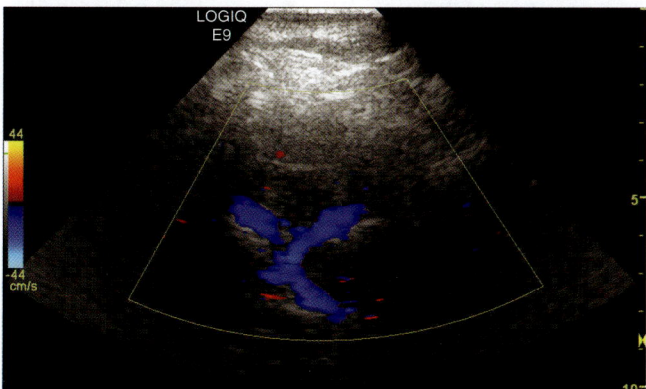

FIG. 38.12 Color Doppler image obtained using the suboccipital approach to visualize the Y created by the confluence of the vertebral arteries to form the basilar artery. Blood flow is away from the transducer, as displayed in blue. The right vertebral artery is on the left side of the image, and the left vertebral artery is on the right side. The basilar artery is deep to the vertebral arteries.

SD signal. Additionally, it is important to remember that the CD image is displayed in only two dimensions; consequently, tortuous intracranial arteries often cannot be displayed along their entire length as a continuous pathway.

INTERPRETATION OF TRANSCRANIAL DOPPLER IMAGING

Proper identification of the intracranial vasculature is, of course, the first step in evaluating the TCD examination. GS imaging should first be used to identify anatomic or bony landmarks (when appropriate), followed by CD imaging to visualize intracranial vasculature blood flow. Each TCD window provides access to specific arteries. The identification of those arteries are based on the following:

1. *Depth of the sample volume.* The sample volume depth is measured in millimeters (mm) and is the distance from the face of the ultrasound transducer to the middle of the SD gate. The SD gate should be kept large (5 to 10 mm) for an optimal signal-to-noise ratio. Depth ranges at which the intracranial arteries are located from each TCD window are listed in Table 38.1. Artery depths vary with each individual, but in most adults, the artery in question will fall within these ranges. Midline is in the range of 70 to 80 mm in most adults.
2. *Angle of the transducer.* The angle of the transducer is important, as different arteries can be insonated at the same depth from the same acoustic window. The operator's position at the patient's head enables the best perception of the transducer-artery angle because it permits orientation of the ultrasound transducer relative to the body's axes and planes.
3. *Blood flow direction.* The normal direction of blood flow in the intracranial arteries relative to the ultrasound transducer is listed in Table 38.1. From the different acoustic windows, SD waveforms may demonstrate blood flow direction away from, toward, or in both directions (bidirectional) from the transducer. If the direction of blood flow is reversed from the established norm, it can be assumed that the artery is functioning as a collateral channel, or it is due to an anatomic variant.
4. *Spatial relationship.* Understanding the spatial relationship of each artery to the others is necessary to properly identify the intracranial arteries. Using the t-ICA bifurcation as a guide, the location of the intracranial arteries is determined with greater technical ease.
5. *Traceability of an artery.* The operator should be able to trace the anatomic route of the artery in a stepwise fashion by increasing or decreasing the depth setting of the SD gate. The SD gate should be moved slowly along the path of the vessel to thoroughly assess its entire length, using the CD display as a guide.
6. *Adjacent anatomic structures.* Using the anatomic structures visualized on GS imaging as a guide to correctly identify the intracranial arteries is especially important. It is the major advantage of using the TCD imaging technique versus the nonimaging TCD.

TABLE 38.1 Intracranial Arterial Identification Criteria

Window/Artery	Depth (mm)	Mean Velocity (cm/sec)	Direction[a]
Transtemporal			
MCA	30–67	62 ± 12	Toward
ACA	60–80	50 ± 11	Away
t-ICA	55–67	39 ± 9	Toward
PCA	60–75	39 ± 10	Toward
PCoA	60–75	36 ± 15	Toward, away
Transorbital			
Ophthalmic	40–60	21 ± 5	Toward
ICA siphon	60–80	47 ± 14	Bi, away, toward
Suboccipital			
Vertebral	60–85	38 ± 10	Away
Basilar	>85	41 ± 10	Away
Submandibular			
ICA	35–80	37 ± 9	Away

[a]Relative to the ultrasound transducer.
ACA, Anterior cerebral artery; *Bi,* bidirectional; *ICA,* internal carotid artery; *t-ICA,* terminal internal carotid artery; *MCA,* middle cerebral artery; *PCA,* posterior cerebral artery; *PCoA,* posterior communicating artery.

Standard interpretation criteria for TCD examinations have been reported in the literature.[7,29,41] These criteria were previously developed using nonimaging TCD, although they have subsequently been applied to TCD imaging. The same measurements are obtained in both techniques, but TCD imaging permits the identification of structural landmarks that elevates the accuracy of the examination by providing visual confirmation of correct SD waveform sampling locations.

Physiologic Factors

The evolution of TCD imaging has made it apparent that important underlying physiologic variables, in addition to pathology, affect blood flow velocities within the intracranial arterial system.[29,41] Therefore, it is important that the operator be aware of the factors that can influence intracranial hemodynamics to interpret each case on an individual basis.[42]

Age. The most important factor influencing intracranial arterial velocity measures obtained in a TCD examination is patient age.[43] Several investigators have reported lower velocities levels in individuals with increasing age.[23,29,41–43] The downward trend in intracranial arterial velocities is most likely multifactorial, possibly due to changes in cardiac output, age-related decrease in cerebral perfusion, decreases in metabolic demands, and/or elevated hematocrit levels.[44]

Sex. Women between 20 and 60 years of age demonstrate higher flow velocities than men, by an estimated 10% to 15%.[29,43–46] Possible explanations for these differences are lower levels of hematocrit found in women, intracranial arteries of women may be smaller in diameter, and/or women having higher hemispheric cerebral blood flow than men.[29,43] It is important to note that there are thought to be no detectable velocity differences between genders after age 70 years.[29]

Hematocrit. Hematocrit (Hct) is the percent of red blood cells by volume in whole blood and is a major determinant of blood viscosity. Blood viscosity, or the thickness, is an important factor that influences intracranial arterial velocities, as blood hematocrit and viscosity levels are inversely related to intracranial arterial blood flow velocity. It has been reported that a decrease in Hct levels from 40% to 30% can cause velocity increases by up to 20%.[47] A clinical example of this is demonstrated in patients with anemia (Hct less than 30%), in which elevated intracranial arterial velocities are expected. If anemia is the cause of elevated velocities, increased velocities should be seen in all intracranial arteries. Focal or localized velocity increases suggest a different cause.

Carbon Dioxide Reactivity. Changes in arterial carbon dioxide (CO_2) partial pressure (P_{CO_2}) have a direct effect relationship on cerebral blood flow and intracranial arterial velocities. Alteration of cerebral vascular resistance and changes in TCD signals result from changes at the level of the arteriolar channels. Clinical examples include hyperventilation (deficient CO_2 in the blood known as hypocapnia), which causes a decrease in MCA mean velocity and an increase in PI. Conversely, hypoventilation (excess CO_2 in the blood referred to as hypercapnia) causes an MCA mean velocity increase and decrease in PI. This information suggests that general changes in the intracranial arterial velocities caused by CO_2 reactivity must be taken into account when interpreting TCD data.

Heart Rate and Cardiac Output. Intracranial arterial velocities are a reflection of an individual's heart rate. Therefore most experienced TCD examiners caution against obtaining SD waveforms during times of cardiac rhythm fluctuations. Fluctuations can occur when the patient is yawning, agitated, experiencing pain, or in any other situation causing a change in heart rate. To this end, any cardiac arrhythmia will be reflected in the TCD SD waveform. If a change in the patient's heart rate is suspected as a cause of an abnormality, several SD waveform tracings should be obtained. To compensate for extreme cases of bradycardia or tachycardia, ultrasound instrumentation such as SD sweep speed or PRF may need to be adjusted. Changes resulting from cardiac output not associated with hemodilution have little effect on the cerebral blood flow if autoregulation is intact. This suggests that TCD velocities should be theoretically independent of small changes in cardiac output. Data on the relationship between cardiac output and intracranial arterial velocities are limited, and further investigation in this area is necessary.[47]

Many parameters are involved in the accurate interpretation of TCD data. Each patient must be considered individually because of the variety of physiologic factors that affect intracranial arterial hemodynamics (Box 38.2).

> **BOX 38.2 Physiologic Factors That Influence Intracranial Arterial Hemodynamics by Location**
>
> **Proximal to the Circle of Willis**
> Patient age
> Amount and location of extracranial arterial obstruction
> Hematocrit level
> Cardiac output
>
> **At the Level of the Circle of Willis**
> Vessel diameter
> Blood viscosity
> Blood flow Turbulence
>
> **Distal to the Circle of Willis**
> Infarction
> Intracranial arteriovenous malformations
> Elevated intracranial pressure
> Change in partial pressure of carbon dioxide (P_{CO_2})

The parameters that affect the intracranial velocities can be categorized into those factors that are (1) proximal to the circle of Willis, (2) at the level of the circle of Willis, and (3) distal to the circle of Willis.

Normal Intracranial Velocities

As mentioned previously, interpretation of a TCD examination is performed through analysis of intracranial arterial SD waveforms. Parameters most commonly derived from SD waveforms are mean flow velocity (time-averaged peak velocities), pulsatility index, and resistive index. Furthermore, qualitative information regarding intracranial hemodynamics can be derived using SD waveform morphology.[7] Peak systolic velocity and end-diastolic velocity can also be used, although they are done so less commonly. Each institution must decide which velocity measure to report and adjust its diagnostic criteria accordingly.

Vessel depths, mean velocities, and normal direction of blood flow relative to the ultrasound transducer for the intracranial arteries from each TCD window are listed in Table 38.1. Although somewhat controversial, it is customary to assume a zero-degree angle (no angle correction) when performing TCD examinations.

The **mean flow velocity (MFV)** is calculated during TCD imaging examinations and is based on the time average of the outline velocity (maximum velocity envelope). The velocity envelope is a trace of the peak velocities as a function of time. Therefore the MFV can be estimated by positioning the horizontal cursor at the velocity location on the SD tracing where the area below the peak velocity and above the cursor are equal to the area below the cursor and above the peak velocity envelope in diastole (Fig. 38.13). Because this measure is an average of the velocities within an SD tracing, and thereby takes into account more physiologic information, it is less affected by changes in central cardiovascular factors (heart rate, peripheral resistance, etc.) than are systolic and/or diastolic values. Therefore MFV diminishes interindividual variation.

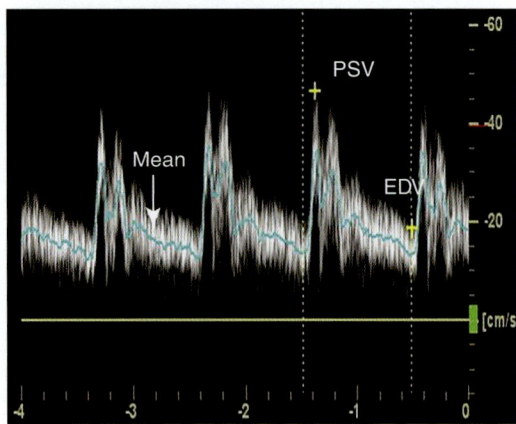

FIG. 38.13 **A spectral Doppler waveform obtained from the middle cerebral artery.** The manually placed electronic calipers mark the peak systolic velocity (PSV) and the end-diastolic velocity (EDV). The mean flow velocity *(blue line)* is an automated tracing by the ultrasound system applied through each cycle of systole and diastole.

Furthermore, due to the physiologic factors that can influence intracranial arterial blood flow, velocity measures vary between each individual (although the most commonly reported measure of MFV is based on average velocities and is used to reduce this).[23] Differences between intracranial arterial velocities are more important than the absolute values recorded from an individual. The most useful TCD results are derived through a comparison of MFVs from different sample volume depths within the same artery and also from different arteries within an individual.[7,29,41,42] General observations of MFVs in the intracranial arteries are as follows:
- Velocities are highest in the MCA.
- ACA velocity greater than 25% of the MCA velocity suggests a hypoplastic ACA. The ACA may also be stenotic, serving as a collateral vessel, or there may be an MCA distribution infarction.
- Velocities in the anterior circulation are higher than in the posterior circulation.

In the asymptomatic adult patient, side-to-side asymmetry should be minimal. Any difference less than 20 cm/sec between two contralateral segments should be considered within normal physiologic range.[48] Others have reported a minimum of 30% asymmetric difference is suggestive of disease.[7] If a significant side-to-side difference is noted during the examination, velocity measurements should be repeated in the side with the lower velocities. Slight changes in the transducer-to-artery angle from what was previously used can reduce the side-to-side differences found on the initial examination. If a significant MFV discrepancy is still observed after multiple remeasures, the examination should be interpreted as abnormal. Additionally, asymmetries in the intracranial vertebral arteries make it difficult to interpret asymmetric velocities from these arteries unless the differences are in a focal vessel segment.

In addition to velocity information, pulsatility index and resistive index can be obtained from SD waveforms. These measures are the most commonly used parameters to provide information regarding intracranial resistance.

The **pulsatility index (PI)** was first described in an attempt to quantify SD waveforms during the evaluation of lower extremity arterial disease.[49] Most imaging systems automatically calculate the PI with each Doppler display using the following formula derived from Gosling and colleagues[49]:

$$PI = \frac{\text{Peak systolic velocity} - \text{End-diastolic velocity}}{\text{Mean flow velocity}}$$

When using the PI measure, the resistance encountered with each cardiac cycle is considered. For example, dampened blood flow distal to an obstruction will have a decreased PI (diastolic velocity greater than 50% to 60% of peak systolic). SD waveforms obtained proximal to a high resistive lesion (i.e., increased intracranial pressure [ICP]) will have increased PI (pulsatile spectral waveform). Normal PI is in the range of 0.6 to 1.1. Elevated PIs are also seen in cases of elevated ICP and decreased cerebral perfusion due to diminished diastolic velocities.[50] Conversely, diminished PI values are seen in arteries supplying arteriovenous malformations, as well as distal to a severe extracranial or intracranial stenosis.

The **resistive index (RI)**, first described by Pourcelot and colleagues, is another measure of arterial resistance within the intracranial arterial system.[51] Similar to PI, the RI is automatically calculated on most imaging systems using the following formula:

$$RI = \frac{\text{Peak systolic velocity} - \text{End-diastolic velocity}}{\text{Peak systolic velocity}}$$

The normal range of RI values is 0.49 to 0.63. Elevated RI values have also been used as indicators for elevated ICP and have been positively associated with many other pathologic conditions, including hydrocephalus.[51,52]

In addition to the quantitative information gained from the SD tracing, analysis of the SD waveforms can provide information regarding intracranial hemodynamics qualitatively. These findings can be compared with the contralateral side to determine whether differences in intracranial hemodynamics exist within that segment. Proximal to a significant stenosis, dampened waveforms (characterized by normal systolic and diastolic flow but diminished in magnitude) are seen. Within a stenosis, a spike in waveform amplitude with an increase in acceleration, as well as diminished diastolic flow, are typically seen. Artifacts such as CD and SD signal aliasing may also be present. Distal to an area of significant stenosis, SD waveforms are often described as "blunted." Blunted waveforms are characterized by flattened or delayed systolic flow, as well as diminished size.

It is important to note that spectral broadening is a common observation in SD waveforms obtained during TCD imaging; however, it should not be interpreted as turbulent flow. It is caused by the large size of the SD gate. SD gate size used during TCD imaging is typically larger than what is used while performing extracranial or peripheral arterial SD imaging. In fact, the sample volume often includes the entire cross-sectional lumen of an intracranial artery and any small branches that may be present. Therefore even though spectral broadening may be used as a diagnostic criterion for moderate degrees of stenosis in the extracranial carotid arteries, it is not helpful in refining the TCD interpretation.

Last, bilateral symmetric disease may be difficult to diagnose by TCD imaging, as a comparison between the same segments of the ipsilateral and contralateral could demonstrate no significant differences. To aid in detection, the correct identification of intracranial arteries, knowledge of normal velocity ranges, familiarity with the technique's limitations, and an understanding of how cerebral hemodynamics are affected by different physiologic factors are essential for accurate interpretation of TCD examinations. It is imperative that each institution develop a TCD imaging protocol that defines the standard examination (arteries to be evaluated from each window, the number of images, both CD and SD, to be obtained from each artery, etc.). This protocol must include the technique, clinical applications, indications for a complete and/or limited examination, and interpretation criteria. A standard complete examination typically includes evaluation of the right and left sides, acquiring Doppler information from both the anterior and posterior intracranial arterial systems.

CLINICAL APPLICATIONS

Vasospasm

Cerebral vasospasm (vasoconstriction of the cerebral arteries) is a serious complication that occurs following SAH in 50% to 70% of cases and is a significant cause of morbidity and mortality.[53] SAH affects between 25,000 and 30,000 individuals in the United States annually, with an incidence of approximately 30% to 70%.[54,55] The most common cause of SAH is leakage of blood from intracranial cerebral aneurysms into the subarachnoid space. Common sites for intracranial aneurysm formation are the ACoA, the MCA, and the PCoA. Vasospasms manifest clinically as decreased levels of consciousness, headaches, and focal neurologic signs.[42]

The primary pathologic condition associated with vasospasm is vasoconstriction of cerebral arteries, causing a decreased lumen diameter.[54] Blood flow velocity is inversely related to the cross-sectional area of the arterial lumen; thus elevated flow velocities are detectable with TCD imaging. A pressure drop distal to the narrowed arterial segment can also be seen with TCD. Compensatory mechanisms within the intracranial arteries account for pressure changes and maintain cerebral blood flow via collateral circulations and cerebral autoregulation. When ICP is increased, or the vasomotor reserve exhausted, cerebral blood flow is reduced to critical levels, resulting in ischemia or infarction. Therefore accurate detection is critical, as this will lead to earlier and more effective patient management.[56]

TCD examinations are most commonly performed bedside in the intensive care unit (ICU). Important technical features when studying a patient with vasospasm associated with SAH are as follows:

- The operator must be properly positioned at the patient's bedside so transducer angle adjustments can be made while still maintaining the ability to adjust instrumentation settings on the ultrasound machine.
- Headphones are helpful because high-velocity signals associated with vasospasm can be difficult to appreciate in the presence of extraneous background noise.
- If possible, the locations of the transtemporal windows should be marked on the patient's skin for subsequent examinations to be performed at the same location, thereby increasing the reliability of comparisons.
- If possible, repeat or follow-up examinations should be performed by the same operator to eliminate errors associated with interobserver variability.

In some patients, a surgical head dressing may need to be removed to access the transtemporal window. Sterile ultrasound gel should be used if the transducer is placed near a wound. TCD recording is possible through a burr hole, but output power levels should be decreased because there is no bone to cause attenuation of the Doppler signal. TCD imaging in this group of patients can be challenging because of patient cooperation, changes in cardiovascular and cerebral hemodynamics, and less than optimal testing conditions in the ICU. Furthermore, clip artifacts may mask localized segments of increased velocity.

The current gold standard for diagnosing vasospasms is cerebral digital subtraction angiography or computed tomography angiography; however, these cannot be performed bedside and add risks associated with ionizing radiation exposure and being invasive.[57] Vasospasm is detectable with TCD imaging 2 to 5 days after SAH.[58] Therefore, a prespastic TCD examination before day 2 is typically ordered to provide valuable baseline information for comparisons with repeat examinations monitoring the rate of vasospasm development. This also provides a guide for subsequent imaging, as vessels in spasm are small and can be difficult to locate. The TCD examination should be performed daily or every other day for 2 weeks, recording the highest velocity obtained in each artery; however, the frequency of follow-up studies will vary depending on clinical symptoms and vasospasm degree. Although a complete TCD examination is preferred, it is not always possible in this population.

In addition to velocity measurements within the spastic arterial segment, a cervical ICA signal is obtained at a depth of 45 to 60 mm (without angle adjustment) to calculate a hemispheric ratio. The P_{CO_2}, Hct, and blood pressure of the patient are obtained at the time of each TCD examination, as these may affect intracranial arterial blood flow velocities. The time and the date of the examination are also documented for graphing of velocity as a function of time to illustrate the time course of a patient's vasospasm. Over the time of 1 day post-SAH, an elevation of greater than 65 cm/sec or 20% increase in flow velocity is suggestive of vasospasm.[59]

Velocity criteria are generally accepted for vasospasm diagnosis. Most commonly, MFVs of up to 120 cm/sec suggest mild angiographic stenosis (25% to 50% diameter reduction) and are indicative of mild vasospasm.[60] MFVs 120 to 200 cm/sec suggest moderate angiographic stenosis (50% diameter reduction) and are indicative of moderate vasospasm. MFVs greater than 200 cm/sec suggest severe angiographic stenosis (diameter reduction >50%) and are indicative of severe vasospasm.[60] Patients with MFVs greater than 200 cm/sec are at risk for reduced cerebral blood flow that can initiate ischemic processes. A form of this is known as delayed ischemia deficit and typically occurs when a severe vasospasm causes vessel lumen to narrow less than 1 mm.[7] A rapid increase in MFV (65 cm/sec or 20% per day) days after SAH is associated with poor prognosis.[7,23]

The MCA/ICA (distal extracranial ICA) mean velocity ratio, also known as the Lindegaard ratio, may also be used to determine vasospasm.[61] This is a hemispheric ratio that accounts for possible falsely elevated MFV values due to increases in flow volume. The ratio increases with severe spasms resulting from increased MCA velocity with maintained ICA velocity, as well as with reduced blood flow volume in the ipsilateral extracranial ICA caused by elevated cerebral vascular resistance. Lindegaard ratio values greater than six indicate severe vasospasm, values three to six indicate moderate vasospasm, and values less than three are suggestive of hyperemia.

The sensitivity for diagnosing vasospasm by TCD depends on the skill of the operator, the presence of a good transtemporal window, anatomic consistency, a good transducer-to-artery angle, the location and severity of the vasospasm, the presence of proximal hemodynamically significant lesions, physiologic parameters (increased ICP, blood pressure fluctuations, Pco_2 variations, Hct, etc.), the diagnostic criteria used, and the cooperation of the patient. In general, however, the use of TCD for the detection of vasospasm is regarded with high sensitivity and specificity within both anterior and posterior circulation.[62] A review of the literature has reported sensitivity and specificity values up to 94% and 100%, respectively, for the detection of MCA vasospasm.[23] However, sensitivity and specificity levels begin to diminish as vasospasm location becomes more distal.[29] It is important to note that a negative TCD examination does not exclude vasospasm. Sources of error include (1) a tortuous or aberrant artery, (2) distal branch vasospasm, (3) increased ICP, and/or (4) a reduction in flow volume (with or without infarction).

Diagnosis of Intracranial Disease

Among its ability to detect and monitor vasospasm, TCD imaging has the ability to acquire real-time physiologic information noninvasively, which aids in the detection of multiple other intracranial arterial vascular pathologies. However, it is important to remember that the arterial vasculature system is a closed system that preserves pressures within it, allowing pathology within an artery to cause significant effects elsewhere. For this reason, one must be cognizant of hemodynamic changes associated with intracranial (and extracranial) disease to accurately assess the intracranial vasculature.

Stenosis. Atherosclerotic plaque lesions cause narrowing of the arterial lumen. Intracranial atherosclerosis is estimated to cause 10% of transient ischemic attacks and strokes, making detection critical.[63] Stenosis within the ICA siphon, vertebral arteries, and the proximal segments of the MCA, ACA, PCA, basilar arteries, and the proximal (P1) segment of the PCA can be reliably detected using TCD imaging.[63,64]

Intracranial arterial stenoses cause characteristic alterations in the Doppler signal (audio and visually on SD waveforms), including focal increases in MFV, local turbulence, prestenotic decrease in MFV and increase in PI, poststenotic drop in MFV, and an increase in MFV and/or reversal of flow in collateral vessels.[41] Stenoses may also produce low-frequency enhancements around the baseline (bruit) or band-shaped enhancements symmetric with and parallel to the baseline (musical murmur). Changes can also be identified using CD imaging, such as vessel narrowing, turbulent flow, and color aliasing.

Implementation of a standardized TCD imaging protocol has been reported to enhance the reliably of significant intracranial stenoses.[65]

Velocity criteria for diameter reduction diagnosis have been reported for each of the intracranial vessels, but a general consensus on their standardization has not been made.[7] This is due to the many physiologic nonvascular variables (age, Hct, etc.) that can alter MFV. Furthermore, the high level of tortuosity and anatomic variation that exists within arteries of the posterior circulation has caused the reliability measures of the anterior circulation to be, in general, higher.[29,54] Because of the level of MFV variability among individuals, most investigators agree that a focal MFV increase of 30% or greater should raise suspicion of arterial narrowing.[7] Intracranial stenoses are most commonly found in the MCA and the internal carotid siphon. Cerebral tissue perfusion status can also have a considerable impact on intracranial velocity profiles. Patients with central MCA stenosis without infarction demonstrate increased MCA MFV; however, the same patient with a cerebral infarction will demonstrate diminished MCA MFV because of decreased perfusion through the infarcted outflow bed.

Occlusion. TCD imaging demonstrates high levels of sensitivity and specificity (approximately 90%) for the detection of cerebral vessel occlusion.[66] Furthermore, it can also be used with high levels of accuracy to follow the progression of a known occlusion. This is typically done to gauge the effectiveness of treatment.[63] Occlusion should be suspected in the absence of flow if it is at the location and depth of a specific cerebral artery, provided the acoustic window being used allows adequate imaging. The adequacy of an acoustic window can be confirmed by obtaining a signal from a different vessel using that same window. Without an appropriate acoustic window, occlusion detection is very difficult. The absence of blood flow should be documented using both SD and CD imaging. Additional findings of elevated MFVs in collateral vessels will support the diagnosis of cerebral artery occlusion.

Collateral Pathways. The TCD examination is able to reveal intracranial arterial collateral patterns in patients with intracranial or extracranial arterial stenosis or occlusion. These pathways are typically inactive under normal conditions but open when flow-limiting lesions cause a pressure gradient between two anastomosing arterial systems. The direction of collateral flow is dependent on the direction of collateralization, as the flow travels away from the donor artery to the recipient vessel(s).[67,68] Knowing this allows for their accurate identification. Further, the donor artery tends to demonstrate an increase in MFV.[63] Unlike focal increases in MFV found in arterial stenoses, collateral pathways contain diffuse velocity increases throughout the length of the artery.

Three common collateral pathways identifiable by TCD are (1) the ACoA, providing a channel from hemisphere to hemisphere; (2) the PCoA, providing a channel between the posterior and anterior circulation; and (3) the ophthalmic artery, providing a channel from the extracranial ECA to the intracranial ICA. Findings of collateral flow have been reported as markers of pathology with high levels of sensitivity and specificity for the ACoA (both 100%) and the PCoA (85% and 95%, respectively), compared with angiography.[63]

The most commonly found collateral pathway in response to significant extracranial disease is prominent flow within the ACoA. TCD findings of this collateral pathway include (1) elevated MFV in the contralateral ACA; (2) a turbulent SD signal with increased MFV at midline (resultant from high-velocity blood flow through the small ACoA); and (3) reversal of blood flow direction in the ipsilateral ACA (known as anterior cross-filling).

Similarly, prominent flow discovered in the PCoA suggests collateral communication between the anterior and posterior circulation systems of the circle of Willis.[29] Under normal conditions, flow within the PCoA is not typically detectable using TCD imaging. Using a transtemporal approach, the direction of flow in the PCoA is dependent on collateralization, anterior to posterior collateral flow is demonstrated away from the transducer, and posterior to anterior collateral flow is demonstrated toward the transducer. The SD waveform of posterior to anterior collateralization may demonstrate a slight delay in systolic acceleration and is often found in individuals with significant bilateral extracranial carotid artery disease. Conversely, a delay in acceleration time of the SD waveforms will not be evident in circumstances of anterior to posterior collateralization.

The third most common collateral pathway, the ophthalmic artery, can be detected using TCD imaging as it carries blood from the ECA to the ICA. This finding is characterized by blood flow reversal and a low-resistance SD signal in the ophthalmic artery. While imaging via the transorbital window, the blood flow direction will appear to be traveling away from the transducer. Reversed ophthalmic artery flow is typically suggestive of severe ICA stenosis or occlusion.

Subclavian Steal. **Subclavian steal syndrome** is caused by stenosis or occlusion of the left subclavian, innominate, or right subclavian artery proximal to the vertebral artery origin, causing hypoperfusion of the posterior circulation. A

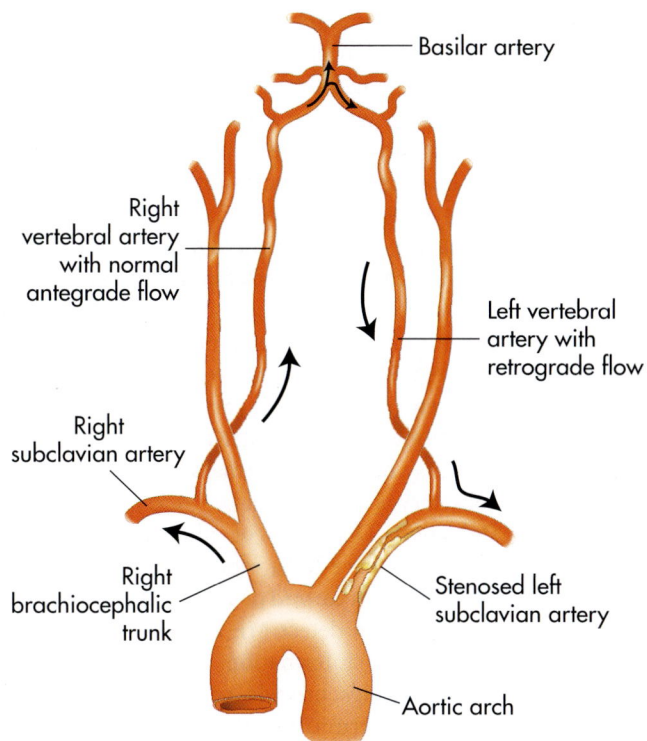

FIG. 38.14 **Subclavian steal.** A narrowing of the left subclavian artery proximal to the vertebral artery causes a pressure drop that may lead to retrograde flow in the left vertebral artery. This change in direction can be visualized in the extracranial or intracranial vertebral arteries.

clinical finding consistent with subclavian steal is a systolic pressure differential greater than 20 mm Hg between brachial blood pressures (with the subclavian or innominate artery obstruction located on the side with the lower pressure). This is caused by an upper extremity pressure gradient resulting in reversal vertebral artery flow (Fig. 38.14). Subclavian steal is especially common during exercise, and when this occurs, the vertebral artery becomes a major collateral pathway to the upper extremity by "stealing" blood from the basilar artery. Retrograde vertebral artery flow causes the patient to experience neurologic symptoms of brainstem ischemia.

If subclavian steal is suspected, a standard TCD examination should be performed with special attention paid to the direction of blood flow and velocities in the vertebral and basilar arteries. Under normal circumstances, blood flows away from the transducer (suboccipital approach) in the vertebrobasilar system. Flow towards the transducer in a vertebral and/or the basilar artery is suggestive of a steal. Often the retrograde flow direction is found only in the vertebral artery, suggesting the possibility of a vertebral-to-vertebral artery steal.

In the absence of retrograde flow at rest or bidirectional (alternating) flow, the upper extremity demonstrating the lower brachial pressure should be stressed to reduce outflow resistance, thereby revealing the hemodynamics of a potentially latent steal. The baseline examination and the subsequent changes in SD waveforms that occur after arm exercise or after occlusive hyperemia are then recorded and labeled as such. To perform postocclusive reactive hyperemia, a blood pressure cuff is applied to the ipsilateral arm with the suspected stenosis/occlusion. The ipsilateral vertebral artery SD signal is located and monitored during the inflation of the arm cuff. The blood pressure cuff is inflated (greater than 30 mm Hg above systolic) for approximately 3 minutes, and any changes in the SD signals are noted. Next, the cuff is rapidly deflated while changes in vertebral artery blood flow direction and velocity are recorded. This procedure should be repeated while monitoring the contralateral vertebral and basilar arteries. A 5- to 10-minute rest period is usually sufficient for the return of baseline arterial hemodynamics between evaluations. Resting basilar artery blood flow is rarely affected but may become abnormal if the contralateral feeding vertebral artery is also diseased.

Microemboli Detection. Detection of microemboli (ME), both gaseous and solid, have been reported during routine TCD testing in patients with carotid or cardiac disease.[54] TCD imaging is not only able to detect ME but can also provide location and quantitative information. Although typically asymptomatic, ME findings provide supplementary information for prognostic determinations when assessing stroke risk.[54] Microemboli monitoring is performed in the MCA, typically in the trunk (depth 45 to 55 mm), using SD. The presence of circulating ME causes irregularities on the SD signal, which are referred to as high-intensity transient signals (HITS) (Fig. 38.15).[69] A proper SD gain setting is critical to detect ME and should be reduced so that HITS are not masked by noise within the SD window. The ME rate is reported as the number of HITS observed on the SD waveform per hour, with a minimum imaging requirement of 15 to 20 minutes. In 1995 the Consensus Committee of the Ninth International Cerebral Hemodynamic Symposium proposed minimal identification criteria for establishing microembolic signals.[70] An individual SD microembolic signal must have the following four features:
- Transient microembolic signal, usually lasting less than 300 microseconds (μsec).
- Microembolic signal amplitude is at least three decibels higher than the background blood flow signal.
- Unidirectional SD waveform signal.
- The microembolic signal is accompanied by a "snap," "chirp," or "moan" on the audio output.

A second International Consensus Group in 1998 supported the previous consensus and went on to establish recommendations for specific ultrasound parameters and interpretation criteria for ME detection.[71]

Microembolic signals have been detected in symptomatic and asymptomatic individuals with high-grade ICA stenosis, prosthetic cardiac valves, myocardial infarction, atrial fibrillation, aortic arch atheroma, fat embolization syndrome, and/or retinal or general cerebral vascular disease. In addition, these signals occur in coronary catheterization, coronary angioplasty, direct current cardioversion, cerebral angiography, carotid endarterectomy, carotid angioplasty, and cardiopulmonary bypass.[63]

Multiple studies have reported TCD imaging to be an effective method of identifying both symptomatic and asymptomatic individuals with hemodynamically significant ICA stenosis who are at higher risk of stroke.[72-74] To this end, TCD imaging can play an important role in providing information to justify an ICA revascularization procedure.[74-76]

The detection of cerebral ME by TCD imaging offers diagnostic information and informs patient management decisions in those with cerebrovascular disease. High levels of interobserver agreement suggest ME detection by TCD is sufficiently reproducible for use in the clinical setting. Finally, adding the potential advantage of ME detection to TCD monitoring must be balanced with known limitations.

Predicting Stroke in Sickle Cell Disease. TCD imaging is used in the pediatric population most commonly as a screening technique for stroke risk in children with sickle cell disease. Pediatric sickle cell disease is characterized by chronic hemolysis, causing low circulating hemoglobin. This leads to fibrous proliferation of the intracranial intima and associated inflammation of the endothelium with subsequent stenosis. As a result, sickle cell anemia is the highest risk of first-ever stroke, with the incidence in children with sickle cell anemia thought to be as high as 11% by age 20 years.[37,54] Cerebral infarction and stroke is associated with an occlusion vasculopathy involving the t-ICA, proximal MCA, and ACA.[37] TCD imaging enables detection of intracranial endothelium inflammation and stenosis by findings increased MFV in focal areas, with the goal of early detection decreasing the risk of stroke.

Criteria for the detection of sickle cell disease using TCD imaging have been established and are well defined in the literature.[77,78] MFVs between 171 to 199 cm/sec are indicative

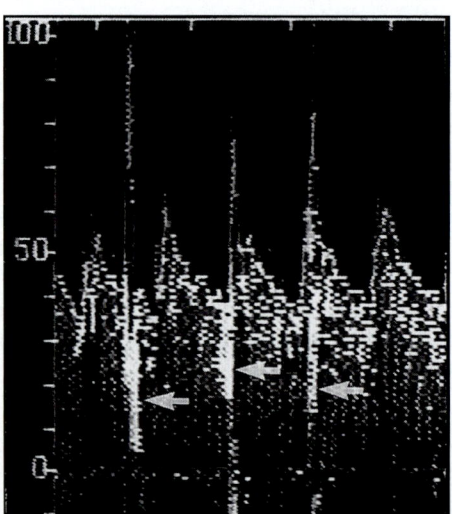

FIG. 38.15 Microemboli *(arrows)* cause irregularities, referred to as high-intensity transient signals, to appear in the spectral Doppler waveform obtained from a middle cerebral artery.

of conditional sickle cell disease and typically warrant further follow-up examinations. MFVs greater than 200 cm/sec on two consecutive TCD examinations suggests a 30% decrease in circulating hemoglobin and a 40% risk of stroke within the next 3 years.[42] This typically warrants a blood transfusion to reduce the chance of stroke.[42] TCD imaging diagnostic criteria of sickle cell disease has been reported with high levels of sensitivity (86%) and specificity (91%) compared with angiographic imaging.[63] This has been supported by a randomized trial which reported up to a 92% decrease in stroke in children with sickle cell who underwent TCD imaging.[79]

Currently, the National Heart, Lung, and Blood Institute, among other consensus groups and guidelines, recommend screening all children with sickle cell anemia between the ages of 2 to 16 years.[80] Therefore, sickle cell screening TCD examinations are common and have established screening criteria.[81] Furthermore, it has been found that siblings of children suffering from sickle cell disease are also at an increased risk of stroke and commonly present for screening examinations.[82] Last, follow-up examinations of high-risk children are also common, as the Second Stroke Prevention Trial in Sickle Cell Anemia (STOP 2) reported that elevated MFV and subsequent stroke is an ongoing risk in children.[83]

Technical adjustments when evaluating children with TCD imaging include using a smaller sample volume size (5 to 6 mm), applying different depth ranges for the intracranial arteries (dependent upon patient age), and adjusting PRF settings to accommodate increased intracranial arterial velocities (Fig. 38.16).

Posttrauma Brain Injury. Traumatic brain injury (TBI) is a major cause of morbidity and mortality. A somewhat innovative use of TCD imaging is the evaluation of cerebral perfusion following TBI. Because TCD imaging is noninvasive and portable, applications in TBI evaluation are common in the emergency department (ED) or ICU to complement computed tomography imaging for the assessment of cerebral perfusion.[84] Degree of neurologic function following TBI depends partially on the extent of cerebral damage, making knowledge of cerebral perfusion critical for patient management decisions.[85] Within the first 48 hours following TBI, diminished intracranial arterial MFVs are present as cerebral hypoperfusion occurs, followed by an increase in MFVs between 48 and 120 hours post-TBI.[23] Early findings of cerebral hypoperfusion allow earlier treatment to increase blood flow to the brain, thereby increasing the degree of neurologic function upon recovery. One study defined MFVs less than 30 cm/sec obtained via TCD imaging as abnormally low cerebral perfusion in adults presenting to the ED with TBI.[86] The investigators found that TCD results were available in approximately 18 minutes and were comparable with invasive cerebral monitoring information, which was not available until approximately 4 hours after ED admission.

Cerebral Circulatory Arrest

An increase in ICP causes compression of the intracranial arteries and impedes brain perfusion leading to cerebral circulatory arrest (CCA), also known as brain death, if prolonged.[59] Once ICP has risen to the level of causing cerebral perfusion less than 70 mm Hg, changes in intracranial arterial pulsatility can be observed, making increased pulsatility the earliest sign of increased ICP.[63] TCD imaging has the ability to detect and quantify these pulsatility changes, but it cannot make this diagnosis alone and is typically used in conjunction with other testing.[87,88] This application is not part of a standard TCD examination and is used only in circumstances of suspected elevated ICP or CCA.

As mentioned, the first detectable sign of elevated ICP is increased pulsatility in the intracranial arteries. If ICP continues to increase, a reduction in diastolic flow will be

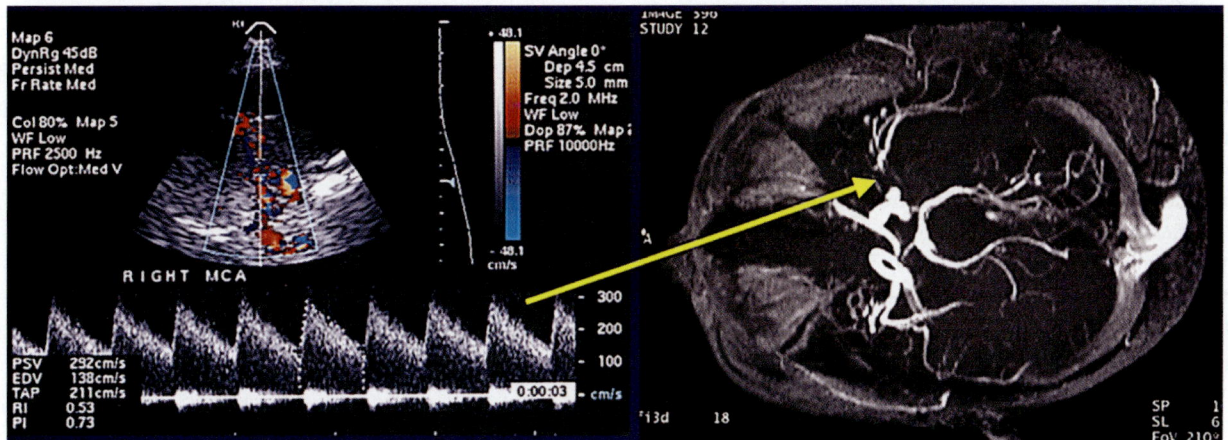

FIG. 38.16 Color and spectral Doppler image obtained during transcranial Doppler imaging, and the corresponding magnetic resonance angiography image of an 8-year-old patient with sickle cell disease. The mean flow velocity of the middle cerebral artery is greater than 200 cm/sec and corresponds to intracranial arterial narrowing *(arrow)*.

observed, followed by diminished MFVs.[63] If ICP levels become severely high, diastolic flow will be absent, followed by bidirectional flow (also known as reverberating or oscillating flow, characterized by a reversed diastolic component); only small systolic peaks will be visualized until, eventually, no flow is detectable.[37,63] Imaging protocols and interpretation guidelines for the determination of CCA have been proposed.[7] TCD imaging's ability to confirm CCA has been well documented and is considered to be fairly accurate, as multiple meta-analyses report combined sensitivities of 89% and specificities of 99%.[89-91]

Intracranial Venous Evaluation. TCD imaging has allowed investigators to begin exploring the intracranial venous system. Although studies investigating TCD's use in the evaluation of intracranial veins are limited, multiple applications have been proposed.[23] One such use is providing information regarding ICP, as venous MFV measures have been reported as a reliable parameter that is directly associated with ICP.[50] Furthermore, TCD imaging has been investigated in its use for evaluating intracranial venous flow direction in individuals with multiple sclerosis.[92] Applications for the detection of intracranial venous thrombosis have also been suggested.[63]

Several instrument adjustments are important when evaluating intracranial venous blood flow. The ultrasound evaluation of normal intracranial veins produces low-amplitude, pulsatile SD signals. Therefore CD, SD PRF, and wall filter settings should be significantly reduced to acquire high-quality intracranial venous Doppler signals.

Intraoperative Use of Transcranial Doppler Technology

TCD can provide noninvasive monitoring of cerebral blood flow during surgery, allowing detection of velocity fluctuations or MEs in real-time. If an abnormality is detected, it can be immediately addressed to reduce the risk of intraoperative ischemic cerebral complications and subsequent injury. Intraoperative TCD monitoring is typically performed during procedures involving the carotid artery, most commonly carotid artery stenting and carotid endarterectomy.[93]

Before the procedure, optimized waveforms of the MCA bilaterally should be obtained for recording throughout the operation. Typically this is done using a transtemporal approach. Because the patient's indication is most often severe extracranial ICA disease, baseline TCD waveforms may appear abnormal (blunted peak systolic wave component) on the ipsilateral side of the stenosed ICA.[93] It is important that the preprocedural (baseline) waveform be thoroughly evaluated to understand the hemodynamics of that individual patient.

During the procedure, the MCA is monitored for changes in (1) MFV/flow volume and (2) the occurrence of ME disturbances on the TCD waveform. When monitoring MFV, it is important to remember that occlusive devices are typically placed in the ICA distal to the area being operated to protect cerebral circulation from debris. When this occurs, an expected dramatic drop in MCA MFV will occur in individuals without adequate collateral pathways or an incomplete circle of Willis.[93] As described previously, ME can be detected in TCD waveform as HITS. These are commonly seen throughout all stages of the procedure; however, a dramatic increase in their frequency warrants attention.

Another intraoperative application of TCD is cerebral hemodynamics monitoring during coronary artery bypass graft placement in patients with concomitant ICA disease.[94] This, however, is a fairly new application that is in need of further investigation.[29]

ADVANTAGES AND LIMITATIONS OF TRANSCRANIAL DOPPLER IMAGING

TCD imaging has several advantages and limitations (Box 38.3) compared with the nonimaging technique. However, advances in TCD imaging technology and the discovery of new knowledge through TCD imaging research will reduce its limitations while maximizing the advantages, leading to optimal and high-quality evaluation of intracranial hemodynamics.

Large advantages of TCD imaging include its noninvasive, portable, and cost-effective nature. It also does not require ionizing radiation. Furthermore, it is largely tolerated by patients and is therefore commonly used when other radiographic imaging is contraindicated. Since its inception in 1982, TCD imaging's clinical utility has been well described with established interpretation criteria, which can provide both diagnostic and prognostic information.

Another advantage to TCD imaging is the ability to visualize anatomic landmarks to guide the examination and ensure the proper identification of the intracranial arteries. This instills confidence in the operator and leads to improved reliability. For those inexperienced in TCD, CD

BOX 38.3 Limitations of Transcranial Doppler Imaging

- Operator inexperience
- User dependent—inter- and intraoperator variability
- Improper instrument control settings
- Uncooperative patient or patient movement
- Absent or poor transtemporal window
- Anatomic variations
- Arterial misidentification
- Distal branch disease
- Distal basilar artery
- Misinterpretation of collateral channels or vasospasm as stenosis
- Arterial displacement by intracranial mass

imaging has the ability to lessen the learning curve for the performance of a quality examination. Additionally, TCD imaging enables identification of the large M2 branches, accurate identification of contralateral arteries (if a transtemporal window can be located only on one side), easy visualization of collateral pathways, ease in following tortuous vessels, and the identification of the vertebral confluence in many patients. Imaging also provides a method to document the location from which the SD waveform is derived, which becomes important during repeat examinations as it decreases interobserver variance in departments with multiple operators and/or interpreters. This is also beneficial when quality improvement is desired.

The main limitation of TCD imaging is its heavy operator dependence. For inexperienced operators, this can cause low levels of intra- and interobserver reliability. Therefore is imperative that the operator have an in-depth knowledge of intracranial anatomy and physiology, as well as a sound understanding of Doppler imaging principles for proper TCD imaging to be performed. A high-quality TCD examination requires appropriate manipulation of more instrument controls than are used during the nonimaging technique in extracranial cerebrovascular sonographic imaging. For example, the distal basilar artery is difficult to visualize using CD because of the large beam width required when CD imaging is employed. The operator must recognize that SD imaging uses a smaller beam diameter, making it more sensitive to detect low-flow states. Therefore the basilar artery can often be followed further distal by increasing the SD gate (sample volume) depth and continuing to follow the course of the basilar artery, as would be done in a nonimaging examination, using the SD waveforms as a guide. Furthermore, the larger beam width associated with CD imaging also hampers penetration of the temporal bone in circumstances of a small transtemporal acoustic window.

Diagnostic Pitfalls

Sources of error that arise during the TCD examination while detecting intracranial arterial disease are as follows:

- Misinterpreting collateral channels or vasospasm as stenosis. Vasospasm typically involves several arteries, and the velocities change with time.
- Technical limitations of evaluating distal branch disease (stenosis or occlusion).
- Misinterpretation of a tortuous or displaced MCA (by hematoma or tumor) as occlusion.
- Mislabeling vessels due to anatomic variability (location, asymmetry, tortuosity), especially in the vertebrobasilar system.
- Technical difficulty evaluating the distal basilar artery.
- Poor-quality arteriography or angiography, leading to inaccurate correlations with TCD imaging results.

TCD imaging offers new and important advantages to the TCD examination. Using appropriate anatomic landmarks and proper instrument controls increases the accuracy and reproducibility of intracranial arterial hemodynamics evaluations. Box 38.4 includes guidelines for TCD imaging. Among others, these will lead to high-quality and accurate examinations. Additional tips to address common technical challenges during TCD imaging examinations are included in Table 38.2. PD imaging offers technical advantages while imaging small intracranial arteries with slower blood flow, as well as intracranial arteries located at unfavorable angles relative to the insonated ultrasound beam (Fig. 38.17). Future technology may offer improved visualization of the intracranial circulation by advances in PD imaging, three-dimensional ultrasound imaging, and contrast-enhanced imaging technologies. Recent advances in TCD imaging technology include an automated TCD imaging system, which has been found to reliably detect MCA blood flow

---

BOX 38.4 Transcranial Doppler Imaging Guidelines

- Obtain a patient medical history, focusing on risk factors, symptoms, and current medications associated with cerebrovascular (specifically intracranial) disease.
- Review the patient's chart or electronic medical record (EMR) to obtain laboratory values (hematocrit, intracranial pressure, blood pressure, heart rate, cardiac output) relevant to intracranial arterial disease.
- Review the patient's chart or EMR for any relevant prior imaging pertaining to the evaluation of intracranial hemodynamics (TCD imaging, arteriography, angiography) to serve as a baseline for comparison the current examination.
- Know the status of the extracranial vessels.
- Understand intracranial arterial anatomy, physiology, and pathology.
- Understand how color Doppler and spectral Doppler instrument controls affect each other, and the effect they will have on the displayed image.
- Use the color/power Doppler display as a guide to ensure that spectral Doppler waveform information is obtained at the correct location.
- Use a large spectral Doppler gate (5–10 mm) with a zero-degree angle.
- Be aware of spectral Doppler waveform morphology.
- Compare spectral Doppler waveforms obtained in the anterior and posterior circulations and in the left and right hemispheres.
- Establish institutional diagnostic criteria for each of the various clinical applications of TCD imaging.

TABLE 38.2	Transcranial Color Doppler Imaging: Technical Hints	
Challenge	Possible Explanations	Action
Absent or poor-quality spectral Doppler or color Doppler signal	• Absent acoustic window • Window not located • Poor patient positioning • Intracranial disease (occlusion or stenosis)	1. Undergo a systematic search for a better acoustic window. A TCD window may be located by repositioning the transducer, changing the angle of insonation, adjusting spectral Doppler gate depth, or modifying color Doppler settings. 2. Check technical settings to ensure maximum output power is being used, especially when imaging via the transtemporal window. Adjusting the color gain/PRF settings may also prove valuable when searching for an acoustic window. 3. Utilize power Doppler to identify low-flow states. 4. Add more ultrasound gel to maintain good transducer-to-skin contact. 5. Use a lower-frequency transducer 6. Reposition the patient, especially from the suboccipital approach. 7. Use headphones to eliminate extraneous noise, to detect subtle spectral Doppler signals.
Multiple spectral Doppler signals	• Large spectral Doppler gate size • Anatomic variation • Overlapping vessel	1. Decrease spectral Doppler gate size. 2. Search for a better acoustic window by repositioning the transducer or changing the angle of the insonation. 3. Use gray-scale imaging to identify bony anatomical landmarks to confirm correct location.
Background noise in spectral Doppler signal	• Improper gain settings • Improper placement of spectral Doppler gate	1. Adjust spectral Doppler gain to optimize waveform by minimizing background noise. 2. Carefully adjust the angle of insonation to improve the signal-to-noise ratio. 3. Change spectral Doppler gate depth by small increments to improve signal quality.
Artifact in spectral Doppler signal	• Patient movement • Transducer movement • Inadequate amount of ultrasound gel	1. Take the time to put the patient at ease or answer any questions to minimize movement. 2. Minimize transducer movement by properly adjusting the operator's position (arm resting on examination table). 3. Adjust spectral Doppler gain settings to optimize waveform by minimizing background noise. 4. Carefully adjust the angle of insonation to improve the signal-to-noise ratio. 5. Change spectral Doppler gate depth by small increments to improve signal quality.
Spectral Doppler or color Doppler aliasing	• Detected frequency is exceeding the Nyquist limit	1. Increase PRF settings. 2. Decrease the zero baseline to increase the display of the scale in one direction.
"I am lost." Possible explanations: not following examination protocol, patient movement, unusual acoustic window, anatomic variations, or intracranial pathology		1. Undergo a systematic search for a better acoustic window. A TCD window may be located by repositioning the transducer, changing the angle of insonation, adjusting spectral Doppler gate depth, or modifying color Doppler settings. 2. Locate the anatomic landmarks specific to the acoustic window being used. 3. Locate the landmark of the t-ICA bifurcation spectral Doppler signal, and use it to locate the other arteries when imaging via the transtemporal approach. 4. Follow the examination protocol. 5. Remember that a patient's physiologic factors and any extracranial vessel disease may affect intracranial spectral Doppler waveforms (velocity and morphology). 6. Take the time to put the patient at ease or answer any questions to minimize movement. 7. Remember the limitations of TCD imaging.

PRF, Pulse repetition frequency; *TCD*, transcranial color Doppler; *t-ICA*, terminal internal carotid artery.

with high levels of accuracy, without the need of a formally trained operator.[95]

Currently, TCD imaging is used to provide real-time, noninvasive physiologic information of the intracranial arterial system in a wide variety of cerebrovascular applications. These include cerebral hematoma, intracranial arterial stenosis or occlusion, acute ischemic stroke, cerebral microembolization, vasospasm, subclavian steal, sickle cell disease, and the evaluation of cerebral perfusion following a TBI and intraoperatively.

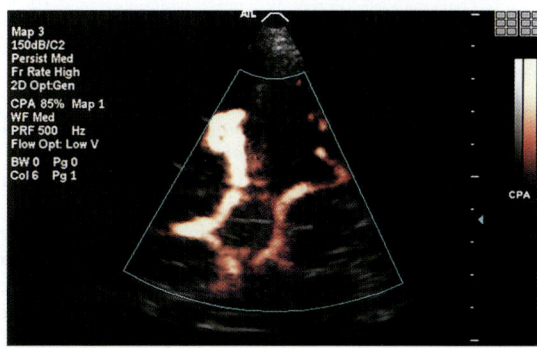

FIG. 38.17 Power Doppler image of the intracranial arteries. Power Doppler imaging is helpful when trying to locate low-flow stats such as those in the small intracranial arteries. Power Doppler imaging does not account for flow directionality and is therefore also useful when imaging arteries unfavorable angles relative to the insonated ultrasound beam.

Key Pearls

- Transcranial Doppler (TCD) imaging was first used as a method to detect cerebral arterial vasospasm after subarachnoid hemorrhage but has since been integrated into a wide variety of clinical applications.
- Blood supply to the brain is provided by the internal carotid (anteriorly) and vertebral (posteriorly) arteries, both of which originate extracranially and terminate intracranially.
- The circle of Willis is composed of the A1 segments of the two anterior cerebral arteries, anterior communicating arteries, posterior communicating arteries, the terminal portions of the internal carotid arteries (ICAs), and the P1 segments of the two posterior cerebral arteries.
- The circle of Willis provides communication between the internal carotid, external carotid, and vertebrobasilar systems.
- The circle of Willis provides multiple communications between intracranial arteries and collateral pathways to ensure cerebral perfusion remains intact and the brain is adequately perfused with oxygenated blood, even in the presence of flow-limiting lesions.
- Four windows are commonly used to perform TCD imaging: the transtemporal, transorbital, suboccipital, and submandibular.
- Proper identification of the intracranial vasculature is the first step in the TCD examination. GS imaging should first be used to identify anatomic or bony landmarks (when appropriate), followed by color doppler (CD) imaging to visualize the blood flow within the intracranial vasculature.
- Changes in arterial carbon dioxide (CO_2) partial pressure (P_{CO_2}) have a direct effect relationship on cerebral blood flow and intracranial arterial velocities.
- Parameters most commonly derived from spectral doppler (SD) waveforms are mean flow velocity (time-averaged peak velocities), pulsatility index, and resistive index.
- Cerebral vasospasm (vasoconstriction of the cerebral arteries) is a serious complication that occurs in an estimated two-thirds of individuals following a subarachnoid hemorrhage and is a significant cause of morbidity and mortality.
- The primary pathologic condition associated with vasospasm is the vasoconstriction of cerebral arteries, leading to a decreased lumen diameter.
- Intracranial arterial stenoses cause characteristic alterations in Doppler signals (audio and visually on SD waveforms), including focal increases in mean flow velocity (MFV), local turbulence, prestenotic decrease in MFV and increase in pulsatility index (PI), poststenotic MFV reduction, and increase in MFV and/or reversal of flow in collateral vessels.
- Subclavian steal syndrome is caused by a stenosis or occlusion of the left subclavian, innominate, or right subclavian artery proximal to the origin of the vertebral artery that causes hypoperfusion of the posterior circulation.
- Microembolic signals have been detected in asymptomatic and symptomatic individuals with high-grade ICA stenosis, prosthetic cardiac valves, myocardial infarction, atrial fibrillation, aortic arch atheroma, fat embolization syndrome, and retinal or general cerebrovascular disease.
- Because of its noninvasive and portable nature, TCD imaging is commonly used in the emergency department or intensive care unit to assess cerebral perfusion in patients with traumatic brain injury in combination with computed tomography.

REFERENCES

1. Aaslid R, Markwalder TM, Nornes H. Noninvasive transcranial Doppler ultrasound recording of flow velocity in basal cerebral arteries. *J Neurosurg.* 1982;56:769–774.
2. Saba L, Raz E, Anzidei M, et al. Differences in plaque morphology and correlation of stenosis at the carotid artery bifurcation and the carotid siphon. *Am J Roentgenol.* 2013;201:1108–1114.
3. Chen XY, Lam WW, Ng HK, et al. The frequency and determinants of calcification in intracranial arteries in Chinese patients who underwent computed tomography examinations. *Cerebrovasc Dis.* 2006;21:91–97.
4. de Weert TT, Cakir H, Rozie S, et al. Intracranial internal carotid artery calcifications: association with vascular risk factors and ischemic cerebrovascular disease. *Am J Neuroradiol.* 2009;30:177–184.
5. Rose DZ, Jindal G, Mullen MT. Extracranial vertebral artery stenosis. In: Litt H, Mohler ER, eds. *Atlas of Vascular Medicine: A Case-Based Approach to Current Management.* New York: Demos Medical Publishing; 2012.
6. Vrselja Z, Brkic H, Mrdenovic S, et al. Function of circle of Willis. *J Cerebral Blood Flow Metabol.* 2014;34:578–584.
7. Barlinn K, Alexandrov AV. Transcranial Doppler sonography. In: AbuRahma AF, Bandyk DF, eds. *Noninvasive Vascular Diagnosis: a Practical Guide to Therapy.* New York: Springer; 2013:133–155.
8. Sinha I, Ghosal AK, Basu R, et al. Variation in the pattern of circle of Willis in human brain—a morphological study and review. *Al Ameen J Med Sci.* 2014;7:13–19.
9. Alfano JM, Kolega J, Natarajan SK, et al. Intracranial aneurysms occur more frequently at bifurcation sites that typically experience higher hemodynamic stresses. *Neurosurgery.* 2013;73:497–505.
10. Dimmick SJ, Faulder KC. Normal variants of the cerebral circulation at multidetector CT angiography. *Radiographics.* 2009;29:1027–1043.
11. Tarulli E, Sneade M, Clarke A, et al. Effects of circle of Willis anatomic variations on angiographic and clinical outcomes of coiled anterior communicating artery aneurysms. *Am J Neuroradiol.* 2014;35:1551–1555.

12. Castro MA, Putman CM, Sheridan MJ, et al. Hemodynamic patterns of anterior communicating artery aneurysms: a possible association with rupture. *Am J Neuroradiol.* 2009;30:297–302.
13. de Rooij NK, Velthuis BK, Algra A, et al. Configuration of the circle of Willis, direction of flow, and shape of the aneurysm as risk factors for rupture of intracranial aneurysms. *J Neurol.* 2009;256:45–50.
14. Tarulli E, Fox AJ. Potent risk factor for aneurysm formation: termination aneurysms of the anterior communicating artery and detection of A1 vessel asymmetry by flow dilution. *Am J Neuroradiol.* 2010;31:1186–1191.
15. Flores BC, Scott WW, Eddleman CS, et al. The A1-A2 diameter ratio may influence formation and rupture potential of anterior communicating artery aneurysms. *Neurosurgery.* 2013;73:845–853.
16. Loukas M, Louis RG, Childs RS. Anatomical examination of the recurrent artery of Heubner. *Clin Anat.* 2006;19:25–31.
17. Dzierżanowski J, Szarmach A, Słoniewski P, et al. The posterior communicating artery: morphometric study in 3D angio-computed tomography reconstruction. The proof of the mathematical definition of the hypoplasia. *Folia Morphologica.* 2014;73:286–291.
18. van der Lugt A, Buter TC, Govaere F, et al. Accuracy of CT angiography in the assessment of a fetal origin of the posterior cerebral artery. *Eur Radiol.* 2004;14:1627–1633.
19. Lo WB, Ellis H. The circle before Willis: a historical account of the intracranial anastomosis. *Neurosurgery.* 2010;66:7–18.
20. Ferguson GG. Physical factors in the initiation, growth, and rupture of human intracranial saccular aneurysms. *J Neurosurg.* 1972;37(6):666–677.
21. Alexandrov AV, Sloan MA, Tegeler CH, et al. Practice standards for transcranial Doppler (TCD) ultrasound. Part II. Clinical indications and expected outcomes. *J Neuroimaging.* 2012;22(3):215–224.
22. Aaslid R. *The Doppler principle applied to measurement of blood flow velocity in cerebral arteries. In: Transcranial Doppler Sonography.* Vienna: Springer; 1986:22–38.
23. White H, Venkatesh B. Applications of transcranial Doppler in the ICU: a review. *Intens Care Med.* 2006;32:981–994.
24. Bioeffects Committee of the American Institute of Ultrasound in Medicine. American Institute of Ultrasound in Medicine consensus report on potential bioeffects of diagnostic ultrasound executive summary. *J Ultrasound Med.* 2008;27:503–515.
25. ter Haar G. Ultrasound bio-effects and safety considerations. *Translational Neurosonol.* 2015;36:23–30.
26. Nelson TR, Fowlkes JB, Abramowicz JS. Ultrasound biosafety considerations for the practicing sonographer and sonologist. *J Ultrasound Med.* 2009;28:139.
27. Rajajee V. Ultrasound in the neurointensive care unit. In Jankowich M, Gartman E, eds. *Ultrasound in the Intensive Care Unit.* New York: Springer; 2015:323–354.
28. Alexandrov AV, Sloan MA, Wong LK, et al. Practice standards for transcranial Doppler ultrasound: part I—test performance. *J Neuroimaging.* 2007;17:11–18.
29. Purkayastha S, Sorond F. Transcranial Doppler ultrasound: technique and application. *Semin Neurol.* 2012;32:411–420.
30. Nedelmann M, Stolz E, Gerriets T, et al. Consensus recommendations for transcranial color-coded duplex sonography for the assessment of intracranial arteries in clinical trials on acute stroke. *Stroke.* 2009;40:3238–3244.
31. American College of Radiology. AIUM practice guideline for the performance of a transcranial Doppler ultrasound examination for adults and children. *J Ultrasound Med.* 2012;31:1489.
32. Fujioka KA, Gates DT, Spencer MP. A comparison of transcranial color Doppler imaging and standard static pulsed wave Doppler in the assessment of intracranial hemodynamics. *J Vasc Technol.* 1994;18:29–35.
33. Jones AM, Seibert JJ, Nichols FT, et al. Comparison of transcranial color Doppler imaging (TCDI) and transcranial Doppler (TCD) in children with sickle-cell anemia. *Pediatr Radiol.* 2001;31:461–469.
34. McCarville MB, Li C, Xiong X, et al. Comparison of transcranial Doppler sonography with and without imaging in the evaluation of children with sickle cell anemia. *Am J Roentgenol.* 2004;183:1117–1122.
35. Soetaert AM, Lowe LH, Formen C. Pediatric cranial Doppler sonography in children: non-sickle cell applications. *Curr Prob Diagn Radiol.* 2009;38:218–227.
36. Neish AS, Blews DE, Simms CA, et al. Screening for stroke in sickle cell anemia: comparison of transcranial Doppler imaging and nonimaging US techniques 1. *Radiology.* 2002;222:709–714.
37. Kirsch JD, Mathur M, Johnson MH, et al. Advances in transcranial Doppler US: imaging ahead. *Radiographics.* 2013;33:E1–E14.
38. Bazan R, Braga GP, Luvizutto G, et al. Evaluation of the temporal acoustic window for transcranial Doppler in a multi-ethnic population in Brazil. *Ultrasound Med Biol.* 2015;41(8):2131–2134.
39. Kwon JH, Kim JS, Kang DW, et al. The thickness and texture of temporal bone in brain CT predict acoustic window failure of transcranial Doppler. *J Neuroimaging.* 2006;16:347–352.
40. Naqvi J, Yap KH, Ahmad G, et al. Transcranial Doppler ultrasound: a review of the physical principles and major applications in critical care. *Int J Vasc Med.* 2013;2013:1–13.
41. Kassab MY, Majid A, Farooq MU, et al. Transcranial Doppler: an introduction for primary care physicians. *J Am Board Fam Med.* 2007;20:65–71.
42. Venkatesh B, Shen Q, Lipman J. Continuous measurement of cerebral blood flow velocity using transcranial Doppler reveals significant moment-to-moment variability of data in healthy volunteers and in patients with subarachnoid hemorrhage. *Crit Care Med.* 2002;30(3):563–569.
43. Tegeler CH, Crutchfield K, Katsnelson M, et al. Transcranial Doppler velocities in a large, healthy population. *J Neuroimaging.* 2013;23(23):466–472.
44. Fu CH, Yang CC, Kuo TB. Age-related changes in cerebral hemodynamics and their correlations with cardiac autonomic functions. *Neurol Res.* 2006;28:871–876.
45. Brouwers PJ, Vriens EM, Musbach M, et al. Transcranial pulsed Doppler measurements of blood flow velocity in the middle cerebral artery: reference values at rest and during hyperventilation in healthy children and adolescents in relation to age and sex. *Ultrasound Med Biol.* 1990;16:1–8.
46. Martin PJ, Evans DH, Naylor AR. Transcranial color-coded sonography of the basal cerebral circulation. Reference data from 115 volunteers. *Stroke.* 1994;25:390–396.
47. Ogoh S, Lericollais R, Hirasawa A, et al. Regional redistribution of blood flow in the external and internal carotid arteries during acute hypotension. *Am J Physiol.* 2014;306:R747–R751.
48. Schmidt EA, Piechnik SK, Smielewski P, et al. Symmetry of cerebral hemodynamic indices derived from bilateral transcranial Doppler. *J Neuroimaging.* 2003;13:248–254.
49. Gosling RG, Dunbar G, King DH, et al. The quantitative analysis of occlusive peripheral arterial disease by a non-intrusive ultrasound technique. *Angiology.* 1971;22:52–55.
50. Bellner J, Romner B, Reinstrup P, et al. Transcranial Doppler sonography pulsatility index (PI) reflects intracranial pressure (ICP). *Surg Neurol.* 2004;62:45–51.
51. Westra SJ, Lazareff J, Curran JG, et al. Transcranial Doppler ultrasonography to evaluate need for cerebrospinal fluid drainage in hydrocephalic children. *J Ultrasound Med.* 1998;17:561–569.
52. de Oliveira RS, Machado HR. Transcranial color-coded Doppler ultrasonography for evaluation of children with hydrocephalus. *Neurosurg Focus.* 2003;15:1–7.
53. Jabbarli R, Gläsker S, Weber J, Taschner C, Olschewski M, Velthoven VV. Predictors of severity of cerebral vasospasm caused by aneurysmal subarachnoid hemorrhage. *J Stroke Cerebrovasc Dis.* 2013;22:1332–1339.
54. Willie CK, Colino FL, Bailey DM, et al. Utility of transcranial Doppler ultrasound for the integrative assessment of cerebrovascular function. *J Neurosci Methods.* 2011;196:221–237.
55. Oyama K, Criddle L. Vasospasm after aneurysmal subarachnoid hemorrhage. *Crit Care Nurse.* 2004;24:58–67.
56. Simpson DM, Gracies JM, Graham HK, et al. Therapeutics and Technology Assessment Subcommittee of the American

Academy of Neurology Assessment: botulinum neurotoxin for the treatment of spasticity (an evidence-based review): report of the Therapeutics and Technology Assessment Subcommittee of the American Academy of Neurology. *Neurology*. 2008;70:1699-1706.
57. Naqvi Jawad, et al. Transcranial Doppler ultrasound: a review of the physical principles and major applications in critical care. *Int J Vasc Med*. 2013
58. Kincaid MS, Souter MJ, Treggiari MM, et al. Accuracy of transcranial Doppler ultrasonography and single-photon emission computed tomography in the diagnosis of angiographically demonstrated cerebral vasospasm: clinical article. *J Neurosurg*. 2009;110:67-72.
59. Tsivgoulis G, Alexandrov AV, Sloan MA. Advances in transcranial Doppler ultrasonography. *Curr Neurol Neurosci Rep*. 2009;9:46-54.
60. Dietrich C, van Lieshout J, Fischer I, et al. Transcranial doppler ultrasound, perfusion computerized tomography, and cerebral angiography identify different pathological entities and supplement each other in the diagnosis of delayed cerebral ischemia. *Acta Neurochir Suppl*. 2020;1:155-160.
61. Lindegaard KF, Grolimund P, Aaslid R, et al. Evaluation of cerebral AVMs using transcranial Doppler ultrasound. *J Neurosurg*. 1986;65:335-344.
62. Mastantuono Jean-Mathieu, et al. Transcranial Doppler in the diagnosis of cerebral vasospasm: an updated meta-analysis. *Crit Care Med*. 2018;46(10):1665-1672.
63. Sloan MA, Alexandrov AV, Tegeler CH, et al. Assessment: transcranial Doppler ultrasonography report of the Therapeutics and Technology Assessment Subcommittee of the American Academy of Neurology. *Neurology*. 2004;62:1468-1481.
64. Feldmann E, Wilterdink JL, Kosinski A, et al. The stroke outcomes and neuroimaging of intracranial atherosclerosis (SONIA) trial. *Neurology*. 2007;68:2099-2106.
65. Zhao L, Barlinn K, Sharma VK, et al. Velocity criteria for intracranial stenosis revisited: an international multicenter study of transcranial Doppler and digital subtraction angiography. *Stroke*. 2011;42:3429-3434.
66. Thorpe Samuel G, et al. Decision criteria for large vessel occlusion using transcranial Doppler waveform morphology. *Frontiers in Neurology*. 2018;9:847.
67. Molina CA, Alexandrov AV, Demchuk AM, et al. Improving the predictive accuracy of recanalization on stroke outcome in patients treated with tissue plasminogen activator. *Stroke*. 2004;35:151-156.
68. Kucinski T, Koch C, Eckert B, et al. Collateral circulation is an independent radiological predictor of outcome after thrombolysis in acute ischaemic stroke. *Neuroradiology*. 2003;45:11-18.
69. Huang Glen, et al. Transcranial Doppler emboli monitoring for infective endocarditis. *J Neuroimaging*. 2020;30(4):486-492.
70. Spensor MP. Basic identification criteria of Doppler microembolic signals. Consensus Committee of the Ninth International Cerebral Hemodynamic Symposium. *Stroke*. 1995;26:1123.
71. Ringelstein EB, Droste DW, Babikian VL, et al. Consensus on microembolus detection by TCD. *Stroke*. 1998;29:725-729.
72. Markus HS, Droste DW, Kaps M, et al. Dual antiplatelet therapy with clopidogrel and aspirin in symptomatic carotid stenosis evaluated using doppler embolic signal detection the clopidogrel and aspirin for reduction of emboli in symptomatic carotid stenosis (CARESS) trial. *Circulation*. 2005;111:2233-2240.
73. Wong KS. CLAIR study investigators: Clopidogrel plus aspirin versus aspirin alone for reducing embolisation in patients with acute symptomatic cerebral or carotid artery stenosis (CLAIR study): a randomised, open-label, blinded-endpoint trial. *Lancet Neurol*. 2010;9:489-497.
74. Markus HS, King A, Shipley M, et al. Asymptomatic embolisation for prediction of stroke in the Asymptomatic Carotid Emboli Study (ACES): a prospective observational study. *Lancet Neurol*. 2010;9:663-671.
75. Ritter MA, Dittrich R, Thoenissen N, et al. Prevalence and prognostic impact of microembolic signals in arterial sources of embolism. *J Neurol*. 2008;255:953-961.
76. King A, Markus HS. Doppler embolic signals in cerebrovascular disease and prediction of stroke risk a systematic review and meta-analysis. *Stroke*. 2009;40:3711-3717.
77. Lee MT, Piomelli S, Granger S, et al. Stroke Prevention Trial in Sickle Cell Anemia (STOP): extended follow-up and final results. *Blood*. 2006;108:847-852.
78. Adams RJ. Stroke prevention in sickle cell disease (STOP) study guidelines for transcranial Doppler testing. *J Neuroimaging*. 2001;11:354-362.
79. Adams R, McKie VC, Hsu L, et al. Prevention of a first stroke by transfusions in children with sickle cell anemia and abnormal results on transcranial Doppler ultrasonography. *N Engl J Med*. 1998;339:5-11.
80. Eckrich MJ, Wang WC, Yang E, et al. Adherence to transcranial Doppler screening guidelines among children with sickle cell disease. *Pediatr Blood Cancer*. 2013;60:270-274.
81. Krejza J, Mariak Z, Melhem ER, et al. A guide to the identification of major cerebral arteries with transcranial color Doppler sonography. *Am J Roentgenol*. 2000;174:1297-1303.
82. Driscoll MC, Hurlet A, Styles L, et al. Stroke risk in siblings with sickle cell anemia. *Blood*. 2003;101:2401-2404.
83. Adam RJ, Brambilla D. Optimizing primary stroke prevention in sickle cell anemia (STOP II) Trial Investigators. *N Engl J Med*. 2005;353:2769-2778.
84. Bouzat P, Oddo M, Payen JF. Transcranial Doppler after traumatic brain injury: is there a role? *Curr Opin Crit Care*. 2014;20:153-160.
85. Maas AI, Stocchetti N, Bullock R. Moderate and severe traumatic brain injury in adults. *Lancet Neurol*. 2008;7:728-741.
86. Ract C, Le Moigno S, Bruder N, et al. Transcranial Doppler ultrasound goal-directed therapy for the early management of severe traumatic brain injury. *Intensive Care Med*. 2007;33:645-651.
87. Lao AY, Sharma VK, Tsivgoulis G, et al. Effect of body positioning during transcranial Doppler detection of right-to-left shunts. *Eur J Neurol*. 2007;14:1035-1039.
88. López-Navidad A, Caballero F, Domingo P, et al. Early diagnosis of brain death in patients treated with central nervous system depressant drugs. *Transplantation*. 2000;70:131-135.
89. De Freitas GR, Andre C. Sensitivity of transcranial Doppler for confirming brain death: a prospective study of 270 cases. *Acta Neurol Scand*. 2006;113:426-432.
90. Monteiro LM, Bollen CW, van Huffelen AC, et al. Transcranial Doppler ultrasonography to confirm brain death: a meta-analysis. *Intensive Care Med*. 2006;32:1937-1944.
91. Alexandrov AV, Grotta JC. Arterial reocclusion in stroke patients treated with intravenous tissue plasminogen activator. *Neurology*. 2002;59:862-867.
92. Zamboni P, Menegatti E, Galeotti R, et al. The value of cerebral Doppler venous haemodynamics in the assessment of multiple sclerosis. *J Neurol Sci*. 2009;282:21-27.
93. Bates MC. Use of TCD in monitoring patients during carotid artery stenting. In: AbuRahma AF, Bandyk DF, eds. *Noninvasive Vascular Diagnosis: A Practical Guide to Therapy*. New York: Springer; 2013:189-199.
94. Rudolph JL, Sorond FA, Pochay VE, et al. Cerebral hemodynamics during coronary artery bypass graft surgery: the effect of carotid stenosis. *Ultrasound Med Biol*. 2009;35:1235-1241.
95. Han SJ, Rutledge WC, Englot DJ, et al. Presto 1000: a novel automated transcranial Doppler ultrasound system. *J Clin Neurosci*. 2015;22(11):1771-1775.

CHAPTER 39

Peripheral Arterial Evaluation

Kevin R. Volz

OBJECTIVES

On completion of this chapter, you should be able to:
- Describe the anatomy encountered during an arterial duplex examination
- Understand arterial physiology as it relates to the development of peripheral arterial disease
- Recognize the risk factors associated with peripheral arterial disease
- Discuss the changes that occur to segmental pressures and pulse volume waveforms in the presence of occlusive arterial disease
- Outline proper instrument control settings used during arterial duplex imaging
- Describe the characteristics of arterial spectral Doppler signals obtained during arterial duplex imaging
- Discuss the imaging characteristics associated with arterial narrowing

OUTLINE

Anatomy Associated With Peripheral Arterial Testing 1111
   Lower Extremity 1111
   Upper Extremity 1112
Arterial Physiology 1112
Arterial Pathophysiology 1113
   Peripheral Arterial Disease 1113
Indirect (Physiologic) Arterial Testing 1114
Segmental Doppler Pressures 1114
Arterial Stress Testing 1116
Digit Pressures 1116
Plethysmography Testing 1117
Pulse Volume Recordings 1117
Other Indirect Arterial Testing 1117
Arterial Duplex Imaging 1118
   Lower Extremity 1119
Upper Extremity 1120
Interpretation 1120
Bypass Graft Surveillance 1122
Dialysis Access Grafts 1123
Aneurysms and Pseudoaneurysms 1124
Guidelines for Evaluation 1126

KEY TERMS

Ankle-brachial index (ABI)
Anterior tibial artery (ATA)
Axillary artery
Brachial artery
Claudication
Common femoral artery
Femoral artery
Dorsalis pedis artery (DPA)
Innominate artery
Ischemic rest pain
Peripheral arterial aneurysms
Peroneal artery
Popliteal artery
Posterior tibial artery (PTA)
Profunda femoris artery
Pseudoaneurysm
Radial artery
Raynaud phenomenon
Subclavian artery
Thoracic outlet syndrome
Tibial-peroneal trunk
Toe-brachial index (TBI)
Ulnar artery

In its advent, noninvasive testing was used to offer objectivity in the diagnosis of peripheral arterial disease (PAD). Today's ultrasound and oscillometric technology allow clinicians to acquire both anatomic and physiologic information while evaluating patients with PAD. Capabilities have advanced from simple oscillometric measurements to segmental pressures, pulse volume recordings, stress testing, and direct evaluation of arteries by duplex imaging. This has allowed indications for its use to be expanded. Further, the current noninvasive evaluation is tailored to patients' specific needs depending on clinical presentation and suspected pathology.

PAD affects an estimated 6.5 million people in the United States over the age of 40.[1] In 2016, this resulted in 1.6 million office visits and 11,000 emergency visits.[1] This results in an estimated $84 to $380 billion annual healthcare costs.[2] PAD can present with a wide variety of symptoms, but may also remain asymptomatic even in patients with advanced stages.[3] Therefore the physical examination alone has poor sensitivity and specificity.[3] Only approximately 10% of individuals with PAD present with the classic symptom of intermittent claudication, while 50% present with non-specific leg symptoms other than claudication.[4] Further, an estimated 40% of patients

| BOX 39.1 | Purposes of Noninvasive Arterial Testing |

- Provide objective documentation of arterial disease severity
- Aid in diagnosis of exercise-induced pain caused by occlusive arterial disease
- Supplement clinical judgment regarding foot ulcer and amputation site healing
- Evaluate pulsatile masses (aneurysms, pseudoaneurysms)
- Evaluate suspected arterial trauma
- Evaluate surrounding arterial anatomy
- Evaluate angioplasty/stent placement (planning and follow-up)
- Establish a baseline study before operative reconstruction
- Provide postoperative monitoring, including bypass and dialysis graft surveillance

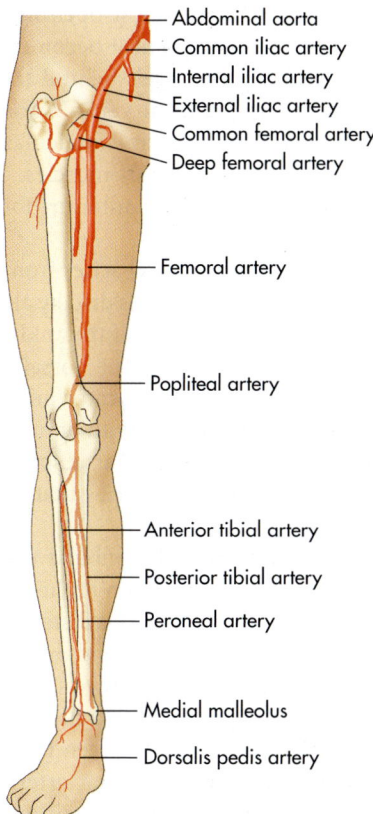

FIG. 39.1 Arteries of the lower extremity.

with PAD have no symptoms.[4] Noninvasive arterial evaluations complement a patient history and physical examination. It has become a valuable tool for many patients and their physicians to confirm suspected diagnoses and detect arterial occlusive disease in the asymptomatic patient. Further, noninvasive testing stages disease severity and is used longitudinally to monitor disease progression and response to treatment (Box 39.1).

Noninvasive arterial testing consists of two different types of ultrasound technology: (1) indirect and (2) direct testing or duplex imaging. Although indirect tests and peripheral arterial duplex imaging are discussed separately in this chapter, a combination of tests from both categories is typically used in combination to obtain a more holistic depiction of disease.

ANATOMY ASSOCIATED WITH PERIPHERAL ARTERIAL TESTING

The peripheral arterial system is made up of arteries, arterioles, and capillaries in the most distal portion. The main function of the arterial system is to transport oxygen-rich blood from the heart to perfuse organs and tissues throughout the body. After exiting the left ventricle of the heart, blood travels through the central arteries until it reaches the arteries of the periphery. The peripheral arteries located in the upper and lower extremities transport blood to the arterial system microcirculation. Blood enters the arterioles, then capillaries which make arterial microcirculation. After the capillaries, blood exits the arterial system and enters the venous system for its return to the heart.

The wall of an artery consists of three layers: (1) tunica intima (innermost), (2) tunica media (middle), and (3) tunica adventitia (outermost). The tunica media layer primarily consists of smooth muscle and connective tissue and provides the vessel with structure and support.

Lower Extremity

The descending aorta is the continuation of the aorta beyond the aortic arch. The descending aorta is divided into the thoracic and abdominal sections. The thoracic portion terminates at the aortic opening in the diaphragm, where the abdominal aorta begins at the approximate level of the twelfth thoracic vertebra as it passes through the aortic hiatus of the diaphragm. At the approximate level of the fourth lumbar vertebra, the abdominal aorta bifurcates to become the right and left common iliac arteries (Fig. 39.1). Each common iliac artery bifurcates into an internal and external iliac artery. The internal iliac artery (hypogastric) perfuses the pelvis, while the external iliac artery continues distally to supply blood to the lower extremity. The external iliac artery terminates at the level of the inguinal ligament where it becomes the common femoral artery.

The **common femoral artery (CFA)** originates beneath the inguinal ligament and travels distally in proximity to the common femoral vein. In the distal portion of the groin, the CFA bifurcates into the femoral and profunda femoris (deep femoral) arteries. The **profunda femoris artery** is located posterior and lateral to the femoral artery. It begins at the CFA bifurcation and terminates in the lower third of the thigh. The profunda femoris artery travels deep within the leg in close association with the profunda femoris vein to perfuse the muscles of the thigh and hip. The **femoral artery (FA)** originates from the CFA bifurcation and travels through the adductor (Hunter) canal and continues along the length of the medial thigh in close proximity to the femoral vein. The proximal FA begins superficial to the profunda femoris artery but dives deep in the distal portion of the thigh. The FA terminates at the opening of the adductor magnus muscle, at which point it becomes the popliteal artery. The **popliteal artery** travels behind the knee in the popliteal fossa with the popliteal vein. Major branches of the popliteal artery are the sural and genicular arteries that perfuse the popliteal fossa and calf muscles. The popliteal artery terminates distally into the anterior tibial artery and the tibioperoneal trunk.

The **anterior tibial artery (ATA)** arises from the popliteal artery in the proximal calf and travels distally along the lateral calf into the anterior compartment of the ankle. At this level, it courses superficial and becomes the dorsalis pedis artery. The **dorsalis pedis artery (DPA)** is located on the dorsal foot. At its distal portion, the DPA joins with branches of the posterior tibial artery to form the plantar arch. Arising off the plantar arch are the metatarsal arteries that divide into the digital branch arteries.

The **tibial-peroneal trunk** (tibial-fibular trunk) begins in the proximal calf from the bifurcation of the popliteal artery. The tibial-peroneal trunk briefly travels distally until its bifurcation into the posterior tibial artery and the peroneal artery. The **posterior tibial artery (PTA)** travels down the medial calf in the posterior compartment, parallel to the posterior tibial veins. The PTA terminates between the ankle and the heel into the medial and lateral plantar arteries. The **peroneal artery** is located deep within the calf and travels with the peroneal veins near the medial aspect of the fibula, parallel and deep to the PTA. The peroneal artery terminates in the distal third portion of the calf. Its branches communicate with branches of the PTA and ATA.

Upper Extremity

The ascending aorta originates from the left ventricle. The transverse aortic arch is located in the superior mediastinum and is formed as the aorta ascends and curves posteroinferiorly from right to left. This occurs superior to the left mainstem bronchus. Three main branches arise from the superior convexity of the arch in its normal configuration. The first is the **innominate artery** (brachiocephalic), which divides into the right subclavian and the right common carotid artery. Next, the left common carotid artery arises, followed by the left subclavian artery (Fig. 39.2).

The **subclavian artery** originates at the inner border of the scalenus anterior muscle in close proximity to the subclavian vein and travels beneath the clavicle to the outer border of the first rib. Here it becomes the axillary artery. Major branches of the subclavian artery are the vertebral artery, thyrocervical trunk, costocervical trunk, internal mammary artery, and dorsal scapular artery. The **axillary artery** is a continuation of the subclavian artery, which begins at the outer border of the first rib and travels through the axilla in close association with the axillary vein. The axillary artery terminates at the lower border of the tendon of the teres major muscle where it becomes the brachial artery. The **brachial artery** travels near and parallel to the paired brachial veins along the medial portion of the upper arm. The brachial artery typically terminates

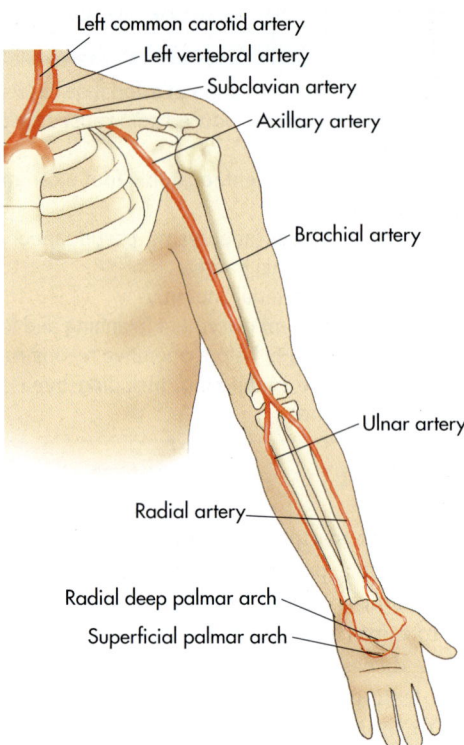

FIG. 39.2 Arteries of the upper extremity.

just below the antecubital fossa into the radial and ulnar arteries, but anatomic variations in this area are common.

The **radial artery** begins at the brachial artery bifurcation and travels distally along the lateral forearm. At the level of the palm, the radial artery terminates to form the deep palmar arch. The **ulnar artery** originates at the brachial artery bifurcation and travels distally along the medial forearm. At the level of the palm, the ulnar artery terminates to form the superficial palmar arch. Both palmar arches supply blood to the digital arteries.

ARTERIAL PHYSIOLOGY

The arterial portion of the circulatory system transports oxygenated, nutrient-rich blood from the heart to the various organs and tissues of the body. On cardiac contraction, the left ventricle ejects a stroke volume of arterial blood into the arterial system. Contraction of the left ventricle applies significant pressure to the ejected blood, creating a large amount of kinetic energy for the blood within the arterial system. The arterial system is characterized as a closed, high-pressure system. Being a closed system preserves the amount of kinetic energy within it. High levels of kinetic energy allow arterial blood to travel far distances within the arterial system quickly and efficiently.

In general, artery diameter decreases distally in the periphery. Vessel diameter has the greatest effect on flow volume and consequently directly influences arterial hemodynamics. Artery diameter and blood flow resistance are inversely related, meaning as the diameter of an artery decreases, arterial resistance increases. To this end, when a constant blood flow volume exists, a decrease in artery diameter will result in an increase in arterial blood flow velocity, as conveyed by Bernoulli's principle (velocity = flow/area). Blood flow velocity is represented as *peak systolic velocity* (PSV) and *end-diastolic velocity* (EDV), typically measured in centimeters per second (cm/sec). Arterial PSV increases can be used as a marker for arterial pathology. Arterial occlusive disorders, such as PAD, cause a reduction in arterial lumen causing PSV elevation in the area of diminished diameter. Detection of PSV increase is used to diagnose, stage, and categorize arterial diseases. This is the main principle on which noninvasive testing relies. Measuring true lumen diameter compared to residual lumen diameter can also be used to detect arterial disease. This is known as a diameter reduction measurement.

ARTERIAL PATHOPHYSIOLOGY

PAD and other occlusive disorders are characterized by a reduction in arterial lumen diameter. Arterial lumen reduction causes an increase in arterial resistance and prevents optimal blood volume to flow through the afflicted segment(s) of the vessel. The result is an inadequate supply of arterial blood to the muscles and/or tissues of the body. When in use, muscle tissue requires more arterial perfusion to meet increased oxygen demand. Therefore, using muscles that are perfused by an artery affected by PAD will cause symptoms arising from muscle tissue oxygen deficiency. This is common in the lower extremities, as muscles require increased perfusion during ambulation. The inability to receive extra arterial blood required for muscle use is known as intermittent claudication. Intermittent claudication is characterized by muscle pain (cramp, ache, numbness, and/or fatigue) during use, which subside on rest. The classic presentation of intermittent claudication is in the calf muscles presenting during ambulation. In severe circumstances, arterial perfusion is diminished to the point at which it can no longer meet the oxygen demands of tissues, even while at rest. This results in tissue ischemia and death, which may present as tissue ulceration or gangrene.

Atherosclerosis is the primary disease process leading to PAD.[5] Atherosclerosis is characterized as the buildup of atherosclerotic plaque on the arterial endothelium as a result of excess lipids present in the blood. Over time, the plaque hardens, while continual buildup reduces the lumen area. Atherosclerosis can also cause an arterial embolism, which can occur when plaque dislodges from the arterial wall and propagates distally in the arterial system. Emboli can travel to the brain resulting in stroke or can lodge in the extremities and occlude small vessels, causing ischemia.

Peripheral Arterial Disease

Treatments. Treatment methods for PAD aim to decrease patient symptoms and improve prognosis by preventing the risk of further cardiovascular events. Treatments can be categorized into three types: (1) medical management/conservative, (2) endovascular, and (3) surgical.

The first goal of conservative treatments is to reduce controllable risk factors for PAD such as tobacco use and poor diet through lifestyle modification. Exercise is also recommended, as evidence has demonstrated this leads to increased walking ability both in range and degree of pain, as compared with non-exercising PAD sufferers.[6] Medical management can also be implemented using pharmacologic agents, but this generally results in only mild to moderate improvement of symptoms. Common types of agents prescribed are anticoagulants, antiplatelets, antihypertensives, and lipid-lowering agents.[7]

Endovascular treatments aim to revascularize limbs afflicted with PAD. Endovascular procedures are becoming a popular treatment strategy, as they are much less invasive than other surgical options. Here, a catheter is introduced into the arterial system, typically in the FA at the groin, and is advanced to the site of the atherosclerotic lesion, where a variety of revascularization methods can be performed. Common types of endovascular revascularization interventions are percutaneous transluminal angioplasty (increases artery diameter in cases of focal lesions), endograft placements (for aneurysm repair), atherectomy (removes plaque), and thrombin injections (for pseudoaneurysm treatment). Although the long-term effects of endovascular revascularizations are debated, it is often the default interventional approach, followed by surgical intervention in case of failure.[8]

Surgical interventions, like endovascular interventions, mainly focus on revascularizing the afflicted limb but are typically more invasive. The most common vascular surgical intervention is bypass graft surgery. Bypass graft surgery creates a new arterial conduit to provide blood flow with an alternative route. This conduit is anastomosed with the affected artery proximal and distal to the atherosclerotic lesion. A variety of bypass graft types can be used ranging from native vessels to synthetic materials. Other common revascularization surgical interventions are thrombectomy (removal of a thrombus or embolus) and endarterectomy (surgical removal of plaque and the intima and media layers of an artery). In severe cases of PAD, the goal of vascular surgical intervention is to prevent further disease progression. The most common form is limb amputation.

It is important for sonographers practicing arterial imaging to understand the different PAD treatment strategies. Familiarization with types of medical management is beneficial while obtaining patient histories. Furthermore, many of the aforementioned endovascular surgical interventions, such as percutaneous angioplasty, thrombin injections, and some bypass graft placements, are performed under ultrasound guidance. Occasionally, sonographers will be asked to assist in these surgeries to perform the ultrasound guidance imaging. If this occurs, an understanding of the surgery and why it is being performed will allow the sonographer to more effectively assist the vascular surgeon by providing accurate and relevant information.

Risk Factors and Symptoms of Peripheral Arterial Disease. Several risk factors have been associated with peripheral occlusive arterial disease, some of which are controllable and others uncontrollable. Controllable risk factors include diabetes mellitus, hyperlipidemia, hypertension, tobacco use, and poor diet. Uncontrollable risk factors include increasing age, genetic predisposition (family history of atherosclerosis), documented atherosclerosis in the coronary and/or carotid system, gender (males at a higher risk than females), and thrombophilia.[9]

Symptoms of lower extremity occlusive arterial disease include claudication and rest pain. **Claudication** is defined as exercise-induced muscular discomfort due to a lack of arterial muscle perfusion. Most commonly, this is walking-induced pain in the calf, thigh, hip, or buttock. Most patients describe claudication as a cramping or aching in the muscles of their legs as they walk or exercise, which is relieved after 2 to 5 minutes of rest. As PAD progresses, the distance afflicted individuals are able to walk before the onset of symptoms decreases. In more severe cases, perfusion is so diminished that muscles are unable to obtain an adequate amount of oxygenated blood even when not being used. This is known as *rest pain*. Further disease progression from this point can result in tissue loss, ulceration, gangrene, and critical limb ischemia, leading to limb amputation.

In a large recent study investigating patients with PAD, 1% to 2% required amputation.[10] In more severe cases, 8.4% of patients with critical limb ischemia required amputation.[10] Beyond amputation, PAD pathophysiologic processes cause a decrease in quality of life and mobility loss.[11]

Ischemic rest pain points to critical ischemia of the distal limb. Typical patient complaints include discomfort in the toes while lying down, which often awakens them from sleep, with relief found by placing the affected limb in a dependent position. This permits gravity to assist in delivering blood flow to the foot.

Physical signs of peripheral occlusive arterial disease are elevation pallor, dependent rubor, ischemic ulcers, gangrene, bruits, and decreased peripheral pulses (femoral, popliteal, dorsalis pedis, posterior tibial, axillary, brachial, radial, and ulnar). Pulses are compared with the contralateral side and are graded on a scale from 0 to 3+; 0 = no pulse, 1+ = questionable pulse, 2+ = weak pulse, and 3+ = normal pulse. Additional physical findings include a decrease in temperature (poikilothermia), loss of skin integrity, and/or hair loss at the affected site.[3]

In the acute stages of arterial occlusion or arterial occlusive disease, common manifestations include pain, pallor, decreased peripheral pulses, paresthesias, paralysis, and a localized decrease in skin temperature.[9]

INDIRECT (PHYSIOLOGIC) ARTERIAL TESTING

Segmental Doppler Pressures

The objective of segmental Doppler testing is to obtain systolic blood pressures at multiple levels of the extremities. This provides a quantitative value that offers physiologic information from the segment of the vessel from which it is obtained. Pressures are compared with others obtained at different segments (levels) within the ipsilateral or contralateral limb to determine disease severity and relative location. Segmental Doppler pressures are often repeated longitudinally to monitor disease progression over time. This testing is also able to differentiate arterial disease from other disorders, such as neurologic or musculoskeletal diseases, as these symptoms often overlap.

Before beginning the examination, the patient should rest for 15 minutes to allow blood pressure to stabilize and legs to recover from walking to the examination room. During this time, the patient's chart can be reviewed and history obtained. The patient's history should focus on risk factors of PAD, documenting current severity and location of symptoms, and a history of any past arterial testing, diagnoses, or interventions. Knowledge of prior vascular intervention is imperative, as pressure cuffs should not be placed over graft or stent placements.

Segmental pressures are obtained with the patient in the supine position, with the legs at the same level as the heart. This prevents hydrostatic pressure (gravity-induced) artifact. While performing segmental pressure testing on the lower extremities, blood pressure cuffs are placed bilaterally on the upper arm (brachial pressure), proximal thigh, low thigh (above the knee), calf (below the knee), and ankle just above the medial malleoli. Using a flow detector (continuous wave Doppler transducer), an audible and visual Doppler waveform is obtained at the level of the ankle. Ankle pressures are obtained in the PTA and DPA. Proximal thigh, low thigh, and calf pressures are then recorded using the strongest distal Doppler signal (PTA or DPA). This is done bilaterally.

To accurately obtain systolic pressures, each cuff is independently inflated from 20 to 30 mm Hg above systolic pressure, then slowly deflated. As cuff pressure decreases, the systolic pressure recorded at that cuff location is the pressure at which the audible and/or visual arterial Doppler signal returns. If no distal Doppler signals are noted (no measurable blood flow or occlusion of the distal vessels), thigh pressures can be obtained using the Doppler signal from the popliteal artery.

A continuous wave (CW) Doppler instrument is used to perform segmental limb pressures. An 8-MHz CW transducer can be used for most patients. If the Doppler signal is attenuated due to vessel depth, a 4-MHz CW transducer may be necessary to improve penetration. A generous amount of ultrasound gel should be used to ensure adequate transducer-to-skin contact. The CW transducer should insonate at an angle of 45 to 60 degrees for optimal Doppler signals. Transducer pressure applied to the skin must maintain good contact but cannot be excessive, as it may obliterate the Doppler signal.

To obtain pressures comparable with direct intraarterial measurements, the blood pressure cuff must have a width 20% greater than the diameter of the limb. The cuff should fit snug, but not too tight as to occlude the artery being investigated. It is also important that the bladder of the cuff be placed directly over the artery to ensure accurate compression. In situations where the width of the cuff is small compared with the girth of the limb, the pressure in the cuff may not be completely transmitted to the arteries, resulting in falsely elevated values. Therefore, falsely elevated pressures may exist in obese patients. Conversely, proximal thigh pressures may be falsely decreased in extremely thin patients, as pressure cuffs may be too large. The cuff-to-limb ratio should be kept in mind when the patient's legs are abnormally large or small.

In a healthy individual, pressure measurements will increase from the ankle to the proximal thigh because of the relationship between constant cuff width and the increase in limb size. Blood pressure cuffs with bladders that measure 12 × 40 cm should be used to obtain ankle and calf pressures, whereas cuffs with longer bladders (12 × 55 cm) should be used for proximal and distal thigh pressures. This may vary depending on institutional protocol.

After all lower extremity pressures are obtained bilaterally, brachial pressures are obtained in both arms, using a Doppler signal from the brachial artery at the antecubital fossa. If a difference of ≥20 mm Hg occurs between arms, an arterial obstruction of the innominate, subclavian, axillary, or proximal brachial artery is suspected on the side with the lower systolic pressure. In the absence of this discrepancy (a healthy subclavian artery is assumed), brachial pressures provide a baseline measure with which lower extremity pressures can be compared.

The proximal thigh pressure should be at least 30 mm Hg greater than the brachial pressure. This is due to cuff size artifact rather than an actual increase in intraarterial pressure. A proximal thigh pressure equal to or less than the brachial pressures suggests disease at or proximal to the FA. While comparing pressure measurements within a limb, there should be no more than a 20 mm Hg pressure gradient between adjacent segments. A ≥20 mm Hg pressure gradient between adjacent cuff placements is abnormal and indicates intercurrent disease. A significant pressure gradient (≥20 mm Hg) between the proximal and distal thigh cuffs suggests disease of the FA. Disease of the distal FA, the popliteal artery, or both is suspected if a significant pressure gradient is present between the low thigh and calf. Disease of the tibial arteries is suspected if a ≥20 mm Hg pressure gradient is present between the calf and ankle. Similarly, pressure measurements obtained at the same level in the contralateral limb also should not differ by more than 20 mm Hg. Like brachial pressures, a 20 mm Hg discrepancy is suggestive of arterial disease at, or proximal to the segment with the lower systolic pressure. When interpreting segmental pressures, it may be difficult to localize disease in the presence of multilevel pathology. Proximal arterial obstruction or stenosis can cause a significant pressure gradient that may mask distal disease. Additionally, segmental pressure gradients are unable to distinguish between arterial stenosis and occlusion.

Because systemic pressures vary by the individual, and from examination to examination, absolute pressures are not used to categorize or monitor disease progression. Instead, all pressures are divided by the highest brachial pressure and expressed as a ratio. This is known as the pressure index (PI). Although PIs are reported at each level that pressures are obtained, the most commonly used are those obtained at the level of the ankle (from the PTA or DPA). This is known as the **ankle-brachial index (ABI),** and it is one of the most commonly ordered segmental pressure examinations.

The American College of Cardiology and the American Heart Association have published standardized guidelines for the interpretation of ABI studies.[12] Normal ABI results range from 1.00 to 1.40. ABI values of greater than 1.40 indicate arterial calcification and vessel noncompressiblity.[12] Although this finding is not able to accurately assess limb perfusion, it is associated with an increased risk of serious cardiovascular events and mortality.[13] ABI values between 0.91 and 0.99 are considered borderline. If borderline ABI values are found in a patient with suspected PAD, further testing is warranted.[14] ABI values of 0.90 or less are abnormal and suggestive of disease.[12] This is the most commonly used ABI threshold for PAD detection, which has been found to have a sensitivity and specificity of greater than 90%.[3,13-16] The value of the ABI correlates to disease severity, with a high risk of amputation when ABI values are less than 0.50.[3] ABI values can be separated into four categories representative of patient symptoms (Table 39.1). Most clinical symptoms and associated ABIs fit into these four categories, but there tends to be overlap between groups. While conducting longitudinal ABI monitoring, it has been reported that a decrease in ABI values of greater than 0.15 is significant and is suggestive of PAD progression.[16]

Modest variability in ankle pressures is expected in the healthy patient due to normal physiologic variations and/or observer variability.[17]

As mentioned previously, lower extremity pressures may be falsely elevated because of medial calcinosis and/or medial sclerosis which causes arteries to become noncompressible during pressure measurements. This is suspected when pressure indices exceed 1.40 and is most commonly seen in the diabetic population.[3,12,18] When this occurs toe pressures and pulse volume recordings should be obtained since these tests are not affected by a noncompliant arterial wall. In the presence of noncompressible vessels, they are able to provide valuable information of ischemia to assist in the patient evaluation.

An alternative to the four-cuff lower extremity segmental pressures method, a three-cuff approach may be used. The three-cuff method is performed in the same way as the four-cuff, but with only a single blood pressure cuff placed in the thigh. This method requires less time but is not able to discriminate between inflow disease and FA disease since only

TABLE 39.1	Interpretation of Ankle-Brachial Pressure Index
Clinical Presentation	**Ankle-Brachial Index**
Normal	>0.90
Claudication	0.50–0.89
Rest pain	0.21–0.49
Tissue loss	<0.21

one thigh pressure is obtained. As a result, the four-cuff technique is preferred and more commonly used.

Segmental pressure measurements in the lower extremity tend to underestimate the extent of the disease. Reasons for underestimation include the following: (1) narrowing of the arterial lumen must be significant enough to cause a pressure change (inability to detect very mild disease), (2) proximal disease may mask distal disease, and (3) calcified vessels may falsely elevate pressures. The purpose of indirect testing, however, is to provide information regarding overall limb hemodynamics, instead of the status of an individual vessel. Vessel-specific information is obtained using direct (duplex imaging) testing. Therefore the data provided by pressure measurements from indirect testing are used in combination with findings from direct testing to provide a holistic representation of extremity perfusion.

Segmental pressure testing can also be performed in the upper extremity, but it is less common. Stenosis and/or obstruction of upper extremity inflow arteries (innominate, subclavian) can occur, but in general arterial disease in the upper extremity is much less prevalent than in the lower extremity. Arterial embolization (cardiac origin) is another reason for upper extremity testing. Small emboli in the presence of atrial fibrillation (AFib) or aortic valve disease can cause ischemic symptoms in the fingers and hands. Upper extremity segmental pressures are performed using three blood pressure cuffs placed on the upper arm, forearm, and wrist. Upper arm pressures are obtained with the CW transducer on the brachial artery. Forearm and wrist pressures are obtained using the distal radial or ulnar artery. Just as in the lower extremity, pressures are obtained bilaterally, with a pressure gradient of greater than 20 mm Hg between adjacent and contralateral segments being suggestive of disease.

Arterial Stress Testing

In individuals without occlusive arterial disease, blood perfusion will increase to muscles during exercise to meet elevated oxygen demands. This is facilitated by a decrease in peripheral vascular resistance. However, in individuals suffering from intermittent claudication, the increased perfusion to muscles used during ambulation is not achieved. Yet, these individuals may experience no symptoms while at rest (normal resting ABIs) if resting systolic pressure is sufficient to meet muscle tissue oxygen demands while not in use. An alternative explanation for normal resting ABIs in the presence of PAD is collateral vessel development. Collateral vessels form when perfusion is inadequate. In some instances, collateral vessel formation is able to provide adequate perfusion while at rest but is not be able to sufficiently meet elevated oxygen demands during ambulation. These patients should be stressed with exercise testing to reduce peripheral resistance, thereby increasing the pressure gradient across arterial segments to unmask hemodynamically significant lesions. The goal of this type of testing is to induce claudication symptoms so a determination of PAD severity can be made.

Contraindications to lower extremity arterial stress testing include forms of cardiac disease, severe pulmonary disease, severe hypertension, inability to walk on a treadmill, and in cases of calcified (noncompressible) vessels (unreliable pressure measurements; the use of pulse volume recordings may be helpful in some patients). If the patient is unable to safely use a treadmill, performing calf raises is an alternative method to induce claudication symptoms.

Arterial stress testing begins by first obtaining bilateral brachial and ankle pressures at rest. Cuffs are then left in place as exercise testing is performed on a treadmill at 1.5 to 2 miles per hour on a 10% to 12% grade (this may vary by institution and should be documented in the patient's report to ensure appropriate testing reproducibility and comparison). After walking for 5 minutes, or until symptoms develop that prevent further exercise, brachial and ankle pressures are quickly obtained. A brachial pressure is obtained unilaterally on the side with the higher resting pressure. Ankle pressures are obtained bilaterally using the artery (posterior tibial or dorsalis pedis) that demonstrated the highest resting pressure in each limb (i.e., the PTA may be used in one limb while the DPA is used on the other). In total, this yields three locations at which postexercise pressures are recorded. These pressures should be obtained within 2 minutes following exercise, then repeated every 2 minutes for 10 minutes, or until pressure values return to baseline (resting). The time it takes for symptoms to onset during exercise, symptom location, total walking time, and pressure values obtained at each location and time point are documented. These are used to monitor changes in an individual upon repeat examination.

The magnitude of ankle pressure decrease following exercise and the time required for the ankle pressure to return to baseline reflect the severity of the underlying arterial disease. In general, ankle pressures that fall after exercise and return to baseline within 5 minutes are suggestive of single-segment occlusive disease. Multisegment arterial disease is typically associated with reduced ankle pressures that persist for greater than 10 minutes after exercise. If ankle pressures are unchanged or improved (elevated) after exercise, underlying arterial disease can be excluded as a cause of the patient's symptoms. Of note, this does not rule out the presence of arterial disease. Arterial disease may still be present but is just not the reason for patient symptoms.

Digit Pressures

Toe pressures are a more accurate method of evaluating distal limb and foot perfusion in individuals with falsely elevated limb pressures. Toe pressures may also be used to determine whether there is an obstructive disease involving the pedal arch and digital arteries. A digital cuff is placed at the base of the hallux (big toe), and its blood pressure is obtained by placing a photoplethysmography sensor on the distal portion of the toe. Similar to the ABI, a **toe-brachial index (TBI)** is reported. A toe pressure is commonly accepted as normal with a TBI ≥ 0.80. TBIs are a more sensitive method for PAD detection; however, they demonstrate similar clinical utility as compared with ABIs in the presence of suspected peripheral occlusive arterial disease.[19]

Plethysmography Testing

Plethysmography testing measures changes in blood volume as a method to obtain arterial waveforms. Two types of plethysmography testing are typically used for indirect testing of the peripheral arterial system: pulse volume recordings and photoplethysmography. These are most often used in conjunction with other indirect testing measures, such as segmental pressures. Although plethysmography testing does not directly measure blood pressure within the limb, it provides valuable information regarding overall limb perfusion for an accurate representation of disease.

Pulse Volume Recordings

Pneumoplethysmography, more commonly known as pulse volume recording (PVR), is used to measure changes in segmental limb volume that occur with each cardiac cycle. This can be performed in the upper or lower extremity. PVRs are obtained using blood pressure cuffs at the same levels as segmental pressure testing. Each cuff is independently inflated between 20 and 30 mm Hg above systolic pressure and slowly deflated. As the cuff deflates, changes in limb volume are represented visually as a PVR waveform. These waveforms are interpreted qualitatively, with a normal waveform demonstrating a rapid rise (acceleration) to a sharp peak during systole, followed by a slower fall (deceleration) during diastole (Fig. 39.3). The downslope of a normal PVR waveform contains a dicrotic notch that reflects the brief period of retrograde flow that occurs in arteries during diastole.

Occlusive arterial disease causes changes in PVR waveform amplitude and contour. Sequential changes in the waveform that occur with progressive occlusive arterial disease are first represented with the loss of the dicrotic notch, followed by a delayed upslope (elevated acceleration time), blunted peak (more rounded), and equalization of upslope and downslope time (Fig. 39.4). PVR waveforms displaying no pulse amplitude (flatline) suggest severe arterial occlusive disease.

The PVR waveform obtained in the calf normally has a greater amplitude than the thigh PVR waveform due to cuff

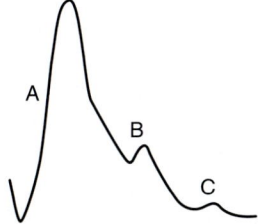

FIG. 39.3 A normal pulse volume recording (PVR) from the lower extremity. Note the rapid rise (acceleration) to a sharp peak during systole (A) and the slower fall (deceleration) during diastole (C). The downslope of a normal PVR contains a dicrotic notch (B) that reflects the brief period of retrograde blood flow in the arteries during diastole.

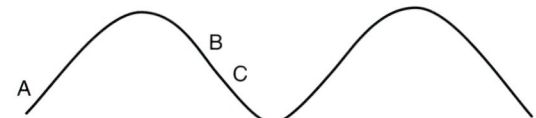

FIG. 39.4 A waveform in the presence of arterial occlusive disease, which causes changes in amplitude and contour of the pulse volume recording. Initially is the absence of the dicrotic notch, followed by (B), followed by a slower upslope (elevated acceleration time) (A), a blunted (more rounded) peak, until finally the downslope (deceleration) time (C) equalizes to the upslope (acceleration) time.

artifact. If the amplitude of the calf PVR waveform is less than or equal to that of the thigh, FA disease should be suspected.

PVRs provide important information and are usually performed in addition to segmental pressure measurements. A discrepancy often occurs between PVR waveforms and segmental pressures when arteries demonstrate noncompressibility (systolic PI > 1.40). In this situation, PVR waveforms provide the only accurate way to obtain information regarding overall limb hemodynamics.

Photoplethysmography. Photoplethysmography (PPG) testing detects cutaneous microcirculation arterial pulses, which are visually represented as a PPG waveform. This form of indirect arterial testing infrared light transmitted into the capillary beds where it reflects off circulating red blood cells, back to a receiver on the PPG probe. This is a very sensitive measure of perfusion and is therefore typically used on the digits, or in situations of severe arterial disease such as wound healing and ischemia. Interpretation of PPG waveforms is qualitative, using the same criteria as PVR waveforms. Also similar to PVR, PPG waveforms are typically obtained in complement to other arterial tests by providing supplementary information of arterial microcirculation.

Other Indirect Arterial Testing

Thoracic Outlet Syndrome. Thoracic outlet syndrome (TOS) is characterized as the compression of neural and/or vascular structures by bone, ligament, or muscular obstacles at the thoracic outlet. This results in ischemic reactions when in certain positions, most commonly when raising the arms. This is known as true TOS and can present with symptoms that resemble claudication of the legs, that is, cramping or pain in the muscles of the arm that is relieved by rest or change in position. Hand wasting (loss of muscle volume in the hand) of the affected side may also be seen in true TOS. Vascular TOS can be related to impingement, but also presents with some types of vascular stenosis, occlusion, or aneurysm. To verify flow reduction, PPG sensors are placed on the index or middle finger bilaterally to obtain PPG waveforms representing distal upper extremity perfusion. Even if symptoms are unilateral, PPG waveforms are always obtained bilaterally for comparison with the contralateral side. The patient is positioned upright with the arms at rest in the lap while a resting (baseline) PPG waveform is obtained. The patient is then asked to perform a series of maneuvers while PPG waveforms are assessed for changes resultant from the impingement of vascular structures. These maneuvers include head to the left, head to the right, exaggerated military position (chest pushed out with arms at the side), military position with the head to the right, and military position with the head to the left. Last, the patient is asked to take the position that causes the onset of symptoms. Maneuvers may vary based on the patient's symptoms or the laboratory protocol. Any decrease, abnormality, or absence of PPG waveforms indicates a flow-reducing position.

It is important to note that a brief resting period should occur between positional maneuvers. If a positive finding of TOS is discovered with the patient in a certain position, a hyperemic response to that limb will occur following relaxation when blood flow is restored to the limb. If time is not taken for this hyperemic to diminish, PPG waveforms obtained in subsequent positions may be falsely elevated.

Raynaud Phenomenon. Primary **Raynaud phenomenon** is characterized as intermittent digital ischemia in response to cold or emotional stress, causing patients to present with color changes (white or blue) in the digits. This can occur in the upper or lower extremity. Secondary Raynaud phenomenon is caused by vascular occlusion or stenosis in the digits, also occurring in response to cold or emotional stress. The key to treatment is identification of the underlying cause of symptoms, whether they are due to vascular blockage or a vasospastic reaction. In the upper extremity, segmental Doppler pressures and PVR waveforms are obtained in the upper arm, forearm, wrist, and digits, bilaterally. Pressure gradients greater than 20 mm Hg compared with the contralateral arm indicate arterial obstruction (typically the subclavian artery) on the side with the lower systolic pressure. No more than a 10 to 15 mm Hg difference should be observed between adjacent segments on the ipsilateral arm. Normal digital pressures will be within 20 mm Hg of the brachial pressure. Typically, PPG sensors are used to obtain digital pressures.

Another test used to evaluate hand perfusion is Allen's test. This evaluates flow within the superficial and deep palmar arch. Allen's test is performed by placing PPG sensors on the thumb and fifth digit of the hand being examined. Normal flow (baseline) is recorded before occluding the radial and ulnar arteries at the wrist using thumb pressure. Adequate pressure has been applied when waveforms become absent (flatline). Thumb pressure on the radial artery is then released. If normal flow does not return, the palmar arch is not intact between the superficial and the deep system. If normal flow returns, both arteries are again occluded, and this is repeated releasing pressure on the ulnar artery while looking for the same results.

Amputation and Ulcer Evaluation. Indirect arterial testing is helpful to predict the likelihood of skin lesion healing. This is especially helpful in the diabetic population, who often present with ulcerations on the foot. Ankle pressures less than 70 mm Hg or ABI values less than 0.50 suggest the presence of significant ischemia and yield a low probability of wound healing.[20] Similarly, toe pressures less than 45 mm Hg or TBI values less than 0.30 have been found to be predictors of poor wound healing and/or amputation.[20,21] PVR and PPG waveforms can also be used to assess the prognosis of wound healing, as the absence of a pulsatile waveform suggests a poor probability.

In cases where limb amputation is required, the goal is to preserve as much tissue as possible.[22] Therefore, the appropriate amputation level must be determined, as this is accepted to be the most important factor to ensure successful amputation wound healing.[23] Although there is no clear consensus on the criteria for determining amputation level, noninvasive testing can be used to assist in this decision. Segmental pressures are commonly used, but a lack of definitive literature does not allow for their routine use or standardized guideline.[24] Furthermore, in diabetic individuals systolic pressures may be falsely elevated and amputation sites may fail to heal, even though pressures appear to be adequate. PVR and PPG waveforms may add information to aid in the selection of amputation level, especially in diabetic patients with calcified vessels.[3]

Prediction of healing after forefoot and toe amputations is less precise, and guidelines for this have not yet been largely accepted, although some evidence suggests preamputation toe pressures are superior to other duplex measures, including ABI, as a prognostic marker for healing.[22,25]

Noninvasive tests including segmental pressures, Doppler waveforms analysis, PVRs, and PPGs are also used to assess perfusion following amputation. Perfusion information collected at the most distal portion of the amputated limb can provide physiologic information regarding amputation wound healing. This is often done repeatedly to monitor healing progression and evaluate the health of the remaining portion of the limb.

In summary, indirect methods of peripheral arterial system evaluation provide much useful information about overall limb hemodynamics. However, these techniques are limited by an inability to establish the exact location of disease, inability to detect disease that causes minor changes, and difficulties in differentiating the level and extent (stenosis vs. occlusion) of disease. Due to these limitations, indirect tests are typically used in conjunction with direct testing (duplex imaging) to provide a holistic representation of limb perfusion.

ARTERIAL DUPLEX IMAGING

Arterial duplex imaging provides direct anatomic information through the use of gray-scale (GS) imaging. Physiologic information is also attainable with the utilization of color and spectral Doppler (SD) imaging. Compared with angiography, duplex imaging has demonstrated high levels of agreement, and 85% to 90% sensitivity and greater than 95% specificity to detect stenosis greater than 50% sensitivities from 85% to 90%, and specificities greater than 95%, for the detection of greater than 50% arterial diameter reduction.[3,26,27] Furthermore, no significant differences were reported in duplex imaging's ability to detect lesions above or below the knee.[3,27]

Duplex imaging, however, does not provide information regarding overall limb hemodynamics and is therefore often used in combination with physiologic (indirect) testing to provide a holistic representation of limb perfusion. Duplex imaging is able to distinguish a stenosis from an occlusion, determine length of the diseased segment, and evaluate patency of distal vessels. Arterial duplex imaging is also used to evaluate results of vascular interventions (angioplasty, stent placement) by aiding in the diagnosis of aneurysm or pseudoaneurysm and monitoring postoperative status.

Color Doppler (CD) imaging provides a guide for accurate placement of the SD gate (sample volume) so accurate arterial SD waveforms are obtained. Additionally, CD imaging reduces the time required to perform an examination, as it enables visual identification of blood flow disturbances, aiding in the detection of arterial stenoses. When using CD to guide the examination, it is imperative for an accurate examination that technical parameters are set appropriately (e.g., pulse repetition frequency, color gain, frame rate).

The GS image and CD display are helpful to recognize anatomic variations and locating plaque and calcification, but are not accurate in determining the amount of arterial narrowing. The percent of narrowing in an artery is determined using information from the SD waveform. SD waveforms are obtained using a small-sized gate (sample volume) placed within the center of the lumen while maintaining a 60-degree angle to the vessel walls. If a 60-degree angle cannot be maintained, it is important to document the angle used during the examination to ensure reproducibility and comparison of future examinations. Waveforms obtained with angles greater than 60 degrees should not be used because of inherent error. Representative SD signals are recorded from standard sites along the peripheral arteries, which will vary by institution. When arterial stenosis is suspected, the SD gate should be swept through the color display at the area in question. This is done to detect focal increases in velocity or blood flow disturbances. If a stenotic area is found, additional SD waveforms should be obtained proximal to, within, and distal to the narrowed segment. Documentation of this is necessary for an accurate interpretation, as it provides key information regarding the extent of stenosis and severity of disease.

It is imperative that each institution develops an arterial imaging protocol that defines the standard examination (e.g., arteries to be evaluated and the location of Doppler samples). This protocol must include information about the technique, clinical applications, indications for a complete and/or limited examination and interpretation criteria. A standard complete examination for arterial occlusive disease usually includes transverse and longitudinal GS images, along with CD/SD duplex images from multiple segments of each artery examined.

Lower Extremity

Peripheral arterial duplex imaging of the lower extremities begins in the abdomen with the evaluation of the aortic bifurcation. A low-frequency transducer (2.0 to 3.5 MHz) provides optimal imaging during this portion of the examination. The aortic bifurcation is typically best visualized with the patient in a decubitus position turned to the left side while using a longitudinal scanning approach from the front of the right iliac crest. Visualization of the aortic bifurcation can be further enhanced by requesting patients take nothing by mouth the morning of the examination. The distal aorta and the origin of both common iliac arteries can typically be visualized fairly easily, allowing for the evaluation of all three vessels.

The patient is then positioned supine to evaluate the remainder of the lower extremity arterial vasculature. At this point, a higher-frequency linear-array transducer (5 to 10 MHz) should be used for the remainder of the examination. The transducer should be placed between the iliac crest and the umbilicus to image the internal and external iliac arteries. If difficulty is encountered locating the iliac arteries, locate the femoral arteries at the level of the groin and follow them proximally.

Next, the CFA is located at the level of the groin and evaluated in the longitudinal plane. The CFA should be followed distally until its bifurcation into the femoral and profunda femoris arteries (Fig. 39.5). At this location, the femoral and profunda femoris artery origins are evaluated. The FA is then followed distally and imaged along the medial portion of the thigh. In the distal thigh, the FA becomes the popliteal artery, which travels through the popliteal fossa. Using a posterior scanning approach, evaluation of the popliteal artery is performed in a longitudinal plane.

Following the popliteal artery distally, the origin of the ATA is visualized diving deep in the proximal calf. The ATA can be followed for only a short distance with this approach. The remainder of the vessel can be located distally by placing the transducer on the lateral calf and following it to the level of the ankle. The tibial-peroneal trunk extends into the calf from the popliteal artery, distal to the origin of the ATA. The posterior tibial and peroneal arteries can be visualized by placing the transducer on the medial calf. The peroneal artery is located deep to, and runs parallel with, the PTA. These vessels can be located above the malleolus and followed proximally. The DPA is located very superficially on the dorsum of the foot between the navicular and intermediate cuneiform

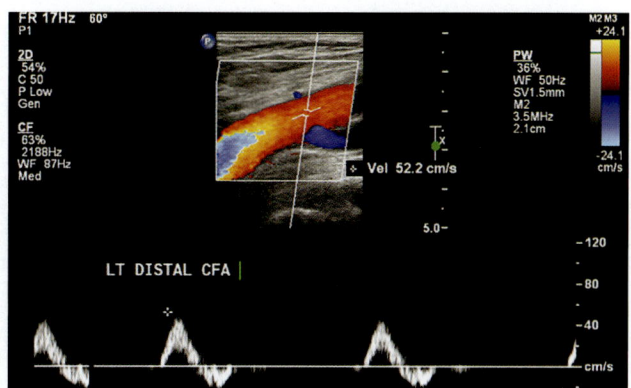

FIG. 39.5 Color and spectral Doppler image of the common femoral artery (CFA) at its bifurcation into the femoral artery and profunda femoris arteries.

bones. To visualize, place the probe sagittally between the extensor longus tendons on top of the foot. Finding the pulse of this artery can also aid in locating (Fig. 39.6).

Upper Extremity

Arteries of the upper extremity are also evaluated with arterial duplex imaging. The patient is positioned supine with the arms relaxed at the sides. A higher-frequency linear-array transducer (5 to 10 MHz) should be used to conduct GS imaging and Doppler evaluations. The subclavian artery should be evaluated using both a supraclavicular and an infraclavicular approach to ensure thorough inspection of the vessel is performed. Segments of the subclavian artery may not be visualized because of acoustic shadowing artifact caused by the overlying clavicle. Beginning in the proximal portion of the axilla, the subclavian vein becomes the axillary artery. The axillary artery may be evaluated from an infraclavicular approach or from the axilla depending on patient anatomy (Fig. 39.7). The scanning approach that provides the best imaging should be used while performing the axillary artery evaluation. Moving distal, the axillary artery is followed as it becomes the brachial artery in the proximal portion of the arm. For the remainder of the examination, a higher-frequency linear-array transducer (>10 MHz) can be used if available. The brachial artery should be followed and evaluated along the length of the upper arm until its bifurcation into the radial and ulnar arteries near the level antecubital fossa. The radial and ulnar arteries are evaluated in a longitudinal plane along the length of the forearm. These vessels are superficial and may become very small at the wrist.

Changes in arterial blood flow to the arms may be related to intermittent compression of the proximal arteries (TOS). Therefore, patients should be sitting with arms relaxed and alongside the body. Arterial Doppler signals should be recorded in the proximal brachial artery at rest and can be monitored during positional maneuvers when compression disorders are suspected.

Interpretation

Arterial duplex imaging examination of the lower extremities focuses on answering a number of important questions (Box 39.2). One large advantage of duplex imaging is its ability to provide SD waveforms, from which morphology and velocity analysis can be performed. In healthy vessels of the periphery, the morphology of an arterial SD waveform is triphasic (Fig. 39.8).[28] The characteristics of a triphasic waveform are a high-velocity forward flow component during systole (ventricular contraction), followed by a brief reversal of flow in early diastole (result of peripheral resistance), and a final low-velocity forward flow phase in late diastole (elastic recoil of the vessel wall). In the presence of a hemodynamically significant stenosis, the reversal of flow component of the waveform will be absent due to high peripheral resistance.

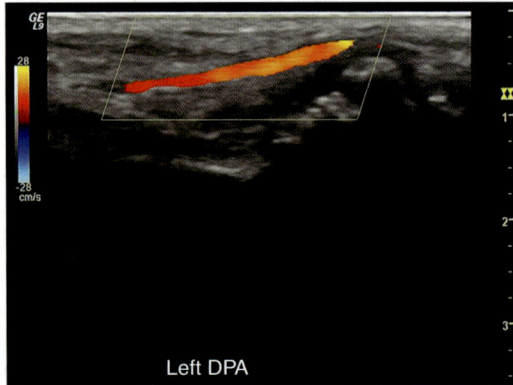

FIG. 39.6 Color Doppler image of a normal dorsalis pedis artery (DPA) in the left foot.

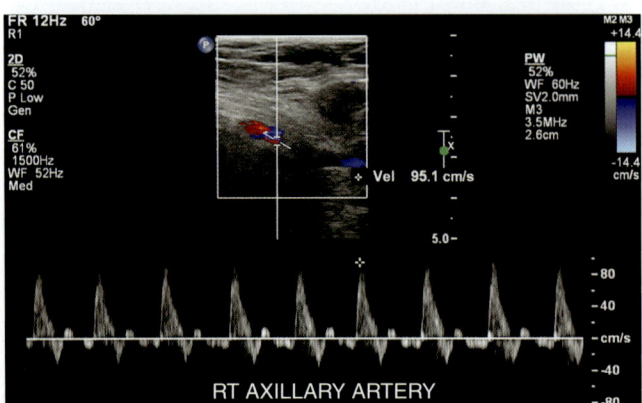

FIG. 39.7 Color and spectral Doppler image demonstrating a normal triphasic waveform in the axillary artery.

BOX 39.2	Essential Questions for Arterial Duplex Imaging

- Is disease present in the extremity?
- Is the disease a stenosis, occlusion, AVF, aneurysm, or pseudoaneurysm?
- What is the location of the narrowing? What is the extent and severity?
- What is the location of the occlusion? What is the extent of the occlusion? Is collateral flow identified near or around the occlusion?
- Is there adequate inflow into the leg?
- Is an outflow vessel identified?
- Is an adequate superficial vein identified that may be used as an arterial conduit?
- Is an AVF identified? What is the location of the fistula?
- Is a patent arterial aneurysm identified? What is the location of the aneurysm and its dimensions?
- Is a pseudoaneurysm identified? What are its location and dimensions? Is the neck of the pseudoaneurysm identified? What is the vessel of origin?
- Is an existing stent or bypass graft patent, or is there stenosis or occlusion? What is the extent of disease? Is an endoleak present?

AVF, Arteriovenous fistula.

CD imaging also aids in the identification of significant arterial narrowing. Color aliasing, color persistence (continuous signal), and color bruit (tissue vibration caused by severe blood flow disturbance) findings are all indicative of a blood flow abnormality, such as turbulence, which is a finding consistent with PAD. These characteristics can also be seen in the SD waveform in the form of spectral broadening (Fig. 39.9).

While evaluating a stenotic region, it is important to obtain GS and CD/SD duplex images proximal to, within, and distal to the stenosis. Proximal to the stenosis, SD waveform size (PSV) is typically diminished and blunted, with a loss of reversal component. Within the stenotic area, waveform amplitude is increased, with turbulent flow present (represented as aliasing on CD and spectral broadening on SD). Distal to the stenosis, turbulent flow is again seen, along with diminished SD waveform amplitude and prolonged waveform upslope with loss of reversal component (Figs. 39.10 to 39.12). Although helpful in the detection of arterial stenosis, SD waveform morphology and CD information provide minimal aid in determining the degree of arterial lumen narrowing.

Quantitative measures of PSV and EDV are obtained from SD waveforms to complement qualitative information provided from the analysis of waveform morphology. PSVs and waveform morphology are used in combination to determine the degree of stenosis and can be characterized into five categories: (1) No increase in PSV relative to the adjacent segment and no waveform abnormalities are normal and suggest no stenosis; (2) no increase in PSV relative to the adjacent segment, but flow disturbances are noted on CD or SD, is suggestive of 1% to 19% vessel narrowing; (3) an increase in PSV from 30% to 100% relative to the adjacent segment is suggestive of 20% to 49% vessel narrowing; (4) an increase in PSV greater than 100% relative to the adjacent segment is

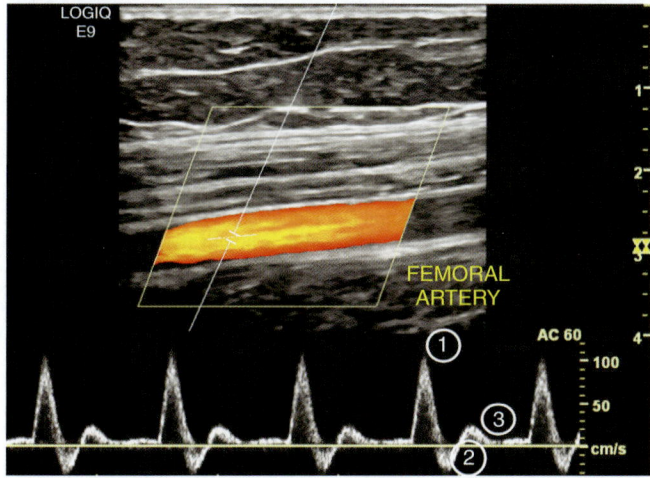

FIG. 39.8 A normal color and spectral Doppler image of the femoral artery. The triphasic spectral Doppler signal demonstrates (1) a rapid upstroke (acceleration) to peak systole, (2) reversal of blood flow component during early diastole, and (3) a forward flow component during late diastole.

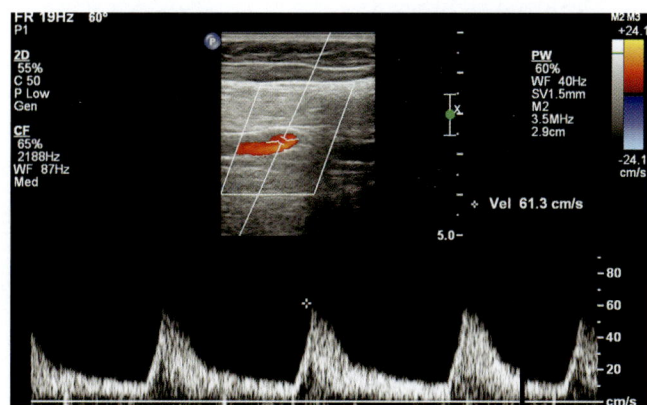

FIG. 39.10 Color and spectral Doppler image of spectral waveforms obtained proximal to a hemodynamically significant stenosis. Peak systolic velocity is approximately 60 cm/sec and the waveform morphology is abnormal, as peaks are diminished and blunted with the absence of the reversal of flow component.

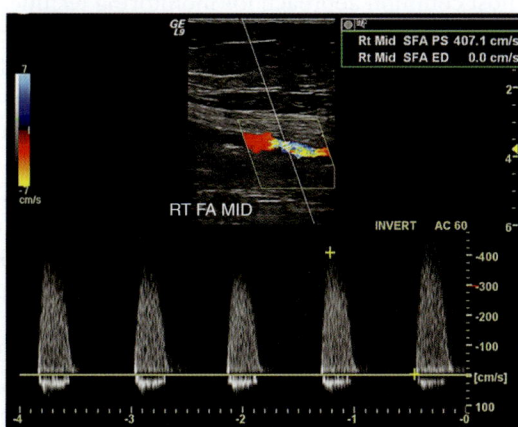

FIG. 39.9 Color and spectral Doppler image of a severe stenosis in the femoral artery (FA). Turbulent flow is demonstrated by color aliasing in the color Doppler display and the presence of spectral broadening in the spectral Doppler waveforms. Turbulent flow can be suggestive of significant arterial lumen narrowing. These qualitative findings are consistent with the elevated peak systolic velocity of 407 cm/sec derived from spectral Doppler waveform analysis.

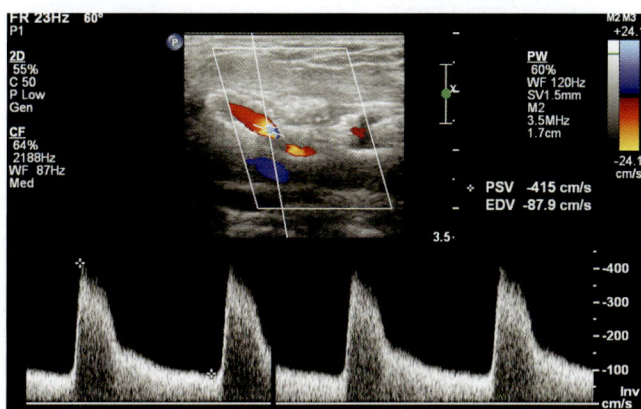

FIG. 39.11 Color and spectral Doppler image demonstrating spectral waveforms obtained within a hemodynamically significant stenosis. Peak systolic velocity (PSV) is elevated at greater 400 cm/sec and the waveform morphology is abnormal, as amplitude is increased with the presence of spectral broadening. Aliasing can also be seen on the color display, suggestive of turbulent flow and/or elevated blood flow velocities. *EDV*, End-diastolic velocity.

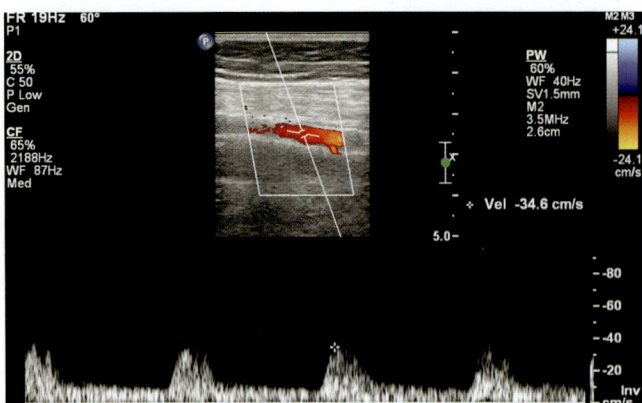

FIG. 39.12 Color and spectral Doppler image demonstrating spectral waveforms obtained distal to a hemodynamically significant stenosis. Peak systolic velocity is approximately 30 cm/sec and the waveform morphology is abnormal, as peaks are diminished with a prolonged upslope and absence of the reversal of flow component. Spectral broadening is also demonstrated in the spectral Doppler waveform and is suggestive of turbulent flow.

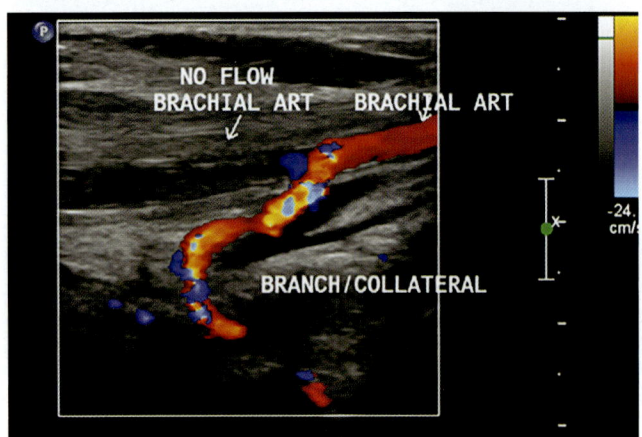

FIG. 39.13 Color Doppler image of a brachial artery occlusion with collateral branch.

suggestive of 50% to 99% vessel narrowing; and (5) no identifiable signal by CD or SD is suggestive of 100% vessel narrowing or occlusion.[29] In the presence of an occlusive lesion, CD may reveal collaterals near the blocked segment (Fig. 39.13). Power Doppler imaging can improve visualization of high-grade stenoses, especially in vessels running parallel to the skin. EDVs can also be used to assist in the determination of arterial stenosis, as values greater than 40 cm/sec suggest the presence of a hemodynamically significant lesion.[30]

In summary, the three major changes in the SD arterial waveform that occur as a result of hemodynamically significant stenoses are (1) increase in PSVs (>100%); (2) marked spectral broadening caused by turbulence; and (3) loss of reversal of blood flow during diastole. All GS, CD, and SD findings should be compiled and documented into a concise and clear report for accurate physician interpretation. Limitations to the examination should also be documented in this report. Common limitations of the lower extremity arterial duplex examination are listed in Box 39.3.

BOX 39.3 Limitations of the Lower Extremity Arterial Duplex Imaging Examination

- Nonvisualization of the iliac system due to overlying bowel gas or increased body habitus
- Shadowing due to vessel calcification
- Imaging of the popliteal trifurcation
- Difficulty evaluating lesions distal to high-grade stenoses due to low flow velocities in these segments

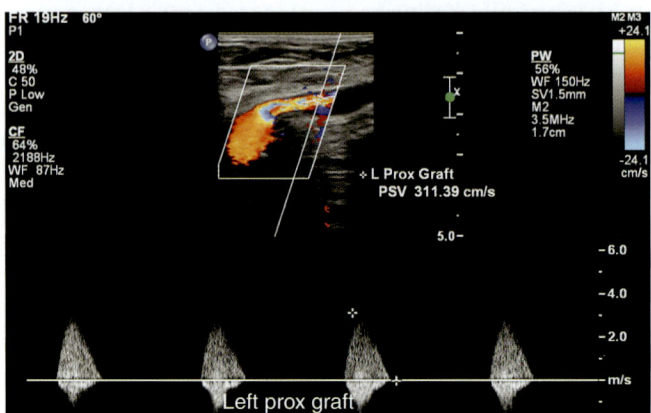

FIG. 39.14 Color and spectral Doppler image with spectral waveforms obtained in the area of narrowing within a in situ bypass graft. Spectral waveforms demonstrate elevated peak systolic velocity (PSV) at approximately 300 cm/sec, along with the presence of spectral broadening.

Bypass Graft Surveillance

Bypass graft patency can be significantly prolonged if developing atherosclerotic lesions are detected and treated before causing thrombosis within the graft. To this end, it has been reported that reintervention directed by duplex imaging has enabled the 5-year patency rate of bypass grafts to reach nearly 80%.[31] Recent evidence and subsequent guidelines have resulted in a combination of ABIs and duplex imaging as the most common approach for monitoring technical adequacy, hemodynamic function, and development of postimplantation lesions[12,32,33] (Fig. 39.14). Graft abnormalities, such as myointimal stenosis, retained valve cusps, arteriovenous fistulas (AVFs), degenerative aneurysmal formation, and low-flow states, can be detected with arterial duplex imaging, even in the absence of symptoms.[34] A graft surveillance program should identify bypass grafts at risk for occlusion, provide information on the mechanism of failure (Fig. 39.15), and direct decisions of intervention to reduce the incidence of graft failure and reintervention.

To accurately evaluate bypass grafts with arterial duplex imaging, it is important to know the location and type of graft before beginning the study. The technique is similar to the GS and CD/SD duplex evaluation of native arteries. The entire length of the bypass graft should be evaluated, along with the native inflow and outflow vessels while also paying close attention to the proximal and distal graft anastomoses.

The timing and frequency of bypass graft surveillance will vary by surgeon and by scenario (e.g., type of graft, location, and patient health status). Some suggest performing an examination after the operation before the patient is discharged from the hospital to establish a baseline. Follow-up examinations for bypass graft monitoring are typically performed at approximately 6-week, 3-month, and then at 3- to 6-month intervals for the first postoperative year.[30] After the first year, surveillance typically occurs on an annual basis. If graft surveillance detects a stenosis, more frequent evaluations may be performed to follow graft integrity more closely.

Findings of PSV greater than 180 cm/sec or a velocity ratio greater than 2 (calculated by dividing the PSV of a graft segment by the PSV in the adjacent proximal segment) are considered abnormal and suggestive of a stenotic area within the bypass graft.[30] Furthermore, PSVs greater than 300 cm/sec, EDVs greater than 20 cm/sec, and a velocity ratio greater than 3.5 suggest graft diameter reduction of greater than 70% and warrant the need for reintervention.[35] In cases of a failing graft (approaching occlusion), low PSVs (<40 cm/sec) may be seen.[30,35]

Arterial duplex imaging plays an important role in the follow-up of patients with lower extremity arterial bypass grafts. Identification of arterial lesions during the preocclusive phase is critical for prolonging the patency of the graft. Likewise, evaluation of peripheral arterial stents is performed in a similar way. The entire portion of the stent, including the segments of the artery proximal and distal to its placement, are evaluated with color and SD to ensure no areas of focal velocity increases exist that suggest a diameter reduction within the stent.

Dialysis Access Grafts

Dialysis grafts (autogenous or synthetic) are typically placed in the forearm to create an AVF in patients undergoing hemodialysis. Dialysis grafts can exist in a variety of ways; the Brescia-Cimino AVF is a direct connection of the radial artery and the cephalic vein. Other direct connections include the cephalic vein to the brachial artery (Fig. 39.16), the basilic vein to the brachial artery, and the basilic vein to the ulnar artery. Dialysis grafts can also be created using a synthetic graft interposed between the artery and the vein (straight or loop graft). These can be placed in the lower or upper arm or in the upper leg. They are usually easily identifiable under the surface of the skin and produce a thrill when palpated. The most common complications associated with these grafts are failure of autologous vein access to mature, thrombus formation, venous outflow obstruction causing venous hypertension and limb edema, venous anastomotic stenosis, pseudoaneurysm, hematoma (Fig. 39.17), perigraft fluid collection, arterial anastomotic stenosis (Fig. 39.18), and arterial steal syndrome resulting in hand ischemia.[36]

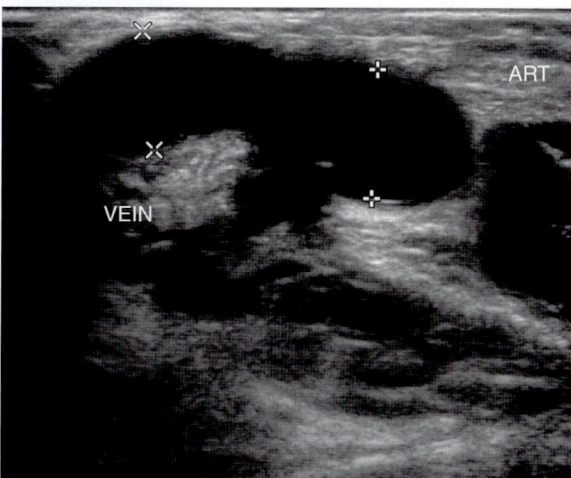

FIG. 39.16 Gray-scale image of a dialysis fistula created between the cephalic vein and the brachial artery.

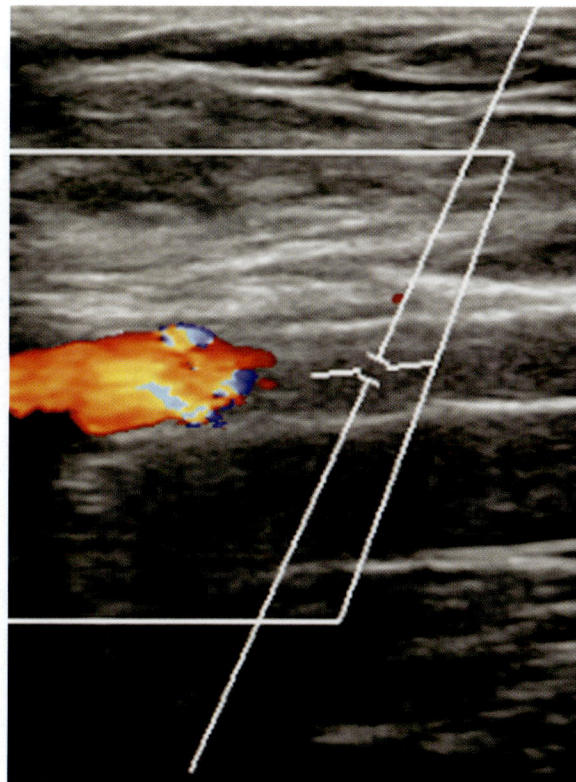

FIG. 39.15 An occluded femoral-popliteal synthetic conduit bypass graft in a patient with progressing claudication, as indicated by the absence of color flow entering the graft.

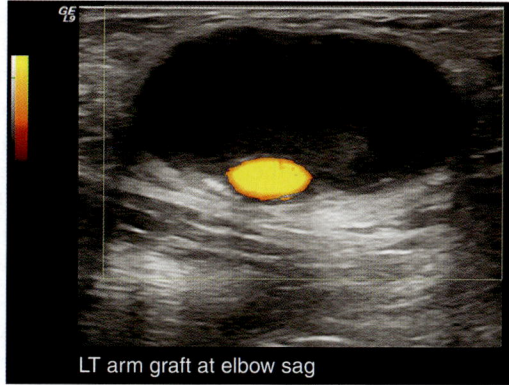

FIG. 39.17 Power Doppler image of a hematoma seen after dialysis. Flow is seen in the graft posterior to the hematoma. The patient presented with a palpable mass.

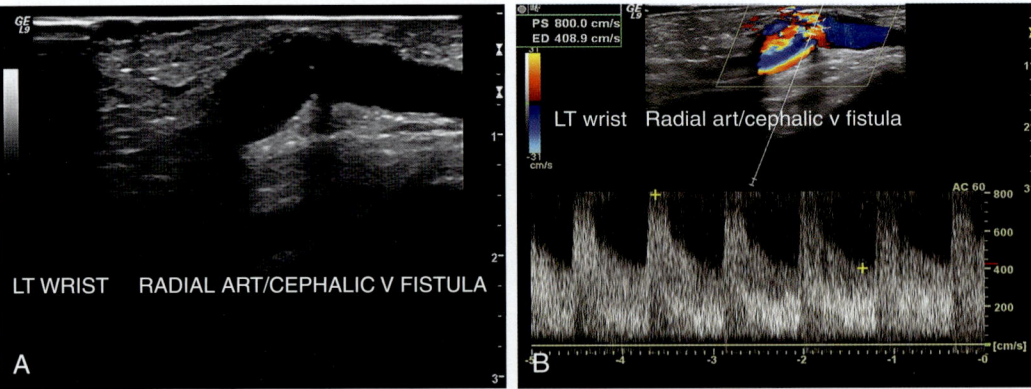
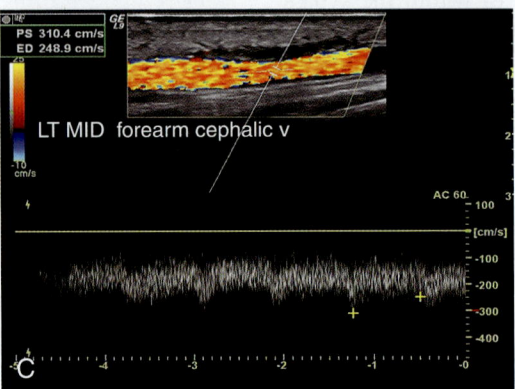

FIG. 39.18 **Brescia-Cimino graft.** (A) Gray-scale image of the radial artery and cephalic vein connection. (B) Color and spectral Doppler image of a stenosis at the anastomotic site between the artery and vein. Peak systolic velocity is 800 cm/sec. (C) Color and spectral Doppler image demonstrating flow in the distal cephalic vein portion of the dialysis graft, which reveals a normal flow velocity of 310 cm/sec.

The failure rate of dialysis grafts has been found to be as high as 40% in the first year.[36] Therefore, sonographic evaluation of dialysis grafts is a common method of surveillance, as recommended by the National Kidney Foundation Kidney Disease Outcomes Quality Initiative (KDOQI).[36,37]

Patients are referred for evaluation and mapping of veins before access placement or because of inadequate dialysis, suspicion of a steal, stenosis, thrombosis, or pseudoaneurysm. The duplex examination should capture SD waveforms and PSVs throughout the native arterial system, graft, and venous outflow system, with close attention being paid to each anastomosis. The examination should also include the evaluation of stenosis and/or thrombus presence within the graft and the native circulation. Healthy access grafts will demonstrate an increased flow velocity that has continuous forward diastolic flow and notable spectral broadening. These velocities will be slightly lower approaching the venous portion of the graft. Peak systolic velocities are typically 200 cm/sec or higher in healthy grafts (Fig. 39.19). A decrease in PSV between 100 and 200 cm/sec is suggestive of an abnormality (usually outflow stenosis). Flow volume measurements within the dialysis graft should be obtained using SD waveforms. KDOQI guidelines suggest that a dialysis graft is abnormal and potentially in need of repair when flow volumes are less than 600 mL/min.[38] Lack of SD signals and intraluminal echoes suggest graft occlusion. An ultrasound surveillance program for early

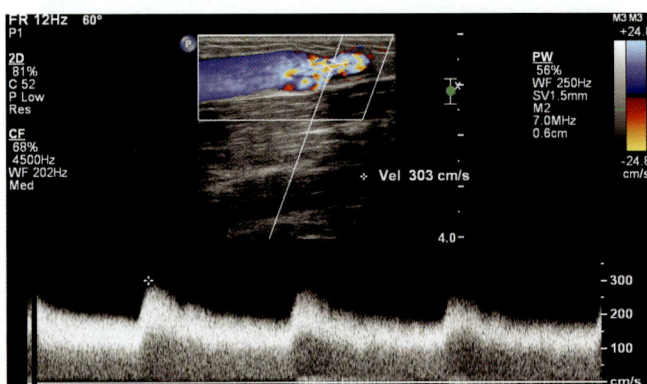

FIG. 39.19 Color and spectral Doppler image of a dialysis graft demonstrating high-velocity flow (~300 cm/sec) through the graft. High flow velocities within these grafts are a normal finding and in general are suggestive of a healthy and mature graft.

detection and treatment of dialysis access graft issues has demonstrated to prolong graft patency while reducing hospitalizations and related health care costs.[39,40]

Aneurysms and Pseudoaneurysms

Arterial duplex imaging has become a valuable tool for evaluating patients with known or suspected aneurysms and pseudoaneurysms in the extremities. Arterial duplex imaging is able to differentiate aneurysms, pseudoaneurysms, perigraft fluid collections, and hematomas, while also providing information about size, location, extent, site of communication, and the potential presence of intraluminal thrombus.

Peripheral arterial aneurysms are most commonly present in the popliteal artery.[41] Although not likely to rupture, peripheral arterial aneurysms can be limb threatening because of their potential to cause embolism.[42-44] Evaluation of peripheral arterial aneurysms by duplex imaging is the recognized noninvasive modality for determining size, extent, position, patency, and associated arterial blood flow dynamics.[45] To accurately measure the size (length and width) of an aneurysm, the artery should be evaluated in both longitudinal and transverse imaging planes. CD should also be used to distinguish the false from the true lumen of the artery (Fig. 39.20). Duplex aneurysm evaluations are often repeated to monitor aneurysm size to ensure it is not progressing.

A **pseudoaneurysm** is a perivascular collection (hematoma) containing pulsatile flow entering through a communication with an artery or a graft. A tract (neck) of variable length connects the native vessel to the blood flow collection. Pseudoaneurysms may occur as a result of trauma, at vascular anastomoses, in angioaccess grafts, or at puncture sites (usually following cardiac catheterization).

Pseudoaneurysms can be unilocular or multilocular and may partially contain thrombus. Pseudoaneurysms occur in variable sizes, with size changing throughout each cardiac cycle. Pseudoaneurysms located in the groin and communicating with the FA occur in 0.2% to 5% as a result of diagnostic procedures, and up to 8% as a result of vascular interventions.[46] Although spontaneous thrombosis of pseudoaneurysms has been reported in the literature, fatal spontaneous hemorrhage of pseudoaneurysms has also occurred.[47-49] An increased risk of rupture is present in pseudoaneurysms measuring greater than 3 cm.

Sonographically, swirling blood within the fluid collection is often visualized on CD imaging (Fig. 39.21). CD imaging also helps identify the neck of the pseudoaneurysm.

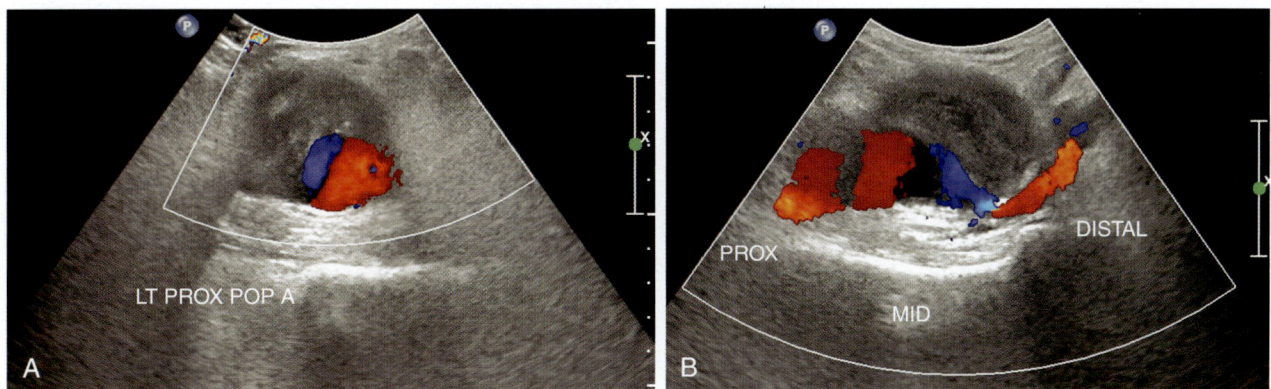

FIG. 39.20 A popliteal artery (PopA) aneurysm imaged with color Doppler in the transverse (A) and longitudinal (B) planes. Color Doppler helps distinguish the false from the true lumen.

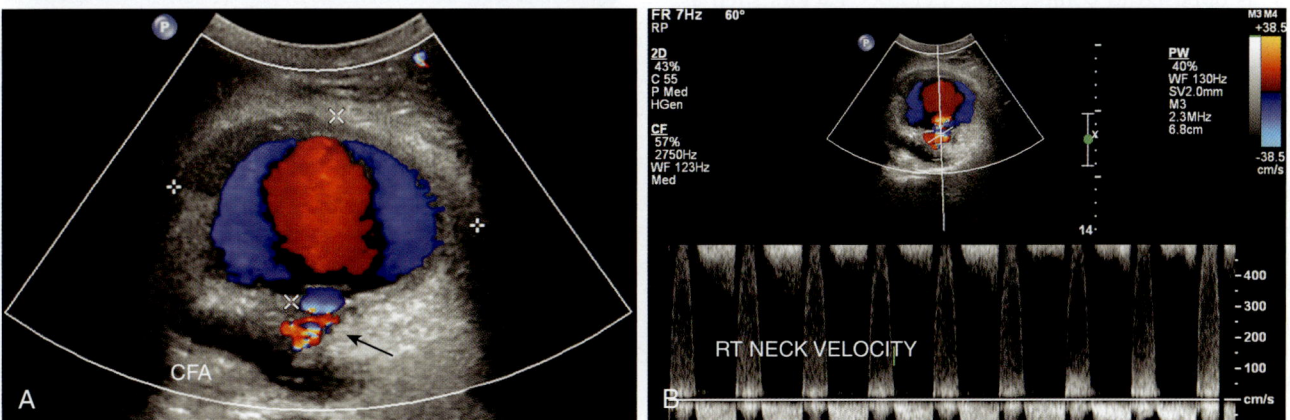

FIG. 39.21 A large pseudoaneurysm located in the groin originating from the common femoral artery (CFA). (A) The swirling of blood can be visualized using color Doppler imaging. The tract or "neck" *(arrow)* can also be seen connecting the pseudoaneurysm to the native vessel (the CFA). (B) Color and spectral Doppler duplex image, demonstrating spectral Doppler waveforms obtained within the neck of the pseudoaneurysm. To-and-fro (bidirectional) flow pattern with elevated velocities is seen, which are expected characteristics of pseudoaneurysm neck blood flow.

Identification of the neck is critical when attempting ultrasound-guided compression therapy, as CD enables the visualization of the vessel of origin, important when planning surgical intervention. SD waveforms obtained from the pseudoaneurysm neck demonstrates a to-and-fro (bidirectional) pattern (see Fig. 39.21). During systole, blood flows from the native artery into the pseudoaneurysm; during diastole, blood return to the native artery. Finally, the size (length, width, and depth) of the pseudoaneurysm should be measured.

Treatment of pseudoaneurysms is commonly accomplished using compression therapy or ultrasound-guided thrombin injection. Compression therapy may be attempted if the neck of the pseudoaneurysm can be clearly identified on arterial duplex imaging. Once identified, pressure is applied to the skin using the ultrasound transducer with the goal of impeding blood flow into the pseudoaneurysm. Compression cycles of 15 to 20 minutes are commonly performed, with progress evaluated between cycles. In most cases, it will take at least 30 to 60 minutes before successful thrombosis of a pseudoaneurysm is achieved. It is extremely important not to occlude blood flow in the native artery. To ensure this does not occur, distal blood flow in the lower extremities should be monitored during compression cycles.

As an alternative to ultrasound compression therapy, an ultrasound-guided thrombin injection can be performed for pseudoaneurysm treatment. As thrombin is injected, its effects are continuously monitored with CD imaging. Thrombin injection is stopped when blood flow is no longer documented (visualized on CD). In addition, distal pulses and other signs suggestive of arterial blood flow impedance are closely monitored.

In a review investigating pseudoaneurysm treatment techniques, it was determined that ultrasound-guided thrombin injections were more effective in achieving primary thrombosis of the pseudoaneurysm.[50] However, this technique was also found to be associated with higher rates of complications, as opposed to compression therapy.[50] Factors such as size, location, and patient health status may also influence the method of treatment implemented.

GUIDELINES FOR EVALUATION

Peripheral arterial testing provides valuable information by addressing specific questions during disease detection and monitoring (Table 39.2). Through duplex testing, anatomic and physiologic information can be obtained and interpreted to provide a holistic representation of peripheral arterial perfusion.

Performing high-quality and complete examinations is essential to the diagnostic value of these tests. The best peripheral arterial evaluation will be achieved by proper attention to detail. Major areas of focus when performing a peripheral arterial evaluation are summarized in Box 39.4. Attention to these technical areas and interpretation details will ensure the best peripheral arterial evaluation.

TABLE 39.2 Evaluation Guidelines Based on Clinical Presentation

Clinical Presentation	Questions	Noninvasive Test
Initial visit	Is disease present? How severe is the process? What segments are involved?	Resting segmental pressures, pulse volume tracings, exercise testing (select patients)
Focal problems	Is pulsatile mass an aneurysm or a pseudoaneurysm? What is the size/location of the aneurysm?	Duplex imaging
Before angioplasty	What is the location of the lesion? Is it a stenosis or an occlusion? What is the length of the disease segment? What is the status of the runoff vessels?	Duplex imaging
After angioplasty	Was the angioplasty successful? What is the degree of improvement?	Pressure measurements and duplex imaging
Bypass graft	Is the bypass graft patent? What is the degree of improvement? Is the graft at risk for failure?	Pressure measurements and duplex imaging

BOX 39.4 Arterial Evaluation Guidelines

- Take a patient history.
- Be familiar with arterial anatomy, physiology, and pathology.
- When measuring ankle pressures, always use the highest brachial pressure to calculate an ankle-brachial index.
- When performing arterial duplex imaging, optimize the grayscale image.
- Understand how each color control affects the image and how the controls affect each other.
- Use a longitudinal imaging plane to obtain color Doppler information, and use it as a guide to obtain the spectral Doppler waveforms.
- Use a small Doppler sample volume size and a 60-degree angle. If needed an angle <60 degrees can be used but must be documented. Waveforms obtained from angles >60 degrees are inaccurate
- Be aware of Doppler spectral waveform velocity and configuration.
- Establish institutional acquisition protocols, interpretation and diagnostic criteria.

Key Pearls

- Noninvasive arterial testing is made up of two different types of ultrasound technology: (1) indirect (oscillometric) and (2) direct testing (duplex imaging).
- The peripheral arterial system is made up of arteries, arterioles, and capillaries in the most distal portion.
- The peripheral arteries are located in the upper and lower extremities and transport blood to the microcirculation of the arterial system, made up of the arterioles and capillaries. After the capillaries, blood exits the arterial system and enters the venous system for return to the heart.
- In general, arterial diameter size decreases the farther they are located in the periphery.
- As the diameter of an artery decreases, arterial resistance increases.
- Peripheral arterial disease, and other occlusive disorders, are characterized by a reduction in arterial lumen diameter.
- The inability to receive the extra-arterial blood required for muscle use is known as intermittent claudication.
- Atherosclerosis is the primary disease process that leads to PAD.
- Atherosclerosis can also cause arterial embolism, which can occur when plaque dislodges from the arterial wall and propagates distally in the arterial system.
- In severe cases, peripheral perfusion is so diminished that muscles are unable to obtain an adequate amount of oxygenated blood even when not in use. This is known as rest pain. Further disease progression from this point can result in tissue loss, ulceration, gangrene, and critical limb ischemia, leading to limb amputation.
- Ischemic rest pain points to critical ischemia of the distal limb.
- Physical signs of peripheral occlusive arterial disease are elevation pallor, dependent rubor, ischemic ulcers, gangrene, bruits, and decreased peripheral pulses (femoral, popliteal, dorsalis pedis, posterior tibial, axillary, brachial, radial, and ulnar).
- The objective of segmental Doppler testing is to obtain systolic blood pressures at different levels of the extremities.
- Two types of plethysmography testing are typically used for indirect testing of the peripheral arterial system: pulse volume recordings and photoplethysmography.
- Thoracic outlet syndrome is characterized as the compression of neural and/or vascular structures by bone, ligament, or muscular obstacles at the thoracic outlet, causing ischemic reactions when the patient presents in certain positions.
- Primary Raynaud phenomenon is characterized as intermittent digital ischemia in response to cold or emotional stress, causing patients to present with color changes (white or blue) in the digits of the upper or lower extremity.
- Secondary Raynaud phenomenon is caused by vascular occlusion or stenosis of the fingers or toes and can occur in response to cold or emotional stress.
- Duplex imaging is able to distinguish a stenosis from an occlusion, determine the length of the diseased segment, evaluate the patency of distal vessels, and evaluate results of vascular interventions (angioplasty, stent placement) by aiding in the diagnosis of aneurysm or pseudoaneurysm and monitoring patients' postoperative course with continual bypass graft surveillance.
- Peripheral arterial duplex imaging of the lower extremities begins in the abdomen with the evaluation of the aortic bifurcation into the iliac arteries.
- Arteries of the upper extremity can also be evaluated with arterial duplex imaging, although lower extremity evaluations are more common in clinical practice.
- The patency of bypass grafts can be significantly prolonged if developing atherosclerotic lesions are corrected before causing a thrombosis within the graft.
- Peripheral arterial aneurysms most commonly present in the popliteal artery.
- A pseudoaneurysm is a perivascular collection (hematoma) containing pulsatile flow entering it through a communication with an artery or graft.

REFERENCES

1. Virani SS, Alonso A, Benjamin EJ, Bittencourt MS, Callaway CW, Carson AP, et al. Heart disease and stroke statistics—2020 update: a report from the American Heart Association. *Circulation.* 2020;141(9):e139–e596.
2. Barnes JA, et al. Epidemiology and risk of amputation in patients with diabetes mellitus and peripheral artery disease. *Arterioscler Thromb Vasc Biol.* 2020;40(8):1808–1817.
3. Tendera M, Aboyans V. Bartelink, et al: ESC guidelines on the diagnosis and treatment of peripheral artery diseases. *Eur Heart J.* 2011;32:2851–2906.
4. Firnhaber JM, Powell CS. Lower extremity peripheral artery disease: diagnosis and treatment. *Am family physician.* 2019;99(6):362–369.
5. Conte SM, Peter RV. Peripheral arterial disease. *Heart, Lung Circulation.* 2018;27(4):427–432.
6. Lane R, et al. Exercise for intermittent claudication. *Cochrane Database Syst Rev.* 2017;12
7. Bevan GH, White Solaru KT. Evidence-based medical management of peripheral artery disease. *Arterioscler thromb Vasc Biol.* 2020;40(3):541–553.
8. Aboyans V, et al. ESC Guidelines on the diagnosis and treatment of peripheral arterial diseases 2017. *Eur Heart J.* 2018;39(9):763–816.
9. Goss SE. In: Beckner JM, ed. *SDMS National Certification Exam (NCER) registry review series—vascular sonography/technology.* Plano, TX: Society of Diagnostic Medical Sonography; 2009.
10. Long CA, et al. Incidence and Factors Associated With Major Amputation in Patients With Peripheral Artery Disease: Insights From the EUCLID Trial. *Circulation: Cardiovasc Qual Outcomes.* 2020;13(7):e006399.
11. McDermott MM. Lower extremity manifestations of peripheral artery disease: the pathophysiologic and functional implications of leg ischemia. *Circ Res.* 2015;116:1540–1550.
12. Anderson JL, Halperin JL, Albert N, et al. Management of patients with peripheral artery disease (compilation of 2005 and 2011 ACCF/AHA guideline recommendations): a report of the American College of Cardiology Foundation/American Heart Association Task Force on Practice Guidelines. *J Am Coll Cardiol.* 2013;61:1555–1570.
13. Schaper NC, Andros G, Apelqvist J, et al. Diagnosis and treatment of peripheral arterial disease in diabetic patients with a foot ulcer. A progress report of the International Working Group on the Diabetic Foot. *Diabetes Metab Res Rev.* 2012;28:218–224.

14. Aboyans V, Criqui MH, Abraham P, et al. Measurement and interpretation of the ankle-brachial index: a scientific statement from the American Heart Association. *Circulation*. 2012;126:2890-2909.
15. Begelman SM, Jaff MR. Noninvasive diagnostic strategies for peripheral arterial disease. *Cleve Clin J Med*. 2006;73:S22.
16. Nicoloff AD, Taylor Jr LM, Sexton GJ, et al. Homocysteine and progression of atherosclerosis study investigators: relationship between site of initial symptoms and subsequent progression of disease in a prospective study of atherosclerosis progression in patients receiving long-term treatment for symptomatic peripheral arterial disease. *J Vasc Surg*. 2002;35:38-46.
17. Casey S, et al. The reliability of the ankle brachial index: a systematic review. *J Foot Ankle Res*. 2019;12(1):1-10.
18. Rooke TW, Hirsch AT, Misra S, et al. ACCF/AHA focused update of the guideline for the management of patients with peripheral artery disease (updating the 2005 guideline). *Vasc Med*. 2011;16(452):2011.
19. Herraiz-Adillo Á, et al. The accuracy of toe brachial index and ankle brachial index in the diagnosis of lower limb peripheral arterial disease: A systematic review and meta-analysis. *Atherosclerosis*. 2020.
20. Brownrigg JRW, et al. Performance of prognostic markers in the prediction of wound healing or amputation among patients with foot ulcers in diabetes: a systematic review. *Diabetes/metabolism Res Rev*. 2016;32:128-135.
21. Norgren L, Hiatt WR, Dormandy JA, et al. Inter-society consensus for the management of peripheral arterial disease. *Int Angiology*. 2007;26:81-157.
22. Caruana L, Formosa C, Cassar K. Prediction of wound healing after minor amputations of the diabetic foot. *J Diabetes Complications*. 2015;29:834-837.
23. Bonham P. Measuring toe pressures using a portable photoplethysmograph to detect arterial disease in high-risk patients: an overview of the literature. *Ostomy Wound Manage*. 2011;57:36-44.
24. Conte MS, et al. Global vascular guidelines on the management of chronic limb-threatening ischemia. *Eur J Vasc Endovasc Surg*. 2019;58(1):S1-S109.
25. Stone PA, et al. Toe pressures are superior to duplex parameters in predicting wound healing following toe and foot amputations. *Ann Vasc Surg*. 2018;46:147-154.
26. Martinelli O, et al. Duplex ultrasound versus CT angiography for the treatment planning of lower-limb arterial disease. *J ultrasound*. 2020;1:1-9.
27. Collins R, Cranny G, Burch J, et al. A systematic review of duplex ultrasound, magnetic resonance angiography and computed tomography angiography for the diagnosis and assessment of symptomatic, lower limb peripheral arterial disease. *Health Technol Assess*. 2007;11:20.
28. Kim ESH, et al. Interpretation of peripheral arterial and venous Doppler waveforms: A Consensus Statement from the Society for Vascular Medicine and Society for Vascular Ultrasound. *Vasc Med*. 2020;25(5):484-506.
29. Strandness Jr DE. Peripheral arterial system. In: Strandness Jr DE, ed. *Duplex scanning in vascular disorders*. ed 3. Philadelphia: Lippincott Williams & Wilkins; 2002:118-143.
30. Hodgkiss-Harlow KD, Bandyk DF. Interpretation of arterial duplex testing of lower-extremity arteries and interventions. *Semin Vasc Surg*. 2013;26:95-104.
31. Bandyk DF, Schmitt DD, Seabrook GR, et al. Monitoring functional patency of in situ saphenous vein bypasses: the impact of a surveillance protocol and elective revision. *J Vasc Surg*. 1989;9:286-296.
32. Mohammed K, et al. Systematic review and meta-analysis of duplex ultrasound surveillance for infrainguinal vein bypass grafts. *J Vasc Surg*. 2017;66(6):1885-1891.
33. Olin JW, et al. Performance measures for adults with peripheral artery disease 2010. *Circulation*. 2010;122(24):2583-2618.
34. Bui TD, Mills JL, Ihnat DM, et al. The natural history of duplex-detected stenosis after femoropopliteal endovascular therapy suggests questionable clinical utility of routine duplex surveillance. *J Vasc Surg*. 2012;55:346-352.
35. Zierler RE, et al. The Society for Vascular Surgery practice guidelines on follow-up after vascular surgery arterial procedures. *J Vasc Surg*. 2018;68(1):256-284.
36. Back MR, Bandyk DF. *Role of duplex ultrasound in dialysis access surveillance. Noninvasive vascular diagnosis*. London: Springer; 2013:395-406.
37. Schwab S, Besarab A, Beathard G, et al. NKF-DOQI clinical practice guidelines for vascular access. *Am J Kidney Dis*. 1997;30: S150-S191.
38. KDOQI Clinical practice guidelines for vascular access. *Am J Kidney Dis*. 2006;48:S176-S247.
39. Dossabhoy NR, Ram SJ, Nassar R, et al. Stenosis surveillance of hemodialysis grafts by duplex ultrasound reduces hospitalizations and cost of care. *Semin Dialysis*. 2004;18:550-557.
40. Sands JJ, Ferrell LM, Perry MA. The role of color flow Doppler ultrasound in dialysis access. *Semin Nephrol*. 2002;22:195-201.
41. Bearse JR. Duplex ultrasound findings of popliteal artery aneurysms with acute limb ischemia. *J Diagn Med Sonogr*. 2014; 30:314-319.
42. Cervin A, Wanhainen A, Björck M. Popliteal aneurysms are common among men with screening detected abdominal aortic aneurysms, and prevalence correlates with the diameters of the common iliac arteries. *Eur J Vasc Endovasc Surg*. 2020;59(1):67-72.
43. Cervin A, et al. Treatment of popliteal aneurysm by open and endovascular surgery: a contemporary study of 592 procedures in Sweden. *Eur J Vasc Endovasc Surg*. 2015;50(3):342-350.
44. Ravn H, Bergqvist D, Björck M. Nationwide study of the outcome of popliteal artery aneurysms treated surgically. *Br J Surg*. 2007;94(8):970-977.
45. Wright LB, Matchett WJ, Cruz CP, et al. Popliteal artery disease: diagnosis and treatment 1. *Radiographics*. 2004;24:467-479.
46. Kleczynski P, Rakowski T, Dziewierz A, et al. Ultrasound-guided thrombin injection in the treatment of iatrogenic arterial pseudoaneurysms: single-center experience. *J Clin Ultrasound*. 2014;42:24-26.
47. Zhou C, Langlois NE, Byard RW. Femoral artery pseudoaneurysm and sudden death. *J Forensic Sci*. 2012;57:254-256.
48. Yasim A, Kabalci M, Eroglu E, et al. Complication of hemodialysis graft: anastomotic pseudoaneurysm: a case report. *Transpl Proc*. 2006;38:2816-2818.
49. Mlekusch W, Haumer M, Mlekusch I, et al. Prediction of iatrogenic pseudoaneurysm after percutaneous endovascular procedures 1. *Radiology*. 2006;240:597-602.
50. Tisi PV, Callam MJ. Treatment for femoral pseudoaneurysms. *Cochrane Library*. 2013;11:1-24.

CHAPTER 40

Peripheral Venous Evaluation

Kevin R. Volz

OBJECTIVES

On completion of this chapter, you should be able to:
- Describe the anatomy encountered during a venous duplex imaging examination
- Understand venous physiology as it relates to the development of peripheral venous disease
- List the risk factors, signs, and symptoms of venous disease
- Outline the proper instrument control settings used during venous duplex imaging
- Describe the characteristics of venous Doppler signals obtained during venous duplex imaging
- Describe the imaging characteristics of a normal venous system
- Discuss the imaging characteristics associated with deep vein thrombosis and venous reflux

OUTLINE

Anatomy for Peripheral Venous Duplex Imaging 1130
   Lower Extremity 1130
   Upper Extremity 1133
Venous Physiology 1134
Venous Pathology and Treatments 1134
   Deep Venous Thrombosis 1134
   Venous Insufficiency 1136
Technical Aspects of Venous Duplex Imaging 1137
Gray-Scale Imaging and Compression Maneuvers 1137
Doppler 1140
Interpretation of Venous Duplex Imaging 1140
Combined Diagnostic Approach 1145
Venous Reflux Imaging 1145
Vein Mapping 1146
Other Pathology 1147
Controversies in Venous Duplex Imaging 1147
Complete Versus Limited Examination 1147
Unilateral Versus Bilateral 1148
Bilateral Deep Vein Thrombosis Symptoms 1148
Calf Vein Imaging 1149
Emergent Venous Duplex Imaging 1149
Sonographic Assessment of Pulmonary Embolism 1149
Imaging Guidelines 1150

KEY TERMS

Anterior tibial veins (ATVs)
Augmentation
Axillary vein
Baker cyst
Basilic vein
Brachial veins
Cephalic vein
Common femoral vein (CFV)
Common iliac vein
Deep vein thrombosis (DVT)
External iliac vein
External jugular vein (EJV)
Femoral vein
Gastrocnemius (sural) veins
Great saphenous vein (GSV)
Innominate vein
Internal iliac vein
Internal jugular vein (IJV)
Perforating veins
Peroneal veins
Popliteal vein
Posterior arch vein
Posterior tibial vein (PTV)
Profunda femoris vein
Pulmonary embolism (PE)
Radial veins
Respiratory phasicity
Small saphenous vein (SSV)
Soleal sinuses
Spontaneous flow
Subclavian vein
Ulnar veins
Valves
Varicose veins
Venous thromboembolism (VTE)

Peripheral venous disease may be categorized as an acute or a chronic process and can present in the upper and lower extremities. Ultrasound technology enables dynamic, non-ionizing, and portable imaging to be acquired in real time, making it an ideal radiologic modality for the interrogation of venous pathology. Among these advantages is its ability to perform color Doppler (CD) and spectral Doppler (SD) imaging, providing the capability to evaluate both the anatomy and physiologic processes of the venous system. To this end, ultrasound imaging is tasked with conducting a variety of venous imaging examinations, spanning multiple areas of the body.

Venous pathology can take many forms; however, deep vein thrombosis (DVT) has a high prevalence and is arguably the most medically concerning. Characterized by a thrombus, or blood clot, in a deep vein(s), DVT can occur peripherally in the upper and lower extremities, although more commonly within the deep veins of the legs. Although the exact incidence or prevalence of DVT in the United States is unknown due to many going undetected, 857,000 cases are estimated to occur annually.[1] The concerning nature of this disease arises from a complication that can occur when a thrombus dislodges from the venous lumen and propagates to the arteries of the lungs. This is known as a pulmonary embolism (PE) or venous thromboembolism (VTE) when describing both the DVT and PE. VTE is the third most common cardiovascular disorder in the United States behind myocardial infarction and stroke, with approximate lifetime risk of 1 in 12 adults in the United States, and maintains a fairly high mortality rate.[1-5] Thus a timely and accurate diagnosis of DVT is imperative.

The signs and symptoms of DVT are common and nonspecific, meaning they may have several other possible causes (e.g., musculoskeletal disorders, ruptured Baker cyst, cellulitis), making a DVT diagnosis based on solely on signs and symptoms unreliable. This, coupled with the criticality of an accurate DVT diagnosis, has caused the peripheral venous duplex examination to become one of the most commonly ordered vascular sonograms.

Besides a PE, other less severe complications of DVT can often result. Postthrombotic syndrome (PTS) consists of chronic leg pain, inflammation, redness, and ulcers. Deep and superficial venous insufficiency, varicose veins, and recurrent DVT are also common manifestations of PTS. Ultrasound imaging is also often used for the evaluation of these DVT complications. Therefore it is necessary to understand and recognize the presentation of a wide variety of venous diseases because the versatility and advantages of ultrasound imaging make it the radiologic modality that is most often initially used for venous pathology detection and evaluation.

ANATOMY FOR PERIPHERAL VENOUS DUPLEX IMAGING

The peripheral venous portion of the circulatory system is located in the upper and lower extremities and consists of the deep, superficial, and perforating (communicating) veins. The main function of the peripheral venous system is to return deoxygenated blood from organs and body tissues back to the heart. In the periphery, deoxygenated blood leaving the capillaries enters the venules of venous microcirculation. From the venules, venous blood drains into the superficial veins and from there to the deep veins. Perforating veins provide a channel between superficial and deep veins.

Like arteries, veins are made up of three layers: (1) tunica intima (innermost), (2) tunica media (middle), and (3) tunica adventitia (outermost). However, these layers differ from those of the arteries in that the venous tunica media layer is poorly developed. The tunica media is the muscular layer of the lumen, and it provides the vessel with stability. As a result, veins are more elastic and less rigid than arteries.

The presence of venous **valves** is another unique feature of the venous system. Venous valves are bicuspid and unidirectional folds that arise from the tunica intima. These valves serve to maintain antegrade venous blood flow (from the peripheral to central veins, toward the heart). These one-way valves are necessary due to the effects placed upon blood flow within the peripheral veins from hydrostatic pressure. Hydrostatic pressure, also known as gravitational pressure when standing upright, is defined as the pressure placed on a fluid in a column as a result of gravity. Because the heart is located above many of the peripheral veins, the blood traveling upward in the peripheral venous system must flow against the pressure placed on it from the weight of the column of blood that exists above it. Accordingly, the further a point within a peripheral vein is from the heart, the more opposing hydrostatic pressure the blood in it must overcome. For this reason, venous valves increase in quantity in the distal portions of the lower extremities.

Lower Extremity

Deep Veins. As the name suggests, lower extremity deep veins are located deep within the muscles of the legs and serve as the primary route of drainage for the leg (Fig. 40.1). Consequently, deep veins are typically larger than superficial veins because they must support a larger blood volume.

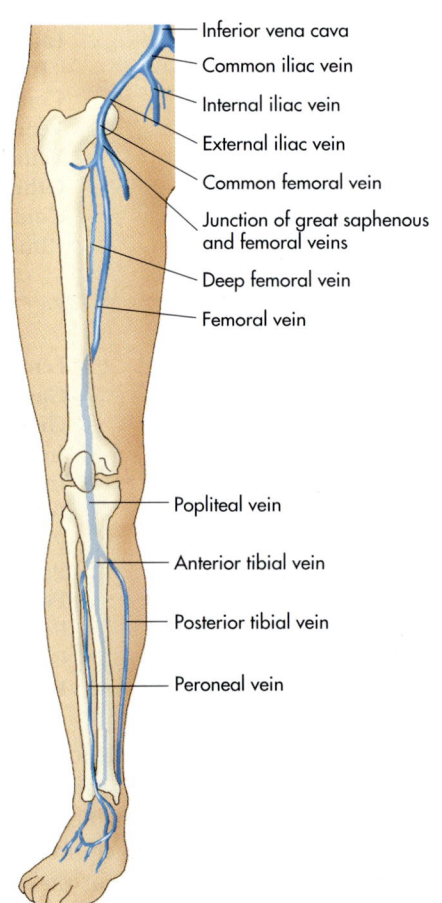

FIG. 40.1 Lower extremity deep veins.

Lower extremity deep veins also have corresponding arteries located in close proximity to them.

Beginning distally, the **anterior tibial veins (ATVs)** are a set of paired veins that drain blood from the dorsum of the foot (dorsalis pedis veins) and the anterior compartment of the calf. Originating near the tibia at the level of the ankle, the ATVs are located anterior to the interosseous membrane, as they ascend the lower leg with the anterior tibial artery. Ultimately the ATVs join the posterior tibial veins (PTVs) to form the popliteal vein.

The **posterior tibial veins (PTVs)** are a set of paired veins that drain the posterior compartment of the lower leg and originate from the plantar veins (superficial and deep) of the foot. The PTVs ascend along the medial calf beginning at the level of the medial malleolus, parallel to the posterior tibial artery. In the proximal calf, the PTVs combine with the peroneal veins to form the tibial-peroneal trunk, just before uniting with ATVs to form the popliteal vein.

The **peroneal veins** (also known as the fibular veins) are another set of paired veins that drain blood from the lateral compartment of the lower leg. The peroneal veins parallel the path of the PTVs, located deep to the soleus and gastrocnemius muscles along the fibula. Also traveling with the peroneal veins is the peroneal artery (also known as the fibular artery). In the proximal calf, the peroneal veins join the PTVs to form the tibial-peroneal trunk.

The final deep veins of the lower leg are the **soleal sinuses** and the **gastrocnemius (sural) veins**. These veins are located deep within the muscular compartments of the soleus and gastrocnemius muscles, respectively. The soleal sinuses are large reservoirs of venous blood that drain to the PTVs or peroneal veins. The gastrocnemius veins are a set of paired veins that, accompanied by the gastrocnemius artery, ascends the leg in the medial and lateral gastrocnemius muscles before draining directly into the popliteal vein.

The **popliteal vein** drains the blood of the lower leg and originates from the confluence of the ATVs with the peroneal and PTVs (tibial-peroneal trunk). The popliteal vein is located in the popliteal fossa (area behind the knee), in close proximity to the popliteal artery. In the lower popliteal fossa, the popliteal vein is medial and superficial to the artery. As they ascend the popliteal space, the popliteal vein remains superficial but moves lateral to the artery. The popliteal vein and artery continue to ascend until they pass through the adductor canal (Hunter canal) at the approximate level of the knee joint. Here they become the femoral vein (FV) and artery. A duplicated popliteal vein has been reported in up to 40% of the population.[6]

The **femoral vein (FV)** originates from the popliteal vein in the distal thigh at the hiatus of the adductor magnus muscle, at the level of the adductor (Hunter) canal. The FV is accompanied by the femoral artery, to which it courses deep throughout the medial thigh. The FV terminates in Scarpa's (femoral) triangle at its confluence with the deep profunda femoris (deep femoral) vein. A duplicated FV is present in up to an estimated 41% of the population.[7] Recognition and thorough evaluation of a duplicated FV system is imperative because 20% of all lower extremity DVTs are isolated to the FV.[8] Furthermore, one study reported duplicated or triplicated popliteal and FVs were not documented on repeat evaluation.[9] It is important to note that the FV is often referred to as the *superficial FV*. This nomenclature began as a method of differentiating the FV from the profunda femoris (also referred to as the deep FV). However, adding *superficial* to the name brought about confusion among clinicians. This resulted in DVTs located in the FV being left untreated because they were mistakenly thought to be within the superficial system. In 2004 an international interdisciplinary committee of physicians met to discuss issues regarding terminology of the lower limb veins. The committee concluded that the word *superficial* be omitted and only the term *femoral vein* be used.[10] Furthermore, accreditation organizations, including the Intersocietal Accreditation Commission (IAC) strongly recommend omitting *superficial* when referring to the FV.[11] Similarly, the same revised nomenclature is applied to the femoral artery.

The **profunda femoris vein**, also known as the deep FV, drains the deep muscles of the proximal thigh. Similar to other deep veins of the leg, the profunda femoris travels in proximity to the profunda femoris artery. The profunda femoris vein ascends the upper leg until it joins the FV to form the common FV. The confluence of these two veins is distal to the bifurcation of the common femoral artery.

The **common femoral vein (CFV)** is formed by the confluence of the FV and profunda femoris vein. The CFV also receives the great saphenous vein (GSV) at the level of the saphenofemoral junction. The CFV lies in the Scarpa triangle, medial to the common femoral artery. The CFV terminates at the level of the inguinal ligament, where it becomes the external iliac vein.

The **external iliac vein** originates at the level of the inguinal ligament as a continuation of the CFV. The external iliac ascends parallel to the external iliac artery before it joins the internal iliac vein to become the common iliac vein. The **internal iliac vein** travels with the internal iliac artery and serves to drain the pelvis before it joins the external iliac vein.

The **common iliac vein** is formed by the confluence of internal and external iliac veins. Further proximal, the union of the right and left common iliac veins forms the inferior vena cava (IVC). The left common iliac vein is oriented obliquely and lies medial to the left common iliac artery. While they ascend, the left common iliac vein must cross beneath the right iliac artery to join the right common iliac vein at their confluence to form the IVC. This anatomic feature of the left common iliac vein crossing beneath the right iliac artery causes mild compression of the vein and has been cited as the reason for slightly greater prevalence of left-side DVT. Continued compression can result in the venous entrapment disorder known as May-Thurner syndrome, which is characterized by the compression of the left common iliac vein by the right common iliac artery. If vein narrowing is identified, left common iliac vein stenting may be necessary to ensure its patency and prevent DVT formation. The right common iliac vein is shorter than the left and is oriented vertically as it ascends posterior and then lateral to its companion artery.

Superficial Veins. The superficial veins of the lower extremities are superficial to the deep veins, located between two layers of superficial fascia in the subcutaneous tissue. The function of superficial veins is to drain blood from the tissues and transport it to the deep system. These veins transport far less blood volume than deep veins and are therefore typically smaller in size. Unlike deep veins, the veins of the superficial venous system are not paired with an artery. Superficial veins also do not travel through muscle tissue; therefore muscle contraction plays a minimal role in the movement or pumping of blood against hydrostatic pressure under which it is placed. To counteract this, venous valves that aid in maintaining antegrade venous flow are more prevalent in the veins of the superficial system than the deep because they play a much more significant role. This is also why venous insufficiency, which is caused by malfunctioning venous valves, is much more common in the superficial system.

The **great saphenous vein (GSV)**, also known as the long saphenous vein, originates on the dorsum of the foot and travels anterior to the medial malleolus and ascends the anteromedial side of the calf and thigh. In the proximal thigh the GSV terminates as it joins the CFV at what is known as the saphenofemoral junction (Fig. 40.2). The GSV is the longest vein in the body and has between 10 and 20 valves. Because of its length, this vein is often harvested for use as an arterial graft. The **small saphenous vein (SSV)**, also known as the lesser saphenous vein, originates on the dorsum of the foot, travels posterior to the lateral malleolus, and ascends along the midline of the posterior calf. The SSV terminates as it joins the popliteal vein in the popliteal fossa (Fig. 40.3). The level of entry of the SSV into the popliteal vein is variable; it has even been visualized to enter the FV in the midthigh. The SSV has approximately 6 to 12 valves.

The **posterior arch vein** (vein of Leonardo) arises posterior to the medial malleolus and courses parallel and posterior to the GSV before it terminates into the GSV just below the knee. It also communicates with the PTV, mainly through the Cockett perforator located in the gaiter area (region above the medial malleolus) of the leg. The posterior arch vein drains blood from the medial ankle.

Perforating Veins. Perforating veins connect the superficial to the deep venous system. Perforating veins originate in the superficial fascia and penetrate the deep fascia. Like other veins, they contain one-way valves that permit unidirectional flow from superficial to deep. Many perforators exist throughout the lower extremity, with a greater number in the calf than thigh. Common perforators are Cockett, Boyd, Dodd, and Hunterian. Cockett perforators largely communicate with the

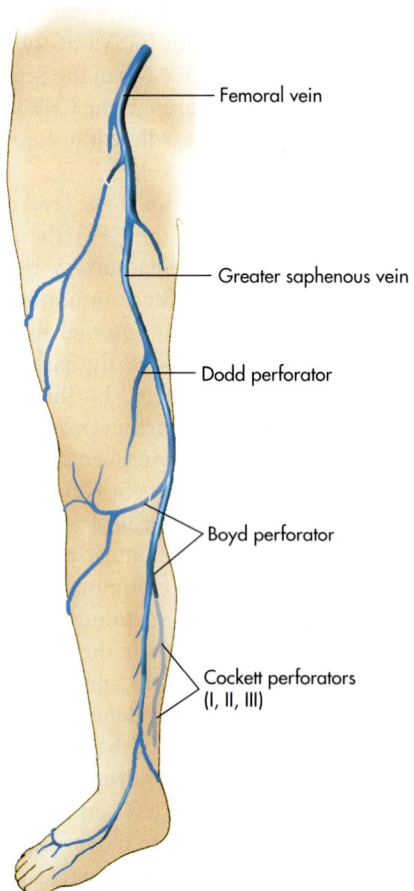

FIG. 40.2 Great saphenous vein and perforators. The great saphenous vein is a superficial vein that travels along the anteromedial portion of the thigh and calf. Many perforators join the great saphenous vein.

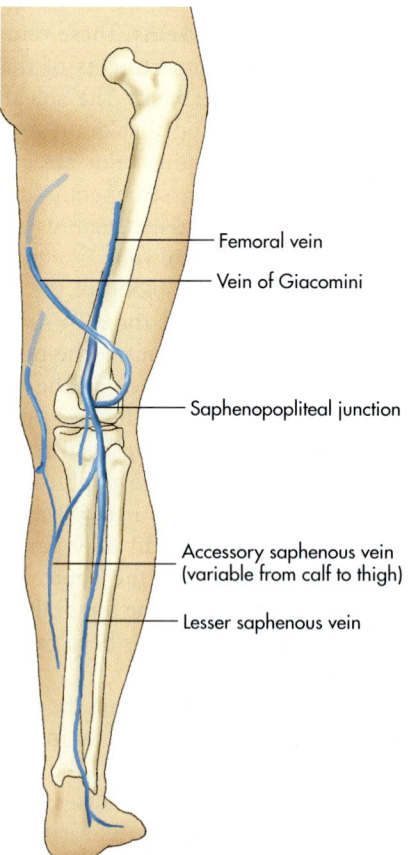

FIG. 40.3 The small saphenous vein, also referred to as the lesser saphenous vein, is a superficial vein that travels along the midline portion of the posterior calf. The small saphenous vein typically drains into the popliteal vein in the popliteal fossa.

posterior arch vein and are found in the lower leg. Boyd perforators are located around the level of the knee, Dodd in the distal thigh, and Hunterian in the proximal thigh.

Upper Extremity

Deep Veins. Like the deep veins of the lower extremity, the deep veins of the upper extremity are located within the musculature of the arms, travel in close association with a corresponding artery, and serve to transport deoxygenated blood from the superficial to central venous system (Fig. 40.4).

Beginning distally, the deep and superficial palmar venous arches in the hands form the paired sets of the radial and ulnar veins. This occurs on the lateral and medial sides of the arm, respectively. These veins are the primary source of venous drainage for the hand. The paired **radial veins** accompany the radial artery, and the paired **ulnar veins** accompany the ulnar artery as they ascend the forearm. Near the level of the antecubital fossa, the radial and ulnar veins join to form the brachial veins.

The **brachial veins** are a paired set of veins that originate from the confluence of the radial and ulnar veins near the antecubital fossa. From this location, the brachial veins ascend the upper arm on each side of the brachial artery. Just proximal to the axilla, at the inferior border of teres major, the brachial veins join the basilic vein and form the axillary vein.

The **axillary vein** is a single vein accompanied by the axillary artery, which originates from the confluence of the basilic and brachial veins in the upper arm. It drains blood from the upper arm supplied by the brachial, basilic, and cephalic veins, as well as the lateral portion of the thorax and the axilla. The axillary vein terminates beneath the clavicle at the outer border of the first rib, where it becomes the subclavian vein.

The **subclavian vein** is a continuation of the axillary vein. Accompanied by the subclavian artery, it extends from the outer border of the first rib to the inner end of the clavicle. Here it joins the internal jugular vein (IJV) to form the innominate (brachiocephalic) vein. The subclavian vein is also joined by the external jugular vein (EJV), just distal to its anastomosis with the IJV. The subclavian vein is located deep to the clavicle and is inferior and anterior to the subclavian artery.

The **innominate vein** (brachiocephalic vein) is formed by the confluence of the subclavian and IJVs. This is the most proximal vein of the upper extremity peripheral venous system, as the right and left innominate veins join just below the first rib to form the superior vena cava of the central venous system. Although present on both sides, the right and left innominate vary greatly. The superior vena cava terminates in the right atrium of the heart, located to the right of midline. Therefore the right innominate vein is considerably shorter than the left because it is in closer proximity to the right atrium. Furthermore, the right innominate vein courses almost vertically downward and is located superficial and to the right of the innominate artery. The right innominate vein receives the right vertebral, internal mammary, and inferior thyroid veins. As mentioned, the left innominate vein is longer than the right because it must travel across midline from the left to the right side of the chest, where it joins the right innominate vein to form the superior vena cava. The left innominate vein courses beneath the sternum at a slight downward angle and receives the left vertebral, internal mammary, inferior thyroid, and left superior intercostal veins.

The **external jugular vein (EJV)** drains many outer structures of the head and face. Originating in the parotid gland, the EJV courses down the neck posterior to the mandible before it crosses the sternomastoid muscle and terminates into the subclavian vein, just distal to its confluence with the IJV.

The **internal jugular vein (IJV)** drains the majority of the cerebral vessels and portions of the face. The IJV originates at the base of the skull in the jugular foramen and courses down the neck just lateral to the internal and then common carotid artery. At its termination, it joins with the innominate vein to form the superior vena cava.

Superficial Veins. In the upper extremity, the superficial venous system drains venous blood into the deep system for its return to the heart (Fig. 40.5). The superficial veins are located between two layers of superficial fascia but outside of the deep investing fascia.

The **cephalic vein** begins on the lateral side of the dorsum of the hand and travels along the outer border of the biceps muscle and deltopectoral groove. The cephalic vein penetrates the deep fascia at variable levels to join the axillary vein just deep to the clavicle. The **basilic vein** originates on the medial side of the dorsum of the hand. The basilic vein is large and courses medially along the inner side of the biceps

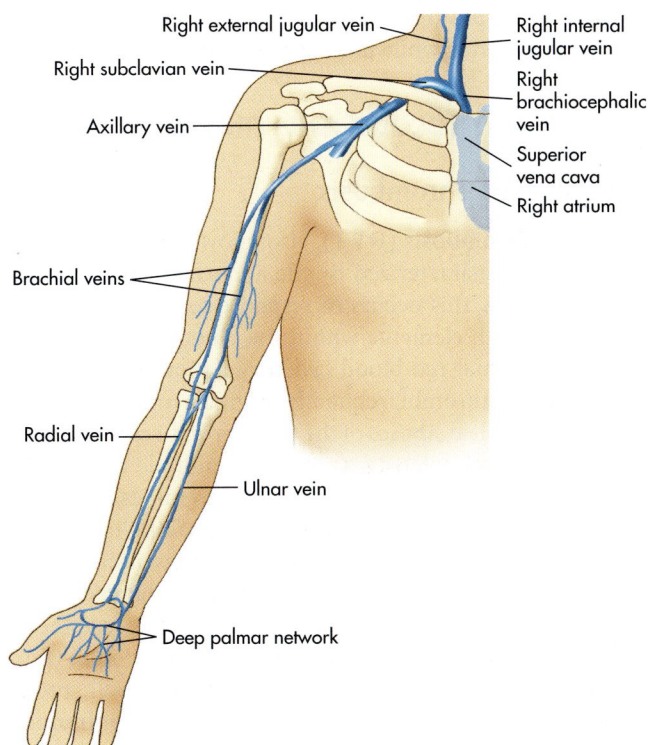

FIG. 40.4 Upper extremity deep veins.

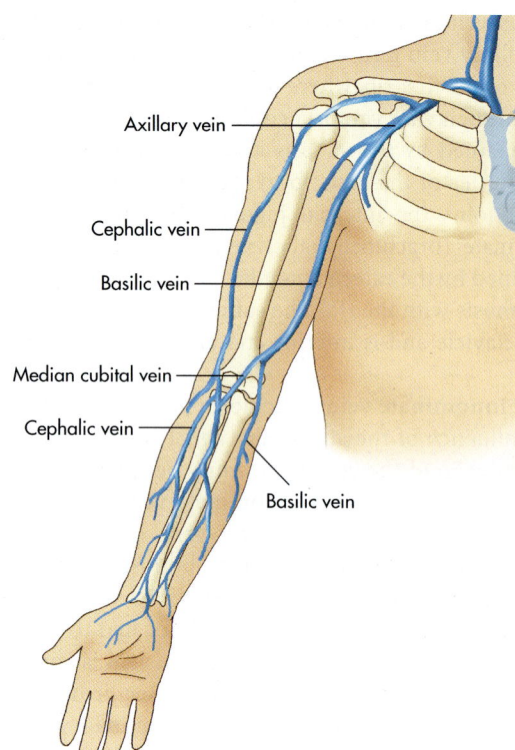

FIG. 40.5 Upper extremity superficial veins.

muscle until it pierces the deep fascia and joins the brachial veins in the upper arm.

VENOUS PHYSIOLOGY

Veins function to return deoxygenated blood to the heart once it has passed through the arterial system and capillaries (microcirculation). The arterial system is characterized as a closed, high-pressure system. Cardiac contractions apply a significant amount of kinetic energy on the arterial system, creating a pressure gradient that forces oxygenated blood through the arteries of the body and then into microcirculation, consisting of arterioles and capillaries. While in microcirculation, blood flow encounters a large amount of hemodynamic resistance due to the reduction in vessel diameter. To overcome this resistance, much of the kinetic energy supplied by the heart is exhausted. The kinetic energy of blood exiting microcirculation present within the venules is greatly reduced, with a pressure of approximately 10 mm Hg.[12] For this reason, the venous system is characterized as a low-pressure system and why normal venous flow is nonpulsatile.

Instead of the heart, the venous system relies on the muscles surrounding the veins to propel blood forward. Contraction of the peripheral muscles mimic the heart as it relates to application of kinetic energy to the venous system. Upon contraction, the muscle will tighten and squeeze the vein within it, propelling venous blood in an antegrade direction. This is made possible by the elasticity of vein walls. In the lower extremity, this is known as the calf muscle pump, which aids in venous blood flow during ambulation. Similarly, the diaphragm contracts and descends, causing intraabdominal pressure to rise during inhalation. This pressure increase compresses a distal portion of the IVC and impedes venous outflow from the legs. With expiration, the diaphragm rises, causing intra-abdominal pressure to decrease and allowing venous flow from the legs to increase toward the IVC. For this reason, normal venous flow changes with respiration. This is called respiratory phasicity.

The other components aiding in antegrade venous flow complementing muscle contraction are the venous valves. Venous valves prevent retrograde. The shape and positioning of these valves along the lumen of the vessel are such that the force of the antegrade flow causes them to open; however, when functioning properly, retrograde flow that occurs between contractions causes the valves to close, preventing significant retrograde flow.

The venous system contains approximately two-thirds of the body's total blood volume at any given time. Veins do not contain a fully developed tunica media (muscular layer of the lumen) as arteries do, resulting in vein walls to be more elastic, making them to appear in a variety of shapes. The cross-sectional shape of a vein is determined by transmural pressure. Transmural pressure is equal to the difference between the pressure inside the vein (intravascular) and the external pressure (interstitial pressure) placed upon the vein from surrounding tissue. Transmural pressure is also referred to as wall tension. Therefore a vein experiencing low transmural pressure will partially collapse and take on an elliptical appearance in a transverse plane, whereas a vein experiencing high transmural pressure will appear more rounded when imaged transversely. In the lower extremities, high transmural pressure is expected when standing or in a reverse Trendelenburg position, whereas a low transmural pressure is normally exhibited while in a supine position.

VENOUS PATHOLOGY AND TREATMENTS

Deep Venous Thrombosis

Deep vein thrombosis (DVT), also known as a thrombus or blood clot, is characterized by the abnormal coagulation of red blood cells. This occurs in response to a wide variety of stimuli in which elements within the blood become altered, causing abnormal red blood cell coagulation, resulting in a thrombus. Leg thrombi frequently originate on venous valves or within the soleal sinuses of the calf. Thrombi can be isolated to a single vein or extensive (present in multiple veins). DVT can occur in the upper and/or lower extremities, but upper extremity DVTs are much less common, making up between 4% and 10% of DVT findings.[13] DVTs can present in an acute or chronic stage and must be appropriately characterized as such because management may greatly differ between them.

Venous thromboembolism (VTE) is a condition in which a venous thrombus dislodges from the vein wall, propagates to the arteries of the lungs, and causes a **pulmonary embolism (PE)**. VTE is the third most common cardiovascular disorder in the United States, resulting in more than

1,220,000 cases annually.[4,13] VTE also maintains a high mortality rate of approximately 19% annually.[14,15]

Because of its high prevalence and life-threatening potential, venous duplex examinations are often used as a diagnostic tool for the detection of DVT. In suspected cases of thrombosis, venous duplex imaging has emerged as the imaging modality of choice, due to its superiority in accuracy over other noninvasive techniques (nonimaging Doppler, impedance plethysmography), and unlike venography has no associated risks. Symptoms commonly associated with DVT and PE are listed in Box 40.1.

Risk Factors. In 1856 Rudolph Virchow presented classic concepts on the causes of thrombus formation within the venous system, which are still largely accepted today.[16] The three factors associated with thrombus formation (Virchow triad) are (1) a hypercoagulable state, (2) venous stasis (blood pools in the veins), and (3) vein wall injury (endothelium of the vein is damaged, exposing the subendothelium to blood, which triggers platelet adhesion and aggregation, promoting blood coagulation). The interplay of these three factors creates the most likely setting for the development of DVT. A more extensive list of common DVT risk factors can be found in Box 40.2.

Acute Deep Venous Thrombosis. Acute DVT is typically defined as a thrombus that is no more than 1 week old. Acute thrombi are characterized by a soft or spongy appearance and may or may not envelop the entire cross section of the vein. Acute DVTs may be symptomatic or asymptomatic. Severe symptoms of lower extremity DVT include phlegmasia alba dolens (swollen, painful white leg) and phlegmasia cerulea dolens (swollen, painful cyanotic leg). Both of these affect arterial inflow and are limb threatening. More common symptoms include pain, warmth, erythema (redness), and edema. Acute DVTs are low in density, which causes their sonographic appearance to be low in echogenicity, or anechoic. Distention of the vein or visualization of the thrombus itself may also be seen.

Because of their soft nature, acute thrombi are more likely to dislodge from the vein wall and propagate, causing the risk of PE to be heightened in acute DVT cases. The risk of PE is further increased with the proximal location of the DVT. Therefore management of acute DVT is typically much more aggressive than that of chronic DVT, with the goal of dissolving or removing the thrombus. Management can be done in a variety of ways.

Conservative treatments consist of elevation, compression stockings, and/or bed rest. However, medical management is most commonly used to treat acute DVT by anticoagulation or antiplatelet agent administration, and/or thrombolytic therapy. Anticoagulation agents can be administered orally, intravenously, or subcutaneously and aim to prevent further clot development by affecting coagulation factors. Common anticoagulants include heparin, warfarin, and Lovenox. Antiplatelet agents prevent further clot formation by decreasing platelet aggregation. Common antiplatelet medications include aspirin, thienopyridines, and ticlopidine. Thrombolytic therapy is used to dissolve or break down an existing thrombus, known as thrombolysis. Common thrombolytic agents include tissue plasminogen activators (tPAs), urokinase, and streptokinase. In more severe cases, a variety of surgical interventions collectively referred to as a venous thrombectomy can be performed to remove the thrombus. Surgical placement of an IVC filter can also be done, which prevents propagating thrombi from reaching the lungs.

Chronic Deep Venous Thrombosis. DVTs older than 1 week are characterized as chronic. Unlike acute DVT, chronic thrombi are more dense and often calcific. As a result, chronic DVTs are more conducive for visualization via sonographic imaging and are typically echogenic, and also cause diffuse wall thickening. Chronic DVTs typically adhere firmly to the vessel wall and therefore do not present a large risk of

---

BOX 40.1 Symptoms and Signs Associated With Deep Vein Thrombosis and Pulmonary Embolism

Deep Vein Thrombosis
- Persistent calf, leg, or arm swelling
- Pain or tenderness of the leg (usually the posterior calf) or arm-shoulder region
- Venous distention
- Increased temperature and redness
- Superficial venous dilation
- Homan sign (calf discomfort on passive dorsiflexion)

Superficial Venous Thrombosis
- Local erythema
- Tenderness or pain
- Palpable subcutaneous "cord"

Pulmonary Embolus
- Dyspnea (shortness of breath)
- Chest pain
- Hemoptysis (spitting up blood)
- Sweating
- Cough

BOX 40.2 Risk Factors for Deep Vein Thrombosis

- Age (>40 years old)
- Malignancy (cancer)
- Previous deep venous thrombosis or pulmonary embolism
- Immobilization (bed rest, paralysis of legs, extended travel)
- Fracture of the pelvis, hip, or long bones
- Myocardial infarction, stroke
- Congestive heart failure or respiratory failure
- Pregnancy and postpartum
- Oral contraceptives and hormone replacement therapy
- Extensive dissection at major surgery (especially orthopedic surgery)
- Trauma (multiple)
- Hereditary factors (antithrombin deficiency, protein C and protein S deficiencies)
- Obesity
- Central venous lines, pacemakers
- Intravenous drug abuse

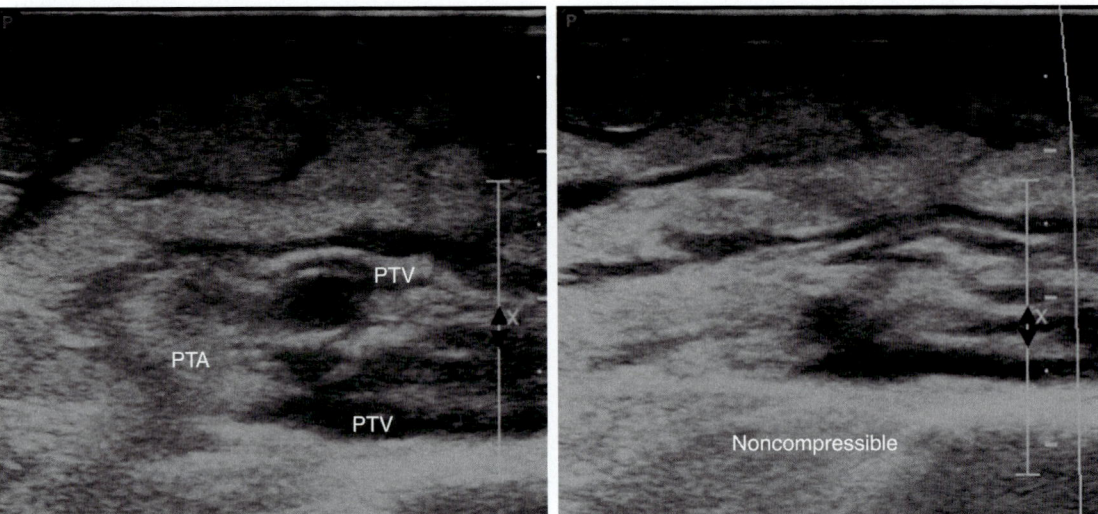

FIG. 40.6 Gray-scale image showing edema present in the tissues surrounding and superficial to a chronically thrombosed pair of posterior tibial veins (PTVs). The posterior tibial artery (PTA) is seen located between the two PTVs.

propagation and PE. Chronic DVTs are often obstructive and can cause the formation of collateral vessels and varicose veins. Individuals with chronic DVT typically present with symptoms that involve the entire extremity, such as edema (Fig. 40.6), hyperpigmentation (brown discoloration), limb heaviness, varicose veins, and, in more severe cases, venous ulcerations.

Severe chronic DVTs can lead to a process known as PTS, which is caused by increased ambulatory venous pressure, also known as venous hypertension. Venous hypertension occurs when venous blood is unable to overcome hydrostatic pressure, resulting in blood stasis within the lower leg. Treatment options for chronic DVT are similar to those used in acute DVT; however, chronic DVT management tends to be more conservative because PE occurrence is low. Therefore the typical focus of treatments is to diminish patient symptoms through limb elevation, compression stockings, and in some cases bed rest.

If left untreated, increasing venous hypertension will lead to ulceration. Venous hypertension can be a result of the venous obstruction (chronic DVT) and/or incompetent venous valves. Over time, the presence of a thrombus on or around venous valves can damage the valves' structure, causing them to become incompetent. This leads to deep venous insufficiency and subsequent venous hypertension. In addition, varicose veins may develop. **Varicose veins** are dilated, elongated, tortuous superficial veins. Primary varicose veins are congenital, stemming from an inherent weakness of venous walls, and occur without coexisting deep venous disease. Secondary varicose veins occur secondary to pathology (chronic DVT) of the deep venous system.

Superficial Venous Thrombosis. A clot formation that exists in the superficial venous system is known as a superficial venous thrombosis (SVT). These are typically found in the GSV and SSV but can present in any superficial vein and also varicose veins. Just as in the deep system, a common location for SVT is on or around venous valves. For this reason, the presence of chronic SVT can cause valvular incompetence, leading to insufficiency of the superficial venous system. Unlike chronic DVTs, symptoms of SVTs are typically localized to the area in which they are located. Common SVT symptoms include localized erythema and tenderness. In some cases they can be palpated as a hard subcutaneous "cord." Treatment for SVT typically includes limb elevation, compression stockings, and application of heat to the afflicted area.

Venous Insufficiency

Venous insufficiency, also known as venous reflux, is caused by incompetent venous valves, often secondary to chronic thrombus. Competent valves aid venous blood in overcoming hydrostatic pressure, allowing it to flow in an antegrade direction. In their absence, venous blood is not able to efficiently overcome the force of opposing hydrostatic pressure, resulting in retrograde flow within the vein and venous stasis with associated venous hypertension. Venous insufficiency can occur in the deep or superficial system and in perforating vessels. This can be caused by previous DVT that has damaged the venous valves and rendered them incompetent. Venous reflux can also develop in veins that have experienced high levels of hydrostatic pressure for prolonged periods. This typically occurs from pregnancy or standing for extended time. Genetic predisposition also increases the likelihood of venous reflux development. Venous reflux is common; one review states that lower extremity venous insufficiency and subsequent varicose veins is the seventh most common indication for referral in the United States, with the overall prevalence estimated to be as high as 25%, occurring more frequently in women than men.[17-21] Symptoms of venous insufficiency include chronic leg swelling, induration (hard, firm, almost leather-like appearance of the skin around the ankles), varicose veins, and venous stasis ulcerations in severe cases. Superficial venous insufficiency noninvasive treatment options include limb elevation and compression stockings. Invasive treatments consist of surgical intervention, including ultrasound-guided endovenous ablation, varicose vein phlebectomies, and sclerotherapy. All interventions aim to reduce venous pressure in the afflicted limb.

TECHNICAL ASPECTS OF VENOUS DUPLEX IMAGING

While performing venous duplex examinations, patient care should always be the first priority. Appropriate measures must be taken to ensure the safety of patients while they are being transported to the examination room and while being transferred to the ultrasound bed. It is critical in cases of suspected acute DVT, extra care be taken while moving the patient, being cognizant of the potential for thrombus dislodgement. In circumstances in which patient mobility is limited, the venous duplex may need to be completed with the patient remaining in the location in which they are restricted (hospital bed, wheelchair, etc.). Care should also be taken while positioning patients to ensure their comfort while still maintaining a position that is conducive to optimal imaging. Consideration should also be paid to proper scanning ergonomics.

Before any ultrasound examination, the sonographer must also complete a review of the patient's chart. Any pertinent information should be noted, with special attention being paid to any previous imaging studies. This can be done efficiently by way of electronic health records (EHRs).

In addition to reviewing the patient's EHR, the sonographer should take a thorough patient history, focusing on risk factors, signs, and symptoms (if present) of venous disease. If the patient is symptomatic, this helps in locating the area for careful evaluation during the venous duplex examination. It is critical that the sonographer is able to differentiate venous versus arterial symptomatology, as well as those associated with acute versus chronic disease. In addition, in the upper extremity, documentation of previous venous catheter placement is critical. Finally, the venous duplex imaging examination is explained to the patient.

Appropriate positioning of the patient is critical because it allows for optimal images to be obtained. While imaging lower extremity veins, patients are evaluated in the supine reverse Trendelenburg (head elevated) position to leverage increased transmural pressure. This position promotes venous distention and optimizes visualization of the veins, while the patient remains in an ergonomically friendly position for the sonographer. The leg being imaged is externally rotated, with the knee slightly flexed. While imaging the veins of the upper extremity, the patient is evaluated in the supine position, unless contraindicated. The arm is positioned at the side of the patient with his or her head turned away from the side being examined. Once the patient is in the proper position, imaging can begin. Venous duplex examinations consist of two main components: (1) gray-scale (GS) imaging with compression maneuvers, and (2) CD and SD evaluation.

A higher-frequency (5- to 7.5-MHz) linear array transducer is used to perform upper and lower extremity venous duplex examinations. In cases of increased body habitus or the presence of large amounts of edema where more penetration is needed, a lower-frequency (3- to 5-MHz) curvilinear or sector transducer can be used. Insonating frequencies above what is indicated here may be used, keeping in mind the trade-off between image resolution and soundwave attenuation.

Gray-Scale Imaging and Compression Maneuvers

While conducting the GS imaging and compression maneuver portion of the venous duplex imaging examination, the transverse view is used to locate the veins and is mandatory for an accurate examination and interpretation. The transverse view allows visualization of multiple venous segments and of the entire lumen (lumina) of the vein(s) during compression maneuvers.

Veins can be distinguished from arteries by the characteristics listed in Box 40.3. In the absence of pathology, veins will change in size with respiration and collapse when light to moderate pressure is applied to the skin using the transducer. If a vein's associated artery is deformed by the compression maneuver, the sonographer knows that adequate pressure has been applied to compress the vein. During each compression maneuver, the vein is observed to confirm that the anterior and posterior portions of the vein walls coapt, or touch. This demonstrates the absence of intraluminal materials, such as thrombi. The lumen of the vein should reopen with the release of transducer pressure. The amount of transducer pressure necessary to compress the vein varies with its location and the patient's body habitus. Presence of pathology, such as edema, may also cause a variation in the amount of pressure needed to produce vein compressibility. Intuitively, veins located close to the surface of the skin require less pressure to compress compared with veins that exist deeper. Peripheral veins are followed distally along the length of the upper and/or lower extremity in a transverse plane, with transducer pressure being applied to the limb approximately every width of the transducer's footprint to confirm closure. It is important that the transducer is not lifted from the surface of the

---

BOX 40.3 Imaging Characteristics of Normal Veins and Arteries in the Lower Extremity

Veins
- Vessel walls collapse with light or moderate pressure by the transducer on the skin.
- Phasic low-velocity Doppler signals augment with distal limb compression.
- Common femoral vein changes in size with respiration.

Arteries
- Vessel does not collapse with light pressure by the transducer on the skin.
- Triphasic high-velocity Doppler signal is seen.
- Pulsation of vessel walls is present.

skin, because this ensures the entire length of each vessel is evaluated. Following this technique along the pathway of the peripheral venous system will provide the best results when performing venous duplex imaging examinations.

In the lower extremity, imaging begins by locating the CFV at the level of the inguinal crease. The CFV typically has a large diameter at this location and is easy to locate compared with the smaller veins located distally in the leg. Here, the compressibility of the CFV is evaluated. The transducer is then moved slightly distal to visualize the proximal GSV at the level of the saphenofemoral junction. Here the CFV and GSV compressibility is evaluated using compression maneuvers (Fig. 40.7). If superficial thrombophlebitis is suspected, the GSV should be evaluated for SVT using compression maneuvers along its entire length. The GSV is superficial in the leg and may be compressed by the weight of the transducer on the skin. If the GSV is not visualized, reduce transducer pressure to ensure the vein is not being inadvertently compressed. This can be avoided by adding more gel to the leg, which will maintain optimal imaging while requiring less transducer pressure on the skin.

A large venous valve, which can often be seen during GS imaging, is located in the proximal portion of the GSV just distal to its confluence with the CFV. Therefore it is important to investigate the compressibility of the proximal GSV during venous duplex imaging, because this site is at an elevated risk of thrombus formation. Thrombus formation at this level can easily extend or propagate into the deep system.

Moving the transducer distally from the saphenofemoral junction along the path of the CFV, the origin of the FV and the profunda femoris vein are visualized. The origins of these veins are evaluated with compression maneuvers. Compressibility of the profunda femoris vein origin can typically be achieved in the absence of pathology, but it varies among patients. In circumstances where profunda femoris vein depth prevents accurate compression maneuvers, it can be evaluated using CD to document patency. As the profunda femoris vein is followed distally, it will course deep and is not able to be visualized past the proximal/midportion of the thigh.

The FV is followed and evaluated using compression maneuvers from its origin through the entire length of the thigh. The FV can be difficult to coapt in the distal thigh because of its depth as it prepares to enter the adductor canal. The distal FV may be imaged with compression maneuvers from the medial portion of the distal thigh, by compressing the vein inward toward the femur. If FV compression is not achievable by transducer pressure alone, the nonscanning hand can be used to apply compression to the posterior thigh while simultaneously applying transducer pressure on the medial thigh.

Next, the popliteal vein is evaluated using a posterior approach, with the patient's knee rotated externally. If this technique does not provide optimal imaging, the patient can also be placed in a decubitus position or in a position with the foot elevated to eliminate extrinsic compression of the vein. The popliteal vein should be evaluated proximally to the distal portion of the FV and then distally to the proximal calf veins. This is done in the transverse plane while performing compression maneuvers. Although venous aneurysms are rare vascular anomalies, popliteal venous aneurysms occur more frequently than in other locations and may be visualized during venous duplex imaging. While evaluating the entire length of the popliteal vein, the SSV can be visualized arising from the popliteal vein at the level of the saphenopopliteal junction. Similar to the GSV, the SSV is typically only evaluated with compression maneuvers if SVT is suspected.

The paired calf veins (posterior tibial and peroneal) are evaluated in the same manner as the aforementioned veins (transverse view), along the entire length they are visualized. The posterior tibial and peroneal veins are usually imaged best by placing the transducer in a transverse plane along the medial calf. The PTVs are located in the distal leg near the medial malleolus and are followed proximally in the calf. The peroneal

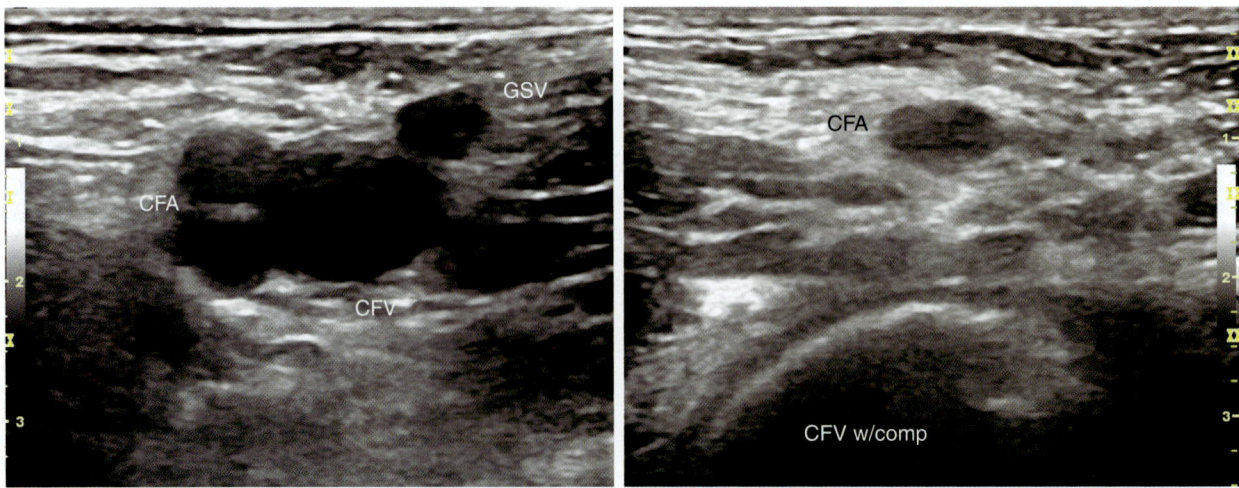

FIG. 40.7 A dual transverse gray-scale image of a common femoral vein (CFV) without compression *(left)* and with compression *(right)* at the level of the saphenofemoral junction. On the right, the CFV and great saphenous vein (GSV) demonstrate normal compressibility with compression. The common femoral artery (CFA) is also seen.

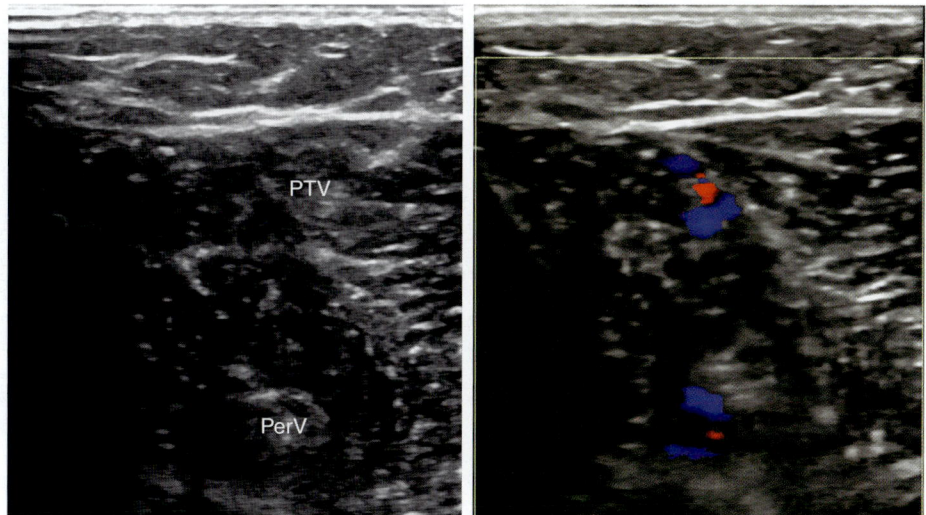

FIG. 40.8 Dual transverse gray-scale *(left)* and color Doppler *(right)* images of the posterior tibial veins (PTV) and peroneal veins (PerV) in the lower calf. The peroneal veins can be seen deep to the PTVs, just anterior to the fibula. The accompanying arteries of the PTVs and peroneal veins can be seen in red, in between the paired veins in blue.

veins are located deep to the PTVs and travel near the fibula (Fig. 40.8). The posterior tibial and peroneal veins run parallel and can typically be visualized in the same plane.

The ATVs are small and can be located by placing the transducer on the lateral aspect of the proximal calf in a transverse plane. The ATVs are located medial to the fibula in the proximal calf and travel just superior to the interosseous membrane, gradually moving in the direction of the tibia in the distal calf. Because of their difficulty to image, coupled with being an uncommon location for thrombus formation, the ATVs are typically evaluated only with compression maneuvers if symptoms are focal in its region.[22]

In addition to the paired calf veins, two sets of muscular calf veins may be visualized: the gastrocnemius and soleus calf veins. The paired gastrocnemius veins can be visualized in the proximal calf as they join the popliteal vein. The gastrocnemius veins are located within the muscles of the posterior calf and are easily compressed when transducer pressure is applied. The soleal sinuses are deeper in the posterior calf and empty into the PTV or peroneal veins.

In the upper extremities, imaging begins with the evaluation of the IJV. Using a lateral approach, the IJV is imaged in a transverse plane along its route in the neck. In the absence of thrombus, the IJV can usually be compressed by applying transducer pressure to the skin. Caution must be taken to not compress the IJV for prolonged amounts of time. To this end, many institutions have adopted alternative methods for compressing the IJV. One way this is done is by tilting the patient's head up, which will typically cause the IJV to compress. Another method, known as the sniff method, is performed by having the patient take a quick breath in through the nose, causing the IJV to temporarily collapse. This has become a popular method of assessing IJV compressibility. If IJV compression cannot be attained through these methods and the lumen is echo free, CD and/or SD evaluation can be helpful alternatives. Evaluate the entire length of the IJV able to be visualized carefully for intraluminal echoes. Often after indwelling lines or catheters are removed, partial thrombus may be noted in the IJV. If an indwelling line or catheter is in place, special attention should be paid while imaging this area, because the use of compressive techniques will be limited. In the presence of central lines, thrombus formation is most often visualized near the line or by its tip.

The subclavian and innominate veins are evaluated next from either a supraclavicular or an infraclavicular approach. Both should be investigated during the upper extremity examination to determine which approach provides the best image quality based on the patient's anatomic variation. In this area, mirror imaging artifacts and/or shadowing artifacts may occur because of the anterior location of the clavicle. A lower-frequency transducer with a small footprint may also aid visualization of these veins and reduce unwanted artifacts. Similar to the IJV, the sniff method is often used to evaluate compressibility of subclavian and innominate veins because the effectiveness of compression maneuvers may be limited due to vessel depth and overlying anatomy. The SVC may also be visualized while imaging this area from a supraclavicular approach. However, a suprasternal approach may be needed depending on patient anatomy.

Next, an infraclavicular approach is typically used to image the distal portion of the subclavian vein and the proximal portion of the axillary vein. These veins are imaged in a transverse plane and can be evaluated via compression maneuvers. Moving distally into the axilla, evaluation of the remaining portion of the axillary vein can be completed. Repositioning the patient's arm may allow easier access to the axilla region.

The cephalic and basilic veins can be seen joining the axillary vein on the lateral and medial side of the arm, respectively. Similar to the superficial veins of the lower extremity, they are often inadvertently compressed from transducer pressure. These veins are not typically evaluated unless specifically indicated by patient symptoms. The cephalic and basilic veins are commonly examined during vein mapping studies, which will be explained in greater detail later in this chapter.

After evaluation of the axillary vein, compression maneuvers continue in the paired brachial veins. This begins in the proximal portion of the upper arm and extends their entire length to the approximate level of the antecubital fossa.

Near the antecubital fossa, the radial and ulnar veins can be visualized as they travel the length of the lateral and medial forearm, respectively. Although they are often small in diameter, they can usually be evaluated without much difficulty. The forearm veins should compress from transducer pressure. The radial and ulnar veins can often be followed to the wrist level.

Doppler

Evaluation of the veins in the upper and lower extremities by Doppler is done after the completion of the GS imaging/compression maneuver portion of the examination. CD and SD dual images of the veins being evaluated should be obtained in a longitudinal plane. The CD scale should be reduced to ensure that thrombus visualization is not compromised. The SD scale should also be reduced to allow for optimal interrogation of low-velocity venous SD signals. Angle correction of the SD signal is not necessary during venous duplex imaging, as discrete velocity values do not provide any clinical information and are therefore not acquired. Instead, the pattern or morphology of the venous SD waveform provides clinically relevant information regarding the state of the vein being examined.

In the lower extremities, dual CD and SD waveform images should be obtained from the CFV, profunda femoris vein, FV, and popliteal vein. The number and location(s) of images obtained in each vein vary among institutions. CD and SD images should also be obtained in any other vein(s) that are clinically indicated. Dual CD and venous SD waveform images should be obtained both with and without augmentation. Augmentation is competed by squeezing or applying a burst of pressure to the patient's limb, distal to the location where the SD waveform is being obtained. Distal augmentation should always be performed using the nonscanning hand to ensure a consistent image is acquired throughout the augmentation maneuver. Performing augmentation forces venous blood proximally, which is visually represented as an increase in flow volume on CD and as a spike on the SD waveform (Fig. 40.9). Last, when conducting a unilateral venous duplex imaging examination, the compressibility and CD/SD signals of the contralateral CFV, at the level of the saphenofemoral junction, should also be documented.

During the Doppler evaluation of the upper extremities, CD/SD images should be acquired in the SVC, IJV, innominate, subclavian, and axillary veins, with and without augmentation. The number and location(s) of images obtained in each vein vary among institutions. Brachial, radial, ulnar, cephalic, and basilic veins are typically evaluated only with Doppler when indicated by patient symptoms. Finally, when evaluating the veins of the upper extremity, it may be helpful to compare Doppler signals from the contralateral side. If the upper extremity venous duplex examination is unilateral, compressibility and Doppler signals of the contralateral IJV and/or subclavian veins should be documented.

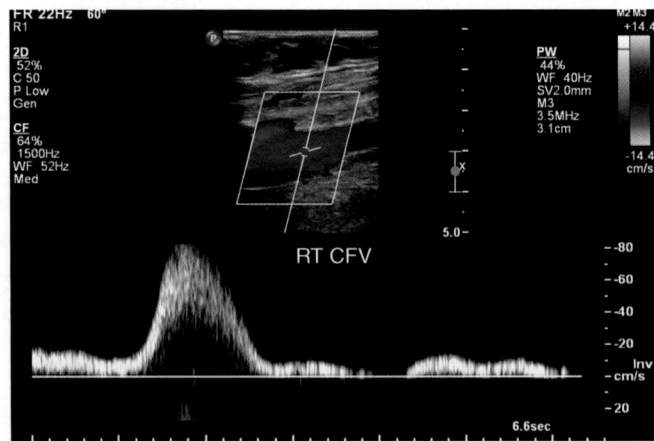

FIG. 40.9 Longitudinal color and spectral Doppler image of the common femoral vein (CFV) demonstrating a normal response to a distal augmentation.

While examining the upper or lower extremity, extra images are necessary in the presence of pathology. In the presence of a thrombus, GS images should be obtained to allow for examination of its echogenicity, which aids in the determination of thrombus age. Longitudinal GS and CD images may also be necessary in order to determine whether the thrombus is partially or totally occluding the vein. In addition, in the presence of SVT, a longitudinal GS image may be required to determine the proximity of the thrombus to the deep system. General tips for performing venous duplex imaging are listed in Table 40.1. The best quality and most reliable examination will be obtained by careful attention to venous anatomy and imaging technique.

INTERPRETATION OF VENOUS DUPLEX IMAGING

It is imperative that each institution develops a venous imaging protocol that defines the standard examination. This protocol must include the technique, clinical applications, indications for a complete and/or limited examination, and interpretation criteria. The interpretation criteria for venous duplex imaging for determining the presence of DVT or SVT are based on three components (Table 40.2): (1) the vein is free of echogenic material; (2) the vein fully coapts while applying transducer pressure on the skin (Fig. 40.10); and (3) the vein is patent, demonstrating a normal venous SD signal (Fig. 40.11).

The following are the characteristics of a normal venous SD signal from a lower extremity:
- *Spontaneous:* **Spontaneous flow** is continuous and present without augmentation maneuvers (usually not found in calf veins).
- *Phasicity:* **Respiratory phasicity** means that blood flow velocity changes with respiration (usually not found in calf veins).

CHAPTER 40 Peripheral Venous Evaluation

TABLE 40.1 Venous Duplex Imaging Tips

Challenge	Action
Nonvisualization of veins	Veins can collapse easily from transducer pressure, particularly superficial veins. If a vein is not be visualized, reduce pressure applied by the transducer. Reducing transducer pressure on the skin decreases extraluminal pressure and allows visualization of the vein from the correct anatomic position.
Veins do not compress	If a vein segment appears patent but does not compress, transducer pressure may be applied from a different site on the skin or by repositioning the patient. Often an adjacent bone or tendon prevents compression of the vein. Having the patient exhale while compressing may also be beneficial.
Pressure assessment	Adequate pressure to compress a vein has been applied if the adjacent artery is slightly deformed by the compression maneuver.
Imaging plane	Transverse imaging is initially performed to evaluate all vein segments for venous pathology in gray-scale (GS) mode. Longitudinal color Doppler (CD)/spectral Doppler (SD) imaging is then performed as multiple veins or vein segments are commonly missed if imaging only in a longitudinal plane.
Imaging limitations	Obesity, extensive edema, leg wounds, calcified arteries, anatomic structures (clavicle), and casts may limit the venous duplex imaging study or affect the quality of the examination. Use transducers of different frequency, and use different imaging planes, to improve visualization of the veins. Color and spectral Doppler may also provide useful information.
Color Doppler limitations	CD may obscure a partially occluding thrombus. When evaluating the vein in the longitudinal plane, visualization of this thrombus type depends on the angle of the imaging plane and an accurate setting of the CD scale and CD gain.
Venous Doppler	Angle correction is not necessary during venous duplex imaging. The peak velocity value does not provide any clinically useful information. Instead, the SD waveform morphology is interrogated. SD signals are obtained in the longitudinal plane with appropriate SD scale and gain settings.
Upper extremities	During upper extremity imaging, use of CD to help locate central veins; the central veins should have a pulsatile and phasic signal; compare Doppler signals from the right and left sides; be aware of mirror imaging artifact caused by the clavicle.

TABLE 40.2 Interpretation Criteria of Venous Duplex Imaging

Gray Scale/Compression	Doppler Signal	Color Doppler
Normal		
No intraluminal echoes, free of echogenic material Vein fully coapts with external compression	Spontaneous, phasic, antegrade flow, augments with distal compression (pulsatile in some upper and central veins)	Color fills entire lumen
Abnormal: Partially Occlusive Thrombus		
Vein lumen partially filled with echoes Vein partially coapts with external compression	May be normal or abnormal (see below for abnormal)	Defect in color as it is displayed around thrombus; may appear normal if thrombus is small or color Doppler scale and gain settings are inappropriate
Abnormal: Occlusive Thrombus		
Vein filled with intraluminal echoes (veins may appear normal in circumstances of acute thrombus) Vein does not coapt with external compression	Absence of spectral Doppler signal, continuous signal, absent or reduced phasicity, and the lack of pulsatility in certain upper extremity and central veins	Absence of color

- *Augmentation:* Blood flow velocity increases with distal limb compression or with the release of proximal limb compression (limited in the upper extremity examination).
- *Pulsatility* (only in the upper extremity veins): Pulsatile signals should be present in the jugular, subclavian, innominate, and SVC because of retrograde transmission of right atrial pressure and movement artifact from cardiac contractions.

Loss of phasicity in a vein helps to identify proximal obstruction. Similarly, the absence or decrease in **augmentation** provides information about a possible distal obstruction. This is true in the peripheral venous system. Normal SD

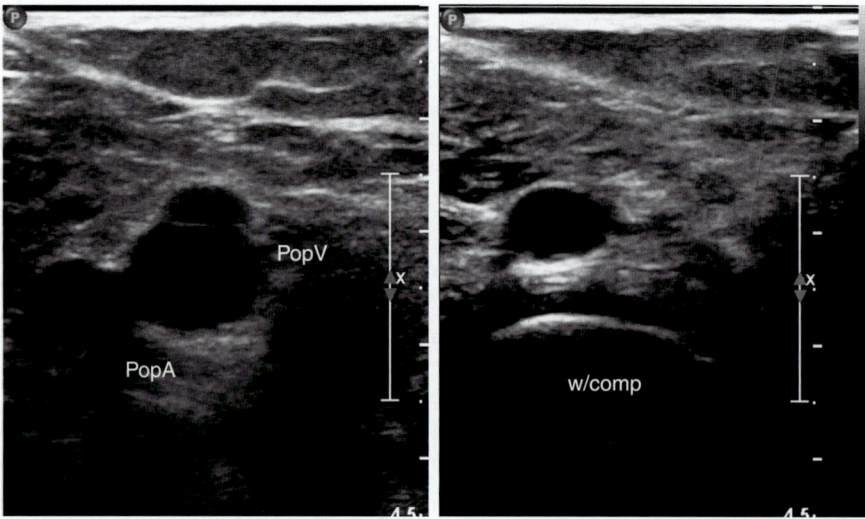

FIG. 40.10 Dual transverse gray-scale images of the popliteal vein (PopV) without *(left)* and with *(right)* applied compression. With compression, the popliteal vein fully coapts, suggesting the absence of venous thrombus. The popliteal artery (PopA) can be seen deep to the popliteal vein.

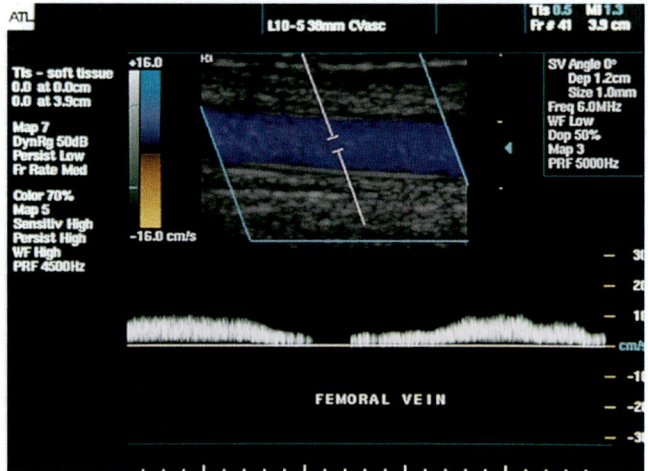

FIG. 40.11 Color and spectral Doppler image of a normal femoral vein in a longitudinal plane. The venous spectral Doppler waveform demonstrates low velocity and the phasic characteristics of a normal venous signal. Note that color fills the entire lumen of the vein when a low color scale is used.

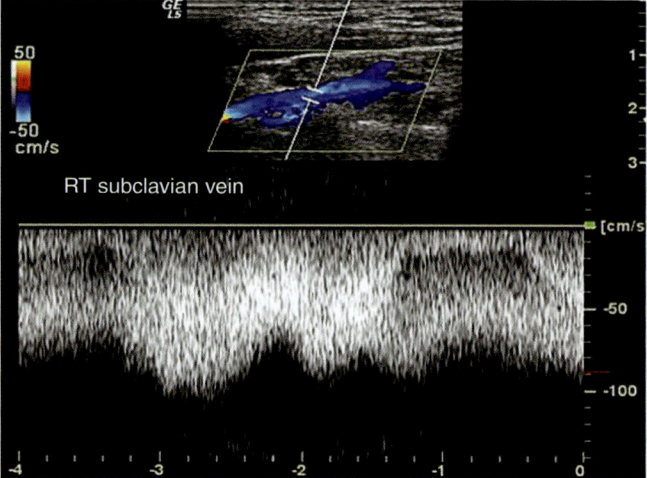

FIG. 40.12 Color and spectral Doppler image demonstrating normal phasic flow found in the subclavian vein.

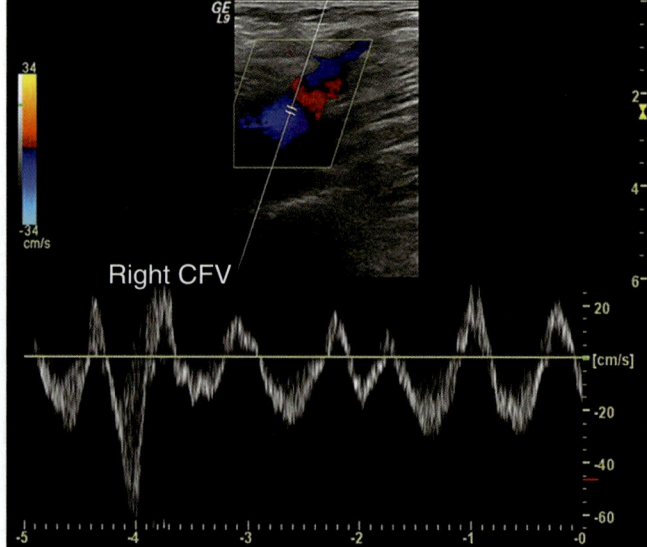

FIG. 40.13 Pulsatile spectral Doppler waveforms obtained from the common femoral vein (CFV) in a patient with congestive heart failure. An augmentation can be seen within the erratic flow.

signals from the central venous system are pulsatile (due to proximity of the right side of the heart) with a phasic respiratory variation superimposed on the venous velocity pattern (Fig. 40.12). Lack of pulsatility in the central veins suggests venous obstruction. Dissimilarly, extremely pulsatile signals in the central and/or peripheral veins can be an indication of congestive heart failure (Fig. 40.13).

It is important to remember that the most significant diagnostic criterion during venous imaging for thrombus detection is the vein's ability to coapt. To ensure adequate pressure was used during the examination, look at the effects that the external compression had on the vein's associated artery, if present. Adequate pressure was used if the artery is deformed during the compression maneuver.

If the vein does not fully coapt and the lumen is echo free, try repositioning the extremity. Having the patient exhale while performing compression may also aid in vein coaptation. If the vein still does not coapt, remember that thrombus visualization is variable. In the acute stages, the thrombus can be anechoic (Fig. 40.14); at other times the thrombus may be echogenic and blend into the surrounding tissue (Fig. 40.15). This is consistent with a chronic thrombus. CD imaging may also be used to visualize a thrombus by the reduction or absence of a CD signal. CD is also helpful in determining if a thrombus is partially or fully occlusive. In partially occlusive thrombi, color is seen flowing around the thrombus within the lumen of the vein (Fig. 40.16). Color flow will be absent in the presence of a fully occlusive clot.

The degree of thrombus echogenicity should be documented to aid in determining its age. Thrombus echogenicity can be variable; mixed degrees of echogenicity can be present within a single lesion (Fig. 40.17). Therefore this information should be combined with previous imaging examinations,

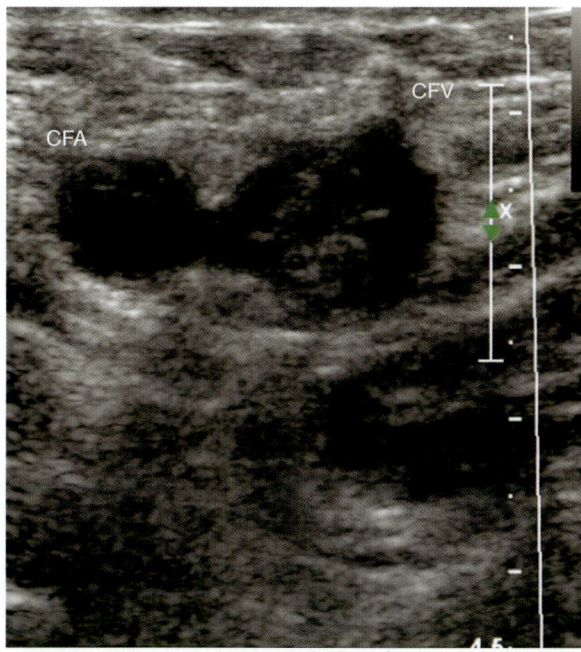

FIG. 40.14 Transverse dual gray-scale image of the common femoral vein (CFV) with transducer pressure being applied on the skin. The vein walls do not coapt; however, no intraluminal echoes are seen. This is suggestive of acute thrombosis. The common femoral artery (CFA) is also visualized medial to the CFV.

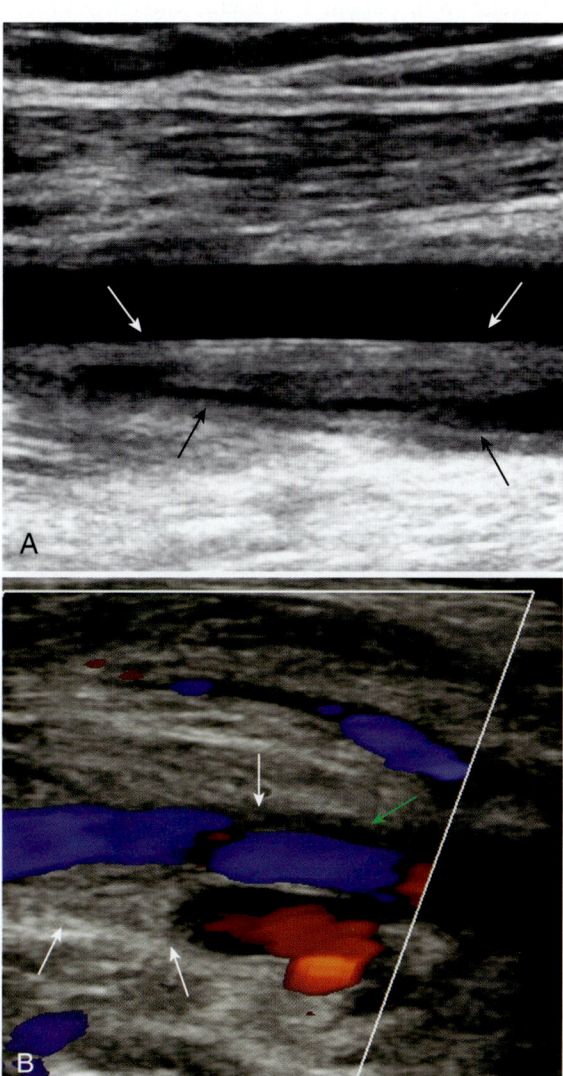

FIG. 40.16 (A) Longitudinal gray-scale image of a popliteal vein containing a partially occlusive thrombus along its posterior wall *(arrows)*. (B) Color Doppler image in which blood flow can be seen traveling around the thrombus *(arrows)* within the lumen of the vein.

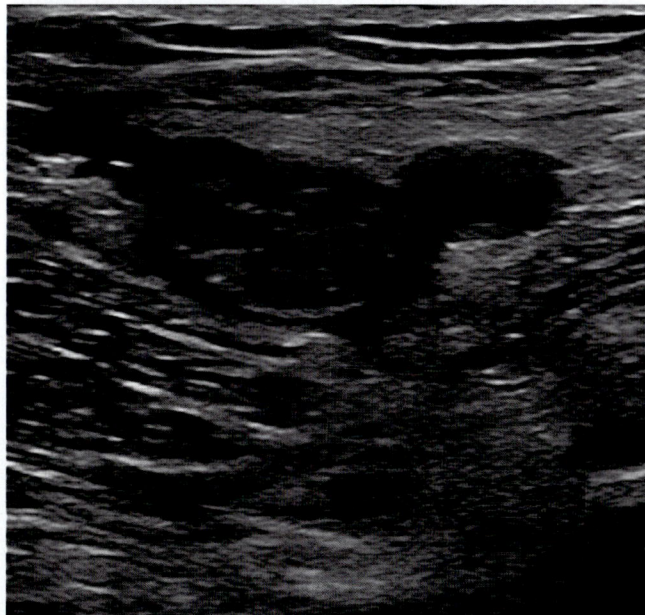

FIG. 40.15 The common femoral artery and vein are visualized in a gray-scale transverse view with transducer pressure being applied on the skin. The vein walls do not coapt, and echogenic material fills the lumen of the vein, suggestive of chronic thrombosis.

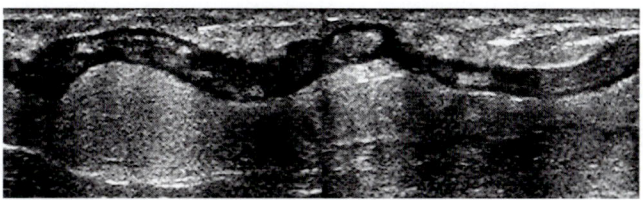

FIG. 40.17 Longitudinal gray-scale image of the basilic vein demonstrating venous thrombosis of mixed echogenicity.

patient history, and symptoms to enable the most accurate estimation of age.

A free-floating thrombus may also be visualized, moving freely within the lumen (Fig. 40.18). When this phenomenon occurs, the compression technique is not performed at that level on the limb. Compression should be limited for the rest of the examination, and CD be used to confirm patency because the risk of PE is much greater from free-floating thrombi.

In follow-up studies, the resolution of a thrombus varies dramatically from patient to patient. This largely depends on the course of management because treatment is typically individualized to each patient. Complete resolution of an extensive clot may occur at 3 months, 6 months, 1 year, or never. Recanalization of veins often occurs, characterized by blood flowing through small channels within or around the thrombus. This can be documented using CD.

Consistency of findings on GS imaging, by compression technique, and with CD and/or venous SD waveforms will limit errors when interpreting venous duplex imaging examinations. However, many pitfalls are involved in the interpretation of these examinations. Proper technique is essential to minimize these errors. If inconsistencies from previous studies are found, technical and equipment adjustments should be considered before the final interpretation (Table 40.3).

A meta-analysis and systematic review examining 100 studies and more than 10,000 cases reported that, compared with venography, venous duplex imaging demonstrated a high sensitivity (94%) and specificity (93%).[23] The same review found that the use of combined GS and CD imaging increased sensitivity in the proximal (96%) and distal (71%) regions.[23] Furthermore, the use of triplex imaging (GS, CD, and SD) increased sensitivity in the distal region (72%) and remained approximately the same in the proximal region (96%).[23] However, it is important to note that the distribution and magnitude of DVT may vary depending on the type of patient.

Evaluation of the calf veins is becoming easier with the advent of newer and improving ultrasound technology. Small veins can now be evaluated with better sensitivity than in the past. Rising sensitivities and specificities are due to better resolution obtained with the use of state-of-the-art imaging systems and CD imaging in most patients (Fig. 40.19).

After the venous duplex examination is complete, it is the responsibility of the sonographer to compile the results of the sonogram into a preliminary report for physician interpretation. Reports must be clear and concise and contain all pertinent information of the duplex study. For this reason, sonographers performing venous imaging examinations must be well informed of the anatomy, presentations of various pathologic findings, and proper imaging techniques, to provide accurate and optimal results. In addition, findings that may be considered emergent, namely acute DVT, must be recognized by the sonographer and relayed to a physician in a timely manner to ensure the safety of the patient.

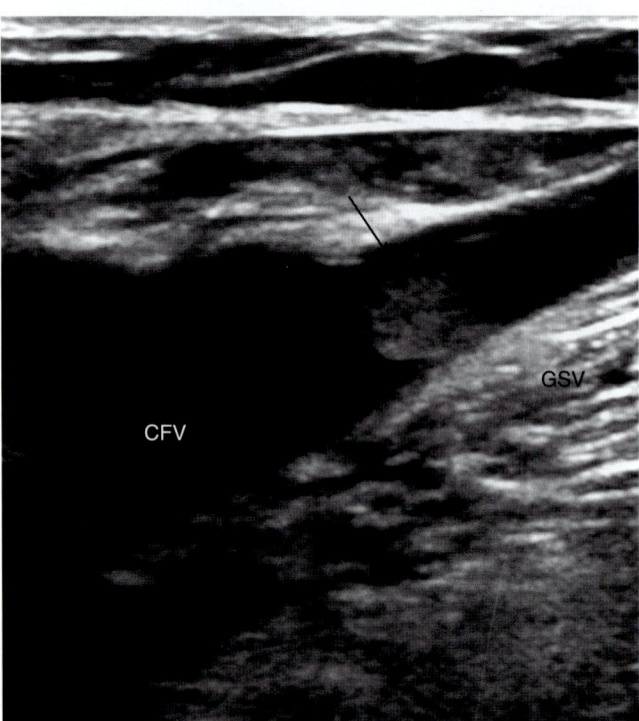

FIG. 40.18 Gray-scale image of the common femoral vein (CFV) and great saphenous vein (GSV). A free-floating thrombus is visualized *(arrow)* within the lumen of the GSV.

TABLE 40.3	Technical Adjustments for Venous Duplex Imaging When Thrombus Is Not Suspected
Challenge	**Action**
Vein does not compress; lumen is echo free	*Technique:* Move the transducer on the skin to attempt compression from a different angle in the transverse plane, check for adequate pressure (marked by deformation of the adjacent artery while being applied), have the patient exhale while applying pressure.
	Patient position: Repositioning the patient's extremity often results in ability to compress the vein.
	Anatomy: At times, the depth of the vessel and the surrounding tissue may make full vein coaptation impossible.
Vein compresses; lumen is filled with echoes	*Equipment:* Gain settings too high. Harmonic imaging should be performed.
	Technique: Use the correct transverse plane to make sure that there is complete coaptation of the venous lumen.

COMBINED DIAGNOSTIC APPROACH

While performing a venous duplex imaging examination for the detection of thrombus, the sonographer must combine other methods of diagnostics, if available. Additional information from previous studies or a patient history facilitates an optimal venous imaging study. The sonographer must use his or her knowledge of pathophysiology while taking a patient's history and evaluating the patient's signs and symptoms. This may give insight to possible findings or indicate areas that should be paid close attention to while performing the sonogram. Similarly, previous imaging studies should also be reviewed to provide a larger perspective on the patient's disease progression. The review of previous imaging studies should not be restricted only to sonograms. All forms of imaging, specifically venogram studies, can provide valuable information that can aid in performing a venous duplex examination.

Beyond imaging, laboratory values such as D-dimer assays have been found to be highly sensitive for diagnosing DVT and is the most routinely used clinical biomarker.[24] Unfortunately, D-dimer assays possess very low specificity. Consequently, a negative result confidently excludes a DVT, whereas a positive result requires additional testing, most commonly venous duplex imaging.[25] The assays measure D-dimer, which is a fibrin-specific degradation product that detects cross-linked fibrin resulting from endogenous fibrinolysis.[26] Elevated D-dimer levels can be the result of DVT or SVT presence; therefore this test alone cannot differentiate the two. This explains its low specificity and why subsequent imaging studies are needed to determine the exact thrombus location, extent, and severity.

VENOUS REFLUX IMAGING

The purpose of venous reflux testing is to identify the presence and the location of incompetent venous valves. When venous valves become incompetent, venous blood flow is unable to fully overcome hydrostatic pressure within the vein, and incompetent venous valves which are no longer closing properly results in retrograde venous flow, often referred to as venous reflux.

Performing a reflux examination begins by explaining the examination to the patient. A patient history is taken focusing on risk factors, signs, and symptoms of venous disease, especially any history of DVT. If the patient has not had one recently, a complete lower extremity DVT study should be done before reflux testing to rule out any preexisting pathology. The examination is performed with the patient in a reverse Trendelenburg or standing position, to promote distention of the venous system. A reverse Trendelenburg position is more frequently used because it is a more ergonomically friendly scanning approach and is more comfortable for the patient, while still maintaining adequate venous distention. The knee of the leg being examined should be slightly bent with the leg rolled to the side to allow for adequate access to the medial thigh and calf for imaging.

Evaluation of venous reflux by duplex imaging is performed using a high-frequency (7- to 10-MHz) linear-array imaging transducer. Although venous valves may be visualized, the GS image is not used for determining valvular incompetence. The absence or presence of venous reflux is measured from the venous SD waveform. This is done by obtaining a SD waveform while simultaneously performing a distal augmentation maneuver. On augmentation a spike in venous flow velocity is seen on the spectral waveform as the blood is being pushed antegrade (toward the heart). In the presence of reflux, retrograde flow (reflux) is demonstrated immediately following the augmentation (Fig. 40.20).

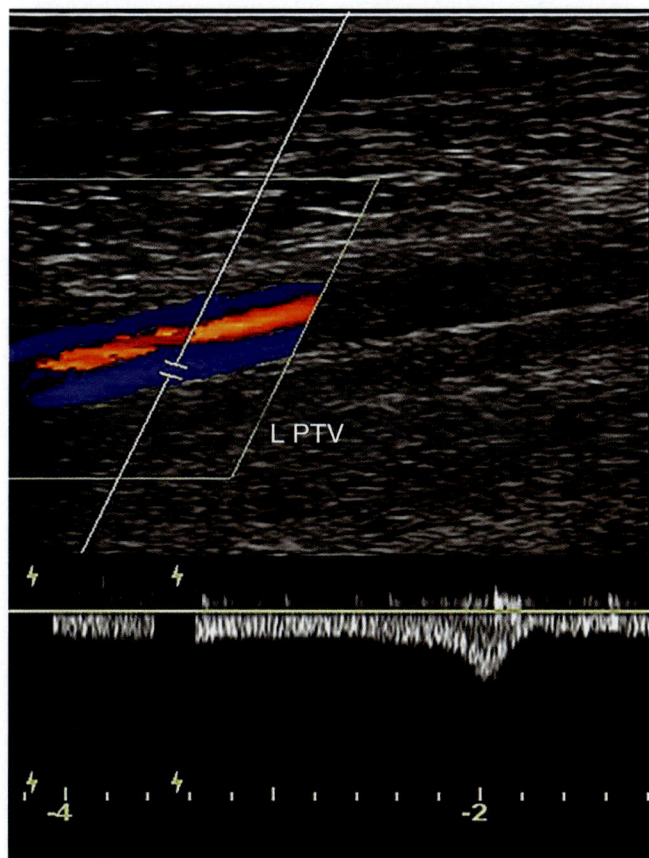

FIG. 40.19 Longitudinal color and spectral Doppler image in the lower calf demonstrating the flow within the posterior tibial veins (PTVs) and associated artery.

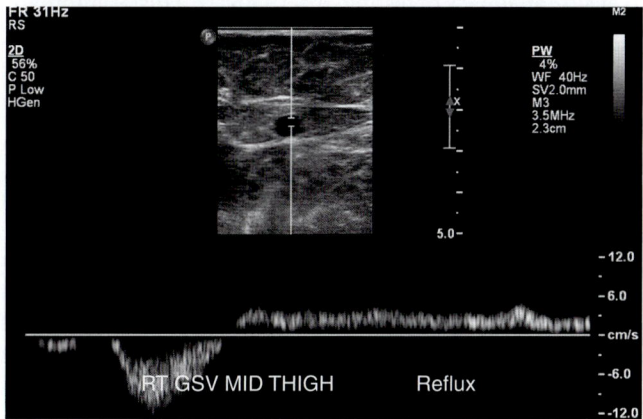

FIG. 40.20 Spectral Doppler waveform obtained from the great saphenous vein (GSV) during a venous reflux test. Antegrade blood flow after distal augmentation is seen below the baseline, followed by the reversal of blood (retrograde) flow above the baseline. This is suggestive of venous reflux.

Retrograde flow is due to the presence of incompetent venous valves that are unable to keep venous blood flowing in an antegrade direction. Absence of retrograde blood flow indicates competent valves. The amount of retrograde flow can be measured to provide a quantified value representing the extent of reflux at that location. Values of what constitutes reflux vary among institutions; however, guidance has been developed indicating presence of reflux disease when retrograde flow occurs 1 second or greater in the FV and PV, or 500 ms or greater in any other deep veins or perforator veins.[27] Augmentation maneuvers are performed to evaluate the deep and superficial veins of the lower extremity; however, special attention is paid to the GSV and SSV. These veins are relatively long and contain a large number of valves making them more susceptible to reflux. Each vein is evaluated at multiple locations to provide information regarding the valvular competence throughout the entirety of the vessel. If visualized, perforating veins should also be evaluated for reflux. Reflux testing in perforating veins is done by augmenting proximally on the limb (as opposed to distally). Depending on the institution, reflux testing may also be required in varicose veins. Once reflux testing is complete, anteroposterior (AP) diameter measurements should be acquired at multiple locations on transverse images of any veins demonstrating reflux. Vein diameter measurements are used in determining treatment method. If reflux exists within large enough veins, the physician may elect to perform a venous ablation. Ablations can be done using laser or radiofrequency technology and are performed in the GSV, SSV, or perforating veins.

Reports for reflux examinations should include the veins and the locations within each vein where reflux is demonstrated. Vein diameter measurements, along with other vein characteristics such as depth, tortuosity, and location, should be clearly stated because certain characteristics may contraindicate surgical intervention.

Venous reflux examinations are technically difficult to perform because one must operate the imaging system, hold the transducer on the patient's leg, and augment the patient's distal limb to test for reflux. Two examiners may be necessary to ensure adequacy of testing. Alternatively, a distal automatic cuff compression-release device can be used. This uses a cuff compression-release device located on the leg distal to the transducer, and it ensures adequate and reproducible compression pressure and timing of augmentation release.

VEIN MAPPING

The purpose of superficial vein mapping is to determine a vein's suitability for use as a bypass conduit, or arteriovenous fistula for dialysis access. Documentation of a vein's anatomic route, size, and tortuosity provides physicians with valuable information regarding a vein's utility to be used as an arterial conduit. This avoids surgically exposing inadequate veins, which decreases operative time, associated health care costs, and risk of wound complications from unnecessary incisions.[28]

Vein mapping examinations are performed by imaging the superficial veins of the upper and/or lower extremities. The cephalic and basilic veins are imaged in the upper extremities and the GSV and SSV in the lower extremities. A high-frequency (7- to 10-MHz) linear-array transducer provides the best resolution for imaging. Maintaining light transducer pressure on the skin is critical because superficial veins are easily compressible and may be inadvertently compressed from transducer pressure. The patient is imaged in a supine reverse Trendelenburg position to promote venous distention. A tourniquet may also be used in the upper extremities to promote venous distention.

While performing a lower extremity vein mapping examination, imaging begins at the level of the groin by locating the GSV at the saphenofemoral junction, in a transverse plane. The GSV is then imaged transversely as it travels distally along the anteromedial side of the thigh and calf. Images are taken at multiple locations throughout the length of the vein to provide an accurate representation of its size. The amount and locations of image acquisition will vary among institutions. In many cases, the GSV has many branches. The presence of branches, including the amount, size, and location, should also be documented because this may be a contraindication for use. In each of the images acquired, the diameter of the GSV should be measured in an AP fashion. Lateral diameter measurements should not be performed, because slight compression of the vein from transducer pressure may result in a falsely inflated diameter measure. As a general rule, vascular surgeons can use vessels that measure 2.5 mm or larger, but this may vary based on surgeon preference.[29] Institutional protocols should include acceptable vessel diameters. Imaging of the GSV should be done bilaterally. The SSV is evaluated in the same fashion as the GSV. The SSV extends posterior to the lateral malleolus and terminates at variable levels of the popliteal vein. Documentation should be made of its tortuosity, presence of branches, and AP diameter measurements. SSV imaging should also be done bilaterally.

While performing an upper extremity vein mapping examination, imaging begins at the level of the shoulder. The distal portion of the axillary vein is identified in the upper arm, from which the cephalic and basilic vein can be seen joining it on the lateral and medial aspects of the arm, respectively. These veins should be imaged in their entirety throughout the upper arm and forearm. Imaging should be done in a transverse plane to allow for AP diameter measurements to be made. Just as in the lower extremity, tortuosity and presence of branches should be reported.

The patency of the superficial veins being examined must also be confirmed while performing an upper or lower extremity vein mapping. This is done using the compression technique. Additional findings that should also be documented include the presence of thickened walls, calcification, recanalization, and stenotic valves. If requested by the physician, mark the vein's path and its branches on the skin using an indelible marker. When marking the skin, make sure that the vein is centered in the ultrasound image, and use a small blunt-ended object (ball point pen, pen cap, etc.) to press the skin just hard enough to leave a small mark.

OTHER PATHOLOGY

A **Baker cyst** is a common finding, defined as a collection of synovial fluid in the popliteal fossa as a result of excess synovial fluid in the knee. Excess synovial fluid can be subsequent to any type of arthritis, more commonly osteoarthritis and rheumatoid arthritis, or to trauma such as cartilage tears. Baker cysts can be unilateral or bilateral. Symptoms mimic those of DVT, with swelling and tightness behind the knee being common. A Baker cyst can also cause severe pain in the upper calf in cases which the cyst ruptures and dissects into the upper calf muscles. The goals while imaging this pathology are to prove a widely patent popliteal vein to rule out DVT, evaluate the popliteal artery to rule out aneurysm, and visualize the fluid collection separate from these structures (Fig. 40.21). These cysts tend to be crescent shape and can be anechoic or complex as the result of hemorrhage or infection. CD can be useful to further confirm it is an avascular structure, as well as confirm patency of the popliteal vein.

Abscesses, cellulitis, and hematomas (Fig. 40.22) can cause focal areas of redness and swelling that may mimic symptoms of DVT or SVT. Proving that there is DVT in the deep venous system is the first goal in these cases; evaluating the symptomatic area to rule out an SVT is secondary. Small fluid collections within the tissue or muscle planes may be seen with these types of tissues. Symptoms mimicking a thrombus may arise from a recent trauma to that area; therefore a thorough patient history can prove helpful in these circumstances.

Lymph nodes in the groin and in the areas of the common femoral or external iliac vein can be confused with findings of a DVT. Enlarged echogenic lymph nodes take on a similar appearance to that of a chronic DVT (Fig. 40.23). Visualizing these structures in transverse and sagittal plane will exclude them from venous pathology. Enlarged lymph nodes should be documented. Color may be seen flowing in from the hilum. Nodes can be enlarged as a result of infection or as an early sign of lymphoma.

CONTROVERSIES IN VENOUS DUPLEX IMAGING

Complete Versus Limited Examination

Why examine the entire leg in a symptomatic patient? The standard technique for venous duplex imaging of the lower extremity in symptomatic patients has been to evaluate the

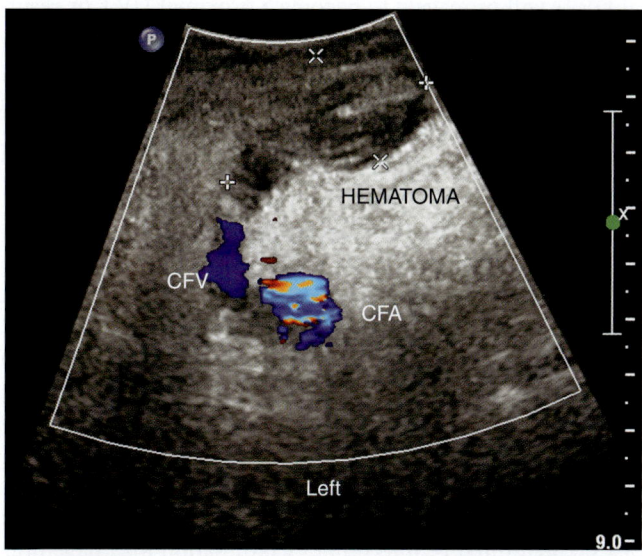

FIG. 40.22 Gray-scale image of a large hematoma located in the groin of a patient who underwent trauma to that area. The duplex examination was ordered to rule out deep vein thrombosis. Color Doppler imaging should be used to demonstrate the absence of flow within the hematoma. The common femoral vein (CFV) and common femoral artery (CFA) are visualized deep to the hematoma.

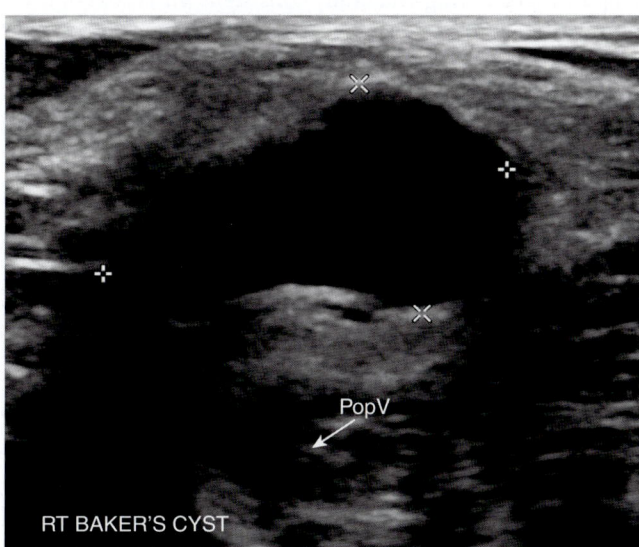

FIG. 40.21 Transverse gray-scale image of a Baker cyst located in the popliteal fossa. The popliteal vein (PopV) can be seen deep to the large Baker cyst slightly compressed (arrow).

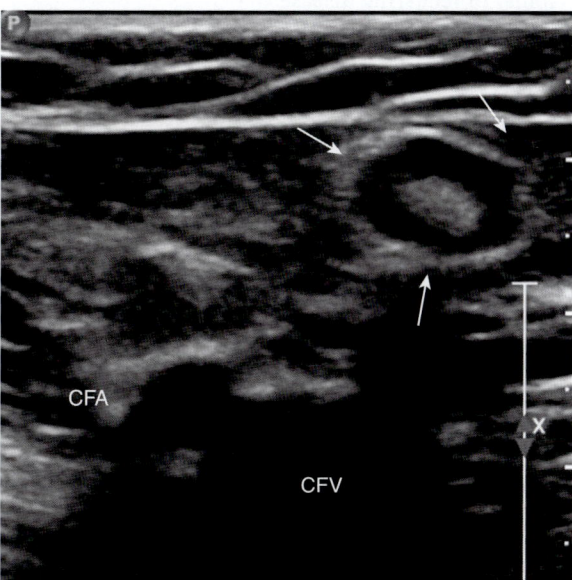

FIG. 40.23 Transverse gray-scale image depicting a large lymph node (arrows) located in the groin of a patient with an elevated white blood cell count. This finding is often confused with chronic deep vein thrombosis in the common femoral vein (CFV). *CFA*, Common femoral artery.

veins from the level of the inguinal ligament to, and including, the calf veins. However, a limited venous duplex of the lower extremity generally involves only imaging the common femoral and popliteal veins. Existing studies have demonstrated that up to 99% of acute DVTs will involve the common femoral and/or the popliteal vein.[30] Therefore it has been suggested that a "two-point" venous duplex examination in symptomatic patients would detect a clot in a high percentage of cases while significantly reducing examination time.[30] On the contrary, similar studies have reported conflicting results, advocating for a more extensive evaluation of the lower limb venous vasculature.[31,32] Furthermore, an estimated 10% of distal DVTs will propagate to become a proximal DVT or result in PE.[33-35] The largest driver for completing limited studies is to reduce examination time. One study compared the amount of time to complete limited and complete unilateral venous duplex examinations, reporting a reduction of approximately 10 minutes when completing the limited examination.[30] Reduction in scan time to this extent could prove beneficial because it could reduce health care expenditures and decrease patient wait time.

Studies investigating the use of a limited venous duplex examination in the emergency department (ED) have reported high levels of sensitivities ranging from 89% to 100% when acute DVT was suspected.[36-39] Unfortunately, these studies used very small sample sizes, so no definitive statements can be made.

Current recommendations state that a complete venous duplex imaging examination should be performed in most cases. The limited venous duplex examination may have utility in symptomatic, critically ill, or symptomatic patients with limited mobility but should not be performed when screening patients who are at a high risk for DVT. To this end, the American College of Chest Physicians guidelines outline several recommended protocols dependent upon the patient's probability of recurring disease.[40]

Unilateral Versus Bilateral

Why examine the asymptomatic leg in a patient with unilateral symptoms? In the past, when venography was the accepted diagnostic test for DVT, only the symptomatic limb was evaluated for the presence of thrombosis. A choice to perform a unilateral study stemmed from the rationale that therapy for the presence of a DVT bilaterally would rarely differ from that of the therapy in situations of a unilateral DVT. Furthermore, the incidence of a contralateral DVT in an asymptomatic limb is low.[41]

On the contrary, it has been customary to study bilateral lower extremities when vascular laboratories used nonimaging Doppler and plethysmographic techniques. However, these examinations required information from bilateral limbs because results and interpretation relied on the comparison of venous hemodynamics from the ipsilateral to contralateral limb.

One retrospective study advocates the use of imaging only the afflicted limb, because 1.8% (n=435) of venous examinations reviewed found DVT contralaterally to the symptomatic limb.[42] A similar study retrospectively reviewed bilateral venous duplex imaging examinations in symptomatic patients, finding acute DVT in 248 of 1694 cases.[43] Of these cases, acute DVT never occurred in the asymptomatic limb if the symptomatic limb was normal.[43] These investigators recommend that patients with unilateral symptoms undergo unilateral venous duplex imaging only, because it improves cost efficiency and treatment would not have been altered regardless of the findings.[43] This was further supported in a study that discovered in cases of bilateral DVT, patient treatment was altered in only 0.8% occurrences as a result of discovering the contralateral DVT.[44]

This topic remains somewhat controversial in the literature nowadays because some advocate imaging of only the symptomatic limb in an attempt to increase vascular laboratory efficiency.[45-49] Others maintain that a significant number of DVTs occur bilaterally and that this, along with the minimal scan time and nonionizing nature of ultrasound imaging, should always warrant bilateral lower extremity imaging.[50-52] Further still, investigators have suggested the appropriateness of bilateral imaging depends upon the status of the patient; it is safe for low-risk individuals to undergo unilateral examinations, whereas high-risk individuals, such as those with malignancies or inpatients with limited mobility, should undergo bilateral imaging.[53] Currently, the recommendation to image the contralateral extremity only if DVT is visualized in the symptomatic extremity is largely accepted. This will document the patency of the FV (for percutaneous placement access of vena cava filters) and the presence of any DVT that may prove to be helpful in follow-up studies. A protocol for this clinical situation should be established by each institution.

Bilateral Deep Vein Thrombosis Symptoms

Why perform venous duplex imaging in patients with bilateral leg symptoms? It has been suggested in the literature that symptoms presenting bilaterally consistent with those of DVT are more likely to be caused by a systemic disease process, as opposed to the presence of two separate DVTs. For example, bilateral edema of the lower extremity may have cardiac disease as the dominant cause of the leg swelling. Other causes of bilateral lower extremity symptoms similar to those of DVT may include peripheral arterial disease, venous stasis, trauma, or a venous entrapment disorder.

To this end, a prospective study examined 50 cases reporting bilateral DVT symptoms; however, none (0%) were diagnosed with DVT.[54] The investigators of this study suggest that DVT in patients with bilateral symptoms is rare and that venous duplex imaging should not be performed if the patient's medical history indicates a more likely alternative cause.[54]

On the contrary, a retrospective study examined 324 cases of patients presenting with bilateral DVT symptoms.[55] On duplex imaging, 19 of the 324 individuals (17%) were found to have bilateral lower extremity DVTs.[55] The investigators of this study concluded that their findings supported the use of bilateral venous duplex imaging in the presence of bilateral symptoms.[42] Similar to conclusions outlined in the previous section, current recommendations encourage that the patient be evaluated on an individualized basis, and the decision to perform bilateral imaging based upon the patient's risk factors for DVT.[56]

Calf Vein Imaging

Why examine the calf veins in patients at high risk for developing DVT or in patients suspected of having DVT? This controversy centers on three distinct points:

1. It is thought that calf veins are difficult to image in many patients and cannot be assessed at a high level of accuracy. This has been initially documented in several past studies and meta-analyses.[57-59] However, with improvements of ultrasound technology, modern ultrasound equipment has adequate resolution and additional technical settings available to the sonographer, making calf vein imaging significantly less complicated than it was once thought to be.[25] Along these lines, other studies have reported more favorable results in the ability to detect deep calf vein thrombosis.[60]
2. Physicians often do not treat isolated calf thrombosis because VTE is thought of as unlikely, and the majority of calf vein DVTs will resolve spontaneously without causing symptoms.[35,61-63] A review of the literature finds the risk of PE to be 0% to 1.5% while patients are not being anticoagulated.[64-67] However, the prevalence of deep calf vein thrombosis has been reported much higher than previously thought, with some findings suggesting its presence in up to approximately 50% of patients, making this a potentially more widespread concern.[68] Current recommended follow-up guidelines when calf DVT is detected is to get repeat imaging if the patient does not present with symptoms.[25,63]
3. Patients can be followed serially with venous duplex imaging to evaluate thrombus propagation, which has been reported to occur in as low as 3.8% of cases.[66] However, a controversy in this area also exists in the literature because some studies maintain that the frequency of calf DVT propagation to adjacent veins is unknown.[69,70] Moreover, other studies have suggested 9% to 21% of distal DVTs will propagate into the proximal deep system,[42,71] although a retrospective study reported the majority of patients ordered for repeat imaging never actually returned for the scan.[72]

Knowledge of venous anatomy and use of proper imaging techniques are critical for the direct evaluation of the calf. Advances in ultrasound technology have improved GS resolution, which aids in a venous duplex imaging examination's capability of adequately visualizing calf veins. To this end, other studies have reported a sensitivity of 85% and 99% specificity for detecting DVT in the calf veins.[73] Furthermore, calf muscle venous thrombosis (defined as the presence of thrombus in the gastrocnemius or soleal veins) was found to be fairly sensitive (88% to 92%), although less specific (64% to 95%) compared with venography in older studies, prior to the advent of modern ultrasound features.[74,75] CD and SD imaging is also beneficial in their interrogation. Evaluation of the calf veins adds approximately 10 minutes to the examination of the lower extremity and provides the clinician with the option to initiate treatment. In addition, even in circumstances where a calf DVT is found but does not result in treatment, its finding may provide an explanation for a patient's symptoms and will be documented for future imaging studies.

Based on recent evidence reported in the relevant literature, in 2018 a multidisciplinary consensus meeting was convened, consisting of representatives from the Society of Radiologists, Society for Vascular Ultrasound, and the American College of Radiologists to establish guidelines for the diagnosis of DVT using duplex ultrasound. As a result, this committee recommended performing a complete examination of the leg, with images acquired from the inguinal ligament extending to the ankle, performing compression maneuvers at 2-cm intervals and including the tibial and calf veins as part of the assessment.[25]

Emergent Venous Duplex Imaging

In cases of suspected DVT, is it justified to use the on-call sonographer to perform an emergent venous duplex imaging examination? Point of care ultrasound (POCUS) has become increasingly popular for use in the ED for detection of DVT. With appropriate training, physicians or other ED practitioners are able to detect proximal DVT with a high degree of accuracy.[76] In 2017 the American College of Emergency Physicians reported guidelines listing POCUS as a core emergency ultrasonographic application.[77]

Eliminating the need for on-call sonographers will result in significant financial savings and reduction in patient wait time to receive the scan. Due to the high volume of venous duplex imaging examinations ordered daily, performing additional scans off hours increases a vascular laboratory's volume even further, causing a physical and financial strain. One study that implemented of a protocol aimed to reduce the number of emergent DVT duplex scans in their vascular lab using patient symptomatology reported the ability to reduce off-hour call-ins by 89%, which resulted in approximately $17,000 in hospital savings from reduced sonographer compensation.[78] In large, two methods of POCUS for DVT detection have been used, the two-point POCUS and three-point POCUS. The two-point POCUS examines compressibility of the CFV and popliteal vein, whereas the three-point POCUS examines FV in addition to the CFV and popliteal vein.[38,39,79-82] A meta-analysis comparing the two approaches concluded no significant differences, reporting high levels of sensitivity and specificity of DVT detection for both (sensitivity: 91%, specificity: 98%; sensitivity: 91%, specificity: 95%, respectively).[83]

Sonographic Assessment of Pulmonary Embolism

Why examine the lower extremities with venous duplex imaging if the patient has signs and symptoms of a PE?

Clinicians not wishing to order pulmonary arteriography or other more invasive procedures, including ionizing imaging, have determined that if venous duplex imaging detects DVT in patients suspected of PE, anticoagulation therapy may be initiated.[84] Because most pulmonary emboli originate from the lower extremity, using venous duplex imaging to clarify an indeterminate lung scan may also help to confirm clinically suspected PE. Since 2000, the volume of ultrasound examinations performed to evaluate DVT has increased and now exceeds that of computed tomography (CT) for the same purpose.[85] However, it has been reported that duplex imaging revealed DVT in only 80% of patients with confirmed PE.[86] Therefore a negative venous duplex imaging study of the legs does not exclude a PE diagnosis, and further work-up in these patients is necessary. Venous duplex imaging should not be used as the first or only diagnostic test for the diagnosis of pulmonary embolus.

IMAGING GUIDELINES

Performing high-quality venous duplex imaging examinations in a thorough manner is essential if it is to have diagnostic value. Venous duplex examinations must possess accuracy as well as reproducibility among the sonographers of a particular vascular laboratory or institution. For this reason, quality assurance measures must be in place to ensure correct diagnostic information is being provided. By comparing venous duplex imaging study results with results of a gold standard such as venography, sonographers are held accountable for the results that they provide.

Optimal examinations are achieved by attention to detail while scanning, and incorporating the information obtained from the patient's history and symptoms with the knowledge of venous anatomy and pathology that is possessed. Recent multidisciplinary committee guidance recommends differing patient management strategies in the presence of DVT dependent upon patient symptoms, reemphasizing the need for a thorough understanding patient history, and expected sonographic findings based upon presenting symptoms. Imaging guidelines are listed in Box 40.4, which, if followed, will ensure a high-quality venous duplex examination while maintaining excellent patient care.

BOX 40.4 Venous Duplex Imaging Guidelines

- Take a patient history.
- Be familiar with venous anatomy, physiology, and pathology.
- Optimize the gray scale.
- Use only a transverse view for compression technique.
- Use a longitudinal view to obtain color Doppler images.
- Use a longitudinal view to obtain Doppler signals. Use a large Doppler sample volume size and a low-velocity scale.
- Upper extremities: Document pulsatility in the Doppler signal, and compare the right and left sides.
- Establish institutional diagnostic criteria based on published, peer-reviewed guidelines.

Key Pearls

- Deep vein thrombosis (DVT) is characterized by thrombus, or blood clot, in a deep vein(s), caused by abnormal coagulation of red blood cells. DVT can occur in both the upper and lower extremities.
- Postthrombotic syndrome consists of chronic leg pain, inflammation, redness, and ulcers.
- The peripheral venous portion of the circulatory system is located in the upper and lower extremities and consists of the deep, superficial, and perforating (communicating) veins located within them.
- The main function of the peripheral venous system is to return deoxygenated blood from organs and body tissues to the heart. In the periphery, deoxygenated blood leaving the capillaries enters the venules of venous microcirculation.
- Venous valves are a unique feature to the venous system; they are bicuspid and unidirectional folds that arise from the tunica intima.
- Hydrostatic pressure, also known as gravitational pressure when standing upright, is defined as the pressure placed on a fluid in a column as a result of gravity.
- Venous valves increase in quantity in the distal portions of the lower extremities.
- Lower extremity deep veins are located deep within the muscles of the legs and serve as the primary route of drainage for the leg.
- The superficial veins of the lower extremities are superficial to the deep veins, located between two layers of superficial fascia in the subcutaneous tissue. Superficial veins serve to drain blood from the tissues and transport it to the deep system.
- The veins of the superficial venous system are not paired with an artery.
- The deep veins of the upper extremity are located within the musculature of the arms, travel in close association with a corresponding artery, and serve to transport deoxygenated blood from the superficial to central venous system.
- The venous system relies on muscles surrounding the veins to propel blood forward.
- Venous thromboembolism is a condition in which a venous thrombus dislodges from the vein wall, propagates to the arteries of the lungs, and causes a pulmonary embolism.
- The three factors associated with thrombus formation (Virchow triad) are (1) a hypercoagulable state, (2) venous stasis (blood pools in the veins), and (3) vein wall injury (endothelium of the vein is damaged, exposing the subendothelium to blood and triggering platelet adhesion and aggregation, which promotes blood coagulation).
- Acute DVT is typically defined as a thrombus no more than a week old.

- Severe chronic DVTs can lead to a process known as postthrombotic syndrome, caused by increased ambulatory venous pressure, also known as venous hypertension.
- Venous hypertension can be a result of the venous obstruction (chronic DVT) and/or incompetent venous valves.
- Varicose veins are dilated, elongated, tortuous superficial veins.
- A clot formation that exists in the superficial venous system is known as a superficial venous thrombosis.
- Venous insufficiency, also known as venous reflux, is caused by incompetent venous valves.
- The purpose of venous reflux testing is to identify the presence and the location of incompetent venous valves.
- The purpose of superficial vein mapping is to determine a vein's suitability for use as a bypass conduit or arteriovenous fistula for dialysis access.
- A Baker cyst is a common finding, defined as a collection of synovial fluid in the popliteal fossa as a result of excess synovial fluid in the knee.

REFERENCES

1. Virani SS, et al. Heart disease and stroke statistics—2020 update: a report from the American Heart Association. *Circulation*. 2020:E139–E596.
2. Bell EJ, Lutsey PL, Basu S, et al. Lifetime risk of venous thromboembolism in two cohort studies. *Am J Med*. 2016;129(339): e19–e339.
3. Liew A, Douketis J. Initial and long-term treatment of deep venous thrombosis: recent clinical trials and their impact on patient management. *Expert Opin Pharmacother*. 2013;14(4):385–396.
4. Heit JA. Epidemiology of venous thromboembolism. *Nat Rev Cardiol*. 2015;12(8):464–474.
5. Varaki ES, et al. Peripheral vascular disease assessment in the lower limb: a review of current and emerging non-invasive diagnostic methods. *Biomed Eng Online*. 2018;17(1):61.
6. Malgor RD, Labropolous N. Diagnosis and follow-up of varicose veins with duplex ultrasound: how and why? *Phlebology*. 2012;27(Suppl 1):10–15.
7. Paraskevas P. Femoral vein duplication: incidence and potential significance. *Phlebology*. 2011;26(2):52–55.
8. Liu GC, Ferris EJ, Reifsteck JR, et al. Effect of anatomic variations on deep venous thrombosis of the lower extremity. *Am J Roentgenol*. 1986;146:845–848.
9. Simpson WL, Krakowsi DM. Prevalence of lower extremity venous duplication. *Indian J Radiol Imaging*. 2010;20(3):230.
10. Kachlik D, Pechacek V, Musil V, et al. Information on the changes in the revised anatomical nomenclature of the lower limb veins. *Biomed Pap*. 2010;154:93–97.
11. Intersocietal Accreditation Commission (IAC) vascular testing standards: venous disease. https://intersocietal.org/wp-content/uploads/2021/11/IACVascularTestingStandards2021.pdf.
12. Porth CM. *Disorders of blood flow and blood pressure. Essentials of Pathophysiology: Concepts of Altered Health States*. Philadelphia: Lippincott Williams & Wilkins; 2004.
13. Cote LP, et al. Comparisons between upper and lower extremity deep vein thrombosis: a review of the RIETE registry. *Clin Appl Thrombosis/Hemostasis*. 2017;23(7):748–754.
14. Minges KE, Bikdeli B, Wang Y, Attaran RR, Krumholz HM. National and regional trends in deep vein thrombosis hospitalization rates, discharge disposition, and outcomes for Medicare beneficiaries. *Am J Med*. 2018;131:1200–1208.
15. Minges KE, Bikdeli B, Wang Y, et al. National trends in pulmonary embolism hospitalization rates and outcomes for adults aged ≥65 years in the United States (1999 to 2010). *Am J Cardiol*. 2015;116:1436–1442.
16. Virchow R. Neuer fall von todlicher emboli der lungenarterie. *Virchows Arch Pathol Anat*. 1856;10:225–231.
17. Fan CM. Venous pathophysiology. *Semin Intervent Radiol*. 2005;22:157.
18. Callam MJ. Epidemiology of varicose veins. *Br J Surg*. 1994;81: 167–173.
19. Kaplan RM, et al. Quality of life in patients with chronic venous disease: San Diego population study. *J Vasc Surg*. 2003;37(5): 1047–1053.
20. Hamdan A. Management of varicose veins and venous insufficiency. *Jama*. 2012;308(24):2612–2621.
21. Taengsakul N, et al. Inflammatory responses in varicose veins surgery: conventional venous stripping vs endovenous radiofrequency ablation (EV-RFA). *J Vasc Endovasc Ther*. 2019;4(1):9.
22. AbuRahma AF, Bergan JJ. *Noninvasive vascular diagnosis: a practical guide*. ed 2. New York: Springer; 2007.
23. Goodacre S, Sampson F, Thomas S, et al. Systematic review and meta-analysis of the diagnostic accuracy of ultrasonography for deep vein thrombosis. *BMC Med Imaging*. 2005;5:6.
24. Liederman Z, Chan N, Bhagirath V. Current challenges in diagnosis of venous thromboembolism. *J Clin Med*. 2020;9(11):3509.
25. Needleman L, et al. Ultrasound for lower extremity deep venous thrombosis: multidisciplinary recommendations from the Society of Radiologists in Ultrasound Consensus Conference. *Circulation*. 2018;137(14):1505–1515.
26. Wells PS, Anderson DR, Rodger M, et al. Evaluation of D-dimer in the diagnosis of suspected deep-vein thrombosis. *N Engl J Med*. 2003;349:1227–1235.
27. Gloviczki P, et al. The care of patients with varicose veins and associated chronic venous diseases: clinical practice guidelines of the Society for Vascular Surgery and the American Venous Forum. *J Vasc Surg*. 2011;53(5):2S–48S.
28. Linni K, Mader N, Aspalter M, et al. Ultrasonic vein mapping prior to infrainguinal autogenous bypass grafting reduces postoperative infections and readmissions. *J Vasc Surg*. 2012;56:126–133.
29. Linni K, Aspalter M, Mader N, et al. Preoperative duplex vein mapping (DVM) reduces costs in patients undergoing infrainguinal bypass surgery: results of a prospective randomised study. *Eur J Vasc Endovasc Surg*. 2012;43:561–566.
30. Pezzullo JA, Perkins AB, Cronan JJ. Symptomatic deep vein thrombosis: diagnosis with limited compression US. *Radiology*. 1996;198:67–70.
31. Aurshina A, et al. Clinical role of the "venous" ultrasound to identify lower extremity pathology. *Ann Vasc Surg*. 2017;38:274–278.
32. Heit, JA., et al. Trends in the incidence of deep vein thrombosis and pulmonary embolism: a 35-year population-based study. *Blood*. 2006;108(11):1488.
33. Righini M, Galanaud J-P, Guenneguez H, et al. Anticoagulant therapy for symptomatic calf deep vein thrombosis (CACTUS): A randomised, double-blind, placebo-controlled trial. *Lancet Haematol*. 2016;3:e556–e562.
34. Robert-Ebadi H, Righini M. Should we diagnose and treat distal deep vein thr Current challenges in diagnosis of venous thromboembolism ombosis? *Hematology*. 2017:231–236.
35. Righini M, Paris S, Le Gal G, Laroche JP, Perrier A, Bounameaux H. Clinical relevance of distal deep vein thrombosis. Review of literature data. *Thromb Haemost*. 2006;95:56–64.
36. Frazee BW, Snoey ER, Levitt A. Emergency department compression ultrasound to diagnose proximal deep vein thrombosis. *J Emerg Med*. 2001;20:107–112.
37. Blaivas M, Lambert MJ, Harwood RA, et al. Lower-extremity Doppler for deep venous thrombosis—can emergency physicians be accurate and fast? *Acad Emerg Med*. 2000;7:120–125.

38. Jacoby J, et al. Can emergency medicine residents detect acute deep venous thrombosis with a limited, two-site ultrasound examination? *J Emerg Med*. 2007;32(2):197–200.
39. Jang T, et al. Resident-performed compression ultrasonography for the detection of proximal deep vein thrombosis: fast and accurate. *Academic Emerg Med*. 2004;11(3):319–322.
40. Bates SM, et al. Diagnosis of DVT: antithrombotic therapy and prevention of thrombosis: American College of Chest Physicians evidence-based clinical practice guidelines. *Chest*. 2012;141(2):e351S–e418S.
41. Bressollette L, Nonent M, Oger E, et al. Diagnostic accuracy of compression ultrasonography for the detection of asymptomatic deep venous thrombosis in medical patients: the TADEUS project. *Thromb Haemost*. 2001;86:529–533.
42. Garcia ND, Morasch MD, Ebaugh JL, et al. Is bilateral ultrasound scanning of the legs necessary for patients with unilateral symptoms of deep vein thrombosis? *J Vasc Surg*. 2001;34:792–797.
43. Strothman G, Blebea J, Fowl RJ, Rosenthal G. Contralateral duplex scanning for deep venous thrombosis is unnecessary in patients with symptoms. *J Vasc Surg*. 1995;22:543–547.
44. Le Gal G, et al. Is it useful to also image the asymptomatic leg in patients with suspected deep vein thrombosis? *J Thrombosis Haemost*. 2015;13(4):563–566.
45. Sheiman RG, McArdle CR. Bilateral lower extremity US in the patient with unilateral symptoms of deep venous thrombosis: assessment of need. *Radiology*. 1995;194:171–173.
46. Miller N, Obrand D, Tousignant L, et al. Venous duplex scanning for unilateral symptoms: When do we need a contralateral evaluation? *Eur J Vasc Endovasc Surg*. 1998;15:18–23.
47. Nix ML, Troillett RD, Nelson CL, et al. Is bilateral duplex examination necessary for unilateral symptoms of deep vein thrombosis? *J Vasc Tech*. 1991;15:296–298.
48. Love M, Blebea J, Strothman G, et al. Bilateral duplex scanning for deep venous thrombosis is unnecessary in symptomatic patients. *J Vasc Tech*. 1996;20:217–220.
49. Naidich JB, Torre JR, Pellerito JS, et al. Suspected deep venous thrombosis: is US of both legs necessary? *Radiology*. 1996;200:429–431.
50. Lohr JM, Hasselfeld KA, Byrne MP, et al. Does the asymptomatic limb harbor deep venous thrombosis? *Am J Surg*. 1994;168:184–187.
51. Prandoni P, Lensing AW, Piccioli A, et al. Ultrasonography of contralateral veins in patients with unilateral deep-vein thrombosis. *Lancet*. 1998;352:786.
52. Pennell RC, Mantese VA, Westfall SG. Duplex scan for deep vein thrombosis—defining who needs an examination of the contralateral asymptomatic leg. *J Vasc Surg*. 2008;48(2):413–416.
53. Sheiman RG, Weintraub JL, McArdle CR. Bilateral lower extremity US in the patient with bilateral symptoms of deep vein thrombosis: assessment of need. *Radiology*. 1995;196:379–381.
54. Lemech LD, Sandroussi C, Makeham V, et al. Is bilateral duplex scanning necessary in patients with symptoms of deep venous thrombosis? *Aust N Z J Surg*. 2004;74:847–851.
55. Beller E, et al. Prevalence and predictors of alternative diagnoses on whole-leg ultrasound negative for acute deep venous thrombosis. *BMC Med Imaging*. 2020;20(1):1–7.
56. Forbes K, Stevenson AJM. The use of power Doppler ultrasound in the diagnosis of isolated deep venous thrombosis of the calf. *Clin Radiol*. 1998;53:752–754.
57. Gottlieb RH, Widjaja J, Mehra S, et al. Clinically important pulmonary emboli: does calf vein US alter outcomes? *Radiology*. 1999;211:25–29.
58. Zhang Y, et al. The rate of missed diagnosis of lower-limb DVT by ultrasound amounts to 50% or so in patients without symptoms of DVT: A meta-analysis. *Medicine*. 2019;98(37).
59. Gottlieb RH, Voci SL, Syed L, et al. Randomized prospective study comparing routine versus selective use of sonography of the complete calf in patients with suspected deep venous thrombosis. *Am J Roentgenol*. 2003;180:241–245.
60. Gaitini D. Current approaches and controversial issues in the diagnosis of deep vein thrombosis via duplex Doppler ultrasound. *J Clin Ultrasound*. 2006;34:289–297.
61. Kearon C, Akl EW, Ornelas J, et al. Antithrombotic therapy for VTE disease. *Chest*. 2016;149:315–352.
62. Gunawansa N, Gunawardena T. Management of isolated distal deep vein thrombosis. A persistent conundrum? *Acta Angiologica*. 2020;26(2):65–71.
63. Sule AA, Chin TJ, Handa P, et al. Should symptomatic, isolated distal deep vein thrombosis be treated with anticoagulation? *Int J Angiology*. 2009;18:83.
64. Schwarz T, Schmidt B, Beyer J, et al. Therapy of isolated calf muscle vein thrombosis with low-molecular-weight heparin. *Blood Coagul Fibrinolysis*. 2001;12:597–599.
65. Schwarz T, Buschmann L, Beyer J, et al. Therapy of isolated calf muscle vein thrombosis: a randomized, controlled study. *J Vasc Surg*. 2010;52:1246–1250.
66. Palareti G, Cosmi B, Lessiani G, et al. Evolution of untreated calf deep-vein thrombosis in high risk symptomatic outpatients: the blind, prospective CALTHRO study. *Thromb Haemost*. 2010;104:1063–1070.
67. Robert-Ebadi H, Righini M. Management of distal deep vein thrombosis. *Thrombosis Res*. 2017;149:48–55.
68. Heller, T, et al. Isolated calf deep venous thrombosis: prevalence, clinical characteristics and implications for ultrasound evaluation. 2020. ResearchSquare.com.
69. Wang C, Wang J, Weng L, et al. Clinical significance of muscular deep-vein thrombosis after total knee arthroplasty. *Chang Gung Med J*. 2007;30:41.
70. Macdonald PS, Kahn SR, Miller N, et al. Short-term natural history of isolated gastrocnemius and soleal vein thrombosis. *J Vasc Surg*. 2003;37:523–527.
71. Nguyen KP, et al. Prospective study comparing the rate of deep venous thrombosis of complete and incomplete lower extremity venous duplex ultrasound examinations. *J Vasc Surg: Venous Lymphatic Disord*. 2019;7(6):882–888.
72. Henry JC, Satiani B. Calf muscle venous thrombosis a review of the clinical implications and therapy. *Vasc Endovasc Surg*. 2014;48:396–401.
73. Ohgi S, Tachibana M, Ikebuchi M, et al. Pulmonary embolism in patients with isolated soleal vein thrombosis. *Angiology*. 1998;49:759–764.
74. Krünes U, Teubner K, Knipp H, et al. Thrombosis of the muscular calf veins—reference to a syndrome which receives little attention. *VASA Z Gefasskrankheiten*. 1998;27:172–175.
75. García JP, et al. Comparison of the accuracy of emergency department-performed point-of-care-ultrasound (POCUS) in the diagnosis of lower-extremity deep vein thrombosis. *J Emerg Med*. 2018;54(5):656–664.
76. Ultrasound guidelines emergency, point-of-care and clinical ultrasound guidelines in medicine. *Ann Emerg Med*. 2017;69:e27–e54.
77. Langan EM, Coffey CB, Taylor SM, et al. The impact of the development of a program to reduce urgent (off-hours) venous duplex ultrasound scan studies. *J Vasc Surg*. 2002;36:132–136.
78. Adhikari S, et al. Isolated deep venous thrombosis: implications for 2-point compression ultrasonography of the lower extremity. *Ann Emerg Med*. 2015;66(3):262–266.
79. Farahmand S, et al. The accuracy of limited B-mode compression technique in diagnosing deep venous thrombosis in lower extremities. *Am J Emerg Med*. 2011;29(6):687–690.
80. Theodoro D, et al. Real-time B-mode ultrasound in the ED saves time in the diagnosis of deep vein thrombosis (DVT). *Am J Emerg Med*. 2004;22(3):197–200.
81. Kline JA, et al. Emergency clinician–performed compression ultrasonography for deep venous thrombosis of the lower extremity. *Ann Emerg Med*. 2008;52(4):437–441.
82. Lee JH, Sun HL, Seong JY. Comparison of 2-point and 3-point point-of-care ultrasound techniques for deep vein thrombosis at the emergency department: a meta-analysis. *Medicine*. 2019;98(22).

83. Rosen MP, Sheiman RG, Weintraub J, McArdle C. Compression sonography in patients with indeterminate or low probability lung scans: lack of usefulness in the absence of both symptoms of deep vein thrombosis and thromboembolic risk factors. *AJR Am J Roentgenol*. 1996;166:285–289.
84. Sheiman RG, McArdle CR. Clinically suspected pulmonary embolism: use of bilateral lower extremity US as the initial examination—a prospective study. *Radiology*. 1999;21:75–78.
85. Wang I, Davenport MS, Kazerooni EA. Imaging trends in acute venous thromboembolic disease: 2000 to 2015. *J Am Coll Radiology*. 2017;14(9):1151–1160.
86. Fard MN, Mostaan M, Zahed Pour Anaraki MR. Utility of lower-extremity duplex sonography in patients with venous thromboembolism. *J Clin Ultrasound*. 2001;29:92–98.

PART VII

Gynecology

Chapter 41 Normal Anatomy and Physiology of the Female Pelvis
Chapter 42 Sonographic and Doppler Evaluation of the Female Pelvis
Chapter 43 Pathology of the Uterus
Chapter 44 Pathology of the Ovaries
Chapter 45 Pathology of the Adnexa
Chapter 46 Role of Ultrasound in Evaluating Female Infertility

CHAPTER 41

Normal Anatomy and Physiology of the Female Pelvis

Sandra L. Hagen-Ansert

OBJECTIVES

On completion of this chapter, you should be able to:
- Name the major landmarks of the bony pelvis and external genitalia
- Identify the sonographically significant muscles of the pelvic cavity
- Describe the pelvic organs and their functions
- Describe the major ligaments of the uterus and ovaries
- Discuss the physiology of the menstrual cycle and describe hormonal changes that occur during the various ovulatory and endometrial phases
- Describe the development of the ovum and its passage from the ovary into the uterus
- Define the function of the corpus luteum

OUTLINE

Pelvic Landmarks 1159
    External Landmarks 1159
    The Bony Pelvis 1159
    The Pelvic Cavity and Perineum 1160
Muscles of the Pelvis 1160
    The Abdominal Wall 1161
    Muscles of the False Pelvis 1161
    Muscles of the True Pelvis 1161
Bladder and Ureters 1161
Vagina 1162

Uterus 1162
    Normal Anatomy 1162
    Endometrium 1165
    Uterine Ligaments 1165
    Positions of the Uterus 1166
Fallopian Tubes 1167
Ovaries 1167
    Position and Size of the Ovaries 1167
    Normal Anatomy 1168
    Ovarian Ligaments 1169

Pelvic Vasculature 1169
Physiology 1170
    The Menstrual Cycle 1170
    Follicular Development and Ovulation 1170
    Endometrial Changes 1172
    Abnormal Menstrual Cycles 1174
Pelvic Recesses and Bowel 1174

KEY TERMS

Amenorrhea
Anteflexed
Anteverted
Broad ligaments
Cardinal ligament
Coccygeus muscles
Corpus luteum
Dysmenorrhea
Estrogen
False pelvis
Follicle-stimulating hormone (FSH)
Gonadotropin
Gonadotropin-releasing hormone (GnRH)
Iliacus muscles
Iliopectineal line

Levator ani
Luteinizing hormone (LH)
Menarche
Menopause
Menorrhagia
Menses
Mesosalpinx
Mesovarium
Obturator internus muscles
Oligomenorrhea
Oocyte
Ovarian ligaments
Ovum
Perimetrium
Piriformis muscles
Polymenorrhea

Premenarche
Progesterone
Psoas major muscle
Rectouterine recess (pouch)
Retroflexed
Retroverted
Round ligaments
Space of Retzius
Striations
Suspensory (infundibulopelvic) ligament
True pelvis
Uterosacral ligament
Vesicouterine recess (pouch)

Understanding the anatomy and physiology of the female genital organs is important for understanding the pathophysiology of the female pelvis. Many pelvic landmarks, ligaments, and muscular structures within the pelvis are important to know in order to differentiate normal reproductive organs from muscular and vascular structures (Fig. 41.1). This chapter presents a discussion of the normal anatomy and physiology of the female genital organs. The sonographer needs to know the significant muscular structures and pelvic ligaments because a basic understanding of these structures is essential for performing an adequate pelvic ultrasound examination.

Two approaches are used to evaluate the female pelvis sonographically: transabdominal and transvaginal. A transabdominal approach requires a full urinary bladder for use as an acoustic window and typically necessitates the use of a 3.5 to 5 MHz transducer for adequate penetration. A transvaginal examination performed with an empty bladder allows the use of a higher-frequency transducer, typically 7.5 to 10 MHz. It is generally recommended that a complete pelvic examination should consist of a transabdominal scan followed by a transvaginal examination. The transabdominal scan offers a wider field of view for a general screening of the pelvic anatomy. The transvaginal examination will usually offer a more detailed study of the pelvic structures and organs but is limited in its field of view and depth of penetration. The approach used will depend on the patient's age and sexual status. Transvaginal examinations are typically contraindicated in minors who are not sexually active. Transvaginal examinations are not contraindicated for the non–sexually active adult female who has had a previous gynecologic examination or has used tampons and consents to the procedure.

When using a transabdominal scanning technique, a distended urinary bladder is optimal. An adequately filled bladder will tilt the uterus posteriorly and push the bowel up and out of the pelvic cavity into the lower abdominal cavity, making visualization of the uterine fundus and adnexa easier. An overly distended bladder, on the other hand, will often push the uterus too far posteriorly, making the pelvic structures difficult to see. An overdistended bladder may also cause compression and distortion of the pelvic organs. If the bladder appears overly distended, throwing the pelvic structures too deep, it may be necessary to have the patient partially or fully void. Because overdistention can alter the true lie of the pelvic organs, it is advised to look at the pelvis from a variety of windows—full, empty, and transvaginally—before making a final assessment.

When transvaginal ultrasound is used to evaluate the pelvic structures, the patient should empty her bladder completely before the transvaginal transducer is inserted into the vaginal canal. With the urinary bladder empty, the uterus and iliac vessels become the primary landmarks used to evaluate and image the pelvic organs.

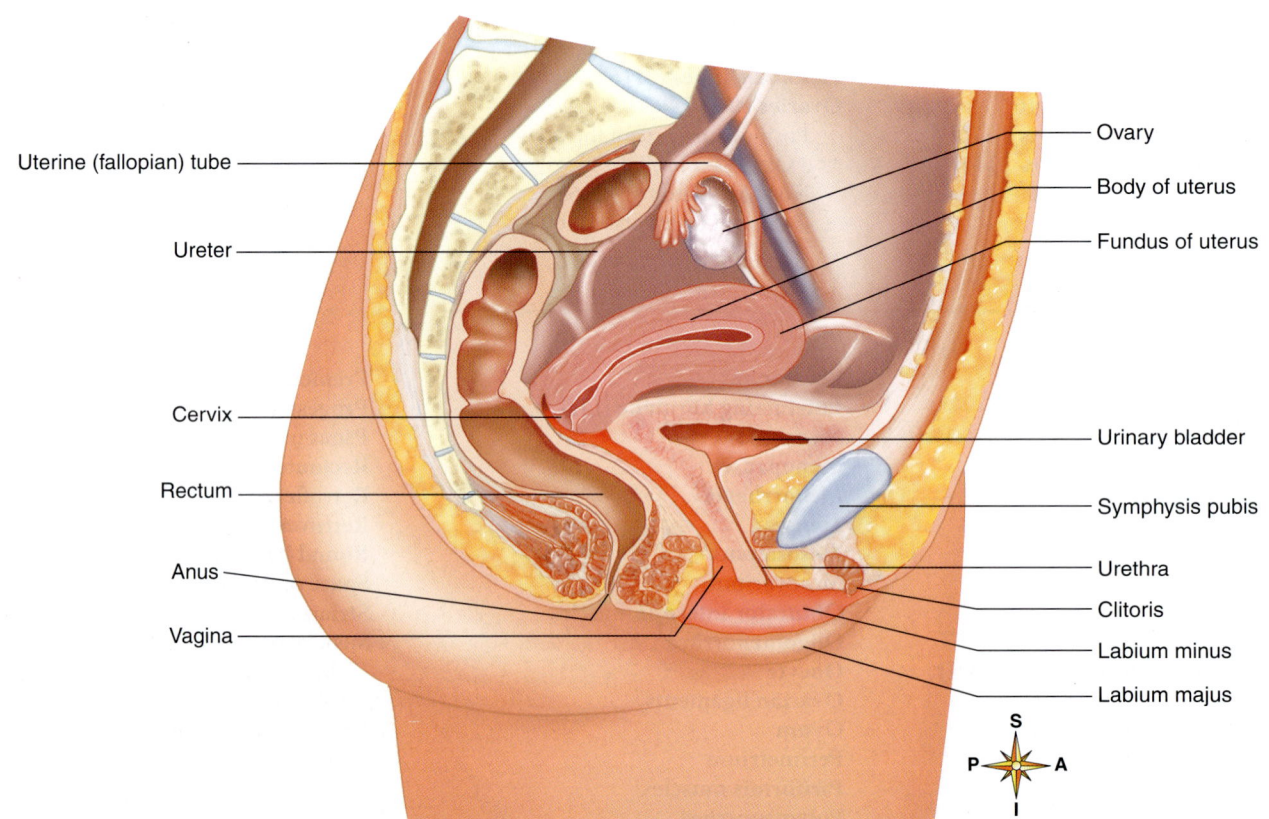

FIG. 41.1 Many pelvic landmarks, ligaments, and muscular structures within the pelvis are important to know in order to differentiate normal reproductive organs from muscular and vascular structures.

PELVIC LANDMARKS

External Landmarks

The external genitalia in the female, also known as the *vulva* or the *pudendum*, consist of the mons pubis, labia majora, labia minora, clitoris, urethral opening, and vestibule of the vagina (Fig. 41.2A). The vagina itself is the part of the female genitalia that forms a canal from the orifice through the vestibule to the uterine cervix. It is behind the bladder and in front of the rectum. These external structures are important to recognize when using translabial and transvaginal scanning techniques. The mons pubis is a pad of fatty tissue and thick skin that overlies the symphysis pubis and is covered by pubic hair after puberty. The labia are folds of skin at the opening of the vagina, with labia majora being the thicker external folds and labia minora being the thin folds of skin between the labia majora. The clitoris is located anterior to the urethra and is usually partially hidden between the labia majora. Posterior to the clitoris, the urethral opening and vestibule of the vagina can normally be identified between the labia minora. The most posterior orifice is the anus.

The Bony Pelvis

The bony pelvis consists of four bones: two innominate (coxal) bones, the sacrum, and the coccyx. The innominate bones make up the anterior and lateral margins of the bony pelvis, and the sacrum and coccyx form the posterior wall. Anatomically, the pelvis is divided into two continuous compartments (true and false pelvis) by an oblique plane that passes through the pelvic brim. (Fig. 41.2B) This plane of division passes from the superior border of the sacrum to the superior margin of the pubic symphysis and corresponds to the **iliopectineal line** (Fig. 41.2C). The **false pelvis**, also known as the greater or major pelvis, is located above the

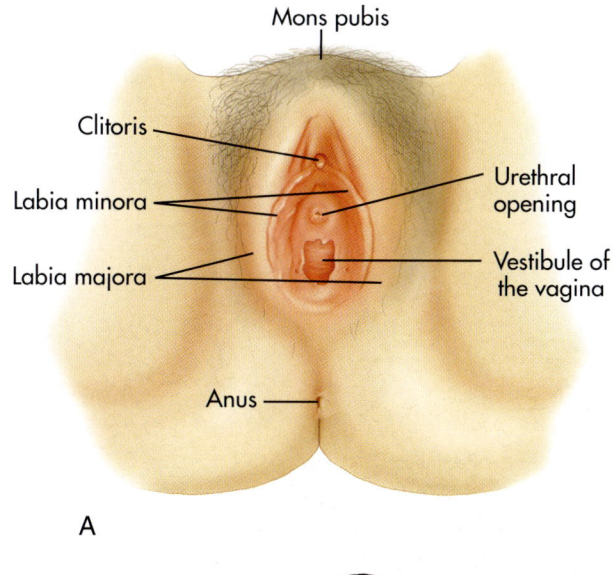

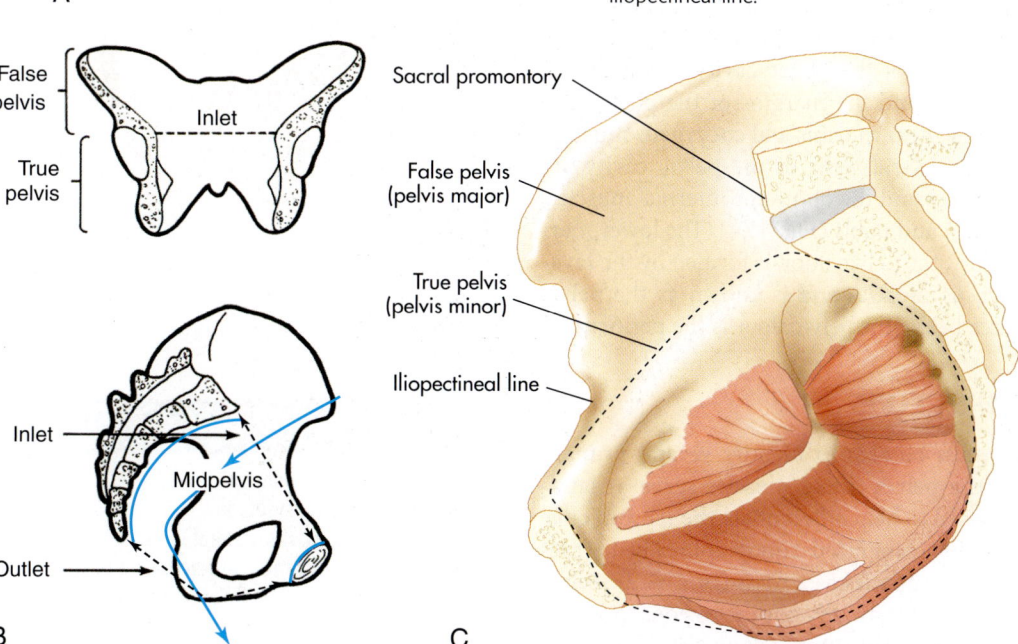

FIG. 41.2 (A) The external genitalia in the female, also known as the *vulva* or the *pudendum*, consist of the mons pubis, labia majora, labia minora, clitoris, urethral opening, and vestibule of the vagina. (B) Anatomically, the pelvis is divided into two continuous compartments (true and false pelvis) by an oblique plane that passes through the pelvic brim. (C) This plane of division passes from the superior border of the sacrum to the superior margin of the pubic symphysis and corresponds to the iliopectineal line.

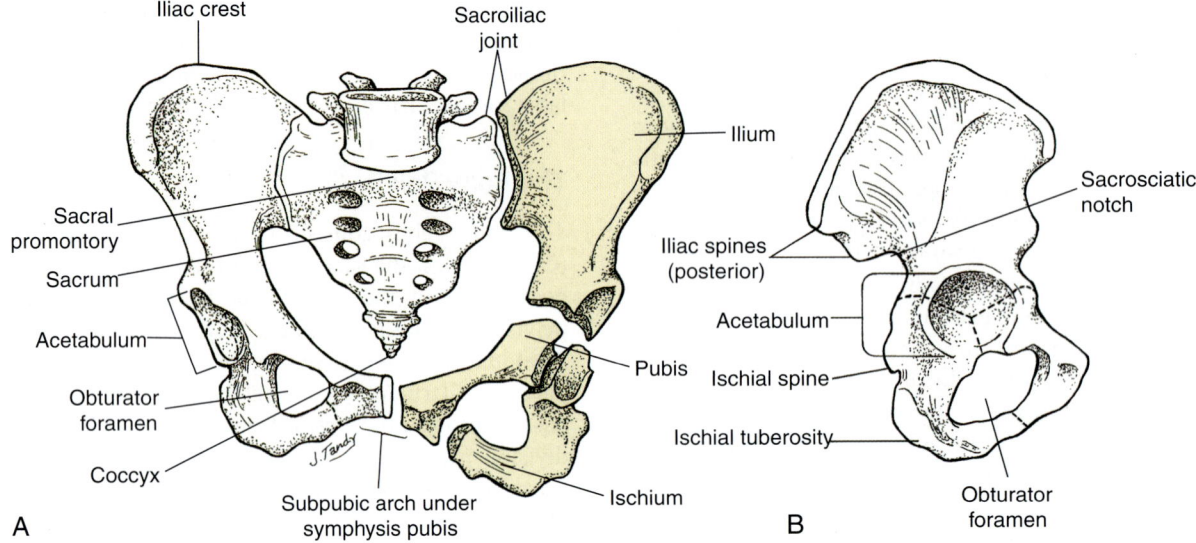

FIG. 41.3 The posterior wall of the pelvic cavity is formed by the sacrum and coccyx, and the margins of the posterolateral wall are formed by the piriformis and coccygeus muscles. The anterolateral walls of the pelvic cavity are formed by the hip bones and the obturator internus muscles, which rim the ischium and pubis.

BOX 41.1 Pelvic Cavity

- Posterior: occupied by rectum, colon, and ileum
- Anterior: occupied by bladder, ureters, ovaries, fallopian tubes, uterus, and vagina

---

brim. The false pelvis communicates with the abdominal cavity superiorly and with the pelvic cavity inferiorly. The **true pelvis**, also known as the lesser or minor pelvis, is the area below the pelvic brim.

The Pelvic Cavity and Perineum

The true pelvis, situated inferior to the caudal portion of the parietal peritoneum, is considered the pelvic cavity (Box 41.1). The posterior wall of the pelvic cavity is formed by the sacrum and coccyx, and the margins of the posterolateral wall are formed by the piriformis and **coccygeus muscles** (Fig. 41.3). The anterolateral walls of the pelvic cavity are formed by the hip bones and the obturator internus muscles, which rim the ischium and pubis (Fig. 41.4). The lower margin of the pelvic cavity, the pelvic floor, is formed by the **levator ani** and coccygeus muscles and is known as the pelvic diaphragm. The area below the pelvic floor is the perineum.

MUSCLES OF THE PELVIS

The sonographer must be able to identify several primary muscle groups in the pelvis. These muscles serve as landmarks that may be used to help differentiate the reproductive organs and should be recognized sonographically to prevent misidentifying the muscles as a mass (Box 41.2). Pelvic muscles vary in shape but typically appear hypoechoic with characteristic hyperechoic **striations** when viewed in their

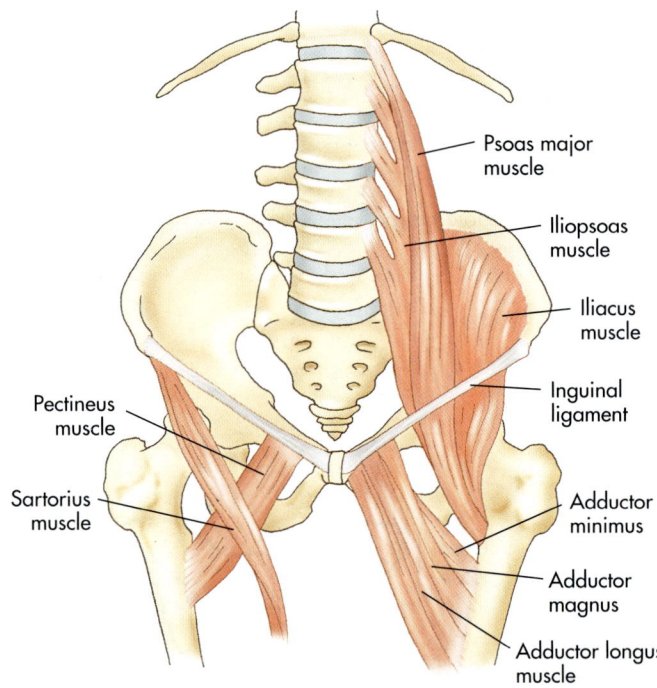

FIG. 41.4 Anterior diagram of the psoas major muscle extending from the abdominal cavity into the false pelvis. The iliacus muscle joins the psoas muscle to form the iliopsoas muscle along the sidewall of the false pelvis.

BOX 41.2 Pelvic Muscles

- Psoas major: pelvic sidewall
- Iliacus: pelvic sidewall
- Piriformis: posterolateral wall
- Obturator internus: anterolateral pelvic sidewall
- Levator ani: pelvic floor (diaphragm)
- Coccygeus: posterior pelvic floor (diaphragm)

long axis. The pelvic muscles are easiest to locate and identify sonographically if classified by region. The major pelvic muscles can be differentiated as muscles of the abdominal wall, those running through the false pelvis, and those found within the true pelvis.

The Abdominal Wall

The muscles of the anterior abdominal wall extend superiorly from the xiphoid process to the symphysis pubis inferiorly. These muscles include the paired rectus abdominis muscles anteriorly and the external oblique, internal oblique, and transversus abdominis muscles anterolaterally.

Muscles of the False Pelvis

Muscles of the false pelvis include the psoas major and iliacus muscles (see Fig. 41.4). The **psoas major muscles** originate at the transverse process of the lumbar vertebrae and descend inferiorly through the false pelvis on the pelvic sidewalls. In the false pelvis, they join with the **iliacus muscles** to form the iliopsoas muscles. The iliopsoas muscles pass anterior to the hip and insert into the lesser trochanters on the posterior aspect of the femurs. Note that the iliopsoas muscles pass outside the pelvic bones and do not enter the true pelvis.

Muscles of the True Pelvis

The muscles found within the true pelvis include the piriformis muscles, obturator internus muscles, and muscles of the pelvic diaphragm (Fig. 41.5). The **piriformis muscles** are flat, triangular muscles that arise from the anterior sacrum and pass through the greater sciatic notch on the posterior aspect of the innominate bone to insert into the superior aspect of the greater trochanter of the femur. The **obturator internus muscles** are triangular sheets of muscle that arise from the anterolateral pelvic wall and surround the obturator foramen. They pass out of the pelvic cavity through the lesser sciatic foramen, where they insert into the superior aspect of the greater trochanter of the femur. The pelvic diaphragm is formed by the levator ani and coccygeus muscles and makes up the floor of the true pelvis (see Fig. 41.5C). The levator ani is a group of three muscles that extend across the pelvic floor like a hammock. This group of muscles consists of the pubococcygeus muscles, the iliococcygeus muscles, and the puborectalis muscles. The pubococcygeus muscles are the most anterior and medial of the three levator ani muscles. They extend from the pubic bones anteriorly to the coccyx posteriorly and surround the urethra, vagina, and rectum. The iliococcygeus muscles extend from the anterolateral pelvic wall to the coccyx posteriorly. The puborectalis muscles arise from the lower part of the pubic symphysis and surround the lower part of the rectum, forming a sling. The levator ani, in addition to forming the floor of the pelvis, has an important role in rectal and urinary continence.

BLADDER AND URETERS

The urinary bladder is located in the anterior portion of the pelvic cavity, posterior to the pubic symphysis

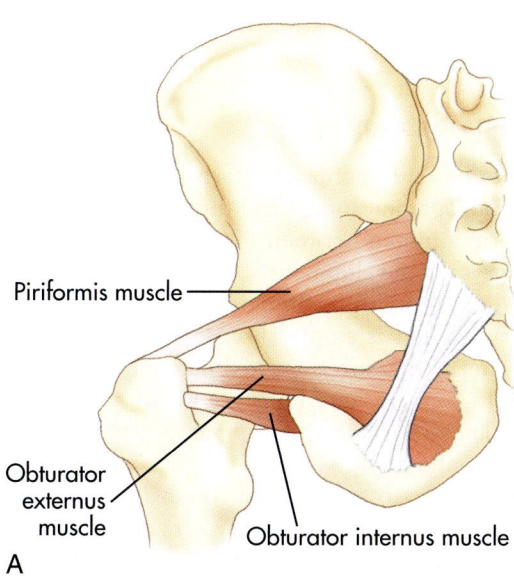

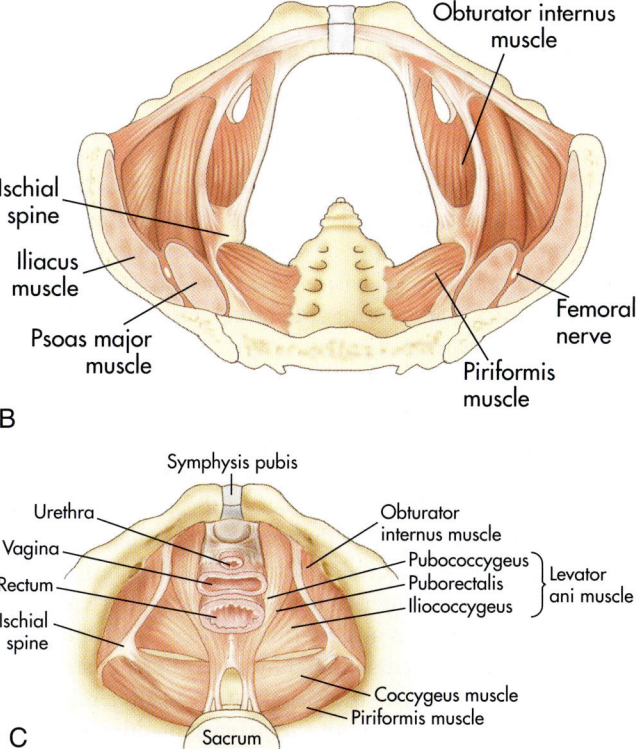

FIG. 41.5 (A) Posterior view of the piriformis and obturator internus muscles. (B) Pelvic cavity viewed from above. The piriformis and obturator internus muscles pass out from the pelvis through the sciatic foramina to attach to the greater tuberosity of the femur. (C) The floor of the pelvis is formed by the coccygeus and levator ani muscles (as viewed from above).

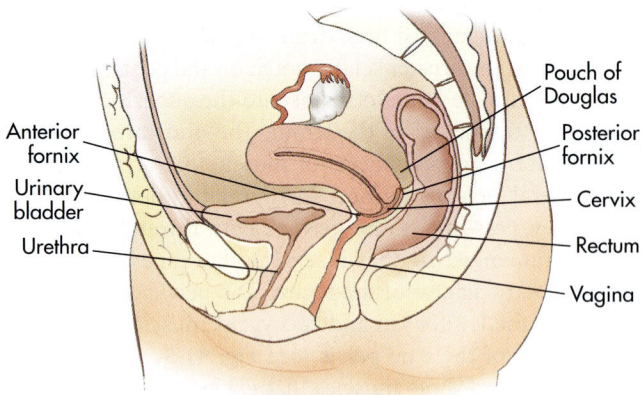

FIG. 41.6 Lateral view of the pelvis demonstrating the relationship of the anterior and posterior fornices to the cervix and vagina.

BOX 41.3 Bladder

- Apex: located posterior to pubic bones
- Base: anterior to vagina, superior surface related to uterus
- Neck: rests on upper surface of urogenital diaphragm; inferolateral surfaces relate to retropubic fat, obturator internus, levator ani muscles, and pubic bone

---

BOX 41.4 Ureters

- Cross the pelvic inlet anterior to bifurcation of common iliac arteries
- Run anterior to internal iliac arteries and posterior to the ovaries
- Run anteriorly and medially under the base of the broad ligament, where they are crossed by the uterine artery
- Run anterior and lateral to the upper vagina to enter the posteroinferior bladder

---

(Fig. 41.6 and Box 41.3). The function of the bladder is to collect and store urine until it empties through the urethra. When the bladder is empty or only slightly filled, it remains entirely within the true pelvis; as it becomes distended, it rises up behind the lower anterior abdominal wall and pushes the peritoneum away from the wall.

The ureters are the two tubes that carry urine from the kidneys to the urinary bladder (Box 41.4). As the ureters descend inferiorly from the kidneys, they run anteriorly and medially, passing anterior to the psoas major muscles, behind the peritoneum, and along the lateral aspect of the cervix and upper portion of the vagina, where they enter the bladder at the trigone (Fig. 41.7). As the ureters descend from the retroperitoneal cavity, they pass anterior to the internal iliac arteries and posterior to the ovaries and uterine arteries. The ureters are not normally visualized sonographically (unless obstructed) but may be identified by the visualization of ureteral jets in the posteroinferior portion of the urinary bladder as it fills. The ureteral jets are identified by a swirling of urine, which is easily identified with color Doppler. The urinary bladder and ureters are discussed in detail in Chapter 15. Pregnancy, uterine fibroids, ovarian masses, or distal ureteral calculi can lead to compression and dilation of the ureters, resulting in hydronephrosis.

VAGINA

The vagina is a collapsed muscular tube that extends from the external genitalia to the cervix of the uterus. It lies posterior to the urinary bladder and urethra and anterior to the rectum and anus (Fig. 41.8). It is normally directed upward and backward, forming a 90-degree angle with the uterine cervix. It measures approximately 9 cm in length and is longest along its posterior wall (Box 41.5). The vaginal canal is a potential space in which the anterior and posterior walls usually touch. It is the passageway for the products of menstruation and is easily distended during sexual intercourse and childbirth. The vagina has a mucous membrane lining its muscular walls. This membrane receives secretions from the vaginal wall, the mucous glands of the cervix (around ovulation), and the vestibular glands of the vagina (during sexual excitement).

The uterine cervix protrudes into the upper portion of the vaginal canal, forming four archlike recesses called *fornices* (Fig. 41.9). The posterior vaginal wall attaches higher on the cervix, and the fornices are blind pockets formed by the inner surface of the vaginal walls and the outer surface of the cervix. It is a continuous ring-shaped space with the posterior fornix running deeper than its anterior counterpart. This design eases the use of the transvaginal probe and concomitant visualization of the cervix and uterus.

UTERUS

Normal Anatomy

The uterus and vagina are derived from the embryonic müllerian (paramesonephric) ducts as they elongate, fuse, and form a lumen between the seventh and twelfth weeks of embryonic development. The uterus is pear shaped and is the largest organ in the normal female pelvis when the urinary bladder is empty (Box 41.6). The average menarcheal uterus measures approximately 6 to 8 cm in length and 3 to 5 cm in anteroposterior and transverse dimensions. The size of the uterus varies with age and parity (Box 41.7 and Table 41.1).

The uterus consists of a fundus, body, and cervix (Fig. 41.10). The fundus is the widest and most superior portion of the uterus. At the lateral borders of the fundus are the cornua, where the fallopian tubes enter the uterine cavity. The body, or corpus (Box 41.8), lies between the fundus and the cervix and is the largest portion of the uterus. The uterine cavity is centrally located within the pelvis and is a potential space for fluid to accumulate, allowing for dynamic changes during the menstrual cycle and pregnancy. The cervix (Box 41.9) is the lower cylindrical portion of the uterus

CHAPTER 41 Normal Anatomy and Physiology of the Female Pelvis

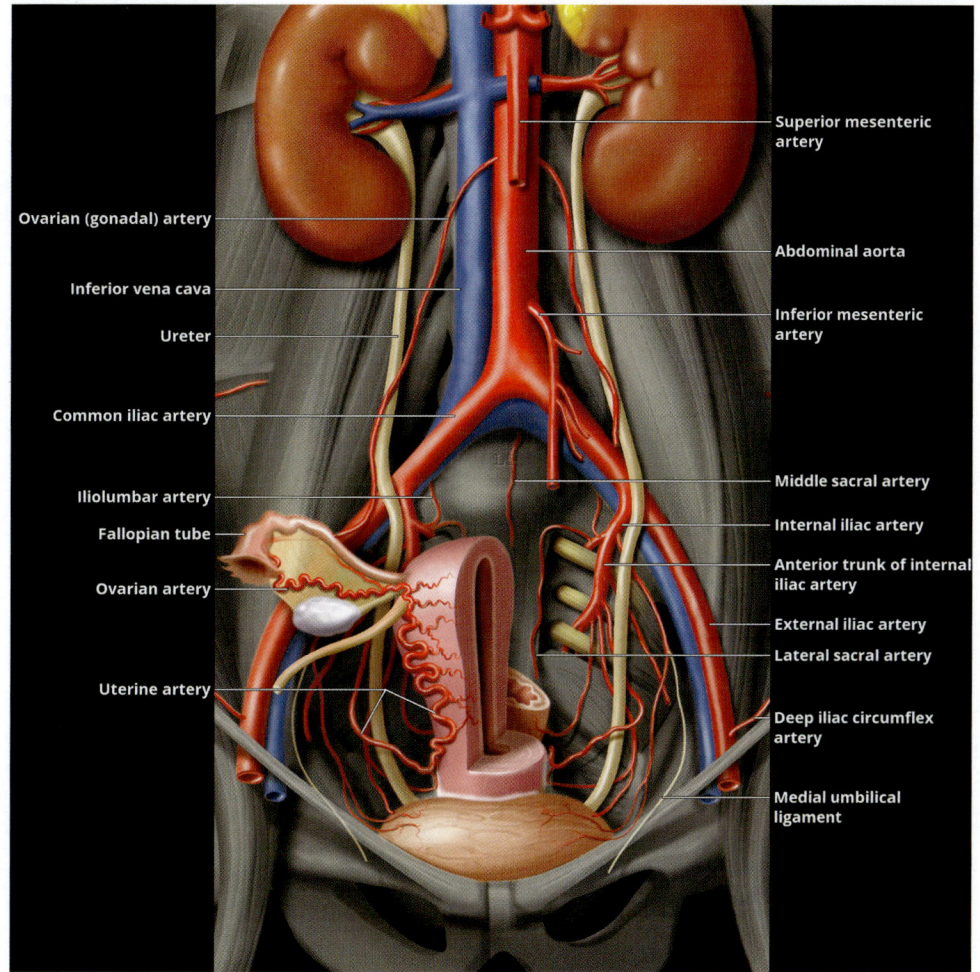

FIG. 41.7 The ureters are the two tubes that carry urine from the kidneys to the urinary bladder. As the ureters descend inferiorly from the kidneys, they run anteriorly and medially, passing anterior to the psoas major muscles, behind the peritoneum, and along the lateral aspect of the cervix and upper portion of the vagina, where they enter the bladder at the trigone. As the ureters descend from the retroperitoneal cavity, they pass anterior to the internal iliac arteries and posterior to the ovaries and uterine arteries.

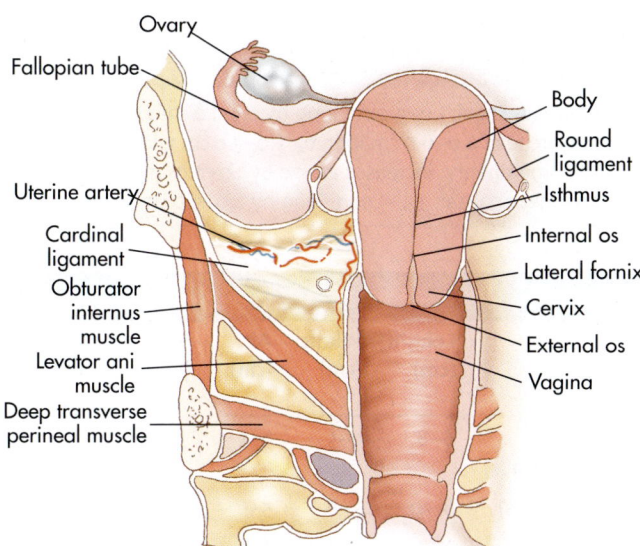

FIG. 41.8 Coronal view of the vagina, cervix, and uterus. The vagina is a collapsed muscular tube that extends from the external genitalia to the cervix of the uterus. It lies posterior to the urinary bladder and urethra and anterior to the rectum and anus.

BOX 41.5	Vagina

- Extends upward and backward from the vulva
- Upper half lies above pelvic floor
- Lower half lies within perineum
- Area of vaginal lumen surrounding the cervix is divided into four fornices
- Arterial supply is from vaginal and uterine arteries; drains into the internal iliac vein

that projects into the vaginal canal (Fig. 41.11). The surface of the cervix is divided into an exocervix and an endocervix (see Fig. 41.10). The exocervix is a squamous epithelium continuous with the vagina. The surface of the endocervix is made up of columnar cells, which excrete mucus. The cervix is constricted at its upper end by the internal os and at its lower end by the external os. The isthmus is the outer transition point between the body of the uterus and the cervix. This is the point where the uterus bends anteriorly (anteversion) or posteriorly (retroversion) with an empty bladder.

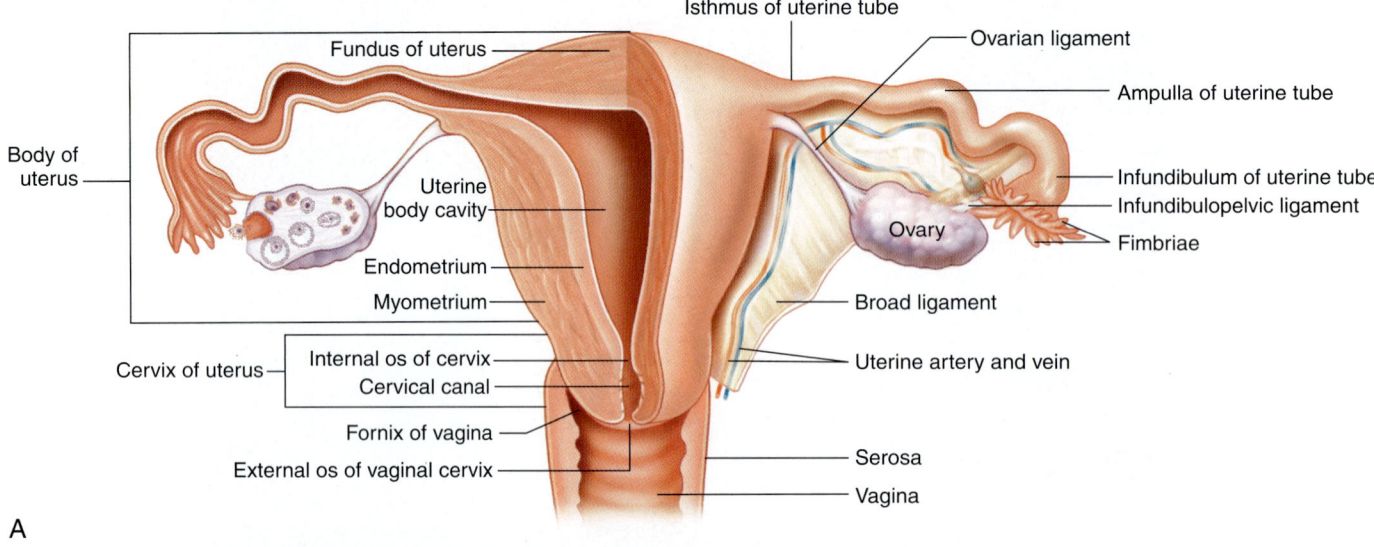

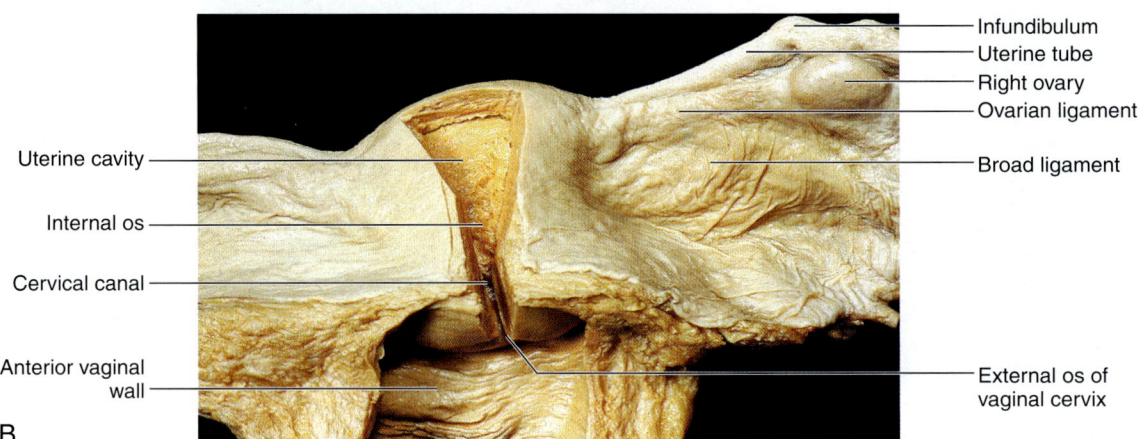

FIG. 41.9 The uterine cervix protrudes into the upper portion of the vaginal canal, forming four archlike recesses called *fornices.*

BOX 41.6 Uterus

- Hollow, pear-shaped organ
- Divided into fundus, body, and cervix
- Usually anteflexed and anteverted
- Covered with peritoneum except anteriorly below the os, where peritoneum is reflected onto bladder
- Supported by levator ani muscles, cardinal ligaments, and uterosacral ligaments
- Round ligaments hold uterus in anteverted position

BOX 41.7 Uterine Size

- Premenarcheal: 1.0–3.0 cm long by 0.5–1.0 cm wide
- Menarcheal: 6.0–8.0 cm long by 3.0–5.0 cm wide
- With multiparity: increases in size by 1.0–2.0 cm
- Postmenopausal: 3.5–5.5 cm long by 2.0–3.0 cm wide

TABLE 41.1 Uterine Size

	Length (cm)	Width (cm)	AP (cm)	Volume (mL)	Cervix/Corpus Ratio
Adult (nulliparous)	6–8	3–5	3–5	30–40	1:2
Adult (parous)	8–10	5–6	5–6	60–80	1:2
Postmenopausal	3–5	2–3	2–3	14–17	1:1

AP, Anteroposterior.
From Standring S, ed. Gray's Anatomy. New York: Churchill Livingstone; 2009.

The uterine wall consists of three histologic layers: the serosa or **perimetrium**, the myometrium, and the endometrium. The external layer, the serosa, reflects on the anterior surface of the uterus at the isthmus. The muscular middle layer, the myometrium, is the thickest layer of the uterus and is primarily a smooth muscle that is longitudinal and circular (Box 41.10). The mucous membrane, glandular tissue lining the uterine cavity is the endometrium.

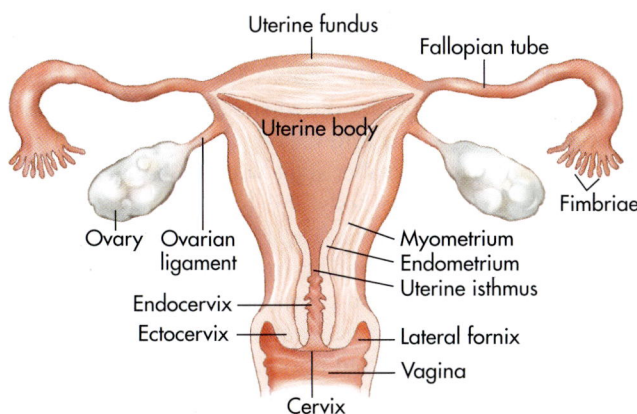

FIG. 41.10 The uterus consists of a fundus, body, and cervix. The fundus is the widest and most superior portion of the uterus. At the lateral borders of the fundus are the cornua, where the fallopian tubes enter the uterine cavity. The body, or corpus, lies between the fundus and the cervix and is the largest portion of the uterus.

BOX 41.8	Body of the Uterus

- Posterior to the vesicouterine pouch and the superior surface of the bladder
- Anterior to the rectouterine pouch (of Douglas), the ilium, and the colon
- Medial to the broad ligaments and uterine vessels
- Uterine cavity is funnel shaped in coronal plane; "slitlike" in sagittal plane

BOX 41.9	Cervix

- Projects into vaginal canal
- Endocervix: cervical canal; communicates with uterine cavity by the internal os; the vagina by the external os
- Exocervix: continuous with the vagina

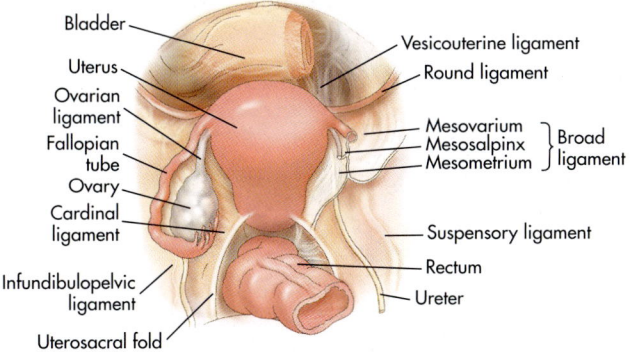

FIG. 41.11 The uterus is supported in its midline position by paired broad ligaments, round ligaments, uterosacral ligaments, and cardinal ligaments.

Endometrium

The endometrium consists primarily of two layers: the superficial functional layer (zona functionalis) and the deep basal layer (zona basalis). The functional layer is a superficial layer of glands and stroma (supporting tissue) that sheds with

BOX 41.10	Layers of the Uterus

- Perimetrium: serous outer layer of the uterus; serosa
- Myometrium: muscular middle layer of the uterus composed of thick, smooth muscle supported by connective tissue
- Endometrium: inner mucous membrane, glandular portion of the uterine body

BOX 41.11	Uterine Ligaments

- Broad: lateral aspect of uterus to pelvic sidewall
- Mesovarium: posterior fold of the broad ligament; encloses the ovary
- Mesosalpinx: upper fold of the broad ligament; encloses the fallopian tube
- Round: fundus to anterior pelvic sidewalls; hold uterus forward
- Cardinal: extend across the pelvic floor laterally; firmly support the cervix
- Uterosacral: extend from uterine isthmus downward, alongside the rectum to the sacrum; firmly support the cervix
- Suspensory: extend from lateral aspect of ovary to the pelvic sidewall
- Ovarian: extend medially from the ovary to the uterine cornua

menses. The basal layer is a thin layer of the blind ends of endometrial glands that regenerates a new endometrium after menses. The endometrium changes dynamically in response to the cyclic hormonal flux of ovulation and varies in sonographic appearance and histologic structure, depending on the patient's menstrual status and the period of life in which it is studied.

Uterine Ligaments

The uterus is supported in its midline position by paired broad ligaments, round ligaments, uterosacral ligaments, and cardinal ligaments (Fig. 41.11 and Box 41.11). The **broad ligaments** are a double fold of peritoneum that drapes over the fallopian tubes, uterus, and ovaries (Fig. 41.12). They extend from the lateral sides of the uterus to the sidewalls of the pelvis. The broad ligaments provide a small amount of support for the uterus and contain the uterine blood vessels and nerves. The upper fold of the broad ligament, known as the **mesosalpinx**, encloses the fallopian tube as it extends from the cornua of the uterus. The posterior portion of the broad ligament that is drawn out to enclose the ovary is the **mesovarium**.

The **round ligaments** are fibrous cords that occur in front of and below the fallopian tubes between the layers of the broad ligaments. These two cords commence on each side of the superior aspect of the uterus, course upward and lateral to the inguinal canal, insert into the labia majora, and help to hold the uterine fundus and body in a forward position. The cervix is the only portion of the uterus that is firmly supported. It is fixed in position by the **cardinal ligament** and uterosacral ligament. The cardinal ligaments are a continuation of the broad ligaments that extend across the pelvic floor laterally. The uterosacral ligaments originate at the lateral uterine isthmus and extend downward along the sides of the rectum to the third and fourth bones of the sacrum.

Positions of the Uterus

The position of the uterus is variable. The average uterine position is considered to be anteverted and anteflexed. The uterine position is described as **anteverted** when the cervical canal forms a 90-degree or smaller angle with the vaginal canal and as **anteflexed** when the body and fundus of the uterus are curved forward on the cervix (Fig. 41.13 and Box 41.12). In the nulliparous female, the round ligaments help to hold the uterus in an anteverted, anteflexed position. In multiparous females, the entire uterus may tip backward rather than forward and is described as a **retroverted** position. The term *retroverted* is used to describe the uterine position when the cervical canal forms an angle less than 90 degrees with the vaginal canal.

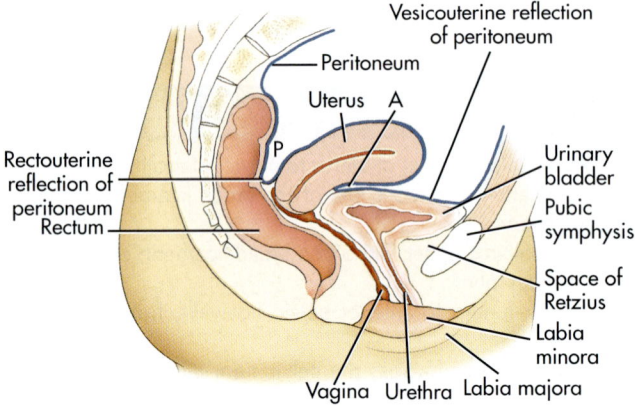

FIG. 41.12 The peritoneum drapes over the uterine fundus and body to divide the pelvis into anterior *(A)* and posterior *(P)* sections. The peritoneum extends laterally from the uterus, forming the broad ligaments and creating the mesosalpinx as it folds over the fallopian tubes. The mesovarium is another fold of the peritoneum, which forms posterior to the broad ligament as it folds over the ovary.

BOX 41.12	Uterine Positions

- Anteversion: most common position; fundus and body bent forward toward the cervix (degree of anteversion is dependent on bladder distention)
- Dextroversion or levoversion: normal variant in absence of pelvic masses
- Retroversion: entire uterus tilted posteriorly
- Retroflexion: fundus and body bent backward toward the cervix

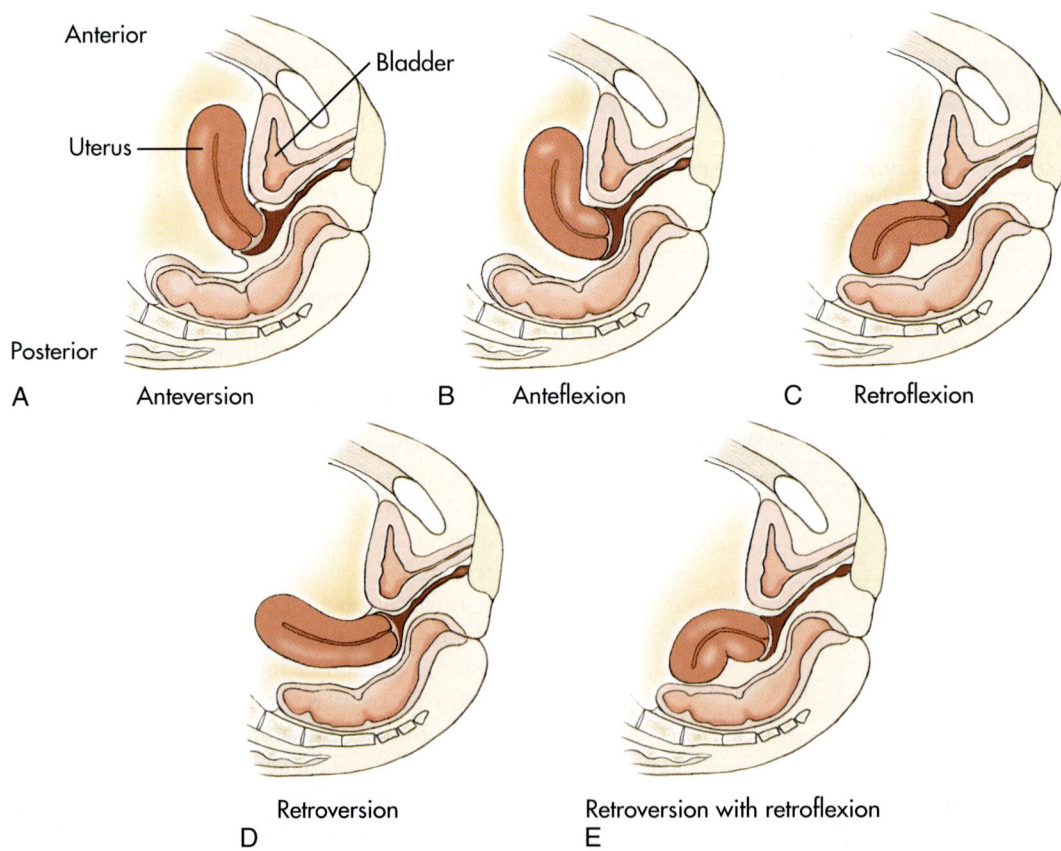

FIG. 41.13 The uterus may be found in one of several positions: (A) anteversion (entire uterus tipped forward); (B) anteflexion (body and fundus folded anteriorly toward the cervix); (C) retroflexion (body and fundus folded posteriorly on the cervix); (D) retroversion (entire uterus tilted backward); (E) retroversion with retroflexion (entire uterus tilted backward with fundus and body folded posteriorly on the cervix).

The uterine fundus or body may also curve backward on the cervix, and this position is described as **retroflexed**. It is not uncommon to see a uterus that has variations of version and flexion. For example, a common variation from the average uterine position is retroverted and retroflexed. Another variation from the normal uterine position is for the entire uterus to tilt to the right (dextro) or to the left (levo) of midline. Abnormal dropping of the uterus (uterine prolapse) occurs if the uterine ligaments and pelvic floor muscles are weak, allowing the uterus to protrude into the vagina. It is also important to recognize that filling of the bladder will affect uterine position. A full urinary bladder will tip the average anteverted, anteflexed uterus backward.

FALLOPIAN TUBES

The fallopian tubes, or oviducts, are coiled, muscular tubes that open into the peritoneal cavity at their lateral end. They are approximately 10 to 12 cm in length and 1 to 4 mm in diameter (Box 41.13). The fallopian tubes lie superior to the utero-ovarian ligaments, round ligaments, and tubo-ovarian blood vessels. They are contained in the upper margin of the broad ligament and extend from the cornua of the uterus laterally, where they curve over the ovary.

The fallopian tubes are divided into four anatomic portions (Fig. 41.14): infundibulum (lateral segment), ampulla (middle segment), isthmus (medial segment), and interstitial portion (segment that passes through the uterine cornua).

The interstitial portion is the narrowest segment of the fallopian tube. The tube widens as it extends laterally, with the infundibulum being the wide, trumpet-shaped, lateral portion. The infundibulum is often referred to as the fimbriated end of the fallopian tube because it contains fringelike extensions, called *fimbriae*, that move over the ovary, directing the ovum into the fallopian tube after ovulation. The ampulla is the longest and most coiled portion of the fallopian tube and is the area in which fertilization of the ovum most often occurs because it is the most distensible region of the tube. The innermost region of the fallopian tube, with its mucosal layer, runs directly into the mucosal layer of the uterus (the endometrium). The continuous nature of the endometrium and the endocervical canal can act as a pathway for organisms, infection, and hemorrhage because it is the most distensible.

The normal fallopian tubes are difficult to distinguish sonographically from surrounding ligaments and vessels. Doppler interrogation may help differentiate prominent blood vessels from the fallopian tubes.

OVARIES

Position and Size of the Ovaries

The ovaries are almond-shaped structures, measuring approximately 3 cm long in a menarcheal female (Table 41.2 and Box 41.14). They usually lie posterior to the uterus at the level of the cornua (Fig. 41.15). They are suspended from the posterior aspect of the broad ligament in a fold of peritoneum

BOX 41.13	Fallopian Tubes

- Infundibulum: funnel-shaped lateral tube that projects beyond the broad ligament to overlie the ovaries; "free edge" of the funnel has fimbriae (finger-like projectors draped over the ovary)
- Ampulla: widest part of the tube, where fertilization occurs
- Isthmus: hardest part; lies just lateral to the uterus
- Interstitial portion: pierces the uterine wall at the cornua
- Length: 12 cm; blood is supplied by ovarian arteries and veins

TABLE 41.2	Normal Ovarian Volume by Menstrual Status			
Group	Mean Volume (cm³)	Standard Deviation	No. of Ovaries Evaluated	95% Confidence Interval (cm³)[a]
Premenarcheal	3.0	2.3	32	0.2–9.1
Menstruating	9.8	5.8	866	2.5–21.9
Postmenopausal	5.8	3.6	100	1.2–14.1

[a]Calculated on the basis of cube root values, then transformed back to cubic centimeters.

From Cohen HL, Tice HM, Mandel FS. Ovarian volumes measured by US: bigger than we think. *Radiology*. 1990;177:189.

BOX 41.14	Ovaries

- Almond shaped
- Attached at posterior aspect of the broad ligament by mesovarium
- Lie in ovarian fossa
- Fossa is bounded by external iliac vessels, ureter, and obturator nerve
- Dual blood supply; receives blood from ovarian artery and uterine artery
- Blood drained by ovarian vein into inferior vena cava on the right and into renal vein on the left

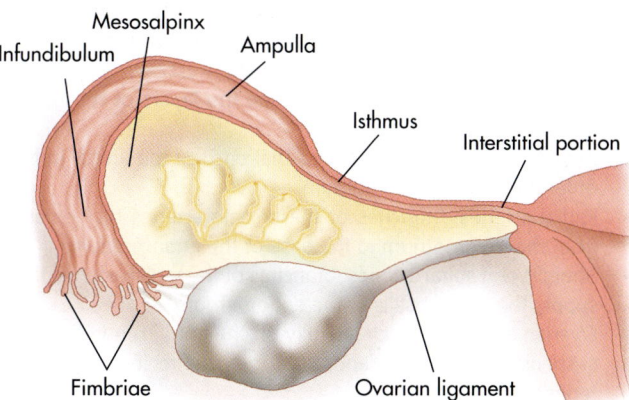

FIG. 41.14 The fallopian tube showing the fimbriae, infundibulum, ampulla, isthmus, and interstitial portions.

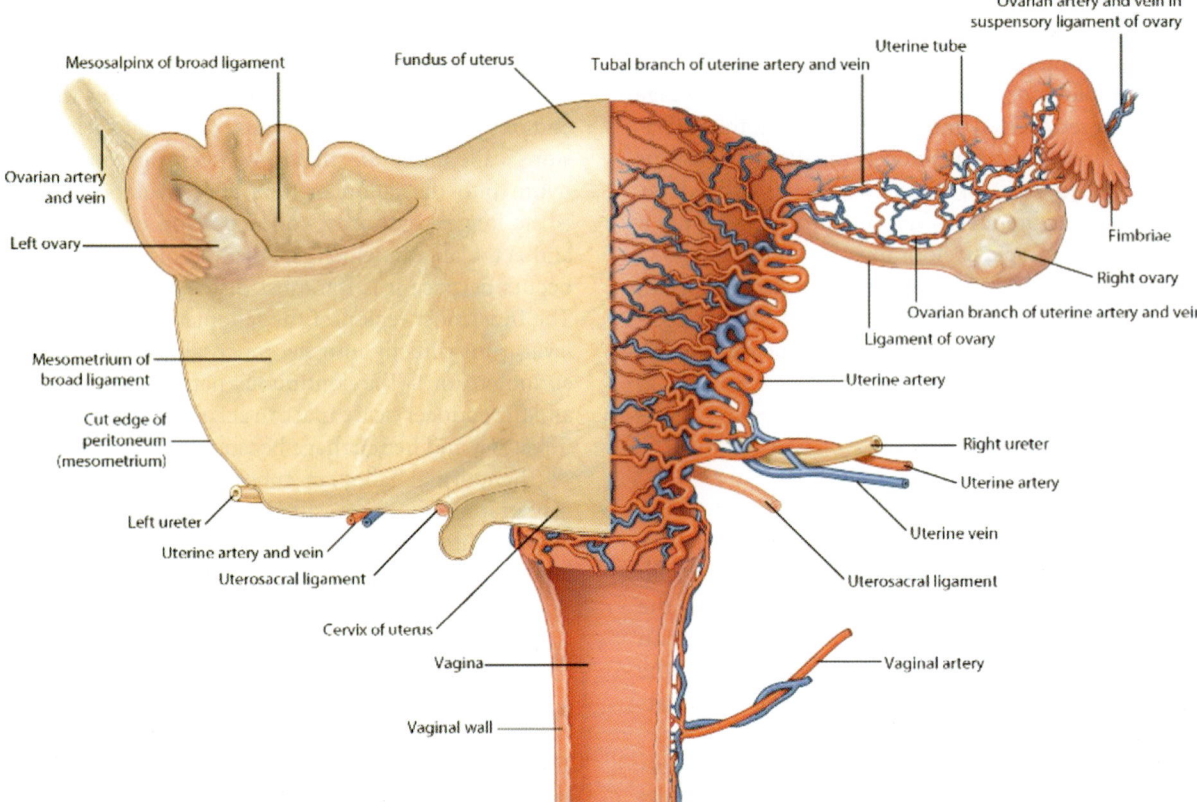

FIG. 41.15 The ovaries are almond-shaped structures, measuring approximately 3 cm long in a menarcheal female. They usually lie posterior to the uterus at the level of the cornua. They are suspended from the posterior aspect of the broad ligament in a fold of peritoneum called the mesovarium. The ovaries are usually located medial to the external iliac vessels and anterior to the internal iliac vessels and ureter.

called the mesovarium. The ovaries are usually located medial to the external iliac vessels and anterior to the internal iliac vessels and ureter (Box 41.15). The ovarian arteries have a double supply of blood. The primary blood supply to the ovaries is from the ovarian arteries, which arise from the lateral aspect of the abdominal aorta, below the renal arteries. The ovarian artery anastomoses with the uterine artery, providing additional blood to the ovary (Box 41.16).

Normal Anatomy

The ovaries consist of an outer layer or cortex, which surrounds the central medulla (Fig. 41.16). The cortex consists primarily of follicles in varying stages of development and is covered by a layer of dense connective tissue, the tunica albuginea. The tunica albuginea is surrounded by a single, thin layer of cells known as the *germinal epithelium*. The central medulla is composed of connective tissue containing blood, nerves, lymphatic vessels, and some smooth muscle at the region of the hilum.

The ovaries produce the reproductive cell, the **ovum**, and two known hormones: **estrogen**, secreted by the follicles, and **progesterone**, secreted by the **corpus luteum**. These steroidal hormones are responsible for producing and maintaining secondary gender characteristics and for preparing the uterus for implantation of a fertilized ovum; they are also responsible for development of mammary glands in the female.

BOX 41.15 Variable Positions of the Ovaries

- Anterior to the internal iliac artery and vein
- Medial to the external iliac artery and vein
- Ellipsoid shape with long axis oriented vertically
- Location highly variable as ligaments loosen, especially after pregnancy

BOX 41.16 Pelvic Vasculature

- External iliac arteries: medial psoas border
- External iliac veins: medial and posterior to the arteries
- Internal iliac arteries: posterior to ureters and ovaries
- Internal iliac veins: posterior to arteries
- Uterine arteries and veins: between the layers of the broad ligaments, lateral to the uterus
- Arcuate arteries: arclike arteries that encircle the uterus in the outer third of the myometrium
- Radial arteries: branches of the arcuate arteries that extend from the myometrium to the base of the endometrium
- Straight and spiral arteries: branches of the radial arteries that supply the zona basalis of the endometrium
- Ovarian arteries: branch laterally off the aorta, run within the suspensory ligaments, and anastomose with the uterine arteries
- Ovarian veins: the right vein drains into the inferior vena cava directly, and the left vein drains into the left renal vein

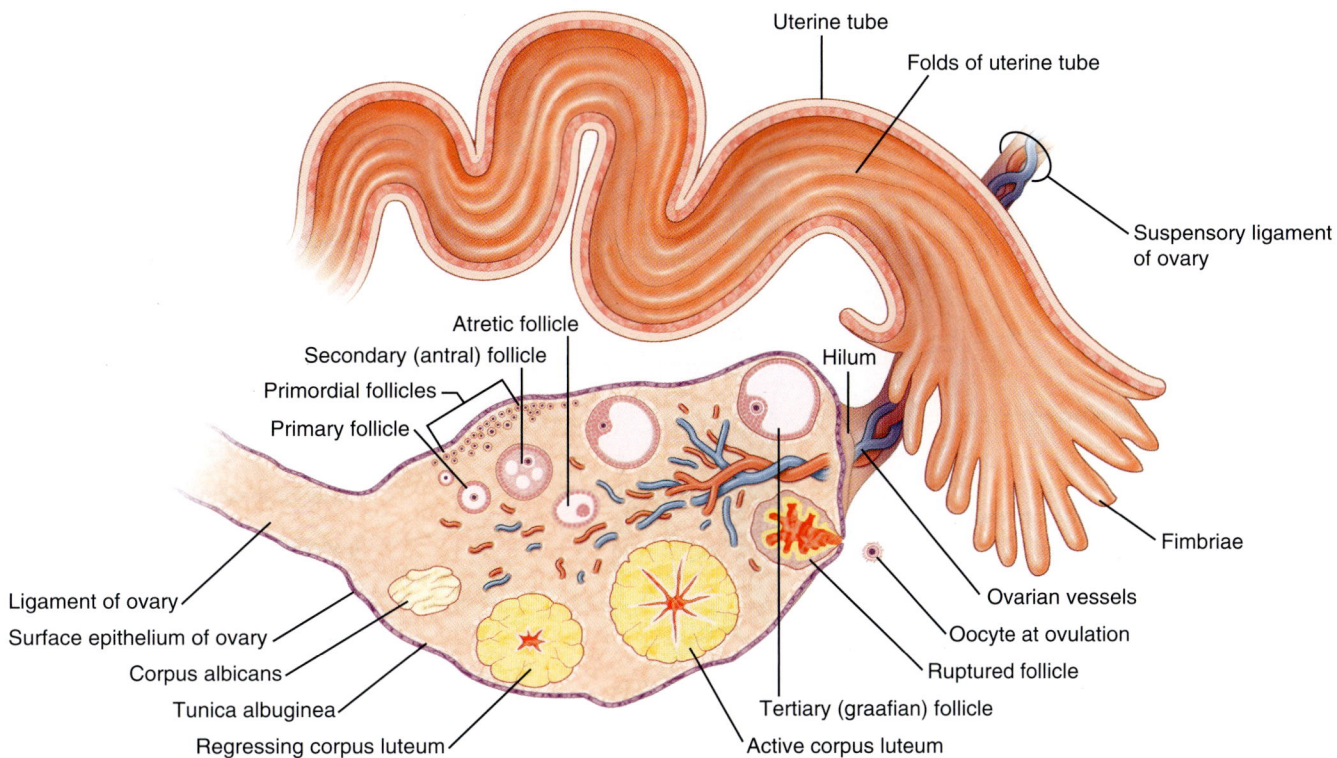

FIG. 41.16 The ovaries consist of an outer layer or cortex, which surrounds the central medulla. The cortex consists primarily of follicles in varying stages of development and is covered by a layer of dense connective tissue, the tunica albuginea. The tunica al albuginea is surrounded by a single, thin layer of cells known as the *germinal epithelium*. The central medulla is composed of connective tissue containing blood, nerves, lymphatic vessels, and some smooth muscle at the region of the hilum.

Ovarian Ligaments

The ovaries are supported medially by the **ovarian ligaments**, originating bilaterally at the cornua of the uterus, and laterally by the **suspensory (infundibulopelvic) ligament**, extending from the infundibulum of the fallopian tube and ovary to the sidewall of the pelvis. The ovary is also attached to the posterior aspect of the broad ligament via the mesovarium (see Fig. 41.15).

PELVIC VASCULATURE

The common iliac arteries course anterior and medial to the psoas muscles, providing blood to the pelvic cavity and lower extremities. The common iliac arteries normally bifurcate into the external and internal iliac (hypogastric) arteries at the level of the superior margin of the sacrum (Fig. 41.17; see Box 41.16). The external iliac arteries course along the pelvic brim and continue inferiorly as the common femoral arteries, supplying blood to the lower extremities. The internal iliac arteries extend into the pelvic cavity, along the posterior wall, and provide multiple branches that perfuse the pelvic structures, including the urinary bladder, uterus, vagina, and rectum. The ovarian veins follow a slightly different course, as the left ovarian vein drains into the left renal vein, and the right ovarian vein drains directly into the inferior vena cava.

Blood is supplied to the uterus by the uterine artery, which arises from the anterior branch of the internal iliac artery (Fig. 41.18). From the internal iliac artery, the uterine artery crosses above and anterior to the ureter, extending medially in the base of the broad ligament to the uterus at the level of the cervix. The uterine artery is tortuous and spirals up the sides of the uterus within the broad ligament to the cornua, where it courses laterally to anastomose with the ovarian artery. The uterine artery gives off many branches that perforate the serosa and carry blood to the myometrium. These branches anastomose extensively anteriorly and posteriorly within the myometrium, forming arcuate (arclike) vessels that encircle the uterus. The arcuate vessels can often be identified sonographically as anechoic tubular structures in the outer third of the myometrium.

Blood is supplied to the endometrium by the radial arteries, which "radiate" from the arcuate arteries within the myometrium. The radial arteries extend through the myometrium to the base of the endometrium, where straight and spiral arteries branch off the radial arteries to supply the zona basalis of the endometrium. The spiral arteries will lengthen during regeneration of the endometrium after menses to traverse the endometrium and supply the zona functionalis. Blood from the spiral arteries is shed during menses. The pelvic vessels supply blood to the functional layer of the endometrium.

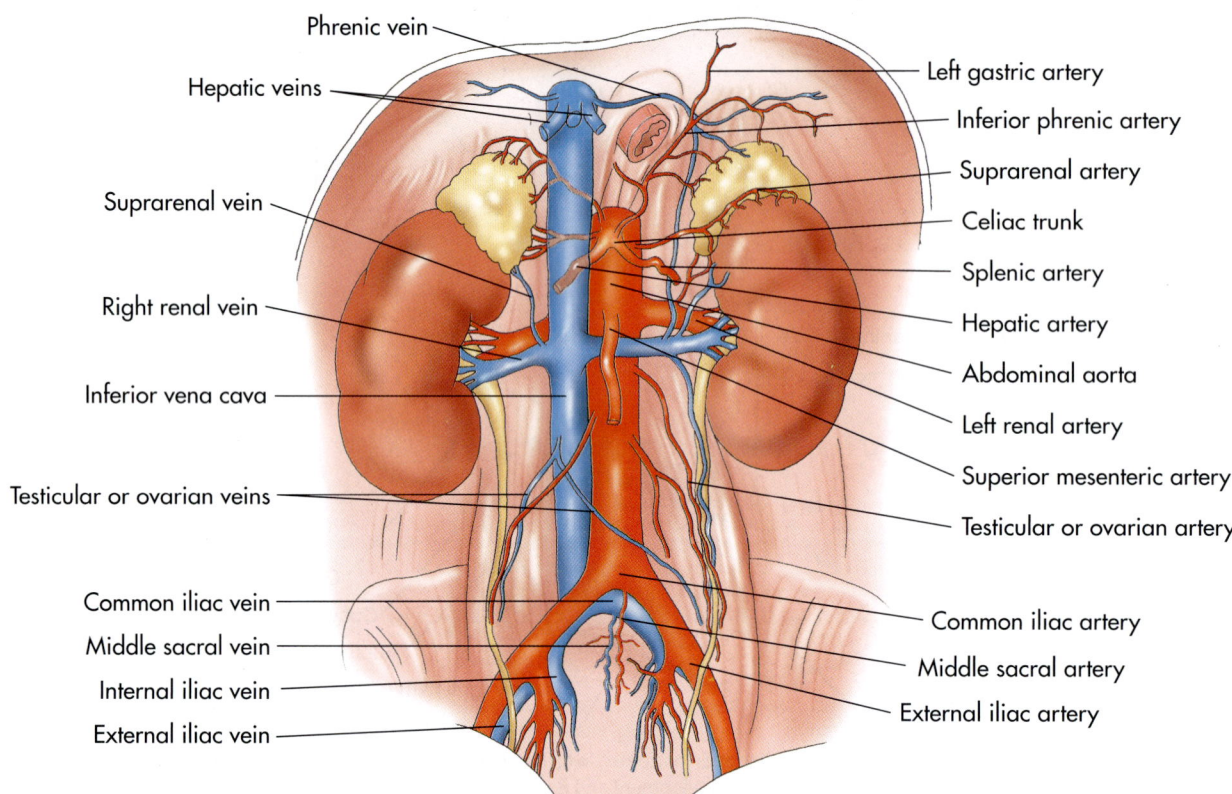

FIG. 41.17 Blood is supplied to the pelvic cavity by the external and internal iliac arteries; the iliac veins drain the pelvis. The ureter enters the pelvis and courses anterior to the internal iliac artery to empty into the posterior base of the bladder.

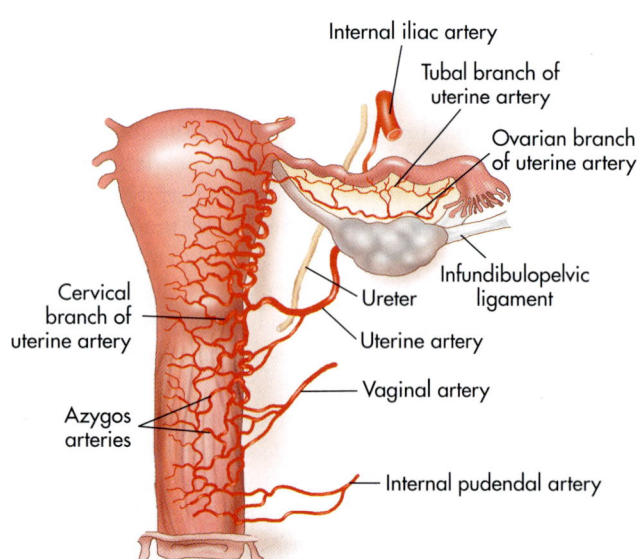

FIG. 41.18 Blood is supplied to the uterus and vagina by the uterine artery (arising from the internal iliac artery) and the vaginal artery (arising from the uterine artery). The ovaries receive blood from branches of the uterine artery and from the ovarian arteries arising from the abdominal aorta.

PHYSIOLOGY

The Menstrual Cycle

A female's reproductive years begin around 11 to 13 years of age at the onset of menses (menstruation) and end around age 50, when menses ceases. The average menstrual cycle is approximately 28 days in length, beginning with the first day of menstrual bleeding (Box 41.17). The length of the menstrual cycle can, however, vary considerably from one woman to another.

Menstrual status is described using the terms *premenarche*, *menarche*, and *menopause*. **Premenarche** is the physiologic status of prepuberty, the time before the onset of menses. **Menarche** is the state after reaching puberty in which menses occurs normally every 28 days. **Menopause** refers to the cessation of menses. The menstrual cycle is regulated by the hypothalamus and is dependent on the cyclic release of estrogen and progesterone from the ovaries.

Follicular Development and Ovulation

During the menarcheal years, an ovum is released once a month by one of the two ovaries. This process is known as ovulation. Ovulation normally occurs midcycle on about day 14 of a 28-day cycle. It is speculated that ovum release alternates between the two ovaries: one month from the right, the next month from the left. All ova begin development during embryonic life and remain in suspended animation within a preantral follicle as an immature **oocyte** until the onset of menarche. Each female ovary contains approximately 200,000 oocytes at the time of birth. Some of these oocytes will mature and be released from the ovaries during ovulation, whereas others will degenerate.

The process of ovulation is regulated by the hypothalamus within the brain. When a girl reaches puberty, the hypothalamus begins the pulsatile release of the **gonadotropin-releasing hormones (GnRHs)**, which stimulate the anterior pituitary gland to secrete varying levels of **gonadotropins** (primarily **follicle-stimulating hormone [FSH]** and **luteinizing hormone [LH]**).

Secretion of FSH by the anterior pituitary gland causes the ovarian follicles to develop during the first half of the menstrual cycle. This phase of the ovulatory cycle, known as the *follicular phase*, begins with the first day of menstrual bleeding and continues until ovulation on day 14 (Fig. 41.19). As the ovarian follicles grow, they fill with fluid and secrete increasing amounts of estrogen. Although typically five to eight preantral follicles will begin to develop, only one usually reaches maturity each month. This mature follicle is known as a *graafian follicle* and typically measures 2 cm right before ovulation. As the estrogen level in the blood rises with follicle development, the pituitary gland is inhibited from further production of FSH and begins to secrete LH. The luteinizing hormone level will typically increase rapidly 24 to 36 hours before ovulation in a process known as the *LH surge*. This surge is often used as a predictor for timing ovulation for conception.

> **BOX 41.17 The Menstrual Cycle**
>
> **Menstruation**
> - Days 1–14
>
> **Proliferative Phase**
> - Days 5–14
> - Corresponds to the follicular phase of ovarian cycle
> - Thin endometrium
> - Estrogen level increases as ovarian follicles develop
> - Increasing estrogen levels cause uterine lining to regenerate and thicken
> - Ovulation occurs on day 14
>
> **Secretory Phase**
> - Days 15–28
> - Corresponds to the luteal phase of ovarian cycle
> - Ruptured follicle becomes corpus luteum
> - Corpus luteum secretes progesterone
> - Endometrium thickens
> - If no pregnancy, estrogen and progesterone decrease

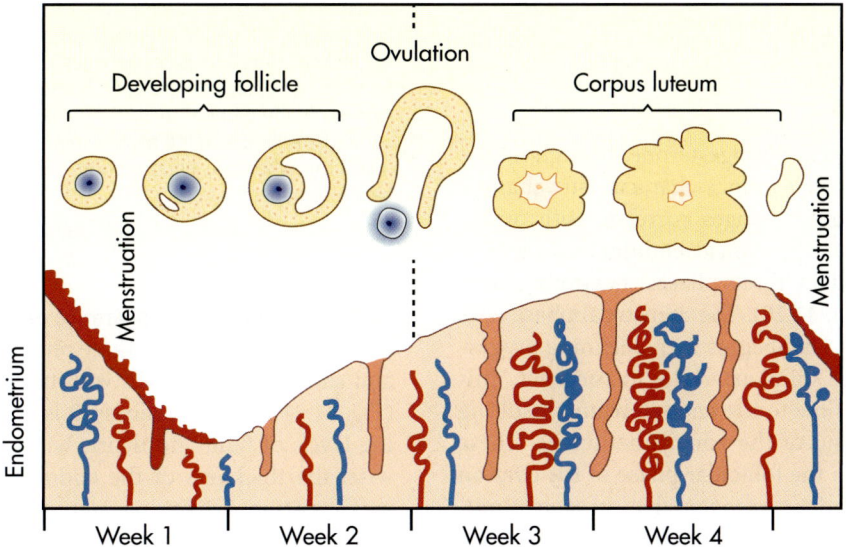

FIG. 41.19 The average menstrual cycle is approximately 28 days, beginning with the first day of bleeding. As the menstrual lining is shed, the pituitary gland begins to secrete follicle-stimulating hormone (FSH), which causes five to eight preantral ovarian follicles to develop. As the ovarian follicles grow, they fill with fluid and secrete increasing amounts of estrogen. This estrogen stimulates the superficial layer of the endometrium to regenerate and grow. As the estrogen level in the blood rises, the pituitary gland is inhibited from further production of FSH and begins to secrete luteinizing hormone (LH). The LH surges 24 to 36 hours before ovulation and is accompanied by a smaller FSH surge that triggers ovulation on about day 14. Ovulation occurs as the follicle ruptures, releasing the mature ovum. After ovulation, the cells lining the ruptured ovarian follicle begin to multiply and create the corpus luteum. The corpus luteum immediately begins to secrete progesterone. Progesterone causes the spiral arteries and endometrial glands to enlarge as the endometrium prepares for implantation should conception occur. Without conception, the corpus luteum degenerates 9 to 11 days after ovulation, causing progesterone levels to decline. Declining progesterone levels cause the spiral arterioles to constrict, resulting in decreasing blood flow to the endometrium with ischemia and shedding of the zona functionalis. As menstruation occurs, the menstrual cycle begins again.

LH level usually reaches its peak 10 to 12 hours before ovulation. It is the LH surge, accompanied by a smaller FSH surge, that triggers ovulation on about day 14.

Ovulation is the explosive release of an ovum from the ruptured graafian follicle. Rupture of the follicle is associated with small amounts of fluid in the posterior cul-de-sac midcycle. Some women can tell when they are ovulating because at midcycle they have pain, typically a dull ache on either side of the lower abdomen lasting a few hours. The term *mittelschmerz*, from the German word meaning "middle pain," is often used to describe this sensation. After ovulation, the ovary enters the luteal phase. This phase begins with ovulation and is about 14 days in length. It is interesting to note that the luteal phase does not usually vary in length. When a menstrual cycle is shorter or longer than 28 days, it is the follicular phase that is altered. Menstruation almost always occurs 14 days after ovulation. During the luteal phase, the cells in the lining of the ruptured ovarian follicle begin to multiply and create the corpus luteum, or yellow body. This process, known as *luteinization*, is stimulated by the LH surge. The corpus luteum immediately begins to secrete progesterone. Nine to 11 days after ovulation, the corpus luteum degenerates, causing progesterone levels to decline. As progesterone levels decline, menstruation occurs and the cycle begins again. Should conception and implantation occur, the human chorionic gonadotropin (hCG) produced by the zygote causes the corpus luteum to persist, and it will continue to secrete progesterone for three more months until the placenta takes over. Box 41.17 summarizes the phases of the menstrual cycle.

Endometrial Changes

Varying levels of estrogen and progesterone throughout the course of the menstrual cycle induce characteristic changes in the endometrium. These changes correlate with ovulatory cycles of the ovary. The typical endometrial cycle is identified and described in three phases, beginning with the menstrual phase (Fig. 41.20). The menstrual phase lasts approximately 1 to 5 days and begins with declining progesterone levels, causing the spiral arterioles to constrict. This causes decreased blood flow to the endometrium, resulting in ischemia and shedding of the zona functionalis. These first 5 days coincide with the follicular phase of the ovarian cycle. As the follicles produce estrogen, the estrogen stimulates the superficial layer of the endometrium to regenerate and grow. This phase of endometrial regeneration, called the *proliferative phase*, will last until luteinization of the graafian follicle around ovulation. With ovulation and luteinization of the graafian follicle, the progesterone secreted by the ovary causes the spiral arteries and endometrial glands to enlarge. This will prepare the endometrium for implantation, should conception occur. The endometrial phase after ovulation, referred to as the *secretory phase*, extends from approximately day 15 to the onset of menses (day 28). The secretory phase of the endometrial cycle corresponds to the luteal phase of the ovarian cycle.

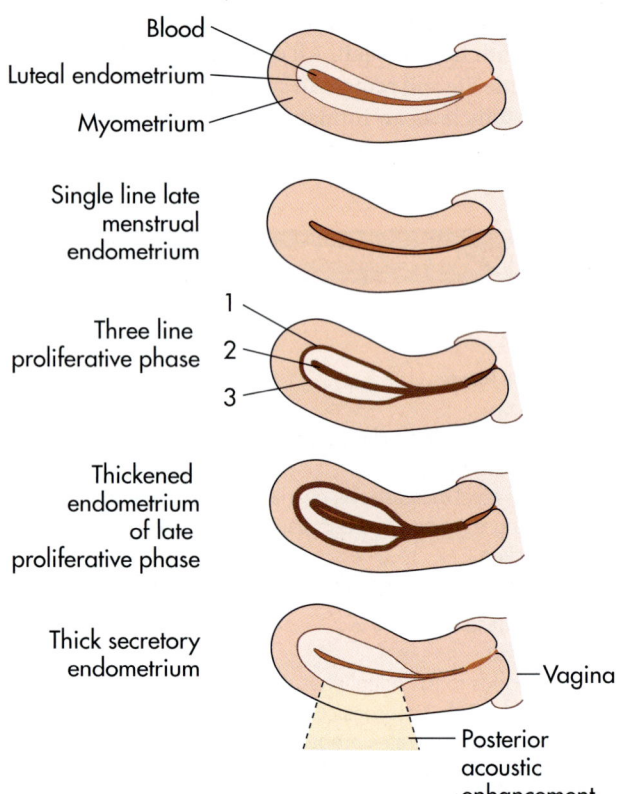

FIG. 41.20 Cyclic changes in the endometrium. The menstrual cycle begins with approximately 5 days of bleeding. During menses, varying levels of fluid and debris may be seen within the uterine cavity. The thickness of the endometrium decreases with menstruation, becoming a thin echogenic line during the early proliferative phase. As regeneration ensues, the endometrium thickens and appears hypoechoic with a "three-line" sign. The outer echogenic line surrounding the hypoechoic functionalis represents the zona basalis, and the central echogenic line represents the uterine cavity. As ovulation nears, the endometrium becomes isoechoic with the myometrium. The secretory phase occurs after ovulation, when the endometrium reaches its thickest dimension and becomes hyperechoic.

The sonographic appearance of the endometrium changes dramatically among the three phases of the endometrial cycle and should be correlated with the patient's menstrual status (Fig. 41.21). During menses, it is not uncommon to see varying levels of fluid and debris within the uterine cavity; likewise, the thickness of the endometrium will decrease with menstruation, becoming a thin echogenic line during the early proliferative phase. As regeneration of the endometrium occurs during the proliferative phase, the endometrium will thicken to an average of 4 to 8 mm in the proliferative phase, when measured as a double layer from anterior to posterior. The endometrium characteristically appears hypoechoic with the appearance of the "three-line" sign. The three echogenic lines seen in the proliferative endometrium represent the zona basalis anteriorly and posteriorly, with the central line representing the uterine cavity. Right before ovulation, the endometrium averages 6 to 10 mm and becomes isoechoic with the myometrium. After ovulation, during the secretory phase, the endometrium reaches its thickest dimension,

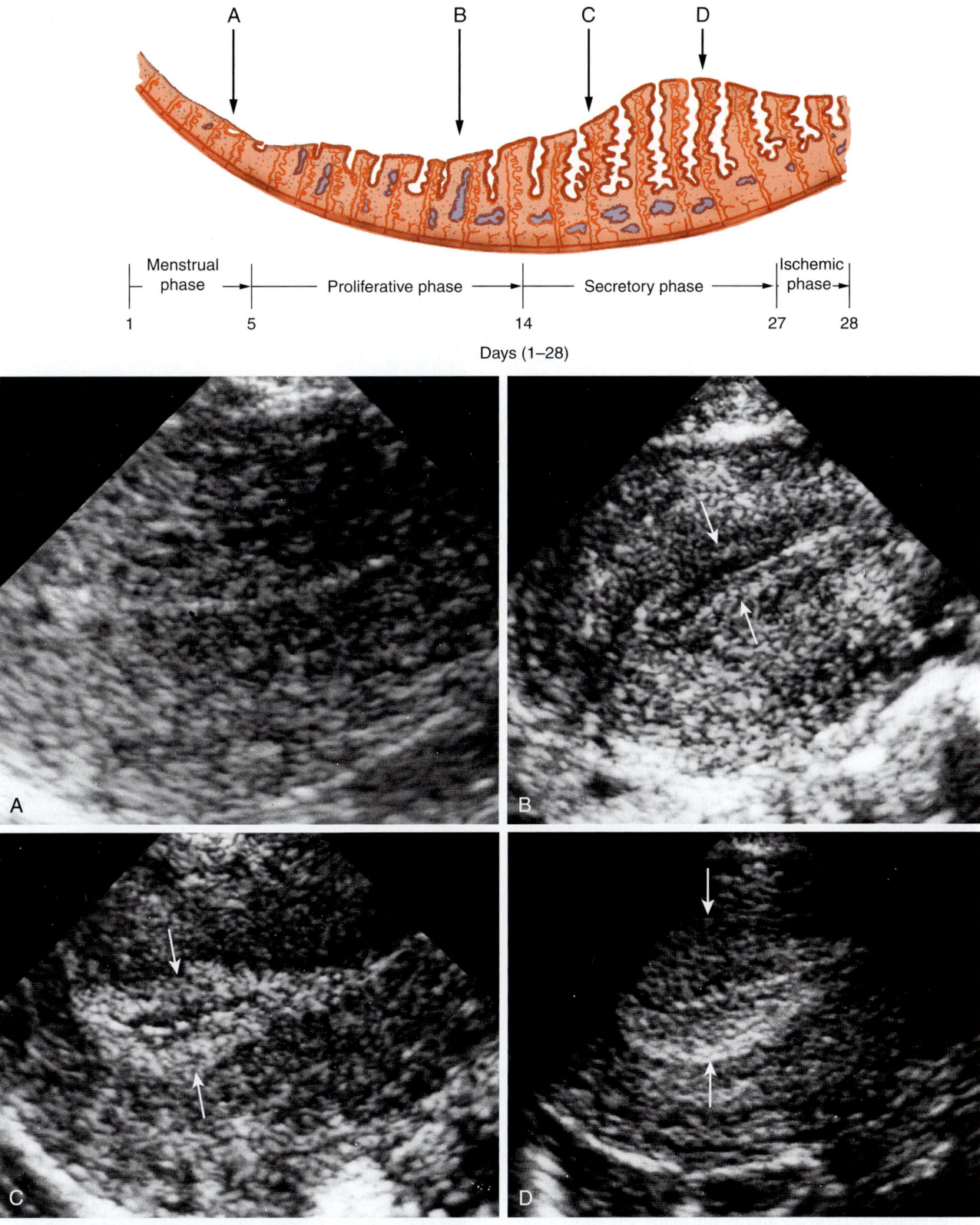

FIG. 41.21 The sonographic appearance of the endometrium changes dramatically among the three phases of the endometrial cycle and should be correlated with the patient's menstrual status. (A) During menses, it is not uncommon to see varying levels of fluid and debris within the uterine cavity; likewise, the thickness of the endometrium will decrease with menstruation, becoming a thin echogenic line during the early proliferative phase. As regeneration of the endometrium occurs during the proliferative phase, the endometrium will thicken to an average of 4 to 8 mm in the proliferative phase, when measured as a double layer from anterior to posterior. (B) The endometrium characteristically appears hypoechoic with the appearance of the "three-line" sign. The three echogenic lines seen in the proliferative endometrium represent the zona basalis anteriorly and posteriorly, with the central line representing the uterine cavity. (C) Right before ovulation, the endometrium averages 6 to 10 mm and becomes isoechoic with the myometrium. (D) After ovulation, during the secretory phase, the endometrium reaches its thickest dimension, averaging 7 to 14 mm, and becomes echogenic, blurring the three-line appearance.

averaging 7 to 14 mm, and becomes echogenic, blurring the "three-line" appearance. The endometrium in anovulatory patients (e.g., those on the birth control pill, postmenopausal patients) will usually appear as a thin, echogenic line. Postmenopausal patients who are not on hormone replacement therapy (HRT) should have an endometrial thickness of less than 5 mm. Postmenopausal patients on HRT or taking tamoxifen (a drug used as adjuvant palliative therapy to help in the prevention of breast cancer) may demonstrate normal endometrial thicknesses of up to 8 mm.

Abnormal Menstrual Cycles

Several terms are used to describe abnormal menstrual cycles and should be familiar to the sonographer. The term **menorrhagia** is used to describe abnormally heavy or long periods and is often associated with uterine fibroids, intrauterine contraceptive devices (IUDs), or hormonal imbalances. Persistent menorrhagia can lead to anemia. The term **oligomenorrhea** describes abnormally short or light periods and is often associated with polycystic ovary syndrome (PCOS). Oligomenorrhea can also be caused by emotional and physical stress, chronic illnesses, tumors that secrete estrogen, poor nutrition and eating disorders (e.g., anorexia nervosa), and heavy exercise. **Polymenorrhea** is when the menstrual cycle occurs at intervals of less than 21 days.

Many patients report **dysmenorrhea** or painful periods. Dysmenorrhea is often associated with endometriosis.

The term **amenorrhea** refers to the absence of menstruation. Amenorrhea is considered primary when menarche is delayed beyond 18 years of age and secondary when cessation of uterine bleeding occurs in women who have previously menstruated. Amenorrhea may be due to a congenital vaginal or cervical stenosis or may result from infection, trauma, ovarian dysfunction, or other endocrine disturbances that affect ovarian function, such as pituitary disease.

PELVIC RECESSES AND BOWEL

The peritoneal cavity contains two potential spaces formed by the caudal portion of the parietal peritoneum (Box 41.18). These potential spaces are sonographically significant in that fluid may accumulate or pathology may be present in these locations. The **vesicouterine recess (pouch)**, or anterior cul-de-sac, is located anterior to the fundus of the uterus between the urinary bladder and the uterus and the **rectouterine recess (pouch)**, or posterior cul-de-sac, is located posterior to the uterus between the uterus and the rectum (Fig. 41.22). The rectouterine pouch is often referred to as the *pouch of Douglas* and is normally the most inferior and most posterior region of the peritoneal cavity. One additional area that is sonographically significant is the retropubic space (also called the **space of Retzius**). It can be identified between the anterior bladder wall and the pubic symphysis. This space normally contains subcutaneous fat, but a hematoma or abscess in this location may displace the urinary bladder posteriorly.

It is normal to observe a small accumulation of free fluid throughout the menstrual cycle in the posterior cul-de-sac. The greatest quantity of free fluid in the cul-de-sac normally occurs immediately after ovulation when the mature follicle ruptures. A small amount of fluid in the posterior cul-de-sac is considered normal; however, there is no sonographic means of confirming that the fluid is related to ovulation. Hemorrhage or infection within the fluid may be related to a ruptured cyst, ascites, a ruptured corpus luteum cyst, ectopic pregnancy, or pelvic inflammatory disease.

BOX 41.18	Pelvic Recesses

- Vesicouterine pouch: anterior cul-de-sac; anterior to the fundus between the uterus and bladder
- Rectouterine pouch: posterior cul-de-sac; posterior to the uterine body and cervix, between the uterus and rectum
- Retropubic space: space of Retzius; between bladder and symphysis pubis

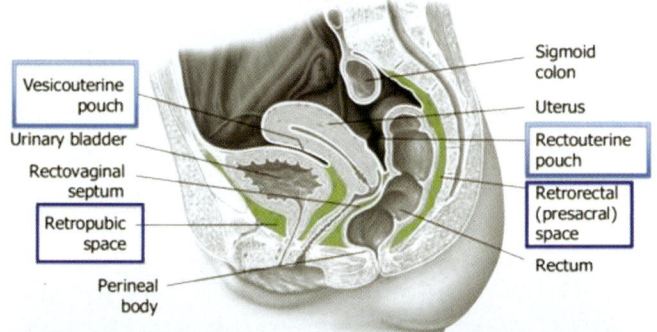

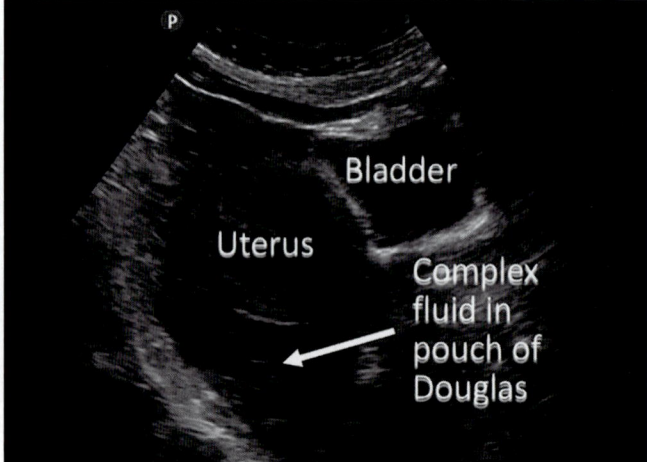

FIG. 41.22 The peritoneal cavity contains two potential spaces formed by the caudal portion of the parietal peritoneum. (A) The vesicouterine recess (pouch), or anterior cul-de-sac, is located anterior to the fundus of the uterus between the urinary bladder and the uterus. (B) The rectouterine recess (pouch), or posterior cul-de-sac, is located posterior to the uterus between the uterus and the rectum.

Key Pearls

- Many pelvic landmarks, ligaments, and muscular structures within the pelvis are important to know to differentiate normal reproductive organs from muscular and vascular structures.
- A transabdominal approach requires a full urinary bladder for use as an acoustic window and typically necessitates the use of a 3.5- to 5-MHz transducer for adequate penetration.
- A transvaginal examination performed with an empty bladder allows the use of a higher-frequency transducer, typically 7.5 to 10 MHz.
- The lower margin of the pelvic cavity, the pelvic floor, is formed by the levator ani and coccygeus muscles and is known as the pelvic diaphragm.
- The muscles found within the true pelvis include the piriformis muscles, obturator internus muscles, and muscles of the pelvic diaphragm.
- The pelvic diaphragm is formed by the levator ani and coccygeus muscles and makes up the floor of the true pelvis.
- The vagina is a collapsed muscular tube that extends from the external genitalia to the cervix of the uterus.
- The uterine cervix protrudes into the upper portion of the vaginal canal, forming four archlike recesses called *fornices*.
- The uterus consists of a fundus, body, and cervix.
- The uterine wall consists of three histologic layers: the serosa or perimetrium, the myometrium, and the endometrium.
- The endometrium consists primarily of two layers: the superficial functional layer (zona functionalis) and the deep basal layer (zona basalis).
- The uterus is supported in its midline position by paired broad ligaments, round ligaments, uterosacral ligaments, and cardinal ligaments.
- The position of the uterus is variable. The average uterine position is considered to be anteverted and anteflexed.
- In multiparous females, the entire uterus may tip backward rather than forward and is described as a retroverted position.
- The uterine fundus or body may also curve backward on the cervix, and this position is described as retroflexed.
- The fallopian tubes are divided into four anatomic portions: infundibulum (lateral segment), ampulla (middle segment), isthmus (medial segment), and interstitial portion (segment that passes through the uterine cornua).
- The ovaries are usually located medial to the external iliac vessels and anterior to the internal iliac vessels and ureter.
- The ovaries produce the reproductive cell, the ovum, and two known hormones: estrogen, secreted by the follicles, and progesterone, secreted by the corpus luteum.
- The ovaries are supported medially by the ovarian ligaments, originating bilaterally at the cornua of the uterus, and laterally by the suspensory (infundibulopelvic) ligament, extending from the infundibulum of the fallopian tube and ovary to the sidewall of the pelvis.
- The left ovarian vein drains into the left renal vein, and the right ovarian vein drains directly into the inferior vena cava.
- Menstrual status is described using the terms *premenarche*, *menarche*, and *menopause*.
- Varying levels of estrogen and progesterone throughout the course of the menstrual cycle induce characteristic changes in the endometrium.
- The vesicouterine recess (pouch), or anterior cul-de-sac, is located anterior to the fundus of the uterus between the urinary bladder and the uterus, and the rectouterine recess (pouch), or posterior cul-de-sac, is located posterior to the uterus between the uterus and the rectum.

BIBLIOGRAPHY

Abrahams PH, Spratt JD, Loukas M, VanSchoor A. *Abrahams' and McMinn's Clinical Atlas of Human Anatomy*. ed 8. Philadelphia: Elsevier; 2020.

AIUM. Practice guideline for the performance of an ultrasound examination of the female pelvis. *J Ultrasound Med*. 2020;9999:1–7.

AIUM/IUGA. Practice parameter for the performance of urogynecological ultrasound examinations: developed in collaboration with the ACR, the AUGS, the AUA, and the SRU. *J Ultrasound Med*. April 2019;38(4):851–864.

Bakos O, Lundkvist O, Bergh T. Transvaginal sonographic evaluation of endometrial growth and exture in spontaneous ovulatory cycles—a descriptive study. *Hum Reprod*. 1993;8:799–806.

Callen PW. *Ultrasonography in obstetrics and gynecology*. ed 6. Philadelphia: Elsevier; 2017.

Kelley LL, Petersen CM. *Sectional Anatomy for Imaging Professionals*. ed 4. St. Louis: Mosby; 2018.

Lyons EA, Gratton D, Harrington C. Transvaginal sonography of normal pelvic anatomy. *Radiol Clin North Am*. 1992;30:663–669.

Naftalin J, Jurkovic D. The endometrial-myoetrial junction: a fresh look at a busy crossing. *Ultrasound Obstet Gynecol*. 2009;34:1–11.

Rosen DJ, Ben-Jun I, Arbel Y, et al. Transvaginal ultrasonographic quantitative assessment of accumulated cul-de-sac fluid. *Am J Obstet Gynecol*. 1992;166:542–544.

Rumack CM, Wilson SR, Charboneau JW. *Diagnostic ultrasound*. ed 3. St Louis: Elsevier; 2005.

Snell RS. *Snell's Clinical Anatomy by Regions*. ed 10. Philadelphia: Lippincott Williams & Wilkins; 2022.

CHAPTER 42

Sonographic and Doppler Evaluation of the Female Pelvis

Sandra L. Hagen-Ansert

OBJECTIVES

On completion of this chapter, you should be able to:
- Demonstrate how to take a patient history specific to a pelvic ultrasound examination
- Discuss the indications and contraindications for transabdominal and transvaginal scans
- Name the important muscles in the pelvic cavity
- Describe the scan orientation for transabdominal and transvaginal ultrasonography
- Describe both the sonographic technique for evaluating the uterus and adnexal area and their sonographic appearances
- Discuss quantitative Doppler measurements

OUTLINE

Patient Preparation and History 1177
Performance Standards for the Ultrasound Examination 1177
Sonographic Technique 1177
   Transabdominal Ultrasonography 1178
   Transvaginal Ultrasonography 1183
Sonographic Evaluation of the Pelvis 1189
   Bony Pelvis 1189
   Muscles of the Pelvis 1189
   Pelvic Vascularity 1190
   Uterus 1192
   Endometrium 1195
Fallopian Tubes 1196
Ovaries 1197
Rectouterine Recess and Bowel 1198
Sonohysterography 1199
Three-Dimensional Ultrasound 1199

KEY TERMS

Arcuate vessels
Cornu, cornua
Coronal plane
Early proliferative phase
Endometrium
Internal os
Late proliferative phase
Menarche
Menopause
Menstruation
Myometrium
Pourcelot resistive index
Premenarche
Premenopause
Pulsatility index (PI)
S/D ratio
Secretory (luteal) phase
Sonohysterography
Translabial (transperineal)

Ultrasonography is an important diagnostic tool for the evaluation of pelvic anatomy and pathology both in adult and in pediatric populations. The noninvasive nature of sonography, its high-resolution imaging capabilities, and its ability to separate fluid from soft tissue structures in multiple imaging planes have proven to be clinically useful.

In the pediatric population, transabdominal (TA) ultrasound is used in a variety of clinical circumstances, including the evaluation of ambiguous genitalia, pelvic masses, and disorders of puberty. It is also used to further evaluate pelvic or lower abdominal pain that may result from appendicitis.

The size, location, contour, vascularity, and physiologic state of pelvic organs are easily obtained using both TA and transvaginal (TV) ultrasound. The information obtained complements the clinical evaluation and aids the process of forming differential considerations.

Color and spectral Doppler have evolved to play a role in assessing normal and pathologic blood flow. Sonohysterography can provide more detailed evaluation of the endometrium. Sonography also plays an important role in guiding interventional procedures.

The role of the sonographer is to gather the clinical history, identify the referring physician's indications for the study (working diagnosis), review the previous imaging results, and tailor the ultrasound examination to each patient. Critical thinking by the sonographer produces valid, reliable, and reproducible results that are the basis of an effective diagnostic medical sonographic practice.

PATIENT PREPARATION AND HISTORY

A complete history is critical in order to tailor the ultrasound examination and correlate ultrasound findings with the proper differential consideration. It is useful for the sonographer to use a routine patient questionnaire requesting the following information: date of last menstrual period, gravidity, parity, physiologic menstrual status, hormone regimen, symptoms, history of cancer, family history of cancer, past pelvic surgeries, laboratory tests, previous Papanicolaou (Pap) smear or biopsy results, and pelvic examination findings. A review of previous examinations (ultrasound, computed tomography, magnetic resonance imaging, positron emission tomography) should be done before the start of the ultrasound examination to determine whether a mass was previously present and to assess if there has been any change in size or internal characteristics.

The patient's menstrual status is described by using the terms *premenarche*, *menarche*, and *menopause*. **Premenarche** is the physiologic status of prepuberty, the time before the onset of menses. **Menarche** is the state after reaching puberty in which menses occur normally every 21 to 28 days. Perimenopause, or **premenopause**, is a transitional stage of 2 to 10 years before complete cessation of the menstrual cycle. This is the stage of gradually declining estrogen during which menstrual cycles may become shorter, longer, or irregular. **Menopause** is when menses have ceased permanently, generally agreed to be defined as 1 year without menses.

After the clinical history has been taken, the sonographer should carefully explain the examination to the patient. If both the TA and TV examinations are going to be performed, the patient should be instructed that the pelvic ultrasound examination will be performed in two parts. The first is the TA approach, in which the transducer is carefully scanned across her lower abdomen after warm gel has been applied, and the second is the TV approach, which is an internal ultrasound and similar to a pelvic examination. The sonographer should tell the patient that she will be allowed to empty her bladder completely after the first part of the examination is completed. After receiving a brief explanation of the entire ultrasound examination, the patient is placed in the supine position. Ideally the scanning should be performed on a gynecologic ultrasound examination table, which can be modified for the TV examination.

By understanding all of the patient's clinical history and by talking and listening to the patient, the sonographer can gain a perspective as to what questions the ultrasound examination needs to answer and can tailor a plan of how to accomplish this. Once the scanning begins, the sonographer adds the information gained to develop a clinical and diagnostic image for each patient.

PERFORMANCE STANDARDS FOR THE ULTRASOUND EXAMINATION

Four major organizations have determined standards for the pelvic ultrasound examination: the Society of Diagnostic Medical Sonography, the American Institute of Ultrasound in Medicine (AIUM), the American Congress of Obstetricians and Gynecologists, and the American College of Radiology (ACR). These organizations can be investigated by visiting their websites. This chapter uses the standards set by the ACR as its primary example. The ACR Standard for the Performance of Ultrasound Examination of the Female Pelvis outlines the following guidelines when performing a pelvic ultrasound examination:

1. Ultrasound examination of the pelvis should be performed only when there is a valid medical reason.
2. The lowest possible ultrasonic exposure settings should be used to gather the necessary information. The AIUM Bioeffects Committee identified ultrasound intensity (free-field spatial peak, temporal average [SPTA]) of $100\,mW/cm^2$ as the intensity below which no significant biologic effects in mammalian tissues exposed in vivo have been confirmed.
3. All relevant structures (anatomy and pathology) should be identified by the TA and TV approaches; in most cases both techniques are used unless contraindicated.
4. Alternatively, a transperineal, also known as translabial, approach can be useful in patients who are not candidates for TV scanning. Such patients might include those with suspected rupture of membranes in pregnancy or uterine prolapse.

The ACR also sets standards for personnel, protocols, documentation, equipment, quality control, and quality improvement.

SONOGRAPHIC TECHNIQUE

The female pelvis is routinely evaluated with at least one of two ultrasound techniques: TA and TV (Box 42.1). The TA examination is performed from the anterior abdominal wall using a curvilinear, or sector, transducer with frequencies of up to 5 MHz. TA scans typically use the distended urinary bladder as a "sonic" window to identify the uterus and adnexa as an overview of the other pelvic structures. However, if the protocol is to do a TA study in conjunction with a TV study, not all institutions begin with the urinary bladder fully distended. Even when the urinary bladder is only partially distended or is empty, a TA scan may still help as an overview to the pelvic structures.

The TV examination is performed with the patient's bladder empty, using higher transducer frequencies of 7.5 MHz or more. These higher frequencies have better near-field focusing and resolution, which permit greater detail and characterization of the uterus and adnexa.

TA and TV sonography are complementary techniques, and both are used extensively in evaluation of the female pelvis. Anatomy and pathology should be identified in at least

> **BOX 42.1 Pelvic Ultrasound Examination**
>
> **Uterus**
> - Vagina and uterus serve as anatomic landmarks
> - Document the following:
>   Uterine size, shape, and orientation
>   Endometrium
>   Myometrium
>   Cervix
> - Vagina serves as a landmark for the cervix and lower uterine segment
> - Uterine length measured in the long axis from the fundus to the cervix
> - Anteroposterior depth of the uterus measured in the long axis from its anterior to posterior walls, perpendicular to the length
> - Width measured from the transaxial or coronal view
> - Cervical diameters (length and width) can be obtained (usually performed in pregnancy)
> - Endometrium analyzed for thickness and echogenicity
> - Myometrium and cervix evaluated for contour changes, echogenicity, and masses
>
> **Adnexa (Ovaries and Fallopian Tubes)**
> - Ovaries should be identified anterior to the internal iliac (hypogastric) vessels
> - Document the following:
>   Size, shape, contour, and echogenicity
>   Position relative to the uterus
> - Ovarian size determined by measuring the length of the long axis with the anteroposterior dimension measured perpendicular to the length
> - Ovarian width measured in the transaxial or coronal view
> - Ovarian volume may be calculated
>
> **Cul-de-sac**
> - Evaluate cul-de-sac for the presence of free fluid or a mass
> - If a mass is detected, document its size, position, shape, echographic pattern (cystic, solid, or complex), and its relationship to the ovaries and uterus
> - Differentiate normal loops of bowel from a mass

two orthogonal planes, usually *sagittal* and *axial* or *coronal* and *transverse*, using both techniques (Fig. 42.1).

When a mass is found on sonography, the following features should be characterized:
- Location (uterine or extrauterine)
- Size
- External contour (well-defined, ill-defined, or irregular borders)
- Internal consistency (cystic, complex, predominantly cystic, complex, predominantly solid, or solid)

Ultrasound scanning equipment usually has built-in presets to optimize visualization techniques. These can be fine-tuned, and each ultrasound laboratory can develop its own unique techniques. Included are the use of harmonic imaging (cleanup on the anterior noise in fluid-filled structures), compound scanning (improved echo texture), and a variety of penetration and resolution capabilities. Sonographers need to be aware of these techniques and their capabilities to improve diagnostic imaging and avoid artifacts that can lead to an inaccurate diagnosis.

Transabdominal Ultrasonography

The TA approach visualizes the entire pelvis to provide a global overview. The TA technique may be limited in patients who are obese and unable to fill their urinary bladders, older patients who are unable to fill due to incontinence issues, or in patients with a retroverted uterus. This technique gives a less optimal characterization of adnexal masses because of distance from the transducer and interference from the bowel.

For an initial study of the female pelvis, it is recommended that a TA study be made, especially if the patient has not had a previous ultrasound. The TA examination is performed with a distended urinary bladder. Instruction should be given to the patient to drink at least 32 oz of fluid 1 hour before examination time and not to empty her bladder before the scheduled appointment. The full bladder displaces the bowel and any gas it contains from the field of view and flattens the anteflexed uterus slightly so it is more perpendicular to the transducer angle. The distended bladder also becomes an acoustic window to view pelvic anatomy and pathology and serves as a "cystic" reference. The bladder is considered optimally full when it covers the fundus of the normal-sized uterus (Fig. 42.2). Over-distention of the bladder may compromise the sonographic evaluation and compress, distort, and displace anatomy (see Fig. 42.2D). When this occurs, imaging may be repeated after the patient partially empties the bladder.

In most average-size patients, the anatomic survey is usually performed with a transducer frequency range of 3.5 to 5 MHz. If the ovaries lie anteriorly, the use of a higher-frequency transducer may be preferable. If the patient is obese, the lower-frequency transducer may be used. The TA examination is best initiated by identifying the urinary bladder and evaluating its walls and lumen. It is important to definitely identify the urinary bladder to rule out the possibility of a midline cystic, complex mass, or free fluid, which can inadvertently be mistaken for the bladder. The patient may even feel that she has a full bladder if a large mass is pushing against the urinary bladder. The bladder shape may be helpful because a well-distended bladder typically has a triangular or elongated shape on midline scans. If there is any question as to whether a cystic structure in the pelvis represents the bladder, it can be confirmed by having the patient void or by checking for ureteral jets entering the bladder.

The uterus should then be identified in its long axis. This may not be in a true anatomic sagittal plane because the uterus can normally deviate toward either the right or the left. A somewhat oblique angulation through the distended bladder may be necessary to visualize the entire uterus and cervix. Anatomic orientation is correct for longitudinal scans

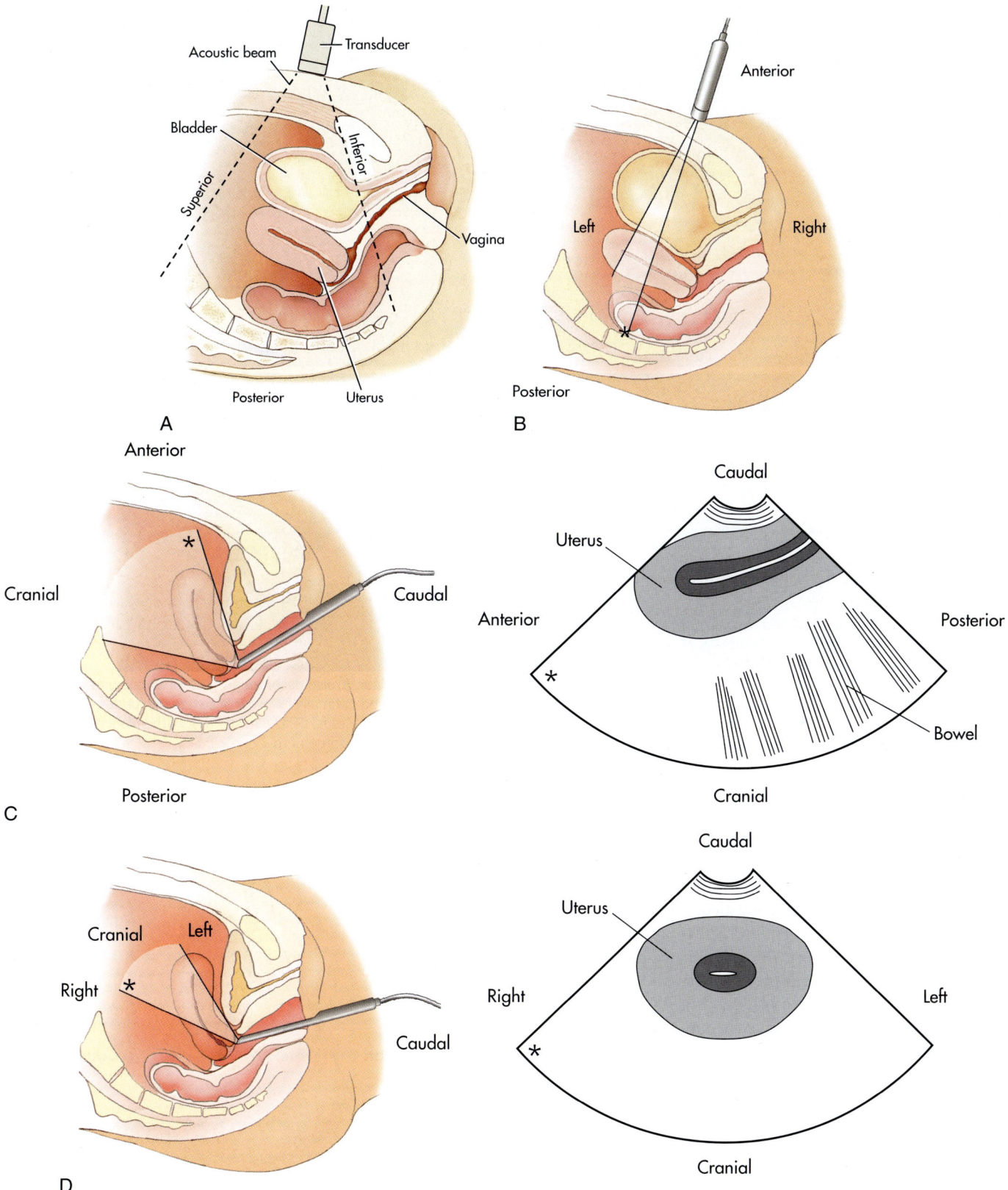

FIG. 42.1 (A) Sagittal plane/transabdominal approach illustrates how transabdominal pelvic sonography may be performed from an anterior approach using the fully distended urinary bladder as the acoustic window. (B) Transverse plane is 90 degrees to the longitudinal plane. The right of the patient is located on the left side of the image. (C) Transvaginal sagittal plane. The notch of the transducer is along the top surface of the handle, so the beam is projected in the midline anteroposterior aspect of the body. (D) Transvaginal coronal plane. The notch of the transducer is rotated toward the sonographer so the beam may image the uterus in a coronal view.

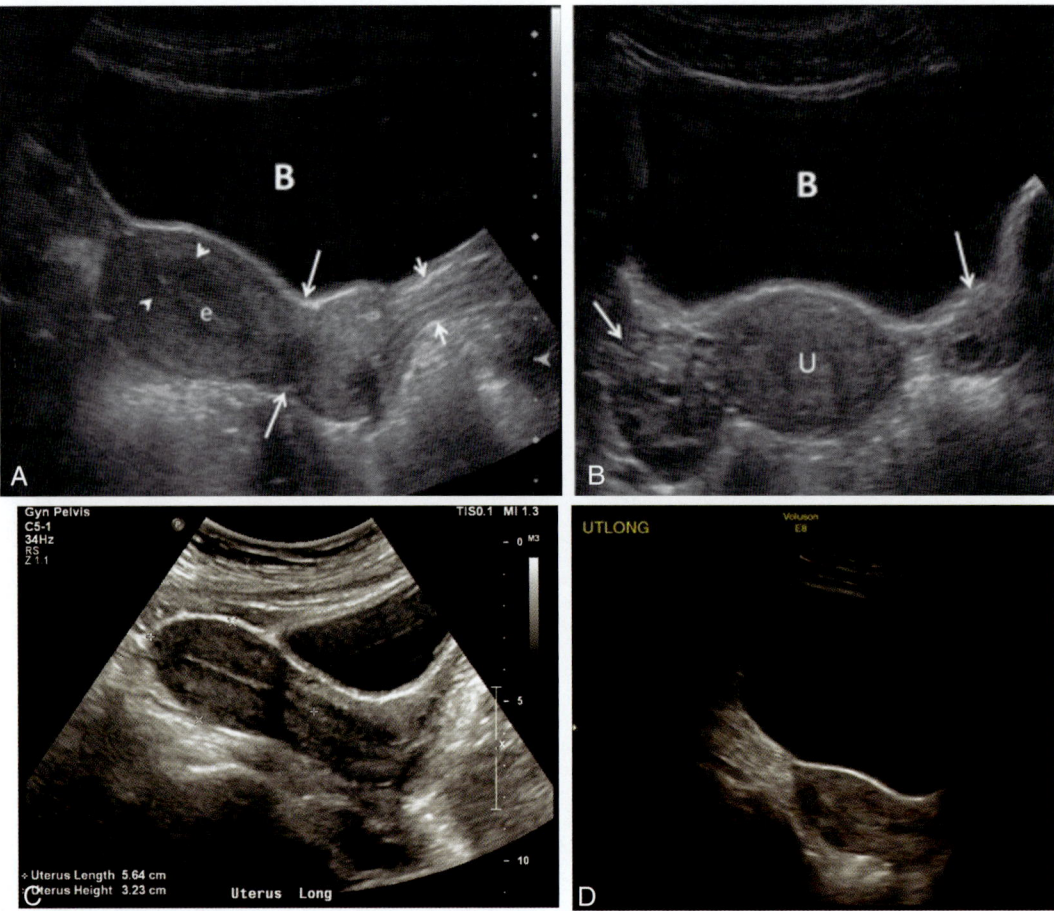

FIG. 42.2 Transabdominal sagittal (A) and transverse (B) images. The distended bladder (B) also becomes an acoustic window to view pelvic anatomy and pathology and serves as a "cystic" reference. The bladder is considered optimally full when it covers the fundus of the normal-sized uterus (U). (C) The bladder is distended but does not cover the fundus of the uterus. (D) Overdistention of the bladder may compromise the sonographic evaluation and compress, distort, and displace anatomy. *e*, Endometrium.

(Fig. 42.3) when the left side of the screen represents cephalic anatomy (toward the patient's head) and the right side of the screen represents caudal anatomy (toward the patient's feet). Once the long axis has been established, parallel sagittal scans are then obtained to the right and left to evaluate the uterine margins and the adnexa. The adnexal area may be imaged by scanning obliquely from the contralateral side and scanning through the fluid-filled bladder. In many instances, the adnexal area can be visualized by scanning directly over the adnexal area. Gentle pressure with the transducer on the pelvic area may be necessary to bring the area of interest within the focal zone. The iliac vessels can be used as a landmark to identify the lateral adnexal borders.

By identifying the true sagittal plane of the uterus and cervix and then rotating the transducer 90 degrees, the axial or axial-coronal (transverse) images can be obtained. Again, angulation from the contralateral side or direct visualization may help to image the adnexa. Anatomic correlation is correct for axial scans when the left side of the screen correlates with the right side of the patient (Fig. 42.4). Applying gentle pressure on the transducer or placing the free hand on the abdomen helps move overlying bowel gas to bring the area

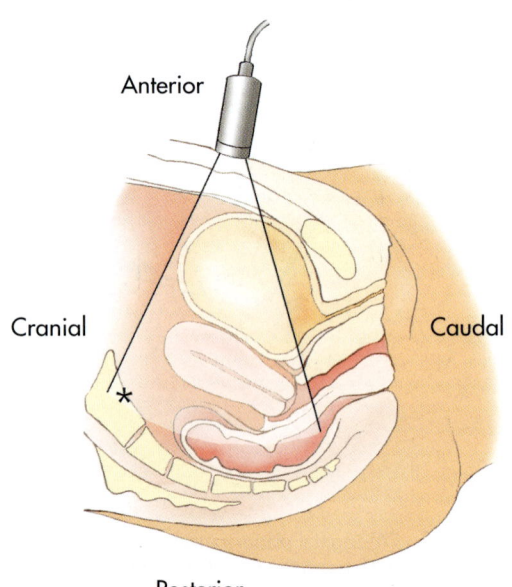

FIG. 42.3 The long axis may not be in a true anatomic sagittal plane because the uterus can normally deviate toward either the right or the left. A somewhat oblique angulation through the distended bladder may be necessary to visualize the entire uterus and cervix.

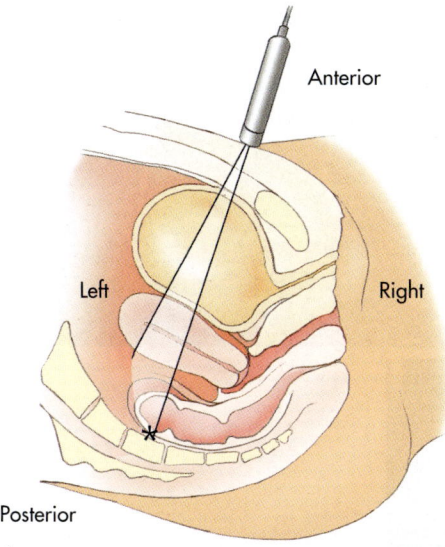

> BOX 42.2 Transabdominal Pelvic Ultrasound Protocol
>
> Survey the pelvic area before images are recorded.
>
> **Longitudinal**
> *Midline:* distended urinary bladder, uterus, endometrium, cervix, vagina
> Measure length of uterus from the fundus to the cervix
> *Angle right of midline:* bladder, uterus, area of right ovary
> *Angle left of midline:* bladder, uterus, area of left ovary
> Look at both right and left adnexal areas in true pelvis (iliacus muscle is lateral border)
>
> **Transverse**
> *Low:* distended urinary bladder, vagina, cervix
> *Mid:* bladder, body of uterus, endometrium; look for ovaries
> *High:* fundus of uterus, endometrium; look for ovaries lateral to cornu of uterus

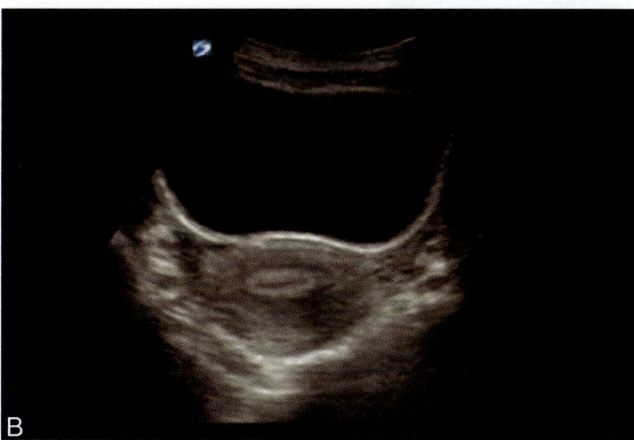

FIG. 42.4 (A) Identify the true sagittal plane of the uterus and cervix, then rotate the transducer 90 degrees to obtain the axial or axial-coronal (transverse) images. Angulation from the contralateral side or direct visualization may help to image the adnexa. Anatomic correlation is correct for axial scans when the left side of the screen correlates with the right side of the patient. (B) Transabdominal image of the distended urinary bladder and uterus. Note the bright endometrial cavity.

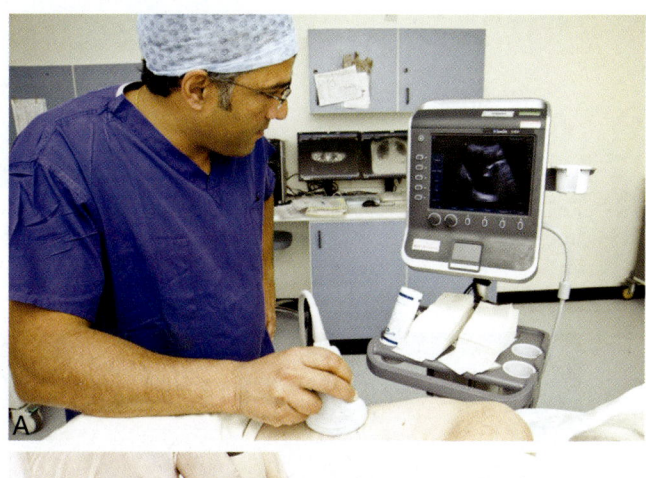

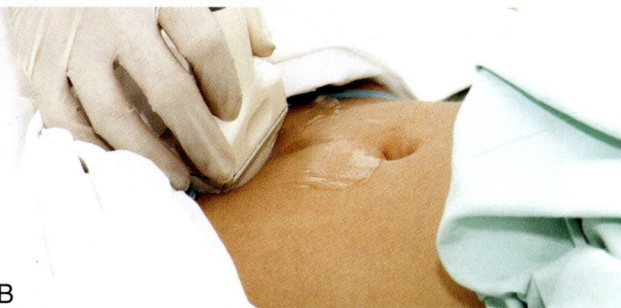

FIG. 42.5 Transabdominal examination of the pelvis includes both sagittal (A) and transverse (B) images.

of interest within the focal zone. The ovaries tend to travel cephalad with increasing bladder distention and may come to lie superior to the uterine fundus. When this occurs, it may be necessary to have the patient empty her bladder before the examination can be completed.

Documentation and scanning techniques should be methodical and become routine for viewing by both the sonographer and the physician. A routine protocol consists of longitudinal and transverse scans of the uterus (including the **myometrium** and **endometrium**), cervix, rectouterine recess (cul-de-sac), right adnexa, and left adnexa (Box 42.2; Figs. 42.5–42.8). Measurements of normal structures and pathology are made in the length, width, and depth dimensions. Additional information may be obtained by the Doppler evaluation of all pelvic anatomy and pathology.

If pathology is present, documentation of the right upper quadrant (Morison's pouch and subphrenic area) and bilateral renal areas must be obtained. The evaluation of these areas demonstrates the presence or absence of free fluid, hydronephrosis (either renal in origin or as a secondary result of a pelvic mass), or anatomic variants related to pelvic findings.

It is important to have adequate bladder filling for all TA examinations. The examination routinely begins with a TA examination to look for large masses, fluid collections, or any obvious abnormalities. The survey of the pelvis is made to identify the uterus and ovaries. Then scan both the right and left flanks, and document the sagittal and transverse views of the liver–right kidney interface and the spleen–left kidney interface.

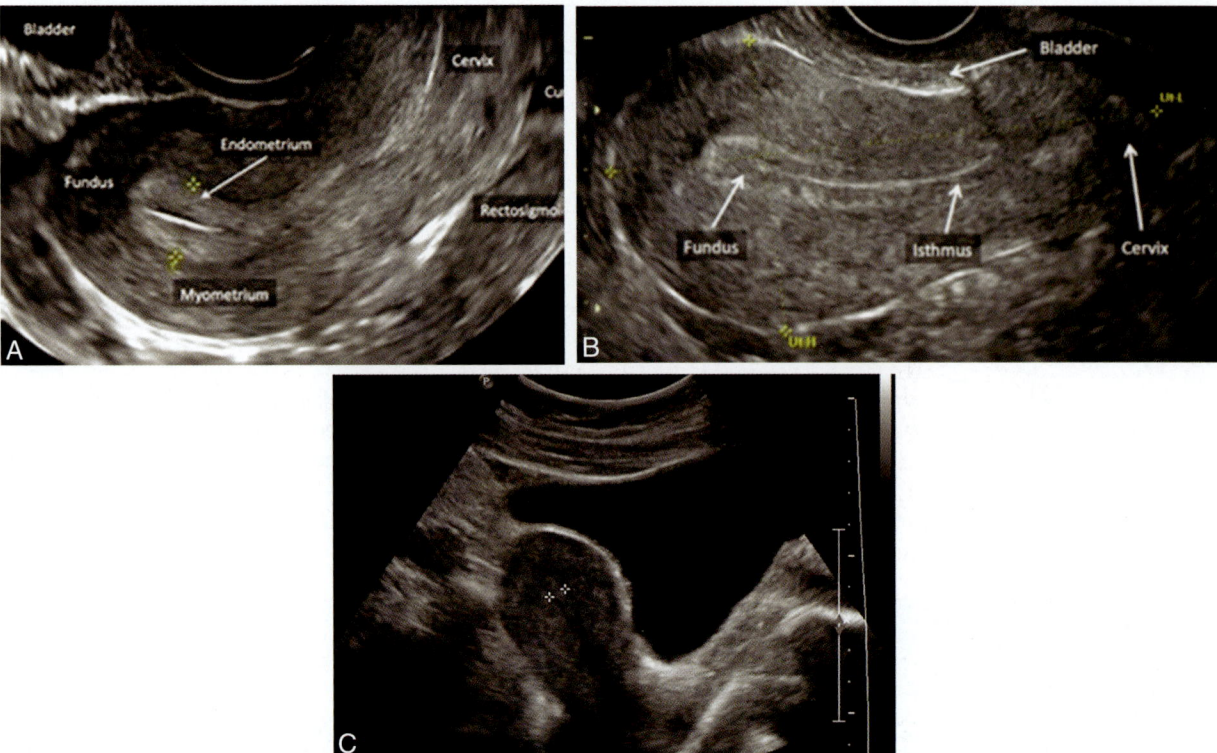

FIG. 42.6 (A) The sagittal scan of the uterus should include the cervix, body, and fundus. (B) The long axis of the uterus is measured from the cervix to the fundus of the uterus. (C) The endometrial cavity should be measured.

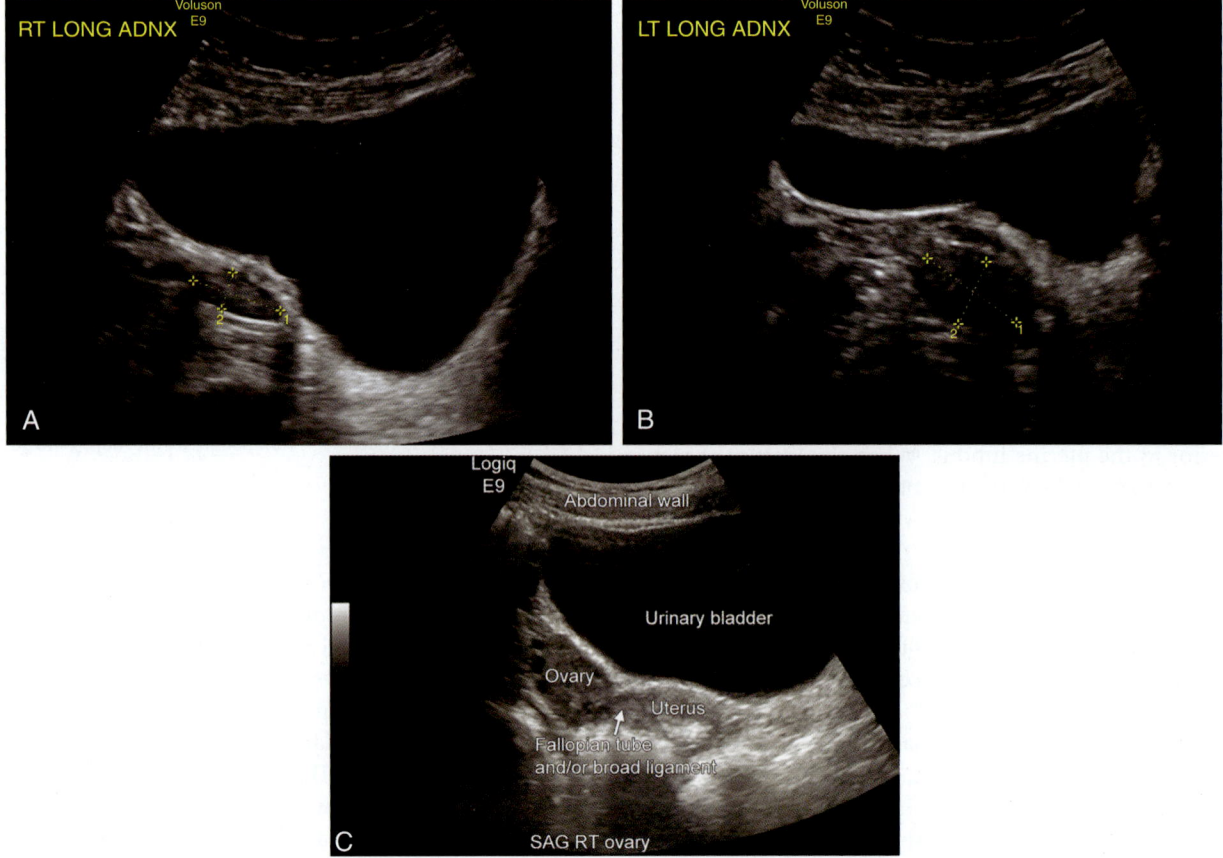

FIG. 42.7 Sagittal image to the right of midline shows the bladder with the right ovary (A) and left ovary (B) posterior. The ovarian length and depth are measured. (C) Sagittal image to the left of midline shows the left ovary posterior to the urinary bladder.

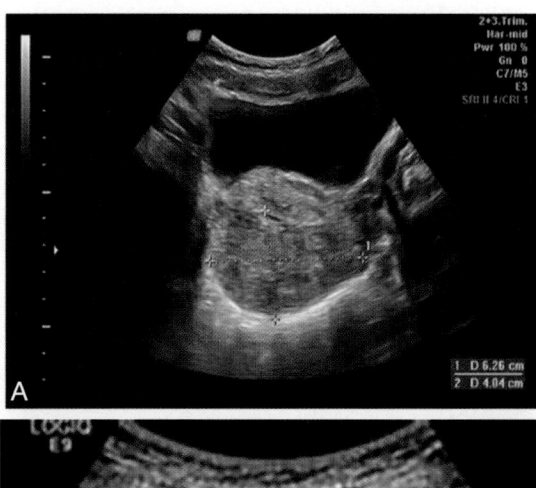

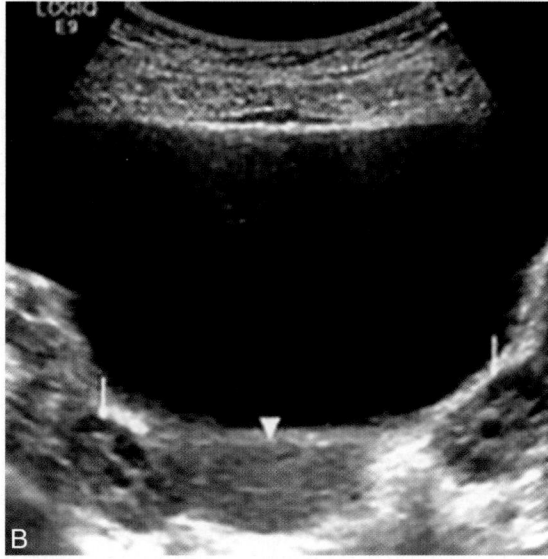

FIG. 42.8 (A) Transabdominal approach to transverse images of the distended urinary bladder and uterus. The measurement is made of the width and depth of the uterus. (B) Transverse image of the ovaries *(long arrow)* and uterus *(arrowhead)*.

Transvaginal Ultrasonography

The inclusion of the TV transducer in standard gynecologic sonography protocols has vastly improved the effectiveness of the pelvic examination. This examination allows the sonographer and physician a better visual survey by shortening the distance from the transducer to the ovaries, uterus, and adnexal regions. The resolution of pelvic structures has improved, and the ability to zoom in on smaller objects has been enhanced. This advance in technology brings with it more frequent detection of small tissue differences.

Patient Instructions. After the TA study is completed, the patient is asked to empty her bladder completely. If the bladder is very full from all the fluids ingested before the examination, the patient may void and think the bladder is "empty" because it had been difficult to hold so much urine during the TA examination. Ask the patient to wait a few seconds after her bladder has been emptied and try to void again; this technique is usually successful in completely emptying the bladder. If the bladder is not completely empty, reverberation artifacts may obscure crucial structures, and problem areas may be pushed too far away from the transducer. This is also an opportune time to reiterate the TV procedure, obtain a verbal consent, and answer any questions the patient may have.

An adequate explanation of the procedure is essential. Many patients are apprehensive at any mention of an "internal" examination, and the referring physician may not have explained the possibility of having one. It is important to explain why it is necessary to perform the TV examination and to stress that the examination is a simple, usually painless procedure and that only part of the probe is inserted. Many laboratories require a verbal or written consent from the patient and examiner for the TV examination. If the examiner is a male, it is essential to have a female staff member in the room during the examination to act as a chaperone.

TV sonography is performed using transducer frequencies of 7.5 MHz or more. These higher frequencies have better near-field resolution, which often permits greater detail of the uterus and adnexal anatomy. The primary disadvantage of high-frequency TV ultrasound is the limited field of view and penetration (8 to 10 cm) because of the high frequency of the transducer and limited movement of the probe within the vagina. TV is often the preferred method of evaluation because it provides optimal visualization of the pelvic organs, and it should always be performed in women with suspected endometrial disorders, a strong family history of ovarian cancer, or a suspected pelvic mass. Contraindications include patient refusal, lack of patient tolerance (usually secondary to intense pelvic pain), and age, both premenarchal and menopausal. It is not recommended that a TV examination be performed in patients who have never been sexually active, have an intact hymen, or have a narrow vaginal canal. If a patient experiences discomfort with an attempted insertion of the transducer, the examination should be discontinued.

Probe Preparation. The TV transducer is prepared with coupling gel on the transducer face and then covered with a sterile probe cover (Fig. 42.9). Currently, most institutions are using latex-free probe covers to prevent allergic reactions in latex-sensitive patients. Instruct the patient that only a short portion of the end of the transducer is introduced into the vaginal canal, because the length of the probe can be intimidating. After the protective sheath has been put on, any air bubbles should be eliminated to prevent artifacts. A sterile external lubricant is then applied to the outside of the probe cover. This provides lubrication for insertion of the probe and is especially important in older women. If the examination is performed on an infertility patient, the use of water to lubricate the transducer is preferred because water does not have a negative effect on sperm mobility.

Examination Technique. After the patient has completely voided, she is asked to undress from the waist down, given a gown, and covered with a sheet. The patient position should be supine, knees gently flexed, and hips elevated slightly on a pillow or folded sheets and feet flat on the table, approximately shoulder length apart. The head and shoulders are slightly elevated with a pillow. A slightly reversed Trendelenburg position may be helpful in lowering the pelvic organs to enhance visualization and detect free intraperitoneal fluid that gravitates to the posterior cul-de-sac. Current ultrasound

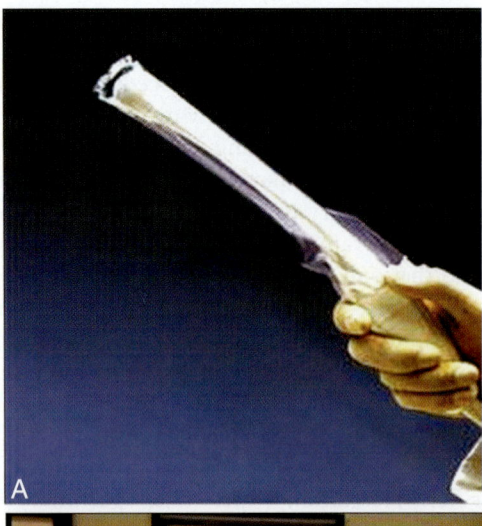

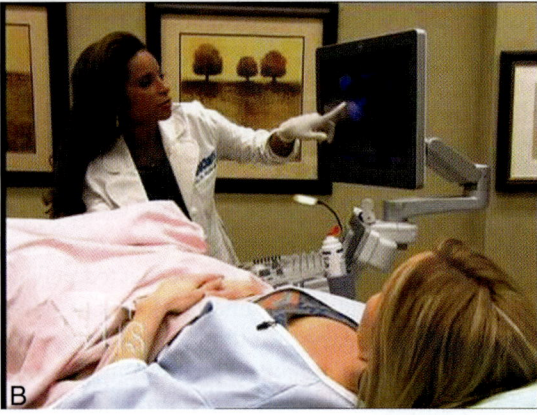

FIG. 42.9 (A) The transvaginal transducer is prepared with coupling gel on the transducer face and then covered with a sterile probe cover. (B) It is important that the patient's buttocks be at the end of the table with the patient's heels in the stirrups. This elevation is necessary to provide adequate mobility of the transducer handle. Being able to easily position the patient, cart, ultrasound equipment, and sonographer chair enhances the ergonomic position and reduces musculoskeletal stress on the sonographer.

scanning tables allow the lower section to be dropped with stirrups added to provide for ease of patient positioning. It is important that the patient's buttocks be at the end of the table with the patient's heels in the stirrups (see Fig. 42.9). This elevation is necessary to provide adequate mobility of the transducer handle. Being able to easily position the patient, cart, ultrasound equipment, and sonographer chair enhances the ergonomic position and reduces musculoskeletal stress on the sonographer. The height adjustment of the scanning table may permit the sonographer to sit or stand during the TV examination. The use of a chair with arms to rest on takes the strain off the examiner's shoulder and elbow.

Scan Orientation. The most accepted method of orientation used during TV scanning is such that the left side of the screen corresponds to the cephalic and right side of the patient, and the right side of the screen corresponds to the caudal and left side of the patient (Fig. 42.10). This method of orientation is the same one for radiography and conventional ultrasound. Residual fluid in the bladder is a helpful orientation landmark and should always appear in the right upper corner of the screen in the sagittal plane. For an anteverted uterus, the cervix would be seen on the right side of the screen, and the fundus of the uterus is found on the left side of the screen. In the case of a retroverted uterus, the cervix would be seen on the left with the fundus on the right.

Scanning Planes. When inserting the transducer in the sagittal plane, the flat part of the transducer is along the top surface of the handle so that the beam is projected in the midline anteroposterior aspect of the body. From the sagittal plane, the transducer is limited in motion because of the vagina. True parasagittal planes are never obtained, but angulation from this central point is considered sagittal imaging (Fig. 42.11A). As in the TA examination, oblique angulation is often necessary to visualize the entire uterus and cervix. It is often necessary to advance the transducer slightly, angling anterior to visualize the fundus, and then withdraw slightly, away from the external os, while angling posterior to see the cervix and rectouterine recess (see Fig. 42.11B). The uterus is surveyed by scanning from the midline to the right and left. Angulation and tilting of the transducer direct the sound beam to visualize the adnexa in an oblique sagittal plane. Applying manual external pressure (either by the sonographer or the patient) to the outer abdominal wall may help displace the bowel and bring the ovaries into the focal zone, helping to visualize and delineate the borders of the ovaries.

When the transducer is rotated 90 degrees from the sagittal plane, image orientation represents the **coronal plane** (see Fig. 42.11C). Rotating the transducer 360 degrees is possible. If the uterus is retroverted, better resolution may be obtained by inverting the transducer 180 degrees. The image should be inverted to properly document the retroverted uterus. It may also help to rotate the transducer 180 degrees in the coronal plane to better image the left ovary. The sonographer should check the orientation to guarantee that the left side of the screen represents the right side of the patient and again invert the image as necessary.

A helpful technique for locating the ovary is to first obtain a coronal image of the uterine fundus and then to angle the probe out to the **cornua** and ovarian ligament. Once this region is identified, the ovary can usually be identified by slowly sweeping the beam anteriorly and posteriorly.

By sweeping from the cervix through the lower, mid, and fundal portions of the uterus, the entire organ can be evaluated and measurements can be taken. For an anteverted uterus, the sweep will be posterior to anterior. A retroverted uterus will be anterior to posterior.

Scan Technique. The orientation of the TV probe is controlled by probe rotation and angulation. The probe can be rotated up to 90 degrees, angled or pointed in any direction, and inserted or withdrawn to allow structures to be placed in the focal zone of the transducer rotation (Box 42.3; Fig. 42.12). Varying the depth of the transducer may optimize the imaging of a structure in that field of view. Movement of the transducer is centered around the *introitus* (opening of the vagina). Any tilting movement of the transducer handle produces reciprocal motion at the probe tip. Rotation of the probe along its long axis provides 360-degree longitudinal visualization of the pelvis. Pushing or pulling the probe can

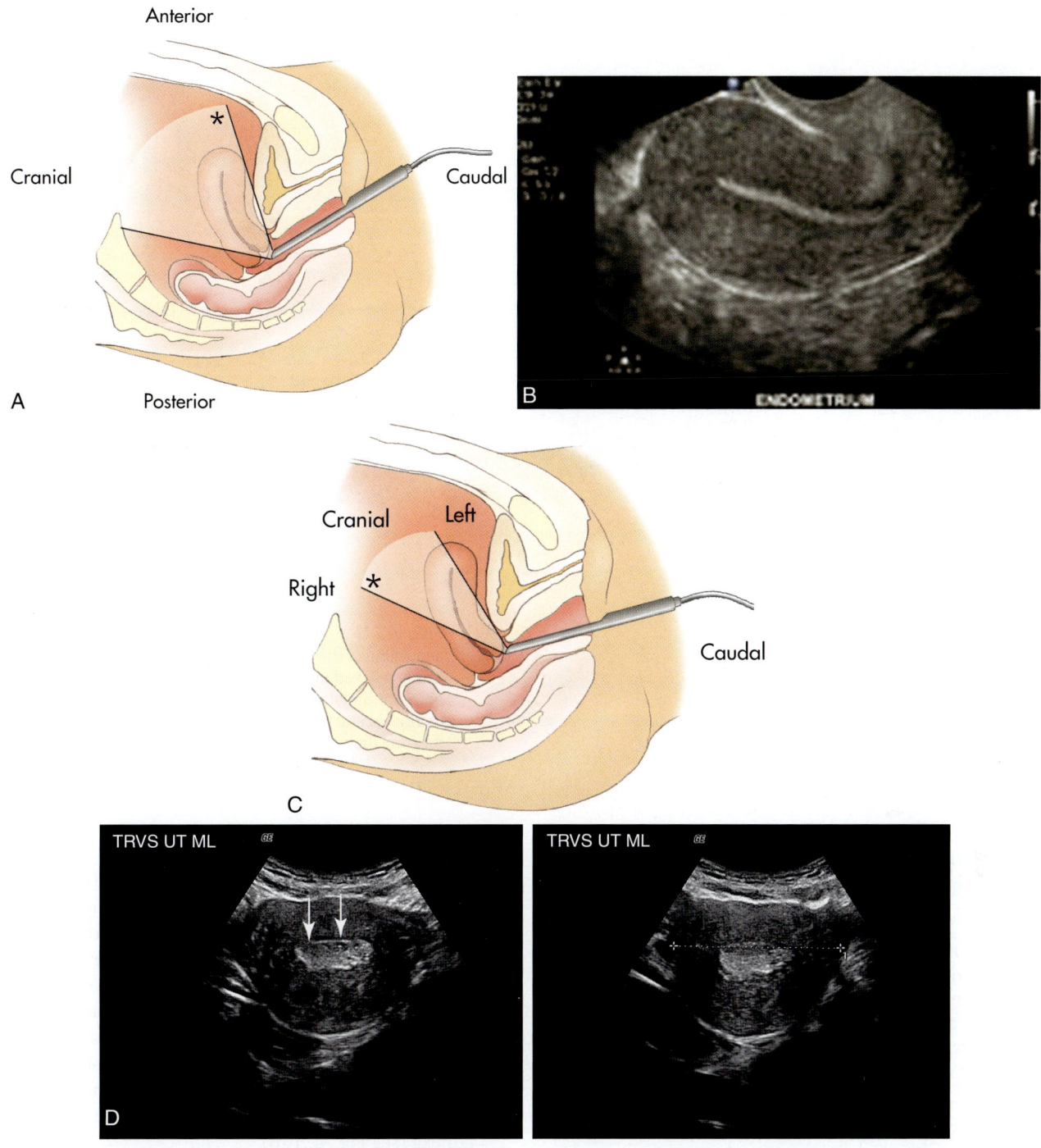

FIG. 42.10 (A) Transvaginal sagittal plane. The notch of the transducer is along the top surface of the handle, so the beam is projected in the midline anteroposterior aspect of the body. (B) The bladder is emptied, so only the uterine cavity and endometrial canal are seen. (C) Transvaginal coronal plane. The notch of the transducer is rotated toward the sonographer so the beam may image the uterus in a coronal view. (D) Coronal views of the uterus with the endometrial canal centrally located.

bring the tip close to a region of interest and provide a method of indirect palpation, allowing evaluation of focal tenderness or fixation.

The insertion of the transducer into the vagina should be done in real-time as the sonographer watches the anatomy, because real-time appears to ensure proper orientation. The probe may be inserted or guided by the patient, sonographer, or physician. It should not be inserted beyond the external cervical os. To maintain patient dignity and privacy, the patient should be properly draped at all times, and all practitioners who will be observing the examination should be present from the beginning of the examination.

Scan Protocol. Before recording any images, a complete pelvic survey should be performed. This survey is performed by slowly sweeping the beam in a sagittal plane from the midline through both adnexa to the lateral pelvic sidewalls. The probe

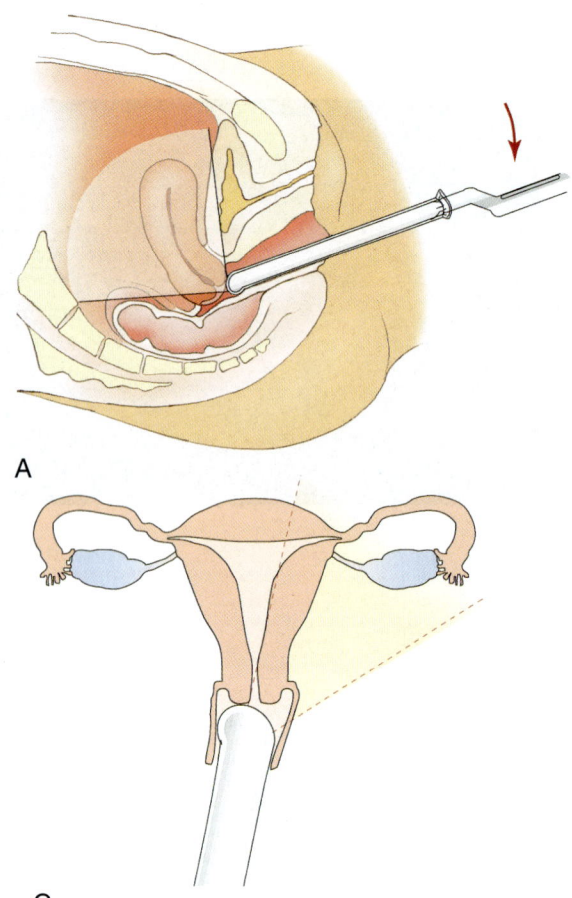

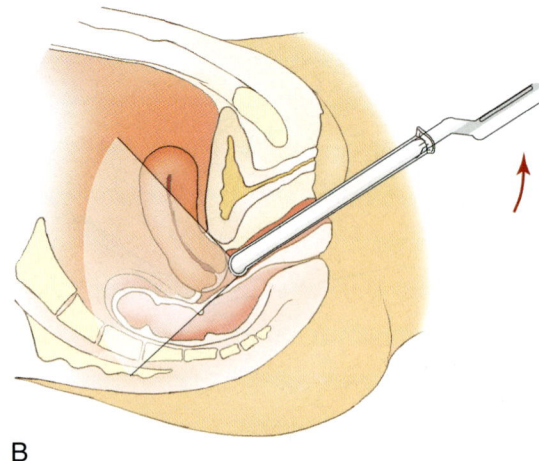

FIG. 42.11 (A) Transvaginal sagittal plane with anterior angulation of the probe to better visualize the fundus of a normal anteflexed uterus. (B) Transvaginal sagittal scanning with posterior angulation to better visualize the cervix and rectouterine recess. (C) The probe is rotated 90 degrees to record the axial (transverse) images.

| BOX 42.3 | Transvaginal Scanning Pelvic Protocol |

Survey the pelvic area before images are made.

Sagittal: Uterus
Image the uterus from cervix to fundus, endometrial cavity: measure the long axis.
Angle slowly to right of uterus.
Angle slowly to left of uterus.
Pull probe out slightly to image cervix.

Coronal: Uterus
Rotate transducer 90 degrees; image uterine fundus, body, and cervix with endometrial canal.
Look for free fluid surrounding uterine cavity.

Sagittal: Ovaries
Follow the fundus of the uterus to the area of the cornu to image the ovaries; the internal iliac vessels serve as their posterior border. Color imaging may be used to separate vascular structures from the ovary. Look for follicles surrounding the periphery of the ovary.
Measure long axis.

Coronal: Ovaries
Rotate transducer 90 degrees once sagittal plane of ovary is obtained.
Measure width and depth.

is then rotated to the coronal plane, and the beam is swept from the cervix to the fundus of the uterus. The survey will orient the sonographer to the relative positions of the uterus and ovaries and identify any obvious masses. After the survey, standard views are obtained. These include the following:
- *Sagittal plane.* Cervix, endocervical canal, posterior cul-de-sac, uterus (midline, right, and left), endometrium, right ovary and adnexa, and left ovary and adnexa (Fig. 42.13A).
- *Coronal plane.* Vagina, cervix and posterior cul-de-sac, uterine corpus and endometrium, uterine fundus and endometrium, right ovary and adnexa, and left ovary and adnexa (see Fig. 42.13B).

Length, width, and axial measurements of the uterus and ovaries should be documented. The thickness of the endometrium should be measured in the sagittal plane (Fig. 42.14). By sweeping side to side through the endometrium, the thickest portion can be identified, and any areas of focal irregularity can be evaluated. It may be helpful either to zoom or to decrease the field of view to obtain an accurate measurement. Do not include any internal fluid in the endometrium measurement. Additional views of pathology or areas indicated should be obtained and measured in three dimensions.

Obtaining the standard images indicates that the entire organ and regions imaged have been carefully assessed in real time in two orthogonal planes. Any pathology or variant from

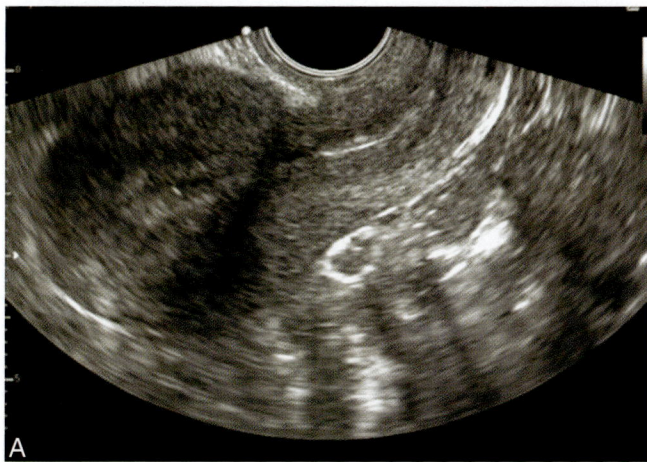

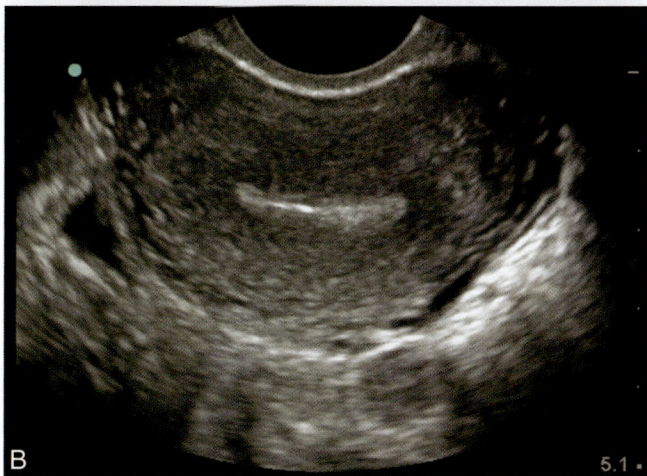

FIG. 42.12 (A) With transvaginal imaging, oblique angulation is often necessary to visualize the entire uterus and cervix. It is often necessary to advance the transducer slightly, angling anterior to visualize the fundus, and then withdraw slightly, away from the external os, while angling posterior to see the cervix and rectouterine recess. (B) When the transducer is rotated 90 degrees from the sagittal plane, image orientation represents the coronal plane. The coronal plane should image the uterine fundus, body, and cervix with the endometrial stripe. This is the fundus of the uterus. The probe is angled caudally to image the miduterine cavity. The width of the uterus is measured at the widest points. The probe is angled slightly more caudal to image the lower uterine segment. The probe is withdrawn slightly to image the cervix.

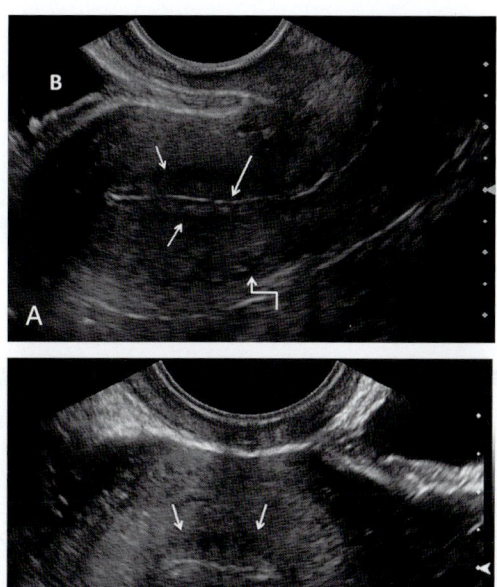

FIG. 42.13 (A) Sagittal plane. Cervix, endocervical canal, posterior cul-de-sac, uterus. (B) Coronal plane of the uterine corpus and endometrium.

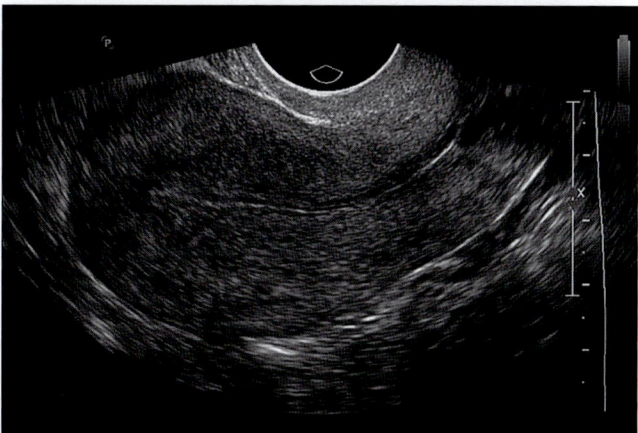

FIG. 42.14 The thickness of the endometrium should be measured in the sagittal plane.

normal must be assessed and appropriate images recorded. Color flow Doppler, power Doppler, and pulsed Doppler are added to the examination, depending on the clinical situation and pathology demonstrated on gray scale.

Translabial (transperineal) sonography provides an alternative technique to TV scanning in the event that TV is contraindicated. The most common scenarios would be premature rupture of membranes, in which one would want to avoid contact with prolapsed membranes, cervical incompetence, and uterine prolapse. A 4.5- to 9-MHz sector transducer is covered with a sterile probe cover and placed at the vaginal introitus and oriented in the direction of the vagina. Partial bladder filling may assist visualization of the cervix. Transperineal sonography is technically more challenging. Rectal gas and the pubic symphysis may obscure visualization and the identification of anatomic landmarks. These limitations can be overcome by elevation of the hips (as in TV scanning), better application of the transducer on the perineum, or changes in the orientation of the probe. The TV probe may also be placed at the vaginal introitus or slightly inserted within. This can assist in imaging the lower cervical area and distal vagina. If the TV transducer is already well within the vaginal vault, withdraw the transducer to visualize the lower cervix (Fig. 42.15).

Disinfecting Technique. The use of an intracavitary device requires the prevention of cross contamination between patients, and high-level disinfection is a requirement of the Centers for Disease Control and Prevention. After completing the TV examination, the sterile probe cover should be removed. This can be done by using the gloved scanning

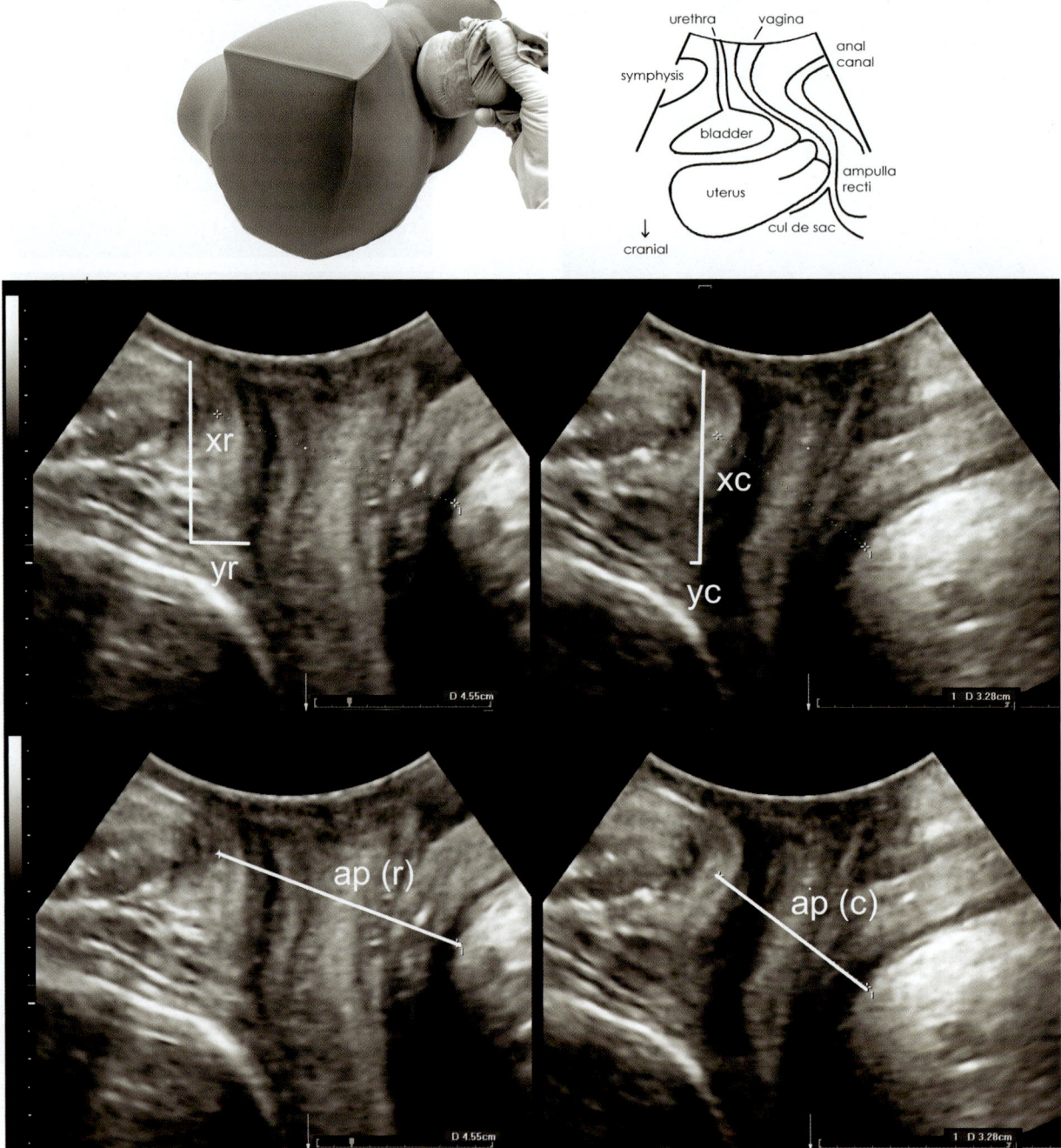

FIG. 42.15 Translabial (transperineal) sonography provides an alternative technique to transvaginal scanning in the event that TV is contraindicated. Partial bladder filling may assist visualization of the cervix. The TV probe may also be placed at the vaginal introitus or slightly inserted within. This can assist in imaging the lower cervical area and distal vagina. If the transvaginal transducer is already well within the vaginal vault, withdraw the transducer to visualize the lower cervix. *B*, Bladder; *PS*, pubic symphysis; *V*, vagina.

hand to slide the probe cover off into the glove, removing the glove, and disposing of both into the waste container. The transducer should then be wiped clean with the organization's approved disinfectant (be sure to read the vendor's recommendation for cleaning transducers) or pre-cleaned with an enzymatic sponge, and then dried with a towel. High-level disinfection can be achieved by either a liquid soak process, such as Cidex OPA, glutaraldehyde, or hydrogen peroxide, or by automated high-level disinfection, now available in the Trophon device. For liquid soaking, the transducer should be soaked in a disinfectant between uses for at least the minimum recommended amount of time from the equipment manufacturer (10 to 20 minutes). Disinfection for extended times can cause damage or degradation to the transducer face. Most disinfectants are now non-glutaraldehyde based (e.g., Cidex OPA) and care should be taken when handling these caustic chemicals. Staff members must wear gloves, and some manufacturers recommend the use of safety goggles. There are various safety "stations" that are commercially available that contain the required venting for this toxic chemical.

Emergency eyewash stations should be available within the facility. After the transducer has been soaked in a Cidex-type solution (high-grade disinfectant), it is important to rinse the transducer with water and dry it before appropriate storage. It is advisable to contact the probe manufacturer if the manual does not provide information regarding the type of disinfectant and immersion time limit.

For automated high-level disinfection with the Trophon device, follow the pre-cleaning method as identified by the central processing team of your organization. Dry the transducer probe, load the probe into the Trophon device according to the manufacturer's directions, and commence the automated cycle of 7 minutes. On removal from the Trophon device, the probe is wiped clean and prepared for storage.

SONOGRAPHIC EVALUATION OF THE PELVIS

Bony Pelvis

Ultrasound is essentially absorbed by bone. The shadow is produced because no sound is returned to the transducer because it is virtually all absorbed. The bony pelvis resembles a ring or funnel in shape. Anteriorly, the pubic symphysis is formed by the articulation of the pubic bones with each other. The TA study is begun just superior or cephalad to this midline landmark. Posteriorly, the sacroiliac joint on either side forms the connection between the os ilium and the sacrum. Sonographically, the sacrum may appear as a bright line with an overlying bowel shadow (Fig. 42.16). This is more apparent in infants, children, and thin patients.

Muscles of the Pelvis

The filled urinary bladder displaces the bowel and acts as an acoustic window for evaluating three major groups of muscles: obturator internus, pelvic floor (levator ani and coccygeus), and iliopsoas (Fig. 42.17). Pelvic muscles may be mistaken for ovaries, fluid collections, or masses. A symmetric bilateral arrangement indicates that they are muscles. The rectus abdominis muscles insert on the pubic rami and are paired parasagittal straps in the abdominal wall; they appear as hypoechoic structures with echogenic striations. The rectus sheath separates the sonographic appearance of the rectus abdominis muscle from surrounding fat and bowel as a bright linear echogenic reflector (Fig. 42.18).

Obturator Internus Muscles. In the lesser or true pelvis, the urinary bladder, reproductive organs, levator ani, and obturator internus muscles can be identified. Sonographically,

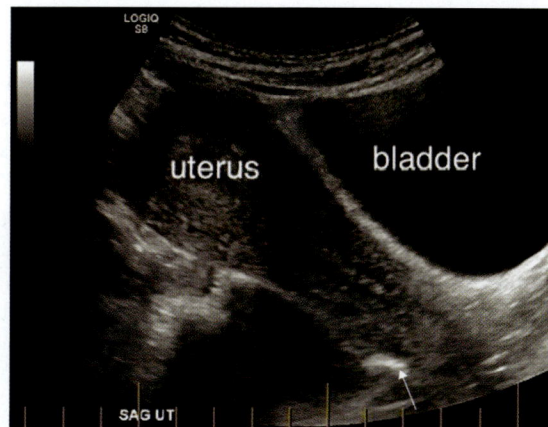

FIG. 42.16 Sonographically, the sacrum may appear as a bright line with an overlying bowel shadow *(arrow)*.

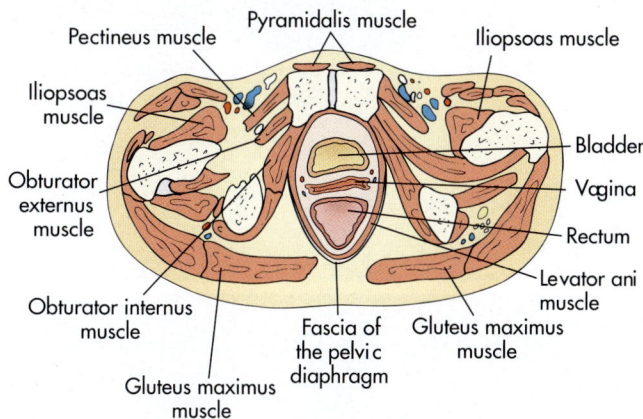

FIG. 42.17 The filled urinary bladder displaces the bowel and acts as an acoustic window for evaluating three major groups of muscles: obturator internus, pelvic floor (levator ani and coccygeus), and iliopsoas.

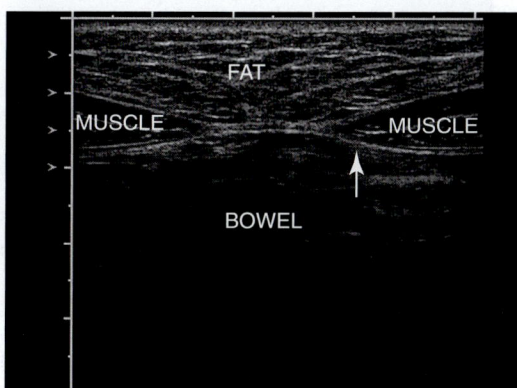
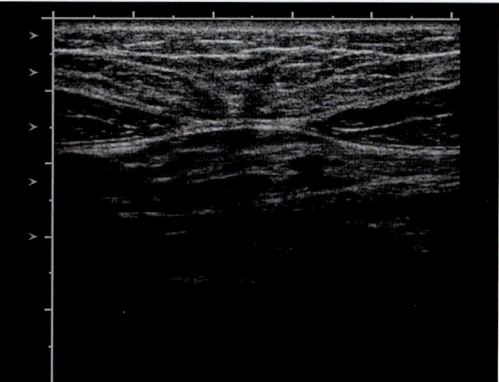

FIG. 42.18 The rectus abdominis muscle is visualized with a 14-MHz linear transducer. The rectus sheath *(arrow)* separates the muscle from surrounding fat and bowel.

sections of the obturator internus muscle are seen at the posterior lateral corners of the bladder at the level of the vagina and cervix. This muscle is hypoechoic, ovoid, and surrounded by the obturator fascia, which serves as a tendinous attachment for the levator ani muscle (Fig. 42.19).

Pelvic Floor Muscles. The levator ani muscle is best visualized sonographically in a transverse plane with caudal angulation at the most inferior aspect of the bladder. It is a hypoechoic, hammock-shaped area that is medial, caudal, and posterior to the obturator internus (Fig. 42.20). The two other muscles of the lesser pelvis, the coccygeus and piriformis, are located deep, cranially, and posteriorly. They are not routinely visualized on ultrasound examination and are not distinguished from other surrounding muscles. The piriformis muscles are located on either side of the midline posterior to the upper half of the uterine body and fundus. This is the most common muscle to be mistaken for the ovary.

Iliopsoas Muscles. The iliopsoas muscles can be seen in the greater pelvis. The iliopsoas muscle is a combination of the iliacus muscle and the psoas major. The psoas major originates bilaterally at the paravertebral lumbar region and courses caudally. The iliacus muscle is contiguous with and arises posterior to the psoas major at the level of the superior two-thirds of the iliac fossa. Together, they form the iliopsoas muscle, which continues in the caudal direction, coursing anterolaterally to its insertion on the lesser trochanter of the femur.

The sonographic appearance of this muscle varies greatly depending on its development. On ultrasound examination, the iliopsoas muscle is discretely marginated and hypoechoic (Fig. 42.21). The bright echogenic line representing the interposed fascial sheath can often determine the separation of the iliacus and psoas muscles. Both longitudinal and transverse images may be obtained through the urinary bladder midline with lateral angulation. Transvaginally, the positions of these muscles are deep and beyond the field of view.

Pelvic Vascularity

Pelvic vascularity can easily be evaluated using real-time and Doppler imaging. The use of color Doppler techniques (color flow, power, and pulsed) permits the vessel to be localized, allows the sample gate to be placed exactly in the area of interest, and reduces examination time (Fig. 42.22).

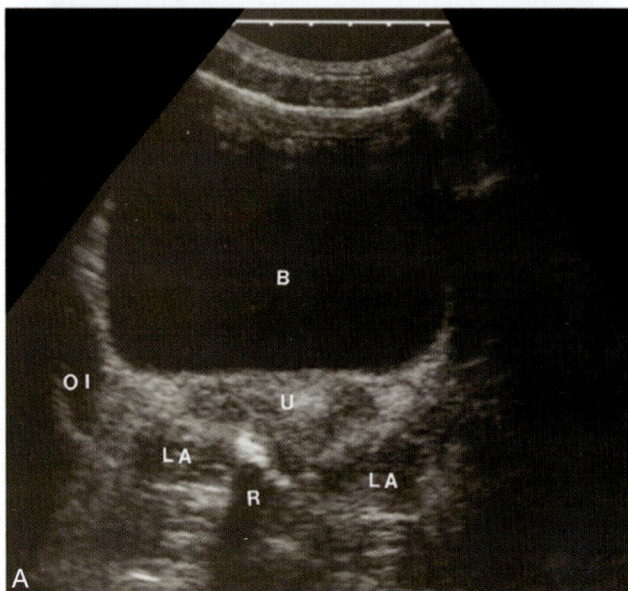
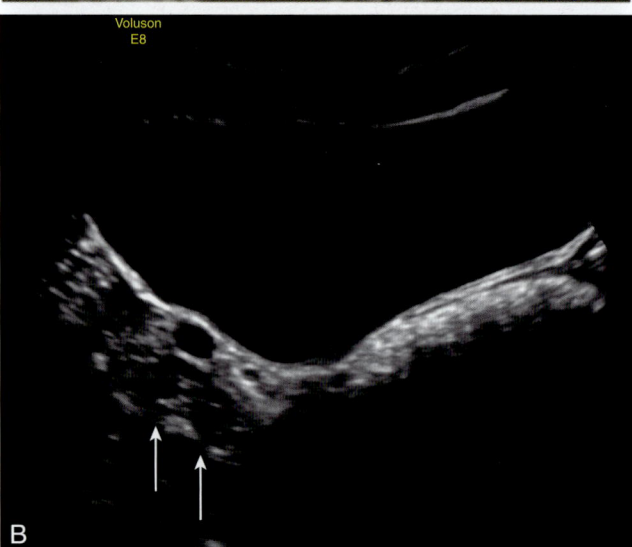

FIG. 42.19 (A) Sections of the obturator internus (OI) muscle are seen at the posterior lateral corners of the bladder at the level of the vagina and cervix. This muscle is hypoechoic, ovoid, and surrounded by the obturator fascia, which serves as a tendinous attachment for the levator ani (LA) muscle. (B) Sagittal image of the obturator internus muscle *(arrows)*. Angle the transducer through a distended bladder from the contralateral side to demonstrate these muscles. *B*, Bladder; *R*, rectum; *U*, uterus.

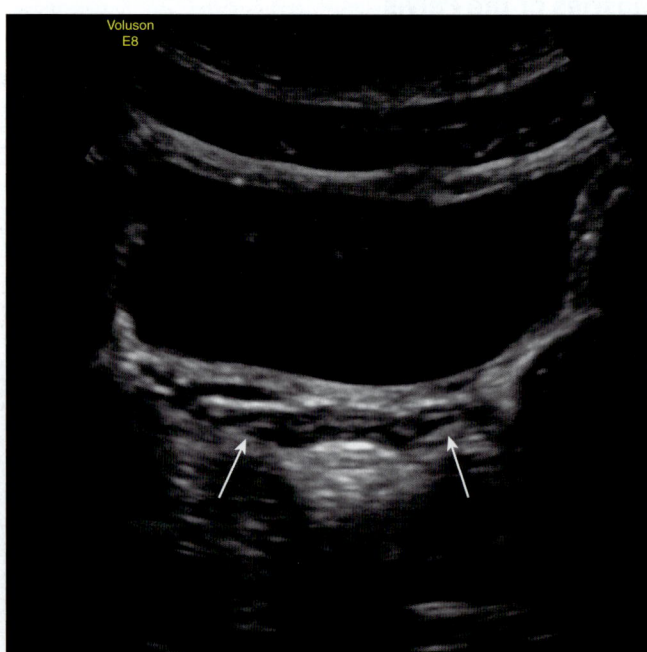

FIG. 42.20 The levator ani muscle *(arrows)* is visualized with the transabdominal sector transducer as hypoechoic, hammock-shaped muscles medial, caudal, and posterior to the obturator internus. Angle from the most superior aspect of the urinary bladder caudally to demonstrate these muscles.

The quantitative waveform is displayed and analyzed in one of the following indices:

S/D ratio (or A/B ratio) (A = peak systolic and B = end diastolic)
Pourcelot resistive index (RI) (A − B/A)
Pulsatility index (PI) (A − B/mean)

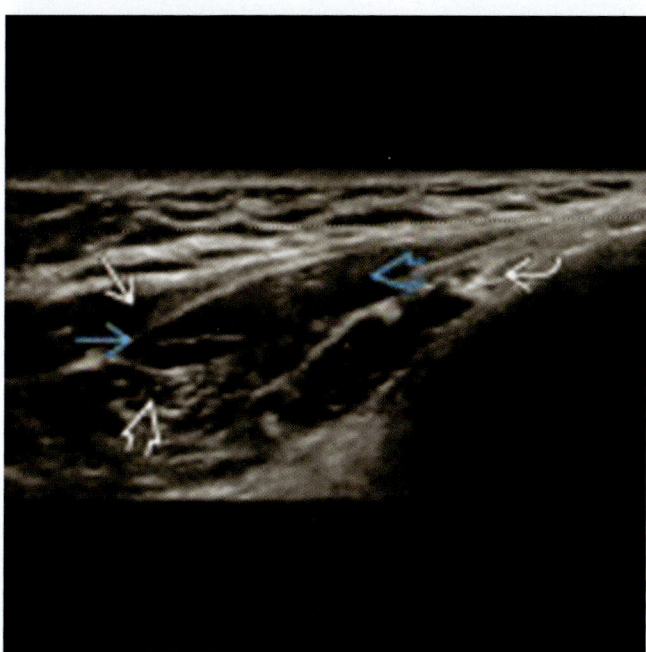

FIG. 42.21 The iliacus muscle is contiguous with and arises posterior to the psoas major at the level of the superior two-thirds of the iliac fossa. Together, they form the iliopsoas muscle, which continues in the caudal direction, coursing anterolaterally to its insertion on the lesser trochanter of the femur.

Because the Doppler velocities are assessed as ratios, the waveform values are angle independent. (Remember that to obtain accurate Doppler velocities, it is critical to have the Doppler as parallel to the flow as possible; however, when ratios are determined, the difference in flow between systole and diastole is assessed and the angle is therefore not as critical.)

Imaging with TA and TV ultrasound, the internal iliac vessels can almost always be visualized and used as a landmark for the lateral pelvic wall and ovary. This vessel is commonly seen lateral and deep to the ovary. The internal iliac vessel has classic characteristic blood flow, demonstrating parabolic flow with an even distribution of velocities throughout the waveform (Fig. 42.23A). The pulsatility and slow movement of blood flow can often be appreciated on gray-scale imaging. It is important to differentiate the vessels from an ovarian cyst because of its proximity to the ovary. If uncertain, the sonographer can use Doppler technique or rotate on the structure to elongate a vessel into a tube.

The arteries may be noted anterior to the veins in the pelvis. To assess the uterine vessels, the sonographer interrogates just lateral to the cervix and lower uterine segment at the level of the **internal os**. Uterine flow in the non-pregnant female usually shows a resistive pattern with an RI of 0.88 in the proliferative phase, decreasing slightly beginning the day before ovulation (see Fig. 42.23B–C).

The vagina has two sources of blood. The anterior surface of the vagina and cervix is supplied with blood from a branch off the uterine artery before it reaches the uterus. The posterior surface of the vagina is supplied with blood from a branch off the internal iliac vessel (see Fig. 42.22).

The ovary receives its blood supply from the aorta. The ovarian arteries also have a tortuous course from the lateral posterior border of the ovary to anastomose, with the uterine

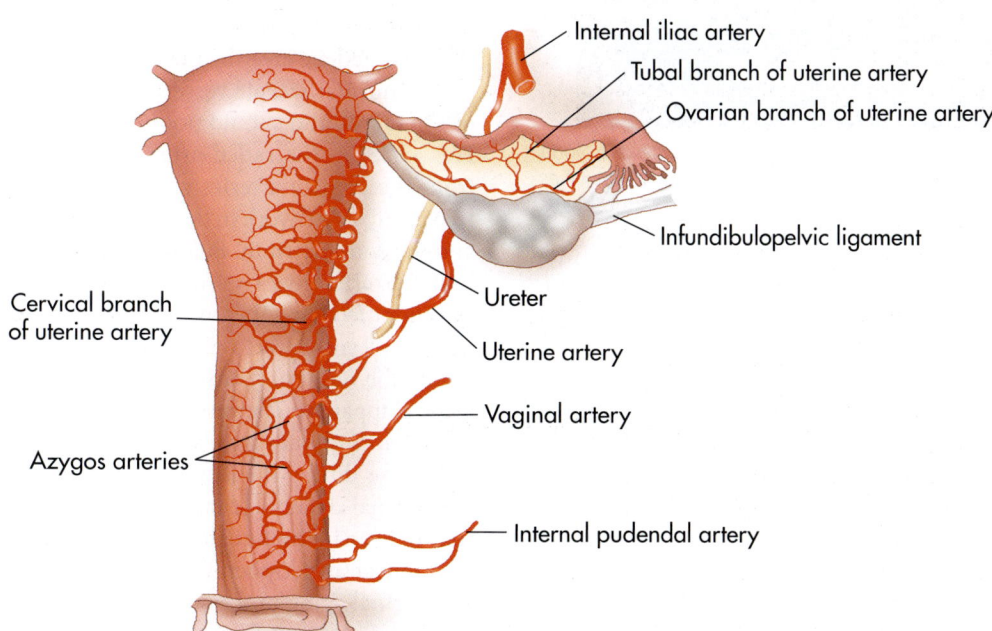

FIG. 42.22 The uterine and vaginal arteries supply blood to the uterus; the ovaries receive blood from the branches of the uterine artery and from the ovarian arteries arising from the abdominal aorta.

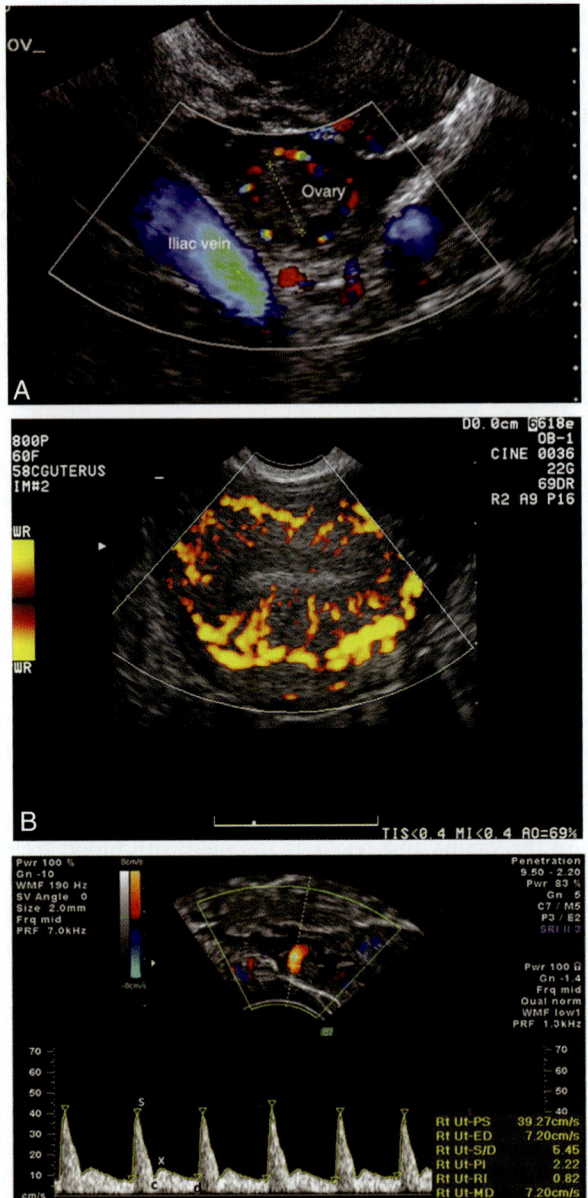

FIG. 42.23 (A) The internal iliac vessel has classic characteristic blood flow, demonstrating parabolic flow with an even distribution of velocities throughout the waveform. (B) Transvaginal coronal view of the uterus with power Doppler that outlines the vascularity of the uterine cavity. The arcuate arteries are in the periphery of the uterine myometrium. (C) Uterine flow in the nonpregnant female usually shows a resistive pattern with a resistive index of 0.88 in the proliferative phase, decreasing slightly beginning the day before ovulation.

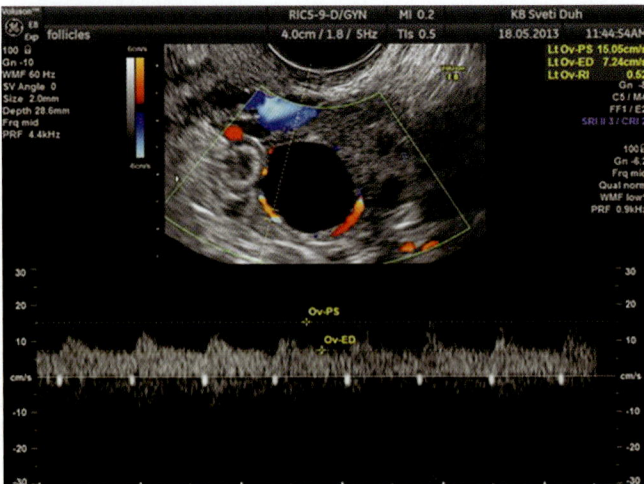

FIG. 42.24 A low-velocity, highly resistive flow pattern is shown during the follicular phase of the menstrual cycle.

artery in the broad ligament adjacent to the cornual area (see Fig. 42.22). This is considered the ovarian branch of the uterine artery, which is the most consistent and successful area for assessing ovarian Doppler flow. The blood flow of the functional ovary varies with the menstrual cycle. The changes in RI are thought to be a result of hormone-mediated changes in vessel wall compliance, allowing increased blood flow to the ovary in the late follicular and early luteal phases. A low-velocity, highly resistive flow pattern is shown during the follicular phase of the menstrual cycle (Fig. 42.24). At ovulation, the maximal velocity increases and the RI decreases. The RI reaches 0.44±0.004, and 4 to 5 days later it rises slightly before menstruation. The non-resistive flow pattern during ovulation probably results from the neovascularization of the follicle and subsequent corpus luteum. A normal pregnancy causes persistent low-resistive corpus luteal flow throughout the first trimester.

Uterus

The uterine muscle consists of three layers, and the outer serosa of the uterus is not visualized sonographically (Fig. 42.25A). The middle layer is the myometrium of the uterus. This layer should have a homogeneous echotexture with smooth-walled borders. Any areas of increased or decreased echotexture should be noted and measured. The inner layer is the endometrium. This layer is thin, compact, and relatively hypovascular. The endometrium is hypoechoic and surrounds the relatively echogenic endometrial stripe, creating a subendometrial halo. The thin outer layer is separated from the intermediate layer by the **arcuate vessels**.

The normal arcuate vessels are often seen in the periphery of the uterus and should not be mistaken for pathology (see Fig. 42.25B). The radial arteries arise as multiple branches from the arcuate arteries and travel centrally to supply the rich capillary network in the deeper layers of the myometrium and the endometrium. Before entering the endometrium, the radial arteries give rise to the straight and spiral arteries of the endometrium. These vessels are most often demonstrated between 1 and 3 weeks after the onset of the last menses. Just before the onset of menses and during menses, these vessels are less apparent. The vasodilating actions of estrogens on the uterus during mid-cycle and the vasoconstricting hormonal influences during the late luteal phase before menses explain the normal dynamic changes of these vessels. Calcifications may be seen in the arcuate arteries in postmenopausal women and appear as peripheral linear echoes with shadowing. This is a normal aging process that may be accelerated in diabetic patients. Echogenic foci in the inner layer of the myometrium, which are usually non-shadowing, are thought to represent dystrophic calcification related to previous instrumentation. Although they are of no clinical significance, they should be

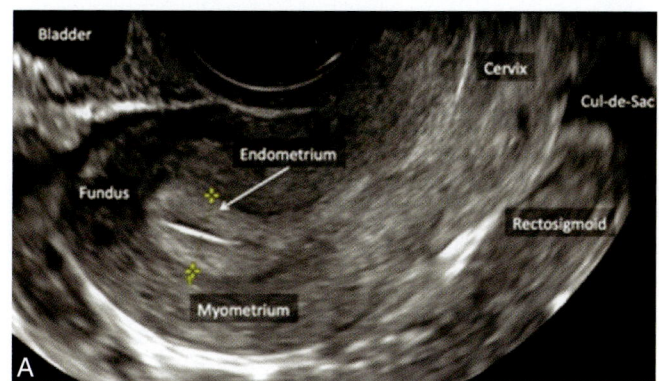

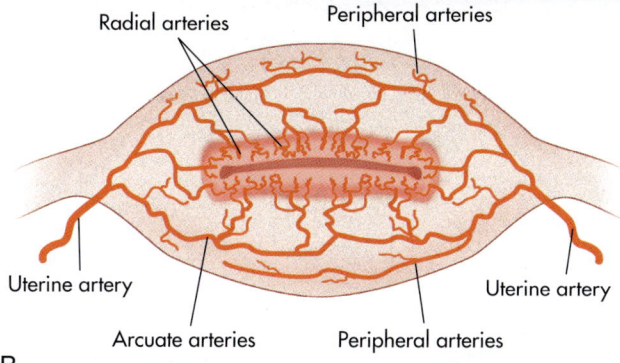

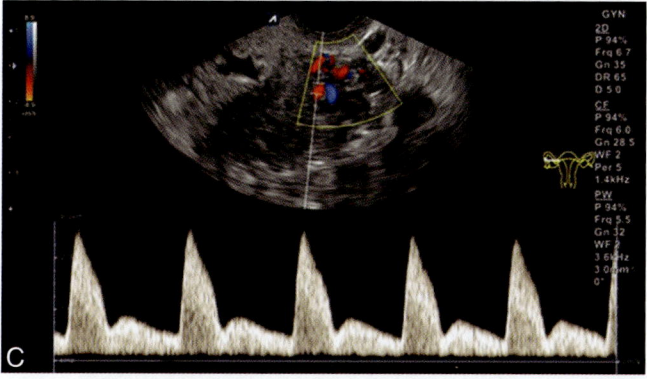

FIG. 42.25 (A) Transvaginal sagittal image of the uterine layers. The uterine muscle consists of three layers, and the outer serosa of the uterus is not visualized sonographically. The middle layer is the myometrium of the uterus. This layer should have a homogeneous echotexture with smooth-walled borders. Any areas of increased or decreased echotexture should be noted and measured. The inner layer is the endometrium. This layer is thin, compact, and relatively hypovascular. The endometrium is hypoechoic and surrounds the relatively echogenic endometrial stripe, creating a subendometrial halo. The thin outer layer is separated from the intermediate layer by the arcuate vessels. (B) The blood is supplied to the uterus from the uterine artery, which bifurcates into the arcuate artery, radial arteries, and peripheral arteries. These vessels are tortuous and have many anastomotic sites. (C) The normal arcuate vessels are often seen in the periphery of the uterus. The Doppler waveform usually shows a high-velocity, high-resistance pattern.

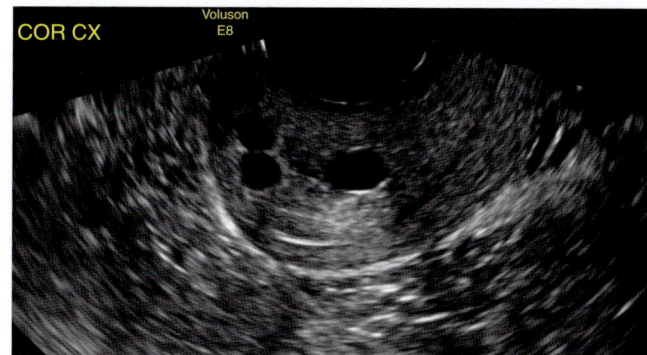

FIG. 42.26 Transvaginal coronal view of the cervix with multiple Naboth cysts.

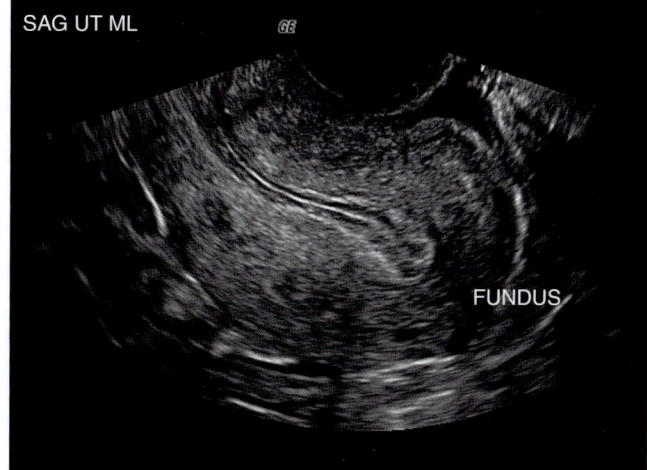

FIG. 42.27 Transvaginal sagittal image of the retroflexed uterus.

distinguished from calcified leiomyomas. Uterine perfusion (the vascular blood flow within the myometrium) can be assessed by Doppler sonography of the uterine arteries. The Doppler waveform usually shows a high-velocity, high-resistance pattern (see Fig. 42.25C).

The body of the uterus is separated from the cervix by the isthmus at the level of the internal os and is identified by the narrowing of the canal. Tissue echogenicity surrounding the cervical canal should appear homogeneous. One can frequently visualize cervical inclusion cysts, known as nabothian cysts, near the endocervical canal. These are generally less than 1 to 2 cm wide and are anechoic smooth-walled structures with acoustic enhancement posteriorly; they are of no clinical significance and generally are not measured (Fig. 42.26).

The cervix is fixed in the midline, but the uterine body is mobile and may lie obliquely on either side of the midline. Flexion refers to the axis of the uterine body relative to the cervix, whereas version refers to the axis of the cervix relative to the vagina. The uterus is usually anteverted and anteflexed. The uterus may also be retroflexed when the body is tilted posteriorly or retroverted when the entire uterus is tilted backward (Fig. 42.27).

The fundus of a retroverted or retroflexed uterus is difficult to assess by TA sonography. It may appear hypoechoic because it is situated a distance from the transducer and may mimic a mass in the rectouterine space. This can be confused for a fibroid. TV sonography is close to the posteriorly located fundus and is much better for assessing the retroverted or retroflexed uterus. As discussed earlier, it is necessary to use all three motions of the TV transducer to optimize the image. The true "lie" of the uterus is seen transvaginally with an empty bladder.

The TA technique is the best way to measure the cervical-fundal dimension of the uterus in the longitudinal plane. Oblique angulation may be necessary to elongate and measure the entire length of the longitudinal plane of the uterus. Its length is always measured from the distal end of the fundus to the distal end of the cervix (Fig. 42.28). Either TA or TV scanning technique may be used to measure the width and anteroposterior dimensions of the uterus (Fig. 42.29). Because of the proximity of the uterus to the broad ligament and surrounding vessels, it may be difficult to delineate the lateral borders of the uterus. Color Doppler technique or changing post-processing controls may help delineate these borders.

The size and shape of the normal uterus vary throughout life and are related to age, hormonal status, and parity. Neonatally, the uterus is pear shaped secondary to maternal hormonal stimulation (Fig. 42.30). Prepubertally, the cervix occupies

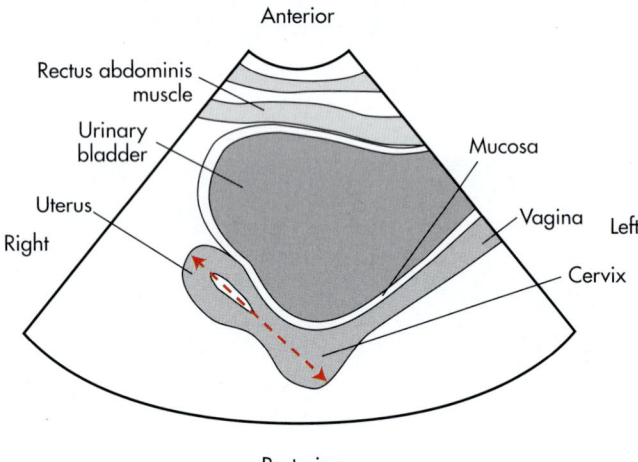

FIG. 42.28 The length of the uterus is measured on the longitudinal image from the fundus to the cervix.

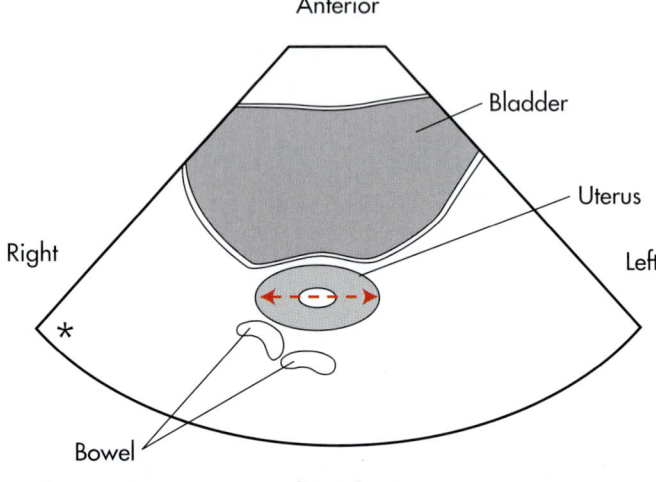

FIG. 42.29 The width of the uterus is measured on the transverse image at the widest diameter of the body.

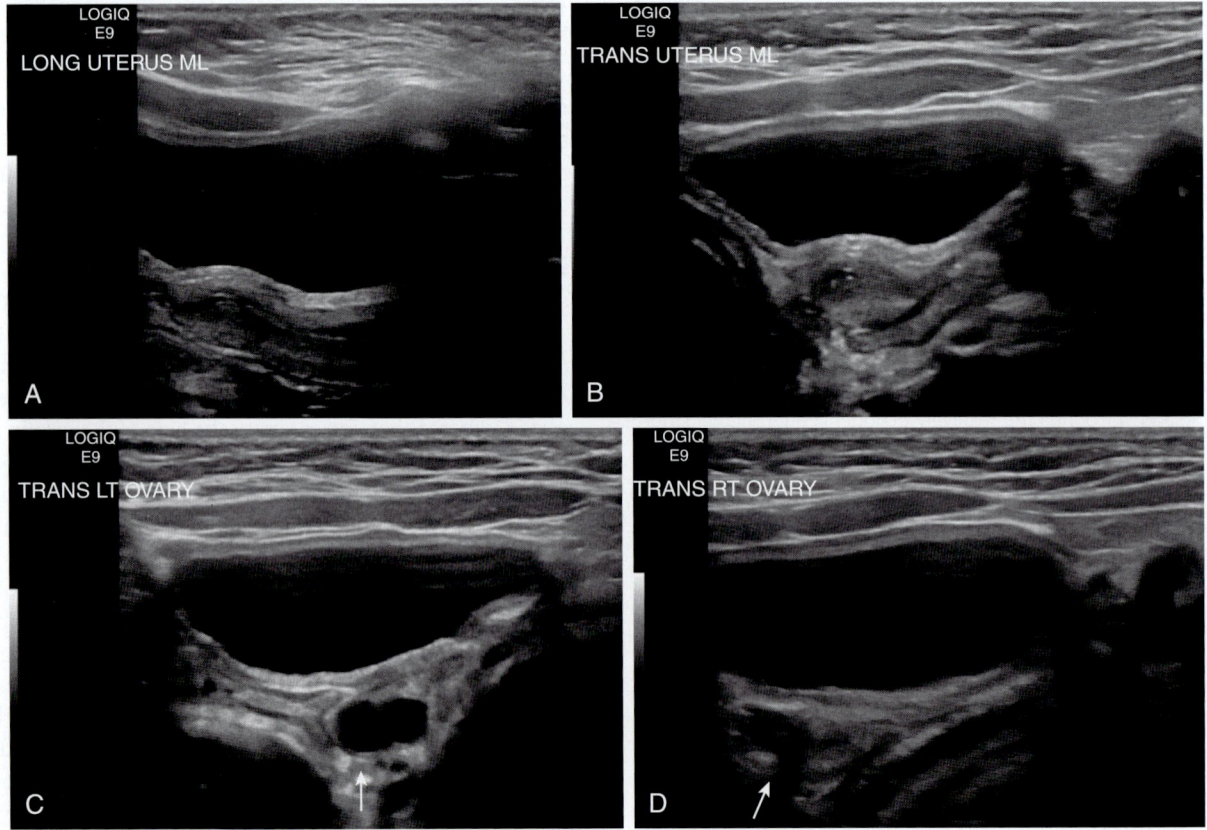

FIG. 42.30 **Neonatal uterus at 12 weeks.** (A) Longitudinal image of the distended bladder and normal uterus posterior. (B) Transverse image of the bladder and uterus. (C) Transverse image of the left ovary *(arrow)*. (D) Transverse image of the right ovary *(arrow)*.

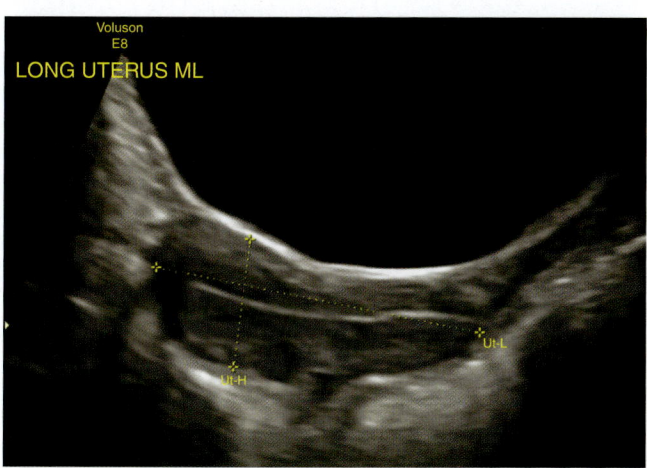

FIG. 42.31 Transabdominal sagittal scan of a 6-year-old prepubertal uterus. The cervix occupies two-thirds of the entire uterine length but loses the pear shape of a neonatal uterus.

two-thirds of the uterine length, and the uterus is about 1 to 3 cm in length and 0.5 to 1 cm in width and diameter (Fig. 42.31). The nulliparous cervix occupies one-third of the uterine length and is about 6 to 8 cm in length and 3 to 5 cm in width and diameter; add 2 cm for multiparous dimensions. The postmenopausal cervix occupies two-thirds of the uterine length. The uterus is about 3 to 5 cm in length and 2 to 3 cm in width and diameter.

Endometrium

Sonographic images of the endometrium disclose a characteristic appearance at each phase of the menstrual cycle (Fig. 42.32). To optimally visualize and discern the endometrium, TV scanning is performed.

The sonographic appearance of the endometrial canal is seen as a thin echogenic line as a result of specular reflections from the interface between the opposing surfaces of the endometrium. The endometrium consists of a superficial functional layer and a deep basal layer.

During **menstruation** (days 1 to 4), the endometrial canal appears as a hypoechoic central line representing blood and tissue and reaching 4 to 8 mm, including the basal layer (Fig. 42.33A). This is surrounded by a hyperechoic basal endometrial echo. If menstrual flow is heavy, the entire endometrial cavity can appear anechoic. During this phase of early menses, acoustic enhancement posterior to the endometrium may appear. As menses progress (days 3 to 7), the hypoechoic echo that represented blood disappears and the endometrial stripe is a discrete thin hyperechoic line, which is usually only 2 to 3 mm (see Fig. 42.33B).

In the **early proliferative phase** (days 5 to 9), the endometrial canal appears as a single thin stripe. The functionalis layer is seen as a hyperechoic halo encompassing it. The basalis layer of the endometrium represents the thin surrounding hyperechoic outermost echo. This complex creates the three-line sign (see Fig. 42.33C). Early in the proliferative phase (days 5 to 9), the endometrial complex is thin, measuring 6 mm, and becomes thicker, 10 mm, from days 10 to 14 before ovulation. The thin surrounding hyperechoic layer of endometrium represents the innermost layer of the

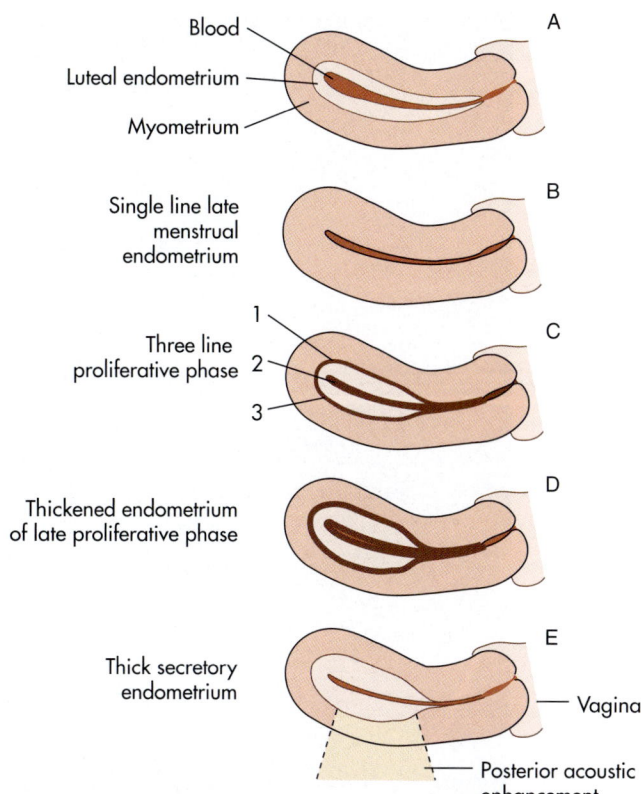

FIG. 42.32 Endometrial changes through a normal menstrual cycle. (A) Endometrium (days 1–4) of early menses. The hypoechoic central cavity represents blood and tissue. This is surrounded by a hyperechoic endometrial echo. (B) Endometrium (days 3–7) as menses progress. The hypoechoic area that represented blood is sloughed. (C) Proliferative phase (days 5–9) endometrium presents as the three-line sign. The thin endometrial center cavity is surrounded by a hypoechoic halo (the functionalis). The thin surrounding echogenic layer represents the basalis. (D) The endometrium of the late proliferative phase (days 10–14) increases in thickness and echogenicity, representing the basalis. (E) The secretory endometrium is at its greatest thickness and echogenicity with posterior acoustic enhancement.

myometrium and is not included in the measurement. In the **late proliferative phase** (days 10 to 14), ovulation occurs (see Fig. 42.33D).

During the **secretory (luteal) phase** (days 15 to 28), the endometrium is at its greatest thickness and echogenicity with posterior enhancement (see Fig. 42.33E). The posterior enhancement is thought to be attributable to the increased vascularity of the endometrium. The functionalis layer becomes isoechoic with the basalis layer. The endometrial complex measures 7 to 14 mm during the secretory phase.

The endometrial thickness is measured from the highly reflective interface of the basalis layer of the endometrium and myometrium in the sagittal view. This sonographic measurement includes both the anterior and posterior layers of the endometrium (see Fig. 42.33D). The surrounding hypoechoic area represents the innermost layer of myometrium and is not included in the measurement. Similarly, fluid presenting within the endometrial cavity should not be included in the measurement of the endometrial complex (Fig. 42.34). With the use of electronic calipers and TV scanning, measurements of endometrial thickness have been found to be within 1 mm of measurements from pathology examinations.

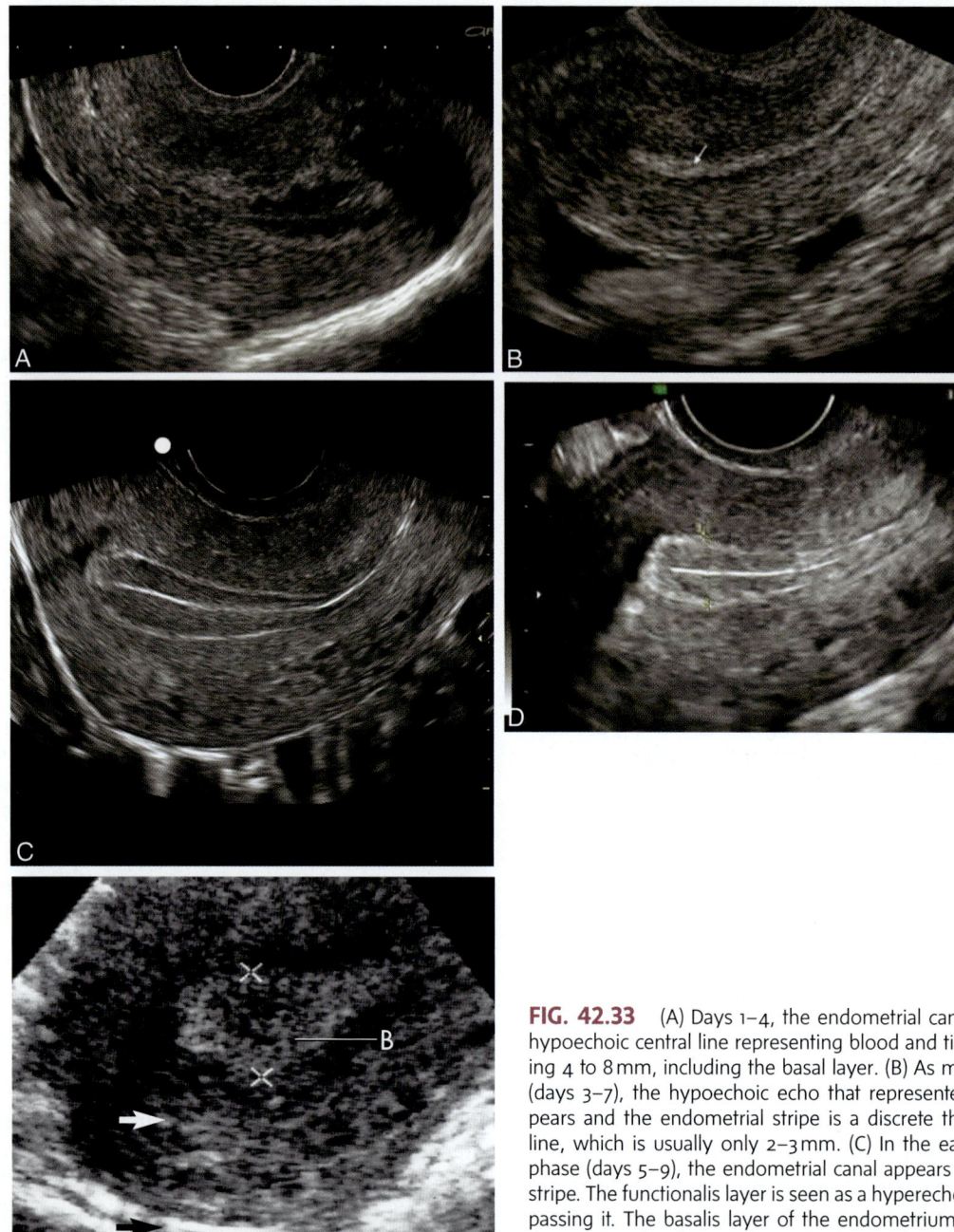

FIG. 42.33 (A) Days 1–4, the endometrial canal appears as a hypoechoic central line representing blood and tissue and reaching 4 to 8 mm, including the basal layer. (B) As menses progress (days 3–7), the hypoechoic echo that represented blood disappears and the endometrial stripe is a discrete thin hyperechoic line, which is usually only 2–3 mm. (C) In the early proliferative phase (days 5–9), the endometrial canal appears as a single thin stripe. The functionalis layer is seen as a hyperechoic halo encompassing it. The basalis layer of the endometrium represents the thin surrounding hyperechoic outermost echo. This complex creates the three-line sign. (D) In the late proliferative phase (days 10–14), ovulation occurs. (E) During the secretory (luteal) phase (days 15–28), the endometrium is at its greatest thickness and echogenicity with posterior enhancement.

In all stages of a female's life, the normal measurement of the endometrium varies depending on hormonal status. In an infant, the endometrium may appear thick and echogenic because of maternal hormonal stimulation. In the childbearing ages, the endometrium varies between 4 and 14 mm. During menopause the endometrium becomes atrophic because it is no longer hormonally stimulated. Sonographically, the postmenopausal endometrial complex is seen as a thin echogenic line measuring less than 8 mm, unless the patient takes hormone therapy. The literature varies for postmenopausal values of the non-hormonally stimulated endometrium. The generally accepted range is between 4 and 10 mm. Patients with postmenopausal bleeding and an endometrial double-layer thickness greater than 5 mm should have further evaluation.

Fallopian Tubes

The normal fallopian tube can be difficult to identify by TA or TV sonography unless it is surrounded by or filled with fluid (dilated). Developmental abnormalities are rare. The normal fallopian tube is a tubular structure, approximately 8 to 10 mm in width, running posterolateral from

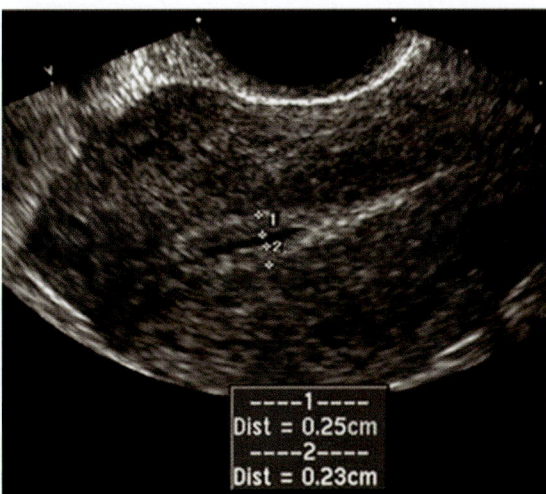

FIG. 42.34 **Transvaginal sagittal image.** Fluid presenting within the endometrial cavity should not be included in the measurement of the endometrial complex.

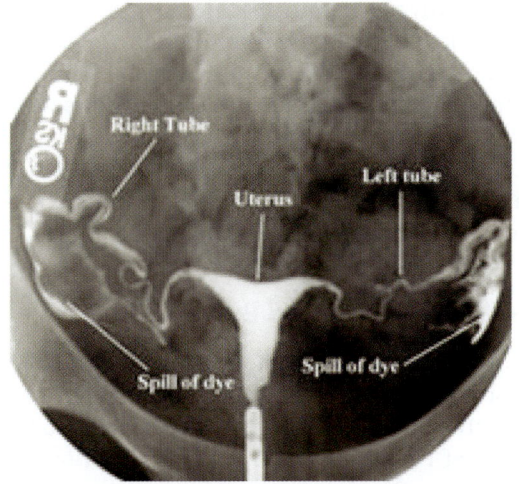

FIG. 42.35 **Hysterosalpingogram of the uterus and fallopian tubes.** The normal fallopian tube is a tubular structure approximately 8 to 10 mm in width and running posterolateral from the uterus to near the ovaries.

the uterus to near the ovaries (Fig. 42.35). It is divided into intramural, isthmic, infundibular, and ampullary portions. In the transverse view transabdominally, or the coronal view transvaginally, the fallopian tube region can be followed laterally from either side of the cornua at the fundal level of the uterus to the ovaries. The high resolution of TV scanning allows improved visualization of the fallopian tube. It is not unusual to visualize the region of the proximal tube and surrounding ligaments. If the tubes are distended with or surrounded by a sufficient amount of fluid, they can be easily outlined by the contrasting fluid. The tubes are easily seen with obstruction by the presence of free fluid, blood, or pus (see Chapter 45).

Ovaries

The sonographic approach to evaluate the ovary is often initially performed transabdominally. The TA approach is especially important when the ovary is in an obscure location (i.e., high in the pelvis) so as to determine a general location to interrogate transvaginally. TA evaluation is also necessary to evaluate a large adnexal mass and determine its origin. The ovary is very mobile and can move considerably in the pelvis, depending on bladder volume and whether women have had a previous pregnancy. Uterine location influences the position of the ovaries. The ovaries are elliptical in shape, with the long axis usually oriented vertically. TV scanning is superior for characterizing the ovary and its contents and for visualizing ovaries that are not visible transabdominally.

Typically, the ovary is located just lateral to the uterus and anteromedial to the internal iliac vessels, which can be used as a landmark to localize the ovary. Transvaginally, the ovaries are easiest to locate in the coronal plane lateral to the cornua (Fig. 42.36). However, it is not uncommon to find the ovaries located above the uterus or posterior in the rectouterine cul-de-sac area.

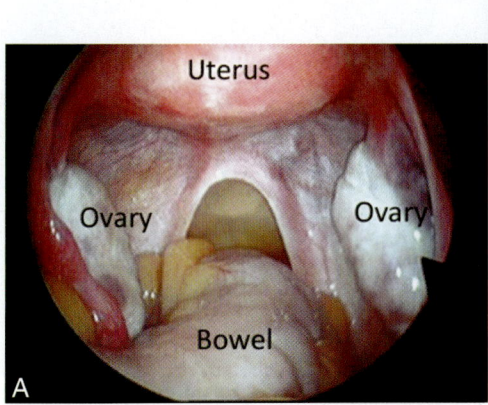
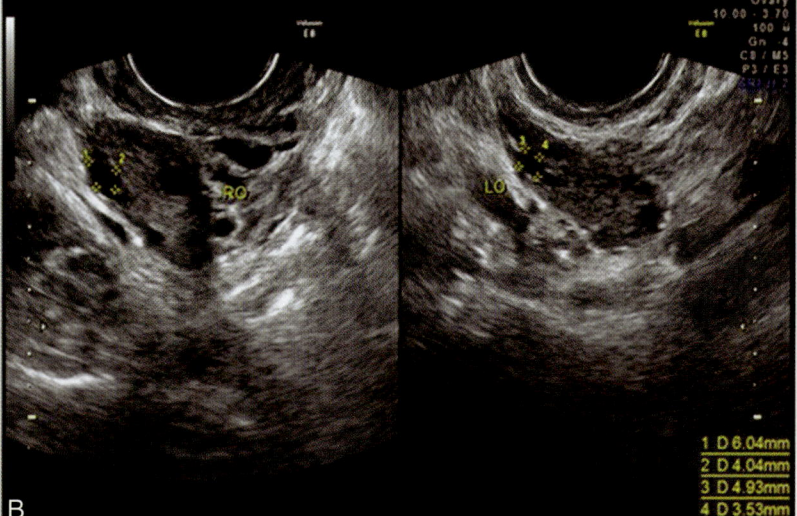

FIG. 42.36 (A) Gross specimen of the pelvic cavity shows the relationship of the ovaries to the uterus. (B) Transvaginal images of the right ovary (RO) and left ovary (LO) with sonolucent follicles.

Sonographically, the normal ovary appears as an ovoid medium-level echogenic structure; follicular cysts may be seen peripherally in the cortex. The appearance of the ovary changes with age and the menstrual cycle. During the proliferative phase, many follicles develop and increase in size until about day 8 or 9 of the menstrual cycle. This is caused by stimulation of follicle-stimulating hormone and luteinizing hormone. At that time, one follicle becomes dominant and increases in size to about 2 to 2.5 cm at the time of ovulation. The other follicles become atretic. If the fluid is not reabsorbed in the non-dominant follicles, a follicular cyst develops.

Following ovulation, the corpus luteum develops and, if fertilization has not occurred, involutes before menstruation. Sonographically, these cysts are unilocular, anechoic structures with well-defined thin walls and posterior acoustic enhancement. Corpus luteum cysts may have a thicker wall and a peripheral rim of color around the wall on color Doppler.

The best sonographic marker for the ovary is identification of a follicular cyst, which has the classic appearance of being thin walled and anechoic with through-transmission posteriorly. The normal range in diameter of a mature graafian follicle is 1.8 to 2.4 cm. These cysts may be present in normal premenarchal, menstruating, and menopausal ovaries.

The ovary is measured in the sagittal or longitudinal plane at its longest length and anteroposterior dimension (Fig. 42.37). In transverse or coronal scans, the width is measured at the widest point. With the use of color Doppler technique, a vessel and a cyst can easily be distinguished. Because of the variability in shape, ovarian volume is considered the best method for determining ovarian size. The volume of the ovary is calculated using the formula for a prolate ellipse: $0.523 = $ length $\times$ thickness $\times$ width. The mean volume for a premenarchal ovary is 3 cm^3, with an upper limit of 8 cm^3; for a normal menstruating ovary, 9.8 cm^3, with an upper limit of 21.9 cm^3; and for a postmenopausal ovary, 5.8 cm^3, with an upper limit of 8 cm^3.

Because of its smaller size and lack of follicles, the postmenopausal ovary may be difficult to see on ultrasound. Scanning must be done slowly to look for peristalsis, so that stationary loops of the bowel are not mistaken for the ovary.

Changes in imaging parameters (e.g., decreased frame averaging) may also help. The absence of a uterus following hysterectomy may also make it more difficult to visualize the ovaries. A difference in size of one ovary greater than twice the volume of the contralateral ovary should be considered abnormal. Small anechoic cysts (less than 3 cm in diameter) may be seen in some postmenopausal ovaries. These may disappear or change in size over time. Surgery is generally recommended for postmenopausal women who have cysts greater than 5 cm and for those who have cysts containing septations or solid nodules.

Occasionally, echogenic ovarian foci are seen in the normal ovary. These are usually tiny (1 to 3 mm) and are non-shadowing foci, which can be peripheral or diffuse. They are thought to represent inclusion cysts and associated calcifications. These are insignificant findings and do not need further follow-up. Focal calcifications may occasionally be seen and are thought to be a stromal reaction to previous hemorrhage or infection. The calcifications are suggested for follow-up to rule out an early neoplasm.

The ovarian arteries arise from the aorta laterally, slightly inferior to the renal arteries. After giving off branches to the ovary, they continue to anastomose with the branches of the uterine artery. The ovarian veins leave the ovarian hilum and communicate with the uterine plexus of veins. The right ovarian vein drains into the inferior vena cava, and the left ovarian vein drains directly into the left renal vein.

Rectouterine Recess and Bowel

The rectouterine recess (posterior cul-de-sac) is the most posterior and inferior reflection of the peritoneal cavity. It is located between the rectum and uterus and is also known as the pouch of Douglas (Fig. 42.38). The posterior cul-de-sac

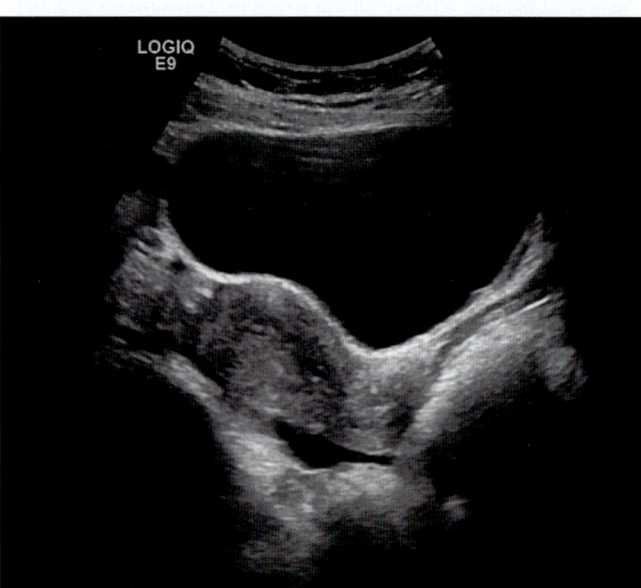

FIG. 42.38 The rectouterine recess (posterior cul-de-sac) is the most posterior and inferior reflection of the peritoneal cavity. It is located between the rectum and uterus and is also known as the pouch of Douglas.

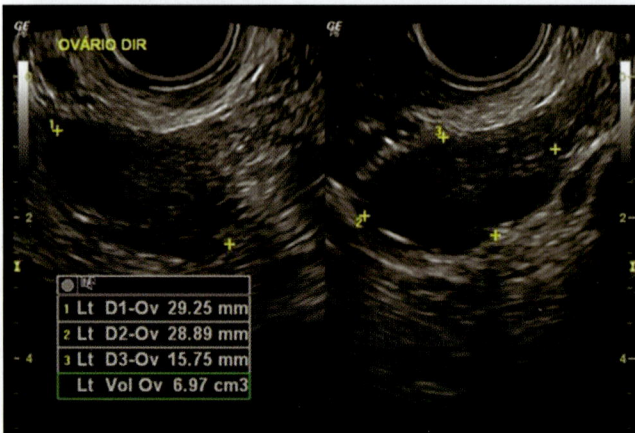

FIG. 42.37 The ovary is measured in the sagittal or longitudinal plane at its longest length and anteroposterior dimension.

is frequently the initial site for intraperitoneal fluid collection. In asymptomatic women, small amounts of fluid can normally be seen in the cul-de-sac during all phases of the menstrual cycle. Possible causes include follicular rupture and retrograde menstruation. Pathologic fluid collections may be seen in association with ascites, blood from ruptured ectopic pregnancy or hemorrhagic cyst, or pus resulting from an infection. TV scanning is better at demonstrating echoes within the fluid and helping to identify the type of fluid along with the clinical indications.

Gas- and fluid-filled bowel loops are poorly defined, echo-free mobile structures that usually demonstrate peristalsis under observation. Solid material in the bowel is hyperechoic and may produce shadowing, as does gas. An empty bowel can look like an irregular bullseye with a thin, sharp, hypoechoic outline on a cross section. When rectal gas obscures the cul-de-sac and it is necessary to differentiate a mass from bowel, a saline or water enema may delineate the rectosigmoid, posterior uterus, and cul-de-sac in a TA view.

Fluid-filled small bowel loops can appear cystic, but they are easily identified by their swirling activity demonstrated on real-time imaging. Fluid may accumulate in the small bowel with rapid oral hydration. The movements of bowel outlining the ovary often aid a TV search for ovaries. Immobile, dilated, or distorted bowel should be investigated further.

Sonohysterography

Sonohysterography, also known as *saline-infused sonography* (SIS) or *hysterosonography*, involves the instillation of sterile saline solution into the endometrial cavity. This technique is used to further evaluate the endometrium when it exceeds the normal thickness or shows focal areas of thickening and polyps are suspected. The patient is prepared in the same manner as for a pelvic examination. The physician inserts a sterile speculum, and the cervix is cleansed with an antiseptic solution. A very small catheter (5 to 7 Fr) filled with saline solution or contrast medium (Albunex) is inserted into the uterine cavity to the level of the uterine fundus. The catheter should be prefilled with saline before insertion to minimize air artifact. The speculum is removed with the catheter in place, and the TV transducer is inserted into the vagina. A hysterosalpingography catheter may have a balloon to prevent retrograde leakage of saline into the vagina. Use fluid to inflate the balloon to minimize air artifact in the lower uterine segment. The balloon should be placed as close to the internal os as possible. The tip of the catheter may be localized on ultrasound, and then 10 to 15 mL of sterile normal saline is injected to distend the endometrial cavity while under continuous sonographic evaluation.

The uterus is surveyed with ultrasound in sagittal and coronal planes to delineate the entire endometrial cavity (Fig. 42.39). Appropriate images are recorded, or cine clips may be recorded in the sagittal and coronal planes. This technique is clinically useful to outline the endometrial cavity to determine the presence of polyps, tumors, or hyperplasia.

In addition, the **cornu** of the uterus may be demonstrated with the interstitial area of the fallopian tube. The examination is contraindicated in patients with pelvic inflammatory disease.

The procedure is usually performed on premenopausal women between days 6 and 10, or soon after the cessation of bleeding in women with irregular cycles. Postmenopausal women who are not on sequential hormone replacement can have the procedure performed at any time. In most cases, there is no special patient preparation. Prophylactic antibiotic can be given for women with chronic pelvic inflammatory disease and women with a history of mitral valve prolapse or other cardiac disorders.

Three-Dimensional Ultrasound

Three-dimensional (3D) ultrasound is now an accepted additional technology in ultrasound that allows imaging from volume sonographic data rather than conventional planar data. Volume data are generally obtained by acquiring many slices of conventional ultrasound data, identifying the location of the slices in space, and reconstructing them into a volume. That data (voxels) can then be viewed as a 3D object and displayed using a variety of formats to rotate and view the images from different angles for optimal visualization of anatomy and pathology. An additional approach to acquiring volume data is to use multidimensional arrays. Display of 3D data has improved greatly. Currently the most common methods include multiplanar display of perpendicular slices through the volume and volume rendering. The display can be optimized to emphasize soft tissue or be changed to optimize vessels. Volume editing can be performed to eliminate or mask structures that obscure the areas of interest. Archived volume data may be further reviewed after the patient examination has been completed, permitting the reviewer to "rescan" the patient in the computer workstation. Volumes often require significant storage media and currently may be stored on magnetic optical disks, CD-ROMs, or hard drives, or transferred to computer networks with Internet capabilities.

The AIUM guidelines regarding 3D sonography state that because it is still a developing technology, its role is that of an adjunct to, not a replacement for, two-dimensional ultrasound. Continued clinical applications will show that the most promise for 3D ultrasound in the pelvis is its ability to provide unique planes for improved evaluation of organs, tubal morphology, tumor invasion, accurate volume estimation, and guidance for invasive procedures. Sonohysterography also benefits from volume scanning. The exact location of a polyp, fibroid, or adhesion is readily identified (Fig. 42.40).

As the 3D technology becomes available in many more clinical sites, additional benefits will be identified. Four-dimensional ultrasound data are another new technology that allows 3D imaging in a real-time mode versus computerized imaging post-capture. These technologies are exciting areas in development along with efforts to improve resolution and application.

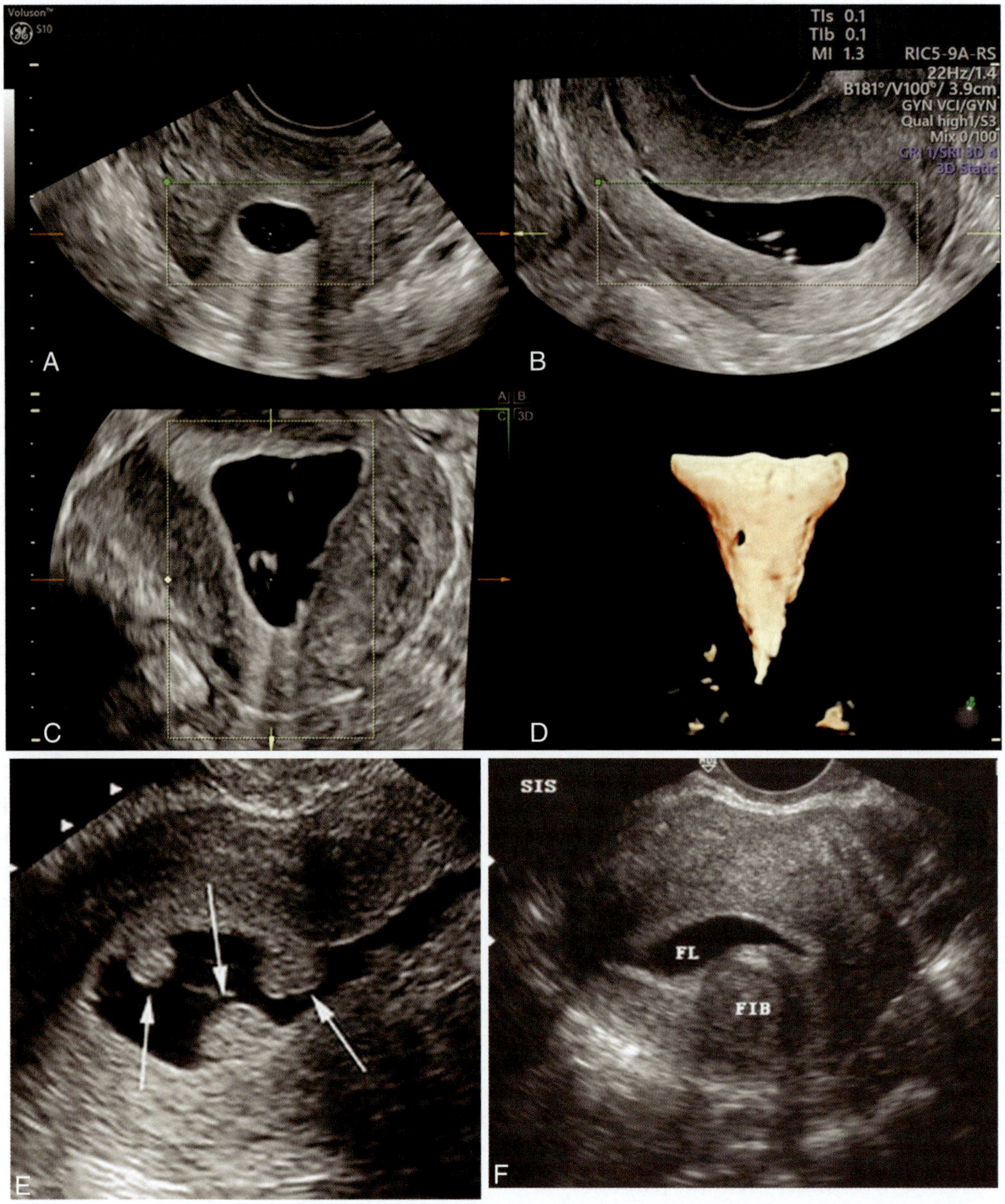

FIG. 42.39 Sonohysterography, also known as *saline-infused sonography* (SIS) or *hysterosonography*, involves the instillation of sterile saline solution into the endometrial cavity. Coronal (A, C–D) and sagittal (B) images of the fluid filled endometrial cavity. (E) Multiple polyps are noted within the endometrial cavity. (F) The fibroid (FIB) impinges into the saline infused endometrial cavity. Note the posterior shadow from the fibroid. *FL*, Fluid.

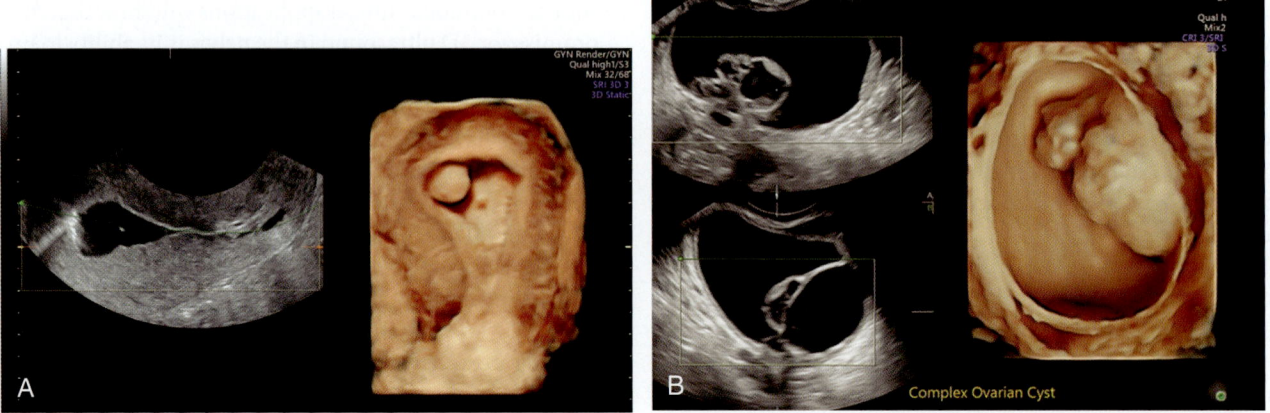

FIG. 42.40 Three-dimensional ultrasound allows imaging from volume sonographic data rather than conventional planar data. (A) Uterine polyp. (B) Complex ovarian cyst.

Key Pearls

- The sonographer should use a routine patient questionnaire requesting the following information: date of last menstrual period, gravidity, parity, physiologic menstrual status, hormone regimen, symptoms, history of cancer, family history of cancer, past pelvic surgeries, laboratory tests, previous Pap or biopsy results, and pelvic examination findings.
- The patient's menstrual status is described by using the terms *premenarche, menarche,* and *menopause.*
- If both the transabdominal (TA) and transvaginal (TV) examinations are going to be performed, the patient should be instructed that the pelvic ultrasound examination will be performed in two parts.
- Anatomy and pathology should be identified in at least two orthogonal planes, usually *sagittal* and *axial* or *coronal* and *transverse,* using both techniques.
- When a mass is found on sonography, the following features should be characterized: location (uterine or extrauterine), size, external contour (well-defined, ill-defined, or irregular borders), and internal consistency (cystic, complex, predominantly cystic, complex, predominantly solid, or solid).
- The filled urinary bladder displaces the bowel and acts as an acoustic window for evaluating three major groups of muscles.
- The ovary receives its blood supply from the aorta.
- The anterior surface of the vagina and cervix is supplied with blood from a branch off the uterine artery before it reaches the uterus. The posterior surface of the vagina is supplied with blood from a branch off the internal iliac vessel.
- The uterine muscle consists of three layers: the outer serosa layer, the myometrium, and the endometrium.
- The normal arcuate vessels are often seen in the periphery of the uterus.
- The radial arteries arise as multiple branches from the arcuate arteries and travel centrally to supply the rich capillary network in the deeper layers of the myometrium and the endometrium.
- The body of the uterus is separated from the cervix by the isthmus at the level of the internal os and is identified by the narrowing of the canal.
- The uterus is usually anteverted and anteflexed. The uterus may also be retroflexed when the body is tilted posteriorly or retroverted when the entire uterus is tilted backward.
- Sonographic images of the endometrium disclose a characteristic appearance at each phase of the menstrual cycle.
- The normal fallopian tube is a tubular structure approximately 8 to 10 mm in width and running posterolateral from the uterus to near the ovaries.
- Typically, the ovary is located just lateral to the uterus and anteromedial to the internal iliac vessels.
- The rectouterine recess (posterior cul-de-sac) is the most posterior and inferior reflection of the peritoneal cavity.
- The posterior cul-de-sac, or pouch of Douglas, is frequently the initial site for intraperitoneal fluid collection.
- Sonohysterography is used to further evaluate the endometrium when it exceeds the normal thickness or shows focal areas of thickening and polyps are suspected.

BIBLIOGRAPHY

ACR-ACOG-AIUM-SPR-SRU. Practice parameter for the performance of ultrasound of the female pelvis. *ACR Res* 27. 2019.

Callen PW. *Ultrasonography in obstetrics and gynecology.* ed 7. Philadelphia: Elsevier; 2022.

Cohen HL, Tice HM, Mandel FS. Ovarian volumes measured by US: bigger than we think. *Radiology.* 1990;177:189.

Cullinan JA, Fleischer AC, Kepple DM, et al. Sonohysterography: a technique for endometrial evaluation. *Radiographics.* 1995;15:501–514.

Hall R. *Pelvic ultrasound imaging: a case-based approach.* Elsevier; 2021.

Rumack C, Levine D. *Diagnostic ultrasound.* ed 5. Elsevier; 2022.

CHAPTER 43

Pathology of the Uterus

Sandra L. Hagen-Ansert

OBJECTIVES

On completion of this chapter, you should be able to:
- Define the pathologies discussed in this chapter and describe their causes, clinical signs, and sonographic findings
- Explain sonohysterography and the indications for performing the procedure
- Identify the role of Doppler in evaluating pelvic pathology
- Differentiate among the types of intrauterine contraceptive devices and describe the sonographic appearance of each

OUTLINE

Pathology of The Vagina And Cervix 1203
   The Vagina 1203
   The Vaginal Cuff 1203
   Rectouterine Recess 1203
   Cervix 1203
Pathology of the Uterus 1207
   Normal Variations of the Uterus 1207
   Leiomyomas 1207

Uterine Calcifications 1210
Adenomyosis 1212
Arteriovenous Malformations 1216
Uterine Leiomyosarcoma 1216
Pathology of the Endometrium 1217
   Sonohysterography 1218
   Endometrial Hyperplasia 1220
   Endometrial Polyps 1220
   Endometritis 1221
   Synechiae 1222

Endometrial Carcinoma 1223
   Small Endometrial Fluid Collections 1224
   Large Endometrial Fluid Collections 1225
Intrauterine Contraceptive Devices 1225
   Lost Intrauterine Device 1225

KEY TERMS

Adenomyosis
Cervical polyp
Cervical stenosis
Dysmenorrhea
Ectocervix
Endometrial carcinoma
Endometrial hyperplasia
Endometrial polyps

Endometritis
Gartner duct cyst
Hematometra
Hydrometra
Intramural leiomyoma
Intrauterine contraceptive device (IUCD)
Leiomyoma

Metrorrhea
Nabothian cyst
Pyometra
Squamous cell carcinoma
Submucosal leiomyoma
Subserosal leiomyoma

Sonography is traditionally applied in the female pelvis to delineate the size, texture, vascularity, and structure of pelvic anatomy. The examination may also supply information on the morphology of malfunctioning organs that seem normal on pelvic examination. Small, nonpalpable submucosal myomas or polyps may cause abnormal bleeding. The localization of intrauterine contraceptive devices (IUCDs) may be assessed by pelvic ultrasound examination. The homogeneity of the myometrium is assessed, and the thickness of the endometrial cavity is measured, in addition to the length and width of the uterus and cervix. Both transabdominal and transvaginal sonography are important in these evaluations. Transabdominal imaging furnishes a survey of anatomy, whereas transvaginal imaging provides better characterization of internal architecture of the vagina, cervix, and uterus. Color and spectral Doppler sonography can also play a role in assessing normal and pathologic blood flow, as well as identify vessels separate from fluid-filled structures. Newer techniques include sonohysterography, a process in which a small catheter, placed under ultrasound guidance, introduces sterile saline into the endometrial canal to provide a detailed evaluation of an intracavitary, endometrial, or submucosal lesion. Additionally, three-dimensional (3D) ultrasound now provides us with coronal representation of the uterus. Other imaging modalities used to evaluate pelvic anatomy and pathology include magnetic resonance imaging (MRI) and computed tomography (CT). These two modalities are particularly useful in the staging of malignant disease.

PATHOLOGY OF THE VAGINA AND CERVIX

The Vagina

The vagina runs anterior and caudal from the cervix, between the bladder and rectum (Fig. 43.1). Occasionally, sonography is used to characterize a vaginal mass, such as a **Gartner duct cyst**. These are the most common cystic lesions of the vagina and usually are found incidentally during sonographic examination (Fig. 43.2). The most common congenital abnormality of the female genital tract is an imperforate hymen that results in obstruction. Obstruction of the uterus or the vagina may result in an accumulation of fluid (hydrometra), blood (hematometra), or pus (pyometra).

Solid masses of the vagina are rare. As with carcinoma of the cervix, sonography is not used for diagnosis of carcinoma of the vagina, but it may play a role in staging. When found, the lesion is usually vaginal adenocarcinoma or rhabdomyosarcoma. The lesions appear as a solid mass, occasionally with areas of necrosis. Translabial scanning may be used to best evaluate the vaginal area (see Chapter 42).

The Vaginal Cuff

A vaginal cuff is seen in hysterectomy patients after surgery. The upper size limit of a normal vaginal cuff is 2.1 cm. If the cuff is larger than this or contains a well-defined mass or areas of high echogenicity, it should be regarded with suspicion for malignancy, especially in the patient who has a previous history of cancer. Nodular areas in the vaginal cuff may be due to post-irradiation fibrosis.

Rectouterine Recess

The rectouterine recess (posterior cul-de-sac) is the most posterior and inferior reflection of the peritoneal cavity (see Fig. 43.1). It is located between the rectum and uterus and is also called the pouch of Douglas. Because of its location, it is frequently the site of intraperitoneal fluid collections. As little as 5 mL of fluid has been detected by transvaginal sonography. Fluid in the cul-de-sac is a normal finding in asymptomatic women and can be seen during all phases of the menstrual cycle. Pathologic fluid collections may be associated with ascites, blood resulting from a ruptured ectopic pregnancy, hemorrhagic cyst, or pus resulting from an infection. Pelvic abscesses and hematomas can also occur in the cul-de-sac. Sonographic characteristics help to differentiate these findings (Fig. 43.3).

Cervix

Benign Conditions. Transvaginal sonography should be utilized to obtain high-quality images of the cervical area. The cervix lies posterior to the bladder between the lower uterine segment and the vaginal canal (see Fig. 43.1). The cervical canal extends from the internal os where it joins the uterine cavity, to the external os, which projects into the vaginal vault. It is a cylindrical portion of the uterus that enters the vagina and measures 2 to 4 cm in length. Transvaginal scanning of the cervix is performed after the patient empties her bladder.

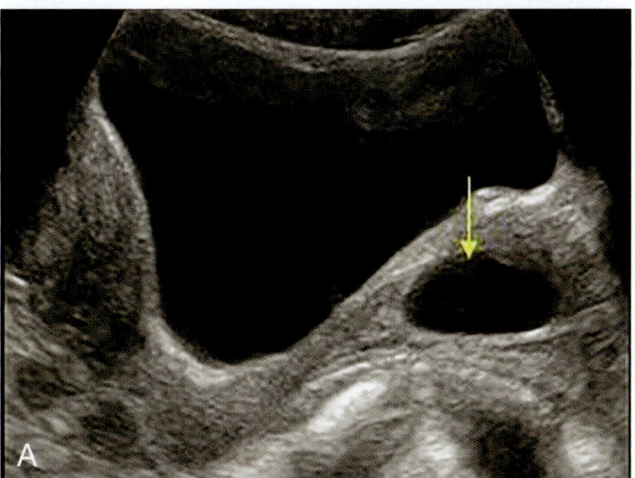

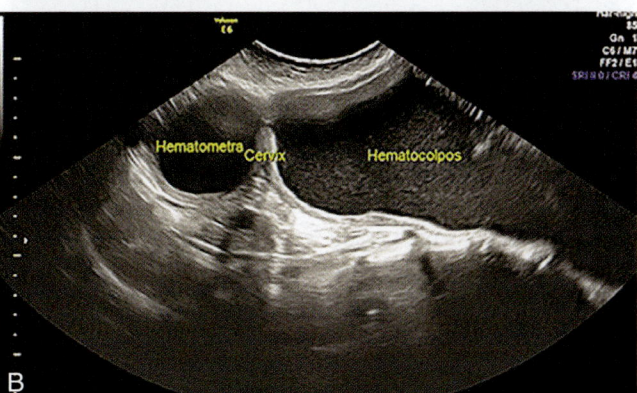

FIG. 43.2 (A) Gartner duct cysts are the most common cystic lesions of the vagina and usually are found incidentally during sonographic examination. (B) The most common congenital abnormality of the female genital tract is an imperforate hymen that results in obstruction that may result in an accumulation of fluid (hydrometra), blood (hematometra), or pus (pyometra).

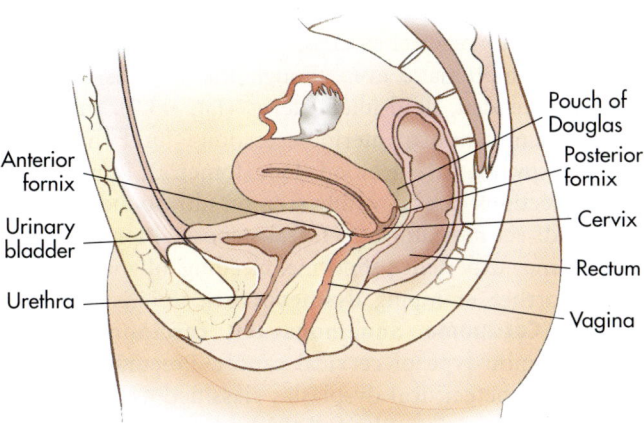

FIG. 43.1 Lateral view of the pelvis demonstrating the relationship of the pelvic organs to the bladder and pouch of Douglas.

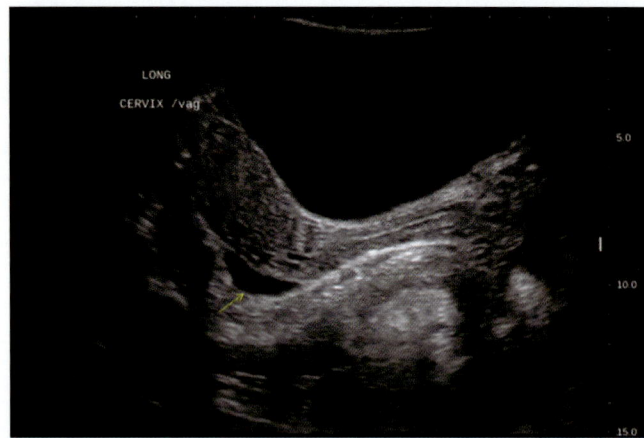

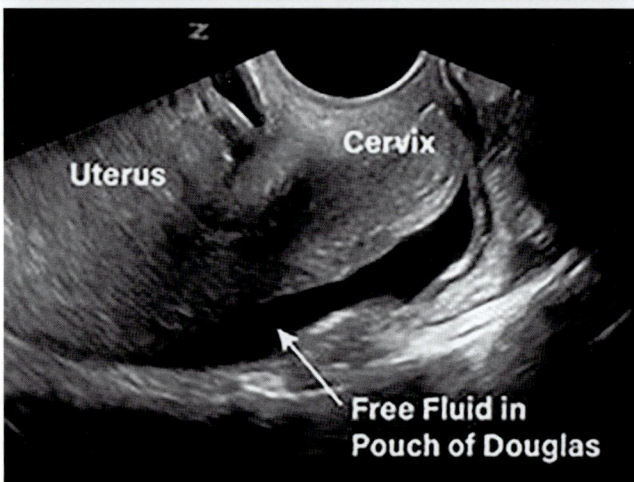

FIG. 43.3 The rectouterine recess (posterior cul-de-sac) is the most posterior and inferior reflection of the peritoneal cavity and is located between the rectum and uterus (also called the pouch of Douglas). Because of its location, it is frequently the site of intraperitoneal fluid collections. Pathologic fluid collections may be associated with ascites, blood resulting from a ruptured ectopic pregnancy, hemorrhagic cyst, or pus resulting from an infection.

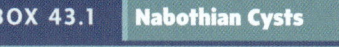

BOX 43.1	Nabothian Cysts

Benign cysts in cervix
Chronic inflammatory retention cysts
Asymptomatic

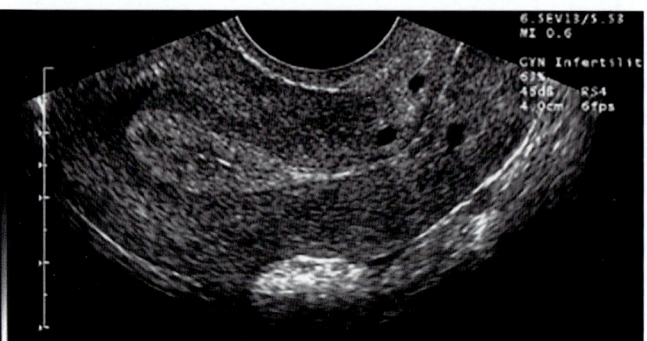

FIG. 43.4 On sonographic evaluation, nabothian cysts appear along the cervical canal as discrete, round, fluid-filled anechoic structures, usually measuring less than 2 cm; they may be multiple, as seen in this transvaginal image.

The transducer is inserted into the vagina with the patient supine, knees gently flexed, and hips elevated on a pillow. After the uterine cavity has been examined, the probe should be slowly pulled back slightly to image the internal and external cervical os. In the sagittal view, the handle of the transducer is slowly moved upward or back to better image the cervix (see Chapter 42). With gentle rotation and angulation of the transducer, coronal images are also obtained.

The most common finding is the presence of **nabothian cysts** (Box 43.1), which result from chronic cervicitis and are seen frequently in middle-aged women. This cyst results from an obstructed dilated transcervical gland and is also called epithelial inclusion cyst.

On sonographic evaluation, these lesions appear along the cervical canal as discrete, round, fluid-filled anechoic structures, usually measuring less than 2 cm; they may be multiple (Fig. 43.4). Occasionally, nabothian cysts may have internal echoes that may be caused by hemorrhage or infection.

Cervical polyps may present clinically with irregular bleeding. This benign condition arises from the hyperplastic protrusion of the epithelium of the endocervix or **ectocervix**. Chronic inflammation is the most likely factor. The polyps may be pedunculated, projecting out of the cervix, or broad-based, and ultrasound may or may not see cervical polyps, depending on their location (Fig. 43.5). Women in their late middle age are more likely to develop polyps.

A small percentage of leiomyomas (myoma tumors) occur in the cervix (Fig. 43.6). When the myomas are small, the patient is asymptomatic, but as the mass enlarges, bladder or bowel obstruction may result. The myoma may be pedunculated and prolapse into the vaginal canal. Sonography may assist in determining the location of the stalk and the thickness of the stalk. Fluid infusion with sonohysterography enhances this visualization.

Cervical stenosis is an acquired condition with obstruction of the cervical canal at the internal or external os, resulting from radiation therapy, previous cone biopsy, postmenopausal cervical atrophy, chronic infection, laser or cryosurgery, or cervical carcinoma. The menopausal patient may be asymptomatic even though the stenosis can produce a distended, fluid-filled uterus (Fig. 43.7), the result of an accumulation of uterine secretions, fluid (hydrometra), pus (pyometra), or blood (hematometra). Intracavitary fluid collections can be readily seen on ultrasound and may be an indirect indicator of cervical stenosis. Premenopausal patients may experience abnormal bleeding, oligomenorrhea or amenorrhea, cramping, **dysmenorrhea**, or infertility.

Cervical Carcinoma. Squamous cell carcinoma is the most common type of cervical cancer. Precursors to this disease are the cervical dysplasias classified as mild, moderate, or severe. When the full thickness of the epithelium is composed of undifferentiated neoplastic cells, the lesion is referred to as carcinoma in situ. The detection of these

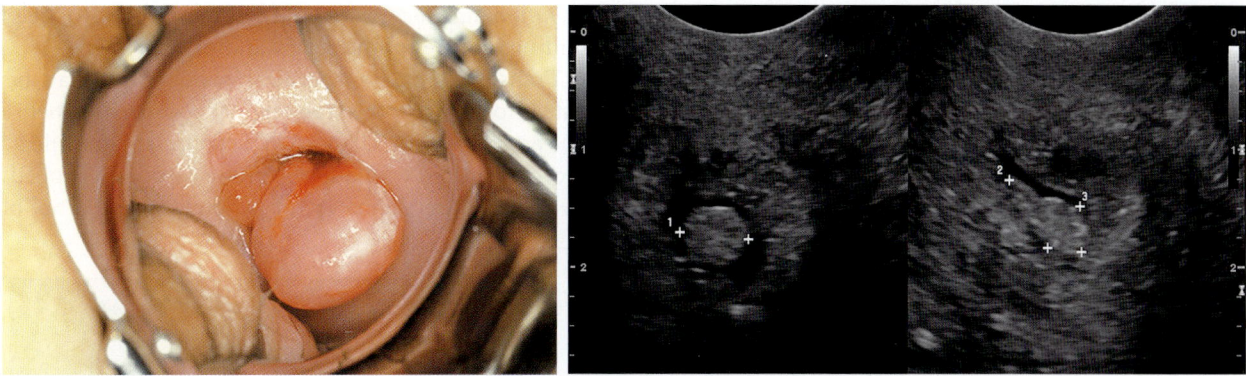

FIG. 43.5 The cervical polyps may be pedunculated, project out of the cervix, or be broad based; ultrasound may or may not detect them depending on their location.

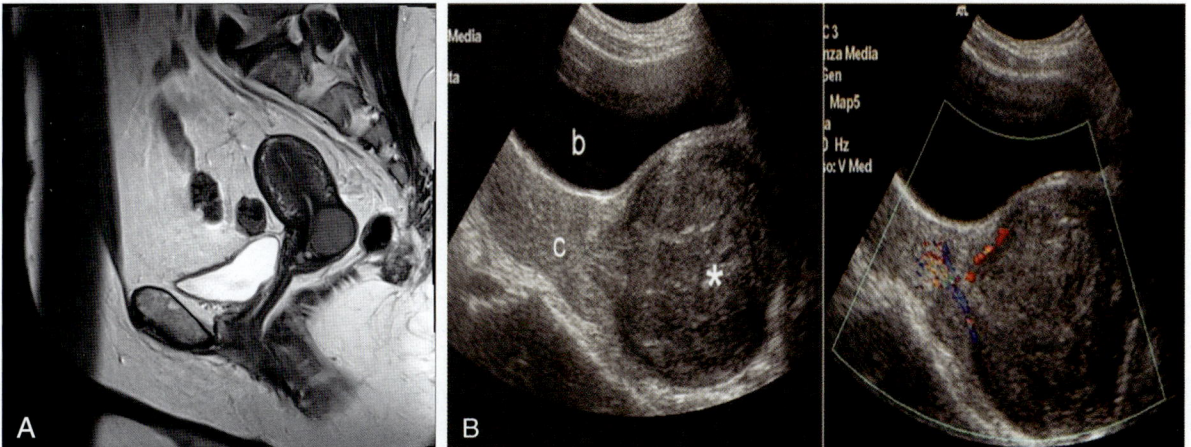

FIG. 43.6 (A) Magnetic resonance image of a small cervical leiomyoma. (B) A large intracavitary pedunculated myoma *(asterisk)* protrudes into the vagina from the cervical os. *b*, Bladder; *c*, cervix.

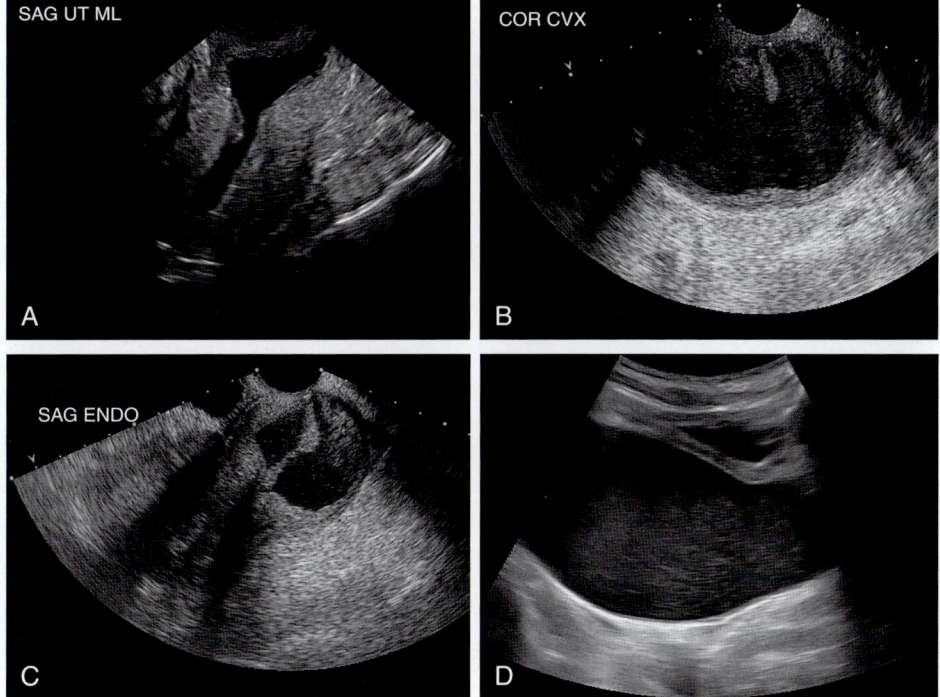

FIG. 43.7 (A–C) A 63-year-old asymptomatic woman on cyclic hormone replacement therapy demonstrates a large endometrial fluid collection. She underwent dilation for cervical stenosis, and bloody fluid was drained. (D) Hematometrocolpos presents as a moderately echogenic collection in the cervical area.

abnormalities is attributed to screening with Papanicolaou (Pap) smears because most of the early lesions are asymptomatic. Advanced cervical cancer is usually evident clinically (Box 43.2 and Fig. 43.8). Sonography may demonstrate a solid retrovesical mass, which may be indistinguishable from a cervical myoma. Transvaginal and translabial ultrasound may demonstrate bladder, ureteral, vaginal, or rectal involvement and may be used in staging cervical cancer. CT and MRI are preferable, however, because they are superior methods for staging and evaluating lymphatic spread. Areas of increased echogenicity or hypoechoic areas with an irregular outline signify changes compatible with cervical carcinoma (Fig. 43.9). Multiple cystic areas within a solid cervical mass are a rare cervical neoplasm arising from the endocervical glands termed *adenoma malignum* or *minimal deviation adenocarcinoma*. Ultrasound is also helpful in guiding biopsies of the cervix and vagina.

Translabial or transperineal sonography may be used instead of or with the transvaginal approach to help define the cervical area. A 5.0 to 7.5 MHz sector or curvilinear transducer is covered with a sterile probe cover and applied to the vestibule of the vagina in the sagittal plane. Partial bladder

BOX 43.2	Cervical Carcinoma

Affects women of menstrual age
Clinical findings: Vaginal discharge or bleeding
Sonographic findings: Retrovesical mass, obstruction of ureters, invasion of bladder

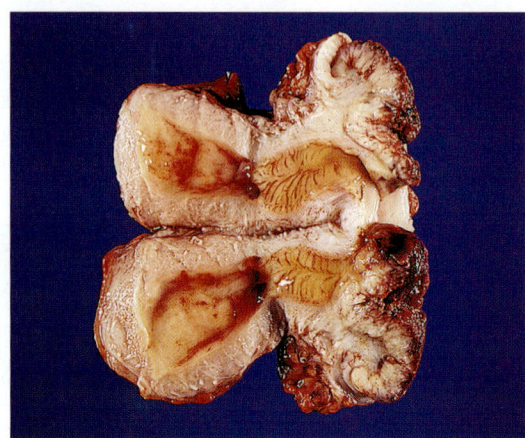

FIG. 43.8 Gross pathologic findings of cervical squamous cell carcinoma.

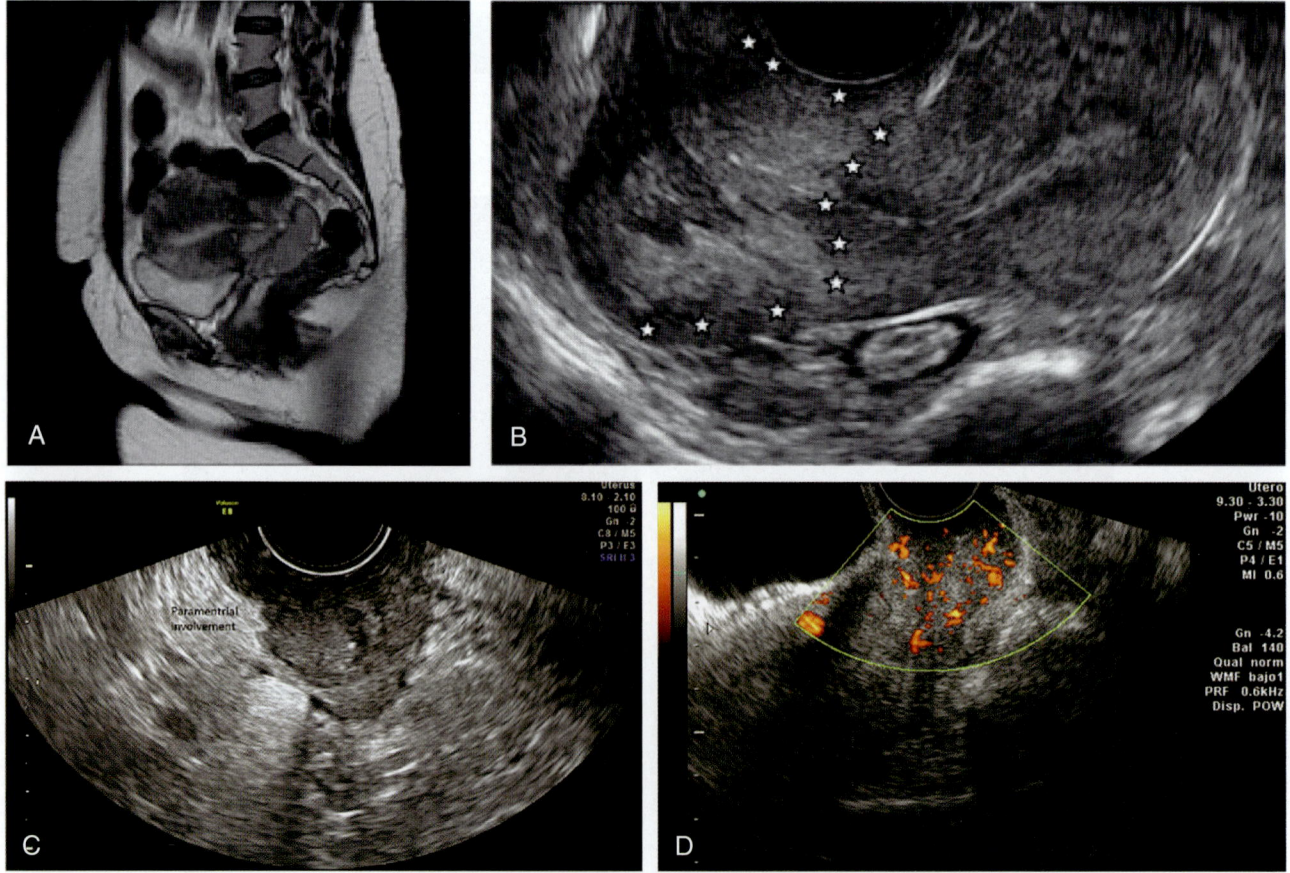

FIG. 43.9 Magnetic resonance (A–B) and transvaginal ultrasound (C) images of the lower uterine segment. The cervical area is enlarged and hypoechoic with decreased through transmission. (D) Color Doppler demonstrates increased vascularity in the mass. Sonography may demonstrate a solid retrovesical mass, which may be indistinguishable from a cervical myoma.

filling may assist visualization of the cervical area. Rotation of the transducer obliquely in a counterclockwise direction shows the coronal images and defines the second plane for visualization. Positioning the patient with the hips elevated, as in the transvaginal approach, helps to displace pelvic gas and identify anatomy. Limitations can be overcome by elevation of the hips, better application of the transducer to the perineum, or changes in the orientation of the probe.

PATHOLOGY OF THE UTERUS

The uterus lies in the true pelvis between the urinary bladder anteriorly and the rectosigmoid colon posteriorly (see Fig. 43.1). Uterine position is variable and changes with the degrees of bladder and rectal distention. The body of the uterus may lie obliquely on either side of the midline, which may mimic a mass on physical examination. Flexion refers to the axis of the uterine body relative to the cervix. Version refers to the axis of the cervix relative to the vagina. The uterus is usually anteverted and anteflexed. It may also be retroflexed (when the body tilts posteriorly) or retroverted (when the uterine fundus tilts backward) (Fig. 43.10). Transvaginal sonography has proven to be excellent for assessing the retroverted or retroflexed uterus because the transducer is close to the posteriorly located fundus. The size and shape of the normal uterus are related to age, hormonal status, and parity.

Common differential considerations for pathology of the uterus are seen in Box 43.3.

Normal Variations of the Uterus

Ultrasound is the first clinical examination ordered to evaluate the enlarged uterus. There are common variations of uterine morphology, the bicornuate—or "two-horned uterus"—and the didelphic uterus, that can be visualized with great specificity with sonography. These developmental variations are discussed in detail in the pediatric chapter. A detailed examination can reveal the endometrium in each horn, identify pathology, or document pregnancy (Fig. 43.11).

Leiomyomas

Leiomyomas, commonly called myomas, are the most common gynecologic tumors, occurring in approximately 20% to 30% (or greater depending on the reference source) of women over 30 years old. They are more common in African American women.

Myoma tumors are composed of spindle-shaped, smooth muscle cells arranged in a *whorl-like* pattern with variable amounts of fibrous connective tissue, which can degenerate into a number of different histologic subtypes (Fig. 43.12). The tumors consist of nodules of myometrial tissue

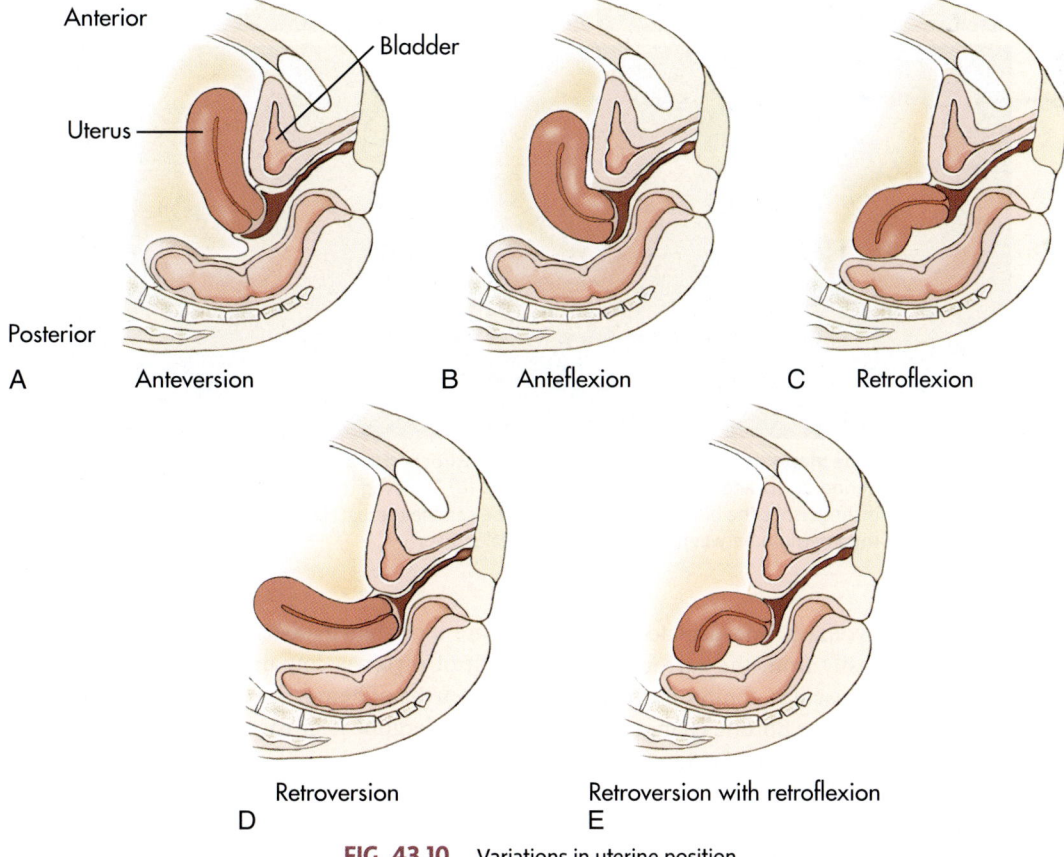

FIG. 43.10 Variations in uterine position.

BOX 43.3 Differential Considerations for the Uterus

Enlarged Uterus
Pregnancy
Postpartum
Leiomyoma
Adenomyosis
Bicornuate or didelphic uterus

Uterine Tumor
Leiomyoma
Carcinoma

Thickened Endometrium
Early intrauterine pregnancy
Endometrial hyperplasia
Retained products of conception or incomplete abortion
Trophoblastic disease
Endometritis

Adhesions
Polyps
Inflammatory disease
Endometrial carcinoma

Endometrial Fluid
Endometritis
Retained products of conception
Pelvic inflammatory disease
Cervical obstruction

Endometrial Shadowing
Gas (abscess)
Intrauterine device
Calcified myomas or vessels
Retained products of conception

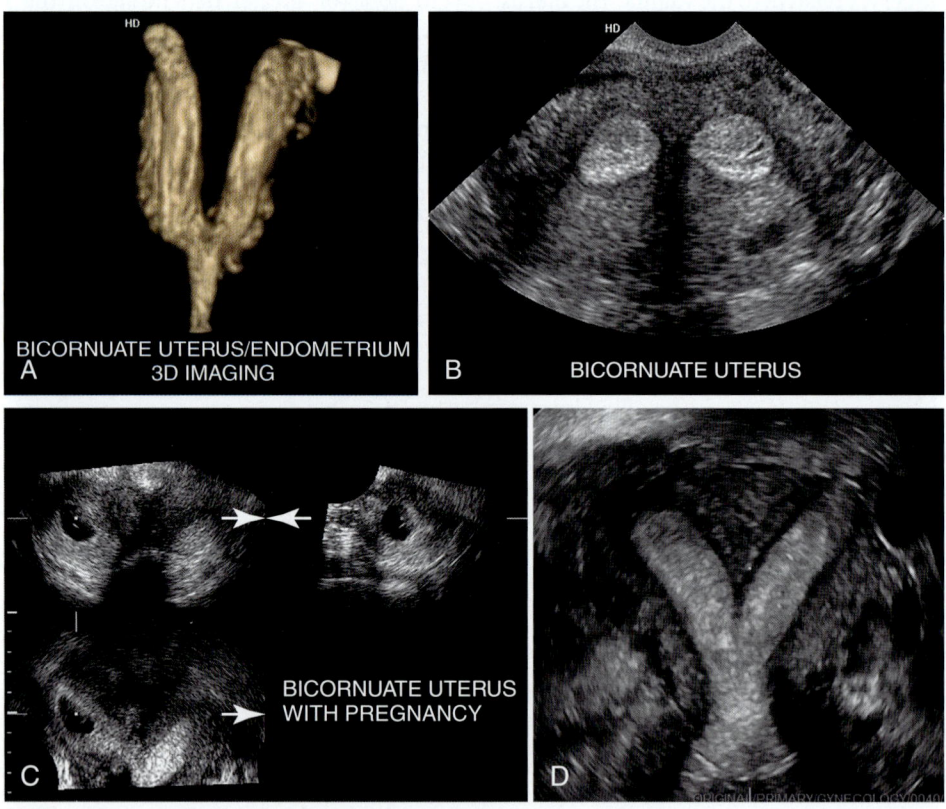

FIG. 43.11 Bicornuate uterus. (A) Three-dimensional (3D) reconstruction of a bicornuate uterus that clearly demonstrates the two uterine horns and echogenic endometrium. (B) Transvaginal image of the bicornuate uterus. (C–D) 3D rendering distinguishes the bicornuate uterus from the septate uterus. Here the fundus is intact and there is a large wedge of myometrium between the two endometrial stripes.

and are usually multiple. The myoma is encapsulated with a pseudocapsule and separates easily from the surrounding myometrium. With atrophy and vascular compromise as a result of outgrowing their blood supply, fibrotic changes and degeneration of the myomas can occur. Liquefaction, necrosis, hemorrhage, and ultimate calcification may take place. Hyalinization (development of an albuminoid mass in a cell or tissue) occurs most often, making the myomas appear more lucent or hypoechoic than the myometrium. Ten percent of myomas contain calcification, and a similar number have areas of hemorrhage. Other myomas contain tissue that has undergone necrosis and liquefaction and become myxoid in texture.

Myomas are estrogen dependent and may increase in size during pregnancy, although about half of all myomas show little change during pregnancy. Myomas identified in the first

CHAPTER 43 Pathology of the Uterus

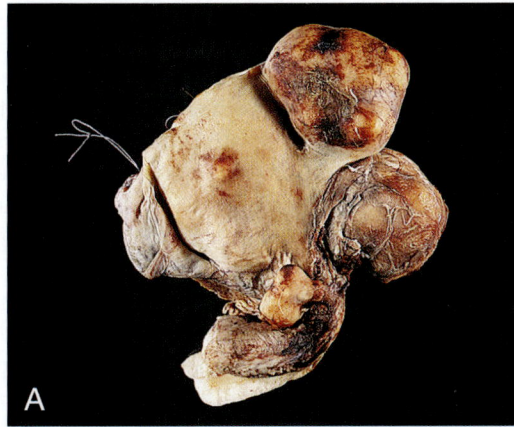

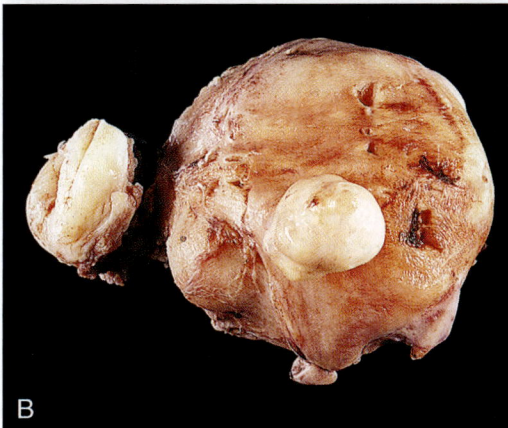

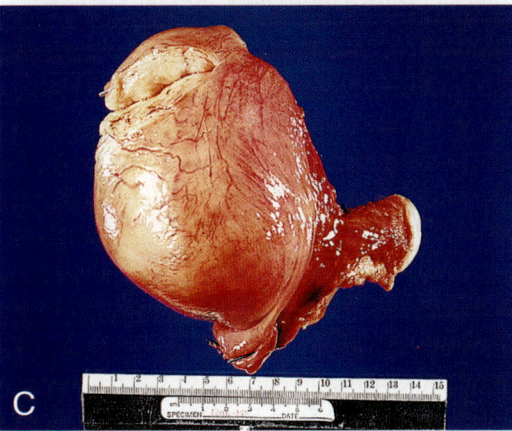

FIG. 43.12 Gross pathologic findings. (A) A uterine cavity with multiple subserosal myoma tumors arising from its walls. (B) A uterus with the encapsulated leiomyoma in the submucosal area. (C) A pedunculated subserosal myoma of the uterus.

BOX 43.4 Characteristics of Leiomyomas

Most common pelvic tumor
Smooth muscle cell composition
Fibrosis occurs after atrophic or degenerative changes
Degeneration occurs when myomas outgrow their blood supply; calcification
May be pedunculated
Clinical findings: enlarged uterus, profuse and prolonged bleeding, pain

BOX 43.5 Uterine Locations of Leiomyomas

Submucosal
Disruption into endometrial cavity—heavy bleeding; infertility

Intramural
Within myometrium—may enlarge to cause pressure on adjacent organs; infertility or recurrent pregnancy loss

Subserosal
Arise from myometrium, project exophytically—may enlarge to cause pressure on adjacent organs

Clinically, myomas cause uterine irregularity and enlargement with the sensation of pelvic pressure and sometimes pain. Patterns of irregular bleeding, menometrorrhagia, or heavy menstrual bleeding (menorrhagia) are the primary clinical problems. Myomas may contribute to infertility by distorting the fallopian tube or endometrial cavity; if located in the lower uterine segment or cervix, the tumor may interfere with normal vaginal delivery. Because of the increased estrogen during pregnancy, the tumor may grow and bleed within, causing pain. Box 43.4 summarizes the characteristics of leiomyomas.

Leiomyomas can affect any portion of the uterine wall; however, the tumor may also be uncommonly found in the lower uterine segment, the cervix, and in the broad ligament. Leiomyomas are either **submucosal leiomyomas** (displacing or distorting the endometrial cavity with subsequent irregular or heavy menstrual bleeding), **intramural leiomyomas** (confined to the myometrium, the most common type), or **subserosal leiomyomas** (projecting from the peritoneal surface of the uterus). Sometimes, subserosal leiomyomas become pedunculated and appear as extrauterine masses (Box 43.5).

The signs and symptoms of leiomyomas depend on their size and location (Fig. 43.13). Submucosal myomas may erode into the endometrial cavity and cause irregular or heavy bleeding, which may lead to anemia. Fertility may be affected by submucosal or intramural myomas, which may impede sperm flow, prevent adequate implantation, or cause recurrent miscarriages. It is particularly important to diagnose submucosal leiomyomas because they are a well-established cause of dysfunctional uterine bleeding, infertility, and spontaneous abortion. Small submucosal leiomyomas may be removed hysteroscopically.

trimester are associated with an elevated risk of pregnancy loss, and this risk is higher in patients with multiple myomas. They rarely develop in postmenopausal women, and most stabilize or decrease in size following menopause because of a lack of estrogen stimulation. They may increase in size in postmenopausal patients who are undergoing hormone replacement therapy. Tamoxifen has also been reported to cause growth in leiomyomas. A rapid increase in myoma size, especially in a postmenopausal patient, should raise the level of concern for a neoplasm.

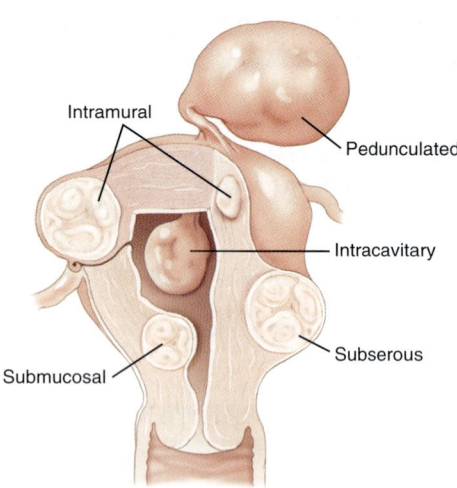

FIG. 43.13 Various locations of fibroid tumors found within the uterine cavity.

Uncommonly, a pedunculated subserosal lesion develops a long stalk and is migratory; it can implant into the blood supply of the broad ligament, omentum, or the bowel mesentery. Transvaginal sonography is often helpful in showing the uterine origin of the mass and identifying the stalk. Occasionally, a pedunculated myoma becomes adherent to surrounding structures and develops an auxiliary blood supply.

Sonographic Findings. Leiomyomas have variable sonographic appearances. The earliest sonographic finding of myomas is the demonstration of uterine enlargement or irregular uterine wall contour with a heterogeneous myometrial texture pattern. The sonographer should also look for contour distortion along the interface between the uterus and the bladder (Fig. 43.14). The myoma alters the normal homogeneous myometrium. Discrete myomas usually are hypoechoic but can be hyperechoic if they contain dense fibrous tissue. Bright clusters of echoes occur with calcific deposits and produce typical distal acoustic shadowing (Fig. 43.15). Some myomas demonstrate an area of acoustic attenuation without a discrete mass, making it impossible to estimate size. The attenuation is thought to be caused by dense fibrosis within the substance of the tumor. The ultrasound technique and gain controls often must be manipulated to provide increased penetration, or a lower frequency may be necessary to fully evaluate the uterus. If extensive calcification is present, the uterus and adnexa may be difficult to image because of shadowing. In such cases, transvaginal imaging is helpful in visualizing the ovaries. Myomas as small as 0.5 cm can be detected by transvaginal sonography and their relationship to the endometrial cavity defined precisely. Larger myomas cause heterogeneous uterine enlargement and may be better outlined by transabdominal sonography.

The sonographic study should include measurement of the uterus in three dimensions: (1) cervix to fundus, (2) widest anteroposterior diameter, and (3) widest transverse diameter at fundus diameter (Fig. 43.16). The texture of the myoma (calcific, complex, or anechoic), size, and location are described. Individual myomas are measured if they are discrete. The shape of the endometrial complex and its thickness are also described; alterations in the endometrial border will be evident if a myoma is present (Fig. 43.17). This is especially important in women with a history of abnormal bleeding. Myomas can be associated with endometrial infection or cancer. Blood debris and polyps can artifactually widen the endometrium; therefore, definitive diagnosis of the cause of abnormal bleeding might require an endometrial biopsy or sonohysterography.

Cystic degeneration of myomas causes lucencies that are well visualized with transvaginal sonography. Cystic degeneration can occur during pregnancy and cause pain. Doppler should be used to assess the vascularity of myomas as a possible predictor of growth. Sonography shows thin vessels with low-velocity flow within myomas. In cases of cystic degeneration, these vessels with low-velocity flow are not seen. Giant leiomyomas with multiple cystic spaces resulting from edema have also been described.

Although ultrasound is used to identify myomas in women with abnormal bleeding, uterine enlargement, or infertility, MRI—with its tissue differentiation characteristics—can be more sensitive for evaluating the exact location, size, and number of myomas.

Treatment of Myomas. The decision to treat or not treat myomas depends on the clinical state of the patient. In the case of infertility and a submucosal myoma, surgery by myomectomy is generally the treatment of choice. In cases of menorrhagia, women now have several choices. The least invasive treatment is hormonal suppression to stop bleeding. Several newer techniques are also now available. Endometrial ablation uses radiofrequency, microwaves, freezing, or heating ablative technology to ablate or remove the endometrium and any small surrounding myomas. Uterine artery embolization is another method utilized to obstruct blood flow to large myomas. Small plastic particles are injected into the blood supply to the myoma to terminate flow. The myoma eventually becomes necrotic. High-intensity focused ultrasound (HIFU) involves the application of "therapeutic" sonic waves to the uterus and myoma. The myoma is ablated by heating the tissue and causing tissue death. Currently, only MRI-guided HIFU is approved in the United States. Ultrasound-guided HIFU is approved and in use in several European countries, Russia, and China.

Other Uterine Masses. A common error among new sonographers is mistakenly identifying all round, large uterine masses as myomas. Color Doppler is crucial in making the distinction. Other uterine masses that may mimic a myoma can include endometrial carcinoma, leiomyosarcoma, or metastatic spread from the ovary into the uterus, such as clear cell cancer. The uterine mass will be highly vascularized, which is the key feature that distinguishes the mass from a benign fibroid.

Uterine Calcifications

Myomas are the most common cause of uterine calcifications. A less common cause is arcuate artery calcification in

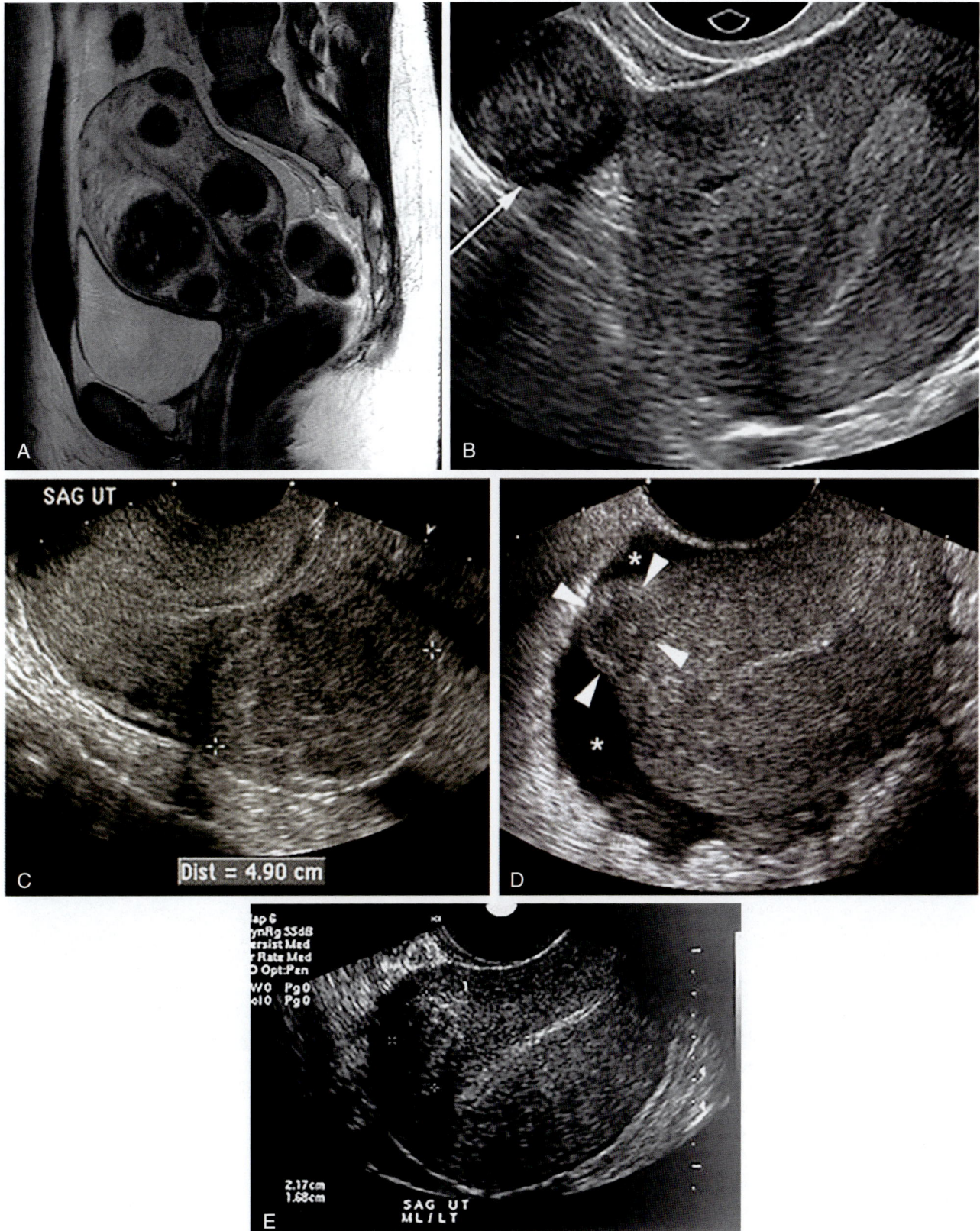

FIG. 43.14 A myoma alters the normal homogeneous myometrium. Discrete myomas usually are hypoechoic but can be hyperechoic if they contain dense fibrous tissue. **(A)** Magnetic resonance image of multiple myomas throughout the uterus. **(B)** Pedunculated myoma. **(C–E)** Intramural myomas.

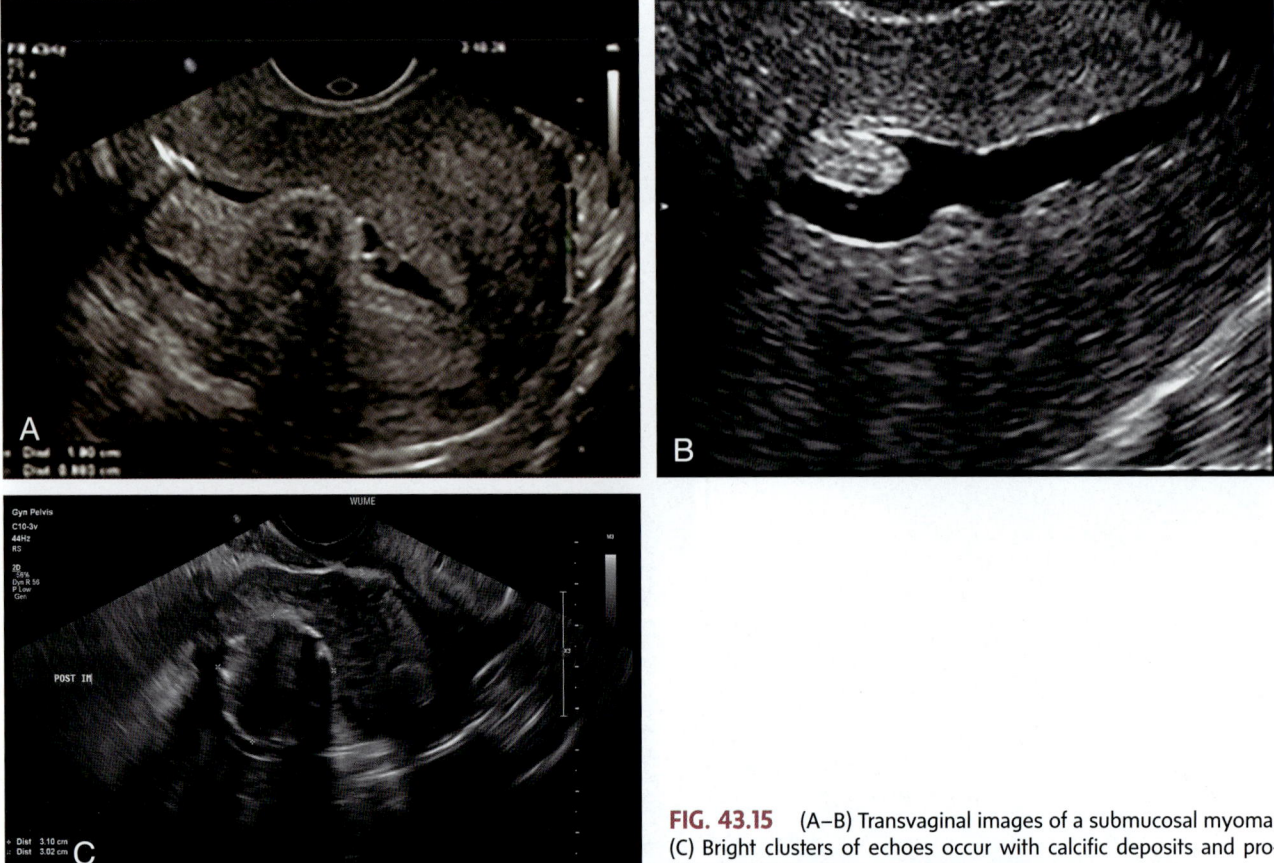

FIG. 43.15 (A–B) Transvaginal images of a submucosal myoma. (C) Bright clusters of echoes occur with calcific deposits and produce typical distal acoustic shadowing.

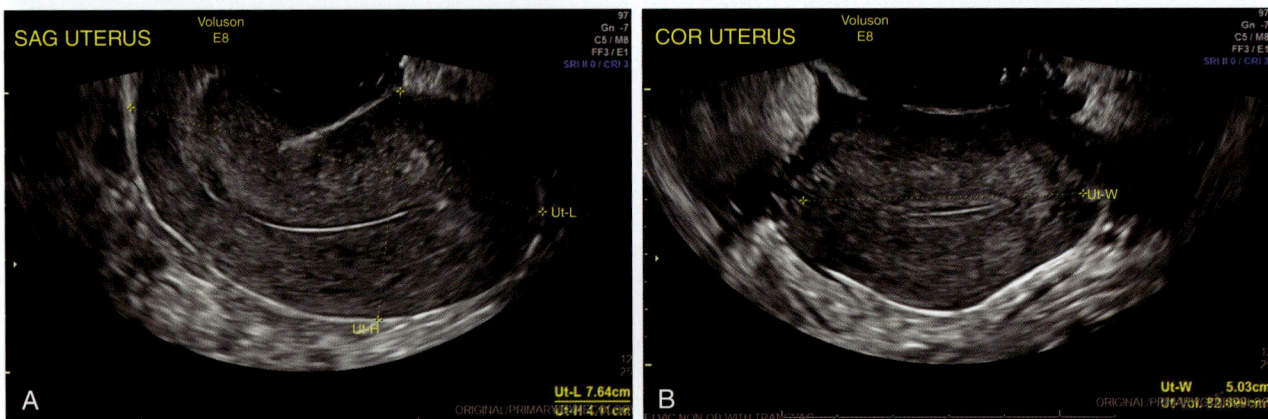

FIG. 43.16 Transvaginal images of the uterus for measurement. (A) Sagittal image should measure the uterus at the longest point from the fundus to the cervix. (B) Coronal image at the level of the fundus measures the anteroposterior dimension and the width of the uterus.

the periphery of the uterus. These calcifications are thought to occur as a consequence of calcific sclerosis within these vessels and can indicate underlying disease, such as diabetes mellitus, hypertension, and chronic renal failure. Such calcifications have been termed *Monckeberg arteriosclerosis* and appear in arteries throughout the body (Fig. 43.18);

Sonographic Findings. Calcifications may occur as focal areas of increased echogenicity with shadowing or may appear as a peripheral echogenic rim (Fig. 43.19).

Adenomyosis

Adenomyosis is a benign disease, commonly diffuse, with global infiltration of the endometrium, which sonographically presents as a bulky enlarged uterus without focal mass. Adenomyosis is the ectopic occurrence of endometrial tissue within the myometrium and is more common in the posterior aspect. On occasion, adenomyosis may be focal with discrete masses or be identified with adenomyomas in the

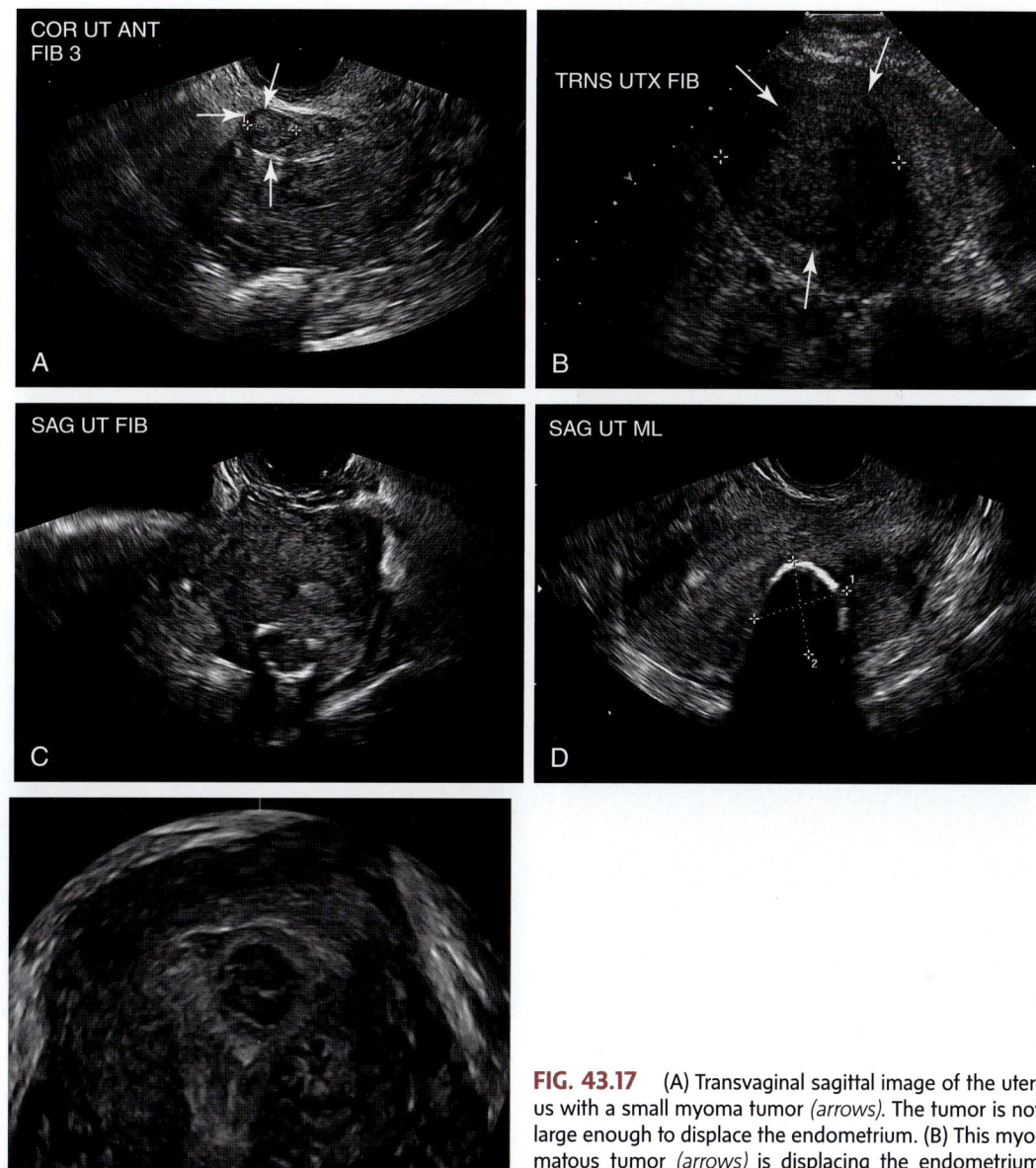

FIG. 43.17 (A) Transvaginal sagittal image of the uterus with a small myoma tumor *(arrows)*. The tumor is not large enough to displace the endometrium. (B) This myomatous tumor *(arrows)* is displacing the endometrium posteriorly. (C) Moderate size myoma with calcification. (D) Calcified rim of the fibroid with complete shadowing posterior. (E) 3D rendering of the intracavity myoma.

FIG. 43.18 (A) Color Doppler image of normal arcuate artery flow within the periphery of the uterus. (B) Transvaginal sagittal view of the uterus with peripheral echogenic foci in the region of Monckeberg arteriosclerosis.

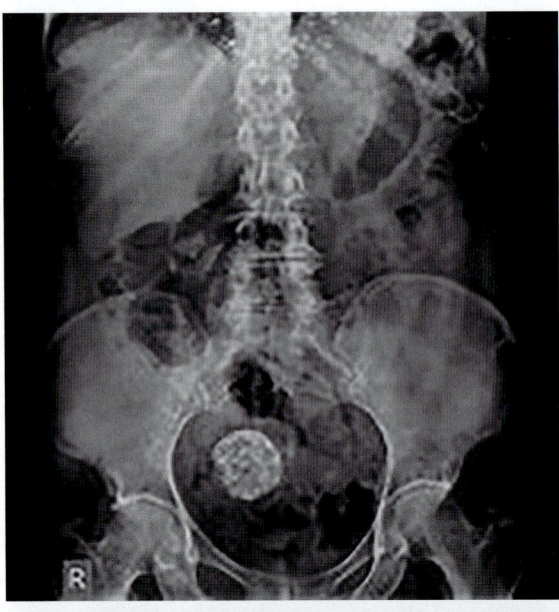

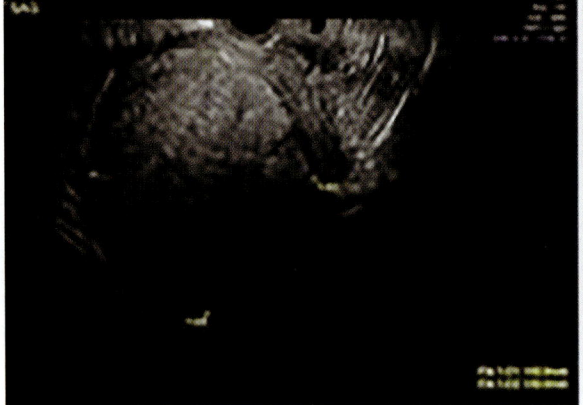

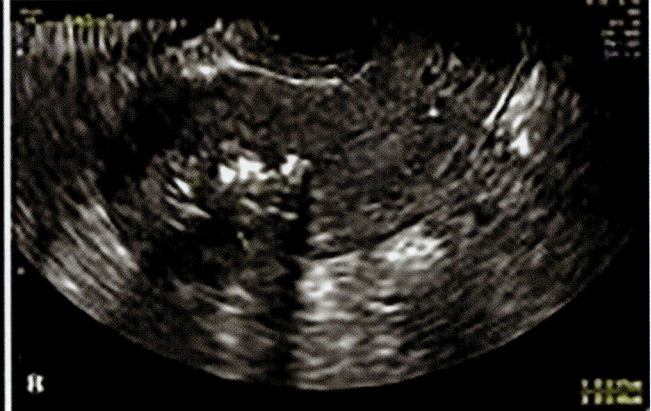

FIG. 43.19 Calcifications within a myoma may occur as focal areas of increased echogenicity with shadowing or may appear as a peripheral echogenic rim.

wall of the uterus. The exact cause is unknown, but the most commonly accepted theory suggests that a compromise of the natural barrier between the endometrium and myometrium occurs—commonly from uterine surgery—allowing the growth of ectopic endometrial bands and stroma within the uterine myometrium. The tissue penetration usually reaches a depth of at least 2.5 mm from the basal layer of the endometrium. Adenomyosis may arise from multiple pregnancies and deliveries with subsequent uterine shrinking. Elevated estrogen levels may also promote the growth of myometrial islands of endometrial tissue.

Adenomyosis is often classified into diffuse and focal forms. The more common form is diffuse adenomyosis. It represents a reactive hypertrophy of the myometrial muscle, which produces uterine enlargement but usually not to the extent seen with leiomyomas. Focal adenomyosis is sometimes called *adenomyoma*, referring to isolated implants that typically cause reactive hypertrophy of the surrounding myometrium and produce diffuse uterine enlargement. Less common than the diffuse form, focal adenomyosis (adenomyoma) lacks a hypoechoic border that is seen with fibroids, not endometriosis. Adenomyosis can be appropriately managed with hormone therapy.

Clinically, both adenomyosis and endometriosis are identical with respect to structure and function, but they are usually regarded as separate and distinct processes. Patients with adenomyosis are often multiparous and older than patients with endometriosis. The patient presents with heavy, painful abnormal menses, and on physical examination, the uterus is found to range from normal to three times normal size and is globular in contour, boggy, and somewhat tender.

An estimated 60% of women with adenomyosis experience abnormal uterine bleeding (hypermenorrhea), prolonged/profuse uterine bleeding (menorrhagia), or irregular, acyclic bleeding (**metrorrhea**). Approximately 25% of patients with adenomyosis also suffer from pelvic pain during menstruation (dysmenorrhea). Currently, only 10% to 20% of adenomyosis cases are correctly diagnosed before surgery. This low rate is thought to exist because many adenomyosis patients are asymptomatic in the absence of other uterine pathology, and its presence may be overshadowed by associated pathology, such as leiomyomas, endometriosis, or endometrial polyps.

Sonographic Findings. Sonographically, the diagnosis of adenomyosis may be challenging, especially if there are concurrent findings, such as adenomyoma or fibroids.

The most common presentation of extensive adenomyosis is diffuse uterine enlargement, thickening of the posterior myometrium, indistinct border between the endometrium and myometrium (Fig. 43.20), and myometrial cysts. Typically, adenomyosis involves the inner two-thirds of the myometrium, where a slight decrease in echo content of the involved areas may be observed (Fig. 43.21).

Hemorrhage in the islands of endometrial tissue appears as small hypoechoic myometrial cysts. This has previously been described as a *Swiss cheese* or *honeycomb* pattern. Lesions of this size are at the limit of ultrasound resolution. The fluid nature of these lesions produces increased posterior acoustic enhancement rather than the degree of attenuation that is normally seen posterior to the uterus. Further evaluation using signal processing (preprocessing and post-processing) is helpful to better distinguish the contour and border differentiation of any coexisting pathology, such as leiomyomas. Doppler studies have also proven helpful in differentiating uterine pathology, as color flow studies of uterine masses show that myomas and sarcomas typically demonstrate a feeding artery, but adenomyosis rarely demonstrates feeding arteries.

Calcifications resulting from prior instrumentation are seen along the inner myometrium and cervix. Localized adenomyomas may be seen by transvaginal sonography as inhomogeneous, circumscribed areas in the myometrium, having indistinct margins and containing anechoic lacunae (see Fig. 43.21). They may be difficult to distinguish from leiomyomas, as these two conditions frequently occur together.

Adenomyosis is not always reliably diagnosed by ultrasonography, and caution is advised because these findings are similar in appearance to uterine myomas, muscular hypertrophy, myometrial contractions, endometritis, endometrial carcinoma, and the presence of increased endometrial secretions. The presence of myomas has been shown to limit the ability to diagnose the severity of adenomyosis. Although not reliably diagnosed by ultrasonography, adenomyosis is well characterized by MRI, which currently is thought by many to be the best technique for the presurgical diagnosis of adenomyosis. The MRI hallmark is the appearance of diffuse or focal widening of the junctional zone or the appearance of an indistinctly bordered myometrial mass (Fig. 43.22).

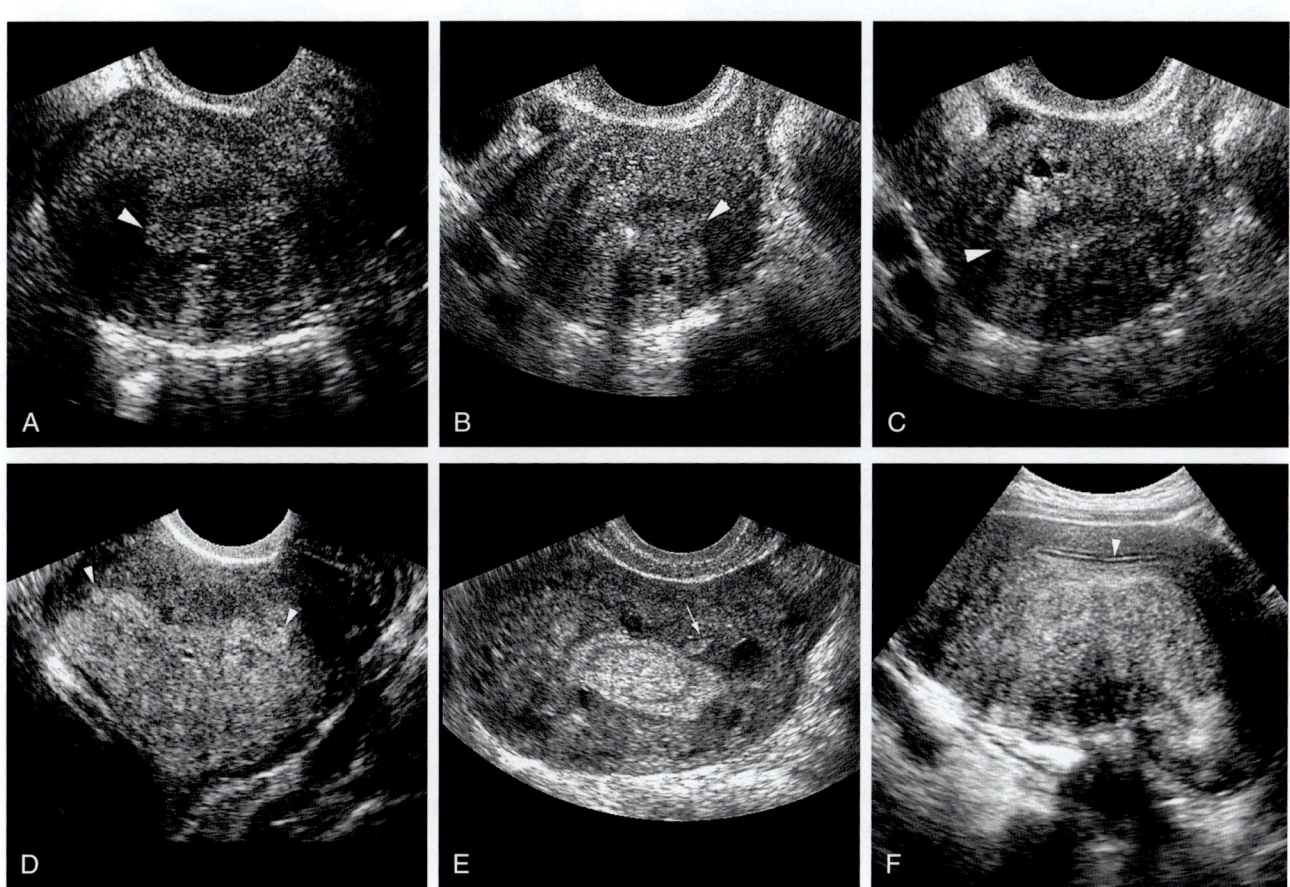

FIG. 43.20 Adenomyosis on transvaginal scans: spectrum of appearances. (A) Subendometrial cyst *(arrowhead)*. (B) Cysts with heterogeneity in both anterior and posterior myometrium. (C) Cysts with heterogeneity in anterior myometrium. (D) Myometrial heterogeneity with ill-defined endometrial borders *(arrowheads)*. (E) Multiple subendometrial cysts and echogenic nodule *(arrow)*. (F) Large area of myometrial heterogeneity producing a focal mass effect and displacing endometrium *(arrowhead)*. This may mimic a fibroid.

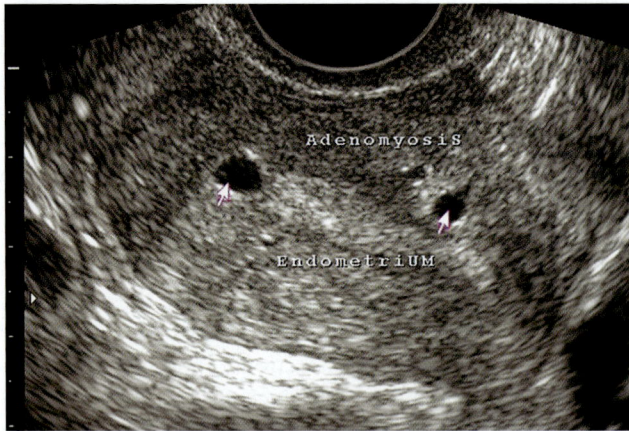
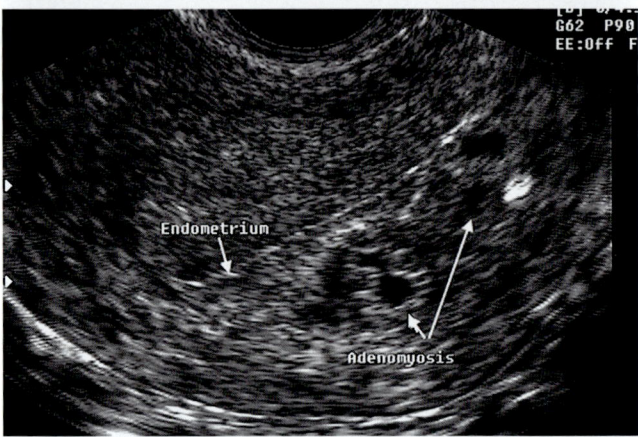

FIG. 43.21 Typically, adenomyosis involves the inner two-thirds of the myometrium, where a slight decrease in echo content of the involved areas may be observed.

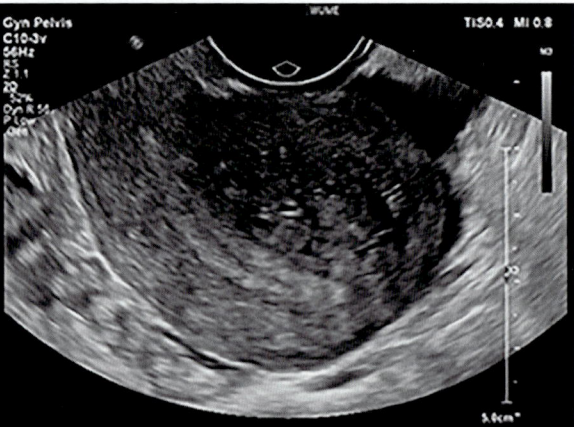
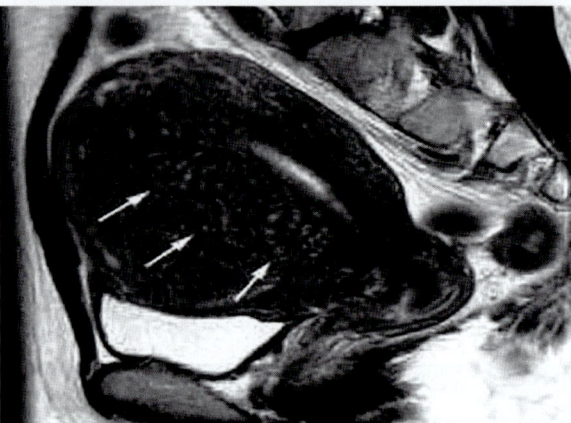
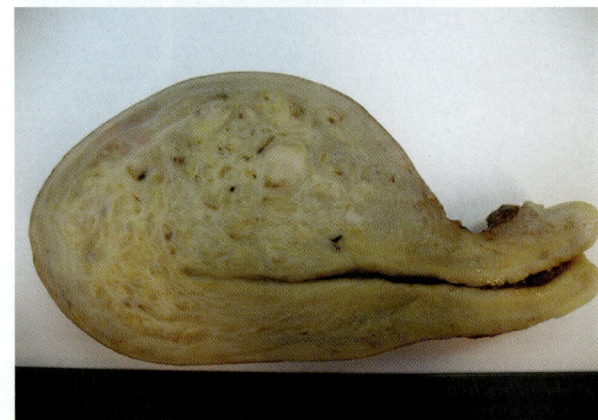

FIG. 43.22 Adenomyosis is well characterized by magnetic resonance imaging (MRI), which currently is believed by many to be the best technique for the presurgical diagnosis of adenomyosis. The MRI hallmark is the appearance of diffuse or focal widening of the junctional zone or the appearance of an indistinctly bordered myometrial mass.

Arteriovenous Malformations

Uterine arteriovenous malformations consist of a vascular plexus of arteries and veins without an intervening capillary network. They are rare, usually involving the myometrium and rarely the endometrium. They can be congenital, but most are teratogenic (acquired) resulting from pelvic trauma, surgery, and gestational trophoblastic neoplasia. Clinically, women of childbearing years have metrorrhagia with blood loss and anemia. Diagnosis is critical because dilation and curettage may lead to catastrophic hemorrhaging.

Sonographic Findings. Sonographically, serpiginous, anechoic structures are seen within the pelvis. Uterine arteriovenous malformations may appear as subtle myometrial inhomogeneity, tubular spaces within the myometrium, intramural uterine mass, endometrial or cervical mass, or sometimes as prominent parametrial vessels. Color Doppler is diagnostic to show blood flow within the anechoic structures (Fig. 43.23). There may be a florid colored mosaic pattern with apparent flow reversals and areas of color aliasing. Spectral Doppler shows high-velocity, low-resistance arterial flow coupled with high-velocity venous flow, with an arterial component. Treatment and confirmation include angiography with embolic therapy.

Uterine Leiomyosarcoma

Leiomyosarcoma is rare, accounting for 1% of all uterine malignancies. The tumors originate from the myometrium or the endometrial lining, are highly aggressive, and have a poor prognosis. Benign leiomyomas and leiomyosarcomas may occur in the same patient, though the two are genetically distinct and different structures (Box 43.6). The most common

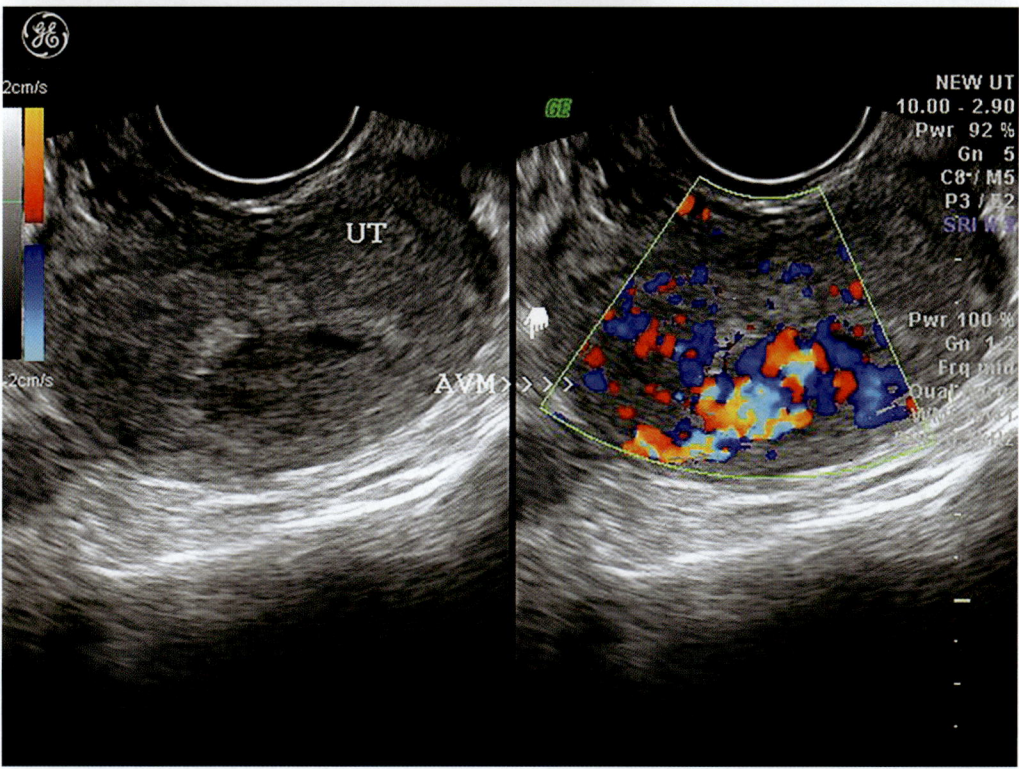

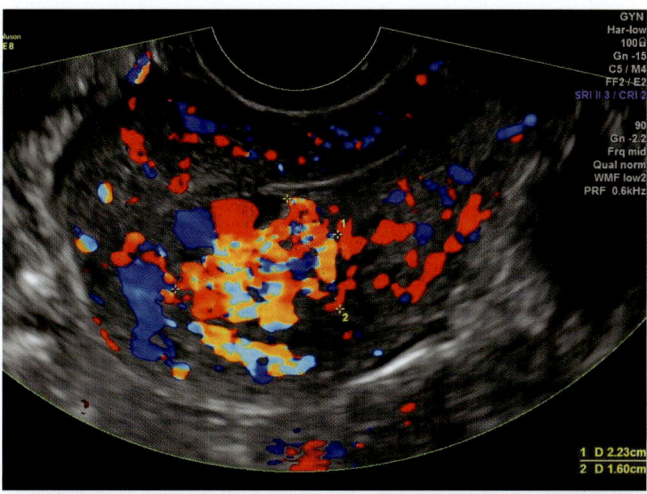

FIG. 43.23 Uterine arteriovenous malformations may appear as subtle myometrial inhomogeneity, tubular spaces within the myometrium, intramural uterine mass, endometrial or cervical mass, or sometimes as prominent parametrial vessels. Color Doppler is diagnostic to show blood flow within the anechoic structures.

| BOX 43.6 | Leiomyosarcoma |

- Rare, solid tumor arising from the myometrium or endometrium
- Commonly in fundus of uterus
- Most common in women 40–60 years of age
- Rapid growth
- *Sarcoma botryoides:* very rare condition in children characterized by grapelike clusters of tumor mass

presentation is abnormal vaginal bleeding, pelvic pain, and an enlarged uterus. Occasionally, patients are asymptomatic.

Sonographic Findings. Leiomyosarcoma may resemble myomas or endometrial carcinoma with features of solid or mixed-solid and cystic texture (Fig. 43.24). Clinically, the rapid enlargement of a solid uterine mass in the perimenopausal or postmenopausal patient raises concern about the development of a malignancy.

PATHOLOGY OF THE ENDOMETRIUM

The endometrial canal is the landmark for the identification of the long axis of the uterus. The echogenicity of the endometrial tissue is compared with the homogeneous, medium-level echogenicity of the middle layer of the myometrium. A hypoechoic layer of inner myometrium surrounds the endometrium. Progressive thickening and increased reflectivity of the endometrium occurs in the majority of patients until it is shed during menstruation. In the immediate preovulatory and postovulatory periods (approximately 2 days), an additional inner hypoechoic layer appears secondary to edema.

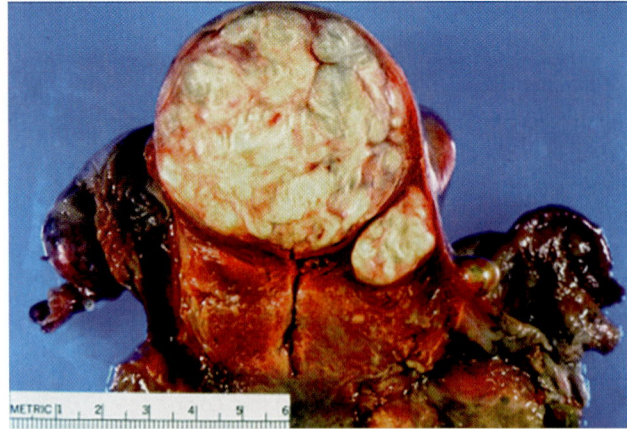

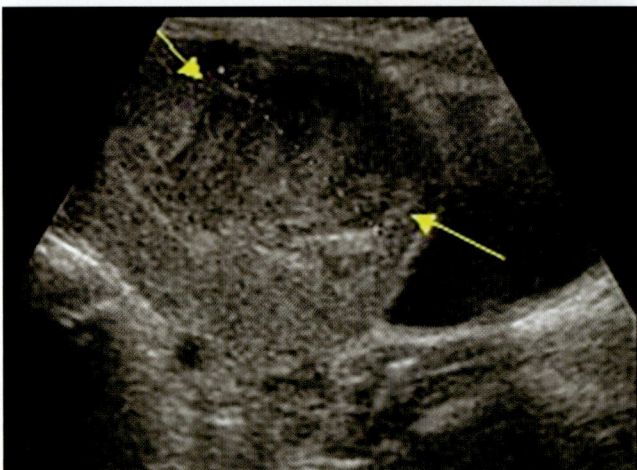

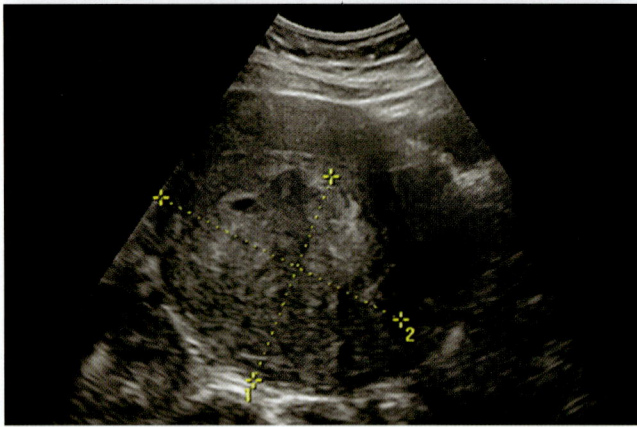

FIG. 43.24 Leiomyosarcomas originate from the myometrium or the endometrial lining. Leiomyosarcoma may resemble myomas or endometrial carcinoma with features of solid or mixed-solid and cystic texture.

TABLE 43.1	Endometrial Thickness Related to Phases of Menstrual Cycle
Phase of Menstrual Cycle	Endometrial Thickness[a] (mm)
Menstrual	2–3
Early proliferative	4–6
Periovulatory	6–8
Secretory	8–15

[a]Measured as full thickness, anteroposterior, from outer border to outer border of hypoechoic interface.
Data from Goldberg BB, Kurtz AB. *Ultrasound Measurements.* St Louis: Mosby–Year Book; 1990.

The endometrium should be measured perpendicular to the long axis of the uterus. The calipers should be placed at the maximum anterior to posterior diameter of the outer borders, from echogenic border to echogenic border. The hypoechoic halo surrounding the endometrium should not be included in the measurement because this represents the inner compact layer of myometrium. Fluid, if present, should not be included in endometrial measurements (Table 43.1). Additionally, the American Institute of Ultrasound in Medicine pelvic sonography guidelines recommend a 3D reconstruction of the uterus and endometrium when clinically indicated for endometrial pathology (also for uterine anomalies and IUCD localization).

Improved resolution with transvaginal sonography is better able to image and see subtle abnormalities within the endometrium. Knowledge of the normal sonographic appearance of the endometrium allows for earlier recognition of the pathologic conditions where the endometrium is thickened, irregular, or poorly defined. An abnormally thick endometrium results from a variety of conditions, including early intrauterine pregnancy, gestational trophoblastic disease, endometrial hyperplasia, secretory endometrium, estrogen replacement therapy, polyps, or endometrial carcinoma. Many endometrial pathologies, such as hyperplasia, polyps, and carcinoma, can cause abnormal bleeding, especially in the postmenopausal patient.

Disorders of the endometrium may also occur in menopausal patients with breast cancer who are receiving tamoxifen therapy. This is a partial estrogen receptor antagonist used in postmenopausal women with estrogen receptor–positive breast cancer. The effects on the uterus include epithelial metaplasia, hyperplasia, and even carcinoma. In these patients, transvaginal scanning may show thickened, irregular cystic endometrium. These patients frequently have biannual serial ultrasound examinations of their uterus and endometrium. A biopsy is performed in suspicious cases.

Sonohysterography

Sonohysterography (saline-infused sonography) has been shown to be of great value in further evaluating the abnormally thickened endometrium. By distending the endometrial cavity with saline, the examiner can distinguish endometrial growths and abnormalities. After performing routine transvaginal examination to orient the sonographer to the patient's anatomy and pathology, the doctor should explain the procedure to the patient and obtain consent. A sterile speculum is inserted into the vagina, and the cervix is cleansed with an antiseptic solution. A hysterosalpingography catheter is inserted into the uterine cavity beyond the cervical os. The catheter is prefilled with sterile saline before insertion to minimize air artifact. The speculum is removed and the transvaginal transducer is inserted into the vagina. The catheter is identified in the endometrial cavity by locating the saline-filled balloon, and the saline is slowly injected through the catheter under sonographic visualization. The uterus is scanned systematically in sagittal and coronal planes to delineate the entire endometrial cavity. Appropriate images are obtained under the direction of the physician performing the procedure. A sweep of the fluid-filled endometrium in both planes can be captured on cine clips to further document the presence of any pathology.

In premenopausal women, the procedure is performed in the midmenstrual cycle, usually between days 6 and 10. This will prevent the possibility of disrupting an early pregnancy and prevent blood clots artifactually filling some of the endometrial cavity. For women with irregular cycles, the procedure is performed soon after the cessation of bleeding, if possible. In postmenopausal women, the procedure can be performed at any time or shortly after the monthly bleeding period if they are on sequential hormone replacement therapy. The procedure is not performed in women with acute pelvic inflammatory disease (PID). In most cases there is no special patient preparation. Prophylactic antibiotics are given to women with chronic PID and to women with a history of mitral valve prolapse or other cardiac disorders.

Sonographic Findings. Sonographically, after the saline is injected, the endometrial canal fills with saline and the borders are clearly identified (Fig. 43.25). Any projections or

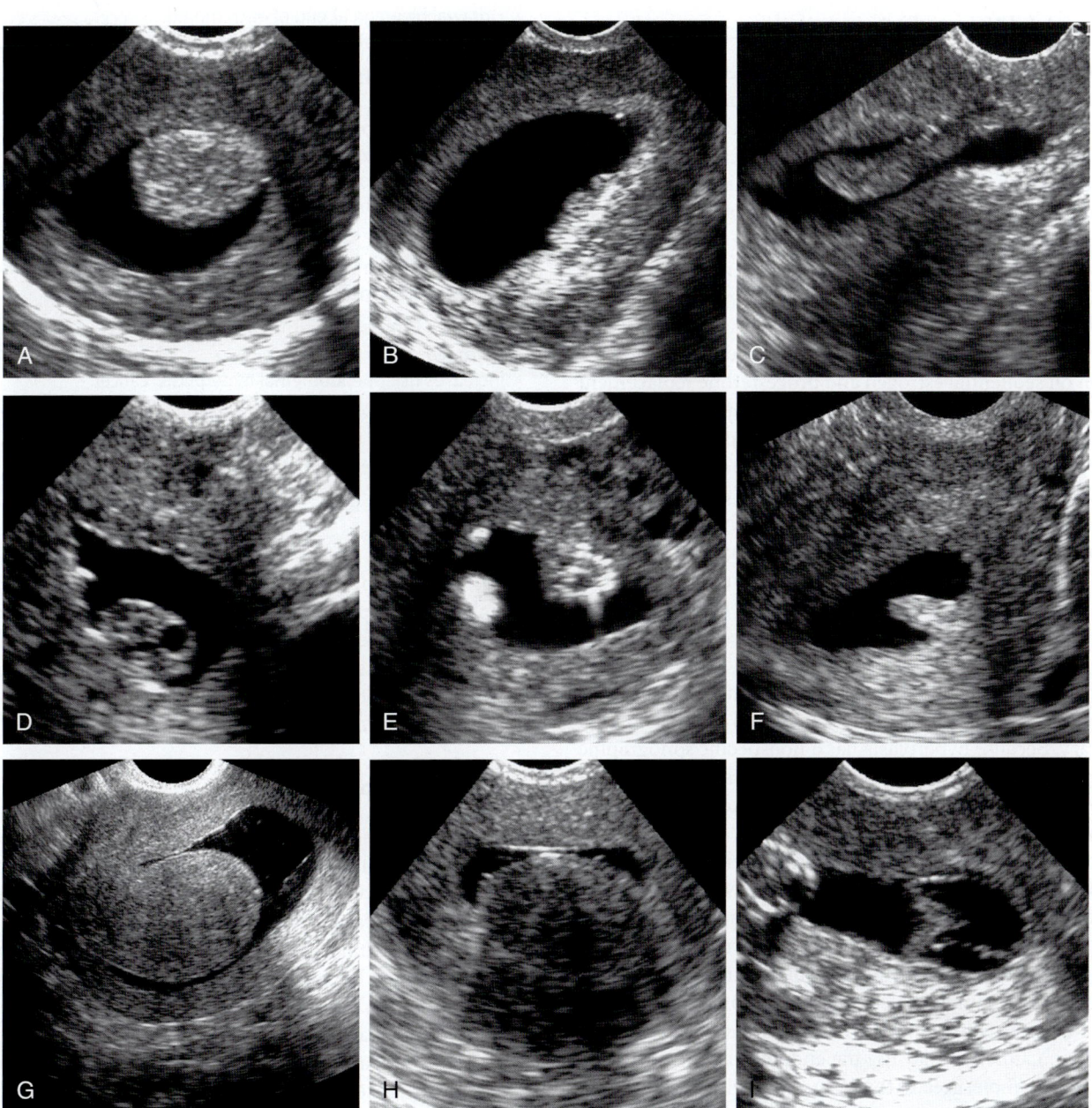

FIG. 43.25 Sonohysterograms. (A) Well-defined, round echogenic polyp. (B) Carpet of small polyps. (C) Polyp on a stalk. (D) Polyp with cystic areas. (E) Small polyp. (F) Small polyp. (G) Hypoechoic submucosal fibroid. (H) Hypoechoic attenuating submucosal fibroid. (I) Endometrial adhesions. Note bridging bands of tissue within the fluid-filled endometrial canal.

BOX 43.7	Endometrial Hyperplasia

Follows prolonged endogenous or exogenous estrogenic stimulation
May be precursor of endometrial cancer
Sonographic findings: abnormal thickening of endometrium

filling defects can be delineated and confirmed in the sagittal and coronal planes. By using color Doppler, a vascular pedicle can be identified in polyps. The clinician carefully removes the catheter while injecting a small amount of the saline to help distinguish the cervical area.

Endometrial Hyperplasia

Endometrial hyperplasia (Box 43.7) is the most common cause of abnormal uterine bleeding in both premenopausal and postmenopausal women. Hyperplasia develops from unopposed estrogen stimulation. It appears as thickening of the endometrium. In premenopausal women, if the endometrium measures more than 14 mm (double thickness), hyperplasia is suggested. The optimal time period for this assessment in a woman still having menses is day 6 through day 10, after bleeding and before the endometrium is again stimulated. In asymptomatic postmenopausal women, 8 mm (double thickness) is the upper limit of normal. However, women on sequential estrogen and progesterone replacement regimens may have endometrial thickness up to 15 mm during the estrogen phase; the thickness decreases after progesterone is added. Ideally a woman using sequential hormones should be studied at the beginning or end of her hormone cycle, when the endometrium is theoretically at its thinnest. Common hormonal regimens in menopausal women are listed in Box 43.8. Hyperplasia is less common during the reproductive years, but it may occur with persistent anovulatory cycles, with polycystic ovarian disease, and in obese women with increased production of endogenous estrogens. Hyperplasia may also be seen in women with estrogen-producing tumors, such as granulose cell tumors and thecomas of the ovary. Because hyperplasia has a nonspecific sonographic appearance, an endometrial biopsy is necessary for diagnosis. Sonohysterography can also be performed to evaluate the internal structure of the endometrial canal.

Most women with postmenopausal uterine bleeding are experiencing endometrial atrophy. On transvaginal sonography, an atrophic endometrium is thin, measuring less than 5 mm. If the postmenopausal patient has irregular bleeding and a thickened endometrium, this may warrant a sonohysterography procedure or an endometrial biopsy. Ultrasound is used to help the clinician triage which patients are candidates for biopsy. Clinicians may use the endometrial measurement alone (for example, greater than 5 to 8 mm without bleeding), or they may use symptoms as their criteria (for example, less than 5 to 8 mm with bleeding).

Sonographic Findings. The endometrium is usually diffusely thick and echogenic with well-defined margins

BOX 43.8	Common Hormonal Regimens in Menopausal Women

1. No hormones.
2. Unopposed estrogen (usually Premarin). If uterus is present, unopposed estrogen is associated with increased risk for endometrial hyperplasia or carcinoma.
3. Continuous/combined estrogen and progesterone (Premarin and Provera). This combination produces endometrial atrophy after 3–6 months. Usually, there is no risk of endometrial cancer; however, women may have "breakthrough" bleeding during the month or annoying progesterone side effects (i.e., irritability, depression, bloating, and breast tenderness).
4. Sequential estrogen and progesterone (Premarin first half then Provera second half of month). Women have predictable withdrawal bleeding at end of each month.

In the United States, regimens 2 and 4 are most commonly used.

Beneficial Effects
Estrogen
Alleviates menopausal symptoms (hot flashes, night sweats, painful intercourse)
Reduces risk of osteoporosis, vertebral and hip fractures
Reduces risk of heart attacks, strokes

Progesterone
Produces endometrial atrophy; reduces risk of endometrial hyperplasia/cancer

Negative Effects
Estrogen
Increases risk of endometrial hyperplasia/cancer

Progesterone
Increases risk of breast cancer
Irritability, depression, breast tenderness in some women

(Fig. 43.26). Focal or asymmetric thickening can occur. Small cysts representing dilated cystic glands may be seen within the endometrium. Although cystic changes within a thickened endometrium are more frequently witnessed in benign conditions, they can also be observed in endometrial carcinoma.

Endometrial Polyps

Patients with **endometrial polyps** can be asymptomatic, or they may present with uterine bleeding. Histologically, polyps are overgrowths of endometrial tissue covered by epithelium. They contain a variable number of glands, stroma, and blood vessels. Approximately 20% of endometrial polyps are multiple. They may be pedunculated, be broad based, or have a thin stalk. They typically cause diffuse or focal endometrial thickening and are more frequently seen in perimenopausal and postmenopausal women. In menstruating women, they may be associated with menometrorrhagia or infertility. In postmenopausal women, especially those being investigated for bleeding, the major differential considerations are hyperplasia, submucosal myomas, or, less commonly, endometrial carcinoma.

the endometrial cavity (Fig. 43.27). Cystic areas representing histologically dilated glands may be seen within a polyp. A feeding artery in the pedicle may be identified with color Doppler, especially with the newer systems that have sensitive power Doppler or high-definition flow. Individual polyps are better visualized when outlined by intracavitary fluid. Sonohysterography is a valuable technique when transvaginal sonography is unable to differentiate an endometrial polyp from a submucosal leiomyoma. Color Doppler sonohysterography can be particularly useful in discriminating polyps from submucosal myomas based on the presentation of feeding vessels. Polyps present most often with one primary feeding vessel, whereas myomas typically have multiple microvessels arising from the inner myometrium.

Endometritis

Endometrial thickening or fluid may indicate endometritis (Box 43.9). **Endometritis** is an infection within the endometrium of the uterus. It occurs most often in association with PID, in the postpartum state, or following instrumentation of the uterus. In patients with pelvic infection, the uterus is the conduit for infectious spread to the tubes and adnexa. Postpartum patients may develop endometritis after prolonged labor, vaginitis, premature rupture of the membranes, or retained products of conception. Clinically, the patient has intense pelvic pain.

Sonographic Findings. Sonographically, the endometrium appears prominent, irregular, or both, with a small amount of endometrial fluid (Fig. 43.28). Pus may be demonstrated in the cul-de-sac as echogenic particles or debris. Enlarged ovaries with multiple cysts and indistinct margins may be seen secondary to periovarian inflammation. Dilation of the fallopian tube shows fluid-filled tubular shapes in a folded configuration and well-defined echogenic walls. A thickened tubal wall (5 mm or more) indicates acute disease. These should be distinguished from a fluid-filled bowel by gentle compression on the pelvic wall to look for peristalsis or movement in the bowel lumen.

As the infection worsens, periovarian adhesions may form and fuse the inflamed tube and ovary, called the *tubo-ovarian complex*. Further progression results in a tubo-ovarian abscess that appears as a complex multiloculated mass with septations, irregular shaggy margins, and scattered internal echoes. There can be posterior enhancement and a fluid-debris level. Gas bubbles are present in rare cases; however, these also are observed in normal postpartum patients. In the immediate postpartum period, the presence of retained tissue is difficult to distinguish from inflammatory debris or blood clots. The sonographic appearance can be similar to that of other adnexal masses, so clinical correlation is important. Sonography can also be useful in following the response to antibiotic therapy or in guided transvaginal aspirations and drainage. If the aspirate is purulent, catheter drainage is used. In chronic PID, fibrosis and adhesions may make identification of pelvic organs difficult. Torsion of the tube is uncommon, but it occurs in association with chronic hydrosalpinx.

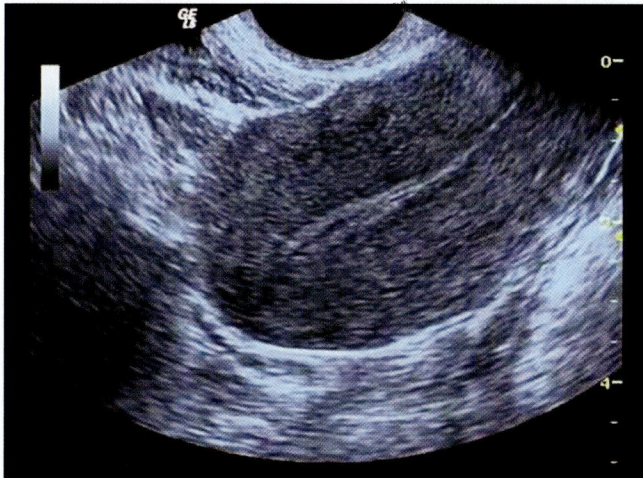

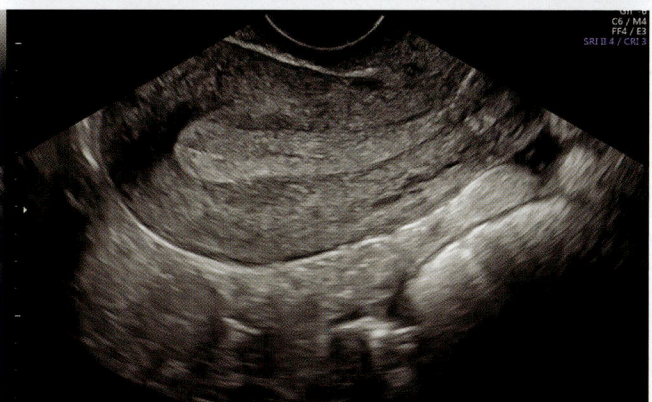

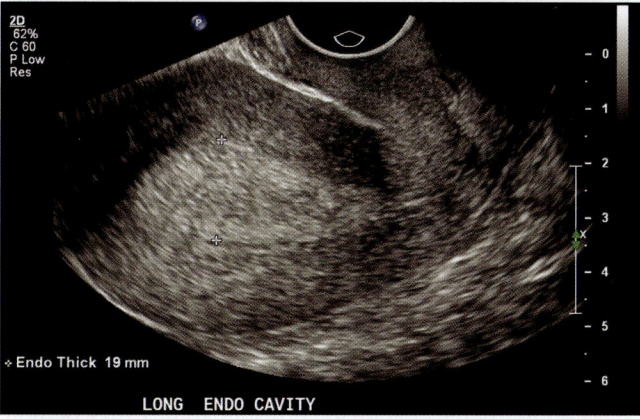

FIG. 43.26 Endometrial hyperplasia is the most common cause of abnormal uterine bleeding in both premenopausal and postmenopausal women. In premenopausal women, if the endometrium measures >14 mm (double thickness), hyperplasia is suggested. In asymptomatic postmenopausal women, 8 mm (double thickness) is the upper limit of normal. However, women on sequential estrogen and progesterone replacement regimens may have endometrial thickness up to 15 mm during the estrogen phase; the thickness decreases after progesterone is added.

Sonographic Findings. Sonographically, polyps appear toward the end of the luteal phase and are represented by a hypoechoic or isoechoic region within the hyperechoic endometrium. They initially may appear as nonspecific echogenic endometrial thickening. The polyp may be diffuse or focal and may also appear as a round echogenic mass within

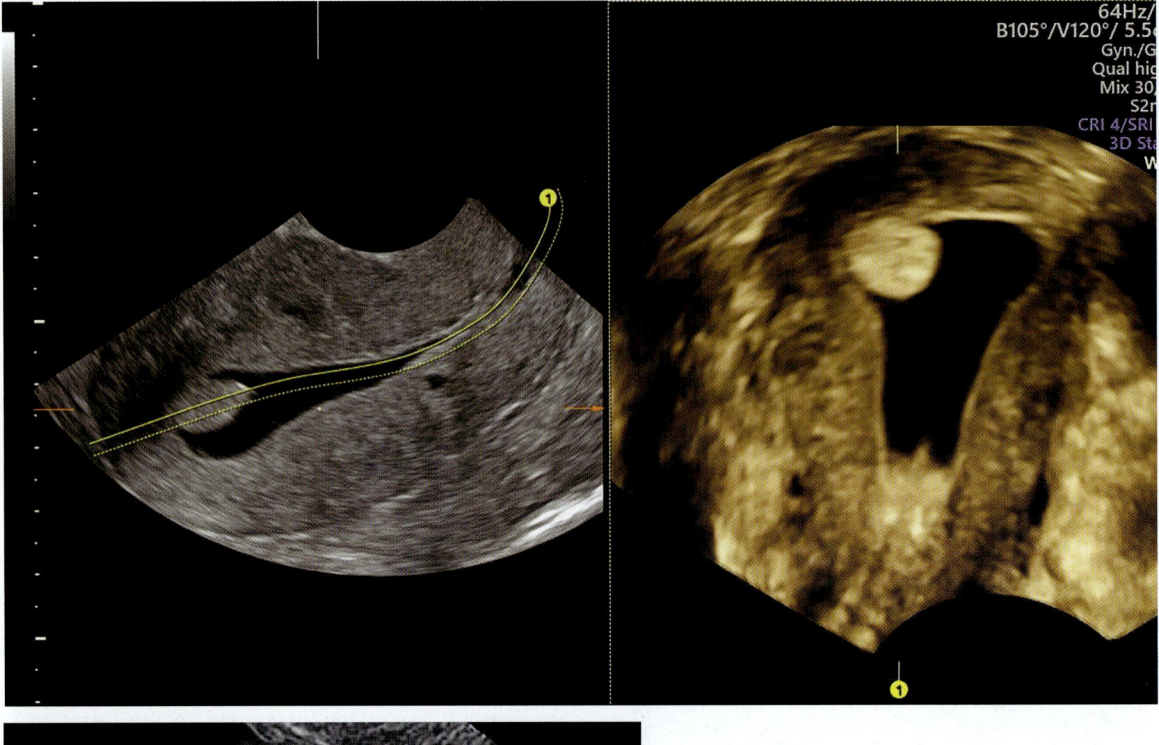

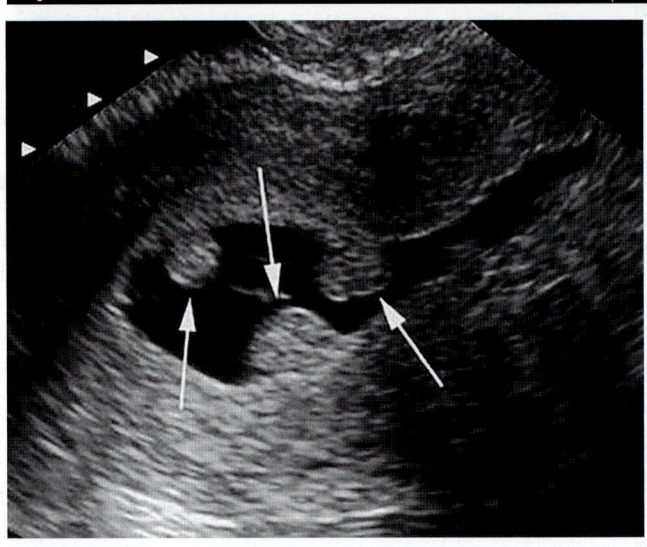

FIG. 43.27 Sonographically, polyps appear toward the end of the luteal phase and are represented by a hypoechoic or isoechoic region within the hyperechoic endometrium. They initially may appear as nonspecific echogenic endometrial thickening. The polyp may be diffuse or focal and may also appear as a round echogenic mass within the endometrial cavity. Saline infusion will help define the border of the polyp.

BOX 43.9	Endometritis

- Inflammation of the endometrium
- *Clinical findings:* low back pain and fever; lower abdominal pain; dysmenorrhea; menorrhagia; sterility; constipation
- *Sonographic findings:* endometrium appears prominent or irregular; pus may be seen in the cul-de-sac; enlarged ovaries with multiple cysts secondary to periovarian inflammation; dilated fallopian tubes

Synechiae

Intrauterine synechiae (endometrial adhesions, Asherman syndrome) are found in women with posttraumatic or postsurgical histories, including uterine curettage. Synechiae can cause infertility or recurrent pregnancy loss.

Sonographic Findings. Ultrasonography may demonstrate bright echoes within the endometrial cavity in this condition. The diagnosis is difficult unless fluid is distending the endometrial cavity (Fig. 43.29). This is best identified during the secretory phase when the endometrium is more hyperechoic. Synechiae are more easily observed in the gravid uterus, where they appear as a hyperechoic band traversing the uterus from anterior to posterior.

Sonohysterography is an excellent technique for demonstrating adhesions and should be performed in cases of suspected adhesions. Adhesions appear as bridging bands of tissue that distort the cavity or as thin, undulating membranes that connect from one side of the uterus to the other. Thick, broad-based adhesions may prevent distention of the uterine cavity. Adhesions can be divided under hysteroscopy.

CHAPTER 43 Pathology of the Uterus   1223

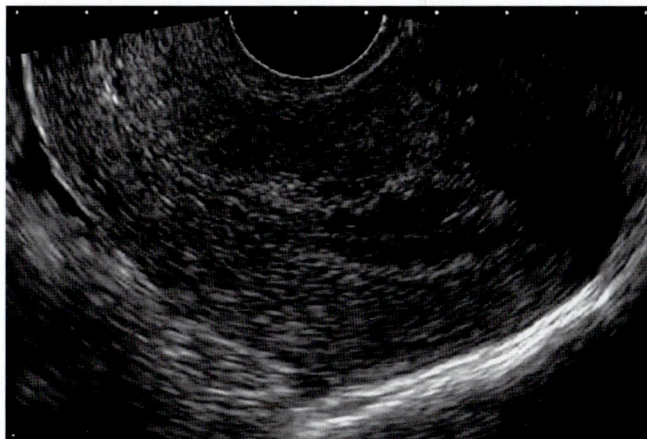

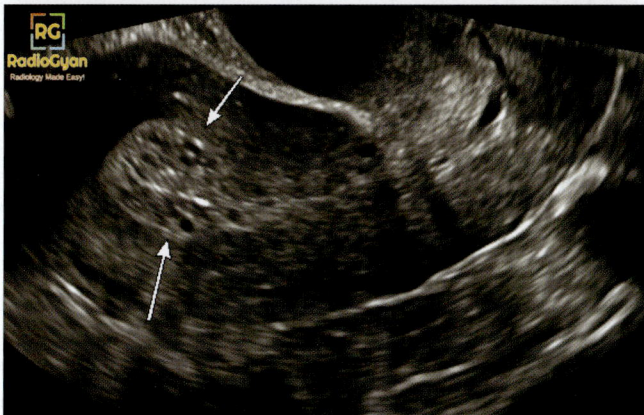

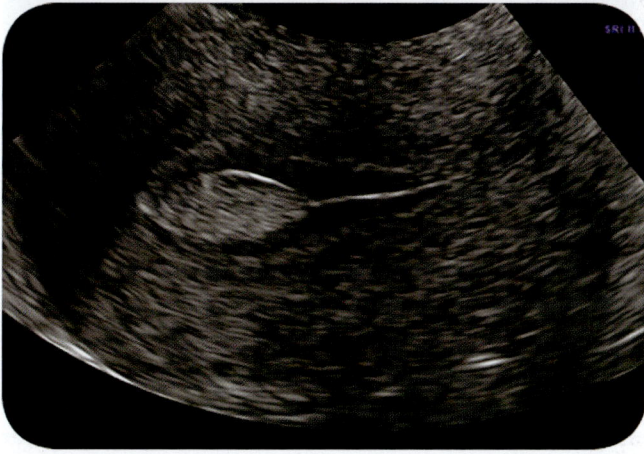

FIG. 43.28 Sonographically, the endometrium appears prominent, irregular, or both, with a small amount of endometrial fluid.

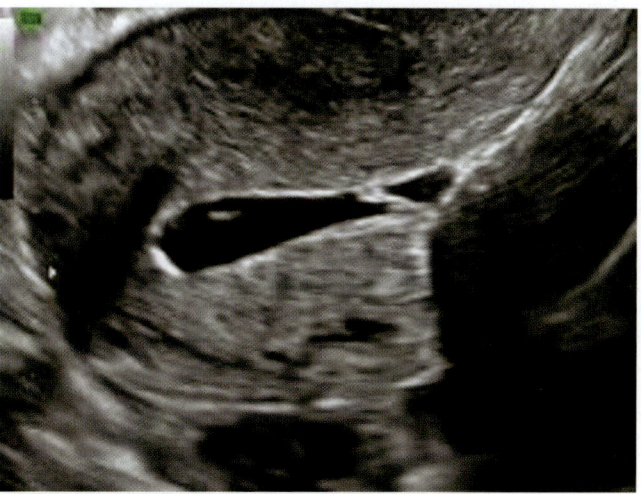

FIG. 43.29 **Sonography may demonstrate bright echoes within the endometrial cavity.** The diagnosis of synechiae is difficult unless fluid is distending the endometrial cavity. This is best identified during the secretory phase when the endometrium is more hyperechoic.

change of endometrial carcinoma is a thickened endometrium. An abnormally thick endometrium is also associated with endometrial hypertrophy and polyps.

Recent studies of patients with postmenopausal bleeding show that an endometrial thickness (double layer) of less than 5 mm reliably excludes significant endometrial abnormality.[1-3] At present, most investigators believe biopsies should be performed for all symptomatic patients. In the future, however, transvaginal ultrasonography may be used to follow symptomatic patients with normal endometrial thickness for whom biopsy is contraindicated or who do not wish to undergo an invasive procedure.

Although increased endometrial thickness is an early finding in endometrial carcinoma, enlargement with lobular contour of the uterus and mixed echogenicity are correlated with more advanced stages of the disease. The risk of malignancy increases with the presence of a large endometrial fluid collection or clinical symptoms, such as abdominal pain or bleeding.

Sonographic Findings. Transvaginal examination is help-ful in screening for early changes of endometrial hyperplasia or carcinoma by accurately measuring endometrial thickness. Sonographically, a thickened endometrium (greater than 4 to 5 mm, and this value varies institution to institution) should be considered cancer until proven otherwise (Fig. 43.30). Demonstration of myometrial invasion is clear evidence for endometrial carcinoma. Transvaginal ultrasonography demonstrates myometrial invasion as thickening and irregularity of the central endometrial interface with echogenic or hypoechoic patterns combined with infiltration of hyperdense structures in the myometrium (Box 43.10). Cystic changes within the endometrium are more commonly seen in endometrial atrophy, hyperplasia, and polyps but can also be seen with carcinoma. Endometrial masses containing numerous vascular branches with color imaging should also raise the level of suspicion for carcinoma.

Endometrial Carcinoma

Endometrial carcinoma is the most common gynecologic malignancy in North America, and its incidence has been rising. Most endometrial malignancies are adenocarcinomas occurring in postmenopausal patients. The most common clinical presentation is uterine bleeding, although only 10% of women with postmenopausal bleeding will have endometrial carcinoma. There is a strong association with replacement estrogen therapy. In the premenopausal woman, anovulatory cycles and obesity are also considered risk factors. The earliest

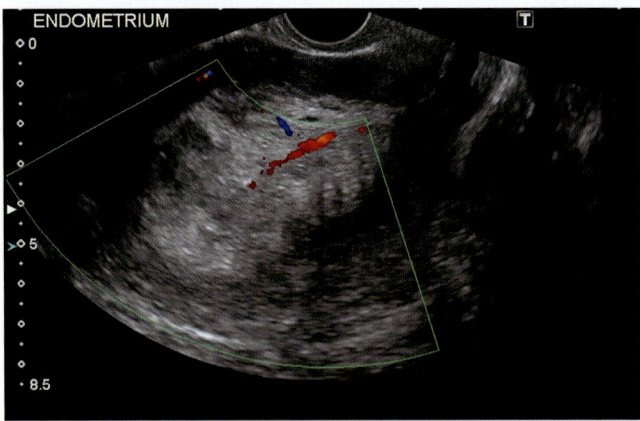

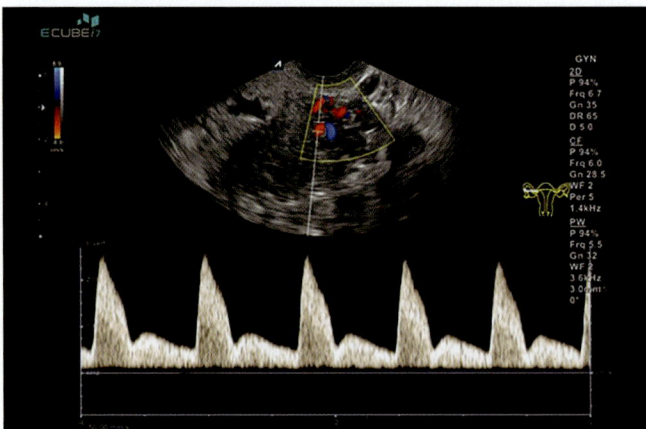

FIG. 43.31 Pulsed Doppler is used to evaluate the resistive index (RI = peak systolic − end diastolic/peak systolic) or pulsatility index (PI = peak systolic − end diastolic/mean). Low-resistance flow (RI < 0.4) has been found in patients with endometrial carcinoma and high-resistance flow (RI > 0.5) in normal or benign endometria.

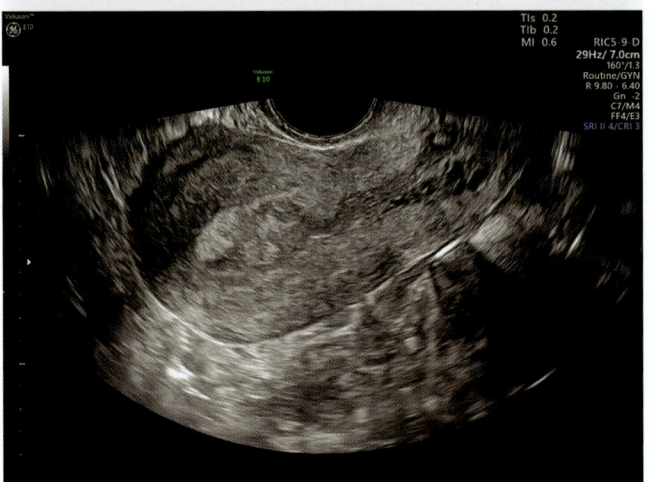

FIG. 43.30 Transvaginal examination is helpful in screening for early changes of endometrial hyperplasia or carcinoma by accurately measuring endometrial thickness. Sonographically, a thickened endometrium (>4 to 5 mm, and this value varies institution to institution) should be considered cancer until proven otherwise. Transvaginal ultrasonography demonstrates myometrial invasion as thickening and irregularity of the central endometrial interface with echogenic or hypoechoic patterns combined with infiltration of hyperdense structures in the myometrium.

BOX 43.10 Endometrial Carcinoma

Associated with estrogen stimulation
Clinical findings: postmenopausal bleeding
Sonographic findings: prominent endometrial complex; enlarged uterus with irregular areas of low-level echoes

---

Endometrial carcinoma may obstruct the endometrial canal, resulting in **hydrometra** or **hematometra**. The level of myometrial invasion (superficial versus deep) also can be detected by transvaginal ultrasonography, although contrast-enhanced MRI is more sensitive. Intactness of the subendometrial halo (the inner layer of myometrium) usually indicates superficial invasion, whereas obliteration of the halo is indicative of deep invasion. MRI is also valuable in evaluating extrauterine extension and involvement of lymph nodes.

Tamoxifen, a nonsteroidal antiestrogen compound, is widely used for adjuvant therapy in premenopausal and postmenopausal women with breast cancer and has secondary effects on the endometrium. Various new medications have been developed for the postmenopausal woman, including Aromasin, Evista, and Femara. An increased risk of endometrial carcinoma, hyperplasia, and polyps has been reported in patients on tamoxifen therapy. On sonography, tamoxifen-related endometrial changes are nonspecific and similar to those described in hyperplasia, polyps, and carcinoma. Because it may be difficult to distinguish the endometrial-myometrial border in many of these patients, sonohysterography is valuable.

Sonography may be helpful in staging carcinoma and in distinguishing between tumors limited to the uterus (stages I and II) and those with extrauterine extension (stages III and IV). Both MRI and CT are useful in staging by demonstrating lymphadenopathy and distant disease (stages III or IV). Endometrial biopsy is usually required for a definite diagnosis.

Doppler Evaluation. The role of color and spectral Doppler in the diagnosis of endometrial carcinoma is controversial. Doppler ultrasonography of the uterine artery may help distinguish between benign and malignant endometrial thickening. Pulsed Doppler is used to evaluate the resistive index (RI = peak systolic − end diastolic/peak systolic) or pulsatility index (PI = peak systolic − end diastolic/mean). The technique of this examination is discussed in Chapter 42. Low-resistance flow (RI less than 0.4) has been found in patients with endometrial carcinoma and high-resistance flow (RI greater than 0.5) in normal or benign endometria (Fig. 43.31). If a PI is used, the cutoff is 1. Intratumoral neovascularity is a more sensitive marker of endometrial carcinoma than resistive index alone.

Small Endometrial Fluid Collections

Small endometrial fluid collections also occur with ectopic pregnancy, endometritis, degenerating myomas, and recent abortion.

Sonographic Findings. Transvaginal sonography, with its improved resolution, sometimes shows tiny endometrial fluid collections not seen on transabdominal scans. These small endometrial fluid collections (less than 2 mL) are common in women during the menstrual phase of the cycle. They are seen in postmenopausal women, especially during the menstrual phase in women taking sequential hormones. In a uterus with a fluid collection, the anteroposterior diameter of the fluid should be subtracted from the endometrial measurement for a true assessment of endometrial thickness (Fig. 43.32).

Large Endometrial Fluid Collections

Large endometrial fluid collections should be regarded with suspicion. Obstruction of the cervical os results in the accumulation of secretions, blood, or both in the uterus. Before menstruation, the accumulation of secretions is referred to as hydrometrocolpos. Following menstruation, hematometrocolpos results from the presence of retained menstrual blood. The obstruction may be congenital, imperforate hymen (most common), vaginal septum, vaginal atresia, or a rudimentary uterine horn. Hydrometra and hematometra may also be acquired as a result of cervical stenosis from endometrial or cervical tumors or from post-irradiation fibrosis. They may also be caused by uterine, cervical, tubal, or ovarian carcinoma. Hyperplasia and polyps also cause endometrial fluid collections, so these collections also indicate increased risk of endometrial carcinoma. However, large amounts of endometrial fluid also are associated with benign conditions, such as congenital anomalies or cervical stenosis from prior instrumentation or childbirth.

The patient typically complains of abdominal pain and has an enlarged abdominal mass. She may or may not have vaginal bleeding. The presence of fever suggests infection of the blood collection. Laboratory results show an elevated white blood cell count. In simple hematometra, the uterine cavity returns to normal promptly after dilation and curettage. **Pyometra** is more likely to occur with uterine cancer. Abnormal development of the vagina or uterus may result in a cystic uterine or vaginal collection of mucus in children. When menstruation begins, the collection consists of blood.

Sonographic Findings. The sonographic picture of large endometrial cavity fluid collections is that of a centrally cystic, round, moderately enlarged uterus. This may contain echogenic material if pus or blood is present (Fig. 43.33).

INTRAUTERINE CONTRACEPTIVE DEVICES

Lost Intrauterine Device

Intrauterine contraceptive devices (IUCDs) are devices placed in the uterine cavity during menses for the purpose of birth control. Proper placement is verified by weekly digital palpation of the string in the cervix, performed by the patient. If the patient does not feel the string in the cervix, the IUCD may have been expelled or more likely the string has fallen off or retracted into the uterus. A pregnancy test is performed. If it is negative, the gynecologist explores the uterine cavity with a sterile hooked probe. If no string is found or if the pregnancy test is positive, an ultrasound examination is performed.

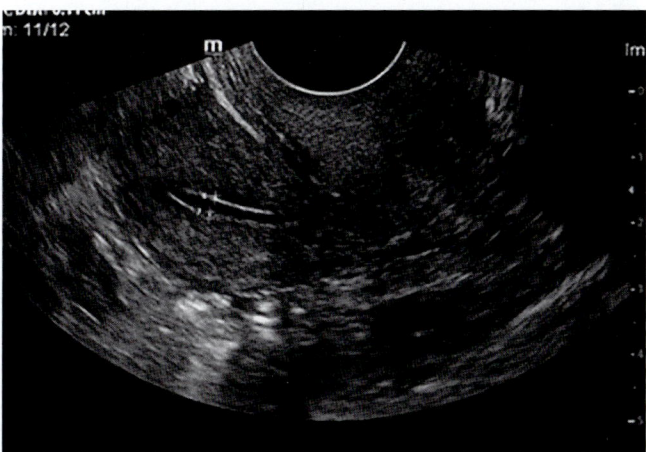
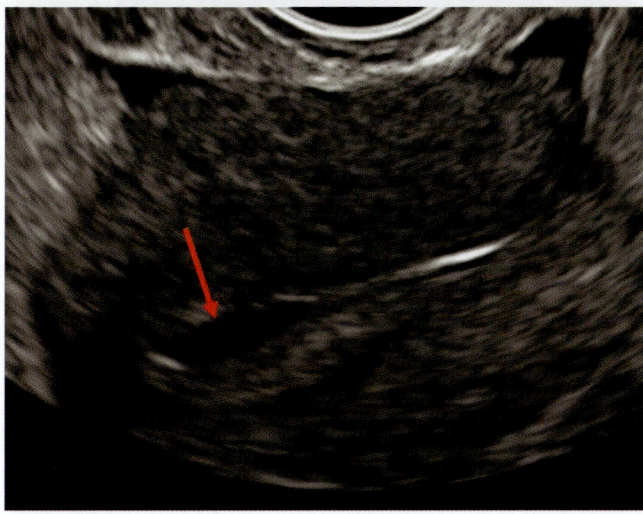

FIG. 43.32 In a uterus with a fluid collection, the anteroposterior diameter of the fluid should be subtracted from the endometrial measurement for a true assessment of endometrial thickness.

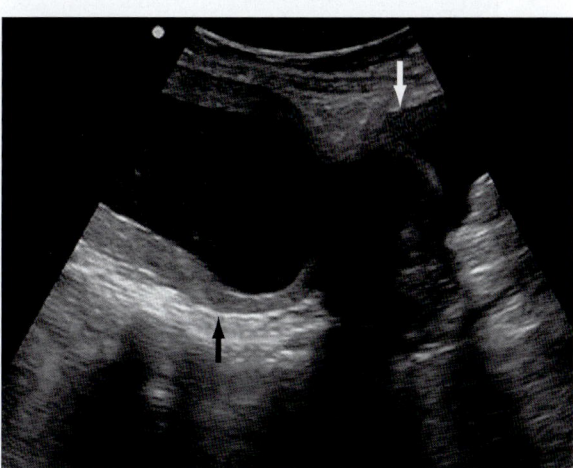

FIG. 43.33 Hematometra: the endometrial cavity is distended with blood, most commonly associated with cervical stenosis. Hematometra can also develop after uterine surgery such as endometrial ablation or dilation and curettage.

Sonography can demonstrate malposition, perforation, and incomplete removal of the IUCD. Eccentric position of an IUCD from midline suggests myometrial penetration. If the IUCD is not observed during sonography, a radiograph should be done. The IUCD may be difficult to see with coexisting intrauterine abnormalities, such as blood clots or an incomplete abortion. In the first trimester, the IUCD can usually be removed safely under ultrasound guidance. After the first trimester, an IUCD is very difficult to visualize. Patients with IUCDs are at increased risk for ectopic pregnancy and PID. In these women, tubo-ovarian abscess may be unilateral; more commonly, though, it is bilateral.

Sonographic Findings. Transabdominal and transvaginal scanning demonstrate the IUCD. The sonographic appearance of an IUCD varies according to the components of the device (Fig. 43.34). The most commonly used IUCDs

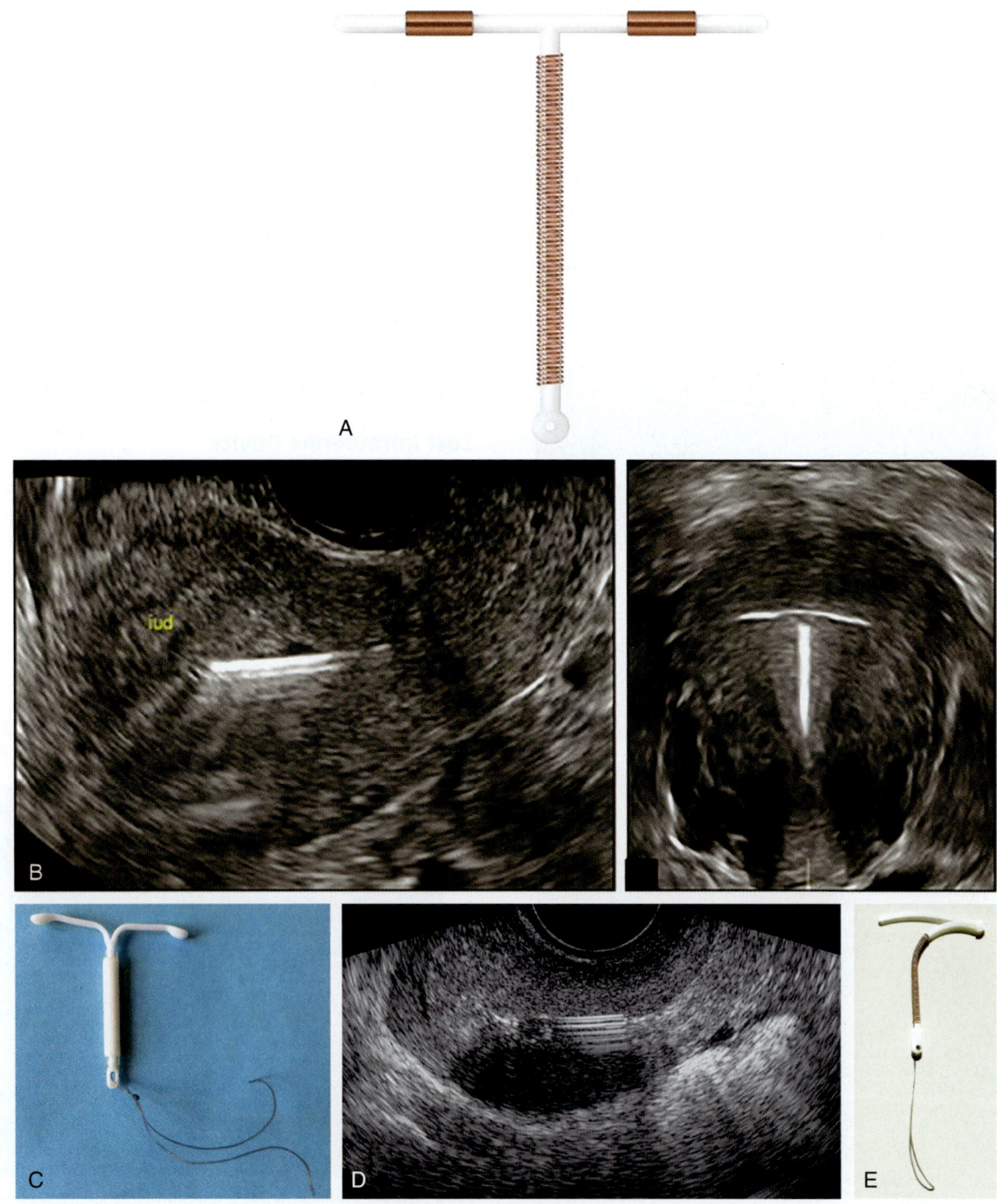

FIG. 43.34 Paraguard (A–B), a T-shaped flexible plastic wrapped in copper, and Mirena (C–D), a T-shaped flexible plastic that releases low amounts of progestin to act as an additional measure to prevent pregnancy. (E–F) Copper 7 is shaped like a 7, with a copper wire spiraled around the vertical shaft.

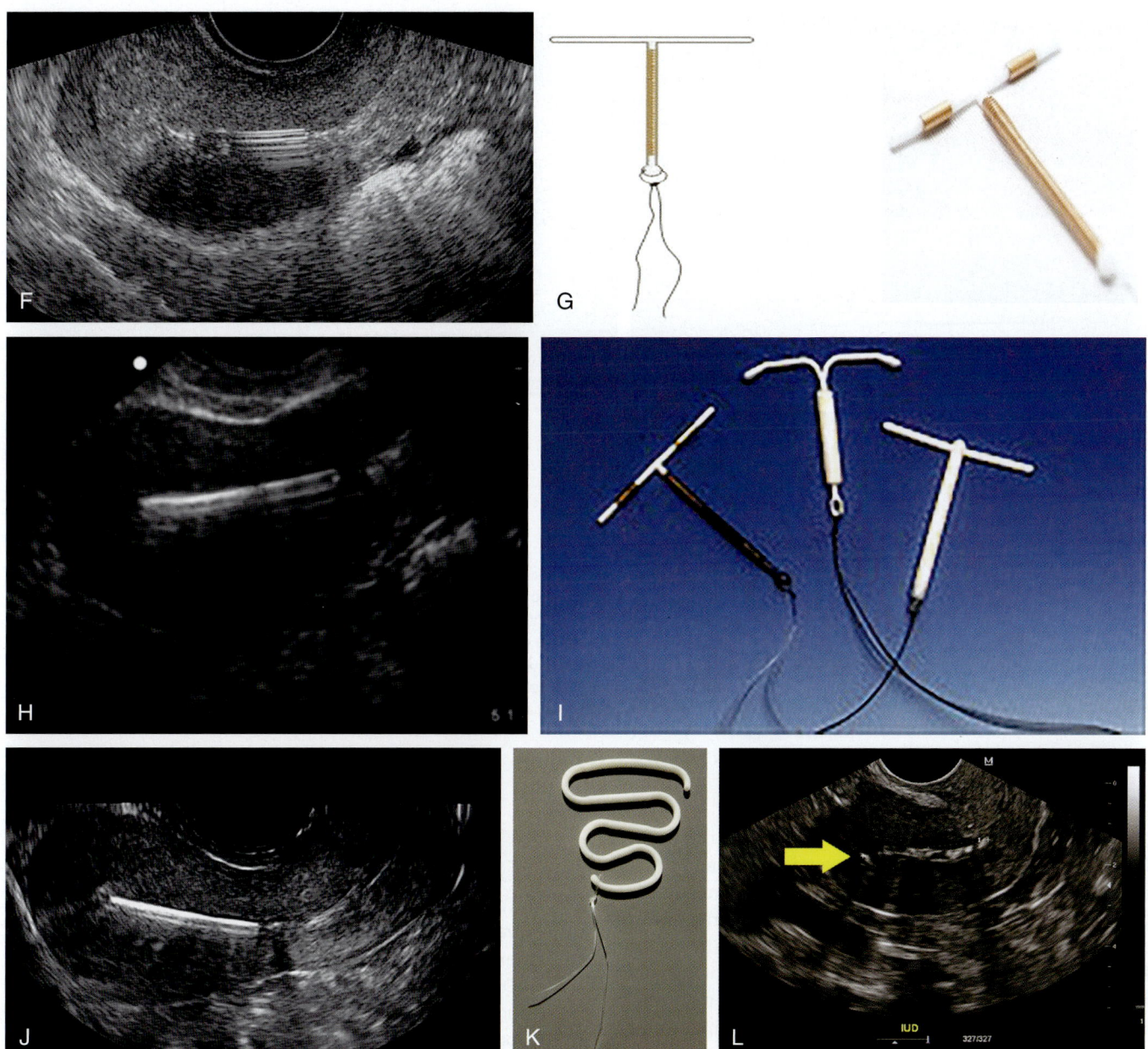

FIG. 43.34, Cont'd (G–H) Tatum T with copper wire spiraled along the vertical shaft. (I–J) Progestasert contains a drug reservoir along the vertical shaft with a suspension of progesterone and barium sulphate in silicone medical fluid. (K–L) Lippes Loop is a serpentine intrauterine contraceptive device.

are currently the Paraguard—a T-shaped flexible plastic wrapped in copper—and the Mirena—a T-shaped flexible plastic that releases low amounts of progestin to act as an additional measure to prevent pregnancy. Traditionally, the metal-containing devices appear as highly echogenic linear structures in the endometrial cavity within the uterine body. Do not confuse them with the normal, central endometrial echoes. The newer plastic polymer hormone-releasing Mirena appears only mildly echogenic and may be difficult to appreciate when visualizing for the first time. For this reason, it is important to ask the patient what type of IUCD she has. An analysis of in vivo and in vitro transabdominal images of the many types of IUCDs previously used in the United States found that the shafts of all of them appeared as a double line. This is because of entrance-exit reflections of sound waves when scanned perpendicular to the uterine cavity with high-resolution equipment. Posterior shadowing occurs when the ultrasound beam is entirely interrupted. This requires that the scanning plane be placed perpendicular to the IUCD. The development of 3D scanning has greatly enhanced our ability to fully demonstrate IUCD position by displaying the coronal plane. This acquisition is highly recommended for all IUCD localization examinations.

The Copper 7, the Tatum T, and Progestasert are T-shaped, and the Lippes loop is serpentine. Occasionally, a thick midcycle endometrium obscures the bright IUCD echo when

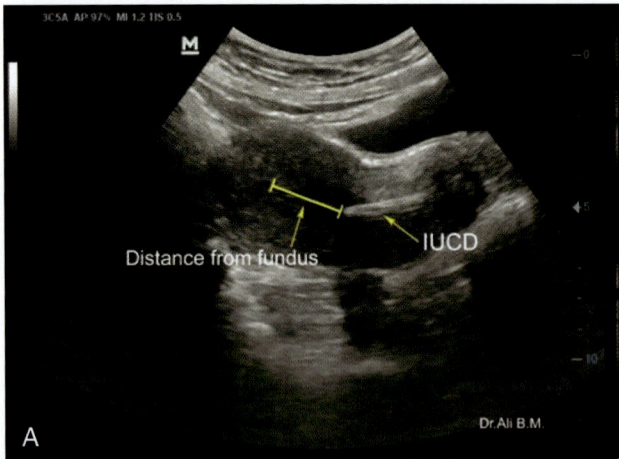
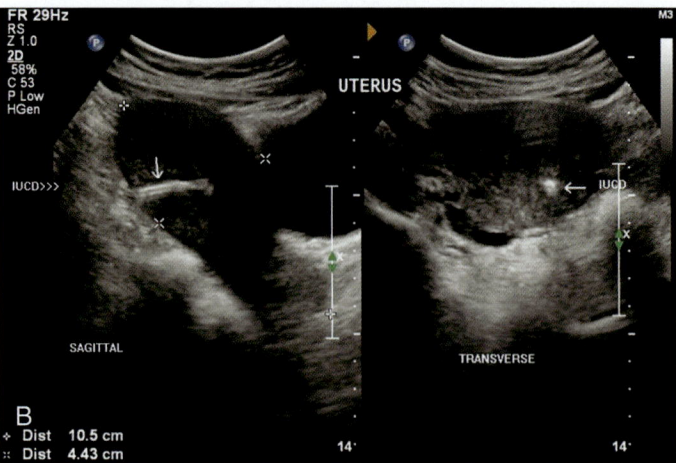
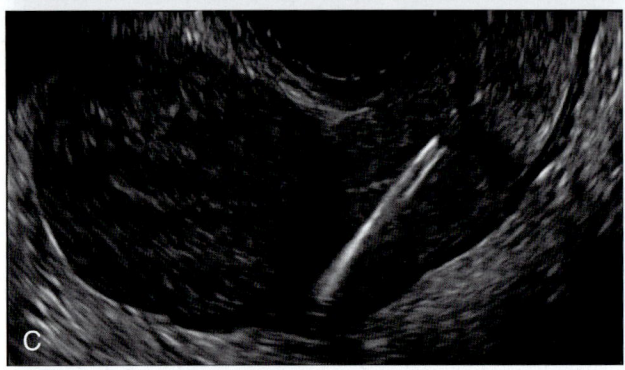

FIG. 43.35 Proper placement of the intrauterine contraceptive device (IUCD) should be within the endometrial cavity. (A) Device not inserted far enough into the cavity. (B) Perforation of the uterus by an intrauterine contraceptive device (IUCD) almost always occurs at the time of insertion. The displaced IUCD may not be suspected until an abscess or painful bowel involvement occurs. (C) An IUCD displaced caudally in the lower uterine segment, approaching the cervix, should be reported to the clinician.

transabdominal ultrasonography is used. If no intrauterine IUCD is identified on ultrasound examination and the pregnancy test is negative, a thin metal probe is inserted into the uterine cavity to mark it, and abdominal x-ray films are obtained to search for the IUCD in an extrauterine location. Perforation of the uterus by an IUCD almost always occurs at the time of insertion. The displaced IUCD may not be suspected until an abscess or painful bowel involvement occurs (Fig. 43.35). If the IUCD is displaced caudally in the lower uterine segment, approaching the cervix, this should be reported to the clinician. The IUCD may not be effective in this location and may be at risk for being expelled.

When a pregnancy is present, either transabdominal or transvaginal ultrasound examination demonstrates both gestational age and the location of the IUCD. Occasionally, a string is visible in the external os of a pregnant uterus. Approximately 50% of pregnancies abort on extraction of the IUCD. With transvaginal scanning, the location of the IUCD can be detected relative to the sac, and it may be possible to predict which pregnancy will be disrupted. IUCDs are always external to fetal membranes.

ACKNOWLEDGMENT

The author recognizes Candace Goldstein for her contribution to this chapter in the previous edition.

Key Pearls

- The Gartner duct cyst is the most common cystic lesion of the vagina and usually is found incidentally during sonographic examination.
- Obstruction of the uterus or the vagina may result in an accumulation of fluid (hydrometra), blood (hematometra), or pus (pyometra).
- The most common finding in the cervix is the presence of nabothian cysts.
- Cervical polyps may present clinically with irregular bleeding. This benign condition arises from the hyperplastic protrusion of the epithelium of the endocervix or ectocervix.
- A small percentage of leiomyomas (myoma tumors) occur in the cervix.
- Squamous cell carcinoma is the most common type of cervical cancer.
- Common variations of uterine morphology, the bicornuate—or "two-horned uterus"—and the didelphic uterus, may be seen with sonography imaging.
- Leiomyomas, commonly called myomas, are the most common gynecologic tumors in women over 30 years old.
- Myomas are the most common cause of uterine calcifications. A less common cause is arcuate artery calcification in the periphery of the uterus.

- Adenomyosis is a benign disease, commonly diffuse, with global infiltration of the endometrium, which sonographically presents as a bulky enlarged uterus without focal mass.
- Uterine arteriovenous malformations consist of a vascular plexus of arteries and veins without an intervening capillary network.
- Endometrial hyperplasia is the most common cause of abnormal uterine bleeding in both premenopausal and postmenopausal women.
- Patients with endometrial polyps can be asymptomatic, or they may present with uterine bleeding.
- Endometritis is an infection within the endometrium of the uterus. It occurs most often in association with pelvic inflammatory disease, in the postpartum state, or following instrumentation of the uterus.
- Intrauterine synechiae (endometrial adhesions, Asherman syndrome) are found in women with posttraumatic or postsurgical histories, including uterine curettage.
- Most endometrial malignancies are adenocarcinomas occurring in postmenopausal patients.
- Before menstruation, the accumulation of secretions is referred to as hydrometrocolpos. Following menstruation, hematometrocolpos results from the presence of retained menstrual blood.
- Intrauterine contraceptive devices are devices placed in the uterine cavity during menses for the purpose of birth control.

REFERENCES

1. Carlson Jr JA, et al. Clinical and pathologic correlation of endometrial cavity fluid detected by ultrasound in the postmenopausal patient. *Obstet Gynecol.* 1991;77:119.
2. Goldstein SR, et al. Endometrial assessment by vaginal ultrasonography before endometrial sampling in patients with postmenopausal bleeding. *Am J Obstet Gynecol.* 1990;163:119.
3. Karlsson B, Granberg S, Wikland M, et al. Endovaginal ultrasonography of the endometrium in women with postmenopausal bleeding: a Nordic multicenter study. *Am J Obstet Gynecol.* 1995;172:1488–1494.

BIBLIOGRAPHY

AIUM, ACR, ACOG, SPR, SRU. AIUM practice guideline for the performance of ultrasound examination of the female pelvis. *J Ultrasound Med.* 2014;33(6):1122–1130.

AIUM, ACOG, ACR. AIUM standard for the performance of saline infusion sonohysterography. *J Ultrasound Med.* 2003;22(1):121–126.

Andreotti RF. The sonographic diagnosis of adenomyosis. *Ultrasound Q.* 2005;213:167.

Arger PH. Endovaginal ultrasound in postmenopausal patients. *Radiol Clin North Am.* 1992;30:759.

Callen PW. *Ultrasonography in obstetrics and gynecology.* ed 6, Philadelphia: Elsevier; 2017.

Cohen HL, Tice HM, Mandel FS. Ovarian volumes measured by US: bigger than we think. *Radiology.* 1990;177:189.

Cullinan JA, Fleischer AC, Kepple DM, et al. Sonohysterography: a technique for endometrial evaluation. *Radiographics.* 1995;15:501–514.

Kliewer MA, Hertzberg BS, George Y, et al. Acoustic shadowing from uterine leiomyomas: sonographic-pathologic correlation. *Radiology.* 1995;196:99.

Lee EJ. Sonographic findings of uterine polypoid adenomyomas. *Ultrasound Q.* 2004;20:2.

Murase E, Siegelman ES, Outwater EK, et al. Uterine leiomyomas: histopathologic features, MR imaging findings, differential diagnosis, and treatment. *Radiographics.* 1999;19:1170.

Occhipinti K, Jutcher R, Rosenblatt R. Sonographic appearance and significance of arcuate artery calcification. *J Ultrasound Med.* 1991;10(2):97–100.

Polat P, Suma S, Kantarcy M, et al. Color Doppler US in the evaluation of uterine vascular abnormalities. *Radiographics.* 2002;22:47.

Rumack CM, Levine D. *Diagnostic Ultrasound,* vol 1, ed 5. St Louis: Elsevier; 2018.

Tamai K. MRI imaging findings of adenomyosis: correlation with histopathologic features and diagnostic pitfalls. *Radiographics.* 2005;25:21.

Valsky DV, Cohen SM, Hochner-Celnikier D, et al. The shadow of the intrauterine device. *J Ultrasound Med.* 2006;25:613.

Varner RE, et al. Endovaginal sonography of the endometrium in postmenopausal women. *Obstet Gynecol.* 1991;78:195.

CHAPTER 44

Pathology of the Ovaries

Sandra L. Hagen-Ansert

OBJECTIVES

On completion of this chapter, you should be able to:
- Describe the effects of hormones on the ovarian cycle
- State the characteristics of the simple ovarian cyst and a functional ovarian cyst
- Discuss the sonographic findings of the common cystic and complex ovarian masses, common solid ovarian masses, and ovarian neoplasms
- List the characteristics of the ovarian syndromes discussed in this chapter
- Discuss the benign pelvic masses found in neonates and adolescent girls
- Differentiate between mucinous and serous types of tumors
- Explain the Doppler parameters used in ovarian torsion

OUTLINE

Anatomy of the Ovaries 1231
  Normal Sonographic Appearance 1231
Sonographic Evaluation of the Ovaries 1234
  Simple Cystic Masses 1234
  Complex Masses 1234
  Solid Tumors 1235
  Doppler of the Ovary 1236
Benign Adnexal Cysts 1236
  Functional Ovarian Cysts 1236
  Ovarian Syndromes 1237
  Other Benign Ovarian Cysts 1239
Endometriosis 1242
Ovarian Torsion 1243

Sonographic Evaluation of Ovarian Neoplasms 1244
Ovarian Carcinoma 1244
  Doppler Findings in Ovarian Cancer 1245
Epithelial Tumors 1246
  Mucinous Cystadenoma 1247
  Mucinous Cystadenocarcinoma 1247
  Serous Cystadenoma 1247
  Serous Cystadenocarcinoma 1248
  Other Epithelial Tumors 1249
Germ Cell Tumors 1250
  Teratoma 1250

  Immature and Mature Teratomas 1251
  Dysgerminoma 1252
  Endodermal Sinus Tumor 1252
Stromal Tumors 1252
  Fibroma and Thecoma 1254
  Granulosa 1255
  Sertoli-Leydig Cell Tumor 1255
  Arrhenoblastoma 1256
  Metastatic Disease 1256
Carcinoma of the Fallopian Tube 1257
Other Pelvic Masses 1257

KEY TERMS

Androgen
Corpus luteum cyst
Cystadenocarcinoma
Cystadenoma
Dermoid tumor
Endometriosis
Estrogen
Follicular cyst

Functional cyst
Mucinous cystadenocarcinoma
Mucinous cystadenoma
Ovarian carcinoma
Ovarian torsion
Paraovarian cyst
Polycystic ovarian syndrome (PCOS)
Pulsatility index (PI)

Resistive index (RI)
Serous cystadenocarcinoma
Serous cystadenoma
Simple ovarian cyst
Surface epithelial-stromal tumors
Theca-lutein cysts

Sonography is clinically useful to characterize adnexal masses, evaluate abnormal bleeding, assess infertility, monitor follicular growth, perform transvaginal needle aspiration and biopsy, and screen for ovarian carcinoma. Both transabdominal and transvaginal sonography are important in these evaluations. Transabdominal imaging furnishes a global survey of anatomy, whereas transvaginal imaging provides better characterization of internal architecture of the ovary, vascular anatomy, and adnexal area. It is important to note that information from the clinical pelvic examination is required for optimal interpretation of the sonographic studies, thus necessitating good communication between the referring physician and the sonologist.

A woman will ovulate nearly 400 times in her reproductive life, and a quarter of a million follicles will be stimulated to varying degrees during this time. It is not surprising that an organ as dynamic as the ovary can form more than 100 different types of tumors, both benign and malignant. These masses are described on the sonographic examination as primarily cystic, complex, or predominantly solid. However, the final diagnosis is left to the pathologist on surgical excision. Precise diagnosis on the basis of sonography alone is highly predictive, although not conclusive until the surgery. The primary role of sonography is to indicate the need for surgical or medical intervention.

ANATOMY OF THE OVARIES

The ovaries are paired, almond-shaped structures situated one on each side of the uterus close to the lateral pelvic wall (Fig. 44.1). The ovaries can vary in position and are influenced by the uterine location and the ligament attachments. In the anteflexed midline uterus, the ovaries are usually identified laterally or posterolaterally. When the uterus lies to one side of the midline, the ipsilateral ovary often lies superior to the uterine fundus. In a retroverted uterus, the ovaries tend to be lateral and superior, near the uterine fundus. When the uterus is enlarged, the ovaries tend to be displaced more superiorly and laterally. Following hysterectomy, the ovaries tend to be located more medially and directly superior to the vaginal cuff. They can be located high in the pelvis or in the cul-de-sac. Superiorly or extremely laterally placed ovaries may not be visualized by the transvaginal approach because they are out of the field of view. Ovaries are ellipsoid in shape, with their craniocaudad axes paralleling the internal iliac vessels, which lie posterior and serve as a reference point.

Normal Sonographic Appearance

The normal ovary has a homogeneous echotexture, exhibiting a central, more echogenic medulla. Small anechoic or cystic follicles may be seen peripherally in the cortex (Fig. 44.2). The appearance of the ovary varies with age and the menstrual cycle (Fig. 44.3). During the reproductive years, three phases are recognized sonographically during each menstrual cycle. Many follicles develop during the early proliferative phase and increase in size until about day 8 or 9 of the menstrual cycle. This is due to stimulation by both follicle-stimulating hormone (FSH) and luteinizing hormone (LH). At that time,

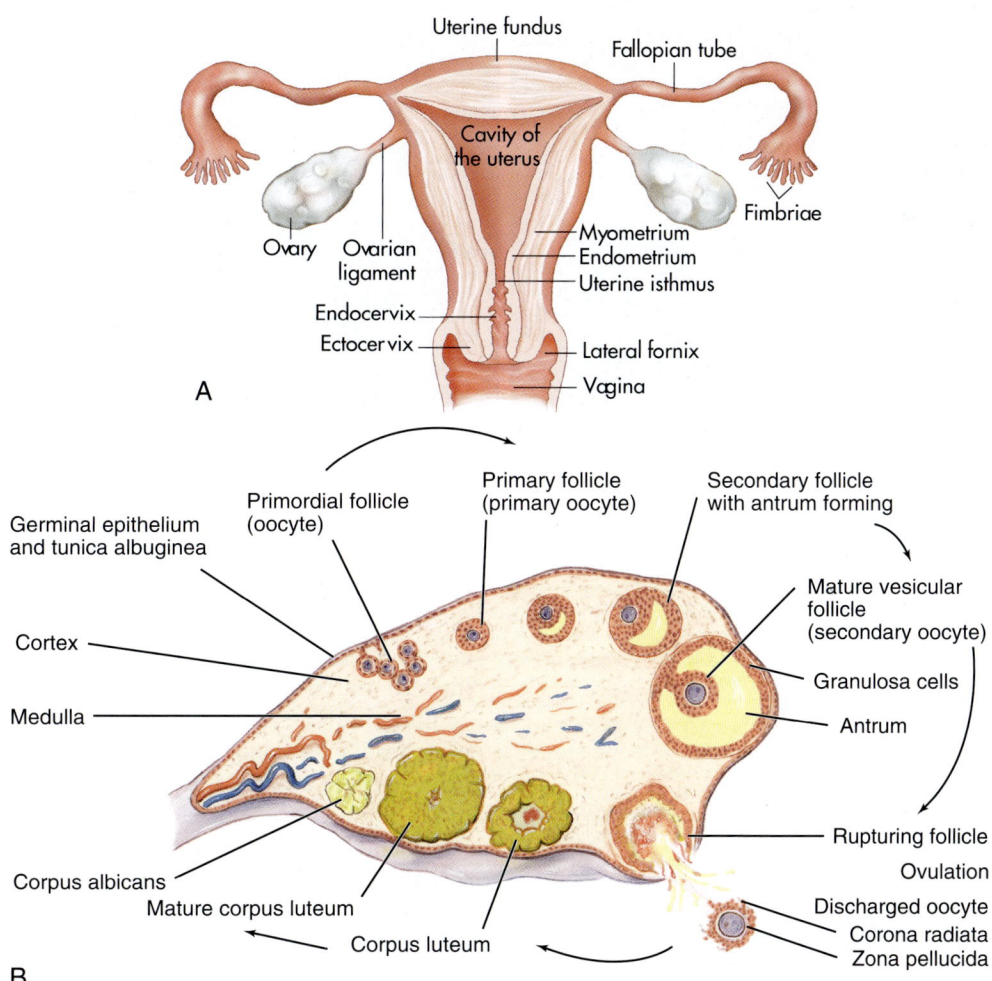

FIG. 44.1 (A) Normal anatomy of the female pelvis. Note the relationship of the ovaries to the lateral walls of the uterus and the position of the fallopian tubes to the ovaries. (B) Detailed anatomy of the ovary.

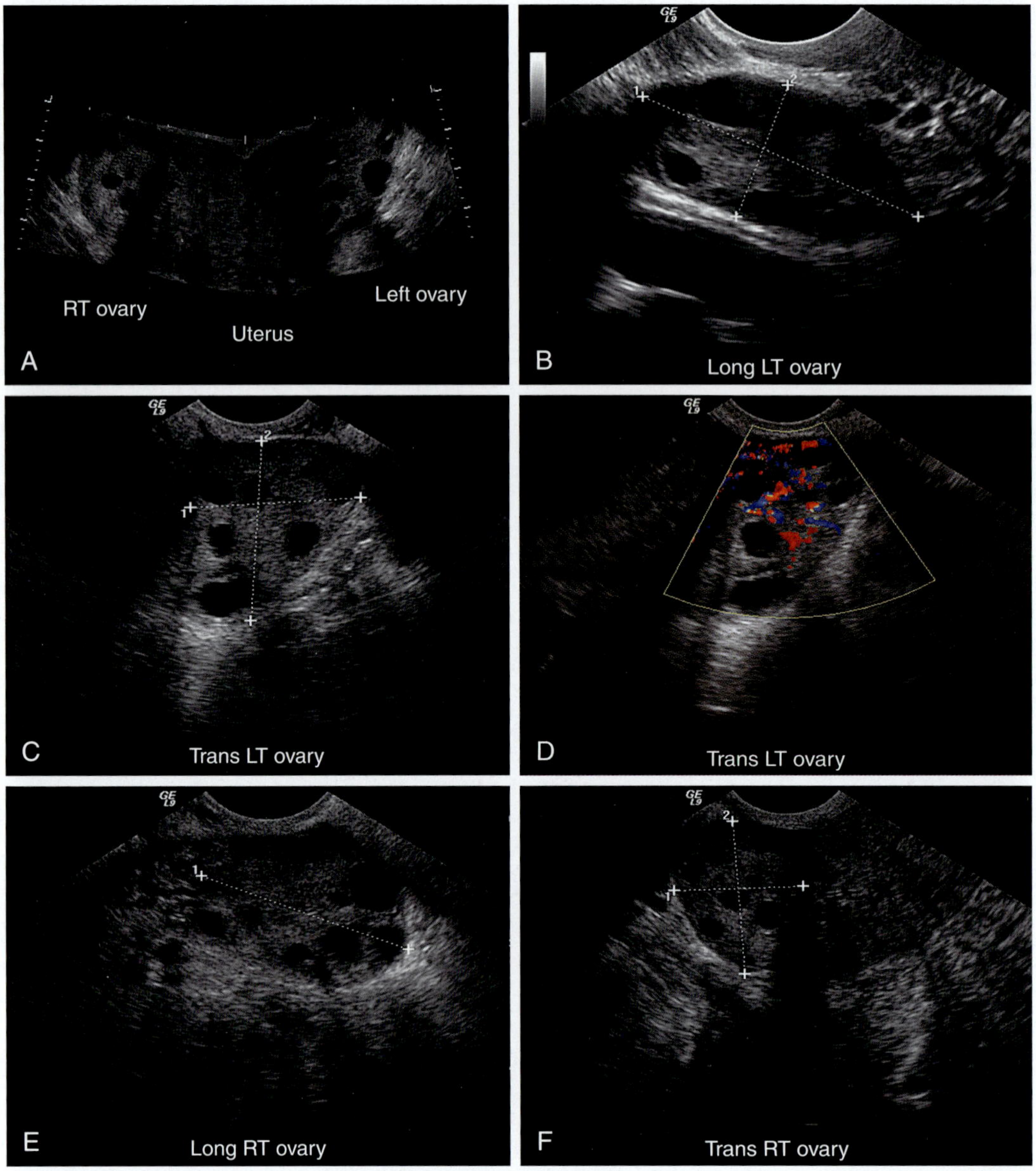

FIG. 44.2 **Normal transvaginal image of the ovaries with multiple follicles.** (A) Both ovaries are well seen with multiple follicles. (B) Long left ovary. (C) Transverse left ovary. (D) Normal color Doppler of the ovary. (E) Long right ovary. (F) Transverse right ovary.

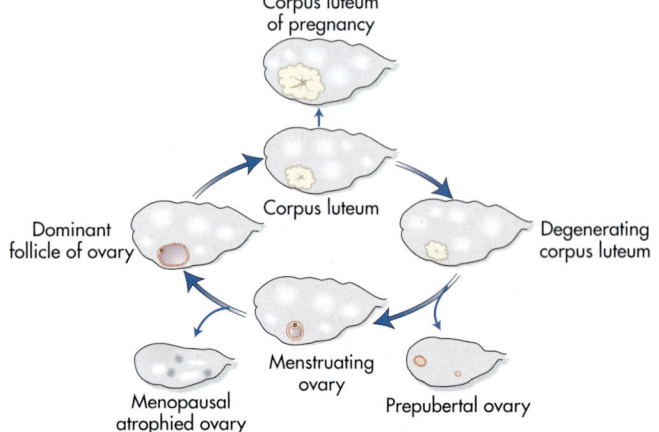

FIG. 44.3 Cyclic changes of the normal ovary.

one follicle becomes dominant, reaching up to 2 to 2.5 cm at the time of ovulation. The cumulus oophorus may occasionally be detected as an eccentrically located, cystlike, 1-mm internal mural protrusion. Although visualization of the cumulus indicates a mature follicle and imminent ovulation, no reproducible sonographic sign is reliable. The other follicles become atretic. A follicular cyst develops if the fluid in the nondominant follicles is not reabsorbed. Usually, the dominant follicle disappears immediately after rupture at ovulation (Fig. 44.4). Occasionally the follicle decreases in size and develops a wall that appears *crenulated* (scalloped). Fluid in the cul-de-sac commonly occurs after ovulation and peaks in the early luteal phase. Following ovulation in the luteal phase, a mature corpus luteum develops and may be identified sonographically as a small hypoechoic or isoechoic

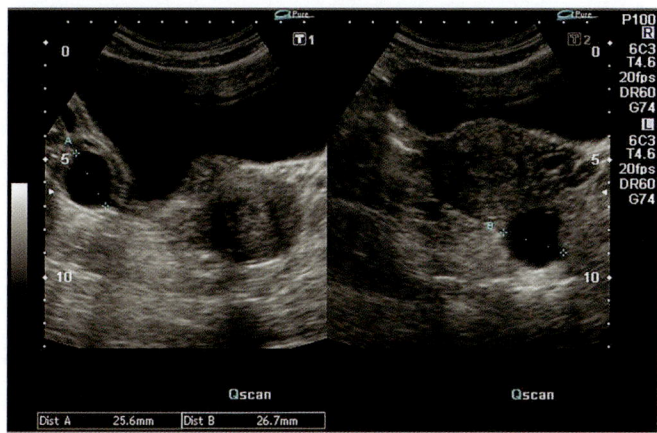

FIG. 44.4 A follicular cyst develops if the fluid in the nondominant follicles is not reabsorbed. Usually, the dominant follicle disappears immediately after rupture at ovulation.

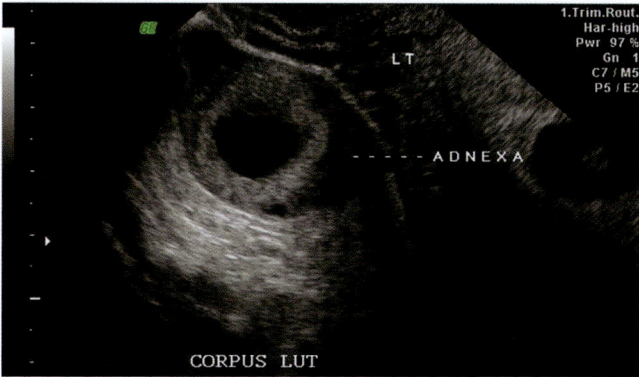

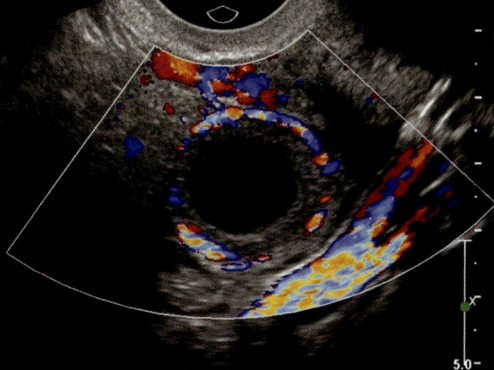

FIG. 44.5 Following ovulation in the luteal phase, a mature corpus luteum develops and may be identified sonographically as a small hypoechoic or isoechoic structure peripherally within the ovary. It may appear irregular with echogenic crenulated walls and contain low-level echoes. Less frequent appearances include a typical "ring" color Doppler pattern around the wall of an isoechoic corpus luteum. In the absence of fertilization, the corpus luteum begins to undergo involutional changes on postovulatory day 8 or 9 and disappears shortly before or with the onset of menstruation.

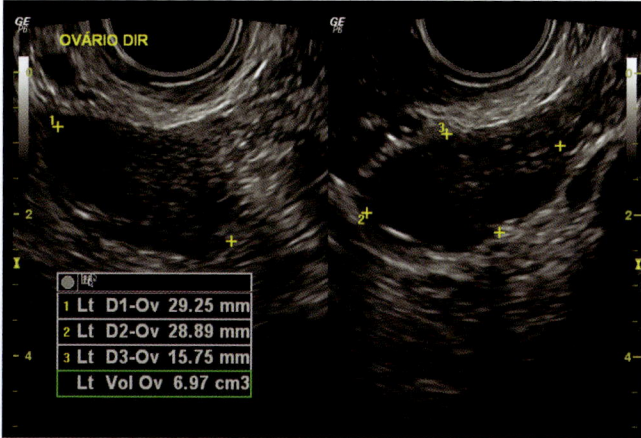

FIG. 44.6 Because of the variability in ovarian shape and size, the volume measurement is the best method for determining overall ovarian size. The volume measurement is based on the prolate ellipse formula (0.523 × length × width × height).

structure peripherally within the ovary. It may appear irregular with echogenic crenulated walls and contain low-level echoes (Fig. 44.5). Less frequent appearances include a typical ring color Doppler pattern around the wall of an isoechoic corpus luteum. In the absence of fertilization, the corpus luteum begins to undergo involutional changes on postovulatory day 8 or 9 and disappears shortly before or with the onset of menstruation.

Multiple small, punctate, echogenic foci are commonly seen in the normal ovary. These foci are reported to be a common finding with transvaginal examination. They are generally very small (1 to 2 mm) and located in the periphery. The foci are nonshadowing and can be multiple. A possible source of these foci of specular reflections is from the walls of tiny unresolved cysts below the spatial resolution of ultrasound. More central punctate echogenic foci represent stromal reaction to previous hemorrhage or infection. Because they do not indicate significant underlying disease, no follow-up is necessary.

Following menopause, the ovary atrophies and the follicles disappear with increasing age. For this reason, the postmenopausal ovary may be difficult to visualize sonographically because of the smaller size and lack of discrete follicles. A stationary loop of the bowel may mimic a small shrunken ovary, so scanning must be done slowly to look for peristalsis in the bowel. After a hysterectomy, the ovaries can be difficult to visualize with ultrasound. The use of both transabdominal and transvaginal approaches increases the chance of visualization.

Because of the variability in ovarian shape and size, the volume measurement is the best method for determining overall ovarian size (Fig. 44.6). The volume measurement is based on the prolate ellipse formula (0.523 × length × width × height). In the menstruating adult female, a normal ovary may have a volume as large as 22 mL,[3] with a mean ovarian volume of 9.8 ± 5.8 mL. An ovarian volume of more than 8 mL is definitely considered abnormal for the postmenopausal patient. An ovarian volume more than double that of the opposite side should also be considered abnormal, regardless of the actual size. Three-dimensional (3D) ultrasound may provide the most accurate method of ovarian volume measurement by allowing accurate determination of the ovarian long axis and objective calculation of stromal and cystic volume components. Further development in this technology will define future applications.

SONOGRAPHIC EVALUATION OF THE OVARIES

Simple Cystic Masses

An ovary's function is to mature oocytes until ovulation under the influence of LH and FSH hormone from the pituitary. At the same time, the ovary synthesizes **androgens** (male hormones) and converts them to **estrogens** (female hormones). Finally, it produces progesterone after ovulation to sustain early pregnancy until the placenta can do so at 10 to 12 weeks of gestation.

Usually, only one follicle enlarges from 3 mm to approximately 24 mm over about 10 days in the mid- and late-follicular phases of the cycle. This is followed by ovulation. The resulting corpus luteum or an abnormal unruptured follicle can persist as a simple or complex cystic structure from 1 to 10 cm in size. These so-called functional cysts may produce discomfort or delayed menses but can be observed to regress within 8 weeks with serial ultrasound studies. Surgical intervention may be considered if a cyst greater than 6 cm persists more than 8 weeks.

Ultrasound-guided needle aspiration has become another option for reducing recurrent **simple ovarian cysts** in carefully selected cases. Most ovarian masses are simple cysts, most of which are benign. Sonographic criteria for a simple cyst include a thin, smooth wall, anechoic contents, and acoustic enhancement (Fig. 44.7). In premenopausal women, these cysts usually are functional. The differential considerations of simple adnexal cysts include functional cyst, paraovarian cyst, cystadenoma, cystic teratoma, endometrioma, and rarely tubo-ovarian abscess (Box 44.1).

Small anechoic cysts may be seen in postmenopausal ovaries. They can disappear or change in size over time. Serial sonographic studies can monitor the size and document any changes. Surgery is generally recommended for postmenopausal cysts greater than 5 cm and for those containing internal septations or solid nodules (Fig. 44.8).

Complex Masses

Any simple cyst that hemorrhages as it involutes may appear as a complex mass (Box 44.2). In patients of reproductive age,

BOX 44.1	Common Cystic or Homogeneous Ovarian Masses

- Follicular cyst
- Corpus luteum cyst of pregnancy
- Cystic teratoma
- Paraovarian cyst
- Hydrosalpinx
- Endometrioma (low-level echoes)
- Hemorrhagic cyst

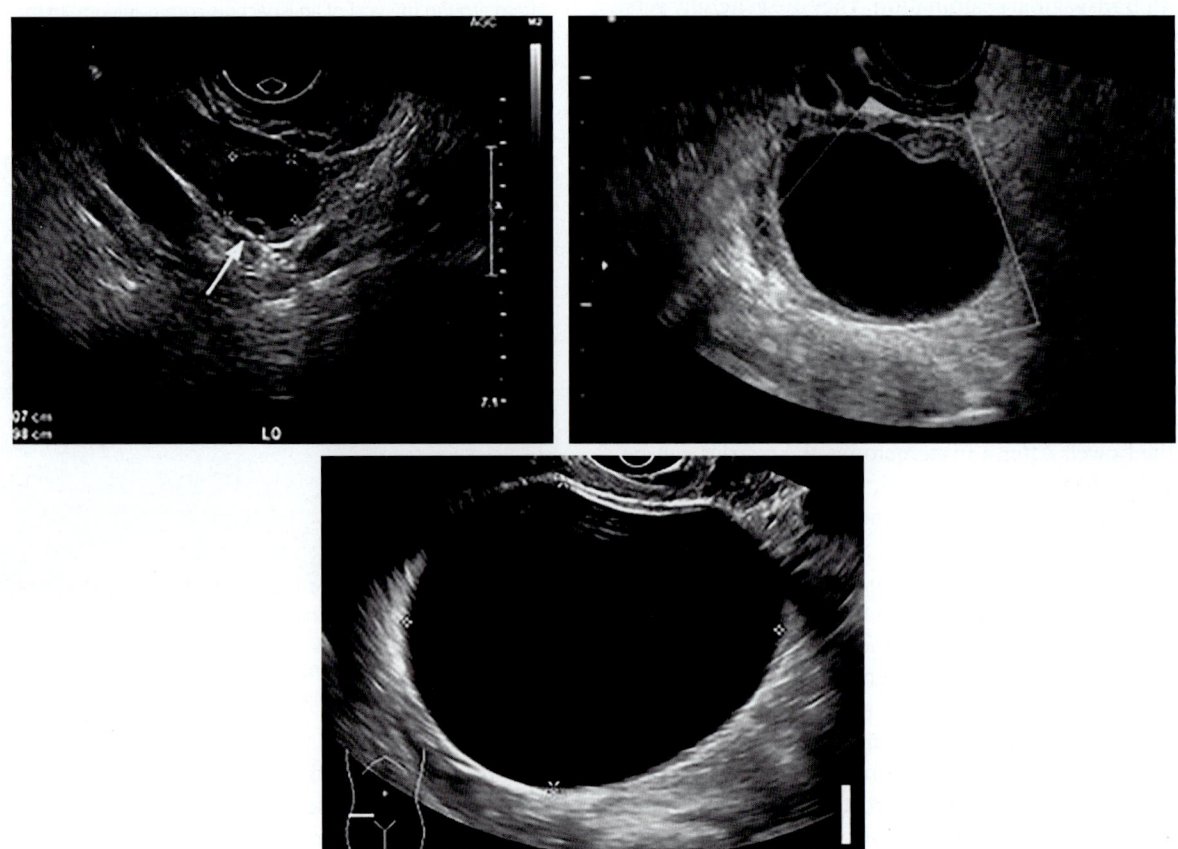

FIG. 44.7 The majority of ovarian masses are simple cysts, most of which are benign. Sonographic criteria for a simple cyst include a thin, smooth wall, anechoic contents, and acoustic enhancement.

CHAPTER 44 Pathology of the Ovaries

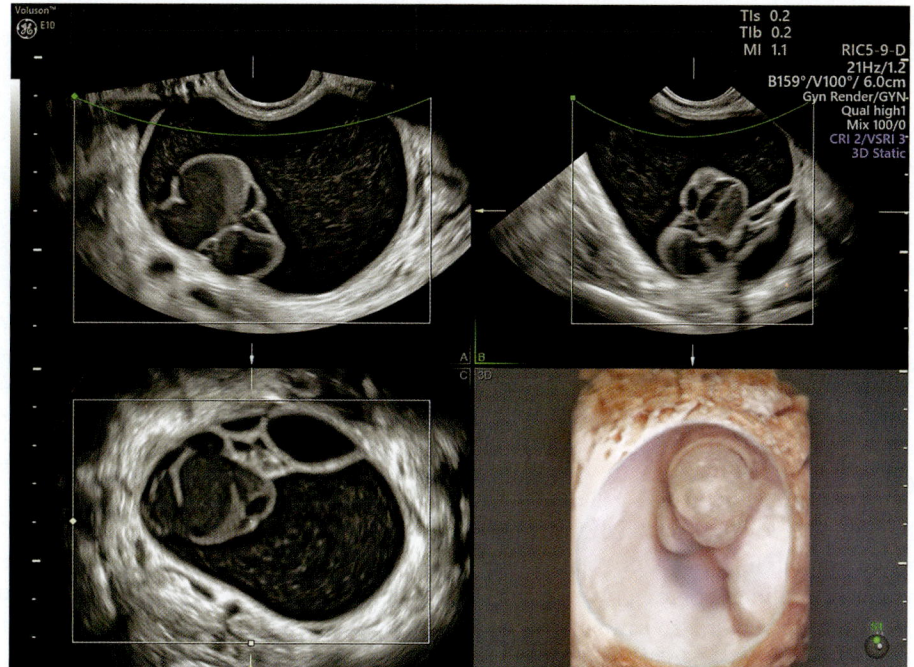

FIG. 44.8 Surgery is generally recommended for postmenopausal cysts greater than 5 cm and for those containing internal septations or solid nodules.

> **BOX 44.2   Common Complex Masses**
>
> - Cystadenoma
> - Dermoid cyst
> - Tubo-ovarian abscess
> - Ectopic pregnancy
> - Granulosa cell tumor

the classic differential considerations of a complex adnexal mass are ectopic pregnancy, endometriosis, and pelvic inflammatory disease (PID) (Fig. 44.9). Dermoids and other benign tumors can appear similarly.

Solid Tumors

Mixed solid to cystic ovarian masses are typical of all the epithelial ovarian tumors; the most common are the serous types: **cystadenoma** and **cystadenocarcinoma**. During the peak fertile years, only 1 in 15 is malignant; this ratio becomes 1 in 3 after age 40 years.

The more sonographically complex the tumor, the more likely it is to be malignant, especially if associated with ascites. The epithelium of serous tumors is tubal in type, and there may be one or multiple cysts. One-fourth of them are bilateral, and most occur in women over age 40. They are large and often fill the pelvic cavity.

The differential considerations of a solid-appearing adnexal mass include pedunculated fibroid, dermoid, fibroma, thecoma, granulosa cell tumor, Brenner tumor, and metastasis. Tubo-ovarian abscess, ovarian torsion, hemorrhagic cysts, and ectopic pregnancy also may appear solid. Solid adnexal masses are often difficult to diagnose because normal ovarian size varies widely. However, as previously noted, an ovary with a volume double that of the opposite side is generally considered abnormal. When a solid mass is found, care should be taken to identify a connection with the uterus to differentiate an ovarian lesion from a pedunculated fibroid

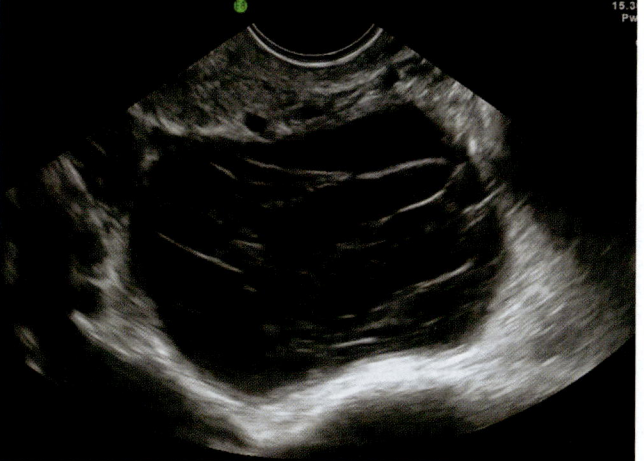

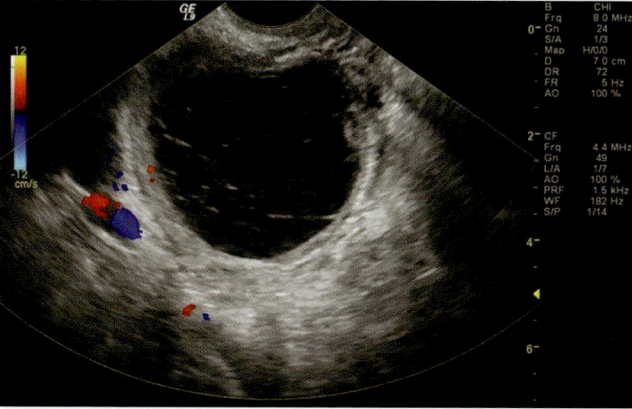

FIG. 44.9 Any simple cyst that hemorrhages as it involutes may appear as a complex mass. There may be various patterns of hemorrhage within the cyst as the blood clots and become more hyperechoic.

BOX 44.3	Common Solid Masses

- Solid teratoma
- Adenocarcinoma
- Arrhenoblastoma
- Fibroma
- Dysgerminoma
- Torsion

(Box 44.3). The use of color Doppler can be helpful, as color can be used to identify a vascular pedicle between the uterus and the mass, as can often be identified with pedunculation.

Doppler of the Ovary

When any abnormality of the ovary is detected, Doppler examination should be performed. In the case of a suspected cystic lesion, color Doppler helps differentiate a potential cyst from adjacent vascular structures. Color also can be used to localize flow to further determine flow velocity with pulsed Doppler, which can be obtained on all ovarian masses. Pulsed Doppler interrogation of the adnexal branch of the uterine artery, the ovarian artery, or intratumoral flow is performed to determine the resistive index (RI) or pulsatility index (Fig. 44.10). Patients with normal menstrual cycles are best scanned in the first 10 days of the cycle to avoid confusion with normal changes in intraovarian blood flow because high diastolic flow occurs in the luteal phase.

A debate in the literature exists regarding the value of an RI in distinguishing between benign and malignant adnexal masses. The largest study in the literature uses a cutoff of greater than 0.4 as a normal RI in a nonfunctioning ovary.[7] Other investigators employ a pulsatility index of greater than 1 as normal.[1,5] Intratumoral vessels, low-resistance flow, and absence of a normal diastolic notch in the Doppler waveform are signs that may be worrisome for malignancy. In addition, abnormal waveforms can be seen in inflammatory masses, metabolically active masses (including ectopic pregnancy), and corpus luteum cysts. The most significant problem in using an RI is that it is not a sensitive indicator of malignancy. One study found a low RI in only 25% of malignant lesions.[8]

The color Doppler central distribution of the small arteries within an ovarian mass may be important in malignancy. Two pulsed Doppler indices have been analyzed, comparing the relative amount of diastolic to systolic components of their arterial waveforms. The **pulsatility index (PI)** is calculated as peak systolic velocity minus end-diastolic velocity divided by the mean velocity. The **resistive index (RI)** is the peak systolic velocity minus the end-diastolic velocity divided by the peak systolic velocity. Although these indices have different cutoff values, increased diastolic flow suggests neovascularity and the likelihood of malignancy. The cutoff value for the PI is 1, and the value for the RI is 0.4, with malignancy considered more likely below and benign disease more likely above these values. Inflammatory masses, active endocrine tumors, and trophoblastic disease (ectopic pregnancies) may give low indices, thus mimicking cancer.

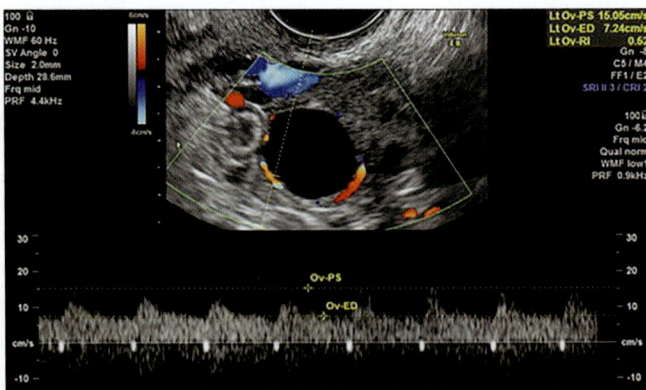

FIG. 44.10 Pulsed Doppler flow with normal low resistance is demonstrated in this simple ovarian cyst. Color also can be used to localize flow to further determine flow velocity with pulsed Doppler, which can be obtained on all ovarian masses.

A mass showing a complete absence or minimal diastolic flow (very elevated RI and PI values) is usually benign. A diastolic notch in early diastole may also signify benign disease. This finding is not often noted, and its absence has no diagnostic value.

The PI and RI values may vary considerably in the fertile patient during the menstrual cycle, complicating the pulsed Doppler analysis. In the first 7 days, the flow to the ovaries has the greatest resistance with the lowest diastolic flow, and the indices are at their highest. Later in each cycle, the diastolic flow increases, particularly to the dominant ovary, and may lower the indices sufficiently to falsely suggest a malignant process. A Doppler study can be performed at any time during the cycle. If the indices are in the benign range, they do not need to be repeated. However, if a suspicious mass is present and the indices suggest possible malignancy and are expected to affect management, a repeat study should be performed to confirm the abnormal indices in the first week of another cycle.

BENIGN ADNEXAL CYSTS

Functional Ovarian Cysts

Functional cysts result from the normal function of the ovary. They are the most common cause of ovarian enlargement in young women. Functional cysts include follicular, corpus luteum, hemorrhagic, and theca-lutein cysts. Hormonal therapy is sometimes administered to suppress a cyst. Most cysts measure less than 5 cm in diameter and regress during the subsequent menstrual cycle. A follow-up sonographic examination in 6 weeks usually documents change in size.

Follicular Cysts. A **follicular cyst** forms when a mature follicle fails to ovulate or involute post-ovulation (Box 44.4). These cysts are usually unilateral, asymptomatic, and less than 2 cm in size, but they can be as large as 20 cm in diameter. They regress spontaneously and are frequently detected incidentally on sonographic examinations.

Corpus Luteum Cysts. **Corpus luteum cysts** result from failure of resorption or excess bleeding into the corpus luteum. These cysts usually are less than 4 cm in diameter and are unilateral. They are prone to hemorrhage and rupture. The presenting feature is often pain. If the ovum is fertilized, the corpus luteum continues as the corpus luteal cyst of pregnancy during the first trimester of pregnancy, when maximum size is reached by 10 weeks, and resolution occurs by 12 to 16 weeks (Box 44.5).

Sonographic Findings. Because of the hemorrhagic nature of these cysts, they usually appear as complex masses with central blood clot and echogenic septations (Fig. 44.11). This appearance is difficult to distinguish from ectopic pregnancy and endometriosis. They may exhibit posterior acoustic enhancement, depending on the content.

Duplex Doppler reveals prominent diastolic flow in corpus luteum cysts. This low-velocity waveform is present throughout the luteal phase of the cycle. They may also have a peripheral rim of color around the wall of color Doppler, sometimes termed the "ring of fire."

Hemorrhagic Cysts. Internal hemorrhage may occur in follicular cysts or, more commonly, in corpus luteal cysts. The patient may present with an acute onset of pelvic pain.

Sonographic Findings. The sonographic picture is variable depending on the amount of hemorrhage, clot formation, and time passed since hemorrhage (Fig. 44.12). The internal characteristics are better visualized by transvaginal scanning, but transabdominal scanning should also be performed for a global view. An acute hemorrhagic cyst is usually hyperechoic and may mimic a solid mass. It usually has a smooth posterior wall and shows posterior acoustic enhancement indicating its cystic component. Diffuse low-level echoes may be seen but are more commonly seen in endometriomas. As time goes on, the internal pattern becomes more complex. The clotted blood becomes more echogenic and may show a fluid level. Echogenic free intraperitoneal fluid in the cul-de-sac can help confirm the diagnosis of a ruptured or leaking hemorrhagic cyst. This may mimic a ruptured ectopic pregnancy, so it is critical to know if the patient has a positive pregnancy test.

Theca-Lutein Cysts. **Theca-lutein cysts** are the largest of the functional cysts and appear as very large, bilateral, multiloculated cystic masses. They are associated with high levels of human chorionic gonadotropin. They are seen most frequently associated with gestational trophoblastic disease (30%). Similar cysts occur in normal pregnancies, especially multiple gestations, and in some patients being treated with infertility drugs, particularly Pergonal (Box 44.6). These cysts may undergo hemorrhage, rupture, and torsion (Fig. 44.13).

Ovarian Syndromes

Ovarian Hyperstimulation Syndrome. Ovarian hyperstimulation syndrome is a frequent iatrogenic complication of ovulation induction. This hyperstimulation can result in mild, moderate, and severe forms. In the mild form, the patient presents with pelvic discomfort but no significant weight gain. The ovaries are enlarged but measure less than 5 cm in diameter (Fig. 44.14). The patient has severe pelvic pain, abdominal distention, and notably enlarged ovaries with severe hyperstimulation, measuring greater than 10 cm in

---

BOX 44.4 Follicular Cysts

- Occur when a dominant follicle does not succeed in ovulating and remains active though immature
- Usually unilateral
- Thin-walled, translucent, watery fluid; may project above or within surface of the ovary
- May grow 1–8 cm
- Usually disappear spontaneously by resorption or rupture
- *Clinical findings:* asymptomatic to dull, adnexal pressure and pain, abnormal ovarian function, torsion of the ovary resulting in severe pain
- *Sonographic findings:* simple cyst

BOX 44.5 Corpus Luteum Cysts

- Result from hemorrhage within a persistently mature corpus luteum
- Filled with blood and cystic fluid
- May grow 1–10 cm in size
- May accompany intrauterine pregnancy
- *Clinical findings:* irregular menstrual cycle, pain, mimic ectopic pregnancy, rupture
- *Sonographic findings:* "cystic" type of lesion; may have internal echoes secondary to hemorrhage and increased color

---

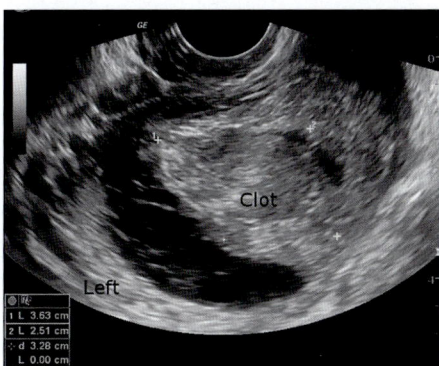 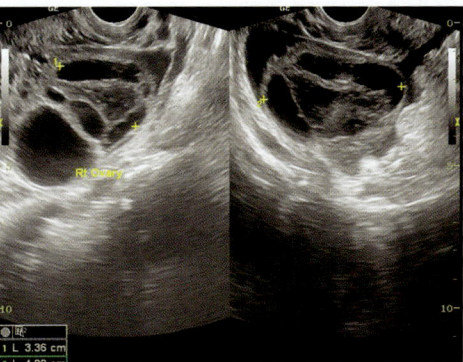 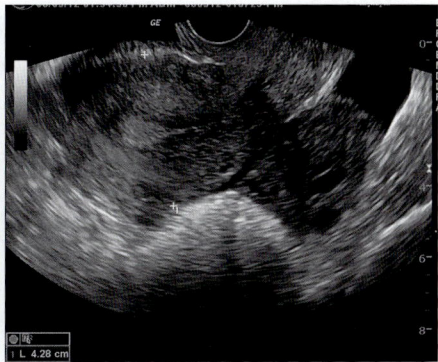

FIG. 44.11 **Corpus luteum cysts result from failure of resorption or from excess bleeding into the corpus luteum.** These cysts usually are <4 cm in diameter and unilateral. They are prone to hemorrhage, clot, and rupture.

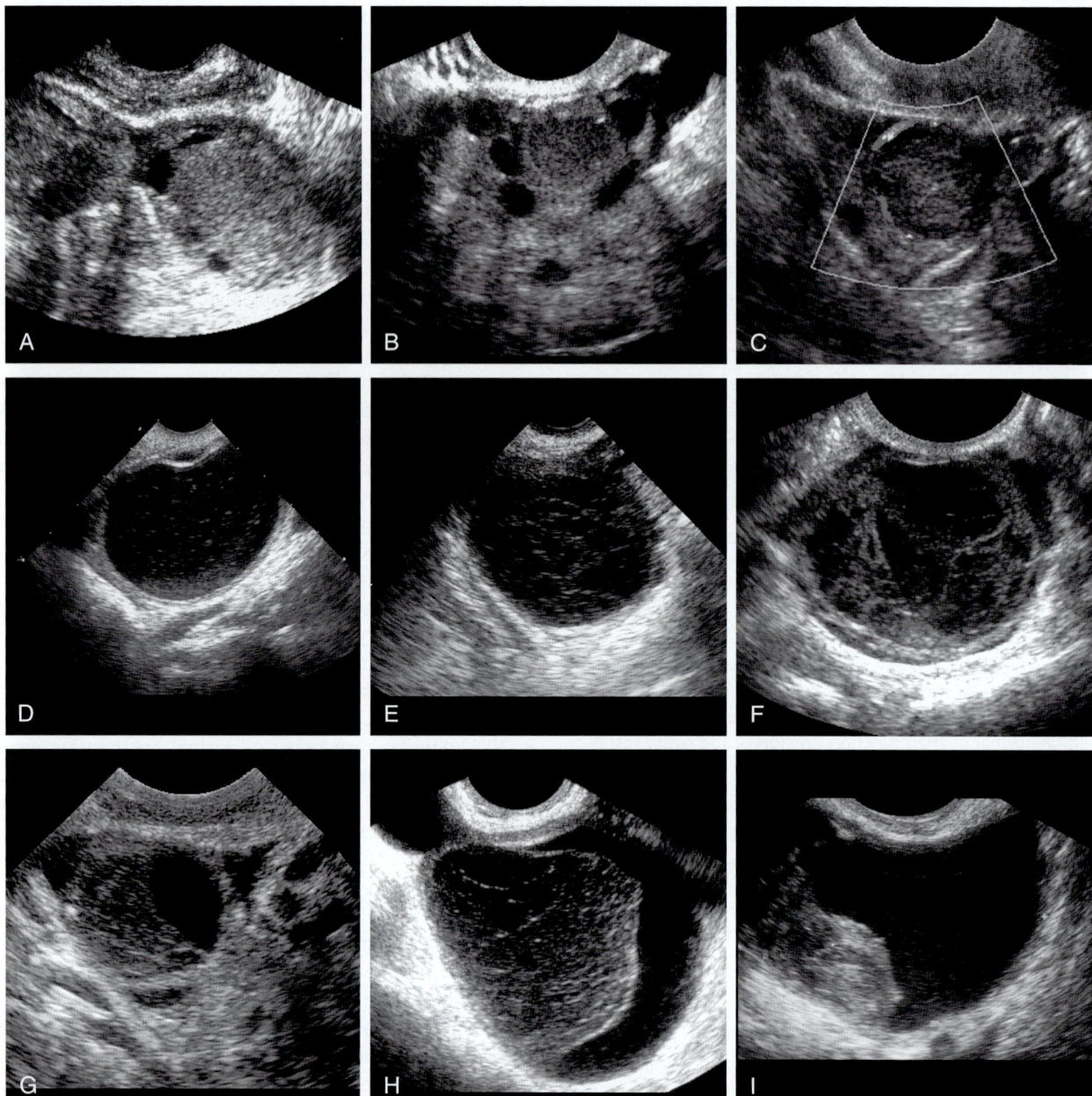

FIG. 44.12 Hemorrhagic cysts on transvaginal scans: spectrum of appearances. (A) Acute hyperechoic hemorrhagic cyst. (B) Acute hemorrhagic cyst mimicking a solid lesion. (C) Color Doppler shows peripheral ring of vascularity but no vascularity within the cyst. (D) Large cyst containing multiple internal low-level echoes. (E) Reticular pattern of internal echoes and septations within the cyst. (F) Reticular pattern. (G–I) Variations in clot retraction. The clot in part I suggests a solid mass; however, lack of color Doppler flow supports its benign nature.

BOX 44.6 Theca-Lutein Cysts

- Large, bilateral, multiloculated cysts
- Associated with high levels of human chorionic gonadotropin
- Seen in 30% of patients with trophoblastic disease
- *Clinical findings:* nausea and vomiting
- *Sonographic findings:* multilocular cysts in both ovaries

diameter. There can also be associated ascites, pleural effusions, and numerous large, thin-walled cysts throughout the periphery of the ovary. When treated, this condition usually resolves within 2 to 3 weeks.

Polycystic Ovarian Syndrome. Polycystic ovarian syndrome (PCOS), which includes Stein-Leventhal syndrome (infertility, oligomenorrhea, hirsutism, and obesity), is an endocrine disorder associated with chronic anovulation (Box 44.7). An imbalance of LH and FSH results in abnormal estrogen and androgen production. The serum LH level is high, and the FSH level is low. An elevated LH/FSH ratio is characteristic. Pathologically, the ovaries are rounded, usually two to five times normal size, with an increased number of follicles. Clinically, PCOS encompasses a spectrum of findings from hyperandrogenism in lean, normally menstruating women to obese women with severe hirsutism and oligomenorrhea or amenorrhea, as originally described by Stein and Leventhal.

| BOX 44.7 | Polycystic Ovarian Syndrome |

- Includes Stein-Leventhal syndrome
- Bilaterally enlarged polycystic ovaries
- Occurs in late teens through twenties
- May have endocrine imbalance
- Spectrum of ultrasound appearances
- *Clinical findings:* amenorrhea, obesity, infertility, hirsutism
- *Sonographic findings:* multiple tiny cysts around the periphery of the ovary; ovary may be normal size or enlarged

Manifestations of unopposed estrogenic hyperplasia and endometrial carcinoma occur in a significant proportion of patients, so long-term follow-up is recommended. PCOS is a common cause of infertility and a higher-than-usual rate of early pregnancy loss.

Sonographic Findings. On sonography, the ovaries appear normal or enlarged with echogenic stroma (Fig. 44.15). Multiple small follicles are seen, often bilaterally, in the size range of 5 to 8 mm. The reported number of immature follicles varies in the literature from 11 to less than 15. The ovaries have a more rounded shape, with the follicles usually located peripherally, commonly referred to as the "string of pearls." Small cysts of variable size can also occupy both the subcapsular and stromal parts of the ovary. The multitude of these small cysts contributes to the enlarged size of the ovary. Transvaginal sonography is more sensitive for detecting these small follicles than is transabdominal scanning. The diagnosis of PCOS is usually made biochemically, but sonography is useful. Serial studies show the follicles persist because ovulation does not occur.

Ovarian Remnant Syndrome. Infrequently, a cystic mass may be seen in a patient who has a history of bilateral oophorectomy. This usually results in a technically difficult surgery (because of adhesions), in which a small amount of residual ovarian tissue has been unintentionally left behind. The residual ovarian tissue can become functional and produce cysts with a thin rim of ovarian tissue in the wall.

Other Benign Ovarian Cysts

Peritoneal Inclusion Cysts. Peritoneal inclusion cysts are lined with mesothelial cells and are formed when adhesions trap peritoneal fluid around the ovaries, resulting in a large adnexal mass. Clinically, most patients have pelvic pain or a pelvic mass.

Sonographic Findings. Peritoneal inclusion cysts (benign cystic mesothelioma) are multiloculated cystic adnexal masses. The diagnosis must include the presence of an intact ovary either within or on the margin of the cyst. The fluid may contain echoes resulting from hemorrhage or

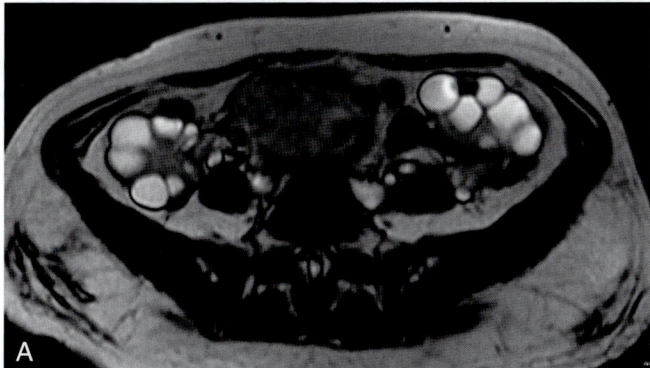
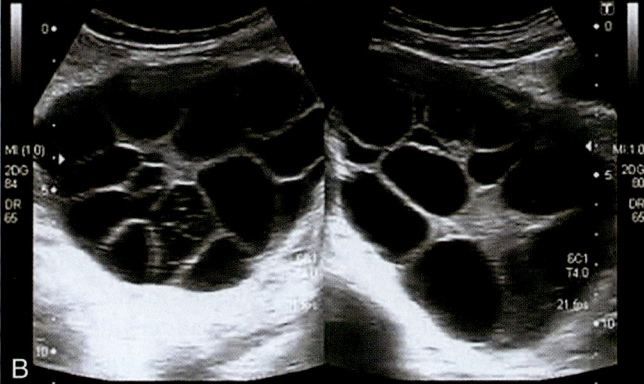

FIG. 44.13 Theca-lutein cysts are the largest of the functional cysts and appear as very large, bilateral, multiloculated cystic masses. They are associated with high levels of human chorionic gonadotropin. Magnetic resonance (A) and ultrasound (B) images of the multiloculated cysts.

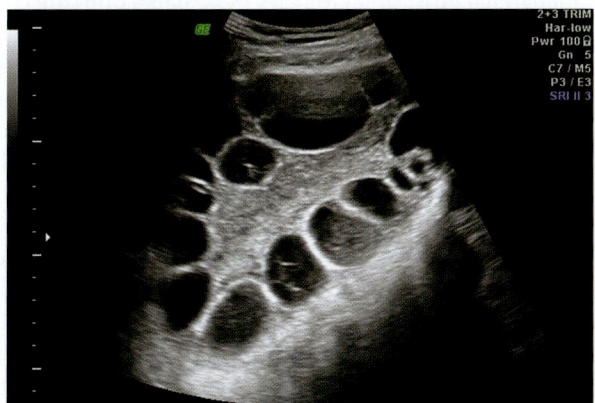
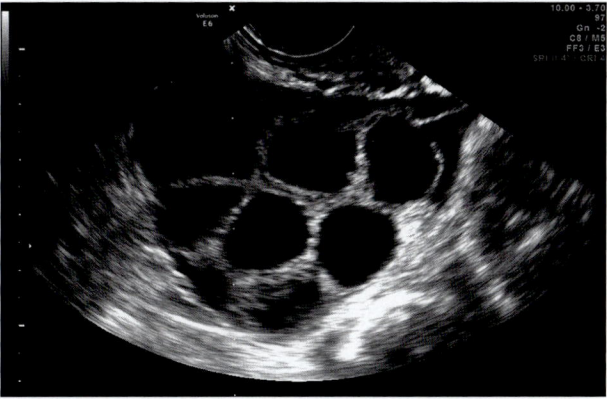

FIG. 44.14 Ovarian hyperstimulation syndrome is a frequent iatrogenic complication of ovulation induction. This hyperstimulation can result in mild, moderate, and severe forms. In the mild form, the ovaries are enlarged but measure <5 cm in diameter. With severe hyperstimulation, the patient has severe pelvic pain, abdominal distention, and notably enlarged ovaries, measuring >10 cm in diameter.

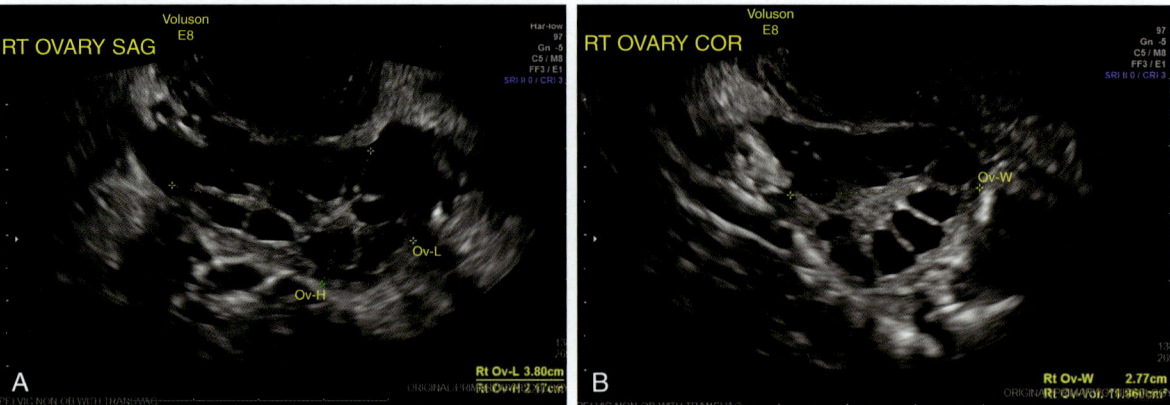

FIG. 44.15 Polycystic ovarian syndrome. (A) The right ovary is enlarged with prominent follicles around the periphery of the outer margin. (B) The left ovary is likewise enlarged with the "string of pearls" enlarged follicles.

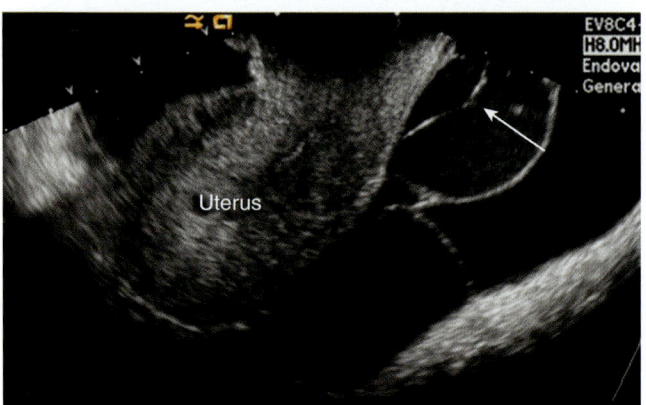

FIG. 44.16 Peritoneal inclusion cyst. Transabdominal scan shows multiple fluid-filled cystic areas with linear septations *(arrow)* representing adhesions attached to normal ovary.

BOX 44.8	Paraovarian Cysts

- Usually simple
- Can bleed or torse
- Wolffian duct remnants
- Ten percent of all adnexal masses
- Located in broad ligament
- *Clinical findings:* asymptomatic
- *Sonographic findings:* simple cyst adjacent to ovary

proteinaceous fluid (Fig. 44.16). Predominantly these occur in premenopausal women with a history of abdominal surgery. The cyst may also occur in patients with a history of trauma, PID, or endometriosis. The risk of recurrence after surgical resection is 30% to 50%. Do not confuse this condition with hydrosalpinx, which appears as a tubular or ovoid cystic structure with visible folds, where the ovary lies outside the cystic structure.

Paraovarian Cysts. **Paraovarian cysts** account for approximately 10% of adnexal masses (Box 44.8). They arise from the broad ligament and usually are of mesothelial or paramesonephric origin. They may occur at any age but are more common in the third and fourth decades of life. A specific diagnosis of a paraovarian cyst is possible only by demonstrating a normal ipsilateral ovary close to, but separate from, the cyst. The cyst may undergo hemorrhage, torsion, or rupture similar to other cystic masses.

Sonographic Findings. Paraovarian cysts have thin, deformable walls that are not surrounded by ovarian stroma. They are difficult to distinguish from ovarian cysts and may contain small nodular areas and occasionally have septations. Paraovarian cysts vary in size and can become large enough to extend into the upper abdomen. Paraovarian cysts can arise anywhere in the adnexal structures, and if they fill the pelvis, their point of origin may not be clear (Fig. 44.17). Their size does not change with the hormonal cycle.

Fluid Collections in Adhesions. Fluid collections in adhesions can create cystic structures of odd shapes throughout the abdomen. Omental cysts tend to be higher in the abdomen, and urachal cysts are midline in the anterior abdominal wall peritoneum above the bladder (Fig. 44.18). Any tumor may have cystic elements, and the sonographer should demonstrate if the tumor is a simple cyst or a complex mass.

Benign Cysts in Fetuses and Adolescents. Small simple cysts (1 to 7 mm) normally occur in fetuses and newborn girls because of stimulation by maternal hormones. In premenarchal girls, small follicles (less than 9 mm) are common. Larger cysts also are seen in otherwise healthy premenarchal girls. These may be followed closely if they are regressing, as long as the child's growth and development appear normal. Occasionally, ovarian cysts produce symptoms of precocious puberty in young girls. These may arise spontaneously or in association with other hormonal derangements.

Simple Cysts in Postmenopausal Women. Palpable ovaries in postmenopausal women are of concern. However, the cause of ovarian enlargement is often a simple adnexal cyst. In postmenopausal women, small (up to 3 cm) simple cysts of the ovaries are seen in approximately 15% of patients. These cysts commonly change in size and often disappear completely.

Most ovarian malignancies are epithelial in origin, and most are cystic. In the past, the occurrence of any ovarian cyst in a postmenopausal woman was considered abnormal and

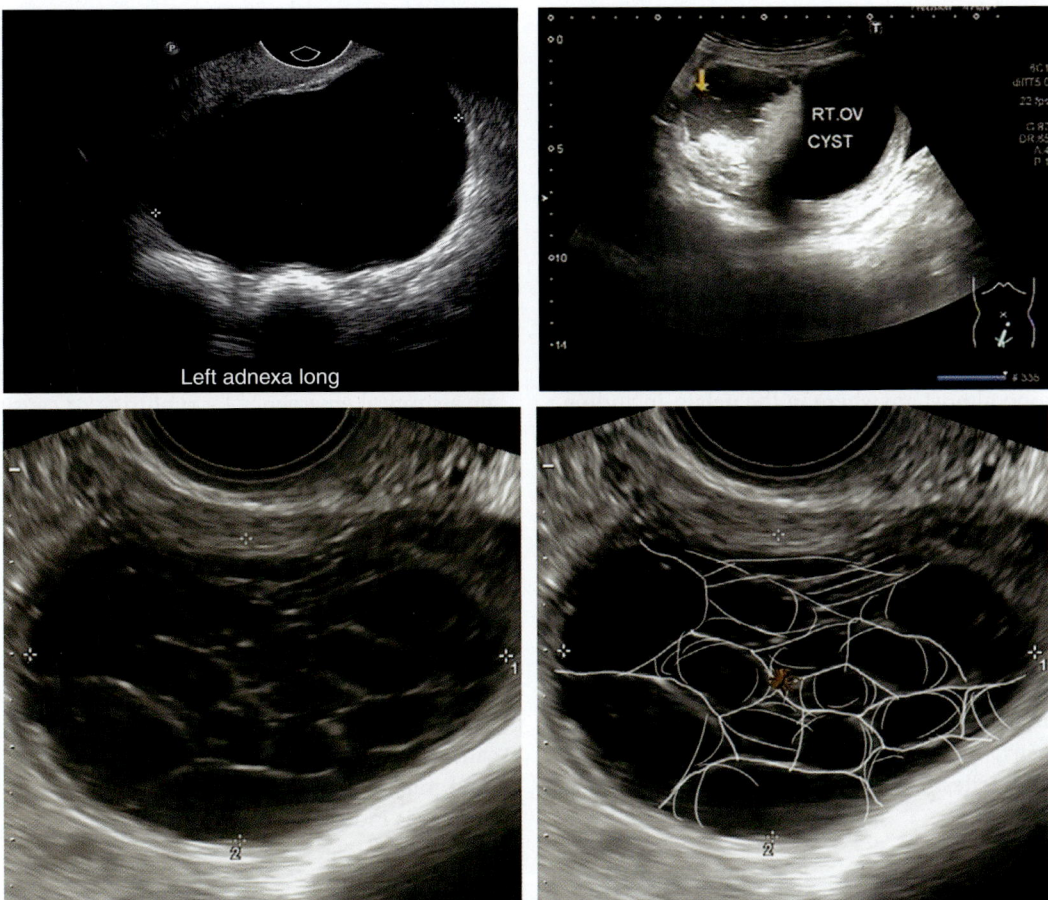

FIG. 44.17 Paraovarian cysts have thin, deformable walls that are not surrounded by ovarian stroma. They are difficult to distinguish from ovarian cysts and may contain small nodular areas and occasionally have septations. Paraovarian cysts vary in size and can become large enough to extend into the upper abdomen.

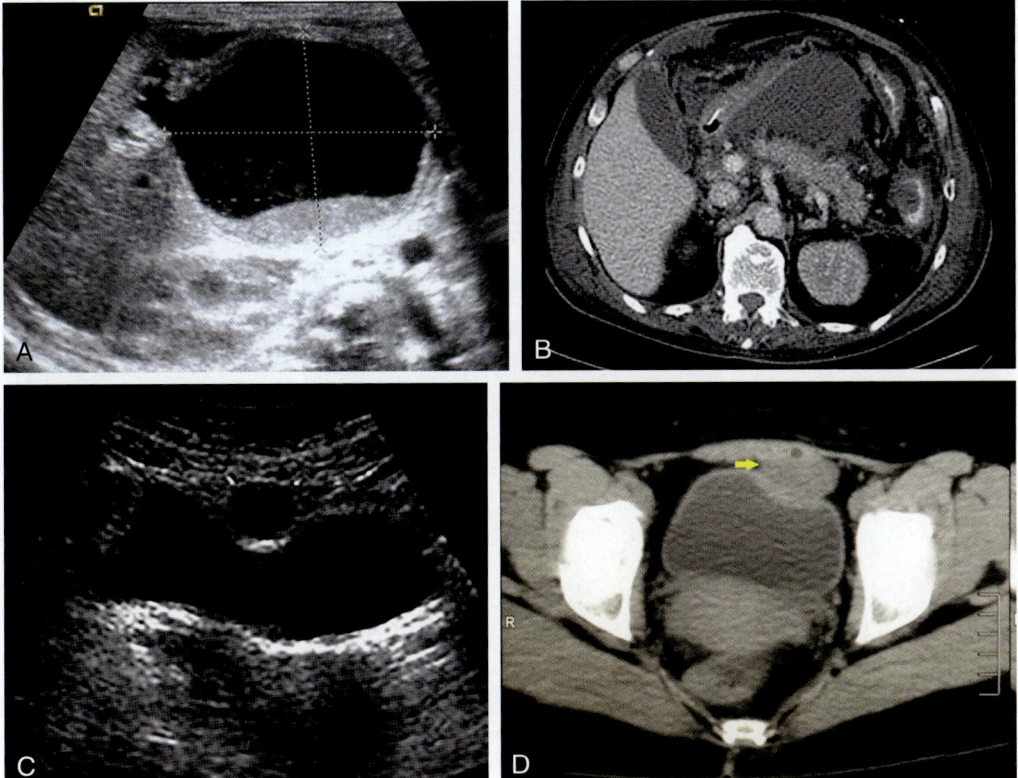

FIG. 44.18 Fluid collections in adhesions can create cystic structures of odd shapes throughout the abdomen. Omental cysts (A–B) tend to be higher in the abdomen, and urachal cysts (C–D) are midline in the anterior abdominal wall peritoneum above the bladder.

an indication for surgery. However, several retrospective studies have evaluated simple ovarian cysts and concluded that simple cystic lesions of the ovary, especially cysts less than 5 cm in diameter, are not likely to be malignant. It has therefore been recommended that if the RI is normal (greater than 0.4), these simple adnexal cysts should be followed sonographically rather than surgically removed.

ENDOMETRIOSIS

Endometriosis is a common condition in which functioning endometrial tissue is present outside the uterus. The ectopic tissue can be found almost anywhere in the pelvis, including the ovary, fallopian tube, broad ligament, the external surface of the uterus, and scattered over the peritoneum, cul-de-sac, and even the bladder. The endometrial tissue cyclically bleeds and proliferates. In the diffuse form, this leads to disorganization of the pelvic anatomy with an appearance similar to PID or chronic ectopic pregnancy. Two forms of endometriosis have been described: diffuse and localized (endometrioma). The diffuse form is more common, consists of endometrial plantings within the peritoneum, and is rarely diagnosed by sonography. The localized form consists of a discrete mass called an *endometrioma*, or *chocolate cyst*, and can frequently be found in multiple sites. The patient with an endometrioma is usually asymptomatic.

There are two possible explanations for endometriosis. The first is that the chronic reflux of menstrual fluid through the tubes and into the pelvis may, in some women, produce implantation and proliferation of endometrial cells with cyclic bleeding. The second theory involves the evolution of endometrial activity in susceptible cells that retain the embryonic capacity to differentiate in response to chronic irritation (e.g., by menstrual fluid) or hormonal stimulation. The resulting tissue bleeds and proliferates in response to cyclic hormones, producing pain, scarring, and distortion of adherent pelvic organs and endometrium-lined collections of blood known as endometriomas in the ovary. These may become moderately enlarged and create a surgical emergency by rupturing or causing the ovary to twist on the vessels that supply it (torsion). Further discussion of endometriosis may be found in Chapter 45.

Sonographic Findings. Endometriosis may appear as bilateral or unilateral ovarian cysts with patterns ranging from anechoic to solid, depending on the amount of blood and its organization (Fig. 44.19). The ovaries are typically adherent to the posterior surface of the uterus or stuck in the cul-de-sac and may be intimately associated with the rectosigmoid colon and difficult to define. Obscured organ borders and multiple irregular cystic masses also suggest either disseminating cancer or pelvic infection, and the clinical picture and serial sonographic studies determine when and if exploratory surgery is indicated.

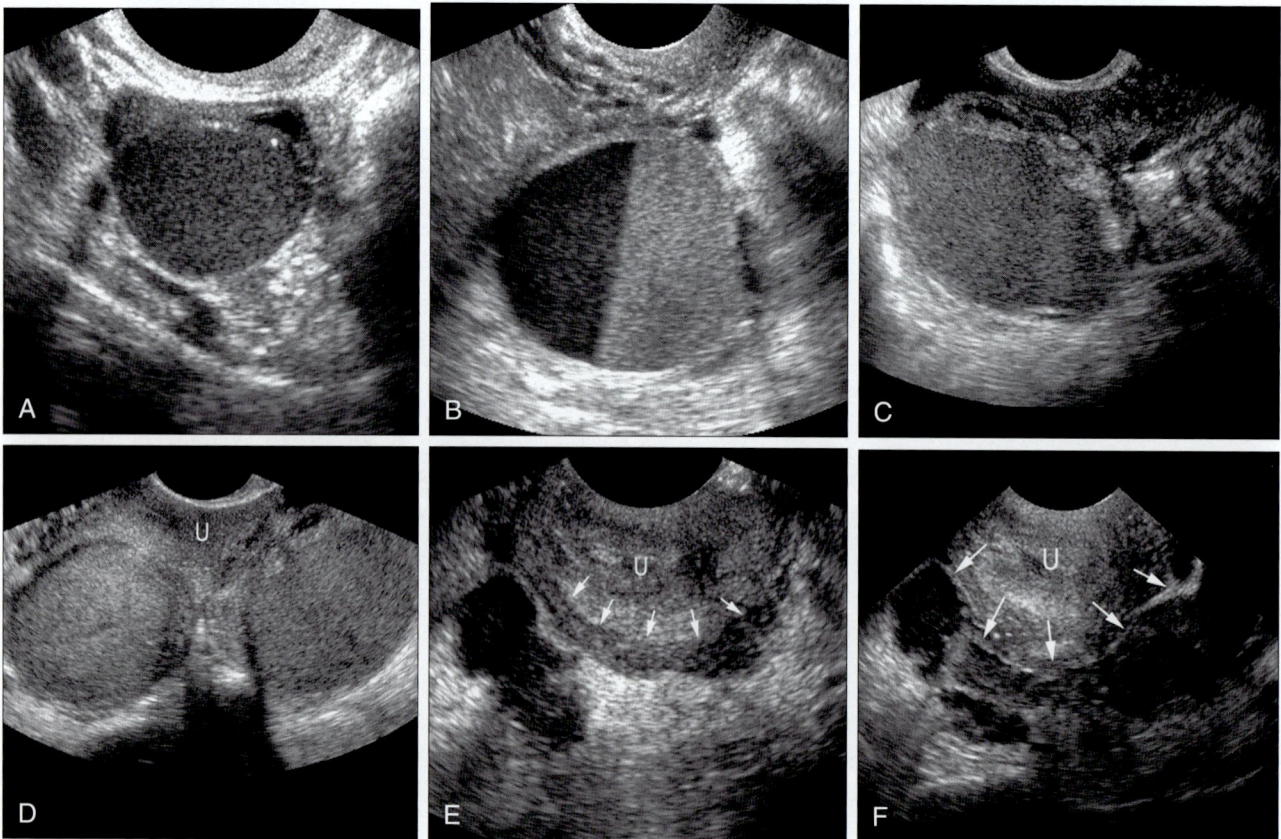

FIG. 44.19 Endometriosis: spectrum of appearances. Transvaginal scans. Images (A–D) show uniform low-level echoes within a cystic ovarian mass. (A) Typical peripheral echogenic foci. (B) A fluid-filled level. (C) Avascular marginal echogenic nodules. (D) Bilateral disease. (E) Endometriotic plaque on the posterior surface of the uterus *(arrows)* filling the pouch of Douglas (F; *arrows*). *U,* Uterus.

BOX 44.9 Ovarian Torsion

- Usually associated with a mass
- Hypoechoic, enlarged ovary, with or without peripheral follicles
- Absent blood flow on Doppler examination
- Free fluid in cul-de-sac
- Surgical emergency

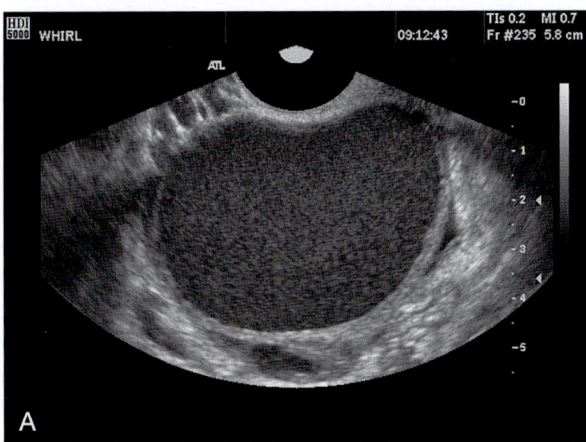
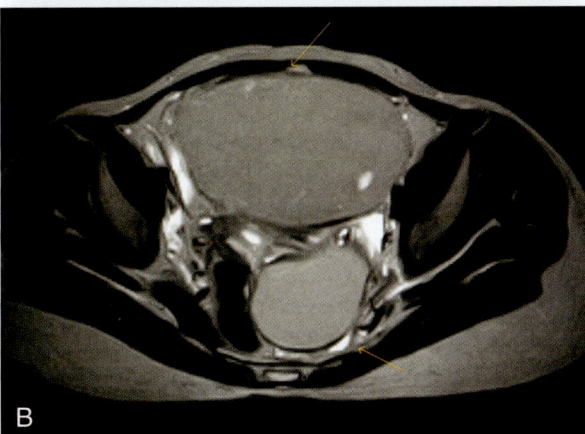

FIG. 44.20 The endometrioma is a well-defined unilocular or multilocular, predominantly cystic mass containing diffuse homogeneous, low-level internal echoes. (A) Ultrasound of the well-defined endometrioma "chocolate cyst." (B) Magnetic resonance image of a patient with bilateral endometrioma cysts.

The endometrioma is a well-defined unilocular or multilocular, predominantly cystic mass containing diffuse homogeneous, low-level internal echoes (Fig. 44.20). It is better characterized on transvaginal scanning. Occasionally a fluid-fluid level can be seen. Small linear hyperechoic foci may be present in the wall and are thought to be cholesterol deposits accumulating in the cyst wall. Clinical symptoms help to differentiate endometriosis from a hemorrhagic ovarian cyst, ovarian neoplasm, or tubo-ovarian abscess.

OVARIAN TORSION

Torsion of the ovary is caused by partial or complete rotation of the ovarian pedicle on its axis. Torsion usually occurs in childhood and adolescence and is common in association with adnexal masses. **Ovarian torsion** produces an enlarged edematous ovary, usually greater than 4 cm in diameter. The classically described appearance is of multiple tiny follicles around a hypoechoic mass, but the most common presentation is that of a completely solid adnexal mass. Free fluid often is present in the pelvis. Doppler examination usually reveals absent blood flow to the torsed ovary (Box 44.9). Occasionally, however, blood flow can be detected to torsed ovaries. This is thought to be the result of the ovary's dual blood supply or venous thrombosis, leading to symptoms before arterial thrombosis occurs.

Ovarian torsion is an unusual but serious problem because it accounts for 3% of gynecologic operative emergencies. Ovarian torsion is an acute abdominal condition requiring prompt diagnosis and surgical intervention. The ovarian pedicle partially or completely rotates on its axis, compromising the lymphatic and venous drainage. This causes edema and eventual loss of arterial perfusion with subsequent infarct. Torsion typically involves not only the ovary but also frequently the fallopian tube. It may also be seen in women during the fertile years and even occurs during pregnancy in 20% of the cases. Torsion may present at any time in female life, from childhood to the postmenopausal period. Occasionally the lead point is an ovarian mass. Once torsion has occurred, there is a 10% increased incidence of torsion occurring in the contralateral adnexa. Torsion of a normal ovary usually occurs in children and younger females with mobile adnexa, preexisting ovarian cyst or mass, or pregnancy.

Clinically, acute severe unilateral pain is typically the presenting symptom in patients with torsion. Intermittent pain may precede the acute pain by weeks. These symptoms can be mimicked by many other pelvic or lower abdominal processes, and therefore quite frequently, torsion is part of a differential diagnostic list. The patient may also have fever, nausea, and vomiting. More than 50% of patients feel a palpable mass. The right ovary is three times more likely to torse than the left.

Sonographic Findings. As a general rule, ovarian torsion is unlikely when the ovary is normal in size and texture with sonography. The torsed ovary is typically enlarged and heterogeneous in appearance, owing to edema, hemorrhage, or necrosis (Fig. 44.21). There is often a lead mass, but in some cases, this mass is not appreciated because it is mixed in with the necrosis and hemorrhage of the torsed mass. Torsed masses are often large (greater than 4 cm in diameter), vary in appearance from cystic to solid, and vary in echogenicity from relatively anechoic to markedly hyperechoic. A palpable mass may be present. Torsion occurs more frequently on the right side, and the pain may mimic acute appendicitis.

The differentiation of torsion from other adnexal masses is often impossible unless there is clinical suspicion. The sonographic picture varies, depending on the duration and degree of vascular compromise. The ovary is enlarged and may have multiple cortical follicles. Free fluid in the cul-de-sac is a common finding. Color and spectral Doppler may show

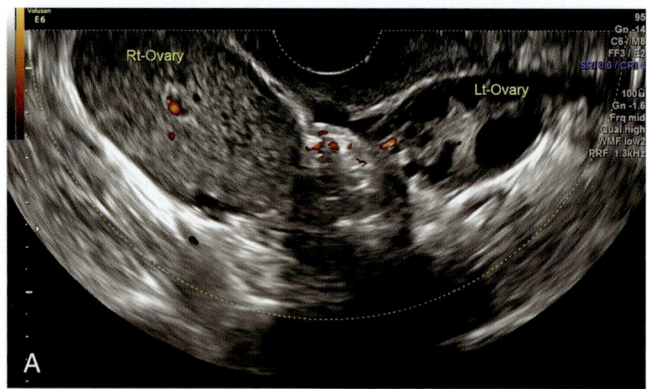

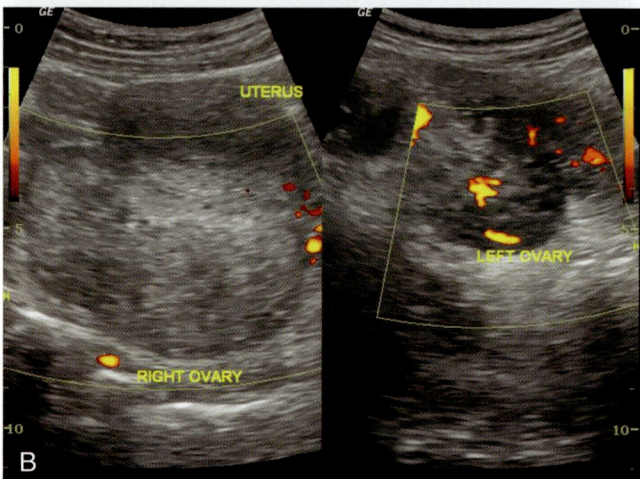

FIG. 44.21 The torsed ovary is typically enlarged and heterogeneous in appearance, owing to edema, hemorrhage, or necrosis. Torsed masses are often large (>4 cm in diameter), vary in appearance from cystic to solid, and vary in echogenicity from relatively anechoic to markedly hyperechoic. (A) Note the size discrepancy between the enlarged right ovary and the normal size left ovary. (B) There is decreased blood flow to the right ovary as compared to the left.

absent flow in the affected ovary. However, Doppler findings may vary on the degree and chronicity of the torsion and whether or not there is an associated adnexal mass. If torsion is intermittent, a "hyperemic" increased diastolic flow during the times when torsion is not present may be seen. This could be related to the dual ovarian arterial blood supply from the ovarian artery and ovarian branches of the uterine artery. Different appearances include target, ellipsoid, or tubular structures with internal heterogeneous echoes. Doppler may show the presence of circular, coiled twisted vessels, known as the *whirlpool sign*. The presence of arterial or venous flow or both does not exclude the diagnosis of torsion. Comparison with the appearance of morphology and flow patterns in the contralateral ovary helps in the evaluation.

SONOGRAPHIC EVALUATION OF OVARIAN NEOPLASMS

Sonographic screening finds adnexal cysts in 1% to 15% of postmenopausal women. Only 3% of ovarian cysts less than 5 cm are malignant. Therefore it is recommended that a cyst greater than 5 cm be surgically removed. In the postmenopausal woman, the ovaries are enlarged; if a mass is seen, it may be mixed texture to solid with papillae within. Well-defined anechoic lesions are more likely to be benign, whereas lesions with irregular walls, thick irregular septations, mural nodules, and solid echogenic elements favor malignancy. Doppler examination shows a low-resistive pattern. Extension beyond the ovary into the omentum or peritoneum and liver metastases should be evaluated. Malignant ascites may also be present. Unilocular or thinly septated cysts are more likely to be benign. Multilocular, thickly septated masses and masses with solid nodules are more likely to be malignant. In advanced stages, peritoneal carcinomatosis with malignant ascites and peritoneal implants can be seen.

Any change in ovarian echogenicity or volume of more than 20 mL should be considered suspicious. In postmenopausal women, the ovaries become atrophic and often do not have follicles. Thus the ovary can be difficult to identify. Only women receiving hormone replacement therapy continue to have normal-sized ovaries. Abnormal ovaries suggestive of malignancy are defined as enlarged echogenic ovaries (more than twice the size of normal ovaries or greater than 2 standard deviations above the norm [for the woman's age]).

Although ultrasound can identify masses and subtle changes in ovaries, it is not often able to distinguish benign from malignant. Doppler imaging has been studied to determine whether it can detect the neovascularity of malignant masses. Pulsed Doppler imaging is then performed to analyze the vascular component. The person who evaluates the soft tissue from the margins of the abnormal ovary or mass must take care so that the sample volume does not obtain flow patterns from adjacent normal structures.

OVARIAN CARCINOMA

Ovarian cancer is often detected by a combination of physical examination and laboratory and imaging findings. Every year **ovarian carcinoma** kills more women than cancer of the uterine cervix and body combined and is the fourth leading cause of cancer death. Ovarian carcinoma is the leading cause of death from gynecologic malignancy (25%) in the United States. Sixty percent of the ovarian malignancies occur in women between 40 and 60 years of age. New chemotherapeutic and surgical techniques have done little to decrease mortality rates, so continued efforts are being directed at developing methods of early diagnosis. The 5-year survival rate is 50% (stages I through IV). If the cancer is found early (stage I), the survival greatly improves to 93%; however, less than 20% of all ovarian cancer is found at this stage.

Ovarian malignancy is a "silent" cancer. Because of its relative absence of symptoms early in the disease, ovarian cancer commonly is not detected until advanced, either having spread beyond the capsule but still within the pelvis (stage II) or into the abdomen (stage III). At the time of initial detection, 50% of women present with stage III spread. The adnexal finding on physical examination is variable, ranging from almost "normal" to slightly enlarged firm irregular ovaries to pelvic masses. In advanced disease, ascites and omental masses may be palpated. The blood chemistry test CA 125 is helpful in some patients but has been disappointing as a screening test because of its inability to detect many cases of ovarian cancer. It has many false-positive and false-negative results, and elevated levels are found in only 50% of stage III ovarian cancer patients. If a baseline level is known, however, such as for patients who have undergone resection of primary ovarian cancer, then an elevated follow-up level has greater significance.

Clinical symptoms include vague abdominal pain, swelling, indigestion, frequent urination, constipation, and weight change (ascites). Ovarian cancer can present as either a complex, cystic, or solid mass, but it is more likely predominantly cystic; as many as 20% are bilateral. Differential diagnoses include endometriosis, hemorrhagic ovarian cyst, ovarian torsion, PID, and benign ovarian neoplasms (e.g., serous cystadenoma, mucinous cystadenoma, dermoid, fibroma, and thecoma). An exophytic fibroid or a non-gynecologic mass may also appear in the adnexa and resemble an ovarian neoplasm. The likelihood of malignancy is increased by the greater the amount of solid tissue in a complex ovarian mass and the presence of complex ascites.

The size of the ovarian mass, age of the patient, and ultrasound characteristics of the mass relate directly to its potential for being malignant. Masses less than 5 cm in their longest axis are much more likely to be benign, whereas masses larger than 10 cm are more likely to be malignant. Increasing patient age also correlates with an increased incidence of malignancy. The primary clinical problem with this disease is the asymptomatic and undetectable nature of the cancer in the earliest stages. Often the patient will seek medical attention after ascites has initiated abdominal distention.

The incidence of ovarian cancer is greatly increased in women who have had breast and colon cancer. This appears to be primarily related to genetic mutations in the BRCA1 and BRCA2 genes and less commonly in the MSH2 and MLH1 genes. The strongest risk factor is a family history of ovarian or breast cancer. Women with carcinoma of the breast have an increased risk of developing ovarian cancer, and women with ovarian cancer are three to four times more likely to develop breast cancer. Other risk factors include increasing age, nulliparity, infertility, uninterrupted ovulation, and late menopause. About 3% to 5% of women with a family history of ovarian cancer will have a hereditary ovarian cancer syndrome. The three main hereditary syndromes associated with ovarian cancer are the breast-ovarian, nonpolyposis colorectal, and site-specific ovarian cancer syndrome. They have an earlier age of onset than do other ovarian cancers.

Ovarian cancer arises primarily from epithelial tumors (60% to 70%), including serous cystadenocarcinoma (50%), endometrioid tumor similar to endometrial adenocarcinoma (15% to 30%), mucinous cystadenocarcinoma (15%), clear cell carcinoma (5%), Brenner tumor (2.5%), and undifferentiated tumor (less than 5%).[4] Germ cell tumors contribute 15% to 30% of the malignancies and are more common in girls and young women (age 4 to 27 years); they include mature teratoma, dysgerminoma, immature teratoma, transdermal sinus tumor, malignant mixed germ cell tumor, choriocarcinoma, and embryonal carcinoma. Metastases (5% to 10%) and stromal tumors (5%) are the remaining tumors that contribute to ovarian cancer.

On laparotomy, the cancer is classified into one of the following stages:

Stage I: Limited to ovary
  a. Limited to one ovary
  b. Limited to two ovaries
  c. Positive peritoneal lavage (ascites)
Stage II: Limited to pelvis
  a. Involvement of the uterus/fallopian tubes
  b. Extension to other pelvic tissues
  c. Positive peritoneal lavage (ascites)
Stage III: Limited to abdomen-intraabdominal extension outside pelvis/retroperitoneal nodes/extension to small bowel/omentum
Stage IV: Hematogenous disease (liver parenchyma)/spread beyond abdomen

Sonographic Findings. Sonographically, ovarian cancer usually presents with an adnexal mass (Figs. 44.22 and 44.23). Although sonography can detect morphologic characteristics of the tumor, it cannot (with the exception of dermoid cysts) histologically distinguish benign from malignant tumors. In general, well-defined, smooth-bordered anechoic lesions are more likely to be benign. Lesions with irregular walls, thick, irregular septations, mural nodules, and solid echogenic elements are frequently malignant. Mixed cystic and solid masses are the most frequent presentation of the common epithelial tumors of the ovary. Ascites, extension to adjacent organs, peritoneal implants, lymphadenopathy, and hepatic metastases support the diagnosis of malignant disease.

Doppler Findings in Ovarian Cancer

Abnormal tumor vascularity and abnormal RI or PI are also worrisome for malignancy. The results of the many studies using Doppler are quite variable. It is difficult to compare studies because of many factors, such as the lack of standardization of equipment, technical settings and techniques, and differences in various patient populations. Absence of flow within a lesion usually indicates a benign lesion. This is based on the premise that malignant masses will have high diastolic flow because of internal neovascularization, which can be seen on spectral Doppler waveforms. Malignant tumor growth is dependent on angiogenesis with the development of abnormal tumor vessels. This leads to decreased vascular resistance and higher diastolic flow velocity.

Contrast imaging in ultrasound will enable us to image the anatomic area better and give the physician more confidence in determining whether an examination is abnormal or normal. It might allow us to distinguish between benign and malignant lesions. Vascular contrast agents consist of surfactant-coated or encapsulated gas microbubbles less than 10 μm in diameter. These agents are injected into the bloodstream

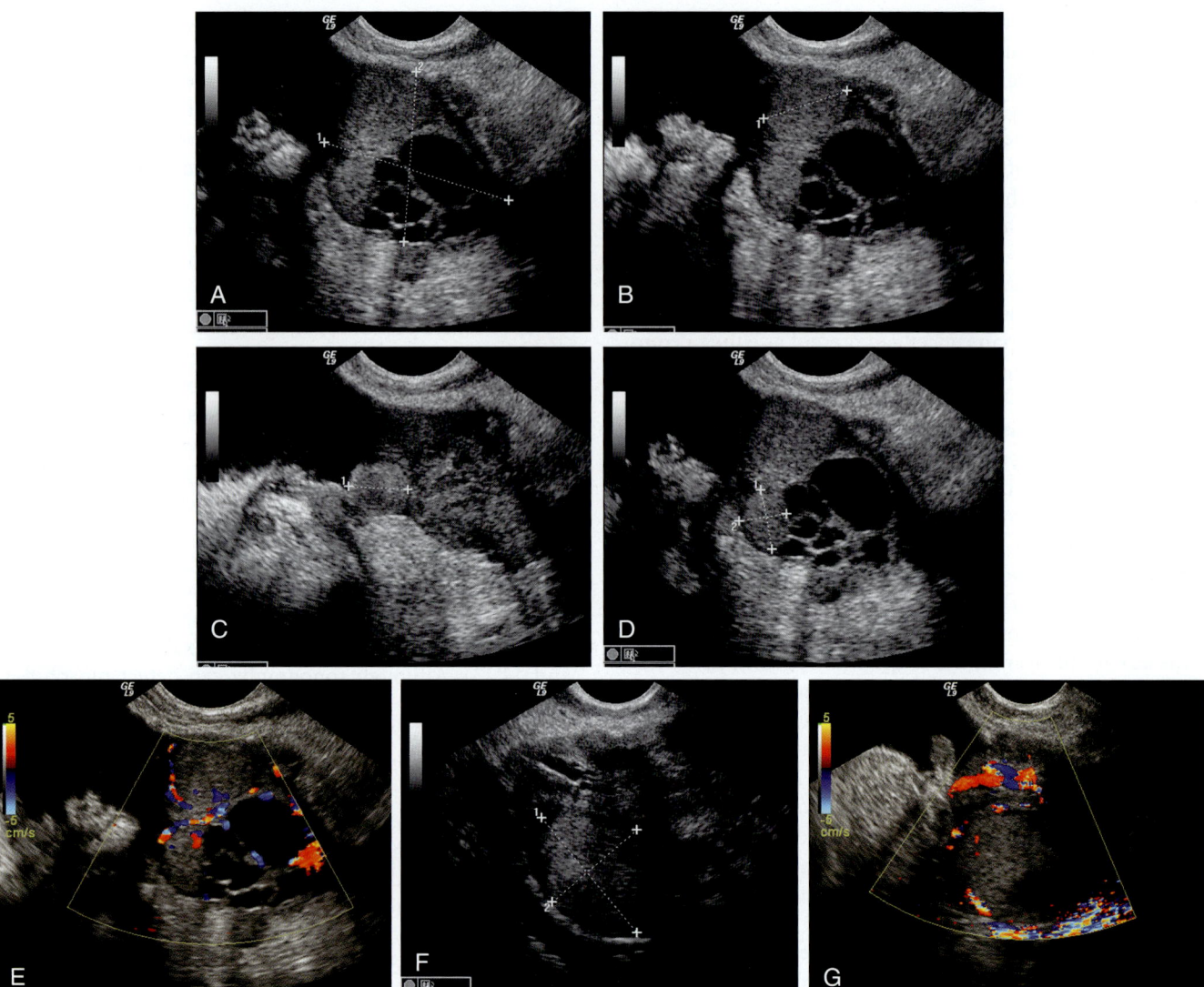

FIG. 44.22 Ovarian carcinoma with bilateral metastases. (A) Transverse left adnexa shows large complex mass. (B) Transverse left adnexa. (C) Transverse left adnexa shows nodule superior to uterine fundus. (D) Transverse left adnexa shows uterus, mass, ovaries, and vascular structures. (E) Color Doppler of increased vascular flow. (F) Right transverse of large mass. (G) Increased vascularity demonstrated with color Doppler.

via a peripheral vein and then circulate through the body. The vascular contrast agent Echovist, used to diagnose ovarian malignancies, shows increased brightness of power Doppler signal and the amount of recognizable vascular areas after contrast administration. The contrast agent enhancement was significantly higher in malignant than benign adnexal masses. There was also an increase in the number of recognizable vessels after contrast agent administration. Contrast agent uptake times were significantly shorter in malignant than benign tumors. For differentiation of benign from malignant tumors, the kinetic properties of the contrast agent, such as uptake and washout times, have significant potential in diagnosis.

EPITHELIAL TUMORS

Gynecologic tumors that arise from the surface epithelium and cover the ovary and the underlying stroma are termed **surface epithelial-stromal tumors**. This group accounts for 65% to 75% of all ovarian neoplasms and 80% to 90% of all ovarian malignancies. The two most common types are serous and mucinous tumors. Serous tumors are the most common and constitute 30% of all ovarian neoplasms. Mucinous tumors account for 20% to 25% of ovarian neoplasms. The benign or low-malignancy potential form is termed *adenoma*, and the malignant form is termed *adenocarcinoma*. The prefix *cyst* is added if the lesion is cystic, and *fibroma* is added if the tumor is more than 50% fibrous. Mucinous tumors are less frequently bilateral than are the serous type.

Metastatic spread is primarily intraperitoneal, although direct extension to surrounding structures and lymphatics is not uncommon. Hematogenous spread usually occurs late in the course of the disease.

Sonographic Findings. Serous and mucinous tumors vary greatly in size but can be very large. They often fill the

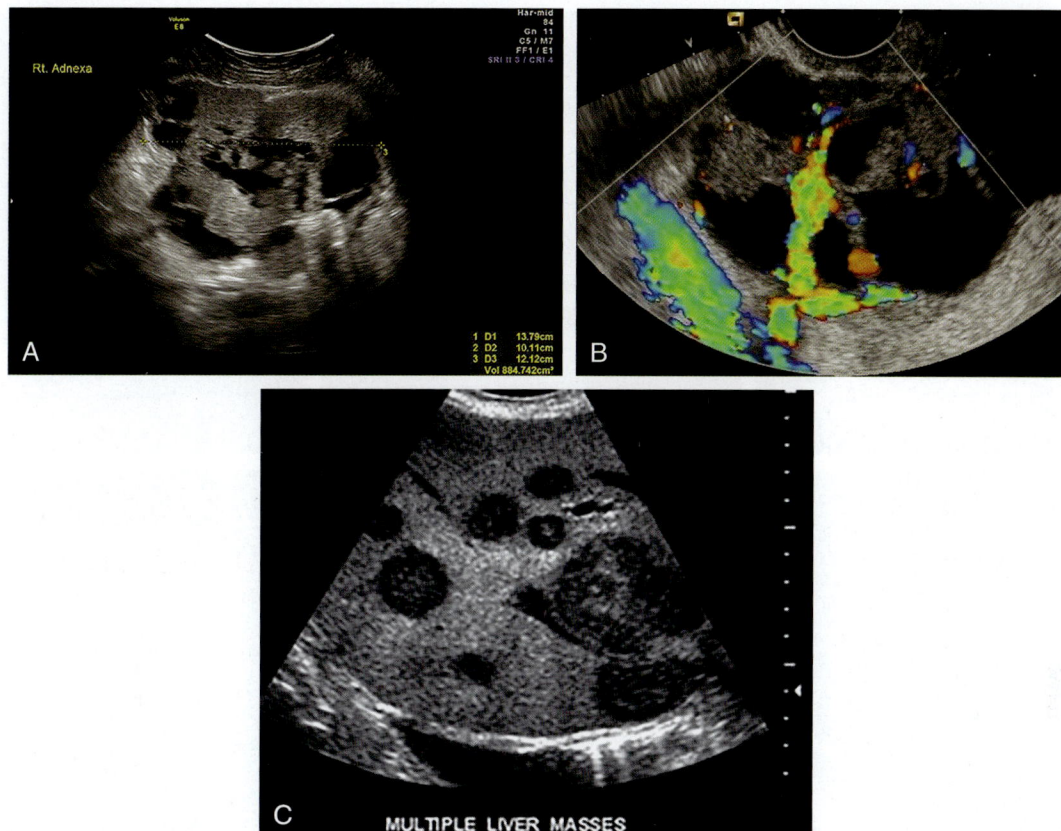

FIG. 44.23 **Sonographically, ovarian cancer usually presents with an adnexal mass.** Lesions with irregular walls, thick, irregular septations, mural nodules, and solid echogenic elements are frequently malignant. (A) Mixed cystic and solid masses are the most frequent presentation of the common epithelial tumors of the ovary. (B) Increased color flow is present. (C) Ascites, extension to adjacent organs, peritoneal implants, lymphadenopathy, and hepatic metastases support the diagnosis of malignant disease.

pelvis and extend into the abdomen. Serous tumors are generally smaller than mucinous tumors (Fig. 44.24).

Mucinous Cystadenoma

Mucinous cystadenoma is a type of epithelial tumor that is lined by the mucinous elements of the endocervix and bowel. It constitutes 20% to 25% of all benign ovarian neoplasms. When benign, it is a mucinous cystadenoma; when malignant, it is a cystadenocarcinoma. This type of tumor is usually found in girls and women between 13 and 45 years of age. A reported 80% to 85% of mucinous tumors are benign. These tumors can be large, measuring 15 to 30 cm in diameter, and weigh more than 100 pounds. They can fill the entire pelvis and abdomen. The tumor is usually benign and unilateral (5% bilateral) (Box 44.10).

Sonographic Findings. In 75% of patients with mucinous tumors, ultrasound examination shows simple or septate thin-walled multilocular cysts (Fig. 44.25). They often contain internal echoes with compartments differing in echogenicity caused by the mucoid material in the dependent portions.

Mucinous Cystadenocarcinoma

Mucinous cystadenocarcinoma most frequently occurs in women 40 to 70 years old and accounts for 5% to 10% of all primary malignant ovarian neoplasms; 15% to 20% are bilateral when malignant (Box 44.11); 10% occur in menopausal women. These tumors can also become very large and are more likely than the benign form to rupture. If the tumor ruptures, it is associated with pseudomyxoma peritoneum. This causes loculated ascites with mass effect.

Sonographic Findings. On examination, malignant cysts tend to have thick, irregular walls and septations with papillary projections and echogenic material (Figs. 44.26 and 44.27). They generally have a sonographic appearance similar to that of serous cystadenocarcinomas.

Penetration of the tumor capsule or rupture may lead to the mucoid ascites that appears as hypoechoic fluid with bright punctate echoes. This condition, known as pseudomyxoma peritonei, can be seen in mucinous cystadenomas and cystadenocarcinomas or mucinous tumors of the appendix and colon. It may contain multiple septations and low-level echogenic material that fills much of the pelvis and abdomen.

Serous Cystadenoma

Serous cystadenoma is the second most common benign tumor of the ovary (after the dermoid cyst) and represents 20% to 25% of all benign ovarian neoplasms (Fig. 44.28). This tumor is usually unilateral (20% are bilateral) (Box 44.12).

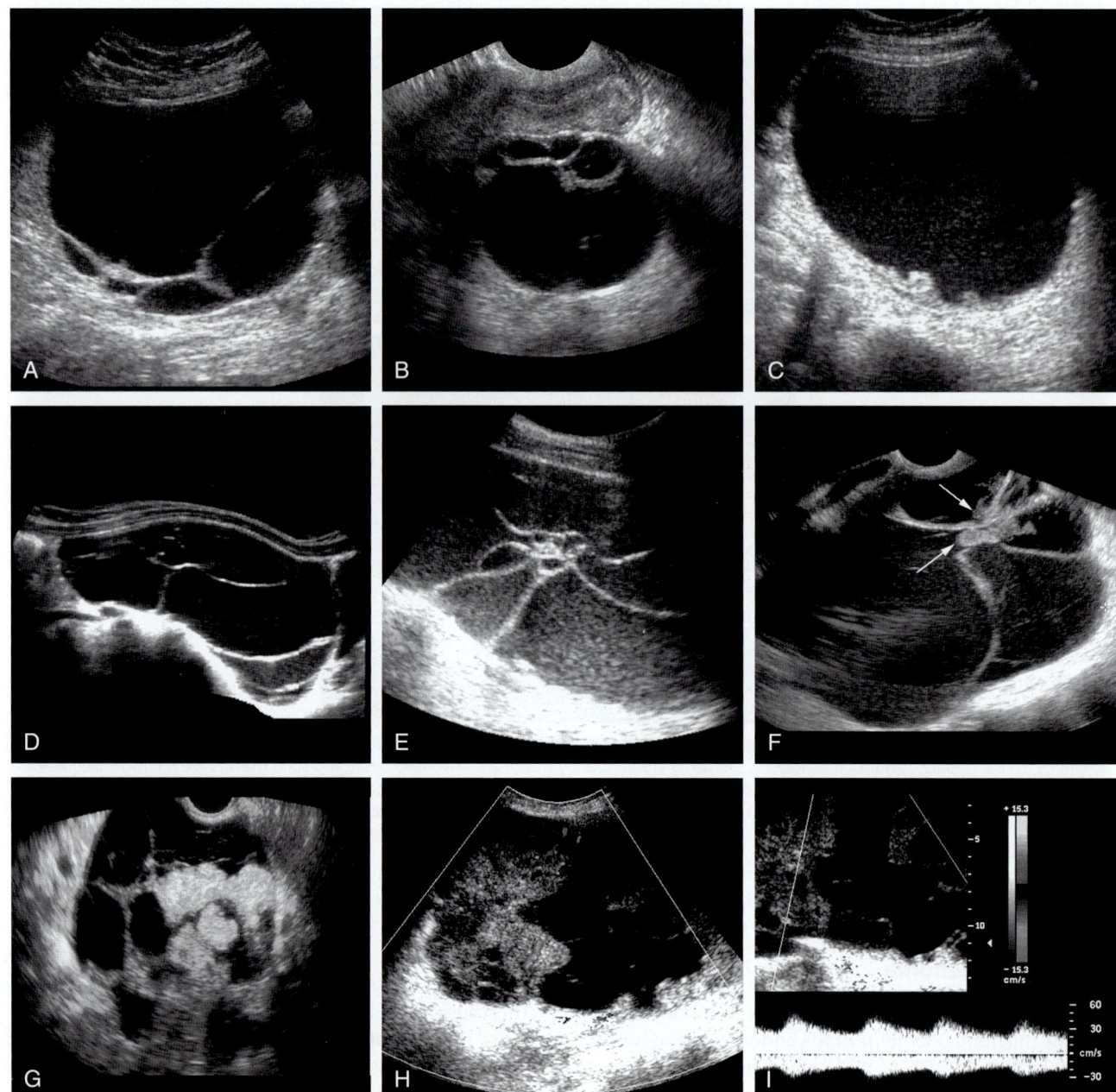

FIG. 44.24 Epithelial ovarian neoplasms: spectrum of appearances. (A–C) Serous cystadenomas. (A) Septations within this cystic mass are fairly thin. (B) Thicker septations. (C) Septations in low-level echogenic particles and small mural nodules. (D–E) Mucinous cystadenomas. (F) Mucinous cystadenocarcinoma. Large size and septations are characteristic; septal nodularity is marked in part F *(arrows)*. (G–I) Images in a single patient with a serous cystadenocarcinoma. Extensive nodularity shows vascularity confirming the morphologic suspicion of a malignant mass. There is high diastolic flow resulting in a low resistive index.

BOX 44.10	Mucinous Cystadenoma

- Unusually large (15–30 cm)
- Most common cystic tumor
- Usually unilateral
- Cyst filled with sticky, gelatin-like material
- Multilocular cystic spaces
- Benign type more common than malignant
- *Clinical findings:* pressure, pain, increased abdominal girth
- *Sonographic findings:* simple or septate thin-walled multilocular cysts

Sonographic Findings. Serous tumors are usually unilocular or multilocular with thin septations (Fig. 44.29). They are smaller than the mucinous cysts (up to 20 cm); borders are irregular with a loss of capsular definition. Multilocular cysts contain a small amount of solid tissue in chambers of varying size with occasional internal septum or mural nodules.

Serous Cystadenocarcinoma

Serous cystadenocarcinoma constitutes 60% to 80% of all ovarian carcinomas. More than half of these tumors are bilateral.

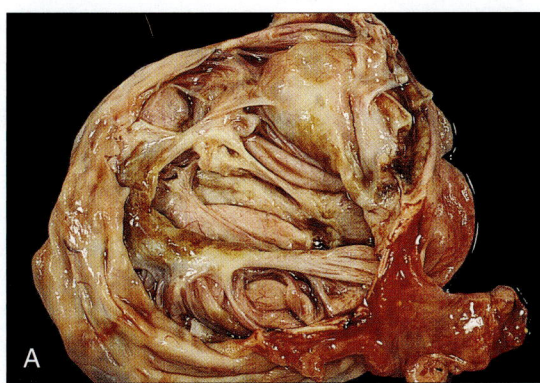

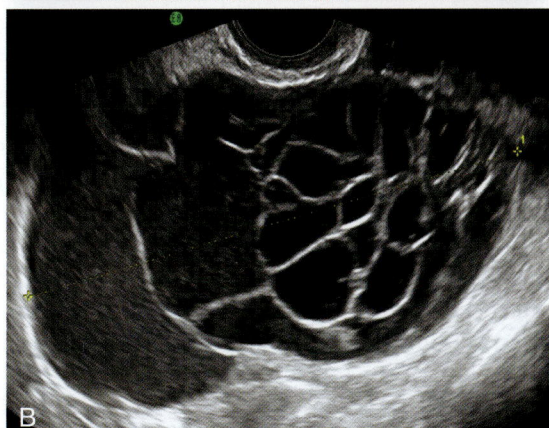

FIG. 44.25 **Mucinous cystadenoma.** (A) Gross pathology of a mucinous cystadenoma of the intestinal type. (B) Ultrasound shows multiple simple or septate thin-walled multilocular cysts.

BOX 44.11 **Mucinous Cystadenocarcinoma**

- Bilateral
- May occur in menopausal women (10%)
- Large, likely to rupture—ascites
- *Clinical findings:* pelvic pressure, pain when ruptured
- *Sonographic findings:* ascites appears as hypoechoic fluid with bright punctate echoes; thick, irregular walls and septations

---

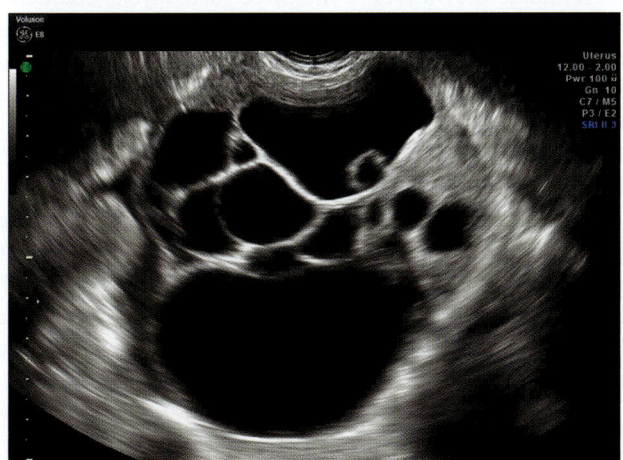

FIG. 44.26 Mucinous cystadenocarcinoma is demonstrated as a large septated mass with thick, irregular walls and numerous septations. Mucoid material is found within the cysts that represent cellular debris or blood.

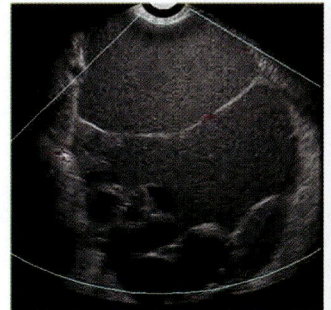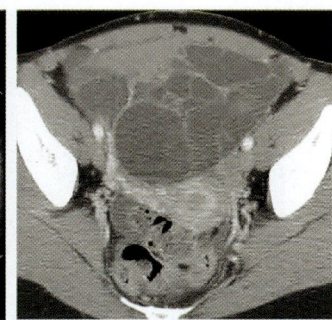

FIG. 44.27 **Mucinous cystadenocarcinoma.** Ultrasound *(left)* and computed tomographic *(right)* images of the large mass. These tumors can also become very large and are more likely than the benign form to rupture. If the tumor ruptures, it is associated with pseudomyxoma peritoneum. This causes loculated ascites with mass effect.

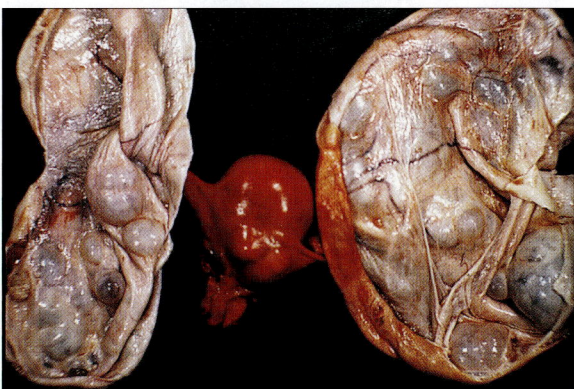

FIG. 44.28 **Serous cystadenoma.** Gross pathology of the lesion that demonstrates the multiple small cystic areas within the mass.

BOX 44.12 **Serous Cystadenoma**

- Usually unilateral
- Smaller than mucinous cysts
- Multilocular cysts with septations
- *Clinical findings:* pelvic pressure, bloating
- *Sonographic findings:* multilocular cyst—may have nodule

Sonographic Findings. Serous cystadenocarcinomas are smaller than mucinous cysts, but they still may be quite large, with irregular borders and a loss of capsular definition (Box 44.13). The tumor may be accompanied by bilateral ovarian enlargement. Multilocular cysts contain chambers of varying size with septated, internal papillary projections. Calcifications may be present. Solid elements or bilateral tumors suggest malignancy (Fig. 44.30). Ascites forms secondary to peritoneal surface implantation and is frequently seen. The tumor may spread to the lymph nodes (e.g., periaortic, mediastinal, and supraclavicular).

Other Epithelial Tumors

Less common varieties of epithelial tumors are endometrioid, clear cell, Brenner (transitional cell), and undifferentiated

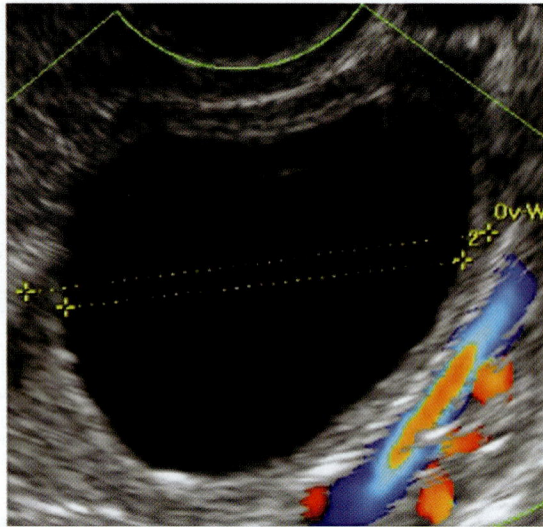

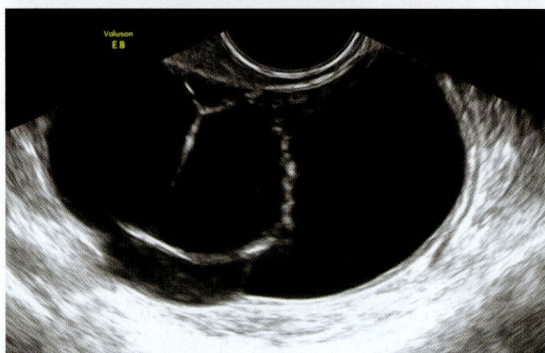

FIG. 44.29 Serous cystadenoma tumors are usually unilocular or multilocular with thin septations. They are smaller than the mucinous cysts (up to 20 cm); borders are irregular with a loss of capsular definition. Multilocular cysts contain a small amount of solid tissue in chambers of varying size with occasional internal septum or mural nodules.

BOX 44.13 Serous Cystadenocarcinoma

- External papillary mass adhesions and infection lead to bilateral involvement
- Loss of capsular definition and tumor fixation; calcifications
- Peritoneal implants; ascites; metastases to omentum, lymph nodes, liver, and lungs
- Clinical findings: pelvic fullness, bloating
- Sonographic findings: cystic structure with septations or papillary projections; internal and external papillomas usually present

---

carcinoma. Endometrioid tumors are nearly all malignant and are the second most common epithelial malignancy. Approximately 25% to 30% are bilateral and occur most frequently postmenopausal; peak age ranges from 50 to 60 years. Clear cell tumors are considered to be of müllerian duct origin and a variant of the endometrioid carcinoma. Clear cell tumors are nearly always malignant and are bilateral about 20% of the time. Peak age ranges from 50 to 70 years. Transitional cell tumor, also known as *Brenner tumor*, is uncommon. The Brenner tumor is found in 1.5% to 2.5% of patients; peak age ranges from 40 to 70 years. It is nearly always benign, and 6% to 7% are bilateral; 30% are associated with cystic neoplasms in the ipsilateral ovary.

Sonographic Findings. These types of epithelial tumors cannot be distinguished sonographically; however, they are more frequently found unilaterally. They are usually small and present as a nonspecific, complex, predominantly cystic mass (Fig. 44.31). Occasionally the tumor may contain hemorrhage or necrosis. The Brenner tumors are hypoechoic, solid masses that may contain calcifications in the outer wall. They are composed of dense fibrous stroma and appear similar to ovarian fibromas and thecomas.

GERM CELL TUMORS

Germ cell tumors are derived from the primitive germ cells of the embryonic gonad. They account for 15% to 20% of ovarian neoplasms, with approximately 95% being benign cystic teratomas. Besides teratomas, germ cell tumors include dysgerminoma, embryonal cell carcinoma, choriocarcinoma, and transdermal sinus tumor. These types are rare, occur mainly in adolescents, and are the most common ovarian malignancy in this age group. Germ cell tumors often occur as mixed tumors with elements of two or three varieties of germ cell tumors. They are associated with elevated alpha-fetoprotein (AFP) and human chorionic gonadotropin levels.

Clinical symptoms include pelvic or abdominal pain and a palpable mass (average diameter is 15 cm). The germ cell tumor is usually unilateral; 40% of tumors will calcify. The tumor ranges in texture from homogeneously solid (3%), predominantly solid (85%), to predominantly cystic (12%).

Teratoma

Dermoid Tumors. Dermoid tumors are the most common ovarian neoplasm, constituting 20% of ovarian tumors. Up to 15% are bilateral. About 80% occur in women of childbearing age, but they may occur at any age. They are composed of well-differentiated derivatives of the three germ layers: ectoderm, mesoderm, and endoderm. In 10% of cases, the tumor is diagnosed during pregnancy. A rare dermoid that is composed of thyroid tissue is termed a *stroma ovarii* (thyroid tissue) and may produce insuppressible thyrotoxicosis. Malignant degeneration into squamous cell carcinoma is uncommon (2%) in teratomas, usually in older women.

Sonographic Findings. Dermoids have a spectrum of sonographic appearances, depending on which elements (ectoderm, mesoderm, or transderm) are present. Teeth, bones, and fat can be seen on plain films (Box 44.14). Clinical findings include abdominal mass or pain secondary to torsion or hemorrhage.

Sonography may demonstrate one of several patterns: (1) a completely cystic mass, (2) a cystic mass with a very echogenic nodule along the mural wall representing a "dermoid plug," (3) a fat-fluid level, (4) high-amplitude echoes with shadowing (e.g., teeth or bone), or (5) a complex mass

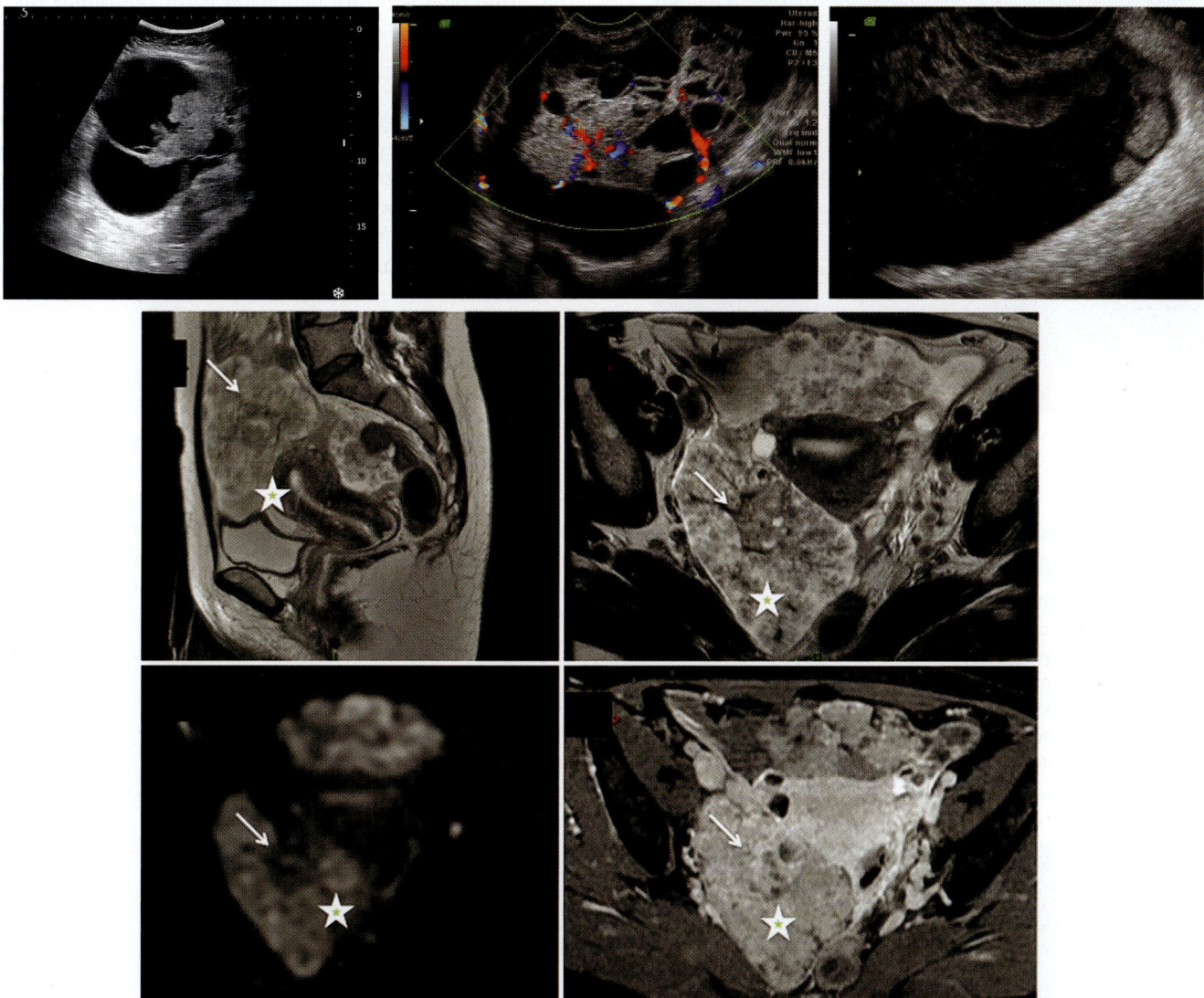

FIG. 44.30 Serous cystadenocarcinomas are smaller than mucinous cysts, but they still may be quite large, with irregular borders and a loss of capsular definition. The tumor may be accompanied by bilateral ovarian enlargement. Multilocular cysts contain chambers of varying size with septated, internal papillary projections. Calcifications may be present. Solid elements or bilateral tumors suggest malignancy.

with internal septations (Fig. 44.32). Echogenic dermoids are often confused with bowel, as the mass may have characteristics similar to those of complex bowel tissue with shadowing posterior. If a palpable pelvic mass is present that is not identified on sonography, an echogenic dermoid must be considered, and further imaging is usually performed. Indentation on the bladder wall will be a clue that a pelvic mass is present. The calcification within the pelvic cavity is also shown on the radiograph (Fig. 44.33).

The expression "tip of the iceberg" refers to a mixture of matted hair and sebum-producing ill-defined acoustic shadowing that obscures the posterior wall of the lesion. "Dermoid mesh" refers to multiple linear hyperechoic interfaces floating within the cyst and represent hair.

Acute hemorrhage into an ovarian cyst or an endometrioma may be so echogenic that it resembles a dermoid or a dermoid plug. Posterior sound enhancement is usually seen where a dermoid plug usually causes attenuation. Other pitfalls include a pedunculated fibroid or an appendicolith in a perforated appendix.

Immature and Mature Teratomas

Immature teratomas are uncommon and occur in girls and young women 10 to 20 years. These are rapidly growing, solid malignant tumors with many tiny cysts. AFP is elevated in 50% of patients. The tumor is unilateral and small in size, although it may grow to a larger dimension.

Sonographic Findings. On examination, the texture of immature teratomas ranges from cystic to complex; the teratoma usually is solid with internal echoes. Calcifications are commonly seen (Fig. 44.34).

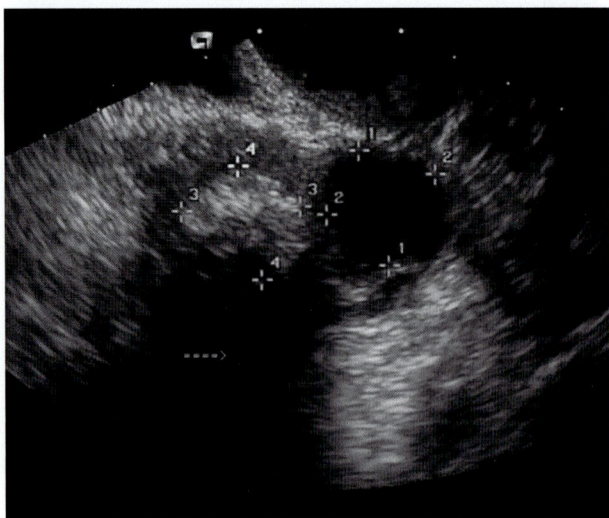

FIG. 44.31 Transitional cell tumor, also known as *Brenner tumor*, is uncommon. This tumor is usually unilateral and quite small in size and present as a nonspecific, complex, predominantly cystic mass.

BOX 44.14 Dermoid Tumors

- Size ranges from small to 40 cm
- Unilateral, round to oval mass
- Contains fatty, sebaceous material, hair, cartilage, bone, teeth
- *Clinical findings:* asymptomatic to abdominal pain, enlargement, and pressure; pedunculated, subject to torsion
- *Sonographic findings:* cystic/complex/solid mass, echogenic components; acoustic shadowing

---

Dysgerminoma

Dysgerminoma is a rare malignant germ cell tumor that is bilateral in 15% of cases. The mass constitutes 1% to 2% of primary ovarian neoplasms and 3% to 5% of ovarian malignancies. An entirely solid ovarian mass in a woman less than 30 is usually a dysgerminoma. The dysgerminoma and the serous cystadenoma are the two most common ovarian neoplasms seen in pregnancy.

Sonographic Findings. Dysgerminoma is a hyperechoic solid mass with areas of hemorrhage and necrosis on ultrasound examination. It may show a speckled pattern of calcifications (Fig. 44.35). In a postmenopausal patient, a fibroma or thecoma is most likely.

Endodermal Sinus Tumor

Endodermal sinus tumors are rare, rapidly growing tumors also called *yolk sac tumors*. The lesion usually occurs in women under 20 and is almost always unilateral. Increased serum AFP may be seen. Endodermal sinus tumor has a poor prognosis and is the second most common malignant ovarian germ cell neoplasm after dysgerminoma. The sonographic appearance is similar to that of the dysgerminoma.

STROMAL TUMORS

Sex-cord stromal tumors typically are solid adnexal masses that arise from the sex cords of the embryonic gonadal or

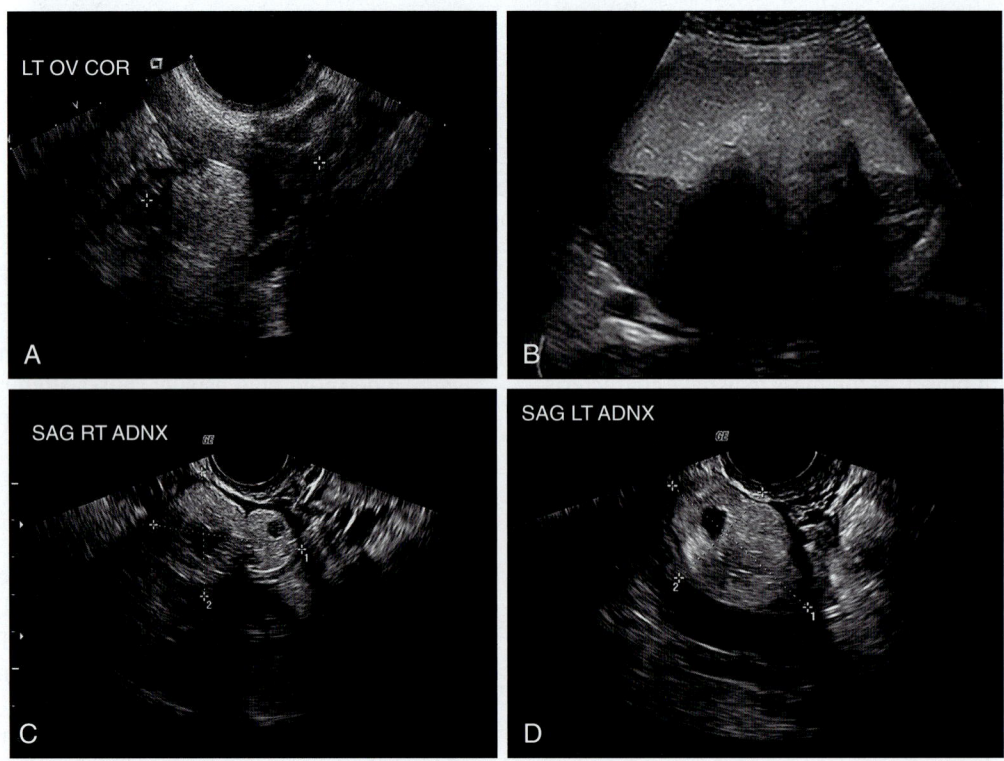

FIG. 44.32 **Dermoid tumor.** Spectrum of appearances on sonography. (A) Complex dermoid with an echogenic mural nodule. (B) Solid dermoid with calcification and shadowing. (C) Calcification and shadowing are shown in this complex dermoid tumor. (D) Complex pattern of a dermoid tumor.

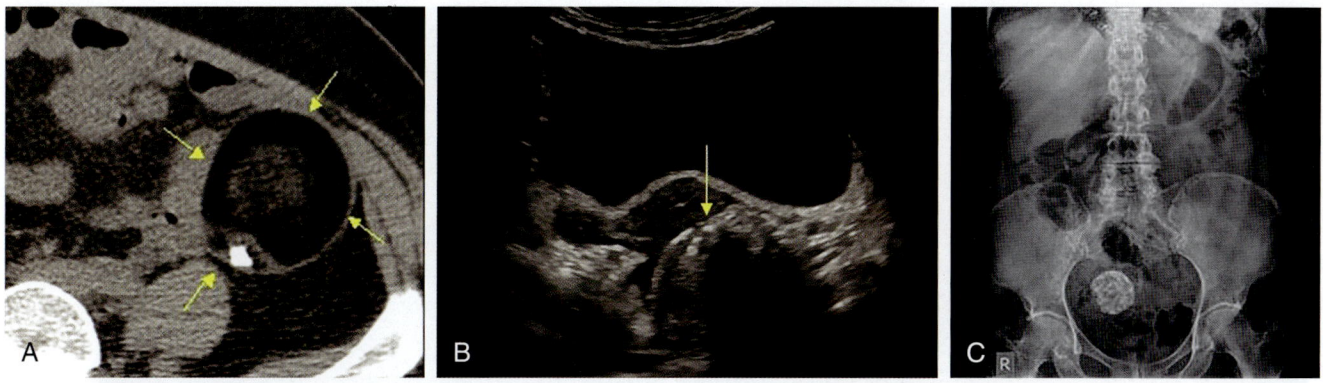

FIG. 44.33 (A) Computed tomography image of the calcified dermoid tumor. (B) Ultrasound image of a dermoid tumor with high-amplitude echoes with shadowing (e.g., teeth or bone). (C) Radiograph of the calcified dermoid tumor.

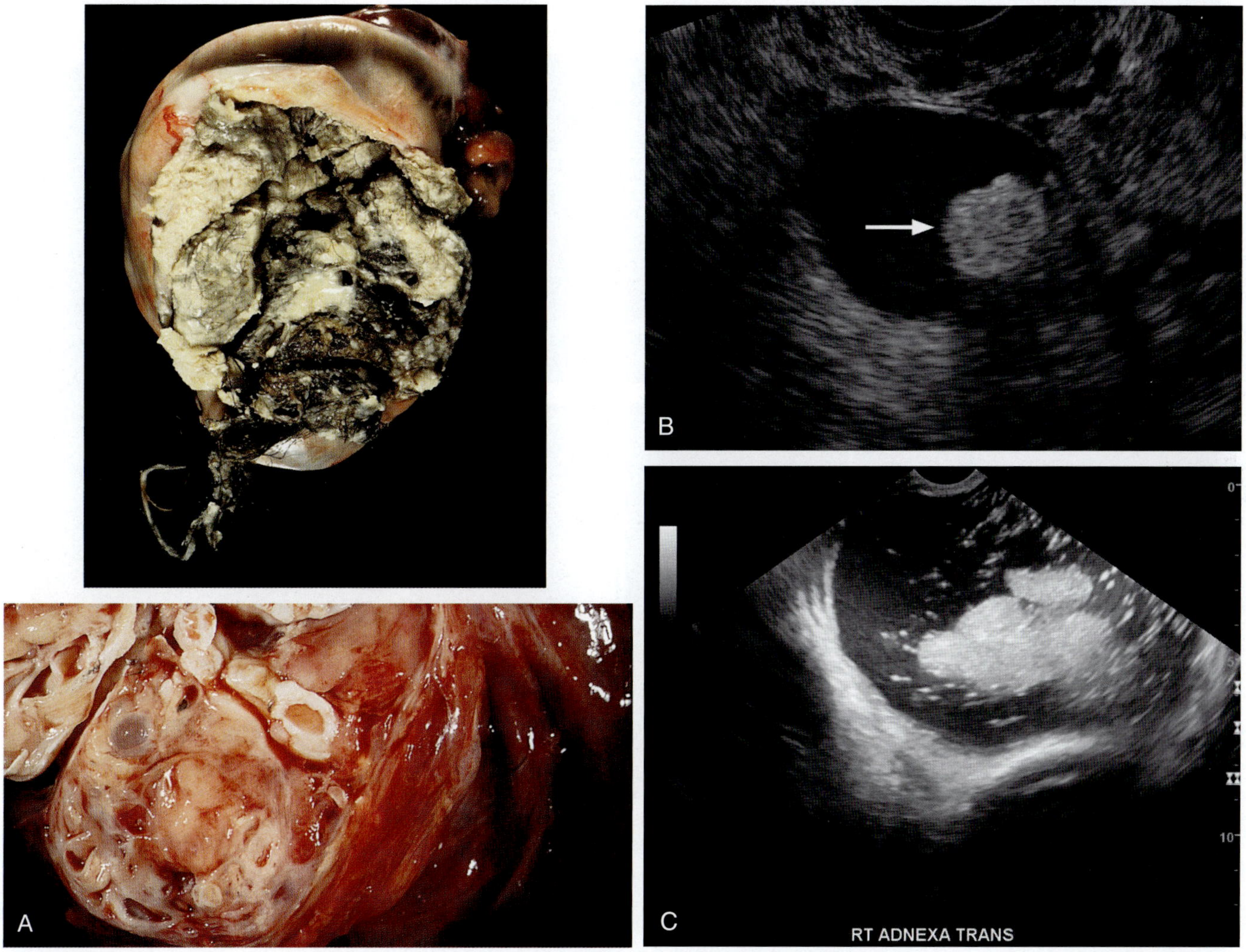

FIG. 44.34 (A) Gross pathology of an immature teratoma tumor. (B–C) The ultrasound texture of immature teratomas ranges from cystic to complex; the teratoma usually is solid with internal echoes. Calcifications are commonly seen.

ovarian stroma. This category includes granulosa cell tumor, thecoma, fibroma, and Sertoli-Leydig cell tumors (androblastoma). This group accounts for 5% to 10% of all ovarian neoplasms and 2% of all ovarian malignancies. Thecomas and fibromas are the most common of these. They are benign solid hypoechoic adnexal masses that occur in middle-aged women.

Sonographic Findings. Stromal tumors are often so hypoechoic as to appear cystic, but there is lack of through-transmission (Fig. 44.36).

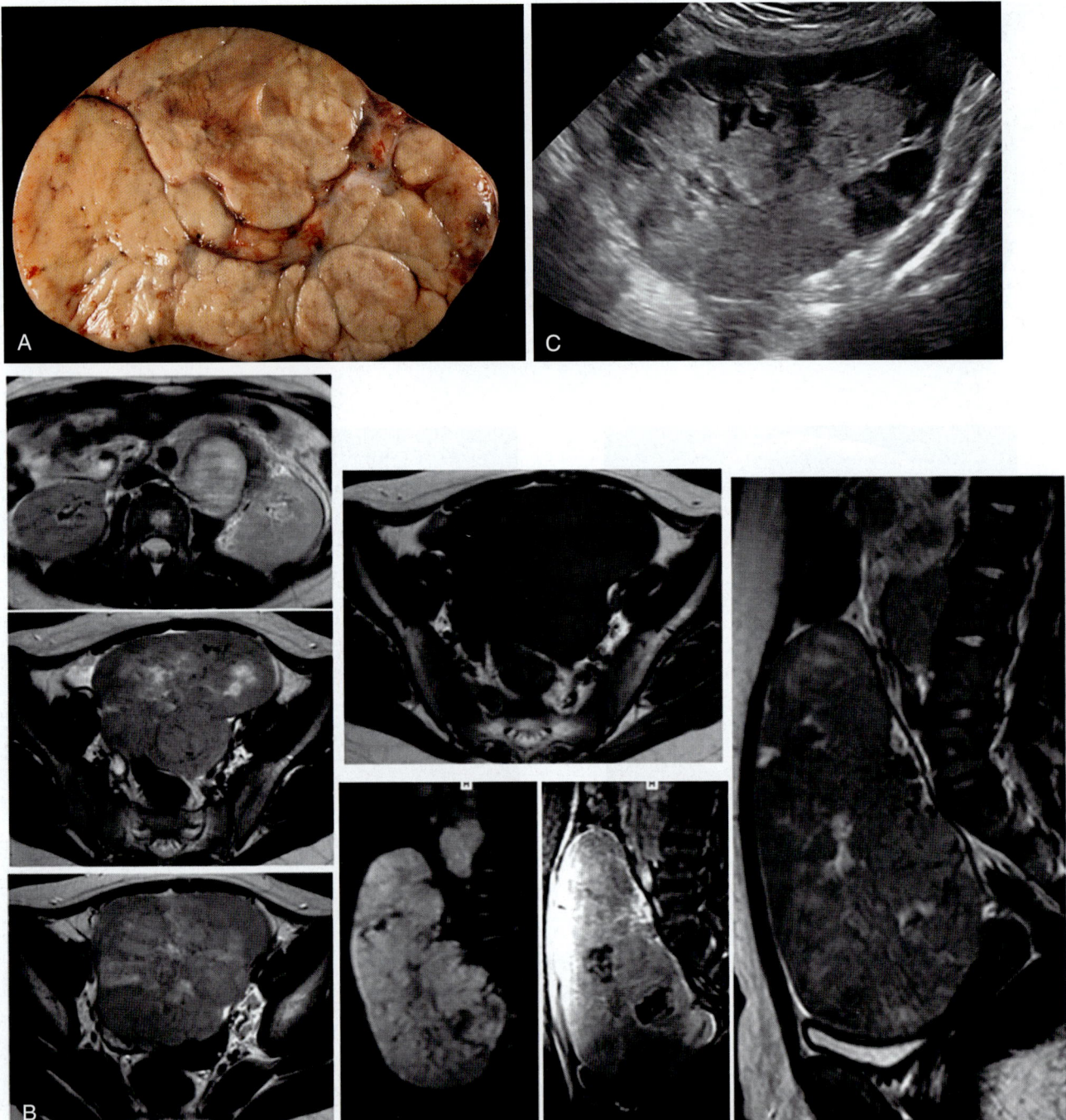

FIG. 44.35 Dysgerminoma is a hyperechoic solid mass with areas of hemorrhage and necrosis on ultrasound examination. It may show a speckled pattern of calcifications. (A) Gross anatomy. (B) Magnetic resonance images of the tumor. (C) Large tumor in the right adnexal area.

Fibroma and Thecoma

Both fibroma and thecoma tumors arise from the ovarian stroma and are pathologically similar (Fig. 44.37). Tumors with an abundance of thecal cells are called thecomas, and those with an abundance of fibrous tissue are called fibromas. Thecomas are usually benign and unilateral, comprising 1% of all ovarian neoplasms, and 70% occur in postmenopausal women. They frequently show signs of estrogen production.

Fibromas comprise 4% of ovarian neoplasms. Unlike thecomas, they are rarely associated with estrogen production. Clinical signs include lack of symptoms if the tumor is small; if large, increasing pressure and pain are apparent. Ascites has been reported in up to 50% of patients with fibromas larger than 5 cm in diameter. Associated ascites along with pleural effusion, termed *Meigs' syndrome*, occurs in 1% to 3% of patients with fibroma, but it is not specific, as it can occur with other ovarian neoplasms as well. The tumor is found in postmenopausal women. Fibromas occurring with basal cell nevus syndrome are commonly bilateral and calcified and occur in women with a mean age of 30 years.

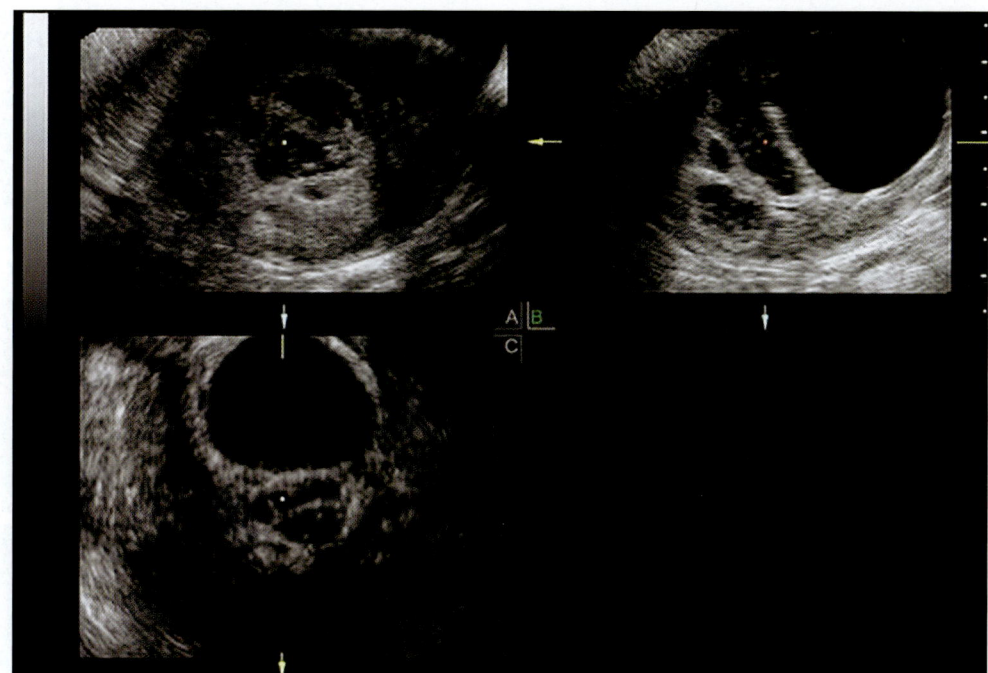

FIG. 44.36 Stromal tumors are often so hypoechoic as to appear cystic, but there is lack of through-transmission.

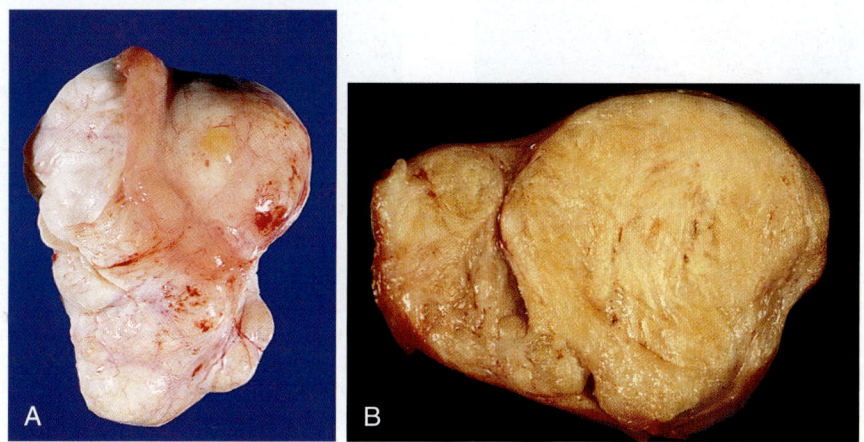

FIG. 44.37 (A) Gross pathology of a fibroma. (B) Gross pathology of a thecoma.

Sonographic Findings. Fibromas are usually unilateral (90%) and range from small to melon size, with a variable sonographic appearance. A hypoechoic mass with posterior attenuation is seen from the homogeneous fibrous tissue. The larger tumors are pedunculated and prone to torsion, edema, and cystic degeneration (Fig. 44.38).

Granulosa

A granulosa is a feminizing neoplasm composed of cells resembling the graafian follicle. It is the most common hormone-active estrogenic tumor of the ovary but is rarely found (1% to 3%). It is more common after menopause (50%) but is also seen in the reproductive ages (45%) and in adolescence (5%). Clinical symptoms of estrogen production may include precocious puberty or vaginal bleeding and full breasts. Pain, pressure, and fullness may also be present. The tumor may twist on itself to cause torsion or rupture, leading to Meigs' syndrome. Malignant transformation is rare, but when it occurs, the lesion spreads via the lymphatics and bloodstream.

Sonographic Findings. On examination, adult granulosa cell tumors have a variable appearance. A mass without torsion is similar to an endometrioma or cystadenoma, with low-level homogeneous echoes; if torsion occurs, a multilocular cyst containing blood or fluid is seen (Fig. 44.39). The solid masses may have an echogenicity similar to that of uterine fibroids. The size may range up to 40 cm in diameter; the mass is usually unilateral. Endometrial glandular hyperplasia may be apparent. Metastases are uncommon and appear as peritoneal-based masses.

Sertoli-Leydig Cell Tumor

Sertoli-Leydig cell tumors (also called *androblastomas*) are rare. They generally occur in women under 30 years and

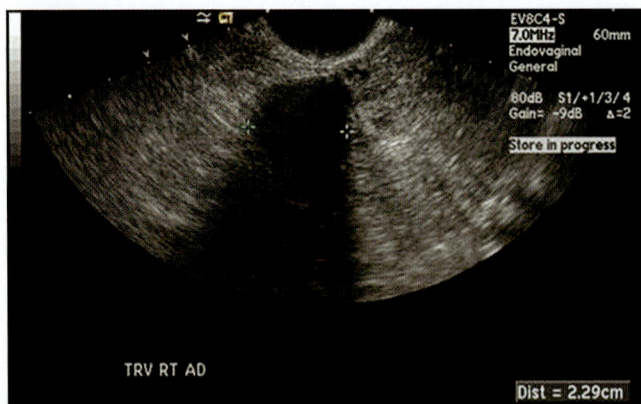

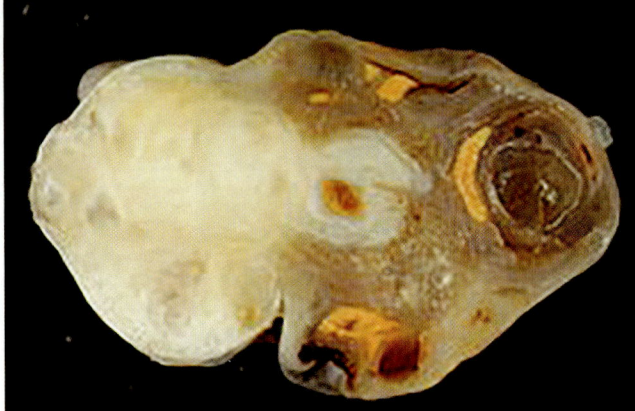

FIG. 44.38 Fibromas are usually unilateral (90%) and range from small to melon size, with a variable sonographic appearance. A hypoechoic mass with posterior attenuation is seen from the homogeneous fibrous tissue. The larger tumors are pedunculated and prone to torsion, edema, and cystic degeneration.

constitute less than 0.5% of ovarian neoplasms. Almost all are unilateral, and malignancy occurs in 10% to 20% of these tumors. Clinically, symptoms of virilization occur in about 30% of patients. Occasionally, these tumors may be associated with estrogen production.

Sonographic Findings. Sonographically, the tumor usually appears as a solid hypoechoic mass (Fig. 44.40).

Arrhenoblastoma

Arrhenoblastoma is a masculinizing ovarian tumor that occurs in females 15 to 65 years of age, with a peak incidence at 25 to 45 years. Clinical features are the same as for other pelvic masses, with the addition of amenorrhea and infertility. This mass may undergo malignant transformation in 22% of patients.

Sonographic Findings. The tumor is a solid mass with cystic components; it is lobulated and well encapsulated. In 95% of patients, the mass is unilateral, and the size ranges from 2 to 30 cm.

Metastatic Disease

The ovaries are more involved with metastatic disease than any other pelvic organ, and these metastases often

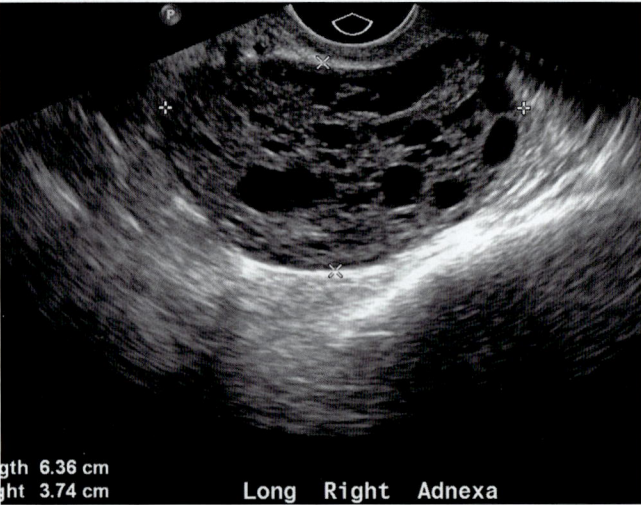

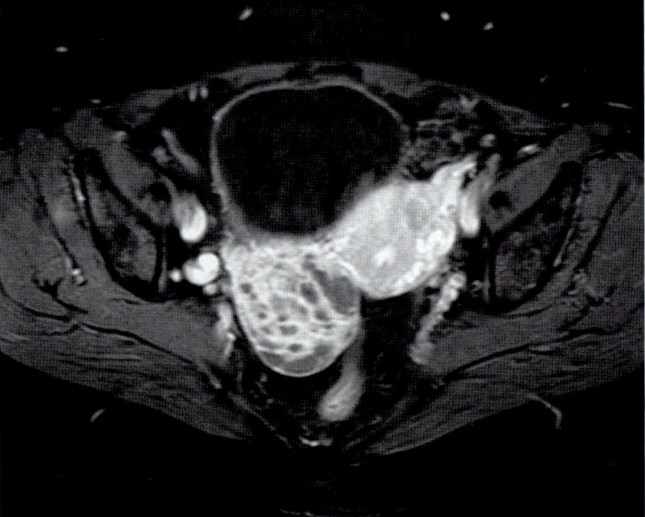

FIG. 44.39 Adult granulose cell tumors have a variable appearance. A mass without torsion is similar to an endometrioma or cystadenoma, with low-level homogeneous echoes; if torsion occurs, a multilocular cyst containing blood or fluid is seen.

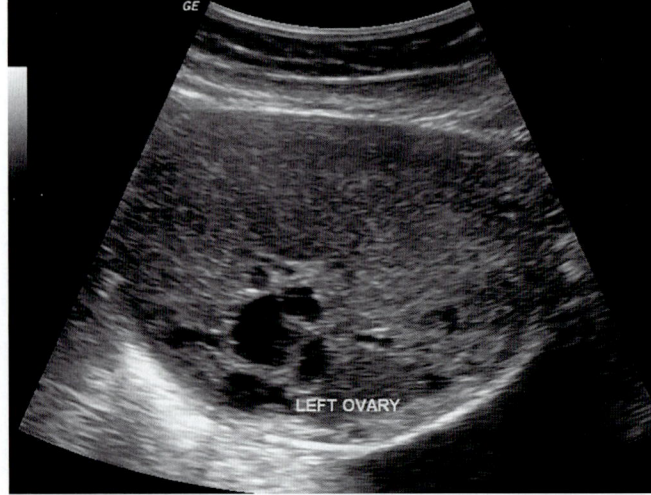

FIG. 44.40 Sertoli-Leydig cell tumors (also called *androblastomas*) are rare. Sonographically, the tumor usually appears as a solid hypoechoic mass.

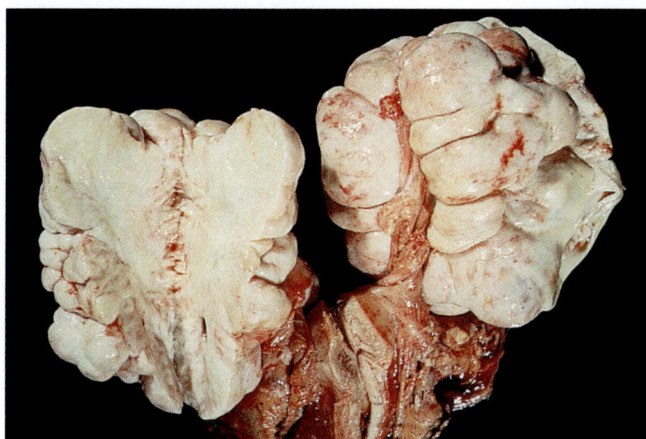

FIG. 44.41 Gross pathology of a Krukenberg tumor.

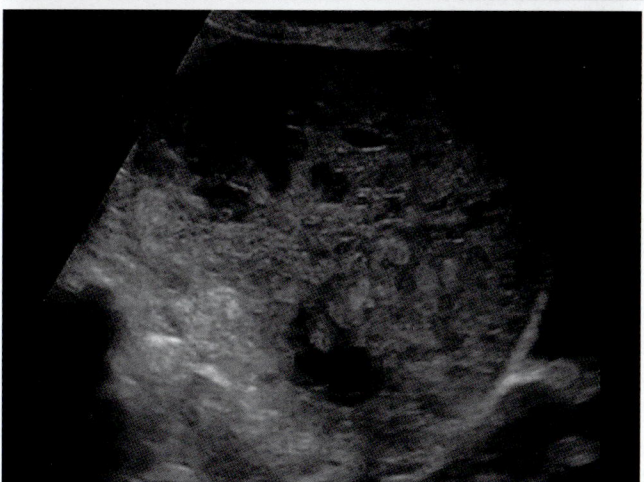

FIG. 44.42 **Krukenberg tumor.** Metastatic disease to the ovaries frequently is bilateral and is often associated with ascites. Metastases are usually completely solid or solid with a "moth-eaten" cystic pattern that occurs when they become necrotic.

mimic the appearance of advanced stages II to III primary ovarian cancer. Approximately 5% to 10% of ovarian neoplasms are metastatic in origin. Metastatic cancer can arise from the breast, upper gastrointestinal tract, and other pelvic organs by direct extension or lymphatic spread. Krukenberg tumors are "drop" metastases to the ovaries from the gastrointestinal tract, primarily from the stomach, but also from the biliary tract, gallbladder, and pancreas (Fig. 44.41). These masses are typically solid. Cystic metastatic masses appear to result more commonly from rectosigmoid colon cancers. Regardless of the site of origin, when there are metastases to the ovaries, these malignancies are often widespread, with metastasis to the peritoneum (including ascites) and the mesentery. The ovary is a common site of metastasis from carcinoma of the bowel (Krukenberg tumor), breast, and endometrium and from melanoma and lymphoma.

Sonographic Findings. Metastatic disease to the ovaries is frequently bilateral and often associated with ascites (Fig. 44.42). Metastases are usually completely solid or solid with a "moth-eaten" cystic pattern that occurs when they become necrotic. Lymphoma involving the ovary is usually diffuse and disseminated and is also frequently bilateral. Sonographically, the mass appears as a solid hypoechoic tumor similar to lymphoma elsewhere in the body.

CARCINOMA OF THE FALLOPIAN TUBE

Carcinoma of the fallopian tube is the least common (less than 1%) of all gynecologic malignancies. Adenocarcinoma is the most common histologic finding. It occurs most frequently in postmenopausal women with pain, vaginal bleeding, and a pelvic mass. The tumor usually involves the distal end, but it may involve the entire length of the tube.

Sonographic Findings. Sonographically, carcinoma of the fallopian tube appears as a sausage-shaped, complex mass, with cystic and solid components often with papillary projections. The clinical and sonographic findings are similar to those of ovarian carcinoma.

OTHER PELVIC MASSES

Not all pelvic masses are gynecologic in origin. Pelvic kidneys, omental cysts, distended impacted feces in the rectosigmoid colon, a distended bladder, hydroureters, colonic cancer or masses, diverticular abscesses, and retroperitoneal masses can all be identified by ultrasound examination. In addition, the use of ultrasound in detecting an ectopic pregnancy has been well documented. A flexible combination of transvaginal and transabdominal scanning can define the location, size, consistency, and source of adnexal masses. It is of key importance to distinguish solid ovarian masses from pedunculated myomas by identifying the uterine connection and searching for an ovary. Any fluid present in the pelvis can outline dependent portions of the pelvic organs by tilting the patient, using a transvaginal approach, or both. Large palpable tumors rising out of the pelvis are best viewed with transabdominal technique.

Sonography is useful in defining symptomatic or palpable masses, as described previously. It allows the surgeon to observe functional-appearing cysts without resorting to immediate surgery and plan a surgical exploration and treatment strategy when necessary. Obvious signs of malignancy, such as sonolucent liver metastases or nodular peritoneum outlined by ascites, assist in the preoperative assessment. With current equipment, excellent resolution is available, and the experienced sonographer may frequently identify the tumor by its texture if the clinical context is understood. However, histologic diagnosis is the job of the pathologist.

ACKNOWLEDGMENT

The author acknowledges the work of Candace Goldstein on this chapter in the previous edition.

Key Pearls

- The ovaries are paired, almond-shaped structures situated one on each side of the uterus close to the lateral pelvic wall.
- The ovaries can vary in position and are influenced by the uterine location and the ligament attachments.
- The normal ovary has a homogeneous echotexture, which may exhibit a central, more echogenic medulla. Small anechoic or cystic follicles may be seen peripherally in the cortex.
- A follicular cyst develops if the fluid in the nondominant follicles is not reabsorbed.
- An ovary's function is to mature oocytes until ovulation under the influence of luteinizing hormone and follicle-stimulating hormone from the pituitary.
- The majority of ovarian masses are simple cysts, most of which are benign.
- Mixed solid to cystic ovarian masses are typical of all the epithelial ovarian tumors; the most common are the serous types: cystadenoma and cystadenocarcinoma.
- The more sonographically complex the tumor, the more likely it is to be malignant, especially if associated with ascites.
- The differential considerations of a solid-appearing adnexal mass include pedunculated fibroid, dermoid, fibroma, thecoma, granulosa cell tumor, Brenner tumor, and metastasis. Tubo-ovarian abscess, ovarian torsion, hemorrhagic cysts, and ectopic pregnancy also may appear solid.
- Pulsed Doppler interrogation of the adnexal branch of the uterine artery, the ovarian artery, or intra-tumoral flow is performed to determine the resistive index or pulsatility index.
- A mass showing a complete absence or minimal diastolic flow (very elevated resistive index and pulsatility index values) is usually benign.
- Functional cysts include follicular, corpus luteum, hemorrhagic, and theca-lutein cysts.
- Theca-lutein cysts are the largest of the functional cysts and appear as very large, bilateral, multiloculated cystic masses. They are associated with high levels of human chorionic gonadotropin and are seen most frequently in association with gestational trophoblastic disease.
- Ovarian hyperstimulation syndrome is a frequent iatrogenic complication of ovulation induction.
- Polycystic ovarian syndrome (PCOS), which includes Stein-Leventhal syndrome (infertility, oligomenorrhea, hirsutism, and obesity), is an endocrine disorder associated with chronic anovulation.
- Paraovarian cysts arise from the broad ligament and usually are of mesothelial or paramesonephric origin.
- Omental cysts tend to be higher in the abdomen, and urachal cysts are midline in the anterior abdominal wall peritoneum above the bladder.
- Endometriosis is a common condition in which functioning endometrial tissue is present outside the uterus.
- The localized form of endometriosis consists of a discrete mass called an *endometrioma*, or *chocolate cyst*, and can frequently be found in multiple sites.
- Torsion of the ovary is caused by partial or complete rotation of the ovarian pedicle on its axis.
- Ovarian torsion is an acute abdominal condition requiring prompt diagnosis and surgical intervention.
- Ovarian lesions with irregular walls, thick irregular septations, mural nodules, and solid echogenic elements favor malignancy. Malignant ascites may also be present.
- Ovarian cancer can present as either a complex, cystic, or solid mass, but it is more likely predominantly cystic; as many as 20% are bilateral.
- Mucinous cystadenoma is a type of epithelial tumor lined by the mucinous elements of the endocervix and bowel. It constitutes 20% to 25% of all benign ovarian neoplasms. When benign, it is a mucinous cystadenoma; when malignant, it is a cystadenocarcinoma.
- Mucinous cystadenocarcinoma most frequently occurs in women aged 40 to 70 years and accounts for 5% to 10% of all primary malignant ovarian neoplasms.
- Serous cystadenoma is the second most common benign tumor of the ovary (after the dermoid cyst) and represents 20% to 25% of all benign ovarian neoplasms.
- Serous cystadenocarcinoma constitutes 60% to 80% of all ovarian carcinomas.
- Germ cell tumors include teratomas, dysgerminoma, embryonal cell carcinoma, choriocarcinoma, and transdermal sinus tumor.
- Tumors with an abundance of thecal cells are called thecomas, and those with an abundance of fibrous tissue are called fibromas.
- The ovaries are more involved with metastatic disease than any other pelvic organ, and these metastases often mimic the appearance of advanced stages II to III primary ovarian cancer.
- Krukenberg tumors are "drop" metastases to the ovaries from the gastrointestinal tract, primarily from the stomach, but also from the biliary tract, gallbladder, and pancreas.

BIBLIOGRAPHY

Ackerman S, Irshad A, Lewis M, et al. Ovarian cystic lesions: a current approach to diagnosis and management. *Radiol Clin North Am.* 2013;51(6):1067–1085.

Amor F, Alcazar JL, Vaccaro H, et al. GI-RADS reporting system for ultrasound evaluation of adnexal masses in clinical practice: a prospective multicenter study. *Ultrasound Obstet Gynecol.* 2011;38(4):450–455.

Brown DL, Dudiak Kzm, Laing FC. Adnexal masses: US characterization and reporting. *Radiology*. 2010;254(2):342–354.

Brown DL, Frates MC, Muto MG, et al. Large calcifications in ovaries otherwise normal on ultrasound. *Ultrasound Obstet Gynecol*. 2007;29(4):438–442.

Crum CP, McKeon FD, Xian W. The oviduct and ovarian cancer; causality, clinical implications, and targeted prevention. *Clin Obstet Gynecol*. 2012;55:24–35.

McDermott S, Oei TN, Iyer VR, et al. MR imaging of malignancies arising in endometriomas and extraovarian endometriosis. *Radiographics*. 2012;32(3):845–863.

Paladini D, Testa A, Van Holsbeke C, et al. Imaging in gynecological disease: clinical and ultrasound characteristics in fibroma and fibrothecoma of the ovary. *Ultrasound Obstet Gynecol*. 2009;34(2):188–195.

Patel MD. Pitfalls in the sonographic evaluation of adnexal masses. *Ultrasound Q*. 2012;28(1):29–40.

Shaaban AM, Rezvani M, Elsayes KM, et al. Ovarian malignant germ cell tumors: cellular classification and clinical and imaging features. *Radiographics*. 2014;34(3):777–801.

Timor-Tritsch IE, Goldstein SR. The complexity of a "complex mass" and the simplicity of a simple cyst. *J Ultrasound Med*. 2005;24(3):255–258.

Valentin L. Use of morphology to characterize and manage common adnexal masses. *Best Pract Res Clin Obstet Gynecol*. 2004;18(1):71–89.

Wang S, Johnson S. Prediction of benignity of solid adnexal masses. *Arch Gynecol Obstet*. 2012;285(3):721–726.

Zeligs KP, Javitt MC, Barner R, et al. Atypical ovarian calcifications associated with bilateral borderline ovarian tumors. *J Ultrasound Med*. 2013;32(6):1059–1061.

CHAPTER 45

Pathology of the Adnexa

Sandra L. Hagen-Ansert

OBJECTIVES

On completion of this chapter, you should be able to:
- List the causes of and risk factors for pelvic inflammatory disease
- Describe the sonographic findings of salpingitis, pyosalpinx, tubo-ovarian abscess, endometrioma, and adenomyosis
- Identify the locations of endometrial implants in the body
- Explain the development of endometritis in the postpartum patient
- Discuss the role of ultrasound in pelvic inflammatory disease

OUTLINE

Pelvic Inflammatory Disease 1260
    Salpingitis, Hydrosalpinx, and Pyosalpinx 1261
    Tubo-ovarian Abscess 1263

Peritonitis 1264
Endometritis 1266
Endometriosis and Endometrioma 1267

Interventional Ultrasound 1270
Postoperative Uses of Ultrasound 1271

KEY TERMS

Adenomyosis
Endometrioma
Endometriosis
Endometritis
Hydrosalpinx

Myometritis
Oophoritis
Parametritis
Pelvic inflammatory disease (PID)
Periovarian inflammation

Pyosalpinx
Salpingitis
Tubo-ovarian abscess (TOA)
Tubo-ovarian complex

Pelvic inflammatory disease (PID) and endometriosis are diffuse disease processes of the female pelvic cavity. Most commonly, PID is caused by sexually transmitted diseases, including gonorrhea and chlamydia. Although uncommon, PID can also be caused by a ruptured appendix and peritonitis. PID and endometriosis have very different clinical presentations and pathologies. However, early in the disease, the clinical presentation of both endometriosis and PID is nonspecific and may mimic functional bowel disease.

PID is an inclusive term that refers to all pelvic infections (e.g., endometritis, salpingitis, hydrosalpinx, pyosalpinx, **periovarian inflammation**, **tubo-ovarian complex**, and tubo-ovarian abscess). The infection usually occurs bilaterally and may be found in the endometrium (**endometritis**), the uterine wall (**myometritis**), the uterine serosa and broad ligaments (**parametritis**), the ovary (**oophoritis**), and the most common location, the oviducts (**salpingitis**) (Fig. 45.1). Sonography has limited value during acute PID or at early onset when inflammatory changes have not yet begun to manifest. In cases of chronic PID, ultrasound can identify dilated fallopian tubes (hydrosalpinx or pyosalpinx), abscess, and complex intraperitoneal fluid.

Endometriosis is the presence of endometrial glands or stroma in abnormal locations. It occurs most commonly in two forms: adenomyosis of the uterus and endometriosis of the adnexa. In most cases, endometriosis is diagnosed clinically and is not detectable by sonography. When identified sonographically, it presents as an adnexal mass or masses (endometriomas) of variable echogenicity, shape, and size.

PELVIC INFLAMMATORY DISEASE

The occurrence of PID is becoming more common. PID occurs in 11% of young women during reproductive age, with a peak incidence at 20 to 24 years, affecting 750,000 American women each year. The increased incidence in younger populations may be due to the immaturity of the cervix and consequent higher risk of sexually transmitted infections. Risk factors include early sexual contact, multiple sexual partners, history of sexually transmitted disease, previous history of

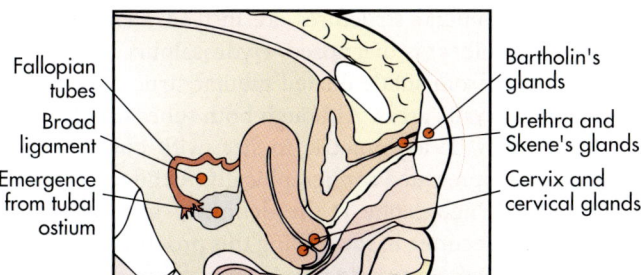

FIG. 45.1 Pelvic inflammatory disease may be found in the endometrium, the uterine wall, the uterine serosa and broad ligaments, the ovary, and the fallopian tubes.

> **BOX 45.1 Pelvic Inflammatory Disease**
>
> - Inflammatory disease (acute or chronic); infection spreads to pelvis
> - Large, palpable, bilateral complex mass; ovary may be seen separate from mass
> - Free fluid in cul-de-sac
> - Doppler image shows increased vascularity and diastolic flow
> - Associated with infertility and endometritis

> **BOX 45.2 Sonographic Findings of Pelvic Inflammatory Disease**
>
> - *Endometritis:* thickening or fluid in the endometrium
> - *Periovarian inflammation:* enlarged ovaries with multiple cysts, indistinct margins
> - *Salpingitis:* nodular thickening, irregularity of tube with diverticula
> - *Pyosalpinx or hydrosalpinx:* fluid-filled irregular fallopian tube with or without echoes
> - *Tubo-ovarian abscess:* complex mass with septations, irregular margins, and internal echoes; usually in cul-de-sac

PID, use of an intrauterine contraceptive device (IUCD), and douching (douching may push bacteria into the upper genital tract). Although sexually transmitted diseases such as gonorrhea and chlamydia are the most common forms of infection, other routes of infection are possible, such as direct extension from appendiceal, diverticular, or postsurgical abscess collections that have ruptured into the pelvis, the string from an IUCD, or puerperal and postabortion complications. Other types of invasive instrumentation procedures in the pelvic cavity may leave the route more open to bacterial invasion. PID is usually found as a bilateral collection of fluid and pus within the pelvic cavity, except when it is caused by direct extension of an adjacent inflammatory process, in which case it is most commonly unilateral (Box 45.1).

Infrequently, particularly in patients with PID resulting from gonorrhea, a pelvic infection may travel upward through the right flank, causing a perihepatic inflammation. The pain may mimic liver, gallbladder, or right renal pain. Perihepatic inflammation can be detected sonographically by scanning along the liver margin and identifying a hypoechoic rim between the liver and the adjacent ribs. This perihepatic inflammation is called the Fitz-Hugh–Curtis syndrome.

Sexually transmitted PID is spread via the mucosa of the pelvic organs through the cervix into the uterine endometrium (endometritis) and out the fallopian tubes (acute salpingitis) to the area of the ovaries and peritoneum. As the tube becomes obstructed, it fills with pus (pyosalpinx). In the setting of extensive PID, the margins of the ovaries and other pelvic structures can become difficult to distinguish from each other.

The bacterial infection may arise from *Chlamydia trachomatis* and *Neisseria gonorrhoeae*. Other bacteria that have been found in PID patients include aerobes (*Streptococcus* species, *Escherichia coli, Haemophilus influenzae*), anaerobes (*Bacteroides, Peptostreptococcus,* and *Peptococcus*), *Mycobacterium tuberculosis, Actinomycetes* species in IUCD users, and herpesvirus hominis type 1.

If the pregnancy test result is positive in a woman with previously treated PID, a careful evaluation of the adnexa is indicated, even if a normal intrauterine pregnancy is detected. From the previous fallopian tube damage, the incidence of an ectopic pregnancy is significantly increased. The possibility of a rare heterotopic pregnancy (a concomitant intrauterine and extrauterine pregnancy) increases in this patient.

Clinically, patients may present with intense pelvic pain and tenderness described as dull and aching, with constant vaginal discharge. Other symptoms include fever, pain in the right upper abdomen, painful intercourse, and irregular menstrual bleeding. A history of infertility may also be present. Laboratory tests may show an elevated white blood cell count in PID, particularly when caused by a chlamydial infection. The patient may be asymptomatic, or the disease may produce only minor symptoms, even though it can seriously damage the reproductive organs. A palpable mass may be present on clinical examination. Current criteria of the Centers for Disease Control and Prevention for diagnosing PID include pelvic or lower abdominal pain and one or more of the following: cervical motion tenderness, uterine tenderness, or adnexal tenderness.

The sonographic findings may be normal early in the course of the disease (Box 45.2). As the disease progresses or becomes chronic, a variety of findings may occur. Differential considerations may include hematoma, dermoid cyst, ovarian neoplasm, and endometriosis.

Salpingitis, Hydrosalpinx, and Pyosalpinx

Salpingitis is inflammation of a fallopian tube (Fig. 45.2). This condition may be acute, subacute, or chronic. Clinical signs may range from asymptomatic to pelvic fullness or discomfort or a low-grade fever. An obstructed tube filled with serous secretions is a **hydrosalpinx**; this can occur as a result of PID, endometriosis, or postoperative adhesions. The sonographer should look closely at the fundal uterus to search for prominent or enlarged fallopian tubes. The dilated tube may show a pointed beak at the swollen end of the tube near the isthmus where the tube enters the uterus. If the dilated tube becomes infected, it is called **pyosalpinx**. The likelihood of recurrent infection and ectopic pregnancy increases significantly. Infected or hemorrhagic pelvic fluid may also be present. Infection can obscure normal tissue planes, making anatomy unclear. Severe pain requires gentle use of ultrasound probes in acute PID, and in some cases, a full bladder for transabdominal study is intolerable (Table 45.1).

▶ **Sonographic Findings.** Sonographically, the normal fallopian tube is generally not visualized unless fluid surrounds it. If outlined by ascitic fluid, it is a thin, less than 5-mm hypoechoic tissue band originating from the uterine fundus and can be imaged in an axial-coronal view. The sonographer can try to follow the dilated fallopian tube as it enters the cornu of the uterus (at the fundus). Careful oblique angulations of the transducer are necessary to trace the pathway of the tube. If fluid, pus, or products of conception (POCs) fill the tube, detection is easier. A pathologic state is probable if the lumen is outlined and shows irregularity and multiple diverticula.

If distinct tubular structures are instead seen, hydrosalpinx (dilated tubes) is diagnosed. Hydrosalpinx has variable presentations, from subtle dilated tubular structures to massive tortuous cystic areas. Although both tubes may be damaged, they may be asymmetric in size, with only the more dilated tube appreciated sonographically. Although contrast-enhanced salpingography is the definitive test, ultrasound appears to be accurate in identifying this process, particularly when performed transvaginally. Hydrosalpinx may present as echogenic fluid or fluid-debris levels (Fig. 45.3), indicating infection (pyosalpinx).

Severe and chronic pyosalpinx often contains thick, echogenic mucoid pus, which does not transmit sound as well as serous fluid or blood. A pyosalpinx may appear as a complex mass. A transvaginal examination is particularly useful for identifying the tubular nature and folds of the dilated tube, thus avoiding the mistaken diagnosis of a mass. Careful coronal scanning and rotation of the probe will help the sonographer to discern a dilated tube from an adnexal cyst.

Acute salpingitis is evident as a thick-walled nodular hyperemic tube (Fig. 45.4). The dilated tubes usually surround the ovaries like two lunar crescents encircling the posterior surface of the uterus and filling the cul-de-sac.

The sonographer should be sure not to confuse the dilated tube with a dilated ureter or prominent vessel. Occasionally, prominent blood vessels may be present in the adnexa. Although these may initially be misinterpreted as a hydrosalpinx, color or pulsed Doppler imaging will show blood flow in an adnexal blood vessel and no flow in a hydrosalpinx. Evaluation of the kidneys for possible hydronephrosis and trying to trace the dilated ureter to the bladder should help. The ovaries may be difficult to delineate because of surrounding tissue, edema, and pus. In addition to hydrosalpinx or pyosalpinx, sonographic findings of PID include fluid in the cul-de-sac (Fig. 45.5), mild uterine enlargement, and endometrial fluid or thickening. Transabdominal and transvaginal sonography can reveal the presence of pelvic

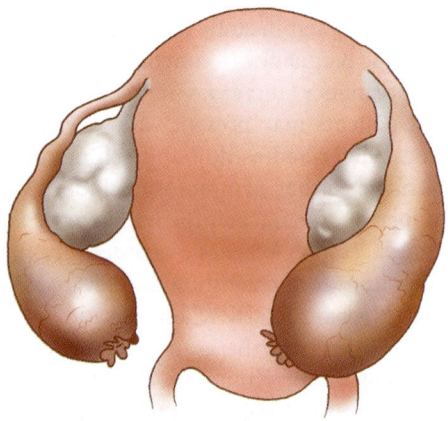

FIG. 45.2 Salpingitis is an inflammation of the fallopian tubes that causes nodular dilation. This infection may be unilateral or bilateral.

TABLE 45.1	Salpingitis, Hydrosalpinx, and Pyosalpinx		
	Description	Clinical Findings	Sonographic Findings
Salpingitis	Inflammation of fallopian tube Acute, subacute, or chronic	Asymptomatic to pelvic fullness or discomfort Low-grade fever	Dilated tube Tortuous
Hydrosalpinx	Obstructed tube filled with serous secretions Occurs secondary to PID, endometriosis, or postoperative adhesions	Asymptomatic to pelvic fullness or discomfort Low-grade fever	Walls become thin secondary to dilation Appearance of multicystic or fusiform mass Follow dilated tubes from fundus of uterus Look for pointed "beak" at swollen end of tube near isthmus Bilateral Ampullary portion more dilated than interstitial part of tube
Pyosalpinx	Retained pus in oviduct with inflammation	Asymptomatic to pelvic fullness or discomfort Low-grade fever	May appear as complex mass Pus within dilated tube very thick Transmission and echogenic–poor sound

PID, Pelvic inflammatory disease.

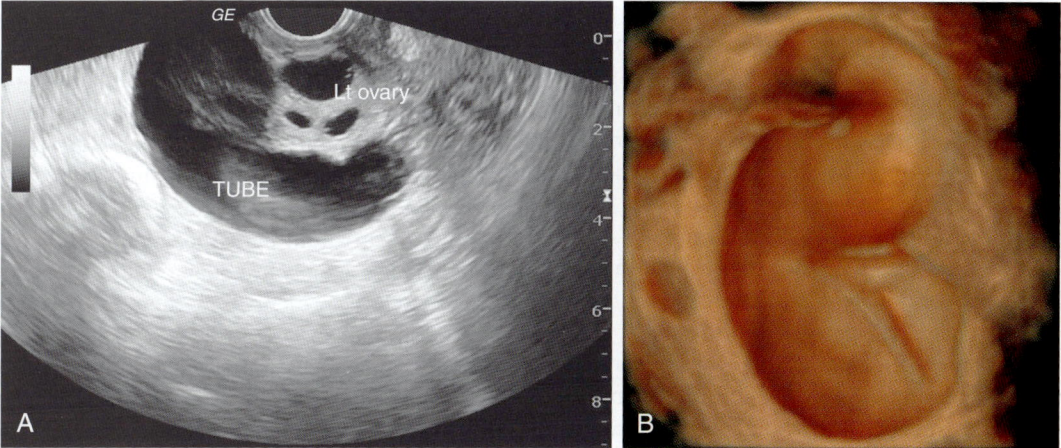

FIG. 45.3 (A) Hydrosalpinx. Patient presented with abdominal pain, status post-hysterectomy, and right oophorectomy 5 years prior. A serpiginous, mostly anechoic structure abuts the left ovary. Fluid accumulates from tubal secretions. (B) Three-dimensional rendering of the hydrosalpinx demonstrates the dilation and curvature of the tube.

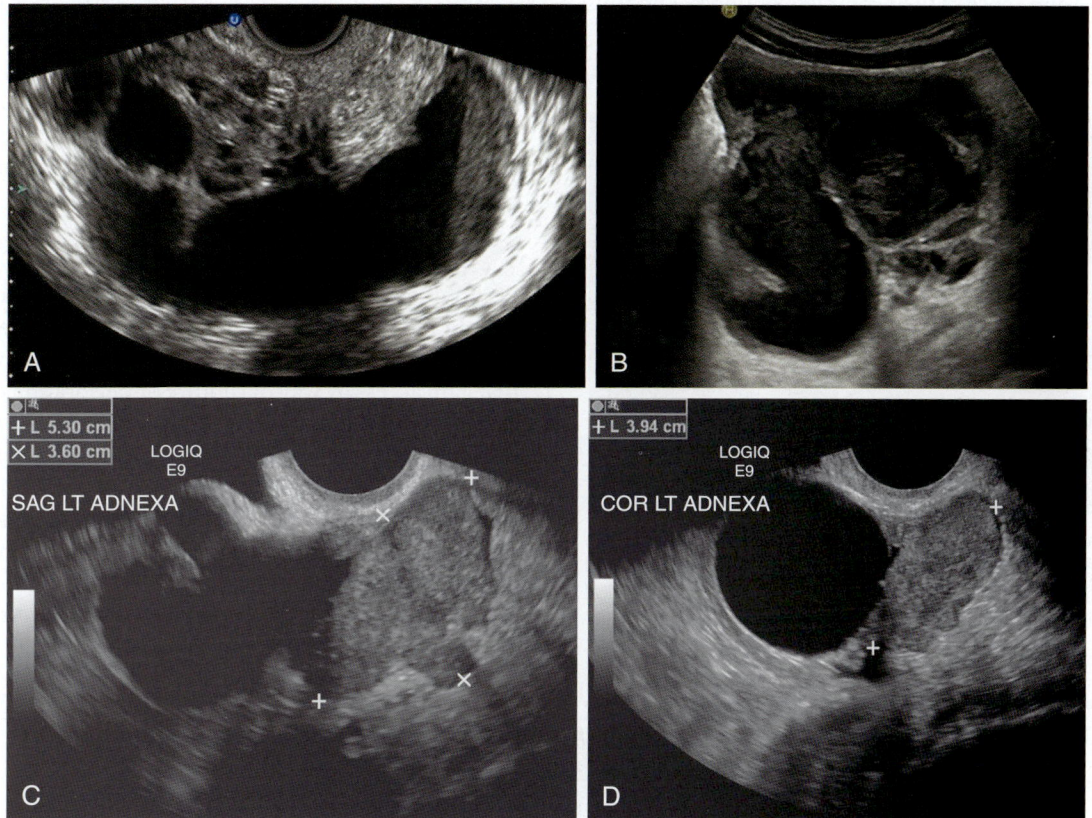

FIG. 45.4 (A) Pyosalpinx. In the presence of infection, the fallopian tube fills with pus, which is seen as low-level echoes and thick walls. (B) Acute salpingitis. The tube is enlarged and distended with pus appearing as complex echoes within. Note the thick walls. (C–D) Hydrosalpinx. This 81-year-old patient presented with left lower leg swelling. Computed tomography confirmed left common iliac vein thrombosis. Ultrasound demonstrated a left hydrosalpinx with adjacent mass, possibly within the fallopian tube. Surgical pathology confirmed a left hydrosalpinx with adjacent ovarian serous adenocarcinoma.

intraperitoneal fluid in the cul-de-sac. Pelvic fluid may frequently have internal echoes, septations, and fluid levels, a sign that the fluid is not simple but rather may be infected or hemorrhagic (Fig. 45.6).

Any simple cyst that hemorrhages may appear as a complex mass. In patients of reproductive age, the classic differential diagnosis of a complex adnexal mass is hemorrhagic cyst, ectopic pregnancy, endometrioma, and PID. Dermoids and other benign tumors can appear in a similar fashion.

Tubo-ovarian Abscess

The adhesive, edematous, and inflamed serosa may further adhere to the ovary and/or other peritoneal surfaces, which distorts anatomy. As the infection worsens, periovarian adhesions may form. The ovary cannot be separated from the inflamed dilated tube and is called the tubo-ovarian complex. In trying to determine whether an adnexal mass is separate from the ovary, gentle pushing with the transvaginal transducer can be used to identify separate or contiguous movement. Periovarian adhesions fuse the inflamed ovary and tube, and the ovary cannot be separated from the tube. This causes a further loculation of pus known as a **tubo-ovarian abscess (TOA)**. This may be unilateral abscess or bilateral and appears as a complex mass in the posterior cul-de-sac.

The tubo-ovarian complex or abscess usually responds well to antibiotic treatment without the need for surgical drainage. Serial ultrasound images during treatment allow observation of resolution and can indicate which patients need prolonged intravenous antibiotics and which patients may benefit more from removal of the involved tissue. Sonographic guidance can be used to assist in percutaneous or transvaginal drainage, for culture and sensitivity or complete drainage, and thus hasten recovery.

Sonographic Findings. A pelvic abscess is usually a complex mass in the cul-de-sac that distorts pelvic anatomy (Fig. 45.7). It can involve the ovary alone or the fallopian tube and ovary as a tubo-ovarian abscess. The TOA appears as a complex multiloculated mass with variable septations, irregular margins, and scattered internal echoes. The ovaries are often difficult to recognize as separate from the mass because of surrounding tissue, edema, and pus (Fig. 45.8). As noted, TOAs usually are bilateral, but they may be unilateral if an IUCD is present or if there is direct extension from an abdominal abscess. There is usually posterior acoustic enhancement. Occasionally a fluid-debris level or gas may be seen within the mass. Gas within the abscess may appear as hyperechoic punctate echoes that exhibit a comet tail shadowing effect. Drainage of the collection of pus may be done with interventional sonography (Fig. 45.9). Recognizable ovarian tissue may be identified within the inflammatory mass by transvaginal sonography.

The sonographic appearance may be indistinguishable from other adnexal masses, and clinical correlation is necessary for the correct diagnosis. The transvaginal approach is helpful in assessing the extent of the disease. Dilated tubes, periovarian inflammatory change, and the internal characteristics of TOAs are better defined with transvaginal scanning.

Peritonitis

Peritonitis is inflammation of the peritoneum, the serous membrane lining the abdominal cavity and covering the viscera. This inflammation is caused by infectious organisms that gain access by way of rupture or perforation of the viscera or associated structures, via the female genital tract, by piercing the abdominal wall, via the bloodstream or lymphatic vessels, via surgical incisions, or by failure to practice antiseptic techniques during surgery. If the infectious process spreads to involve the bladder, ureter, bowel, and adnexal area, it becomes pelvic peritonitis.

Sonographic Findings. If the abscess collection has gas-forming bubbles within, it may be difficult to delineate

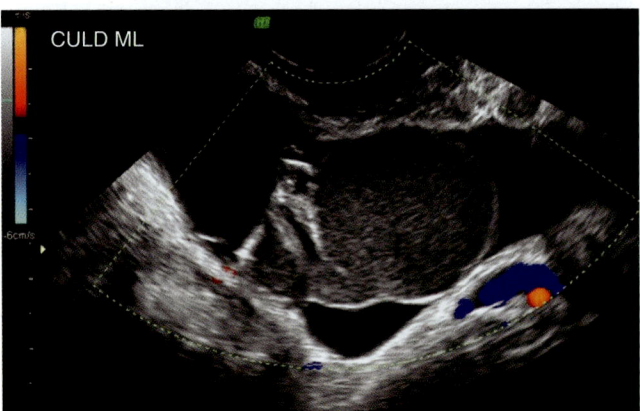

FIG. 45.5 Peritoneal pseudocyst with hemorrhagic mesothelial cyst. Patient presented with right lower quadrant pain for 2 weeks. Ultrasound suggests free fluid with mass and septations in the cul-de-sac. Surgical pathology confirmed a peritoneal pseudocyst with hemorrhagic mesothelial cyst.

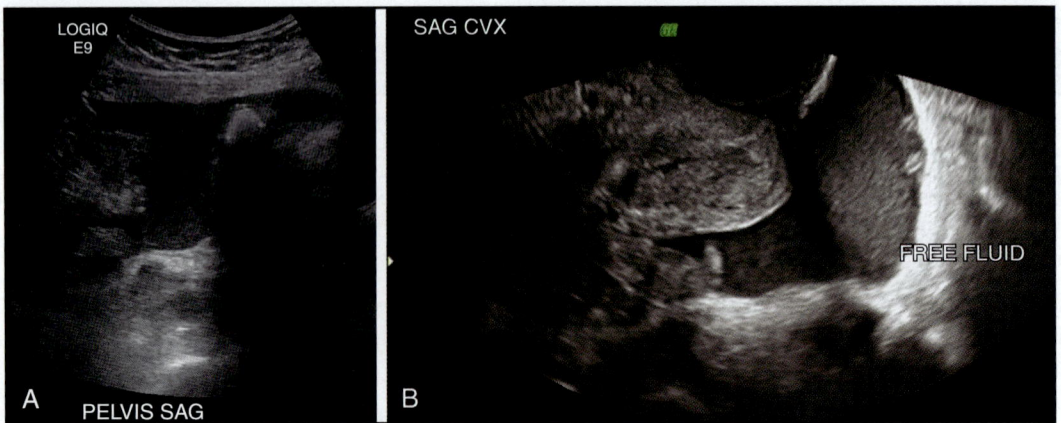

FIG. 45.6 (A) Pelvic fluid. Fluid in the pelvis from malignant ascites; this patient had primary carcinomatosis and endometrial adenocarcinoma. (B) Free fluid in cul-de-sac. This patient has free fluid in the cul-de-sac in addition to retained products of conception in the uterus. Low-level echoes within the fluid suggest blood or cellular debris.

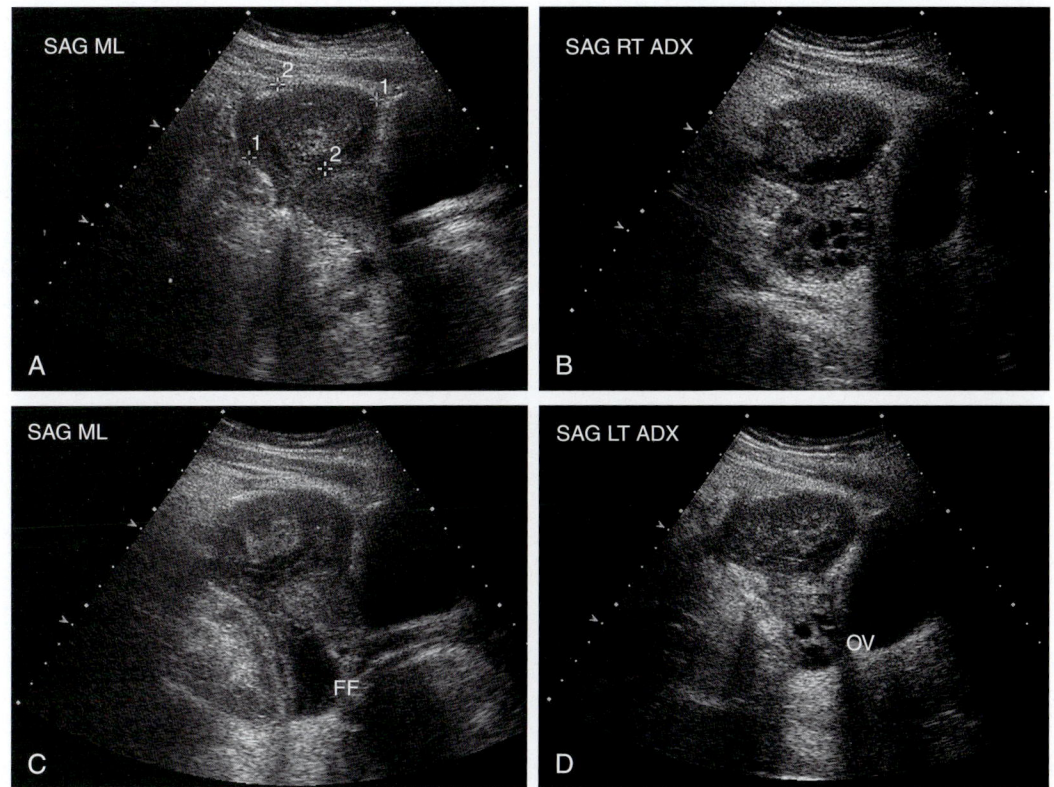

FIG. 45.7 (A) Transabdominal midline sagittal image of the bladder, uterus, and complex mass that is displacing the uterus anteriorly. (B) The scan over the right adnexal area shows the uterus with the right ovary posterior. The bladder is seen inferiorly. (C) The scan over the midline of the pelvis demonstrates the mass posterior to the uterus. Free fluid (FF) is seen adjacent to the complex mass. (D) The scan over the left adnexal area shows the left ovary (OV) and uterus.

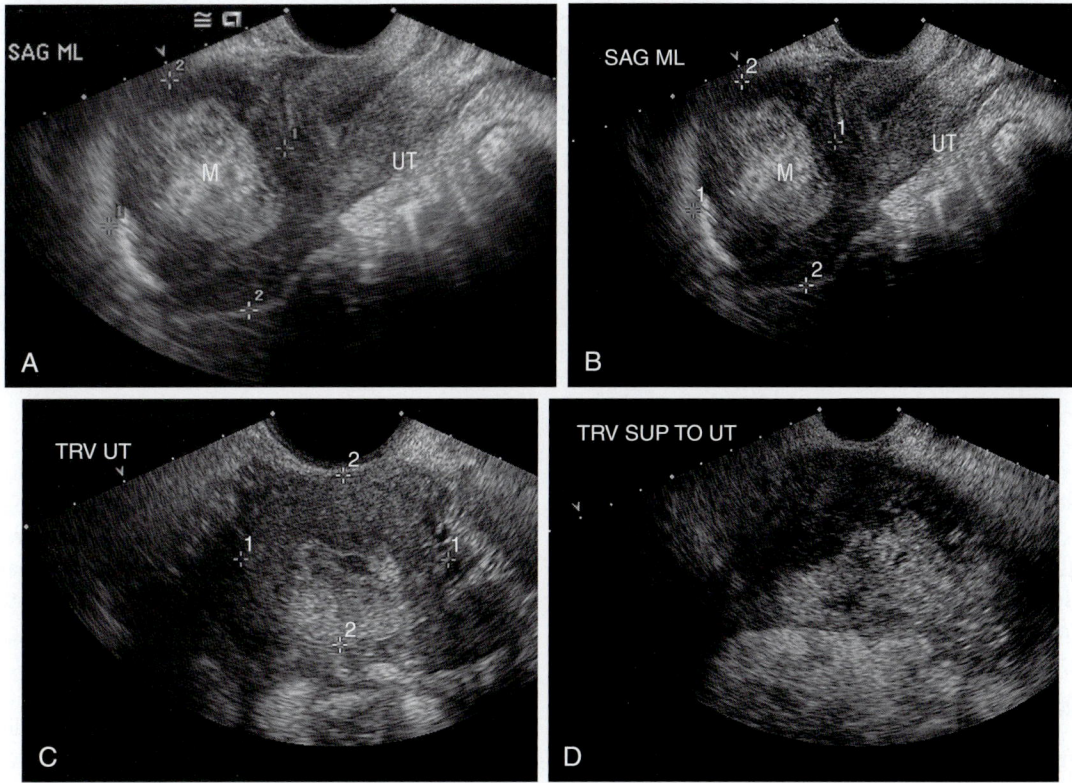

FIG. 45.8 (A) Transvaginal sagittal midline image of the uterus (UT) with a large complex echogenic mass (M) adjacent to the uterine cavity. (B) The complex mass (M) is clearly separate from the uterus (UT). (C) Transvaginal image of the uterus. (D) Transvaginal image superior to the uterine fundus shows the complex mass.

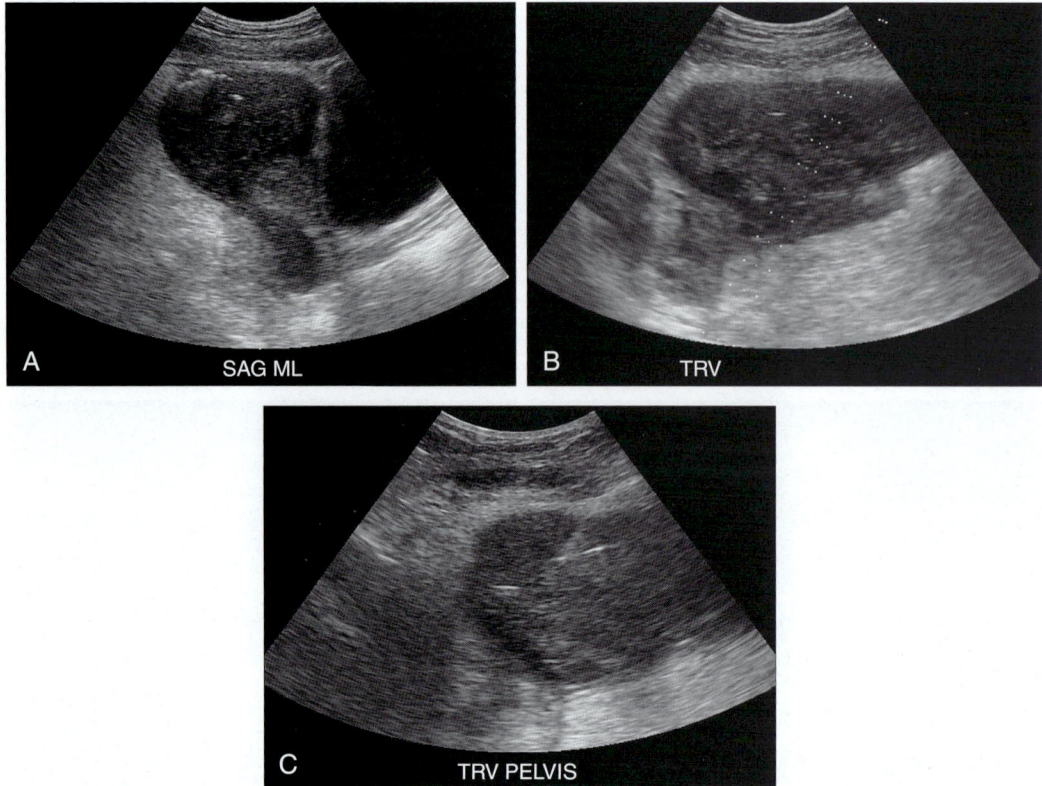

FIG. 45.9 (A) Transabdominal sagittal midline image of the pelvis shows the distended urinary bladder, the complex mass anterior to the uterus. (B) Transabdominal transverse image over the complex mass. (C) A drainage catheter is inserted into the mass.

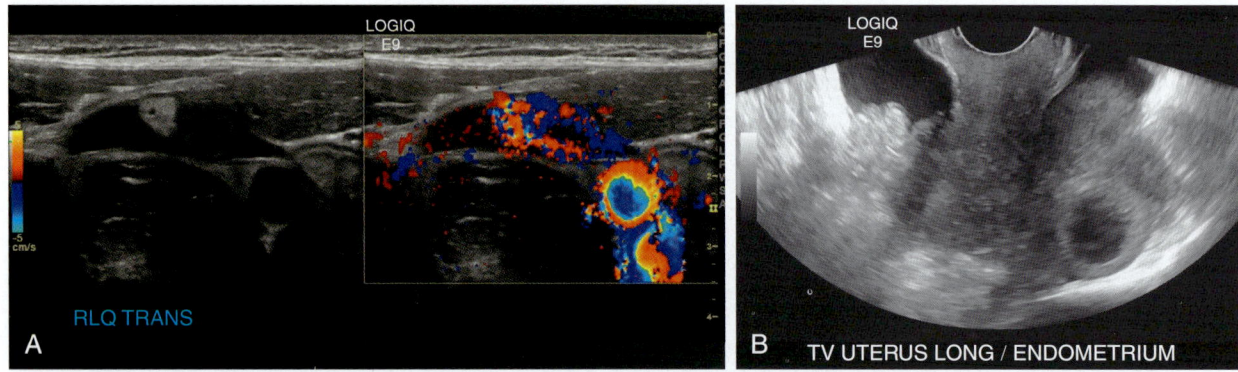

FIG. 45.10 (A) Free fluid associated with acute appendicitis. A moderate amount of free fluid can be seen associated with an inflamed appendix. (B) Free fluid can be seen anterior and posterior to the uterus, secondary to a right ovarian torsion.

well with sonography because the beam is reflected from the area of interest. The sonographer should look for loculated areas of fluid within the pelvis, the paracolic gutters, and mesenteric reflections (Fig. 45.10). Evaluation of the space between the right kidney and liver and the left kidney and spleen should also include a check for fluid.

ENDOMETRITIS

Endometritis, infection of the endometrium, can be divided into obstetric and nonobstetric cases; it can be acute or chronic (Fig. 45.11). Nonobstetric infection is associated with either PID or gynecologic instrumentation. Obstetric cases occur in the immediate postpartum period. Endometritis is the most common cause of fever in the postpartum patient. Postpartum fever is considered a temperature greater than 101°F (38°C) on any 2 of the first 10 days postpartum (excluding the initial 24-hour period). Clinical presentation includes fever, uterine/adnexal tenderness, and bleeding.

Sonographic Findings. On sonography, the endometrium may appear thick; contain fluid, air, or clot; or appear normal (Fig. 45.12). The endometrium is considered normal in size up to 20 mm. A measurement of greater than 20 mm should raise the suspicion of endometritis, hemorrhage, or retained POCs. The risk for endometritis goes up with premature rupture of membranes, retained clot or POCs, and prolonged labor.

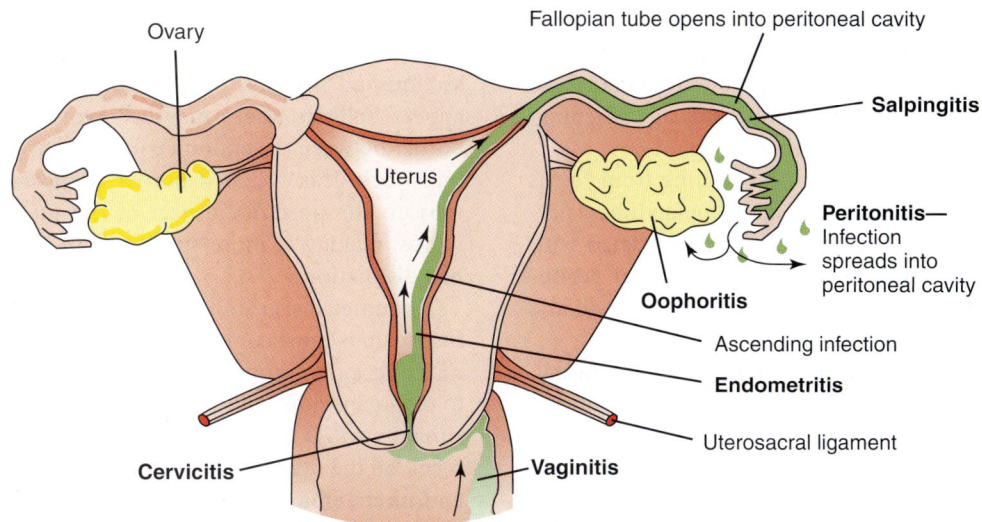

FIG. 45.11 Endometritis, infection of the endometrium, can be divided into obstetric and nonobstetric cases; it can be acute or chronic.

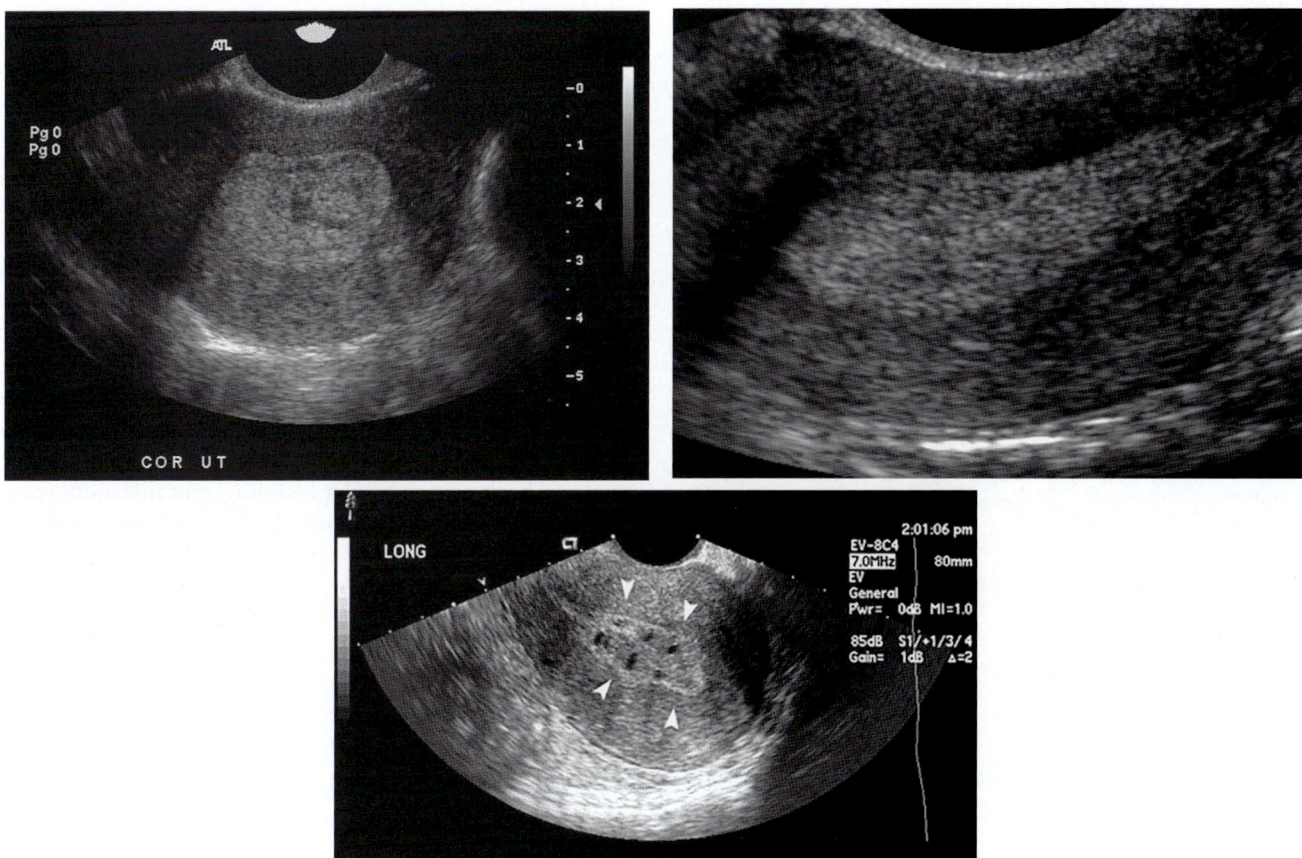

FIG. 45.12 On sonography, the endometrium may appear thick; contain fluid, air, or clot; or appear normal. The endometrium is considered normal in size up to 20 mm. A measurement of >20 mm should raise the suspicion of endometritis, hemorrhage, or retained products of conception.

ENDOMETRIOSIS AND ENDOMETRIOMA

Endometriosis is one of the most common gynecologic diseases. It is defined as the presence of functioning endometrial tissue in abnormal locations. The ectopic tissue can be found almost anywhere in the body, including the ovaries, fallopian tubes, broad ligaments, the external surface of the uterus, and scattered over the peritoneum, bowel, or bladder, especially in the dependent parts of the pelvis or cul-de-sac (Fig. 45.13). The incidence of endometriosis is found in up to

15% of premenopausal women. It affects women in their third to fourth decade of life and is dependent on normal hormonal stimulation. Clinical findings include severe dysmenorrhea, chronic pelvic pain from peritoneal adhesions and bleeding, or dyspareunia (Table 45.2).

The cause may arise from peritoneal seeding from retrograde travel of endometrial cells through fallopian tubes (perhaps through the contractions of the uterus associated with the menstrual cycle), metaplastic transformation of peritoneal epithelium into endometrial tissue, or through traumatic spread from uterine surgery or amniocentesis.

Endometriosis has two forms: internal and external. Internal endometriosis occurs within the uterus (adenomyosis). External endometriosis is outside the uterus and may be found in the pouch of Douglas; surface of the ovary, fallopian tube, and uterus broad ligaments; or rectovaginal septum.

The more common form of endometriosis is the external, or indirect, form. The disease process for the external form varies in extent from small foci to widespread sheets of tissue to focal discrete masses. The endometrial tissue in endometriosis cyclically bleeds and proliferates as stimulated by changes in hormonal influence. Though the true prevalence of endometriosis is unknown (as most cases are asymptomatic), it is estimated that 5.5 million women in North America are currently affected.

The second, less common, form of endometriosis, known as the internal or direct form, is called **adenomyosis**. Endometrial cells begin to grow into the uterine body, invading the junctional zone and the myometrium. The clinical symptoms of adenomyosis are heavy menstrual bleeding, painful menses, and uterine enlargement. Adenomyosis is most common in women who have had uterine surgery, including cesarean section and myomectomy. Sonographically, the uterus may appear bulbous, there may be myometrial "cysts," and the border between the endometrium and myometrium becomes indistinct. This "blurred border" appearance is more common in the posterior aspect of the uterus. Magnetic resonance imaging is more specific than ultrasound in making this distinction.

Endometriosis can be either diffuse or localized. The diffuse form is most common and is rarely diagnosed by sonography because the implants are so small. The diffuse form leads to disorganization of the pelvic anatomy with an appearance similar to PID or chronic ectopic pregnancy. The localized form, on the other hand, consists of a discrete mass called an **endometrioma**, or "chocolate cyst." Patients with endometriomas are usually asymptomatic, and the cysts can frequently be multiple and have a unique sonographic appearance. They may become moderately enlarged and create a surgical emergency by rupturing or causing the ovary to twist on the vessels that supply it and cause torsion.

Two possible explanations for the cause of endometriosis are presented. The first is that the chronic retrograde flow of menstrual fluid through the tubes and into the pelvis may produce implantation and proliferation of endometrial cells with cyclic bleeding. This is the "transtubal migration" theory. The second theory involves the evaluation of endometrial activity in susceptible cells that retain the embryonic capacity to differentiate in response to hormonal stimulation. The resulting tissue bleeds and proliferates with the resultant production of pain, scarring, and endometrium-lined collections of blood known as endometriomas.

Endometriosis may occur in any menstruating female. Clinical symptoms include painful periods (dysmenorrhea) or painful intercourse (dyspareunia); lower abdominal, pelvic, and back pain; irregular bleeding; and infertility secondary to adhesions and fibrosis. Differential diagnosis would include hemorrhagic ovarian cyst, TOA, cystic ovarian neoplasm, solid ovarian tumor, or ectopic pregnancy. Clinically, most women with an acute hemorrhagic cyst or abscess present with acute pelvic pain, whereas women with an endometrioma are asymptomatic or have more chronic discomfort associated with their menses.

Symptoms depend on the location and extent of the disease, but there is no direct relationship between the extent

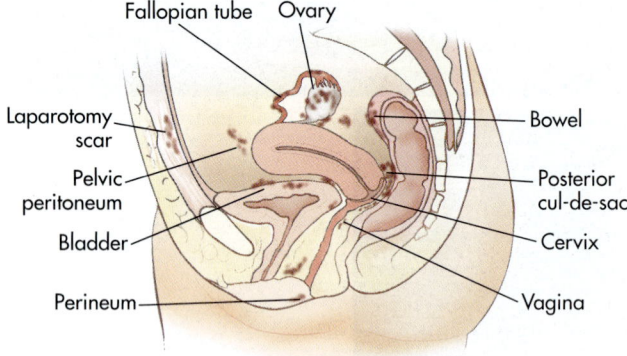

FIG. 45.13 Possible pelvic sites of endometriosis.

TABLE 45.2	Endometriosis	
Description	**Clinical Findings**	**Sonographic Findings**
Presence of functional ectopic endometrial glands and stroma outside the uterine cavity	Not distinctive Complaints of dysmenorrhea with pelvic pain Premenstrual dyspareunia Sacral backache during menses Infertility	Bilateral or unilateral ovarian cysts Cysts are anechoic to solid, depending on amount of blood Ovaries adherent to posterior uterus or in cul-de-sac; difficult to define Obscured organ borders Focal mass is endometrioma ("chocolate cyst") with low-intensity echoes and acoustic enhancement

of disease and severity of symptoms. Patients can be asymptomatic if the condition is confined to the ovaries, or they can suffer severe pain if it is widespread. Although typically associated with infertility, endometriosis may be identified in a pregnant patient by evidence of an endometrioma.

Sonographic Findings. Diffuse endometriosis, the more common form, is rarely detected sonographically unless a focal mass, an endometrioma, is present. Endometriomas may appear as bilateral or unilateral ovarian masses with patterns ranging from anechoic (rare) to solid, depending on the amount of blood and its state of organization (Fig. 45.14). The ovaries typically adhere to the posterior surface of the uterus or are stuck in the cul-de-sac and may be difficult to define. Obscured organ borders and multiple irregular cystic masses are also suggestive of either disseminating cancer or pelvic infection.

An endometrioma often appears as a well-defined, predominantly cystic mass with transabdominal ultrasound, but, with transvaginal ultrasound, uniform internal echoes are usually evident. The most common presentation is termed a *chocolate cyst* because of the presence of low-level echoes (secondary to internal bleeding and organization) and acoustic enhancement. The echogenicity of endometriomas can vary from cystic to solid, and their size varies widely from less than 1 cm to more than 10 cm in diameter. The masses are the result of multiple episodes of bleeding. Fluid-fluid levels and internal septations are frequently noted. Some endometriomas are multiloculated, often with varied internal echo

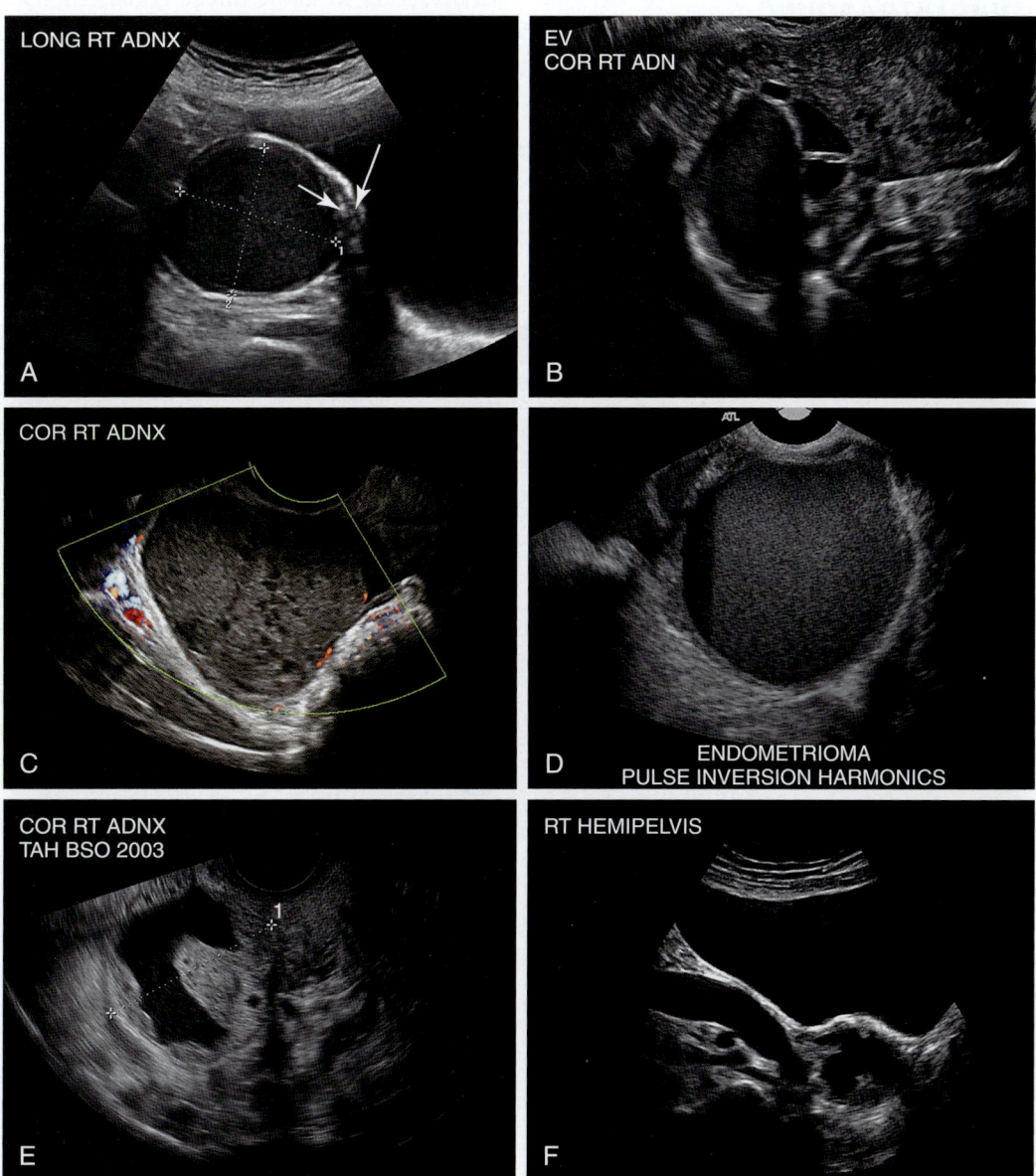

FIG. 45.14 (A) Transvaginal sagittal view of the uterus demonstrates endometrial calcification *(arrows)* with shadowing in a 34-year-old woman with pelvic fullness. (B) The transvaginal coronal image shows a complex mass in the right adnexal area. (C) Color Doppler imaging shows increased flow in the pelvic vessels surrounding the endometrioma. (D) A different patient with a large endometrioma that is completely filled with low-level homogeneous echoes ("chocolate cyst"). Transvaginal coronal image (E) and sagittal transabdominal image (F) of the right adnexa in a patient with a dilated right hydroureter.

patterns and interconnecting loculations. Endometriomas may be multiple and present in both adnexa. Endometriomas can have a similar appearance to inflammation (abscess), trophoblastic tissue (ectopic pregnancy), and dermoids.

Other appearances include an enlarged multicystic ovary with a thick wall and internal septations or a cyst with fluid-debris levels (because of different degrees of organization of the hemorrhage). Small linear hyperechoic foci may be present in the cyst wall and are thought to be caused by cholesterol deposits accumulating in the cyst wall. Endometriomas may also demonstrate microcalcification. Ovarian abscesses or hemorrhagic ovarian cysts may demonstrate sonographic appearances similar to endometriomas; however, the clinical picture is usually different.

INTERVENTIONAL ULTRASOUND

Ultrasound-guided percutaneous biopsy and abscess drainage have become valuable diagnostic and therapeutic procedures (see Chapter 18). Interventional biopsy has also decreased patient costs by obviating the need for surgery and a lengthy hospital stay. Contraindications to needle biopsy include uncorrectable coagulopathy, lack of a safe biopsy route, and an uncooperative patient. A patient's bleeding history can be evaluated with a platelet count, international normalized ratio, prothrombin time, and partial thromboplastin time. Evaluation of the patient's use of aspirin, Coumadin, or heparin should also be used to screen for an increased risk of bleeding. If these values are abnormal, the procedure should be delayed if deemed necessary after consulting with the patient's doctor. Transabdominal or transvaginal guidance is used for aspiration of benign-appearing cysts. Transvaginal drainage is helpful in TOAs; other pelvic abscesses, such as appendicitis and diverticulitis; and drainage of postoperative fluid collections (Fig. 45.15). Transrectal drainage can be used for deep pelvic abscesses. Transvaginal sonography is also used to obtain biopsies for benign and malignant pelvic masses and to drain recurrent malignant collections. Biopsy kits can be used with the transvaginal transducers to allow direct visualization of the region of interest.

Ultrasonically guided needle drainage of abscesses and stable hematomas, either through the abdominal wall or the vagina, is diagnostic and therapeutic. Recurrent tumor masses may be biopsied in a similar fashion. The transvaginal ultrasound and needle guide make entering the anterior or posterior cul-de-sacs safer and easier for pelvic fluid aspiration, biopsies, or radiation needle placement.

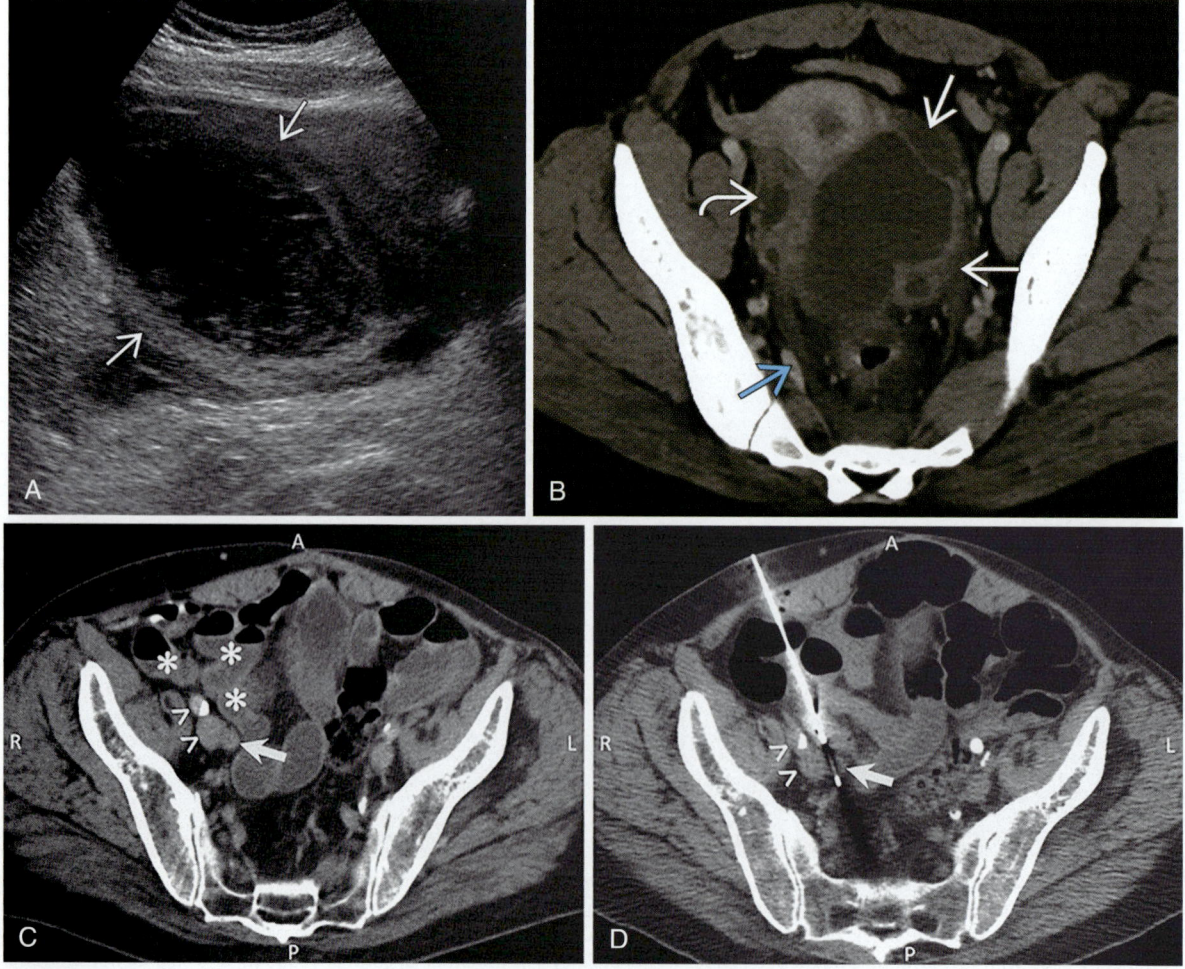

FIG. 45.15 (A) Ultrasound of inflamed fallopian tube. (B) Computed tomographic percutaneous biopsy of tubo-ovarian abscess. (C) The tubo-ovarian abscess is localized prior to the insertion of the needle (D).

POSTOPERATIVE USES OF ULTRASOUND

Pain and the development of a pelvic mass after pelvic surgery can indicate complications, such as postoperative bleeding, hematomas, or abscess formation. Postoperative ultrasound can be used to distinguish a distended bladder from an abnormal fluid collection at the operative site. The ability to palpate specific structures with the transvaginal probe and avoid the abdominal wound is valuable in determining the site of pain in a postoperative pelvis. Resolving hematomas often appear to be of a solid consistency and can be followed as they recede.

An expert combination of transvaginal and transabdominal techniques is essential as new gynecologic applications of ultrasound continue to be found for screening, diagnosis, and therapy of pelvic pathology in a female patient. The inclusion of translabial and the perineal approaches to gynecologic imaging allows another field of view for the sonographer to evaluate the pelvic structures. Three-dimensional imaging will surely add additional understanding of ovarian pathologies.

Key Pearls

- Pelvic inflammatory disease (PID) is caused by sexually transmitted diseases, including gonorrhea and chlamydia. PID can also be caused by a ruptured appendix and peritonitis.
- PID is an inclusive term that refers to all pelvic infections (e.g., endometritis, salpingitis, hydrosalpinx, pyosalpinx, periovarian inflammation, tubo-ovarian complex, and tubo-ovarian abscess).
- Endometriosis is the presence of endometrial glands or stroma in abnormal locations. It occurs most commonly in two forms: adenomyosis of the uterus and endometriosis of the adnexa.
- Sexually transmitted PID is spread via the mucosa of the pelvic organs through the cervix into the uterine endometrium (endometritis) and out the fallopian tubes (acute salpingitis) to the area of the ovaries and peritoneum.
- An obstructed tube filled with serous secretions is a hydrosalpinx; this can occur due to PID, endometriosis, or postoperative adhesions.
- If the dilated tube becomes infected, it is called pyosalpinx.
- The adhesive, edematous, and inflamed serosa may adhere to the ovary and/or other peritoneal surfaces, which distorts anatomy. As the infection worsens, periovarian adhesions may form. The ovary cannot be separated from the inflamed dilated tube and is called the tubo-ovarian complex.
- Peritonitis is the inflammation of the peritoneum, the serous membrane lining the abdominal cavity and covering the viscera.
- Endometritis is the most common cause of fever in the postpartum patient.
- An endometrioma often appears as a well-defined, predominantly cystic mass with transabdominal ultrasound, but, with transvaginal ultrasound, uniform internal echoes are usually evident.

BIBLIOGRAPHY

American College of Radiography. ACR Appropriateness Criteria for Diagnostic Imaging: Acute Pelvic Pain in the Reproductive Age Group. 2015. www.acr.org.

Asch E, Levin D. Variations in appearance of endometriomas. *J Ultrasound Med Q*. 2007;26:993–1002.

Benjaminov O, Atri M. Sonography of the abnormal fallopian tube. *Am J Roentgenol*. 2004;183(3):737–742.

Burney RO, Giuduce LC. Pathogenesis and pathophysiology of endometriosis. *Fertil Steril*. 2012;98:511–519.

Cacciatore B, Leminen A, Ingman-Friberg S, et al. Transvaginal sonographic findings in ambulatory patients with suspected pelvic inflammatory disease. *Obstet Gynecol*. 1992;80:912–916.

Callen P. *Ultrasonography in obstetrics and gynecology*. ed 6. Philadelphia: Elsevier; 2017.

Chamie LP, Blasbalg R, Pereira RM, et al. Findings of pelvic endometriosis at transvaginal US, MR imaging and laparoscopy. *Radiographics*. 2011;31(4):E77–E100.

Cicchiello LA, Hamper UM, Scoutt LM. Ultrasound evaluation of gynecologic causes of pelvic pain. *Obstet Gynecol Clin North Am*. 2011;38:85–114.

Guidice LC. Endometriosis. *N Engl J Med*. 2010;362(25):2389–2398.

Haggerty CL, Ness RB. Diagnosis and treatment of pelvic inflammatory disease. *Women's Health*. 2008;4:383–397.

Horrow MM, Rodgers SK, Naqvi S. Ultrasound of pelvic inflammatory disease. *Ultrasound Clin*. 2007;2(2):297–309.

Koninckx PR, Ussia A, Adamyan L, et al. Deep endometriosis: definition, diagnosis, and treatment. *Fertil Steril*. 2012;98:564–571.

Patel MD, Feldstein VA, Chen DC, et al. Endometriomas: diagnostic performance of US. *Radiology*. 1999;210:739–745.

Rezvani M, Shaaban AM. Fallopian tube disease in the nonpregnant patient. *Radiographics*. 2011;31(2):527–548.

Soper DE. Pelvic inflammatory disease. *Obstet Gynecol*. 2010;116:419–428.

Timor-Tritsch IE, Lerner JP, Monteagudo A, et al. Transvaginal sonographic markers of tubal inflammatory disease. *Ultrasound Obstet Gynecol*. 1998;12:56–66.

# CHAPTER 46

Role of Ultrasound in Evaluating Female Infertility

Carol Mitchell, Barbara Trampe, and Dan Lebovic

OBJECTIVES

On completion of this chapter, you should be able to:
- Define *infertility* and list its treatment options
- List the female pelvic organs to be imaged in an infertility workup
- State anatomic variations or pathologies that need to be defined when imaging an infertility patient
- List complications that may occur because of infertility treatments

OUTLINE

Evaluating the Cervix 1272
Evaluating the Uterus 1273
    Congenital Uterine Anomalies 1273
Evaluating the Endometrium 1274
Evaluating the Fallopian Tubes 1275
Evaluating the Ovaries 1276

Peritoneal Factors 1277
Treatment Options 1277
    Ovulation Induction Therapy 1277
    Monitoring the Endometrium 1277
    In Vitro Fertilization and Embryo Transfer 1278
    Intrauterine Insemination 1278

Complications Associated With Assisted Reproductive Technology 1278

KEY TERMS

Assisted reproductive technology (ART)
Embryo transfer
Human chorionic gonadotropin (hCG)

Intrauterine insemination
In vitro fertilization (IVF)
Ovarian hyperstimulation syndrome (OHSS)

Ovulation induction therapy
Subfertility

Ultrasound has come to play an important role in the management and guidance of treatment for the infertile patient. By definition, infertility is the inability to conceive within 12 months with regular coitus (or within 6 months for those 35 years or older).[1,2] It is estimated that infertility affects 1 in 7 couples in America. Approximately 30% of infertility cases are attributable to the male or female alone, and the remaining 40% are combined male/female or unexplained factors.[2] Infertility can be grouped into cervical, endometrial/uterine, tubal, ovulatory, peritoneal, and male factor causes.[3] Male factor causes of infertility are an inadequate number of motile sperm (5th percentile, 10 million) and decreased motility of sperm, obstruction of the spermatic ducts or vas deferens, and scrotal varicoceles. This chapter focuses on female factors, including discussing cervical, uterine/endometrial, tubal, ovulatory, and peritoneal causes of infertility.

As reproductive technologies continue to advance, it is important for the sonographer to be aware of the different treatment plans and the role that ultrasound plays in evaluating the infertile patient because many of these patients will come to the ultrasound appointment very knowledgeable about their procedures. The sonographer should be compassionate toward each patient's situation.

EVALUATING THE CERVIX

The role of the cervix in fertility is to provide a nonhostile environment to harbor sperm.[3] The cervix does this with glands that secrete mucus and crypts that hold the sperm. Ultrasound can evaluate the cervical length during pregnancy to assess for cervical incompetence. However, in the nongravid uterus, both the length of and any opening in the cervix are difficult to assess. Hysterosalpingography (HSG) can be used to evaluate the internal os diameter. A diameter less than 1 mm by HSG may indicate cervical stenosis.[3] Nabothian cysts within the cervix can appear demonstrable but rarely, if ever, play a role in **subfertility**. Subfertility is a condition in which pregnancy can be conceived without medical intervention but may take longer than average to achieve.

EVALUATING THE UTERUS

When evaluating the uterus of the infertility patient, the sonographer has two main objectives: (1) to assess the structural anatomy and (2) to assess the endometrium. Assessing for structural anatomy refers to evaluating the uterine shape (i.e., unicolis, bicornuate, congenital malformations) (Fig. 46.1) and evaluating echogenicity. Is the uterus uniform in echogenicity? Are there any masses suggestive of submucosal fibroids that may impede implantation of the fertilized egg (Fig. 46.2)? When assessing the endometrium, the sonographer wants to evaluate the endometrial stripe thickness and echogenicity characteristics and any intracavitary lesions.

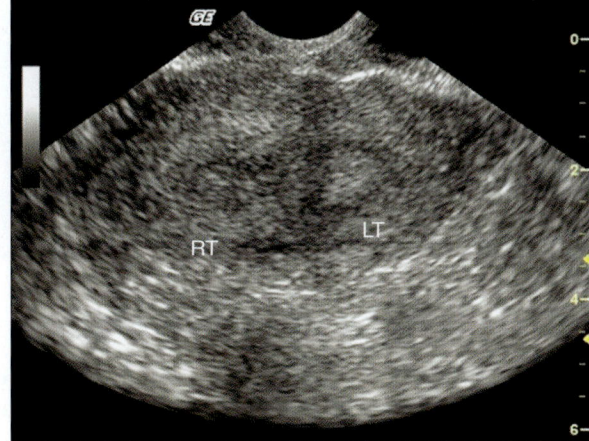

FIG. 46.1 Bicornuate uterus. *LT,* Left; *RT,* right.

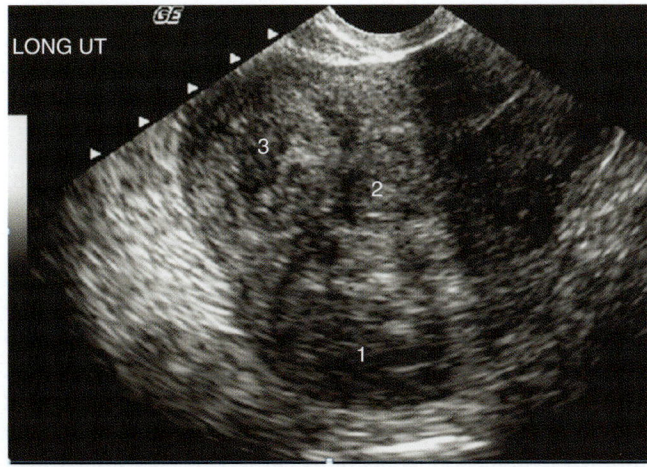

FIG. 46.2 Longitudinal transvaginal image of the uterus with multiple fibroids *(1, 2, 3).*

Congenital Uterine Anomalies

It is estimated that congenital uterine anomalies occur in 6.7% of women in the general fertile population.[4,5] Congenital uterine anomalies result from defects in müllerian duct development, fusion, or resorption and are associated with renal anomalies except for arcuate or septate uteri. Although nine descriptive terms[6,7] are used to describe uterine anomalies, this chapter discusses only those that ultrasound is best suited to evaluate. The congenital anomalies most easily assessed with ultrasound are a septate or bicornuate uterus and uterus didelphys. Although these three entities are difficult to accurately confirm with ultrasound, ultrasound is good at depicting the two endometrial interfaces in the transverse plane. This finding should alert the sonographer to further evaluate the pelvic anatomy for two versus one cervix and vagina. Didelphys or bicornuate uterus is associated with a higher rate of fertility complications such as fetal malposition, preterm labor/delivery, and miscarriage.

A uterine anomaly associated with a high incidence of infertility is the septate uterus. This congenital anomaly presents with two uterine cavities and a single fundus. In this case, the septum presumably causes a problem for implantation. If the pregnancy implants along the septum, the pregnancy may be at an increased risk of failure because of inadequate blood supply from the septum. For these patients, the septum can be removed hysteroscopically to improve implantation and fertility success (no nonrandomized trial published to date), so this is an important diagnosis to make and offer counseling on surgical management.

On ultrasound, the septate uterus appears as two endometrial cavities without a fundal notch compared with the bicornuate and didelphys uterus, which have two endometrial cavities, a wide uterine body, and a fundal notch (see Fig. 46.1). The septate uterus should not be confused with a uterine cavity filled with myomatous tumors, as shown in Fig. 46.2.

The T-shaped uterus is another uterine anomaly to evaluate. This congenital anomaly is caused by exposure to diethylstilbestrol in utero. Diethylstilbestrol was a medication given to women to treat for threatened abortion from 1950 to 1970. The T-shaped uterus also is at risk for cervical incompetence, and there is no treatment known for this type of congenital anomaly. Because many uteruses imaged will not fit completely into one of these categories, the anatomy needs to be described as thoroughly as possible and may not be given a label immediately. Magnetic resonance imaging and HSG are other imaging methods that may be offered to better evaluate the wide range of uterine anomalies.

Three-dimensional ultrasound imaging allows the coronal plane to be viewed. The coronal plane has afforded a diagnostic opportunity that two-dimensional imaging was unable to obtain. Fig. 46.3 demonstrates the standard two-dimensional images of a septate uterus as well as the three-dimensional coronal plane. Note that in the coronal plane, the diagnosis of septate uterus becomes apparent. Three-dimensional ultrasound imaging can offer images of the uterine contour and

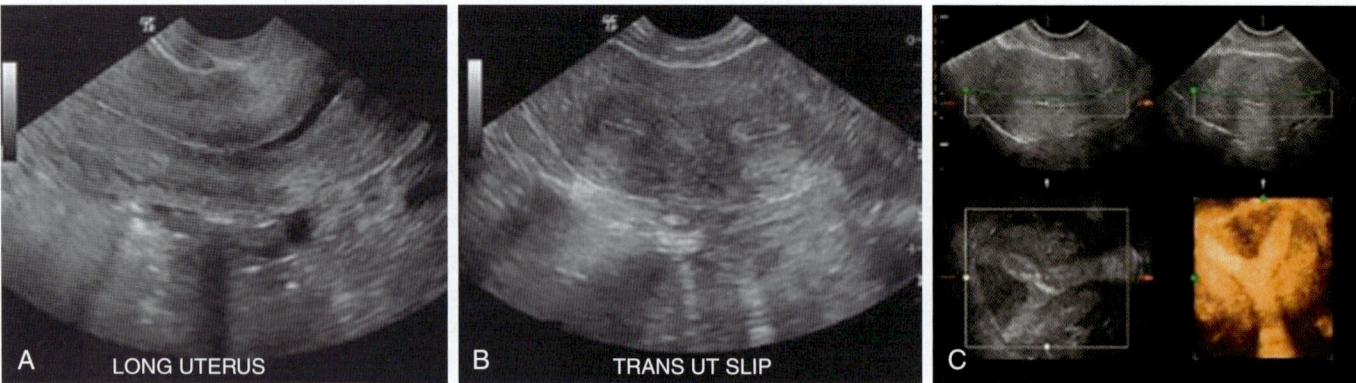

FIG. 46.3 (A) Longitudinal image of the uterus. (B) Transverse image of the uterus. (C) Three-dimensional reconstruction of the same patient demonstrating a septate uterus.

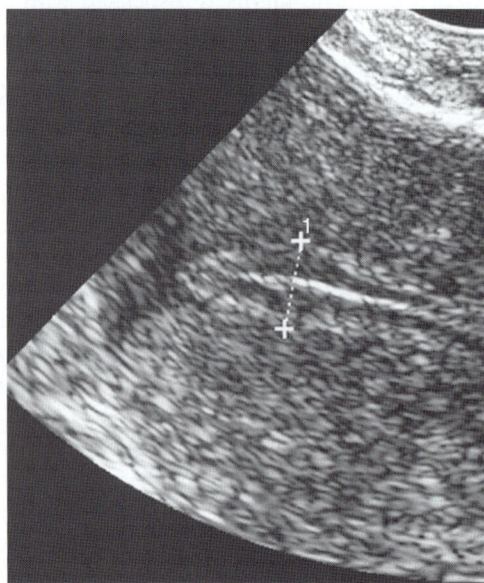

FIG. 46.4 Longitudinal image of the proliferative endometrium.

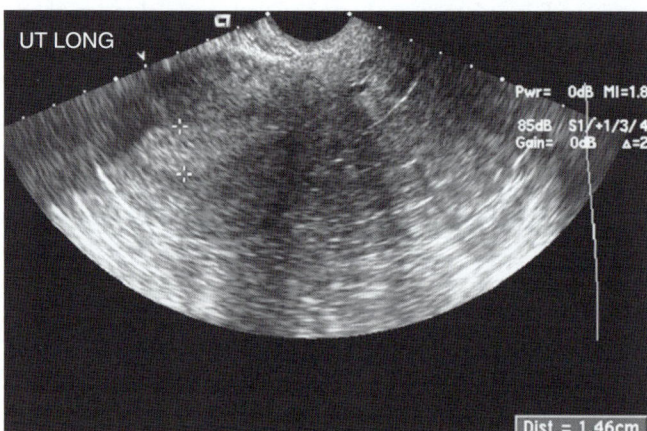

FIG. 46.5 Longitudinal image of the secretory endometrium.

the entire endometrial cavity that are on par with the diagnostic accuracy of magnetic resonance imaging to diagnose müllerian anomalies.[4,8,9]

EVALUATING THE ENDOMETRIUM

The endometrium can be measured throughout the menstrual cycle to look for appropriate changes.[10] The endometrial lining encompasses the thickness of both anterior and posterior endometrial layers in the sagittal plane. During the first half of the menstrual cycle, the mucosa begins to proliferate because of increasing estrogen levels. On ultrasound examination, the proliferative endometrial phase is seen as a triple line sign consisting of the hypoechoic mucosa and the echogenic interface where they meet in the central plane of the uterus (Fig. 46.4). After ovulation, progesterone is secreted by the corpus luteum. This secretion of progesterone begins the secretory phase of the endometrial cycle. During the secretory phase, the endometrium becomes thickened and very echogenic due to stromal edema, and there is loss of the triple line sign (Fig. 46.5). A thickness of at least 6 mm appears to represent a central threshold for achieving pregnancy.[11] If not enough progesterone is produced in the luteal phase, the endometrial lining may be thinner than expected on ultrasound evaluation. This lack of progesterone production has been referred to as "luteal phase deficiency" (LPD), although this entity itself causing infertility has not been substantiated. Moreover, there is no reproducible, clinically accepted standard to diagnose LPD to differentiate fertile from infertile women. The endometrial appearance/thickness has particular importance when monitoring for infertility treatment with subsequent embryo transfer.[12]

Other things that can make the endometrium appear irregular or more echogenic than normal are submucosal fibroids, polyps, and adhesions. Saline infusion sonography (SIS) can be used in these situations to further delineate the anatomic structure of the endometrium. SIS can demonstrate fibroids and polyps by outlining the endometrial cavity.[13] Fibroids tend to have a broad base and are more isoechoic to the uterine myometrium. They also tend to have circumferential flow around them (Figs. 46.6 and Fig. 46.7). Polyps tend to have a uniform hyperechoic appearance, a narrow base attachment to the endometrium (a stalk), and a vascular pedicle feeding them (Fig. 46.8). Fibroids and polyps can potentially impede

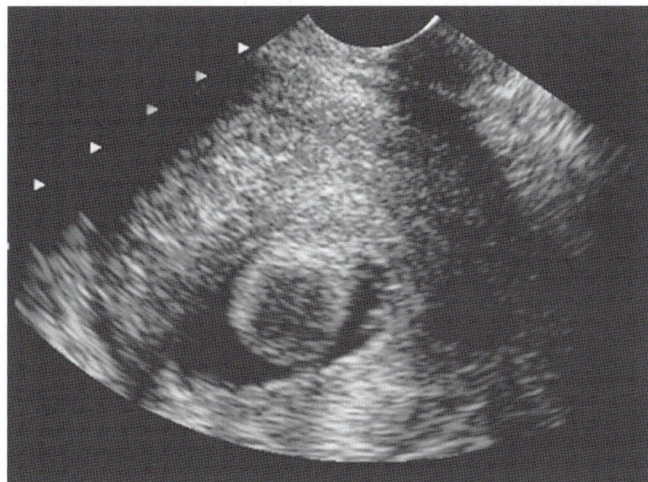

FIG. 46.6 Submucosal fibroid with saline infusion sonography.

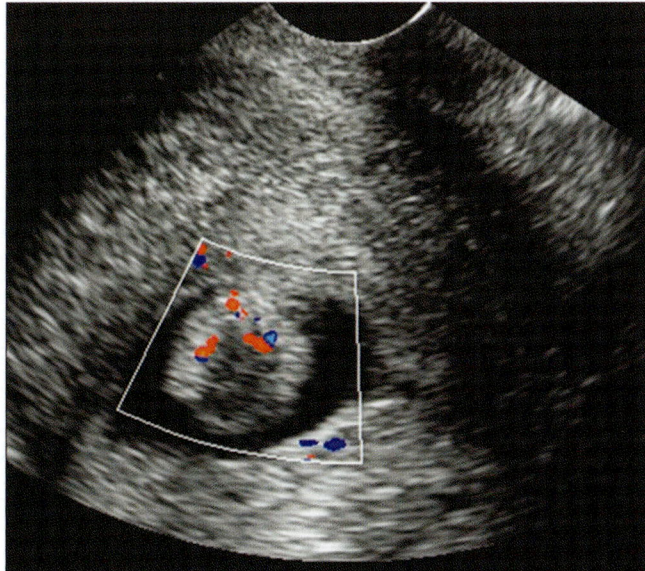

FIG. 46.7 Submucosal fibroid with saline infusion sonography and color Doppler showing circumferential flow.

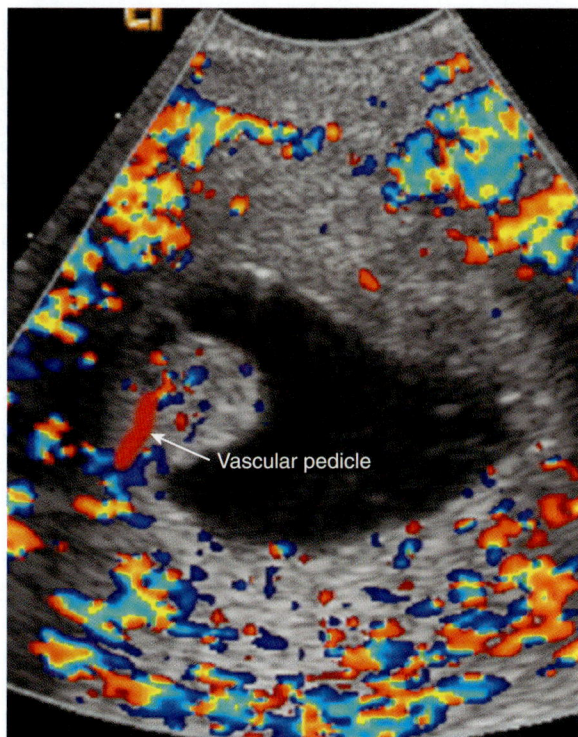

FIG. 46.8 Polyp with saline infusion sonography; color Doppler shows the vascular pedicle.

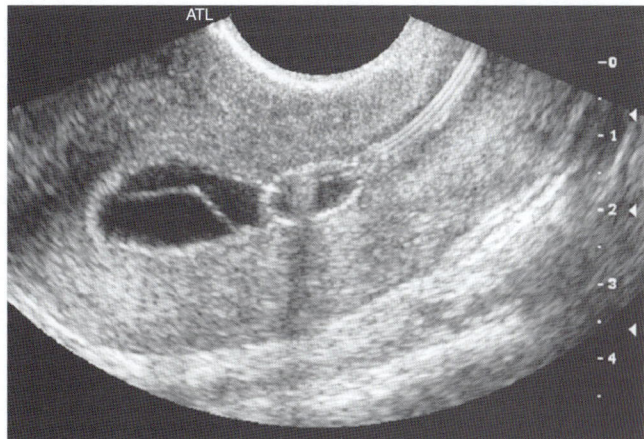

FIG. 46.9 Uterine synechia with saline infusion sonography.

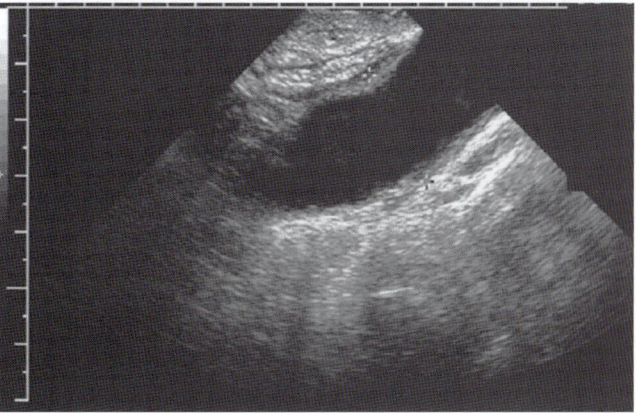

FIG. 46.10 Hydrosalpinx.

implantation, and therefore if found, they can be removed to enhance fertility. SIS can also be used to evaluate the uterine cavity for synechiae, which are scars or adhesions from uterine trauma and/or infections (Fig. 46.9). Synechiae are typically seen on ultrasound as linear strands of tissue extending from one wall of the uterine cavity to the other.[14]

EVALUATING THE FALLOPIAN TUBES

The fallopian tubes can be examined by ultrasound[15] for hydrosalpinx and to assess patency. A hydrosalpinx is a fallopian tube containing fluid (Fig. 46.10). On ultrasound, this appears as multiple cystic tubular structures in the adnexa. Hydrosalpinx is associated with a 50% reduction in pregnancy rate and a doubling of the spontaneous miscarriage rate. Removing such damaged tubes can dramatically improve in vitro fertilization (IVF) success. Tubal patency is assessed by injecting saline mixed with air to produce bubbles instilled into the tube and looking for spillage of such echogenic fluid into the cul-de-sac or using contrast to evaluate for spillage. Before performing a saline or contrast study of the fallopian tubes, it is recommended that the sonographer perform a transvaginal ultrasound to assess pelvic anatomy. The transvaginal examination allows the sonographer to see where the ovaries are in relation to the uterus and to assess for mobility of the tube and ovary. This is done by using probe pressure and hand palpation of the lower abdomen. After performing the transvaginal ultrasound, an SIS is recommended to evaluate the structure of the endometrial cavity. Because of the expense of contrast imaging, most centers prefer to start with a saline injection to evaluate a tube patency and then, if it is indeterminate, move on to air instillation or contrast imaging. Ideally, a catheter is placed in the cervical canal to perform a saline infusion assessment of the fallopian tube. At this point, the catheter's balloon tip is inflated with the minimal amount of saline required to maintain its location. Afterward, and with the vaginal transducer in place, 10 to 30 mL of sterile saline is injected to assess for patency. If saline is inconclusive, air can be injected to induce echogenic bubbles. The approximate position of the fallopian tube will be between the ovary and the cornu. The sonographer is looking for spillage of saline or air around the ovary or into the posterior cul-de-sac. If this is seen, patency is inferred. If no spillage is noted and the patient complains of pain during injection, it may be because the tube is blocked. Obstruction of the fallopian tube can be caused by adhesions or transient muscle spasm within the proximal tube.

Before the use of ultrasound to assess for patency, there were two nonsurgical methods: the Rubin's test and HSG. The Rubin's test involves insufflation of the fallopian tube with carbon dioxide gas, and HSG involves inserting a catheter through the cervix and then injecting contrast medium to assess the uterine cavity and fallopian tube anatomy under fluoroscopic imaging. A surgical method used to evaluate the fallopian tubes is laparoscopic chromopertubation.

EVALUATING THE OVARIES

During the ovarian follicular phase, several antral follicles in the ovary are less than 5 mm in diameter (Fig. 46.11).

A follicle is selected to develop into a dominant follicle in response to follicle-stimulating hormone (FSH). The dominant follicle will grow at a rate of approximately 1 to 3 mm/day until it reaches an average diameter of 22 mm (Fig. 46.12). Luteinizing hormone (LH) rises just before ovulation and can also be found in the patient's urine and is the hormone detected in ovulation predictor kits. Once a follicle reaches a mean diameter of 22 mm, the dominant follicle will rupture. Rupture may be associated with an increase or decrease in size. Sonographic findings associated with ovulation are echoes within the fluid left behind (corpus luteum cyst) or free fluid in the peritoneal cavity. However, the best predictor of ovulation is a serum progesterone level of at least 3 ng/mL.

One condition that can inhibit the release of FSH and LH is polycystic ovary syndrome (PCOS). PCOS often occurs with the diagnostic triad of (1) oligoovulation, (2) hyperandrogenism, and (3) polycystic ovaries. With PCOS, follicles begin to grow but do not develop normally. In this syndrome, the immature follicles continue to produce estrogen and androgen. This production of estrogen and androgen inhibits the pituitary gland's function and prevents normal ovulation. This is due to the pituitary gland producing more LH than FSH, which causes the follicles to remain in an arrested state of development, leading to no mature oocyte being released. Women with PCOS may often present with irregular bleeding and a thickened endometrium due to the chronic exposure to estrogen. Because of the chronic elevations of androgens, some women may reveal hirsutism.[3]

Sonographic Findings. A polycystic appearing ovary typically presents as a round ovary with multiple (≥25) small immature follicles on the periphery.[16] Usually, these follicles are 2 to 9 mm in diameter. This sonographic finding has been described as the "string of pearls" sign (Fig. 46.13), with the periphery of the ovary representing the neck and the multiple small cysts around the outside representing a string of pearls. When evaluating for PCOS, transvaginal sonography is the preferred method and is more sensitive for detecting this syndrome.[17]

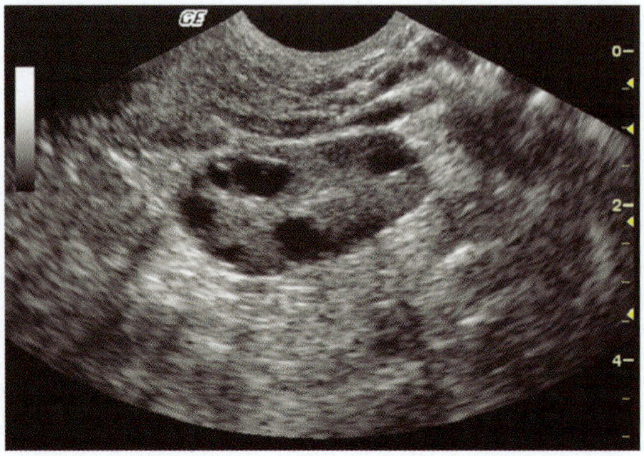

FIG. 46.11 Ovarian follicular phase.

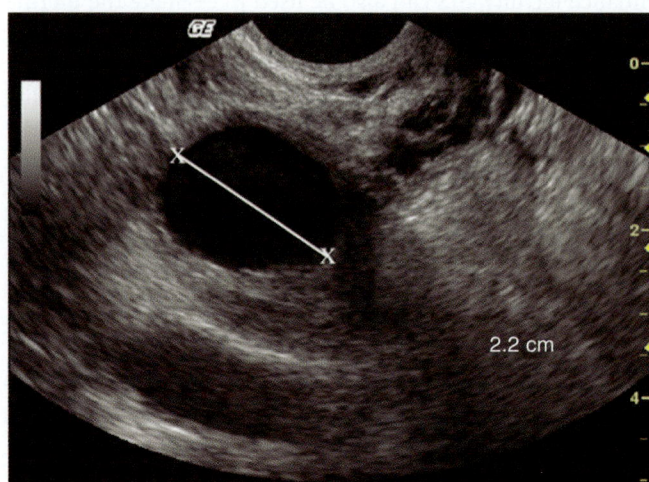

FIG. 46.12 Dominant follicle.

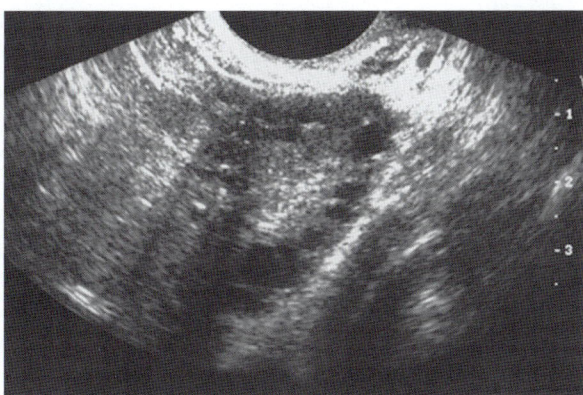

FIG. 46.13 Polycystic ovary and the "string of pearls" sign.

PERITONEAL FACTORS

Peritoneal factors may cause as many as 10% to 13% of infertility cases.[2] Peritoneal factors include adhesions and endometriosis. Adhesions are bands of scar tissue that can obstruct the fimbriated end of the fallopian tube. Sometimes fluid will collect in between these adhesions, resulting in a peritoneal inclusion cyst. Endometriosis is caused by the ectopic placement of endometrial tissue outside the uterus. A common site of endometriosis is the ovaries, and often there is additional peritoneal disease. The gold standard for evaluating pelvic adhesions and endometriosis is laparoscopy.[3]

Endometriosis involving the ovary can lead to the formation of endometriomas, which are blood-filled cysts with endometrial tissue lining the cyst wall. They range in size from smaller than 1 cm to larger than 10 cm on rare occasions. Endometriomas typically have a characteristic sonographic appearance with homogeneous low-amplitude internal echoes. Ultrasound is 93% sensitive and 96% specific for diagnosing endometriomas.[18]

TREATMENT OPTIONS

Ovulation Induction Therapy

Ovulation induction therapy is a treatment in which ovarian stimulation is achieved in a controlled setting. The first step in this process is to obtain a baseline transvaginal ultrasound of the ovaries to rule out an ovarian cyst and assess for the presence of a dominant follicle. If a cyst measuring greater than 15 mm is detected, it could represent persistent follicular activity that could interfere with response to ovarian stimulation medication. The presence of follicular activity may be further evaluated by correlating the sonographic findings with serum estradiol levels. If serum estradiol is elevated and a large ovarian cyst is present, oral contraceptives may be indicated to suppress further follicular activity before starting ovarian stimulation therapy or simply waiting for the subsequent menstrual cycle. This is also an optimal time to assess for any intracavitary masses (polyp, fibroid) because the lining of the uterus is usually at its thinnest during the early proliferative phase.

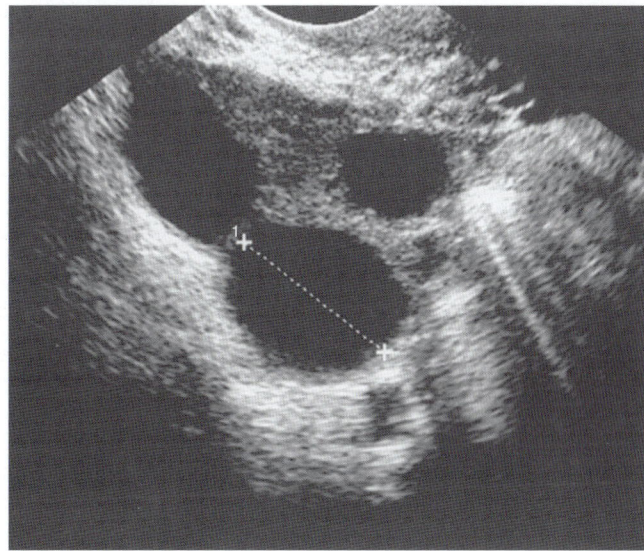

FIG. 46.14 Enlargement of multiple ovarian follicles.

Ovulation induction therapy is usually accomplished by administering oral clomiphene citrate (Clomid), oral aromatase inhibitors (e.g., letrozole), or injectable human menopausal gonadotropins. The administration of these medications is expected to result in the enlargement of multiple follicles compared with a single dominant follicle from a naturally occurring menstrual cycle. Once therapy has started, ultrasound monitors the number and size of follicles, typically during days 10 to 14 (follicular phase) of the menstrual cycle. When evaluating the number and size of follicles, the sonographer must count and measure all follicles greater than 1 cm in longitudinal and transverse planes (Fig. 46.14). The optimal mean measurement of a mature follicle is 20 mm.[19,20] During this time, though not essential, ultrasound can be correlated with the serum estradiol levels to determine whether the follicular growth corresponds with adequate estradiol (E2) production. Correctly measuring the follicles is important because **human chorionic gonadotropin (hCG)**, a substitute for LH, may need to be given subcutaneously to trigger ovulation.

One method of evaluating ovarian reserve (decrease in quantity of the ovarian follicle pool) is a sonographic antral follicle count (AFC).[20,21] During the early follicular phase of the menstrual cycle, the numbers of follicles sized 2 to 6 mm from both ovaries are added to give a total AFC. High AFC values generally represent an abundance of antral follicles and thus predict a vigorous response to hormonal induction, whereas low AFC values (less than 5) foreshadow lower pregnancy rates.

Monitoring the Endometrium

The endometrium is also evaluated during ovarian stimulation by assessing the thickness and echogenicity pattern of the endometrial cavity. A normal endometrial response associated with ovarian stimulation is an increasing thickness from 2 to 3 mm to 12 to 14 mm. To measure the endometrial thickness, the sonographer should image the uterus transvaginally

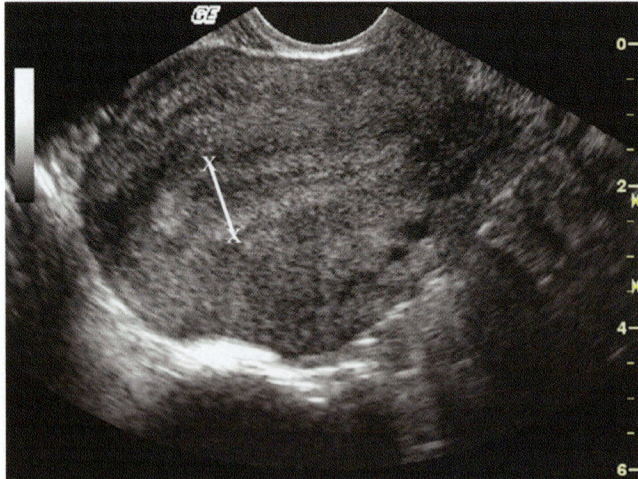

FIG. 46.15 Endometrial measurement.

and in the longitudinal/sagittal plane. Calipers should measure from the anterior endometrial interface to the posterior endometrial interface (Fig. 46.15). This is referred to as the *double-layer thickness*. Also important to evaluate is the echogenicity pattern. A normal pattern is trilaminar. This would be similar to the echographic pattern of the periovulatory endometrium. A thin endometrium (less than 6 mm in diameter) and an abnormal echographic pattern have been associated with decreased fertility.

In Vitro Fertilization and Embryo Transfer

In vitro fertilization (IVF) is a method of fertilizing the human oocyte outside the body. Mature oocytes are collected and mixed in a dish with a sample of sperm. The resulting embryo(s) is then placed into the uterine cavity. The treatment plan for IVF consists of ovarian monitoring, needle aspiration of oocytes, incubation of oocytes, fertilization, and transferring the embryo(s) into the uterus. The ovarian monitoring is performed as described in the ovarian induction therapy section but with greater assertiveness, with one difference: instead of evaluating for two optimal follicles, several follicles are identified before triggering final oocyte maturation with hCG. Oocyte retrieval is accomplished by transvaginal ultrasound guidance.

Transvaginal sonography is used as a guide to locate the ovaries and provide easy access to the follicles containing oocytes. The transvaginal transducer is covered with a protective sheath (e.g., transducer cover), and the needle guide is attached. Sterile gel should be placed inside the tip of the protective sheath. If using an ultrasound machine with needle guide software, the sonographer turns on the needle guide function. This function shows a stippled line where the needle will go in relation to the image. Once the transducer is prepared, it is inserted into the vagina and the ovary imaged. A 35-cm, 17-gauge echotip needle is placed in the guide and introduced transvaginally following the outlined needle path, and under ultrasound imaging, one will see the needle tip go into the desired follicle. Some centers prefer using a scored needle tip, which is more easily seen on ultrasound.

Once the needle tip is in the follicle, the fluid in the follicle is aspirated with the intention that the oocyte is within this aspirate. Occasionally the ovum may be stuck to a wall; some clinicians may use a buffer solution injected into the follicle to flush out the cavity. The solution is then reaspirated to maximize the potential for ovum retrieval.

Once the oocytes are retrieved, they are fertilized in a dish and incubated for a few days before embryo transfer into the uterus. **Embryo transfer** is done by transabdominal ultrasound guidance with a full bladder serving as a fluid-filled interface between the probe and uterine lining. Ultrasound is first used to map the endometrial cavity. This can be done by using the trace function on the ultrasound machine and tracing the endometrial interface from the cervix to the apex of the fundus to determine the length of the uterine cavity. Optimal placement of the embryo is considered to be within 2 cm of the apex of the fundal region of the endometrium, so the clinician needs to know the length of the uterine cavity to ensure proper placement of the embryo. After the endometrium is mapped, using transabdominal ultrasound guidance, a catheter is inserted through the cervix and placed within 2 cm of the fundus of the uterine cavity. The embryo is then released, and a transfer air bubble is often visible on ultrasound after the embryo is released from the catheter. After embryo transfer, the catheter is checked under a stereomicroscope to ensure that all embryos have been transferred.

Intrauterine Insemination

Intrauterine insemination is a technique used to treat male factor or unexplained infertility. With intrauterine insemination, a catheter containing washed sperm is placed into the uterine fundus. The sperm preparation may be from a donor, and this is referred to as donor insemination. Ultrasound is rarely used to guide this procedure.

COMPLICATIONS ASSOCIATED WITH ASSISTED REPRODUCTIVE TECHNOLOGY

Complications associated with **assisted reproductive technology (ART)** include **ovarian hyperstimulation syndrome (OHSS)**, multiple gestations, and ectopic pregnancy. OHSS is a syndrome that presents sonographically as enlarged ovaries (5 to 10 cm) with multiple cysts, abdominal ascites, and in severe cases, pleural effusions, leg edema, hypotension, and polycythemia (Fig. 46.16). This syndrome is often seen in younger patients who have undergone aggressive superovulation induction. This syndrome is more common in patients with a history of PCOS and can be graded based on patient symptoms. In mild cases of OHSS, patients complain of lower abdominal pain and back pain.

Patients who undergo in vitro fertilization are at an increased risk for having multiple gestations. It is estimated that about 30% of in vitro fertilization pregnancies result in a multiple gestation. The concern with multiple gestations is that if there are two or more fetuses, there is an increased risk of fetal or neonatal morbidity and mortality.

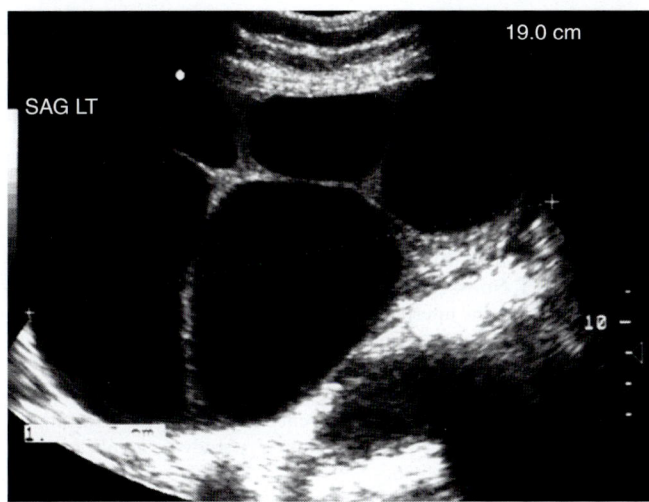

FIG. 46.16 Enlarged ovary with multiple cysts in a patient with ovarian hyperstimulation syndrome.

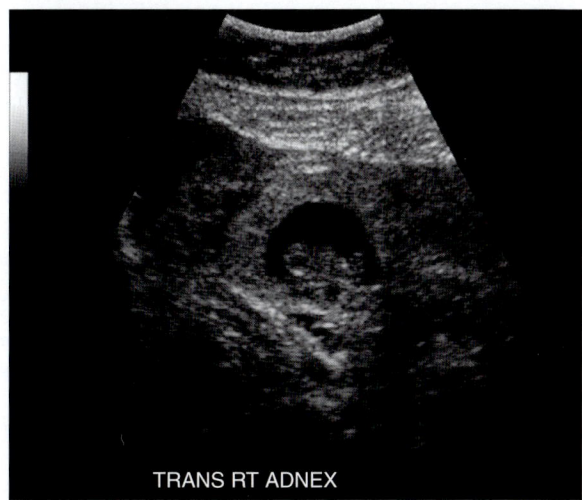

FIG. 46.18 Live heterotopic pregnancy in the same patient shown in Fig. 46.17.

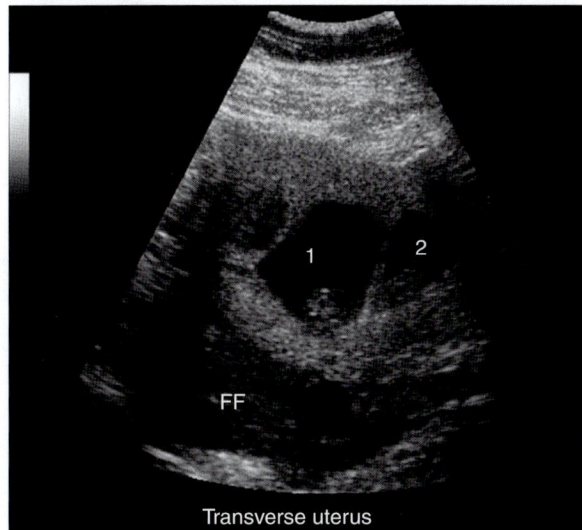

FIG. 46.17 Intrauterine twin pregnancy. *FF*, Free fluid.

Therefore pregnancies with three or more fetuses are often counseled about fetal reduction options. Fetal reduction is performed under ultrasound guidance by injecting potassium chloride into the fetal chest/heart.

Patients who undergo assisted reproductive technologies are at an increased risk for ectopic pregnancy. An ectopic pregnancy is a pregnancy that is implanted outside of the uterus. These patients are also at risk for having a heterotopic pregnancy. A heterotopic pregnancy is an ectopic pregnancy coexisting with an intrauterine pregnancy (Figs. 46.17 and Fig. 46.18). This used to be a rare occurrence (1:4000). However, with the advancement in ART, the estimated occurrence is 1:100 in this patient population.[22] The incidence of a heterotopic pregnancy with an intrauterine multiple gestation is 1:10,000, but in the ART patient subgroup, this risk may increase to 1:100.[22] When an intrauterine pregnancy is visualized in this patient population, it is important to carefully image the adnexa, not just for ovarian pathology but also to evaluate for a heterotopic pregnancy.

Key Pearls

Ultrasound has come to play an important role in the management and guidance of treatment for the infertile patient.

- One method of evaluating ovarian reserve (decrease in quantity and possibly quality of the ovarian follicle pool) is a sonographic antral follicle count.
- It is estimated that infertility affects one in seven couples in the United States.
- The congenital uterine anomalies most easily assessed with ultrasound are a septate or bicornuate uterus and uterus didelphys. On ultrasound, the septate uterus appears as two endometrial cavities without a fundal notch compared with the bicornuate and didelphys uterus.
- The endometrium can be measured throughout the menstrual cycle to look for appropriate changes.
- Saline infusion sonography can be used to help delineate polyps, fibroids, or adhesions.
- The fallopian tubes can be examined by ultrasound for hydrosalpinx and to assess patency.
- Ultrasound can be used to assess for follicular recruitment and signs of ovulation.
- Peritoneal factors may be the cause for as many as 25% of infertility cases.
- Endometriosis involving the ovary can lead to the formation of endometriomas, which are blood-filled cysts with endometrial tissue lining the cyst wall.

REFERENCES

1. Practice Committee of the American Society for Reproductive Medicine. Fertility evaluation of infertile women: a committee opinion. *Fertil Steril*. 2021;116(5):1255–1265.
2. Lindsay TJ, Vitrikas KR. Evaluation and treatment of infertility. *Am Fam Physician*. 2015;91(5):308–314. Erratum: *Am Fam Physician*. 2015;92 (6):437.
3. Thurmond AS. Imaging of female infertility. *Radiol Clin North Am*. 2003;41(4):757–767.

4. Faivre E, Fernandez H, Deffieux X, Gervaise A, Frydman R, Levaillant JM. Accuracy of three-dimensional ultrasonography in differential diagnosis of septate and bicornuate uterus compared with office hysteroscopy and pelvic magnetic resonance imaging. *J Minim Invasive Gynecol.* 2012;19(1):101–106.
5. Saravelos SH, Cocksedge KA, Li TC. Prevalence and diagnosis of congenital uterine anomalies in women with reproductive failure: a critical appraisal. *Hum Reprod Update.* 2008;14(5):415–429.
6. Davis AJ, Reindollar RH. The new ASRM müllerian anomaly classification: a picture is worth one thousand words. *Fertil Steril.* 2021;116(5):1253–1254.
7. The American Fertility Society classifications of adnexal adhesions distal tubal occlusion, tubal occlusion secondary to tubal ligation, tubal pregnancies, müllerian anomalies and intrauterine adhesions. *Fertil Steril.* 1988;49(6):944–955.
8. Pfeifer SM, Attaran M, Goldstein J, et al. ASRM müllerian anomalies classification 2021. *Fertil Steril.* 2021;116(5):1238–1252.
9. Benacerraf BR, Abuhamad AZ, Bromley B, et al. Consider ultrasound first for imaging the female pelvis. *Am J Obstet Gynecol.* 2015;212(4):450–455.
10. Ghi T, Casadio P, Kuleva M, et al. Accuracy of three-dimensional ultrasound in diagnosis and classification of congenital uterine anomalies. *Fertil Steril.* 2009;92(2):808–813.
11. Campbell S. Ultrasound evaluation in female infertility: part 2, the uterus and implantation of the embryo. *Obstet Gynecol Clin North Am.* 2019;46(4):697–713.
12. Craciunas L, Gallos I, Chu J, et al. Conventional and modern markers of endometrial receptivity: a systematic review and meta-analysis. *Hum Reprod Update.* 2019;25(2):202–223.
13. Liu KE, Hartman M, Hartman A, Luo ZC, Mahutte N. The impact of a thin endometrial lining on fresh and frozen-thaw IVF outcomes: an analysis of over 40 000 embryo transfers. *Hum Reprod.* 2018;33(10):1883–1888.
14. Groszmann YS, Benacerraf BR. Complete evaluation of anatomy and morphology of the infertile patient in a single visit; the modern infertility pelvic ultrasound examination. *Fertil Steril.* 2016;105(6):1381–1393.
15. Hajishafiha M, Zobairi T, Zanjani VR, Ghasemi-Rad M, Yekta Z, Mladkova N. Diagnostic value of sonohysterography in the determination of fallopian tube patency as an initial step of routine infertility assessment. *J Ultrasound Med.* 2009;28(12):1671–1677.
16. Teede HJ, Misso ML, Costello MF, Dokras A, Laven J, Moran L, Piltonen T, Norman RJ. International PCOS Network. Recommendations from the international evidence-based guideline for the assessment and management of polycystic ovary syndrome. *Fertil Steril.* 2018;110(3):364–379.
17. Takahashi K, Nishigaki A, Eda Y, Yamasaki H, Yoshino K, Kitao M. Transvaginal ultrasound is an effective method for screening in polycystic ovarian disease: preliminary study. *Gynecol Obstet Invest.* 1990;30(1):34–36.
18. Nisenblat V., Bossuyt P.M.M., Farquhar C., Johnson N., Hull M.L. Imaging modalities for the non-invasive diagnosis of endometriosis. Cochrane Database Syst Rev 2016;2: CD009591.
19. Campbell S. Ultrasound evaluation in female infertility: part 1, the ovary and the follicle. *Obstet Gynecol Clin North Am.* 2019;46(4):683–696.
20. Klenov V, Van Voorhis B. Ultrasound in infertility treatments. *Clinical Obstetrics and Gynecology.* 2017;60(1):108–120.
21. Coelho Neto MA, Ludwin A, Borrell A, et al. Counting ovarian antral follicles by ultrasound: a practical guide. *Ultrasound Obstet Gynecol.* 2018;51(1):10–20.
22. Barnhart KT. Clinical practice. Ectopic pregnancy. *N Engl J Med.* 2009;361(4):379–387.

PART VIII

Obstetrics

Chapter 47 The Role of Sonography in Obstetrics
Chapter 48 Clinical Ethics for Obstetric Sonography
Chapter 49 The Early Embryonic Stage of the First Trimester
Chapter 50 First-Trimester Complications
Chapter 51 Sonography of the Second and Third Trimesters
Chapter 52 Obstetric Measurements and Gestational Age
Chapter 53 Fetal Growth Assessment by Sonography
Chapter 54 Sonography and High-Risk Pregnancy
Chapter 55 Prenatal Diagnosis of Congenital Anomalies
Chapter 56 Placenta
Chapter 57 The Umbilical Cord
Chapter 58 Amniotic Fluid and Fetal Membranes
Chapter 59 Fetal Face and Neck
Chapter 60 Fetal Neural Axis
Chapter 61 The Fetal Thorax
Chapter 62 The Fetal Anterior Abdominal Wall
Chapter 63 The Fetal Abdomen
Chapter 64 Fetal Urogenital System
Chapter 65 Fetal Skeleton

CHAPTER 47

The Role of Sonography in Obstetrics

Sandra L. Hagen-Ansert

OBJECTIVES

On completion of this chapter, you should be able to:
- Discuss indications for obstetric sonography
- Analyze the differences among standard, limited, and specialized obstetric sonography examinations
- List maternal risk factors that increase the chances of producing a fetus with congenital anomalies
- Recount important questions to ask the patient before beginning the obstetric sonography examination
- Describe the biologic effects of diagnostic medical ultrasound energy and related patient safety
- Describe the steps of the first-, second-, and third-trimester sonography protocols
- List fetal anatomy visualization required as part of the standard second-trimester examination
- Discuss the use of sonography as a diagnostic and screening test

OUTLINE

Indications for Obstetric Sonography 1284
Classification of Fetal Ultrasound Examinations 1285
Patient History 1286
  Gravidity and Parity 1286
  Clinical Dates 1287
  Nägele's Rule 1287
  Maternal Risk Factors 1287
The Safety of Ultrasound 1288
The Safety of Doppler for the Obstetric Patient 1288
Guidelines for First-Trimester and Standard Second- and Third-Trimester Obstetric Sonography Examinations 1289
  Documentation 1289
  Equipment Specifications 1289
  Quality Control 1289
  First-Trimester Protocol 1289
  Second- and Third-Trimester Protocol 1290
Diagnostic and Screening Aspects of Obstetric Sonography Examinations 1292

KEY TERMS

Abruptio placentae
Amniocentesis
Amnion
Anencephaly
Aneuploidy
Cerclage
Cervix
Chorion
Corpus luteum
Ductus venosus
Embryo
Gestational (menstrual) age
Gestational sac
Gravidity
Hydatidiform mole
Incompetent cervix
Intrauterine growth restriction (IUGR)
Macrosomia
Maternal serum alpha-fetoprotein (MSAFP)
Nuchal translucency (NT)
Oligohydramnios
Parity
Placenta previa
Polyhydramnios
Quad screen
Trimesters
Umbilical cord
Yolk sac
Zygote

Sonography is the primary tool for evaluating the developing fetus during pregnancy. The visualization of pregnancy with sonography has revolutionized obstetrics. Obstetric sonography allows the clinician to assess the development, growth, and well-being of the fetus. When an abnormal condition is recognized prenatally, obstetric management may be altered to provide optimal care for the fetus and mother. Conditions that were once detected only at delivery are now diagnosed early in pregnancy and monitored with sonography. Prenatal diagnosis has led to prenatal treatments performed under ultrasound visualization. Sharing sonographic images and diagnostic results facilitates prenatal parental education and counseling. Although obstetric sonography is popular in many aspects of our culture, including books, television, and family gatherings, its value lies in its medical use.

The sonographer performing fetal studies must understand both sonographic and obstetric principles to accurately and thoroughly compile pertinent information and provide an optimal sonographic assessment of the fetus. Fetal sonography should be performed only when there is a valid medical reason and using the lowest possible ultrasound energy exposure settings to gain the necessary diagnostic information. The sonographer is responsible to obstetric patients and clinicians to provide competent, safe, and appropriate examinations.

Practice parameters are guidelines produced by the American College of Radiology (ACR), the American Institute of Ultrasound in Medicine (AIUM), the Society of Maternal Fetal Medicine (SMFM), and the American College of Obstetricians and Gynecologists (ACOG) that recommend specific components of a standard obstetric sonography examination. Sonographers must strive during each examination to meet the recommended requirements. In addition, components may be altered or added to serve the patient's interests or the referring clinician. It is often the responsibility of the sonographer, under the general direction of a physician, to apply knowledge, competence, and critical thinking to determine and perform additional appropriate examination components based on the specific indication for the study and the clinical history of the mother.

Following recommendations, the sonographer should establish a systematic scanning protocol that encompasses all criteria indicated in the guidelines. An organized approach to scanning ensures completeness and reduces the risk of missing a detectable obstetric or fetal concern.

This chapter describes the medical indications for obstetric sonography examinations and the types of obstetric examinations performed, summarizes practice parameter guidelines, reviews the safety of ultrasound in obstetrics, and describes maternal risk factors and history that may alter examination protocols.

INDICATIONS FOR OBSTETRIC SONOGRAPHY

The sonographer needs to be aware of the indications for obstetric sonography and to understand the medical complications associated with each indication. Recommended indications for obstetric sonography examinations are incorporated into diagnosis codes and billing codes. The AIUM, ACR, ACOG, SMFM, and Society of Radiologists in Ultrasound (SRU) first defined these indications in 2018. Current practice guidelines include first-trimester obstetric sonography and second- and third-trimester obstetric sonography. These indications are listed in Boxes 47.1 and 47.2. An additional explanation for these indications is provided in the following paragraphs.

BOX 47.1 Indications for First-Trimester Sonography

- To confirm the presence of an intrauterine pregnancy
- Confirmation of cardiac activity
- Estimation of gestational (menstrual) age
- Diagnosis or evaluation of multiple gestations, including determination of chorionicity
- To evaluate a suspected ectopic pregnancy
- To define the cause of vaginal bleeding
- Evaluation of pelvic pain
- As an adjunct to chorionic villous sampling, embryo transfer, or localization and removal of an intrauterine device
- To assess for certain fetal anomalies, such as anencephaly, in patients at high risk
- To screen for fetal aneuploidy by measuring the nuchal translucency when part of a screening program
- To evaluate suspected gestational trophoblastic disease
- To evaluate maternal pelvic or adnexal masses or uterine abnormalities

---

BOX 47.2 Indications for Second- and Third-Trimester Sonography

- Screen for fetal anomalies
- Evaluation of fetal anatomy
- Estimation of gestational age
- Evaluation of suspected multiple gestation
- Evaluation of cervical length
- Evaluation of fetal growth
- Significant discrepancy between uterine size and clinical dates
- Determination of fetal presentation
- Evaluation of fetal well-being
- Evaluation of suspected amniotic fluid abnormalities
- Evaluation for premature rupture of membranes and/or premature labor
- Evaluation of vaginal bleeding
- Evaluation of abdominal or pelvic pain
- Evaluation of suspected placental abruption
- Evaluation of suspected fetal death
- Follow-up evaluation of a fetal anomaly
- Follow-up evaluation of placental appearance and location, including suspected placenta previa, vasa previa, and abnormally adherent placenta
- Adjunct to amniocentesis or other procedure
- Adjunct to external cephalic version
- Evaluation of suspected gestational trophoblastic disease
- Evaluation of pelvic mass
- Evaluation of suspected uterine abnormality

---

1. Estimation of **gestational (menstrual) age** for patients with uncertain clinical dates or verification of dates for patients who undergo scheduled elective repeat cesarean delivery, indicated induction of labor, or elective termination of pregnancy. Sonographic confirmation of dating permits proper timing of cesarean delivery or labor induction to avoid premature delivery.
2. Evaluation of fetal growth, for example, when the patient has an identified cause for uteroplacental insufficiency,

such as severe preeclampsia, chronic hypertension, chronic renal disease, or severe diabetes mellitus, or for other medical complications of pregnancy in which fetal malnutrition (e.g., **intrauterine growth restriction [IUGR]**, or **macrosomia**) is suspected. Measuring fetal growth by sonography at 2- to 4-week intervals permits assessing the impact of a complicating condition of the fetus and guides pregnancy management.

3. Vaginal bleeding of undetermined cause in pregnancy. Sonography often allows the determination of the source of bleeding and the status of the fetus.
4. Serial evaluation of cervical length in pregnant women with increased risk for recurrent preterm birth or primary preterm birth.
5. Evaluation of abdominal or pelvic pain in pregnancy that may be associated with ectopic pregnancy, **abruptio placentae**, or maternal appendicitis, gallstones, renal calculi, pelvic mass, or other conditions.
6. Determination of fetal presentation when the presenting part cannot be adequately determined in labor or the fetal presentation is variable in late pregnancy. Accurate knowledge of presentation guides management of delivery.
7. Suspected multiple gestation based on detection of more than one fetal heartbeat pattern, fundal height larger than expected for dates, or prior use of fertility drugs. Pregnancy management may be altered in multiple gestation.
8. Adjunct to **amniocentesis**, chorionic villous sampling (CVS), and other invasive pregnancy procedures. Sonography permits guidance to the intended target.
9. Significant discrepancy between uterine size and clinical dates. Sonography permits accurate dating and detection of such conditions as **oligohydramnios** and **polyhydramnios**, along with multiple gestation, IUGR, and anomalies.
10. Evaluation of pelvic mass. Sonography can detect the location and nature of the mass and can aid in diagnosis.
11. **Hydatidiform mole** suspected based on clinical signs of hypertension, proteinuria, or the presence of ovarian cysts felt on pelvic examination or failure to detect fetal heart tones with a Doppler ultrasound device after 12 weeks. Sonography permits accurate diagnosis and differentiation of this neoplasm from fetal death.
12. Adjunct to cervical **cerclage** placement. Sonography aids in timing and proper cerclage placement for patients with **incompetent cervix**.
13. Suspected ectopic pregnancy, or pregnancy that occurs after tuboplasty or prior ectopic gestation. Sonography is a valuable diagnostic aid for this complication.
14. Evaluation of suspected fetal death. Rapid diagnosis enhances optimal management.
15. Suspected uterine abnormality (e.g., clinically significant leiomyomas; congenital structural abnormalities, such as bicornuate uterus or uteri didelphys). Serial surveillance of fetal growth and state enhances fetal outcome.
16. Evaluation of fetal well-being. Biophysical evaluation for fetal well-being after 28 weeks of gestation may include assessment of amniotic fluid, fetal tone, body movements, breathing movements, and heart rate patterns.
17. Evaluation of suspected amniotic fluid abnormalities such as suspected polyhydramnios or oligohydramnios. Confirmation of the diagnosis and identification of the condition's cause in certain pregnancies are necessary.
18. Suspected abruptio placentae. Confirmation of diagnosis and extent of abruption assists in clinical management.
19. Adjunct to external version from breech to vertex presentation. The visualization provided by sonography facilitates performance of this procedure.
20. Estimation of fetal weight and presentation in premature rupture of the membranes or premature labor. Information provided by sonography guides management decisions on timing and method of delivery.
21. Evaluation following maternal serum biochemical marker results. Elevated **maternal serum alpha-fetoprotein (MSAFP)** increases the risk for open defects such as neural tube defects. Other biochemical markers in the first trimester or **quad screen** biochemistry in the second trimester may indicate increased risk for certain obstetric or fetal conditions.
22. Follow-up observation of identified fetal anomaly. Sonographic assessment of progression or lack of change may assist in clinical management.
23. Follow-up evaluation of placenta location for suspected **placenta previa**.
24. Evaluation for those with a history of previous congenital anomaly. Detection of recurrence may be facilitated, or psychological benefit to patients may result from reassurance of no recurrence.
25. Evaluation of fetal condition in late registrants for prenatal care. Assessment of gestational age and fetal size assists in pregnancy management decisions for this group.
26. Assessment of findings that may increase the risk of **aneuploidy**.
27. Screening for fetal anomalies by measuring the nuchal translucency or visualization of fetal structural anomalies.

CLASSIFICATION OF FETAL ULTRASOUND EXAMINATIONS

The four practice guidelines define the major types of sonographic examinations performed in the first trimester, second and third trimesters of pregnancy, using the terms *limited*, *standard*, and *specialized* or *detailed*. In practice, the examinations may also be referred to by the current procedure terminology (CPT) code most commonly used for billing of the examinations. The major types of obstetric sonography examinations are listed in Box 47.3 and are described in the following sections.

The first-trimester examination (CPT code 76801) is performed before 13 weeks and 6 days of gestation. The examination includes the uterus, the **cervix**, the maternal adnexa, and the gestational sac and embryo. The pregnancy is dated based on embryonic size, and fetal heart motion is documented if these findings are present. Uterine anomalies and

BOX 47.3	Most Common Obstetric Sonography Examinations

- First-trimester examination (CPT 76801)
- First-trimester nuchal translucency (CPT 76813)
- Standard obstetric examination—routine, "low-risk" (CPT 76805)
- Limited obstetric examination (CPT 76815)
- Follow-up obstetric examination (CPT 76816)
- Specialized obstetric examination (CPT 76811)
- Fetal biophysical profile with NST (CPT 76819)

CPT, Current procedure terminology; *NST*, non–stress testing.

pelvic masses associated with pregnancy are more easily seen in first-trimester examinations. The chorionicity and amnionicity of multiple gestations should be documented at this time as well. An examination of fetal anatomy should also be performed during first-trimester examinations.

The first-trimester risk assessment examination (CPT code 76813) is known as the **nuchal translucency (NT)** examination. This examination is performed only when women choose first-trimester screening tests for aneuploidy. The examination includes measurement of fetal crown-rump length and NT using standard criteria. In some centers, the examination may also include visualization of the fetal nasal bone and other risk assessment parameters. Sonographers who perform these examinations must demonstrate competence in the standardized measurement of NT and must participate in an ongoing quality-monitoring program.

The standard obstetric sonography examination (CPT code 76805) is typically performed during the second trimester, around 18 weeks of gestational age. The standard examination includes an evaluation of gestational age by fetal biometry, fetal number, fetal presentation, placental position, cardiac activity, amniotic fluid volume, and a fetal anatomic survey, including all of the elements specified in the guidelines. The standard examination may include the maternal cervix and adnexa when clinically appropriate. If the cervix cannot be visualized, a transvaginal scan may be considered when evaluation or measurement of the cervix is needed.

The limited obstetric sonography examination (CPT code 76815) is used when the answer to a specific acute clinical question when an immediate impact on management is anticipated and when time or other constraints make performance of a standard ultrasound examination impractical or unnecessary. A specific clinical question such as presentation of the fetus, placental location, cervical length, amniotic fluid volume, or verification of fetal heart motion is required. If a limited examination is done on a woman without a previous standard obstetrical ultrasound, a subsequent standard or detailed ultrasound exam should be performed when appropriate.

A repeat obstetric sonography examination (CPT code 76816) is similar to a standard obstetric examination and typically includes biometry to evaluate fetal growth and reevaluation of anatomy that may or may not have been well visualized on the standard examination. The repeat obstetric examination is done when a previous standard obstetric examination has been recorded and the second examination is ordered for the same indication.

The specialty obstetric sonography examination (CPT code 76811) is also known as a detailed fetal anatomic sonogram. It is performed when an anomaly is suspected based on maternal history, biochemistry, or the results of a previous obstetric sonogram, when there is a known fetal growth disorder, or when there is increased risk for a fetal condition. The specialty obstetric sonography examination includes all components of the standard examination plus a more in-depth view of fetal anatomy. The specialty examination typically includes additional views of the fetal heart and may include color Doppler views of the heart. The specialty examination may include additional views of the extremities and a focus on areas of anomalous or expected findings associated with the patient history. The specialty obstetric sonography examination is typically performed in referral centers by physicians and sonographers with specific expertise in high-risk obstetrics. A consensus report on the detailed fetal anatomic examination was developed in 2018 by representatives from AIUM, ACOG, ACR, the SMFM, the American College of Osteopathic Obstetricians and Gynecologists (ACOOG), the SRU, and the Society of Diagnostic Medical Sonography (SDMS).

Additional CPT codes are used for transvaginal obstetric examinations, multiple gestations, fetal echocardiography, three-dimensional (3D)/four-dimensional (4D) examinations, biophysical profiles, and invasive procedures. Sonographers performing obstetric sonography must know the components required for each type of examination. Health care compliance regulations require that the billing or CPT code must match the examination performed.

PATIENT HISTORY

The sonographer should ask the patient several important questions before beginning the obstetric sonography evaluation. Both open-ended questions such as "Do you have concerns?" and closed questions such as "When was your last normal period?" are used in gathering important patient information.

Gravidity and Parity

Key obstetric history of the patient is summarized using gravidity (G) and parity (P). The sonographer should recognize this clinical description of the pregnant patient. **Gravidity** is the number of pregnancies, including the present one. **Parity** is reported using a numeric system that describes all possible pregnancy outcomes. The letter "P" followed by four numbers in sequence, P0000, is commonly used. The numbers represent, in order, full-term deliveries, premature births and stillborns, early pregnancy loss or termination, and living children. For instance, a G4P2103 describes a patient undergoing her fourth pregnancy. She has had two full-term deliveries, one premature birth, no early pregnancy losses, and three living children.

Clinical Dates

The sonographer first tries to determine the clinical dates of the pregnancy. It is important to document the clinical date reported by the patient and the date determined by the earliest sonographic examination. An accurate clinical date facilitates correlation of obstetric measurements with the expected gestational age.

The first date of the last normal menstrual period (LMP or LNMP) is the standard way to date a pregnancy in the United States. Human pregnancy lasts 266 days plus or minus 10 days. If conception occurs on day 14 from the LNMP, the pregnancy duration from LNMP is 280 days or 40 weeks. Pregnancy is divided into **trimesters** of approximately 13 weeks. A pregnant woman is in the first trimester until 13 weeks and 6 days of gestational age, and in the second trimester from 14 weeks to 26 weeks and 6 days of gestational age. The third trimester begins at 27 weeks of gestational age and lasts until term.

In reality, the assessment of gestational age is often not precise. Many women have irregular periods, conceive within 3 months of ceasing birth control pills when ovulation is irregular, or do not record dates. Even with a known menstrual date, conception may occur from day 6 to day 27, a difference of 3 weeks in gestational age as determined by sonography. Physicians may use clinical parameters such as uterine size and growth or ovulation indications to estimate pregnancy dates. Gestational age provides an estimate of how long a patient has been pregnant, but the exact date that labor will begin cannot be determined owing to the variable length of human pregnancy.

The sonographer first asks the patient the first day of her last normal menstrual period. If the patient does not remember the date (LNMP), the sonographer may ask for the expected delivery date (EDD). The sonographer should also ask if previous sonographic examinations were performed before 20 weeks and the estimated date of delivery determined by the earliest sonographic examination. *The sonographer should not change the EDD or "redate" the pregnancy once an earlier sonogram has established gestational age.*

Dates established by sonography performed in the first or second trimester typically take precedence over menstrual dates when the discrepancy is greater than 7 days in the first trimester or greater than 10 days in the second trimester. Sonography may be considered to confirm menstrual dates if there is gestational age agreement within a week by crown-rump length or within 10 days by second-trimester fetal biometry. The pregnancy should not be dated by sonographic measurements in the third trimester, and dates should not be changed after they have been calculated from an early examination. It is ultimately the responsibility of the obstetrician who is following the pregnancy to determine the clinical gestational age.

Nägele's Rule

The EDD may be calculated using Nägele's rule (Box 47.4). According to this method, the EDD is derived by subtracting 3 months from the LNMP and adding 7 days. For example,

> **BOX 47.4 Nägele's Rule**
>
> EDD = LNMP − 3 months + 7 days
> LNMP = EDD − 3 months + 7 days

EDD, Estimated date of delivery; *LNMP*, last normal menstrual period.

an LNMP of 10/17 would result in an EDC of 7/24 (10/17 − 3 months = 7/17 + 7 days = 7/24). A sonographer familiar with this rule may determine EDD or LNMP when the patient verbally reports only one. Commercial date wheels simplify this method to determine the due date and assign fetal age at the time of the sonography study.

Maternal Risk Factors

Sonographers need to ask if the patient has latex allergies. Many sonography laboratories use only latex-free materials to prevent allergic reactions. It is also important to ask if the patient has experienced supine hypotension (i.e., difficulty lying on her back during pregnancy) and to caution the patient to report any sense of warmth, dizziness, or syncope experienced during the sonography examination.

The sonographer needs to know if the patient is currently taking any medication or has experienced clinical problems with the pregnancy, such as bleeding, decreased fetal movement, or pelvic pain. If the patient has had problems with previous pregnancies, such as a spontaneous preterm birth, fibroids, fetal macrosomia or growth restriction, structural or chromosomal fetal anomalies, this information must be documented. Finally, the sonographer needs to know if the patient has maternal risk factors for anomalies that may impact the examination or interpretation.

Factors that may affect the risk of producing a fetus with congenital anomalies include increased maternal age, first- or second-trimester maternal serum biochemistry values, first-trimester increased NT, maternal disease (e.g., diabetes mellitus, systemic lupus erythematosus), and a pregnant uterine cavity that is too small or too large for dates. Other risk factors include a previous child born with a chromosomal disorder or exposure to a known teratogenic drug or infectious agent known to cause birth defects. Some anomalies are caused by a reduced or increased number of fetal chromosomes. These anomalies, the most common of which is Down syndrome, trisomy 21, are called *aneuploidies*. Other anomalies are thought to have both genetic and environmental causes. For example, neural tube defects have a genetic component but are influenced by the maternal environment, especially a lack of adequate folic acid before pregnancy and during the early embryonic period. Assessment of maternal risk may include discussing genetic and family history; environmental triggers, such as maternal disease and nutrition; and available testing. Genomic technologies have created multiple options for prenatal testing to screen and diagnose fetal anomalies. It is important that women are educated about their options early in pregnancy to choose the level of testing/detection that is acceptable to themselves and their families. Genetic counselors are trained to assist patients in determining risks before or during pregnancy. With adequate pre-pregnancy counseling and environmental factor control, some anomalies may be prevented.

THE SAFETY OF ULTRASOUND

Ultrasound imaging has been used in pregnancy since the 1950s without apparent side effects. The first studies conducted to determine the safety of ultrasound in pregnancy were small and were hampered by imprecise dosimetry and poorly matched control groups. Physicists and researchers have made tremendous strides in defining the variables of importance in terms of bioeffects and the types of tissue interactions and damage that may occur. Using human epidemiology studies, animal experiments, and in vitro studies of tissue and cells, scientists continue to study the safety of ultrasound, but challenges remain. Existing human studies are not large enough to document small increases in normally occurring anomalies that may occur as the result of sonography. Similarly, it is difficult to determine potential long-term effects of prenatal ultrasound imaging. Animal experiments and therapeutic applications document that high-intensity ultrasound may modify biologic structures and functions. Studies in pregnancy with animals and humans have suggested possibilities of growth differences (reduction in animals), increased non–right-handedness, and delayed speech.

The major biologic effects of ultrasound are believed to be thermal (a rise in temperature) and mechanical forces, including cavitation (production and collapse of gas-filled bubbles). Sonographers can minimize thermal effects during obstetric examinations by not staying in one spot, especially over fetal bone, for long periods of time and by extending the focus of the beam as deeply into the body as is reasonable to obtain adequate images. Cavitation is dependent on the presence of preexisting gas within the tissue and is not an issue in the fetus. Sonographers who work with newborns may choose to be cautious of long examinations through newborn lungs filled with gas.

The AIUM has a committee of scientists, clinicians, sonographers, and engineers who regularly review and summarize information regarding bioeffects. The AIUM adopted three statements in 2007 and reapproved such in 2019 (Prudent Use and Clinical Safety, Prudent Use in Pregnancy, and Statement on Measurement of the Fetal Heart Rate) that read as follows:

Diagnostic ultrasound has been in use since the late 1950s. Given its known benefits and recognized efficacy for medical diagnosis, including use during human pregnancy, the American Institute of Ultrasound in Medicine herein addresses the clinical safety of such use: No independently confirmed adverse effects caused by exposure from present diagnostic ultrasound instruments have been reported in human patients in the absence of contrast agents. Biological effects (such as localized pulmonary bleeding) have been reported in mammalian systems at diagnostically relevant exposures, but the clinical significance of such effects is not known. Ultrasound should be used by qualified health professionals to provide medical benefit to the patient. Ultrasound exposures during examinations should be as low as reasonably achievable (ALARA).

The AIUM advocates the responsible use of diagnostic ultrasound and strongly discourages the nonmedical use of ultrasound for entertainment purposes. Using ultrasound to view the fetus, obtain images of the fetus, or determine the fetal sex is inappropriate and contrary to responsible medical practice. Qualified health professionals should use ultrasound to provide medical benefit to the patient.

When attempting to obtain fetal heart rate with a diagnostic ultrasound system, AIUM recommends using M-mode first because the time-averaged acoustic intensity delivered to the fetus is lower with M-mode than with spectral Doppler. If this is unsuccessful, use spectral Doppler only briefly (4 to 5 heartbeats) and keep the thermal index (TIS for soft tissues in the first trimester, TIB for bone after 10 weeks) as low as possible, preferably below 1 in accordance with the ALARA principle.

In summary, sonographers should recognize that there are theoretical effects of ultrasound energy on the fetus, and it is the responsibility of sonographers to be knowledgeable regarding bioeffects and to use ALARA principles to minimize fetal exposure.

Appropriate use of ALARA during pregnancy requires that sonographers do the following:

1. Monitor the output displays on their machine, especially the thermal index (TI). Keep both the mechanical index (MI) and the TI as low as possible and well under 1. Use TIS for soft tissue during the early first trimester and TIB for bone after 10 weeks of gestational age. The TIB should be under 0.7 (preferably under 0.5) at all times. If the TIB is higher than 0.7, decrease the power used.
2. Move frequently and do not dwell on a single portion of the fetus for any length of time, especially when there is bone in the near field of the image. A sonographer should not dwell on the fetal facial profile—if there is a medical indication to take multiple images, move in and out of that area allowing time for the tissue to cool if needed.

THE SAFETY OF DOPPLER FOR THE OBSTETRIC PATIENT

Doppler ultrasound provides a noninvasive method to assess the physiology and pathophysiology of fetal and maternal circulations when such examinations are required for diagnosis. In most cases, pulsed wave Doppler rather than continuous wave Doppler is used in the fetus. Doppler may be used to detect flow in the maternal vessels (uterine artery), the fetal vessels (umbilical artery and vein, aorta and inferior vena cava, renal arteries, and cerebral vessels), the fetal **ductus venosus**, the fetal heart, and the placenta. Doppler interrogation is an important part of fetal echocardiography examinations and aids in diagnosing fetal heart defects. Specific applications of Doppler in obstetrics are presented in the respective chapters.

Doppler is a higher ultrasound energy level, and these examinations may require prolonged dwell times. It is extremely important that sonographers using Doppler energy in pregnancy are proficient in the examinations so that they are completed as quickly as possible. The thermal index must be monitored closely during Doppler examinations. The TIS should be used at earlier than 10 weeks' gestation, and the TIB should be used at 10 weeks gestation or later when bone ossification is evident. In the first trimester, it is best to utilize M-Mode recordings to document the fetal heart rate.

The benefits of Doppler imaging most likely outweigh the risks when specific indications require Doppler interrogation. Fetal sonography with or without Doppler should be performed only when there is a valid medical reason, and the lowest possible ultrasonic exposure settings should be used to obtain the necessary diagnostic information.

GUIDELINES FOR FIRST-TRIMESTER AND STANDARD SECOND- AND THIRD-TRIMESTER OBSTETRIC SONOGRAPHY EXAMINATIONS

In the late 1980s, in response to concerns about variability in quality and practices, obstetric examination parameters were introduced by professional organizations. The practice parameters have been updated multiple times. The societies collaborate on the clinical aspects of their statements and include identical wording related to classification and specifications for examinations. Portions of their statements, including information related to physician qualifications, procedure documentation, quality control, background, and clinical recommendations, differ between organizations.

The purpose of the current practice parameters is to provide practitioners with information regarding the criteria for a complete examination. These documents are often cited as a legal standard, although this use was not intended. Although it is not possible to detect all fetal anomalies with sonography, adherence to practice parameters and referral of any suspicious studies for further evaluation will optimize the possibilities of detection.

All sonographers should strive to consistently meet or exceed minimum standards during every obstetric sonographic examination. Quality standards include the components of the examination protocol and the qualifications of personnel performing the examination, documentation, equipment specifications, fetal safety, quality control, infection control, and patient education concerns.

Although no mechanism exists to ensure technical competence, the standard of practice for personnel in sonography is national board certification in the major areas of practice, including obstetrics and gynecology. The purpose of certification or registry is to assure the public that the person performing sonography has the necessary knowledge, skills, and experience to provide this service.

Documentation

Documentation guidelines recommend maintaining a permanent record that includes the measurements and anatomic findings. Images of all appropriate areas, both normal and abnormal, should be recorded. Measurements should accompany variations from normal size. The images also should be labeled with the patient's name, date, facility identification, exam date, and side (right or left) of the anatomic site imaged. Fetal echocardiography is often stored in a real-time format for future reference and review. The availability of real-time sonography equipment with transabdominal and transvaginal transducers is essential to confirm fetal life and to permit the sonographer to view fetal anatomy and movements and to obtain the biometric parameters used to determine fetal age and growth. A written report by the physician should outline the study's findings and must be maintained in the patient medical records. Retention of the ultrasound examination should be consistent both with clinical needs and with relevant legal and local health care facility requirements.

Equipment Specifications

The obstetrical ultrasound examinations should be conducted with real-time ultrasound instrumentation, using a transabdominal and/or transvaginal approach. Real-time cine loops are necessary to confirm the presence of fetal life through observation of cardiac activity and fetal movement.

Transducer frequency selection and equipment settings should balance optimal imaging resolution and penetration. Generally, 3 to 5 MHz curved array abdominal transducers allow sufficient penetration in most patients while providing adequate resolution. The sector array and linear array transducer may also be useful to define specific anatomy. The lower frequency transducer may be necessary to provide adequate penetration for abdominal imaging in obese patients. In the first trimester, a 5 MHz abdominal transducer or a 5 to 10 MHz or greater transvaginal transducer may provide superior resolution while still allowing adequate penetration.

The lowest possible exposure setting should be used according to the ALARA principle. Policies and procedures related to patient information, infection control, quality control, and safety should be developed and implemented in every laboratory. Policies typically address personnel and patient safety and may address musculoskeletal injury concerns for the sonographer. A monitor mounted on the wall for patient viewing provides ergonomic protection for the sonographer in obstetric laboratories.

Quality Control

The Policies and procedures related to quality control, patient education, infection control, and safety should be developed and implemented in accordance with the *AIUM Standards and Guidelines for the Accreditation of Ultrasound Practices*. The ultrasound equipment performance monitoring should also be in accordance with the AIUM Standards and Guidelines.

First-Trimester Protocol

Indications for first-trimester sonography are shown in Box 47.1. A transabdominal or transvaginal transducer may be used to examine the first-trimester embryo and fetus. If a transabdominal examination is not definitive, a transvaginal or transperineal examination is required. A transabdominal examination may provide an overview of the entire pelvic cavity and enable the sonographer to image the uterus from the cervix to the fundus, evaluate the ovaries and adnexal areas for abnormal collections of fluid or a mass, and look for the presence of free fluid. The transvaginal transducer provides a more limited view of the pelvic cavity but allows excellent visualization of the **embryo, yolk sac, amnion, chorion**, and **gestational sac**.

Sample Protocol

1. The uterus and adnexa should be evaluated for the presence of a gestational sac.
   - If a gestational sac is seen, its location (intrauterine or extrauterine) should be noted.
   - The gestational sac should be recorded when the embryo is not identified during the **zygote** or implantation stage of pregnancy. Caution must be used in diagnosing a gestational sac without a yolk sac or embryo because intrauterine fluid collections may appear similar.
   - The presence or absence of a yolk sac and an embryo should be noted.
   - The crown-rump length is the most accurate measurement of gestational age during the first trimester and should be recorded when an embryo is present.
2. Presence or absence of cardiac activity should be documented with real-time or M-mode.
   - Cardiac motion is usually seen when the embryo is 7 mm or greater in length.
   - The fetal heart rate is much faster than the mother's heart rate. According to fetal development stages, the fetal heart rate changes; early in embryologic development, the heart rate is slow (90 beats/min). The rate may go up to 180 beats/min in the middle of the first trimester before returning to 120 to 160 beats/min throughout the pregnancy.
3. Fetal number should be documented.
   - Count only the embryo and yolk sac to determine multiple pregnancies. The membrane structure and the number of amniotic and chorionic membranes should be documented in all multiple pregnancies. The chorionicity is most reliably documented during the first trimester.
4. A fetal anatomy survey should be performed as many structural anomalies have been diagnosed during the first trimester. A first-trimester fetal anatomy survey cannot replace the second-trimester survey, however.
5. During late first trimester (11 to 14 weeks), an NT measurement may be performed according to standard criteria for women desiring to assess their risk for fetal aneuploidy.
   - Guidelines for NT measurement:
     a. The margins of the NT edges must be clear enough for proper placement of the calipers.
     b. The fetus must be in the midsagittal plane.
     c. The image must be magnified so that it is filled by the fetal head, neck, and upper thorax.
     d. The fetal neck must be in a neutral position, not flexed or hyperextended.
     e. The amnion must be seen as separate from the NT line.
     f. The + calipers on the ultrasound must be used to perform the NT measurement.
     g. Electronic calipers must be placed on the inner to inner border of the nuchal line space with none of the horizontal crossbar itself protruding into the space.
     h. The calipers must be placed perpendicular to the long axis of the fetus.
     i. The measurement must be obtained at the widest space of the NT.
6. The uterus, adnexal structures, and cul-de-sac should be evaluated.
   - It is important to document the texture of the ovaries and the presence of **corpus luteum** or other adnexal masses.
   - Document the presence, size, and location of leiomyomatous masses within the uterus. Note the inhomogeneous uterine texture of the leiomyomatous growth that may be stimulated by the hormonal changes of pregnancy.
   - Document the presence, location, appearance, and size of adnexal masses
   - Evaluate the cul-de-sac for the presence or absence of fluid.
   - Uterine anomalies should be documented.

Second- and Third-Trimester Protocol

The indications for second- and third-trimester sonography are shown in Box 47.2. Practice parameters for the second- and third-trimester ultrasound examination, which include a biometric and anatomic survey of the fetus, suggest the following:

1. Fetal cardiac motion, fetal number, presentation, and activity should be documented.
   - In multiple gestations, the following individual studies should be performed on each fetus: amnionicity, chorionicity, comparison of fetal sizes, estimation of amniotic fluid (increased, decreased, or normal) on each side of the membrane, and fetal sex (when visualized).
   - An abnormal heart rate and/or rhythm should be documented.
2. A qualitative or semiquantitative estimate of amniotic fluid volume should be reported. Abnormal fluid amounts should be described.
   - In early pregnancy, amniotic fluid is produced by the placenta; the fetal kidneys begin to produce urine, which contributes to the production and replacement of amniotic fluid as the fetus swallows and urinates. The fluid increases in volume until the 34th week of gestation.
   - Experienced observers may subjectively estimate amniotic fluid volume. Semiquantitative methods may be

used, including the four-quadrant amniotic fluid index (AFI), the single deepest pocket, and the two-diameter pocket.
- Excessive fluid is termed *hydramnios (polyhydramnios)*; too little fluid is called *oligohydramnios*.
3. Placental localization, appearance, and relationship to the internal cervical os should be recorded. The **umbilical cord** should be imaged, and the number of vessels should be evaluated when possible. The placental cord insertion site should be documented when technically possible.
    - The placental position early in pregnancy may not correlate well with the location at the time of delivery. Transvaginal imaging may help visualize the internal os and the position of the placenta in relation to the cervix.
    - An overdistended maternal urinary bladder or a contraction in the lower uterine cavity can give a false impression of placenta previa.
    - Transvaginal or transperineal imaging may be necessary to document cervical length if there are risk factors for spontaneous preterm birth when the cervix appears shortened or if there is a history of uterine contractions. Transvaginal cervical length measurements may be used for screening in low-risk pregnancies.
    - A velamentous placental cord insertion that crosses the internal os of the cervix is vasa previa, a condition that has a high risk of fetal mortality if not diagnosed before labor.
4. Gestational (menstrual) age should be assessed by sonographic biometry. Crown-rump length measured during the first trimester is the most accurate method to assess gestational age. During the second and third trimesters, multiple sonographic parameters can be used to estimate gestational age. The variability of these measurements increases as the pregnancy progresses. If the clinical gestational age and sonographic parameters demonstrate significant discrepancies, the possibility of fetal growth abnormalities, such as macrosomia or IUGR, is suggested. Biometric parameters that may be used include the following:
    - Biparietal diameter (BPD) is measured in an axial plane at the level of the thalami and the cavum septi pellucidi or columns of the fornix. The cerebellar hemispheres should not be visible in this scanning plane. The biparietal measurement is taken from the outer edge to the inner edge of the skull. (NOTE: The head may normally be more rounded [brachycephaly] or elongated [dolichocephaly], which will make measurement of the head circumference more accurate than measurement of the BPD.)
    - Head circumference is measured at the same level as BPD, around the outer perimeter of the calvarium. Head circumference is not affected by head shape.
    - Femur length, that is, the length of the femoral diaphysis is reliably measured after the 14th week of gestation. The long axis of the femoral shaft is most accurately measured with the beam of insonation being perpendicular to the shaft, excluding the distal femoral epiphysis.
    - Abdominal circumference is measured on a transverse view at the level of the junction of the umbilical vein and the portal sinus. Circumference should be measured at the skin line on a true transverse view of the fetal abdomen, where the portal sinus, fetal stomach, and umbilical vein are visible. Abdominal circumference or average abdominal diameter is used with other biometric parameters to estimate fetal weight and may allow detection of intrauterine growth restriction or macrosomia.
5. Fetal weight may be estimated by obtaining measurements such as the biparietal diameter, head circumference, abdominal circumference or average abdominal diameter, and femoral diaphysis length. Results from various prediction models can be compared to fetal weight percentiles from published nomograms.
    - If previous studies have been performed, appropriateness of growth should be documented.
    - The best fetal weight estimates may yield significant errors. Sonographic measurements taken 2 to 4 weeks apart may determine interval growth.
    - Even the best fetal weight prediction methods can yield errors as high as ± 15%. Many factors may influence this variability (patient population, the number and type of anatomic parameters being measured, technical factors that affect the resolution of ultrasound images, and the weight range being studied).
6. Evaluation of maternal anatomy, including uterine, adnexal, and cervical evaluations, should be performed to document the presence, location, and size of uterine or adnexal masses, which may complicate obstetric management. Normal maternal ovaries may not be imaged during the second and third trimesters. If the cervix cannot be visualized, a transperineal or transvaginal scan may be considered when evaluation of the cervix is needed.
7. Fetal anatomy may be adequately assessed after 18 weeks of gestation. It may be possible to document normal structures prior to this time, although some structures can be difficult to visualize due to fetal size, position, movement, abdominal scars, or increased maternal abdominal wall thickness. The sonographer should note the reason when anatomy is not seen because of technical limitations. A follow-up examination may be ordered.

The practice guidelines recommend that the following anatomy be documented during a standard obstetric sonography examination. A more detailed fetal anatomic examination may be necessary if an abnormality or suspected abnormality is found on the standard examination. Documentation and images of the required anatomy should be retained. Anatomic areas to be assessed are listed in Box 47.5 and include the following:
1. Head, face, and neck:
    - Cerebellum
    - Choroid plexus
    - Cisterna magna
    - Lateral cerebral ventricles

- Midline falx
- Cavum septi pellucidi
- Upper lip
- A measurement of the nuchal fold may be helpful during specific age intervals to assess the risk of aneuploidy.

2. Chest/heart:
   - Four-chamber view of the fetal heart
   - Left ventricular outflow tract
   - Right ventricular outflow tract
   - Three vessel view
3. Abdomen:
   - Stomach (presence, size, and situs)
   - Kidneys
   - Urinary bladder
   - Umbilical cord insertion into the fetal abdomen
   - Umbilical cord; number of vessels
4. Spine:
   - Cervical, thoracic, lumbar, and sacral spine
5. Extremities:
   - Arms and legs
6. Sex:
   - In multiple pregnancies and when medically indicated

DIAGNOSTIC AND SCREENING ASPECTS OF OBSTETRIC SONOGRAPHY EXAMINATIONS

Obstetric sonography examinations are both diagnostic and screening tests. Diagnostic tests can give definitive information about a clinical question or the presence or absence of a finding. Obstetric sonography examinations are typically diagnostic with respect to fetal heart motion, fetal number, fetal biometry, fetal presentation, location of the placenta, presence of a maternal pelvic or adnexal mass, and major disruptions of fetal anatomy such as **anencephaly**.

Obstetric sonography may also diagnose other fetal problems, but, in general, it is considered a screening test for detection of fetal anomalies. A screening test does not provide a definitive diagnosis but indicates whether the patient or pregnancy is at greater or lesser risk. In other words, an obstetric sonography examination with normal findings may reduce the risk of that fetus having an anomaly but does provide certainty that the fetus is not affected.

The sensitivity of routine sonography in detecting fetal anomalies has been analyzed in multiple studies. It is generally agreed that sensitivity depends on many factors, including maternal habitus, the expertise of the sonographers and physicians responsible for the study, the patient's risk level, the number and timing of sonography examinations, and the type of anomaly. Sensitivity tends to be higher for defects of the central nervous and urinary systems and lower for defects of the heart and great vessels. Sensitivity is higher in tertiary care centers and with specialty obstetric examinations. Maternal obesity is known to have an impact on sonographic visualization of anatomy. In one review of 36 studies involving more than 900,000 fetuses, overall sensitivity for detecting fetal anomalies by obstetric sonography was 40.4%, and the range was 13.3% to 82.4%.

> **BOX 47.5 Essential or Minimal Elements of a Standard Examination of Fetal Anatomy**
>
> - Head, face, and neck
>   - Cerebellum
>   - Choroid plexus
>   - Cisterna magna
>   - Lateral cerebral ventricles
>   - Midline falx
>   - Cavum septi pellucidi
>   - Upper lip
>   - Measurement of the nuchal fold may be helpful during specific age intervals (approximately 16–20 weeks' gestational age) to assess the risk of aneuploidy)
> - Chest
> - Heart: document size and position, four-chamber view of the fetal heart, the left and right ventricular outflow tracts, and the three-vessel view
>   - Abdomen
>   - Stomach (presence, size, and situs)
>   - Kidneys
>   - Urinary bladder
>   - Umbilical cord insertion site into the fetal abdomen
>   - Umbilical cord vessel number
> - Spine: cervical, thoracic, lumbar, and sacral spine
> - Extremities: presence of legs and arms, hands and feet
> - Sex: in multiple gestations and when medically indicated

Patients must be counseled about the limitations of obstetric sonography. This counseling should inform patients that screening examinations do not detect all anomalies, that false-positive findings are possible, and that the sensitivity of sonography is not certain in any situation.

Key Pearls

- Obstetric sonography allows the clinician to assess the development, growth, and well-being of the fetus.
- The sonographer performing fetal studies must understand both sonographic and obstetric principles to accurately and thoroughly compile pertinent information and provide an optimal sonographic assessment of the fetus.
- Fetal sonography should be performed only when there is a valid medical reason and using the lowest possible ultrasound energy exposure settings to gain the necessary diagnostic information.
- Practice parameters are guidelines produced by the American College of Radiology (ACR), the American Institute of Ultrasound in Medicine (AIUM), and the American College of Obstetricians and Gynecologists (ACOG) that recommend specific components of a standard obstetric sonography examination.
- The sonographer needs to be aware of the indications for obstetric sonography and to understand the medical complications associated with each indication.
- The standard obstetric sonography examination (CPT code 76805) is typically performed during the second trimester around 18 weeks' gestational age.

- The standard examination includes an evaluation of gestational age by fetal biometry, fetal number, fetal presentation, placental position, cervical length, cardiac activity, amniotic fluid volume, fetal anatomic survey, and maternal pelvic anatomy survey, including all of the elements specified in the guidelines.
- The specialty obstetric sonography examination includes all components of the standard examination plus a more in-depth view of fetal anatomy, including a complete fetal heart evaluation, extremities to include fingers and toes, and/or specific areas of suspected abnormal anatomy development.
- Key obstetric history of the patient is summarized using gravidity (G) and parity (P). Gravidity is the number of pregnancies, including the present one. Parity is reported using a numeric system that describes all possible pregnancy outcomes.
- The first date of the last normal menstrual period (LMP or LNMP) is the standard way to date a pregnancy in the United States.
- Factors that may affect the risk of producing a fetus with congenital anomalies include increased maternal age, first- or second-trimester maternal serum biochemistry values, first-trimester increased nuchal translucency, maternal disease (e.g., diabetes mellitus, systemic lupus erythematosus), and a pregnant uterine cavity that is too small or too large for dates.
- Ultrasound exposures during examinations should be as low as reasonably achievable (ALARA).
- Doppler ultrasound provides a noninvasive method to assess the physiology and pathophysiology of fetal and maternal circulations when such examinations are required for diagnosis.

ACKNOWLEDGMENT

The author acknowledges the contributions of Jean Lea Spitz to this chapter in the previous edition.

BIBLIOGRAPHY

Abramsky L, Fletcher O. Interpreting information: what is said, what is heard- a questionnaire study of health professional and members of the public. *Prenat Diagn*. 2002;22:1188m.

Practice parameter for the performance of limited obstetric ultrasound examinations by advanced clinical providers. 2018. https://onlinelibrary.wiley.com/doi/full/10.1002/jum.14677.

AIUM-ACR-ACOG-SMFM-SRU Practice parameter for the performance in standard diagnostic obstetric ultrasound examinations, 2018. https://onlinelibrary.wiley.com/doi/full/10.1002/jum.14831.

American College of Obstetricians and Gynecologists practice bulletin number 101: ultrasonography in pregnancy. *Obstet Gynecol*. 2009;113:451–461.

American College of Radiology. *Practice guideline for the performance of obstetric ultrasound: ACR practice guidelines and technical standards, 2007*. Reston, VA: American College of Radiology; 2007: 1025-1033. www.acr.org.

American Institute of Ultrasound in Medicine. Consensus report on potential bioeffects of diagnostic ultrasound: executive summary. *J Ultrasound Med*. 2008;27:503–516.

American Institute of Ultrasound in Medicine. AIUM Practice parameter for the performance of detailed second- and third-trimester diagnostic obstetric ultrasound examinations. *J Ultrasound Med*. 2019;38:3093–3100.

Andrist LS, Schroedter W. Editors: Standards for assurance of minimum entry-level competence for the diagnostic ultrasound professional *J Diagn Med Ultrasound*. 2001;17:307–311.

Bernacerraf, BR, Minton KK, Benson CB, et al. Proceedings: Beyond ultrasound first forum on improving quality of ultrasound imaging in obstetrics and gynecology, 2018. https://europepmc.org/article/med/29297609.

Bhide A, Acharya G, Bilardo CM, et al. ISUOB practice guidelines: use of Doppler ultrasonography in obstetrics. *Ultrasound Obstet Gynecol*. 2013;41:233–239.

Chasen ST, Kalish RB, Chervenak FA. Basic versus detailed sonography: what do we miss? *J Ultrasound Med*. 2009;28:1015–1018.

Crane JP, LeFevre ML, Winborn RC, et al. A randomized trial of prenatal ultrasonographic screening: impact on the detection, management, and outcome of anomalous fetuses, RADIUS Study Group. *Am J Obstet Gynecol*. 1994;171:392–399.

Dashe JS, McIntire DD, Twickler DM. Maternal obesity limits the ultrasound evaluation of fetal anatomy. *J Ultrasound Med*. 2009;28:1025–1030.

Ewigman BG, Crane JP, Frigoletto FD, et al. Effect of prenatal ultrasound screening on perinatal outcome, RADIUS Study Group. *N Engl J Med*. 1993;329:821–827.

Hershkovitz R, Sheiner E, Mazor M. Ultrasound in obstetrics: a review of safety. *Eur J Obstet Gynecol Reprod Biol*. 2002;101:15.

Levi S. Ultrasound in prenatal diagnosis: polemics around routine ultrasound screening for second trimester fetal malformations. *Prenat Diagn*. 2002;22:285–295.

Rados C: FDA cautions against ultrasound keepsake images. *FDA Consumer Magazine*, Washington, DC: U.S. Food and Drug Administration Office of Public Affairs; 2004.

Salvesen KA, Lees C, Abramowicz J, et al. Safe use of Doppler ultrasound during the 11 to 13 +6 week scan: is it possible? *Ultrasound Obstet Gynecol*. 2011;37:625–628.

Szabo TL, Lewin PA. Ultrasound transducer selection in clinical imaging practice. *J Ultrasound Med*. 2013;32(4):573–582.

Mieghem V, Hindryckx A, Van Calsteren K. Early fetal anatomy screening: who, what, when, and why? *Curr Opin Obstet Gynecol*. 1997;10(1).

Wax J, Minkoff H, Johnson A, et al. Consensus report on the detailed fetal anatomic ultrasound examination indications, components, and qualifications. *J Ultrasound Med*. 2014;33(2):189–195.

CHAPTER 48

Clinical Ethics for Obstetric Sonography

Jean Lea Spitz

OBJECTIVES

On completion of this chapter, you should be able to:
- Identify multiple sources of moral beliefs in a pluralistic society
- Differentiate morality from ethics
- Describe the application of nonmaleficence, beneficence, justice, veracity, and autonomy in various settings where sonographic examinations are performed
- Define the principle of beneficence in clinical ethics
- Define the principle of respect for autonomy in clinical ethics
- Identify beneficence-based obligations to the fetal patient
- Identify ethical issues in competence and referral in sonography examinations
- Identify ethical issues in routine obstetric sonography screening
- Identify ethical issues in disclosure of results in sonographic examinations
- Identify ethical issues in the confidentiality of findings

OUTLINE

Morality and Ethics Defined 1294
History of Medical Ethics 1295
Principles of Medical Ethics 1295
Nonmaleficence 1295
Beneficence 1296
Autonomy 1296
Veracity and Integrity 1297
Justice 1298
Confidentiality of Findings 1298

KEY TERMS

Autonomy
Beneficence
Confidentiality
Ethics
Informed consent
Integrity
Justice
Morality
Nonmaleficence
Respect for persons
Veracity

Ethical codes are important regulators in health care. Patient trust is built on the expectation that health care professionals will follow established ethical principles and guidelines. Medical ethics promotes excellence and protects patients by encouraging practitioners to reflect on, communicate, and demonstrate optimal care.

Sonographers have ethical responsibilities to their patients and colleagues. The principles of nonmaleficence, beneficence, autonomy, respect for persons, veracity and integrity, and justice must be implemented in the sonography laboratory to ensure ethical practice. Sonographers who regularly participate in ethical discussions and discourse within their environment may best meet these requirements. The Society of Diagnostic Medical Sonography (SDMS) has adopted a code of ethics for sonographers. This code includes elements consistent with principles of nonmaleficence, beneficence, autonomy, veracity, justice, and confidentiality.

MORALITY AND ETHICS DEFINED

Ethics is a systematic reflection on and analysis of morality. **Morality** concerns right and wrong conduct (what we ought or ought not to do) and good and bad character (the kinds of persons we should become and the virtues we should cultivate in doing so). Morality reflects duties and values. Freedom and autonomy are integral to morality because they allow people to express values. All aspects of morality, duties, values, and rights are important in the clinical ethics of sonography practice.

In a pluralistic, multicultural society such as the United States, moral beliefs and behaviors vary widely. People learn morality through personal experiences, family traditions, and normative behavior within communities, ethnic and racial groups, or geographic regions. Religions disagree about conduct and character, and religious ethics provides an inadequate foundation for professional ethics in a culturally diverse society. National identity and history also contribute to beliefs, as do the laws of the states and the federal government. These many sources of moral beliefs can sometimes cause conflict. Health care providers with good intentions may disagree among themselves or with patients on moral directions. When these disagreements are discussed and analyzed, a collaborative and ethical resolution of the conflict can be achieved. This type of discussion, reflection, and discourse on morality constitutes ethics.

Whereas morality has to do with protecting cherished values, ethics is a discipline of study that seeks to articulate clear, consistent, coherent, and practical guidelines for conduct and character. Ethics tries to answer the key question, "What is good?" To be applicable to a medical context such as sonography, ethics must transcend moral pluralism by offering an approach with minimal ties to any substantive prior belief about moral conduct and character. This is what philosophical ethics attempts to do because it requires only a commitment to the results of rational discourse in which all substantive commitments about what morality is are open to question. Every such substantive moral claim requires intellectual justification in the form of rigorous ethical analysis and argument. Therefore, philosophical ethics properly serves as the foundation for medical ethics, especially in an international context.

HISTORY OF MEDICAL ETHICS

Medical ethics has evolved since the beginning of civilization when health care knowledge was shared orally, and healers exemplified a community's moral code. Prince Hammurabi of Babylon recorded the responsibilities of health care providers in 1727 BCE, and early Hindu writers at about the same time cautioned healers to treat patients with respect, gentleness, and dignity. Fundamental principles of Western medical ethics were first recorded in ancient Greece in about the 5th century BCE. Hippocrates cautioned his students, "Primum non nocere," which famously means, "First, do no harm." In ethics, this is known as the *ethical principle of nonmaleficence*. Hippocrates' teachings emphasize choosing treatment based on the knowledge that would best benefit patients, treating patients as one would treat family members, upholding confidentiality, and practicing personal piety.

Ethical norms, elements, and principles were refined through the centuries. Thomas Percival (1740–1805) wrote a treatise that substantially changed medical ethics. Previously, a patient was someone who paid for treatment, but Percival redefined *patient* as anyone needing care. He also foresaw a team approach in health care and public health. Percival emphasized patient care provided by all professionals and ordered competitive or professional interests as secondary to the patient's needs.

Modern medical ethics was codified after the Nuremberg trials, which judged the atrocities done in medical experimentation by Nazi doctors. The judges in the Nuremberg trial issued a verdict that included a section on permissible human experimentation. That section, which became known as the Nuremberg code, was incorporated into regulatory policy in the United States. The same protections were adopted internationally and published within the Helsinki report in 1964. The Nuremberg code emphasized individual rights and autonomy and has become a key element of modern ethics.

Basic principles of medical ethics have been incorporated into research regulations, professional codes, and clinical practices worldwide. The ethical codes of various professional groups may differ slightly in definition and emphasis, but the basic principles of autonomy, justice, beneficence, nonmaleficence, integrity, and respect for persons are universal.

The *Code of Ethics for the Profession of Diagnostic Medical Sonography* has been adopted and is maintained by the SDMS.

PRINCIPLES OF MEDICAL ETHICS

Nonmaleficence

The principle of **nonmaleficence** directs the sonographer not to cause harm. Application of the principle of nonmaleficence requires the sonographer to obtain appropriate education and clinical skills to ensure competence in performing each required examination. Ensuring an appropriate level of competence imposes a rigorous standard of education and continuing education. Problems result when obstetric sonographers do not maintain a baseline level of competence in the techniques and interpretation of sonographic imaging: (1) They may cause unnecessary harm to the pregnant woman or fetal patient, for example, from mistaken impressions of fetal anomalies that in turn lead to unnecessary anxiety or testing; and (2) they may undermine the **informed consent** process regarding the management of pregnancy by reporting incompletely or inaccurately to the physician, who in turn reports misinformation to the pregnant woman.

Sonographers need to be accountable for and participate in regular assessment and review of protocols, equipment, procedures, and results to ensure that patients are not harmed by outdated procedures or poorly functioning equipment. Appropriate oversight and approval of protocols by research or hospital committees contribute to patient safety. Protocols and diagnostic criteria should be established by peer review. Sonographers may contribute to the safety of patients by sharing with others and publishing peer-reviewed information about mistakes made or lessons learned.

The sonographer must practice emergency procedures and ensure patient safety in all procedures and circumstances. Sonographers must refrain from substance abuse or any activity that may alter their judgment or ability to provide safe and effective patient care.

Because ultrasound energy poses a theoretical risk to the fetus, the principle of nonmaleficence requires sonographers to perform only medically indicated examinations and perform all examinations in keeping with the concept of ALARA, an energy exposure that is *as low as reasonably achievable*, to obtain the desired results. Sonographers should not perform obstetric ultrasound examinations for entertainment purposes.

Sonographers need to read the current medical literature to stay abreast of new developments related to patient safety. Sonographers should not perform ultrasound examinations without medical benefit.

Beneficence

Protections for patients and subjects based on the ethical principle of nonmaleficence only partially explain what is in the patients' interests because medicine, and therefore sonography, seeks to benefit patients, not simply avoid harming them. The use of obstetric ultrasound, like other medical interventions, must be justified by the goal of seeking the greater balance of clinical "goods" over "harms," not simply avoiding harm to the patient at all cost. This ethical principle is called **beneficence** and is a more comprehensive basis for sonography ethics than nonmaleficence.

Goods and harms must be defined and balanced from a rigorous clinical perspective. The goods that obstetric sonography should seek for patients include preventing early or premature death (not preventing death at all costs); preventing and managing disease, injury, and handicapping conditions; and alleviating unnecessary pain and suffering. Pain and suffering are unnecessary and therefore represent clinical harms to be avoided when they do not contribute to seeking the good of the beneficence-based clinical judgment. *Pain* is a physiologic phenomenon involving central nervous system processing of tissue damage. *Suffering* is a psychological phenomenon involving blocked intentions, plans, and projects. Pain often causes suffering, but one can suffer without being in pain.

The principle of beneficence obligates the obstetric sonographer to seek the greatest benefit in the care of pregnant patients. Beneficence encourages sonographers to go beyond the minimum standard protocol and to seek additional images and information if achievable and in the best interests of patients. Beneficence requires sonographers to focus on small comforts for patients, respecting their privacy, and including their family on request. Kindness and attention to small details minimize suffering caused by frustration or anger. Beneficence, like nonmaleficence, requires competency, knowledge, and excellent sonographic skills to ensure that the patient and the fetus receive the greatest benefit from the examination.

Fetal interests in sonography are understood exclusively in terms of beneficence. This principle explains the moral (as distinct from legal) status of the fetus as a patient and generates ethical obligations owed by physicians and sonographers to the fetus. In the technical language of beneficence, the sonographer has beneficence-based obligations to the fetal patient to protect and promote fetal interests and those of the child it will become, as these are understood from a rigorous clinical perspective. The clinical good to be sought for the fetal patient includes preventing premature death, disease, handicapping conditions, and unnecessary future pain and suffering. Therefore, it is appropriate to refer to fetuses as patients, except when a patient elects to terminate her pregnancy.

In clinical practice, beneficence may be balanced against other ethical principles. A health professional's duty of beneficence may suggest one course of action, and the patient may choose another. In these cases, beneficence must be balanced by respecting a person's autonomy. On occasion, the principles of veracity and integrity may conflict with beneficence when truth-telling causes undue stress and complications. The principle of justice or fair distribution of benefits may conflict with beneficence for individual patients who need extra resources. Fortunately, in most situations, it is in the patients' best interests to respect their autonomy, tell the truth, and distribute benefits justly.

Autonomy

In the 21st century, **autonomy**, or the right to self-determination, has become a key ethical principle. **Respect for persons** incorporates both respect for the autonomy of individuals and the requirement to protect those with diminished autonomy. Patients, including pregnant women, have their own perspective on their interests, which should be respected as much as the clinician's perspective on patients' interests. A patient's perspective on her interests is shaped by wide-ranging and sometimes idiosyncratic values and beliefs. *Autonomy* refers to a person's capacity to formulate, express, and carry out value-based preferences. The ethical principle of respect for autonomy obligates the sonographer to acknowledge the integrity of a patient's values and beliefs and her value-based preferences; to avoid interfering with the expression or implementation of these preferences; and, when necessary, to assist in their expression and implementation. This principle generates the autonomy-based obligations of the sonographer.

Informed consent is an autonomy-based right. Each health professional has autonomy-based obligations regarding the informed consent process. This process must include discourse about what sonography examinations can and cannot detect, the sensitivity and frequency of false-negative and false-positive results of the sonography techniques employed, and the difficult and sometimes uncertain interpretation of sonographic images. In the face of medical uncertainty about the clinical good and harm of routine ultrasound, the sonographer must inform pregnant patients about that uncertainty and allow them to make their own choices about how that uncertainty should be managed. In routine examinations, informing the woman of the possibility of confronting an anomaly that will lead her to decide whether to terminate the pregnancy or take it to term is also important.

As the protocols and options for gaining medical information regarding potential fetal anomalies increase and risk assessment becomes more individualized, requirements are increased for patient education that is sufficient for informed choice. Genetic counselors, patient educators, sonographers, and physicians often work together to counsel women regarding their options and choices.

The sonographer respects the patient's autonomy by providing a detailed explanation of the examination, including appropriate choices such as the right to view the screen or to learn the gender of the fetus. Respect for maternal autonomy dictates responding frankly to requests from the pregnant woman for information about the gender of the fetus. As part of the disclosure process, the pregnant woman should be made aware of the uncertainties of ultrasound gender identification. The sonographer can use their own experience to help the pregnant woman understand these uncertainties. A second choice that may be presented during obstetric examinations is the choice to view the images. This choice concerns the phenomenon of apparent bonding of pregnant women and their families to the fetus as a result of seeing the sonographic images. Such bonding often enriches pregnancies that will be taken to term, but at other times can complicate decisions to terminate a pregnancy.

A current ethical issue is the nonmedical use of sonography to videotape or photograph "baby pictures." Nothing is intrinsically wrong with the practice if it is a side product of a legitimate ultrasound examination. However, when videotaping or photography is performed to generate revenue, this practice trivializes medical sonography and may result in harm because problems that could be diagnosed may be missed. Dwelling on the fetal profile or face for entertainment purposes is contrary to ALARA and the principle of nonmaleficence. It is the responsibility of sonographers to ensure that women have the information necessary to make informed choices.

It is an autonomy-enhancing strategy for a woman to be allowed to insert a vaginal probe herself to make the experience more comfortable and less threatening. It is also a sonographer's obligation to respect a patient's right to refuse a procedure.

Maternal interests are protected and promoted by the sonographer's autonomy-based and beneficence-based obligations to the pregnant woman. Fetuses are incapable of having their own perspective on their interests because the immaturity of their central nervous system renders them incapable of having the requisite values or beliefs. Thus there can be no autonomy-based obligations to the fetus. The pregnant woman also has beneficence-based obligations to the fetal patient when the pregnancy will be taken to term. She is expected to protect and promote the fetal patient's interests and those of the child it will become. However, when a pregnant woman elects to have an abortion, these obligations do not exist. A sonographer with moral objections to abortion should keep two things in mind: First, the moral judgment and decision of the pregnant woman to end her pregnancy should not be criticized or commented on in any way; her autonomy demands respect as shown by the sonographer and the physician being neutral to her judgment and decision. Second, the sonographer is free to follow his or her conscience and to withdraw from further involvement with patients who elect abortion. As a matter of office policy, physicians should respect this important matter of individual conscience on the part of the sonographer.

Veracity and Integrity

Telling the truth is an ethical practice that most sonographers have been taught from a young age. Yet, on occasion, most of us will tell "white lies" in kindness or to escape unwanted consequences. The universal acceptance and even cultural preference in some countries for white lies is evidence of the difficulty of adhering to the veracity principle. **Veracity** means truthfulness. **Integrity** means adherence to moral and ethical principles. Integrity is related to the word *integrate*, meaning "to bring together." In terms of honesty, integrity means that there is no difference between what you think, what you say, and what you do: They all come together in ethical behavior.

In medical care, patients properly rely for their protection on their clinicians' personal and professional integrity. A crucial aspect of that integrity on the part of physicians is willingness to refer to specialists when the limits of their own knowledge are being approached. Integrity should also be one of the fundamental virtues of sonographers and thus a standard for judging professional character. Similar to other virtues, such as self-sacrifice and compassion, integrity directs sonographers to focus primarily on the patient's interests as a way to blunt mere self-interest. Sonographers must avoid conflicts of interest and situations that exploit others, create unreasonable expectations, or misrepresent information.

Veracity concerning abilities and limitations is essential among sonographers. If a practitioner asks a sonographer to perform an examination that he or she is not competent to do, the sonographer must be truthful about his or her limitations to protect the patient. A sonographer asked by a patient or a colleague must accurately represent their level of competence, education, and credentials.

Premature disclosure of the results of an abnormal sonographic examination raises significant clinical ethical issues for sonographers. Sonographers are justified in disclosing findings of normal anatomy directly to the pregnant woman. When images reveal abnormal findings, sonographers must not act "dumb" or tell the patient they do not know what they see. Veracity is upheld by telling the patient in a nonalarming way the procedure for diagnosis, that "multiple eyes need to look at some of the images," and that the physician will determine the results. Disclosure of and discussion about abnormal findings by sonographers is inappropriate because it is not in the patient's best interest. If the disclosure and the discussion are to respect and enhance maternal autonomy and avoid unnecessary psychological harm to the pregnant woman, the discussion should occur in a setting where the alternatives and choices available to manage the pregnancy are presented. Sonographers cannot, by training or by experience, claim the clinical competence to engage in such discussions. Physicians can and therefore should.

Sonographers must strive to supply patients and colleagues with complete and accurate information. The sonographer's integrity is an essential safeguard for the patient's autonomy. At times, the sonographer will need to become an advocate, even a vigorous advocate, to disclose information to a patient. In such cases, sonographers must address their concerns not to the patient but the practitioner involved. Failure to make patient disclosures undermines professional integrity and the moral authority of health care professionals. When the sonographer disagrees with the clinical judgment of his or her supervising physician, professional communication and discussion of the matter need to occur. Such conversations enhance the best interests of the health care team and the patient.

Justice

Justice is the ethical principle that requires fair distribution of benefits and burdens; an injustice occurs when a benefit to which a person is entitled is withheld or when a burden is unfairly imposed. Justice means simply that sonographers must strive to treat all patients equally. In practical terms, justice requires that translators be used when necessary to ensure adequate and appropriate communication with all patients. Sonographers should ensure that disabled patients have access to reasonable accommodations and pathways and that obese patients have comfortable chairs, gowns, and stretchers. Children, adults, and geriatric patients need to feel equally welcome and cared for within the sonography laboratory.

Justice is served when protocols are standardized. Men and women with similar symptoms should receive similar tests and interventions. If a group is denied services or is asked to assume an undue burden to obtain care provided to others, justice is not being served.

Justice and autonomy are the ethical principles that determine the timing of obstetric sonography examinations. The information obtained from a sonogram enhances women's choices. It is an injustice to provide this information to some women and not to others. For this reason, recommendations are made that all women be offered risk assessment for anomalies during the first trimester. Sonography results, such as risk for an abnormality, are relevant to the woman's decision about whether she will seek an abortion. In pregnancies taken to term, sonography enhances a pregnant woman's autonomy. The timing of the information is also relevant if anomalies are detected, and she does not choose abortion, as she may begin to prepare herself for the decisions that she will confront later regarding management of the anomalies in the intrapartum and postpartum periods. Providing requested information early in pregnancy permits a pregnant woman ample time to deal with psychological and practical issues before she must confront decisions.

The principle of justice implies that health care professionals should act in accordance with the best interest of the community. As health care costs increase, insurance costs skyrocket, and bankruptcy becomes associated with chronic illness, the societal aspects of medical justice are receiving more attention. The traditional focus of medical ethics is the individual patient. In some cases, however, the costs and benefits of treating one patient may place an undue burden on others. An individual ethical focus may conflict with a society's focus when an individual uses a disproportionate amount of health care without paying for it. This forces others to pay for the service—a burden that society accepts if the service is considered essential. However, as the benefit of the service decreases, as in experimental protocols, or as the cost of the service increases, the conflict grows. If the resources used are not replaced, others may be deprived of similar services. The solution to such conflicts is not clear politically, socially, or ethically. However, what is clear is that the community aspect of justice will receive more attention in the future. Sonographers can support community interests by performing only medically indicated procedures prescribed by a clinician.

CONFIDENTIALITY OF FINDINGS

Confidentiality concerns the obligation of caregivers to protect clinical information about patients from unauthorized access. The obligation of confidentiality derives from the principles of beneficence (patients will be more forthcoming) and respect for autonomy (patients' privacy rights are protected). Others, including the pregnant woman's spouse and/or sex partner and family, should be understood as third parties to the patient–sonographer relationship. Diagnostic information about a woman's pregnancy is confidential. It can be justifiably disclosed to third parties *only* with the pregnant woman's *explicit permission*. Federal regulations, including the Health Insurance Portability and Accountability Act (HIPAA), determine acceptable conditions for releasing confidential information. To prevent awkward situations, sonographers and their supervising physicians should establish policies and procedures that reflect the ethics of confidentiality.

The ethics of confidentiality when the pregnant woman is younger than 18 years of age should be the same as when the patient is 18 years of age or older. The law, however, may complicate matters because pregnancy does not emancipate a minor in every jurisdiction, and different jurisdictions give different levels of protection to the privacy of the physician–patient relationship when the patient is younger than 18 years of age.

ACKNOWLEDGMENTS

The author acknowledges the work of Frank A. Chervenak and Laurence B. McCullough on this chapter in the previous edition.

Key Pearls

- Patient trust is built on the expectation that health care professionals will follow established ethical principles and guidelines.
- Medical ethics promotes excellence and protects patients by encouraging practitioners to reflect on, communicate, and demonstrate optimal care.
- The principles of nonmaleficence, beneficence, autonomy, respect for persons, veracity and integrity, and justice must be implemented in the sonography laboratory to ensure ethical practice.
- Application of the principle of nonmaleficence requires the sonographer to obtain appropriate education and clinical skills to ensure competence in performing each required examination.
- Sonographers need to be accountable for and participate in regular assessment and review of protocols, equipment, procedures, and results to ensure that patients are not harmed by outdated procedures or poorly functioning equipment.
- The sonographer must practice emergency procedures and ensure patient safety in all procedures and circumstances.
- The principle of nonmaleficence requires sonographers to perform only medically indicated examinations and perform all examinations in keeping with ALARA, an energy exposure that is as low as reasonably achievable, to obtain the desired results.
- The goods that obstetric sonography should seek for patients include preventing early or premature death (not preventing death at all costs); preventing and managing disease, injury, and handicapping conditions; and alleviating unnecessary pain and suffering.
- Beneficence encourages sonographers to go beyond the minimum standard protocol and to seek additional images and information if achievable and in the best interests of patients.
- The ethical principle of respect for autonomy obligates the sonographer to acknowledge the integrity of a patient's values and beliefs and her value-based preferences; to avoid interfering with the expression or implementation of these preferences; and, when necessary, to assist in their expression and implementation.
- Veracity means truthfulness. Integrity means adherence to moral and ethical principles.
- If a practitioner asks a sonographer to perform an examination that he or she is not competent to do, the sonographer needs to be truthful about his or her limitations to protect the patient.
- Sonographers are justified in disclosing findings of normal anatomy directly to the pregnant woman.
- Veracity is upheld by telling the patient in a nonalarming way the procedure for diagnosis, that "multiple eyes need to look at some of the images," and that the physician will determine the results.
- Justice means simply that sonographers must strive to treat all patients equally.
- The obligation of confidentiality derives from the principles of beneficence (patients will be more forthcoming) and respect for autonomy (patients' privacy rights are protected).

BIBLIOGRAPHY

American College of Obstetricians and Gynecologists. Practice bulletin no. 77: screening for fetal chromosomal anomalies. *Obstet Gynecol.* 2007;109:217–227.

Annas G, Grodin M, eds. *The Nazi doctors and the Nuremberg code: human rights in human experimentation.* New York: Oxford University Press; 1992.

Beauchamp TL, Childress JF. *Principles of biomedical ethics.* ed. 6, New York: Oxford University Press; 1997.

Beauchamp TL, McCullough LB. *Medical ethics: the moral responsibilities of physicians.* Englewood Cliffs, NJ: Prentice-Hall; 1984.

Benn PA, Chapman AR. Practical and ethical considerations of noninvasive prenatal diagnosis. *J Am Med Assoc.* 2009;301:2154–2156.

Boodt CL. A historical review of the SDMS code of ethics. *J Diagn Med Sonogr.* 2004;20:238.

Campbell S. Ultrasound scanning in pregnancy: the short-term psychological effects of early real time scans. *J Psychosomat Obstet Gynecol.* 1986;1:57.

Chervenak FA, McCullough LB. Perinatal ethics: a practical method of analysis of obligations to mother and fetus. *Obstet Gynecol.* 1985;66:442–446.

Chervenak FA, McCullough LB. Ethics in obstetric ultrasound. *J Ultrasound Med.* 1989;8:493–497.

Chervenak FA, McCullough LB, Chervenak JL. Prenatal informed consent for sonogram (PICS): an indication for obstetric ultrasound. *Am J Obstet Gynecol.* 1989;161:857–860.

Chervenak FA, McCullough LB, Sharma G, et al. Enhancing patient autonomy with risk assessment and invasive diagnosis: an ethical solution to a clinical challenge. *Am J Obstet Gynecol.* 2008; 199(19e):1–19e.4.

Dunn CM, Chadwick GL. *Protecting study volunteers in research: a manual for investigative sites.* ed. 2, Boston: Thomson Centerwatch; 2002.

Eddy DM. Clinical decision making: from theory to practice: The individual vs society: is there a conflict? *J Am Med Assoc.* 1991; 265:1446–1450.

Eddy DM. Clinical decision making: from theory to practice. The individual vs society: resolving the conflict. *J Am Med Assoc.* 1991;265:2399–2401.

Ewigman BG, Crane JP, Frigoletto FD, et al. Effect of prenatal ultrasound screening on perinatal outcome, RADIUS study group. *N Engl J Med.* 1993;329:821–827.

McCullough LB. Methodological concerns in bioethics. *J Med Phil.* 1986;11:17–37.

McCullough LB, Chervenak FA. *Ethics in obstetrics and gynecology.* New York: Oxford University Press; 1994.

Purtilo R. *Ethical dimensions in the health professions.* ed. 2, Philadelphia: Saunders; 1993.

Skupski DW, Chervenak FA, McCullough LB. Is routine ultrasound screening for all patients? *Clin Perinatol.* 1994;21:707–722.

Society of Diagnostic Medical Sonography. Code of ethics for the profession of diagnostic medical sonography. http://www.sdms.org/about/who-we-are/code-of-ethics.

CHAPTER 49

The Early Embryonic Stage of the First Trimester

Sandra L. Hagen-Ansert

OBJECTIVES

On completion of this chapter, you should be able to:
- Describe the early development of the embryo and its sonographic appearance at different gestational ages
- Explain the clinical roles of first-trimester maternal serum biochemistry
- Define the sonographic characteristics of the yolk sac, embryo, amnion and chorion, and gestational sac
- Describe the sonographic measurements performed in the first trimester and the goals of first-trimester sonography

OUTLINE

Overview of the First Trimester 1301
    Embryologic Age and Gestational Age 1301
    Normal Pregnancy Progression 1301
Maternal Serum Analysis in Early Pregnancy 1303
Transvaginal Sonographic Technique and Evaluation 1305

Embryology of the First Trimester 1305
Fetal Period (Weeks 9–14) 1306
    Visualization of the Embryo: 6 to 10 Weeks of Gestational Age 1310
Determination of Gestational Age 1313
    Mean Gestational Sac Size 1314
    Crown-Rump Length 1315
First-Trimester Complications 1316

Positive hCG Without Intrauterine Fluid Collection or Adnexal Mass 1316
Positive hCG With Intrauterine Fluid Collection Without Yolk Sac or Embryo; No Adnexal Mass 1316
First-Trimester Risk Assessment 1316
    First-Trimester Risk Assessment Sonography Techniques 1317

KEY TERMS

Amniotic cavity
Chorionic cavity
Chorionic villi sampling (CVS)
Crown-rump length (CRL)
Decidua basalis
Decidua capsularis

Double decidual sac sign
Embryonic period
Gestational age
Hematopoiesis
Human chorionic gonadotropin (hCG)
Intrauterine pregnancy (IUP)

Mean sac diameter (MSD)
Primary yolk sac
Secondary yolk sac
Yolk stalk
Zygote

Transvaginal ultrasound evaluation of the first-trimester pregnancy is an important component of prenatal care. The ultrasound examination may diagnose conditions that require intervention, and even in "normal" intrauterine pregnancies (IUPs) the exam may provide patients and clinicians with information that influences clinical management. Information about multiple pregnancies, uterine anomalies, and pelvic masses that are readily visualized during the first trimester may be more difficult to obtain later.

Aspects of prenatal fetal screening and diagnosis are shifting from second trimester to first trimester. First-trimester aneuploidy screening protocols have higher detection rates than second-trimester tests. Genomic technology allows screening of cell-free fetal deoxyribonucleic acid (DNA) in early pregnancy. The current standard of care suggests offering aneuploidy screening during the first trimester to all obstetric patients and, where available, offering diagnostic genetic testing through **chorionic villi sampling (CVS)** between 11 and 13 weeks. Fetal anatomy has not been routinely assessed until the second trimester, but recent studies have demonstrated the possibility of detecting many structural anomalies earlier. In the morbidly obese gravida, assessment of fetal anatomy through transvaginal sonography in the late first trimester may be an improvement over second-trimester scanning.

Although the ability to image the first-trimester pregnancy with ultrasound may seem routine, the potential for false-positive and false-negative diagnoses for any given pathology is substantial. Extreme care should be taken when evaluating the first-trimester pregnancy sonographically.

OVERVIEW OF THE FIRST TRIMESTER

Embryologic Age and Gestational Age

It is especially important to have a clear understanding of terminology when discussing embryology. Embryologists state time in *conceptual age*, also known as *embryologic age*, with conception as the first day of pregnancy. Clinicians and sonographers use **gestational age**, also known as *menstrual age*, to date the pregnancy, with the first day of the last menstrual period (LMP) as the beginning of gestation. Thus the gestational age would add 2 weeks onto the conceptual age. For 12 days after conception, during the implantation process, the conceptus is called a *zygote*. From the time of implantation until the end of the 10th week menstrual age, the conceptus is called an *embryo*. After the first 10 weeks, the embryo is called a *fetus*.

Normal Pregnancy Progression

Except when specifically noted, dates in this chapter reflect menstrual/gestational age rather than embryologic age. Menstrual age refers to the length of time calculated from the first day of the LMP, to the point at which the pregnancy is being assessed. During a 28-day menstrual cycle, a mature ovum is typically released at day 14. The ovum is swept into the distal fallopian tube via fimbriae; fertilization occurs within this region 1 to 2 days after ovulation. Meanwhile, the follicle that released the mature ovum hemorrhages and collapses to form the corpus luteum, which begins to secrete progesterone and estrogen (Fig. 49.1).

The fertilized conceptus that is now referred to as a zygote undergoes rapid cellular division to form the 16-cell morula. Further cell proliferation brings the morula to the blastocyst stage. The blastocyst contains trophoblastic cells and the "inner cell mass," which forms the embryo. The trophoblastic cells begin to secrete **human chorionic gonadotropin (hCG)** that is absorbed within the tubes and stimulates maternal pregnancy responses.

The hCG causes the uterine endometrium to convert to decidua, a glycogen-rich mucosa that nourishes the early pregnancy. The blastocyst typically enters the uterus 4 to 5 days after fertilization. Implantation into the uterine decidua is completed within 12 days after fertilization. During implantation, proteolytic enzymes produced by the trophoblasts "eat into" decidual tissue, creating spaces for trophoblastic cell proliferation. Blood pools

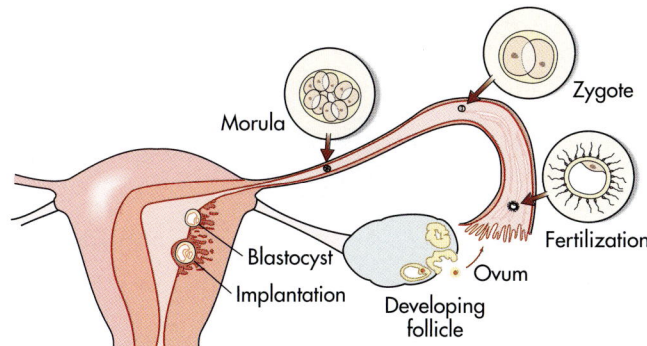

FIG. 49.1 Fertilization takes place in the upper third of the fallopian tube as the zygote begins its development and moves toward the uterine cavity. Diagram illustrates the zygote stage from conception through implantation.

known as *lacunae* that form as maternal capillaries erode nourish the proliferating trophoblastic cells. A primitive blood exchange network between mother and conceptus is formed, and the lacunae and trophoblastic cells develop into a mature placental/maternal circulation complex that will sustain the pregnancy. By the end of the implantation process, the zygote has buried itself within one wall of the uterus. The implantation process sometimes results in light vaginal bleeding about the same time as the expected menstrual period.

When implantation is complete, the trophoblast has formed primary villi, which initially encircle the early gestational sac. Within the conceptus, the inner cell mass matures into the bilaminar embryonic disk, the future embryo, and the primary yolk sac (Fig. 49.2). At approximately 23 days of menstrual age, the **primary yolk sac** is pinched off by the extraembryonic coelom, forming the **secondary yolk sac**. The secondary yolk sac is the yolk sac seen sonographically throughout the first trimester (Fig. 49.3). The amniotic and chorionic cavities also develop and evolve during this period of gestation. Note the gestational sac should be visible by transvaginal ultrasound at 5 weeks, and the yolk sac may be visible from 5.5 weeks throughout the first trimester. The embryo is usually seen at 6 weeks, and the amnion is visualized at approximately 7 weeks.

The embryonic phase occurs from the fourth to the ninth weeks (Fig. 49.4). It is during this phase that all major internal and external structures begin to develop (Table 49.1). The cardiovascular system undergoes rapid development, with the initial heartbeat occurring at approximately 5 to 6 weeks. The embryo's appearance changes from a flat, disk-like configuration to a C-shaped structure, and it develops a human-like appearance. During this period of embryogenesis, the **crown-rump length (CRL)** develops rapidly, measuring 35 mm by the end of the 10th week.

The last 3 weeks of the first trimester (weeks 10 to 12) constitute the beginning of the fetal period. During the fetal period, growth of the organs and structures formed during the embryonic period continues. At this stage, the fetal head is disproportionately larger than the rest of the fetus, constituting one half of the CRL (Fig. 49.5). As the fetus grows,

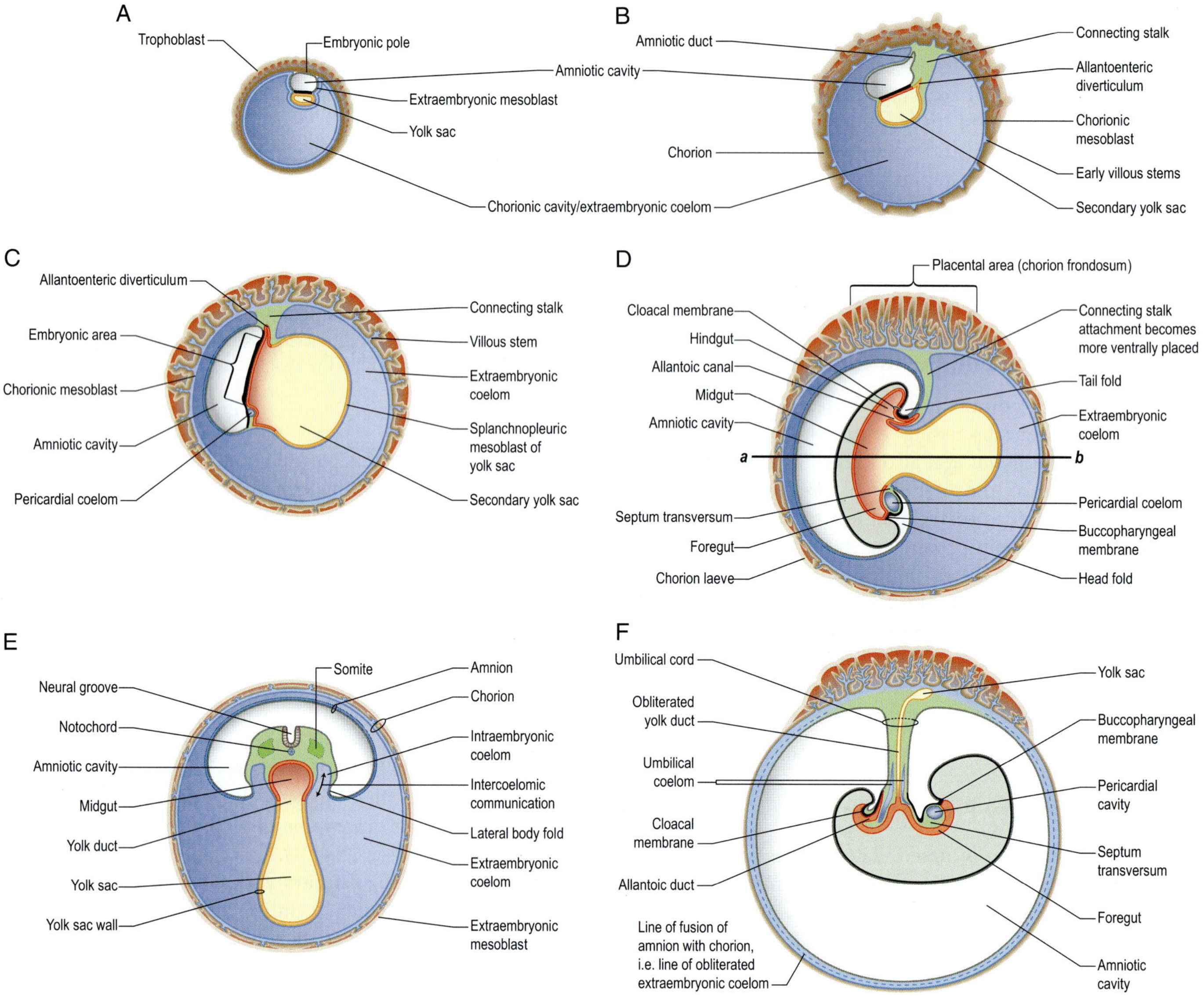

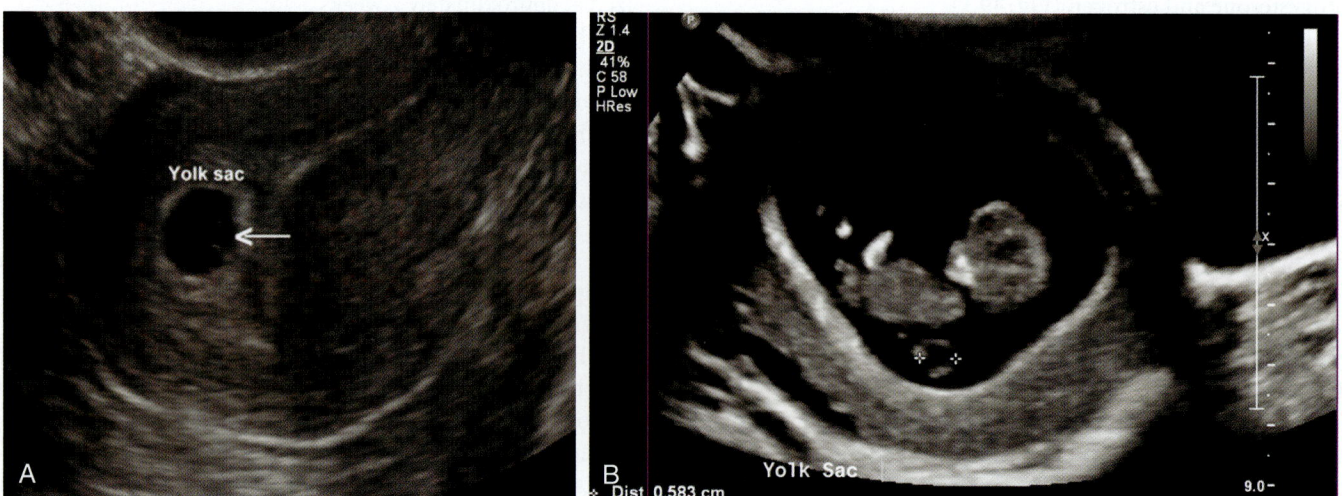

FIG. 49.2 When implantation is complete, the trophoblast has formed primary villi, which initially encircle the early gestational sac. Within the conceptus, the inner cell mass matures into the bilaminar embryonic disk, the future embryo, and the primary yolk sac. At approximately 23 days of menstrual age, the primary yolk sac is pinched off by the extraembryonic coelom, forming the secondary yolk sac.

FIG. 49.3 The secondary yolk sac is the yolk sac seen sonographically throughout the first trimester.

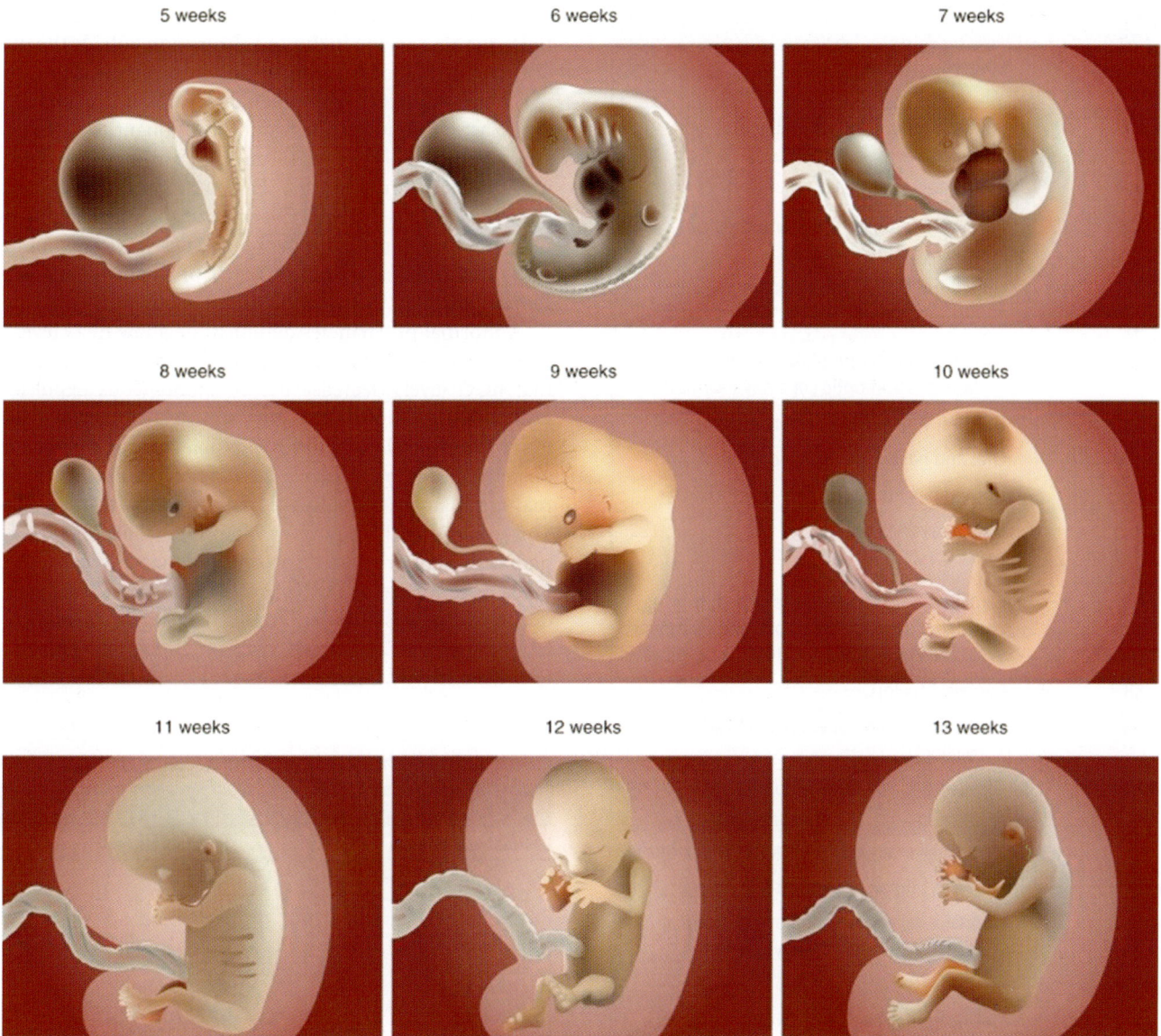

FIG. 49.4 The embryonic phase occurs from the fourth to the ninth weeks. During this phase, all major internal and external structures begin to develop.

body growth accelerates, and this proportionality becomes less pronounced. Fetal anatomy is fully developed in the late first trimester, and the goal of sonography at this stage includes anomaly detection.

MATERNAL SERUM ANALYSIS IN EARLY PREGNANCY

Maternal serum biochemistry values can be very useful in evaluation of the early pregnancy. A direct relationship exists in early pregnancy between the sonographic findings and quantitative serum hCG levels. Gestational sac size and hCG levels increase proportionately until 10 menstrual weeks, at which time the gestational sac is approximately 45-mm **mean sac diameter (MSD)**, and an embryo should be easily detected by transabdominal or transvaginal sonography.

Quantitative hCG levels in viable IUPs, nonviable IUPs, and ectopic pregnancies have considerable overlap. In general, a normal gestational sac is expected to be visible when the hCG level is greater than 1000 mIU/mL (Second International Standard) to 2000 mIU/mL (Table 49.2). The sonographer must be aware that when the hCG value is greater than the 2000 or even 3000 mIU/mL level, and the gestational sac is not seen by transvaginal ultrasound within the uterus, a normal IUP is not fully excluded; an ectopic pregnancy may be considered. However, a single hCG measurement in a woman with a pregnancy of unknown location does not reliably distinguish a normal IUP from a failed IUP or ectopic pregnancy. If the women is hemodynamically stable, there is little risk in delaying treatment by a few days in a woman with ectopic pregnancy and no adnexal mass on ultrasound. The patient should be reevaluated in 7 to 10 days to confirm if a viable pregnancy is present.

TABLE 49.1		Normal Embryonic Development
Menstrual Age	CRL (mm)	Embryonic Observations
Week 5		Prominent neural folds and neural groove are recognizable.
Day 36		Heart begins to beat.
Week 6		Anterior and posterior neuropores close and neural tube forms.
Day 41		Upper and lower limb buds are present.
Day 42	4.0	
Day 46		Paddle-shaped hand plates are present; lens pits and optic cups have formed.
Day 48		Cerebral vesicles are distinct.
Day 50		Oral and nasal cavities are confluent.
Day 52		Upper lip is formed.
Day 54		Digital rays are distinct.
Day 56	16.0	
Week 9		Cardiac ventricular septum is closed; truncus arteriosus divides into aorta and pulmonary trunk; kidney collecting tubules develop.
Day 58		Eyelids develop.
Day 64		Upper limbs bend at elbows; fingers are distinct.
Week 10		Glomeruli form in metanephros.
Day 73		Genitalia show some female characteristics but are still easily confused with male genitalia.
Day 80		Face has human appearance.
Day 82		Genitalia have male and female characteristics but still are not fully formed.
Day 84	55.0	
Month 7		Ossification is complete throughout vertebral column.
Month 8		Ossification centers appear in distal femoral epiphysis.

CRL, Crown-rump length.
From Neiman HL. Sonoembryology. In Nyberg DA, et al, editors. *Transvaginal Ultrasound*. St Louis: Mosby–Year Book; 1990.

Ectopic pregnancies demonstrate a lower hCG level than IUPs, perhaps owing to limited absorption outside the uterus. The rate of rise or increase in hCG during early pregnancy may help to detect ectopic pregnancies. The normal IUP at less than 7 weeks demonstrates doubling of quantitative maternal serum hCG levels every 3.5 days, or an increase of 66% in hCG levels within 48 hours. If this normal rate of increase is not seen, there is a greater chance that the pregnancy is ectopic. However, some ectopic pregnancies will show a normal rate of increase, and some normal pregnancies will show a reduced rate.

Abnormal pregnancies demonstrate a low hCG level relative to gestational sac development, and it has been shown that hCG levels decrease before spontaneous expulsion of nonviable gestations. Sonographers need to review quantitative hCG levels whenever possible before first-trimester obstetric examinations are performed, because physicians may correlate hCG levels with the gestational sac appearance. This is particularly important when vaginal bleeding or pelvic pain is present or when an ectopic pregnancy is suspected.

At 9 to 10 weeks, hCG levels plateau and subsequently decline while gestation continues. In pregnancies where the fetus is trisomy 21 (Down syndrome), the hCG levels plateau later and decrease much more slowly. Levels of hCG are

TABLE 49.2	Beta–Human Chorionic Gonadotropin Levels During Pregnancy
Menstrual Weeks	hCG Levels (mIU/mL)
3	0–5
4	5–426
5	18–7340
6	1080–56,500
7–8	7650–229,000
10–12	25,700–288,000

Human chorionic gonadotropin rates typically decrease after the first trimester, when the placenta takes over. Even if levels rise, failure of the levels to double every few days is not a good sign, and the pregnancy may end in miscarriage. If the test is low or borderline, a repeat test will be ordered in a few days.

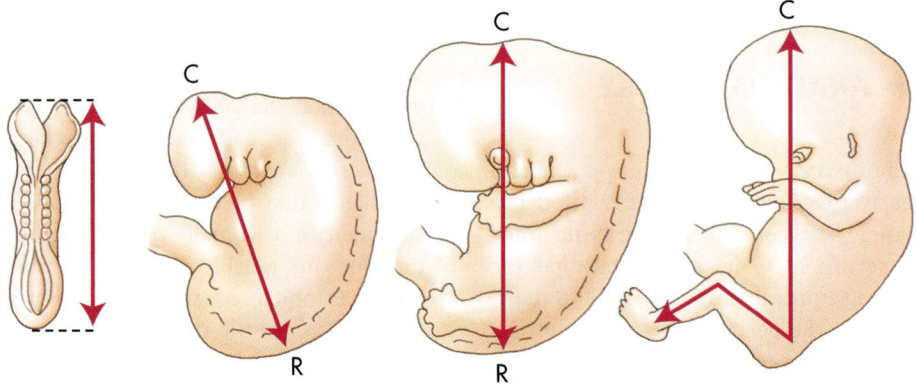

FIG. 49.5 The relationship of neural tube development to crown-rump length in the first trimester. Note the size of the embryo's head relative to the body. At the beginning of the fetal period in the late first trimester, the embryo's head measures almost half of the crown-rump length.

increased in these pregnancies compared with normal pregnancies, and the difference increases as gestation advances. Consequently, increased hCG levels can be used as a screening marker for Down syndrome during the first and second trimesters. Increased hCG is not a strong marker and does not have sufficient sensitivity to be used by itself in screening for Down syndrome. It is combined with other independent markers to enhance detection. The hCG is a component of first-trimester risk assessment and a component of triple-screen and quad-screen testing performed during the second trimester. The sensitivity of hCG for Down syndrome assessment is improved by measurement of the free beta subunit. Both total hCG and free beta hCG are used for aneuploidy screening in the United States.

Pregnancy-associated plasma protein–A (PAPP-A), also known as pappalysin-1, is an insulin-like growth factor produced by trophoblastic (placental) cells during pregnancy. It is involved in proliferative growth processes such as bone and tissue formation. Maternal serum PAPP-A increases with advancing gestation. In trisomy 21–affected pregnancies, PAPP-A levels are initially lower than in normal pregnancies, but the difference decreases with increasing gestational age. Decreased values of maternal serum PAPP-A may be a marker for Down syndrome during the first trimester but are not useful in the second trimester. Currently, PAPP-A analysis at 9 to 11 weeks of gestational age is the strongest biochemical marker for Down syndrome. However, PAPP-A is not sensitive enough to be used by itself and is combined with hCG levels for serum biochemistry screening or with hCG and sonographic markers for combined screening. Some studies project an association between PAPP-A levels in early pregnancy and pregnancy pathology such as growth restriction, preterm labor, and preeclampsia.

Genomic techniques allow fragments of fetal DNA, cell-free fetal DNA, that originate primarily from the placenta to be found in maternal serum and analyzed from 9 weeks of gestation. The cell-free DNA screening tests have very high detection rates for trisomy 21, but false-positive and false-negative results have been reported. The positive predictive value of the tests varies depending on the prevalence of the condition and risk level of the mother. Before or after cell-free DNA screening, there is substantial value in first-trimester ultrasound screening for structural fetal anomalies.

TRANSVAGINAL SONOGRAPHIC TECHNIQUE AND EVALUATION

First-trimester obstetric sonography has evolved rapidly with the high-definition transvaginal transducers, which allow the gravid uterus and adnexa to be visualized with improved resolution by allowing higher frequencies and transducer placement closer to anatomic structures compared with transabdominal scanning. With transvaginal transducers, the pelvic anatomy is imaged in both sagittal and coronal/semicoronal planes. Such coronal imaging of the pelvis is unique within sonography, and the images should not be misconstrued as transverse sections.

Although transvaginal sonography has gained overall acceptance within the medical community because of its improved image quality, transabdominal and transperineal sonography should not be overlooked. The transabdominal approach allows visualization of a larger field of anatomy, which is important when specific anatomic relationships are in question. For instance, the size, extent, and anatomic relationships of a large pelvic mass with surrounding structures can be determined only with transabdominal techniques. In many labs, the transabdominal approach is used first while the patient has a full bladder (Fig. 49.6). This is followed by the detailed transvaginal exam after the bladder is completely emptied. In addition, when necessary, the transperineal approach may be used to visualize the cervix. Three-dimensional sonography may also be performed in the first trimester in those patients who may require better visualization of specific anatomical detail. The use of pulsed Doppler analysis during the first trimester is not recommended and should be performed only when there are clear benefits.

Embryology of the First Trimester

The first 4 weeks of early development are not clearly visible with transvaginal ultrasound. During this period after fertilization, the foundation is begun with the development of the primary yolk sac, the primitive streak, neurulation, intraembryonic coelom, primitive cardiovascular system, and chorionic villi are formulated. Although the pregnancy implants in the decidua on one side of the uterine cavity approximately 1 week after fertilization, it may not be visible on ultrasound for at least another 2 weeks (Fig. 49.7). The variability of determining gestational age by ultrasound is approximately ±0.5 weeks.

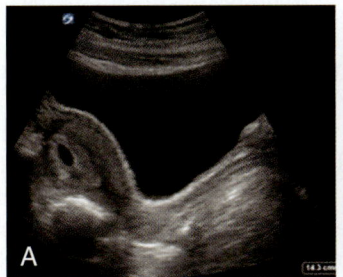 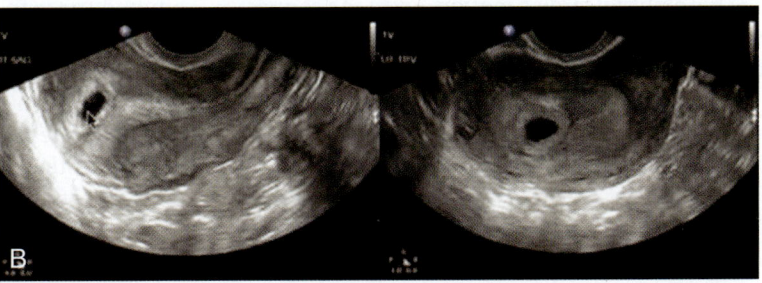

FIG. 49.6 (A) In many labs, the transabdominal approach is used first while the patient has a full bladder. (B) This is followed by the detailed transvaginal exam after the bladder is completely emptied.

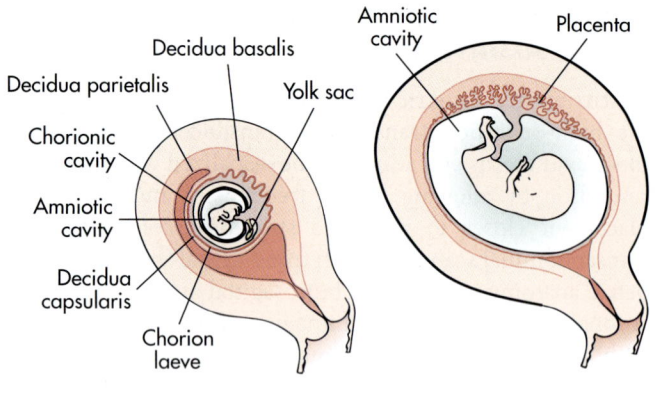

FIG. 49.7 Relation of the fetal membranes and the wall of the uterus. (A) End of the second month. Note the yolk sac in the chorionic cavity between the amnion and chorion. At the embryonic pole, the villi have disappeared (chorion laeve). (B) End of the third month. The amnion and chorion have fused and the uterine cavity is obliterated by fusion of the chorion laeve and the decidua parietalis.

> **BOX 49.1 Sonographic Features of a Typical Gestational Sac**
>
> - Shape: round or oval.
> - Position: fundal or middle portion of uterus; a center position relative to endometrium (double decidual sac or intradecidua finding).
> - Contour: smooth.
> - Wall (trophoblastic reaction): echogenic.
> - Internal landmarks: yolk sac typically present when gestational sac is >12 mm; embryo present when gestational sac is >25 mm.

Week 4. During the fourth week of growth, there is significant development of the embryotic body, with the formation of the primordium of the brain from the previously formed neural tube, the oropharyngeal membrane, and the foregut. Also during the fourth week, hematopoietic cells begin to colonize the newly forming liver. The primordial heart begins to develop and contract. At this point, as the embryo folds in both the cephalocaudal and lateral directions, the intraembryonic coelom is divided by the septum transversum, which becomes the diaphragm. This septum transversum divides the primordial body cavities into the cranial pericardial cavity and the caudal peritoneal cavity. The maxilla and mandible begin to form. The forebrain prominence results in the "C-shaped" curve of the embryo. The limb buds appear at the end of the fourth week.

Week 5. During the fifth week of embryonic development, the **intrauterine pregnancy (IUP)** can be visualized well with transvaginal ultrasound. There is marked accelerated growth, with the head growth outpacing the other embryonic structures. The face begins to take form, and the future kidneys are noted by the development of the mesonephric ridges. The embryonic heart develops into a four-chambered structure.

At 5.5 weeks' gestation, the primitive yolk sac gradually reduces in size to become the secondary yolk sac. The MSD should measure 6 mm. The yolk sac may be used as a landmark to image the embryo/cardiac motion, given the connection between the yolk sac and embryo.

Week 6. The sixth week shows further differentiation of the limb buds. The primordial ears and eyes develop. Now the fetal liver occupies the majority of the abdominal cavity. The intestines exceed the growth of the abdominal cavity, which causes physiologic herniation of the intestines into the umbilical cord. Spontaneous movements and reflex responses to touch are now present.

An embryo should be seen on transvaginal ultrasound at 6 weeks' gestational age, when the MSD is greater than 10 mm (Box 49.1). The embryo appears as a 1- to 4-mm echogenic structure within the gestational sac. The fluttering motion inside the embryo represents cardiac activity.

Week 7. The seventh week of development shows further growth of the limbs, hands, and feet. The central nervous system is divided into the prosencephalon (forebrain), mesencephalon (midbrain), and rhombencephalon (hindbrain); the lateral ventricles are a single ventricle at this stage because the midline falx cerebri has not yet developed.

At 7 weeks the embryo is 10 mm in length and the amnion should become visible around the embryo, as the **amniotic cavity** enlarges with fluid between the embryo and the amniotic membrane and chorionic cavity.

Week 8. Week 8 marks the final week of embryonic development. At this point, the heart is fully developed (pulmonary veins; tricuspid, mitral, pulmonary and aortic valves; coronary arteries; interventricular septum; and inferior and superior vena cava). Near the end of the eighth week the choroid plexus begins to fold inward and the falx cerebri develops to divide the single ventricle into two lateral ventricles. The face forms over the weeks 5 to 8. By the end of the eighth week, the mandibular, maxillary, and nasal processes have merged in the midline, and the primary and secondary palates have fully fused to produce the two palatal shelves of the definitive palate. By 8 weeks the embryo is 16 mm in length, and the individual anatomic body parts may be visualized by transvaginal ultrasound.

FETAL PERIOD (WEEKS 9–14)

At 9 weeks, nearly half of the fetus is composed of the fetal head. Weeks 9 through 12 demonstrate a marked acceleration in body growth. At 10 weeks the hindbrain develops and the cerebellum takes form. The corpus callosum begins to take form at the 12th week and continues through the second trimester. The male and female genitalia begin to differentiate between the 10- to 12-week period. The intestines begin to return to the abdominal cavity in the 10th week, with a full return by the end of the 11th week. Palate fusion occurs in the 10- to 12-week period. Primary ossification centers appear by 12 weeks. The upper limbs are nearly at their relative length at 12 weeks, while the lower limbs have reached their final relative length. Between 9 and 12 weeks the fetal kidneys

TABLE 49.3	First-Trimester Ultrasound Findings		
Gestational Weeks	Ultrasound Findings	Mean Sac Diameter (mm)	Crown-Rump Length (mm)
4.3–5.0	Possible small gestational sac Possible double decidual sac sign Possible intradecidual sac sign		
5.1–5.5	Definite gestational sac	2	
5.5–6.0	Yolk sac	6	
>6.0	Embryo identified with cardiac motion (90–115 beats/min)	10	3
6.5	Crown-rump length	14	5
7.0–8.0	Cephalad and caudal poles identified Amnion	18–22	11–16
8.0–9.0	Limbs buds appear Head seen as separate from body	26	17–23
9.0–10.0	Fetal movement is seen Fetal rhombencephalon is seen Nuchal translucency is seen		23–32

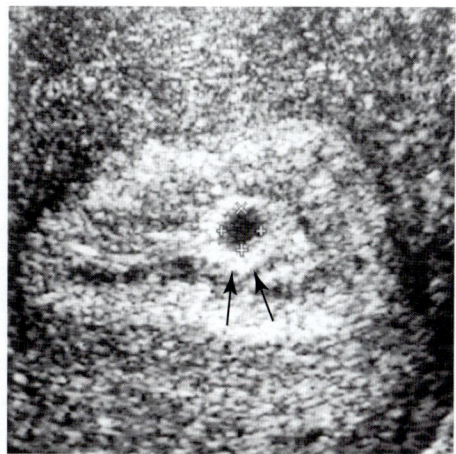

FIG. 49.8 The early gestational sac is seen embedded in the decidual basalis on one side of the endometrial cavity. The *arrows* point to the decidua capsularis.

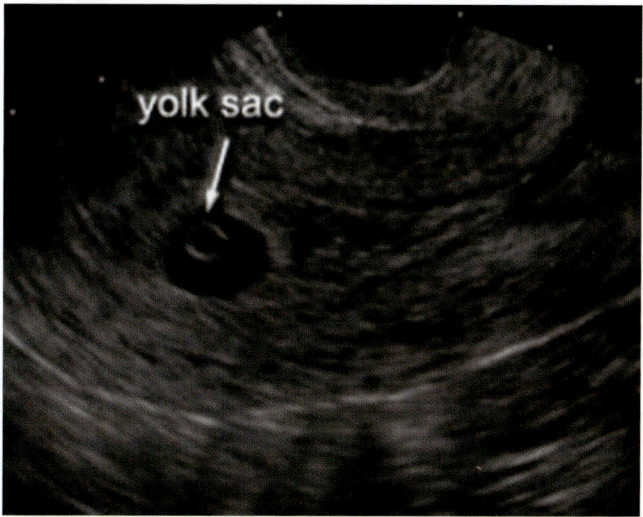

FIG. 49.9 In a normal pregnancy the yolk sac is the first structure that is sonographically identifiable within a gestational sac and should be seen when the mean sac diameter is greater than 6.0 mm or at 5.5 weeks' gestation.

begin urine production and excretion into the amniotic fluid. Weeks 13 and 14 demonstrate more fetal growth. Limb movements are coordinated at 14 weeks.

Gestational Sac. The sonographic finding that is definitive for a gestational sac is an anechoic fluid collection containing a yolk sac or an embryo with cardiac activity (Table 49.3). This fluid collection appears as a 2- to 3-mm sac with an echogenic ring having a sonolucent center Normally the sac is located in the central echogenic uterus, which corresponds to the decidua. The echogenic ring represents the chorion and decidua capsularis. The anechoic center represents the chorionic cavity. The circumferential echogenic rim seen surrounding the gestational sac represents trophoblastic tissue and the associated decidual reaction. The echogenic ring around the gestational sac can be divided embryologically into several components. The portion on the myometrial or burrowing side of the conceptus is known as the **decidua basalis**. The villi covering the developing embryo are referred to as the **decidua capsularis** (see Fig. 49.7). The interface between the decidua capsularis and the echogenic, highly vascularized decidua on the opposite wall of the endometrial cavity forms the **double decidual sac sign**, which has been reported to be a reliable sign of an early intrauterine gestation. The gestational sac is eccentrically placed in relation to the endometrial cavity, secondary to its implantation (Fig. 49.8). At this gestation, the MSD should measure 2 mm.

Yolk Sac. In a normal pregnancy the yolk sac is the first structure that is sonographically identifiable within a gestational sac and should be seen when the MSD is greater than 6.0 mm or at 5.5 weeks' gestation (Fig. 49.9). The secondary or sonographic yolk sac has essential functions in embryonic development, including (1) provision of nutrients to the developing embryo, (2) **hematopoiesis**, and (3) development of embryonic endoderm, which forms the primitive gut.

The yolk sac appears as a circular structure and measures 2 to 6 mm in diameter throughout the first trimester. The diameter of the yolk sac should be measured from inner border to inner border. If the yolk sac is abnormal in appearance, too small or too large, calcified, misshapen, or highly echogenic, it may be representative of pending loss or fetal abnormality. The yolk sac may be used as a landmark to image the embryo, given the connection between the yolk sac and embryo.

Initially, the yolk sac is attached to the embryo via the yolk stalk, but with amniotic cavity expansion, the yolk sac, which lies between the amniotic and chorionic membranes, detaches from the yolk stalk at approximately 8 weeks of gestation (Fig. 49.10).

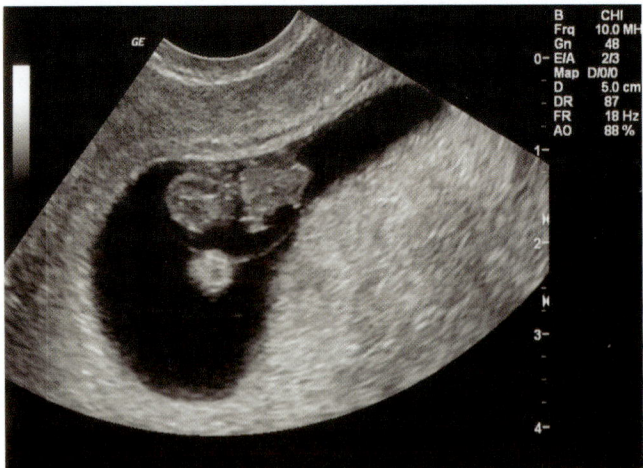

FIG. 49.10 Initially, the yolk sac is attached to the embryo via the yolk stalk, but with amniotic cavity expansion, the yolk sac, which lies between the amniotic and chorionic membranes, detaches from the yolk stalk at approximately 8 weeks of gestation.

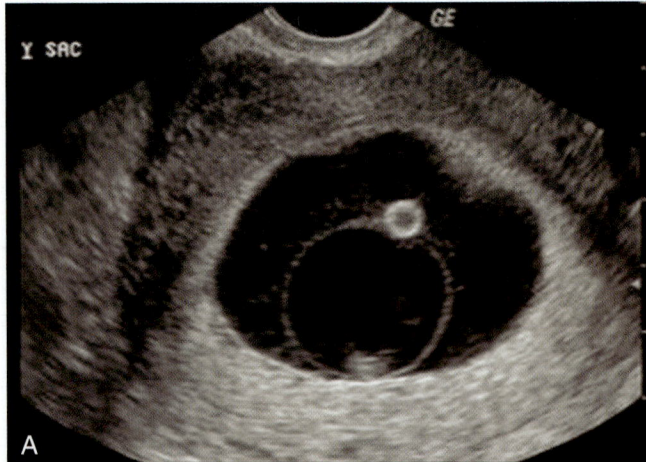

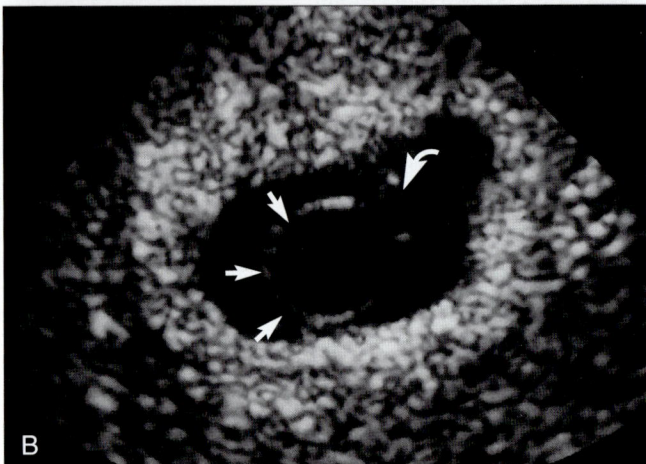

FIG. 49.11 The normal diameter of the yolk sac should not exceed 6 mm. Enlarged yolk sacs may have ominous outcomes.

Visualization of the yolk sac predicts a viable pregnancy in more than 90% of cases. Conversely, failure to visualize the yolk sac, with a minimum of 12 mm MSD, using transvaginal sonography, should provoke suspicion of abnormal pregnancy. Transabdominal studies have shown that the yolk sac should be seen within MSDs of 10 to 15 mm and should always be visualized with an MSD of 20 mm.

The growth rate of the yolk sac has been reported to be approximately 0.1 mm/mL of growth of the MSD when the MSD measures less than 15 mm, and 0.03 mm/mL of growth of the MSD through the first trimester. The normal diameter of the yolk sac should not exceed 6 mm. Enlarged yolk sacs may have ominous outcomes (Fig. 49.11).

The number of yolk sacs is consistent with the number of amnion membranes (Fig. 49.12). In twin pregnancies, one yolk sac signifies a monochorionic, monoamniotic pregnancy, whereas two yolk sacs signify a diamniotic, monochorionic or a diamniotic, dichorionic pregnancy. Double yolk sacs have been reported in singleton pregnancies without effect.

Typically, the yolk sac resorbs and is no longer seen sonographically by 12 weeks. Persistent yolk sac does occur. A persistent yolk sac may be visualized at the placental umbilical cord insertion, where the amniotic and chorionic membranes are fused.

Embryo. The early embryo often is not identified with transvaginal ultrasound until the heart motion is detected at approximately 5.5 to 6 weeks, when the CRL is approximately 3 mm. The embryonic heartbeat should be seen in a viable embryo when the CRL is greater than 4 mm. At this stage, the embryo is seen between the secondary yolk sac and the immediate gestational sac wall. Because the amniotic cavity is still relatively small, it appears that no space lies between the yolk sac and embryo (Fig. 49.13). As pregnancy progresses, the amniotic cavity grows in size, and the corresponding space between the embryo and the yolk sac, which is located outside the amniotic sac, increases.

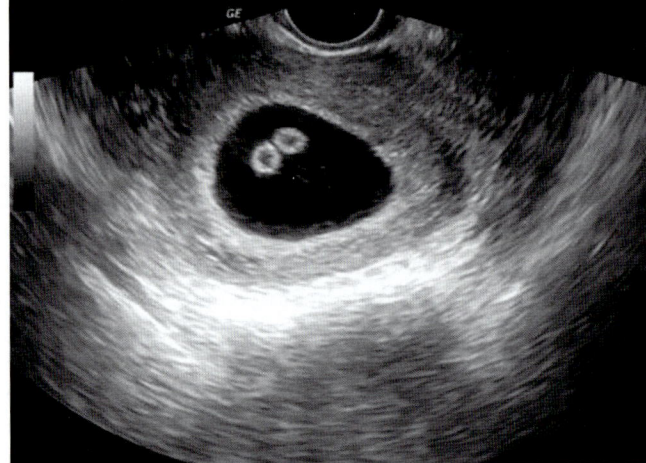

FIG. 49.12 The number of yolk sacs is consistent with the number of amnion membranes. In twin pregnancies, one yolk sac signifies a monochorionic, monoamniotic pregnancy, whereas two yolk sacs signify a diamniotic, monochorionic or a diamniotic, dichorionic pregnancy.

Between the fifth and sixth weeks of gestation, identification of the amniotic membrane may not be possible using transabdominal techniques. Using transvaginal transducers, the amniotic membrane that separates the amniotic cavity and **chorionic cavity** is routinely seen after 5.5 weeks. Although with normal gain settings the chorionic cavity (extraembryonic coelom) may appear sonolucent, increased overall gain settings may fill the fluid with low-level echoes. This appearance corresponds to increased density of the chorionic cavity fluid in relation to the amniotic fluid (Fig. 49.14). The chorionic cavity is the initial dumping ground for embryonic waste. Later the placenta takes over the process of waste removal, the amniotic cavity expands, and the chorionic cavity decreases in size. Fusion of the membranes (i.e., chorioamniotic fusion) occurs at approximately 14 to 15 weeks.

At the beginning of the sixth week of gestation, the embryonic disk folds into a C-shaped embryo (Fig. 49.15). While embryonic

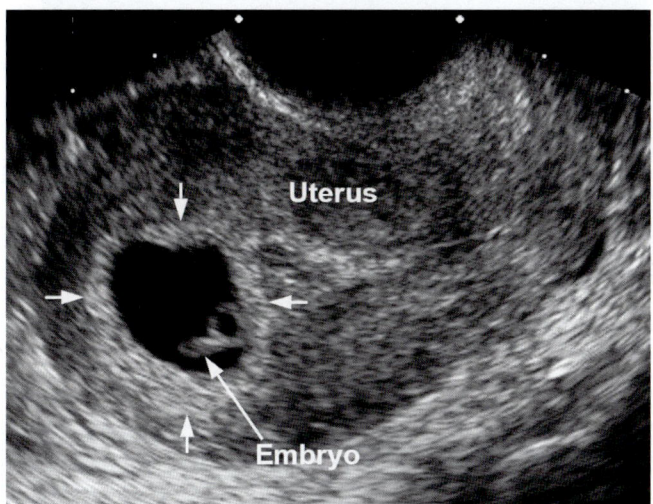

FIG. 49.13 The early embryo often is not identified with transvaginal ultrasound until the heart motion is detected at approximately 5.5 to 6 weeks, when the crown-rump length is approximately 3 mm.

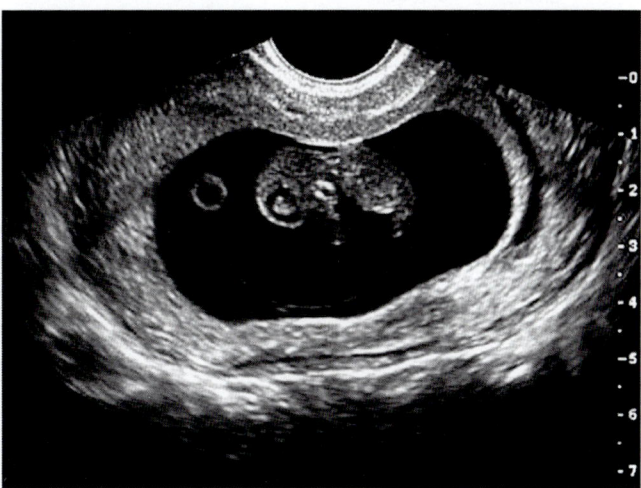

FIG. 49.14 The fluid in the extraembryonic coelom between the chorion and the amnion has low-level echoes and greater density compared with the amniotic fluid.

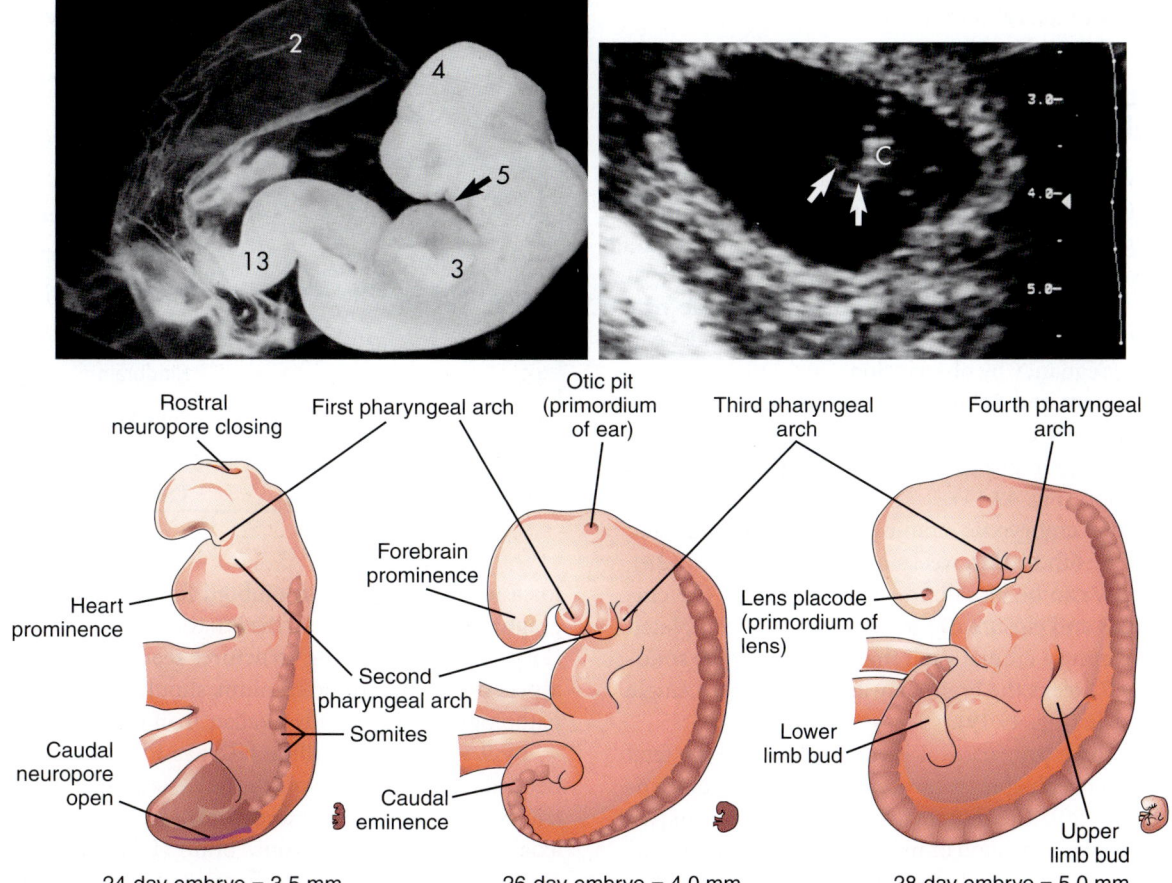

FIG. 49.15 At the beginning of the sixth week of gestation, the embryonic disk folds into a C-shaped embryo.

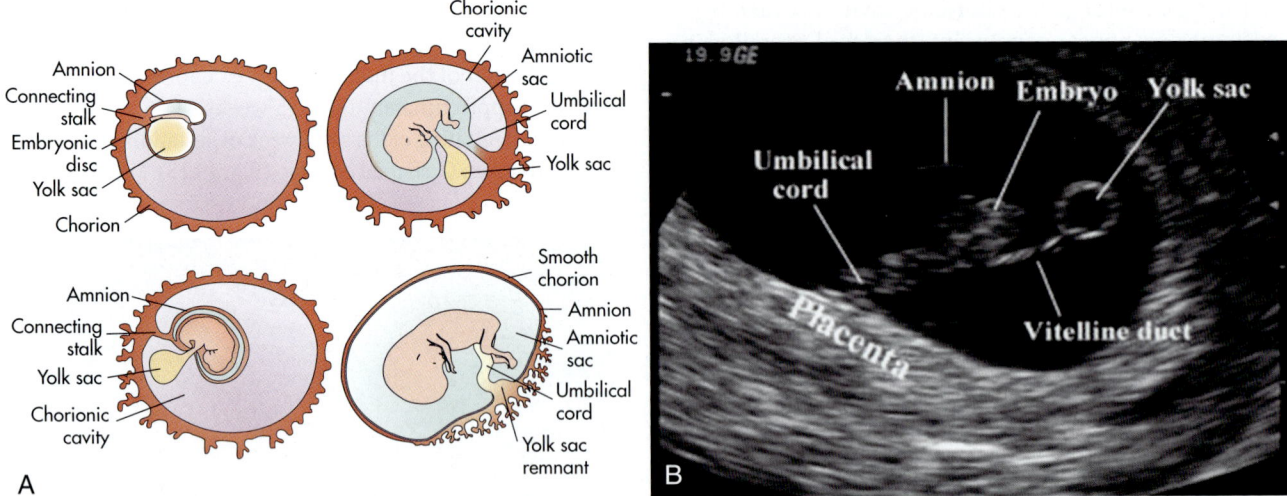

FIG. 49.16 (A) Schematics of the development of amnion, yolk sac, and embryo. (B) Sonogram of a transverse axis through the embryonic abdomen at approximately 8 weeks, demonstrating amniotic membrane, vitelline duct, umbilical cord, yolk sac, and embryo.

folding continues, the embryonic head, caudal portions, and lateral folds form, resulting in constriction or narrowing between embryo and yolk sac, creating the **yolk stalk**. During embryonic folding, the dorsal aspect of the yolk sac is incorporated into the embryo, developing the foregut, midgut, and hindgut and forming the entire gastrointestinal tract, liver, biliary tract, and pancreas. The yolk stalk, connecting stalk, and allantois are brought together by the expanding amnion, which covers the three structures forming the umbilical cord (Fig. 49.16).

Visualization of the Embryo: 6 to 10 Weeks of Gestational Age

The time between 4 and 10 weeks of gestation is considered the **embryonic period**. A distinct pattern of development occurs through the embryonic and fetal periods and is outlined in Tables 49.1 and 49.4. The appearance of the embryo changes so rapidly and is so characteristic during the first trimester that the experienced sonographer or sonologist can often date the pregnancy by observation.

Embryonic Cranium and Spine. The spine closes at approximately the sixth week of gestation. The developing spine may be visualized sonographically as parallel echogenic lines at 6 weeks of gestation (Fig. 49.17).

Although the embryonic cranium undergoes dramatic changes from the 6th to 10th weeks of gestation. (Fig. 49.18), specific anatomy can be visualized sonographically. The cranial neural folds and closure of the neuropore are completed by 7 weeks, forming a cranial vault that is recognizable sonographically. At 7 weeks the brain may appear to have a single fluid-filled vesicle (Fig. 49.19).

By 8 weeks, three primary vesicles are seen within the fetal brain: the prosencephalon, mesencephalon, and rhombencephalon (Fig. 49.20). The rhombencephalon divides into two segments: the cephalic portion or metencephalon, and the caudal component or myelencephalon. Once the rhombencephalon divides with its corresponding flexure, the cystic rhomboid

TABLE 49.4	Appearance of Embryonic Structures
Menstrual Week of Appearance	**Structure**
4–5	Gestational sac
5	Yolk sac
5.5–6	Fetal heartbeat
6	Fetal pole
7	Single ventricle
7.5	Spine
7.5	Lower limbs
8	Upper limbs
9	Falx
9	Body movements
9.2	Limb movements
9.5	Midgut herniation
9.5	Choroid plexus
9.5	Hindbrain
12	Fingers
12	Jaw
12.5	Toes

fossa forms. The cystic rhomboid fossa can be imaged sonographically routinely from the 8th to the 10th week of gestation (Fig. 49.21). This cystic structure, seen within the posterior aspect of the embryonic cranium, should not be confused with pathology, such as Dandy-Walker malformation.

By 9 weeks, the midline falx has formed and the prominent echogenic choroid plexus tissue is seen in the lateral ventricles. The cerebral falx and choroid plexus may be seen in axial views of the embryonic brain (Fig. 49.22). Sonolucent cerebrospinal fluid can be demarcated around the choroid plexus. The lateral ventricles completely fill the cerebral vault

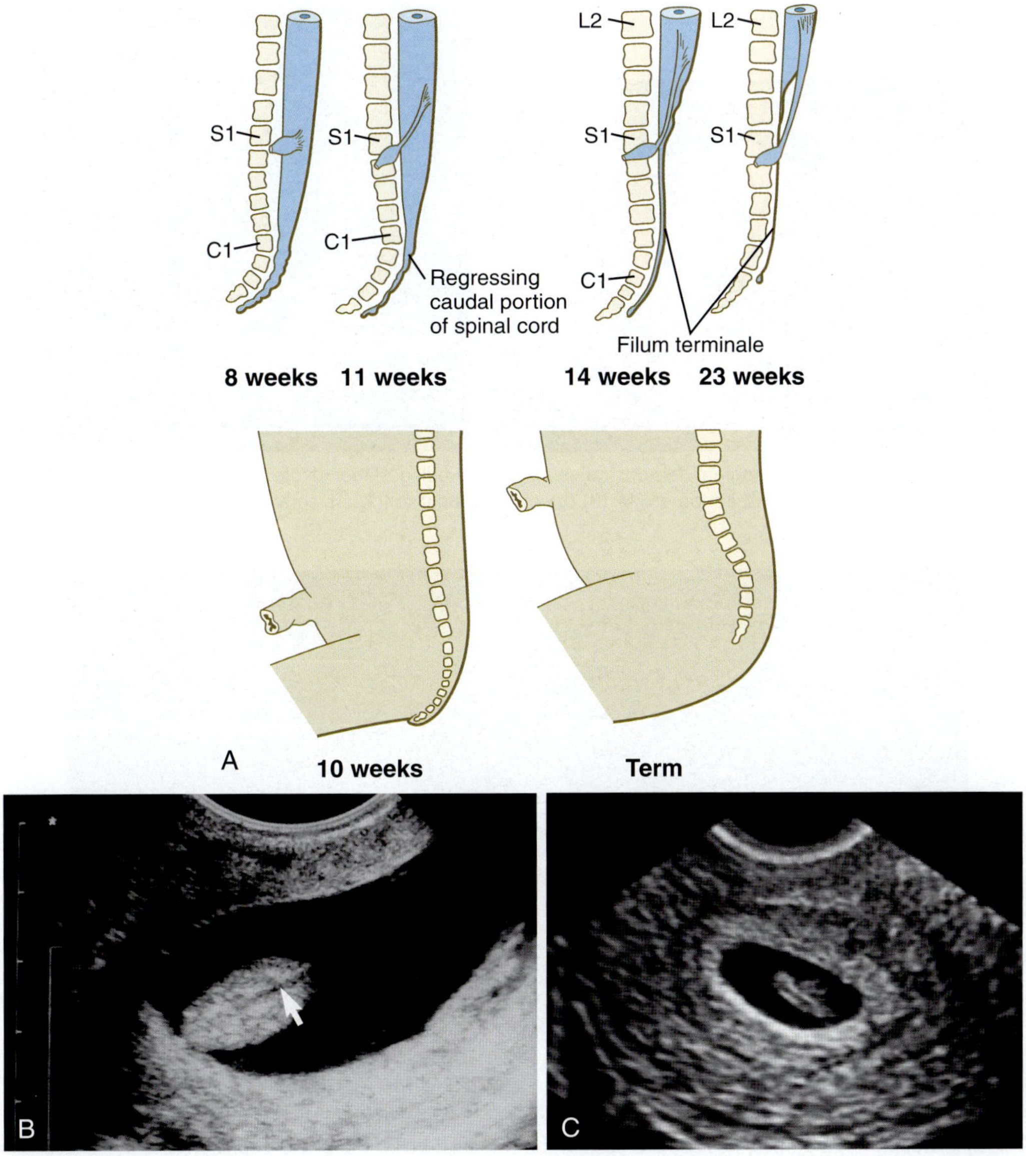

FIG. 49.17 (A) The fetal spine closes around the sixth week of gestation. (B) Sonogram of an 8-week embryo demonstrating parallel echogenic lines with the sonolucent center representing spine. (C) Similar image demonstrating early spinal formation.

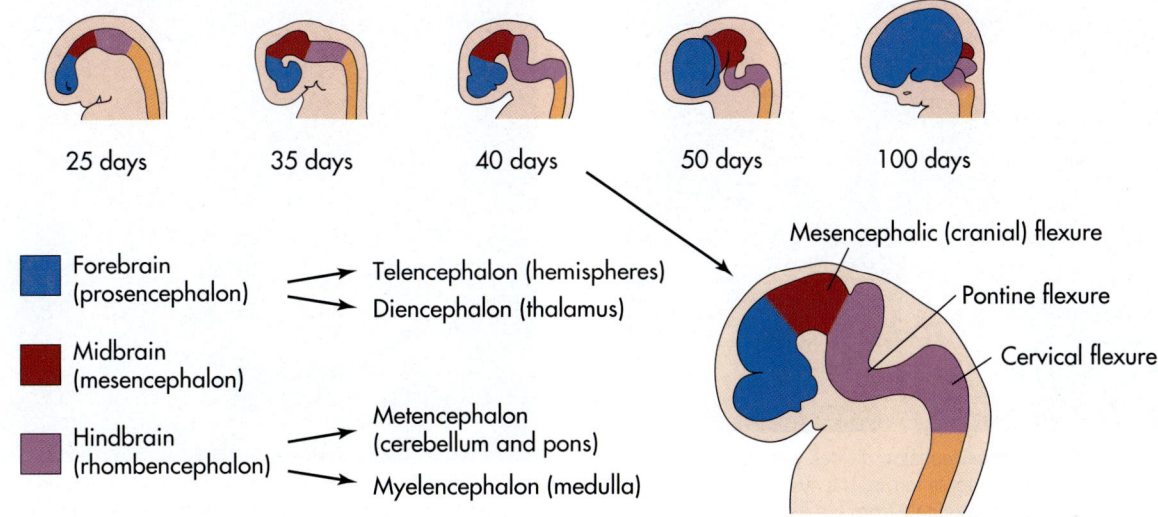

FIG. 49.18 Embryonic development of the brain.

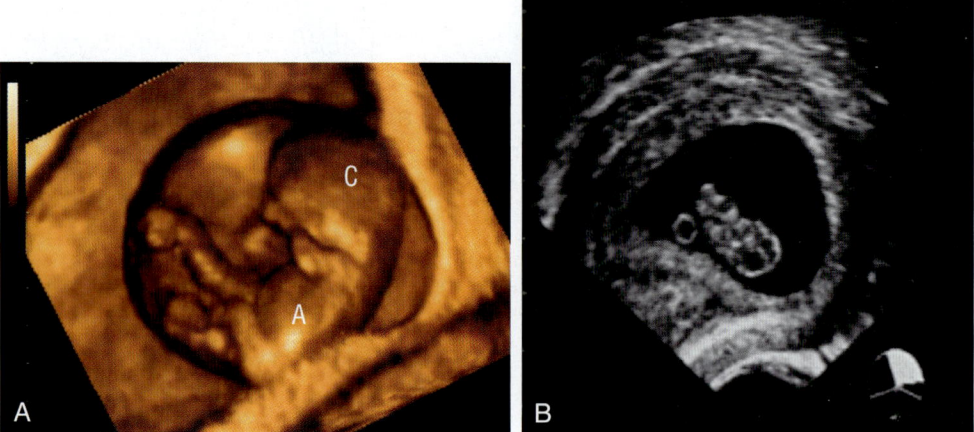

FIG. 49.19 (A) Three-dimensional sonogram demonstrating a 7- to 7.5-week gestation. Note the morphologic distinction between the embryonic cranium (C) and the embryonic abdomen (A). (B) Two-dimensional sonogram showing the same gestational age.

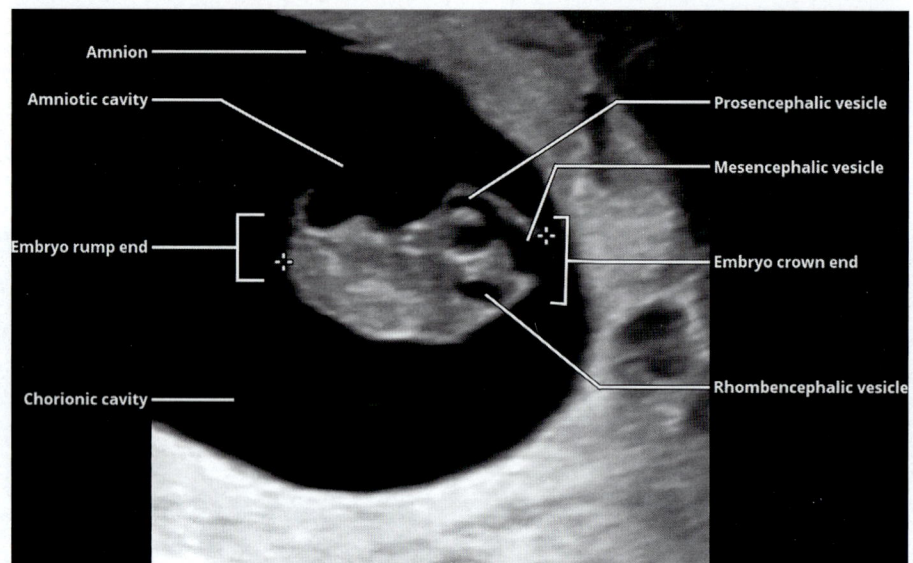

FIG. 49.20 By 8 weeks, three primary vesicles are seen within the fetal brain, the prosencephalon, the mesencephalon, and the rhombencephalon.

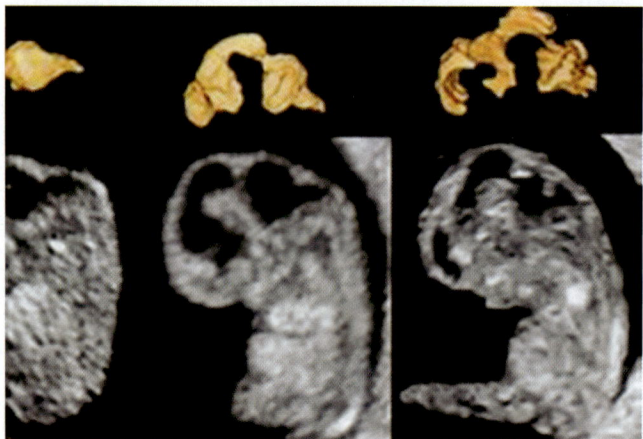

FIG. 49.21 Once the rhombencephalon divides with its corresponding flexure, the cystic rhomboid fossa forms. The cystic rhomboid fossa can be imaged sonographically routinely from the 8th to the 10th week of gestation.

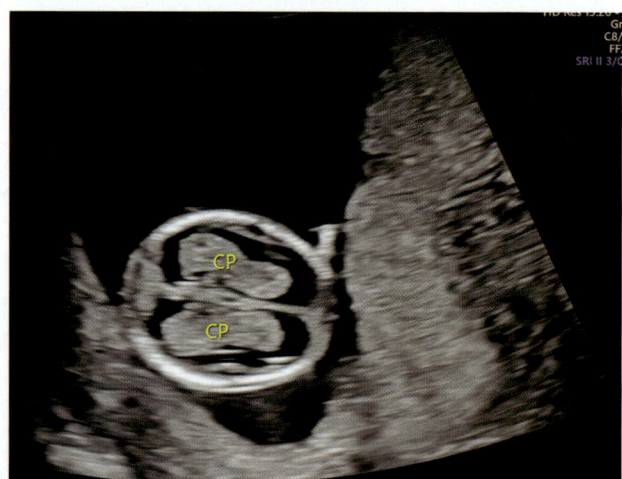

FIG. 49.22 By 9 weeks, the midline falx has formed and the prominent echogenic choroid plexus tissue is seen in the lateral ventricles. The cerebral falx and choroid plexus may be seen in axial views of the embryonic brain.

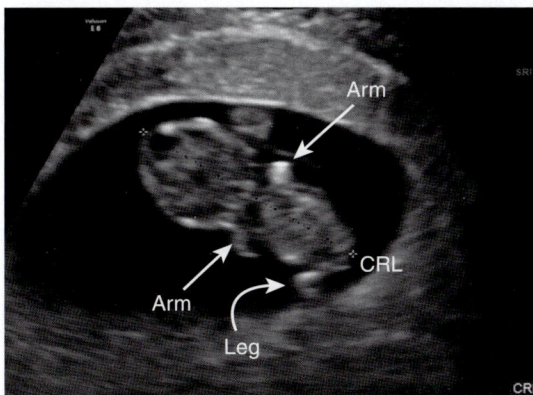

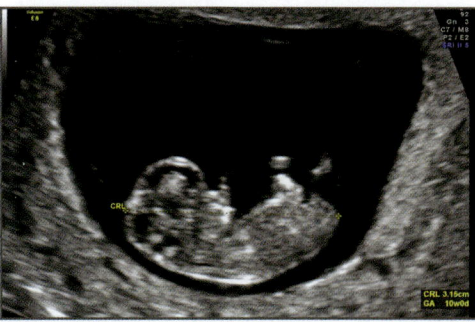

FIG. 49.24 By the ninth week, the maxilla and the mandible are noted as brightly echogenic structures; further bony palate development may be visualized from the 10th week.

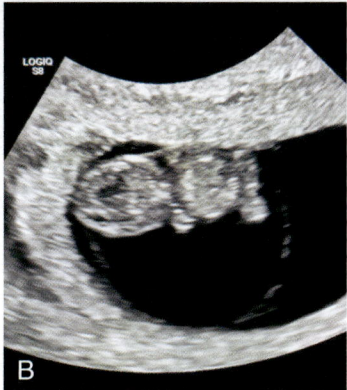

FIG. 49.23 Sonographically, the limb buds may be detected from the seventh week on; however, the limbs are not routinely identified until calcification of the long bones, which begins at 10 weeks.

at this time. Although the cerebral hemispheres may be seen at approximately 9 weeks of gestation, the hemispheric brain tissue is relatively small compared with the rest of the brain. Cerebral brain tissue develops rapidly at the beginning of the second trimester.

At 10 weeks, further evolution of the cerebellum, medulla, and medulla oblongata encloses the rhomboid fossa to form the primitive fourth ventricle and part of the cerebral aqueduct of Sylvius. The cerebellum is fused, and the brain structure is completed shortly thereafter.

Limb Development. Sonographically, the limb buds may be detected from the seventh week on; however, the limbs are not routinely identified until calcification of the long bones, which begins at 10 weeks (Fig. 49.23). Fingers and toes also may be identified by transvaginal sonography at 10 weeks' gestation.

Skeletal Ossification. Calcification of the clavicle begins at approximately 8 weeks, followed by ossification of the mandible, palate, vertebral column, and neural arches. Frontal cranial bones begin to calcify at 9 weeks, followed by long bones. Palate fusion occurs late in the first trimester. Sonographically, the embryonic face typically is difficult to see with diagnostic detail. By the ninth week, the maxilla and the mandible are noted as brightly echogenic structures; further bony palate development may be visualized from the 10th week (Fig. 49.24).

Physiologic Herniation of Bowel. The anterior abdominal wall is developed by 6 weeks of gestation. Simultaneously, the primitive gut is formed as a result of incorporation of the dorsal yolk sac into the embryo. The midgut, derived from the primitive gut, develops and forms the majority of the small bowel, cecum, ascending colon, and proximal transverse colon. Because the midgut is in direct communication with the yolk sac, the amniotic cavity expansion pulls the yolk sac away from the embryo, forming the yolk stalk.

As amniotic expansion occurs, the midgut elongates faster than the embryo is growing, causing the midgut to herniate into the base of the umbilical cord. Until approximately 10 weeks of gestation, the midgut loop continues to grow and rotate before it descends into the fetal abdomen at approximately the 11th week.

Sonographically, this transition of the bowel with the base of the umbilical cord can readily be visualized (Fig. 49.25). The small bowel appears as an echogenic mass within the base of the umbilical cord; little echogenic bowel is seen within the embryonic or fetal abdomen. After 12 weeks of gestation, the echogenic umbilical cord mass is no longer visualized and the bowel is seen within the fetal abdomen. It is important that this normal embryologic event not be confused with pathologic processes, such as omphalocele or gastroschisis.

Embryonic Heart. The heart is the first organ to function within the embryo. The embryonic heart starts beating at approximately 35 days (5 to 5.5 weeks), when the endocardial heart tubes fuse to form a single heart tube. Complex embryogenesis occurs to fully develop all cardiac structures by the eighth week. If possible, the sonographer should document the situs of the heart.

Embryonic cardiac activity should always be seen by 46 menstrual days, or when the CRL is greater than 4 mm. Embryonic heart rates vary with gestation age and should be documented with a real time cine clip or M-mode tracing (Fig. 49.26). Six-week embryonic heart rates of 90 to 110 increase to rates of 120 to 140 at 9 weeks, with further increase to rates of 130 to 160 at 12 weeks (Table 49.5).

DETERMINATION OF GESTATIONAL AGE

It is widely accepted that the most accurate pregnancy dating is obtained via first-trimester sonography. Two parameters for sonographic gestational dating may be used: MSD and CRL.

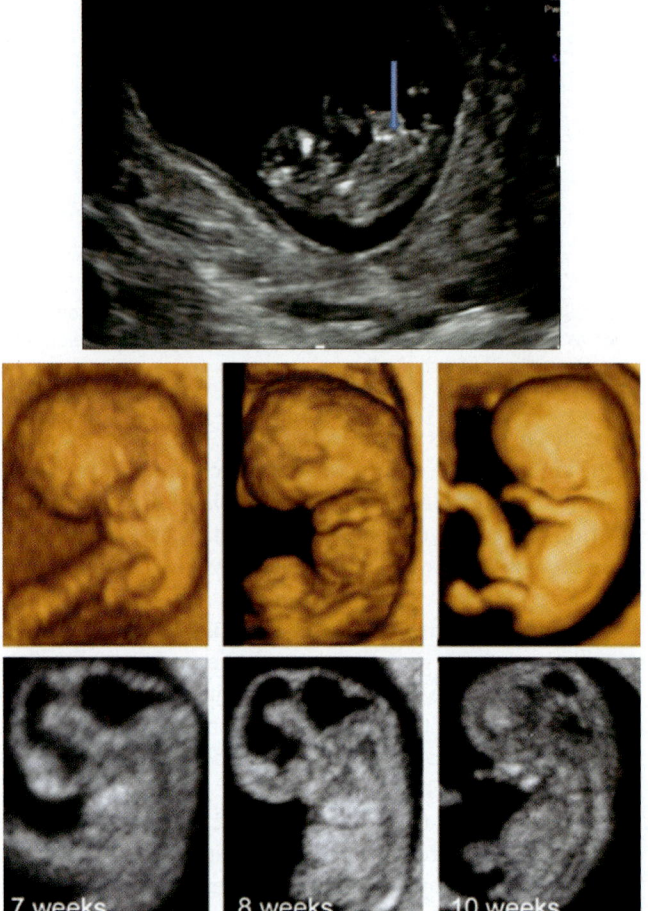

FIG. 49.25 As amniotic expansion occurs, the midgut elongates faster than the embryo is growing, causing the midgut to herniate into the base of the umbilical cord. Until approximately 10 weeks of gestation, the midgut loop continues to grow and rotate before it descends into the fetal abdomen at approximately the 11th week.

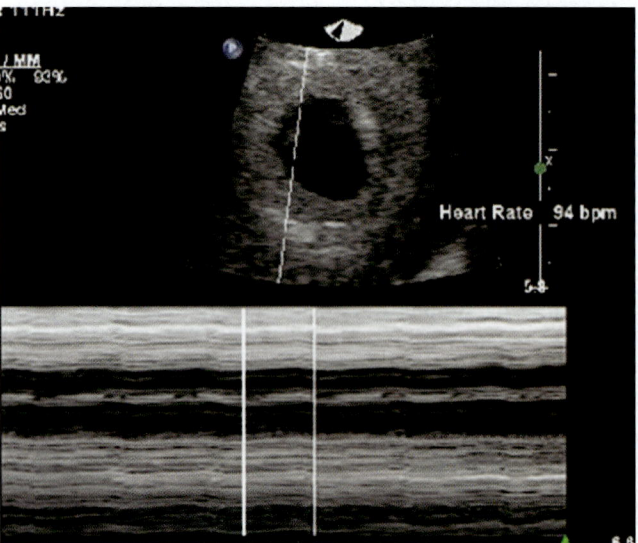

FIG. 49.26 Embryonic cardiac activity should always be seen by 46 menstrual days, or when the crown-rump length is >4 mm. Embryonic heart rates vary with gestation age and should be documented with a real-time cine clip or M-mode tracing.

TABLE 49.5	First-Trimester Fetal Heart Rates
Gestational Age (Weeks)	Mean Fetal Heart Rate (Approximate Beats/Min)
5	92–109
6	112–136
7	112–140
8	126–160
9	126–150
10	126–150
11	120–150
12	125–160

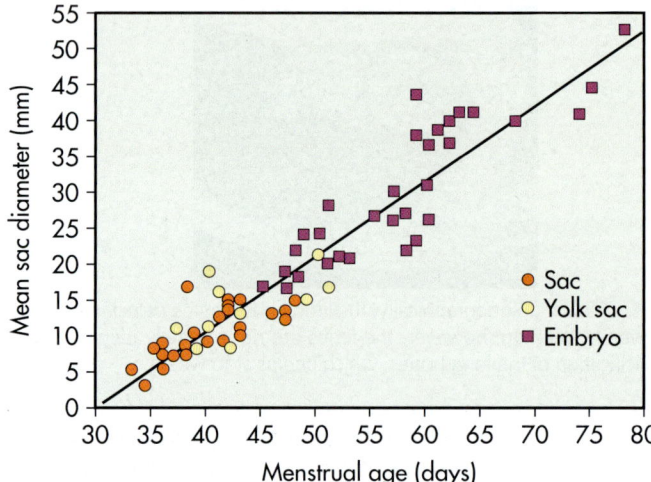

FIG. 49.27 Growth of gestational sac, yolk sac size, and embryo length in relation to mean sac diameter and menstrual days.

Mean Gestational Sac Size

Mean gestational sac size correlates closely with menstrual age during early pregnancy (Fig. 49.27). As a rule, the gestational sac size remains accurate through the first 8 weeks of gestation. Sonographically, the gestational sac size or MSD is determined by calculating the average sum of the lateroposterior, transverse, and sagittal of the gestational sac. These measurements are obtained in both sagittal and coronal/semicoronal sonographic planes. When measuring the MSD, the sonographer should measure only the gestational sac fluid space, not including the echogenic decidua (Fig. 49.28).

To calculate MSD, the following formula should be used:

Length (mm) + Width (mm) + Height (mm)/3 = MSD
MSD (mm) + 30 = Menstrual age (days)
Menstrual age (days)/7 = Menstrual age (weeks)

It is important to note that precise standard deviations for gestational sac size have not been determined, although linear regression analysis demonstrates excellent correlation of MSD and menstrual age.

Crown-Rump Length

Determination of first-trimester gestational dates by direct measurement of the embryo using the CRL was first reported in 1975. This produced gestational dating standard deviations of plus or minus 5 to 7 days, by far the most accurate dating parameters within obstetric biometry. Hadlock and colleagues reevaluated CRL data using modern equipment and determined gestational age standard deviation to be plus or minus 8% throughout the first trimester—essentially unchanged from the original data (Fig. 49.29).

Once the embryo is visible, the most accurate way to assign gestational age is the CRL. CRL measurements can be obtained as early as 6 weeks using transvaginal sonography. There is a 95% accuracy in the CRL measurement, with a confidence range of approximately +0.5 week. Visualization of embryonic heart motion is a marker signifying the beginning of CRL measurements.

CRLs are considered the most accurate method for dating through 12 weeks of gestation. After this time, the fetus begins to curl into the fetal position, making measurement of length more difficult (Fig. 49.30). From 13 weeks on, second-trimester biometric measurements, such as biparietal diameter and femur length, are used for pregnancy dating. The ultrasound dates for the pregnancy are determined by the earliest measurement of the embryo or fetus. Once the estimated delivery date is set, it should not be changed during later ultrasound examinations.

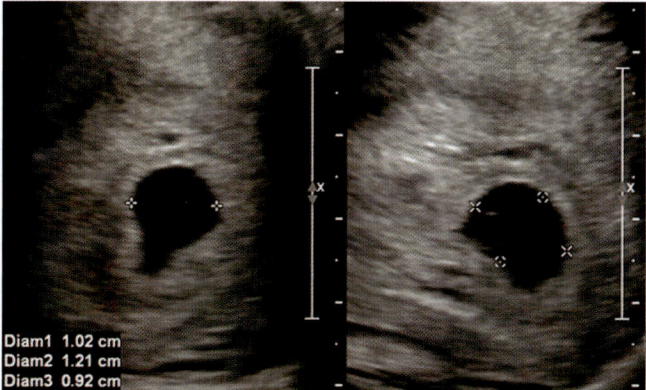

FIG. 49.28 As a rule, the gestational sac size remains accurate through the first 8 weeks of gestation. Sonographically, the gestational sac size or mean sac diameter is determined by calculating the average sum of the lateroposterior, transverse, and sagittal measurements of the gestational sac.

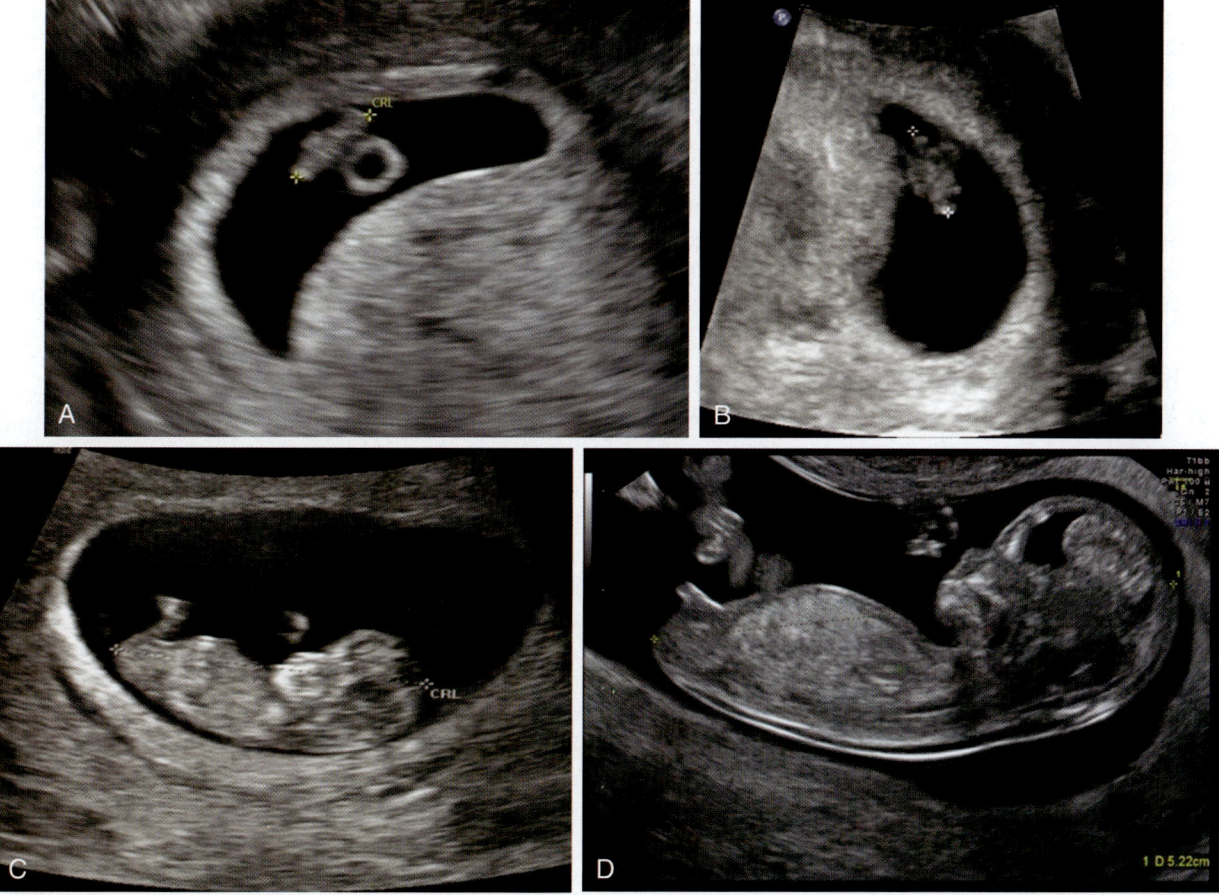

FIG. 49.29 Once the embryo is visible, the most accurate way to assign gestational age is the crown-rump length (CRL). CRL measurements can be obtained as early as 6 weeks using transvaginal sonography.

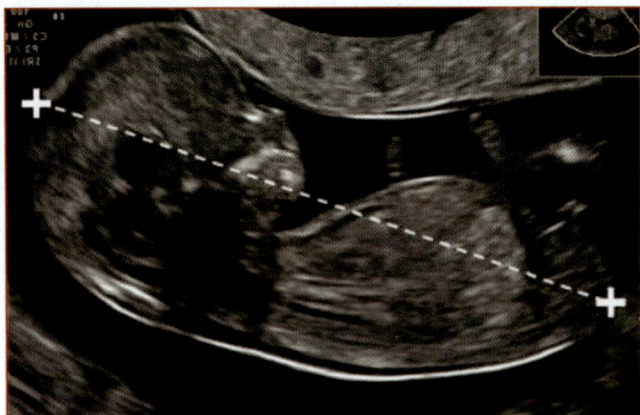

FIG. 49.30 Crown-rump length is considered the most accurate method for dating through 12 weeks of gestation. After this time, the fetus begins to curl into the fetal position, making measurement of length more difficult.

FIRST-TRIMESTER COMPLICATIONS

Positive hCG Without Intrauterine Fluid Collection or Adnexal Mass

When a pregnant patient presents with a positive hCG level but the transvaginal ultrasound shows neither an intrauterine fluid collection or adnexal abnormality, the thought is that a pregnancy may exist in an unknown location. It may be one of three reasons: (1) the patient is pregnant, but the LMP dates are incorrect, (2) there is a failed IUP, or (3) an ectopic pregnancy may be present. Remember not to rely on a single hCG level. Although the recommended hCG level is 1000 to 2000 mIU/mL, an hCG level greater than 2000 or 3000 mIU/mL in conjunction with a sonogram demonstrating no intrauterine gestational sac does not exclude a normal IUP. This patient should be rescanned in 2 to 7 days to see if a clear image of the gestational sac may be visualized. Follow-up testing with at least one additional sonogram and hCG measurement should be made.

Positive hCG With Intrauterine Fluid Collection Without Yolk Sac or Embryo; No Adnexal Mass

If a patient presents with a positive pregnancy test and the transvaginal ultrasound shows an intrauterine fluid collection with a yolk sac or embryo, the fluid could represent an early gestational sac, fluid from blood or secretions, or a cyst within the decidua. Fluid from a gestational sac should be seen within the decidua, whereas fluid from an ectopic pregnancy is seen within the uterine cavity. Decidual cysts may be seen in patients with a normal IUP or ectopic pregnancy.

FIRST-TRIMESTER RISK ASSESSMENT

Women may choose before birth to seek information regarding chromosomal anomalies in the fetus that they are carrying. There are many reasons to seek this information. Prior knowledge provides the opportunity to connect with support groups, to learn about resources and treatments, to choose a delivery hospital that can meet special medical needs, perhaps to find out about special needs adoptions, to choose further testing such as fetal echocardiography, or to choose pregnancy termination.

Women may choose not to seek this information, participate in noninvasive screening tests to determine the level of individual risk, or have an invasive and definitive diagnostic test. There is not a right or wrong choice; the choice is up to the individual woman and her family.

Invasive obstetric techniques allow definitive diagnosis of chromosomal anomalies, including trisomy 21. CVS may be performed between 10 and 14 weeks. Amniocentesis may be performed at 16 weeks. With both techniques, cells from the conceptus are obtained, cultured, and analyzed for chromosomal number and distribution. These diagnostic techniques are definitive but invasive and carry a risk of fetal loss of approximately 1 loss per 300 procedures when done by experienced physicians.

Because chromosomal anomalies are relatively rare, performing invasive procedures on every woman who wants additional information may lead to an unacceptable procedure-related loss of normal fetuses. Offering noninvasive screening tests initially directs women at higher risk toward invasive testing.

Screening for aneuploidy initially focused on maternal age alone. Because the risk for Down syndrome at age 35 is 1:200 (approximately the same as the reported amniocentesis-related risk in the 1980s), women older than age 35 were offered amniocentesis. However, younger women have many more babies than older women, and although their risk is lower, 75% to 80% of Down syndrome babies in the United States are born to women younger than 35 years of age.

When CVS became available, there was an incentive to move prenatal screening and diagnosis of aneuploidy into the first trimester. Performing these tests in the first trimester provides earlier reassurance for more than 95% of patients and earlier diagnosis for affected pregnancies. The results can be obtained before the pregnancy is visible, and when termination is chosen, it is 7 times safer when performed in the first trimester. First-trimester testing also allows more time for counseling and additional options for testing.

The current standard for first-trimester risk assessment is the combined test using maternal age, the nuchal translucency (NT) measurement, and biochemistry analyses of hCG and PAPP-A. The combined first-trimester test has a higher detection rate (at the same false-positive rate) than maternal age alone, triple screen, or quad screen. It is important to note that none of the first-trimester markers should be used alone for risk assessment. The combination of multiple markers is required. Risk assessment markers are incorporated into examinations when women choose to have aneuploidy screening tests and when the combination test, including serum biochemistry and NT, is performed.

Cell-free DNA screening tests are available from 9 weeks of gestational age and have a very high detection rate, but the cost-effectiveness of these tests is not clear and results must be verified by amniocentesis or CVS.

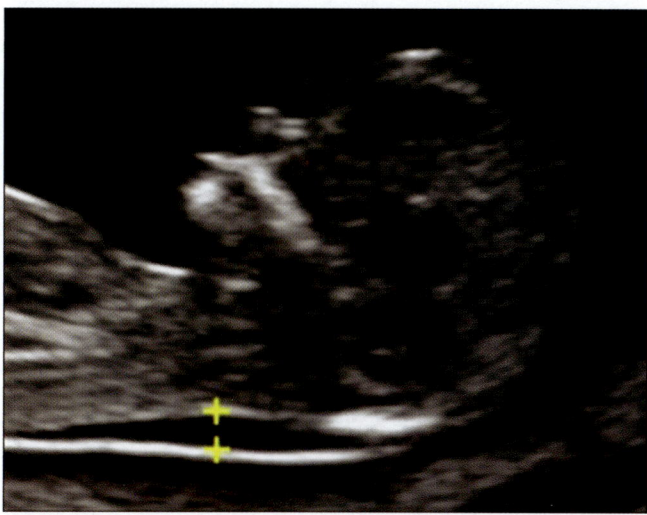

FIG. 49.31 The normal first-trimester fetus has a small pocket of fluid along its back known as the nuchal translucency.

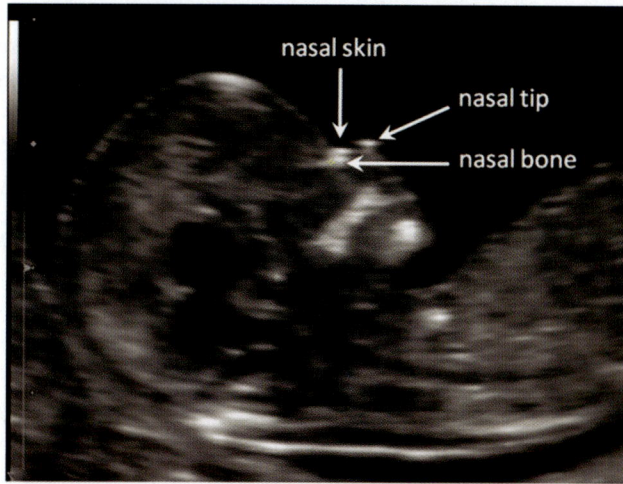

FIG. 49.32 Nasal bone imaging is a useful adjunct to nuchal translucency and serum biochemistry.

BOX 49.2	Nuchal Translucency (NT) Measurement Criteria

- The margins of the NT edges are clear.
- The fetus is in a midsagittal plane.
- The fetus occupies the majority of the image.
- The fetal head is in a neutral position.
- The fetus is observed away from the amnion.
- (+) Calipers are used.
- Horizontal crossbars are placed correctly on the inner surface of the border of the lucency.
- Calipers are placed perpendicular to the long axis of the fetus.
- The measurement is taken at the widest NT space.

First-Trimester Risk Assessment Sonography Techniques

Nuchal Translucency Measurements. The normal first-trimester fetus has a small pocket of fluid along its back that is known as the NT (Fig. 49.31). Measurement of the NT is a component of first-trimester risk assessment. The NT must be measured in a standardized way (Box 49.2), and measurement techniques need to be monitored and continually assessed to ensure that accurate risks based on these measurements are given to women and their families.

To participate in NT measurements and first-trimester risk assessment, sonographers and sonologists must demonstrate competency to measure the NT. The Perinatal Quality Foundation Nuchal Translucency Quality Review program (https://ntqr.perinatalquality.org/default.aspx) and the Fetal Medicine Foundation USA (http://www.fetalmedicineusa.com) provide credentialing and ongoing quality monitoring in the United States.

Nasal Bone. Absence of the fetal nasal bone in late first-trimester sonography is associated with trisomy 21. Nasal bone imaging is a useful adjunct to NT and serum biochemistry (Fig. 49.32). Many laboratories will incorporate the presence or absence of the fetal nasal bone into their risk algorithm and will provide to women a risk adjusted for nasal bone. A small

 Key Pearls

- Embryologists state time in conceptual age, also known as embryologic age, with conception as the first day of pregnancy.
- Clinicians and sonographers use gestational age, also known as menstrual age, to date the pregnancy, with the first day of the last menstrual period as the beginning of gestation.
- For 12 days after conception, during the implantation process, the conceptus is called a zygote. From the time of implantation until the end of the 10th week of menstrual age, the conceptus is called an embryo. After the first 10 weeks, the embryo is called a fetus.
- Gestational sac size and human chorionic gonadotropin (hCG) levels increase proportionately until 10 menstrual weeks, at which time the gestational sac is approximately 45 mm mean sac diameter (MSD), and an embryo should be easily detected by transabdominal or transvaginal sonography.
- The normal sonographic features of a gestational sac include a round or oval shape; a fundal position in the uterus, or an eccentrically placed position in the middle portion of the uterus; smooth contours; and a decidual wall thickness greater than 3 mm.
- A yolk sac should be seen when the MSD is greater than 6 mm. An embryo should be seen when the MSD is greater than 10 mm.
- Crown-rump lengths are considered the most accurate method for dating through 12 weeks of gestation.
- Chorionic villi sampling may be performed between 10 and 14 weeks. Amniocentesis may be performed at 16 weeks.
- The triple screen includes measurement of hCG, estriol, and alpha-fetoprotein. The quad screen involves measurement of hCG, estriol, alpha-fetoprotein, and inhibin.
- The current standard for first-trimester risk assessment is the combined test using maternal age, the nuchal translucency measurement, and biochemistry analyses of hCG and pregnancy-associated plasma protein–A.
- The normal first-trimester fetus has a small pocket of fluid along its back that is known as the nuchal translucency.

nose and midface hypoplasia are well-known components of the Down syndrome phenotype. It is important to note these characteristics and to look for the fetal nasal bone in both first- and second-trimester examinations.

ACKNOWLEDGMENT

The author recognizes Jean Lea Spitz for contributions to this chapter in the previous edition.

BIBLIOGRAPHY

Abuhamad A. Technical aspects of nuchal translucency measurement. *Semin Perinatol*. 2005;29:376–379.

Ackerman TE, Levi CS, Lyons EA, et al. Decidual cyst: transvaginal sonographic sign of ectopic pregnancy. *Radiology*. 1993;189:727–731.

AIUJM-ACR-ACOG-SMFM-SRUP. Practice parameter for the performance of standard diagnostic obstetric ultrasound examinations. *J Ultrasound Med*. 2018;2018:999-1-12.

Bateman BG, Nunley WC, Kolp LA, et al. Vaginal sonography findings and hCG dynamics of early intrauterine and tubal pregnancies. *Obstet Gynecol*. 1990;75:421–427.

Bohm-Velez M, Mendelson EB. Endovaginal sonography: applications, equipment and technique. In: Nyberg DA, Hill LM, Bohm-Velez M, eds. *Endovaginal ultrasound*. St Louis: Mosby; 1992.

Bowerman RA. Sonography of fetal midgut herniation: normal size criteria and correlation with crown-rump length. *J Ultrasound Med*. 1993;5:251–254.

Bromley B, Harlow BL, Laboda LA. Small sac size in the first trimester: a predictor of poor fetal outcome. *Radiology*. 1991;178:375–377.

Callen P. *Ultrasonography in obstetrics and gynecology*. ed 6, Philadelphia: Elsevier; 2017.

D'Alton MD, Cleary-Goldman J. Additional benefits of first trimester screening. *Semin Perinatol*. 2005;29:405–411.

Doubilet PM, Benson CB, Bourne T, et al. Early first trimester diagnostic criteria for nonviable pregnancy. *N Engl J Med*. 2013; 369:1442–1451.

Doubilet PM, Benson CB. Further evidence against the reliability of the hCG discriminatory level. *J Ultrasound Med*. 1637-2011;30

Doubilet PM, Benson CB. Double sac sign and intradecidual sign in early pregnancy: interobserver reliability and frequency of occurrence. *J Ultrasound Med*. 2013;32:1207–1214.

Doubilet PM, Benson CB. The "appearing twin": undercounting of multiple gestations on early first trimester sonograms. *J Ultrasound Med*. 1998;17:199–203.

Hadlock FP, Shah YP, Kanon DJ, Lindsay JV. Fetal crown-rump length: reevaluation of relation to menstrual age (5–18 weeks) with high resolution real time US. *Radiology*. 1992;182:501–505.

Hertzberg BS, Mahony BS, Bowie JD. First trimester fetal cardiac activity: sonographic documentation of a progressive early rise in heart rate. *J Ultrasound Med*. 1988;7:573–575.

Laboda LA, Estroff JA, Benaceraff BR. First trimester bradycardia: a sign of impending fetal loss. *J Ultrasound Med*. 1989;8:561–563.

Lindsay DJ, Lovett IS, Lyons EA, et al. Yolk sac diameter and shape at endovaginal ultrasound: predictors of pregnancy outcome in the first trimester. *Radiology*. 1992;183:115–118.

Moore KL, Persaud TVN. *The developing human: clinically oriented embryology*, ed 8. Philadelphia: Elsevier; 2008.

Nyberg DA, Filly RA, Mahony BS, et al. Early gestation: correlation of hCG levels and sonographic identification. *Am J Roentgenol*. 1985;144:951–954.

Nyberg DA, Mack LA, Harvey D, et al. Value of the yolk sac in evaluating early pregnancies. *J Ultrasound Med*. 1988;7:129–135.

Rizk B, Tan SL, Morcos S, et al. Heterotopic pregnancies after in vitro fertilization and embryo transfer. *Am J Obstet Gynecol*. 1991;164:161–164.

Rosen T, D'Alton MD. Down syndrome screening in the first and second trimesters: what do the data show? *Semin Perinatol*. 2005;29:367–375.

Rosen T, D'Alton ME, Platt LD, et al. First trimester ultrasound assessment of the nasal bone to screen for aneuploidy. *Obstet Gynecol*. 2007;110:399–404.

Schats R, Jansen CAM, Wladimiroff JW, et al. Embryonic heart activity: appearance and development in early human pregnancy. *Br J Obstet Gynecol*. 1990;97:989–994.

Timor-Tritsch IE, Farine D, Rosen MG. A close look at early embryonic development with high-frequency transvaginal transducer. *Am J Obstet Gynecol*. 1988;159:676–681.

Timor-Tritsch IE, Fuchs KM, Monteagudo A, D'Alton ME. Performing a fetal anatomy scan at the time of the first trimester screening. *Obstet Gynecol*. 2009;113:402–407.

CHAPTER 50

First-Trimester Complications

Sandra L. Hagen-Ansert

OBJECTIVES

On completion of this chapter, you should be able to:
- Describe viable and nonviable pregnancy with appropriate terminology
- List sonographic features of failed pregnancy
- Describe sonographic findings of retained products of conception
- Explain the clinical and sonographic findings in ectopic pregnancy
- Discuss the normal range for fetal cardiac rhythm
- Describe the cranial abnormalities seen in the first trimester
- Distinguish among normal bowel herniation, gastroschisis, and omphalocele
- Explain the sonographic findings with cystic hygroma in the first trimester
- Name the types of umbilical cord masses that may be seen with ultrasound
- Differentiate between a hemorrhagic corpus luteum cyst and other ovarian masses
- Discuss the difference between a fibroid and uterine contraction on sonography

OUTLINE

Criteria for Viability and Nonviability 1320
First-Trimester Bleeding and Sonographic Appearances 1320
    Placental Hematomas and Subchorionic Hemorrhage 1320
    Absent Intrauterine Sac 1320
    Gestational Sac Without an Embryo or Yolk Sac 1322
    Criteria for Abnormal Sac 1322
    Anembryonic Pregnancy (Blighted Ovum) 1323
    Gestational Trophoblastic Disease 1323
Abnormal or Absent Cardiac Activity 1326
    Absent Cardiac Activity 1327
    Embryonic Bradycardia and Tachycardia 1327
Embryonic Development of Yolk Sac and Amnion 1327
    Embryonic Oligohydramnios and Growth Restriction 1327
    Embryonic Yolk Sac Evaluation 1327
    Amnion Evaluation 1327
Ectopic Pregnancy 1327
    Sonographic Findings in Ectopic Pregnancy 1328
    Adnexal Mass With Ectopic Pregnancy 1330
    Heterotopic Pregnancy 1332
    Interstitial Pregnancy 1332
    Cervical Pregnancy 1332
    Ovarian Pregnancy 1333
Diagnosis of Embryonic Abnormalities in the First Trimester 1333
    Nuchal Translucency 1333
    Cardiac Anomalies 1334
    Cranial Anomalies 1334
    Abdominal Wall Defects 1338
    Obstructive Uropathy 1339
    Cystic Hygroma 1339
    First-Trimester Umbilical Cord Cysts 1340
First-Trimester Pelvic Masses 1340
    Ovarian Masses 1340
    Uterine Masses 1340

KEY TERMS

Acrania
Anembryonic pregnancy (blighted ovum)
Anencephaly
Bowel herniation
Cephalocele
Complete abortion
Corpus luteum cyst
Cystic hygroma
Ectopic pregnancy
Failed pregnancy
Gastroschisis
Gestational trophoblastic disease
Heterotopic pregnancy
Holoprosencephaly
Incomplete abortion
Interstitial pregnancy
Pseudogestational sac
Turner syndrome
Ventriculomegaly
Yolk sac

The first trimester consists of a series of complex, sequential events that make up the early stage of embryonic development. Interruption in development may lead to complications in the embryonic period. Approximately 15% of clinically recognized pregnancies are spontaneously miscarried. The loss rate may be even higher for early pregnancies that are not clinically recognized. The most common presentation for complications is vaginal spotting or frank bleeding, which occurs in nearly 25% of patients during the early stage of pregnancy. In many cases, bleeding is inconsequential, resulting from implantation of the conceptus into the decidualized endometrium. However, if bleeding is accompanied by severe pain, uterine contractions, or a dilated cervix, the pregnancy is unlikely to progress. Patients benefit from early transvaginal examination to carefully investigate the uterine cavity for the presence of an embryo, a fetal heartbeat, a yolk sac, or retained products of conception.

A threatened abortion covers a wide range of conditions based on the stage of development and the sonographic appearance of the products of conception. *Threatened abortion* is a term used for pregnancies of fewer than 20 weeks when the patient has a viable embryo, documented fetal heartbeat, and vaginal bleeding. The diagnosis of *threatened abortion* is made when the cervix is long and closed in a patient with vaginal bleeding. At least 50% of pregnant women with these complications will go on to spontaneously lose or "abort" the pregnancy. Specific terminology has been adopted to describe the complications of these pregnancies. *Embryonic demise*, or **failed pregnancy**, is used when there is clear evidence of a nonviable embryo (absence of cardiac activity). *Blighted ovum*, or *anembryonic pregnancy*, is used to describe a uterus containing a gestational sac but no visible embryo. *Pregnancy of unknown location* (PUL) refers to the patient who has a positive urine or serum pregnancy test but presents with no intrauterine nor ectopic pregnancy visualized on transvaginal ultrasound.

Other conditions that may present clinically as a threatened abortion are ectopic pregnancy and gestational trophoblastic disease. Knowledge of the quantitative level of serum human chorionic gonadotropin (hCG) is necessary to make this diagnosis and should be correlated with the sonographic appearance.

CRITERIA FOR VIABILITY AND NONVIABILITY

Historically the diagnosis of pregnancy failure has relied upon several diagnostic criteria: the absence of cardiac activity at a certain crown-rump length (CRL), the absence of a visible embryo at a certain mean sac diameter (MSD), or the absence of an appreciable embryo by a point in time. These criteria were reviewed by the Society of Radiologists in Ultrasound (SRU), whose consensus paper was published in the *New England Journal of Medicine* (NEJM) in October 2013. The SRU believed that the previous studies which determined these threshold values were based on very small patient populations and that the criteria were at risk for increased false-positive results. These criteria reflect their attempt to increase the specificity to 100% and give a positive predictive value of close to 100%. The goal was to prevent erroneously diagnosing nonviability and preventing surgical or medical intervention that damages a true viable pregnancy. See the criteria in Boxes 48.1 and 48.2.

FIRST-TRIMESTER BLEEDING AND SONOGRAPHIC APPEARANCES

Placental Hematomas and Subchorionic Hemorrhage

The embryonic placenta, or frondosum, may become detached, resulting in the formation of a hematoma, which typically causes vaginal bleeding. Most of these hemorrhages are contiguous with a placental edge. Although no risk factors have been associated with first-trimester placental separation, it has been reported to have a 50% or greater fetal loss rate. Although the prognosis seems to depend on the size of the hematoma, no specific volumes have been correlated in the first trimester with fetal outcomes. That said, improved outcomes do seem to be consistent with smaller hematomas.

Sonographically, placental hematomas may be difficult to distinguish from subchorionic hemorrhages. Patients who present with placental hematomas generally do not have symptoms, bleeding, or spotting because the bleed is within the chorionic sac and has no communication with the endometrium.

Subchorionic Hemorrhage. The most common occurrence of bleeding in the first trimester is from subchorionic hemorrhage. These low-pressure bleeds result from the process of implantation of the fertilized ovum into the endometrial cavity and myometrial wall. The hemorrhage is found between the myometrium and the margins of the gestational sac and may or may not be associated with the placenta. This finding can help to distinguish a subchorionic hemorrhage from abruptio placentae, which generally occurs in the second trimester and may present as a lucency posterior to the placenta. Clinical findings may include bleeding, spotting, or uterine cramping. If the hemorrhage becomes large enough, this can lead to spontaneous pregnancy loss (SPL).

Sonographic Findings. The appearance of bleeding varies with the stage of its organization. An early bleed may appear slightly echogenic as the red blood cells actively fill the area of hemorrhage. With time, the hemorrhage becomes more anechoic and may be seen between the uterine wall and the fetal membrane (Fig. 50.1). Color flow Doppler will demonstrate the avascular nature of the hemorrhage. Patients may present with active vaginal bleeding, and the subchorionic bleed is easily seen by ultrasound adjacent to the gestational sac. Other patients may have no bleeding yet have a subchorionic lucency that can be seen with imaging. Patients may be symptomatic with a large subchorionic bleed, or asymptomatic with a small subchorionic bleed, perhaps only seen with transvaginal imaging.

Absent Intrauterine Sac

Sonography is routinely used to evaluate for the presence or absence of an intrauterine gestational sac. For example, if the patient presents with a positive pregnancy test with a normal sonographic appearance of the uterus but the endometrial complex shows no sign of a gestational sac, the differential diagnosis would include a very early intrauterine pregnancy, a nondeveloping pregnancy, or possible ectopic pregnancy.

Characteristics for the sonographic diagnosis of an absent intrauterine sac include an empty uterus with no evidence of an endometrial fluid collection (early gestational sac), absence of adnexal masses or free fluid, and positive beta-hCG levels. Clinical findings may be characterized by bleeding and cramping. Correlation between the serum beta-hCG level and uterine findings can be used to confirm whether the sonographic indications of a first-trimester pregnancy have

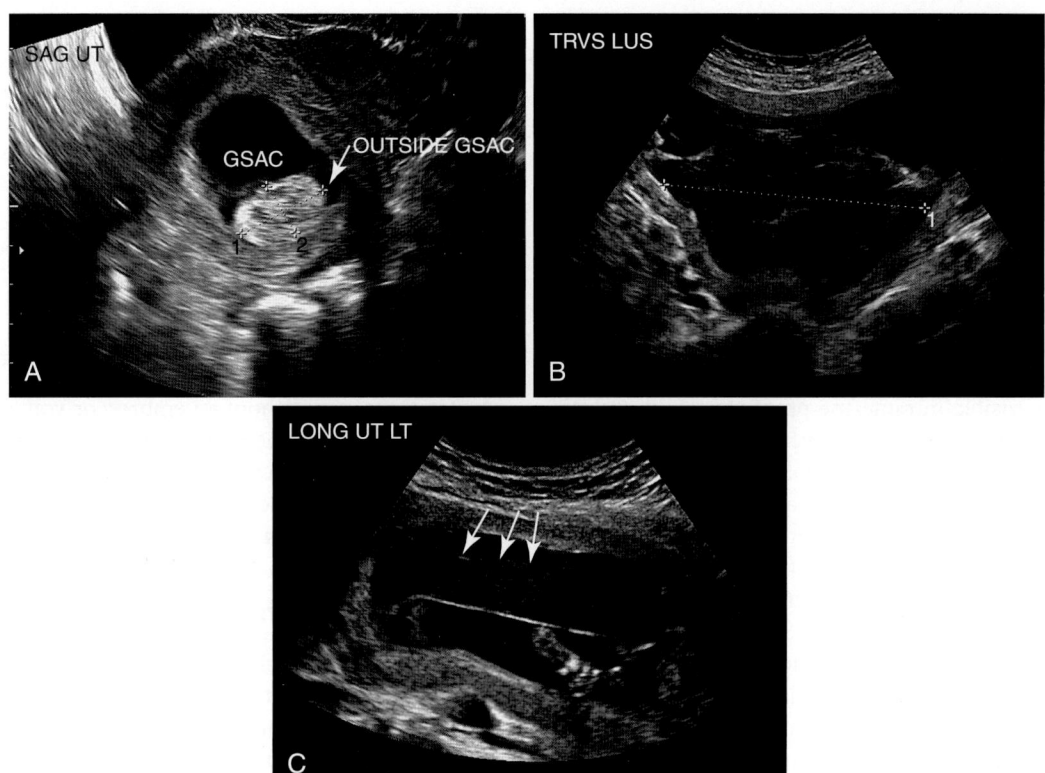

FIG. 50.1 Subchorionic hemorrhages are shown at 8 weeks' gestation (A), 14 weeks' gestation (B), and 16 weeks' gestation (C). Note the separation of the anterior placenta from the uterine wall *(arrows)*. *GSAC*, Gestational sac; *LUS*, lower uterine segment; *UT*, uterus.

TABLE 50.1	Terminology and Diagnostic Tests Used Early in the First Trimester of Pregnancy
Terminology	**Comments**
Viable	A pregnancy is viable if it can potentially result in a liveborn baby.
Nonviable	A pregnancy is nonviable if it cannot possibly result in a liveborn baby. Ectopic pregnancies and failed intrauterine pregnancies are nonviable.
Intrauterine pregnancy of uncertain viability	A woman is considered to have an intrauterine pregnancy of uncertain viability if transvaginal ultrasonography shows an intrauterine gestational sac with no embryonic heartbeat (and no findings of definite pregnancy failure).
Pregnancy of unknown location	A woman is considered to have a pregnancy of unknown location if she has a positive urine or serum pregnancy test and no intrauterine or ectopic pregnancy is seen on transvaginal ultrasonography.
Diagnostic Tests	
Human chorionic gonadotropin (hCG)	Serum hCG concentration is measured with the use of the World Health Organization 3rd or 4th International Standard.
	A positive serum pregnancy test is defined by a serum hCG concentration above a positivity threshold (5 mIU/mL).
Pelvic ultrasonography	Minimum quality criteria include transvaginal assessment of the uterus and adnexa and transabdominal evaluation for free intraperitoneal fluid and a mass high in the pelvis; oversight provided by an appropriately trained physician; scans performed by providers and interpreted by physicians, all of whom meet at least minimum training or certification standards for ultrasonography, including transvaginal ultrasonography; and scanning equipment permitting adequate visualization of structures early in the first trimester.

been met. Recall that the gestational sac is identified sonographically at 4 to 5 weeks' gestation. The sac grows approximately 1 mm per day in the first trimester. The yolk sac should be visualized transvaginally when the gestational sac reaches 8 mm in size, and the embryo *must* be visualized when the MSD measures 25 mm. The normal embryo grows at a rate of 1 mm/day. Cardiac activity is visible by 5.5 to 6.5 weeks (Table 50.1). Failure to observe these developmental markers suggests a pregnancy of "uncertain viability" (PUV). Applying the SRU criteria, pregnancy failure can be definitively stated when the embryo is 7 mm or greater without a heartbeat or the MSD is 25 mm but no embryo is visible.

In the case of pregnancy loss (**complete abortion**), serial hCG levels demonstrate successive decline. Caution should be taken when a positive pregnancy test and an empty uterus are seen, given the possibility that an early normal intrauterine pregnancy between 3 and 5 weeks' gestation may be present. Consequently, serial hCG levels should always be obtained and followed for appropriate rise or decline.

If the endometrium is abnormally thick or irregularly echogenic, the differential diagnosis includes intrauterine blood, retained products of conception after an incomplete spontaneous loss, a decidual reaction associated with an ectopic pregnancy, or decidual changes resulting from an early but not yet visible intrauterine pregnancy. **Incomplete spontaneous abortion** may show several sonographic findings, ranging from an intact gestational sac with a nonviable embryo to a collapsed gestational sac that is grossly misshapen (Fig. 50.2). Women who are clinically undergoing a spontaneous abortion or who have had an elective termination often require follow-up sonography to determine whether retained products of conception are present. Sonographic signs of retained products may be subtle; a thickened endometrium greater than 8 mm and increased vascularization of the endometrial complex with color Doppler are strongly predictive. The presence of visible embryonic parts, a gestational sac, or an embryonic disk is obvious evidence of retained products of conception (Fig. 50.3). It sometimes can be difficult to distinguish retained products of conception from blood clots. Quantitative hCG levels, which do not decline normally, a thickened endometrium, and increased vascular flow will provide discriminating evidence for retained products. Patients most often present with persistent bleeding after SPL, dilation and curettage, or being prescribed misoprostol for uterine evacuation.

Gestational Sac Without an Embryo or Yolk Sac

A gestational sac without an embryo or yolk sac on sonography may represent one of three conditions: (1) a normal early intrauterine pregnancy of less than 5 weeks, (2) an abnormal intrauterine pregnancy, or (3) a pseudogestational sac in a patient with an ectopic pregnancy.

Criteria for Abnormal Sac

The gestational sac should be imaged consistently by both transabdominal and transvaginal sonography when its mean diameter is 5 mm, which corresponds to a gestational age of 4 to 5 weeks. Transvaginal sonography may demonstrate the sac

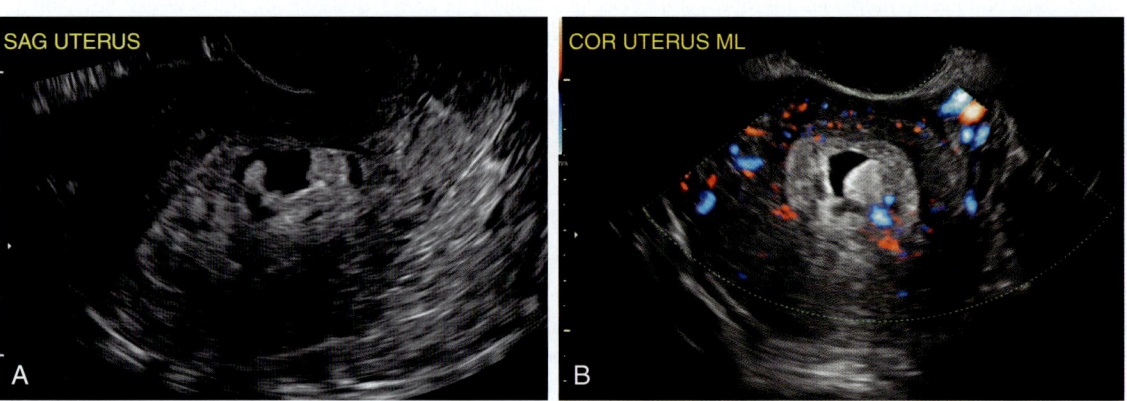

FIG. 50.2 Transvaginal scan of a patient who presented with fever, pain, and bleeding secondary to an abortion 2 days previously. The endometrial cavity is distended, with retained products of conception casting small shadows into the myometrial cavity. (A) Sagittal uterus. (B) Coronal uterus.

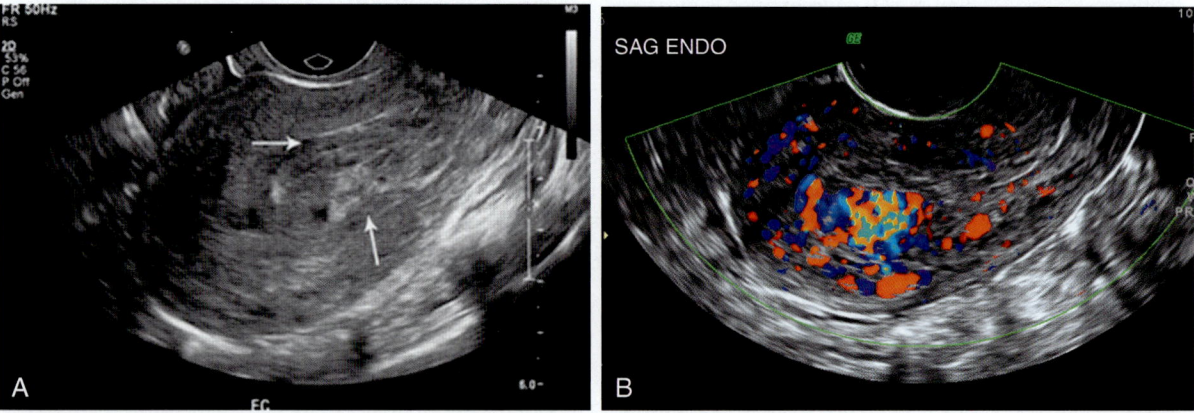

FIG. 50.3 Sonographic signs of retained products may be subtle; a thickened endometrium greater than 8 mm and increased vascularization of the endometrial complex with color Doppler are strongly predictive. The presence of visible embryonic parts, a gestational sac, or an embryonic disk is obvious evidence of retained products of conception.

as early as 4 weeks, when it measures 2 to 3 mm. At this early size the "sac" can be described only as an intrauterine fluid collection. This cannot be definitively called a gestational sac until there is further growth and a **yolk sac** can be identified. Measuring the gestational sac at this early stage provides a baseline for monitoring appropriate interval growth. Caution should be used in evaluating these early stages of pregnancy to allow for the possibility that a patient may have inaccurate dates for their last menstrual period. Sequential scanning can document appropriate interval growth of 1 mm per day. Lack of appropriate growth indicates an abnormally growing gestational sac or a pregnancy of unknown viability.

Regarding gestational sac values, a gestational sac may be seen as early as 4.3 weeks, the *threshold level*, and must be seen by 5.2 weeks, the *discriminatory level*. Given the new pregnancy failure criteria, absence of a gestational sac at this stage would also be termed PUV and follow-up ultrasound would be ordered.

Transvaginal sonography is the ideal method to examine the early gestational sac. When the sac measures 8 mm or greater, a definitive yolk sac should be demonstrated. The yolk sac can be expected to grow 0.1 mm per 1 mm of MSD growth, up to 15 mm. When the gestational sac measures 25 mm, an embryo with cardiac activity must be seen. Follow-up examination in 7 to 10 days is recommended if the findings are indeterminate.

Anembryonic Pregnancy (Blighted Ovum)

By definition, **anembryonic pregnancy**, or **blighted ovum**, is a gestational sac in which the embryo fails to develop or stops developing at such an early stage that it is imperceptible by ultrasound (see Table 50.1). The trophoblastic tissue may continue to proliferate despite the failed embryonic growth, the gestational sac will continue to grow, and hCG levels may continue to rise, although not at the expected rate. The typical sonographic appearance of anembryonic pregnancy is a large, empty gestational sac that does not demonstrate a yolk sac, an amnion, or an embryo (Fig. 50.4). The MSD increases by 1.13 mm/day in a normal gestation, but the growth rate of an abnormal sac is only 0.70 mm/day. Therefore abnormal sac growth can be diagnosed when the MSD fails to increase by 0.6 mm/day. In subsequent repeat studies, the sonographer evaluates growth size of the sac, presence of the yolk sac, development of an embryo, and presence or absence of cardiac activity. Box 50.1 outlines several sonographic intrauterine findings associated with abnormal pregnancies. The SRU criteria for failed pregnancy in the presence of an empty sac is an MSD of 25 mm without an embryo.

Gestational Trophoblastic Disease

Gestational trophoblastic disease is a proliferative disease of the trophoblast that occurs after an abnormal conception. It represents a spectrum of disease from a relatively benign

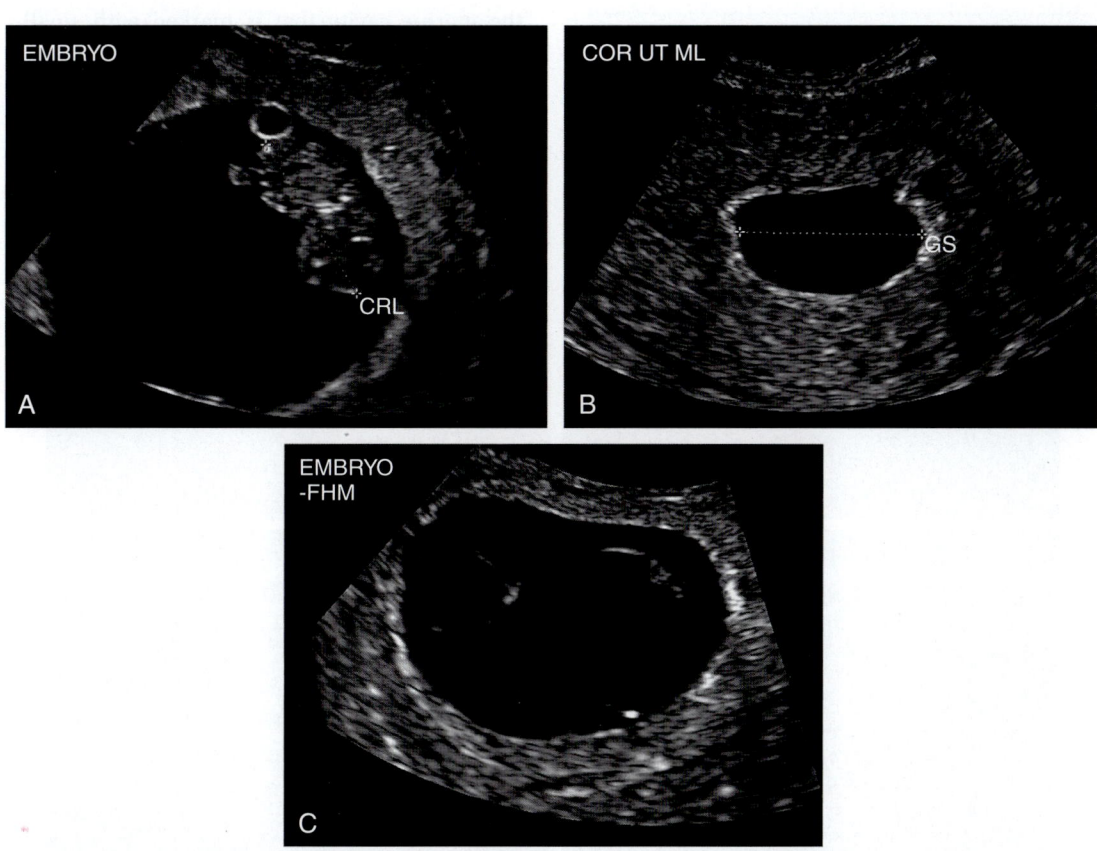

FIG. 50.4 (A) Transvaginal image demonstrating a normal embryo and yolk sac. (B) Large, empty 6-week gestational sac that does not contain yolk sac, amnion, or embryo. This is consistent with anembryonic pregnancy. (C) Large, empty gestational sac *(at right)* with an abnormal yolk sac.

> **BOX 50.1** **Sonographic Findings of Gestational Sacs Associated With Abnormal Intrauterine Pregnancies**
>
> **Embryo**
> - Absence of cardiac motion in embryos ≥5 mm
> - Absence of cardiac motion after 6.5 menstrual weeks
>
> **Yolk Sac and Amnion**
> - Large yolk sac or amnion without a visible embryo
> - Calcified yolk sac
>
> **Large Gestational Sac**
> - >18 mm lacking a viable embryo
> - >8 mm lacking a visible yolk sac
>
> **Shape**
> - Irregular or misshapen
>
> **Position**
> - Cornual, low, or hour-glassing through cervical os
>
> **Trophoblastic Reaction**
> - Irregular
> - Absent double decidual sac finding
> - Thin trophoblastic reaction <2 mm
> - Intratrophoblastic venous flow
>
> **Growth**
> - Gestational sac growth of <0.6 mm/day
> - Absent embryonic growth
>
> **Human Chorionic Gonadotropin Correlation**
> - Discrepancy in sac size with levels
>
> From Nyberg DA, Laing FC. First trimester. In Nyberg DA, Hill LM, Bohm-Velez M, et al, editors. *Transvaginal Ultrasound*. St Louis: Mosby–Year Book; 1992.

form called hydatidiform (partial, complete, or coexistent) mole to a more malignant form called an invasive mole, or choriocarcinoma. The clinical hallmark of gestational trophoblastic disease is vaginal bleeding in the first or early second trimester. Serum levels of beta-hCG are dramatically elevated and are often greater than 100,000 IU/mL. The patient may also experience symptoms of hyperemesis gravidarum or preeclampsia. Maternal serum alpha-fetoprotein levels will be notably low in pregnancies complicated by a complete hydatidiform mole.

In the United States, gestational trophoblastic disease affects approximately 1 out of every 1000 pregnancies. Associations with women younger than age 20 and older than age 40 with molar pregnancy have been reported. Molar pregnancies are divided into two categories: partial and complete. A partial mole is karyotypically abnormal, usually triploid, and commonly occurs when a normal egg is fertilized by two sperm. Fetal parts may develop concurrently with abnormal trophoblastic tissue. In contrast, genetic studies indicate that a complete hydatidiform mole has a normal diploid karyotype of 46XX, which is usually entirely derived from the father. Complete moles occur when an egg without a nucleus is fertilized by one normal sperm. Trophoblastic tissue proliferates, but no fetal parts ever develop.

Sonographic Findings. The sonographic appearance of molar pregnancy varies with gestational age. The characteristic "snowstorm" appearance of a hydatidiform mole, which includes a moderately echogenic soft tissue mass filling the uterine cavity that is marked with small cystic spaces representing hydropic chorionic villi, may not be apparent initially but will present with advancing time (Fig. 50.5).

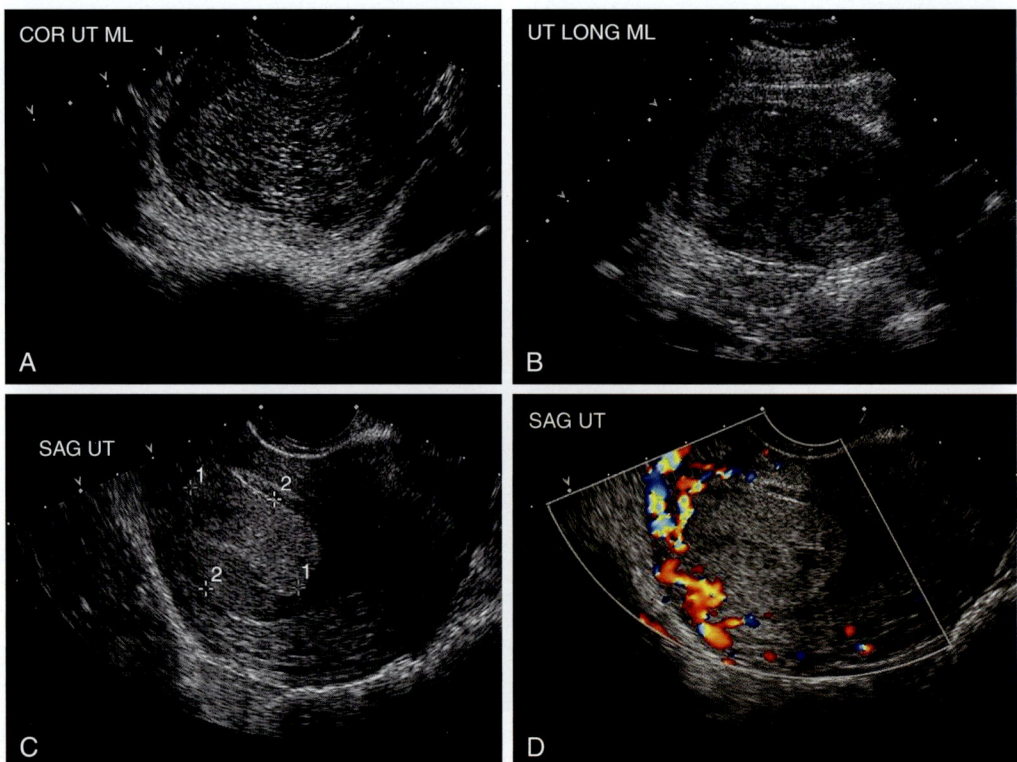

FIG. 50.5 Transvaginal coronal (A–B) and sagittal (C–D) images of the pregnant uterus in a patient who presented larger than appropriate for dates and with bleeding. The uterus is filled with tiny grape-like clusters of tissue, which represent a hydatidiform mole.

The appearance of first-trimester molar pregnancy may simulate a missed abortion, **incomplete abortion**, blighted ovum, or hydropic degeneration of the placenta associated with missed abortion (Fig. 50.6).

On transvaginal sonography, the abnormal-appearing choriodecidual or trophoblastic reaction consists of a distorted sac shape with a thin, weakly echogenic or irregular choriodecidual reaction and absence of a double decidual sac when the MSD exceeds 10 mm. There is usually no sign of a viable embryo, and the early developing placenta exhibits multiple abnormal trophoblastic changes. The sonographic examination may reveal a uterus that is larger in size than dates and filled with a heterogeneous complex pattern ("cluster of grapes") along with bilateral adnexal fullness that may represent ovarian enlargement of theca lutein cysts. The trophoblastic reaction may also be seen as a small echogenic mass filling the uterine cavity without the characteristic vesicles. Typically, remarkable increased blood flow is seen with color Doppler, and spectral Doppler shows low-resistive waveforms with high diastolic flow.

The primary treatment of molar pregnancy is uterine curettage followed by serial monitoring of serum hCG levels and possibly methotrexate administration. Serum hCG level decreases toward normal within 10 to 12 weeks after evacuation. The reported incidence of residual disease after curettage is approximately 20%. The use of sonography for direct visualization of the uterine content to ensure complete evacuation during the curettage procedure has been shown to substantially reduce the incidence of residual gestational trophoblastic disease.

A partial mole on sonography has an identifiable placenta, although the placental tissue is grossly enlarged and engorged with cystic spaces, which represent the hydropic villi. An embryo or embryonic tissue may also be identified, but often the embryo is abnormal and is aborted in the first trimester. In later stages of pregnancy (>12 weeks), careful analysis should be performed to look for structural defects because triploid fetuses usually exist with a partial mole. This includes trisomies 13, 18, and 21.

Bilateral theca lutein cysts have been reported in as many as half of molar pregnancies. Enlarged ovaries may rupture or torse, causing extreme pain for the patient. Theca lutein cysts are well demonstrated on sonography as enlarged ovaries with multiple cystic areas throughout (Fig. 50.7).

Malignant forms of trophoblastic disease include invasive mole and choriocarcinoma. An invasive hydatidiform mole

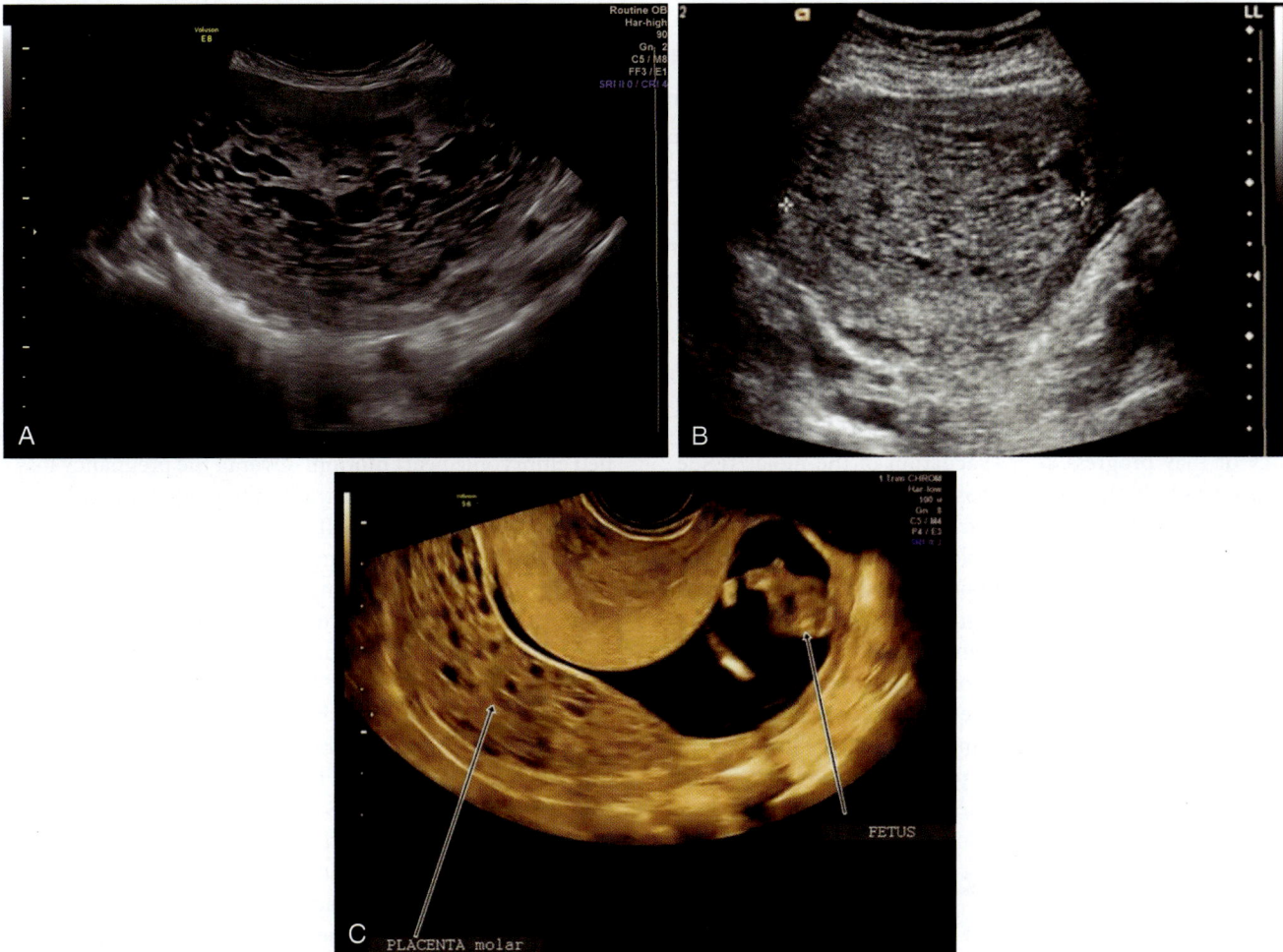

FIG. 50.6 Partial hydatidiform mole with coexisting fetus. The lower uterine fundus demonstrates a small but relatively normal area of placenta *(upper right)* and a large area of cystic and solid components consistent with hydatidiform mole. Between the two placentas is an amniotic cavity with fetal parts.

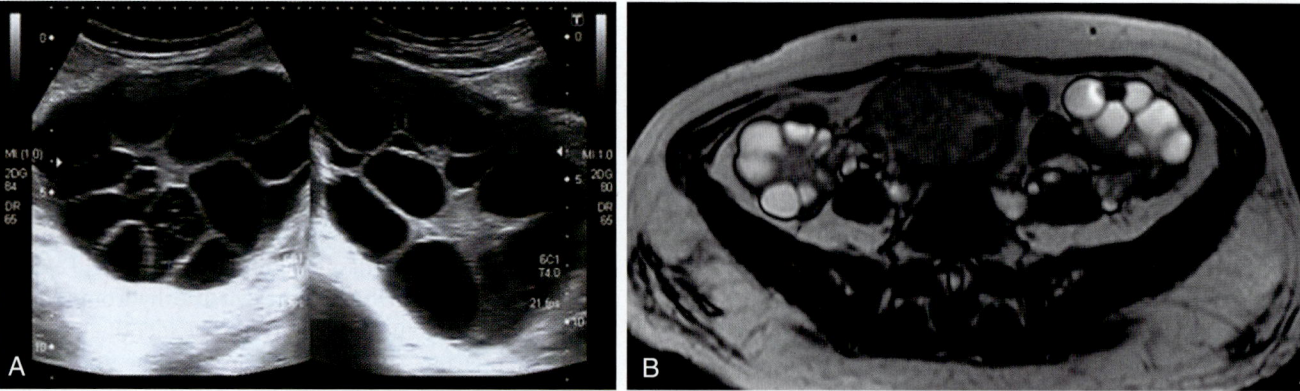

FIG. 50.7 (A) Theca lutein cysts are well demonstrated on sonography as enlarged ovaries with multiple cystic areas throughout. (B) Magnetic resonance imaging of theca lutein cysts.

TABLE 50.2	Guidelines for Transvaginal Ultrasonographic Diagnosis of Pregnancy Failure in a Woman With an Intrauterine Pregnancy of Uncertain Viability[a]
Findings Diagnostic of Pregnancy Failure	**Findings Suspicious for, but Not Diagnostic of, Pregnancy Failure[b]**
Crown-rump length of ≥7 mm and no heartbeat	Crown-rump length of <7 mm and no heartbeat
Mean sac diameter of 25 mm and no embryo	Mean sac diameter of 16–24 mm and no embryo
Absence of embryo with heartbeat ≥2 weeks after a scan that showed a gestational sac without a yolk sac	Absence of embryo with heartbeat 7–13 days after a scan that showed a gestational sac without a yolk sac
Absence of embryo with heartbeat ≥11 days after a scan that showed a gestational sac with a yolk sac	Absence of embryo with heartbeat 7–10 days after a scan that showed a gestational sac with a yolk sac
	Absence of embryo >6 weeks after last menstrual period
	Empty amnion (amnion seen adjacent to yolk sac, with no visible embryo)
	Enlarged yolk sac (>7 mm)
	Small gestational sac in relation to the size of the embryo (<5 mm difference between mean sac diameter and crown-rump length)

[a]Criteria are from the Society of Radiologists in Ultrasound Multispecialty Consensus Conference on Early First Trimester Diagnosis of Miscarriage and Exclusion of a Viable Intrauterine Pregnancy, October 2012.
[b]When there are findings suspicious for pregnancy failure, follow-up ultrasonography at 7–10 days to assess the pregnancy for viability is generally appropriate.

occurs when the hydropic villi of a partial or complete mole invade the uterine myometrium and may further penetrate the uterine wall. This may occur along with the molar pregnancy or may progress after evacuation of the molar tissue has occurred. If this occurs postoperatively, it is referred to as *persistent trophoblastic disease*. Clinically, the patient presents with continued heavy bleeding and highly elevated hCG levels. The sonographic appearance shows an enlarged uterus with multiple focal areas of grape-like clusters throughout.

Choriocarcinoma is a malignant form of trophoblastic disease that occurs in 2% to 3% of molar pregnancies. This tumor is fast-growing and commonly metastasizes to the lungs, liver, and brain. Clinical symptoms include vaginal bleeding, in addition to dyspnea, abdominal pain, and neurologic symptoms, depending on where the metastasis has spread.

ABNORMAL OR ABSENT CARDIAC ACTIVITY

Sonographic differentiation of normal and abnormal appearances of first-trimester pregnancy may be subtle. Distinguishing viable from nonviable gestations is crucial, and demonstration of a living embryo does not necessarily mean a normal outcome. Recent data prospectively looking at 556 pregnancies between 6 and 13 weeks' gestation identified embryonic heart motion.[1] Overall the pregnancy loss rate after identification of an intrauterine pregnancy with positive cardiac motion was 8.8%. If sonographic abnormalities were detected (subchorionic hematoma being the most frequent), the loss rate was 15.2% compared with 8.8% when sonogram findings were normal. It is of interest that the loss rate after a normal sonogram was similar in symptomatic (10.6%) and asymptomatic patients (9.1%).[1]

Identifying an intrauterine pregnancy with cardiac activity is the first conclusive sonographic sign of viability. With transvaginal sonography, a living embryo should be detected when the MSD reaches 25 mm. Other sonographic appearances allow the ultrasound clinician to differentiate normal and abnormal findings within the early gestational period: cardiac rate, gestational sac growth, and yolk sac size and appearance. More than one sonogram may be necessary to establish a normal pregnancy. Sonographic signs are discussed throughout this chapter and are outlined in Table 50.2.

Absent Cardiac Activity

Absence of cardiac activity in the first trimester is the most critical sign for viability of the pregnancy. The heart tube is formed between 3.5 and 5 weeks of conception. If the embryo is visible by sonography but cardiac activity cannot be documented, the prognosis is poor. Caution should be used in interpreting any case that involves a question regarding the accuracy of menstrual dating and in which heart motion is not yet visible by sonography. Usually by the time the embryonic sac measures 9 mm, the presence of cardiac activity is noted. Other studies have noted that with transvaginal sonography, when the CRL measures 4 mm, the embryo should demonstrate cardiac function, although the SRU criteria state that pregnancy failure is diagnosed at a CRL of 7 mm without cardiac function.

Recall that between 6 and 7 weeks' gestation, the embryo and yolk sac are close in proximity and can be viewed as contiguous structures. After 7 weeks, these structures diverge from one another. Scans should be made with the highest possible transducer frequency to image with the greatest accuracy. The transducer should be very carefully swept through the gestational sac to image the embryo, cardiac motion, and yolk sac (Fig. 50.8). Once cardiac activity is seen, M-mode should be used to record the actual heart rate.

Embryonic Bradycardia and Tachycardia

Variations in embryonic cardiac rate during the first trimester range between 90 and 170 beats/min (see Table 50.1). Embryonic cardiac rates of less than 90 beats/min at any gestational age within the first trimester have been shown to have a poor prognostic finding. In fact, no reported embryo has survived beyond the second trimester with this finding. The fetus with a heart rate greater than 170 beats/min shows signs of tachycardia, which may lead to heart failure and fetal hydrops (pleural effusion, pericardial effusion, and ascites).

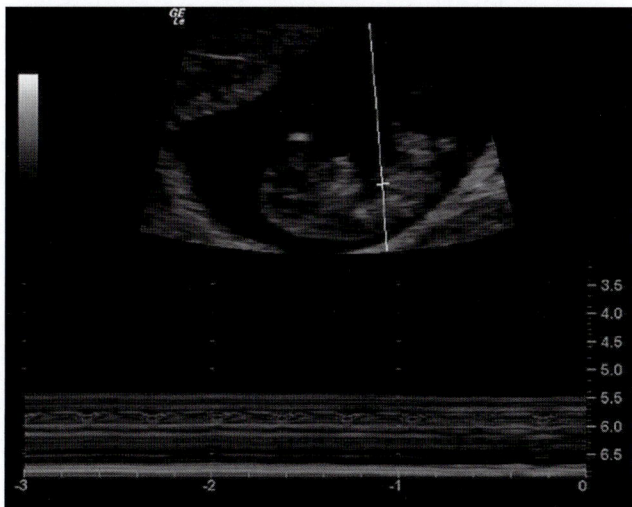

FIG. 50.8 The transducer should be very carefully swept through the gestational sac to image the embryo, cardiac motion, and yolk sac. Once cardiac activity is seen, M-mode should be used to record the actual heart rate.

EMBRYONIC DEVELOPMENT OF YOLK SAC AND AMNION

Embryonic Oligohydramnios and Growth Restriction

Growth delay and oligohydramnios within the first trimester have poor outcomes. If the gestational sac measures 5 mm less than the CRL, embryonic oligohydramnios may be suspected, and demise is highly probable.

Embryonic growth restriction can be determined only by relative sonographic dating, either by reliable menstrual history or by growth delay of the embryo or gestational sac in relation to serial sonograms. Chromosome abnormalities, such as triploidy, have been associated with embryonic growth restriction and embryonic oligohydramnios.

Embryonic Yolk Sac Evaluation

The size and appearance of the yolk sac should be evaluated in the first trimester. Expected yolk sac growth is 0.3 mm/day. A normal yolk sac has a maximal diameter of 5.5 mm between 5 and 10 weeks' gestation. An enlarged yolk sac (7 mm or greater) has an increased risk for SPL. If the yolk sac is abnormal in appearance, too large or too small for gestational age, calcified, misshapened, or highly echogenic, the patient should be watched for early pregnancy failure. If cardiac activity is present, the pregnancy should be followed carefully with ultrasound for continued embryonic growth.

Amnion Evaluation

The amnion is best visualized with transvaginal sonography between the fifth and seventh weeks of gestation. The side-by-side appearance of the amnion and the yolk sac is described as the "double bleb sign." The amnion should appear as the thinner of the two concentric structures. The embryonic disk lies between the amnion and the yolk sac. Abnormal development is suggested when the thickness and echogenicity of the amnion approach that of the yolk sac. The mean amniotic sac diameter should be approximately equal to the CRL. Pregnancy exhibiting an MSD greater than 25 mm without an embryo is consistent with anembryonic pregnancy or *failed pregnancy*.

ECTOPIC PREGNANCY

Ectopic pregnancy is one of the most emergent diagnoses made with sonography. An ectopic pregnancy is pregnancy located outside the central/fundal location of the uterus. Approximately 10% of maternal deaths are related to ectopic pregnancy. The occurrence of ectopic pregnancy also has an effect on the future fertility of a patient and increases the risk of a repeat ectopic pregnancy. The incidence of ectopic pregnancy has increased in recent years. Associated risk factors include the rise in the incidence of pelvic infections, the use of intrauterine contraceptive devices (IUCDs), fallopian tube surgeries, infertility treatments, and a history of ectopic pregnancy.

Clinical findings of pain are nonspecific and may vary. Pelvic pain has been reported in 97% of patients, although pain may be consistent with other pathologic processes, such as appendicitis or pelvic inflammatory disease. The classic clinical findings associated with ectopic pregnancy are vaginal bleeding, an empty uterus, the presence of an adnexal mass, and a positive pregnancy test. These clinical findings are found in nearly 45% of patients.

Pathologically, tubal ectopic pregnancy is diagnosed by the invasion of trophoblastic tissue within the fallopian tube mucosa. This causes the bleeding often associated with ectopic pregnancy, which may cause hematosalpinx, hemoperitoneum, or both.

Ectopic pregnancy occurs within the fallopian tube in approximately 95% of cases. Other sites, such as the ovary, broad ligament, peritoneum, cervix, and cornua, account for the remaining cases (Fig. 50.9). When an ectopic pregnancy is found in the interstitial portion of the fallopian tube near the uterine cornu, the risk for massive hemorrhage with rupture that may lead to hysterectomy or even death is increased.

Correlating clinical findings with sonographic findings in ectopic pregnancy is imperative for diagnosis. Specific assays for hCG allow the sonographer/sonologist to discern the sonographic findings. Beta-hCG is quantified from maternal blood by two preparations: the First International Reference Preparation (1st IRP) or the Second International Standard (2IS). It is crucial that the sonographer understands which hCG assay a particular institution or laboratory is using. Quantification of hCG is directly correlated with gestational age throughout the first trimester. In general, the 1st IRP has hCG quantities double those of the 2IS.

Given the complexities of hCG testing, it is vital that the sonographer have a good understanding of the discriminatory level of hCG and sonographic findings. The discriminatory level of hCG in pregnancy should be thought of as a minimum level of hCG in normal intrauterine or ectopic pregnancy. Using transvaginal techniques, the hCG discriminatory level for detecting an intrauterine pregnancy has been shown to be 800 to 1000 IU/L based on the 2IS and 1000 to 2000 IU/L based on the 1st IRP.

If discriminatory levels of beta-hCG are met or surpassed and no intrauterine gestational sac is seen, an ectopic pregnancy should be suspected. Caution should be taken if beta-hCG levels are less than discriminatory levels. Ectopic gestations do not produce hCG at normal levels (hCG levels double every 2 days) and 90% of ectopic gestations are not viable and so may not reflect typical correlation between gestational age and hCG levels. Ectopic pregnancy may have a similar appearance to an early intrauterine pregnancy. Thus in nonemergent cases, serial beta-hCG levels are preferred because trending of these levels would demonstrate a continuing pregnancy if hCG levels increase normally, whereas decreasing hCG levels may indicate missed or incomplete abortion.

Sonographic Findings in Ectopic Pregnancy

The sonographic appearances of ectopic pregnancy have been well documented with both transabdominal and transvaginal techniques (Fig. 50.10). The most important finding when

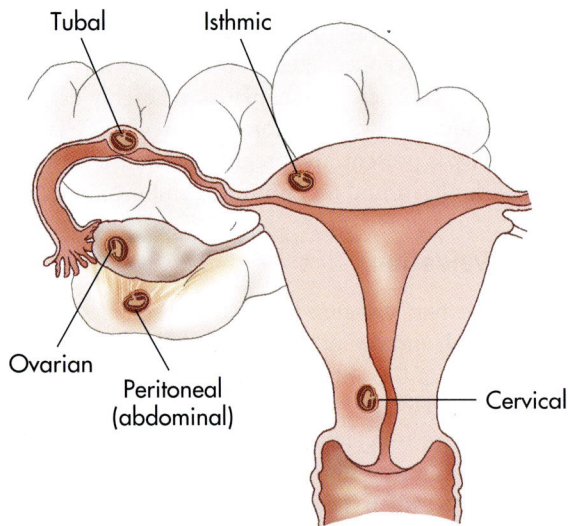

FIG. 50.9 Potential sites for ectopic pregnancy.

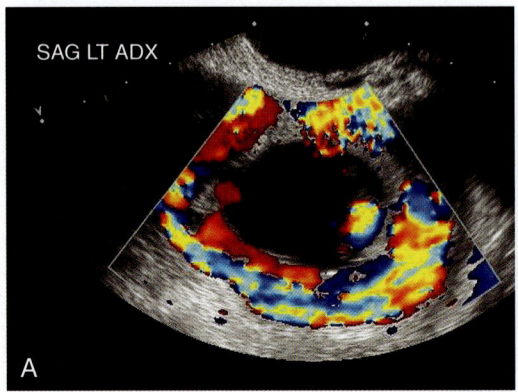
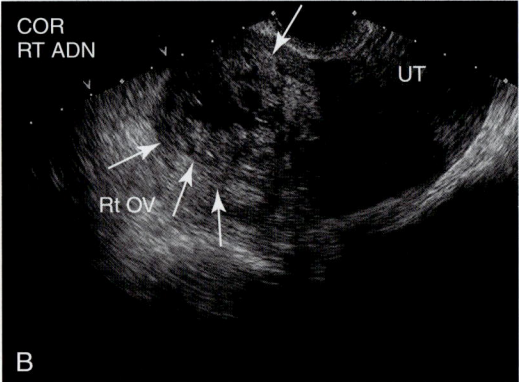

FIG. 50.10 (A) Sagittal sonogram demonstrating high-velocity color flow in the left adnexa that surrounded the ectopic gestational sac. Other images demonstrated an empty uterus with normal endometrial canal. (B) Coronal sonogram demonstrating uterus (UT) and right ovary (Rt OV), with an echogenic concentric ring and embryo seen centrally with fetal heart motion consistent with ectopic pregnancy. *Arrows*, Decidua/trophoblastic villi.

scanning for ectopic pregnancy is to determine whether there is a normal intrauterine gestation (reducing the probability of an ectopic pregnancy) or whether the uterine cavity is empty and an adnexal mass is present (Table 50.3). The expectation of visualizing a normal intrauterine gestation is directly correlated with beta-hCG levels. Although the visualization of an intrauterine gestational sac that includes embryonic heart motion firmly makes the diagnosis of intrauterine pregnancy, earlier gestations (5 to 6 weeks) may not demonstrate these findings.

As many as 20% of patients with ectopic pregnancy demonstrate an intrauterine sac-like structure known as the **pseudogestational sac**. Although it is challenging, differentiating between normal early gestation and a pseudogestational sac is possible (Fig. 50.11) by using the following guidelines: (1) pseudogestational sacs do not contain a living embryo or yolk sac; (2) pseudogestational sacs are centrally located within the endometrial cavity, unlike the burrowed gestational sac, which is eccentrically placed; and (3) homogeneous level echoes are commonly observed in pseudogestational sacs, unlike in normal gestational sacs. The presence of a yolk sac positively indicates an intrauterine gestation. These findings are commonly observed using transvaginal ultrasound.

TABLE 50.3	First-Trimester Pelvic Mass	
Condition	**Sonographic Findings**	**Differential Considerations**
Corpus luteum cyst	>5 cm in size Internal septations and debris (secondary to hemorrhage) Increased vascularity surrounding corpus luteum	Dermoid Ovarian cancer
Uterine leiomyoma	Increased hormone stimulation growth May compress gestational sac Various sonographic patterns: hypoechoic, echogenic, isoechoic when compared with myometrium Increased size causes uterine endometrial deformity	Uterine contractions Dermoid

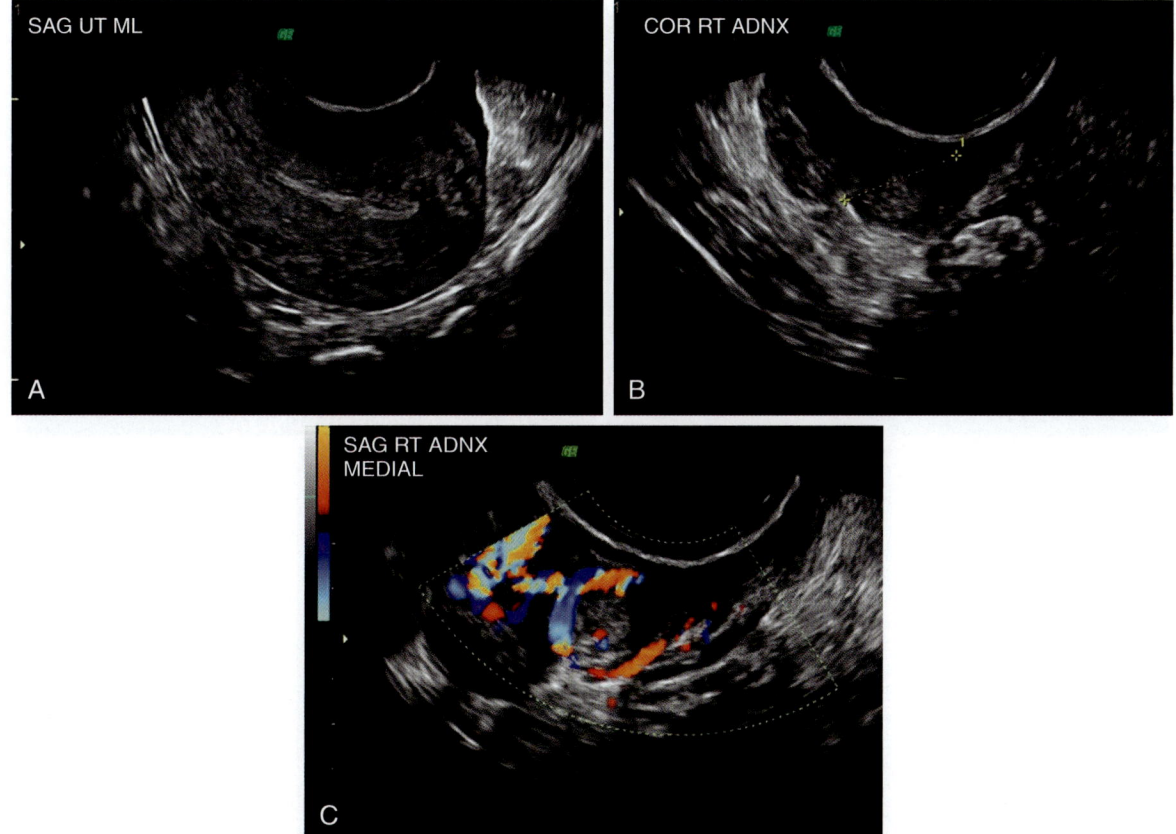

FIG. 50.11 A patient in her first trimester presented in the emergency department with elevated human chorionic gonadotropin levels, bleeding, and pelvic pain. (A) Sagittal midline transvaginal image shows the uterus without an embryo. (B) Coronal images of the right adnexa demonstrate the ectopic gestational sac. (C) Sagittal image of the right adnexa shows an ectopic gestational sac within the adnexal area.

Color Doppler imaging and spectral analysis may be helpful in distinguishing a normal sac from a pseudogestational sac with the demonstration of peritrophoblastic flow associated with intrauterine pregnancy. Typically, peritrophoblastic flow demonstrates a low-resistance (high-diastolic) pattern, with fairly high peak velocities (approximately 20 cm/sec). The decidual cast of the endometrium, as seen in the pseudogestational sac, typically demonstrates a high-resistance pattern (low-diastolic component) with low peak velocities.

Examining the adnexa sonographically is critical in the evaluation of ectopic pregnancy. Identification of a live embryo within the adnexa is most specific for ectopic gestation. Unfortunately, this occurs approximately only 25% of the time. It is important to note that only approximately 10% of live ectopic pregnancies are identified using transabdominal sonography (Fig. 50.12).

Identification of an extrauterine sac within the adnexa is one of the most frequent findings of ectopic pregnancy. It has been reported that more than 71% of patients with ectopic pregnancy demonstrate an extrauterine sac or ring, although this study did include living extrauterine ectopic fetuses.[2] The extrauterine gestational sac has sonographic appearances and characteristics similar to those of the intrauterine gestational sac. Extrauterine gestational sacs often demonstrate a thickened echogenic ring, separate from the ovary, which represents trophoblastic tissue or chorionic villi, and there is a possibility that the embryo or yolk sac will be seen (Fig. 50.13).

Color flow imaging and Doppler waveforms may also help to diagnose extrauterine gestational sacs. One study reported color flow detection in and around 95 of 106 ectopic gestations with a Doppler resistive index of less than 0.40.[3] The positive predictive value of this technique was 96.8%, with sensitivity and specificity of 89.3% and 96.3%, respectively.[3] Other studies must be performed to correlate these criteria.

Adnexal Mass With Ectopic Pregnancy

The risk of ectopic pregnancy can be greater than 90% when an intrauterine gestation is absent and there is a corresponding adnexal mass. Complex adnexal masses, aside from extrauterine gestational sacs, often represent hematoma within the peritoneal cavity, which is usually contained within the fallopian tube (hematosalpinx) or broad ligament. In early gestational ectopic pregnancy, a hematoma may be the only sonographic sign of ectopic pregnancy. However, it should be distinguished from an ovarian cyst, such as the corpus luteum, which is typically hypoechoic. A hemorrhagic corpus luteum cyst may mimic an extrauterine gestational sac or a distal hematosalpinx.

Often, ovarian processes, such as corpus luteal cysts and endometriomas, can be differentiated based on their location within the ovary, and one can often visualize surrounding ovarian tissue. Although this does not rule out the rare ovarian ectopic gestation, correlation with beta-hCG should help to differentiate the two.

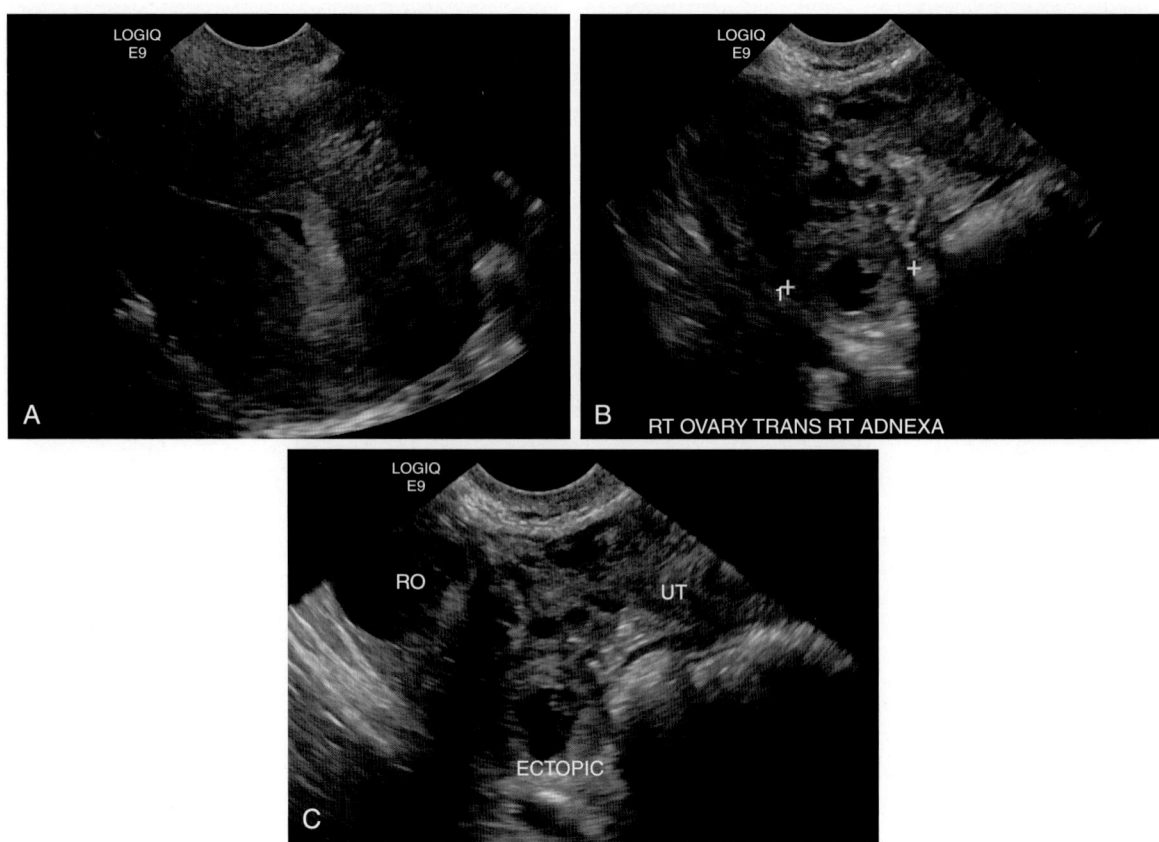

FIG. 50.12 (A) Longitudinal scan depicting an empty uterus, fluid in the cul-de-sac, and a ring-like cystic mass anterior to the uterus, representing an ectopic gestational sac. (B–C) Transverse representations of ectopic gestational sacs. In part C, the ectopic sac is in close proximity to the uterine wall. *RO*, Right ovary; *U*, uterus.

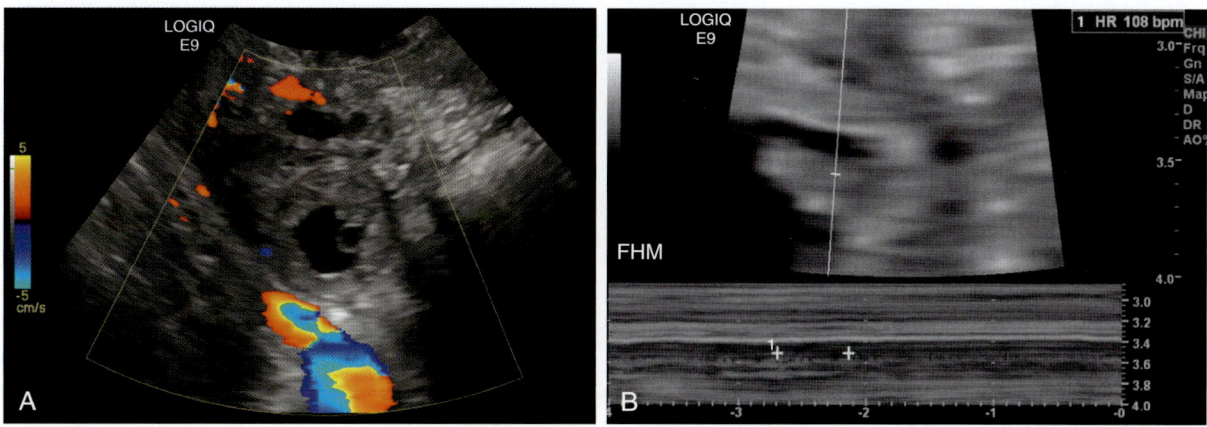

FIG. 50.13 Coronal section demonstrating empty uterus and a right adnexal mass with an echogenic ring and a sonolucent center consistent with a gestational sac. This is consistent with ectopic pregnancy with extrauterine sac. (B) M-mode through the fetal heart demonstrated a heart rate of 108 beats/min.

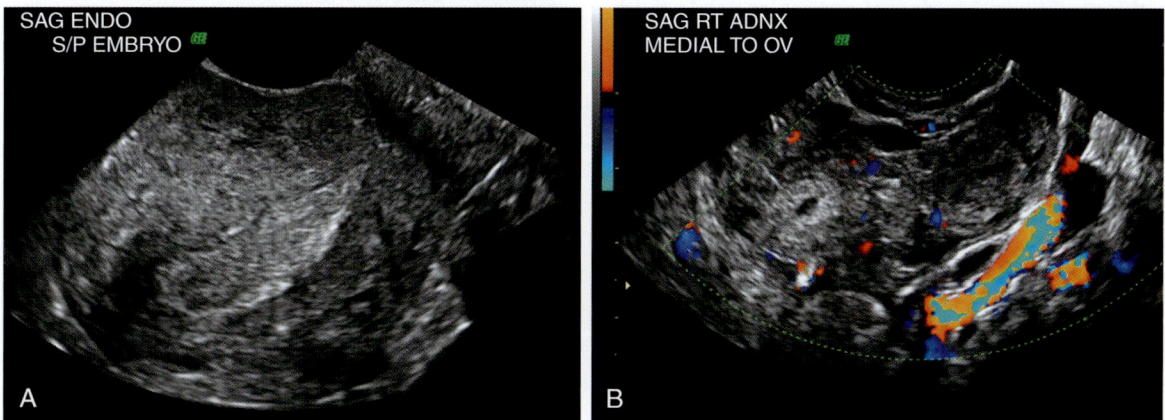

FIG. 50.14 This patient presented with onset of right-sided pain 5 weeks and 2 days after in vitro fertilization embryo transfer. The endometrium is empty, with no signs of an intrauterine gestational sac. (B) Right adnexal mass medial to the ovary represented the ectopic pregnancy.

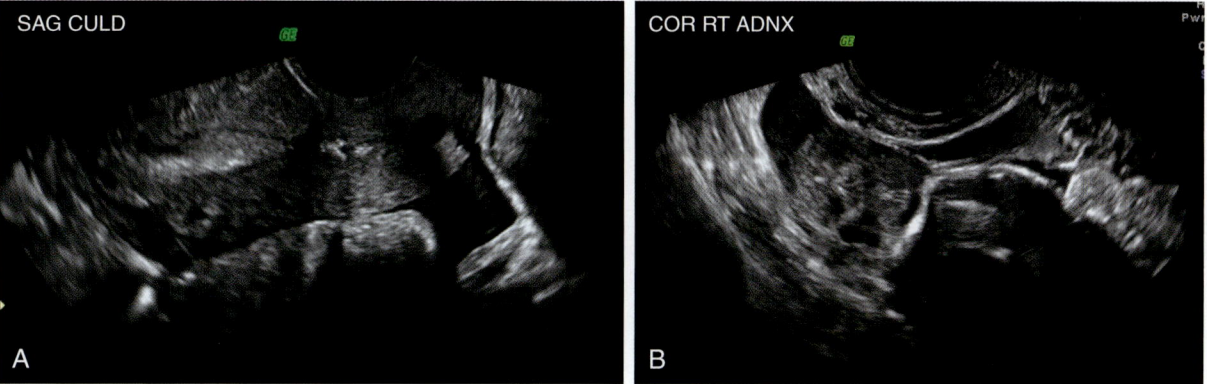

FIG. 50.15 Free fluid in a patient with an ectopic pregnancy. (A) Patient presented with a 5-week, 2-day ectopic pregnancy with a small amount of free fluid in the cul-de-sac. (B) Free fluid in the right adnexa surrounding the ectopic pregnancy, which represented a hemoperitoneum.

It has been reported that approximately 80% of patients with ectopic pregnancy demonstrate at least 25 mL of blood within the peritoneum, caused by blood escaping from the distal tube (fimbria). Approximately 60% of women with an ectopic pregnancy demonstrate intraperitoneal fluid, using transvaginal sonography (Fig. 50.14). Studies have correlated an increased risk of ectopic pregnancy with moderate to large quantities of free intraperitoneal fluid and an associated adnexal mass.[4]

The presence of echogenic free fluid has been shown to be highly specific for hemoperitoneum and to be highly correlated with ectopic pregnancy. A 92% risk of ectopic pregnancy with echogenic free fluid has been reported,[5] with 15% of cases demonstrating echogenic free fluid as the only sonographic finding (Fig. 50.15). When fluid is present, the sonographer should also look at the abdominal gutters and the right and left upper quadrants to evaluate the extent/volume of fluid present. The combination of an adnexal mass and free pelvic fluid is the most precise sonographic correlation in the diagnosis of ectopic pregnancy.

Although intrauterine and adnexal findings are crucial in diagnosing ectopic pregnancy, it is clear that the described sonographic findings vary in their presentation. One report states that 52.5% of cases with ectopic pregnancy could not accurately demonstrate an adnexal mass or masses.[6] Of that 52.5%, less than half (25.5%) were overshadowed by coexisting findings, such as bowel segments that were echogenic or had isoechoic acoustic properties that did not allow sonographic demarcation of tissue from surrounding ovary or adnexa.[6] Another study demonstrated that in 74% of ectopic pregnancies, a confident diagnosis was made of an intrauterine pregnancy using transvaginal techniques and that 26.3% of ectopic pregnancies had a normal transvaginal sonogram at initial presentation.[7] A normal transvaginal sonogram as defined in this study had no adnexal masses or pelvic fluid identified and no evidence of intrauterine gestation. These findings reiterate the need for meticulous scanning when looking for evidence of ectopic pregnancy and for an understanding of the limitations of all ultrasound techniques.

Heterotopic Pregnancy

Fortunately, simultaneous intrauterine and extrauterine pregnancies are extremely uncommon, even in patients undergoing an infertility work-up. The sonographic observer should be aware that ovulation induction and in vitro fertilization with embryo transfer lead not only to a higher risk of **heterotopic pregnancy** but also to an overall increase in ectopic pregnancies, including bilateral ectopic pregnancies (Table 50.4).

Interstitial Pregnancy

Interstitial pregnancy, or cornual pregnancy, is potentially the most life-threatening of all ectopic gestations (see Table 50.4). This is because of the location of the ectopic pregnancy, which lies in the segment of the fallopian tube that enters the uterus. This site involves the parauterine and myometrial vasculature, creating life-threatening hemorrhage when rupture occurs. Interstitial pregnancies have been reported to occur in approximately 2% of all ectopic pregnancies. Sonographic identification of an interstitial ectopic pregnancy is difficult, but it has been described as an eccentrically placed gestational sac within the uterus that has an incomplete myometrial mantle surrounding the sac (Fig. 50.16). Some institutions measure the myometrial thickness and follow these implantations carefully for evidence of myometrial thinning and uterine rupture.

Cervical Pregnancy

Cervical pregnancy has a reported incidence of 1 in 16,000 pregnancies. Sonographic demonstration of a gestational sac within the cervix suggests a cervical pregnancy, although a spontaneous abortion may have a similar appearance. Several

TABLE 50.4	Normal Versus Ectopic Pregnancy
Condition/Sonographic Findings	Differential Considerations
Empty uterus	Normal early IUP (3–4 weeks) Recent spontaneous abortion
Normal IUP Yolk sac present Burrowed gestational sac eccentrically positioned in uterus (usually in the fundus) No internal echoes seen within the gestational sac Peritrophoblastic flow around sac Low-resistive flow pattern	
Ectopic Pregnancy With Pseudogestational sac	
"Intrauterine" sac-like structure	Intrauterine debris
Yolk sac not present	Incomplete spontaneous abortion
Pseudosac seen in central location in uterus	Intrauterine blood
Homogeneous echoes within pseudosac No peritrophoblastic flow High-resistive pattern	
Ectopic Pregnancy	
Pseudogestational sac	Incomplete spontaneous abortion
Extrauterine sac in adnexa with thickened echogenic ring Gestational sac or yolk sac	Intrauterine blood or fluid in cul-de-sac
Heterotopic Pregnancy Simultaneous IUP and ectopic pregnancy (see findings above for IUP and ectopic pregnancy)	Normal IUP and pelvic mass
Interstitial Pregnancy Found in segment of fallopian tube Rupture with hemorrhage Eccentric intrauterine gestational sac with incomplete myometrial mantel surrounding sac	Ectopic pregnancy Pelvic mass
Nonviable IUP Pseudogestational sac of ectopic pregnancy	Embryo, no cardiac motion/nonliving IUP Embryo, cardiac motion/living IUP

IUP, Intrauterine pregnancy.

sonographic features can help to make the distinction between true cervical pregnancy and spontaneous loss "in situ." An established cervical pregnancy demonstrates a concentric shape with decidual reaction and increased color Doppler flow around the trophoblast. In contrast, SPL appears as a misshapen sac, possibly hour-glassing (the hour-glass sign)

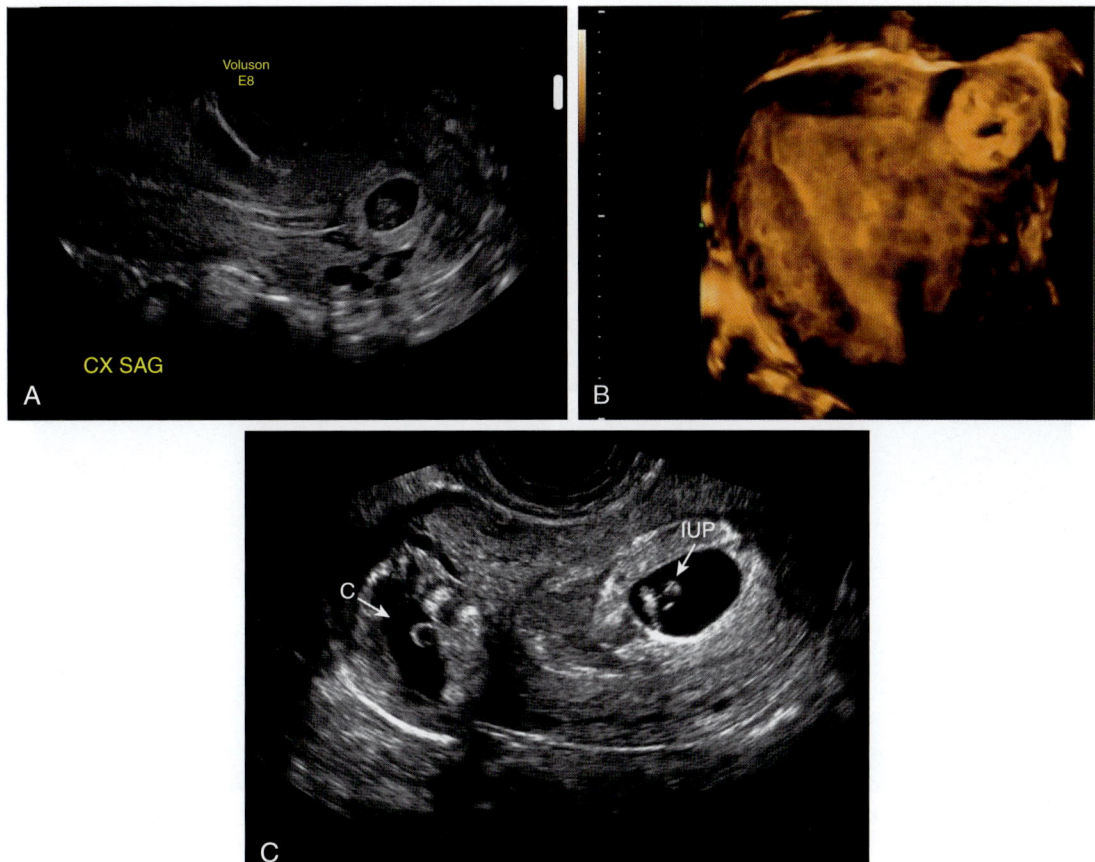

FIG. 50.16 Pregnancy of alternate locations. (A) Cervical pregnancy: a well-decidualized gestational sac with intrauterine contents can be seen in the cervical region of the uterus. (B) Three-dimensional coronal view of the uterus showing a left corneal pregnancy. (C) Transvaginal image, coronal projection, showing concurrent intrauterine pregnancy (IUP) and right cornual pregnancy (C).

through the cervical os, with lack of color flow around the decidual ring. Cervical ectopic pregnancies have an increased risk of complete hysterectomy because of uncontrollable bleeding caused by increased vascularity of the cervix. Treatment may include hysterectomy, or if uterine preservation is desired by the patient, methotrexate can be given.

Ovarian Pregnancy

An ovarian pregnancy is also very rare, accounting for less than 3% of all ectopic pregnancies. The sonographic diagnosis of ovarian pregnancy may be difficult; reported cases have demonstrated complex adnexal masses that involve or contain the ovary. Thus distinguishing ovarian pregnancy from a hemorrhagic ovarian cyst or from other ovarian processes needs close correlation with the quantitative beta-hCG level.

DIAGNOSIS OF EMBRYONIC ABNORMALITIES IN THE FIRST TRIMESTER

Normal embryologic processes that are sonographically visible in the first-trimester embryo have been described in Chapter 49. These normal processes should not be mistaken for anomalies, and the sonographer should be aware of the pathology that can be diagnosed in the first trimester. The development of both high-frequency transvaginal transducers and three-dimensional (3D) technology has significantly increased the sensitivity of ultrasound to detect anomalies in the latter portion of the first trimester. These may include monoamniotic twins, conjoined twins, cardiac defects, cystic hygroma, abdominal wall defects, and cranial and spinal defects. Although many abnormalities can be seen at the end of the first trimester, they are more clearly identified as the fetus matures into the second trimester. Other less common abnormalities, such as ectopia cordis, malformations of the skeleton, and complications of multifetal pregnancies, will be discussed in their respective chapters.

Nuchal Translucency

The nuchal translucency is the maximum thickness of the subcutaneous lucency at the back of the neck in an embryo at 11 to 14 weeks' gestation (Fig. 50.17). Fluid collection between the skin and the soft tissue over the spine is now an accepted method of assessing genetic risk between 11 and 13 weeks 6 days of fetal life. Original research linked increased nuchal measurement with trisomy 21, although we now know that increased nuchal translucency may be found with trisomies 13 and 18 and in fetuses with cardiac defects and other genetic syndromes. In addition, high-resolution transducers have

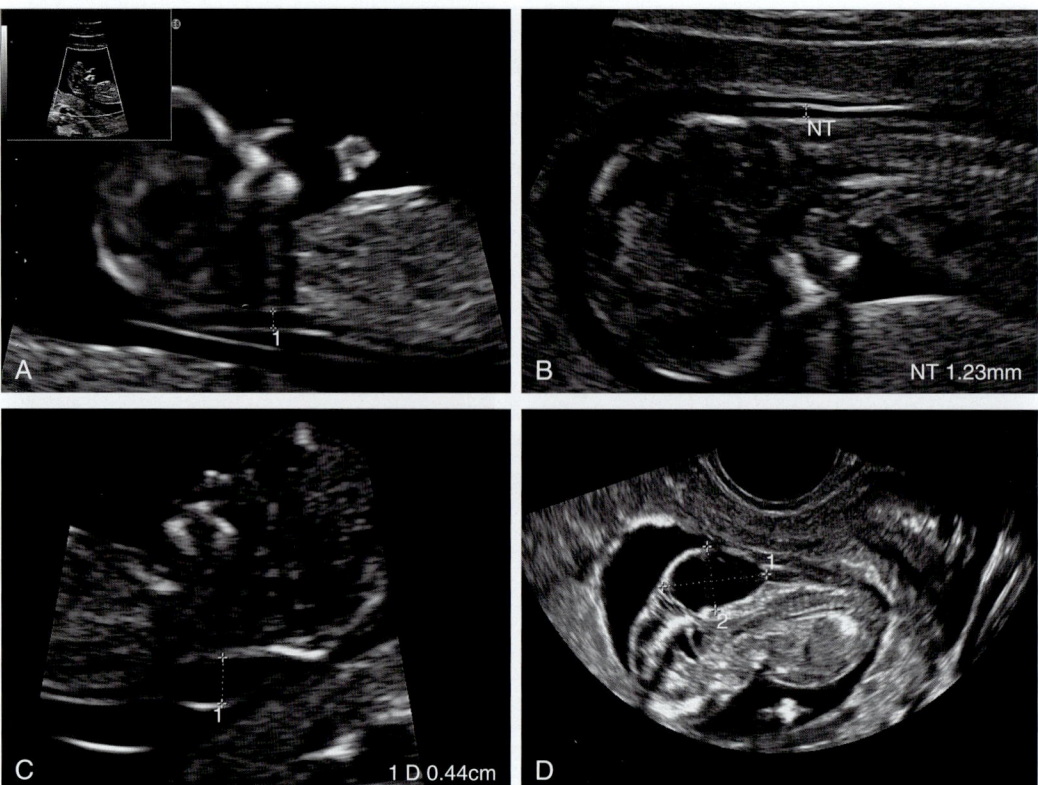

FIG. 50.17 (A) Normal 11-week embryo demonstrating a well-defined neural tube lucency. (B) Normal 12-week embryo lying face down demonstrates nuchal translucency at the back of the neck. (C–D) Abnormal nuchal thickening is demonstrated in these embryos with a cystic hygroma.

lowered the threshold of when we are able to sonographically visualize these anomalies. The nuchal translucency measurement is combined with biochemical markers—free beta-hCG and pregnancy-associated plasma protein–A (PAPP-A)—to assess risk for aneuploidy.

The Fetal Medicine Foundation (FMF) established the following criteria for nuchal measurements, which have become the internationally accepted standard:
- Fetus must be between 11 weeks and 13 weeks 6 days.
- The CRL must be between 45 and 84 mm.
- The sonographer must obtain an optimal image of the midsagittal plane.
- The embryo must be away from the amniotic membrane with the head in a neutral position, with no hyperextension or flexion.

Further research by the FMF has established that we can evaluate first-trimester fetuses for nuchal thickening, presence or absence of nasal bone, tricuspid regurgitation, abnormal flow in the ductus venosus, and possible abnormalities of the hindbrain.

Cardiac Anomalies

Adoption of the first-trimester scan for aneuploidy and advancements in transducer resolution have given us the opportunity to look for cardiac defects at an earlier gestation than ever before. It is now known that there is a strong relationship between increased nuchal translucency and fetuses with cardiac defects. Researchers are reporting the ability to detect a four-chamber view and great vessels as early as 12 weeks. These fetuses are brought back later in gestation to confirm suspected findings. Markers for cardiac defects include increased nuchal translucency, tricuspid regurgitation, and reversal (or absence) of flow in the ductus venosus. Other cardiac associations that can be detected in the first trimester are ectopia cordis and limb body wall complex.

Cranial Anomalies

Although the embryonic head can be sonographically identified by 7 weeks, the cerebral hemisphere continues to evolve throughout the second trimester. The dominant structure seen within the embryonic cranium in the first trimester is the choroid plexus, which fills the lateral ventricles, which in turn fill the cranial vault (Fig. 50.18A). Thus the diagnosis of hydrocephalus in the first trimester is not possible. However, anomalies of cranial organization, such as holoprosencephaly, have been described in the first trimester. The rhombencephalon-hindbrain is a cystic structure appearing in the embryonic cranium within the posterior aspect at 6 to 8 weeks that should not be confused with an abnormality (see Fig. 50.18B). A diagnosis of hydranencephaly has been reported during the first trimester; loss of all intracranial anatomy was sonographically demonstrated. (Hydranencephaly is brain

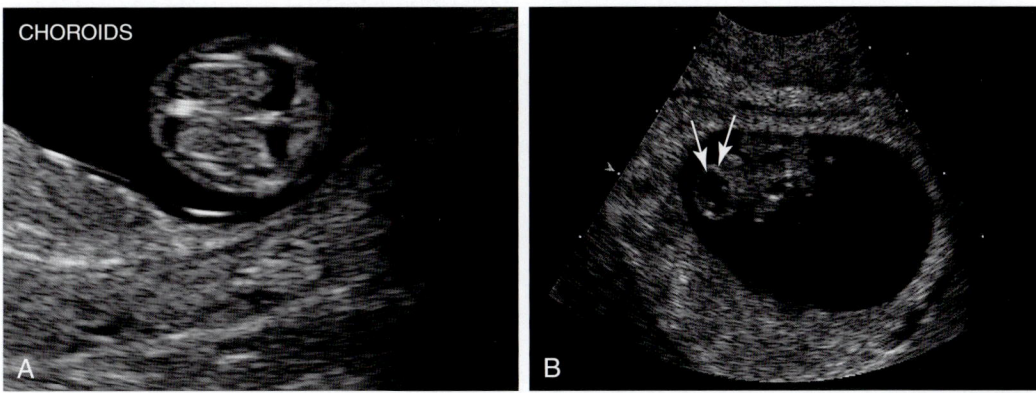

FIG. 50.18 (A) Transvaginal axial scan of the choroid plexus in a first-trimester fetus. (B) Sonogram of an 8.5-week gestation demonstrating the cystic rhombencephalon within the fetal cranium *(arrows)*.

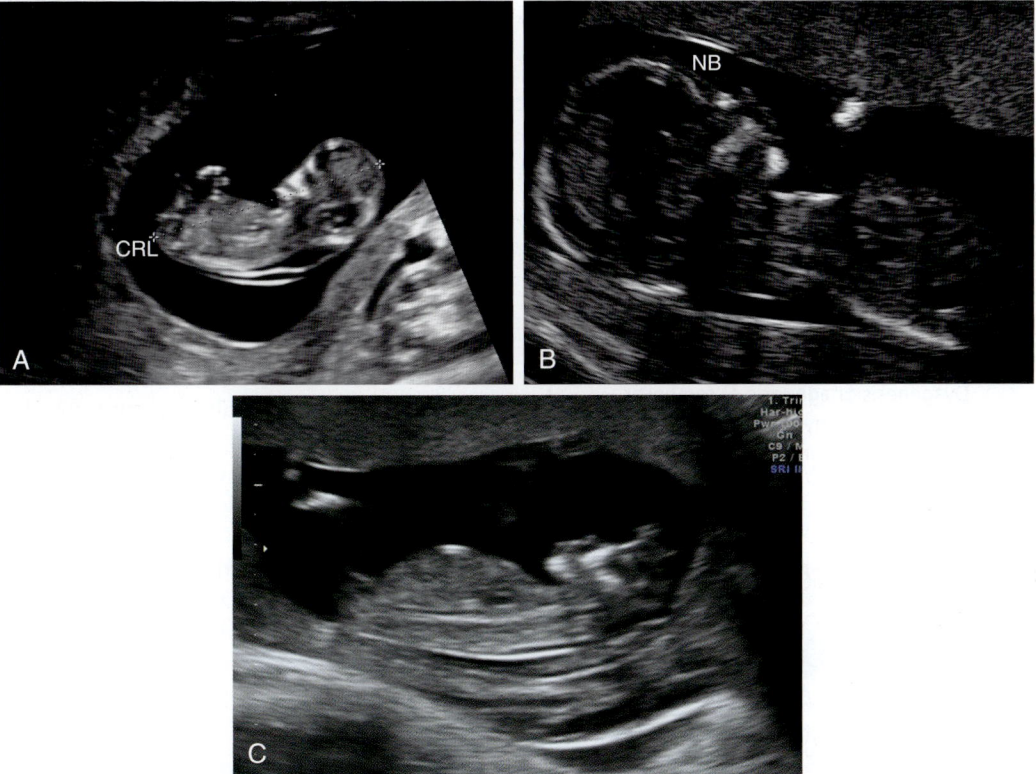

FIG. 50.19 (A) Crown-rump length of a normal 11-week, 5-day fetus with a well-defined cranial cavity. (B) The normal cranial cavity is seen in this 13-week, 5-day fetus. (C) Fetal profile of an anencephalic fetus at 13 weeks. The fetus is lying in a vertex position with the spine down. The face is pointing toward the anterior placenta; the skull is absent from the fetal forehead to the top of the cranium. *NB,* Nasal bone.

necrosis resulting from occlusion of the internal carotid arteries.) In the first trimester, anencephaly should be diagnosed with caution. Reports have shown normal amounts of brain matter seen in the first-trimester embryo with anencephaly, unlike classic sonographic appearances in the second and third trimesters (Fig. 50.19). Ossification of the cranial vault is not complete in the first trimester; the resulting false cranial border definition may give rise to a false-negative diagnosis. Caution is advised if an embryonic cranial abnormality is suspected (Table 50.5). Because traditional cranial anatomy can be visualized after 12 to 14 weeks' gestation, the sonogram should be repeated at this time to confirm or rule out abnormality.

Acrania. The partial or complete absence of the cranium is called **acrania**. It is thought to be the predecessor of anencephaly. Ossification of the cranium begins after 9 weeks. Sonography is able to demonstrate abnormal mineralization of the bony structures: Well-mineralized bone is highly echogenic and is easily imaged with sonography. Acrania has been reported as early as the 12th week of gestation. When this abnormality occurs, the fetus has an abnormally shaped head, referred to as a "Mickey Mouse" head (Fig. 50.20).

Anencephaly. **Anencephaly** is the congenital absence of the brain and cranial vault, with the cerebral hemispheres missing or reduced to small masses. This abnormality may be seen near the end of the first trimester, when there is an

TABLE 50.5	Cranial Anomalies in the First Trimester
Anomaly	Sonographic Findings
Acrania	Abnormal mineralization of bony structures (lack of echogenicity) Abnormally shaped "Mickey Mouse" head
Anencephaly	Absence of cranium superior to orbits with preservation of base of skull and face Brain may project from open cranium
Cephalocele	Midline cranial defect Herniation of brain and meninges
Ventriculomegaly	Dilation of ventricular system without enlargement of the cranium Compression of choroid plexus Increased cerebrospinal fluid Dangling choroid in dilated lateral ventricle
Holoprosencephaly	Failure of prosencephalon to differentiate into cerebral hemispheres and lateral ventricles between fourth and eighth weeks Complete to partial failure of cleavage of prosencephalon Facial dysmorphism Remember, brain appears to be single ventricle until falx cerebri develops after 9 weeks
Dandy-Walker malformation	Sixth to seventh week of gestation Cystic dilation of fourth ventricle Dysgenesis or agenesis of cerebellar vermis and hydrocephaly Elevated tentorium

absence of the cranium superior to the orbits with preservation of the base of the skull and facial features (Fig. 50.21). The brain may be seen as it projects from the open cranial vault.

Cephalocele. A **cephalocele** is a midline cranial defect in which there is herniation of the brain and meninges (Fig. 50.22). The cephalocele may also involve the occipital, frontal, parietal, orbital, nasal, or nasopharyngeal region of the head. The prevalence of the lesion is geographic. In the Western hemisphere, the defect is primarily occipital, whereas in the Eastern hemisphere, the frontal defect is more common.

Ventriculomegaly. Ventriculomegaly, or dilation of the ventricular system without enlargement of the cranium, may be seen near the end of the first trimester, generally after 11 weeks. The normal lateral ventricle is quite prominent in the first trimester and is filled with choroid. Look for compression and thinning of the choroid plexus as increased cerebrospinal fluid accumulates in the ventricular system. The choroid plexus is shown to be "dangling" in the dilated dependent lateral ventricle (Fig. 50.23).

Holoprosencephaly. **Holoprosencephaly** is a malformation sequence that results from failure of the prosencephalon to differentiate into cerebral hemispheres and lateral ventricles between the fourth and eighth gestational weeks. The anomaly ranges from complete to partial failure of cleavage of the prosencephalon with variable degrees of facial dysmorphism. Holoprosencephaly is divided into three types: alobar, semilobar, and lobar. Alobar is the most serious and consists of a single ventricle, a small cerebrum, fused thalami, agenesis of the corpus callosum, and falx cerebri. It is important to remember that before 9 weeks, the normal fetal brain appears to have a single ventricle until the falx cerebri develops after 9 weeks (Fig. 50.24).

Dandy-Walker Malformation. This malformation results from cystic dilation of the fourth ventricle with dysgenesis or complete agenesis of the cerebellar vermis, and frequently

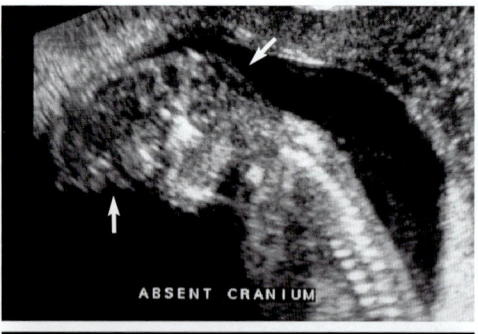
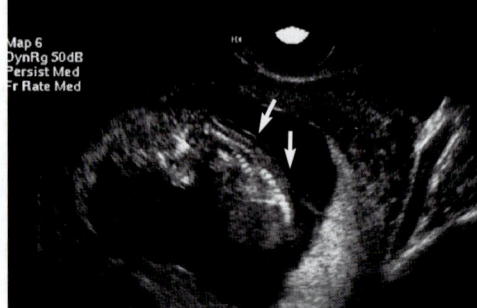

FIG. 50.20 **Acrania.** Patient presented with an elevated maternal serum alpha-fetoprotein level. Note the amnion *(arrows)* along the back of the fetus. Amniotic band syndrome was the probable cause of acrania in this fetus.

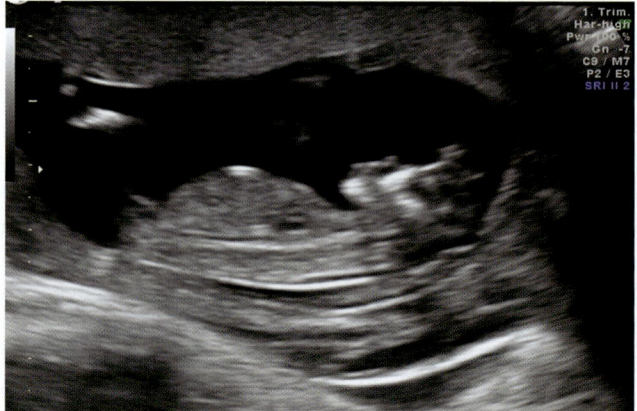

FIG. 50.21 Anencephaly is the congenital absence of the brain and cranial vault, with the cerebral hemispheres missing or reduced to small masses. This abnormality may be seen near the end of the first trimester, when there is an absence of the cranium superior to the orbits with preservation of the base of the skull and facial features.

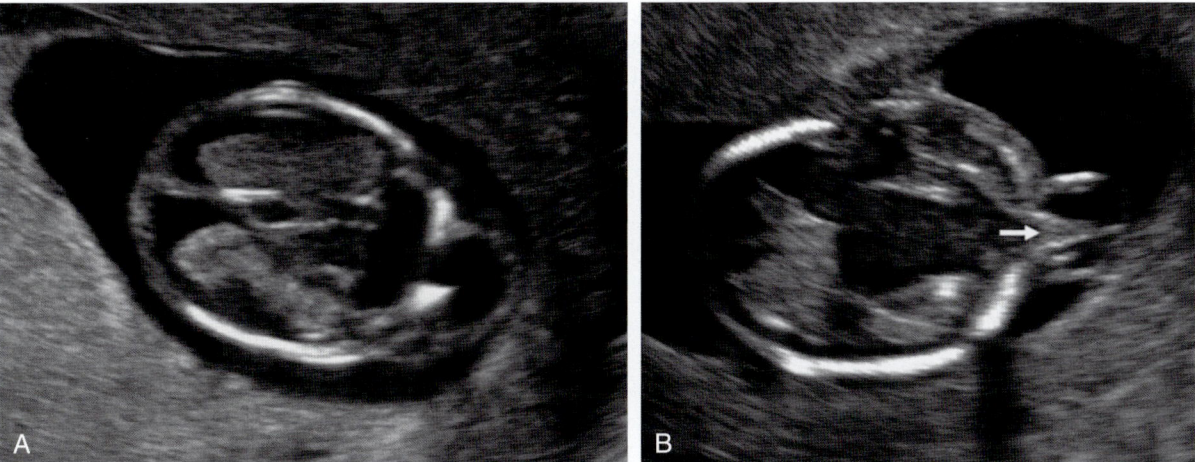

FIG. 50.22 A cephalocele is a midline cranial defect in which there is herniation of the brain and meninges. The cephalocele may also involve the occipital, frontal, parietal, orbital, nasal, or nasopharyngeal region of the head.

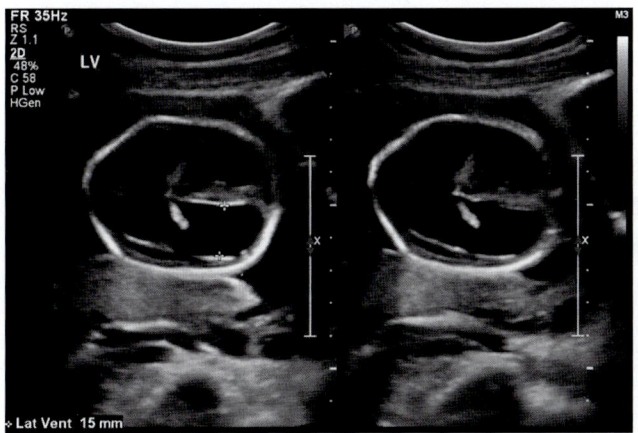

FIG. 50.23 Ventriculomegaly, or dilation of the ventricular system without enlargement of the cranium, may be seen near the end of the first trimester, generally after 11 weeks. The choroid plexus is shown to be "dangling" in the dilated dependent lateral ventricle.

hydrocephaly. The abnormality occurs around the sixth to seventh week of gestation. In the first trimester, sonographic presentation may include a large posterior fossa cyst continuous with the fourth ventricle, an absent cerebellum, and dilated third and lateral ventricles (Fig. 50.25). Dandy-Walker malformation has been reported as early as 11 weeks with transvaginal ultrasound.

Spina Bifida. Spina bifida occurs when the neural tube fails to close after 6 weeks' gestation. Improvements in ultrasound resolution have enhanced our sensitivity to detecting spina bifida, which may be detected at the end of the first trimester. Appearances may include spinal irregularities or bulging within the posterior contour of the fetal spine and extrusion of a mass from the vertebral column. Cranial signs, the lemon sign (scalloping of frontal bones), and the banana sign (curved appearance of the cerebellum) may be appreciated closer to 12 weeks (Fig. 50.26).

New evidence suggests that we may soon be able to evaluate for spina bifida by measuring the fourth ventricle during the 11- to 13.6-week scan.[8] Because the fourth ventricle is usually caudally displaced in spina bifida, the authors sought to measure the hindbrain in the midsagittal view. In normal

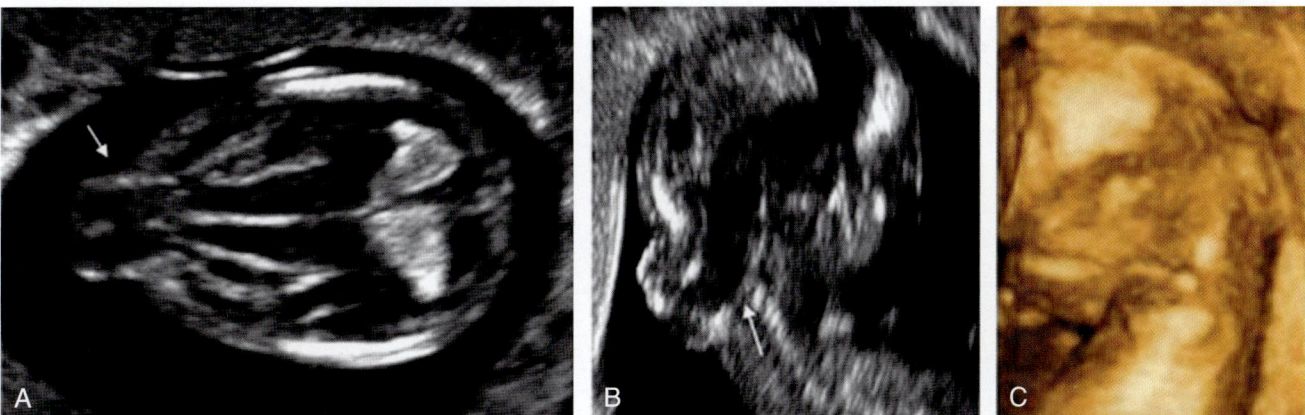

FIG. 50.24 Holoprosencephaly is a malformation sequence that results from failure of the prosencephalon to differentiate into cerebral hemispheres and lateral ventricles between the fourth and eighth gestational weeks.

fetuses, the fourth ventricle appears as an intracranial lucency that is measurable. In this study, the four affected fetuses demonstrated a compressed hindbrain and the intracranial lucency could not be measured. Larger prospective studies are needed to establish the intracranial lucency measurement as a screen for spina bifida.

Abdominal Wall Defects

Although the diagnoses of omphalocele, gastroschisis, and limb–body wall complex have been reported in the first trimester, such diagnoses should be made with care (Fig. 50.27). Abdominal wall defects must be distinguished from normal physiologic midgut herniation. As stated previously, normal **bowel herniation** appears sonographically as an echogenic mass at the base of the umbilical cord between 8 and 12 weeks. Because the liver is never normally herniated into the base of the umbilical cord, any evidence of the liver outside the anterior abdominal wall should be considered abnormal. Although the diagnosis of **gastroschisis** in the first trimester may be more difficult, reports have shown the bowel to be separate from the umbilical cord. Gastroschisis is usually visualized as an anterior wall defect, bowel containing, commonly to the right of the umbilical cord. Omphaloceles may contain abdominal organs and bowel and may protrude into the base of the umbilical cord. Bowel-only **omphaloceles** have been reported to have a high association with chromosomal abnormalities and cannot be differentiated from normal physiologic bowel migration until after 12 weeks.

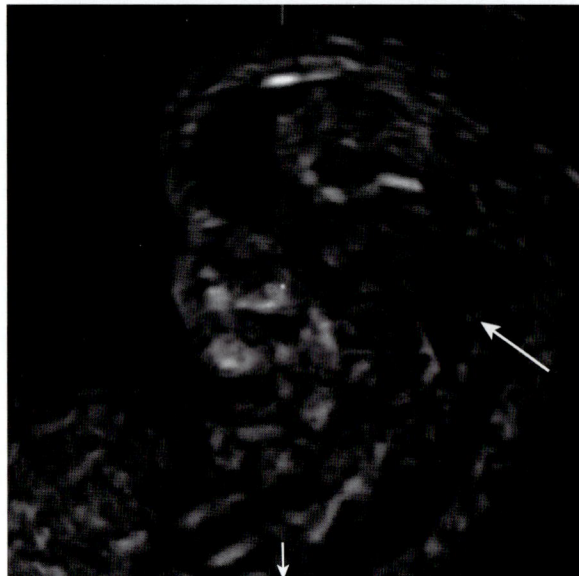

FIG. 50.25 Dandy-Walker cyst. Fetus presents at 11 weeks, 4 days with cystic dilation of the fourth ventricle and cisterna magna *(arrow)*.

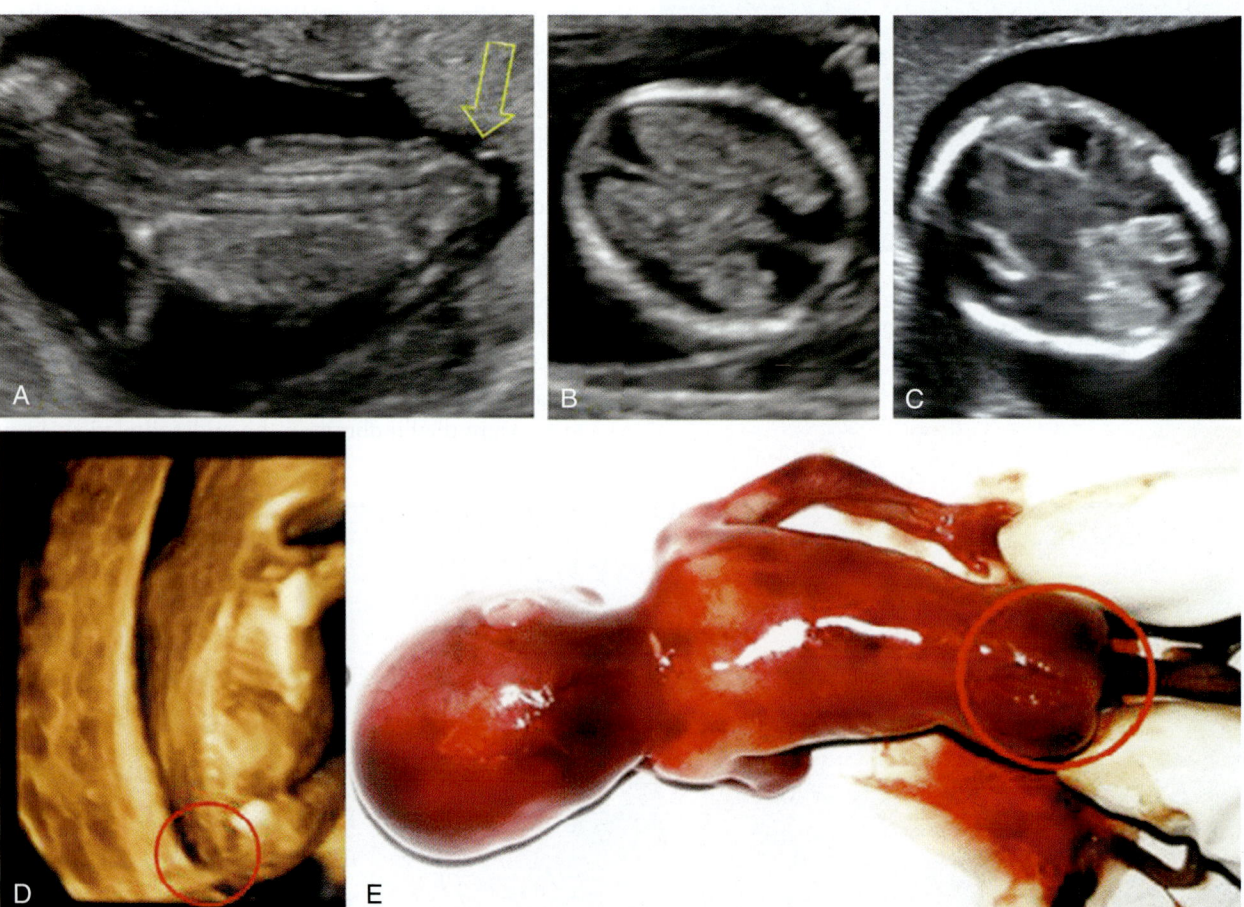

FIG. 50.26 Spina bifida occurs when the neural tube fails to close after 6 weeks' gestation. Cranial signs, the lemon sign (scalloping of frontal bones), and the banana sign (curved appearance of the cerebellum) may be appreciated closer to 12 weeks.

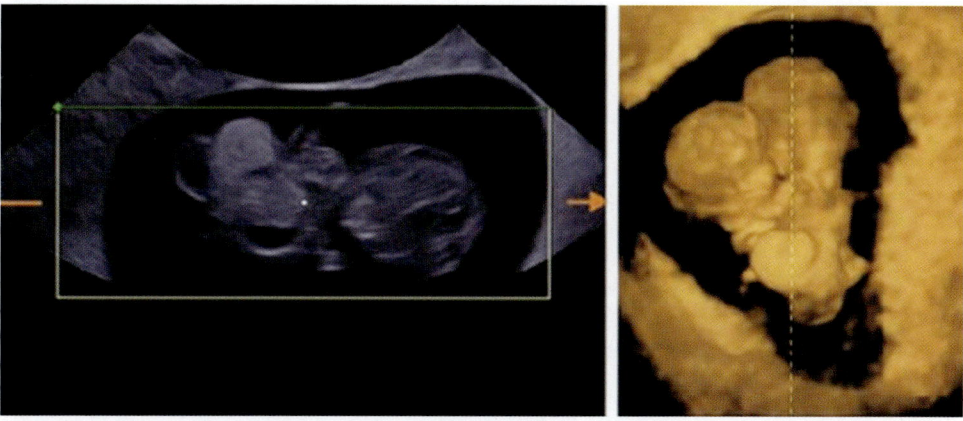

FIG. 50.27 An 11-week fetus with bowel herniation as part of the limb–body wall complex.

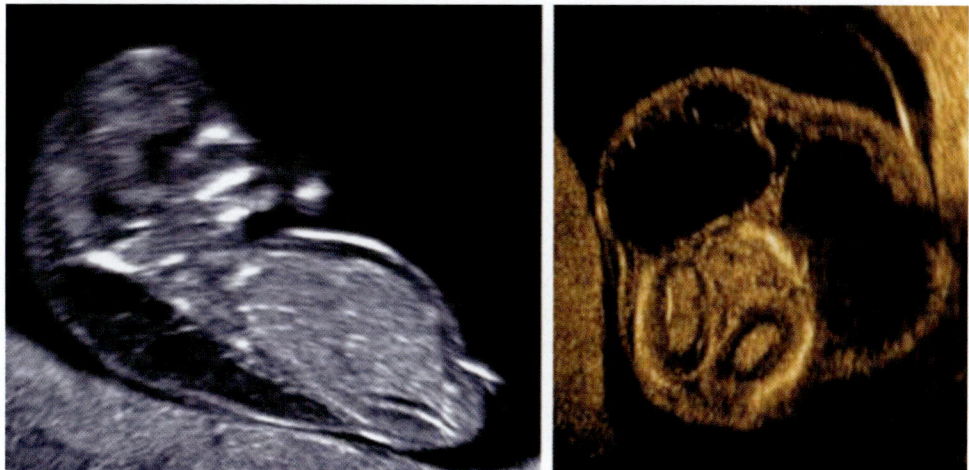

FIG. 50.28 An 11-week fetus demonstrating sonolucent cystic hygroma with nuchal thickening.

The research of Schmidt et al. suggests that measuring normal gut herniation is possible with transvaginal scanning and ought to be in the range of 6- to 9-mm circumference at 8 weeks, decreasing to 5- to 6-mm circumference at 9 weeks. Any gut herniation larger than 6 mm should be considered suspicious and should be followed for resolution after 11 weeks 5 days.[9]

Obstructive Uropathy

The fetal urinary bladder becomes sonographically apparent at 10 to 12 weeks' gestation. Obstructive uropathy, especially when it occurs at the level of the urethra, results in a very large urinary bladder and is well imaged with sonography. The bladder may be large enough to extend out of the pelvis into the fetal abdomen, presenting as a cystic mass, or it may protrude outside the body (bladder exstrophy). Other anomalies reported in the first trimester include bladder outlet obstruction, megacystis, and cloacal anomalies.

Cystic Hygroma

Cystic hygroma is one of the most common abnormalities seen sonographically in the first trimester (Fig. 50.28). Cystic hygromas seen early in fetal life have a high association with chromosomal abnormalities. The most common abnormalities are trisomies 13, 18, and 21. Newer evidence suggests that even if aneuploidy has been ruled out, these fetuses may have other genetic syndromes, deformations, and disruptions.[10] Perinatal risk increases significantly when the nuchal translucency reaches 3.5 mm or greater—the 99th percentile.

In fetuses detected with cystic hygroma in the second and third trimesters, **Turner syndrome** is the most common karyotype abnormality. If the hygroma resolves by 18 weeks and the fetus has a normal targeted ultrasound at 20 to 22 weeks without anomalies, then the perinatal risk is still unknown.

Cystic hygromas visualized in the first trimester may vary in size, but all appear on the posterior aspect of the fetal neck and upper thorax. Soft tissue thickening may also be present and should be considered nuchal thickening. Although cystic hygroma and nuchal thickening may be concordant, differentiation may be difficult. Any posterior neck thickness greater than 3 mm, with or without septations, should be followed. Differentiation between cystic hygroma, encephalocele, cervical meningomyelocele, teratoma, or hemangioma should be assessed. If cystic hygroma or nuchal thickening is seen in the

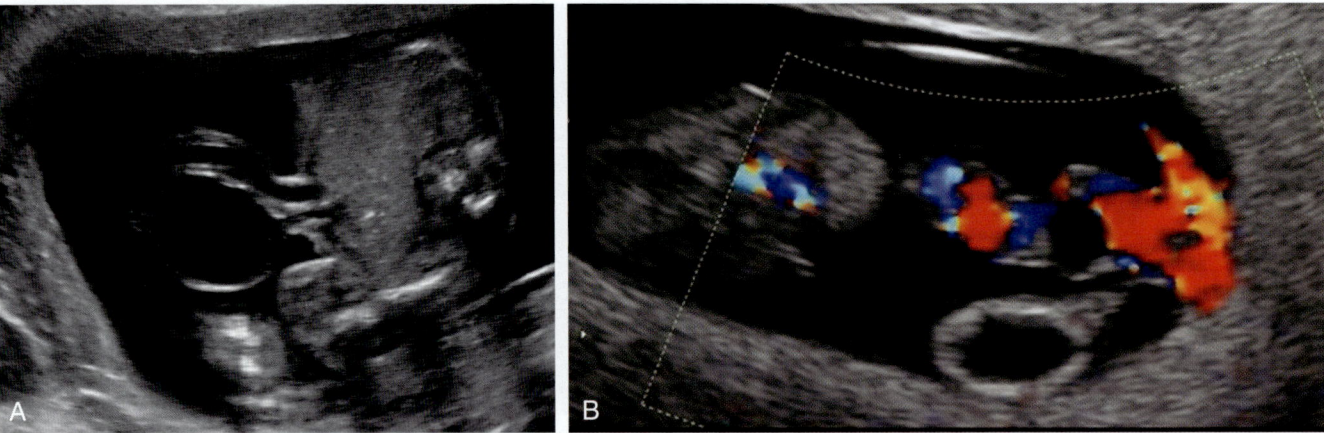

FIG. 50.29 An early gestation demonstrating an umbilical cord cyst. This cyst resolved by 14 weeks' gestation, and the patient went on to normal delivery.

first trimester, genetic counseling and further sonographic monitoring are required.

First-Trimester Umbilical Cord Cysts

Sonographic identification of first-trimester umbilical cord cysts has been reported. One study found a 0.4% incidence of umbilical cord cysts between 8 and 12 weeks' gestation.[11] Cyst size varied with a range of 2.0 to 7.5 mm, and embryos whose cysts resolved by the second trimester progressed to normal delivery. Differential considerations of umbilical cord cysts include (1) amniotic inclusion cysts, (2) omphalomesenteric duct cysts, (3) allantoic cysts, (4) vascular anomalies, (5) neoplasms, and (6) Wharton jelly abnormalities. Umbilical cord cysts that persist through the second trimester or are associated with other abnormalities warrant further investigation and genetic evaluation (Fig. 50.29).

FIRST-TRIMESTER PELVIC MASSES

Ovarian Masses

The **corpus luteum cyst** is the most common ovarian mass seen in the first trimester of pregnancy. Corpus luteum cysts secrete the progesterone necessary to preserve the embryo. The typical corpus luteum cyst measures less than 5 cm in diameter and does not contain septations. Occasionally, corpus luteum cysts are large, measuring more than 10 cm, with internal septations and echogenic debris, which are thought to be secondary to internal hemorrhage (Fig. 50.30). Because of high metabolic activity, color flow imaging may demonstrate a ring of increased vascularity surrounding the corpus luteum, displaying low-resistance (high-diastolic) waveforms on pulsed Doppler imaging. Such findings are similar to decidual flows characterized in ectopic pregnancies but are intraovarian in location (see Table 50.2).

A hemorrhagic corpus luteum cyst cannot always be differentiated from other pathologic cysts, such as ovarian cancer or dermoid (see Fig. 50.30D). As the pregnancy progresses, corpus luteum cysts regress and typically are not seen beyond 16 to 18 weeks' gestation. If ovarian cystic masses persist beyond 18 weeks' gestation or increase in size, surgical removal may be required because benign and malignant processes cannot be distinguished sonographically. A high incidence of torsion of ovarian masses during the second and third trimesters has been reported. All persistent ovarian masses in pregnancy should be followed closely.

Uterine Masses

Uterine leiomyomas, or fibroids, are common throughout pregnancy. If fibroids coexist with a first-trimester pregnancy, the fibroid should be identified in relation to the placenta and cervix. Fibroids may increase in size throughout the first trimester and early second trimester because of estrogen stimulation. A rapid increase in fibroid size may lead to necrosis of the leiomyoma, a degenerating fibroid that may cause significant pain. Myomectomy is generally avoided during pregnancy, owing to the increased vascularity of the uterus and the possibility of marked bleeding. Rapidly growing fibroids may compress the gestational sac, causing spontaneous abortion.

Sonographically, fibroids may be hypoechoic, echogenic, or isoechoic in relation to the myometrium (see Fig. 50.31). They typically cause deformity or displacement of the uterus, endometrium, or both. Fibroids are high-acoustic attenuators that give rise to poor acoustic transmission (see Fig. 50.27). It may be difficult to differentiate fibroid from focal uterine contractions, although preliminary data suggest that color Doppler imaging shows a more hypovascular appearance with uterine contractions than with fibroids. Fibroids may also be differentiated from focal myometrial contractions by observing the focal lesion over time (typically 20 to 30 minutes); the myometrial contraction should disappear, whereas a fibroid persists (see Table 50.2).

ACKNOWLEDGMENT

The author acknowledges the contributions of Candace Goldstein to this chapter in the previous edition.

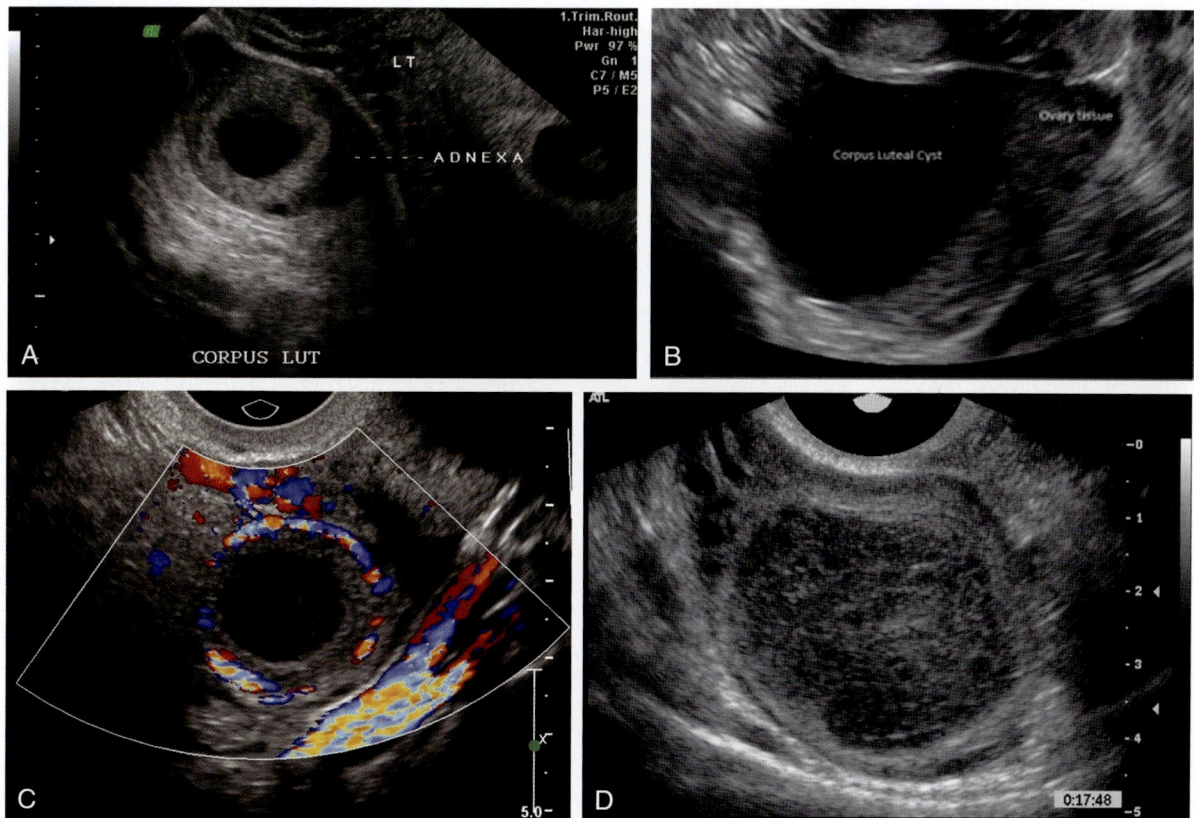

FIG. 50.30 (A–C) The typical corpus luteum cyst measures <5 cm in diameter and does not contain septations. (D) A hemorrhagic corpus luteum cyst cannot always be differentiated from other pathologic cysts, such as ovarian cancer or dermoid.

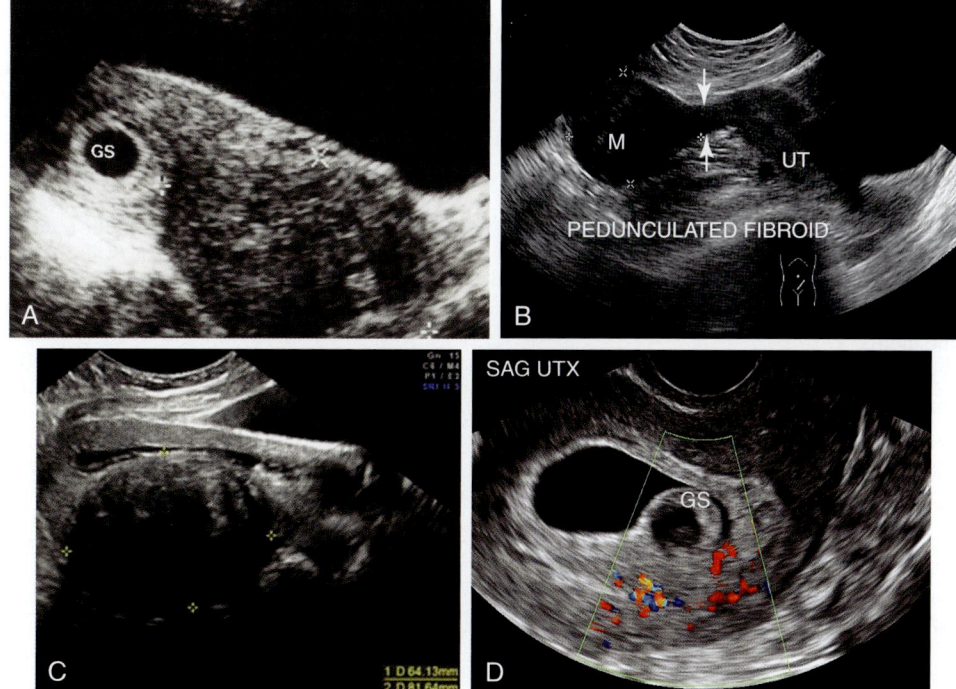

FIG. 50.31 (A) Longitudinal image of a large submucosal fibroid in the first trimester. The sonographer's role is to measure the size of the fibroid, so growth can be monitored, and define the proximity to the gestational sac. In the early stages of pregnancy, a large myoma will occupy a large portion of the uterus. As the pregnancy advances, the myoma may be displaced to the periphery as the fetus grows and distends the intrauterine environment. (B) Pedunculated fibroid. The stalk connecting the uterine corpus to the pedunculated fibroid can be well seen in early stages of pregnancy, prior to the uterine enlargement. (C) Presumably pedunculated fibroids result in less impact on the pregnancy since they do not distort the uterine body or interfere with conception. (D) Other intrauterine masses: "chorionic bump" internal hematoma.

Key Pearls

- The most common presentation for complications is vaginal spotting or frank bleeding, which occurs in nearly 25% of patients during the early stage of pregnancy.
- If bleeding is accompanied by severe pain, uterine contractions, or a dilated cervix, the pregnancy is unlikely to progress.
- *Threatened abortion* and *pregnancy of uncertain viability* are terms used for pregnancies of fewer than 20 weeks when the patient has a viable embryo, documented fetal heartbeat, and vaginal bleeding.
- *Blighted ovum, anembryonic pregnancy*, and *failed pregnancy* are terms used to describe a uterus containing a gestational sac but no visible embryo.
- Characteristics for the sonographic diagnosis of an absent intrauterine sac include an empty uterus with no evidence of an endometrial fluid collection (early gestational sac), absence of adnexal masses or free fluid, and positive beta-human chorionic gonadotropin (hCG) levels.
- Incomplete spontaneous abortion may show several sonographic findings, ranging from an intact gestational sac with a nonviable embryo to a collapsed gestational sac that is grossly misshapen.
- A gestational sac without an embryo or yolk sac on sonography may represent one of three conditions: (1) a normal early intrauterine pregnancy of less than 5 weeks, (2) an abnormal intrauterine pregnancy, or (3) a pseudogestational sac in a patient with an ectopic pregnancy.
- The anembryonic pregnancy, or blighted ovum, is a gestational sac in which the embryo fails to develop or stops developing at such an early stage that it is imperceptible by ultrasound.
- Gestational trophoblastic disease is a proliferative disease of the trophoblast that occurs after an abnormal conception.
- Absence of cardiac activity in the first trimester is the most critical sign for viability of the pregnancy.
- Chromosome abnormalities, such as triploidy, have been associated with embryonic growth restriction and embryonic oligohydramnios.
- An ectopic pregnancy is pregnancy located outside the central/fundal location of the uterus.
- As many as 20% of patients with ectopic pregnancy demonstrate an intrauterine sac-like structure known as the pseudogestational sac.
- The risk of ectopic pregnancy can be greater than 90% when an intrauterine gestation is absent and there is a corresponding adnexal mass.
- The presence of echogenic free fluid has been shown to be highly specific for hemoperitoneum and to be highly correlated with ectopic pregnancy.
- Although the embryonic head can be sonographically identified by 7 weeks, the cerebral hemisphere continues to evolve throughout the second trimester.
- The rhombencephalon-hindbrain is a cystic structure appearing in the embryonic cranium within the posterior aspect at 6 to 8 weeks that should not be confused with an abnormality.
- Ventriculomegaly, or dilation of the ventricular system without enlargement of the cranium, may be seen near the end of the first trimester, generally after 11 weeks.
- Gastroschisis is usually visualized as an anterior wall defect, bowel containing, commonly to the right of the umbilical cord. Omphaloceles may contain abdominal organs and bowel and may protrude into the base of the umbilical cord.
- Obstructive uropathy, especially when it occurs at the level of the urethra, results in a very large urinary bladder and is well imaged with sonography.
- Cystic hygromas seen early in fetal life have a high association with chromosomal abnormalities.
- A hemorrhagic corpus luteum cyst cannot always be differentiated from other pathologic cysts, such as ovarian cancer or dermoid.

REFERENCES

1. Nyberg DA, Filly RA. Predicting pregnancy failure in empty gestational sacs. *Ultrasound Obstet Gynecol*. 2003;21:9–12.
2. Fleisher AC, Pennell RG, McKee MS, et al. Ectopic pregnancy: features at transvaginal sonography. *Radiology*. 1990;174:375–378.
3. Kurjak A, Zalud I, Schulman H. Ectopic pregnancy: transvaginal color Doppler of trophoblastic flow in questionable adnexa. *J Ultrasound Med*. 1991;10:685–689.
4. Thorsen MK, Lawson TL, Aiman EJ, et al. Diagnosis of ectopic pregnancy: endovaginal vs. transabdominal sonography. *AJR Am J Roentgenol*. 1990;155:307–310.
5. Nyberg DA, Hughes MP, Mack LA, Wang KY. Extrauterine findings of ectopic pregnancy at transvaginal US: importance of echogenic fluid. *Radiology*. 1991;178:823–826.
6. Parvey HR, Maklad W. Pitfalls in the transvaginal sonographic diagnosis of ectopic pregnancy. *J Ultrasound Med*. 1993;3:139–144.
7. Russell SA, Illy RA, Damato N. Sonographic diagnosis of ectopic pregnancy with endovaginal probes: what really has changed? *J Ultrasound Med*. 1993;3:145–151.
8. Chaoui R, Benoit B, Mitkowska-Wozniak H, et al. Assessment of intracranial translucency (IT) in the detection of spina bifida at the 11-13 week scan. *Ultrasound Obstet Gynecol*. 2009;34:249–252.
9. Schmidt W, Yarkoni S, Crelin ES, et al. Sonographic visualization of physiologic anterior abdominal wall hernia in the first trimester. *Obstet Gynecol*. 1987;69:911–915.
10. Souka AP, von Kaisenberg CS, Hyett JA, et al. Increased nuchal translucency with normal karyotype. *Am J Obstet Gynecol*. 2005;192:1005–1021.
11. Skibo LK, Lyons EA, Levi CS. First trimester umbilical cord cyst. *Radiology*. 1992;182:719–722.

CHAPTER 51

Sonography of the Second and Third Trimesters

Christina Taff

OBJECTIVES

On completion of this chapter, you should be able to:
- List the components of a standard obstetric examination in the second and third trimesters, recognize and describe the fetal anatomy recommended for review
- Define terminology specific to fetal presentation and fetal situs
- Specify equipment and policies required for facilities performing obstetric sonography
- Describe sonographic techniques used to image specific fetal structures
- Describe normal fetal anatomy visualized in an obstetric sonography examination and variations that may be significant

OUTLINE

A Suggested Protocol 1344
Equipment and Practices 1344
Initial Steps and Examination Overview 1344
    Fetal Presentation 1345
Fetal Anatomy of the Second and Third Trimesters 1348
    The Cranium 1348
    The Face 1352
    The Vertebral Column 1355

The Thorax 1357
The Heart 1359
The Diaphragm and Thoracic Vessels 1360
Fetal Circulation 1362
The Hepatobiliary System and Upper Abdomen 1363
The Gastrointestinal System 1365
The Urinary System 1366
The Genitalia 1368

The Upper and Lower Extremities 1369
Extrafetal Obstetric Evaluation 1371
    The Umbilical Cord 1372
    The Placenta 1373
    The Amniotic Fluid 1374
    The Membranes 1374
    The Cervix 1375
Genetic Sonogram 1375

KEY TERMS

Breech
Corpus callosum
Frontal bossing
Genetic sonogram

Likelihood ratio
Micrognathia
Midline falx
Nomogram

Normal situs
Transverse fetal lie
Trimester
Vertex

The second and third **trimesters** are the ideal time to obtain sonographic images of detailed fetal anatomy. Fetal anatomy may be accurately assessed after 18 weeks of gestation, although structures may be seen earlier in many pregnancies. Technical factors, such as fetal movement, fluid quantity, fetal position, and maternal wall thickness or obesity, may obscure the anatomy and result in less than optimal images throughout pregnancy.

To perform a complete evaluation of the fetus during the second and third trimesters, the sonographer should follow a specific protocol that includes, at a minimum, the components recommended for a standard examination. The practice parameter guidelines for obstetric scanning as outlined by the American Institute of Ultrasound in Medicine (AIUM), the American College of Radiology (ACR), and the American College of Obstetricians and Gynecologists (ACOG) were utilized to create the suggested scanning protocol in this chapter.

This chapter focuses on the fetal anatomy that the sonographer needs to recognize and analyze within a systematic scanning protocol. A sonographer will screen many normal fetuses when performing standard antepartum obstetric examinations during the second or third trimester of pregnancy. A systematic protocol will ensure a comprehensive review of fetal anatomy in each patient. Thoroughness and experience applied to the recommended components and to additional details, such as facial features, open hands, and fetal situs, will maximize the opportunity to detect fetal anomalies.

A SUGGESTED PROTOCOL

The protocol for second- and third-trimester sonography examinations includes a biometric and anatomic survey of the fetus (see Box 51.1). The second- and third-trimester sonography examination often includes the following:

1. Observation of fetal viability by visualization of cardiac motion.
2. Demonstration of presentation (fetal lie).
3. Demonstration of the number of fetuses. In multiple gestations, anatomy images are obtained on each fetus, growth parameters of each fetus are obtained and compared, placenta and membrane structures are assessed, and amniotic fluid levels in each sac are documented.
4. Characterization of the quantity of amniotic fluid as normal or abnormal by subjective visualization or by semiquantitative estimates.
5. Characterization of the placenta, including localization and relationship to the internal cervical os. Placenta previa should be excluded by examination of the lower uterine segment.
6. Visualization of the cervix. Transvaginal or transperineal imaging may be necessary to document cervical length if there are risk factors for spontaneous preterm birth, when the cervix appears shortened, or if there is a history of uterine contractions. Transvaginal cervical length measurements may be used for screening in low-risk pregnancy.
7. Assessment of fetal age through fetal biometry. Fetal growth studies may include a serial growth analysis when serial examinations are performed at intervals that are 2 to 4 weeks apart. Typically, the following fetal measurements are included, and gestational age correlation from each measure is averaged to assess fetal age by sonography:
   - Biparietal diameter
   - Head circumference
   - Femur length
   - Humerus length
   - Abdominal circumference
8. Evaluation of uterus, adnexa, and cervix to exclude masses that may complicate obstetric management. Maternal ovaries may not be visualized during the second and third trimesters of pregnancy.
9. Anatomic survey of the fetus to exclude major congenital malformations. At a minimum, the anatomy specified in Box 51.1 must be visualized. Specialty or repeat studies may be appropriate if anatomy is not well visualized. Technical difficulty in visualizing anatomy should be recorded and images preserved to document visualization of all required components.

The sonographer should establish a systematic scanning protocol encompassing elements of the protocol outlined previously, all criteria of the guidelines, and any additional views requested in the practice environment. A referral for a detailed fetal anatomy examination may be necessary when a fetal anomaly is suspected. An organized approach to scanning ensures completeness and reduces the risk of missing a fetal defect.

EQUIPMENT AND PRACTICES

The second- and third-trimester standard sonography examination requires current two-dimensional real-time sonography equipment with transabdominal and transvaginal capability. Doppler capabilities facilitate evaluation of amniotic fluid volume, the umbilical cord, and specialty evaluations of the fetal heart and other aspects of fetal and maternal circulation. Three-dimensional equipment can record the volume of a targeted anatomic region and represents an advance in imaging technology. The technical advantage of three-dimensional imaging is that it can acquire, manipulate, and display a number of two-dimensional planes within a volume that may not be accessible with traditional real-time imaging. Three-dimensional equipment is currently an adjunct to traditional scanning. Until clinical evidence shows a clear medical advantage, three-dimensional sonography is not considered required equipment.

Practice parameters related to patient education and communication during an examination, competency requirements for sonographers and interpreting physicians, equipment use, scheduling, documentation of results, and image storage specific to obstetric patients must be developed at every facility. Practices that receive ultrasound accreditation from the ACR or the AIUM show improved compliance with published national standards and guidelines. Accreditation is available for fetal echocardiography and for the detailed anatomic examination, as well as for a standard obstetric ultrasound practice.

INITIAL STEPS AND EXAMINATION OVERVIEW

Recognizing normal fetal anatomy is essential to the performance of obstetric sonography. The task of capturing images of standard anatomic planes and organs in a small and mobile fetus poses a considerable challenge for the sonographer. The "eye" and experience required to recognize abnormal structures develop over time.

A key to developing scanning expertise is to become organized and systematic in assessing the fetus, placenta, and amniotic fluid.

BOX 51.1 Second- and Third-Trimester Protocol

- Survey uterus and determine fetal number.
- Observe fetal cardiac activity.
- Determine fetal position(s) and placental location(s).
- Check cervix and lower uterine segment.
- Survey for uterine or adnexal masses.
- Assess amniotic fluid.
- Perform anatomy survey of each fetus.
- Perform biometric measurements of each fetus.

The sonographer should initially determine the position of the fetus in relation to the position of the mother. In determining fetal position and in surveying the uterine contents, the sonographer can systematically move the transducer superior toward the uterine fundus, maintaining a midline path. By angling the probe from side to side, fetal position, cardiac activity, the number of fetuses, the presence of uterine and placental masses, and any obvious fetal anomalies may be recognized and amniotic fluid assessed.

It is important to remember to view cardiac activity at the beginning of each study to ensure that the fetus is alive. If a fetal demise or an obvious anomaly is initially recognized, the sonographer is better prepared to perform the study and involve the physician immediately.

After fetal position is conceptualized, the sonographer determines the left and right sides of the fetus. Being continuously aware of the right and left sides of the fetus is necessary to correctly assess fetal anatomy and situs. Assessment and measurement of the fetus may proceed systematically by moving from fetal head to feet, obtaining anatomy images and measurement at each level. The obstetric sonographer also needs to be prepared to vary this systematic examination and "catch as catch can" when pertinent anatomy presents during fetal movements. The placenta, amniotic fluid, uterus, and adnexa are also examined.

Fetal Presentation

Fetal position may change as a result of fetal movement until actual labor commences. However, fetal position changes less frequently after 34 weeks. Visualizing nonvertex fetal positions after 34 weeks may be predictive of positional difficulties during labor and delivery. An atypical fetal presentation, such as face, brow, or shoulder presentation, will complicate delivery. Similarly, hyperextension of the fetal head may alter obstetric management.

The fetal lie is described in relation to the maternal long axis. Fetuses generally assume a longitudinal, transverse, or oblique lie within the uterus (Fig. 51.1). If the fetus is lying perpendicular to the long axis of the mother, this is described as a **transverse fetal lie**. When the fetus lie is transverse, the sonographer typically reports the position of the fetal head (maternal right or left) and the position of the fetal spine (inferior, superior, anterior, or posterior) (Fig. 51.2). When the fetal lie is oblique, it is generally described by stating which quadrant of the uterus contains the fetal head and the direction and position of the fetal spine. If the fetus is lying longitudinal or parallel to the maternal long axis, this is described as a **vertex** (head down) presentation or **breech** (head up) presentation (Fig. 51.3).

Vertex. A simple method to determine fetal presentation consists of a midline sagittal scan in the lower uterine segment. Immediately cephalad to the symphysis pubis, the

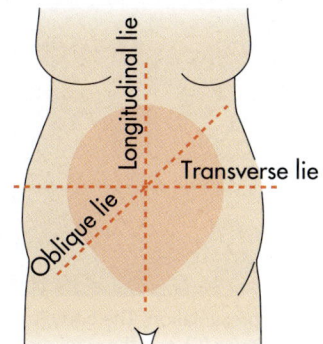

FIG. 51.1 Vectors demonstrating the three major possible axes that a fetus may occupy. Fetal lie does not necessarily indicate whether the vertex or the breech is closest to the cervix.

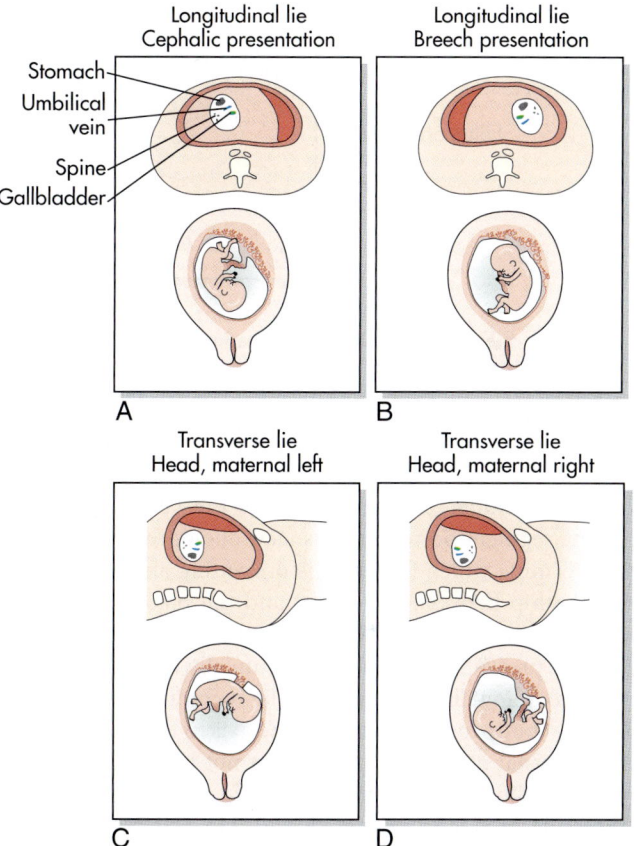

FIG. 51.2 Knowledge of the plane of section across the maternal abdomen (longitudinal or transverse) and the position of the fetal spine and left-side (stomach) and right-side (gallbladder) structures can be used to determine fetal lie and presenting part. (A) This transverse scan of the gravid uterus demonstrates the fetal spine on the maternal right, with the fetus lying with its right side down (stomach anterior, gallbladder posterior). Because these images are viewed looking up from the patient's feet, the fetus must be in longitudinal lie and cephalic presentation. (B) When the gravid uterus is scanned transversely, and the fetal spine is on the maternal left with the right side down, the fetus is in a longitudinal lie and breech presentation. (C) When a longitudinal plane of section demonstrates the fetal body to be transected transversely, and the fetal spine is nearest the uterine fundus with the fetal left side down, the fetus is in a transverse lie with the fetal head on the maternal left. (D) When a longitudinal plane of section demonstrates the fetal body to be transected transversely, and the fetal spine is nearest the lower uterine segment with the fetal left side down, the fetus is in a transverse lie with the fetal head on the maternal right. Although real-time scanning of the gravid uterus quickly allows the observer to determine fetal lie and presenting part, this maneuver of identifying specific right- and left-side structures within the fetal body force one to determine fetal position accurately and to identify normal and pathologic fetal anatomy.

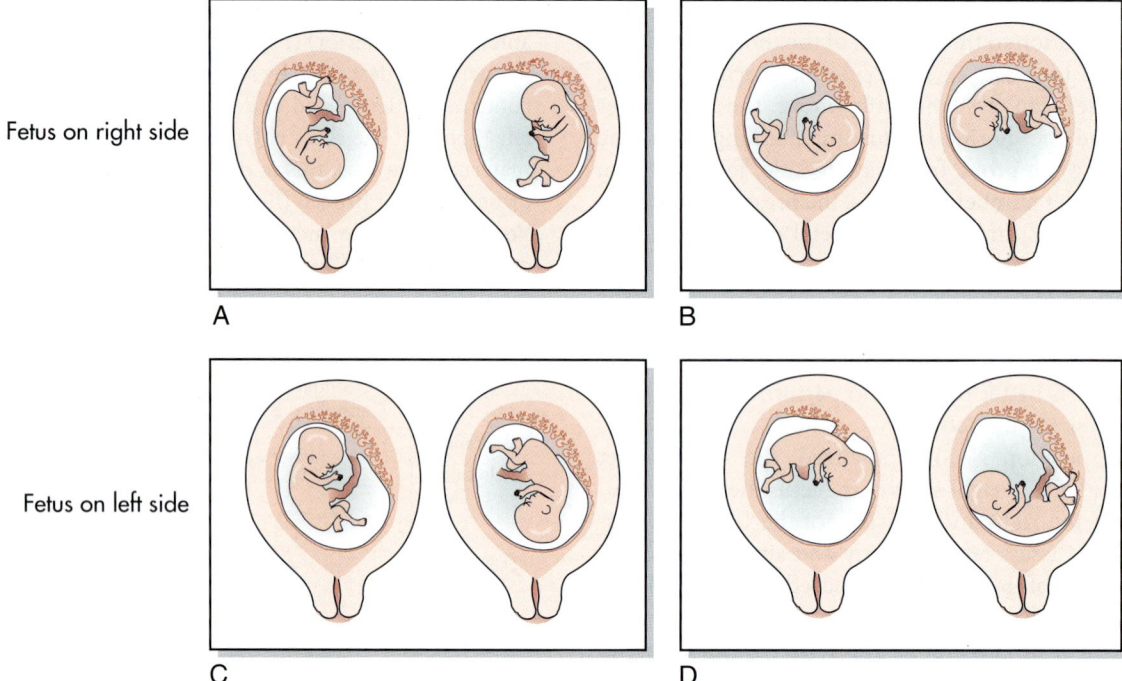

FIG. 51.3 Fetal positions and the method used to differentiate the left side from the right side. (A) Fetus lying on the right side; whether the head is up or down, the left side of the fetus is up or closer to the transducer. (B) Fetus lying on right side in a transverse lie; left side is closer to the transducer. (C) Fetus lying on the left side; whether the head is up or down, the right side is up or closer to the transducer. (D) Fetus lying on left side in a transverse lie; the right side is closer to the transducer.

maternal bladder is visualized with the cervix and lower uterine segment posterior. This view allows the sonographer to determine which fetal part is presenting and to check the relationship between the cervix and the placenta. The fetal head is visualized at this level when the fetus is in a vertex or cephalic presentation. Proceeding fundally, if the fetal body is noted to follow the head, a vertex lie is confirmed (Fig. 51.4). The fetal body may lie in an oblique axis to the right or left of the maternal midline. If the body is not initially recognized in the midline, the sonographer should direct the transducer from side to side to search for the abdomen. Identification of the vertebral column when entering the cranium further delineates the fetal lie. The position of a fetus in vertex position may be described by stating the relationship of the fetal occiput (back of the head) to the maternal pelvis. If the occiput is adjacent to the left anterior portion of the maternal pelvis, the fetal position is left occiput anterior. If the occiput is adjacent to the left lateral portion of the maternal pelvis, this is called left occiput transverse. Similarly, fetuses may be described as left occiput posterior, occiput posterior (OP), right occiput posterior, right occiput transverse, right occiput anterior, or occiput anterior. Fetuses that are occiput anterior (looking straight down) or OP (looking straight up) may present technical difficulties in measuring the fetal head and abdomen and in visualizing fetal cranial anatomy.

Breech. When the lower extremities or buttocks are found to be in the lower uterine segment, and the head is visualized in the uterine fundus, a breech presentation is suspected (Fig. 51.5). In fetuses near term, determination of the specific type of breech lie provides important clinical information for the obstetrician

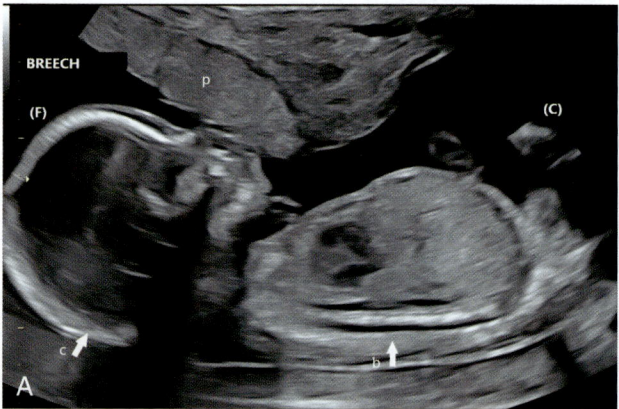

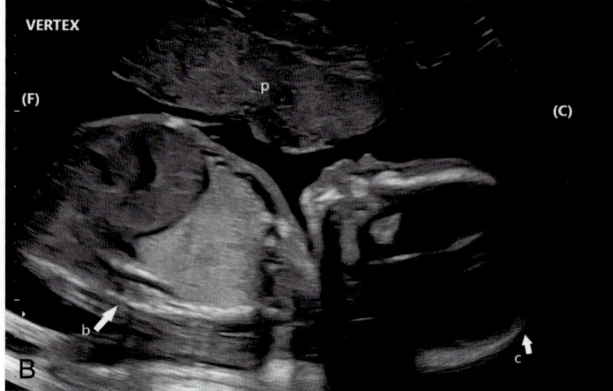

FIG. 51.4 (A) A breech presentation. The body (b) is closest in proximity to the direction of the cervix (C), and the cranium (c) is directed toward the uterine fundus (F). (B) A vertex presentation. The cranium (c) is closest in proximity to the direction of the cervix (C), and the body (b) is directed toward the uterine fundus (F). *p*, Placenta.

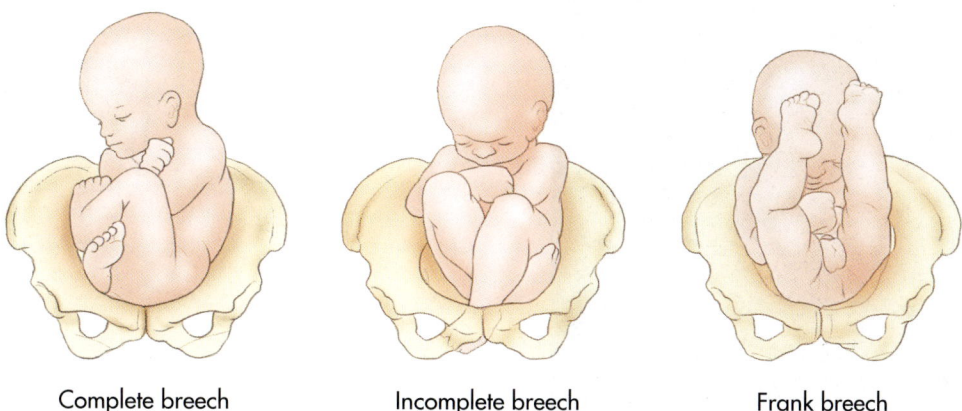

Complete breech   Incomplete breech   Frank breech

FIG. 51.5 **Three possible breech presentations.** The complete breech demonstrates flexion of the hips and knees. The incomplete breech demonstrates intermediate deflexion of one hip and knee (single or double footling). The frank breech shows flexion of the hips and extension of both knees.

planning the safest route of delivery. Some fetuses in a breech position, such as those in a frank breech position with the thighs flexed at the hips and the lower legs extended in front of the body and up in front of the head (Fig. 51.6), may be safely turned, allowing vaginal delivery. Fetuses in other breech lies, such as complete breech (when both the hips and the lower extremities are found in the lower pelvis), need to be delivered by cesarean section. A footling breech is found when the hips are extended and one (single footling) or both feet (double footling) are the presenting parts closest to the cervix. The position of a fetus in breech position may be described by stating the relationship of the fetal sacrum (lower spine) to the maternal pelvis. If the sacrum is adjacent to the left anterior portion of the maternal pelvis, the fetal position is left sacrum anterior. If the sacrum is adjacent to the left lateral portion of the maternal pelvis, this is called left sacrum transverse. Similarly, fetuses may be described as left sacrum posterior, sacrum posterior (SP), right sacrum posterior, right sacrum transverse, right sacrum anterior, or sacrum anterior. When a fetus is in breech presentation, the shape of the head may appear elongated or dolichocephalic, especially in the third trimester.

Transverse. When a transverse cross section of the fetal head or body is noted in the sagittal plane, a transverse lie is suspected (Fig. 51.7). By rotating the transducer perpendicular to the maternal axis, the long axis of the fetus may be observed. When a fetus remains in transverse lie late in pregnancy, it is important to screen for a mass or placenta previa in the lower uterine segment that is preventing the fetus from moving into a vertex or breech position.

Situs. In addition to determining fetal lie, the right and left sides of the fetus need to be conceptualized to ensure **normal situs** (positioning) of fetal organs. Some sonographers memorize this relationship. For example, if the fetus is in a vertex presentation with the fetal spine toward the maternal right side, the right side of the fetus is down, and the left side is up. However, it is more helpful to practice maintaining a mental picture of the fetal body and position throughout the examination, which allows recognition of the fetal right and left sides.

A sonographer may also differentiate the right from left side by identifying anatomic landmarks after an initial

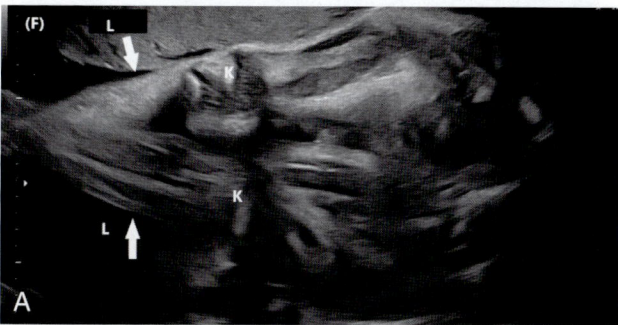

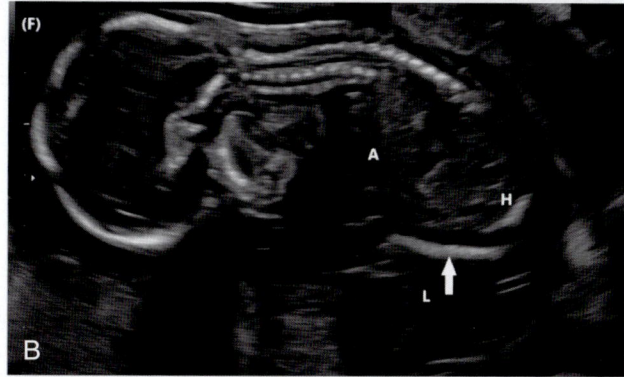

FIG. 51.6 (A) A fetus in a frank breech presentation with both legs extended upward toward the uterine fundus (F). (B) Complete breech presentation with one leg flexed at the hips, with the lower leg (L) and foot positioned under the hips (H). The other leg was in a similar position. *A*, Abdomen; *F*, fundus; *K*, knee; *L*, lower leg.

orientation is verified. For example, if the sonographer initially verifies that the fetal stomach lies on the fetal left side, later in the examination, the fetal right and left may be determined in relation to the stomach. The gallbladder on the right side and the apex of the heart pointing toward the fetal left side may be verified by their relationship to the stomach. The fetal aorta lies slightly to the left of midline, anterior to the spine, and the inferior vena cava is to the right of midline and slightly more anterior to the aorta.

Effective obstetric scanning is founded on the operator's ability to visualize fetal position.

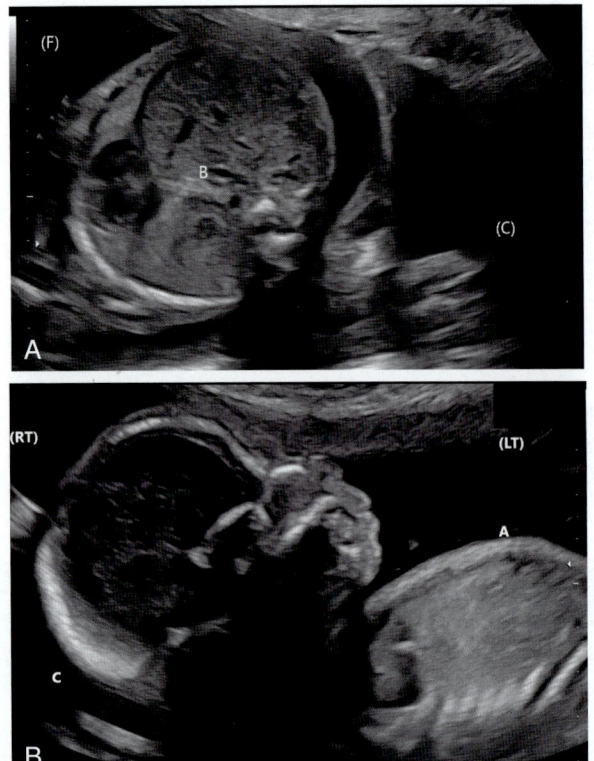
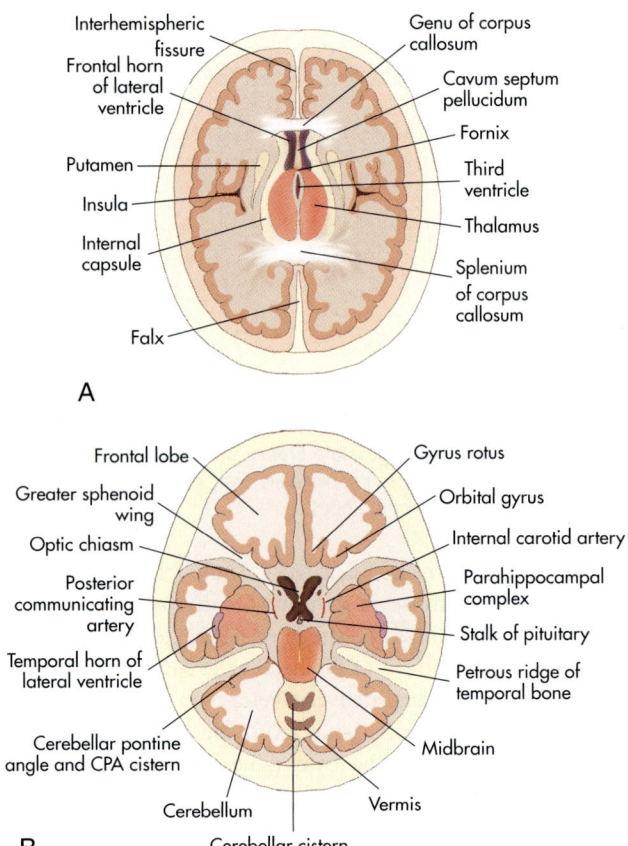

FIG. 51.7 (A) A sagittal scan at the level of the lower uterine segment reveals the fetal body in a transverse position rather than a sagittal or coronal orientation (compare with Fig. 51.4). (B) In the same fetus, by rotating the transducer 90 degrees, the abdomen may be connected to the head to reveal the transverse lie with the head oriented to the maternal right side (RT) and the abdomen (A) to the maternal left side (LT). *B*, Body; *C*, toward cervix; *F*, fundus.

FIG. 51.8 (A) Transverse view of the fetal intracranial anatomy taken at the midsection of the fetal head. (B) Transverse view inferior to part A taken at the level of the cerebellum and vermis.

FETAL ANATOMY OF THE SECOND AND THIRD TRIMESTERS

The Cranium

The sonographer must be adept at recognizing the normal appearances and developmental changes of the fetal brain throughout pregnancy. It is imperative to identify neuroanatomy at specific levels where measurements are obtained, such as a biparietal diameter or posterior fossa, and to screen for malformations in brain development.

By the 12th week of gestation, the cranial bones ossify. It is important to survey the fetal head to check the contour or outline of the skull bones by sweeping the transducer through the cranium from the highest level (roof) in the brain to the skull base. The cranium appears as a circle at the highest levels and as an oval at the ventricular, peduncular, and basal levels. Extracranial masses (e.g., cephaloceles), central nervous system anomalies, skeletal pathology, or fetal death may distort the normal shape of the skull.

Transverse scanning planes are required to evaluate brain anatomy and perform cranial measurements (Fig. 51.8). The transducer is aligned in a longitudinal or sagittal position over the fetus and then is specifically positioned over the fetal head. Rotation of the transducer perpendicular to the sagittal plane generates transverse sections of the brain. Brain anatomy and measurements are assessed in serial transverse planes. A longitudinal or oblique view of the fetal brain may also be used to locate and assess normal anatomy.

Normal fetal brain parenchyma appears hypoechoic because of the small size reflectors and high water content in the tissue. The sulcus and gyrus are more echogenic. The gyral/sulcal pattern of the brain becomes more complex and more prominent as gestational age increases. Branches of the anterior cerebral artery run within the midline sulci and may be seen to pulsate within the echogenic structures.

As pregnancy progresses, brain anatomy may be more difficult to visualize because of increasing calcification of the skull and the position of the fetal head deeper in the pelvis. The calcification of the skull may cause reverberation artifacts in the proximal (near-field) cranial hemisphere that preclude evaluation. Fortunately, most brain anomalies are symmetrical processes, and documentation of the brain may be based on the anatomy seen in the distal hemisphere. In most cases, if there is a defect, it is present bilaterally, even though the anatomy may not be adequately discerned. When a brain anomaly is suspected, and the fetus is in a vertex presentation, use of a transvaginal probe or transperineal scanning may allow better visualization of the skull and brain. Magnetic resonance imaging may also be used to evaluate fetal brain anatomy.

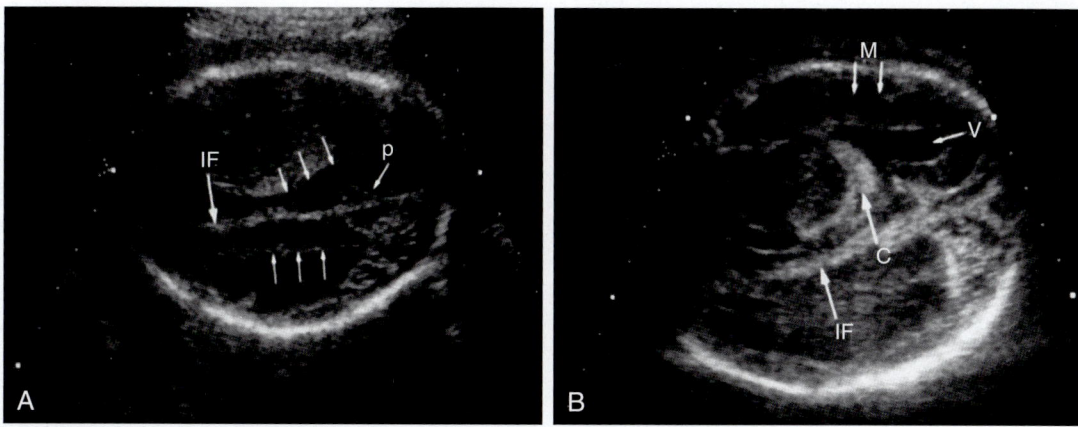

FIG. 51.9 (A) Transverse cross section revealing white-matter tracts *(arrows)* coursing parallel to the interhemispheric fissure (IF) at 26 weeks of gestation. (B) The choroid plexus (C) is located in the proximal or near hemisphere within the ventricular cavity (V). Note the homogeneous appearance of the brain tissue. *M,* Mantle; *P,* peduncles.

Standard obstetric examination guidelines require the sonographer to image and record the cerebellum, the choroid plexus, the cisterna magna, the lateral cerebral ventricles, the midline falx, and the cavum septum pellucidi. It is also suggested that measurement of the nuchal fold may be helpful during a specific age interval to suggest increased risk of aneuploidy. These specific portions of anatomy are described in the following paragraphs in a systematic review of brain structures seen when moving in transverse planes from the roof to the base of the skull.

In a transverse plane, at the most superior level within the skull (Fig. 51.9), the contour of the skull should be round or oval and should have a smooth surface. At this level, the interhemispheric fissure, **midline echo (falx)**, or falx cerebri, is observed as a membrane separating the brain into two equal hemispheres. The midline falx is an important landmark to visualize because its presence implies that separation of the cerebrum has occurred. Lateral and parallel to the midline falx in the superior plane, two linear echoes representing deep venous structures (white matter tracts) are viewed (see Fig. 51.9). It is important to recognize that these white-matter tracts are positioned above the level of the lateral ventricles.

The fetal ventricular system consists of two paired lateral ventricles, a midline third ventricle, and a fourth ventricle adjacent to the cerebellum. The ventricular system contains cerebrospinal fluid (CSF), which coats the brain and spinal cord. Choroid plexus tissue within the lateral ventricles produces the CSF. Choroid plexus tissue is located within the roof of each ventricle, except at the frontal ventricular horns. This spongelike material is echogenic and is very prominent in early pregnancy. Occasionally, small cysts—which are engorged, spongelike cavities—may be seen in normal pregnancy. It is thought that CSF may become trapped during development within the neuroepithelial folds, resulting in the formation of choroid plexus cysts. This commonly represents a normal fetal development, but these cysts are also associated with trisomy 18. As the cerebral hemispheres grow, the ventricular system and the choroid plexus appear to occupy a much smaller portion of the cranium.

From the lateral ventricles, the fluid travels to the third ventricle through the foramen of Monro. From the third ventricle, the fluid travels through the aqueduct of Sylvius to the fourth ventricle. When the fluid reaches the fourth ventricle, it flows into the cerebral and spinal subarachnoid spaces from the interventricular foramina and the foramen of Luschka. CSF then spreads through the cisterns and surrounds the hemispheres along the subarachnoid spaces. After reaching the arachnoid granulations, it is reabsorbed and enters the venous system (e.g., cranial venous sinuses).

The fetal ventricles are important to assess because ventriculomegaly or hydrocephalus (dilated ventricular system) may be a sign of central nervous system abnormalities. Mild ventriculomegaly may also be associated with congenital anomalies. Aqueductal stenosis at the level of the aqueduct of Sylvius is the most common type of fetal hydrocephaly and will result in excess fluid in the lateral and third ventricles. Dilation of the entire system, including the fourth ventricle, is associated with spinal defects.

The lateral ventricles are viewed at a level just below the white-matter tracts (Fig. 51.10). The lumina of the ventricles may be recognized by the bright reflection of their borders and the presence of hyperechoic choroid plexus tissue that fills the cavity of the ventricles early in gestation. The lateral borders of the ventricular chambers are represented as echogenic lines coursing parallel to the midline falx. The lateral ventricle is more easily imaged in the distal hemisphere because of reverberation artifacts in the near field. The ventricular cavity is seen sonographically as a cystic space filled with choroid plexus (Figs. 51.11 and 51.12).

The inferior portion of the lateral ventricles connects with the temporal (inferior) and posterior horns. This portion of the ventricle is called the *atrium of the lateral ventricles.* The choroid plexus is tear shaped. The most inferior portion of the choroid plexus body or glomus marks the site of the atrium. The glomus or body of the choroid plexus will fill the lateral ventricle in a normal pregnancy. If the glomus appears to float or dangle within the cavity, this is a sign of abnormally enlarged or dilated ventricles (ventriculomegaly). Measurements of the atrium portion of the ventricle are clinically practical because the size of this portion remains the same throughout gestation.

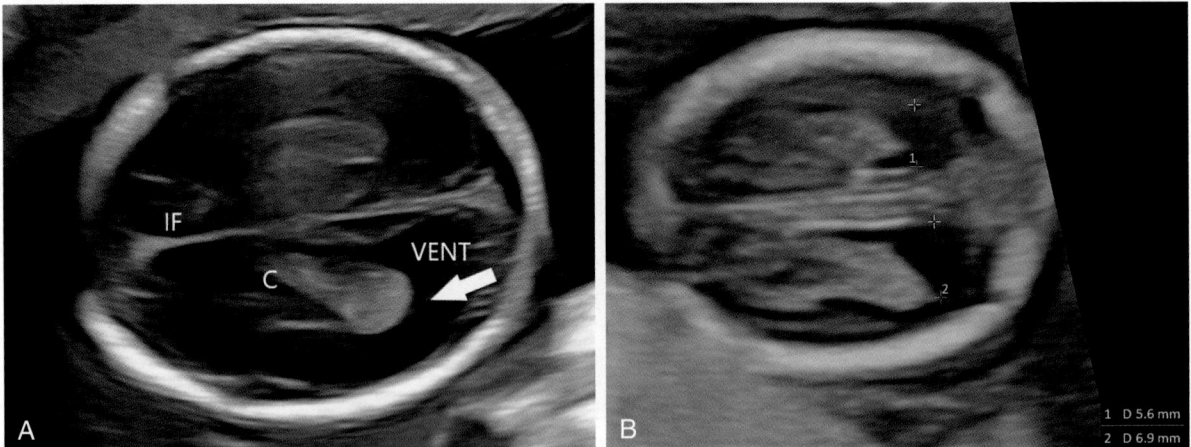

FIG. 51.10 (A) Transverse view demonstrating ventricular atrial diameter representing a normal-size ventricle (Vent). (B) Measurements of the atria of the lateral ventricle diameters that correspond to normal-size ventricles. *C,* Choroid plexus; *IF,* interhemispheric fissure.

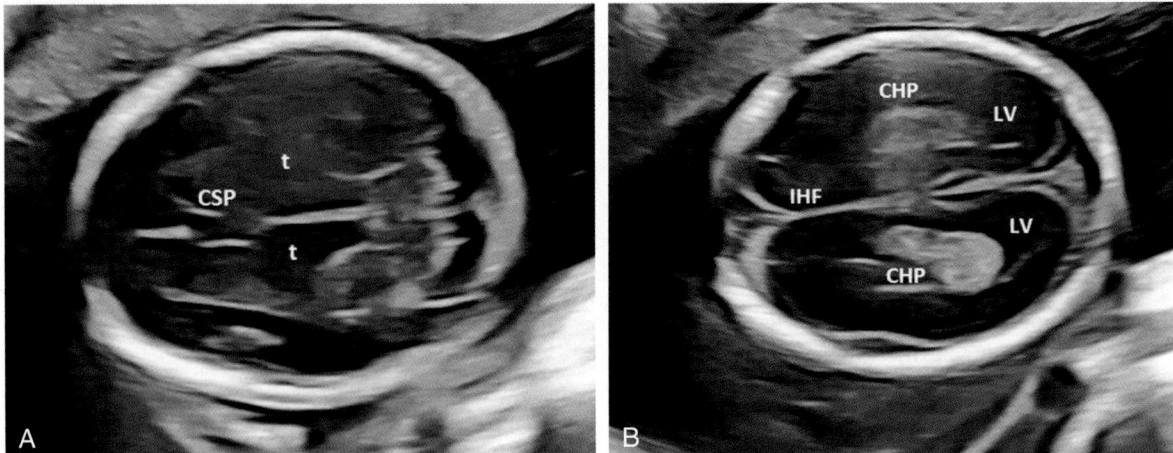

FIG. 51.11 (A) Cranial anatomy at the level of the thalamus (t). Note the contour of the bony calvarium. (B) Cerebral ventricles are seen at this level. The midline echo from the interhemispheric fissure (IHF) is noted. The medial ventricular border and the lateral ventricular borders (LV) are identified. The echogenic choroid plexus (CHP) are demonstrated. *CSP,* cavum septum pellucidum.

When measuring the ventricle, the sonographer locates the atrium and measures directly across the posterior portion, measuring perpendicular to the long axis of the ventricle rather than the falx while placing the calipers at the junction of the ventricular wall and lumen or cavity of the ventricle (see Fig. 51.10). The normal atrium measures 6.5 mm. If the atrium measures greater than 10 mm, this warrants serial imaging and further evaluation.

Moving the transducer slightly inferior to the ventricular atrium identifies the area of the thalami and the ambient cisterns. This is the widest transverse diameter of the skull and is therefore the proper level at which to measure the biparietal diameter and head circumference. The midline brain structures (see Fig. 51.12) include the cavum septum pellucidum (CSP), the midline echo, and the paired thalami lying on either side. The thalamus resembles a heart with the apex projected toward the fetal occiput.

Between the thalami lies the cavity of the third ventricle (see Fig. 51.12). In the same scanning plane, the box-shaped CSP is observed anterior to the thalamus. The CSP is the space between the leaves of the septum pellucidum.

At this transverse level, the frontal horns of the ventricles may be seen as two diverging echo-free structures within the frontal lobes of the brain. The frontal horns are prominent in the presence of ventricular dilation. The **corpus callosum** is an echogenic structure seen in the transverse plane as the band of tissue between the frontal ventricular horns. The corpus callosum can be better appreciated as a linear band in a sagittal view from the top of the fetal head, but this plane is often not accessible in pregnancy.

The ambient cisterns are pulsatile structures vascularized by the posterior cerebral artery bordering the thalamus posteriorly. When scanning laterally in the brain, the temporal lobe is visible, along with evidence of the insula (i.e., the sylvian cistern complex). The insula appears to pulsate because of blood circulation through the middle cerebral artery, which courses through the insula (see Fig. 51.12). The subarachnoid spaces may be seen projecting from the inner skull table.

As the transducer is moved toward the base of the skull, the heart-shaped cerebral peduncles are imaged (Fig. 51.13). Although similar to the thalamus in shape, they are smaller. Pulsations from the basilar artery are observed between the

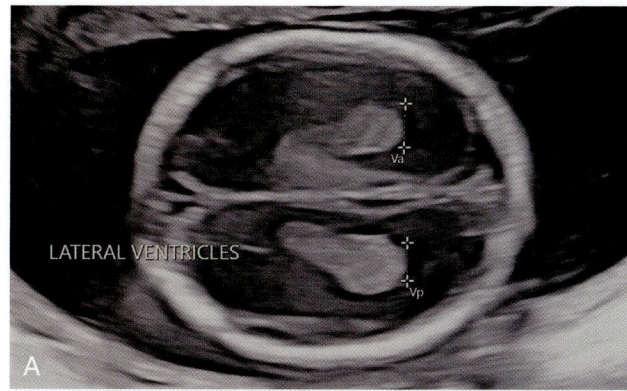

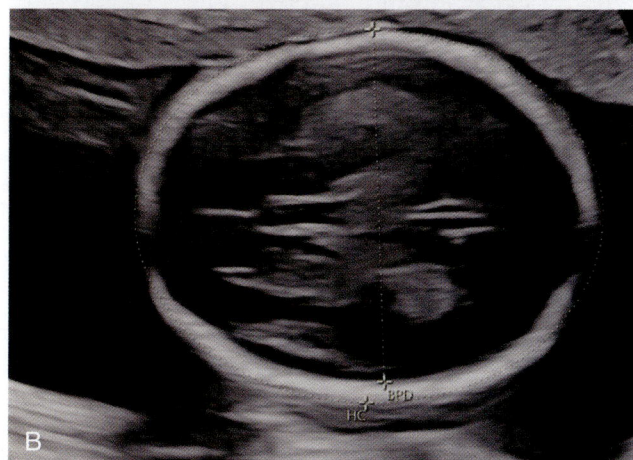

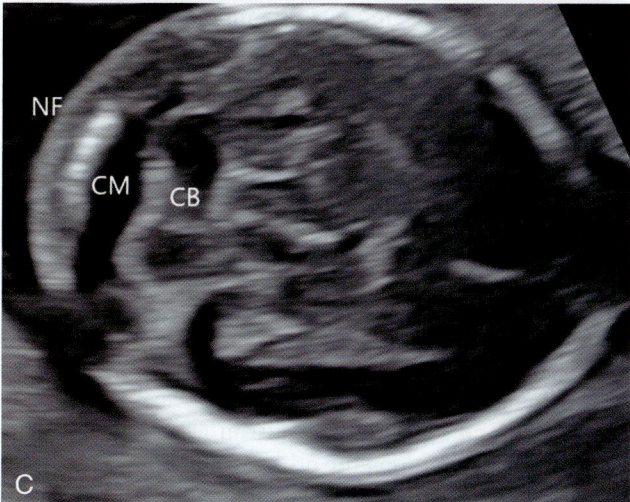

FIG. 51.12 (A) Transverse view at the level of the ventricles. The width of the lateral ventricle is measured from medial to lateral edges. (B) Transverse view slightly inferior to the level of the ventricles, near the thalamus (hypoechoic "heart" structure in the center of the skull). This is the level at which the biparietal diameter and head circumference are measured. (C) Transverse view inferior to the level of part B; the posterior fossa is seen at this level with the cerebellum (CB), cisterna magna (CM), and the nuchal fold (NF) demonstrated.

lobes of the peduncles at the interpeduncular cistern. The circle of Willis may be seen anterior to the midbrain and appears as a triangular region that is highly pulsatile as a result of the midline-positioned anterior cerebral artery and lateral convergence of the middle cerebral arteries. The suprasellar cistern may be recognized in the center of the circle of Willis.

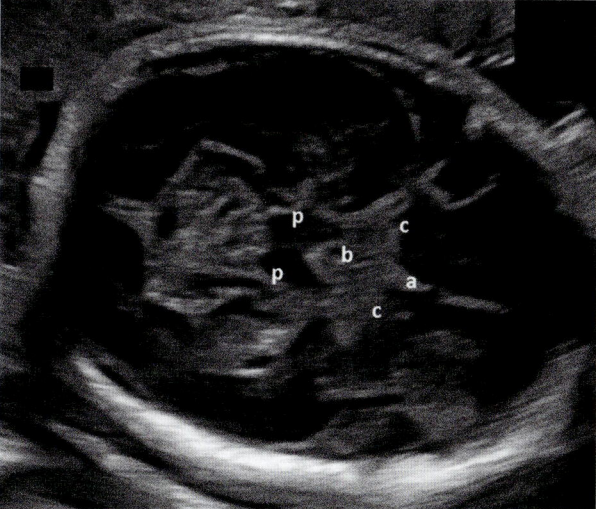

FIG. 51.13 Circle of Willis (c) identified anterior to the cerebral peduncles (p). Arterial pulsations may be observed from the basilar artery (b) and the anterior cerebral artery (a) in real-time imaging. The middle cerebral artery pulsations may be seen at the lateral margins of the circle of Willis.

The *cerebellum* is in back of the cerebral peduncles within the posterior fossa. The cerebellar hemispheres are joined together by the cerebellar vermis (Fig. 51.14). It is important to recognize the usual configuration of the cerebellum because distortion may represent findings suggestive of an open spina bifida. The *banana sign* is the sonographic term that describes the Arnold-Chiari malformation in which the cerebellum may be small or displaced downward into the foramen magnum. Measurements of transverse cerebellar width allow assessment of fetal age and permit necessary follow-up in fetuses with spinal defects and other anomalies of the cerebellum.

The *cisterna magna* (a posterior fossa cistern filled with CSF) lies directly behind the cerebellum (Fig. 51.15). A normal-appearing cisterna magna may exclude almost all open spinal defects. The cisterna magna is almost always effaced (thinned out) or obliterated in fetuses with the Arnold-Chiari malformation changes associated with spina bifida. The cranial changes occur because tethering of the spinal cord resulting from spina bifida pulls brain tissue downward, obliterating the cisterna magna. In patients at low risk of spinal defect, confirmation of a normal posterior fossa suggests the absence of spina bifida. Because evaluation of the fetal spine remains challenging in excluding small spinal defects, cranial findings associated with this disorder may be very helpful in screening for these lesions.

Enlargement of the cisterna magna may indicate a space-occupying cyst, such as a Dandy-Walker malformation or other abnormalities of the posterior fossa. Enlargement is often a normal variant. The normal cisterna magna measures 3 to 11 mm, with an average size of 5 to 6 mm. Measurements of cisterna magna size are obtained by measuring from the vermis to the inner skull table of the occipital bone. Within the cisterna magna space, linear echoes, which are paired, may be observed posteriorly. These echogenic structures represent dural folds that attach the falx cerebelli (see Fig. 51.14).

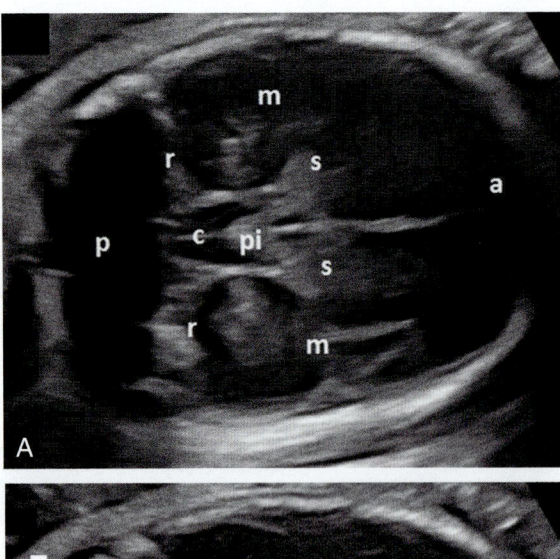

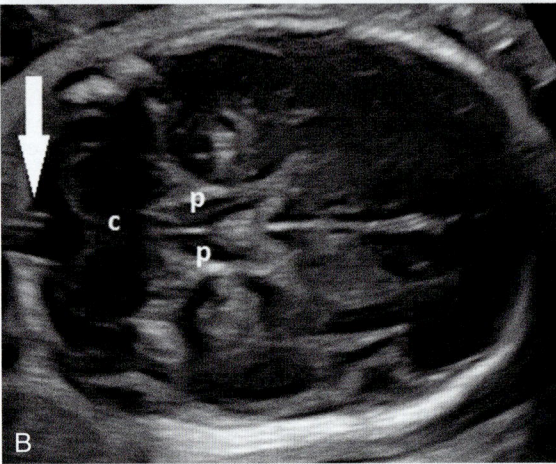

FIG. 51.14 (A) Anatomic depiction at the cerebellar level showing the cerebral peduncles (p) positioned anteriorly to the cerebellum (c). The dural folds that connect the bottom of the falx cerebelli are seen within the cisterna magna *(arrow)*. (B) In the same fetus, at a level slightly below the cerebellar level, the anterior (a), middle (m), and posterior fossae are shown. Note the sphenoid bones (s) and petrous ridges (r). *c*, Suprasellar cistern; *pi*, piarachnoid tissue in the basilar cistern.

In the second trimester, the thickness of the nuchal skin fold is measured in a plane containing the cavum septi pellucidi, the cerebellum, and the cisterna magna. Values of skin thickness of 5 mm or less up to 20 weeks of gestational age are normal. Fetuses with thickened nuchal skin are at increased risk for aneuploidy.

At the base of the skull, the anterior, middle, and posterior cranial fossae are observed (see Fig. 51.14). The sphenoid bones create a V-shaped appearance as they separate the anterior fossa from the middle fossa, with the petrous bones further dividing the fossa posteriorly. At the junction of the sphenoid wings and the petrous bones lies the sella turcica (site of the pituitary gland).

The Face

The architecture and morphology of the fetal face are easily appreciated after the first trimester of pregnancy. Viewing facial behaviors such as fetal yawning, swallowing, and eye movements not only may be enjoyable but may provide insightful clues to fetal well-being and normal facial anatomy.

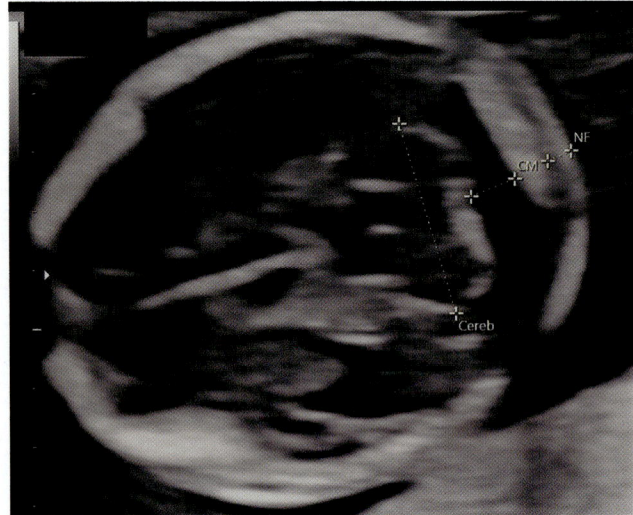

FIG. 51.15 Depiction of a normal cerebellum (Cereb) and cisterna magna (CM) in a normal fetus. At the same level, the skin behind the neck is measured. A normal nuchal skin fold (NF) is shown. This measurement is unreliable after 20 weeks of gestation.

The fetal face may be recognized even in the first trimester of pregnancy, and the gestational age at which the nasal bone first appears may contribute to aneuploidy risk determination. Facial morphology becomes more apparent in the second trimester, but visualization is heavily dependent on fetal positioning, adequate amounts of amniotic fluid, and excellent acoustic windows. Incorporation of three-dimensional ultrasound imaging has enhanced images of facial details and created patient demand for *fetal portraits*.

Fetal Eye Orbits. When scanning inferior to or below the cerebellar plane, the orbits may be visualized. It is important to note that both fetal orbits (and eyes) are present and that the spacing between both orbits appears normal. There are conditions in which eyes may be missing (anophthalmia), fused or closely spaced (hypotelorism), or abnormally widened (hypertelorism).

The fetal orbits are observed and measured in two planes: (1) a coronal scan posterior to the glabellar-alveolar line (Figs. 51.16) and (2) a transverse scan at a level below the biparietal diameter (along the orbitomeatal line) (Fig. 51.17). The individual orbital rings, nasal structures, and maxillary processes can be identified in these views. When the fetus is in an occipitoposterior position (fetal orbits directed up), orbital distances can also be determined. In this view, the orbital rings, lens, and nasal structures may be demonstrated (Fig. 51.18). Measurements of the inner orbital distance should be made from the medial border of the orbit to the opposite medial border, and the outer orbital (or binocular) distance (OOD) should be measured from the lateral border of one orbit to the opposite lateral wall (see Figs. 51.16 to 51.18). **Nomograms** for orbital distance spacing have been published and may confirm impressions of hypertelorism or hypotelorism. Orbital measurements are not used for routine screening because there is a wide range of normal values.

Facial Profile. Views of the fetal forehead and facial profile are achieved by imaging the facial profile (Fig. 51.19). In this

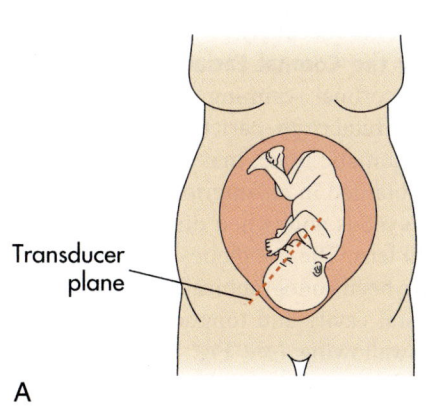
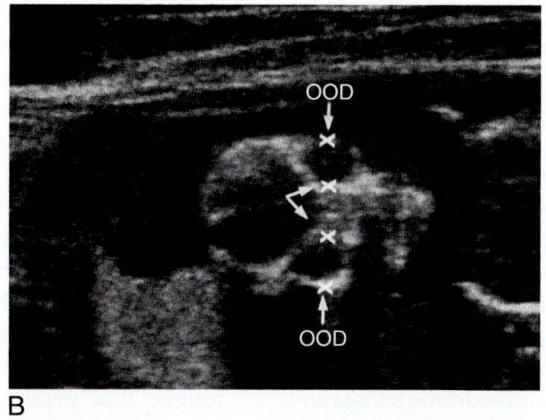

FIG. 51.16 (A) Frontal view. Fetus in a vertex presentation with the fetal cranium in an occipitotransverse position. The transducer is placed along the coronal plane (approximately 2 cm posterior to the glabellar-alveolar line). (B) This sonogram shows the orbits in the coronal view. The outer orbital diameter (OOD) and inner orbital diameter (IOD) *(angled arrows)* are viewed. The IOD is measured from the medial border of the orbit to the opposite medial border *(angled arrows)*. The OOD is measured from the outermost lateral border of the orbit to the opposite lateral border.

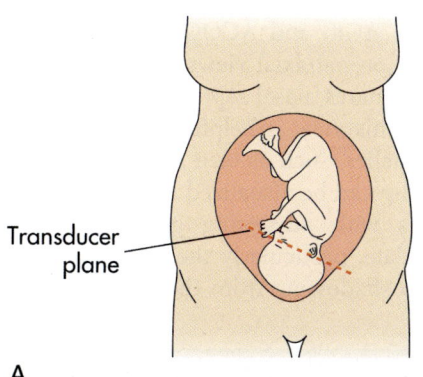
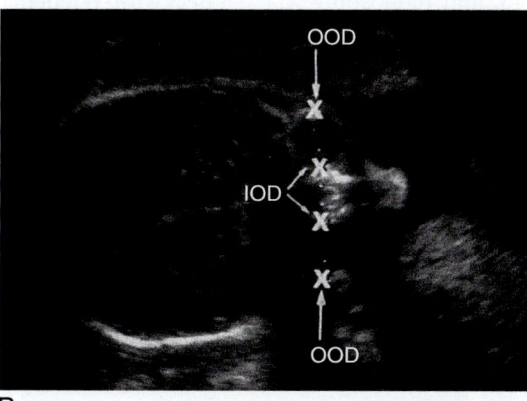

FIG. 51.17 (A) Frontal view demonstrating the fetal cranium in an occipitotransverse position. The transducer is placed along the orbitomeatal line (approximately 2 to 3 cm below the level of the biparietal diameter). (B) Sonogram demonstrating the orbits in the occipitotransverse position. *IOD*, Inner orbital diameter; *OOD*, outer orbital diameter.

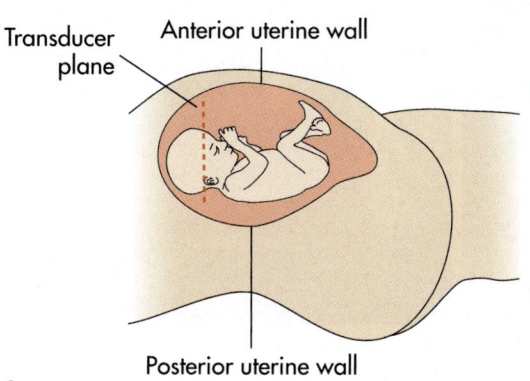
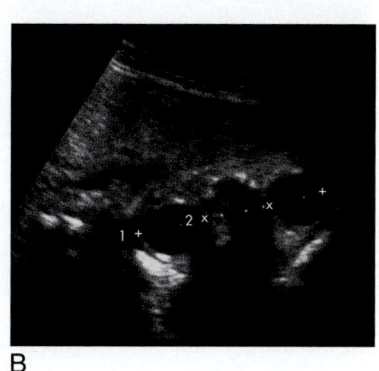

FIG. 51.18 (A) Side view demonstrating the fetus in an occipitoposterior position. The transducer is placed in a plane that transects the occiput, orbits, and nasal processes. (B) Sonogram of the orbits in an occipitoposterior position.

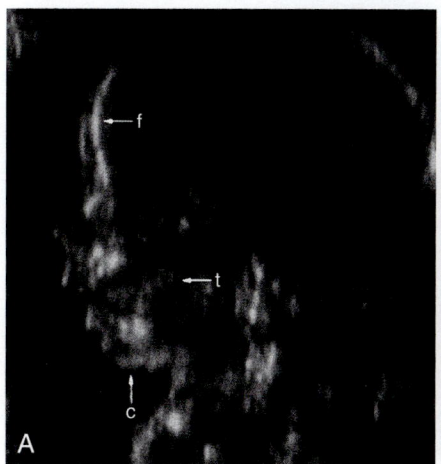
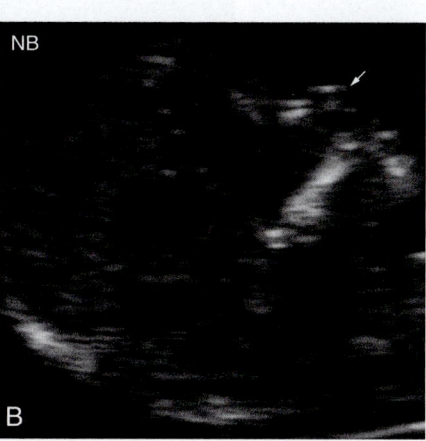

FIG. 51.19 (A) Sagittal view in a 23-week-old fetus showing the contour of the face in profile. Note the smooth surface of the frontal bone (f) and the appearance of the nose and upper and lower lips, tongue (t), and chin (c). (B) The fetal nasal bone is seen as a bright linear echo under the linear skin line echo in this profile of the fetus.

view, the contour of the frontal bone, the nose, the upper and lower lips, and the chin may be assessed. Profile views of the face are useful in assessing the nasal bone; in excluding forehead malformations such as anterior cephaloceles, abnormal slopes, or **frontal bossing**; and in assessing the chin to exclude an abnormally small chin—**micrognathia**. In a normally proportioned face, each of the segments containing the forehead, the eyes and nose, and the mouth and chin forms approximately one-third of the profile.

Nasal Bone. A small nose and midface hypoplasia are recognized components of Down syndrome facies. Studies have shown that the nasal bone is absent during the second trimester in one-quarter to one-third of Down syndrome fetuses and is present in all normal fetuses. An absent nasal bone is also associated with trisomy 18, trisomy 13, and monosomy X. The nasal bone appears as a bright echo parallel to the echogenic skin interface in the superior aspect of the nose (see Fig. 51.19). It is important that the nasal bone be visualized and documented if present in a midline fetal profile in second-trimester examinations. Nomograms are available for measuring the nasal bone during the second trimester. A shortened nasal bone is a risk factor for aneuploidy.

Frontal bossing is a variation of facial structure where the forehead is more prominent than usual. It is seen in skeletal dysplasias. Frontal slanting is the opposite of frontal bossing and is characterized by a forehead that slopes backward. Frontal slanting is seen in microcephaly.

Anatomic Landmarks of the Coronal Facial View. By placing the transducer in a coronal scanning plane, sectioning through the face reveals orbital rings, parietal bones, ethmoid bones, nasal septum, zygomatic bone, maxillae, and mandible (Fig. 51.20). Scans obtained in an anterior plane over the orbits demonstrate the eyelids and, when directed posterior to this plane, the orbital lens. The eye globes, hyaloid artery, and vitreous matter have been sonographically identified.

Fetal Tongue. The oral cavity and tongue are frequently outlined during fetal swallowing (see Fig. 51.19). A large tongue that persistently protrudes outside of the mouth is called macroglossia. Macroglossia is associated with Beckwith-Wiedemann syndrome and with aneuploidies.

Fetal Lips. The most recent revisions of the obstetric guidelines from AIUM, ACR, and ACOG require visualization of the fetal lip. Coronal/axial views of the face help differentiate the nostrils, nares, nasal septum, maxillae, and mandible (Fig. 51.21). This view is helpful in the diagnosis of craniofacial anomalies, such as cleft lip. The soft tissues of the fetal upper lip can be visualized in most fetuses. Visualization improves with advancing gestational age. Visualization of the palate, particularly the hard palate, is more difficult owing to shadowing from the alveolar ridge

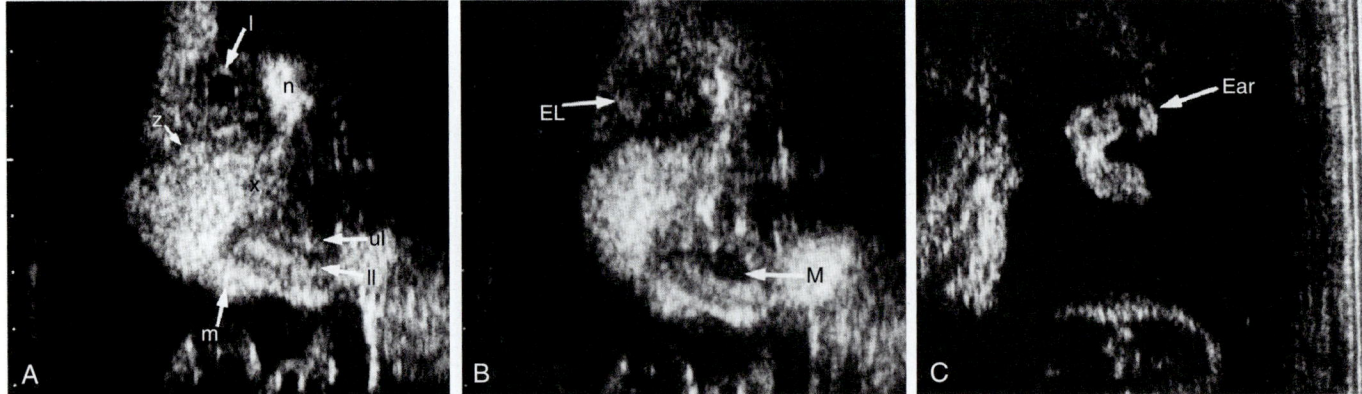

FIG. 51.20 (A) Coronal view showing facial features. (B) In the same fetus, the eyelids (EL) and mouth (M) are shown. (C) In the same fetus, the ear is shown. *l*, Lens; *ll*, lower lip; *m*, mandible; *n*, nasal bones; *ul*, upper lip; *x*, maxilla; *z*, zygomatic bone.

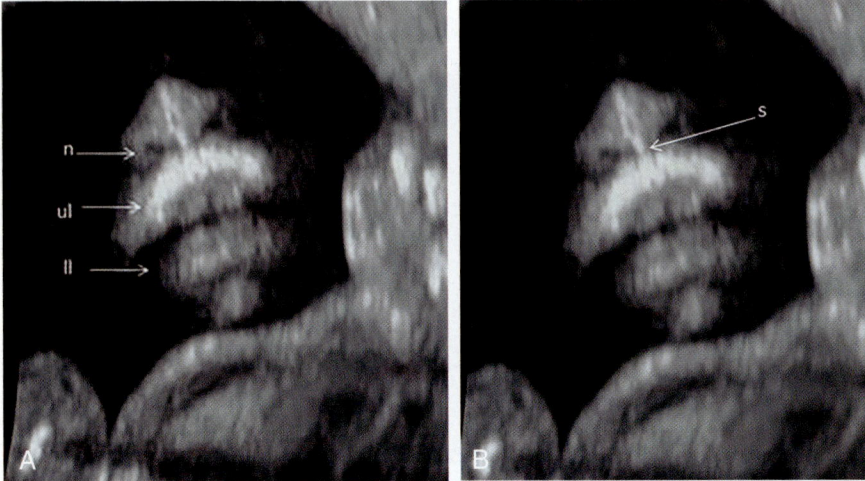

FIG. 51.21 (A) Axial view through the upper (ul) and lower lip (ll) in a fetus with an open mouth. Note the nares (n) and nasal septum (s). This view is used to check for a cleft of the upper lip. (B) In the same fetus, same anatomy viewed with a closed mouth.

and interference by the tongue. Sonographers should strive to diagnose cleft lip in utero, as prenatal classes for parents of these children are associated with faster weight gain, quicker surgical intervention, and better outcomes postnatally. It is important to recognize normal facial landmarks that may also mimic defects.

Fetal Ears. Fetal ears may be defined in the second trimester as lateral protuberances emerging from the parietal bones. Later in pregnancy, the components of the external ear, helix, lobule, and antitragicus (small muscle in the pinna of the ear) may be seen (Fig. 51.22). The semicircular canals and the internal auditory meatus have been sonographically recognized. Low-set ears are difficult to diagnose with ultrasound. Some have suggested that if a plane passing through the lower jaw intercepts the ear, they may be low set. Others have suggested measuring the ears. However, there is a wide range of normal, and visualization of fetal ears has not yet been shown to be sensitive for diagnosis.

Fetal hair is often observed along the periphery of the skull and must not be included in the biparietal diameter measurement (Fig. 51.23).

The Vertebral Column

Standard antepartum obstetric examination guidelines require the sonographer to image and record the cervical, thoracic, lumbar, and sacral spine to better exclude major spinal malformations (e.g., meningomyelocele).

The longitudinal fetal spine is studied in coronal, sagittal, and transverse scanning planes. There are three ossification points in each vertebra. When scanning in the coronal and sagittal planes, only two ossification points are typically seen. In a sagittal section, the spine appears as two curvilinear lines extending from the cervical spine to the sacrum. The normal fetal spine tapers near the sacrum and widens near the base of the skull (Figs. 51.24 to 51.26). This double-line appearance of the spine is referred to as the *railway sign* and is generated by echoes from the posterior and anterior laminae and the spinal cord.

In a transverse plane, three ossification points are visible. The three are spaced equidistant, and the spinal column appears as a closed circle, indicating closure of the neural tube. Three echoes form a circle or equilateral triangle that

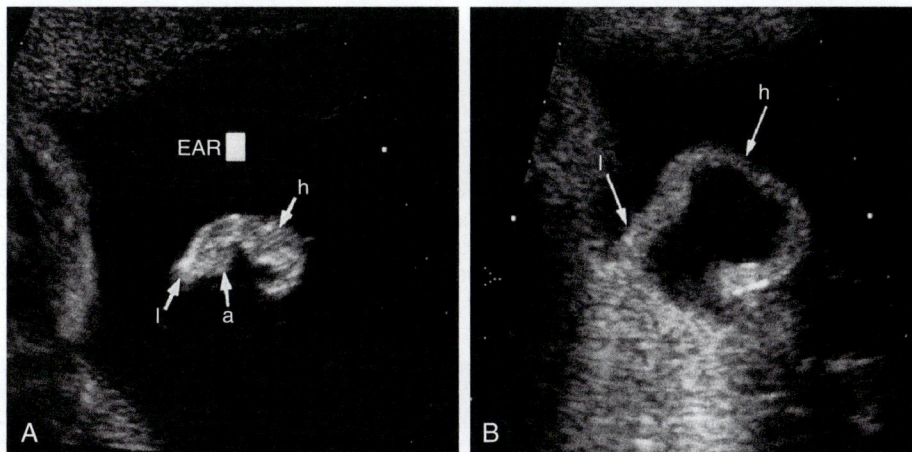

FIG. 51.22 (A) The external ear observed in a 26-week-old fetus showing the helix (h), lobule (l), and antitragicus (a). (B) At 36 weeks of gestation, the lobule (l) and helix (h) are observed.

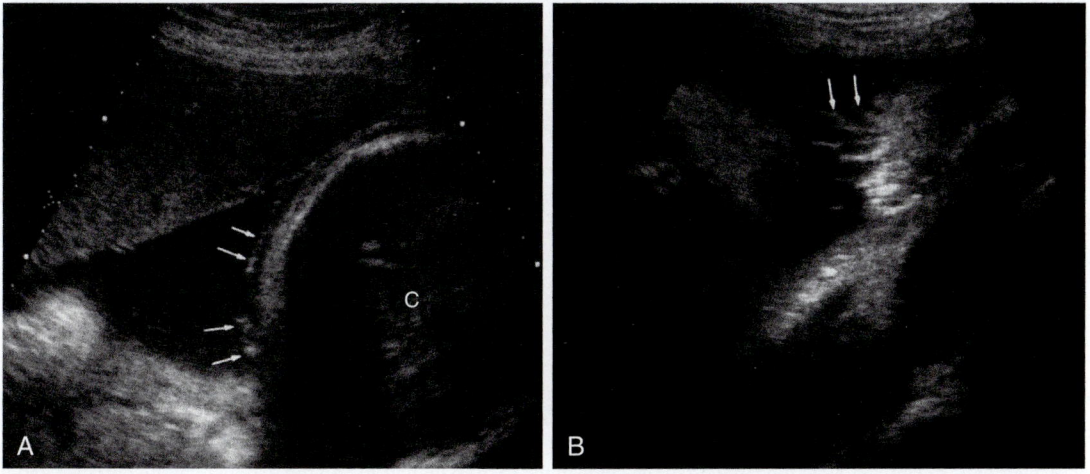

FIG. 51.23 (A) Fetal hair *(arrows)* observed as a series of dots around the periphery of the fetal cranium in a 39-week-old fetus. (B) Long hair *(arrows)* observed in a 34-week-old fetus. *C,* Cranium.

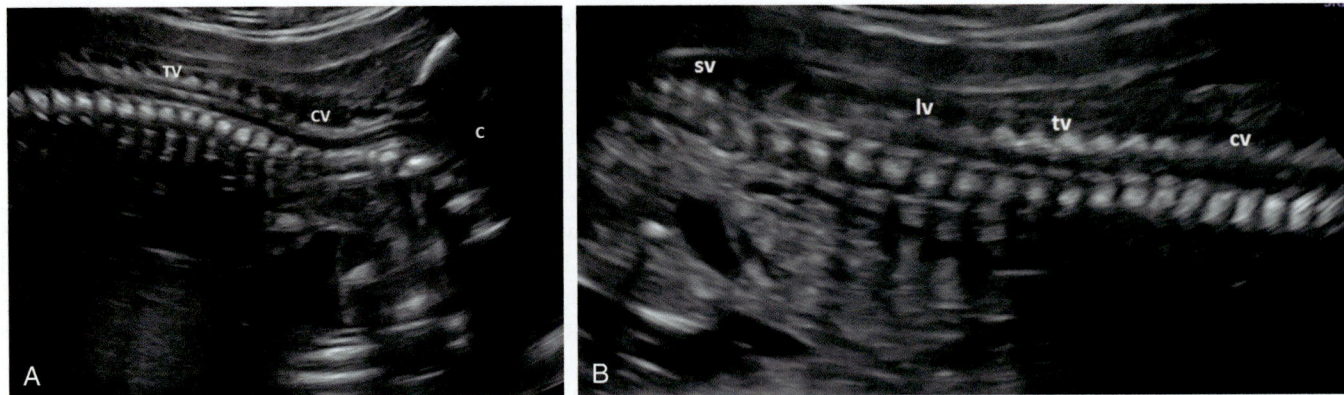

FIG. 51.24 (A) Longitudinal view of the fetal spine outlining the cervical vertebrae (cv) and cranium (c). The thoracic vertebrae (tv) are visualized distally. (B) In the same fetus, the cervical vertebrae (cv), thoracic vertebrae (tv), lumbar vertebrae (lv), and the sacral vertebrae (sv) are seen.

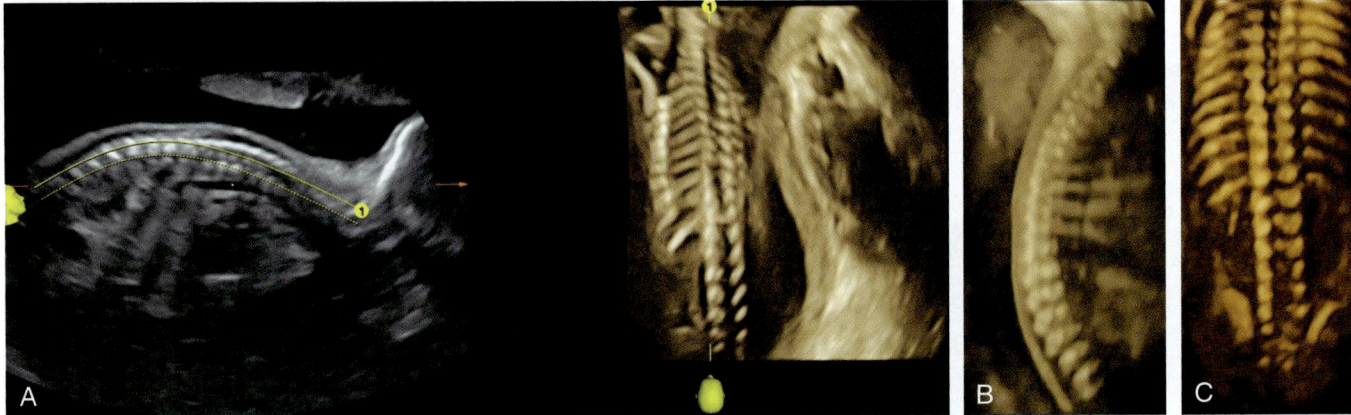

FIG. 51.25 (A) Longitudinal view of the spine is demonstrated and, with the use of four-dimensional (4D) imaging, a coronal view of the fetus is seen demonstrating the parallel nature of the posterior elements. (B) In the same fetus, a 4D view of the spine is manipulated to a longitudinal view to demonstrate the thick skin line seen covering the vertebrae. (C) A 3D rendering in the skeleton view of the fetal spine is manipulated to demonstrate the vertebrae in a coronal view.

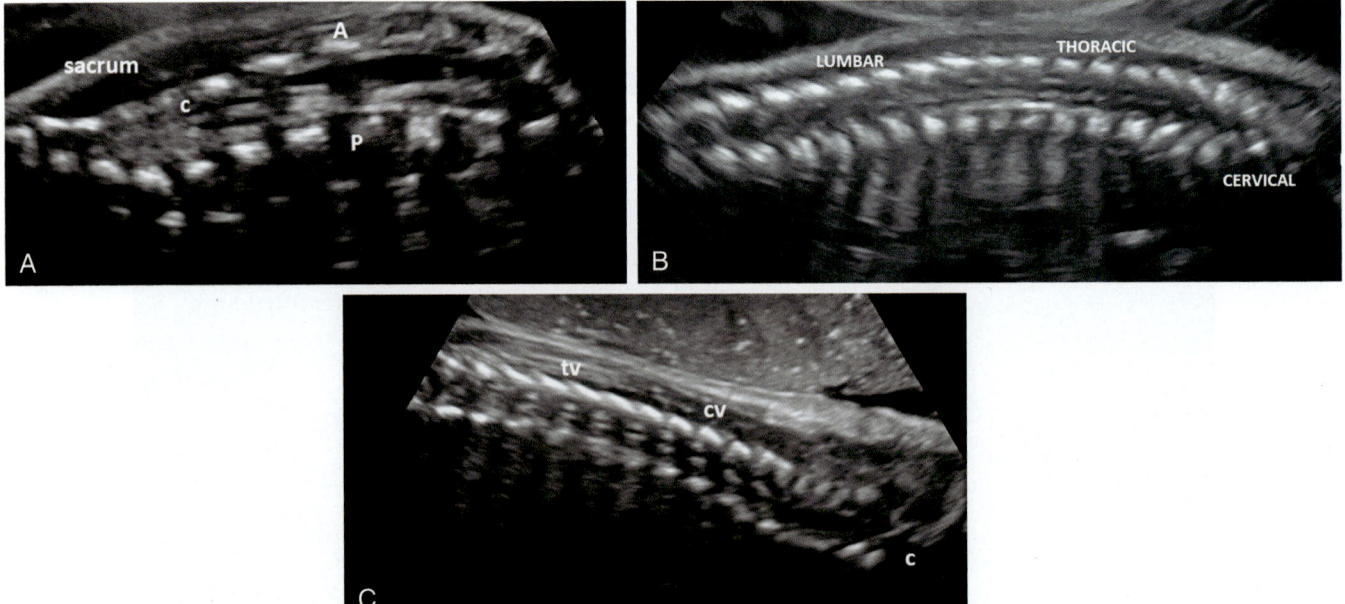

FIG. 51.26 Longitudinal sections of the lumbosacral (A), thoracic (B), and cervical (C) spine in a fetus displaying the anterior (A) and posterior (P) elements, or laminae. Note the tapering of the spine at the sacrum (in part A) and the widening at the entrance into the base of the skull (part C). Between the posterior elements lie the spinal canal and cord (may be seen as a linear echo within the spinal canal). *c*, Cranium; *cv*, cervical vertebrae; *tv*, thoracic vertebrae.

represents the center of the vertebral body and the posterior elements (laminae or pedicles) (Fig. 51.27). These elements should be identified in the normal fetus, whereas the pedicles appear splayed in a V-, C-, or U-shaped configuration in a fetus with a spinal defect.

When evaluating the spine, it is imperative for the sonographer to align the transducer in a perpendicular axis to the spinal elements. Incorrect angles may falsely indicate an abnormality. The spinal muscles and the posterior skin border are viewed adjacent to the circular ring of the ossification centers (see Fig. 51.27). It is important to note the integrity of the skin surface because this membrane is absent in fetuses with open spina bifida. Inspection of the spine is often impossible when the fetus is lying with the spine against the uterine wall. Optimal viewing of the spine occurs when the fetus is lying on its side in a transverse direction with its back a slight distance from the uterine wall. The sonographer may need to ask the mother to turn slightly to encourage the fetus to move away from the uterine wall.

The Thorax

Although the fetus is unable to breathe air in utero, the lungs are important landmarks to visualize within the thoracic cavity. The lungs serve as lateral borders for the heart and are therefore helpful in assessing the relationship and position of the heart in the chest. Fetal breathing movements are also observed at this level. Like all fetal organs, the lungs are subject to abnormal development. Lung size, texture, and location should be assessed routinely to exclude a lung mass.

The fluid-filled fetal lungs are observed as solid, homogeneous masses of tissue bordered medially by the heart, inferiorly by the diaphragm, and laterally by the rib cage (Fig. 51.28). The heart occupies a midline position within the chest; its displacement warrants further study to exclude a possible mass of the lung or a subdiaphragmatic hernia that may alter the position of the heart.

In sagittal views, lung tissue is present superior to the diaphragm and lateral to the heart (see Fig. 51.28). Investigators have attempted to define textural variations of the lung in

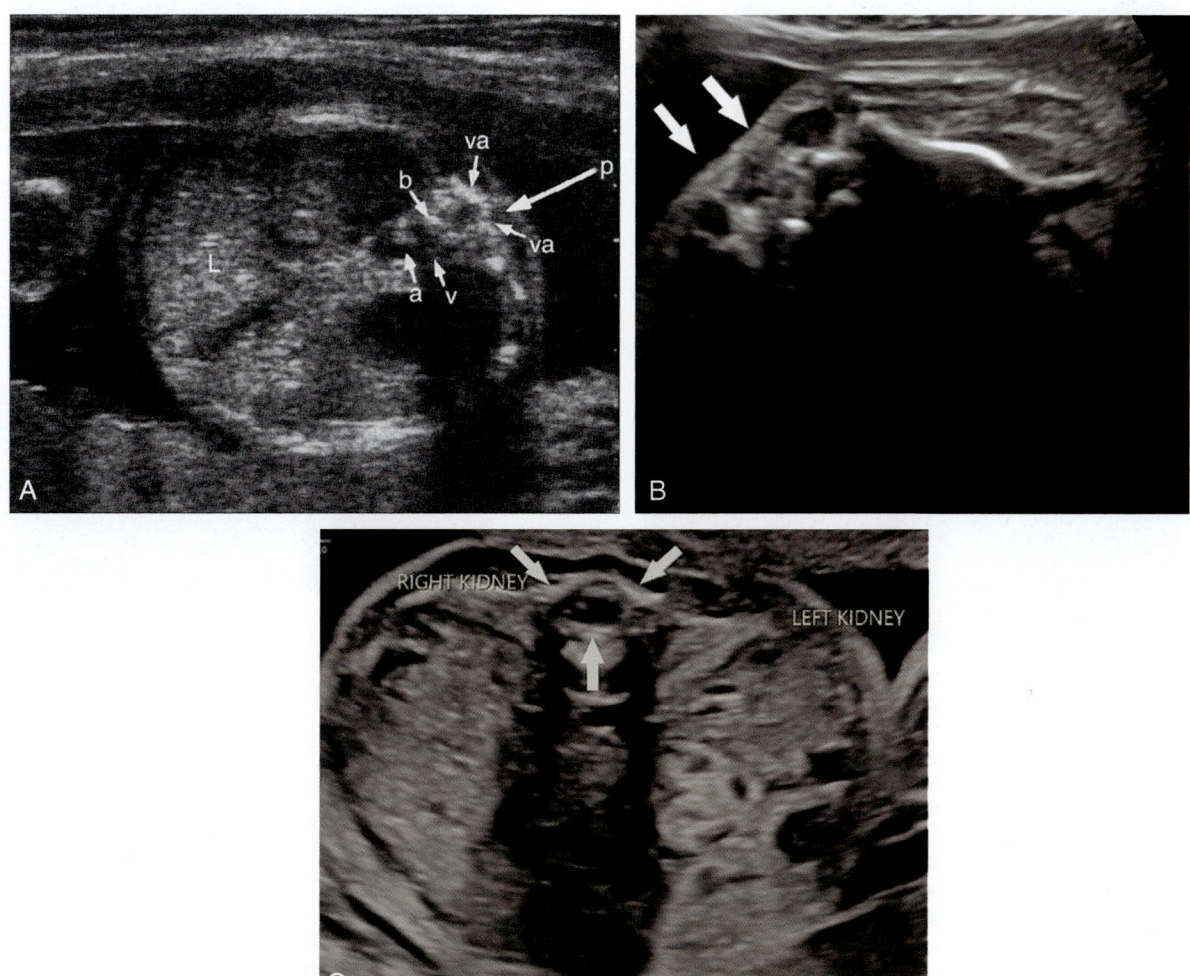

FIG. 51.27 (A) Transverse scans of the vertebral column showing the echogenic ring produced by the vertebral body and posterior elements, or laminae. Thoracic vertebrae with typical landmarks. (B) Sacral vertebra outlined. Note the intact posterior skin wall in this normal fetus. (C) Transverse view through the spine at kidney level demonstrating the closed-circle appearance *(arrows)* of the spine created by the intact vertebral arch. *a*, Aorta; *b*, body; *L*, liver; *p*, posterior vertebral muscles; *v*, vena cava; *va*, vertebral arch or posterior elements.

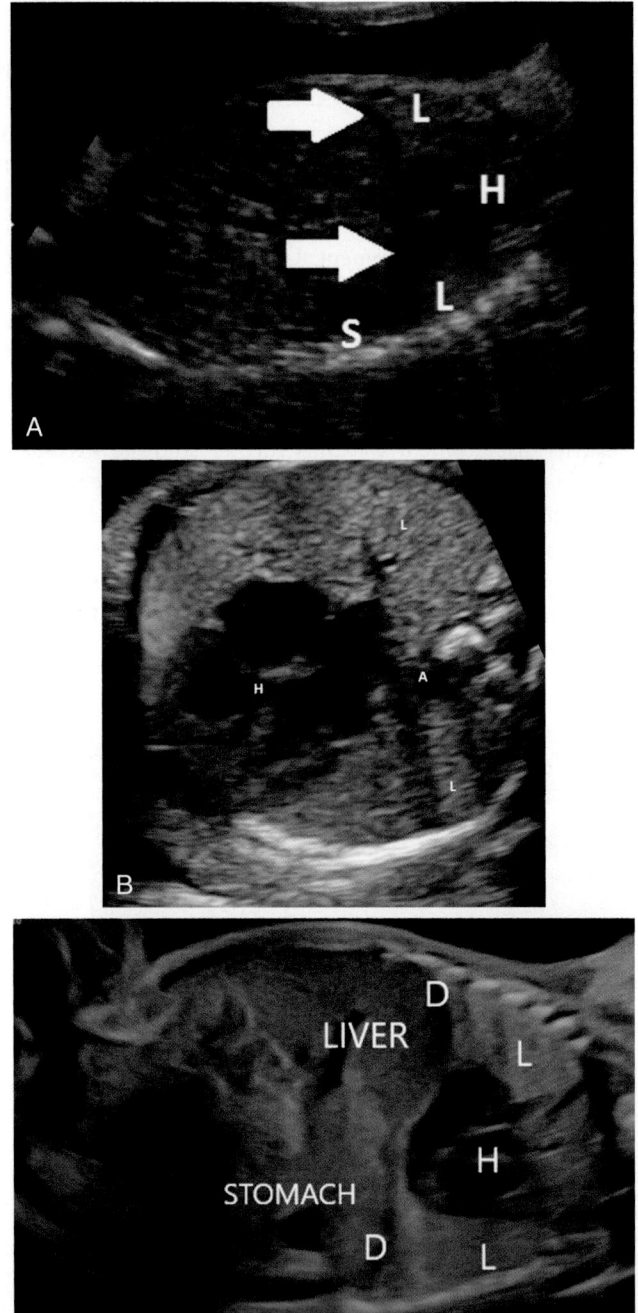

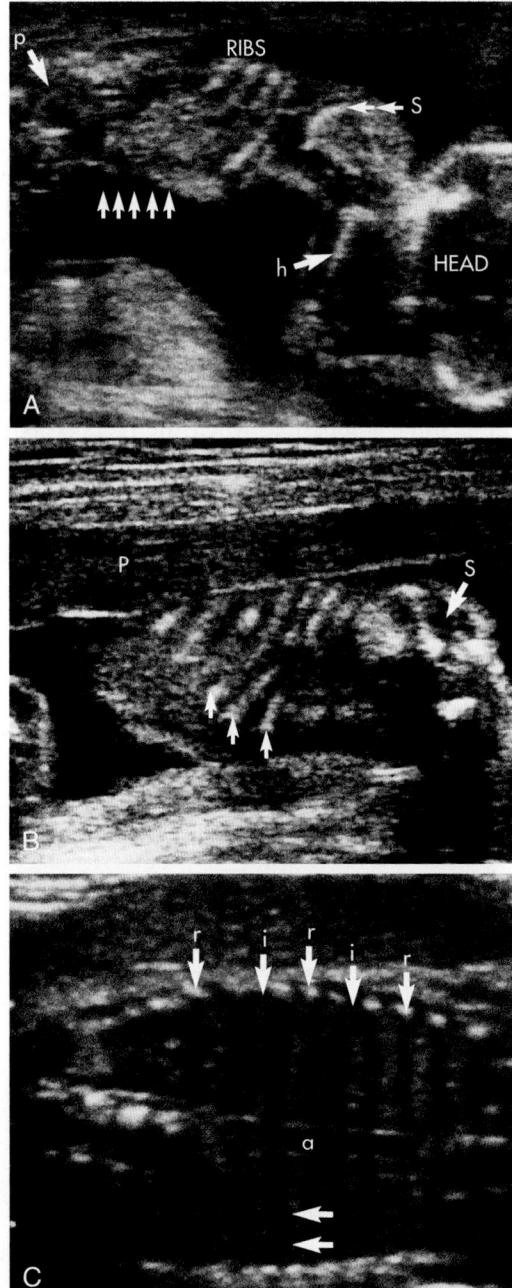

FIG. 51.28 (A) Sagittal scan showing the homogeneous lungs positioned lateral to the heart (H) and superior to the diaphragm *(arrows)*. Note the normal placement of the stomach inferior to the diaphragm. (B) In the same fetus, a transverse section demonstrates the position of the lungs (L) in relationship to the heart. Note the apex of the heart to the left side of the chest. The base of the heart is in the midline and anterior to the aorta (A). Displacement or shifting of the heart should alert the sonographer to search for a mass of the lungs, heart, or diaphragm. (C) In the late third trimester of pregnancy, the lung tissue can be observed and compared with the liver texture. *D*, Diaphragm; *H*, heart.

FIG. 51.29 (A) Sagittal view showing the rib cage, scapula (S), anterior abdominal wall *(arrows)*, and humerus (h) in a fetus in a back-up position. (B) Tangential view depicting the length of the ribs *(arrows)*. (C) Sagittal view of the rib cage. Note that sound waves are unable to pass through the bony rib, resulting in a shadow of echoes *(arrows)* posterior to the ribs (r). Sound passes through the intercostal space (i). *a*, Aorta; *P*, placenta; *p*, pelvis; *S*, shoulder.

comparison with the liver. Fetal lung tissue appears more echogenic than the liver as pregnancy progresses.

The ribs, scapulae, and clavicles are bony landmarks of the chest cavity. Because these structures are composed of bone,

acoustic shadowing occurs posteriorly. Portions of the rib cage may be identified when sections are obtained through the posterior aspects of the spine and rib cage (Fig. 51.29). Oblique sectioning of the ribs reveals the total length of the ribs and floating ribs. On sagittal planes, the echogenic rib interspersed with the intercostal space creates the typical "washboard" appearance of the rib cage (see Fig. 51.29). Sound waves strike the rib and are reflected upward, leaving

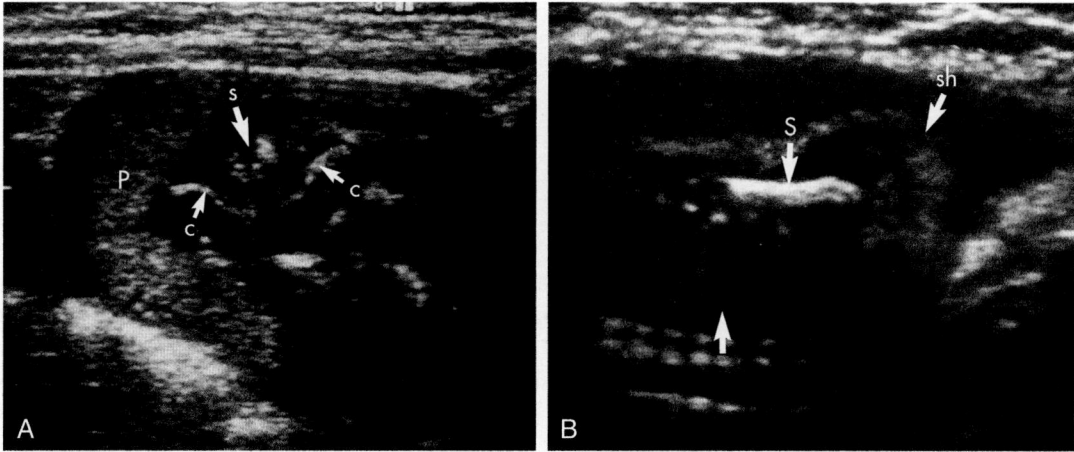

FIG. 51.30 (A) Coronal section of upper thoracic cavity showing the clavicles (c) and spine (s). (B) Sagittal section demonstrating the scapula (S) in relationship to the shoulder (sh) and ribs *(arrow)*. P, Placenta.

the characteristic void of echoes posterior to the bony element, whereas sound waves pass through the intercostal space.

On a transverse cross section through the chest and upper abdomen, the curvature of the rib may be appreciated below the skin. It is important to differentiate the rib from the skin wall, especially when measuring the abdominal circumference. The entire rib cage is impractical to routinely examine, but study of the ribs is warranted in fetuses at risk for congenital rib anomalies (e.g., rib fractures found in osteogenesis imperfecta).

The clavicles are observed in coronal sections through the upper thorax (Fig. 51.30). The clavicular length may aid in determining gestational age. In this same view, the spinal elements, esophagus, and carotid arteries may be seen. The clavicles may also be demonstrated as echogenic dots superior to the ribs. Measurements of the clavicles may be useful in predicting congenital clavicular anomalies. The clavicles may be shortened with aneuploidy.

The scapula may be recognized on sagittal sections as an echogenic linear echo adjacent to the rib shadows, whereas on transverse sections, it is viewed medial to the humeral head (see Fig. 51.30). Oblique views demonstrate the entire length of the scapula. The sternum may be seen in axial sections as a bony sequence of echoes beneath the anterior chest wall.

The Heart

Standard antepartum obstetric examination guidelines require the sonographer to image and record a four-chamber view of the fetal heart and the left and right ventricular outflow tracts. See Chapter 35 for more detailed fetal cardiac anatomy. Many major anomalies of the fetal heart are excluded when cardiac anatomy appears normal in the four-chamber view of the heart. Additional views, including outflow tracts and the three-vessel cranial view, further reduce the risk of cardiovascular anomalies.

The heart lies more transversely in the fetus than in the adult because the lungs are not inflated. The apex of the heart is directed toward the left anterior chest with the right ventricle closest to the chest wall and the left atrium closest to the spine. The four chambers may be seen in a view taken with the beam perpendicular to the septum or in a view with the beam perpendicular to the valves (Fig. 51.31). The four-chamber view may be obtained by angling cephalad after obtaining a transverse view of the fetal abdomen that displays the stomach. In a four-chamber view of the heart, it is important to assess the following:

- Cardiac position, situs, and axis. The apex of the heart should point to the fetal left side.
- Presence of the right ventricle and left ventricle (the right ventricle is found when a line is drawn from the spine to the anterior chest wall and is characterized by the presence of moderator bands).
- Equal-sized ventricles. By the end of pregnancy, the right ventricle may be larger than the left ventricle because it is the chamber that pumps blood through the ductus arteriosus to the descending aorta and to the placenta.
- Presence of equal-sized right and left atria, with the foramen ovale opening toward the left atrium as blood is shunted from the right atrium, bypassing the lungs.
- An interventricular septum that appears uninterrupted. The septum appears wider toward the ventricles and thins as it courses cephalad within the heart.
- Normal placement of the tricuspid and mitral valves. The tricuspid valve inserts lower, or closer to the apex, than the mitral valve. Both valves should open during diastole and close during systole.
- Normal rhythm and rate (120 to 160 beats/min).

Guidelines require that the standard antepartum obstetric examination include views of the ventricular outflow tracts. These views (Fig. 51.32) can document that the aortic and pulmonic outflow tracts are similar in size and appropriate in size for gestational age, that the anterior wall of the aorta is contiguous with the ventricular septum (excludes overriding aorta), and that the great vessels are in normal alignment. These views may provide additional images of the cardiac septum.

An echogenic structure as bright as bone that appears within a cardiac chamber and persists despite changes in transducer position is termed an *echogenic intracardiac focus* (EIF)

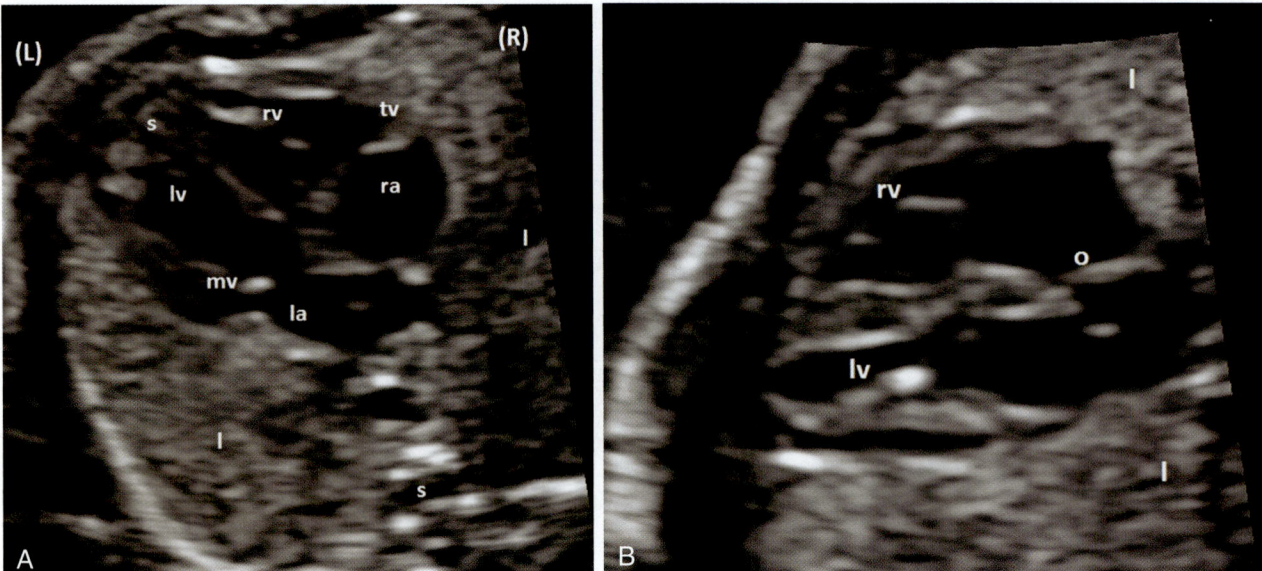

FIG. 51.31 (A) The four-chambered heart view is demonstrated in a 31-week-old fetus with the spine in the 6 o'clock position. The fetal left side is down, and the right side is up. Structures observed are the right (rv) and left (lv) ventricles; the interventricular septum (s), dividing the two ventricular chambers; and the left (la) and right (ra) atria. The foramen ovale allows blood to shunt from the right to left atrium, permitting most of the blood to bypass the lungs. The flap of the foramen ovale is positioned within the left atrium. The atrioventricular valves (mitral and tricuspid) are viewed in systole (closed position). The tricuspid valve (tv) allows blood to move from the right atrium to the right ventricle (rv), and the mitral valve (mv) regulates blood flow from the left atrium to the left ventricle (lv). Note the normal central position of the heart bordered by the lungs (l). The apex of the heart is pointed to the fetal left side (L). When a line is drawn from the spine (S) to the anterior chest wall, the right ventricle is found. (B) In this fetus, the heart is observed in the 5 o'clock position. The fetal left side is down. The lungs (l) are viewed bordering the heart laterally. The muscularity of the interventricular septum *(arrow)* is observed along with the foramen ovale (o), separating the atrial chambers.

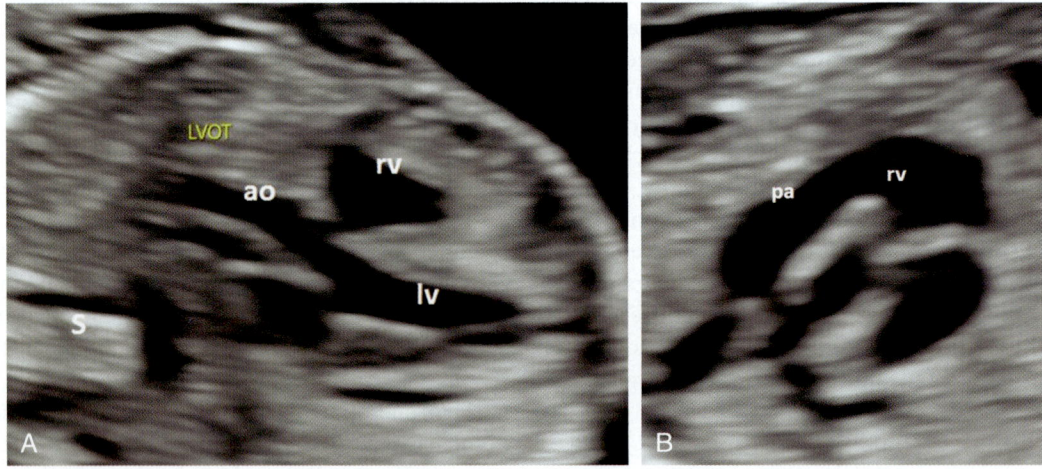

FIG. 51.32 (A) The left ventricular outflow tract (LVOT) is observed as the aorta (ao) exits the left ventricle (lv). (B) The right ventricular outflow tract (RVOT) is observed as the pulmonary artery (pa) exits the right ventricle. The LVOT and RVOT should course perpendicularly to each other. *rv*, Right ventricle; *S*, spine.

(Fig. 51.33). This normal variation appears in many normal pregnancies but is associated with increased risk of aneuploidy and cardiac defects. In fetuses at risk for a cardiac anomaly, including those with an EIF, targeted fetal echocardiography may be recommended to further evaluate the outflow tracts, pulmonic valve and veins, and other complex cardiac relationships beyond the scope of a standard obstetric examination. (For further discussion of normal cardiac anatomy, physiology, and targeted echocardiography, see Chapters 35 and 36.)

The Diaphragm and Thoracic Vessels

The diaphragm is the muscle that separates the thorax and abdomen and is commonly viewed in the longitudinal plane. The diaphragm lies inferior to the heart and lungs and superior to the liver, stomach, and spleen (Fig. 51.34). The diaphragm curves gently toward the thorax. If the diaphragm extends outward toward the abdomen, this may be a sign of increased pressure in the thorax as a result of a thoracic

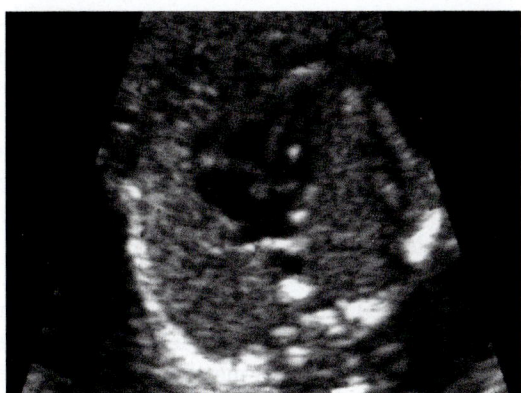

FIG. 51.33 A four-chamber view of the heart showing an echogenic cardiac focus in the left ventricle.

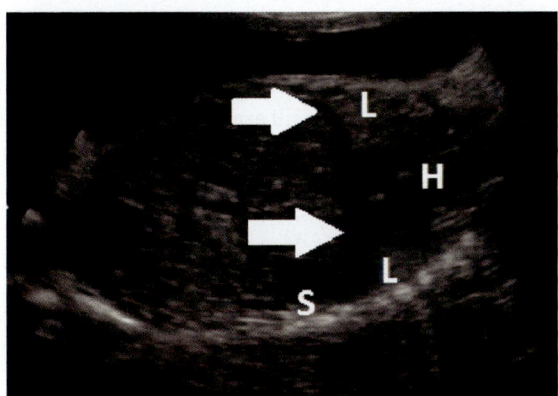

FIG. 51.34 Sagittal scan showing the diaphragm (arrows) separating the thoracic and abdominal cavities. *H*, heart; *L*, liver; *l*, lung; *S*, stomach.

mass or effusion. Sonographically, the diaphragm appears as a sonolucent liner structure separating the thorax from the abdomen.

The diaphragm may be more obvious on the right side because of the strong liver interface but attempts to observe an intact left diaphragm are encouraged because diaphragmatic defects occur on both sides of the diaphragm. The stomach should be viewed inferior to the diaphragm. Although abdominal contents can move into and out of the thoracic cavity with fetal movement, visualization of the stomach inferior to the diaphragm generally excludes a left-side diaphragmatic hernia. If the fetal heart is displaced to the right, this may be a sign of a left-side diaphragmatic hernia.

Vascular structures may be observed within the thoracic cavity and neck. Vessels emanating from the heart are visible within the fetal neck. The carotid arteries (lateral to the esophagus) and the jugular veins (lateral to the carotid arteries) are frequently noted when the fetal neck is extended (Fig. 51.35).

The trachea may be identified as a midline structure in both sagittal and transverse planes. The esophagus and the oropharynx help determine the location of the carotid arteries and are outlined when amniotic fluid is swallowed by the fetus (Fig. 51.36).

The aorta, inferior vena cava, and superior vena cava are routinely observed. The aorta is recognized on sagittal planes as it exits the left ventricle and forms the aortic arch (see Fig. 51.33). The vessels branching cephalad into the brain

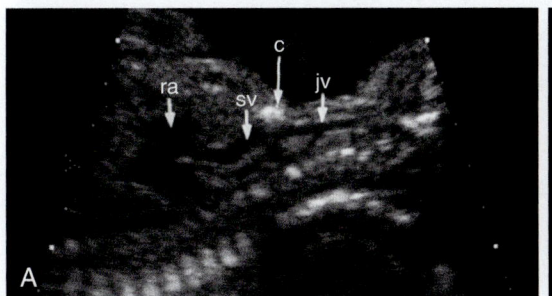 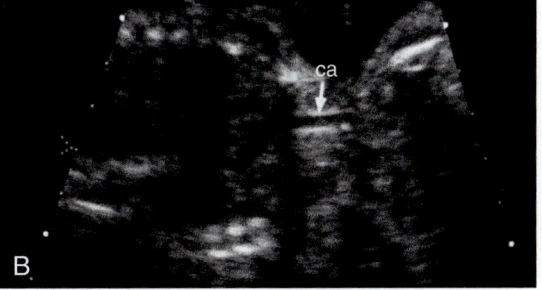

FIG. 51.35 (A) The jugular vein (jv) is observed laterally as it empties into the superior vena cava (sv) with drainage into the right atrium (ra) in a 25-week-old fetus. This sagittal position is helpful in looking for neck masses such as a goiter (enlarged thyroid gland). (B) A carotid artery (ca) is observed in a more medial location coursing cephalad into the brain. *c*, Clavicle.

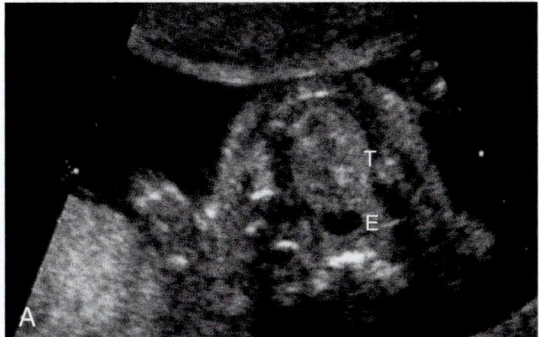 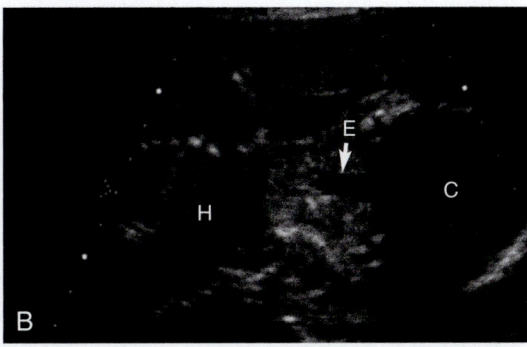

FIG. 51.36 (A) Cross section through the tongue (T) and esophagus (E) or oropharynx in a 24-week-old fetus. Recent swallowing of amniotic fluid by the fetus allows visualization of these structures. (B) Fluid-filled esophagus (E) or oropharynx seen in a longitudinal view. The bolus of swallowed amniotic fluid will travel to the stomach. *C*, Cranium; *H*, heart.

may be observed in the cooperative fetus as they arise from the superior wall of the aortic arch. The innominate artery, left common carotid artery, and left subclavian artery may be identified (Fig. 51.37).

As the vessels course posteriorly, the thoracic aorta and the descending aorta are observed coursing into the bifurcation of the common iliac arteries (Fig. 51.38). The sonographer should recognize the characteristic arterial pulsations from the aorta and its branches. Further divisions of the aorta may be observed as the sonographer views the common iliac vessels, internal iliac vessels, and umbilical arteries that diverge laterally around the bladder (see Fig. 51.41). The external iliac arteries are observed as they enter the femoral arteries. The aorta is observed in a transverse plane to the left of the spine.

The inferior vena cava is identified coursing to the right and parallel with the aorta. Transversely, the inferior vena cava is seen anterior and to the right of the spine. It is important to note that the inferior vena cava appears anterior to the aorta within the chest as the vena cava enters anteriorly at the junction of the right atrium.

The hepatic veins may be imaged in sagittal planes or in cephalad-directed transverse planes. The right, left, and middle hepatic vessels are often delineated and followed as they drain into the inferior vena cava (Fig. 51.39).

Differentiation of a hepatic and portal vessel may be possible by evaluating the thickness of the vessel wall. In general, the walls of the portal vessels are more echogenic than those of hepatic vessels.

Divisions of the inferior vena cava (i.e., renal veins, hepatic veins, and iliac veins) may be observed. When accessing the presence of renal tissue, color mapping of the renal veins is helpful. The superior vena cava may be outlined entering the right atrium from above the heart. By following the superior vena cava into the neck, the jugular veins may be observed.

Fetal Circulation

Fetal oxygenation occurs in the placenta, where small fetal vessels on the surface of the villi are bathed by maternal blood within the intervillous spaces. Fetal basal metabolic rate and

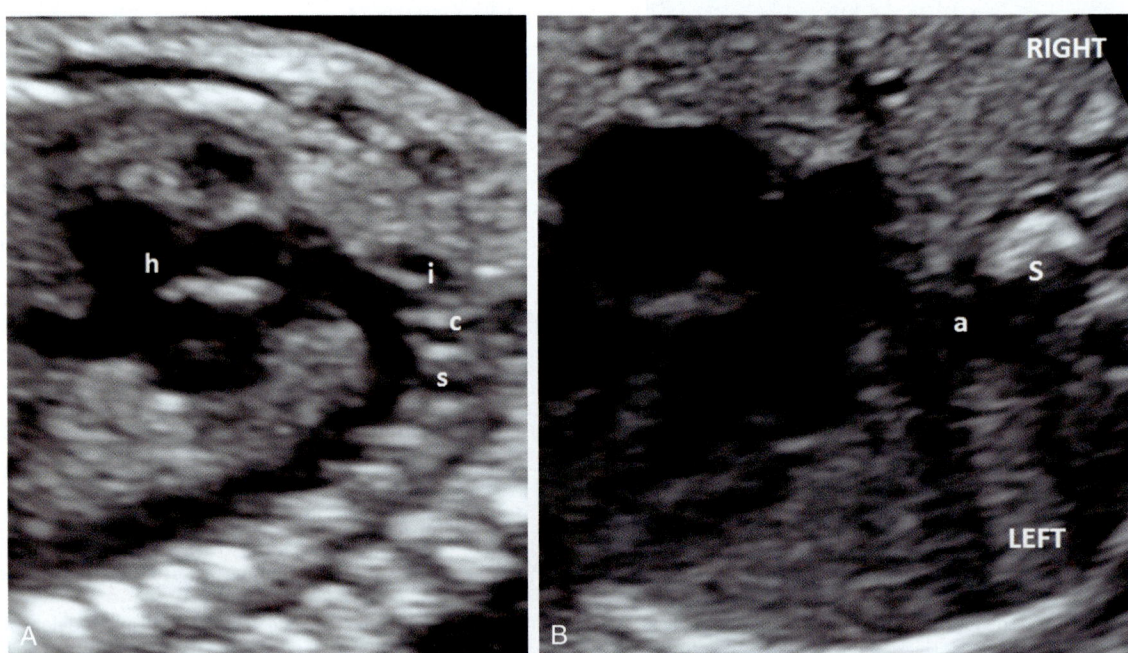

FIG. 51.37 (A) The aortic arch branches are shown in a fetus with an extended neck. (B) Aorta (a) visualized to the left of the spine (S) in a transverse cross section. *c*, Left common carotid artery; *h*, heart; *i*, innominate artery; *s*, left subclavian artery.

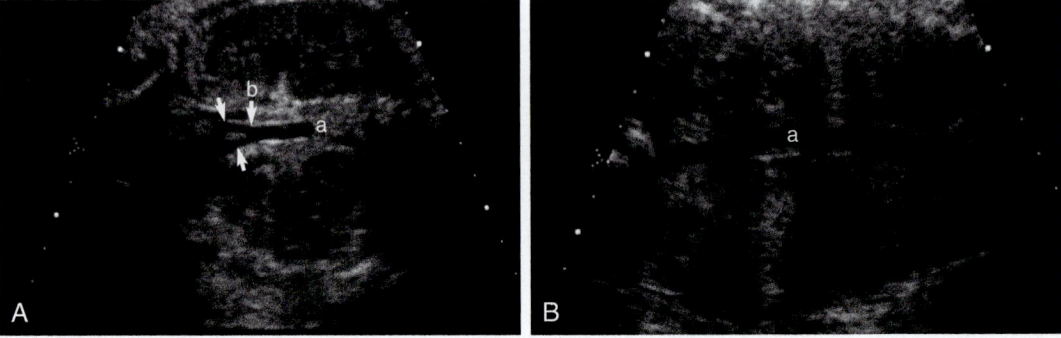

FIG. 51.38 (A) The bifurcation (b) of the aorta (a) into the common iliac arteries *(arrows)* is viewed in a 32-week-old fetus. (B) In the same fetus, a sagittal plane shows the abdominal portion of the aorta.

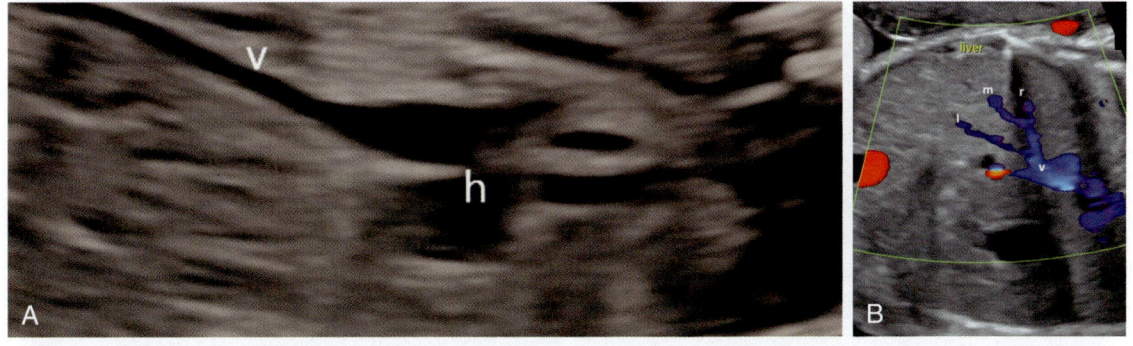

FIG. 51.39 (A) Sagittal view of the inferior vena cava (v) entering the right atrium of the heart (h). (B) The left (l), middle (m), and right (r) hepatic veins are shown emptying into the inferior vena cava (v).

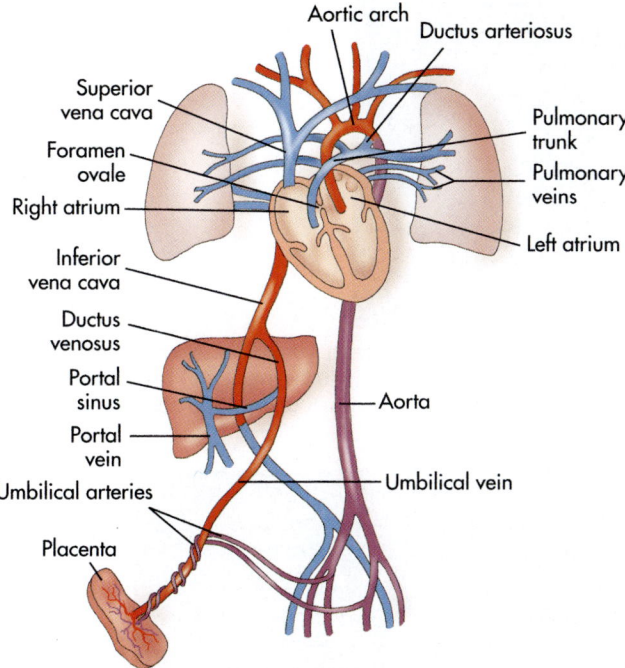

FIG. 51.40 Fetoplacental circulation.

temperature are higher, causing fetal blood levels of essential nutrients to be relatively low compared with maternal blood. Oxygen and nutrients from maternal blood cross by simple diffusion to fetal vessels. Concentrations of waste products, such as urea and creatinine, are higher in fetal blood, and these products diffuse into the maternal circulation.

Fetal circulation differs from postnatal circulation. Fetal circulation bypasses the lungs because the fetal lungs do not oxygenate blood. The ductus arteriosus shunts blood away from the lungs. Fetal circulation shunts oxygenated blood arriving from the placenta away from the abdomen directly to the heart and then to the brain. The hepatobiliary system serves the important function of shunting oxygen-rich blood arriving from the placenta directly to the heart through the ductus venosus (Fig. 51.40).

Oxygenated blood from the placenta flows through the umbilical vein, within the umbilical cord, to the fetal cord insertion, where it enters the abdomen (Fig. 51.41). From the umbilicus, the umbilical vein courses cephalad along the falciform ligament to the liver, where it connects with the left portal vein (Fig. 51.42). The left portal vein courses posteriorly to meet the right anterior and right posterior portal veins (Fig. 51.43). This blood then filters into the liver sinusoids, returning to the inferior vena cava by drainage into the hepatic veins.

A special vascular connection, the ductus venosus, carries oxygen-rich blood from the umbilical vein directly to the inferior vena cava, which empties directly into the right atrium. This blood bypasses the liver. Inferior vena cava blood flows from the right atrium through the left atrium by way of the foramen ovale. This blood bypasses the lungs. Less oxygenated blood from the superior vena cava and a small portion of blood from the inferior vena cava empty into the right atrium and into the right ventricle. The two ventricles pump blood into the systemic circulation at the same time. Blood ejected from the left ventricle flows to the ascending aorta and to the fetal brain. From the right ventricle, the blood courses from the pulmonary artery into the ductus arteriosus and through the descending aorta to provide oxygenated blood to the abdominal organs. Deoxygenated blood exits the fetus through the umbilical arteries, which arise from the fetal iliac arteries. Only 5% to 10% of the blood circulates to the lungs. After birth, the foramen ovale, the ductus venosus, and the ductus arteriosus close; fetal circulation converts to this pattern, as seen throughout the rest of life.

The Hepatobiliary System and Upper Abdomen

The fetal hepatobiliary system includes the liver, portal venous system, hepatic veins and arteries, gallbladder, and bile ducts. Circulation of fetal blood through the ductus venosus in the hepatobiliary system is unique to intrauterine life. The ductus venosus blood flow is a direct link to the fetal heart, and fetal heart failure may be diagnosed by Doppler analysis of flow through the ductus venosus.

The liver is a large organ that fills most of the upper abdomen. The left lobe of the liver is larger than the right lobe because of the large quantity of oxygenated blood flowing through the left lobe. The liver appears pebble-gray and is discerned by its corresponding portal and hepatic vessels. The liver borders may be seen by viewing the diaphragm at

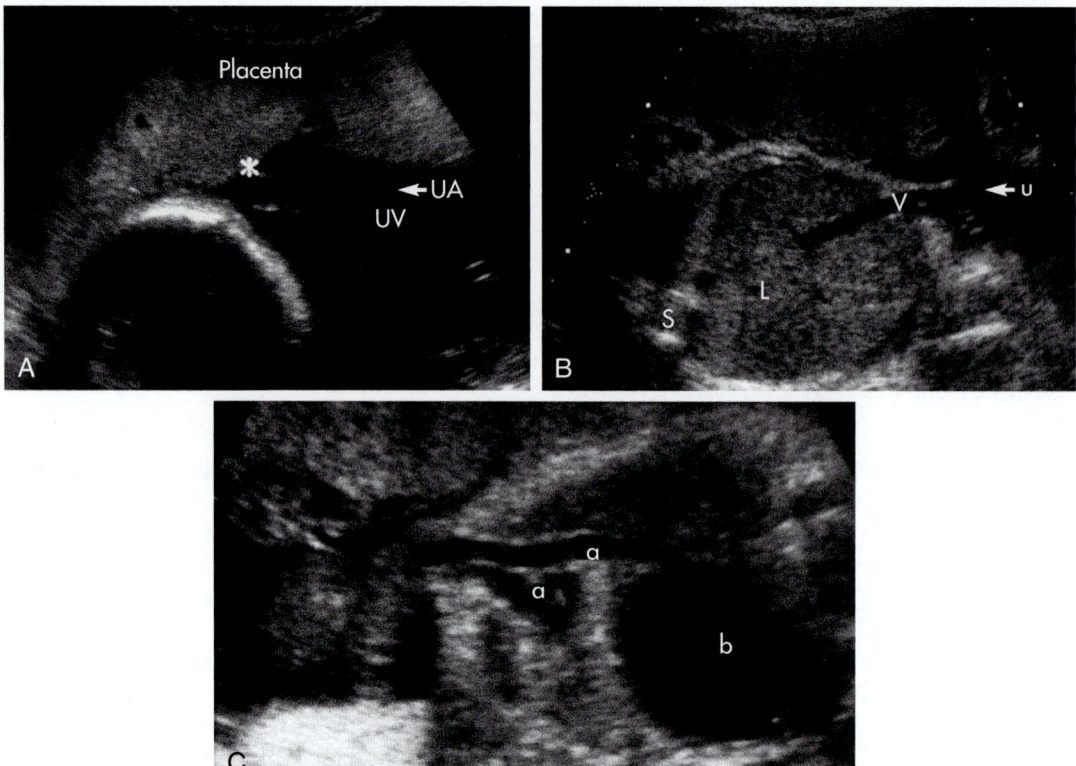

FIG. 51.41 (A) Oxygenated blood leaving the placenta travels through the umbilical vein (UV) to the fetal umbilicus. *Asterisk* denotes placental cord insertion. (B) The umbilical vein (V) after entering at the umbilicus (u) courses cephalad and into the liver (L). (C) The umbilical arteries (a) enter the umbilicus and course laterally around the bladder (b) to meet the common iliac arteries. *S*, Spine; *UA*, umbilical artery.

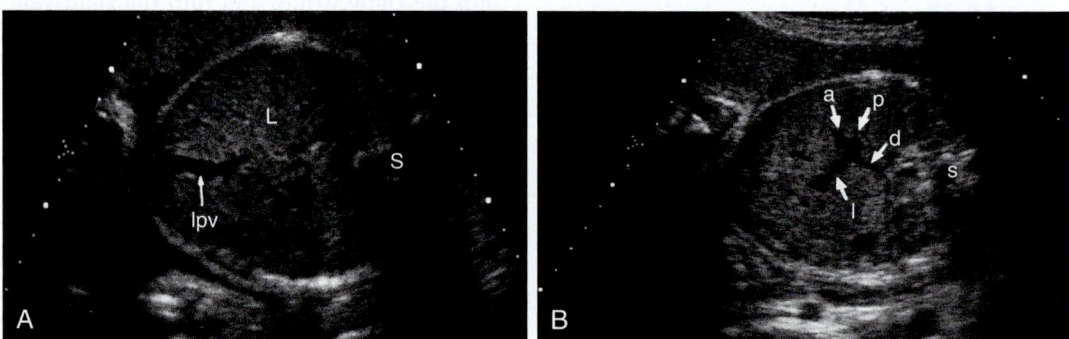

FIG. 51.42 (A) Transverse section of the liver in a 31-week-old fetus outlining the course of the left portal vein (lpv) at its entrance into the liver (L) from the fetal umbilical cord insertion. The left portal vein ascends upward and into the liver tissue. (B) The left portal vein (l) is shown to bifurcate into the portal sinus, right anterior (a), and right posterior (p) portal veins. The ductus venosus (d) is observed before its drainage into the inferior vena cava. *S*, Spine.

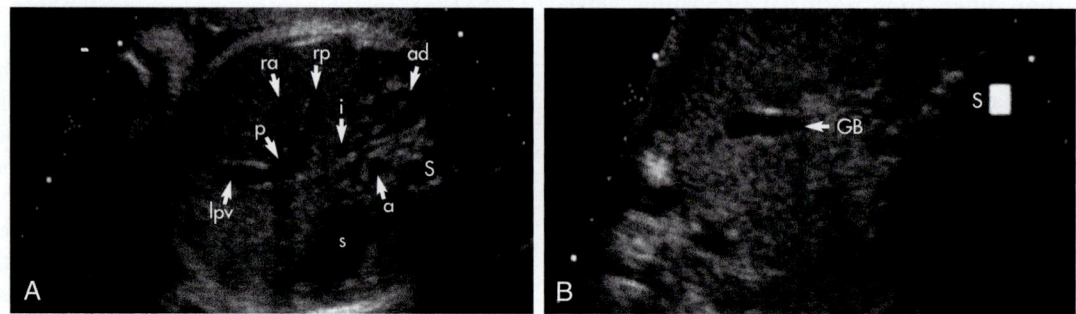

FIG. 51.43 (A) Transverse section of the liver and related structures in a 32-week-old fetus showing the left portal vein (lpv) coursing into the portal sinus (p). The blood then moves into the right anterior (ra) and right posterior (rp) portal veins and ductus venosus. The right adrenal gland (ad), fluid-filled stomach (s), aorta (a), and inferior vena cava (i) are shown. (B) The gallbladder (GB) is viewed in the right upper quadrant of the abdomen in a 32-week-old fetus. The teardrop shape of the gallbladder should be distinguished from the left portal vein. *S*, Spine.

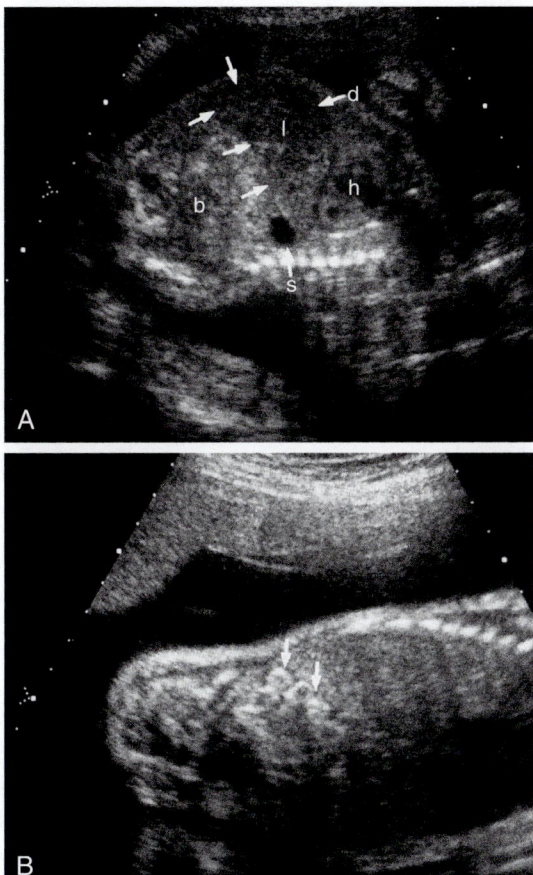

FIG. 51.44 (A) Liver (*l, arrows*) bordered by the diaphragm (*d*) superiorly and the bowel inferiorly in a 29-week-old fetus. (B) Small bowel (*arrows*) pictured as small fluid-filled rings. *b,* Bowel; *h,* heart; *s,* stomach.

the cephalad margin and the small bowel distally in the sagittal plane (Fig. 51.44). The fetal liver is the main storage site for glucose and is very sensitive to disturbances in growth; therefore, this is the site at which abdominal measurements reflect liver size. It is important to check for any collection of fluid around the liver margins because this indicates ascites, that is, fluid retention resulting from anemia, heart failure, or congenital anomalies. Masses of the liver are uncommon but may be detected.

The fetal gallbladder appears as a cone-shaped or teardrop-shaped cystic structure located in the right upper abdomen just below the left portal vein (see Fig. 51.43). The gallbladder should not be misinterpreted as the left portal vein. The left portal vein is a midline vessel that appears more tubular and can be traced back to the umbilical insertion.

The fetal pancreas may be seen posterior to the stomach and anterior to the splenic vein when the fetus is lying with the spine down.

The spleen may be observed by scanning transversely and posteriorly to the left of the stomach (Fig. 51.45). Recognition of the spleen is helpful when assessing the sensitized pregnancy (anti-D) to check for enlargement resulting from increased blood production (hematopoiesis) or to screen for anomalies of the spleen, such as duplication defects.

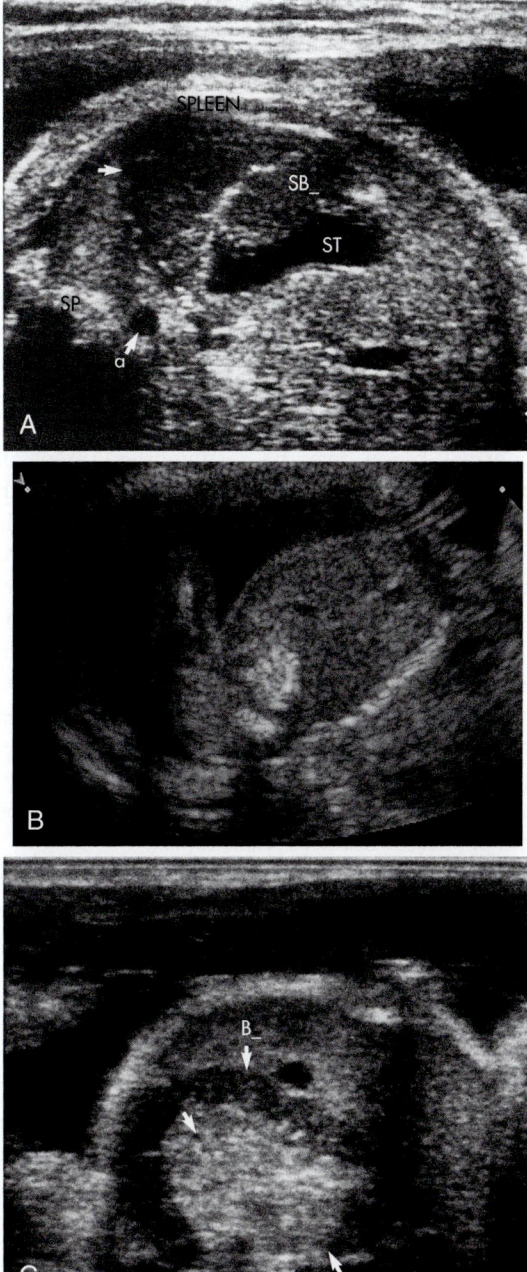

FIG. 51.45 (A) Transverse scan showing the spleen (*arrow*), small bowel (SB), and fluid-filled stomach (ST). (B) Longitudinal view of the fetus demonstrating hyperechoic bowel. (C) Transverse view of the transverse colon (B) and small bowel (*arrows*) in a fetus in a spine-down position. *a,* Aorta; *SP,* spine shadow.

The Gastrointestinal System

The fetal gastrointestinal tract comprises the esophagus, stomach, and small and large intestines (colon). Guidelines for the standard antepartum obstetric examination require the sonographer to image and document the stomach. The esophagus may be recognized after fetal ingestion of amniotic fluid, which may be traced during swallowing into the oral cavity, through the hypopharynx, and as it travels downward toward the stomach (see Fig. 51.36).

The stomach becomes apparent as early as the 11th week of gestation because swallowed amniotic fluid fills the stomach cavity. The full stomach should be seen in all fetuses beyond the 16th week of gestation. Some conditions, such as diminished amounts of amniotic fluid (fetuses with rupture of the membranes) or blockage that prevents the stomach from filling (esophageal atresia), prohibit normal filling of the stomach. On occasion, the stomach has emptied into the small bowel before scanning and is not observed. Repeat studies to confirm the presence of the stomach are warranted. Enlargement of the stomach may occur when a fetus ingests a large quantity of amniotic fluid (non–insulin-dependent diabetic pregnancies) or when a congenital anomaly prohibits normal passage of fluid through the bowel (duodenal atresia).

A normal bowel may be distinguished prenatally by observing characteristic sonographic patterns for each segment. Beyond 20 weeks of gestation, small bowel may be differentiated from large bowel. Small bowel appears to occupy a central position within the lower abdomen, with a cluster appearance of the bowel loops. Peristalsis and even fluid-filled small bowel loops may be observed (see Figs. 51.44 and 51.45).

The large intestine and the ascending, transverse, and descending colon and rectum are identified by their peripheral locations in the lower pelvis (see Fig. 51.45). The large bowel typically contains meconium particles and may measure up to 20 mm in the preterm fetus and even larger near the time of birth or in the postdate fetus.

The echogenicity of the fetal bowel is typically greater than the echogenicity of the fetal liver. If the fetal bowel is as echogenic as fetal bone, this is termed *hyperechoic bowel* (see Fig. 51.45) and is associated with increased risk for aneuploidy and neonatal/childhood pathology.

The Urinary System

Guidelines for the standard obstetric examination require the sonographer to image and document the kidneys and the bladder. The urinary system of the fetus is composed of the kidneys, ureters, and bladder. The adrenal glands are more prominent in the fetus and are seen adjacent to the kidneys.

The kidneys are located on either side of the spine in the posterior abdomen and are apparent as early as the 13th week of pregnancy. The appearance of the developing kidney changes with advancing gestational age. In the second trimester of pregnancy, the kidneys appear as ovoid retroperitoneal structures that lack distinctive borders. The pelvocaliceal center may be difficult to define in early pregnancy, whereas with continued maturation of the kidneys, the borders become more defined, and the renal pelvis becomes more distinct (Fig. 51.46). The renal pelvis appears as an echo-free area in the center of the kidney.

The normal renal pelvis appears to contain a small amount of fluid. This most often represents a normal finding during pregnancy. A measurement of the renal pelvis is typically made in a sagittal view of the fetal kidney when fluid is present. The deepest diameter of the fluid is measured. A renal pelvis that measures greater than 5 mm before 20 weeks of gestational age, greater than 8 mm between 20 and 30 weeks of gestational age, and greater than 10 mm beyond 30 weeks of gestational age is considered abnormal. It is common to see extra fluid within the renal pelvis in fetuses with extra amounts of amniotic fluid and when the mother has a full bladder. Persistent mild bilateral renal pelvis dilation termed *pyelectasis* (Fig. 51.47) has been associated with aneuploidy.

By the third trimester of pregnancy, internal renal anatomy becomes clear with observation of the renal pyramids (lining up in sequence in anterior and posterior rows), the cortex or medulla, and renal margins (perirenal and sinus fat at this age allows clear visualization) (see Figs. 51.45 and 51.46).

The kidneys appear as elliptic structures when scanning in the longitudinal axis and appear circular in their retroperitoneal locations adjacent to the spine in transverse views. Commonly, in a transverse position, the acoustic spine may shadow the bottom or distal kidney. Rotating to the sagittal plane may image the distal kidney. With the fetus in the spine-up or spine-down position, the kidneys are observed lateral to the spine (see Fig. 51.46).

The length, width, thickness, and volume of the kidney have been determined for different gestational ages. This information is useful when a renal malformation is suspected.

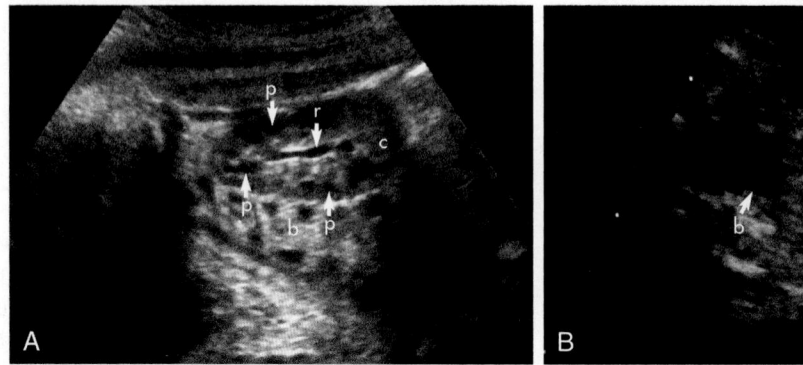

FIG. 51.46 (A) Longitudinal view of the kidney in a 35-week-old fetus showing the renal cortex (c), pelvis, and pyramids (p). The kidney is marginated by the renal capsule, which is highly visible later in pregnancy because of perirenal fat. (B) Sagittal view of the fluid-filled bladder (b) in the pelvis. Note the more cephalic location of the stomach (s) in the upper abdomen. *b*, Bowel; *h*, heart; *L*, liver; *r*, renal pelvis; *arrows*, diaphragm.

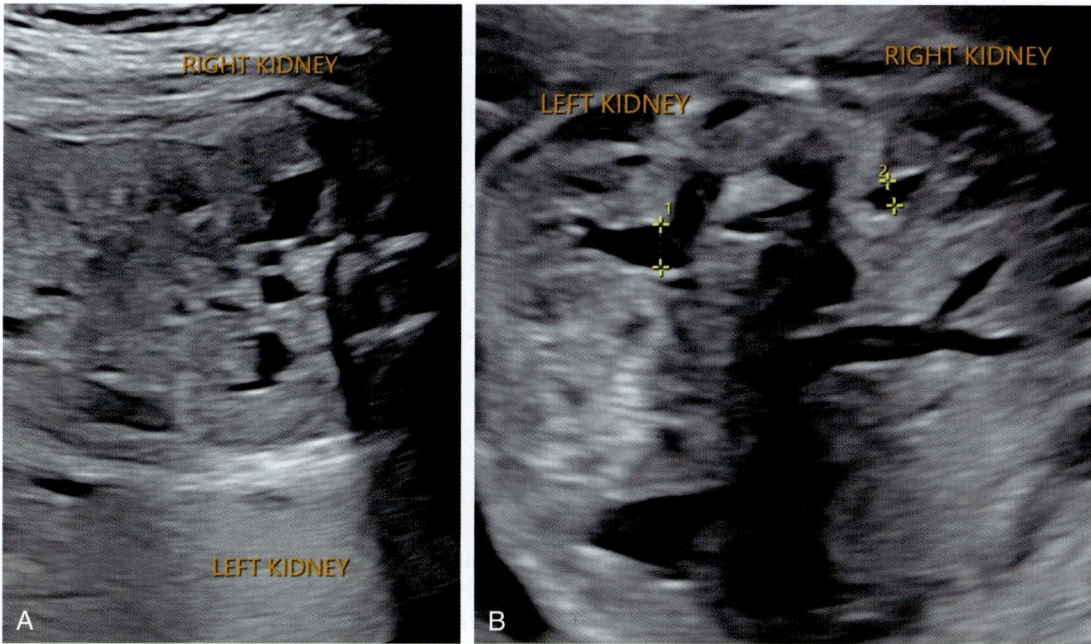

FIG. 51.47 (A) The fetus is lying on its side, the left kidney is seen posterior, and the right kidney anterior with some fluid noted in each renal pelvis. (B) A transverse image demonstrating pyelectasis.

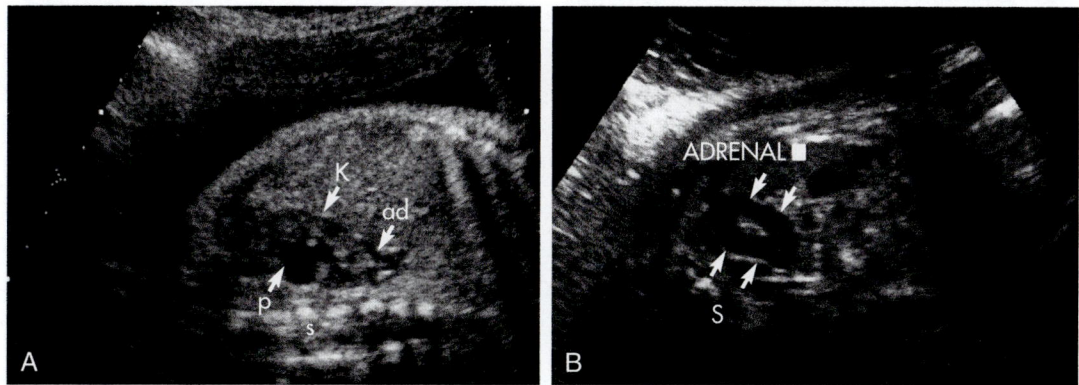

FIG. 51.48 (A) The adrenal gland (ad) is observed in a sagittal view in a 32-week-old fetus. The adrenal is located above the kidney (K) in this spine-down (s) position. The texture of the adrenal gland is similar to that of the kidney; often, when a kidney is missing (agenesis), the adrenal is mistaken for the kidney. (B) The "rice grain" appearance of the adrenal gland *(arrows)* is depicted in this transverse plane in a 36-week-old fetus. Note the dense central interface. *p*, Renal pelvis; *S*, stomach.

The fetal adrenal glands are most frequently observed in a transverse plane just above the kidneys. The adrenals are seen as early as the 20th week of pregnancy and by 23 weeks assume a rice-grain appearance (Fig. 51.48). The center of the adrenal gland appears as a central echogenic line surrounded by tissue that is less echogenic. The central midline interface widens after the 35th week of gestation. The transverse aorta may be used to locate the left adrenal gland because of its proximity to the anterior surface of the gland. Likewise, the inferior vena cava is helpful in isolating the right adrenal gland. Occasionally, the adrenal glands may be identified in sagittal planes, although rib shadowing may interfere with their recognition.

It is important to realize that adrenal glands may normally appear large in utero and should not be confused with the kidneys. The texture of the adrenal gland is similar to that of the kidney; when a kidney is missing (agenesis), the adrenal may be mistaken for the kidney. Nomograms for normal adrenal size are available. Visualization of the renal arteries with color Doppler may be helpful in confirming the presence of kidneys.

At 1 mm, the normal fetal ureter is too small to be recognized. Dilated or obstructed ureters (hydroureter) are readily apparent.

The urinary bladder is visualized in transverse or sagittal sections through the anterior lower pelvis (see Figs. 51.41 and 51.46). The bladder is located in midline and appears as a round, fluid-filled cavity. The size of the bladder varies, depending on the amount of urine contained within the bladder cavity. A fetus generally voids at least once an hour, so failure to see the bladder should prompt the investigator to recheck for bladder filling.

The bladder should be visualized in all normal fetuses. The fetal bladder is an important indicator of renal function. When the bladder and amniotic fluid appear normal, one may assume that at least one kidney is functioning. If one fails to identify the urinary bladder in the presence of oligohydramnios (severe lack of amniotic fluid), one should suspect a renal abnormality or premature rupture of the membranes. In some normal situations, the bladder may not be full because of decreased ingestion of fluid. When the bladder empties in utero, it will typically refill within the time frame of an examination.

Fetal bladder size may appear increased in pregnancies complicated by polyhydramnios (large quantities of amniotic fluid).

The Genitalia

Guidelines for the standard antepartum obstetric examination require the sonographer to image and document the stomach, the kidneys, the bladder, the umbilical cord insertion site, and the number of vessels in the umbilical cord. Documentation of gender is not medically necessary in most pregnancies.

Identification of the male and female genitalia is possible provided the fetal legs are abducted, and a sufficient quantity of amniotic fluid is present. Providing information regarding gender identification is clinically important when a fetus is at risk for a gender-linked disorder such as aqueductal stenosis or hemophilia and in multiple gestations. In multiple pregnancies, there is a medical indication for determining gender as it relates to chorionicity.

Information regarding the gender of the fetus may have significant emotional impact; therefore policies should be established within each department regarding its disclosure. Only sonographers with proven gender detection skills should attempt to provide this information and only with consent of the patient.

When attempting to localize the genitalia, the sonographer should follow the long axis of the fetus toward the hips. The bladder is a helpful landmark within the pelvis by which to identify the anteriorly located genital organs. Tangential scanning planes directed between the thighs are useful in defining the genitalia. The gender of the fetus may be appreciated as early as 12 weeks of gestation. When the fetus is in a breech position, gender may be difficult to determine.

The female genitalia may be seen in a transverse plane. The thighs and labia are identified ventral to the bladder, whereas, in tangential projections, the entire labial folds and often the labia minora are visible (Fig. 51.49). In scans of the perineum obtained parallel to the femora, the shape of the genitalia appears rhomboid (Fig. 51.50). Keep in mind that the labia may appear edematous and swollen owing to circulating maternal hormones. This normal finding should not be confused with the scrotum.

The scrotum and penis are easy to recognize in either scanning plane (Fig. 51.51). The male genitalia may be differentiated as early as the 12th week of pregnancy. The scrotal sac is

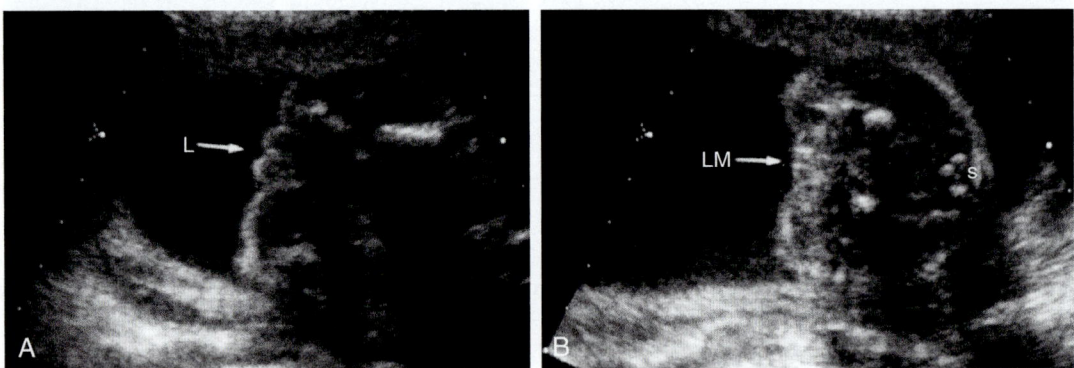

FIG. 51.49 (A) Female genitalia viewed axially in a 23-week-old fetus showing the typical appearance of the labia majora (L). (B) In the same fetus, the labia minora (LM) are represented as linear structures between the labia majora. *s*, Spine.

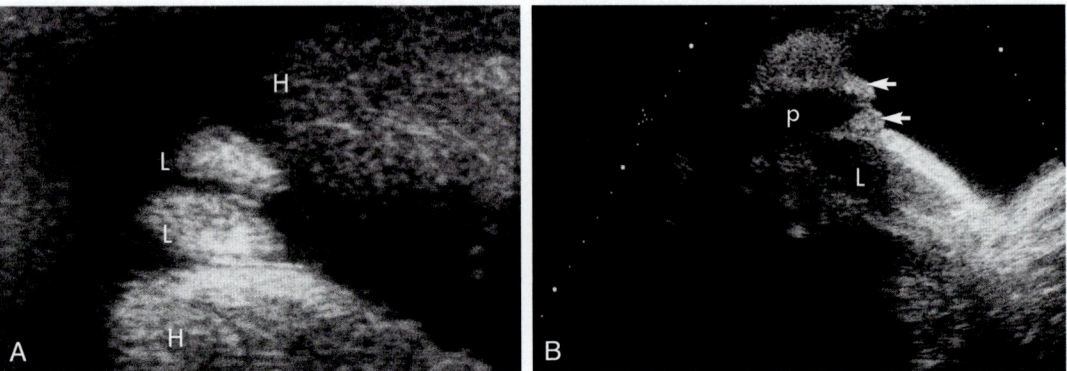

FIG. 51.50 (A) The labia majora (L) are imaged in a sagittal plane. (B) The rhomboid-shaped perineum (p) is shown in a plane that runs parallel to the femur (L). The labia *(arrows)* are observed in a more frontal plane. *H*, Hips.

seen as a mass of soft tissue between the hips with the scrotal septum and testicles. Fluid around the testicles—hydrocele—is a common benign finding during intrauterine life.

The Upper and Lower Extremities

Guidelines for the standard obstetric examination require the sonographer to verify the presence or absence of legs and arms. The fetal limbs are accessible to both anatomic and biometric surveillance. Bones of the upper and lower skeleton have been described extensively, and many nomograms detailing normal growth patterns for each limb have been generated.

Fetal long-bone measurements help assess fetal age and growth and allow detection of skeletal dysplasias and various congenital limb malformations. Short femora and a short humerus are associated with increased risk for aneuploidy. The sonographer may not only measure fetal limb bones but also survey the anatomic configurations of individual bones whenever possible for evidence of bowing, fracture, or demineralization, as seen in several common forms of skeletal dysplasia.

The upper extremity consists of the humerus, elbow, radius, ulna, wrist, metacarpals, and phalanges.

The humerus is found in a sagittal plane by moving the probe laterally away from the ribs and scapula. The long axis of the humerus should be seen lateral to the scapular echo. The cartilaginous humeral head is noted, as is the cartilage at the elbow (Fig. 51.52). The shaft of the humerus should be seen, along with its characteristic acoustic shadow.

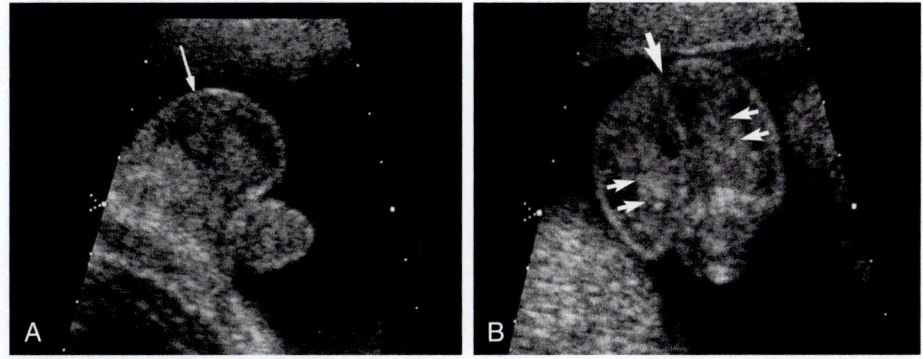

FIG. 51.51 (A) Male genitalia in a 40-week-old fetus showing the scrotum *(arrow)* and phallus. (B) Coronal view of the male genitalia outlining descended testicles *(double arrows)* within the scrotum. Note the scrotal septum *(thick arrow)* and phallus.

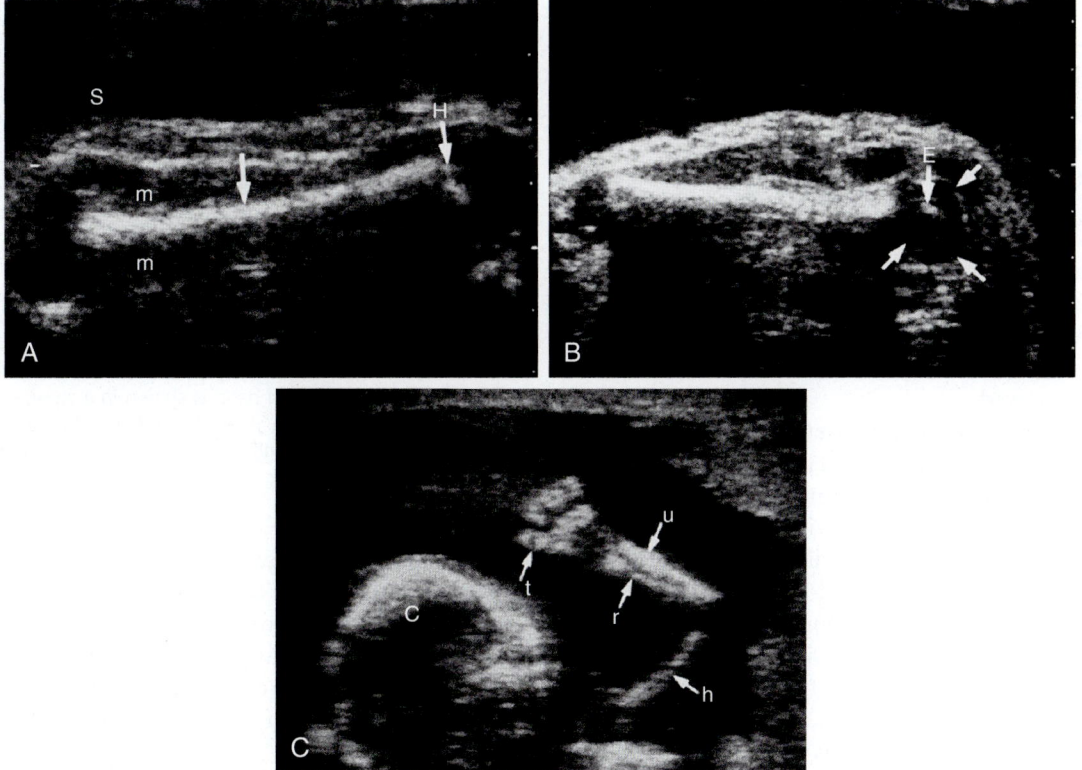

FIG. 51.52 (A) Longitudinal scan of the humeral shaft with the humeral head (H) near the shoulder (s). Note the muscles (m) lateral to the bones and the skin interface (S). (B) Similar section of a humerus in a 39-week-old fetus identifying the proximal humeral epiphysis (E) within the humeral cartilage *(arrows)*. (C) Sagittal image of the fetal humerus (*h*). *C*, Cranium; *r*, radius; *t*, thumb; *u*, ulna.

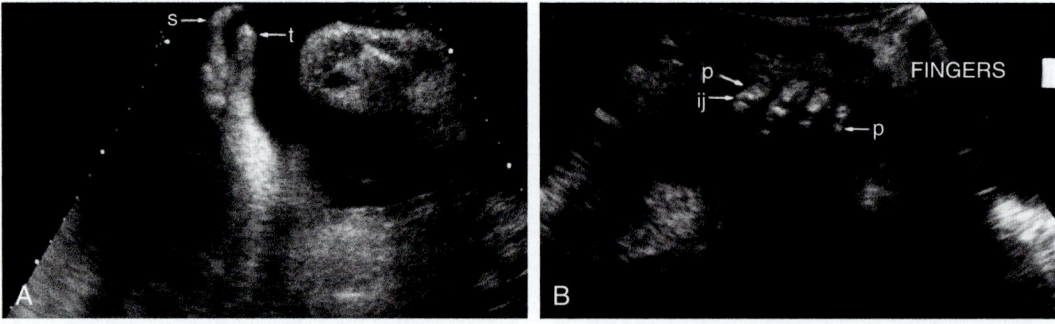

FIG. 51.53 (A) Lateral view of the hand showing the thumb (t) and second finger (s) in a 36-week-old fetus. (B) Curvature of the hand in a 30-week-old fetus showing the phalanges (p) of the second through fifth fingers. The thumb is not imaged in this view because it is located slightly lower. Note the interphalangeal joints (ij) between the phalanges.

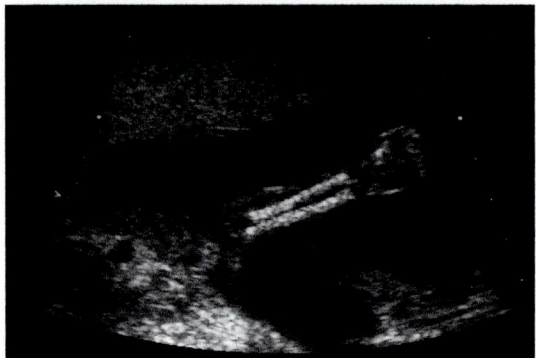

FIG. 51.54 Long section of the forearm; the radius is shorter than the ulna (seen along the posterior forearm). The closed fist is shown with the thumb closest to the anterior surface.

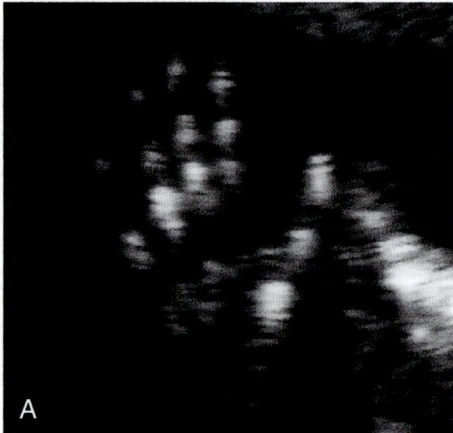
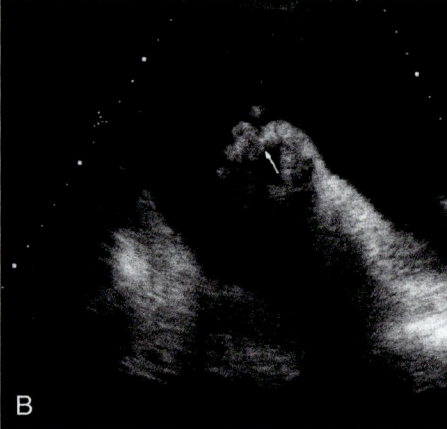

FIG. 51.55 (A) An open hand is shown in a 24-week-old fetus. (B) A closed hand is viewed in a 38-week-old fetus with the thumb crossing in front of the palm of the hand *(arrow)*, with the second through fifth digits identified above the thumb.

The muscles and skin may be noted. Epiphyseal ossification centers may be apparent around the 39th week of pregnancy. In transverse planes, the humerus appears as a solitary bone surrounded by muscle and skin.

By tracing the humerus to the elbow, the radius and ulna are imaged (Fig. 51.53; see also Fig. 51.52). In transverse sections, two bones are seen as echogenic dots, whereas in a sagittal plane, the long axis of each is identified. The laterally positioned ulna projects deeper into the elbow, which is helpful in differentiating this bone from the medially located radius. When the transducer is moved downward, the wrist and hand are observed.

The hands and fingers may be viewed, and it should be noted whether the hands are clenched throughout the examination or if they open and close normally. When the fingers are viewed in the sagittal plane, individual phalanges, interphalangeal joints, metacarpals, and digits may be observed (Figs. 51.54 and 51.55; see also Figs. 51.52 and 51.53). Hand movement counts as a positive demonstration of fetal tone that is one component of the biophysical profile. Individual fingers can often be counted even in the first trimester. It is important to observe the hands if an anomaly is suspected, as in chromosome disorders, such as trisomy 18, in which clenching of the hands is common.

Adequate amounts of amniotic fluid are essential in evaluating the hands or feet. With oligohydramnios, the extremities may be difficult to localize. Fetal position may also prevent adequate visualization of the extremities.

Nomograms have been generated that relate the lengths of the humerus, radius, and ulna to gestational age assessment. These values are also beneficial in diagnosing abnormal developmental growth of the extremities, as seen in certain skeletal dysplasias.

Similar to the upper extremity, the bones of the lower extremity are visualized and measured both for gestational age dating and for detecting limb anomalies. The femur is the most widely measured long bone and can be found by moving the transducer along the fetal body to the fetal bladder. At this junction, the iliac wings are noted. By moving the transducer inferior to the iliac crests, the femoral echo comes into view. With the transducer centered over the femoral echo, one should rotate the probe until the shaft (diaphysis) of the femur is observed. In this view, the cartilaginous femoral head, muscles, and occasionally the femoral artery are noted (Fig. 51.56).

The distal femoral epiphysis is seen within the cartilage at the knee (see Fig. 51.56), and this signifies a gestational age beyond 33 to 35 weeks of gestation. At the tibial end, the proximal tibial epiphyseal center is found after the 35th week of pregnancy (Fig. 51.57). Medially, the tibia and the laterally positioned fibula (see Fig. 51.57) are noted. The tibia is larger than the fibula.

The ankle, calcaneus, and foot are viewed at the most distal point (Fig. 51.58). The diagnosis of clubfeet may be suspected when persistent and abnormal flexion of the ankle is seen. Individual metatarsals and toes are frequently seen (see Fig. 51.58). Like the hands, fetal feet may have malformations, such as extra digits, overlapping, and splaying.

EXTRAFETAL OBSTETRIC EVALUATION

After the fetus has been studied, evaluation of the placenta, amniotic fluid, umbilical cord, and pelvis is recommended.

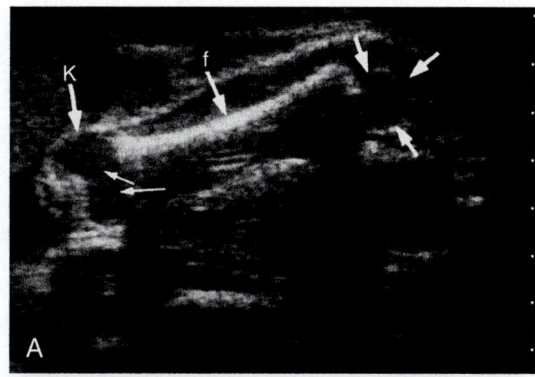
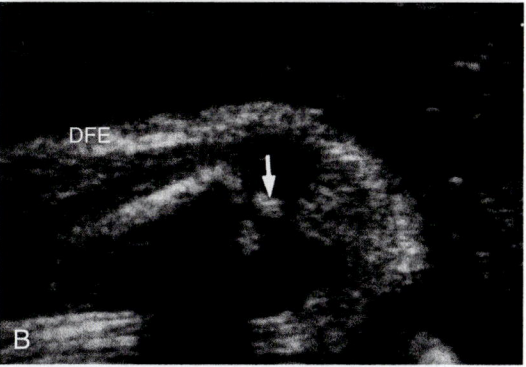

FIG. 51.56 (A) Longitudinal section showing the femoral shaft (f), with the femoral cartilage *(thick arrows)* and epiphyseal cartilage *(thin arrows)* shown at the knee (K). (B) The distal femoral epiphysis *(arrow)* is clearly shown within the epiphyseal cartilage at the knee in a 42-week-old fetus. *DFE,* Distal femoral epiphysis.

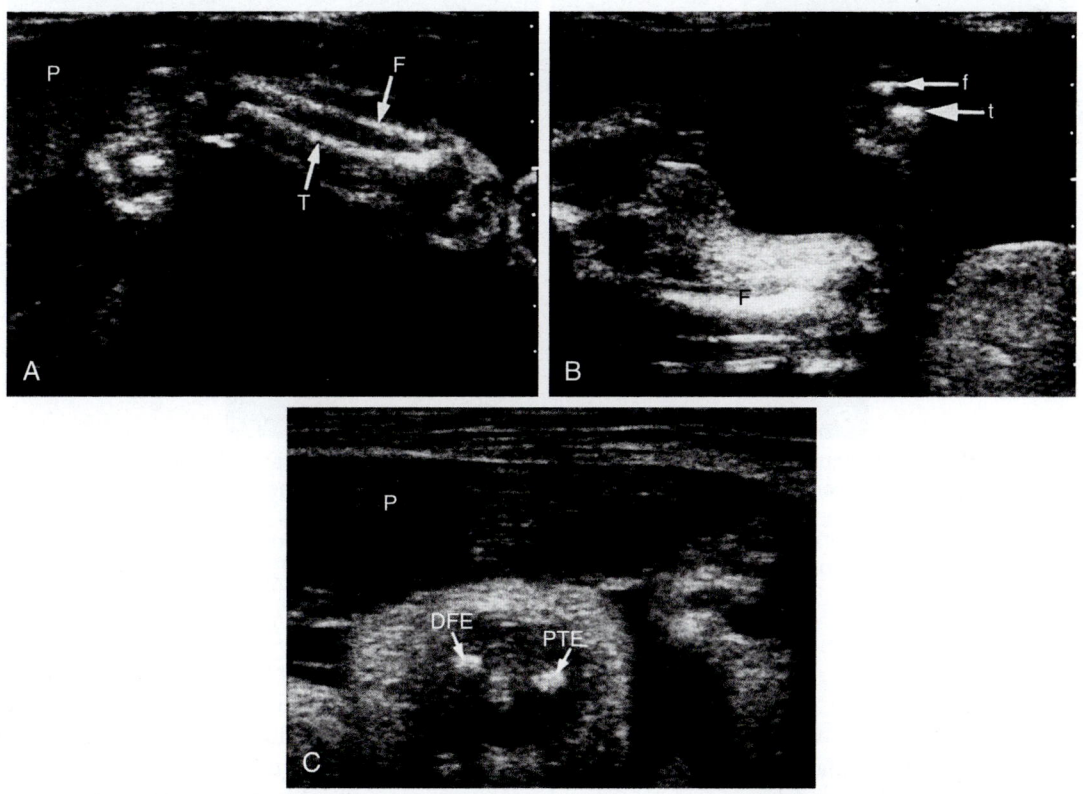

FIG. 51.57 (A) Sagittal view of the medially positioned tibia (T) and the laterally positioned fibula (F). (B) In the same fetus, a transverse cross section reveals the two bones. (C) View of the knee in a 42-week-old fetus showing both the distal femoral epiphysis (DFE) and the proximal tibial epiphysis (PTE). *f,* Opposite femur; *P,* placenta; *t,* tibia.

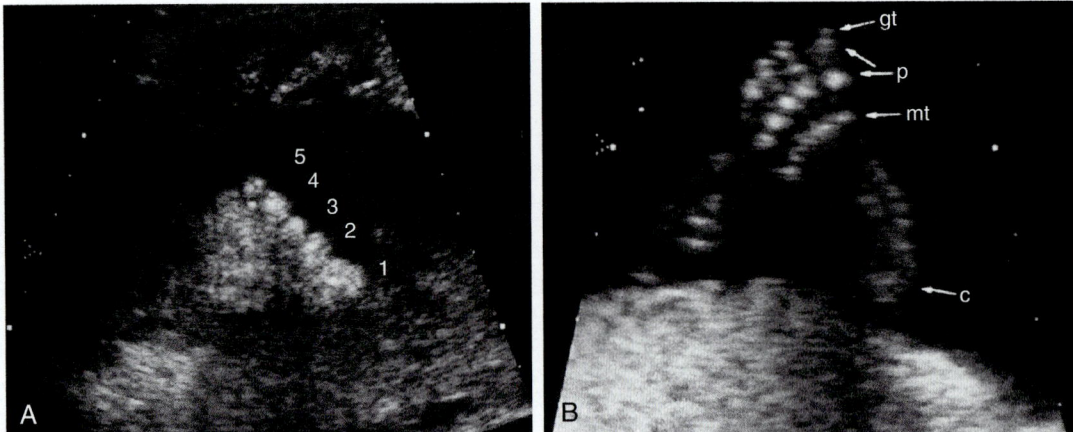

FIG. 51.58 (A) Five toes (1 to 5) viewed on end in a 38-week-old fetus. Note the continuity and shape of each toe. Extra toes, webbing, or clefts are considered abnormal. (B) Plantar foot view in a 20-week-old fetus showing five toes and ossified metatarsals (mt) and phalanges (p). *c*, Calcaneus; *gt*, great toe.

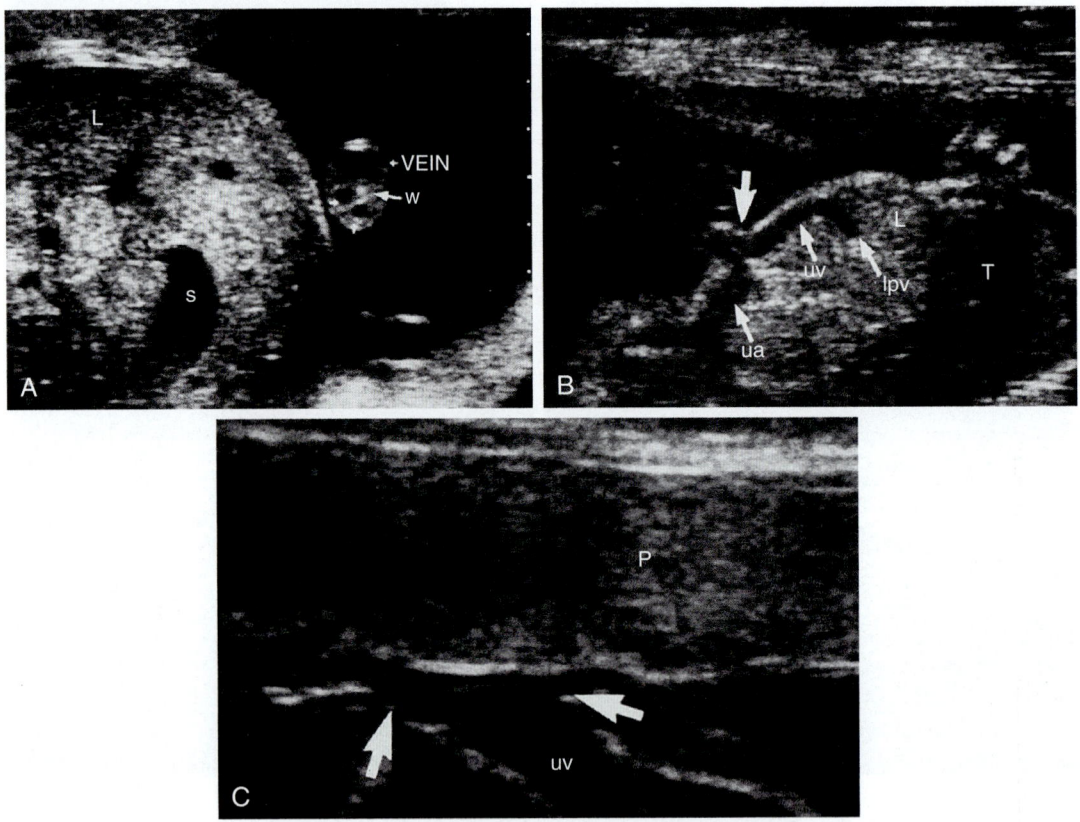

FIG. 51.59 (A) A three-vessel umbilical cord is shown in a transverse plane represented as paired umbilical arteries and a single larger umbilical vein. The vessels are supported by the gelatinous Wharton jelly (w). A cross section of the liver (L) and stomach (s) is in view. (B) Fetal insertion of the umbilical cord into the umbilicus in a sagittal plane *(large arrow)*. The umbilical vein (uv) courses superiorly to enter the liver and becomes the left portal vein (lpv), whereas the umbilical arteries (ua) course posteriorly to join the hypogastric arteries. (C) Placental insertion of the umbilical cord showing the umbilical vein (uv) at this junction *(arrows)*. *P*, Anterior placenta; *T*, thoracic cavity.

The Umbilical Cord

Guidelines for the standard antepartum obstetric examination require the sonographer to image and document the umbilical cord insertion site and the number of vessels in the umbilical cord. The normal human umbilical cord contains an umbilical vein and two umbilical arteries (Fig. 51.59). The umbilical vein transports oxygenated blood from the placenta, whereas the paired umbilical arteries return deoxygenated blood from the iliac arteries of the fetus to the placenta for purification. The umbilical cord is identified at the cord insertion into the placenta and at the junction of the cord into the fetal umbilicus. The arteries spiral with the larger umbilical vein, which is surrounded by Wharton jelly (material that

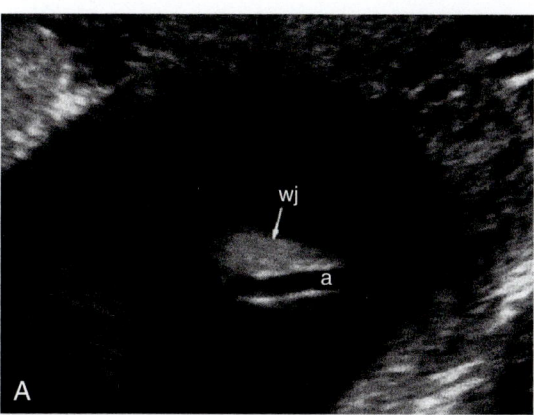 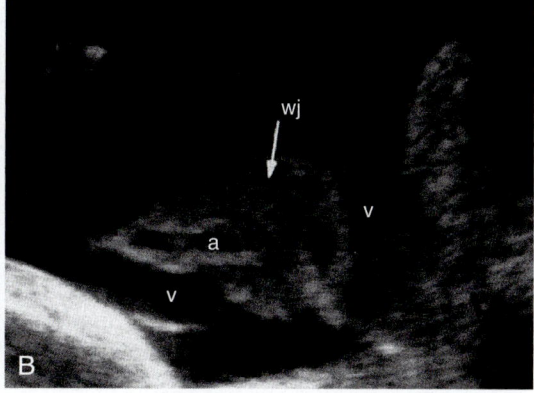

FIG. 51.60 (A) Wharton jelly (wj) observed in a 30-week-old fetus. One of the umbilical arteries (a) is in view. (B) Wharton jelly is present adjacent to one of the umbilical arteries, and the single umbilical vein (v) is observed in a 35-week-old fetus. Wharton jelly is an important structure to recognize in performing cordocentesis procedures when the needle is directed into the cord vessels.

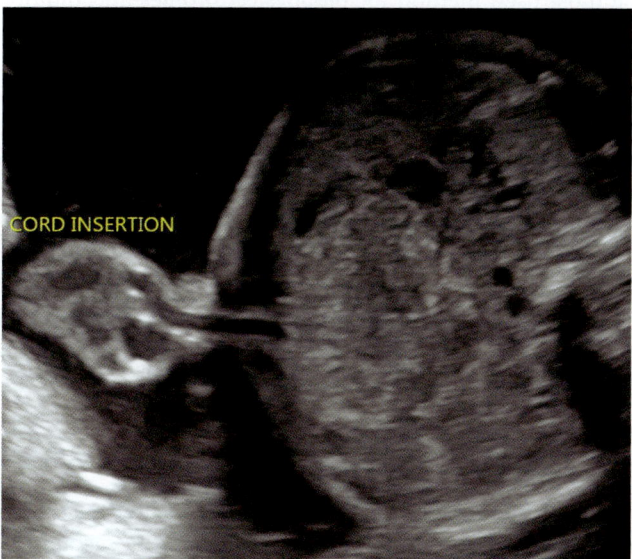

FIG. 51.61 Umbilical cord insertion into the fetal abdomen.

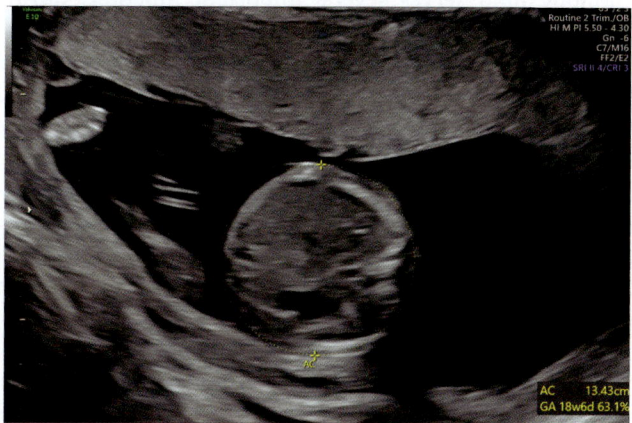

FIG. 51.62 The homogeneous placenta is shown along the anterior wall of the uterus. The fetal abdomen is seen in cross section.

supports the cord) (Fig. 51.60). Absent cord twists may be associated with a poor pregnancy outcome. The cord is easily imaged in both sagittal and transverse sections. The umbilical vein diameter increases throughout gestation, reaching a maximum diameter of 0.9 cm by 30 weeks of gestation.

When cord is seen on both sides of the fetal neck, color Doppler may be used to visualize nuchal cord or encirclement of cord around the fetal neck. Multiple loops of nuchal cord have been identified with color Doppler.

Identification of the placental insertion of the cord is important in choosing a site for amniocentesis and in selecting the appropriate site for other invasive procedures. Rarely, the umbilical insertion is atypically located (velamentous insertion).

Insertion of the cord into the fetal umbilicus should be routinely scrutinized in all fetuses because anterior abdominal wall defects are present at this level. Use of color Doppler imaging at this location may demonstrate two umbilical arteries traveling on either side of the fetal bladder toward the iliac. This image confirms two arteries and aids in three-vessel identification (Fig. 51.61).

The uterus and ovaries should be scrutinized for large masses, such as fibroids or ovarian masses, that may alter pregnancy management. This evaluation may be accomplished by surveying the lateral borders of the uterus from the cervix to the fundus along both lateral margins while following both sagittal and transverse axes.

The Placenta

The main role of the placenta is to permit the exchange of oxygenated maternal blood (rich in oxygen and nutrients) with deoxygenated fetal blood. Maternal vessels coursing posterior to the placenta circulate blood into the placenta, whereas blood from the fetus reaches this point through the umbilical cord.

The substance of the placenta assumes a relatively homogeneous pebble-gray appearance during the first part of pregnancy and is easily recognized with its characteristically smooth borders (Fig. 51.62). The position of the placenta is readily apparent in most obstetric ultrasound studies. The placenta may be located within the fundus of the uterus along the anterior, lateral, or posterior uterine walls (Fig. 51.63), or it may be implanted over or near the cervix. The sonographer should attempt to carefully define the entire length of the placenta and should document both upper and lower margins of this organ.

The placenta may originate close to the fundus and extend along the anterior wall (anterior placenta) or along the posterior uterine wall (posterior placenta). When the placenta appears to lie on both anterior and posterior uterine walls, check for a laterally positioned placenta. By moving the transducer laterally, one should be able to define the lateral placenta.

The Amniotic Fluid

Amniotic fluid serves several important functions during intrauterine life. It allows the fetus to move freely within the amniotic cavity while maintaining intrauterine pressure and protecting the developing fetus from injury. The umbilical cord and membranes, lungs, skin, and kidneys all contribute to the production of amniotic fluid. Fetal urination into the amniotic sac accounts for most of the total volume of amniotic fluid by the second half of pregnancy, and the quantity of fluid is directly related to kidney function. A fetus lacking kidneys or with malformed kidneys produces little or no amniotic fluid. The amount of amniotic fluid is regulated not only by the production of amniotic fluid but also by removal of fluid by swallowing, by fluid exchange within the lungs, and by the membranes and cord. Normal lung development is critically dependent on the exchange of amniotic fluid within the lungs. Inadequate lung development may occur when severe oligohydramnios is present, placing the fetus at high risk for developing small or hypoplastic lungs.

The volume of amniotic fluid increases until the 34th week of gestation and then slowly diminishes. The investigator must be aware of relative differences in amniotic fluid volume throughout pregnancy. During the second and early third trimesters of pregnancy, amniotic fluid appears to surround the fetus and should be readily apparent (Fig. 51.64). From 20 to 30 weeks of gestation, amniotic fluid may appear somewhat generous, although this typically represents a normal amniotic fluid variant. By the end of pregnancy, amniotic fluid is scanty, and isolated fluid pockets may be the only visible areas of fluid. Subjective observation of amniotic fluid volumes throughout pregnancy helps the sonographer determine the norm and extremes of amniotic fluid.

Several semiquantitative methods of estimating amniotic fluid volume have been developed. Measurement of the deepest vertical pocket of fluid in each of the four quadrants of the uterus and measurement of the single deepest pocket in the sac are two such methods. The deepest vertical pocket is the most used method for biophysical profiles and multiple pregnancy examinations.

Amniotic fluid generally appears echo free, although occasionally fluid particles (particulate matter) may be seen. Vernix caseosa (fatty material found on fetal skin and in amniotic fluid late in pregnancy) may be seen within the amniotic fluid.

In accordance with the guidelines for obstetric scanning, every obstetric examination should include an evaluation of amniotic fluid volume. When extremes in amniotic fluid volume (polyhydramnios or oligohydramnios) are found, targeted studies for the exclusion of fetal anomalies are recommended.

The Membranes

The inner membrane (the amnion) and the outer membrane (the chorion) typically are not seen during the second and third trimesters. The amnion is contiguous with the membrane lining the umbilical cord. At the site of umbilical cord

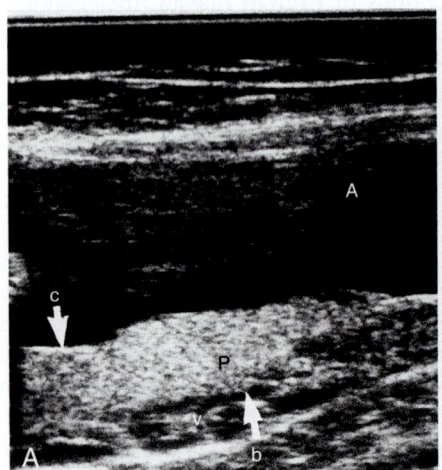 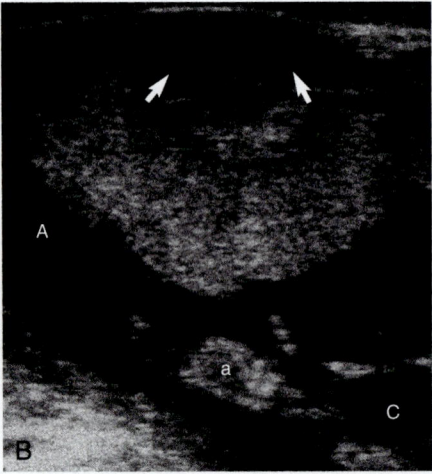 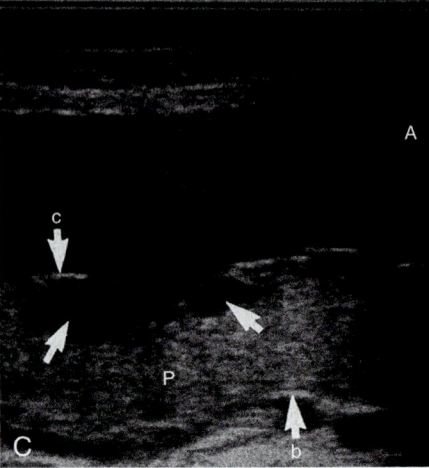

FIG. 51.63 (A) Posterior placenta (P) at 21 weeks of gestation showing the chorionic plate (c), adjacent to the amniotic cavity (A), and the basal plate (b), closest to the maternal (endometrial) vessels (v). (B) Anterior placenta (P) at 14 weeks of gestation with evidence of a Braxton-Hicks contraction *(arrows)*. (C) Posterior placenta at 26 weeks of gestation showing several subchorionic cystic spaces *(arrows)* that represent blood vessels or fibrin deposits. *A*, Amniotic fluid; *a*, fetal abdomen; *b*, basal plate; *C*, fetal cranium; *c*, chorionic plate.

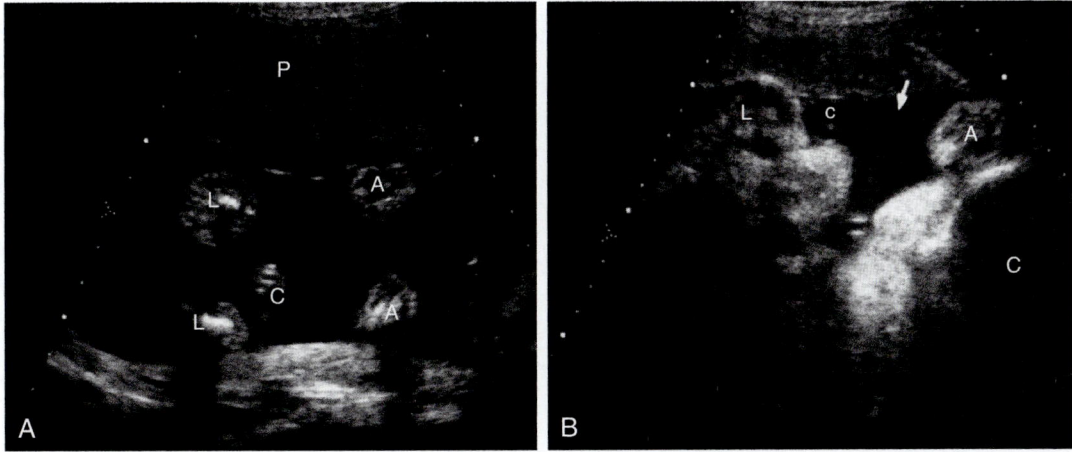

FIG. 51.64 (A) Amniotic fluid in a 20-week pregnancy outlining the legs (L) and arms (A). This is a typical appearance of the abundance of amniotic fluid during this period of pregnancy. (B) Amniotic fluid *(arrow)* in a 35-week pregnancy demonstrating an amniotic fluid pocket *(arrow)* surrounded by fetal parts and the placenta. The amount of amniotic fluid compared with the fetus and placenta is less at this stage of pregnancy. *C*, Cranium; *c*, umbilical cord; *P*, placenta.

insertion into the placenta, the amnion spreads out over the surface of the chorionic surface of the placenta. At the edge of the placenta, the amnion lies over the smooth chorion lining the uterine wall. When there is a break in the amnion, fluid can infuse between the amnion and chorion. If fluid is seen under a membrane floating on top of the placenta and anchored at the placental cord insertion, this is a subamniotic collection. If fluid is seen under a membrane and fluid collection ends at the edge of the placenta, it is a subchorionic collection.

The Cervix

The uterine cervix in pregnancy can be visualized with abdominal scanning when the maternal bladder is partially full; however, transabdominal cervical measurements are not acceptable. Image quality is better, and the cervical measurements reproducible when the cervix is visualized and measured using transvaginal or transperineal imaging. When the cervix appears shortened or funneling is suspected during the abdominal scan, when the patient has risk factors for incompetent cervix or spontaneous preterm birth, when preterm labor is suspected, or whenever a measurement of the cervix is requested, transperineal or transvaginal imaging of the cervix is added to the second-trimester examination. The normal cervix in pregnancy measures 3 cm or longer. The standard criteria for measurement of the cervix are listed in Box 51.2. If the cervix is shortened, or if the internal os appears to have a V or U shape, it may be important to monitor and/or treat.

GENETIC SONOGRAM

A common type of specialized second-trimester obstetric sonography examination is called the **genetic sonogram**. In a genetic sonogram, the patient's individual risk for aneuploidy is adjusted on the basis of sonographic findings. The genetic sonogram includes all elements of the standard obstetric

> **BOX 51.2 Standard Criteria for Measurement of the Cervix**
>
> Measurement is taken on a transvaginal image.
> The transvaginal image is filled primarily with the cervix, and the field of view is optimized for the measurement.
> - The cervix occupies approximately 75% of the image.
> - The bladder area is visible.
>
> The maternal bladder is empty.
> The internal os is seen.
> The external os is seen.
> The endocervical canal is visible throughout.
> Caliper placement is correct.
> - Measure extends from where the walls of the cervix touch at the interior and external os.
> - Calipers do not extend to the outermost edge of the cervical tissue.
> - Calipers extend along the cervical canal.
> - If the cervix is curved, two or more linear measures are taken and added together.
>
> Cervix mobility is considered.
> - The cervix is observed for 3–5 min to watch for shortening or funneling.
> - Apply mild suprapubic or fundal pressure to watch for funneling.

examination with additional attention to anatomic markers for aneuploidy. The markers that are typically evaluated include the nuchal fold, echogenic bowel, humerus length, femur length, EIF, and renal pyelectasis.

Researchers have defined statistical **likelihood ratios** for aneuploidy for each of these *anatomy markers*. For example, a fetus with echogenic bowel may have a risk (or likelihood) for aneuploidy that is increased sixfold. The probability that a fetus with echogenic bowel may have an aneuploidy is six times greater than the probability for a fetus without echogenic bowel. Because these markers are independent and are also independent of age and biochemistry, the probabilities for each element can be multiplied together to determine individual risk.

Patients enter a genetic sonogram with a risk for aneuploidy determined by age or biochemistry. This risk may be increased if a single marker is found by a factor consistent with the likelihood ratio associated with that finding. For example, if a 35-year-old woman enters a genetic sonogram with a risk of 1 in 200 and echogenic bowel is found, the risk can be adjusted, that is, increased, to 1 in 33. If two or more anatomic markers are documented, the risk is increased even further.

Somewhat more controversial is lowering risk by a factor of one-half or more if no anatomic markers are found. For example, a patient at age 35 with an aneuploidy risk of approximately 1 in 200 may have that risk lowered by a factor of one-half or more with a normal sonogram. This patient would be counseled regarding a risk level of approximately 1 in 400.

The genetic sonogram and risk adjustment based on sonographic findings in the second trimester should be limited to centers with specialty expertise and partnered with genetic counselors and resources. The anatomic markers must be interpreted carefully, and experience can eliminate errors associated with assignment of markers such as hyperechoic bowel or EIF that include subjective assessment of echogenicity.

If the patient has had the combined test for aneuploidy risk assessment or a cell-free DNA test during the first trimester, the genetic sonogram should not be used or used only with caution in the second trimester. Because most Down syndrome fetuses are detected by testing in the first trimester, the likelihood of detecting Down syndrome with sonographic factors in the second trimester is greatly reduced. The anatomy markers may still be assessed in relation to fetal issues but should not be used to adjust risk for aneuploidy. For example, echogenic bowel may relate to cystic fibrosis, and an increased nuchal fold may relate to Noonan syndrome. The EIF and other minor markers are not useful for patients who have had first-trimester aneuploidy screening.

ACKNOWLEDGMENT

Mid-South Maternal Fetal Medicine, PC, and Roy Bors-Koefoed, MD, are acknowledged for their contribution of sonographic images to this chapter. The author also acknowledges the work of Jean Lea Spitz on this chapter in the previous edition.

Key Pearls

- Fetal anatomy may be accurately assessed after 18 weeks of gestation, although structures may be seen earlier in many pregnancies.
- To perform a complete evaluation of the fetus during the second and third trimesters, the sonographer should follow a specific protocol that includes, at a minimum, the components recommended for a standard examination.
- The protocol for second- and third-trimester sonography examinations includes a biometric and anatomic survey of the fetus.
- The second- and third-trimester standard sonography examination requires current two-dimensional real-time sonography equipment with transabdominal and transvaginal capability.
- Doppler capabilities facilitate evaluation of amniotic fluid volume, the umbilical cord, and specialty evaluations of the fetal heart and other aspects of fetal and maternal circulation.
- Three-dimensional equipment can record the volume of a targeted anatomic region and represents an advance in imaging technology.

BIBLIOGRAPHY

Abuhamad AZ, Benacerraf BR, Woletz P, Burke BL. The accreditation of ultrasound practices: impact on compliance with minimum performance guidelines. *J Ultrasound Med.* 2004;23:1023–1029.

Benacerraf B. The significance of the nuchal fold in the second trimester fetus. *Prenat Diagn.* 2002;22:798–801.

Bromley B, Benacerraf BR. The genetic sonogram scoring index. *Semin Perinatol.* 2003;27:124–129.

Callen P. *Ultrasonography in obstetrics and gynecology.* ed 6. Philadelphia: Elsevier; 2017.

Chauhan SP, Doherty DD, Magann EF, et al. Amniotic fluid index vs single deepest pocket technique during modified biophysical profile: a randomized clinical trial. *Am J Obstet Gynecol.* 2004;191:661–667.

Cicero S, Bindra R, Rembouskos G, et al. Integrated ultrasound and biochemical screening for trisomy 21 using fetal nuchal translucency, absent fetal nasal bone, free B-hCG and PAPP-A at 11 to 14 weeks. *Prenat Diagn.* 2003;23:306–310.

Filly RA: *The fetal neural axis: a practical approach for identifying anomalous development.* Chicago: The Society of Radiologists in Ultrasound; 1992.

Finberg HJ. Avoiding ambiguity in the sonographic determination of the direction of umbilical cord twists. *J Ultrasound Med.* 1992;11:185–187.

International Society of Ultrasound in Obstetrics and Gynecology: Cardiac screening examination of the fetus: guidelines for performing the "basic" and "extended basic" cardiac scan. *Ultrasound Obstet Gynecol.* 1997;89:227–232.

International Society of Ultrasound in Obstetrics and Gynecology Education Committee: Sonographic examination of the fetal central nervous system: guidelines for performing the "basic examination" and the "fetal neurosonogram," *Ultrasound Obstet Gynecol.* 2007;29:109–116.

Jeanty P, Chervenak F, Grannum P, Hobbins JC. Normal ultrasonic size and characteristics of the fetal adrenal glands. *Prenat Diagn.* 1984;4:21–28.

Jeanty P, Dramaix-Wilmet MS, Elkasan N. Measurement of the fetal kidney growth on ultrasound. *Radiology.* 1982;144:159–162.

Jeanty P, Dramaix-Wilmet MS, VanGansbeke D. Fetal ocular biometry by ultrasound. *Radiology.* 1982;143:513–516.

Jeanty P, Kirkpatrick C, Dramaix-Wilmet MS. Fetal limb growth. *Radiology.* 1981;140:165–167.

Jeanty P, Romero R, Hobbins JC. Vascular anatomy of the fetus. *J Ultrasound Med.* 1984;3:113–122.

Jeanty P, Romero R, Staudach A, Hobbins JC. Facial anatomy of the fetus. *J Ultrasound Med.* 1986;5:607–616.

Mahony BS, Bowie JD, Killam AP, et al. Epiphyseal ossification centers in the assessment of fetal maturity: sonographic correlation with the amniocentesis lung profile. *Radiology.* 1986;159:521–524.

Mahony BS, Callen PW, Filly RA, Hoddick WK. The fetal cisterna magna. *Radiology*. 1984;153:773–776.

Mandell R. Structural genitourinary defects detected in utero. *Radiology*. 1991;178:193–195.

Mayden KL, Tortora M, Berkowitz RL, et al. Orbital diameters: a new parameter for prenatal diagnosis and dating. *Am J Obstet Gynecol*. 1982;144:289–297.

Maymon R, Shulman A, Ariely S, et al. Sonographic assessment of cervical changes during pregnancy and delivery: current concepts. *Eur J Obstet Gynecol Reprod Biol*. 1996;67:149–155.

Merz E. *Ultrasound in obstetrics and gynecology*, vol 1: Obstetrics. New York: Thieme; 2005.

Nicolaides KH, Campbell S, Gabbe SG, Guidetti R. Ultrasound screening for spina bifida: cranial and cerebellar signs. *Lancet*. 1986;2:72–74.

Nicolaides KH, Snijders RJM, Sebire N. *The 11-14 week scan: the diagnosis of fetal anomalies*. London: Informa Healthcare; 1999.

Nyberg DA, Mack LA, Patten RM, Cyr DR. Fetal bowel: normal sonographic findings. *J Ultrasound Med*. 1987;6:3–6.

O'Rahilly R, Muller F, eds. *Human embryology and teratology*, ed 3. New York: Wiley-Liss; 2001.

Pretorius DH, Kallmann CE, Grafe MR, et al. Linear echoes in the fetal cisterna magna. *J Ultrasound Med*. 1992;11:125–128.

Rosen T, D'Alton ME, Platt LD, Wapner R. First-trimester ultrasound assessment of the nasal bone to screen for aneuploidy. *Obstet Gynecol*. 2007;110:399–404.

Sonek JD, McKenna D, Webb D, et al. Nasal bone length throughout gestation: normal ranges based on 3537 fetal ultrasound measurements. *Ultrasound Obstet Gynecol*. 2003;21:152–155.

Spong CY. Prediction and prevention of recurrent spontaneous preterm birth. *Obstet Gynecol*. 2007;110:405–415.

Yeo L, Vintzileos AM. The use of genetic sonography to reduce the need for amniocentesis in women at high-risk for Down syndrome. *Semin Perinatol*. 2003;27:152–159.

Sanders RC *Structural Fetal Abnormalities: The Total Picture*. St. Louis: Elsevier; 2016. ed 3.

Rumack CM, Wilson SR, Charboneau JW, Johnson JA. *Diagnostic Ultrasound*. ed 5. St. Louis: Elsevier; 2018.

CHAPTER 52

Obstetric Measurements and Gestational Age

Sandra L. Hagen-Ansert

OBJECTIVES

On completion of this chapter, you should be able to:
- Discuss gestational sac growth, take measurements, and assess gestational age
- Describe how to perform a crown-rump measurement and evaluate growth
- Measure, calculate the biparietal diameter, head circumference, three-dimensional cranium, abdominal circumference, and extremity measurements
- Assess fetal parameter measurements, proportions, and fetal growth
- Describe when other measurements should be used to provide additional clinical information
- Evaluate the fetal growth time-series for intrauterine growth restriction and growth disturbances

OUTLINE

Gestational Age Assessment: First Trimester 1379
- Gestational Sac Diameter 1379
- Crown-Rump Length 1381
- Embryonic Heart Rate 1382

Gestational Age Assessment: Second and Third Trimesters 1382
- Fetal Measurements 1382
- Abdominal Circumference 1388
- Bone Lengths 1389

Using Multiple Parameters 1390
Fetal Weight Estimation 1391
Other Parameters 1392

KEY TERMS

Anophthalmos
Banana sign
Binocular distance (BiOD or BD)
Biparietal diameter (BPD)
Brachycephaly
Chorionic sac
Crown-rump length (CRL)
Dolichocephaly
Embryonic heart rate (EHR)
Femur length (FL)

Fetal age
Gestational sac
Gestational sac diameter (GSD)
Growth-adjusted sonar age (GASA)
Humeral length
Hypertelorism
Hypotelorism
Intrauterine growth restriction (IUGR)

Last menstrual period (LMP)
Lemon sign
Microphthalmos
Oxycephaly
Small for gestational age (SGA)
Spina bifida

Reliably assessing gestational age and the growth of the fetus has long posed a challenge to all who care for pregnant women. Although not without value, clinical parameters lack the necessary consistency for optimal perinatal care. With recent advances in diagnostic sonography, however, fetal age and growth can be assessed with high accuracy.

The difference between menstrual and fetal age is important to establish in clinical obstetrics. **Fetal age** begins at conception and is also known as *conceptional age*. Conceptional age is restricted to pregnancies in which the actual date of conception is known, as found in patients with in vitro fertilization or artificial insemination. If conceptual age is already known, the menstrual age may be found by adding 14 days to the conceptual age.

Obstetricians date pregnancies in menstrual weeks, calculated from the first day of the **last [normal] menstrual period (LMP)**. This method is called *menstrual age* or *gestational age*. The sonography student must understand that gestational ages are estimated from measurements of fetal parameters and are not the actual age of the parameters. The estimated ages are no more accurate than the measurements taken, and all parameters in a fetus will not result in the same fetal age because fetuses have different body size proportions.

It is clinically important to know the menstrual age of a patient because this information is used for the following reasons:
- In early pregnancy to schedule invasive procedures (chorionic villus sampling and genetic amniocentesis)
- To interpret maternal serum alpha-fetoprotein screening
- To plan date of delivery
- To evaluate fetal growth

Before the use of sonographic determination of fetal growth, menstrual age was calculated by three factors: (1) the menstrual history, (2) physical examination of the fundal height of the uterus, and (3) postnatal physical examination of the neonate. This process was not always reliable if the patient could not recall the date of her last period or if other factors—such as oligomenorrhea, implantation bleeding, use of oral contraceptives, or irregular menstrual cycle—were present.

Because all gestations do not deliver exactly at 40 weeks after LMP, specific terminology has been defined for the relative gestational age at term (Box 52.1).

BOX 52.1	Definitions of "Term" Deliveries, in Weeks (w) and Days (d)
Early term: 37w0d to 38w6d
Full term: 39w0d to 40w6d
Late term: 41w0d to 41w6d
Post-term: 42w0d to delivery

Data from Spong CY. Defining "term" pregnancy: recommendations from the Defining "Term" Pregnancy Workgroup. *JAMA*. 2013; 309:2445–2446.

GESTATIONAL AGE ASSESSMENT: FIRST TRIMESTER

Gestational Sac Diameter

Transvaginal sonography enables visualization and evaluation of intrauterine pregnancies earlier than was previously thought possible. The earliest sonographic finding of an intrauterine pregnancy is thickening of the decidua. Sonographically, this appears as an echogenic, thick filling of the fundal region of the endometrial cavity occurring at approximately 3 to 4 weeks after the normal LMP (Box 52.2, Fig. 52.1).

At approximately 4 weeks of menstrual age, a small hypoechoic area appears in the fundus or midportion of the uterus, known as the *double decidual sac sign*. As the sac embeds further into the uterus, it is surrounded by an echogenic rim and is seen within the choriodecidual tissue. This is known as the chorionic or **gestational sac** (Fig. 52.2).

BOX 52.2	Gestational Sac Measurements

- A distended urinary bladder affects the gestational sac measurement; it changes its shape from round to ovoid or teardrop.
- If the sac is round, measure one GSD diameter inner to inner (all three diameters equal).
- If the sac is ovoid, make two measurements inner to inner, one transverse and the other perpendicular to the length. Take the third GSD inner to inner.
- The three GSD diameters are averaged for the diameter of record.

GSD, Gestational sac.

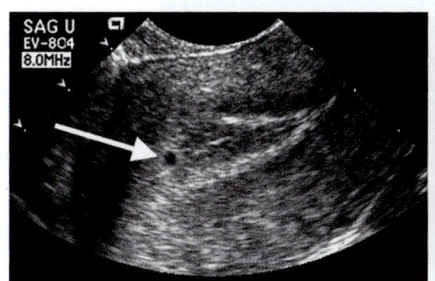 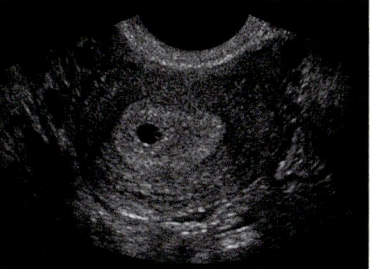 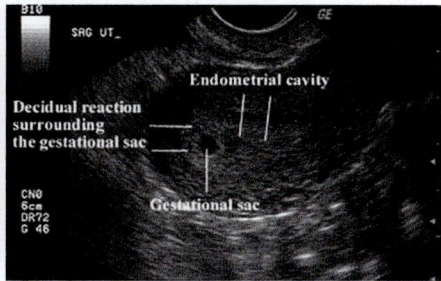

FIG. 52.1 The earliest sonographic finding of an intrauterine pregnancy is thickening of the decidua. Sonographically, this appears as an echogenic, thick filling of the fundal region of the endometrial cavity occurring at approximately 3 to 4 weeks after the last normal menstrual period.

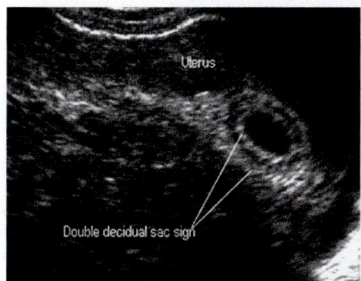 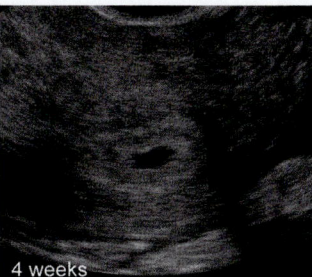 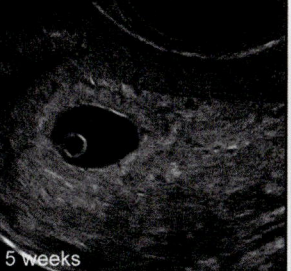 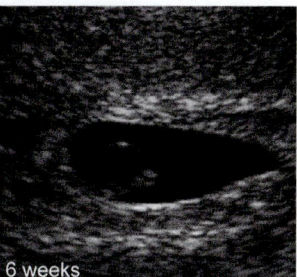

FIG. 52.2 At approximately 4 weeks of menstrual age, a small hypoechoic area appears in the fundus or midportion of the uterus, known as the *double decidual sac sign*. As the sac embeds further into the uterus, it is surrounded by an echogenic rim and is seen within the choriodecidual tissue. This is known as the chorionic or gestational sac.

At 5 weeks after the LMP, the average of the three perpendicular internal diameters of the GSD—calculated as the mean of the anteroposterior diameter, the transverse diameter, and the longitudinal diameter—can provide an adequate estimation of menstrual age (Fig. 52.3). A gestational sac should be seen within the uterine cavity when the β-human chorionic gonadotropin (β-hCG) is above 500 mIU/mL (second international standard). This becomes especially important when evaluating a pregnancy for ectopic implantation.

The sac grows rapidly in the first 10 weeks, with an average increase of 1 mm/day (see Table 52.1). According to one report, a gestational sac growing less than 0.7 mm/day is associated with impending early pregnancy loss. Even the most experienced sonographer may incorporate a measuring error; therefore, the β-hCG test in conjunction with a sonographic evaluation is suggested in a sequential time frame.

A yolk sac should be seen when the gestational sac exceeds 8 mm in mean internal diameter (Fig. 52.4). The yolk sac is a small, spherical structure with an anechoic center within the gestational sac. It provides early transfer of nutrients from the trophoblast to the embryo. It also aids in the early formation of the primitive gut and vitelline arteries and veins and in producing the primordial germ cells. Yolk sac size has not been correlated with gestational age determination. Normal yolk sac size should be less than 6 mm. Yolk sacs greater than 8 mm have been associated with poor pregnancy outcomes and solid, echogenic yolk sacs. Box 52.3 lists sonographic landmarks for early pregnancy.

When the mean **gestational sac diameter (GSD)** exceeds 16 mm, an embryo with definite cardiac activity should be

TABLE 52.1	Gestation Age Calculation by MSD In Early First Trimester
Gestational Age (Weeks)[a]	**MSD**
5.0	2
5.1	3
5.2	4
5.4	5
5.5	6
5.6	7
5.7	8
5.9	9
6.0	10

[a]95.5% confidence level = ±0.5 weeks.
MSD, Mean sac diameter.
Data from Daya S, Woods S, Ward S, et al. Early pregnancy assessment of transvaginal ultrasound scanning. *Can Med Assoc J.* 1991;144(4):441–446.

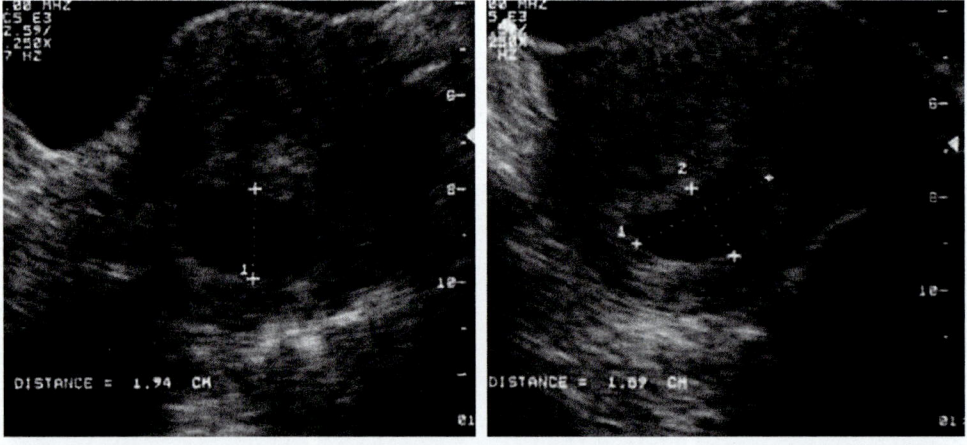

FIG. 52.3 At 5 weeks after the LMP, the average of the three perpendicular internal diameters of the gestational sac—calculated as the mean of the anteroposterior diameter, the transverse diameter, and the longitudinal diameter—can provide an adequate estimation of menstrual age.

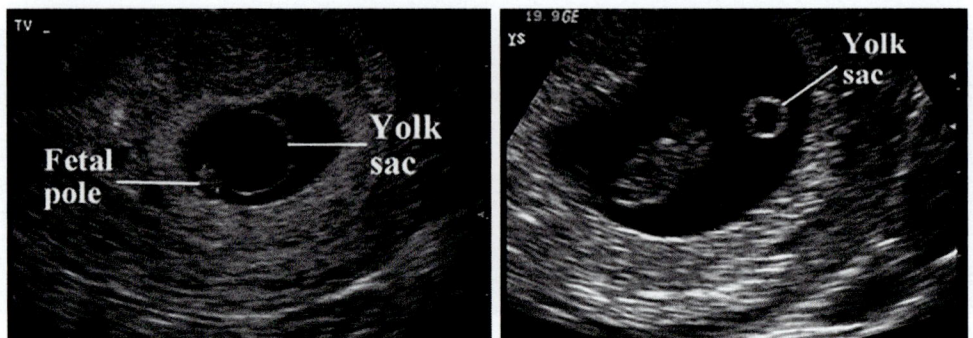

FIG. 52.4 When the gestational sac exceeds 8 mm in mean internal diameter, a yolk sac should be seen. The yolk sac is identified as a small, spherical structure with an anechoic center within the gestational sac.

BOX 52.3	Transvaginal Sonographic Landmarks for Early Pregnancies

- 500 mIU/mL β-hCG = gestational sac seen
- >8 mm gestational sac = yolk sac seen
- >16 mm gestational sac = embryo seen
- <6 mm yolk sac = normal
- >8 mm yolk sac = abnormal
- >7 mm fetal pole = positive cardiac activity

hCG, Human chorionic gonadotropin.

BOX 52.4	Crown-Rump Length (CRL)

- CRL can be measured from 6 to 12 gestational weeks by transvaginal sonography.
- Measurements should be made along the long axis of the embryo from the top of the head (crown) to the bottom of the trunk (rump).
- CRL is the most accurate fetal age measurement.

well visualized with transvaginal scanning. This usually occurs by the 6th menstrual week (Fig. 52.5) but may be as early as the fifth LMP week with transvaginal sonography. The maternal urinary bladder must be filled to create an acoustic window for the transabdominal scanning approach. With this technique, the sac shape can vary secondary to bladder compression, maternal bowel gas, or myomas and should not be misinterpreted as abnormal.

Assessing gestational age using a single gestational sac diameter or even up to three averaged diameters yields an accuracy of only ±2 to 3 weeks in 90% of cases.[1] Accordingly, gestational sac diameter has not been widely used as a determinant of gestational age after more accurate embryonic parameters can be measured (see Chapters 49 and 53).

Crown-Rump Length

With transvaginal sonography, embryonic echoes can be identified as early as 38 to 39 days of menstrual age (Box 52.4). The **crown-rump length (CRL)** is usually 1 to 2 mm at this stage. The embryo is usually located adjacent to the yolk sac. The CRL is the most accurate sonographic technique for establishing gestational age in the first trimester (Fig. 52.6). The reason for this high accuracy is the excellent correlation between fetal length and age in early pregnancy because pathologic disorders minimally affect the growth of the embryo during this time.

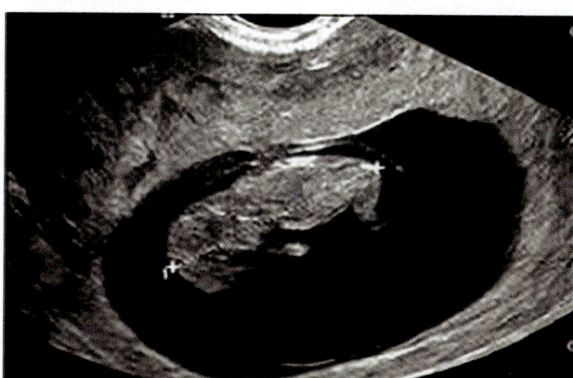
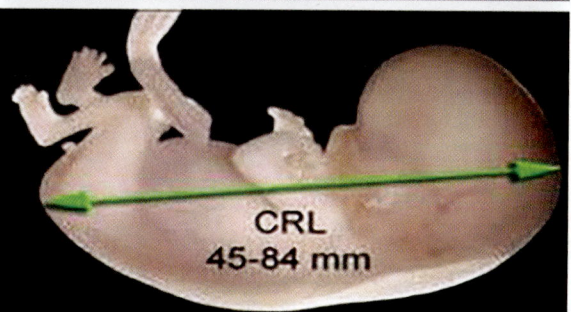

FIG. 52.6 A first trimester crown rump length (CRL) is the most accurate sonographic technique for establishing gestational age in the first trimester.

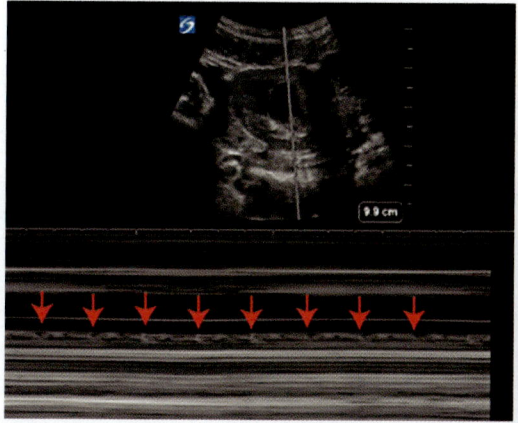
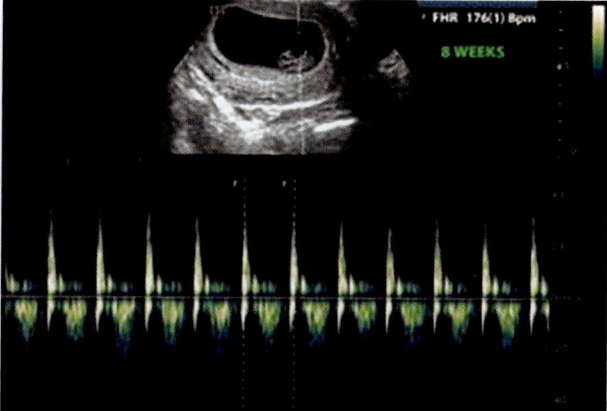

FIG. 52.5 When the mean gestational sac diameter exceeds 16 mm, an embryo with definite cardiac activity should be well visualized with transvaginal scanning. This usually occurs by the sixth menstrual week but may be as early as the fifth last menstrual period week with transvaginal sonography.

The embryo can be measured easily with real-time dynamic imaging. For transabdominal imaging, the mother's bladder should be full to create an acoustic window. The measurement should be taken from the top of the fetal head to the outer fetal rump, excluding the fetal limbs or yolk sac (Table 52.2 and Fig. 52.7). The accuracy is ±5 days with a 95% confidence level. The average of three separate measurements of the CRL may be obtained to determine gestational age.

Cardiac activity should be seen when the CRL exceeds 7 mm, but it may be seen by transvaginal sonography once the CRL reaches 2 mm. It is generally accepted that it is good to follow patients with small CRL and no fetal heartbeat over a few days. In general, the CRL should increase at a rate of 8 mm/day. Occasionally an embryo is seen with no visible cardiac activity and a small CRL for menstrual age. It is advisable to wait a week and rescan to see if the patient spontaneously aborts the products of conception or needs medical intervention, such as a dilation and curettage procedure. Infrequently an appropriate fetal CRL and positive cardiac activity are seen after the week's wait. Why this happens is not known, but experienced sonographers have observed it.

Absence of an embryo by 7 to 8 weeks of gestation is consistent with an embryonic demise or an anembryonic pregnancy. If a nomogram is not readily available to identify gestational age, a convenient formula is: Gestational age (weeks) = CRL (cm)+6. After the twelfth week, CRL is no longer considered accurate because of flexion and extension of the active fetus; therefore, other biometric parameters should be used.

Embryonic Heart Rate

The **embryonic heart rate (EHR)** accelerates linearly during the first month of beating between the 5th and 9th gestational weeks (Fig. 52.8). This linear acceleration correlates well with the embryonic age before the CRL reaches 2.5 cm or before approximately 9.2 LMP weeks. The mean rate of acceleration is 3.3 beats/min per day, 10 beats/min every 3 days, or approximately 100 beats/min between the start of beating until the early ninth week (Box 52.5). The embryonic age in days can be estimated with the following formula:

$$\text{LMP age (days)} = \text{EHR} \times 0.3 + 6\,\text{days}$$

The result of this estimation will be within ±6 days in 95% of normal pregnancies.[2] If the age estimated by the CRL leads the age by EHR by more than 1 week, it may be prognostic for first-trimester failure and warrants follow-up. Because the heart rate is accelerating so rapidly during the embryonic period, accurate M-mode measurements are desirable. The greatest accuracy can be achieved by magnifying the embryo as much as possible and using a fast M-mode tracing to stretch out the heartbeats for more precise cursor placement. The cursors should be carefully placed on identifiable, repeating locations of the M-mode tracing (Fig. 52.9).

GESTATIONAL AGE ASSESSMENT: SECOND AND THIRD TRIMESTERS

Fetal Measurements

In the second trimester, the gestational age parameters extend to the biparietal diameter (BPD), head circumference (HC), abdominal circumference (AC), femur length (FL), and other parameters that may be used. It is critical for the sonographer to know precisely which landmarks are necessary to determine these measurements. Proper gain settings, instrumentation, and fetal lie all influence the accuracy of measurements used to estimate the gestational age.

TABLE 52.2			Gestational Age (GA) Estimation by Crown-Rump Length (CRL)												
GA	CRL	GA	CRL	GA	CRL	GA	CRL	GA	CRL	GA	CRL	GA	CRL	GA	CRL
6.0	5	7.0	10	8.0	16	9.0	24	10.0	33	11.0	44	12.0	56	13.0	70
6.2	6	7.2	11	8.3	18	9.3	26	10.2	35	11.2	46	12.2	58	13.2	72
6.4	7	7.4	12	8.4	19	9.5	28	10.4	37	11.4	49	12.4	62	13.4	76
6.6	8	7.7	14	8.7	21	9.7	30	10.6	39	11.6	51	12.6	64	13.6	79
6.8	9	7.8	15	8.8	22	9.8	31	10.8	41	11.8	53	12.8	67	13.7	80

GA in weeks, CRL in millimeters.
Modified from Robinson HP, Fleming JEE. A critical evaluation of sonar "crown-rump length" measurements. *Br J Obstet Gynecol.* 1975;82:702–710.

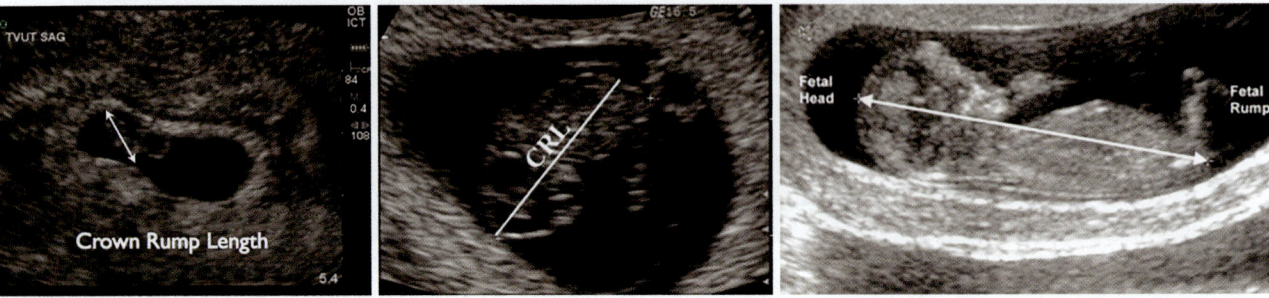

FIG. 52.7 The crown rump length measurement should be taken from the top of the fetal head to the outer fetal rump, excluding the fetal limbs or yolk sac.

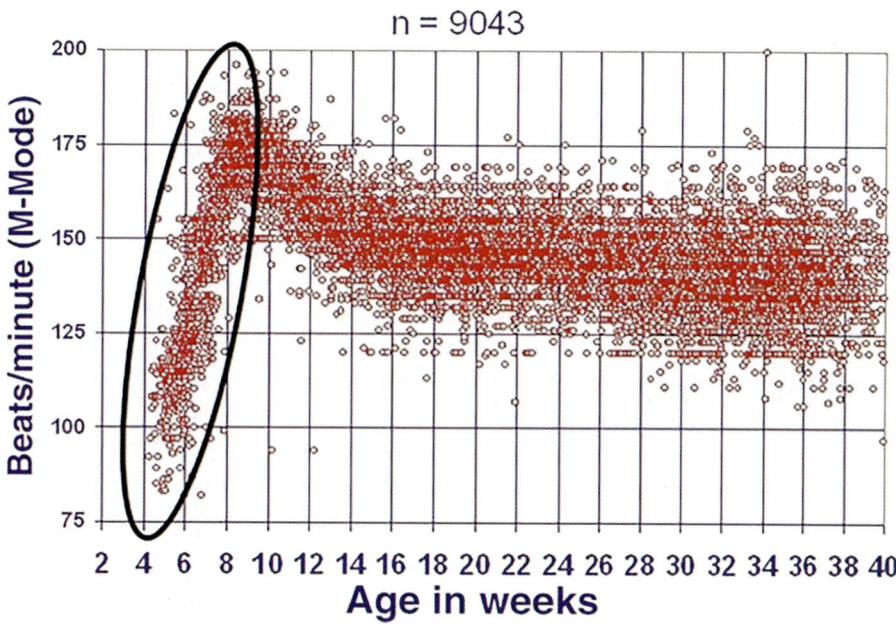

FIG. 52.8 Scatter plot of embryo fetal heart rates calculated by M-mode throughout gestation. Notice the rapid, linear acceleration in the first month from the early fifth week until the early ninth week. The peak heart rate of 175 beats/min (mean, ±25) comes at 9.2 last menstrual period weeks.

BOX 52.5 Embryonic Heart Rate (EHR)

- EHR can be measured by M-mode transvaginal sonography to estimate age from the early fifth to early ninth gestational weeks when the CRL is <25 mm.
- The most accurate EHR measurements can be obtained by enlarging the two-dimensional image and using a fast sweep speed for the M-mode tracing. Measure from repeating distinct points on M-mode.
- The EHR age will be accurate to within ±6 days. An EHR age that trails the CRL age by >6 days may be associated with impending first-trimester failure and warrants follow-up.
- The normal EHR accelerates linearly at 3.3 beats/min/ per day, which is approximately 10 beats every 3 days, or 100 beats in the first month of beating.

CRL, Crown-rump length.

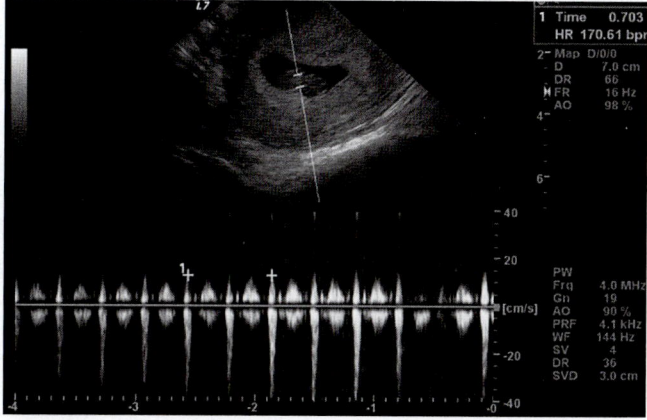

FIG. 52.9 The greatest accuracy can be achieved by magnifying the embryo as much as possible and using a fast M-mode tracing to stretch out the heartbeats for more precise cursor placement. The cursors should be carefully placed on identifiable, repeating locations of the M-mode tracing. This fetal heart measured 170 beats/min.

Biparietal Diameter. In the second trimester, the **biparietal diameter (BPD)** was the first and is the most widely accepted means of measuring the fetal head and estimating fetal age. As the pregnancy enters the third trimester, an accurate measurement of fetal age becomes more difficult to obtain because the fetus begins to drop into the pelvic outlet cavity. The reproducibility of the BPD is ±1 mm (±2 standard deviations). When dating a pregnancy between 17 and 26 weeks of gestation, the predictive value is ±11 days in 95% of the population.[3] After 26 weeks, the correlation of BPD with gestational age decreases because of cranial molding and the increased biologic variability. The predictive value decreases to ±3 weeks in the third trimester. The growth of the fetal skull slows from 3 mm/week in the second trimester to 1.8 mm/week in the third trimester.

When measuring the BPD, it is important to determine the landmarks accurately (Box 52.6, Fig. 52.10). The fetal head should be imaged in a transverse axial section, ideally with the fetus in a direct occiput transverse position. The BPD should be measured perpendicular to the fetal skull at the level of the thalamus and the cavum septi pellucidi. Intracranial landmarks should include the falx cerebri anteriorly and posteriorly, the cavum septi pellucidi anteriorly in the midline and the choroid plexus in the atrium of each lateral ventricle. With real-time sonography, one can identify the middle cerebral artery pulsating in the insula. Once the BPD has been measured, the gestational age may be assessed (Table 52.3).

The head shape should be ovoid, not round (**brachycephaly**) because this can lead to overestimation of gestational age, just as a flattened or compressed head (**dolichocephaly**) can lead to underestimation of gestational age estimated from the BPD measurement. The calipers should be placed from the leading edge of the parietal bone to the leading edge of the opposite parietal bone (i.e., outer edge to inner edge). The parietal bones should measure less than 3 mm each. On the outer edge of the fetal head, the soft tissue should not be included; measuring should begin from the skull bone, excluding the scalp. Gain settings should not be set too high because this can produce a false thickening and incorrect measurement. A reference curve should be applicable to the local population. BPD should not be used to date a pregnancy in cases of severe ventriculomegaly, which may alter the head size and produce macrocephaly, or when microcephaly, skull-altering head lesions, or molding are present. In these cases, other biometric parameters should be used.

If the fetus is too large for an accurate CRL but too early for a BPD with the proper landmarks identified, an approximation of the BPD can be obtained by incorporating the following landmarks: a smooth, symmetric head; visible choroid plexuses; and a well-defined midline echo that is an equal distance from both parietal bones (Fig. 52.11).

Growth-Adjusted Sonar Age. A technique utilized to adjust for the biologic variability of fetal head growth uses the fetus as its own control. Two separate BPD measurements are obtained, the first between 20 and 26 weeks and the second between 31 and 33 weeks. The growth interval was compared with average growth. This technique has been termed **growth-adjusted sonar age (GASA)**.[4] The fetus is then categorized into a small, average, or large growth percentile. The developers of this method claim the use of GASA reduces the

BOX 52.6	Biparietal Diameter (BPD)

- BPD is measured on an axial image of the fetal head at the level of the paired thalami, third ventricle, and cavum septum pellucidum.
- Ensure the head is symmetric and oval.
- Measure from the outer edge of skull to the inner margin of the skull.
- In the third trimester, the BPD is not as accurate in predicting fetal age.

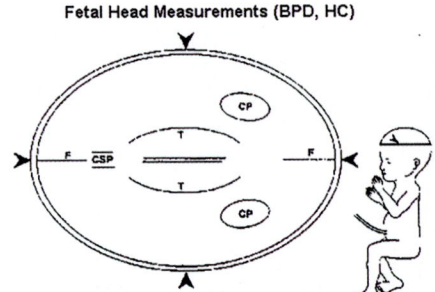
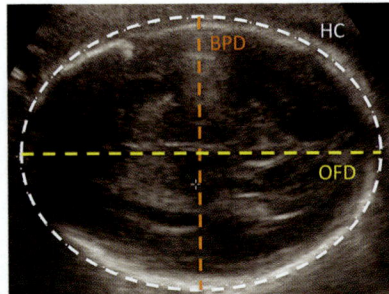
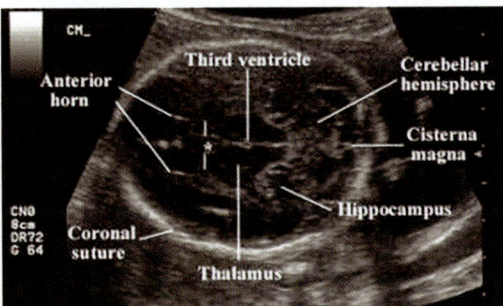

FIG. 52.10 The fetal head should be imaged in a transverse axial section, ideally with the fetus in a direct occiput transverse position. The biparietal diameter should be measured perpendicular to the fetal skull at the level of the thalamus and the cavum septi pellucidi. Intracranial landmarks should include the falx cerebri (F) anteriorly and posteriorly, the cavum septi pellucidi anteriorly in the midline, and the choroid plexus in the atrium of each lateral ventricle. *BPD,* Biparietal diameter; *HC,* head circumference; *OFD,* occipital frontal diameter.

TABLE 52.3		Gestational Age (GA) Estimation by Biparietal Diameter (BPD)													
GA	BPD	GA	BPD	GA	BPD	GA	BPD	GA	BPD	GA	BPD	GA	BPD	GA	BPD
20	13.2	30	15.4	40	17.9	50	20.8	60	24.2	70	28.1	80	32.7	90	38.0
21	13.4	31	15.6	41	18.1	51	21.1	61	24.5	71	28.5	81	33.2	91	38.6
22	13.6	32	15.8	42	18.4	52	21.4	62	24.9	72	29.0	82	33.7	92	39.2
23	13.8	33	16.1	43	18.7	53	21.7	63	25.3	73	29.4	83	34.2	93	39.8
24	14.0	34	16.3	44	19.0	54	22.1	64	25.7	74	29.9	84	34.7	94	40.4
25	14.3	35	16.6	45	19.3	55	22.4	65	26.1	75	30.3	85	35.2	95	41.0
26	14.5	36	16.8	46	19.6	56	22.8	66	26.5	76	30.8	86	35.8	96	41.6
27	14.7	37	17.1	47	19.9	57	23.1	67	26.9	77	31.2	87	36.3	±97	42.0
28	14.9	38	17.3	48	20.2	58	23.5	68	27.3	78	31.7	88	36.9		
29	15.1	39	17.6	49	20.5	59	23.8	69	27.7	79	32.2	89	37.4		

GA in weeks, BPD in millimeters.
From Doublilet PM, Benson CB: Improved prediction of gestational age in the late third trimester. *J Ultrasound Med.* 1993; 12:647–653.

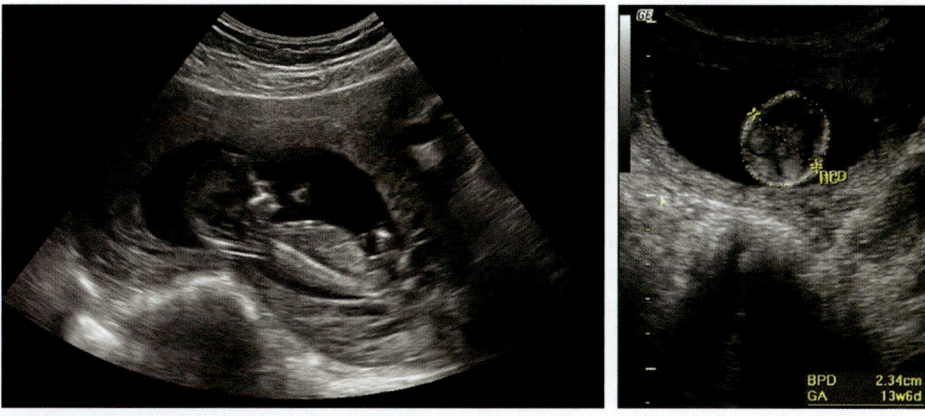

FIG. 52.11 If the fetus is too large for an accurate crown-rump length but too early for a biparietal diameter (BPD) with the proper landmarks identified, an approximation of the BPD can be obtained by incorporating the following landmarks: a smooth, symmetric head; visible choroid plexuses; and a well-defined midline echo that is an equal distance from both parietal bones. *GA,* Gestational age.

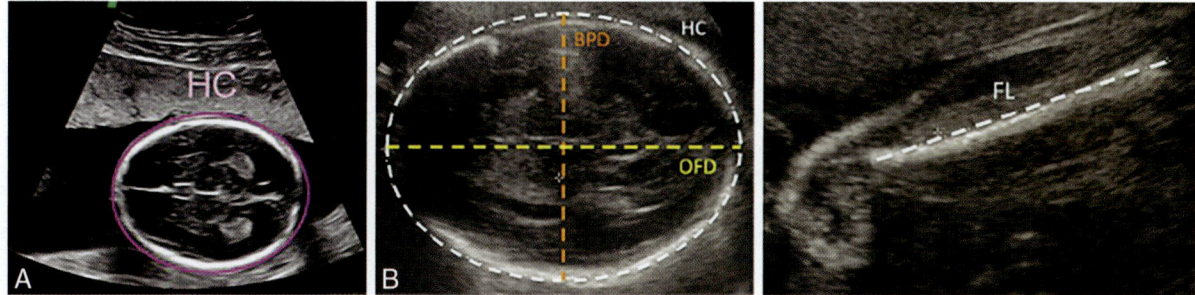

FIG. 52.12 (A) The head circumference (HC) measurement is taken in the transverse plane at the level of the biparietal diameter (BPD) and can be calculated from the same frozen image. The transverse HC is done by elliptical calipers around the outer perimeter of the cranium measuring from the outer border of the occiput to the outer border of the frontal bone. (B) The length of the occipital frontal diameter (OFD) is measured as the longest skull diameter. (C) Measurement of the femur length (FL).

range in gestational age from ±11 days to ±3 days in 90% of fetuses and to ±5 days in approximately 97% of fetuses.[3] Although GASA compensates for the biologic variability in the individual fetus, it does not consider other factors, such as dolichocephaly, brachycephaly, and **oxycephaly** caused by molding, variations in head shape, or the standard error of measurement.

Head Circumference. Prenatal compression of the fetal skull is common. It occurs more often in fetal malpresentation, such as breech, or in conditions of intrauterine crowding, such as multiple pregnancies. The fetal skull can also be compressed in vertex presentations without any obvious reason or as a result of an associated uterine abnormality, such as leiomyoma. The transverse HC is less affected than the BPD by head compression, so the HC is a valuable tool in assessing gestational age (see Box 52.6).

The HC measurement is taken in the transverse plane at the level of the BPD and can be calculated from the same frozen image. Most sonographic equipment has built-in electronic calipers that open to the outline of the fetal head. To measure the widest transverse diameter of the skull manually, the BPD level should be measured from the outer skull, not including the scalp, to the inner table of the distal skull (Fig. 52.12A). Note that the BPD is not the diameter of the outer cranial perimeter. The length of the occipital frontal diameter (OFD) is measured as the longest skull diameter (Box 52.7 and Fig. 52.12B). The transverse HC is done by elliptical calipers around the outer perimeter of the cranium measuring from the outer border of the occiput to the outer border of the frontal bone (Box 52.8). The HC (Table 52.4) can be calculated manually by the following formula:

$$HC = \frac{BPD + OFD \times \pi}{2}$$

Therefore,

$$HC = (BPD + OFD) \times 1.57$$

Cephalic Index. Two frequently noted alterations in head shape are dolichocephaly and brachycephaly. In dolichocephaly, the head is shortened in the transverse diameter (BPD) and elongated in the anteroposterior diameter (OFD) (Fig. 52.13A). In brachycephaly, the head is elongated in the transverse diameter (BPD) and shortened in the anteroposterior diameter (OFD) (see Fig. 52.13B). One can underestimate gestational age from a dolichocephalic head or overestimate with brachycephaly. Because of these variations in fetal head shape, a cephalic index (CI) has been devised to determine the normality of the fetal head shape:

$$CI = BPD/OFD \times 100$$

A normal CI is 80% ±1 standard deviation. The range of normal CI is 75% to 85% (±1 SD ~ 68% of the population). A CI of greater than 85% suggests brachycephaly, and one of less than 75% suggests dolichocephaly. In one case report, the CI changed from a high normal of 83% to a significantly abnormal index of 63% during a 2.5-week period.[5] This change would normally take approximately 7 weeks. Fetal death resulted. The report's authors concluded that an abnormal CI might be an early indication of impending fetal death.

The BPD and transverse HC do not account for changes in the vertical cranial height or diameter (VCD). The VCD is a relatively dynamic parameter because pressure on the vertex of the cranium as the fetus stretches and pushes the head against the uterine wall or maternal pubic bone will compress the VCD and exaggerate the BPD and HC in compensation, often resulting in a CI indicating brachycephaly. Conversely, if the BPD is compressed in dolichocephaly, the VCD will increase to compensate.[6,7] Unfortunately, this fact has been ignored for the most part, but as true three-dimensional

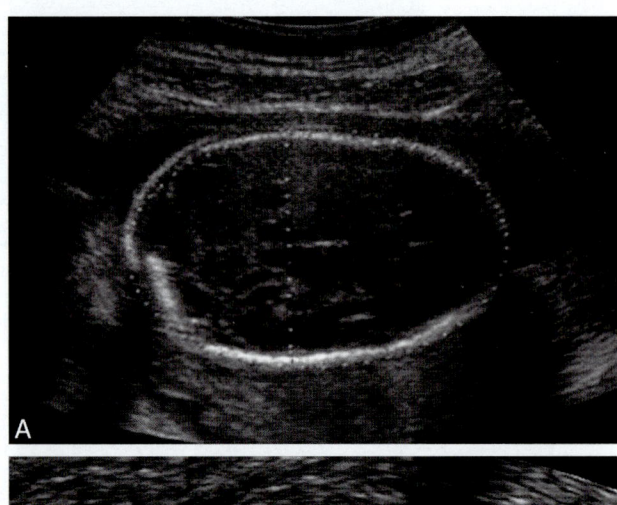

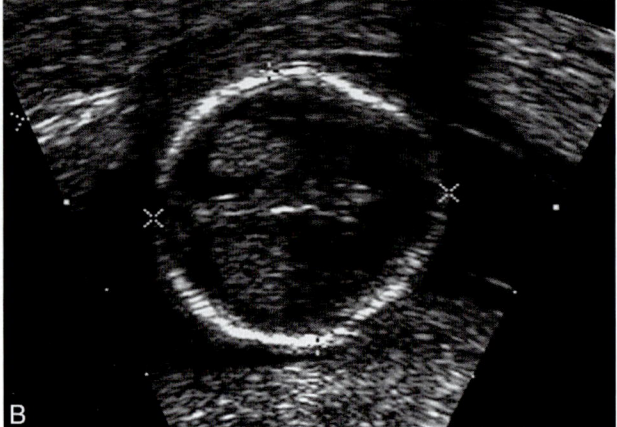

FIG. 52.13 (A) In dolichocephaly, the head is shortened in the transverse diameter (biparietal diameter [BPD]) and elongated in the anteroposterior diameter (occipital frontal diameter [OFD]). (B) In brachycephaly, the head is elongated in the transverse diameter (BPD) and shortened in the anteroposterior diameter (OFD).

BOX 52.7	Occipitofrontal Diameter Measurement

- Use the axial image of the fetal head at the level of the BPD to calculate the occipitofrontal diameter
- Place one caliper in the anterior midline in the middle of the echogenic line of the frontal bone; place the second caliper posteriorly in the middle of the echogenic line of the occipital bone.
- The OFD is used in conjunction with the BPD to take into account the shape of the fetal head.

BPD, Biparietal diameter; *OFD*, occipital frontal diameter.

BOX 52.8	Transverse Head Circumference

- Use the transverse plane at the level of the biparietal diameter to calculate head circumference.
- Place area calipers along the outer margin of the skull to obtain circumference.
- Accurate to ±2 to 3 weeks.

TABLE 52.4	Gestational Age (GA) Estimation by Head Circumference (HC)										
GA	HC	GA	HC	GA	HC	GA	HC	GA	HC	GA	HC
13.4	80	17.0	135	21.3	190	26.6	245	33.3	300	41.6	355
13.7	85	17.3	140	21.7	195	27.1	250	33.9	305	42.4	360
14.0	90	17.7	145	22.2	200	27.7	255	34.6	310		
14.3	95	18.1	150	22.6	205	28.3	260	35.3	315		
14.7	100	18.4	155	23.1	210	28.9	265	36.1	320		
15.0	105	18.8	160	23.6	215	29.4	270	36.8	325		
15.3	110	19.2	165	24.0	220	30.0	275	37.6	330		
15.6	115	19.6	170	24.5	225	30.7	280	38.3	335		
16.0	120	20.0	175	25.0	230	31.3	285	39.1	340		
16.3	125	20.4	180	25.5	235	31.9	290	39.9	345		
16.6	130	20.8	185	26.1	240	32.6	295	40.7	350		

GA in weeks, HC in millimeters.
From: Law RG, MacRe KD. Head circumference as an index of fetal age. *Ultrasound Med.* 1982;1:281–288.

(3D) sonography becomes available, these measurements will come into use.[8]

Coronal View, Vertical Cranial Diameter, and 3D Biparietal Diameter Correction. The coronal view of the fetal head is useful for viewing anatomy and assessing the degree of head molding and biologic changes in shape (Fig. 52.14). 3D ultrasound can produce perpendicular orthogonal planes, which makes it relatively easy to perform this assessment of overall head shape; however, the coronal view is also easily acquired with standard two-dimensional sonographic instruments (Fig. 52.15). The proper coronal view should be perpendicular to the standard transverse HC view passing through the thalamus (Box 52.9).

> **BOX 52.9 Coronal Head Circumference**
>
> - Use the plane perpendicular to the transverse head circumference. This plane should include the thalamus and brainstem.
> - Place area calipers at the mid-edge of the skull to delineate the coronal triangle; the base of the triangle is tangential to the circles around the hippocampal gyri.
> - The height of the triangle is the VCD. The average of the BPD, OFD, and VCD is the 3D-BPD correction for fetal skull molding.
> - The 3D-BPD is accurate to ±1 to 2 weeks.
>
> *BPD*, Biparietal diameter; *OFD*, occipital frontal diameter; *VCD*, vertical cranial diameter.

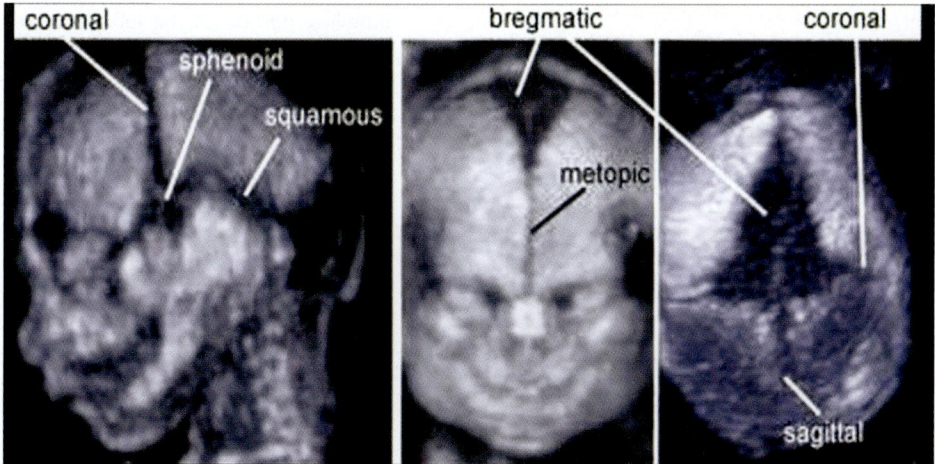

FIG. 52.14 Three-dimensional ultrasound of the fetal skull demonstrates the bones that form the skull and show the interposed sutures and fontanelles.

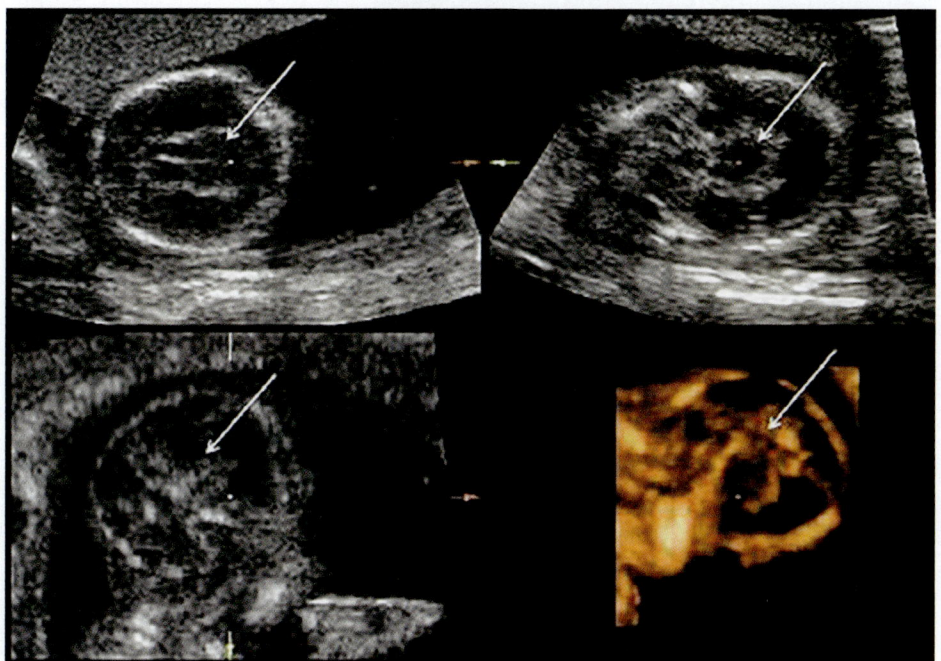

FIG. 52.15 Three-dimensional ultrasound can produce perpendicular orthogonal planes, which makes it relatively easy to perform this assessment of overall head shape; however, the coronal view is also easily acquired with standard two-dimensional sonographic instruments. The proper coronal view should be perpendicular to the standard transverse head circumference view passing through the thalamus.

Abdominal Circumference

The AC is very useful in monitoring normal fetal growth and detecting fetal growth disturbances, such as **intrauterine growth restriction (IUGR)** and macrosomia. It is more useful as a growth parameter than in predicting gestational age.

The fetal abdomen should be measured in a transverse plane at the level of the liver, where the umbilical vein branches into the left portal sinus (Box 52.10). In this plane, the umbilical vein and the portal vein form a J shape. The stomach bubble may be seen at this level on the left side of the fetal abdomen (Fig. 52.16). The abdomen should be more circular than oval because an oval shape may indicate an oblique cut resulting in a false estimation of size. Fetal kidneys usually should not be seen when the proper plane is imaged. The AC may change shape with fetal breathing activity, transducer compression, or intrauterine crowding (as in multiple pregnancies or oligohydramnios) or secondary to fetal position, as in a breech presentation. When discrepancies do occur in AC measurements, multiple measurements should be taken and averaged to ensure accuracy. This is also true for other fetal measurements.

The AC can be measured and calculated with similar instruments used to measure the transverse HC. The calipers should be placed along the external perimeter of the fetal abdomen to include subcutaneous soft tissue. The following formula can be used to calculate the AC:

$$AC = \frac{D_1 + D_2 \times \pi}{2}$$

Therefore,

$$AC = (D_1 + D_2) \times 1.57$$

BOX 52.10	Abdominal Circumference

- The abdominal circumference should be taken from a round transverse image, perpendicular to the fetal spine, with the umbilical portion of the left portal vein midline within the liver.
- The outer margin of the abdominal wall should be traced.
- The abdominal wall measurement is the least accurate for fetal age.

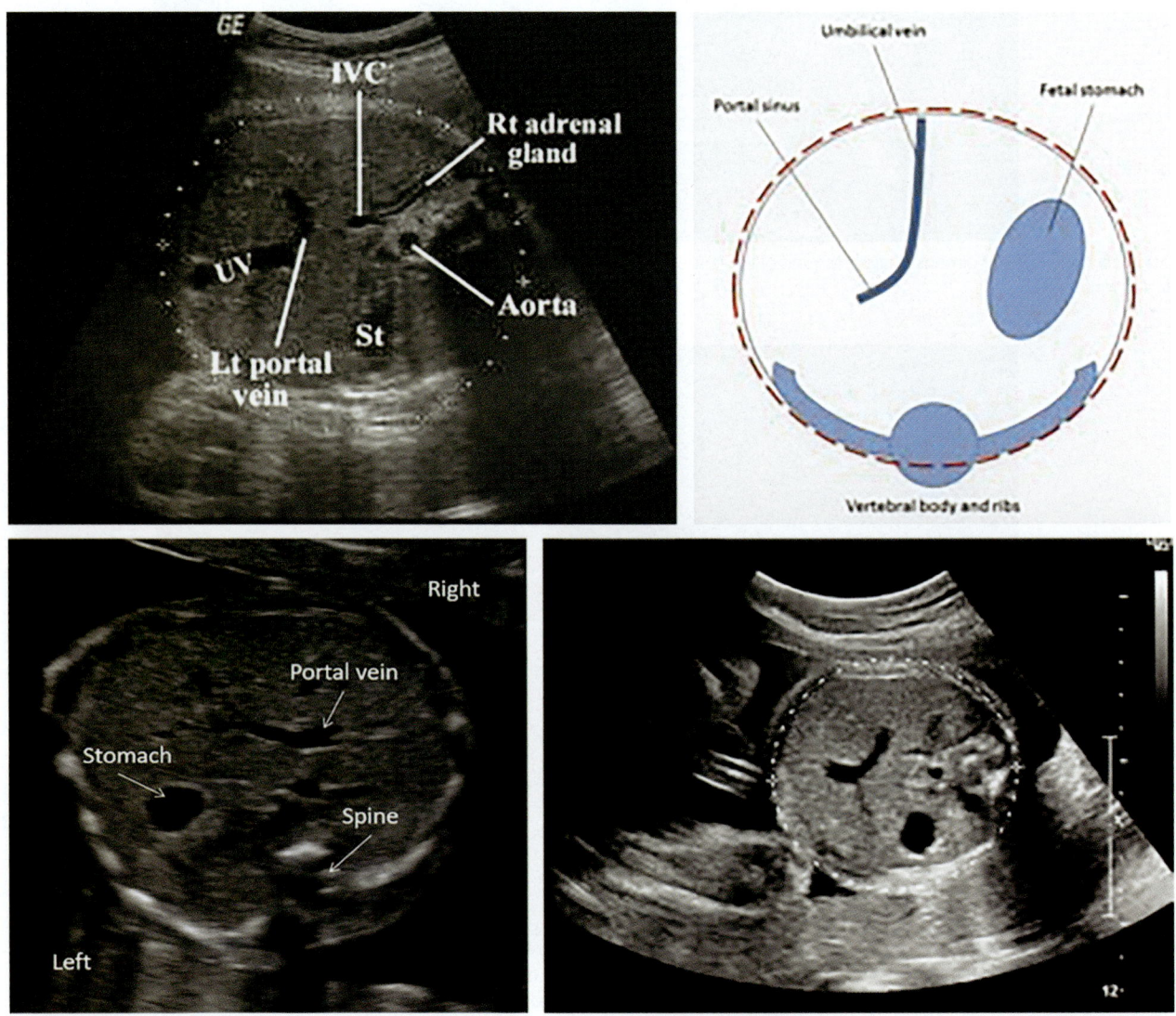

FIG. 52.16 The fetal abdomen should be measured in a transverse plane at the level of the liver, where the umbilical vein branches into the left portal sinus. In this plane, the umbilical vein and the portal vein form a J shape. The stomach bubble may be seen at this level on the left side of the fetal abdomen. *IVC,* Inferior vena cava; *Lt,* left; *Rt,* right; *St,* stomach; *UV,* umbilical vein.

In this equation, D1 is the diameter from the skin line behind the fetal spine to the outer skin line of the anterior abdominal wall, and D2 is the transverse diameter perpendicular to D1. Unlike in the fetal head (HC), there is no consistent relationship between the anteroposterior and transverse diameters of the AC. Sonographers must be sure to measure the AC at the skin line and not to the more obvious rib, spine, and peritoneal echoes.

Of the four basic gestational age measurements, AC has the largest reported variability and is more affected by growth disturbances than the other basic parameters. Later in gestation, the AC correlates more closely with fetal weight than with age.

Bone Lengths

Femur. The most widely measured and easily obtainable of all fetal long bones is the femur. It usually lies at 30 to 70 degrees to the long axis of the fetal body. **Femur length (FL)** is about as accurate as BPD in determining gestational age. FL is an especially useful parameter that can be used to date a pregnancy when a fetal head cannot be measured because of position or when there is fetal head molding or an anomaly (Box 52.11).

The technique for measuring the FL with sonography is fairly simple. First, the lie of the fetus should be determined and the fetal body followed in a transverse section until the fetal bladder and iliac crests are identified. The iliac crests are echogenic and oblique to the fetal spine and on either side of the bladder. The transducer is moved slightly and rotated to visualize the full length of the femur. The ends of the femur should be distinct and blunt, not pointed, and an acoustic shadow should be cast because of the absorption of the sound waves into the bone (Fig. 52.17).

Sonographers measure the femoral diaphysis, which is the calcified portion from end to end. Table 52.5 provides the

> **BOX 52.11** **Femur Measurement**
>
> - The hyperechoic linear structure represents the ossified portion of the femoral diaphysis and corresponds to femoral length measurement from the greater trochanter to the femoral condyles. These are imaged as rounded hypoechoic masses at each end of the diaphysis called the epiphyseal cartilages; they should not be included in the femoral length measurement. Do not include the distal femoral point.
> - The normal femur has a straight lateral border and a curved medial border.
> - Femur length may be used with the same accuracy as biparietal diameter to predict gestational age.
> - Femur length may indicate skeletal dysplasias or intrauterine growth restriction.

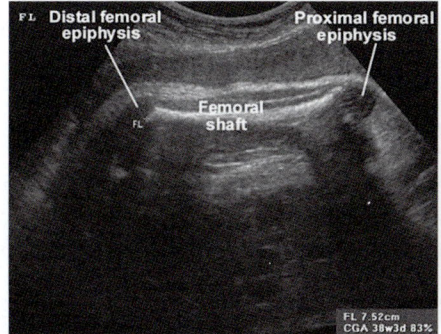 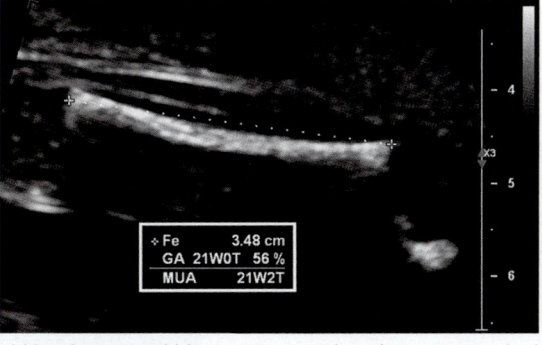 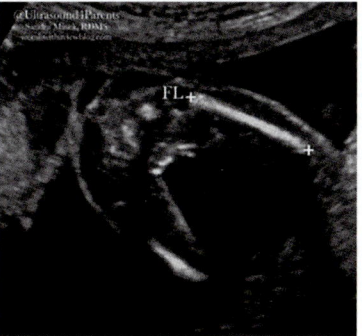

FIG. 52.17 The ends of the femur should be distinct and blunt, not pointed, and an acoustic shadow should be cast because of the absorption of the sound waves into the bone. Measure the femoral diaphysis, which is the calcified portion from end to end. The femoral head is not taken into account even when it is visible.

TABLE 52.5		Gestation Age (GA) Estimation by Femur Length (FL)											
GA	FL	GA	FL	GA	FL	GA	FL	GA	FL	GA	FL	GA	FL
13.7	10	16.2	20	19.1	30	22.5	40	26.6	50	31.4	60	37.1	70
13.9	11	16.4	21	19.4	31	22.9	41	27.0	51	31.9	61	37.7	71
14.2	12	16.7	22	19.7	32	23.3	42	27.5	52	32.5	62	38.3	72
14.4	13	17.0	23	20.1	33	23.7	43	28.0	53	33.0	63	39.0	73
14.6	14	17.3	24	20.4	34	24.1	44	28.4	54	33.6	64	39.8	74
14.9	15	17.6	25	20.7	35	24.5	45	28.9	55	34.1	65	40.3	75
15.1	16	17.9	26	21.1	36	24.9	46	29.4	56	34.7	66	40.9	76
15.4	17	18.2	27	21.4	37	25.3	47	29.9	57	35.3	67	41.6	77
15.8	18	18.5	28	21.8	38	25.7	48	30.4	58	35.9	68	42.0	±78
15.9	19	18.8	29	22.2	39	26.2	49	30.9	59	36.5	69		

GA in weeks, FL in millimeters.
From: Doubilet PM, Benson CB: Improved prediction of gestational age in the later third trimester. *J Ultrasound Med* 1993; 12:647–653.

FL measurement in correlation with the gestational age. The femoral head is not taken into account even when it is visible. After 32 weeks, the distal femoral epiphysis is seen, but it is not included in the FL measurement. Often an echo from the near side of the cartilaginous distal femoral condyles will be seen, called the distal femoral point (DFP), and should not be included in the measure of the diaphysis.

Overestimating the length of the femur by high gain settings or by including the femoral head or distal epiphysis in the measurement is possible. Underestimation can result from using incorrect plane orientation and not obtaining the full length of the bone.

In any routine obstetric evaluation, the femur is usually the only long bone measured, but if there is a 2-week or greater difference between FL and all the other biometric parameters, all fetal long bones should be measured, and a targeted examination of the fetal anatomy should be performed. Three studies found an association between shortened femur and humerus lengths and trisomy.[9-11] Dwarfism is also a possibility. Constitutional hereditary growth factors should also be considered. Other bone lengths are sometimes valuable in assessing gestational age.

Distal Femoral and Proximal Tibial Epiphyseal Ossification Centers. One report has correlated the distal femoral epiphyseal ossification (DFE) and the proximal tibial epiphyseal ossification (PTE) with advanced gestational age.[12] The DFE and PTE appear as a high-amplitude echo that is separate but adjacent to the femur or the tibia. The authors of the report found that the DFE can be identified in gestations greater than 33 weeks and that the PTE is identified in gestations greater than 35 weeks. It is not necessary to measure these ossifications; they are either present or absent. These assessments can be helpful when other growth parameters are compromised because of congenital anomalies or when differentiating an incorrectly dated fetus from a fetus that is **small for gestational age (SGA)** or one with intrauterine growth restriction (IUGR).

BOX 52.12	Tibia and Fibula Measurements

- The tibia is longer than the fibula.
- The fibula is lateral to the tibia and thinner.
- Measure the length point to point.

Tibia and Fibula. The tibia and fibula can be measured by first identifying the femur, then following it below the knee until the two parallel bones can be identified. The tibia can be identified because the tibial plateau is larger than the fine, tapering fibula. The tibia is medial to the fibula (Box 52.12, Fig. 52.18).

Humerus. Humeral length is sometimes more difficult to measure than FL. The humerus is usually found very close to the fetal trunk, but it can exhibit a wide range of motion. The "up side" humerus, or the humerus closest to the transducer, falls in the near-field zone, where detail is not always focused, and the acoustic shadow is less clear. The opposite, or "down side," humerus may be obscured because of the overlying fetal spine or fetal ribs (Box 52.13, Fig. 52.19). The cartilaginous humeral head surface is also acoustically shiny and may produce specular reflections that should not be included in the measurement of the humeral diaphysis. These specular reflections from the cartilaginous head of the humerus are called the proximal humeral point as a corollary to the DFP of the femur. Both the DFP and the proximal humeral point, when observed, will always be on the side of the acoustically shiny cartilage proximal to the transducer.

Radius and Ulna. The radius and ulna can be recognized by following the humerus down until two parallel bones are visualized and then rotating the transducer slightly until the full length of the bones is identified. The forearms are commonly found near the fetal face. The ulna can be distinguished from the radius because it penetrates much deeper into the elbow (Box 52.14, Fig. 52.20). The ulna is larger and anatomically medial.

Using Multiple Parameters

No single parameter is perfect in predicting gestational age, and estimates of fetal age may improve significantly when two or more parameters are averaged. Use of multiple parameter's

BOX 52.13	Humerus Measurement

- Image fetal spine in upper thoracic, lower cervical region.
- Identify scapula, then rotate transducer until long axis of humerus is seen.
- Only humeral shaft (diaphysis) is ossified and is measured; do not include the proximal humeral point.

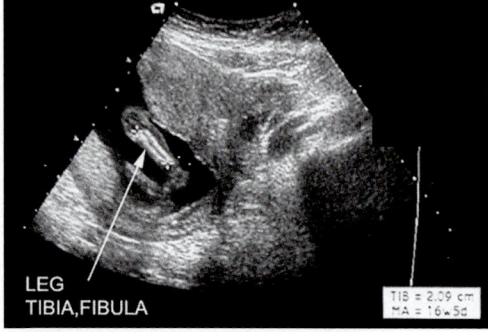 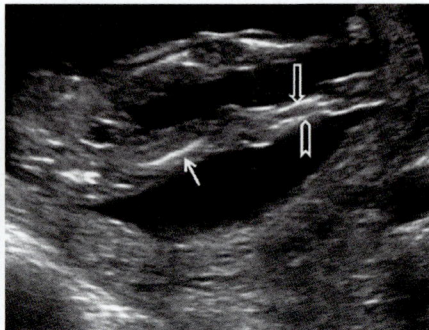

FIG. 52.18 The tibia and fibula can be measured by first identifying the femur, then following it below the knee until the two parallel bones can be identified. The tibia can be identified because the tibial plateau is larger than the fine, tapering fibula. The tibia is located medial to the fibula.

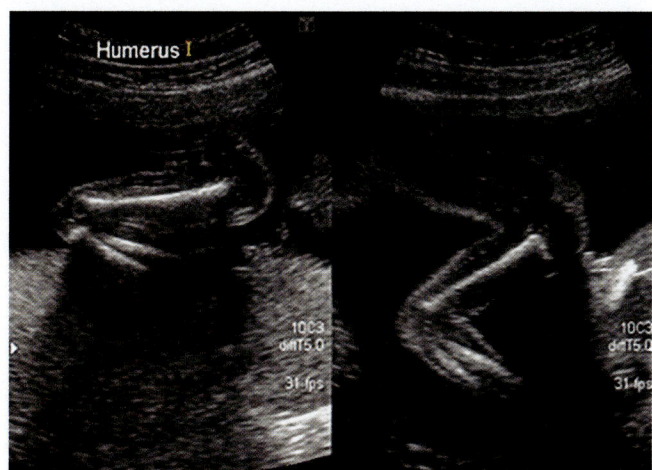

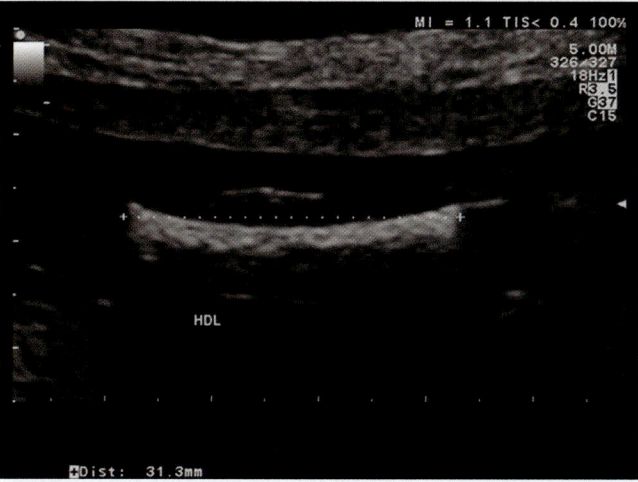

FIG. 52.19 The humerus is usually found very close to the fetal trunk, but it can exhibit a wide range of motion. The "up side" humerus, or the humerus closest to the transducer, falls in the near-field zone, where detail is not always focused, and the acoustic shadow is less clear.

BOX 52.14	Radius and Ulna Measurements

- The ulna is longer than the radius proximally; distally, they are the same.
- Measure length from point to point.

ages averaged in estimating fetal age is appropriate when the fetus is growing normally or in growth assessment time-series studies. Congenital anomalies of the head, abdomen, and skeleton and functional disturbances must be considered before using multiple parameters. In a normal population, the various ages estimated from the parameters of the fetal cranium exhibit about half the variation ($\pm 5\%$ of age), as do the ages from the fetal torso and extremity parameters ($\pm 10\%$ of age).

A birth weight table was developed based on measurements from a group of neonates who had accurate gestational dating using prenatal first-trimester sonography to improve the accuracy of neonatal birth weight percentiles.[13] Prenatally, weight tables are used in conjunction with sonographically estimated fetal weight to help guide obstetric management decisions, especially those concerning the timing of delivery. Fetal weight estimation is a useful parameter in following IUGR fetuses.

A study compared 3D sonographic birth weight predictions with 2D methods and found a significant correlation existed between thigh volume and birth weight at term gestation.[14] Thigh volumes that included the soft tissue mass may represent important markers for fetal growth. The 3D sonography may be an important predictor of growth-restricted fetuses, and the volume measurements may be able to be applied to each fetus to monitor growth.

Fetal Weight Estimation

There have been several methods to obtain the gestational age with sonographic measurements of fetal body parts. Numerous formulas have been published for estimating fetal weight from one or more of these measurements: head (BPD, OFD, or HC), abdomen (AC), and femur (FL) (Table 52.6). The accuracy of fetal weight prediction formulas improves as the number of measured body parts increases up to three, achieving greater accuracy when measurements of the head, abdomen, and femur are used. There is no apparent improvement by adding the thigh circumference as a fourth measurement and no proven benefit from using 3D sonography or MRI.[10]

Even when based on measurements of the head, abdomen, and femur, sonographic fetal weight prediction has a rather wide 95% confidence range of at least $\pm 15\%$.[10] Accuracy appears to be worse in small fetuses weighing less than 1000 g than in larger fetuses (Table 52.7). Weight is less accurate in

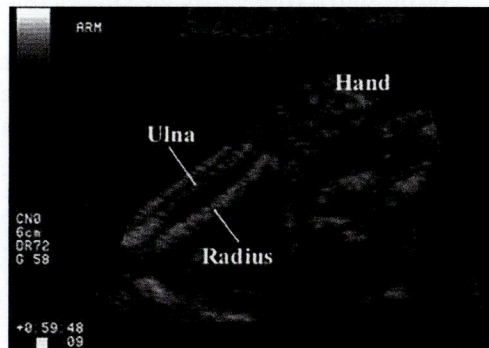 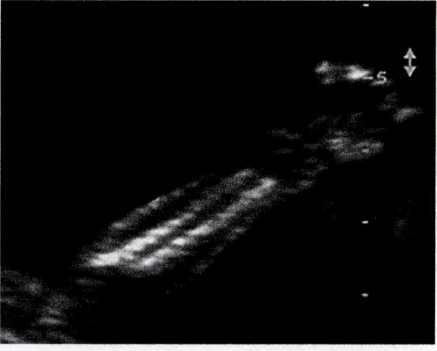

FIG. 52.20 The radius and ulna can be recognized by following the humerus down until two parallel bones are visualized and then rotating the transducer slightly until the full length of the bones is identified. The forearms are commonly found near the fetal face. The ulna can be distinguished from the radius because it penetrates much deeper into the elbow.

diabetic than in nondiabetic mothers. The presence of oligohydramnios or polyhydramnios has no impact on accuracy. Important to note that scan quality has an important effect on the accuracy of the measurements.

TABLE 52.6	Approach to Fetal Weight Estimation
Body Parts Imaged	Formula Used for Weight Estimate
Head, Abdomen, and Femur	
OFD measurable	Formula 1, using corrected BPD in placed of BPD
OFD not measurable	Formula 1
Head and Abdomen	
OFD measurable	Formula 2, using corrected BPD in place of BPD
OFD not measurable	Formula 2
Abdomen and Femur	Formula 3

Formula 1: $\text{Log}_{10}(\text{EFW}) = 1.4787 - 0.003343\ AC \times FL + 0.001837\ BPD^2 + 0.0458\ AC + 0.158\ FL$.
Formula 2: $\text{Log}_{10}(\text{EFW}) = 1.1134 + 0.05845\ AC - 0.000604\ AC^2 - 0.007365\ BPD^2 + 0.00595\ BPD \times AC + 0.1694\ BPD$.
Formula 3: $\text{Log}_{10}(\text{EFW}) = 1.3598 + 0.051\ AC + 0.1844\ FL - 0.0037\ AC \times FL$.
AC, Abdominal circumference; *BPD*, biparietal diameter; *EFW*, estimated fetal weight; *FL*, femur length; *OFD*, occipital frontal diameter.
Data from Hadlock FP, Harrist RB, Carpenter RJ, et al. Sonographic estimation of fetal weight: the value of femur length in addition to head and abdomen measurements. *Radiology.* 1984;150:535–540.

TABLE 52.7	Fetal Weight Percentiles in the Third Trimester		
	Weight Percentiles (g)		
GA (Weeks)	10th	50th	90th
26	570	860	1320
27	660	990	1470
28	770	1150	1660
29	890	1310	1890
30	1030	1460	2100
31	1180	1630	2290
32	1310	1810	2500
33	1480	2010	2690
34	1670	2220	2880
35	1870	2430	3090
36	2190	2650	3290
37	2310	2870	3470
38	2510	3030	3610
39	2680	3170	3750
40	2750	3280	3870
41	2800	3360	3980
42	2830	3410	4060
43	2840	3420	4100

From Doubilet PM Benson CB, Nadel AS, et al. Improved birth weight for neonate developed from gestations dated by early ultrasonography. *J Ultrasound Med.* 1997;16:241–249.

Other Parameters

Numerous other nomograms have been used to correlate almost every aspect of fetal anatomy with gestational age. Among the most interesting of these parameters are the orbits, the cerebellum, the fetal epiphyseal ossification centers, and cranial volume. In general, it can be stated that parameters that normally grow to larger sizes at term will have a more rapid growth trajectory and will generally produce the most accurate fetal age estimates.

Orbits. Another parameter useful in predicting gestational age is the fetal orbit measurements. The orbital diameter (OD), **binocular distance (BiOD or BD)**, and interocular distance (IOD) can be measured. Gestational age can best be predicted from the BiOD. This measure is more strongly related to the BPD and gestational age than are the other orbital parameters. The fetal orbits should be measured in a plane slightly more caudal than the BPD. The orbits are accessible in every head position except the occipitoanterior position (i.e., face looking down). All measurements should be taken from outer border to outer border (Box 52.15, Fig. 52.21). The OD measures a single fetal orbit. The BiOD includes both fetal orbits at the same time, whereas the IOD measures the distance between the two orbits. One view states that (1) both eyes should have the same diameter, (2) the largest diameter of the eyes should be used, and (3) the image should be symmetric. Care should be taken not to underestimate the measurement when there is oblique shadowing from the ethmoid bone. This parameter is especially useful when other fetal growth parameters are affected, such as in ventriculomegaly or skeletal dysplasia. With careful sonographic examinations, the fetus with **hypotelorism, hypertelorism, anophthalmos,** or **microphthalmos** can be diagnosed.

Cerebellum. One study found the fetal cerebellum to be a more accurate reflection of gestational age than the BPD in cases of cranial molding in oligohydramnios, dolichocephaly, breech presentation, or twins or in the presence of a uterine anomaly.[15] The authors of the study claim this is true because the posterior fossa is not affected by any of these conditions. The cerebellum can be measured from the level at which the BPD is obtained by angling back into the posterior fossa to include the full width of the cerebellum. The cerebellum should have a dumbbell or heart shape, depending on the angle of the plane of view.

The widest transverse diameter of the cerebellum should be measured (Box 52.16, Fig. 52.22). Authors have described the **"banana"** and **"lemon" signs** that associate an abnormally shaped cerebellum with detection of fetal **spina bifida**.[16] In the presence of spina bifida, the fetal cerebellum is displaced downward into the foramen magnum, altering its shape to

BOX 52.15	Orbital Measurements

- Orbital diameter increases from 13 mm at 12 weeks to ≥59 mm at term.
- Measure outer-to-outer diameter.
- Measure inner-to-inner diameter.

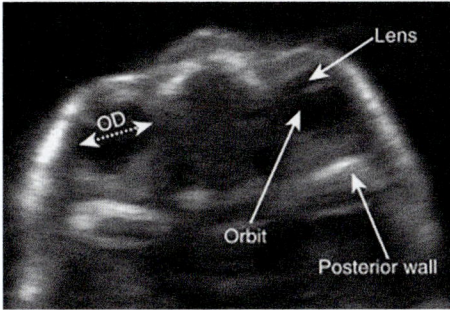 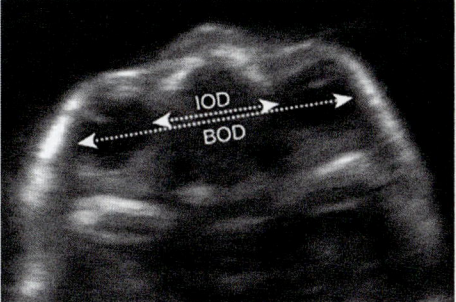 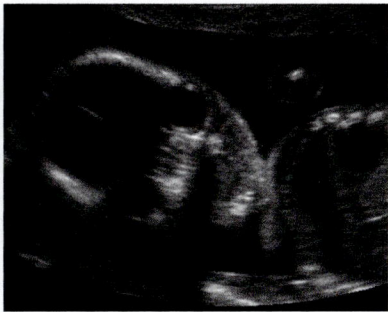

FIG. 52.21 The fetal orbits should be measured in a plane slightly more caudal than the biparietal diameter. The orbits are accessible in every head position except the occipitoanterior position (i.e., face looking down). All measurements should be taken from outer border to outer border. *BOD*, Binocular distance; *IOD*, Interocular distance; *OD*, orbital diameter.

BOX 52.16	Cerebellar Dimensions

- Posterior fossa: in the transaxial image of the head, obtain the biparietal diameter (cavum septi pellucidi and thalamus), then angle the transducer inferior toward the base of the skull to image the posterior fossa.
- Obtain the length of the cerebellum at the level of the cerebellum, vermis, and fourth ventricle.
- Angle the transducer slightly more inferior from the cerebellum to record the cistern magnum and nuchal fold area.
- The depth of the cisterna magna is from the posterior aspect of the cerebellum to the occipital bone measured 5 mm ± 3 mm; measurements >10 mm are abnormal.
- The nuchal fold should measure <3 mm.

Key Pearls

- Obstetricians date pregnancies in menstrual weeks, which are calculated from the first day of the last normal menstrual period (LMP). This method is called *menstrual age* or *gestational age*.
- The earliest sonographic finding of an intrauterine pregnancy is thickening of the decidua. Sonographically, this appears as an echogenic, thick filling of the fundal region of the endometrial cavity occurring at approximately 3 to 4 weeks after the normal LMP.
- At approximately 4 weeks of menstrual age, a small hypoechoic area appears in the fundus or midportion of the uterus, known as the *double decidual sac sign*.
- As the sac embeds further into the uterus, it is surrounded by an echogenic rim and is seen within the choriodecidual tissue. This is known as the chorionic or gestational sac.
- At 5 weeks after the LMP, the average of the three perpendicular internal diameters of the gestational sac (GSD)—calculated as the mean of the anteroposterior diameter, the transverse diameter, and the longitudinal diameter—can provide an adequate estimation of menstrual age.
- The sac grows rapidly in the first 10 weeks, with an average increase of 1 mm/day.
- When the gestational sac exceeds 8 mm in mean internal diameter, a yolk sac should be seen.
- Normal yolk sac size should be less than 6 mm. Yolk sacs greater than 8 mm have been associated with poor pregnancy outcomes.
- When the mean gestational sac diameter (GSD) exceeds 16 mm, an embryo with definite cardiac activity should be well visualized with transvaginal scanning.
- The crown rump length (CRL) is the most accurate sonographic technique for establishing gestational age in the first trimester.
- Cardiac activity should be seen when the CRL exceeds 7 mm, but it may be seen by transvaginal sonography once the CRL reaches 2 mm.
- In the second trimester, the gestational age parameters extend to the biparietal diameter, head circumference, abdominal circumference, femur length, and other parameters that may be used.
- The fetal head should be imaged in a transverse axial section, ideally with the fetus in a direct occiput transverse

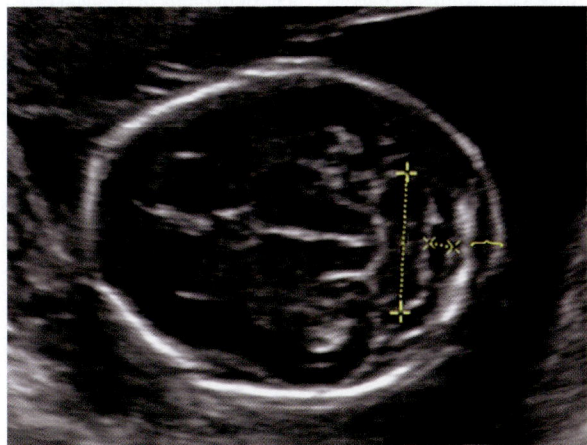

FIG. 52.22 The widest transverse diameter of the cerebellum should be measured (see crossbar with vertical markers). *X*, Foramen magnum.

appear oblong or banana shaped. The frontal bones of the fetal skull also give in to this reduced pressure, collapsing and giving the fetal head a lemon shape. This association is known as the Arnold-Chiari malformation type II.

The fetal cerebellum should not be used as a gestational dating parameter in the presence of a cerebellar or spinal abnormality. A more recent report states that the coronal or other views are just as accurate as long as the transverse width of the cerebellum is measured, especially in fetal heads when the traditional views are unobtainable.[17]

- position. The biparietal diameter (BPD) should be measured perpendicular to the fetal skull at the level of the thalamus and the cavum septi pellucidi. Intracranial landmarks should include the falx cerebri anteriorly and posteriorly, the cavum septi pellucidi anteriorly in the midline, and the choroid plexus in the atrium of each lateral ventricle.
- The head circumference (HC) measurement is taken in the transverse plane at the level of the BPD and can be calculated from the same frozen image. To measure the widest transverse diameter of the skull manually, the BPD level should be measured from the outer skull, not including scalp, to the inner table of the distal skull.
- The coronal view of the fetal head is useful for viewing anatomy and assessing the degree of head molding and biologic changes in shape.
- The fetal abdomen should be measured in a transverse plane at the level of the liver, where the umbilical vein branches into the left portal sinus. In this plane, the umbilical vein and the portal vein form a J shape. The stomach bubble may be seen at this level on the left side of the fetal abdomen.
- Of the four basic gestational age measurements, AC has the largest reported variability and is more affected by growth disturbances than the other basic parameters. Later in gestation, the AC correlates more closely with fetal weight than with age.
- The most widely measured and easily obtainable of all fetal long bones is the femur. Femur length is an especially useful parameter that can be used to date a pregnancy when a fetal head cannot be measured because of position or when there is fetal head molding or an anomaly.
- The accuracy of fetal weight prediction formulas improves as the number of measured body parts increases up to three, achieving greater accuracy when measurements of the head, abdomen, and femur are used.
- The orbital diameter (OD), binocular distance (BiOD or BD), and interocular distance (IOD) can be measured. Gestational age can best be predicted from the BiOD.
- The widest transverse diameter of the cerebellum should be measured. The cerebellum should have a dumbbell or heart shape, depending on the angle of the plane of view.

REFERENCES

1. Hohler CW. Ultrasonic estimation of gestational age. *Clin Obstet Gynecol.* 1984;27:2.
2. DuBose TJ, Cunyus JA, Johnson L. Embryonic heart rate and age. *J Diagn Med Sonogr.* 1990;6:151–157.
3. Sabbagha RE, Tamura RK, Dal Campo S. Fetal dating by ultrasound. *Sem Roentgenol.* 1982;17:3.
4. Sabbagha RE, Hughey M, Depp R. Growth-adjusted sonographic age (GASA): a simplified method. *Obstet Gynecol.* 1978;51:383.
5. Ford K, McGahan J. Cephalic index: its possible use as a predictor of impending fetal demise. *Radiology.* 1982;143:517.
6. Goldberg BB, Kurtz AB. *Atlas of ultrasound measurements.* St. Louis: Mosby–Year Book; 1990.
7. Kurtz AB, Goldberg BB. Fetal head measurements. In: Kurtz AB, Goldberg BB, eds. *Obstetrical measurements in ultrasound: a reference manual.* St. Louis: Mosby; 1988.
8. Dubose TJ. Reliability and validity of three-dimensional fetal brain volumes. *J Ultrasound Med.* 2002;21:709–711.
9. Benacerraf B, Neuberg D, Frigoletto FD. Humeral shortening in second trimester fetuses with Down syndrome. *Obstet Gynecol.* 1991;77:223.
10. Benson CB, Doubilet PM. *Fetal Measurements: Normal and abnormal fetal growth. Diagnostic Ultrasound.* 4th ed. St. Louis: Elsevier; 2011.
11. Rodis JF, et al. Comparison of humerus length with femur length in fetuses with Down syndrome. *Am J Obstet Gynecol.* 1992;165:1051.
12. Chinn D, et al. Ultrasonic identification of fetal lower extremity epiphyseal ossification centers. *Radiology.* 1983;147:815.
13. Doubilet PM, et al. Improved birth weight table for neonates developed from gestations dated by early ultrasonography. *J Ultrasound Med.* 1997;16:241.
14. Lee W, et al. Birthweight prediction by three-dimensional ultrasonographic volumes of the fetal thigh and abdomen. *J Ultrasound Med.* 1997;16:799.
15. Mcleary R, Kuhns L, Barr M. Ultrasonography of the fetal cerebellum. *Radiology.* 1984;151:441.
16. Nicolaides KH, et al. Ultrasound screening for spina bifida: cranial and cerebellar signs. *Lancet.* 1986;1:72.
17. Sarno AP, Rose GS, Harrington RA. Coronal transcerebellar diameter: an alternate view. *Ultrasound Obstet Gynecol.* 1992;2:158.

CHAPTER 53

Fetal Growth Assessment by Sonography

Sandra L. Hagen-Ansert

OBJECTIVES

On completion of this chapter, you should be able to:
- Describe how intrauterine growth restriction may be detected by sonography
- Differentiate between symmetric and asymmetric intrauterine growth restriction
- List which growth parameters should be used to assess intrauterine growth restriction
- Describe how to perform a biophysical profile on a fetus
- Discuss quantitative and qualitative Doppler measurements as applied to obstetrics
- Analyze the significance of macrosomia in a fetus
- Discuss the multiple fetal parameters and calculated ages used to assess the fetal somatic proportions and growth

OUTLINE

Intrauterine Growth Restriction 1395
   Symmetric Intrauterine Growth Restriction 1397
   Asymmetric Intrauterine Growth Restriction 1397
   Small for Gestational Age 1397
Diagnostic Criteria 1397
Biparietal Diameter 1397
Abdominal Circumference 1397
Head Circumference to Abdominal Circumference Ratio 1397
Estimated Fetal Weight 1398
Tests of Fetal Well-Being 1399
   Biophysical Profile 1399
   Nonstress Test 1401
Doppler Sonography 1402
Macrosomia and Large for Gestational Age 1404
   Assessment of the Large for Gestational Age Fetus 1405
   Other Methods for Detecting Macrosomia 1405

KEY TERMS

Biophysical profile (BPP)
Continuous wave (CW) Doppler
Estimated fetal weight (EFW)
Intrauterine growth restriction (IUGR)
Large for gestational age (LGA)
Macrosomia
Nonstress test (NST)
Pulsatility index (PI)
Pulsed wave (PW) Doppler
Resistance index (RI)
Small for gestational age (SGA)
Systolic to diastolic (S/D) ratio

Fetal growth assessment is very important to the perinatologist and obstetric physician. Prior to the sonographic determination of fetal growth, physicians had to rely on their physical assessment of the neonate to determine what occurred during fetal development. The neonate's assessment would determine if the fetus was born preterm (35 to 36 weeks), early term (37 to 38 weeks), full term (39 to 40 weeks), late term (41 weeks), or postterm (after 42 weeks). Clinicians now utilize ultrasound to assess accurate fetal growth by early sonographic dating and subsequent growth series examinations.

Further classification of fetal growth dictated whether the fetal birth weight was appropriate for gestational age, small for gestational age, or large for gestational age or demonstrated restricted intrauterine growth. Fetal growth restriction describes a fetus that is abnormally small for gestational age, which is often the result of placental insufficiency. This chapter covers growth restriction and the fetal monitoring tests available for the growth restricted fetus, which include the nonstress test, biophysical profile, and umbilical artery Doppler evaluation.

INTRAUTERINE GROWTH RESTRICTION

Intrauterine growth restriction (IUGR) is best described as a decreased rate of fetal growth. IUGR complicates 3% to 7% of all pregnancies. It is most commonly defined as a fetal weight at or below 10% for a given gestational age. It often becomes difficult to differentiate the fetus that is constitutionally small (relatively normal but small for gestational age [SGA]) from one that is growth restricted. IUGR (unwell) babies are at a greater risk of antepartum death, perinatal asphyxia, neonatal morbidity, and later developmental problems (Box 53.1).

The most significant maternal factors for IUGR are the history of a previous fetus with IUGR, significant maternal hypertension or smoking, the presence of a uterine anomaly (bicornuate uterus or large leiomyoma), and significant placental hemorrhage (Box 53.2). Constitutional factors such as the sex of the fetus, race of the mother, parity, body mass index, and environmental factors can affect the distribution of normal birth weight in any population.

Before abnormal growth can be diagnosed, the gestational age of the pregnancy must be accurately determined, as presented in Chapter 52. In the prenatal period, an accurate last menstrual period or a first-trimester sonographic age can be used, and both are important for comparison to subsequent sonographic studies for growth assessment. If first-trimester sonography was not performed, then in the second or third trimester, the standard biparietal diameter, head circumference, abdominal circumference, femur length (FL), and other fetal parameters should be used in conjunction with other tests of fetal well-being (e.g., biophysical profile [BPP] and fetal Doppler velocimetry Box 53.3).

The reader should not confuse IUGR with SGA. SGA describes the fetus with a weight below the 10th percentile without reference to the cause. Fetal growth restriction describes a subset of the SGA fetuses with a weight below the 10th percentile as a result of pathologic processes resulting from a variety of maternal, fetal, or placental disorders. The classification of IUGR is based on the morphologic characteristics of the fetuses studied. There are two basic clarifications: symmetric and asymmetric IUGR. The SGA fetus may simply be normal but constitutionally small, but a fetus with IUGR is ill and not following a normal growth trajectory. IUGR is often progressive, with the fetal size lagging further and further behind the expected growth rate.

Symmetric IUGR is usually the result of a first-trimester insult, such as a chromosomal abnormality or infection. This results in a fetus that is proportionately small throughout the pregnancy. Approximately 20% to 30% of all IUGR cases are symmetric. The timing of the pathologic insult is recognized as more important than the actual nature of the underlying pathologic process.

Asymmetric IUGR generally begins in the second or third trimester and usually results from placental insufficiency. This fetus usually shows head sparing at the expense of abdominal and soft tissue growth. The fetal FL exhibits varying degrees of compromise. An early diagnosis of IUGR and close fetal monitoring (BPP, Doppler, and fetal growth evaluation) are of significant help in managing a pregnancy suspected of IUGR. Clinical observations and appropriate actions for IUGR are listed in Box 53.4.

BOX 53.3 Multiple Parameters for IUGR

BPD: imaged in the transverse plane using the cavum septi pellucidi, thalamic nuclei, falx cerebri, and choroid plexus as landmarks. The BPD can be misleading in cases associated with unusual head shapes. Used alone, it is a poor indicator of IUGR.
HC:AC ratio: high false-positive rate for use in screening general population. HC:AC ratio is useful in determining the type of IUGR.
FL:AC ratio: not dependent on knowing gestational age. FL:AC ratio has a poor positive predictive value.
FL: may decrease in size with symmetric IUGR.
AC: measure at level of portal-umbilical venous complex. When growth is compromised, AC is affected secondary to reduced adipose tissue and depletion of glycogen storage in liver. AC is the single most sensitive indicator of IUGR.

AC, Abdominal circumference; *BPD,* biparietal diameter; *FL,* femur length; *HC,* head circumference; *IUGR,* intrauterine growth restriction.

BOX 53.1 Key Points for IUGR

- Oligohydramnios occurs if the fetal urine output is reduced.
- Polyhydramnios develops if the fetus cannot swallow.
- Amniotic fluid pocket <1–2 cm may represent IUGR.
- Not all oligohydramnios is associated with IUGR.

IUGR, Intrauterine growth restriction.

BOX 53.2 Maternal Factors for Intrauterine Growth Restriction

- Previous history of fetus with intrauterine growth restriction
- Significant maternal hypertension
- History of tobacco use
- Presence of uterine anomaly
- Significant placental hemorrhage
- Placental insufficiency

BOX 53.4 Clinical Observations and Actions for Intrauterine Growth Restriction

Clinical signs: decreased fundal height and fetal motion.
Key sonographic markers: grade 3 placenta before 36 weeks or decreased placental thickness.
Sonographer action: alert the physician, determine the cause (maternal history, habits, environmental exposure, viruses, diseases, drug exposure), and carefully evaluate placenta and fetal anatomy with sonography.
Assessment of umbilical artery Doppler for increased resistance to flow: systolic to diastolic ratio >3.0 after 30 weeks after last normal menstrual period is considered abnormal.

Symmetric Intrauterine Growth Restriction

Symmetric growth restriction is characterized by a fetus that is small in all physical parameters (e.g., biparietal diameter [BPD], head circumference [HC], abdominal circumference [AC], and femur length [FL]), which is usually the result of a severe insult in the first trimester. The causes may include low genetic growth potential, intrauterine infection, severe maternal malnutrition, fetal alcohol syndrome, chromosomal anomaly, or severe congenital anomaly. Symmetric IUGR cannot be diagnosed by a single sonographic study because all parameters will have similar growth restriction. To diagnose symmetric IUGR takes two or more growth series over time (at least one month between examinations) so the fetal growth trajectory can be compared and analyzed (Table 52.1).

Asymmetric Intrauterine Growth Restriction

Asymmetric growth restriction is the more common form of IUGR and is usually caused by placental insufficiency. This may be the result of maternal disease, such as diabetes, chronic hypertension, cardiac or renal disease, abruptio placentae, multiple pregnancy, smoking, poor weight gain, drug usage, or uterine anomaly. It should be noted that IUGR fetuses have been born to mothers who have no high-risk factors; therefore, all pregnancies undergoing sonographic examinations should be evaluated for IUGR.

Asymmetric IUGR is characterized by an appropriate BPD and HC and a disproportionately small AC. This reinforces the brain-sparing effect, which states that the last organ to be deprived of essential nutrients is the brain. The BPD and HC may be slightly smaller, but this usually does not happen until the late third trimester.

A proposed third type of IUGR suggests that fetuses with long FL (90th percentile or above) and small AC (at or below the 5th percentile) may be nutritionally deprived, even though their **estimated fetal weight (EFW)** falls at least in the lowest 10%. The theory is that in asymmetric IUGR the fetal length is well preserved, whereas the soft tissue mass is deprived. The FL to AC ratio or ponderal index would be abnormally low. The proponents of this theory claim this occurs in less than 1% of IUGR cases but stress the importance of detection because these cases of IUGR have an EFW within the limits of normal.

Small for Gestational Age

Ultrasound is utilized to discover if a fetus is smaller than normal for their gestational age. The term **small for gestational age (SGA)** is used to describe a neonate or fetus whose birth weight falls below the 10th percentile. The small fetus has been shown to have a compromised fetal growth. The causes for a SGA fetus may include genetic diseases, inherited metabolic disease, chromosome anomalies, or multiple gestations (twins, triplets, and more). The growth restricted pregnancy has an increased risk of perinatal morbidity and mortality, including fetal demise, brain injury, fetal distress, neonatal hypothermia, hypoglycemia, hyperbilirubinemia, and decreased immune function.

Multiple parameters are recommended to determine if the fetus is at risk for growth restriction. These parameters include EFW percentile, amniotic fluid volume, and maternal blood pressure status (normal vs. hypertensive). Benson and Doubilet state that for each week of data on gestation, amniotic fluid volume classification, and maternal blood pressure status, the table presents an EFW range. For a particular fetus, if the EFW is below the lower end of the EFW range, then the fetus can be confidently diagnosed with growth retardation. If the EFW is above the upper end of the range, growth retardation can be excluded with confidence. If the EFW falls within the range, the likelihood of growth retardation is elevated but indeterminate. Doppler of the umbilical and uterine arteries is useful to monitor changes and guide management decisions.

Close fetal monitoring is necessary for the small growth restricted fetus, which includes the nonstress test, the BPP, and the umbilical artery Doppler evaluation.

DIAGNOSTIC CRITERIA

The multiple parameters of IUGR are shown in Box 53.3. Key points of IUGR are listed in Box 53.1.

Biparietal Diameter

The BPD is not a reliable predictor of IUGR for many reasons. The first is the head-sparing theory, which is associated with asymmetric IUGR. Fetal blood is shunted away from other vital organs to nourish the fetal brain, giving the fetus an appropriate BPD (±1 standard deviation) for the true gestational age.

The second problem is the potential alteration in fetal head shape secondary to oligohydramnios. Oligohydramnios is a decreased amount of amniotic fluid often associated with IUGR. Dolichocephaly, or a falsely shortened BPD, can lead to underestimation of the fetal weight, and brachycephaly, or a falsely widened BPD, can lead to overestimation of the EFW. The HC measurement is a more consistent parameter, but a combination of multiple growth parameters (BPD, HC, AC, and FL) at a minimum should be used when diagnosing a fetal growth discrepancy.

Abdominal Circumference

Because of the variability of fetal proportion and size, the AC is a poor predictor of gestational age but is valuable for assessing fetal size. In IUGR, the fetal liver is one of the most severely affected body organs, which, therefore, alters the circumference of the fetal abdomen.

Head Circumference to Abdominal Circumference Ratio

The HC to AC ratio was first developed to detect IUGR in cases of uteroplacental insufficiency. The HC to AC ratio is especially useful in differentiating symmetric and asymmetric

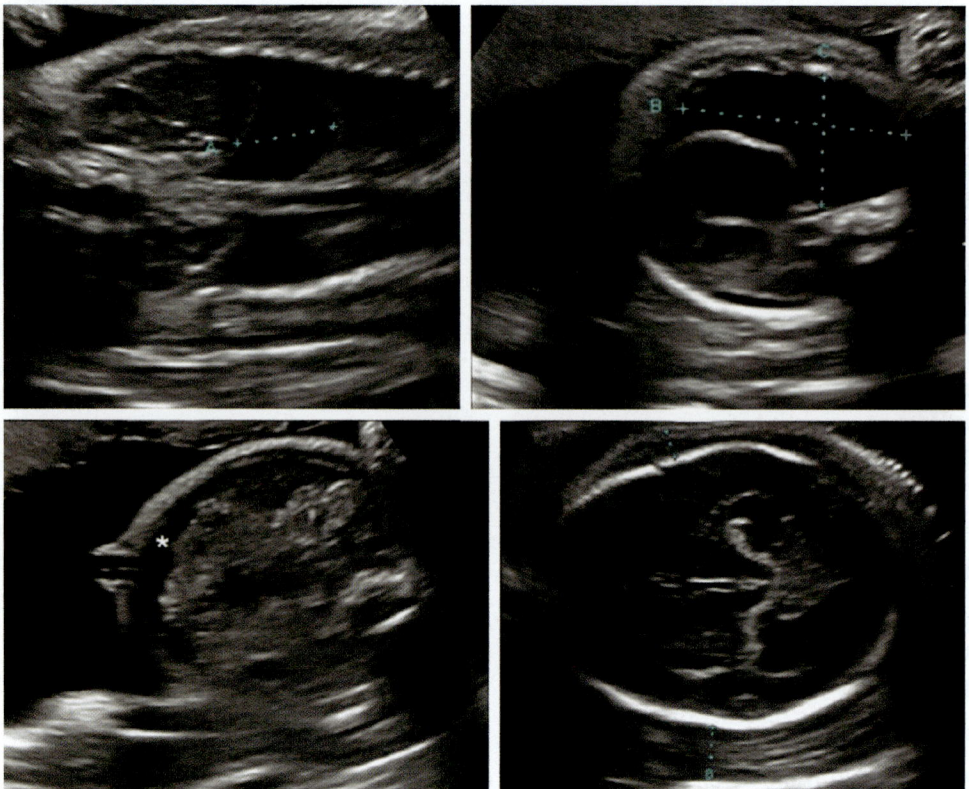

FIG. 53.1 Because of the variability of fetal proportion and size, abdominal circumference is a poor predictor of gestational age but is valuable for assessing fetal size. In intrauterine growth restriction (IUGR), the fetal liver is one of the most severely affected body organs, which therefore alters the circumference of the fetal abdomen. This is a 27-week IUGR fetus with signs of hydrops.

IUGR (Fig. 53.1). For each gestational age, a ratio is assigned with standard deviations. In an appropriate for gestational age (AGA) pregnancy, the ratio should decrease as the gestational age increases.

In the presence of IUGR and with the loss of subcutaneous tissue and fat, the ratio increases. This is counterintuitive because as the fetal AC decreases, the HC:AC ratio increases, and vice versa. The HC:AC ratio is at least two standard deviations above the mean in approximately 70% of fetuses affected with asymmetric IUGR. The HC:AC ratio is not very useful, however, in predicting symmetric IUGR, because the fetal head and fetal abdomen are both equally small. This can be further complicated in cases of fetal infections (TORCH infections), which can produce organomegaly with enlargement of the liver or spleen and the resulting increase in the abdominal circumference in the presence of fetal IUGR.

Estimated Fetal Weight

The most reliable EFW formulas incorporate multiple fetal parameters, such as BPD, HC, AC, and FL. This is important because an overall reduction in the size and mass of these parameters naturally gives a below-normal EFW. An EFW below the 10th percentile is considered by most to be IUGR.

There are numerous formulas for estimating fetal weights. One method uses the BPD and AC to derive the fetal weight, with an accuracy of plus or minus 20%. This formula does not take into consideration HC and FL, which contribute to fetal mass. It also ignores the fact that BPD can be altered slightly because of normal variations in head shape, such as brachycephaly or dolichocephaly. These variations can occur in association with oligohydramnios, which may be found with IUGR.

Another method uses three basic measurements: HC, AC, and FL. The use of the HC instead of the BPD has improved the predictive value to ±15%.

A third method defines three zones of EFW. Each zone has a different prevalence of IUGR. In zone 1, the EFW is above the lower 20% confidence limit and IUGR is ruled out. In zone 3, the EFW is below the lower 0.5% confidence limit and yields an 82% prevalence of IUGR. Patients in this zone should be delivered as soon as lung maturity can be proven. If the EFW is between zone 1 and zone 3, it falls into zone 2, which has a 24% prevalence of IUGR. Patients in this zone should have serial sonograms and fetal heart rate monitoring.

Numerous other growth curves are available, but the one chosen must be appropriate for the population of patients (e.g., sea level versus above sea level). It is also important to remember that symmetric IUGR cannot be diagnosed in a single examination. The interval growth can be plotted on a graph or chart to show the growth sequences. Ethnicity, previous obstetric history, paternal size, fetal gender, and the results of tests of fetal well-being must be considered before IUGR, rather than a healthy SGA, can be diagnosed.

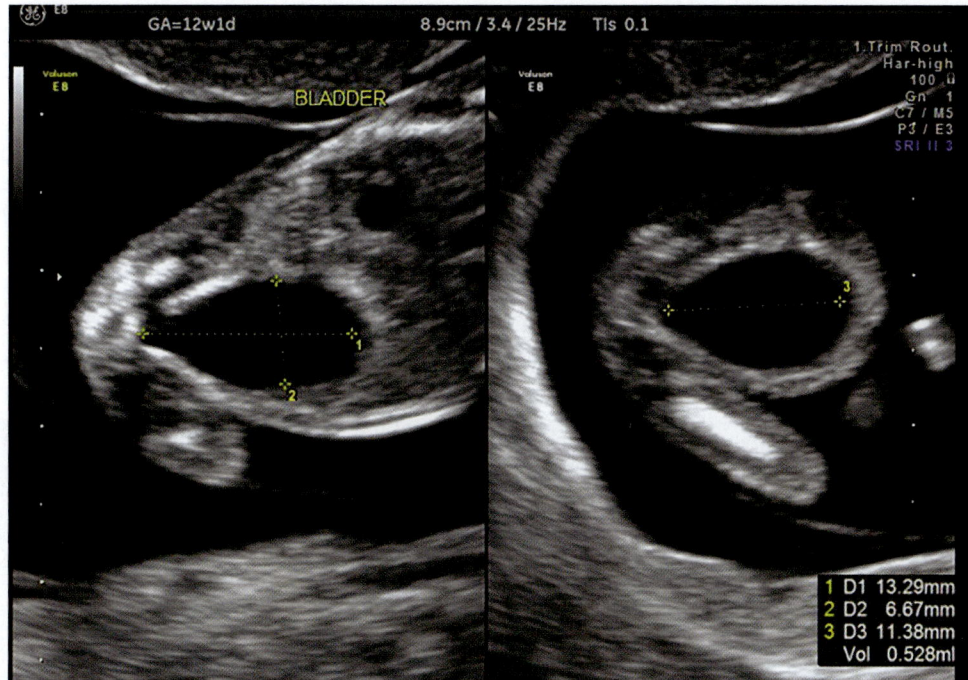

FIG. 53.2 Fetal breathing motion and urine production were the first functional tests to be assessed to determine fetal well-being. The fetal bladder is measured in three dimensions, and the volume is calculated. This is repeated hourly, and the increase is calculated.

TESTS OF FETAL WELL-BEING

Early diagnosis and estimation of fetal well-being are the main problems in managing IUGR. Fetal breathing motion and urine production were the first functional tests to be assessed. The fetal urine production rate was first described in 1973. The fetal bladder was measured in three dimensions, and the volume was calculated (Fig. 53.2). This was repeated hourly, and the increase was calculated. Because of the time and cumbersome technique involved, this method has not been adopted for widespread use.

Biophysical Profile

The **biophysical profile (BPP)** was originally described by Manning and associates in 1980. Since that time, numerous modifications and variations have been contributed by others. The BPP was adapted to form a linear relationship with the assessment of multiple fetal biophysical variables, similar to the Apgar score in the newborn infant or vital signs in the adult. Five biophysical parameters were assessed individually and in combination. Each test had a high false-positive rate that was greatly reduced when all five variables were combined.

The five parameters are as follows:
1. Cardiac nonstress test (NST)
2. Observation of fetal breathing movements (FBM)
3. Gross fetal body movements (FM)
4. Fetal tone (FT)
5. Amniotic fluid volume (AFV)

The BPP has a specified time limit (30 minutes) to observe these parameters (Box 53.5). Each variable is arbitrarily assigned a score of 2 when normal and 0 when abnormal. A

> **BOX 53.5 Biophysical Profile (BPP)**
>
> To determine the BPP, assign a value of 2 points to each of the following:
> - *Fetal breathing movement:* one episode for 30 seconds continuous during a 30-minute observation.
> - *Gross body movement:* at least three discrete body or limb movements in 30 minutes, unprovoked. Continuous movement for 30 minutes should be counted as one movement.
> - *Fetal tone:* active extension and flexion of at least one episode of limbs or trunk.
> - *Fetal heart rate:* also known as the nonstress test. At least two episodes of fetal heart rate changes of 15 beats/min and at least 15 seconds' duration in a 20-minute period.
> - *Amniotic fluid index (AFI):* one pocket of amniotic fluid at least 2 cm in two perpendicular planes or AFI total fluid measures of 5–22 cm.

BPP score of 8 to 10 is considered normal. A score of 4 to 6 has no immediate significance. A score of 0 to 2 indicates either immediate delivery or extending the test to 120 minutes.

Fetal Breathing Movements. A true breathing movement is described as simultaneous inward movement of the chest wall with outward movement of the anterior abdominal wall during inspiration (Fig. 53.3). An alternative area to watch for breathing is the fetal kidney movement in the longitudinal plane. Two points are given if the practitioner notes one episode of breathing lasting 30 seconds within a 30-minute period. If this is absent, no points are given. The fetal central nervous system initiates and regulates the frequency of fetal breathing movements; these patterns vary with sleep-wake cycles.

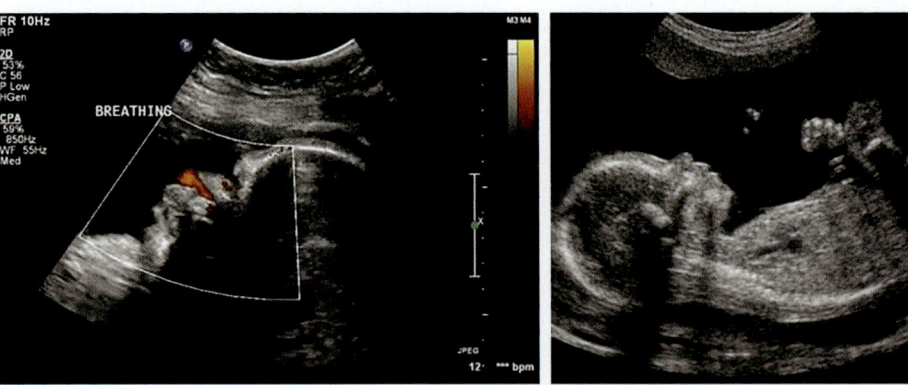

FIG. 53.3 The biophysical profile was adapted to form a linear relationship with the assessment of multiple fetal biophysical variables. A true breathing movement is described as simultaneous inward movement of the chest wall with outward movement of the anterior abdominal wall during inspiration. (*Right image*, Courtesy The Mayo Foundation.)

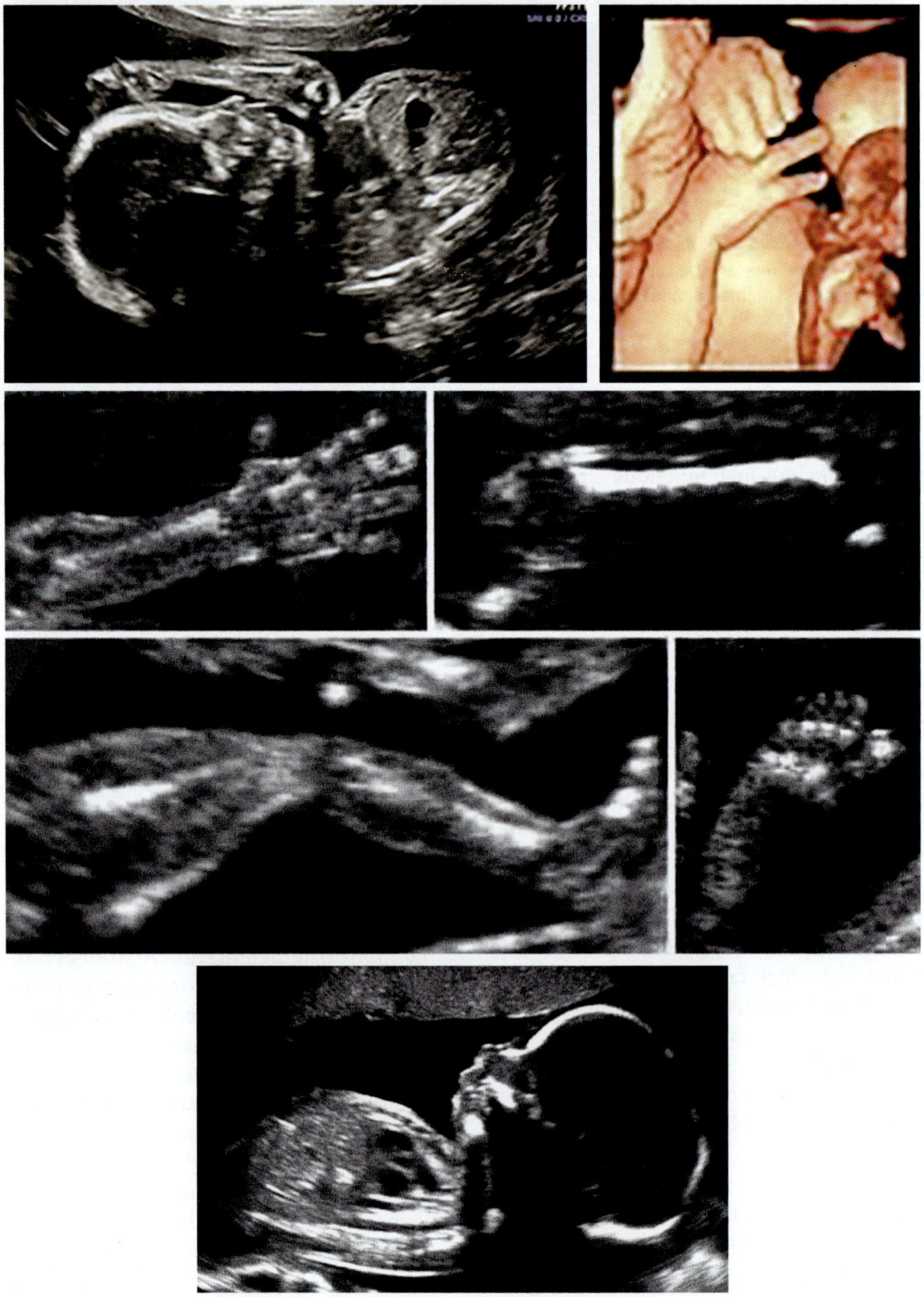

FIG. 53.4 Fetal body and trunk gross movements. At least three definite extremity or trunk movements must be observed within the 30-minute period to score 2 points.

Fetal Body and Trunk Gross Movements. At least three definite extremity or trunk movements must be observed within the 30-minute period to score two points (Fig. 53.4). Fewer than three movements scores zero points. The intact nervous system controls gross fetal body movements; these patterns vary with sleep-wake cycles.

Fetal Tone. Fetal tone is characterized by the presence of at least one episode of extension and immediate return to flexion of an extremity or the spine (Fig. 53.5). One active extension and flexion of an open and closed hand would be a good example of positive fetal tone. Such a movement would score two points. Abnormal fetal tone is noted by a partial extension or flexion of an extremity without a quick return and would score zero points.

Amniotic Fluid Volume. Amniotic fluid volume is related to the fetal-placental unit and is not influenced by the fetal central nervous system. Premature aging of the placenta (grade III) may contribute to oligohydramnios of IUGR syndrome. Evaluation of the four-quadrant amniotic fluid volume is considered normal if the pockets (quadrants) of fluid measure at least 2 cm or more in two planes, and a score of 2 points is given (Fig. 53.6). The transducer must be perpendicular to the center of the pocket of fluid in the center of the screen, and the uterine wall, cord, or fetal parts cannot be included as part of the fluid measurement.

Decreased amniotic fluid may represent IUGR or intrauterine stress, and serial growth parameters may need to be assessed. Fluid that is decreased near term indicates that the baby may need to be delivered earlier than planned. Decreased fluid means the blood is redistributed to the head and the heart; a decrease in renal perfusion and the resulting reductions in urine output cause the AFI to decrease.

Nonstress Test

The **nonstress test (NST)** is done using Doppler to record fetal heart rate and its reactivity to the stress of uterine contraction (Fig. 53.7). The time expended for this portion of the

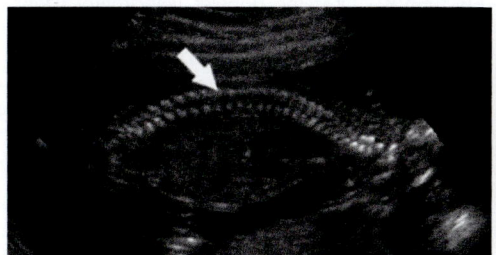
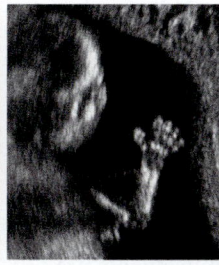
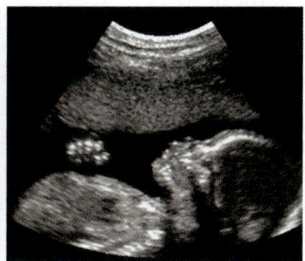

FIG. 53.5 Fetal tone. Fetal tone is characterized by the presence of at least one episode of extension and immediate return to flexion of an extremity or the spine. One active extension and flexion of an open and closed hand would be a good example of positive fetal tone. (*Left image,* Courtesy The Mayo Foundation.)

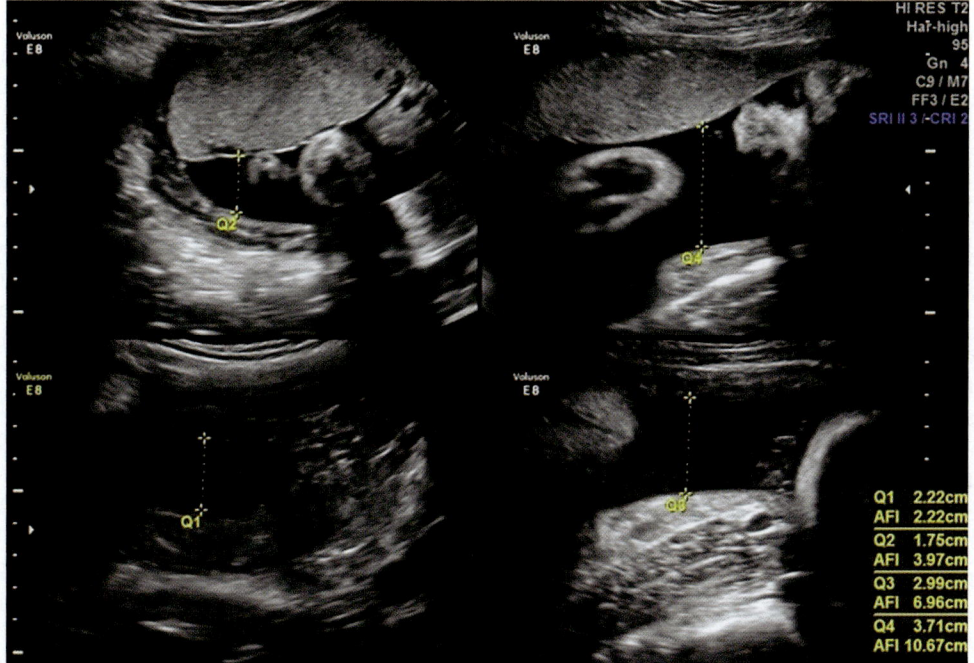

FIG. 53.6 Amniotic fluid volume. Evaluation of the four-quadrant amniotic fluid volume is considered normal if the pockets (quadrants) of fluid measure at least 2 cm or more in two planes and a score of 2 points is given. The transducer must be perpendicular to the center of the pocket of fluid in the center of the screen, and the uterine wall, cord, or fetal parts cannot be included as part of the fluid measurement.

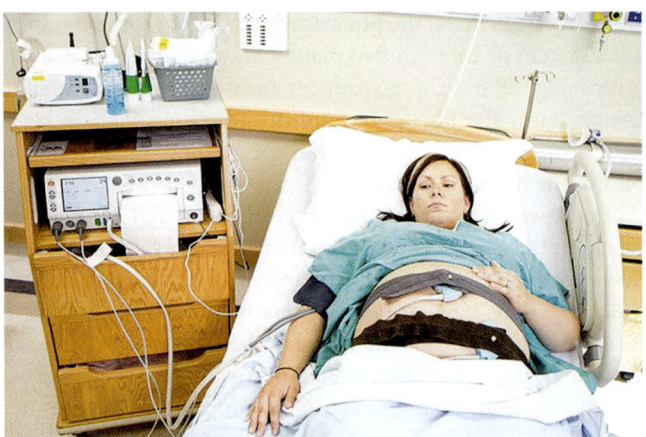

FIG. 53.7 The nonstress test is done using Doppler to record fetal heart rate and its reactivity to the stress of uterine contraction. The time expended for this portion of the examination is usually 40 minutes. Fetal motion is detected as a rapid rise on the recording of uterine activity or the patient noting fetal movements.

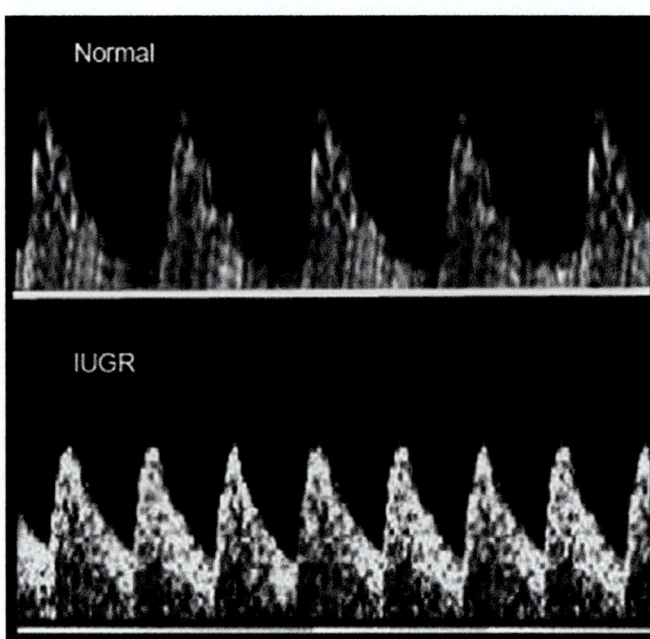

FIG. 53.8 Obstetric Doppler velocimetry (Doppler flow studies) is often used when a fetus has intrauterine growth restriction (IUGR). The waveforms may show that blood flow in the umbilical vessels of the fetus with IUGR is decreased, which would indicate that the fetus may not be receiving enough blood, nutrients, and oxygen from the placenta.

examination is usually 40 minutes. Fetal motion is detected as a rapid rise on the recording of uterine activity or the patient noting fetal movements. The following conditions indicate a reactive, or normal, NST and score of 2 points:
- Two fetal heart rate accelerations of 15 beats/min or more
- Accelerations lasting at least 15 seconds
- Gross fetal movements noted over 20 minutes without late decelerations

These fetal heart accelerations with fetal movements are a positive sign of fetal well-being; late reductions in rate or decelerations indicate a poor prognosis. Zero points are awarded if two fetal heart rate accelerations with gross fetal movements are not seen during a 40-minute period. Forty minutes is arbitrarily used to accommodate the fetal sleep-wake cycles.

The test is considered normal when all the variables monitored by sonography are normal (FBM, FM, FT, AFV) without the performance of the NST.

The goal of the BPP is to find a way to predict and manage the fetus with hypoxia. One study analyzed the BPP variables based on the gradual hypoxia concept. This concept states that dynamic biophysical activities (FT, FM, FBM, and fetal heart rate reactivity) are controlled by neural activity arising in distinct anatomic sites in the brain. These become functional at different stages of development, with the later-developing centers requiring higher oxygen levels. The fetal tone center develops at 7.5 to 8.5 weeks. The fetal movement center develops at nine weeks, and regular diaphragmatic motion develops by 20 to 21 weeks. Heart rate reactivity is the last to occur; it appears by the late second to early third trimester. The hypothesis of gradual hypoxia further supposes that centers that develop later are more sensitive to acute hypoxia. It is therefore expected that the loss of cardiac reactivity and suppression of fetal breathing movements will occur with relatively mild hypoxia. Cessation of FM and eventually loss of FT will occur with progressively more profound hypoxemia.

Doppler Sonography

Obstetric Doppler velocimetry (Doppler flow studies) is often used when a fetus has IUGR. The waveforms may show that blood flow in the umbilical vessels of the fetus with IUGR is decreased, which would indicate that the fetus may not be receiving enough blood, nutrients, and oxygen from the placenta (Fig. 53.8).

Two basic types of Doppler are used in sonography. The simplest technique is continuous wave (CW) Doppler. The second is pulsed wave Doppler. With **CW Doppler**, a single transducer has two separate piezoelectric crystals, one that continuously transmits signals and one that simultaneously receives signals. Because the crystals are either emitting or receiving sound, CW Doppler measures no specific range or depth resolution (i.e., it records all velocities along the designated line of interrogation). No intrauterine imaging is available with CW, but it may be used in conjunction with a real-time sonographic system to locate or confirm a vessel sampling site. CW is limited to the study of superficial vessels because it cannot discriminate between signals arising from different structures along the beam path.

In **pulsed wave (PW) Doppler**, short bursts of ultrasonic energy are emitted at regular intervals. The same piezoelectric crystal both sends and receives the signals, which allows for range or depth discrimination. The depth of the target is calculated from the elapsed time between transmission of the pulse and reception of its echoes, assuming a constant speed of sound in tissue. In pulsed wave Doppler, a sonographer can electronically steer the insonating Doppler beam with the trackball or joystick on the keyboard, along with transducer position and angle manipulations. This permits sampling of vessels at specific anatomic locations.

Doppler, or real-time, ultrasonic energy has not been associated with any ill effect to the mother or the fetus when used at the manufacturer's recommended safety level. US Food and Drug Administration guidelines state that the spatial peak-temporal average intensity (SPTA, a unit used to measure ultrasonic intensity) must be less than 94 milliwatts per square centimeter (mW/cm^2) in situ. Most commercial equipment uses variable acoustic outputs between 1 mW/cm^2 and 46 mW/cm^2. The power output of a given unit should be known before the unit is used on a fetus. Newer sonographic equipment now allows the user to display this information on the screen as the examination is being performed. The mechanical index and thermal index are used to indicate the relative acoustic output intensities. The thermal index is an estimation of the acoustical power that may result in an increase of tissue temperature 1°C. The mechanical index is an indication of the likelihood of causing cavitation, or micro gas bubbles, in the tissues.

Quantitative and Qualitative Measurements. Two main types of measurements can be taken from a Doppler waveform: quantitative and qualitative. Quantitative Doppler flow measurements include blood flow and velocity, whereas qualitative measurements look at the characteristics of the waveform that indirectly approximate flow and resistance to flow. Qualitative measurements include **systolic to diastolic (S/D) ratio**, **resistance index (RI)**, and **pulsatility index (PI)** (Box 53.6). The S/D ratio measures peak systole to end-diastolic blood flow. The resistance index is calculated as systole minus diastole divided by systole. The pulsatility takes the difference between peak systole and end diastole and divides this by the mean of the maximum frequency over the whole cardiac cycle.

Doppler sonography has shown that in fetuses with asymmetric IUGR, vascular resistance increases in the aorta and umbilical artery and decreases in the fetal middle cerebral artery. This reinforces the head-sparing theory, which describes the assurance of blood flow to the fetal brain at the expense of the extremities and the rest of the body (Fig. 53.9).

Increased vascular resistance is reflected by an increased S/D ratio or pulsatility index. Some authors consider an S/D ratio of more than 3.0 in the umbilical artery after 30 weeks to be abnormal, and it is demonstrated by increased resistance in the fetal circulation. The maternal uterine artery S/D ratio should be below 2.6 (Fig. 53.10). A ratio above 2.6 suggests increased vascular resistance and indicates a decreased maternal blood supply to the uterus.

In the umbilical circulation, extreme cases of elevated resistance causing absent or reverse end-diastolic flow velocity waveforms are associated with high rates of morbidity and mortality. One report demonstrated that an SGA fetus with an increased umbilical artery S/D ratio is at much higher risk for poor perinatal outcome than a small fetus with a normal S/D ratio.

> **BOX 53.6 Doppler Measurements**
>
> **Resistive index** = Maximum systolic velocity − Diastolic velocity/systolic velocity
> **Systolic/diastolic ratio** = Maximum systolic velocity/diastolic velocity
> **Pulsatility index** = Maximum systolic velocity − Diastolic velocity/mean velocity
> **Acceleration time** = Time from beginning of systole to peak systole
> **Deceleration time** = Time from peak systole to end diastole

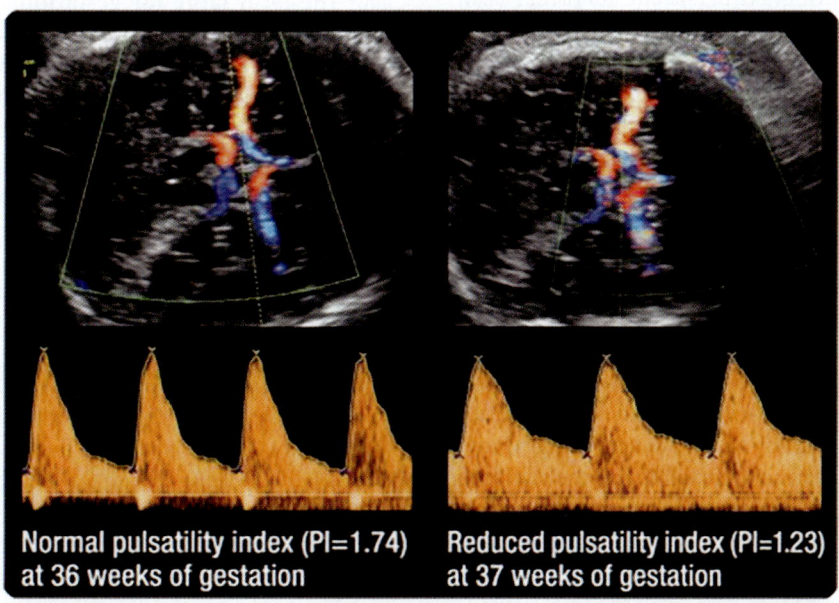

FIG. 53.9 Doppler sonography has shown that in fetuses with asymmetric intrauterine growth restriction vascular resistance increases in the aorta and umbilical artery and decreases in the fetal middle cerebral artery. This reinforces the head-sparing theory, which describes the assurance of blood flow to the fetal brain at the expense of the extremities and the rest of the body.

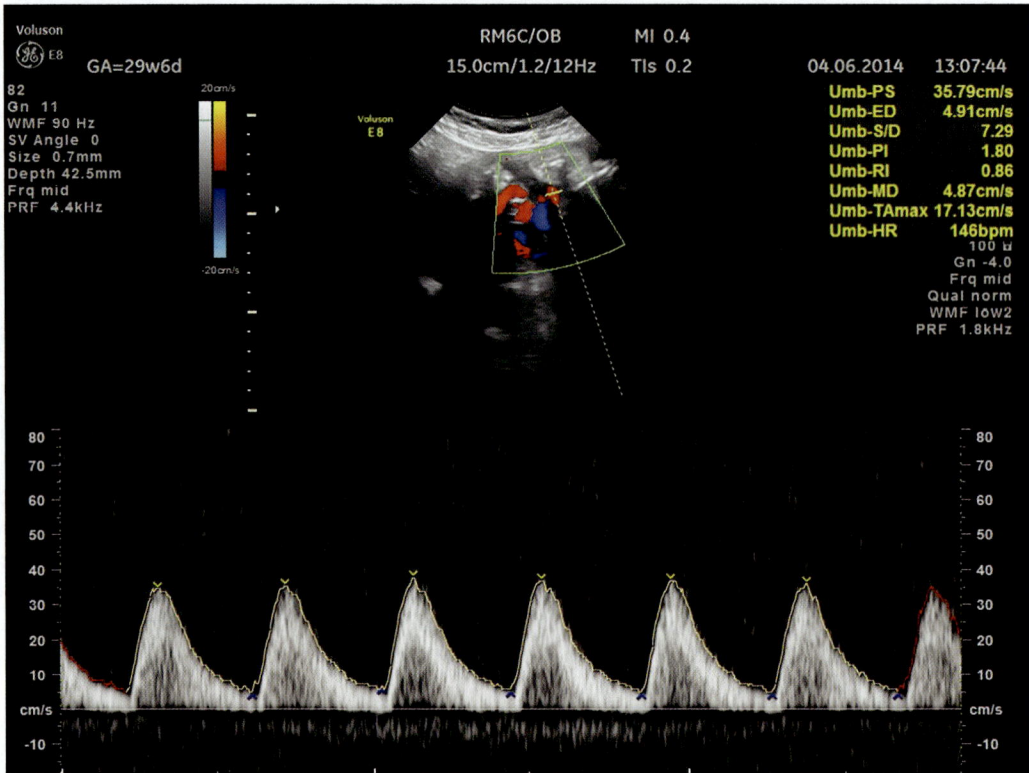

FIG. 53.10 Increased vascular resistance is reflected by an increased systolic to diastolic (S/D) ratio or pulsatility index. This S/D ratio measured abnormal at 7.29. The maternal uterine artery S/D ratio should be <2.6. A ratio >2.6 suggests increased vascular resistance and indicates a decreased maternal blood supply to the uterus.

Abnormal umbilical artery S/D velocity waveforms have been shown to improve with the patient on bed rest in the left lateral position. The patients were closely monitored with serial Doppler, BPP, and fetal growth evaluation. Of 128 pregnant women, 66 (51.5%) reverted to normal flow in 4.5 ±1.5 weeks. Another group (48.5%) exhibited persistent abnormal flow. None of the improved group exhibited fetal distress or perinatal mortality, whereas in the abnormal flow group 24% experienced fetal distress and 13% experienced perinatal mortality. The report of the study proposes that a subset of patients with abnormal Doppler velocimetry improves with bed rest and has a better perinatal outcome, whereas patients with persistent abnormal flow are at risk for poor perinatal outcome.

In conclusion, the best method of solving the puzzle of whether a fetus has IUGR or is constitutionally small is to combine an evaluation of all parameters. A normal umbilical artery, maternal uterine artery, and fetal middle cerebral artery help in evaluating the fetus that is normal, but just small, rather than small secondary to IUGR. The practitioner also must consider the family history of birth weights and ethnicity. For example, it is almost invalid to use the standard EFW growth curves when plotting the fetal growth of a constitutionally small ethnic group, such as some Southeast Asians. A fetus could be labeled as SGA, although its size might be totally appropriate for its heritage. Use of all the fetal surveillance tests (i.e., EFW, AFI, placental grading, BPP, NST) may allow better evaluation of the in utero environment.

MACROSOMIA AND LARGE FOR GESTATIONAL AGE

Macrosomia is traditionally defined as a large neonate with a birth weight of 4000 g or greater, independent of gestational age. The term **large for gestational age (LGA)** describes a neonate with a birth weight above the 90th percentile for estimated gestational age. With respect to delivery, however, any fetus that is too large for the pelvis through which it must pass is macrosomic. Macrosomia has shown to be 1.2 to 2 times more frequent than normal in women who are multiparous, are 35 years or older, have a pre-pregnancy weight of more than 70 kg (154 lb), have a ponderal index in the upper 10%, have pregnancy weight gain of 20 kg (44 lb) or greater, have a postdate pregnancy, or have a history of delivering an LGA fetus.

Macrosomia is also a common result of poorly controlled maternal diabetes mellitus. The frequency of macrosomia in the offspring of mothers with diabetes ranges from 25% to 45%. It is widely accepted that increased levels of glucose and other substrates result in fetal hyperinsulinemia, which promotes accelerated somatic growth. Macrosomic infants of insulin-dependent diabetic mothers are usually heavy and show a characteristic pattern of organomegaly. In addition to adipose tissue, the liver, heart, and adrenals are disproportionately increased in size, which can be reflected by an increased AC. Keep in mind that not all infants of diabetic mothers are larger than average; diabetic mothers with severe vascular disease may in fact be growth restricted.

Malformation syndromes in which the fetus demonstrates an increase in size, with or without organomegaly, is a feature of the following syndromes: Beckwith-Wiedemann, Marshall-Smith, Sotos, and Weaver syndrome.

The macrosomic fetus has an increased incidence of morbidity and mortality as a result of head and shoulder injuries and cord compression. Clavicular fractures, facial and brachial palsies, meconium aspiration, perinatal asphyxia, neonatal hypoglycemia, and other metabolic complications are significantly increased in macrosomic pregnancies.

Clinical considerations of macrosomia should include the genetic constitution (e.g., familial traits) and environmental factors (e.g., maternal diabetes or prolonged pregnancy).

Two terms relating to macrosomic fetuses are *mechanical macrosomia* and *metabolic macrosomia*. Three types of mechanical macrosomia have been identified: (1) fetuses that are generally large, (2) fetuses that are generally large but with especially large shoulders, and (3) fetuses that have a normal trunk but a large head. The first type can result from genetic factors, prolonged pregnancy, or multiparity. The second type is found in the diabetic pregnancy, and the third type can be caused by genetic constitution or pathologic process, such as hydrocephalus. One type of metabolic macrosomia has been identified, which is the group of LGA fetuses based on a standard weight curve appropriate for the population being studied and a normal range extending two standard deviations above the mean.

Assessment of the Large for Gestational Age Fetus

Accurate sonographic prediction of macrosomia would be invaluable to the obstetrician in managing and delivering a fetus with macrosomia. The BPD is not the optimal parameter for prediction of macrosomia. The abdominal circumference is useful as a parameter to assess fetal size, although it is not very predictive of gestational age and not as accurate in the third trimester.

The prenatal diagnosis of macrosomia relies on the EFW. A weight above 4500 g in a nondiabetic mother or a weight above 4000 g in a diabetic mother is suggestive of macrosomia. The EFW above the 90th percentile for gestational age suggests an LGA fetus.

Other Methods for Detecting Macrosomia

In addition to the numerous biometric parameters useful for detecting macrosomia discussed, there are other sonographic observations that can help rule out the possibility of fetal macrosomia. Mothers with diabetes may accumulate more amniotic fluid (polyhydramnios) than nondiabetic patients. The presence of polyhydramnios in the nondiabetic patient could alert the physician to the presence of undiagnosed maternal glucose intolerance. The possibility of a fetal anomaly should not be excluded; polyhydramnios has been associated with open neural tube defects and other conditions that may limit fetal swallowing of amniotic fluid.

The placenta of the macrosomic fetus can become significantly large and thick because it is not immune to the growth-enhancing effects of fetal insulin. A placental thickness greater than 5 cm is considered thick when the measurement is taken at right angles to its long axis.

ACKNOWLEDGMENT

The author acknowledges the contributions of Terry Dubose to this chapter in the previous edition.

Key Pearls

- Intrauterine growth restriction is best described as a decreased rate of fetal growth as measured by ultrasound over time.
- Small for gestational age describes the fetus with a weight below the 10th percentile without reference to the cause.
- Symmetric intrauterine growth restriction (IUGR) is usually the result of a first-trimester insult, such as a chromosomal abnormality or infection.
- Symmetric IUGR generally begins in the second or third trimester and usually results from placental insufficiency.
- There is an association between IUGR and decreased amniotic fluid (oligohydramnios).
- Doppler may show that blood flow in the umbilical vessels of the fetus with IUGR is decreased, which would indicate that the fetus may not be receiving enough blood, nutrients, and oxygen from the placenta.
- Macrosomia is traditionally defined as a birth weight of 4000 g or greater, or above the 90th percentile for estimated gestational age.

BIBLIOGRAPHY

Benson CB, Doubilet PM. *Fetal Biometry and Growth in Callen's Ultrasonography in Obstetrics and Gynecology*. ed 6, Philadelphia: Elsevier; 2017.

Crane JP, Kropa MM. Prediction of intrauterine growth retardation via ultrasonically measured head/abdominal circumference ratios. *Obstet Gynecol*. 1979;54:597.

Hadlock FP, et al. Estimation of fetal weight with the use of head, body, and femur measurements: a prospective study. *Am J Obstet Gynecol*. 1985;15:333.

Manning FA, Platt LP, Sypus L. Antepartum fetal evaluation: development of a biophysical profile. *Am J Obstet Gynecol*. 1980;136:787.

Mehalek K, et al. Comparison of continuous wave and pulsed wave S/D ratios of umbilical and uterine arteries. *Am J Obstet Gynecol*. 1988;72:603.

Phelan JP, et al. Amniotic fluid volume assessment with the four quadrant technique at 36–42 weeks gestation. *J Reprod Fertil*. 1987;32:540.

Sengupta S, et al. Perinatal outcome following improvement of abnormal umbilical artery velocimetry. *Obstet Gynecol*. 1992;78:1062.

Trudinger BJ, et al. Flow velocity waveforms in the material uteroplacental and fetal umbilical placental circulations. *Am J Obstet Gynecol*. 1985;152:155.

CHAPTER 54

Sonography and High-Risk Pregnancy

Carol Mitchell, Barbara Trampe, and Kelsey Doyle

OBJECTIVES

On completion of this chapter, you should be able to:
- Define *high-risk pregnancy*
- Describe the maternal and fetal factors for a pregnancy that are considered high risk
- Discuss the role of sonography in the high-risk pregnancy

OUTLINE

Screening Tests 1406
Maternal Factors in High-Risk Pregnancy 1407
    Advanced Maternal Age 1407
    Immune and Nonimmune Hydrops 1407
    Vaginal Bleeding 1412
Maternal Diseases of Pregnancy 1413
    Diabetes 1413
    Hypertension 1415
    Systemic Lupus Erythematosus 1415
    Other Maternal Disease 1415
Ultrasound in Labor and Delivery 1416
    Preterm Labor 1416
Fetal Factors in High-Risk Pregnancy 1417
    Fetal Death 1417
    Large for Gestational Age 1417
    Small for Gestational Age 1417
Multiple Gestation Pregnancy 1418
    Dizygotic Twins 1419
    Monozygotic Twins 1419
    Anomalies Specific to Twin Pregnancies 1422
    Scanning Multiple Gestations 1423

KEY WORDS

Acardiac anomaly
Advanced maternal age (AMA)
Anasarca
Caudal regression syndrome
Conjoined twins
Detailed fetal anatomic survey ultrasound
Dizygotic
Eclampsia
Fetus papyraceous
Hydrops
Hydrops fetalis
Hyperemesis gravidarum
Maternal serum alpha-fetoprotein
Maternal serum quad screen
Monozygotic
Nonimmune hydrops (NIH)
Oligohydramnios
Polyhydramnios
Preeclampsia
Pregnancy-induced hypertension (PIH)
Premature rupture of membranes (PROM)
Spalding sign
Systemic lupus erythematosus (SLE)
Twin anemia-polycythemia syndrome (TAPS)
Twin-to-twin transfusion syndrome (TTTS)

A high-risk obstetric patient is one who has the potential for or is at an increased risk for an adverse maternal or fetal pregnancy outcome. At its extreme, *adverse* would mean maternal or fetal injury or death. When identifying the high-risk pregnant patient, both the mother and the fetus must be considered. Therefore, this chapter discusses both maternal and fetal high-risk factors.

SCREENING TESTS

Screening tests, as opposed to diagnostic tests, are offered to low-risk populations to identify patients whose risk is high enough for them to be offered diagnostic testing.

There are a variety of tests that can be offered in either the first or second trimester. The first-trimester screen is performed by looking for the pattern of biochemical markers associated with plasma protein A (PAPP-A) and free β-human chorionic gonadotropin (β-hCG). These laboratory values are used in conjunction with an ultrasound (performed between 11 and 14 weeks) to measure the nuchal translucency and the presence of the nasal bone. Based on the patient's PAPP-A and free β-hCG laboratory values, age, nuchal translucency measurement, and the presence or absence of the nasal bone, a more accurate risk calculation can be made for having a child with a chromosomal abnormality, congenital heart defect, skeletal dysplasia, or other syndromes. To offer this screening, sonographers must become certified for first-trimester screening. This requires the sonographers performing the test to take an online course and pass a written test. Upon receiving a passing score, a minimum of three ultrasound evaluations of the nuchal translucency must be evaluated for compliance with the certifying organization before the sonographer is certified to perform the examination. This evaluation is repeated annually. Laboratories performing the first-trimester screen will only accept samples and data from certified sonographers. The advantage to parents with first-trimester screening is that they can evaluate their risk for having a child with a chromosomal or syndromatic abnormality much earlier in pregnancy. They may then choose to undergo additional testing, including noninvasive prenatal testing (NIPT) or invasive testing such as chorionic villus sampling (CVS) or amniocentesis to obtain tissue for chromosomal analysis. Cell-free DNA is an advanced screening NIPT with a much higher detection rate for Down syndrome and trisomy 18 (99%), and trisomy 13 (91%) than the first-trimester screen or the quad screen, which is performed in the second trimester.[1] NIPT can be offered as early as 10 weeks, and because it can also screen for abnormalities with the sex chromosomes, such as Klinefelter syndrome (XXY), triple X syndrome (XXX), and Turner syndrome (XO), it can identify the fetal sex. This test evaluates the chromosomes from small pieces of fetal DNA found within a maternal blood sample. NIPT is usually combined with ultrasound evaluation of the nuchal translucency for additional accuracy. Although this test is currently offered to populations of pregnant women with a high risk of abnormal findings only, it holds promise for the future as an alternative to current screening and invasive testing.

Second-trimester screening can be performed with the maternal serum quad screen laboratory value and/or a detailed fetal anatomic survey ultrasound examination. The **maternal serum quad screen** looks at four serum markers: alpha-fetoprotein (AFP), hCG, unconjugated estriol (uE3), and inhibin-A. If a first-trimester screening was performed, it would not include the AFP testing so it may be recommended to be done as a single test to screen for neural tube defects in the second trimester.

The **detailed fetal anatomic survey ultrasound** is a detailed evaluation of specified fetal anatomy and biometry that can be seen at the time of examination. Most ultrasound departments prefer to perform a detailed fetal anatomic survey examination between 18 and 20 weeks of gestation. This time period is chosen because it often yields the best view of fetal anatomy based on size, and the accuracy of the dating biometry is within 10 to 14 days of the expected date of delivery. The detailed fetal anatomic survey ultrasound examination includes, but is not limited to, the evaluation of the anatomy shown in Table 54.1.

Based on the results of the screening maternal serum quad screen and the detailed fetal anatomic survey ultrasound, patients' risk for having a child with a chromosomal anomaly or neural tube defect can be reassessed. Parents are counseled with this information and can then choose to have NIPT or a diagnostic amniocentesis to obtain fluid for chromosomal analysis, if desired.

MATERNAL FACTORS IN HIGH-RISK PREGNANCY

Advanced Maternal Age

By definition, **advanced maternal age (AMA)** describes a patient who will be 35 or older at the time of delivery. AMA can be an indicator for high-risk pregnancy. For example, the incidence of Down syndrome increases with age. The risk of a 35-year-old woman conceiving a fetus with Down syndrome is 1 in 294, but the risk rises to 1 in 40 at age 40 years.[2] Maternal age alone, however, fails to detect approximately 66% of fetuses with Down syndrome[2] because these babies are being born to younger women without known risk factors for chromosomal abnormalities. In the United States, it is now standard practice to offer AMA women genetic counseling, screening options, or invasive prenatal testing for karyotypic analysis. The American College of Obstetricians and Gynecologists (ACOG) guidelines recommend that maternal serum screening for neural tube defects and Down syndrome be offered to all women.

Immune and Nonimmune Hydrops

Hydrops fetalis is a condition in which excessive fluid accumulates within at least two fetal body cavities. This fluid accumulation may result in **anasarca**, ascites, pericardial effusion, pleural effusion, placental edema, and polyhydramnios. There are two classifications of fetal **hydrops**: immune hydrops and nonimmune hydrops (NIH). By ultrasound evaluation, both types are characterized by extensive accumulation of fluids in fetal tissues or body cavities. NIH is unrelated to the presence of maternal serum immunoglobulin G (IgG) antibody against one of the fetal blood cell antigens.

Immune Hydrops. Blood group isoimmunization is diagnosed on routine antenatal laboratory evaluation, which tests for the presence of a variety of antibodies. Any significant antibodies are evaluated for strength of antibody response, which is reported in a titer format (i.e., 1:4, 1:16). If an antibody titer is detected, the pregnancy should be monitored.

Immune hydrops is initiated by the presence of maternal serum IgG antibody against one of the fetal red blood cell (RBC) antigens in a process known as *sensitization*. An antigen is any substance that elicits an immunologic response such as the production of an antibody to that substance. In pregnancy, this can occur anytime a mother is exposed to RBC antigens different from her own. For example, if a father and fetus are

TABLE 54.1 Components of a Basic and Detailed Fetal Ultrasound

Component	Basic	Detailed
Head and neck	Lateral cerebral ventricles Choroid plexus Midline falx Cavum septi pellucidi Cerebellum Cisterna magna	Third ventricle[a] Fourth ventricle[a] Lateral ventricles[b] Cerebellar lobes, vermis, and cisterna magna[b] Corpus callosum[a] Integrity and shape of cranial vault Brain parenchyma Neck
Face	Upper lip	Profile Coronal face (nose/lips/lens[a]) Palate,[a] maxilla, mandible, and tongue[a] Ear position and size[a] Orbits[a]
Chest Heart and thorax	Cardiac activity Four-chamber view Left ventricular outflow tract Right ventricular outflow tract	Aortic arch Superior and inferior venae cava Three-vessel view Three-vessel and trachea view Lungs Integrity of diaphragm Ribs[a]
Abdomen	Stomach (presence, size, and situs) Kidneys Urinary bladder Cord insertion site into fetal abdomen Umbilical cord vessel number	Small and large bowel[a] Adrenal glands[a] Gallbladder[a] Liver Renal arteries[a] Spleen[a] Integrity of abdominal wall[b]
Spine	Cervical Thoracic Lumbar Sacral spine	Integrity of spine and overlying soft tissue[b] Shape and curvature
Extremities	Legs Arms	Number: architecture and position Hands Feet Digits: number and position[a]
Genitalia	In multiple gestations When medically indicated	Sex[a]
Placenta	Location Relationship to internal os Appearance Placental cord insertion (when possible)	Masses Placental cord insertion Accessory/succenturiate lobe connecting vascular supply to primary placenta[a]
Standard evaluation	Fetal number Presentation Qualitative or semiqualitative estimate of amniotic fluid	
Maternal anatomy	Cervix (transvaginal when indicated) Uterus Adnexa	
Biometry	Biparietal diameter Head circumference Femur length Abdominal circumference Fetal weight estimate	Cerebellum[a] Inner and outer orbital diameters[a] Nuchal thickness (16–20 weeks) Nasal bone measurement (15–22 weeks) Humerus[a] Ulna/radius[a] Tibia/fibula[a]

[a]Performed when medically indicated.
[b]Also included in the basic obstetric examination.
From American Institute of Ultrasound in Medicine (AIUM). 76811 Task Force: consensus report on the detailed fetal anatomic ultrasound examination. J Ultrasound Med. 2014;33:189–195.

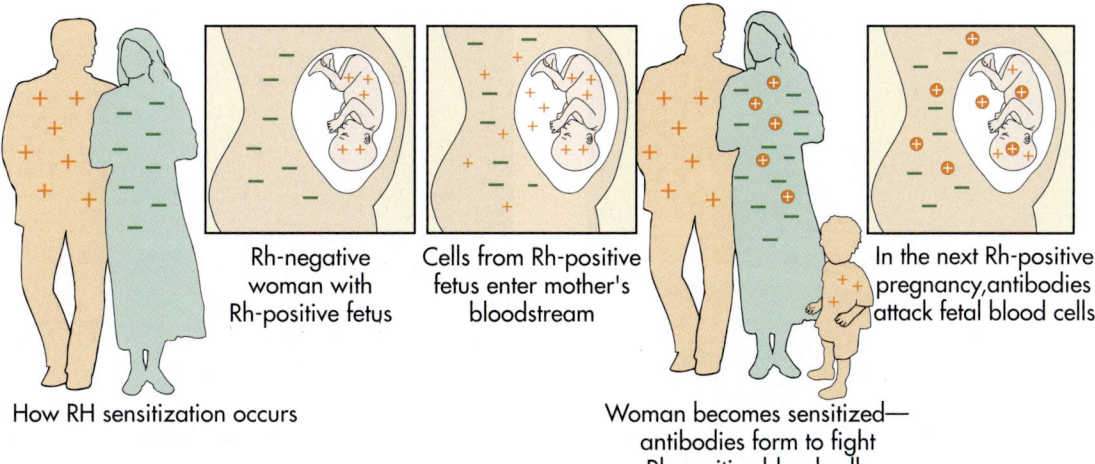

FIG. 54.1 The concept of Rh sensitization.

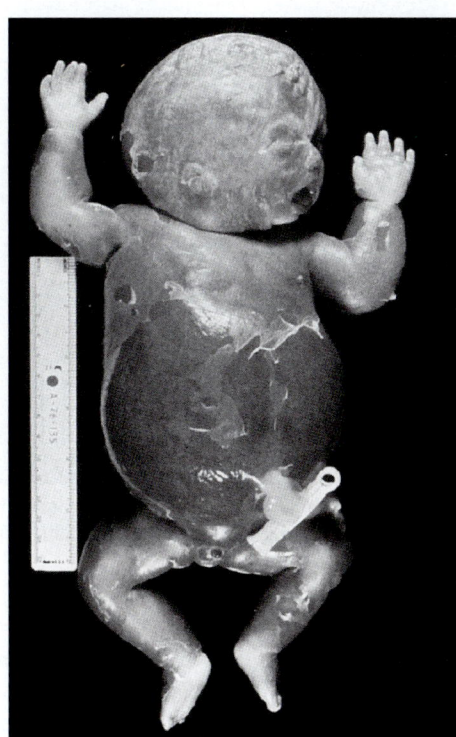

FIG. 54.2 Hydropic, Rh-sensitized fetal demise. Note edema of the extremities and protuberant abdomen.

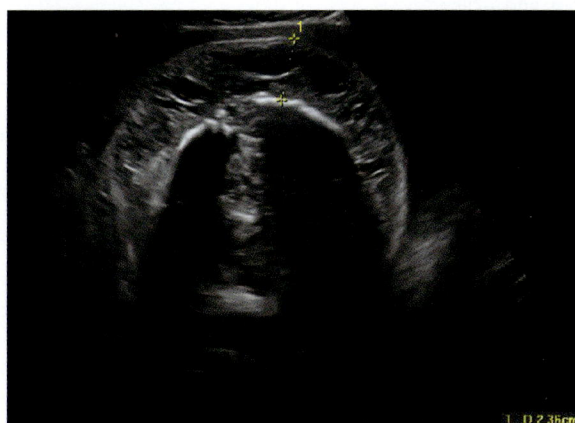

FIG. 54.3 Scalp edema.

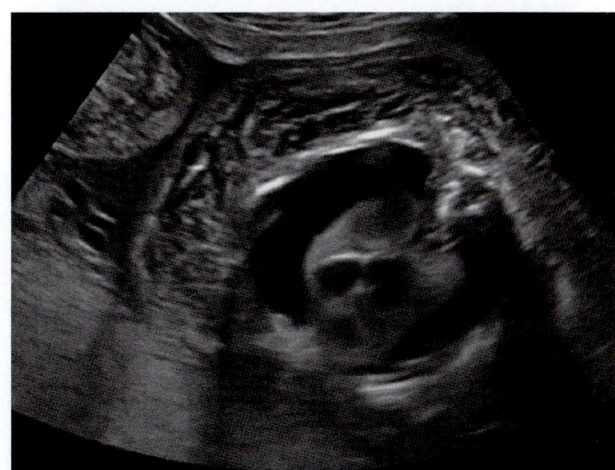

FIG. 54.4 Pleural effusion.

Rh+ and a mother is Rh− and there is a maternal-fetal hemorrhage (mixing of blood), maternal antibodies can be produced against the Rh antigen. In subsequent pregnancies, these antibodies can pass through the placenta and destroy fetal blood cells, resulting in fetal anemia (Fig. 54.1). Today, this condition is rare and can be prevented if RhoGAM is given any time there is potential mixing of the maternal and fetal circulation.

When a sensitized gravid uterus is not treated with RhoGAM, the mother develops an antibody called maternal IgG. This antibody is able to cross the maternal-fetal barrier and enter fetal circulation. It attaches to the fetal RBCs and destroys them in a process called *hemolysis*. Hemolysis can result in fetal anemia, leading to congestive heart failure and hydrops (Fig. 54.2). The severity of fetal anemia can be determined by sonographic surveillance, amniocentesis, and cordocentesis.

Sonographic Surveillance. Sonographic surveillance for an isoimmunized pregnancy should include (but not be limited to) assessment for signs of hydrops. Sonographic findings of hydrops are scalp edema (Fig. 54.3), pleural effusion (Fig. 54.4),

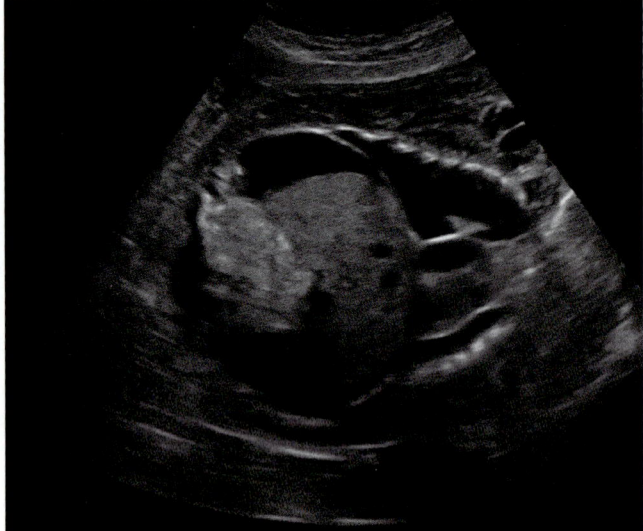

FIG. 54.5 Coronal view of the fetal chest and abdomen with pleural effusion and ascites.

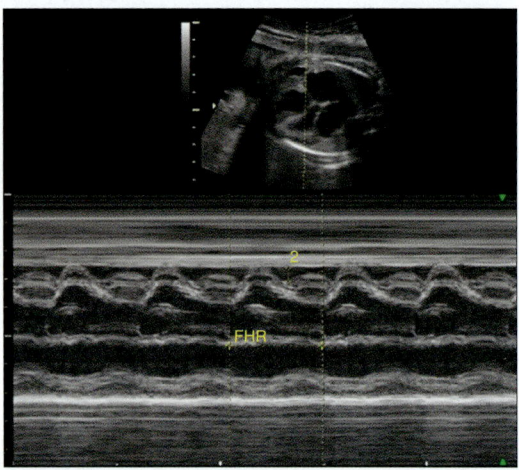

FIG. 54.6 Two-dimensional and M-mode image demonstrating a pericardial effusion.

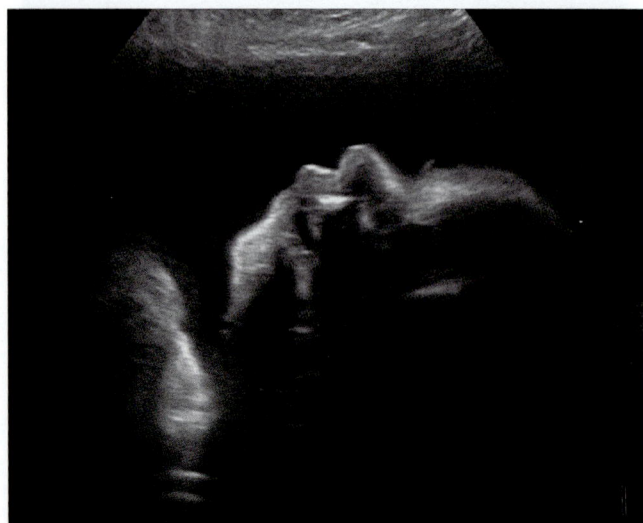

FIG. 54.7 Fetal profile and polyhydramnios.

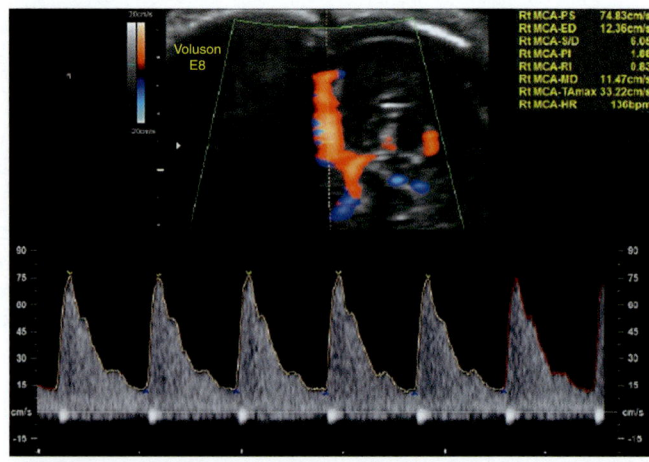

FIG. 54.8 Doppler of the middle cerebral artery.

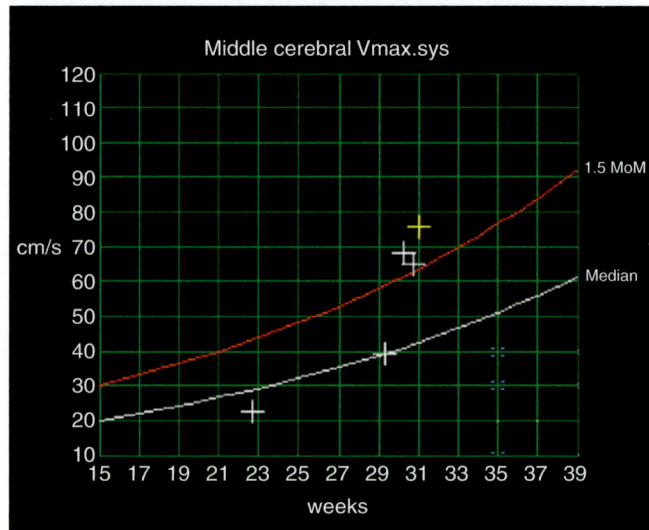

FIG. 54.9 **Middle cerebral blood flow velocity for gestational age.** Note that this fetus is anemic; the velocity is marked by the yellow caliper denoting an elevated velocity for gestational age.

pericardial effusion, ascites (Fig. 54.5), polyhydramnios (Fig. 54.6), pericardial effusion (Fig. 54.7), and thickened placenta. Hydrops can be due to fetal anemia. Another ultrasound tool available to predict fetal anemia is Doppler evaluation of the middle cerebral artery (MCA) (Figs. 54.8 and 54.9). Because there are fewer RBCs with anemia, the viscosity of the blood is decreased. A decrease in viscosity results in a decrease in resistance to flow, which can be detected by an increase in velocity in the MCA. A peak systolic velocity of more than 1.5 multiples of the median is an indicator of severe fetal anemia and requires follow-up evaluation.[3]

Cordocentesis. Cordocentesis is a procedure in which a needle is placed into the fetal umbilical vein to obtain a blood sample. The laboratory evaluates this sample for fetal blood type, hematocrit, and hemoglobin. If indicated, a fetal blood transfusion may be performed. There are two methods of transfusing a fetus. The first, intraperitoneal transfusion, uses ultrasound guidance to place a needle in the peritoneal cavity of the fetus. Blood is transfused into the peritoneal space

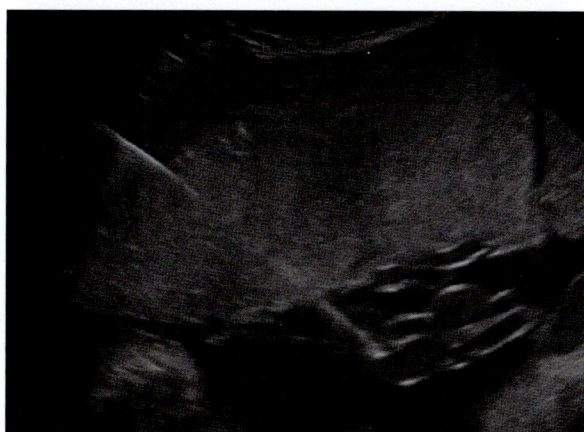

FIG. 54.10 Cordocentesis. Note echogenic needle tip placed in the umbilical vein.

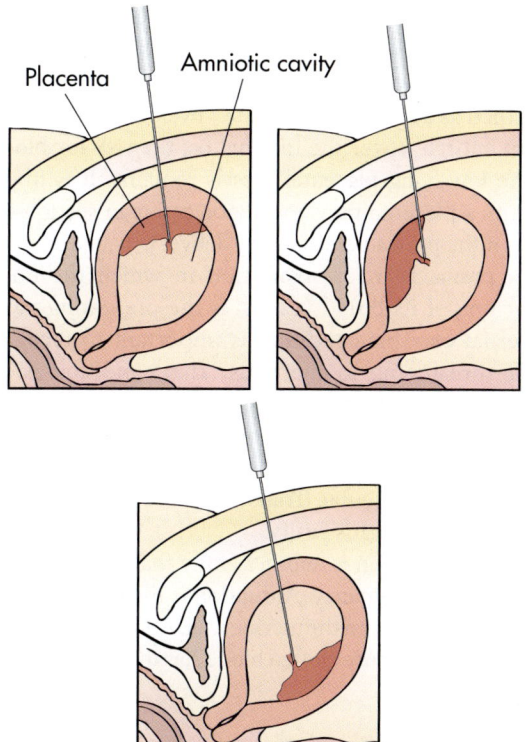

FIG. 54.11 Possible needle paths in cordocentesis depending on the placental position.

BOX 54.1	Disorders Associated With Nonimmune Hydrops

Cardiovascular
Tachyarrhythmia
Complex dysrhythmia
Congenital heart block
Anatomic defects
Cardiomyopathy
Myocarditis
Intracardiac tumors

Chromosomal
Trisomy 21
Turner syndrome
Other trisomies
XX/XY mosaicism
Triploidy

Hematologic
α-Thalassemia
Arteriovenous shunts
In utero closed-space hemorrhage
Glucose-6-phosphate deficiency

Urinary
Obstructive uropathies
Congenital nephrosis
Prune-belly syndrome
Ureterocele

Respiratory
Diaphragmatic hernia
Cystic adenomatoid malformation of the lung
Tumors of the lung

Gastrointestinal
Jejunal atresia
Midgut volvulus
Meconium peritonitis

Liver
Hepatic vascular malformations
Biliary atresia

Infectious
Cytomegalovirus/parvovirus
Syphilis
Herpes simplex
Rubella
Toxoplasmosis congenital hepatitis parvovirus B19

Placenta/Umbilical Cord
Chorioangioma
Fetomaternal transfusion
Placental and umbilical vein thrombosis
Umbilical cord anomalies

Twin Pregnancy
Twin-to-twin transfusion syndrome

where it is slowly absorbed by the fetus. The second method is direct intravascular transfusion via the umbilical vein (cordocentesis). Using ultrasound guidance, a fine needle is directed through the maternal abdomen toward the umbilical vein where it enters the placenta (Figs. 54.10 and 54.11). RBCs are transfused directly into the umbilical vein. This method is preferred because a specimen of fetal blood can be obtained before transfusion to confirm that the fetus is truly anemic and isoimmunized. A specimen can be obtained after transfusion to document that the fetal hematocrit is adequate.

Alloimmune Thrombocytopenia. In a rare circumstance, a mother may develop an immune response to fetal platelets, much as one might develop an immune response to RBCs. When this occurs, she develops antibodies to the fetal platelets. The result can be a fetus with a dangerously low platelet count (thrombocytopenia). Infants born with this condition are at increased risk for intracerebral hemorrhage in utero and spontaneous bleeding. Cordocentesis is performed in these cases to document fetal platelet counts before vaginal delivery is attempted. Ultrasound can also be useful to look for evidence of in utero fetal intracerebral hemorrhage.

Nonimmune Hydrops. Nonimmune hydrops (NIH) describes a group of conditions in which hydrops is present in the fetus but is not a result of fetomaternal blood group incompatibility. Numerous fetal, maternal, and placental disorders are known to cause or be associated with NIH (Box 54.1). The incidence of NIH is approximately 1 in 1700 to 1 in 3000 pregnancies, but NIH accounts for about 3% of fetal mortality.[4] The exact mechanism for why it occurs is unclear, although the same processes described for the hydrops associated with Rh sensitization may apply to NIH.

A variety of maternal, fetal, and placental problems are known to cause or have been found in association with NIH (see Box 54.1). Cardiovascular lesions are the most frequent causes of NIH. Congestive heart failure may result from functional cardiac problems, such as dysrhythmias, tachycardias, and myocarditis, as well as from structural anomalies, such as hypoplastic left heart and other types of congenital heart disease. Obstructive vascular problems occurring outside of the heart, such as umbilical vein thrombosis, and pulmonary diseases, such as diaphragmatic hernia and congenital cystic adenomatoid malformation, can cause NIH. Large vascular tumors functioning as arteriovenous shunts can also result in NIH.

Severe anemia of the fetus is another well-recognized etiology for NIH. Although anemia is not caused by isoimmunization, the result is the same. Severe anemia may occur in a donor twin of a twin-to-twin transfusion syndrome (TTTS), thalassemia, or significant fetomaternal hemorrhage. To make the diagnosis of NIH, isoimmunization is ruled out with an antibody screen.

Sonographic Findings. The fetus may appear similar to a sensitized baby. In addition to ascites, scalp edema and pleural and pericardial effusions may be present. Other abnormal findings may also be present that would indicate the cause of the hydrops. If the hydrops is a result of a cardiac tachyarrhythmia, a heart rate in the range of 200 to 240 is common. If a diaphragmatic hernia is present, bowel will be visible in the chest cavity.

In as many as 46% of all cases, an etiology for NIH cannot be determined.[4] If an etiology is found, treatment is dependent on the cause. As an example, if hydrops results from a tachycardia, medicine can be given to the mother in an attempt to slow the fetal heart rate. Ultrasound can be useful in monitoring the progress of the fetus. Resolution of ascites and gross edema has been documented after the fetal heart was converted to a normal rhythm. If the fetus is anemic because of twin-to-twin transfusion, intrauterine transfusion will not solve the anemia problem because most of the fetal blood is being shunted to the recipient twin (Fig. 54.12). Ultrasound can help the clinician assess how sick the fetus is by indicating the severity of the hydrops, by performing a biophysical profile, and by Doppler evaluation. The clinician can then make an informed choice about when to deliver the fetus.

A thorough examination of the fetus, along with fetal echocardiography, must be carried out because abnormalities of almost every organ system have been described with NIH. In addition to the ultrasound examination, genetic amniocentesis for karyotype is indicated because chromosomal abnormalities have been described as etiologies for NIH. If left unresolved, fetal hydrops has a very poor fetal prognosis and a very high incidence of fetal demise.

Vaginal Bleeding

Vaginal bleeding in the second and third trimesters can be associated with placental anomalies such as placenta previa and placental abruption. Placenta previa is the main cause of third-trimester bleeding. In this condition, the placenta covers the internal cervical os and prohibits the delivery of the fetus (Fig. 54.13). If the cervical os dilates with labor, there is a significant risk of the placenta detaching from the uterus, resulting in maternal hemorrhage as well as loss of oxygen and blood supply to the fetus. Transvaginal sonography is the best way to evaluate the relationship of the cervical os to the placental edge. Early in pregnancy, the placenta is often lying low, but as the uterus grows, the placenta will appear to migrate away from the cervical os. If this distance is less than 2 cm, the condition may be classified as a low-lying placenta.[5] Even though the placenta may not entirely cover the internal os, the risk for blood loss from the low-lying placental vessels remains. It is important to identify a placenta previa so that a cesarean section may be planned if the previa persists until delivery.

Vasa previa is a rare condition in which the umbilical cord, or one of its blood vessels, is the presenting part over the internal os. This condition is important to recognize as it is life-threatening to the fetus. This condition is associated with a velamentous cord insertion or succenturiate lobe. Ultrasound is used to assess for vasa previa by using color Doppler to evaluate any structures near or over the cervical os to see if they are vascular. Transvaginal sonography may also assist in identifying this entity.

Placental abruption is another entity that may cause vaginal bleeding during pregnancy. Abruption is the premature separation of the placenta from the uterine wall. Abruptions can be difficult to diagnose because clotted blood has the same sonographic

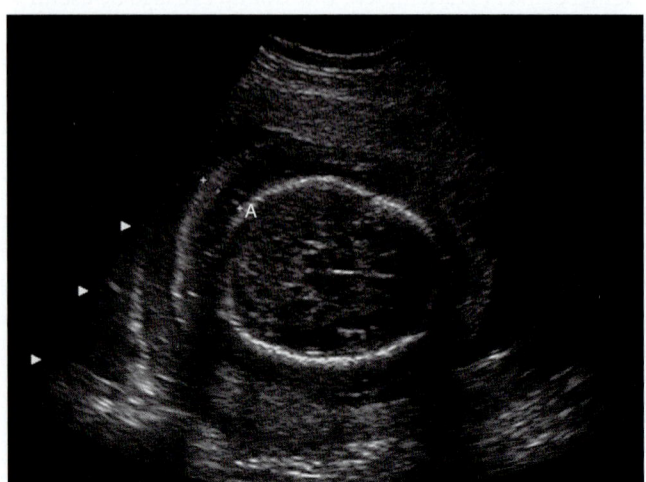

FIG. 54.12 Twin-to-twin transfusion syndrome showing hydropic twin with scalp edema.

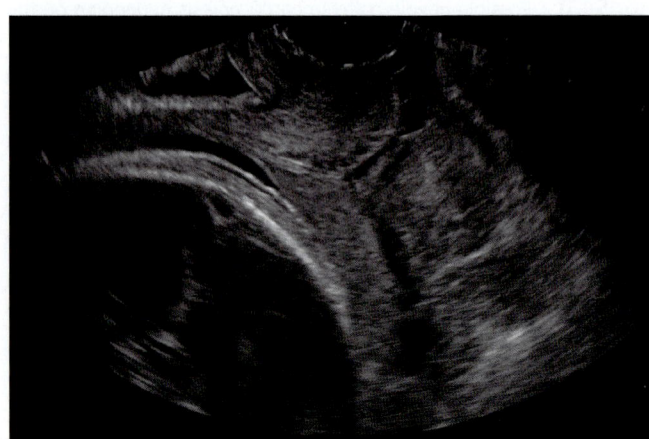

FIG. 54.13 Placenta previa. Note that the placenta is covering the cervical os.

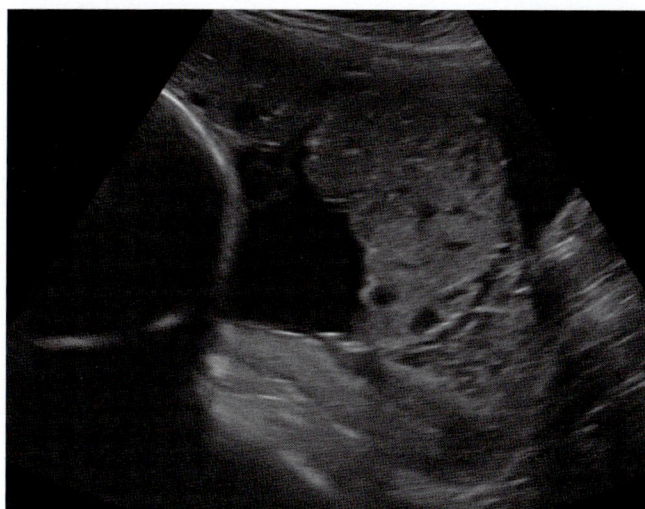

FIG. 54.14 **Placenta accreta.** Note loss of uterine wall in the image, with placenta extending to the maternal bladder. Note the hypoechoic lacunae in the placenta.

appearance as the placental tissue. If bleeding from the abruption has been recent, the sonographer may notice a thin echolucent area between the placenta and the uterus. However, there may be no sonographic signs of an abruption at all.

During normal embryonic implantation, the placental chorionic villi connect directly to the decidua basalis, a membrane formed after fertilization separating the myometrium from the placenta. A defect in the decidua basalis can cause the placenta to adhere directly to the uterine myometrium-placenta accreta, invade the myometrium-placenta increta, or completely invade through the myometrium-placenta percreta. Intrauterine scarring from previous infections or uterine surgeries are risk factors for a poorly developed decidua basalis, as is placenta previa. These abnormal placental attachments can result in serious maternal and fetal complications, including massive hemorrhage, damage to organ structures surrounding the uterus, cesarean-hysterectomy, and maternal or fetal death. The most important factor in reducing these risks is in the diagnosis of the condition so the delivery and surgical teams can prepare for the birth well in advance. The patient should be prepared to receive blood products and consulted about the potential for these complications, including the potential loss of future fertility if the bleeding cannot be controlled and a hysterectomy needs to be performed.

Magnetic resonance imaging has been the diagnostic test of choice until the recent identification of ultrasound findings associated with accreta, increta, and percreta.[5] The decidua basalis appears as a thin hypoechoic area between the uterine and placental surfaces. Loss of this retroplacental clear zone should alert the ultrasound team to evaluate for placental lacunae or distinct vascular channels with turbulent flow seen within the placenta, hypervascularity between uterine and bladder interface or a disruption in this vascular interface, and a thin uterine wall or reduced myometrial thickening. It is now estimated that placenta accreta can be detected in 50% to 80% of cases using these ultrasound screening criteria (Figs. 54.14 and 54.15).

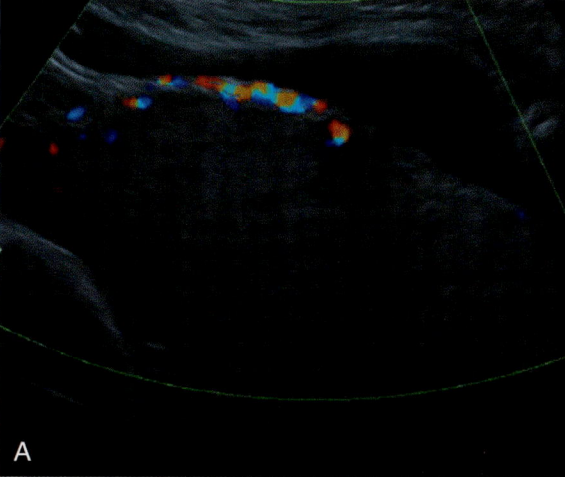
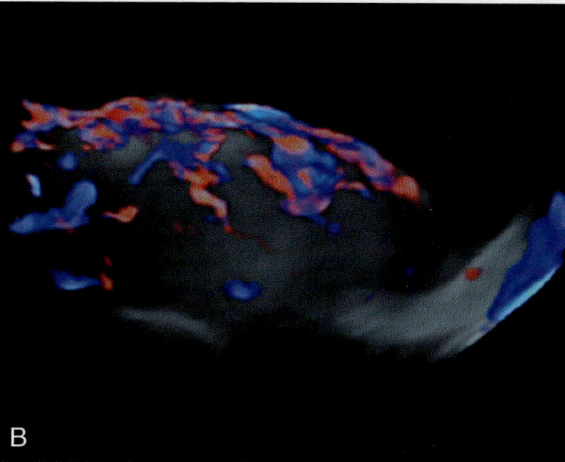

FIG. 54.15 Hypervascularity in the uterine wall in two-dimensional (A) and three-dimensional (B) imaging techniques.

MATERNAL DISEASES OF PREGNANCY

Diabetes

Mothers with insulin-dependent diabetes mellitus are at an increased risk for pregnancy-related complications that include early- and late-trimester pregnancy loss and congenital anomalies (Box 54.2). Diabetic pregnancies may be complicated by frequent hospitalizations for glucose control, serious infections such as pyelonephritis, and problems at the time of delivery. These mothers need to be monitored frequently for adequate nutritional and fluid intake, especially if they are experiencing hyperemesis in the first trimester.

Glucose is the primary fuel for fetal growth. If glucose levels are very high and uncontrolled (which happens in diabetes resulting from not being able to produce enough insulin), the fetus may also become macrosomic. *Macrosomia* is defined as a fetus whose weight is greater than the 90th percentile for gestational age. A macrosomic infant (Figs. 54.16 and 54.17) may become too large to fit through the mother's pelvis at the time of delivery, necessitating a cesarean section. If delivery is accomplished vaginally, the physician may have difficulty delivering the shoulders of the baby after the head has delivered, a condition termed *shoulder dystocia*. Brachial plexus

> **BOX 54.2 Congenital Anomalies in Infants of Diabetic Mothers[6]**
>
> **Skeletal and Central Nervous System**
> Caudal regression syndrome
> Neural tube defects excluding anencephaly
> Anencephaly with or without herniation of neural elements
> Microcephaly
>
> **Cardiac**
> Transposition of the great vessels with or without ventricular septal defect
> Ventricular septal defect
> Atrial septal defect
> Coarctation of the aorta with or without ventricular septal defect
> Cardiomegaly
>
> **Renal**
> Hydronephrosis
> Renal agenesis
> Ureteral duplication
>
> **Gastrointestinal**
> Duodenal atresia
> Anorectal atresia
> Small left colon syndrome
>
> **Other**
> Single umbilical artery

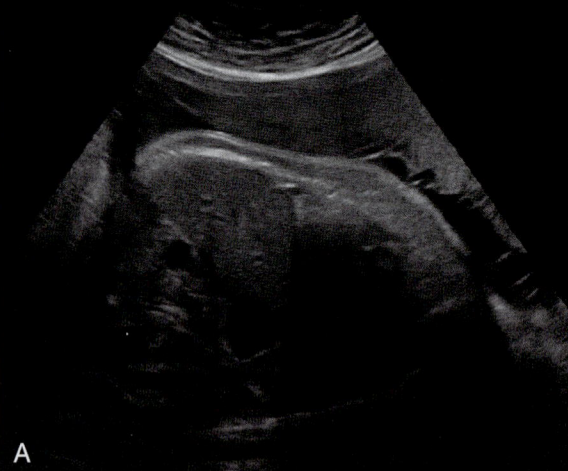

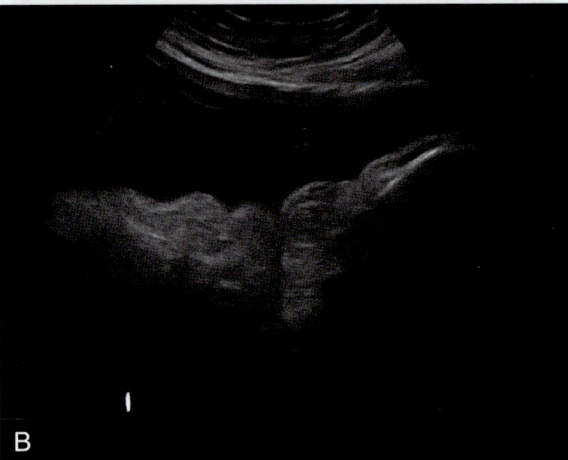

FIG. 54.17 **A macrosomic fetus.** (A) Note the adipose tissue along the chest and abdominal wall. (B) Note the adipose rolls of tissue on the side of the fetus.

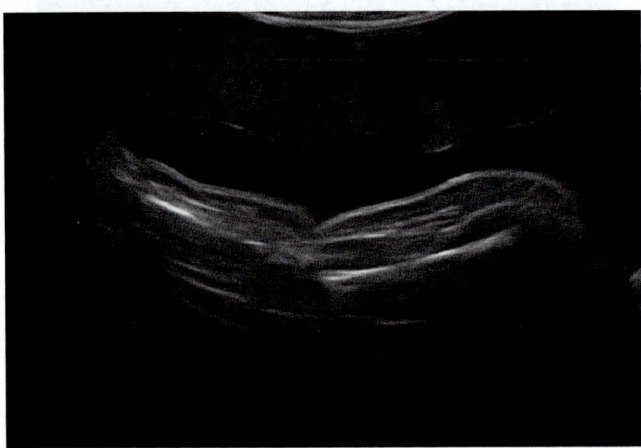

FIG. 54.16 Upper arm in a macrosomic fetus. Note the adipose tissue on the extremity.

nerve injuries may result from the traction placed on the head and neck in attempts to get the remainder of the baby out.

Once delivered, an infant of a diabetic mother may experience problems with glucose control in the nursery, necessitating intravenous glucose administration.

Sonographic Findings. Because correct dating is so important, pregnancy dates should be confirmed with ultrasound. There is an increased risk of early fetal demise, so the presence of a fetal heartbeat should be confirmed before initiating maternal diabetic protocols. There also is an increased risk of third-trimester loss, as well as other pregnancy complications that may necessitate the induction of labor before term when the fetal lung maturity is demonstrated. A diabetic baby delivered preterm may have respiratory distress syndrome and require placement in the high-risk nursery.

Polyhydramnios can be seen with elevated blood sugars and macrosomic fetuses. Polyhydramnios can predispose to premature labor, **premature rupture of membranes (PROM)**, and maternal discomfort. The fetus of a diabetic mother may measure large for gestational age, making late pregnancy dating inaccurate. Increased adipose tissue may be seen on the fetus in utero (see Figs. 54.16 and 54.17). Monthly ultrasounds can give the clinician important information regarding fetal growth. If the estimated fetal weight is greater than 4500 g at term, the clinician will be alert to the problems of dystocia with a vaginal delivery and may prefer cesarean delivery.

Ultrasound plays a very important role in scanning for fetal anomalies. **Caudal regression syndrome** (lack of development of the caudal spine and cord) is seen almost exclusively in diabetic individuals. Other associated anomalies include congenital heart and neural tube defects. In diabetics who have vasculopathy, fetuses may be at risk for fetal growth restriction (FGR). Sonographic findings with this condition may include small-for-gestation growth patterns and an elevated systolic to diastolic (S/D) ratio (peak systolic divided by end-diastolic flow velocity) and may warrant fetal echocardiography.

Hypertension

Hypertension is a medical complication of pregnancy that occurs frequently in high-risk populations. Hypertension places both mother and fetus at risk. Hypertensive pregnancies may be associated with small placentas because of the effect of the hypertension on the blood vessels. If the placenta develops poorly, the blood supply to the fetus may be restricted, possibly leading to growth restriction. Growth-restricted fetuses are at increased risk of fetal distress and death in utero.

There are various forms of hypertensive disease during pregnancy. In the past, the term *toxemia* was used to describe hypertensive disorders, because it was believed that a "toxin" in the mother's bloodstream caused the hypertension. Currently, **pregnancy-induced hypertension (PIH)** is thought to be caused by prostaglandin abnormalities.

The terminology currently used in clinical practice to describe hypertensive states during pregnancy includes (1) PIH (preeclampsia, severe preeclampsia, and eclampsia) and (2) chronic hypertension, which was present before the woman became pregnant. Preeclampsia is a pregnancy condition in which high blood pressure develops with proteinuria (protein in the urine) or edema (swelling). If the hypertension is neglected, the patient may develop seizures that can be life-threatening to both mother and fetus. Severe preeclampsia may develop in some cases and refers to the severity of hypertension and proteinuria. Severe preeclampsia generally indicates that the patient must be delivered immediately. **Eclampsia** represents the occurrence of seizures or coma in a preeclamptic patient. Chronic hypertension is diagnosed in patients in whom high blood pressure is found before 20 weeks of gestation. Chronic hypertension can result from primary essential hypertension or from secondary hypertension (renal, endocrine, or neurologic causes).

Sonographic Findings. The ultrasound team may be called on to perform serial scans for fetal growth and to monitor for the adequacy of amniotic fluid. If fetal growth is falling off the normal growth curve or oligohydramnios occurs, the obstetrician may intervene and deliver the fetus, fearing that intrauterine fetal demise is imminent. Doppler ultrasound can also give the physician information regarding the fetal and maternal circulatory status, which may help determine the pregnancies at risk for developing FGR or fetal hypoxia.

Systemic Lupus Erythematosus

Systemic lupus erythematosus (SLE) is a chronic autoimmune disorder that can affect almost all organ systems in the body. It is most common in women of childbearing age and may cause multiple peripartum complications (e.g., risk of maternal disease flares [25%–65%] and a three to five times higher rate of preeclampsia).[7] The incidence of pregnancy loss has decreased from 43% to 17% in patients with SLE.[7] The placenta is affected by the immune complex deposits and inflammatory responses in the placental vessels and may account for the increased number of spontaneous abortions, stillbirths, and growth-restricted fetuses. The fetal heart must be monitored to rule out congenital heart block (Fig. 54.18) and pericardial effusion.

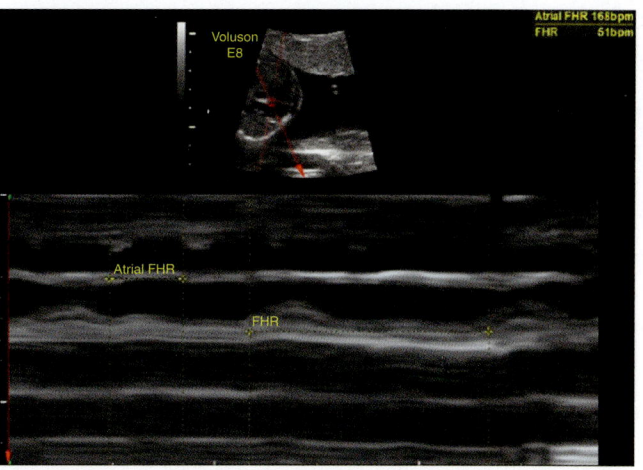

FIG. 54.18 M-mode through the atrial and ventricular wall demonstrating a ventricular heart rate of 51 beats/min and an atrial heart rate of 168 beats/min in a fetus with complete heart block.

Other Maternal Disease

Hyperemesis. Ultrasound can be useful in the workup of excessive vomiting in the pregnant woman. **Hyperemesis gravidarum** exists when a pregnant woman vomits so much that she develops dehydration and electrolyte imbalance. When this occurs, hospitalization with intravenous fluid administration is usually necessary. The physician must ensure that the vomiting results strictly from pregnancy and not another disease, such as gallstones, peptic ulcers, or trophoblastic disease. Trophoblastic disease can easily be ruled out by demonstrating a viable intrauterine pregnancy. Gallstones can be ruled out by careful sonographic examination of the gallbladder. Hyperemesis is also more common for pregnancies with multiple fetuses.

Urinary Tract Disease. Ultrasound can also be useful in the workup of urinary tract disease. Approximately 4% to 6% of pregnant women have asymptomatic bacteriuria. If left untreated, the bacteriuria can develop into pyelonephritis in some women. Although pyelonephritis usually presents with flank pain, fever, and white blood cells in the urine, hydronephrosis is another condition that presents with flank pain. Pregnancy is normally associated with mild hydronephrosis. The hydronephrosis may result from a combination of effects. First, progesterone has a dilatory effect on the smooth muscle of the ureter. Second, the enlarging uterus also compresses the ureters at the pelvic brim, causing a hydronephrosis or obstruction. If a woman presents with more than one episode of pyelonephritis or has continued flank pain, ultrasound examination may provide information as to the etiology.

Adnexal Cysts. Physiologic ovarian cysts may be associated with early pregnancy. These cysts may be large, ranging from 8 to 10 cm, and may be associated with pelvic pain. The cyst should diminish as the pregnancy progresses. If the cyst does not resolve, surgical exploration may be necessary to rule out other ovarian pathologies such as endometriomas, dermoid cysts (Fig. 54.19), and even cancers. Periodic ultrasound examinations are necessary for follow-up of a cyst.

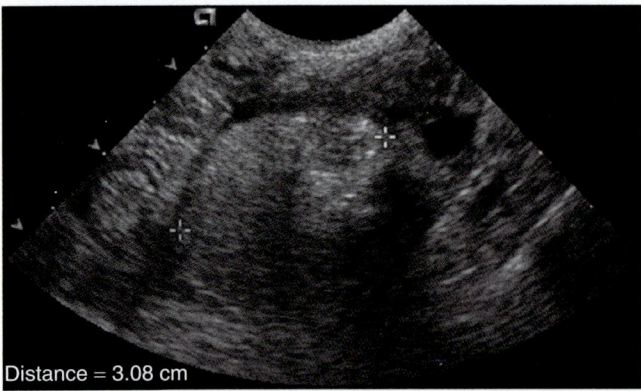

FIG. 54.19 Dermoid cyst.

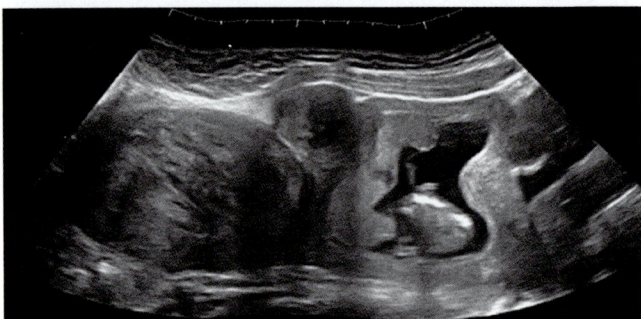

FIG. 54.20 Uterine fibroids.

BOX 54.3	Warning Signs of Preterm Labor[10]

Menstrual-like cramps (constant or intermittent)
Low, dull backache
Pressure (feels like baby is pushing down)
Abdominal cramping (with or without diarrhea)
Increase of change in vaginal discharge (contains mucus or is watery, light, or bloody)
Fluid leaking from the vagina
Feeling poorly
Uterine contractions

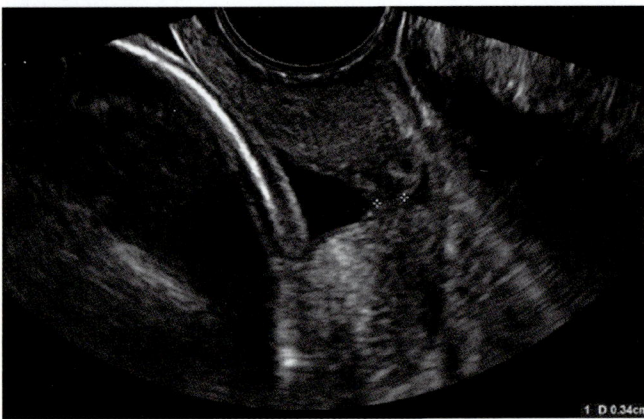

FIG. 54.21 Incompetent cervix in a patient with triplets.

Obesity. Maternal obesity (body mass index of 30 kg/m² or greater) has been associated with an increased incidence of fetal anomalies, including neural tube defects. Obese women start their pregnancy with existing chronic hypertension more often than women who start their pregnancy at a normal weight. Moreover, obese women are at an increased risk for PIH. Likewise, obese women are at an increased risk for severe preeclampsia[5] and stillbirth.[8]

Uterine Fibroids. Pregnant women may periodically present with problems related to uterine fibroids. Fibroids are actually benign tumors of uterine smooth muscle that may be stimulated to excessive growth by the hormones of pregnancy, specifically estrogen. If the growth is very rapid, the fibroid may outgrow its blood supply and undergo necrosis, which may cause pain and premature labor. Ultrasound examination of the uterus in a pregnant woman may detect uterine fibroids (Fig. 54.20). It is important to document the size and location of these fibroids, as they may obstruct a clear pathway for fetal delivery. If the placenta implants over a fibroid, it may lead to poor placental profusion in that area, which can be a cause of FGR.

ULTRASOUND IN LABOR AND DELIVERY

Preterm Labor

Preterm, or premature, labor is the onset of labor before 37 weeks of gestation (Box 54.3). It is an obstetric complication occurring in 9.5% to 11.5% of all pregnancies.[9] Premature infants are at greater risk for having problems such as respiratory distress syndrome, intracranial hemorrhage, bowel immaturity, and feeding difficulties.

Potential etiologies of preterm labor include PROM, intrauterine infection, bleeding, fetal anomalies, polyhydramnios, multiple pregnancy, growth restriction, maternal illness (diabetes or hypertension), incompetent cervix, and uterine abnormalities.

Epidemiologic factors such as socioeconomic class; maternal age, weight, and height; late prenatal care; smoking; coitus; a history of cervical injury or surgery; and a poor previous obstetric history are presumed etiologies as well. Another patient population at increased risk for preterm labor is patients with multiple gestations. In about half of all cases, no cause or association can be identified for the preterm labor.

Sonographic Findings. Ultrasound assessment of the preterm labor patient should include, but not be limited to, amniotic fluid assessment, cervical assessment (Fig. 54.21), fetal number, placental assessment, and detailed fetal anatomic survey ultrasound (see Table 54.1). The sonographer should be aware of the potential causes of preterm labor and tailor the examination accordingly.

Premature Rupture of Membranes. The intrauterine membranes containing the fetus and amniotic fluid are usually intact until the mother is in early labor or they are intentionally ruptured to begin labor. The membranes may rupture and cause the loss of amniotic fluid before labor begins, bringing the mother to a triage center for evaluation of PROM. The amniotic sac containing the fluid protects the fetus from infection, and a disruption of this membrane without ensuing labor is a concern for the potential of infection. The ultrasound staff is often asked to evaluate the amount of amniotic fluid in a pregnancy with a suspicion of PROM. Oligohydramnios, or a decreased amount of amniotic fluid, may be evident and reported to the medical staff to help confirm the diagnosis.

FETAL FACTORS IN HIGH-RISK PREGNANCY

Fetal Death

Intrauterine fetal death is the fifth leading cause of death worldwide.[8] Although the cause of death is undetermined in approximately 76% of the cases,[8] known causes are infection (usually associated with PROM), congenital or chromosomal abnormalities, preeclampsia, placental abruption, diabetes, growth restriction, and blood group isoimmunization, or abnormalities of the placenta or umbilical cord.

Fetal death may occur in any trimester of pregnancy. The overall miscarriage rate, defined as fetal age less than 20 weeks, is reported to be 10% to 26%.[11] In the first trimester, embryonic causes of spontaneous abortion are the predominant etiology. Genetic abnormalities within the embryo are the most common cause of spontaneous abortion. Trisomies are the single largest group of chromosomal anomalies and account for approximately half of all anomalies associated with miscarriage. Approximately 20% of genetic abnormalities are triploidies.

Clinically, first-trimester pregnancy loss may be diagnosed when the patient presents to her physician with vaginal bleeding, cramping, or passage of tissue. Ultrasound examination may reveal a blighted ovum or a fetus with no heart motion. As the pregnancy progresses into the second trimester, pregnancy landmarks become important for determining whether the pregnancy is proceeding normally. Fetal heart tones should be heard with Doppler at approximately 10 to 12 weeks of gestation. At 20 weeks of gestation, the uterine fundal height should have risen to the umbilicus and the uterus should measure approximately 20 cm above the symphysis pubis. The mother should also perceive fetal movements on a daily basis beginning between 16 and 20 weeks of gestation. Failure to achieve any one of these landmarks may prompt the clinician to obtain an ultrasound examination.

As the pregnancy progresses, the clinician will follow the pregnant woman at regular intervals, listening to fetal heart tones and measuring the uterine fundal height at each visit. The mother will be questioned about fetal movements. The absence of a fetal heart rate usually prompts the clinician to obtain an ultrasound examination. Cessation of fetal movements should prompt an immediate search for fetal heart tones. If none are present, ultrasound examination will confirm or rule out intrauterine fetal demise.

Sonographic Findings. Sonographic findings associated with fetal death are (1) absent heartbeat, (2) absent fetal movement, (3) overlap of skull bones (**Spalding sign**), (4) an exaggerated curvature of the fetal spine (Fig. 54.22), and (5) gas in the fetal abdomen. A brief ultrasound examination of the fetus for structural anomalies should be performed and biometry obtained to determine the estimated weight for delivery. Care should be taken and consideration given to the family to not add to their emotional stress during this difficult time.

Large for Gestational Age

When a fetus is measuring large for gestational age, the sonographer is asked to evaluate for fetal macrosomia. Macrosomia is accelerated growth in utero and is defined as an estimated birth weight greater than 4000 g. Macrosomia can be symmetric or asymmetric. Symmetric macrosomia is usually due to prolonged pregnancy or to genetics. Asymmetric macrosomia is often seen in diabetic mothers; the fetus will have an abdominal girth larger relative to head size and length. The significance of macrosomia is that there is increased morbidity associated with it due to birth trauma (birth asphyxia). These findings are usually associated with a fetus whose estimated fetal weight is greater than 4000 to 4500 g (8 lb, 13 oz to 9 lb, 15 oz).

Small for Gestational Age

Small for gestational age can be due to chromosomal anomalies, intrauterine infection (Fig. 54.23), genetics, or placental insufficiency (Figs. 54.24 and 54.25). If chromosomal anomalies are the etiology for the fetus measuring small, growth is often affected symmetrically, meaning that all the fetal measurements will be smaller than expected for gestational age. When placental insufficiency is the cause, fetuses often develop an asymmetric FGR pattern. This pattern results in normal head and limb measurements but with a small abdominal circumference and decreased amniotic fluid. In general, an abdominal circumference or estimated fetal

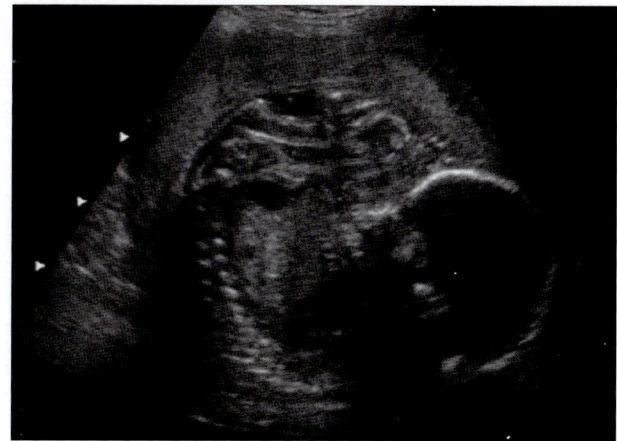

FIG. 54.22 Extreme curvature of the fetal spine in a fetal demise.

weight of less than 10% for gestational age are the parameters used to define assymetric fetal growth restriction.[12] The clinical significance of recognizing a growth-restricted fetus is that these pregnancies are at an increased risk for perinatal morbidity and mortality compared with normal-weight fetuses and neurologic and intellectual impairment when delivered at term. If the FGR fetus is recognized early, bed rest can be instituted in an attempt to increase maternal uterine profusion and potentially increase fetal blood supply. Fetal growth and behaviors can be monitored for signs of worsening profusion, and early delivery can be induced if necessary for fetal well-being. Infants delivered at 34 to 35 weeks of gestation have a better chance of catching up to their peers by 2 years of age than growth-restricted fetuses delivered at term.

MULTIPLE GESTATION PREGNANCY

Ultrasound is an extremely valuable tool in the assessment of multiple gestation pregnancies. It is used to assess the amnionicity and chorionicity, to monitor the growth of the fetuses, and for guidance of diagnostic and therapeutic procedures. The mother with a multiple gestation is at increased risk for obstetric complications, such as **preeclampsia**, third-trimester bleeding, and prolapsed cord. The fetuses are at increased risk of premature delivery and congenital anomalies. As a result, a twin has a four times greater chance of perinatal death than a singleton fetus.[8] Physicians follow multiple gestations closely with ultrasound.

During the first trimester, multiple gestations can be identified by visualizing more than one gestational sac within the uterus. A firm diagnosis should not be made unless a fetal pole can be seen within each sac, regardless of the number of sacs that are seen. In the second and third trimesters, several clinical findings may prompt an ultrasound examination. The patient's uterus may be larger on examination than expected for dates. **Maternal serum alpha-fetoprotein** (MSAFP) screening is performed routinely to detect neural tube defects. By virtue of having two fetuses rather than one, twin pregnancies are associated with elevations of MSAFP. Therefore, a patient with elevated MSAFP may present for a scan to rule out neural tube defects and be found to be carrying twins. The physician may detect two fetal heartbeats or palpate two heads, prompting an ultrasound examination. Finally, the twins may be unsuspected and found serendipitously.

Once a multiple gestation has been identified, a detailed fetal anatomic survey ultrasound examination should be performed to look specifically for fetal sex.[13] In each multiple gestation evaluated by ultrasound, the sonographer needs to evaluate placentation type (Box 54.4). This refers to the number of chorions (chorionicity) and amnions (amnionicity). In a twin pregnancy, this depends on the number of zygotes and,

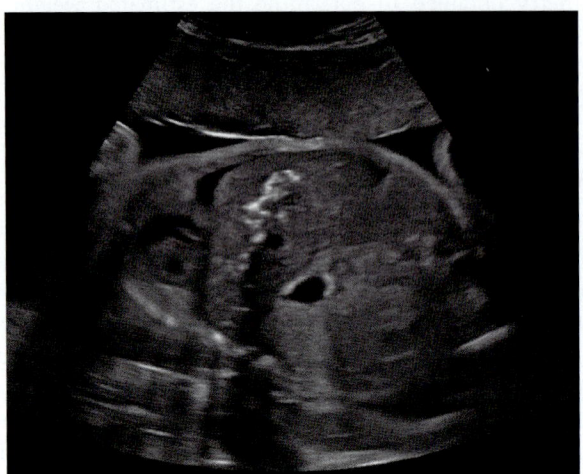

FIG. 54.23 Liver calcifications in a pregnancy affected by cytomegalovirus.

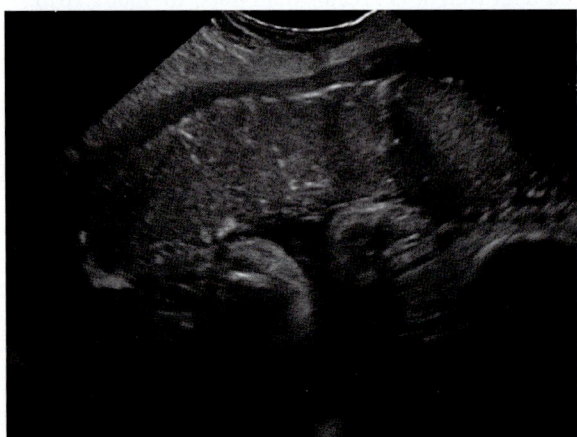

FIG. 54.24 Placental calcifications.

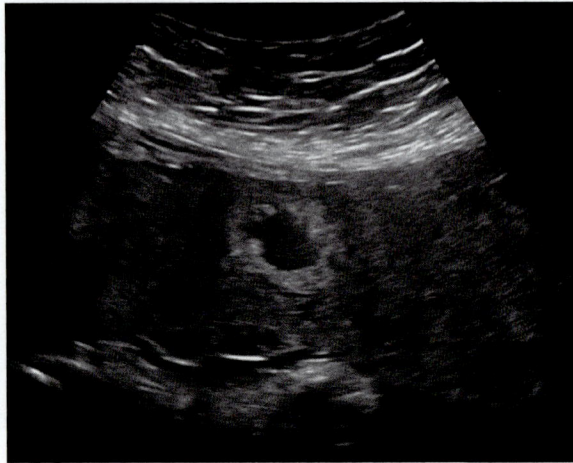

FIG. 54.25 Placental infarct.

BOX 54.4	Types of Placentation[14]

- All *dizygotic* pregnancies are dichorionic/diamniotic.
- Of *monozygotic* pregnancies, 25% are dichorionic (two placentas); the majority (75%) are monochorionic (one placenta).
- In *dichorionic* pregnancies, whether monozygotic or dizygotic, two layers of amnion and two layers of chorion separate the fetuses.

in monozygotic twinning, the timing of zygotic division (Figs. 54.26–54.28).

Dizygotic Twins

There are two types of twins: dizygotic (fraternal) and monozygotic (identical). **Dizygotic** twins arise from two separately fertilized ova. Each ovum implants separately in the uterus and develops its own placenta, chorion, and amniotic sac (diamniotic, dichorionic) (Fig. 54.29). The placentas may implant in different parts of the uterus and be distinctly separate or may implant adjacent to each other and fuse. Although the placentas are fused, their blood circulations remain distinct and separate from each other.

Monozygotic Twins

Monozygotic twins (identical) arise from a single fertilized egg, which divides, resulting in two genetically identical fetuses. Depending on whether the fertilized egg divides early or late, there may be one or two placentas, chorions, and amniotic sacs. If the division occurs early, 0 to 4 days postconception, there will be two amnions and two chorions (dichorionic, diamniotic). If the division occurs at 4 to 8 days,

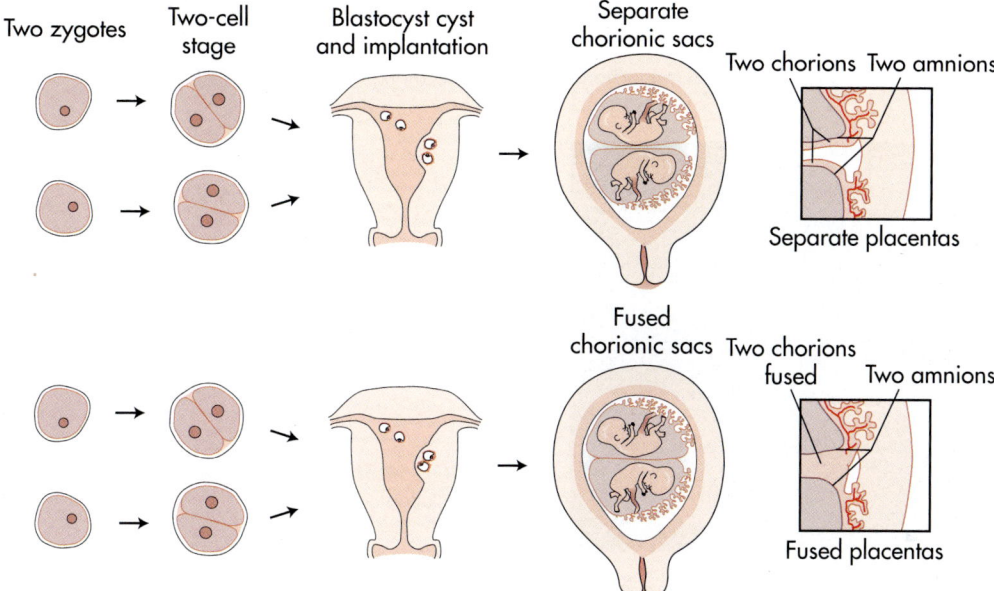

FIG. 54.26 Dichorionicity and diamnionicity of dizygotic twins.

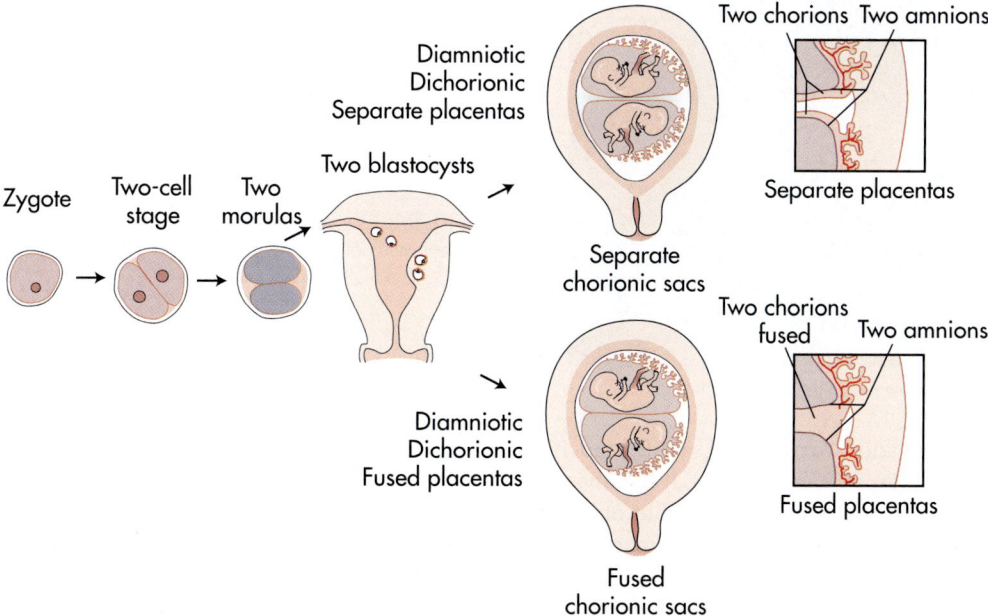

FIG. 54.27 Possible dichorionicity and diamnionicity of monozygotic twins.

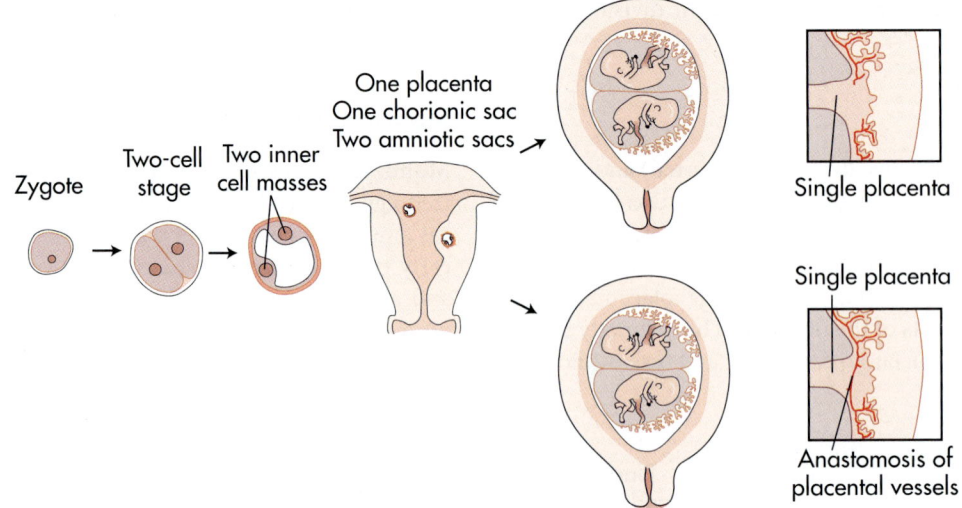

FIG. 54.28 A monochorionic, diamniotic, monozygotic twin gestation.

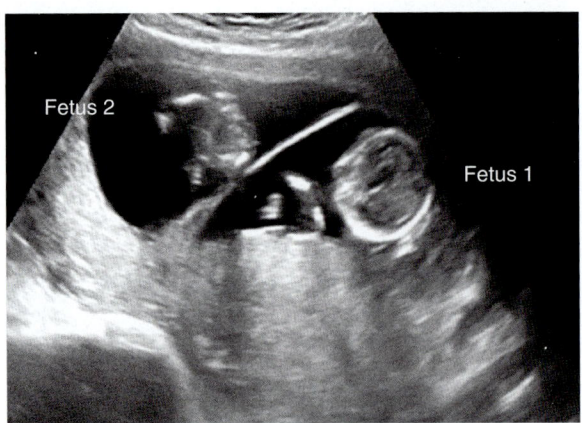

FIG. 54.29 A dichorionic, diamniotic, twin gestation.

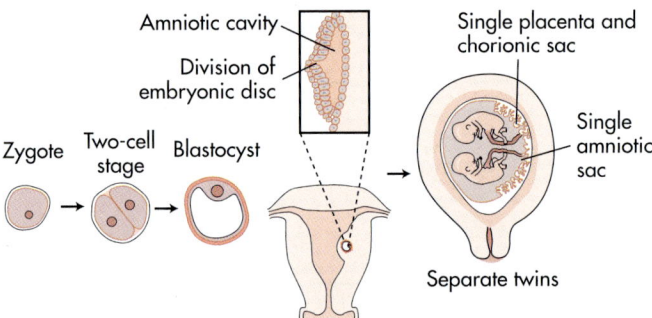

FIG. 54.31 A monochorionic, monoamniotic, monozygotic twin gestation.

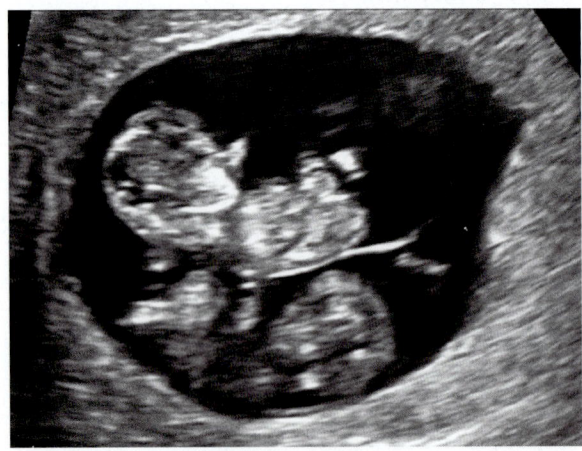

FIG. 54.30 A monochorionic diamniotic twin gestation.

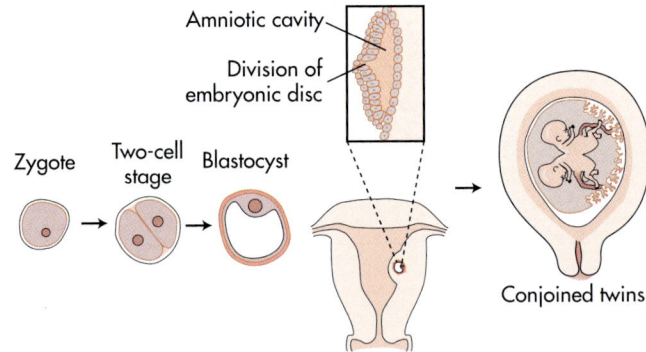

FIG. 54.32 A monochorionic, monoamniotic, monozygotic twin gestation with late division resulting in conjoined twins.

there will be one chorion and two amniotic sacs (monochorionic, diamniotic) (see Figs. 54.27 and 54.30). If the division occurs after 8 days, two fetuses will be present but only one chorion and one amnion (monochorionic, monoamniotic) (Figs. 54.31 and 54.32). If the division occurs after 13 days, the division may be incomplete and **conjoined twins** may result. The twins may be joined at a variety of sites, including

the head, thorax, abdomen, and pelvis (Figs. 54.33 and 54.34). Identification of these membranes is easily achieved with ultrasound in the first trimester and should be noted in the report because monozygotic twins present a very high-risk situation (Figs. 54.35 and 54.36). Frequent ultrasound evaluations of monozygotic twins are performed every 2 weeks beginning at 16 weeks of gestational age to look for signs of complications described below.

Besides an association with an increased incidence of fetal anomalies, if there is only one amniotic sac, the twins

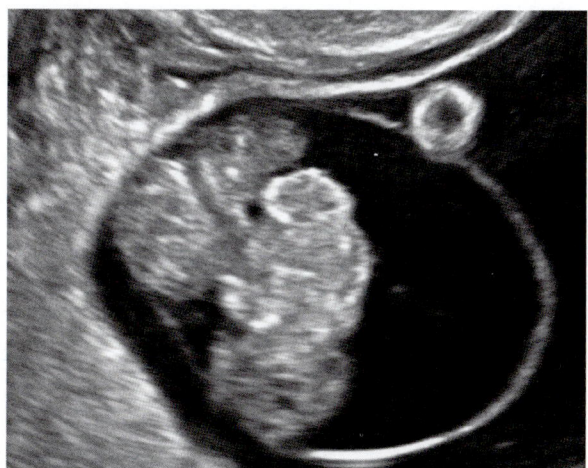

FIG. 54.33 Two-dimensional ultrasound image of conjoined twins.

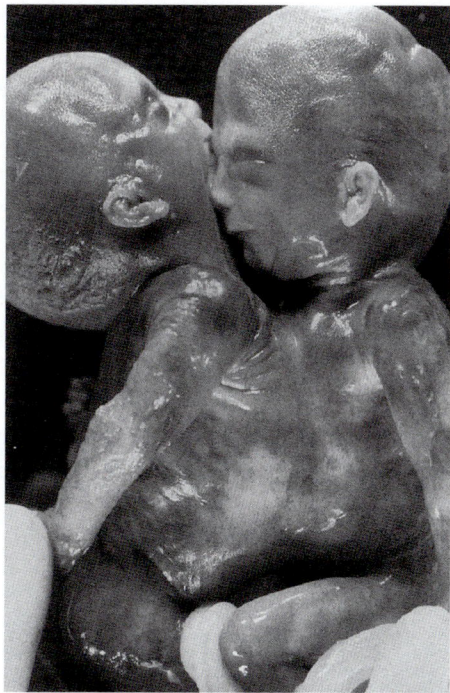

FIG. 54.36 Thoracoabdominal conjoined twins.

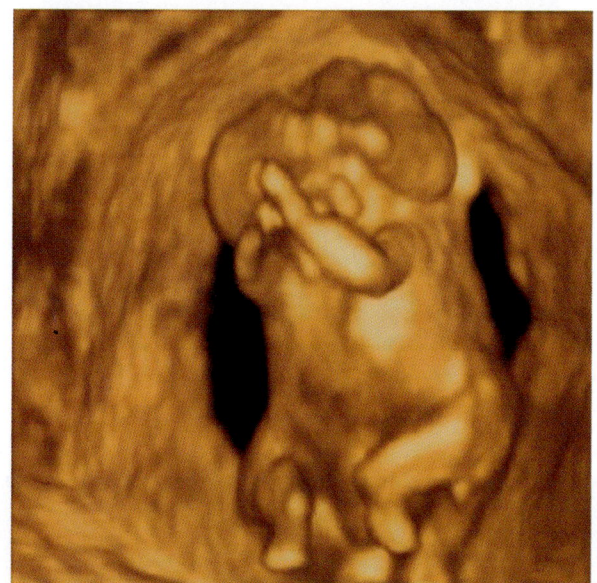

FIG. 54.34 Three-dimensional ultrasound image of conjoined twins.

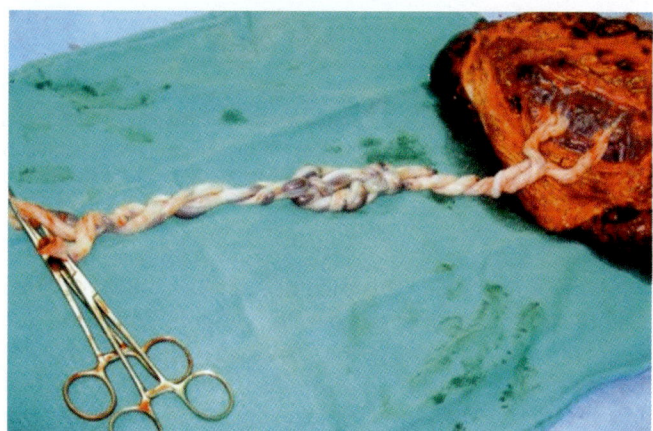

FIG. 54.35 Monochorionic, monoamniotic placenta with two tangled amniotic cords.

may become entangled in their umbilical cords, cutting off their blood supply. In these monochorionic diamniotic pregnancies, only the two layers of amnion separate the twins. Because the circulations of the monozygotic twins communicate through a single placenta, they are at increased risk for two syndromes known as twin anemia-polycythemia syndrome (or TTTS, discussed later in this chapter).

One obstacle to imaging twins is the phenomenon of the vanishing and appearing twin. One twin may die in utero and the other one continue to grow. One study showed that 70% of pregnancies that began with twins ended with a singleton.[15] Many of these losses occur very early and are never detected. Others are detected early when the patient presents with vaginal bleeding in the second trimester and two sacs are visualized, one with a healthy fetus and one with a demised fetus (Fig. 54.37). If the demise occurs very early, complete resorption of both embryo and gestational sac or early placenta may occur. This phenomenon is sometimes referred to as the "vanishing twin," because once reabsorbed, the products of conception of this twin will no longer be seen on ultrasound. If the fetus dies after reaching a size too large for resorption, the fetus is markedly flattened from loss of fluid and most of the soft tissue. This is termed **fetus papyraceous** (Fig. 54.38).

Just as a twin may appear to vanish, one may also "appear." The appearing twin is seen when ultrasound examinations are performed very early in gestation (5 to 6 weeks) and undercounting of the gestational sacs occurs. Undercounting can occur because of a discrepancy in gestational sac size; the locations of the sacs; if the patient is scanned before yolk sacs are seen; in cases of monochorionic, monoamniotic gestation without crown-rump lengths; and failure of the operator to identify a second gestational sac.

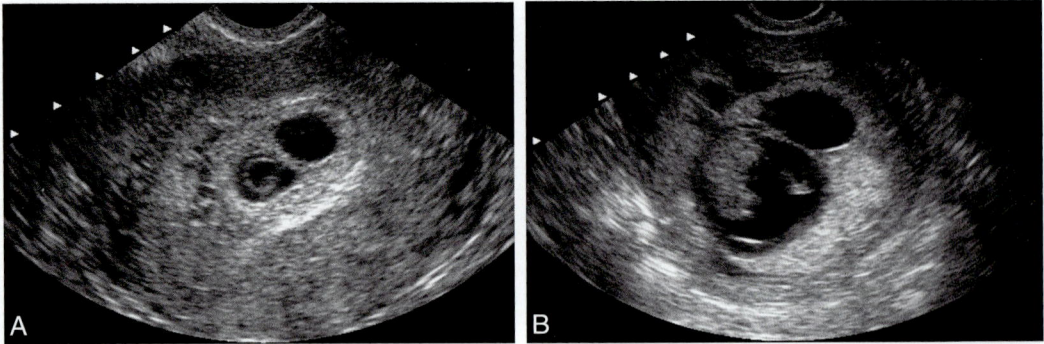

FIG. 54.37 (A) An early twin gestation. (B) Same patient further into pregnancy demonstrates vanishing twin phenomenon.

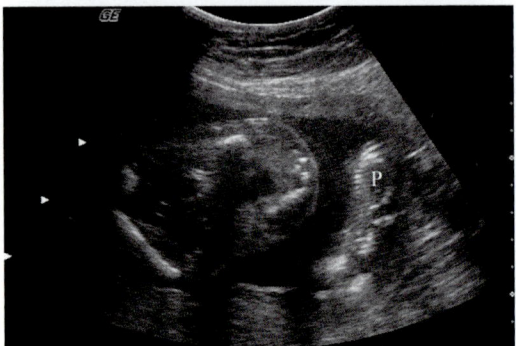

FIG. 54.38 The demise of one twin resulting in a fetus papyraceous (P).

Anomalies Specific to Twin Pregnancies

As stated, multiple gestations have a high rate of anomalies, and a careful search must be performed to rule out birth defects. It is also important for sonographers to understand which abnormalities are unique to multiple gestations they should be screening for. Several abnormalities are specific to multiple gestations. They are poly-oli sequence, TTTS, twin anemia-polycythemia syndrome, **acardiac anomaly**, and conjoined twins.

Poly-Oli Sequence ("Stuck Twin"). Polyhydramnios-oligohydramnios (poly-oli) sequence, also known as "stuck twin" syndrome, is characterized by a diamniotic pregnancy with polyhydramnios in one sac and severe oligohydramnios and a smaller twin in the other sac (Fig. 54.39). This syndrome usually manifests between 16 and 26 weeks of gestation. Most involve monochorionic gestations. Stuck twin syndrome may result from a fetal anomaly in one sac resulting in polyhydramnios, compressing the blood flow in the normal twin's placenta and resulting in oligohydramnios; placental insufficiency in one placenta; and TTTS. When oligohydramnios exists in one sac and polyhydramnios in the other, the small twin may appear stuck in position within the uterus; hence, the term stuck twin. In the event that twin-to-twin transfusion exists, the growth of the twins will be discordant, with the donor twin falling off the growth curve (Fig. 54.40).

Twin-to-twin transfusion syndrome (TTTS) exists when there is a vascular connection within the placenta. The arterial blood of one twin is pumped into the venous system of the other twin. As a result, the donor twin becomes anemic

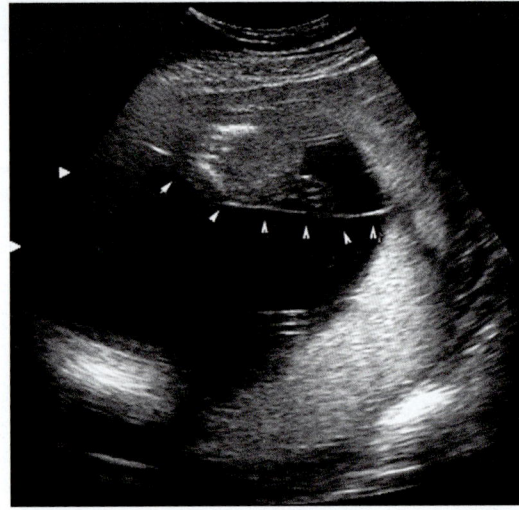

FIG. 54.39 A "stuck twin." *Arrowheads* point to the amnion surrounding the stuck twin.

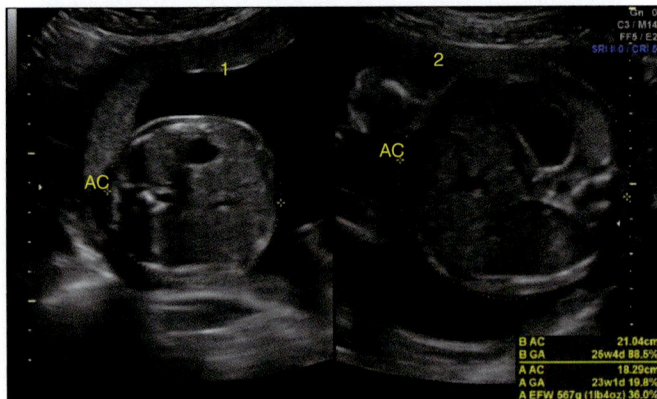

FIG. 54.40 Multiple gestation affected by twin-to-twin transfusion syndrome. Note the size discrepancy between the two fetal abdominal circumferences.

and growth restricted. This twin has less blood flow through its kidneys, urinates less, and develops **oligohydramnios**. The recipient twin, however, gets too much blood flow. The twin may be normal or large in size. This fetus has excess blood flow through its kidneys and urinates too much, leading to **polyhydramnios**. This twin may even go into heart failure and become hydropic.

If TTTS exists, both twins are at risk of dying—the smaller one because its nutritional and oxygen-rich blood supply is severely restricted, and the larger one because of heart failure. Depending on the gestational age, the obstetric specialist may be forced to deliver the fetuses early if it appears one or both of the twins are at risk of dying in utero. Fetal surveillance is increased when growth discordance, oligohydramnios, or polyhydramnios is discovered. Current treatment for TTTS involves the laser occlusion of anastomosing placental vessels using fetoscopy and guided by ultrasound.

Twin anemia-polycythemia syndrome (TAPS) was identified in 2007 as another complication seen in monochorionic pregnancies as a result of a shared placental vascular supply but can also occur spontaneously after laser surgery for TTTS. These twins present without the poly-oli fetus but develop a discordance in intertwin hemoglobin values. One has too little hemoglobin and is anemic whereas the other has too much hemoglobin and is polycythemic.

Acardiac Anomaly. By definition, the acardiac anomaly is a rare anomaly, occurring in monochorionic twins, in which one twin develops without a heart and often without the upper half of the body (Fig. 54.41). It has been suggested that this occurs because of an artery-to-artery connection in the placenta that leads to perfusion of the abnormal twin via the co-twin. The reversed direction of blood flow in the abnormal twin alters the hemodynamic properties needed for normal cardiac formation. On ultrasound, one will see a monochorionic twin gestation with one normal fetus and one fetus with an absent heart. The abnormal twin also has other anomalies such as absent head, absent organs in the thorax and abdomen, and absent or abnormal limbs.

Conjoined Twins. This condition occurs when there is an incomplete division of the embryo after 13 days from conception. Five types of conjoined twins have been described: thoracopagus (joined at the thorax), omphalopagus (joined at the anterior wall), craniopagus (joined at the cranium, syncephalus, conjoined twins with one head), pygopagus (joined at the ischial region), and ischiopagus (attached at the buttocks). On ultrasound, one will see a monochorionic, monoamniotic gestation with two fetuses connected.

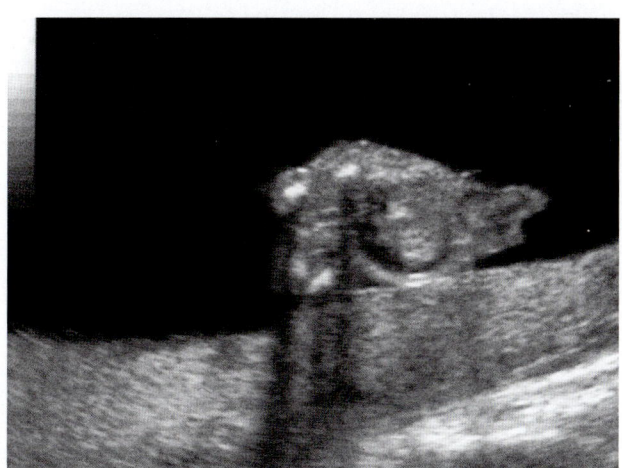

FIG. 54.41 An acardiac, acephalic twin gestation.

Scanning Multiple Gestations

Multiple gestations have many potential risks, so the sonographer must do a complete job of scanning the fetuses. In addition to the anatomy listed in Table 54.1, the ultrasound report should include the following information[13]:
- Definition of amnions and chorions
- Number of sacs
- Number and location of placentas and location of placental cord insertions
- Sex of the fetuses
- Biometric data
- Presence of anomalies

The fetal gestational sacs should be assigned a label (typically an alphabetical letter or number) to consistently identify them in subsequent examinations. The sac and fetus directly over the internal os is labeled A. Sacs above that should be additionally identified by their placental location or additional identifying information such as the left or right side of the uterus. This will be important in future examinations to consistently evaluate the growth of each fetus against its own previous growth, not that of another sibling.

During the first trimester, the sonographer must be careful to analyze the uterine contents for the presence of multiple gestations. Multiple gestations may be initially undercounted in early pregnancies of less than 6 weeks performed with transvaginal ultrasound. After 6 weeks of gestational age, determining pregnancy number is easily accomplished by counting embryos in the uterus. Before 6 weeks the embryo is not consistently visualized and the sonographer must count the gestational sacs and small yolk sacs. An article reported that the frequency of undercounting multiple gestations on a 5.0- to 5.9-week sonogram was highest for monochorionic twins (86%), followed by higher-order gestations (16%), and last by dichorionic twins (11%).[16] The authors of the report reasoned that some of the gestational sacs may differ in size or the yolk sac may be too small to adequately image so early. This may account for the vanishing twin or appearing twin phenomenon.

When scanning multiple gestations, the sonographer should always try to determine whether there are one or two amniotic sacs by locating the membrane that separates the sacs. If two sacs are seen, the pregnancy is known to be diamniotic, but sonography will not be able to indicate whether the twins are identical. As previously noted, both monozygotic and dizygotic twins may have two amniotic sacs.

Documentation of a membrane separating the fetuses confirms the presence of a diamniotic pregnancy. The membrane, composed of amnion with or without chorion, exhibits a characteristic appearance that permits distinction from other membranes of pregnancy. In a twin pregnancy with two separate placentas, the membrane extends between the fetuses obliquely across the uterus from the edge of the placenta to the contralateral edge of the other placenta. If only one placental site exists, the membrane extends between the fetuses away from the central portion of the placental site. The fetus may touch the membrane but does not cross it, and the membrane does not adhere to entrap the fetus. The membrane has no free edge within the amniotic fluid. These features distinguish the normal membrane separating twins from other membranes or membrane-like structures within the amniotic fluid (i.e., uterine synechiae, partial uterine septations, or amniotic bands).

Failure to image the membrane separating the twin fetuses does not reliably predict the presence of a monoamniotic pregnancy. If only one placenta is seen and a membrane cannot be visualized, other features may assist in the prediction of amnionicity, chorionicity, and zygosity. A male and female fetus is dizygotic, diamniotic, and dichorionic. Twin pregnancy with intertwined umbilical cords, conjoined twins, or more than three vessels in the umbilical cord is found in a monozygotic pregnancy that is monoamniotic and monochorionic.

The location of the placenta should be determined. An attempt also should be made to determine the number of placentas. Occasionally, clearly separate placentas may be identified. If two placentas are implanted immediately adjacent to each other and fuse, it may be difficult to determine whether there are one or two placentas. The body of the placenta should be scanned to determine whether a line of separation can be seen.

The twins should each then be scanned for corroboration of dates and size, measuring parameters that include biparietal diameter (BPD), head circumference, abdominal circumference, and femur length.

Dolichocephaly can be common in twin pregnancies as a result of crowding. In dolichocephaly, the BPD is shortened and the occipitofrontal diameter (OFD) is lengthened because of compression. Therefore, the BPD underestimates gestational age with dolichocephaly. The sonographer should always determine the cephalic index (CI) (CI=BPD/OFD×100). CI of less than 75% suggests dolichocephaly. The normal CI is 75% to 85%.

Because the growth of twins is similar to that of singletons early in pregnancy, singleton growth charts are generally used. However, it is important to keep in mind that a fetus from a multiple gestation is usually smaller than a singleton fetus. It is known that twins are smaller in size at birth than singleton fetuses of comparable gestational age. Of concern is the ability to detect growth restriction in one or both fetuses. When attempting to determine whether only one twin is growth restricted, differences between the measurements of the two twins must be examined. A difference in estimated fetal weight of more than 20% has been reported as a predictor of discordance of growth between twins.[15]

The genitalia of the fetuses are important to determine. If there is growth discordance between the twins but one is male and one is female, TTTS cannot exist. If both twins are of the same sex, however, and growth discordance exists, TTTS may be a possibility.

Umbilical cord Doppler may be useful for fetal surveillance. During the fetal cardiac cycle, there is umbilical blood flow during both the pumping (systole) and filling (diastole) phases of the heartbeat. No flow (absent end-diastolic flow)

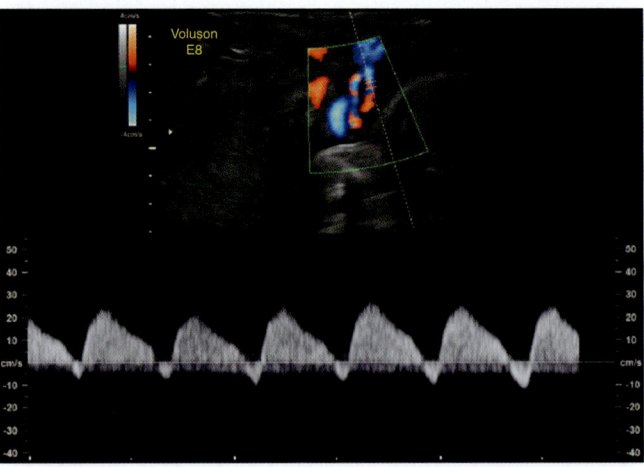

FIG. 54.42 Reversal of diastolic flow in a twin gestation with twin-to-twin transfusion syndrome.

and reverse flow during diastole (reverse end-diastolic flow) (Fig. 54.42) are signs of fetal jeopardy and may prompt the obstetrician to do further fetal well-being testing or even to deliver the fetuses.

One report suggests that most cases of TTTS are identified in the second trimester.[13] Abnormal Doppler studies in twin pregnancies should prompt a search for other findings seen in this syndrome, such as polyhydramnios, stuck twin, or hydrops. When Doppler flow patterns are abnormal, careful follow-up should be used to determine whether shunting exists.

The multifetal pregnancy reduction method has been used on pregnancies of more than four fetuses to improve the survival chances of the remaining fetuses. The procedure is performed toward the end of the first trimester by ultrasound-guided injection of potassium chloride into the thoraxes of the fetuses to be aborted.

ACKNOWLEDGMENTS

The authors acknowledge the contributions of Sandra Hagen-Ansert, Kara L. Mayden-Argo, and Laura J. Zuidema to this chapter in the previous edition.

Key Pearls

- Screening tests are offered to low-risk populations to identify patients whose risk is high enough to be offered diagnostic testing.
- The detailed fetal anatomic survey ultrasound is an extended obstetric examination performed in pregnancies with indications for potential maternal or fetal complications.
- When evaluating the high-risk pregnancy with obstetric ultrasound, the sonographer needs to be aware of maternal and fetal indications for making the pregnancy high risk and needs to be able to apply knowledge and expertise to tailor the examination to the clinical indication.

- Advanced maternal age (AMA) describes a patient who will be 35 or older at the time of delivery. AMA can be an indicator for high-risk pregnancy.
- Hydrops fetalis is a condition in which excessive fluid accumulates within the fetal body cavities. This fluid accumulation may result in anasarca, ascites, pericardial effusion, pleural effusion, placental edema, and polyhydramnios.
- Vaginal bleeding in the second and third trimesters can be associated with placental anomalies such as placenta previa and placenta abruption.
- Mothers with insulin-dependent diabetes mellitus are at an increased risk for pregnancy-related complications that include early- and late-trimester pregnancy loss and congenital anomalies.
- The terminology currently used in clinical practice to describe hypertensive states during pregnancy includes (1) pregnancy-induced hypertension (preeclampsia, severe preeclampsia, and eclampsia) and (2) chronic hypertension, which was present before the woman became pregnant.
- Ultrasound is used to assess the amnionicity and chorionicity, to monitor the growth of the fetuses, and for guidance of diagnostic and therapeutic procedures. The mother with a multiple gestation is at increased risk for obstetric complications, such as preeclampsia, third-trimester bleeding, and prolapsed cord.

REFERENCES

1. Screening for fetal chromosomal abnormalities: ACOG Practice Bulletin Number 226. *Obstet Gynecol*. 2020;136(4):e48–e69.
2. Wax J, Minkoff H, Johnson A, et al. Consensus report on the detailed fetal anatomic ultrasound examination: indications, components, and qualifications. *J Ultrasound Med*. 2014;33(2):189–195.
3. Committee on Practice Bulletins—Obstetrics and the American Institute of Ultrasound in Medicine Practice Bulletin No. 175: Ultrasound in Pregnancy. *Obstet Gynecol*. 2016;128(6):e241–e256.
4. Sparks TN, Thao K, Lianoglou BR, et al. and the University of California Fetal–Maternal Consortium. Nonimmune hydrops fetalis: identifying the underlying genetic etiology. *Genet Med*. 2019;21(6):1339–1344.
5. Reddy UM, Abuhamad AZ, Levine D, Saade GR, et al. Fetal imaging: executive summary of a joint Eunice Kennedy Shriver National Institute of Child Health and Human Development, Society for Maternal-Fetal Medicine, American Institute of Ultrasound in Medicine, American College of Obstetricians and Gynecologists, American College of Radiology, Society for Pediatric Radiology, and Society of Radiologists in Ultrasound Fetal Imaging Workshop. *J Ultrasound Med*. 2014;33(5):745–757.
6. Gabbay-Benziv R, Reece EA, Wang F, Yang P. Birth defects in pregestational diabetes: defect range, glycemic threshold and pathogenesis. *World J Diabetes*. 2015;6(3):481–488.
7. Lateef A, Petri M. Managing lupus patients during pregnancy. *Best Pract Res Clin Rheumatol*. 2013;27(3):435–447.
8. Maslovich M.M., Burke L.M. Intrauterine Fetal Demise. In: StatPearls [Internet]. Nov 5, 2021.
9. Suman V, Luther EE. Preterm Labor. In: StatPearls [Internet]. Jan 2022. https://www.ncbi.nlm.nih.gov/books/NBK536939/.
10. American College of Obstetricians and Gynecologists. Preterm Labor and Birth Frequently Asked Questions, Symptoms and Risk Factors. https://www.acog.org/womens-health/faqs/preterm-labor-and-birth.
11. Dugas C, Slane VH. Miscarriage. In: StatPearls [Internet]. Jun 29, 2021.
12. Fetal Growth Restriction: ACOG Practice Bulletin, Number 227. *Obstet Gynecol*. 2021;137(2):e16–e28.
13. AIUM-ACR-ACOG-SMFM-SRU Practice Parameter for the Performance of Standard Diagnostic Obstetric Ultrasound Examinations. *J Ultrasound Med*. 2018;37(11):E13–E24.
14. Contemporary OB/GYN. The importance of determining chorionicity in twin gestations. February 2, 2013. https://www.contemporaryobgyn.net/view/importance-determining-chorionicity-twin-gestations
15. Doubilet PM, Benson CB. "Appearing twin": undercounting of multiple gestations on early first trimester sonograms. *J Ultrasound Med*. 1998;17:199–203.
16. Doubilet PM. *Sonography of multiple gestations*. Laurel, MD: American Institute of Ultrasound in Medicine; 1997.

CHAPTER 55

Prenatal Diagnosis of Congenital Anomalies

Kelsi Weakley

OBJECTIVES

On completion of this chapter, you should be able to:
- Describe methods of genetic screening testing, including maternal serum markers and cell-free DNA
- Describe methods of diagnostic genetic screening testing, including chorionic villus sampling and amniocentesis
- Describe the ultrasound technique of amniocentesis
- Discuss how anomalies are transmitted genetically
- Detail the prevalence and prognosis of the most common chromosomal anomalies
- Describe the sonographic appearance of chromosomal anomalies

OUTLINE

Chromosomal Disorders 1426
Genetic Screening Tests 1427
    Alpha-Fetoprotein 1427
    Quadruple Screen 1429
    Cell-Free DNA Testing 1429
Diagnostic Screening Testing 1429
    Chorionic Villus Sampling 1429
    Amniocentesis 1430
    Technique of Genetic Amniocentesis 1431

Genetic Amniocentesis and Multiple Gestations 1432
Cordocentesis 1432
First Trimester Screening 1432
    Pregnancy-Associated Plasma Protein A 1432
    Human Chorionic Gonadotropin 1432
Medical Genetics 1433
Chromosomal Abnormalities 1433

Nuchal Translucency 1433
Trisomy 21 1433
Trisomy 18 1436
Trisomy 13 1437
Triploidy 1438
Turner Syndrome 1438

KEY TERMS

Alpha-fetoprotein (AFP)
Amniocentesis
Cell-free DNA (cfDNA)
Cystic hygroma
Hypertelorism

Hypoplasia
Hypotelorism
Intrauterine growth restriction (IUGR)
Micrognathia

Nuchal translucency
Omphalocele
Polydactyly

CHROMOSOMAL DISORDERS

Prenatal ultrasound has become the investigative tool for the obstetrician to access the developing fetus, and it is likely the fetus with an anomaly will be subjected to ultrasound at some point during pregnancy. The sonographer's role is to screen the fetus for any unexpected anomaly and evaluate the fetus at risk. The examination benefits are greatest when the sonographer is adept at detecting congenital anomalies and understands the cause, progression, and prognosis of the most commonly seen congenital anomalies, including chromosomal anomalies.

When a fetal anomaly is found antenatally, a multidisciplinary team approach is ideal when managing the fetus, mother, and family. The fetus may require special monitoring (e.g., serial ultrasound, antenatal testing, additional imaging), delivery postnatal care, and surgery. This multidisciplinary team includes the perinatologist (maternal-fetal medicine specialist), neonatologist (specialist for critically ill infants), sonologist, perinatal sonographer, pediatric surgeons, other pediatric specialists, geneticist, obstetrician, perinatal and pediatric social workers, and other support personnel. Consultation with specialists is recommended when diagnosis is uncertain. Once an anomaly is discovered, these specialists can collaborate to optimize clinical management, prepare the family for the potential need for surgery, provide the patient and family with emotional support and resources, and develop a delivery plan. Most fetuses with major birth defects are delivered in perinatal centers where the specialized physicians, nurses, equipment, treatment, and postnatal surgery are available.

GENETIC SCREENING TESTS

Alpha-Fetoprotein

Alpha-fetoprotein (AFP) is the major protein in fetal serum and is produced by the yolk sac in early gestation and later in pregnancy by the fetal liver. AFP is found in the fetal spine, gastrointestinal tract, liver, and kidneys. This protein is transported into the amniotic fluid by fetal urination and reaches maternal circulation through the fetal membranes (Fig. 55.1). AFP may be measured in the maternal serum (MSAFP) or amniotic fluid (AFAFP).

AFP levels are considered abnormal when elevated or low. Neural tube defects, such as anencephaly and open spina bifida, are common reasons for high AFP levels. In both instances, AFP leaks from the defect to enter the amniotic fluid and then diffuses into the maternal bloodstream (see Fig. 55.1). AFP elevations will not be found in cases where there is closed spina bifida (occulta) because there is no opening to allow leakage into the maternal bloodstream.

Monitoring of AFP is a screening test for neural tube defects and other conditions (Box 55.1). Evaluation is usually based on 2.0 to 2.5 multiples of the median, but false positives do occur. MSAFP screening detects approximately 75% to 90% of open neural tube defects and may also detect up to 85% of abdominal wall defects.[1]

MSAFP levels increase with advancing gestational age and peak from 15 to 18 weeks of gestation (the ideal sampling time). AFAFP, in contrast, decreases with fetal age. A common reason for elevations is incorrect dates. Because AFP levels vary with gestational age, if the fetus is older or younger than expected, AFP levels will be reported as increased or decreased.

Other reasons for elevations are acrania and encephalocele (which may occur in association with Meckel-Gruber syndrome), with AFP leakage from the exposed membranes and tissue. The concentration of AFP correlates with the size of the defect. AFP levels tend to be significantly higher in fetuses with anencephaly than with spina bifida because more tissue is exposed. It is important to remember that approximately 20% of spina bifida lesions are covered by skin, so AFP

BOX 55.1	Reasons for Elevation of Alpha-Fetoprotein and Acetylcholinesterase
Neural Tube Defects Anencephaly Exencephaly (acrania) Encephalocele (including Meckel-Gruber syndrome) Spina bifida Sacrococcygeal teratoma **Abdominal Wall Defects** Omphalocele Gastroschisis Limb–body wall complex Amniotic band syndrome Bladder or cloacal exstrophy Ectopia cordis **Multiple Gestation** Twin with a co-twin death Acardiac twin Fetus papyraceous **Gastrointestinal Obstruction** Annular pancreas Duodenal atresia Esophageal atresia **Renal Anomalies** Congenital nephrosis Hydronephrosis Polycystic kidney disease (including Meckel-Gruber syndrome) Urinary tract obstruction Prune-belly syndrome Urethral atresia **Placental and Cord Abnormalities** Chorioangioma Placental or cord hematoma Umbilical cord hemangioma Hydatidiform mole	**Fetal Heart Failure** Hydrops or ascites Lymphangiectasia Rh isoimmunization **Neck Masses** Cystic hygroma Noonan syndrome (with hygroma) **Liver Disease** Hepatitis Maternal herpes virus (fetal liver necrosis and skin lesions) Hepatocellular carcinoma Hamartoma of liver **Miscellaneous Causes** Incorrect dates Fetal demise Oligohydramnios Unexplained Hereditary overproduction of alpha-fetoprotein Blood in amniotic fluid Chromosome abnormalities (trisomies 18 and 13, Turner syndrome, triploidy) Cystadenomatoid malformation Epignathus Intracranial tumor Pilonidal cyst Skin defects Hydrocephalus Congenital heart defects Viral infections (cytomegalovirus, parvovirus)

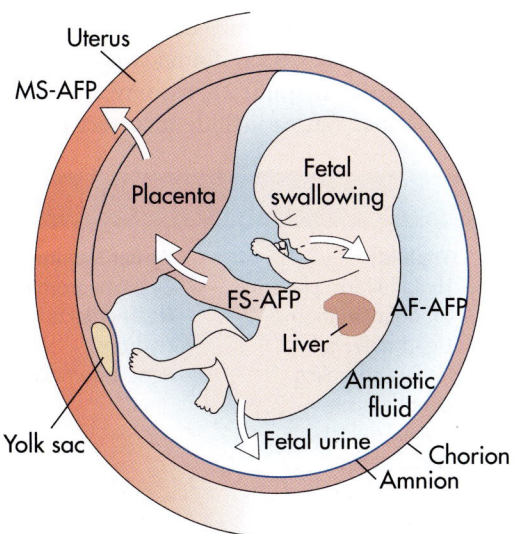

FIG. 55.1 Production and distribution of alpha-fetoprotein (AFP) into its three components: fetal tissues, amniotic fluid (AF), and maternal serum (MS). *FS*, Fetal serum.

elevations will not be detected in serum or amniotic fluid. Sacrococcygeal teratomas are also known to be associated with high AFP levels.

Two common abdominal wall defects, omphalocele and gastroschisis, produce elevations of AFP. With an **omphalocele**, AFP leaks through the membrane encasing the herniated bowel or liver. In gastroschisis, AFP diffuses directly into the serum and amniotic fluid from the herniated bowel, which lacks a covering membrane; thus, AFP levels are higher in a fetus with gastroschisis than in a fetus with an omphalocele.

Other abdominal wall defects cause leakage in the same manner. Bladder or cloacal exstrophy, ectopia cordis (herniation of the heart out of the chest), limb-body wall complex, and amniotic band syndrome are examples of other anomalies that may present with an elevated AFP level.

It is expected that the AFP level in a twin pregnancy will be twice that of a singleton pregnancy because two fetuses make twice the AFP. AFP may be higher than normal in multiple gestations in which there is death of a co-twin (fetus papyraceous) or when one twin is acardiac.

Obstructions of the gastrointestinal tract may cause reduced clearance of AFP. This may explain elevations with anomalies, such as an annular pancreas, esophageal atresia, and duodenal atresia.

A fetus with a kidney lesion may produce increased AFP. In congenital nephrosis, the kidneys excrete extremely high levels of AFP. Polycystic kidneys and urinary tract obstruction may also lead to higher levels of AFP because there is abnormal clearance or filtration of AFP because of kidney maldevelopment and urinary tract leakage.

Placental lesions, such as chorioangiomas, hemangiomas, and hematomas, are responsible for AFP elevations. Placental problems, in general, may explain the prevalence of growth restriction, fetal death, and abruption in patients with unexplained AFP elevations.

In heart failure, faulty diffusion of AFP may lead to an abnormal AFP increase when hydrops, ascites, or lymphangiectasia is present. Severely sensitized fetuses with Rh isoimmunization may have heart failure because of severe anemia. In the fetus with a **cystic hygroma**, obstructed lymph sacs lead to AFP diffusion through the hygroma into the bloodstream and amniotic fluid.

Liver disease in the mother or fetus may cause high AFP levels. Hepatitis, maternal herpes virus, resultant fetal liver necrosis, skin lesions, hepatocellular carcinoma, and fetal liver tumors (hamartomas) are rare causes of elevated AFP.

Other causes include chromosomal abnormalities associated with fetal anomalies or placental problems that permit the abnormal passage of AFP. Fetuses with trisomy 13 or trisomy 18 may also have renal anomalies, neural tube defects, ventral wall defects, or skin lesions that cause elevated AFP levels. Fetuses with Turner syndrome often present with cystic hygromas. In triploidy, abnormal placental molar degeneration leads to increased AFP diffusion.

Cystic adenomatoid malformations cause rises in AFP because of excessive leakage from the lungs. Pilonidal cysts of the back and various skin disorders and tumors, such as epignathus and intracranial lesions, are also associated with high AFP levels. Rarely does the fetus manufacture excessive amounts of AFP as a hereditary condition.

Fetal death is a frequent cause of a high MSAFP level. Pregnancies complicated by oligohydramnios may have higher concentrations of AFP because of less amniotic fluid to diffuse the protein. Contamination of an amniotic fluid specimen by blood may also falsely increase the level of AFP.

In utero viral infections (cytomegalovirus and parvovirus) are reported to permit excessive AFP leakage because the maternal-fetal surface may be irritated and disrupted by inflammation.

Unexplained elevations in MSAFP suggest that the pregnancy is at increased risk for complications and poor outcomes, including low birth weight and stillbirth. Preeclampsia, hypertension, and abruption placentae are other third-trimester complications associated with these elevations.

Mothers with elevated MSAFP values and normal AFAFP values are potentially at risk for other fetal anomalies unrelated to neural tube defects. Hydrocephalus, without a spinal defect (increased cerebrospinal fluid allows increased diffusion), and congenital heart disease (probable altered perfusion of blood flow through placenta) are reported in conjunction with unexplained, non–neural tube defect problems.

Low AFP levels have been found with chromosomal abnormalities, such as trisomy 21, trisomy 18, and trisomy 13 (Box 55.2). Other causes include incorrect patient dates

---

BOX 55.2 Common Sonographic Features of Chromosomal Anomalies

Trisomy 21	Trisomy 18	Trisomy 13	Triploidy	Turner Syndrome
Nuchal thickness	Heart defects	Holoprosencephaly	Hydatidiform placental degeneration	Cystic hygroma
Heart defects	Choroid plexus cysts	Heart defects	Heart defects	Heart defects
Duodenal atresia	Clenched hands	Cleft lip and palate	Renal anomalies	Hydrops
Shortened femurs	Micrognathia	Omphalocele	Omphalocele	Renal anomalies
Mild pyelectasis	Talipes	Polydactyly	Cranial defects	
Mild ventriculomegaly	Renal anomalies	Talipes	Facial defects	
Echogenic bowel	Cleft lip and palate	Echogenic chordae tendineae		
	Omphalocele	Renal anomalies		
	Congenital diaphragmatic hernia	Meningomyelocele		
	Cerebellar hypoplasia	Micrognathia		

(fetus younger than expected), fetal death, hydatidiform moles, spontaneous abortion, and a nonpregnant state. In some cases, the cause may remain unknown.

Amniocentesis may be offered when MSAFP levels are elevated and ultrasound reveals no obvious explanation. Amniotic fluid tests usually include karyotyping for chromosomal abnormalities, AFAFP levels, and acetylcholinesterase. AFAFP is more specific for detecting levels of AFP. Acetylcholinesterase is specific for detecting an open neural tube. Beyond 20 weeks of gestation, acetylcholinesterase is the preferred test because AFP analysis is no longer sensitive.

When AFP is elevated (greater than 3 multiples of the median) and the cranium (ventricles and cisterna magna) and spine appear normal, the risk of the fetus actually having a small spinal defect is approximately halved. Though the risk of miscarriage from amniocentesis is low, it is important to weigh the risk of complication with the possible yield of identifying an abnormality.

Prenatal scanning and amniocentesis are used to evaluate the fetus with a low AFP value to exclude any physical features that may suggest a chromosomal abnormality. Such findings might include choroid plexus cysts, hand anomalies, or cardiac defects.

Quadruple Screen

Another biochemical screening test used in the early second trimester is the quadruple (quad) screen. Formally known as the triple test or triple screen, this biochemical screening test combines three serum markers: AFP, human chorionic gonadotropin (hCG), and unconjugated estriol. This blood test improved the detection rate for trisomy 21 over MSAFP testing alone. Biochemical screening in trisomy 21 fetuses reveals high hCG levels and decreased AFP and estriol levels. Additionally, biochemical screening may suggest trisomy 18 when hCG, AFP, and estriol levels are all decreased. The quad screen added another maternal serum marker, dimeric inhibin A, improving the sensitivity to more than 80% for detecting Down fetuses in women of advanced maternal age.[1] The risk for a neural tube defect or chromosomal problem is calculated for each mother. A patient may elect to undergo ultrasound with or without amniocentesis based on the risk for chromosomal or neural tube defects.

Cell-Free DNA Testing

Fetal **cell-free DNA (cfDNA)** or circulating fetal DNA testing was discovered when the Y chromosome was first isolated from the plasma of pregnant women carrying male fetuses.[2] cfDNA is released from the placenta into maternal circulation and is quantifiable as early as 10 weeks' gestation, with the accuracy of the results increasing with advancing gestation as the ratio of placental to total cfDNA also advances.[2] Marketed as noninvasive prenatal testing, cfDNA is considered more accurate than serum screening tests for aneuploidy and has increased in popularity when examining the risk a patient has for some of the more common chromosomal abnormalities (most notably Down syndrome) and has been incorporated into common practice by many physicians and clinics.[3]

As with any screening test, there are limitations to cfDNA testing. The results are derived from the placenta, which can result in false positives due to placental mosaicism, maternal chromosomal abnormalities, fetal demise, multiple gestation pregnancies, and other factors.[2] With an increase in popularity, the demand for genetic counseling services to explain and interpret these results to physicians and patients has also increased to ensure that the findings are appropriately relayed so that medical decisions regarding pursuing additional diagnostic testing, management, and treatment plans can be discussed.[3]

DIAGNOSTIC SCREENING TESTING

Chorionic Villus Sampling

Chorionic villus sampling (CVS) is an ultrasound-directed biopsy of the placenta or chorionic villi (chorion frondosum). The chorion frondosum is the active trophoblastic tissue that becomes the placenta. Because the chorionic villi are fetal in origin, chromosomal abnormalities may be detected when cells from the villi are grown and analyzed. Other conditions, such as biochemical or metabolic disorders, thalassemia, and sickle cell disease (hemoglobinopathies), may also be diagnosed using chorionic villi.

CVS is an alternative diagnostic test used to obtain a fetal karyotype by culturing fetal cells similar to amniocentesis. The advantages of CVS include the following: (1) it is performed early in pregnancy (10 to 14 weeks), (2) results are typically available within 1 week, and (3) earlier results allow more options for parents.

CVS is performed transcervically or transabdominally (Fig. 55.2). Ultrasound performed before the actual procedure aids in several ways: (1) It determines the relationship between the lie of the uterus and cervix and path of the catheter. Bladder fullness influences this relationship. Filling or emptying the bladder may be necessary to facilitate the

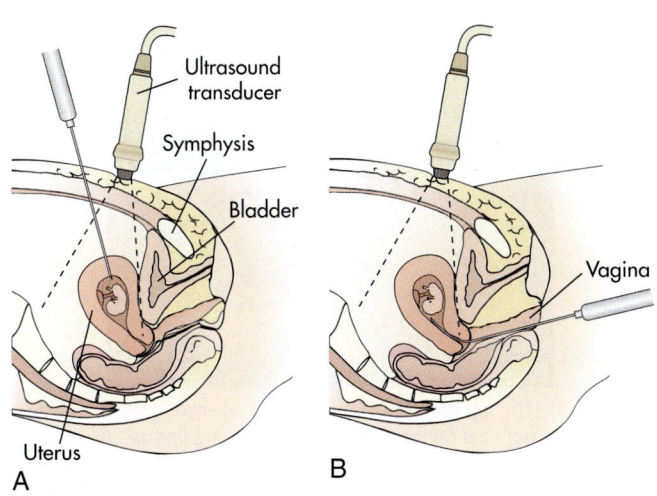

FIG. 55.2 (A) Transabdominal chorionic villus sampling. (B) Transcervical chorionic villus sampling.

catheter route. (2) It assesses the fetus in terms of life, normal morphology, and age. (3) It identifies uterine masses or potential problems that may interfere with passage of the catheter.

Transvaginal CVS is performed in the dorsolithotomy position (pelvic examination position). The sonographer aids the obstetrician in determining the correct route to pass the catheter through the cervix to the placenta. A guiding stylet is initially introduced to check uterine and placental position. A flexible catheter is then introduced and directed into the placental tissue (Fig. 55.3). The placental cells are aspirated through the catheter. The villi are collected and transported to the cytogenetics technician for analysis. Additional retrievals often are necessary. The sonographer should monitor the fetal heart rate and check for procedural bleeding during and and after the procedure.

The transabdominal CVS approach entails using a syringe and needle inserted into the placenta to withdraw the villi. The procedure is performed in a manner similar to amniocentesis (see the discussion of amniocentesis).

The risk of fetal loss because of CVS is approximately 0.05% to 1.0%. There has been some association with limb reduction defects when CVS is performed before 10 weeks of gestation.[4] $Rh_o(D)$ immune globulin (RhoGAM) should be administered to Rh-negative unsensitized women to prevent sensitization problems in subsequent pregnancies. Experienced operators have a higher success rate with lower complication rates; however, due to the increasing popularity of noninvasive prenatal testing testing, the number of invasive procedures has declined.[4]

Amniocentesis

Amniocentesis was first used as a technique to relieve polyhydramnios, to predict Rh isoimmunization, and to document fetal lung maturity. In the mid-1960s, amniocentesis was introduced as a diagnostic invasive procedure used to study fetal cells from amniotic fluid that allowed the analysis of fetal chromosomes (Fig. 55.4). Normal and abnormal chromosomal patterns (Figs. 55.5 and 55.6) could be identified.

Amniocentesis is a test offered to expectant patients at risk (similar to the indications of a CVS) for a chromosomal abnormality or biochemical disorder that may be prenatally detectable.[4] The results are available between 1 and 3 weeks; however, if rapid results are desired, fluorescence in situ

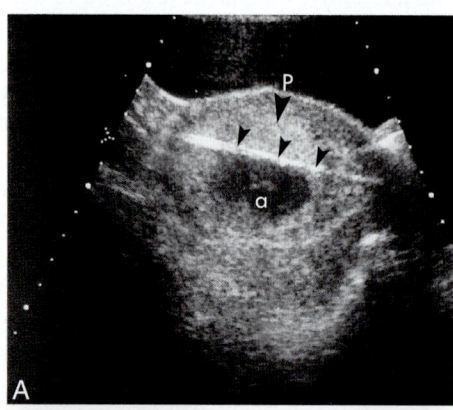
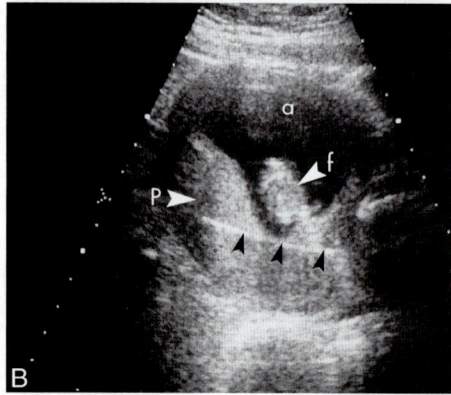

FIG. 55.3 (A) Transcervical chorionic villus sampling at 10 weeks of gestation demonstrating the placement of the sampling catheter *(arrowheads)* within an anterior placenta (P) or chorion frondosum. (B) Transcervical chorionic villus sampling at 11 weeks of gestation showing the placement of the sampling catheter *(arrowheads)* within a posterior placenta (P). Note the fetal abdomen (f) within the amniotic cavity (a).

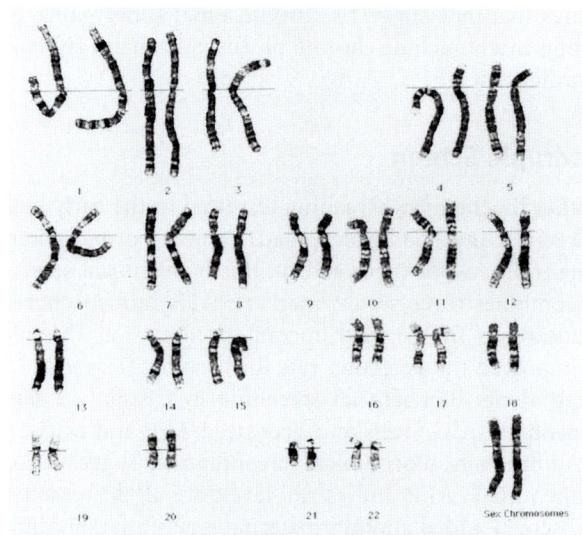

FIG. 55.4 Normal karyotype demonstrating 46 chromosomes in a female fetus (46,XX).

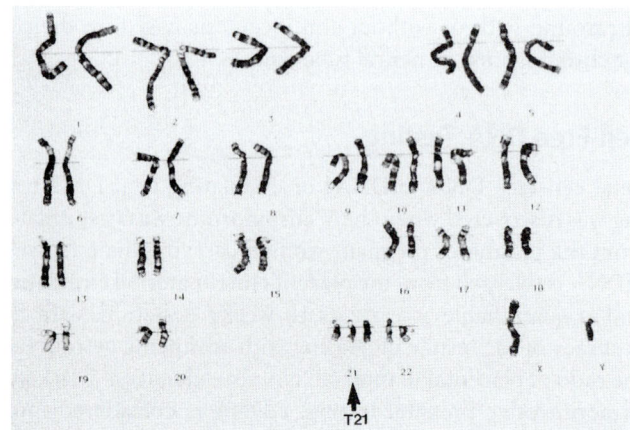

FIG. 55.5 Karyotype of trisomy 21 (Down syndrome) in a male fetus (47,XY,21). Note the extra chromosome at the 21st position *(arrow)*. Note the sex chromosomes indicating a male fetus.

hybridization (FISH) provides a limited analysis within 24 to 48 hours for the most common chromosomal anomalies. The FISH assay most commonly evaluates for numeric abnormalities of chromosomes 21, 13, 18, X, and Y.

Advanced maternal age is a common reason for performing amniocentesis. All pregnant women are at risk for having a child with a chromosomal defect; however, the risk increases as the mother advances in age.

Other indications for genetic amniocentesis include a history of a balanced rearrangement in a parent or previous child with a chromosomal abnormality, a history of an unexplained abnormal AFP level or an abnormal screening test, and a fetus with a known or suspected congenital anomaly.

Amniocentesis for genetic reasons is ideally performed between 15 and 20 weeks of gestation, with common practice waiting until after 16 weeks gestation to minimize some of the associated risks with an unfused amnion which can be seen up to 16 weeks. Amniocentesis may be done as early as 12 weeks; however, it may lead to fetal scoliosis or clubfoot secondary to the reduced amount of amniotic fluid. The rate of miscarriage in early amniocentesis is not clearly defined. Some studies have shown that the loss rate is similar to midtrimester amniocentesis, whereas others have shown a higher loss rate. One study reported the fetal loss rate of midtrimester amniocentesis at 1 in 769.[4] Amniocentesis performed beyond 20 weeks of gestation is possible but may be associated with poor cell growth or may require cells to culture longer delaying the results.

The amniocentesis procedure should include a fetal survey to exclude congenital anomalies. A fetal examination should be performed, and targeted areas of anatomy should be documented to exclude the physical features that would suggest a chromosomal anomaly (e.g., hand clenching, hypoplasia of the fifth middle phalanx, choroid plexus cysts, ventriculomegaly, thickened nuchal fold, cardiac anomalies, omphalocele, spina bifida, or foot anomalies).

The sonographer will also assist the physician in the amniocentesis procedure similar to their role during a CVS, while an amniocentesis is performed exclusively transabdominally. The optimal collection site for amniotic fluid should be away from the fetus, away from the central portion of the placenta, away from the umbilical cord, and near the maternal midline to avoid the maternal uterine vessels and ensure an appropriate sample is obtained.

Technique of Genetic Amniocentesis

Ultrasound-monitored amniocentesis is a technique that allows the continuous monitoring of the needle during the amniocentesis procedure. Using this technique, the maternal skin is prepared with a povidone-iodine solution. The transducer is placed in a sterile cover or sterile glove to allow monitoring on the sterile field during the procedure. Sterile coupling gel may be applied to the maternal skin to ensure good transmission of the sound beam. The amniocentesis site is rescanned to confirm the amniotic pocket, and then the site and pathway for the introduction of the needle are determined. The distance to the amniotic fluid may be measured with electronic calipers, which may be useful in obese patients in whom a longer needle may be necessary. In many instances, a new site is chosen as a result of fetal movement or a myometrial contraction in the proposed site, and the transducer is moved to a new sterile area. On successful identification of the amniocentesis site, a finger is placed between the transducer and the skin to produce an acoustic shadow. The needle is then inserted under continuous ultrasound observation (Fig. 55.7). Inserting the needle in a plane perpendicular to the transducer will allow for a bright reflection of the needle tip so that it can be easily observed (Fig. 55.8) at the edge of the uterine wall and then as it punctures the uterine cavity. When incorrectly directed, the needle may be repositioned through manipulation and angling of the needle tip. Amniotic fluid is aspirated through a syringe connected to the needle hub. Typically, the initial sample of 3 to 5 mL is discarded to assure a clean sample is sent for analysis. Approximately 20 mL of amniotic fluid will be collected for chromosomal analysis and AFP evaluation. In advanced pregnancies, additional amniotic fluid may be required to ensure appropriate analysis can be performed.

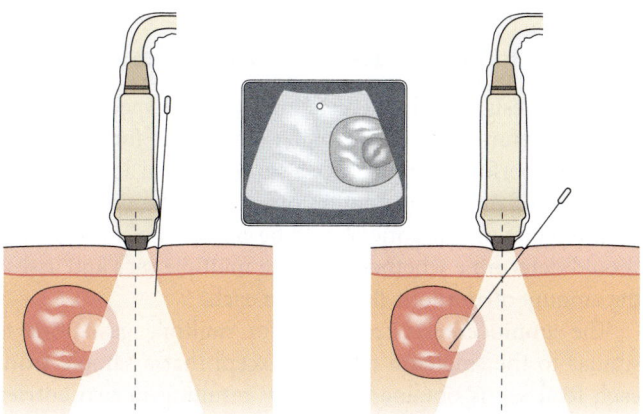

FIG. 55.7 If the needle is inserted parallel to the transducer, only the tip will be represented. If the needle is inserted at an angle with the transducer, the beam will intersect the needle, but it will not demonstrate its tip, which could be in a harmful position. Notice that in both cases the image on the screen is the same. Angling the needle is a dangerous procedure that should be avoided.

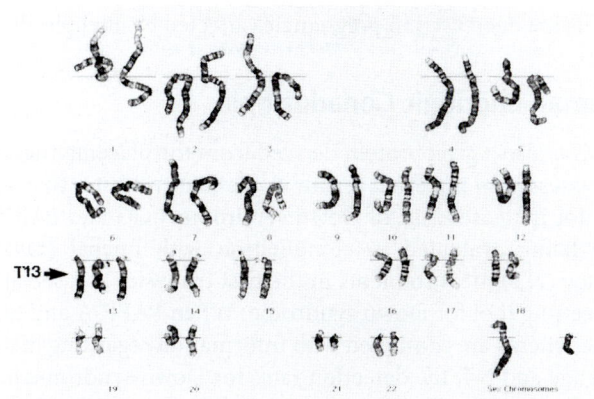

FIG. 55.6 Karyotype of trisomy 13 (47,XY,13) *(arrow)* male fetus.

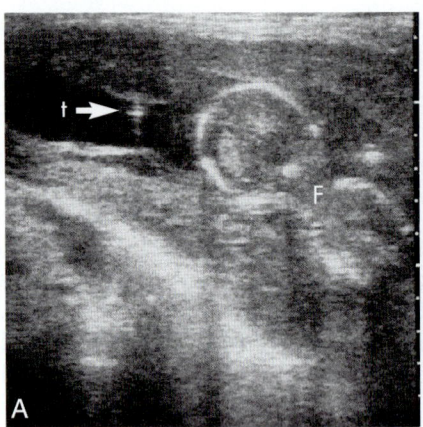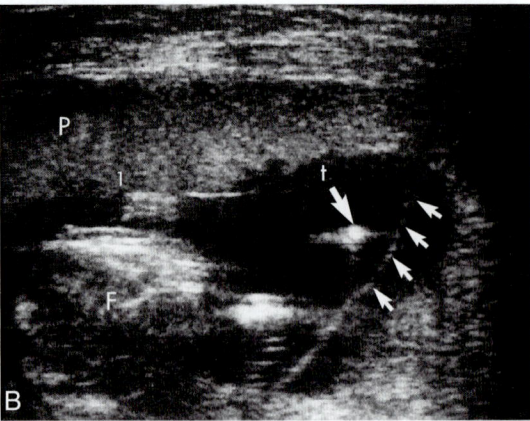

FIG. 55.8 (A) Genetic amniocentesis at 15.6 weeks of gestation using direct visualization method. The needle tip (t) is identified within the amniotic cavity. (B) Genetic amniocentesis at 16 weeks of gestation in a twin pregnancy. The needle tip is identified within the sac above the amniotic membrane *(arrows)*. *1*, Umbilical cord insertion into placenta; *F*, fetus; *P*, placenta.

When amniocentesis is performed because of a known fetal anomaly, acetylcholinesterase and viral studies including toxoplasmosis, other (including syphilis), rubella, cytomegalovirus, and herpes simplex virus may be ordered. This panel is typically referred to as a TORCH panel. Following aspiration of amniotic fluid, the needle is removed from the uterus under sonographic guidance.

After the amniocentesis has been completed, fetal cardiac activity should be identified and documented. If the placenta has been traversed, the site should be monitored for bleeding. The use of cine clips and video recording can allow for continuous recording and documentation of the fetal examination, the amniocentesis, and postamniocentesis ultrasound evaluation. In some cases of advanced gestation, the physician may request a nonstress test after the procedure to monitor for fetal well-being and/or maternal contractions.

The continuous monitoring with ultrasound during amniocentesis is invaluable in cases of oligohydramnios, anterior placental position, and premature rupture of membranes. Ultrasound imaging can help achieve a successful amniocentesis when only small pockets of fluid are available.

Genetic Amniocentesis and Multiple Gestations

Amniocentesis in multiple gestations warrants special consideration. Preliminary sonographic examination for each fetus should be performed to include a survey of fetal anatomy and growth profiles. Determination of whether the pregnancy is monozygotic or dizygotic should be made. The sonographer should determine whether there are multiple sacs and assess the amount of amniotic fluid within each.

The amniocentesis technique for multiple gestations is similar to the singleton method, except that a sample from each fetal sac is obtained, typically resulting in two entries into the uterus. To be certain that amniotic fluid is obtained from each sac, indigo carmine dye can be injected into the first sac after the first sample is obtained. The presence of clear amniotic fluid indicates that the second sac has been penetrated when the second pass is made. Visible dye-stained fluid indicates that the first sac has been penetrated a second time. Documentation of each amniocentesis and meticulous labeling of fluid samples are recommended to ensure delineation between each fetus. Avoiding the placenta in patients who are Rh-negative is desirable. In all Rh-negative patients, RhoGAM is administered within 72 hours of the procedure and may be required again later in pregnancy before delivery.

Cordocentesis

Cordocentesis is another method by which chromosomes are analyzed. Fetal blood is obtained through needle aspiration of the umbilical cord. Karyotype results can be processed within 2 to 3 days; however, the availability of FISH has decreased the need for cordocentesis for chromosomal analysis. Cordocentesis is more commonly used for guidance for transfusions to treat fetal isoimmunization

FIRST TRIMESTER SCREENING

Pregnancy-Associated Plasma Protein A

A first-trimester serum marker used to detect anomalies is pregnancy-associated plasma protein A (PAPP-A). PAPP-A is a glycoprotein derived from the trophoblastic tissue that is then diffused into the maternal circulation. PAPP-A levels increase in maternal serum throughout pregnancy. PAPP-A levels are decreased in pregnancies affected by aneuploidy.

Human Chorionic Gonadotropin

hCG is also a glycoprotein derived from the placenta that can be assessed in maternal serum in the first trimester to evaluate for increased risk of Down syndrome. hCG and PAPP-A are being evaluated in combination with nuchal translucency (NT) measurements in the first trimester as a sensitive screening tool for Down syndrome. When PAPP-A and hCG assessments are combined with information regarding maternal age and NT, the detection rates for Down syndrome have been reported to be 79% to 90%,[4] and the information can be provided to women at a much earlier gestational age.

First-trimester assessment techniques that utilize sonographic evaluation for the detection of aneuploidy are discussed further in Chapter 49.

MEDICAL GENETICS

A normal karyotype consists of 46 chromosomes, 22 pairs of autosomes, and a pair of sex chromosomes (see Fig. 55.4). Aneuploidy is an abnormality of the number of chromosomes. One of the most common aneuploid conditions is Down syndrome, in which an individual has an extra chromosome number 21 (see Fig. 55.5). The cause of trisomy is usually nondisjunction, the failure of normal chromosomal division at the time of meiosis. The cause of nondisjunction is unknown, although there is a strong association with maternal age.

A chromosomal disorder is caused by too much or too little chromosome material. A dominant disorder is a condition caused by a single defective gene (autosomal dominant). It is usually inherited from one parent (who is also affected), but it may arise as a new mutation (spontaneous gene change). An inherited dominant disorder carries a 50% chance that each time pregnancy occurs, the fetus will have the condition. An example of an autosomal dominant condition is osteogenesis imperfecta (types 1 and 4).

A recessive disorder (autosomal recessive) is caused by a pair of defective genes, one inherited from each parent. With each pregnancy, the parents have a 25% chance of having a fetus with the disorder. An example of an autosomal recessive condition is infantile polycystic kidney disease.

Boys inherit X-linked disorders from their mothers. Affected males do not transmit the disorder to their sons, but all of their daughters will be carriers of the disorder. The sons of female carriers each have a 50% chance of being affected, and the daughters each have a 50% chance of being a carrier. Whereas an X-linked gene is located on the female sex chromosome (the X), an autosomal gene is located on one of the numbered chromosomes. An example of an X-linked condition occurring in male fetuses is aqueductal stenosis. Aqueductal stenosis, however, may also occur in females.[4]

A multifactorial condition is an abnormal event that arises because of the interaction of one or more genes and environmental factors. Anencephaly is an example of a multifactorial disorder.

Mosaicism is the occurrence of a gene mutation or chromosomal abnormality in a portion of an individual's cells. It is difficult to predict the types of problems that will occur when mosaicism is found.

CHROMOSOMAL ABNORMALITIES

There is a high prevalence of chromosomal abnormalities in patients referred for second-trimester amniocentesis because of advanced maternal age, abnormal AFP, abnormal quad screen (hCG, AFP, estriol, and inhibin A), or ultrasound detection of multiple fetal anomalies. It is important to become familiar with and search for the physical features (see Box 55.2) that would suggest trisomies 13, 18, and 21, triploidy, and Turner syndrome.

Nuchal Translucency

Nuchal translucency (NT) is the sonographic appearance of the subcutaneous fluid collection on the posterior aspect of the neck of the fetus. An abnormal fluid collection behind the fetal neck has been strongly associated with aneuploidy. This NT has been reported as a late first-trimester finding identified between 11 and 14 weeks of gestation. The NT increases with gestational age, so the NT measurement should be compared with the gestational age or crown-rump length to determine risk for aneuploidy and combined with maternal age and first-trimester serum screening. A thickened NT is associated with chromosomal abnormalities, such as trisomies 13, 18, and 21; triploidy; and Turner syndrome (Fig. 55.9). This first-trimester finding is not a precursor to the development of a cystic hygroma or second-trimester edema. Even in fetuses with normal chromosomes, an increased NT has been associated with an increased incidence of structural defects, such as cardiac, diaphragmatic, renal, and abdominal wall anomalies.[5] In addition to the increased risk of chromosomal abnormality and other anomalies, an increased NT has also been associated with spontaneous miscarriage and perinatal death. The criteria used in measuring the NT are defined in Chapter 49.

Trisomy 21

Trisomy 21, also known as Down syndrome, occurs in 14.2 in 10,000 live births.[6] It is one of the most common chromosomal disorders and is characterized by an extra chromosome number 21. There is an association with advanced maternal age; however, this anomaly may affect infants born to women of all ages. Trisomy 21 is associated with an increased NT, an abnormal first-trimester screen, and an abnormal quad screen.

Infants with trisomy 21 may present with a variety of physical features (Fig. 55.10), including brachycephaly; epicanthal folds (a fold of skin that covers the inner corner of the eye); a flattened nasal bridge; round, small ears; broad neck with extra skin (nuchal fold); and a protruding tongue. Other anomalies that have been associated with Down syndrome

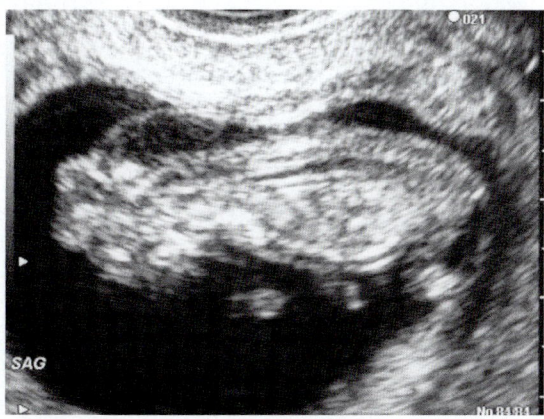

FIG. 55.9 This fetus with trisomy 13 presented with a thickened and septated nuchal translucency and anencephaly in the late first trimester of pregnancy.

include heart defects (septal defects, endocardial cushion defect, tetralogy of Fallot), duodenal atresia, esophageal atresia, anorectal atresia, and omphalocele (Fig. 55.11). Cystic hygroma, nonimmune hydrops, hydrothorax, and echogenic intracardiac foci may also be observed. Skeletal anomalies may be present, including shortened extremities, space between the first and second toes, hypoplasia or absence of the middle fifth phalanx (Fig. 55.12), and clinodactyly of the fifth finger (inward curving). A single palmar (hand) crease may be identified in affected infants.[7]

The prognosis for survival depends on associated anomalies, with heart anomalies a major cause of mortality in infancy. Intellectual disability is always present, with IQ ranges between 25 and 50 in childhood. In addition to heart failure, alimentary defects can also be life threatening. Respiratory problems, eye problems, and premature aging are common.

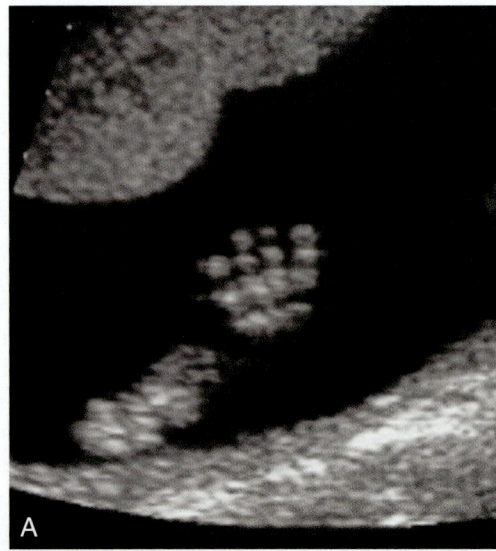
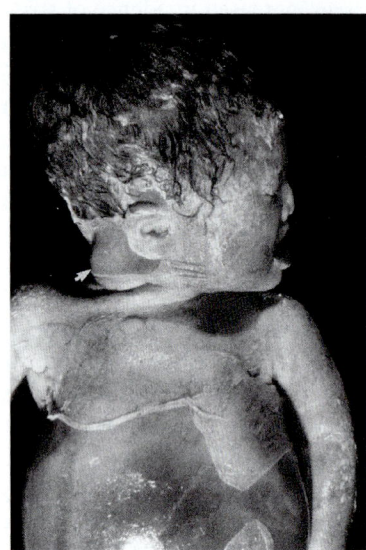

FIG. 55.10 Postmortem photograph of a neonate with trisomy 21 (Down syndrome). Duodenal atresia was found. Note the nuchal thickening *(arrow)*.

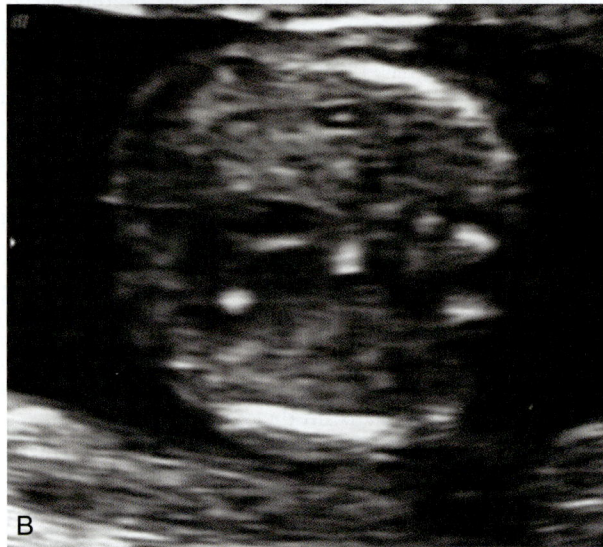

FIG. 55.12 (A) Absent fifth middle phalanx in a fetus with trisomy 21. (B) In the same fetus, an echogenic intracardiac focus is observed.

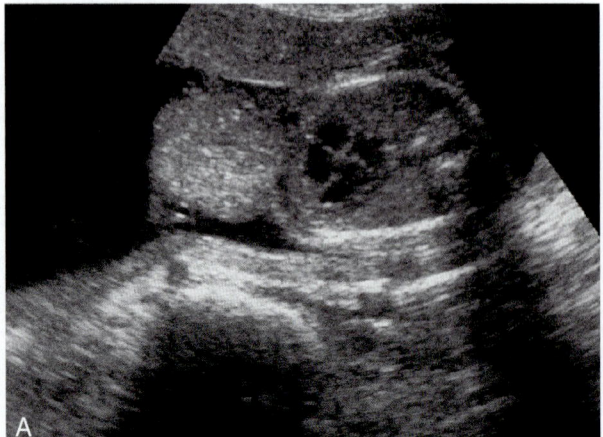
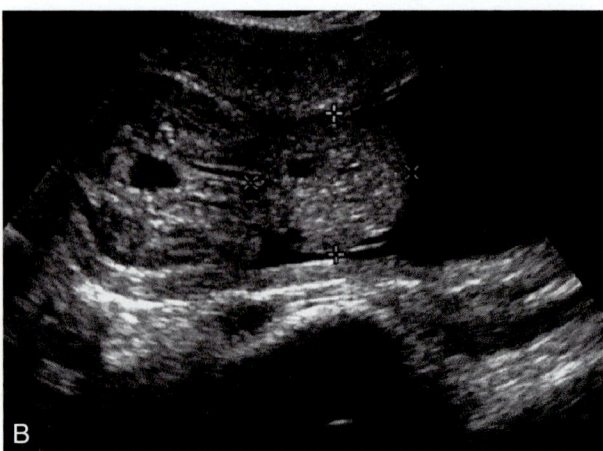

FIG. 55.11 (A) A 22-week-old fetus with tetralogy of Fallot (ventricular septal defect [VSD], overriding aorta, pulmonary stenosis, right ventricular hypertrophy). Only the VSD is appreciated in this four-chamber view. (B) Omphalocele in the same fetus. These findings together are highly suggestive of a chromosomal anomaly.

Sonographic Findings. Ultrasound diagnosis of trisomy 21 is limited because of the subtleness and infrequency of some of the phenotypic expressions. Accuracy of detection in the first trimester can be increased by assessing NT and nasal bone in conjunction with serum screening. Anomalies that may be identified with Down syndrome (Figs. 55.13–55.17) include the following:

- Nuchal fold of 5 mm or greater[8] (see Fig. 55.13)
- Extremity anomalies (hypoplasia of the middle phalanx or clinodactyly of the fifth finger; space between first and second toes)
- Shortened femur or short humerus (less than the 5th percentile)
- Duodenal atresia (see Fig. 55.14)
- Heart defects (see Fig. 55.15) (present in approximately 30% to 40%)
- **Intrauterine growth restriction (IUGR)**
- Mild pyelectasis (≥4 mm in anteroposterior diameter)[8]
- Echogenic bowel (see Fig. 55.16)
- Mild ventriculomegaly
- Echogenic intracardiac focus
- Absence of the nasal bone between 11 and 14 weeks

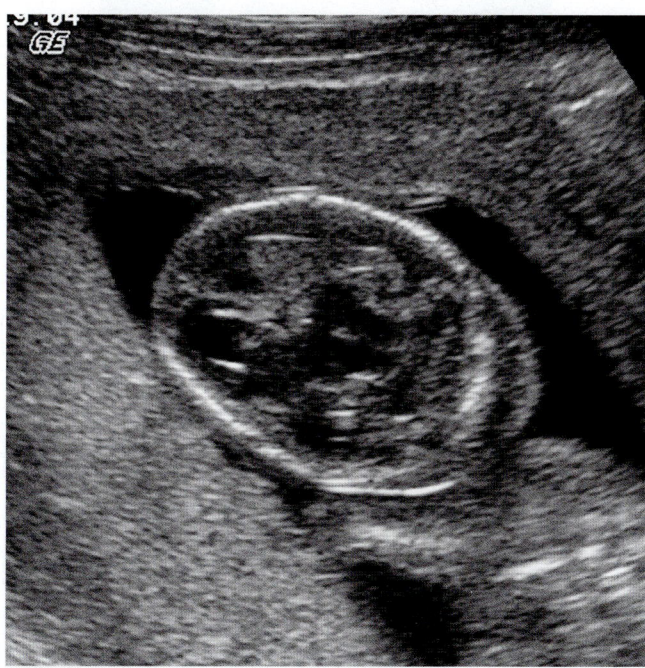

FIG. 55.13 A thickened nuchal fold is seen in a fetus with trisomy 21.

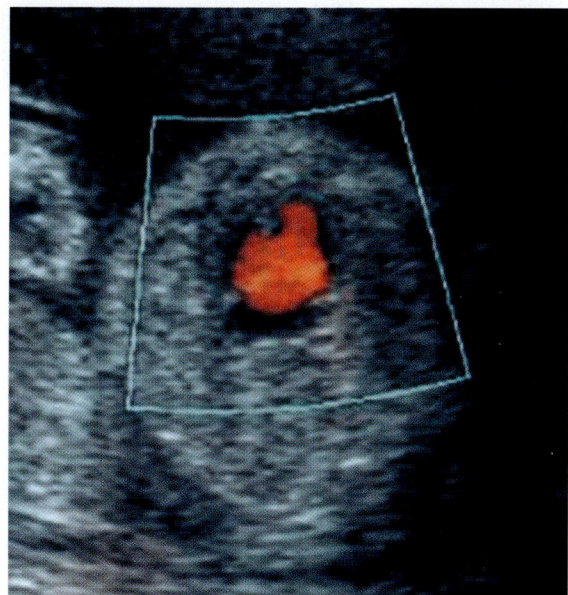

FIG. 55.15 This endocardial cushion defect (atrioventricular canal) presented with an atrial septal defect, ventricular septal defect, and common valve.

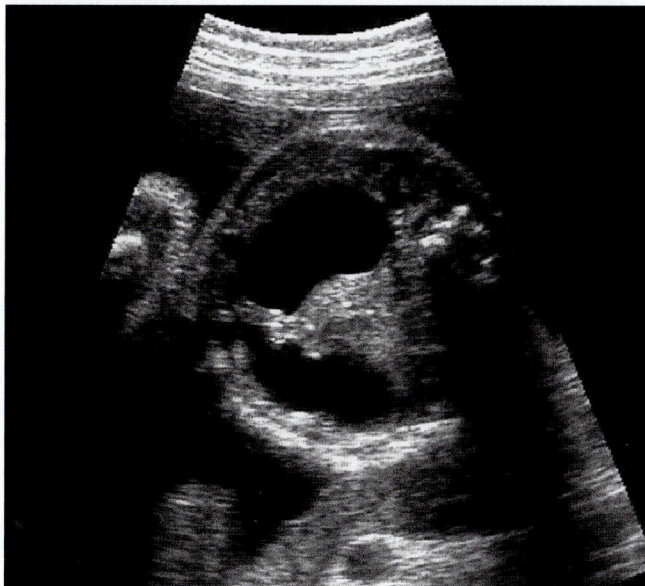

FIG. 55.14 The "double bubble" sign is identified in this case of duodenal atresia. This is a significant finding associated with trisomy 21.

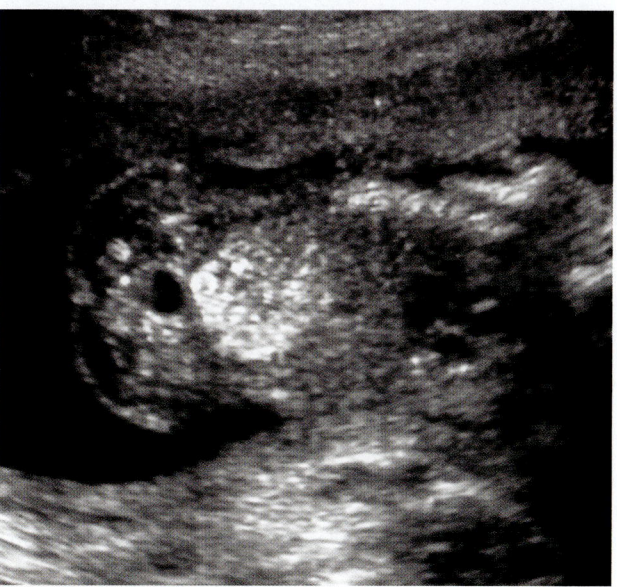

FIG. 55.16 Echogenic bowel, bowel with the same echogenicity as fetal bone, is a subtle finding associated with trisomy 21.

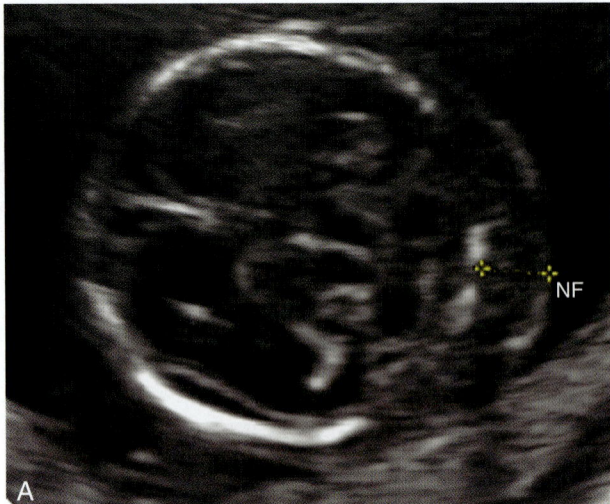
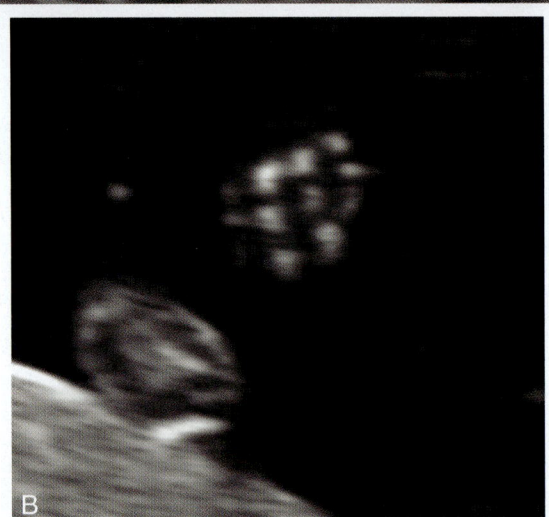
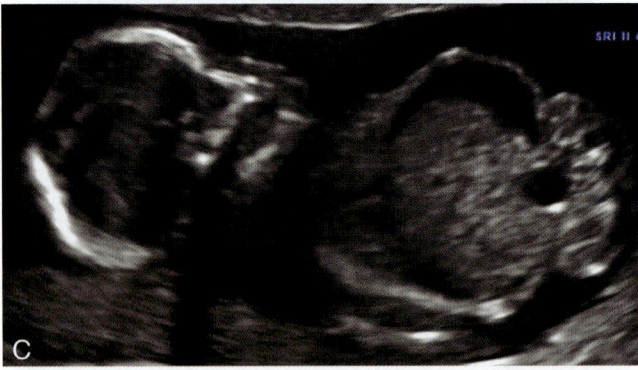

FIG. 55.17 A female with fetus presented at 18 weeks of gestation with increased risk for Down syndrome. Ultrasound revealed an increased nuchal fold (NF; A), clinodactyly of the fifth digit (B), and ascites (C). Amniocentesis confirmed trisomy 21.

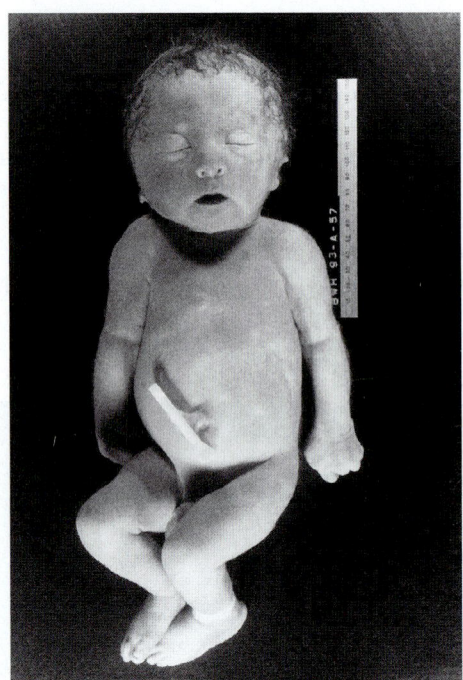

FIG. 55.18 **Neonate with trisomy 18.** Note the clenched hands and rocker-bottom feet. Prenatal ultrasound revealed a supratentorial cyst confirmed after autopsy.

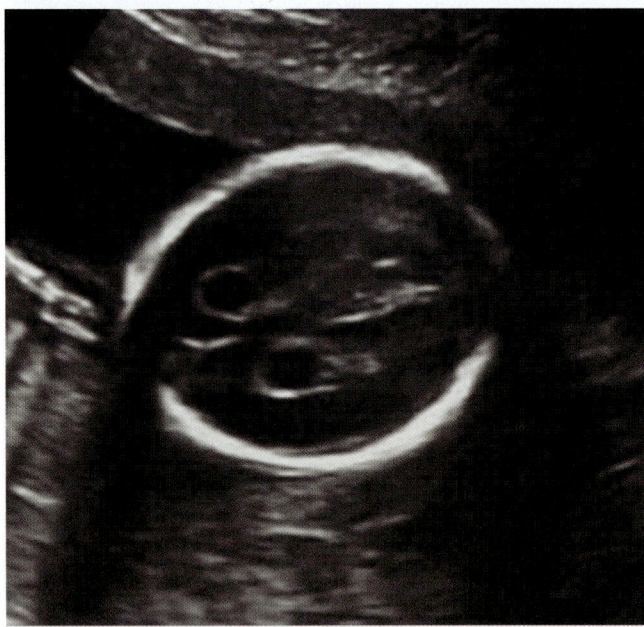

FIG. 55.19 Bilateral choroid plexus cysts were identified in a pregnancy referred for serum screening suggestive of trisomy 18. Amniocentesis confirmed Edwards syndrome.

Trisomy 18

Trisomy 18, also known as Edwards syndrome, is the second most common chromosomal trisomy, occurring in 1 of 8000 live births.[9] This karyotype demonstrates an extra chromosome 18. Trisomy 18 is associated with an abnormal quad screen.

Physical features that have been identified in fetuses with trisomy 18 (Fig. 55.18) include cardiac anomalies, which are present in the majority of fetuses with this chromosomal anomaly. Cranial anomalies that have been identified are dolichocephaly, microcephaly, hydrocephalus, agenesis of the corpus callosum, cerebellar hypoplasia, encephalocele, a strawberry-shaped head, and choroid plexus cysts (Fig. 55.19). Facial abnormalities include low-set ears, **micrognathia**, and cleft lip (Fig. 55.20) and palate. Abnormal extremities identified with trisomy 18 include persistently clenched hands and overlapping digits (Fig. 55.21), talipes, rocker-bottom feet, and radial aplasia. Other anomalies associated with Edwards' syndrome include omphalocele, congenital diaphragmatic hernia (Fig. 55.22), neural tube defects, cystic hygroma, and renal anomalies.

The fetus with trisomy 18 will often spontaneously abort. Infants have profound intellectual disability. It is considered a lethal anomaly, with 90% of infants dying within the first year of life.[9]

Sonographic Findings. Sonographic features of trisomy 18 are evident in 80% of affected fetuses,[10] and, in addition to the features listed previously, may also include polyhydramnios, IUGR, single umbilical artery, and nonimmune hydrops.

Trisomy 13

Trisomy 13, also known as Patau syndrome, occurs in 1 in 6500 births.[11] It is the result of an extra chromosome 13. This extremely severe anomaly consists of multiple anomalies, many of which involve the brain.

The physical features (Fig. 55.23) characteristic of trisomy 13 include holoprosencephaly (Fig. 55.24), a common finding in fetuses with trisomy 13. Other cranial anomalies include agenesis of the corpus callosum and microcephaly. Facial anomalies may be associated with the presence of holoprosencephaly and include **hypotelorism**, proboscis, cyclopia (Fig. 55.25), and nose with a single nostril. Cleft lip and palate (Fig. 55.26), microphthalmia, and micrognathia may also be present. Heart

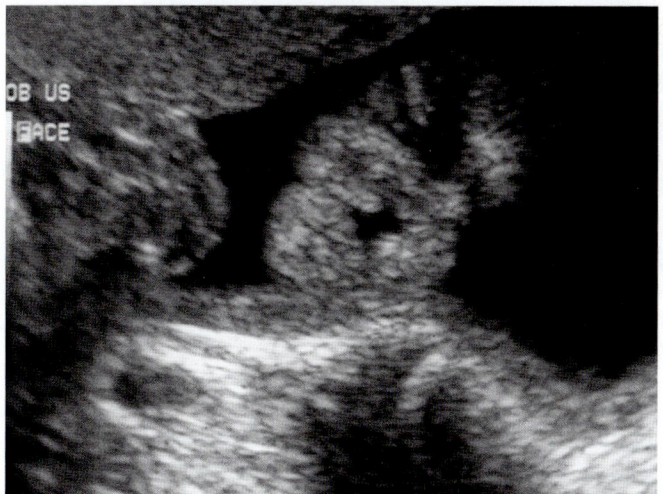

FIG. 55.20 **Cleft lip and palate are associated with aneuploidy.** A median cleft, as in this example, and bilateral clefts carry a greater risk than a unilateral cleft.

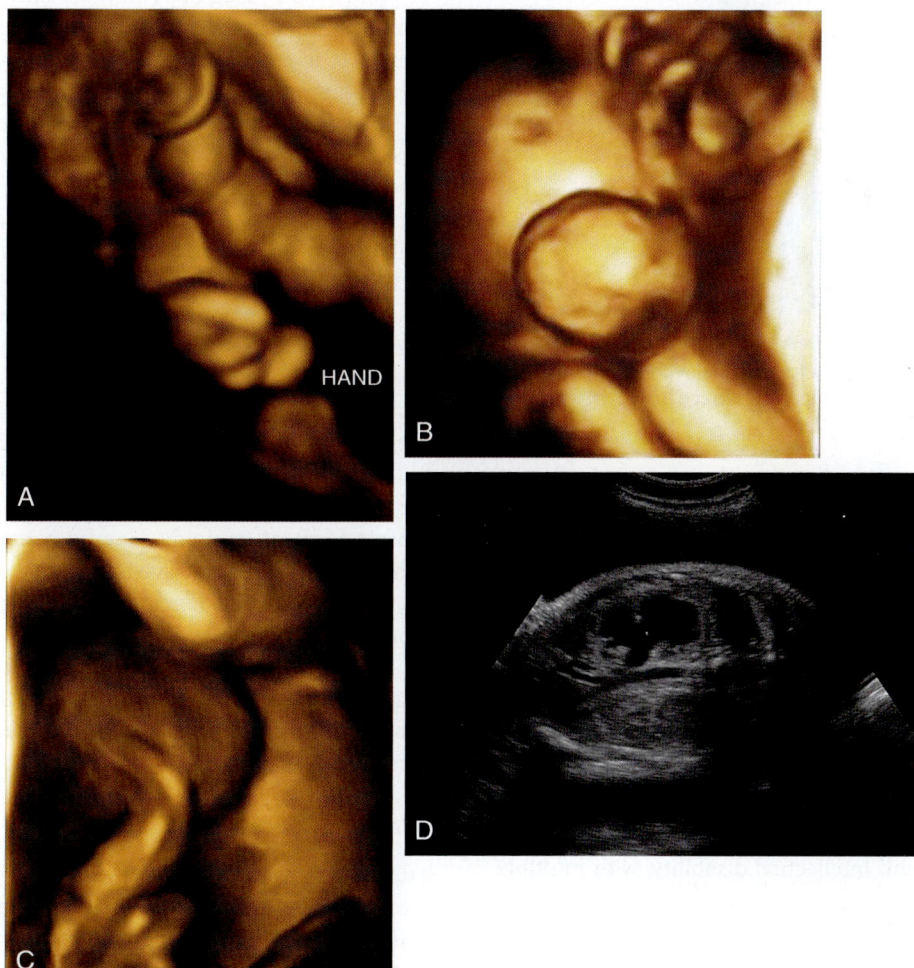

FIG. 55.21 This fetus with trisomy 18 presented with persistently clenched hands (A) and an omphalocele (B). Note that the cord insertion into the abdominal wall defect is consistent with omphalocele (C). Hydronephrosis was also present (D).

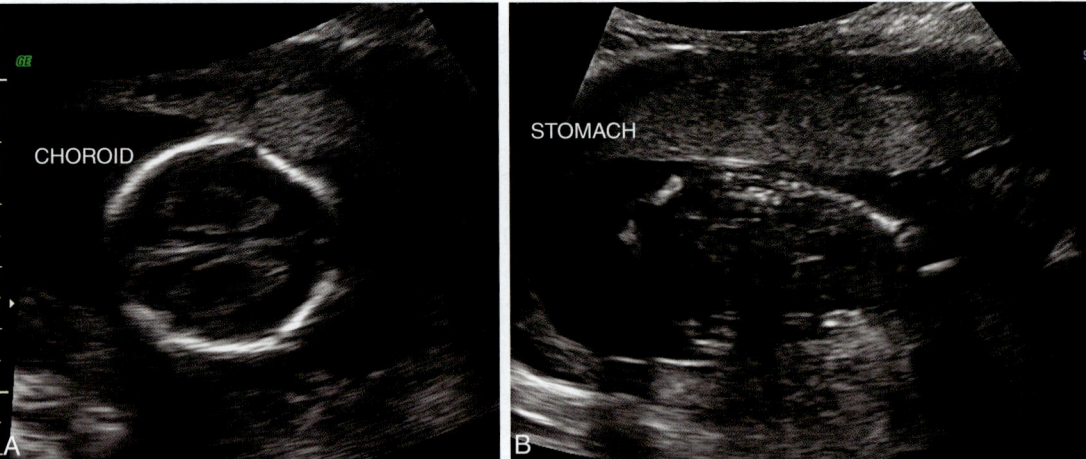

FIG. 55.22 Congenital diaphragmatic hernia (CDH) is associated with aneuploidy, most commonly with trisomy 18. This fetus presented with bilateral choroid plexus cysts (A) and CDH with the stomach evident within the thorax and absence of an intraabdominal stomach (B). A heart defect was also seen. Amniocentesis revealed Edwards syndrome.

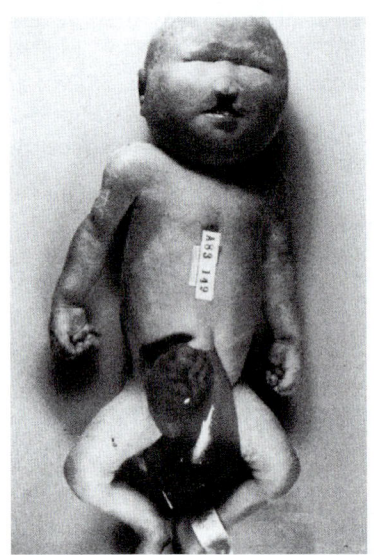

FIG. 55.23 Neonate with trisomy 13. Note the hypotelorism, bilateral cleft lip and palate, bowel-filled omphalocele, and polydactyly of the hands.

defects are present in 90% of fetuses and may include ventricular septal defect, atrial septal defect, and hypoplastic left heart. Other anomalies associated with trisomy 13 include omphalocele, renal anomalies, and meningomyelocele. Associated limb anomalies (Fig. 55.27) include **polydactyly**, talipes, rocker-bottom feet, and overlapping fingers. Cystic hygroma and echogenic chordae tendineae (Fig. 55.28) may also be identified.

The prognosis for trisomy 13 is extremely poor, with 80% of infants dying within the first month and only 5% surviving the first 6 months of life.[11] It is considered a lethal anomaly. Survivors have profound intellectual disability, with multiple deficits and problems.

Sonographic Findings. Sonographic features are evident in 90% of fetuses with trisomy 13.[12] In addition to the features listed previously; trisomy 13 may also be associated with IUGR, single umbilical artery, and polyhydramnios.

Trisomy 18 and Meckel-Gruber syndrome (encephalocele, cystic kidneys, polydactyly) may have a similar sonographic appearance.

Triploidy

Triploidy is the result of a complete extra set of chromosomes. It often occurs as the result of an ova being fertilized by two sperm. It is estimated to occur in 1 in 10,000 live births, although prevalence in utero is much higher.[13]

Physical features of triploidy include heart defects, renal anomalies, omphalocele, and meningomyelocele. Cranial defects associated with triploidy include holoprosencephaly, agenesis of the corpus callosum, hydrocephalus, and Dandy-Walker malformation. Facial anomalies may be present and include low-set ears, **hypertelorism**, cleft lip and palate, and micrognathia. Cryptorchidism, ambiguous genitalia, syndactyly, and talipes may also be observed. Maternal diseases associated with triploidy include preeclampsia and gestational trophoblastic disease; additionally, theca lutein cysts of the maternal ovaries have been identified.[14]

Triploidy is considered a lethal condition, with those surviving the gestational period dying shortly after birth. A mosaic form of triploidy may be compatible with survival, although these infants have intellectual disability.

Sonographic Findings. Sonographic features of triploidy include the previously described findings in addition to severe IUGR and placental changes (hydatidiform degeneration). Oligohydramnios is often present and may hamper adequate visualization of the fetus. In the first trimester of pregnancy, an increased NT may be seen.

Turner Syndrome

Turner syndrome (45,X) is a genetic abnormality marked by the absence of the X or Y chromosome. It is not associated with advanced maternal age. It occurs in 1 of every 2500 live births; however, the prevalence is much higher in spontaneous abortions.[15] Patients may present with an elevated MSAFP when a cystic hygroma is present.

CHAPTER 55 Prenatal Diagnosis of Congenital Anomalies

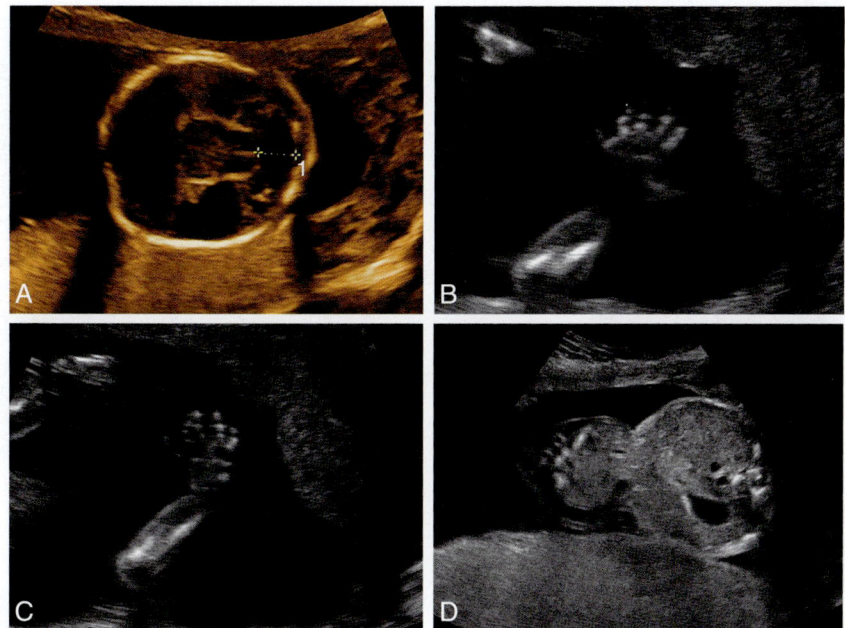

FIG. 55.24 Multiple anomalies were identified in this pregnancy consistent with alobar holoprosencephaly. Amniocentesis confirmed trisomy 13. Ultrasound findings included a single ventricle characteristic of holoprosencephaly, and splaying of the cerebellar hemispheres consistent with a Dandy-Walker malformation was also noted (A). Polydactyly was identified on right (B) and left hands (C), as well as an omphalocele (D).

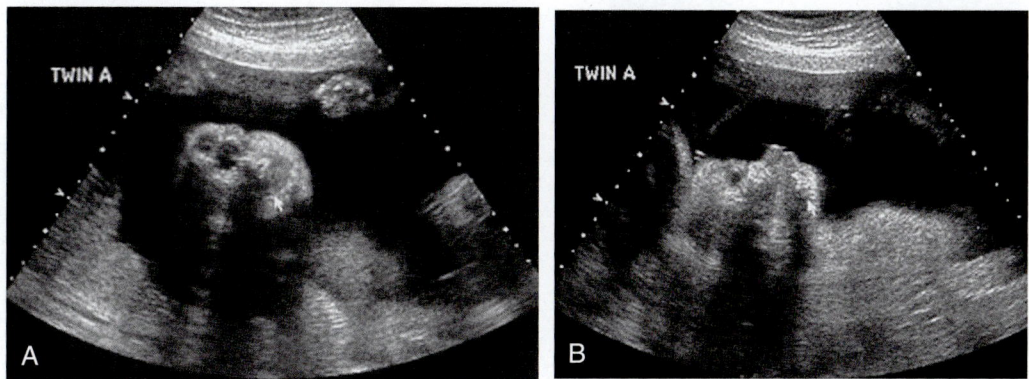

FIG. 55.25 The facial anomalies associated with trisomy 13 include cyclopia (A). The nose was also absent (B).

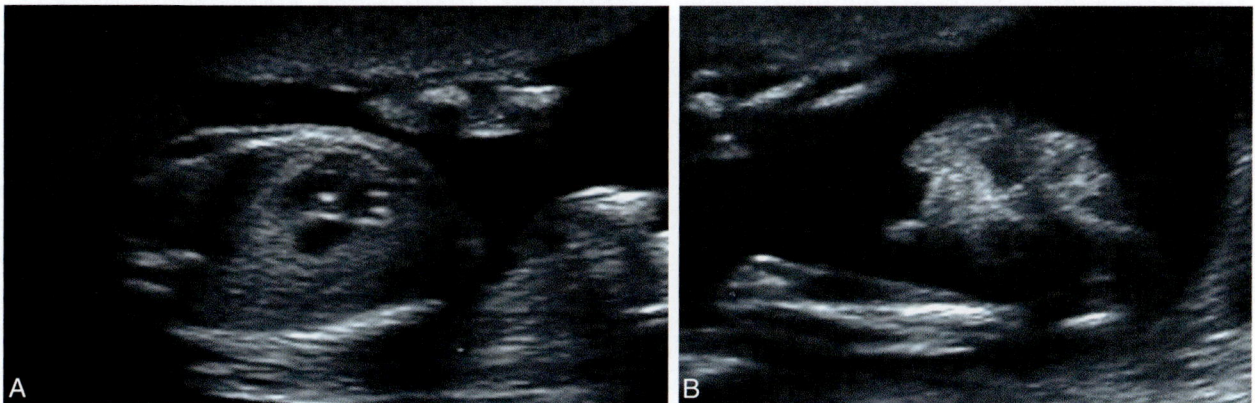

FIG. 55.26 A fetus with trisomy 13 presents with bilateral and multiple echogenic intracardiac foci (A) and a large median cleft lip (B). Holoprosencephaly was also identified.

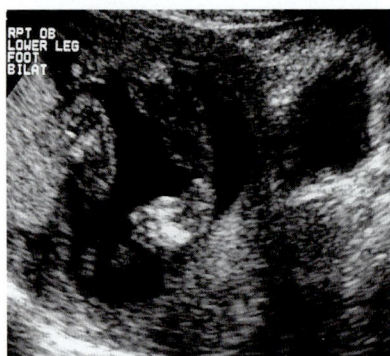

FIG. 55.27 Limb anomalies associated with aneuploidy include talipes (clubfoot).

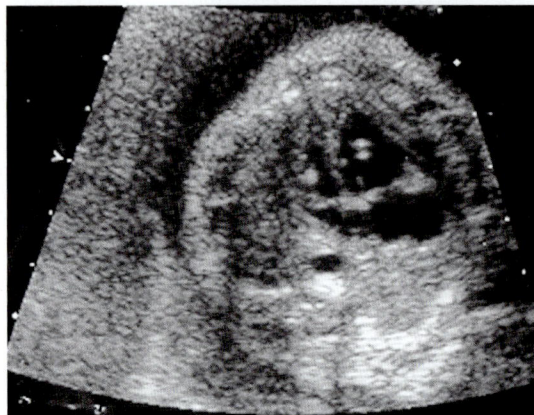

FIG. 55.28 **Isolated echogenic foci may be insignificant.** When in the right ventricle or bilateral as seen in this image, aneuploidy should be considered. Chromosomal analysis revealed trisomy 13.

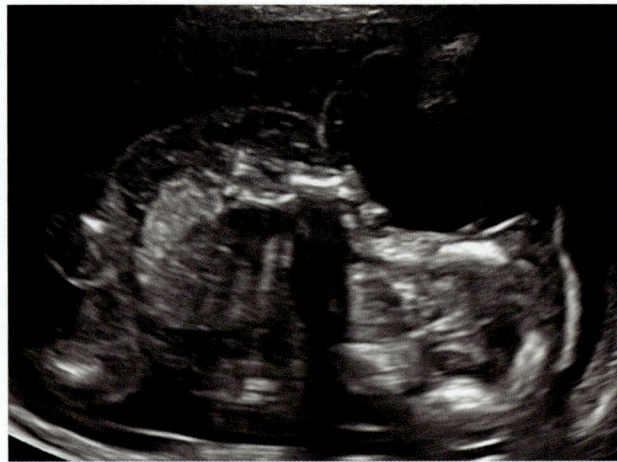

FIG. 55.29 A cystic hygroma and hydrops were identified in a fetus with Turner syndrome.

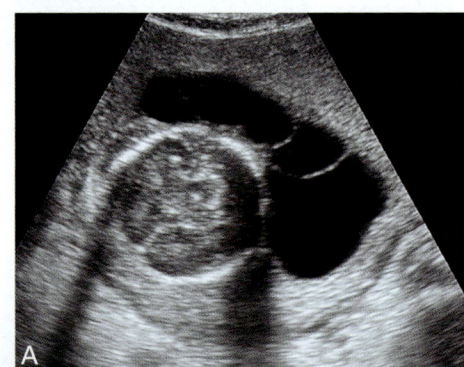

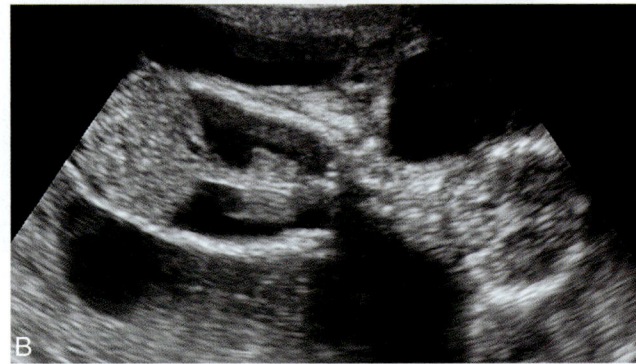

FIG. 55.30 **Turner syndrome.** (A) A septated cystic hygroma is noted in the nuchal region in a 22-week-old fetus. (B) Bilateral pleural effusions and a small amount of ascites were also noted. This fetus died shortly after imaging.

Cystic hygroma (Fig. 55.29) is one of the most pathognomonic findings for this disorder. Other physical features include cardiac anomalies, of which coarctation of the aorta is the most common; however, ventricular septal defects and tetralogy may also be identified.[15] General lymphedema and hydrops may also be present. Renal anomalies, such as horseshoe kidney, renal agenesis, hydronephrosis, and hypoplastic kidney, may coexist. Short femurs are also associated with Turner syndrome.

Most fetuses with Turner syndrome will spontaneously abort. The prognosis is especially grave when the fetus presents with a large cystic hygroma and edema or hydrops (Fig. 55.30). If the hygroma is isolated, it may regress in utero. The prognosis after birth depends on the severity of associated anomalies. Female infants who survive will have immature sexual development, amenorrhea, short stature, a webbed neck, cubitus valgus (abnormal elbow angle), and a shield chest with widely spaced nipples. They may also have poor hearing, and hormone replacement is necessary for sexual development. Children with Turner syndrome usually have typical intelligence.

Sonographic Findings. The previously listed ultrasound findings for Turner syndrome may also include oligohydramnios, especially when severe renal anomalies are present. IUGR has also been seen. Identification of female gender with a cystic hygroma strongly suggests Turner syndrome. In the first trimester, increased NT and fetal tachycardia have been identified.[16]

ACKNOWLEDGMENT

The author acknowledges the contributions of Charlotte G. Henningsen to this chapter in the previous edition.

Key Pearls

- When a fetal anomaly is found antenatally, a multidisciplinary team approach to managing the fetus, mother, and family is preferable because the fetus may need special monitoring (e.g., serial ultrasound), delivery, postnatal care, and surgery.
- The role of genetic testing is to provide noninvasive prenatal testing and invasive testing, which may include screening tests and diagnostic tests, when needed, to identify chromosomal anomalies.
- Alpha-fetoprotein (AFP) is the major protein in fetal serum and is produced by the yolk sac in early gestation and later by the fetal liver.
- Neural tube defects, such as anencephaly and open spina bifida, are common reasons for high AFP levels.
- Two common abdominal wall defects, omphalocele and gastroschisis, produce elevations of AFP.
- Bladder or cloacal exstrophy, ectopia cordis (herniation of the heart out of the chest), limb–body wall complex, and amniotic band syndrome are examples of other anomalies that may present with an elevated AFP level.
- Another biochemical screening test used in the early second trimester is known as the quadruple (quad) screen; this biochemical screening test combines three serum markers: AFP, human chorionic gonadotropin, and unconjugated estriol.
- A relatively newer screening test is noninvasive prenatal screening testing (NIPS) which utilizes cell-free DNA (cfDNA) present in maternal circulation to screen for aneuploidy as well as the sex chromosome.
- Chorionic villus sampling (CVS) is an ultrasound-directed biopsy of the placenta or chorionic villi (chorion frondosum).
- CVS is an alternative test used to obtain a fetal karyotype by the culturing of fetal cells similar to amniocentesis.
- Amniocentesis is a test offered to expectant patients at risk for a chromosomal abnormality or biochemical disorder that may be prenatally detectable.
- The amniocentesis technique for multiple gestations is similar to the singleton method, except that each fetal sac is entered.
- Cordocentesis is another method by which chromosomes are analyzed. Fetal blood is obtained through needle aspiration of the umbilical cord.
- A first-trimester serum marker used to detect anomalies is pregnancy-associated plasma protein A (PAPP-A).
- Human chorionic gonadotropin (hCG) is also a glycoprotein derived from the placenta that can be assessed in maternal serum in the first trimester to evaluate for increased risk of Down syndrome.
- A normal karyotype consists of 46 chromosomes, 22 pairs of autosomes, and a pair of sex chromosomes.
- There is a high prevalence of chromosomal abnormalities in patients referred for second-trimester amniocentesis because of advanced maternal age, abnormal AFP, abnormal quad screen (hCG, AFP, estriol, and inhibin A), or ultrasound detection of multiple fetal anomalies.
- Nuchal translucency has been reported as a late first-trimester finding identified between 11 and 14 weeks of gestation.
- Trisomy 21 is associated with an increased nuchal translucency, an abnormal first-trimester screen, and an abnormal quad screen.
- Trisomy 18 is associated with an abnormal quad screen.
- The physical features characteristic of trisomy 13 include holoprosencephaly, a common finding in fetuses with trisomy 13.
- Physical features of triploidy include heart defects, renal anomalies, omphalocele, and meningomyelocele.
- Turner syndrome (45,X) is a genetic abnormality marked by the absence of the X or Y chromosome. Cystic hygroma is one of the most pathognomonic findings for this disorder. Other physical features include cardiac anomalies, of which coarctation of the aorta is the most common; however, ventricular septal defects and tetralogy may also be identified.
- General lymphedema and hydrops may also be present. Renal anomalies, such as horseshoe kidney, renal agenesis, hydronephrosis, and hypoplastic kidney, may coexist. Short femurs are also associated with Turner syndrome.

REFERENCES

1. Odibo AO, Gray DL, Dicke JM, et al. Revisiting the fetal loss rate after second-trimester genetic amniocentesis: a single center's 16-year experience. *Obstet Gynecol.* 2008;111:589–595.
2. Wagner R, Tse W, Gosemann JH, et al. Prenatal maternal biomarkers for the early diagnosis of congenital malformations: A review. *Pediatr Res.* 2019;86:560–566.
3. Parham L, Michie M, Allyse M. Expanding use of cfDNA screening in pregnancy: current and emerging ethical, legal, and social issues. *Curr Genet Med Rep.* 2017;5:44–53.
4. Tabor A, Alfirevic Z. Update on procedure-related risks for prenatal diagnosis techniques. *Fetal Diagnosis and Therapy.* 2010;27:1–7.
5. Driscoll DA, Gross SJ. Screening for fetal aneuploidy and neural tube defects. *Genet Med.* 2009;11:818–821.
6. Mai C, Kucik JE, Isenburg J, et al. Selected birth defects data from population-based birth defects surveillance programs in the United States, 2006-2010: featuring trisomy conditions. *Birth Defects Res Part A.* 2013;97:709–725.
7. Bromley B, Shipp TD, Lyons J, et al. What is the importance of second-trimester "soft markers" for trisomy 21 after an 11- to 14-week aneuploidy screening scan? *J Ultrasound Med.* 2014;33:1747–1752.
8. Wax JR, Pinette MG, Cartin A, Blackstone J. Second-trimester genetic sonography after first-trimester combined screening for trisomy 21. *J Ultrasound Med.* 2009;28:321–325.
9. Zheng Y, Zhou X-D, Zhu Y-L, et al. Three- and 4-dimensional ultrasonography in the prenatal evaluation of fetal anomalies associated with trisomy 18. *J Ultrasound Med.* 2008;27:1041–1051.
10. Niknejadi M, Ahmadi F, Akhbari F, Parvaneh A. Sonographic findings in partial type of trisomy 18. *Int J Fertil Steril.* 2014;7:349–352.
11. Nyberg DA, Souter VL. Sonographic markers of fetal trisomies: second trimester. *J Ultrasound Med.* 2001;20:655–674.
12. Kroes I, Janssens S, Defoort P. Ultrasound features in trisomy 13 (Patau syndrome) and trisomy 18 (Edwards syndrome) in a consecutive series of 47 cases. *Facts Views Vis OBGyn.* 2014;6:245–249.
13. Engelbrechtsen L, Brondum-Nielsen K, Ekelund C, et al. Detection of triploidy at 11-14 weeks' gestation: a cohort study of 198000 pregnant women. *Ultrasound Obstet Gynecol.* 2013;42:530–535.
14. Chen C-P, Chien S-C, Lin H-H. Prenatal sonographic features of triploidy. *J Med Ultrasound.* 2007;15:175–182.
15. Papp C, Beke A, Mezei G, et al. Prenatal diagnosis of Turner syndrome, report on 69 cases. *J Ultrasound Med.* 2006;25:711–717.
16. Vladareanu R, Tutunaru D, Alexandru B, et al. Ultrasound in prenatal diagnosis of triploidy and Turner syndrome. *Gynaecol Perinatol.* 2006;15:192–201.

CHAPTER 56

Placenta

Mitzi Roberts

OBJECTIVES

On completion of this chapter, you should be able to:
- Describe embryogenesis of the placenta
- List the functions of the placenta
- List and describe imaging techniques and sonographic findings of the placenta
- Identify placental position and describe its importance
- Describe the sonographic findings and clinical significance of placental pathologies
- Recognize placental abruption with diagnostic ultrasound

OUTLINE

Embryogenesis 1443
    Fetal-Placental-Uterine Circulation 1444
    Cordal Attachments 1444
    Placental Implantation 1445
    Membranes 1445
The Amniotic Sac and Amniotic Fluid 1445
The Umbilical Cord 1445
    Sonographic Evaluation of the Umbilical Cord 1446
Sonographic Evaluation of the Normal Placenta 1446
    Placental Position 1448

Doppler Evaluation of the Placenta 1449
Evaluation of the Placenta After Delivery 1450
    Fibrin Deposition 1450
Abnormalities of the Placenta 1450
    Placentomegaly 1451
    Placenta Previa 1451
    Vasa Previa 1452
    Morbidly Adherent Placenta 1452
    Succenturiate Placenta 1454
    Circumvallate/Circummarginate Placenta 1454
    Placental Hemorrhage 1455

Placental Abruption 1455
    Retroplacental Abruption 1456
    Marginal Abruption 1456
    Intervillous Thrombosis 1456
    Placenta Infarcts 1456
Placental Tumors 1456
    Gestational Trophoblastic Disease 1456
    Chorioangioma 1457
    The Placenta in Multiple Gestation 1457

KEY TERMS

Abruptio placentae
Basal plate
Chorion frondosum
Chorionic plate
Chorionic villi
Circumvallate/circummarginate placenta
Decidua basalis

Decidua capsularis
Ductus venosus
Ligamentum venosum
Lower uterine segment (LUS)
Low-lying placenta
Molar pregnancy
Placenta accreta
Placenta increta

Placenta percreta
Placenta previa
Placental migration
Succenturiate placenta
Vasa previa
Wharton jelly

The placenta is a maternal-fetal organ developed during pregnancy. Sonography is used to assess information regarding placental configuration, location, pathology, and maturation. The anatomic components of the placenta are discernible from as early as the seventh or eighth week of gestation. By the end of the first trimester, sonography can determine the location and position and identify specific components of the placenta. The placenta can be effectively evaluated during a second-trimester and third-trimester sonographic examination.

The major role of the placenta is to permit the exchange of oxygenated maternal blood, which is rich in oxygen and nutrients, with deoxygenated and nutrient-depleted fetal blood. Maternal blood flows through the decidual spiral arteries, circulating blood into the intervillous space within the placenta. The umbilical arteries, two of the vessels within the umbilical cord, carry the deoxygenated blood from the fetus to the placenta.

EMBRYOGENESIS

The development of the placenta begins after fertilization when the trophoblastic cells of the blastocyst implant into the uterus. Implantation of the blastocyst occurs 6 to 7 days after fertilization. The enlargement of the trophoblasts helps to anchor the blastocyst to the endometrial lining, or *decidua*. The development of the placenta is seen in the changes in the decidua (Box 56.1).

There are two types of trophoblastic cells. The syncytiotrophoblast is the outer layer of multinuclear cells, and the cytotrophoblast is the inner layer of mononuclear cells (Box 56.2). These cells, along with the extraembryonic mesoderm, make up the chorion of the placenta. The chorion, amnion, yolk sac, and allantois constitute the embryonic or fetal membranes.

The placenta has two components: the maternal portion, the **decidua basalis**, formed from the endometrial surface (Fig. 56.1), and the fetal portion, which develops from the **chorion frondosum**. The major functioning unit of the placenta is the chorionic villus (Fig. 56.2). Within the chorionic villus are the intervillous spaces, which the maternal blood enters. As the embryo and membranes grow, the **decidua capsularis** is stretched. The **chorionic villi** on the associated part of the chorionic sac gradually atrophy and disappear (smooth chorion or chorion laeve). The chorionic villi related to the decidua basalis increase rapidly in size and complexity (villous chorion or chorion frondosum).

The maternal surface of the placenta, which lies contiguous with the decidua basalis, is termed the **basal plate**. The fetal surface, which is contiguous with the surrounding chorion, is termed the **chorionic plate**. The cotyledons are cobblestone in appearance and composed of several main stem villi and their branches. They are covered with a thin layer of the decidua basalis.

During pregnancy, the fetal membranes and placenta perform the following functions and activities: protection, nutrition, respiration, and excretion (Box 56.3). The placental membranes are often called a barrier because a few compounds are unable to cross the placental membranes. At birth, or *parturition*, the placenta and membranes separate from the fetus and are expelled from the uterus as the afterbirth.

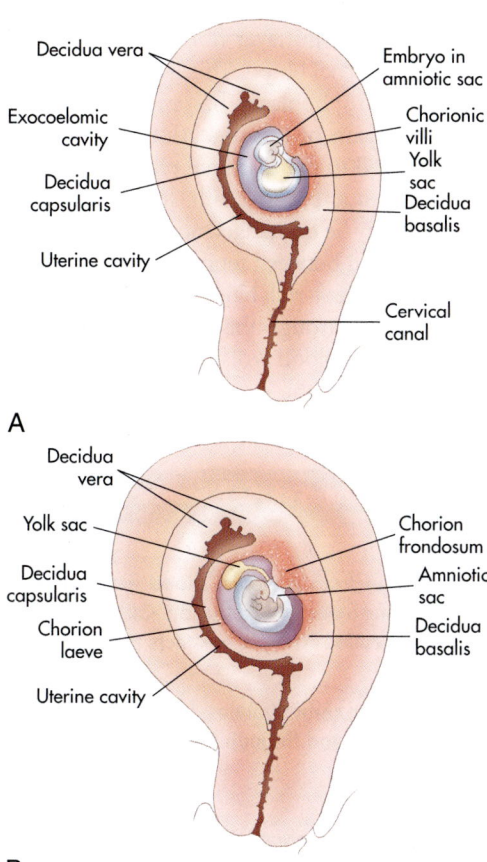

FIG. 56.1 (A) The placenta has two components: the fetal portion, developed from the chorion frondosum (chorionic plate), and a maternal portion, the decidua basalis, formed by the endometrial surface. (B) The chorionic villi gradually atrophy and disappear (chorion laeve). The chorionic villi in the decidua basalis increase rapidly in size and complexity.

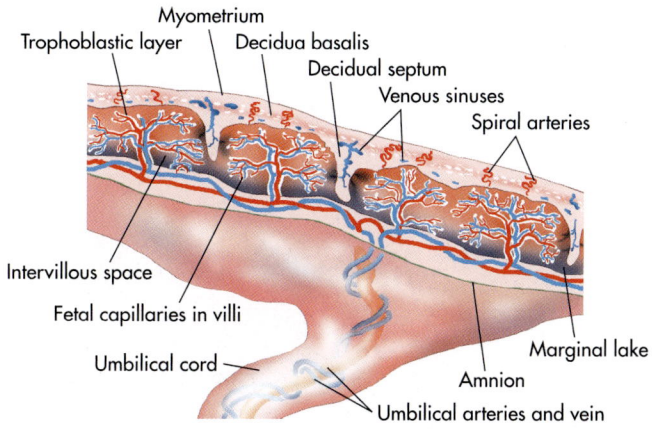

FIG. 56.2 The major functioning unit of the placenta is the chorionic villus. The spiral arteries, venous sinuses, and uterine arteries line the periphery of the placenta.

BOX 56.1 Decidual Changes

Decidua basalis: the decidual reaction that occurs between the blastocyst and the myometrium
Decidua capsularis: the decidual reaction that occurs over the blastocyst closest to the endometrial cavity
Decidua vera (parietalis): the decidua reaction except for the areas beneath and above the implanted ovum

---

BOX 56.2 Fetal Chorion

Chorion frondosum: forms the fetal part of the placenta and contains the villi
Chorion laeve: the nonvillous part of the chorion around the gestational sac
Chorionic plate: the fetal surface of the placenta
Basal plate: the maternal surface of the placenta

Fetal-Placental-Uterine Circulation

Oxygenated maternal blood is brought to the placenta through 80 to 100 end branches of the uterine arteries, the spiral arteries. Maternal blood enters the intervillous space near the central part of each placental lobule, where it flows around and over the surface of the villi. Maternal blood returns to the maternal circulation through the endometrial and then uterine veins. A very thin layer normally separates the fetal blood from the maternal blood. This layer is composed of the capillary wall, the trophoblastic basement membrane, and a thin rim of cytoplasm of the syncytiotrophoblast. The fetal placenta is anchored to the maternal placenta by the cytotrophoblastic shell and anchoring villi. It provides a large area where materials may be exchanged across the placental membrane and interposed between fetal and maternal circulation.

Oxygen- and nutrient-rich blood is carried back to the fetal systemic circulation through the umbilical vein. In the fetal abdomen, some of the blood is distributed to the liver, whereas the rest passes through the ductus venosus into the inferior vena cava and continues to the heart through the right atrium across the foramen ovale and into the left atrium. This oxygen-rich blood then passes into the left ventricle and the ascending aorta and supplies the brain and upper part of the body through the brachiocephalic circulation. Unoxygenated blood from the superior vena cava passes into the right atrium, through the right ventricle, and across the main pulmonary artery. A minor portion of blood from the right ventricle supplies the lungs, whereas the majority of the blood passes through a fetal shunt, the ductus arteriosus, into the aorta arch. This shunt protects the lungs against circulatory overload. The fetal blood continues inferiorly through the descending aorta, internal iliac arteries, and umbilical arteries and into the umbilical cord to return to the placenta for oxygen and nutrient exchange. By term, approximately 40% of the fetal cardiac output is directed through the umbilical circulation.

The placenta is dedicated to the survival of the fetus. Even when exposed to a poor maternal environment (e.g., when the mother is malnourished, ill, smokes, or abuses drugs), the placenta can compensate by becoming more efficient. Unfortunately, there are limits to the placenta's ability to cope with external stressors. Eventually, if multiple or severe enough, these stressors may lead to placental insufficiency, fetal growth restriction, intrauterine death, and pregnancy loss.

During pregnancy, maternal blood volume increases 40% to 50% by term compared with the nonpregnant state. Maternal placental circulation may be affected by maternal conditions that decrease uterine blood flow, such as severe hypertension and renal disease. Intrauterine growth restriction (IUGR) is a fetal change that may be associated with decreased placental flow.

> **BOX 56.3 Functions of the Placenta**
>
> **Respiration**
> Transfer of oxygen from maternal blood across the placental membrane into fetal blood is by diffusion. Carbon dioxide passes in the opposite direction. The placenta acts as "fetal lungs."
>
> **Nutrition**
> Water, inorganic salts, carbohydrates, fats, proteins, and vitamins pass from maternal blood through the placental membrane into fetal blood.
>
> **Excretion**
> Waste products cross membrane from fetal blood and enter maternal blood. Excreted by maternal kidneys.
>
> **Protection**
> Some microorganisms cross the placental border.
>
> **Storage**
> Carbohydrates, proteins, calcium, and iron are stored in placenta and released into fetal circulation.
>
> **Hormonal Production**
> Produced by syncytiotrophoblast of placenta: human chorionic gonadotropin, estrogens, progesterone.

Cordal Attachments

The location of the umbilical cord attachment to the placenta is important. The majority of the time, the umbilical cord inserts on the fetal surface of the placenta more than 3 cm from the margin. Abnormal cord insertions include marginal insertion and velamentous insertion. With a *marginal insertion*, also referred to as a *battledore placenta*, the insertion of the umbilical cord is at or close to the placental margin within less than 2 cm of the edge (less than 10%) (Fig. 56.3). A *velamentous* insertion refers to an umbilical cord that inserts into the fetal membranes and then travels to the placenta within

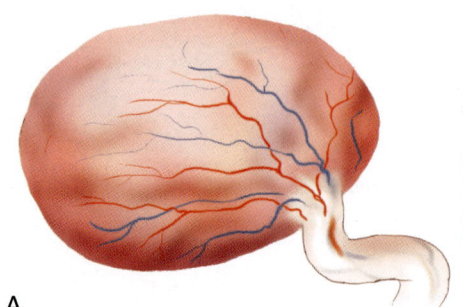
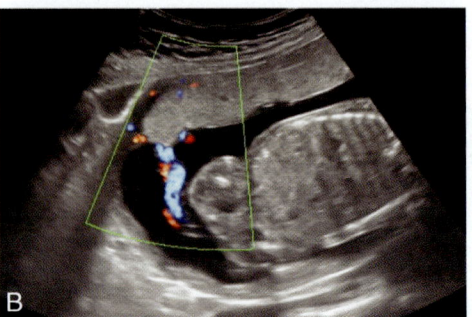

FIG. 56.3 (A) A battledore placenta refers to the insertion of the umbilical cord at the margin of the placenta. (B) This sagittal transabdominal image reveals a marginal cord insertion.

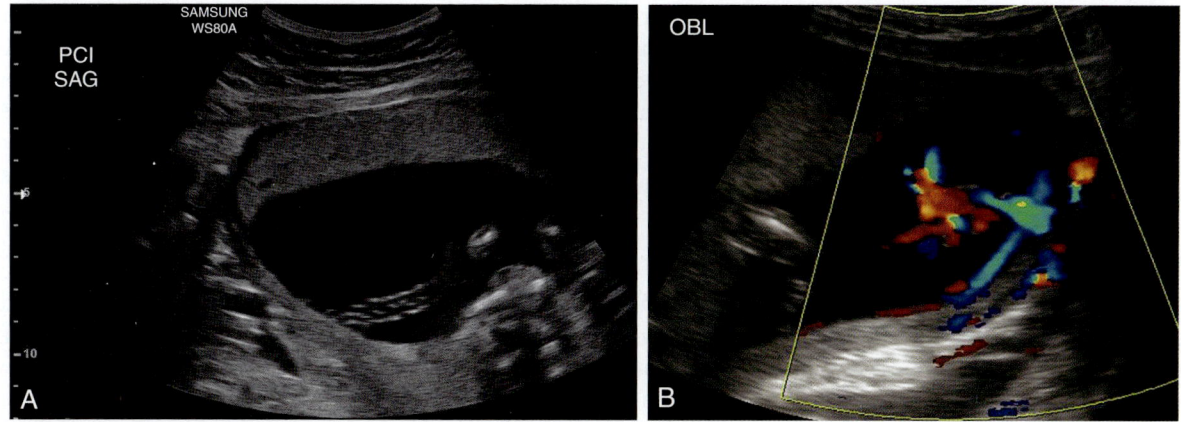

FIG. 56.4 **Velamentous insertions.** (A) Sagittal image of an anterior placenta showing the placental cord inserting into the membranes. (B) Oblique view of uterus with color Doppler demonstrates a velamentous insertion.

the membranes (1%) (Fig. 56.4). These submembranous vessels are fragile and, in a small number of cases (less than 2%), may be associated with significant fetal hemorrhage, especially if the membrane carrying the vessels is positioned across the internal cervical os (vasa previa).

Placental Implantation

Placental location should be documented during the second-trimester sonographic examination. Normally the placenta will be located on the anterior, fundal, posterior, or lateral wall of the uterus. The relationship of the placental edge to the internal cervical os should be evaluated during each sonogram. Occasionally, placental implantation will occur within the lower uterine segment (LUS), resulting in a **placenta previa** or a **low-lying placenta**.

Membranes

The fetal membranes consist of the chorion, amnion, allantois, and yolk sac. The chorion originates from the trophoblastic cells and remains in contact with the trophoblasts throughout pregnancy. The amnion develops at the 28th menstrual day and is attached to the margins of the embryonic disk. As the embryo grows and folds ventrally, the junction of the amnion is reduced to a small area on the ventral surface of the embryo to form the umbilicus.

Expansion of the amniotic cavity occurs with the production of amniotic fluid. Usually, by 16 weeks of gestation, fusion of the amnion with the chorion occurs and will no longer be visualized sonographically as two separate membranes. If the amnion/chorion separation extends beyond 16 weeks of gestation, it may be associated with polyhydramnios, aneuploidy, or prior amniocentesis. Placental hemorrhage may mimic the appearance of amnion/chorion separation on sonogram.

The secondary yolk sac forms after the regression of the primary yolk sac on the ventral surface of the embryonic disk at 28 menstrual days. The yolk sac has a role in transferring nutrients to the embryo during the second and third weeks of gestation while the uteroplacental circulation is developing.

It is connected to the midgut by a narrow yolk stalk. By 5 menstrual weeks, the amniotic sac and secondary yolk sac are pressed together with the embryonic disk between them. This structure is suspended within the chorionic cavity. The yolk sac becomes displaced from the embryo and lies between the amnion and the chorion (see Fig. 56.1). By 9 weeks, the yolk sac has diminished to less than 5 mm in diameter.

THE AMNIOTIC SAC AND AMNIOTIC FLUID

The amnion forms a sac that contains amniotic fluid. This sac surrounds the embryo and forms the epithelial lining of the umbilical cord. Most of the amniotic fluid is derived from the maternal blood by diffusion across the amnion from the decidua parietalis and intervillous spaces of the placenta.

During the second trimester, the fetal kidneys begin to function and secrete urine, contributing to the amniotic fluid volume. The fetus swallows the amniotic fluid, and this cycle continues throughout pregnancy. The amniotic fluid has many functions, including permitting the fetus room to move, assisting in maintaining a constant fetal body temperature, serving as a protective buffer for the fetus, and helping in the formation of the gastrointestinal tract and lung development.

THE UMBILICAL CORD

The umbilical cord forms during the first 5 weeks of gestation. The cord is surrounded by a mucoid connective tissue called **Wharton jelly**. The intestines grow at a faster rate than the abdomen and herniate into the proximal umbilical cord at approximately 7 weeks of gestation and remain there until approximately 10 weeks of gestation. The insertion of the umbilical cord into the ventral abdominal wall is an important sonographic anatomic landmark as this area can reveal abdominal wall defects such as omphalocele, gastroschisis, or limb–body wall complex.

The normal umbilical cord has one large vein and two smaller arteries. A single umbilical artery, also referred to as a "two-vessel cord," is found in approximately 1% of singleton births and 7% of twin gestations. A single umbilical artery may be isolated, but if it is also associated with congenital malformations (renal, cardiac, facial, and musculoskeletal) or aneuploidy, amniocentesis should be offered. There is a reported association with a single umbilical artery and abnormal fetal growth, specifically IUGR. For this reason, a growth ultrasound in the third trimester to evaluate fetal size should be obtained.

Sonographic Evaluation of the Umbilical Cord

The vessels of the cord may be followed with real-time ultrasound from the placenta to the fetal abdomen, and the sonographer should document the umbilical cord insertion into the placenta (Fig. 56.5) and the fetal abdomen. The intraabdominal portion of the umbilical vein courses superiorly. The **ductus venosus** shunts a significant amount of the oxygenated blood from the umbilical vein directly into the inferior vena cava. A portion of the umbilical venous blood also supplies the liver (Fig. 56.6).

Sonographically, the ductus venous appears as a thin intrahepatic channel with echogenic walls branching from the umbilical vein (Fig. 56.7). It lies in the groove between the left lobe and the caudate lobe of the liver. The ductus venosus is patent during fetal life until shortly after birth, when closure occurs. After closure, the remnant of the ductus venosus is known as the **ligamentum venosum**.

The two umbilical arteries carry deoxygenated blood from the fetus to the placenta. They ascend into the umbilical cord and are a branch of the internal iliac arteries. Their normal position extends around the fetal bladder. There are two acceptable ways to document the umbilical arteries. The first approach is to image the fetal pelvis in an axial scanning plane at the level of the fetal bladder. The umbilical arteries will be visible along the lateral aspect of the fetal bladder and then ascend toward the umbilical cord insertion. Color and power Doppler can be used to visualize the umbilical arteries. The second approach is to evaluate a free loop of cord in a short axis plane to visualize the umbilical vein and two smaller arteries. After birth, the umbilical arteries become the superior vesical arteries.

SONOGRAPHIC EVALUATION OF THE NORMAL PLACENTA

The placenta can be identified with sonography as early as 8 menstrual weeks. The placenta assumes a relatively homogenous midlevel gray appearance between 8 and 20 weeks of gestation and is easily recognized with its characteristically smooth borders. After 20 weeks of gestation, placental lakes (anechoic areas) and placental calcification may begin to appear. The thickness of the placenta varies with gestational age, but an anterior-posterior dimension is usually 2 to 3 cm in fetuses greater than 23 weeks of gestation. The thickness of a normal placenta will rarely exceed 4 cm. When evaluating placental thickness, the sonographer should be perpendicular to the uterine wall and measure through the placenta. Enlarged placentas may be associated with TORCH infections, diabetes, hydrops, and congenital anomalies (Fig. 56.8A).

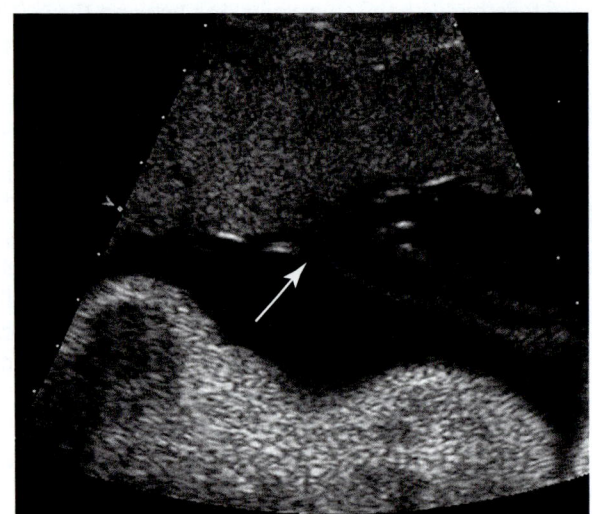

FIG. 56.5 Umbilical cord is seen at placental insertion site *(arrow)*.

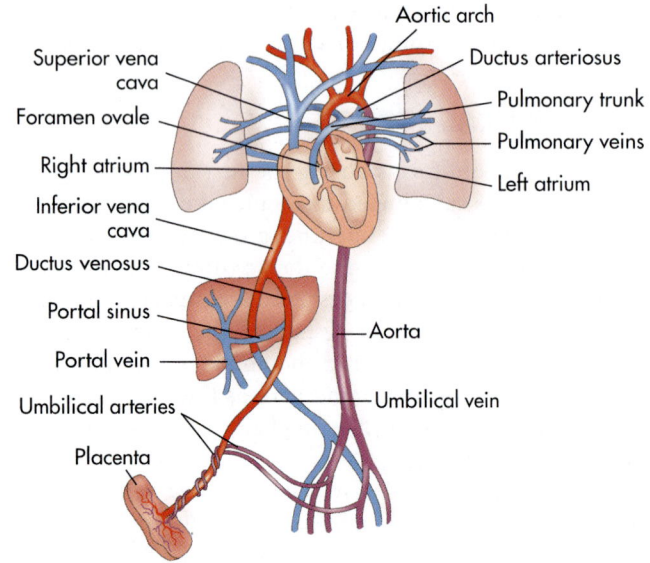

FIG. 56.6 Fetal circulation.

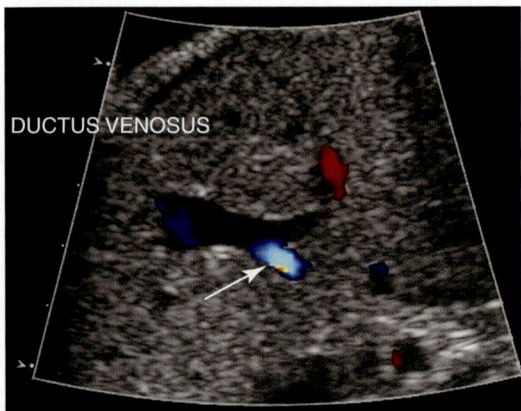

FIG. 56.7 Axial view of fetal abdomen identifies the ductus venosus *(arrow)* as it branches off the umbilical vein.

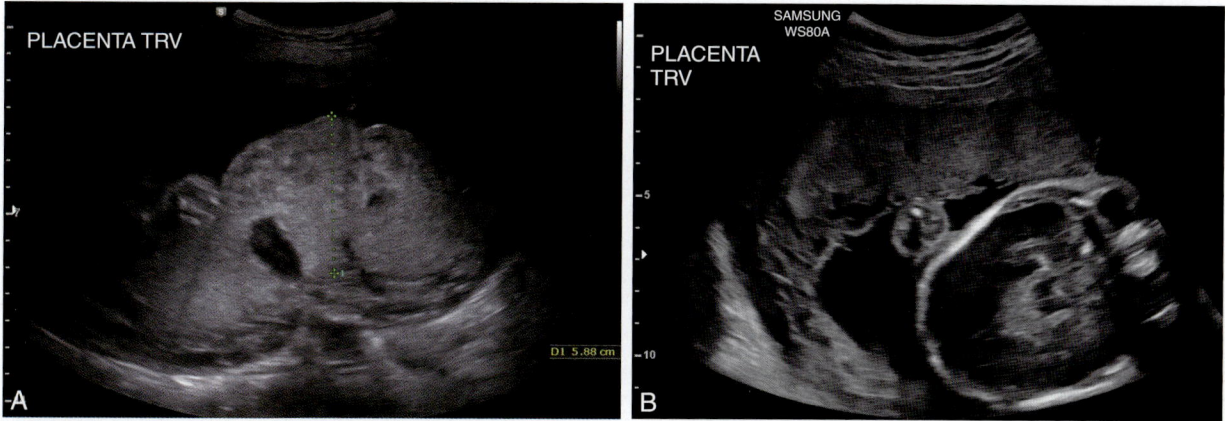

FIG. 56.8 (A) Placentomegaly. The anterior-posterior thickness of the placenta measures 5.88 cm. Calipers should be placed perpendicular to the placental borders. (B) Small placenta. This transverse image of a placenta extended from the maternal right sidewall to the maternal umbilicus. At 28 weeks of gestation, the fetus was growth restricted.

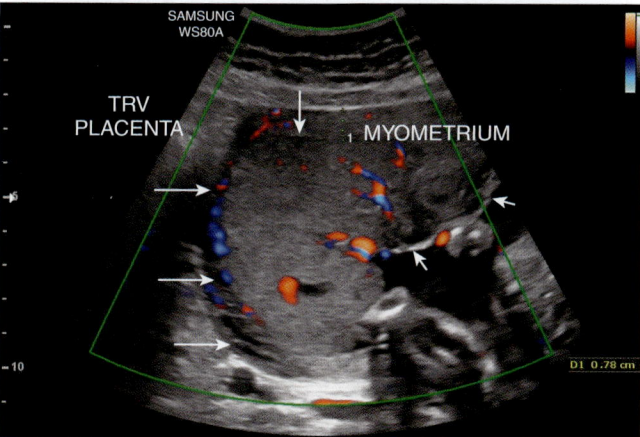

FIG. 56.9 Anterior right sidewall placenta demonstrating a smooth homogeneous sonographic appearance. The chorionic plate *(short arrow)* can be seen on the fetal surface of the placenta, and the basal surface *(long arrows)* can be seen adjacent to the myometrium, which measures 7.8 mm in an anterior-posterior dimension along the anterior uterine wall.

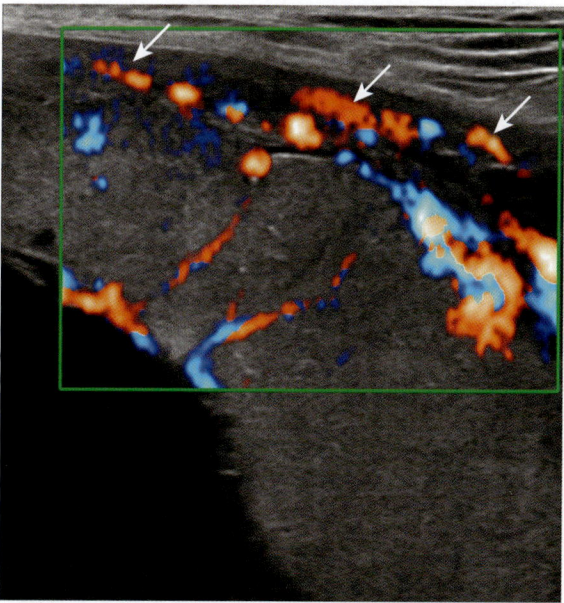

FIG. 56.10 Color Doppler demonstrates the normal vascularity of the chorionic plate, placental vessels, basal area of the placenta, and the maternal blood vessels *(arrow)*.

A small placenta may be associated with IUGR, intrauterine infection, and aneuploidy (see Fig. 56.8B).

The chorionic and basal plate of the placenta are important in assessing normal placental anatomy and evaluating for placental abruption. The fetal surface of the placenta is the chorionic plate that gives rise to the chorionic villi. Sonographically the chorionic plate appears echogenic and is the portion of the placenta that is adjacent to the amniotic cavity (Fig. 56.9). The basal plate or maternal portion of the placenta, which lies at the junction of the myometrium and the substance of the placenta (see Fig. 56.9). Maternal blood vessels reside between the placenta and the myometrium (see Fig. 56.9). This represents normal vascularity, which sonographically appears hypoechoic but can be visualized well with color Doppler. The maternal vessels are more apparent sonographically when the placenta is positioned fundally or posteriorly within the uterus. Blood flow can easily be detected within the placenta with color Doppler (Fig. 56.10).

Placental lakes may also be seen within the placenta. These have been referred to as placental sonolucencies and are most often surrounded by normal placenta (Fig. 56.11). Placental lakes located along the fetal surface may appear to bulge into the amniotic cavity. These areas may change dramatically in shape and size during the course of the ultrasound examination, and with real-time sonography, slow swirling flow can be appreciated.

The placenta is separated from the myometrium by a subplacental venous complex. These veins (basilar and marginal) can become very prominent, especially for lateral and posterior positioned placentas, and should not be confused for a retroplacental or marginal hemorrhage. The myometrium appears slightly less echogenic when compared to the echogenicity of the placenta (see Fig. 56.9). The basilar veins and the myometrium measure as much as 9 to 10 mm in thickness.

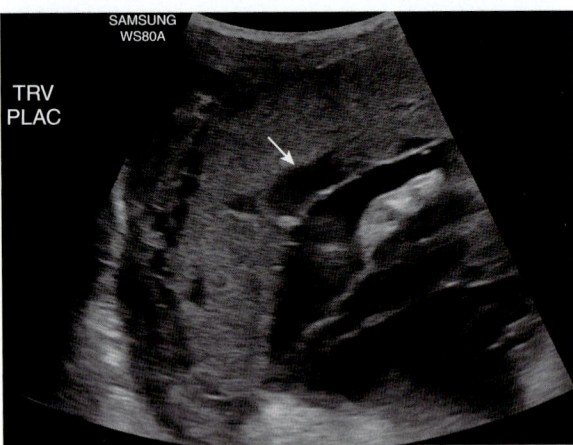

FIG. 56.11 Placental lake seen within this anterior right sidewall placenta at 20 weeks of gestation. Blood flow was visualized under real-time imaging *(arrow)*.

Placental Position

A survey of the placenta transabdominally should always be performed, scanning longitudinally across the uterus from side to side and transversely from inferior to superior. The insertion of the umbilical cord into the placenta should be visualized and described as mid-placental, marginal, or velamentous. The inferior edge of the placenta should be documented to evaluate its relationship to the internal cervical os.

The position of the placenta is readily apparent on most obstetric sonographic examinations. The placental location varies but may be seen along the fundus, anterior, posterior, or lateral uterine wall (Fig. 56.12). Specific names are given to the placenta according to its location, such as fundus of the uterus along the anterior wall *(fundal anterior placenta)* or along the posterior uterine wall *(fundal posterior placenta)*. Occasionally, the placenta may be dangerously low, implanted over or near the cervix (placenta previa) (Fig. 56.13).

The location of the placenta may appear to change dramatically with the development of focal myometrial contractions. These normal contractions of pregnancy should not be confused with a uterine fibroid. Their appearance may distort the uterine contour, but they will resolve with time, and the uterine contour should return to normal (Fig. 56.14). The sonographer should reevaluate the myometrium where the focal myometrial contraction was seen to confirm resolution prior to the end of the examination. Sonographically, a uterine myoma will typically appear as a hypoechoic mass. If the placenta is implanted over a myoma, it may have poor perfusion, which will increase the risk for placental abruption (Fig. 56.15). Color Doppler may be used to document blood flow of the myoma.

For the sonographer to visualize the internal os of the cervix, a sagittal transabdominal image of the **lower uterine segment (LUS)** and cervix should be obtained to evaluate the relationship of the placenta to the internal os (Fig. 56.16). If the maternal bladder is full, a normally implanted placenta may appear to be covering the internal cervical os as a result of the cervix appearing as falsely elongated, resulting in a false impression of a placenta previa. Emptying the maternal

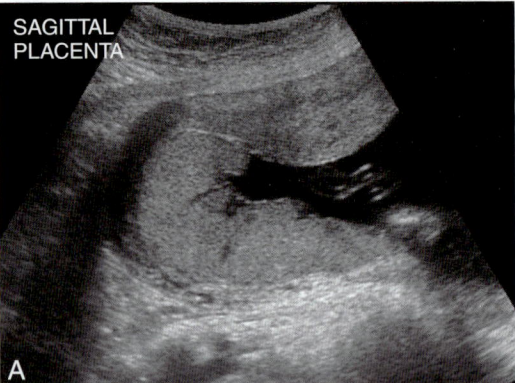

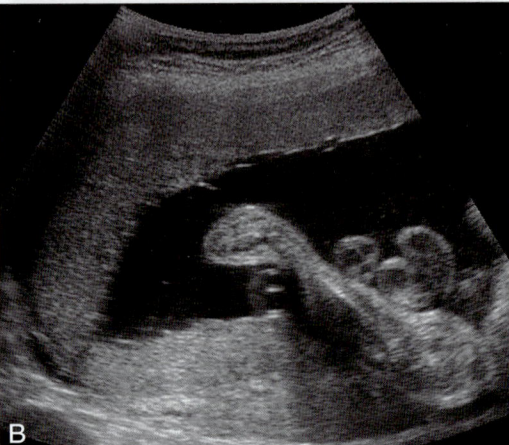

FIG. 56.12 (A) Sagittal view of the uterus reveals a posterior fundal placenta. (B) Transverse view of the uterus demonstrates a right sidewall placenta that extends along the anterior wall of the uterus.

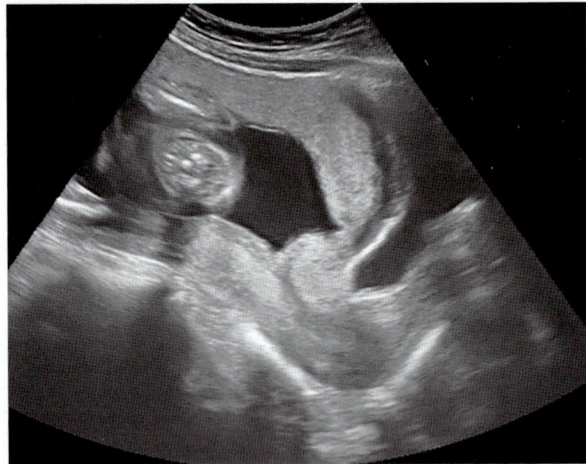

FIG. 56.13 Transabdominal image of placenta and internal cervical os.

bladder reduces the pressure on the LUS and allows the cervix to assume a more normal position. Another method to better demonstrate the internal cervical os when scanning transabdominally is to tilt the patient in a slight Trendelenburg position (head lower than body). This relieves the pressure of the uterus on the LUS.

Transvaginal sonography is the best imaging modality to identify the LUS, especially when evaluating the inferior edge of the placenta. The sonographer should acquire a midline

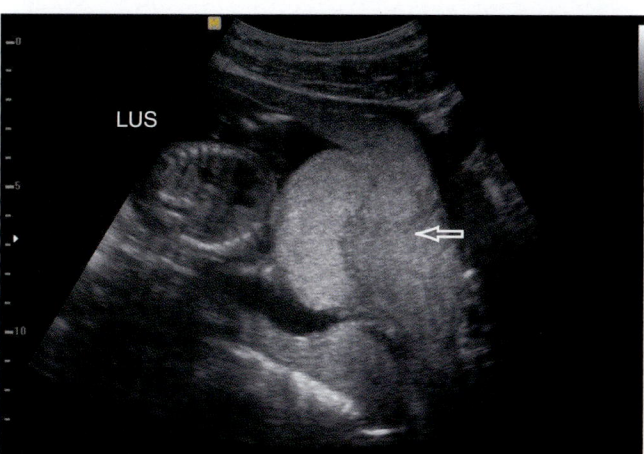

FIG. 56.14 Focal myometrial contraction *(arrow)* is seen distorting the placenta. *LUS,* Lower uterine segment.

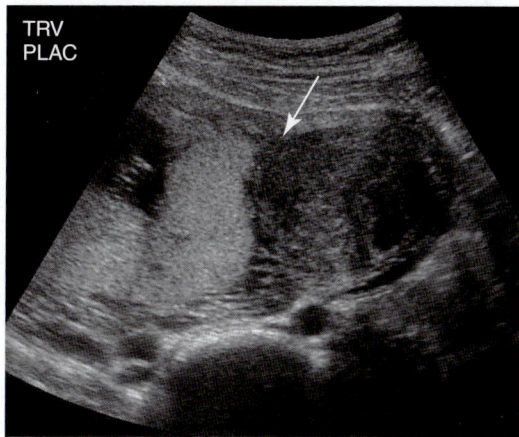

FIG. 56.15 Transverse view of the uterus reveals a hypoechoic uterine myoma *(arrow)*. The left sidewall placenta is implanted on the myoma.

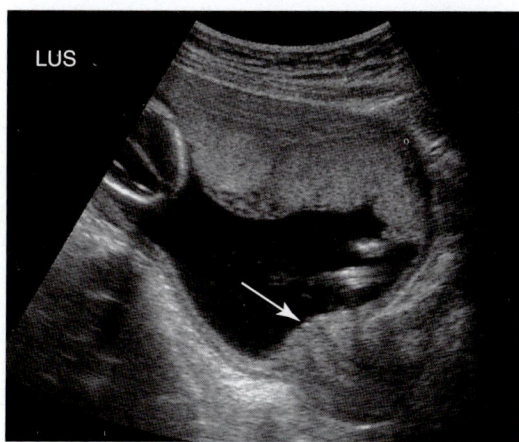

FIG. 56.16 Ultrasound image clearly showing the inferior edge of the placenta away from the internal cervical os *(arrow)*. *LUS,* Lower uterine segment.

sagittal image of the cervix and LUS to display the internal cervical os. Measurement can confirm the distance from the cervix. If transvaginal sonography is not available or possible, the cervix can be evaluated with the transperineal or translabial technique. If a placenta is noted to be in a low-lying position (less than 2 cm from, but not covering, the internal cervical os), a follow-up ultrasound examination should be performed at 32 weeks of gestation.

The concept that the placenta changes its position within the uterine cavity has been termed **placental migration**, implying that the placenta moves and relocates. There are different theories as to why the placenta appears to migrate. One theory suggests that the placenta does not move but rather that the position appears to change because of the physiologic growth and development of the LUS. Another theory postulates that the low blood supply in the LUS causes the placenta in that area to atrophy and disappear, while the areas of rich blood supply toward the fundus and midportion of the uterus cause the placenta to hypertrophy.

Although the majority of placentas that appear to be previas in the early second trimester will not be a previa by the third trimester, there are exceptions. If the placenta is a complete previa in the early second trimester, it is unlikely to change its position drastically. In all likelihood, during the third trimester, such a placenta will remain a complete previa. A placenta previa should not be diagnosed before 20 weeks of gestation.

When the placenta appears to lie on both the anterior and posterior uterine walls, the sonographer needs to scan laterally for a connection that confirms this is a sidewall placenta. If the anterior and posterior placenta does not appear to communicate, it may be a **succenturiate placenta**. A succenturiate, or accessory lobe placenta, is when there are additional placental lobes joined to the main placenta by blood vessels. The sonographer can differentiate the main lobe from the accessory lobe by locating the placental cord insertion site, which will identify the main placenta. There is a slight risk that these connecting blood vessels may rupture or that an extra lobe may be inadvertently left in the uterus after delivery; therefore the clinician should be notified of this finding.

DOPPLER EVALUATION OF THE PLACENTA

Color, power, and pulsed Doppler can be used to assess placental function. Fetal Doppler recordings should be obtained at the lowest energy levels, exposure time should be kept to a minimum, and the thermal index should be less than or equal to 1.0. The sonographer should use color Doppler to better delineate the vessel, magnify the image, and then obtain a pulsed Doppler waveform, optimizing with the correct gate size, placement, gain, and scale. The waveform should be measured and evaluated, and the resistance index, pulsatility index, and Systolic/Diastolic ratio obtained.

The uterine artery sonographically reveals a high-resistance flow pattern in the first trimester, which should become a low-resistance flow pattern in the second trimester. The normal trophoblastic invasion of the spiral arteries produces this low-resistance Doppler waveform pattern. In the first trimester, the flow velocity waveform shows a notched appearance in early diastole. This notch usually disappears by 24 weeks of gestation. In the second trimester, Doppler waveforms of the uterine arteries vary depending on the location of the placenta. The lowest resistance in the uterine arteries is seen on the placental side (Fig. 56.17). Abnormal trophoblastic

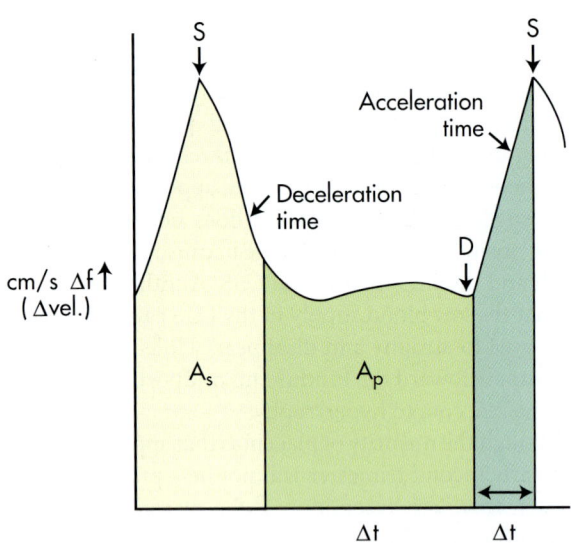

FIG. 56.17 **Waveform analysis.** After 24 weeks, the uterine artery Doppler typically shows a high-flow, low-resistance pattern, particularly for the uterine artery on the same side as the placenta.

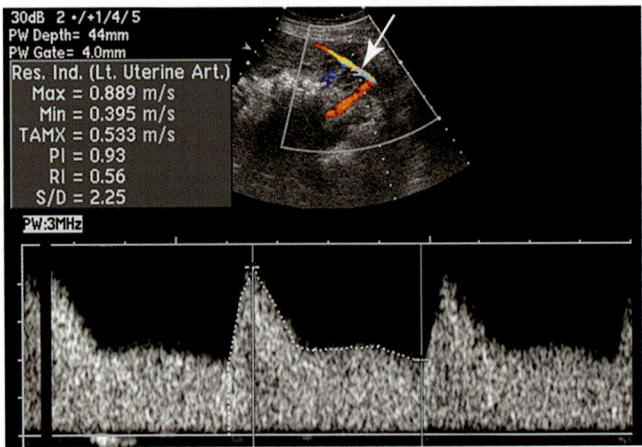

FIG. 56.18 Pulsed Doppler gate is seen *(arrow)* within the uterine artery after it crosses the external iliac artery. Corresponding normal uterine artery waveform is demonstrated.

invasion of the spiral arteries of the maternal uteroplacental circulation is associated with a range of pregnancy complications, including placental insufficiency, IUGR, preeclampsia, and placental abruption.

To acquire a uterine artery Doppler waveform transabdominally, the sonographer should scan in a sagittal scanning plane, superior to the symphysis pubis. The transducer should be moved laterally and manipulated to find the main branch of the uterine artery where it crosses the external iliac artery (Fig. 56.18). Both right and left uterine arteries should be evaluated, and the sonographer should record if they are the placental or nonplacental waveform. The waveform should be measured and evaluated for the presence or absence of a diastolic notch. The umbilical artery can also be evaluated sonographically, and the normal waveform should always have antegrade flow. In a singleton pregnancy, the sonographer should acquire an umbilical artery waveform in a free loop of the cord, making certain that the fetus is in an inactive state. Color Doppler should be used to visualize the umbilical cord vessels and to obtain correct alignment with flow.

EVALUATION OF THE PLACENTA AFTER DELIVERY

The normal-term placenta has several characteristics at delivery. It measures about 15 to 20 cm in diameter, is discoid in shape, weighs about 600 g, and measures less than 4 cm in thickness. The clinician ascertains that the placenta has been delivered intact to avoid complications of postpartum hemorrhage or infection. The amnion and chorion are inspected for color and consistency, with attention to meconium staining or signs of infection. The length of the umbilical cord is measured. Short umbilical cords may result in traction during labor and delivery, leading to tearing of the cord, abruption, or inversion of the uterus. Long umbilical cords are more likely to prolapse, become twisted around the fetus, or tie in true knots.

Fibrin Deposition

Fibrin is a protein derived from fibrinogen. It is found throughout the placenta, but it is most pronounced in the floor of the placenta (in the septa) and increases continuously throughout pregnancy. Fibrin deposits on the villi may increase their mechanical stability; the deposits may result from eddies in the turbulent flow—more flow equals increased fibrin deposits. Fibrin may also be attributed to the regulation of intervillous circulation.

Sonographic Findings. Fibrin deposition (subchorionic) appears as hypoechoic areas beneath the chorionic plate of the placenta. Differential diagnosis of fibrin deposition includes a venous lake or a subchorionic hematoma. A venous lake will have slow flow that can be appreciated with real-time sonography. It may be difficult to distinguish fibrin deposits from a hematoma on ultrasound.

ABNORMALITIES OF THE PLACENTA

The major pathologies seen in the placenta that can adversely affect pregnancy outcome include intrauterine bacterial infections, decreased maternal blood flow to the placenta, and an immunologic attack of the placenta by the mother's immune system. Intrauterine infections can lead to severe fetal hypoxia because of villous edema (fluid buildup within the placenta itself). Most intrauterine infections result from the migration of vaginal bacteria through the cervix into the uterine cavity. Both chronic and acute decreases in blood flow to the placenta can cause IUGR and even demise.

In addition to supplying the fetus with nutrition, the placenta is a barrier between the mother and fetus, protecting the fetus from immune rejection by the mother, a pathologic process that can lead to IUGR or even demise. In addition to these major pathologic categories, many other insults—such as placental separation, cord accidents, trauma, and viral and parasitic infections—can adversely affect pregnancy outcome by affecting the function of the placenta (Table 56.1).

TABLE 56.1	Lesions of the Placenta		
Significance	Incidence	Etiology	Clinical Findings
Intervillous thrombosis	36%	bleeding from fetal vessels	Fetal-maternal hemorrhage
Massive perivillous fibrin deposition	22%	pooling and stasis of blood in intervillous space	None
Infarct	25%	thrombosis of maternal vessel or retroplacental bleed and associated condition	Depends on extent
Subchorionic fibrin	20%	pooling and stasis of blood in subchorionic space	None
Hydatidiform change	<1%: complete mole <1%: partial mole		Predisposes to choriocarcinoma Associated with symptoms of preeclampsia
Chorioangioma	1%	vascular malformation	Usually none, depends on size

BOX 56.4 Placenta Size

Placentomegaly
Maternal diabetes
Maternal anemia
α-Thalassemia
Fetal hydrops
Fetomaternal hemorrhage
Chronic intrauterine infections
Twin-to-twin transfusion syndrome
Congenital neoplasms
Fetal malformations

Small Placenta
Intrauterine growth restriction
Intrauterine infection
Aneuploidy

Placentomegaly

Placentomegaly is an enlarged placenta weighing more than 600 g. Primary causes include maternal and fetal disorders, maternal diabetes, fetal hydrops, and Beckwith-Wiedemann syndrome (Box 56.4). Sonographically, the placenta appears abnormally thick and measures greater than 4 cm in an anterior to posterior dimension (see Fig. 56.8). Measurement should extend from the myometrium to the amniotic fluid junction.

Placenta Previa

Placenta previa is the implantation of the placenta over the internal cervical os. The placenta normally implants in the body or fundus of the uterus; however, in 1 of 200 births, the placenta implants over the cervix or adjacent to the cervix.

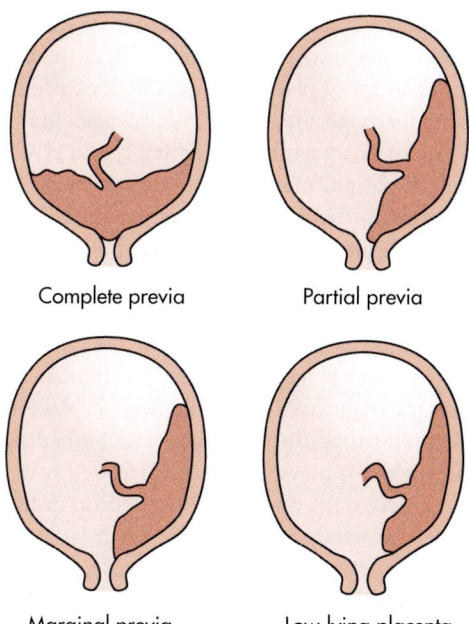

FIG. 56.19 Types of placenta previa.

The risk of placenta previa increases for women with a history of cesarean birth.

The traditional methods of classifying placenta previa included (1) a complete or total previa, (2) a partial previa, (3) a marginal previa, or (4) a low-lying placenta (Fig. 56.19). With complete placenta previa, the placenta completely covers the internal cervical os; a partial previa only partially covers the internal cervical os; with marginal previa, the placental edge just reaches the internal cervical os; and a low-lying placenta is within 2 cm of the internal cervical os. A revised classification system uses only placenta previa (which includes complete, partial, and marginal previa) and low-lying placenta, as it can be extremely difficult to differentiate a partial from a marginal previa. It is important for the sonographer to comment on the location of the edge of the placenta relative to the internal cervical os.

A pregnancy complicated by placenta previa is considered high risk due to the association with life-threatening hemorrhage. During the third trimester of pregnancy, two very important changes occur. First, the LUS is changing, thinning, and elongating in preparation for labor. As the LUS develops, the placental attachment to the lower uterine wall may be disrupted, resulting in bleeding. Second, the cervix softens, and some dilation can occur before the onset of labor. Cervical dilation may also disrupt the attachment of a placenta located over or near the cervical os.

Before 20 weeks of gestation, complete previa may be noted in about 5% of second-trimester pregnancies, with 90% resolving by term with growth of the lower-uterine segment. A good rule of thumb is that if the placenta is covering the cervix but also extends to the uterine fundus in the second trimester, it will usually not be covering the cervix by the third trimester.

Multiple risk factors are associated with placenta previa: advanced maternal age, smoking, cocaine use, prior placental previa, multiparity, abnormal lie (either transverse or breech), multiple gestations, and prior cesarean birth or uterine surgery. Complications of placenta previa include preterm birth, maternal hemorrhage, increased risk of placental invasion, increased risk of postpartum hemorrhage, and IUGR.

Clinically, a patient may present with painless, bright-red vaginal bleeding in the third trimester. About 25% of women will present with bleeding during the first 30 weeks of gestation. Twenty percent of cases are associated with uterine focal myometrial contractions.

Clinical diagnosis is imperative when a patient presents with third-trimester bleeding because the treatment will differ based on the diagnosis. If the diagnosis is placenta previa, the fetus is preterm, and the mother is not bleeding heavily, clinical management may be conservative: bed rest, maternal transfusion if necessary, and close observation until the point where delivery is necessary. Cesarean birth is needed in the majority of complete previa cases (Box 56.5).

Sonographic Findings. Clear documentation of the location of the placenta in relation to the LUS and cervix is required. Sonographic approaches to consider include transabdominal, transvaginal, and transperineal/translabial. Transvaginal approach allows for improved visualization of the cervix and internal cervical os. The transperineal/translabial approach is also useful for evaluating the LUS when the placenta edge needs to be clarified, and transvaginal sonography is unavailable.

The maternal urinary bladder may be used as a landmark to identify the location of the internal cervical os using the transabdominal approach. The sonographer should be cautious about misinterpreting a low-lying placenta covering the internal os secondary to an overdistended bladder. Therefore, evaluation with an empty bladder is warranted to visualize the inferior edge of the placenta in relation to the os.

If the fetus is in a cephalic presentation in the last trimester of pregnancy, the sonographer should examine the fetal head transabdominally in relationship to the posterior wall of the uterus and the mother's sacrum. A distance of less than 1.5 cm indicates there will not be enough room for the placenta between the fetal head and posterior uterine wall (Fig. 56.20).

If there is any question of a placenta previa transabdominally, the patient should be evaluated with transvaginal sonography. The transducer should be prepared as for a transvaginal examination with a protective covering. If the edge of the placenta covers the internal cervical os more than 15 mm,

it will probably not resolve (Fig. 56.21). With a low-lying placenta, the placenta edge is less than 2 cm from the internal cervical os but is not covering the internal cervical os.

Vasa Previa

Vasa previa is a potentially life-threatening fetal complication that occurs in approximately 1 in 2500 deliveries. This condition consists of fetal vessels within fetal membranes lying over or near the cervical os. These vessels are not protected by placenta tissue and are at risk of rupture and a life-threatening hemorrhage. The two most common causes of vasa previa are (1) velamentous insertion of the umbilical cord into placental membranes, which cross over the cervix, and (2) when a succenturiate lobe is present, and the connecting vessels traverse the cervix. When delivery is imminent, the unsupported fetal vessels may tear when the cervix dilates, which can result in exsanguination of the fetus. A rapid cesarean delivery may prevent fetal demise.

Sonographic Findings. Vasa previa is diagnosed with sonography when the implanted fetal umbilical vessels are seen covering the cervix. The vessels appear anechoic with echogenic walls. Color Doppler demonstrates blood flow within the vessels. The vessels are located near or covering the cervical os (Fig. 56.22).

Morbidly Adherent Placenta

Morbidly adherent placenta, previously referred to as an *invasive placenta*, is defined as an abnormal penetration of placental tissue that attaches to the myometrium rather than the decidua. There are three general types of morbidly adherent placenta. With **placenta accreta**, the chorionic villi attach *to* the myometrium without muscular invasion. Placenta accreta occurs in approximately 1 in 2500 deliveries. The risk of placenta accreta increases in patients with placenta previa and a prior cesarean birth. **Placenta increta** is further extension of the chorionic villi *into (in-)* the myometrium. The risk of

BOX 56.5	Predisposing Factors for Abnormal Placental Adherence
Placenta previa	
Chronic endometritis	
Prior cesarean section	
Submucosal leiomyomas	
Uterine scars	
Intrauterine synechiae	

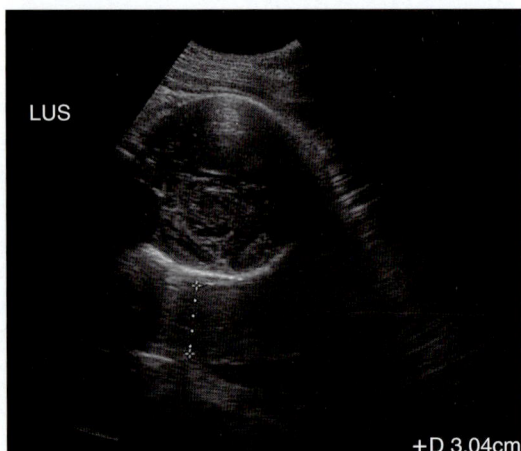

FIG. 56.20 Transabdominally, the lower uterine segment (LUS) in the longitudinal plane shows the placental tissue (30 mm) lying between the maternal sacrum and the fetal head. This woman had a complete placenta previa.

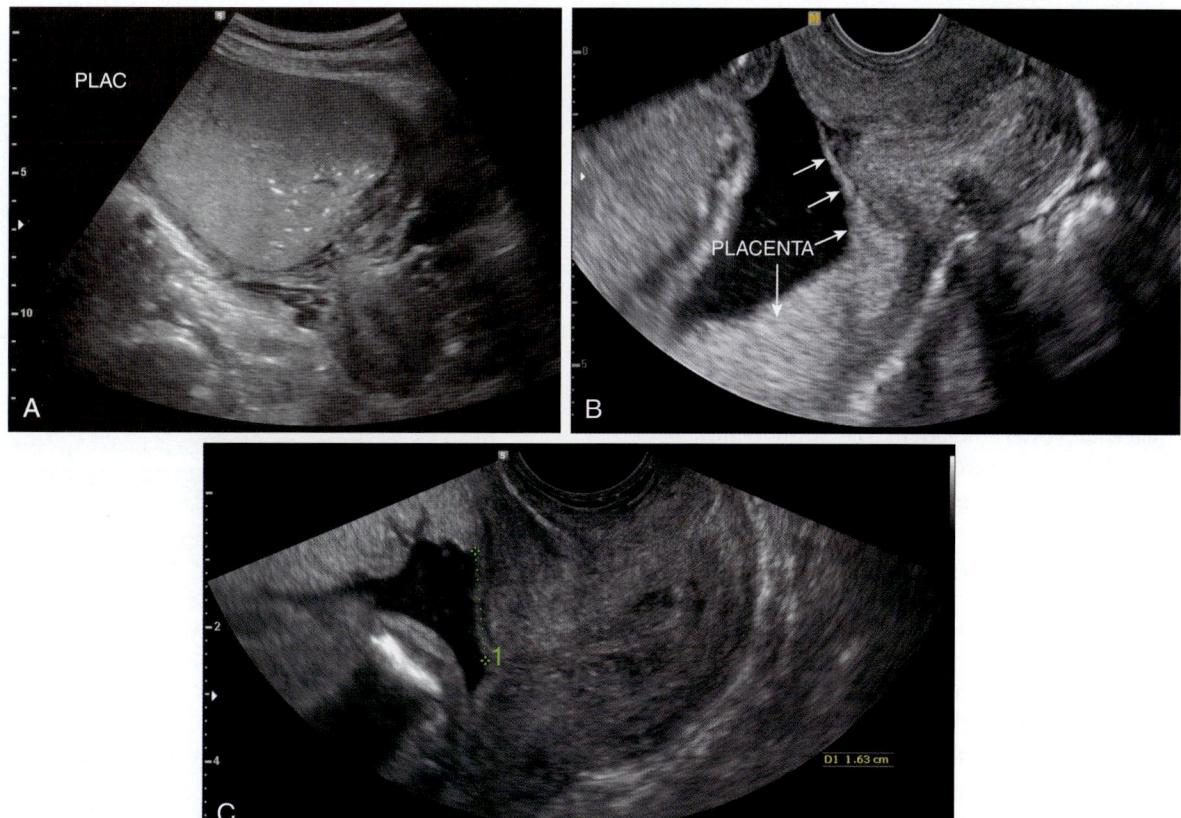

FIG. 56.21 Placenta previa. (A) Complete placenta previa is visualized with a transabdominal approach to evaluate the lower uterine segment. (B) Posterior placenta previa *(single downward arrow)* is visualized with a transvaginal approach covering the posterior lip of the cervix *(three arrows)* and extends across the internal cervical os. (C) The inferior edge of this anterior placenta transvaginally is 1.63 cm away from the internal cervical os, consistent with a low-lying placenta.

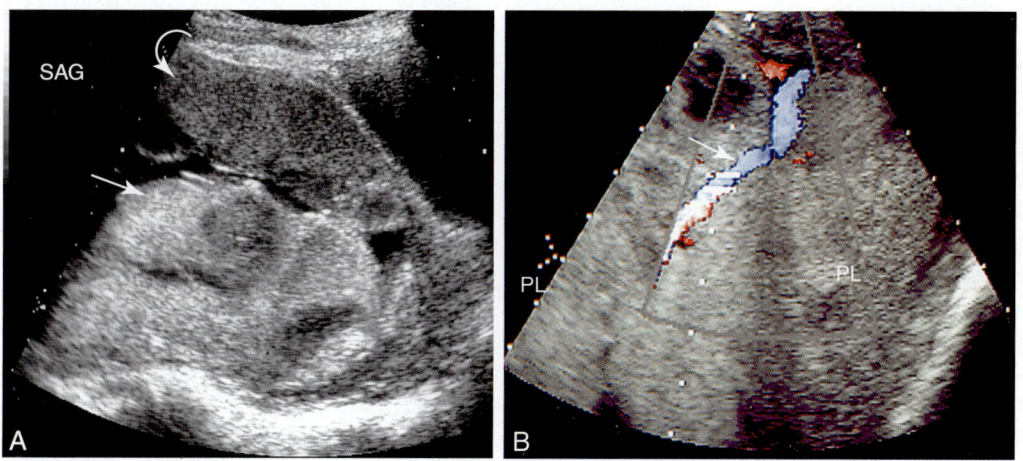

FIG. 56.22 (A) Vasa previa. Transabdominal image of succenturiate lobe anterior *(arrow)* and main placenta posterior *(curved arrow)*. (B) Transvaginal image reveals fetal vessel *(arrow)* crossing cervical os.

increta is 10% to 25% in women with one previous cesarean section when the placenta is implanted over the scar and exceeds 50% in women with placenta previa and multiple cesarean births. **Placenta percreta** is penetration of the chorionic villi *through (per-)* the uterus (Table 56.2).

Placenta increta results from underdeveloped decidualization of the endometrium. The association of placenta previa reflects the thin, poorly formed decidua of the LUS that offers

TABLE 56.2	Morbidly Adherent Placenta	
Type of Bleeding	**Invasion of Chorionic Villi**	**Blood Loss**
Placenta accreta	Superficially to myometrium	Mild
Placenta increta	Deep into myometrium	Moderate
Placenta percreta	Through the myometrium	Severe

Data from http://telpath2.med.utah.edu/WebPath/PLACHTML/PLA-C070.html.

little resistance to deeper invasion by the trophoblast. The previous cesarean scar permits the trophoblastic invasion. High maternal mortality and morbidity rates are associated with placenta increta/percreta, so accurate prenatal diagnosis is critical.

Sonographic Findings. There is usually a loss of the normal hypoechoic retroplacental zone between the placenta and the uterus, anechoic placental vascular lacunae, extreme thinning of the myometrium, bladder wall irregularities, and bulging of the placenta into the wall of the bladder. Color Doppler may display increased peripheral vascularity. Sonographic findings may be limited due to increased abdominal fat, bladder fullness, placenta location, as well as dense placenta vessels noted in the third trimester. A multimodality imaging approach may aid in developing a patient care plan. Magnetic resonance imaging has proven to be very useful when placenta accreta is suspected. The depth of placenta invasion into the myometrium is limited even with advanced imaging techniques.

Almost all cases of morbidly adherent placenta have an anterior placenta previa in a woman with a prior history of cesarean birth. The sonographer should evaluate the placenta previa to look for the loss of the normal hypoechoic retroplacental zone. A transvaginal ultrasound examination should be performed, but the patient should *not* empty her bladder. With an anterior placenta, the probe should be angled toward the maternal urinary bladder to evaluate the uterine-bladder interface (Fig. 56.23). Color Doppler will define vessels that have extended into or to the urinary bladder wall. The perineal scanning approach may also help further define the LUS and the vascularity of the placenta in relation to the maternal bladder.

Succenturiate Placenta

A succenturiate placenta is the presence of one or more accessory lobes connected to the body of the placenta by placental vessels (Fig. 56.24). This occurs in 3% to 6% of pregnancies. Normally, the placenta is oval with a shape that varies somewhat depending on its implantation site. When the placenta develops a secondary lobe or several other smaller lobes, they are called *succenturiate lobes*. These lobes tend to develop infarcts and necrosis in 50% of deliveries. They may create a placenta previa or be retained after delivery. The retention of the succenturiate lobe at delivery may result in postpartum hemorrhage and infection. Rarely, rupture of the connecting vessels may occur during delivery, causing fetal hemorrhage and demise.

Sonographic Findings. A discrete lobe that has "placenta texture" but is separate from the main body of the placenta (Fig. 56.25). Color Doppler will demonstrate communicating vessels between the main placenta and additional lobe. The sonographic appearance and size vary. The placental cord insertion is usually within the main placenta.

Circumvallate/Circummarginate Placenta

A **circumvallate/circummarginate placenta** is the attachment of the placental membranes to the fetal surface of the placenta rather than to the underlying villous placental margin (Fig. 56.26). This abnormality occurs in 1% to 2% of pregnancies. It results in placental villi around the placenta border that is not covered by the chorionic plate. A circumvallate placenta is diagnosed when the placental margin is folded, thickened, or elevated with underlying fibrin and hemorrhage. It is associated with premature rupture of the membranes, preterm labor, IUGR, and placental abruption.

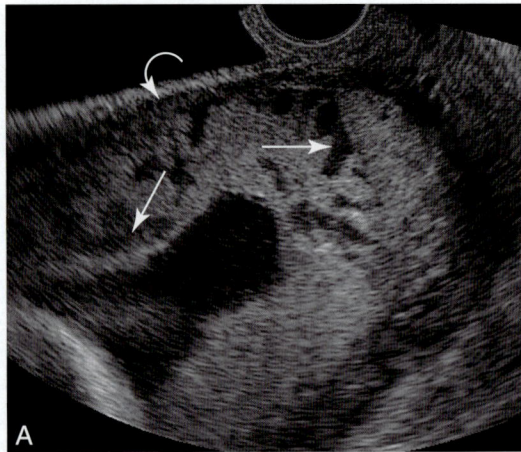
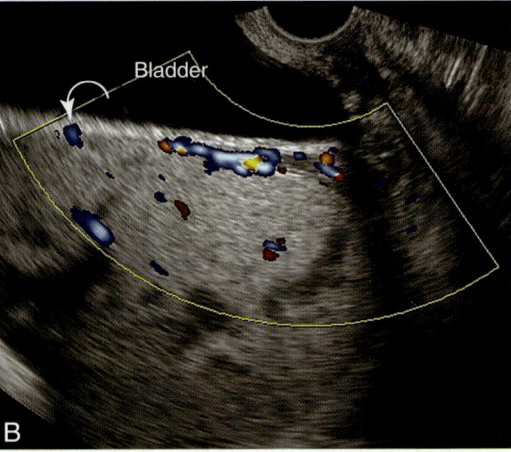

FIG. 56.23 (A) Transvaginal image of placenta and maternal urinary bladder. *Arrows* show hypoechoic vascular lacunae. *Curved arrow* points at loss of the subplacental hypoechoic zone. (B) Color Doppler demonstrates vessels in the thinned subplacental zone *(curved arrow)*.

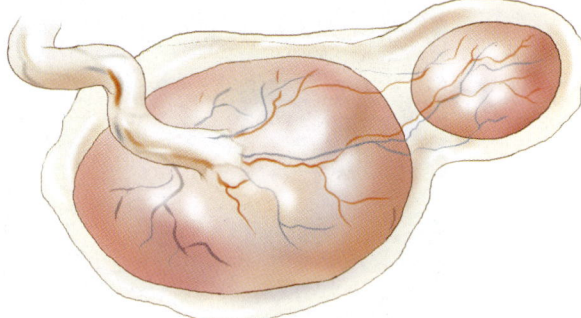

FIG. 56.24 A succenturiate placenta is the presence of one or more accessory lobes connected to the body of the placenta by blood vessels.

Placental Hemorrhage

Hemorrhage may occur within or around the placenta and is more commonly seen than a placental abruption. Placental hemorrhage refers to bleeding from the placenta from any cause. The locations of placental hemorrhage include retroplacental, subchorionic, subamniotic, and intraplacental sites. A hemorrhage seen in the first trimester does not carry the same risk as a hemorrhage in the third trimester. First-trimester hemorrhages are more likely to resolve naturally if bleeding subsides.

▶ **Sonographic Findings.** The sonographic appearance of a placental hemorrhage varies greatly with the location, size, and age of onset of the hemorrhage. A disruption in the normal appearance and size of the placenta will be visualized. If a hemorrhage is present, the echogenicity depends on the age of the hemorrhage; an acute bleed is similar to the echogenicity of the placenta, whereas a subacute and chronic bleed becomes more hypoechoic. The bleed may be retroplacental or subchorionic. Careful analysis should be made from the normal villus attachment of the placenta to the uterine wall to detect an abnormal collection of blood secondary to hemorrhage. The sonographer needs to evaluate the fetal heart rate for all types of abruption, as a poor outcome will be seen when fetal bradycardia is present.

PLACENTAL ABRUPTION

Placental abruption refers to the separation of a normally implanted placenta before delivery of the fetus. Placental abruption is a premature placental detachment and occurs in 1 in 120 pregnancies. Bleeding in the decidua basalis occurs with separation (Fig. 56.27). The mortality rate ranges from 20% to 60% and accounts for 15% to 25% of perinatal deaths. Clinically, the patient may present with any of the following signs: vaginal bleeding, abdominal or back pain, preterm labor, fetal bradycardia or demise, or uterine irritability. The detection of acute abruptions with ultrasound is not sensitive, as the hemorrhage may have the same echogenicity as the placenta. **Abruptio placentae** may be further classified as retroplacental or marginal. With abruption, bleeding into the decidua basalis is apparent. An expanding hematoma can lead to loss of surface area for respiratory and nutrient exchange, placing the fetus at risk for hypoxia and even sudden fetal death.

Maternal hypertension is seen in approximately 50% of severe abruptions associated with fetal demise. Hypertension is chronic in half of these cases; in the other half, it is

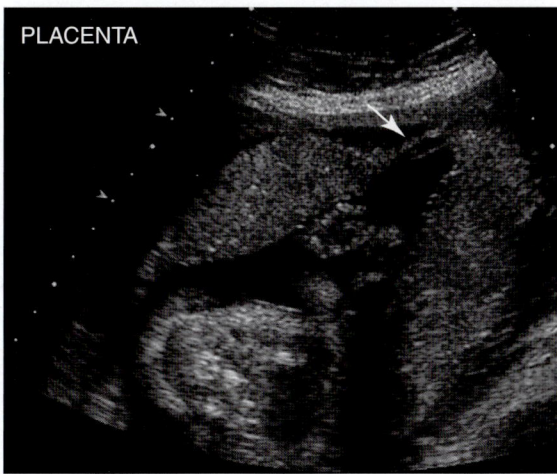

FIG. 56.25 Transverse image of the uterus reveals a left sidewall placenta. Vessels *(arrow)* can be seen connecting the accessory lobe, which is anterior.

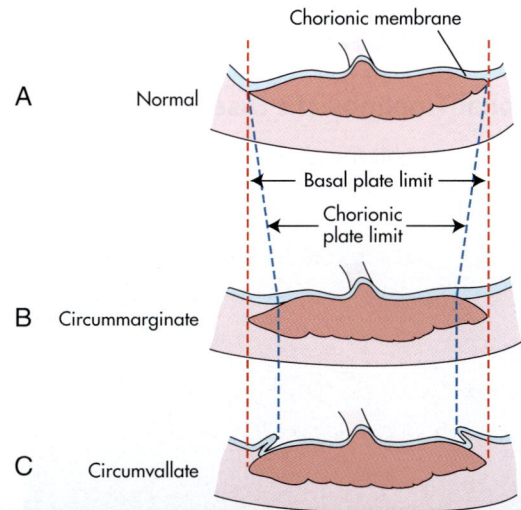

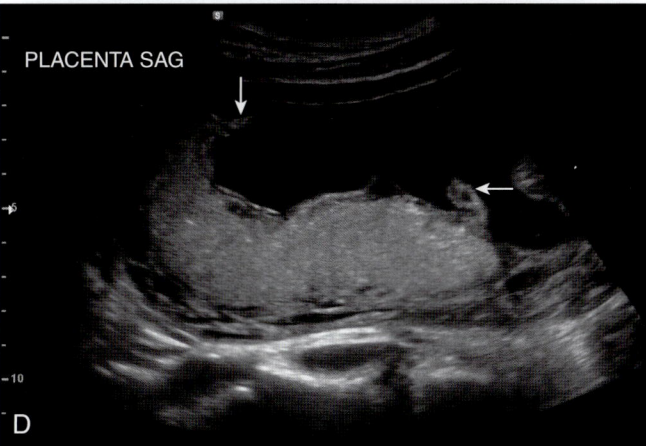

FIG. 56.26 Comparison of extrachorial placentas with a normal placenta. (A) The transition of membranous to villous chorion is at the placental edge. (B) Circummarginate placenta. The transition of membranous to villous chorion occurs central to the edge of the placenta, but the chorionic surface remains smooth. (C) Circumvallate placenta. The chorionic membrane is folding. (D) This posterior fundal placenta reveals that the placental margin is folded *(arrows)*, consistent with a circumvallate placenta.

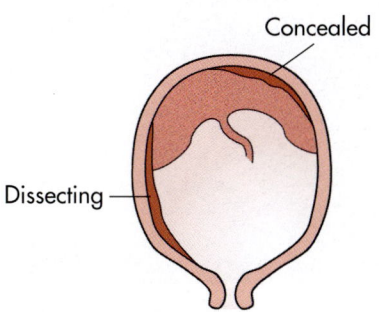

FIG. 56.27 Types of placental abruption.

pregnancy induced. Other risk factors for abruption include a prior abruption, short umbilical cord, uterine anomaly, myomas, abdominal trauma, placenta previa, tobacco use, and cocaine use. The recurrence of placental abruption ranges from 5% to 16% in subsequent pregnancies.

Retroplacental Abruption

Retroplacental abruption results from the rupture of spiral arteries and is a "high-pressure" hemorrhage. It is associated with hypertension and vascular disease and occurs between the placenta and the uterus. Acute sonographic findings may initially appear to be thickening of the placenta. Older hemorrhages tend to be hypoechoic compared with the placenta, and the visual sonographic clue is separation of the placenta from the uterine wall (Fig. 56.28). If the blood remains retroplacental, the patient may have no vaginal bleeding.

Marginal Abruption

Marginal abruptions are the most common type of abruption and are also known as *subchorionic hemorrhage*. This type of hemorrhage results from tears of the marginal veins and represents a "low-pressure" bleed. This arises from the edge of the placenta, dissects beneath the placental membranes, and is associated with little placental detachment. A subchorionic hemorrhage accumulates at the site of the separation from the placenta. A woman may continue to bleed after the initial hemorrhage when blood tracks behind the membranes and through the cervix. This will be old blood and frequently brownish in color. Sonographic imaging along the edge of the placenta aids in the identification of a marginal abruption (Fig. 56.29).

Intervillous Thrombosis

The presence of thrombus within the intervillous spaces occurs in one-third of pregnancies. It results from an intraplacental hemorrhage caused by breaks in the villous capillaries. Usually there is little risk to the fetus, although the condition is associated with Rh sensitivity and elevated alpha-fetoprotein levels from a fetal-maternal hemorrhage.

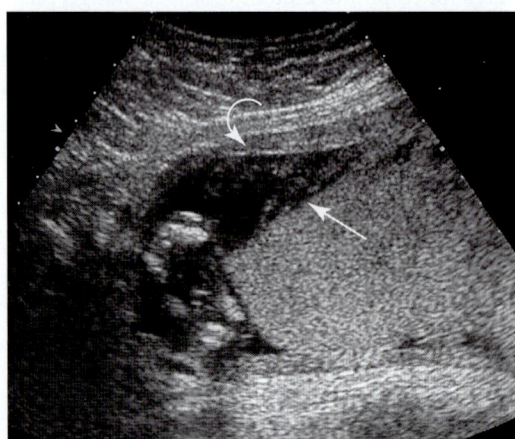

FIG. 56.28 Hypoechoic hematoma is seen separating the placenta *(arrow)* from the uterine wall *(curved arrow)*.

Sonographic Findings. Sonolucencies can be seen within the homogeneous texture of the placenta. These sonolucencies increase with advanced gestational age and indicate maturity of the placenta (Fig. 56.30).

Placenta Infarcts

Placental infarction is a focal discrete lesion caused by ischemic necrosis. Infarcts are common (25% of pregnancies) and are usually small with no clinical significance. Large infarcts may reflect underlying maternal vascular disease. Infarcts within the placenta evolve through acute, subacute, and chronic stages. The majority of infarcts are hypoechoic in the acute stage, and ultrasound may be unable to distinguish from intraplacental hemorrhages. Calcification may occur over time. Maternal floor infarction is a complication of the third trimester; large amounts of fibrin are deposited in and around the maternal plate with extension into the intervillous space and entrapment of chorionic villi.

PLACENTAL TUMORS

Gestational Trophoblastic Disease

Gestational trophoblastic disease, also known as a **molar pregnancy**, encompasses disease processes that originate in

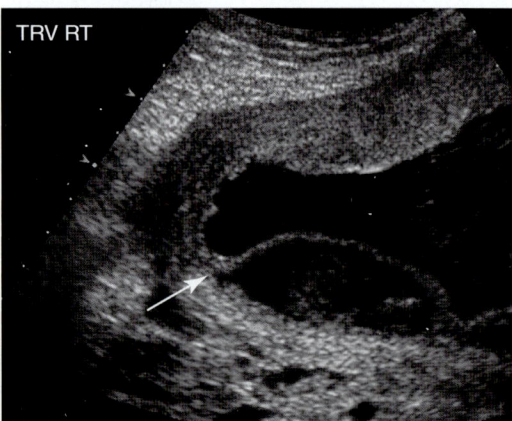

FIG. 56.29 Subchorionic bleed arising from the edge of the placenta *(arrow)*.

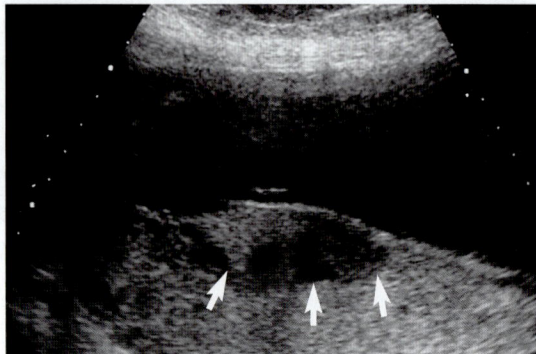

FIG. 56.30 Thrombus within the intervillous spaces occurs in one-third of the pregnancies. The inhomogeneity of the placenta is seen with sonolucent areas within the texture of the placenta *(arrow)*.

the placenta. They may be benign or malignant and include complete or partial mole, choriocarcinoma, and invasive mole. Diagnosis is usually made in the first trimester.

Complete molar pregnancies generally have a diploid karyotype and no fetal tissue. Clinical symptoms include nausea and vomiting (from elevated human chorionic gonadotropin [hCG] levels), vaginal bleeding, and uterine size larger than dates. In this group, 12% to 15% of women will develop malignant gestational trophoblastic disease (choriocarcinoma). Partial or incomplete moles usually have a triploid karyotype, and fetal tissue is often present. Clinically these women may present with vaginal bleeding. Malignancy is diagnosed in 2% to 3% of partial hydatidiform moles. Twinning with a complete mole and fetus is rare, but the fetus will have a normal placenta.

Sonographic Findings. An enlarged uterus, no embryo, and an inhomogeneous intrauterine mass with cystic structures completely filling the uterine cavity are typical sonographic findings (Fig. 56.31). A partial mole is associated with the presence of an abnormal fetus or fetal tissue, and a reduced amount of amniotic fluid is noted. The placenta is thickened with multiple intraplacental cystic spaces (Fig. 56.32). Bilateral ovarian theca lutein cysts are seen secondary to ovarian hyperstimulation related to the elevated hCG hormone levels.

Chorioangioma

A chorioangioma is a benign vascular tumor of the placenta. Second to trophoblastic disease, chorioangioma is the most common tumor of the placenta, occurring in 1% of pregnancies. The tumor is usually small and consists of a benign proliferation of fetal vessels; most are capillary hemangiomas that arise beneath the chorionic plate. Large tumors can act as arteriovenous malformations shunting blood from the fetus, thus causing complications. Fetal complications include polyhydramnios, hydrops, anemia, cardiomegaly, IUGR, and demise. The maternal serum alpha-fetoprotein may be elevated in the amniotic fluid or maternal serum, especially from vascular tumors. Preterm labor is another complication of large chorioangiomas and is thought to be related to polyhydramnios.

Sonographic Findings. Well-circumscribed solid (hyperechoic or hypoechoic) or complex mass is identified protruding from the fetal surface of the placenta (Fig. 56.33). The mass may be located near the umbilical cord insertion site. The majority of these benign tumors are small and incidentally noted at delivery. Those larger than 5 cm are usually detected prenatally and are more likely to have complications. Color Doppler is helpful, although the amount of flow in tumors varies. When a placental mass is seen, associated sonographic findings may be polyhydramnios, hydrops, IUGR, and signs of anemia. Excessive amniotic fluid occurs due to transudation through the wall of abnormal tumor vessels. Differential diagnosis for solid placental masses includes gestational trophoblastic disease, teratoma, or maternal tumor metastases to the placenta.

The Placenta in Multiple Gestation

Monozygotic twins are associated with all three types of membranes: dichorionic/diamniotic (di/di), monochorionic/

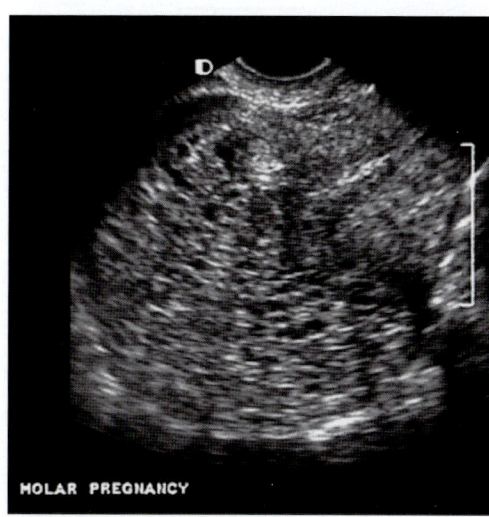

FIG. 56.31 A hydatidiform mole is seen with ultrasound as multiple tiny vesicles throughout the uterine cavity.

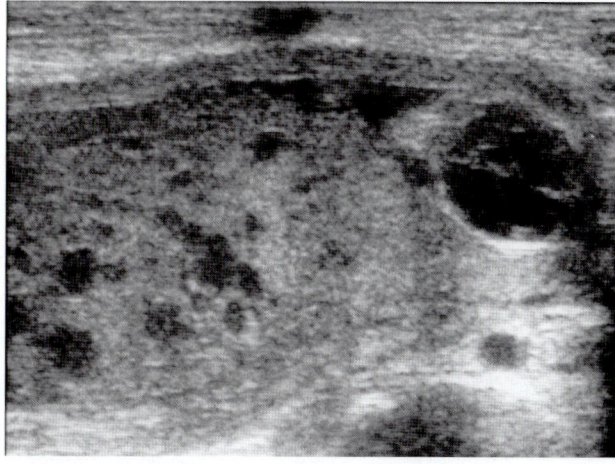

FIG. 56.32 **Partial mole.** Thickened placenta with cystic changes is seen.

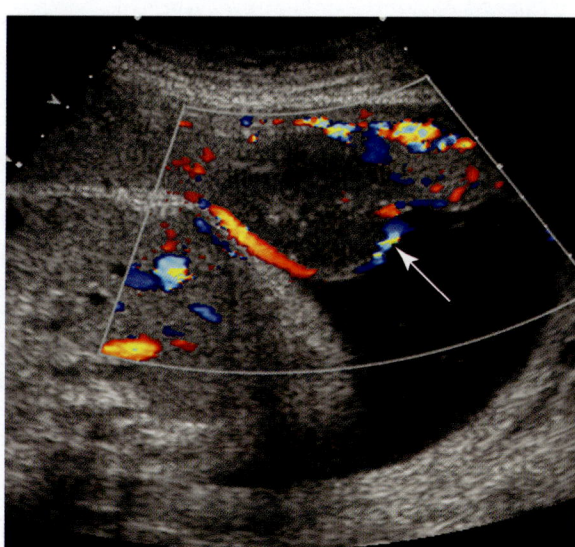

FIG. 56.33 The hypoechoic mass compared with the normal placenta parenchyma is a chorioangioma (arrow). Vascularity is demonstrated with color Doppler.

diamniotic (mono/di), or monochorionic/monoamniotic (mono/mono), depending on when the twinning event occurred. If the membranes are di/di, the pregnancy is probably dizygotic (97% chance), with only a 3% chance of a monozygotic pregnancy. The di/di two placentas can also occur in monozygotic pregnancies when the division occurs during the first 4 days of gestation. If the membranes are mono/di or mono/mono, they are from a monozygotic pregnancy (Box 56.6).

Sonographic Findings. The sonographic appearance of the placenta in a multigestation aligns with sonographic findings in singleton pregnancies. The main differentiation is determining the number of placentas associated with a multigestation pregnancy. A separate placenta may be identified in each gestational sac, or a shared placenta may be identified associated with multiple gestational sacs. A twin peaking or lambda sign located at the level of the placenta and separating membrane indicates separate placentas for each gestation. This sign is seen as a triangular projection of placenta tissue extending into the membrane (Fig. 56.34).

> **BOX 56.6 Multiple Gestation Pregnancies and Placentas**
>
> **Dizygotic (Fraternal Twins)**
> Derived from two zygotes
> Diamniotic/dichorionic/two placentas
> Occurs during first 4 days of gestation
>
> **Monozygotic (Identical Twins)**
> Derived from one zygote
> Diamniotic/dichorionic/two placentas
> Monochorionic/diamniotic/one placenta
> Occurs during first week of gestation
> Monochorionic/monoamniotic/one placenta
> Occurs during second week of gestation
>
> **Risks Involved**
> Monochorionic
>   Placental vascular anastomosis
> Monoamniotic
>   Entanglement of umbilical cord

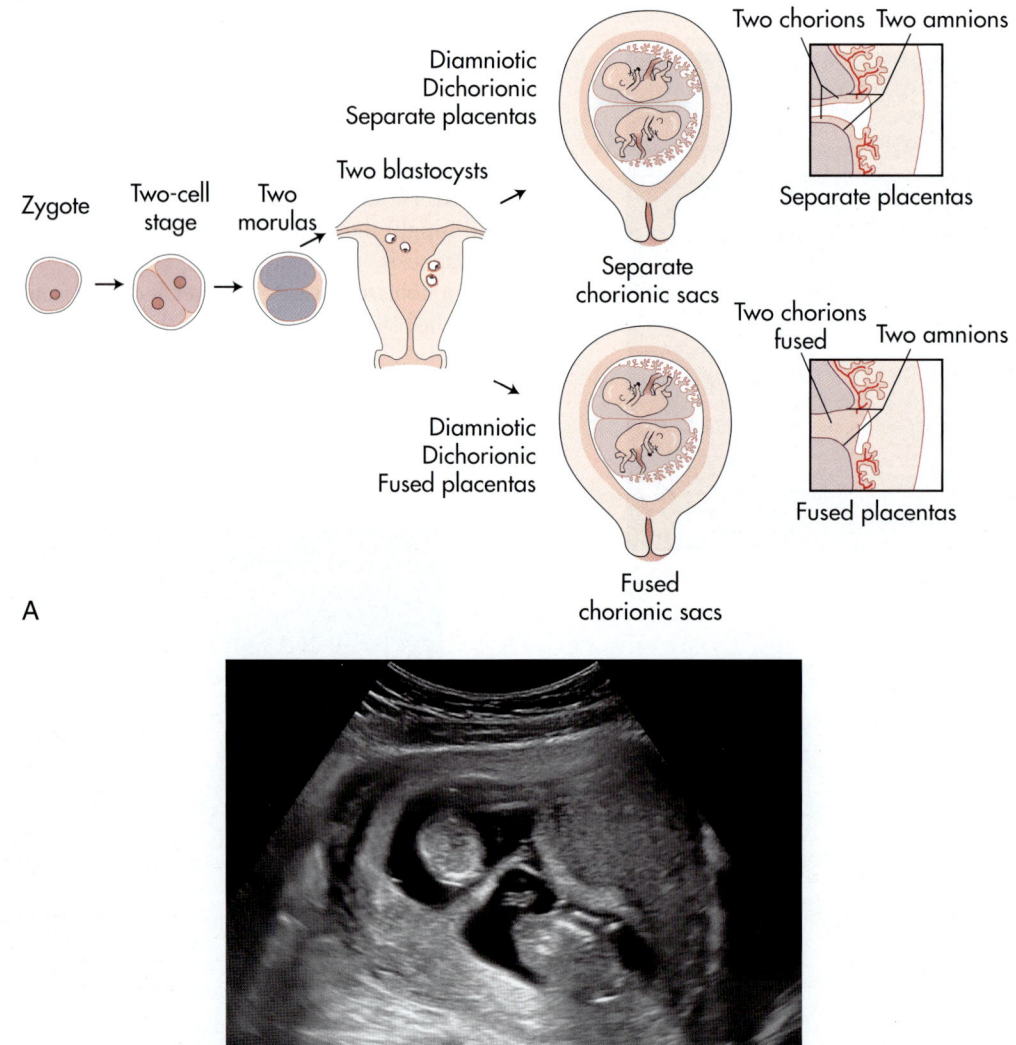

FIG. 56.34 (A) Possible dichorionicity and diamnionicity of monozygotic twins. (B) Twin peaking sign of a dichorionic diamniotic twins.

Key Pearls

- The main role of the placenta is to permit the exchange of oxygenated maternal blood, which is rich in oxygen and nutrients, with deoxygenated and nutrient-depleted fetal blood.
- The placenta has two components: the maternal portion, the decidua basalis, formed from the endometrial surface, and the fetal portion, which develops from the chorion frondosum.
- The maternal surface of the placenta, which lies contiguous with the decidua basalis, is termed the *basal plate*. The fetal surface, which is contiguous with the surrounding chorion, is termed the *chorionic plate*.
- During pregnancy, maternal blood volume increases 40% to 50% by term compared with the nonpregnant state.
- The relationship of the placental edge to the internal cervical os should be evaluated on every ultrasound examination.
- Placental lakes may be seen within the placenta. These have been referred to as placental sonolucencies and are most often surrounded by normal placenta.
- A succenturiate, or accessory lobe placenta, is when additional placental lobes are joined to the main placenta by blood vessels.
- Fibrin deposition (subchorionic) appears as hypoechoic areas beneath the chorionic plate of the placenta.
- Placenta previa is the implantation of the placenta over the internal cervical os.
- Vasa previa is a potentially life-threatening fetal complication that occurs when large fetal vessels run in the fetal membranes across the cervical os.
- With placenta accreta, the chorionic villi attach *to* the myometrium without muscular invasion. Placenta accreta occurs in approximately 1 in 2500 deliveries. Placenta increta is further extension of the chorionic villi into (in-) the myometrium. Placenta percreta is penetration of the chorionic villi through (per-) the uterus.
- A circumvallate/circummarginate placenta is the attachment of the placental membranes to the fetal surface of the placenta rather than to the underlying villous placental margin.
- The locations of placental hemorrhage include retroplacental, subchorionic, subamniotic, and intraplacental sites.
- Placental abruption refers to the separation of a normally implanted placenta before delivery of the fetus.
- Placental infarction is a focal discrete lesion caused by ischemic necrosis.
- Gestational trophoblastic disease, also known as a molar pregnancy, encompasses disease processes that originate in the placenta.
- A chorioangioma is a benign vascular tumor of the placenta.

BIBLIOGRAPHY

Acharya G, Wilsgaard T, Berntsen GKR, et al. Reference ranges for serial measurements of umbilical artery Doppler indices in the second half of pregnancy. *Am J Obstet Gynecol*. 2005;192:3.

Ananth CV, Smulian JC, Vintzileos AM. The association of placenta previa with history of cesarean delivery and abortion: a metaanalysis. *Am J Obstet Gynecol*. 1997;177:1071.

Bader TJ. *Ob/Gyn Secrets*. ed 3. St Louis: Elsevier; 2005.

Ball RH, Buchmeier SE, Longnecker M. Clinical significance of sonographically detected uterine synechiae in pregnant patients. *J Ultrasound Med*. 1997;16:465.

Benirschke K, Kaufmann P, Baergen R. *Pathology of the Human Placenta*. ed 5. New York: Springer; 2006.

Callen P. *Ultrasonography in Obstetrics and Gynecology*. ed 6. Philadelphia: Elsevier; 2017.

Finberg HJ. The "twin peak" sign: reliable evidence of dichorionic twinning. *J Ultrasound Med*. 1992;11:571–577.

Dahmarde H, Parooie F, Salarzaei M. Prenatal diagnosis of placental invasion: a systematic review and meta-analysis on accuracy of ultrasonography and MRI in diagnosis of placental invasion. *J Ultrasound Med*. 2020;36(5):446–461.

da Cunha Castro EC, Popek E. Abnormalities of placenta implantation. *APMIS*. 2018;126:613–620.

Detweiler M, Downs E. Sonographic detection of placenta percreta with associated placenta previa and succenturiate lobe. *J Ultrasound Med*. 2021;37(2):194–199.

Franceschina KM. Sonographic evaluation of a large placental chorangioma. *J Ultrasound Med*. 2017;33(3):246–250.

Gabbe SG, Niebyl JR, Simpson JL, et al. *Obstetrics: Normal and Problem Pregnancies*. ed 5. Philadelphia: Elsevier; 2007.

Gandhi A. Atypical vasa previa in a velamentous cord insertion identified during sonographic examination. *J Ultrasound Med*. 2019;36(1):73–78.

Herrick EJ, Bordoni B. Embryology, placenta. In: *StatPearls*. https://www.ncbi.nlm.nih.gov/books/NBK551634/

Hertzberg BS. Diagnosis of placenta previa during the third trimester: role of transperineal sonography. *Am J Radiol*. 1992;159:83.

Jaffe R, Jauniaux E, Hustin J. Maternal circulation in the first-trimester human placenta: myth or reality? *Am J Obstet Gynecol*. 1997;176:695.

Jauniaux E, Campbell S. Ultrasonographic assessment of placental abnormalities. *Am J Obstet Gynecol*. 1990;163:1650.

Jurkovic D. Transvaginal color Doppler assessment of the uteroplacental circulation in early pregnancy. *Obstet Gynecol*. 1991;77:365.

Elsayes KM, Trout AT, Friedkin AM, et al. Imaging of the placenta: a multimodality pictorial review. *RadioGraphics*. 2009;29(5):1371–1391.

King DL. Placental migration demonstrated by ultrasonography. *Radiology*. 1973;109:167.

Lerner JP, Deane S, Timor-Tritsch IE. Characterization of placenta accreta using transvaginal sonography and color Doppler imaging. *Ultrasound Obstet Gynecol*. 1995;5:198–201.

Lu D. Prenatal diagnosis of placenta previa complicated by placenta percreta. *J Ultrasound Med*. 2019;35(1):70–73.

Miller DA, Chollet JA, Goodwin TM. Clinical risk factors for placenta previa-placenta accreta. *Am J Obstet Gynecol*. 1997;177:210.

Nyberg DA, Cyr DR, Mack LA, et al. Sonographic spectrum of placental abruption. *Am J Roentgenol*. 1987;148:161–164.

Pretorius DH, Chau C, Poeltler DM, et al. Placental cord insertion visualization with prenatal ultrasonography. *J Ultrasound Med*. 1996;15:585–593.

Rathbun KM, Hildebrand JP. Placenta Abnormalities. In: *StatPearls*. https://www.ncbi.nlm.nih.gov/books/NBK459355/.

Rumack CM, Wilson SR, Charboneau JW, Johnson JA. *Diagnostic Ultrasound, vol 2*, ed 5. St. Louis: Elsevier; 2018.

Sepulveda W, Rojas I, Schnapp C, Alcalde JL. Prenatal detection of velamentous insertion of the umbilical cord: a prospective color Doppler ultrasound study. *Ultrasound Obstet Gynecol*. 2003;21:564–569.

Sistrom CL, Ferguson JE. Abnormal membranes in obstetrical ultrasound: incidence and significance of amniotic sheets and circumvallate placenta. *Ultrasound Obstet Gynecol*. 1993;3:249.

Zalel Y, Weisz B, Gamzu R, et al. Chorioangiomas of the placenta sonographic and Doppler flow characteristics. *J Ultrasound Med*. 2002;21(8):909–913.

Zhau Q, Lei XY, Xie Q, Cardoza JD. Sonographic and Doppler imaging in the diagnosis and treatment of gestational trophoblastic disease: a 12-year experience. *J Ultrasound Med*. 2005;24(1):15–24.

CHAPTER 57

The Umbilical Cord

Sandra L. Hagen-Ansert

OBJECTIVES

On completion of this chapter, you should be able to:
- Describe the development and normal anatomy of the umbilical cord
- Predict obstetric problems that may be associated with abnormal umbilical cord dimensions
- Discuss the umbilical cord disorders presented in this chapter, including causes and clinical significance
- Differentiate how the sonographer may distinguish tumors and cysts from a true knot in the umbilical cord

OUTLINE

Development and Anatomy of the Umbilical Cord 1460
    Embryologic Development 1460
    Normal Anatomy 1461
    Sonographic Evaluation of the Umbilical Cord 1461
Abnormal Umbilical Cord Dimensions 1462
Umbilical Cord Masses 1464
    Omphalocele 1466
    Gastroschisis 1466
    Umbilical Herniation 1467
    Omphalomesenteric Cyst 1467
    Hemangioma of the Cord 1467

Hematoma of the Cord 1467
Thrombosis of the Umbilical Vessels 1467
Umbilical Cord Knots 1467
    True Knots of the Cord 1467
    False Knots of the Cord 1468
    Nuchal Cord 1468
Umbilical Cord Insertion Abnormalities 1468
    Marginal Insertion of the Cord (Battledore Placenta) 1468
    Membranous or Velamentous Insertion of the Cord 1469

Vasa Previa and Prolapse of the Cord 1470
    Cord Presentation and Prolapse 1470
    Prematurity 1470
    Multiple Pregnancy 1470
    Obstetric Procedures 1470
Single Umbilical Artery 1470
Varix of the Umbilical Vein 1472
Persistent Intrahepatic Right Umbilical Vein 1472

KEY TERMS

Allantoic duct
Battledore placenta
Ductus venosus
False knots of the umbilical cord
Gastroschisis
Hemangioma of the cord

Membranous or velamentous insertion of the cord
Nuchal cord
Omphalocele
Omphalomesenteric cyst
Single umbilical artery

Superior vesical arteries
True knots of the umbilical cord
Umbilical herniation
Vasa previa
Wharton jelly
Yolk stalk

DEVELOPMENT AND ANATOMY OF THE UMBILICAL CORD

The umbilical cord is the essential link for oxygen and important nutrients for the fetus, the placenta, and the mother. The amnion covers the cord and blends with the fetal skin at the umbilicus. The umbilical cord comprises two arteries and one vein surrounded by gelatinous stroma. Vascular connections within the cord serve a reverse function in the fetus; the vein carries oxygenated blood to the fetus, whereas the two arteries bring venous blood back to the placenta.

The umbilical cord can be clearly visualized with sonography from the eighth gestational week until term. The amniotic membrane covers the fetal surface of the placenta and the multiple vessels that branch from the umbilical vein and arteries. The cord should normally insert into the center of the placenta.

Embryologic Development

The umbilical cord forms during the first 5 weeks of gestation (7 menstrual weeks) as a fusion of the omphalomesenteric

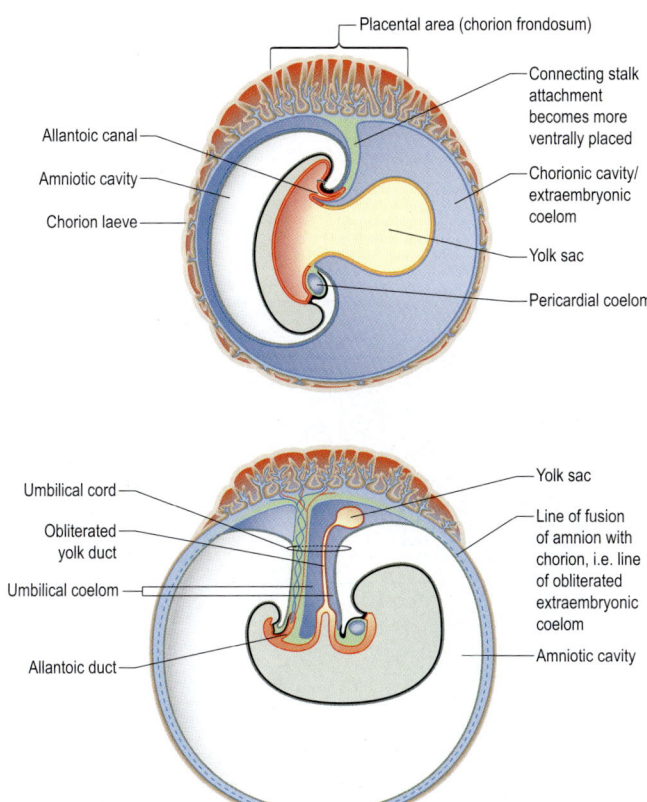

FIG. 57.1 The umbilical cord forms during the first 5 weeks of gestation (7 menstrual weeks) as a fusion of the omphalomesenteric (yolk stalk) and allantoic ducts.

(yolk stalk) and **allantoic ducts** (Fig. 57.1). An outpouching from the urinary bladder forms the urachus, which projects into the connecting stalk to form the allantois. The allantoic vessels become the definitive umbilical vessels. The umbilical cord acquires its epithelial lining as a result of enlargement of the amniotic cavity and envelopment of the cord by the amniotic membrane. The intestines grow at a faster rate than the abdomen; they herniate into the proximal umbilical cord at approximately 7 weeks and remain there until approximately 10 weeks. The insertion of the umbilical cord into the ventral abdominal wall is an important sonographic anatomic landmark because scrutiny of this area will reveal abdominal wall defects, such as omphalocele, gastroschisis, or limb–body wall complex.

Normal Anatomy

The umbilical cord is covered by the amniotic membrane. The cord includes two umbilical arteries and one umbilical vein (Fig. 57.2) and is surrounded by a homogeneous substance called Wharton jelly. **Wharton jelly** is a myxomatous connective tissue that varies in size and may be imaged with high-frequency ultrasound transducers. The diameter of the cord usually measures 1 to 2 cm (variations in cord diameter are usually attributed to Wharton jelly). The normal length of the cord is 40 to 60 cm; it is difficult to assess the length reliably with ultrasound.

The umbilical arteries arise from the fetal internal iliac arteries, course alongside the fetal bladder, and exit the umbilicus to form part of the umbilical cord. The paired umbilical arteries course along the entire length of the cord in a helicoidal fashion surrounding the umbilical vein. The umbilical arteries branch along the chorionic plate of the placenta.

The umbilical vein is formed by the confluence of the chorionic veins of the placenta, with its primary purpose to transport oxygenated blood back to the fetus. The umbilical vein enters the umbilicus and joins the left portal vein as it courses through the liver. The intraabdominal portions of the umbilical vessels degenerate after birth; the umbilical arteries become the lateral ligaments of the bladder, and the umbilical vein becomes the round ligament of the liver.

Sonographic Evaluation of the Umbilical Cord

The umbilical cord has one large vein and two smaller arteries (Fig. 57.3). The umbilical vein transports oxygenated blood from the placenta, and the paired umbilical arteries return deoxygenated blood from the fetus to the placenta for purification. The umbilical cord is identified at the cord insertion into the placenta and at the junction of the cord into the fetal umbilicus (Fig. 57.4). The arteries spiral with the larger umbilical vein, which is surrounded by Wharton jelly. Absent cord twists may be associated with decreased fetal movement and a poor pregnancy outcome (Fig. 57.5).

In the second and third trimesters, the two arteries and the vein can be clearly seen. The number of umbilical arteries can be distinctly identified and should be documented. The three vessels of the cord may be followed with real-time ultrasound as they enter the abdomen and travel toward the liver and iliac arteries (Fig. 57.6). From the left portal vein, umbilical blood may flow through the **ductus venosus** to the systemic veins (inferior vena cava or hepatics), bypassing the liver, or through the right portal sinus to the right portal vein. The ductus venosus forms the conduit between the portal system and the systemic veins.

Sonographically, the ductus venosus appears as a thin intrahepatic channel with echogenic walls. (Fig. 57.7) It lies in the groove between the left lobe and the caudate lobe. The ductus venosus is patent during fetal life until shortly after birth, when transformation of the ductus into the ligamentum venosum occurs in the second week after birth.

The umbilical arteries may be followed caudally from the cord insertion, in their normal path adjacent to the fetal bladder, to the iliac arteries. On sonography, the sonographer may look at the cord in a transverse plane to see one large umbilical vein and two smaller umbilical arteries. Another sonographic approach to viewing the arteries is to look lateral to the fetal bladder in a transverse or coronal plane. The umbilical arteries run along the lateral margin of the fetal bladder and are well imaged with color flow Doppler (Fig. 57.8). In the postpartum stage, the umbilical arteries become the **superior vesical arteries**.

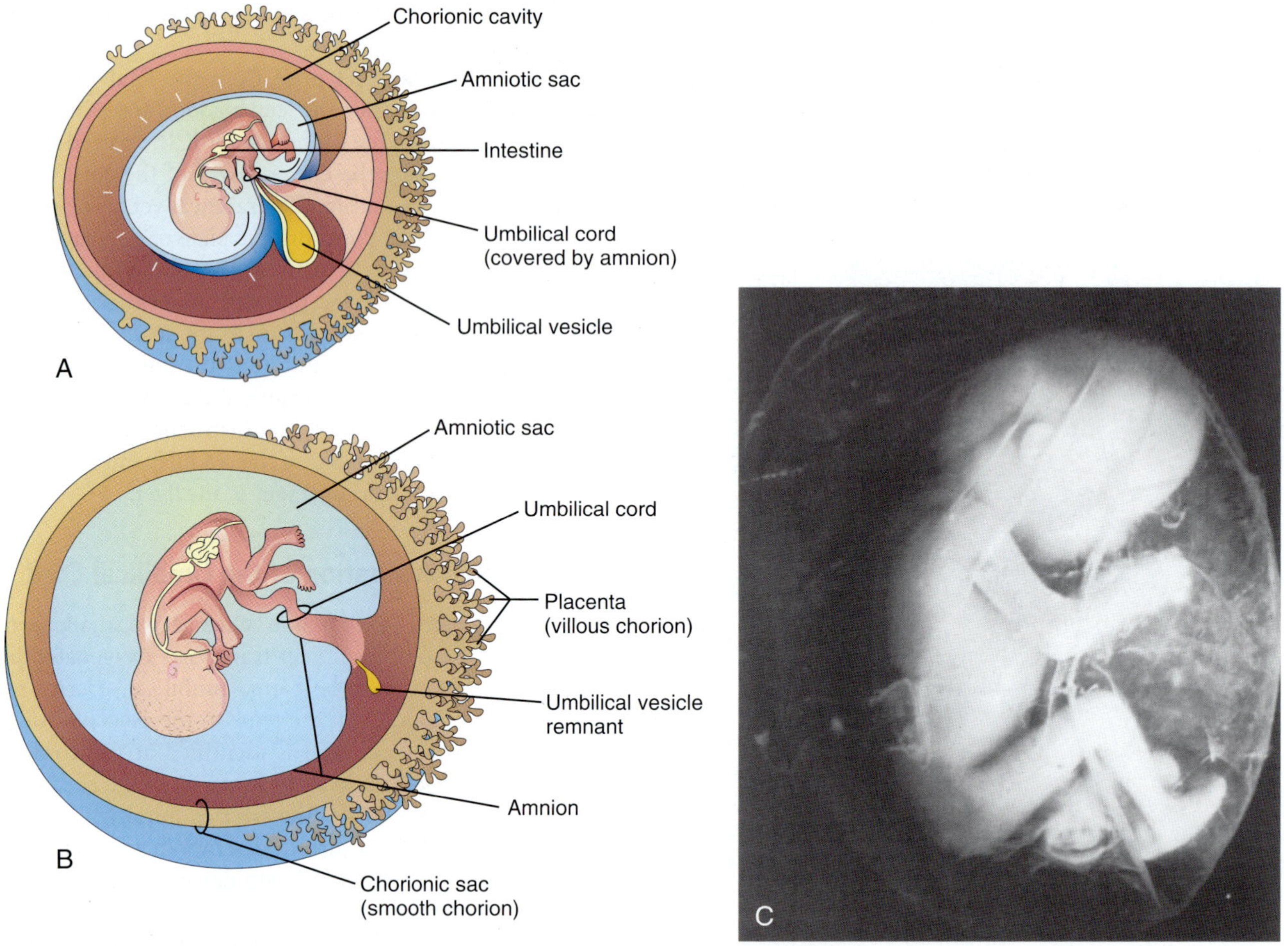

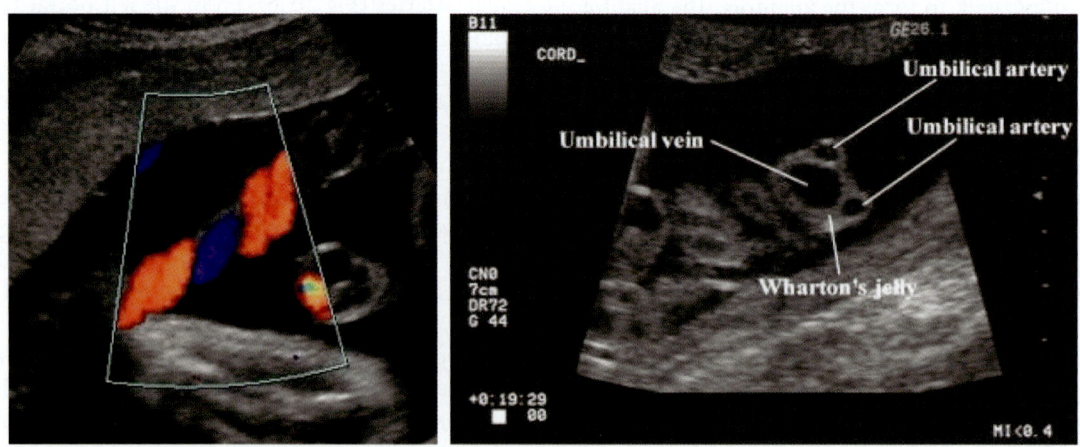

FIG. 57.2 The umbilical cord is covered by the amniotic membrane. The cord includes two umbilical arteries and one umbilical vein and is surrounded by a homogeneous substance called Wharton jelly. The paired umbilical arteries course along the entire length of the cord in a helicoidal fashion surrounding the umbilical vein. The umbilical arteries branch along the chorionic plate of the placenta. The diameter of the cord usually measures 1 to 2 cm. The normal length of the cord is 40 to 60 cm.

FIG. 57.3 The umbilical cord has one large vein and two smaller arteries.

ABNORMAL UMBILICAL CORD DIMENSIONS

Although the umbilical cord varies normally in length and width, researchers have found specific problems associated with a cord that varies from standard dimensions. In the first trimester, the length is approximately the same as the crown-rump length. The normal cord measures 40 to 60 cm in length and is difficult to measure reliably with sonography (Fig. 57.9).

A short umbilical cord measures less than 35 cm in length. This condition is associated with or is predisposed to the following:

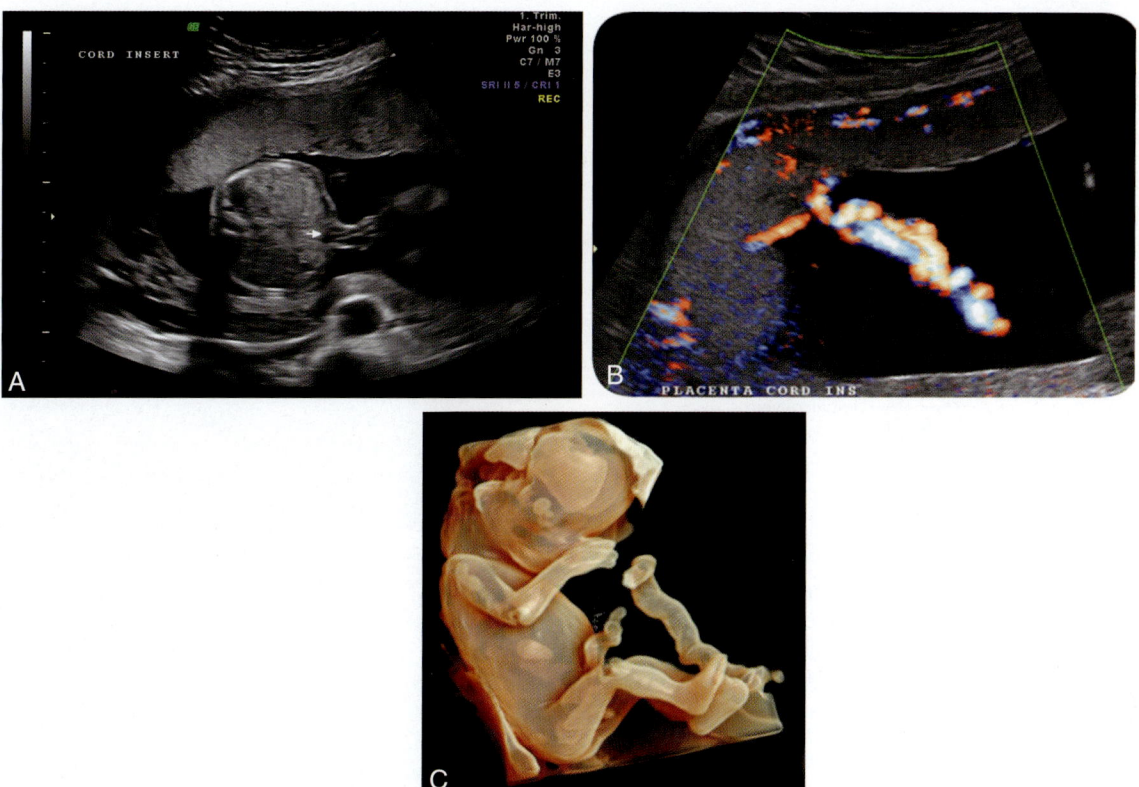

FIG. 57.4 (A) The umbilical cord is identified at the cord insertion into the placenta and at the junction of the cord into the fetal umbilicus. (B) Normal cord insertion into the placenta. (C) Three-dimensional image of the cord insertion.

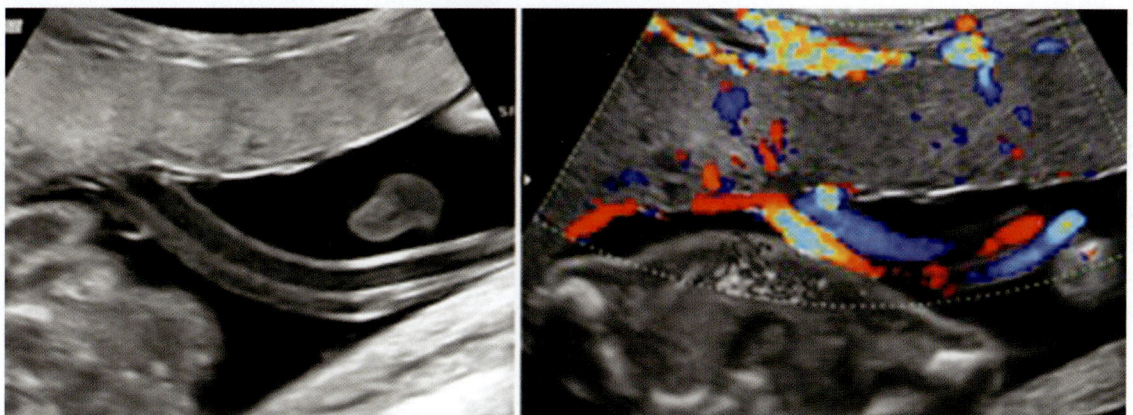

FIG. 57.5 Absent cord twists may be associated with decreased fetal movement and a poor pregnancy outcome.

- Oligohydramnios
- Restricted space (as in multiple gestations)
- Intrinsic fetal anomaly
- Tethering of the fetus by an amniotic band
- Inadequate fetal descent
- Cord compression
- Fetal distress

Coiling of the umbilical cord is normal and is related to fetal activity. The normal cord may coil as many as 40 times, usually to the left and near the fetal insertion site. The helical twisting of the cord can be easily determined by gross pathologic inspection. With the cord held vertically, vessels along the anterior surface that spiral downward from high left to low right, angled like the left side of the letter V, indicate a left helix (Fig. 57.10A). The incidence of a "left" twist of the cord in pregnancy is found at a rate of 7:1. The significance of this is that a fetus with a "right" twist in the cord has a higher incidence of fetal anomalies than one with a left twist (Fig. 57.10C).

The absence of cord twisting is an indirect sign of decreased fetal movement (Fig. 57.11). This event occurs in a small (4.3%) number of deliveries; however, it may lead to increased mortality and morbidity. Other obstetric problems seen with a short umbilical cord include preterm delivery, decreased heart rate during delivery, meconium staining secondary to fetal distress, and fetal anomalies. If the cord

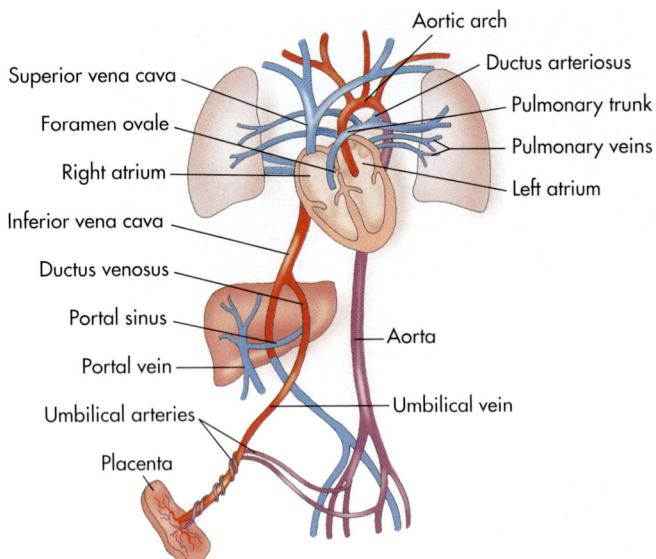

FIG. 57.6 The umbilical vein leaves the placenta to deliver nutrients to the fetus. From the left portal vein, the umbilical blood flows through the ductus venosus to the inferior vena cava or hepatics, or through the right portal sinus to the right portal vein. The iliac arteries drain into the umbilical arteries.

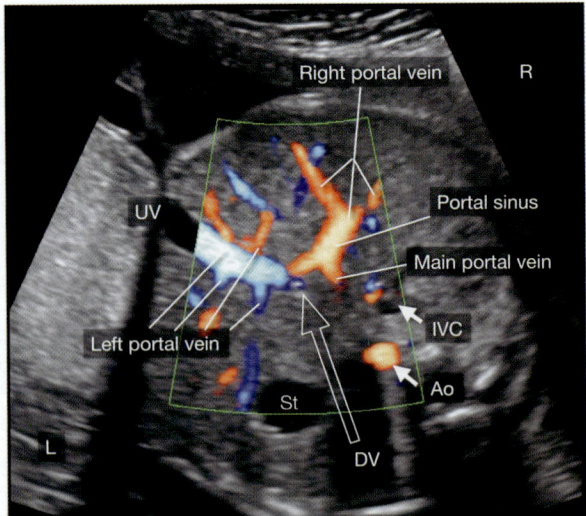

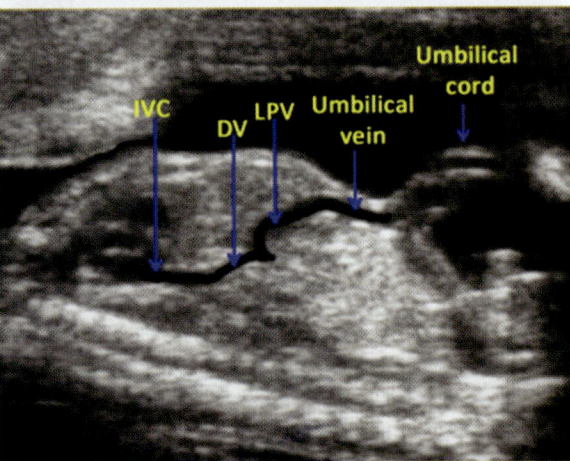

FIG. 57.7 From the left portal vein, umbilical blood may flow through the ductus venosus to the systemic veins (inferior vena cava [IVC] or hepatics), bypassing the liver, or through the right portal sinus to the right portal vein. The ductus venosus forms the conduit between the portal system and the systemic veins. Sonographically, the ductus venosus appears as a thin intrahepatic channel with echogenic walls. It lies in the groove between the left lobe and the caudate lobe. *Ao,* Aorta; *DV,* ductus venosus; *IVC,* inferior vena cava; *LPV,* left portal vein; *St,* stomach; *UV,* umbilical vein.

is completely atretic and the fetus is attached directly to the placenta at the umbilicus, an omphalocele is always present.

It has been theorized that the length of the umbilical cord is determined in part by the amount of amniotic fluid present in the first and second trimesters, and in part by fetal mobility. Therefore, the presence of oligohydramnios, amniotic bands, or limitation of fetal movement for any reason may impede umbilical cord growth.

A long umbilical cord measures longer than 80 cm and may be associated with or predisposed to the following:
- Polyhydramnios
- Nuchal cord (occurs in 25% of deliveries)
- True cord knots (occur in 0.5% of deliveries); may be difficult to distinguish from "false" cord knot or redundancy of cord; true knots cause vascular compromise and fetal demise
- Umbilical cord compression, cord presentation, and prolapse of the cord leading to fetal distress
- Umbilical cord stricture or torsion resulting from excessive fetal motion

The diameter of the umbilical cord measures from 2.6 to 6.0 cm. Variations in cord diameter are usually attributed to diffuse accumulation of Wharton jelly. This condition has been associated with maternal diabetes, edema secondary to fetal hydrops, Rh incompatibility, and fetal demise.

UMBILICAL CORD MASSES

Umbilical cord masses are not very common in the fetus. Many of the "masses" seen on ultrasound may be attributed to focal accumulation of Wharton jelly and may be isolated or associated with an omphalocele or cyst. Cystic masses in

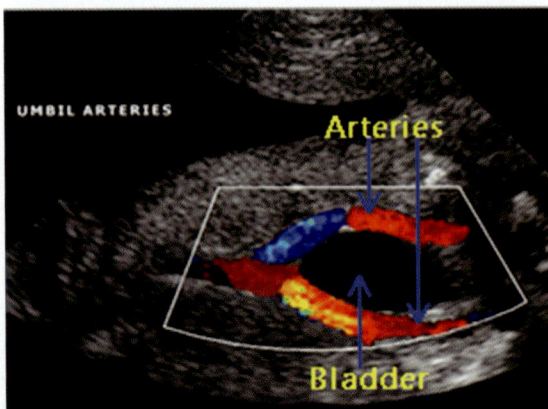

FIG. 57.8 The umbilical arteries run along the lateral margin of the fetal bladder and are well imaged with color flow Doppler.

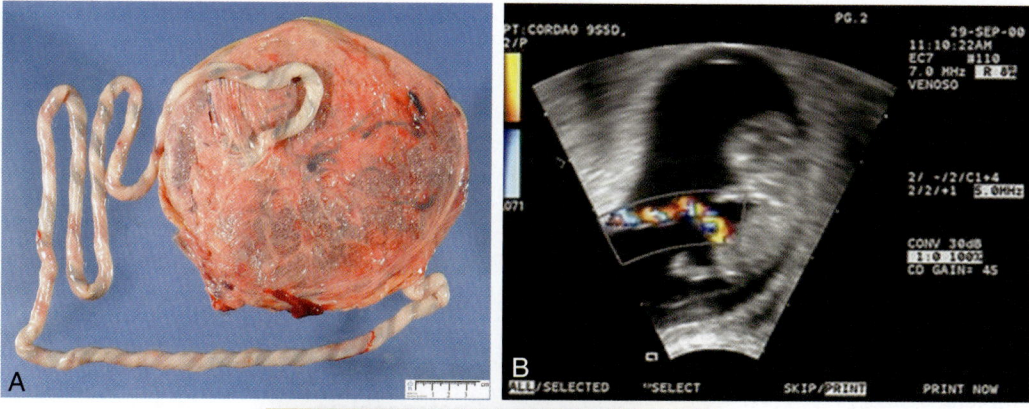

FIG. 57.9 The normal cord measures 40 to 60 cm in length and is difficult to measure reliably with sonography. (A) Gross pathology of a long umbilical cord. (B) Ultrasound image of a short umbilical cord. (C) Three-dimensional reconstruction of a fetus with a short cord.

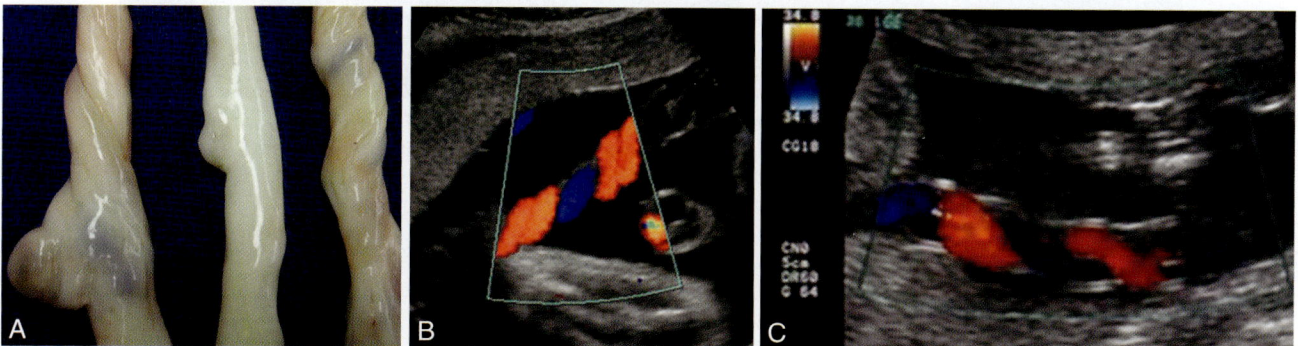

FIG. 57.10 (A) Gross specimens of the left twist, untwist, and right twist of the cord. (B) With the cord held vertically, vessels along the anterior surface that spiral downward from high left to low right, angled like the left side of the letter V, indicate a left helix. The incidence of a "left" twist of the cord in pregnancy is found at a rate of 7:1. (C) A fetus with a "right" twist in the cord has a higher incidence of fetal anomalies than one with a left twist.

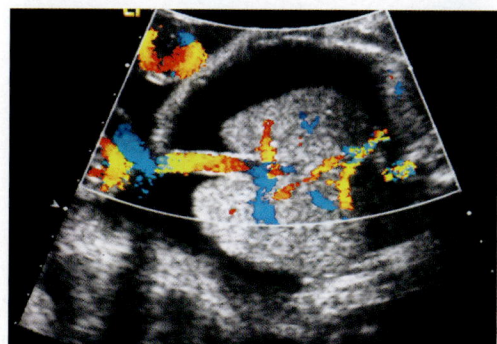

FIG. 57.11 This hydropic fetus showed decreased movement over 24 hours. The cord is shown without its usual twisting and coiling, indicating decreased fetal movement.

the cord are usually omphalomesenteric or allantoic in origin. These are generally small (less than 2 cm), tend to occur near the fetal end of the cord, and resolve by the second trimester. Cysts that persist beyond the first trimester usually are associated with other fetal anomalies and aneuploidy.

Other masses associated with the umbilical cord include the following:
- Omphalocele (cord runs through the middle of this mass as it protrudes from the umbilicus)
- Gastroschisis (mass is usually found to the right of this cord)
- Umbilical herniation
- Teratoma of the umbilical cord

- Aneurysm of the cord
- Varix of the cord (may be intraabdominal)
- Hematoma of the cord (usually iatrogenic—cordocentesis or amniocentesis)
- True knot of the cord
- Angioma of the cord (well-circumscribed echogenic mass that may cause increased cardiac failure and hydrops; alpha-fetoprotein level is increased; associated with a cyst caused by transudation of fluid from a hemangioma)
- Thrombosis of cord secondary to compression or kinking, focal cord mass, true cord knots, velamentous cord insertion, or cord entanglement in monoamniotic twins (commonly seen with fetal demise)

Omphalocele

Omphalocele occurs 1 in 5000 births and results from failure of the intestines to return to the abdomen. The omphalocele is categorized on whether the sac contains liver or only bowel. This hernia may consist of a single loop of bowel, or it may contain most of the intestines (Fig. 57.12). The covering for the hernia sac consists of epithelium derived from the parietal peritoneum and amnion. The umbilical cord inserts into the base of the omphalocele sac.

There is a strong association of omphalocele with aneuploidy; more than half of the fetuses with omphaloceles have additional malformations and chromosomal abnormalities. Trisomy 18 is the most common associated aneuploidy, followed by trisomy 13.

Gastroschisis

Gastroschisis is usually a right paraumbilical defect involving all layers of the abdominal wall and usually measuring 2 to 4 cm. The small bowel always eviscerates through the defect (Fig. 57.13). The loops of bowel are never covered by

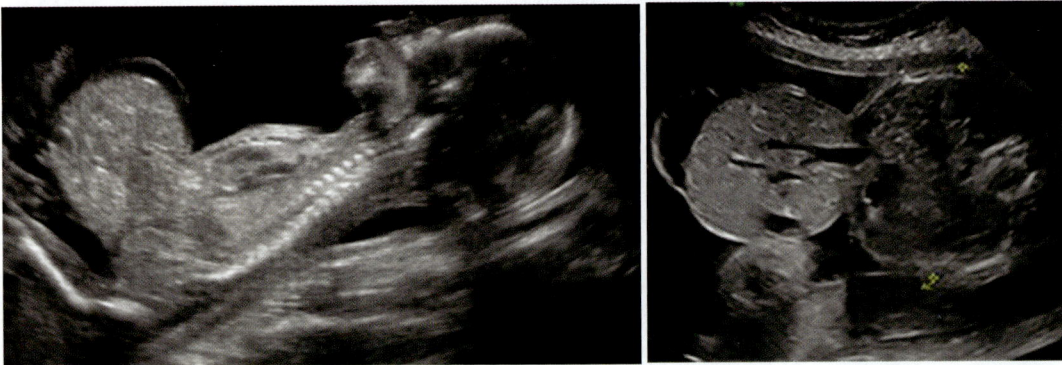

FIG. 57.12 The omphalocele is categorized on whether the sac contains liver or only bowel. This hernia may consist of a single loop of bowel, or it may contain most of the intestine. The covering for the hernia sac consists of epithelium derived from the parietal peritoneum and amnion. The umbilical cord inserts into the base of the omphalocele sac.

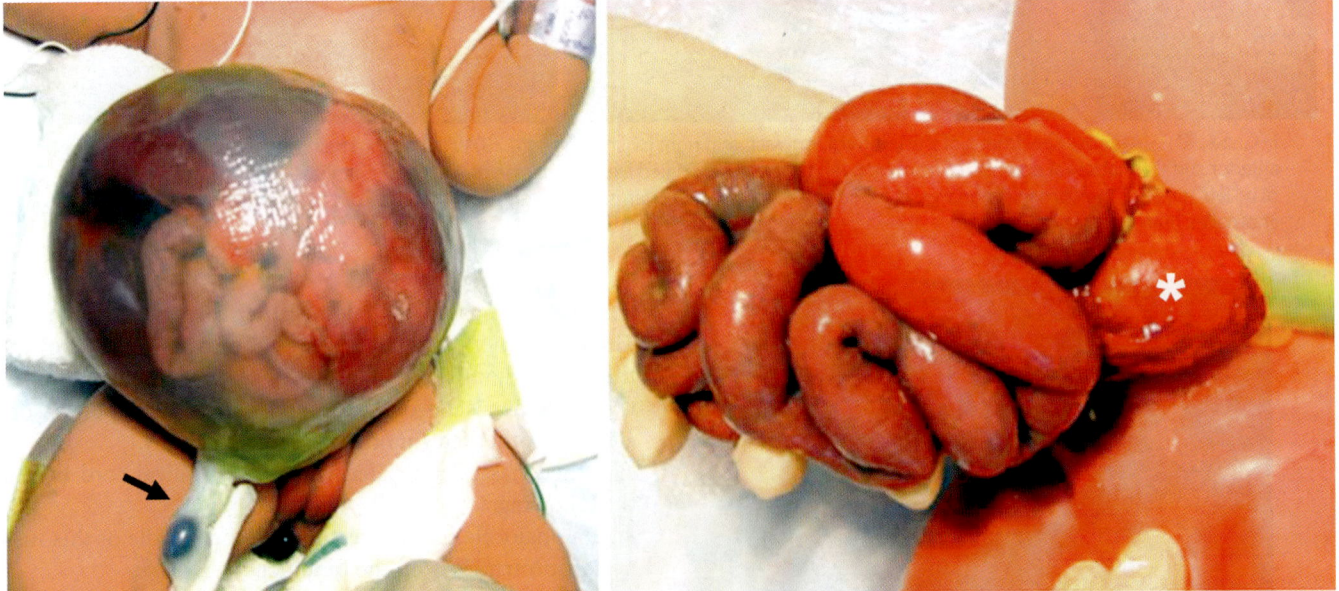

FIG. 57.13 The omphalocele (*left*) is covered by a membrane. Gastroschisis (*right*) is usually a right paraumbilical defect involving all layers of the abdominal wall and usually measuring 2 to 4 cm. The small bowel always eviscerates through the defect. The loops of bowel are never covered by a membrane; thus they are directly exposed to amniotic fluid and elevated alpha-fetoprotein levels. Other organs that may eviscerate are large bowel, stomach, a portion of the gastrointestinal system, and, rarely, liver.

a membrane; thus they are directly exposed to amniotic fluid and elevated alpha-fetoprotein levels. Other organs that may eviscerate are large bowel, stomach, a portion of the gastrointestinal system, and, rarely, liver.

Umbilical Herniation

Umbilical herniation occurs when the intestines return normally to the abdominal cavity and then herniate prenatally or postnatally through an inadequately closed umbilicus (Fig. 57.14).

Omphalomesenteric Cyst

Omphalomesenteric cyst is a cystic lesion of the umbilical cord caused by persistence and dilation of a segment of the omphalomesenteric duct lined by epithelium of gastrointestinal origin. During the third week of early development, the omphalomesenteric duct joins the embryonic gut and the yolk sac. This is closed by the 16th week of gestation; however, in some cases, small vestigial remnants of the duct may be found in normal umbilical cords (Fig. 57.15). The omphalomesenteric cyst is found closer to the fetal cord insertion and may vary in size (up to 6 cm). This condition affects females more frequently than males, at a rate of 5:3. In addition, an associated condition of Meckel diverticulum may be noted.

Hemangioma of the Cord

A **hemangioma of the cord** arises from the transepithelial cells of the vessels of the umbilical cord (Fig. 57.16). Pathologically, this angiomatous nodule is surrounded by edema and myxomatous degeneration of Wharton jelly. The sites of origin are the main vessels of the umbilical cord, and the nodule may involve more than one vessel. This condition is rare; however, when found near the placental end of the cord, the size varies from small to large (up to 15 cm). The fetus may develop nonimmune hydrops.

Hematoma of the Cord

Trauma to the umbilical vessels occasionally may cause extravasation of blood into Wharton jelly. This usually occurs near the fetal insertion of the cord. The umbilical vein is most frequently involved. If the blood clot is new, the mass is hyperechoic on ultrasound; if the clot is old, the mass is hypoechoic and septated. Complications have been reported at rates as high as 47% to 52% with fetal mortality.

Thrombosis of the Umbilical Vessels

Thrombosis of the umbilical vessels is defined as occlusion of one or more vessels of the umbilical cord; primarily it occurs in the umbilical vein (Fig. 57.17). The incidence is higher in infants of diabetic mothers than in infants of nondiabetic mothers. Thrombosis may be primary or may occur secondary to torsion, knotting, looping, compression, or hematoma. The sonographer should look for aneurysmal dilation of the cord and the presence of fetal hydrops. Other maternal factors are phlebitis and arteritis. The prognosis is poor in the fetus with umbilical vein thrombosis.

UMBILICAL CORD KNOTS

True Knots of the Cord

True knots of the umbilical cord have been associated with long cords, polyhydramnios, intrauterine growth

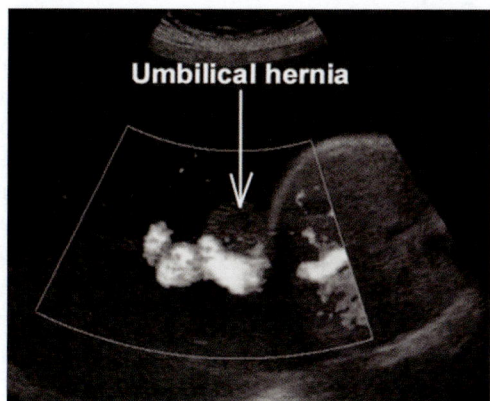

FIG. 57.14 Umbilical herniation occurs when the intestines return normally to the abdominal cavity and then herniate prenatally or postnatally through an inadequately closed umbilicus.

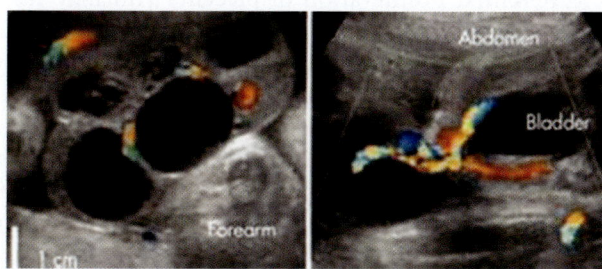

FIG. 57.15 Omphalomesenteric cyst observed in a 34-week fetus.

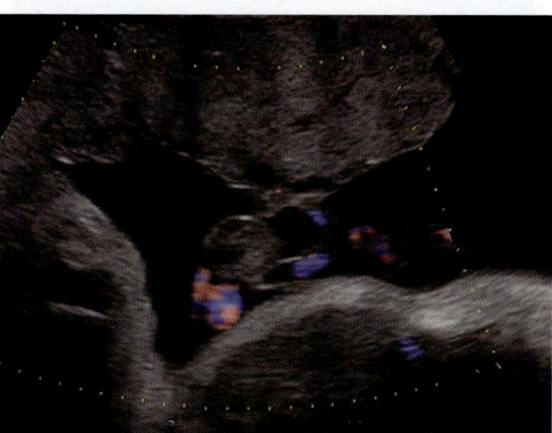

FIG. 57.16 A hemangioma of the cord arises from the transepithelial cells of the vessels of the umbilical cord. Pathologically, this angiomatous nodule is surrounded by edema and myxomatous degeneration of Wharton jelly. (Copyright 2011 Albana Cerekja.)

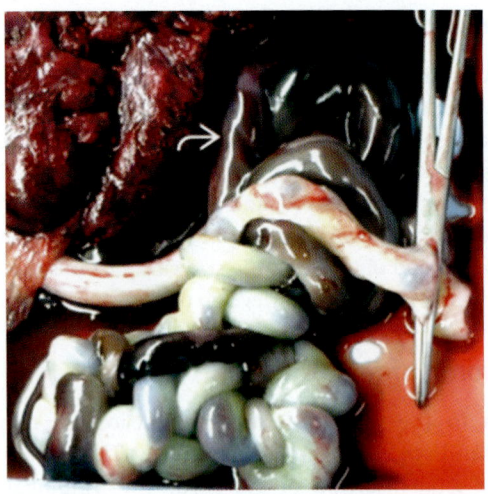

FIG. 57.17 Thrombosis of the umbilical vessels is defined as occlusion of one or more vessels of the umbilical cord; primarily it occurs in the umbilical vein. Thrombosis may be primary or may occur secondary to torsion, knotting, looping, compression, or hematoma.

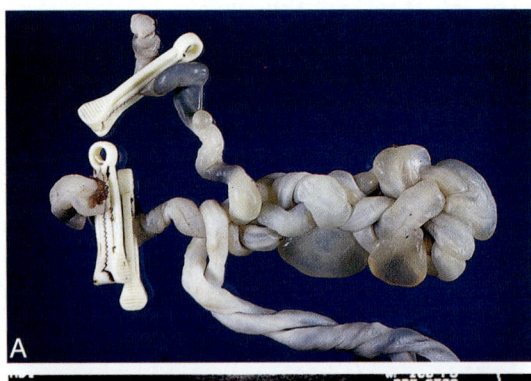

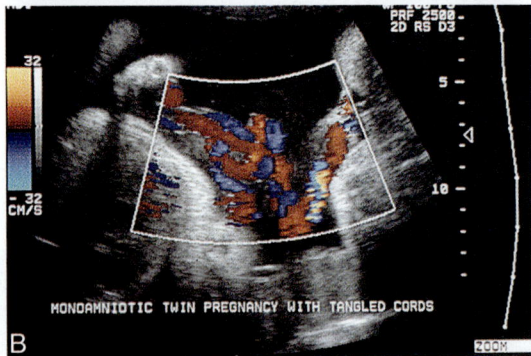

FIG. 57.18 (A) Pathologic specimen of an umbilical cord with multiple knots. (B) Ultrasound image of a monoamniotic twin pregnancy showing multiple knots and tangles within the cord. Doppler flow shows decreased velocity in the blood flow.

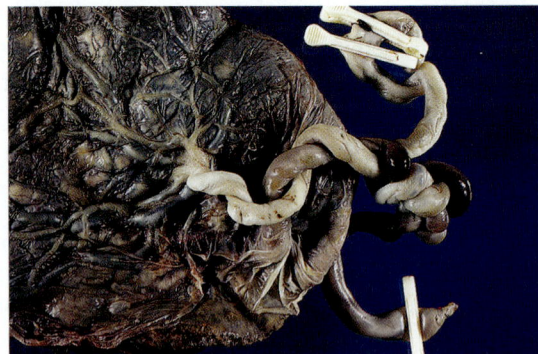

FIG. 57.19 Pathologic specimen of a double placenta with a false knot.

restriction, and monoamniotic twins. The knots may be single or multiple, with increased incidence of congenital anomalies (Fig. 57.18). The mortality rate is 8% to 11%. In these cases, a flattening or dissipation of Wharton jelly is seen, with venous congestion distal to the knot and vascular thrombi within the cord.

The knot may be formed when a loop of cord is slipped over the infant's head or shoulders during delivery. Usually, the umbilical vessels are protected by Wharton jelly and are not constricted enough to cause fetal anoxia in this condition.

Color Doppler is useful for recording absence of blood flow within the umbilical cord. When Doppler is used to image a false knot, flow is not completely constricted but may appear to show constriction secondary to fetal activity and tension on the cord as the fetus moves.

False Knots of the Cord

False knots of the umbilical cord are seen when the blood vessels are longer than the cord. Often they are folded on themselves and produce nodulations on the surface of the cord (Fig. 57.19).

Nuchal Cord

Nuchal cord is the most common cord entanglement in the fetus. Multiple coils may be seen around the fetal neck (Fig. 57.20). A single loop of cord has been reported in more than 20% of deliveries; two loops have been documented in 2.5%. Trouble begins as the fetus descends into the birth canal during delivery and the coils tighten sufficiently enough to reduce the flow of blood through the cord. Fetal heart deceleration, meconium-stained amniotic fluid, and babies requiring resuscitation are seen more frequently when a cord entanglement occurs.

UMBILICAL CORD INSERTION ABNORMALITIES

Marginal Insertion of the Cord (Battledore Placenta)

The differential proliferation of placenta villi may result in eccentric insertion of the umbilical cord into the placenta. The cord implants into the edge of the placenta **(battledore placenta)** instead of into the middle of the placenta (Fig. 57.21). This is significant when the cord is inserted near the internal os because labor may cause the cord to prolapse or be compressed during contractions. The marginal insertion occurs in 2% to 10% of singleton births, 20% of twins, and 18% of pregnancies with a single umbilical artery.

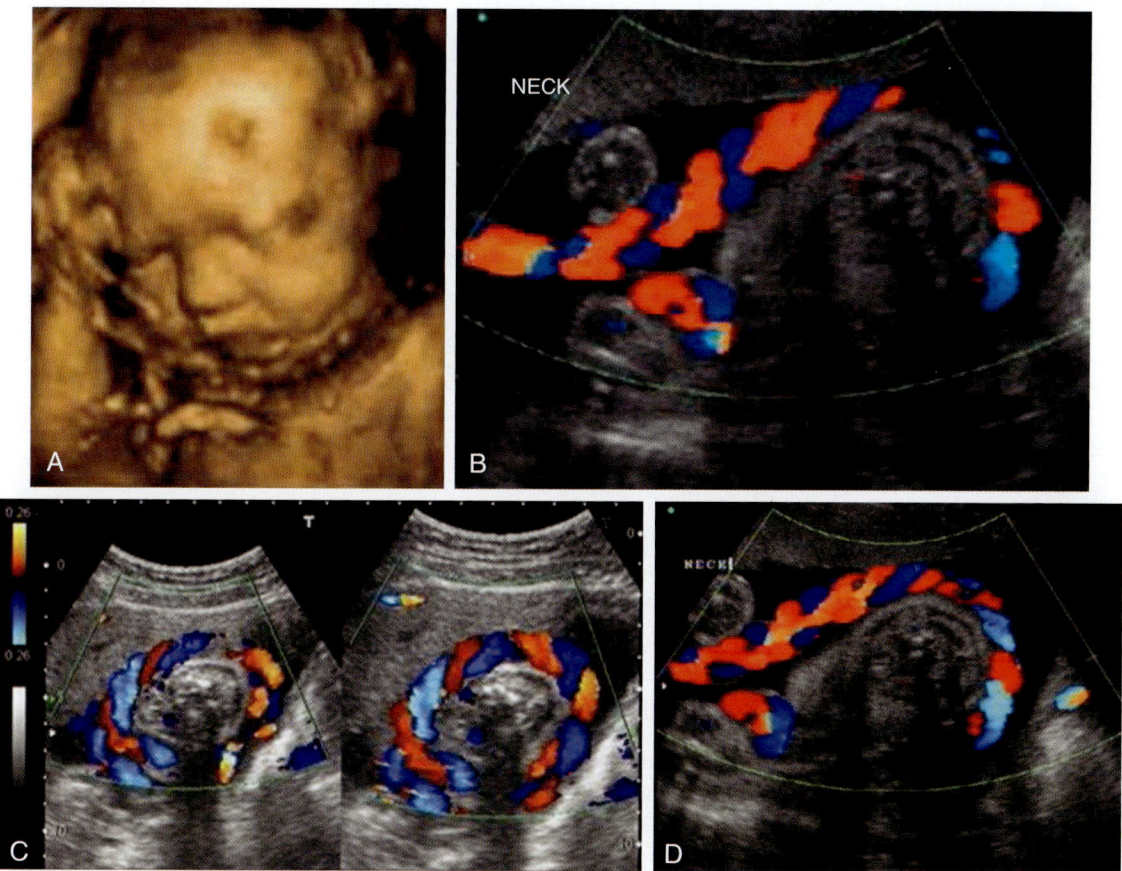

FIG. 57.20 (A) Nuchal cord is well demonstrated by three-dimensional ultrasound. (B–D) Color Doppler is utilized to show the cord as it wraps multiple times around the fetal neck.

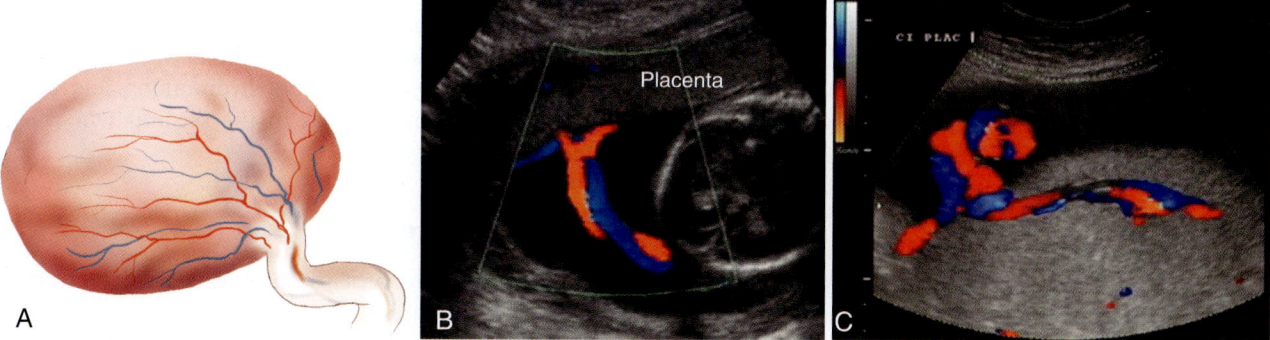

FIG. 57.21 (A) Battledore placenta with insertion of cord at the margin of the placenta. (B–C) Color Doppler shows the marginal insertion of the cord into the edge of the placenta instead of into the middle of the placenta.

Membranous or Velamentous Insertion of the Cord

Membranous or velamentous insertion of the cord occurs when the cord inserts into the membranes before it enters the placenta, rather than inserting directly into the placenta (Fig. 57.22A). This condition occurs in 1% of singleton births, 12% of twins, and 9% of pregnancies with a single umbilical artery. Risk of thrombosis, cord rupture during delivery, or vasa previa is increased.

Velamentous insertion may occur when most of the placental tissue grows laterally, leaving the initially centrally located cord in an area that becomes atretic. Another theory shows a defect in the implantation of the cord that occurs at the site of the trophoblast in front of the decidua capsularis, instead of at the area of trophoblast that forms the placental mass. Implantation occurs in the chorion leave, where the umbilical vessels lie on the membranous surface.

Velamentous umbilical cord insertion is associated with higher risk of low birth weight, small for gestational age, preterm delivery, low Apgar scores, and abnormal intrapartum fetal heart rate pattern.

Associated anomalies occur in less than 10% of pregnancies with velamentous insertion of the cord. These anomalies

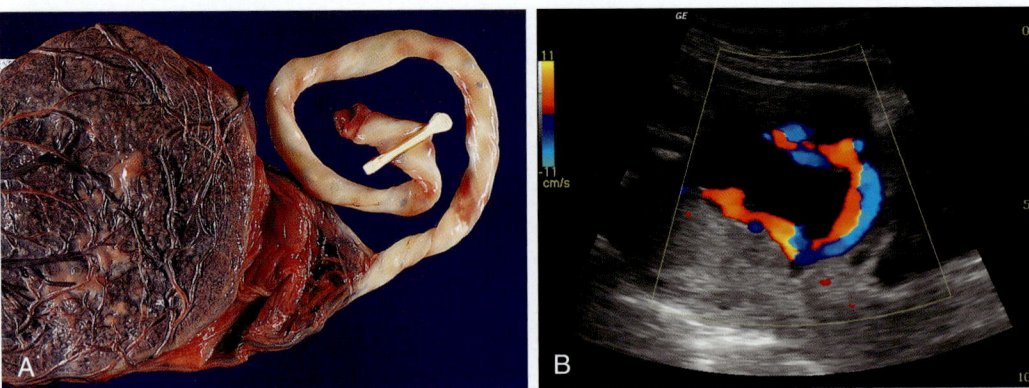

FIG. 57.22 (A) Pathologic specimen of the membranous insertion of the cord into the membranes of the placenta. (B) Color Doppler of the fetus with vasa previa shows the umbilical cord crossing the internal os of the cervix.

include esophageal atresia, obstructive uropathies, congenital hip dislocation, spina bifida, ventricular septal defect, and cleft palate. An increased risk has been reported for intrauterine growth restriction and premature birth.

VASA PREVIA AND PROLAPSE OF THE CORD

Prolapse of the umbilical cord occurs when the cord lies below the presenting part. This condition may exist whenever the presenting part does not fit closely and fails to fill the pelvic inlet; further risk is incurred if the membranes rupture early. Compression of the cord reduces or cuts off the blood supply to the fetus and may result in fetal demise. Abnormal fetal presentation occurs in nearly half of prolapse cord cases. A slightly higher risk is incurred when the fetus is in a transverse or breech presentation.

Vasa previa is defined as the presence of umbilical cord vessels crossing the internal os of the cervix (see Fig. 57.22B). Mortality rates may be high, ranging from 60% to 70% for vaginal delivery. Death results from rupture of the vessels and fetal exsanguination. Color Doppler is the best method of detection in the ultrasound examination. Vasa previa may be due to many factors, including velamentous insertion of the cord, succenturiate lobe of the placenta, or low-lying placenta with marginal insertion of the cord near the internal os.

Cord Presentation and Prolapse

Cord presentation with prolapse of the umbilical cord through the cervix into the vagina occurs in 0.5% of deliveries. An occult prolapse occurs when the cord lies alongside the presenting part. The perinatal mortality rate of 25% to 60% is due to cord compression during vaginal delivery. Conditions predisposing to cord presentation and prolapse are as follows:
- Abnormal fetal presentation
- Nonengagement of the fetus because of prematurity
- Long umbilical cord
- Abnormal bony pelvic inlet
- Leiomyomas
- Polyhydramnios
- Vasa previa
- Velamentous insertion of the cord
- Marginal insertion of the cord in a low-lying placenta
- Incompetent cervix with premature rupture of the membranes

Prematurity

Two factors contribute to failure of the fetus to fill the pelvic inlet cavity: small presenting part and increased frequency of abnormal presentation in premature labor. Fetal mortality rate is high in the premature population secondary to birth trauma and anoxia.

Multiple Pregnancy

Multiple pregnancy factors include failure of adequate adaptation of the presenting part to the pelvis, higher incidence of abnormal presentation, polyhydramnios, and premature rupture of the membranes of the second twin when it is unengaged.

Obstetric Procedures

One-third of cord prolapse problems are produced during obstetric procedures:
- Artificial rupture of membranes
- Disengagement of the head
- Flexion of an extended head
- Version and extraction

SINGLE UMBILICAL ARTERY

A **single umbilical artery** occurs in 0.08% to 1.9% of singleton births and 3.5% of twin pregnancies; it is more frequent in miscarriages and autopsy series (Fig. 57.23). Reports have found single umbilical artery in 18% of pregnancies with marginal insertion of the cord and in 9% with membranous insertion of the cord. The probable cause is atrophy of one of the umbilical arteries in the early development stage. The left umbilical artery is absent a slightly higher percentage of time than the right.

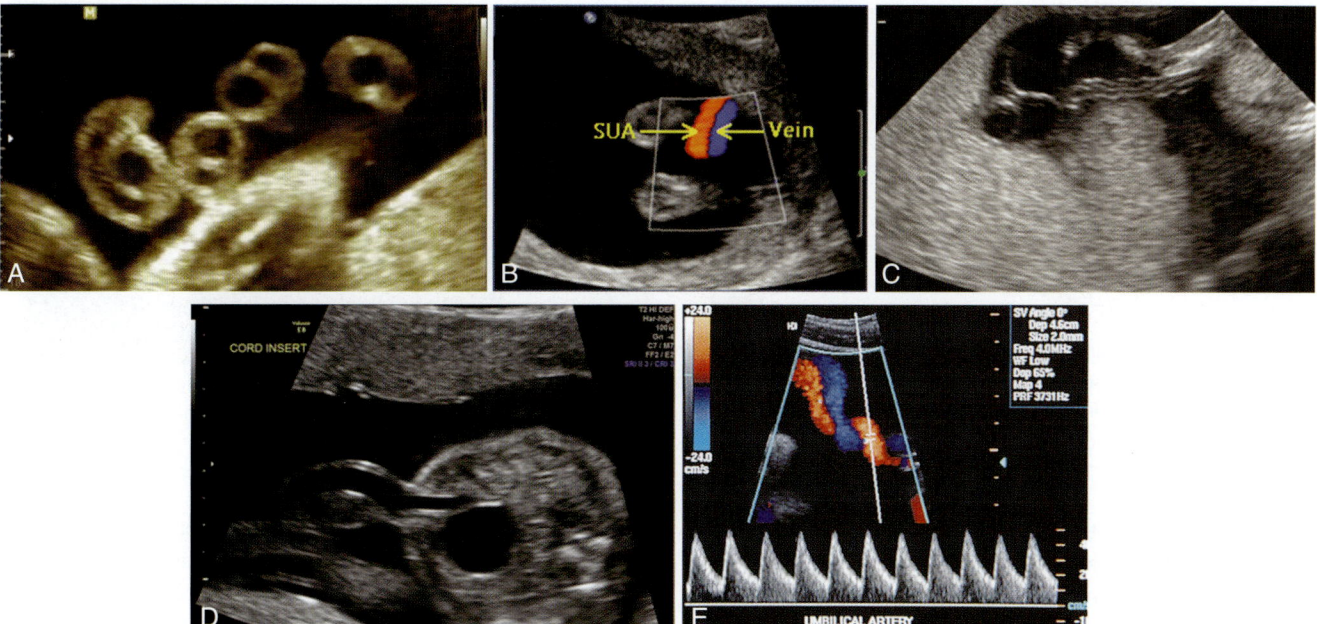

FIG. 57.23 (A–D) A characteristic sonographic finding of the two-vessel cord is disconcordance of the two vessels on cross section. Once the transducer is rotated to record the long-axis view, the two-vessel cord appears straight and noncoiled, although occasionally the single artery may loop around the vein. (E) Spectral Doppler shows normal umbilical artery flow in a fetus with a two-vessel cord. *SUA*, Single umbilical artery.

Single umbilical artery has been associated with the following:
- Congenital anomalies in 20% to 50% of cases
- Increased incidence of intrauterine growth restriction (small placenta)
- Increased perinatal mortality
- Increased incidence of chromosomal abnormalities (trisomies 18, 13, and 21; Turner syndrome; and triploidy)
- Infants with single umbilical arteries have associated anomalies that affect other organ systems, such as the following:
  - Musculoskeletal (23%)
  - Genitourinary (20%)
  - Cardiovascular (19%)
  - Gastrointestinal (10%)
  - Central nervous system (8%)

Multiple studies have investigated normal measurements of the vessels within the umbilical cord. A three-vessel cord showing artery-to-artery difference of more than 50% was defined as hypoplastic umbilical artery. A study of 100 pregnancies found that at between 20 and 36 weeks of gestation, all pregnancies with a single umbilical artery had a transverse umbilical artery diameter greater than 4 mm, and all pregnancies with two umbilical arteries had a transverse umbilical arterial diameter less than 4 mm. In another study, the diameter of the umbilical artery was greater than 50% of that of the umbilical vein in the fetus with a single umbilical artery.

Sonographic detection of a single umbilical artery should prompt the investigation of further fetal anomalies. The incidence of associated anomalies has been reported to range from 25% to 50%. Major anomalies have included cardiac defects, skeletal abnormalities, abdominal wall defects, diaphragmatic hernia, holoprosencephaly, and hydrocephalus. The diagnosis of a single umbilical artery in the second and third trimesters has increased with routine visualization of the number of vessels within the cord. A characteristic sonographic finding of the two-vessel cord is disconcordance of the two vessels on cross section. Once the transducer is rotated to record the long-axis view, the two-vessel cord appears straight and noncoiled, although occasionally the single artery may loop around the vein. Visualization with color of the umbilical artery alongside the bladder may provide further confirmation that only one artery is present.

Another variation that may be seen is discordant size between the two arterial vessels, with one being more

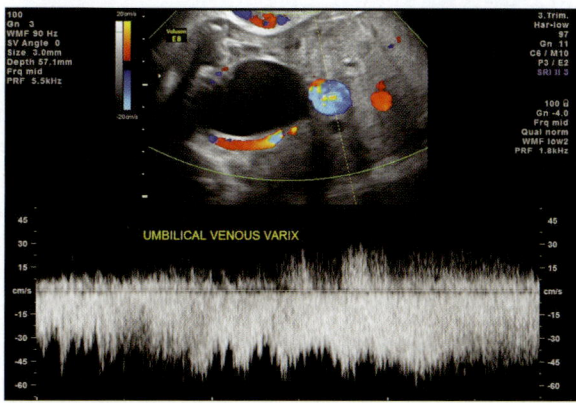

FIG. 57.24 Aneurysm and varix are focal dilations of the umbilical vessels affecting the umbilical artery and vein, respectively. Focal dilation of the umbilical vein is nearly always intraabdominal, but extrahepatic in location. A varix appears on sonography as a dilated intraabdominal, extrahepatic portion of the umbilical vein. Color Doppler shows continuity with the umbilical vein.

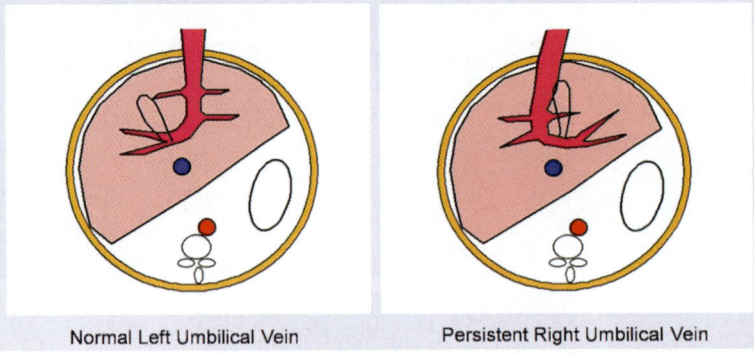
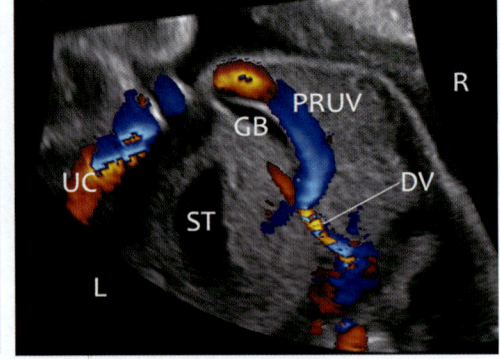

FIG. 57.25 Persistence of the right umbilical vein is rare and may be related to an involution of the left umbilical vein. If it persists, the right umbilical vein enters the right lobe of the liver to join the right portal vein. *DV*, Ductus venosus; *GB*, gallbladder; *PRUV*, persistent right umbilical vein; *ST*, stomach; *UC*, umbilical cord.

hypoplastic than the other. Discordant blood flow would be seen in the umbilical artery Doppler. The resistive index is almost always higher in the smaller artery, and end-diastolic flow may be absent.

Variations in the number of umbilical arteries have been reported. The presence of more than three vessels in the cord has been documented in conjoined twins.

VARIX OF THE UMBILICAL VEIN

Aneurysm and varix are focal dilations of the umbilical vessels affecting the umbilical artery and vein, respectively (Fig. 57.24). Focal dilation of the umbilical vein is nearly always intraabdominal, but extrahepatic in location. A varix appears on sonography as a dilated intraabdominal, extrahepatic portion of the umbilical vein. Color Doppler shows continuity with the umbilical vein. Usually, the prognosis is for a normal outcome in a fetus with a varix of the umbilical vein.

PERSISTENT INTRAHEPATIC RIGHT UMBILICAL VEIN

Persistence of the right umbilical vein is rare and may be related to an involution of the left umbilical vein. If it persists, the right umbilical vein enters the right lobe of the liver to join the right portal vein. At least 50% of patients with this condition have other fetal anomalies as well. On sonography, the umbilical vein curves toward the left-sided stomach rather than toward the liver (Fig. 57.25).

Key Pearls

- The umbilical cord is the essential link for oxygen and important nutrients for the fetus, the placenta, and the mother.
- The umbilical vein transports oxygenated blood from the placenta, and the paired umbilical arteries return deoxygenated blood from the fetus to the placenta for purification.
- The umbilical cord forms during the first 5 weeks of gestation (7 menstrual weeks) as a fusion of the omphalomesenteric (yolk stalk) and allantoic ducts.
- The umbilical cord is covered by the amniotic membrane. The cord includes two umbilical arteries and one umbilical vein and is surrounded by a homogeneous substance called Wharton jelly.
- The umbilical arteries arise from the fetal internal iliac arteries, course alongside the fetal bladder, and exit the umbilicus to form part of the umbilical cord.
- The umbilical vein is formed by the confluence of the chorionic veins of the placenta, with its primary purpose to transport oxygenated blood back to the fetus.
- A short umbilical cord measures less than 35 cm in length and is associated with or is predisposed to the following: oligohydramnios, restricted space (as in multiple gestations), intrinsic fetal anomaly, tethering of the fetus by an amniotic band, inadequate fetal descent, cord compression, fetal distress.
- The normal cord may coil as many as 40 times, usually to the left and near the fetal insertion site.
- A long umbilical cord measures longer than 80 cm and may be associated with or predisposed to the following: polyhydramnios, nuchal cord, true cord knots, umbilical cord compression, cord presentation, prolapse of the cord leading to fetal distress, and umbilical cord stricture or torsion resulting from excessive fetal motion.
- Many of the cord "masses" seen on ultrasound may be attributed to focal accumulation of Wharton jelly and may be isolated or associated with an omphalocele or cyst.
- The omphalocele may consist of a single loop of bowel, or it may contain most of the intestines. The covering for this hernia sac consists of epithelium from the umbilical cord.
- Gastroschisis is usually a right paraumbilical defect involving all layers of the abdominal wall and usually measuring 2 to 4 cm.
- Omphalomesenteric cyst is a cystic lesion of the umbilical cord caused by persistence and dilation of a segment of the omphalomesenteric duct lined by epithelium of gastrointestinal origin.
- Trauma to the umbilical vessels occasionally may cause extravasation of blood into Wharton jelly. This usually occurs near the fetal insertion of the cord.
- Thrombosis of the umbilical vessels is defined as occlusion of one or more vessels of the umbilical cord; primarily it occurs in the umbilical vein.

- The true knot may be formed when a loop of cord is slipped over the infant's head or shoulders during delivery. They have been associated with long cords, polyhydramnios, intrauterine growth restriction, and monoamniotic twins.
- False knots of the umbilical cord are seen when the blood vessels are longer than the cord.
- Nuchal cord is the most common cord entanglement in the fetus.
- The differential proliferation of placenta villi may result in eccentric insertion of the umbilical cord into the placenta. The cord implants into the edge of the placenta (battledore placenta) instead of into the middle of the placenta.
- Membranous or velamentous insertion of the cord occurs when the cord inserts into the membranes before it enters the placenta, rather than inserting directly into the placenta.
- Prolapse of the umbilical cord occurs when the cord lies below the presenting part.
- Vasa previa is defined as the presence of umbilical cord vessels crossing the internal os of the cervix.
- Sonographic detection of a single umbilical artery should prompt the investigation of further fetal anomalies.
- Aneurysm and varix are focal dilations of the umbilical vessels affecting the umbilical artery and vein, respectively.

BIBLIOGRAPHY

Bellotti M, Pennati G, DeGasperi C, et al. Simultaneous measurements of umbilical venous, fetal hepatic, and ductus venosus blood flow in growth-restricted human fetuses. *Am J Obstet Gynecol*. 2004;190:1347–1358.

Bellver J, Lara C, Rossal LP, et al. First-trimester reversed end-diastolic flow in the umbilical artery is not always an ominous sign. *Ultrasound Obstet Gynecol*. 2003;22:652–655.

Bornemeier S, Carpinito LA, Winter TC. Sonographic evaluation of the two-vessel umbilical cord: a comparison between umbilical arteries adjacent to the bladder and cross sections of the umbilical cord. *J Diagn Med Sonogr*. 1996;12:260–265.

Callen P. *Ultrasonography in Obstetrics and Gynecology*. ed 5, Philadelphia: Elsevier; 2008.

Chow JS, Benson CB, Doubilet PM. Frequency and nature of structural anomalies in fetuses with single umbilical arteries. *J Ultrasound Med*. 1998;17:765–768.

Cromi A, Ghezzi F, Duerig P, et al. Sonographic atypical vascular coiling of the umbilical cord. *Prenat Diagn*. 2005;25:1–6.

Di Salvo DN, Benson CB, Laing FC, et al. Sonographic prenatal diagnosis of marginal placental cord insertion: clinical importance. *J Ultrasound Med*. 2002;21:627–632.

Finberg HJ. Avoiding ambiguity in the sonographic determination of the direction of umbilical cord twists. *J Ultrasound Med*. 1992;11:185–187.

Harris RD, Alexander RD. Ultrasound of the placenta and umbilical cord. In: Callen PW, ed. *Ultrasonography in obstetrics and gynecology*. ed 5, Philadelphia: Elsevier; 2008.

Heinonen S, Ryynänen M, Kirkinen P, Saarikoski S. Perinatal diagnostic evaluation of velamentous umbilical cord insertion. *Obstet Gynecol*. 1996;87:112–117.

Kilicdag EB, Kilicdag H, Bagis T, et al. Large pseudocyst of the umbilical cord associated with patent urachus. *J Obstet Gynaecol Res*. 2004;30:444–447.

Marino T. Ultrasound abnormalities of the amniotic fluid, membranes, umbilical cord, and placenta. *Obstet Gynecol Clin North Am*. 2004;31:177–200.

Moore KL, Persaud TVN. *Before We Are Born: Essentials of Embryology and Birth Defects*. ed 7, Philadelphia: Elsevier; 2008.

Oyelese Y, Chavez MR, Yeo L, et al. Three-dimensional sonographic diagnosis of vasa previa. *Ultrasound Obstet Gynecol*. 2004;24:211–215.

Persutte WH, Lenke RR. Transverse umbilical arterial diameter: technique for the prenatal diagnosis of single umbilical artery. *J Ultrasound Med*. 1994;13:763–766.

Petrikovsky B, Schneider E. Prenatal diagnosis and clinical significance of hypoplastic umbilical artery. *Prenat Diagn*. 1996;16:938–940.

Predanic M, Perni SC, Chasen ST, et al. Assessment of umbilical cord coiling during the routine fetal sonographic anatomic survey in the second trimester. *J Ultrasound Med*. 2005;24:185–191.

Predanic M, Perni SC, Chasen ST, et al. Fetal aneuploidy and umbilical cord thickness measured between 14 and 23 weeks' gestational age. *J Ultrasound Med*. 2004;23:1177–1183.

Prucka S, Clemens M, Craven C, et al. Single umbilical artery: what does it mean for the fetus? A case-control analysis of pathologically ascertained cases. *Genet Med*. 2004;6:54–57.

Raio L, Ghezzi F, Cromi A, et al. Sonographic morphology and hyaluronan content of umbilical cords of healthy and Down syndrome fetuses in early gestation. *Early Hum Dev*. 2004;77:1–12.

Ramon Y, Cajal CL, Martinez RO. Prenatal diagnosis of true knot of the umbilical cord. *Ultrasound Obstet Gynecol*. 2004;23:99–100.

Rembouskos G, Cicero S, Longo D, et al. Single umbilical artery at 11-14 weeks' gestation: relation to chromosomal defects. *Ultrasound Obstet Gynecol*. 2003;22:567–570.

Twining P, McHugo JM, Pilling DW. *Textbook of Fetal Abnormalities*. ed 2, London: Churchill Livingstone; 2007.

Woodward PJ, Kennedy A, Sohaey R, et al. *Diagnostic Imaging Obstetrics*. Salt Lake City, UT: Amirsys; 2005.

CHAPTER 58

Amniotic Fluid and Fetal Membranes

Mitzi Roberts

OBJECTIVES

On completion of this chapter, you should be able to:
- Describe how amniotic fluid is derived
- Describe the production of amniotic fluid
- List the functions of amniotic fluid
- Describe methods for assessing amniotic fluid volume
- Determine abnormal volumes of amniotic fluid
- Understand the significance of ruptured membranes
- Describe the significance of amniotic band syndrome
- Differentiate amniotic band syndrome from amniotic sheets with sonography
- Distinguish between immune and nonimmune hydrops
- Identify causes of hydrops
- Recognize the sonographic features of hydrops

OUTLINE

Amniotic Fluid 1474
   Derivation 1474
   Characteristics of Amniotic Fluid 1475
   Assessment of Amniotic Fluid 1475
   Amniotic Fluid Index 1477
   Single Pocket Assessment 1478

Two-Diameter Pocket Assessment 1478
Amniotic Fluid Assessment in Twin Pregnancies 1478
Abnormal Amniotic Fluid Volumes 1479

Fetal Membranes 1481
   Ruptured Fetal Membranes 1482
   Amniotic Band Syndrome 1483
   Amniotic Sheets 1485
Hydrops 1486
   Immune Hydrops 1487
   Nonimmune Hydrops 1488

KEY TERMS

Amniotic band syndrome
Amniotic cavity
Amniotic fluid
Amniotic fluid index (AFI)
Anasarca
Ascites
Asherman syndrome
Chorioamnionitis
Corticosteroid
Edema

Hydramnios
Immune hydrops fetalis (IHF)
Nonimmune hydrops fetalis (NIHF)
Maximum vertical pocket
Oligohydramnios
Pericardial effusion
Pleural effusion
Placental insufficiency
Polyhydramnios

Preterm premature rupture of the membranes (PPROM)
Premature rupture of the membranes (PROM)
Spontaneous premature rupture of the membranes (SPROM)
Subjective assessment
Synechiae
Vernix caseosa

AMNIOTIC FLUID

Amniotic fluid plays a vital role in fetal growth and serves several important functions during intrauterine life. **Amniotic fluid** allows the fetus to move freely within the amniotic cavity while maintaining intrauterine temperature and protecting the developing fetus. Abnormalities of the fluid may interfere with normal fetal development and cause structural abnormalities or may represent an indirect sign of an underlying anomaly.

Derivation

The **amniotic cavity** forms early in fetal life and is filled with amniotic fluid. The fluid surrounds and protects the embryo and, later, the fetus. Amniotic fluid is produced by the umbilical cord, the membranes, lungs, skin, and kidneys. The amount of amniotic fluid present reflects a balance between amniotic fluid production and amniotic fluid removal. The mechanisms of amniotic fluid production and consumption and the composition and volume of amniotic fluid depend on gestational age.

Early in gestation, the main source of amniotic fluid is the amniotic membrane, a thin membrane lined by a single layer of epithelial cells. During this stage of development, water crosses the membrane freely, and the production of amniotic fluid is accomplished by active transport of electrolytes and other solutes by the amnion, with passive diffusion of water following in response to osmotic pressure changes.

As the fetus and placenta mature, amniotic fluid production and consumption change. The change includes movement of fluid across the chorion frondosum and fetal skin, fetal urine output and fetal swallowing, and gastrointestinal absorption. The chorion frondosum (the portion of the chorion that develops into the fetal portion of the placenta) is a site where water is exchanged freely between fetal blood and amniotic fluid across the amnion. Fetal skin is also permeable to water and some solutes to permit a direct exchange between the fetus and amniotic fluid until keratinization occurs at 24 to 26 weeks. Fetal production of urine and the ability to swallow begins between 8 and 11 weeks of gestation. The amount of urine produced is most significant at approximately 18 to 20 weeks of gestation. Fetal urination into the amniotic sac accounts for nearly the total volume of amniotic fluid by the second half of pregnancy. The quantity of fluid is directly related to kidney function and urination. In turn, the fetus swallows amniotic fluid, which is absorbed by the digestive tract.

Characteristics of Amniotic Fluid

Amniotic fluid has the following six functions:
1. Acts as a cushion to protect the fetus
2. Allows embryonic and fetal movements
3. Prevents adherence of the amnion to the embryo
4. Allows symmetric growth
5. Maintains a constant temperature
6. Acts as a reservoir to fetal metabolites before their excretion by the maternal system

Quantity of Fluid. The amount of amniotic fluid is regulated not only by the production of fluid but also by removal of the fluid by swallowing, by fluid exchange within the lungs, the membranes, and the umbilical cord (Fig. 58.1). Normal lung development depends critically on the exchange of amniotic fluid within the lungs. Inadequate lung development may occur when the amount of amniotic fluid is severely low, placing the fetus at high risk for developing small or hypoplastic lungs.

The volume of amniotic fluid increases progressively until about 33 weeks of gestation, with the average increment per week of 25 mL from the 11th to the 15th week and 50 mL from the 15th to 28th week of gestation. In the last trimester, the mean amniotic fluid volume does not change significantly (Box 58.1). The sonographer must be aware of the relative differences in amniotic fluid volume throughout pregnancy. During the second and early third trimester of pregnancy, amniotic fluid appears to surround the fetus and should be readily visible. From 20 to 30 weeks of gestation, amniotic fluid may appear rather generous, although this typically represents a normal amniotic fluid variant. By the end of pregnancy, the amniotic fluid is limited and appears sonographically as isolated fluid pockets. Toward the end of the pregnancy, after 38 weeks of gestation, there is a general decline in the amniotic fluid.

Sonographic Appearance. Amniotic fluid generally appears echo-free, although occasionally, echogenic fluid particles may be seen (Fig. 58.2). The echogenic fluid particles may represent a normal variant, particulate matter, **vernix caseosa**, intraamniotic blood, or intrauterine meconium passage. The term *amniotic sludge* has been used to describe a dense collection of echogenic particles within the fluid at the level of the cervix. The presence of sludge may be related to intrauterine infection and is associated with the risk of preterm premature rupture of membranes (ROM), chorioamnionitis, and preterm delivery. In cases of intrauterine meconium passage, the amniotic fluid may take on an echogenic "snowstorm" appearance.

Assessment of Amniotic Fluid

In accordance with the guidelines for obstetric scanning, every obstetric examination should include a thorough evaluation of amniotic fluid volume. Abnormal amounts of amniotic fluid are described as hydramnios (**polyhydramnios**)

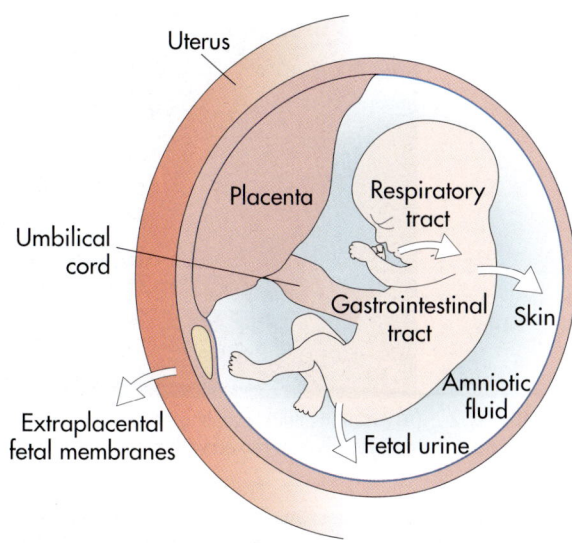

FIG. 58.1 Amniotic fluid formation.

BOX 58.1 Amniotic Fluid Volume Regulation

- Amniotic fluid volume increases rapidly during first trimester
- Fetus swallows fluid; reabsorbed by gastrointestinal tract; recirculates through kidneys
- Increased amniotic fluid production in first trimester
- By 20 weeks of gestation, amniotic fluid volume increases by 10 mL/day
- Amount of fluid produced by fetal urination slightly exceeds amount removed by fetal swallowing; less than 40% of fluid increase originates from other sources

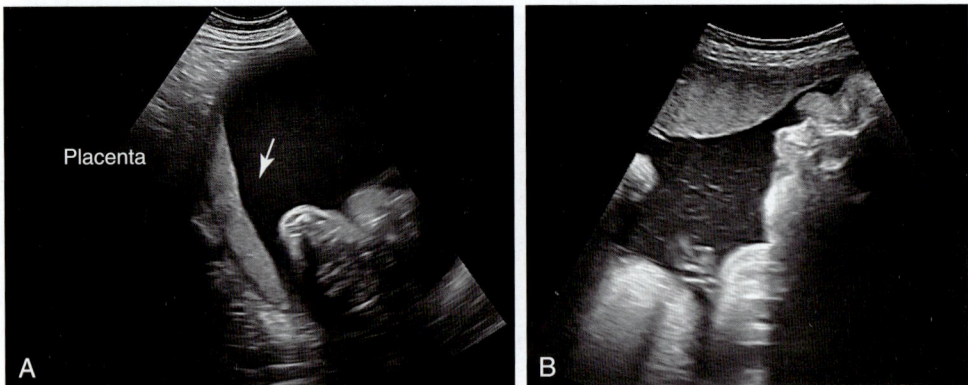

FIG. 58.2 (A) Amniotic fluid revealing echo-free fluid appearance and a flattened placenta due to polyhydramnios. (B) At 37 weeks of gestation, the amniotic fluid is mixed with particulate matter or vernix.

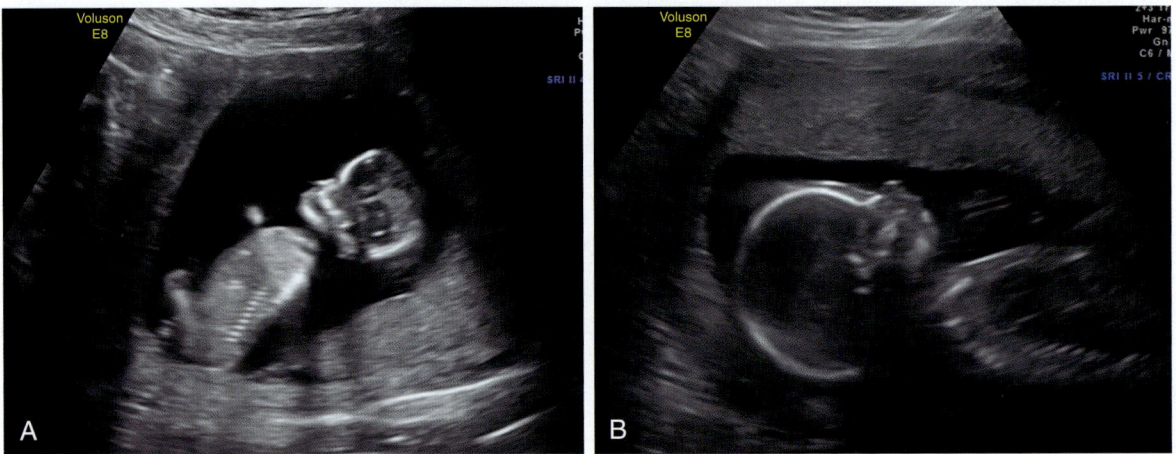

FIG. 58.3 (A) Amniotic fluid around a 13-week-old fetus in a sitting position. (B) Amniotic fluid around an 18-week-old fetus.

and oligohydramnios. **Hydramnios** refers to an increase of amniotic fluid, whereas oligohydramnios refers to a decreased amount of amniotic fluid. When extremes in amniotic fluid volume (hydramnios or oligohydramnios) are found, targeted studies for the exclusion of fetal anomalies are recommended. In some instances, the cause of the abnormal fluid levels may be associated with maternal factors, unknown etiologies, or correlation with fetal weight (small-for-age fetus has decreased amniotic fluid, whereas large-for-age fetus has increased volume of fluid). The amount of amniotic fluid present can be determined in several ways.

Subjective Assessment. Subjective assessment is performed as the sonographer initially scans "through" the entire uterus to determine the visual assessment of the fluid present, fetal position, and the location of the placenta (Fig. 58.3). When amniotic fluid is assessed subjectively, decreased amniotic fluid is identified by an overall sense of crowding of the fetus and obvious lack of amniotic fluid and/or inability to identify any significant pockets of fluid in any sector of the uterus (Fig. 58.4). Excessive fluid is defined subjectively; when there is an obvious excess of fluid, the fetus appears in the most dependent portion of the uterus, or the fetus appears to move excessively for the gestational age (Fig. 58.5). This subjective assessment is

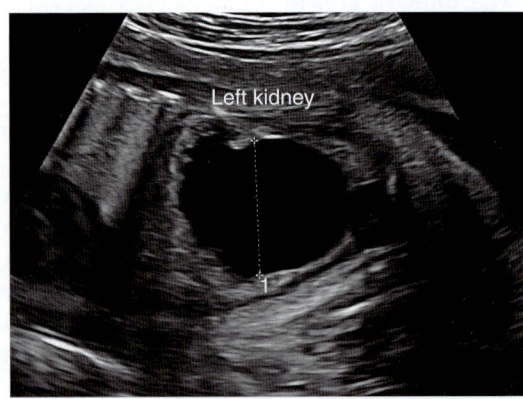

FIG. 58.4 Obvious lack of fluid surrounding this 26-week-old fetus presenting with a bladder outlet obstruction. The left kidney is visualized with severe hydronephrosis.

more successful in the hands of experienced sonographers than in the hands of a beginner. The subjective assessment leads the sonographer to perform a more quantitative method to document the amount of amniotic fluid.

Quantitative Assessment. Several methods are used to calculate an amniotic fluid measurement. Each obstetric center may use one or a combination of the methods. These methods include amniotic fluid index (AFI), single pocket assessment, and two-diameter pocket assessment. Each department should have clear guidelines for sonographers to use when assessing amniotic fluid. These guidelines will help to aid in proper amniotic fluid assessments when multiple sonographers are monitoring the same patient.

Amniotic Fluid Index

The **amniotic fluid index (AFI)** is used most frequently for evaluating and quantifying amniotic fluid volume at different intervals during a pregnancy. The AFI method is both a valid and a reproducible technique. With this method, the uterine cavity is divided into four equal quadrants by two imaginary lines perpendicular to each other (Fig. 58.6). The largest vertical pocket of amniotic fluid, excluding fetal structures, or umbilical cord loops, is measured.

The sonographer should hold the transducer in the sagittal plane and perpendicular to the table (not the curved skin surface) when determining these pockets of fluid. Each quadrant should be evaluated to reflect the most accurate display of fluid. The transducer should be moved until the cord loops and/or fetal structures are not visualized within the pocket of fluid (Fig. 58.7). Care must be taken not to include the thickness of the maternal uterine wall in the measurement or apply too much pressure to the skin, causing the pocket of fluid to appear smaller. Slight adjustment of the gain will aid in the

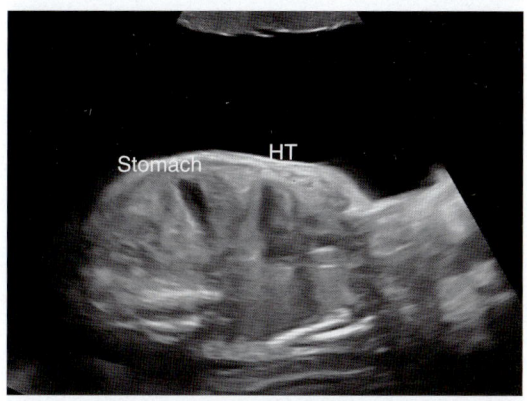

FIG. 58.5 Fetus presenting with severe polyhydramnios at 30 weeks of gestation. *HT*, Heart.

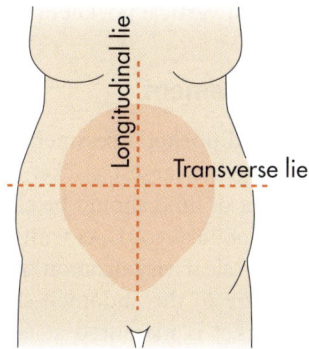

FIG. 58.6 The amniotic cavity is divided into quadrants by two imaginary lines perpendicular to each other. The largest pocket of fluid is measured in each quadrant.

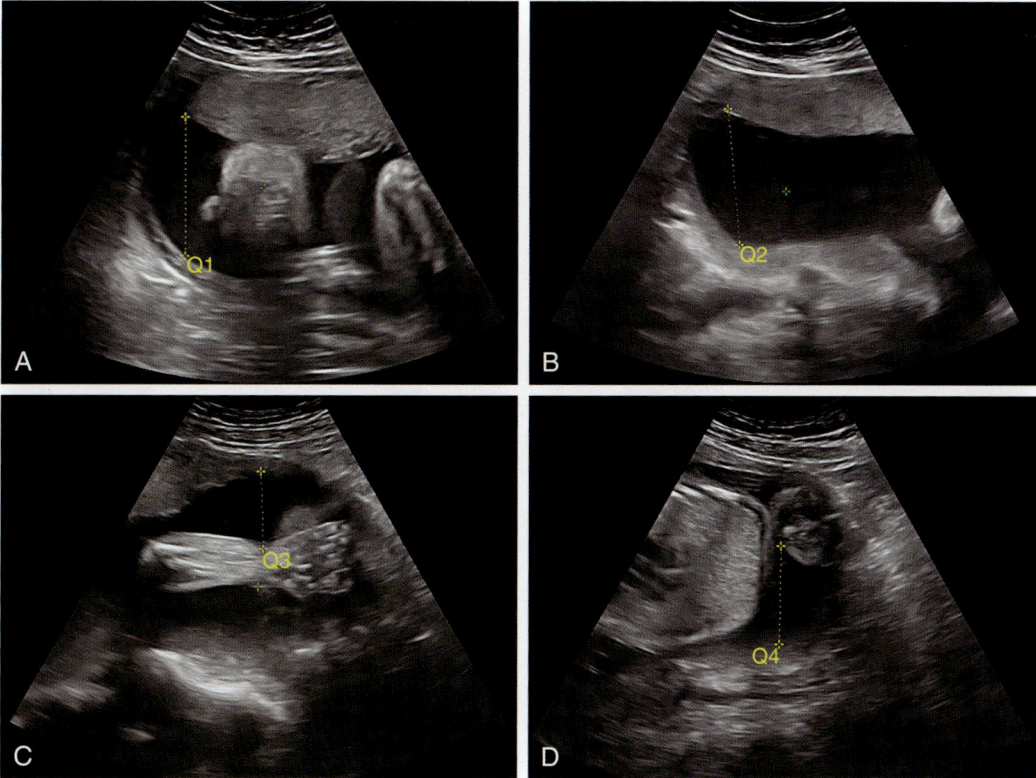

FIG. 58.7 The deepest vertical pocket is measured in each quadrant free of any fetal components.

visualization of the uterine wall or visualization of the umbilical cord within the fluid. Color Doppler technology can be used to document a pocket of fluid free of the umbilical cord or any fetal structures.

Normal values have been calculated for each gestational age (±2 standard deviations). The values are relatively stable after 20 weeks until the end of the third trimester. The AFI peaks late in the third trimester of pregnancy, with a rapid decline near term.

- Normal amniotic fluid correlates with an AFI of 10 to 20 cm.
- Borderline values of 5 to 10 cm indicate low fluid, and values of 20 to 24 cm indicate increased fluid.
- Oligohydramnios correlates with an AFI of less than 5 cm, with the largest vertical pocket measuring 2 cm or less.
- Polyhydramnios correlates with an AFI of greater than 24 cm and the largest vertical pocket of 8 cm or more.

Single Pocket Assessment

The **maximum vertical pocket** assessment of amniotic fluid is done by identifying the largest pocket of amniotic fluid (Fig. 58.8). The pocket of fluid should be clear of fetal structures as well as the umbilical cord. As with the AFI, the gain should be adjusted for clear visualization of the uterine wall, and minimum pressure to the abdomen should be applied. The depth of the pocket is measured at right angles to the uterine contour and placed into three categories:
1. Less than 2 cm, indicating oligohydramnios
2. From 2 to 8 cm, indicating normal amniotic fluid
3. Greater than 8 cm, indicating polyhydramnios

Two-Diameter Pocket Assessment

The two-diameter pocket determination uses the largest pocket of amniotic fluid. The horizontal and vertical dimensions of the maximum vertical pocket are multiplied together to obtain a single volume. A two-diameter pocket of 15 to 50 cm is considered normal (Fig. 58.9).

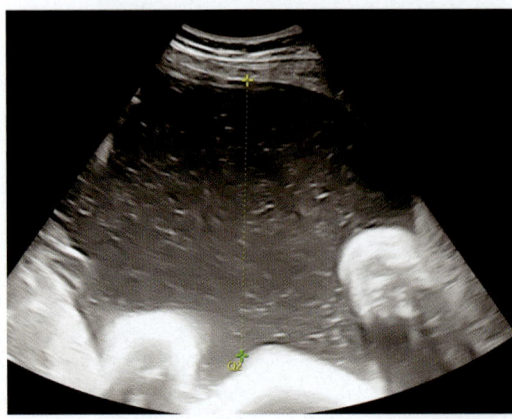

FIG. 58.8 A single largest vertical pocket is noted measuring 18.65 cm.

Amniotic Fluid Assessment in Twin Pregnancies

In twin pregnancies, it is important to assess each sac independently when performing amniotic fluid determinations (Fig. 58.10). Twin pregnancies have a slightly lower median AFI value than singleton pregnancies. However, in polyhydramnios, the largest vertical pocket has been reported to be more accurate (Fig. 58.11). Because the AFI gives an overall assessment of the pregnancy, it does not accurately show differences between sacs. The only method for accurately

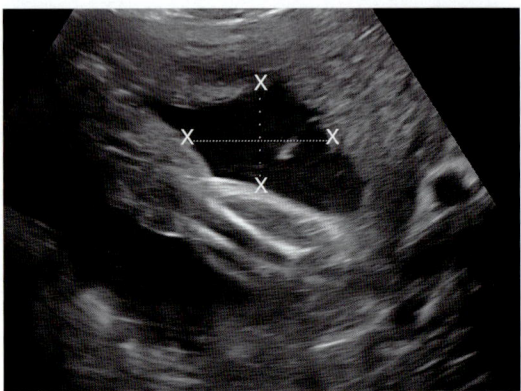

FIG. 58.9 The two-diameter measurement technique.

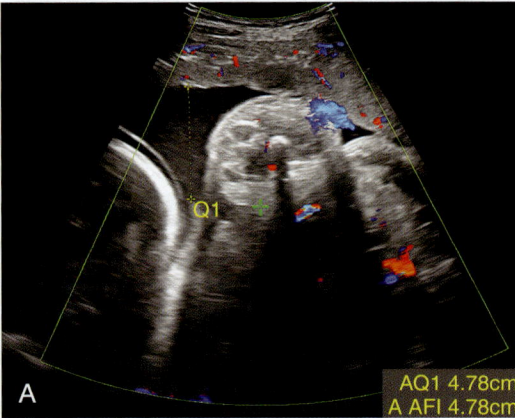

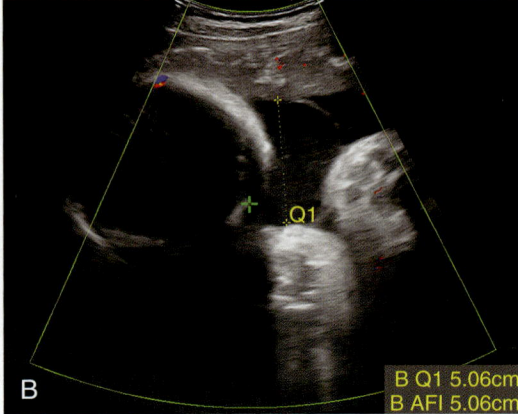

FIG. 58.10 (A) Measurement of the largest vertical pocket of fluid for twin A. Color Doppler is used to ensure the cord is not present within the pocket (+ indicates fetal body of twin A). (B) Measurement of the largest vertical pocket of fluid for twin B. Note the visualization of the dividing membrane (+ indicates fetal head of twin B).

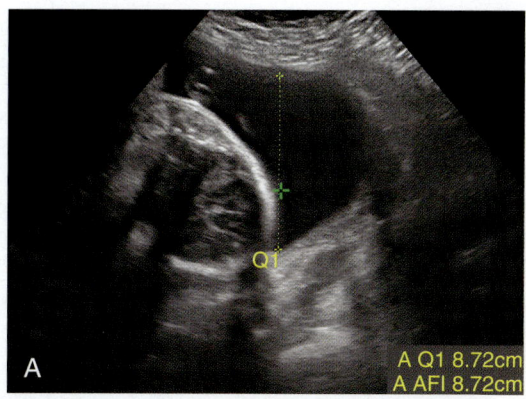 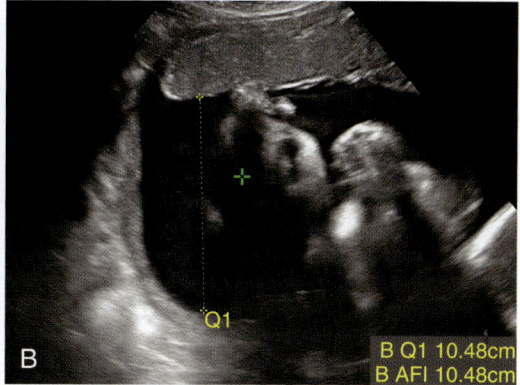

FIG. 58.11 Single vertical pocket measurements are used in this twin pregnancy at 30 weeks of gestation with polyhydramnios.

determining the amount of amniotic fluid is the dye-determined method. It can be used in singleton or multiple gestations. The dye technique requires injection of dye into the sac(s) via amniocentesis; after 20 minutes, another amniocentesis is performed in which 1 mL greater than the injected dye is removed and frozen; and then the fluid/dye mixture is evaluated for the amount of concentrate, which determines the amniotic fluid volume.

Abnormal Amniotic Fluid Volumes

Polyhydramnios. Polyhydramnios (also known as hydramnios) is defined as an amniotic fluid volume of greater than 2000 mL. In addition, the finding of polyhydramnios is associated with increased perinatal mortality and morbidity and maternal complications. By clinical definition, polyhydramnios is an excessive amount of fluid that causes the uterine size to be larger than expected for gestational age. Often the patient will present for a sonographic examination with the clinical finding of uterus larger than dates.

Etiology. The amniotic fluid compartment is in a dynamic equilibrium with the fetal and maternal compartments. In polyhydramnios, the equilibrium shifts so that the net transfer of water is into the amniotic space. As discussed earlier, many factors are involved in the regulation of amniotic fluid volume (e.g., swallowing, urination, uterine-placental blood flow, fetal respiratory movements, and fetal membrane physiology).

Clinical Findings. Increased amniotic fluid volume produces uterine stretching and enlargement that may lead to preterm labor and various other maternal symptoms. In addition, the acute onset of hydramnios may result in painful maternal clinical symptoms, compress other organs or vascular structures, cause hydronephrosis of the kidneys, or produce shortness of breath from compression of the organs on the diaphragm.

Often polyhydramnios may be diagnosed sonographically before it is clinically suspected. Chronic hydramnios characteristically develops between the 28th week of gestation and term. Acute polyhydramnios may develop over a few days or chronically over weeks. Acute polyhydramnios occurs in the second trimester and accounts for only 2% of the cases. Usually, the cause of acute polyhydramnios is congenital anomalies or twin-to-twin transfusion syndrome.

Polyhydramnios is often associated with central nervous system disorders and/or gastrointestinal problems. Central nervous system disorders cause depressed swallowing. With gastrointestinal abnormalities, often a blockage (atresia) of the esophagus, stomach, duodenum, or small bowel results in ineffective swallowing. Fetal hydrops, skeletal anomalies, and some renal disorders (usually unilateral) may also be associated with hydramnios. Other forms of polyhydramnios that cannot be explained by congenital anomalies are considered idiopathic (Box 58.2). Maternal conditions such as diabetes mellitus, obesity, Rh incompatibility, anemia, congestive cardiac failure, and syphilis have been associated with polyhydramnios.

Prognosis. Once polyhydramnios has been diagnosed, the prognosis for pregnancy is guarded. There is increased perinatal mortality and morbidity, as well as increased maternal morbidity and mortality. The mother has an increased risk of developing pregnancy-induced hypertension, preterm labor, or postpartum hemorrhage. Other conditions associated with increased amniotic fluid volume include maternal diabetes mellitus, fetal macrosomia, and Rh isoimmunization. Diabetes mellitus is associated with an increased frequency of hydramnios and represents the most common maternal cause of elevated amniotic fluid volume, especially when poorly controlled.

Sonographic Findings. Serial sonographic examinations are indicated to monitor the progression of amniotic fluid. Amniotic fluid production is a dynamic process. Changes in maternal, fetal, or placental conditions may dramatically affect the AFI.

The visual criteria for polyhydramnios include an obvious discrepancy between the size of the fetus, the size of the uterus, and the amount of amniotic fluid. During the second trimester, the amniotic fluid completely surrounds the fetus; however, as the pregnancy progresses, the fetal parts consume the majority of the uterine space, and therefore the amount of amniotic fluid appears to be less than in the first and second trimesters. Serial scans may be necessary when the amniotic

BOX 58.2	Congenital Anomalies Associated With Polyhydramnios

Gastrointestinal System
Esophageal atresia and/or tracheoesophageal fistula
Duodenal atresia
Jejunoileal atresia
Gastroschisis
Omphalocele
Diaphragmatic hernia
Meckel diverticulum
Congenital megacolon
Meconium peritonitis
Annular pancreas
Pancreatic cyst

Head and Neck
Cystic hygroma
Goiter
Cleft palate
Epignathus

Respiratory System
Cystic adenomatoid malformation
Extralobar sequestration
Primary pulmonary hypoplasia
Congenital pulmonary lymphangiectasia
Asphyxiating thoracic dystrophy
Arrhythmias
Coarctation of the aorta
Myxomas and hemangiomas
Ectopia cordis
Cardiac tumors
Heart anomalies with hydrops

Genitourinary System
Ureteropelvic junction obstruction
Posterior urethral valves
Urethral stenosis
Multicystic kidney disease
Large ovarian cyst
Mesoblastic nephroma
Bartter syndrome
Megacystis microcolon hypoperistalsis syndrome
Thanatophoric dwarf
Camptomelic dwarf
Osteogenesis imperfecta
Heterozygous achondroplasia
Arthrogryposis multiplex
Klippel-Feil syndrome
Nager acrofacial dysostosis
Achondrogenesis

Congenital Infections
Cytomegalovirus
Toxoplasmosis
Listeriosis
Congenital hepatitis

Miscellaneous
Sacrococcygeal teratoma
Cranial teratoma
Cervical teratoma
Congenital sarcoma
Placental chorioangioma
Cavernous hemangioma
Metastatic neuroblastoma
Myotonic dystrophy
Fetal acetaminophen toxicity
Retroperitoneal fibrosis
Multisystem anomalies
Pena-Shokeir syndrome
Cutaneous vascular hemarthrosis
Twin reversed arterial perfusion sequence/acardiac anomaly

From Nyberg DA, Mahony BS, Pretorius DH. *Diagnostic Ultrasound of Fetal Anomalies: Text and Atlas.* St Louis: Mosby–Year Book; 1990.

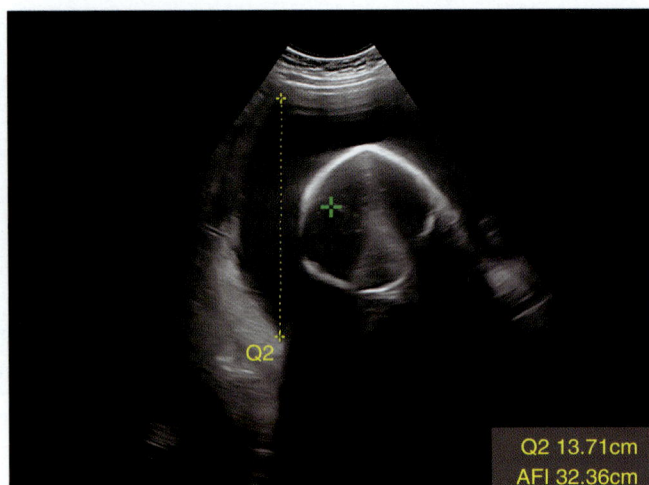

FIG. 58.12 Fetus presenting at 29 weeks of gestation with duodenal atresia. The single vertical pocket measurement of 13.71 cm suggests polyhydramnios. An amniotic fluid index measurement of 32.36 cm supported the findings (+ indicates fetal head).

BOX 58.3	Causes of Oligohydramnios

Nonanomalous Conditions
- Intrauterine growth restriction
- Premature rupture of membranes
- Postdate pregnancy (42 weeks)
- Chorionic villus sampling

Fetal Anomalous Conditions
- Infantile polycystic kidney disease
- Renal agenesis
- Posterior urethral valve syndrome
- Dysplastic kidneys
- Chromosomal abnormalities

fluid appears to be more generous than normal at a particular gestational age. Sonographic signs of polyhydramnios are as follows:
- Appearance of a freely floating fetus within the swollen amniotic cavity (the fetus commonly will be seen lying on his or her back, freely moving in the amniotic fluid)
- Accentuated fetal anatomy as increased amniotic fluid improves image resolution
- AFI equal to or greater than 20 cm.

Polyhydramnios may be further defined as mild when the single largest pocket is greater than 8 cm; moderate, greater than 12 cm; and severe, greater than 16 cm. The AFI may also be further qualified as mild polyhydramnios, greater than 20 cm; moderate, greater than 24 cm; and severe, greater than 25 cm (Fig. 58.12).

Oligohydramnios. *Oligohydramnios* is an overall reduction in the amount of amniotic fluid resulting in fetal crowding and decreased fetal movement. The incidence of oligohydramnios is estimated to be between 0.5% and 5.5% of all pregnancies, depending on the population tested and the criteria used for diagnosis.

Etiology. The development of oligohydramnios may be attributed to one of five causes: congenital anomalies (Box 58.3), intrauterine growth restriction (IUGR), post-term pregnancies, ruptured membranes, and iatrogenesis. Second-trimester oligohydramnios is associated with a poor prognosis, especially if maternal serum alpha-fetoprotein level is concurrently elevated. Maternal conditions associated with oligohydramnios include hypertension, preeclampsia, chronic cardiac or renal disease, connective tissue disorders, and patients receiving indomethacin.

Clinical Findings. The association between IUGR and decreased amniotic fluid (oligohydramnios) is well recognized. Fetal hypoxemia may produce growth restriction and oligohydramnios. There is a fourfold increased risk of growth delay when oligohydramnios is present. Doppler evaluation of the growth-restricted fetus shows abnormal umbilical flow in patients with oligohydramnios.

Placental insufficiency may cause IUGR associated with oligohydramnios. The placental insufficiency produces a redistribution of fetal blood flow away from the kidneys and toward the brain to counterattack the hypoxia. This results in decreased urine output, which decreases fluid volume.

Post-term pregnancy is defined as a gestational age of 42 weeks or more. Oligohydramnios is a common complication of postdate pregnancies (remember the decrease in amniotic fluid production near the end of pregnancy), and it is associated with diminished placental function. It is also associated with arterial redistribution of fetal blood flow with the brain-sparing effect.

Iatrogenic causes of oligohydramnios include medications, insensible fluid loss, maternal intravascular fluid depletion, and prior procedures such as chorionic villus sampling. Medications associated with oligohydramnios include nonsteroidal antiinflammatory drugs, angiotensin-converting enzyme inhibitors, calcium channel blockers, and nitrous oxide. The nonsteroidal drugs are prostaglandin synthetase inhibitors that inhibit renal vascular flow and decrease glomerular filtration. The angiotensin-converting-enzyme inhibitors reduce fetal blood pressure and decrease renal perfusion (see Box 58.3).

Prognosis. The development of oligohydramnios may cause potential complications, such as fetal demise, pulmonary hypoplasia, and various skeletal and facial deformities from the compression of the fetus on the uterine wall. Fetal deformations, such as clubbing of the hands or feet, pulmonary hypoplasia, hip displacement, and phenotypical features of Potter's sequence have been reported. The fetus that presents with oligohydramnios in the second trimester has a higher prevalence of structural malformations than the fetus that presents in the third trimester.

Persistent oligohydramnios in the second trimester carries a poor prognosis regardless of the cause. Severe oligohydramnios with a single pocket measurement of less than 1 cm lasting 14 days after a spontaneous premature rupture of the membranes (PROM) at less than 25 weeks of gestation is associated with an extremely high mortality rate.

Maternal hydration has been shown to improve amniotic fluid for patients with oligohydramnios and in women with normal amniotic fluid volumes. If fetal anomalies or premature ruptured membranes are present, maternal hydration will have little effect. A study was performed to see if maternal hydration would increase the AFI in women with low AFIs. The control group was instructed to drink their normal amount of fluid; the hydration group was instructed to drink 2 L of water in addition to their usual amount of fluid 2 to 4 hours before the posttreatment AFI was determined. The mean posttreatment AFI was significantly greater in the hydration group. The findings suggested that maternal oral hydration increased the amniotic fluid volume in women with decreased fluid levels.

Sonographic Findings. Criteria for oligohydramnios are based on subjective experience and quantitative methods. Oligohydramnios may be defined as a single pocket of fluid with a depth of less than 2 cm or an AFI of less than 5 cm. A gray zone for decreased fluid ranges from 5 to 9 cm when a four-quadrant approach is used. Poor scanning resolution is common in pregnancies complicated by oligohydramnios, and limited anatomy surveys are expected (Fig. 58.13). The sonographer should consider examining the fetus with endovaginal sonography to better define fetal anatomy in an effort to detect the anomaly causing the oligohydramnios.

If the intrauterine membranes are not ruptured and oligohydramnios is present before 28 weeks of gestation, careful evaluation of the fetal renal system should be made by the sonographer to rule out fetal abnormalities such as renal agenesis, infantile polycystic disease, or posterior urethral valve syndrome. If the oligohydramnios is severe in a fetus with posterior urethral valves, the prognosis is typically poor. Identification of the renal area may be difficult to assess in the presence of severe oligohydramnios, and the use of color Doppler to demarcate the renal arteries may be helpful for the sonographer to determine the presence of kidneys.

In the presence of oligohydramnios, care should be taken when evaluating the fetal growth parameters because the fetal head and abdomen can be compressed when the fluid level is low. The lack of surrounding fluid protecting the fetus can result in the circumferences being inaccurately measured by increased transducer pressure on the maternal abdomen. This pressure, in turn, may alter the estimated fetal weight by erroneous measurements. Evaluation of the blood flow in the umbilical cord, the placenta, and the cerebrovascular system with color and Doppler techniques is critical to determine the presence or absence of IUGR.

FETAL MEMBRANES

The primary fetal membranes are known as amnion and chorion. The chorion is derived from the outer layer of the developing blastocyst, specifically the chorion laeve and the chorion frondosum. The amnion is derived from the inner cell mass of the blastocyst and is attached to the embryonic disc at the insertion of the umbilical cord. The chorionic

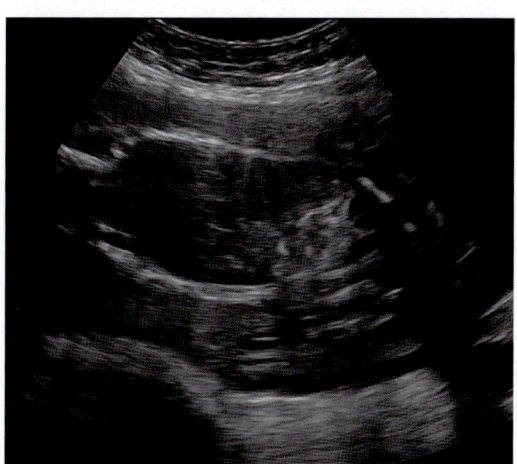

FIG. 58.13 Fetal anatomy is difficult to evaluate due to oligohydramnios.

membrane is always in contact with the developing decidua and is separated from the amnion with fluid early in embryonic development (Fig. 58.14). The amniotic membrane is very thin (0.02 to 0.5 mm) and echogenic. It is mostly seen as a small line; however, under certain circumstances, it can be seen as a circular membrane surrounding the embryo (Fig. 58.15). The amnion can be visualized within the chorionic cavity with endovaginal sonography between 4 and 5 weeks of gestation. The amnion will grow approximately 1 mm/day and fuse with the chorion between 12 and 16 weeks of gestation (Fig. 58.16). The fusion results in the development of the amniotic cavity surrounded by the chorioamniotic membrane. Abnormalities involving the fetal membranes can occur at multiple points in the pregnancy. It is important for sonographers to evaluate the membranes, differentiate membranes from other abnormalities, and identify abnormalities associated with disruptions in the membranes.

Ruptured Fetal Membranes

The tissue makeup of the chorioamniotic membrane consists of several types of cells. The integrity and makeup of the cells aid in the determination of the strength of the membrane. Under normal conditions, the chorioamniotic membranes rupture due to normal cell death activation of enzymes and mechanical forces. Normally the membranes will rupture after the onset of labor. **Premature rupture of the membranes (PROM), preterm premature rupture of the membranes (PPROM),** and **spontaneous rupture of the membranes (SPROM)** describe conditions in which the membranes rupture abnormally, resulting in loss of amniotic fluid and/or oligohydramnios.

Etiology. The ROM too soon, before labor, or both has numerous causes. The cause may be due to normal cell death, activation of enzymes, and mechanical forces present just as in normal cases. Multiple underlying pathologic processes have also been associated with abnormal ruptured membranes. Research has indicated that several other factors may play a role in increasing the risk of abnormal ruptured membranes. Those risks include smokers, history of sexually transmitted disease, African American descent, vaginal bleeding, previous preterm delivery, lower socioeconomic status, presence of intrauterine infection, and pregnancy-related invasive procedures.

Clinical Findings. Patients who are suspected of having ROM clinically present with a sudden leaking of fluid in large or

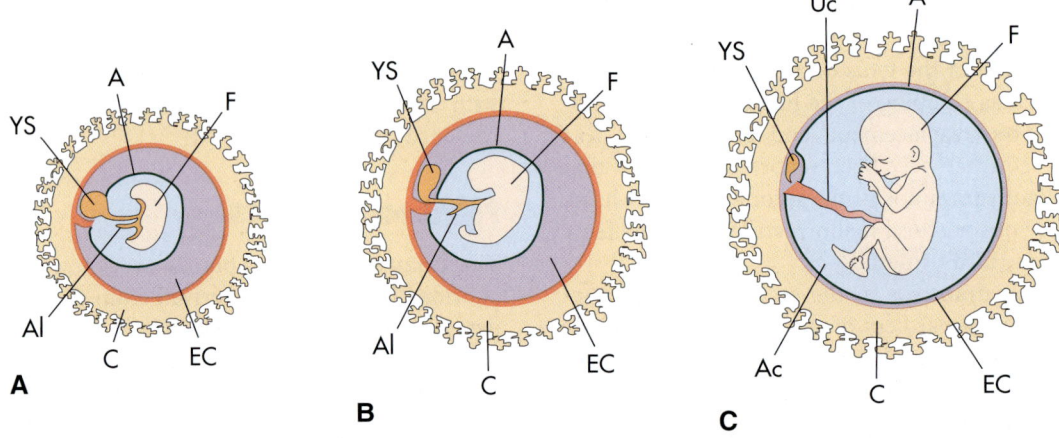

FIG. 58.14 (A) Four-week gestation. The amnion is formed from cells found on the interior of the developing cell mass that is to become the fetus and placenta. (B) Six-week gestation. (C) Eight-week gestation. *A*, amnion; *Ac*, amniotic cavity; *Al*, allantois; *C*, chorion; *EC*, extraembryonic coelom; *F*, fetus; *Uc*, umbilical cord; *YS*, yolk sac.

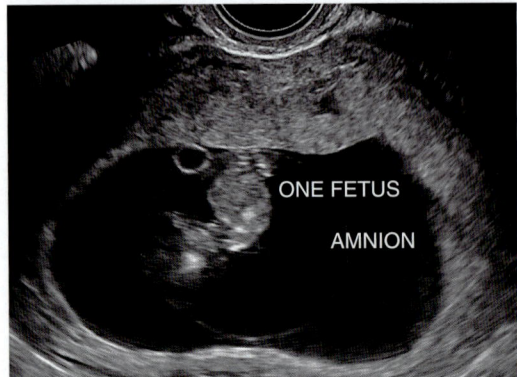

FIG. 58.15 Transverse scan demonstrating the amnion dividing the amniotic cavity and chorionic cavity at 10 weeks of gestation.

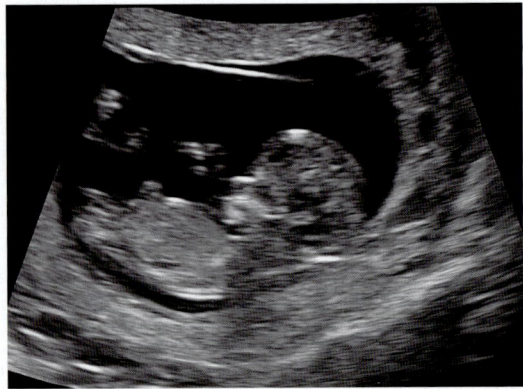

FIG. 58.16 In this image of a 12-week fetus, the amnion can be seen as an echogenic line unattached from the chorion anteriorly.

small amounts. The patient often refers to this symptom as "water break." On physical examination, nitrazine paper and fern test is used as a screening test to determine the presence of amniotic fluid in vaginal secretions. The patient will also be checked for cervical dilation, as well as leaking of fluid with coughing or fundal pressure. It has been documented that an amniocentesis may be performed to inject an indigo carmine dye into the amniotic sac. If the membranes are truly ruptured, the patient will leak blue dye from the vagina. To estimate the amount of amniotic fluid present and evaluate fetal well-being, a sonogram is performed.

Prognosis. The prognosis of a fetus affected by abnormal ruptured membranes is dependent on the fetal gestational age, fetal status, and the ability to control uterine contractions. In general, abnormal rupture of the membranes is associated with preterm delivery (common), fetal and neonatal death, neonatal respiratory distress, prolapsed umbilical cord, chorioamnionitis, and placental abruption. Approximately one-third of all preterm births have been associated with PROM.

Pregnancy management for patients presenting with ROM includes hospitalization, fetal monitoring (nonstress test and biophysical profile [BPP]), bed rest, administration of antibiotics (**chorioamnionitis**), and **corticosteroid** therapy. Although there are variations in treatment for patients presenting with ROM, pregnancy management may include the following:

- Active labor, consistent abnormal fetal heart tracings, evidence of amniotic infection, placental abruption, or cord prolapsed indicates delivery of the fetus.
- If rupture of the membranes occurs at 24 to 33 weeks of gestation, follow-up procedure includes administration of corticosteroids, antibiotics, and delivery at approximately 34 weeks of gestation.
- An amniocentesis is performed to verify fetal lung maturity in cases in which the fetus needs to be delivered before 34 weeks of gestation.
- If the fetus is between 34 and 36 weeks of gestation, antibiotics are usually given, followed by delivery.
- It is common for term patients who experience ROM to move into active labor within 24 hours.

Sonographic Findings. The role of sonography in patients presenting with ROM includes documenting the integrity of the placenta, fetal size, amniotic fluid volume, fetal well-being, and fetal Doppler studies. The information gathered is important in determining pregnancy management. Although not all patients with ROM will present for sonography, it is common for patients to be evaluated sonographically every day to assess fetal well-being and fluid volumes.

The integrity of the placenta, fetal growth, and BPP should be evaluated. Placental abruption is associated with ROM. Sonographers should pay close attention to the retroplacental complex and the anterior-posterior diameter of the placenta. The sonographic appearance of abruptions will vary. However, a few key findings may be helpful in identifying abruption. Those findings include areas of increased diameter, areas of questionable echogenicity, interrupted retroplacental complex, or abnormal continuum of the attachment of the placenta to the uterine wall. Placenta location is essential as well when documenting the integrity of the placenta. Abnormal location of the placenta, such as circumvallate placenta, is associated with placental abruption and oligohydramnios. Documentation of the placenta should be followed by fetal growth measurements. Sonography is not reliable in determining fetal growth day to day; it is usually most reliable when measurements are taken at 2-week intervals. Initial weight and age estimations provided by sonography will help physicians determine pregnancy management, as well as be prepared to advise the mother and other health care providers of vital information for delivery preparation. The longer the pregnancy can be maintained, the more sonography can aid in providing fetal growth information. Along with evaluating the placenta and fetal growth, assessing the fetal well-being plays a significant role in the management of the pregnancy. The fetal well-being should be evaluated sonographically by performing a BPP. These examinations are usually done daily to monitor the fetus for amniotic fluid volumes, fetal breathing movements, fetal tone, and fetal gross body movements. Abnormal results or sudden changes may indicate fetal distress, thus changing the course of pregnancy management.

Patients presenting with ROM may present with oligohydramnios. Oligohydramnios may be defined as a single pocket of fluid with a depth of less than 2 cm or an AFI of less than 5 cm (Fig. 58.17). It has been noted that patients presenting with less than 2 cm of fluid have been associated with intrauterine infections. Although there is increased significance of infection in patients with severe oligohydramnios, other findings should be considered. Other findings associated with intrauterine infection or chorioamnionitis include changes to fetal heart rate (tachycardia) and fetal behavioral states (specifically, lack of fetal breathing). One should also note that maternal clinical symptoms may also be present. Those symptoms include fever, tachycardia, tender uterus, possible abnormal white blood cell count, and abnormal vaginal discharge.

Color and spectral Doppler are used to indicate alterations in blood flow that can help determine the degree of fetal distress. Umbilical artery, umbilical vein, middle cerebral artery (MCA), and ductus venosus blood flow aid in determining fetal distress. In cases of ROM, fetuses are at risk for umbilical cord compression or prolapse. These conditions may first be indicated by variable decelerations on fetal heart monitor tracings as well as lack of fetal movements by the mother. The use of color and spectral Doppler can provide information regarding blood perfusion in the fetus. If compression or prolapse is evident, an amnioinfusion (saline is injected directly into the amniotic sac) may be helpful in decompressing the cord. If the fetus is in continued distress, delivery is indicated.

Amniotic Band Syndrome

Amniotic band syndrome (ABS) is associated with an abnormality in the fetal membranes. It is a common, nonrecurrent cause of various fetal malformations involving the limbs, craniofacial region, and trunk. Numerous synonyms have been documented to describe the disruption of fetal tissue due to the presence of amniotic bands. Synonyms include ADAM

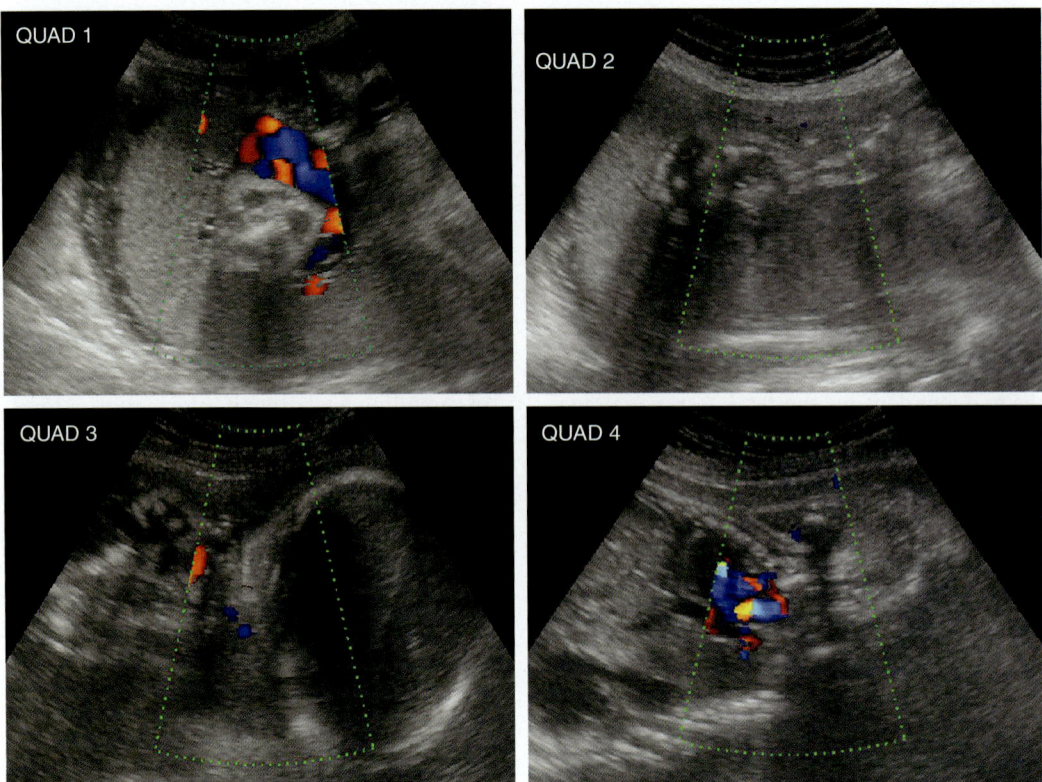

FIG. 58.17 Patient presents at 30 weeks of gestation with rupture of membranes. Amniotic fluid index reveals severe oligohydramnios. Color Doppler was used to ensure anechoic fetal cord was not misrepresented as fluid.

complex (amniotic deformities, adhesion, mutilation), amniotic band sequence, aberrant tissue bands, and congenital constricting bands.

Etiology. The most widely accepted theory for the formation of amniotic bands is that rupture of the amnion during early pregnancy development leads to subsequent entanglement of various embryonic or fetal parts by fibrous mesodermic bands, which emanate from the chorionic side of the amnion. Entrapment of fetal parts by the bands may cause lymphedema, amputations, or slash defects in nonembryologic distributions. The amnion, which is contiguous with the fetal skin at the umbilicus, is thought to protect the fetus from contact with the chorion. When disruption of the amnion occurs, the fetus may adhere to and fuse with the chorion, with subsequent maldevelopment of the subjacent fetal tissue. This theory suggests that when gastroschisis results in exteriorization of the liver, ABS should be strongly considered. The rupture of the amnion may be associated with exposure to teratogens, genetic factors, multifactorial, chorionic villi sampling, and amniocentesis. However, the exact etiology is unknown.

Clinical Findings. Various congenital malformation syndromes are thought to be caused by compression of the fetus by amniotic "bands," which results in developmental abnormalities or fetal death. ABS may represent a milder form of limb–body wall complex and may be predicted by amniotic bands that entangle or amputate fetal parts. Facial clefts, asymmetric encephaloceles, constriction or amputation defects of the extremities, and clubfoot deformities are common findings. The site where the amniotic band cuts across the fetus is usually evident after birth.

Prognosis. The prognosis of a fetus diagnosed with ABS is dependent on the extent of the malformations. There may be minor soft tissue malformation or lethal malformations. Patients should receive counsel on all malformations identified and be given appropriate options. In some cases, intrauterine fetal surgery to remove the bands is an option. These cases are typically limited to fetuses in which the benefit of the surgery outweighs the risks. It is common for bands to be found around the upper and lower extremities. If Doppler evaluation indicates that the band is constricting blood flow to a portion of an extremity, endoscopic intrauterine surgical removal (intrauterine lysis) of the band may be performed to avoid limb dysfunction or amputation.

Sonographic Findings. Sonography can be very useful in determining the extent of malformations of a fetus affected by ABS; however, it should be noted that research indicates that minor deformities may only be identified after birth. Sonographers should first be suspicious of the abnormality if echogenic bands are present within the amniotic cavity (Fig. 58.18). Following the band closely with real-time scanning will allow the sonographer to observe where the band is attached to the uterine wall and what, if any, constriction is placed on the fetus (Fig. 58.19). In addition, careful observation with real-time scanning will allow the sonographer to observe if the fetus is free from the band or if movement is restricted. All extremities and all soft tissues should be closely evaluated to determine whether interference of fetal development or amputation has occurred. Entanglement of the bands around soft tissue is usually seen as an indention of the soft tissue surrounded by edema (Fig. 58.20). The use of

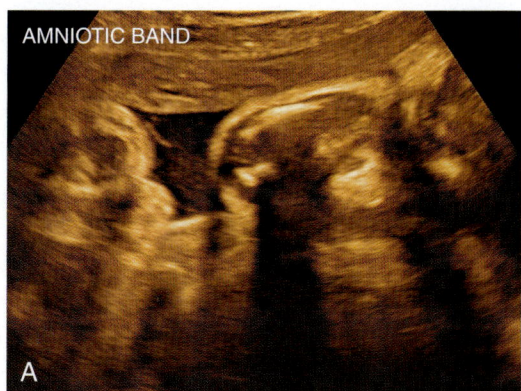
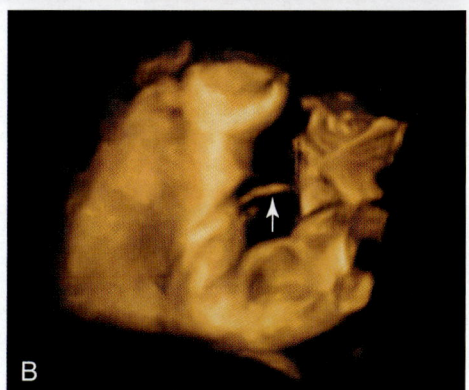

FIG. 58.18 (A) An echogenic band is noted floating in the amniotic fluid. The echogenic band was attached to the wall of the gestational sac. (B) Three-dimensional imaging with reformatting demonstrates the band *(arrow)*.

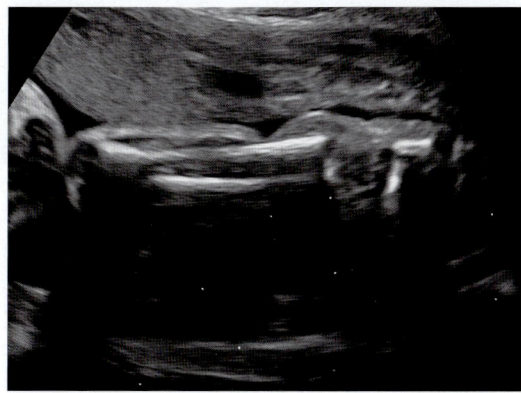

FIG. 58.19 In the same patient seen in Fig. 57.18, the band was followed through the sac and appeared to be attached to the right forearm.

three-dimensional sonography and other advanced techniques has helped to improve the visualization of bony and soft tissue malformations (Fig. 58.21). Other malformations include anencephaly, exencephaly, gastroschisis, limb or digit amputation, facial clefts, encephaloceles, or any slash defect.

Amniotic Sheets

Amniotic sheets, shelves, or folds are identified as echogenic nonfloating bands crossing through the amniotic cavity. They

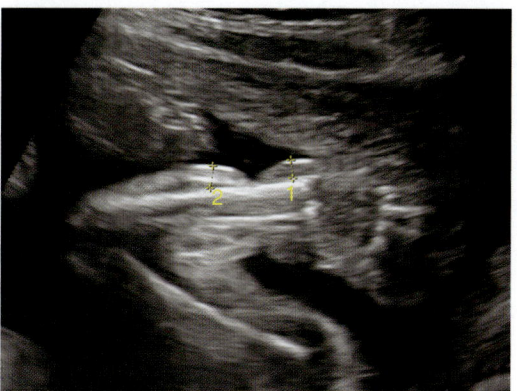

FIG. 58.20 Soft tissue edema is seen in the forearm, where the band is constricting the soft tissue.

are thicker than bands associated with ABS, do not cause fetal malformations, and most likely signify uterine synechiae.

Etiology. The visualization of amniotic sheets is believed to be caused by uterine scars (**synechiae**) from previous instrumentation used in the uterus (usually curettage), cesarean section, or episodes of endometritis. When a pregnancy begins to grow in the uterine cavity, the expanding membranes encounter the scar and wrap around it. The flat portion of the sheet consists of apposed layers of chorion and amnion. The free edge of the sheet is defined by the course of the synechia itself, which may produce a bulbous appearance. Amniotic sheets arise because of redundant amnion-chorion, which may, in turn, be related to bleeding and subchorionic hemorrhages.

Clinical Findings. Patients with a history of endometrial dilation and curettage, intrauterine infections, endometritis, removal of fibroids or endometrial pylons, or prior cesarean section are at risk for developing uterine scars (synechiae). Synechiae have been associated with infertility and miscarriages. Patients who present with uterine synechiae and infertility are often diagnosed with **Asherman syndrome**.

Prognosis. Amniotic sheets are thick muscular tissue bands that are not associated with fetal malformations. Surgical removal of the scars may be indicated for those patients with recurrent pregnancy loss or infertility.

Sonographic Findings. Sonographic findings in patients with amniotic sheets may show a fine echo-dense line in the uterine cavity separated from the uterine wall by an anechoic space. The membrane may completely surround the fetus, or the membrane may be freely mobile in the amniotic cavity. The membranes can appear anywhere in the uterine or cervical cavity. They are seen extending from one side of the uterus to the other, oblique across the uterus, or as multiple echogenic lines (Fig. 58.22). Color and spectral Doppler may be used to aid in the visualization and documentation of maternal blood flow within the synechiae. Amniotic sheets are present in 0.6% of patients having screening obstetric ultrasound examinations. Care should be taken to separate the diagnosis of amniotic sheets from amniotic bands or the circumvallate placenta. In the circumvallate placenta, the chorion and attached amnion

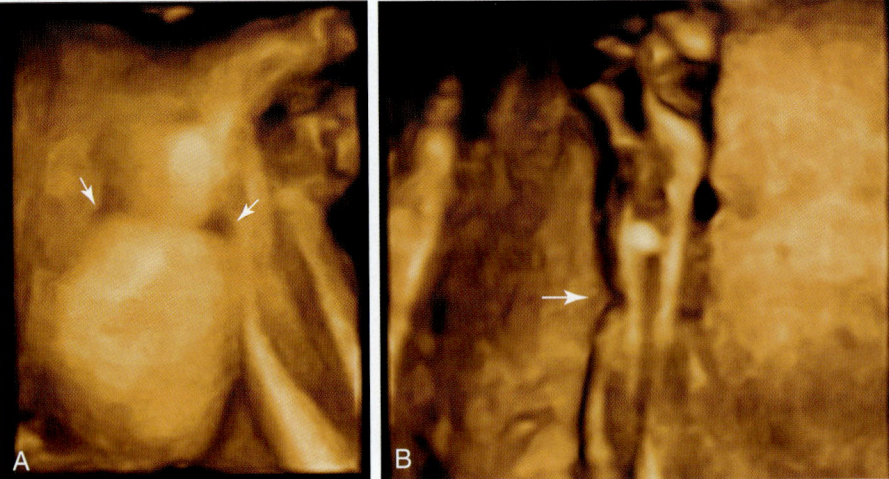

FIG. 58.21 (A) The constriction of the soft tissue is easily seen on four-dimensional evaluation. (B) Additional rendering to the three-dimensional image demonstrates the depth of the constricted soft tissue as it relates to the ulna and radius of the forearm.

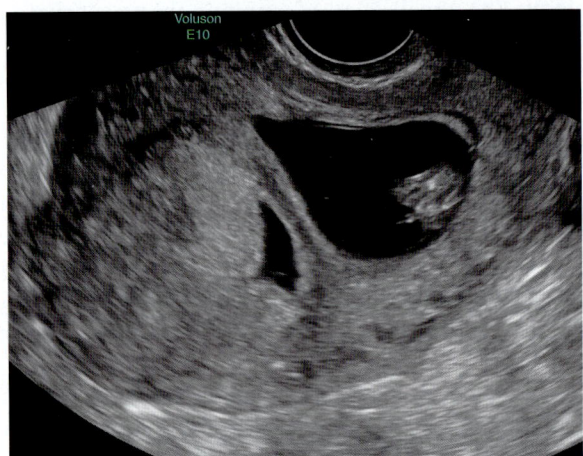

FIG. 58.22 Uterine synechia is visualized traversing the amniotic sac.

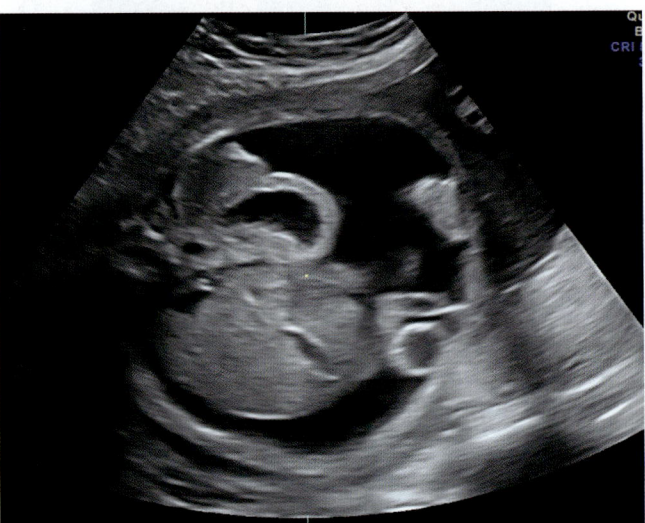

FIG. 58.23 Transverse image of a 30-week-old fetal abdomen demonstrating ascites surrounding the liver and other abdominal organs.

form a raised ridge of tissue at the junction of the chorion and the basal plate. Beyond this ridge, the normal vessels on the fetal surface are absent; after delivery, these redundant membranes are described as being adherent to the fetal surface rather than projecting from it.

Both the circumvallate placenta and amniotic sheets appear as a thick membrane projecting into the amniotic fluid. Circumvallate placental membranes originate from the edge of the fetal surface of the placenta, whereas amniotic sheets attach to the uterine wall itself.

HYDROPS

In cases of hydrops, there is a disparity between the amount of serous fluid being produced and absorbed. This disparity leads to the accumulation of fluid or edema within a fetus and can be represented by pleural effusions, ascites, cardiac effusion, skin edema, or anasarca. Other fetal findings identified with hydrops include an enlarged umbilical cord, polyhydramnios, placental edema, and an enlarged liver and spleen. The fetus, as well as the mother, can be affected by the presence of fetal hydrops. In many cases, fetal hydrops is highly associated with death. Diagnosis and determination of cause are essential in providing proper pregnancy management. Hydrops is categorized as immune related and nonimmune related. Sonographically, hydrops is identified by the presence of abnormal collections of fluid.

- **Ascites** can be seen as anechoic fluid surrounding abdominal and pelvic organs and the umbilical cord insertion (common site of early ascites) (Fig. 58.23). Careful attention should be made not to mistake normal hypoechoic abdominal musculature for ascites (pseudoascites).
- **Pleural effusions** can be seen as anechoic fluid filling the thoracic cavity or outlining the fetal lungs (Fig. 58.24).
- Skin **edema** can appear as increased skin thickening around the skull, neck, extremities, or abdomen. In some reports, a measurement of greater than 5 to 6 mm for soft tissue thickness is used for diagnosis. When skin edema is massive, encasing most of the body, the term **anasarca** is typically used (Fig. 58.25).

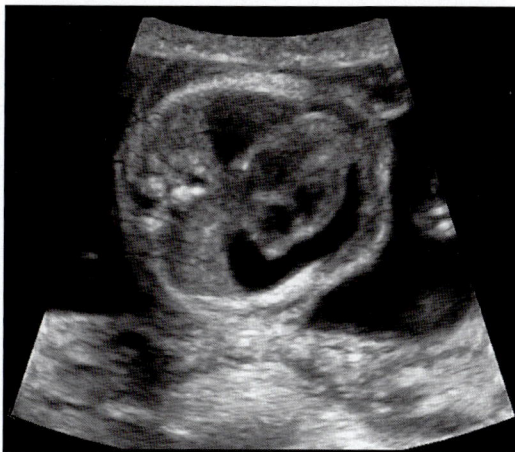

FIG. 58.24 Bilateral pleural effusions seen surrounding the heart and lungs.

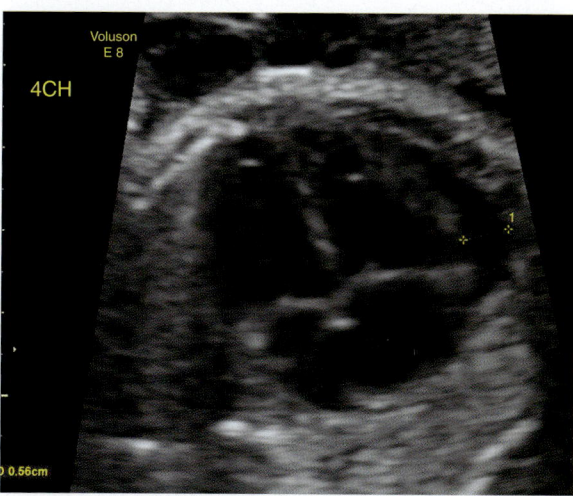

FIG. 58.26 Pericardial effusion is visualized as an anechoic fluid collection lateral to the right atrium and ventricle.

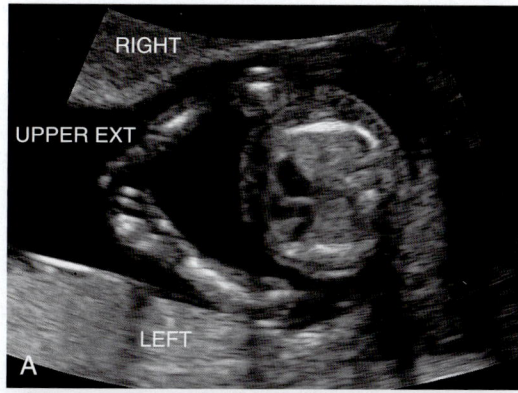
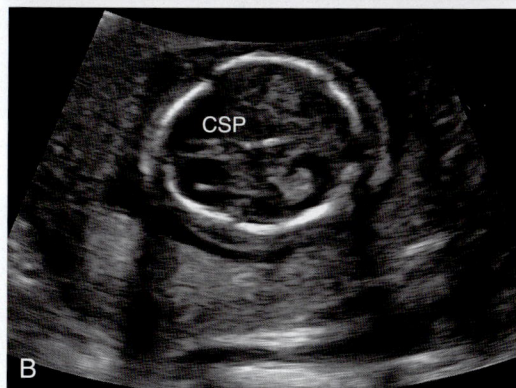

FIG. 58.25 (A) In this 16-week-old fetus, skin edema is noted surrounding the thoracic cavity. (B) In the same fetus, the skin edema is also noted surrounding the skull. *CSP*, Cavum septum pellucidum; *EXT*, extremity.

- **Pericardial effusion** is seen as excess anechoic fluid in the pericardial cavity. Normally a small amount of fluid is noted in this cavity, particularly in the apex. If the fluid collection measures greater than 2 mm, pericardial effusion is considered (Fig. 58.26).
- Placental edema can be identified as a thickened placenta measuring greater than 4 to 4.5 cm in true anterior-posterior diameter.

Maternal clinical presentations include those associated with polyhydramnios in most cases. Those symptoms include preterm labor, PPROM, and supine hypotension syndrome. In a few cases, the maternal clinical symptoms may mimic the clinical features of the hydropic fetus. This is known as *Mirror syndrome, Ballantyne syndrome*, or *pseudotoxemia*. The mother will exhibit features of edema, rapid weight gain, hypertension, and mild proteinuria.

Immune Hydrops

Immune hydrops fetalis (IHF) is associated with alloimmune hemolytic disease (erythroblastosis fetalis) or Rh isoimmunization. Maternal blood sampling and history of a previously affected fetus are extremely important for pregnancy management.

Causes. Immune hydrops is associated with Rh isoimmunization (sensitization or development of antibodies). Maternal blood serum tests are used in the evaluation of antibodies and for blood typing. Maternal blood tests involve evaluating the blood for the presence of Rh-D antigen (positive blood grouping) or the absence of the Rh-D antigen (negative blood grouping). The risk of isoimmunization is not apparent when the mother's blood test results indicate the Rh-D–positive blood group. However, patients presenting with Rh-D–negative blood grouping are at risk for developing antibodies that can attack a fetus that is Rh-D positive. The results of the production of antibodies contribute to fetal anemia progressing into immune hydrops. This typically occurs with the second and subsequent pregnancy due to the lack of sufficient amounts of the Rh antigen to stimulate the maternal immune system.

The risk of the development of hydrops in the second and subsequent pregnancies is increased due to the formation of an immunoglobulin G (IgG) antibody with the first pregnancy. The formation of the IgG antibody resulted from the maternal lymphocytes that were formed during the first pregnancy to recognize Rh-D antigen. If maternal serum blood tests indicate a positive IgG antibody, further evaluation of the blood titers is required. Blood titers aid in determining the level of specific antibodies in the blood. The titers will be evaluated multiple times throughout the pregnancy to determine whether the IgG has crossed into the fetus and is destroying fetal blood cells. If at any point the titer results are greater than 1:16, amniocentesis is performed to evaluate for fetal anemia and severity of fetal hemolysis.

There are multiple types of other blood compatibility and alloimmunizations than those discussed here. Sonographers should understand the possible sonographic features and appropriate follow-up in all patients diagnosed with a form of Rh incompatibility.

Prognosis. In general, the diagnosis of Rh incompatibility, fetal anemia, or hemolytic disorders is associated with high perinatal morbidity. There are a few treatments and preventive measures that can be taken to help reduce poor fetal outcomes. For instance, if maternal blood serum indicates an Rh-D–negative blood group, the mother should be given an anti-D immunoglobulin such as RhoGAM to protect the Rh-positive fetus from the Rh-negative maternal antibodies. The medication is usually given at approximately 28 weeks of gestation and has proven to be successful in decreasing perinatal mortality and morbidity. In cases in which severe fetal anemia is diagnosed, intrauterine blood transfusions are used to help correct the anemia. Research has shown that fetuses treated with blood transfusions before the onset of hydrops have an increased survival rate compared to those with hydrops.

Sonographic Findings. Sonography indicates evidence of ascites, pleural effusion, and/or skin edema. Other findings include a thickened placenta and hydramnios (Fig. 58.27). Fetal ascites may be the first fluid collection to be seen within the fetus (Fig. 58.28). In addition to gray-scale imaging, spectral Doppler analysis of the MCA should be used to monitor the fetus for anemia. Doppler evaluation of the MCA includes recording peak velocity measurements of the artery. The artery should be sampled at the proximal end and at a zero-degree angle. Most facilities obtain velocities from the MCA in the closest proximity to the transducer. It should be noted that research has indicated support for sampling both MCAs. If the peak velocity is 50 cm/sec after 30 weeks of gestation, fetal anemia is mostly indicated (Fig. 58.29). Other forms of measurement are available that calculate the multiples of the mean for the MCA. The MCA should be evaluated every 1 to 2 weeks in fetuses at risk for developing anemia. In addition to recording the velocities of the MCA, a peak systolic measurement of the aorta has also been found to be useful in diagnosing anemia. Peak velocity measurements of the aorta over 1 cm/sec are a clinical finding for anemia. Fetal anemia may be present with or without hydrops. Conclusive evidence of anemia is further evaluated by means of amniocentesis (evaluation of amniotic fluid) or cordocentesis (evaluation for fetal blood via the umbilical cord).

Nonimmune Hydrops

Nonimmune hydrops fetalis (NIHF) describes the presence of abnormal accumulations of fluid in the fetal body and/or skin. It is associated with numerous conditions and causes.

Causes. Nonimmune hydrops may be a sporadic condition or associated with numerous other causes. Cardiac insufficiency is one of the most common causes. Cardiac insufficiency can result from cardiac anomalies or arrhythmias (Fig. 58.30).

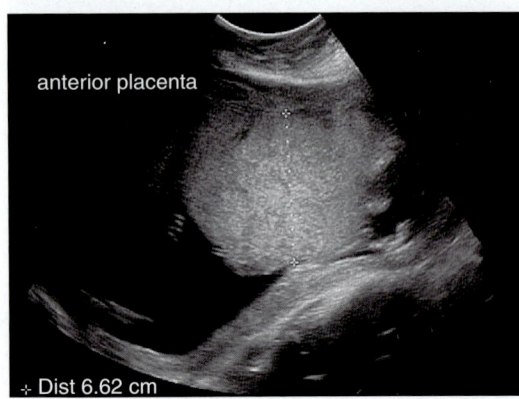

FIG. 58.27 A thickened placenta is identified in a fetus with hydrops. The anterior-posterior diameter of the placenta measured 6.62 cm.

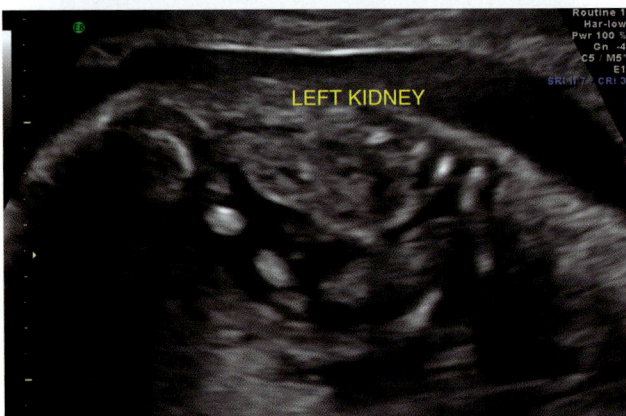

FIG. 58.28 Ascites around the left kidney and intestines.

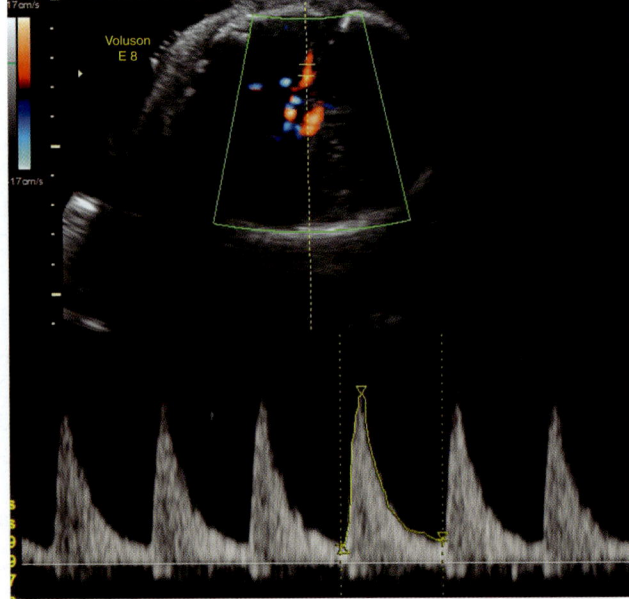

FIG. 58.29 Middle cerebral artery color and spectral Doppler analysis in this anemic fetus indicates abnormal peak velocities.

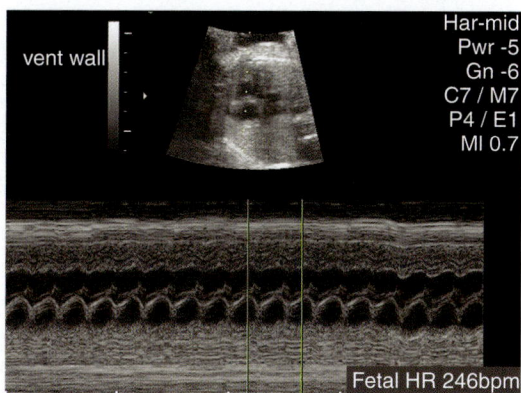

FIG. 58.30 Tachycardia was identified in this patient with a heart rate of 246 beats/min.

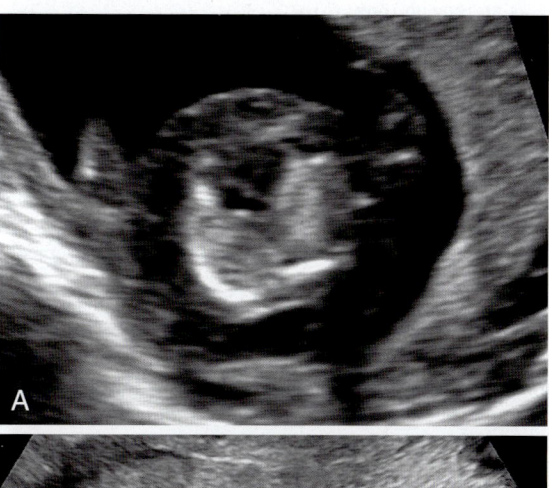

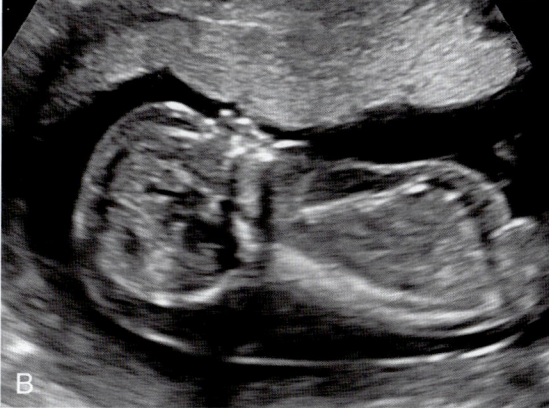

FIG. 58.31 Massive skin edema visualized in this fetus with trisomy 21.

Fetal anomalies associated with decreased venous return to the heart, structural lymphatic obstruction, and hypoproteinuria are other causes.

Prognosis. The prognosis for a fetus presenting with NIHF is poor. It has been noted that the overall mortality rate is 50% to 98%. This varying percentage rate is directly related to the etiology of the hydrops. In some cases of anemia or tachycardia, the cause can be treated, thereby reducing or resolving the hydrops. Laser therapy has been used to treat hydrops in cases of twin-to-twin transfusion syndrome involving NIHF. Fetuses born with NIHF are typically very distressed and require immediate medical attention.

Sonographic Findings. Sonographically all abnormal fluid collections should be documented and measured. The fetus should be thoroughly evaluated for anomalies that may be associated with NIHF. Anomalies that may be present include fetal tumors (heart or liver), cardiac anomalies, cystic adenomatoid malformation of the lung, and chorioangioma of the placenta. Sonographic findings associated with characteristics of trisomy 21 (Fig. 58.31), 45,X, and fetal infections (TORCH) should be documented due to their relationship with NIHF.

ACKNOWLEDGMENT

The author acknowledges Roy Bors-Koefoed, MD, and Christina Taff, BHS, at Mid-South Maternal Fetal Medicine for their contribution of sonographic images for this chapter.

Key Pearls

- Amniotic fluid allows the fetus to move freely within the amniotic cavity while maintaining intrauterine temperature and protecting the developing fetus from injury.
- Amniotic fluid is produced by the umbilical cord, membranes, lungs, skin, and kidneys.
- The amount of amniotic fluid present at any one time reflects a balance between amniotic fluid production and amniotic fluid removal.
- Early in gestation, the major source of amniotic fluid is the amniotic membrane, a thin membrane lined by a single layer of epithelial cells.
- The amount of amniotic fluid is regulated not only by the production of fluid but also by removal of the fluid by swallowing, by fluid exchange within the lungs, and by the membranes and cord.
- Normal lung development depends critically on the exchange of amniotic fluid within the lungs. Inadequate lung development may occur when the amount of amniotic fluid is severely low, placing the fetus at high risk for developing small or hypoplastic lungs.
- In accordance with the guidelines for obstetric scanning, every obstetric examination should include a thorough evaluation of amniotic fluid volume.
- Abnormal amounts of amniotic fluid are described as hydramnios (polyhydramnios) and oligohydramnios.
- The amniotic fluid index (AFI) is used most frequently for evaluating and quantifying amniotic fluid volume at different intervals during a pregnancy.
- In twin pregnancies, it is important to assess each sac independently when performing amniotic fluid determinations.
- Polyhydramnios is often associated with central nervous system disorders and/or gastrointestinal problems.
- Fetal hydrops, skeletal anomalies, and some renal disorders may also be associated with hydramnios.
- Oligohydramnios is an overall reduction in the amount of amniotic fluid resulting in fetal crowding and decreased fetal movement.

- The primary fetal membranes are known as amnion and chorion.
- Premature rupture of the membranes (PROM), preterm PROM (PPROM), and spontaneous rupture of the membranes (SPROM) describe conditions in which the membranes rupture ("water breaks") abnormally, resulting in loss of amniotic fluid and/or oligohydramnios.
- Amniotic band syndrome is associated with an abnormality in the fetal membranes. It is a common, nonrecurrent cause of various fetal malformations involving the limbs, craniofacial region, and trunk.
- Amniotic sheets, shelves, or folds are identified as echogenic nonfloating bands crossing through the amniotic cavity.
- In cases of hydrops, there is a disparity between the amount of serous fluid being produced and absorbed. This disparity leads to the accumulation of fluid or edema within a fetus and can be represented by pleural effusions, ascites, cardiac effusion, skin edema, or anasarca.
- Immune hydrops fetalis is associated with alloimmune hemolytic disease (erythroblastosis fetalis) or rhesus isoimmunization.
- Sonography indicates evidence of ascites, pleural effusion, and/or skin edema.
- Nonimmune hydrops fetalis describes the presence of abnormal accumulations of fluid in the fetal body and/or skin.
- Nonimmune hydrops may be a sporadic condition or associated with numerous other causes. Cardiac insufficiency is one of the most common causes.
- Fetal anomalies associated with decreased venous return to the heart, structural lymphatic obstruction, and hypoproteinuria are other causes.

BIBLIOGRAPHY

Ackerman AN. Accuracy of sonographic amniotic fluid volume assessments in diamniotic dichorionic twin pregnancies a literature review. *J Diagn Med Sonogr.* 2007;23:330–335.

Allen L, Silverman RK, Nosovitch JT, et al. Constriction rings and congenital amputations of the fingers and toes in a mild case of amniotic band syndrome. *J Diagn Med Sonogr.* 2007;23:280–285.

Banks EH, Miller DA. Perinatal risks associated with borderline amniotic fluid index. *Am J Obstet Gynecol.* 1999;180:1461–1463.

Bisset RA, et al. *Differential Diagnosis in Obstetric and Gynecologic Ultrasound.* Philadelphia: Elsevier; 2013.

Blakelock R, Upadhyay V, Kimble R, et al. Is a normally functioning gastrointestinal tract necessary for normal growth in late gestation? *Pediatr Surg Int.* 1998;13:17–20.

Borgida AF, Mills A, Feldman DM, et al. Outcome of pregnancies complicated by ruptured membranes after genetic amniocentesis. *Am J Obstet Gynecol.* 2000;183:937–939.

Brace RA. Physiology of amniotic fluid volume regulation. *Clin Obstet Gynecol.* 1997;40:280–289.

Burton E. Serial evaluation of perinatal uterine synechiae versus amniotic bands. *J Diagn Med Sonogr.* 2004;20:51–56.

Callen P. *Ultrasonography in Obstetrics and Gynecology.* ed 6. Philadelphia: Elsevier; 2017.

Carbillon L, Oury JF, Guerin JM, et al. Clinical biological features of Ballantyne syndrome and the role of placental hydrops. *Obstet Gynecol Surv.* 1997;52(5):310–314.

Croom CS, Banias BB, Ramos-Santos E. Do semiquantitative amniotic fluid indexes reflect actual volume? *Am J Obstet Gynecol.* 1992;167:995–999.

DeLange M, Rouse G. *OB/GYN Sonography: An Illustrated Review.* Pasadena, CA: Davies Publishing; 2004.

Durre S, Nawaz K, MacDonald S, Sabih Z. Hydrops fetalis imaging. 2019. https://emedicine.medscape.com/article/403962-overview.

Entezami M, Albig M, Gasiorek-Wiens A, Becker R. *Ultrasound Diagnosis of Fetal Anomalies.* New York: Thieme; 2011.

Gramellini D, Chiaie D, Piantelli G, et al. Sonographic assessment of amniotic fluid volume between 11 and 24 weeks of gestation: construction of reference intervals related to gestational age. *Ultrasound Obstet Gynecol.* 2001;17:410–415.

Grover J, Mentakis A, Ross MG. Three-dimensional method for determination of amniotic fluid volume in intrauterine pockets. *Obstet Gynecol.* 1997;90:1007–1010.

Hill LM, Krohn M, Lazebnik N, et al. The amniotic fluid index in normal twin pregnancies. *Am J Obstet Gynecol.* 2000;182:950–954.

Horsager R, Nathan I, Leveno KJ. Correlation of measured amniotic fluid volume and sonographic predictions of oligohydramnios. *Obstet Gynecol.* 1994;83:955–958.

Hsich TT, Hung TH, Chen KC, et al. Perinatal outcome of oligohydramnios without associated premature rupture of membranes and fetal anomalies. *Gynecol Obstet Invest.* 1998;45:232–236.

Jazayer A. Premature rupture of membranes. 2018. https://emedicine.medscape.com/article/261137-overview.

Lalicker A, Himmelberg J. Middle cerebral artery Doppler used to detect fetal anemia. *J Diagn Med Sonogr.* 2004;20:94–99.

Magann EF, Chauhan SP, Whitworth NS, et al. Determination of amniotic fluid volume in twin pregnancies: ultrasonographic evaluation versus operator estimation. *Am J Obstet Gynecol.* 2000;182:1606–1609.

Magann EF, Martin Jr JN. Amniotic fluid assessment in singleton and twin pregnancies. *Obstet Gynecol Clin North Am.* 1999;26:579–593.

Magann EF, Nolan TE, Hess LW, et al. Measurement of amniotic fluid volume: accuracy of ultrasonography technique. *Am J Obstet Gynecol.* 1992;167:1533–1537.

Magann EF, Sanderson M, Martin JN, et al. The amniotic fluid index, single deepest pocket, and two-diameter pocket in normal human pregnancy. *Am J Obstet Gynecol.* 2000;182:1581–1588.

Manning FA, Harman CR, Morrison I, et al. Fetal assessment based on fetal biophysical profile scoring IV. An analysis of perinatal morbidity and mortality. *Am J Obstet Gynecol.* 1990;162:703–709.

Medina T, Hill DA. Preterm premature rupture of membranes: diagnosis and management. *Am Fam Physician.* 2006;73:659–664.

Moore KL, Persaud TVN. *The Developing Human: Clinically Oriented Embryology.* 8th ed. Philadelphia: Elsevier; 2018. 11th ed.

Moore TR, Cayle JE. The amniotic fluid index in normal human pregnancy. *Am J Obstet Gynecol.* 1990;162:1168–1173.

Paladini D, Foglia S, Sglavo G, Martinelli P. Congenital constriction band of the upper arm: the role of three-dimensional ultrasound in diagnosis, counseling and multidisciplinary consultation. *Ultrasound of Obstet Gynecol.* 2004;23(5):520–522.

Peipert JF, Donnenfeld AE. Oligohydramnios: a review. *Obstet Gynecol Surv.* 1991;46:325.

Roberts D, Dalziel S. Antenatal corticosteroids for accelerating fetal lung maturation for women at risk of preterm birth. *Cochrane Database Syst Rev.* 2006;19(3):CD004454.

Selam B, Koksal R, Ozcan T. Fetal arterial and venous Doppler parameters in the interpretation of oligohydramnios in post-term pregnancies. *Ultrasound Obstet Gynecol.* 2000;15:403–406.

Sistrom CL, Ferguson JE. Abnormal membranes in obstetrical ultrasound: incidence and significance of amniotic sheets and circumvallate placenta. *Ultrasound Obstet Gynecol*. 1993;3:249.

Smith-Weaver M. Second-trimester findings associated with nonimmune hydrops. *J Diagn Med Sonogr*. 2008;24:93–96.

Stephenson S, Dmitrieva J. *Diagnostic Medical Sonography: Obstetrics and Gynecology*. 4th ed. New York: Lippincott; 2018.

Stringer M, Miesnik SR, Brown L, et al. Rupture of membranes. *Am J Matern Child Nurs*. 2004;29:145–150.

Thompson O, Brown R, Gunnarson G, et al. Prevalence of polyhydramnios in the third trimester in a population screened by first and second trimester ultrasonography. *J Perinat Med*. 1998;26:371–377.

Tskitishvili E, Tomimatsu T, Kanagawa T, et al. Amniotic fluid "sludge" detected in patients with subchorionic hematoma: a report of two cases. *Ultrasound Obstet Gynecol*. 2009;33(4):484–486.

Wang H, Parry S, Macones G, et al. Functionally significant SNP MMP8 promoter haplotypes and preterm premature rupture of membranes (PPROM). *Hum Mol Genet*. 2004;13:2659–2669.

Williams K. Amniotic fluid assessment. *Obstet Gynecol Surv*. 1993;48:795.

Yu D, Wong YM, Cheong Y, et al. Asherman syndrome—one century later. *Fertil Steril*. 2008;89:759–779.

CHAPTER 59

Fetal Face and Neck

Michelle Wilson

OBJECTIVES

On completion of this chapter, you should be able to:
- Discuss basic embryology of the face
- Describe how to sonographically evaluate the fetal face and neck for normal features
- Define the most common face and neck congenital anomalies discovered sonographically in utero

OUTLINE

Embryology of The Fetal Face   1493
    Development of the Lips   1493
    Development of the Nose   1494
    Development of the Mouth   1494
    Development of the Palate   1494
    Development of the Ears   1494
Sonographic Evaluation of the Fetal Face   1495

Abnormalities of the Face and Neck   1496
    Abnormalities of the Forehead, Calvarium, Mandible, and Ear   1496
    Abnormalities of the Orbits   1501
    Abnormalities of the Mid-Face: Nose, Maxilla, Lips, and Palate   1503

Abnormalities of the Oral Cavity   1510
Abnormalities of the Neck   1512
Three-Dimensional Evaluation   1516
Additional Imaging   1517

KEY TERMS

Agnathia
Anotia
Anophthalmia
Arhinia
Beckwith-Wiedemann syndrome
Branchial cleft cyst
Cebocephaly
Cephalocele
Craniosynostosis
Cyclopia
Cystic hygroma (CH)
Dacryocystocele
Epignathus

Encephalocele
Ethmocephaly
Exophthalmia
Fetal goiter
Hemangioma
Hemifacial microsomia
Holoprosencephaly
Hypertelorism
Hypotelorism
Macroglossia
Meloschisis
Microcephaly
Micrognathia

Microphthalmia
Microsomia
Microtia
Otocephaly
Phenylketonuria (PKU)
Pierre Robin syndrome
Proboscis
Strabismus
Teratoma
Thyromegaly
Treacher Collins syndrome
Trigonocephaly
Turner syndrome

Embryological development is often arduous and complex, with facial feature embryogenesis being no exception. The evolution happens early in development, occurring between weeks 4 to 10, and necessitates the coordination and timing of various tissues in order to reach each person's unique facial features. The World Health Organization (WHO) reports approximately 20% of surviving infants with congenital facial disparities have other associated anomalies, with the statistic much higher among stillborn infants.[1]

The WHO also reports congenital anomalies of the face to affect 1 in 500 to 700 births; however, this comes with a wide variance across ethnic, socioeconomic, and geographic groupings.[2] Orofacial clefts have long been recognized as one of the most common facial malformations, and with the assistance of sonographic evaluation, are often discovered prior to delivery.[3] Affecting 1 in every 940 births, an oral cleft abnormality is the most common of these congenital facial anomalies and represents the second most common congenital disability in the United States.[4] However, the highest proportion is seen among Asian populations.[3,4]

As is the case with sonography in general, the detection of subtle facial malformations can depend on the investigator's skill set and ability to thoroughly perform a complete study. Given the nature of sonographic imaging, many detrimental factors may inhibit a thorough and accurate examination of the fetal face, including the position of the fetus, maternal body habitus, presence of uterine pathology, and even the amount of amniotic fluid present. Any facial abnormality should immediately incite clinicians to meticulously search for other defects, as they often occur as signposts of syndromes. This chapter discusses the overall concept of embryological development of the facial features and examines some of the more commonly encountered craniofacial and fetal neck pathologies discovered with sonographic evaluation.

EMBRYOLOGY OF THE FETAL FACE

During the fourth and fifth weeks, the embryo has characteristic external features of the head and neck area in the form of a series of branchial arches, pouches, grooves, and membranes. Their development and evolution require a very precise and complex process with defined and orderly expectations throughout the fetal stage of formation. These structures, referred to as the *branchial apparatus*, bear a resemblance to gills and necessitate all three primary embryonic tissues of the endoderm, mesoderm, and ectoderm working together in sequence to avoid potential disfiguring and devastating facial malformations. The broad spectrum of congenital facial anomalies ranges from cosmetic indiscretions such as cleft lips to potentially life-threatening malformations such as arrhinia and obstructive oropharyngeal **teratomas** and their sequelae.

There are six branchial arches, but only the first four are visible externally (Fig. 59.1A). Neural crest cells migrate into the branchial arches and proliferate, resulting in swelling that demarcates each arch. The neural crest cells develop the skeletal features of the face, and the mesoderm of each arch develops the musculature of the face and neck. The arches are separated by branchial grooves, and each is composed of a core of mesenchymal cells and tissues derived from intraembryonic mesoderm covered by ectoderm. The mesenchyme forms the cartilage, bone, muscle, and blood vessels.

The fusion of five facial prominences must occur to form the lips and nose: frontonasal prominence, a pair of maxillary prominences, and a pair of mandibular prominences. Aberrant anatomical variations affecting the face may occur due to defects involving any of the branchial arches.[5] The first branchial arch develops into the maxillary and mandibular arches, forming the jaw, zygomatic bone, ear, and temporal bone (see Fig. 59.1B). The maxillary prominences arise and grow cranially just inferior to the eyes, and the mandibular prominence grows inferiorly, forming the mandible and squamous components of the temporal bones.[6] The second branchial arch contributes to the hyoid bone. The severity and magnitude of congenital abnormalities of the first and second branchial arches will depend on the extent of the insult, with timing playing a crucial component of its scope, often relating to hypoplasia or even aplasia of these anatomical variations.[7]

Development of the Lips

The complex formation of the facial lips is composed of multiple prominences growing steadily together, with the correct timing being essential to completing the process correctly. The maxillary prominences grow medially between the fifth and eighth weeks, with this growth compressing the medial nasal prominences together towards the midline. The two medial nasal prominences and the two maxillary prominences lateral to them fuse together to form the upper lip (Fig. 59.2). The medial nasal prominences form the medial

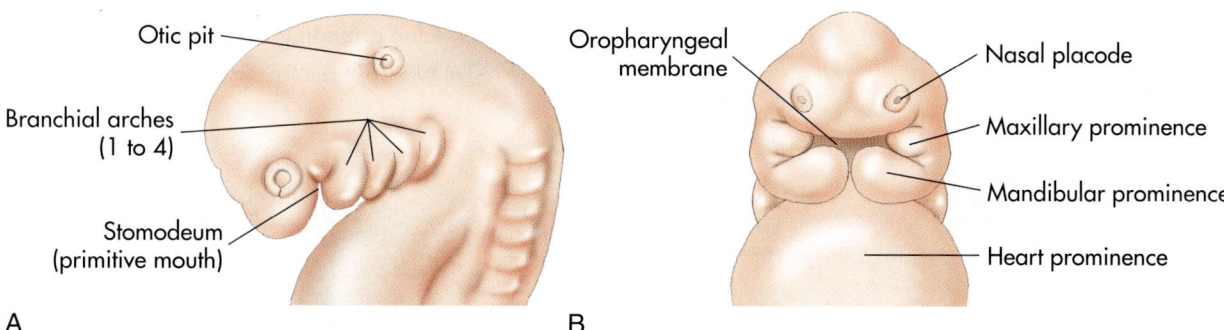

FIG. 59.1 (A) Lateral view of the embryo at 28 days shows four of the six branchial arches, otic pit, and stomodeum. (B) Frontal view of the embryo at 24 days demonstrates the nasal placode, maxillary prominence, and mandibular prominence.

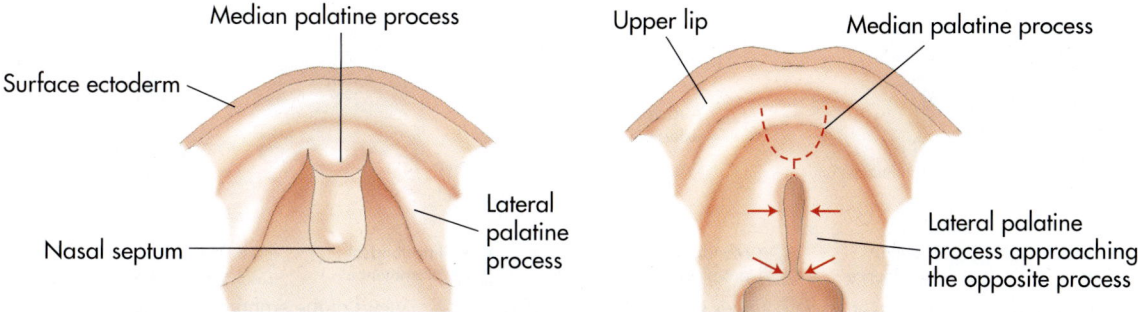

FIG. 59.2 First-trimester development of the roof of the mouth showing formation of the upper lip and palate.

aspect of the lip, which is the origin of the labial component of the lip, the upper incisor teeth, and the anterior aspect of the primary palate. The lateral nasal prominences form the alae of the nose. The maxillary prominences and lateral nasal prominences are separated by the nasolacrimal groove, where the nasolacrimal duct and lacrimal sac reside. The mandibular prominences merge at the end of the fourth to fifth week and form the lower lip and jaw, chin, and mandible.

Development of the Nose

The nose is formed in three parts. The nasal pits are formed as the surface ectoderm thickens into the nasal placodes on each side of the frontal nasal prominence; these placodes then invaginate on either side (Fig. 59.3). The bridge of the nose originates from the frontal prominence, the two medial nasal prominences form the crest and tip of the nose, and the lateral nasal prominences form the sides, or alae. The maxillary prominences then fuse with the nasal prominences and soon after fuse in the midline to form a continuous central structure.

Development of the Mouth

The primitive mouth is an indentation on the surface of the ectoderm (referred to as the *stomodeum*) (see Fig. 59.2). Until 24 to 26 days of gestation, the stomodeum is separated from the pharynx by a membrane that ruptures to place the primitive gut in communication with the amniotic cavity. At approximately the same time, five prominences are identified: the frontal nasal prominence, forming the upper boundary of the stomodeum; the paired maxillary prominences of the first branchial arch, forming the lateral boundaries of the stomodeum; and the paired mandibular prominences, forming the caudal boundary.[8] As these prominences fuse together in the midline, the mouth continues to be separated from the nasal cavity by the palate (Fig. 59.4).

Development of the Palate

The palate forms the roof of the mouth and the floor of the nasal cavity and is divided into the hard palate, located more anteriorly, and the soft palate, which is located more posteriorly. The primary palate begins forming early in the sixth week, with the wedge-shaped mass created by the emergence of the medial nasal prominences between the developing maxillae.[8] As the nose forms, the fusion of the medial nasal prominence with its contralateral counterpart creates the primary palate (becomes the anterior one-third of the definitive palate). The primary palate forms the anterior and midline aspect of the maxilla, which represents a small part of the adult hard palate (Fig. 59.5).

The intermaxillary segment also contributes to the labial component of the philtrum and the upper four incisors. The maxillary prominences expand medially to give rise to the palatal shelves, which continue to advance medially, fusing superior to the tongue. Simultaneously, the developing mandible expands to increase the size of the oral cavity; this allows the tongue to drop out of the way of the growing palatal shelves. The palatal shelves then fuse with each other in the horizontal plane and the nasal septum in the vertical plane, forming the secondary palate. The face and palate complete midline fusion between the sixth and twelfth weeks of gestation.[8]

Development of the Ears

Human ear development is complex and lengthy, commencing around week 4 and extending well beyond the neonatal period into puberty, when the glands of the external canal become

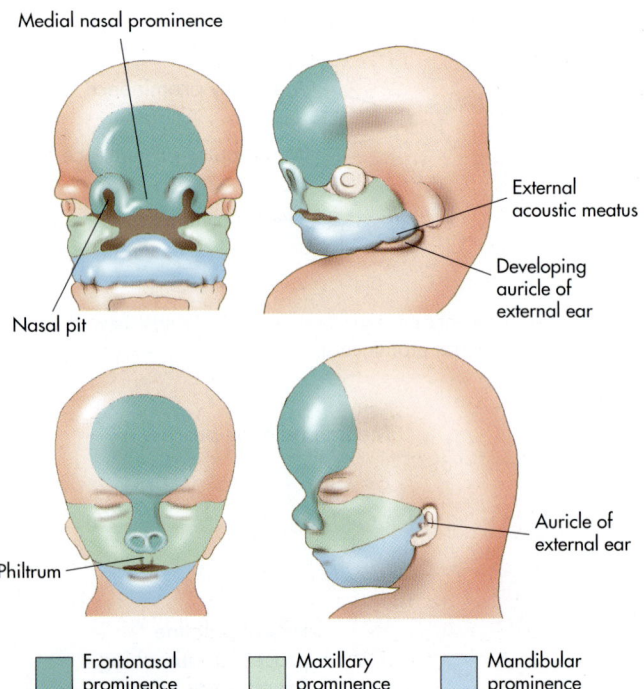

FIG. 59.3 Frontal view of the embryo at 40 days shows the nasal pit and the medial nasal prominence.

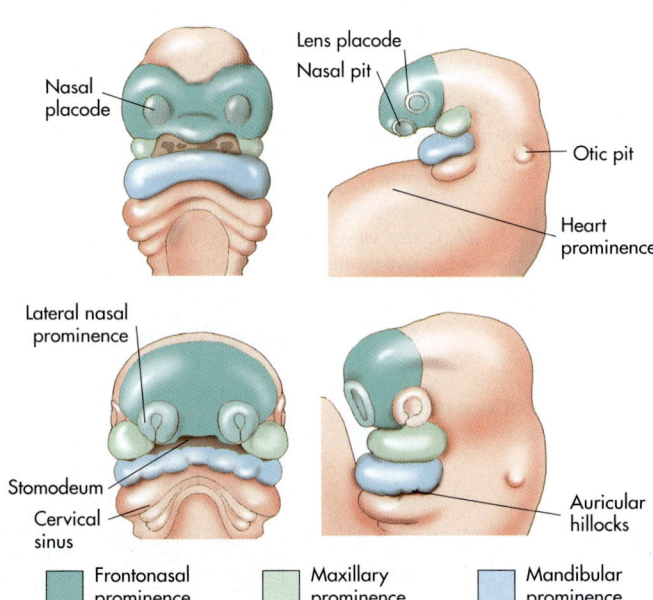

FIG. 59.4 Views of the embryo at 33 days show the stomodeum, lateral nasal prominence, and cervical sinus.

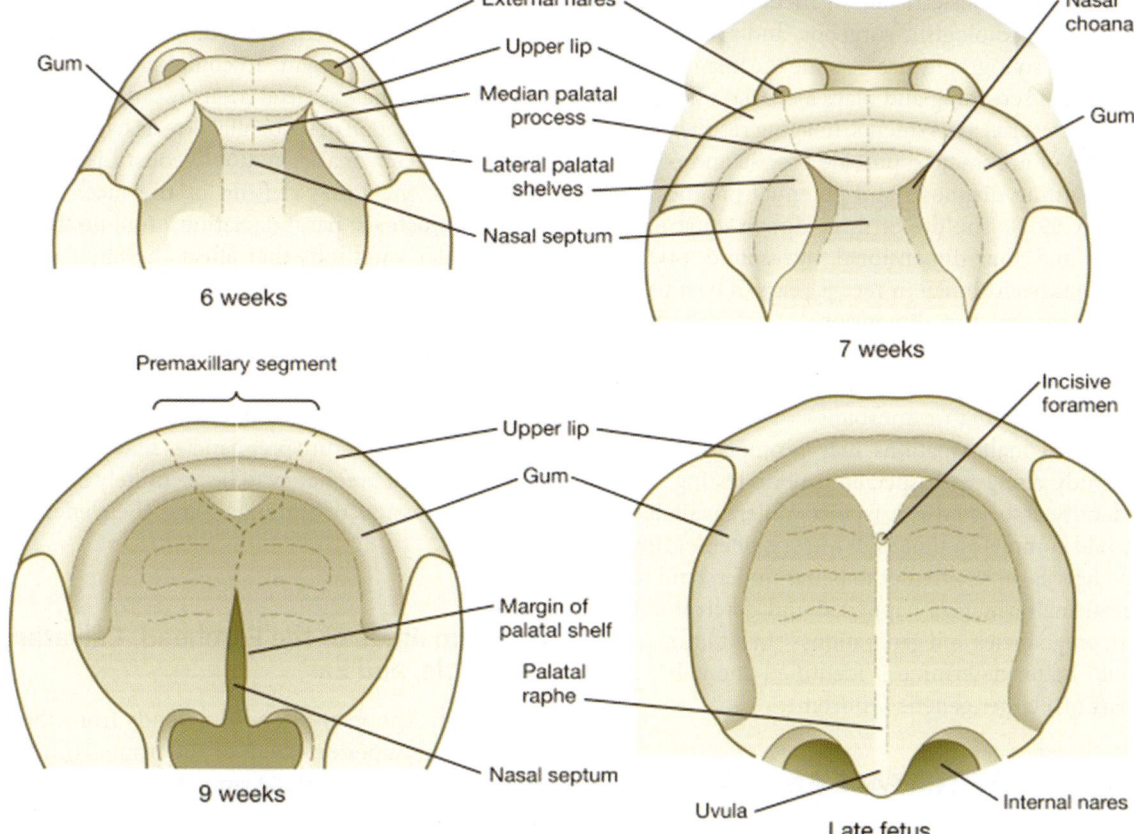

FIG. 59.5 Development of the primary palate.

fully functional.[9] However, for purposes of sonographic evaluation, the pinna, or external ear, embryogenesis is the most relevant for a thorough understanding of external ear development disorders. Around the fifth week, the vestigial gills on each lateral side, external to the fetal cranium, begin widening as the start of the development of the external auditory canal. Around this opening, six tissue thickenings, called hillocks, arise from the branchial arches I and II to fuse and form the basic units of the pinna.[10] The first and second pharyngeal arch apparatus lends the structural foundation for formation of the external ear. By approximately the 20th week, the auricular hillocks enlarge asymmetrically and ultimately coalesce to form a recognizable external ear.[9] They then migrate superiorly to the adult location and overall configuration.

SONOGRAPHIC EVALUATION OF THE FETAL FACE

Given the often-fearful reaction that fetal anomalies in general and especially facial anomalies can carry due to their negative social and psychological impacts, sonographic facial evaluation must be closely scrutinized. Evaluations should be routinely included in all fetal anatomic surveillance studies and with increased analysis when there is a family history of craniofacial malformation or when another congenital anomaly is discovered due to the close association of facial abnormalities with coexisting fetal malformations.[11] Typically, the sonographic evaluation consists of utilizing all three orthogonal

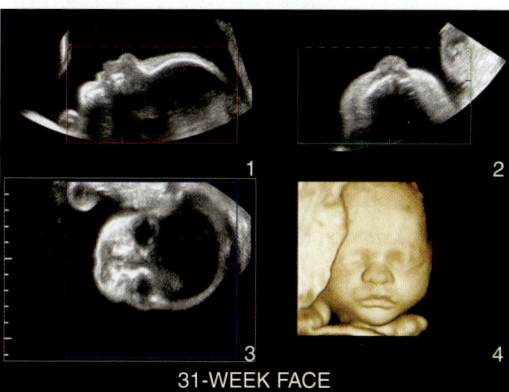

FIG. 59.6 Multiplanar reconstruction through the fetal face displaying three orthogonal planes: (1) sagittal plane, (2) axial plane, (3) coronal plane, and (4) reconstructed facial image.

imaging planes (sagittal, axial, and coronal), as each provides a unique perspective of the three dimensions of organs; however, with the advent of three- and four-dimensional imaging, specific information beyond these planes can often be obtained (Fig. 59.6).

Facial anomalies are heterogeneous and can occur as isolated defects or as part of a larger setting (with global anomalies), as a condition, or as part of a larger syndrome (e.g., orbital fusion and a **proboscis** suggest alobar holoprosencephaly). Often a fetus with congenital facial deformations discovered prenatally will require a multidisciplinary team approach consisting of obstetricians, geneticists, sonographers, pediatricians, radiologists, surgeons, and specific specialty domains.[12] As sonography has become the imaging gold standard in prenatal screening and plays a crucial role in the evaluation and with serial assessments, imaging results necessitate a high level of accuracy to provide precise and correct information regarding diagnosis and potential prognosis to the parents (Box 59.1). The use of three-dimensional ultrasound (3DUS) and four-dimensional ultrasound (4DUS) reconstruction has been shown in recent years to be a useful adjunct to conventional two-dimensional (2D) or bidirectional screening assessment of the fetal face.[13,14]

Worldwide, craniofacial anomalies are a concern for infant mortality and pediatric morbidity.[3,4,15] A family history of craniofacial malformations may prompt a targeted sonographic study along with specific genetic testing in an attempt to identify associated risk factors. When available, a geneticist should complete a thorough history, often of three-generation pedigrees, in an attempt to better understand how the craniofacial malformation happened and determine the risk for future pregnancies and generations.[16] In addition, this exercise should better determine if identified anomalies are isolated or part of a larger genetic syndrome.

ABNORMALITIES OF THE FACE AND NECK

Dysmorphology, or the study of human congenital malformations and syndromes, divides congenital anomalies into three classifications of alterations that occur to typical morphology. A *malformation sequence*, or the process of poor formation of tissue, allows for a chain reaction of defects to occur as normal tissue is not a foundation. A *deformation sequence* gives way to normal tissue development; however, external factors contribute to secondary distortion or deformation. These may occur in a variety of ways, and their scope of effect may be slight to profound, affecting normal tissue growth with exacerbated anatomical variations. Finally, a *disruption sequence* occurs when embryogenesis is disrupted by tissue breakdown or injury from a possible broad spectrum of opportunities, including infectious, mechanical, vascular, or metabolic origin. To complicate the comprehension of congenital anomalies, a fetal anomaly can often only be explained by the combination of sequential defects happening in utero.

Craniofacial malformations constitute a spectrum of anomalies, including clefting of the face, lip, and palates; **craniosynostosis**; nasal deviations; tongue sizes and masses; mandibular variations that affect the chin; **microtia** or ear irregularities; orbital architecture disparities; and many other well-described craniofacial pathologies. Because orofacial anomalies can be isolated events or inclusive of a larger setting of a more severe syndrome, recurrence rates vary. Knowing as much information as possible will better allow the family to understand how future pregnancies may be affected and allow for the current pregnancy to be accurately monitored for possible progression of anomalies and their effects (Boxes 59.2 and 59.3).

Abnormalities of the Forehead, Calvarium, Mandible, and Ear

Forehead. The fetal forehead extends from the hairline (or in utero the superior extent of the frontalis) inferiorly to the area of the superior orbital rim. The forehead in utero often is best appreciated with sonography by evaluation of the profile or in a coronal scanning plane similar to that used when evaluating the fetal lips. The profile plane of section is achieved by a series of midsagittal scans through the face in a lateral to medial and/or medial to lateral fashion. The frontal bone

---

BOX 59.1 Sonographic Points to Remember

- Features of the fetal face can be identified at the end of the first trimester.
- The fetal profile is well imaged with transvaginal sonography beginning late first trimester to early second trimester (make sure adequate amniotic fluid surrounds the face) (see Fig. 59.5).
- The modified coronal view is best for imaging the cleft lip and palate (see Fig. 59.6).
- The maxilla and orbits are well imaged in a true coronal plane.
- The lens of the eye is seen as a small echogenic circle within the orbit (see Fig. 59.7).
- The longitudinal view demonstrates the nasal bones, soft tissue, and mandible (useful to rule out micrognathia, anterior encephalocele, or nasal bridge defects; examine upper lip) (see Fig. 59.8).
- Transverse view shows orbital abnormalities and intraorbital distances (useful to evaluate the maxilla, mandible, and tongue).

BOX 59.2 Questions for the Sonographer Evaluating Facial Profile

- Are the orbits normally spaced?
- Are the nose and nasal bridge clearly imaged; is a proboscis or cebocephaly present?
- Are any periorbital masses apparent?
- Is the upper lip intact?
- Is the tongue normal size?
- Is the chin abnormally small?
- Are the ears of normal size and in normal position?

BOX 59.3 Sonography of the Facial Profile

Use midsagittal scans through the face to assess the following:
- Curvilinear surface with differentiation of forehead, nose, lips, and chin
- Cloverleaf skull: appears as misshapened skull with cloverleaf appearance
- Frontal bossing: may appear as lemon-shaped skull or absent, depressed nasal bridge
- Strawberry-shaped cranium: bulging of frontal bones and wide occiput
- Masses of nose and upper lip: distortion of facial profile (look for cleft lip)

appears as a curvilinear surface with differentiation of the nose, lips, and chin seen inferiorly (Fig. 59.7). This view readily allows for the diagnosis of soft tissue masses projecting from the anterior surface of the fetal face or forehead, depiction of possible bony defects, and appreciation of the relative proportion of the forehead size and shape in comparison to other facial features.

Frontal bossing is sonographically appreciated with the presence of a prominent forehead or heavy brow ridge and may be associated with a depression of the nasal bridge. It is often observed in fetuses with a lemon-shaped skull (from spina bifida) or with a myriad of skeletal dysplasias. Any irregularities in the contour of the forehead should prompt the investigator to search for other malformations as well. When the presence of a calvarial deformation is suspected, a fetal magnetic resonance (MRI) examination is typically ordered to ascertain the anomaly and its involvement or extent into surrounding anatomical structures (Fig. 59.8).

Encephaloceles are rare neural tube defects characterized by a protrusion of the brain and membranes that cover it through an opening or defect of the skull. Sonographic findings of anterior encephaloceles (Fig. 59.9) will typically be readily demonstrated by an abnormal sagittal plane or profile image. Encephaloceles are often accompanied by other craniofacial abnormalities; however, they can also be isolated and small, sometimes causing those in the nasal and forehead regions to go undetected or be very subtle (Fig. 59.10). Off-axis, or non-midline, encephaloceles have also been reported with amniotic band syndrome along with unilateral facial clefting.[17,18] This stresses the importance of sonographically evaluating not only the midline dimension of the fetal face but also the parasagittal or lateral aspects for pathology and using multiple scanning planes.

Congenital forehead hemangiomas should also be evident with sonographic evaluation in the sagittal plane (Fig. 59.11). **Hemangiomas** are benign tumors composed of small blood vessels and are most commonly found on the head and face (80%).[19] A familial history increases the risk factor for hemangioma formation twofold.[20] As with all sonographic studies, any unexpected mass should be investigated with color and or power Doppler to delineate any vascular characteristics, with pulsed wave Doppler being utilized to better characterize vascular flow or even very low flow states. These solid lesions should readily exhibit a higher than expected distinctive

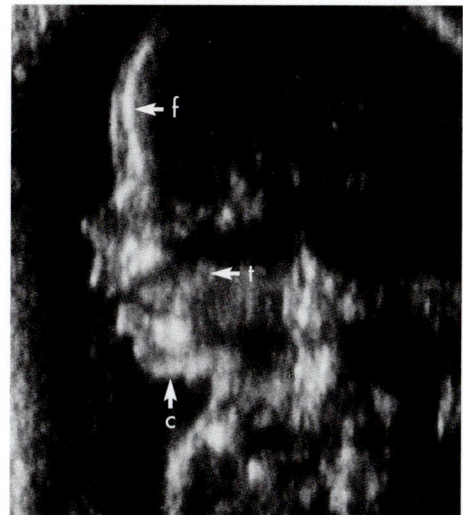

FIG. 59.7 Sagittal view in a 23-week-old fetus showing the contour of the face in profile. Note the smooth surface of the frontal bone (f) and the appearance of the nose, upper and lower lips, tongue (t), and chin (c).

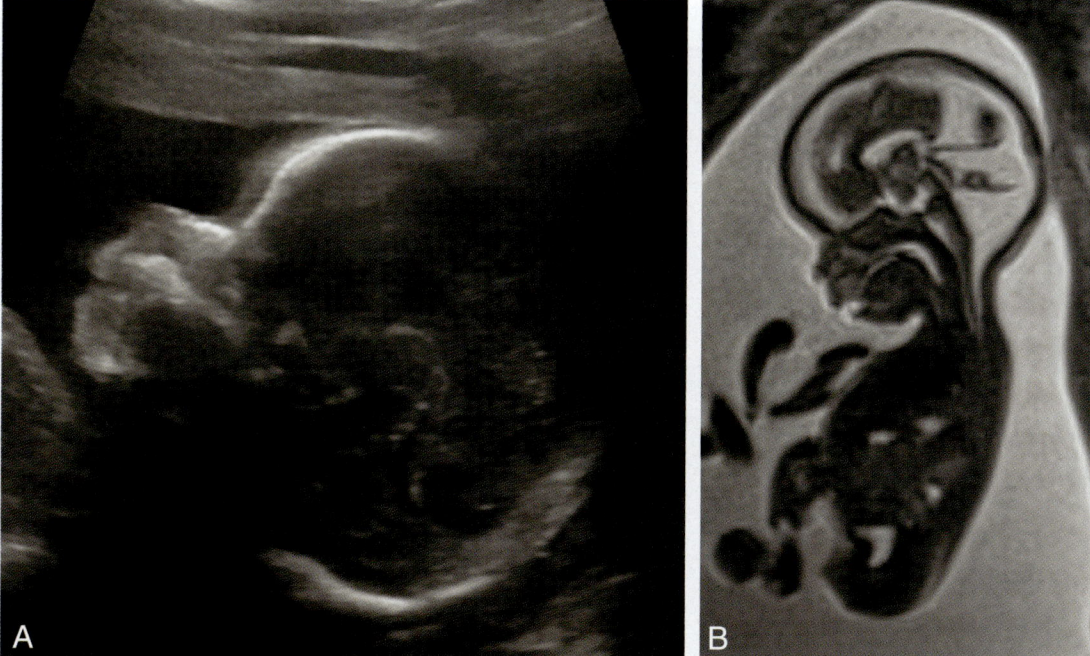

FIG. 59.8 (A) Sagittal view of a 22-week-old fetus diagnosed with frontal bossing. Notice the prominence and exaggerated roundness of the forehead. (B) Corresponding sagittal magnetic resonance image depicting the frontal bossing more readily. Also note micrognathia, pulmonary hypoplasia from a constricted thoracic cavity, a posteriorly displaced tongue in the oropharyngeal cavity, and a large posterior Dandy-Walker malformation.

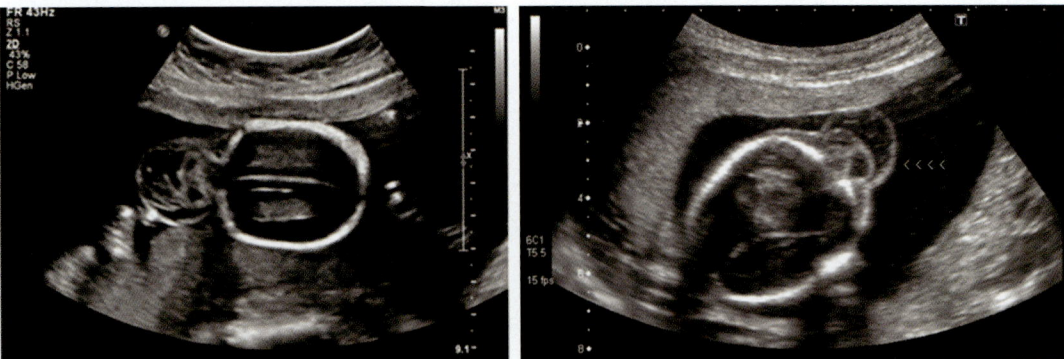

FIG. 59.9 Midline sagittal views of a fetus with an anterior (frontal) encephalocele.

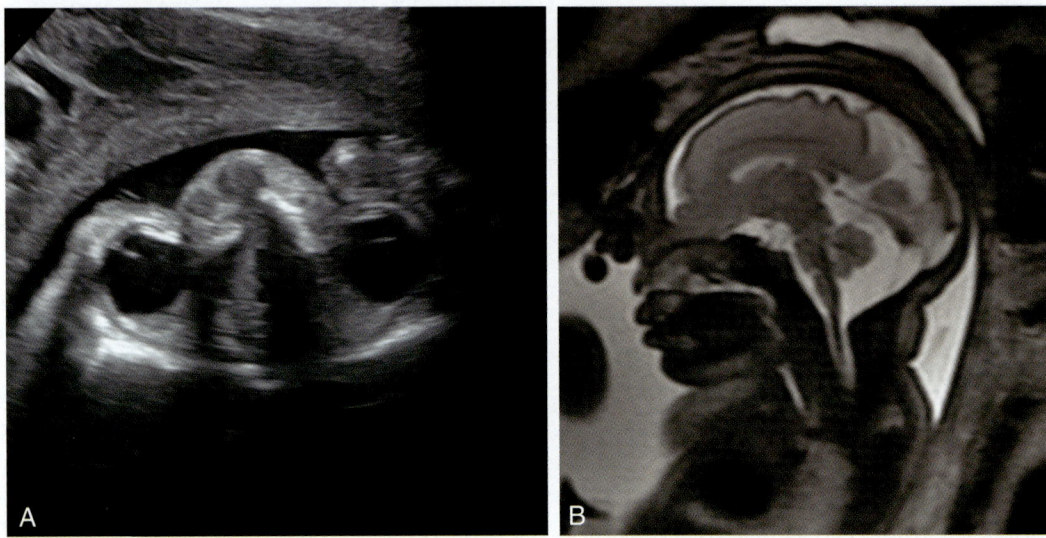

FIG. 59.10 (A) Axial image in a 29-week-old male fetus displaying an anterior frontonasal encephalocele protruding through the nasal cavity *(arrow)*. Notice the eye globe with the circular echogenic lens within both orbits. (B) Corresponding sagittal magnetic resonance image displaying the anterior frontonasal encephalocele *(arrow)*.

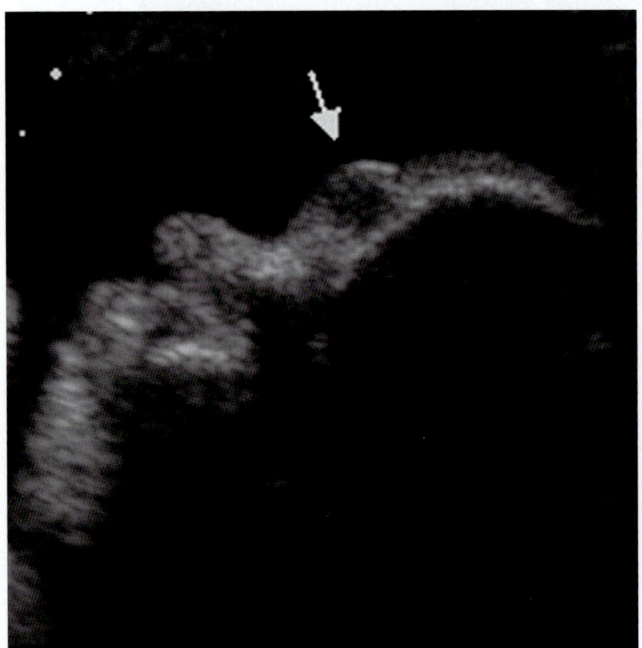

FIG. 59.11 Sagittal image of the fetal profile displaying a soft tissue hemangioma mass overlying the fetal forehead *(arrow)*.

vascularity due to their endothelial origin (Fig. 59.12). A high-resolution transducer in conjunction with 3DUS should be implemented if this abnormality is suspected, as the capillary formation may be more difficult to depict in utero with 2DUS. MRI is a good adjunct imaging tool for fetal hemangiomas as it holds the ability to demarcate vascular shunting more readily than sonography, define the extent of the lesion, and possibly demarcate involvement of other surrounding structures.[21]

Skull. Multiple calvarial malformations may occur in utero, including craniofacial microsomia and craniosynostosis. Craniofacial **microsomia** refers to the underdevelopment or the lack of full development of the anatomical structures on one side of the head and face, thus causing sometimes significant facial asymmetry.[22] Secondary only to cleft lip and palate defects, craniofacial microsomia can vary in extremes from mild asymmetry between the two sides of the face to severe underdevelopment of one facial half, with orbital implications, a partially formed ear, or even a total absence of the ear.[23] Affecting an estimated 1 in 2100 to 1 in 2500 births,[24] craniosynostosis is defined as the premature fusion of any or all six of the cranial sutures causing the fetal cranium to become abnormally shaped. This condition may have variable effects ranging from small premature closures to significant skull and facial deformities.[25] A cloverleaf skull (Kleeblattschädel) appears as an unusually misshapen skull with a cloverleaf appearance in the anterior view (Fig. 59.13). Cloverleaf skull has been associated with numerous skeletal dysplasias (most notably thanatophoric dysplasia) and has been associated with over 100 syndromes as well as occurring as an isolated event.[26] **Trigonocephaly** (premature closure of the metopic suture) may cause the forehead to have an elongated (tall) appearance in the sagittal plane and appear triangular shaped in the axial plane (Fig. 59.14). 3DUS imaging has been shown to be useful in evaluating fetal cranial sutures.

Mandible. Mandibular congenital anomalies are not common; however, when encountered, they often bring challenging predicaments. They range in severity from slight face asymmetry to complete absence of the mandible, known as **otocephaly** (a rare anomaly by which absence of the mandible causes the ears to form closer than expected anteriorly and toward the neck).[27]

Once an incidental finding with sonography, **micrognathia** is now routinely documented when present in the midline fetal profile image (Fig. 59.15). Sonographic demarcation can range from a subtle facial malformation such as a small mandible and receding chin to a much more serious concern in which the mechanical obstruction of the tongue may be present in the upper airway, leading to suffocation (Fig. 59.16). Congenital micrognathia should be suspected when a small chin is subjectively observed and diagnosed when the jaw index (JI) is calculated to be less than 21 (this number is constant across gestational ages after 18 weeks). This measurement is readily obtained and specifically utilized to detect this condition with a 100% sensitivity and 98.1% specificity.[28] The JI is calculated when the anteroposterior (AP) mandibular length is divided by the biparietal diameter (BPD) ×100 (Box 59.4). Another useful measurement in determining

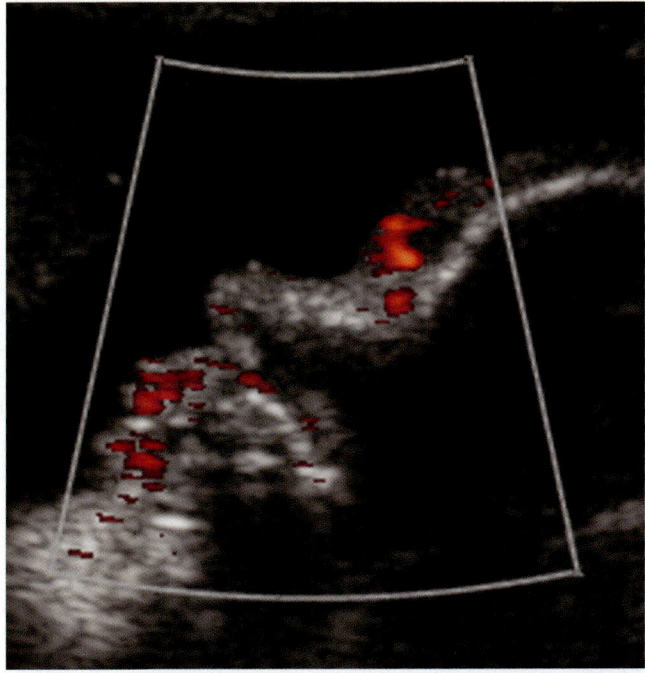

FIG. 59.12 Sagittal image of the fetal face. Color Doppler demonstrates the mass to have vascular flow within, suggesting a hemangioma.

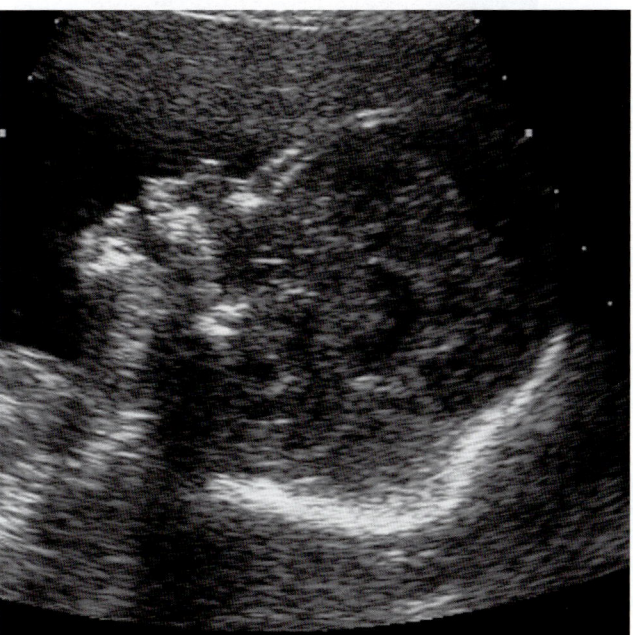

FIG. 59.13 Sagittal view of a fetus with thanatophoric dysplasia with a cloverleaf skull (Kleeblattschädel).

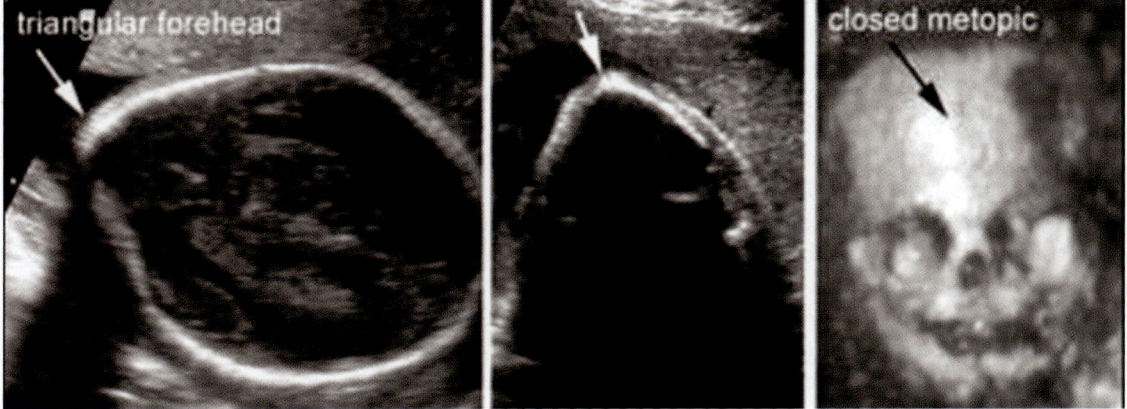

FIG. 59.14 Sagittal view of a fetus with premature closure of the metopic suture, which elongated and flattened the fetal forehead.

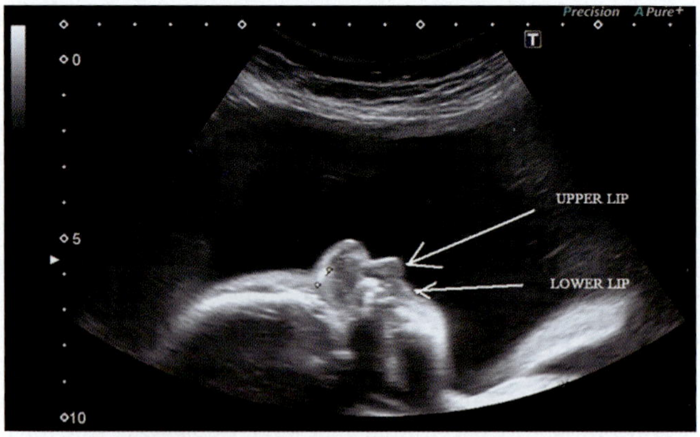

FIG. 59.15 Sagittal view of a fetus with micrognathia.

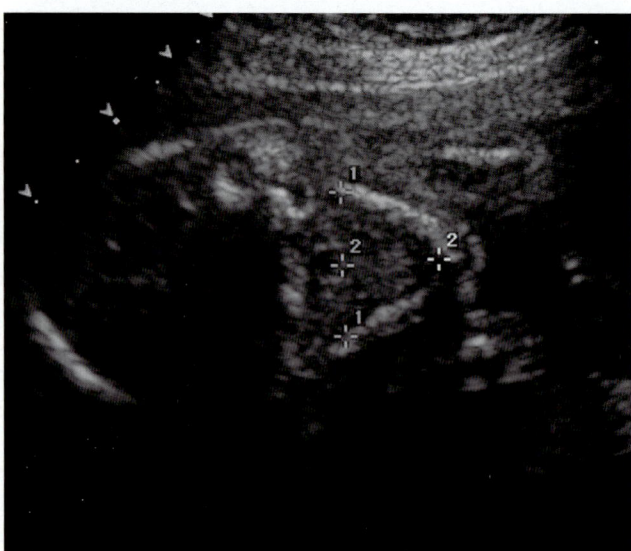

FIG. 59.17 Axial view of a normal fetal mandible demonstrating mandibular width (1) and mandibular anterior-posterior diameter (2).

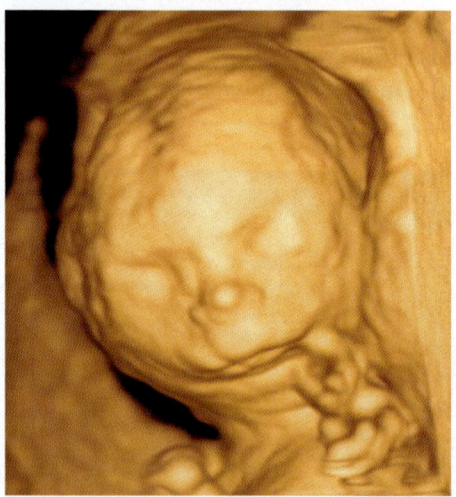

FIG. 59.16 Three-dimensional axial image of a 19-week, 6-day-old male fetus with profound micrognathia and later confirmed Robert syndrome. This patient also had anotia or absence of the ears.

BOX 59.4	Jaw Index Calculation

$$\text{Jaw index} = \frac{\text{Mandibular length (AP)}}{\text{Biparietal diameter}} \times 100$$

AP, Anteroposterior.

proper mandibular growth is the mandibular width, which is obtained in an axial plane (laterally from rami to rami) (Fig. 59.17).

Micrognathia is associated with many conditions, yet all can fit within three broad categories: (1) chromosomal anomalies, such as Edward syndrome (trisomy 18) and triploidy; (2) skeletal dysplasias, in which normal outcomes of bony structures do not form as expected; and (3) primary mandibular disorders such as **Pierre Robin syndrome** and **Treacher Collins syndrome**, in which hypoplasia of the mandible is a concern. All of these conditions carry the potential for a reduced mandibular size, causing its retruded position, which in effect requires the displacement of the tongue and reduction of the oropharyngeal airway and, when severe enough, may lead to upper airway obstruction.[29,30]

Ear. Embryogenesis of the fetal ear is complex, with changes in the size, shape, position, and even orientation of the external anatomy being the first sonographic sign of a possible deformity. The ear can be classified into three distinct areas: the inner (bony and membranous labyrinth and cochlea), middle (space occupying cavity for air, internal layer of the tympanic membrane, and the three ossicles), and exterior portions (auricle, external acoustic meatus and canal, and the external layer of the tympanic membrane). Ear malformations can occur in any of these areas, with changes in the ear's size, shape, or locations causing a possible detrimental situation due to their functionality dependence. The outer or external ear's primary function is resonance and the amplification of sound,[31] with its external location being easily accessible with sonography. The symmetrical arrangement of the two ears helps elicit balance as well as facilitates the localization of sound. As with other facial deformities, external ear disfigurement often carries the possible negative psychological repercussions that most craniofacial anomalies prescribe.

The pinna and auricle of the external fetal ears may be imaged in a parasagittal plane or in a coronal plane, and when suspicion of an abnormality is present, should be imaged in all three orthogonal planes (Fig. 59.18). Ear malformations range in variance from being correctly formed, yet located more inferiorly than expected or malrotated, to being small and not properly formed as anticipated, as is indicative of microtia, to being completely absent **(anotia)** (Fig. 59.19).[32] Biometric nomograms have long been established to correlate ear size with gestational age for both bidimensional and 3DUS evaluations.[14] When placement of the ear appears subjectively lower than usual, a concern for other craniofacial malformations and syndromes should arise.[27]

Several ear malformations may be sonographically observed, such as is noted with Goldenhar syndrome or oculo-auriculo-vertebral spectrum, a form of **hemifacial microsomia** (which typically affects the development of the eye, ear, and spine, causing facial asymmetry) to even severe lateral facial clefting, which has the potential to affect the correct development of the fetal ear.[33] Roberts syndrome typically involves multiple facial abnormalities, including clefting of the lip with or without cleft palate, micrognathia, hypertelorism, and ear abnormalities often accompanied by nasal disfigurement.[34] Nager syndrome affects the first and second branchial arches and is associated with ear deformities, micrognathia, and other upper limb anomalies. Treacher-Collins syndrome affects the development of bones and other tissues in the face and ears and may be observed prenatally.[10,35] Otocephaly may also be sonographically noted as a rare anomaly in which absence of the mandible (**agnathia**) causes the ears to form close together towards the anterior neck, with microstomia and possible hypoplasia or even absence of the tongue (aglossia).[36] Although these syndromes are not common, a thorough investigation of the fetal ear may prevent a subtle or even severe malformation from being undiscovered.

Abnormalities of the Orbits

The sonographic assessment of orbital architecture has become increasingly important in the evaluation of craniofacial anomalies. The anatomical components of the orbits, the utilization of orbital measurements correlated to gestational age, and the role of ultrasound in detecting ocular abnormalities continue to expand as technology continues to improve.[37,38]

Sonographic assessment of the orbits should begin with the basics, including the presence of both eyes and their overall size, to exclude **microphthalmia** (in which the ocular globe is present but the axial length of the eye is at least two standard deviations below the mean for gestational age) and **anophthalmia** (an absent eye) (Fig. 59.20).[39] Masses of the orbit (periorbital) and of the eye (intraocular) should be excluded with meticulous investigation in multiple planes through each of the sockets due to the fact that periorbital masses, such as lacrimal duct cysts (**dacryocystoceles**), dermoids, congenital teratomas, and even hemangiomas, have been reported in the literature (Fig. 59.21).[40–45]

The hyaloid artery, which regresses in the third trimester, is a branch of the primitive dorsal ophthalmic artery. It extends from the optic nerve through the vitreous cavity to the lens to aid in its development (Fig. 59.22). Although typically searched out only in the presence of pathology, the hyaloid artery may be observed within the fetal eye in a laterally approached axial plane.

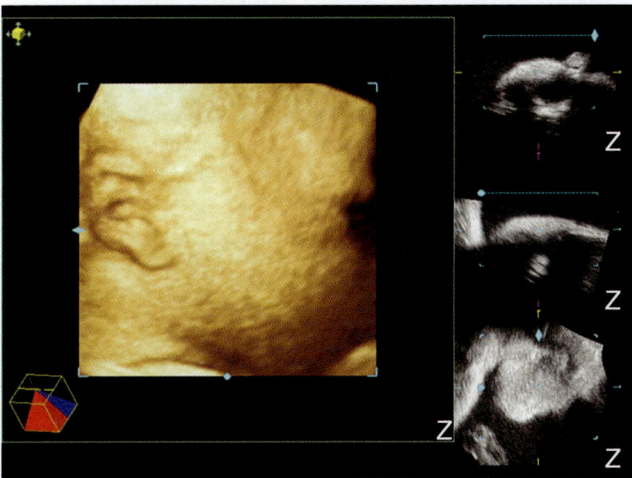

FIG. 59.18 Multiplanar reconstruction of a fetus with the earlobe well seen.

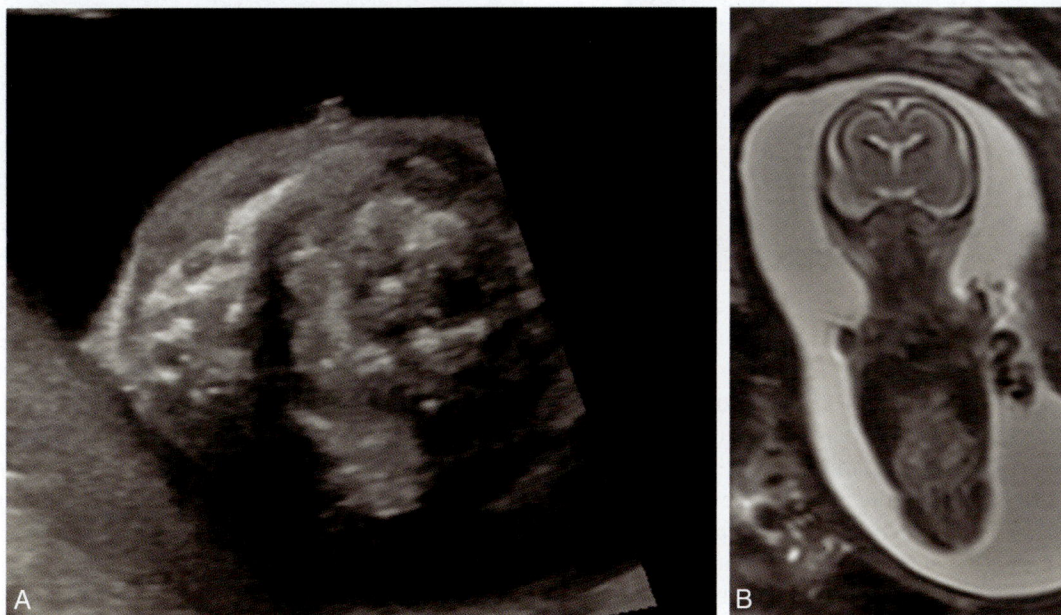

FIG. 59.19 (A) Axial image of a 19-week-old fetus at the level of the pinna. Notice the small dysplastic soft tissue mass where the pinna of the ear should be located. (B) Coronal magnetic resonance image of the same fetus displaying the evident anotia *(arrows)*. A diagnosis of Robert syndrome was found in this fetus.

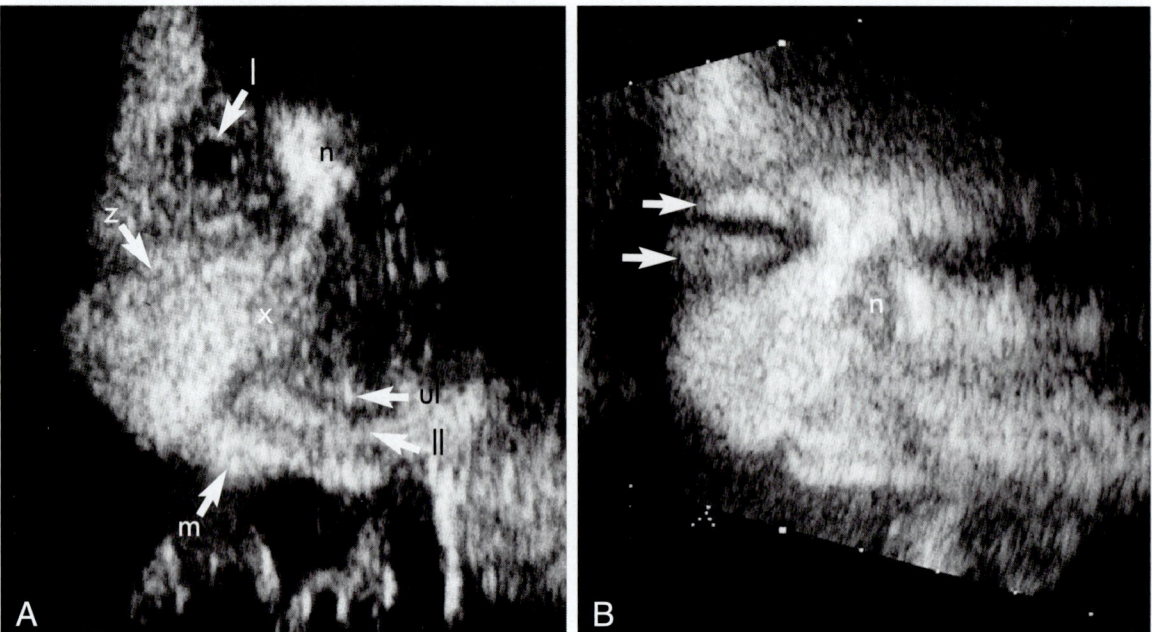

FIG. 59.20 (A) Coronal view showing facial features: lens (l), zygomatic bone (z), maxilla (x), upper lip (ul), lower lip (ll), mandible (m), and nasal bones (n). (B) In a more anterior coronal view of the same fetus, the upper and lower eyelids *(arrows)* and the nose (n) are visible.

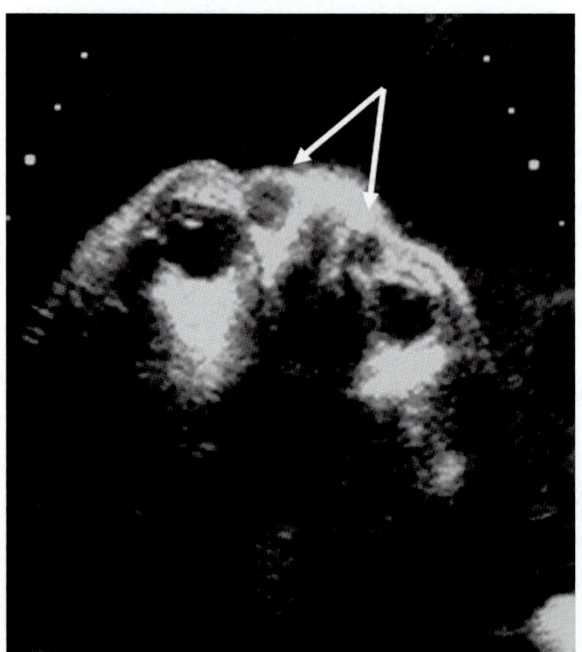

FIG. 59.21 In the transverse plane, bilateral lacrimal duct cysts are seen *(arrows)*.

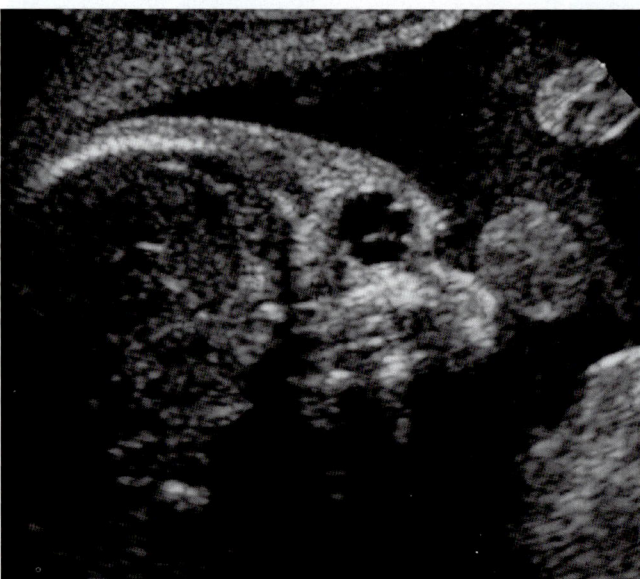

FIG. 59.22 An axial view of the fetal head demonstrates the hyaloid artery seen as a linear structure within the vitreous cavity of the eye.

Transvaginal sonography, due to its detailed resolution, has aided in the detection of first-trimester ocular anomalies and other intracranial abnormalities.[46,47] In addition, an oblique tangential section from the nasal bridge can be used to detect the lens of the eye, which appears as hypoechogenic circular entities within the anterior aspect of the orbits, just lateral to the nose. Using this method, ocular abnormalities have been demonstrated, including **strabismus** (eyes do not properly align while looking at an object), microphthalmia, divergence of lens, **exophthalmia**, and cataracts.

Orbital distance measurements are helpful in the diagnosis of fetal conditions in which hypotelorism or hypertelorism is a feature. Both conditions are associated with other anomalies, and the orbital concern often helps determine which cranial anomaly or genetic syndrome is present. An anatomic and biometric evaluation of the fetal orbits should be attempted in fetuses at risk for abnormal orbital distance (Fig. 59.23).

Hypotelorism. **Hypotelorism** is a condition characterized by decreased distance between the orbits. Hypotelorism is most commonly associated with midline abnormalities such as **holoprosencephaly**; however, it has also been associated with several syndromes and other anomalies, including **microcephaly**, craniosynostoses, and **phenylketonuria (PKU)** (Fig. 59.24).

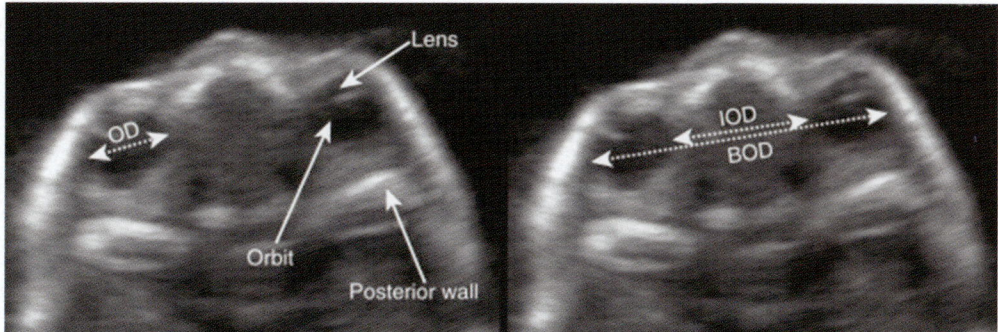

FIG. 59.23 Images through the fetal orbits may allow the correct placement of calipers to measure the outer-to-outer distance of the orbits, sometimes referred to as the binocular distance (BOD), and the inner-to-inner orbital measurement. *IOD,* Interocular distance; *OD,* ocular distance.

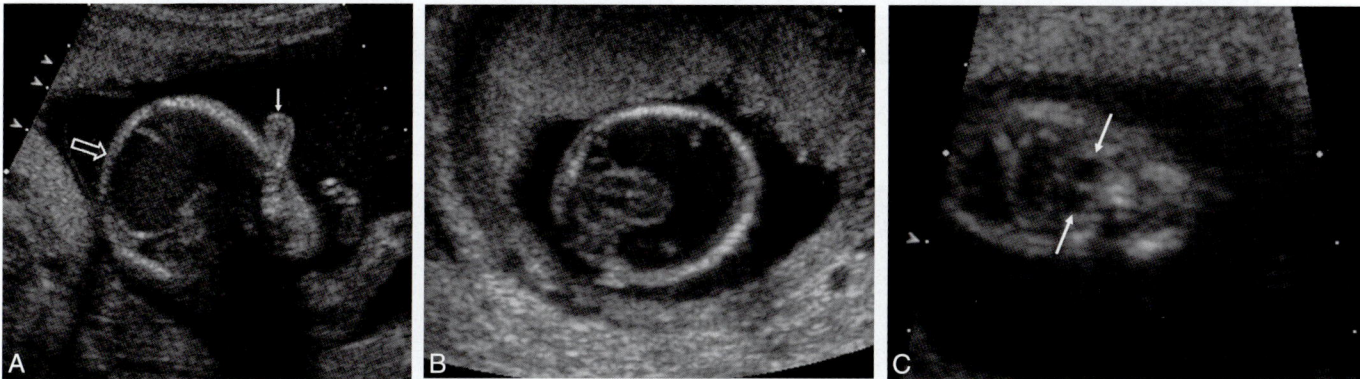

FIG. 59.24 (A) A midline sagittal view of the face in a fetus with holoprosencephaly shows a proboscis *(small arrow)*; a dorsal sac (sometimes seen with holoprosencephaly) can be seen in the posterior fetal cranium *(open arrow)*. (B) An axial view of the same fetus displays the monoventricle seen with holoprosencephaly. (C) Coronal view of the same fetus reveals hypotelorism *(arrows)*.

Obvious hypotelorism will be seen in **ethmocephaly** (proboscis separating narrow-set eyes with an absent nose and microphthalmia) and **cebocephaly** (two separate eyes set close together and a small flat nose with a single nostril) (Fig. 59.25) or may be so severe that a single orbit is demonstrated with a fused or single eye, as is seen in **cyclopia** (Fig. 59.26).

Hypertelorism. **Hypertelorism** is characterized by abnormally wide-spaced orbits. Hypertelorism is found in several abnormal fetal conditions, genetic syndromes, and chromosomal anomalies. Fetuses exposed to phenytoin (an antiepileptic medication to control seizures) during pregnancy may manifest signs of hypertelorism as part of fetal phenytoin syndrome (microcephaly; growth abnormalities; cleft lip and/or palate; and cardiac, genitourinary, central nervous system, and skeletal anomalies). Frontal **cephaloceles** may widen the space between the eyes (Fig. 59.27). In both Pfeiffer syndrome and Apert syndrome, hypertelorism and brachycephaly have been described as a result of abnormal closure of the calvarial sutures (craniosynostosis).[25,48,49] Frontonasal dysplasia (median cleft facial syndrome) was diagnosed in a fetus with ventriculomegaly based on sonographic findings of hypertelorism and cleft lip (Fig. 59.28).[47] Other conditions that manifest with hypertelorism and premature suture closure include Crouzon syndrome, cephalosyndactyly, and acrocephalopolysyndactyly.

Fetal hypertelorism and or hypotelorism is sonographically determined by obtaining measurements of orbital width found with the external canthal distance or the transverse distance between the outermost rims of the left and right orbits (outer to outer measurement). The internal canthal distance may also be determined by obtaining, in the transverse plane, the distance between the innermost rims of the left and right orbits (inner to inner) (Fig. 59.29). Again, these measurements correlate to well-established nomograms for gestational ages.

Abnormalities of the Mid-Face: Nose, Maxilla, Lips, and Palate

The mid-face, which consists of the nose, maxilla, lips, and palate, may be viewed by placing the transducer in a lateral coronal plane or sagittal profile plane and in modified tangential maxillary view or modified coronal view (inferior-superior projection) (Fig. 59.30). In the lateral coronal view, the integrity of the nasal structures in relation to the orbital rings and maxillae can be investigated. In a profile plane, the contour of the nose, upper and lower lips, and chin is observed. In this same parasagittal plane, the transducer should be swept from the most lateral right aspect to the most lateral left aspect of the face to rule out any soft tissue

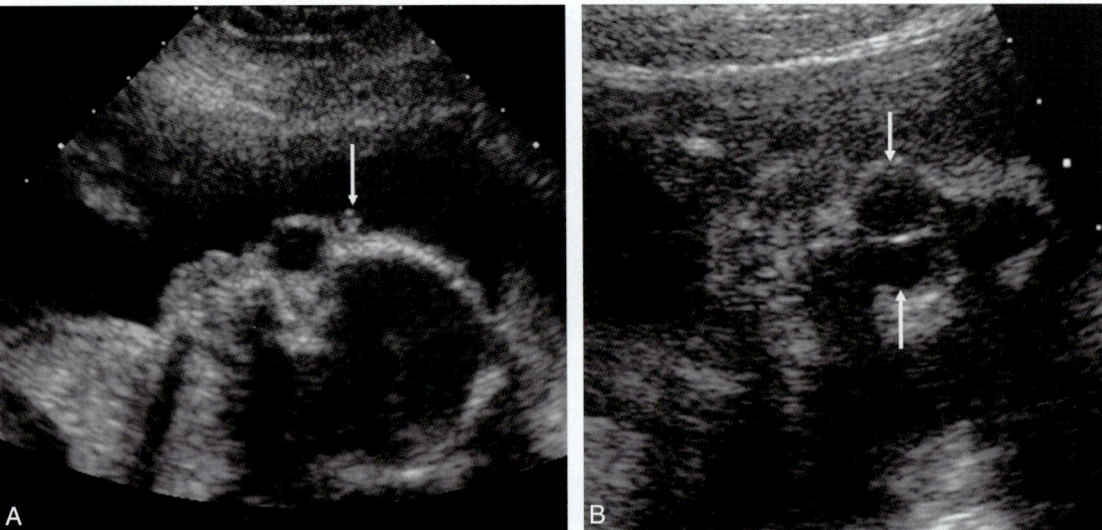

FIG. 59.25 (A) A midline sagittal plane view through the face of a fetus with holoprosencephaly demonstrates cyclopia with a small proboscis *(arrow)* above the central eye. (B) The coronal view of the same fetus shows two asymmetrically sized eyes within one orbit *(arrows)*.

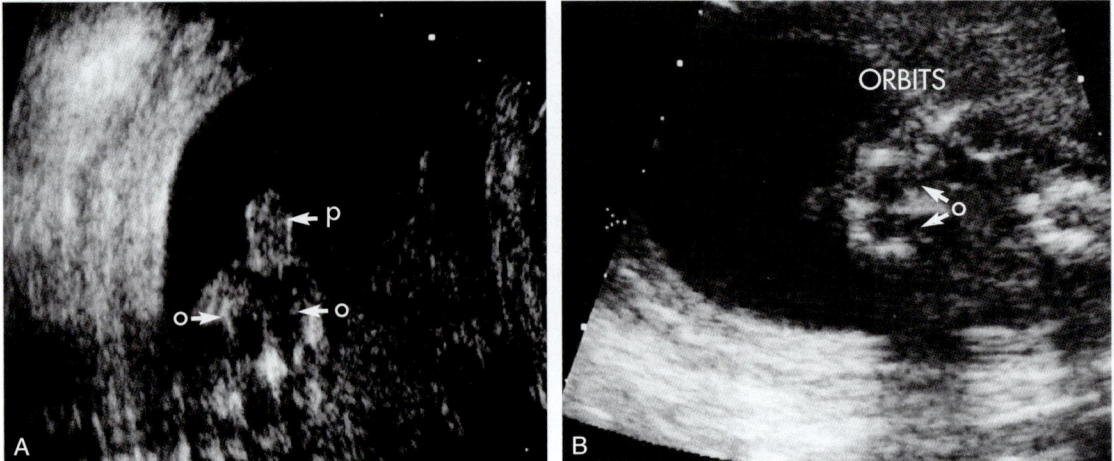

FIG. 59.26 (A) Proboscis (p) observed in a frontal facial view in a midline position above the closely spaced orbits (o) in a 20-week-old fetus with ethmocephaly. (B) In the same fetus, the orbits are observed. A single eye with fused orbits was found. Trisomy 13 was noted after delivery.

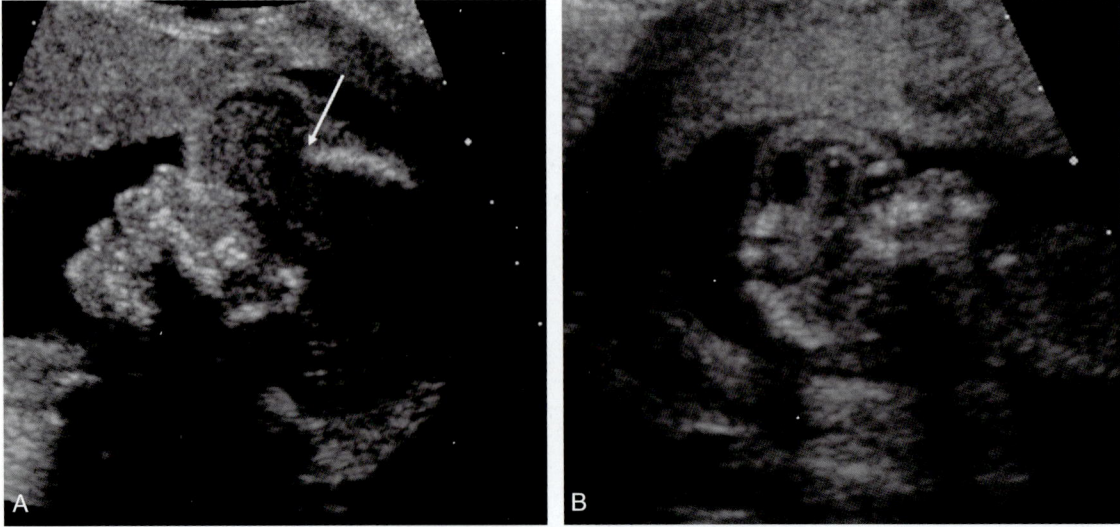

FIG. 59.27 (A) Midline sagittal view of a fetus with an anterior (frontal) encephalocele and delineation of the bony defect *(arrow)*. (B) Midline sagittal image of a large frontal encephalocele that also involved facial structures.

masses or presence of facial clefting defects. This is an important view in assessing the presence or absence of the nose, lips, chin, and integrity of facial skin coverings (Fig. 59.31). Tangential planes, with the transducer angled inferiorly to superiorly through the maxilla, demonstrate the nasal septum and nostril openings, or nares (Fig. 59.32), and the absence of any facial masses or clefting (Fig. 59.33).

Nose. Evaluation of the nasal triad should assess (1) nostril symmetry, (2) nasal septum integrity, and (3) continuity of the upper lip to exclude cleft lip and discontinuity of the soft palate to exclude soft palate clefting. The maxilla marks the posterior border of the nose and is a landmark used in assessing the fetus at risk for premaxillary protuberance, as seen in Roberts syndrome. Besides face, lip, and palate clefting, other congenital anomalies and syndromes contribute to a wide range of possible nasal abnormalities such as holoprosencephaly effects of nasal anomalies ranging from the absence of the nose (**arhinia**) to the presence of a proboscis to a single-nostril nose (cebocephaly) (see Fig. 59.25). The fetal nasal bone may be small or absent with certain chromosomal anomalies, particularly Down syndrome (trisomy 21). Much has been written in the literature about the presence or absence of the fetal nasal bone as a predictor of abnormal karyotypes (Fig. 59.34).[50-56]

Isolated intranasal masses, especially those encountered prenatally via sonographic examination, are very rare, with teratomas having the highest incidence of 1 in 20,000 to 40,000 live births.[57] Teratomas composed of all three germ layers may be found anywhere in the body, yet those of the head and neck account for less than 5% of all teratomas.[58-60] Because they are a germ cell tumor, teratomas may have a variable appearance and size, but they are typically noted as well-circumscribed complex solid masses by sonography. Differential diagnosis for intranasal solid masses includes nasal glioma (encephalocele that has lost its intracranial connection and continuation with meninges), nasal encephalocele, nasal polyp, dermoid cyst, and nasal chondromesenchymal hamartoma (see Fig. 59.10).[58,61]

Midface Hypoplasia. Midface or maxillary hypoplasia results from an underdevelopment or maldevelopment of the middle structures of the face.[62,63] When maxilla-nasal dysplasia affects the anterior aspect of the maxilla and nasal complex, it is specifically termed Binder syndrome.[64,65] The typical appearance includes a flattened and retruded nose, half-moon-shaped nostrils, short columella, and an acute nasolabial angle, resulting in an almost concave midfacial profile.[66] Sonographically,

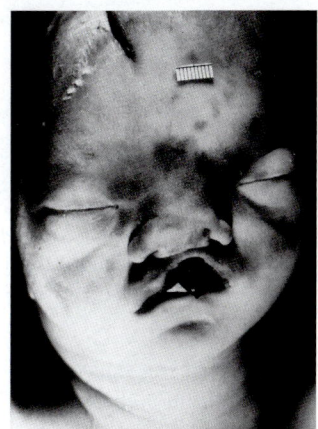

FIG. 59.28 Postmortem image of neonate with median cleft facial syndrome (frontonasal dysplasia). Note the hypertelorism and mass of the upper lip. Other abnormalities observed prenatally include severe ventriculomegaly with a shift of the interhemispheric fissure.

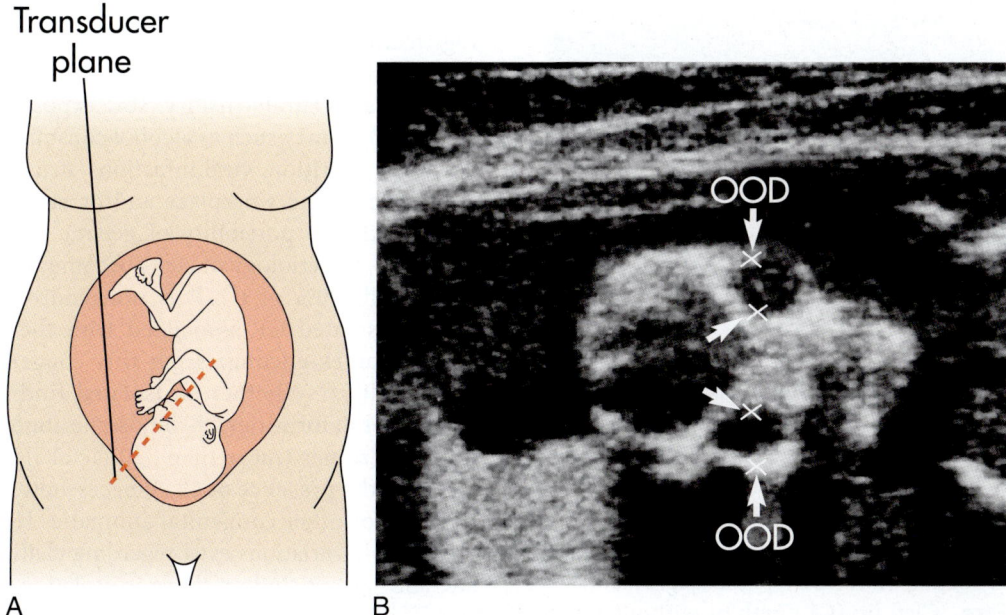

FIG. 59.29 (A) Frontal view demonstrating a fetus in a vertex presentation with the fetal cranium in an occipitotransverse position. The transducer is placed along the coronal plane (approximately 2 cm posterior to the glabella-alveolar line). (B) Sonogram demonstrating the orbits in the coronal view. The outer orbital diameter (OOD) and inner orbital diameter (IOD; *angled arrows*) are noted. The IOD is measured from the medial border of the orbit to the opposite medial border. The OOD is measured from the outermost lateral border of the orbit to the opposite lateral border.

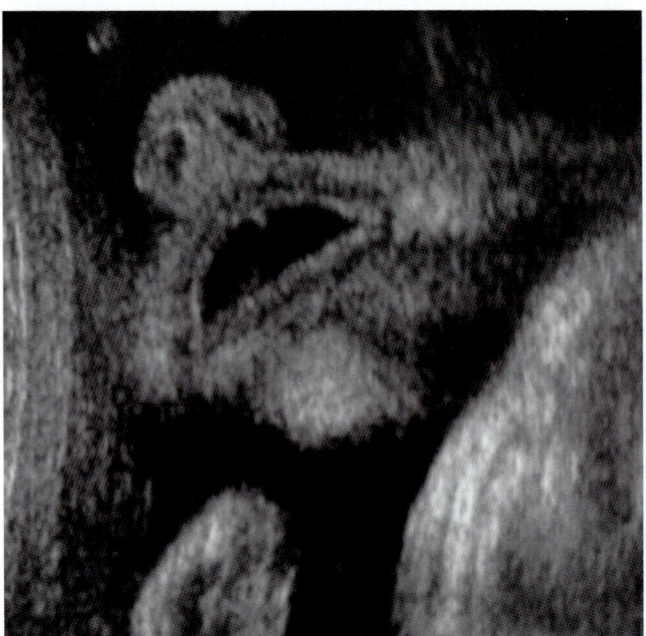

FIG. 59.30 Axial view through the upper lip, lower lip, nares, and the nasal septum. The vermilion tissue of the lips can be differentiated.

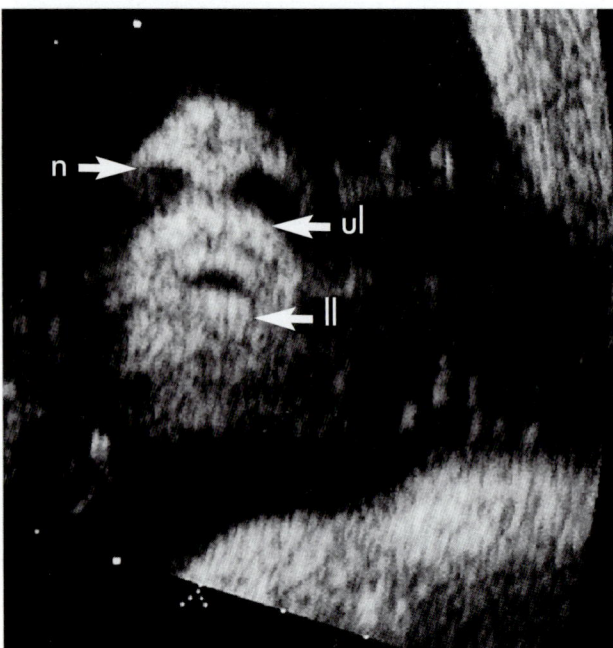

FIG. 59.32 Axial view through the upper (ul) and lower lip (ll) in a fetus with an open mouth. Note the nares (n) and nasal septum. This view is used to check for a cleft of the upper lip.

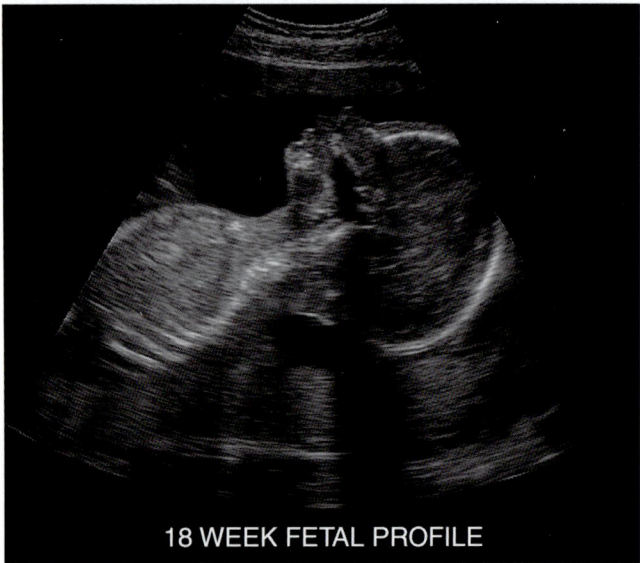

FIG. 59.31 The fetal profile is well seen with amniotic fluid surrounding the face. This is a useful plane to image the forehead, nose, lips, and chin.

this condition in utero is most readily appreciated with the fetal midsagittal profile image (Fig. 59.35).

Midface hypoplasia may be seen in fetuses with chromosome anomalies such as Down syndrome (trisomy 21), craniosynostosis syndromes such as Apert syndrome, and limb and skeletal dysplasias such as achondroplasia, chondrodysplasia punctata, and asphyxiating thoracic dysplasia (Fig. 59.36).[62]

Lip, Palate, and Face. Cleft lip (CL) with or without a cleft palate (CL/P) component is the most common congenital craniofacial anomaly.[4,67] The incidence of CL/P shows racial variation, with the highest risk occurring in the Asian population at 1 per 350 births. Whites have a rate of 1 per 600 births, and African Americans have a rate of 1 per 3000 births.[3,6,68] CL with or without cleft palate (CP) occurs more commonly in males; however, isolated CP is more common in females, and an equal incidence of 0.4 per 1000 live born is found in all races.[69,70] As with most congenital craniofacial abnormalities, facial clefting defects often hold a high psychosocial impact for those affected as well as their families, often requiring a multidisciplinary team approach to provide diagnostic, therapeutic, and psychologic counseling/treatment. Several contributing factors may be involved with orofacial clefting predispositions, including geographic factors, race, family history, sex, exposure to risk factors during pregnancy such as alcohol consumption and tobacco use, poor nutrition, viral infections, drugs, and presence of teratogens at the workplace and/or at home. When combined with the possibility of genetic predispositions and processes, the etiology of clefts becomes multifactorial.[3,71,72]

Overall, 90% of CL/P is nonsyndromic compared to 50% of isolated CP associated with the broad spectrum of syndromes encompassing this congenital craniofacial abnormality.[73] Whether an isolated finding or associated with other deformities, chromosome abnormalities, or various syndromes (more than 350 facial cleft syndromes are known), the presence of CL/P necessitates thorough investigation for other congenital anomalies (Fig. 59.37).[67,74-76]

Multiple variations exist regarding clefting of the lip, palate, and face, including those in isolation and in combination.[77,78] Three main lip classifications are recognized:
1. Unilateral CL, occurring more frequently on the left side in isolation[79]
2. Bilateral CL
3. Median CL

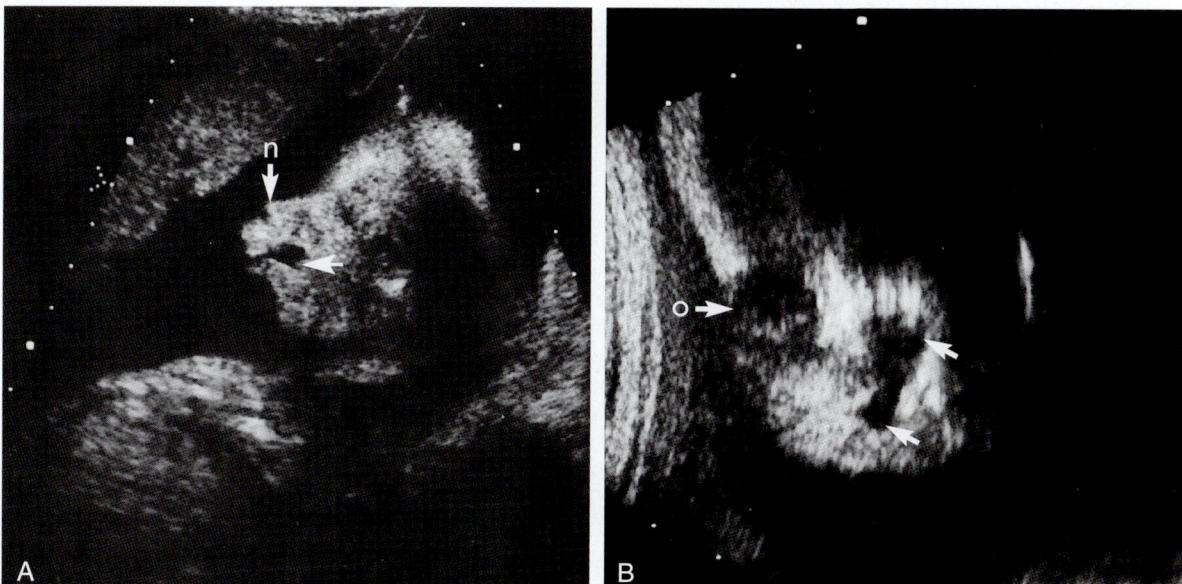

FIG. 59.33 (A) Unilateral cleft lip with clefting defect extending through the palate into the nasal cavity *(arrow)* in a sagittal plane in a 25-week-old fetus. Note the globular appearance of the tissue under the nose (n) (premaxillary protuberance). (B) In the same fetus, the coronal plane illustrates the extent of clefting *(arrows)*. Note the defect extending from the upper lip to the nasal cavity. *O,* Orbit.

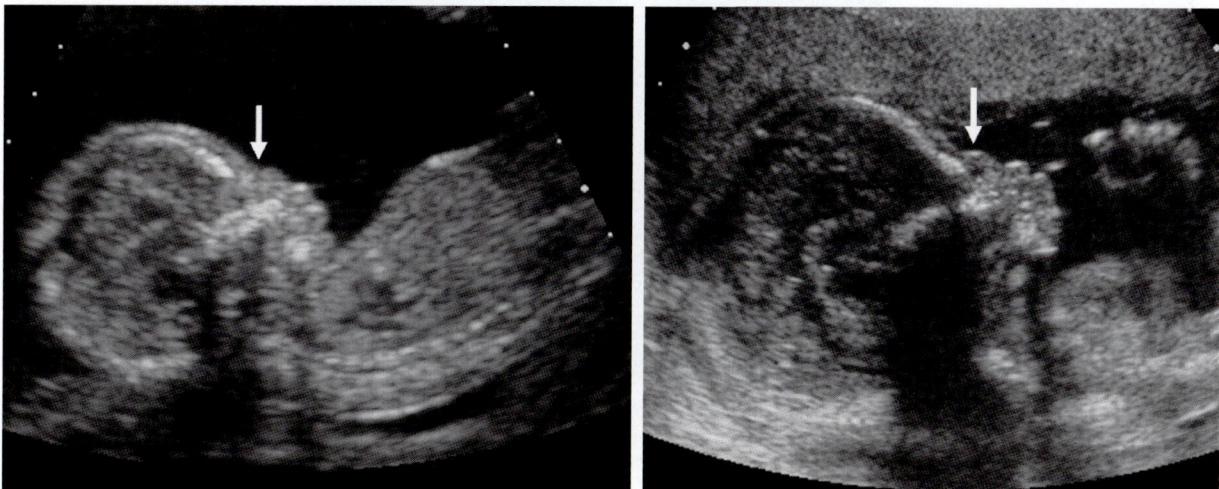

FIG. 59.34 Two fetuses with trisomy 21 showing an absent nasal bone *(arrows)*.

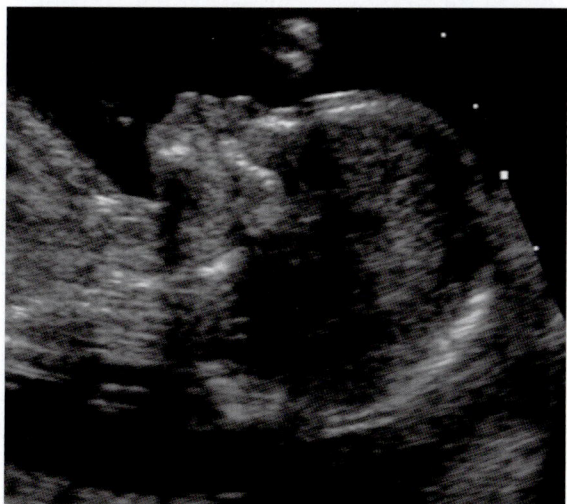

FIG. 59.35 Midline sagittal view of a fetus affected by familial midface hypoplasia.

Failure of fusion of the maxillary and medial nasal prominences or between the palatal processes results in clefts of varying extent, unilaterally or bilaterally. Specifically, CL occurs due to the failure of fusion of the primary and secondary palate, resulting in a cleft defect coursing anteriorly through the upper lip and alveolus to assorted extents. The depth of the cleft may vary from the soft tissue of the lip to a complete cleft of the maxillary bone. CP occurs when the lateral palatine processes fail to fuse at the midline, and CL/P occurs in unison when both fusions are absent.

CP diagnosed alone without any other abnormality is often a challenge with 2D ultrasound due to location; however, the detection rate of CL/P increases, especially in the setting of other congenital abnormalities (Fig. 59.38).[80] Although the distribution for clefts differs by geographic location and ethnicity, it is estimated to be 20% to 25% CL, 40% to 50% CL/P, and 30% to 35% CP.[69] Clefts occur in a ratio of 6:3:1 unilateral

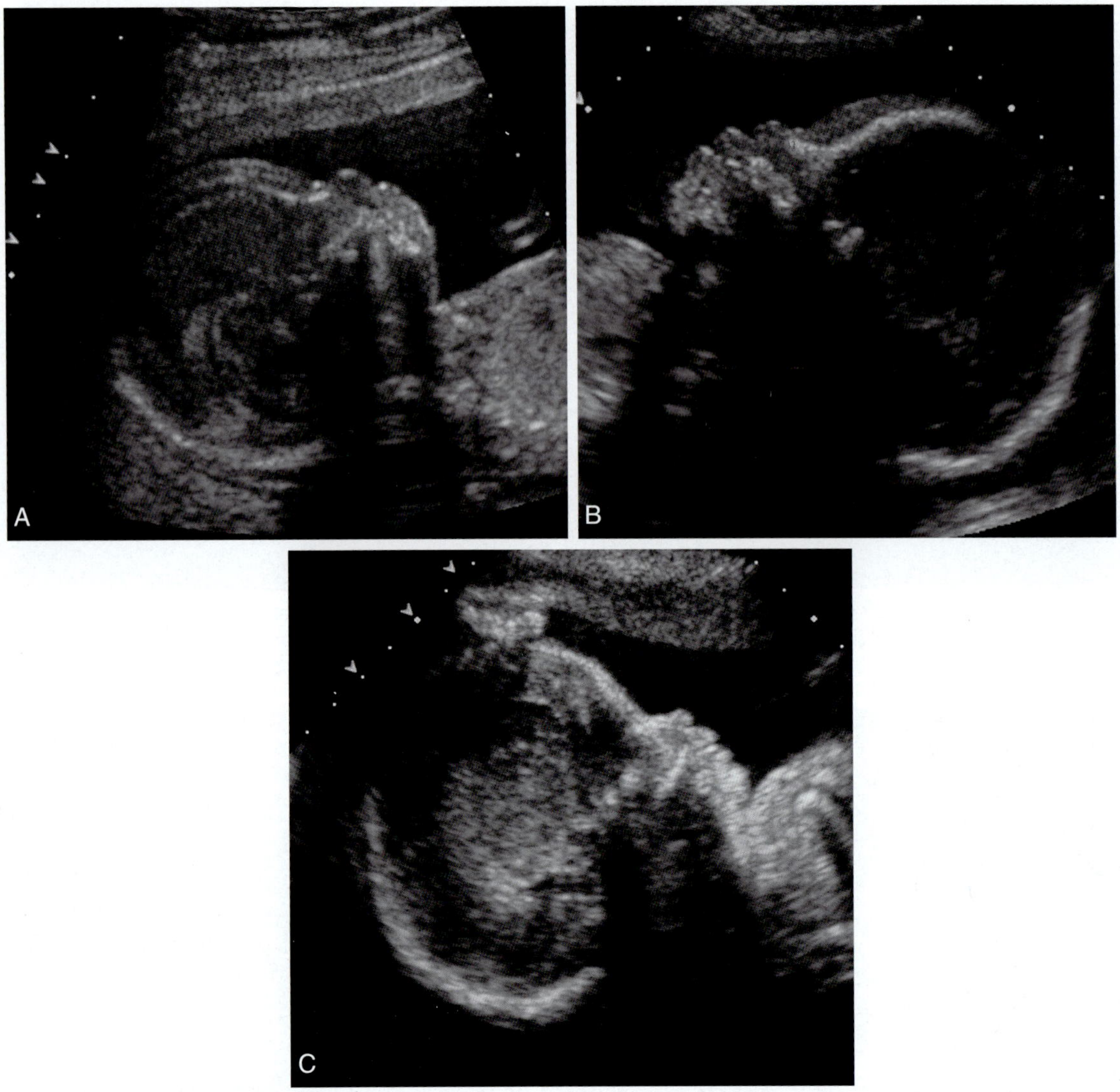

FIG. 59.36 Midline sagittal views. (A) A fetus with trisomy 21 (Down syndrome); note flattened facies. (B) A fetus with a skeletal dysplasia demonstrates mild frontal bossing and midface hypoplasia. (C) A fetus with neonatal progeroid syndrome; note smallness of facial profile compared with the head. Cranial biometry was consistent with gestational age.

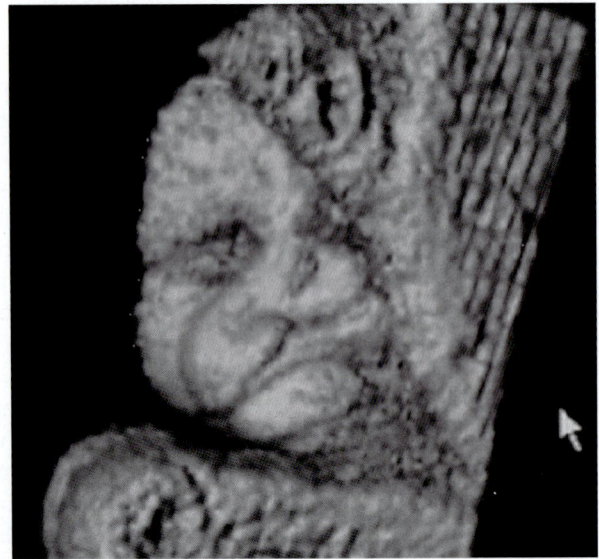

FIG. 59.37 An early three-dimensional image of a median facial cleft seen with holoprosencephaly.

left, unilateral right, and bilateral.[81] When bilateral CL lesions are present, CP is found in up to 85% of neonates. When unilateral, CP may be seen in 70% of infants. Isolated CP is a separate disorder from CL/P.[82] When CP is present, fetal breathing may be observed with color Doppler in both the nasopharynx and the oropharynx. In the presence of a normal palate, color flow should be observed only in the fetal nasopharynx when the mouth is closed (Fig. 59.39).[83] Color flow Doppler may also be used to identify abnormal oral cavity bidirectional blood flow, vessel formation, and oropharynx abnormalities.

Other prenatally detectable clefting conditions include acrocephalopolysyndactyly, amniotic band syndrome, anencephaly, congenital cardiac disease, diastrophic dysplasia, holoprosencephaly, spondyloepiphyseal dysplasia congenita, Meckel-Gruber syndrome, Roberts syndrome, and multiple pterygium syndromes. A premaxillary protrusion or a premaxillary mass suggests the presence of a bilateral CL/P, even when only a unilateral defect is suspected sonographically. This premaxillary mass of tissue may correspond to

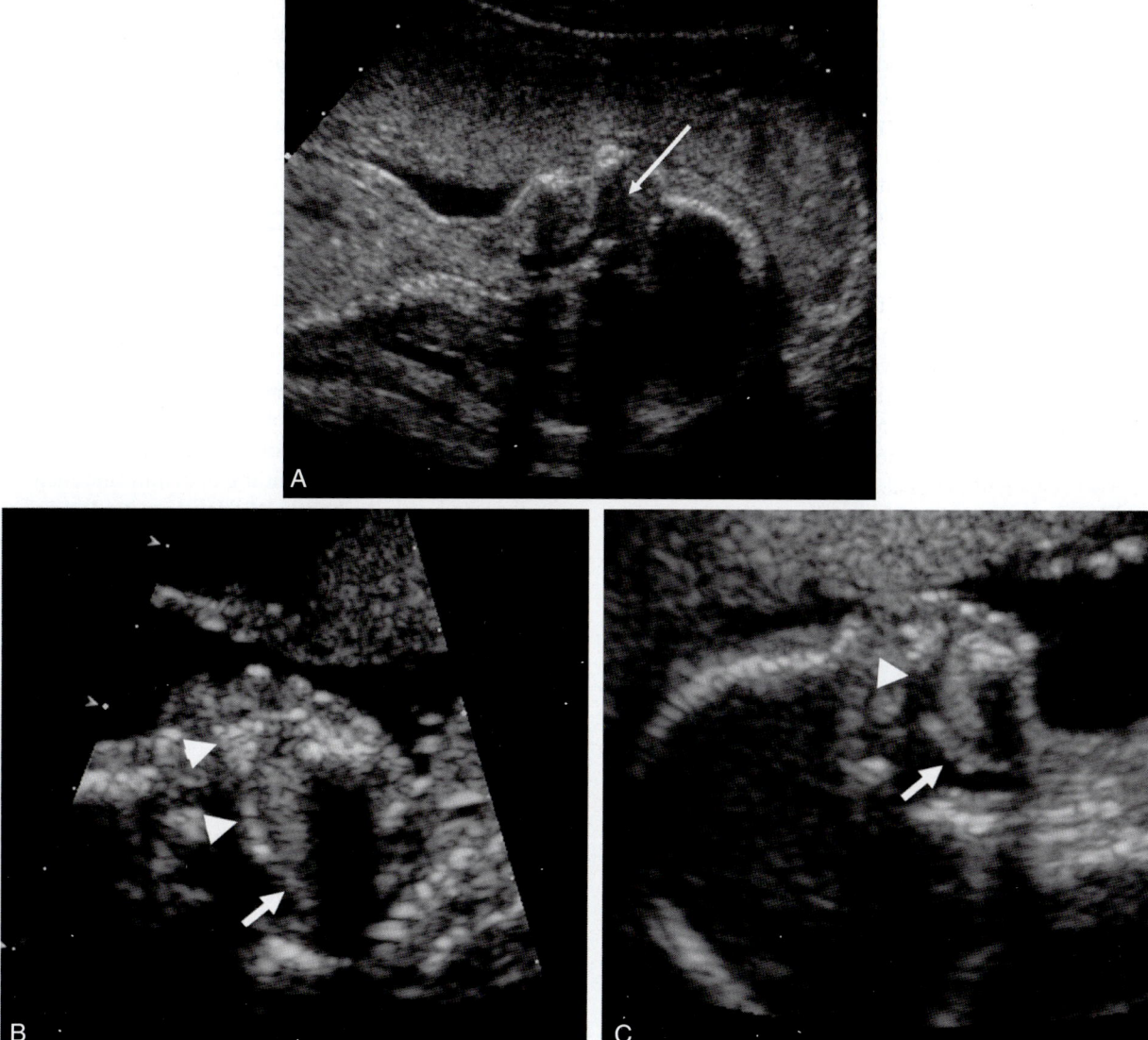

FIG. 59.38 (A) Sagittal image of a fetus with a bilateral cleft lip and palate. Fluid is seen in the common oropharynx-nasopharynx area, suggesting a cleft palate *(arrow)*. (B) Midline sagittal plane of a normal palate in a 29-week-old fetus *(left)* and a 21-week-old fetus *(right)*. The hard palate can be seen adjacent to the fetal tongue *(arrowheads)*, and the fetal soft palate can be visualized between the oropharynx and nasopharynx *(arrows)*. Observation of the fetus while swallowing and moving the mouth may aid in delineation of these structures.

abnormal anterior herniation of the hard palate and teeth caused by defects in the alveolar ridge (Fig. 59.40).

Sonographically, visualization of the hard and soft palates remains a diagnostic challenge due to the considerable bony shadowing by the maxilla, alveolus, and tongue (Box 59.5). The operator should utilize a systematic approach when examining the fetal face for clefts in all three orthogonal planes (Fig. 59.41). The addition of 3DUS and 4DUS reconstruction has been a proven adjunct imaging tool to bidirectional ultrasound assessment of craniofacial anomalies, in particular with facial clefts (Fig 59.42).[80,84]

Facial Clefting. Although encountered less frequently, oblique facial clefts (**meloschisis**) have variations such as the lip and palate and include (1) unilateral, (2) bilateral, and (3) combined with other clefting (possibly lip and/or palate).

Clefts of the face may occur along various facial planes. Defects range from clefting of the lip alone to involvement of the hard and soft palate, which may extend into the nose and, in rare cases, into the orbital socket.[85] Facial clefts may be observed when clefting courses laterally from the corner of the mouth and, in severe cases, may extend to the ear and up into the orbital cavity where preservation or protection of the cornea is a concern. Besides the embryogenic deviation to the formation of the fetal face that may elicit clefting, mechanical impingement may propagate asymmetric facial clefting, such as is seen with amniotic band syndrome.[18,86]

In the setting of lip, palate, nasal, or facial clefting, the challenge exists to preserve normal appearance and functionality. These corrections often require careful planning of their staged reconstruction, entailing multiple surgical corrections beginning in infancy and lasting through adulthood, frequently with less than expected esthetic outcome gratification. However, the goal of these surgeries is not limited to facilitating social integration; their intent is first and foremost to restore functions such as airway patency, feeding abilities, maxillary sinus reconstruction, speech and language acquisition, dental reconstruction, and in extreme cases, orbital structure preservation.[3,85,86] Infants with CL are often able to breastfeed without much difficulty; however, if a CP or facial cleft is also present, securing the proper suction may make sucking suboptimal to nonexistent and may leave the neonate at an increased risk for ear infections, retinal or corneal degradation, and sinus infections.[63,73,80,87]

Frontonasal Dysplasia. Frontonasal dysplasia is a median cleft face syndrome consisting of a range of midline facial defects involving the eyes, forehead, and nose. Abnormalities include ocular hypertelorism, a variable bifid nose, a broad nasal bridge, a midline defect of the frontal bone, and extension of the frontal hairline to form a widow's peak. The cause of frontonasal dysplasia is unknown, and its occurrence is sporadic. Two separated external nares with median CL can occur in patients with a severe form of this dysplasia.

With ultrasound, the primary finding will likely be hypertelorism, with any midline lip/palate/facial clefting being obvious in the coronal and midsagittal profile images or parasagittal images. If one cranial abnormality is found, the sonographer should carefully investigate for additional dysmorphic features (see Fig. 59.41).

Abnormalities of the Oral Cavity

Tongue. In utero, the fetus typically exhibits various behavioral patterns such as swallowing, protrusion and retrusion of the tongue, and hiccupping. Therefore, an abnormal positioning of the tongue may be indicative of a mass of the oral cavity, an obstructive process, or **macroglossia**. Macroglossia can be diagnosed sonographically when tongue protrusion is beyond the teeth or alveolar ridge during a resting state and can be either an isolated finding or syndromic such as is typically noted with **Beckwith-Wiedemann syndrome** (congenital overgrowth of tissues) (Fig. 59.43).[88] Organomegaly is also a feature of this particular syndrome; however, some glycogen storage diseases may also exhibit macroglossia and organomegaly, such as Pompe disease.[89]

Multiple simple cystic lesions of the oral cavity have been found in utero, with the majority of them being benign. Congenital ranulas are rare retention cystic masses caused by

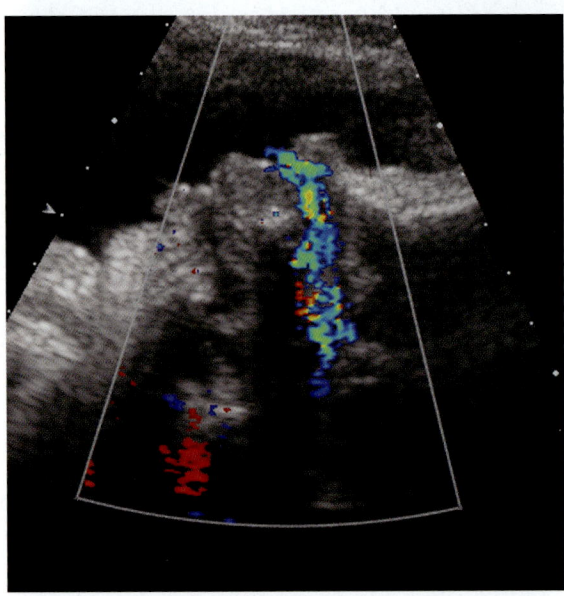

FIG. 59.39 Color Doppler image of fetal breathing in a fetus with a normal palate, demonstrating color seen only in the nasopharynx.

> **BOX 59.5 Sonographic Findings of Cleft Lip and Palate**
>
> - Median cleft lip: caused by incomplete merging of the two medial nasal prominences at the midline
> - Oblique facial cleft: failure of maxillary prominence to merge with the lateral nasal swelling, with exposure of the nasolacrimal duct
> - Complete bilateral cleft lip and palate: large gap in upper lip on modified coronal view; nose is flattened and widened; a premaxillary mass may be present
> - Unilateral complete cleft lip and palate: incomplete fusion of maxillary prominence to the medial prominence on one side; modified coronal view
> - Incomplete cleft: nose is intact; modified coronal view of lip

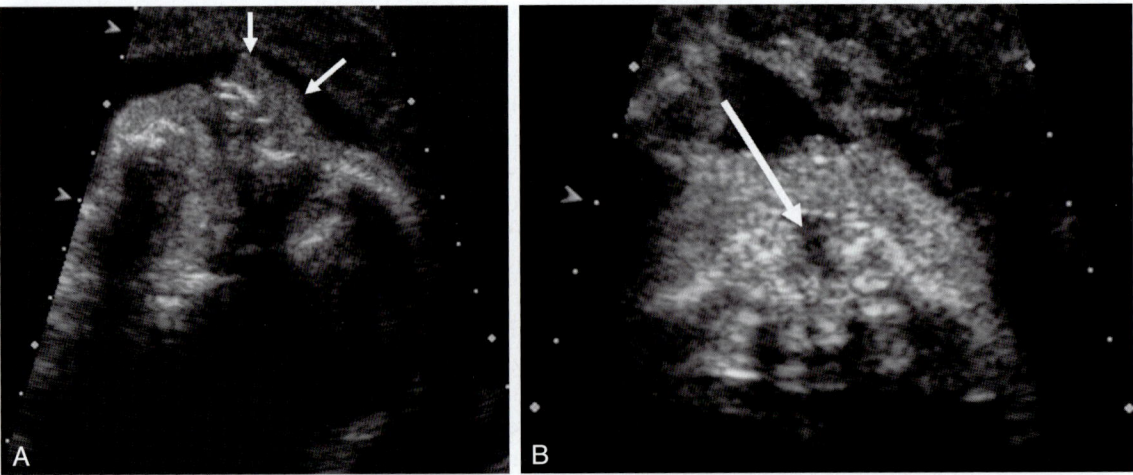

FIG. 59.40 (A) Sagittal image of a fetus with a cleft lip and palate. The fetal profile is distorted by a premaxillary mass *(lower arrow)*. Upper arrow, Fetal nose. (B) Axial view of the maxilla in the same fetus delineates the bony defect of the maxilla *(arrow)*.

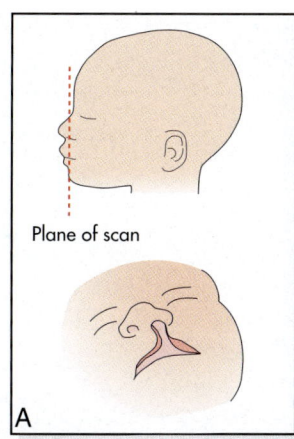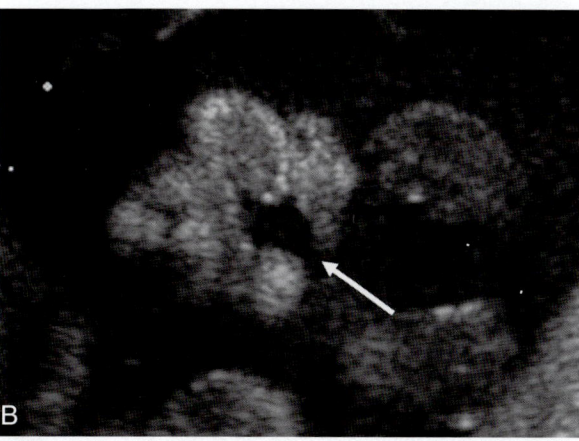

FIG. 59.41 Facial cleft. (A) A plane of section that visualizes clefts of the upper lip. (B) A modified coronal plane demonstrates a unilateral cleft lip *(arrow)*. The cleft extended into the fetal nose, and an associated cleft palate was present.

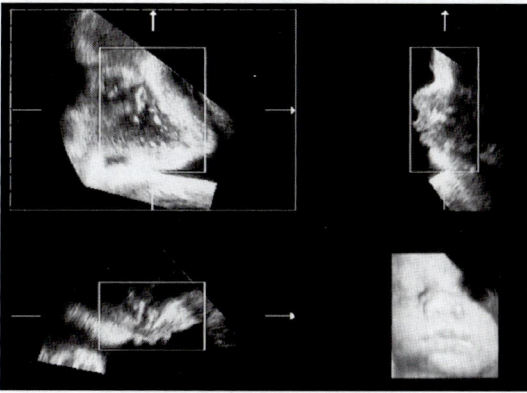

FIG. 59.42 Three-dimensional (3D) reconstruction of the fetal face in a 34-week-old fetus. The x, y, and z axes are aligned to reproduce the 3D image on the *lower right*.

mucous retention that originates at the base of the oral cavity located within the sublingual and submandibular ducts (Fig. 59.44). Ranulas are often small enough to be of no immediate consequence; however, if they become large enough, the mass can cause hypoxia immediately after birth due to upper airway obstruction and restrictive breathing, as well as cause swallowing, speech, and mastication difficulties later in life.[90,91] Ranulas in utero typically appear as unilateral, avascular, cystic lesions located inferior to the tongue, thus displacing the tongue persistently more superiorly in the intraoral cavity than expected.[92,93] If large enough, ranulas may cause macroglossia, making fetal and neonatal swallowing more difficult and potential airway obstruction more serious.

Larynx and Trachea. Due to the pivotal and necessary requirement of oxygen exchange with the pulmonary structures for survival, airway obstructions, whether intrinsic or extrinsic, carry a high neonatal morbidity when compromised.[94] Multiple syndromes have a predilection to intrinsic atresia of the trachea and larynx, and any mass not routinely expected in the oropharynx cavity carries the potential for airway obstruction due to extrinsic compression. Whether

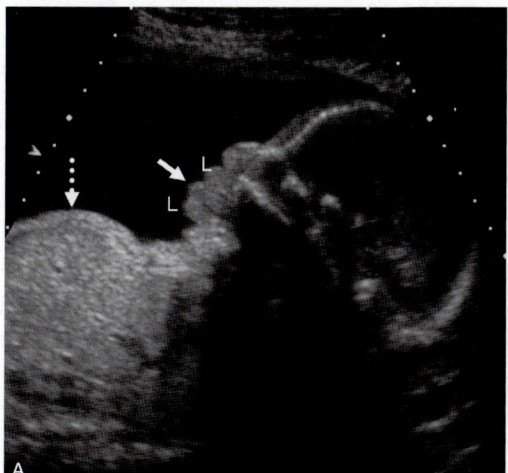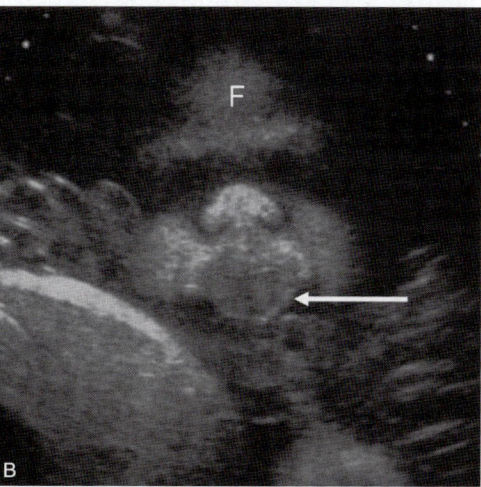

FIG. 59.43 (A) A fetus with Beckwith-Wiedemann syndrome. Note tongue protruding from mouth *(arrow)* between lips (L) and enlarged fetal liver *(dotted arrow)*. (B) Another fetus with Beckwith-Wiedemann syndrome. Coronal view of the fetal face demonstrates a protruding tongue suggesting macroglossia *(arrow)*. The fetal liver was also enlarged in this fetus. F, Forehead.

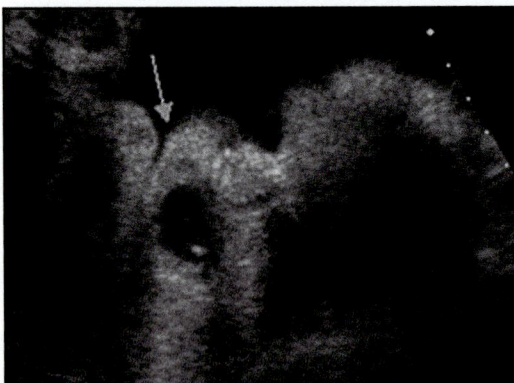

FIG. 59.44 Coronal view of fetal face showing a hypoechoic mass in the fetal mouth. A sublingual cyst was noted to move into and out of the fetal mouth in the sagittal plane *(arrow)*.

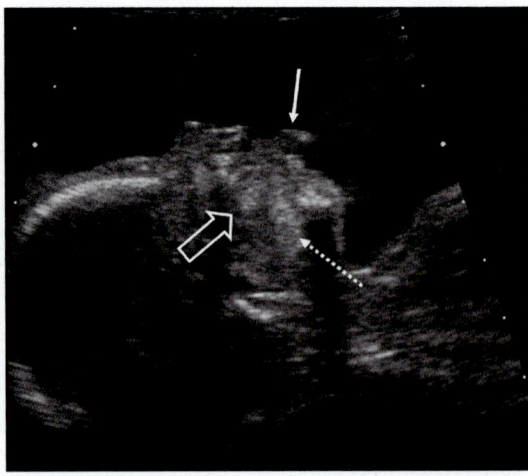

FIG. 59.45 Sagittal view of a fetus with a small epignathus: external portion of the mass *(solid arrow)*, mass erupting from the maxilla *(open arrow)*, and tongue compressed against the lower jaw *(dotted arrow)*.

by maldevelopment or via a congenital neck mass, congenital high airway obstruction syndrome is often a medical emergency quickly attended to postnatally.[95]

Fetal teratomas can be located anywhere in the body and are the most commonly diagnosed congenital tumor noted prenatally; however, they are rare in the oropharynx region.[21] Cured by complete resection in the neonate or even debulking interventions in utero with the fetus, these tumors are typically benign but may have high morbidity and mortality implications depending on their location and size, which can differ dramatically.[96,97]

Sonographically, characteristics of teratomas present as encapsulated cystic, solid, or multiloculated masses with small foci of calcifications being highly suggestive of their presence. They may be found anywhere in the palate, sphenoid, skull base, neck, or pharynx.[98] An **epignathus** is a teratoma located in the oropharynx; due to both their location and often their size, an epignathus may impair swallowing in utero, thus inducing polyhydramnios. As with any compromise in the ability of a fetus to properly swallow, the stomach may also appear smaller or non–fluid filled on sonographic examination (Fig. 59.45).

Isolated oral masses, significant macroglossia, and syndromic forms of macroglossia carry the potential for various respiratory and nutritional issues that may require immediate intervention upon birth (Fig. 59.46).[99] Larger tumors or those that involve the nasopharynx can cause obstruction of the airway, which may require an ex utero intrapartum treatment (EXIT) procedure at delivery. The EXIT procedure is a specialized surgical procedure performed under cesarean section with the fetus still receiving placental oxygenation in which the fetal airway is secure before complete delivery of the fetus is performed. It is utilized to deliver babies with airway compression or obstruction concerns.[28,100] Again, due to the compromised state of the fetus to properly swallow amniotic fluid, the presence of polyhydramnios often accompanies airway obstruction processes.

Abnormalities of the Neck

Congenital anomalies of the neck are not common but, when present, may represent life-threatening conditions due to their obstructive possibilities either by size, location, or both factors present in the upper airway.[101] Neck masses can be large and

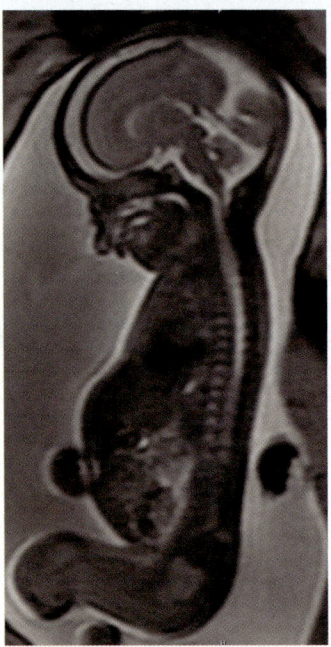

FIG. 59.46 Sagittal magnetic resonance image of a 27-week-old fetus noted to have campomelic dysplasia. Pathology confirmed frontal bossing, cebocephaly, micrognathia with a posteriorly displaced tongue, a bell-shaped chest, and pulmonary hypoplasia due to the small thoracic cavity, along with multiple shortened and dysmorphic long bones.

therefore obvious, as they may cause distortion or displacement of the neck contour and compression of adjacent structures. Congenital lesions in this anatomical area may appear with multiple presentations, being cystic, solid, or a combination of both, as is noted with masses such as teratomas. The most common congenital neck mass is the cystic hygroma.[102] Less common lesions include cervical meningomyelocele, hemangioma, teratoma, goiter, sarcoma, encephalocele, nuchal edema, **branchial cleft cyst**, cystic teratoma, thyroglossal duct cyst, and metastatic adenopathy.

Clinically, a fetal neck mass is cause for concern as when a large tumor exists; delivery of the infant may become complicated, instigating an abnormal hyperextension of the neck or an obstruction. Delivery dystocia (inability to deliver the trunk once the head has been delivered) and obstruction of the fetal airway, may require an EXIT procedure upon delivery.[103] Resection of the tumor or mass is then performed on placental support to allow for a more controlled delivery process and an increase in the chances of postnatal survival.[104,105]

Fetal Cystic Hygroma. Fetal **cystic hygromas** (CHs) are considered a congenital lymphatic malformation and result from an abnormal formation of the lymphatic system.[106] Normally, the upper lymphatic vessels empty into two sacs lateral to the jugular veins (jugular lymph sacs) that communicate with the jugular veins and form the right lymphatic duct and thoracic duct (Fig. 59.47). Failure of the lymphatic system to properly connect with the venous system results in distention of the jugular lymph sacs and accumulation of lymph in fetal tissue. This leads to either a single or often multiple multiloculated lymph-filled cavities around the neck; often, a dense midline septum divides the hygroma (Fig. 59.48). This abnormal collection of lymph in the newly formed lymph cavities may become so extreme as to lead to fetal hydrops and even fetal death.[107] About 75% of CHs involve the neck (usually arising from the posterior aspect of the neck bilaterally and less likely originating from the anterior or lateral surfaces). Up to 20% involve the axillae, with the retroperitoneum and intraabdominal organs, limbs, and bones accounting for 2% each and the mediastinum occurrence being approximately 1%.[108,109] When discovered early in pregnancy, CH is associated with chromosomal aneuploidies 50% of the time; therefore, identification should be accompanied by a thorough anatomical survey.[107,108,110]

CHs may be small or large and may regress with time, as alternate routes of lymph drainage may eventually develop.[111] When the resolution of a CH is noted in utero, webbing of the neck and swelling of the extremities may be appreciated after birth (Fig. 59.49).[112] Although CHs can occur in isolation, these classic features are frequently seen in neonates with **Turner syndrome** (45,X),[106] in which females are of short stature and sterile, as they only develop ovarian streaks instead of fully functional ovarian tissue (Fig. 59.50).

CHs are often found with accompanying edema, pericardial effusions, pleural effusions, edema of the thoracic and abdominal skin, ascites, anasarca, and limb edema, which, combined with the fluid overload, may lead to fetal hydrops (Fig. 59.51). In the most extreme cases, CHs accompanied by fetal hydrops carry a 100% mortality rate, as heart failure commonly results in intrauterine death (Fig. 59.52).[113,114]

An obstructed lymphatic system can have presentations not classic for multiseptic cystic collections and can, in fact, become almost infiltrative into the facial sinuses and oropharyngeal spaces (Fig. 59.53). The differential diagnosis considerations for CH include meningomyelocele, encephalocele, nuchal

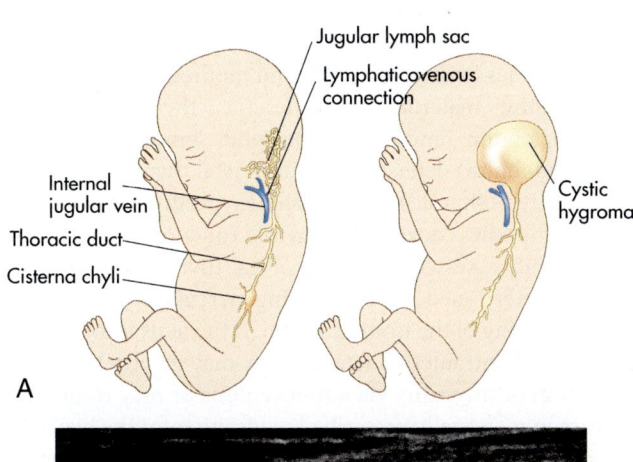

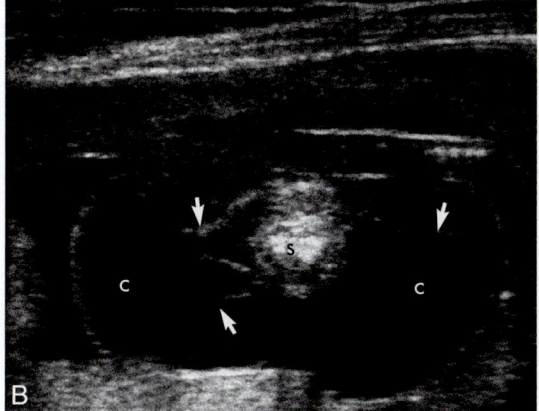

FIG. 59.47 (A) Lymphatic system in a normal fetus *(left)* with a patent connection between the jugular lymph sac and the internal jugular vein, and a cystic hygroma and hydrops from a failed lymphaticovenous connection *(right)*. (B) Transverse plane of the neck demonstrating a larger posterolateral septated cystic mass. *Arrows* depict multiple septations. *c*, Body of cystic hygroma.

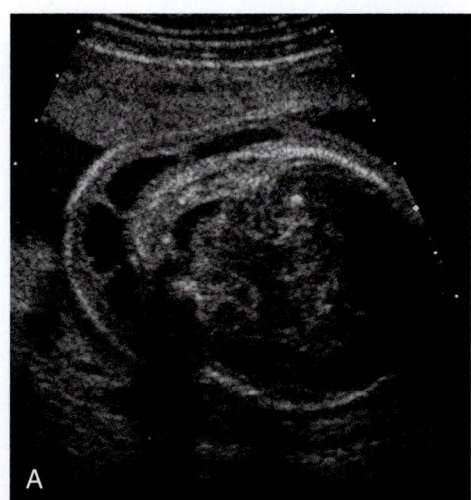

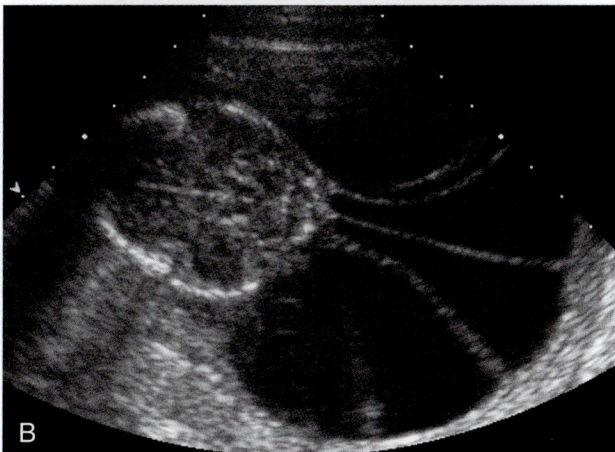

FIG. 59.48 (A) Transverse view of the neck demonstrating a small cystic hygroma. (B) The large septated compartments seen in a fetus with a large cystic hygroma.

edema, branchial cleft cyst, cystic teratoma, hemangioma, and thyroglossal duct cyst (Fig. 59.54). If the posterior neck skin appears thick without significant fluid-filled areas, this may represent a thickened nuchal fold, as seen with other chromosomal anomalies such as Down syndrome (trisomy 21).

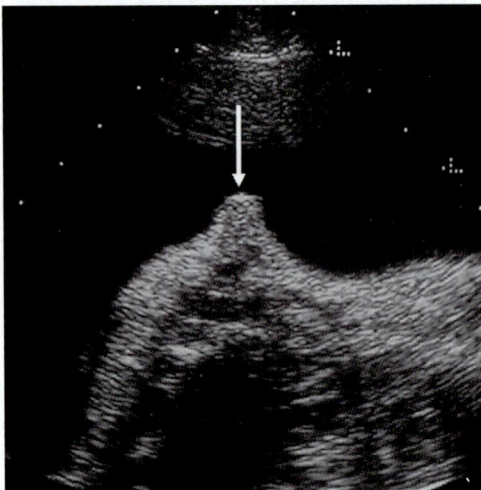

FIG. 59.49 Transverse view of the fetal neck demonstrates the remaining "webbing" from resolution of a cystic hygroma *(arrow)*.

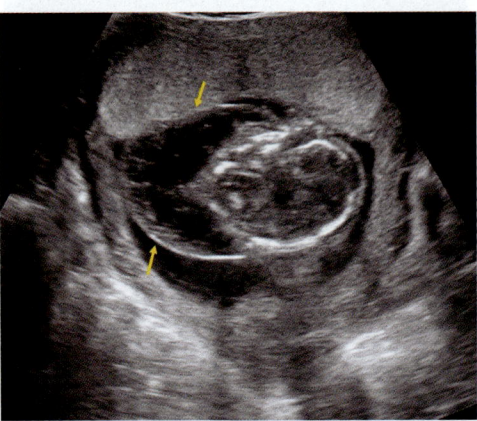

FIG. 59.50 Transverse plane of the neck demonstrating a large posterolateral cystic mass representing a cystic hygroma in a fetus with Turner syndrome. Note the multiple septations within the hygromas.

A multitude of other congenital cystic lesions of the neck may be encountered sonographically in the fetus and can be located anywhere from the oral cavity to the lower mediastinum. These typically display the same sonographic characteristics of simple cysts found in other areas of the body and may be solitary or multicystic and thin walled or thicker walled, have internal echoes from layering debris or hemorrhage, should display through transmission with no internal vascular flow, and may be microcystic or macrocystic. Most frequently encountered cystic lesions are foregut duplication cysts, thymic cysts, branchial pouch remnant cysts, and lymphatic malformations.

Fetal Goiter. Whenever maternal thyroid disease is present, the fetal thyroid should be evaluated, as maternal Graves disease is the most common cause of **fetal goiters**, with the transplacental transfer of thyroid-stimulating hormone receptor antibody.[115] Although fetal goiters are not common, with an occurrence rate estimated to be 1 in 40,000 births, a fetal goiter carries potential for peril in its actual physical size as a space-occupying entity causing possible compression upon surrounding structures and airway and/or swallowing complications.[116] Goiters also hold the possibility for thyroid dysfunction and its potential for neurological impairment and life-threatening attributes.[117] Whether the goiter can be attributed to fetal hyperthyroidism or hypothyroidism is an essential clinical diagnosis to correctly manage the implications that accompany thyroid dysfunction. In the presence of hyperthyroidism, maternal Graves disease accounts for 85% to 90% of the dysfunction and may result in poor outcomes for both the fetus and mother.[117,118]

Circulating maternal antibodies (i.e., thyroid-stimulating immunoglobulin and/or thyrotrophic binding inhibiting immunoglobulin) determine whether fetal thyroid function is inhibited (hypothyroid) or stimulated (hyperthyroid). However, if both antibodies coexist, fetal thyroid function cannot be easily or readily assessed accurately. Fetal thyroid function may then be determined by performing percutaneous umbilical blood sampling of the umbilical vein. If the fetus is found to be hypothyroid, intrauterine fetal therapy may involve the weekly instillation of thyroxine via amniocentesis or may result in an increase in maternally prescribed medication for the hyperthyroid fetus, as these medications promptly cross the placenta.

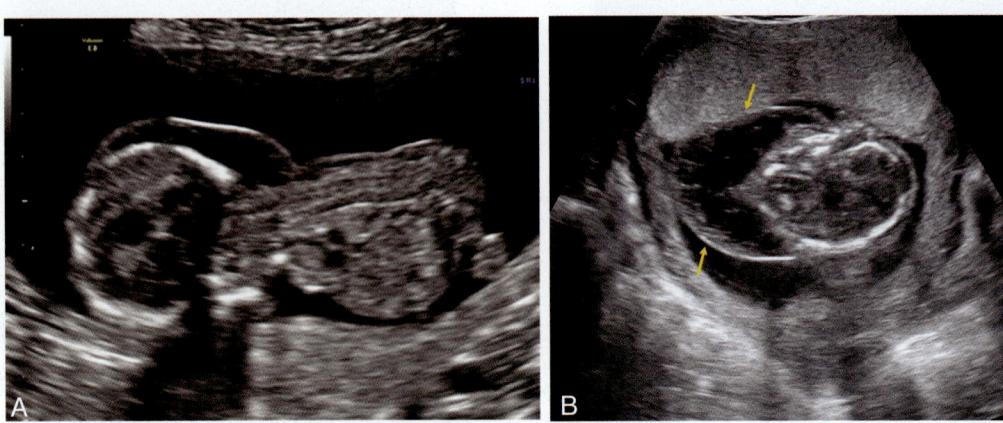

FIG. 59.51 (A) Fifteen-week-old fetus with a large cystic hygroma that extends to include most of the fetal trunk. (B) Limb edema in a fetus with cystic hygroma and generalized anasarca.

A fetal goiter may cause **thyromegaly** (an enlarged thyroid gland) which typically appears sonographically as a hyperechogenic, symmetric (bilobed), solid, homogeneous mass arising from the anterior base of the fetal neck (Fig. 59.55). Once identified, serial sonographic assessments should be performed to document size and vascularity, proximity to and possible impingement on the trachea (accurate measurements of the trachea should be documented), and the presence of fetal swallowing. If less swallowing than expected is noted in a given time period, assessment of amniotic fluid and the presence of fluid in the stomach should be assessed for possible swallowing impairment. A quantitative measurement of the thyroid gland width and circumference should be obtained and matched to established nomograms for gestational age.[115] Follow-up sonographic examinations should include assessment of fetal thyroid size (to include quantitative measurements), measurements of the trachea, signs of fetal tachycardia (if the fetus is hyperthyroid), presence of swallowing, fluid in the stomach, and a quantitative amniotic fluid volume.

Teratoma. Cervical teratomas, similar to epignathus, are not common and are usually unilaterally located anteriorly.[95,119] They may have complex sonographic (intermingled cystic and solid components) patterns similar to teratomas of other organs (Fig. 59.56). They can typically be differentiated from other neck lesions such as lymphatic malformations by their larger solid components and calcifications often noted heterogeneously throughout.[21] Color Doppler may also help to differentiate this mass from atypical cystic hygromas or other more cystic congenital masses.

Neuroblastomas may also be a differential diagnosis for a solid congenital fetal neck mass. Similar to the sonographic presentation of a cervical teratoma, they are less likely to occur in this region and should prompt the targeted search for fetal liver metastases and maternal considerations such as the presence of hypertension and catecholamine metabolites.[21,103]

The cervical neck region can be a challenge to assess with sonography, especially when amniotic fluid is decreased when the fetus is in an unfavorable position or when the neck is in close proximity to the placenta. Nonetheless, evaluation of the neck should be routinely performed with every anatomical survey as lesions in this area are generally a concern in and of themselves; however, due to their location, they also become a therapeutic dilemma with the potential for upper airway obstruction and cardiovascular management being at the forefront. Box 59.6 lists questions the sonographer should ponder regarding fetal neck masses.

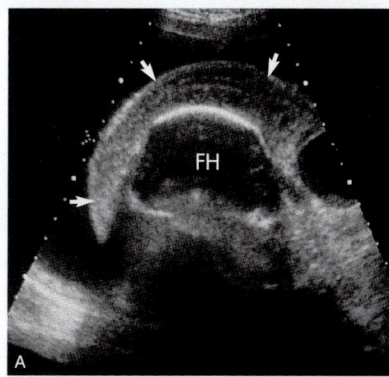
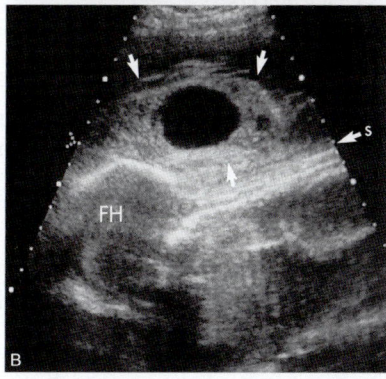

FIG. 59.52 (A) In the fetus shown in Fig. 59.25, at 26 weeks of gestation fetal movements were decreased, prompting ultrasound evaluation, which revealed a fetal demise. Note the helmet-like appearance of the scalp edema *(arrows)*. (B) In the same fetus, sagittal views revealed the posterolateral cystic hygroma *(arrows)* caused by lymphangiectasia from heart failure. Tetralogy of Fallot was revealed on autopsy. *FH*, Fetal head; *s*, spine.

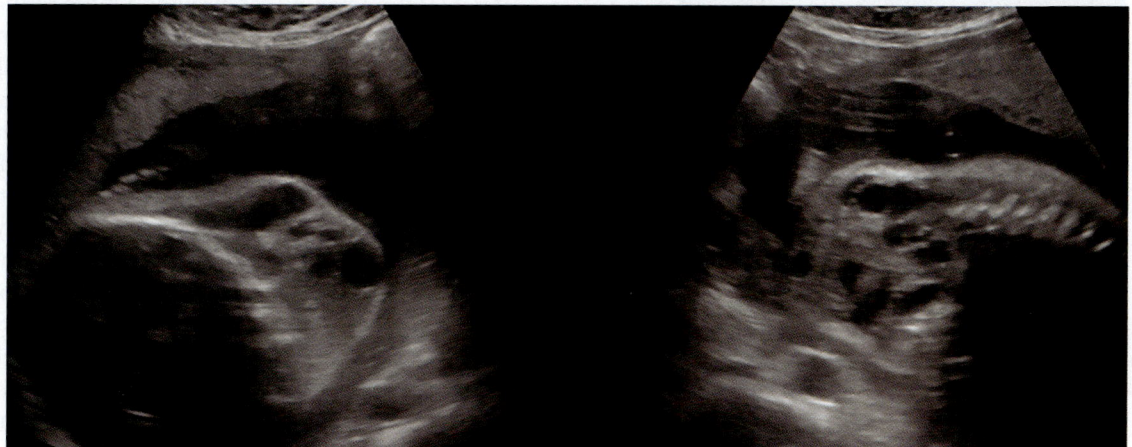

FIG. 59.53 (A) Split-screen displaying sonographic images of a multiloculated cystic mass infiltrating into cranial facial spaces in a 29-week-old male fetus. The left image is an axial plane at the level of the neck. The right image is the same pathology in a sagittal plane. No other abnormalities were identified on this fetus. (B) Coronal magnetic resonance image of the same fetus displaying the left lateral macrocystic hygroma involving the oral cavity, the mandible, and the lateral aspect of the fetal face and neck, including displacement of the fetal ear.

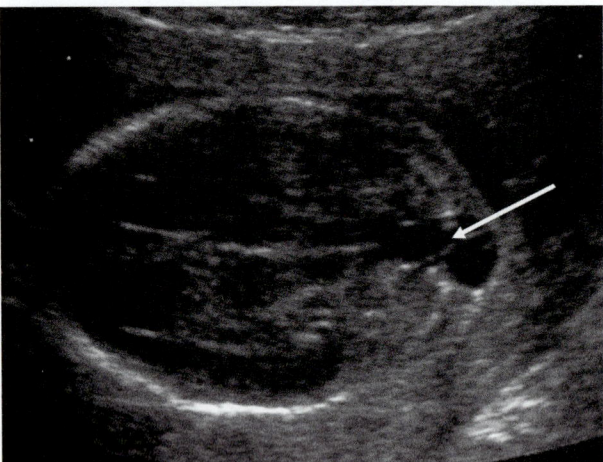

FIG. 59.54 A fetus with a small encephalocele that could be mistaken for a small cystic hygroma. Identification of a bony defect suggests an encephalocele *(arrow)*.

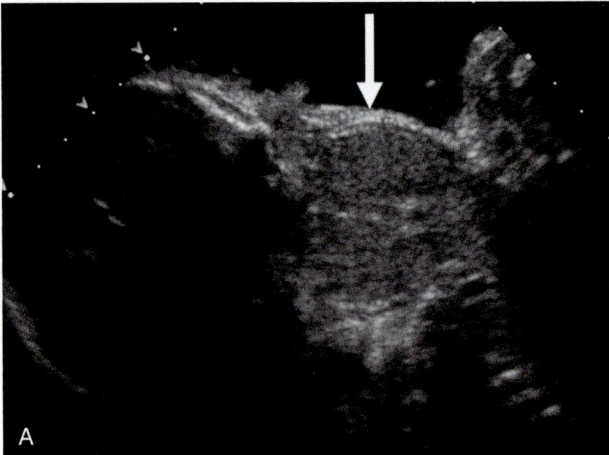

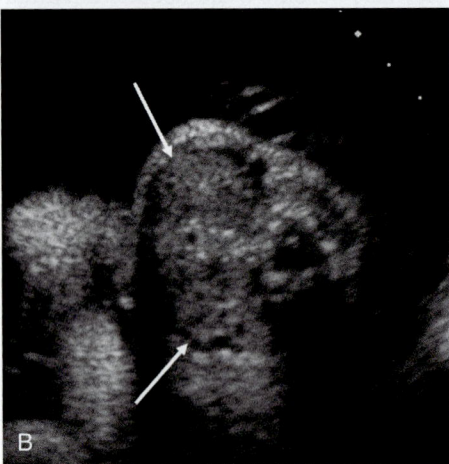

FIG. 59.55 (A) Axial image of the fetal neck, which reveals the bilobed enlarged fetal thyroid gland *(arrow)*. (B) A coronal view of the same fetus with the enlarged thyroid gland *(arrows)*.

Three-Dimensional Evaluation

3DUS and 4DUS have held critical roles and continue to influence both clinical decision making as well as the parental emotional implications it holds regarding craniofacial anomalies. The additions of external workstations, static volume sweeps, matrix

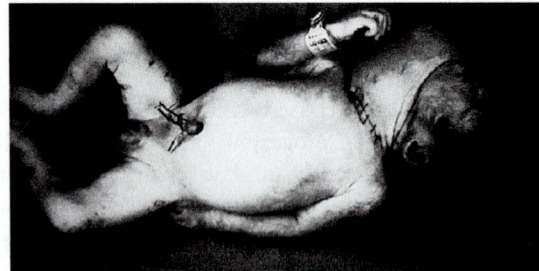

FIG. 59.56 A large teratoma was found to arise from the posterior neck of this neonate. Multiple ultrasound studies demonstrated the mass to be complex in texture.

BOX 59.6	Questions for the Sonographer Evaluating a Fetal Neck Mass

- What is the position of the mass (anterior, posterior, lateral, or midline)?
- Is it a unilateral or bilateral lesion?
- What are the Doppler properties? (Hemangiomas have arterial and venous characteristics.)
- Is there polyhydramnios?
- Is heart failure or hydrops present?
- Are there coexisting anomalies?
- Is there hyperextension of the neck, which may suggest the presence of a neck mass or iniencephaly (fusion of occiput to spine)?

transducers, and streamlined equipment with onboard technological software have brought rapidly improving technology that has become more feasible to even the rural settings.

3DUS imaging is a well-documented diagnostic tool often used to detect craniofacial abnormalities and their extent of involvement with surrounding structures in both the setting of screening examinations as well as more in-depth targeted or focused studies and diagnostic procedures.[14] By utilizing rendered and multiplanar displays comprised of volumes of data (voxels) that have been stored during the examination, 3DUS/4DUS imaging can provide a more rounded and concise concept of the extent of anomalies and how they relate to surrounding structures that may be impinged upon or obstructed.[14] Accurate 3DUS analysis of morphology can help the practitioner identify and describe the pathology and relate it to a syndromic entity, if present. However, the 3DUS ultrasound image is often a direct result of the quality of the bidirectional or 2DUS imaging study, meaning if suboptimal scanning parameters were encountered during the 2DUS screening examination, such as oligohydramnios, they will also play a negative factor in the 3DUS assessment. 3DUS/4DUS also holds the same requisite parameters in that the sonographer must be competent in their sonographic skill set to obtain quality images and the acquisition of excellent volume datasets for offline analysis.[120]

3DUS visualizes soft tissue structures more optimally than bidimensional ultrasound—that is, the ears, nose, mouth, mandible, eyelids, and the hard and the soft palates—providing additional valuable information for both the parents and clinical team preparing to provide care to the fetus postnatally (see

Fig. 59.18). In fact, 3DUS morphological analysis of the ears is often very revealing and accurate due to the clear and detailed visualization, with hard palate interrogation probably providing better definition compared to 2DUS (see Fig. 59.16).[121] Without doubt, visualization of the soft palate is formidably enhanced with 3DUS compared to bidimensional ultrasound due to its curved anatomical arrangement, which results in neighboring tissues casting shadowing artifacts, making diagnostic decisions and analysis of soft palate clefts of the alveolar ridge of the maxilla worth the additional imaging efforts of 3DUS.[120–122]

Prenatal 3DUS of craniofacial anatomy should include visualization of the tip of the nose, nostrils, upper and lower lips, hard and soft palates, orbital components, both ears, and the fetal profile (Fig. 59.57). The eyes are visible in a bidimensional ultrasound axial approach, as discussed earlier; however, 3DUS might improve analysis of biometric anomalies and the anatomy of the eyes, lenses, and orbits when used as a secondary tool.[123] An axial acquisition seems to render the best results, but sagittal acquisition planes are often used in the setting of prone fetuses. Prenatal biometric nomograms have been established by 3DUS to analyze microphthalmia.[124]

When searching for facial anomalies or associated syndromes, investigation of the fetal profile is a fundamental part of the morphological evaluation, and 3DUS assessment is no different. Analysis of nasal bone length, prefrontal thickness, the frontomaxillary facial angle, maxilla-nasion-mandible angle, nose length (distance between nasion at the intersection of the frontal bones and nasal bones and upper anterior corner of maxilla), nose protrusion, philtrum length, and facial height (distance from nasion to lower anterior corner of the mandible) are all possible with optimal fetal positions and conditions.

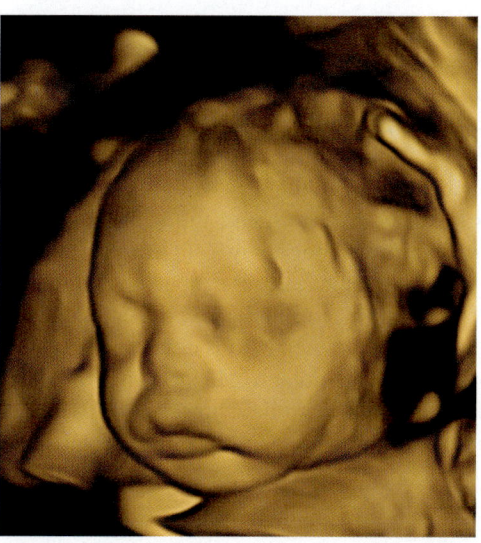

FIG. 59.57 Three-dimensional sonographic rendered image of a 22-week-old fetal face. Notice the micrognathia readily displayed.

Additional Imaging

MRI in utero has been proven to be a fantastic adjunct examination in conjunction with sonography and is a beneficial diagnostic tool to aid with the more difficult diagnosis of facial clefting and fetal oropharyngeal masses.[21,25,62,125–128] MRI can provide a larger field of view, provides great detail of soft tissue entities, does not expose the fetus to radiation, and has the ability to visualize in great detail fluid-filled structures including the nasal passages, vascular structures, and oropharyngeal cavity (Fig. 59.58). As an accessory imaging tool, MRI holds the ability to often determine the extent of congenital

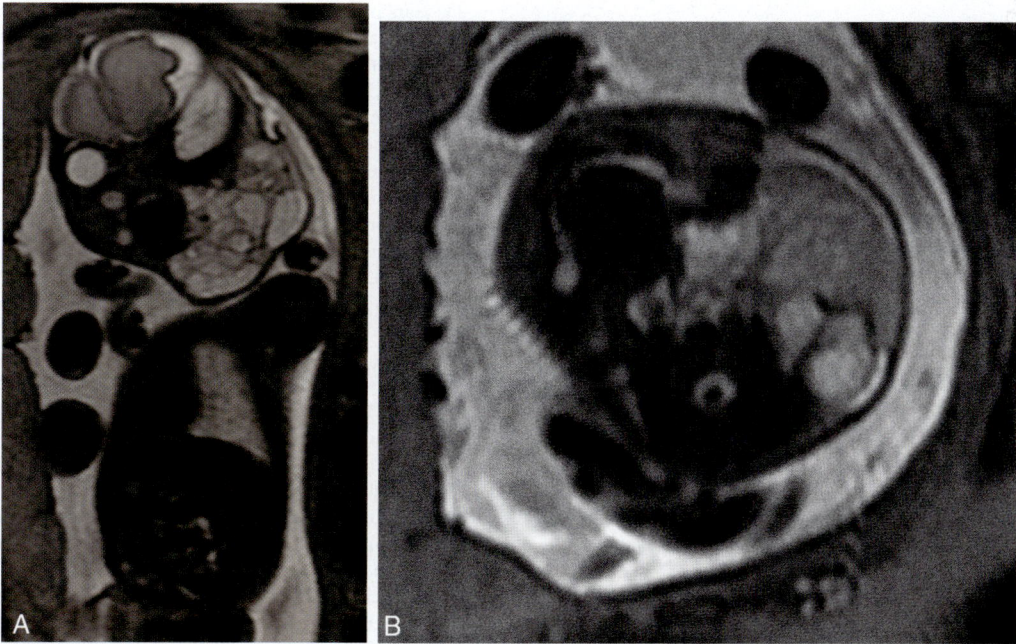

FIG. 59.58 (A) Axial magnetic resonance imaging (MRI) of a 29-week-old fetus. The hard palate is well noted and intact; however, a large macrocystic hygroma is noted on the midline and to the left lateral aspect of the fetal face. Note the detail in the relationship of adjacent anatomy and the detail of the entirety of the lesion. (B) Coronal MRI image of the same fetus displaying the left lateral macrocystic hygroma involving the oral cavity, the mandible, and the lateral aspect of the fetal face and neck, including displacement of the fetal ear.

abnormalities better than sonography, distinguish motion of the mass in relation to the surrounding anatomy, and verify airway obstruction or potential obstructions with continued fetal growth (due to the detail of proximal anatomical structures).[125,128,129] MRI, however, does have a few disadvantages, including the high cost, the very real potential for fetal motion artifacts and, for many patients, inducing maternal claustrophobia. Computed tomography (CT) imaging may also be utilized to add diagnostic features of specific anomalies in utero, in particular, oral masses and proximal osseous visualization or bone involvement when MRI is not available as a secondary imaging option. CT, similar to MRI, also has the ability to provide 3D reconstruction models; however, CT is less likely to be used in the fetal setting due to its radiation exposure.

Key Pearls

- Features of the fetal face can be identified at the end of the first trimester.
- The fetal profile is well imaged with transvaginal sonography beginning late first trimester to early second trimester (make sure adequate amniotic fluid surrounds the face).
- The modified coronal view is best for imaging the cleft lip and palate.
- The maxilla and orbits are well imaged in a true coronal plane.
- The lens of the eye is seen as a small echogenic circle within the orbit.
- The longitudinal view demonstrates the nasal bones, soft tissue, and mandible (useful to rule out micrognathia, anterior encephalocele, or nasal bridge defects; examine the upper lip).
- Transverse view shows orbital abnormalities and intraorbital distances (useful to evaluate the maxilla, mandible, and tongue).

REFERENCES

1. World Health Organization (WHO). Craniofacial anomalies and 2 associated birth defects. Global registry and database on craniofacial anomalies, Report of a WHO Registry Meeting on Craniofacial Anomalies. Geneva: WHO; 2020:15–33.
2. World Health Organization (WHO) Human Genomics in Global Health, 2020. International Collaborative Research on Craniofacial Anomalies. Geneva: WHO; 2020.
3. van der Hoek-Snieders HEM, van den Heuvel AJML, van Os-Medendorp H, Kamalski DMA. Diagnostic accuracy of fetal MRI to detect cleft palate: A meta-analysis. *Eur J Pediatr*. 2020;179(1):29–38.
4. Ansari A, Bordoni B. Embryology, Face. In: StatPearls. https://www.ncbi.nlm.nih.gov/books/NBK545202/.
5. Hsuan K, Tung-Yao C, Lussier EC, et al. Multidisciplinary team approach to the prenatal management of orofacial clefts: A single center cohort study in Taiwan. *Sci Rep Nat*. 2020;10(1).
6. Avhad R, Sar R, Tembhurne J. Presurgical management of unilateral cleft lip and palate in a neonate: a clinical report. *J Prosthet Dent*. 2014;112(3):676–679.
7. Johnson JM, Moonis G, Green GE, et al. Syndromes of the first and second branchial arches, part 2: syndromes. *AJNR*. 2011;32:230–237.
8. Nagarajan M, Sharbidre KG, Bhabad SH, Byrd SE. MR imaging of the fetal face: comprehensive review. *Radiographics*. 2018;38(3):962–980.
9. Johnson JM, Moonis G, Green GE, Carmody R, Burbank HN. Syndromes of the first and second branchial arches, part 1: embryology and characteristic defects. *AJNR*. 2011;32:14–19.
10. Wright GC. Development of the human external ear. *J Am Acad Audiol*. 1997;8:379–382.
11. Mai CT, Isenburg JL, Canfield MA, et al. National population-based estimates for major birth defects, 2010-2014. *Birth Defects Res*. 2019;111:1420–1435.
12. Menzel MB, Lawrence AK, Rubio EI, Bulas DI. Team counseling in prenatal evaluation: The partnership of the radiologist and genetic counselor. *Pediatr Radiol*. 2018;48(4):457–460.
13. Alshabanah RF, Alshahrani SS, Almohayya TS, Alahmari EM. The accuracy of three-dimensional ultrasound imaging in detection of lip and palate clefts. *Egypt J Hospital Medicine*. 2017;69(4):2308–2314.
14. Bäumler M, Bigorre M, Faure J. Radiological evaluation of the fetal face using three-dimensional ultrasound imaging. *Rep Med Imaging*. 2012;5:103–113.
15. Farhan TM, Al-Abdely BA, Abdullateef AN, Jubair AS. Craniofacial anomaly association with the internal malformations in the pediatric age group in Al-Fallujah City, Iraq. *Biomed Res Int*. 2020;2020:4725141.
16. Yoon AJ, Pham BN, Dipple KM. Genetic screening in patients with craniofacial malformations. *J Pediatr Genet*. 2016;5(4):220–224.
17. Schüttauf RC, Hellebrekers BWJ. Fetal ingestion of an amniotic band: How rare is it. *Case Rep Perinat Med*. 2015;4(1):49–50.
18. Schramm C, Rohrbach JM, Reinert S, et al. Amniotic bands as a cause of congenital anterior staphyloma. *Graefe's Archive for Clinical and Experimental Ophthalmology*. 2013;251(3):959–965.
19. Lee JW, Chung HY. Capillary malformations (portwine stains) of the head and neck: natural history, investigations, laser, and surgical management. *Otolaryngol Clin North Am*. 2018;51(1):197–211.
20. Kawaguchi A, Kunimoto K, Inaba Y, et al. Distribution analysis of infantile hemangioma or capillary malformation on the head and face in Japanese patients. *J Dermatol*. 2019;46(10):849–852.
21. Rubio EI. Imaging of the fetal oral cavity, airway and neck. *Ped Radiol*. 2020;51:1122–1133.
22. Parameswaran A, Ramanathan M. Hemifacial microsomia. *J Ind Orthod Soc*. 2018;52:155–166.
23. Sanjana M, Manikandan S, Maheshwari U, Parameswaran R, Vijayalakshmi D. An interdisciplinary management of severe facial asymmetry due to hemifacial microsomia. *Contemp Clin Dent*. 2020;11:387–394.
24. Nazzaro A, Della Monica M, Lonardo F, et al. Prenatal ultrasound diagnosis of a case of Pfeiffer syndrome without cloverleaf skull and review of the literature. *Prenat Diagn*. 2004;24:918–922.
25. Rubio EI, Blask A, Bulas DI. Ultrasound and MR imaging findings in prenatal diagnosis of craniosynostosis syndromes. *Pediatr Radiol*. 2016;46(5):709–718.
26. Fish D, Lima D, Reber D. Cranial remolding orthoses. In: Webster JB, Murphy DP, eds. *Atlas of Orthoses and Assistive Devices*. ed 5. Philadelphia: Elsevier; 2019:359–375.
27. Wei J, Ran S, Yang Z, et al. Prenatal ultrasound screening for external ear abnormality in the fetuses. *BioMed Res Int*. 2014;2014:4357564.
28. Tay SY, Krishnasarma R, Mehta D, Mehollin-Ray A, Chandy B. Predictive factors for perinatal outcomes of infants diagnosed with micrognathia antenatally. *Ear Nose Throat J*. 2021;100(1).
29. Almajed A, Viezel-Mathieu A, Gilardino M, et al. Outcome following surgical interventions for micrognathia in infants with Pierre Robin sequence: a systematic review of the literature. *Cleft Palate Craniofac J*. 2017;54:32–42.
30. Bianchi A, Betti E, Badiali G, Ricotta F, Marchetti C, Tarsitano A. 3D computed tomographic evaluation of the upper airway space of patients undergoing mandibular distraction osteogenesis for micrognathia. *Acta Otorhinolaryngol Ital*. 2015;35(5):350–354.

31. Georgakopoulos B, Zafar Gondal A. Embryology, Ear Congenital Malformations. 2021. In: StatPearls. https://www.ncbi.nlm.nih.gov/books/NBK545256/
32. Saikia R, Bordoloi UKR. A study of congenital malformations of the external ear. *J. Evid. Based Med. Healthc.* 2016;3(81):4383–4388.
33. De Golovine S, Wu S, Hunter JV, et al. Goldenhar syndrome: a cause of secondary immunodeficiency? *All Asth Clin Immun.* 2012;8:10.
34. Borjas-Lucio CG, Briones-Bernal BL, Tello Gutiérrez HE, González JV. Roberts syndrome: an isolated case. *Medicina Universitaria.* 2017;19(75):98–99.
35. Rai A, Nandimath KR, Sattur AP, Naikmasur VG. Nager's acrofacial dysostosis. *J Orofac Sci.* 2013;5:138–142.
36. Díaz del Arco C, Agustín A, Alarcón A. Agnathia-microstomia-synotia syndrome (otocephaly). *Autopsy and Case Reports.* 2020:10.
37. Bojikian KD, de Moura CR, Tavares IM, Leite MT, Moron AF. Fetal ocular measurements by three-dimensional ultrasound. *J AAPOS.* 2013;17(3):276–281.
38. Sukonpan K, Vorapong P. A biometric study of the fetal orbit and lens in normal pregnancies. *J Clin Ultrasound.* 2009;37:69–74.
39. Verma AS, Fitzpatrick DR. Anophthalmia and microphthalmia. *Orphanet J Rare Dis.* 2007;2:47.
40. Castro PT, Matos AP, Werner H, Lopes J, Ribeiro G, Araujo EJ. Evaluation of fetal nasal cavity in bilateral congenital dacryocystocele: 3D reconstruction and virtual navigation by magnetic resonance imaging. *Ultrasound Obstet Gynecol.* 2020;55(1):141–143.
41. Nair AG, Mulay K, Honavar SG. Congenital teratoma of the orbit: a rare tumor. *J Pediatr Ophthalmol Strabismus.* 2015;52(2):128.
42. Miranda-Rivas A, Villegas VM, Nieves-Melendez JR, De La Vega A. Congenital dacryocystocele: sonographic evaluation of 11 cases. *J AAPOS.* 2018;22(5):390–392.
43. Kim YH, Lee YJ, Song MJ, Han BH, Lee YH, Lee KS. Dacryocystocele on prenatal ultrasonography: diagnosis and postnatal outcomes. *Ultrasonography.* 2015;34(1):51–57.
44. Gujar SK, Gandhi D. Congenital malformations of the orbit. *Neuroimaging Clin North Am.* 2011;21(3):585–602.
45. Yazici Z, Kline-Fath BM, Yazici B, Rubio EI, Calvo-Garcia MA, Linam LE. Congenital dacryocystocele: prenatal MRI findings. *Pediatr Radiol.* 2010;40(12):1868–1873.
46. Searle A, Shetty P, Melov SJ, Alahakoon TI. Prenatal diagnosis and implications of microphthalmia and anophthalmia with a review of current ultrasound guidelines: two case reports. *J Med Case Rep.* 2018;12(1):250.
47. Dharmasena A, Keenan T, Goldacre R, Hall N, Goldacre MJ. Trends over time in the incidence of congenital anophthalmia, microphthalmia and orbital malformation in England: database study. *Br J Ophthalmol.* 2017;101(6):735–739.
48. Greig AV, Wagner J, Warren SM, Grayson B, McCarthy JG. Pfeiffer syndrome: analysis of a clinical series and development of a classification system. *J Craniofac Surg.* 2013;24(1):204–215.
49. Weber B, Schwabegger AH, Vodopiutz J, et al. Prenatal diagnosis of Apert syndrome with cloverleaf skull deformity using ultrasound, fetal magnetic resonance imaging and genetic analysis. *Fetal Diagn Ther.* 2010;27(1):51–56.
50. Du Y, Ren Y, Yan Y, Cao L. Absent fetal nasal bone in the second trimester and risk of abnormal karyotype in a prescreened population of Chinese women. *Acta Obstet Gynecol Scand.* 2018;97(2):180–186.
51. Papasozomenou P, Athanasiadis AP, Zafrakas M, et al. Fetal nasal bone length in the second trimester: comparison between population groups from different ethnic origins. *J Perinat Med.* 2016;44(2):229–235.
52. Kagan KO, Sonek J, Berg X, et al. Facial markers in second- and third-trimester fetuses with trisomy 18 or 13, triploidy or Turner syndrome. *Ultrasound Obstet Gynecol.* 2015;46(1):60–65.
53. Tomai XH, Phan TH. Fetal nasal bone length at 19-26 weeks' gestation in Vietnam. *J Obstet Gynaecol Res.* 2016;42(10):1245–1249.
54. Tournemire A, Groussolles M, Ehlinger V, et al. Prenasal thickness to nasal bone length ratio: effectiveness as a second or third trimester marker for Down syndrome. *Eur J Obstet Gynecol Reprod Biol.* 2015;191:28–32.
55. Vos FI, De Jong-Pleij EA, Bakker M, et al. Nasal bone length, prenasal thickness, prenasal thickness-to-nasal bone length ratio and prefrontal space ratio in second- and third-trimester fetuses with Down syndrome. *Ultrasound Obstet Gynecol.* 2015;45(2):211–216.
56. Moreno-Cid M, Rubio-Lorente A, Rodríguez MJ, et al. Systematic review and meta-analysis of performance of second-trimester nasal bone assessment in detection of fetuses with Down syndrome. *Ultrasound Obstet Gynecol.* 2014;43(3):247–253.
57. Yeo WX, Tan KK. Diagnosis and surgical management of congenital intranasal teratoma in a newborn: A rare case report. *Case Rep Otolaryngol.* 2018;2018:4.
58. Van Wyhe R, Chamata E, Hollier L. Midline craniofacial masses in children. *Semin Plastic Surg.* 2016;30(4):176–180.
59. Bahgat M, Bahgat Y, Bahgat A. Oropharyngeal teratoma, a rare cause of airway obstruction in neonates. *BMJ Case Rep.* 2012;2012 bcr20120065800.
60. Chakravarti A, Shashidhar TB, Naglot S, Sahni JK. Head and neck teratomas in children: a case series. *Ind J Otolaryngol Head Neck Surg.* 2011;63:193–197.
61. Tirumandas M, Sharma A, Gbenimacho I, et al. Nasal encephaloceles: a review of etiology, pathophysiology, clinical presentations, diagnosis, treatment, and complications. *Childs Nerv Syst.* 2013;29(5):739–744.
62. Blask AR, Rubio EI, Chapman KA, Lawrence AK, Bulas DI. Severe nasomaxillary hypoplasia (binder phenotype) on prenatal US/MRI: An important marker for the prenatal diagnosis of chondrodysplasia punctata. *Pediatr Radiol.* 2018;48(7):979–991.
63. Levaillant J-M, Nicot R, Benouaiche L, Couly G, Rotten D. Prenatal diagnosis of cleft lip/palate: the surface rendered oropalatal (SROP) view of the fetal lips and palate, a tool to improve information-sharing within the orofacial team and with the parents. *J Craniomaxillofac Surg.* 2016;44:835–842.
64. Deshpande S, Juneja M. Binder's syndrome (maxillonasal dysplasia) different treatment modalities: Our experience. *Ind J Plast Surg.* 2012;45(1):62–66.
65. Cuillier F, et al. Maxillo-nasal dysplasia (Binder syndrome): antenatal discovery and implications. *Fetal Diagn Ther.* 2005;20:301–305.
66. Seyhan T, Kircelli BH, Caglar B. Correction of septal and midface hypoplasia in maxillonasal dysplasia (Binder's syndrome) using high-density porous polyethylene. *Aesthetic Plast Surg.* 2009;33(4):661–665.
67. Zheng W, Li B, Zou Y, Lou F. The prenatal diagnosis and classification of cleft palate: The role and value of magnetic resonance imaging. *Eur Radiol.* 2019;29(10):5600–5606.
68. Nicot R, Rotten D, Opdenakker Y, et al. Fetal dental panorama on three-dimensional ultrasound imaging of cleft lip and palate and other facial anomalies. *Clin Oral Investig.* 2019;23(4):1561–1568.
69. Smarius B, Loozen C, Manten W, Bekker M, Pistorius L, Breugem C. Accurate diagnosis of prenatal cleft lip/palate by understanding the embryology. *World J Methodol.* 2017;7(3):93–100.
70. Mulliken JB. The changing faces of children with cleft lip and palate. *N Engl J Med.* 2004;351:745–747.
71. Dămăşaru E, Nicolae C, Caraiane A, Bordeianu I. Cleft lip with or without cleft palate: its incidence at birth. *Int J Med Dent.* 2019;9:256–260.
72. Reiter R, Brosch S, Lüdeke M, et al. Genetic and environmental risk factors for submucous cleft palate. *Eur J Oral Sci.* 2012;120:97–103.
73. Hens K, Hens G. Pregnancy termination in the case of an orofacial cleft: an investigation of the concept of reproductive autonomy. *Cleft Palate Craniofac J.* 2020;57:1134–1139.
74. Fuchs F, Burlat J, Grosjean F, et al. A score-based method for quality control of fetal hard palate assessment during routine second-trimester ultrasound examination. *Acta Obstet Gynecol Scand.* 2018;11:1300–1308.

75. Mishra S, Sabhlok S, Panda PK, et al. Management of midline facial clefts. *J Maxillofac Oral Surg.* 2015;14:883–890.
76. Marazita ML. The evolution of human genetic studies of cleft lip and cleft palate. *Annu Rev Genomics Hum Genet.* 2012;13 263-283 11.
77. Yu Y, Yao J. Classification of cleft lip and palate. In: Yao J, Xu J, eds. *Atlas of Cleft Lip and Palate & Facial Deformity Surgery.* Singapore: Springer; 2020.
78. Allori AC, et al. Classification of cleft lip/palate: then and now. *Cleft Palate Craniofac J.* 2017;54(2):175–188.
79. Jamilian A, Lucchese A, Darnahal A, et al. Cleft sidedness and congenitally missing teeth in patients with cleft lip and palate. *Progr Orthodonts.* 2016;17:1–4.
80. Martínez-Ten P, Sepulveda W, Wong AE, Tonni G. The role of 2D/3D/4D ultrasound in the prenatal assessment of cleft lip and palate. In: Tonni G, Sepulveda W, Wong A, eds. *Prenatal Diagnosis of Orofacial Malformations.* Springer; 2017.
81. Fraser FC. The genetics of cleft lip and cleft palate. *Am J Hum Genet.* 1970;22:336–352.
82. Desai BB, Patel DP, Sinha SV, Jain M, Patel RN, Bhanat ST. Correlating causative factors in cleft lip and palate patients: An epidemiological study. *J Cleft Lip Palate Craniofac Anomal.* 2019;6:11–16.
83. Lu Y, Yang T, Luo H, et al. Visualization and quantitation of fetal movements by real-time three-dimensional ultrasound with live X-Plane imaging in the first trimester of pregnancy. *Croat Med J.* 2016;57(5):474–481.
84. Vezzetti E, et al. Diagnosing cleft lip pathology in 3D ultrasound: a landmarking-based approach. Image Analysis. *Stereology.* 2016;35:53–65.
85. Binet A, et al. Complete bilateral Tessier's facial cleft number 5: surgical strategy for a rare case report: SRA. *Surg Radiol Anat.* 2019;41(5):569–574.
86. Muraskas JK, McDonnell JF, Chudik RJ, Salyer KE, Glynn L. Amniotic band syndrome with significant orofacial clefts and disruptions and distortions of craniofacial structures. *J Pediatr Surg.* 2013;38(4):635–638.
87. Portier-Marret N, Hohlfeld J, et al. Complete bilateral facial cleft (Tessier 4) with corneal staphyloma: a rare association. *J Pediatr Surg.* 2008;43(10).
88. Kadouch DJM, et al. Surgical treatment of macroglossia in patients with Beckwith-Wiedemann syndrome: a 20-year experience and review of the literature. *Int J Oral Maxillofac Surg.* 2012;41:300–308.
89. Staretz-Chacham O, Lang TC, LaMarca ME, Krasnewich D, Sidransky E. Lysosomal storage disorders in the newborn. *Pediatrics.* 2009;123(4):1191–1207.
90. Esmer AC, Has R, Yüksel A, Kalelioğlu I. Prenatal diagnosis of congenital ranula: case report. *Turk J Obstet Gynecol.* 2013;10:256–259.
91. Harrison JD. Modern management and pathophysiology of ranula: literature review. *Head Neck.* 2010;32(10):1310–1320.
92. George MM, Mirza O, Solanki K, Goswamy J, Rothera MP. Serious neonatal airway obstruction with massive congenital sublingual ranula and contralateral occurrence. *Ann Med Surg (Lond).* 2015;4(2):136–139.
93. Gul A, Gungorduk K, Yildirim G, Gedikbasi A, Ceylan Y. Prenatal diagnosis and management of a ranula. *J Obstet Gynaecol Res.* 2008;34(2):262–265.
94. Mong A, Johnson AM, Kramer SS, et al. Congenital high airway obstruction syndrome: MR/US findings, effect on management, and outcome. *Pediatr Radiol.* 2008;38(11):1171–1179.
95. Peiró JL, Sbragia L, Scorletti F. Management of fetal teratomas. *Pediatr Surg Int.* 2016;32(7):635–647.
96. Maddali MM, Al Balushi FKA, Waje ND. Elephant trunk–like teratoma of the face with compromised airway in an infant with complex congenital cardiac defects. *A & A Case Rep.* 2016;6(3):52–55.
97. Posod A, Griesmaier E, Brunner A, Pototschnig C, Trawoger R, Kiechl-Kohlendorfer U. An unusual cause of inspiratory stridor in the newborn: congenital pharyngeal teratoma: a case report. *BMC Pediatr.* 2016:16.
98. Chauhan DS, Guruprasad Y, Inderchand S. Congenital nasopharyngeal teratoma with a cleft palate: case report and a 7 year follow up. *J Maxillofac Oral Surg.* 2011;10:253–256.
99. Simmonds JC, Patel AK, Mildenhall NR, Mader NS, Scott AR. Neonatal macroglossia. *Cleft Palate Craniofac J.* 2018;55:1122–1129.
100. Jiang S. Ex utero intrapartum treatment (EXIT) for fetal neck masses: a tertiary center experience and literature review. 2020. https://data.mendeley.com/datasets/6t2psy2bj9/1
101. Gupta A, Maddalozzo J, Win Htin T, Shah A, Chou PM. Spindle cell rhabdomyosarcoma of the tongue in an infant: a case report with emphasis on differential diagnosis of childhood spindle cell lesions. *Pathol Res Pract.* 2004;200(7-8):537–543.
102. Doğer E, Ceylan Y, Çakıroğlu AY, Çalışkan E. Prenatal diagnosis and management of a fetal neck mass. *J Turk Ger Gynecol Assoc.* 2015;16(2):118–120.
103. Güzelmansur I, Aksoy HT, Hakverdi S, Seven M, Dilmen U, Dilmen G. Fetal cervical neuroblastoma: prenatal diagnosis. *Case Rep Med.* 2011;2011:529749.
104. Tonni G, De Felice C, Centini G, Ginanneschi C. Cervical and oral teratoma in the fetus: a systematic review of etiology, pathology, diagnosis, treatment and prognosis. *Arch Gynecol Obstet.* 2010;282(4):355–361.
105. Lazar DA, Cassady CI, Olutoye OO, et al. Tracheoesophageal displacement index and predictors of airway obstruction for fetuses with neck masses. *J Pediatr Surg.* 2012;47(1):46–50.
106. Noia G, Pellegrino M, Masini L, et al. Fetal cystic hygroma: the importance of natural history. *Eur J Obstet Gynecol Reprod Biol.* 2013;170:407–413.
107. Shimura M, Ishikawa H, Nagase H, et al. Predicting the intrauterine fetal death of fetuses with cystic hygroma in early pregnancy. *Congenit Anom (Kyoto).* 2018;58(5):167–170.
108. Chen YN, Chen CP, Lin CJ, Chen SW. Prenatal ultrasound evaluation and outcome of pregnancy with fetal cystic hygromas and lymphangiomas. *J Med Ultrasound.* 2017;25(1):12–15.
109. Wassef M, Blei F, Adams D, et al. Vascular anomalies classification: recommendations from the International Society for the Study of Vascular Anomalies. *Pediatrics.* 2015;136(1):e203–e214.
110. Malone FD, Ball RH, Nyberg DA. First-trimester septated cystic hygroma. Prevalence, natural history, and pediatric outcome. *Obstet Gynecol.* 2005;106:288–294.
111. Gedikbasi A. Multidisciplinary approach in cystic hygroma: prenatal diagnosis, outcome, and postnatal follow up. *Pediatr Int.* 2009;51:670–677.
112. Rosati P, Guariglia L. Prognostic value of ultrasound findings of fetal cystic hygroma detected in early pregnancy by transvaginal sonography. *Ultrasound Obstet Gynecol.* 2000;16(3):245–250.
113. Munteanu O, Cîrstoiu MM, Filipoiu FM, et al. Morphological and ultrasonographic study of fetuses with cervical hygroma. A cases series. *Romanian J Morphol Embryology.* 2016:57.
114. Ali MK, Abdelbadee AY, Shazly SA, Othman ER. Hydrops fetalis with cystic hygroma: a case report. *Middle East Fertil Soc J.* 2012;17:134–135.
115. Gietka-Czernel M, Dębska M, Kretowicz P, Jastrzębska H, Zgliczyński W. Increased size and vascularisation, plus decreased echogenicity, of foetal thyroid in two-dimensional ultrasonography caused by maternal Graves disease. *Endokrynol Pol.* 2014;65(1):64–68.
116. Delay F, Dochez V, Biquard F, et al. Management of fetal 570 goiters: 6-year retrospective observational study in three prenatal 571 diagnosis and treatment centers of the pays de Loire perinatal network. *J Matern Fetal Neonatal Med.* 2018;4:1–191.
117. Iijima S. Current knowledge about the in utero and peripartum management of fetal goiter associated with maternal Graves' disease. *Eur J Obstet Gynecol Reprod Biol.* 2019;3:100027.
118. De Groot L, Abalovich M, Alexander EK, et al. Management of thyroid dysfunction during pregnancy and postpartum: an Endocrine Society clinical practice guideline. *J Clin Endocrinol Metab.* 2012;97:2543–2565.

119. Cilingir IU, Sayın NC, Erzincan SG, et al. Rapidly growing cervical teratoma: fetal death during delivery. *J Pediatr Neonat Individ Med.* 2017;6(2):E060228.
120. Lituania M, Tonni G. Bifid uvula and familial stickler syndrome diagnosed prenatally before the sonographic "equals sign" landmark. *Arch Gynecol Obstet.* 2013;288(3):483–487.
121. Wong HS, Tait J, Pringle KC. Viewing of the soft and the hard palate on routine 3-D ultrasound sweep of the fetal face: feasibility study. *Fetal Diagn Ther.* 2008;24(2):146–154.
122. Tonni G, Grisolia G. Fetal uvula: navigating and lightening the soft palate using HDlive. *Arch Gynecol Obstet.* 2013;288(2):239–244.
123. Roy-Lacroix ME, Moretti F, Ferraro ZM, et al. A comparison of standard two-dimensional ultrasound to three-dimensional volume sonography for routine second-trimester fetal imaging. *J Perinatol.* 2017;37:380–386.
124. Gaëlle AG, Hossu G, Banasiak C, et al. Optimization of fetal biometry with 3D ultrasound and image recognition (EPICEA): protocol for a prospective cross-sectional study. *BMJ Open.* 2019;9(12).
125. Rubio EI, Blask AR, Badillo AT, Bulas DI. Prenatal magnetic resonance and ultrasonographic findings in small-bowel obstruction: imaging clues and postnatal outcomes. *Pediatr Radiol.* 2017;47(4):411–421.
126. Kline-Fath BM, Bahado-Singh R, Bulas DI. *Fundamental and Advanced Fetal Imaging: Ultrasound and MRI.* Lippincott Williams & Wilkins; 2015.
127. Moreira NC, Ribeiro V, Teixeira J, et al. Visualization of the fetal lip and palate: is brain-targeted MRI reliable? *Cleft Palate Craniofac J.* 2013;50:513–519.
128. Anilawan S, Rubio EI, Blask AR, Loomis JM, Bulas DI. Normal size of the fetal adrenal gland on prenatal magnetic resonance imaging. *Pediatr Radiol.* 2020;50(6):840–847.
129. Milic A, Blaser S, Robinson A, et al. Prenatal detection of microtia by MRI in a fetus with trisomy 22. *Pediatr Radiol.* 2006;36:706–710.

CHAPTER 60

Fetal Neural Axis

Tanya Nolan

OBJECTIVES

On completion of this chapter, you should be able to:
- Describe the embryology of the neural tube fetal brain development
- Discuss the anomalies that can occur in the fetal head and spine
- Recognize the sonographic appearance of fetal head and spine anomalies

OUTLINE

Embryology 1522
Anencephaly 1523
Acrania 1524
Cephalocele 1525
Spina Bifida 1527
Dandy-Walker Malformation 1531

Holoprosencephaly 1531
Agenesis of the Corpus Callosum 1535
Aqueductal Stenosis 1536
Vein of Galen Aneurysm 1537
Choroid Plexus Cysts 1537

Porencephalic Cysts 1538
Schizencephaly 1538
Hydranencephaly 1538
Ventriculomegaly (Hydrocephalus) 1540
Microcephaly 1542

KEY TERMS

Acrania
Alobar holoprosencephaly
Anencephaly
Anomaly
Cebocephaly
Cyclopia

Cystic hygroma
Holoprosencephaly
Hydranencephaly
Hydrocephalus
Macrocephaly
Meningocele

Meningomyelocele
Myeloschisis
Spina bifida
Spina bifida occulta
Ventriculomegaly

EMBRYOLOGY

The central nervous system (CNS) arises from the ectodermal neural plate at approximately 18 to 23 days gestation.[1] The cephalic portion of the neural plate will differentiate into the primitive brain, and the caudal portion will form the spinal cord. As the neuropore folds and closes, three brain vesicles develop in the rostral cavity of the neural tube. These brain vesicles include the prosencephalon, mesencephalon, and rhombencephalon. The prosencephalon differentiates into the forebrain, the mesencephalon develops into the midbrain, and the rhombencephalon becomes the hindbrain. Unfused cranial and caudal neuropores will eventually close between 24 to 26 weeks of gestation.[2] If the neural tube fails to fuse within 3 to 4 weeks of gestation, several malformations may be manifest, including anencephaly, encephalocele, and spina bifida.[3]

At the end of the third week, the cephalic end of the neural tube will bend into the shape of a C (cephalic flexure), with the area of the mesencephalon having a very prominent bend. The brain then folds back on itself, and by the beginning of the fifth week another prominent bend, the cervical flexure, appears between the hindbrain and the spinal cord. The brain that originally was composed of three parts has now further divided into five parts. The prosencephalon divides into the telencephalon, which becomes the cerebral hemispheres, and the diencephalon, which eventually develops into the epithalamus, thalamus, hypothalamus, and infundibulum. The rhombencephalon also subdivides into the metencephalon, which ultimately becomes the cerebellum and pons, and the myelencephalon, which transforms into the medulla. The fundamental organization of the brain is represented in these five divisions that persist into adult life.

The primitive spinal cord divides into two regions. The alar plate region matures into the sensory region of the cord, and the basal plate region develops into the motor region of the cord. These regions further subdivide into specialized functions. During the first trimester, the spinal cord and the vertebral column extend the length of the body. After this, the growth of the spinal cord lags behind that of the vertebral column and the posterior portion the body grows beyond both vertebral column and spinal cord. At birth, the spinal cord terminates at the level of the third lumbar vertebra, although by adulthood, the cord will end at the level of the second lumbar vertebra.[4]

Neural function begins at 6 weeks of gestation and commences with primitive reflex movement at the level of the face and neck. By 12 weeks of gestation, sensitivity has spread across the surface of the body except at the back and top of the head. The fetus begins to have defined periods of activity and inactivity at the end of the fourth month. Between the fourth and fifth months, the fetus can grip objects and is capable of weak respiratory movements. At 6 months of gestation, the fetus displays the sucking reflex, and by about 28 weeks, significant changes in brain wave patterns have occurred.[5]

A wide range of defects may affect the fetal spine and/or brain. The remainder of this chapter presents anomalies of the CNS (Table 60.1). Correctly identifying anomalies of the fetal head and spine can be a complex task. Some of the distinguishing characteristics that help to define specific anomalies are listed in Table 60.2.

ANENCEPHALY

Anencephaly may also be known as aprosencephaly or atelencephaly. It is the most common neural tube defect. The etiology of anencephaly is widely unknown and multifactorial with both environmental and genetic variables. Anencephaly may result from a syndrome, such as Meckel-Gruber (i.e., cystic kidneys, occipital encephalocele and/or polydactyly [postaxial], microcephaly, microphthalmia, cleft palate, and genitourinary anomalies), or a chromosomal abnormality, such as trisomy 13 and trisomy 18. Risk is increased in patients with diabetes mellitus, including those whose disorders are well controlled. Environmental and dietary factors, including hyperthermia, folate and vitamin deficiencies, and teratogenic levels of zinc, may also increase the prevalence of neural tube defects. Other teratogens associated with neural tube defects include valproic acid, methotrexate, and aminopterin. Another cause of neural tube defects is amniotic band syndrome, which may manifest with clefting defects.[6,7]

Overall, the estimated prevalence of anencephaly is reported as 3 per 10,000 births. Due to its complicated etiology, incidence varies markedly among geographic locations, gender, ethnicity, and environmental exposures. A recurrence risk of 2% to 5% for subsequent pregnancies has been documented for a woman with a history of a prior pregnancy with an open neural tube defect. The recurrence risk can be reduced by 50% to 70% with use of folic acid supplements beginning 1 month before pregnancy.[6,8]

Anencephaly, which means absence of the brain, is caused by a failure of the rostral end of the neural tube to close.[5] During early development, a relatively normal brain forms, but it lacks both the calvarium and meninges. In time, mechanical and chemical influences of amniotic fluid on the exposed brain cause the brain to disintegrate and both cerebral hemispheres and skull fail to fully develop. As result, the base of the skull and facial structures are preserved, but there is a complete or partial absence of the cranium. The brainstem also remains but without the presence of a cerebrum, cerebellum, and basal ganglia. The remnant brain is

TABLE 60.1	Anomalies Most Frequently Associated With Ventriculomegaly
Anomaly	Distinguishing Characteristics
Spina bifida	Deformed cranium "lemon" sign; usually disappears in third trimester Obliteration of cisterna magna Open spinal defect
Cephalocele	Open cranial defect; usually occipital skull base Obliteration of the cisterna magna Occasional lemon sign
Holoprosencephaly	Absent/incomplete midline Single ventricular cavity Facial anomalies
Dandy-Walker complex	Midline posterior fossa cyst Defect in cerebellar vermis
Agenesis of corpus callosum	Absent cavum septi pellucidi Elevated third ventricle Interhemispheric cyst/lipoma
Arachnoid/glioependymal cyst	Intracranial cyst with regular contours displacing/compressing cortex
Porencephaly	Intracranial cyst with jagged outline often communicating with lateral ventricles
Schizencephaly	Clefts in cortical mantle
Intracranial hemorrhage	Echogenic/complex mass in lateral ventricles/brain parenchyma
Microcephaly	Small head
Vascular malformations	Fluid-filled lesion with blood flow at Doppler examination
Craniostenosis	Abnormal skull shape
Lissencephaly	Absent/reduced cerebral convolutions
Infection	Intracranial/periventricular echogenicities

From Nyberg D. *Diagnostic Imaging of Fetal Anomalies*, Philadelphia: Lippincott Williams & Wilkins; 2003.

TABLE 60.2 Differential Considerations for Central Nervous System Anomalies

Anomaly	Sonographic Findings	Differential Considerations	Distinguishing Characteristics
Anencephaly	Absence of brain and cranial vault Froglike appearance Cerebrovasculosa	Microcephaly Acrania Cephalocele	No calvarium above vault orbits
Cephalocele	Extracranial mass Bony defect in calvarium	Cystic hygroma	Defect in skull
Dandy-Walker malformation	Posterior fossa cyst Splaying of cerebellar hemispheres	Arachnoid cyst Cerebellar hypoplasia	Cerebellar hemispheres will be splayed
Vein of Galen aneurysm	Midline cystic structure Turbulent Doppler flow	Arachnoid cyst Porencephalic cyst	Doppler flow in the cystic space
Porencephalic cyst	Cyst within brain parenchyma No mass effect Communication with ventricle	Arachnoid cyst Cyst communicating with ventricle	No mass effect
Hydranencephaly	Absence of brain tissue Fluid-filled brain Absent or partially absent falx	Hydrocephaly Holoprosencephaly	Lack of intact falx No rim of brain tissue

covered by a thick membrane called angiomatous stroma or cerebrovasculosa.

Anencephaly is a lethal disorder, with up to 50% of cases resulting in fetal demise. The remainder die at birth or shortly thereafter. Because of the severity of this disorder, early diagnosis is preferred. Prenatal diagnosis is often made with ultrasound following referral for elevated maternal serum alpha-fetoprotein levels that occur because of the absence of skull and exposed tissue. Sonographic diagnosis of anencephaly during the first and second trimesters of pregnancies has approached 100%.[6,7]

Sonographic Findings. Anencephaly may be detected with ultrasound as early as 10 to 14 weeks of gestation. The brightly echogenic calvarium is missing beyond the forehead, and normal-appearing orbits and facial structures are retained. Variable amounts of disorganized brain tissue remain atop of the head, including mostly brainstem. The crown-rump length may be normal because degeneration of the fetal brain is progressive, leading to a reduction in the crown-rump length with advancing gestation. Second-trimester identification of anencephaly is more obvious.[6,8]

Sonographic features of anencephaly include the following:
- Absence of the brain and cranial vault (Fig. 60.1)
- Rudimentary brain tissue characterized as the cerebrovasculosa (Fig. 60.2)
- Bulging fetal orbits, giving the fetus a froglike appearance (Fig. 60.3)

Other sonographic findings associated with anencephaly include polyhydramnios, which is commonly seen but may not be present until after 26 weeks of gestation. Echogenic amniotic fluid is best evaluated transvaginally or with increased overall gain. Coexisting spina bifida and/or craniorachischisis may be identified in fetuses with anencephaly. Additional anomalies include cleft lip and palate, hydronephrosis, diaphragmatic hernia, cardiac defects, omphalocele, gastrointestinal defects, and talipes.[6,8]

When severe, microcephaly may be confused with anencephaly, although the presence of the cranium should aid in a definitive diagnosis. Other defects that may mimic anencephaly include cephalocele (brain herniation) and amniotic band syndrome (usually asymmetric cranial defects).[6]

ACRANIA

Acrania, or exencephaly, is the precursor for anencephaly and manifests as the absence of cranial bones in the presence of complete, although abnormal, development of the cerebral hemispheres. This **anomaly** occurs at the beginning of the fourth gestational week, when the mesenchymal tissue fails to migrate and bone does not form over the cerebral tissues.

Acrania may be confused with anencephaly, although the presence of significant brain tissue and the lack of a froglike appearance should establish the diagnosis. Other disorders that may mimic acrania include hypophosphatasia and osteogenesis imperfecta, both of which result in hypomineralization of the cranium. Identification of additional findings, such as long bone fractures, should help to distinguish these disorders from acrania.

Acrania is readily detected in the first trimester during nuchal translucency screenings. A fetus presents on ultrasound with a wide and irregular shaped head that lacks echogenic calvarium surrounding the brain. Sonographic landmarks for fetal head evaluation, appropriate for gestational age, are also difficult to decipher. Within the coronal plane, the cerebral hemispheres surrounded by amniotic fluid give the fetal head a bilobed appearance. This bilobed brain is best identified in the first trimester and has been described as a "Mickey Mouse" appearance.[8]

Sonographic Findings. Sonographic features of acrania include the following:
- The presence of brain tissue without the presence of a calvarium (Fig. 60.4)

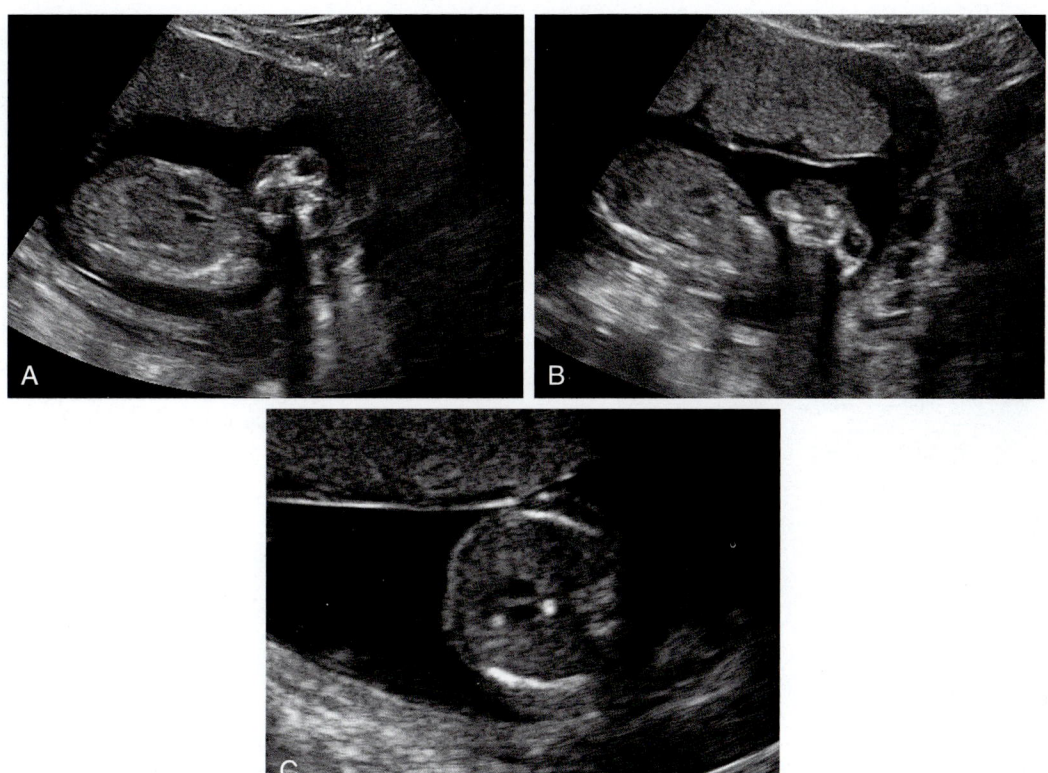

FIG. 60.1 (A) An anencephalic fetus; absence of the brain and calvarium is identified. Note the froglike appearance. (B) A profile of the anomaly. (C) Echogenic foci were noted in the heart; amniocentesis revealed trisomy 13.

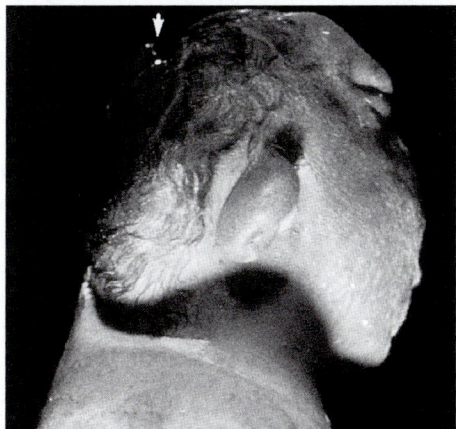

FIG. 60.2 Postmortem image of anencephaly. The *arrow* points to the rudimentary brain (cerebrovasculosa).

- Disorganization of brain tissue
- Prominent sulcal markings (Figs. 60.5–60.7)

Acrania may be associated with other anomalies, including spinal defects, cleft lip and palate, talipes, cardiac defects, and omphalocele. Acrania has also been associated with amniotic band syndrome (see Fig. 60.4B).

CEPHALOCELE

A cephalocele is a neural tube defect in which the brain, meninges, or both herniate through a defect in the calvarium. These malformations are classified according to their anatomic herniation and may occur in the occipital, frontal, temporal, and parietal regions of the fetal head. *Encephalocele* is the term used to describe herniation of the meninges and brain through the defect; *cranial meningocele* describes the

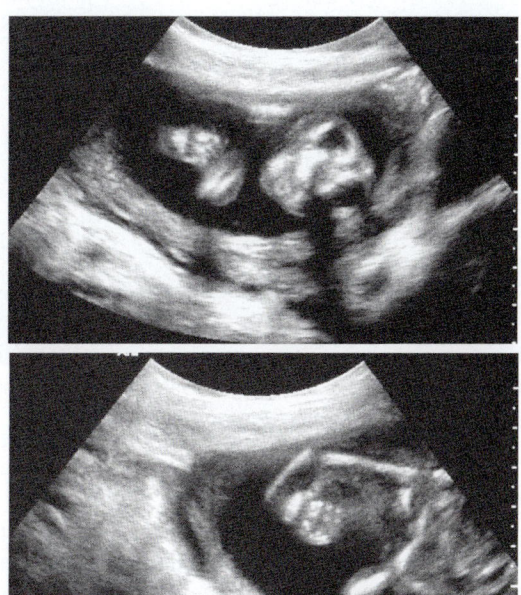

FIG. 60.3 Anencephaly was identified in a fetus with a radial ray defect and tetralogy of Fallot. A chromosomal anomaly was suspected.

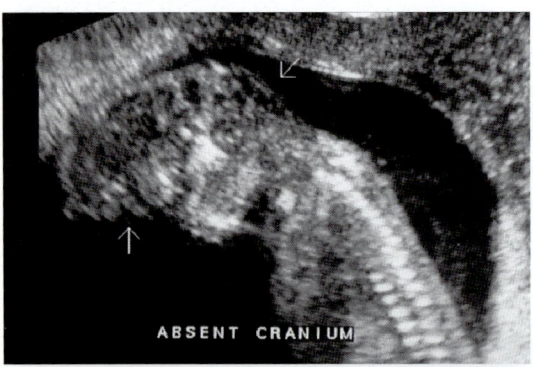

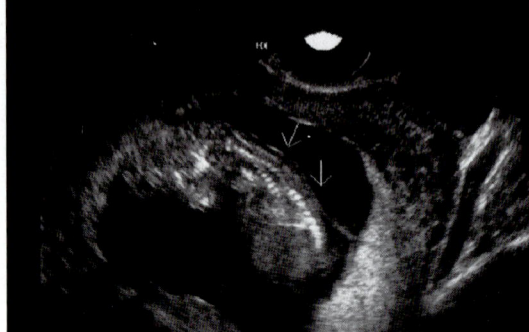

FIG. 60.4 **Acrania.** The patient presented with an elevated maternal serum alpha-fetoprotein. Note the amnion *(arrows)* along the back of the fetus. Amniotic band syndrome was the probable cause.

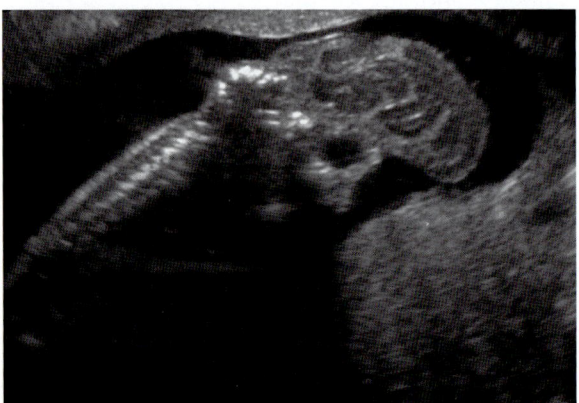

FIG. 60.5 Sagittal view of a fetus with acrania with prominent sulcal markings.

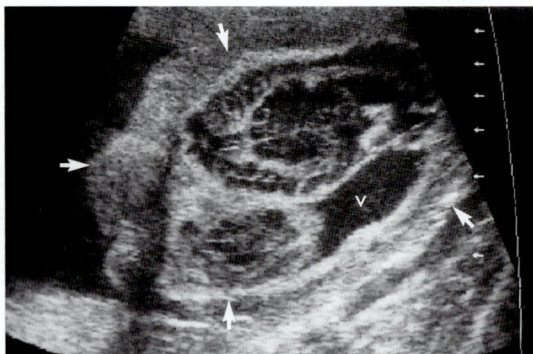

FIG. 60.6 Transverse view of a fetus showing the disorganized and freely floating brain tissue *(arrows)*. The brain anatomy is enhanced because of the absence of skull bones. Note the herniated ventricle (v) and sulcal markings.

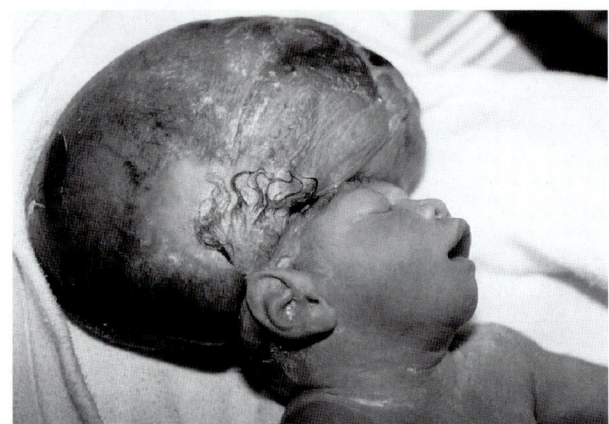

FIG. 60.7 Same neonate shown in Fig. 60.6, with acrania shortly after birth. The infant died within a few hours.

herniation of only meninges (Fig. 60.8). Overall, cephaloceles occur at a rate of 0.8 per 10,000 live births. Meningoceles are considered 10 times less common than encephaloceles. The incidence of different categorizations of cephalocele vary dependent on geographic location. The majority of cephaloceles in Europe and North America are occipital and posterior. Maternal serum alpha fetoprotein levels are likely within the low-risk range because the majority of encephaloceles are closed defects.[9,10]

The prognosis for the infant with a cephalocele varies based on the size, location, involvement of other brain structures, and the presence of intracranial or extracranial malformations and microcephaly. Fetal death is common because of severe associated malformations and/or the inability to repair the defect. A giant encephalocele occurs when the protrusion is larger than the head from which it arises. Giant encephaloceles pose a significant surgical challenge. In addition, both preterm delivery and fetal growth restriction increase the risk for infant mortality. An infant with an isolated cranial meningocele has a chance of normal mentation; however, disabilities are common among surviving children.[9,10]

Sonographic Findings. The sonographic appearance of a cephalocele depends on the location, size, and involvement of brain structures. Cephaloceles are classified as occipital cephaloceles when the defect lies between the lambdoid suture and the foramen magnum; parietal cephaloceles occur between the bregma and the lambda; and anterior cephaloceles lie between the anterior aspects of the ethmoid bone. Anterior cephaloceles are further classified into frontal and basal varieties. The frontal cephaloceles are always external lesions that occur near the root of the nose. Basal cephaloceles are internal lesions that occur within the nose, the pharynx, or the orbit.

Most encephaloceles are diagnosed during the first trimester. The occipital lobes are most common in a posterior encephalocele, and the cerebellum may be present in very low posterior encephaloceles (Fig. 60.9). The fetus often demonstrates a significantly smaller head circumference (HC) and biparietal

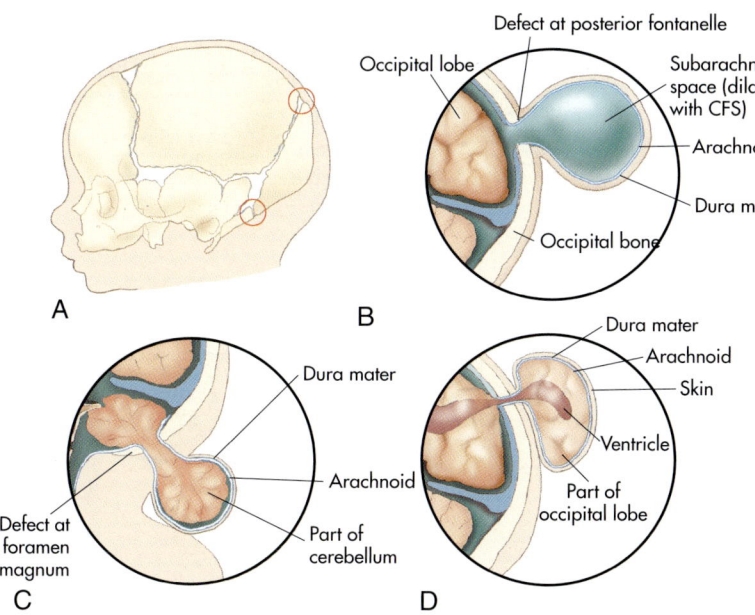

FIG. 60.8 **Cranium bifidum (bony defect in the cranium) and various types of herniation of the brain and/or meninges.** (A) A newborn with a large protrusion from the occipital region of the skull. The upper circle indicates a cranial defect at the posterior fontanelle, and the lower circle indicates a cranial defect near the foramen magnum. (B) Meningocele consisting of a protrusion of the cranial meninges that is filled with cerebrospinal fluid. (C) Meningoencephalocele consisting of a protrusion of part of the cerebellum that is covered by meninges and skin. (D) Meningohydroencephalocele consisting of a protrusion of the part of the occipital lobe that contains part of the posterior horn of a lateral ventricle.

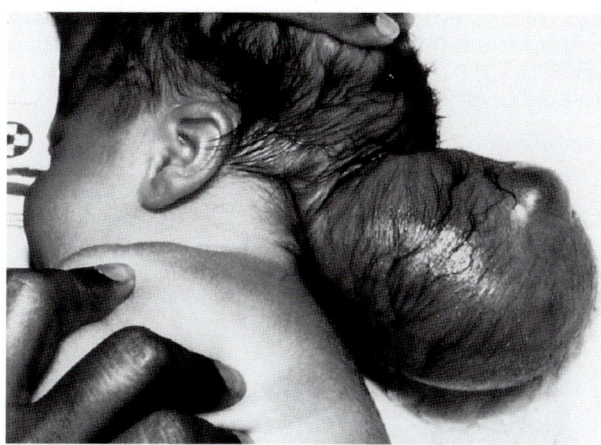

FIG. 60.9 Neonate with a posterior occipital encephalocele.

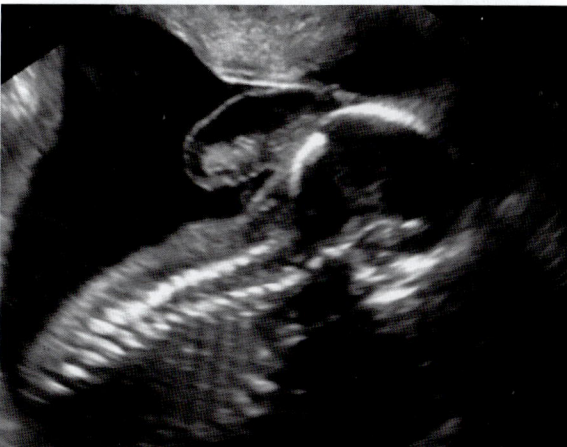

FIG. 60.10 **Encephalocele.** The sac protruding from the cranium contains fluid and solid components.

diameter (BPD) when compared with the expected fetal age, and use of three-dimensional (3D) ultrasound in orthogonal planes and tomographic imaging assists in demonstrating the location, extent, and evidence of intracranial anatomy.

Sonographic features of cephaloceles include the following:
- An extracranial mass (Fig. 60.10), which may be fluid filled (cranial meningocele) or contain solid components (encephalocele)
- A bony defect in the skull
- Ventriculomegaly, which is more commonly identified with an encephalocele
- Smaller than expected HC and/or BPD

Another sonographic finding associated with cephaloceles is polyhydramnios. Coexisting anomalies include microcephaly, agenesis of the corpus callosum (ACC), facial clefts, spina bifida, cardiac anomalies, and genital anomalies. Chromosomal anomalies and syndromes have been identified with cephaloceles, including trisomy 13 and Meckel-Gruber syndrome, which is an autosomal recessive disorder characterized by encephalocele, polydactyly, and polycystic kidneys (Fig. 60.11). Other syndromes linked with cephalocele include Chemke, cryptophthalmos, Knobloch, dyssegmental dysplasia, von Voss, Roberts, and Walker-Warburg. Cephaloceles located off midline are usually the result of amniotic band syndrome and may be further distinguished by associated limb anomalies and abdominal wall defects.

Cephaloceles must be distinguished from other midline masses and may be confused with **cystic hygromas**, although they lack a cranial defect. Anencephaly may be difficult to distinguish from encephaloceles of significant size, and the presence of the cranial vault with encephalocele should establish the diagnosis. Frontal encephaloceles may be difficult to distinguish from a facial teratoma.[10]

SPINA BIFIDA

Spina bifida encompasses a wide range of vertebral defects that result from failure of neural tube closure and incomplete fusion of the vertebral arches. The meninges and neural elements may

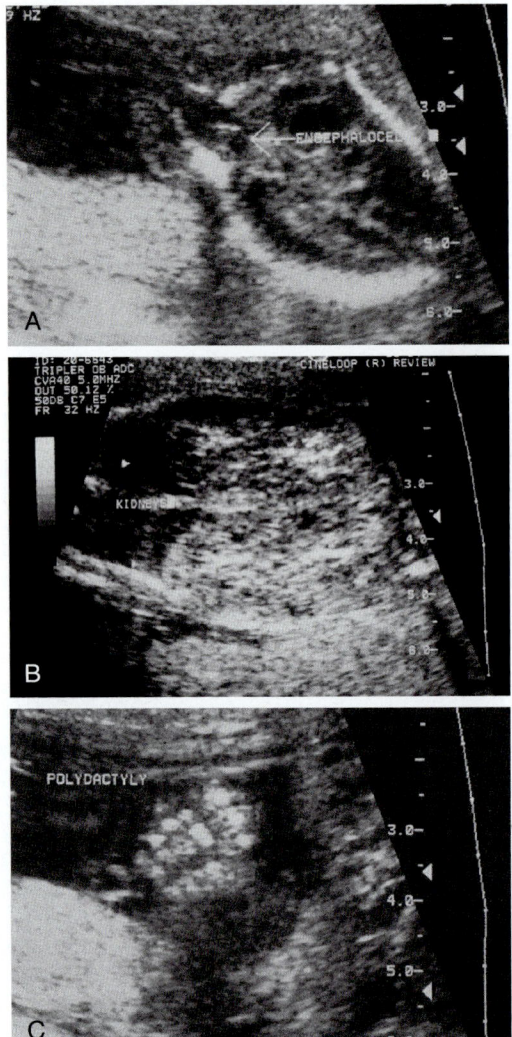

FIG. 60.11 Encephalocele as part of Meckel-Gruber syndrome. (A) Brain tissue herniating from the occipital region. (B) Large echogenic kidneys consistent with autosomal recessive polycystic kidney disease. (C) Polydactyly was noted on the hands.

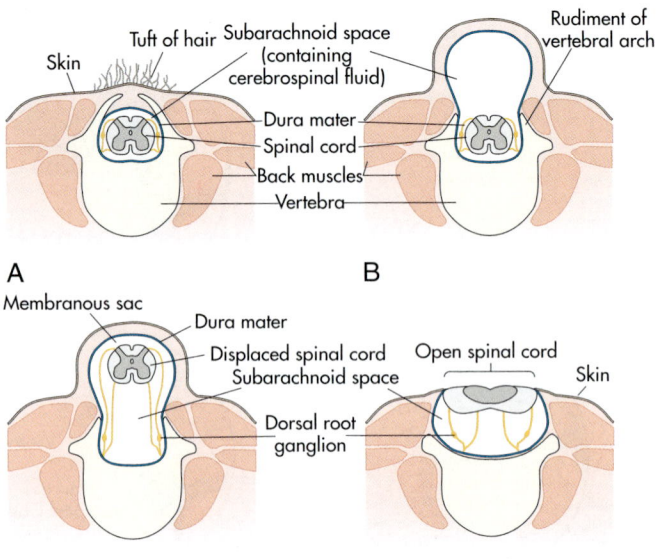

FIG. 60.12 Various types of spina bifida and commonly associated malformations of the nervous system. (A) Spina bifida occulta. Approximately 10% of people have this vertebral defect in L5 and/or S1. It usually causes no back problems. (B) Spina bifida with meningocele. (C) Spina bifida with meningomyelocele. (D) Spina bifida with myeloschisis. The types illustrated in parts B through D are often referred to collectively as *spina bifida cystica* because of the cystic sac that is associated with them.

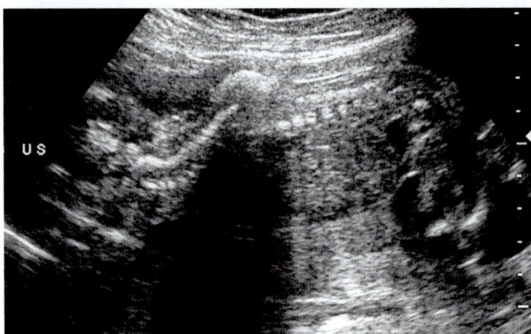

FIG. 60.13 A large spinal defect at the thoracic level is seen in the fetus. The prognosis was extremely poor.

protrude through this defect. The defect may occur anywhere along the vertebral column but most commonly occurs along the lumbar and sacral regions. Spina bifida etiology is complex with genetic, environmental, and/or drug-use factors. The incidence of this defect has declined as a result of campaigning by the US Public Health Service, which encourages women to increase their intake of folic acid before becoming pregnant, and the subsequent mandate by the Food and Drug Administration to add folic acid to cereal grain products. The estimated incidence in the United States is 3.50 per 10,000 live births.

The term *spina bifida* means that there is a cleft or opening in the spine (Fig. 60.12). The two main categories of spina bifida include *spina bifida aperta* (open) and *spina bifida occulta* (closed). These two main categories are further divided based on whether the skin covers the defect, a herniated sac is present, and if there are multiple components found within the herniated sac. When covered with skin or hair, it is referred to as **spina bifida occulta**, an anomaly that is associated with a normal spinal cord and nerves and normal neurologic development. Spina bifida occulta is extremely difficult to detect in the fetus. Because the defect is covered by skin, the maternal serum alpha-fetoprotein level will be normal.

Spina bifida aperta has three clinical forms: meningocele, myelomeningocele, and myeloschisis. When the defect involves only protrusion of the meninges, it is termed a **meningocele**. More commonly, the meninges and neural elements protrude through the defect, called a **meningomyelocele**. The most severe form of spina bifida is termed **myeloschisis** (rachischisis). Myeloschisis (Fig. 60.13) is a significantly large and severe defect including multiple adjacent vertebrae. Several variants include an adipose tissue component in addition to meningeal and/or neural components and are termed lipomyelomeningocele and lipomeningocele. Open neural tube defects are commonly associated with increased maternal serum alpha-fetoprotein.

Spina bifida is also associated with varying degrees of neurologic impairment, which may include minor anesthesia, paraparesis, or death. Life-long mobility impairments result from denervation of the sensory and motor nerves at and below the spinal deformity. Fetuses with myelomeningoceles often present with cranial defects associated with the Arnold-Chiari (type II) malformation, which is identified in 90% of patients. The Arnold-Chiari II malformation invariably presents with hydrocephalus caused by the cerebellar vermis being displaced into the cervical canal. This changes the shape of the cerebellum, giving it a "banana" appearance, and leads to obliteration of the cisterna magna. In addition, caudal displacement of the cranial structures causes scalloping of the frontal bones of the skull, making the fetal head resemble a lemon, decreasing the size of the BPD.

Management of a fetus with spina bifida usually includes serial ultrasound examinations to monitor progression and extent of ventriculomegaly and to follow fetal growth. Fetuses may be delivered early for ventricular shunting, usually by cesarean section to preserve as much motor function as possible. Intrauterine surgery is considered for nonlethal conditions aimed to ameliorate the effect of advancing age on neuromuscular development and reverse hindbrain herniations. In addition to management of the actual defect, attention to any hydrocephalus, urinary tract anomalies or dysfunction, and orthopedic issues may be part of the long-term care required for this child. Risks incurred with this procedure include premature delivery, maternal morbidity, and fetal mortality. Early and accurate diagnosis is relevant for pregnancy management including planned delivery, postnatal surgery, and/or open or laparoscopic intrauterine fetal surgery, if available. Three-dimensional sonographic imaging can assist in identifying the upper level of the defect, which predicts neurologic function and mortality. In affected fetuses, 3D imaging is also useful in demonstrating the architecture of the ventricular system and cisterna magna.

Sonographic Findings. Evaluation of spina bifida during the first trimester screening shares many characteristics with the second trimester assessment. However, during early gestation, the sonographer should focus on the indirect versus the direct characteristics of spina bifida. At the time of the second trimester evaluation, sonographic imaging must include a focused methodical survey of the fetal spine in both sagittal and transverse planes (Fig. 60.14). The normal fetal spine should demonstrate the posterior ossification centers completing a spinal circle. Unfortunately, the survey of the fetal spine may be impeded when the spine is down, the fetus is in the breech position, oligohydramnios is present, or in cases of maternal obesity which precludes adequate visualization.

Direct sonographic features of spina bifida include the following:
- Splaying of the posterior ossification centers with a V or U configuration (Fig. 60.15)
- Protrusion of a saclike structure that may be anechoic (meningocele) or contain neural elements (myelomeningocele) (Fig. 60.16)
- A cleft in the skin (Fig. 60.17)

After a spinal defect has been identified, the level and extent of the defect, the presence or absence of neural

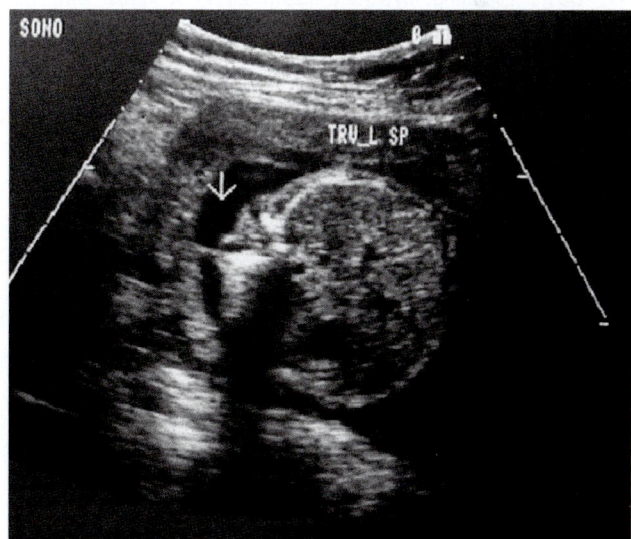

FIG. 60.15 Meningomyelocele with spinal splaying appearing as a V.

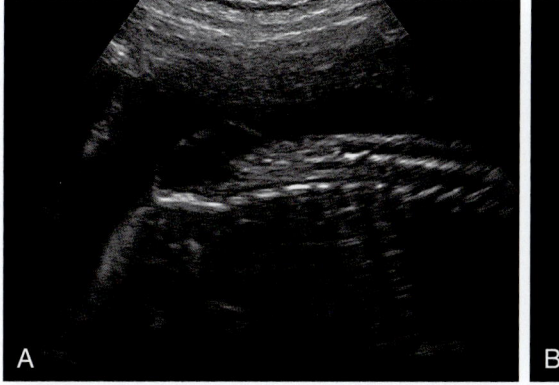
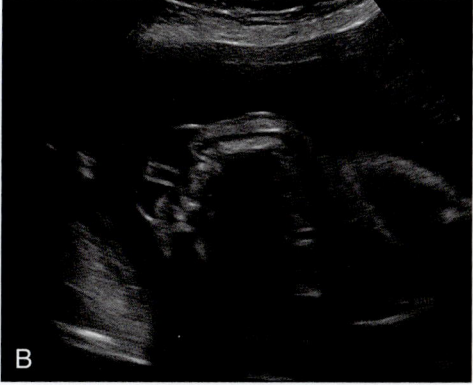

FIG. 60.14 Sagittal (A) and transverse (B) views of the fetal spine demonstrate this defect in the lumbar region consistent with a myelomeningocele.

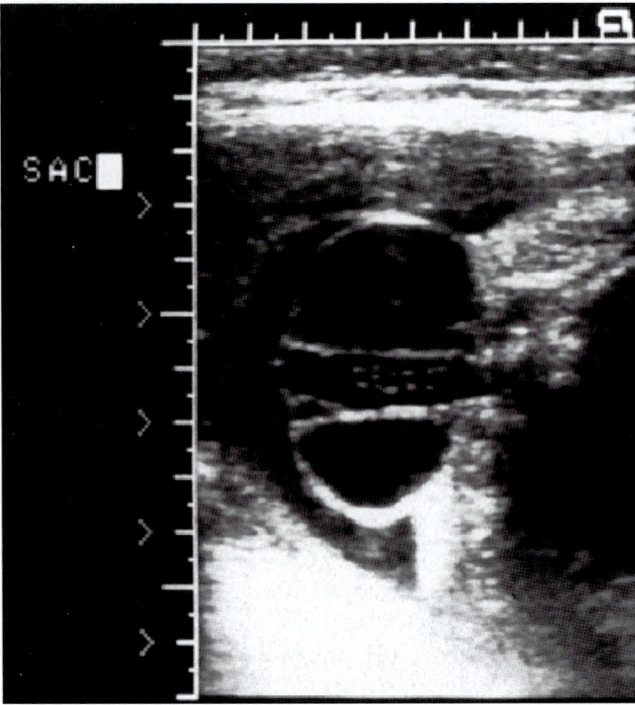

FIG. 60.16 **Meningomyelocele identified in a fetus with mild ventriculomegaly.** Note the neural elements protruding into the sac.

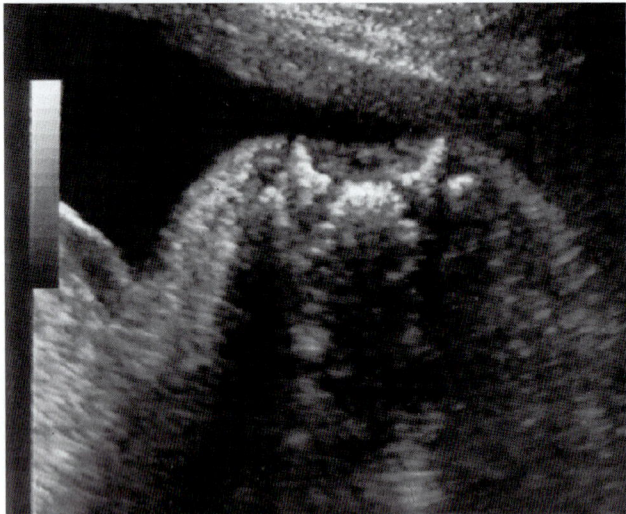

FIG. 60.17 Spina bifida with a U-shaped configuration and an open cleft in the skin.

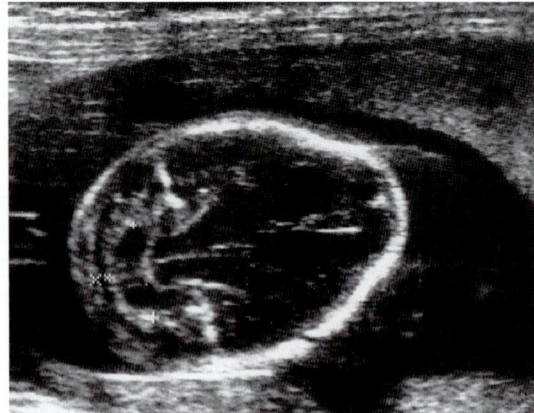

FIG. 60.18 Abnormally shaped cerebellum "banana" sign in a 21-week fetus with a lumbosacral meningomyelocele. Note the lemon-shaped frontal bones consistent with frontal bossing.

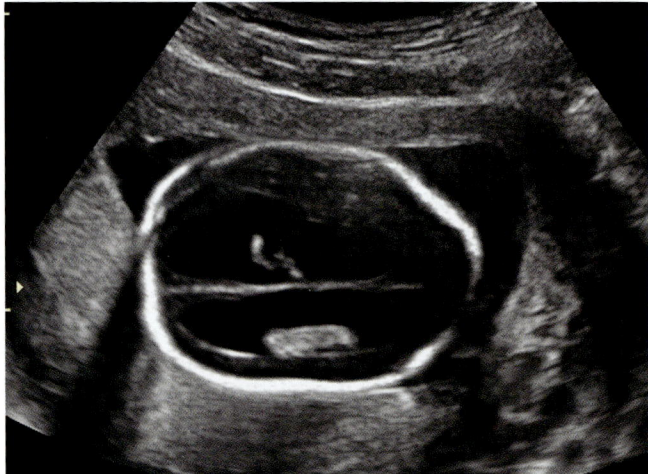

FIG. 60.19 **Ventriculomegaly in a fetus with a myelomeningocele.** The frontal bones clearly demonstrate the scalloping that is seen with the "lemon" sign.

elements contained in the protruding sac, and associated intracranial findings should be documented.

Indirect sonographic cranial findings include the following:
- Flattening of the frontal bones, giving the head a "lemon" shape (Fig. 60.18)
- Small BPD and HC.
- Obliteration of the cisterna magna and nonvisualization of the fourth ventricle
- Inferior displacement of the cerebellar vermis, giving the cerebellum a rounded, "banana" shape (see Fig. 60.18)
- Ventriculomegaly (Figs. 60.19 and 60.20)

The "lemon" sign is nonspecific for spina bifida, and similar head shapes have been described with other CNS malformations, such as encephalocele, and with non-CNS malformations, such as thanatophoric dysplasia. This appearance may also be indistinguishable from the "strawberry" sign described in association with trisomy 18. Other sonographic findings associated with spina bifida include talipes, cephaloceles, cleft lip and palate, hypotelorism, heart defects, and genitourinary anomalies. Spina bifida has also been associated with multiple syndromes and chromosomal anomalies, including trisomy 18. Fetuses exposed to teratogens, such as valproic acid (Fig. 60.21), carbamazepine, methotrexate, and aminopterin, are also at greater risk for developing spina bifida. Maternal diabetes, maternal obesity, hyperthermia, and folic acid deficiency have been associated with spina bifida. A family history of spina bifida or anencephaly is also a significant risk factor for the occurrence of spina bifida.[11-14]

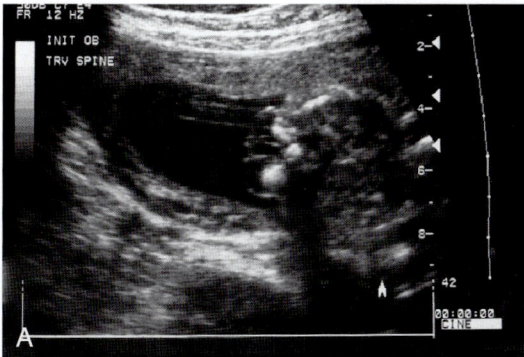
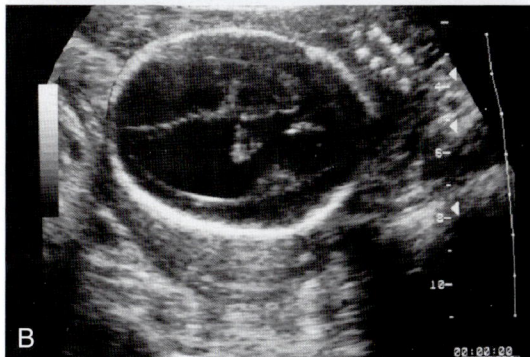

FIG. 60.20 (A) A fetus at 24.6 weeks of gestation with a meningomyelocele. Neural elements were identified in the sac. (B) A significant amount of ventricular dilation was identified within the fetal head.

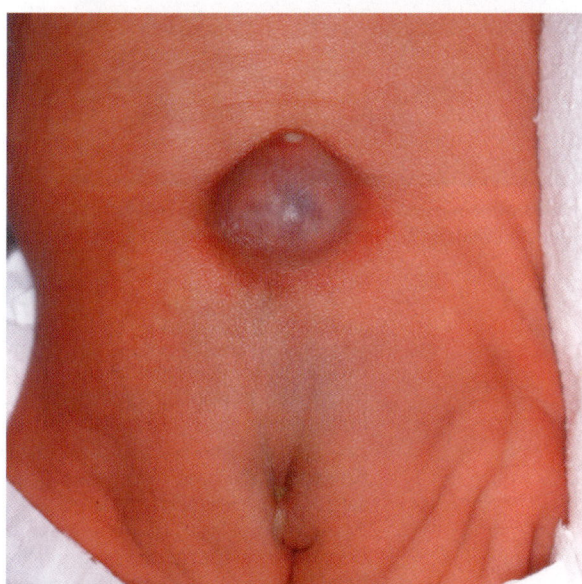

FIG. 60.21 A neonate with a lumbar myelomeningocele.

DANDY-WALKER MALFORMATION

Dandy-Walker malformation (DWM) is a complex malformation affecting both the posterior fossa and cerebellum. It manifests with agenesis or hypoplasia of the cerebellar vermis with resulting dilation of the fourth ventricle and enlargement of the posterior fossa. This rare condition occurs in approximately 1 in 10,000 to 30,000 births, and hydrocephaly is seen in 80% of cases. Development of the cerebellar vermis begins during the 9th week of gestation; however, communications between the fourth ventricle and the cisterna magna are not complete until the 18th week of gestation. Because of this, diagnosis of agenesis and hypoplasia of the cerebellar vermis should not be made before the 18th week of gestation.[15,16]

DWM is associated with other intracranial anomalies approximately 50% of the time. These include ventriculomegaly, ACC, aqueductal stenosis, holoprosencephaly, microcephaly, **macrocephaly**, encephalocele, gyral malformations, heterotopias, and lipomas. Other common associated anomalies include cardiac anomalies, polycystic kidneys, and facial clefts. Chromosomal anomalies that may be associated with DWM include trisomies 13, 18, and 21 and triploidy. DWM has been associated with several syndromes, including Meckel-Gruber syndrome, Walker-Warburg syndrome, and Aicardi syndrome, and has been linked with congenital infection and maternal diabetes.[15,16]

The prognosis for DWM depends on the presence or absence of associated anomalies and on the degree of hypoplasia of the cerebellar vermis because this correlates with the severity of intellectual disability. Mortality depends highly on other anomalies. Many infants with isolated DWM have a subnormal IQ, although some may have normal function.[15]

Sonographic Findings. Both axial and sagittal images of the posterior fossa should be used to differentiate DWM from other posterior fossa abnormalities such as mega cisterna magna, vermian hypoplasia, and Blake pouch cyst. The vermis is easily distinguished in the median plane because it is highly echogenic in comparison with the cerebellar hemispheres.[16]

Sonographic features of DWM include the following:
- A posterior fossa cyst that can vary considerably in size (Fig. 60.22)
- Splaying of the cerebellar hemispheres as a result of complete or partial agenesis of the cerebellar vermis
- An enlarged cisterna magna (>10 mm in axial plane at the level of the transcerebellar diameter) caused by the cerebellar vermis anomaly and posterior fossa cyst
- Ventriculomegaly (≥10 mm) (Fig. 60.23)

Other differential diagnoses to consider include an arachnoid cyst, but identification of the splayed cerebellar hemispheres may help to confirm DWM. Cerebellar hypoplasia should also be ruled out when the cisterna magna is enlarged; however, confirming the small cerebellum aids in the diagnosis of DWM.[15,16]

HOLOPROSENCEPHALY

Holoprosencephaly encompasses a range of abnormalities resulting from abnormal cleavage of the prosencephalon (forebrain) during the fourth week of embryogenesis. As a result, there is a lack of separation between the two cerebral hemispheres of varying degrees. The incidence is 1 in 10,000 live births, although the incidence in aborted fetuses is 1 in 250, which promotes holoprosencephaly as the most common forebrain malformation in humans.[17,18] Holoprosencephaly has been associated with chromosomal anomalies in up to 50% of

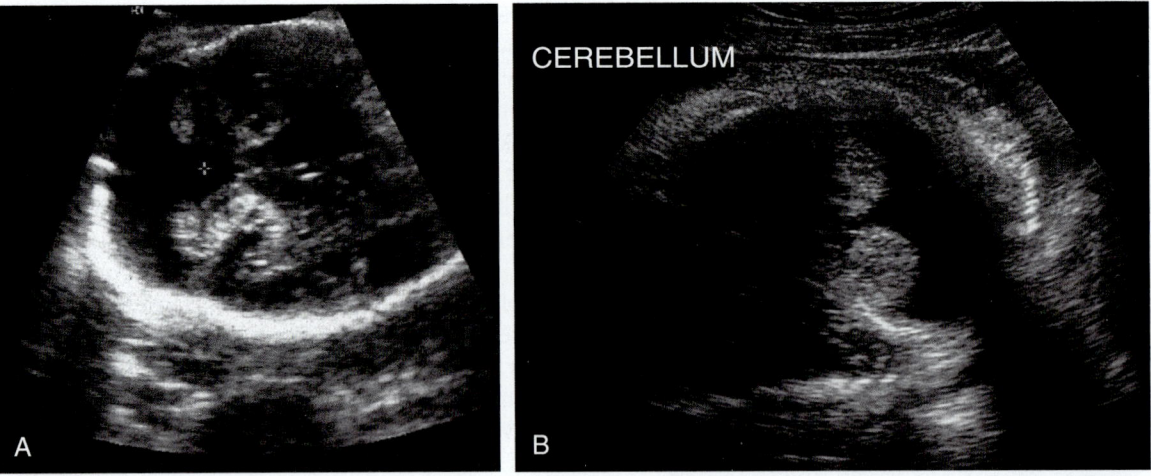

FIG. 60.22 (A) Dandy-Walker cyst. Note the splayed cerebellar hemispheres. (B) This Dandy-Walker malformation was not associated with ventriculomegaly; amniocentesis revealed normal chromosomes.

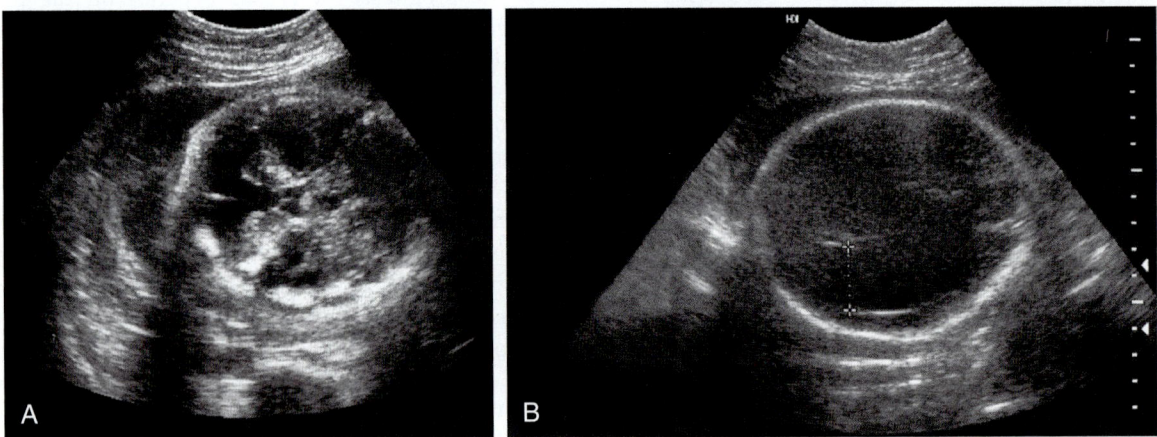

FIG. 60.23 This patient had a history of elevated maternal serum alpha-fetoprotein. Follow-up in a maternal fetal center for a history of hydrocephalus revealed a Dandy-Walker malformation (A) and ventriculomegaly (B). The fetus was 30 weeks and 4 days, with a head size typical of 36 weeks of gestation.

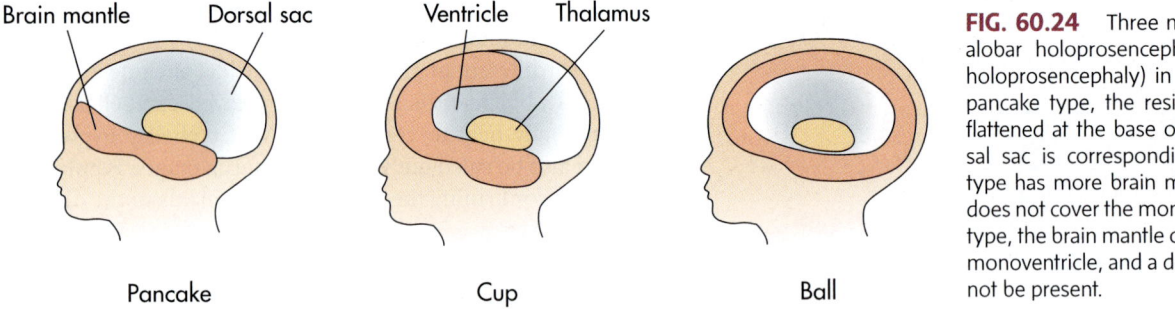

FIG. 60.24 Three morphologic types of alobar holoprosencephaly (and semilobar holoprosencephaly) in sagittal view. In the pancake type, the residual brain mantle is flattened at the base of the brain. The dorsal sac is correspondingly large. The cup type has more brain mantle present, but it does not cover the monoventricle. In the ball type, the brain mantle completely covers the monoventricle, and a dorsal sac may or may not be present.

cases; however, it may also be a sporadic event or may be associated with syndromes, genetic factors, and teratogens.[17-19]

Three forms of holoprosencephaly are known. The most severe form is classified as alobar, the intermediate form as semilobar, and the mildest form as lobar. Identification of the specific form depends on the degree of failed hemispheric division. Approximately two-thirds of cases are alobar holoprosencephaly.[18,19]

Alobar holoprosencephaly is characterized by a singular monoventricle brain tissue that is small and may have a cup, ball, or pancake configuration (Fig. 60.24); fusion of the thalamus; and absence of the interhemispheric fissure, cavum septum pellucidum, corpus callosum, optic tracts, and olfactory bulbs. Semilobar holoprosencephaly presents with a singular ventricular cavity with partial formation of the occipital horns, partial or complete fusion of the thalamus,

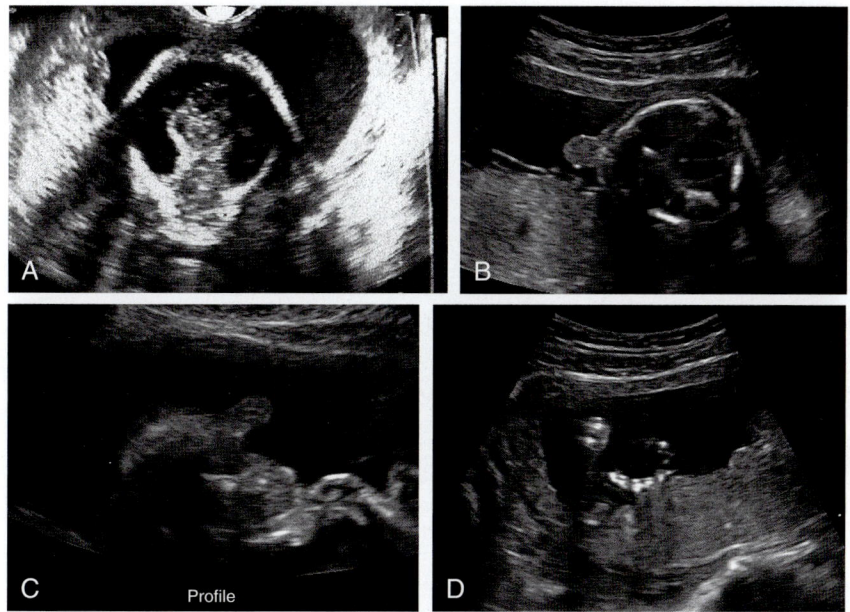

FIG. 60.25 Holoprosencephaly. (A) C-shaped monoventricle. (B) A different fetus with a proboscis. (C) Note the abnormal-appearing profile. (D) Polydactyly was also identified on all four extremities, suggesting the possibility of trisomy 13.

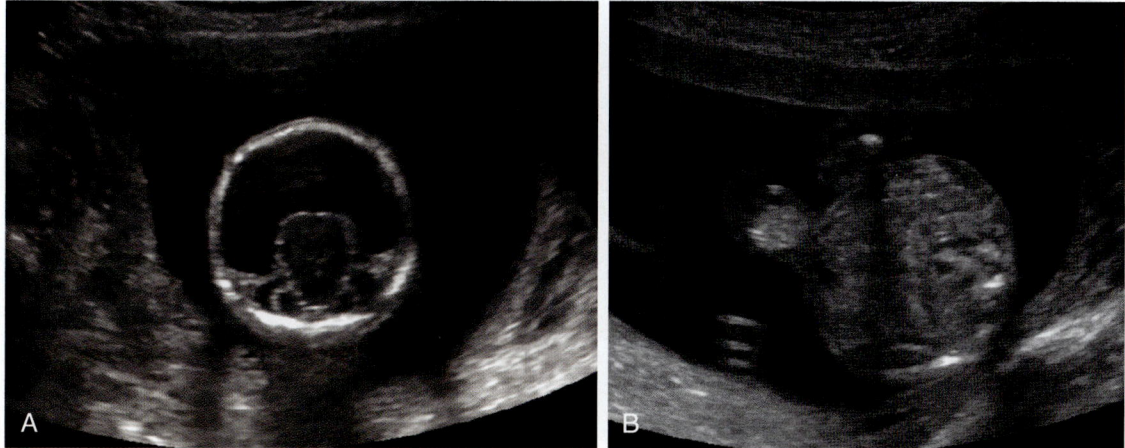

FIG. 60.26 (A) Holoprosencephaly. C-shaped ventricle that is grossly distended, preventing the visualization of the compressed brain tissue. (B) A small omphalocele is also visualized, suggestive of a chromosomal abnormality.

a rudimentary falx and interhemispheric fissure, and absent corpus callosum, cavum septum pellucidum, and olfactory bulbs. In lobar holoprosencephaly, almost complete division of the ventricles is seen with a corpus callosum that may be normal, hypoplastic, or absent, although the cavum septum pellucidum will still be absent.[17]

The cause of holoprosencephaly varies. It is frequently sporadic but has been associated with chromosomal anomalies, most specifically trisomy 13 (Fig. 60.25); however, trisomy 18, monosomy 18p syndrome, and triploidy have been identified, along with anomalies of chromosomes 7, 3, and 11. Rare familial patterns have been transmitted in autosomal dominant and autosomal recessive forms. Multiple syndromes have also been associated with holoprosencephaly, including Meckel-Gruber syndrome, Aicardi syndrome, Fryns syndrome, and hydrolethalus syndrome. Teratogens reported to produce holoprosencephaly include alcohol, phenytoin, retinoic acid, maternal diabetes, and congenital infection. Holoprosencephaly has also been associated with radiation exposure and, in rare instances, with the use of oral contraceptives and aspirin during the first trimester.[17-19]

The prognosis for holoprosencephaly is considered uniformly poor. In its most severe forms, fetuses die at birth or shortly thereafter. In the least severe form, survival is possible, although usually with severe intellectual disability.

Sonographic Findings. Sonographic features of holoprosencephaly include the following:
- A common C-shaped ventricle that may or may not be enlarged (Fig. 60.26)
- Brain tissue with a horseshoe shape as it surrounds the monoventricle (Fig. 60.27)
- Fusion of the thalamus with absence of the third ventricle
- Absence of the interhemispheric fissure
- A dorsal sac with expansion of the monoventricle posteriorly

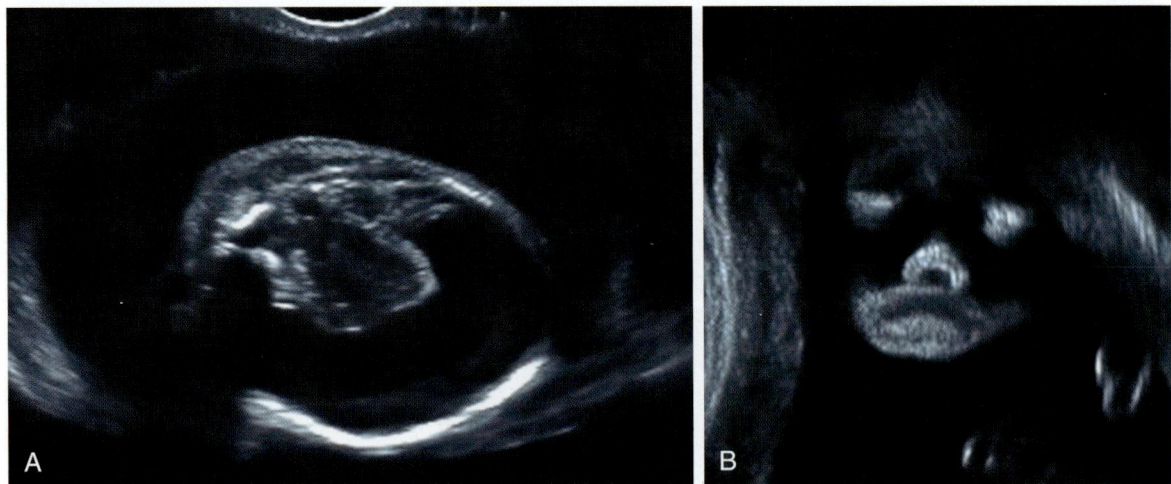

FIG. 60.27 (A) Holoprosencephaly demonstrating surrounding brain tissue and the fused thalami. (B) Evaluation of the face demonstrated protuberant eyes with a normally placed nose with a single nostril. Amniocentesis revealed a normal karyotype.

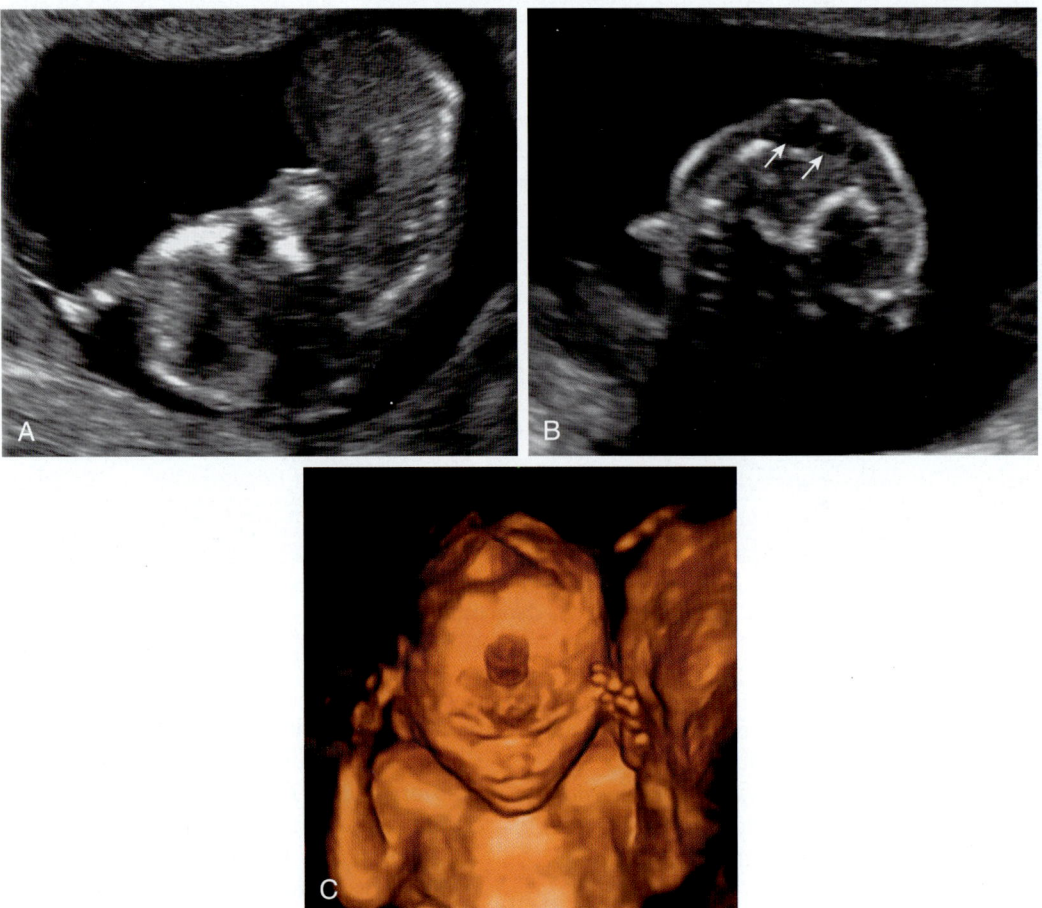

FIG. 60.28 **Facial abnormalities seen in fetuses with holoprosencephaly.** (A) Absent nose noted on profile. (B) Microphthalmia with hypotelorism. (C) A proboscis.

- Absence of the corpus callosum
- Absence of the cavum septum pellucidum

Holoprosencephaly has been diagnosed sonographically during first trimester screening with failure to identify the characteristic butterfly shape of the choroid plexus in the transaxial view.[18] Facial abnormalities may not be visualized during this time, but severe facial abnormalities are frequently present, especially with the most severe forms of holoprosencephaly (Figs. 60.28 and 60.29). The facial anomalies identified include **cyclopia**, hypotelorism (Fig. 60.28B), an absent nose, a flattened nose with a single nostril, and proboscis (Figs. 60.28C, 60.30B, and 60.31). **Cebocephaly** consists of the combination of hypotelorism with a normally placed nose with a single nostril. Ethmocephaly consists of

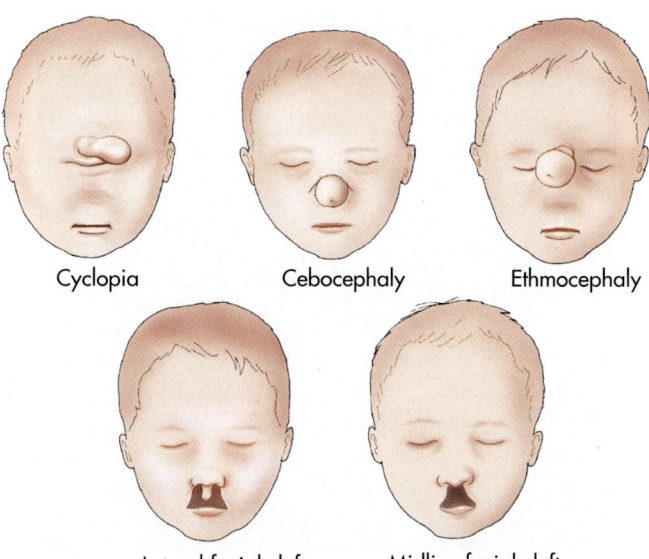

FIG. 60.29 Facial features of holoprosencephaly. Normal facial features in contrast with the variable facial features of holoprosencephaly. In cyclopia, the proboscis projects from the lower forehead superior to one median orbit, and the nose is absent. Ethmocephaly is very similar to cyclopia but has two narrowly placed orbits with a proboscis and absent nose. In cebocephaly, a rudimentary nose with a single nostril and hypotelorism are present. Hypotelorism may occur with a median cleft lip or a bilateral cleft lip.

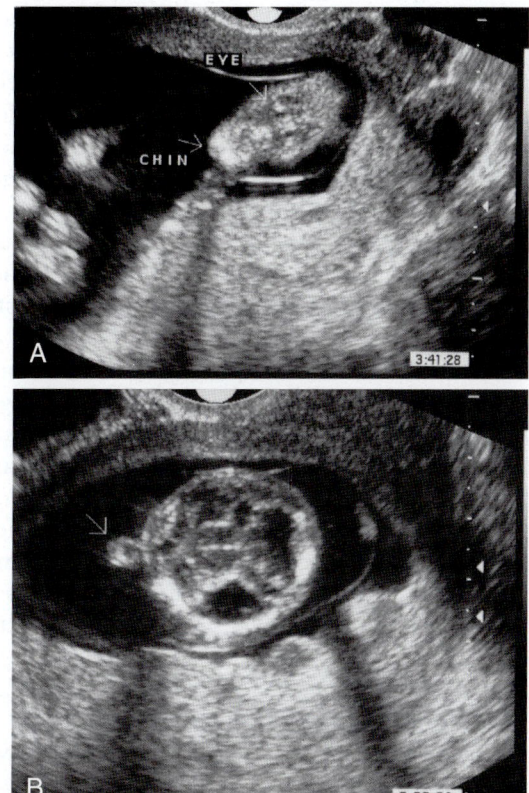

FIG. 60.30 (A) A fetus with trisomy 13 demonstrates small eyes with hypotelorism. (B) In the same fetus, a proboscis *(arrow)* is seen above the orbits.

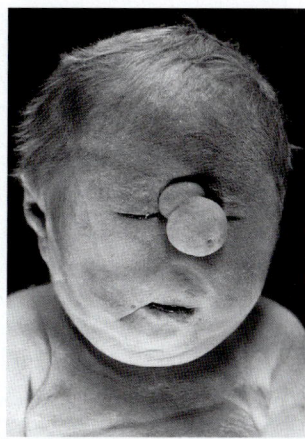

FIG. 60.31 Postmortem image of a neonate with ethmocephaly. Note the proboscis and hypotelorism. The mouth appears normal. A common ventricle and absent optic and ophthalmic nerves were found. The chromosomes were consistent with trisomy 13.

severe hypotelorism with a proboscis superior to the eyes. In addition, facial clefts may be present, with median or bilateral clefting most commonly observed. Therefore the face is an excellent predictor of malformations associated with the brain.[17-19]

Other sonographic findings associated with holoprosencephaly include hydrocephaly, microcephaly, polyhydramnios, and intrauterine growth restriction. In addition, renal cysts or dysplasia, omphalocele, cardiac defects, spina bifida, talipes, and gastrointestinal anomalies have been identified in the presence of holoprosencephaly. Chromosomal anomalies must also be considered if holoprosencephaly is present, especially trisomy 13.[17-19]

AGENESIS OF THE CORPUS CALLOSUM

The corpus callosum is a fibrous white matter tract that connects the cerebral hemispheres and aids in cognition and neurologic functions. Dysgenesis of the corpus callosum is rare and includes a range of complete to partial absence of the callosal fibers that cross the midline, forming a connection between the two hemispheres. Development of the corpus callosum begin at approximately 8 weeks of gestation and is completed at approximately 18 to 19 weeks.[20]

The cause of ACC is somewhat unclear but is thought to involve a vascular disruption or inflammatory lesion before 12 weeks. Cases of ACC, also known as callosal agenesis, are sporadic. It may be associated with other CNS malformations, including hydrocephalus, gyral anomalies, heterotopias, DWM, and holoprosencephaly.[21] Genetic causes have been identifiable in 20% to 45% of cases.[22] It may be transmitted in an autosomal dominant or autosomal recessive manner, and X-linked syndromes have also been identified. Chromosomal anomalies that may accompany ACC include trisomies 21, 13, and 18 and triploidy; multiple syndromes have been associated with ACC, including Aicardi, Apert, Opitz, and Joubert syndromes,

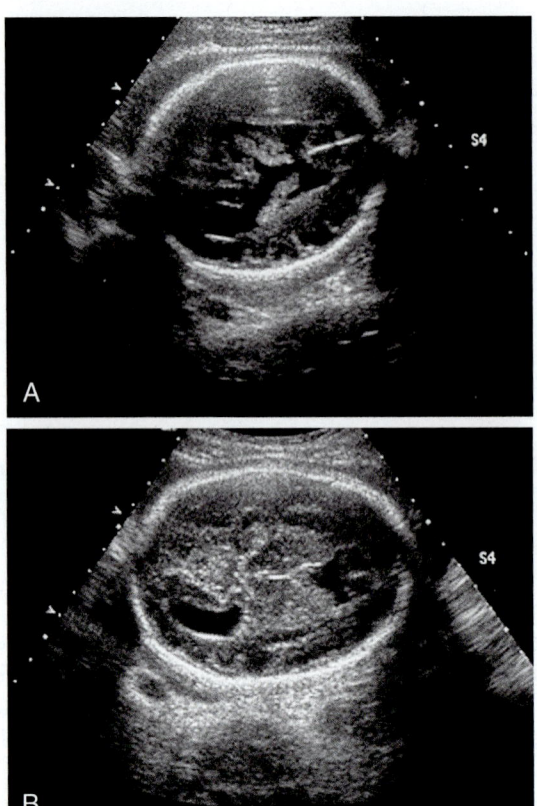

FIG. 60.32 (A) Agenesis of the corpus callosum is diagnosed in this fetus with an absent cavum septum pellucidum. (B) The occipital horn of the lateral ventricle also appears dilated.

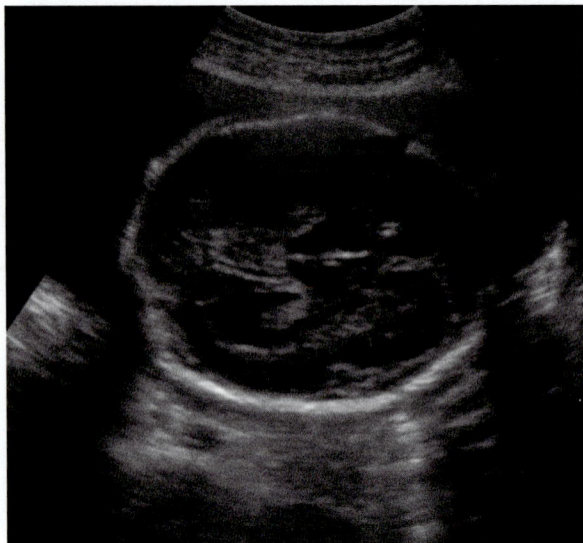

FIG. 60.33 Agenesis of the corpus callosum demonstrates dilated occipital horns which measured 13 mm and absence of the cavum septum pellucidum in a fetus with trisomy 18.

to name a few. Maternal diseases such as diabetes, infection, and alcohol abuse are also contributing factors. In addition, extracranial anomalies are associated with ACC. The prognosis for ACC depends largely on the high incidence of associated anomalies, many of which carry a poor prognosis. As an isolated event, ACC may be asymptomatic or may be associated with intellectual disability and/or seizures.[21]

Sonographic Findings. Sonographic features of ACC (Figs. 60.32 and 60.33) include the following:
- Absence of the corpus callosum
- Elevation and dilation of the third ventricle
- Widely separated lateral ventricular frontal horns with medial indentation of the medial walls
- Dilated occipital horns (colpocephaly), giving the lateral ventricles a teardrop shape
- Absence of the cavum septum pellucidum

Isolated ACC may go undetected prenatally, and absence of the cavum septum pellucidum with enlarged ventricles may be the only sonographic signs. Sonographic findings associated with ACC include other CNS and chromosomal anomalies and syndromes, as described earlier. Other abnormalities associated with ACC include cardiac malformations, diaphragmatic hernia, lung agenesis or dysplasia, and absent or dysplastic kidneys.[21]

AQUEDUCTAL STENOSIS

Aqueductal stenosis results from obstruction, atresia, or stenosis of the aqueduct of Sylvius causing ventriculomegaly. Due to its narrow diameter, the Sylvian aqueduct is the most common location for intraventricular blockage of cerebral spinal fluid (CSF). In cases of aqueductal stenosis, the shape of the aqueduct opening changes to form a funnel-like structure with a posterior stenosis. Because the aqueduct of Sylvius connects to the third and fourth ventricles, enlargement of the lateral ventricles and the third ventricle in the presence of a normal fourth ventricle is common.[23]

Aqueductal stenosis may be congenital or acquired, idiopathic, or secondary to a known etiology.[23] Although many anomalies are sporadic in nature, aqueductal stenosis may result from intrauterine infection, such as cytomegalovirus, rubella, and toxoplasmosis. Cranial masses and ventricular hemorrhage are other contributing factors to acquired obstruction. Primary aqueductal stenosis is usually X-linked and has an autosomal recessive inheritance.

The prognosis for aqueductal stenosis is considered poor and varies with associated anomalies. Approximately 90% of survivors have an IQ less than 70. Infants with X-linked aqueductal stenosis are profoundly intellectually disabled.

Sonographic Findings. Sonographic features of aqueductal stenosis include the following:
- Ventricular enlargement of the lateral ventricles, which may be severe (Fig. 60.34)
- Third ventricular dilation, with macrocephaly
- Flexion and adduction of the thumb (seen in the X-linked form)

VEIN OF GALEN ANEURYSM

An aneurysm of the vein of Galen, also known as a vein of Galen malformation, is a rare arteriovenous malformation. The vein will be enlarged and will communicate with normal-appearing arteries resulting in a high-flow complex lesion.[24]

Vein of Galen aneurysm (VAGA) is considered sporadic, is predominant in males, and comprises less than 1% of all cerebral arteriovenous malformations. Early diagnosis is critical because systemic shunting may lead to cardiac failure, hydrops, and perinatal death. VAGA can be associated with neurologic damage, which may result from ischemia, hemorrhage, or a mass effect.[24]

The prognosis for VAGA is generally poor, especially when associated with hydrops and/or cardiac failure. When symptoms present later in older children and young adults, the prognosis is generally good. Embolization is the primary treatment.

Evaluation of VAGA with 3D power Doppler has proven to be a useful tool in characterizing vascular anatomic features before planned delivery and neonatal treatment.[24]

Sonographic Findings. Sonographic features of VAGA include the following:
- A cystic space that may be irregular in shape and is located midline and posterosuperior to the third ventricle
- Turbulent flow with Doppler evaluation

Other sonographic findings associated with VAGA include fetal cardiomegaly and nonimmune hydrops. Ventriculomegaly with resultant macrocephaly may also develop.

VAGA may be confused with arachnoid cysts, which are very rare and may occur anywhere within the brain. Doppler evaluation of an arachnoid cyst will reveal no blood flow within the structure. Porencephalic cysts should also be listed in the differential considerations; however, these may be distinguished by the absence of blood flow and by communication of this cyst with the ventricle.

CHOROID PLEXUS CYSTS

Choroid plexus cysts (CPCs) are round or ovoid anechoic structures found within the choroid plexus. These cysts are common, occurring with a frequency of 0.18% to 3.6%.[25] CPCs contain cerebrospinal fluid and cellular debris that have become trapped within the neuroepithelial folds.

CPCs are usually isolated findings that resolve between 25 and 33 weeks of gestation without any other associated anomalies. However, CPCs have been related to fetal aneuploidy, particularly trisomy 18 (Fig. 60.35). The risk for aneuploidy

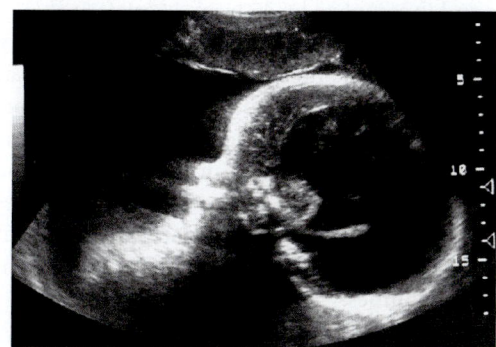

FIG. 60.34 A sagittal image of a fetus with severe hydrocephaly that was thought to result from aqueductal stenosis.

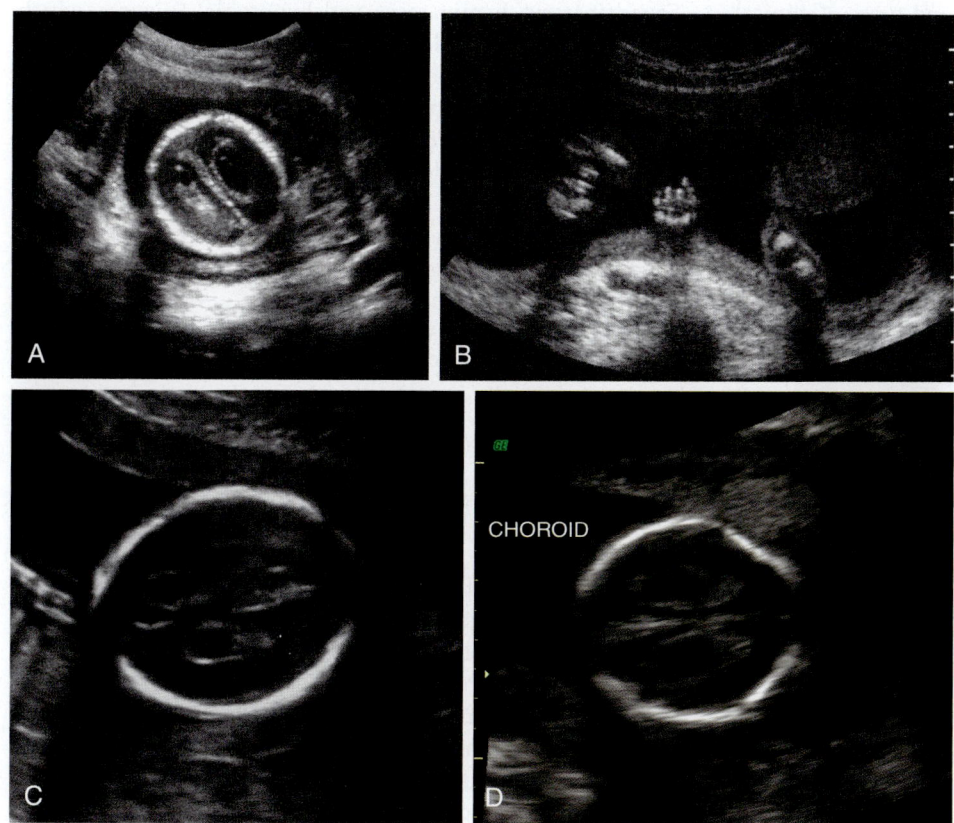

FIG. 60.35 (A) Bilateral choroid plexus cysts are observed in this fetus with trisomy 18. (B) The same fetus also had a heart defect and these persistently clenched hands. (C) Bilateral choroid plexus cysts. (D) Choroid plexus cysts associated with trisomy 18.

increases depending on the type and size of the CPCs present.[26]

Sonographic Findings. Sonographic features of CPCs include the following:
- Cysts within the choroid plexus
- Unilateral or bilateral cysts (see Fig. 60.35)
- Solitary or multiple
- Unilocular or multilocular
- Enlargement of the ventricle with a large cyst

Careful sonographic survey for anomalies that might suggest aneuploidy should follow identification of a CPC to include nuchal fold measurement, meticulous survey of the heart, and a survey of the feet and hands to look for abnormal posturing and polydactyly. Amniocentesis for karyotyping may be offered, especially when other factors that may increase the risk for aneuploidy are considered, including maternal age, abnormal triple screen, and other ultrasound findings.

PORENCEPHALIC CYSTS

Porencephalic cysts, also known as porencephaly, are cysts filled with cerebrospinal fluid that communicate with the ventricular system or subarachnoid space. They may result from hemorrhage, infarction, delivery trauma, or inflammatory changes in the nervous system. Porencephalic cysts are reported to occur 3.5 per 100,000 live births.[27] The affected brain parenchyma undergoes necrosis, brain tissue is resorbed, and a cystic lesion remains.

Porencephalic cysts are not associated with fetal anomalies. However, postnatal problems may include seizures, developmental delays, motor deficits, visual and sensory problems, and hydrocephalus. The varied severity and types of clinical presentation depend upon the size and sites of the lesions. For example, frontal lobe cysts are associated with psychosis, and cerebral hemisphere cysts have been associated with seizures.[27]

Sonographic Findings. The sonographic features of porencephalic cysts include the following:
- A cyst within the brain parenchyma without mass effect
- Communication of the cyst with the ventricle or subarachnoid space (Fig. 60.36)

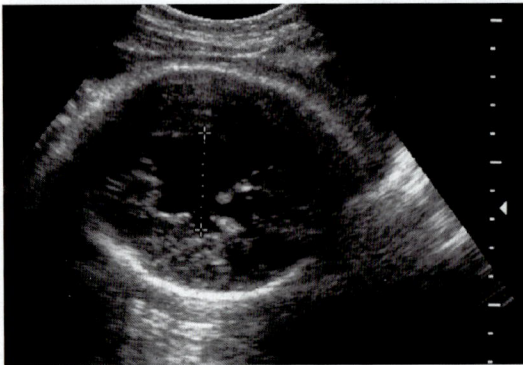

FIG. 60.36 This patient with a history of hydrocephalus seen on ultrasound examination was referred at 32 weeks of gestation to a fetal diagnostic center. A porencephalic cyst was identified communicating with the lateral ventricle. Ventriculomegaly was also noted. The patient was counseled that this finding carried a poor prognosis.

- Reduction in size of the affected hemisphere, which may cause a midline shift and contralateral ventricular enlargement

Porencephalic cysts may be confused with arachnoid cysts (see Fig. 60.40), although the lack of a mass effect seen with porencephaly may aid in differentiating the two.

SCHIZENCEPHALY

Schizencephaly is a very rare disorder characterized by clefts of anomalous gray matter within the cerebral cortex. The clefts may be unilateral or bilateral and typed as open lip or closed lip, depending on whether the cleft has a communication between the subpial space and lateral ventricle. Most defects are noted in the area of the sylvian fissure, and they are considered the result of abnormal neuron migration. The majority of neural migration occurs between 8 and 16 weeks' gestation and is complete by 25 weeks' gestation.[28]

The cause of schizencephaly may result from either genetic or acquired causes. The literature has revealed some association between schizencephaly and the genetic mutation of the EMX2.[28] Schizencephaly has also been linked with multiple assaults during pregnancy which include vascular incidents (e.g., hypotension), congenital infections (e.g., cytomegalovirus), and drugs (e.g., cocaine and warfarin).[29] Patients may present as asymptomatic, as oligosymptomatic, or with severe neurologic disabilities.[28]

The prognosis for patients with schizencephaly varies, ranging from mild to severe outcomes. Open-lip lesions and bilateral clefts carry a worse prognosis. Long-term effects include blindness; motor deficits, which may include spastic quadriparesis; hemiparesis; and hypotonia. Seizures, which may be uncontrollable, intellectual disability, and language impairment are also possible. Hydrocephalus may be progressive, requiring shunt placement.[29]

Sonographic Findings. Sonographic features of schizencephaly include the following:
- A fluid-filled cleft in the cerebral cortex extending from the lateral ventricle to the subarachnoid space (Fig. 60.37)
- Echogenic cleft edges
- Observation of ventriculomegaly

Schizencephaly is associated with other intracranial malformations, including the absence of the septum pellucidum and corpus callosum, ventriculomegaly, and optic nerve hypoplasia.[28]

HYDRANENCEPHALY

Hydranencephaly is a rare brain abnormality characterized by destruction of the cerebral hemispheres by occlusion of the internal carotid arteries, which occurs after the brain and ventricles have fully formed. Brain parenchyma is destroyed and is replaced by cerebrospinal fluid. Because the posterior communicating arteries are preserved, the midbrain and cerebellum are present, and the basal ganglia, choroid plexus, and thalamus may be spared.[30] Hydranencephaly is reported to occur 1 in 10,000 births and found within 0.2% of infant autopsies.[31]

Several factors have been associated with vascular insults, including both intrauterine infections (i.e., toxoplasmosis, cytomegalovirus, and other viral infections) and exposure to toxins (i.e., smoking and cocaine use).[31] Brain ischemia may result from maternal hypotension, twin-to-twin embolization, or vascular agenesis. Hydranencephaly may also be associated with polyhydramnios. No coexisting structural or chromosomal anomalies are associated.

The prognosis for hydranencephaly is grave (Fig. 60.38), with death occurring at birth or shortly thereafter; however, some long-term survivors have been reported.[31]

Sonographic Findings. Sonographic features of hydranencephaly include the following:
- Absence of normal brain tissue with almost complete replacement by cerebrospinal fluid (Fig. 60.39)
- Absent or partially absent falx
- Presence of the midbrain, basal ganglia, and cerebellum
- Possible identification of the choroid plexus
- Possible occurrence of macrocephaly

Hydranencephaly may be confused with severe hydrocephaly, although the presence of an intact falx and surrounding rim of brain parenchyma may help to differentiate hydrocephaly

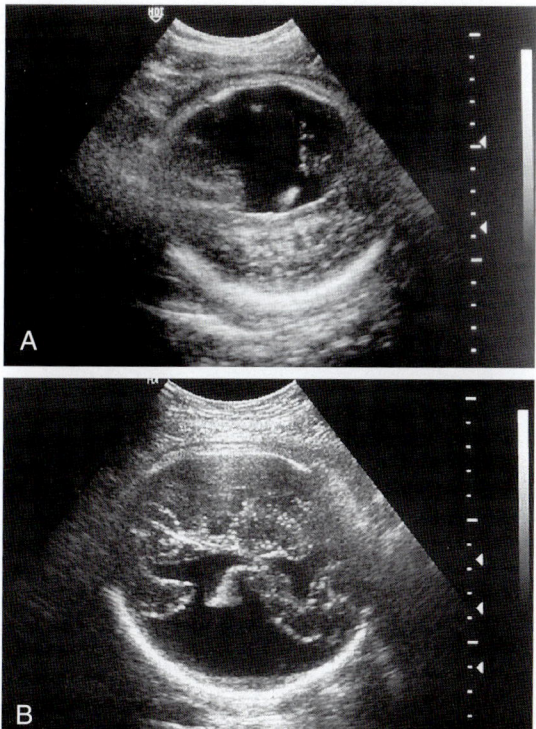

FIG. 60.37 This patient came for an initial ultrasound at 32 weeks of gestation for late prenatal care. The ultrasound revealed hydrocephaly, and the patient was referred to a maternal-fetal center, where the diagnosis of schizencephaly was made based on the cleft that extends to the calvarium. This diagnosis was confirmed at birth with computed tomography.

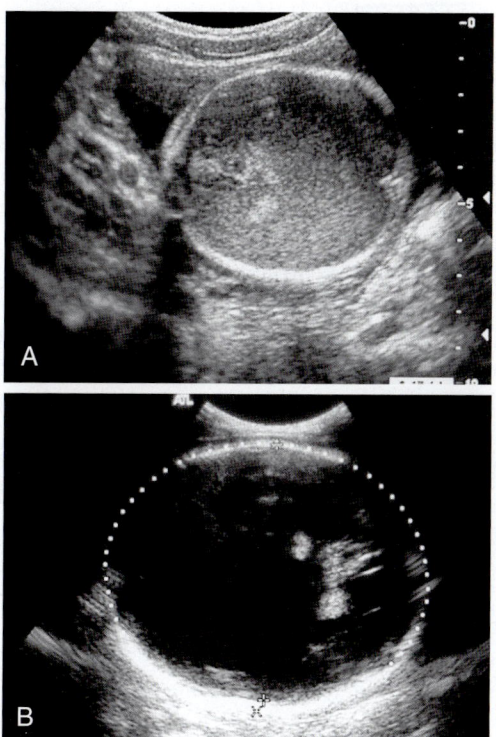

FIG. 60.38 (A) Hydranencephaly was suspected in this patient with poorly controlled diabetes. The low-level echoes seen in this image of the fetal head swirled on real-time examination. (B) Follow-up examinations revealed a grossly enlarged head with little identified brain tissue and replacement of low-level echoes by anechoic fluid. The woman presented to labor and delivery near term with absence of movement, and fetal demise was confirmed with ultrasound.

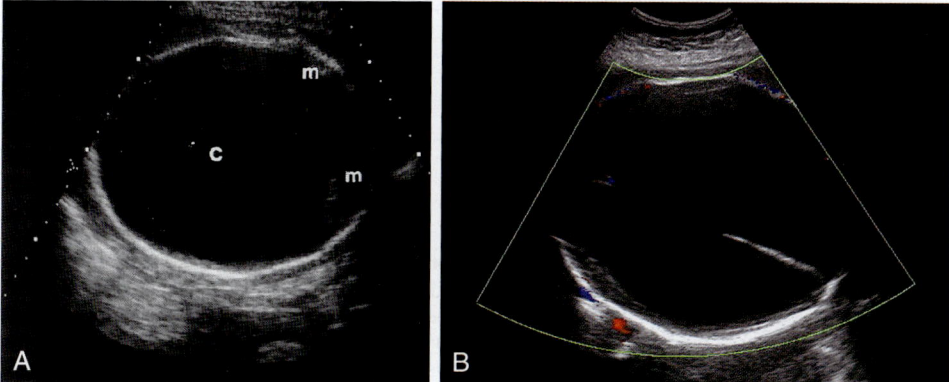

FIG. 60.39 (A) Hydranencephaly (c) in a fetus at 33 weeks of gestation showing a massive collection of cerebrospinal fluid. Note the brain tissue in the occipital region (m). (B) In a different fetus at 37 weeks of gestation, hydranencephaly is identified. The head measurements were greater than the 95th percentile, so the infant was delivered by cesarean section.

from hydranencephaly. Holoprosencephaly with severe ventriculomegaly may have a similar appearance. However, these three anomalies have extremely poor outcomes.[30]

VENTRICULOMEGALY (HYDROCEPHALUS)

Ventriculomegaly is a common finding and refers to dilation of the ventricles within the brain. Ventriculomegaly may be categorized as mild (10 to 12 mm), moderate (13 to 15 mm), or severe (>15 mm).[32] **Hydrocephalus** occurs when ventriculomegaly is coupled with enlargement of the fetal head. Enlargement of the ventricles occurs with obstruction of cerebrospinal fluid flow. This obstruction may be caused by a ventricular defect, such as aqueductal stenosis, and is referred to as *noncommunicating hydrocephalus*. The obstruction may be noted outside of the ventricular system, such as with an arachnoid cyst (Fig. 60.40), and is referred to as *communicating hydrocephalus* (Fig. 60.41). Rarely, ventriculomegaly results from overproduction of cerebrospinal fluid by a choroid plexus papilloma.

Mild to moderate ventriculomegaly has approximately a 1% incidence rate. It may be associated with several underlying CNS abnormalities, infections, and genetic disorders. Many of the abnormalities linked with ventricular dilation were discussed earlier in this chapter and include aqueductal stenosis, arachnoid cysts, and VAGAs. Common causes of ventriculomegaly include spina bifida and encephaloceles. DWM, ACC, lissencephaly, schizencephaly, and holoprosencephaly may also present with hydrocephalus. Intracranial neoplasms, such as a teratoma, may also cause ventricular dilation. Ventriculomegaly may be associated with musculoskeletal anomalies, such as thanatophoric dysplasia and achondroplasia. Approximately 5% of all cases are reported to result from congenital fetal infections, such as cytomegalovirus, toxoplasmosis, Zika virus, and parainfluenza (Fig. 60.42).[32]

Another 5% of fetuses with isolated mild to moderate ventriculomegaly have an abnormal karyotype, most commonly trisomy 21. Ventriculomegaly has also been identified in trisomies 13 and 18. Other syndromes associated with ventriculomegaly include Meckel-Gruber syndrome, Apert syndrome, Roberts syndrome, hydrolethalus, Walker-Warburg

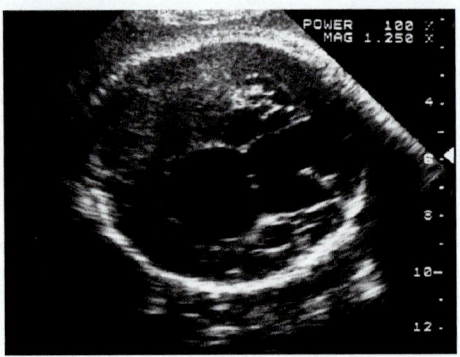

FIG. 60.40 Multiple arachnoid cysts identified in this fetal head.

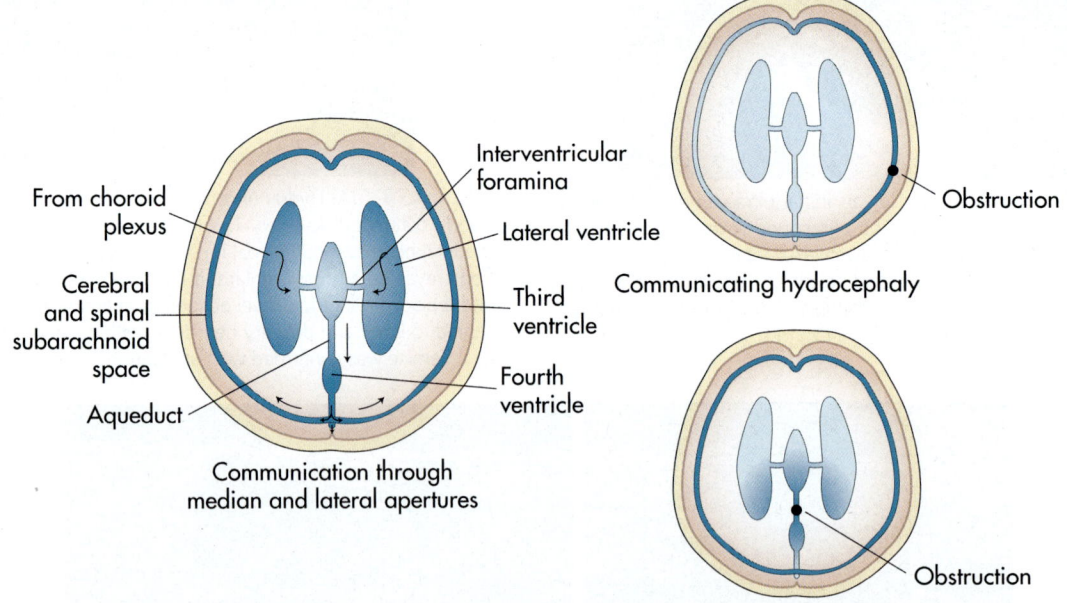

FIG. 60.41 The course of the cerebrospinal fluid and its obstruction in hydrocephaly. Normally, the cerebrospinal fluid from the choroid plexuses flows through the interventricular foramina to the third ventricle, aqueduct, fourth ventricle, median and lateral apertures, and spinal and cerebral subarachnoid space. It is then taken into the venous system (e.g., the cranial venous sinuses). Obstruction occurs within the ventricular system (e.g., at the aqueduct) in noncommunicating hydrocephaly (i.e., the ventricles and the subarachnoid space do not communicate). Obstruction occurs outside the ventricular system (e.g., in the cranial subarachnoid space) in communicating hydrocephaly (i.e., the ventricles and the subarachnoid space communicate).

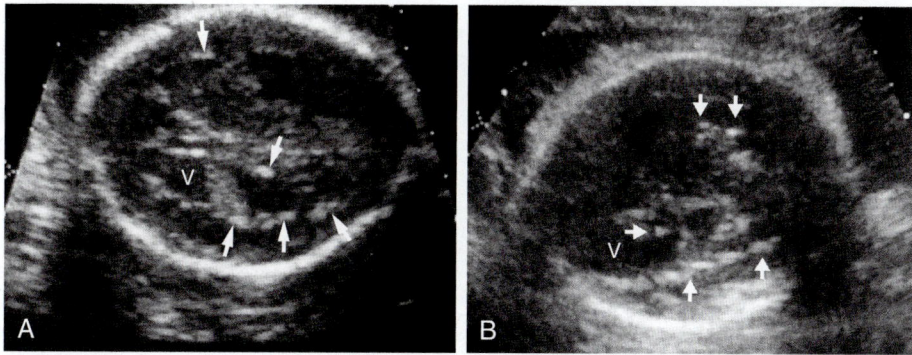

FIG. 60.42 (A) Periventricular calcifications *(arrows)* and ventriculomegaly (v) in a 20-week-old fetus. An infectious cause was suspected. All testing had proved negative. (B) In the same fetus at 30 weeks of gestation, persistent periventricular calcifications *(arrows)* with ventriculomegaly were observed. No other anomalies or complications were present.

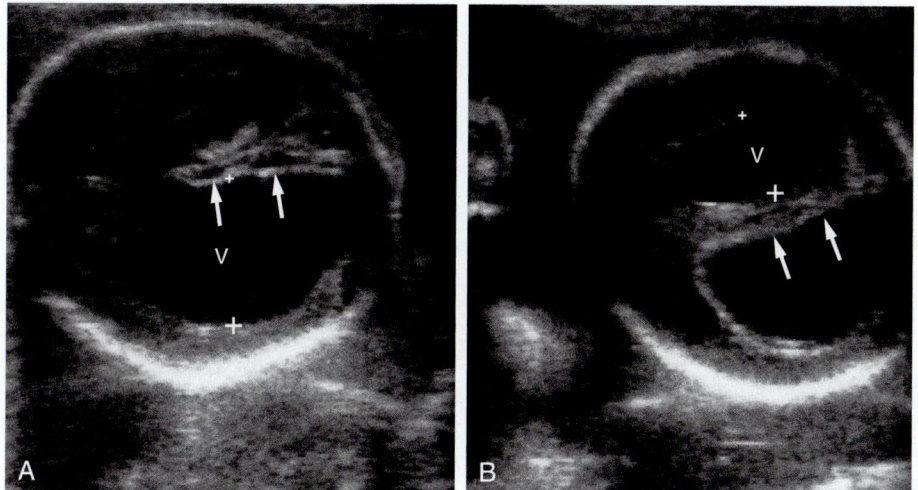

FIG. 60.43 (A) Ventriculomegaly observed in the distal cranial hemisphere in a 25-week-old twin fetus with severe growth restriction. The ventricle measured 28 mm in diameter. *Arrows,* Interhemispheric fissure. (B) In the same fetus, the proximal ventricle (V) is displayed measuring 17 mm in diameter. Note the asymmetry between ventricles, suggesting a shift of the interhemispheric fissure *(arrows)* and porencephaly. The larger distal ventricle represents the actual porencephalic cyst, whereas the smaller ventricle has dilated in response to the infarction. Premature delivery occurred at 26 weeks of gestation because of chronic twin-to-twin transfusion syndrome in a monochorionic pregnancy. The twin depicted in these figures died shortly after birth. Autopsy confirmed the occurrence of the porencephalic event as an end result of severe shunting of blood within the placental cotyledons.

syndrome, Smith-Lemli-Opitz syndrome, nasal-facial-digital syndrome, and Albers-Schönberg disease.[32]

Ventriculomegaly may be unilateral (50% to 60%) or bilateral (40% to 50%), and asymmetry of the lateral ventricles is common. Unilateral ventriculomegaly, especially when isolated and mild, may have a good prognosis. Approximately 7% to 10% of mild ventriculomegaly fetuses are found to have other structural abnormalities after birth.[32]

Fetal ventriculomegaly typically progresses from the occipital horns into the temporal and then the frontal ventricular horns. Ventriculomegaly may be quantitated by measuring the ventricular atrium across the glomus of the choroid plexus. A ventricle is considered dilated when its diameter exceeds 10 mm. The proximal ventricle may be difficult to adequately image because of reverberation artifacts from the calvarium. Transvaginal technique may be used to further clarify the defect when the fetus is in a vertex position.

The mortality rate for fetuses with hydrocephalus is high. The prognosis depends largely on the presence and severity of associated anomalies, fetal infection, and extent of ventricular dilation. The prognosis is improved in those with isolated ventriculomegaly. Survivors may require ventricular shunting to improve survival and intellectual outcome.[32]

Sonographic Findings. Sonographic features of ventriculomegaly include the following:
- Lateral ventricular enlargement exceeding 10 mm (Fig. 60.43)
- A "dangling choroid" sign as the gravity-dependent choroid plexus falls into the increased ventricular space (Fig. 60.44)

- Possible dilation of the third and fourth ventricles
- Fetal head enlargement when biparietal and HC measurements exceed those for the established gestational age
- Serial sonographic examinations over time should assess the progression, stabilization, and resolution of fetal ventriculomegaly. In approximately 16% of cases, ventricular dilation is progressive.[32] In addition, the fetus should also be surveyed for associated anomalies. Obstetric management may include amniocentesis to rule out chromosomal anomalies and laboratory tests to rule out congenital infection. The fetus should also be surveyed for defects involving the face, heart, kidneys, abdominal wall, thorax, and limbs. In the absence of other abnormalities, fetal therapy for shunt placement may be an option. Cesarean delivery may also be necessary because of the large size of the fetal head.

Severe hydrocephaly may be confused with hydranencephaly and holoprosencephaly. Documenting a complete falx and the presence of the choroid plexus in the lateral ventricles, as well as separate third and fourth ventricles, may help to differentiate severe ventriculomegaly from other anomalies.

MICROCEPHALY

Microcephaly is an abnormally small head that is at least 2 standard deviations below the mean, resulting in reduced brain size. Some experts have increased the cutoff to 3 standard deviations in that there is a high false-positive rate and 2% of the population with normal to borderline cognitive capacity may be located within a range of 2 standard deviations.[33] Microcephaly is categorized according to whether it occurs before or after neuronal migration. Premigrational microencephaly is linked to genetic disorders, and postmigrational microencephaly is associated with late gestation ischemia, infection, trauma, teratogens, and genetic disorders.[34] Genetically, microencephaly may result from inherited autosomal dominant or autosomal recessive pattern and may also occur with chromosomal aberrations and various brain anomalies. Teratogens linked with microcephaly include congenital infection (Zika, rubella, toxoplasmosis, cytomegalovirus), maternal alcohol abuse, heroin addiction, mercury poisoning, maternal phenylketonuria, radiation, and hypoxia.

The prognosis for fetuses with microcephaly depends to a degree on the cause. It is usually associated with neurologic deficits.

Sonographic Findings. Sonographic diagnosis of microcephaly depends on an accurate assessment of fetal age. BPD, occipitofrontal diameter, and HC should be used when evaluating for microcephaly. In addition, ratios comparing the head perimeter with abdominal perimeter and the head perimeter with femur length are also useful. Impaired cranial growth should coincide with appropriate growth of the abdominal circumference and femur length. Serial measurements for a fetus at risk for microcephalus should be performed at monthly intervals. Because microcephaly may manifest later in the pregnancy, diagnosis before 24 weeks of gestation may be impossible.

Sonographic features of microcephaly include the following:
- Small BPD (Fig. 60.45)
- Small HC
- Abnormal HC/abdomen circumference and HC/femur length ratios
- A sloping forehead may be noted in the profile view

Other sonographic findings associated with microcephaly may include disorganized brain tissue and ventriculomegaly. A thorough search for evidence of an associated anomaly

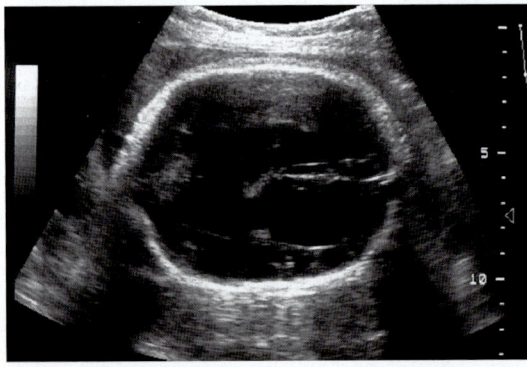

FIG. 60.44 **Ventriculomegaly caused by spina bifida.** The anterior choroid plexus "dangles" into the posterior ventricle.

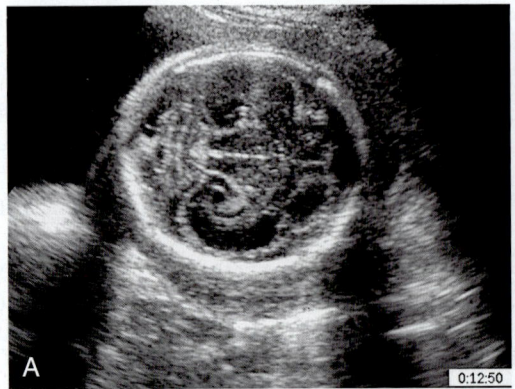 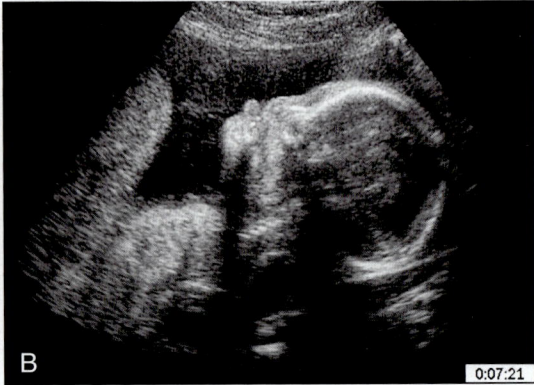

FIG. 60.45 (A) Microcephaly is demonstrated in this fetus with semilobar holoprosencephaly. (B) In the same fetus, the profile shows the small head; the fetus also had a bilateral cleft lip.

should ensue, including careful investigation of the fetal heart. Cerebral calcifications may be identified with congenital infection. A fetus with an encephalocele may have microcephaly caused by the amount of brain tissue protruding outside the calvarium. Other cranial anomalies associated with microcephaly include porencephaly, ACC, craniosynostosis, holoprosencephaly, lissencephaly, schizencephaly, macrogyria, microgyria, agyria, and Kleeblattschädel defect. Microcephaly has been associated with trisomies 13, 18, 21, and 22 and with triploidy. Numerous syndromes have been linked with microcephaly, including Meckel-Gruber syndrome, Pena-Shokeir syndrome, and Neu-Laxova syndrome.

ACKNOWLEGMENT

The author recognizes the contributions of Charlotte Henningsen to this chapter in the previous edition.

Key Pearls

- Anencephaly, also known as aprosencephaly or atelencephaly, is the most common neural tube defect. Anencephaly, which means absence of the brain, is caused by failure of closure of the neural tube at the cranial end.
- Acrania, also known as exencephaly, is a lethal anomaly that manifests as absence of the cranial bones with the presence of complete, although abnormal, development of the cerebral hemispheres.
- A cephalocele is a neural tube defect in which the meninges alone or the meninges and brain herniate through a defect in the calvarium.
- *Encephalocele* is the term used to describe herniation of the meninges and brain through the defect; *cranial meningocele* describes the herniation of only meninges.
- Spina bifida encompasses a wide range of vertebral defects that result from failure of neural tube closure. The meninges and neural elements may protrude through this defect.
- Dandy-Walker malformation is a defect that may have varying degrees of severity. It manifests with agenesis or hypoplasia of the cerebellar vermis with resulting dilation on the fourth ventricle and enlargement of the posterior fossa.
- Holoprosencephaly encompasses a range of abnormalities resulting from abnormal cleavage of the prosencephalon (forebrain). Three forms of holoprosencephaly are known. The most severe form is classified as alobar, the intermediate form as semilobar, and the mildest form as lobar.
- The cause of agenesis of the corpus callosum is somewhat unclear but is thought to involve a vascular disruption or inflammatory lesion before 12 weeks.
- Aqueductal stenosis results from obstruction, atresia, or stenosis of the aqueduct of Sylvius causing ventriculomegaly.
- An aneurysm of the vein of Galen, also known as a vein of Galen malformation, is a rare arteriovenous malformation.
- Choroid plexus cysts are round or ovoid anechoic structures found within the choroid plexus.
- Porencephalic cysts, also known as porencephaly, are cysts filled with cerebrospinal fluid that communicate with the ventricular system or subarachnoid space.
- Schizencephaly is a very rare disorder characterized by clefts in the cerebral cortex.
- Hydranencephaly is a rare brain abnormality characterized by destruction of the cerebral hemispheres by occlusion of the internal carotid arteries.
- Ventriculomegaly refers to dilation of the ventricles within the brain. Hydrocephalus occurs when ventriculomegaly is coupled with enlargement of the fetal head.
- Microcephaly is an abnormally small head that is 2 standard deviations below the mean.

REFERENCES

1. Dmitrieva J. Sonographic assessment of the fetal head. In: Stephensen SR, Dmitrieva J, eds. *Diagnostic Medical Sonography: Obstetrics and Gynecology*. 4th ed. Philadelphia: Lippincott Williams & Wilkins; 2018:467–494.
2. Fotos J, Olson R, Kenekar S. Embryology of the brain and molecular genetics of the central nervous system malformation. *Seminars in Ultrasound, CT, and MRI*. 2011;32(3):159–166.
3. Stephensen SR. Sonographic signs of fetal neural tube and central nervous system defects. *JDMS*. 2003;19(6):347–357.
4. Long BW, Rollins JH, Smith BJ. *Merrill's Atlas of Radiographic Positioning and Procedures*. 14th ed. St. Louis: Elsevier; 2020:163–176.
5. Moore KL, Persaud TVN. *The Developing Human*. 11th ed. Philadelphia: Elsevier; 2019.
6. Moore L. Anencephaly. *J Diagn Med Sonogr*. 2010;26:286–289.
7. Cope HL, Garrett ME, Ashley-Koch A. Ancencephaly: insights for genetic counseling. *J Prenat Perinat Psychol Health*. 2019;33(3):189–206.
8. Monteagudo A. Exencephaly-anencephaly. *Am J Obstet Gynecol*. 2020;223(6):B5–B8.
9. Kanesen D, Rosman A, Kandasamy R. Giant occipital encehpalocele with Chiari malformation type 3. *J Neurosci Rural Pract*. 2018;9(4):619–621.
10. Monteagudo A. Posterior encephalocele. *Am J Obstet Gynecol*. 2020;223(6):B9–B12.
11. Tamas-Csaba S, Lorand D, Klara B, Sebastian SR, Gergo R, Zsuzsanna P. Study of spina bifida occulta based on age, sex and localization. *ARS Medica Tomitana*. 2019;25(3):95–99.
12. Buyukkurt S, Binokay F, Seydaoglu G, et al. Prenatal determination of the upper lesion level of spina bifida with three-dimensional ultrasound. *Fetal Diagn Ther*. 2013;33:36–40.
13. Crytzer TM, Cheng YT, Bryner MJ, et al. Impact of neurological level and spinal curvature on pulmonary function in adults with spina bifida. *J Pediatr Rehabil Med*. 2018;11(4):243–254.
14. Sepulveda W, Wong AE, Sepulveda F, et al. Prenatal diagnosis of spina bifida: from intracranial translucency to intrauterine surgery. *Childs Nerv Syst*. 2017;33:1083–1099.
15. Li DZ, Liao C. Monozygotic twins discordant for Dandy-Walker malformation. *Fetal Diagn Ther*. 2009;25:141–143.
16. Monteagudo A. Dandy-Walker Malformation. *Am J Obstet Gynecol*. 2020;223(6):B38–B41.
17. Diawara FM, Diallo M, Camara M, Traore M. Sonographic detection of holoprosencephaly with cyclopia and proboscis. *J Diagn Med Sonogr*. 2010;26:28–31.
18. Monteagudo A. Holoprosencephaly. *Am J Obstet Gynecol*. 2020;223(6):B13–B16.
19. Ionescu CA, Vladareanu S, Tudorache S, et al. The wide spectrum of ultrasound diagnosis of holoposencephaly. *Medical Ultrasonography*. 2019;21(2):163–169.

20. Bayram AK, Kutuk MS, Doganay S, et al. An analysis of 109 fetuses with prenatal diagnosis of complete agenesis of corpus callosum. *NeurolSciences*. 2020;41:1521–1529.
21. Santo S, D'Antonio F, Homfray T, et al. Counseling in fetal medicine: agenesis of the corpus callosum. *Ultrasound Obstet Gynecol*. 2012;40:513–521.
22. Hoffman J, Hutny M, Sztuba K, Paprocka J. Corpus callosum agenesis: An insight into the etiology and spectrum of symptoms. *Brain Sciences*. 2020;19(9):625.
23. Cinalli G, Spennato P, Nastro A, et al. Hydrocephalus in aqueductal stenosis. *Childs Nerv Syst*. 2011;27:1621–1642.
24. Mohan R, Nayyar R, Ryder L, et al. Vein of Galen aneurysm. *Australas J Ultrasound Med*. 2016;19(2):75–77.
25. Sasani M, Afsharian R, Sasani H, et al. A large choroid plexus cyst diagnosed with magnetic resonance imaging in utero: a case report. *Cases J*. 2009 2.1:7098.
26. Petrikovsky BM, Terrani MD, Sichinava LG. Natural history and clinical significance of multiple cysts in a single choroid plexus. *Journal of Diagnostic Medical Sonography*. 2018;34(6):481–483.
27. Pepe F, Marchese G, Pepe GG, et al. Pregnancy in an asymptomatic woman with porencephalic and arachnoid cysts. *Case Rep Obstet Gynecol*. November 2020:1–3.
28. Braga VL, da Costa MDSMD, Riera R, et al. Schizencephaly: a review of 734 patients. *Pediatric Neurology*. 2018;87:23–29.
29. Dyson L, Carlan SJ, Busowski J, Rasmussen O. Unilateral type II schizencephaly: prenatal diagnosis and review. *J Diagn Med Sonogr*. 2012;28:128–130.
30. Sepulveda W, Cortes-Yepes H, Wong AE, et al. Prenatal sonography in hydranencephaly: Findings during the early stages of the disease. *J Ultrasound Med*. 2012;31(5):799–804.
31. Omar AT, Minalo MKA, Rommualdo R, et al. Hydranencephaly: clinical features and survivorship in a retrospective cohort. *World Neurosurg*. 2020;144:589–596.
32. Fox NS, Monteagudo A, Kuller J, et al. Mild fetal ventriculomegaly: Diagnosis, evaluation, and management. *Am J Obstet Gynecol*. 2018;219(1):B2–B9.
33. Pavone P, Pratico A, Ruggieri M, Rizzo R, et al. Resuming the obsolete term "small head" when microcephaly occurs without cognitive impairement. *Neurological Sciences*. 2017;38(9):1723–1725.
34. Leibovitz Z, Lerman-Sagie T. Diagnostic approach to microencephaly. *Eur J Paediatr Neurol*. 2018;22(6):934–943.

CHAPTER 61

The Fetal Thorax

Sandra L. Hagen-Ansert

OBJECTIVES

On completion of this chapter, you should be able to:
- Describe the development of the thoracic cavity
- List the normal sonographic features of the thorax and diaphragm
- Describe the development and consequences of pulmonary hypoplasia
- Differentiate between solid and cystic lesions of the lung
- Discuss the sonographic findings in a diaphragmatic hernia

OUTLINE

Embryology of the Thoracic Cavity 1545
Normal Sonographic Characteristics 1545
   Size 1546
   Position 1546
   Texture 1547
   Respiration 1547
Abnormalities of the Thoracic Cavity 1548
Abnormalities of the Lungs 1548
Abnormalities of the Diaphragm 1555

KEY TERMS

Asphyxiating thoracic dystrophy
Bronchogenic cyst
Congenital bronchial atresia
Congenital cystic adenomatoid malformation (CCAM)
Congenital diaphragmatic hernia (CDH)
Foramen of Bochdalek
Foramen of Morgagni
Lymphangiectasia
Pleural effusion (hydrothorax)
Pulmonary hypoplasia
Pulmonary sequestration

The detection of thoracic defects is important because such lesions may compromise fetal breathing and require surgery in the immediate neonatal period. Lung and diaphragm disorders are discussed in this section. Heart abnormalities may also cause devastating secondary compression effects (pulmonary hypoplasia) and are discussed in Chapters 35 and 36.

EMBRYOLOGY OF THE THORACIC CAVITY

One of the important determinants of whether the fetus can survive as a neonate in the air-filled, ex utero environment is the adequacy of biochemical and structural development and maturity of the lungs. Adequacy of pulmonary development is probably the single most important determinant of fetal viability, and pulmonary immaturity is the major reason why fetuses younger than 24 weeks of gestation are generally considered nonviable.

In early development, mesenchymal buds from the early trachea form and penetrate the masses destined to become the lungs. The bronchi, bronchioles, alveolar ducts, and alveoli are developed through multiple divisions and budding. Between 16 and 20 weeks, the normal number of bronchi has formed. Between 16 and 24 weeks, a dramatic increase in the number and complexity of air spaces and vascular structures has occurred. After 24 weeks, another important developmental phenomenon occurs: progressive flattening of the epithelial cells lining the air spaces, which allows closer apposition of capillaries to the fluid-filled air space lumen and results in further development of the air-blood barrier necessary for efficient gas exchange after birth.

Breathing movements that occur before birth result in the aspiration of fluid into the lungs. The lungs at birth are about half filled with fluid derived from the amniotic cavity, tracheal glands, and lungs. The fluid present in the lungs at birth clears by three routes: (1) through the mouth and nose, (2) into the pulmonary capillaries, and (3) into the lymphatics and the pulmonary vessels.

NORMAL SONOGRAPHIC CHARACTERISTICS

The fetal thorax is examined by the sonographer in both the transverse and coronal or parasagittal planes. The normal thoracic cavity is symmetrically bell shaped, with the ribs forming the lateral margins, the clavicles forming the upper margins, and the diaphragm forming the lower margins. The lungs serve as the lateral borders for the heart and lie superior to the diaphragm. The diaphragm may be observed on sonography as an echogenic smooth hypoechoic muscular margin between the fetal liver or spleen and the lungs (Box 61.1).

Size

The thorax is normally slightly smaller than the abdominal cavity (Fig. 61.1). The ratio (thoracic circumference to abdominal circumference) has been reported to remain constant throughout pregnancy (0.94 ± 0.05). Extreme variations in thoracic size should signal the sonographer to look for other anomalies. In the presence of oligohydramnios,

> **BOX 61.1 Sonography of the Normal Fetal Chest**
>
> - Transverse, coronal, and/or parasagittal
> - Evaluate chest: size, shape, symmetry
> - Evaluate heart: position, size, rate, pericardial fluid
> - Evaluate pulmonary texture
> - Centrally positioned mediastinum

resultant pulmonary hypoplasia may be seen with a reduction in overall thoracic size. Chest circumference measurements are made in the transverse plane at the level of the four-chamber view of the heart (see Fig. 61.1C).

A fetus with a significant narrow diameter of the chest may have **asphyxiating thoracic dystrophy**. Several syndromes may be associated with this finding, including thanatophoric dwarfism. The best ultrasonic determination for predicting pulmonary hypoplasia is the chest area (CA) minus the heart area (HA) times 100 divided by the CA:

$$\frac{(CA - HA \times 100)}{CA}$$

The cardiothoracic ratio is fairly constant throughout gestation, with a mean value of 0.45 at 17 weeks and 0.50 at term (Fig. 61.2). Cardiomegaly is present when the cardiothoracic ratio is greater than two standard deviations. The C/A ratio may also be present in cases of reduced chest volume rather than an enlarged heart; thus it is important to compare the measure of the chest circumference to gestational age nomogram.

Position

The central portion of the thorax is occupied by the mediastinum, with most of the heart positioned in the midline and left chest. The apex of the heart should be directed toward the

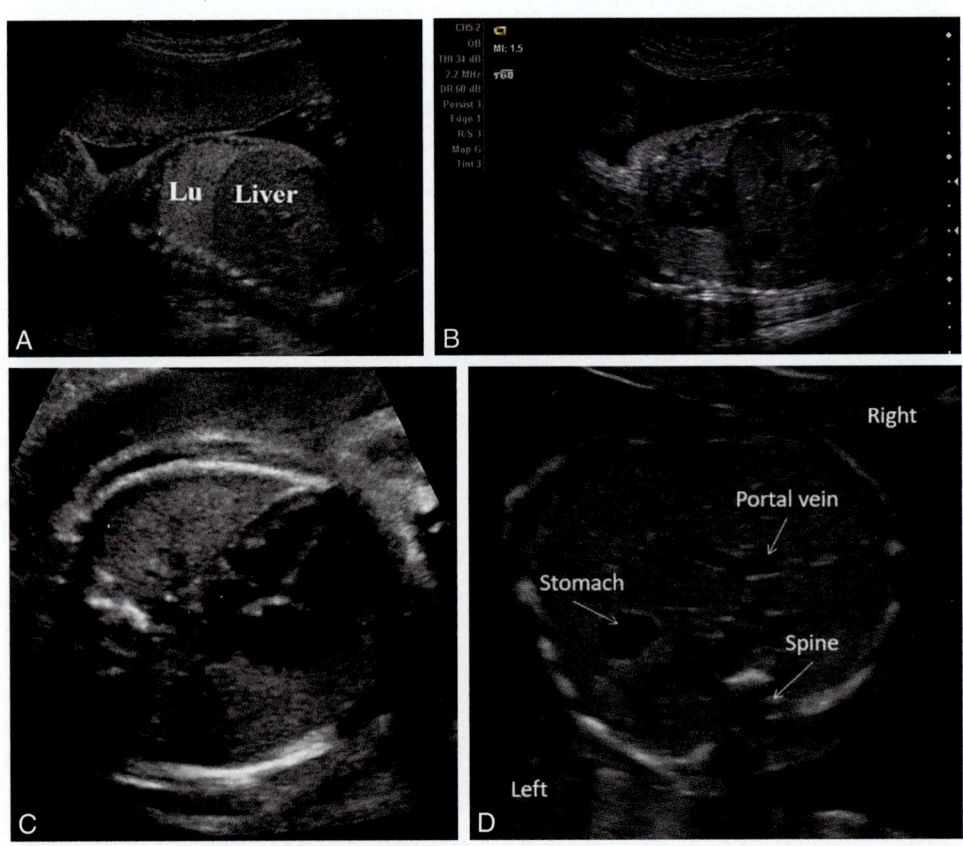

FIG. 61.1 The thorax is normally slightly smaller than the abdominal cavity. (A) Fetal thorax and abdomen from the right sagittal view. (B) Fetal thorax, with heart and abdomen from the left sagittal view. (C) Chest circumference measurements are made in the transverse plane at the level of the four-chamber view of the heart. (D) Abdominal circumference measurements are made at the level where the umbilical vein branches into the portal sinus and forms a J shape.

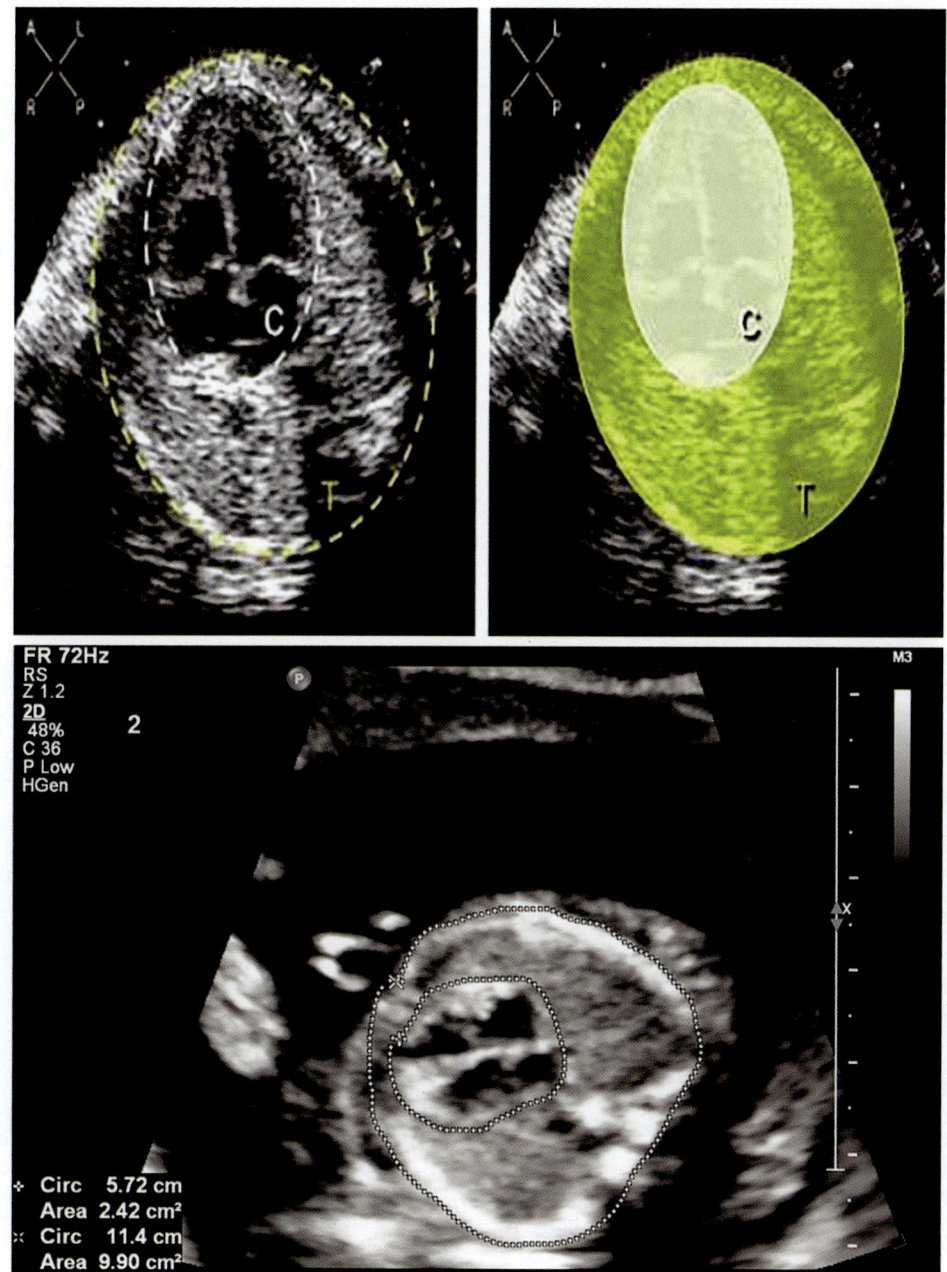

FIG. 61.2 The cardiothoracic ratio is fairly constant throughout gestation, with a mean value of 0.45 at 17 weeks and 0.50 at term.

spleen; the base of the heart lies horizontal to the diaphragm (Fig. 61.3). The location of the heart is important to document in a routine sonographic examination because detection of abnormal position may indicate the presence of a chest mass, pleural effusion, or cardiac malformation.

Texture

The fetal lungs appear homogeneous on sonography with moderate echogenicity. Early in gestation, the lungs are similar to or slightly less echogenic than the liver (Fig. 61.4), and, as gestation progresses, a trend toward increased pulmonary echogenicity relative to the liver is observed. Overlying ribs and acoustic enhancement produced by blood in the heart are two important problems that may complicate the exact determination of echogenicity of the lungs. Color Doppler may be used to outline the vascular pattern within the lungs. Ultrasound cannot be used to assess lung maturity.

Respiration

Fetal breathing becomes more prominent in the second and third trimesters. The mature fetus spends almost one-third of its time breathing. Fetal breathing movements are documented if characteristic seesaw movements of the fetal chest or abdomen are sustained for at least 20 seconds. Fetal breathing movements are considered absent if no such fetal activity is noted during the 20-minute observation period.

Color flow Doppler may be used to detect fetal breathing through the nostrils. The fetal facial profile should be obtained with the nose clearly demonstrated; as color is turned on, flow disturbance movement may be seen to flow from the nostrils (Fig. 61.5).

The biophysical profile used by many obstetricians to assess fetal well-being uses the respiration pattern as a factor in its scoring. Fetal respiration may vary in response to maternal activities and substance ingestion; it is stimulated by increased sugar doses and is decreased by smoking.

ABNORMALITIES OF THE THORACIC CAVITY

Abnormalities of the Lungs

To exclude pleural masses, a thorough investigation of lung texture and homogenicity is necessary. Lung masses are separate from the heart and are located above the level of the diaphragm. Lesions of the lungs may be cystic, solid, or complex (Fig. 61.6).

When evaluating the fetus for a lung mass, the sonographer should assess the following: position of the fetal heart, orientation of the cardiac axis, and measurement of the thoracic circumference (which can be evaluated with a thoracic/abdominal ratio growth chart). Cardiac axis may be evaluated in a four-chamber heart view (see Chapter 35) by estimating the angle at which the intraventricular septum crosses the spine at the anterior chest wall. The normal cardiac axis ranges from 22 to 75 degrees (average, 45 degrees). Deviation from the normal axis may suggest the presence of an intrathoracic mass. Measurements of thoracic circumference may aid in estimating the size of the thoracic cavity and may predict an abnormally small chest cavity and secondary pulmonary hypoplasia. Nomograms for thoracic circumference are available (Table 61.1). These data vary from the more recent data of Laudy and Wladimiroff, especially during the end of the last

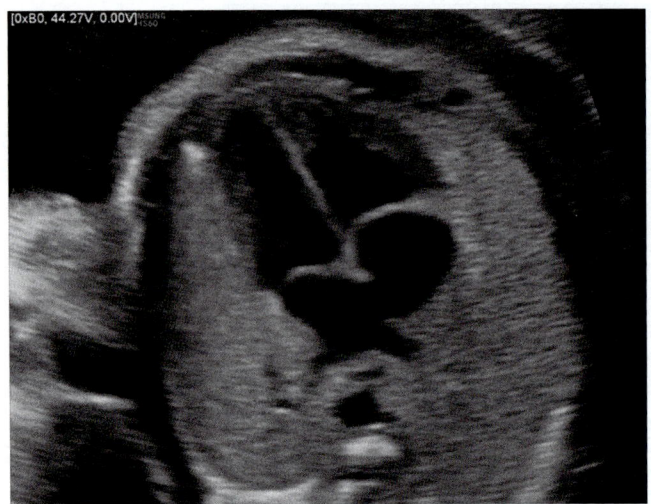

FIG. 61.3 The central portion of the thorax is occupied by the mediastinum, with most of the heart positioned in the midline and left chest. The apex of the heart should be directed toward the spleen; the base of the heart lies horizontal to the diaphragm.

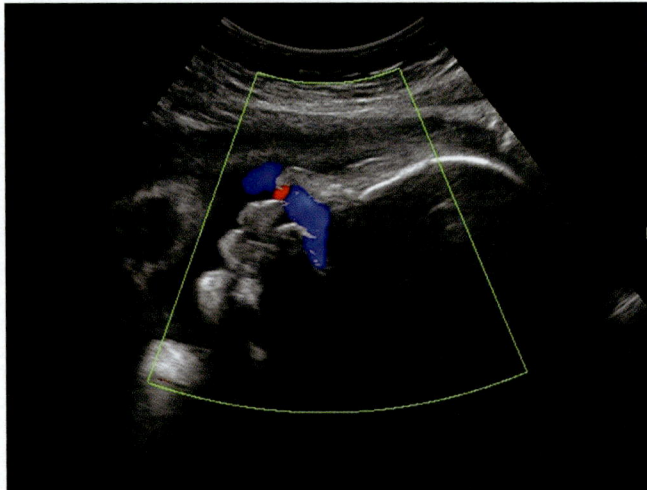

FIG. 61.5 Color flow Doppler may be used to detect fetal breathing through the nostrils. The fetal facial profile should be obtained with the nose clearly demonstrated; as color is turned on, flow disturbance movement may be seen to flow from the nostrils.

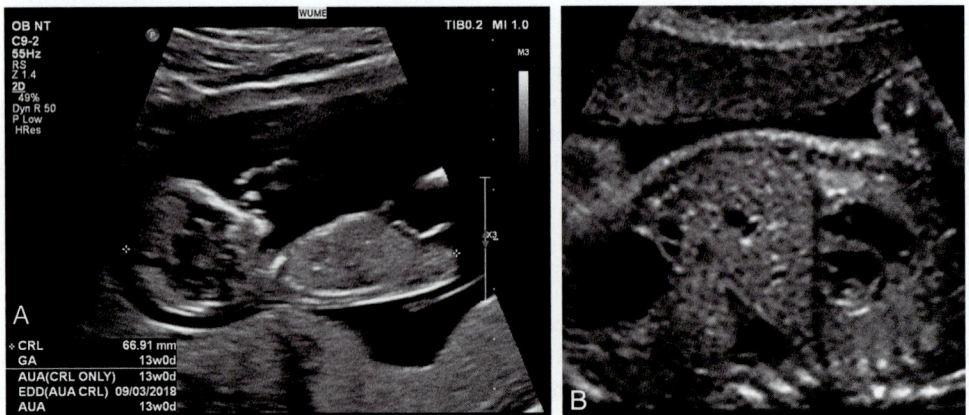

FIG. 61.4 **The fetal lungs appear homogeneous on sonography with moderate echogenicity.** (A) Early in gestation, the lungs are similar to or slightly less echogenic than the liver. (B) As gestation progresses, a trend toward increased pulmonary echogenicity relative to the liver is observed.

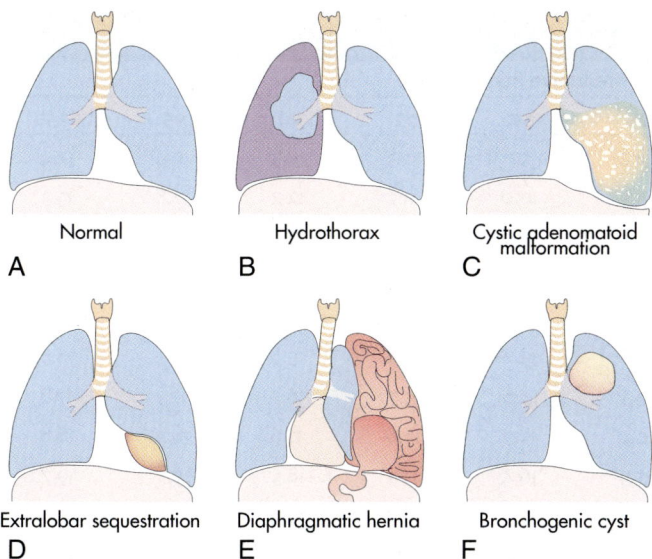

FIG. 61.6 Thoracic masses and mass effect. (A) Normal thorax. The lungs have convex margins anterolaterally. (B) Hydrothorax. Anechoic pleural fluid displaces the lungs away from the chest wall and compresses the lungs. (C) Cystic adenomatoid malformation. An intrapulmonary mass of variable echogenicity may shift the mediastinum and create hydrops. (D) Bronchopulmonary extralobar sequestration. A spherical or triangular echogenic mass is evident in the inferior portion of the thorax or upper abdomen. (E) Diaphragmatic hernia. A complex mass (usually on the left side) creates mediastinal shift. Peristalsing bowel in the thorax provides convincing evidence of the diagnosis. Displaced stomach or scaphoid abdomen is an ancillary finding. (F) Bronchogenic cyst. If it causes bronchial compression, a simple cyst near the mediastinum or appearing centrally in the lung may produce a mediastinal shift.

trimester.[1] Methods for measuring the lung include length, area, and volume, with the use of three-dimensional ultrasound. The right lung volume is slightly greater than the left.

When the heart position and axis vary from the normal position, the sonographer should look closely for any abnormality that may be the cause of such displacement (i.e., pleural mass or diaphragmatic hernia). Fetal echocardiography is beneficial for excluding cardiac involvement, and evaluation of an intact diaphragm is necessary to exclude diaphragmatic hernia. Abnormalities in cardiac rhythm and fetal hydrops may be present in fetuses with lung masses caused by compression of venous return and cardiac failure. Pleural effusions are commonly found in conjunction with lung masses.

The lungs will not grow or develop properly when a small uterine cavity results from severe oligohydramnios, when the chest cavity is abnormally small, when the balance between tracheal and airway pressure and fluid volume is inadequate, or when the fetus is unable to practice breathing movements.

A mass within the thoracic cavity may have detrimental effects on lung development. The heart and mediastinal structures may be displaced from the normal position, and the lung may be compressed and destroyed. These effects may lead to pulmonary hypoplasia.

Pulmonary Hypoplasia. Pulmonary hypoplasia is caused by a decrease in the numbers of lung cells, airways, and alveoli, with a resulting decrease in organ size and weight. This reduction in lung volume leads to small, inadequately developed lungs. A decreased ratio of lung weight to body weight is a consistent method of diagnosing pulmonary hypoplasia. This condition most commonly occurs after prolonged oligohydramnios or secondary to a small thoracic cavity caused by a structural or chromosomal abnormality.

Pulmonary hypoplasia may occur when amniotic fluid volume is extremely reduced. Kidney abnormalities (bilateral renal agenesis, bilateral multicystic renal disease, severe renal obstruction [e.g., posterior urethral valve syndrome], unilateral renal agenesis with contralateral multicystic renal development or severe obstruction, and infantile polycystic kidney disease) result in lethal pulmonary hypoplasia. Pulmonary hypoplasia may also occur in fetuses with severe intrauterine growth restriction and early rupture of the membranes.

Masses within the thoracic cavity, including pleural effusion, diaphragmatic hernia (and eventration), cystic adenomatoid malformation (CAM) of the lung, bronchopulmonary sequestration, and other large cysts and tumors of the lung and thorax, may lead to pulmonary hypoplasia. Cardiac defects, some skeletal dysplasias, central nervous system disorders, and chromosomal trisomies (13, 18, and 21) may manifest with pulmonary hypoplasia. A small percentage of infants have pulmonary hypoplasia with no fetal or uterine problem.

Unilateral pulmonary agenesis or hypoplasia is a rare anomaly that is often associated with other fetal malformations. An absent lung should be considered in the differential diagnosis of every fetus with a mediastinal shift and apparent chest mass, especially when it is seen in conjunction with other defects, such as esophageal abnormalities.

The prognosis for infants with pulmonary hypoplasia is grave, with 80% dying after birth. The severity of pulmonary hypoplasia depends on when pulmonary hypoplasia occurred during pregnancy, its severity, and its duration (Box 61.2). Other factors, such as pulmonary fluid dynamics, fetal breathing movements, and hormonal influences, may contribute to pulmonary hypoplasia.

Sonographic Findings. Various methods used to determine the presence of pulmonary hypoplasia include thoracic measurements, various lung measurements, estimation of lung volume, Doppler studies of the pulmonary arteries, and assessment of fetal breathing activity. The sonographer may be able to check for pulmonary hypoplasia by measuring the thoracic circumference at the level of the four-chamber heart view, excluding the skin and subcutaneous tissues. A thoracic circumference less than the fifth percentile suggests the possibility of pulmonary hypoplasia. The sonographer should understand that this measurement may not be helpful in conditions in which an intrathoracic mass compresses lung tissue and yet the thoracic circumference remains normal (i.e., diaphragmatic hernia, pleural effusion, and CAMs). The sonographer should also look for the finding of small echogenic lungs because they lie lateral to the cardiac chambers in the fetus with pulmonary hypoplasia (Fig. 61.7).

Cystic Lung Masses. Lung cysts are echo-free masses that replace normal lung parenchyma. Lung cysts may vary in size, ranging from small, isolated lesions to large cystic masses that

TABLE 61.1	Fetal Thoracic Circumference Measurements								
Gestational Age (Weeks)	No. Fetal Measurements	Predictive Percentiles							
		2.5	5	10	25	50	75	90	95	97.5
16	6	5.9	6.4	7.0	8.0	9.1	10.3	11.3	11.9	12.4
17	22	6.8	7.3	7.9	8.9	10.0	11.2	12.2	12.8	13.3
18	31	7.7	8.2	8.8	9.8	11.0	12.1	13.1	13.7	14.2
19	21	8.6	9.1	9.7	10.7	11.9	13.0	14.0	14.6	15.1
20	20	9.5	10.0	10.6	11.7	12.9	13.9	15.0	15.5	16.0
21	30	10.4	11.0	11.6	12.6	13.7	14.8	15.8	16.4	16.9
22	18	11.3	11.9	12.5	13.5	14.6	15.7	16.7	17.3	17.8
23	21	12.2	12.8	13.4	14.4	15.5	16.6	17.6	18.2	18.8
24	27	13.2	13.7	14.3	15.3	16.4	17.5	18.5	19.1	19.7
25	20	14.1	14.6	15.2	16.2	17.3	18.4	19.4	20.0	20.6
26	25	15.0	15.5	16.1	17.1	18.2	19.3	20.3	21.0	21.5
27	24	15.9	16.4	17.0	18.0	19.1	20.2	21.3	21.9	22.4
28	24	16.8	17.3	17.9	18.9	20.0	21.2	22.2	22.8	23.3
29	24	17.7	18.2	18.8	19.8	21.0	22.1	23.1	23.7	24.2
30	27	18.6	19.1	19.7	20.7	21.9	23.0	24.0	24.6	25.1
31	24	19.5	20.0	20.6	21.6	22.8	23.9	24.9	25.5	26.0
32	28	20.4	20.9	21.5	22.6	23.7	24.8	25.8	26.4	26.9
33	27	21.3	21.8	22.5	23.5	24.6	25.7	26.7	27.3	27.8
34	25	22.2	22.8	23.4	24.4	25.5	26.6	27.6	28.2	28.7
35	20	23.1	23.7	24.3	25.3	26.4	27.5	28.5	29.1	29.6
36	23	24.0	24.6	25.2	26.2	27.3	28.4	29.4	30.0	30.6
37	22	24.9	25.5	26.1	27.1	28.2	29.3	30.3	30.9	31.5
38	21	25.9	26.4	27.0	28.0	29.1	30.2	31.2	31.9	32.4
39	7	26.8	27.3	27.9	28.9	30.0	31.1	32.2	32.8	33.3
40	6	27.7	28.2	28.8	29.8	30.9	32.1	33.1	33.7	34.2

Measurements in centimeters.
From Chitkara U, Rosenberg J, Chervenak FA, et al. Prenatal sonographic assessment of the fetal thorax: normal values. *Am J Obstet Gynecol.* 1987;156:1069–1074.

BOX 61.2	Pulmonary Hypoplasia

- Reduction in lung volume resulting in small, inadequately developed lungs
- Occurs from prolonged oligohydramnios or secondary to small thoracic cavity
- Look for chromosome anomalies, renal anomalies, intrauterine growth restriction, premature rupture of membranes, masses within thoracic cavity

may cause notable shifts of intrathoracic structures. Simple cysts may be surgically excised after delivery (Box 61.3).

Bronchogenic Cysts. The most common lung cyst detected prenatally is the **bronchogenic cyst**. Bronchogenic cysts occur as a result of abnormal budding of the foregut and lack any communication with the trachea or bronchial tree. They typically occur within the mediastinum or lung; infrequently they are seen inferior to the diaphragm.

Sonographic Findings. Sonographically, bronchogenic cysts appear as small well-circumscribed masses with no evidence of a mediastinal shift or heart failure (Fig. 61.8). Amniotic fluid volume is within the normal range.

Pleural Effusion (Hydrothorax). An accumulation of fluid within the pleural cavity that may appear as an isolated lesion or secondary to multiple fetal anomalies is called a **pleural effusion** or **hydrothorax** (see Fig. 61.6B). The most common reason for a pleural effusion is chylothorax occurring as a right-side unilateral collection of fluid secondary to a malformed thoracic duct. Hydramnios often accompanies chylothorax resulting from esophageal compression. Fetal hydrothorax can be unilateral or bilateral. When it is bilateral, it occurs about equally on the right and left sides.

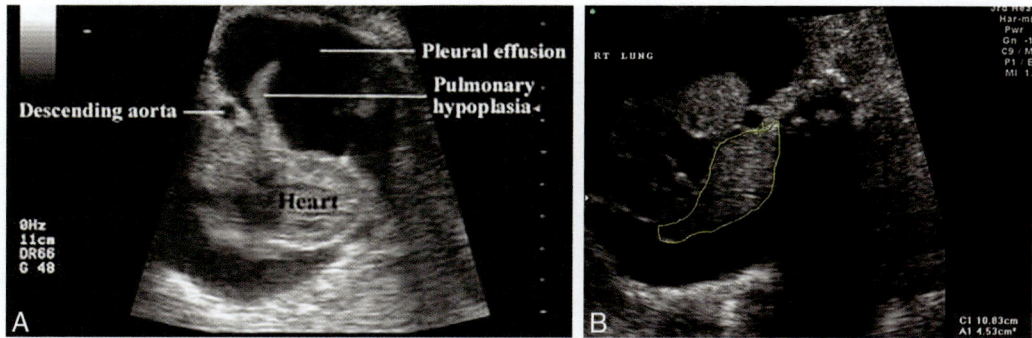

FIG. 61.7 The sonographer should look for the finding of small echogenic lungs as they lie lateral to the cardiac chambers in the fetus with pulmonary hypoplasia. The presence of pleura effusion is evident.

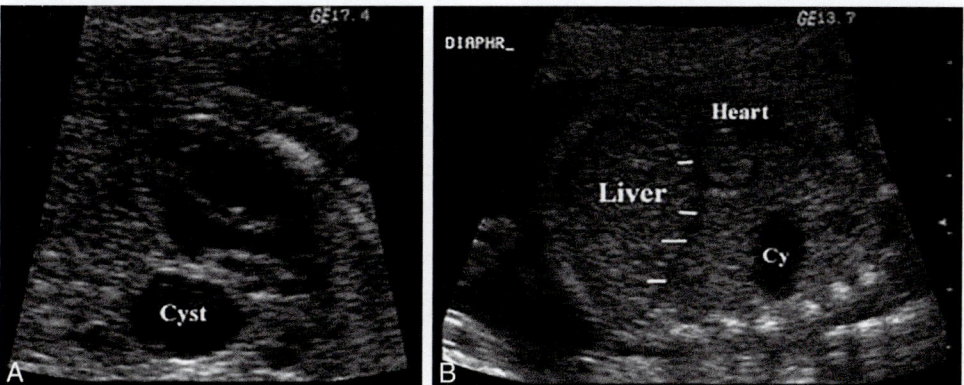

FIG. 61.8 Sonographically, bronchogenic cysts appear as small well-circumscribed masses with no evidence of a mediastinal shift or heart failure.

BOX 61.3 Cystic Lung Masses

- Bronchogenic cysts: most common; unilocular or multilocular cysts usually within mediastinum or lung; normal amniotic fluid
- Pleural effusions: hydramnios accompanies chylothorax (esophageal compression); may result from immune or nonimmune causes or congestive heart failure; may occur with cardiac mass; lymphangiectasia, cystic adenomatoid malformation, sequestration, hernia; compression of lung tissue; shift of mediastinal structures

---

Pleural effusions may result from immune (e.g., Rh hemolytic disease) or nonimmune causes or from congestive heart failure. Effusions may also occur in fetuses with chromosomal abnormalities (e.g., trisomy 21) and in fetuses with a cardiac mass. Other reasons for pleural effusions include **lymphangiectasia**, CAMs, bronchopulmonary sequestration, diaphragmatic hernia, hamartoma, atresia of the pulmonary vein, and other, unknown causes.

Sonographic Findings. Sonographically, pleural effusions appear as echo-free peripheral masses on one or both sides of the fetal heart (Fig. 61.9). The effusions conform to the thoracic cavity and often compress lung tissue. The lung appears to float in the fluid. Pleural fluid is rarely encountered before the 15th week of gestation, except in association with Down or Turner syndrome. Compression of lung parenchyma may cause pulmonary hypoplasia, which often represents a life-threatening consequence for the neonate.

The presence of a pleural effusion may cause a shift in mediastinal structures, compression of the heart, and inversion of the diaphragm. The shape of the lung appears normal in the presence of a pleural effusion. Once a pleural effusion has been discovered, a careful search for lung, cardiac, and diaphragmatic lesions should be attempted. Likewise, evaluation for signs of hydrops (ascites, scalp edema, and tissue edema) should be performed. Correlation with clinical parameters is warranted to exclude immunologic causes of pleural effusion.

The mortality rate for the infant with a pleural effusion approaches 50%; the prognosis is poorer with associated hydrops. When the pleural effusion is large, lung development is impaired, which may result in pulmonary hypoplasia. Some neonatologists advocate draining a large pleural collection (thoracentesis) by placing a thoracoamniotic shunt within the pleural space. This approach attempts to allow for lung growth when it is performed during the second trimester of pregnancy. Thoracentesis may be performed to determine whether the lung has the ability to reexpand once the fluid is removed, thus excluding pulmonary hypoplasia, lessening the effects of hydramnios, and obtaining a fetal karyotype using lymphocytes from the aspirated lung fluid.

Solid Lung Masses. Solid tumors of the fetal lungs, appearing as echo-dense masses in the lung tissue, have been reported

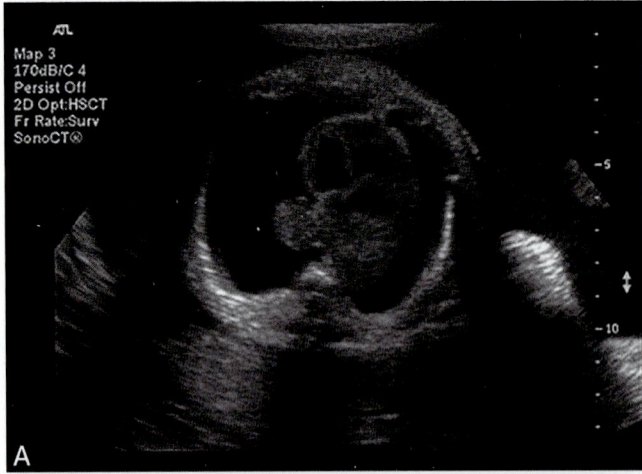
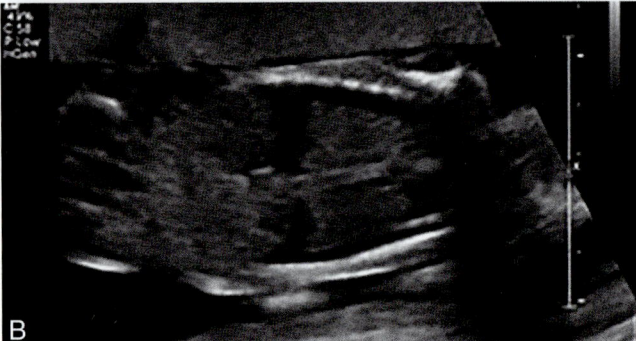

FIG. 61.9 Sonographically, pleural effusions appear as echo-free peripheral masses on one or both sides of the fetal heart. The effusions conform to the thoracic cavity and often compress lung tissue. The lung appears to float in the fluid.

BOX 61.4	Sonographic Findings in Sequestration

- Echogenic solid mass resembling lung tissue
- Rarely occurs below diaphragm
- Associated with hydrops and polyhydramnios, diaphragmatic hernia, gastrointestinal anomalies
- Normal intra-abdominal anatomy

by ultrasound. Pulmonary sequestration and certain types of CAMs appear as solid lung masses (see Fig. 61.6) (Box 61.4).

Pulmonary Sequestration. Pulmonary sequestration is a supernumerary lobe of the lung, separated from the normal tracheobronchial tree. In **pulmonary sequestration**, extra pulmonary tissue is present within the pleural lung sac (intralobar) or is connected to the inferior border of the lung within its own pleural sac (extralobar). This probably develops from a separate outpouching of the foregut or by separation of a segment of the developing lung from the tracheobronchial tree. This extra lung tissue is nonfunctional and receives its blood supply from the systemic circulation. The arterial supply is usually derived from the thoracic aorta, with venous drainage into the vena cava.

Sonographic Findings. Sonographically, an echo-dense solid mass resembling lung tissue is observed, usually in the lower lobe of the lung (Fig. 61.10). A majority of

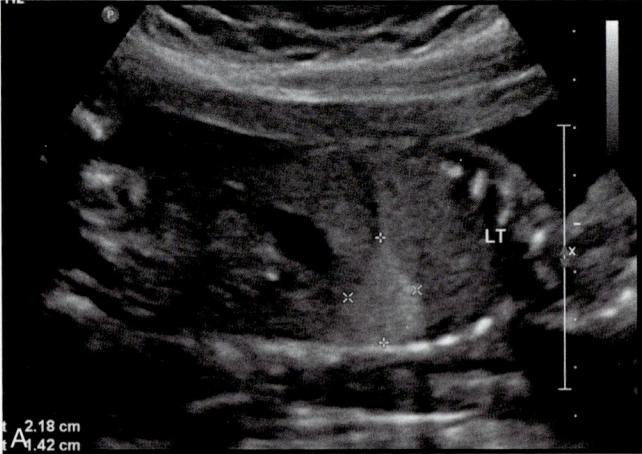
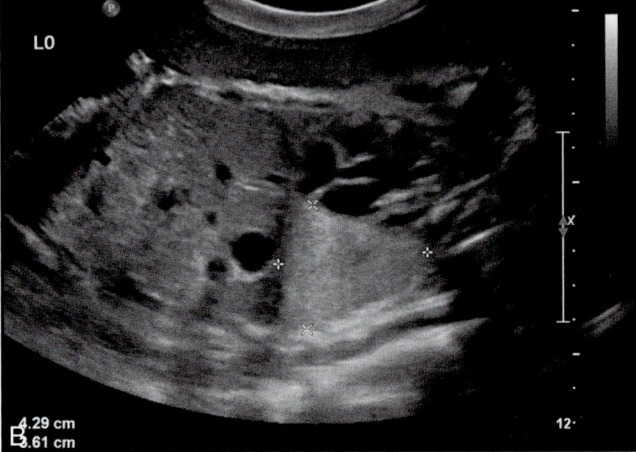

FIG. 61.10 Pulmonary sequestration. Sonographically, an echo-dense solid mass resembling lung tissue is observed, usually in the lower lobe of the lung. A majority of extralobar defects occur on the left side and rarely below the diaphragm.

extralobar defects occur on the left side and rarely below the diaphragm. Intralobar lesions are spherical, and extralobar sequestration appears as a cone-shaped or triangular mass. These lesions may resemble a cystic adenomatoid (type II) malformation. Color Doppler may aid the sonographer in viewing this anomalous circulation. A hypoplastic lung may be observed on the affected side. Hydrops is a frequent finding. Other associated anomalies are diaphragmatic hernia and gastrointestinal and lung anomalies (pulmonary hypoplasia). The prognosis for intralobar sequestration is highly favorable, whereas extralobar sequestration carries a poor prognosis because of associated anomalies and hydrops.

Congenital Cystic Adenomatoid Malformation. Congenital cystic adenomatoid malformation (CCAM) is a multicystic mass within the lung consisting of primitive lung tissue and abnormal bronchial and bronchiolar-like structures (Fig. 61.11). CCAM, one of the bronchopulmonary foregut malformations, results from an embryogenetic alteration in the developing lung during the first 8 to 9 gestational weeks. The lesion may involve one or more lobes of the lung or an entire lung or, in rare cases, may be bilateral. The malformation may communicate with the bronchial tree.

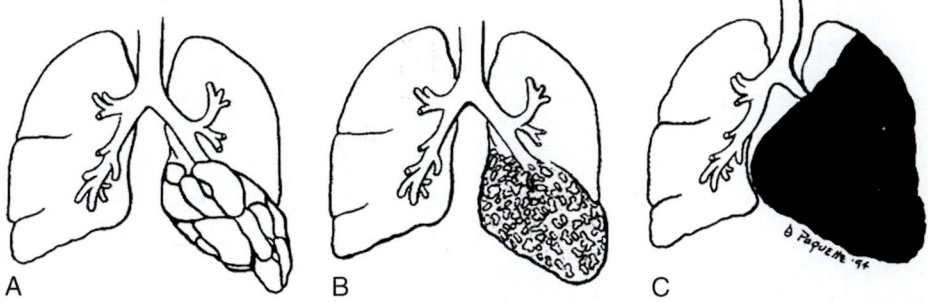

FIG. 61.11 Congenital cystic adenomatoid malformation (CCAM) is a multicystic mass within the lung consisting of primitive lung tissue and abnormal bronchial and bronchiolar-like structures. There are three classifications: type I, 50% of postnatal cases (A); type II, 40% of postnatal cases and associated with congenital anomalies (B); and type III, 10% of postnatal cases and linked to poor prognosis (C).

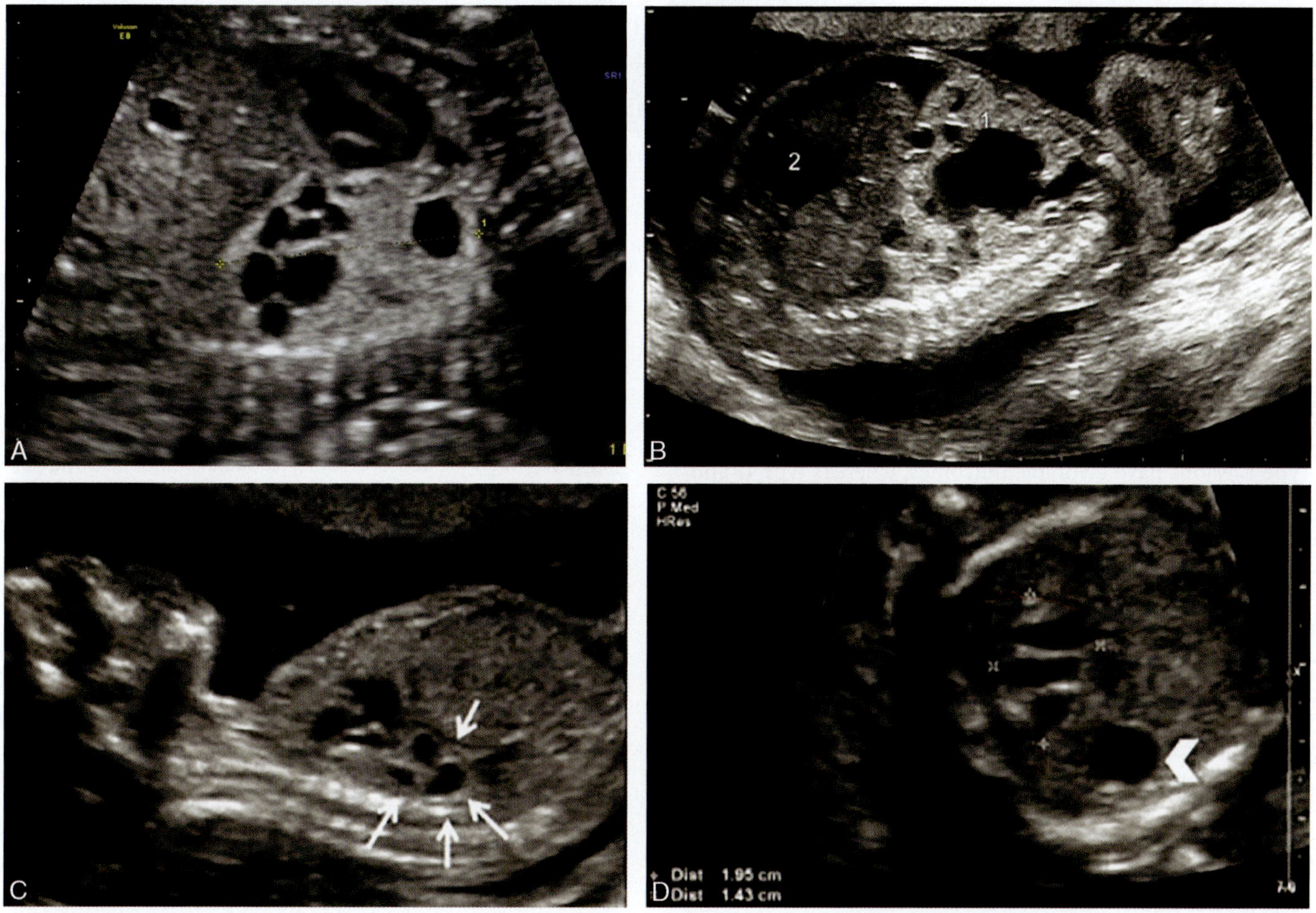

FIG. 61.12 (A) In congenital cystic adenomatoid malformation type I (macrocystic), one or more large cysts replace normal lung tissue (single or multiple cysts measuring >2 to 10 cm). (B–D) Type II (macrocystic with a microcystic component) lesions consist of multiple small cysts (<1 cm).

The cysts within the mass may be large or small, with a variable texture that may be solid, mixed, or cystic in appearance. Most lesions are unilateral and do not favor either lung.

Three forms of CAM are known. In CCAM type I (macrocystic), one or more large cysts replace normal lung tissue (single or multiple cysts measuring more than 2 cm and up to 10 cm) (Fig. 61.12A). Type I is found in 50% of postnatal cases with a favorable outcome. Type II (macrocystic with a microcystic component) lesions consist of multiple small cysts (less than 1 cm) (see Fig. 61.12B). Type II lesions are associated with fetal and/or chromosomal abnormalities in 25% of cases. These anomalies may include renal agenesis, pulmonary anomalies, and diaphragmatic hernia. Type III (microcystic) malformations are characterized as bulky, large, noncystic lesions appearing as echo-dense masses of the entire lung lobe (Fig. 61.13). When a shift of mediastinal structures occurs,

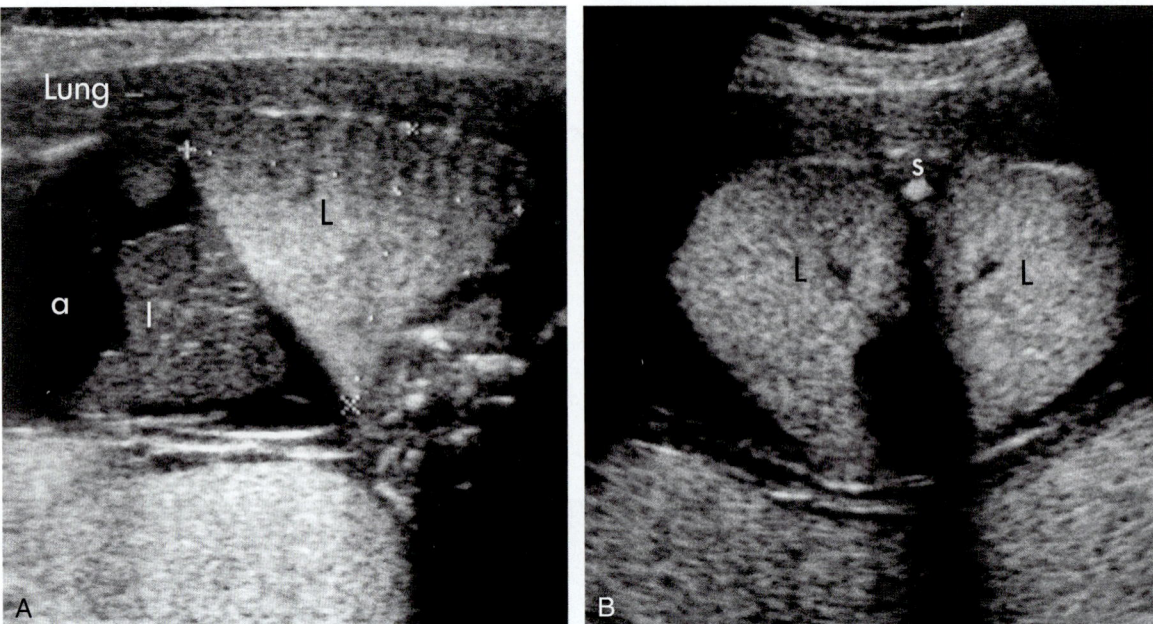

FIG. 61.13 (A) Echogenic lung (L, in calipers) in a 21-week-old fetus with severe hydrops. The opposite lung appeared similar in texture. Oligohydramnios and episodes of bradycardia were evident. *a*, Ascites; *l*, liver. (B) In the same fetus, both echogenic lungs (L) are viewed. Laryngeal or tracheal agenesis was suspected. It is believed that excess lung fluid is manufactured by the abnormal lung. *S*, Spine.

lung compression may occur and nonimmune hydrops may develop. Hydramnios may be observed secondary to esophageal compression, preventing normal fetal swallowing. This lesion is the least common with a poor prognosis.

Differentiation among the types of CAMs is imperative because prognosis varies depending on the type of lesion. Type I lesions have favorable outcomes, whereas type II and III lesions have poor prognoses.

Sonographic Findings. When a cystic or solid lung mass has been identified, the sonographer should attempt to do the following:
- Determine the number(s) and size(s) of cystic structure(s)
- Check for presence or absence of a mediastinal shift
- Identify and assess the size of the lungs
- Look for fetal hydrops
- Exclude cardiac masses
- Search for other fetal anomalies

Based on these findings, an appropriate prognosis and management plan may be instituted (Box 61.5).

A review of the spontaneous improvement of these thoracic masses in utero indicates the following[2]:
- Sonographically detected fetal chest masses may result in pathologically proven thoracically derived lesions or may resolve, some without sequelae.
- The mass lesions may change in size and echogenicity.
- Sonograms of fetuses with CAM may be normal in the first and second trimesters and only later may show abnormalities on ultrasound.
- The presence of polyhydramnios, hydrops, or notable cardiac deviation predicts poor outcome more accurately than the lesion type.

Congenital Bronchial Atresia. Congenital bronchial atresia is a rare pulmonary anomaly that results from the focal

> **BOX 61.5 Sonographic Findings in Cystic Adenomatoid Malformations**
>
> - Type I: single or multiple large cysts 2 cm in diameter; good prognosis after resection of affected lung
> - Type II: multiple small cysts, less than 1 cm in diameter, echogenic; high incidence of other congenital anomalies (renal, gastrointestinal)
> - Type III: large, bulky, noncystic lesions producing mediastinal shift; poor prognosis

obliteration of a segment of the bronchial lumen. It is found most commonly in the left upper lobe and appears on ultrasound as an echogenic pulmonary mass lesion. In normal fetuses, the bronchi are not visualized. If a fetal main stem or segmental bronchus can be seen on sonography, this is probably because it is fluid-filled and abnormal.

Other Complex Lung Masses. The internal components of complex lung masses are cystic and solid and appear heterogeneous. At times, compressed adjacent thoracic organs further complicate determination of the type of lesion (pleural effusion surrounding lungs and heart). Congenital dilation of the bronchial tree may have both cystic and solid characteristics.

Congenital lobar emphysema is lobar overinflation of the lung without destruction of alveolar septa. It usually occurs in the upper left or middle lobe and is located within the normal pleural envelope. This condition may appear identical to microcystic CCAM, presenting as a large solid mass.

Laryngeal and tracheal atresia is an uncommon finding in utero. The sonographic findings show enlarged, bilateral, symmetrically distended echogenic fetal lungs due to fluid distention of tiny air spaces within the lung tissue (Fig. 61.14).

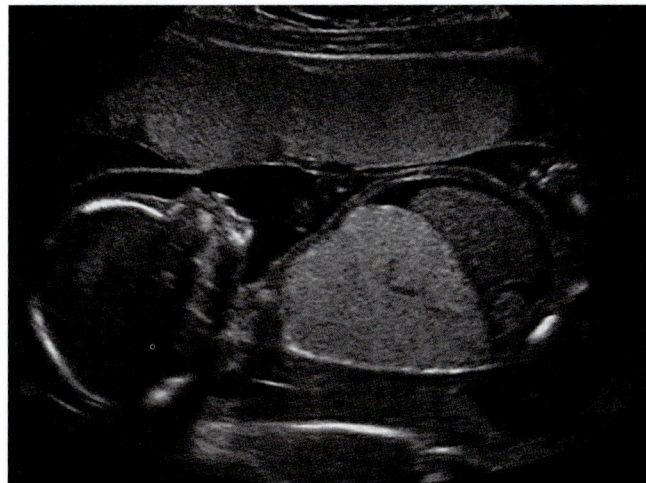

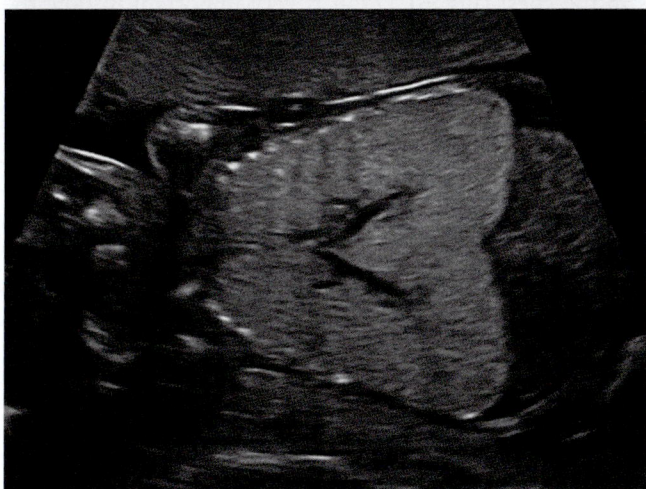

FIG. 61.14 Tracheal atresia. The sonographic findings show enlarged, bilateral, symmetrically distended echogenic fetal lungs due to fluid distention of tiny air spaces within the lung tissue. Fetal ascites is usually present without other findings of hydrops.

The heart may be displaced anteriorly in the midline and may appear engulfed by the prominent lung fields. The trachea and bronchi may be fluid filled. Fetal ascites is usually present without other findings of hydrops. Polyhydramnios may be seen secondary to esophageal compression. Oligohydramnios has also been reported as a result of cardiac compromise or diminished lung fluid efflux into the amniotic space.

Abnormalities of the Diaphragm

The diaphragm is an important muscle separating the thoracic cavity from the abdomen. The diaphragm is specifically studied in fetuses at risk for congenital defects of the diaphragm when there is a shift in the cardiac silhouette, or when atypical structures are found in the fetal chest. In the normal fetus, the diaphragm should appear as a curvilinear hypoechoic structure coursing anteriorly to posteriorly (Fig. 61.15). The fetal stomach and liver should be identified caudal to the diaphragm, with the lungs and heart positioned cephalad. Failure to recognize these normal relationships should prompt the sonographer to search for diaphragmatic defects.

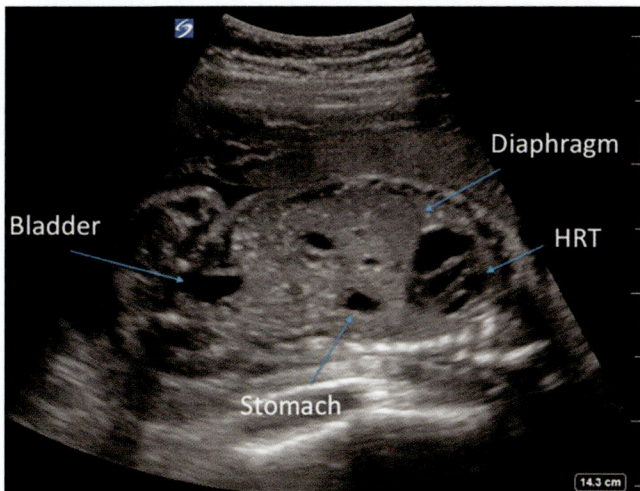

FIG. 61.15 In the normal fetus, the diaphragm should appear as a curvilinear hypoechoic structure coursing anteriorly to posteriorly. The fetal stomach and liver should be identified caudal to the diaphragm, with the lungs and heart (HRT) positioned cephalad.

Congenital Diaphragmatic Hernia. Congenital diaphragmatic hernia (CDH) is a herniation of the abdominal viscera into the chest that results from a congenital defect in the fetal diaphragm. It is a sporadic defect, occurring in 1 per 2000 to 1 per 5000 births. The muscular diaphragm forms between the 6th and 14th weeks of gestation as a result of a chain of events involving the fusion of four structures: (1) septum transversum (future central tendon), (2) pleuroperitoneal membranes, (3) dorsal mesentery of the esophagus (future crura), and (4) body wall. Normally, the primitive diaphragm is intact by the end of the eighth menstrual week. The most posterior aspect of the diaphragm, derived from the body wall, is the part of the diaphragm that forms last and is most commonly defective.

During the embryologic phase, when the gut is moving back into the abdominal cavity (around 10 to 12 weeks), sufficient intraabdominal pressure may be produced, so that if fusion of the primitive diaphragmatic structures is incomplete, abdominal viscera can herniate into the thorax.

The diaphragmatic hernia permits the abdominal organs to enter the fetal chest (Fig. 61.16). The most common type of diaphragmatic defect occurs posteriorly and laterally in the diaphragm (herniation through the **foramen of Bochdalek**). This hernia is usually found on the left side of the diaphragm, and in left-side organs (stomach, spleen, and portions of the liver) enters the chest through the opening. The abnormally positioned abdominal organs shift the heart and mediastinal structures to the right side of the chest. Usually the stomach is in the chest near the heart, instead of below the diaphragm. In left-side hernias, the sonographer should look for the stomach, portions of the small and large intestines, and the left lobe of the liver and spleen in the thoracic cavity. Peristalsis of the bowel loops may be seen within the thoracic cavity (Box 61.6).

Diaphragmatic hernias may occur anteriorly and medially in the diaphragm, through the **foramen of Morgagni**, and may communicate with the pericardial sac. In anteromedial defects, the heart may be normally positioned but surrounded

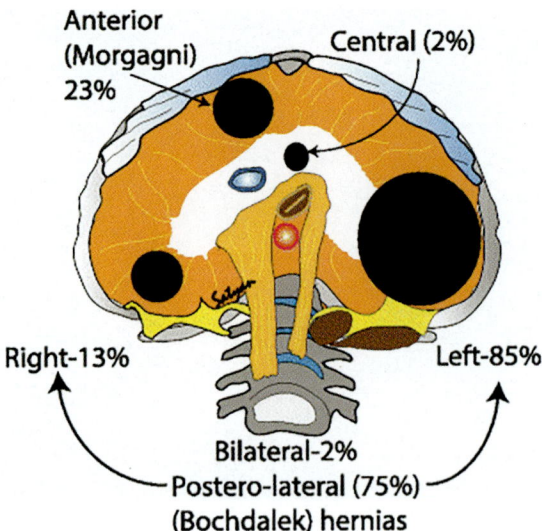

FIG. 61.16 The most common type of diaphragmatic defect occurs posteriorly and laterally in the diaphragm (herniation through the foramen of Bochdalek). Diaphragmatic hernias may occur anteriorly and medially in the diaphragm, through the foramen of Morgagni, and may communicate with the pericardial sac.

BOX 61.6 Sonographic Criteria Suggestive of a Diaphragmatic Hernia

- Shift of the heart and mediastinal structures (right shift in left-side defects; left shift in right-side defects)
- Mass within the thoracic cavity (liver, stomach, spleen, and large bowel in left-side defects; liver, gallbladder, intestines in right-side defects)
- Small abdominal circumference resulting from herniated abdominal structures
- Obvious diaphragm defect
- Hydramnios
- More than 50% have structural anomalies or chromosomal abnormalities
- Structural defects include cardiovascular (tetralogy of Fallot and others), genitourinary (renal agenesis, cystic dysplasia, and ureteropelvic junction obstruction), central nervous system (holoprosencephaly, hydrocephalus, and spinal anomalies), clubbed feet, hemivertebrae and absent ribs, genital (ambiguous genitalia and others), and gastrointestinal (imperforate anus, annular pancreas, and absence of the gallbladder)
- Growth restriction suggests associated anomalies
- Abdominal circumference less than the fifth percentile and the liver in the chest indicate poor prognosis (see Teixeira et al.)

---

by pleural fluid, while the fetal stomach may be located in its normal position in the abdomen. Thinning of the diaphragm (eventration) may give rise to sonographic characteristics similar to those of diaphragmatic hernias.

Defects on the right side of the diaphragm allow the right-side abdominal viscera (liver, gallbladder, intestines) to enter the chest. As a consequence of herniated abdominal organs, the lungs are compressed and may become hypoplastic.

The size of the diaphragmatic defects can be variable, ranging from small to large to complete absence of both diaphragms. The smaller defects are difficult to diagnose in utero. Hydrops usually is not present with left-side CDHs unless associated fetal malformations are present. The presence of pulmonary hypoplasia and pulmonary hypertension is the real issue that results from the size of the hernia. The pulmonary arteries become hypertrophied and thickened, resulting in pulmonary hypertension that after birth leads to persistent fetal circulation. Bilateral hernias are very unusual and more difficult to detect with sonography because the degree of cardiomediastinal shift may not be evident. The heart may be slightly displaced anteriorly and superiorly, and the stomach may be found in the left chest.

Sonographic Findings. On sonographic examination, a *left-side CDH* is usually found when the cardiac silhouette is displaced to the right and an ectopic stomach is in the chest (Fig. 61.17). It is very important to note the cardiomediastinal shift to make the diagnosis of a hernia. The apex of the heart will be abnormally shifted, depending on the size of the CDH defect. The small bowel and colon are commonly intrathoracic but are often collapsed and difficult to identify specifically if peristalsis is not present. The sagittal image of the fetus may allow visualization of the diaphragm, depending on how large the defect is. The fetal lung may be small and compressed.

A portion of the liver herniates into the chest in approximately two-thirds of cases, and the presence or absence of intrathoracic liver is important to note because it is associated with a poorer outcome. Color flow may be useful in demarcating the portal vasculature within the liver to ascertain whether the tissue is truly liver or not. Box 61.7 lists the sonographic features of left congenital hernia.

In a *right-side diaphragmatic hernia*, the sonographer will see the liver in the chest, possibly a collapsed bowel, and the heart deviated far to the left. The stomach alignment will be abnormal, but inferior to the diaphragm and moved to the right. Color may help to trace the portal vasculature in the liver as it lies within the chest cavity. The gallbladder may also herniate into the thoracic cavity and appear as a solitary "cystic" mass in the lung. A small amount of ascitic fluid adjacent to the liver may be present with right-side hernias. Pleural fluid is not usually associated with other chest masses, except in sequestration. At birth, respiration may be severely compromised, which may result in death of the newborn.

The amniotic fluid may be normal unless the bowel is obstructed with resulting polyhydramnios. The placenta is normal; the abdominal circumference will be abnormally small. Careful scanning before 18 weeks of gestation is important to identify the normal contour of the diaphragm on sagittal and coronal views. A small defect may not show abnormalities early in the gestational period.

The prognosis is poor for the fetus if the CDH is detected before birth; if the stomach is found in the chest, especially if it is dilated; if the left side of the heart is underdeveloped; or if congenital heart disease is present. The primary cause of death is pulmonary hypoplasia. If the diagnosis is made before 25 weeks of gestation and polyhydramnios is present, the survival rate is low.

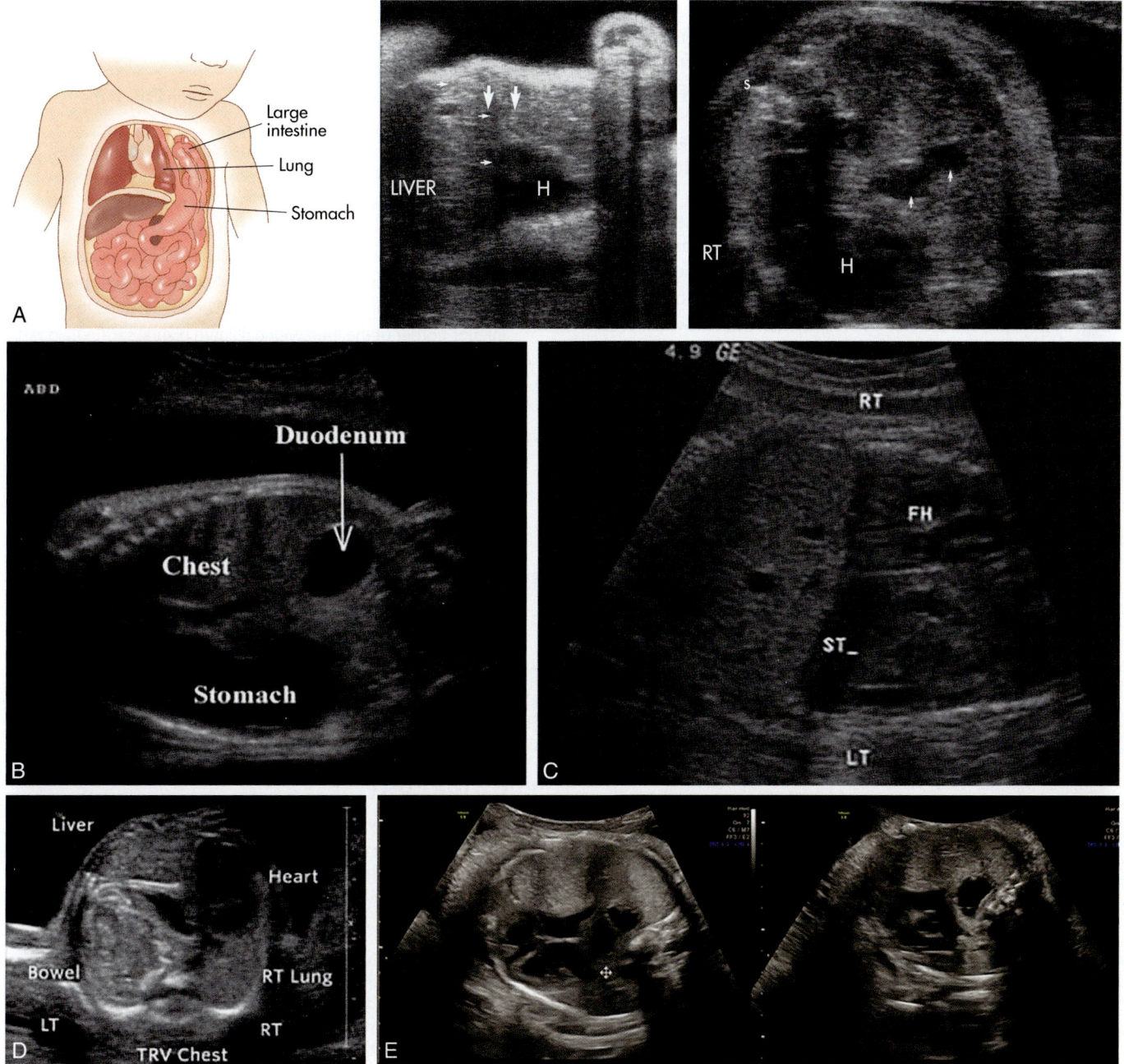

FIG. 61.17 (A) Hernia of intestinal loops and part of the stomach into the pleural cavity. The heart and mediastinum are pushed to the right, whereas the left lung is compressed. (B) Long-axis views of the stomach projecting into the thoracic cavity. (C–E) Transverse views of the bowel projecting into the thoracic cavity. *FH*, Fetal heart; *H*, heart; *S*, spine; *ST*, stomach.

BOX 61.7	Sonographic Features of Left Congenital Hernia

- Intrathoracic stomach
- Displaced cardiac apex
- Cardiomediastinal shift is critical in making the diagnosis
- Intrathoracic liver (look for portal venous flow)
- Small right lung
- Small left ventricle of heart
- Evaluate for chromosomal abnormalities

Frequently associated abnormalities include cardiac malformations (20%), central nervous system malformations (30%), renal anomalies, vertebral defects, pulmonary hypoplasia, and facial clefts. In addition, chromosome abnormalities (trisomy 18 and 21) have been associated with diaphragmatic hernia.

It is important to note that when a diaphragmatic hernia is present, the stomach may not be filled when there is concomitant oligohydramnios or if the fetus is swallowing abnormally. The only clue to a diaphragmatic hernia in this situation may be evidence of a solid mass in the chest. Peristalsis within the herniated intestines confirms the diagnosis. When the sonographer is unable to demonstrate the stomach bubble in the normal anatomic location after repeated observations, a search for a diaphragmatic hernia should be attempted.

Lung and mediastinal masses, particularly CAMs, may be difficult to distinguish from diaphragmatic hernias. The normally positioned peritoneal organs should aid in differentiating between these two conditions.

At birth, most infants with CDH have pulmonary hypoplasia and secondary respiratory insufficiency. The mortality rate is high (75%) because of the increased frequency of coexisting fetal congenital anomalies. The extracorporeal membrane oxygenation procedure has provided such babies with severe diaphragmatic hernias a chance for survival immediately after delivery. This procedure canalizes the carotid artery (while occluding the opposite carotid artery) in an effort to bypass the pulmonary circulation to provide an opportunity for the lung tissue to mature before circulation demands are in place.

Key Pearls

- Adequacy of pulmonary development is probably the single most important determinant of fetal viability, and pulmonary immaturity is the major reason why fetuses younger than 24 weeks of gestation are generally considered nonviable.
- Breathing movements that occur before birth result in the aspiration of fluid into the lungs.
- The fluid present in the lungs at birth clears by three routes: (1) through the mouth and nose, (2) into the pulmonary capillaries, and (3) into the lymphatics and the pulmonary vessels.
- The thorax is normally slightly smaller than the abdominal cavity.
- Chest circumference measurements are made in the transverse plane at the level of the four-chamber view of the heart.
- The fetal lungs appear homogeneous on sonography with moderate echogenicity.
- The mature fetus spends almost one third of its time breathing. Fetal breathing movements are documented if characteristic seesaw movements of the fetal chest or abdomen are sustained for at least 20 sec.
- When evaluating the fetus for a lung mass, the sonographer should assess the following: position of the fetal heart, orientation of the cardiac axis, and measurement of the thoracic circumference.
- The lungs will not grow or develop properly when a small uterine cavity results from severe oligohydramnios, when the chest cavity is abnormally small, when the balance between tracheal and airway pressure and fluid volume is inadequate, or when the fetus is unable to practice breathing movements.
- Pulmonary hypoplasia is caused by a decrease in the numbers of lung cells, airways, and alveoli, with a resulting decrease in organ size and weight.
- Masses within the thoracic cavity, including pleural effusion, diaphragmatic hernia (and eventration), cystic adenomatoid malformation of the lung, bronchopulmonary sequestration, and other large cysts and tumors of the lung and thorax, may lead to pulmonary hypoplasia.
- The most common lung cyst detected prenatally is the bronchogenic cyst.
- An accumulation of fluid within the pleural cavity that may appear as an isolated lesion or secondary to multiple fetal anomalies is called a pleural effusion or hydrothorax.
- Pulmonary sequestration and certain types of cystic adenomatoid malformations appear as solid lung masses.
- In pulmonary sequestration, extra pulmonary tissue is present within the pleural lung sac (intralobar) or is connected to the inferior border of the lung within its own pleural sac (extralobar).
- Congenital cystic adenomatoid malformation is a multicystic mass within the lung consisting of primitive lung tissue and abnormal bronchial and bronchiolar-like structures.
- Congenital diaphragmatic hernia is a herniation of the abdominal viscera into the chest that results from a congenital defect in the fetal diaphragm.

REFERENCES

1. Laudy JA, Wladimiroff JW. The fetal lung. 2. Pulmonary hypoplasia. *Ultrasound Obstet Gynecol.* 2000;16:482–494.
2. Budorick NE, Pretorius DH, Leopold GR, Stamm ER. Spontaneous improvement of intrathoracic masses diagnosed in utero. *J Ultrasound Med.* 1992;11:653–662.

BIBLIOGRAPHY

Bahlmann F, Merz E, Hallermann C, et al. Congenital diaphragmatic hernia: ultrasonic measurement of fetal lungs to predict pulmonary hypoplasia. *Ultrasound Obstet Gynecol.* 1999;14:162–168.

Bootstaylor BS, Filly RA, Harrison MR, et al. Prenatal sonographic predictors of liver herniation in congenital diaphragmatic hernia. *J Ultrasound Med.* 1995;14:515–520.

Bromley B, Parad R, Estroff JA, Benacerraf BR. Fetal lung masses: prenatal course and outcome. *J Ultrasound Med.* 1995;14:927–936.

Bunduki V, Ruano R, de Liva MM, et al. Prognostic factors associated with congenital cystic adenomatoid malformation of the lung. *Prenat Diagn.* 2000;20:459–464.

Callen P. *Ultrasonography in Obstetrics and Gynecology.* ed 5. Philadelphia: Elsevier; 2008.

Cass DL, Crombleholme TM, Howell LJ, et al. Cystic lung lesions with systemic arterial blood supply: a hybrid of congenital cystic adenomatoid malformation and bronchopulmonary sequestration. *J Pediatr Surg.* 1997;32:986–990.

Cosmi EV, Aneschi MM, Cosmi E, et al. Ultrasonographic patterns of fetal breathing movements in normal pregnancy. *Int J Gynaecol Obstet.* 2003;80:285–290.

De Santis M, Masini L, Nois G, et al. Congenital cystic adenomatoid malformation of the lung: antenatal ultrasound findings and fetal-neonatal outcome. Fifteen years of experience. *Fetal Diagn Ter.* 2000;15:246–250.

Enns G, Cox VA, Goldstein RB, et al. Congenital diaphragmatic defects and associated syndromes, malformations, and chromosome anomalies: a retrospective study of 60 patients and literature review. *Am J Med Genet.* 1998;79:215–225.

Ishikawa S, Kamata S, Usui N, et al. Ultrasonographic prediction of clinical pulmonary hypoplasia: measurement of the chest/trunk-length ratio in fetuses. *Pediatr Surg Int.* 2003;19:172–175.

Johnson A, Callan NA, Bhutank VK, et al. Ultrasonic ratio of fetal thoracic to abdominal circumference: an association with fetal pulmonary hypoplasia. *Am J Obstet Gynecol.* 1987;157:764–769.

Johnson AM, Hubbard AM. Congenital anomalies of the fetal/neonatal chest. *Semin Roentgenol.* 2004;39:197–214.

La Torre R, Cosmi E, Anceschi MH, et al. Preliminary report on a new and noninvasive method for the assessment of fetal lung maturity. *J Perinat Med.* 2003;31:431–434.

Laudy JA, Wladimiroff JW. The fetal lung. I. Developmental aspects. *Obstet Gynecol.* 2000;16:284–290.

Mayden KL, Tortora M, Chervenak FA, Hobbins JC. The antenatal, sonographic detection of lung masses. *Am J Obstet Gynecol.* 1984;148:349–351.

Merz E, Miric-Tesanic D, Bahlmann F, et al. Prenatal sonographic chest and lung measurements for predicting severe pulmonary hypoplasia. *Prenat Diagn.* 1999;19:614–619.

Osada H, Iitsuka Y, Masua K, et al. Application of lung volume measurement by three-dimensional ultrasonography for clinical assessment of fetal lung development. *J Ultrasound Med.* 2002;21:841–847.

Ruano R, Benachi A, Aubry MC, et al. Prenatal sonographic diagnosis of congenital hiatal hernia. *Prenat Diagn.* 2004;24:26–30.

Song MS, Yoo SJ, Smallhorn JF, et al. Bilateral congenital diaphragmatic hernia: diagnostic clues at fetal sonography. *Ultrasound Obstet Gynecol.* 2001;17:255–258.

Teixeira J, Sepulveda W, Hassan J, et al. Abdominal circumference in fetuses with congenital diaphragmatic hernia: correlation with hernia content and pregnancy outcome. *J Ultrasound Med.* 1997;16:407–410.

Usui N, Kamata S, Sawai S, et al. Outcome predictors for infants with cystic lung disease. *J Pediatric Surg.* 2004;39:603–606.

Vintzileos AM, Campbell WA, Rodis JF, et al. Comparison of six different ultrasonographic methods for predicting lethal fetal pulmonary hypoplasia. *Am J Obstet Gynecol.* 1989;161:606–612.

Winters WD, Effmann EL, Nghiem HV, et al. Congenital masses of the lung: changes in cross-sectional area during gestation. *J Clin Ultrasound.* 1997;25:372–377.

CHAPTER 62

The Fetal Anterior Abdominal Wall

Sandra L. Hagen-Ansert

OBJECTIVES

On completion of this chapter, you should be able to:
- Describe the embryology of the abdominal wall
- Define and describe the anterior abdominal wall abnormalities discussed in this chapter
- List the sonographic findings for an omphalocele and for a gastroschisis
- Identify the fetal anomalies in pentalogy of Cantrell
- Explain the sonographic findings in a fetus with amniotic band syndrome

OUTLINE

Embryology of the Abdominal Wall 1560
Sonographic Evaluation of the Fetal Abdominal Wall 1562
Abnormalities of the Anterior Abdominal Wall 1562
Omphalocele 1562
Gastroschisis 1565
Amniotic Band Syndrome 1566
Beckwith-Wiedemann Syndrome 1566
Bladder and Cloacal Exstrophy 1567
Pentalogy of Cantrell, Ectopia Cordis, and Cleft Sternum 1568
Limb–Body Wall Complex 1570

KEY TERMS

Amniotic band syndrome
Beckwith-Wiedemann syndrome
Cloacal exstrophy
Gastroschisis
Limb–body wall complex
Omphalocele
Pentalogy of Cantrell

Sonography has proven to be very effective for detecting anterior abdominal wall defects in utero. These defects occur during the first trimester as the midgut elongates and migrates into the umbilical cord. The midgut usually returns into the abdominal cavity by the 11th week of gestation. When this fails to occur, an abdominal wall defect is formed. The two most common defects are omphalocele and gastroschisis. Less common defects are ectopia cordis, limb–body wall complex, and cloacal exstrophy.

EMBRYOLOGY OF THE ABDOMINAL WALL

By the end of the fifth week of development, an embryo is a flat disk consisting of three layers: ectoderm, mesoderm, and endoderm. In the sixth week, a process called *folding* helps the embryo to transform itself into a cylindrical shape (Fig. 62.1). This transformation is a critical part of the process of closing the abdominal wall.

As the embryo folds at the cranial end, the base of the yolk sac is partially incorporated as the foregut, which later develops as the pharynx, lower respiratory system, esophagus, stomach, duodenum (proximal to the opening of the bile duct), liver, pancreas, gallbladder, and biliary duct system (Fig. 62.2).

The growth of the neural tube causes the embryo to fold at the caudal end, incorporating part of the yolk sac as the hindgut, which turns into the cloaca. It also causes the connecting stalk (located at the tail) to move to the ventral surface of the embryo, incorporating the allantois into the umbilical cord. The derivatives of the hindgut are the distal part of the transverse colon, the descending colon, the sigmoid colon, the rectum, the superior portion of the anal canal, the epithelium of the urinary bladder, and most of the urethra (Fig. 62.3).

The sides of the embryo fold, leading to the formation of the lateral and anterior abdominal wall. The midgut is the primordium of the small intestines (including most of the duodenum), cecum, vermiform appendix, ascending colon, and the right half to two-thirds of the transverse colon. The connection of the yolk sac and body stalk will form the umbilical cord at

CHAPTER 62 The Fetal Anterior Abdominal Wall

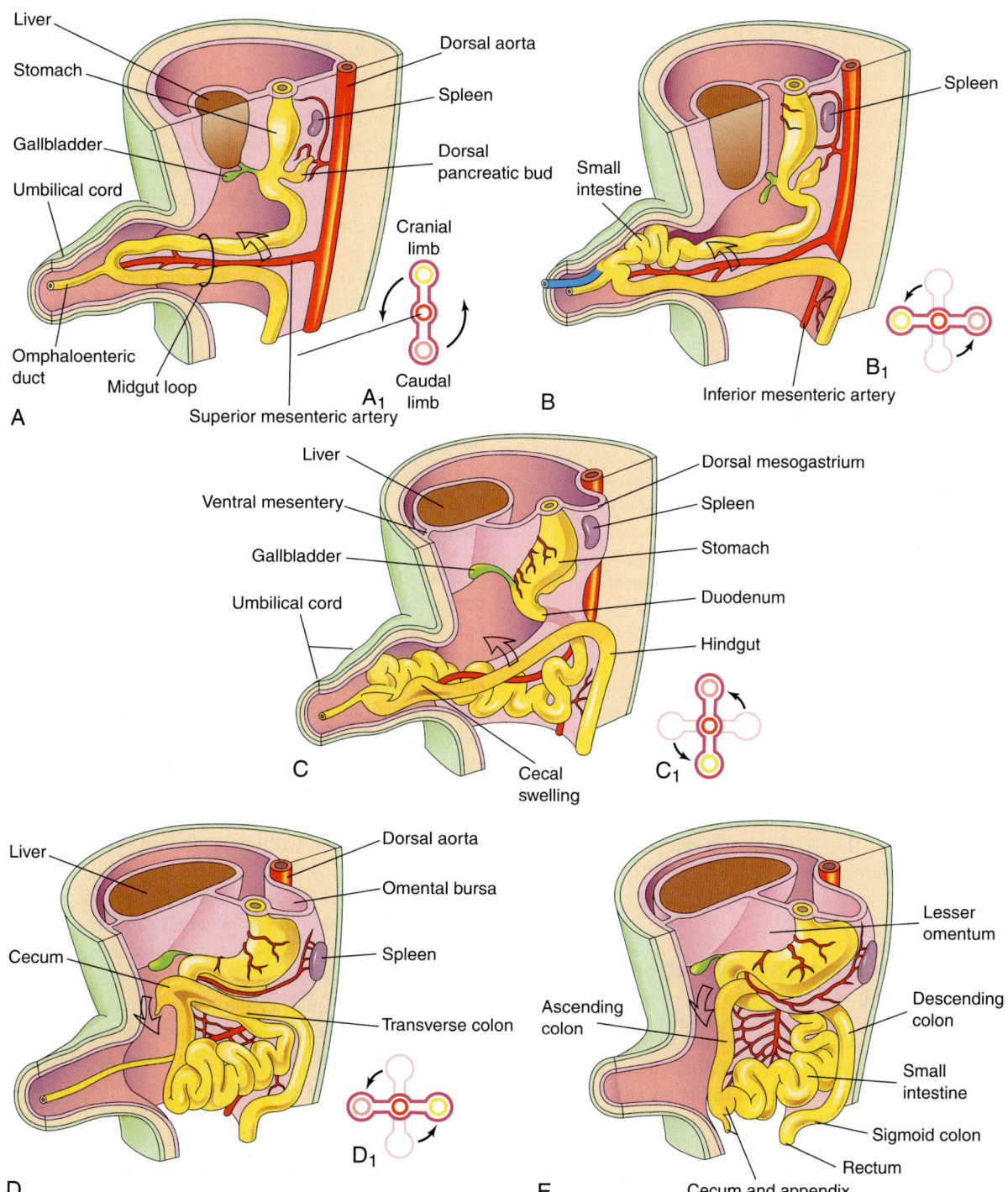

FIG. 62.1 By the end of the fifth week of development, an embryo is a flat disk consisting of three layers: ectoderm, mesoderm, and endoderm. In the sixth week, a process called *folding* helps the embryo to transform itself into a cylindrical shape.

the ventral region of the embryo. Expansion of the amniotic cavity will cover the umbilical cord by the amnion. Fusion of the midline begins during the seventh week of development and is completed by the eighth week.

The umbilical veins drain the placenta, body stalk, and the evolving abdominal wall. During the seventh week, the hepatic bud enlarges, and the right umbilical vein atrophies. The proximal portion of the left umbilical vein between the subhepatic portion and the common cardinal vein also atrophies. Branches of the aorta now replace the nutritive function of the umbilical veins with respect to the developing abdominal wall. The superior mesenteric artery is formed from the right omphalomesenteric artery.

Umbilication hernia of the bowel occurs during the eighth week of development as the midgut extends to the extraembryonic coelom in the proximal portion of the

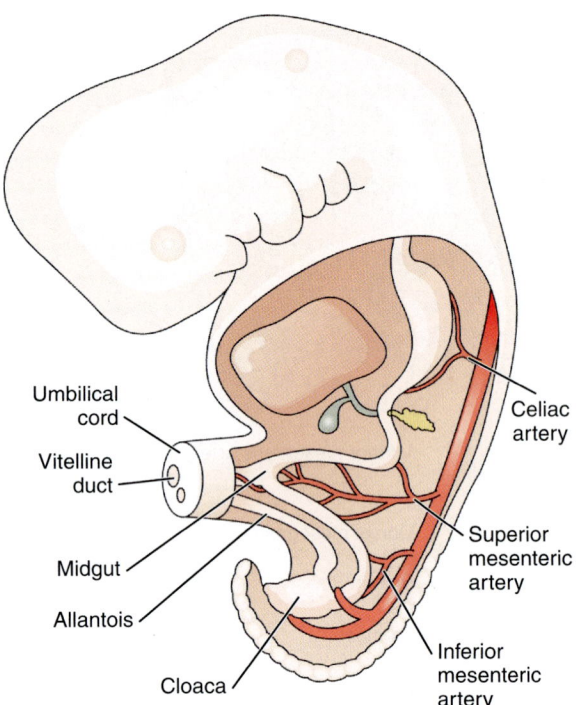

FIG. 62.2 As the embryo folds at the cranial end, the base of the yolk sac is partially incorporated as the foregut, which later develops as the pharynx, lower respiratory system, esophagus, stomach, duodenum (proximal to the opening of the bile duct), liver, pancreas, gallbladder, and biliary duct system.

umbilical cord. The midgut grows faster than the abdominal cavity at this stage because of the increased size of the liver and kidneys. Thus the herniation develops. The intestines return to the abdominal cavity by the 12th week of gestation.

SONOGRAPHIC EVALUATION OF THE FETAL ABDOMINAL WALL

It should be possible to detect abdominal wall defects in utero because the defects form early in embryologic development. It is very important to image the cord insertion site and the fetal anterior abdominal wall to evaluate for the presence or absence of such defects. If the urinary bladder and pelvis are evaluated closely, the diagnosis of bladder and cloacal exstrophy may also be made with sonography. The most common types of abdominal wall defects are gastroschisis, omphalocele, and umbilical hernia. Other types of abdominal ventral wall defects include ectopia cordis, pentalogy of Cantrell, bladder and cloacal exstrophy, amniotic band syndrome, and the limb–body wall complex. The following questions should be routinely answered:

1. Is a limiting membrane present?
2. What is the relation of the umbilical cord to the defect?
3. Which organs are eviscerated?
4. Is the bowel normal in appearance?
5. Are other fetal malformations evident?

ABNORMALITIES OF THE ANTERIOR ABDOMINAL WALL

Abdominal wall defects cause distortion of the normal contour of the ventral or anterior surface of the fetal abdomen. Table 62.1 summarizes the typical sonographic features and associated conditions of fetal abdominal wall defects.

The most common abdominal wall defects, omphalocele, umbilical hernia (a form of omphalocele), and gastroschisis, will be presented. The incidence of omphaloceles is approximately 1 in 4000 live births. Overall, gastroschisis has an incidence of 12 per 10,000, although only rarely are affected infants born to older mothers. The role of the perinatal team is to distinguish among these lesions because clinical management, associated anomalies, delivery, and postnatal surgical survival vary, depending on the specific type of abdominal wall defect. Box 62.1 outlines what the sonographer should investigate to distinguish between omphalocele and gastroschisis.

Omphalocele

During the 8th to 12th weeks of development, the fetal bowel normally migrates into the umbilical cord from the abdominal cavity. This normal embryologic herniation of the bowel permits the development of the intra-abdominal organs and allows necessary bowel rotation. Because of the lack of space within the abdominal cavity and the large fetal liver and kidneys, the bowel is forced from the abdomen and into the extraembryonic coelom of the umbilical cord. This herniation permits the bowel to rotate around the superior mesenteric artery. These herniated loops of bowel normally return and rotate into position within the abdominal cavity by the 12th week of pregnancy. When bowel loops fail to return to the abdomen, a bowel-containing omphalocele occurs (Fig. 62.4).

An **omphalocele** develops when there is a midline defect of the abdominal muscles, fascia, and skin that results in herniation of intra-abdominal structures into the base of the umbilical cord. This herniation is covered by a membrane that consists of the amnion and peritoneum. The alpha-fetoprotein (AFP) level may be slightly elevated or within normal limits. Omphaloceles are characterized as two types: (1) those that contain the liver within the sac and (2) those that contain a variable amount of bowel without liver.

Fetuses with an omphalocele that contains only a bowel have a higher risk for chromosomal abnormalities and other anomalies (Fig. 62.5). Bowel within the omphalocele develops because the intestine fails to return to the abdomen (primitive body stalk remains). A liver omphalocele represents a developmental defect in abdominal wall closure. This type of omphalocele affects the abdominal wall muscles, fascia, and skin. Liver omphaloceles may contain a bowel and demonstrate a relatively large abdominal wall defect in comparison with the abdominal diameter (Fig. 62.6).

The prognosis for infants with an omphalocele varies according to the extent of the primary defect and associated structural and chromosomal abnormalities. Perinatal

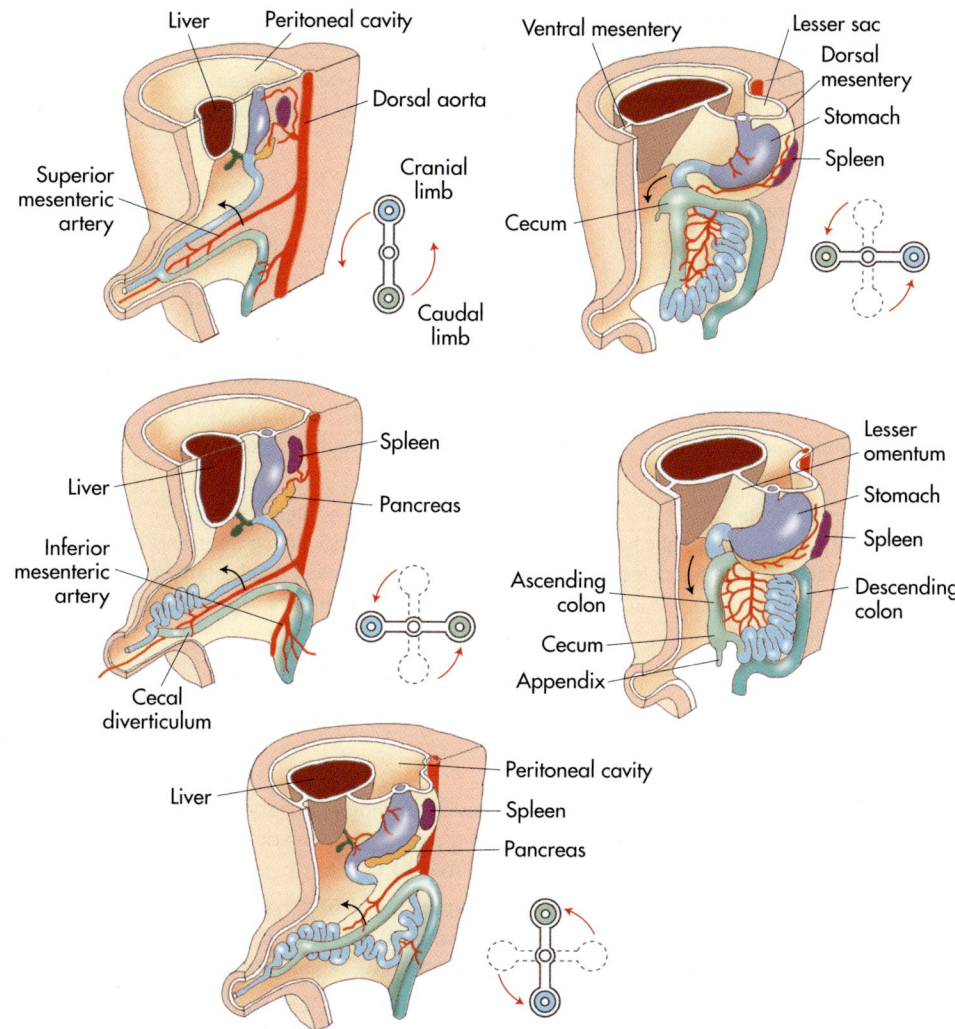

FIG. 62.3 **Development and rotation of the midgut from the 6th to 11th week.** The midgut is the primordium of the small intestines, cecum, appendix, ascending colon, and right half to two-thirds of the transverse colon. The connection of the yolk sac and body stalk will form the umbilical cord at the ventral region of the embryo.

mortality rate approaches 80% when more than one fetal abnormality exists, and almost all infants die when there is a chromosomal or major heart defect. Without other anomalies, the mortality rate is approximately 10% with an isolated omphalocele.

The mode of delivery for fetuses with an omphalocele varies according to the type of omphalocele and other anomalies. The obstetrician may elect vaginal delivery when a chromosomal abnormality and other major anomalies predict no chance for survival.

Sonographic Findings. The sonographic signs of an omphalocele are as follows:

- Central abdominal wall defect with evisceration of the bowel or a combination of liver and bowel into the base of the umbilical cord. Color flow imaging may aid in viewing the continuity of the umbilical cord into the omphalocele. The stomach may be involved (see Fig. 62.6). Bowel omphaloceles appear echogenic and must be distinguished from umbilical hernia (covered by skin and fat).
- Membrane consisting of the peritoneum and amnion forms the omphalocele sac encasing the herniated organs.
- Umbilical hernias may be confused with liver omphaloceles; however, a normal cord insertion suggests hernia.
- Ascites may coexist with an omphalocele.
- Hydramnios is found in one-third of fetuses.
- Associated anomalies (50% to 70%) include complex cardiac disease (30% to 50%) and gastrointestinal, neural tube, and genitourinary tract anomalies (polycystic kidneys with a small omphalocele may indicate trisomy 13).
- Omphaloceles may occur concurrently with diaphragmatic hernia.
- Chromosomal anomalies occur in 35% to 60% of omphaloceles. Most common are trisomies 13 and 18. Omphaloceles may be found with trisomy 21, Turner syndrome, and triploidy.
- When scoliosis is found, consider limb–body wall complex (or body-stalk anomaly), a lethal disorder, which also includes severe cranial defects (acrania, encephalocele),

TABLE 62.1 Typical Features of Ventral Wall Defects and Associated Conditions

Defect	Description	Sonographic Features	Other Anomalies
Gastroschisis	Paraumbilical defect	Typically only bowel is eviscerated; occasionally other organs, but almost never the liver	Associated anomalies are uncommon; high rate of bowel-related complications
Omphalocele	Midline defect, contained by membrane	Variable	High risk of other anomalies and/or aneuploidy
Extracorporeal liver	Typically large	When isolated without other detectable anomalies, risk of aneuploidy is very low; however, high rate of cardiac anomalies	
Intracorporeal liver	Typically small	>50% risk of aneuploidy when detected prenatally	
Beckwith-Wiedemann syndrome	Syndromic condition	Macroglossia; omphalocele; visceromegaly	Omphalocele is typically intracorporeal liver type
Pentalogy of Cantrell	Omphalocele Anterior diaphragmatic hernia Distal partial sternal defect Pericardial defect Cardiac defect	May appear only as high omphalocele; pleural effusion, even transient, is highly suggestive of diaphragmatic hernia in this situation	None
Absent sternum	Absent sternum	Dynamic heart covered by skin	Rare; usually isolated
Ectopia cordis	Thoracic defect of sternum and skin	Dynamic heart not covered by skin	Rare; high rate of cardiac and other defects; may be associated with high omphalocele
Bladder exstrophy	Eviscerated urinary bladder	Nonvisualization of urinary bladder; soft tissue mass of anterior abdominal wall may be subtle	Increased risk of fetal aneuploidy
Cloacal exstrophy	Eviscerated cloaca with two hemibladders	Nonvisualization of urinary bladder; in one variation, ileal prolapse produces "elephant trunk" appearance	Severe, complex anomaly
Limb–body wall complex	Multiple anomaly condition	Bizarre, complex defect with ventral wall defect, close attachment to placenta, cranial defects, scoliosis	100% lethal but no risk of aneuploidy

From Nyberg DA, McGahan JP, Pretorius DH, et al, editors. *Diagnostic Ultrasound of Fetal Anomalies: Text and Atlas*. Philadelphia: Lippincott Williams & Wilkins; 2003.

BOX 62.1 Differentiation of Omphalocele From Gastroschisis

The sonographer should investigate the following to differentiate an omphalocele from a gastroschisis:
- Look for the presence of a membrane; gastroschisis does not have one.
- Look at the umbilical cord; the cord goes through the omphalocele, whereas gastroschisis is found to the right of the cord.
- Determine which organs are eviscerated.
- Determine whether the bowel is normal in texture.
- Look for other anomalies because omphaloceles often occur with chromosomal abnormalities.

---

facial clefts, extensive abdominal wall defect of the chest, and abdomen and limb defects. Abnormal fusion of the amnion and chorion extends as a sheet from the cord and adheres to the fetus and placenta.

- Amniotic band syndrome may represent a milder form of limb–body wall complex and may be predicted by amniotic bands (fibrous tissue strands) that entangle or amputate fetal parts. Facial clefts, asymmetric encephaloceles, constriction or amputation defects of the extremities, and clubfoot deformities are common findings. Uterine sheets (synechiae) should not be confused with amniotic bands.
- Pentalogy of Cantrell is considered when a large omphalocele, diaphragmatic hernia, ectopia cordis (evisceration of heart), and other heart defects are observed.
- Consider bladder or cloacal exstrophy when a low omphalocele is observed. Other anomalies may include anal atresia, spina bifida, and lower-limb defects.
- When organomegaly and macroglossia are observed, Beckwith-Wiedemann syndrome is suspected (occurs in 12% of infants with an omphalocele).

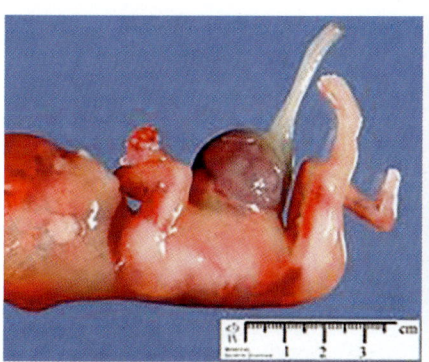 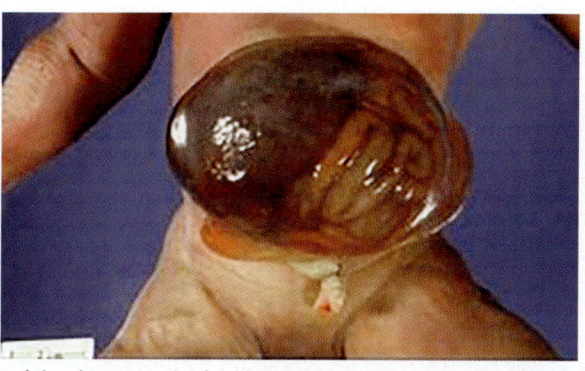 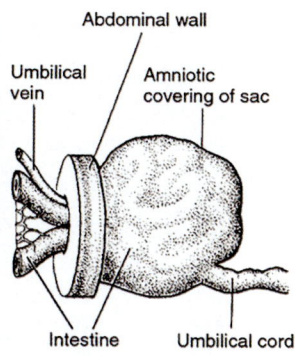

FIG. 62.4 During the 8th to 12th weeks of development, the fetal bowel normally migrates into the umbilical cord from the abdominal cavity. Because of the lack of space within the abdominal cavity and the large fetal liver and kidneys, the bowel is forced from the abdomen and into the extraembryonic coelom of the umbilical cord. These herniated loops of bowel normally return and rotate into position within the abdominal cavity by the 12th week of pregnancy. When bowel loops fail to return to the abdomen, a bowel-containing omphalocele occurs.

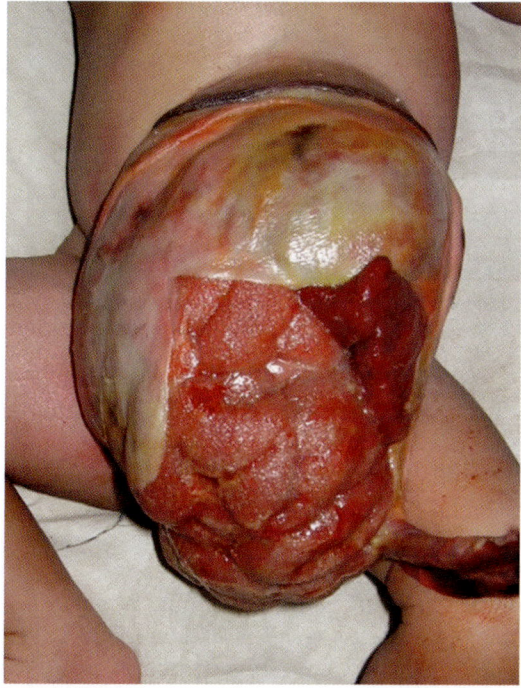

FIG. 62.5 Fetuses with an omphalocele that contains only a bowel have a higher risk for chromosomal abnormalities and other anomalies.

Gastroschisis

Gastroschisis is a small periumbilical defect that nearly always is located to the right of the umbilicus. The insertion of the umbilical cord is normal in fetuses with gastroschisis. This abnormality is an opening in the layers of the abdominal wall with evisceration (herniation) of the bowel and small bowel (Fig. 62.7). Other organs that may be involved in the herniation include the large bowel, the stomach, occasionally portions of the genitourinary system, and rarely the liver. Gastroschisis does not have a covering membrane as is found in omphalocele defects. AFP levels are significantly higher in gastroschisis compared with an omphalocele because of the exposed bowel. The occurrence of gastroschisis is 1.75 to 2.5 in 10,000 live births. It has been found more frequently in males.

It is thought that gastroschisis is a consequence of atrophy of the right umbilical vein or a disruption of the omphalomesenteric artery. Gastroschisis defects are usually not known to be genetically transmitted, although the recurrence risk for gastroschisis has been estimated at 3.5%.

Although coexisting anomalies are rare with gastroschisis, associated gastrointestinal problems may be of considerable medical consequence to the infant. This defect prevents the occurrence of normal bowel rotation, and intestinal atresia or stenosis may ensue because of ischemia (compression of mesenteric vessels or bowel torsion). Ischemia may cause bowel perforation or meconium peritonitis.

The obstetrician usually prefers to deliver the infant by cesarean section to prevent bowel damage and contamination from a vaginal delivery. The prognosis for the infant with uncomplicated gastroschisis is excellent. Surgical repair usually occurs within hours of delivery; with extensive defects, reconstruction is performed in stages using Silastic sheets.

Sonographic Findings. The sonographer may be able to detect gastroschisis after 12 weeks of gestation. The patient usually has a notably elevated maternal serum AFP level. As the sonographer evaluates the area of umbilical cord insertion, multiple loops of the bowel (small bowel and often colon) may be seen outside the abdominal cavity in the area of the cord. The cord is normally inserted into the abdominal wall, and the defect is almost always to the right of the umbilical cord insertion. The edges of the bowel are irregular and free floating without a covering membrane, as is seen with an omphalocele (Fig. 62.8). Ascites is not present in the abdominal cavity.

The sonographic appearance of gastroschisis is as follows:
- Right paraumbilical defect of abdominal wall, rarely a left-side defect.
- Free-floating herniated small bowel. Large bowel, stomach, gallbladder, urinary bladder, and pelvic organs may be involved. When organs other than small or large bowel are seen, body stalk anomalies should be suspected.
- A herniated bowel may be mildly dilated with a bowel wall thickening (chemical peritonitis because of irritation by urine within amniotic fluid) (Fig. 62.9). Dilation may be

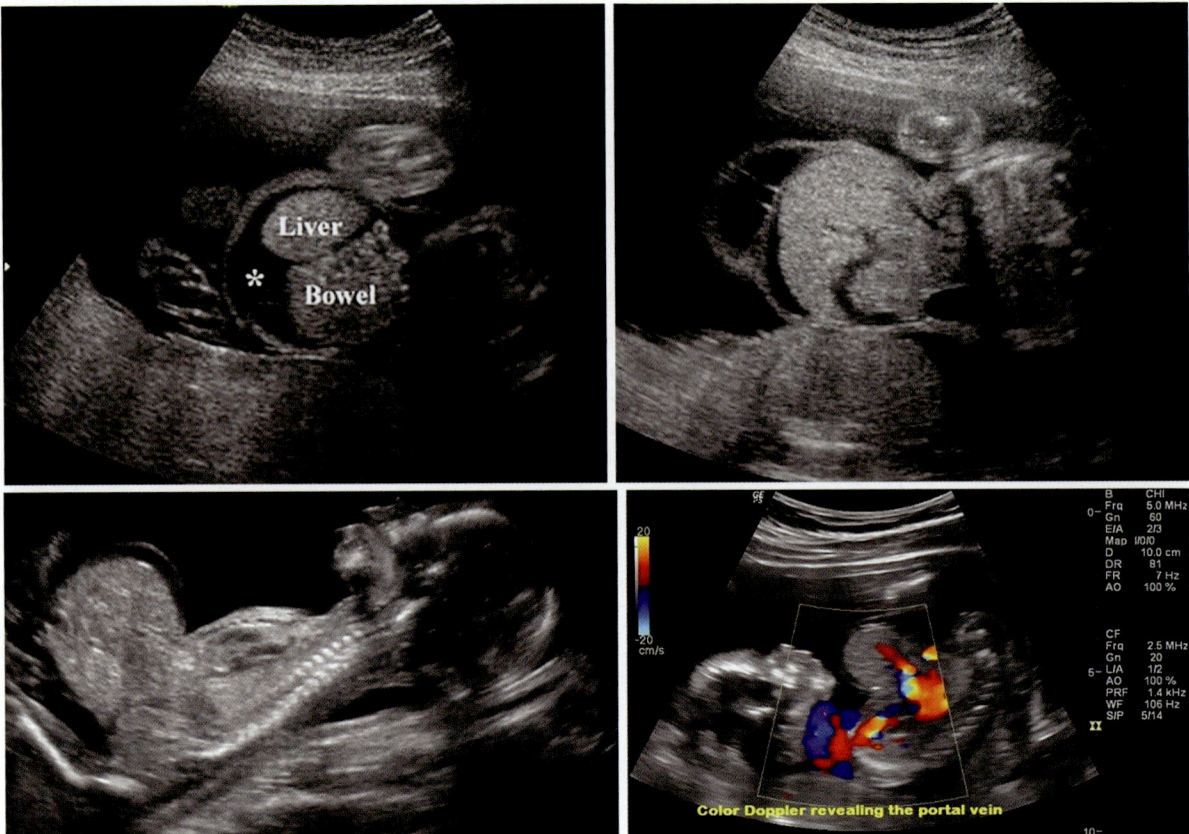

FIG. 62.6 **A liver omphalocele represents a developmental defect in abdominal wall closure.** This type of omphalocele affects the abdominal wall muscles, fascia, and skin. Liver omphaloceles may contain a bowel and demonstrate a relatively large abdominal wall defect in comparison with the abdominal diameter.

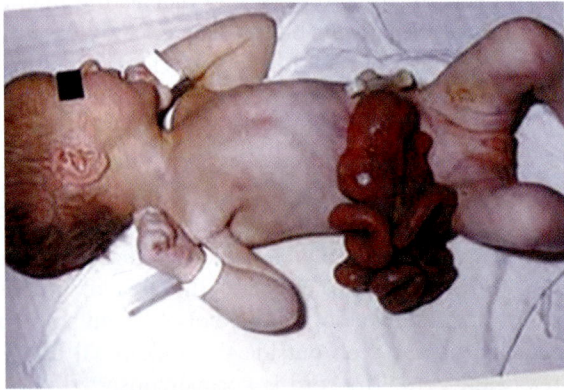

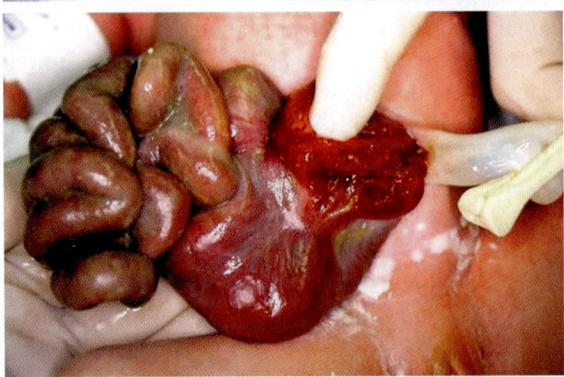

FIG. 62.7 Gastroschisis is a periumbilical defect that nearly always is located to the right of the umbilicus. This abnormality is an opening in the layers of the abdominal wall with evisceration (herniation) of the bowel and, infrequently, the stomach and genitourinary organs but rarely the liver.

seen in herniated portions of the bowel or within the fetal abdominal cavity.
- Notably dilated bowel may suggest infarction or bowel atresia.
- Hydronephrosis, bladder deviation, and exstrophy may be observed.
- Consider amniotic band syndrome amputations when clefting of the face or encephalocele is found. Severe body wall defects may be seen in gastroschisis with secondary band formation.

Amniotic Band Syndrome

Amniotic band syndrome is the rupture of the amnion, which leads to entrapment or entanglement of the fetal parts by the "sticky" chorion. This may cause amputation or defects in random sites. Early entrapment by the bands may lead to severe craniofacial defects and internal malformations (Fig. 62.10). Late entrapment leads to amputations or limb restrictions. The prevalence of this syndrome is low, occurring in 7.8 per 10,000 births. Anomalies associated with amniotic band syndrome include anomalies of the limbs, cranium, face, thorax, spine, abdominal wall (gastroschisis, omphalocele, bladder exstrophy), and perineum.

Beckwith-Wiedemann Syndrome

Beckwith-Wiedemann syndrome is a rare group of disorders having in common the coexistence of an omphalocele,

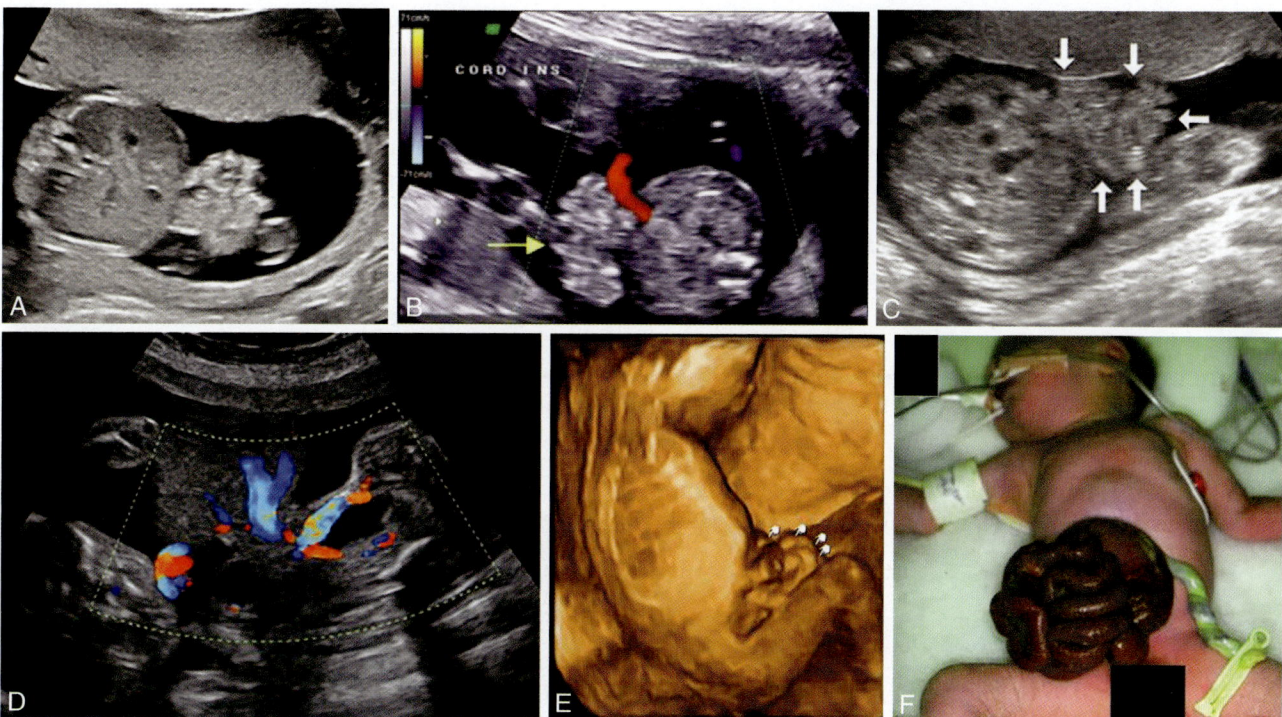

FIG. 62.8 (A–F) In gastroschisis, multiple loops of the bowel (small bowel and often colon) may be seen outside the abdominal cavity in the area of the cord. The cord is normally inserted into the abdominal wall, and the defect is almost always to the right of the umbilical cord insertion. The edges of the bowel are irregular and free floating without a covering membrane, as is seen with an omphalocele. (C–D, Courtesy Marcos Antonio Velasco Sanchez, copyright 2011.)

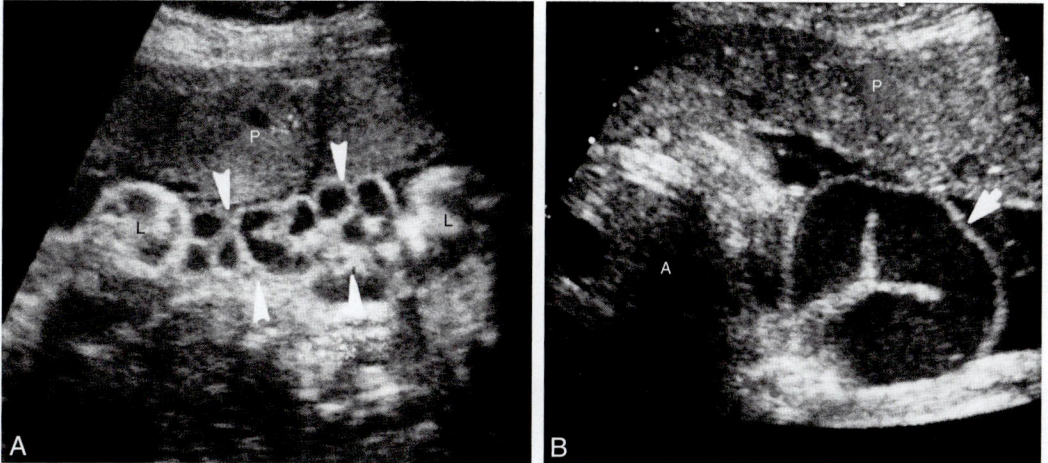

FIG. 62.9 (A) Gastroschisis showing herniated bowel *(arrowheads)* in the amniotic cavity. Cesarean section was performed at 36 weeks of gestation because of a nonreactive nonstress test with variable decelerations and absent breathing. A small-for-gestational-age infant with left-side gastroschisis was delivered. (B) Isolated bowel segment *(arrow)* observed in another fetus with gastroschisis at 29 weeks of gestation. Bowel dilation (29 mm) and obstruction (meconium ileus) are shown. Note the haustral markings within the obstructed bowel. *A*, Abdomen; *L*, limb; *P*, placenta.

macroglossia, and visceromegaly. Most of the cases are sporadic. Beckwith-Wiedemann syndrome is characterized by macrosomia, macroglossia, visceromegaly, embryonic tumors (i.e., Wilms tumor, hepatoblastoma, neuroblastoma, and rhabdomyosarcoma), an omphalocele, neonatal hypoglycemia, and ear creases. Sonographic findings usually note the presence of an omphalocele, growth acceleration, macroglossia, and visceromegaly (Fig. 62.11). In the third trimester, polyhydramnios may be present.

Bladder and Cloacal Exstrophy

Bladder exstrophy is characterized by a defect in the lower abdominal wall and anterior wall of the urinary bladder (Fig. 62.12). The everted bladder becomes exposed on the lower abdominal wall. The anomaly may be mild or severe (accompanied by an omphalocele, inguinal hernia, undescended testes, and anal problems). **Cloacal exstrophy** is rare and more complex than bladder exstrophy. This condition occurs early in development with involvement of the primitive gut and persistent cloaca. It results in exstrophy of the bladder in which two hemibladders are separated by intestinal mucosa.

Sonographic Findings. With bladder exstrophy, the normal urinary bladder is not visible on sonographic evaluation. Instead, a soft tissue mass, representing the exposed bladder mucosa, may be seen on the surface of the lower abdominal wall (Fig. 62.13). In addition, an anterior abdominal wall defect may be the primary ultrasound finding of cloacal exstrophy.

Pentalogy of Cantrell, Ectopia Cordis, and Cleft Sternum

The **pentalogy of Cantrell** is rare and is the association of a cleft distal sternum, diaphragmatic defect, midline anterior ventral wall defect, defect of the apical pericardium with communication into the peritoneum, and an internal cardiac defect. A high or superumbilical omphalocele is usually the primary finding of pentalogy of Cantrell (Fig. 62.14). If the diaphragmatic defect is large enough to produce a diaphragmatic hernia, displacement of the heart and mediastinum may be observed, but the sternal and pericardial defects are not well seen. The presence of pericardial effusion may be found. Pentalogy of Cantrell may be associated with various cardiac defects, cleft lip (may also have cleft palate), encephalocele, exencephaly, and sirenomelia. In the first trimester, cystic hygroma may be present. This has also been associated with trisomies 13 and 18 and 45,X (Turner syndrome).

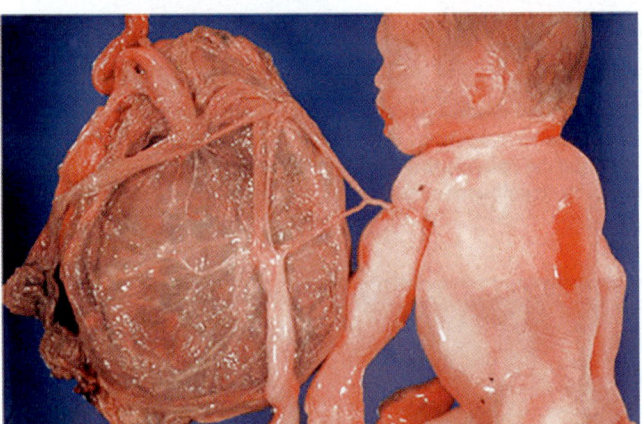

FIG. 62.10 Amniotic band syndrome is the rupture of the amnion, which leads to entrapment or entanglement of the fetal parts by the "sticky" chorion. This may cause amputation or defects in random sites. Anomalies associated with amniotic band syndrome include those of the limbs, cranium, face, thorax, spine, abdominal wall (gastroschisis, omphalocele, bladder exstrophy), and perineum.

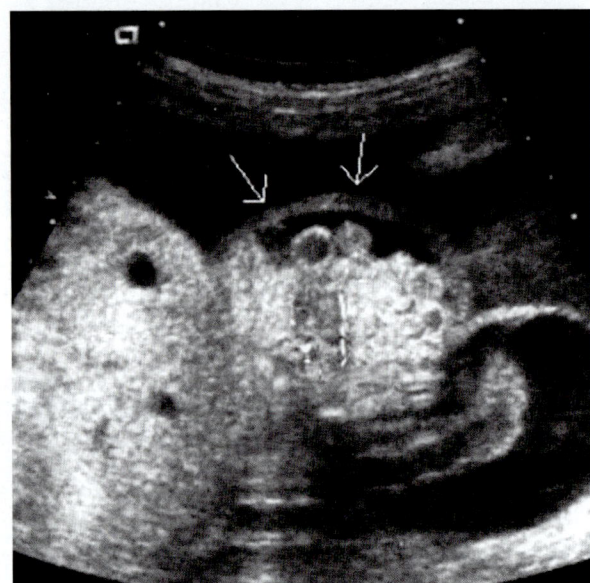

FIG. 62.11 Beckwith-Wiedemann syndrome is a rare group of disorders having in common the coexistence of an omphalocele *(arrows)*, macroglossia, and visceromegaly.

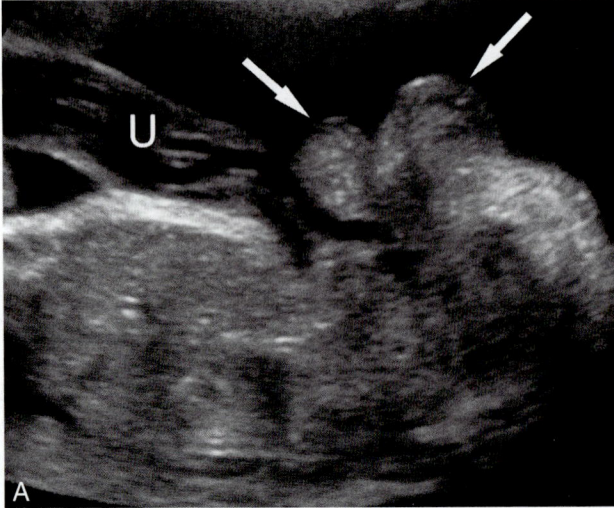

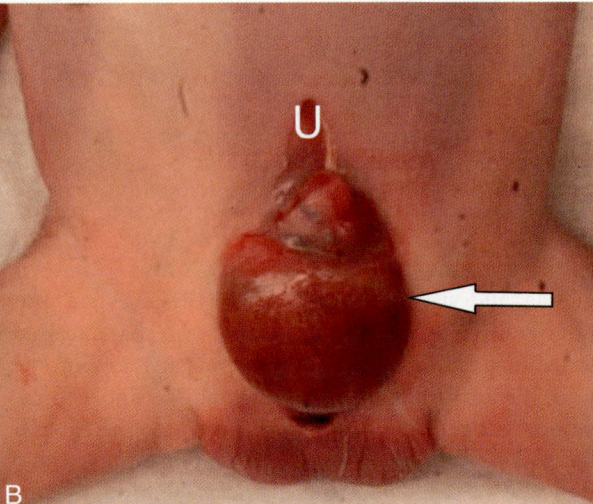

FIG. 62.12 Bladder exstrophy is characterized by a defect in the lower abdominal wall and anterior wall of the urinary bladder. The everted bladder becomes exposed on the lower abdominal wall *(arrows)*. *U*, Umbilical cord/umbilicus.

In ectopia cordis, the exposed heart presents outside the chest wall through a cleft sternum (Fig. 62.15). The most dramatic finding is the presence of a heart outside the thoracic cavity; a portion or all of the heart may protrude through the

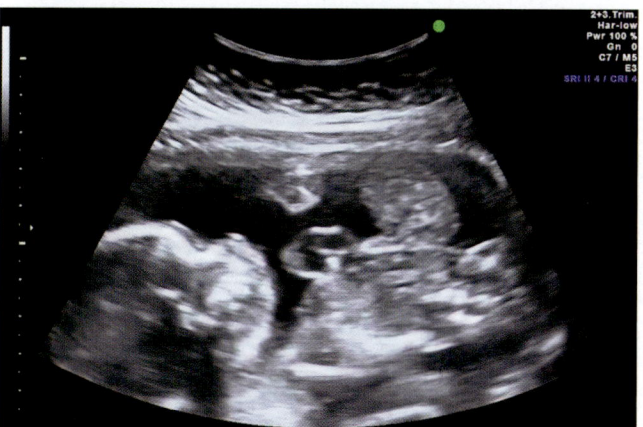

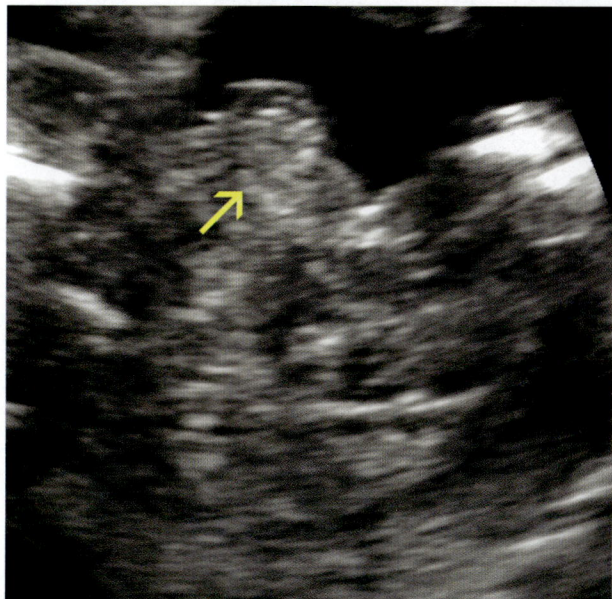

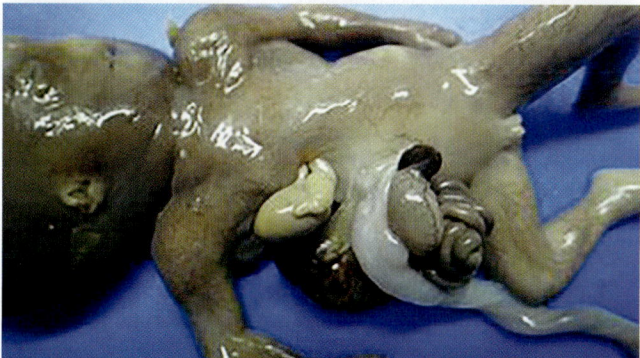

FIG. 62.13 With bladder exstrophy, the normal urinary bladder is not visible on sonographic evaluation. Instead, a soft tissue mass, representing the exposed bladder mucosa, may be seen on the surface of the lower abdominal wall.

FIG. 62.14 In pentalogy of Cantrell there is a cleft distal sternum, diaphragmatic defect, midline anterior ventral wall defect, defect of the apical pericardium, and cardiac defects.

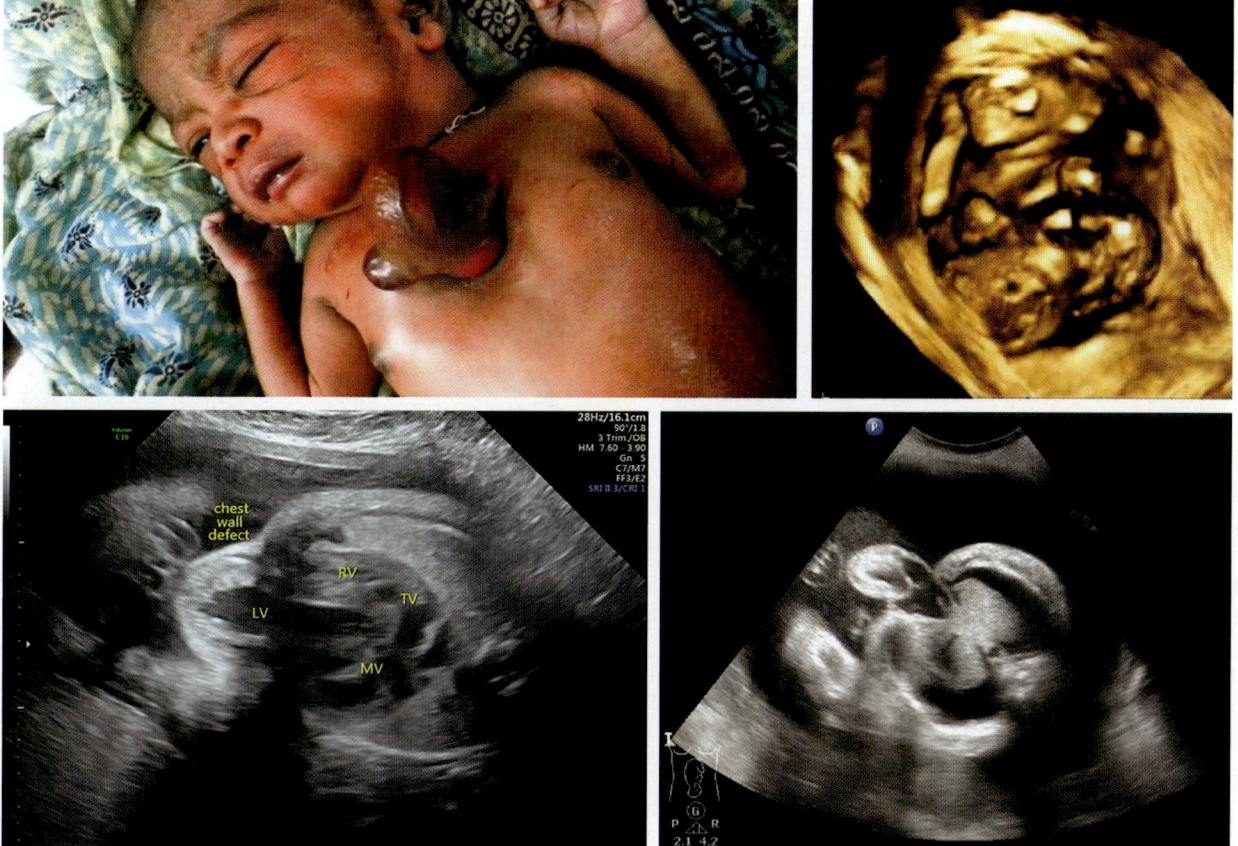

FIG. 62.15 In ectopia cordis, the exposed heart presents outside the chest wall through a cleft sternum. The most dramatic finding is the presence of a heart outside the thoracic cavity; a portion or all of the heart may protrude through the defect in the sternum. *LV*, Left ventricle; *MV*, mitral valve; *RV*, right ventricle; *TV*, tricuspid valve. (Courtesy Jaypraksh Shah Ahmedabad.)

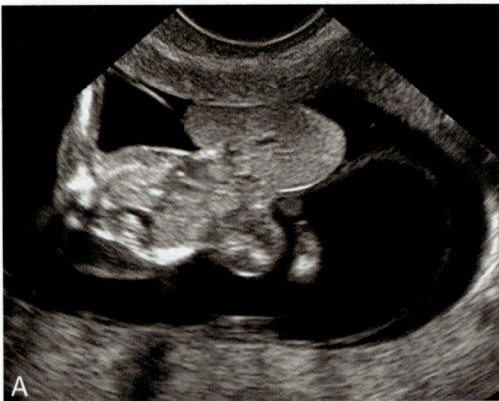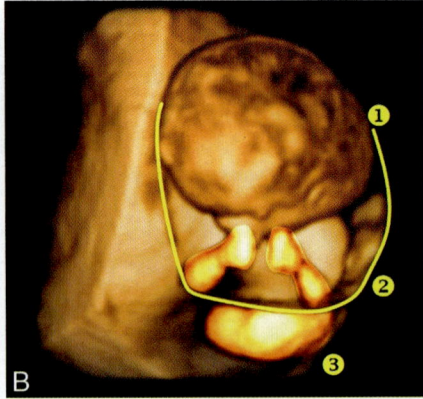

FIG. 62.16 (A–B) The limb–body wall complex anomaly is associated with large cranial defects (exencephaly or encephalocele); facial cleft; body wall complex defects involving the thorax, abdomen, or both; and limb defects. Other anomalies include scoliosis and various internal malformations. The limb–body wall complex occurs with the fusion of the amnion and chorion; the amnion does not cover the umbilical cord normally but extends as a sheet from the margin of the cord and is continuous with both the body wall and the placenta. *1*, Amnion; *2*, hands (not affected); *3*, liver.

defect in the sternum. Anomalies most frequently associated with ectopia cordis include an omphalocele, cardiovascular malformations, and craniofacial defects.

A cleft sternum may be either partial or absent without ectopia cordis and is typically a superior or total cleft. Dramatic pulsations of the anterior chest wall occur from the heart beating against the chest without the presence of the sternum to protect it. This condition is associated with vascular malformations, including cavernous hemangiomas and an omphalocele.

Sonographic Findings. On sonographic examination, the heart may be seen to lie outside the normal thoracic cavity or bulge through the defective sternum. It is common to see pericardial and pleural effusions. Differential considerations include body stalk anomaly, amniotic band syndrome, and isolated ectopia cordis. The prognosis depends on many factors, including the extent of the defect and the size of the thoracic cavity that allows surgical intervention to place the heart back into the chest.

Limb–Body Wall Complex

The **limb–body wall complex** anomaly is associated with large cranial defects (exencephaly or encephalocele); facial cleft; body wall complex defects involving the thorax, abdomen, or both; and limb defects. Other anomalies include scoliosis and various internal malformations. The limb–body wall complex occurs with the fusion of the amnion and chorion; the amnion does not cover the umbilical cord normally but extends as a sheet from the margin of the cord and is continuous with both the body wall and the placenta. Left-side body wall defects are 3 times more common than right-side defects.

Sonographic Findings. On ultrasound examination, the defects are large and involve the abdomen and thorax (Fig. 62.16). The eviscerated organs form a complex, bizarre-appearing mass entangled with membranes. The umbilical cord is short and adherent to the placental membranes.

Key Pearls

- By the end of the fifth week of development, an embryo is a flat disk consisting of three layers: ectoderm, mesoderm, and endoderm. In the sixth week, a process called *folding* helps the embryo to transform itself into a cylindrical shape. This transformation is a critical part of the process of closing the abdominal wall.
- Umbilication hernia of the bowel occurs during the eighth week of development as the midgut extends to the extraembryonic coelom in the proximal portion of the umbilical cord. During the 8th to 12th weeks of development, the fetal bowel normally migrates into the umbilical cord from the abdominal cavity.
- It is very important to image the cord insertion site and the fetal anterior abdominal wall to evaluate for the presence or absence of such abdominal wall defects.
- Abdominal wall defects cause distortion of the normal contour of the ventral or anterior surface of the fetal abdomen.
- The three most common abdominal wall defects are the omphalocele, umbilical hernia (a form of omphalocele), and gastroschisis.
- Rarer abdominal wall defects include ectopia cordis, pentalogy of Cantrell, limb–body wall complex, amnion rupture sequence, and bladder and cloacal exstrophy.
- An omphalocele develops when there is a midline defect of the abdominal muscles, fascia, and skin that results in herniation of intra-abdominal structures into the base of the umbilical cord.
- Omphaloceles are characterized as two types: (1) those that contain the liver within the sac and (2) those that contain a variable amount of bowel without liver.
- Fetuses with an omphalocele that contains only a bowel have a higher risk for chromosomal abnormalities and other anomalies.
- Gastroschisis is a periumbilical defect that nearly always is located to the right of the umbilicus. Gastroschisis is an

opening in the layers of the abdominal wall with evisceration (herniation) of the bowel and, infrequently, the stomach and genitourinary organs but rarely the liver.
- Gastroschisis defects are small (2–4 cm in size) and are located next to the normal cord insertion. In the majority of cases, the defect is positioned to the right of the umbilical cord.
- Amniotic band syndrome is the rupture of the amnion, which leads to entrapment or entanglement of the fetal parts by the "sticky" chorion.
- Beckwith-Wiedemann syndrome is characterized by macrosomia, macroglossia, visceromegaly, embryonic tumors (i.e., Wilms tumor, hepatoblastoma, neuroblastoma, and rhabdomyosarcoma), an omphalocele, neonatal hypoglycemia, and ear creases.
- Bladder exstrophy is characterized by a defect in the lower abdominal wall and anterior wall of the urinary bladder.
- The pentalogy of Cantrell is rare and is the association of a cleft distal sternum, diaphragmatic defect, midline anterior ventral wall defect, defect of the apical pericardium with communication into the peritoneum, and an internal cardiac defect.
- In ectopia cordis, the exposed heart presents outside the chest wall through a cleft sternum.
- The limb–body wall complex anomaly is associated with large cranial defects (exencephaly or encephalocele); facial cleft; body wall complex defects involving the thorax, abdomen, or both; and limb defects.

BIBLIOGRAPHY

Barnewolt CT. Congenital abnormalities of the gastrointestinal tract. *Semin Roentgenol.* 2004;39(2):263–281.

Bonilla-Musoles F, Machado LE, Bailao LA, et al. Abdominal wall defects: two- versus three-dimensional ultrasonographic diagnosis. *J Ultrasound Med.* 2001;20(4):379–389.

Chen CP, Lin SP, Hwu YM, et al. Prenatal identification of fetal overgrowth, abdominal wall defect, and neural tube defect in pregnancies achieved by assisted reproductive technology. *Prenat Diagn.* 2004;24(5):396–398.

Davenport M, Haugen S, Greenough A, et al. Closed gastroschisis: antenatal and postnatal features. *J Pediatr Surg.* 2001;36(12):1834–1837.

Fong KW, Toi A, Hornberger LK, et al. Detection of fetal structural abnormalities with US during early pregnancy. *Radiographics.* 2004;24(1):157–174.

Gibbin C, Touch S, Broth RE, et al. Abdominal wall defects and congenital heart disease. *Ultrasound Obstet Gynecol.* 2003;21(4):334–337.

Hossain GA, Islam SM, Mahmood S, et al. Abdominal wall defect: a case report and review. *Mymensigh Med J.* 2003;12(1):64–68.

Kiliedag EB, Kilieday H, Bagis T, et al. Large pseudocyst of the umbilical cord associated with patent urachus. *J Obstet Gynecol Res.* 2004;30(6):444–447.

Leon G, Chedrau P, San Miguel G. Prenatal diagnosis of Cantrell's pentalogy with conventional and three-dimensional sonography. *J Matern Fetal Neonatal Med.* 2002;12(3):209–211.

Salihu HM, Boos R, Schmidt W. Omphalocele and gastroschisis. *J Obstet Gynaecol.* 2002;22(5):489–492.

Salvesen KA. Fetal abdominal wall defects—easy to diagnose—and then what? *Ultrasound Obstet Gynecol.* 2001;18(4):301–304.

Wu JL, Fang KH, Yeh GP, et al. Using color Doppler sonography to identify the perivesical umbilical arteries: a useful method in the prenatal diagnosis of omphalocele-exstrophy-imperforate anus-spinal defects complex. *J Ultrasound Med.* 2004;23(9):1211–1215.

CHAPTER 63

The Fetal Abdomen

Sandra L. Hagen-Ansert

OBJECTIVES

On completion of this chapter, you should be able to:
- Describe the development of the digestive system and list the unique features of the fetal abdomen
- Describe normal development of the stomach and the importance of its sonographic visualization
- Define abnormalities of the fetal gastrointestinal tract and hepatobiliary system and describe their sonographic findings

OUTLINE

Embryology of the Digestive System 1572
- The Foregut 1573
- The Midgut 1574
- Malformations of the Midgut 1575
- The Hindgut 1576

Sonographic Evaluation of the Abdominal Cavity 1576
- Gastrointestinal System 1576

Hepatobiliary System 1579

Abnormalities of the Hepatobiliary System 1580
- Liver 1580
- Situs Inversus 1581
- Pseudoascites 1581
- Gallbladder 1582
- Pancreas 1583
- Spleen 1583

Abnormalities of the Gastrointestinal Tract 1584
- Esophagus, Stomach, and Duodenum 1584
- Bowel 1586

Miscellaneous Cystic Masses of the Abdomen 1590

KEY TERMS

Anorectal atresia
Asplenia
Choledochal cyst
Cholelithiasis
Cystic fibrosis
Duodenal atresia
Duodenal stenosis
Esophageal atresia

Esophageal stenosis
Gastroschisis
Haustral folds
Hemopoiesis
Hirschsprung disease (megacolon)
Jejunoileal atresia
Meckel's diverticulum
Meconium ileus

Omphalocele
Partial situs inversus
Peristalsis
Polysplenia
Pseudoascites
Situs inversus
VACTERL

The fetal abdominal organs—liver, biliary system, spleen, stomach, kidneys, and colon—are well formed by the second trimester. The following differences between the fetal and neonatal/pediatric abdomen have been noted:

- The umbilical arteries and veins provide important anatomic landmarks for fetal abdominal anatomy and measurements.
- The ductus venosus is patent and serves as a conduit between the portal veins and systemic veins.
- The proportions of the fetal body differ from those in the pediatric abdomen. The fetal abdomen is larger relative to body length, and the liver occupies a larger volume of the fetal abdomen.
- The fetal pelvic cavity is small; therefore, the urinary bladder, ovaries, and uterus lie in the abdominal cavity.
- The apron of the greater omentum is small, contains little fat, and remains unfused in the fetus. Fetal ascites may therefore separate the omental leaves.

EMBRYOLOGY OF THE DIGESTIVE SYSTEM

The primitive gut forms during the fourth week of gestation as the dorsal part of the yolk sac is incorporated into the embryo during folding (Fig. 63.1). The primitive gut is divided into three sections: foregut, midgut, and hindgut (Fig. 63.2).

The Foregut

The derivatives of the foregut are the pharynx, lower respiratory system, esophagus, stomach, part of the duodenum, liver and biliary apparatus, and pancreas (Fig. 63.3).

Esophagus. The esophagus is short in the beginning, but it rapidly lengthens as the body grows, reaching its final length by the seventh week (see Fig. 63.3). The *tracheoesophageal septum* partitions the trachea from the esophagus. **Esophageal atresia**, usually associated with a tracheoesophageal fistula, results from abnormal deviation of the tracheoesophageal septum in a posterior direction. When this occurs, amniotic fluid cannot pass to the intestines for absorption and hydramnios results.

Esophageal stenosis is the narrowing of the esophagus, usually in the distal third portion. This occurs from incomplete recanalization of the esophagus during the eighth week of development.

Stomach. The stomach appears as a fusiform dilation of the caudal part of the foregut. During the fifth and sixth weeks, the dorsal border (greater curvature) grows faster than the ventral border (lesser curvature) (see Fig. 63.3). The stomach is suspended from the dorsal wall of the abdominal cavity by the dorsal mesentery or dorsal mesogastrium. The dorsal

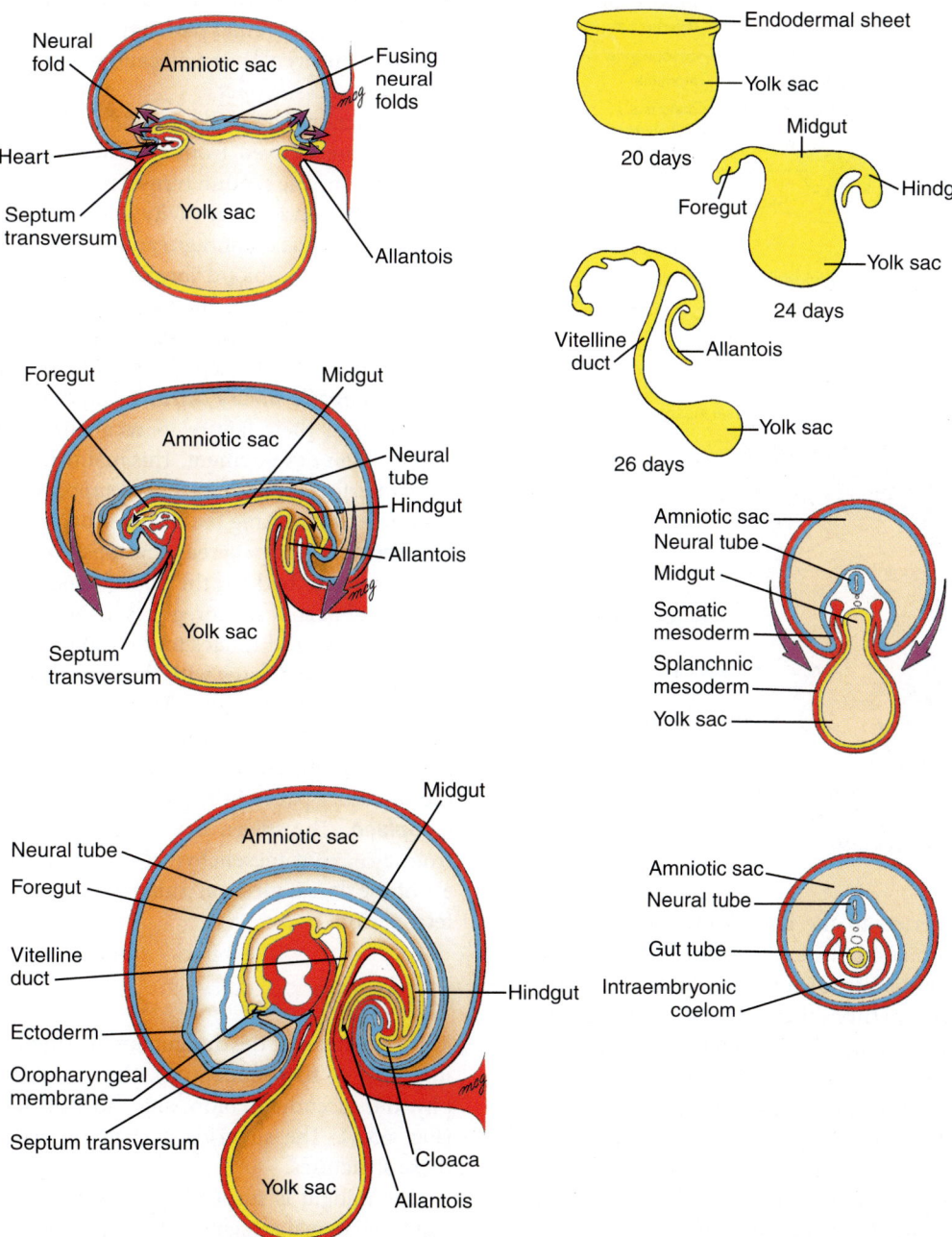

FIG. 63.1 The primitive gut forms during the fourth week of gestation as the dorsal part of the yolk sac is incorporated into the embryo during folding.

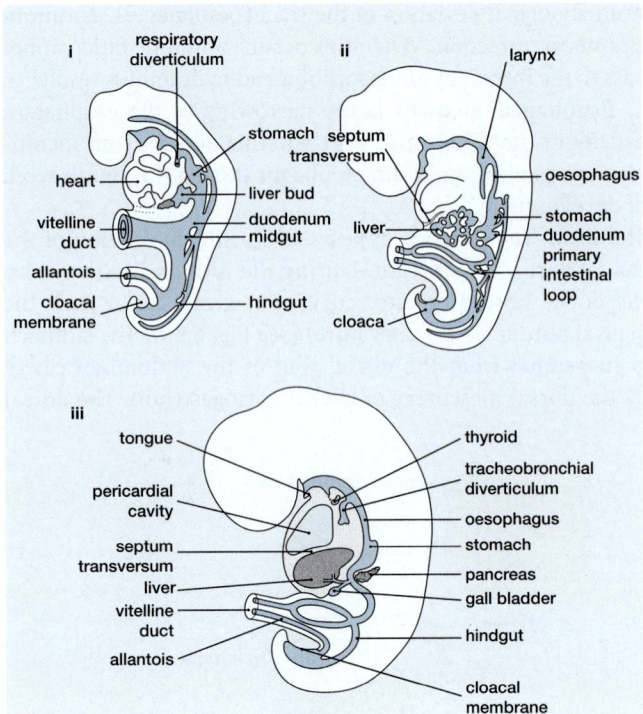

FIG. 63.2 The primitive gut is divided into three sections: foregut, midgut, and hindgut.

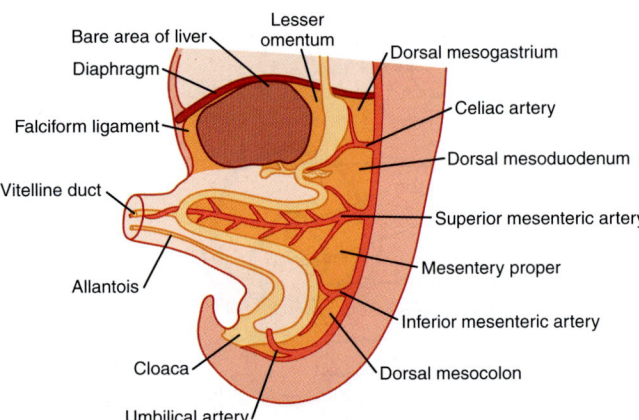

FIG. 63.3 The derivatives of the foregut are the pharynx, lower respiratory system, esophagus, stomach, part of the duodenum, liver and biliary apparatus, and pancreas.

mesogastrium is carried to the left during rotation of the stomach and the formation of a cavity known as the omental bursa or lesser sac of the peritoneum. The lesser sac communicates with the main peritoneal cavity or greater peritoneal sac through a small opening called the epiploic foramen.

Duodenum. The duodenum develops from the caudal part of the foregut and the cranial part of the midgut. The two parts grow rapidly and form a C-shaped loop that rotates to the right, where it comes to lie primarily in the retroperitoneum. The junction of the two embryonic parts of the duodenum in the adult is just distal to the entrance of the common bile duct. The duodenum is supplied by branches of the celiac trunk and the superior mesenteric artery (see Fig. 63.3).

During the fifth and sixth weeks, the lumen of the duodenum becomes partly or totally occluded (depending on the proliferation of its lining of epithelial cells). Normally the duodenum is recanalized by the end of the eighth week. Partial or complete failure of this process results in either **duodenal stenosis** (narrowing) or **duodenal atresia** (blockage). Usually, the third or fourth parts of the duodenal are affected.

Liver and Biliary System. The liver, gallbladder, and biliary ducts arise as a bud from the most caudal part of the foregut in the fourth week (see Fig. 63.3). The hepatic diverticulum grows between the layers of the ventral mesentery, where it rapidly enlarges and divides into two parts. The liver grows rapidly and intermingles with the vitelline and umbilical veins, divides into two parts, and fills most of the abdominal cavity. The large cranial part is the primordium of the parenchyma of the liver. The small caudal part gives rise to the gallbladder and cystic duct.

The hemopoietic cells, Kupffer cells, and connective tissue cells are derived from the mesenchyme in the septum transversum. The septum transversum is a mass of mesoderm between the pericardial cavity and the yolk stalk. It forms a major part of the diaphragm and the ventral mesentery.

Hemopoiesis (blood formation) begins during the sixth week and accounts for the large size of the liver between the seventh and ninth weeks of development. By the twelfth week, bile formation by the hepatic cells has begun.

Extrahepatic Biliary Atresia. Blockage of the bile ducts results from their failure to recanalize following the solid stage of their development. This malformation may also result from interference with the blood supply of the ducts resulting from infection during the fetal period.

Pancreas. The pancreas develops from the dorsal and ventral pancreatic buds of the endodermal cells that arise from the caudal part of the foregut (see Fig. 63.3). When the duodenum grows and rotates to the right, the ventral bud is carried dorsally and fuses with the dorsal bud. The ducts of the two pancreatic buds join. The combined duct becomes the main pancreatic duct that opens with the bile duct into the duodenum. The proximal part of the duct may persist as the accessory pancreatic duct.

Spleen. The spleen is a lymphatic organ that is derived from a mass of mesenchymal cells located between the layers of the dorsal mesogastrium. The spleen is lobulated in the fetal period.

The Midgut

The derivatives of the midgut are the small intestines (including most of the duodenum), the cecum and cloaca exstrophy, the ascending colon, and most of the transverse colon (Fig. 63.4). The superior mesenteric artery supplies all of these structures.

The midgut is suspended from the abdominal wall by an elongated dorsal mesentery. It communicates with the yolk sac via the yolk stalk. While the midgut lengthens and forms a midgut loop, it herniates outside the abdomen into the proximal part of the umbilical cord. Usually, by the 10th or 11th week, this midgut herniation returns to the abdomen and undergoes further rotation resulting from the decrease in size of the liver and kidneys and the growth of the abdominal cavity.

After the intestines return to the abdominal cavity, they enlarge, lengthen, and assume their final positions. Their mesenteries are pressed against the posterior abdominal wall. At this time, the ascending colon and descending colon become retroperitoneal. Likewise, the duodenum and most of the pancreas also become retroperitoneal structures. At the same time, the small intestines form a new line of attachment that extends from where the duodenum becomes retroperitoneal to the ileocecal junction. The mesentery of the transverse colon fuses with the dorsal mesogastrium to form the posterior wall of the inferior part of the omental bursa. The sigmoid colon retains its mesentery, but it is shorter than in the early fetus.

Malformations of the Midgut

Omphalocele and Gastroschisis. Omphalocele and gastroschisis are defects that occur when the midgut fails to return to the abdominal cavity from the umbilical cord during the 10th week (Fig. 63.5). In an **omphalocele**, coils of the intestine protrude from the umbilicus and are covered by a transparent sac of amnion. The umbilical cord pierces the central part of the omphalocele. Conversely, a **gastroschisis** is a condition

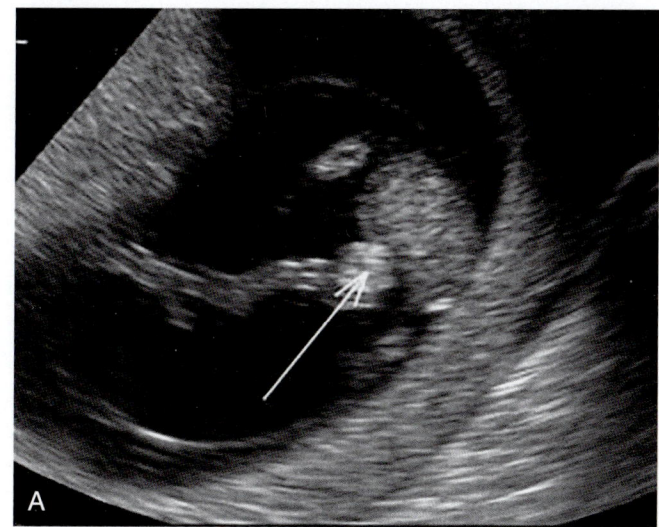

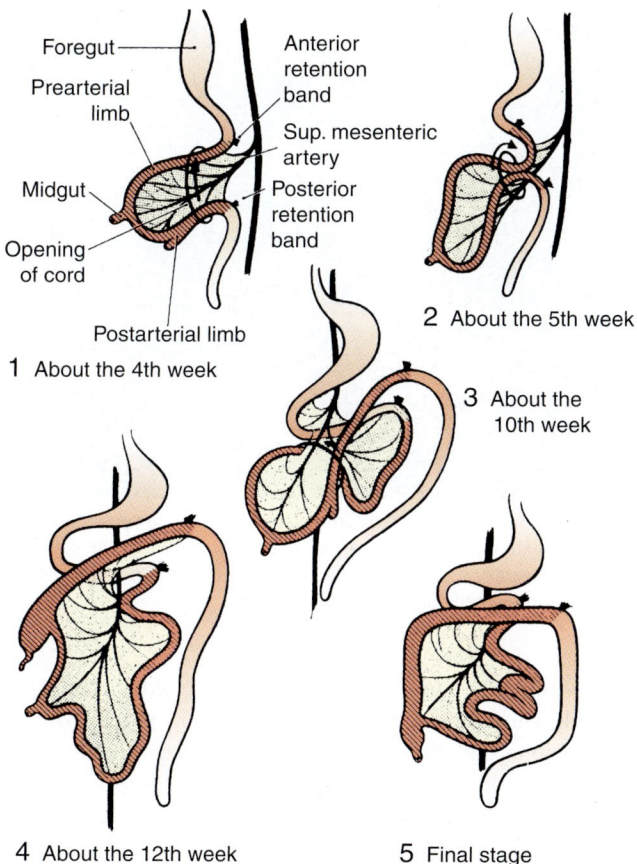

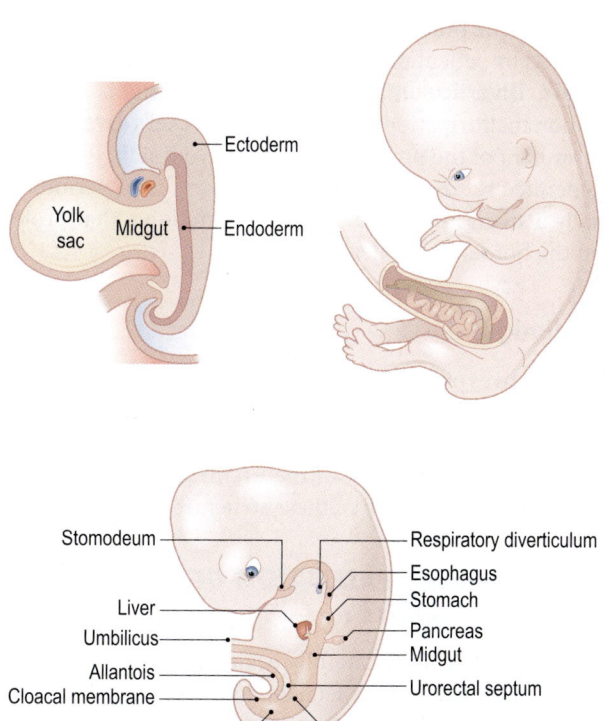

FIG. 63.4 (A) The midgut is suspended from the abdominal wall by an elongated dorsal mesentery. It communicates with the yolk sac via the yolk stalk. While the midgut lengthens and forms a midgut loop, it herniates outside the abdomen into the proximal part of the umbilical cord. Usually, by the 10th or 11th week, this midgut herniation returns to the abdomen and undergoes further rotation resulting from the decrease in size of the liver and kidneys and the growth of the abdominal cavity. (B) The derivatives of the midgut are the small intestines (including most of the duodenum), the cecum and cloaca exstrophy, the ascending colon, and most of the transverse colon. The superior mesenteric artery supplies all of these structures.

FIG. 63.5 Omphalocele and gastroschisis are defects that occur when the midgut fails to return to the abdominal cavity from the umbilical cord during the 10th week. In an omphalocele, coils of the intestine protrude from the umbilicus and are covered by a transparent sac of amnion. The umbilical cord pierces the central part of the omphalocele. Conversely, a gastroschisis is a condition in which the bowel or organs are free floating from the midline defect.

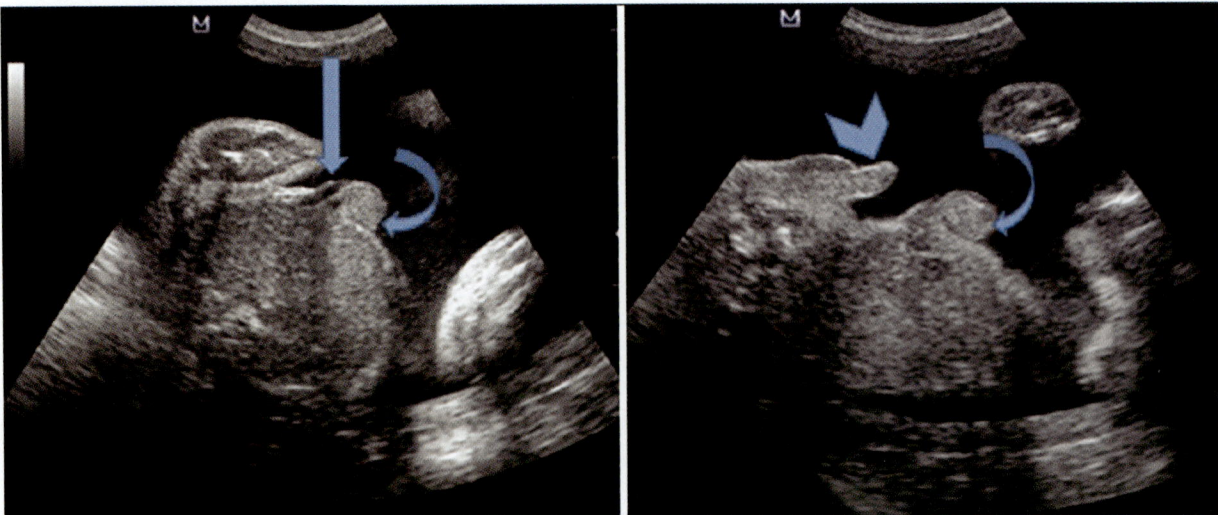

FIG. 63.6 The hernia differs from an omphalocele in that the protruding mass (omentum or loop of bowel) is visualized *(curved arrow)*. The hernia is covered by subcutaneous tissue and skin *(straight arrow)*.

in which the bowel or organs are free floating from the midline defect. The gastroschisis is usually located to the right of the umbilical cord. (See Chapter 62 for further discussion of omphalocele and gastroschisis.)

Umbilical Hernia. When the intestines return, normally to the abdominal cavity and then herniate either prenatally or postnatally through an inadequately closed umbilicus, an umbilical hernia forms. The hernia differs from an omphalocele in that the protruding mass (omentum or loop of bowel) is covered by subcutaneous tissue and skin (Fig. 63.6).

Meckel's Diverticulum. Meckel's diverticulum is the most common malformation of the midgut. **Meckel's diverticulum** is a remnant of the proximal part of the yolk stalk that fails to degenerate and disappear during the early fetal period. It is usually a small finger-like sac, about 5 cm long, that projects from the border of the ileum (Fig. 63.7).

The Hindgut

The derivatives of the hindgut are the left part of the transverse colon, the descending colon, the sigmoid colon, the rectum, the superior portion of the anal canal, the epithelium of the urinary bladder, and most of the urethra. The inferior mesenteric artery supplies all of these structures (see Fig. 63.2).

SONOGRAPHIC EVALUATION OF THE ABDOMINAL CAVITY

The sonographer must carefully evaluate the gastrointestinal system during the routine fetal anatomy sonographic examination. The stomach, liver, vascular structures, cord insertion, small bowel, and colon should be clearly identified.

Gastrointestinal System

Stomach. The stomach should be identified as a fluid-filled structure in the *left* upper quadrant inferior to the diaphragm. A marked variation in the size of the stomach can be seen,

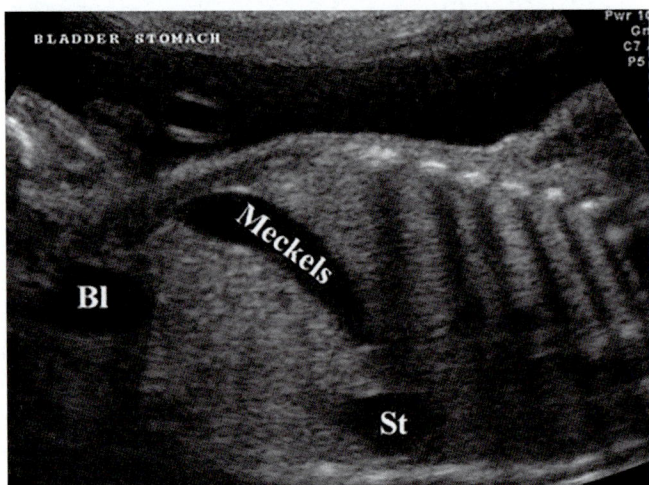

FIG. 63.7 Meckel's diverticulum is a remnant of the proximal part of the yolk stalk that fails to degenerate and disappear during the early fetal period. It is usually a small finger-like sac, about 5 cm long, that projects from the border of the ileum.

even within the same fetus. Most fetuses older than 14 to 16 weeks should have fluid in their stomach (Fig. 63.8). If no fluid is apparent, the stomach should be reevaluated in 20 to 30 minutes to rule out the possibility of a central nervous system problem (swallowing disorders), obstruction, oligohydramnios, or atresia. If fluid is still not noted during the sonographic evaluation, the fetus may be reexamined the following day or week to see if there has been a change in the size of the stomach. Esophageal anomalies are the least common problem for nonvisualization of the stomach.

The fluid within the stomach should be anechoic with linear rugae in the normal fetus. Echogenic debris may sometimes be seen along the dependent wall of the stomach that may represent vernix, protein, or intraamniotic hemorrhage (Fig. 63.9). The presence of an echogenic mass in the fetal stomach in a patient who demonstrates clinical or sonographic evidence of placental abruption should raise the possibility

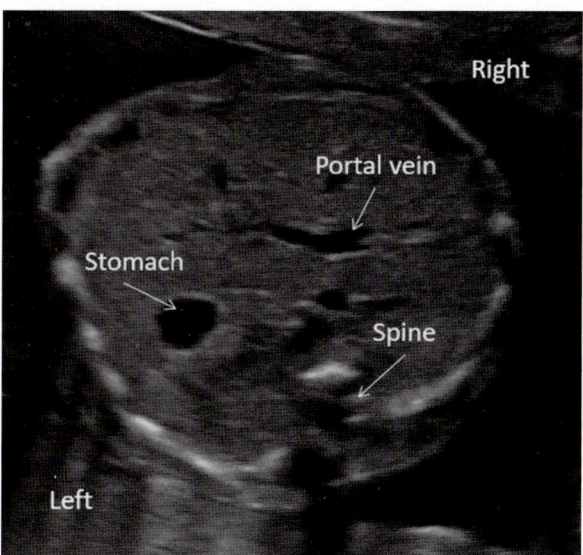

FIG. 63.8 The stomach should be identified as a fluid-filled structure in the left upper quadrant inferior to the diaphragm. A marked variation in the size of the stomach can be seen, even within the same fetus. Most fetuses older than 14 to 16 weeks should have fluid in the stomach.

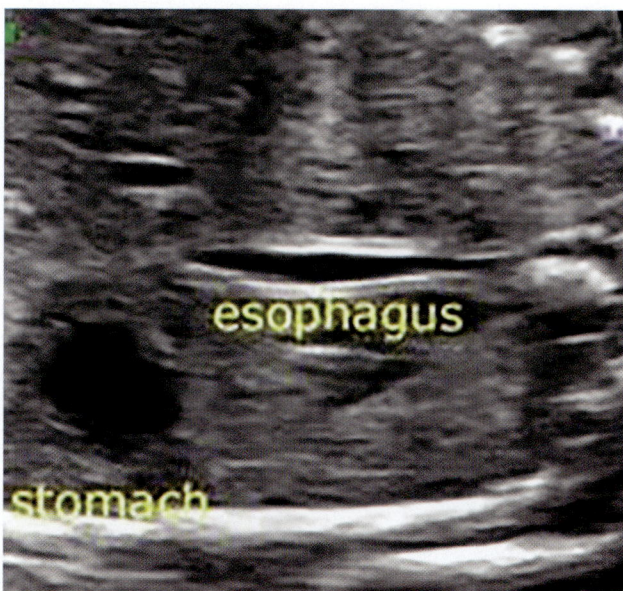

FIG. 63.10 The normal esophagus can be visualized in the thorax during the second and third trimesters as two or more parallel echogenic structures.

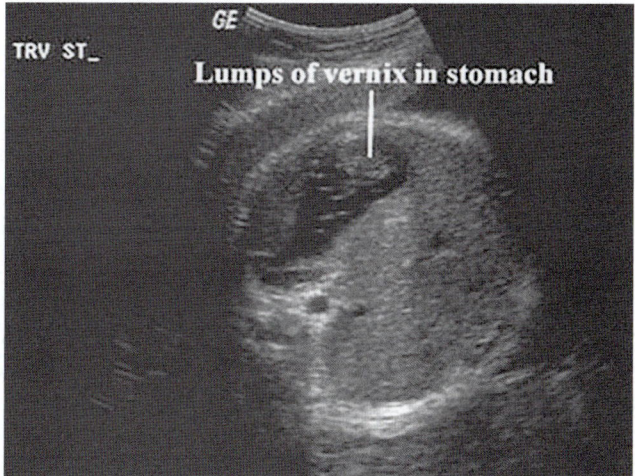

FIG. 63.9 Echogenic debris may sometimes be seen along the dependent wall of the stomach that may represent vernix *(arrow)*, protein, or intra-amniotic hemorrhage.

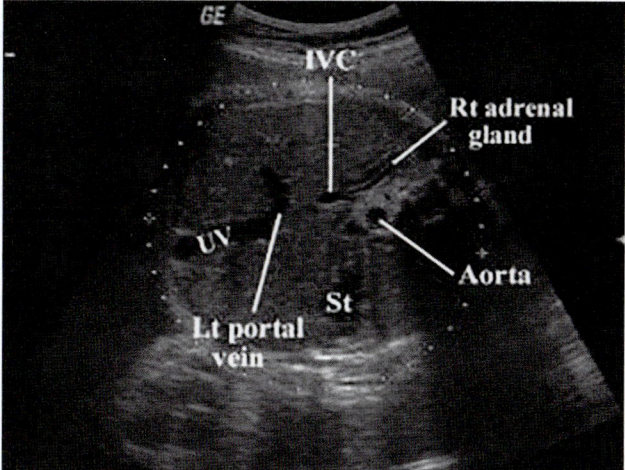

FIG. 63.11 The abdominal circumference is measured at the level of the portal sinus and the umbilical portion of the left portal vein, which has a "hockey stick" appearance on the sonogram. *IVC,* Inferior vena cava; *St,* stomach; *UV,* umbilical vein.

of hematoma formation associated with an intraamniotic hemorrhage.

Although the fetal stomach is usually located on the left of the abdomen, there are conditions in which the stomach will be seen in the right upper quadrant (**situs inversus**). The fetal position must be identified, followed by the identification of the right and left sides of the fetus. If the fetus is in a vertex presentation with the spine up, the aorta and stomach both should be seen to the left of the spine.

Esophagus. The normal esophagus can be visualized in the thorax during the second and third trimesters as two or more parallel echogenic lines (multilayered pattern) (Fig. 63.10). Sometimes it is possible to see fluid in the esophagus as the fetus swallows the amniotic fluid.

Abdominal Circumference. The abdominal circumference is measured at the level of the portal sinus and the umbilical portion of the left portal vein, which has a "hockey stick" appearance on the sonogram (Fig. 63.11). Be careful to avoid oblique scanning of the abdomen that may lead to an incorrect diameter-circumference measurement. The abdomen should be round, not oval. The pressure of the transducer should not compress the abdominal cavity.

Umbilical Cord Insertion. In the fetus, the umbilical vein courses cephalically in the free, inferior margin of the falciform ligament. It joins the umbilical portion of the left portal vein at the caudal margin of the left intersegmental fissure of the liver (Fig. 63.12). The insertion of the umbilical cord

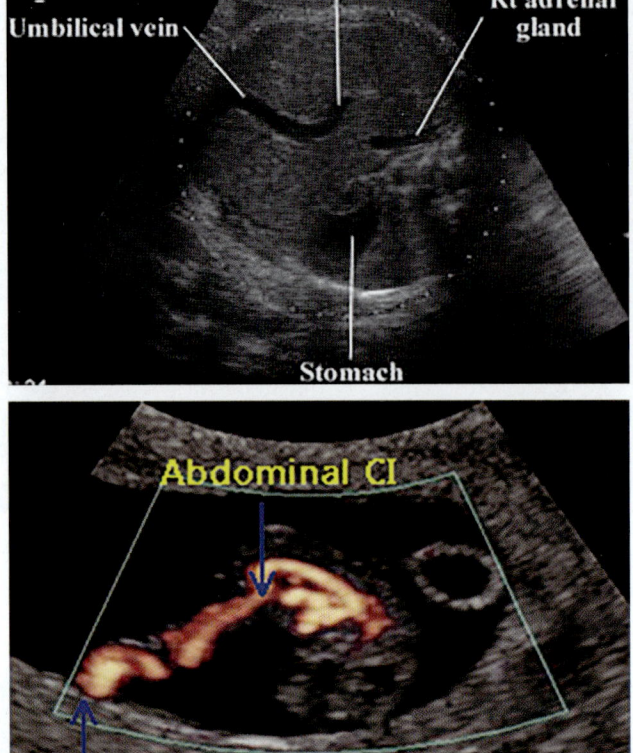
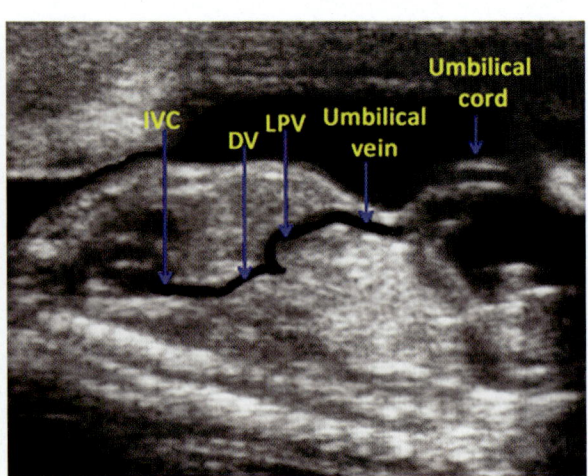

FIG. 63.12 The umbilical vein courses cephalically in the free, inferior margin of the falciform ligament. It joins the umbilical portion of the left portal vein at the caudal margin of the left intersegmental fissure of the liver. The insertion of the umbilical cord must be imaged with color because it inserts into both the fetal abdomen and the placenta. *CI*, Cord insertion; *DV*, ductus venosus; *IVC*, inferior vena cava; *LPV*, left portal vein.

must be imaged with color because it inserts into both the fetal abdomen and the placenta. Visualization of the umbilical cord insertion site must be made to rule out the presence of an omphalocele, gastroschisis, hernia, or mass formation. After birth, the umbilical vein collapses and ultimately becomes the ligamentum teres hepatis.

Bowel. Movement of the gastric musculature begins in approximately the fourth to fifth month of gestation. The sonographic appearance of the bowel varies with menstrual age. The fetus is capable of swallowing sufficient amounts of amniotic fluid to permit visualization of the stomach by 11 menstrual weeks. In the second trimester, this movement and fetal swallowing result in the delivery of increased amniotic fluid volume distally into the small bowel and colon, where fluid and nutrients are reabsorbed. After the 15th to 16th week, meconium begins to accumulate in the distal part of the small intestine as a combination of desquamated cells, bile pigments, and mucoproteins.

Until the mid-second trimester, the small bowel lumen is quite difficult to demonstrate and appears as an ill-defined area of increased echogenicity in the mid to lower abdomen. The distinction of the large bowel from the small bowel is possible after 20 menstrual weeks. The region of the small bowel can be seen because it is slightly hyperechoic compared with the liver and may appear mass-like in the central abdomen and pelvis (Fig. 63.13). The hyperechoic appearance could be secondary to reflections from the walls of collapsed loops of the small bowel or from mesenteric fat between the loops. This hyperechoic appearance of the small bowel persists throughout the pregnancy. As the pregnancy progresses, the hyperechoic area becomes less prominent, and the small bowel is located more centrally in the abdomen than the colon. After 27 weeks, **peristalsis** of the normal small bowel is increasingly observed. The normal diameter of the small bowel lumen is less than or equal to 5 mm, with a length of 15 mm near term.

The colon is seen near the end of the second trimester as a long tubular hypoechoic structure with well-defined walls. The **haustral folds** of the colon help to differentiate it from the small bowel. In early gestation, haustral folds appear as thin linear echoes within the lumen of the colon; later, the colon diameter increases, and the folds become longer and thicker. Normal measurements of the colon diameter range from 3 to 5 mm at 20 weeks to 23 mm or larger at term. The colon is more peripheral than the small bowel. Hypoechoic echoes from the meconium may be seen within the lumen. The colon does not have peristalsis like the small bowel.

After 14 weeks of gestation, the lipid is absorbed from the fetal colon, and the remaining contents collect in the colon as meconium. The meconium within the lumen of the colon

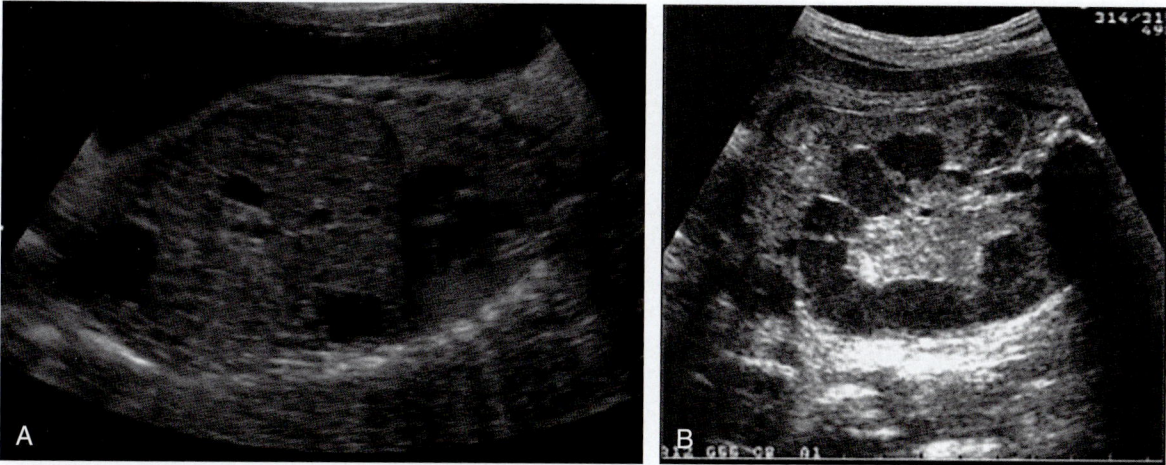

FIG. 63.13 (A) The region of the small bowel *(arrow)* can be seen because it is slightly hyperechoic compared with the liver and may appear mass-like in the central abdomen and pelvis. (B) The colon is seen near the end of the second trimester as a long tubular hypoechoic structure with well-defined walls. The haustral folds of the colon help to differentiate it from the small bowel.

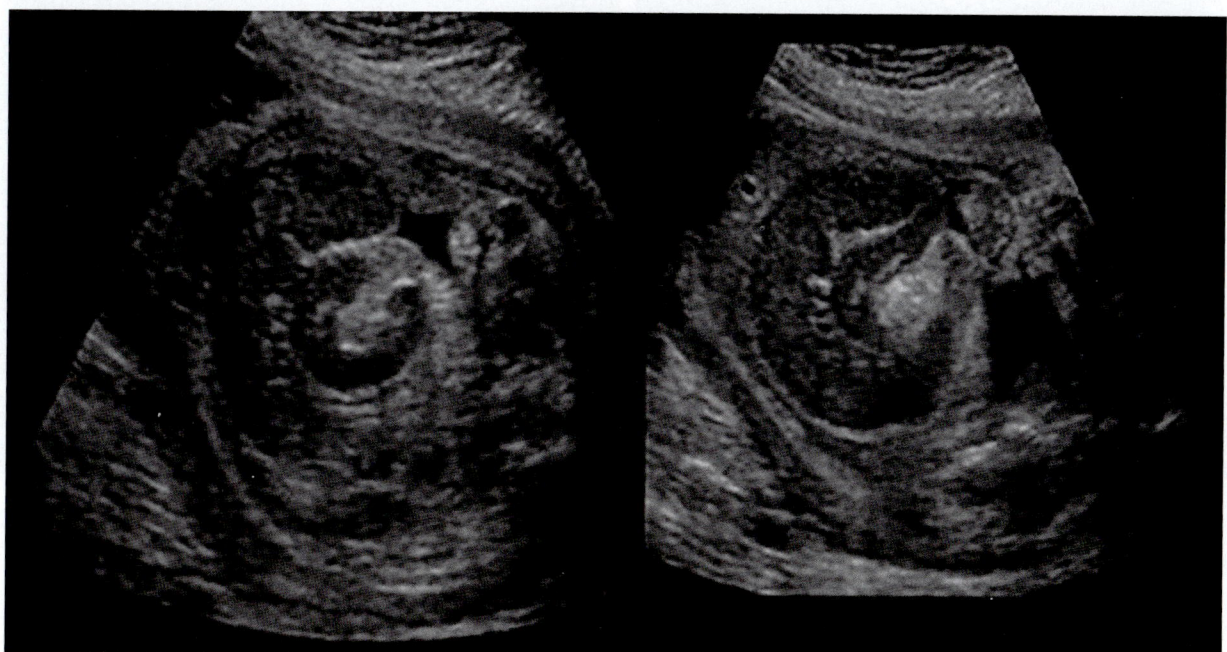

FIG. 63.14 After 14 weeks of gestation, the lipid is absorbed from the fetal colon, and the remaining contents collect in the colon as meconium. The meconium increases slightly in echogenicity as the fetus grows nearer to term delivery.

appears hypoechoic relative to the fetal liver and compared with the bowel wall. This is the point where the normal colon can be mistaken for an abnormally dilated small bowel or other pathologic processes, including renal cysts and pelvic masses. This pitfall is more prominent when the meconium has a more sonolucent appearance than usual (reflective of increased water content). The meconium increases slightly in echogenicity as the fetus grows nearer to term delivery (Fig. 63.14).

Hepatobiliary System

Liver. The fetal liver is relatively large compared with the other intraabdominal organs and occupies most of the upper abdomen in the fetus. It accounts for 10% of the total weight of the fetus at 11 weeks and 5% of the total weight at term. The hepatic veins and fissures are formed by the end of the first trimester (Fig. 63.15A). The left lobe of the liver is larger than the right in utero secondary to the greater supply of oxygenated blood. This, of course, reverses after birth.

Gallbladder. The normal gallbladder may be seen sonographically after 20 weeks of gestation. Both the gallbladder and portal-umbilical vein appear as oblong fluid-filled structures on the transverse view of the fetal abdomen through the liver (see Fig. 63.15B). The gallbladder is distinguished by its location to the right of the portal-umbilical vein and as an oblong, more oval structure than the "tubular" intrahepatic umbilical vein.

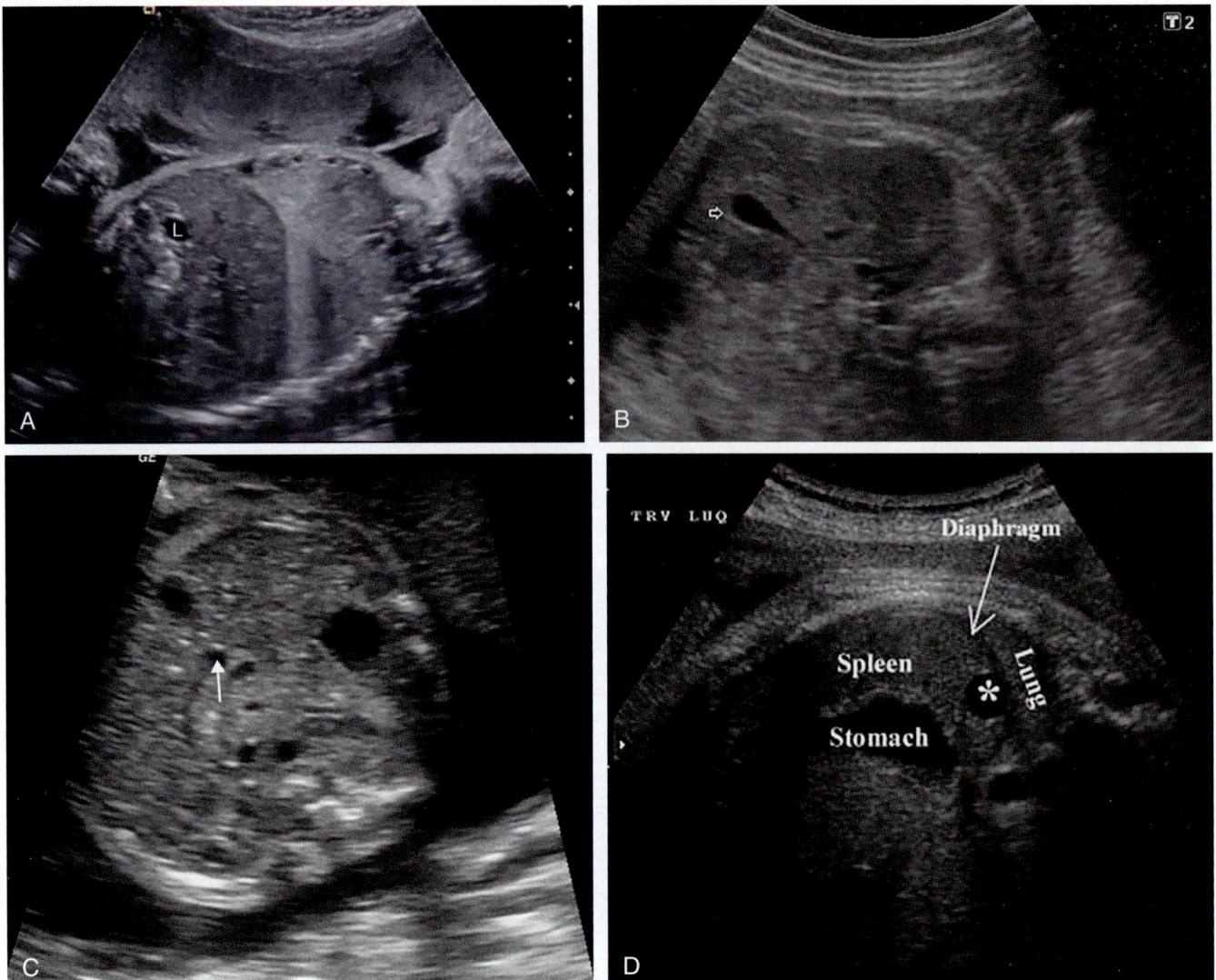

FIG. 63.15 (A) The fetal liver (L) is relatively large compared with the other intraabdominal organs and occupies most of the upper abdomen in the fetus. (B) Both the gallbladder and portal-umbilical vein appear as oblong fluid-filled structures on the transverse view of the fetal abdomen through the liver. (C) The pancreas *(arrow)* lies in the retroperitoneal cavity anterior to the superior mesenteric vessels, aorta, and inferior vena cava. (D) The spleen is imaged on a transverse plane posterior and to the left of the fetal stomach.

Pancreas. The normal fetal pancreas has been seen in utero, but it is more difficult to routinely recognize because of the lack of fatty tissue within the gland. It lies in the retroperitoneal cavity anterior to the superior mesenteric vessels, aorta, and inferior vena cava (see Fig. 63.15C).

Spleen. The spleen is homogeneous in texture, similar in echogenicity to the kidney, and slightly less echogenic than the liver. It increases in size during gestation. The spleen is imaged on a transverse plane posterior and to the left of the fetal stomach (see Fig. 63.15D).

ABNORMALITIES OF THE HEPATOBILIARY SYSTEM

Anomalies of the liver, gallbladder, pancreas, and spleen are rare. Detection of abnormal morphology is beneficial because many lesions may be clinically undetected in the newborn period.

Liver

Although involved in several congenital anomalies (diaphragmatic hernia, omphalocele as presented in Chapter 62), the fetal liver is rarely affected by isolated hepatic lesions. Liver parenchymal cysts and hemangiomas of the liver have been reported. The liver enlarges in fetuses with Rh-immune disease in response to increased hematopoiesis (red blood cell production in the liver).

Liver tumors, hamartoma, and hepatoblastoma are uncommon and may be observed prenatally. Other tumors seen with sonography include hepatic teratoma, adenoma, or metastases from neuroblastoma. Although a rare tumor, hemangioendothelioma is the most common, symptomatic, vascular hepatic tumor of infancy and may cause nonimmune hydrops in the fetus (Fig. 63.16A).

Sonographic Findings. Most of these tumors appear as hypoechoic solid masses within the liver, although cystic

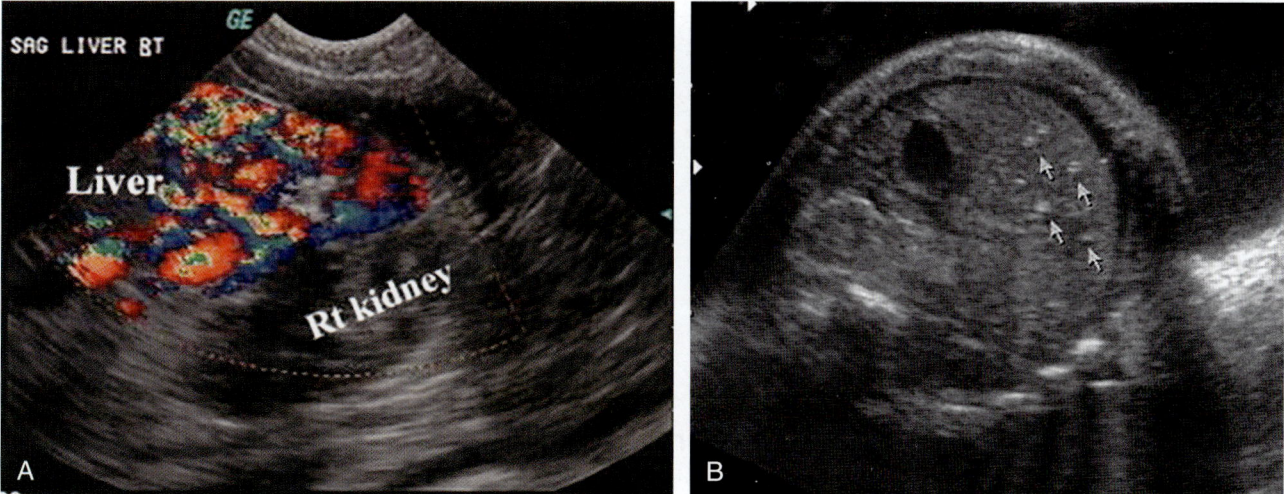

FIG. 63.16 (A) Hemangioendothelioma is a rare vascular hepatic tumor of infancy and may cause nonimmune hydrops in the fetus. (B) Liver calcification may be observed as an isolated echogenic focus. This calcification is usually a benign finding; rarely, it may be a hemangioma, multiple foci secondary to infection (transplacental infections, cytomegalovirus, toxoplasmosis), or hepatic necrosis from ischemia.

components have also been reported as mixed with the solid masses. About 5% of benign and malignant liver tumors are calcified.

Liver calcification may be observed as an isolated echogenic focus. This calcification is usually a benign finding; rarely, it may be a hemangioma, multiple foci secondary to infection (transplacental infections, cytomegalovirus, toxoplasmosis), or hepatic necrosis from ischemia. (see Fig. 63.16B) If multiple calcifications are seen within the liver, other organs such as the brain and spleen may also be affected.

Situs Inversus

Situs inversus may present as a total reversal of the thoracic and abdominal organs or as a partial reversal (mirror image of some organs) (Fig. 63.17). **Partial situs inversus** is a more severe disorder and may develop in two different combinations of organ reversals. In partial situs inversus, the thoracic viscera are usually reversed, and the abdominal viscera may or may not be reversed. Occasionally, partial situs inversus may involve the abdominal organs only without affecting the heart position in the left chest. Partial situs is divided into asplenia and polysplenia.

The infant with total situs inversus usually has a normal outcome. About 20% may have Kartagener syndrome (immotile cilia, bronchiectasis). The mortality rate for partial situs inversus is extremely high, with death occurring in 90% to 95% with asplenia syndrome and 80% with polysplenia syndrome.

Asplenia. Asplenia (absence of the spleen) is represented by an abnormally positioned stomach and gallbladder (more midline position), a more centrally positioned liver, and an abnormal positioning of the aorta and inferior vena cava on the same side. **Polysplenia** (more than one spleen) is represented by a transposition of the liver, spleen, and stomach and by an absence of the gallbladder. There is interruption of the inferior vena cava, and the azygos vein is directly posterior to the heart and in front of the spine. At least two spleens are present along the greater curvature of the stomach (which is on the right side). Heart block is common in polysplenia syndrome. In polysplenia-asplenia, the normal size spleen is not seen on sonography between the stomach and left kidney on the transverse abdominal image.

The cause of situs inversus is unclear, but it is thought to occur early in embryogenesis before normal laterality determination (before 3 weeks). Cardiac malformations are particularly common (99%) in asplenia syndrome and are seen with less frequency in polysplenia syndrome (90%). Cardiac defects include endocardial cushion defects, hypoplastic left heart (Fig. 63.18), and transposition of the great vessels.

Sonographic Findings. Sonographically, these signs may be observed:
- Total situs inversus (right-side heart axis and aorta; transposition of liver, stomach, and spleen; left-side gallbladder).
- Partial situs inversus (right-side stomach, left-side liver). Dextrocardia with normal stomach position.
- Other anomalies to check for include gastrointestinal, genitourinary, and neural tube defects.

Pseudoascites

There are many causes of pseudoascites in the fetus. Gastrointestinal obstruction with bowel perforation may present as meconium peritonitis and ascites. The nongastrointestinal causes include immune and nonimmune hydrops, urinary tract obstruction, congenital infection, and some abdominal tumors.

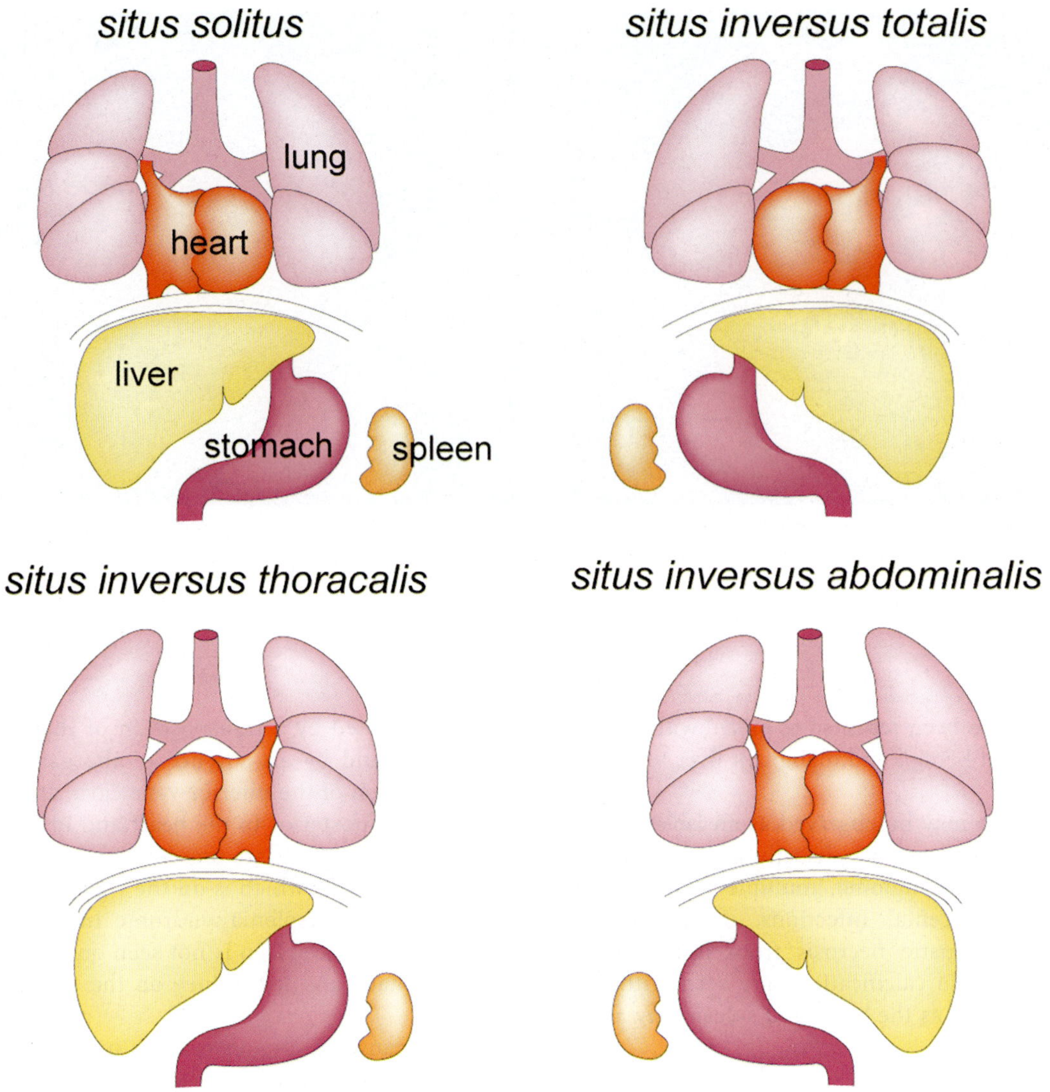

FIG. 63.17 Situs solitus demonstrates the normal thoracic and abdominal organs. Situs inversus may present as a total reversal of the thoracic and abdominal organs or as a partial reversal (mirror image of some organs). Partial situs inversus is a more severe disorder and may develop in two different combinations of organ reversals. In partial situs inversus, the thoracic viscera are usually reversed, and the abdominal viscera may or may not be reversed.

Pseudoascites occurs when a sonolucent band near the fetal anterior abdominal wall is commonly identified during routine obstetric examinations in the fetus over 18 weeks of gestation (Fig. 63.19). This band results from normal musculature surrounding the abdominal wall. True ascites is identified within the peritoneal recesses and is interspaced between loops of the small bowel (which then causes the bowel loops to appear more echogenic), whereas pseudoascites is always confined to an anterior fetal abdomen and is centrally located. Furthermore, **pseudoascites** never outlines the falciform ligament like true ascites.

Gallbladder

Anomalies of the gallbladder may be detected using prenatal sonographic techniques. **Cholelithiasis** (gallstones) may be identified in the fetus when calcifications are found within the gallbladder. These gallstones resolve spontaneously in utero or in the childhood period (Fig. 63.20).

A **choledochal cyst** (dilation of the common bile duct) may be diagnosed when a cystic mass is identified adjacent to the fetal stomach and gallbladder (Box 63.1). Choledochal cysts may be confused with malformations of the stomach or bowel or duodenal atresia. The sonographer should remember that the gallbladder is more anterior than the duodenum, and thus a cystic mass attached to the bile duct near the gallbladder would make the mass more likely a choledochal cyst. Choledochal cysts may be associated with intermittent biliary obstruction and severe biliary cirrhosis; therefore, early diagnosis is important. (See Chapter 25 for further information.)

Agenesis of the gallbladder occurs in approximately 20% of patients with biliary atresia. The absence of the

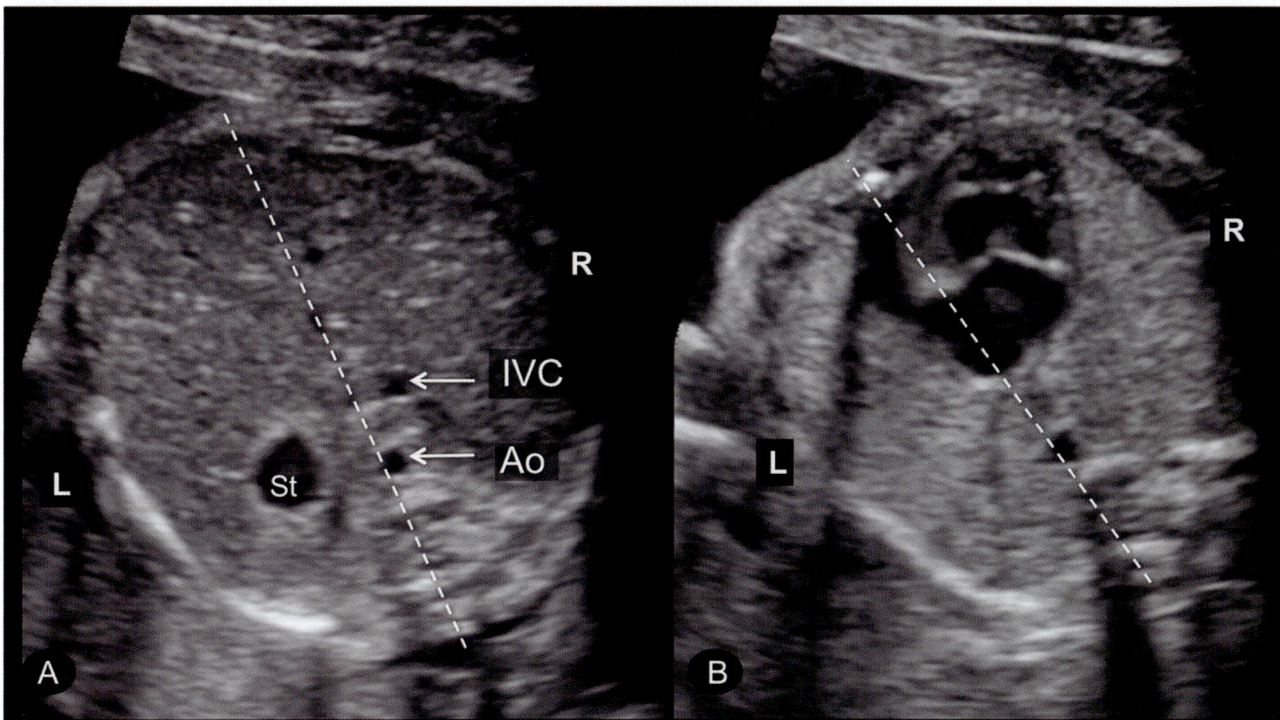

FIG. 63.18 Partial situs inversus shows the aorta (Ao) and heart to the right of midline. The stomach (St) and liver (L) are on the left. *IVC*, Inferior vena cava.

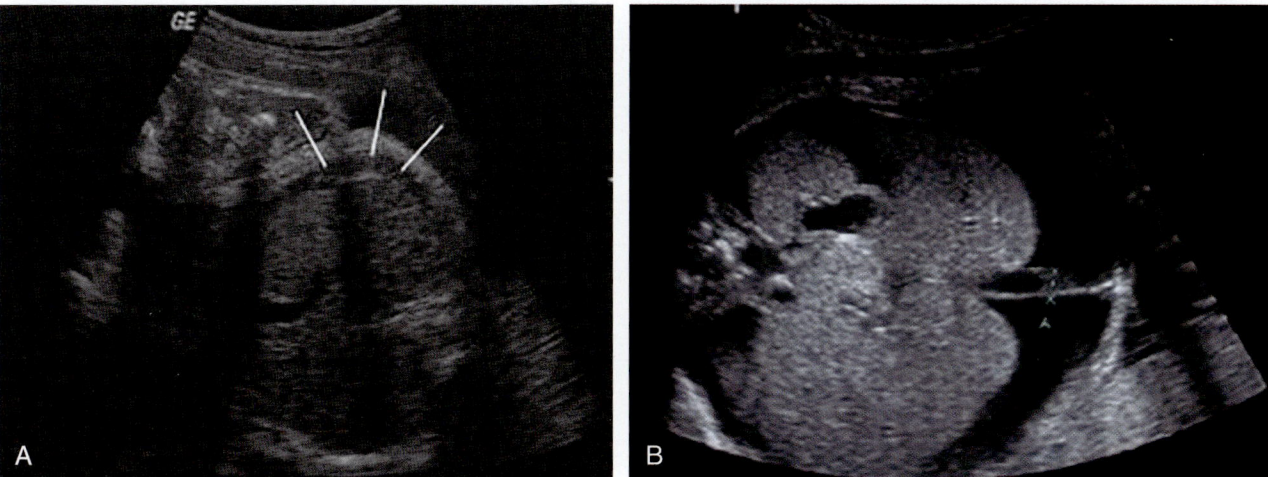

FIG. 63.19 (A) Pseudoascites occurs when a sonolucent band near the fetal anterior abdominal wall is commonly identified during routine obstetric examinations in the fetus over 18 weeks of gestation. (B) Fetus with ascites outlining the falciform ligament.

gallbladder also can occur in association with polysplenia and rare multiple anomaly syndromes. The ability to visualize the fetal gallbladder routinely increases with gestational age.

Pancreas

Pancreatic cysts are uncommon but, when present, may appear as midline anechoic cystic masses in the fetal abdomen.

Spleen

Evaluation of the fetal spleen for exclusion of splenic anomalies is possible. Asplenia (absence of the spleen) may be amenable to antenatal identification, and in association with congenital heart disease, the polysplenia-asplenia syndrome should be considered.

Congenital splenic cysts are rare but have been reported in utero. Enlargement of the spleen (splenomegaly) may be seen on the ultrasound examination. The spleen, like the liver, may

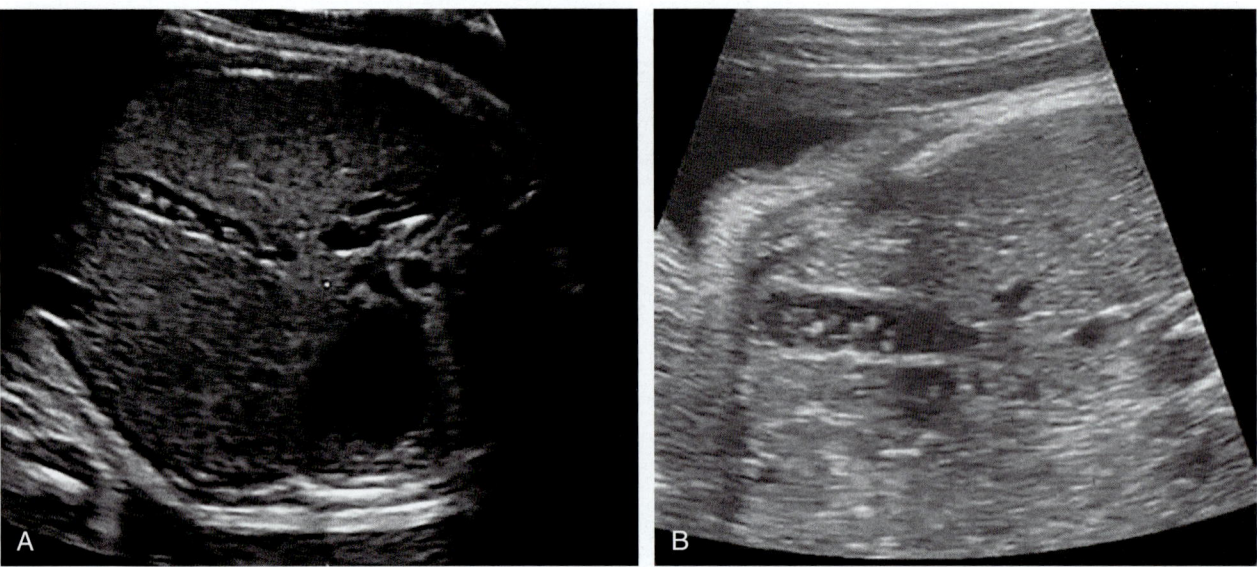

FIG. 63.20 Fetal gallstones. (A) Transverse image of a fetus with gallstones. (B) Small calcifications without shadowing were seen in the fetal ultrasound in the gallbladder.

> **BOX 63.1 Sonographic Criteria for Choledochal Cyst**
>
> - Close proximity of the cyst to the neck of the gallbladder
> - An ovoid right upper quadrant cyst with an entering bile duct
> - A cyst and gallbladder that enlarge as gestation progresses
> - Absence of peristaltic activity in the cyst

From Schwartz H, et al. Choledochal cyst in a second trimester fetus. *J Diagn Med Sonogr.* 1989;1:10.

> **BOX 63.2 Causes of Nonvisualization of the Stomach**
>
> - Esophageal atresia or tracheoesophageal fistula
> - Diaphragmatic hernia
> - Facial cleft
> - Central nervous system disorder
> - Other swallowing disorders
> - Oligohydramnios from other causes

From Schwartz H, et al. Choledochal cyst in a second trimester fetus. *J Diagn Med Sonogr.* 1989;1:10.

---

enlarge in fetuses with Rh-immune disease. Nomograms are available to detect hepatomegaly and splenomegaly.

ABNORMALITIES OF THE GASTROINTESTINAL TRACT

The majority of gastrointestinal malformations are correctable after birth; consequently, recognition of a gastrointestinal anomaly before delivery may prevent the complications of dehydration, bowel necrosis, and respiratory difficulties that occur when these lesions are unsuspected before delivery. Box 63.2 lists the causes of nonvisualization of the stomach. The fetal bowel can be altered by a number of pathologic processes. A bowel obstruction results in proximal bowel dilation, which is characteristically recognized as one or more tubular structures within the fetal abdomen. Dilated bowel loops are generally sonolucent in texture but may be normal or increased in echogenicity. The most reliable criterion for diagnosing a dilated bowel is the bowel diameter rather than the sonographic appearance. One should be careful not to mistake a dilated ureter for a dilated loop of the bowel. Most cases of bowel dilation do not become evident on sonography until after 20 weeks of gestation. Polyhydramnios commonly accompanies obstruction of the gastrointestinal tract, and this rarely develops before 20 weeks of gestation as a result of a gastrointestinal cause.

Esophagus, Stomach, and Duodenum

The normal upper esophagus may be seen after amniotic fluid is swallowed. This fluid passes from the esophagus into the fetal stomach. Obstruction of the normal swallowing sequence may occur because of an atretic or obstructive process. Atresias develop when a portion of the bowel grows and infarcts; this can occur anywhere in the gastrointestinal tract. A membrane covering the lumen and intestinal loops enlarges above the obstruction, and bowel loops below the atresia are narrowed (stenotic). This enlargement of the bowel proximal to the obstruction is readily apparent on ultrasound. Blockage results in the backup of amniotic fluid and hydramnios.

Esophageal atresia is a congenital blockage of the esophagus resulting from the faulty separation of the foregut into its respiratory and digestive components (Fig. 63.21). The most common form occurs in conjunction with a fistula, communicating between the trachea and esophagus (tracheoesophageal fistula), which allows the passage of amniotic fluid into the stomach. Gastric secretions may contribute to stomach fluid. In some instances, however, a fistula is not present, fluid does not reach the stomach, and the stomach will not be

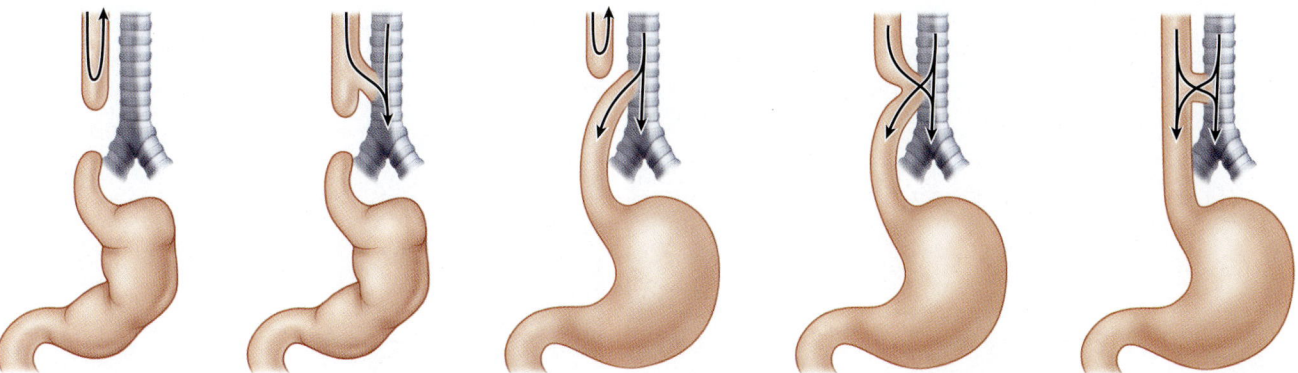

FIG. 63.21 Esophageal atresia is a congenital blockage of the esophagus resulting from the faulty separation of the foregut into its respiratory and digestive components. There are five types of esophageal atresia.

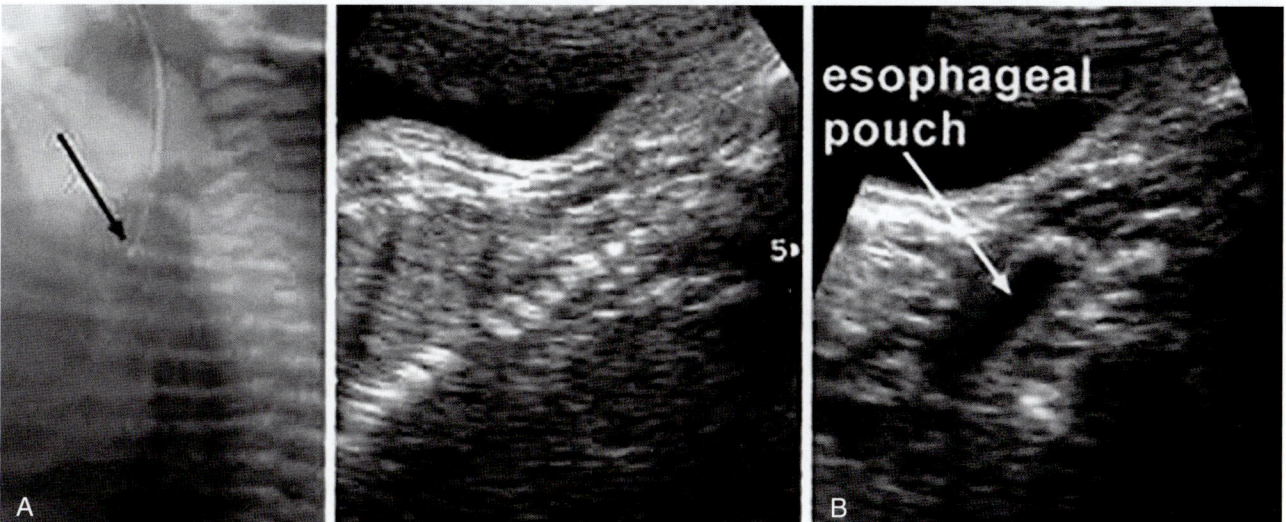

FIG. 63.22 (A) A fluid-filled stomach should be seen by 14 weeks of gestation; if the stomach is not seen, wait 30 minutes and rescan to see if the stomach fills with fluid. A small or absent stomach may indicate a fistula is present. (B) In esophageal atresia, fluid may collect in the esophageal pouch if a fistula is not present.

visualized by ultrasound. The combination of polyhydramnios and an absent stomach over repeated studies may be suggestive of esophageal atresia. Esophageal atresia will not be diagnosed in the majority of cases because of a tracheoesophageal fistula.

Esophageal atresia occurs in 1 in 2500 live births. The sonographer may observe the absent stomach and hydramnios (Fig. 63.22A). However, in more than half of the cases, the stomach is present because a fistula is usually present that leads to fluid filling the stomach. Hydramnios may exist from impaired reabsorption of swallowed fluid and may be associated with esophageal atresia, but it usually does not develop until the third trimester. The upper neck sign has been observed as an additional finding in a patient with esophageal atresia. A fluid-filled, blind-ending esophagus during fetal swallowing has been noted in a 22-week fetus (see Fig. 63.22B).

Coexisting anomalies are common in 50% to 70% of fetuses with esophageal atresia. The most commonly observed anomaly is **anorectal atresia** (others include vertebral defects, heart defects, and renal and limb anomalies [**VACTERL**]). Growth restriction is present in 40% of the cases. Chromosomal trisomies (18 and 21) are reported in association. Survival depends on the presence of associated congenital anomalies. Further discussion is found in Chapter 65, Skeletal Anomalies.

Duodenal atresia is a blockage of the duodenal lumen by a membrane that prohibits the passage of swallowed amniotic fluid. Atresia or narrowing of the bowel segment below the obstruction occurs. In duodenal atresia, the amniotic fluid fails to move beyond the obstruction, and consequently, amniotic fluid backs up in the duodenum and stomach.

Sonographic Findings. Two echo-free structures (stomach and duodenum) are found in the upper fetal abdomen, and they communicate. This sonographic appearance is termed the *double bubble sign* (Fig. 63.23, Box 63.3). Hydramnios is almost always seen with duodenal atresias later in pregnancy. Most cases of duodenal atresia are found distal to the ampulla and often coexist with annular pancreas.

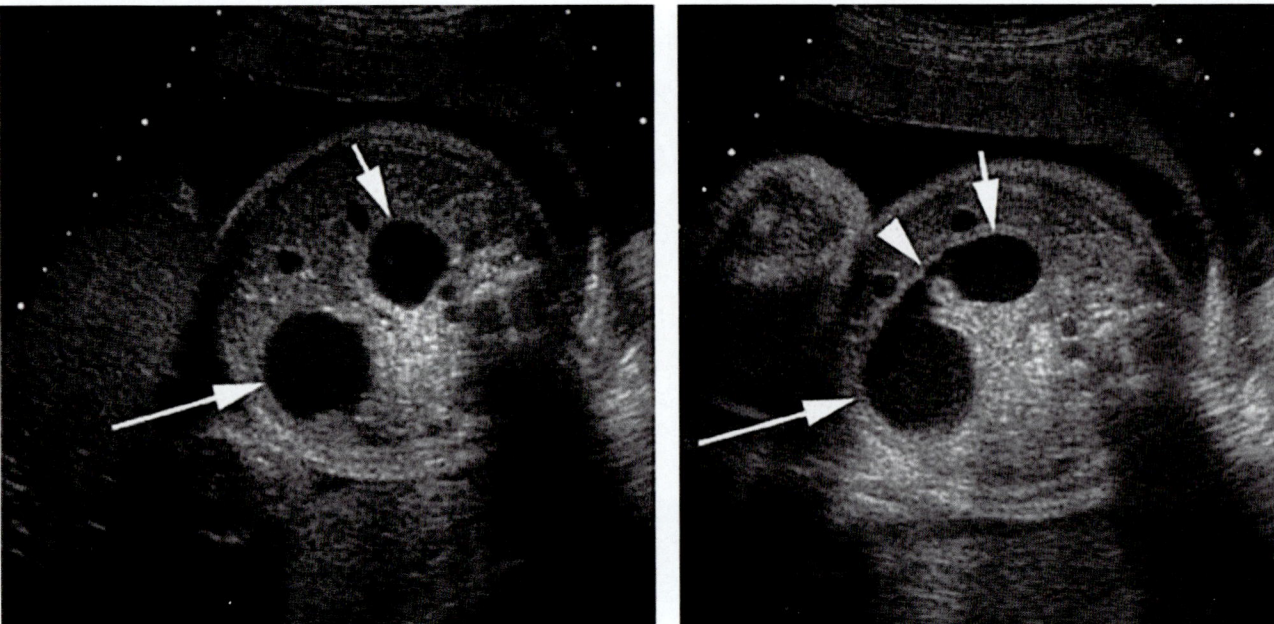

FIG. 63.23 In duodenal atresia, the amniotic fluid fails to move beyond the obstruction, and consequently, amniotic fluid backs up in the duodenum and stomach. The "double bubble" sign is noted *(arrows)*.

BOX 63.3 Causes of Double Bubble

- Duodenal atresia
- Duodenal stenosis
- Annular pancreas
- Ladd bands
- Proximal jejunal atresia
- Malrotation
- Diaphragmatic hernia

From Schwartz H, et al. Choledochal cyst in a second trimester fetus. *J Diagn Med Sonogr.* 1989;1:10.

About 30% of fetuses with duodenal atresia have trisomy 21 (Down syndrome). Cardiovascular anomalies are frequent, and therefore fetal echocardiography is invaluable in excluding cardiac lesions. Anomalies occur in approximately 50% of infants with duodenal atresia. Genitourinary anomalies (horseshoe kidney, ectopic kidneys) may coexist with this condition. Other gastrointestinal abnormalities, such as imperforate anus and atresia of the small bowel, may be present. Esophageal atresia may also be found.

Symmetric growth restriction commonly occurs in fetuses with duodenal atresia. Amniotic fluid alpha-fetoprotein values are commonly elevated in fetuses with duodenal atresia caused by faulty swallowing. Infants with duodenal atresia require immediate surgery after birth to connect the stomach to the jejunum, thus bypassing the obstruction.

Bowel

Intestinal Obstructions. Atresia or stenosis of the jejunum, ileum, or both, and small bowel atresia are slightly more common than duodenal atresia; it occurs in 1 in 3000 to 5000 live births and is thought to be secondary to a vascular accident, sporadic, or secondary to volvulus or gastroschisis. Various fetal malformations may also occur with maternal drug usage. The entire length of the bowel is subject to obstruction. Blockage of the jejunum and ileal bowel segments (**jejunoileal atresia** or stenosis) appears as multiple cystic structures (more than two) proximal to the site of atresia within the fetal abdomen. Because these structures are high in the abdomen, hydramnios may be present. The general rule is that the more distal the obstruction, the less severe the hydramnios, and the later it will develop. The causes of fetal small-bowel obstruction include malrotation, atresias, volvulus, peritoneal bands, and cystic fibrosis. The dilated bowel loops may be isolated or may be associated with other anomalies, ascites, or meconium peritonitis. Meconium peritonitis may lead to ascites, intra-abdominal calcifications, meconium cysts, dilated loops of bowel, and polyhydramnios.

The sequence of change in fetal bowel obstruction has four steps: (1) bowel obstruction, (2) dilated loops of bowel, (3) bowel rupture, and finally (4) meconium peritonitis.

Sonographic Findings. Sonographically, intestinal obstructions appear as cystic bowel loops that are discontinuous with the stomach (Fig. 63.24). It is important to remember that bowel loops may be identified in the third trimester of pregnancy. It has been reported that the normal fetal colon progressively increased in diameter after 23 weeks of gestation, although it never exceeded 18 mm in a preterm fetus. Fetal intestinal obstruction should be suspected when clear cystic structures are found in the pelvis. In some instances, echoes within the bowel may be identified in intestinal obstructions but may also represent normal meconium patterns. Vascular restriction may lead to obstruction secondary to a gastroschisis.

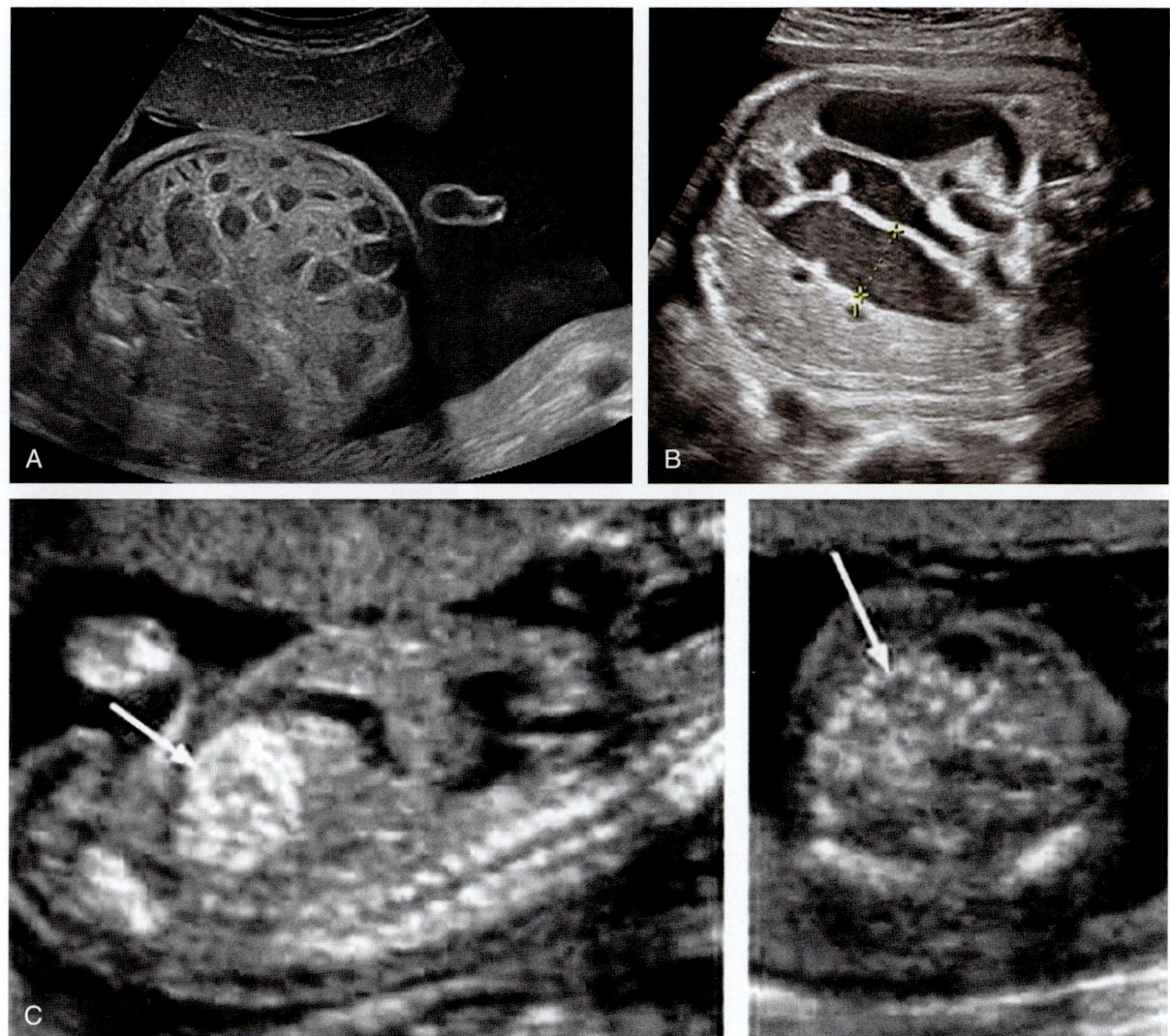

FIG. 63.24 (A–B) Sonographically, intestinal obstructions appear as cystic bowel loops that are discontinuous with the stomach. (C) Meconium peritonitis may lead to intra-abdominal calcifications (*arrows*).

Meconium Ileus. **Meconium ileus** is a small-bowel disorder marked by the presence of thick meconium in the distal ileum. Meconium ileus is the earliest manifestation of cystic fibrosis, occurring in 10% to 15% of patients, and is the third most common form of neonatal bowel obstruction after atresia and malrotation. Most cases of meconium ileus occur in newborns with cystic fibrosis. Infants with **cystic fibrosis** have multiple medical problems, including pancreatic disease and respiratory problems resulting from long-standing lung disease. Cystic fibrosis is an autosomal recessive condition.

Meconium begins to accumulate in the fetal bowel in the second trimester, at which time it can be seen sonographically as tiny echogenic reflections within the peristaltic small bowel (Fig. 63.25A). Because the colon does not exhibit peristalsis in utero, the meconium remains suspended at the rectum. The anal sphincter prevents the passage of meconium (meconium plug) into the amniotic fluid unless the fetus is stressed or traumatized.

Sonographic Findings. With meconium ileus, the ileum dilates because of impacted meconium (which appears echogenic) (see Fig. 63.25B). Increased production of mucus by the gastrointestinal organs and electrolyte imbalance explains the overproduction of meconium (characteristic of cystic fibrosis). It is important to realize that the normal small bowel may appear echogenic during the second trimester of pregnancy. Other fetal conditions have been associated with echogenic small bowel (cytomegalovirus and trisomy 21). Meconium peritonitis may occur secondary to the perforation of an obstructed bowel. An inflammatory response occurs because of leakage of the bowel contents, which may cause fibrosis of tissue and calcifications. A pseudocyst may develop because of chronic meconium peritonitis (Box 63.4).

Other Small Bowel Obstructions. Rarer small-bowel obstructions, chloridorrhea (life-threatening diarrhea in the newborn), and megacystis-microcolon intestinal hypoperistalsis syndrome (absence of peristalsis), may be observed during

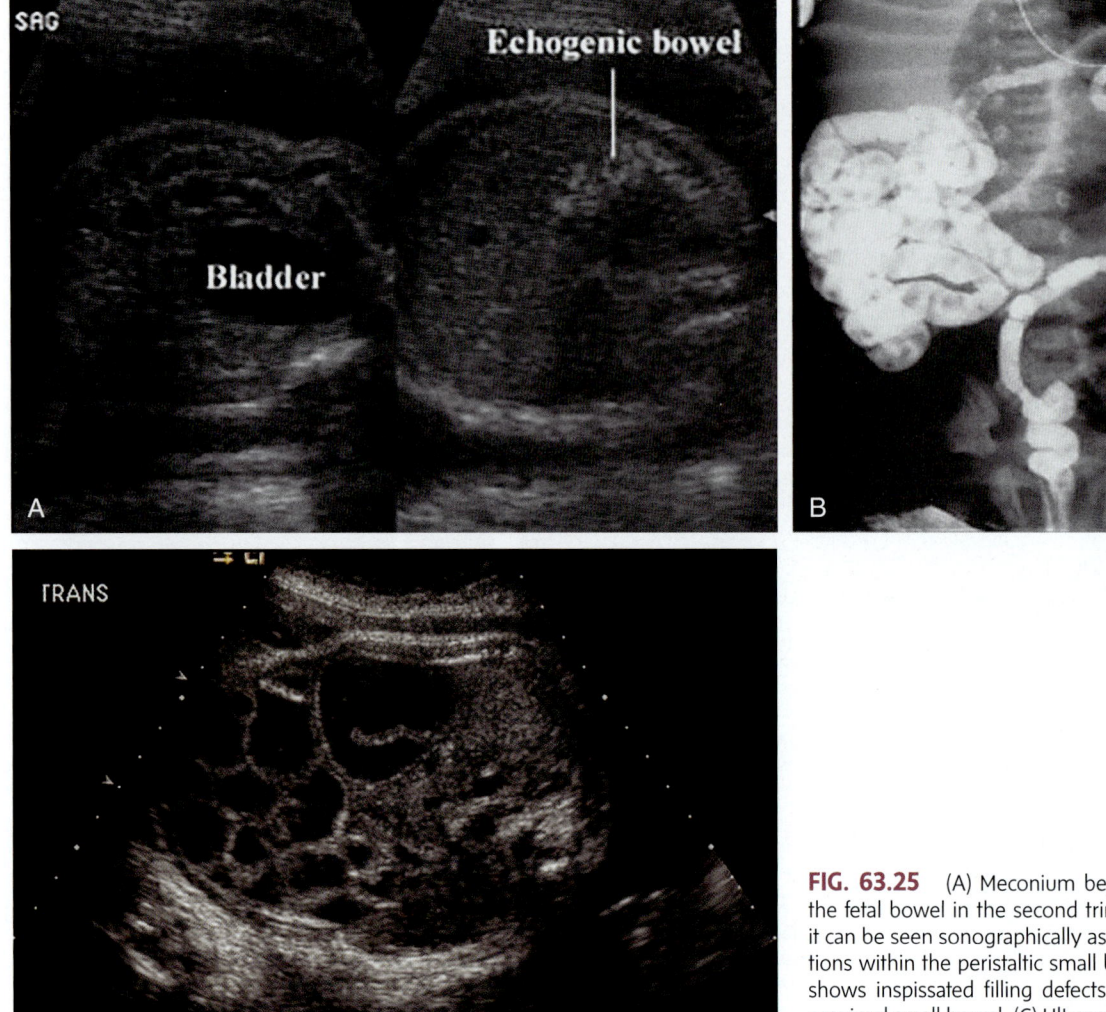

FIG. 63.25 (A) Meconium begins to accumulate in the fetal bowel in the second trimester, at which time it can be seen sonographically as tiny echogenic reflections within the peristaltic small bowel. (B) Radiograph shows inspissated filling defects of meconium in the proximal small bowel. (C) Ultrasound demonstrates the meconium ileus within the small bowel.

BOX 63.4	Pitfalls in the Diagnosis of Meconium Ileus

- Significant dilation of the meconium-filled ileum in the meconium ileus can look like the colon in shape, size, and location.
- More proximal small bowel may have the features of active peristalsis and fluid-filled contents.
- Do not be distracted by the difference in diameter between the proximal and distal small bowel when making a diagnosis of small-bowel obstruction or meconium ileus.

From Schwartz H, et al. Choledochal cyst in a second trimester fetus. *J Diagn Med Sonogr.* 1989;1:10.

pregnancy. In the latter, bladder dilation and hydronephrosis are characteristic findings in predominantly female fetuses. Amniotic fluid volume is typically normal to increased. Obstruction may also be present when gastroschisis is present. Obstructions of the large intestine diagnosed prenatally include anorectal atresia and Hirschsprung disease.

Anorectal Atresia. Anorectal atresia presents as a complex disorder of the bowel and genitourinary tract. Imperforate anus (a finding in anorectal atresia) is a disorder that occurs when a membrane covers the anus prohibiting the expulsion of meconium. Anorectal atresia may present as part of the VACTERL association or in caudal regression. The prognosis is poor with anorectal atresia because of associated anomalies. Incontinence of both bowel and bladder is common in the infant.

Sonographic Findings. Anorectal atresia may be diagnosed sonographically by observing dilated colon and calcified meconium. Amniotic fluid is typically normal or may be decreased when there are associated renal problems.

Hirschsprung Disease. Hirschsprung disease (megacolon) is a congenital disorder in which there is abnormal innervation of the large intestine.

Sonographic Findings. This condition is difficult to diagnose prenatally but may be suspected when dilated bowel loops are observed (Fig. 63.26).

Meconium Peritonitis. Meconium peritonitis is a condition that may arise when the fetus has a sterile chemical peritonitis secondary to in utero bowel perforation. Hydramnios is present in 65% of fetuses with meconium peritonitis. A complication may result in the formation of a meconium pseudocyst as the inflammatory reaction seals the perforation.

▶ **Sonographic Findings.** On ultrasound examination, calcifications are seen on the peritoneal surfaces or in the scrotum via the processus vaginalis. The ascitic fluid may also be echogenic. It is unusual to see calcification in the meconium ileus in a fetus with cystic fibrosis.

Hyperechoic Bowel. Hyperechoic bowel is a subjective impression of an unusually echogenic bowel, typically seen during the second trimester. The cause of hyperechoic bowel may be due to decreased water content, alterations of meconium, or both. The decreased water content may be secondary to hypoperistalsis, given that fluid is normally resorbed by the small bowel.

▶ **Sonographic Findings.** The significance of hyperechoic bowel varies with its location in the small bowel or colon, menstrual age, and degree of echogenicity (Box 63.5). The degree of hyperechogenicity may be compared with the iliac wing of the fetus. There are three gradations of the degree of hyperechogenicity of the bowel:
- Grade 1: mildly echogenic and typically diffuse
- Grade 2: moderately echogenic and typically focal
- Grade 3: very echogenic, similar to that of bone structures

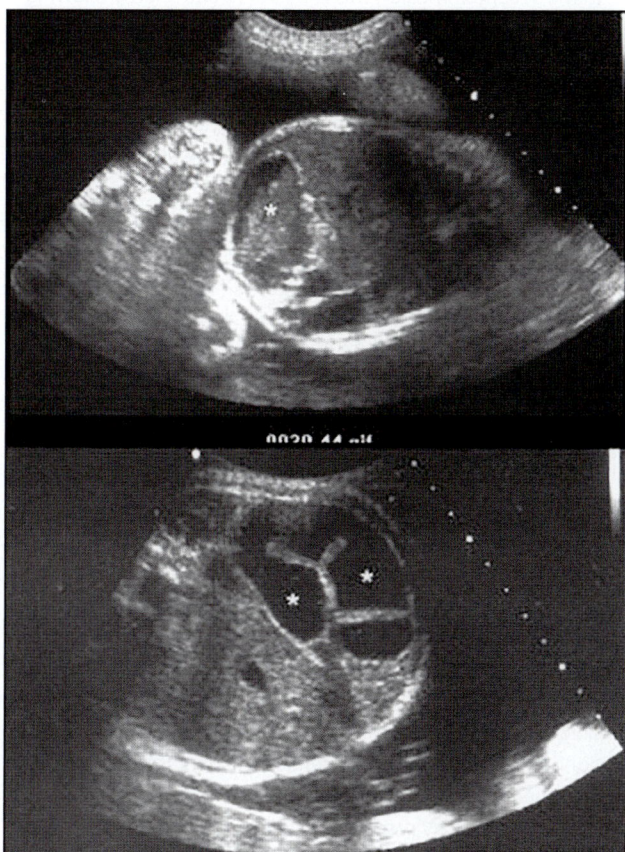

FIG. 63.26 Hirschsprung disease (megacolon) is a congenital disorder in which there is abnormal innervation of the large intestine.

BOX 63.5	Causes of Echogenic Areas in the Fetal Abdomen

Calcified
- Peritoneal calcification: meconium peritonitis, hydrometrocolpos
- Intraluminal meconium calcification: anorectal atresia, small bowel atresia; rarely isolated without bowel obstruction
- Parenchymal: liver, splenic, adrenal, ovarian cyst
- Cholelithiasis: gallbladder

Noncalcified
- Echogenic meconium
- Intraabdominal extrathoracic pulmonary sequestration
- Tumors
- Adrenal hemorrhage

From Nyberg DA, Neilsen IR. Abdomen and gastrointestinal tract. In Nyberg DA, McGahan JP, Pretorius DH, et al, editors. *Diagnostic imaging of fetal anomalies,* Philadelphia: Lippincott Williams & Wilkins; 2003.

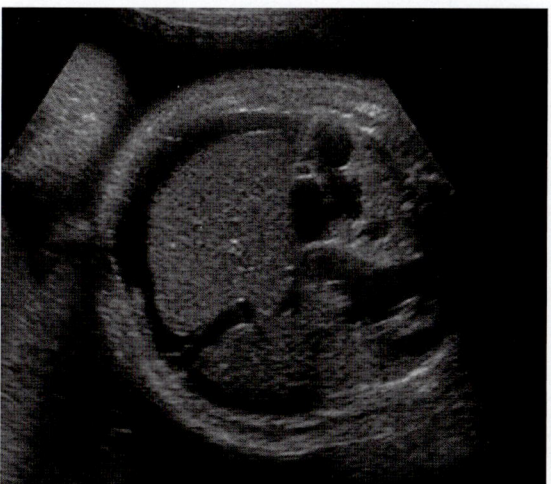 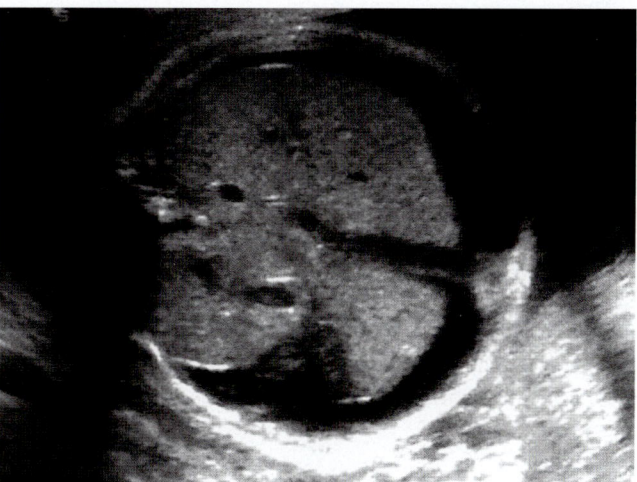

FIG. 63.27 Ascites usually outlines the falciform ligament and umbilical vein. When ascites is associated with hydrops fetalis, pleural effusions, and pericardial effusion, integumentary edema is often observed.

Ascites. True ascites in the fetal abdomen is always abnormal. In the fetus, the ascitic fluid collects between the two leaves of unfused omentum, resulting in a cyst-like appearance in the abdomen (Fig. 63.27). The prognosis is poor in nonimmune hydrops. Other conditions that may cause ascites to develop include bowel perforation or urinary ascites secondary to bladder rupture.

Sonographic Findings. Ascites usually outlines the falciform ligament and umbilical vein. When ascites is associated with hydrops fetalis, pleural effusions, and pericardial effusion, integumentary edema will often be observed.

MISCELLANEOUS CYSTIC MASSES OF THE ABDOMEN

Cystic masses of the lower fetal abdomen may be observed prenatally. It is important for the sonographer to determine the size of the mass, determine its precise location, and identify resultant compression of other organ systems (hydronephrosis, hydroureter, fetal hydrops).

When a cystic mass is discovered, attempts should be made to determine the characteristics of the mass. A description of the mass should include the components of the structure, such as (1) an echo-free versus an echo-filled mass, (2) the presence or absence of septations, and (3) coexisting fetal anomalies. The sonographer should systematically investigate all abdominal organ systems to determine the anatomic origin of the mass. The hepatic system (liver, gallbladder, spleen, and pancreatic areas) should be evaluated along with the gastrointestinal system (esophagus, stomach, and intestines) and genitourinary system (kidneys, ureters, and bladder).

Occasionally, cysts arise from the urachus (dilation of remnant allantoic stalk between umbilicus and bladder), fetal ovary, or omentum. Ovarian and omental cysts are generally isolated and well circumscribed. Determination of the fetal gender is beneficial when an ovarian mass is suspected. If abdominal masses are large, they may occupy the entire lower fetal pelvis, making a specific intrauterine diagnosis impossible.

> ### Key Pearls
>
> - Meckel's diverticulum is the most common malformation of the midgut. Meckel's diverticulum is a remnant of the proximal part of the yolk stalk that fails to degenerate and disappear during the early fetal period.
> - The stomach should be identified as a fluid-filled structure in the *left* upper quadrant inferior to the diaphragm.
> - The normal esophagus can be visualized in the thorax during the second and third trimesters as two or more parallel echogenic lines.
> - The abdominal circumference is measured at the level of the portal sinus and the umbilical portion of the left portal vein, which has a "hockey stick" appearance on the sonogram.
> - In the fetus, the umbilical vein courses cephalically in the free, inferior margin of the falciform ligament. It joins the umbilical portion of the left portal vein at the caudal margin of the left intersegmental fissure of the liver.
> - In the second trimester, this movement and fetal swallowing result in the delivery of increased amniotic fluid volume distally into the small bowel and colon, where fluid and nutrients are reabsorbed. After the 15th to 16th week, meconium begins to accumulate in the distal part of the small intestine as a combination of desquamated cells, bile pigments, and mucoproteins.
> - The colon is seen near the end of the second trimester as a long tubular hypoechoic structure with well-defined walls. The haustral folds of the colon help to differentiate it from the small bowel.
> - The meconium within the lumen of the colon appears hypoechoic relative to the fetal liver and compared with the bowel wall.
> - The fetal liver is relatively large compared with the other intraabdominal organs and occupies most of the upper abdomen in the fetus.
> - The normal gallbladder may be seen sonographically after 20 weeks of gestation.
> - The spleen is homogeneous in texture, similar in echogenicity to the kidney, and slightly less echogenic than the liver. It increases in size during gestation.
> - Liver tumors, hamartoma, and hepatoblastoma are uncommon and may be observed prenatally. Other tumors seen with sonography include hepatic teratoma, adenoma, or metastases from neuroblastoma.
> - Situs inversus may present as a total reversal of the thoracic and abdominal organs or as a partial reversal (mirror image of some organs).
> - In partial situs inversus, the thoracic viscera are usually reversed, and the abdominal viscera may or may not be reversed.
> - Asplenia (absence of the spleen) is represented by an abnormally positioned stomach and gallbladder (more midline position), a more centrally positioned liver, and an abnormal positioning of the aorta and inferior vena cava on the same side.
> - Polysplenia (more than one spleen) is represented by a transposition of the liver, spleen, and stomach and by an absence of the gallbladder.
> - True ascites is identified within the peritoneal recesses and is interspaced between loops of the small bowel (which then causes the bowel loops to appear more echogenic), whereas pseudoascites is always confined to an anterior fetal abdomen and is centrally located.

- Cholelithiasis (gallstones) may be identified in the fetus when calcifications are found within the gallbladder.
- A choledochal cyst (dilation of the common bile duct) may be diagnosed when a cystic mass is identified adjacent to the fetal stomach and gallbladder.
- Agenesis of the gallbladder occurs in approximately 20% of patients with biliary atresia.
- The fetal bowel can be altered by a number of pathologic processes. A bowel obstruction results in proximal bowel dilation, which is characteristically recognized as one or more tubular structures within the fetal abdomen.
- Obstruction of the normal swallowing sequence may occur because of an atretic or obstructive process. Atresias develop when a portion of the bowel grows and infarcts; this can occur anywhere in the gastrointestinal tract.
- Enlargement of the bowel proximal to the obstruction is readily apparent on ultrasound. Blockage results in the backup of amniotic fluid and hydramnios.
- The most common form of esophageal atresia occurs in conjunction with a fistula, communicating between the trachea and esophagus (tracheoesophageal fistula), which allows the passage of amniotic fluid into the stomach.
- Coexisting anomalies are common in 50% to 70% of fetuses with esophageal atresia. The most commonly observed anomaly is anorectal atresia (others include vertebral defects, heart defects, and renal and limb anomalies [VACTERL]).
- Duodenal atresia is a blockage of the duodenal lumen by a membrane that prohibits the passage of swallowed amniotic fluid.
- About 30% of fetuses with duodenal atresia have trisomy 21 (Down syndrome).
- Atresia or stenosis of the jejunum, ileum, or both, and small bowel atresia are slightly more common than duodenal atresia.
- Meconium ileus is a small-bowel disorder marked by the presence of thick meconium in the distal ileum.
- Meconium begins to accumulate in the fetal bowel in the second trimester, at which time it can be seen sonographically as tiny echogenic reflections within the peristaltic small bowel.
- Meconium peritonitis is a condition that may arise when the fetus has a sterile chemical peritonitis secondary to in utero bowel perforation.
- Hyperechoic bowel is a subjective impression of an unusually echogenic bowel, typically seen during the second trimester.
- True ascites in the fetal abdomen is always abnormal.

BIBLIOGRAPHY

Barnewolt CE. Congenital abnormalities of the gastrointestinal tract. *Semin Roentgenol.* 2004;39(2):263-281.

Bethune M, Bell R. Evaluation of the measurement of the fetal fat layer, interventricular septum, and abdominal circumference percentile in the prediction of macrosomia in pregnancies affected by gestational diabetes. *Ultrasound Obstet Gynecol.* 2003;22(6):586-590.

Boito SM, Laudy JA, Stuijk PC, et al. Three-dimensional US assessment of hepatic volume, head circumference, and abdominal circumference in healthy and growth-restricted fetuses. *Radiology.* 2002;223(3):661-665.

Brautverg A, Blaas M, Salvasen KA, et al. Fetal duodenal obstructions: increased risk of prenatal sudden death. *Ultrasound Obstet Gynecol.* 2002;20:439-446.

Bronshtein M, Gover A, Zimmer EZ. Sonographic definition of the fetal situs. *Obstet Gynecol.* 2002;99(6):1129-1130.

Callen DW, ed. *Ultrasonography in Obstetrics and Gynecology.* ed 5. Philadelphia: Saunders; 2008.

Centini G, Rosignoli L, Kenanidis A, et al. Prenatal diagnosis of esophageal atresia with the pouch sign. *Ultrasound Obstet Gynecol.* 2003;21(5):494-497.

Chinn DH, Filly RA, Callen PW. Ultrasonic evaluation of fetal umbilical and hepatic vascular anatomy. *Radiology.* 1982;144:153.

Gul A, Tekoglu G, Aslan H, et al. Prenatal sonographic features of esophageal and ileal duplications at 18 weeks of gestation. *Prenat Diagn.* 2004;24(12):969-971.

Haratz-Rubinstein N, Sherer DM. Prenatal sonographic findings of congenital duplication of the cecum. *Obstet Gynecol.* 2003;101(5 Pt 2):1085-1087.

Hill LM. Ultrasound of fetal gastrointestinal tract. In: Callen PW, ed. *Ultrasonography in Obstetrics and Gynecology.* ed 5. Philadelphia: Elsevier; 2008.

Ji EK, Lee EK, Kwon TH. Isolated echogenic foci in the left upper quadrant of the fetal abdomen: are they significant? *J Ultrasound Med.* 2004;23(4):483-488.

Kalache KD, et al. The upper neck pouch sign: a prenatal sonographic marker for esophageal atresia. *Ultrasound Obstet Gynecol.* 1998;11:138.

Kamata S, Nose K, Sawai T, et al. Fetal mesenchymal hamartoma of the liver: report of a case. *J Pediatr Surg.* 2003;38(4):639-641.

Lawrence MJ, Ford WD, Furness ME, et al. Congenital duodenal obstruction: early antenatal ultrasound diagnosis. *Pediatr Surg Int.* 2000;16:342-345.

McEwing R, Hayward C, Furness M. Foetal cystic abdominal masses. *Australas Radiol.* 2003;47(2):101-110.

Moore KL, Persaud TVN, eds. *The Developing Human.* ed 8. Philadelphia: Elsevier; 2008.

Parulekar SG. Sonography of the normal fetal bowel. *J Ultrasound Med.* 1991;10:211.

Pretorius DH. Tracheoesophageal fistula in utero (twenty-two cases). *J Ultrasound Med.* 1987;6:509.

Rumack CM, Wilson SR, Charboneau JW, eds. *Diagnostic Ultrasound.* ed 3. St Louis: Elsevier; 2005.

Sase M, Asada M, Okuda M, et al. Fetal gastric size in normal and abnormal pregnancies. *Ultrasound Obstet Gynecol.* 2002;19:467-470.

Schmidt W. Sonographic measurements of the fetal spleen. *J Ultrasound Med.* 1985;4:667.

Yoshizato T, Satoh S, Taguchi T, et al. Intermittent "double bubble" sign in a case of congenital pyloric atresia. *Fetal Diagn Ther.* 2002;17(6):334-338.

CHAPTER 64

Fetal Urogenital System

Mitzi Roberts

OBJECTIVES

On completion of this chapter, you should be able to:
- Discuss the development of the urogenital and genital system
- Describe the sonographic appearance of the fetal kidneys and bladder
- Detail the complications of renal agenesis
- Describe the sonographic findings associated with abnormalities of the kidney
- Differentiate renal cystic disease
- Distinguish between different types of urinary obstruction
- Identify congenital malformations of the genital system

OUTLINE

Embryology and Development of the Urogenital System 1593
   Embryology 1593
   Development of the Kidneys 1593
   Development of the Urinary Bladder 1595
   Development of the External Genitalia 1595

Sonographic Evaluation of the Urogenital System 1595
   Kidneys 1595
   Ureters, Bladder, and Urethra 1596
   Genitalia 1596
   Amniotic Fluid 1599

Sonographic Findings Suggesting Abnormalities of the Urogenital System 1599
   Dilation of Any Component of the Urinary Tract 1599
   Appearance of Hydronephrosis in Only One Pole of the Kidney 1599
   Renal Cyst 1600
   Enlarged Echogenic Kidneys 1600
   Kidney Not Seen 1600
   Bladder Not Seen 1600
   Anechoic, Tortuous Pelvic Mass 1600
   Dilated Posterior Urethra 1600
   Abnormal Amniotic Fluid Volume 1600

Abnormalities of the Urinary Tract 1601

Congenital Malformations of the Kidneys 1601
   Renal Agenesis 1601
   Horseshoe Kidneys 1602
   Renal Ectopia 1603
   Exstrophy of the Bladder 1603
   Urachal Abnormalities 1604

Renal Cystic Disease 1605
   Infantile Polycystic Kidney Disease 1605
   Multicystic Dysplastic Kidney Disease 1606
   Adult Dominant Polycystic Kidney Disease 1607
   Obstructive Cystic Dysplasia 1608

Obstructive Urinary Tract Abnormalities 1608
   Hydronephrosis 1609
   Ureteropelvic Junction Obstruction 1610
   Ureterovesical Junction Obstruction 1610
   Posterior Urethral Valve Obstruction 1611
   Anterior Urethral Valves 1612
   Prune-Belly Syndrome 1614

Other Urinary Anomalies 1615
   Ureterocele 1615
   Renal Tumors 1615

Congenital Malformations of the Genital System 1616
   Hydrocele 1617
   Undescended Testicles 1617
   Ambiguous Genitalia 1617

Other Pelvic Masses 1618
   Hydrometrocolpos 1618
   Fetal Ovarian Cyst 1618

KEY TERMS

Cloacal exstrophy
Cryptorchidism
Epispadias
Fetal hydronephrosis
Hermaphroditism
Horseshoe kidney
Hydrometrocolpos
Hydroureters
Hypospadias

Infantile polycystic kidney disease (IPKD)
Megacystis
Megaureter
Multicystic dysplastic kidney disease (MDKD)
Ovarian cyst
Pelvic kidney
Posterior urethral valve
Potter sequence

Potter syndrome
Prune-belly syndrome
Pyelectasis
Renal agenesis
Urachal cyst
Ureterocele
Ureteropelvic junction (UPJ)
Ureterovesical junction (UVJ)
Urethral atresia

Prenatal sonography aids in the diagnosis of many anomalies of the genitourinary system. A complete sonographic examination includes evaluation of both kidneys, documentation of the urinary bladder, and assessment of amniotic fluid. Abnormalities of the genitourinary system may be discovered incidentally during the complete obstetric sonogram evaluation. For example, in the presence of oligohydramnios, the sonographer may identify abnormalities of the kidneys or bladder, which may have led to the diminished production of amniotic fluid. Maternal history of drug usage or renal disease is also associated with an increased risk of urogenital fetal malformations as listed in Table 64.1.

EMBRYOLOGY AND DEVELOPMENT OF THE UROGENITAL SYSTEM

Embryology

Embryologically and functionally, the urogenital system can be divided into two parts: the urinary system and the genital system. Both systems develop from the intermediate mesoderm, and the excretory ducts of both systems initially enter a common cavity called the cloaca. While the embryo bends and folds in the horizontal plane during the fourth week, the intermediate mesoderm forms a longitudinal mass on both sides of the aorta called the *urogenital ridge*. Both the urinary and genital systems develop from the mesoderm in these ridges. The part of the urogenital ridge that gives rise to the urinary system is known as the nephrogenic cord or nephrogenic ridge. The part that gives rise to the genital system is known as the gonadal ridge or *genital ridge*. The urinary system develops first.

TABLE 64.1	Potential Urogenital Fetal Malformations Associated With Maternal Drug or Chemical Use
Drug	**Fetal Malformations**
Amitriptyline	Micrognathia, limb reduction, swelling of hands and feet, urinary retention
Amobarbital	NTDs, cardiac defects, severe limb deformities, congenital hip dislocation, polydactyly, clubfoot, cleft palate, ambiguous genitalia, soft tissue, deformity of neck
Caffeine	Musculoskeletal defects, hydronephrosis
Cocaine	Spontaneous abortion, placental abruption, prematurity, IUGR, possible cardiac defects, skull defects, genitourinary anomalies
Imipramine	NTDs, cleft palate, renal cysts, diaphragmatic hernia
Sulfonamide	Limb hypoplasia, foot defects, urethral obstruction

Modified from Nyberg DA, Mahony BS, Pretorius DH. *Diagnostic ultrasound of fetal anomalies: text and atlas.* St Louis: Mosby–Year Book; 1990.
IUGR, Intrauterine growth restriction; *NTDs*, neural tube defects.

The sex of the fetus is determined at the time of fertilization, but there is no morphologic indication of sex until the seventh week of development. Early embryogenesis shows similar development in both sexes. The gonads are derived from the gonadal ridges and are the first parts of the genital system to undergo development. As the genital ridge enlarges and frees itself from the mesonephros by developing a mesentery, the male ridge becomes the mesorchium and the female the mesovarium. At the same time, the coelomic epithelium covering the primitive gonads proliferate and form the primary sex cords. The primary sex chords grow into the mesenchyme of the developing gonads. The primordial germ cells originate in the wall of the yolk sac and migrate into the embryo and enter the primary sex cords to give rise to the ova and sperm.

Development of the Kidneys

There are three sets of excretory organs that develop in the embryo: the pronephros, mesonephros, and metanephros. Only the third set remains as the permanent kidneys (Fig. 64.1). The first pair of "kidneys," *pronephros*, are rudimentary and nonfunctional. The second pair of "kidneys," *mesonephroi*, function for a short time during the early fetal period and degenerate after they are replaced by the metanephros or permanent kidneys.

The permanent kidneys (metanephros) begin to develop early in the fifth week while the mesonephroi are still developing (Fig. 64.2). Urine formation begins toward the end of the first trimester, around the 11th to 12th gestational week, and continues actively throughout fetal life. Urine is excreted into the amniotic cavity and forms a major part of the amniotic fluid. The kidneys do not need to function in utero because the placenta eliminates waste from the fetal blood. The kidneys must be able to assume their waste excretion role after birth.

The permanent kidneys develop from two different sources: (1) the metanephric diverticulum or ureteric bud and (2) the metanephric mesoderm (Fig. 64.3). The ureteric

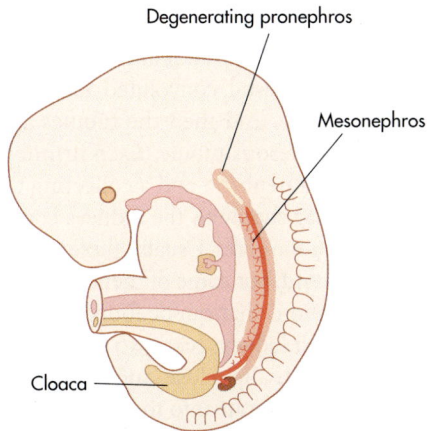

FIG. 64.1 Five-week embryo showing three sets of kidneys that developed in the embryo. The pronephros is rudimentary and nonfunctional. The mesonephros functions for 2 weeks and then degenerates. The metanephros develops into the permanent kidney.

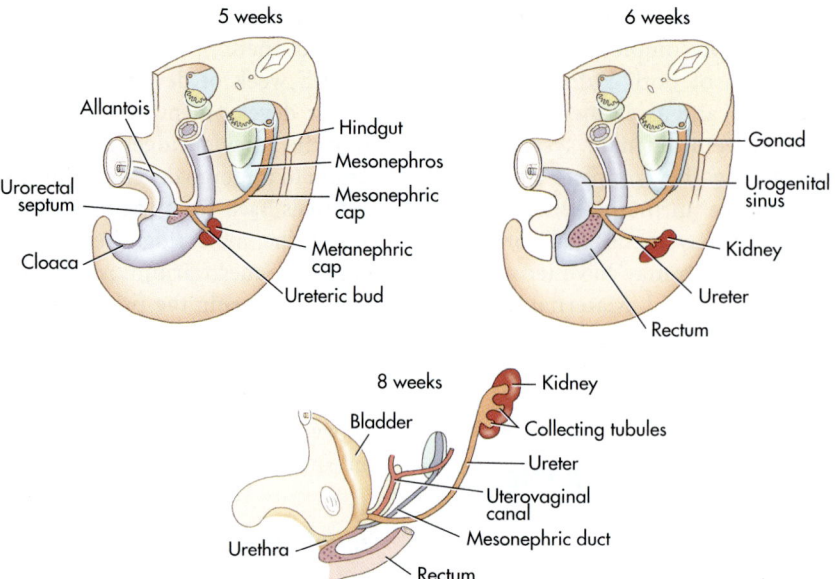

FIG. 64.2 Early embryologic development of the urinary system.

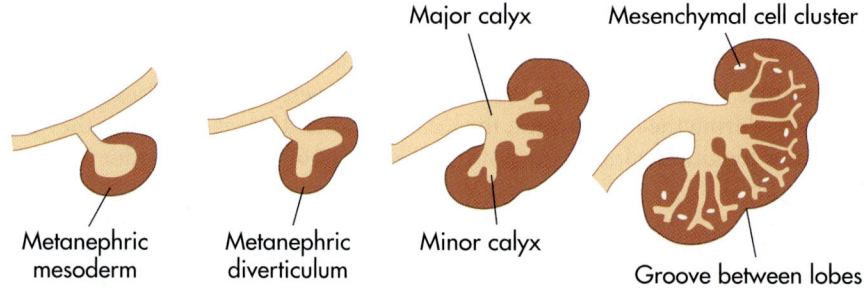

FIG. 64.3 Developing kidney in weeks 5 through 8.

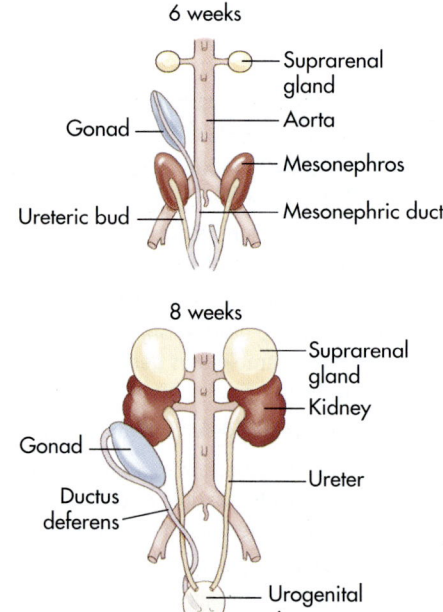

FIG. 64.4 The kidneys begin in the pelvis with gradual migration into the abdomen.

bud gives rise to the ureter, renal pelvis, calyces, and collecting tubules. The collecting tubule is also derived from the ureteric bud. The major and minor calyces are developed from these collecting tubules.

The ends of the tubules form metanephric vesicles. The ends of these tubules are invaginated by an ingrowth of the fine blood vessels, the glomerulus, to form a double-layered cup called the glomerular capsule or Bowman capsule. The renal corpuscle (glomerulus and capsule) and its associated tubules form a nephron. Each distal convoluted tubule contacts an arched collecting tubule, and then the tubules become confluent, forming a uriniferous tubule. Each uriniferous tubule consists of two parts: a nephron and a collecting tubule.

The arterial vascular supply to the kidneys comes from the arteries that arise from the aorta. Usually, these vessels disappear when the kidneys ascend, but some of them may persist, which accounts for the variations that can be found in the renal arteries. At least 25% of adult kidneys have two to four renal arteries.

The kidneys initially lie close together in the pelvis. Gradually, the kidneys migrate into the abdomen and become separated from one another (Fig. 64.4). They normally complete this migration by the ninth week of gestation. In some cases, one of the kidneys may remain in the pelvic cavity while the other migrates into the posterior flank of the abdomen.

With sonography, the identification of a **pelvic kidney** may be seen with adequate bladder dilation and may appear in females as a pelvic mass.

Development of the Urinary Bladder

The fetal urinary bladder is derived from the hindgut derivative known as the urogenital sinus (see Fig. 64.2). The caudal ends of the mesonephric ducts open into the cloaca, and parts of them are gradually absorbed into the wall of the urinary bladder. This development causes the ureters (derived from the ureteric buds) and the mesonephric ducts to enter the bladder separately.

Although the kidneys migrate upward, the orifices of the ureters move cranially, and the primordia of the ejaculatory ducts (derived from the mesonephric ducts) move toward one another and enter the prostatic part of the urethra. The epithelium of the female urethra and most of the epithelium of the male urethra is derived from the endoderm of the urogenital sinus.

Development of the External Genitalia

Although the early development of the external genitalia is similar for both sexes, distinguishing sexual characteristics begin during the ninth week and external genital organs are fully differentiated by the 12th week of gestation (Fig. 64.5). In the fourth week, a genital tubercle develops at the cranial end of the cloacal membrane. Labioscrotal swellings and urogenital folds develop on either side of this membrane. The genital tubercle elongates to form a phallus, which is similar in both sexes. The hormonal changes cause further development of the male and female reproductive system (Fig. 64.6).

Development of the Male External Genitalia. The fetal testes produce androgens that cause the masculinization of the external genitalia. The phallus elongates to form the penis. This sonographic finding is known as the "turtle" sign. The urogenital folds fuse on the ventral surface of the penis to form the spongy urethra. The labioscrotal swellings grow toward the median plane and fuse to form the scrotum. The line of fusion of the labioscrotal folds is called the scrotal raphe.

Development of the Female External Genitalia. Both the urethra and vagina open into the urogenital sinus, the vestibule of the vagina. The urogenital folds become the labia minora, the labioscrotal swellings become the labia majora, and the phallus becomes the clitoris.

SONOGRAPHIC EVALUATION OF THE UROGENITAL SYSTEM

Kidneys

The kidneys should be evaluated by assessing their anatomy, texture, and size. With transvaginal sonography, the fetal kidneys have been documented as early as 9 weeks of gestation. By 12 weeks of gestation, at least 86% of the fetal kidneys may be imaged. The fetal kidneys and bladder may be seen sonographically by 13 weeks of gestation. The kidneys appear as bilateral hyperechoic structures in the paravertebral regions. At approximately 15 weeks of gestation, the overall echogenicity will decrease, and the renal pelvis may

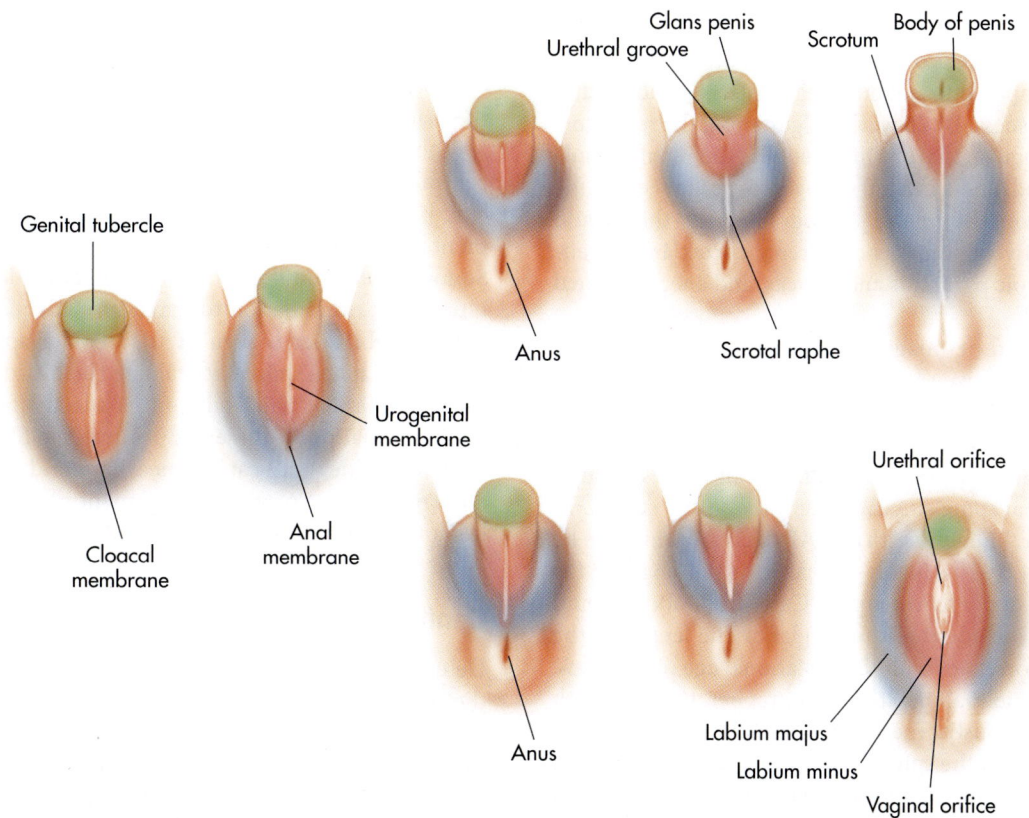

FIG. 64.5 Sexual characteristics begin to develop during the 9th week and are fully differentiated by the 12th week.

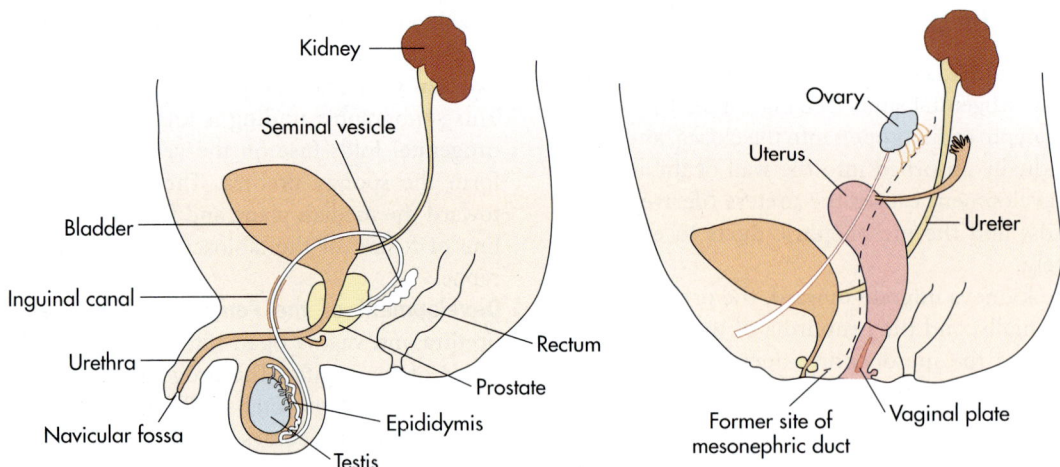

FIG. 64.6 Hormonal changes cause further development of the male and female reproductive systems.

> **BOX 64.1 Sonographic Evaluation of the Urogenital System**
>
> - Bladder: assess presence and size
> - Kidneys: assess presence, number, position, and appearance (texture)
> - Collecting system: assess if normal or dilated; if dilated, look for level and cause of obstruction, whether it is unilateral or bilateral
> - Fetal sex

appear as sonolucent areas within the central kidney. As the fetal age advances, fat deposits in the perinephric and sinus regions become visible. Beginning at 18 weeks of gestation, kidneys should be documented in all fetuses sonographically. Between 18 and 20 weeks of gestation, the kidneys are slightly hyperechoic compared to surrounding tissues (i.e., bowel and paravertebral tissues). By 25 weeks of gestation, the renal cortex can be distinguished from the medulla, the renal capsule is clearly outlined, and a central echogenic area is seen in the renal sinus region (Box 64.1). Sonographically, this would appear as a relatively homogeneous renal cortex and parenchyma, hypoechoic pyramids and calyces, and anechoic renal pelvis (Fig. 64.7).

The kidneys can be imaged in the sagittal, transverse, or coronal planes. The size of the fetal kidneys may be assessed by measuring the length, width, and height (anterior-posterior [AP] diameter) of the kidney (Table 64.2). In both the sagittal and transverse view, the kidneys can be best visualized with the fetal spine situated anteriorly on the screen. In the sagittal plane, kidney length and AP measurements can be obtained (Fig. 64.8). This involves measuring the length of the kidney from the upper to lower pole. Careful attention should be made not to include the adrenal gland. The length of the kidney closely correlates with the gestational age of the fetus. The transverse view allows the sonographer to view both kidneys simultaneously. The kidneys are circular structures lying on each side of the spine. In this view, both kidneys can be evaluated and compared for echogenicity, width size, and renal pelvis size. The renal pelvis, if visible, may be measured in the AP diameter when the fetal spine is toward the maternal anterior wall (Fig. 64.9). The upper limit of normal is 4 mm up to the third trimester and 7 mm from the third trimester until term. A small amount of urine may be seen in the renal pelvis in the normal fetus. On coronal images, the kidneys are bordered medially by the psoas muscles and superiorly by the hypoechoic adrenal glands.

Ureters, Bladder, and Urethra

In normal conditions, the fetal bladder is well visualized as an anechoic structure in the fetal pelvis (see Box 64.1). The fetal ureters and urethra are typically not seen. The ureter visualized sonographically as an anechoic fluid structure at the renal pelvis in normal conditions with the ureters measuring less than 1 mm to 2 mm in diameter. Urine jets may be seen in the bladder where the ureters enter.

The bladder is imaged as a rounded echo-free area located centrally in the pelvis (see Fig. 64.7B–D). There is no specific bladder measurement usually applied; however, documentation of the bladder filling and emptying is important. Sonographers should identify the fetal bladder early in the ultrasound examination to make sure adequate fluid is present. If no bladder is seen or the bladder appears too large, the sonographer should reevaluate the bladder at the end of the examination. This is due in part to the fact that the fetal bladder usually takes at least 30 minutes to fill and empty. The normal bladder wall can be measured and should be thin in a normal fetus. Normal measurement of the wall is 2 mm or less and is best measured at the level of the umbilical artery.

Genitalia

Determination of the fetal sex should be documented with the presence of other abnormalities or in cases in which the external organ does not meet the sonographic criteria for a male or female. Therefore, it is extremely important that the sonographer use specific sonographic criteria when determining the sex of the fetus. The inability to visualize the penis

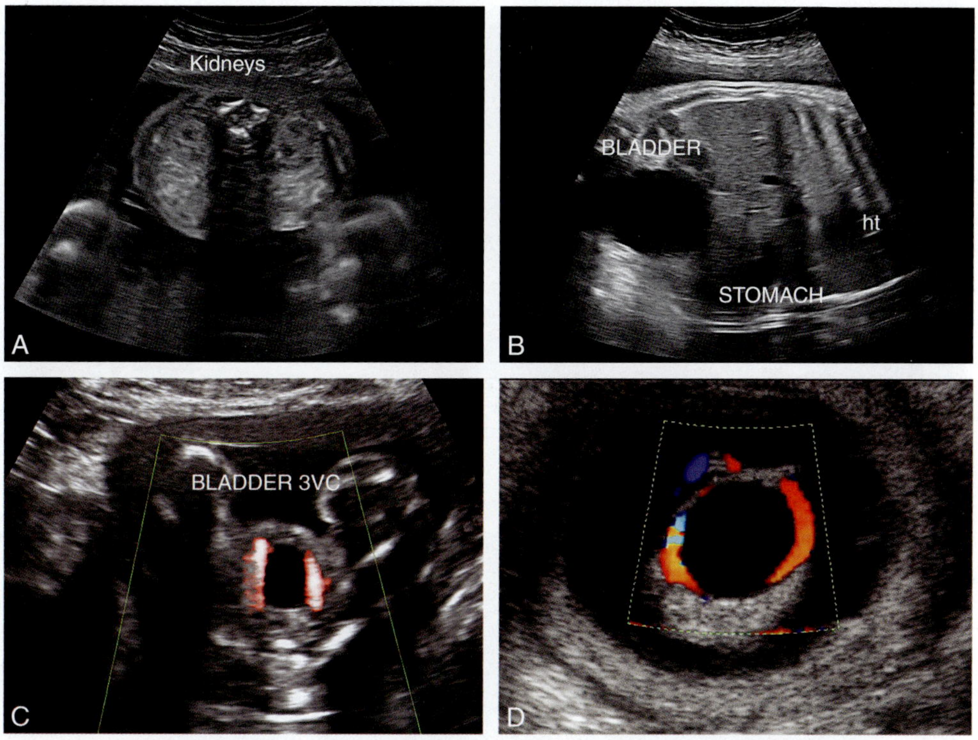

FIG. 64.7 (A) Normal kidneys in the transverse view located on either side of the fetal spine. The anterior position of the spine provides optimal resolution for evaluating the kidneys. (B) The anechoic bladder is noted caudal in the fetal body as it relates the anechoic fetal stomach. (C) The bladder is noted lying between, low within the pelvis. Color Doppler reveals arterial blood flow on each side of the bladder, supporting the findings of a three-vessel cord (3VC). (D) An obstructed fetal bladder is noted in an early second-trimester fetus. Color Doppler reveals the presence of a three-vessel cord. *ht*, Heart.

TABLE 64.2	Kidney Dimensions: Normal Values											
Age (Weeks)	Kidney Thickness (mm)			Kidney Width (mm)			Kidney Length (mm)			Kidney Volume (cm³)		
	5th	50th	95th	5th	50th	95th	5th	50th	95th	5th	50th	95th
16	2	6	10	6	10	13	7	13	18	—	0.4	2.6
17	3	7	11	6	10	14	10	15	20	—	0.6	2.8
18	4	8	12	6	10	14	12	17	22	—	0.7	2.9
19	5	9	13	7	10	14	14	19	24	—	0.9	3.1
20	6	10	13	7	11	15	15	21	26	—	1.1	3.3
21	6	10	14	8	12	15	17	22	28	—	1.4	3.6
22	7	11	15	8	12	16	19	24	29	—	1.7	3.9
23	8	12	16	9	13	17	21	26	31	—	2.1	4.3
24	9	13	17	10	14	18	22	28	33	0.3	2.5	4.7
25	10	14	18	11	15	19	24	29	34	0.8	3.0	5.2
26	11	15	19	12	16	19	25	31	36	1.3	3.5	5.7
27	11	15	19	12	16	20	27	32	37	1.9	4.1	6.3
28	12	16	20	13	17	21	28	33	38	2.5	4.7	6.9
29	13	17	21	14	18	22	29	35	40	3.2	5.4	7.6
30	14	18	22	15	19	23	31	36	41	3.9	6.1	8.3
31	14	18	22	16	20	24	32	37	42	4.6	6.8	9.0
32	15	19	23	17	20	24	33	38	43	5.4	7.5	9.7
33	16	20	23	17	21	25	34	39	44	6.1	8.3	10.5
34	16	20	24	18	22	26	35	40	45	6.8	9.0	11.2
35	17	21	25	18	22	26	35	41	46	7.4	9.6	11.8
36	17	21	25	19	23	27	36	41	47	8.1	10.2	12.4
37	18	22	26	19	23	27	37	42	47	8.6	10.8	13.0
38	18	22	26	19	23	27	37	43	48	9.0	11.2	13.4
39	19	23	27	19	23	27	38	43	48	9.4	11.6	13.8
40	19	23	27	19	23	27	38	44	49	9.6	11.8	14.0

From Romero R, et al. *Prenatal diagnosis of congenital anomalies.* Norwalk, CT: Appleton & Lange; 1988.

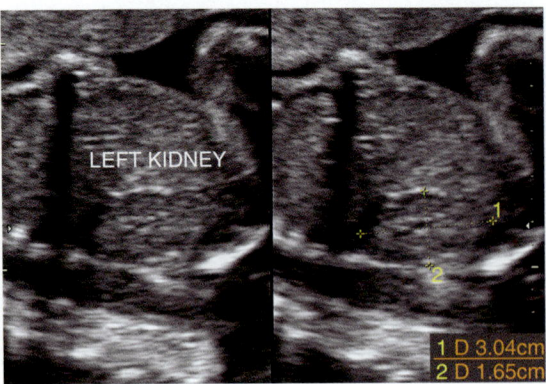

FIG. 64.8 A length measurement of the left kidney is 3.04 cm. This is in normal range for the 30-week-old fetus. The length of a normal kidney reflects the approximate gestational age of the fetus.

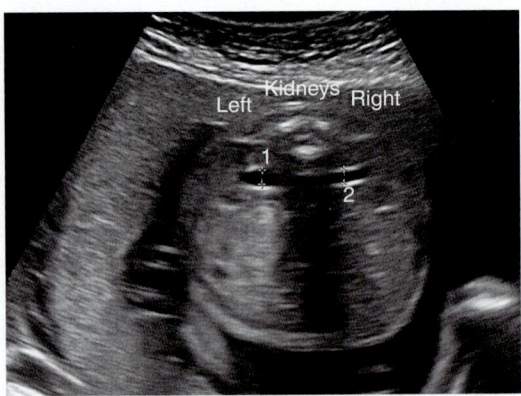

FIG. 64.9 A normal amount of fluid is noted within the renal pelvis. Anterior-posterior diameters reflect the amount of pyelectasis.

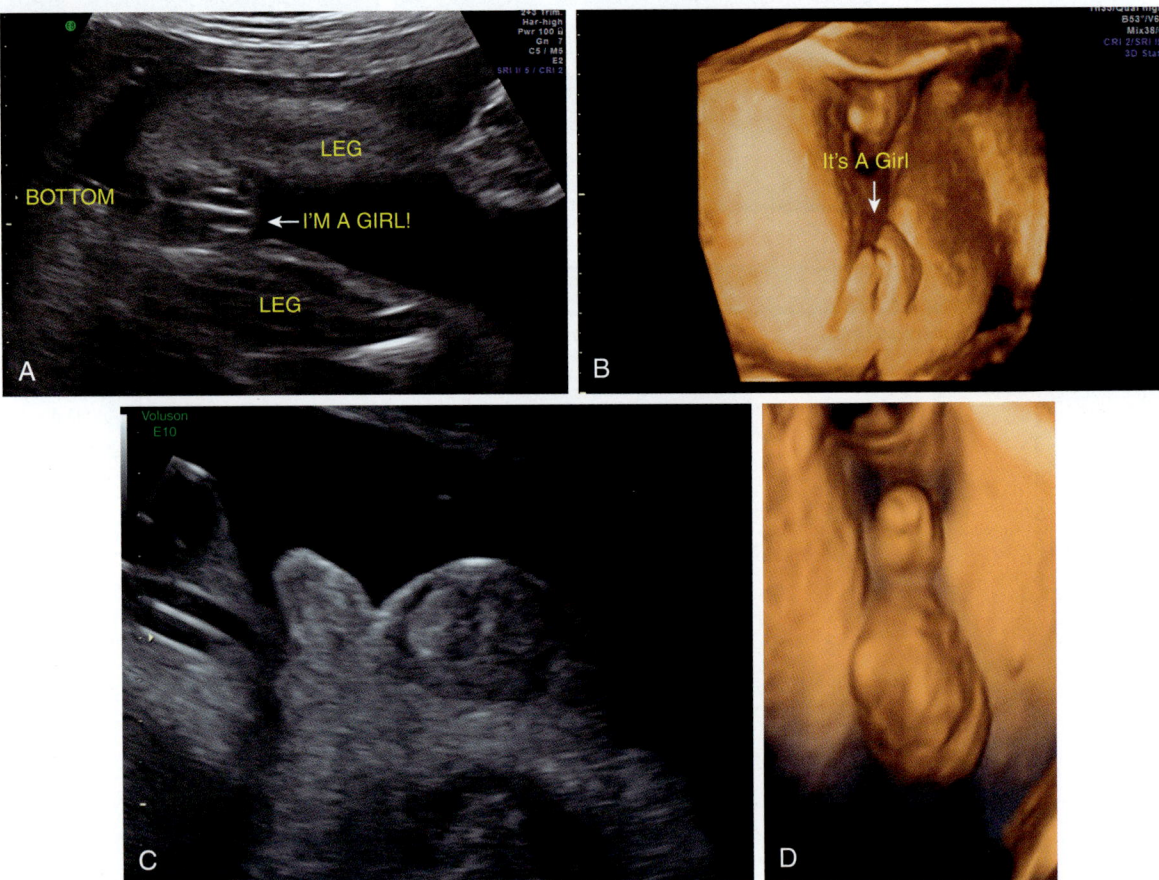

FIG. 64.10 (A) Echogenic lines of the labia majora and labia minora reflect the "hamburger" sign in this female fetus. (B) Use of three- and four-dimensional (3D/4D) technology aids in the visualization of the female genitalia. (C) The scrotum and penis of this male fetus are clearly appreciated. (D) Use of 3D/4D technology aids in the visualization of the male genitalia.

and scrotum should not be used as the determining factor to identify a female fetus.

In the majority of fetuses, the external genitalia can be differentiated in the second trimester. In the first trimester, differentiation is hard to determine due to the protrusion of the external genital tubercle. The genital tubercle will appear the same in the male and female fetus. In the second trimester, identification of the female fetus should only be determined when the major and minor labia are seen. Visualization of the labia is often called the "hamburger" sign (Fig. 64.10A). The male fetus in second trimester is determined by the visualization of the penis and scrotal sac, also known as the "turtle" sign (see Fig. 64.10C). The testes are not visible within the scrotal sac until approximately 28 weeks of gestation. The use of three-dimensional (3D) or four-dimensional (4D) imaging has proven helpful as well (see Fig. 64.10B and D).

Amniotic Fluid

Amniotic fluid is a critical marker in the assessment of renal function. The fetal kidneys begin to excrete urine after the 11th week but do not become the major contributor of fetal urine (and hence of amniotic fluid volume) until 14 to 16 weeks of pregnancy. Therefore, the observation of normal amniotic fluid volume before this time will not exclude the possibility of **renal agenesis** (absent kidneys).

SONOGRAPHIC FINDINGS SUGGESTING ABNORMALITIES OF THE UROGENITAL SYSTEM

In this section, several sonographic findings are listed that suggest abnormalities of the urogenital system. Detail descriptions of each pathology mentioned will follow on later pages. This section is intended to stimulate the sonographer's mind into thinking through any abnormality that may be seen and documenting images specifically related to the abnormality. Sonographers should be encouraged to critically think through their images and document supporting evidence that would aid in diagnosis.

Dilation of Any Component of the Urinary Tract

Obstructions of the urinary system may originate anywhere along the urinary tract. The sonographic features of the dilation include anechoic enlargement of the affected area (Fig. 64.11A). The consequences and sonographic findings of an obstruction depend on the origin of the blockage. For example, in fetuses with a urethral obstruction, such as complete posterior urethral valve obstruction, urine is unable to pass through the urethra and into the amniotic fluid. Consequently, urine backs up in the posterior urethra, bladder, and ureters and often extends to the kidneys (hydronephrosis).

If dilation of the renal collecting system is present, either hydronephrosis or reflux should be considered. Complete sonographic evaluation of the kidney, ureter, and bladder should be made to help determine the level of the obstruction causing the dilation. The level of obstruction is determined by the degree of dilation of the renal pelvis and ureter. When the entire renal collecting system is involved, a simple hydronephrosis is usually the cause. Ureteropelvic junction obstruction shows dilation of the renal pelvis, whereas ureteric dilation suggests either a ureterovesical junction obstruction or reflux (see Fig. 64.11B). Ureterovesical reflux may also cause bilateral hydronephrosis. When the hydronephrosis is bilateral, the possibility of bladder outlet obstruction should be considered. The sonographer should look for dilated ureters, thickened (hypertrophied) bladder wall, and dilation of the posterior urethra (see Fig. 64.11C). The renal parenchyma should be made in the presence of hydronephrosis. If an echogenic cortex is present with subcapsular cysts, secondary renal dysplasia and poor function of the affected kidney may be present. In cases of urethral obstruction and bilateral renal dysplasia, oligohydramnios is typically noted after 16 weeks of gestation.

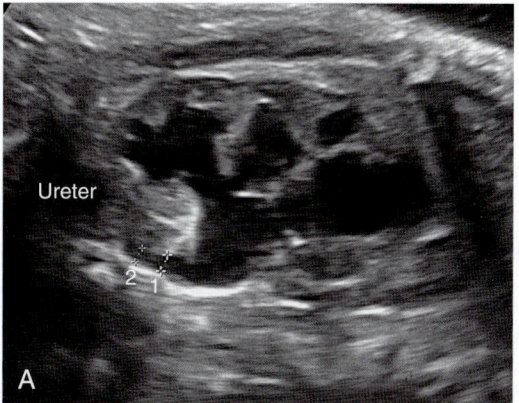
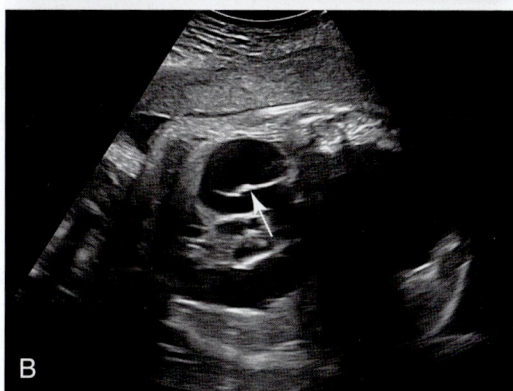
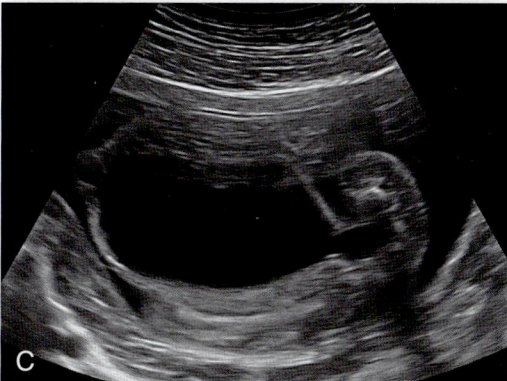

FIG. 64.11 (A) The kidney in this fetus reflects dilation of ureter, renal pelvis, and calyces. (B) Image of a dilated tortuous ureter. (C) The signature keyhole sign is noted in this enlarged bladder and urethra.

Appearance of Hydronephrosis in Only One Pole of the Kidney

Duplication of the renal collecting system is common. It usually occurs in females and typically is not diagnosed in utero. The duplication occurs during embryology in which two ureteral buds are formed. The term *moiety* is often used to describe the two parts of the kidney. The degree of duplication will vary: two renal pelves are noted with two ureters each entering the bladder, two renal pelves join to form one ureter, and two renal pelves with two ureters that join in the abdominopelvic cavity before bladder insertion.

In most cases, the upper pole is susceptible to obstruction whereas the lower pole is susceptible to reflux. In utero, the sonogram may reveal an enlarged kidney; however, the presence of hydronephrosis located high in the kidney rather than mid is an indication of possible obstruction related to duplication. The bladder should be carefully examined for the presence of a ureterocele. Ureteroceles are commonly associated with duplicated collecting systems and appear as an anechoic cystic structure within the bladder.

Renal Cyst

The cause and sonographic appearance of fetal renal cysts vary. Careful assessment of the kidneys includes comparison of both kidneys as well as distinguishing cyst from hydronephrosis. For example, a multicystic kidney may be seen with a large central cyst and multiple small noncommunicating peripheral cysts. Hydronephrosis involving the calyces can be differentiated from the multicystic kidney by verifying communication among the cysts. A single large cyst most likely represents a simple renal cyst.

Enlarged Echogenic Kidneys

When the kidneys appear enlarged and echogenic, the sonographer should consider a form of polycystic disease, trisomy 13, or Meckel-Gruber syndrome. In cases of congenital polycystic diseases, a thorough review of family history should be completed. In infantile polycystic renal disease, oligohydramnios may be present, whereas normal amniotic fluid volumes are seen with adult polycystic disease. In cases of syndrome association, a complete obstetric sonogram will most likely reveal other findings related to the syndrome.

Kidney Not Seen

Kidneys should be visualized at the same level on each side of the spine in the transverse view. If either kidney is not visualized, the sonographer should evaluate for a pelvic kidney or absence of one or both kidneys. A pelvic kidney may be visualized with a thorough evaluation of the fetal pelvis. Renal agenesis may involve one or both kidneys. In unilateral renal agenesis the contralateral kidney is usually quite large because of compensating for the absent kidney. If both kidneys are absent, the bladder will not be seen, the stomach will not be seen, and severe oligohydramnios is evident beginning in the second trimester. Early in the first trimester, the oligohydramnios may not be apparent, and the stomach may be visible. The use of color Doppler aids in determining the location of the renal vessels leading into the kidney or lack of kidney.

Bladder Not Seen

Failure to observe the bladder may indicate a severe renal abnormality when accompanied by oligohydramnios. When obstruction occurs at the level of the urethra, the bladder wall becomes hypertrophied. The presence of ureteral jets may be assessed in the fetus to rule out obstruction. Using color Doppler over the area of the bladder, near the base, will aid in the visualization of ureteral jets. The presence of ureteral jets streaming into the bladder indicates that the ureter is not obstructed.

Anechoic, Tortuous Pelvic Mass

When the ureters are pathologically dilated, they become visible as tortuous cystic masses in the midportion of the lower fetal pelvis. Abnormally dilated ureters are referred to as **hydroureters** and may be traced into the kidney and bladder (see Fig. 64.11B). Careful attention should be made not to mistake the dilated ureter for bowel. In cases of unilateral ureter obstruction, the amniotic fluid will most likely be low to normal; however, if both ureters are obstructed, oligohydramnios will be present.

Dilated Posterior Urethra

Dilation of the posterior urethra is highly suspicious for an obstructive process, such as posterior urethral valve syndrome, known as the *key bladder sign* on sonography, as the dilated bladder has the shape of a keyhole superior to the obstructed urethra (see Fig. 64.11C). Both kidneys will appear with severe hydronephrosis (late stages may appear with dysplastic changes), oligohydramnios will be present, the stomach will not be seen, and both ureters will be dilated. The **posterior urethral valve** occurs only in male fetuses and is manifested by the presence of a valve in the posterior urethra.

Abnormal Amniotic Fluid Volume

Amniotic fluid volume is a significant factor in predicting outcome. Box 64.2 lists common renal abnormalities. In fetuses with severe renal disease, amniotic fluid is reduced, and in the most severe malformations, it is virtually absent. When severe oligohydramnios is found, usually both kidneys or ureters and the urethra are malformed. Unilateral obstructions may yield a normal amount of amniotic fluid because the contralateral kidney produces urine. Conversely, hydramnios may be present with some renal disorders, such as mesoblastic nephroma and unilateral renal obstruction.

BOX 64.2 Renal Abnormalities

Renal agenesis
Multicystic renal dysplasia
Congenital hydronephrosis
Renal duplication
Pelvic kidney
Horseshoe kidney
Infantile polycystic kidney disease
Adult polycystic kidney disease
Meckel-Gruber syndrome

ABNORMALITIES OF THE URINARY TRACT

Renal malformations may be divided into two categories: (1) those involving congenital malformation and (2) those resulting from an obstructive process (see Box 64.2). The consequences of renal malformations vary depending on the type of lesion and extent of obstruction (Fig. 64.12). The recognition of urinary tract anomalies is of significant clinical concern because several fetal conditions are incompatible with life. Recognition of lethal or treatable renal anomalies is necessary to ensure appropriate clinical and therapeutic management.

CONGENITAL MALFORMATIONS OF THE KIDNEYS

Renal Agenesis

Etiology. Complete absence of the kidney(s) is known as renal agenesis. This condition occurs when the ureteric buds fail to develop or when they degenerate before they can induce the metanephric mesoderm to form nephrons.

Clinical Findings and Prognosis. Prognosis is dependent on unilateral or bilateral involvement of the kidneys as well as associated abnormalities. In the diagnosis of renal agenesis, acquiring a complete clinical history and a thorough examination of all fetal structures is critical. Family members should be screened for renal abnormalities to rule out the possibility of autosomal dominant inheritance. Clinical history should include documentation of possible cocaine usage and maternal diabetes. Both have been linked to renal agenesis.

Bilateral renal agenesis is a lethal disorder due to renal insufficiency and hypoplasia of the lungs. The absence of amniotic fluid plays a role in the underdevelopment of the fetal lungs. In cases of unilateral agenesis, the presence of at least one functioning kidney contributes to excellent survival rates. Therefore, unilateral agenesis carries a good prognosis, especially with appropriate urologic follow-up. Bilateral agenesis occurs in 1 in 3000 to 1 in 10,000 births and the male-to-female ratio is 2.5:1. Unilateral agenesis is more common and has been estimated to occur in 1 in 600 to 1000 births with a male-to-female ratio of 1:1.

Bilateral renal agenesis is often referred to as **Potter syndrome**. Infants born with bilateral renal agenesis exhibit Potter facies (flat nose, recessed chin, abnormal ears, and wide-set eyes) and abnormal or malpositioned limbs. These deformities are caused by the lack of amniotic fluid. Under normal conditions amniotic fluid protects the fetus from the walls of the uterus allowing fetal structures such as the extremities to open and close. In cases of oligohydramnios, the uterine walls place pressure on the fetus and the fetal extremities are typically held in limited positions, leading to abnormal development.

Other fetal anomalies found in association with bilateral renal agenesis include cardiac defects and musculoskeletal disorders (sirenomelia, absent radius and fibula, anomalies of the digits, sacral agenesis, diaphragmatic hernia, and cleft palate). Central nervous system anomalies include hydrocephalus, meningocele, cephalocele, holoprosencephaly, anencephaly, and microcephaly. Gastrointestinal anomalies include duodenal atresia, imperforate anus, tracheoesophageal fistula, malrotation, and omphalocele. The sonographer should understand that most of these malformations are not detected prenatally because of poor visualization resulting from anhydramnios (complete lack of amniotic fluid). Unilateral agenesis may be associated with uterine anomalies in females and testicular hypoplasia, agenesis, or **hypospadias** in males. It should also be noted that there is a high incidence of abnormalities in the functioning kidney, specifically vesicoureteral reflux.

Sonographic Findings. Sonographic findings are dependent on unilateral or bilateral renal agenesis. In both cases, the kidney or kidneys are not visualized (Figs. 64.13 and 64.14). Careful examination of the abdominopelvic region must be completed to rule out a possible ectopic or pelvic kidney. Color Doppler can be used to delineate the renal vessels and the attachment to the aorta in the area of the kidneys. In the renal fossa of the absent kidney(s), the adrenal gland may mimic the kidney. The adrenal gland will appear hypoechoic with an echogenic center and in a flattened or lying-down position.

In bilateral renal agenesis, the kidney(s) and bladder are not visualized sonographically (Box 64.3; see Fig. 64.14). Nonvisualization of the anechoic urinary bladder during 1 hour of consistent scanning has been considered a sonographic sign of bilateral renal agenesis. The lack of urine being produced results in oligohydramnios. In the early stages of renal agenesis (before 15 to 18 weeks), amniotic fluid may be visible as it is produced from other fetal sources.

In unilateral renal agenesis, the contralateral kidney may be hypertrophied to compensate for the absent kidney (see Fig. 64.13B). Therefore, the length of the kidney present will

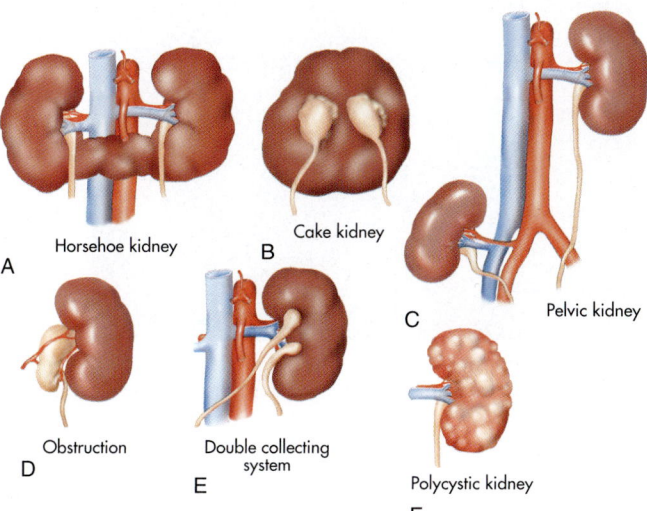

FIG. 64.12 Variations of the kidney. (A) Horseshoe kidney shown as two kidneys connected by an isthmus anterior to the aorta and inferior vena cava. (B) "Cake" kidney that has failed to divide with a double collecting system. (C) Pelvic kidney with one kidney in the normal retroperitoneal position. (D) Extrarenal pelvis. (E) Double collecting system. (F) Polycystic kidney.

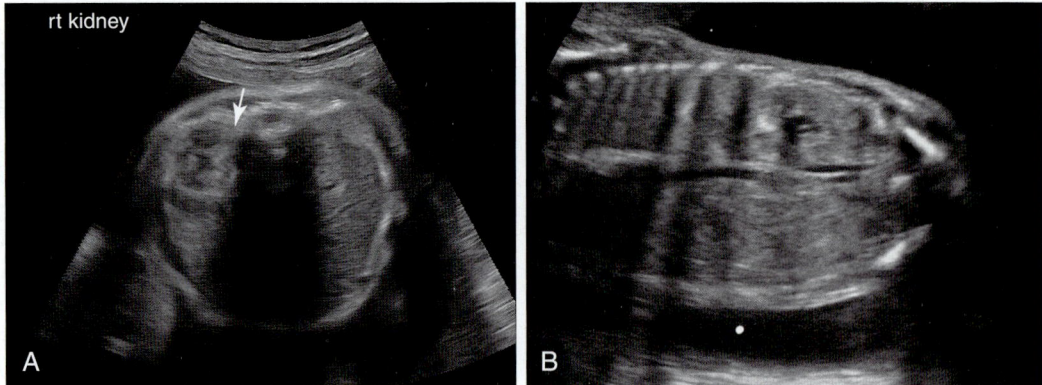

FIG. 64.13 (A) Transverse view of the fetal kidneys in this 31-week-old fetus reveals visualization of the right kidney without visualization of the left kidney at the same level. (B) This sagittal view of the same fetus supports the empty renal fossa on the left.

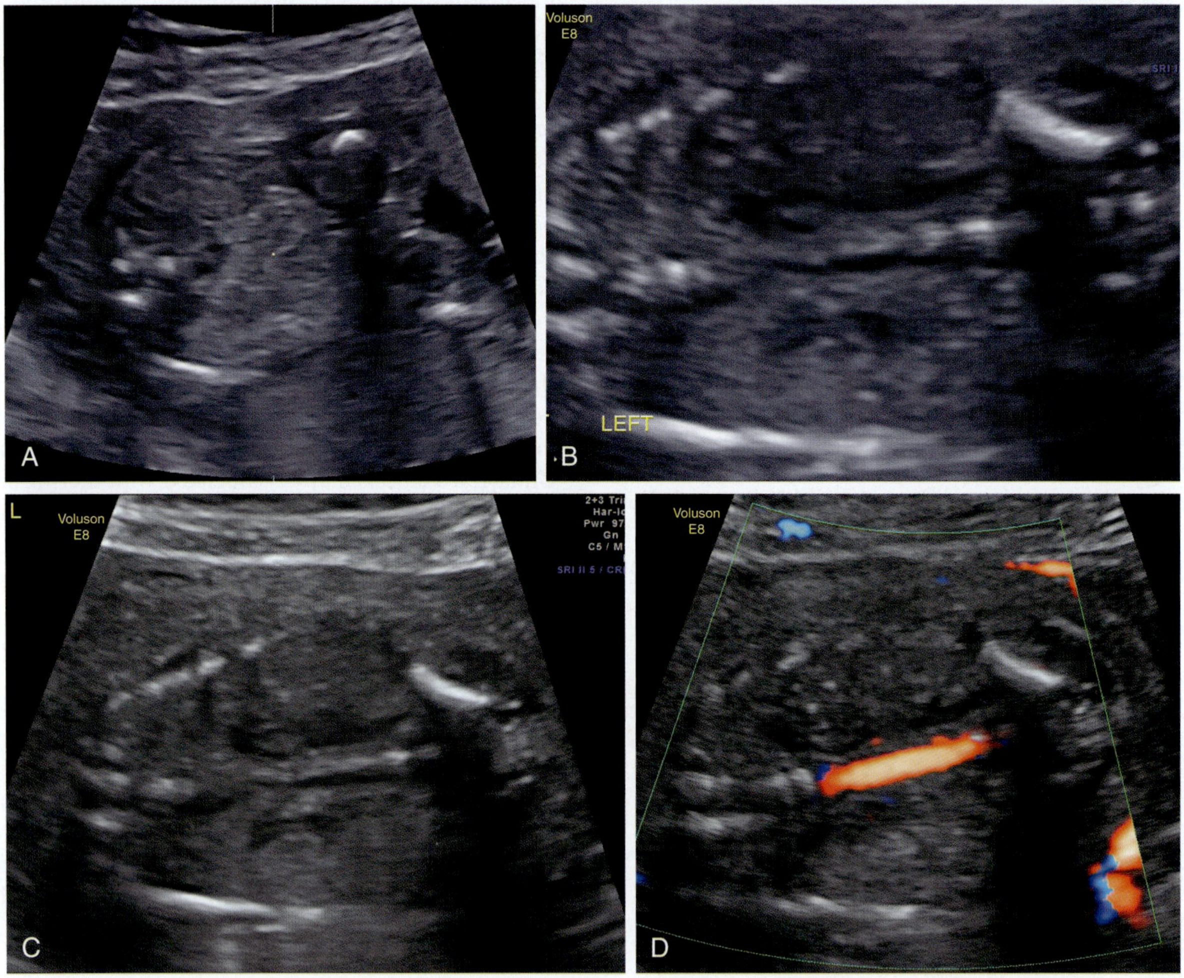

FIG. 64.14 (A) Transverse image of the abdomen does not demonstrate the right and left kidney. (B) Coronal image of the fetal abdomen demonstrating nonvisualization of the kidneys. (C) The adrenal glands appear hypoechoic and flat in the coronal image. (D) Use of Doppler at the level of the renal arteries demonstrates absence of both renal arteries.

be greater than the gestational age. The bladder will be visualized, and adequate amounts of amniotic fluid are produced.

Horseshoe Kidneys

Etiology. A **horseshoe kidney** forms when the inferior poles of the kidney fuse while they are in the pelvis. This fusion may occur in 1 to 4 in 1000 births and is 2 to 3 times more common in males (see Fig. 64.12).

Clinical Findings and Prognosis. Horseshoe kidneys may be found as an isolated anomaly or in associated with other anomalies or syndromes. The frequency of horseshoe kidneys is approximately 1 in 450 births. Isolated horseshoe kidneys carry a good prognosis. Renal conditions, such as kidney stones,

> **BOX 64.3** **Sonographic Findings in Renal Agenesis**
>
> - Severe oligohydramnios after 13–15 weeks of menstrual age
> - Persistent absence of urine in fetal bladder (observe for period of 1 hour)
> - Failure to visualize kidneys or renal arteries (use color flow to outline renal arteries)
> - Abnormally small thorax

Difficulties arise when oligohydramnios is present or when fetus is in breech presentation. Be careful not to mistake bowel or adrenal gland for kidneys. An empty bladder may be due to other impaired renal function problems.

urinary tract infections, hydronephrosis, and reflux, are often associated with horseshoe kidneys.

The presence of other abnormalities is uncommon. Central nervous system disorders, cardiac abnormalities, and/or urogenital abnormalities have been documented. The incidence of trisomy 18 and 45,X has also been noted. The presence of other abnormalities directly affects the outcome of the fetus.

Sonographic Findings. The horseshoe kidney is the fusion of the lower poles of both kidneys. In general, horseshoe kidneys are difficult to diagnosis in utero. The bridge of tissue connecting the lower poles must be demonstrated for accurate diagnosis. In a transverse image of the fetal abdomen with the spine down, a connecting isthmus may be seen anterior to the aorta. In the sagittal and coronal views, clear delineation of the inferior pole of the kidney is not well seen and the kidneys may appear oblique.

Renal Ectopia

Etiology. As discussed, the kidneys initially lie remarkably close in the pelvis. Gradually they migrate into the abdomen and become separated from one another. They normally complete this migration by the ninth week of gestation. In some cases, one of the kidneys may remain in the pelvic cavity while the other migrates into the posterior flank of the abdomen.

Clinical Findings and Prognosis. Ectopic kidney(s) occurs when the kidney lies outside of its normal position in the renal fossa, usually in the area of the pelvis (see Fig. 64.12). Occasionally, crossed ectopia will occur. In crossed ectopia, both kidneys may be fused or appear to be fused because they are located on the same side of the body (considered a form of horseshoe kidney). The crossed-fused ectopic kidney lies on the opposite side of the abdomen relative to its ureteral insertion into the bladder. The kidneys are usually fused together and are usually found on the right side of the abdomen. In rare incidences, the kidney may be located in the thoracic cavity and more commonly on the left side.

Prognosis for ectopic kidneys is based on acquired complications or in association with other anomalies. Ectopic kidneys can have complications of dilation or dysplasia. Associated anomalies include skeletal, cardiovascular, gynecologic, and gastrointestinal abnormalities.

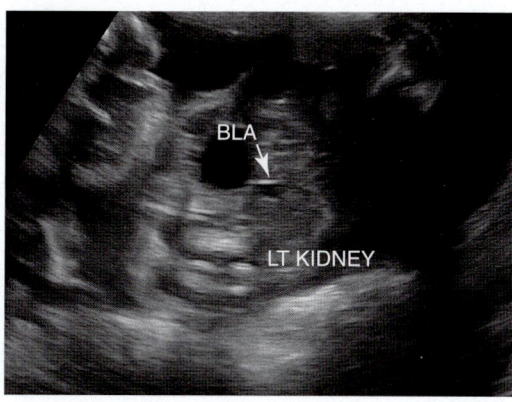

FIG. 64.15 The left kidney was not seen in its normal location in this 23-week-old fetus. Further evaluation of the fetus identified the left kidney adjacent to the bladder in the lower pelvis.

Sonographic Findings. Sonography will demonstrate absence of the kidney in its normal position, with the adrenal gland filling the space of the renal fossa. The abnormally located kidney will typically be smaller and rotated obliquely or horizontal. If the kidney is located in the pelvis, it is typically found lying superior to the bladder or adjacent to the iliac wing (Fig. 64.15). In cases of crossed-fused ectopic kidneys, both kidneys will appear on the same side demonstrating an enlarged bilobed kidney.

Exstrophy of the Bladder

Etiology. Exstrophy of the bladder is characterized by the protrusion of the posterior wall of the urinary bladder, which contains the trigone of the bladder and the ureteric orifices. It is caused by the defective closure of the inferior part of the anterior abdominal wall during the fourth week of gestation. As a result, no muscle or connective tissue forms in the anterior abdominal wall to cover the urinary bladder, resulting in the bladder forming external to the abdominal wall.

Clinical Findings and Prognosis. Exstrophy of the bladder occurs primarily in males, with an incidence of 1 in 30,000 births. It is most likely of sporadic occurrence and isolated. Laboratory markers will reveal an elevated maternal serum alpha-fetoprotein. Genitalia malformations are commonly seen, such as undescended testes or anterior displaced scrotum and a small penis with **epispadias** in males or a cleft clitoris in females. Multiple surgical procedures are required to correct the bladder abnormality as well as other associated genital anomalies. In the majority of cases urinary continence is restored.

Sonographic Findings. A fluid-filled bladder is not visualized in the presence of normal kidneys and normal amniotic fluid levels. A small irregular mass representing the everted atrophied bladder is identified in the lower abdomen below the umbilical cord insertion (Fig. 64.16). The abdominal umbilical cord insertion site appears abnormally. A sagittal view of the abdominal pelvic region of the fetus will reveal and anterior mass that appears as a mound of soft tissue. Transverse view of the pelvic bones will demonstrate widening

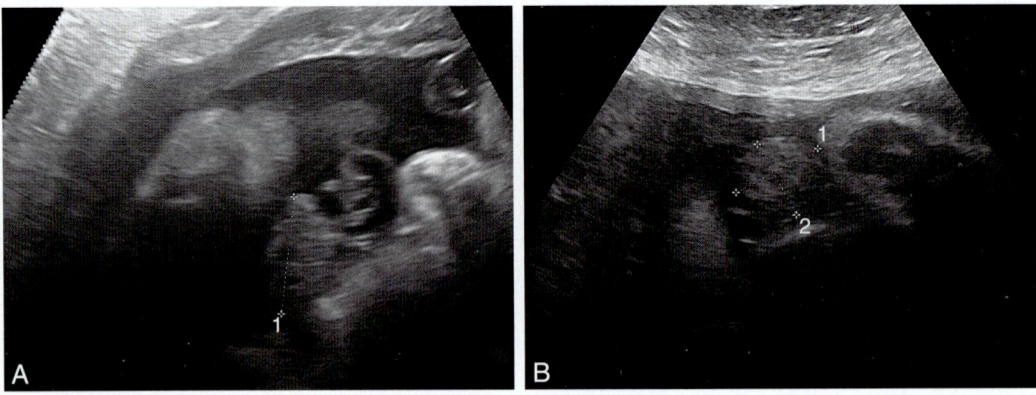

FIG. 64.16 (A) A 33-week-old female fetus presents with a soft tissue mass anterior to the area of the bladder. (B) The mass was seen in both sagittal and transverse views. No bladder was documented sonographically. Patient presented with bladder exstrophy at birth.

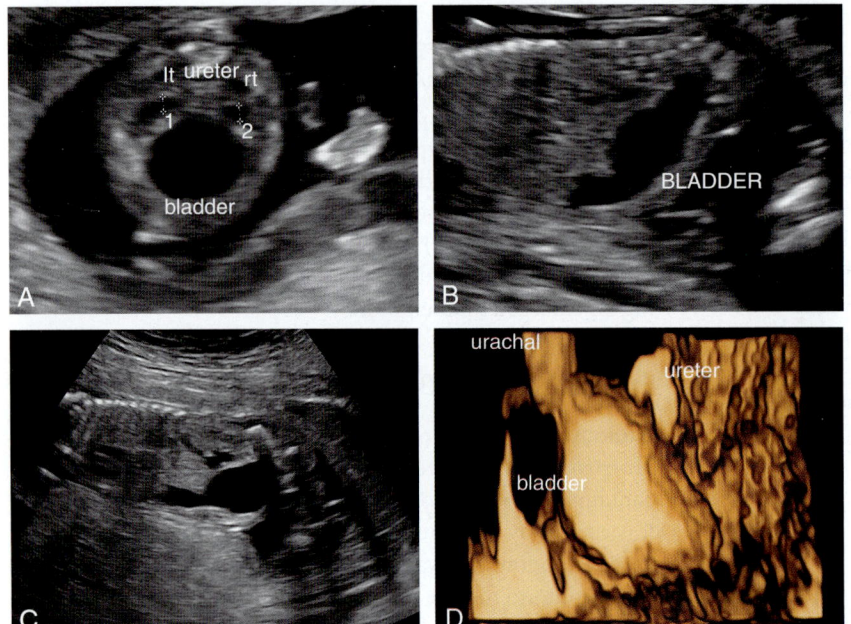

FIG. 64.17 (A) Transverse image showing bilateral pyelectasis as well as an enlarged bladder at the level of the kidneys. (B) On sagittal view, the bladder appeared abnormal in shape with the cranial end becoming narrow. (C) Continuous scanning of the bladder indicated a change in shape and size of the abnormal bladder with fetal urination. (D) With the aid of 3D/4D technology the diagnosis of a urachal abnormality was clearly seen.

of the iliac crest. **Cloacal exstrophy** should be differentiated from exstrophy of the bladder. Sonographic findings related to the bladder are similar. However, with cloacal exstrophy the large and small intestines are included in the anterior wall mass and multiple other anomalies are visualized.

Urachal Abnormalities

Etiology. The urinary bladder is continuous with the allantois during embryonic development. The allantois regresses to become a fibrous cord known as the urachus. The urachus extends from the apex of the bladder to the umbilicus. If the lumen of the allantois persists while the urachus forms, a urachal fistula will develop resulting in urine draining from the bladder into the umbilicus. If only a small part of the lumen of the allantois persists, it is called a **urachal cyst** or *vesicoallantoic cyst*. If a larger portion of the lumen persists, it may cause a urachal sinus to develop. The term *patent urachus* is often used to describe a urinary sinus that opens at the umbilicus or into the urinary bladder.

Clinical Findings and Prognosis. Urachal abnormalities are sporadic in occurrence and uncommon. If seen, urachal anomalies are more common in males. An association with posterior urethral valves and prune-belly syndrome has been documented. After the fetus is born, urine discharge or drainage from the umbilicus is frequently noted. Rupture of a urachal cyst may occur in utero into the cord or amniotic fluid. In either case, the urachal remnant is surgically removed.

Sonographic Findings. Sonographically, an anechoic cyst is usually seen within the base of the umbilical cord. The cyst can be visualized communicating with the bladder. The amniotic fluid level and kidneys typically appear normal. Hydronephrosis has been noted as the result of reflux in patients with urachal abnormalities. A cystic mass is seen superior to the bladder and will change size along with emptying of the bladder (Fig. 64.17). For instance, the cystic mass may become larger as the fetus urinates from the bladder because of reflux into the allantoic canal.

RENAL CYSTIC DISEASE

Renal cystic disease is a heterogeneous group of heritable, developmental, and acquired disorders. The diseases have been categorized in many ways: Potter classification or **Potter sequence** is used to describe diseases that are associated with renal failure, oligohydramnios, and Potter facies (Box 64.4); dividing the diseases into groups of hereditary versus nonhereditary; and dividing the diseases by dysplastic kidney, hereditary cyst, and nondysplastic nonhereditary cyst. Several very rare syndromes associated with renal cystic disease, as outlined in Table 64.3, are included in some classifications by not in others. This section details numerous types of renal cystic disease without using a classification system.

Infantile Polycystic Kidney Disease

Etiology. Infantile polycystic kidney disease (IPKD), also called autosomal recessive polycystic kidney disease (ARPKD), is an autosomal recessive congenital disorder that affects both fetal kidneys and liver. The disorder is characterized by the development of small cysts in both kidneys and liver cysts. The cysts in the kidney are thought to be caused by tubular malformation and ectasia of the collecting ducts. The distal collecting ducts are typically affected more than the proximal ducts. The malformation results in cystic dilation of the renal tubules (1 to 2 mm) usually arranged in a symmetric pattern leading to overall enlargement of the kidneys. The formation of the cysts results in tubulointerstitial damage resulting in tubular and fibrosis. Renal failure will occur due to the replacement of normal tissue by enlarged nonfunctioning collecting tubules.

Clinical Findings and Prognosis. IPKD has varying presentations, affects 1 in 40,000 to 50,000 births, and is associated with a 25% recurrence rate. Varying presentations include both perinatal form and the juvenile form. In view of the high recurrence rate and dismal prognosis in severe IPKD, recognition of this defect is important. IPKD may occur as part of a genetic syndrome, such as Meckel-Gruber syndrome or trisomy 13. The most severe forms of IPKD are found prenatally and are associated with renal failure, oligohydramnios, and absence of the urinary bladder. Renal enlargement may result in complete filling of the abdominal cavity. Prognosis depends on the severity of the disease. Most fetuses diagnosed in utero will be stillborn or death will occur early in the neonatal period due to renal failure and lung hypoplasia. It is rare for a fetus to survive the first year of life.

Sonographic Findings. The collecting tubules of the kidney are microscopically dilated. Sonographically, individual cysts are not identified. The kidneys appear massively enlarged due to the hundreds of dilated tubules (Fig. 64.18). Enlargement of the kidneys may not occur until the 24th week of gestation; therefore, serial studies of at-risk fetuses are recommended. It is not uncommon for the kidneys to measure above the 90th percentile in length and width. This enlargement will lead to abdominal circumference that is large for the gestational age.

Enhanced renal tissue echogenicity is characteristic because of the multiple interfaces created by the dilated cystic tubules. Oligohydramnios and a small or absent bladder are present. The oligohydramnios may not be evident until after 15 to 18 weeks of gestation. Liver cysts and fibrosis may or may not be visualized.

BOX 64.4 Renal Cystic Disease

Potter Type I: Sonographic Findings in Infantile Polycystic Kidney Disease
- Progressive renal enlargement
- Echogenic renal parenchyma
- Empty bladder and oligohydramnios

Potter Type II: Sonographic Findings in Adult Multicystic Dysplastic Kidney Disease
- Multiple noncommunicating cysts of variable size
- No distinct renal pelvis
- No distinct renal parenchyma
- Renal size may be normal, hypoplastic, or enlarged
- Severe oligohydramnios if bilateral

Potter Type III: Sonographic Findings in Adult Polycystic Kidney Disease
- Large kidneys with hyperechoic parenchyma
- Size may be asymmetric
- Genetic link

Potter Type IV: Sonographic Findings in Obstructive Cystic Disease
- Small, echogenic kidneys
- Cortical peripheral cysts
- Bilateral disease: keyhole bladder, bilateral hydronephrosis, thick-walled bladder, severe oligohydramnios

---

TABLE 64.3 Syndromes Associated With Cystic Renal Disease

Syndrome	Clinical Findings
Meckel-Gruber syndrome	Large echogenic kidneys, polydactyly, encephalocele
Patau syndrome (trisomy 13)	Large echogenic kidneys, polydactyly, holoprosencephaly, facial clefting
Beckwith-Wiedemann syndrome	Large echogenic kidneys, macrosomia, hepatosplenomegaly, macroglossia, omphalocele
Jeune syndrome	Echogenic kidneys, dwarfism, small thorax
Short rib polydactyly syndrome	Large echogenic kidneys, dwarfism, polydactyly, small thorax
Laurence-Moon syndrome (Bardet-Biedl syndrome)	Cystic kidneys, hypotonicity, limb contractures, congenital cataracts, hypoplastic corpus callosum, heterotopias

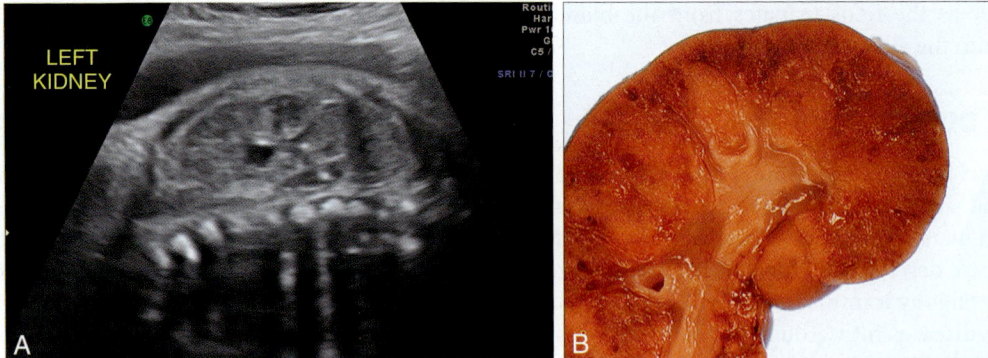

FIG. 64.18 Autosomal recessive polycystic kidney disease. (A) The left kidney is enlarged with increased echogenicity at 29 weeks of gestation. (B) Gross pathology of the disease showing microscopic cysts. (From Rumack C, Wilson S, Charboneau W. *Diagnostic ultrasound*, ed 3. St Louis: Elsevier; 2005.)

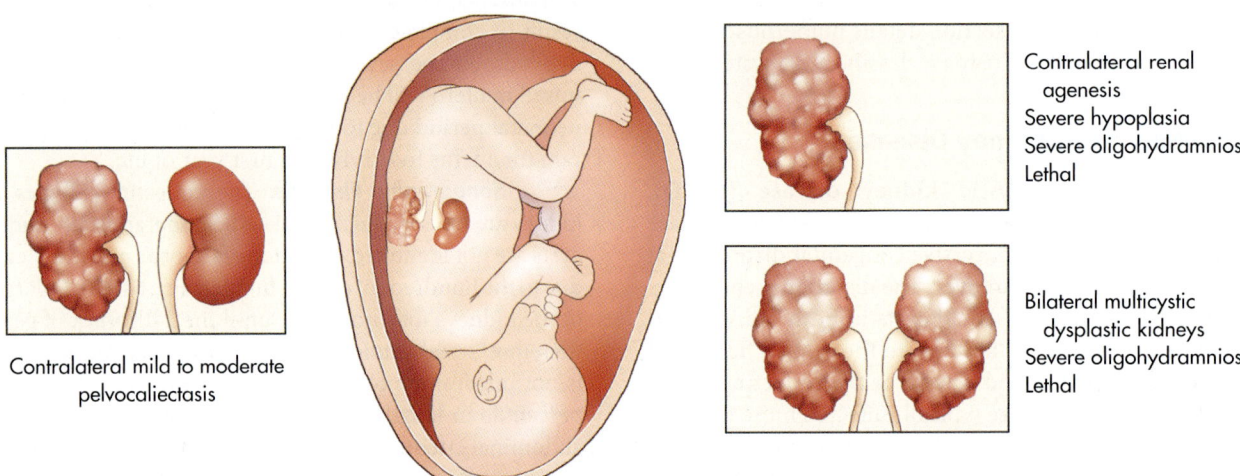

FIG. 64.19 Multicystic dysplastic kidney disease may be unilateral, bilateral, or associated with contralateral renal agenesis. Although the affected kidney typically produces very little urine, it may change in size throughout gestation. Because the contralateral kidney is the only potentially functional kidney, it must be examined carefully.

Multicystic Dysplastic Kidney Disease

Etiology. Congenital **multicystic dysplastic kidney disease (MCDK)** is characterized by multiple, smooth-walled, nonfunctioning, noncommunicating cysts of variable size and number. The renal tissue is replaced by cysts of varying sizes found throughout the kidney. The lack of renal tissue results in a nonfunctional kidney. Between the cysts, renal stroma may be present; however, normal renal tissue is absent. The entire kidney or only a portion of the kidney may be affected. The ureter and renal pelvis may be atretic and the renal artery is hypoplastic or absent. MCDK is thought to result from early obstruction uropathy or abnormal development of the metanephric mesoderm and the ureteric bud.

Clinical Findings and Prognosis. MCDK is the most common form of renal cystic disease in childhood and represents one of the most common abdominal masses in the neonate. The incidence is 1 of 3000 births and is often found more in males than females. Research has also concluded a link with maternal diabetes.

Most cases are unilateral; however, nearly one quarter of the cases are bilateral. Associated fetal abnormalities have been identified. The abnormalities may involve the contralateral kidney, heart, central nervous system, extremities, and gastrointestinal system. Many syndromes have also been identified in associations with MCDK. Meckel-Gruber, Apert, Zellweger, and short rib polydactyly only represent a few of the syndromes.

The prognosis for infants with multicystic kidney disease varies based on the prenatal findings (Fig. 64.19). In isolated cases of unilateral involvement, the disease will regress with time and disappear, or a small collection of cysts with a calcified border will be present in the renal fossa. If the kidney appears to be interfering with other organs such as bowel it can be surgically removed. If only a segment of the kidney is involved renal insufficiency may result. When both kidneys are found to be multicystic, and oligohydramnios and an absent bladder are expected, a lethal condition exists for the neonate. This is also true when one kidney is multicystic and the other absent.

Sonographic Findings. Typically, during the anatomy sonogram between 18 and 20 weeks of gestational age, the fetus with multicystic renal dysplasia will present with at least one kidney, demonstrating multiple cysts of varying size that may affect a part or the entire kidney (Fig. 64.20). The cysts typically start at the periphery and appear small. Over time,

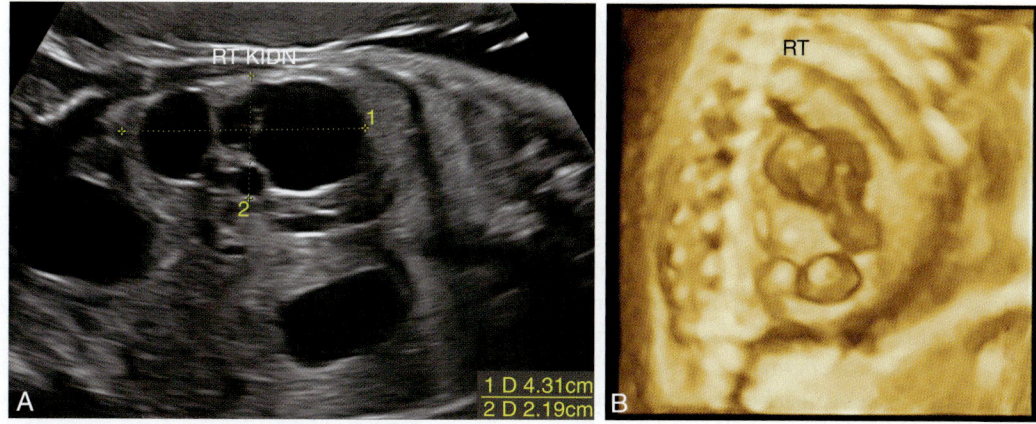

FIG. 64.20 (A) A unilateral multicystic dysplastic kidney is identified with multiple cysts of varying sizes throughout the kidney. The kidneys are enlarged, measuring 4.31 cm for this 28-week-old fetus. (B) The cysts are clearly seen using three-dimensional technology. The lack of communication between the cysts communicating helps differentiate it from hydronephrosis.

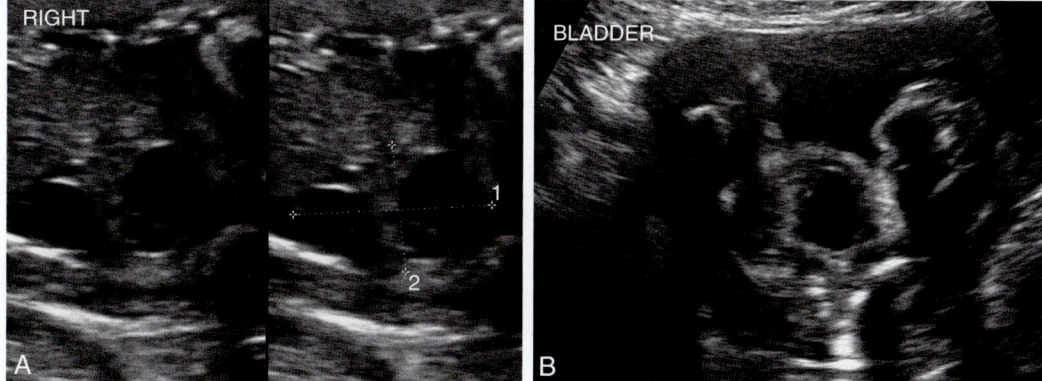

FIG. 64.21 (A) Enlarged cysts in this case of multicystic dysplastic kidney prevents clear delineation the borders of the kidney. (B) Only one kidney in this fetus is affected; therefore visualization of a normal bladder is clear.

the cyst enlarges and more cysts will develop in the hilum. Echogenic stroma may be visible between the cysts. The overall size of the kidney may be enlarged, resulting in possible enlargement of the abdominal circumference. Kidney borders are difficult to define because of the distorted renal outline and absence of significant renal parenchyma (Fig. 64.21A). If only one kidney is affected, the contralateral kidney may be enlarged because of compensatory hypertrophy. The contralateral kidney should be carefully evaluated for renal anomalies. The bladder and amniotic fluid volume are usually within normal limits (see Fig. 64.21B). In the presence of bilateral MCKD, sonographic findings include oligohydramnios and absence of the bladder. The progression of the disease will result in decreased size of the nonfunctioning kidney. The reduction in size may not be evident until after birth.

Adult Dominant Polycystic Kidney Disease

Etiology. Congenital adult (autosomal) dominant polycystic kidney disease (ADPKD) is associated with cystic dilation of the nephrons and on the collecting tubule walls in both kidneys. It is thought to be caused by a defective gene that does not allow for normal epithelial cell development. This results in cystic development of the cortex and medulla.

The cysts typically do not enlarge or impair renal function until adulthood.

Clinical Findings and Prognosis. ADPKD has an incidence of 1 in 1000 births and is the most common of the hereditary renal cystic diseases, with a recurrence risk of 50%. The manifestations of the disease typically develop in adulthood; however, the disease may be diagnosed in a fetus when there is a family history of polycystic kidneys, liver, or both. Conversely, visualization of bilateral enlargement of the kidneys may prompt a renal and liver workup in the parents to exclude this disorder. Associated anomalies include cysts (liver, spleen, and pancreas), cardiac malformations, pyloric stenosis, and skeletal anomalies. Extrarenal cysts are typically only identified in the adult.

Prognosis for prenatal diagnosis of ADPKD is dependent on the progression of cyst development, leading to renal failure. In some cases, the cyst development is rapid with renal failure apparent at birth and in other cases the cyst development is slow with progression to hypertension and ultimately end-stage renal failure. If a sibling has been affected, the outcome may be easier to predict. Renal dialysis with eventual renal transplant is required in cases of bilateral renal failure.

Sonographic Findings. The sonographic appearance is similar to autosomal recessive polycystic renal disease.

In both diseases, the kidneys are symmetrically enlarged and echogenic. ADPKD is nearly always associated with bilateral kidney involvement. The bladder is usually present and amniotic fluid volume is normal. The corticomedullary junction may appear accentuated or indistinct (Fig. 64.22). Occasionally, macroscopic cysts within the echogenic kidneys are seen.

The rarity of diagnosing ADPKD in utero often leads to the diagnosis of other diseases presenting with similar sonographic findings. The appearance of bilateral echogenic kidney enlargement may be found in association with a syndrome, such as Beckwith-Wiedemann syndrome. This syndrome presents with visceromegaly of many organs (Fig. 64.23). The urinary bladder is usually present. The corticomedullary junction may appear accentuated or be indistinct. Meckel-Gruber syndrome is associated with the presence of bilateral renal cystic disease and additional anomalies such as encephalocele, polydactyly, and severe oligohydramnios.

Obstructive Cystic Dysplasia

Etiology. In obstructive cystic dysplasia, renal dysplasia occurs secondary to kidney obstruction in the first or early second trimester of pregnancy. The long-standing obstruction leads to the development of fibrosis and cystic replacement of the renal tissue (Fig. 64.24). Unilateral disease can be caused by a ureteropelvic or ureterovesical junction obstruction. Severe obstruction from a ureterocele can cause dysplasia in an upper pole of a duplex kidney. Bilateral obstructive dysplasia is caused by severe bladder outlet obstruction, usually **urethral atresia** or posterior urethral valves.

Clinical Findings and Prognosis. The incidence is 1 in 8000 births, although this is difficult to determine because only a small number of obstructive kidneys progress to renal dysplasia. Due to the variety of causes of this disease anomaly, associations are variable. The prognosis is dependent on unilateral or bilateral involvement. Bilateral involvement would indicate a poor outcome due to renal failure and lung hypoplasia. Unilateral involvement may vary from normal outcome to dependent on associated anomalies or the presence of anomalies affecting the functioning kidney.

Sonographic Findings. Early sonographic findings may only be hydronephrosis or hydroureter depending on the level of obstruction. The kidney will most likely appear enlarged during this time. Early signs of dysplasia include the presence of hydronephrosis with cortical cysts. The cortical cyst will not communicate with the anechoic, cyst-like appearance of the hydronephrosis. As the kidney slowly stops functioning, the renal cortex becomes completely dysplastic and replaced with the multiple cortical cysts. The dysplastic kidney will appear small and echogenic with cortical peripheral cysts (Fig. 64.25). If only one kidney is affected, the bladder and amniotic fluid level will be within normal limits. If the disease is bilateral, a bladder outlet obstruction (keyhole bladder) may be apparent, as well as severe oligohydramnios.

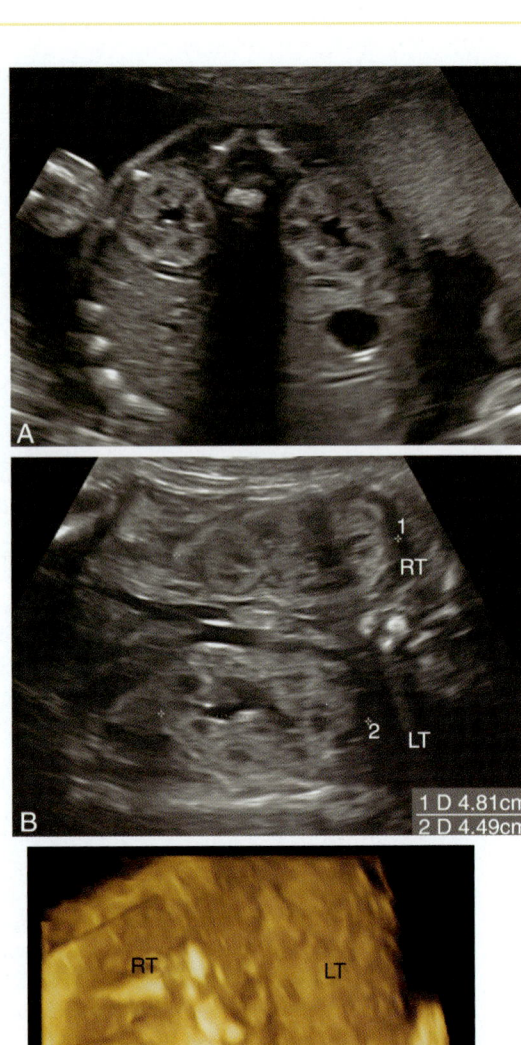

FIG. 64.22 (A) This 25-week-old female fetus presented with a known family history of adult polycystic kidney disease (including mother). The transverse view of the kidneys demonstrates symmetric enlarged echogenic kidneys. (B) In a follow-up sonogram at 35 weeks of gestation, the enlargement is clearly seen in the longitudinal images. The kidneys measure 4.81 cm and 4.49 cm. (C) The use of advanced technology aids in visualizing the kidneys.

OBSTRUCTIVE URINARY TRACT ABNORMALITIES

The urinary tract may be obstructed at the junction of the ureter entering the renal pelvis (**ureteropelvic junction [UPJ]**), at the junction of the ureter where it enters the

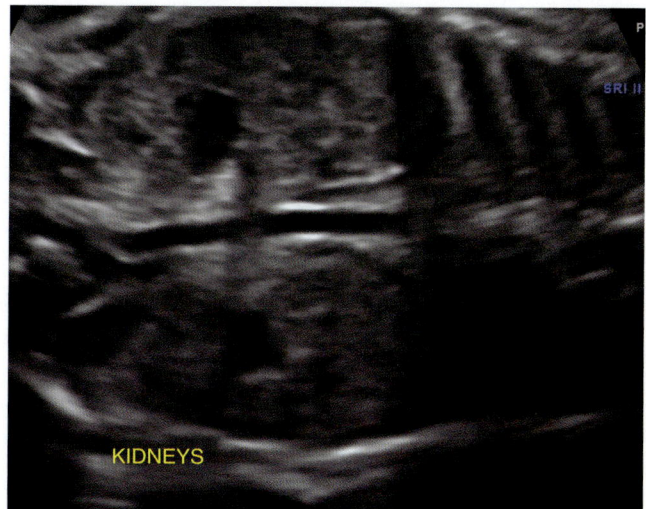

FIG. 64.23 Bilateral renal enlargement of the kidneys in a 30-week-old fetus with Beckwith-Wiedemann syndrome. Both kidneys occupy more than half of the abdomen.

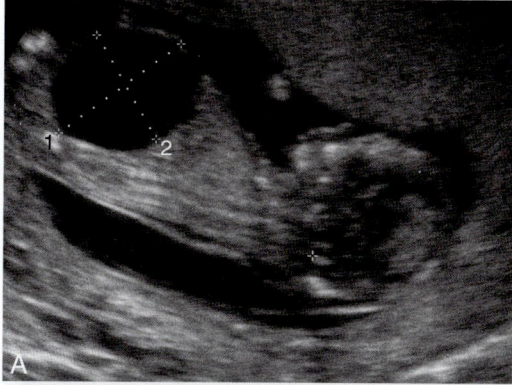

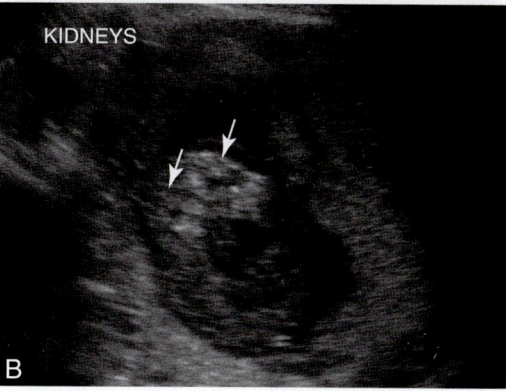

FIG. 64.25 (A) Bladder outlet obstruction was suspected in this 14-week-old fetus. (B) The kidneys were later seen as very small and echogenic. Renal dysplasia was a result of the early onset of obstruction that led to renal compromise.

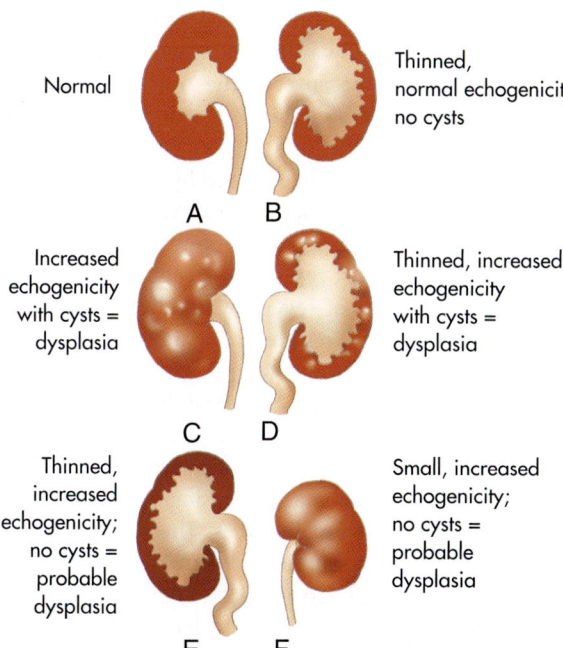

FIG. 64.24 Renal parenchymal responses to obstruction. (A) In distal urinary tract obstruction without reflux, the kidneys may remain normal. (B) Pyelocaliectasis may thin the renal parenchyma. (C) Cystic dysplasia may occur with renal cysts and fibrosis (increased echogenicity) and cease to function (lack of pyelocaliectasis). (D) Cystic dysplasia may occur with persistent pyelocaliectasis. (E) Increased renal echogenicity with visible cysts suggests but is not diagnostic of dysplasia. (F) A small, echogenic kidney without pyelocaliectasis is also suggestive but not diagnostic of dysplasia.

bladder (**ureterovesical junction [UVJ]**), or at the level of the urethra (**megacystis**). The amount and degree of obstruction will depend on the gestational age at which the obstruction began (see Fig. 64.24). If the obstruction is early, a multicystic kidney may develop. If the obstruction occurs in the first or second trimester, cystic dysplasia may result. Late obstruction produces hydronephrosis. The term *pelviectasis* is commonly used in conjunction with hydronephrosis. **Pyelectasis** refers to dilation of the renal pelvis without dilation of the calyces, and hydronephrosis refers to dilation of the renal pelvis and calyces.

Hydronephrosis

Etiology. Dilation of the renal pelvis occurs in response to a blockage of urine at some junction in the urinary system. Hydronephrosis commonly occurs when there is an obstruction in the ureter, bladder, or urethra. Hydronephrosis is generally the result of an obstruction at a lower level in the urinary tract. **Fetal hydronephrosis** may occur as a unilateral or bilateral process. Unilateral renal hydronephrosis commonly results from an obstruction at the junction of the renal pelvis and the ureter.

Clinical Findings and Prognosis. Fetal hydronephrosis is the most common fetal anomaly. Findings suggesting hydronephrosis include an abnormal intrapelvic AP diameter measurement. Although this measurement will fluctuate with gestational age, if the measurement is greater than 4 to 4.5 mm before the third trimester or greater than 7 mm after the third trimester, the kidney should be followed with serial examinations (Box 64.5). Also, if the measurement exceeds one-third of the renal diameter, follow-up should be considered. In cases in which pyelectasis is diagnosed, the fetus should be

> **BOX 64.5 Anterior-Posterior Diameter Measurement of the Renal Pelvis**
>
> - Intrapelvic diameter >7 mm is considered mild hydronephrosis
> - Intrapelvic diameter measuring 7–15 mm is considered moderate hydronephrosis
> - Intrapelvic diameter measuring >15 mm is considered marked dilation or severe hydronephrosis

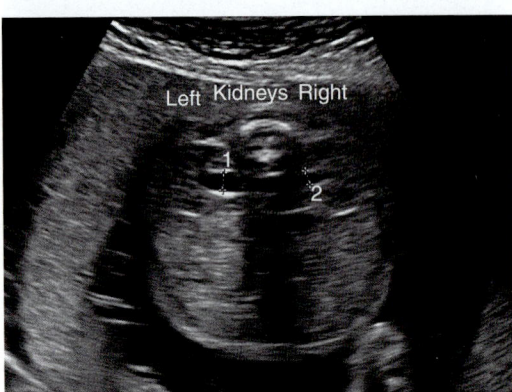

FIG. 64.26 Mild pyelectasis is noted in both kidneys in this fetus diagnosed with Down syndrome.

carefully examined for anomalies associated with aneuploidy. Mild pyelectasis is a common feature associated with Down syndrome (Fig. 64.26).

The prognosis of a fetus with hydronephrosis is dependent on the severity and cause. When considering severity without relating to cause or dysplasia, mild hydronephrosis has been found to resolve antenatally or postnatally without surgical intervention. Cases of moderate to severe hydronephrosis have resolved antenatally and postnatally; however, surgical correction is common. In cases in which the hydronephrosis is related to a specific cause and no dysplasia is evident, surgical correction is required. In some cases of a fetus with unilateral obstructions of the urinary tract, early delivery of the fetus may be warranted to salvage the normal kidney. The common finding of renal dysplasia following obstruction is represented by cystic changes within the renal tissue. Renal dysplasia often leads to renal failure of all or part of the kidney.

Sonographic Findings. The sonographic appearance of urinary tract obstruction varies depending on the site and extent of blockage (Fig. 64.27). A true cross-sectional plane through the mid renal pelvis must be obtained for measuring the AP diameter of the anechoic pelvis. A transverse view of the abdomen with the spine located anteriorly is optimal. Oblique or off-axis images will lead to erroneous measurements.

The dilated anechoic renal pelvis is centrally located and distended with urine. If only the pelvis is seen, the term *pyelectasis* is used. Hydronephrosis will be identified with a dilation of the renal pelvis and calyces. The sonographic appearance of the surrounding parenchymal tissue will appear within normal limits; however, depending on the degree of dilation the parenchyma may appear thin. If dysplasia is evident, cystic replacement of the renal tissue will be evident.

Based on the severity and cause of the hydronephrosis, the bladder and amniotic fluid level will vary. Further investigation into the sonographic findings associated with these causes will follow in the next section.

Ureteropelvic Junction Obstruction

Etiology. UPJ obstructions occur at the junction between the renal pelvis and ureter. The obstruction results in a backup of urine into the renal pelvis and calyces. The causes of UPJ obstruction include abnormal bends or kinks in the ureter, adhesions, abnormal valves in the ureter, abnormal outlet shape at the ureteropelvic junction, or absence of the longitudinal muscle that is imperative to the normal excretion of urine from the kidney.

Clinical Findings and Prognosis. UPJ obstruction is the most common reason for hydronephrosis in the neonate. It is more common in males and is usually unilateral. Only half of these disorders are found during early childhood; therefore, early prenatal detection may improve long-term renal function. UPJ obstruction is usually a unilateral defect, and amniotic fluid remains normal because of the normal contralateral kidney. Bilateral UPJ obstruction is uncommon. Anomalies associated with this disorder may involve the presence of a urinoma. Prognosis for UPJ is determined by the degree of renal impairment caused by the obstruction. Serial sonograms are performed to document progression of obstruction as well as amniotic fluid levels. Most cases do not require early delivery unless there is evidence of severe bilateral obstruction with oligohydramnios. Following birth, neonates will typically receive antibiotics and a complete urologic examination.

Sonographic Findings. Sonographically, a collection of anechoic urine is located medially within the renal pelvis communicating with the calyces (caliectasis) (Fig. 64.28). The renal pelvis may take on a "bullet shape" appearance surrounded by dilated or normal calyces. The renal cortex, ureter, bladder, and amniotic fluid are usually normal in cases of unilateral involvement. Ureteropelvic junction obstruction may be severe, leading to distended calyces and renal cortex reduction. In cases of severe obstruction, the affected kidney should be evaluated for sonographic features associated with dysplasia.

Ureterovesical Junction Obstruction

Etiology. UVJ obstruction commonly presents with dilation of the lower end of the ureter. The obstruction leads to the backup of urine in the kidney (hydronephrosis) and an enlarged urine-filled ureter (megaureter). **Megaureter** may result from a primary ureteral defect (stenotic ureteral valves or fibrosis) or occur secondary to obstruction at another level (causing reflux or backward flow of urine). In most cases, the cause is the distal portion of the ureter being aperistaltic (primary megaureter). Under normal conditions, constant muscular contractions of the ureter are responsible for moving

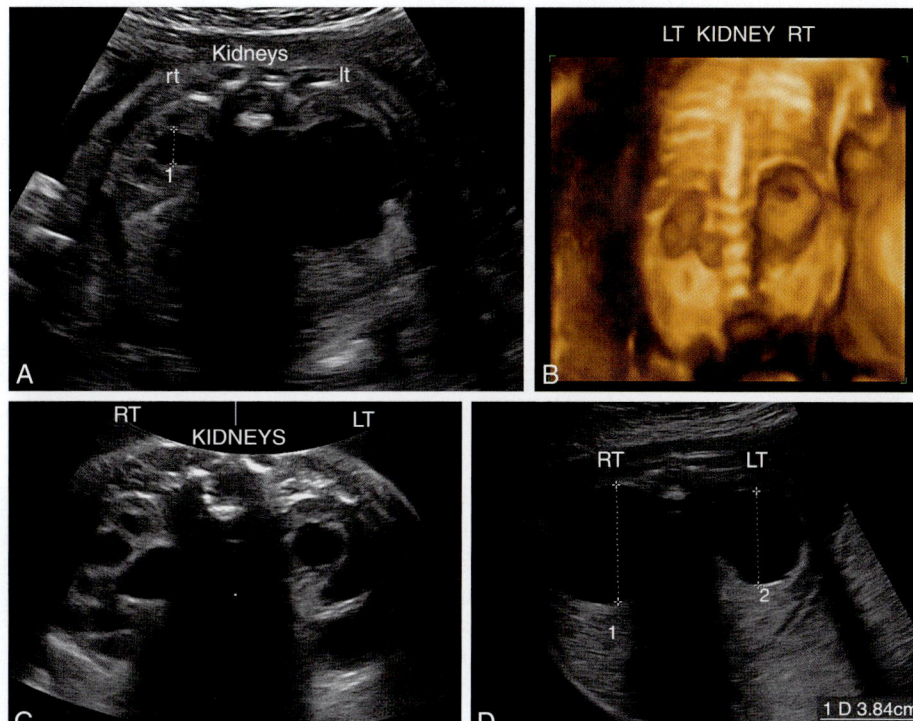

FIG. 64.27 (A) Mild hydronephrosis is noted in the right kidney and severe hydronephrosis is seen in the left kidney. (B) Use of three-dimensional technology clearly identifies the round cystic structure in the renal pelvis connecting to ureters. (C) In this case of hydronephrosis, the renal pelvis and connecting calyces are seen. (D) This fetus presents with bilateral severe hydronephrosis. Notice the thinning of the renal tissue.

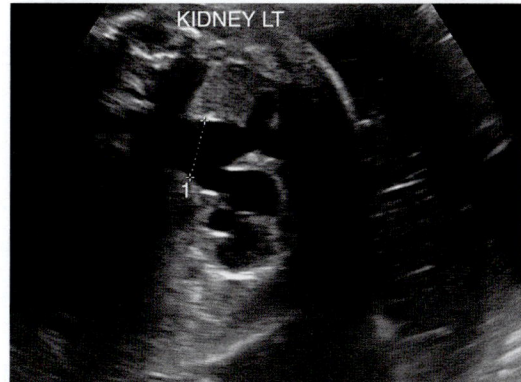

FIG. 64.28 The renal pelvis and calyces are clearly seen connecting. Identifying the connection between the pelvis and calyces should be used to differentiate the anechoic areas from renal cysts.

the urine from the kidney to the bladder. If a segment of the ureter is aperistaltic, it lacks the ability to compress those muscles. The constant contractions are disrupted, leading to the inability of urine to be moved into the bladder at a constant normal rate. UVJ obstruction has also been found to result from an ectopic ureterocele within the bladder, causing obstruction of the upper pole of the kidney.

Clinical Findings and Prognosis. UVJ obstruction is more common in males, is usually unilateral, and is of sporadic incidence. Bilateral involvement has been reported. It is not uncommon for other abnormalities to be found in the affected kidney. Duplication of the renal collecting system is common and may be diagnosed prenatally. In approximately 25% of cases, the contralateral kidney will present with anomalies.

Other fetal anomalies have been reported in some cases but are not specific. One of the most important components in the diagnosis of UVJ obstruction is to determine whether the obstruction is associated with retrograde flow of urine from the bladder back to the ureter (reflux). Unfortunately, definitive diagnosis is only made after delivery with the aid of a voiding cystourethrogram (VCU) examination.

The prognosis for infants with UVJ obstruction is good regardless of whether it associated with a refluxing ureter or a nonrefluxing ureter. Like other renal obstructions, the prognosis is dependent on the degree of renal impairment caused by the obstruction. Surgical correction may be required in some cases to help prevent further renal damage.

Sonographic Findings. The affected kidney is visualized with anechoic dilation of the renal pelvis and tortuous fluid-filled dilated ureter (Fig. 64.29). Careful attention should be made to differentiate dilated bowel from the dilated ureter. If the ureter is dilated it should appear anechoic, whereas the bowel will appear with low-level echoes. The bladder and amniotic fluid volume are normal in cases involving only one kidney. If both kidneys are affected, the amniotic fluid volume may be reduced.

If renal duplication is identified, a dilated upper renal pole is observed with a normal lower pole. In cases of reflux, sonography may reveal changes in the AP diameter measurements of the renal pelvis. These changes may represent the presence of reflux.

Posterior Urethral Valve Obstruction

Etiology. Posterior urethral valve (PUV) obstruction results in hydronephrosis, hydroureters, or dilation of the bladder

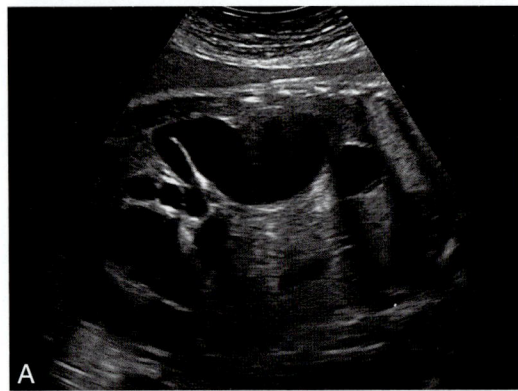
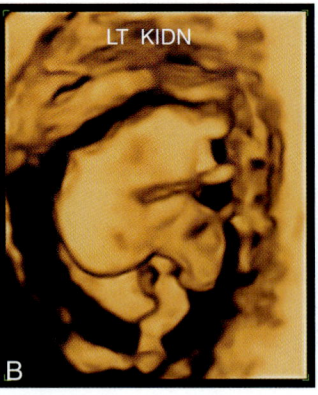

FIG. 64.29 (A) The dilated renal pelvis is seen communicating with a dilated tortuous renal ureter in this example of ureterovesical junction obstruction. (B) Three-dimensional imaging further supports the degree of dilation of the renal pelvis and ureter.

and posterior urethra (Fig. 64.30). The obstruction is produced by an abnormal congenital membrane within the posterior urethra. The membrane is thought to be valvelike and derived from Wolffian duct tissue. The congenital malformation results in the inability of urine to pass through the urethra and into the amniotic fluid. The degree of obstruction can be complete, partial, or intermittent.

Clinical Findings and Prognosis. PUV obstruction is considered the most common urethral anomaly and, in males, is the most common cause of infravesical obstruction. The obstruction causes a backup of urine in the bladder, ureter, and, in the most severe cases, the kidneys. Obstruction is apparent throughout the pregnancy leading to impaired renal function and dysplasia. Fetal renal function may be assessed by aspirating urine from an obstructed bladder (Fig. 64.31). Cystic dysplasia and poor renal function are suggested when sodium, chloride, and osmolality are unusually elevated. The prognosis is typically poor in cases of complete obstruction due to the high association of renal failure and pulmonary hypoplasia when oligohydramnios is present. When the urinary tract is completely blocked, severe oligohydramnios and the Potter sequence occur. A fetus surviving birth commonly develops chronic renal failure. Intrauterine therapeutic procedures have been utilized. Intrauterine decompression of an obstructed urinary tract (posterior urethral valve syndrome), which includes draining of the bladder and adding fluid to the amniotic sac, has been performed to relieve the obstruction and allow expansion of the lungs to prevent pulmonary hypoplasia. In some cases, an indwelling bladder shunt is inserted to relieve the obstruction; this has improved chances for survival in some cases (Fig. 64.32). The shunt drains the blocked urine into the amniotic fluid, allowing the fetal lungs to develop. Bladder rupture and kidney rupture have occurred in cases where the pressure from the obstruction was too high. In those cases, fetal ascites or perirenal uromas may develop. The prognosis for patients with partial and intermittent obstruction depends on the severity of renal function and associated oligohydramnios.

Sonographic Findings. Sonographic features most seen with PUV obstruction include severe bladder dilation, massive hydronephrosis with dysplastic changes seen in the renal tissue, dilated tortuous ureters, and oligohydramnios.

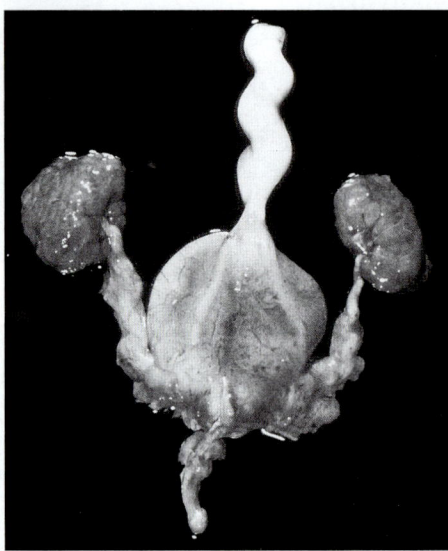

FIG. 64.30 Pathologic specimen of obstructed urinary tract showing bladder enlargement, hydroureters, and bilateral hydronephrosis in posterior urethral valve syndrome.

The bladder wall is severely thickened with a dilated posterior urethra—the keyhole sign (Fig. 64.33A). If the kidneys have become dysplastic, the sonographic features include an anechoic dilated bladder that occupies the abdomen, mild hydronephrosis, and small echogenic kidneys (Fig. 64.34). It is possible for the bladder to rupture in utero due to the pressure of the fluid. In these cases, ascites or hydrops is present; the bladder appears normal in size, there is moderate hydronephrosis, and there is little to no amniotic fluid. Intermittent PUV obstruction may occur with a normal amount of amniotic fluid. Diminishing fluid volume and increased hydronephrosis may prompt early delivery.

Anterior Urethral Valves

Etiology. It is a congenital defect resulting in obstruction of the anterior urethral valve in males. Valves are in multiple locations in the anterior urethra. An exact cause of obstruction is unclear; however, in some cases, it is thought to be caused by abnormal tissue growth, dilated periurethral glands, and proximal and distal urethra formation failure.

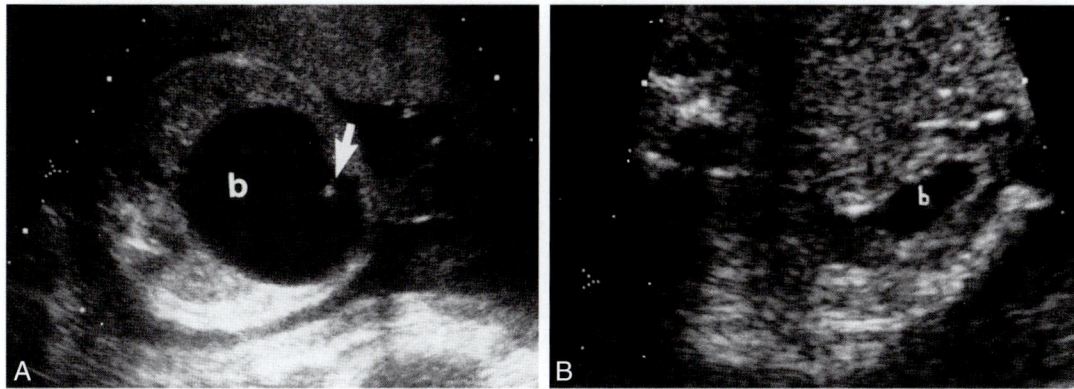

FIG. 64.31 (A) In this fetus, bladder aspiration was performed to assess kidney function. Note the needle *(arrow)* within the bladder (b). (B) After urine aspiration, decompression of the bladder occurred. Note the thickened bladder wall. Laboratory analysis of osmolality, sodium, potassium, and chloride indicates favorable renal function. Bilateral reflux was diagnosed after birth.

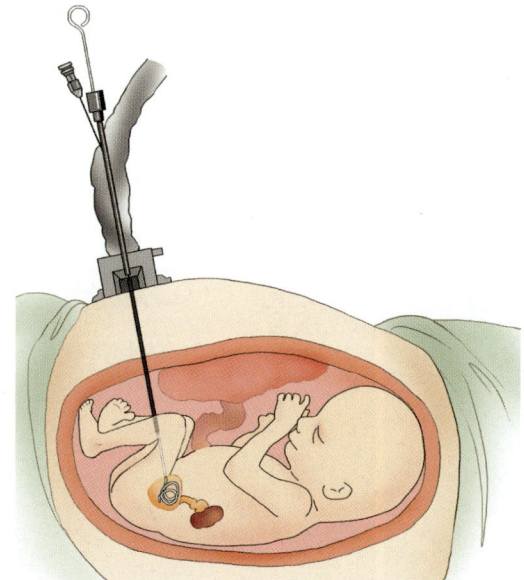

FIG. 64.32 Initial steps in a bladder shunt procedure.

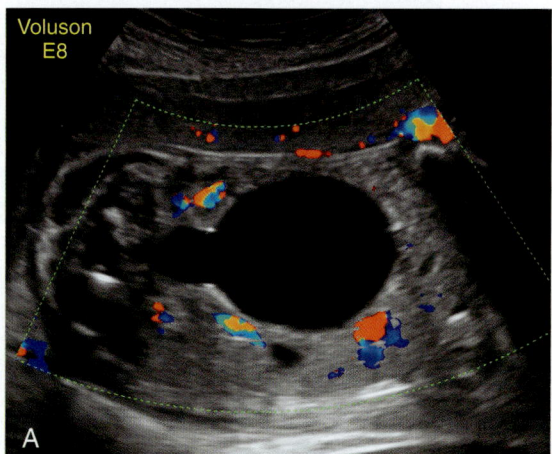

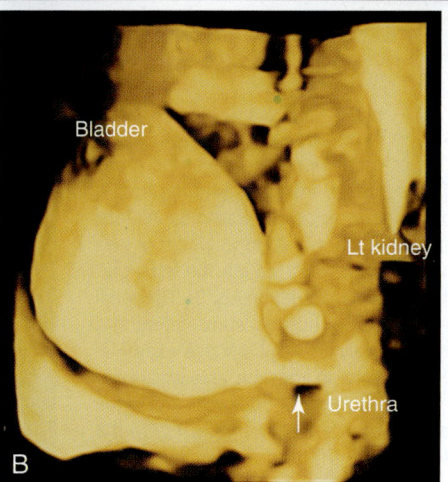

FIG. 64.33 (A) The keyhole sign is clearly depicted in this fetus with posterior urethral valve obstruction. (B) Advanced technology enables the sonographer to view the enlarged bladder in relation to the kidney and ureter.

Clinical Findings and Prognosis. Anterior urethral valves are rare and may be found as an isolated finding or in conjunction with a diverticulum. The degree of obstruction varies owing to a range of clinical findings such as bilateral hydronephrosis with dilated ureters, end-stage renal disease, and bladder rupture. Most cases present after birth with clinical symptoms of a weak urinary stream. VCU examinations are used to make the definite diagnosis. Prognosis is good with endoscopic resection of the abnormal valve. Other surgeries may be required if other abnormalities are identified. However, like other obstructed lesions, the prognosis will vary depending on the degree of renal impairment.

Sonographic Findings. Dilated anechoic urethra is seen proximal to the valve. The valve is usually not appreciated in obstetric examinations. Use of 3D/4D technology can be extremely helpful in determining the extent of the obstruction within the urethra. The obstruction may be complete, partial, or intermittent (Fig. 64.35). The amount of amniotic fluid present as well as dilation of the collecting system and ureter will vary from normal to severe. The obstruction may not be apparent until late in gestation.

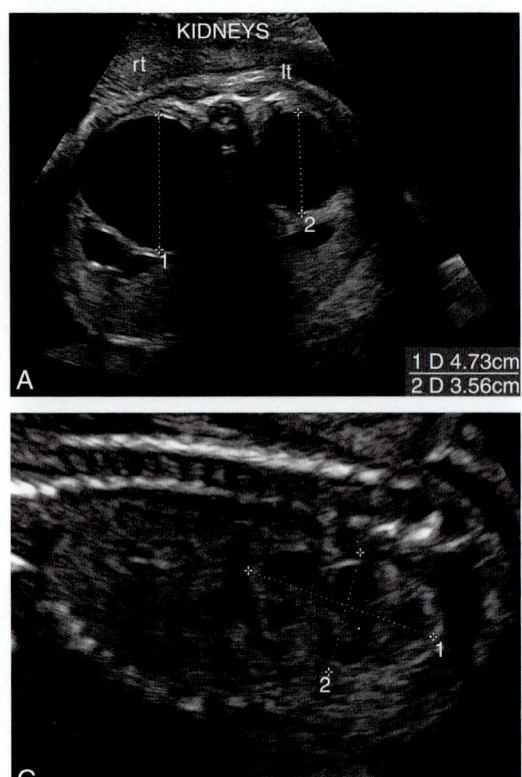
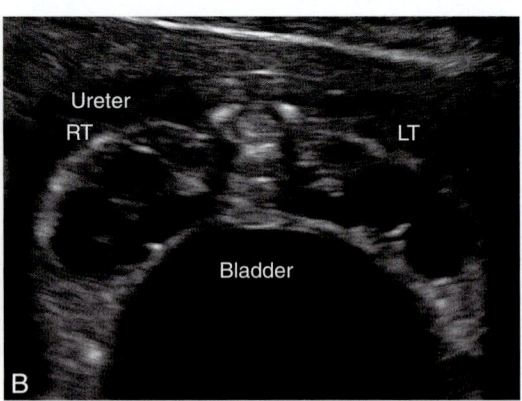

FIG. 64.34 (A) The kidneys will both appear with severe hydronephrosis in the early stages of posterior valve obstruction. (B) The severe hydronephrosis will eventually lead to cystic replacement of renal tissue. (C) Once dysplasia occurs the renal function is impaired, resulting in small echogenic kidneys.

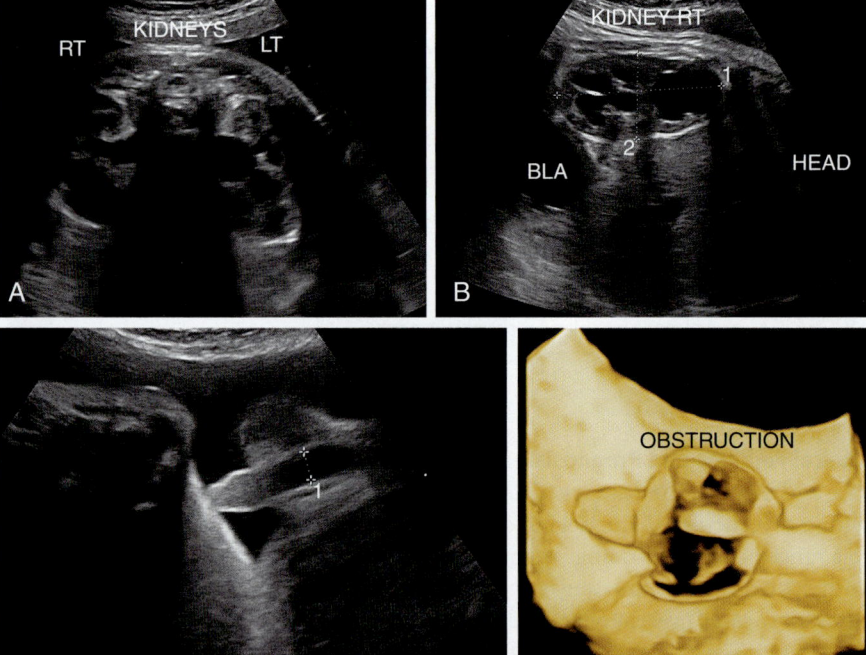

FIG. 64.35 A male fetus presented with a rare case of obstructed anterior urethral valves. Previous sonograms did not indicate hydronephrosis, an abnormal bladder, or polyhydramnios. All fetal structures appeared normal up to 36 weeks of gestation. (A) At 38 weeks of gestation the fetus presented with bilateral hydronephrosis. (B) The renal parenchyma appeared normal surrounding the dilated pelvis and calyces. (C) On close examination of the male penis, an anechoic area was noted within the penis, suggesting obstruction of urine flow at the distal end of the urethra. (D) With the aid of 3D technology the obstruction was clearly identified. Anterior urethral valve obstruction was diagnosed on delivery.

Prune-Belly Syndrome

Etiology. **Prune-belly syndrome** is recognized by three features: cryptorchidism, agenesis or hypoplasia of abdominal wall muscle, and dilation of the collecting system. It is thought to result from an embryologic defect of the mesoderm or a urethral obstruction malformation complex. Hypoplasia of the abdominal muscles is thought to be caused by the dilation of the collecting system.

Clinical Findings and Prognosis. Prune-belly syndrome is often referred to as Eagle-Barrett syndrome. It is a rare condition seen mostly in males. The association with males is

> **BOX 64.6 Sonographic Findings in Prune-Belly Syndrome**
>
> - Absent abdominal musculature
> - Undescended testes
> - Large urinary bladder
> - Dilated prostatic urethra
> - Dilated and tortuous ureters
> - Kidneys can be normal, hydronephrotic, or dysplastic

thought to be due to the complex development of the male urethra. The prognosis is dependent on renal function. In cases in which normal amniotic fluid levels are apparent, the prognosis is typically good. However, most cases are associated with early obstruction, which leads to renal dysplasia and hypoplasia of the lungs. Other anomalies that may also be present and that can affect the prognosis are microcolon, intestinal malrotation, and cardiac anomalies.

Sonographic Findings. The bladder appears anechoic, large, and thin walled. The prostatic urethra in males may be enlarged, mimicking the features of PUV obstruction, but the keyhole appearance may not be seen. Both kidneys appear with hydronephrosis with possible dysplasia. The ureters are dilated and tortuous. The ureters may appear as numerous cystic lesions within the distended abdominal cavity. Oligohydramnios is usually apparent. The abdomen is extremely distended compared with the small thoracic cavity. The sonographic documentation of absent or hypoplastic abdominal muscles, as well as undescended testicles, is often difficult (Box 64.6).

OTHER URINARY ANOMALIES

Ureterocele

Etiology. A **ureterocele** is a cystic dilation of the intravesical (bladder) segment of the distal ureter. Ureteroceles are commonly found in cases of duplex collecting systems and are associated with upper pole moiety. The ureter attached to the ureterocele in a duplex collecting system drains the upper pole of the kidney as it enters the bladder in a more medial and caudal position (ectopic ureter). The ureter typically inserts into an ectopic location on the bladder and can easily become obstructed. The lower pole of the duplicated kidneys is more prone to reflux and the upper pole more prone to obstruction. The hydronephrotic, nonfunctioning upper pole may cause downward displacement of the lower pole calyces.

Clinical Findings and Prognosis. Females are more likely to present with ureteroceles in the presence of renal duplication. Ureteroceles can occur with normal renal collecting system development. In those cases males are more likely to be affected. Ureteroceles may also appear bilaterally. The prognosis for an infant diagnosed with an isolated ureterocele and good renal function is excellent with surgical correction. In cases of duplication where the upper pole has become impaired, surgical removal of the upper pole (partial nephrectomy) and the attached accessory ureter is required. Resection or drainage of the ureterocele is also required.

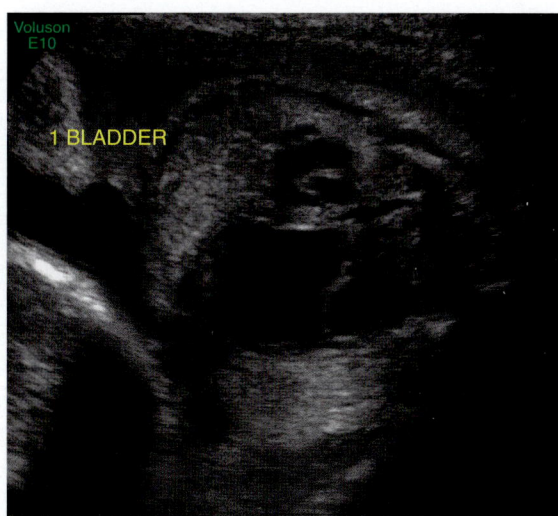

FIG. 64.36 An anechoic mass surrounded by an echogenic rim is identified as a ureterocele in this patient with an obstructed upper pole of the right kidney.

Sonographic Findings. The sonographic appearance of a ureterocele is that of an anechoic cyst surrounded by a thin echogenic membrane within the bladder (Fig. 64.36). It is best visualized when the bladder is somewhat full. If the bladder is empty, the ureterocele may be mistaken for a small bladder, and in cases in which the bladder is too full, the ureterocele may be compressed. The bladder should be evaluated multiple times throughout the examination.

In cases of duplication, the kidney will typically appear with hydronephrosis of the upper pole. It is not uncommon to see urine collected in the lower pole due to reflux (Fig. 64.37A–B). The ureter associated with the ureterocele is commonly dilated, tortuous, and connected to the bladder in an abnormal location. A duplication abnormality is associated with the splitting of the embryologic buds resulting in possible duplication of the renal vessels. The use of color Doppler can aid in this finding (see Fig. 64.37C–D). The amniotic fluid level is typically normal.

Renal Tumors

Tumors of the fetal kidney are rare. It is often difficult to differentiate lung, liver, renal, and adrenal tumors in utero.

Etiology. The most common renal tumor is a mesoblastic nephroma. Also known as a hamartoma, it is a benign tumor that consists of a collection of oddly arranged tissue indigenous to the area (Fig. 64.38). Wilms' tumor is a malignant tumor thought to be derived from abnormal renal cells and is more commonly seen in females (Fig. 64.39). A neuroblastoma of the adrenal gland is a malignant tumor that develops from nerve tissue in the adrenal gland.

Clinical Findings and Prognosis. Although renal and adrenal tumors are rare, there is an associated risk of tumor development in Beckwith-Wiedemann, Perlman, and Drash syndromes. In cases of mesoblastic nephroma, the opposite kidney is usually normal and, therefore, with surgical

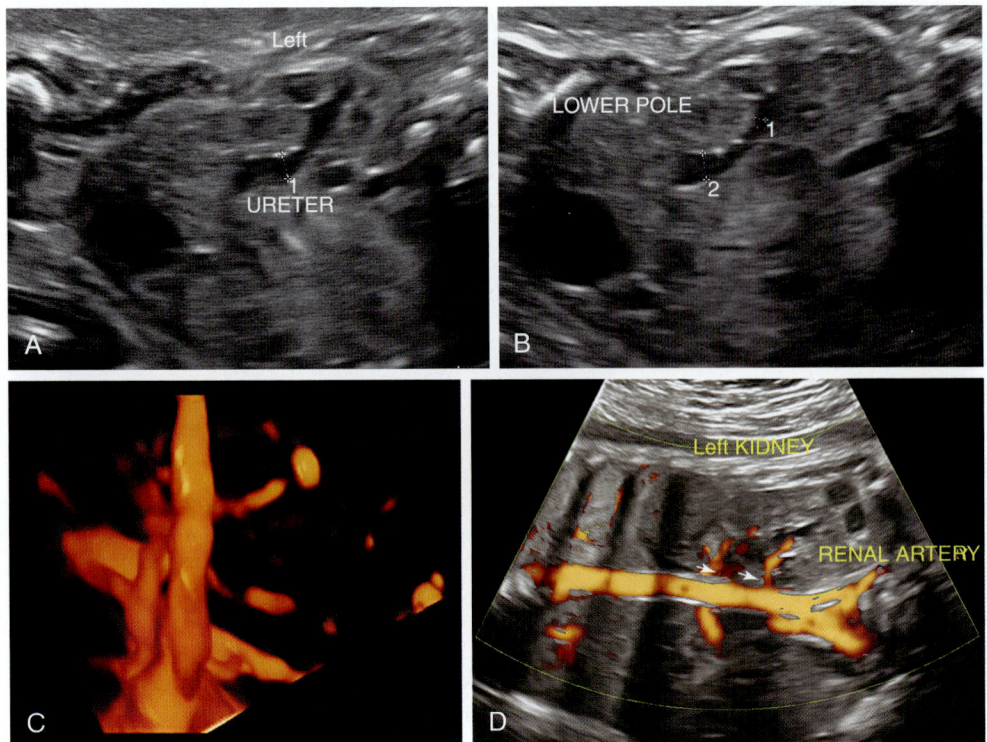

FIG. 64.37 (A) In this image of the upper pole of the left kidney, a slightly dilated renal pelvis and ureter are seen exiting the kidney. (B) In the same kidney, a slightly dilated renal pelvis and ureter are seen exiting the lower pole of the left kidney. (C) Power Doppler and three-dimensional technology were used to visualize the renal arteries. Two left renal arteries were imaged. They were each traced to the left kidney; one entered at the upper pole and the other at the lower pole. (D) A coronal view with power Doppler easily identified the duplicated renal arteries.

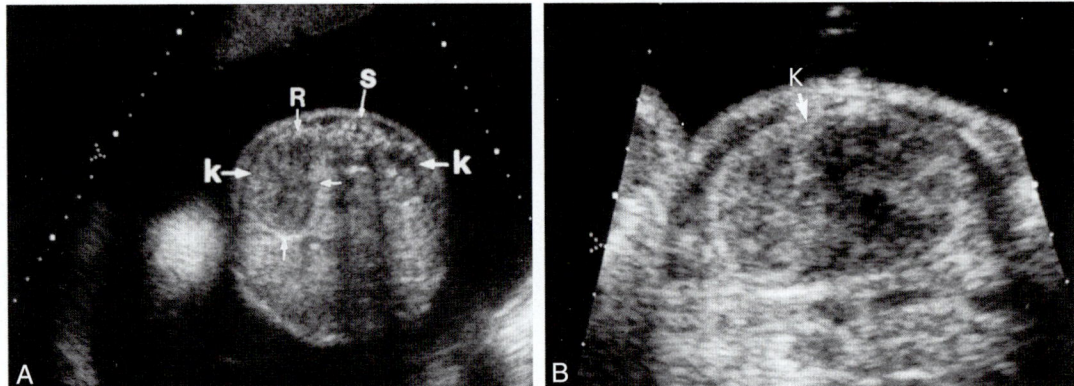

FIG. 64.38 (A) Mesoblastic nephroma in a 32-week-old fetus showing obvious enlargement of the right (R) kidney (k, arrows) compared with the left kidney (k). Hydramnios was observed. (B) In the same fetus the encapsulated and solid appearance of the nephroma (K) was observed. The nephroma was removed within few days after birth. S, Spine.

removal of the affected kidney, prognosis is excellent. Tumors typically appear more commonly in males and are benign. The prognosis for Wilms' tumor is good with early resection. Neuroblastomas usually present in the third trimester and occur more often on the right side. If the mass is solid it will likely metastasize to the liver in utero. If the mass is large or metastases are evident fetal hydrops is likely to develop. Polyhydramnios is a typical finding with these tumors; therefore, the patient may undergo therapeutic amnioreductions to prevent preterm labor or as a result of maternal clinical symptoms.

Sonographic Findings. Masses in the kidney should be suspected when the contour of the kidney is distorted or replaced by a mass and the pelvicaliceal echoes are absent (Box 64.7). Polyhydramnios and enlarged abdominal circumference measurements are typical manifestations.

CONGENITAL MALFORMATIONS OF THE GENITAL SYSTEM

Although congenital malformations of the genital system are rare, the sonographic team may be requested to determine the sex of the fetus when a sex-linked disorder is considered (e.g., hemophilia or aqueductal stenosis). Because these conditions usually occur in male fetuses, identification of male genitalia aids in counseling and diagnostic testing. Likewise, the

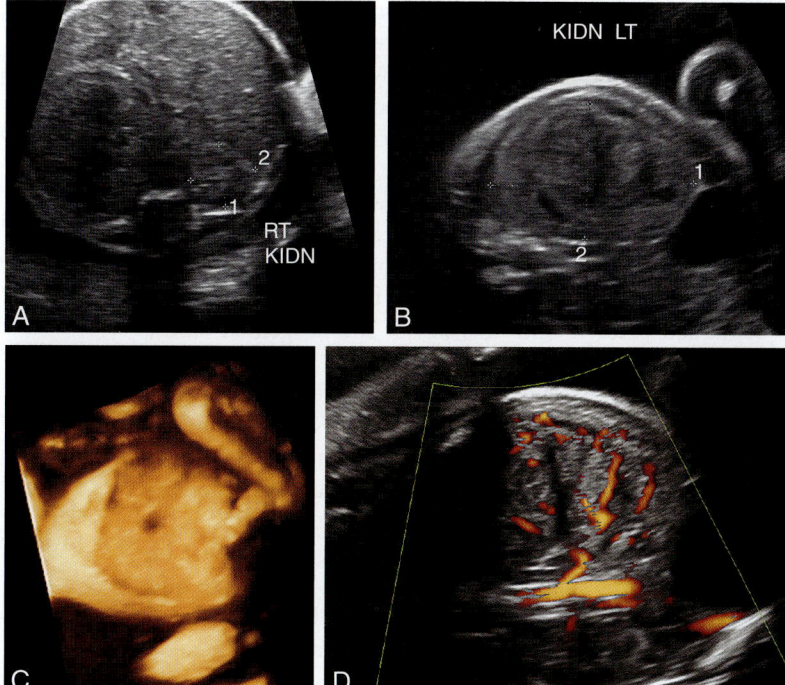

FIG. 64.39 (A) This fetus presented with a solid abdominal mass in the area of the left kidney. The right kidney appears within normal limits. (B) The left kidney could not be clearly seen. The solid mass was large and extended from the stomach to the fetal bladder. (C) Rendering of the mass determined that the mass was inferior to the diaphragm. (D) Color Doppler revealed internal vascularity within the mass. On delivery a biopsy of the mass revealed Wilms tumor.

BOX 64.7	Sonographic Findings of Renal Tumors

- Mesoblastic nephromas: large, single, solid masses originating from the kidney that appear isoechoic or hyperechoic to kidney parenchyma
- Wilms tumor: solid or partially cystic
- Neuroblastoma: varying echo patterns (usually echogenic) with diffuse vascularity and possibly liver metastasis

demonstration of abnormal fetal genitalia may be indicative of syndromes of the endocrine and genital systems. In the female, positive identification of the labia is as essential to the diagnosis as demonstration of the penis and scrotum is in the male.

Hydrocele

Etiology. Hydrocele occurs in the male fetus and is seen as an accumulation of serous fluid surrounding the testicle, resulting from a communication with the peritoneal cavity.

Clinical Findings and Prognosis. Hydroceles may occur as unilateral or bilateral and are generally benign. They can be identified as simple or complex. Complex hydroceles have been identified secondary to hemorrhage, infarction, or torsion of the testes. In the majority of cases of simple hydroceles the testes are normal and the hydrocele will resolve after birth. Hydroceles have been reported in cases of hydrops.

Sonographic Findings. Simple hydroceles appear as anechoic fluid surrounding or partially surrounding the testes. Echogenicities present within the fluid are indicative of a complex hydrocele.

Undescended Testicles

Etiology. The gonads eventually descend from the abdomen to the pelvis. As this occurs, a diverticulum of the peritoneum, the processus vaginalis, protrudes through the anterior abdominal wall to form the primordium of the inguinal canal. The processus vaginalis is attached to a ligament that extends from the caudal pole of the gonad to the labioscrotal swelling.

In the male, the testes remain near the deep inguinal rings until the 28th week. They descend through the inguinal canals and enter the scrotum before birth. If the descent is interrupted or stopped, the testes will remain located within the inguinal canal; this is referred to as undescended testes or **cryptorchidism**. The distal part of the processus vaginalis persists as the tunica vaginalis of the testis. In the female, the ligament attaches to the uterus to form the ovarium ligament and the round ligament.

Clinical Findings and Prognosis. Undescended testicles are associated with risk of torsion and development of cancer. However, the risks are significantly lowered if the testes are surgically placed within the scrotum sac early in childhood.

Sonographic Findings. The scrotal sac will appear void of testicular tissue. Small amounts of anechoic fluid will likely be evident in the scrotum. In utero, diagnosis of the testes within the inguinal canal is difficult.

Ambiguous Genitalia

Etiology. *Ambiguous genitalia* refers to the sonographic inability to delineate fetal sex. Several congenital malformations are associated with this finding. Malformations typically result from chromosomal defects or abnormal hormone levels and include the following:

- *True **hermaphroditism***. This is a rare condition in which both ovarian and testicular tissues are present. The internal and external genitalia are variable. Most fetuses will have a normal karyotype, but some are mosaics (46,XX/46,XY). Determination of fetal sex may be critical in establishing a correct diagnosis.
- *Female pseudohermaphrodites*. The female fetus with pseudohermaphroditism has a 46,XX karyotype. The most common cause is congenital virilizing adrenal hyperplasia that causes masculinization of the external genitalia (enlarged clitoris, abnormalities of the urogenital sinus, and partial fusion of the labia majora).
- *Male pseudohermaphrodites*. The male fetus with pseudohermaphroditism has testes and a 46,XY karyotype. There are variable external and internal genitalia depending on the development of the penis and genital ducts.

Clinical Findings and Prognosis. The sonographer must be careful diagnosing ambiguous genitalia because penile and clitoral size may vary in the normal fetus. Genetic amniocentesis is needed for karyotyping to determine the genetic makeup. Chromosomal abnormalities associated with ambiguous genitalia include trisomy 13, triploidy, certain deletions, and translocation. Other associations include cloacal malformation and adrenogenital syndrome. Surgery may be required to repair associated abnormalities or for cosmetic concerns.

Sonographic Findings. Sonographically, the key signs to investigate for sex are absent. In many cases, an abnormally small penis is hard to differentiate from the enlarged clitoris, and a bifid scrotum may appear as enlarged labia (Fig. 64.40).

OTHER PELVIC MASSES

Hydrometrocolpos

Etiology. Obstruction of the uterus and vagina resulting in collections of fluid is referred to as **hydrometrocolpos**. The obstruction results from numerous causes such as atresia of the vagina or cervix, imperforate hymen, or abnormal membranes within the vaginal lumen.

Clinical Findings and Prognosis. Hydrometrocolpos has been noted in conjunction with a double uterus and septated vagina (vagina divided by a septum into two components), cloacal malformations, renal agenesis, and as part of a syndrome. The fluid collection may be so large that it extends into the abdominal cavity or may cause compression of the ureters and hydronephrosis of the kidneys. The prognosis is dependent on other abnormalities present; however, the malformation itself can be surgically corrected.

Sonographic Findings. Hydrometrocolpos appears as a hypoechoic cyst-like ovoid mass posterior to the bladder around the uterus. These masses may be predominantly cystic, may contain midlevel echoes, or may have fluid-debris levels. Echoes within these masses may result from mucous secretions.

Fetal Ovarian Cyst

Etiology. The ovarian mass results from maternal hormonal stimulation and is usually benign. The cysts typically represent normal functional ovarian cysts.

Clinical Findings and Prognosis. Ovarian cysts represent the most common cystic mass in female fetuses. They range

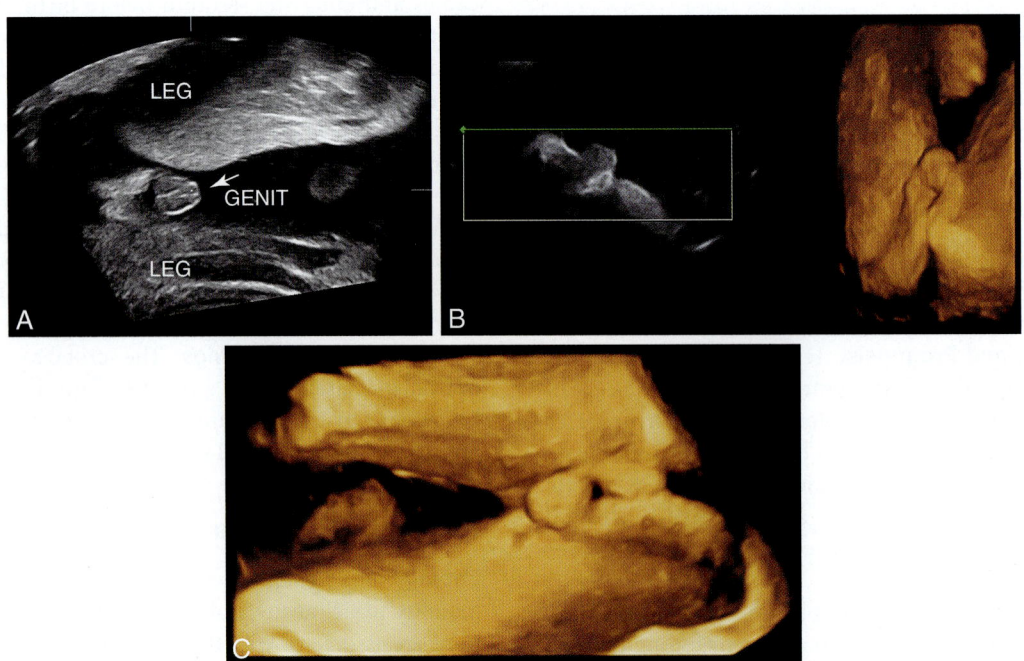

FIG. 64.40 (A) A clear delineation of external genitalia could not be made in this third-trimester fetus. (B–C) Further evaluation with advanced technology did not provide additional information regarding clear support of male or female external genitalia.

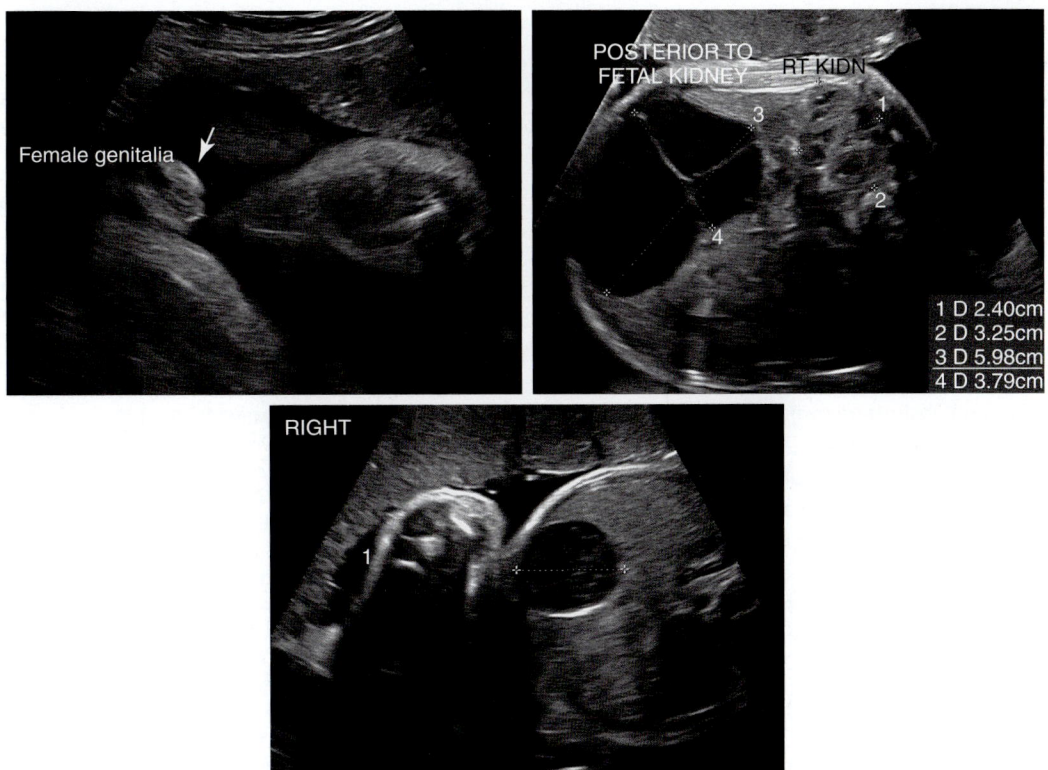

FIG. 64.41 Ovarian cysts may appear anechoic or hypoechoic. If the cyst is associated with hemorrhage or torsion, sonographic features may include a complex or solid appearance.

in size from small to large and are usually located on one side of the abdomen or lower pelvis. They can be unilateral or bilateral and often confused with other masses. Differential considerations would include a mesenteric cyst, a urachal cyst, or an enteric duplication. Most cysts will regress either in utero or during the postnatal period. However, complications have been documented. The mass may twist on itself, which may lead to torsion, rupture, or intestinal obstruction. Treatment depends on associated complications.

Sonographic Findings. An ovarian cyst may appear anechoic or hypoechoic. If the cyst is associated with hemorrhage or torsion, sonographic features may include a complex or solid appearance (Fig. 64.41).

ACKNOWLEDGMENT

The author acknowledges Roy Bors-Koefoed, MD, and Christina Taff, BHS, RDMS, for their contribution of images to this chapter.

Key Pearls

- The fetal kidneys should be evaluated by assessing their anatomy, texture, and size.
- The fetal kidneys and bladder may be seen by 13 weeks of gestation.
- In normal conditions, the fetal bladder is well visualized as an anechoic structure in the fetal pelvis. The fetal ureters and urethra are typically not seen.
- Determination of the fetal sex should be documented with the presence of other abnormalities or in cases in which the external organ does not meet the sonographic criteria for a male or female.
- Obstructions of the urinary system may originate anywhere along the urinary tract.
- Dilation of the posterior urethra is highly suspicious for an obstructive process, such as posterior urethral valve syndrome, known as the key bladder sign on sonography.
- Renal malformations may be divided into two categories: (1) those involving congenital malformation and (2) those resulting from an obstructive process.
- Complete absence of the kidney(s) is known as renal agenesis. Bilateral renal agenesis is often referred to as Potter syndrome.
- A horseshoe kidney forms when the inferior poles of the kidney fuse while they are in the pelvis.
- Exstrophy of the bladder is characterized by the protrusion of the posterior wall of the urinary bladder, which contains the trigone of the bladder and the ureteric orifices.
- Infantile polycystic kidney disease or autosomal recessive polycystic kidney disease is an autosomal recessive congenital disorder that affects both fetal kidneys and liver.
- Congenital multicystic dysplastic kidney disease is characterized by multiple, smooth-walled, nonfunctioning, noncommunicating cysts of variable size and number.

- In obstructive cystic dysplasia, renal dysplasia occurs secondary to kidney obstruction in the first or early second trimester of pregnancy.
- The urinary tract may be obstructed at the junction of the ureter entering the renal pelvis (ureteropelvic junction), at the junction of the ureter where it enters the bladder (ureterovesical junction), or at the level of the urethra (megacystis).
- Hydronephrosis commonly occurs when there is an obstruction in the ureter, bladder, or urethra.
- Ureteropelvic junction obstructions occur at the junction between the renal pelvis and ureter.
- Ureterovesical junction obstruction commonly presents with dilation of the lower end of the ureter.
- Posterior urethral valve obstruction results in hydronephrosis, hydroureters, or dilation of the bladder and posterior urethra.
- Prune-belly syndrome is recognized by three features: cryptorchidism, agenesis or hypoplasia of abdominal wall muscle, and dilation of the collecting system.
- A ureterocele is a cystic dilation of the intravesical (bladder) segment of the distal ureter.
- The most common renal tumor is a mesoblastic nephroma.
- Hydrocele occurs in the male fetus and is seen as an accumulation of serous fluid surrounding the testicle, resulting from a communication with the peritoneal cavity.
- If the descent of the testes is interrupted or stopped, the testes will remain located within the inguinal canal; this is referred to as undescended testes or cryptorchidism.
- True hermaphroditism is a rare condition in which both ovarian and testicular tissues are present.
- The female fetus with pseudohermaphroditism has a 46,XX karyotype.
- The male fetus with pseudohermaphroditism has testes and a 46,XY karyotype.
- Obstruction of the uterus and vagina resulting in collections of fluid is referred to as hydrometrocolpos.

BIBLIOGRAPHY

Anderson NG, et al. Detection of obstructive uropathy in the fetus: predictive value of sonographic measurements of renal pelvic diameter at various gestational ages. *Am J Roentgenol.* 1995;164:719.

Anderson NG, Allan RB, Abbott GKD. Fluctuating fetal or neonatal renal pelvis: marker of high-grade vesicoureteral reflux. *Pediatr Nephrol.* 2004;19(7):749–753.

Apocalypsa GT, Oliverira EA, Rabelo EA, et al. Outcome of apparent ureteropelvic junction obstruction identified by investigation of fetal hydronephrosis. *Int Urol Nephrol.* 2003;35(4):441–448.

Ayers E. Incidental sonographic finding of bilateral ureteroceles. *J Diagn Med Sonogr.* 2006;22(2):123–126.

Baker A, Goepfert M, Whitney E. Multicystic dysplastic kidney and sonography: a case report. *J Diagn Med Sonogr.* 2016;33(2):120–123.

Bateman GA, Giles WK, Enland SL. Renal venous Doppler sonography in preeclampsia. *J Ultrasound Med.* 2004;23(12):1607–1611.

Benaceraf BR. *Ultrasound of Fetal Syndromes.* ed 2. Philadelphia: Elsevier; 2007.

Berg S, Michael K. Imperforate anus with renal ectopia. *J Diagnostic Medical Sonography.* 2008;24(1):34–48.

Berkowitz RL, et al. Fetal urinary tract obstruction: what is the role of surgical intervention in utero? *Am J Obstet Gynecol.* 1982; 144:367.

Berrocal T, Lopez-Pereira P, Arjonilla A, Gutierrez J. Anomalies of the distal ureter, bladder and urethra in children: embryologic, radiologic and pathologic features. *Radiographics.* 2002;22: 1139–1164.

Birewar S, Zawada ET. Jr: Early onset polycystic kidney disease: how early is early? *S D J Med.* 2003;56(11):465–468.

Bisset RA, Khan AN, Thomas NB. *Differential Diagnosis in Obstetric and Gynecologic Ultrasound.* Philadelphia: WB Saunders; 2002.

Bobrowski RA, et al. In utero progression of isolated renal pelvis dilation. *Am J Perinatol.* 1997;14:423.

Borrelli AL, Borrelli P, Di Domenico A, et al. The incidence of chromosomal anomalies in fetuses affected by mild renal pyelectasis. *Minerva Ginecol.* 2004;56(2):137–140.

Callen P. *Ultrasonography in Obstetrics and Gynecology.* ed 6. Philadelphia: Elsevier; 2017.

Celik H, Kefeli M, Tosun M, et al. Congenital mesoblastic nephroma prenatal diagnosis by sonography. *J Diagn Med Sonogr.* 2009;25:112–115.

Chitty LS, Altman DG. Charts of fetal size: kidney and renal pelvis measurements. *Prenat Diagn.* 2003;23(11):891–897.

Curtis MR, et al. Prenatal ultrasound characterization of the suprarenal mass: distinction between neuroblastoma and subdiaphragmatic extralobar pulmonary sequestration. *J Ultrasound Med.* 1997;16:75.

DeVore GR. The value of color Doppler sonography in the diagnosis of renal agenesis. *J Ultrasound Med.* 1995;14:443.

Eckoldt F, Heling KS, Woderich R. Posterior urethral valves: prenatal diagnostic signs and outcome. *Urol Int.* 2004;73(4):296–301.

Entezami M, Albig M, Gasiorek-Wiens A, Becker R. *Ultrasound Diagnosis of Fetal Anomalies.* New York: Thieme; 2004.

Guthrie JD. Prenatal diagnosis of posterior urethral valves. *J Diagn Med Sonogr.* 2007;23:123–125.

Ismaili K, Ayni FE, Martin Wissing K, et al. Long-term clinical outcome of infants with mild and moderate fetal pyelectasis: validation of neonatal ultrasound as a screening tool to detect significant nephrouropathies. *J Pediatr.* 2004;144(6):759–765.

John U, Kahler C, Schultz S, et al. The impact of fetal renal pelvic diameter on postnatal outcome. *Prenat Diagn.* 2004;24(8):591–595.

Kaneshiro NK: Potter syndrome. https://medlineplus.gov/ency/article/001268.htm.

Kibar Y, Coban H, Irkilata HC, et al. Anterior urethral valves: an uncommon cause of obstructive uropathy in children. *J Pediatr Urol.* 2007;3(5):350–353.

Kohler M, Pease PW, Upadhayay V. Megacystis-microcolon-intestinal hypoperistalsis syndrome (MMIHS) in siblings: case report and review of the literature. *Eur J Pediatr Surg.* 2004;14(5):362–367.

Lonergan GJ, Rice RR, Suarez ES. Autosomal recessive polycystic kidney disease: radiologic-pathologic correlation. *Radiographics.* 2000;20:837–855.

Maizels M, Alpert SA, Houston JT, et al. Fetal bladder sagittal length: a simple monitor to assess normal and enlarged fetal bladder size, and forecast outcome. *J Urol.* 2004;172(S Pt 1): 1995–1999.

Mali VP, Prabhakaran K, Loh D. Anterior urethral valves. *Asian J Surg.* 2006;29(3):165–169.

Mazza V, Di Monte I, Pati M, et al. Sonographic biometrical range of external genitalia differentiation in the first trimester of pregnancy: analysis of 2593 cases. *Prenat Diagn.* 2004;24(9):677–684.

Nyberg DA, McGahan JP, Pretorius DH, eds. *Diagnostic Ultrasound of Fetal Anomalies: Text and Atlas.* Philadelphia: Lippincott Williams & Wilkins; 2003.

Odibo AO, Raab E, Elovitz M, et al. Prenatal mild pyelectasis: evaluating the thresholds of renal pelvic diameter associated with normal postnatal renal function. *J Ultrasound Med.* 2004;23(4):513–517.

Pinette MG, Wax JR, Blackstone J. Normal growth and development of fetal external genitalia demonstrated by sonography. *J Clin Ultrasound*. 2003;31(9):465–472.

Rumack CM, Wilson SR, Charboneau JW, Johnson JA. *Diagnostic Ultrasound*, vol 2, 5th ed, St. Louis: Elsevier; 2018.

Rushton HG, Parrott TS, Woodard JR, Walther M. The role of vesicostomy in the management of anterior urethral valves in neonates and infants. *J Urol*. 1987;138(1):107–109.

Sanders RC *Structural Fetal Abnormalities: The Total Picture*. ed 3. St Louis: Elsevier; 2016.

Schoellnast H, Lindbichler F, Riccabona M. Sonographic diagnosis of urethral anomalies in infants the value of perineal sonography. *J Ultrasound Med*. 2004;23:769–776.

Souzada MC, Oliverira EA, Pereira AK, et al. Diagnostic accuracy of postnatal renal pelvic diameter as a predictor of uropathy: a prospective study. *Pediatr Radiol*. 2004;34(10):798–804.

Stephenson S. *Diagnostic Medical Sonography: Obstetrics and Gynecology*. ed 4. New York: Lippincott; 2017.

Tanzer PJ, Butwin AN. Prenatal diagnosis of urinary tract dilation: a case study. *J Diagn Med Sonogr*. 2018;34(3):238–241.

Toiviainen-Salo S, Garel L, Grignon A, et al. Fetal hydronephrosis: is there hope for consensus? *Pediatr Radiol*. 2004;34(7):519–529.

Vijayaraghavan SB, Nirmala AB. Complete duplication of urinary bladder and urethra: prenatal sonographic features. *Ultrasound Obstet Gynecol*. 2004;24(4):464–466.

Woodard PJ, Kennedy A, Sohaey R, et al. EXPERTddx: obstetrics. Amirsys. 2009.

CHAPTER 65

Fetal Skeleton

Kelsi Weakley

OBJECTIVES

On completion of this chapter, you should be able to:
- Describe in detail the embryology of the fetal skeleton
- Describe the variety of musculoskeletal anomalies that can occur in the fetus
- Differentiate sonographically among the most common skeletal dysplasias
- List limb abnormalities and the anomalies that are associated with and unique to specific defects

OUTLINE

Embryology of the Fetal Skeleton 1622
Abnormalities of the Skeleton 1622
   Sonographic Evaluation of Skeletal Dysplasias 1623
   Thanatophoric Dysplasia 1624
   Achondroplasia 1626
   Achondrogenesis 1626
   Osteogenesis Imperfecta 1626
Congenital Hypophosphatasia 1628
Diastrophic Dysplasia 1628
Camptomelic Dysplasia 1629
Roberts Syndrome 1629
Short-Rib Polydactyly Syndrome 1630
Jeune Syndrome 1631
Ellis–van Creveld Syndrome 1631
Caudal Regression Syndrome/Sirenomelia 1631
VACTERL Association 1632
Postural Anomalies 1632
Arthrogryposis Multiplex Congenita 1632
Other Limb Abnormalities 1633

KEY TERMS

Achondrogenesis
Achondroplasia
Craniosynostosis
Heterozygous achondroplasia
Homozygous achondroplasia
Hypophosphatasia
Osteogenesis imperfecta
Polydactyly
Thanatophoric dysplasia

EMBRYOLOGY OF THE FETAL SKELETON

The majority of the musculoskeletal system forms from the primitive mesoderm arising from mesenchymal cells that are the embryonic connective tissue. These cells arise from different regions of the body. The vertebral column and ribs arise from the somites, and the limbs arise from the lateral plate mesoderm. The formation of the head is more complex in that the cranial bones that form the roof and base of the skull arise from mesenchymal cells of the primitive mesoderm, but the facial bones actually arise from mesenchymal cells arising from the neural crest, which is ectodermal in origin. The skeleton initially appears as cartilaginous structures that later undergo ossification.

Limb development begins the 26th or 27th day after conception with the appearance of upper limb buds. Lower extremity development begins 2 days later. Although the stages of development for the upper and lower extremities are the same, lower extremity development continues to lag behind that of the upper extremities. Initially the limbs have a paddle shape with a ridge of thickened ectoderm, known as the apical ectodermal ridge, at the apex of each bud. Digital rays begin to differentiate from the apical ectodermal ridge around day 41 through a process of cell death of the ridge between the digits. The fingers are distinctly evident by day 49, although they are still webbed, and by the eighth week of development the fingers are longer. The development of the feet and toes is essentially complete by the ninth week, although the soles of the feet are still turned inward at this time.

Anomalies of the skeletal system often result from genetic factors, although the cause may be unknown or be the result of environmental factors, including drug or mechanical effects.

ABNORMALITIES OF THE SKELETON

Skeletal dysplasia is the term used to describe abnormal growth and density of cartilage and bone, and the incidence is 3 in

10,000 births, with a significantly greater incidence in stillbirths.[1] This grouping of disorders is characterized by abnormal shape, growth, and integrity of the skeletal system. Although the prenatal diagnosis can be challenging, routine ultrasound in conjunction for familial history and other assessments of risk can prove beneficial to diagnosing these conditions. There are more than 450 types of skeletal anomalies,[1] and not all of them are amenable to sonographic detection. The perinatal team may be able to isolate a skeletal dysplasia when abnormal skeletal structures are observed, such as bone shortening or hypomineralization. Dwarfism is the condition of a disproportionately short stature; it occurs secondary to a skeletal dysplasia.

Skeletal dysplasias are considered rare, and many are considered incompatible with life. What determines whether these conditions are potentially lethal is the assessment for the presence of pulmonary hypoplasia as a result of a skeletal dysplasia limiting the ability to intubate or provide adequate ventilation once the neonate is born. The lethal forms characteristically are extremely severe in their prenatal appearance, as with severe micromelia. Nonlethal skeletal dysplasias tend to manifest in a milder form. The sonographer should become familiar with the sonographic characteristics of the more common skeletal dysplasias that can be diagnosed in utero.

There are multiple anomalies of the musculoskeletal system that may be identified with ultrasound. Many of these osteochondrodysplasias have similar features, although often there are distinguishing features that can lead to a diagnosis. The primary focus should be on identifying those features suggestive of lethality. A list of short-limb skeletal dysplasias, ultrasound characteristics, and their distinguishing features are listed in Table 65.1.

Sonographic Evaluation of Skeletal Dysplasias

The patient whose fetus is at risk for a skeletal dysplasia is commonly referred to a maternal-fetal center for genetic counseling and a targeted ultrasound. Although many skeletal dysplasias are inherited, sporadic occurrences and new mutations do occur, so it is important to screen for skeletal dysplasias as part of every obstetric ultrasound examination. Most prenatally diagnosed skeletal dysplasias occur in association with polyhydramnios or other fetal anomalies or when there is a risk for recurrence.

When a skeletal dysplasia is suspected, the protocol of the obstetric ultrasound examination should be adjusted to include the following criteria:
1. Assess limb shortening. All long bones should be measured. A skeletal dysplasia is suspected when limb lengths are more than 2 standard deviations below the mean (Tables 65.2 and 65.3).
2. Assess bone contour. Thickness, assessment for abnormal bowing or curvature, fractures, and a ribbon-like appearance should be performed.
3. Estimate degree of ossification. Decreased attenuation of the bones with decreased shadowing suggests hypomineralization. Special attention should be focused toward this assessment of the cranium, spine, ribs, and long bones.

TABLE 65.1 Osteochondrodysplasia Findings

Anomaly	Sonographic Findings	Distinguishing Characteristics
Thanatophoric dysplasia	Severe micromelia Macrocephaly Cloverleaf skull Narrow thorax	Cloverleaf skull
Achondrogenesis	Severe micromelia Macrocephaly Poor ossification of spine, skull Short thorax	Decreased ossification Severity of limb shortening
Achondroplasia	Rhizomelia Macrocephaly Trident hands	Rhizomelic shortening Trident hands
Camptomelic dysplasia	Hypoplastic fibulas Long bone bowing Micrognathia Small thorax Talipes	Fibular hypoplasia Bowing affects lower extremities
Osteogenesis imperfecta (type II)	Severe micromelia Generalized hypomineralization Narrow thorax Multiple fractures	Normal head size Hypomineralization of skull Multiple fractures
Short-rib polydactyly syndrome	Micromelia Narrow thorax Facial cleft Polydactyly	Facial anomalies Polydactyly
Hypophosphatasia	Mild limb shortening Narrow thorax Limb fractures and bowing	Hypomineralization of skull Fractures

4. Evaluate the thoracic circumference and shape. A long, narrow chest or a bell-shaped chest may be indicative of specific dysplasias.
5. Survey for coexistent hand and foot anomalies, such as talipes and polydactyly.
6. Evaluate the face and profile for facial clefts, frontal bossing, micrognathia, hypertelorism, and other facial anomalies that may be associated with skeletal dysplasias.
7. Survey for other associated anomalies, such as hydrocephaly, heart defects, and nonimmune hydrops.

The manifestation of skeletal dysplasias varies based on the specific dysplasia, and three-dimensional ultrasound may aid in the diagnosis. First trimester assessment may present with an increased nuchal translucency, which increases the risk for lethality,[2] and chorionic villus sampling may provide important diagnostic information regarding the type of skeletal dysplasia. In addition, long bones are affected in different patterns (Fig. 65.1) according to the dysplasia. Rhizomelia is shortening of the proximal bone segment (humerus and femur). Mesomelia refers to shortening of the middle segments (radius/ulna and tibia/fibula). Micromelia describes the shortening of the entire extremity. Sonographic examination of the long bones should include an assessment to

TABLE 65.2	Length of the Bones of the Leg: Normal Values (mm)					
	Tibia Percentile			Fibula Percentile		
Week	5th	50th	95th	5th	50th	95th
12	—	7	—	—	6	—
13	—	10	—	—	9	—
14	7	12	17	6	12	19
15	9	15	20	9	15	21
16	12	17	22	13	18	23
17	15	20	25	13	21	28
18	17	22	27	15	23	31
19	20	25	30	19	26	33
20	22	27	33	21	28	36
21	25	30	35	24	31	37
22	27	32	38	27	33	39
23	30	35	40	28	35	42
24	32	37	42	29	37	45
25	34	40	45	34	40	45
26	37	42	47	36	42	47
27	39	44	49	37	44	50
28	41	46	51	38	45	53
29	43	48	53	41	47	54
30	45	50	55	43	49	56
31	47	52	57	42	51	59
32	48	54	59	42	52	63
33	50	55	60	46	54	62
34	52	57	62	46	55	65
35	53	58	64	51	57	62
36	55	60	65	54	58	63
37	56	61	67	54	59	65
38	58	63	68	56	61	65
39	59	64	69	56	62	67
40	61	66	71	59	63	67

From Jeanty P, Romero R, editors. *Obstetrical Ultrasound.* New York: McGraw-Hill; 1984.

TABLE 65.3	Length of the Bones of the Arm: Normal Values (mm)					
	Ulna Percentile			Radius Percentile		
Week	5th	50th	95th	5th	50th	95th
12	—	7	—	—	7	—
13	5	10	15	6	10	14
14	8	13	18	8	13	17
15	11	16	21	11	15	20
16	13	18	23	13	18	22
17	16	21	26	14	20	26
18	19	24	29	15	22	29
19	21	26	31	20	24	29
20	24	29	34	22	27	32
21	26	31	36	24	29	33
22	28	33	38	27	31	34
23	31	36	41	26	32	39
24	33	38	43	26	34	42
25	35	40	45	31	36	41
26	37	42	47	32	37	43
27	39	44	49	33	39	45
28	41	46	51	33	40	48
29	43	48	53	36	42	47
30	44	49	54	36	43	49
31	46	51	56	38	44	50
32	48	53	58	37	45	53
33	49	54	59	41	46	51
34	51	56	61	40	47	53
35	52	57	62	41	48	54
36	53	58	63	39	48	57
37	55	60	65	45	49	53
38	56	61	66	45	49	54
39	57	62	67	45	50	54
40	58	63	68	46	50	55

From Jeanty P, Romero R, editors. *Obstetrical Ultrasound.* New York: McGraw-Hill; 1984.

define whether there is segmental shortening or micromelia, because this will aid in the diagnosis. Three-dimensional evaluation may provide further definition of the abnormality.

Thanatophoric Dysplasia

Thanatophoric dysplasia is the most common lethal skeletal dysplasia and occurs in 1 in 20,000 to 40,000 live births (Fig. 65.2).[3] The term *thanatophoric* comes from the Greek word *thanatos*, which means *death personified*. The two main subdivisions of thanatophoric dysplasia are types I and II. Type I is characterized by short, curved femurs and flat vertebral bodies. Type II is characterized by straight, short femurs, flat vertebral bodies, and a cloverleaf skull. Most cases of thanatophoric dysplasia are sporadic occurrences and the result of mutations in the fibroblast growth factor receptor 3 *(FGFR3)* gene. Prenatal molecular analysis can aid in making the definitive diagnosis.

The prognosis for thanatophoric dysplasia is extremely grim. It is considered a lethal anomaly, with most infants dying shortly after birth as a result of pulmonary hypoplasia, which results from the narrow thorax.

Sonographic Findings. The sonographic features of thanatophoric dysplasia include the following:
- Severe micromelia (Fig. 65.3A–B), especially of the proximal bones (rhizomelia)
- Cloverleaf deformity (Kleeblattschädel skull), which occurs as a result of premature **craniosynostosis** and may be associated with agenesis of the corpus callosum
- Narrow thorax with shortened ribs (see Fig. 65.3C–D)

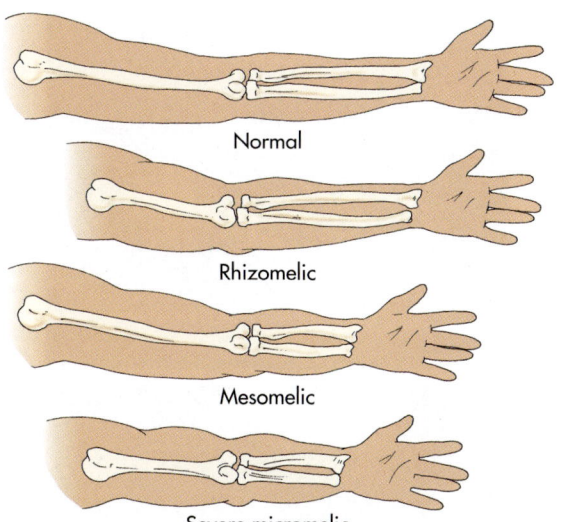

FIG. 65.1 Varieties of short-limb dysplasia according to the affected bones. Rhizomelic dysplasia is characterized by shortening of the proximal long bones (humerus and femur). Mesomelic dysplasia is described as shortening of the distal extremities (radius/ulna and tibia/fibula). Severe micromelia produces shortening of both proximal and distal extremities.

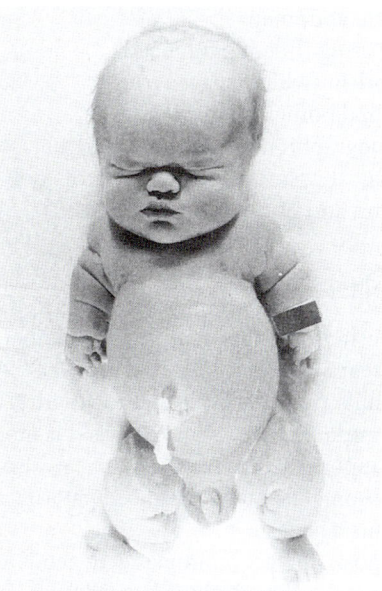

FIG. 65.2 Thanatophoric neonate.

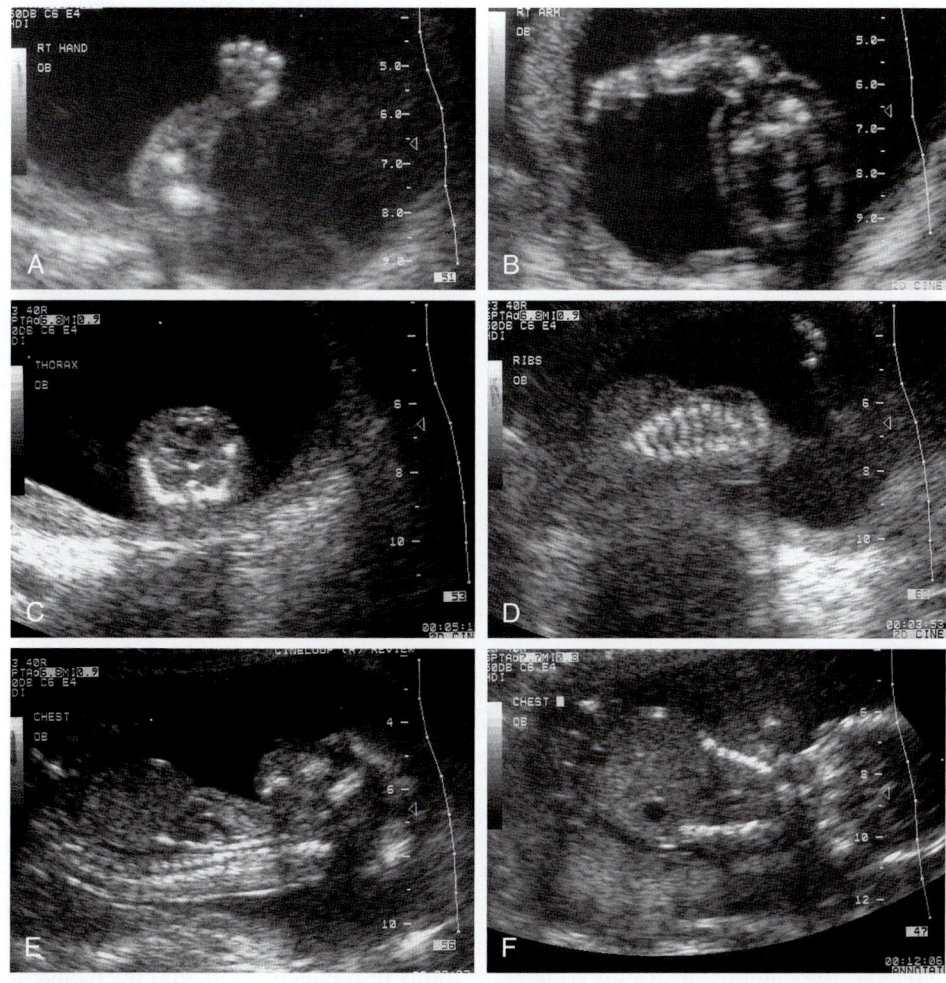

FIG. 65.3 **Lethal skeletal dysplasia consistent with thanatophoric dysplasia at a gestational age of 18 weeks, 1 day.** (A–B) The right arm demonstrates micromelia. The lower extremities were also short, with the femurs measuring a gestational age of 14 weeks. (C) The thorax was very narrow. (D) The ribs were short. The abdomen was protuberant (E) and compared with the narrow thorax (F) gives the appearance of a champagne cork.

- Protuberant abdomen
- Frontal bossing (bulging forehead)
- Hypertelorism (widely spaced eyes)
- Flat vertebral bodies (platyspondyly)

Other sonographic findings that may be associated with thanatophoric dysplasia include severe polyhydramnios, hydrocephalus, and nonimmune hydrops.

Achondroplasia

Achondroplasia is the most common nonlethal skeletal dysplasia and occurs in approximately 1 in 10,000 to 30,000 live births.[4] It results from decreased endochondral bone formation, which produces short, squat bones. It is most commonly the result of a spontaneous mutation but can also be transmitted in an autosomal fashion. Advanced paternal age increases the risk for this dysplasia.

The prognosis for achondroplasia depends on the form. **Heterozygous achondroplasia**, inherited from one parent, has a good survival rate with normal intelligence and a normal life span. Health problems may include neurologic complications that may require orthopedic or neurologic surgical intervention. **Homozygous achondroplasia**, inherited from two parents, is considered lethal, with most infants dying shortly after birth from respiratory complications. With this form, sonographic findings are more severe and include a narrow thorax.

Sonographic Findings. The sonographic features of achondroplasia may not be evident until after 22 weeks of gestation, when biometry becomes abnormal. Ultrasound-guided chorionic villus sampling may aid in the diagnosis in the first trimester for parents with this genetic disorder, and amniocentesis may also be used. Sonographic findings include the following:
- Rhizomelia
- Macrocephaly
- Trident hands (short proximal and middle phalanges)
- A depressed nasal bridge
- Frontal bossing
- Mild ventriculomegaly may be identified

Achondrogenesis

Achondrogenesis is a rare, lethal skeletal dysplasia occurring in 1 in 40,000 births[5] and is caused by cartilage abnormalities that result in abnormal bone formation and hypomineralization. The two types of achondrogenesis are types I (Parenti-Fraccaro) and II (Langer-Saldino). Type I is considered more severe and is transmitted in an autosomal recessive mode, whereas type II is less severe, is more common, and is the result of a spontaneous mutation.

The prognosis for achondrogenesis is grim. It is a lethal abnormality with infants either being stillborn or dying shortly after birth from pulmonary hypoplasia.

Sonographic Findings. The sonographic features (Figs. 65.4–65.6) of achondrogenesis include the following:
- Severe micromelia
- Decreased or absent ossification of the spine

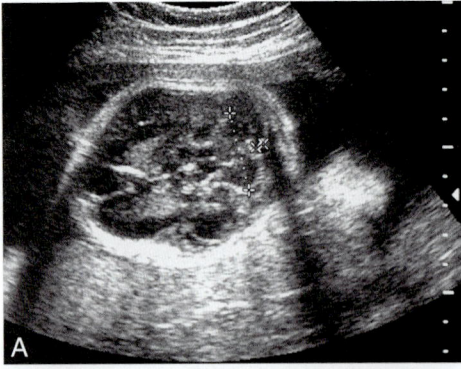
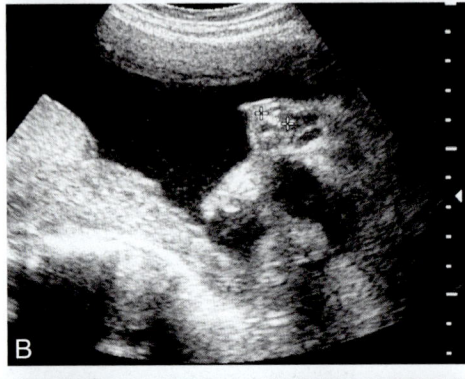
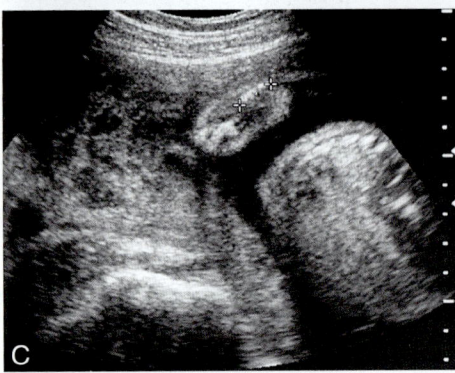

FIG. 65.4 (A) This fetus at 24 weeks of gestation presented with decreased ossification that was noted in the spine and calvarium, which was compressible. Severe micromelia is evidenced in the femur (B) and humerus (C), where the measurement was consistent with 13 weeks of gestation. Achondrogenesis was diagnosed following delivery, and the baby died shortly thereafter.

- Macrocephaly
- Short trunk
- Short thorax and short ribs
- Micrognathia
- Polyhydramnios
- Hydrops possibly identified

Osteogenesis Imperfecta

Osteogenesis imperfecta is a rare disorder of collagen production leading to brittle bones, blue sclera, and manifestations in the teeth, skin, and ligaments. It has been linked to mutations in the *COL1A1* and *COL1A2* genes.[6] There are four classifications, types I to IV. Types I and IV are the mildest forms, and it would be unlikely that a diagnosis would be

CHAPTER 65 Fetal Skeleton   1627

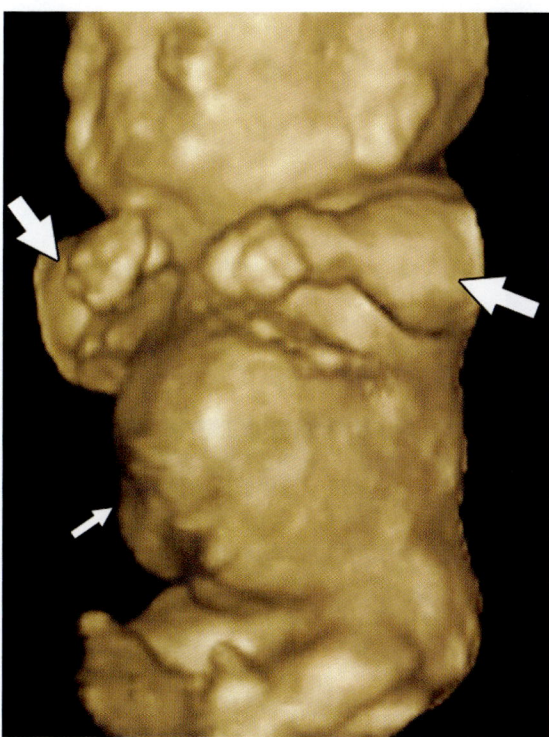

FIG. 65.5 Three-dimensional fetus at 17 weeks of gestation with achondrogenesis type II demonstrating foreshortening of limbs *(large arrows)* and protuberant abdomen *(small arrow)*.

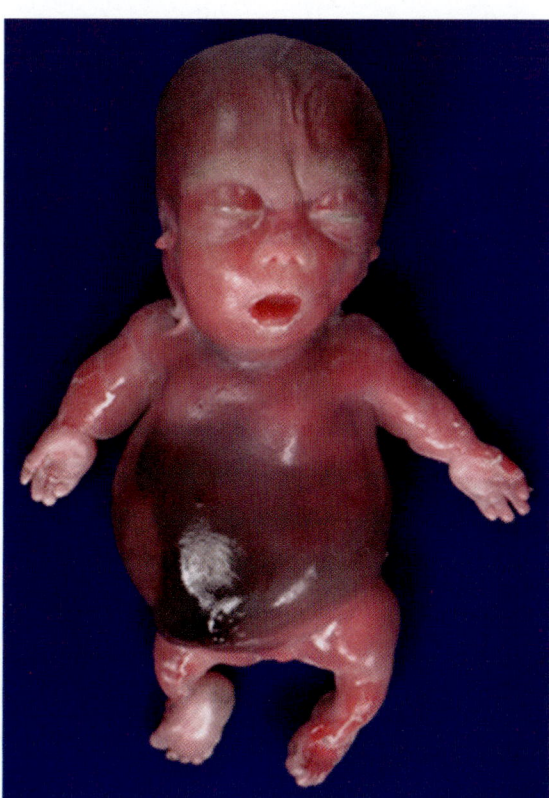

FIG. 65.6 Postmortem image of neonate with achondrogenesis type II demonstrating short barrel-shaped trunk, distended abdomen, and micromelia.

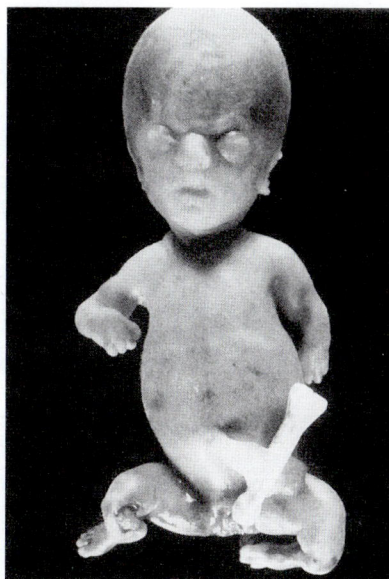

FIG. 65.7 Postmortem image of neonate with osteogenesis imperfecta (type II).

made in utero. Types I and IV are transmitted in an autosomal dominant fashion. Type III is a severe form that may be transmitted in an autosomal dominant or autosomal recessive manner. Type II (Fig. 65.7) is considered the most severe form of osteogenesis imperfecta, having a lethal outcome. It is inherited in an autosomal dominant or autosomal recessive fashion or may result from a spontaneous mutation.

The prognosis for osteogenesis imperfecta depends on the type. Children with types I and IV may have multiple fractures during childhood and may be short. Type I children may also have kyphoscoliosis and deafness. Because of the severity of the brittle bones and multiple fractures, osteogenesis imperfecta type III may produce significant disabilities with progressive deformities of the long bones and spine. Infants with type II usually die shortly after birth because of respiratory complications.

Sonographic Findings. Osteogenesis imperfecta has presented with an increased nuchal translucency in the first trimester of pregnancy. Other more specific sonographic features of osteogenesis imperfecta type II include the following:
- Generalized hypomineralization of the bones, especially the calvarium (Fig. 65.8)
- Multiple fractures of the long bones, ribs, and spine (Figs. 65.9 and 65.10)
- Narrow thorax (see Fig. 65.8A)
- Micromelia

In addition to these findings, brain structures are clearly visualized because of the hypomineralization of the calvarium. The calvarium will also be compressible. The multiple fractures that have occurred during the course of pregnancy may leave the bones bowed, thickened, and sharply angulated. Polyhydramnios may also be evident.

The sonographic features of osteogenesis imperfecta type III are similar to those of type II, although it is less severe.

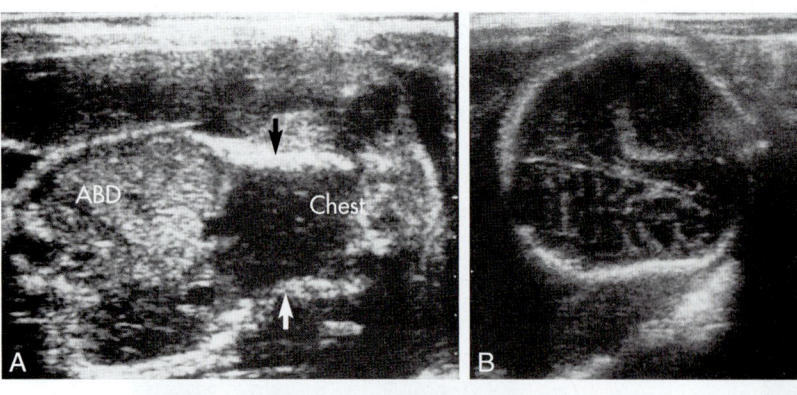

FIG. 65.8 Fetus with osteogenesis imperfecta (type II). (A) A small thoracic cavity *(arrows)* is shown. (B) Hypomineralization of the skull is evident. Note the improved resolution of brain anatomy because of the lack of calvarial calcification. *ABD,* Abdomen.

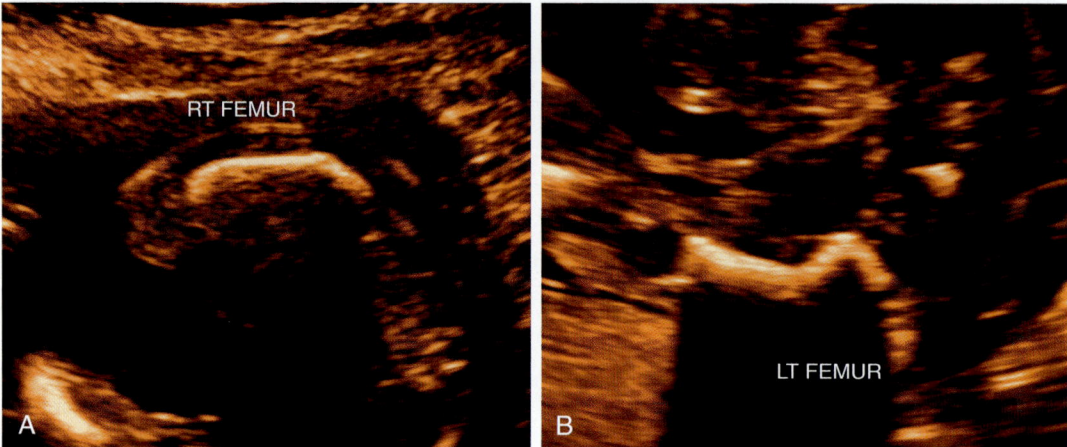

FIG. 65.9 Images of both femurs in a 20-week fetus. (A) The right femur is bowed and fractured and demonstrates significant bowing consistent with a healing fracture (B). Other long bones were also bowed and/or fractured. There was also a beaded appearance of the ribs. Osteogenesis imperfecta type II was confirmed at delivery.

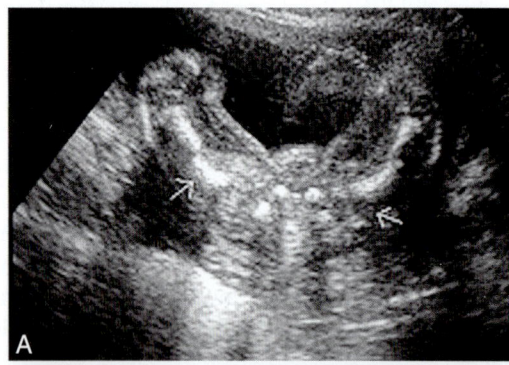
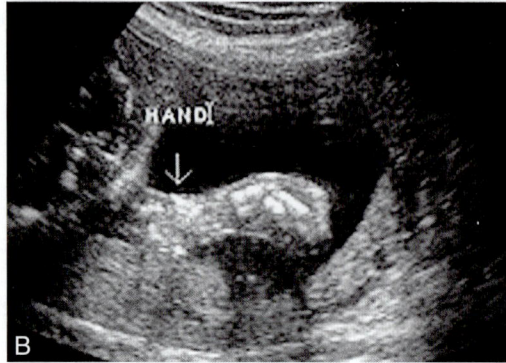

FIG. 65.10 (A) Bilateral fractured femora in a fetus with osteogenesis imperfecta (type II). (B) In the same fetus, fractures of the ulna and radius are visible.

Congenital Hypophosphatasia

Congenital **hypophosphatasia** is a condition that presents with diffuse hypomineralization of the bone caused by an alkaline phosphatase deficiency. It is an inherited condition transmitted in an autosomal recessive manner. Congenital hypophosphatasia may have features similar to osteogenesis imperfecta and achondrogenesis. Diagnosis can be confirmed with alkaline phosphatase assay, which can be achieved through fetal blood sampling or chorionic villus sampling, or through DNA analysis.

Congenital hypophosphatasia is a lethal disorder, with death usually occurring shortly after birth as a result of respiratory complications.

Sonographic Findings. The sonographic features of congenital hypophosphatasia include the following:
- Diffuse hypomineralization of the bones
- Moderate to severe micromelia
- Extremities that may be bowed, fractured, or absent
- Poorly ossified cranium with well-visualized brain structures
- Small thoracic cavity

Diastrophic Dysplasia

Diastrophic dysplasia is a rare disorder characterized by micromelia, talipes, cleft palate, micrognathia, scoliosis, short

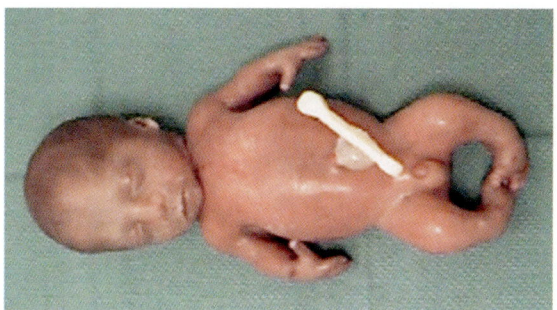

FIG. 65.11 Postmortem image of a fetus with diastrophic dysplasia.

stature, earlobe deformities, and hand abnormalities (Fig. 65.11). It is inherited in an autosomal recessive pattern, and the mutation has been mapped to the long arm of chromosome 5. It has been reported with a significant increased frequency in the Finnish population.

The prognosis for diastrophic dysplasia is variable. There is an increase in infant mortality because of respiratory complications related to the micrognathia and kyphoscoliosis. This is not a lethal disorder, with most patients having a normal life span and normal intelligence. Adult height is usually less than 4 feet, and orthopedic abnormalities can cause significant disabilities.

Sonographic Findings. The sonographic features of diastrophic dysplasia include the following:
- Micromelia (Fig. 65.12)
- Talipes
- Fixed abducted thumb (hitchhiker thumb; see Fig. 65.12B)
- Scoliosis
- Talipes (clubfoot)
- Micrognathia (small chin)
- Cleft palate

Camptomelic Dysplasia

Camptomelic (bent bone) dysplasia is a group of lethal skeletal dysplasias that are characterized by bowing of the long bones. This rare, short-limbed dysplasia usually occurs as a spontaneous mutation, but camptomelic dysplasia is also inherited in an autosomal recessive pattern.

Camptomelic dysplasia is considered a lethal anomaly, with most infants dying in the neonatal period because of pulmonary hypoplasia. Infants surviving the neonatal period usually die within the first year of life, have respiratory and feeding problems, are developmentally delayed, and are intellectually disabled.

Sonographic Findings. The sonographic features of camptomelic dysplasia include the following:
- Bowing of the long bones with the lower extremities affected most severely (Figs. 65.13 and 65.14)
- Small thorax
- Hypoplastic fibulas
- Hypoplastic scapulae
- Hypertelorism
- Cleft palate

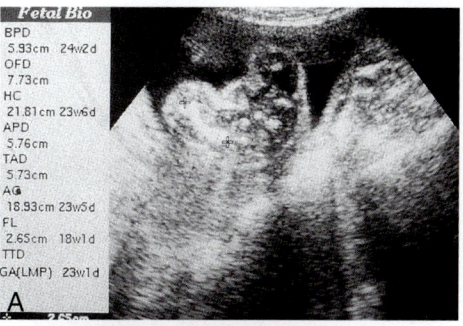
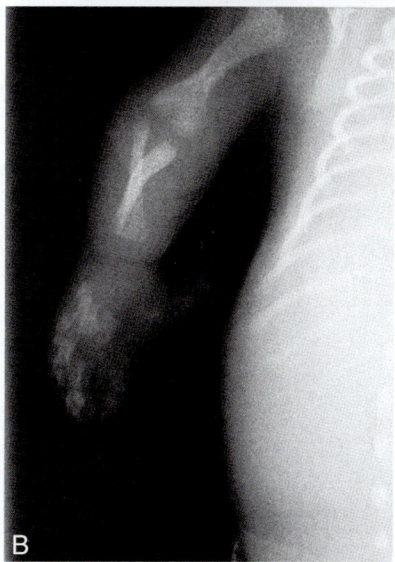

FIG. 65.12 **Diastrophic dysplasia imaged at 23 weeks, 1 day.** (A) Micromelia is demonstrated in this femur measuring 18 weeks, 1 day. The thoracic circumference was also small. (B) Postmortem radiograph demonstrates the "hitchhiker thumb."

- Micrognathia
- Talipes (Figs. 65.15 and 65.16)
- Hydrocephalus
- Polyhydramnios
- Hydronephrosis

Roberts Syndrome

Roberts syndrome is a rare autosomal recessive disorder characterized by phocomelia and facial anomalies. It is also known as a pseudothalidomide syndrome. Roberts syndrome may present with associated chromosomal abnormalities.

The prognosis for Roberts syndrome is poor. Stillbirth and infant mortality are common. Survivors are growth restricted and have severe intellectual disability.

Sonographic Findings. The sonographic features of Roberts syndrome include the following:
- Phocomelia, with the upper extremities more severely affected
- Bilateral cleft lip and palate
- Hypertelorism
- Microcephaly
- Cardiovascular, renal, and gastrointestinal anomalies

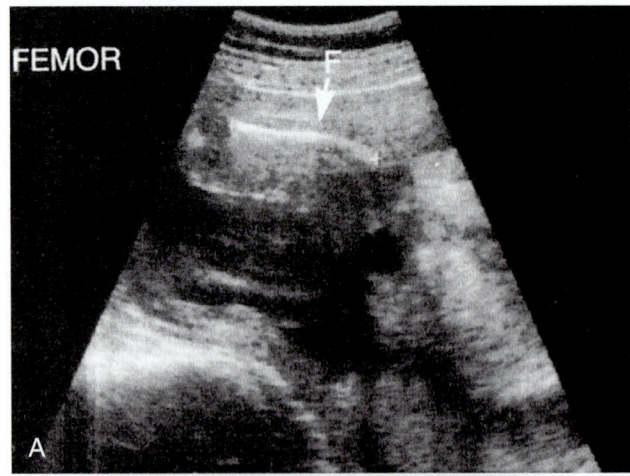
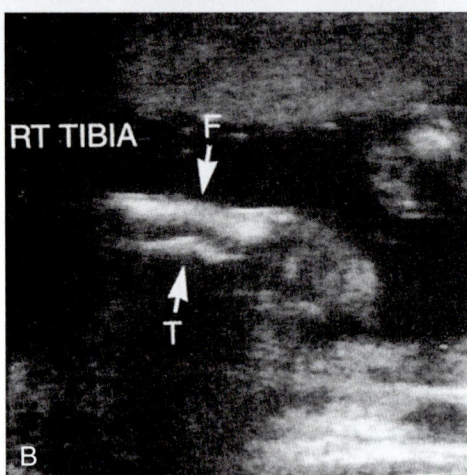

FIG. 65.13 (A) Camptomelic dysplasia and Swyer syndrome in a 20-week-old fetus with femoral bowing (F) found bilaterally. The femoral lengths were normal. (B) In the same fetus, the tibias (T) were short and hypoplastic with sharp anterior bowing of the midshaft of the bone. Distal bowing was also observed. The fibulas (F) were hypoplastic and bowed. The upper extremities were normal in length without bowing or angulation. Bilateral hydronephrosis was observed. Examination of the neonate and radiologic findings (see Fig. 65.12) confirmed the diagnosis of camptomelic dysplasia. Gonadal dysgenesis (female internal and external genitalia with a male karyotype) was consistent with Swyer syndrome. The neonate had other characteristic signs of the disorder, including tall and narrow hypomineralized ischial bones, absent pubic bone ossification, receding chin, hypoplastic cervical vertebrae, elongated clavicles, hypoplastic scapulae, and flexion abnormalities of the feet.

Short-Rib Polydactyly Syndrome

Short-rib polydactyly syndrome is a lethal skeletal dysplasia characterized by short ribs, short limbs, and **polydactyly**, with a prevalence of 1 in 200,000 births. There have been four primary types of this dysplasia defined, which are inherited in an autosomal recessive manner. Type I is also known as Saldino-Noonan syndrome, type II is also known as Majewski syndrome, and type III is known as Naumoff syndrome. Type IV, Beemer-Langer dysplasia, was included in this group of short-rib dysplasias in the 1992 International Classification of Osteochondrodysplasias, and there have been a total of seven types of short-rib polydactyly syndrome classified in the literature.

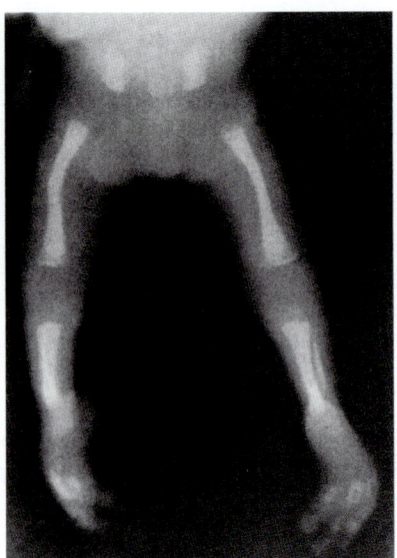

FIG. 65.14 Radiograph of neonate shown in Fig. 65.13 with camptomelic dysplasia and Swyer syndrome. The radiograph demonstrates the lower extremity deformities, including anterior lateral bowing of the femurs at the midshaft. Both tibias are short, with sharp anterior bowing at midshaft and mild bowing at the distal ends. The fibulas are hypoplastic and bowed. Minimal ischial ossification and absent mineralization of the pubic bone are shown.

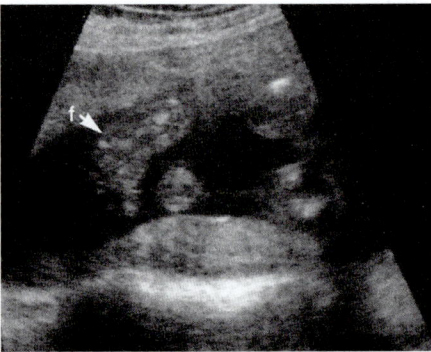

FIG. 65.15 In the fetus with camptomelic dysplasia and Swyer syndrome, as shown in Figs. 65.13 and 65.14, abnormal plantar flexion of the feet is shown. The feet (f) are notably supinated, with curvature to the soles of the feet. The toes are plantarflexed, with the great toes separated by flexion.

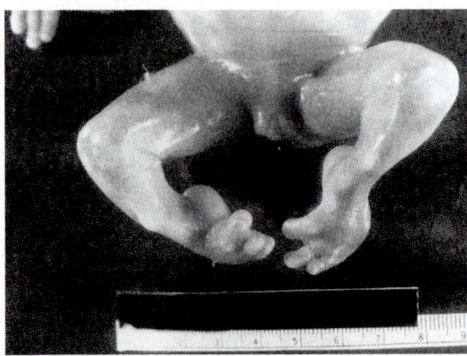

FIG. 65.16 Postmortem image of the neonate shown in Figs. 65.13 to 65.15 with camptomelic dysplasia and Swyer syndrome. Note the markedly angulated lower legs with protrusion of the tibia anteriorly at the midshaft. The fibulas were hypoplastic and bowed. The feet, as shown in Fig. 65.15, are abnormally rotated with prominent heels (rocker-bottom feet).

Short-rib polydactyly syndrome is considered a lethal anomaly. Most infants die shortly after birth as a result of pulmonary hypoplasia.

Sonographic Findings. Common sonographic features of short-rib polydactyly syndrome include the following:
- Narrow thorax with short ribs
- Polydactyly (Fig. 65.17)
- Micromelia
- Midline facial cleft

Other sonographic findings associated with short-rib dysplasias include anomalies of the central nervous system, cardiovascular system, and genitourinary tract. Polyhydramnios may also be identified. Saldino-Noonan and Naumoff syndromes are usually not associated with cleft lip and palate, and polydactyly may not always be present in Beemer-Langer dysplasia.

Jeune Syndrome

Jeune syndrome, also known as asphyxiating thoracic dysplasia, is a skeletal dysplasia characterized by a very narrow thorax. The prevalence of Jeune syndrome is 1 in 100,000 births,[7] and it is inherited in an autosomal recessive manner. Two types of Jeune syndrome have been described, and there is a range of severity, with the most severe form resulting in death because of pulmonary hypoplasia, which results from the narrow thorax.

Sonographic Findings. The sonographic features of Jeune syndrome include the following:
- Small thorax
- Rhizomelia
- Renal dysplasia
- Polydactyly (less common)

Ellis–van Creveld Syndrome

Ellis–van Creveld syndrome, also known as chondroectodermal dysplasia, is a rare skeletal dysplasia with an increased frequency in the Amish community. It is inherited in an autosomal recessive pattern.

Ellis–van Creveld syndrome may present with a narrow thorax, causing pulmonary hypoplasia, and heart defects, the most common of which is the atrial septal defect. Approximately half of these patients will die during infancy from cardiorespiratory complications. Other features identified with this syndrome include abnormal teeth, hypoplastic nails, and thin hair. Survivors have normal intellect and are short in stature.

Sonographic Findings. The sonographic features of Ellis–van Creveld syndrome include the following:
- Limb shortening
- Narrow thorax
- Polydactyly (see Fig. 65.17)
- Heart defects (50%)

Caudal Regression Syndrome/Sirenomelia

Caudal regression syndrome (CRS) is rare and includes a range of malformations of the caudal end of the neural tube. Sirenomelia is a very rare anomaly in which there is fusion of the lower extremities. Sirenomelia had been traditionally considered an extreme form of CRS, but it is currently thought to be a separate disorder. Sirenomelia has a male prevalence of 3 to 1.[8]

The cause of CRS is not completely understood, although it has been associated with diabetes. Genetic factors have also been linked with this disorder. Vascular hypoperfusion is thought to be a causative factor in sirenomelia, with a single umbilical artery commonly associated that may divert blood flow to the caudal end. Sirenomelia is also associated with diabetes, in addition to monozygotic twinning and teratogens including cocaine and isotretinoin.[8]

The prognosis for CRS depends on the severity and the associated anomalies. Neurologic and orthopedic evaluations with their interventional techniques can help to reduce and correct deformities and minimize disabilities. Sirenomelia is considered a lethal anomaly because of the severe renal anomalies that result in oligohydramnios and pulmonary hypoplasia.

Sonographic Findings. Sonographic features of CRS include the following:
- Sacral agenesis (Fig. 65.18)
- Talipes
- Abnormal lumbar vertebrae, pelvic abnormalities, and contractures or decreased movement of the lower extremities may also be seen

Sonographic features of sirenomelia include the following:
- Variable fusion of the lower extremities (Fig. 65.19)
- Bilateral renal agenesis

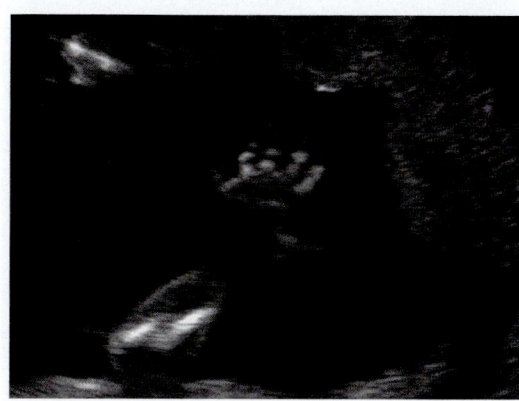

FIG. 65.17 Polydactyly of the fetal hands is identified.

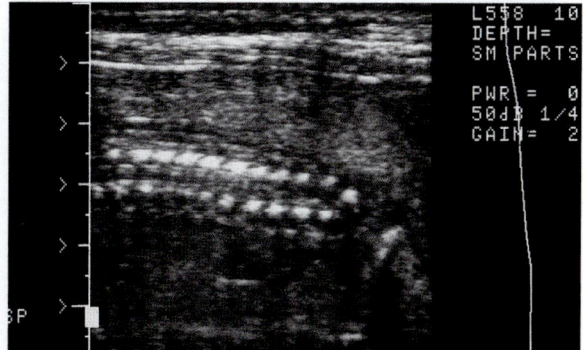

FIG. 65.18 Sacral agenesis noted at 21 weeks of gestation. Note the lack of tapering usually seen in the lumbosacral area.

- Oligohydramnios
- Single umbilical artery

When severe oligohydramnios is present, a confident diagnosis with ultrasound may be difficult. Amnioinfusion, three-dimensional sonography, and magnetic resonance imaging may be used to evaluate the severity of anomalies.

VACTERL Association

The VACTERL association is a group of anomalies that may occur together. In this sporadic group of anomalies, *v*ertebral defects, *a*nal atresia, *c*ardiac anomalies, *t*racheo*e*sophageal fistula, *r*enal anomalies, and *l*imb dysplasia may occur in combination. For the VACTERL association to be considered, three of these features must be identified. A single umbilical artery may also be identified. When the VACTERL association is seen with accompanying hydrocephalus, it has been termed *VACTERL-H syndrome*. The VACTERL association with concurrent sirenomelia has also been reported.

Postural Anomalies

The normal development of the fetus requires movement. There are multiple events that can cause a decrease in fetal movement, including oligohydramnios, multiple gestations, and congenital uterine anomalies. Decreased movement may also be due to an abnormality of the fetal nerves, connective tissue, or musculature. These fetal conditions may not only cause a decrease or absence of fetal movement, but they may also result in abnormal contractures and postural deformities.

Arthrogryposis Multiplex Congenita

Arthrogryposis multiplex congenita is a condition marked by severe contractures of the extremities because of abnormal innervation and disorders of the muscles and connective tissue. It represents a group of disorders that may be inherited or sporadic.

Sonographic Findings. The sonographic findings for arthrogryposis include the following:
- Rigid extremities (Fig. 65.20)
- Flexed arms
- Hyperextension of the knees
- Clenched hands
- Talipes (see Fig. 65.20B)

Polyhydramnios or oligohydramnios may accompany this anomaly, as can anomalies of the central nervous system. Other defects that may be associated include facial and renal anomalies. In addition, fetal seizures have been identified in fetuses with arthrogryposis.

Lethal Multiple Pterygium Syndrome. Lethal multiple pterygium syndrome is characterized by webbing across the joints and multiple contractures. It is usually inherited in an autosomal recessive fashion; however, an X-linked mode of inheritance has also been reported.

Sonographic Findings. The sonographic findings for pterygium syndrome include the following:
- Limb contractures
- Webbing across joints
- Cystic hygroma

Micrognathia, renal anomalies, hydrops, and polyhydramnios are also associated with this syndrome.

Pena-Shokeir Syndrome. Pena-Shokeir syndrome is characterized by abnormal joint contractures, facial abnormalities, polyhydramnios, intrauterine growth restriction, and

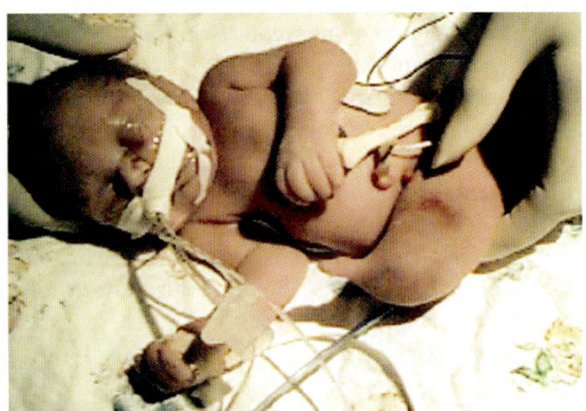

FIG. 65.19 A neonate with sirenomelia. Note the fusion of the lower extremities. There was also bilateral renal agenesis, and the infant died shortly after birth. This was a twin pregnancy, and the other infant was normal.

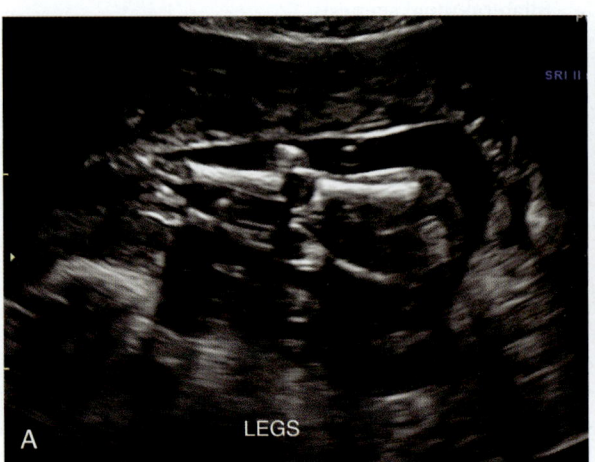 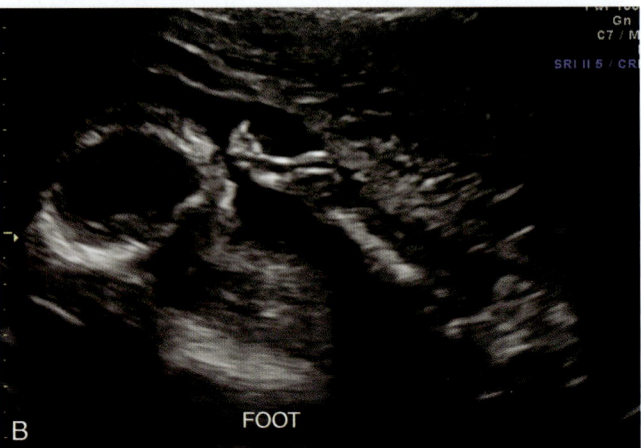

FIG. 65.20 (A) Rigid extremities. (B) Talipes (clubfoot). Both images demonstrate sonographic findings related to arthrogryposis.

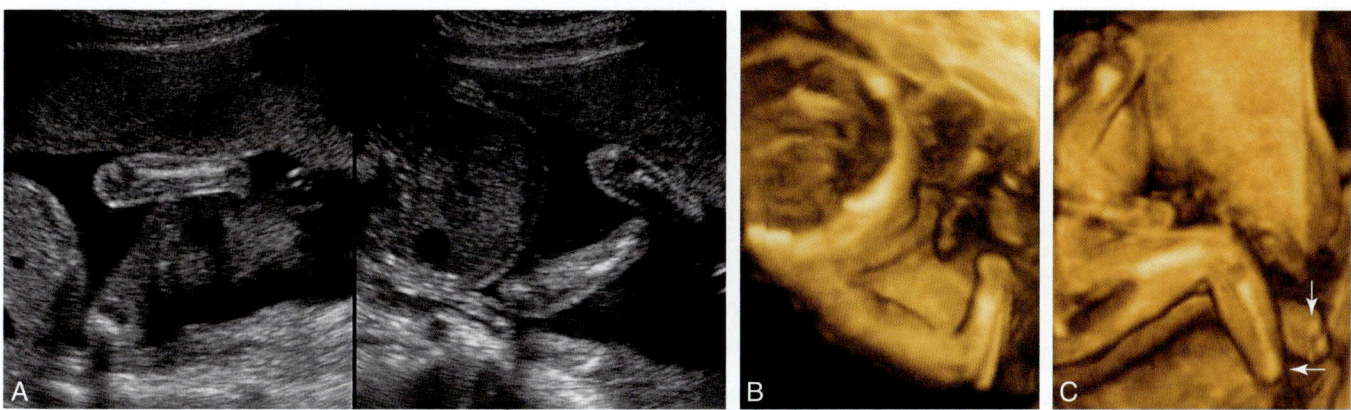

FIG. 65.21 **A fetus at 20 weeks of gestation with acheiropodia (symmetric absence of the hands and feet) of unknown etiology.** (A) Two-dimensional image demonstrating the arms with no hands. (B) A three-dimensional image of the arm showing the absence of the hand. (C) A three-dimensional image of the legs showing absence of the feet.

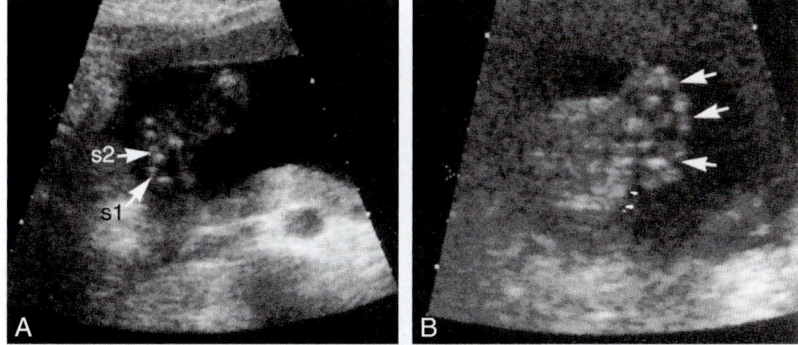

FIG. 65.22 (A) Polysyndactyly in a fetus with Carpenter syndrome. There was webbing (syndactyly) of the first and second toes (s1) and of the third and fourth toes (s2). Six toes were present (polydactyly). (B) In the same fetus, scans of the toes *(arrows)* show malalignment of the phalanges. Other sonographic findings included craniosynostosis, ventriculomegaly, and umbilical hernia.

pulmonary hypoplasia. This syndrome may be inherited in an autosomal recessive manner or as a sporadic occurrence. Pena-Shokeir syndrome and trisomy 18 have similar features, so karyotyping should be offered.

Sonographic Findings. The sonographic findings of Pena-Shokeir include the following:
- Limb abnormalities such as contractures, clenched hands, talipes, and rocker-bottom feet
- Facial abnormalities, including micrognathia and cleft palate
- Polyhydramnios and hydrops may also be identified

OTHER LIMB ABNORMALITIES

Hand and foot abnormalities may occur with skeletal dysplasias, as part of a chromosomal syndrome, or as an isolated event. Amputation defects may be identified as total or partial absence and may be associated with amniotic band syndrome. Congenital absence of one or more extremities (amelia) may be observed prenatally (Fig. 65.21).

Hand anomalies may include missing digits, fused digits (syndactyly) (Fig. 65.22), or a split hand (lobster-claw deformity) (Fig. 65.23). Extra digits (polydactyly) may be isolated or part of a syndrome or chromosomal anomaly (Figs. 65.22 to 65.26). Overlapping digits (clinodactyly) and clenched hands (Fig. 65.25B) may also be a feature of a syndrome or chromosomal anomaly.

Radial ray defects include hypoplasia or aplasia of the radius and thumb. Radial ray defects (Fig. 65.27) are associated with

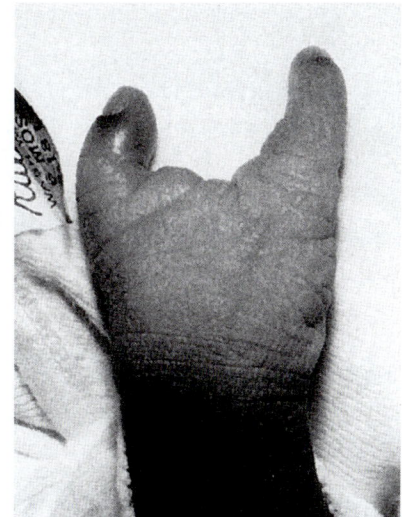

FIG. 65.23 Pathologic specimen showing a split-hand deformity (ectrodactyly).

chromosomal anomalies, such as trisomies 13 and 18 and the VACTERL association. Numerous syndromes have also presented with an absent or hypoplastic radius and thumb, including Holt-Oram syndrome and thrombocytopenia with absent radii syndrome (Fig. 65.28). Ulnar ray anomalies can also occur.

Clubfoot, also known as talipes, describes deformities of the foot and ankle. It occurs in approximately 1 in 1000 live

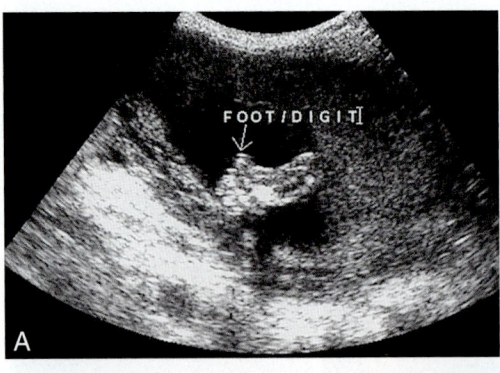
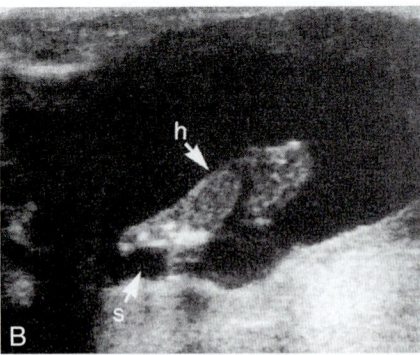

FIG. 65.24 (A) Polydactyly is identified in the foot of a fetus. (B) The foot of a fetus with trisomy 18 was split (ectrodactyly). Note the splaying of the toes (s) and malalignment of the metatarsals. Coexisting anomalies included a septal cardiac defect, bilateral choroid plexus cysts, polydactyly, hydramnios, and growth restriction. Autopsy was declined. *h*, Heel.

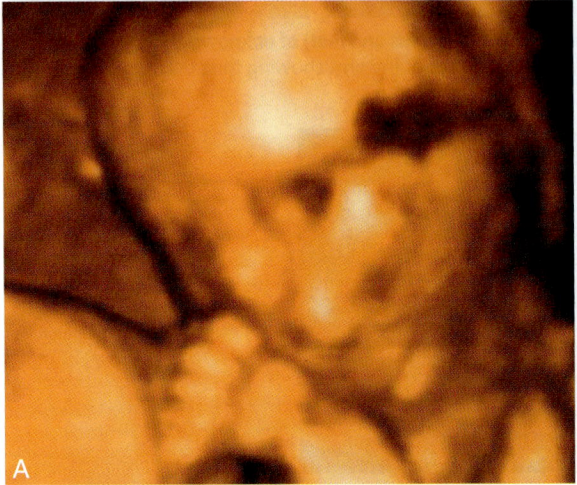
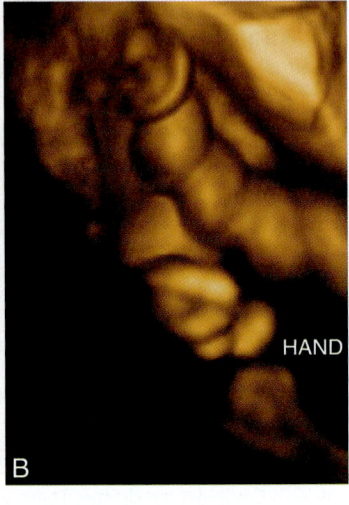

FIG. 65.25 (A) Polydactyly (six fingers) was noted in a fetus with multiple congenital anomalies, including holoprosencephaly and cleft lip. Trisomy 13 was confirmed with amniocentesis. (B) A different fetus with clenched hands and overlapping digits in which chromosomal analysis revealed trisomy 18.

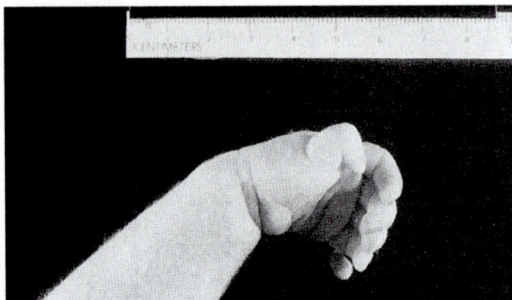

FIG. 65.26 Polydactyly of the hand in a neonate.

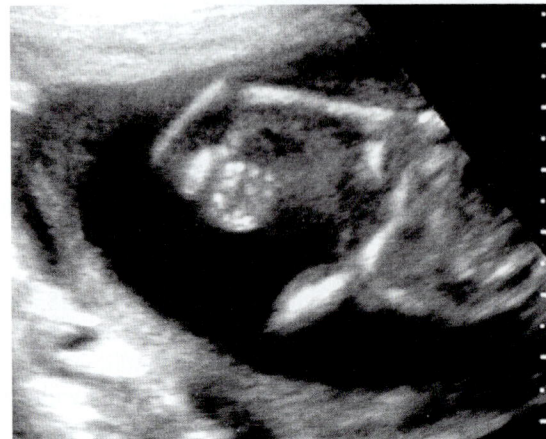

FIG. 65.27 A radial ray defect in a fetus that also presented with anencephaly and tetralogy of Fallot. A chromosomal anomaly was suspected.

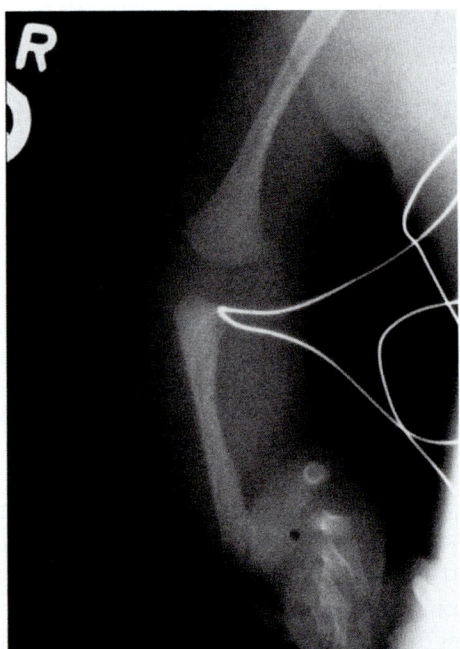

FIG. 65.28 A radiograph of a neonate with thrombocytopenia with absent radii syndrome. Note the absence of the radius in the arm and the turned-back hand.

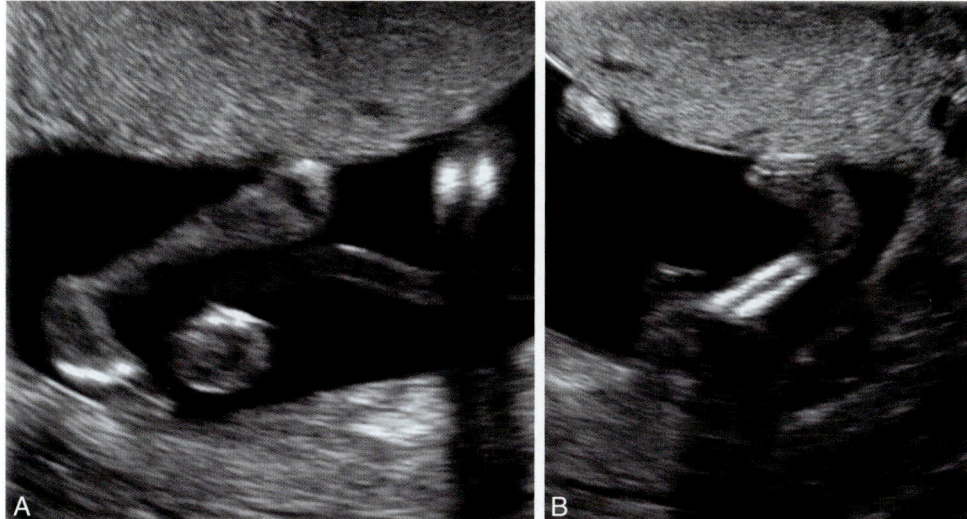

FIG. 65.29 Bilateral talipes is identified in this fetus. The right (A) and left (B) feet are both noted to be medially inverted. Multiple other anomalies were noted suggestive of aneuploidy.

births.[9] There is a male predominance, and half of the cases of clubfoot are unilateral.

The majority of cases of talipes are idiopathic and isolated findings. Talipes may be associated with chromosomal anomalies, syndromes, musculoskeletal disorders, and spina bifida. It has also been associated with exposure to tubocurarine, sodium aminopterin, and lead poisoning. Clubfoot has also been identified with oligohydramnios and in multiple gestations. Because of the numerous anomalies that may be identified, karyotyping should be offered.

Clubfoot may be identified sonographically when there is persistent abnormal inversion of the foot perpendicular to the lower leg (Fig. 65.29).

Rocker-bottom foot is characterized by a prominent heel and a convex sole. It has been associated with multiple syndromes and chromosomal anomalies, especially trisomy 18.

ACKNOWLEDGMENT

The author acknowledges the contributions of Charlotte G. Henningsen to this chapter in the previous edition.

Key Pearls

- Skeletal dysplasia is the term used to describe abnormal growth and density of cartilage and bone.
- Dwarfism is the condition of a disproportionately short stature; it occurs secondary to a skeletal dysplasia.
- When a skeletal dysplasia is suspected, the protocol of the obstetric ultrasound examination should be adjusted to include the following criteria: (1) assess limb shortening; (2) assess bone contour; (3) estimate degree of ossification; (4) evaluate the thoracic circumference and shape; (5) survey for coexistent hand and foot anomalies, such as talipes and polydactyly; (6) evaluate the face and profile for facial clefts, frontal bossing, micrognathia, hypertelorism, and other facial anomalies that may be associated with skeletal dysplasias; (7) survey for other associated anomalies, such as hydrocephaly, heart defects, and nonimmune hydrops.
- The two main subdivisions of thanatophoric dysplasia are types I and II. Type I is characterized by short, curved femurs and flat vertebral bodies. Type II is characterized by straight, short femurs, flat vertebral bodies, and a cloverleaf skull.
- Achondroplasia results from decreased endochondral bone formation, which produces short, squat bones.
- Achondrogenesis is a rare, lethal skeletal dysplasia occurring in 1 in 40,000 births and is caused by cartilage abnormalities that result in abnormal bone formation and hypomineralization.
- Osteogenesis imperfecta is a rare disorder of collagen production leading to brittle bones, blue sclera, and manifestations in the teeth, skin, and ligaments.
- Congenital hypophosphatasia is a condition that presents with diffuse hypomineralization of the bone caused by an alkaline phosphatase deficiency.
- Diastrophic dysplasia is a rare disorder characterized by micromelia, talipes, cleft palate, micrognathia, scoliosis, short stature, earlobe deformities, and hand abnormalities.
- Camptomelic (bent bone) dysplasia is a group of lethal skeletal dysplasias that are characterized by bowing of the long bones.
- Roberts syndrome is a rare autosomal recessive disorder characterized by phocomelia and facial anomalies.
- Short-rib polydactyly syndrome is a lethal skeletal dysplasia characterized by short ribs, short limbs, and polydactyly.
- Jeune syndrome, also known as asphyxiating thoracic dysplasia, is a skeletal dysplasia characterized by a very narrow thorax.
- Ellis-van Creveld syndrome, also known as chondroectodermal dysplasia, is a rare skeletal dysplasia with an increased frequency in the Amish community.

- Caudal regression syndrome is rare and includes a range of malformations of the caudal end of the neural tube.
- Sirenomelia is a very rare anomaly in which there is fusion of the lower extremities.
- The VACTERL association is a group of anomalies that may occur together. In this sporadic group of anomalies, vertebral defects, anal atresia, cardiac anomalies, tracheoesophageal fistula, renal anomalies, and limb dysplasia may occur in combination.
- Arthrogryposis multiplex congenita is a condition marked by severe contractures of the extremities because of abnormal innervation and disorders of the muscles and connective tissue.
- Lethal multiple pterygium syndrome is characterized by webbing across the joints and multiple contractures.
- Pena-Shokeir syndrome is characterized by abnormal joint contractures, facial abnormalities, polyhydramnios, intrauterine growth restriction, and pulmonary hypoplasia.
- Hand and foot abnormalities may occur with skeletal dysplasias, as part of a chromosomal syndrome, or as an isolated event.

REFERENCES

1. Nelson DB, Dashe JS, McIntire DD, Twickler DM. Fetal skeletal dysplasias: Sonographic indices associated with adverse outcomes. *J Ultrasound Med*. 2014;33:1085–1090.
2. Bilder A. Prenatal sonographic detection of skeletal dysplasias: a case of multiple pterygium syndrome, or Escobar syndrome. *J Diagn Med Sonogr*. 2014;30:205–210.
3. Tsai PY, Chang CH, Yu CH, et al. Thanatophoric dysplasia: role of 3-dimensional sonography. *J Clin Ultrasound*. 2009;37:31–34.
4. Horton WA, Hall JG, Hecht JT. Achondroplasia. *Lancet*. 2007;370:162–172.
5. Taner MZ, Kurdoglu M, Taskiran C, et al. Prenatal diagnosis of achondrogenesis type I: a case report. *Cases J*. 2008;1:406.
6. Chitty LS, Griffin D. Prenatal diagnosis of skeletal dysplasias. *Fetal Matern Med Rev*. 2008;19(2):135–164.
7. Rahmani R, Sterling CL, Bedford HM. Prenatal diagnosis of Jeune-like syndromes with two-dimensional and three-dimensional sonography. *J Clin Ultrasound*. 2012;40:222–226.
8. Dosedla E, Kalafusova M, Calda P. Sirenomelia apus after trimethoprim exposure: first-trimester ultrasound diagnosis—a case report. *J Clin Ultrasound*. 2012;40:594–597.
9. Bakalis S, Sairam S, Homfray T, et al. Outcome of antenatally diagnosed talipes equinovarus in an unselected obstetric population. *Ultrasound Obstet Gynecol*. 2002;20:226–229.

GLOSSARY FOR VOLUME 2

abdominal circumference (AC) a fetal measurement at the level of the stomach, left portal vein, and left umbilical vein

abruptio placenta premature detachment of a normally situated placenta after the twentieth week of gestation

acardiac anomaly rare anomaly in monochorionic twins in which one twin develops without a heart and often without an upper half of the body

achondrogenesis lethal autosomal recessive short-limb dwarfism marked by long bone and trunk shortening, decreased echogenicity of the bones and spine, and flipper-like appendages

achondroplasia defect in the development of cartilage at the epiphyseal centers of the long bones producing short, square bones

acrania condition associated with anencephaly in which there is complete or partial absence of the cranial bones

adenomyosis benign invasive growth of the endometrium into the muscular layer of the uterus

advanced maternal age (AMA) when a woman is age 35 years or older at the time of delivery

afterload aortic arterial pressure and vascular resistance the ventricle must overcome to eject blood or any resistance against which the ventricles must pump to eject its volume

age range analysis (ARA) fetal parameters' size and proportionality expressed as age

allantoic duct elongated duct that contributes to the development of the umbilical cord and placenta during the first trimester

alobar holoprosencephaly most severe form of holoprosencephaly characterized by a single common ventricle and malformed brain; orbital anomalies range from fused orbits to hypotelorism, with frequent nasal anomalies and clefting of the lip and palate

alpha-fetoprotein protein manufactured by the fetus, which can be studied in amniotic fluid and maternal serum; elevations may indicate fetal anomalies (neural tube, abdominal wall, gastrointestinal), multiple gestations, or incorrect patient dates; decreased levels may be associated with chromosomal abnormalities

amaurosis fugax transient or complete loss of vision in one eye

amenorrhea absence of menstruation

amniocentesis transabdominal removal of amniotic fluid from the amniotic cavity using ultrasound

amnion innermost thin, transparent fetal membrane that holds the fetus suspended in amniotic fluid

amniotic band syndrome multiple fibrous strands of amnion that develop in utero that may entangle fetal parts to cause amputations or malformations of the fetus

amniotic cavity cavity in which the fetus exists; forms early in gestation; fills with amniotic fluid to protect the fetus

amniotic fluid produced by the umbilical cord and membranes, the fetal lung, skin, and kidney

amniotic fluid index (AFI) quantitative estimate of amniotic fluid and an indicator of fetal well-being; measured by evaluating the four quadrants of the uterus with the transducer perpendicular to the table in the deepest vertical pockets without fetal parts

anasarca severe generalized massive edema throughout the body often seen with fetal hydrops

androgen substance that stimulates the development of male characteristics, such as the hormones testosterone and androsterone

anembryonic pregnancy (blighted ovum) ovum without an embryo

anencephaly neural tube defect characterized by the lack of development of the cerebral and cerebellar hemispheres and cranial vault; incompatible with life

aneuploidy having an abnormal number of chromosomes

anomaly an abnormality or congenital malformation

anophthalmia absent eyes

anorectal atresia complex disorder of the bowel and genitourinary tract

anteflexed position of the uterus when the uterine fundus bends forward toward the cervix

anterior cerebral artery (ACA) smaller of the two terminal branches of the internal carotid artery

anterior communicating artery (ACoA) short vessel that connects the anterior cerebral arteries at the interhemispheric fissure

anterior tibial artery begins at the popliteal artery and travels down the lateral calf in the anterior compartment to the level of the ankle

anterior tibial veins drain blood from the dorsum of the foot and anterior compartment of the calf

anteverted refers to the position of the uterus when the uterus is tipped slightly forward so the cervix forms a 90-degree angle or less with the vaginal canal; most common uterine position

aortic stenosis abnormal development of the cusps of the aortic valve that results in thickened and domed leaflets

aphasia inability to communicate by speech or writing

arcuate vessels small vessels found along the periphery of the uterus

arhinia absence of the nose

ascites abnormal serous fluid collection found in the abdomen or pelvis

Asherman syndrome acquired uterine condition characterized by the presence of intrauterine scars or synechiae

asphyxiating thoracic dystrophy significantly narrow diameter of the chest in a fetus

asplenia no development of splenic tissue

assisted reproductive technology (ART) technologies used to assist the infertility patient to become pregnant; includes ovulation induction therapy, in vitro fertilization and embryo transfer, and intrauterine insemination

ataxia gait disturbance

atrioventricular block occurs when the transmission of the electrical impulse from the atria to the ventricles is blocked

atrioventricular node derived from cells in the walls of the sinus venosus and atrioventricular canal

atrioventricular septal defect (AVSD) failure of the endocardial cushion to fuse; defect providing communication between the ventricles, between the atria, or between the atria and ventricles

atrioventricular valves cardiac valves located between the atria and ventricle; tricuspid valve is between the right atrium and right ventricle while the mitral valve is between the left atrium and left ventricle

augmentation blood flow velocity increasing with distal limb compression or with the release of proximal limb compression

autonomy self-governing or self-directing freedom and especially moral independence; the right of persons to choose and to have their choices respected

average age (AA) average of multiple fetal parameters' ages

axillary artery continuation of the subclavian artery

axillary vein begins where the basilica vein joins the brachial vein in the upper arm and terminates beneath the clavicle at the outer border of the first rib

basilar artery (BA) formed by the union of the two vertebral arteries

basilic vein originates on the small finger side of the dorsum of the hand and enters the brachial veins in the upper arm

battledore placenta marginal or eccentric insertion of the umbilical cord into the placenta

Beckwith-Wiedemann syndrome group of disorders having in common the coexistence of an omphalocele, macroglossia, and visceromegaly

beneficence bringing about good by maximizing benefits and minimizing possible harm

Bernoulli equation measures the pressure gradient across the orifice using blood flow velocities; three components are present: convective acceleration, flow acceleration, and viscous friction

bicuspid aortic valve congenital abnormality that causes two of the three aortic leaflets to fuse, resulting in a two-leaflet valve instead of the normal three leaflets; may lead to aortic stenosis and/or insufficiency

biparietal diameter (BPD) fetal transverse cranial diameter at the level of the thalamus and cavum septum pellucidum

blood flow velocity profiles factors that affect blood flow, including the shape and size of the vessel or chamber it is traveling through, wall characteristics, the timing within the cardiac cycle, flow rate, and the viscosity of the blood

bowel herniation normal bowel protrusion outside the abdominal cavity at between 8 and 12 weeks of gestation

brachial artery continuation of the axillary artery

brachycephaly fetal head that is relatively wide in the transverse diameter and shortened in the anteroposterior diameter

bradycardia heart rate less than 60 beats/min

branchial cleft cyst cystic defect that arises from the primitive branchial apparatus

Braxton Hicks contractions intermittent painless uterine contractions that may occur every 10 to 20 minutes

breech position of the fetal head toward the fundus of the uterus

broad ligament broad fold of peritoneum draped over the fallopian tubes, uterus, and ovaries; extends from the sides of the uterus to the pelvic sidewall, dividing the pelvis from side to side and creating the vesicouterine pouch anterior to the uterus and posterior to the rectouterine pouch

bronchogenic cyst most common lung cyst detected prenatally

bruit noise caused by tissue vibration produced by turbulence that causes flow disturbance

bulbus cordis part of the developing heart that forms the right ventricle

cardiac output product of stroke volume and heart rate

cardiac tamponade condition occurring when the intrapericardial pressure increases to the point of compromising systemic venous return to the right atrium

cardinal ligament wide bands of fibromuscular tissue arising from the lateral aspects of the cervix and inserting along the lateral pelvic floor; a continuation of the broad ligament that provides rigid support for the cervix; also called the transverse cervical ligaments

caudal regression syndrome lack of development of the caudal spine and cord that may occur in the fetus of diabetic mother

cebocephaly form of holoprosencephaly characterized by a common ventricle, fusion of the orbits with one or two eyes present, and a proboscis (maldeveloped cylindrical nose)

cephalic vein begins on the thumb side of the dorsum or the hand and joins the axillary vein just below the clavicle

cephalocele protrusion of the brain from the cranial cavity

cerclage encircling tissues with a ligature, wire, or loop

cerebral vasospasm vasoconstriction of the arteries

cerebrovascular accident (CVA) loss of blood flow to part of the brain that damages brain tissue

cervical polyp hyperplastic protrusion of the epithelium of the cervix

cervical stenosis acquired condition with obstruction of the cervical canal

cervix the lower, narrow end of the uterus that forms a canal between the uterus and vagina

Chlamydia trachomatis bacterium that causes a variety of diseases, including genital infections

choledochal cyst cystic growth within the common bile duct

chorioamnionitis bacterial infection of the fetal membranes usually caused by an upward movement of infection from the vagina

chorion extraembryonic membrane that, in early development, forms the outer wall of the blastocyst

chorion frondosum outer surface of the chorion

chorionic cavity surrounds the amniotic cavity; contains the yolk sac

chorionic plate in the placenta, the portion of the chorion attached to the uterus

chorionic villi vascular projections from the chorion

circle of Willis polygonal vascular ring at the base of the brain

circumvallate placenta cup-shaped placenta with raised edges that exposes an area of fetal surface encircling the site of umbilical cord insertion

claudication walking-induced muscular discomfort of the calf, thigh, hip, or buttock

cloacal exstrophy complex malformation involving lower limb anomalies, spinal defect, anal atresia, and lower abdominal wall defect below the cord insertion; involves exstrophy of the bladder and protrusion of the intestines

coarctation of the aorta narrowing of the aortic arch; may be discrete, long-segment, or tubular; most commonly occurs as a shelf-like protrusion in the isthmus of the arch or at the site of the ductal insertion near the left subclavian artery

coccygeus muscles one of two muscles in the pelvic diaphragm; located on the posterior pelvic floor where it supports the coccyx

collateral pathway occurs when one vessel becomes obstructed; smaller side branches of the vessel provide alternative flow pathways

color Doppler displays intracavitary blood flow in shades of red, blue, yellow, green depending on the velocity, direction, and extent of turbulence

color flow mapping (CFM) form of pulsed wave Doppler in which the energy of the returning echoes is displayed as an assigned color that is superimposed on the B-mode image to allow simultaneous visualization of anatomy and flow dynamics; by convention, flow toward the transducer is displayed as shades of red; the flow away from the transducer is seen as shades of blue

common carotid artery (CCA) arises from the aortic arch on the left side and from the innominate artery on the right side

common femoral vein (CFV) formed by the confluence of the profunda femoris and the superficial femoral vein; also receives the greater saphenous vein

common iliac vein formed by the confluence of the internal and external femoral veins

complete abortion completed removal of all products of conception, including the placenta

confidentiality holding information in confidence; respect for privacy

congenital bronchial atresia pulmonary anomaly that results from the focal obliteration of a segment of the bronchial lumen

congenital cystic adenomatoid malformation (CCAM) abnormality in the formation of the bronchial tree with secondary overgrowth of mesenchymal tissue from arrested bronchial development

congenital diaphragmatic hernia (CDH) opening in the pleuroperitoneal membrane that develops in the first trimester

conjoined twins twins that are physically joined at birth; occur when the egg divides after 13 days of gestation

constrictive pericarditis chronic pericardial disease condition in which the pericardium may become thickened and inelastic, which in turn limits the ventricular filling, leading to chronic biventricular diastolic dysfunction, right-sided heart failure, and low systemic output

continuity principle principle stating that energy cannot be created or destroyed, only transferred from one form to another

continuous murmur cardiac murmur beginning in systole and continuing without interruption through the time of the second heart sound into all or part of diastole

continuous wave Doppler transducer delivering continuous pulses out and back; it constantly transmits and receives, with no specific pulse duration or sample volume area

cor triatriatum condition in which the left atrial cavity is portioned into two components; pulmonary veins drain into an accessory left atrial chamber proximal to the true left atrium

cornu, cornua horn-like projection; refers to the fundus of the uterus where the fallopian tube arises

coronal horizontal plane through the longitudinal axis of the body to image structures from anterior to posterior

corpus luteum anatomic structure on the surface of the ovary consisting of a spheroid of yellowish tissue that grows within the ruptured ovarian follicle after ovulation; acts as a short-lived endocrine organ that secretes progesterone to maintain the decidual layer of the endometrium should conception occur

corpus luteum cyst small yellow endocrine structure that develops within a ruptured ovarian follicle and secretes progesterone and estrogen; prevents menses if fertilization occurs; may persist until the sixteenth to eighteenth week of pregnancy

corrected transposition of the great arteries connection of the right atrium and left atrium to the morphologic left and right ventricle, respectively; the positions of the great arteries are transposed

corticosteroids drug administered to pregnant women to help accelerate fetal lung maturity

costal margin lower boundary of the thorax formed by the cartilages of the seventh through tenth ribs and the ends of the eleventh and twelfth cartilages

craniosynostosis early ossification of the calvarium with destruction of the sutures; hypertelorism is frequently found in association; sonographically, the fetal cranium may appear brachycephalic

crossed renal ectopia occurs when the kidney is located on the opposite side of its ureteral orifice

crown rump length (CRL) most accurate measurement for determining gestational age; performed in the first trimester

cryptorchidism failure of the testes to descend into the scrotum

cyclopia severe form of holoprosencephaly characterized by a common ventricle, fusion of the orbits with one or two eyes present, and a proboscis (maldeveloped cylindrical nose)

cystadenocarcinoma malignant tumor that forms cysts

cystadenoma benign adenoma containing cysts

cystic fibrosis mucous buildup within the lungs and other areas of the body

cystic hygroma fluid-filled structure, often with septations, initially surrounding the neck but may extend upward to the head or laterally to the body; dilation of jugular lymph sacs because of improper drainage of the lymphatic system into the venous system

dacryocystocele cystic dilation of the lacrimal sac at the nasocanthal angle

decidua basalis villi on the maternal side of the placenta or embryo; unites with the chorion to form the placenta

decidua capsularis part of the decidua that surrounds the chorionic sac

deep femoral vein (DFV) travels with the profunda femoris artery to unite with the superficial femoral vein to form the common femoral vein

depolarization electrical activity that triggers contraction of the heart muscle

dermoid tumor benign tumor comprised of hair, muscle, teeth, and fat

dextrocardia heart position in the right chest with the apex pointed to the right of the thorax

dextroposition heart position in the right chest with the cardiac apex pointed medially or to the left

diamniotic multiple pregnancies with two amniotic sacs

diastole part of the cardiac cycle in which the ventricles fill with blood; the tricuspid and mitral valves are open during this time, and the aortic and pulmonic valves are closed

diastolic murmur begins with or after the time of the second heart sound and ends at or before the time of the first heart sound

dichorionic multiple pregnancies with two chorionic sacs

dilated cardiomyopathy dilation and reduced contractility of the left ventricle or both the left and right ventricles

diplopia double vision

dizygotic twins that arise from two separately fertilized ova

dolichocephaly fetal head is relatively narrow in the transverse plane and elongated in the anteroposterior plane

Doppler effect change in the frequency of waves (through sound, light, etc.) that occurs as the source and observer change in motion relative to each other (away or toward)

Doppler frequency red blood cells move from a lower frequency sound source at rest toward a higher frequency sound source; change in frequency is called the Doppler shift in frequency

dorsalis pedis artery continuation of the anterior tibial artery on the top of the foot

double decidual sac sign interface between the decidua capsularis and the echogenic, highly vascular endometrium

ductal constriction occurs when flow is diverted from the ductus secondary to tricuspid or pulmonic atresia or secondary to maternal medications given to stop early contractions

ductus arteriosus communication between the aorta and pulmonary artery that is patent during fetal development

ductus venosus smaller, shorter, and posterior of the two branches into which the umbilical vein divides after entering the abdomen; empties into the inferior vena cava

duodenal atresia complete blockage at the pyloric sphincter

duodenal stenosis narrowing of the pyloric sphincter

dysarthria difficulty with speech because of impairment of the tongue or muscles essential to speech

dysmenorrhea pain associated with menstruation

dysphagia inability or difficulty in swallowing

Ebstein anomaly of the tricuspid valve abnormal displacement of the septal leaflet of the tricuspid valve toward the apex of the right ventricle; right ventricle above the leaflet becomes the "atrialized" chamber

eclampsia coma and seizures in the second- and third-trimester patient secondary to pregnancy-induced hypertension

ectocervix portion of the canal of the uterine cervix lined with squamous epithelium

ectopic pregnancy pregnancy outside the uterus

edema fluid in body tissues

electrocardiography method of recording the electrical activity generated by the heart muscle

embryo stage of early fetal development between the second and eighth weeks

embryo transfer technique that follows in vitro fertilization in which the embryo is placed into the uterus through the cervix

embryonic heart rate (HER) heart rate before the early ninth week of gestation

endocardium inner layer of the heart wall

endometrial carcinoma malignancy characterized by abnormal thickening of the endometrial cavity

endometrial hyperplasia condition that results from estrogen stimulation to the endometrium without the influence of progestin; frequent cause of bleeding

endometrial polyp pedunculated or sessile well-defined mass attached to the endometrial cavity

endometrioma localized tumor of endometriosis most frequently found in the ovary, cul-de-sac, rectovaginal septum, and peritoneal surface of the posterior wall of the uterus

endometriosis condition that occurs when functioning endometrial tissue invades other sites outside the uterus

endometritis infection within the endometrium of the uterus

endometrium inner lining of the uterine cavity that appears echogenic to hypoechoic on ultrasound depending on the menstrual cycle

epicardium outer layer of the heart wall

epignathus teratoma located in the oropharynx

epispadias abnormal congenital opening of the male urethra on the top side of the penis

esophageal atresia congenital hypoplasia of the esophagus; usually associated with a tracheoesophageal fistula

esophageal stenosis narrowing of the esophagus, usually in the distal third segment

estimated fetal weight incorporation of all fetal growth parameters (biparietal diameter, head circumference, abdominal circumference, femur, and humeral length)

estrogen steroidal hormone secreted by the theca interna and granulosa cells of the ovarian follicle that stimulates the development of the female reproductive structures and secondary sexual characteristics; promotes the growth of the endometrial tissue during the proliferative phase of the menstrual cycle; the female hormone produced by the ovary

ethics study of what is good and bad and of moral duty and obligation; systematic reflection on and analysis of morality

exophthalmia abnormal protrusion of the eyeball

external carotid artery (ECA) smaller of the two terminal branches of the common carotid artery

exudative accumulative fluid in a cavity

false knots of the umbilical cord nodulations on the surface of the cord that occurs when blood vessels are longer than the cord and fold over themselves

false pelvis portion of the pelvis found above the brim; also called the greater or major pelvis

femur length (FL) measurement of the femoral diaphysis

fetal age begins at the time of conception; also known as conceptional age

fetal cystic hygroma malformation of the lymphatic system that leads to single or multiloculated lymph-filled cavities around the neck

fetal goiter enlargement of the thyroid gland

fetal hydronephrosis dilated renal pelvis

fetus papyraceous fetal death that occurs after the fetus has reached a certain growth that is too large to resorb into the uterus

fibrous pericardium outer sac of the pericardium

follicle-stimulating hormone (FSH) hormone secreted by the anterior pituitary gland that stimulates growth and maturation of graafian follicles in the ovary

follicular cyst benign cyst within the ovary that may occur and disappear on a cyclic basis

foramen of Bochdalek diaphragmatic defect that occurs posterior and lateral in the diaphragm; usually found on the left side

foramen of Morgagni diaphragmatic hernia that occurs anterior and medial in the diaphragm that may communicate with the pericardial sac

foramen ovale opening between the free edge of the septum secundum and the dorsal wall of the atrium

frequency number of cycles per second that a periodic event or function undergoes per unit of time

frequency shift change or shift in received sound waves from the initial transmitted sound waves or pulse

frontal bossing protrusion or bulging of the forehead that results from hydrocephalus

Gartner duct cyst small cyst within the vagina

gastrocnemius veins paired veins that lie in the medial and lateral gastrocnemius muscles; terminate into the popliteal vein

gastroschisis abnormality of the abdominal wall in which the bowel, without a covering membrane, protrudes outside of the wall

gestational (menstrual) age length of time from conception to birth

gestational sac diameter (GSD) used in the first trimester to estimate appropriate gestational age with menstrual dates

gestational sac structure normally found within the uterus containing the developing embryo

gestational trophoblastic disease condition in which trophoblastic tissue overtakes the pregnancy and propagates throughout the uterine cavity

gonadotropin hormonal substance that stimulates the function of the testes and the ovaries; in females follicle stimulating hormone and luteinizing hormone are gonadotropins

gonadotropin-releasing hormone (GnRH) hormone secreted by the hypothalamus that stimulates the release of the follicle-stimulating hormone and luteinizing hormone by the anterior pituitary gland

gravidity (G) total number of pregnancies

greater saphenous vein (GSV) originates on the dorsum of the foot and ascends anterior to the medial malleolus and along the anteromedial side of the calf and thigh; joins the common femoral vein in the proximal thigh

growth-adjusted sonar age (GASA) method by which the fetus is categorized into small, average, or large growth percentiles

haustral folds sacculations of the colon caused by longitudinal bands that are shorter than the gut

hemangioma of the cord vascular tumor within the umbilical cord

hematometra obstruction of the uterus and/or the vagina characterized by an accumulation of blood

hematopoiesis production and development of blood cells

hemifacial macrosomia abnormal smallness of one side of the face

hemiparesis unilateral partial or complete paralysis

hemodynamics study of the forces involved with blood flow and circulation

hemopoiesis formation of blood

hermaphroditism condition in which both ovarian and testicular tissues are present

heterotopic pregnancy simultaneous intrauterine and extrauterine pregnancy

heterozygous achondroplasia short-limb dysplasia that manifests in the second trimester of pregnancy; conversion abnormality of cartilage to bone affecting the epiphyseal growth centers; extremities are notably shortened at birth, with normal trunk and frequent enlargement of the head

Hirschsprung disease (megacolon) congenital disorder in which there is abnormal innervation of the large intestine

holoprosencephaly congenital defect caused by an extra chromosome, which causes a deficiency in the forebrain; a range of abnormalities from abnormal cleavage of the forebrain

homozygous achondroplasia short-limbed dwarfism affecting fetuses of achondroplastic parents

horseshoe kidney forms when the inferior poles of the kidney fuse while they are in the pelvis

human chorionic gonadotropin (hCG) hormone secreted by the trophoblastic cells (developing placental cells) of the blastocyst; laboratory test indicates pregnancy when values are elevated

humeral length measurement from the humeral head to the distal end of the humerus

hydatidiform mole polycystic mass in which the chorionic villi have undergone cystic degeneration, resulting in rapid growth of the uterus with hemorrhage

hydramnios increased amount of amniotic fluid

hydranencephaly congenital absence of the cerebral hemispheres because of an occlusion of the carotid arteries; midbrain structures are present, and fluid replaces cerebral tissue

hydrocephalus ventriculomegaly in the neonate; abnormal accumulation of cerebrospinal fluid within the cerebral ventricles, resulting in compression and frequently destruction of brain tissue

hydrometra obstruction of the uterus and/or vagina characterized by an accumulation of fluid

hydrometrocolpos collection of fluid in the vagina and uterus

hydrops (hydrops fetalis) abnormal accumulation of fluid or edema found in at least two fetal areas

hydrops fetalis fluid occurring in at least two areas: pleural effusion, pericardial effusion, ascites, or skin edema

hydrosalpinx fluid within the fallopian tube

hydroureters dilated ureters

hyperemesis gravidarum excessive vomiting that leads to dehydration and electrolyte imbalance

hypertelorism abnormally wide-spaced orbits usually found in conjunction with congenital anomalies and mental retardation

hypertrophic cardiomyopathy hypertrophied, non-dilated left ventricle in the absence of another cardiac or systemic disease capable of producing hypertrophy

hypophosphatasia congenital condition characterized by decreased mineralization of the bones resulting in ribbon-like and bowed limbs, underossified cranium, and compression of the chest; early death often occurs

hypoplasia underdevelopment of a tissue, organ, or body

hypoplastic left heart syndrome underdevelopment of the left ventricle with aortic and/or mitral atresia; the left ventricle is extremely thickened compared with the right ventricle

hypoplastic right heart syndrome underdevelopment of the right ventricular outflow tract secondary to pulmonary stenosis; tricuspid atresia is often present

hypospadias abnormal congenital opening of the male urethra on the undersurface of the penis

hypotelorism abnormally closely spaced orbits; association with holoprosencephaly, chromosomal, central nervous system disorders, and cleft palate

iliacus muscle paired triangular, flat muscles that cover the inner curved surface of the iliac fossae; they arise from the iliac fossae and join the psoas muscles to form the lateral walls of the pelvis

iliopectineal line bony ridge on the inner surface of the ilium and pubic bones that divides the true and false pelvis; also called the pelvic brim or linear terminalis

immune hydrops accumulation of abnormal fluid collections caused by rhesus incompatibility

in vitro fertilization (IVF) method of fertilizing the human ova outside the body by collecting the mature ova and placing them in a dish with a sample of sperm

incompetent cervix inadequate ability to perform the function or action normal to the cervix

incomplete abortion retained products of conception

infantile polycystic kidney disease (IPKD) autosomal recessive disease that affects the fetal kidneys and liver; the kidneys are enlarged and echogenic on ultrasound

informed consent providing complete information and ensuring comprehension and voluntary consent by a patient or subject to a required or experimental medical procedure

innominate artery first branch artery from the aortic arch

innominate veins right vein: courses vertically downwards to join the left innominate vein below the first rib to form the superior vena cava; left vein: longer than right, courses from left chest to the right beneath the sternum to join the right innominate vein

integrity adherence to moral and ethical principles

intensity murmurs, both systolic and diastolic, varying from grade 1 to grade 6; grade 1 murmur is very faint with possible progression to grade 6 murmur, which is exceptionally loud and heard with the stethoscope

internal carotid artery (ICA) arises from the common carotid artery to supply the anterior brain and meninges; larger of the two terminal branches of the common carotid artery

internal os inner surface of the cervical os\menarche state after reaching puberty in which menses normally occur every 21 to 28 days

interstitial pregnancy pregnancy occurring in the fallopian tube near the cornu of the uterus; also known as corneal pregnancy

intramural leiomyoma most common type of leiomyoma

intrauterine contraceptive device (IUCD) device inserted into the endometrial cavity to prevent pregnancy

intrauterine growth restriction (IUGR) decreased rate of fetal growth; may be symmetric (all growth parameters are small) or asymmetric (may be caused by placental problems; head measurements correlate with dates, body disproportionately smaller); usually a fetal weight below the 10th percentile for a given gestational age; usually considered as malnourished or abnormal

intrauterine insemination introduction of semen into the uterus by mechanical or instrumental means rather than by sexual intercourse

intrauterine pregnancy (IUP) when a gestational sac contains either a yolk sace or an embryo/fetal pole with fetal heart activity and located in the uterus

ischemic rest pain implies critical ischemia (lack of blood) of the distal limb when the patient is at rest

jejunoileal atresia blockage of the jejunum and ileal bowel segments that appears as multiple cystic structures within the fetal abdomen

justice ethical principle that requires fair distribution of benefits and burdens; an injustice occurs when a benefit to which a person is entitled is withheld or when a burden is unfairly imposed

large for gestational age (LGA) fetus measures larger than dates (diabetic fetus)

last menstrual period (LMP) first day of the LMP is used as the start date for human pregnancies

leiomyoma most common benign gynecologic tumor in women during their reproductive years

lesser saphenous vein originates on the dorsum of the foot and ascends posterior to the lateral malleolus and runs along the midline of the posterior calf; terminates as it joins the popliteal vein

levator ani one of two muscles of the pelvic diaphragm that stretch across the floor of the pelvic cavity like a hammock, supporting the pelvic organs and surrounding the urethra, vagina, and rectum; muscle group consists of the pubococcygeus, iliococcygeus, and puborectalis

levocardia normal position of the heart in the left chest with the cardiac apex pointed to the left

levoposition condition in which the heart is displaced further toward the left chest, usually in association with a space-occupying lesion

ligamentum venosum fetal communication between the caudate and left lobes of the liver connecting the left branch of the portal vein to the inferior vena cava

limb–body wall complex anomaly with large cranial defects, facial cleft, large body wall defects, and limb abnormalities

lipomatous hypertrophy thickening seen along the superior/inferior interatrial septum

luteinizing hormone (LH) hormone secreted by the anterior pituitary gland that stimulates ovulation and then induces luteinization of the ruptured follicle to form the corpus luteum

lymphangiectasia dilation of a lymph node

macrocephaly enlargement of the fetal cranium as a result of ventriculomegaly

macroglossia hypertrophied tongue

macrosomia birth weight greater than 4000 g or above the 90th percentile for estimated gestational age

malignant primary cardiac tumors tumors such as angiosarcoma, rhabdomyosarcoma, mesothelioma, fibrosarcoma, and synovial fibrosarcoma

maternal serum alpha-fetoprotein (MsAFP) antigen present in the fetus; the maternal serum is tested between 15 and 22 weeks of gestation to detect abnormal levels; can also be tested directly from the amniotic fluid during amniocentesis

maternal serum quad screen blood test conducted during the second trimester (15 to 22 weeks) to identify pregnancies at a higher risk of chromosomal anomalies (trisomy 21 and 18) and neural tube defects

maximum vertical pocket method to determine the amount of amniotic fluid; pocket less than 2 cm may indicate oligohydramnios and greater than 8 cm polyhydramnios; used more often in multiple-gestation pregnancy

mean sac diameter (MSD) sonographic measurement of the gestational sac

mean velocity based on the time average of the outline velocity (maximum velocity envelope)

Meckel diverticulum remnant of the proximal part of the yolk stalk

meconium ileus small bowel disorder marked by the presence of thick echogenic meconium in the distal ileum

megacystis level of the urethra at which the urinary tract may become obstructed

megaureter dilation of the lower end of the ureter; common presentation of ureterovesical junction obstruction

Meig syndrome benign tumor of the ovary associated with ascites and pleural effusion

membranous or velamentous insertion of the cord cord that inserts into the membranes before it enters the placenta

menarche onset of menstruation and the commencement of cyclic menstrual function; usually occurs between 11 and 13 years of age

meningocele open spinal defect characterized by protrusion of the spinal meninges

meningomyelocele open spinal defect characterized by protrusion of the meninges and spinal cord through the defect, usually within a meningeal sac

menopause permanent cessation of menses
menorrhagia abnormally heavy or long periods
menses periodic flow of blood and cellular debris that occurs during menstruation
menstrual age calculated from the first day of the last normal menstrual period; if conceptual age is already known, menstrual age may be found by adding 14 days to the conceptual age
menstruation elimination of the thickened lining of the uterus (endometrium) from the body through the vagina
mesocardia atypical location of the heart in the middle of the chest with the cardiac apex pointing toward the midline of the chest
mesometrium portion of the broad ligament below the mesovarium, composed of the layers of peritoneum that separate to enclose the uterus
mesosalpinx upper portion of the broad ligament that enclosed the fallopian tubes
mesovarium posterior portion of the broad ligament that is drawn out to enclose and hold the ovary in place
metrorrhea irregular, acyclic bleeding
microcephaly head smaller than the body
micrognathia abnormally small chin; commonly associated with other fetal anomalies
microphthalmia small eyes
midaxillary line runs vertically from a point midway between the anterior and posterior axillary folds
midclavicular line lies in the median plane over the sternum
middle cerebral artery (MCA) large terminal branch of the internal carotid artery
midline echo (the flax) linear echoes located centrally in the fetal head that are produced by the borders of the opposing cerebral hemispheres
mitral atresia abnormal development of the mitral leaflet; may lead to development of hypoplastic left ventricle; also called congenital mitral stenosis
mitral regurgitation leaking of blood from the left ventricle into the left atrium during systole; occurs when the mitral leaflet is thickened and deformed and unable to close properly
monoamniotic multiple pregnancies with one amniotic sac
monozygotic twins that arise from a single fertilized egg that divides to produce two identical fetuses
morality protection of cherished values that relate to how persons interact and live in peace
mucinous cystadenocarcinoma malignant tumor of the ovary with multilocular cysts
mucinous cystadenoma benign tumor of the ovary that contains thin-walled multilocular cysts
multicystic dysplastic kidney disease multiple cysts replace normal renal tissue throughout the kidney; usually causes renal obstruction
murmur relatively prolonged series of auditory vibrations of varying intensity (loudness), frequency (pitch), quality, configuration, and duration; produced by structural changes and/or hemodynamic events in the heart or blood vessels
myocardium thickest muscle in the heart wall
myometritis infection within the myometrium of the uterus
myometrium middle layer of the uterine cavity that appears homogeneous with sonography
myxoma common benign tumor of the heart
nabothian cyst benign tiny cyst within the cervix
necrosis death of areas of tissue
nomogram representation of the relationship between numerical variables in the form of graphs, diagrams, or charts
nonimmune hydrops (NIH) group of conditions in which hydrops is present in the fetus but not as a result of fetomaternal blood group incompatibility
non-immune hydrops accumulation of abnormal fluid collections not caused by rhesus incompatibility
nonmaleficence refrain from harming oneself or others
normal situs typical position of the abdominal organs with the liver and inferior vena cava on the right, stomach on the left, and the apex of the heart directed toward the left hip
nuchal cord umbilical cord wrapped around the fetal neck
nuchal lucency increased thickness in the nuchal fold area in the back of the neck associated with trisomy 21
nuchal translucency collection of fluid that extends behind the fetal neck and along the spine in the first trimester
obturator internus muscle triangular sheet of muscle that arises from the anterolateral pelvic wall and surrounds the obturator foramen; it passes through the lesser sciatic foramen and inserts into the medial aspect of the greater trochanter of the femur; serves to rotate and abduct the thigh
oculodentodigital dysplasia underdevelopment of the eyes, fingers, and mouth
oligohydramnios too little amniotic fluid; associated with intrauterine growth restriction, renal anomalies, premature rupture of membranes, postdate pregnancy, and other factors; fluid measures lower than 5th percentile of the amniotic fluid index
oligomenorrhea abnormally light menstrual periods
omphalocele anterior abdominal wall defect in which abdominal organs (liver, bowel, stomach) are atypically located within the umbilical cord; highly associated with cardiac, central nervous system, renal, and chromosomal anomalies; abnormality of the abdominal wall in which bowel and liver, both covered by a membrane, protrude outside the wall
omphalomesenteric cyst cystic lesion of the umbilical cord
oocyte incompletely developed or immature ovum
oophoritis infection within the ovary
ophthalmic artery first branch of the internal carotid artery
osteogenesis imperfecta metabolic disorder affecting the fetal collagen system that leads to varying forms of bone disease; intrauterine bone fractures, shortened long bones, poorly mineralized calvaria, and compression of the chest found in type II forms
otocephaly underdevelopment of the jaw that causes the ears to be located close together toward the front of the neck
ovarian carcinoma malignant tumor of the ovary that may spread beyond the ovary and metastasize to other organs via the peritoneal channels
ovarian cyst may be found in the fetus; results from maternal hormone stimulation and is usually benign
ovarian hyperstimulation syndrome (OHSS) syndrome that presents sonographically as enlarged ovaries with multiple cysts, abdominal ascites, and pleural effusions; occasionally seen in patients who have undergone ovulation induction after administration of follicle-stimulating hormone or a gonadotropin releasing hormine analogue followed by human chorionic gonadotropin
ovarian ligament paired ligament that extends from the inferior-medial pole of the ovary to the uterine cornua; also called the utero-ovarian ligament

ovarian torsion partial or complete rotation of the ovarian pedicle on its axis

ovulation induction therapy controlled ovarian stimulation, usually accomplished by administering oral clomiphene citrate (Clomid), oral aromatase inhibitors (i.e., letrozole), or injectable human menopausal gonadotropins

ovum female egg

oxycephaly, acrocephaly malformed cranial vault with a high or peaked appearance and a vertical index above 77; caused by premature closure of the coronal, sagittal, and lambdoidal sutures

papillary fibroelastoma small noncancerous tumor that arises on aortic or mitral valve tissue

parametritis infection within the uterine serosa and broad ligaments

paraovarian cyst cystic structure that lies adjacent to the ovary

parity (P) number of live births

partial anomalous pulmonary venous return condition in which the pulmonary veins do not all enter into the left atrial cavity

partial situs inversus condition in which only the heart or the abdominal organs are reversed (dextrocardia or liver on the left, stomach on the right)

pelvic inflammatory disease (PID) all-inclusive term that refers to all pelvic infections

pelvic kidney occurs when the kidney does not migrate upward into the retroperitoneal space

pentalogy of Cantrell rare anomaly with five defects: omphalocele, ectopic heart, lower sternum, anterior diaphragm, and diaphragmatic pericardium

perforating veins connect the superficial and deep venous systems

pericardial effusion—abnormal collection of fluid surrounding the heart greater than 2 mm

pericardium sac surrounding the heart with reflections off the great arteries

perimetrium serous membrane enveloping the uterus; also called the serosa

periovarian inflammation enlarged ovaries with multiple cysts and indistinct margins

peristalsis movement of the bowel

peroneal artery posterior lateral branch of the tibial-peroneal trunk in the lower extremity just distal to the popliteal fossa

peroneal veins drain blood from lateral compartment of the lower leg

Pierre Robin syndrome micrognathia and abnormal smallness of the tongue, usually with a cleft palate

piriformis muscle flat, pyramidal muscle arising from the anterior sacrum, passing through the greater sciatic notch to insert into the superior aspect of the greater trochanter of the femur; rotates and abducts the thigh

Proximal isovelocity surface area (PISA) method in echocardiography, an estimate of the area of an orifice through which blood flows

placenta accreta growth of the chorionic villi to the myometrium; it does not penetrate through the myometrium

placenta increta growth of the chorionic villi deep into the myometrium

placenta migration movement of the placenta as the uterus enlarges

placenta percreta growth of the chorionic villi through the myometrium to the uterine serosa

placenta previa placenta implantation that encroaches upon the lower uterine segment; the placenta presents first in late pregnancy, and bleeding is inevitable

placental insufficiency inability of the placenta to adequately provide adequate blood/nutrient supply to the fetus to underlying maternal disease, such as hypertension or diabetes or caused by extensive placenta abruption

platycephaly flattening of the skull

pleural effusion (hydrothorax) accumulation of fluid within the thoracic cavity

pleural effusion abnormal fluid collection in the thoracic cavity

polycystic ovarian syndrome (PCOS) endocrine disorder associated with chronic anovulation

polydactyly anomalies of the hands or feet in which there is an addition of a digit; may be found in association with certain skeletal dysplasias

polyhydramnios too much amniotic fluid; associated with central nervous system disorder, gastrointestinal anomalies, fetal hydrops, skeletal anomalies, renal disorders, and other factors; fluid measures greater than 95th percentile of the amniotic fluid index

polymenorrhea abnormally frequent recurrence of the menstrual cycle; a menstrual cycle of less than 21 days

polysplenia more than one spleen; associated with cardiac malformations

popliteal artery begins at the opening of the adductor magnus muscle and travels behind the knee in the popliteal fossa

popliteal vein originates from the confluence of the anterior tibial veins with the posterior and peroneal veins

posterior arch vein main tributary of the greater saphenous vein

posterior cerebral artery (PCA) originates from the terminal basilar artery and courses anteriorly and laterally

posterior communicating artery (PCoA) courses posteriorly and medially from the internal carotid artery to join the posterior cerebral artery

posterior tibial veins originate from the plantar veins of the foot and drain blood from the posterior compartment of the lower leg

posterior urethral valve occurs only in male fetuses; is manifested by the presence of a valve in the posterior urethra

postmenopause period of life after menopause

post-term fetus born later than the 42-week gestational period

Potter sequence renal diseases other than renal agenesis that result in renal failure and facial or structure abnormalities caused by oligohydramnios

Potter syndrome group of findings associated with oligohydramnios and renal failure or bilateral renal agenesis; includes abnormally positioned extremities, wide-set eyes, low-set ears, and broad nasal bridge

Pourcelot resistive index Doppler measurement that takes the highest systolic peak minus the highest diastolic peak divided by the highest systolic peak

preeclampsia complication of pregnancy characterized by increasing hypertension, proteinuria, and edema; also known as pregnancy-induced hypertension

preload degree that muscle fiber stretches prior to contraction (end diastole)

premature atrial contractions (PACs), premature ventricular contractions (PVCs) benign condition that arises from the electrical impulses generated outside the cardiac pacemaker (sinus node); immature development of the electrical pacing system causes irregular heartbeats scattered throughout the cardiac cycle

premature rupture of membranes (PROM) pregnancy in which the amniotic bag has ruptured, labor has not begun, and the pregnancy is beyond 37 weeks of gestation

premenarchal time period in young girls before the onset of menstruation

pressure half time (PHT) time required for the transmitral pressure gradient to decrease by half

pressure exertion of force upon a surface by an object or fluid it is in contact with or the force per unit area

preterm fetus born earlier than the standard 38- to 42-week gestational period

preterm premature rupture of membranes (PPROM) pregnancy in which the amniotic bag has ruptured, labor has not yet begun, and the pregnancy is less than 37 weeks of gestation

primary yolk sac first site of formation of red blood cells that will nourish the embryo

proboscis cylindrical protuberance of the face that in cyclopia or ethmocephaly represents the nose

profunda femoris artery posterior and lateral to the superficial femoral artery

progesterone steroidal hormone produced by the corpus luteum that helps prepare and maintain the endometrium for the arrival and implantation of an embryo

proliferative phase (early) days 5 to 9 of the menstrual cycle; the endometrium appears as a single thin stripe with a hypoechoic halo encompassing it, creating the "three-line sign"

proliferative phase (late) days 10 to 14 of the menstrual cycle; ovulation occurs; the endometrium increases in thickness and echogenicity

prune-belly syndrome dilation of the fetal abdomen secondary to severe bilateral hydronephrosis and fetal ascites; fetus also has oligohydramnios and pulmonary hypoplasia

pseudoaneurysm well-defined collection of blood and connective tissue outside the vessel wall; typically results from a contained rupture of the aortic wall; perivascular collection (hematoma) that communicates with an artery or a graft and has the presence of pulsating blood entering the collection

pseudoascites sonolucent band near the fetal anterior abdominal wall from the abdominal wall muscles in the fetus older than 18 weeks of gestation

pseudogestational sac decidual reaction that occurs within the uterus in a patient with an ectopic pregnancy

psoas major muscle paired muscles that originate at the transverse process of the lumbar vertebrae and extend inferiorly through the false pelvis on the pelvic sidewall, where it unites with the iliacus muscle to form the iliopsoas muscle before inserting into the lesser trochanter of the femur

pulmonary embolism (PE) blockage of the pulmonary circulation by foreign matter

pulmonary hypoplasia small, underdeveloped lungs with resultant reduction in lung volume; secondary to prolonged oligohydramnios or as a consequence of a small thoracic cavity

pulmonary sequestration extra pulmonary tissue present within the pleural lung sac (intralobar) or connected to the inferior border of the lung within its pleural sac (extralobar)

pulmonary stenosis abnormal pulmonary valve characterized by thickened, domed leaflets that restrict the amount of blood flowing from the right ventricle to the pulmonary artery to the lungs

pulsatility index (PI) Doppler measurement of peak systole minus peak diastole divided by the mean systole minus peak diastole divided by the mean

pulsed wave Doppler transducers send and receive ultrasound pulses at timed intervals so that the location of where the sample volume is positioned can be known

pyelectasis dilated renal pelvis without involvement of the calyces

pyometra obstruction of the uterus and/or the vagina characterized by an accumulation of pus

pyosalpinx retained pus within the inflamed fallopian tube

radial artery branch of the brachial artery that runs parallel to the ulnar artery in the forearm

reactive hyperemia alternative method to stress the peripheral arterial circulation

rectouterine recess (pouch) area in the pelvic cavity between the rectum and the uterus that is likely to accumulate free fluid; also known as the posterior-cul-de-sac and the pouch of Douglas

renal agenesis failure of the renal system to develop

repolarization begins just before the relaxation phase of cardiac muscle activity

resistive index (RI) peak systolic velocity minus the end diastolic velocity divided by the peak systolic velocity

respect for persons incorporates both respect for the autonomy of individuals and the requirement to protect those with diminished autonomy

respiratory plasticity blood flow velocity changes with respiration

retroflexed refers to the position of the uterus when the uterine fundus bends posteriorly upon the cervix

retroverted refers to the position of the uterus when the entire uterus is tipped posteriorly so the angle formed between the cervix and vaginal canal is greater than 90 degrees

Rh blood group system of antigens that may be found on the surface of red blood cells; when the Rh antigen is present, the blood type is Rh positive; when the Rh antigen is absent, the blood type is Rh negative; a pregnant woman who is Rh negative may become sensitized by the blood of an Rh-positive fetus, and in subsequent pregnancies, if the fetus is Rh positive, the Rh antibodies produced in maternal blood may cross the placenta and destroy fetal cells, causing erythroblastosis fetalis

rhabdomyoma benign cardiac tumor; most common tumor in children with tuberous sclerosis

reversible ischemic neurologic deficit (RIND) stroke that lasts more than 24 hours and settles within a week; important warning sighs for the development of cerebral infarction

round ligaments paired ligaments that originate at the uterine cornua, anterior to the fallopian tubes, and course anterolaterally within the broad ligament to insert into the fascia of the labia majora; they hold the uterus forward in its anteverted position

S/D ratio difference between peak systole and end diastole

salpingitis infection within the fallopian tubes

secondary yolk sac formed at 23 days when the primary yolk sac is pinched off by the extra embryonic coelom

secretory (luteal) phase days 15 to 28 of the menstrual cycle; the endometrium is at its greatest thickness and echogenicity with posterior enhancement

semilunar valves pocket-like structures attached at the point at which the pulmonary artery and the aorta leave the ventricles

septum primum first part of the atrial septum to grow from the dorsal wall of the primitive atrium and fuses with the endocardial cushion

septum secundum muscular flap that is semilunar in shape and grows downward from the upper wall of the atrium immediately to the right of the septum primum and ostium secundum

serous cystadenocarcinoma second most common benign tumor of the ovary

serous pericardium inner sac of the pericardium with two layers: visceral and parietal

simple ovarian cyst smooth, well-defined cystic structure entirely filled with fluid

single umbilical artery high association of congenital anomalies with single umbilical artery

single ventricle congenital anomaly in which there are two atria but only one ventricular chamber

sinoatrial node forms in the wall of the sinus venosus near its opening into the right atrium; later, it is incorporated into the right atrium with the right horn of the sinus venosus

situs inversus complete reversal of the heart and abdominal organs

small for gestational age (SGA) normal but small fetus; measures smaller than dates

soleal sinuses large venous reservoirs that lie in the soleus muscle and empty into the posterior tibial or peroneal veins

sonohysterography technique that uses a catheter inserted into the endometrial cavity; saline or contrast is inserted to fill the endometrial cavity to demonstrate abnormalities within the cavity or uterine tubes; also known as saline-infused sonography

space of Retzius located between the anterior bladder wall and the pubic symphysis; contains extraperitoneal fat

Spalding sign overlapping of the skull bones; indicates fetal death

spectral Doppler ultrasound form of ultrasound display in which the spectrum of flow velocities is represented graphically on the y-axis and time on the x-axis; both pulsed wave and continuous wave Doppler are displayed in this manner

spina bifida neural tube defect of the spine in which the dorsal vertebrae (vertebral arches) fail to fuse together, allowing the protrusion of meninges and/or spinal cord through the defect

spina bifida occulta closed defect of the spine without protrusion of meninges or spinal cord; not detectable by alpha-fetoprotein analysis

spontaneous flow present without augmentation

spontaneous premature rupture of membranes (SPROM) pregnancy in which the amniotic bag ruptures with labor or just after labor begins

squamous cell carcinoma most common type of cervical cancer

sternal angle angle between the manubrium and the body of the sternum; also known as the angle of Louis

strabismus eye disorder in which optic axes cannot be directed to the same object

striations parallel longitudinal lines commonly seen in muscle tissue when imaged sonographically; appear as hyperechoic parallel lines running in the long axis of the hypoechoic muscle tissue

stroke volume volume of blood ejected by the ventricles with each contraction

subclavian artery originates at the inner border of the scalenus anterior and travels beneath the clavicle to the outer border of the first rib to become the axillary artery

subclavian steal syndrome characterized by symptoms of brainstem ischemia associated with a stenosis or occlusion of the left subclavian, innominate, or right subclavian artery proximal to the origin of the vertebral artery

subclavian vein continuation of the axillary vein joins the internal jugular vein to form the innominate vein

subfertility diminished reproductive capacity

subjective assessment sonographer surveys uterine cavity to determine visual assessment of amniotic fluid present

submandibular window transducer is placed at the angle of the mandible and angled slightly medially and cephalad toward the carotid canal

submucosal leiomyoma type of leiomyoma found to deform the endometrial cavity and cause heavy or irregular menses

suboccipital window transducer is placed on the posterior aspect of the neck inferior to the nuchal crest

subpulmonic stenosis occurs when a membrane or muscle bundle obstructs the outflow tract into the pulmonary artery

subserosal leiomyoma type of leiomyoma that may become pedunculated and appear as an extrauterine mass

succenturiate placenta one or more accessory lobes connected to the body of the placenta by blood vessels

superficial femoral artery (SFA) courses the length of the thigh through Hunter canal and terminates at the opening of the adductor magnus muscle

superficial femoral vein (SFV) originates at the hiatus of the adductor magnus muscle in the distal thigh and ascends through the adductor (Hunter) canal

superior vesical arteries after birth, the umbilical arteries become the superior vesical arteries

suprasternal notch superior margin of the manubrium sterni; lies opposite the lower border of the body of the second thoracic vertebra

supravalvular pulmonic stenosis abnormal narrowing in the main pulmonary artery superior to the valve opening

supraventricular tachyarrhythmias abnormal cardiac rhythm above 200 beats/min with a conduction rate of 1:1

surface epithelial-stromal tumors gynecologic tumors that arise from the surface epithelium and cover the ovary and the underlying stroma

suspensory (infundibulopelvic) ligament paired ligaments that extend from the infundibulum of the fallopian tube and the lateral aspect of the ovary to the lateral pelvic wall; also called the infundibulopelvic ligament

synechiae scars within the uterus secondary to previous gynecologic surgery

systemic lupus erythematosus (SLE) inflammatory disease involving multiple organ systems; a fetus of a mother with SLE may develop heart block and pericardial effusion

systole part of the cardiac cycle in which the ventricles are pumping blood through the outflow tract into the pulmonary artery or the aorta; the mitral and tricuspid valves are closed

systolic murmur begins with or after the time of the first heart sound and ends at or before the time of the second heart sound

tachycardia fetal heart rate more than 200 beats/min

takotsubo cardiomyopathy acute cardiac syndrome characterized by transient left ventricular regional wall motion abnormalities, chest pain and/or dyspnea, ST segment elevations, and minor elevations in cardiac enzymes

targeted ultrasound detailed fetal ultrasound performed in pregnancies with indications for fetal or maternal complications

teratoma solid tumor

tetralogy of Fallot most common form of cyanotic heart disease characterized by a high, membranous ventricular septal defect, a large, anteriorly displaced aorta, pulmonary stenosis, and right ventricular hypertrophy

thanatophoric dysplasia lethal short-limb dwarfism characterized by a notable reduction in the length of the long bones, pear-shaped chest, soft tissue redundancy, and frequently cloverleaf skull deformity and ventriculomegaly

theca-lutein cysts multilocular cysts that occur in patients with hyperstimulation

thoracic outlet syndrome changes in arterial blood flow to the arms may be related to intermittent compression of the proximal arteries (or neural and venous structures)

transient ischemic attack (TIA) brief, stroke-like event that resolves over minutes to hours

TORCH acronym originally coined from the first letters of toxoplasmosis, rubella, cytomegalovirus, and herpes virus type 2; the "o" stands for other transplacental infections

total anomalous pulmonary venous return (TAPVR) condition in which the pulmonary veins do not return at all into the left atrial cavity; the veins may return into the right atrial cavity or a chamber posterior to the left atrial cavity

translabial across or through the labia

transorbital window transducer is placed on the closed eyelid

transperineal across or through the perineum

transposition of the great arteries abnormal condition that exists when the aorta is connected to the right ventricle, and the pulmonary artery is connected to the left ventricle; atrioventricular valves are normally attached and related

transtemporal window transducer is placed on the temporal bone cephalad to the zygomatic arch anterior to the ear

transudative fluid that passes through a membrane

transverse fetal lie indicates fetus is lying transversely in the uterus, horizontal, or perpendicular to the maternal sagittal axis

Treacher Collins syndrome underdevelopment of the jaw and cheek bone and abnormal ears

tricuspid atresia interruption of the growth of the tricuspid leaflet that begins early in cardiac embryology

trigonocephaly premature closure of the metopic suture

trimester division of pregnancy into three 13-week segments

true knots of the umbilical cord formed when a loop of cord is slipped over the fetal head or shoulders during delivery

true pelvis pelvic cavity found below the brim of the pelvis; also called the minor or lesser pelvis

truncus arteriosus congenital heart lesion in which only one great artery arises from the base of the heart; the pulmonary trunk, the systemic arteries, and the coronary arteries arise from this single great artery

tubo-ovarian abscess (TOA) infection that involves the fallopian tube and the ovary

tubo-ovarian complex fusion of the inflamed dilated tube and ovary

Turner syndrome non-lethal genetic abnormality in which the chromosomal composition is 45XO instead of the normal 46XX or XY

twin-twin transfusion syndrome monozygotic twin pregnancy with single placenta and arteriovenous shunt within the placenta; the donor twin becomes anemic and growth restricted with oligohydramnios; the recipient twin may develop hydrops and polyhydramnios

ulnar artery branch of the brachial artery that runs parallel to the radial artery in the forearm

umbilical cord connecting lifeline between the fetus and placenta; contains two umbilical arteries and one umbilical vein encased in Wharton jelly

umbilical herniation failure of the anterior abdominal wall to close completely at the level of the umbilicus

urachal cyst small part of the lumen of the allantois that persists while the urachus forms

ureterocele congenital outpouching of the distal ureter into the bladder

ureteropelvic junction junction of the ureter entering the renal pelvis; most common site of obstruction

ureterovesical junction junction where the ureter enters the bladder

urethral atresia massively distended bladder (prune belly)

uterosacral ligaments posterior portion of the cardinal ligament that extends from the cervix to the sacrum

uterus didelphys double uterus and double vagina

VACTERL vertebral defects, heart defects, renal and limb abnormalities

valves folds of the intima that temporarily close to permit blood flow in one direction only

varicose veins dilated, elongated, tortuous superficial veins

vasa previa occurs when the umbilical cord vessels cross the internal os of the cervix

velocity speed with which something moves in a given direction

ventricular septal defect defect in the ventricular septum that provides communication between the right and left chambers of the heart; most common congenital lesion

ventriculomegaly abnormal accumulation of cerebrospinal fluid within the cerebral ventricles resulting in dilation of the ventricles; compression of developing brain tissue and brain damage may result; commonly associated with additional fetal anomalies

ventriculomegaly dilation of the ventricular system without enlargement of the cranium

veracity truthfulness, honesty

vernix caseosa fatty material found on fetal skin and in amniotic fluid late in pregnancy

vertebral artery branch of the subclavian artery

vertex indicates that the fetus is positioned head down in the uterus

vertigo sensation of objects moving about

vesicouterine recess (pouch) area in the pelvic cavity between the urinary bladder and the uterus; also known as the anterior-cul-sac

volume amount of space occupied by a three-dimensional object as measured in cubic units such as cubic centimeters or milliliters

Wharton jelly myxomatous connective tissue that surrounds the umbilical vessels and varies in size

xiphisternal joint junction between the xiphoid and the sternum

xiphoid lowest point of the sternum

yolk sac circular structure within the gestational sac between the chorion and the amnion that is seen on ultrasound between 4 and 10 weeks of gestation; supplies nutrition, facilitates waste removal and is the origin of early hematopoietic stem cells in the embryo

yolk stalk umbilical duct connecting the yolk sac with the embryo

zygote fertilized ovum resulting from union of male and female gametes

ILLUSTRATION CREDITS

Figure 21.55
Adam A, et al. *Grainger & Allison's Diagnostic Radiology: A Textbook of Medical Imaging*, 7th ed. Elsevier; 2021.

Figure 2.39A
Aehlert B. *Mosby's Comprehensive Pediatric Emergency Care.* Elsevier; 2007.

Figure 35.20B
Anderson DF, Bissonnette JM, Faber JJ, Thornburg KL. Central shunt flows and pressures in the mature fetal lamb. *Am J Physiol.* 1981;241:H60-H66.

Figure 62.8F
Arensman RM. *Pediatric Surgery*, ed 2. Landes Bioscience; 2009.

Figure 63.10A
AWHONN. *Core Curriculum for Neonatal Intensive Care Nursing*, 6th ed. Elsevier; 2021. Courtesy V. Becker, Pathologisches Institut der Universität, Erlangen, Germany.

Figure 21.45
Balleyguier C, et al. Breast pain and imaging. *Diagnost Intervent imaging.* 2015;96(10):1009-16.

Figure 8.21A
Banasik JL. *Pathophysiology*, 7th ed. Elsevier; 2022.

Figure 1.6B
Bassett LW, et al. *Breast Imaging*. Elsevier; 2011. Courtesy B. Goldberg, Philadelphia.

Figure 11.8, 62.2
Becker JM, Stucchi AF. *Essentials of Surgery*. Elsevier; 2006.

Figure 21.50A
Berg WA, Jessica Leung. *Diagnostic Imaging: Breast*, 3rd ed. Elsevier; 2019.

Figures 8.1, 9.37
Black JM, Hawks JH. *Medical-Surgical Nursing: Clinical Management for Positive Outcomes*, ed 8. Elsevier; 2008.

Figure 11.5
Black JM, Matassarin-Jacobs E, editors. *Luckmann and Sorensen's Medical-Surgical Nursing*, ed 4. Saunders; 1993.

Figure 21.13
Bland K, et al. *The Breast: Comprehensive Management of Benign and Malignant Diseases*, 5th ed. Elsevier; 2018.

Figure 43.24A
Bogani G, et al. Morcellation of undiagnosed uterine sarcoma: a critical review. *Crit Rev Oncol/Hematol.* 2016;98:302-8.

Figure 43.3B
Bowra J, et al. *Emergency Ultrasound Made Easy*, 3rd ed. Elsevier; 2022.

Figure 63.21
Bradley PA, et al. *Elsevier's Canadian Comprehensive Review for the NCLEX-RN Examination*, 2nd ed. Elsevier; 2022.

Figures 1.21, 32.4A
Broaddus VC, et al. *Murray & Nadel's Textbook of Respiratory Medicine*, 7th ed. Elsevier; 2022.

Figure 32.28A
Brown D, Edwards H, Seaton L, Buckley T. *Lewis's medical-Surgical Nursing: Assessment and Management of Clinical Problems*, 4th ed. Elsevier; 2015.

Figure 33.24A
Buja LM, Butany J. *Cardiovascular Pathology*, 4th ed. Elsevier; 2016.

Figure 1.37A–B
Callen P. *Ultrasonography in Obstetrics and Gynecology*, 5th ed. Elsevier; 2008.

Figure 33.35
Cameron JL, Cameron AM. *Current Surgical Therapy*, 13th ed. Elsevier; 2020.

Figure 49.17A
Carlson BM. *Human Embryology and Developmental Biology*, 6th ed. Elsevier; 2019.

Figure 19.1
Carlson KK. *AACN Advanced Critical Care Nursing*. Elsevier; 2009.

Figure 22.32A
Cetani F, et al. Parathyroid Carcinoma. *Front Horm Res.* 2019;51:63-76.

Figure 53.9
Cetin I, et al. Evaluation of fetal growth and fetal well-being. *Semin Ult CT MR.* 2008;29(2):136-46.

Figure 4.13A
Chabner D-E. *Language of Medicine*, 12th ed. Elsevier; 2021.

Figure 33.10C–F
Chandrashekar Y, Westaby S, Narula J. Mitral stenosis. *Lancet.* 2009;374:1273.

Figure 1.9A
Cheng C. *Handbook of Vascular Motion*. Elsevier; 2019.

Figure 59.39A
Chervenak FA, et al. Fetal cystic hygroma: cause and natural history. *N Engl J Med.* 1983;309(14):822-5.

Figure 33.1
Chikwe J, et al. The surgical management of mitral valve disease. *Br J Cardiol.* 2004;11:42-9.

Figure 44.14
Cicchiello LA, et al. Ultrasound evaluation of gynecologic causes of pelvic pain. *Obstet Gynecol Clin North Am.* 2011;38(1):85-114.

Figures 35.19B, 49.20, 52.14, 63.16B
Coady AM, Bower S. *Twining's Textbook of Fetal Abnormalities*, 3rd ed. Elsevier; 2015.

ILLUSTRATION CREDITS

Figure 35.20
Cohen MS. Clarifying anatomical complexity: diagnosing heterotaxy syndrome in the fetus. *Prog Pediatr Cardiol.* 2006;22(1):61-70.

Figure 35.6
Colville TP. *Clinical Anatomy and Physiology for Veterinary Technicians*, 2nd ed. Mosby; 2008.

Figure 61.12B, 63.8
Copel JA, et al. *Obstetric Imaging: Fetal Diagnosis and Care*, 2nd ed. Elsevier; 2018.

Figure 1.36B
Correas J-M, et al. Ultrasound-based imaging methods of the kidney-recent developments. *Kidney Int.* 2016;90(6):1199-1210.

Figure 1.2
Craig M. *Essentials of Sonography and Patient Care*, 3rd ed. Elsevier; 2013.

Figure 35.32
Curry RA, Tempkin BB. *Sonography: Introduction to Normal Structure and Function*, 4th ed. Elsevier; 2016.

Figure 61.2
Curry RA, Tempkin BB. *Sonography: Introduction to Normal Structure and Function*, 5th ed. Elsevier; 2021.

Figures 8.43B, 9.24A, 9.29, 9.33A, 9.44, 9.50D, 9.51A, 9.52C, 9.53C, 9.55, 9.57, 10.19, 10.28, 10.37, 10.51, 10.54, 12.22, 12.23, 12.27, 12.29, 12.31, 12.32A, 12.34A, 12.35, 12.36, 12.40B, 11.21A, 11.21C, 19.16C, 22.8, 22.14, 22.17, 22.18, 22.20, 22.24, 22.26, 22.30, 22.32, 25.12, 25.17, 25.19A, 25.22, 25.26, 26.14, 26.19, 27.26, 27.35, 27.37, 44.21, 44.24, 44.29, 44.30, 44.31, 44.34
Damjanov I, Linder J. *Pathology: A Color Atlas*. Mosby; 2000.

Figure 1.7
de Jong MR. *Craig's Essentials of Sonography and Patient Care*, 4th ed. Elsevier; 2018.

Figures 1.34, 49.23A
de Jong, MR. *Sonography Scanning: Principles and Protocols*, 5th ed. Elsevier; 2021.

Figure 1.5
Dempsey PJ. The history of breast ultrasound. *J Ultrasound Med.* 2004;23:887–894.

Figure 42.15A
Dietz HP. Ultrasound in the assessment of pelvic organ prolapse. *Clin Obstet Gynaecol.* 2019;54:12-30.

Figures 43.14A, 43.22B
Dighe M, et al. *Abdominal Imaging: Case Review Series*. Elsevier; 2022.

Figure 35.11A–H
Dijkema EJ, et al. Diagnosis, imaging and clinical management of aortic coarctation. *Heart (British Cardiac Society).* 2017;103(15):1148-1155.

Figures 30.4, 30.5, 30.10B
Drake RL, et al. *Gray's Anatomy for Students*, 3rd ed. Elsevier; 2015.

Figures 41.15, 41.16
Drake RL, et al. *Gray's Atlas of Anatomy*, 2nd ed. Elsevier; 2015.

Figure 11.3B
Drake RL, Vogl W, Mitchell AWM. *Gray's Anatomy for Students*. Churchill Livingstone; 2005.

Figure 35.33A
Drose JA. *Fetal Echocardiography*, 2nd ed. Elsevier; 2010.

Figure 8.32
Elefteriades JA, Farkas EA. Thoracic aortic aneurysm clinically pertinent controversies and uncertainties. *J Am Coll Cardiol.* 2010;55(9):841-57.

Figure 43.5A
Elsevier. *Buck's Step-By-Step Medical Coding*. Elsevier; 2021.

Figure 32.21
Elsevier. *Medical Assistant: Cardiopulmonary Systems, Vital Signs, Electrocardiography and CPR, Module D*, 2nd ed. Elsevier; 2016.

Figure 49.14
England, MA. *Colour Atlas of Life before Birth*. Elsevier; 1983.

Figure 1.22B
Ettinger SJ, et al. *Textbook of Veterinary Internal Medicine: Diseases of the Dog and Cat, Volume 2*, 8th ed. Elsevier; 2017;1083-2182.

Figure 11.3A
Federle MP, et al. *Imaging Anatomy: Chest, Abdomen, Pelvis*, 2nd ed. Elsevier; 2017.

Figure 10.51A
Feldman M, et al. *Sleisenger and Fortran's Gastrointestinal and Liver Disease*, ed 11. Elsevier; 2021.

Figure 41.21
Fleischer AC, Kepple DM. Benign conditions of the uterus, cervix, and endometrium. In: Nyberg DA, Hill LM, Bohm-Velez M, et al, eds. *Transvaginal Ultrasound*. Mosby–Year Book; 1992.

Figure 63.11
Fliegauf M, et al. When cilia go bad: cilia defects and ciliopathies. *Nat Rev Mol Cell Biol.* 2007;8(11):880-93.

Figure 10.46
Floch MH. *Netter's Gastroenterology*, 3rd ed. Elsevier; 2020.

Figure 13.36A
Franklin IJ, et al. *Essentials of Clinical Surgery*, 2nd ed. Elsevier; 2013.

Figure 1.1B
Frentzel-Beyme B. Vom Echolot zur Farbdopplersonographie. *Der Radiologe.* 2005;45(4):363–370.

Figure 32.3A
Fretwell D, et al. Epidural intravascular injection detection by transthoracic echocardiography. *J Cardiovasc Vasc Anesth.* 2020;34(5):1288-1291.

Figure 19.25B
Gabbe SG, et al. *Obstetrics: Normal and Problem Pregnancies*, 7th ed. Elsevier; 2017.

Figure 63.5
Gilbert-Barness E. *Potter's Pathology of the Fetus, Infant, and Child*. Elsevier; 2007.

Figure 33.23A-C
Gilbert-Barness E, Debich-Spicer DE. *Handbook of Pediatric Autopsy Pathology*. Humana Press; 2005.

Figure 1.19A
Gil-Rodrigo A, et al. Diploma on ultrasound training and competency for intensive care and emergency medicine: Consensus document of the Spanish Society of Anesthesia (SEDAR), Spanish Society of Internal Medicine (SEMI) and Spanish Society of Emergency Medicine (SEMES). *Revista Espanola de Anestesiologia y Reanimacion*. 2021;68(10):610-612.

Figure 26.9
Goldman L. *Cecil Medicine*, 23rd ed. Elsevier; 2009.

Figure 12.7
Gregg JA, et al. Pancreas divisum: results of surgical intervention, *Am J Surg*. 1983;145:488–492.

Figure 19.25A
Griffith JF, et al. *Diagnostic Ultrasound. Musculoskeletal*. 2nd ed. Elsevier; 2019.

Figure 63.2
Griffiths M. *Crash Course Gastrointestinal System*, 4th ed. Elsevier; 2016.

Figure 16.3
Haaga JR. *CT and MRI of the Whole Body*, 5th ed. Elsevier; 2009.

Figure 43.6A-B
Haaga JR, Boll DT. *CT and MRI of the Whole Body*, 6th ed. Elsevier; 2017.

Figures 49.26, 49.28
Hadlock FP, et al. Fetal crown-rump length: reevaluation of relation to menstrual age (5-18 weeks) with high-resolution real-time US. *Radiology*. 1992;182(2):501-5.

Figure 8.62A
Hall S, Stephens J. *Crash Course Anatomy and Physiology*, 5th ed. Elsevier; 2019.

Figure 63.4B
Haller JD, Morgenstern L. Anomalous rotation and fixation of the left colon: embryogenesis and surgical management. *Am J Surg*. 1964;108:331.

Figure 6.2A
Harmon D. *Perioperative Diagnostic and Interventional Ultrasound*. Elsevier; 2008.

Figure 1.3
Harmon D. *Perioperative Diagnostic and Interventional Ultrasound*. Elsevier; 2008. Courtesy B. Goldberg, Chairman of the Archives Committee of the Association for Medical Ultrasound, www.aium.org.

Figure 1.28
Hawes RH, et al. *Endosonography*, 3rd ed. Elsevier; 2015.

Figures 15.52, 15.53, 21.29, 27.33, 27.38, 27.39, 25.13, 28.13B, 28.13B, 28.16, 28.18, 55.13, 55.20, 55.25A-B, 55.28, 60.13, 60.32A-B, 60.38A-B, 60.45A-B, 65.4A-C, 65.8A-B, 65.22A
Henningsen C. *Clinical Guide to Ultrasonography*. Elsevier; 2004.

Figures 4.20B, 28.3, 49.27
Herlihy BL. *The Human Body in Health and Illness*, 4th ed. Elsevier; 2011.

Figure 10.33B
Herring w. *Learning Radiology: Recognizing the Basics*, 3rd ed. Elsevier; 2016.

Figure 43.2A-B
Hertzberg BS, Middleton WD. *Ultrasound: The Requisites*, 3rd ed. Elsevier; 2016.

Figures 57.13, 62.15A
Holcomb GW, et al. *Holcomb and Ashcraft's Pediatric Surgery*, 7th ed. Elsevier; 2020.

Figures 4.15, 4.22, 4.25B, 9.30, 9.33
Hombach-Klonisch S, et al. *Sobotta Clinical Atlas of Human Anatomy*. Elsevier; 2019.

Figure 12.6
Ignatavicius DD, Workman ML. *Medical-Surgical Nursing: Patient-Centered Collaborative Care*, ed 8. Elsevier; 2016.

Figure 21.51
Ikeda DM, Miyake KK. *Breast Imaging: The Requisites*, 3rd ed. Elsevier; 2017.

Figure 9.40
Jong EC, Stevens DL. *Netter's Infectious Diseases*, 2nd ed. Elsevier; 2022.

Figures 4.20A, 9.4A-D, 10.35A, 12.3, 43.4, 43.6C-D, 44.13B, 45.15A-B, 53.5B, 62.16B, 63.12B
Kamaya A, et al. *Diagnostic Ultrasound for Sonographers*. Elsevier; 2019.

Figure 42.15B
Kamisan A, et al. Does pregnancy affect pelvic floor functional anatomy? A retrospective study. *Eur J Obstet Gynecol Reprod Biol*. 2021;259:26-31.

Figure 33.20A-D
Kaplan JA, et al. *Kaplan's Cardiac Anesthesia: For Cardiac and Noncardiac Surgery*, 7th ed. Elsevier; 2017.

Figure 57.10A
Kaplan C. Gross examination of the placenta. *Surg Pathol Clin*. 2013;6(1):1-26.

Figure 30.13C
Kasel AM, et al. Standardized imaging for aortic annular sizing: implications for transcatheter valve selection. *JACC Cardiovasc Imaging*. 2013;6(2):249-62.

Figures 31.3, 31.4, 31.5, 31.6, 31.10, 31.14, 31.15, 31.16, 31.17, 31.19, 31.21
Kisslo JA, et al. *Basic Doppler Echocardiography*. Elsevier; 1986.

Figure 1.27B
Kitai T, et al. Optimal timing of surgery for patients with active infective endocarditis. *Cardiol Clin.* 2021;39(2):197-209.

Figure 42.36A
Klatt EC. *Robbins and Cotran Atlas of Pathology*, 4th ed. Elsevier; 2021.

Figures 7.28A–C, 7.29A–E, 7.33
Kremkau FW. *Principles and Pitfalls of Real-Time Color-Flow Imaging.* In Bernstein EF, editor. *Vascular Diagnosis*, ed 4. Elsevier; 1993.

Figure 1.26
Kremkau FW. *Sonography: Principles and Instruments*, 9th ed. Elsevier; 2016.

Figure 7.27C
Kremkau FW. *J Vasc Technol.* 1991;15:265–266.

Figure 7.31
Kremkau FW. *Principles and Instrumentation.* In Merritt CRB, editor: *Doppler Color Imaging.* Elsevier; 1992.

Figures 7.25; 7.27B
Kremkau FW. Doppler principles. *Semin Roentgenol.* 1992;27:6–16.

Figure 7.6
Kremkau FW, Taylor KJ. Artifacts in ultrasound imaging. *J Ultrasound Med.* 1986;5(4):227-37.

Figures 33.9C–D
Kumar V, Abbas A, Fausto N. *Robbins & Cotran's Pathologic Basis of Disease*, ed 10. Elsevier; 2018.

Figure 10.27A
Kumar V, et al. *Robbins Essentials of Pathology.* Elsevier; 2021.

Figures 4.5, 8.49, 8.59A, 15.16A
Lampignano JP, Kendrick LE. *Bontrager's Textbook of Radiographic Positioning and Related Anatomy*, 10th ed. Elsevier; 2021.

Figure 52.10A
Landon M, et al. *Gabbe's Obstetrics: Normal and Problem Pregnancies*, 8th ed. Elsevier; 2021.

Figure 30.28
Lang RM, et al. *ASE's Comprehensive Echocardiography*, 2nd ed. Elsevier; 2016.

Figures 1.35A, 19.16, 33.14A–C, 33.15
Lang RM, et al. *ASE's Comprehensive Echocardiography*, 3rd ed. Elsevier; 2022.

Figure 21.43
Larribe M, et al. Breast cancers with round lumps: correlations between imaging and anatomopathology. *Diagnost Intervent Imaging* 2014;95(1):37-46.

Figure 21.34
Lawrence R, Lawrence R. *Breastfeeding: A Guide for the Medical Profession*, 9th ed. Elsevier; 2022.

Figure 42.9A–B
Legato MJ. *The Plasticity of Sex: The Molecular Biology and Clinical Features of Genomic Sex, Gender Identity and Sexual Behavior.* Elsevier; 2020. Courtesy Dr. Rodriguez-Wallberg, Karolinska University Hospital, Stockholm.

Figures 4.30A–B, 22.3
Leonard P. *Quick & Easy Medical Terminology*, 9th ed. Elsevier; 2020.

Figure 12.43C
Lester SC. *Diagnostic Pathology: Intraoperative Consultation*, 2nd ed. Elsevier; 2018.

Figures 10.4A, 16.3A
Levine RM. *Textbook of Gastrointestinal Radiology*, 5th ed. Elsevier; 2021.

Figures 1.36C, 41.7
Lockhart ME, et al. *Diagnostic Ultrasound: Vascular.* Elsevier; 2019.

Figure 35.13B
Lockwood CJ, et al. *Creasy and Resnik's Maternal-Fetal Medicine: Principles and Practice*, 8th ed. Elsevier; 2019.

Figure 35.19A
Lockwood CJ, et al. *Creasy and Resnik's Maternal-Fetal Medicine: Principles and Practice*, 8th ed. Elsevier; 2019. Courtesy I.R. Tessler.

Figure 13.2
Lyons VT. *Netter's Essential Systems-Based Anatomy.* Elsevier; 2022.

Figure 4.13B
Magowan B, et al. *Clinical Obstetrics & Gynaecology*, 4th ed. Elsevier; 2019.

Figure 32.15, 33.32A
Mann DL, Zipes DP, Libby P, et al, eds. *Braunwald's Heart Disease: A Textbook of Cardiovascular Medicine*, 10th ed. Elsevier; 2015:186. Courtesy B.E. Bulwer.

Figure 35.33B
Martin RJ, et al. *Fanaroff and Martin's Neonatal-Perinatal Medicine: Diseases of the Fetus and Infant*, 10th ed. Elsevier; 2015.

Figure 35.18
Martin RJ, et al. *Fanaroff and Martin's Neonatal-Perinatal Medicine: Diseases of the Fetus and Infant*, 11th ed. Elsevier; 2020.

Figure 49.30
Maternal Fetal Medicine Foundation, Washington, DC.

Figure 1.32
Mattoon JS, et al. *Small Animal Diagnostic Ultrasound*, 4th ed. Elsevier; 2021.

Figure 63.12C
Mavrides E, Moscoso G, Carvalho JS, et al. The anatomy of the umbilical, portal and hepatic venous systems in the human fetus at 14-19 weeks of gestation. *Ultrasound Obstet Gynecol.* 2001;18:598.

Figure 61.8
Mayden KL, et al. Cystic adenomatoid malformation in the fetus: ultrasound evaluation, *Am J Obstet Gynecol.* 1984;148:349.

Figure 42.21
McCarthy CJ, et al. *Specialty Imaging: Acute and Chronic Pain Intervention*. Elsevier; 2020.

Figures 1.20, 1.25A
McGahan J, et al. *Fundamentals of Emergency Ultrasound*. Elsevier; 2020.

Figure 13.17A
McGee S. *Evidence Based Physical Diagnosis*, 3rd ed. Elsevier; 2012.

Figure 6.2B
Mclean A, Huang S. *Critical Care Ultrasound Manual*. Elsevier; 2013.

Figure 4.25A
McMinn R. *Last's Anatomy: Regional and Applied*, 9th ed. Elsevier; 2020.

Figures 63.25B, 63.26A
Merrow AC. *Diagnostic Imaging: Pediatrics*, 3rd ed. Elsevier; 2017.

Figure 44.18C
Merrow AC, Hariharan S. *Imaging in Pediatrics*. Elsevier; 2018.

Figure 1.1A
Mikla VI, Mikla VV. *Medical Imaging Technology*. Elsevier; 2014.

Figure 33.24B
Miller DV, Revelo MP. *Diagnostic Pathology: Cardiovascular*, 2nd ed. Elsevier; 2018.

Figure 19.20
Mitchell RN, Halushka MK. Blood vessels. In Kumar V, et al, editors. *Robbins & Cotran Pathologic Basis of Disease*, 10th ed. Elsevier; 2021:485–526.

Figure 33.2
Monin J, et al. Functional assessment of mitral regurgitation by transthoracic echocardiography using standardized imaging planes: diagnostic accuracy and outcome implications. *J Am Coll Cardiol*. 2005;46(2):302–309.

Figures 49.15B, 57.2, 62.1
Moore KL, et al. *Before We Are Born: Essentials of Embryology and Birth Defects*, 10th ed. Elsevier; 2020.

Figure 50.6A
Moore KL, et al. *Before We Are Born: Essentials of Embryology and Birth Defects*, 10th ed. Elsevier; 2020. Courtesy M.S. Patel and F. Gaillard, Radiopaedia.com.

Figure 49.4
Moore KL, et al. *The Developing Human: Clinically Oriented Embryology*, 11th ed. Elsevier; 2020.

Figures 11.11, 28.1
Moses KP. *Atlas of Clinical Gross Anatomy*, 2nd ed. Elsevier; 2013.

Figure 21.4A
Norman AW, Henry H. *Hormones*, 3rd ed. Elsevier; 2015.

Figure 1.22A, 42.13, 50.29A, 62.13, 63.26B
Norton ME, et al. *Callen's Ultrasonography in Obstetrics and Gynecology*, 6th ed. Elsevier; 2017.

Figure 43.22C
Nucci MR. *Gynecologic Pathology: A Volume in Foundations in Diagnostic Pathology*, 2nd ed. Elsevier; 2020.

Figure 55.23
Nyberg DA, et al. *Diagnostic Ultrasound of Fetal Anomalies: Text and Atlas*. Elsevier; 1990.

Figure 1.6A
Nyborg WL. Biological effects of ultrasound: development of safety guidelines. Part I: personal histories. *Ultrasound Med Biol*. 2000;26(6):911-64.

Figures 10.33A, 10.34A
Odze RD, Goldblum JR. *Odze and Goldblum Surgical Pathology of the GI Tract, Liver, Biliary Tract, and Pancreas*, 3rd ed. Elsevier; 2015.

Figure 34.22
Oh JK. *The Echo Manual*, ed 3, 2006. Courtesy Mayo Foundation for Medical Education and Research.

Figure 32.3B
Otto CM, et al. *Echocardiography Review Guide: Companion to the Textbook of Clinical Echocardiography*, 4th ed. Elsevier; 2020.

Figure 1.17
Otto CM. *Textbook of Clinical Echocardiography*, 5th ed. Elsevier; 2013.

Figures 1.35B, 30.27, 32.6A, 33.30
Otto CM. *Textbook of Clinical Echocardiography*, 6th ed. Elsevier; 2018.

Figures 33.18, 33.25, 33.31
Otto CM. *The Practice of Clinical Echocardiography*, 6th ed. Elsevier; 2022.

Figure 33.13
Otto CM. *Valvular Heart Disease*. Elsevier; 2004.

Figure 33.32B
Oxorn DC, Otto CM. *Intraoperative and Interventional Echocardiography Atlas of Transesophageal Imaging*, 2nd ed. Elsevier; 2018.

Figure 10.1B
Pandey P, et al. Updates in hepatic oncology imaging. *Surg Oncol*. 2017;26(2):195–206.

Figures 8.15, 11.6, 22.28, 30.3B, 30.12, 30.13B, 34.1
Patton KT, Thibodeau GA. *Anatomy & Physiology*, 8th ed. Elsevier; 2013.

Figure 4.21, 41.9
Patton KT, Thibodeau GA. *Anatomy & Physiology*, 10th ed. Elsevier; 2019.

Figures 2.7, 4.1, 4.3, 13.4, 13.5
Patton KT, Thibodeau GA. *The Human Body in Health & Disease*, 6th ed. Elsevier; 2013.

Figure 30.23, 41.1
Patton KT, Thibodeau GA. *The Human Body in Health & Disease*, ed 7. Elsevier; 2018.

Figure 4.16
Patton KT, Thibodeau GA. *Mosby's Handbook of Anatomy and Physiology*. Elsevier; 2000.

Figures 1.15, 1.33A–B
Pellerito JS, Polak JF. *Introduction to Vascular Ultrasonography*, 7th ed. Elsevier; 2020.

Figures 41.2B, 41.3
Perry S, et al. *Maternal Child Nursing Care*, 6th ed. Elsevier; 2018.

Figure 53.4B
Polin RA, et al. *Fetal and Neonatal Physiology*, 5th ed. Elsevier; 2017.

Figure 10.2
Polin RA, et al. *Fetal and Neonatal Physiology*, 6th ed. Elsevier; 2022.

Figure 1.14
Pomeroy, L. *Encyclopedia of Materials: Technical Ceramics and Glasses*. Elsevier; 2021.

Figures; 2.28A–B, 2.18B, 2.23B–C
Potter PA, Perry AG. *Fundamentals of Nursing*, 7th ed. Elsevier; 2013.

Figure 10.3
Quick CRG, et al. *Essential Surgery: Problems, Diagnosis, and Management*, 5th ed. Elsevier; 2014.

Figures 43.9A–B, 50.6B
Raman S, et al. *ExpertDDX. Abdomen and Pelvis*, 2nd ed. Elsevier; 2017.

Figure 16.10
Ramirez, PT, et al. *Principles of Gynecologic Oncology Surgery*. Elsevier; 2019.

Figure 35.13A
Resnik R, et al. *Creasy Y Resnik, Medicina Materno-Fetal: Principios Y Práctica*. Elsevier; 2020. Courtesy Irving R. Tessler, MD.

Figures 1.4A–B
Roelandt JR. Seeing the invisible: a short history of cardiac ultrasound. *Eur J Echocardiogr*. 2000;1:811.

Figure 33.33A
Roman MJ, et al. Prognostic significance of the pattern of aortic root dilation in the Marfan syndrome. *J Am Coll Cardiol* 1993;22:1470–1476.

Figure 10.42A
Rosai J. *Rosai and Ackerman's Surgical Pathology*, 10th ed. Elsevier; 2011:984.

Figure 19.3
Rothrock JC. *Alexander's Care of the Patient in Surgery*, 13th ed. Elsevier; 2007.

Figures 21.30, 21.41A–B, 21.43A–B, 21.44A–B, 26.4, 28.10 A–B, 28.11A, 28.13A, 28.14, 29.14, 29.11A–F, 29.17D, 29.19A–G, 29.24, 43.20, 43.25, 43.35A–I, 44.8A–C, 44.9, 44.15, 44.20, 60.21, 64.18B
Rumack CM, et al. *Diagnostic Ultrasound*, 4th ed. Elsevier; 2011.

Figure 63.24A–B
Rumack CM, et al. *Diagnostic Ultrasound: Obstetrics and Gynecology*, 4th ed. Elsevier; 2014.

Figures 1.31, 10.39A, 22.23, 52.10B, 52.10C, 61.7, 62.12, 63.23
Rumack CM, Levine D. *Diagnostic Ultrasound*, 5th ed. Elsevier; 2018.

Figure 13.36B
Sabiston DC, et al. *Sabiston Textbook of Surgery: The Biological Basis of Modern Surgical Practice*, 19th ed. Elsevier; 2012. Courtesy M.H. Schreiber, The University of Texas Medical Branch.

Figure 63.3
Sadler TW. *Langman's Medical Embryology*, 8th ed. Philadelphia: Lippincott Williams & Wilkins; 2000:273.

Figure 45.11
Salvo SG. *Mosby's Pathology for Massage Therapists*, 4th ed. Mosby, 2018.

Figure 63.1
Schoenwolf GC, et al. *Larsen's Human Embryology*, 6th ed. Elsevier; 2022.

Figure 10.43B
Shackelford RT, et al. *Shackelford's Surgery of the Alimentary Tract*, 6th ed. Elsevier; 2007.

Figure 34.7
Sharp JT, Bunnell IL, Holand JF, et al. Hemodynamics during induced cardiac tamponade in man. *Am J Med*. 1960;25:640.

Figure 44.1B
Shiland BJ, et al. *Medical Assistant Endocrine, Skeletal, and Reproductive Systems, Pediatrics, and Geriatrics, Module F*, 2nd ed. Elsevier; 2010.

Figure 10.58B
Shiomi H, et al. Modified double-guidewire technique using a unique double-lumen sphincterotome for difficult biliary cannulation. *VideoGIE*. 2020;6(3):124-128.

Figure 33.34A–B
Sidawy AN, Perler B. *Rutherford's Vascular Surgery and Endovascular Therapy*, 9th ed. Elsevier; 2019.

Figure 6.10
Siddiqui IA, et al. Cross-sectional imaging of the metal-on-metal hip prosthesis: the London ultrasound protocol. *Clin Radiol*. 2013;68(8):e472-8.

Figure 35.5
Silvestri LA, Silvestri AE. *Saunders Comprehensive Review for the NCLEX-PN® Examination*, 8th ed. Elsevier; 2022.

Figure 10.1C, 8.63B
Soni N, et al. *Point of Care Ultrasound*. Elsevier; 2015.

Figures 4.14, 6.9, 30.3, 43.3A, 53.4A
Soni NJ, et al. *Point of Care Ultrasound*, 2nd ed. Elsevier; 2020.

Figure 32.5
Sorantin E, Heinzl, B. What every radiologist should know about paediatric echocardiography. *Eur J Radiol*. 2014;83(9):1519–1528.

Figures 14.1B, 49.2A–F, 57.1
Standring S. *Gray's Anatomy: The Anatomical Basis of Clinical Practice*, 42nd ed. Elsevier; 2021.

Figures 9.3B–C
Sugarbaker PH. Toward a standard of nomenclature for surgical anatomy of the liver. *Neth J Surg*. 1988;PO:100.

Figure 7.23A–E
Taylor KJW, Holland S. Doppler US. Part 1. Basic principles, instrumentation, and pitfalls. *Radiology*. 1990;174:297–307.

Figure 50.26A–C
Torigian DA, Ramchandani P. *Radiology Secrets Plus*. Elsevier; 2016.

Figure 8.17, 8.35
Townsend CM. *Sabiston Textbook of Surgery*, 18th ed. Elsevier; 2008.

Figures 9.7A, 62.5
Townsend CM, et al. *Sabiston Textbook of Surgery: The Biological Basis of Modern Surgical Practice*, 21st ed. Elsevier; 2022.

Figure 4.12A
Tublin ME. *Imaging in Urology*. Elsevier; 2018.

Figure 12.47A
Union for International Cancer Control (UICC). TNM Classification of Malignant Tumours, 8th ed. UICC; 2017.

Figure 30.13
Urden LD, et al. *Critical Care Nursing: Diagnosis and Management*, 9th ed. Elsevier; 2022.

Figure 21.53
Washington CM, Leaver DT. *Principles and Practice of Radiation Therapy*, 4th ed. Elsevier; 2016.

Figure 11.3A
Waugh A, Grant A. *Ross and Wilson Anatomy and Physiology in Health and Illness*, 12th ed. Elsevier; 2014.

Figures 33.19A–B
Willett DL, et al. Assessment of aortic regurgitation by transesophageal color Doppler imaging of the vena contracta: validation against an intraoperative aortic flow probe. *J Am Coll Cardiol*. 2001;37(5):1450-5.

Figure 4.29
Williams P, et al. *Gray's Anatomy*, 38th edition. Elsevier; 1995.

Figure 21.10A
Williams S, et al. *Fundamentals of Mammography*, 3rd ed. Elsevier; 2022.

Figure 1.36D
Wing E, Schiffman FJ. *Cecil Essentials of Medicine*, 10th ed. Elsevier; 2022. Courtesy S.E. Litwin, University of Utah, Salt Lake City.

Figures 1.27A, 1.36A, 51.17, 57.25A, 63.22B
Woodward PJ, et al. *Diagnostic Imaging: Obstetrics*, 3rd ed. Elsevier; 2016.

Figure 62.7
Wyllie R, et al. *Pediatric Gastrointestinal and Liver Disease*, 6th ed. Elsevier; 2021.

Figure 36.55A, 62.26
Van Hoorn JH. Pentalogy of Cantrell: two patients and a review to determine prognostic factors for optimal approach. *Eur J Pediatr*. 2008;167(1): 29–35.

Figure 12.44
Yeo CJ. *Shackelford's Surgery of the Alimentary Tract*, 8th ed. Elsevier; 2019.

Figures 2.3, 2.4, 2.6A, 2.38
Young AP. *Kinn's the Administrative Medical Assistant: An Applied Learning Approach*, 7th ed. Elsevier; 2011.

Figure 42.35
Yune HY, et al. Hysterosalpingography in infertility. *Am J Roentgenol Radium Ther Nucl Med*. 1974;122:642-651.

Figure 10.14
Zaheer A, Raman SP. *Diagnostic Imaging: Gastrointestinal*, 4th ed. Elsevier; 2022.

Figure 1.25B
Zimmerman J, Rotta AT. *Fuhrman and Zimmerman's Pediatric Critical Care*, 6th ed. Elsevier; 2022.

Figure 1.23
Zipes DP, et al. *Braunwald's Heart Disease: A Textbook of Cardiovascular Medicine*, 11th ed. Elsevier; 2019.

Figure 33.18C
Zoghbi WA, et al. Recommendations for evaluation of the severity of native valvular regurgitation with two-dimensional and Doppler echocardiography. *J Am Soc Echocardiogr*. 200316(7):777–802.

INDEX

Note: Page numbers followed by b indicate boxed material; those followed by f indicate figures; those followed by t indicate tables.

A

Abdomen
  FAST scan of, 563f
  fetal, 1572, 1590b–1591b
    cystic masses of, 1590–1591
    ultrasound, 1408t
  pain in, 84, 85t
  pseudopulsatile masses of, 195
  quadrants of, 88f
  regions of, 99f
  trauma to, 561–563
  ultrasound protocols for, 134–141, 134f
  viscera of, 88–89, 89f
Abdominal abscesses, 420–421, 423f
Abdominal aorta, 172, 173f, 174f, 178t
  branches of, 179–180
    anterior, 179–180
      celiac trunk, 179–180, 179f
      inferior mesenteric artery, 184, 184f
      superior mesenteric artery, 180–182, 183f
    dorsal, 187
    lateral, 185–187
  coronal plane of, 173, 176f
  Doppler flow patterns in, 212–214, 212b, 213f
  longitudinal plane of, 172–178, 175f, 176f
  longitudinal scans of, 130f, 131f, 140–141
  measurement of, 174–178, 177f
  size of, 176–178
  sonographic evaluation of, 172, 174b
  subcostal view of, 911f
  transverse plane of, 174, 177f
  transverse scans, 135–140, 136f, 137f, 138f, 139f
Abdominal aortic aneurysms, 188–193, 189f, 190f
  classification of, 190–191, 191f
  descriptive terms for, 191–192, 192f
  epigastric pain and, 569–570, 569f, 570f
  features of, 189b
  graft repair of, 194–195, 196f
  growth rate of, 190t
  risk factors for, 188, 190b
  symptoms of, 188–190, 190t
Abdominal cavity, 88–92
  abdominal muscles, 90–92, 90f
  abdominal wall, 89–90, 90f
  diaphragm, 88–89
  sonographic evaluation of, 1576–1580
    gastrointestinal system, 1576–1579
    hepatobiliary system, 1579–1580
  visceral organs of, 88–89
Abdominal circumference, 1291, 1577, 1577f
Abdominal cysts, 426, 427f
Abdominal hernias, 432, 432f
Abdominal muscles, 90–92, 90f
Abdominal pain
  acute, 767–775, 768f
  in children, 767–775, 768f
  description of, 84, 85t
Abdominal planes, 104–105, 104f
  body sections, 105, 105b, 105f
Abdominal quadrants, 104–105, 104f

Abdominal regions, 104–105, 104f
Abdominal scanning
  abnormalities in, 131
  clinical considerations before
    documentation, 125
    general abdominal examination, 125
    patient positions, 125, 125f
    scanning techniques, 125
    transducer positions, 126–128, 129f
    transducer selection, 125–126, 126f, 127f
    written order for examination, 125
  criteria for adequate scan in, 134, 135f
  Doppler evaluation, 141–146, 209–217
  fasting before, 125
  labeling scans, 124
  patient breathing technique tip in, 124
  sectional anatomy and, 102, 105–122, 122b
    in longitudinal plane, 104, 108–122
      at aorta and superior mesenteric artery level, 109, 121f
      at inferior vena cava, left lobe of the liver, and pancreas level, 109, 120f
      at liver, caudate lobe, and psoas muscle, 109, 119f
      at liver, duodenum, and pancreas level, 109, 120f
      at liver, gallbladder, and right kidney level, 108–109, 118f
      at liver, inferior vena cava, pancreas, and gastroduodenal artery level, 109, 120f
      at liver and gallbladder level, 108–109, 118f
      at right lobe of the liver level, 108, 117f
    in transverse plane, 104–108
      at bifurcation of aorta level, 108, 112f
      caudate lobe and celiac axis, 106–107, 108f
      at caudate lobe level, 106, 107f
      at dome of the liver level, 106–108, 106f
      at external iliac arteries level, 108, 113f
      at external iliac veins level, 108, 113f
      at female pelvis level, 108, 116f
      at gallbladder and right kidney level, 107, 110f
      at liver, gallbladder, and right kidney level, 107, 111f
      at male pelvis level, 108, 114f
      at right lobe of the liver level, 107, 112f
      at superior mesenteric artery and pancreas level, 107, 109f
Abdominal sonography, 129
Abdominal wall, 89–90, 90f, 434b
  anatomy of, 413–419, 414f–415f, 416f, 1161
  embryology of, 1560–1562, 1561f, 1562f, 1563f
  fetal, 1562
  hernia of, 432–434, 432f, 433f
  masses of, 428
  neoplasms of, 432
  pathology of, 428–434
  regions of, 105f
  sonographic evaluation of, 413–419, 414f–415f, 416f
Abdominal wall defects, 1338–1339, 1339f
Abdominopelvic cavity, 88–102

Abdominopelvic membranes and ligaments, 95–98, 96f
Abduction
  of hip joint, 853
  of scanning arm, 74f, 76
ABI. *see* Ankle-brachial index
Abortion
  complete, 1322
  incomplete spontaneous, 1322, 1322f
  threatened, 1320
Abruptio placentae, 1285, 1455
Abscesses
  abdominal, 420–421, 423f
  amebic, 264t, 266–267, 269f
  biloma, 425, 425f
  breast, 658t, 664, 664f
  definition of, 420
  gas-containing, 421–422, 423f
  lesser-sac, 423, 424f
  in liver transplantation patients, 593, 595f
  neck, 705–706, 706f
  pancreatic, 369t, 375–377
  in pancreatic transplantation patients, 633, 634f
  pelvic, 425–426, 425b, 426f
  pyogenic, 264t, 265–266, 267f
  in renal transplantation patients, 616, 619f
  splenic, 342–344, 345f, 346f
  subphrenic, 423–424, 424f
  tubo-ovarian, 1261b, 1263–1264
  ultrasound-guided draining and collection of, 534–535, 559
Absent cardiac activity, 1327, 1327f
Absorption, 12, 393
ACA. *see* Anterior cerebral artery
Acalculous cholecystitis, 294t–295t, 297, 300f
Acardiac anomaly, 1423, 1423f
Acceptance, illness and, 60
Accessory fissures, 239
Accessory spleen, 329, 331f
Acetabular notch, 853
Acetabulum, 851
  bony and cartilaginous, 854
Achilles tendon, 736, 749, 750f, 751b
Achondrogenesis, 1623t, 1626, 1626f, 1627f
Achondroplasia, 1623t, 1626
Acidic solution, 83
Acidosis, 83
Acini, 645–646
Acini cells, 360–361
ACKD. *see* Acquired cystic kidney disease
Acoustic emission, 514–515, 515f
Acoustic impedance, 11t, 12, 13f
Acoustics, 10–14, 11f, 11t
Acquired cystic disease of dialysis, 454t–458t
Acquired cystic kidney disease (ACKD), 460–461
Acquired immunodeficiency syndrome (AIDS)
  sonographic findings in, 471, 471f, 472f
  spleen in, 344
ACR FORM breast disease, 658
Acrania, 1335, 1336f, 1336t, 1524
  sonographic findings in, 1524, 1526f
Acromioclavicular joint, 744f

I-1

ACTH. *see* Adrenocorticotropic hormone
Acute appendicitis, 403–405, 404*t*, 406*f*
Acute cholecystitis, 293, 297*f*
  complications of, 296–297, 299*f*
  right upper quadrant pain in, 567–568, 568*f*
  sonographic findings in, 296, 298*f*, 299*f*
Acute glomerulonephritis, 454*t*–458*t*, 470
Acute hepatitis, 243*t*, 246, 246*f*
Acute interstitial nephritis, 470–471, 471*f*
Acute liver failure, 584–585
Acute mastitis, 663–664, 663*f*
Acute pancreatitis, 369–371, 369*t*, 370*f*
  extrapancreatic fluid collections and edema, 371–372, 372*f*
  sonographic findings in, 370–371, 371*f*
Acute pelvic pain, 578–579
Acute pyelonephritis, 806
Acute renal failure, 454*t*–458*t*, 473
Acute tubular necrosis (ATN), 473
  in renal transplantation patients, 615–616, 618*f*
  sonographic findings in, 473–474, 474*f*
Addison disease, 497, 499–500, 502*t*
Adduction, of hip joint, 853
Adenocarcinoma
  macrocystic, 380
  pancreatic, 638
  pancreatic ductal, 381, 384*f*, 385*f*
Adenoma, 775
  adrenal, 503–504, 504*f*
  cortical, 500–501
  follicular, 692, 693*f*
  gallbladder, 294*t*–295*t*, 305, 308*f*
  hepatic, 250*f*, 269–270, 273*f*
  liver cell, 271*t*
  parathyroid, 702–703
  renal, 454*t*–458*t*
  thyroid, 692, 694*f*
Adenomatoid malformation, congenital cystic, 1552–1554, 1553*f*
  sonographic findings in, 1554, 1554*b*
  type I, 1553–1554, 1553*f*
  type II, 1553–1554
  type III, 1553–1554, 1554*f*
Adenomatous tumors, renal, 468, 470*f*
Adenomyomas, 1212–1214
Adenomyomatosis of gallbladder, 294*t*–295*t*, 304, 307*f*
Adenomyosis, 1212–1216, 1260
  sonographic findings in, 1214
  transvaginal scanning of, 1212–1216
ADHD. *see* Attention-deficit/hyperactivity disorder
Adhesions
  female infertility and, 1277
  fluid collections in, 1240, 1241*f*
Administrative controls, 73–74
Adnexa
  interventional ultrasound of, 1270, 1270*f*
  pathology of, 1260, 1271*b*
    endometriosis and endometriomas, 1267–1270, 1268*f*, 1269*f*
    endometritis, 1266–1267, 1267*f*
    pelvic inflammatory disease, 1260–1266, 1261*b*, 1261*f*
    peritonitis, 1264–1266, 1266*f*
    salpingitis, hydrosalpinx, and pyosalpinx, 1261–1263, 1262*f*, 1262*t*, 1263*f*, 1264*f*
  postoperative ultrasound for, 1271
  tubo-ovarian abscesses, 1261*b*, 1263–1264
  ultrasound examination of, 1178*b*

Adnexal cysts, 1415, 1416*f*
Adnexal masses
  with ectopic pregnancy, 1330–1332, 1331*f*
  resistive index and, 1236
Adolescents
  benign ovarian cysts in, 1240
  special needs of, 58
ADPKD. *see* Autosomal dominant polycystic kidney disease
Adrenal cortex, 497
Adrenal cysts, 502–503, 502*f*, 503*f*
Adrenal glands, 88
  anatomy of, 494, 494*f*
  fetal ultrasound, 1408*t*
  neonatal/pediatric, 494
    adrenal hemorrhages, 796*t*
    anatomy of, 794, 794*f*
    hydronephrosis, 796*t*
    pathology of enlargement of, 796*t*
      adrenal hemorrhages, 796*t*, 807, 808*f*
      hydronephrosis, 796*t*
      prune belly syndrome, 796*t*, 801–802
      renal cystic disease, 804–805, 804*f*
      renal vein thrombosis, 807, 807*f*
    sonographic evaluation of, 497–498, 498*f*, 499*f*, 791
    vascular supply of, 496–497
Adrenal hemorrhage
  description of, 503, 503*f*
  neonatal/pediatric, 796*t*, 807, 808*f*
Adrenal medulla, 497
  neonatal, 795*f*
  tumors, 505–506
Adrenal neuroblastoma, 505–506, 506*f*, 810*f*
Adrenal tumors, 503–505
  malignant, 504, 504*f*
Adrenocorticotropic hormone (ACTH), 497
Adrenogenital syndrome, 500, 502*t*
Advanced maternal age (AMA), 1407
AED. *see* Automated external defibrillation
AFC. *see* Antral follicle count
Afferent arterioles, 437
AFP. *see* Alpha-fetoprotein
Afterload, 903–904, 910
Agenesis
  corpus callosum, 840–841, 841*f*, 1523*t*, 1535–1536
    sonographic findings in, 1536, 1536*f*
  liver, 239
  pancreatic, 359
  splenic, 327–329
Aging, 57
Agnathia, 1500–1501
AHW. *see* Anterior horn width
AI. *see* Aortic insufficiency
AIDS. *see* Acquired immunodeficiency syndrome
Airborne precautions, 54
Airborne transmission, of infections, 50
AIUM. *see* American Institute of Ultrasound in Medicine
Alanine aminotransferase (ALT), 228, 228*t*, 230
ALARA principle, 1288
Albumin, 228, 231
Alcoholic cirrhosis, 247*f*
Aliasing, 24
  color Doppler, 160, 161*f*, 162*f*
  definition of, 156
  elimination of, 159*b*
  range-ambiguity artifact values and, 157*t*
  reduction of, 159*b*
  spectral Doppler, 156

Alimentary tract, 389–390, 390*f*
Alkaline phosphatase, 228, 228*t*, 231
Alkaline solution, 83
Alkalosis, 83
Allantoic ducts, 1460–1461
Alloimmune thrombocytopenia, 1411
Alobar holoprosencephaly, 843, 843*f*, 1532–1533, 1532*f*
Alpha angle, Graf's, 860–866, 862*b*, 862*f*
Alpha cells, 361
Alpha-fetoprotein (AFP), 531–532
  prenatal diagnosis of congenital anomalies, 1427–1429, 1427*b*, 1427*f*, 1428*b*
ALT. *see* Alanine aminotransferase
AMA. *see* Advanced maternal age
Amaurosis fugax, 1072
Ambiguous genitalia, 1617–1618, 1618*f*
Amebic abscess, 264*t*, 266–267, 269*f*
Amenorrhea, 1174
American College of Radiology (ACR), Standard for the Performance of Ultrasound Examination of the Female Pelvis, 1177
American College of Radiology Sonography Descriptive Form, 658, 658*t*
American Institute of Ultrasound in Medicine (AIUM), 6
  pelvic ultrasound standards, 1177
  shoulder imaging recommendations, 744
American Registry for Diagnostic Medical Sonography (ARDMS), 4, 6
American Society of Echocardiography (ASE), 6
Ammonium, 229
Amniocentesis, 1285
  prenatal diagnosis of congenital anomalies, 1430–1431, 1430*f*, 1431*f*
Amnion, 1289–1290, 1443*f*, 1462*f*
  embryonic development of, 1327
  evaluation of, 1327
  sonographic findings of, in abnormal intrauterine pregnancies, 1324*b*
Amniotic band syndrome, 1564, 1566, 1568*f*
  amniotic fluid and, 1483–1485
  fetal membranes and, 1483–1485, 1485*f*, 1486*f*
Amniotic cavity, 1308–1310, 1474
Amniotic fluid, 1374, 1375*f*, 1599
  abnormal volumes, 1479–1481
    oligohydramnios, 1480–1481, 1480*b*, 1481*f*
    polyhydramnios, 1479–1480, 1480*b*, 1480*f*
  amniotic band syndrome, 1483–1485
  amniotic fluid index, 1477–1478, 1477*f*
  assessment of, 1475–1477
    quantitative, 1476–1477
    subjective, 1476, 1476*f*, 1477*f*
  characteristics of, 1475, 1475*b*, 1475*f*, 1476*f*
  derivation, 1474–1475
  fetal membranes and, 1474, 1489*b*–1490*b*
  single pocket assessment, 1478, 1478*f*
  twin pregnancies, assessment in, 1478–1479, 1478*f*, 1479*f*
  two-diameter pocket assessment, 1478, 1478*f*
  volume, abnormal, 1600, 1600*b*
Amniotic sac, 1443*f*, 1462*f*
Amniotic sludge, 1475
A-mode transducers, 528, 529*f*
Amplitude, 11–12
Amplitude modulation (A-mode), 17, 18*f*
Ampulla of Vater, 282
Amputation, 1118

Amylase, 360–361, 361t
  diseases that affect, 361t, 362, 362t
  urine, 362
Amyloid cardiomyopathy, 992, 994f
Amyloidosis, 339–340, 339f
Anaplastic carcinoma, 697, 697f
Anasarca, 1407
Anastomosis, 206
  stenosis at, 1124f
Anatomic directions, 132–134, 135f
Anatomy, 80, 101b
Androgen, 1234
Anechoic, 130, 133f
Anembryonic pregnancy, 1320, 1323, 1323f, 1324b
Anemia
  autoimmune hemolytic, 341
  hemolytic, 341
  sickle cell
    description of, 340
    illustration of, 340f
    stroke in, 1102, 1103f
Anencephaly, 1292, 1335, 1336f, 1336t, 1523–1524
  differential considerations for, 1524t
  sonographic findings in, 1524, 1525f
Aneuploidies, 1285, 1287–1288
Aneurysms
  arterial duplex imaging of, 1124–1126, 1125f
  cervical carotid system, 1078
  definition of, 971
  false, 190–191, 191f, 974t
  fusiform, 191, 192f
  graft repair complications, 194–195, 196f
  iliac, 195
  inflammatory aortic, 192
  mycotic, 192
  popliteal artery, 1125f
  saccular, 191, 192f
  sinus of Valsalva, 974, 976f
  sonographic findings of, 192, 193b, 193f
  splanchnic, 185–187, 185f, 195
  thoracic, 195
  true, 190–191, 191f, 974t
  vein of Galen, 1537
Angiogram, ultrasound, 516f
Angiolipomas, 454t–458t, 469f
Angiomyolipoma, renal, 467, 469f, 624
Angle of incidence, 6
Angle of reflection, 6
Anisotropy, 741, 741f, 743t
Ankle, 749–750, 750t
Ankle-brachial index (ABI), 1115, 1115t
Annotation, 656–658, 656f, 657b, 657f, 658t
Annular pancreas, 360, 361f
Anophthalmia, 1501
Anophthalmos, 1392
Anorectal atresia, 1585, 1588
Anotia, 1500, 1501f
Anteflexion, 1166f, 1207f
Anterior, 132
Anterior abdominal wall
  abnormalities of, 1562–1571, 1564b, 1564t
    amniotic band syndrome, 1566, 1568f
    Beckwith-Wiedemann syndrome, 1566–1567, 1568f
    bladder and cloacal exstrophy, 1567–1568, 1568f, 1569f
    limb-body wall complex, 1570–1571, 1570f
    pentalogy of Cantrell, ectopia cordis, and cleft sternum, 1568–1570, 1569f

Anterior abdominal wall (Continued)
    fetal, 1560, 1570b–1571b
    muscles of, 1161f
Anterior cerebral artery (ACA), 1089–1090
Anterior communicating artery (ACoA), 1090
Anterior horn width (AHW), 830, 831f
Anterior pararenal space, 92, 492, 492b, 493f
Anterior/posterior direction, 132
Anterior tibial artery, 1112
Anterior tibial veins (ATVs), 1130f, 1131
Anterior urethral valves, 1612–1614, 1614f
Anteversion, 1162–1163, 1166f, 1207f
Antiradial plane, 657
Antral follicle count (AFC), 1277
Aorta
  abdominal, 172, 173f, 174f, 178t
    dorsal branches of, 187
    lateral branches of, 185–187
  abdominal scanning of, at bifurcation level, 108, 112f
  abnormalities, 971–979, 973f
  anatomy of, 971
  ascending, 172
  atherosclerosis of, 974, 977f
  descending, 172
  Doppler flow patterns in, 145, 212–214, 212b, 213f
  fetal circulation, 1446f
  pathology of, 187–195, 187f
    tumors, 978–979, 978f
  retroperitoneum and, 494f, 496
  root of, 171, 172f
  sections of, 171–172
  sections/segments of, 971
  sonographic evaluation of, 179–180, 179f
Aortic aneurysms, 971–974
  abdominal, 188–193, 189f, 190f
    classification of, 190–191, 191f
    descriptive terms for, 191–192, 192f
    epigastric pain and, 569–570, 569f, 570f
    features of, 189b
    graft repair of, 194–195, 196f
    growth rate of, 190t
    risk factors for, 188, 190b
    symptoms of, 188–190, 190t
  aortic ectasia versus, 187
  causes of, 971–974
  diagnosis of, 972–973
  fusiform, 191, 192f
  rupture of, 192–193, 192f
  sonographic findings of, 192, 193b, 193f
Aortic arches, 901, 901f, 1008–1009, 1009b, 1009f
  Doppler measurements, 1014t
  extracranial cerebrovascular imaging, 1070
  fetal circulation, 1446f
  interrupted, 1056–1057
  oblique long axis view of, 1026–1029, 1027f, 1028f
Aortic branches, 901, 901f
Aortic dissection, 193–194, 194f, 195f, 572–573, 572f
  causes of, 572, 572b
  classification of, 974
  clinical findings for, 572–573, 573t
  complications of, 974
  DeBakey and Stanford classification of, 974, 974f
  imaging of, 973
  sonographic findings of, 573, 574f
  type I, 974, 974f, 975f
  type II, 974, 974f, 975f
  type III, 974, 974f, 976f

Aortic ectasia, 187
Aortic insufficiency (AI), 956, 963–966, 963t
Aortic regurgitation, 963, 963t, 964f, 965f, 966f
Aortic root motion, 989, 991f
Aortic sclerosis, 967
  types of, 966
Aortic stenosis, 964t, 966–970, 966f, 967f, 969b, 969f, 970b, 970f, 972t, 1050–1052
  critical, 1050, 1051f
  subvalvular/supravalvular, 1050–1052, 1051f, 1052f
Aortic ulcer, penetrating, 977, 977f
Aortic valve, 901, 901f
  atherosclerosis of, 968f
  bicuspid, 966–967, 968f
  Doppler measurements, 1014t
  M-mode imaging of, 935f, 945–946, 946f, 950f
  unicuspid, 967f
Aortic valve area (AVA), 967
Aphasia, 1072
Apical transducer location, 918, 919f
Apical views
  two-chamber, 933, 938b, 940f, 941f, 944f
  four-chamber, 572f, 911, 911f, 912f, 921f, 922b, 922f, 941f, 943f
    right heart, 938b
  five-chamber, 922b, 932–938, 936f, 937f, 938b
  for color flow mapping, 932–938, 944f
  long-axis, 938b
  for pericardial effusion, 1036f
  two-dimensional, 932–938, 936f, 937f, 938b
Apical window, 924b
Apocrine metaplasia, 661
Aponeuroses, 736
Aponeurosis tissue, 735f
Appendectomy, 777
Appendiceal abscess, 781f
Appendicitis
  acute, 403–405, 404t, 406f
  pediatric, 776–781, 777f, 780f, 781f
  retrocecal, 404
  right lower quadrant pain in, 573t, 574–575, 576f
Appendicoliths, 404, 779, 781f
Appendix
  abnormalities of, mucocele, 404t, 405–408, 408f
  normal, 779f
  sonographic evaluation of, 398, 404–405, 407f
Appendix testis, 710f
Aqueductal stenosis, 829, 1536, 1537f
Arachnoid cysts, 845–846, 846f, 1523t, 1540f
Arachnoid mater, 873–875
Architectural distortion, 658
Arcuate arteries, 436
  calcifications of, 1192–1193
  neonatal, 793
  in renal allograft, 611
Arcuate vessels, 1192–1193, 1193f
ARDMS. see American Registry for Diagnostic Medical Sonography
Areola, 645
Arhinia, 1505
Arnold-Chiari malformation, 839–840, 840f
  type II, 1392–1393
Arrhenoblastoma, 1256
Arrhythmia
  causes of, 35
  definition of, 35
  fetal, 1012–1013

ART. *see* Assisted reproductive technology
Arterial duplex imaging, 1118–1126
  interpretation of, 1120–1122, 1120*b*, 1121*f*, 1122*b*, 1122*f*
    aneurysms and pseudoaneurysms, 1124–1126, 1125*f*
    bypass graft surveillance, 1122–1123, 1122*f*, 1123*f*
    dialysis access grafts, 1123–1124, 1123*f*, 1124*f*
    lower extremity, 1119–1120, 1119*f*, 1120*f*
    upper extremity, 1120, 1120*f*
Arterial occlusive disease, 1117, 1117*f*
Arterial stress testing, 1116
Arterial system, 1134
Arterial testing, indirect, 1114–1118
Arterial thrombosis, 633–634, 635*f*, 636*f*
Arteries, 171
  anatomy of, 1111
  femoral, 178*t*
  layers of, 171, 171*f*
  lower extremity, 1111–1112, 1111*f*
  upper extremity, 1112, 1112*f*
  veins *versus*, 1134
Arterioles, 437
Arteriosclerosis, 187–188, 188*f*
Arteriovenous fistulas (AVFs), 482–483, 484*f*, 589, 617*f*
Arteriovenous malformations (AVMs), 1216, 1217*f*
Arthrogryposis multiplex congenita, 1632–1633, 1632*f*
Artifacts, 147, 165*b*
  attenuation, 153–156
    enhancement and, 156, 156*f*, 157*f*
    shadowing and, 153–156, 155*f*
  color Doppler, 160–163
    aliasing and, 160, 161*f*, 162*f*
    mirror image, shadowing, clutter, and noise and, 160–163, 162*f*, 163*f*
  definition of, 147
  musculoskeletal imaging, 740–743, 741*f*, 742*f*, 743*t*
  propagation of, 147–153
    grating lobes and, 151, 153*f*
    mirror image and, 149, 151*f*
    range ambiguity and, 151–152, 154*f*
    refraction and, 149, 152*f*
    reverberation and, 148–149, 149*f*, 150*f*, 151*f*
    section thickness and, 148, 148*f*
    speckle and, 148, 149*f*
    speed error and, 151, 154*f*
  reverberation, 129, 132*f*, 149*f*
  spectral Doppler, 156–160
    aliasing and, 156, 159*b*
    mirror image and, 160, 160*f*
    noise and, 160, 160*f*
    Nyquist limit and, 156–159, 157*t*, 158*f*, 159*b*, 159*f*
    range ambiguity and, 157*t*, 159–160
    speed error, 743, 743*t*
  types of, 129
As low as reasonably achievable (ALARA) principle, 1091
Ascariasis, 318, 319*f*
Ascending aorta, 172

Ascites, 96, 408
  after liver transplantation, 605, 605*f*
  fetal, 1589*f*, 1590
  hydrops and, 1486–1487
  inflammatory, 420, 422*f*
  malignant, 420, 422*f*
  pancreatic, 374–375
  peritoneal, 419–420, 421*f*, 422*f*
  ultrasound-guided draining of, 559
ASD. *see* Autism spectrum disorder
ASE. *see* American Society of Echocardiography
Aspartate aminotransferase (AST), 228, 228*t*, 230
Asphyxia, neonatal, 814
Asphyxiating thoracic dystrophy, 1546
Aspiration, of renal masses, 449–450, 452*t*
Asplenia, 1581
Assisted reproductive technology (ART), 1278–1279, 1279*f*
AST. *see* Aspartate aminotransferase
Ataxia, 1072
Atherosclerosis
  aortic, 974, 977*f*
  description of, 187, 188*f*, 480
Atherosclerotic disease, 1076–1077, 1077*f*, 1078*f*
ATN. *see* Acute tubular necrosis
Atoms, 81
Atresia
  laryngeal, 1554–1555
  tracheal, 1554–1555, 1555*f*
Atretic common bile duct, 771
Atrial septal defect, 1036–1038, 1037*f*
  ostium primum, 1037–1038, 1037*f*, 1038*f*
  ostium secundum, 1037, 1037*f*
  sinus venosus septal defect, 1037*f*, 1038, 1038*f*
Atrial systole, 901*b*
Atrialized chamber, 1043
Atrioventricular block, 1064–1066, 1064*f*
Atrioventricular canal
  division of, 1009
  partitioning of, 1010*f*
Atrioventricular node, 1010
Atrioventricular septal defect (AVSD), 1041–1043, 1041*f*
Atrioventricular valves, 902
Atrium
  of lateral ventricles, 815, 816*f*
  primitive, 1010*f*
Atrophy
  renal, 454*t*–458*t*, 472
  splenic, 336
Attention-deficit/hyperactivity disorder (ADHD), 763*t*
Attenuation
  artifacts associated with, 153–156
    enhancement and, 156, 156*f*, 157*f*
    shadowing and, 153–156, 155*f*
  description of, 12*t*, 14, 14*f*
Attenuation effects, 669
ATVs. *see* Anterior tibial veins
Audio signals, 920–923
Augmentation, 1140*f*
  lower extremity, 1140–1141
  upper extremity, 1140
Autism spectrum disorder (ASD), 763*t*, 831–832
Autoimmune hemolytic anemia, 341
Automated external defibrillation (AED), 66, 66*f*
Automated whole breast ultrasound, 678–681, 679*f*

Autonomy, 1296–1297
Autosomal dominant polycystic disease, 377
Autosomal dominant polycystic kidney disease (ADPKD), 378*t*, 461, 1607–1608, 1608*f*, 1609*f*
  neonatal/pediatric, 805
  sonographic findings in, 461–462, 462*f*
Autosomal recessive polycystic kidney disease (ARPKD), 461
  neonatal/pediatric, 804*f*, 805*f*
AVA. *see* Aortic valve area
AVFs. *see* Arteriovenous fistulas
AVMs. *see* Arteriovenous malformations
AVSD. *see* Atrioventricular septal defect
Axial imaging, 1177–1178
Axial resolution, 13–14, 13*f*
Axilla, 645, 645*f*
Axillary artery, 1112, 1120, 1120*f*
Axillary vein, 1133
Azimuthal resolution, 13–14

B

BA. *see* Basilar artery
Back muscles, 91
Bacteremia, 332–333
Bacterial cholangitis, 315, 318*f*
Baker, Donald, 8–10, 10*f*
Baker cyst, 579, 580*f*, 739, 1147, 1147*f*
Ballantyne syndrome, 1487
Banana sign, 1351, 1392–1393, 1530*f*
Banding, 157*f*
Bandwidth, 13
Barber, Frank, 8–10
Bare area, 219, 220*f*, 417
Barlow maneuver, 859, 859*f*
Barrier devices, 54
Basal ganglia, neonatal, 818, 819*f*
Basal plate, 1443, 1443*b*
Baseline, 26
Baseline shift, 156–160
Basic ultrasound imaging, 123, 146*b*
Basilar artery (BA), 1089
Basilic vein, 1140
"Basket sign," 464, 464*f*
Battledore placenta, 1444–1445
B-cell tumor, 381, 384*f*
Beckwith-Wiedemann syndrome, 1510, 1511*f*, 1566–1567, 1568*f*
  pediatric, 773, 807–808
  sonographic findings of, 1564*t*
Bed rest, 48–49
Bedpans, 48–49, 48*f*
Beemer-Langer dysplasia, 1630
Bell clapper deformity, 720
Beneficence, 1296
Benign conditions, breast, 659–660
Benign lesions, thyroid gland, 691–693, 693*f*
Benign ovarian cysts
  in adolescents, 1240
  paraovarian cysts, 1240, 1240*b*, 1241*f*
  peritoneal inclusion cysts, 1239–1242, 1240*f*
  simple cysts in postmenopausal women, 1240–1242
Benign testicular masses, 726–728, 727*f*
Benign tumors
  hepatic, 268–269
  liver, pediatric, 773–775
  renal, 467, 469*f*, 488–490

Benign tumors (Continued)
    adenomatous tumors, 468, 470f
    angiomyolipoma, 467, 469f
    lipomas, 454t–458t, 468, 470f
    oncocytoma, 468, 470f
    splenic, 349, 350f
Bernoulli equation, 913–914, 914f
Beside ultrasound, 63–64, 63f, 64f
Beta angle, Graf's, 860–866, 862b, 862f
Beta cells, 361
Bezoars, gastric, 399–400, 400t, 401f
Biceps tendon, 736, 736f
    sonographic evaluation of, 744, 744f, 745f
    subluxation/dislocation of, 751, 751f
Bicornuate uterus, 1208f, 1273f
Bicuspid aortic valve, 966–967, 968f, 973, 1033, 1050, 1050f
Bifid renal pelvis, 436–437, 446
Bilateral pararectal space, 496, 496f
Bilateral venous duplex imaging, 1148
Bile, 83, 230, 230f
Bile ducts, 282, 282f
    cholangitis and, 315–318
    sonographic evaluation of, 289, 292f, 293f
Bile leaks, 604, 604f
Bile pigments, 230
Biliary atresia, neonatal, 771, 771t, 772f
Biliary cirrhosis, 247f
Biliary dilation, 568, 569f
Biliary ductal ischemia, 597–598
Biliary neoplasms, intrahepatic, 318
Biliary obstructions, 312, 313f
    distal, 259, 261t, 262f
    extrahepatic, 312–313, 313f
    proximal, 258–259, 261t, 262f
Biliary system, 281, 322b–323b
    anatomy of, 281–285, 282f
    laboratory data regarding, 285
    pathology of, 289–308, 294t–295t
        cholelithiasis, 294t–295t, 300, 301f, 302f, 303f, 304f
        gallbladder carcinoma, 306–308, 309f, 310f
        gallbladder disease, 290–293
        gallbladder torsion, 299–300
        gallbladder wall thickening, 293, 296b, 296f
        sludge, 290–293, 294t–295t, 295f
    pediatric, 765, 765b, 766f
    physiology of, 285
    sonographic evaluation of, 285–289, 290b
        bile ducts, 289, 292f, 293f
        gallbladder, 284f, 286f, 287–289, 290f, 291f, 292f
        protocol, 285–287, 289f, 290f
        transverse scans of, 134
    ultrasound protocol for, 289t
    vascular supply of, 285
Biliary tree pathology, 308–321
    ascariasis, 318, 319f
    Caroli disease, 310, 311f
    cholangiocarcinoma, 318–321, 319f, 320f
    cholangitis, 315–318
    dilated biliary ducts, 311–312, 312f
    hemobilia, 315, 317f
    intrahepatic biliary neoplasms, 318
    metastases, 321
    pneumobilia, 315, 317f

Bilirubin, 285
    definition of, 225
    detoxification of, 229
    direct-acting, 229, 229t
    indirect-acting, 229, 229t
    liver function tests, 231
Biloma, 425, 593, 594f, 604, 604f
Biometry, fetal ultrasound, 1408t
Biophysical profile (BPP), 1399–1401, 1399b
    amniotic fluid volume, 1401, 1401f
    fetal body and trunk gross movements, 1400f, 1401
    fetal breathing movements, 1399, 1400f
    fetal tone, 1401, 1401f
Biopsy, 543–548, 543f, 544f, 545f, 546f, 547f, 548f
    after renal transplants, 555, 555f
    breast, large-core needle, 676
    complications of, 539–540, 539f
    contraindications for, 531, 531f
    core, 533, 533f, 534f
    indication for, 530–531, 531f
    kidney, 554–555, 555f
    liver, 552–553, 552f, 553f, 554f
    lung, 556–557, 556f
    musculoskeletal, 557–558, 557f, 558f
    neck nodes and masses, 557
    pancreatic, 553–554
    pelvic mass, 558
    prostate, 558, 558f, 559f
    renal, 548f, 555f, 615, 616f, 617f
    retroperitoneal lymph nodes, 555–556, 556f
    thyroid, 557, 557f
Biopsy gun, 533
Biparietal diameter (BPD), 1291, 1383, 1384b, 1384f, 1384t, 1385f
BI-RADS. see Breast Imaging Reporting and Data System
Bladder, 89
    as acoustic window, 1189, 1189f
    anatomy of, 86, 437, 1161–1162, 1162b, 1163f
    development of, 1595
    distended, 1178, 1266f
    exstrophy of, 1564t, 1567–1568, 1568f, 1569f
    extrophy of, 1603–1604, 1604f
    fetal
        not seen, 1600
        sonographic evaluation of, 1596
    neonatal/pediatric
        anatomy of, 794–795, 795f
        sonographic evaluation of preparation for, 792
    sonographic evaluation of, 451–453, 1177, 1179f, 1182f
    tumors of, 486–487, 488f
Bladder diverticulum, 485, 488f
Bladder-flap hematoma, 430
Bladder outlet obstruction, neonatal/pediatric, 801–802, 802f
Bleeding, first-trimester, 1320–1326
    abnormal sac criteria, 1322–1323
    absent intrauterine sac, 1320–1322, 1321t, 1322f
    anembryonic pregnancy, 1323, 1323f, 1324b
    gestational sac without embryo or yolk sac, 1322
    gestational trophoblastic disease, 1323–1326, 1324f, 1325f, 1326f
    placental hematomas, 1320
    subchorionic hemorrhage, 1320, 1321f
Blighted ovum, 1320

Bliss, William Roderic, 7, 8f
Blood
    composition of, 81, 82f
    functions of, 81–83
    in urine, 437–438
Blood-borne precautions, 55
Blood flow
    direction of, in transcranial color Doppler imaging, 1096
    physiology of, 908
    principles of, 905–907, 905f
    velocity of, 910, 910f
Blood flow analysis, 209–210
Blood glucose, 361t, 362
Blood pressure
    definition of, 36
    in gastrointestinal assessment, 84
    measurement of, 36, 36f, 37b, 37f
Blood pressure cuff, 36, 37f
Blood urea nitrogen (BUN), 229, 439
Blood vessels, 1008, 1008f
Blunt trauma
    abdomen, 767
    FAST scan in, 563–567, 563b, 563f, 564b, 564f, 565f
        sonographic findings of, 564–566, 566f
    splenic, 345–348, 350f
B-mode transducers, 528, 529f
Bochdalek, foramen of, 1555, 1556f
Body cavities, 88, 88f
Body fluids, sonographer exposure to, 67
Body mechanics
    definition of, 38
    patient transfer and, 38–39
Body systems, 81–88, 82t
Bones
    hip, 851, 851f
    nasal, 1317–1318, 1317f
Bony pelvis, 1159–1160, 1159f, 1189
Bosniak classification, of cysts, 449, 452t, 458–459
Bouffard position, 747f
Bowel, 1174–1175
    fetal
        abnormalities of, 1586–1590
        sonographic evaluation of, 1578–1579, 1579f
    herniation of, 1561–1562, 1565–1566, 1567f
    hyperechoic, 1589, 1589b
    layers of, 394, 394b
    physiologic herniation of, 1313, 1314f
    sonographic evaluation of, 1198–1199, 1198f
Bowel herniation, 1338, 1339f
Bowel ischemia, 606–607, 607f
Bowel omphaloceles, 1563, 1566f
Bowman capsule, 437
Boyle, Robert, 6
BPD. see Biparietal diameter
BPP. see Biophysical profile
Brachial artery, 1112
Brachial pressures, 1115
Brachial veins, 1133
Brachiocephalic artery, 901
Bradycardia
    definition of, 35
    embryonic, 1327
    fetal, 1012
Brain death, 1103
Brainstem, neonatal, 818–819
Branchial apparatus, 1493

Branchial cleft cysts, 705, 705f, 1512
Breast, 643, 680b–681b
  abscesses of, 658t, 664, 664f
  anatomy of, 645–652
    clock face method, 656f
    lymphatic drainage of, 651, 651f
    male, 651–652, 652b, 652f
    normal, 645–648, 645f, 646f, 647f, 648f
    quadrant method, 656f
    vascular supply, 649–650, 650f
  augmentation of, 666–671, 666f, 667f
  biopsy of, large-core needle, 676
  clinical evaluation of patient with problem, 659b
  dense, 648, 649f
  evaluation of, 652–658
    clinical assessment, 654
    diagnostic breast interrogation, 654
    interventional breast procedures, 654
    screening, 652, 653b
    targeted *versus* whole breast scan, 654
  fatty, 648–649, 649f
  interventional procedures, 654
  lumps in, 654
  parenchymal patterns, 648–649, 649f
  pathology of, 658–666
    abscesses, 658t, 664, 664f
    acute mastitis, 663–664, 663f
    chronic mastitis, 664
    cystosarcoma phyllodes, 658t, 675, 675f
    diabetic mastopathy, 666
    fat necrosis, 658t, 664, 665f
    fibroadenoma, 658t, 661–662, 662f
    fibrocystic changes, 658t
    fibrocystic dysplasia/fibrocystic changes, 660–661, 661f
    hematoma, 664–665
    intraductal papilloma, 658t, 665–666, 666f
    lipomas, 658t, 665, 665f
    lymphoma, 676
    metastatic disease, 676
    pregnant and/or lactating patient, 662
    seroma/lymphocele, 665, 665f
  physiology of, 644–645
  sonographic evaluation of, 654–658
    automated whole breast ultrasound, 678–681, 679f
    elastography, 679–681, 679f, 680f
    patient positioning for, 655, 655f
    technique for, 655–656, 655f, 656f
  ultrasound-guided interventional procedures in, 676
    large-core needle biopsy, 676
    preoperative needle wire localization, 676, 676f
  zones of, 657f
Breast cancer, 644, 671
  in males, 651–652, 652b, 652f
  mammographic findings in, 653–654, 653b, 653t, 654b
  risk factors for, 644b
  screening for, 652, 653b
  signs and symptoms of, 653b
  types of
    colloid/mucinous carcinoma, 675
    comedocarcinoma, 672, 672f
    ductal carcinoma in situ, 671, 671f
    inflammatory carcinoma, 673, 674f

Breast cancer *(Continued)*
    invasive ductal carcinoma, 672
    invasive lobular carcinoma, 673, 674f
    medullary carcinoma, 673, 675f
    Paget disease, 654–655, 673, 673f
    papillary carcinoma, 672–673, 672f
    scirrhous carcinoma, 674–675
    tubular carcinoma, 674
Breast cysts
  description of, 659
  sonographic evaluation of, 659–660
Breast hematoma, 664–665
Breast Imaging Reporting and Data System (BI-RADS), 653
  categories of mammographic masses, 653t
Breast implants
  complications of, 667–668, 667f
  extracapsular, 669, 669f
  intracapsular, 668, 669f
  ruptured, 668–669, 669f
Breast masses
  in males, 652f
  sonographic characteristics of, 669–671
    attenuation effects, 669
    compressibility, 669
    internal echo pattern, 669
    margins, 669, 670f
    mobility, 669
    orientation, 669
    shape, 669
    vascularity, 671
  vascularity, 657–658
Breast self-examination (BSE), 652, 653b
Breathing, by patient
  in abdominal scanning, 124
  extreme shortness of breath, 570–572
Breech, 1346–1347, 1347f
Brescia-Cimino graft, 1124f
Brightness modulation (B-mode), 17–18, 18f
Broad ligaments, 1165, 1166f
Bronchial atresia, congenital, 1554
Bronchogenic cysts, 1550, 1551f
Brown, Tom, 7
Bruit, 1072
B-scanners, 7–8
BSE. *see* Breast self-examination
Budd, George, 256–257
Budd-Chiari syndrome, 258
  liver findings in, 258t
  sonographic findings in, 258, 259f
Buffers, 83
Bulbus cordis, 1009
Bull's eye (target) lesion, 266
Bull's eye sign, 406f
BUN. *see* Blood urea nitrogen
Bundle of His, 903
Bursa, 738–739, 738f, 740t
Bursitis, 72
Bypass graft surveillance, 1122–1123, 1122f, 1123f

C

CA. *see* Celiac axis
CA 125 test, 1244–1245
"Cake" kidney, 1601f
Calcifications
  arcuate arteries, 1192–1193
  dermoid tumors, 1253f
  intratendinous, 753f

Calcifications *(Continued)*
  periventricular, 1541f
  urinary tract, 479, 480f
  uterine, 1210–1212, 1213f
Calcitonin, 682–683
Calcium, serum, 700–701
Calf vein imaging, 1149
  duplex imaging, 1149
  evaluation of, 1149
Calyx, 436–437
Camptomelic dysplasia, 1623t, 1629, 1630f
Candidiasis
  hepatic, 264t, 266, 267f
  hepatosplenic, 344
Capillaries, 171
Capsular arteries, 710–711, 711f
Carbohydrates, 227
Carbon dioxide reactivity, 1097
Carcinoma, 671
  anaplastic, 697, 697f
  cervical, 1204, 1206b, 1206f
  cholangiocarcinoma, 318–321, 319f, 320f
  colloid, 675
  colorectal, 520f
  endometrial, 1223–1224, 1224b, 1224f
  fallopian tube, 1257
  follicular, 694–696, 696f
  gallbladder, 306–308, 309f, 310f
  gastric, 400t, 401–402, 402f
  ovarian, 1244–1246, 1246f, 1247f
  parathyroid, 703–704
  transitional cell, 454t–458t, 464–466
Cardiac abnormalities, 1058–1062
  cardiosplenic syndromes, 1060–1062
  congenital vena cava to left atrial communication, 1059–1060
  cor triatriatum, 1059, 1059f
  ectopia cordis, 1062, 1062f
  single ventricle, 1058–1059, 1058f, 1059f
  total anomalous pulmonary venous return, 899, 1060, 1060f, 1061f
Cardiac anomalies, 1334
Cardiac arrest, 66
Cardiac axis, 1018f
Cardiac cycle, 901–903, 902f, 909–910, 909f
Cardiac enlargement, 1034–1036
Cardiac malposition, 1033, 1035f
Cardiac masses, 1005b
  definition of, 995
  normal variants *versus*, 995, 998b
  subacute bacterial endocarditis, 1000–1006, 1004f, 1005f
  thrombus, 998–1000, 1003f
  vegetations, 1000–1006, 1004f, 1005f
Cardiac nerves, 903
Cardiac orifice, 390
Cardiac output (CO), 910, 914, 990b, 1097, 1097b
Cardiac structures, M-mode imaging of, 920, 943–952, 950b
  aortic valve, 935f, 945–946, 946f, 950f
  interventricular septum, 946, 951f
  left atrium, 945–946, 950f
  left ventricle, 946, 951f
  mitral valve, 943–944, 950f
  normal measurements, 950t
  pulmonary valve, 950–952, 951f
  tricuspid valve, 946
Cardiac tamponade, 982–983, 984f, 985b, 985f

Cardiac tumors, 1058
  categories of, 995–998, 999f
  lipomatous hypertrophy, 998, 1001f
  malignant primary, 998, 1002f
  myxomas, 998, 999f
  papillary fibroelastoma, 998, 1000f
  rhabdomyoma, 998, 1001f
Cardinal ligaments, 1165, 1165f
Cardiomyopathy, 1005b, 1034–1036, 1036f
  amyloid, 992, 994f
  categories of, 985–986
  definition of, 985–986
  dilated, 986–993, 988b, 988f, 989f, 990b, 990f, 991f, 992b
  eosinophilic, 992, 993f
  hypertrophic, 993–995, 996f, 997b, 997f
  idiopathic restrictive, 992
  infiltrative, 990–992, 992b
  ischemic, 989
  nonischemic, 989
  predictors of, 992b
  prognosis of, 990
  restrictive, 990–992, 992b
  Takotsubo, 993
Cardiopulmonary resuscitation (CPR), 66–67, 66f
Cardiosplenic syndromes, 1060–1062
Cardiovascular system, embryology of, 1008–1010
Caroli disease, 310, 311f
Carotid artery disease, 1082–1083
Carotid artery stenting, 1083–1084, 1084f
Carotid body tumors, 1078, 1079f
Carotid duplex imaging, 1070f
  after stent placement or endarterectomy, 1083–1084, 1084f
  aneurysms, 1078
  atherosclerotic disease, 1076–1077, 1077f, 1078f
  carotid body tumors, 1078, 1079f
  dissection, 1078, 1079f
  fibromuscular dysplasia, 1078–1079
  interpretation of, 1079–1082, 1080t, 1081f, 1082b
  intraoperative use of, 1083
  normal findings of, 1074–1076, 1074f, 1075f
  procedure, 1073–1074, 1073f
  pseudoaneurysms, 1078
  technical aspects of, 1072–1079
  three-dimensional, 1084–1085, 1085f
Carotid intima-media thickness, 1081
Carotid pulse, 35, 36f
Carotid sheath, 1070
Carotid siphon, 1088, 1094
Carpal tunnel
  definition of, 72
  sonographic evaluation of, 748, 749f
Carpal tunnel syndrome (CTS), 755–757, 756b, 756f
Carpenter syndrome, 1633f
Cartilage interface sign, 752
Catheters, urinary, 43–44, 44f
Cat-scratch disease, 769, 770f
Cauda equina, 873, 874f, 875–876, 876f
  normal pulsatile movement of, 879–880, 880f
Caudal direction, 132–134
Caudal pancreatic artery, 180, 359
Caudal regression syndrome (CRS), 1414, 1631–1632, 1631f, 1632f

Caudate lobe
  abdominal scanning of, 106–107, 108f
  at celiac axis level, 106–107, 108f
  description of, 221
  at liver and psoas muscle level, 106, 107f
Caudate nucleus, 818, 819f
Caudothalamic groove, 818, 819f, 827
Caudothalamic notch, 818
Cavernous hemangioma
  contrast-enhanced imaging of, 518, 520f
  hepatic, 268, 271t, 272f
Cavernous transformation, of portal vein, 214, 260t
Cavum septum pellucidum, 816, 826
Cavum vergae, 816
CBD. see Common bile duct
CBE. see Clinical breast examination
CCA. see Common carotid artery
CCAM. see Congenital cystic adenomatoid malformation
CDH. see Congenital diaphragmatic hernia
Cebocephaly, 1503, 1534–1535, 1535f
Celiac axis (CA)
  abdominal transverse scanning of, at level of caudate lobe, 106–107, 108f
  Doppler flow patterns in, 212–214, 212b, 213f
  pancreas and, 358f, 359
Celiac trunk, 179–180, 179f
Cell-free DNA testing, prenatal diagnosis of congenital anomalies, 1429
Cells, 81
Centesis catheter, 534, 534f
Central nervous system anomalies, in fetus, embryology of, 1522
Centripetal arteries, 711, 711f
Cephalic direction, 132–134
Cephalic index, 1385, 1386f
Cephalic vein, 1124f, 1133–1134
Cephalocele, 1336, 1336t, 1337f, 1503, 1523t, 1525–1526, 1527f
  differential considerations for, 1524t
  sonographic findings in, 1526, 1527f, 1528f
Cerclage placement, 1285
Cerebellum, 1351
  fetal, 1392, 1393b, 1393f
  neonatal, 819, 820f
Cerebral circulatory arrest, 1103–1104
Cerebral hemispheres, neonatal, 817
Cerebral vasospasm, 1099
Cerebrospinal fluid (CSF), neonatal, 816, 817f
Cerebrovascular accident
  costs associated with, 1069
  risk factors for, 1070
  warning signs and symptoms of, 1071–1072, 1072b
Cerebrovascular evaluation
  extracranial, 1069, 1085b
    anatomy for imaging in, 1070–1071
  intracranial, 1087, 1107b
    anatomy for imaging in, 1088–1090, 1088f
    physiology in, 1090
Cerebrovascular system, neonatal, 819
Cerebrum
  hemispheres of, 817
  neonatal, 817–818, 818f
Certification, in ultrasound, 6
Cervical canal, 1443f
Cervical carcinoma, 1204, 1206b, 1206f

Cervical carotid system aneurysms, 1078
Cervical leiomyoma, 1204, 1205f
Cervical polyps, 1204
Cervical pregnancy, 1332–1333
Cervical stenosis, 1204, 1205f
Cervix, 1162, 1165b, 1375, 1375b
  coronal view of, 1163f
  female infertility and, 1272–1273
  lateral view of, 1162f
  pathology of, 1203–1207
    benign conditions, 1203–1204, 1203f, 1204b
    cervical carcinoma, 1204, 1206b, 1206f
  transvaginal scanning of, 1187f, 1193f
CEUS. see Contrast-enhanced ultrasound imaging
ceVUS. see Contrast-enhanced voiding urosonography
CFM. see Color flow mapping
CFV. see Common femoral vein
Chest, fetal ultrasound, 1408t
CHF. see Congestive heart failure
CHI. see Contrast harmonic imaging
Chiari, Hans, 256–257
Chiari malformations, 821, 839
Children
  abuse of, 763t
  acute abdominal pain in, 767
  cat-scratch disease in, 769, 770f
  cholangitis in, 769
  choledocholithiasis in, 767
  cirrhosis in, 768–769
  critically ill, 763t
  cystic fibrosis in, 769
  fatty liver in, 768–769
  food allergies in, 763t
  obesity in, 763t
  pancreatic disease in, 769
  pancreatitis in, 767
  portal hypertension in, 768–769
  special needs of, 58–59
  splenic disease in, 769
  splenic sequestration syndrome in, 767
  splenomegaly in, 769f
  trauma in, 767
Chlamydia trachomatis, 1261
Choking, 65–66, 65b, 65f
Cholangiocarcinoma, 318–321, 319f, 320f
Cholangiopathy, 602f
Cholangitis, 315–318, 769
Cholecystectomy, 285
Cholecystitis, 293–299, 297b
  acalculous, 294t–295t, 297, 300f
  chronic, 294t–295t, 300
  clinical findings for, 573t
  emphysematous, 294t–295t, 296–297
  gangrenous, 294t–295t, 297, 300f
  hyperplastic, 303–306, 306f, 307f
Cholecystokinin, 289, 393
Choledochal cysts, 308–311
  fetal, 1582, 1584b
  pediatric, 771t, 772, 773f
  sonographic findings in, 294t–295t, 308, 310f, 311f
Choledocholithiasis
  in children, 767
  description of, 294t–295t, 313, 316f, 597–598
Cholelithiasis, 294t–295t, 300, 301f, 302f, 303f, 304f
  fetal, 1582, 1584f
  right upper quadrant pain in, 567–568, 568f
  sonographic findings in, 300–303, 302f, 304f, 305f

Cholesterolosis, 303–304, 306f
Chorioamnionitis, 1483
Chorioangioma, placental tumors, 1457, 1457f
Choriocarcinoma, 728t, 1326
Chorion, 1289–1290
Chorion frondosum, 1443, 1443b, 1443f
Chorion laeve, 1443b, 1443f
Chorionic cavity, 1308–1309, 1462f
Chorionic or gestational sac, 1379
Chorionic plate, 1443, 1443b
Chorionic sac, 1462f
Chorionic villi, 1443, 1443f
Chorionic villus sampling (CVS), 1300–1301
    prenatal diagnosis of congenital anomalies, 1429–1430, 1429f, 1430f
Choroid plexus, neonatal, 816, 817f, 825–826
Choroid plexus cysts, 844–845, 845f, 1537–1538, 1537f
    subependymal cysts versus, 845
Chromosomal abnormalities, congenital heart disease and, 1032, 1032t
Chromosomal disorder, 1433
Chronic cholecystitis, 294t–295t, 300
Chronic granulomatous disease, 264t, 266, 268f
Chronic hepatitis, 243t, 246, 247f
Chronic kidney disease (CKD), 474
Chronic liver failure, 584–585
Chronic lymphocytic leukemia, 728t
Chronic pancreatitis, 369t, 372–373, 373f
Chronic pyelonephritis, 806–807
Chronic renal failure, 454t–458t
Circle of Willis, 1088f, 1089, 1351f
    transtemporal approach to, 1092–1093, 1092f
Circulation
    coronary, 906–907
    fetal
        description of, 1010–1012
        illustration of, 1011f
    neonatal, 1012f
Circulatory system, 81–83, 170–171
Circumvallate/circummarginate placenta, 1454, 1455f
Cirrhosis, 246–248, 247f
    in children, 768–769
    intrahepatic portal hypertension and, 251
    liver transplantation for, 584–585, 584f
    pathology of, 584f
    sonographic findings in, 243t, 246–248, 248f
Cisterna magna, 816, 1351
Cisterns, neonatal, 816
CKD. see Chronic kidney disease
"Clapper-in-the-bell" sign, 755–756
Claudication, 1114
Clear cell tumors, 1249–1250
Cleft lip/palate, 1506, 1507f, 1508f, 1509f, 1510b, 1510f, 1511f, 1512f
Cleft sternum, 1568–1570, 1569f
Clicks, 905
Clinical breast examination (CBE), 652, 653b
Clinical laboratory orientation, 124–125
Clinical sonography, foundations of, 3, 27b
Cloacal exstrophy, 1564t, 1567–1568, 1568f, 1569f, 1603–1604
Clock face method, 656, 656f
C-loop of duodenum, 356–358, 358f
Closed dysraphic associations, 880–881, 881t
Closed spinal dysraphism, 880–881
Cloverleaf skull, 1498–1499, 1499f

Clubfoot, 1633–1635, 1635f
Clutter, 160–163, 162f, 163f
CO. see Cardiac output
Coagulopathy, 532
Coarctation of aorta, 1032t, 1048, 1055–1056, 1057f
Coccygeus muscles, 94f, 1160, 1160f
Coccyx, 876, 877f
Code of Ethics for the Profession of Diagnostic Medical Sonography, 1295
Colitis, 410f
Collateral circulation, 252–253, 252f, 254f, 255t, 256t
Collateral pathways, 1071, 1100–1101
Colloid carcinoma, 675
Colon
    sonographic evaluation of, 398–399, 399f
    tumors of, 409–412
"Color blooming" artifacts, 515–516
Color box size, 715t
Color Doppler imaging, 24–25, 26f, 211–212
    of acoustic emission, 514–515, 515f
    of arteriovenous malformations, 1216
    artifacts of, 160–163
        aliasing and, 160, 161f, 162f
        mirror image, shadowing, clutter, and noise and, 160–163, 162f, 163f
    carotid duplex
        procedure, 1073
        of tortuous arteries, 1075–1076, 1076b, 1076f
        of vertebral arteries, 1081
    of collateral circulation, 252–253, 254f, 255t, 256t
    color flow, 912, 912f
    contrast-enhanced
        of renal artery flow, 512f
        of renal artery stenosis, 521, 521f
        of right renal artery, 512f
    of ovaries, 1236, 1236f
    of pancreatic mass, 553–554
    of pelvic vascularity, 1190
    principles of, 912, 912f, 913f
    of renal transplantation complications, 555, 555f
    of scrotum, 715t, 718
        epididymo-orchitis, 718
        hematoceles, 726
        torsion, 710f, 722f
        tubular ectasia of the rete testis, 726–728
        varicoceles, 722–723, 724f
    of spleen, 335–336, 336f
    of testes, 716f
    transorbital approach, 1094, 1094f
    venous, 1147f
Color flow Doppler, 24, 1015, 1015f
Color flow imaging
    of renal artery flow, 512f
    of single ventricle, 1059f
Color flow mapping (CFM)
    apical view for, 933–936, 944f
    examination, 919–920, 922b, 922f
    M-mode, 920, 943–952, 950b
    parasternal views
        long-axis, 920f, 922b, 925–928, 927f
        short-axis, 922b, 929–931, 931f, 932f, 933f, 934f
    right parasternal window for, 928, 930f
    subcostal view for, 938, 948b
    suprasternal view for, 939–943

Colostomies, 47
Colpocephaly, 840–841
Columns of Bertin, 444, 446f
Comedocarcinoma, 672, 672f
Comet tail artifacts, 148–149, 150f, 742, 742f
Common atria, 1042
Common bile duct (CBD), 282, 282f
    atretic, 771
    pancreas and, 358f, 359
    pediatric, 765, 765b, 766f
    right upper quadrant pain and, 568, 569f
    sonographic evaluation of, 289, 292f, 293f
    stones of, 313
    stricture of, 259
Common carotid artery (CCA), 1070, 1070f
Common femoral artery, 178t, 611, 1111–1112, 1143f
Common femoral vein (CFV), 1131
    venous duplex imaging of, 1147f
Common hepatic artery, 179–180, 180f
    color Doppler technique for, 255t
    pancreas and, 359
Common hepatic duct, 282, 282f
Common iliac arteries, 178–179, 178f, 178t
Common iliac vein, 1131
Communicating hydrocephalus, 829, 1540, 1540f
Communication, sonographers and, 5b, 550
Compartments
    intraperitoneal, 417–418, 418f, 419f
    lower abdominal, 418–419, 419f
    pelvic, 418–419, 419f
    perihepatic, 417–418
    psoas, 495, 495f
    upper abdominal, 417–418, 418f
Complete atrioventricular septal defect, 1041–1043, 1042f
Complete blood count, 83
Complete duplication, 447, 450f, 451f
Complex cysts
    breast, 658t, 659b, 660, 661f
    renal, 458, 459b, 459f, 460f
Complex lung masses, 1554–1555
Complicated cyst, in breast, 659b
Compound imaging, 540, 715t
Compression, 10
Compression therapy, 1125–1126
Computed tomography (CT), 103–104, 103t
    abdominal trauma on, 562
    of calcified dermoid tumor, 1253f
    fusion technology and, 540, 540f, 541f
    noncontrast, 439
Conceptional age, 1378
Conduction system, of heart
    development of, 1010
    electrical, 903, 903f
    mechanical, 903–904
Confidentiality, of findings, 1298
Confluence of splenic and portal veins, 107
Congenital anomalies
    of face, 1492
    prenatal diagnosis of, 1426, 1441b
        chromosomal abnormalities, 1433–1441
            nuchal translucency, 1433, 1433f
            triploidy, 1438
            trisomy 13, 1437–1438, 1438f, 1439f, 1440f
            trisomy 18, 1436–1437, 1436f, 1437f, 1438f
            trisomy 21, 1433–1436, 1434f, 1435f, 1436f
            Turner syndrome, 1438–1441, 1440f

Congenital anomalies (Continued)
    chromosomal disorders, 1426–1427
    diagnostic screening tests, 1429–1432
        amniocentesis, 1430–1431, 1430f, 1431f
        chorionic villus sampling, 1429–1430, 1429f, 1430f
        cordocentesis, 1432
        genetic amniocentesis, 1431–1432, 1431f, 1432f
        multiple gestations, genetic amniocentesis and, 1432
    first trimester screening, 1432–1433
        human chorionic gonadotropin, 1432–1433
        pregnancy-associated plasma protein A, 1432
    genetic screening tests, 1427–1429
        alpha-fetoprotein, 1427–1429, 1427b, 1427f, 1428b
        cell-free DNA testing, 1429
        quadruple screen, 1429
    medical genetics, 1433
    scrotal, 728t, 730–732
    splenic, 327–329, 331f
    uterus, 1273–1274, 1273f, 1274f
Congenital bronchial atresia, 1554
Congenital cystic adenomatoid malformation (CCAM), 1552–1554, 1553f
    sonographic findings in, 1554, 1554b
    type I, 1553–1554, 1553f
    type II, 1553–1554
    type III, 1553–1554, 1554f
Congenital diaphragmatic hernia (CDH), 1555–1558, 1556b
Congenital heart disease, 1065b–1066b
    atrioventricular septal defect, 1041–1043, 1041f
    cardiac abnormalities, 1058–1062
        single ventricle, 1058–1059, 1058f, 1059f
    cardiac enlargement, 1034–1036
    cardiac malposition terms, 1033, 1035f
    cardiac tumors, 1058
    cardiosplenic syndromes, 1060–1062
    chromosomal abnormalities and, 1032, 1032t
    congenital vena cava to left atrial communication, 1059–1060
    cor triatriatum, 1059, 1059f
    ectopia cordis, 1062, 1062f
    familial risks of, 1033
    fetal echocardiography of, 1008
    four-chamber view of, 1033, 1034f
    great vessel abnormalities, 1054–1058
        coarctation of the aorta, 1055–1056, 1057f
        ductal constriction, 1057
        interrupted aortic arch, 1056–1057
        transposition of the great arteries, 1054, 1054f, 1055f
        truncus arteriosus, 1054–1055, 1055f, 1056f
    incidence of, 1007, 1033
    left ventricular inflow disturbance, 1048–1050
    left ventricular outflow tract disturbance, 1050–1054
        aortic stenosis, 1050–1052
        bicuspid aortic valve, 1033, 1050, 1050f
        hypoplastic left heart syndrome, 1052–1054, 1052f, 1053f
        mitral regurgitation, 1050
    prenatal evaluation of, 1033
    right ventricular inflow disturbance, 1043–1045
    right ventricular outflow disturbance, 1045–1048
    single ventricle, 1058–1059, 1058f, 1059f

Congenital heart disease (Continued)
    total anomalous pulmonary venous return, 1060, 1060f, 1061f
Congenital hepatic cysts, 264
Congenital hydrocephalus, 829
Congenital hypophosphatasia, 1628
Congenital lobar emphysema, 1554
Congenital mesoblastic nephroma, 796t
Congenital mitral stenosis, 1048–1050, 1048f, 1049f
Congenital spherocytosis, 340, 341f
Congenital vena cava to left atrial communication, 1059–1060
Congestive heart failure (CHF), 1076, 1077f, 1142f
Congestive splenomegaly, 338b, 339
Conjoined twins, 1419–1420, 1421f, 1423
Conn syndrome, 500–501, 502t
Consent
    form, 33f, 543
    patient, 32, 33f
    verbal, 32
    written, 32
Constrictive pericarditis, 983–985, 986b, 986f, 987f
Contact precautions, 54
Continuity equation
    aortic stenosis assessments using, 971b
    description of, 915, 915f
    mitral stenosis assessments using, 960–961, 961f
Continuity principle, 915
Continuous murmur, 905
Continuous wave (CW) Doppler, 23, 25f
    aortic regurgitation, 963–964
    description of, 913, 913f
    echocardiography, 923, 923f
    hypertrophic cardiomyopathy evaluations, 995, 997f
    mitral regurgitation, 956, 957f
    transducers for, 913f
Continuous wave probe, 923, 924f
Contrast-enhanced ultrasound imaging (CEUS), 511
    focal nodular hyperplasia, 518, 520f
    harmonic imaging for, 515–516
    hepatic blood flow, 517
    hepatic tumors, 517f, 518, 518f, 519f, 520f, 521f
    intermittent imaging and, 516
    liver metastases, 520f
    organ transplants and, 523–524
    pancreatic applications of, 523
    renal masses, 522, 522f
    splenic applications of, 522–523
Contrast-enhanced voiding urosonography (ceVUS), 795–796, 797f
Contrast harmonic imaging (CHI), 515–516
Conus medullaris, 873, 874f, 878–879, 879b, 879f
Cooper's ligaments, 645–646, 647f
Copper 7, 1227–1228
Cor triatriatum, 1059, 1059f
Coracohumeral ligament, 738f
Cordis, ectopia, 1564t
Cordocentesis, 1410–1411, 1411f
    prenatal diagnosis of congenital anomalies, 1432
Core biopsy, needles for, 533, 533f, 534f
Coronal imaging, transvaginal, 1186, 1186b, 1187f
Coronal plane
    abdominal, 104–105
    neonatal head examination, 822f, 823t, 824–827, 824f
Coronary circulation, 906–907

Corpus callosum
    agenesis of, 840–841, 841f, 1523t, 1535–1536
        sonographic findings in, 1536, 1536f
    neonatal, 818, 818f
Corpus luteum, 1168, 1198
Corpus luteum cysts, 1236–1237, 1237b, 1237f, 1329t, 1340, 1341f
    hemorrhagic, 1237, 1238f
    sonographic findings in, 1237, 1237f
Cortex, 792
    adrenal, 497
    renal, 436, 444
Corticomedullary differentiation, 792
Corticosteroid therapy, 1483
Costal margin, 891–892
Costophrenic sinus, 892
Couinaud's system, of hepatic nomenclature, 219–220, 220b, 221f
Courvoisier sign, 289, 292f
CPR. see Cardiopulmonary resuscitation
Craig, Marveen, 69
Cranial cavity, 88
Cranial direction, 132–134
Cranial meningocele, 1525–1526
Craniostenosis, 1523t
Craniosynostosis, 1496, 1624
Cranium
    embryonic
        anomalies of, 1334–1338, 1335f, 1336t
        sonographic findings of, 1310–1313, 1311f, 1312f
    fetal, 1348–1352, 1348f, 1349f, 1350f, 1351f, 1352f
Cranium bifidum, 1527f
Crass position, 746f
Creatinine (Cr), 438–439
Creatinine clearance, 439
Cremasteric artery, 712
Cremasteric muscle, 712
Crepitus, 754
Crisscross view, 1021, 1022b, 1022f
Critical aortic stenosis, 1050, 1051f
CRL. see Crown-rump length
Crohn's disease, 404t, 409, 409f
Crossed-fused renal ectopia, 448–449, 451f, 452f, 800, 803f
Cross-talk, 160
Crown-rump length (CRL), 1301, 1304f, 1315, 1315f, 1316f, 1381–1382, 1381b, 1381f, 1382f, 1382t
CRS. see Caudal regression syndrome
Crus of diaphragm, 106, 107f
Crying patients, 57
Cryptorchidism, 1617
    neonatal/pediatric, 730–732, 731f
Crystals, piezoelectric, 12–13, 13f
CSF. see Cerebrospinal fluid
CT. see Computed tomography
CTS. see Carpal tunnel syndrome
Cubital tunnel, 72
Cuffs, blood pressure, 36, 37f
Cul-de-sac
    fluid, 1198f
    sonographic evaluation of, 578
    ultrasound examination of, 1178b
Culling, 332
Curie, Paul-Jacques, 6
Curie, Pierre, 6

Curved array transducer, 16–17, 125, 127f, 128f
Cushing syndrome, 502, 502t
Cushions, 78
Cushman, Richard, 7
CVS. see Chorionic villus sampling
Cyanosis, 38
Cyclopia, 1503, 1504f, 1534–1535, 1535f
Cyst(s)
  abdominal, 426, 427f
  adrenal, 502–503, 502f, 503f
  arachnoid, 845–846, 846f, 1523t, 1540f
  Baker, 579, 580f, 1147, 1147f
  Bosniak classification of, 449, 452t, 458–459
  branchial cleft, 705, 705f, 1512
  bronchogenic, 1550, 1551f
  choledochal, 308–311
    fetal, 1582, 1584b
    pediatric, 771t, 772, 773f
    sonographic findings in, 294t–295t, 308, 310f
  choroid plexus, 844–845, 845f, 1537–1538, 1537f
    subependymal cysts versus, 845
  complex, renal, 458, 459b, 459f, 460f
  corpus luteum, 1236–1237, 1237b, 1237f, 1329t, 1340, 1341f
    hemorrhagic, 1237, 1238f
    sonographic findings in, 1237, 1237f
  developmental, of neck, 704–707
  duplication, 399, 400f, 400t
  echinococcal, 264t, 267–268, 270f
  epididymal, 717t, 722, 723f
  follicular, 1198, 1231–1233, 1233f
  Gartner duct, 1203, 1203f
  glioependymal, 1523t
  hepatic, 260–262, 264t
  intratesticular, 727, 727f
  kissing, 459, 460f
  masses within, 468–470, 470f
  medullary, 454t–458t
  mesenteric, 426, 427f
  nabothian, 1193, 1193f, 1204, 1204b, 1204f, 1205f
  pancreatic, 1583
  paraovarian, 1240, 1240b, 1241f
  peribiliary, 264, 265f
  peritoneal, 426
  peritoneal inclusion, 1239–1242, 1240f
  renal
    simple, 453, 459f
      sonographic findings in, 453–458
    sinus parapelvic, 454t–458t, 459–460
  simple, hepatic, 262–264, 264t, 265f
  splenic, 337t, 348–349, 349f, 1583–1584
  subependymal, 845
  sublingual, 1512f
  theca-lutein, 1237, 1238b, 1239f
  thyroglossal duct, 704–705, 705f
  tunica albuginea, 718
  urachal, 427, 427f
  von Hippel-Lindau, 454t–458t, 460
Cystadenocarcinomas
  mucinous, 1247, 1248b, 1249f
  ovarian, 1247
  serous, 1248–1249, 1249b, 1250b, 1251f
Cystadenomas
  mucinous, 382f, 1247, 1248b, 1249f
  ovarian, 1235
  serous, 1249b, 1250f, 1252f

Cystic adenomatoid malformation
  AFP and, 1428
  congenital, 1552–1554, 1553f
    sonographic findings in, 1554, 1554b
    type I, 1553–1554, 1553f
    type II, 1553–1554
    type III, 1553–1554, 1554f
Cystic degeneration of myomas, 1210
Cystic duct, 282f, 283
Cystic fibrosis
  in children, 769
  meconium ileus and, 1587
  pancreatic lesions, 377, 379f
Cystic hygroma
  AFP and, 1428
  cephaloceles versus, 1527
  fetal, 1513–1514, 1513f, 1514f, 1515f, 1516f
  first-trimester, 1339–1340, 1339f
  Turner syndrome, 1440, 1440f
Cystic lesions
  hepatic, 262–265, 264t
  neonatal, 844–846
  pancreatic, 377, 378t
Cystic masses
  abdomen, fetal, 1590–1591
  left upper quadrant, 396
  lung, 1549–1550, 1551b
  ovarian, 1234, 1234b, 1234f, 1235f
Cystic medial necrosis, 193–194
Cystic pancreatic neoplasms, 377–381
Cystic rhombencephalon, 1335f
Cystitis, 485–486
Cystosarcoma phyllodes, 658t, 675, 675f
Cytopathology, 538–539

D

da Vinci, Leonardo, 6
Dacryocystoceles, 1501
Dandy-Walker malformation, 841–842, 841f, 1336, 1336t, 1338f, 1523t, 1531
  differential considerations for, 1524t
  sonographic findings in, 1531, 1532f
  sonographic findings of, 841, 842f
"Dangling choroid" sign, 1541
DCIS. see Ductal carcinoma in situ
DDH. see Developmental displacement of the hip
De Quervain disease, 72
De Quervain tendinitis, 754
De Quervain thyroiditis, 699
DeBakey model, 194, 194f
Decibel (dB) unit, 11–12, 12t
Decidua basalis, 1307, 1443f, 1443f
Decidua capsularis, 1307, 1443, 1443b, 1443f
Decidua vera (parietalis), 1443b, 1443f
Decidual septum, 1443f
Deciduas basalis, 1443
Dedication, 5b
Deep flexor tendon, 736f
Deep structures, 134
Deep vein thrombosis (DVT), 1130, 1134–1136, 1147f
  bilateral symptoms, 1148–1149
  complications of, 1130
  diagnostic approach to, 1145
  risk factors for, 1135b
  signs and symptoms of, 1130, 1135b
Deep veins
  lower extremity, 1130–1131, 1130f
  upper extremity, 1133–1134, 1133f

Deferential artery, 712
Deformation sequence, 1496
Delta cells, 361
Denial, illness and, 60
Depth gain compensation (DGC), 21–22
Dermal sinus, 883, 885f
Dermoid cyst, 1416f
Dermoid tumors, 1250–1251, 1252b, 1252f, 1253f
Descending aorta, 172, 1111
Desmoid tumor, 432, 432f
Detailed fetal anatomic survey ultrasound, 1407
Detoxification
  bilirubin, 229
  drug, 230
  hormone, 230
  liver, 229–230, 229t
Developmental cysts, of neck, 704–707, 705f
Developmental displacement of the hip (DDH), 857–867
  abnormal, 858
  Barlow maneuver for, 859, 859f
  causes of, 866–867
  genetic factors, 867
  hormonal factors, 866
  incidence of, 866
  mechanical factors, 866–867
  Ortolani maneuver for, 859, 859f
  physical examination for, 858–859, 859f
  signs of, 859f
  sonographic findings of
    coronal/flexion view, 855, 856f, 859–860, 861f
    coronal/neutral view, 855, 855f, 856b, 859, 860f
    dynamic Harcke technique, 862–863, 865f
    follow-up, 866, 866f, 867f
    Graf checklist, 856b
    linear-array transducer for, 854, 854b
    modified Graf technique, 860–866, 862b, 862f, 863f, 863t, 864f
    overview of, 854
    positioning for, 855
    preparation for, 854–855
    static femoral head coverage measurement with, 862, 865f
    static Graf technique, 860–866, 862b, 862f, 863f, 863t, 864f
    techniques used in, 860–866
    transverse/flexion view, 855–856, 857f, 858f, 860, 861f
    transverse/neutral view, 857, 860
  treatment of, 866, 866f, 867f
Dextrocardia, 1033, 1035f
Dextroposition, 1033, 1035f
Dextroversion, 1035f
DGC. see Depth gain compensation
Diabetes, 1413–1415
  type 1, pancreatic transplantation for, 586
Diabetic mastopathy, 666
Diagnostic breast interrogation, 653–654
Diagnostic medical ultrasonography, 4
Diagnostic peritoneal lavage (DPL), 562, 562f
Dialysis, description of, 585–586
Dialysis access grafts, 1123–1124, 1123f, 1124f
Diaphragm, 88–89, 90f
  abnormalities of, 1555–1558, 1555f
  anatomy of, 88
  longitudinal scans of, 141, 141f
  thoracic vessels and, fetal, 1360–1362, 1361f, 1362f, 1363f

Diaphragmatic crura, 172
  anatomy of, 444, 445f, 494, 494f
  sonographic evaluation of, 498, 500f
Diaphragmatic hernia
  right-side, 1556
  sonographic criteria of, 1556b
Diarrhea, 84–86, 85t
Diastematomyelia, 872, 879–880, 883, 885f
Diastole, 909, 926–928
Diastolic measurement, 36
Diastolic murmur, 905
Diastrophic dysplasia, 1628–1629, 1629f
Diffuse disease, 340–342
  autoimmune hemolytic anemia, 341
  cirrhosis, 243t, 246–248, 247f
  congenital spherocytosis, 340, 341f
  fatty infiltration, 243–244, 244b
  glycogen storage disease, 243t, 248–249, 250f
  granulocytopoietic abnormalities, 342
  Hand-Schüller-Christian disease, 342
  hemochromatosis, 243t, 249, 250f
  hemolytic anemia, 341
  hepatitis, 244–246
    acute, 243t, 246, 246f
    chronic, 243t, 246, 247f
  hepatocellular, 243
  Letterer-Siwe disease, 342
  myeloproliferative disorders, 342, 343f
  polycythemia vera, 341
  reticuloendotheliosis, 342
  sickle cell anemia, 340
  thalassemia, 341–342, 343f
  thyroid gland, 698–700, 699f, 700f
Diffuse orchitis, 717t
Digestive system, 84f
  embryology of, 1572–1576, 1573f, 1574f
Digital subtraction angiography, 1083
Dilated biliary ducts, 311–312, 312f
Dilated posterior urethra, 1600
Dilation, lower gastrointestinal, 403, 404t, 405f
Diplopia, 1072
Direct-acting bilirubin, 229, 229t
Disbelief, illness and, 60
Discriminatory level, 1323
Disinfection technique, 1187–1189
Dislocation
  neonatal hip, 857, 858f
  shoulder biceps tendon, 751, 751f
Disruption sequence, 1496
Dissecting aneurysm, 194, 194f
Dissection, carotid artery, 1078, 1079f
Distal cholangiocarcinoma, 321, 322f
Distal direction, 132–134
Distal femoral and proximal tibial epiphyseal ossification centers, 1390
Disturbed flow, 905
Diverticulum, 408–409
Dolichocephaly, 1424
Dome of liver, 106–108, 106f
Dominant disorder, 1433
Donald, Ian, 7
Doppler, Christian Johann, 6
Doppler angle, 23
Doppler effect, 6, 22–23, 22f, 23f, 910–911, 911f
Doppler flow patterns
  in abdominal vessels, 212–214, 212b
  aorta, 212–214, 212b, 213f
  cardiac, 920, 922f

Doppler flow patterns (Continued)
  celiac axis, 212–214, 212b, 213f
  hepatic artery, 212–214, 212b, 213f
  inferior vena cava and hepatic veins, 214, 214b, 215f
  portal vein, 214, 214b, 215f
  renal artery, 212b, 214, 214f
  renal vein, 214, 214b, 215f
  splenic artery, 212–214, 212b, 213f
  superior mesenteric artery, 212b, 213f, 214
Doppler frequency shift, 910–911, 910f, 911f
Doppler interrogation, 253
Doppler quantitation, 924, 924t
Doppler sample volume, 210
Doppler shift, 23, 1091
Doppler sonography, fetal growth assessment, 1402–1404, 1402f
  quantitative and qualitative measurements, 1403, 1403b, 1403f, 1404f
Doppler spectral analysis
  of intracranial carotid arterial system, 1090–1091
  venous reflux imaging, 1145–1146, 1145f
Doppler ultrasound, 22–28
  abdominal
    scanning techniques, 145–146, 145f
    techniques, 209–217
      blood flow analysis, 209–210
  artifacts in, 147, 165b
  cirrhosis, 248, 249f
  color flow, 24
  for echocardiography, 920
    audio signals and spectral display of Doppler signals, 920–923
    continuous-wave Doppler, 923, 923f
    Doppler examination, 924, 924b
    Doppler quantitation, 924, 924t
    normal cardiac Doppler flow patterns, 920, 922f
    pulsed wave Doppler, 923, 923f
  endometrial carcinoma, 1224, 1224f
  examination, 925–943, 925f, 926f, 927b
  left parasternal window for, 928, 930f
  lower extremity veins, 1140
  methods of, 211–212, 212f
  optimization of, 25–28
  ovaries, 1236, 1236f, 1245–1246
  parasternal short-axis window for, 922–923, 928, 932f, 935f
  pitfalls in, 970–971, 971f, 972f
  portal hypertension, 252, 253b
  right parasternal window for, 928, 930f
  segmental pressures, 1114–1116, 1115t
  spectral, 945b
  subcostal window for, 924b, 938–939
  suprasternal window for, 941–943, 949f
  technical considerations, 970–971, 971f, 972f
  venous, 1142f
Doppler waveform analysis, abdominal techniques, 210
Dorsal aortic branches, 187
Dorsal cavity, 88, 88f
Dorsal direction, 132
Dorsal pancreatic artery, 359
Dorsalis pedis artery, 1112
Dorsiflexion, 750
Double bubble sign, 1585, 1586b, 1586f
Double decidual sac sign, 1307, 1379, 1379f

Double-layer thickness, 1277–1278
Double-outlet right ventricle, 1032t, 1046
Douglas, pouch of, 564, 566f, 1174
Down syndrome, 1032, 1042
  absent nasal bone in, 1505, 1507f
  midface hypoplasia and, 1506, 1508f
DPL. see Diagnostic peritoneal lavage
Drainage
  of abscess, 534–535, 559
  of ascites, 559
Drains, 46–47
Dressings, 46–47
Dromedary hump, 444, 446t
Droplet precautions, 54
Droplet transmission, of infections, 50
Drug detoxification, 230
Duct of Santorini, 358–359
Duct of Wirsung, 358–359, 358f
Ductal arch view, 1026–1029, 1027f, 1028f
Ductal carcinoma in situ (DCIS), 671, 671f
Ductal constriction, 1057
Ductography, of breast, 676, 677f
Ductus arteriosus, 1010
  fetal circulation, 1446f
Ductus venosus, 1288, 1446, 1461
  fetal circulation, 1446f
Duke University, 10
Duodenal atresia, 1574, 1585
Duodenal bulb, 390
Duodenal stenosis, 1574
Duodenum
  abdominal scanning of, at level of liver and pancreas, 109, 120f
  abnormalities of, 1584–1586
  C-loop of, 356–358, 358f
  embryology of, 1574
  segments of, 390, 392f
  sonographic evaluation of, 396–397, 397f
Duplex collecting, 446t
Duplication cysts, 399, 400f, 400t
Dura mater, 873–875
Dussik, Karl, 7, 7f
DVT. see Deep vein thrombosis
Dynamic range, 22
Dysarthria, 1072
Dysgerminoma, 1252, 1254f
Dysmenorrhea, 1174, 1204
Dysphagia, 1072
Dysplasia
  frontonasal, 1503, 1505f, 1510
  thanatophoric, 1499f
Dyspnea, 38
Dysrhythmias
  atrioventricular block, 1064–1066, 1064f
  ectopy, 1062–1063
  fetal, 1062–1066, 1062t, 1063f
  supraventricular tachyarrhythmias, 1063–1064, 1064f
Dysuria, 86, 87t

E

Ear
  abnormalities of, 1500–1501, 1501f
  development of, 1494–1495
Early proliferative phase, 1195
Ebstein anomaly, 1043–1045, 1044f
EBV. see Epstein-Barr virus
ECA. see External carotid artery

Echinococcal cyst, 264t, 267–268, 270f
Echinococcus, 348–349
Echocardiography, 920, 952b
  cardiac protocol for, 927b
  constrictive pericarditis, 983–985, 986b, 986f, 987f
  definition of, 4
  Doppler applications and technique, 920–925
    audio signals and spectral display of Doppler signals, 920–923
    cardiac Doppler flow patterns, 920, 922f
    continuous-wave Doppler, 923, 923f
    Doppler examination, 924, 924b
    Doppler quantitation, 924, 924t
    pulsed wave Doppler, 942f
  examination for, 925–943, 925f, 926f, 927b
  pericardial disease, 980–985
  pericardial effusion, 981–982, 981f, 981t, 982f, 983f
  positioning for, 927b
  subcostal views, 938–939, 948b
  techniques, 916
  transducers for, 918–919, 919f
  two-dimensional, 917–919, 917f, 918f
Echogenic, 130, 133f
Echogenic intracardiac focus (EIF), 1359–1360
Echogenic kidneys, enlarged, 1600
Eclampsia, 1415
ECMO. *see* Extracorporeal membrane oxygenation
Ectasia
  aortic, 187
  neonatal/pediatric, 804–805
Ectocervix, 1204
Ectopia
  renal, 448–449, 451f, 452f, 800, 803f
  testicular, 730
Ectopia cordis, 1062, 1062f, 1564t, 1568–1570, 1569f
Ectopic kidneys, 448–449, 451f, 452f
Ectopic pancreatic tissue, 359
Ectopic pregnancy, 1257, 1327–1333, 1328f
  adnexal mass with, 1330–1332, 1331f
  human chorionic gonadotrophin levels in, 1303
  sonographic findings in, 1328–1330, 1328f, 1329f, 1329t, 1330f, 1331f
Ectopic ureterocele, 450
  neonatal/pediatric, 797–798, 801f
  sonographic findings, 450–453
Ectopy, 1062–1063
Ectrodactyly, 1633f
Edler, Inge, 7, 8f
Edwards syndrome. *see* Trisomy 18
Efferent arteriole, 437
EFW. *see* Estimated fetal weight
EHR. *see* Embryonic heart rate
EIF. *see* Echogenic intracardiac focus
Ejaculatory ducts, 710
EJV. *see* External jugular vein
Elastography, 679–681, 679f, 680f
  assessment, in children, 768–769, 769f
  thyroid gland applications of, 698, 698f
Elderly, special needs of, 57–58
Electrical conduction system, 903, 903f
Electrocardiography, 904, 904f
Ellis-van Creveld syndrome, 1631

Embryo, 1289–1290, 1301
  aortic arches in, 1009f
  gestational sac without, 1322
  sonographic findings of
    at 6 to 10 weeks of gestational age, 1310–1313, 1310t
      embryonic cranium and spine, 1310–1313, 1311f, 1312f
      embryonic heart, 1313, 1314f, 1314t
      limb development, 1313, 1313f
      physiologic herniation of bowel, 1313, 1314f
      skeletal ossification, 1313, 1313f
    in abnormal intrauterine pregnancies, 1324b
    during fetal period, 1308–1310, 1309f, 1310f
Embryo in amniotic sac, 1443f
Embryo transfer, 1278
Embryogenesis, spine and, 871–872
Embryologic age, 1301
Embryology
  abdominal wall, 1560–1562, 1561f, 1562f, 1563f
  cardiovascular system, 1008–1010
  definition of, 80
  digestive system, 1572–1576, 1573f
  of face, 1493–1495, 1493f
  of neural axis, 1522–1523
  thoracic cavity, 1545
Embryonal cell carcinoma, 728t
Embryonic abnormalities, 1333–1340
  abdominal wall defects, 1338–1339, 1339f
  cardiac anomalies, 1334
  cranial anomalies, 1334–1338, 1335f, 1336t
  cystic hygroma, 1339–1340, 1339f
  first-trimester umbilical cord cysts, 1340, 1340f
  nuchal translucency, 1333–1334, 1334f
  obstructive uropathy, 1339
Embryonic bradycardia, 1327
Embryonic demise, 1320
Embryonic development, 1304t, 1311f
Embryonic heart, 1313, 1314f, 1314t
Embryonic heart rate (EHR), 1382, 1383b, 1383f
Embryonic oligohydramnios, 1327
Embryonic period, 1310
Embryonic tachycardia, 1327
Emergency medical situations, 65–67
  cardiopulmonary resuscitation, 66–67, 66f
  choking, 65–66, 65b, 65f
Emergent ultrasound procedures, 561, 581b
  abdominal trauma assessment, 561–563
  in acute pelvic pain, 578–579
  in appendicitis, 573t, 574–575, 576f
  in epigastric pain, 568–570
  in extremity swelling and pain, 579–581, 580f
  in flank pain caused by urolithiasis, 573–574, 573t
  in paraumbilical hernia, 573t, 575–578, 576f, 577f
  in pericardial effusion, 570–571, 571f, 572f
  in right upper quadrant pain, 567–568
  in scrotal trauma and torsion, 579, 579f, 580f
Emesis basins, 49, 49f
Emotional stability, 5b
Emphysematous cholecystitis, 294t–295t, 296–297
Emphysematous pyelonephritis, 478, 479f
Employment, 5–6
Encephalocele, 1497, 1498f, 1504f, 1525–1526, 1527f, 1568
  Meckel-Gruber syndrome and, 1528f
  occipital, 1527f

Endarterectomy, 1083–1084, 1084f
End-diastolic velocity, 1112–1113
Endemic goiter, 691
Endocardial cushion, 1048
Endocardium, 896
Endocrine, 360
Endodermal sinus tumors, 1252
Endometrial canal, 1185f, 1195, 1196f
Endometrial carcinoma, 1223–1224, 1224b, 1224f
Endometrial fluid, 1223f, 1224–1225
Endometrial fluid collections
  large, 1225, 1225f
  small, 1224–1225, 1225f
Endometrial hyperplasia, 1220, 1220b, 1221f
Endometrial polyps
  description of, 1220–1221
  sonographic findings in, 1221, 1222f
Endometriomas, 1243, 1243f, 1267–1270, 1268f, 1269f
Endometriosis, 1242–1243, 1242f, 1260, 1267–1270, 1268f, 1268t, 1269f
  female infertility and, 1277
  pelvic sites of, 1268f
  sonographic findings in, 1242, 1242f, 1243f, 1268t, 1269–1270
Endometritis, 1221–1222, 1222b, 1260, 1261b, 1261f, 1266–1267, 1267f
Endometrium, 1165
  blood supply to, 1169
  changes in, 1172–1174, 1172f, 1173f
  female infertility and
    evaluation of, 1274–1275, 1274f, 1275f
    monitoring of, 1277–1278
  measurement of, 1186, 1218, 1218t
  pathology of, 1217–1225
    carcinoma, 1223–1224, 1224b, 1224f
    endometritis, 1221–1222, 1222b
    hyperplasia, 1220, 1220b, 1221f
    intrauterine synechiae, 1222–1223, 1223f
    large endometrial fluid collections, 1225, 1225f
    small endometrial fluid collections, 1224–1225, 1225f
    polyps, 1220–1221, 1222f
  sonographic evaluation of, 1195–1196, 1195f
  sonohysterography of, 1218–1220, 1219f
  thickness of, 1218t
  transabdominal pelvic ultrasound of, 1181
Endovascular aneurysm repair, 523f, 524
Endovascular graft, 196f
End-to-side hepaticojejunostomy, 588
Enhancement, 156, 156f, 157f
  definition of, 156
  increased through-transmission, 130, 133f
Enteric isolation, 55
Environment cleanliness, 57
Environmental control, 47–48, 47f, 48f
Enzymes, hepatic, 228–229, 228t
Eosinophilic cardiomyopathy, 992, 993f
Ependymitis, 847–848
Epicardium, 896
Epicondylitis, 72, 72f
Epididymal cysts, 717t, 722
Epididymis
  description of, 709
  enlarge, 718t
  sonographic evaluation of, 709f
Epididymitis, 579f, 717t, 719, 719f

Epididymo-orchitis, 718
Epidural hemorrhages, 835
Epigastric hernias, 433
Epigastric pain, 568-570, 573t
Epigastrium, 219, 564
Epignathus, 1512, 1512f
Epineurium, 739
Epiploic foramen, 98, 99f
Epispadias, 1603
Epithelial ovarian tumors
　mucinous cystadenocarcinoma, 1247, 1248b, 1249f
　mucinous cystadenoma, 1247, 1248b, 1249f
　serous cystadenocarcinomas, 1248-1249, 1249b, 1250b, 1251f
　serous cystadenomas, 1249b, 1249f, 1250f, 1252f
Epstein-Barr virus (EBV), 623
Ergonomic exam tables, 78
Ergonomics
　definition of, 68
　economics of, 77-78
　history of, 68-70
　industry awareness/changes and, 72-74
　work practice changes and, 74-77, 76f, 77f
　work-related musculoskeletal disorders (WRMSDs), 70, 71f
　workstation setup, 78-79, 79f
EROA. see Estimated regurgitant orifice area
Erythrocytes, 83, 332
Erythropoiesis, 83
Esophageal stenosis, 1573
Esophagus
　anatomy of, 390, 390f
　atresia of, 1584-1585, 1585f
　fetal
　　abnormalities of, 1584-1586, 1585f
　　embryology of, 1573
　　sonographic evaluation of, 1577, 1577f
　vascular anatomy of, 392, 394f
Estimated fetal weight (EFW), 1397
Estimated regurgitant orifice area (EROA), 955-956
Estrogen, 497, 1168, 1220b, 1234
ESWL. see Extracorporeal shockwave lithotripsy
Ethics, for obstetric sonography, 1294, 1299b
　confidentiality of findings, 1298
　defined, 1294-1295
　medical
　　history of, 1295
　　principles, 1295-1298
Ethmocephaly, 1503, 1504f, 1534-1535, 1535f
Euthyroid, 685
Ex utero intrapartum treatment (EXIT) procedure, 1512
Exam tables, ergonomic, 78
Excitation contraction coupling, 904
Excretion, urinary, 438
Exencephaly, 1568
Exercise, 77, 77f
Exocoelomic cavity, 1443f
Exocrine, 360
Exophthalmia, 1502
Exophthalmos, 698-699
Explicit permission, 1298
Exstrophy, bladder, 1564t, 1567-1568, 1568f, 1569f
Extension, 853
External carotid artery (ECA), 1070-1071, 1075

External genitalia
　development of, 1595, 1595f, 1596f
　female, 1159, 1159f, 1595
　male, 1595
External iliac arteries, 108, 113f, 612f, 1169, 1170f
External iliac veins, 108, 113f, 1131
External jugular vein (EJV), 1133
External oblique muscle, 90, 90f
Extracorporeal liver, 1564t
Extracorporeal membrane oxygenation (ECMO)
　description of, 767, 821
　in neonates, 835
Extracorporeal shockwave lithotripsy (ESWL), 483-485
Extracranial carotid system, 1070f
Extracranial cerebrovascular evaluation, 1069, 1085b
　anatomy, 1070-1071
Extrahepatic biliary atresia, 1574
Extrahepatic biliary obstructions, 312-313, 313f
Extrahepatic mass, 259, 261t, 263f
Extrapancreatic fluid collections, 371-372, 372f
Extraperitoneal hematomas, 430, 431f
Extrarenal pelvis, 444-445, 446t, 448f
Extratesticular cystic mass, 718t
Extratesticular masses, 718t, 722
Extreme shortness of breath, 570-572
Extremities
　fetal ultrasound, 1408t
　swelling of, 579-581, 580f
Eye, protection for, 56

F
Face, fetal, 1352-1355, 1492, 1518b. see also Facial profile, fetal
　abnormalities of, 1496-1518
　congenital anomalies of, 1492
　coronal facial view, anatomic landmarks of, 1354, 1354f
　　fetal ears, 1355, 1355f
　　fetal lips, 1354-1355, 1354f
　　fetal tongue, 1354
　embryology of, 1493-1495, 1493f
　facial profile, 1352-1354, 1353f
　fetal eye orbits, 1352, 1353f
　nasal bone, 1354
　sonographic evaluation of, 1495-1496, 1495f, 1496b
　　additional imaging, 1517-1518, 1517f
　　three-dimensional, 1516-1517, 1517f
　ultrasound, 1408t
Face shield, 56
Facial clefting, 1508f, 1509-1510, 1511f
Facial profile, fetal
　abnormalities of, 1496-1518, 1496b
　　ear, 1500-1501, 1501f
　　face, 1506-1509
　　forehead, 1496-1498, 1497f, 1498f, 1499f
　　larynx, 1511-1512, 1512f
　　lip, 1506-1509, 1508f, 1509f
　　mandible, 1499-1500, 1500b, 1500f
　　mid-face, 1503-1510, 1506f, 1507f
　　neck, 1512-1516
　　nose, 1505-1506, 1507f
　　orbits, 1501-1503, 1502f, 1503f
　　palate, 1506-1509, 1508f, 1509f, 1510f
　　skull, 1498-1499, 1499f
　　tongue, 1510-1511, 1511f, 1512f
　　trachea, 1511-1512, 1512f
　sonography of, 1496b

Falciform ligament (FL), 98, 106, 221-223, 222f
Fallopian tubes, 93f, 1167, 1167b, 1167f
　carcinoma of, 1257
　female infertility and, 1275-1276, 1275f
　sonographic evaluation of, 579, 1196-1197, 1197f
　ultrasound examination of, 1178b
False aneurysm, 190-191, 191f, 974t
False lumen, 1078
False-negative hydronephrosis, 477-478
False pelvis, 93f, 94, 94f, 495, 1159-1160, 1159f
　anatomy of, 492
　muscles of, 1160f, 1161
False-positive hydronephrosis, 477, 478b
Falx cerebri, 815
Fan, 126
Fasciculi, 739
FAST. see Focused assessment with sonography for trauma
Fat necrosis, 658t, 664, 665f
Fats, 227-228
　retroperitoneal, 506
　subcutaneous, 646, 647f
Fatty breast, 648-649, 649f
Fatty infiltration, 243-244, 244b
　causes of, 244b
　focal, 244, 245f
　sonographic findings in, 244, 244f, 245f
Fatty liver, 243-244, 244b
　in children, 768-769
　description of, 227-228, 608
Fear, illness and, 60
Fecalith, 404
Female infertility
　evaluation of, 1272, 1279b
　　cervix, 1272-1273
　　endometrium, 1274-1275, 1274f, 1275f
　　fallopian tubes, 1275-1276, 1275f
　　ovaries, 1276-1277, 1276f, 1277f
　　uterus, 1273, 1273f
　peritoneal factors in, 1277
　treatment options for, 1277-1278
　　endometrial monitoring, 1277-1278, 1278f
　　intrauterine insemination, 1278
　　ovulation induction therapy, 1277, 1277f
　　in vitro fertilization and embryo transfer, 1278
Female pelvis, 92, 1157, 1175b, 1201b
　abdominal scanning at level of, 108, 116f
　bladder, 1161-1162, 1162b, 1163f
　blood supply to, 1191-1192
　bowel, 1174-1175, 1174b
　endometrial changes and, 1172-1174, 1172f, 1173f
　follicular development and ovulation and, 1170-1172, 1171f
　landmarks of, 1158f, 1159-1160
　　bony pelvis, 1159-1160, 1159f
　　external, 1159, 1159f
　　pelvic cavity and perineum, 1160, 1160b, 1160f
　muscles of, 1160-1161, 1160b
　recesses, 1174-1175
　ureters, 1161-1162, 1162b, 1163f
　vasculature of, 1168b, 1169, 1169f, 1170f
Female pseudohermaphrodites, 1618
Femoral arteries, 178t, 1111-1112
　Doppler image of, 1121f
　narrowing of, 1121f
　stenosis in, 1121f

Femoral head, 851, 852f
  coverage of, 854
Femoral veins, 1130f, 1131, 1142f
Femur length (FL), 1389, 1389b, 1389f, 1389t
Fetal age, 1378
Fetal capillaries in villi, 1443f
Fetal circulation, 1010–1012, 1011f, 1012f, 1446f
Fetal death, 1417, 1417f
Fetal echocardiography, 1008, 1030b
  color flow Doppler, 1015, 1015f
  ductal and aortic arch views, 1026–1029, 1027f, 1028f
  evaluation, 1017–1030
  four-chamber view, 1017–1021, 1018b, 1019f, 1020f, 1021f
  instrumentation, 1013
  landmarks, 1016–1017, 1016f, 1017f, 1018f
  left and right ventricular outflow tracts
    crisscross view, 1021, 1022b, 1022f
    five-chamber view, 1021, 1021b, 1022f
    long-axis view, 1022–1023, 1023b, 1023f, 1024f, 1025f, 1026f
    short-axis view, 1023–1026, 1026b, 1026f, 1027f
  motion mode imaging, 1013, 1014f, 1014t
  pulsed Doppler, 1014, 1014f, 1014t
  risk factors indicating, 1012–1013
  three-dimensional imaging, 1015, 1015f
  three-vessel view, 1029–1030, 1029f
  transducer requirements, 1013, 1013f
Fetal growth assessment, by sonography, 1395, 1405b
  diagnostic criteria, 1396b, 1397–1399
    abdominal circumference, 1397
    biparietal diameter, 1397
    estimated fetal weight, 1398
    head circumference to abdominal circumference ratio, 1397–1398, 1398f
  fetal well-being, tests of, 1399–1404, 1399f
    biophysical profile, 1399–1401, 1399b
    Doppler sonography, 1402–1404, 1402f
    nonstress test, 1401–1402, 1402f
  intrauterine growth restriction, 1395–1397, 1396b
  macrosomia and large for gestational age, 1404–1405
Fetal heart rate, 1012
Fetal lobulation, 444–445, 446t, 447f
Fetal measurements, 1382–1388
  biparietal diameter, 1383, 1384b, 1384f, 1384t, 1385f
    growth-adjusted sonar age, 1384–1385
  cephalic index, 1385
  coronal view, vertical cranial diameter, and 3D biparietal diameter correction, 1387, 1387b, 1387f
  head circumference, 1384b, 1385, 1385f, 1386b, 1386t
Fetal membranes, 1481–1486, 1482f
  amniotic band syndrome, 1483–1485, 1485f, 1486f
  amniotic fluid and, 1474, 1489b–1490b
  amniotic sheets, 1485–1486, 1486f
  ruptured, 1482–1483, 1484f
Fetal period (weeks 9-14), 1306–1313
  embryo during, 1308–1310, 1309f, 1310f
  gestational sac during, 1307–1310, 1307f, 1307t
  yolk sac during, 1307–1308, 1307f, 1308f

Fetal presentation, sonography of second and third trimesters, 1345–1348, 1345f, 1346f
  breech, 1346–1347, 1347f
  situs, 1347
  transverse, 1347, 1348f
  vertex, 1345–1346, 1346f
Fetal thoracic circumference measurements, 1550t
Fetor hepaticus, 229
Fetus, 1301
  abdominal wall of, 1562
  diaphragm of, abnormalities of, 1555–1558, 1555f
  heart of
    crisscross view of, 1021, 1022b, 1022f
    five-chamber view of, 1021, 1021b, 1022f
    four-chamber view of, 1017–1021, 1018b, 1019f, 1020f, 1021f
Fetus papyraceous, 1421, 1422f
Fibrinogen, 81
Fibroadenoma, 658t, 661–662, 662f
Fibrocystic dysplasia/fibrocystic changes, 660–661, 661f
Fibroelastoma, papillary, 998, 1000f
Fibroids, 1340, 1341f
  submucosal, 1275f
  uterine, 1273f, 1274–1275
    various locations, 1210f
Fibrolipomas, 883, 883f, 884f, 885f
Fibromas, 1254–1255, 1256f
Fibromuscular dysplasia (FMD), 480–481, 1078–1079
Fibrosarcomas, 507
Fibrosis, retroperitoneal, 509–510, 509f
Fibrous pericardium, 980, 981f
Fibula, fetal measurement, 1390, 1390b, 1390f
Field of view, 22
Filum terminale, 873, 876, 877f, 880, 880b, 880f
Fimbriae, 1167
Fine-needle aspiration (FNA), 532–533
  needles for, 532–533, 533f
First-degree heart block, 1065
First trimester pregnancy
  complications during, 1316, 1319, 1342b
    abnormal or absent cardiac activity, 1326–1327, 1326t
    bleeding, 1320–1326
      abnormal sac criteria, 1322–1323
      absent intrauterine sac, 1320–1322, 1321t, 1322f
      anembryonic pregnancy, 1323, 1323f, 1324b
      gestational sac without embryo or yolk sac, 1322
      gestational trophoblastic disease, 1323–1326, 1324f, 1325f, 1326f
      placental hematomas, 1320
      subchorionic hemorrhage, 1320, 1321f
    embryonic abnormalities, 1333–1340
      abdominal wall defects, 1338–1339, 1339f
      cardiac anomalies, 1334
      cranial anomalies, 1334–1338, 1335f, 1336f
      cystic hygroma, 1339–1340, 1339f
      nuchal translucency, 1333–1334, 1334f
      obstructive uropathy, 1339
      umbilical cord cysts, 1340, 1340f
    embryonic development of yolk sac and amnion, 1327
    pelvic masses, 1329t, 1340
    positive hCG with intrauterine fluid collection without yolk sac or embryo, 1316

First trimester pregnancy (Continued)
    positive hCG without intrauterine fluid collection or adnexal mass, 1316
  early embryonic stage, 1300, 1317b
  embryology of, 1305–1306, 1306b, 1306f
  gestational age assessment, 1379–1382
    crown-rump length, 1381–1382, 1381b, 1381f, 1382f, 1382t
    embryonic heart rate, 1382, 1383b, 1383f
    gestational sac diameter, 1379–1381, 1379b, 1379f, 1380f, 1380t, 1381b, 1381f
  gestational age determination, 1313–1316
  overview of, 1301–1303
  risk assessment, 1316–1318
  sonography during, indications for, 1284b, 1289–1290
  transvaginal sonographic technique and evaluation during, 1305–1306, 1305f
  at 6 to 10 weeks of gestational age, 1310–1313, 1310t
    embryonic cranium and spine, 1310–1313, 1311f, 1312f
    embryonic heart, 1313, 1314f, 1314t
    limb development, 1313, 1313f
    physiologic herniation of bowel, 1313, 1314f
    skeletal ossification, 1313, 1313f
  fetal period (weeks 9-14), 1306–1313
    embryo during, 1308–1310, 1309f, 1310f
    gestational sac during, 1307–1310, 1307f, 1307t
    yolk sac during, 1307–1308, 1307f, 1308f
Fissures
  liver, 221–223, 222f, 239
  neonatal, 817–818, 818f
Fistula
  arteriovenous, 482–483, 484f, 589, 617f
  dialysis, 1123f
  pancreatic, 636, 637f
Five-chamber view
  apical, 922b, 932–938, 936f, 937f, 938b
  of left and right ventricular outflow tracts, 1021, 1021b, 1022f
  of ventricular septal aneurysm, 1040f
FL. see Falciform ligament
Flank pain, 573–574, 573t
Flat flow velocity profile, 905–906
Flexion, 853
"Floating gallstones," 303, 305f
Flow cytometry, 538–539
Fluid collections
  in adhesions, 1240, 1241f
  endometrial
    large, 1225, 1225f
    small, 1224–1225, 1225f
  pleural, 559
  retroperitoneal, 508–509
  scrotal, 718t
  ultrasound-guided, 534–535
Fluid-fluid level, 130
FMD. see Fibromuscular dysplasia
FNA. see Fine-needle aspiration
FNH. see Focal nodular hyperplasia
Focal banding, 156, 157f
Focal brain necrosis, 837–838
Focal enhancement, 156, 157f
Focal fatty infiltration, 244, 245f
Focal fatty sparing, 244, 245f

Focal hepatic disease, 260–265, 264t
Focal nodular hyperplasia (FNH), 268–269, 272f
  contrast-enhanced ultrasound imaging of, 518, 520f
  liver findings, 271t
Focal orchitis, 717t
Focal pyelonephritis, 806f
Focal sparing, 608
Focal zone, 13–14, 22, 22f
Focused assessment with sonography for trauma (FAST), 563f
  in blunt trauma, 563–567, 563b, 563f, 564b, 564f, 565f
  in parenchymal injury, 566–567, 567f
Foley catheter, 43–44
Follicle-stimulating hormone (FSH), 1171, 1231–1233
Follicular adenomas, 692
Follicular carcinoma, 694–696
Follicular cysts
  description of, 1231–1233, 1233f
  ovarian, 1231–1233, 1233f
Follicular development, 1170–1172, 1171f
Fontanels, 814, 815b, 815f
  anterior, 822f, 824, 824f
Food allergies, 763t
Foot, ulcers of, 1118
Foramen of Bochdalek, 1555, 1556f
Foramen of Monro, 816
Foramen of Morgagni, 1555–1556, 1556f
Foramen ovale, 1014t
  fetal circulation, 1446f
Foramen secundum, 1009, 1010f
Ford Motor Company, 69
Foregut, 1573–1574, 1574f
Forehead, abnormalities of, 1496–1498, 1497f, 1498f, 1499f
Formed elements, 81
Fornices, 1162, 1164f
Fossa ovale, 1010
Fossa ovalis, 1037
Four-chamber view
  apical, 572f, 921f, 922b, 922f, 941f, 943f
    right heart, 938b
  of congenital heart disease, 1033, 1034f
  of cor triatriatum, 1059f
  of critical aortic stenosis, 1051f
  of Ebstein anomaly, 1043–1045, 1044f
  of fetal heart, 1017–1021, 1018b, 1019f, 1020f, 1021f
  of fetus, 1017–1021, 1018b, 1019f, 1020f, 1021f
  of hypoplastic left heart, 1053f
  of membranous septal defect, 1040f
  of mitral and tricuspid valves, 1014f
  of ostium primum atrial septal defect, 1038f
  of rhabdomyomas, 1058f
  of single ventricle, 1058–1059, 1058f, 1059f
  subcostal, 939f, 947f
  of total anomalous pulmonary venous return, 1060f
  of transposition of the great arteries, 1054f
Four-chambered heart, 1009, 1010f
Four-dimensional ultrasound, 20–21, 20f
Fourth ventricle, neonatal, 827
Fracture bedpan, 48, 48f
Frame rate, 18
Frank dislocation, 860
Frank-Starling law of the heart, 903

Free-hand techniques, 535–536
  one-person, 536f
  two-person, 535f
Frequency, 12, 12t
Frequency shift, 22
Fresnel, Augustin, 6
Frontal bossing, 1352–1354, 1497, 1497f
Frontonasal dysplasia, 1503, 1505f, 1510
Fry, William, 7
FSH. see Follicle-stimulating hormone
Full-thickness rotator cuff tears, 752, 753b, 753f
Functional cysts, 1236
  corpus luteum cysts, 1236–1237, 1237b, 1237f
  follicular cysts, 1236, 1237b
  hemorrhagic cysts, 1237, 1238f
  theca-lutein cysts, 1237, 1238b, 1239f
Fundus
  description of, 390, 1162–1163
  illustration of, 1166f
  transvaginal scanning of, 1186, 1186f, 1193
Fused crossed renal ectopia, 448
Fusiform aneurysm, 191, 192f
Fusion technology, 540–542, 540f, 541f, 542f

G
Gain, 21–22, 21f, 26, 715–716, 715t
Galactoceles, 663, 663f
Galactography, of breast, 676, 677f
Galeazzi sign, 858–859, 859f
Galenic venous malformation, 845, 846f
Galilei, Galileo, 6
Gallbladder, 88, 89f
  abdominal scanning of
    at level of liver, 108–109, 118f
    at level of liver and right kidney transverse, 107, 111f
    at level of liver and right kidney longitudinal, 107, 111f
    at level of right kidney, 107, 111f
  anatomy of, 282f, 283
    variations in, 283f, 285, 287f
  double, 288f
  fetal
    abnormalities of, 1582–1583
    sonographic evaluation of, 1579
  laboratory data of, 285
  longitudinal scans of, 141
  pathology of, 289–308, 294t–295t
    carcinoma, 306–308, 309f, 310f
    cholelithiasis, 294t–295t, 300, 301f, 302f, 303f, 304f
    gallbladder disease, 290–293
    porcelain gallbladder, 294t–295t, 303, 305f
    sludge, 290–293, 294t–295t, 295f
    torsion, 299–300
    wall thickening, 293, 296b, 296f
  pediatric, 765–766, 765b, 765f
  physiology of, 285
  removal of, 285
  septations of, 288f
  sonographic evaluation of, 284f, 286f, 287–289, 290f, 291f, 292f
Gallbladder wall, thickening of, 293, 296b, 296f
Gallstones
  in children, 767
  fetal, 1582, 1584f
  floating, 303, 305f
  in hepatic duct, 262f

Gallstones (Continued)
  pancreatitis and, 370
  sonographic findings of, 296, 298f, 299f
Galton, Sir Francis, 6
Gangrenous cholecystitis, 294t–295t, 297, 300f
Garrett, William, 7–8
Gartner duct cyst, 1203, 1203f
GASA. see Growth-adjusted sonar age
Gas-containing abscesses, 421–422, 423f
Gastric bezoars, 399–400, 400t, 401f
Gastric carcinoma, 400t, 401–402, 402f
Gastric tumors, 400–401
Gastrin, 393
Gastrinoma, 381, 384f
Gastrocnemius muscle, 735f, 755f
Gastrocnemius veins, 1139
Gastroduodenal artery (GDA), 179–180, 180f
  abdominal scanning of
    at gallbladder and right kidney level, 107, 110f
    at level of liver, inferior vena cava, and pancreas, 109, 120f
  pancreas and, 359
Gastroesophageal junction, 395, 396f
Gastrohepatic ligament, 390
Gastrointestinal (GI) system, 83–86
  assessment of, 84
  diseases and disorders of, 84–86, 85t
  fetal, 1365–1366, 1365f, 1576–1579
  normal findings for, 84
Gastrointestinal (GI) tract
  anatomy of, 389–393, 390f, 411b–412b
  fetal, abnormalities of, 1584–1590, 1584b
    bowel, 1586–1590
    esophagus, stomach, duodenum, 1584–1586, 1585f
  pathology of, 399–412, 400t
    acute appendicitis, 403–405, 404t, 406f
    Crohn's disease, 404t, 409, 409f
    duplication cysts, 399, 400f, 400t
    gastric bezoars, 399–400, 400t, 401f
    gastric carcinoma, 400t, 401–402, 402f
    leiomyomas, 400, 400t, 401f
    leiomyosarcoma, 400t, 402, 403f, 404t
    lymphoma, 400t, 402, 402f, 404t
    Meckel's diverticulitis, 404t, 408–409
    metastatic disease, 400t, 402, 403f
    mucocele, 404t, 405–408, 408f
    obstruction and dilation, 403, 404t, 405f
    polyps, 400, 400t, 401f
  physiology and laboratory data of, 393–394
  sonographic evaluation of, 394–399, 396f
    appendix, 398
    colon, 398–399, 399f
    duodenum, 396–397, 397f
    layers of bowel and, 394, 394b
    small bowel, 397–398, 398f
    stomach, 395–396, 396f
  vascular anatomy of, 392–393, 394f
Gastrophrenic ligament, 390
Gastroschisis, 1338, 1466–1467, 1466f, 1562, 1564t, 1565–1566, 1566f, 1575–1576, 1575f
  left-side, 1567f
  omphalocele versus, 1562, 1564b
  sonographic findings in, 1565, 1567f
Gastrosplenic ligament, 326, 328f, 390, 418, 418f
Gate, 23–24
Gaucher disease, 332, 340

G-cell tumors, 381, 384f
GDA. see Gastroduodenal artery
Gender pronouns, 62t
Genetic amniocentesis, prenatal diagnosis of congenital anomalies, 1431–1432, 1431f, 1432f
Genital ridge, 1593
Genitalia
 external female, 1159, 1159f
 fetal, 1368–1369, 1368f, 1369f
  ultrasound, 1408t
 sonographic evaluation of, 1596–1598, 1598f
Genitourinary pathology, 797f
Genitourinary system, 86–88
Germ cell tumors, 507–508, 728, 1250–1252
 dysgerminoma, 1252, 1254f
 endodermal sinus tumors, 1252
 sonographic findings in, 728–730, 729f
 teratomas
  dermoid tumors, 1250–1251, 1252b, 1252f, 1253f
  immature and mature, 1251–1252, 1253f
Germinal epithelium, 1168
Germinal matrix, 818, 832
Germinal matrix-intraventricular hemorrhages (GM-IVHs), 832, 833b
Gerota fascia, 92, 436, 492
Gestational age, 814t, 1284–1285, 1301, 1378
 determination of, first trimester, 1313–1316
  crown-rump length, 1301, 1304f, 1315, 1315f, 1316f
  mean gestational sac size, 1314, 1314f, 1315f
Gestational sac, 1289–1290
 abnormal
  absent intrauterine sac, 1320–1322, 1321t, 1322f
  criteria, 1322–1323
  sonographic findings associated with, 1324b
  without embryo or yolk sac, 1322
 sonographic findings of, during fetal period, 1307–1310, 1307f, 1307t
Gestational sac diameter (GSD), 1379–1381, 1379b, 1379f, 1380f, 1380t, 1381b, 1381f
Gestational trophoblastic disease, 1323–1326, 1324f, 1325f, 1326f, 1456–1457, 1457f
Gilbreth, Frank, 69
Gilbreth, Lillian, 69
Glioependymal cyst, 1523t
Glisson's capsule, 221–223
Globulins, 81, 231
Glomerulus, 437
Gloves
 removing, 52
 standard precautions and, 56, 56f
Glucagon, 361, 361t
Glucocorticoids, 497
Glucose, 362
Gluteus maximus, 115f, 853
Gluteus medius, 853
Gluteus minimus, 853
Glycogen storage disease, 243t, 248–249, 250f
GM-IVHs. see Germinal matrix-intraventricular hemorrhages
Goiters, 683
 endemic, 691
 fetal, 1514–1515, 1516f
 nontoxic simple, 691, 691t
Gonadal artery, 186
Gonadal veins, 203–204

Gonadotropin-releasing hormones (GnRHs), 1171
Gowns
 donning, 54
 standard precautions and, 57
Graafian follicles, 1171–1172
Graf's alpha angle, 860–866, 862b, 862f
Graf's beta angle, 860–866, 862b, 862f
Graft, aortic, 194–195, 196f
Granulocytes, 83
Granulocytopoietic abnormalities, 342
Granulomas, sperm, 726, 726f
Granulomatous disease, chronic, 264t, 266, 268f
Granulomatous mastitis, 663
Granulosas, 1255, 1256f
Grating lobes, 151, 153f
Graves disease, 698–699
 hyperthyroidism caused by, 685, 685b
 sonographic findings in, 699, 699f
Gravidity, 1286
Gray scale, 17–18
Gray-scale harmonic imaging (GSHI), 516f, 1137–1140
Great pancreatic artery, 180
Great vessels
 abnormalities of, 1054–1058
  coarctation of the aorta, 1055–1056, 1057f
  ductal constriction, 1057
  interrupted aortic arch, 1056–1057
  transposition of the great arteries, 1054, 1054f, 1055f
  truncus arteriosus, 1054–1055, 1055f, 1056f
 anatomy of, 894–901, 895f, 896f
Greater omentum, 97, 97f, 390, 413–414, 416f
Greater sac, 97, 98f, 414, 416f
Greater saphenous vein (GSV), 1132
Greater trochanter, 851
Grey Turner sign, 188, 375
Griffith, James, 8
Gross anatomy, 80
Growth-adjusted sonar age (GASA), 1384–1385
Growth restriction, 1327
GSD. see Gestational sac diameter
GSHI. see Gray-scale harmonic imaging
GSV. see Greater saphenous vein
Gutters, 99–100, 414
Guyon canal, 748, 749f
Gynecomastia, 651–652, 652f
Gyrus, 817

H
Hamartoma
 mesenchymal, 775
 of spleen, 349–351
"Hamburger" sign, 1598, 1598f
Hammurabi, Prince, 1295
Hand, 747–749
 anomalies, 1633, 1633f, 1634f
Hand sanitizers, 53, 53b
Hand-Schüller-Christian disease, 342
Hand washing, 52–53, 53b
Harmonic imaging (HI), 18–20, 19f, 515–516, 540
 gray-scale, 516f
 intermittent imaging and, 516
Hartmann pouch, 285
Hashimoto thyroiditis, 700, 700f
Haustra, 390–391
Haustral folds, 1578, 1579f

HCC. see Hepatocellular carcinoma
hCG. see Human chorionic gonadotropin
Head and neck, fetal ultrasound, 1408t
Health Insurance Portability and Accountability Act (HIPAA), 32, 62–63, 1298
Heart
 aortic arch and branches, 901, 901f
 aortic valve, 901, 901f, 935f, 945–946, 946f, 950f
 apical views of, 919f, 922b
 auscultation of valves of, 904–905, 905f
 cardiac cycle, 901–903, 901b, 902f
 development of, 1009–1010, 1009f, 1010f
 electrical activity of, 904, 904f
 electrical conduction system, 903, 903f
 embryonic, 1313, 1314f, 1314t
 FAST scan of chambers of, 564, 564f
 fetal, 1359–1360, 1360f, 1361f
  crisscross view of, 1021, 1022b, 1022f
  five-chamber view of, 1021, 1021b, 1022f
  four-chamber view of, 1017–1021, 1018b, 1019f, 1020f, 1021f
 Frank-Starling law of, 903
 great vessels of, 894–901, 895f, 896f
 heart wall linings, 896–897, 897f
 interatrial septum, 897, 897f
 interventricular septum, 900, 900f, 946, 951f
 intracardiac pressures and volumes, 909–910, 909f
 left atrium, 894, 899, 899f, 945–946, 950f
 left ventricle, 946, 951f
 mechanical conduction system, 903–904
 mitral valve, 899, 899f, 900f, 943–944, 950f
 M-mode imaging of, 920, 943–952, 950b
 pericardial sac, 895f, 896
 pulmonary trunk, 898, 898f
 pulmonary valve, 898, 898f
 right atrium, 897, 897f
 subcostal view of, 564f
 thorax and, fetal ultrasound, 1408t
 tricuspid valve, 897, 897f
Heart failure, AFP and, 1428
Heart rate
 fetal, 1012
 intracranial arterial velocities and, 1097, 1097b
Heart sounds, 904–905
Height-adjustable stools, 78
Heimlich maneuver
 definition of, 65
 techniques of, 65
Heister valve, 285
Hemangioblastoma, 377
Hemangioendothelioma, infantile, 774–775, 775t
Hemangiomas, 1497–1498, 1498f, 1499f
 cavernous
  contrast-enhanced imaging of, 518, 520f
  hepatic, 268, 271t, 272f
 of cord, 1467, 1467f
 hepatic, 608
 liver, 519f
Hemangiosarcoma, splenic, 352
Hematoceles, 579, 717t, 725–726
Hematochezia, 85t, 86
Hematocrit, 83, 332–333, 438, 1097
Hematomas
 bladder-flap, 430
 of cord, 1467
 extraperitoneal, 430, 431f
 intramural, 977, 977f
 intramuscular, 580f, 738f

Hematomas (Continued)
  in liver transplantation patients, 598, 603f
  in Morison's pouch, 539f
  in pancreatic transplantation patients, 636
  placental, 1320
  in renal transplantation patients, 620-621, 624f
  scrotal, 714f, 717t
  splenic, 347-348, 348f, 349f, 566f
  subfascial, 430
Hematometrocolpos, 1205f, 1225
Hematopoiesis, 326, 337b, 1307
Hematuria, 438
Hemianopsia, 1072
Hemifacial microsomia, 1500-1501
Hemihypertrophy, 773
Hemiparesis, 1072
Hemobilia, 315, 317f
Hemochromatosis, 243t, 249, 250f
Hemodynamics, 915ba
  Bernoulli equation, 913-914, 914f
  cardiac cycle, 909-910, 909f
  cardiac output, 910, 1097
  in cardiac tamponade, 985b
  color Doppler imaging, 912, 912f, 913f
  continuity principle, 915
  continuous wave Doppler, 913, 913f
  definition of, 908
  Doppler effect, 910-911, 911f
  Doppler frequency shift, 910-911, 910f, 911f
  extracranial arterial, 1071
  pulsed wave Doppler, 911-912, 911f
  right atrial pressure, 914, 914f
  stroke volume, 910, 914
  terminology associated with, 908
Hemoglobin, 83, 332, 438
Hemolysis, 1409
Hemolytic anemia, 341
Hemoperitoneum, 563
Hemopoiesis, 1574
Hemorrhage, 399, 426
  adrenal
    description of, 503, 503f
    illustration of, 503f
    neonatal/pediatric, 796t, 807, 808f
  epidural, 835
  intracerebellar, 834-835, 837f
  intracranial, 832-836, 833b, 1523t
  intraparenchymal, 566, 834, 836f
  intraventricular, 816, 833-834, 833f, 834f, 835f
  retroperitoneal, 508, 508f
  subchorionic, 1320, 1321f
Hemorrhagic corpus luteum cysts, 1237, 1238f
Hemorrhagic cysts, 1237, 1238f
Hemorrhagic pancreatitis, 369t, 375, 376f
Hemosiderin, 332
Henry, Walter, 8
Hepatic adenoma, 250f, 269-270, 273f
Hepatic arteries, 223, 225f
  anomalies in, 242-243
  Doppler observations of, 256t
  sonographic findings of, 260t
Hepatic artery
  Doppler flow patterns in, 212-214, 212b, 213f
  pseudoaneurysms of, 597, 601f
  stenosis of, after liver transplantation, 596, 599f
  thrombosis of, after liver transplantation, 596, 600f
Hepatic blood flow, 517
Hepatic candidiasis, 264t, 266, 267f

Hepatic congestion, passive, 259-260, 261t, 263f
Hepatic cyst, 260-262, 264t, 608
Hepatic duct, 262f, 282, 282f
Hepatic flexure, 390-391
Hepatic hemangiomas, 775
Hepatic tumors, 268-280, 271t
  benign, 268-269
  contrast-enhanced evaluation of, 517f, 518, 518f, 519f, 520f, 521f
  malignant, 270-280
    hepatocellular carcinoma, 270-271, 271t, 274f, 275f
    lymphoma, 271t, 274-280, 277f
    metastatic disease, 271-274, 271t, 276f
Hepatic vasculature technique, 255t
Hepatic veins (HV), 204-206, 205f, 223, 226f
  abdominal scanning of
    at level of caudate lobe, 106, 107f
    at level of inferior vena cava, pancreas, and superior mesenteric vein, 106f
  characteristics of, 223-225, 227f
  Doppler flow patterns in, 145, 146f, 214, 214b, 215f
  sonographic findings of, 198, 205f, 206f
  stenosis and thrombosis of, after liver transplantation, 594, 595f, 596f
Hepatitis, 244-246
  A, 245-246
  acute, 243t, 246, 246f
  B, 245-246
  C, 245-246, 605-606
  chronic, 243t, 246, 247f
  neonatal, 770, 771f, 771t
Hepatobiliary system
  abnormalities of, 1580-1584
  embryology of, 1574
  physiology and laboratory data of, 225-231
  sonographic evaluation of, 1579-1580
  upper abdomen and, fetal, 1363-1365, 1364f, 1365f
Hepatoblastoma, 773, 774f
Hepatocellular carcinoma (HCC), 270-271, 271t, 274f, 275f
  after liver transplantation, 605, 605f
  contrast-enhanced ultrasound imaging of, 518, 519f
  pediatric, 774
Hepatocellular disease, 228t
  definition of, 225-226
  obstructive disease versus, 225-226
Hepatocytes, 229
Hepatofugal flow, 209, 231
Hepatopetal flow, 209, 231
Hepatorenal recess, 420, 422f
Hepatosplenic candidiasis, 344
Hermaphroditism, true, 1618
Hernia
  abdominal, 432-434, 432f, 433f
  bowel, 1561-1562, 1565-1566, 1567f
  congenital diaphragmatic, 1555-1558, 1556b
  epigastric, 433
  incarcerated, 575
  inguinal, 577f
  left congenital, 1557b
  paraumbilical, 573t, 575-578, 576f, 577f
  reducible, 575
  scrotal, 723-725, 725f
  spigelian, 433
  strangulated, 575
  umbilical, 1563

Hertz, Hellmuth, 7, 8f
Hertz (Hz), 10, 12t
Heterogeneous, 130, 133f
Heterogeneous testicular tumor, 730f
Heterotopic pregnancy, 1279, 1279f, 1332, 1332t
Heterozygous achondroplasia, 1626
HI. see Harmonic imaging
HIFU. see High-intensity focused ultrasound
High-intensity focused ultrasound (HIFU), 1210
High-risk pregnancy
  sonography and, 1406, 1424b-1425b
    fetal factors, 1417-1418
      fetal death, 1417, 1417f
      large for gestational age, 1417
      small for gestational age, 1417-1418, 1418f
    maternal diseases of pregnancy, 1413-1416
      adnexal cysts, 1415
      diabetes, 1413-1415, 1414b, 1414f
      hyperemesis, 1415
      hypertension, 1415
      obesity, 1416
      systemic lupus erythematosus, 1415
      urinary tract disease, 1415
      uterine fibroids, 1416
    maternal factors, 1407-1413
      advanced maternal age, 1407
      alloimmune thrombocytopenia, 1411
      immune and nonimmune hydrops, 1407-1412
      nonimmune hydrops, 1411
      vaginal bleeding, 1412-1413, 1412f, 1413f
    multiple gestation pregnancy, 1418-1424, 1418b
    screening tests, 1406-1407, 1408t
    ultrasound in labor and delivery, 1416-1417
  systemic lupus erythematosus, 1064f
Hilar cholangiocarcinoma, 318
Hilus, 436
Hindgut, 1574f, 1576
Hip
  anatomy of, 851-854
  bones of, 851, 851f
  ligaments of, 853
  movements of, 853, 854f
  muscles of, 853
  stability of, 854
HIPAA. see Health Insurance Portability and Accountability Act
Hippocrates, 1295
Hirschsprung disease, 1588, 1589f
His, bundle of, 903
Histology, 80
History, 1177
Hodgkin lymphoma, 274-280, 351
Holmes, Joseph, 7
Holoprosencephaly, 842-843, 1336, 1336t, 1337f, 1502, 1503f, 1504f, 1523t, 1531-1533, 1532f, 1533f
  alobar, 843, 843f
  definition of, 842
  lobar, 843, 844f
  semilobar, 843, 843f, 1542f
  sonographic findings in, 1533, 1533f, 1534f, 1535f
Homeostasis, 81, 438
Homogeneous, 130, 133f
Homozygous achondroplasia, 1626
Hormone detoxification, 230

Hormone replacement therapy (HRT), 1172–1174
   description of, 1205f
   in menopausal women, 1220b
Horseshoe kidney, 446t, 448–449, 452f, 1601f, 1602–1603
Howry, Douglass, 7, 8f
HPS. *see* Hypertrophic pyloric stenosis
HRT. *see* Hormone replacement therapy
HSG. *see* Hysterosalpingography
Human chorionic gonadotropin (hCG), 1277, 1301
   in ectopic pregnancy, 1303
   prenatal diagnosis of congenital anomalies, 1432–1433
Humerus, fetal measurement, 1390, 1390b, 1391f
HV. *see* Hepatic veins
Hyaloid artery, 1502f
Hydatidiform mole, 1285, 1323–1324, 1324f, 1325f
Hydranencephaly, 837, 843–844, 1538–1539
   differential considerations for, 1524t
   sonographic findings in, 843–844, 845f, 1539, 1539f
Hydrocele, 579f, 710f, 714f, 720, 1617
   idiopathic, 726f
   sonographic appearance of, 717t
Hydrocephalus, 829–832, 1540–1542.
         see also Ventriculomegaly
   acquired, 829
   communicating, 829, 1540, 1540f
   congenital, 829
   definition of, 829
   description of, 814
   Doppler measurements in, 830–831, 831f
   extra-axial spaces in, 831–832, 832b, 832f
   increased intracranial pressure and, 830
   neonatal, 829–832
   noncommunicating, 1540, 1540f
   pericallosal artery in, 831f
   posthemorrhagic, 829
   ventricular measurements, 830
   ventriculoperitoneal shunt for, 829, 829f
Hydrocephaly, 1540f
Hydrometra, 1224
Hydrometrocolpos, 1618
Hydromyelia, 883, 885f
Hydronephrosis, 474–475
   causes of, 475b
   false-negative, 477–478
   false-positive, 477, 478b
   fetal, 1609–1610
      clinical findings in, 1609–1610, 1610b, 1610f
      etiology of, 1609
      in one pole of kidney, 1599–1600
      prognosis, 1609–1610
      sonographic findings in, 1610, 1611f
   neonatal/pediatric, 796t
   nonobstructive, 477
   obstructive, 454t–458t, 475–476, 477f
   urinary tract obstruction, 474, 475f, 476f
Hydrops, 1486–1489, 1486f, 1487f
   immune, 1487–1488, 1488f
   nonimmune, 1488–1489, 1489f
Hydrops fetalis, 292f, 1407
Hydrosalpinx, 1261–1263, 1262f, 1262t, 1263f, 1264f
   infertility and, 1275–1276, 1275f
Hydrothorax, 1550–1551
Hydroureters, 1600

Hypercalcemia, 372
Hypercapnia, 1097
Hyperechoic bowel, 1366, 1589, 1589b
Hyperemesis gravidarum, 1415
Hyperglycemia, 227
Hyperlipidemia, 372
Hyperparathyroidism
   primary, 702–704, 703f
   secondary, 704
Hyperplasia
   adrenal, 497
   endometrial, 1220, 1220b, 1221f
   nodular, 690–691, 692f
Hyperplastic cholecystosis, 303–306, 306f, 307f
Hypertelorism, 1392, 1503, 1504f, 1505f
Hypertension, 84, 1415
   dissection caused by, 1079f
Hypertensive nephropathy, 454t–458t, 471
Hyperthyroidism, 685, 685b
Hypertrophic cardiomyopathy, 993–995, 996f, 997b, 997f
Hypertrophic pyloric stenosis (HPS), 777t, 783–787, 783f, 784f, 785f, 786f, 787f
Hypoalbuminemia, 228
Hypocapnia, 1097
Hypoechoic, 130, 133f
Hypoechoic lesion, 718t
Hypoechoic masses, differential considerations for, 728t
Hypoglycemia, 227
Hypomotility, 779
Hypophosphatasia
   congenital, 1628
   sonographic findings in, 1623t
Hypoplasia
   midface, 1505–1506, 1507f, 1508f
   renal, 445–446
Hypoplastic left heart syndrome, 1052–1054, 1052f, 1053f
Hypoplastic right heart syndrome, 1045, 1045f
Hypospadias, 1601
Hypotelorism, 1392, 1502–1503, 1503f, 1534–1535, 1535f
Hypotension, 84
Hypothalamus, neonatal, 818
Hypothyroidism, 685
Hypoxia, neonatal, 814
Hypoxic-ischemic injury lesions, 836–838
Hysterosalpingography (HSG), 1272–1273

I

IA. *see* Iliac arteries
IAE. *see* Induced acoustic emission
ICA. *see* Internal carotid artery
IHF. *see* Immune hydrops fetalis
IJV. *see* Internal jugular vein
ILC. *see* Invasive lobular carcinoma
Ileostomies, 47
Iliac aneurysm, 195
Iliac arteries (IA), 108, 113f, 172, 173f, 174f, 178t, 1169, 1170f
Iliac fossa, 492b, 495
Iliac veins, 108
Iliacus muscle, 94, 495f, 1161
Iliofemoral ligament, 853
Iliopectineal line, 1159–1160, 1159f
Iliopsoas muscle, 94, 494f, 495f, 1160f, 1190–1192, 1191f

Illness, patient reactions to, 60–61
IMA. *see* Inferior mesenteric artery
Image resolution, 13–14
Immune and nonimmune hydrops, 1407–1412
Immune hydrops, 1407, 1409f
   cordocentesis, 1410–1411, 1411f
   sonographic surveillance, 1409–1410, 1409f, 1410f
Immune hydrops fetalis (IHF), 1487–1488, 1488f
Imperforate anus, 803f
In vitro fertilization, 1278
Incarcerated hernia, 575
Inclusion cysts, peritoneal, 1239–1242, 1240f
Incompetent cervix, 1285
Incomplete atrioventricular septal defect, 1041, 1042f
Incomplete duplication, 446
Increased intracranial pressure, 830
Independence, 5b
Indirect-acting bilirubin, 229, 229t
Indirect arterial testing, 1114–1118
Induced acoustic emission (IAE), 514–515, 515f
Infant head, 813, 847b–848b
Infant hip, 850, 869b
Infantile hemangioendothelioma, 774–775, 775f
Infantile polycystic kidney disease (IPKD), 1605–1606, 1606f
Infarction
   renal, 454t–458t, 481–482
   splenic, 337t, 344–345, 347f
Infection
   after liver transplantation, 593, 595f
   after pancreatic transplantation, 633, 634f
   after renal transplantation, 616, 619f
   neural axis, 1523t
   nosocomial, 50
   renal, 478, 479f, 616, 619f
   splenic, 344, 344f, 347f
   urinary tract, neonatal/pediatric, 806–807
Infection prevention, 49–53, 50f, 51f
   nosocomial infection and, 50
   standard precautions and, 49–53, 50f, 51f
Infectious disease, of liver, 265–268
Inferior direction, 132–134
Inferior mediastinum, 892, 893b
   illustration of, 892
Inferior mesenteric artery (IMA), 184, 184f
   abdominal scanning of, at liver, gallbladder, and right kidney level, 107, 111f
   sonographic evaluation of, 184–195
Inferior mesenteric vein, 209
   sonographic findings of, 198
Inferior vena cava (IVC), 195–206, 197f, 198f, 199f
   abdominal scanning of
      at level of caudate lobe, 106, 107f
      at level of hepatic vein, pancreas and superior mesenteric vein, 109, 121f
      at level of left lobe of the liver and pancreas, 109, 120f
      at level of liver, pancreas, and gastroduodenal artery, 109, 120f
   abnormalities, 198–199
   anatomy of, 92, 195–197
   anterior tributaries to, 204–206
   color Doppler technique for, 255t
   congenital left atrial communication with, 1059, 1060f
   diagnostic criteria for, 260t

Inferior vena cava (IVC) (Continued)
    dilation or compression of, 198–199, 201f
    Doppler flow patterns in, 214, 214b, 215f
    Doppler ultrasound of, 146, 256t
    fetal circulation and, 1010, 1446f
    hepatic portion of, 198
    lateral tributaries to, 199–204
    longitudinal scans of, 141, 198
    pancreatic portion of, 198
    renal vein obstruction, 202–203
    retroperitoneum and, 496
    small bowel (lower) segment of, 198
    sonographic findings of, 198–204, 200f, 201f, 202f
    stenosis of, after liver transplantation, 594, 595f, 596f
    thrombosis of, 199–204
    tributaries of, 197
    tumors of, 198
Inferior vena cava filters, 199–204, 203f
Infertility
    female. see Female infertility
    male, 724f
Infiltrating, 131, 133f
Infiltrating carcinomas, 671
Infiltrative cardiomyopathy, 990–992, 992b
Inflammatory aortic aneurysm, 192
Inflammatory ascites, 420, 422f
Inflammatory carcinoma, 673, 674f
Inflammatory reaction, 660
Informed consent, 1295–1296
Infracristal defects, 1038–1039
Infrapatellar tendon bursa, 738f
Infrasound, 11t
Infraspinatus tendon, 745, 747f
Infundibulum, 1167, 1167f
Inguinal canal, 100–101, 100f
Inguinal hernia, 577f
Inguinal ligament, 90–91
Initiative, 5b
Injuries
    parenchymal, 566–567, 567f
    in sonography, 70–72, 71f, 71t
Innominate artery, 1070, 1112
Innominate veins, 1133
INR. see International normalized ratio
Inspissated bile, 770
Instrumentation
    fetal echocardiography, 1013
    pulse-echo, 21–22, 21f
    transcranial color Doppler imaging, 1091
Insulin, 361t
Insulinoma, 381, 383f, 384f
Integrity, 1297–1298
Intellectual curiosity, 5b
Intensity, 11–12
Interatrial septum, 897
Interface, 12
Intermittent imaging, 516
Internal carotid artery (ICA), 1070, 1071f, 1088, 1088f
    diagnostic criteria for, 1080, 1080t
    hemodynamics of, 1071
    occlusion of, 1077, 1078f, 1080–1081
    stenosis of, 1080, 1081f
Internal iliac arteries, 1169
Internal iliac vein, 1131
Internal jugular vein (IJV), 1133

Internal oblique muscle, 90, 90f
Internal os, 1191
International normalized ratio (INR), 532
Interrupted aortic arch, 1056–1057
Interstitial nephritis, acute, 454t–458t, 470–471
Interstitial pregnancy, 1332, 1333f
Intertubercular plane, 105
Interventional ultrasound, of adnexa, 1270f
Interventricular septum, 900, 900f
    description of, 1023
    M-mode imaging of, 946, 951f
Intervertebral disks, 873, 874f
Intervillous space, 1443f
Intervillous thrombosis, 1456, 1456f
Intestinal obstructions, 1586–1587, 1587f
Intestine, 1462f
Intima-media thickness, 1081
Intracerebellar hemorrhage, 834–835, 837f
Intracorporeal liver, 1564t
Intracranial arteries
    anatomy of, 1088–1090, 1088f
    identification of, 1096t
    occlusion of, 1100
    stenosis of, 1100
    velocities
        normal, 1096t, 1097–1099, 1098f
        physiologic factors, 1096–1097
Intracranial cerebrovascular evaluation, 1087, 1107b
    anatomy for imaging in, 1088–1090, 1088f
    physiology in, 1090
Intracranial hemorrhage, 1523t
Intracranial venous evaluation, 1104
Intraductal papillary mucinous neoplasms, 379–380, 382f
Intraductal papilloma, 658t, 665–666, 666f
Intrahepatic biliary neoplasms, 318
Intrahepatic cholangiocarcinoma, 319–320, 321f
Intrahepatic ducts, 136
Intrahepatic masses, 260–262
Intrahepatic vessels and ducts, 223–225
Intraluminal transducer, 17, 17f
Intramural benign gastric tumors, 400–401
Intramural hematoma, 977, 977f
Intramural leiomyomas, 1209, 1209b
Intrapancreatic obstruction, 312, 314f
Intraparenchymal hemorrhage, 566, 834, 836f
Intraperitoneal compartments, 417–418, 418f, 419f
Intraperitoneal organ, 326
Intratesticular cysts, 727, 727f
Intratesticular varicocele, 724f
Intrauterine contraceptive devices (IUCDs), 1225–1228, 1226f–1227f
Intrauterine growth restriction (IUGR), 1284–1285, 1388, 1395–1397, 1396b
    asymmetric, 1397
    small for gestational age, 1397
    symmetric, 1397
Intrauterine insemination, 1278
Intrauterine pregnancy (IUP), 1306
    abnormal
        cardiac activity and, 1326
        sonographic findings associated with, 1324b
    assisted reproductive technology and, 1279, 1279f
Intrauterine sac, absent, 1320–1322, 1321t, 1322f
Intrauterine synechiae, 1222–1223, 1223f
Intravenous (IV) injection, 513

Intravenous (IV) therapy
    definition of, 41–42
    patient care and, 41–43, 41f, 42f, 43f
Intravenous urography (IVU), 573
Intraventricular hemorrhage (IVH), 816, 833–834, 833f, 834f, 835f
Intrinsic factor, 83
Intussusception, 777t, 781–783, 782f, 783f
Invasive ductal carcinoma, 672
Invasive lobular carcinoma (ILC), 673, 674f
IPKD. see Infantile polycystic kidney disease
Irregular borders, 131, 133f
Ischemic cardiomyopathy, 989
Ischemic rest pain, 1114
Islet cell tumors, nonfunctioning, 381, 384f
Islet cells
    metastasis of, 605f
    transplantation of, 627
Islets of Langerhans, 359, 361
Isoechoic, 131
Isolation precautions, 53–55, 53b
Isovolumetric contraction, 901b
Isovolumic contraction, 909
Isthmus
    of fallopian tubes, 1167f
    thyroid, 683, 684f
IUCDs. see Intrauterine contraceptive devices
IUGR. see Intrauterine growth restriction
IUP. see Intrauterine pregnancy
IVC. see Inferior vena cava
IVH. see Intraventricular hemorrhage
IVU. see Intravenous urography
Izumi, Kato, 8–10
Izumi, T., 8–10

J

Jastrzebowski, Wojciech, 68
Jaundice, 83
    bilirubin elevations in, 229
    gallbladder disease and, 290–293
    neonatal, 770
    nonobstructive, 770
    obstructive, 770
Jaw index, 1499, 1500b
Jejunoileal atresia, 1586
Jeune syndrome, 1631
Joint, hip, 851–853, 853f
Joint effusions, of hip, 867–868, 868f
Joint Review Committee on Education in Cardiovascular Technology (JRC-CVT), 6
Joint Review Committee on Education in Diagnostic Medical Sonography (JRC-DMS), 6
JRC-CVT. see Joint Review Committee on Education in Cardiovascular Technology
JRC-DMS. see Joint Review Committee on Education in Diagnostic Medical Sonography
Junctional fold, 287–289
Junctional parenchymal defects, 444, 446f, 447f
Justice, 1298
Juxtamedullary lipoma, 884f

K

Kager's fat pad, 751f
Kasai, Chihiro, 8–10
Kasai portoenterostomy, 771–772

KDOQI. *see* Kidney Disease Outcomes Quality Initiative
Key bladder sign, 1600
Kidney(s), 88
   agenesis of, 445–446, 449f
   anatomy of, 86, 435–437, 436f
   ectopic, 448–449, 451f, 452f
   fetal
      congenital malformations of, 1601–1605
      development of, 1593–1594, 1593f, 1594f
      not seen, 1600
      sonographic evaluation of, 1595–1599, 1597f, 1597t, 1598f
   function of, 438
   medullary sponge, 454t–458t, 462, 479, 480f
   neonatal/pediatric
      anatomy of, 792–793, 793f, 810b–811b
      hydronephrosis, 796t
      pathology of enlargement of, 796, 796t, 797t
         adrenal hemorrhages, 796t, 807, 808f
         hydronephrosis, 796t
         prune belly syndrome, 796t, 801–802
         renal cystic disease, 804–805, 804f
         renal vein thrombosis, 807
      sonographic evaluation of, 792–793, 793f, 794f
   physiology of, 438–439
   secondary malignancies of, 466, 468f, 469f
   sonographic evaluation of, 439–444, 766f
      patient position and technique in, 439, 440f, 441f, 442f
      renal medulla, 444
      renal parenchyma, 440–441, 442f, 443f
      renal vessels, 441–444, 443f, 444f, 445f
   transverse scans of, 141, 144f
   ultrasound-guided biopsy of, 554–555, 555f
   variants of, 444, 446f
      columns of Bertin, 444, 446f
      extrarenal pelvis, 444–445, 446t, 448f
      fetal lobulation, 444–445, 446t, 447f
      junctional parenchymal defects, 444, 446f, 447f
      sinus lipomatosis, 444, 447f
Kidney disease, chronic, 474
Kidney Disease Outcomes Quality Initiative (KDOQI), 1123–1124
Kilohertz (kHz), 10
Kissing cysts, 459, 460f
Klatskin tumor, 320–321, 322f
Kleeblattschädel, 1498–1499, 1499f
Knobology, 126
Kossoff, George, 7–8
Krause, Walter, 8
Krukenberg tumors, 1256–1257, 1257f

L

Labeling scans, 124
Labia majora, 1159, 1159f
Labia minora, 1159, 1159f
Labor and delivery
   preterm labor, 1416–1417
   ultrasound in, 1416–1417
Laboratory orientation, 124–125
Laboratory tests
   pancreatic, 361, 362t
   renal disease, 438–439
   thyroid function, 685–686, 686t
   ultrasound-guided, 531–532

Labrum, acetabular, 851–853
Lactating patient, breast imaging in, 649, 650f, 662
Lactic acid dehydrogenase, 230–231
Lacunae, 1301
Laminar flow, 23, 905
Langevin, Paul, 6
Large for gestational age (LGA), 1404, 1417
Large intestine, 89, 93f. *see also* Bowel
   anatomy of, 392, 395f
   vascular anatomy of, 390–391, 393f, 395f
Large-core needle biopsy, ultrasound-guided, 676
Larynx, abnormalities of, 1511–1512, 1512f
Last menstrual period (LMP), 1378
Late proliferative phase, 1195
Lateral arcuate ligament, 89
Lateral direction, 132
Lateral resolution, 13–14
Lateral rotation, 853
Lateral ventricles
   atrium (trigone) of, 815, 816f
   neonatal, 816f, 824–825
Lateroconal fascia, 492–493, 493f
LCIS. *see* Lobular carcinoma in situ
Left atrial appendage, 1000
Left atrium, 894, 899, 899f
   congenital vena cava communication, 1059–1060
   development of, 1009
   fetal circulation, 1446f
   M-mode imaging of, 945–946, 950f
Left congenital hernia, 1557b
Left crus of diaphragm, 89, 89f
Left gastric artery, 180
Left hepatic artery, 180, 255t
Left hepatic vein, 223, 255t
Left hypochondrium, 219
Left kidney, abdominal scanning at level of spleen and, 109, 122f
Left lateral decubitus compression, 778
Left lateral decubitus position, 239
Left lobe of liver, 219f, 221
   abdominal scanning at level of inferior vena cava, pancreas, and, 109, 120f
   transverse scanning of, 143f
Left lower quadrant (LLQ), 88, 88f
Left parasternal window for Doppler, 928, 930f
Left portal vein, 206, 208f, 223, 224f, 255t
Left renal artery (LRA), 185, 441, 444f
Left renal vein (LRV), 200–202, 204f, 441, 445f
Left subclavian artery, 901
Left upper quadrant (LUQ), 88, 88f, 396
Left ventricle, 894, 900
   dilation of, 988f
   formation of, 1009
   M-mode imaging of, 946, 951f
Left ventricular inflow disturbance, 1048–1050
Left ventricular outflow tract disturbance, 1050–1054
   aortic stenosis, 1050–1052
   bicuspid aortic valve, 1033, 1050, 1050f
   in hypertrophic cardiomyopathy, 993–995, 997b
   hypoplastic left heart syndrome, 1052–1054, 1052f, 1053f
Left ventricular outflow tracts, 914
   crisscross view, 1021, 1022b, 1022f
   five-chamber view of, 1021, 1021b, 1022f
   long-axis view of, 1022–1023, 1023b, 1023f, 1024f, 1025f, 1026f
   short-axis view of, 1023–1026, 1026b, 1026f, 1027f

Left ventricular thrombus, 988, 989f
Left ventricular volumes, 990b
Left-sided valvular heart disease, 953, 978b–979b
   aortic atherosclerosis, 974, 977f
   aortic dissection, 973–974
   aortic insufficiency, 956, 963–966, 963t
   aortic regurgitation, 963, 963t, 964f, 965f, 966f
   aortic stenosis, 964t, 966–970, 966f, 967f, 969b, 969f, 970b, 970f
   aortic tumors, 978–979, 978f
   intramural hematoma, 977, 977f
   mitral regurgitation, 953–957, 954f, 955b, 955f, 956f, 957f, 958f
   mitral stenosis. *see* Mitral stenosis
   penetrating aortic ulcer, 977, 977f
   pseudoaneurysm, 973
   sinus of Valsalva, 974, 976f
Lehman, Stauffer, 7, 9f
Leiomyoma, 1207–1210, 1209f
   cervical, 1204, 1205f
   characteristics of, 1209b
   gastrointestinal, 400, 400t, 401f
   intramural, 1209, 1209b, 1210f
   submucosal, 1209, 1209b
   subserosal, 1209, 1209b, 1210f
   uterine, 1209, 1209b
      first-trimester, 1329t
      locations of, 1209, 1209b, 1210f
      sonographic findings in, 1210, 1211f, 1212f, 1213f
      treatment of, 1210
Leiomyosarcoma
   colon, 409–412, 411f
   gastrointestinal
      upper, 400t, 402, 403f, 404t
   primary retroperitoneal tumor and, 507, 507f
   uterine, 1216–1217, 1217b
Lemon sign, 1392–1393, 1530
Lenticulostriate vasculopathy, 838
Lesser omental bursa, 418
Lesser omentum, 97, 390, 414
   pancreas and, 358f, 359
Lesser sac
   abscesses of, 423, 424f
   description of, 97, 414
   illustration of, 416f
Lesser saphenous vein, 1132, 1132f
Lesser trochanter, 851
Lethal multiple pterygium syndrome, 1632
Letterer-Siwe disease, 342
Leukemia
   lymphatic, 83
   myelogenous, 83
   testicular, 730
Leukocytes, 83, 438
Leukocytosis, 333, 420
Leukopenia, 333
Leukopoiesis, 83
Levator ani muscles, 1160, 1160f, 1190, 1190f
Levocardia, 1033, 1035f
Levoposition, 1033
Levoversion, 1035f
LGA. *see* Large for gestational age
Lienorenal ligament, 328f, 390
Lifting, 38

Ligaments
  hip joint, 853
  liver, 221–223, 222f
  peritoneal, 98, 99f
  sonographic appearance of, 737–738, 738f, 740t
  vertebral column, 873
Ligamentum arteriosum, 898
Ligamentum teres, 98, 221–223
Ligamentum venosum, 106, 107f, 221–223, 222f, 1446
Likelihood ratios, 1375
Limb abnormalities, 1633–1635, 1633f, 1634f, 1635f
Limb development, 1313, 1313f
Limb-body wall complex, 1564t, 1570–1571, 1570f
Lindegaard ratio, 1100
Line density parameters, 715t, 716, 716f
Linea alba, 90f, 91
Linea semilunaris, 90, 419
Linear-array transducers, 16, 17f, 854, 854b, 1146
Linens, 50
"Linguine" sign, 667–668, 668f
Lip, abnormalities of, 1506–1509, 1508f, 1509f
Lipases, 361t, 362
Lipoma
  breast, 658t, 665, 665f
  juxtamedullary, 884f
  renal, 454t–458t, 468, 470f
  spinal, 882, 883f
Lipomatous hypertrophy, 998, 1001f
Lipomyelomeningocele, 885f
Lipoproteins, 227–228
Lips, development of, 1493–1494, 1493f
Lissencephaly, 1523t
Lister, Joseph, 49
Liver, 88, 89f, 218, 277b–280b
  abdominal scanning of
    at level of caudate lobe and psoas muscle, 107, 119f
    at level of duodenum and pancreas, 109, 120f
    at level of gallbladder, 108–109, 118f
    at level of gallbladder, right kidney, and longitudinal, 107, 111f
    at level of inferior vena cava, pancreas, and gastroduodenal artery, 109, 120f
  anatomy of, 219–225, 219f, 220f
    ligaments and fissures, 221–223, 222f
    lobes of, 219–223
    vascular supply, 221, 222f, 223–225
  bile and, 230, 230f
  biopsy of, ultrasound-guided, 552–553, 552f, 553f, 554f
  detoxification functions of, 229–230, 229t
  dome of, 106–108, 106f
  extracorporeal, 1564t
  FAST scan of, 564, 565f
  fatty, 243–244, 244b, 608
  fetal
    abnormalities of, 1580–1581, 1581f
    embryology of, 1574
    sonographic evaluation of, 1579, 1580f
  hepatic versus obstructive disease, 225–226
  intracorporeal, 1564t
  metabolic functions of, 227–229
  metastases to, 520f
  pathology of, 239–280
    developmental anomalies, 239–243
    diffuse parenchymal abnormalities, 258–260, 261t

Liver (Continued)
  focal hepatic disease, 260–265, 264t
  infectious disease, 265–268
  vascular flow abnormalities
    Budd-Chiari syndrome. see Budd-Chiari syndrome
    diagnostic criteria for imaging, 260t
    portal hypertension. see Portal hypertension
  pediatric, 765, 765b, 765f
  physiology of, 225, 227b
  segmental anatomy of, 220b, 221f
  sonographic evaluation of, 231–239, 232f, 233f, 234f
    anatomy and texture in, 234–235
    assessment criteria in, 233, 235f
    diagnostic criteria for, 260t
    in lateral decubitus plane, 239
    in sagittal plane, 235–239, 236f–237f, 238f
    in transverse plane, 239, 240f–241f, 242f
    ultrasound protocol for, 233–234, 235t
  vascular supply, 221, 222f, 223–225
Liver calcifications, in pregnancy affected by cytomegalovirus, 1418f
Liver cell adenoma, 271t
Liver disease, 585
  AFP and, 1428
Liver function tests, 230–231
Liver hemangioma, 519f
Liver Imaging Reporting & Data Systems (LI-RADS) system, 518
Liver omphaloceles, 1566f
Liver parenchyma
  diffuse abnormalities of, 258–260, 261t
  longitudinal scans of, 141
  sonographic findings, 590
Liver transplantation
  allograft
    Doppler evaluation of, 589
    evaluation of, 588–590, 589f
    postoperative imaging of, 590, 592f
    rejection of, 593
  biopsy after, 590, 593f, 594f
  cadaveric liver donation for, 586–587, 587f
  for cirrhosis, 584–585, 584f
  complications of
    abscesses, 593, 595f
    ascites, 605
    bile leaks, 604, 604f
    biliary, 597–598, 602f, 603f
    biloma, 604, 604f
    bleeding, 598, 603f
    bowel ischemia, 606–607, 607f
    cholangiopathy, 602f
    fatty liver, 608
    hematomas, 598, 603f
    hepatic artery pseudoaneurysms, 597, 601f
    hepatic artery stenosis, 596, 599f
    hepatic artery thrombosis, 596, 600f
    hepatic cysts, 608
    hepatic hemangioma, 608
    hepatic vein stenosis and thrombosis, 594, 595f, 596f
    hepatitis C recurrence, 605–606, 606f
    hepatocellular carcinoma, 605, 605f
    infarction and necrosis, 597, 601f
    infection, 593, 595f
    inferior vena cava stenosis, 594, 595f, 596f

Liver transplantation (Continued)
  intrahepatic abscesses, 593, 595f
  intrahepatic ductal dilation with stones, 603f
  islet cell metastasis, 605f
  lymphoceles, 604
  metastatic disease, 605, 605f
  pneumobilia, 608, 609f
  portal vein thrombus and stenosis, 594–596, 597f, 598f
  portal venous gas, 606–607, 607f
  rejection, 593
  seromas, 600, 604f
  surveillance for, 590–593, 593f, 594f
  cost of, 585–586
  criteria for, 584–585
  Doppler imaging of, 589–590
  expanded criteria donors for, 586
  history of, 584–585
  living donor for, 587–588, 588f
  Milan criteria for, 585
  Model for End-stage Liver Disease scale for, 585
  parenchymal biopsy after, 590, 593f, 594f
  Pediatric End-Stage Liver Disease scale for, 585
  rejection of, 593
  sonographic findings in, 590, 591f
  surgical technique of, 586–588
  waiting list for, 585
Liver tumors, pediatric, benign, 774–775, 775t, 776f
Living donor liver transplantation, 587–588, 588f
LLQ. see Left lower quadrant
Lobar dysmorphism, 444–445, 446t
Lobar holoprosencephaly, 843, 844f
Lobular carcinoma in situ (LCIS), 673
Lobular neoplasia, 673
Loculated mass, 131, 133f
Loeffler endocarditis, 992, 993f
Long-axis view
  apical, 938b
  of atrioventricular septal defect, 1041f
  ductal and aortic arch, 1026–1029, 1027f, 1028f
  of left ventricular outflow tracts, 1022–1023, 1023b, 1023f, 1024f, 1025f, 1026f
  parasternal
    of aortic stenosis, 1051f
    for color flow mapping, 922b, 925–928, 927f
    of congenital mitral stenosis, 1048f
    two-dimensional, 926–928, 927f
Longitudinal plane, abdominal, 104
Longitudinal scanning
  abdominal, 108–122, 128–129, 130f, 131f
  protocols for, 140–141
  transabdominal pelvic, 1178–1181
Longus colli muscle, 683, 684f
Loop of Henle, 437
Lower abdominal compartments, 418–419, 419f
Lower abdominal pain, 573t
Lower extremity
  arterial duplex imaging of, 1119–1120, 1119f, 1120f
  deep veins of, 1130–1131, 1130f
  fetal, 1369–1371, 1369f, 1370f, 1371f, 1372f
  superficial veins of, 1132–1133, 1132f
  venous duplex imaging of
    examination, 1146
    tips for, 1141t

Lower gastrointestinal tract
  acute appendicitis, 403–405, 404t, 406f
  Crohn's disease, 404t, 409, 409f
  Meckel's diverticulitis, 404t, 408–409
  mucocele, 404t, 405–408, 408f
  obstruction and dilation, 403, 404t, 405f
Lower urinary tract, 450, 453b, 453t
Lower uterine segment (LUS), 1448
Ludwig, George, 7
Lumason, 514
Lumbar artery, 187
Lumbar myelomeningocele, 1531f
Lumbar puncture, failed, 886f
Lumbosacral spine, neonatal, 878f
Lung
  anatomy of, 892–894, 893f, 894f, 895f
  fetal
    abnormalities of, 1548–1555, 1549f, 1550t
      cystic lung masses, 1549–1550, 1551b
      pleural effusions. see Pleural effusions
      pulmonary hypoplasia, 1549, 1550b, 1551f
      solid masses, 1551–1554
        congenital bronchial atresia, 1554
        congenital cystic adenomatoid malformation, 1552–1554, 1553f, 1554f
        pulmonary sequestration, 1552, 1552b, 1552f
  ultrasound-guided biopsy of, 556–557, 556f
Lung masses
  complex, 1554–1555
  solid, 1551–1554
    congenital bronchial atresia, 1554
    congenital cystic adenomatoid malformation, 1552–1554, 1553f, 1554f
    pulmonary sequestration, 1552, 1552b, 1552f
Lupus nephritis, 454t–458t, 471
LUQ. see Left upper quadrant
LUS. see Lower uterine segment
Luteal phase deficiency (LPD), 1274
Luteinization, 1172
Luteinizing hormone (LH), 1171–1172, 1231–1233
Lymph nodes
  abnormal, 651f
  normal, 651f
  para-aortic, 494–495, 494f, 498–499, 500f, 501f
  retroperitoneal
    ultrasound-guided biopsy of, 555–556, 556f
    visualization of, 550f
Lymph vessels, 326
Lymphadenopathy, 498, 706–707, 706f
  cervical, 706–707
Lymphangiectasia, 1551
Lymphangioma, 351, 351f
Lymphatic leukemia, 83
Lymphatic system
  of breast, 651, 651f
  in fetus, 1513, 1513f
Lymphoceles, 428–430, 430f, 604, 621–622, 625f, 636, 665, 665f
Lymphocytes, 83
Lymphoma, 676
  colon, 409, 410f
  gastrointestinal
    lower, 402–412, 404t, 406f
    upper, 400t, 402, 402f
  hepatic, 271t, 274–280, 277f
  mesentery, 428, 429f

Lymphoma (Continued)
  omentum, 428, 429f
  renal, 454t–458t, 466, 467f
  retroperitoneal, 506–507, 507f
  splenic, 351, 352f
  testicular, 730
  thyroid gland, 697–698, 698f
Lymphoscintigraphy, of breasts, 677–681, 678f

M
Macro movement, 126
Macrocephaly, 1531
Macroglossia, 1510
Macronodular cirrhosis, 246, 247f
Macrosomia, 1284–1285, 1404, 1413–1414
"Magic triangle," 78–79, 79f
Magnetic resonance angiography (MRA), 1083
Magnetic resonance imaging (MRI), 103t, 104
  of breasts, 652, 676–677, 677f
  fusion technology and, 540, 540f, 541f
  of kidneys, 439
  of tendons, 733–734
Main lobar fissure, 221–223, 290f
Main portal vein, 223, 224f, 255t
Main pulmonary artery, 1010
Majewski syndrome, 1630
Major calyces, 436–437
Male infertility, 724f
Male pelvic cavity, 94–95
Male pelvis, 108, 115f
Male pseudohermaphrodites, 1618
Male urethral discharge, 87
Male urinary hesitancy, 87
Malformation sequence, 1496
Malignant ascites, 420, 422f
Malignant primary cardiac tumors, 998, 1002f
Malignant tumors. see also Carcinoma
  adrenal, 504, 504f
  gastrointestinal, 401–402
  hepatic, 270–280
    hepatocellular carcinoma, 270–271, 271t, 274f, 275f
    lymphoma, 271t, 274–280, 277f
    metastatic disease, 271–274, 271t, 276f
  parapancreatic, 386–388, 386f
  pediatric, 773–774
  renal
    renal cell carcinoma. see Renal cell carcinoma
    squamous cell carcinoma, 454t–458t, 466, 467f
    transitional cell carcinoma, 454t–458t, 464–466
  spleen, 351–354
  testicular, 728–730, 728t
  thyroid gland, 693–698, 695f
Malpighian corpuscles, 330
Mammary layer, 645, 645f, 646f
Mammography
  benign gynecomastia on, 651–652, 652f
  BI-RADS categories of masses on, 653t
  breast cancer on
    males, 651–652, 652b, 652f
    signs of, 653b
  dense breast on, 648, 649f
  difficult or compromised, 653–654, 654b
  fatty tissue on, 648–649, 649f
  screening, 653–654, 653b, 653t, 654b
Mandible, abnormalities of, 1499–1500, 1500b, 1500f

Marfan syndrome, 193–194, 974
Marginal abruption, 1456, 1456f
Marginal insertion, placenta, 1444–1445
Marginal lake, 1443f
Masks
  oxygen, 45–46, 46f
  standard precautions and, 56
Mass(es)
  abdominal wall, 428
  adnexal
    with ectopic pregnancy, 1330–1332, 1331f
    resistive index and, 1236
  breast. see Breast masses
  cystic. see Cystic masses
  extrahepatic, 259, 261t, 263f
  extratesticular, 718t, 722
  liver, 552–553, 554f
  mesenteric, 426t
  neck
    developmental, 704–707
    ultrasound-guided biopsy of, 557
  omental, 426, 426t
  ovarian
    complex, 1234–1235, 1235b, 1235f
    first-trimester, 1340, 1341f
    simple cystic, 1234, 1234b, 1234f, 1235f
  pancreatic, 553–554
  pelvic, 1257–1258
    biopsy, 558
    first-trimester, 1329t, 1340
  peritoneal, 426t
  pseudopulsatile abdominal, 195
  retroperitoneal, 555–556
  scrotal, 718t, 723f
  testicular
    benign, 726–728, 727f
    malignant, 728–730, 728t
  uterine, 1340
Mastitis
  acute, 663–664, 663f
  chronic, 664
Mastodynia, 660
Mastoid fontanel, 821
Maternal anatomy, fetal ultrasound, 1408t
Maternal diseases of pregnancy, 1413–1416
  adnexal cysts, 1415
  diabetes, 1413–1415, 1414b, 1414f
  hyperemesis, 1415
  hypertension, 1415
  obesity, 1416
  systemic lupus erythematosus, 1064f, 1415
  urinary tract disease, 1415
  uterine fibroids, 1416
Maternal serum alpha-fetoprotein (MSAFP), 1285
  multiple gestation pregnancy and, 1418
Maternal serum quad screen, 1407
Maxillary prominences, 1493–1494
Maximum vertical pocket, 1478
MCA. see Middle cerebral artery
McBurney's point, 398, 398f, 777f, 778f
McBurney's sign, 403
MCDK. see Multicystic dysplastic kidney
MCL. see Medial collateral ligament
Mean flow velocity, 1097
Mean gestational sac size, 1314, 1314f, 1315f
Mean pressure gradient, 959
Mechanical conduction system, 903–904
Mechanical index (MI), 516

Mechanical macrosomia, 1405
Meckel-Gruber syndrome, 1528f
Meckel's diverticulitis, 404t, 408-409
Meckel's diverticulum, 408-409, 408f, 1576, 1576f
Meconium ileus, 1587, 1588b, 1588f
Meconium peritonitis, 1589
Medial arcuate ligament, 89
Medial collateral ligament (MCL), 738, 738f
Medial rotation, 853
Medial/lateral direction, 132
Median nerve, 739t
 compression of, 756-757, 756b
 illustration of, 739f
Mediastinum, 892
 inferior, 892, 893b
 superior, 893b
Mediastinum testis, 710, 710f
Medical ethics
 history of, 1295
 principles, 1295-1298
Medulla, 436, 497
Medulla oblongata, neonatal, 819
Medulla tumor, 502t
Medullary carcinoma
 of breast, 673, 675f
 of thyroid gland, 696-697, 697f
Medullary cystic disease, 454t-458t, 462-463
 nephronophthisis and, 463, 463f
Medullary nephrocalcinosis, neonatal/pediatric, 807f
Medullary pyramids
 description of, 440, 443f
 neonatal/pediatric, 792, 793f
Medullary sponge kidney, 454t-458t, 479
Mega cisterna magna, 842
Megacolon, 1588
Megacystis, 1608-1609
Megahertz (MHz), 10
Megaureter, 1610-1611
Meigs' syndrome, 1254
Melanoma, metastatic disease from, 555f
Membranes, fetal, 1374-1375
Membranous septal defect, 1038-1040, 1040f
Menarche, 1170, 1177
Meninges
 neonatal, 815, 816f
 spinal cord, 873-876, 874f, 877f
Meningocele, 883-885, 1528
Meningomyelocele, 1528, 1529f, 1530f
Menopause, 1170
 definition of, 1177
 hormonal regimens for women in, 1220b
Menorrhagia, 1174
Menses, endometrium and, 1164, 1172
Menstrual age, 1378. see also Gestational age
Menstrual cycle, 1170, 1171b, 1171f
 abnormal, 1174
 endometrial changes during, 1172
 endometrial thickness related to phases of, 1218t
Menstruation, 1170, 1171b, 1195, 1196f. see also Menstrual cycle
Mesenchymal hamartoma, 775
Mesenteric cysts, 426, 427f
Mesentery, 96-97, 97f, 390, 414
 lymphoma, 428, 429f
 pathology of, 426-428, 426t
Mesoblastic nephroma, 1615, 1616f
 congenital, 796t, 809

Mesocardia, 1033, 1035f
Mesocaval shunt, 256-257, 257f
Mesonephroi, 1593
Mesosalpinx, 1165
Mesothelium, 95
Mesovarium, 1165, 1166f
Metabolic macrosomia, 1405
Metabolism, 81, 227-229
Metastatic disease, 676
 adrenal glands, 504-505, 505f
 biliary tree, 321
 gastrointestinal, 400t, 402, 403f
 hepatic, 271-274, 271t, 276f, 520f
 from melanoma, 555f
 pancreas, 386
 peritoneal, 427-428, 429f
 splenic, 352-354, 353f
 testicular, 730
Methicillin-resistant *Staphylococcus aureus* (MRSA), 52
Metrorrhea, 1214
Meyers, Russell, 7
"Mickey Mouse" sign, 289
Micro movement, 126
Microcalcifications, 669, 693-694
Microcephaly, 1502, 1523t, 1542-1543
 sonographic findings in, 1542-1543, 1542f
Microemboli detection, 1102, 1102f
Micrognathia, 1352-1354, 1499-1500, 1500f
Microlithiasis, testicular, 727-728, 728f
Micronodular cirrhosis, 246, 247f
Microphthalmia, 1501
Microphthalmos, 1392
Microsomia
 craniofacial, 1498-1499
 hemifacial, 1500-1501
Microtia, 1496
Midaxillary line, 891-892
Midbrain, 819
Middle cerebral artery (MCA), 1089, 1093
 Doppler spectral waveform from, 1098f
 right, 1093f
Middle hepatic vein, 223, 255t
Mid-face, abnormalities of, 1503-1510, 1506f, 1507f
Midface hypoplasia, 1505-1506, 1507f, 1508f
Midgut, 1574f
 development and rotation of, 1563f
 embryology of, 1574-1575, 1575f
 malformations of, 1575-1576
Midgut malrotation, 784
Midsternal line, 891-892
Mineralocorticoids, 497
Minor calyces, 436-437
Mirizzi syndrome, 312, 314f
Mirror image artifacts
 color Doppler, 160-163, 162f, 163f
 description of, 149, 151f
 spectral Doppler, 160, 160f
Mirror syndrome, 1487
Mirror-image artifacts
 description of, 129
 illustration of, 132f
Mitral annular calcification, 957-958
Mitral atresia, 1049-1050, 1049f
Mitral regurgitation, 930f, 995, 1050

Mitral stenosis
 causes of, 957-963
 congenital, 1048-1050, 1048f, 1049f
 degenerative, 957-958
 echocardiographic evaluation of, 959
 hemodynamic measurements of, 959
 management of, 963
 pathophysiology of, 958-963, 958f, 959f
 percutaneous mitral balloon valvuloplasty for, 963
 rheumatic, 957-959, 958f
 severity assessments, 954, 955b, 959
 severity of, 960t
 treatment of, 963t
Mitral valve, 899, 899f, 900f
 fetal circulation and, 1010-1011
 M-mode imaging of, 943-944, 950f
 normal Doppler measurements, 1014t
 "parachute," 1048
 regurgitation of. see Mitral regurgitation
 stenosis of. see Mitral stenosis
Mitral valve area, 954f, 960, 961b, 961f
Mitral valve disease
 anatomy of, 953-963, 954f
 mitral regurgitation, 953-957, 954f, 955b, 955f, 956f, 957f, 958f
Mittelschmerz, 1172
M-mode imaging, 18, 19f
 of cardiac structures, 920, 943-952, 950b
  aortic valve and left atrium, 935f, 945-946, 950f
  interventricular septum, 946, 951f
  left ventricle, 946, 951f
  mitral valve, 943-944, 950f
  normal measurements, 950t
  pulmonary valve, 950-952, 951f
  tricuspid valve, 946
 color flow mapping, 920, 943-952, 950b
 fetal, 1013, 1014f, 1014t
 of hypertrophic cardiomyopathy, 997b
 of hypoplastic left heart syndrome, 1053
 of mitral stenosis, 959, 960f
Model for End-stage Liver Disease (MELD) scale, 585
Modified coronal plane, 827
Molar pregnancy, 1456-1457
Molecular imaging agents, 514
Molecules, 81
Monckeberg's arteriosclerosis, 1210-1212
Monocytes, 83
Mononucleosis, 341
Morality, 1294-1295
Morbidly adherent placenta, 1452-1454, 1453t, 1454f
Morgagni, foramen of, 1555-1556, 1556f
Morison's pouch, 98, 108-109, 417, 418f, 436
 FAST scan of, 563f, 564, 565f, 566f
 hematoma in, 539f
Mosaicism, 1433
Mouth, development of, 1494, 1494f
MPV. see Main portal vein
MRI. see Magnetic resonance imaging
MRSA. see Methicillin-resistant *Staphylococcus aureus*
MSAFP. see Maternal serum alpha-fetoprotein
Mucinous cystadenocarcinoma, 1247, 1248b, 1249f
Mucinous cystadenoma, 382f

Mucinous cystadenomas, 1247, 1248b, 1249f
Mucinous cystic neoplasms, 377–379
Mucocele, 404t, 405–408, 408f
Mucosa, 390, 782–783
Multicentricity, 671
Multicultural patients, 59
Multicystic dysplastic kidney disease (MDKD), 1606–1607, 1606f, 1607f
   neonatal/pediatric, 796t, 802–803, 803f
   sonographic findings in, 454t–458t, 461f, 462
Multicystic encephalomalacia, 837
Multielement transducer, 16, 16f
Multifactorial condition, 1433
Multifocality, 671
Multinodular goiter (MNG), 683, 690–691, 691t, 692f
Multiple gestation pregnancy, 1418–1424, 1418b, 1419f, 1420f
   anomalies specific to twin pregnancies, 1422–1423
   dizygotic twins, 1419, 1420f
   genetic amniocentesis and, prenatal diagnosis of congenital anomalies, 1432
   monozygotic twins, 1419–1421, 1420f, 1421f, 1422f
   placental tumors, 1457–1459, 1458b, 1458f
   scanning, 1408t, 1423–1424, 1424f
Murmurs, 905
Murphy sign, 296
Muscle(s)
   abdominal, 90–92, 90f
   back, 91
   false pelvis, 1160f, 1161
   hip, 853
   pelvis, 1160–1161, 1160b, 1189–1192, 1190f
   sonographic appearance of, 740t
   transvaginal scanning of endometrium during, 1195f
   types of, 735, 735f
Muscle tears, 754–755, 755f
Muscularis propria, 408–409
Musculoskeletal system, 733
   anatomy of, 734–740, 735f, 756b–757b
   artifacts, 740–743, 741f, 742f, 743t
   pathology of, 751–757
      carpal tunnel syndrome, 755–757, 756b, 756f
      muscle tears, 754–755, 755f
      shoulder biceps tendon subluxation/dislocation, 751, 751f
      tendinitis, 753–754, 753f, 754b, 754f
   sonographic appearance and evaluation, 740, 743–751
      Achilles tendon, 736, 749, 750f, 751b
      bursa, 738–739, 738f
      carpal tunnel, 748, 749f
      ligaments, 737–738, 738f, 740t
      muscles, 735, 735f, 740t
      nerves, 739, 739f, 739t, 740t
      rotator cuff, 744, 744b
         biceps tendon, 744, 744f, 745f
         indications for, 749b
         infraspinatus tendon, 745, 747f
         subscapularis tendon, 744, 745f
         supraspinatus tendon, 744–745, 746f
      tendons, 736–737, 736f, 737f, 740t
   work-related disorders of. see Work-related musculoskeletal disorders
Mycotic aneurysm, 192

Myelin, 739
Myeloceles, 883–885
Myelogenous leukemia, 83
Myelomeningocele, 1531f
Myeloproliferative disorders, 342, 343f
Myeloschisis, 883–885, 1528, 1528f
Myocarditis, 1034–1036
Myocardium, 896
Myoma, calcifications within, 1214f
Myometritis, 1260
Myometrium, 1181, 1192f, 1443f
Myxedema, 685
Myxomas, 998, 999f

N

Nabothian cysts, 1193, 1193f, 1204, 1204b, 1204f, 1205f
Nägele's rule, 1287, 1287b
Naked tuberosity sign, 752
Namekawa, Koroku, 8–10
Nasal bone, 1317–1318, 1317f
Nasal cannula, 45
Nasal pits, 1494, 1494f
Nasogastric (NG) tubes, 43, 44f
National Certification Examination for Ultrasound, 6
National patient safety standards, 544
Naumoff syndrome, 1630
Nausea, 85t, 86
NCCT. see Noncontrast computed tomography
Neck
   fetal, 1492, 1518b
      abnormalities of, 1496–1518
      embryology of, 1493–1495, 1493f
   twisting of, 75–76
Neck masses
   developmental cysts, 704–707, 705f
   fetal, 1512, 1516b
   miscellaneous, 704–707, 705f
   ultrasound-guided biopsy of, 557
Neck nodes, 557
Necrosis
   acute tubular. see Acute tubular necrosis
   focal brain, 837–838
   papillary, 454t–458t, 471–472
Necrotizing enterocolitis (NEC), 787–788, 787f
Needle biopsy, large-core, 676
Needle tips, finding, 550–551, 551f
Needles
   attached to transducer, 536–538, 536f
   for core biopsy, 533, 533f, 534f
   deviation of, 551–552, 551f, 552f
   for fine-needle aspiration, 532–533, 533f
Neonatal abdomen, 788b
   examination of, preparation for, 762–764, 762t, 763b
   pathology of
      liver tumors, 774, 775t, 776f
         benign, 773
         malignant, 773–774
      neonatal jaundice, 770
   sonographic evaluation of, 766
      biliary system, 765, 765b, 766f
      liver, 765, 765b, 765f
      normal measurements, 765b
      pancreas, 764, 764f, 764t
      portal vein, 765b, 765f
      spleen, 765b, 766f, 767f

Neonatal abdomen (Continued)
   surgical conditions, 775–787
      appendicitis, 776–781, 777f, 780f, 781f
      hypertrophic pyloric stenosis, 777t, 783–787, 783f, 784f, 785f, 786f, 787f
      intussusception. see Intussusception
Neonatal brain
   acquired lesions of
      epidural hemorrhages, 835
      extracorporeal membrane oxygenation for, 835
      focal brain necrosis, 837–838
      germinal matrix/subependymal hemorrhages, 833, 833f
      hypoxic-ischemic injury lesions, 836–838
      intracerebellar hemorrhage, 834–835, 837f
      intracranial hemorrhage, 832–836, 833b
      intraparenchymal hemorrhage, 834, 836f
      intraventricular hemorrhage, 833–834, 833f, 834f, 835f
      lenticulostriate vasculopathy, 838
      periventricular leukomalacia, 837, 838f, 839f
      subependymal cysts, 833
   anatomy of, 814–819
      basal ganglia, 818, 819f
      brainstem, 818–819
      cerebellum, 819, 820f
      cerebrovascular system, 819
      cerebrum, 817–818, 818f
      cisterns, 816
      fontanels, 814, 815b, 815f
      meninges, 815, 816f
      ventricular system, 815–817, 817f
   congenital malformations of
      cystic lesions, 844–846
      destructive lesions, 843–844
      neural tube defects, 838–842
         agenesis of corpus callosum, 840–841, 841f
         Arnold-Chiari malformation, 839–840, 840f
         Dandy-Walker malformation, 841–842, 841f
         disorders of diverticulation and cleavage, 842–843
   examination preparation of, 819–821
   focal necrosis of, 837–838
   infections of, 846–848
      congenital, 846–847, 847f
Neonatal head, 813, 847b–848b
Neonatal head examination, 821–829, 821b, 822t
   coronal plane, 822f, 823t, 824–827, 824f
   modified coronal plane, 827
   parasagittal views of, 825t, 827–828
   posterior fossa study, 828, 828f
   sagittal plane, 825t, 826f, 827–828, 827f
   three-dimensional neurosonography for, 821–824
Neonatal hepatitis, 770, 771f, 771t
Neonatal hip
   anatomy of, 851–854
   classification of, 863t
   movements of, 853, 854f
   pathology of
      developmental displacement of the hip. see Developmental displacement of the hip
      dislocation and subluxation of, 857–858, 858f
   sonographic findings of, 851–854
Neonatal intensive care unit (NICU), 762t

Neonatal jaundice, 770, 771t
Neonatal spine, 871, 887b
  anatomy of, 872, 872f
  embryogenesis and, 871–872
  pathology of, 880–883
    diastematomyelia and hydromyelia, 883, 885f
    lipoma, 882, 883f
    myelomeningoceles, 883–885, 885f
    tethered spinal cord, 881–883, 882f
  sonographic evaluation of, 871, 875–880, 878f
Neoplasia, lobular, 673
Neoplasms. see also Adenocarcinoma; Carcinoma
  endocrine pancreatic, 381–386, 383f
  parapancreatic, 386–388, 386f
Nephritis
  acute interstitial, 454t–458t, 470–471
  lupus, 454t–458t, 471
Nephroblastoma, 467. see also Wilms tumor
Nephroblastomatosis, 807–808
Nephrocalcinosis, medullary, 463f, 479, 481f
Nephroma
  congenital mesoblastic, 809
  mesoblastic, 1615, 1616f
Nephronophthisis, 463, 463f
Nephrons, 436–437
Nephropathy
  hypertensive, 454t–458t, 471
  sickle cell, 454t–458t, 471
Nerve(s), 739, 739f, 739t, 740t
  cardiac, 903
  sciatic, 739t
  sonographic appearance, 739, 739f, 739t, 740t
  vertebral column, 872f, 873
Nerve roots, spinal, 873
Neural axis, fetal, 1522, 1543b
Neural tube defects, 838–842
  agenesis of corpus callosum, 840–841, 841f
  Arnold-Chiari malformation, 839–840, 840f
  Dandy-Walker malformation, 841–842, 841f
Neuroblastoma, 773
  adrenal, 505–506, 506f, 807–808, 808f, 809f, 810f
  neonatal/pediatric, 808f, 809–810, 809f, 810f
  pediatric, 274–280
Neuroectodermal tissue, 505
Newton, Isaac, 6
Niemann-Pick disease, 340
Nightingale, Florence, 30
NIH. see Nonimmune hydrops
Nimura, Yasuhara, 8–10
Nodular hyperplasia, 268–269, 271f, 272f, 690–691
Nodular thyroid disease, 690–691, 690f, 691t, 692f
Noise
  as artifact, 156, 157f
  color Doppler, 160–163, 162f, 163f
  spectral Doppler, 160, 160f
Nomograms, fetal eye orbits, 1352
Nonalcoholic steatohepatitis, 768–769
Noncommunicating hydrocephalus, 1540, 1540f
Noncontrast computed tomography (NCCT), 439
Non-Hodgkin lymphoma, 351
Nonimmune hydrops (NIH), 1411, 1411b
  sonographic findings, 1412, 1412f
Nonimmune hydrops fetalis (NIHF), 1488–1489, 1489f
Nonischemic cardiomyopathy, 989
Nonmaleficence, 1295–1296
Nonobstructive hydronephrosis, 477

Nonobstructive jaundice, 770
Nonresistive vessels, 210
Nonstress test (NST), 1401–1402, 1402f
Nontoxic (simple) goiter, 691, 691t
Nose
  abnormalities of, 1505–1506, 1507f
  development of, 1494, 1494f
Nosocomial infection, 50
Nuchal translucency, 1286, 1433, 1433f
  embryonic abnormalities and, 1333–1334, 1334f
  first trimester, measurement, 1317, 1317b, 1317f
Nuclear medicine scintigraphy, 701, 702f
Nucleus, 81
Nyquist limit
  color Doppler artifacts and, 160, 161f
  definition of, 156–159, 715–716
  pulsed wave Doppler and, 911–912
  spectral Doppler artifacts and, 156–159, 157t, 158f, 159b, 159f
Nyquist sampling limit, 24

O

Obesity, 1416
  childhood, 763t
Obstetric measurements and gestational age, 1378, 1379b, 1393b–1394b
  gestational age assessment
    first trimester, 1379–1382
    second and third trimester, 1382–1394
Obstetric sonography
  classification of, 1285–1286, 1286b
  clinical ethics for, 1294, 1299b
    confidentiality of findings, 1298
    defined, 1294–1295
    history of, 1295
    principles, 1295–1298
  diagnostic and screening aspects of, 1292–1293
  Doppler for, 1288–1289
  examination guidelines, 1289–1292
    documentation in, 1289
    equipment specifications, 1289
    first-trimester protocol, 1284b, 1289–1290
    quality control, 1289
    second- and third-trimester protocol, 1284b, 1290–1292, 1292b
  indications for, 1284–1285, 1284b
  patient history, 1286–1288
    clinical dates, 1287
    gravidity and parity, 1286
    maternal risk factors, 1287–1288
    Nägele's rule, 1287, 1287b
  role of, 1283, 1292b–1293b
  safety of, 1288
Obstructions
  biliary. see Biliary obstructions
  bladder outlet, neonatal/pediatric, 801–802, 802f
  intestinal, 1586–1587, 1587f
  lower gastrointestinal, 403, 404t, 405f
  ureteral, 802
  ureteropelvic junction, neonatal/pediatric, 799, 800f, 802
  urinary tract. see Obstructive urinary tract abnormalities
Obstructive cystic dysplasia, 1608, 1609f
Obstructive disease
  definition of, 225–226
  hepatic disease versus, 225–226

Obstructive hydronephrosis, 454t–458t, 475–476, 477f
Obstructive jaundice, 770
Obstructive urinary tract abnormalities, 1608–1615
  anterior urethral valves, 1612–1614, 1614f
  hydronephrosis. see Hydronephrosis
  posterior urethral valve (PUV) obstruction, 1611–1612, 1612f, 1613f, 1614f
  prune belly syndrome, 796t, 801–802
  ureteropelvic junction (UPJ) obstruction, 1610, 1611f, 1612f
  ureterovesical junction (UVJ) obstruction, 1610–1611, 1612f
Obstructive uropathy, 1339
Obturator internus muscles, 1161, 1161f, 1189–1190, 1190f
Occipital encephalocele, 1527f
Occlusion
  internal carotid artery, 1077, 1078f, 1080–1081
  intracranial arteries, 1100
Occupational Safety and Health Act (OSHA), 69
OHS. see Ovarian hyperstimulation syndrome
Oligohydramnios, 1285, 1422, 1480–1481, 1480b, 1481f
  embryonic, 1327
Oligomenorrhea, 1174
Omental cysts, 426–427, 427f
Omentum, 97
  lymphoma, 428, 429f
  pathology of, 426–428, 426t
  tumors of, 428, 430f
Omoto, Ryozo, 8–10
Omphaloceles, 1338, 1428, 1466, 1466f, 1562–1565, 1565f, 1566f, 1575–1576, 1575f
  bowel, 1563, 1566f
  gastroschisis versus, 1562, 1564b
  liver, 1566f
  sonographic findings in, 1563–1565, 1564t, 1566f
Omphalomesenteric cyst, 1467, 1467f
Oncocytoma, 468, 470f
123-ABC method, 657
Oocyte, 1170–1171
Oophoritis, 1260
Open spinal dysraphism, 883–886, 885f, 886f
Ophthalmic artery, 1088, 1094, 1094f
Optison, 513
Oral cavity, abnormalities of, 1510–1512
Orbits
  abnormalities of, 1501–1503, 1502f, 1503f
  fetal, 1392, 1392b, 1393f
Orchiopexy, 730
Orchitis, 717t
Organ Procurement and Transplantation Network (OPTN), 584–585
Organ transplants, 523–524
Organelles, 81
Organism, from atom to, 81
Organomegaly, 1510
Ortolani maneuver, 859, 859f
OSHA. see Occupational Safety and Health Act
Ossification, skeletal, 1313, 1313f
Osteochondral plate sign, 862, 863f
Osteochondrodysplasia, 1623t
Osteogenesis imperfecta, 1623t, 1626–1628, 1627f, 1628f
Ostium primum atrial septal defect, 1037–1038, 1037f, 1038f

Ostium secundum atrial septal defect, 1037, 1037f
Ostomy, 47
Otocephaly, 1499
Ovarian carcinoma, 1244–1246, 1246f, 1247f
Ovarian cysts
  benign, 1239–1242
    in adolescents, 1240
      paraovarian cysts, 1240, 1240b, 1241f
      peritoneal inclusion, 1239–1242, 1240f
      simple cysts in postmenopausal women, 1240–1242
  complex, 1234–1235, 1235b, 1235f
  fetal, 1618–1619, 1619f
  functional, 1236
    corpus luteum cysts, 1236–1237, 1237b, 1237f
    follicular cysts, 1236, 1237b
    hemorrhagic cysts, 1237, 1238f
    theca-lutein cysts, 1237, 1238b, 1239f
  hemorrhagic, 1237, 1238f
Ovarian follicles, multiple, 1277f
Ovarian hyperstimulation syndrome (OHSS), 1237–1239, 1239f, 1278, 1279f
Ovarian ligaments, 1168f, 1169
Ovarian masses
  complex, 1234–1235, 1235b, 1235f
  first-trimester, 1340, 1341f
  simple cystic, 1234, 1234b, 1234f, 1235f
Ovarian neoplasms, 1244
Ovarian pregnancy, 1333
Ovarian remnant syndrome, 1239
Ovarian tumors
  epithelial, 1246–1250, 1248f
    mucinous cystadenocarcinoma, 1247, 1248b, 1249f
    mucinous cystadenoma, 1247, 1248b, 1249f
    serous cystadenocarcinomas, 1248–1249, 1249b, 1250b, 1251f
    serous cystadenomas, 1249b, 1250f, 1252f
  solid, 1235–1236, 1236b
Ovaries
  anatomy of, 1168, 1169f, 1231–1234, 1231f
  blood supply to, 1191–1192
  cyclic changes of, 1172f, 1232f
  Doppler ultrasound of, 1236, 1236f
  female infertility and, 1276–1277, 1276f, 1277f
  ligaments of, 1168f, 1169
  pathology of, 1230, 1258b
    endometriosis, 1242–1243, 1242f
    epithelial tumors. *see* Epithelial ovarian tumors
    fluid collections in adhesions, 1240, 1241f
    functional cysts. *see* Functional cysts
    germ cell tumors. *see* Germ cell tumors
    ovarian carcinoma, 1244–1246, 1246f, 1247f
    ovarian hyperstimulation syndrome, 1237–1239, 1239f
    ovarian remnant syndrome, 1239
    paraovarian cysts, 1240, 1240b, 1241f
    polycystic ovarian syndrome, 1238–1239, 1239b, 1240f
    simple cysts in postmenopausal women, 1240–1242
    stromal tumors, 1252–1257, 1255f
  peritoneal inclusion cysts, 1239–1242, 1240f
  position and size of, 1167–1168, 1167b, 1167t, 1168b, 1168f
  sonographic evaluation of, 578, 1191f, 1197–1198, 1197f, 1231–1233, 1232f, 1233f

Ovaries *(Continued)*
  complex masses, 1234–1235, 1235b, 1235f
  ovarian neoplasms, 1244
  simple cystic masses, 1234, 1234b, 1234f, 1235f
  solid tumors, 1235–1236, 1236b
  transvaginal, 1186b, 1197–1198, 1197f, 1198f
  volume measurements, 1233
  torsion, 1243–1244, 1243b, 1244f
  ultrasound examination of, 1178b
Ovulation, 1170–1172, 1171f, 1231–1233
Ovulation induction therapy, 1277, 1277f
Ovum, 1168
Oximetry, 36–37, 38f
Oxygen masks, 45–46, 46f
Oxygen therapy, 45–46, 45f, 46f

P
P wave, 904, 904f
Packet size, 715t, 717
PACS. *see* Premature atrial contractions
Paget disease, 654–655, 673, 673f
Pain
  abdominal
    acute, 767–775, 768f
    in children, 767–775, 768f
    description of, 84, 85t
  defined, 1296
  epigastric, 568–570, 573t
  flank, 573–574, 573t
  gallbladder disease and, 290–293
  lower abdominal, 573t
  pelvic, acute, 578–579
  right lower quadrant, 573t, 574–575
  right upper quadrant, 567–568, 573t
  scrotal, 720f
  thoracic, 573t
Palate
  abnormalities of, 1506–1509, 1508f, 1509f, 1510f. *see also* Cleft lip/palate
  development of, 1494, 1495f
Pampiniform plexus, 712
Pan Scanner, 8f
Pancreas, 88, 89f, 355, 387b
  abdominal scanning of
    at level of liver, inferior vena cava, and gastroduodenal artery, 109, 120f
    at level of liver and duodenum, 109, 120f
    at level of superior mesenteric artery, 107, 109f
  abscesses, 369t, 375–377
  adenocarcinoma of, 381, 384f, 385f
  anatomy of, 356–360, 356f, 357f
  annular, 360, 361f
  biopsy of, 553–554
  body of, 358, 358f
  congenital anomalies, 359–360
  Doppler imaging of, 631f
  ectopic tissue, 359
  endocrine function of, 361, 361t
  exocrine function of, 360–361, 361t
  fetal
    abnormalities of, 1583
    embryology of, 1574
    sonographic evaluation of, 1580, 1580f
  head of, 356–358, 356f, 357f, 360
    pancreatic landmark, 363–364, 364b
    size of, 359

Pancreas *(Continued)*
  inflammation of, 371f, 767
  laboratory tests, 361, 362t
  masses of, 553–554
  neck of, 356f, 358
    pancreatic landmark, 363–364, 364b
  neoplasms of, 381–386, 383f
    endocrine pancreatic, 381–386
  pancreatitis. *see* Pancreatitis
  parenchyma of, 629–630
  pathology of, 368–388
    cystic lesions, 377, 378t
    metastatic disease, 386
    neoplasms, 377–381, 379t
      parapancreatic, 386–388, 386f
  physiology of, 360–361, 361t
  size of, 359
  sonographic evaluation of, 362–368, 362t
    contrast-enhanced, 523
    normal characteristics of, 363, 363b, 363f
    pancreatic duct, 367, 368f
    pediatric, 764, 764f, 764t
    in sagittal plane, 366–367, 367f, 368f
    technique for, 363–368, 363f, 364f
    in transverse plane, 364–366, 366f
    windows for visualization, 364, 365f
  tail of, 358, 358f
    pancreatic landmark, 363–364, 364b
  transplantation of. *see* Pancreatic transplantation
  transverse scans of, 136–138, 143f
  ultrasound-guided biopsy of, 553–554
  vascular and ductal landmarks, 359
  vascular supply of, 358f, 359
  walled-off fluid collections, 373–374
Pancreas divisum, 359, 360f
Pancreatic ascites, 374–375
Pancreatic cyst(s), 1583
  after pancreatic transplantation, 637–638
  in autosomal dominant polycystic kidney disease, 378t
Pancreatic disease
  laboratory values for, 361, 362t
  metastatic, 386
Pancreatic duct, 282, 358–359, 358f
  acute pancreatitis and, 369–371, 369t, 370f
  as pancreatic landmark, 364b, 367, 368f
  sonographic evaluation of, 367, 368f
Pancreatic ductal adenocarcinoma (PDAC), 523
Pancreatic lipomatosis, 769
Pancreatic neuroendocrine tumor, 377
Pancreatic pseudocysts, 374, 375f, 376f
  after pancreatic transplantation, 636, 637f
  locations of, 374
  sonographic findings in, 377, 377f
Pancreatic transplantation
  allograft for
    computed tomography of, 632f
    Doppler imaging of, 628–629
    evaluation of, 627–629, 629f
    perfusion of, 629f
    postoperative imaging of, 630
    rejection of, 632f, 633, 633f
  biopsy of, 630–632, 632f
  cadaveric pancreas for, 624–625, 629f
  complications of
    abscesses, 633, 634f
    adenocarcinoma, 638

Pancreatic transplantation *(Continued)*
    arterial thrombosis, 633–634, 635*f*, 636*f*
    biopsy-related, 630–632
    cysts, 637–638
    fistula, 636, 637*f*
    hematomas, 636
    infection, 633, 634*f*
    lymphoceles, 636
    pancreatic artery stenosis, 634–635, 637*f*
    pancreatic vein stenosis, 634–635, 637*f*
    pancreatitis, 633, 634*f*
    posttransplant lymphoproliferative disorder, 638, 638*f*
    pseudoaneurysm, 635–636
    pseudocysts, 636, 637*f*
    rejection, 632*f*, 633, 633*f*
    seromas, 636
    surveillance for, 630–632, 632*f*
    venous thrombosis, 633–634, 635*f*, 636*f*
  cost of, 586
  criteria for, 586
  history of, 586
  islet cells, 627
  kidney transplantation with, 586
  rejection of, 632*f*, 633, 633*f*
  simultaneous pancreas-kidney transplant with, 586
  sonographic findings of, 629–630, 630*f*, 631*f*
  surgical technique of, 624–627
  for type 1 diabetes, 586
Pancreaticoduodenal arteries, 358*f*, 359
Pancreatitis, 368–373
  acute. *see* Acute pancreatitis
  after pancreatic transplantation, 633, 634*f*
  in children, 767
  complications of, 373
    chronic pancreatitis, 369*t*, 372–373, 373*f*
    pancreatic abscesses, 369*t*, 375–377
    walled-off pancreatic fluid collections associated with, 373–374, 374*f*
  definition of, 368–373
  epigastric pain with, 568–569, 569*f*, 573*t*
  hemorrhagic, 369*t*, 375, 376*f*
  phlegmonous, 369*t*, 375, 376*f*
Papillary carcinoma
  of breast, 672–673, 672*f*
  of thyroid gland, 694, 695*f*
Papillary fibroelastoma, 998, 1000*f*
Papillary necrosis, 454*t*–458*t*, 471–472
Para-aortic lymph nodes
  anatomy of, 494–495, 494*f*
  sonographic evaluation of, 498–499, 500*f*, 501*f*
Parabolic flow velocity profile, 905–906
Paracolic gutters, 99–100, 100*f*
Paralytic ileus, 403
Parametritis, 1260
Paraovarian cysts, 1240, 1240*b*, 1241*f*
Parapancreatic neoplasms, 386–388, 386*f*
Parapelvic cysts, 454*t*–458*t*, 459–460
Pararectal space, bilateral, 496, 496*f*
Parasternal transducer location, 919*f*
Parasternal views
  Doppler ultrasound, 928
    two-dimensional, 929–931, 935*f*
  long-axis
    of aortic stenosis, 1051*f*
    for color flow mapping, 922*b*, 926–928, 927*f*
    of congenital mitral stenosis, 1048*f*

Parasternal views *(Continued)*
    Doppler window, 920*f*, 924, 927*b*
    with patient in left lateral decubitus position, 936–937, 936*f*, 945*b*, 945*f*
    two-dimensional, 925–926, 927*b*, 928*b*, 928*f*, 929*f*
  of pulmonary stenosis, 1047*f*
  right, for Doppler, 927*b*, 928
  short-axis
    for color flow mapping, 922*b*, 929–931, 931*f*, 932*f*, 933*f*, 934*f*
    Doppler ultrasound, 928, 932*f*, 935*f*
Paratenon, 736–737
Parathyroid adenomas, 703*f*
Parathyroid carcinoma, 703–704
Parathyroid glands, 682, 707*b*
  anatomy of, 684*f*, 700, 701*f*
  embryology of, 700
  nuclear medicine of, 686
  pathology of, 702–704, 703*f*
  physiology and laboratory data of, 700–701
  scintigraphy of, 686, 686*f*
  sonographic evaluation of, 701–702
Parathyroid hormone (PTH), 700–701
Parathyroid hyperplasia, 703, 704*f*
Paraumbilical hernia, 573*t*, 575–578, 576*f*, 577*f*
Parenchyma
  injuries to, 566–567, 567*f*
  liver
    diffuse abnormalities of, 258–260, 261*t*
    longitudinal scans of, 141
    sonographic findings, 590
  renal
    angiomyolipoma and, 480*f*
    biopsy, 555
    junctional defects, 444, 446*f*, 446*t*, 447*f*
    sonographic evaluation of, 440–441, 442*f*, 443*f*
Parenchymal patterns, 648–649, 649*f*
Parietal epicardium, 980, 981*f*
Parietal peritoneum, 95, 562, 1174
Parity, 1286
Partial anomalous pulmonary venous return, 1036
Partial situs inversus, 1581, 1583*f*
Partial thromboplastin time (PTT), 532
Partial-thickness rotator cuff tears, 752, 752*b*, 752*f*
Parvus-tardus, 483*f*
Passive hepatic congestion, 259–260, 261*t*, 263*f*
Patau syndrome. *see* Trisomy 13
Patent ductus arteriosus, 1011–1012
Patent urachus, 804, 804*f*, 1604
Pathology
  in abdominal scanning, identifying, 131
  definition of, 80
Patient(s)
  breathing by
    in abdominal scanning, 124
    extreme shortness of breath, 570–572
  transfer techniques for, 38–40
    in assisting patients from the scanning stretcher into the wheelchair, 40, 41*f*
    body mechanics and, 38–39
    in moving patients toward the head of a stretcher, 39–40
    in moving patients up in bed, 39, 40*f*
    in stretcher transfer, 39, 39*f*
    in turning patients, 40
    in wheelchair transfer, 39, 39*f*

Patient breathing technique tip, 124
Patient care. *see also* Patient-focused care
  emergency medical situations. *see* Emergency medical situations
  equipment for, 57
  evaluating patient reactions to illness, 60–61
  infection prevention, 49–53, 50*f*, 51*f*
  for patients with tubes and tubing, 40–47, 41*f*
    catheters, 43–44, 44*f*
    colostomies and ileostomies, 47
    intravenous therapy, 41–43, 41*f*, 42*f*, 43*f*
    nasogastric tubes, 43, 44*f*
    ostomy, 47
    oxygen therapy, 45–46, 45*f*, 46*f*
    wounds, drains, and dressings, 46–47
  professionalism and, 61
  for special needs patients, 57–60
  during strict bed rest, 48–49
  for terminal patients, 60–61
  transfer techniques for, 38–40
Patient care partnership, 61
Patient consent, 32, 33*f*
Patient privacy, 32
Patient refusal, 32, 33*f*
Patient-centered care, 30–35
Patient-focused care, 61
Patients' Bill of Rights, 61
PCAs. *see* Posterior cerebral arteries
PCoA. *see* Posterior communicating artery
PCOS. *see* Polycystic ovarian syndrome
Peak systolic velocity, 1112–1113
Peau d'orange, 654–655
Pectoralis muscle, 645*f*, 648
Pediatric abdomen, 788*b*
  conditions that affect, 775–787
    appendicitis, 776–781, 777*f*, 780*f*, 781*f*
    hypertrophic pyloric stenosis, 777*t*, 783–787, 783*f*, 784*f*, 785*f*, 786*f*, 787*f*
  examination of, preparation for, 762–764, 762*t*, 763*b*
  pathology of
    liver tumors, 773–775
      benign, 773
    neonatal jaundice, 770, 771*t*
  sonographic evaluation of, 765*b*
    biliary system, 765, 765*b*, 766*f*
    liver, 765, 765*b*, 765*f*
    normal measurements, 765*b*
Pediatric End-Stage Liver Disease (PELD) scale, 585
Pediatric hip, 850, 869*b*
Pediatric patients. *see also* Adolescents; Children
  special needs of, 58–59
Pedicles, 873
Peliosis, 769
Pelvic abscesses, 425–426, 425*b*, 426*f*
Pelvic cavity, 92–95, 92*f*, 1160, 1161*f*
  blood supply to, 1170*f*
  FAST scan of, 564, 565*f*
  sonographic evaluation of, 1197*f*
Pelvic cyst, 154*f*
Pelvic floor muscles, 1190, 1190*f*
Pelvic fluid, 567
Pelvic girdle, 851, 851*f*
Pelvic inflammatory disease (PID), 1260–1266, 1261*b*, 1261*f*
  peritonitis, 1264–1266, 1266*f*
  salpingitis, hydrosalpinx, and pyosalpinx, 1261–1263, 1262*f*, 1262*t*, 1263*f*, 1264*f*

Pelvic inflammatory disease (PID) *(Continued)*
  sonographic findings in, 1261*b*, 1262
  tubo-ovarian abscesses, 1261*b*, 1263–1264
Pelvic kidney, 1594, 1601*f*
Pelvic landmarks, 1158*f*, 1159–1160
  bony pelvis, 1159–1160, 1159*f*
  external, 1159, 1159*f*
  pelvic cavity and perineum, 1160, 1160*b*, 1160*f*
Pelvic mass, 1618–1619
  anechoic tortuous, 1600
Pelvic masses, 1257–1258
  biopsy, 558
  first-trimester, 1329*t*, 1340
Pelvic muscles, 1160–1161, 1160*b*, 1189–1192, 1189*f*
Pelvic pain, acute, 578–579
Pelvic recesses, 1174–1175, 1174*b*
Pelvic retroperitoneum, 495–496, 496*f*
Pelvic ultrasound, 1158
  of bony pelvis, 1189, 1189*f*
  of bowel and rectouterine recess, 1198–1199, 1198*f*
  of fallopian tubes, 1178*b*
  of ovaries, 1197–1198, 1197*f*
  patient preparation and history for, 1177
  of pelvic muscles, 1189–1192, 1189*f*
  performance standards for, 1177
  three-dimensional, 1199–1201, 1200*f*
Pelvis
  acute pain in, 578–579
  false. *see* False pelvis
  female. *see* Female pelvis
  male, 108, 115*f*
  muscles of, 1160–1161, 1160*b*
  neonatal/pediatric, 763*b*
  sonographic evaluation of. *see* Pelvic ultrasound
  ultrasound-guided biopsy of, 558
  vasculature of, 1168*b*, 1169, 1169*f*, 1170*f*
Pena-Shokeir syndrome, 1632–1633
Penetrating aortic ulcer, 977, 977*f*
Pennate patterns, 734
Pentalogy of Cantrell, 1568–1570, 1569*f*
  fetus with, 1062*f*
  sonographic findings in, 1564, 1564*t*, 1570
Percival, Thomas, 1295
Percutaneous mitral balloon valvuloplasty, 963
Perforating veins, 1132–1133
Peribiliary cysts, 264, 265*f*
Pericardial disease, 980–985, 1005*b*
  cardiac tamponade, 571, 982–983, 984*f*, 985*b*, 985*f*
  constrictive pericarditis, 983–985, 986*b*, 986*f*, 987*f*
  pericardial effusion. *see* Pericardial effusion
Pericardial effusion, 1036, 1036*f*
  echocardiography of, 981–982, 981*f*, 981*t*, 982*f*, 983*f*
  extreme shortness of breath and, 570–571, 571*f*, 572*f*
  fluid estimations for, 981–982, 981*t*
  hydrops and, 1487
  size of, 981*t*, 982*f*
  with supraventricular tachyarrhythmias, 1064*f*
  transthoracic echocardiography of, 981, 981*f*
Pericardial sac, 88, 563, 895*f*, 896
Pericarditis, constrictive, 983–985, 986*b*, 986*f*, 987*f*
Pericardium, 896
  fibrous, 980, 981*f*
  serous, 980, 981*f*

Periductal mastitis, 663
Perihepatic compartments, 417–418
Perimetrium, 1164
Perineum, 94, 1160
Perineurium, 739
Periovarian inflammation, 1260
Peripheral arterial disease (PAD)
  pathophysiology of, 1113–1114
  physiology of, 1112–1113
  risk factors for, 1113–1114
  symptoms of, 1110–1111, 1113–1114
  treatment of, 1113
Peripheral arterial evaluation, 1110, 1127*b*
  anatomy associated with
    lower extremity, 1111–1112, 1111*f*
    upper extremity, 1112, 1112*f*
  guidelines for, 1126–1127, 1126*b*, 1126*t*
  indirect testing, 1114–1118
  purpose of, 1111*b*
Peripheral venous evaluation, 1129, 1150*b*–1151*b*
Perirenal space, 92, 491–493, 492*b*, 492*f*, 493*f*
Peristalsis, 393, 1578
Peritoneal cavity, 96, 1174, 1174*f*
  anatomy of, 413–414, 414*f*–415*f*, 416*f*, 434*b*
    intraperitoneal compartments, 417–418, 418*f*, 419*f*
    intraperitoneal location, 414–417, 417*f*, 418*f*
    lower abdominal and pelvic compartments, 418–419, 419*f*
  pathology of, 419–426
    abscess formation and pockets in abdomen and pelvis, 420–421, 423*f*
    ascites, 419–420, 421*f*, 422*f*
  sonographic evaluation of, 413–419, 414*f*–415*f*, 416*f*
Peritoneal cysts, 426
  inclusion cysts, 1239–1242, 1240*f*
Peritoneal lavage, 562, 562*f*
Peritoneal ligaments, 98, 99*f*
Peritoneal pseudocyst, 1264*f*
Peritoneal recesses, 99
Peritoneum, 95–96, 95*f*, 96*f*, 1166*f*
  definition of, 413–414
  metastases to, 427–428
  pathology of, 426–428, 426*t*
  tumors of, 428, 430*f*
Peritonitis, 422–423, 1264–1266, 1266*f*
Periventricular calcifications, 1541*f*
Periventricular leukomalacia (PVL), 837, 838*f*, 839*f*
Peroneal artery, 1112
Peroneal veins, 1131, 1139*f*
Perseverance, 5*b*
Persistent intrahepatic right umbilical vein, 1472–1473, 1472*f*
Persistent trophoblastic disease, 1325–1326
Personal protective equipment (PPE), 55–57, 73–74, 75*f*
pH, urine, 438
Phagocytosis, 332
Phalen sign, 756
Phenylketonuria (PKU), 1502
Pheochromocytoma, 502*t*, 505, 505*f*
Phlegmasia alba dolens, 1135
Phlegmasia cerulea dolens, 1135
Phlegmonous pancreatitis, 369*t*, 375, 376*f*
Photoplethysmography, 1117
Phrenic arteries, 185

Phrenocolic ligament, 326, 328*f*
Phrygian cap, 285, 288*f*
PHT. *see* Portal hypertension
Physiology, 80
Pia mater, 873–875
PID. *see* Pelvic inflammatory disease
Pierre Robin syndrome, 1500
Piezoelectricity, 6
Piriformis muscle, 94*f*, 1161
Pitting, 332
Placenta, 1373–1374, 1373*f*, 1374*f*, 1442, 1459*b*. *see also* Embryogenesis
  abnormalities of, 1450–1455, 1451*t*
    circumvallate/circummarginate placenta, 1454, 1455*f*
    morbidly adherent placenta, 1452–1454, 1453*t*, 1454*f*
    placenta previa, 1451–1452, 1451*f*, 1452*b*, 1452*f*, 1453*f*
    placental hemorrhage, 1455
    placentomegaly, 1451, 1451*b*
    succenturiate placenta, 1454, 1454*f*, 1455*f*
    vasa previa, 1452, 1453*f*
  amniotic sac and amniotic fluid, 1445
  Doppler evaluation of, 1449–1450, 1450*f*
  embryogenesis, 1443–1445, 1443*b*, 1443*f*
    cordal attachments, 1444–1445, 1444*f*, 1445*f*
    fetal-placental-uterine circulation, 1444
    membranes, 1445
    placental implantation, 1445
  evaluation after delivery, 1450
  fibrin deposition, 1450
  fetal circulation, 1446*f*
  fetal ultrasound, 1408*t*
  functions of, 1444*b*
  hematomas, 1320
  normal, sonographic evaluation of, 1446–1449, 1447*f*, 1448*f*
    placental position, 1448–1449, 1448*f*, 1449*f*
  placental abruption, 1455–1456, 1455*f*
    intervillous thrombosis, 1456, 1456*f*
    marginal abruption, 1456, 1456*f*
    placental infarct, 1456
    retroplacental abruption, 1456, 1456*f*
  placental tumors, 1456–1459
    chorioangioma, 1457, 1457*f*
    gestational trophoblastic disease, 1456–1457, 1457*f*
    multiple gestation, 1457–1459, 1458*b*, 1458*f*
  umbilical cord, 1445–1446
    sonographic evaluation of, 1446, 1446*f*
Placenta accreta, 1413*f*, 1452–1453, 1453*t*
Placenta increta, 1452–1453, 1453*t*
Placenta percreta, 1452–1453, 1453*t*
Placenta previa, 1285, 1445, 1451–1452, 1451*f*, 1452*b*, 1452*f*, 1453*f*
Placental abruption, 1412–1413
Placental calcifications, 1418*f*
Placental edema, hydrops and, 1487
Placental hemorrhage, 1455
Placental infarct, 1418*f*, 1456
Placental insufficiency, 1481
Placental lesions, AFP and, 1428
Placental sonolucencies, 1447
Placentomegaly, 1447*f*, 1451, 1451*b*
Planimetry, for mitral valve area evaluations, 961
Plantar flexion, 750
Plaque, common carotid artery, 1077*f*

Plasma, 81
Plethysmography, 1117
Pleural effusions, 1409f, 1550–1551
 hydrops and, 1486–1487
 sonographic findings in, 1551, 1552f
Pleural fluid, 559
Plug flow, 210
Pneumobilia, 315, 317f, 608, 609f
Pneumocystis carinii, 268, 270f
Pneumothorax, 529
Polycystic kidney disease, 454t–458t, 461
 AFP and, 1428
 autosomal dominant. *see* Autosomal dominant polycystic kidney disease
 autosomal recessive. *see* Autosomal recessive polycystic kidney disease
 infantile, 454t–458t
Polycystic liver disease, 264–265, 264t, 266f
Polycystic ovarian syndrome (PCOS), 1238–1239, 1239b, 1240f, 1276, 1277f
Polycystic renal disease, autosomal recessive, 796t, 804–805
Polycythemia, 341
Polycythemia vera, 341
Polydactyly, 1630, 1631f, 1633f, 1634f
Polyhydramnios, 1285, 1410f, 1414, 1422, 1479–1480, 1480b, 1480f
 anencephaly and, 1524
 cephaloceles and, 1527
Polyhydramnios-oligohydramnios (poly-oli) sequence, 1422–1423, 1422f
Polymenorrhea, 1174
Polyorchidism, 731–732
Polyps, 400, 400t, 401f
 cervical, 1204
 endometrial, 1220–1221, 1274–1275, 1275f
  sonographic findings in, 1221, 1222f
 gallbladder, 304
Polysplenia, 327–329, 1581
Polysyndactyly, 1633f
Pons, neonatal, 819
Popliteal artery
 aneurysms of, 1125f
 description of, 1111–1112
 illustration of, 158f
Popliteal nerve, 739t
Popliteal vein, 1131, 1132f
 evaluation of, 1138
Porcelain gallbladder, 294t–295t, 303, 305f
Porencephalic cyst, 844
 sonographic findings in, 844
Porencephalic cysts, 1538
Porencephaly, 837, 1523t
 differential considerations for, 1524t
Porta hepatis
 description of, 282
 illustration of, 283f
 obstruction of, 312, 315f, 316f
 ultrasound protocol for, 233–234, 235t
Portal caval shunts, 254–257, 257f
Portal hypertension (PHT), 249–258
 in children, 768–769
 indications for, 251b
 portal caval shunts and, 254–257, 257f
 secondary to portal vein thrombosis, 253–258, 256f
 sonographic evaluation of
  collateral circulation, 252–253, 254f, 255t, 256f

Portal hypertension (PHT) *(Continued)*
 diagnostic criteria for, 260t
 Doppler interrogation, 253
 Doppler technique in, 252, 253b, 336f
 patient preparation and positioning for, 251–252, 252b
 vascular ultrasound contrast agents and, 517
 venous, 250–251, 251b, 252f, 252t
Portal sinus, fetal circulation, 1446f
Portal triad, 223f, 289, 292f
Portal vein, 206, 207f, 223, 223f
 characteristics of, 223–225, 227f
 Doppler flow patterns in, 214–217, 214b, 215f
 fetal circulation, 1446f
 pancreas and, 356–359, 357f
 pediatric, 765b, 765f
 sonographic findings of, 206, 208f, 209f, 260t
 stenosis, after liver transplantation, 594–596, 597f, 598f
 thrombosis of, 253–258, 256f, 594–596, 597f, 598f
Portal venous gas, 606–607, 607f
Portal venous hypertension, 209
Portal venous system
 anomalies in, 242–243
 Doppler ultrasound of, 146, 146f
 inferior mesenteric vein, 209
 splenic vein, 206–207
 superior mesenteric vein, 207–209
Portal-splenic confluence, 356–358
Posakony, Gerald J., 7, 8f
Positioning
 for abdominal scanning, 125, 125f
 Bouffard position, 747f
 for breast evaluation, 655, 655f
 for carotid duplex imaging, 1072
 Crass position, 746f
 for echocardiography, 927b
 for kidney evaluation, 439, 440f, 441f, 442f
 for portal hypertension, 251–252, 252b
 for scrotum evaluation, 712–713, 712b
 for spleen evaluation, 334–336
 for venous duplex imaging, lower extremity, 1137
Posterior arch vein, 1132
Posterior bimanual compression, 778–779
Posterior cerebral arteries (PCAs), 1090
Posterior communicating artery (PCoA), 1090, 1094, 1094f
Posterior direction, 132
Posterior fossa, studies of, 828, 828f
Posterior pararenal space, 92, 492b, 492f, 495
Posterior tibial artery, 1112
Posterior tibial veins, 1131, 1136f, 1139f
Posterior triangle, 94
Posterior urethral valve, 1600
 illustration of, 802f
 neonatal/pediatric
  bladder outlet obstruction and, 801–802
  sonographic findings in, 796t
 obstruction, 1611–1612, 1612f, 1613f, 1614f
Posthemorrhagic hydrocephalus, 829
Postoperative ultrasound, 1271
Postthyroidectomy neck sonography, 707
Posttransplant lymphoproliferative disorder (PTLD), 607–608
 in pancreatic transplantation patients, 638, 638f
 in renal transplantation patients, 623, 628f

Posttrauma brain injury, 1103
Postural anomalies, 1632
Potter facies, 804–805
Potter sequence, 1605
Potter syndrome, 1601
Pouch of Douglas, 564, 566f, 1162f, 1174, 1198–1199, 1198f, 1203, 1204f
Pourcelot resistive index, 1191
Power, 11–12, 12t, 26–27
Power Doppler imaging, 25, 27f
 vascular ultrasound contrast agents with, 513f
Power output, 21
PPE. *see* Personal protective equipment
P-R interval, 904
Precocious puberty, 810–811
Preeclampsia, 1415
 multiple gestation pregnancy, 1418
Pregnancy. *see also* Obstetric sonography
 anembryonic, 1320, 1323, 1323f, 1324b
 breast imaging in, 649, 650f, 662
 cervical, 1332–1333
 early, maternal serum analysis in, 1303–1305, 1304t
 ectopic, 1257, 1327–1333, 1328f
  adnexal mass with, 1330–1332, 1331f
  human chorionic gonadotrophin levels in, 1303
  sonographic findings in, 1328–1330, 1328f, 1329f, 1329t, 1330f, 1331f
 failed, 1320, 1327
 first-trimester. *see* First trimester pregnancy
 heterotopic, 1279, 1279f, 1332, 1332t
 interstitial, 1332, 1333f
 intrauterine. *see* Intrauterine pregnancy
 maternal diseases of, 1413–1416
  adnexal cysts, 1415
  diabetes, 1413–1415, 1414b, 1414f
  hyperemesis, 1415
  hypertension, 1415
  obesity, 1416
  systemic lupus erythematosus, 1064f, 1415
  urinary tract disease, 1415
  uterine fibroids, 1416
 molar, 1324
 multiple gestation. *see* Multiple gestation pregnancy
 normal progression, 1301–1303, 1301f, 1302f, 1303f, 1304f, 1304t
 second trimester. *see* Second trimester pregnancy
 third trimester. *see* Third trimester pregnancy
Pregnancy-associated plasma protein-A (PAPP-A), 1305
 prenatal diagnosis of congenital anomalies, 1432
Pregnancy-induced hypertension (PIH), 1415
Preload, 910
Premature atrial contractions (PACs), 1062–1063
Premature rupture of membranes (PROM), 1414, 1482
Premature ventricular contractions (PVCs), 1062–1063
Premenarche, 1170, 1177
Premenopause, 1177
Preoperative needle wire localization, 676, 676f
Presacral space, 496
Pressure, 908
Pressure amplitude, 12t

Pressure half-time (PHT), 960–961, 961f, 962f
Preterm infants, 814t
Preterm labor, 1416–1417, 1416b
    premature rupture of membranes, 1416–1417
    sonographic findings, 1408t, 1416, 1416f
Preterm premature rupture of the membranes (PPROM), 1482
Prevesical space, 495
PRF. see Pulse repetition frequency
Primary hyperparathyroidism, 702–704, 703f
Primary yolk sac, 1301
Primitive atrium, 1009, 1010f
Primitive ventricle, 1010f
Privacy, patient, 32
Proboscis, 1503f, 1504f, 1534f
Professionalism, 61
Profunda femoris artery, 1111–1112
Profunda femoris vein, 1131
Progesterone, 1168, 1220b
Projectile vomiting, 784
Proliferative phase, 1171b, 1172, 1195, 1196f
PROM. see Preterm premature rupture of the membranes
Pronephros, 1593
Propagation artifacts, 147–153
    grating lobes and, 151, 153f
    mirror image and, 149, 151f
    range ambiguity and, 151–152, 154f
    refraction and, 149, 152f
    reverberation and, 148–149, 149f, 150f, 151f
    section thickness and, 148, 148f
    speckle and, 148, 149f
    speed error and, 151, 154f
Prostate gland, 558, 558f, 559f
Prostate-specific antigen (PSA), 531–532
Proteins
    liver production of, 228
    urinary, 438
Prothrombin time (PT), 231, 532
Proximal isovelocity surface area (PISA), 954, 957f
    in mitral stenosis, 954, 957f
Proximal/distal direction, 132–134
Prune-belly syndrome, 796t, 801–802, 1614–1615, 1615b
Pseudoaneurysms, 482–483, 484f
    arterial duplex imaging of, 1124–1126, 1125f
    carotid duplex imaging of, 1078
    computed tomography of, 973, 973f, 974f
    definition of, 597, 635–636, 973
    description of, 190–191, 191f
    Doppler imaging of, 145
    hepatic artery, 597, 601f
    in pancreatic transplantation patients, 635–636
    in renal transplantation patients, 620
Pseudoascites, 1581–1582, 1583f
Pseudocysts. see also Cyst(s)
    pancreatic. see Pancreatic pseudocysts
    peritoneal, 1264f
    uriniferous, 427
Pseudodissection, 573
Pseudogestational sac, 1329, 1329f
Pseudomyxoma peritonei, 405, 407–408
Pseudopulsatile abdominal masses, 195
Pseudotoxemia, 1487
Psoas compartment, 495, 495f
Psoas muscles, 94, 495, 495f
    psoas major, 107, 109f, 495f, 1160f, 1161
PT. see Prothrombin time

PTH. see Parathyroid hormone
PTT. see Partial thromboplastin time
Pudendal artery, 712
Pudendum, 1159
Puerperal mastitis, 663
Pulmonary capillary wedge, 909
Pulmonary embolism (PE), 1134–1135, 1135b, 1149–1150
Pulmonary hypertension, 988–989
Pulmonary hypoplasia, 1549, 1550b, 1551f
Pulmonary sequestration, 1552, 1552b, 1552f
Pulmonary stenosis, 1032, 1046–1047, 1047f
    sonographic findings of, 1046–1047, 1047f
    supravalvular, 1048, 1048f
Pulmonary trunk, 898
    fetal circulation, 1446f
Pulmonary valve, 898, 898f, 950–952, 951f
Pulmonary veins
    fetal circulation, 1446f
Pulmonic valve, 1014t
Pulsatility, 1141
Pulsatility index (PI), 1098, 1191, 1403
    definition of, 1236
    ovaries and, 1236
Pulse, 84
    measurement of, 35, 35f, 36f
Pulse duration, 13
Pulse oximetry, 36–37, 38f
Pulse repetition frequency (PRF), 27, 151–152, 253b, 923
    Nyquist limit and, 156–159, 158f, 911–912
    parameters for scrotum evaluation, 715t
Pulse volume recordings, 1117, 1117f
Pulsed wave Doppler, 23–24, 1014, 1014f, 1014t, 1402–1403
    apical four-chamber view with, 911, 911f
    description of, 145, 911–912
    echocardiography, 923, 923f
    hypertrophic cardiomyopathy evaluations, 995, 997f
    illustration, 1014f
    Nyquist limit and, 911–912
    transducers used in, 911, 911f
Pulsed wave transducer, 923
Pulse-echo display modes, 17–18
Pulse-echo instrumentation, 17–22, 21f
PVCs. see Premature ventricular contractions
PVL. see Periventricular leukomalacia
Pyelectasis, 1366, 1610
Pyelonephritis
    acute, 806
    chronic, 806–807
    emphysematous, 478, 479f
    xanthogranulomatous, 454t–458t, 478–479, 480f
Pyloric canal, 390, 783
Pyloromyotomy, 784
Pylorus, description of, 390, 392f
Pyocele, 720, 726f
Pyogenic abscess, 264t, 265–266, 267f
Pyogenic infection, 430–432
Pyometra, 1225
Pyonephrosis, 454t–458t, 478, 479f
Pyosalpinx, 1261–1263, 1262f, 1262t, 1263f, 1264f
Pyramidal lobe, 683
Pyramids, medullary, 440, 443f
Pythagoras, 6
Pyuria, 438

Q
QRS complex, 904
Quad screen, 1285
Quadrant method, 656f, 657
Quadratus lumborum muscle, 492–493, 495f
Quadruple screen, prenatal diagnosis of congenital anomalies, 1429

R
Rachischisis, 1528, 1528f
Radial artery, 1112
Radial nerve, 739t
Radial plane, 657
Radial pulse, 35, 35f
Radial ray defects, 1633, 1634f
Radial veins, 1133
Radiography, 104
Radius, fetal measurement, 1390, 1391b, 1391f
Railway sign, 1355
Ramazzini, Bernardino, 68
Range ambiguity
    propagation, 151–152, 154f
    spectral Doppler, 157t, 159–160
Rarefaction, 10
RAS. see Renal artery stenosis
Raynaud phenomenon, 1118
RBCs. see Red blood cells
RCC. see Renal cell carcinoma
Reaching, 77
Reactive lymph nodes, 779, 781f
Real-time imaging, 18
Recessive disorder, 1433
Recovery, illness and, 60
Rectouterine pouch, 94
Rectouterine recess, 1174, 1198–1199, 1198f, 1203, 1203f, 1204f
Rectovesical spaces, 495
Rectus abdominis muscles, 90, 91f, 419, 420f, 1189, 1189f
Rectus sheath, anatomy of, 90, 1189, 1189f
Recurrent rami, 710–711, 711f
Red blood cells (RBCs), 83
Red pulp, of spleen, 330, 332f
Reducible hernia, 575
Reflection, 12, 12f
Refractile shadowing, 742–743, 742f, 743f
Refraction, 12, 149, 152f
Refusal, 30
    patient, 32, 33f
Reid, John, 8–10
Reidel lobe, 234–235
Rejection, 22
    liver transplantation, 593
    pancreatic transplantation, 632f, 633, 633f
    renal transplantation, 615–616, 618f
Renal adenomatous tumors, 468, 470f
Renal agenesis, 445–446, 449f, 1601–1602, 1602f, 1603b
Renal angiomyolipoma, 467, 469f
Renal anomalies, 445–447, 448f, 797–798
    horseshoe kidney, 448–449, 452f
    renal agenesis, 445–446, 449f
    renal ectopia, 448–449, 451f, 452f
Renal arteries, 185–187, 185f
    accessory, 623f
    Doppler flow patterns in, 212b, 214, 214f
    occlusion, 214
    sonographic findings of, 186, 186f, 187f

Renal arteriography, 481–482, 481*f*, 482*f*, 483*f*
Renal artery stenosis (RAS), 195, 197*f*, 480–481
    after renal transplantation, 622*f*
    contrast-enhanced evaluation of, 521, 521*f*
    sonographic findings in, 481–482, 481*b*, 481*f*, 482*f*, 483*f*
Renal atrophy, 454*t*–458*t*, 472
    sonographic findings in, 472–473, 473*f*
Renal biopsy, 548*f*, 555*f*
Renal capsule, 466–467
Renal cell carcinoma (RCC), 454*t*–458*t*, 464
    in children, 810–811
    in renal transplantation patients, 622–623, 626*f*
    sonographic findings in, 464–466, 464*f*, 465*f*, 466*b*, 466*f*
Renal corpuscle, 437
Renal cortex, 436–437, 444
Renal cystic disease, 453, 454*t*–458*t*, 458*b*, 1605–1608, 1605*b*, 1605*t*
    autosomal dominant polycystic kidney disease. *see* Autosomal dominant polycystic kidney disease
    autosomal recessive polycystic kidney disease. *see* Autosomal recessive polycystic kidney disease
    medullary cystic disease, 454*t*–458*t*, 462–463
    multicystic dysplastic kidney. *see* Multicystic dysplastic kidney
    polycystic kidney disease. *see* Polycystic kidney disease
    renal cysts associated with renal tumors, 460–461
    simple, 453, 459*f*
    sinus parapelvic, 454*t*–458*t*, 459–460
Renal cysts, 1600
    artifactual range-ambiguity echoes within, 154*f*
    complex, 458, 459*b*, 459*f*, 460*f*
    in renal transplantation patients, 624
    simple, 453, 459*f*
Renal disease, 468–470
    acquired immunodeficiency syndrome and, 454*t*–458*t*, 471, 471*f*, 472*f*
    acute interstitial nephritis, 470–471
    cystic. *see* Renal cystic disease
    hypertensive nephropathy, 454*t*–458*t*, 471
    laboratory tests for, 438–439
    lupus nephritis, 454*t*–458*t*, 471
    papillary necrosis, 454*t*–458*t*, 471–472
    renal atrophy, 454*t*–458*t*, 472
    sickle cell nephropathy, 454*t*–458*t*, 471
Renal ectopia, 448–449, 451*f*, 452*f*, 800, 803*f*, 1603, 1603*f*
Renal failure, 473
    acute, 454*t*–458*t*, 473, 585–586
    causes of, 473*b*
    chronic, 454*t*–458*t*, 473
    dialysis for, 585–586
    renal transplantation for, 585–586
    signs and symptoms of, 585–586
Renal hilum, 436
Renal hypoplasia, 445–446
Renal infarction, 454*t*–458*t*, 481–482
Renal infection, 478, 479*f*
Renal lymphoma, 454*t*–458*t*, 466, 467*f*
Renal masses
    aspiration of, 449–450, 452*t*
    complex, 458, 459*b*, 459*f*, 460*f*
    evaluation of, 449
    sonographic evaluation of, 522, 522*f*
    ultrasound-guided biopsy of, 554, 555*f*

Renal medulla, 444
Renal neoplasms, 463–464
Renal parenchyma
    angiomyolipoma and, 480*f*
    biopsy, 555
    junctional defects, 444, 446*f*, 446*t*, 447*f*
    sonographic evaluation of, 440–441, 442*f*, 443*f*
Renal pelvis, 436–437
Renal pyramids, 436
Renal sinus, 436–437
Renal sinus lipomatosis, 454*t*–458*t*
Renal stones. *see* Urolithiasis
Renal transplantation
    allograft for
        evaluation of, 610–611, 610*f*, 611*f*, 612*f*, 613*f*
        perfusion of, 611*f*
        postoperative imaging of, 613–615
        rejection of, 615–616, 618*f*
    autotransplantation, 610
    biopsy after, 615, 615*f*, 616*f*, 617*f*
    cadaveric kidney for, 608–609, 610*f*
    complications of
        abscesses, 616, 619*f*
        acute tubular necrosis, 615–616, 618*f*
        angiomyolipoma, 624
        biopsy-related, 615, 615*f*, 616*f*, 617*f*
        hematomas, 620–621, 624*f*
        infarction, 620, 623*f*
        infection, 616, 619*f*
        lymphoceles, 621–622, 625*f*
        necrosis, 620, 623*f*
        posttransplant lymphoproliferative disorder, 623, 628*f*
        pseudoaneurysms, 620
        rejection, 615–616, 618*f*
        renal artery stenosis and thrombosis, 619–620, 622*f*
        renal cell carcinoma, 622–623, 626*f*
        renal cysts, 623–624
        renal vein stenosis and thrombosis, 617–619, 621*f*
        seromas, 621, 625*f*
        transitional cell carcinoma, 623, 627*f*
        urinary obstruction, 616–617, 620*f*
        urinary stones, 616–617, 620*f*
        urine leak, 622, 626*f*
        urinomas, 622, 626*f*
    criteria for, 585–586
    history of, 585–586
    living donor kidney for, 609–610
    pancreas transplantation with, 586
    reasons for needing, 585–586
    rejection of, 615–616, 618*f*
    for renal failure, 585–586
    simultaneous pancreas-kidney transplant with, 586
    sonographic findings of, 612–613, 613*f*, 614*f*
    surgical technique of, 608–610
    ultrasound contrast agents and, 523–524
    ultrasound-guided biopsy after, 555, 555*f*
Renal tumors
    benign, 467, 469*f*, 488–490
        adenomatous tumors, 468, 470*f*
        angiomyolipoma, 467, 469*f*
        lipoma, 454*t*–458*t*, 468, 470*f*
        oncocytoma, 468, 470*f*
    fetal, 1615–1616, 1616*f*, 1617*b*, 1617*f*
    lymphoma, 454*t*–458*t*, 466, 467*f*
    renal cell carcinoma. *see* Renal cell carcinoma

Renal tumors *(Continued)*
    renal cysts associated with, 460–461
    squamous cell carcinoma, 454*t*–458*t*, 466, 466*f*, 467*f*
    Wilms tumor. *see* Wilms tumor
Renal variants
    columns of Bertin, 444, 446*f*
    dromedary hump, 444, 446*t*
    extrarenal pelvis, 444–445, 446*t*, 448*f*
    fetal lobulation, 444–445, 446*t*, 447*f*
    sinus lipomatosis, 444, 447*f*
Renal vein thrombosis, 807, 807*f*
Renal veins, 199–203, 203*f*, 438
    Doppler flow patterns in, 214, 214*b*, 215*f*
    left, 200–202, 204*f*
    obstruction of, 202–203
    renal transplantation complications of, 617–619, 621*f*
    right, 202–203, 204*f*
    stenosis of, 617–619, 621*f*
    thrombosis of, 202–203, 204*f*, 617–619, 621*f*, 807
Renunculi, 444, 446*f*, 447*f*, 792
Resistance, 12
Resistive index (RI), 210, 589, 1098, 1403
    definition of, 1236
    ovaries and, 1236
    urinary tract obstruction and, 476–478
Resistive vessels, 210
Resolution
    axial, 13–14
    azimuthal, 13–14
    lateral, 13–14
Resonance, 148–149
Resource organizations, 6
Respect for persons, 1296
Respiration, 84
    assessment of, 37–38
    definition of, 37–38
Respiratory phasicity, 1140
Restrictive cardiomyopathy, 990–992, 992*b*
Rete testis, 709, 709*f*
Reticuloendothelial system (RES), 326, 330, 514
Reticuloendotheliosis, 342
Retrocecal appendicitis, 404
Retrofascial space, 492*b*, 495, 495*f*
Retroflexion, 1166*f*, 1207*f*
Retromammary layer, 645, 645*f*, 646*f*
Retroperitoneal abscess, 508–509, 509*f*
Retroperitoneal fat, 506
Retroperitoneal fibrosis, 509–510, 509*f*
    with aneurysms, 192
Retroperitoneal fluid collections, 508–509
Retroperitoneal lymph nodes
    ultrasound-guided biopsy of, 555–556, 556*f*
    visualization of, 550*f*
Retroperitoneal spaces, 91*f*, 92, 492*f*
Retroperitoneal tumor
    primary, 506–508, 507*f*
    secondary, 508
Retroperitoneum, 435–437, 491, 510*b*
    anatomy of, 491–497, 492*b*, 492*f*, 493*f*
        adrenal glands, 494, 494*f*
        anterior pararenal space, 492, 492*b*, 493*f*
        diaphragmatic crura, 494, 494*f*
        iliac fossa, 492*b*, 495
        para-aortic lymph nodes, 494–495, 494*f*
        pelvic retroperitoneum, 495–496, 496*f*
        perirenal space, 491–493, 492*b*, 492*f*, 493*f*

Retroperitoneum (Continued)
  posterior pararenal space, 492b, 492f, 495
  retrofascial space, 492b, 495, 495f
  pathology of, 499–510
    adrenal cortical syndromes, 499–502, 502t
    adrenal cysts, 502–503, 502f, 503f
    adrenal hemorrhage, 503, 503f
    adrenal medulla tumors, 505–506
    adrenal tumors, 503–505
    primary retroperitoneal tumor, 506–508, 507f
    retroperitoneal fat, 506
    retroperitoneal fibrosis, 509–510, 509f
    retroperitoneal fluid collections, 508–509
    secondary retroperitoneal tumor, 508
  physiology and laboratory data of, 497
  sonographic evaluation of, 497–499
    adrenal glands, 497–498, 498f, 499f
    diaphragmatic crura, 498, 500f
    para-aortic lymph nodes, 498–499, 500f, 501f
    pitfalls in, 498
  vascular supply for, 496–497
Retroplacental abruption, 1456, 1456f
Retropubic space, 1174
Retroversion, 1166f, 1207f
Retrovesical space, 418–419
Reverberation, 742, 742f
Reverberation artifacts, 129, 132f, 148–149, 149f, 150f, 151f
Reverse isolation, 55
Reversible ischemic neurologic deficit (RIND), 1072
Rhabdomyoma, 998, 1001f, 1058, 1058f
Rhabdomyosarcomas, 507
Rheumatic fever, 957
Rheumatic heart disease
  aortic stenosis caused by, 967, 968f
  mitral stenosis caused by, 958–959, 958f
Rhombencephalon, 1522
Right atrial pressure, 914
Right atrium, 897, 897f, 1009, 1010f
  fetal circulation, 1446f
Right crus of diaphragm, 89, 89f
Right gastric artery, 179–180
Right hepatic artery, 180, 255t
Right hepatic vein, 223, 255t
Right hypochondrium, 88, 219
Right kidney
  abdominal scanning of
    at level of gallbladder, 107, 111f
    at level of liver and gallbladder longitudinal, 107–109, 111f, 118f
    power Doppler imaging with vascular UCA of, 513f
    transverse scanning of, 140f
Right lobe of liver, 219f, 220–221
  longitudinal scanning of, 108, 117f
  transverse scanning of, 107, 112f, 142f
Right lower quadrant (RLQ)
  description of, 88f
  pain in, 573t, 574–575
Right middle cerebral artery, 1093f
Right parasternal window, 927b, 928, 948b
Right portal vein (RPV), 206, 208f, 223, 224f
  color Doppler technique for, 255t
Right renal artery (RRA), 185
  color Doppler imaging with vascular ultrasound contrast agents of, 512f
  sonographic findings in, 186, 186f, 443f

Right renal vein (RRV), 202–203, 204f, 441–444, 444f
Right upper quadrant (RUQ), 88, 88f, 567–568, 573t
Right ventricle, 898, 898f
  anterior view of, 892f
  fetal circulation and, 1010
Right ventricular inflow disturbance, 1043–1045
Right ventricular outflow disturbance, 1045–1048
Right ventricular outflow tracts
  crisscross view, 1021, 1022b, 1022f
  five-chamber view of, 1021, 1021b, 1022f
  long-axis view of, 1022–1023, 1023b, 1023f, 1024f, 1025f, 1026f
  short-axis view of, 1023–1026, 1026b, 1026f, 1027f
Right-side diaphragmatic hernia, 1556
RIND. see Reversible ischemic neurologic deficit
Ring-down artifacts, 148–149, 151f
Roberts syndrome, 1500–1501, 1629–1630
Robinson, David, 7–8
Rock, 127–128
Rolled nipple technique, 656
Root, aortic, 171, 172f
Rotate motion, 128
Rotator cuff
  injuries to, 72
  minimum shoulder views of, 744b
  sonographic evaluation of, 744, 744b
    biceps tendon, 744, 744f, 745f
    indications for, 748b
    infraspinatus tendon, 745, 747f
    subscapularis tendon, 744, 745f
    supraspinatus tendon, 744–745, 746f
  tears of, 751–753, 751f
    full-thickness, 752, 753b, 753f
    partial-thickness, 752, 752b, 752f
Round ligaments, 1165–1166
Roux-en-Y procedure, 587f
RPV. see Right portal vein
RRA. see Right renal artery
RRV. see Right renal vein
Rubin's test, 1276
Rugae, 390
RUQ. see Right upper quadrant
Rushmer, Robert, 8–10

S

Saccular aneurysm, 191, 192f
Sacral hiatus, 873f
Sacrococcygeal teratomas
  AFP and, 1427–1428
Sacrum, 873, 873f
Safety, national patient standards for, 544
Sagittal imaging
  of female pelvis, 1184
  of hepatic structures, 235–239, 236f–237f, 238f
  in neonatal head examination, 825t, 826f, 827–828, 827f
  of pancreas, 366–367, 367f, 368f
  transabdominal, 1178–1180, 1179f, 1180f
  transvaginal, 1186, 1186b, 1186f, 1193f
Sagittal plane, abdominal, 104
Saldino-Noonan syndrome, 1630
Salpingitis, 1260–1263, 1262f, 1262t, 1263f, 1264f
Sample volume, 920, 1096
"Sandwich sign," 428
Sarcoma, 671

Satomura, Shigeo, 8–10
Scale, 26
Scalp edema, 1409f
Scan window, 125
Scanning, 124
  criteria for adequate scans, 134, 135f
Scattering, 12, 13f
Schizencephaly, 1523t, 1538, 1539f
Sciatic nerve, 739t
Scintigraphy, 770
Scirrhous carcinoma, 674–675
Sclerosing cholangitis, 315, 318f
Sclerotherapy, 1136–1137
Scoliosis, 1563–1564
Screening
  breast, 652, 653b
  mammography, 653–654, 653b, 653t, 654b
Scrotal cavity, 87t, 94–95
Scrotum
  anatomy of, 709–713, 709f, 710f, 731b–732b
  pathology of, 717–732
    congenital anomalies, 728t, 730–732
    epididymo-orchitis, 718
    extratesticular masses, 718t, 722
    hematomas, 714, 714f
    hernias, 723–725, 725f
    hydroceles, pyoceles, and hematoceles, 725–726, 726f
    lymphoma and leukemia, 728t, 730
    masses, 718t
    sperm granulomas, 726, 726f
    torsion, 710f, 720, 722f
    trauma, 717–722, 718f
    varicoceles, 717t, 722–723
  sonographic evaluation of
    patient positioning and scanning protocol, 712–713, 712b, 713f, 713t
    technical considerations for, 713–717, 714f, 715t
  swollen, 87t
  technical considerations for, 713–717, 714f
  testicular masses
    benign, 726–728, 727f
    malignant, 728–730, 728t
  torsion, 579, 579f, 580f
  trauma, 579, 579f, 580f
  vascular supply of, 710–712, 711f, 712b
SDMS. see Society of Diagnostic Medical Sonography
Second trimester pregnancy
  gestational age assessment, 1382–1394
    abdominal circumference, 1388–1389, 1388b, 1388f
    bone lengths, 1389–1390
    fetal measurements, 1382–1388
    fetal weight estimation, 1391–1392, 1392t
    multiple parameters, 1390–1391
    parameters, 1392–1394
  indications for, 1284b, 1290–1292, 1292b
  sonography of, 1343
Secondary hyperparathyroidism, 704
Secondary retroperitoneal tumor, 508
Secondary yolk sac, 1301, 1302f
Second-degree heart block, 1065–1066
Secretin, 393
Secretory phase
  description of, 1171b, 1172
  endometrium during, 1195, 1196f

Section thickness artifacts, 148, 148f
Sectional anatomy, 102
Sector array transducer, 134–135
Sector phased-array transducer, 16, 17f
Segmental Doppler pressures, 1114–1116, 1115t
Semilobar holoprosencephaly, 843, 843f, 1532–1533, 1532f, 1542f
Semilunar valves, 902–903
Seminoma, 728–729, 728t, 729f
Sensitization, 1407–1409
Sentinel node procedure, of breasts, 677–681, 678f
Sepsis, generalized, 420
Septa testis, 710
Septal defects
  atrial, 1036–1038, 1037f
    ostium primum, 1037–1038, 1037f, 1038f
    ostium secundum, 1037, 1037f
    sinus venosus septal defect, 1037f, 1038, 1038f
  atrioventricular, 1041–1043, 1041f
  ventricular, 1038–1041, 1038f, 1039f
    incidence of, 1032t, 1033
    membranous septal defect, 1038–1040, 1040f
    muscular defect, 1040–1041
Septicemia, 430–432
Septum primum, 1009, 1010f
Septum secundum, 1009, 1010f
Seroma
  after liver transplantation, 600, 604f
  after pancreatic transplantation, 636
  after renal transplantation, 621, 625f
  breast, 665, 665f
  definition of, 600
  muscle, 754
Serosa, 398
Serous cystadenocarcinomas, 1248–1249, 1249b, 1250b, 1251f
Serous cystadenoma, 1249b, 1249f, 1250f, 1252f
Serous cystic tumors, 377, 380f, 381f
Serous pericardium, 980, 981f
Sertoli-Leydig cell tumors, 1255–1256, 1256f
Serum albumin, 81, 228t
Serum amylase, 362
Serum calcium, 700–701
Serum creatinine, 439
Sestamibi parathyroid scan, 701
Sex hormones, 497
SGA. *see* Small for gestational age
Shadowing
  attenuation, 153–156, 155f
  causes of, 314–315
  color Doppler, 160–163, 162f, 163f
  definition of, 129, 153–156
  endometrial, 1208b
  example of, 131, 133f
  refractile, 742–743, 742f, 743f
  sonographic findings in, 314–315, 317f
Shone complex, 1048, 1049f
Short bowel syndrome, 787–788
Short-axis view
  of left and right ventricular outflow tracts, 1023–1026, 1026b, 1026f, 1027f
  parasternal
    for color flow mapping, 922b, 929–931, 931f, 932f, 933f, 934f
    Doppler window, 922–923, 931b, 931f, 932f, 933f, 934f
    of pulmonary stenosis, 1047f

Short-rib polydactyly syndrome, 1623t, 1630–1631, 1631f
Shoulder biceps tendon, 751, 751f
Shoulder dystocia, 1413–1414
Sickle cell anemia
  description of, 340
  illustration of, 340f
  stroke in, 1102–1103, 1103f
Sickle cell crisis, 340
Sickle cell nephropathy, 454t–458t, 471
Side lobes, 129, 132f, 151
Silicone breast implants
  low propagation speed in, 154f
  ruptured, 668, 669f
Simple call button, 34, 34f
Simple cysts
  in breast, 658t, 659, 659b, 660f
  hepatic, 262–264, 264t, 265f, 608
  ovarian
    in postmenopausal women, 1240–1242
    sonographic evaluation of, 1234, 1234b, 1234f, 1235f
  renal, 454t–458t
Simultaneous pancreas-kidney transplant (SPK), 586
Single photon emission computed tomography (SPECT), of breasts, 677–681, 678f
Single umbilical artery, 1470–1472, 1471f
Single ventricle, 1058–1059, 1058f, 1059f
Sinoatrial node, 1010
Sinus lipomatosis, 444, 447f
Sinus of Valsalva aneurysm, 974, 976f
Sinus venosus septal defect, 1037f, 1038, 1038f
Sinuses of Valsalva, 903, 974
Sirenomelia, 1631–1632, 1631f, 1632f
Situs ambiguous, 327–329
Situs inversus, 327–329, 1035f, 1577, 1581, 1582f
  partial, 1581, 1583f
  sonographic findings in, 1581
Situs solitus, 327–329, 1035f, 1582f
Skeletal dysplasia, 1622–1623, 1635b–1636b
  achondrogenesis, 1623t, 1626, 1626f, 1627f
  achondroplasia, 1623t, 1626
  arthrogryposis multiplex congenita, 1632–1633, 1632f
  camptomelic dysplasia, 1623t, 1629, 1630f
  caudal regression syndrome, 1631–1632, 1631f, 1632f
  congenital hypophosphatasia, 1628
  diastrophic dysplasia, 1628–1629, 1629f
  Ellis-van Creveld syndrome, 1631
  Jeune syndrome, 1631
  limb abnormalities, 1633–1635, 1633f, 1634f, 1635f
  osteogenesis imperfecta, 1623t, 1626–1628, 1627f, 1628f
  Roberts syndrome, 1629–1630
  short-rib polydactyly syndrome, 1623t, 1630–1631, 1631f
  sonographic evaluation of, 1623–1624, 1624t, 1625f
  thanatophoric dysplasia, 1623t, 1624–1626, 1625f
Skeleton, fetal, 1622, 1635b–1636b
  abnormalities of, 1622–1633. *see also* Skeletal dysplasia
  embryology of, 1622
Skin edema, hydrops and, 1486–1487

Skull. *see also* Cranium
  fetal, abnormalities of, 1498–1499, 1499f
  neonatal, 815f
Slice thickness, 13–14
Slide motion, 127
Sludge, 290–293, 294t–295t, 295f
Small for gestational age (SGA), 1390, 1397, 1417–1418, 1418f
Small intestine, 89, 89f. *see also* Bowel
  anatomy of, 390, 392f, 393f
  sonographic evaluation of, 399f
  vascular anatomy of, 392, 395f
Small saphenous vein (SSV), 1132
Society for Vascular Ultrasound (SVU), 6
Society of Diagnostic Medical Sonography (SDMS), 6
  sonographer's shoulder complaints received by, 69
Soldner, Richard, 8
Soleal sinuses, 1131
Solid lung masses, 1551–1554
  congenital bronchial atresia, 1554
  congenital cystic adenomatoid malformation, 1552–1554, 1553f, 1554f
  pulmonary sequestration, 1552, 1552b, 1552f
Somer, Jan, 8
Sonar, 7
Sonazoid, 514–515
Sonographers, 4
  commitments of, 30–35
  essentials of patient care for, 29, 67b
  in interventional procedures, 548–550, 549f, 550f
  physical health of, 5b
  qualities of, 5b
  resource organizations for, 6
  role of, 4–6
  training of, 129
Sonography
  career in, 5–6
  definition of, 4
  of second and third trimesters, 1343, 1376b
    diaphragm and thoracic vessels, 1360–1362, 1361f, 1362f, 1363f
    equipment and practices, 1344
    extrafetal obstetric overview, 1371–1375
      amniotic fluid, 1374, 1375f
      cervix, 1375, 1375b
      membranes, 1374–1375
      placenta, 1373–1374, 1373f, 1374f
      umbilical cord, 1372–1373, 1372f, 1373f
    fetal anatomy, 1348–1371
      cranium, 1348–1352, 1348f, 1349f, 1350f, 1351f, 1352f
      face, 1352–1355
    fetal circulation, 1362–1363, 1363f, 1364f
    fetal presentation, 1345–1348, 1345f, 1346f
    gastrointestinal system, 1365–1366, 1365f
    genetic sonogram, 1375–1376
    genitalia, 1368–1369, 1368f, 1369f
    heart, 1359–1360, 1360f, 1361f
    hepatobiliary system and upper abdomen, 1363–1365, 1364f, 1365f
    initial steps and examination overview, 1344–1348
    suggested protocol, 1344, 1344b
    thorax, 1357–1359, 1358f, 1359f

Sonography *(Continued)*
　　upper and lower extremities, 1369–1371, 1369f, 1370f, 1371f, 1372f
　　urinary system, 1366–1368, 1366f, 1367f
　　vertebral column, 1355–1357, 1356f, 1357f
Sonohysterography, 1199, 1200f
　　of endometrium, 1218–1220, 1219f
Sonolucent, 130
SonoVue, 514, 517
Sound
　　measurement of, 11–12
　　propagation through tissue, 12
　　velocity of, 10
Sound frequency ranges, 11t
Sound theory, 6–10
Space of Retzius, 1174
Spalding sign, 1417
Spallanzani, Lazzaro, 6
Spaulding's classification system, 51–52, 51t, 52f
Special needs patients, 57–60
　　adolescent patients, 58
　　crying/upset patients, 57
　　elderly patients, 57–58
　　multicultural patients, 59
　　pediatric patients, 58–59
Specific gravity, 438
Speckle
　　algorithms for reduction of, 715t
　　description of, 148, 149f
Spectral analysis, 23, 24f, 922–923, 923f
Spectral analysis waveform, 922–923
Spectral broadening, 23, 212, 1098–1099
Spectral Doppler analysis
　　of renal artery flow, 512f
　　scrotal, 713
Spectral Doppler artifacts, 156–160
　　aliasing and, 156, 159b
　　mirror image and, 160, 160f
　　noise and, 160, 160f
　　Nyquist limit and, 156–159, 157t, 158f, 159b, 159f
　　range ambiguity and, 157t, 159–160
Speed error artifacts, 743, 743t
Speed error propagation, 151, 154f
Sperm granulomas, 726, 726f
Spermatic cord
　　description of, 710
　　torsion of, 579, 720, 721f, 722f
Spermatoceles, 717t, 722
Spherocytosis, congenital, 340, 341f
Sphincter of Oddi, 283
Spiculation, 669, 670f
Spigelian fascia, 419
Spigelian hernia, 433
Spina bifida, 1337–1338, 1338f, 1392–1393, 1523t, 1527–1529, 1528f
　　sonographic findings in, 1529, 1529f, 1530f, 1531f
Spina bifida aperta, 880, 1528
Spina bifida cystica, 1528f
Spina bifida occulta, 880, 1528, 1528f
Spinal canal, 88, 871, 875, 875f
Spinal cord
　　anatomy of, 873, 874f
　　anterior position of, 879
　　injury, 886–887, 886f
　　meninges of, 873–875, 874f
　　primitive, 1523

Spinal cord *(Continued)*
　　sonographic appearance of, 875, 875f
　　tethered, 871, 881–883, 882f
Spinal degeneration, 72
Spinal dysraphism, lumbosacral stigmata associated with, 887b
Spinal nerve roots, 873
Spine. *see also* Vertebral column
　　embryonic, 1310–1313, 1311f, 1312f
　　fetal ultrasound, 1408t
　　neonatal. *see* Neonatal spine
Spiral arteries, 1443f
Splanchnic aneurysm, 185–187, 185f, 195
Spleen, 88, 325, 333b, 335f, 353b
　　abdominal scanning of, at level of left kidney, 109, 122f
　　abscesses of, 337t, 342–344, 346f
　　accessory, 329, 331f
　　agenesis, 327–329
　　anatomy of, 326–327
　　　normal, 326, 327f, 328f
　　　relational, 326, 331f
　　　size, 326, 329f
　　　vascular supply, 326, 330f
　　atrophy, 336
　　congenital anomalies of, 327–329, 331f
　　diffuse disease, 340–342, 340f, 341f
　　displacement of, 326–327
　　fetal
　　　abnormalities of, 1583–1584
　　　embryology of, 1574
　　　sonographic evaluation of, 1580, 1580f
　　functions of, 332, 332b
　　hematoma, 566f
　　infarction, 337t, 344–345, 347f
　　infection, 344, 344f, 347f
　　laboratory data of, 332–333
　　longitudinal scans of, 141
　　nonvisualization of, 336
　　pathology of, 336
　　　acquired immunodeficiency syndrome, 344
　　　benign primary tumors, 349–351, 350f
　　　congestion, 337b, 337t
　　　cysts, 337t, 348–349, 349f
　　　diffuse disease, 340, 341f
　　　hamartoma, 349, 351f
　　　hematoma, 347–348, 348f, 349f
　　　infarction, 337t, 344–345
　　　malignant primary tumors, 351–354
　　　storage disease, 339–340, 339f
　　　trauma, 337t, 345–348, 347f, 350f
　　pediatric, 765b, 766f, 767f
　　physiology of, 329–333
　　pulp of, 329
　　sonographic evaluation of, 333–336
　　　normal texture and patterns in, 333–334, 334f
　　　patient position and technique in, 334–336, 335f
　　size in, 333, 333f, 337t
　　transverse scanning of, 139, 139f, 141
　　wandering, 327
Splenic artery, 106, 106f, 109, 180, 326
　　Doppler flow patterns in, 212, 212b, 213f
　　pancreas and, 358f, 359
　　sonographic evaluation of, 181f, 182f
Splenic flexure, 390–391
Splenic hilum, 326, 330f
Splenic sequestration syndrome, 767–775

Splenic vein, 106–108, 106f, 206–207
　　anatomy of, 326, 330f
　　color Doppler technique for, 255t
　　pancreas and, 358, 358f
　　sonographic findings of, 206, 210f
Splenomegaly, 326, 336–338, 336f, 337t, 338b, 338f, 338t, 339f, 342f
　　in adolescents, 769f
　　congestive, 338b, 339
　　patterns, 339f
　　sonographic evaluation of, 337t, 499, 501f
Splenorenal ligament, 326, 328f, 418, 418f
Split-hand deformity, 1633f
Sponge kidney, medullary, 454t–458t, 462, 479, 480f
Spontaneous abortion, 1322, 1322f
Spontaneous flow, 1140–1141
Spontaneous rupture of the membranes (SPROM), 1482
Squamous cell carcinoma
　　cervical, 1204–1206, 1206f
　　renal, 454t–458t, 466, 466f, 467f
Standard evaluation, fetal ultrasound, 1408t
Standard precautions, 49–53, 50f, 51f
Starzl, Thomas, 585
Static Graf technique, 860–866, 862b, 862f, 863f, 863t, 864f
Stein-Leventhal syndrome, 1238–1239
Stepladder sign, 668, 669f
Sternal angle, 891–892
Sternocleidomastoid muscles, 683, 684f
Sternum, absent, 1564t
Stoma, 47
Stomach, 88, 89f, 219, 220f
　　anatomy of
　　　normal, 390, 391f
　　　vascular, 392, 394f
　　antrum of, 367, 368f
　　fetal
　　　abnormalities of, 1584–1586
　　　embryology of, 1573–1574
　　　sonographic evaluation of, 1576–1577, 1577f
　　sonographic evaluation of, 395–396, 397f
Stools, height-adjustable, 78
Storage disease, 339–340, 339f
Strabismus, 1502
Strangulated hernia, 575
Strap muscles, 683, 684f
Stress testing, arterial, 1116
Stressors, 81
Stretches, 77f
Striations, 1160–1161
Strict isolation, 55
Strictures, ureteral, 450
Stroke volume, 910, 914, 990b
Stroma ovarii, 1250–1251
Stromal tumors, 1252–1257, 1255f
Strutt, John William, 6
Stuck twin. *see* Polyhydramnios-oligohydramnios (poly-oli) sequence
Subacute bacterial endocarditis, 1000–1006, 1004f, 1005f
Subacute (de Quervain) thyroiditis, 699–700
Subarachnoid space, 816
Subcapsular collections, 424–425, 425f
Subchorionic hemorrhage, 1320, 1321f, 1456
Subclavian artery, 162f, 1112
Subclavian steal syndrome, 1081f, 1101, 1101f

Subclavian vein, 1133
Subcostal plane, 105
Subcostal transducer location, 918, 919f
Subcostal view
　for color flow mapping, 938, 948b
　for Doppler, 924b, 938–939
　transducer position, 938–939, 948b
　two-dimensional, 938, 938b, 948f
Subcostal window, 924b, 938–939
Subcutaneous fat, 646, 647f
Subcutaneous layer, 645, 645f, 646f
Subependyma, cysts of, 833, 845
Subfascial hematoma, 430
Subfertility, 1272–1273
Subhepatic lesion, 414
Subhepatic spaces, 99f
Sublingual cysts, 1512f
Subluxation
　of neonatal hip, 857–858, 858f
　of shoulder biceps tendon, 751, 751f
Submandibular window
　intracranial arterial identification criteria, 1096t
　for transcranial color Doppler imaging, 1095–1096
Submucosa, 390
Submucosal leiomyomas, 1209, 1209b
Suboccipital window, 1095, 1095f
Subphrenic abscesses, 423–424, 424f
Subphrenic space, 98, 99f, 219
Subpulmonic stenosis, 1047–1048, 1047f
Subscapularis tendon, 744, 745f
Subserosal leiomyomas, 1209, 1209b, 1210f
Subvalvular aortic stenosis, 966, 967f, 1050–1052, 1051f, 1052f
Subvalvular pulmonary stenosis, 1047f
Succenturiate lobes, 1454
Succenturiate placenta, 1449, 1454, 1454f, 1455f
Suffering, 1296
Sulcus, 817
Superficial flexor tendon, 736f
Superficial inguinal ring, 90
Superficial structures, 134
Superficial veins
　lower extremity, 1132–1133, 1132f
　mapping of, 1146
　upper extremity, 1134f
Superficial venous thrombosis, 1136
Superior mesenteric artery (SMA), 180–182, 183f
　abdominal scanning of
　　at level of aorta, 109, 121f
　　at level of pancreas, 107, 109f
　Doppler flow patterns in, 212b, 213f, 214
　longitudinal scans of, 141
　pancreas and, 358f, 359
　sonographic evaluation of, 182–184, 183f
Superior mesenteric vein (SMV), 207–209
　pancreas and, 356, 357f, 358, 365f
　sonographic findings of, 198, 211f
Superior vena cava
　congenital left atrial communication with, 1059–1060, 1060f
　fetal circulation, 1446f
　fetal circulation and, 1010
Superior vesical arteries, 1461
Superior/inferior direction, 132–134
Supine, 132
Support cushions, 78
Supracolic compartment, 99f

Supracristal defects, 1038–1039
Suprapancreatic obstruction, 312, 314f
Suprarenal veins, 204–206
Suprascapular nerve, 739t
Supraspinatus tendon
　sonographic evaluation of, 746f
　tears of, 752
Suprasternal notch, 891–892, 948b
Suprasternal notch view, 924b, 949f
Suprasternal transducer location, 918, 919f
Suprasternal views
　for color flow mapping, 940–941, 949f
　for Doppler, 941–943, 949f
　transducer position, 949f
　two-dimensional, 939–940, 948b, 948f
Supravalvular aortic stenosis, 966, 966f, 1050–1052, 1051f, 1052f
Supravalvular pulmonary stenosis, 1048, 1048f
Supraventricular tachyarrhythmias, 1063–1064, 1064f
Supravesical space, 418–419
Surgery, for hypertrophic pyloric stenosis, 787–788, 787f
Suspensory ligament, 1169
Sweep motion, 127
Swelling
　extremity, 579–581, 580f
　scrotum, 87t
Swyer syndrome, 1630f
Sylvian fissure, 818f
Syncope, 1072
Synechiae
　intrauterine, 1222–1223, 1223f
　uterine, 1275f
Synovial sheath, 736, 736f
Systemic lupus erythematosus (SLE), 1064f, 1415, 1415f
Systole, 909, 926–928
Systolic measurement, 36
Systolic murmur, 905
Systolic to diastolic (S/D) ratio, 1191, 1403

T

T wave, 904
T$_3$. see Triiodothyronine
T4. see Thyroxine
Tachyarrhythmias, supraventricular, 1063–1064, 1064f
Tachycardia, 84
　definition of, 35
　embryonic, 1327
　fetal, 1012
Tail of Spence, 645
Takotsubo cardiomyopathy, 993
Talipes. see Clubfoot
Tamoxifen, 1224
Tardus-parvus, 481, 483f
Target sign, 404
　double, 783
Tatum T, 1227–1228
Taylor, Frederick Winslow, 68
TCC. see Transitional cell carcinoma
Teardrop/noose sign, 667–668, 668f
Technical aptitude, 5b
TEE. see Transesophageal echocardiography
Temporal resolution, 18
Tendinitis, 72, 753–754, 753f, 754b, 754f
　acute, 753–754
　de Quervain, 754
　sonographic features of, 755t

Tendons, 736–737, 736f, 737f
Tenosynovitis, 72, 753–754, 754f
Tentorium cerebelli, 815
Teratogens, 1533
Teratoma, 508
　dermoid tumors, 1250–1251, 1252b, 1252f, 1253f
　fetal neck, 1515, 1516b, 1516f
　immature and mature, 1251–1252, 1253f
Teres minor tendon, 747, 747f, 748f
Terminal ductal lobular units (TDLUs), 645–646, 646f
Terminal patients, 60–61
Testes, 709
　enlarged, 718t
　hypoechoic band in, 718t
　undescended. see Cryptorchidism
Testicular arteries, 710–711, 712b
Testicular duplication, 731–732
Testicular ectopia, 730
Testicular masses, benign, 726–728, 727f
　malignant, 728–730, 728t
Testicular microlithiasis, 728, 728f
Testicular vein, 712
Tethered spinal cord, 871, 881–883, 882f
Tetralogy of Fallot, 1045–1046, 1046f
TGC. see Time gain compensation
Thalamo-occipital distance (TOD), 830, 831f
Thalamus, neonatal, 818, 819f
Thalassemia, 341–342, 343f
Thanatophoric dysplasia, 1499f, 1623t, 1624–1626, 1625f
Theca-lutein cysts, 1237, 1238b, 1239f, 1325, 1326f
Thecomas, 1254–1255, 1255f
Thermal index (TI), 1288
Third trimester pregnancy
　gestational age assessment, 1382–1394
　　abdominal circumference, 1388–1389, 1388b, 1388f
　　bone lengths, 1389–1390
　　fetal measurements, 1382–1388
　　fetal weight estimation, 1391–1392, 1392t
　　multiple parameters, 1390–1391
　　parameters, 1392–1394
　indications for, 1284b, 1290–1292, 1292b
　sonography of, 1343
Third ventricle, neonatal, 815–816, 825–826
Third-degree heart block, 1065–1066
Thompson's test, 750
Thoracentesis, 543
Thoracic aneurysms, 195
Thoracic cavity, 88, 88f
　abnormalities of, 1548–1558
　　diaphragm, 1555–1558, 1555f
　　lung, 1548–1555, 1549f, 1550t
　anatomy of, 891–892, 892f, 893b, 906b–907b
　embryology of, 1545
Thoracic circumference measurements, fetal, 1550t
Thoracic outlet syndrome (TOS), 72, 1117–1118
Thoracic pain, 573t
Thorax, 891–892, 892f
　fetal, 1357–1359, 1358f, 1359f, 1545, 1558b.
　　see also Thoracic cavity
　sonographic characteristics of, 1545–1548, 1546b
　　position, 1546–1547, 1548f
　　respiration, 1547–1548, 1548f
　　size, 1546, 1546f, 1547f
　　texture, 1547, 1548f

Threatened abortion, 1320
Three-dimensional (3D) imaging
  echocardiography, 916–917
  of female pelvis, 1199–1201, 1200f
  fetal echocardiography, 1015, 1015f
  gray-scale harmonic imaging with vascular UCA, 516, 516f
  for lost intrauterine contraceptive devices, 1225–1228, 1226f–1227f, 1228f
  of ovaries, 1233
  of scrotum, 710f, 713f
Three-dimensional ultrasound (3DU), 20–21, 20f
Threshold level, 1323
Threshold parameters for scrotum evaluation, 715t
Thrombocytes, 83
Thrombocytopenia, 333
Thrombolytic therapy, 1135
Thrombosis
  after pancreatic transplantation, 633–634, 635f, 636f
  inferior vena cava, 199–204, 260t
  renal veins, 202–203, 204f, 617–619, 621f, 805–806
  of umbilical vessels, 1467, 1468f
Thrombus, cardiac, 998–1000, 1003f
Thyroglossal duct cysts, 705, 705f
Thyroid gland, 682, 707b
  anatomy of, 683–684, 684f
    relational, 683–684, 684f
    size, 683, 684t
  aplasia, 690
  blood supply of, 684
  congenital abnormalities of, 690
  ectopic, 690
  elastography of, 698, 698f
  embryology of, 683
  pathology of, 690–700
    benign lesions, 691–693, 693f
    diffuse thyroid disease, 698–700
    malignant lesions, 693–698, 695f
    nodular thyroid disease, 690–691, 690f, 692f
  physiology and laboratory data of, 684–686, 685b
  sonographic evaluation of, 686–690, 687f, 688f, 689f, 690f
  ultrasound-guided biopsy of, 557, 557f
Thyroid inferno, 699
Thyroid metastasis, 698
Thyroiditis, 699
  de Quervain, 699
  Hashimoto, 700, 700f
Thyroid-stimulating hormone (TSH), 684–685
Thyromegaly, 1514, 1516f
Thyrotoxic crisis, 699
Thyrotoxicosis, 683
Thyroxine (T_4), 682–683
TIA. see Transient ischemic attack
Tibia, fetal measurement, 1390, 1390b, 1390f
Tibial-peroneal trunk, 1112
Ticlopidine, 1135
Time gain compensation (TGC), 21–22, 124, 231–232, 439
Time-of-flight artifacts, 743, 743f
Tinel sign, 756
"Tip of the iceberg," 1251
TIPS. see Transjugular intrahepatic portosystemic shunt
Tissue
  definition of, 81
  propagation of sound through, 12

Tissue characterization, 209
Tissue Doppler imaging, 995
Tissue plasminogen activators (tPAs), 1135
Tissue-specific ultrasound contrast agents, 514–515, 515f
TOAs. see Tubo-ovarian abscesses
Toe pressures, 1115
Toe-brachial index (TBI), 1116–1117
Tongue, abnormalities of, 1510–1511, 1511f, 1512f
TORCH, 770
Torsion
  gallbladder, 299–300
  ovarian, 1243–1244, 1243b, 1244f
  scrotal, 579, 579f, 580f, 717t, 720, 722f
Tortuous arteries, 1075–1076, 1076b, 1076f
Tortuous pelvic mass, anechoic, 1600
TOS. see Thoracic outlet syndrome
Total anomalous pulmonary venous return (TAPVR), 899, 1060, 1060f, 1061f
Toxemia, 1415
Toxic goiter, 691, 691t
Trachea, abnormalities of, 1511–1512, 1512f
Tracheoesophageal septum, 1573
Transabdominal (TA) ultrasonography, 1158, 1178–1181, 1181b
  levator ani muscles, 1190, 1190f
  longitudinal, 1178–1181, 1194, 1194f
  obturator internus muscles, 1189–1190, 1190f
  of ovaries, 1231–1234
  patient preparation and history for, 1178–1181
  pelvic vascularity, 1181f, 1190, 1192f
  protocol for, 1181b, 1185
  sagittal imaging, 1178–1180, 1179f, 1180f
    of distended bladder, 1179f, 1180f
  transverse, 1179f, 1180f
  of tubo-ovarian abscess, 1263–1264, 1265f, 1266f
  of uterus
    longitudinal, 1178–1181
    sagittal, 1181f, 1182f
    transverse, 1183f
Transcranial Doppler (TCD) imaging, 1087–1088
  advantages of, 1104–1107
  applications of, 1087–1088, 1088b, 1099–1104
  of brain death, 1103
  of collateral pathways, 1100–1101
  diagnostic pitfalls of, 1105–1107, 1107f
  guidelines for, 1105b
  interpretation of, 1096–1099
  intracranial disease diagnosed using, 1100–1103
  intracranial venous evaluation by, 1104
  intraoperative use of, 1104
  limitations of, 1104–1107, 1104b
  sickle cell disease examination, 1102–1103, 1103f
  technical aspects of, 1090–1096
    hints on, 1106t
    instrumentation, 1091
    technique, 1091–1096, 1092f
      submandibular window, 1095–1096
      suboccipital window, 1095, 1095f
      transorbital window, 1094, 1094f
      transtemporal window, 1092–1094, 1092f, 1093f, 1094f
    vasospasm diagnosis using, 1099–1100
Transducer(s)
  cable management, 76–77
  continuous-wave Doppler, 913f

Transducer(s) *(Continued)*
  curved-array, 16–17
  definition of, 14–15
  Doppler frequency shift and, 25
  for echocardiography, 918–919, 919f
  gripping pressure, 74–75
  intraluminal, 17, 17f
  linear-array, 16, 17f, 854, 854b
  multielement, 16, 16f
  needles attached to, 536–538, 536f
  for neonatal head examination, 820
  placement for transcranial color Doppler, 1092
  positions of
    in abdominal scanning, 126–128, 129f
    cardiac protocol and, 927b
    in echocardiography, 918–919, 919f
    radial/antiradial, 657
  prepping, 544–546, 545f, 546f
  pulsed wave Doppler, 911, 911f, 923, 923f
  requirements for fetal echocardiography, 1013
  sector phased-array, 16, 17f
  selection of, 14–17, 14f, 15f
    in abdominal scanning, 125–126, 126f, 127f
  transvaginal, 1180–1181, 1305
  types of, 14
Transducer angle, 1096
Transesophageal echocardiography (TEE), 916–917
Transfer, of patient, 38–40
  in assisting patients from the scanning stretcher into the wheelchair, 40, 41f
  body mechanics and, 38–39
  in moving patients toward the head of a stretcher, 39–40
  in moving patients up in bed, 39, 40f
  in stretcher transfer, 39, 39f
  in turning patients, 40
  in wheelchair transfer, 39, 39f
Transient ischemic attack (TIA), 1071
Transitional cell carcinoma (TCC), 454t–458t, 464–466, 623, 627f
Transitional cell tumors, 1249–1250, 1252f
Transjugular intrahepatic portosystemic shunt (TIPS), 257, 257f, 517
Translabial sonography, 1187, 1206–1207
Transmediastinal artery, 711, 711f
Transmission, abnormal structures affecting, 134b
Transorbital approach, 1094, 1094f, 1096t
Transorbital window, 1094, 1094f
Transperineal approach, 1177
Transperineal sonography, 1187, 1206–1207
Transplant patient, sonographic techniques in, 583, 638b
Transplantation, 523–524
  liver. see Liver transplantation
  pancreatic. see Pancreatic transplantation
  renal. see Renal transplantation
  team-based approach to, 584
  waiting list for, 584
Transposition of the great arteries, 1054, 1054f, 1055f
  corrected, 1054
  sonographic findings in, 1054, 1055f
Transpyloric plane, 88, 105
Transtemporal approach
  bony landmarks from, 1092–1093, 1092f, 1093f
  intracranial arterial identification criteria, 1096t
  for transcranial Doppler, 1092–1094, 1092f, 1093f, 1094f

Transtemporal window, 1092–1094, 1092f, 1093f, 1094f
Transtesticular artery, 711
Transvaginal transducers, 126, 128f, 1305
Transvaginal (TV) ultrasonography, 1158, 1183–1189
  of adenomyosis, 1212–1216
  of cervix
    benign conditions, 1203–1204, 1203f, 1204b
    cervical carcinoma and, 1204, 1206b, 1206f
  disinfection technique, 1187–1189
  endometrial hyperplasia, 1220, 1220b, 1221f
  of endometriomas, 1267–1270, 1268f, 1269f
  of endometrium, 1195–1196, 1195f, 1196f
    carcinoma, 1223–1224, 1224b, 1224f
    endometritis, 1221–1222, 1222b
  examination technique, 1183–1184
  of fallopian tubes, 1196–1197, 1197f
  first trimester, 1305–1306, 1305f
    at 6 to 10 weeks of gestational age, 1310–1313, 1310t
      embryonic cranium and spine, 1310–1313, 1311f, 1312f
      embryonic heart, 1313, 1314f, 1314t
      limb development, 1313, 1313f
      physiologic herniation of bowel, 1313, 1314f
      skeletal ossification, 1313, 1313f
    fetal period (weeks 9-14), 1306–1313
      embryo during, 1308–1310, 1309f, 1310f
      gestational sac during, 1307–1310, 1307f, 1307t
      yolk sac during, 1307–1308, 1307f, 1308f
  of ovaries, 1186b, 1197–1198, 1197f
    dermoid tumors, 1250–1251, 1252b, 1252f, 1253f
    hemorrhagic corpus luteum cysts, 1237, 1238f
    hemorrhagic cysts, 1237, 1238f
    ovarian hyperstimulation syndrome, 1237–1239, 1239f
    simple cystic masses, 1234, 1234b, 1234f, 1235f
    torsion, 1243–1244, 1243b, 1244f
  paraovarian cysts, 1240, 1240b, 1241f
  patient instructions for, 1183
  of pelvic inflammatory disease, salpingitis, hydrosalpinx, and pyosalpinx, 1261–1263, 1262f, 1262t, 1263f, 1264f
  pelvic vascularity, 1181f, 1190, 1192f
  of peritonitis, 1264–1266, 1266f
  polyps, 1220–1221, 1222f
  probe preparation for, 1183, 1184f
  protocol, 1186b
  scan orientation, 1184, 1185f
  scanning planes, 1184
  scanning techniques, 1184–1185
  small endometrial fluid collections, 1224–1225, 1225f
  technique, 1187–1189, 1188f
  of uterine leiomyosarcoma, 1216–1217, 1217f
  of uterus
    coronal, 1186, 1186b, 1187f
    with hypoechoic myoma, 1206f
    sagittal, 1186, 1186b, 1186f, 1193f, 1197f
Transverse fetal lie, 1345, 1345f
Transverse pancreatic artery, 180
Transverse plane, 88
  abdominal, 104, 106–108
  of abdominal aorta, 174, 177f

Transverse scanning
  abdominal, 128. see also Abdominal scanning
  of abdominal aorta, 138–139, 138f
  of biliary system, 134
  of gallbladder, 141, 144f
  of hepatic structures, 239, 240f–241f, 242f
  of pancreas, 136–138, 364–366, 366f
  protocols for, 135–140, 136f, 137f
  of spleen, 139, 139f, 141
  suprasternal notch view, 949f
Transversus muscle, 90, 90f
Trauma
  abdominal, 561–563
  blunt. see Blunt trauma
  scrotal, 579, 579f, 580f, 717–722, 718f
  splenic, 337t, 345–348, 347f, 350f
Treacher Collins syndrome, 1500
Tricuspid annular plane systolic excursion (TAPSE), 988–989, 990f
Tricuspid regurgitation, 988–989, 990f, 1045f
Tricuspid valve, 897, 897f
  atresia of, 1043, 1043f
  Ebstein anomaly of, 1043–1045, 1044f
  fetal circulation and, 1010
  M-mode imaging of, 946
  normal Doppler measurements, 1014t
Trigger finger, 72
Trigonocephaly, 1498–1499
Triiodothyronine (T_3), 682–683
Trimesters, 1287
Triploidy, 1438
Trisomy 13, 1032, 1437–1438, 1438f, 1439f, 1440f
  sonographic findings in, 1535f
Trisomy 18, 1032, 1436–1437, 1436f, 1437f, 1438f
Trisomy 21, 1433–1436, 1434f, 1435f, 1436f
Trophoblastic layer, 1443f
Trophoblastic reaction, 1324b
True aneurysm, 190–191, 191f
True hermaphroditism, 1618
True pelvis
  description of, 1159–1160
  illustration of, 94, 1161f
  muscles of, 1161, 1161f
Truncus arteriosus, 1054–1055, 1055f
  partitioning of, 1009
  sonographic findings in, 1055, 1056f
Trunk twisting, 75f, 77
Tuberous sclerosis, 454t–458t, 460, 805
Tubes and tubing, 40–47, 41f
  catheters, 43–44, 44f
  colostomies and ileostomies, 47
  drains, 46–47
  dressings, 46–47
  intravenous therapy, 41–43, 41f, 42f, 43f
  nasogastric tubes, 43, 44f
  ostomy, 47
  oxygen therapy, 45–46, 45f, 46f
  wounds, 46–47
Tubo-ovarian abscesses (TOAs), 1261b, 1263–1264
Tubo-ovarian complex, 1221, 1260
Tubular carcinoma, 674
Tumor(s). see also Carcinoma; Neoplasms
  abdominal, 772–775
  adrenal, 503–505
    neonatal/pediatric, 807–811
  adrenal medulla, 505–506
  bladder, 486–487, 488f

Tumor(s) (Continued)
  cardiac. see Cardiac tumors
  carotid body, 1078, 1079f
  dermoid, 1250–1251, 1252b, 1252f, 1253f
  endodermal sinus, 1252
  epithelial ovarian, 1246–1250, 1248f
  gastrointestinal, 401–402
  intrahepatic biliary, 318
  Krukenberg, 1256–1257, 1257f
  liver, 773–775, 774t
    benign, 773
    malignant, 773–774
  medulla, 502t
  mesentery, 428, 430f
  omentum, 428, 430f
  ovarian
    solid, 1235–1236, 1236b
    sonographic evaluation of, 1244
  peritoneal, 428, 430f
  retroperitoneal
    primary, 506–508, 507f
    secondary, 508
  Sertoli-Leydig cell, 1255–1256, 1256f
  splenic, 337t
    benign, 349–351
    malignant, 351–354
  uterine, 1207–1208
Tunica adventitia, 171, 171f, 1111
Tunica albuginea
  cysts of, 722
  description of, 710
Tunica intima, 171, 171f, 1111
Tunica media, 171, 171f, 1111
Tunica vaginalis, 710, 710f
Turbulent flow, 23
Turner syndrome, 1032, 1339, 1438–1441, 1440f, 1513, 1514f
Twin anemia-polycythemia syndrome (TAPS), 1420–1421, 1423
Twin pregnancy, intrauterine, 1279, 1279f
"Twinkling" artifact, 160–163, 163f
Twinkling sign, 485, 485f
Twin-to-twin transfusion syndrome (TTTS), 1412f, 1422, 1422f
Two-dimensional imaging
  ability to conceptualize, 5b
  apical views, 932–938, 936f, 937f, 938b
  echocardiography, 917–919, 917f, 918f
  parasternal long-axis views, 925–926, 927b, 928b, 928f, 929f
  subcostal views, 938, 938b, 948f
  suprasternal views, 939–940, 948b, 948f

U

UCAs. see Ultrasound contrast agents
Ulcerative colitis, 410f
Ulna, fetal measurement, 1390, 1391b, 1391f
Ulnar artery, 1112
Ulnar nerve, 739t
Ulnar veins, 1133
Ultrasonic Institute, 7–8, 9f
Ultrasound, 14, 103, 103t
  annotation of images, 128–129
  certification for, 6
  criteria for identifying abnormal structures, 134b
  definition of, 4, 10
  efficiency in patient care, 34–35

Ultrasound *(Continued)*
  explanation of, 31–32
  historical overview of sound theory and, 6–10
  postoperative uses of, 1271
  principles of, 10–28
    acoustics, 10–14, 11*f*, 11*t*
    harmonic imaging, 18–20, 19*f*
    pulse-echo display modes, 17–18
    system controls for image optimization, 21–22
    three-dimensional and four-dimensional ultrasound, 20–21, 20*f*
    transducer selection, 14–17, 14*f*, 15*f*
  protocols used in
    abdominal survey, 134–135, 134*f*
    biliary system, 289*t*
    liver, 233–234, 235*t*
    longitudinal scans, 140–141
    porta hepatis, 233–234, 235*t*
    transverse scans, 135–140, 136*f*, 137*f*, 138*f*, 139*f*
  resource organizations for, 6
  systems
    ergonomic, 73, 73*f*
    illustration of, 130*f*
  terminology, 129–131, 130*f*
Ultrasound angiogram, 516*f*
Ultrasound contrast agents (UCAs), 511
  abdominal applications of, 511, 524*b*
  clinical applications of, 517–524
    hepatic applications, 517–521
    organ transplants, 523–524
    pancreatic applications of, 523
    renal applications, 521–522
    splenic applications, 522–523
  modes of, 515–516, 516*f*
  types of, 511–515
    tissue-specific, 514–515, 515*f*
    vascular, 511–514, 512*f*, 513*f*, 513*t*, 514*t*
Ultrasound first, 761–762
Ultrasound-guided procedures, 529–530, 529*f*, 530*f*, 531*f*, 559*b*
  abscess drainage and fluid collection, 534–535, 559
  advantage of, 529, 530*f*
  ascites drainage, 559
  in breast, 676
    large-core needle biopsy, 676
    preoperative needle wire localization, 676, 676*f*
  deviation of needles, 551–552, 551*f*, 552*f*
  equipment and techniques of, 532–535, 533*f*, 534*f*, 535*f*
  finding the needle tips, 550–551, 551*f*
  fusion technology and, 540–542, 540*f*, 541*f*, 542*f*
  growth in, 528–529
  laboratory tests, 531–532
  limitations of, 529–530, 530*f*
  methods for, 535–538, 535*f*, 536*f*, 537*f*, 538*f*
    free-hand techniques, 535–536, 535*f*, 536*f*
    needles attached to transducer, 536–538, 536*f*
  new applications of, 559–560
  pleural fluid collections, 559
  sonographer's role in, 548–550, 549*f*, 550*f*
Umbilical arteries, 1443*f*
  fetal circulation, 1446*f*
Umbilical cord, 1291, 1372–1373, 1372*f*, 1373*f*, 1443*f*, 1460, 1472*b*–1473*b*

Umbilical cord *(Continued)*
  abnormal dimensions, 1462–1464, 1464*f*, 1465*f*
  development and anatomy of, 1460–1462
    embryologic development, 1460–1461, 1461*f*
    normal anatomy, 1461, 1462*f*
    sonographic evaluation, 1461, 1462*f*, 1463*f*, 1464*f*
  insertion, 1577–1578, 1578*f*
  insertion abnormalities, 1468–1470
    marginal insertion of the cord (Battledore placenta), 1468, 1469*f*
    membranous or velamentous insertion of the cord, 1469–1470, 1470*f*
  knots, 1467–1468
    false, 1468, 1468*f*
    nuchal cord, 1468, 1469*f*
    true, 1467–1468, 1468*f*
  masses, 1464–1467
    gastroschisis, 1466–1467, 1466*f*
    hemangioma of the cord, 1467, 1467*f*
    hematoma of the cord, 1467
    omphalocele, 1466, 1466*f*
    omphalomesenteric cyst, 1467, 1467*f*
    thrombosis of the umbilical vessels, 1467, 1468*f*
    umbilical herniation, 1467, 1467*f*
  persistent intrahepatic right umbilical vein, 1472–1473, 1472*f*
  prolapse of, 1470, 1470*f*
    cord presentation with prolapse, 1470
    multiple pregnancy, 1470
    obstetric procedures, 1470
    prematurity, 1470
  single umbilical artery, 1470–1472, 1471*f*
  varix of umbilical vein, 1471*f*, 1472
  vasa previa and prolapse of the cord, 1470, 1470*f*
    cord presentation with prolapse, 1470
    multiple pregnancy, 1470
    obstetric procedures, 1470
    prematurity, 1470
Umbilical cord cysts, first-trimester, 1340, 1340*f*
Umbilical cord Doppler, 1424
Umbilical hernia, 1563, 1576, 1576*f*
Umbilical herniation, 1467, 1467*f*
Umbilical vein, fetal circulation, 1446*f*
Umbilical vein catheter, 770
Umbilical vesicle, 1462*f*
Uncinate process, 356–358, 356*f*
Undescended testis, 1617
Unilateral venous duplex imaging, 1140
United Network for Organ Sharing (UNOS), 584
Upper abdominal compartments, 417–418, 418*f*
Upper extremity
  arterial duplex imaging of, 1120, 1120*f*
  arteries of, 1112, 1112*f*
  fetal, 1369–1371, 1369*f*, 1370*f*, 1371*f*, 1372*f*
  venous duplex imaging of, tips for, 1141*t*
Upper gastrointestinal tract, 399–402, 400*t*
  duplication cysts, 399, 400*f*, 400*t*
  gastric bezoars, 399–400, 400*t*, 401*f*
  gastric carcinoma, 400*t*, 401–402, 402*f*
  leiomyomas, 400, 400*t*, 401*f*
  lymphoma, 400*t*, 402, 402*f*
  metastatic disease, 400*t*, 402, 403*f*
  polyps, 400, 400*t*, 401*f*
Upward graded compression, 778
Urachal abnormalities, 1604–1605, 1604*f*

Urachal cysts, 427, 427*f*, 1604
Ureter(s), 450, 453*b*, 453*f*, 1161–1162, 1162*b*, 1163*f*
  anatomy and physiology of, 86, 437
  narrowing of, 450, 453*b*
  sonographic evaluation of, 1596
  strictures of, 450, 453*b*
Ureteral jet phenomenon, 476–478, 477*f*, 478*f*, 574, 575*f*
Ureterocele, 450, 453*f*, 1599–1600, 1615, 1615*f*, 1616*f*
  ectopic, 450
  neonatal/pediatric, 797–798, 801*f*
  sonographic findings, 450–453
Ureteropelvic junction (UPJ), 1599, 1608–1609
  obstructions, 1610, 1611*f*, 1612*f*
  neonatal/pediatric, 799–800
  sonographic findings in, 799–800
Ureterovesical junction (UVJ), 1599, 1608–1609
  obstruction, 1610–1611, 1612*f*
Urethra
  anatomy of, 86, 437, 710
  sonographic evaluation of, 1596
Urethral atresia, 1608
Urethral discharge, 87, 87*t*
Urinals, 48–49, 48*f*
Urinalysis, 438, 573–574
Urinary anomalies, 1615–1616
Urinary bladder. *see* Bladder
Urinary hesitancy, 87*t*
Urinary incontinence, 86, 87*t*
Urinary obstruction, 616–617, 620*f*
Urinary stones, 616–617, 620*f*
Urinary system, 435, 488*b*–490*b*. *see also* Bladder; Genitourinary system; Kidney(s); Urinary tract
  anatomy of, 86, 86*f*, 435–438, 436*f*
  contrast evaluation of, 795–796
  dysfunction of, 86–88
  fetal, 1366–1368, 1366*f*, 1367*f*
  laboratory data of, 438–439
  lower urinary tract, 450, 453*b*, 453*f*
  pathology of, 453, 453*b*
    arteriovenous fistulas and pseudoaneurysms, 482–483, 484*f*
    bladder diverticulum, 485, 488*f*
    bladder tumors, 486–487, 488*f*
    cystitis, 485–486
    renal infarction, 454*t*–458*t*, 481–482
    renal infection, 478, 479*f*
  physiology of, 438–439
  sonographic evaluation of, 439–444
    normal texture and patterns, 439, 439*f*, 440*f*, 441*f*, 442*f*
    renal anomalies, 445–447, 448*f*
    in renal variants, 444, 446*f*
      columns of Bertin, 444, 446*f*
      dromedary hump, 444, 446*t*
      extrarenal pelvis, 444–445, 446*t*, 448*f*
      fetal lobulation, 444–445, 446*t*, 447*f*
      junctional parenchymal defects, 444, 446*f*, 447*f*
      sinus lipomatosis, 444, 447*f*
  urinary tract calcifications, 479, 480*f*
  vascular supply for, 437–438, 437*f*
Urinary tract
  abnormalities of, 1601, 1601*f*
  calcifications, 479, 480*f*
  dilation of, 1599, 1599*f*

Urinary tract dilation (UTD), 791, 798–799, 798t, 799f, 800f
  classification, 798–802
Urinary tract disease, 1415
Urinary tract obstruction (UTO), 474, 475f, 476f
  AFP and, 1428
Urine amylase, 362
Urine leak, 622, 626f
Urine pH, 438
Uriniferous pseudocysts, 427
Urinoma, 427, 428f, 508, 622, 626f, 802f
Urogenital fetal malformations, 1593t
Urogenital ridge, 1593
Urogenital system, fetal, 1592, 1619b–1620b
  abnormalities of, 1599–1601
  development of, 1593–1595
  embryology of, 1593
  sonographic evaluation of, 1595–1599, 1596b
Urolithiasis, 483–485, 573–574
  clinical findings for, 573–574, 573t
  sonographic findings in, 485, 485f, 486f, 487f, 574, 575f
Uterine artery, 1169, 1170f
Uterine artery embolization, 1210
Uterine cavity, 1225, 1443f
Uterine fibroids, 1416, 1416f
Uterine leiomyoma, 1209
  characteristics of, 1209b, 1210
  first-trimester, 1329t
  locations of, 1209b
Uterine masses, 1340
Uterine synechiae, 1275f
Uterosacral ligaments, 1165–1166
Uterus, 89, 93f
  anatomy of, 1162–1164, 1164b, 1164t, 1165b, 1165f
    layers of, 1164, 1165b
    size of, 1162, 1164b, 1165f
  bicornuate, 1207, 1208f, 1273f
  blood supply to, 1169, 1191–1192
  calcifications, 1210–1212, 1213f
  congenital anomalies, 1273–1274, 1273f, 1274f
  coronal view of, 1163f
  leiomyomas, 1207–1208
    characteristics of, 1209b, 1210
    locations of, 1209b
    treatment of, 1210
  leiomyosarcoma, 1216–1217, 1218f
  ligaments of, 1165–1166, 1165b, 1165f, 1166f
  measurement of, 1212f
  pathology of, 1207–1217, 1207f, 1208b, 1228b–1229b
    adenomyosis, 1212–1216, 1215f, 1216f
    arteriovenous malformations, 1216, 1217f
    differential considerations for, 1207
    enlarged uterus, 1207
    uterine leiomyosarcoma, 1216–1217, 1218f
  positions of, 1166–1167, 1166b, 1166f, 1207f
  sonographic evaluation of, 578, 578f, 1177–1189, 1178b
    three-dimensional ultrasound, 1199–1201, 1200f
    transabdominal, 1195f
      longitudinal, 1178–1180, 1195f
      sagittal, 1181f, 1182f
      transverse, 1183f
    transvaginal, 1186, 1187f, 1192–1195, 1194f
      coronal, 1186, 1186b, 1187f

Uterus (Continued)
    with hypoechoic myoma, 1206f
    sagittal, 1186, 1186b, 1186f, 1193f
  tumors, 1207–1208
  variations of, 1207, 1207f
  width of, 1186, 1187f, 1194f

V

VACTERL association, 1572, 1632
VACTERL syndrome, 881
VACTERL-H syndrome, 1632
Vagina, 1159, 1162, 1163b, 1163f, 1164f
  blood supply to, 1170f, 1191, 1192f
  coronal view of, 1163f
  pathology of, 1203, 1203f
Vaginal artery, 1170f
Vaginal bleeding, 1412–1413, 1412f, 1413f
Vaginal cuff, 1203
Valves, venous, 1130
Valvulae conniventes, 390
Valvular aortic stenosis, 966–967
Vanishing twin, 1421
Varicoceles, 717t, 722–723, 724f
Varicose veins, 1136
Varix of umbilical vein, 1471f, 1472
Vas deferens, 710
Vasa previa, 1412, 1444–1445, 1452, 1453f, 1470, 1470f
Vasa vasorum, 171
Vascular malformations, 1523t
Vascular supply
  for biliary system, 285
  for breast, 649–650, 650f
  for liver, 223–225
  of pancreas, 358f, 359
  for retroperitoneum, 496–497
  for scrotum, 710–712, 711f, 712b
  for spleen, 326, 330f
  for urinary system, 437–438, 437f
Vascular system, 169, 170f, 215b–217b
  inferior mesenteric vein, 209
  splenic vein, 206–207
  superior mesenteric vein, 207–209
Vascular ultrasound contrast agents, 511–514, 512f, 513f, 513t, 514t
  hepatic blood flow and, 517
  3D gray-scale harmonic imaging and, 516f
Vasospasm, 1099–1100
Vegetations, cardiac, 1000–1006, 1004f, 1005f
Vein(s), 171
  deep
    lower extremity, 1130–1131, 1130f
    upper extremity, 1133–1134, 1133f
  functions of, 1134
  physiology of, 1134
Vein mapping, 1146–1147
Vein of Galen aneurysm, 1537
  differential considerations for, 1524t
  sonographic findings in, 1537
Velamentous insertion, placenta, 1444–1445, 1445f
Velocity
  definition of, 908
  of propagation, 10
  of sound, 10–11
Vena contracta, 957b, 957f, 958f
Venous disease
  risk factors for, 1135, 1135b
  symptoms of, 1135b

Venous duplex imaging, 1130–1134
  anatomy for, 1130–1134
    lower extremity, 1130–1133, 1130f
    upper extremity, 1133–1134, 1133f
  controversies of, 1147–1150
    bilateral symptoms, 1148–1149
    calf vein imaging, 1149
    complete versus limited examination, 1147–1148
    emergent venous duplex imaging, 1149
    pulmonary embolism assessments, 1149–1150
    unilateral versus bilateral, 1148
  guidelines for, 1150–1151, 1150b
  interpretation of, 1140–1144, 1141t, 1142f, 1143f, 1144f, 1145f
    criteria for, 1140, 1141t
    technical adjustments for, 1144t
    tips for, 1141t
  technical aspects of, 1137–1140
    lower extremity, 1137b, 1138f
Venous insufficiency, 1136–1137
Venous reflux, 1136–1137
Venous reflux imaging, 1145–1146, 1145f
Venous sinuses, 1443f
Venous thromboembolism (VTE), 1134–1135
Venous thrombosis, 633–634, 635f, 636f
Venous valves, 1130
Ventral, 132
Ventral cavity, 88
Ventral direction, 132
Ventricles. see also Lateral ventricles; Left ventricle; Right ventricle
  formation of, 1009, 1010f
Ventricular diastole, 901b
Ventricular ejection, 906
Ventricular index, 830, 830f, 830t
Ventricular septal defects, 1038–1041, 1038f, 1039f
  incidence of, 1032t, 1033
  membranous septal defect, 1038–1040, 1040f
  muscular defect, 1040–1041
Ventricular system, neonatal, 815–817, 817f
Ventriculitis, 847
Ventriculomegaly, 1336, 1336t, 1337f, 1540–1542. see also Hydrocephalus
  anomalies associated with, 1523t
  definition of, 829
  meningomyelocele and, 1530f
  myelomeningocele and, 1530f
  sonographic findings in, 1541f, 1542, 1542f
Ventriculoperitoneal shunt, 766, 829, 829f
Venturi mask, 45–46
Veracity, 1297–1298
Verbal consent, 32
Vernix caseosa, 1475
Vertebrae, 872–873, 872f, 875, 875f
Vertebral arch, 872
Vertebral arteries, 1071, 1075f
Vertebral column
  anatomy of, 872, 872f
  fetal, 1355–1357, 1356f, 1357f
Vertebral foramen, 872, 872f
Vertebrobasilar system, 1089
Vertigo, 1072
Verumontanum, 710
Vesicoallantoic cyst, 1604
Vesicoureteral reflux, 799
Vesicouterine pouch, 94, 1174b

Vidoscan, 8
Villi, 390
Virchow, Rudolph, 1135
Virchow triad, 1135
Virtual beam-forming artifacts, 163, 164b, 164f, 164t
Viscera, abdominal, 88
Visceral peritoneum, 95–96, 413–414
Vital signs, 35–38, 63
 definition of, 35
 homeostasis and, 81
Vitamin K, 81, 228
Volar, 748
Volume, 908
Vomiting, 85t, 86
 basins for, 49
 projectile, 784
von Gierke disease, 248
Von Hippel-Lindau cysts, 454t–458t, 460
Von Hippel-Lindau disease, 805
Von Hippel-Lindau syndrome, 377–381, 378f
Vulva, 1159

W

Wall echo shadow (WES) sign, 300, 301f
Wall filter, 27–28, 589–590, 589f, 715t
Walled-off pancreatic fluid collections, 373–374, 374f
Wandering spleen, 327
Waterhouse-Friderichsen syndrome, 502, 502t
Wave, 10
Wavelength, 12, 12f
Wavy-line sign, 667–668, 668f
WBCs. see White blood cells
WES sign. see Wall echo shadow (WES) sign
Wharton jelly, 1445, 1461
Wheelchair transfer, 39, 39f
Whirlpool sign, 1243–1244
White blood cells (WBCs), 83
White coat hypertension, 36
White pulp, of spleen, 330, 332f
Wild, John, 7
Williams syndrome, 966, 1051
Wilms tumor, 199–204, 274–280, 773
 neonatal/pediatric, 467, 773, 807–808
 sonographic findings in, 454t–458t, 468f, 469f
Work-related musculoskeletal disorders (WRMSDs)
 definition of, 70, 78b
 economics of, 77–78
 history of, 69
 incidence of, 69
 industry awareness/changes and, 72–74
 mechanisms of injury in, 70–72, 71f, 72f
 OSHA and, 69–70
 risk factors for, 70, 71f
 surveys of, 70, 71t
 types of, 72, 72f
 work practice changes and, 74–77, 76f, 77f
 workstation setup, 78–79, 79f
Workstation setup, 78–79, 79f
World Health Organization (WHO), 532
Wounds, patient care and, 46–47
Wrists, 747–749
 carpal tunnel and, 748, 749f
 flexion and extension, 75
Written consent, 32
WRMSDs. see Work-related musculoskeletal disorders

X

Xanthogranulomatous pyelonephritis, 478–479, 480f
Xiphisternal joint, 891–892
X-linked disorders, 1433

Y

Yolk sac, 1289–1290, 1443f
 embryonic development of, 1327
 embryonic evaluation, 1327
 gestational sac without, 1322
 sonographic findings of
  in abnormal intrauterine pregnancies, 1324b
  during fetal period, 1307–1308, 1307f, 1308f
 tumors of. see Endodermal sinus tumors
Yolk stalk, 1309–1310, 1460–1461

Z

Zygote, 1290, 1301